Additional Resources for LPN/LVN Success—

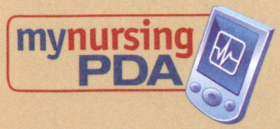 **mynursing PDA**

Provides accurate, informed support for clinical decision making at point of care

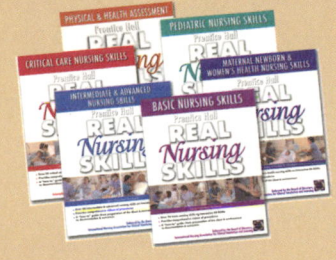

Prentice Hall Real Nursing Skills

The volumes in this series consist of procedures and rationales demonstrated in hundreds of realistic video clips, animations, illustrations, and more!

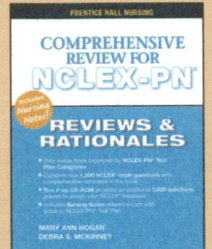

Prentice Hall Nursing: Reviews & Rationales, Comprehensive Comprehensive Review for the NCLEX-PN®
Hogan, McKinney

A concentrated review of core content and hundreds of practice NCLEX-PN® questions with comprehensive rationales.

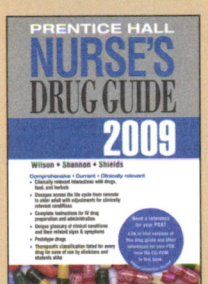

Prentice Hall Nurse's Drug Guide
Wilson, Shannon, and Shields

This annual reference is the most complete source for drug administration information and the only source to identify prototype drugs.

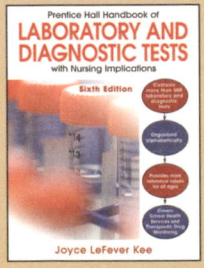

Prentice Hall Handbook of Laboratory Tests & Diagnostic Procedures, 6th Edition
Kee

Provides easy access to information on laboratory and diagnostic tests, emphasizing reference values and normal findings, purposes, procedures, clinical problems and drug effects, factors affecting test results, nursing implications and client teaching.

NLN Practice Tests
www.nlnlinetesting.org/demos.html

- Course specific, nationally standarized tests available
- Two 50-item practice exams available in online format to simula NCLEX® environment
- Instantly scored with rationales
- Students can share results with instructors

For more information and purchasing options on these and other Pearson products visit www.mynursingkit.com

Brief Table of Contents

Your steps to success.

 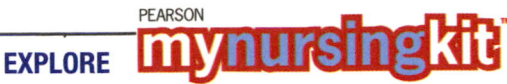
STEP 1: Register

All you need to get started is a valid email address and the access code below. To register, simply:

1. Go to **www.mynursingkit.com**.

2. Click "**Students**" under "**First-time users.**"

3. Find the appropriate book cover. Cover must match the textbook edition being used for your class.

4. Click "**Register**" beside your book cover.

5. Read the **License Agreement** and **Private Policy**. If you accept, click "**I Accept.**"

6. Leave "**No**" selected under "**Do you have a Pearson account?**"

7. Using a coin scratch off the silver coating below to reveal your access code. Do not use a knife or other sharp object, which can damage the code.

8. Enter your access code in lowercase or uppercase, without the dashes.

9. Follow the on-screen instructions to complete registration.

During registration, you will establish a personal login name and password to use for logging into the Website. You will also be sent a registration confirmation email that contains your login name and password. Be sure to save this email.

Your Access Code is:

Note: If there is no silver foil covering the access code, it may already have been redeemed, and therefore may no longer be valid. In that case, you can purchase access online using a major credit card. To do so, go to www.mynursingkit.com. click "Students" under "First Time Users," find the cover of your textbook, then click "Buy Access," and follow the on-screen instructions.

STEP 2: Log in

1. Go to **www.mynursingkit.com** and click "**Students**" under "**Returning Users.**"

2. Find the appropriate book cover. Click on "**Login**" next to your book cover.

3. Enter the login name and password that you created during registration. If unsure of this information, refer to your registration confirmation email.

4. Click "**Login.**"

Got technical questions?

Customer Technical Support: To obtain support, please visit us online anytime at http://247pearsoned.custhelp.com where you can search our knowledgebase for common solutions, view product alerts, and review all options for additional assistance.

SITE REQUIREMENTS

For the latest updates on Site Requirements, go to www.mynursingkit.com. Click "**Students**" under "**Returning Users**". Pick your book and click "**Login**". Click on "**Need help**" at bottom of page for site requirements and other frequently asked questions.

Important: Please read the Subscription and End-User License agreement, accessible from the book website's login page, before using the *mynursingkit* website. By using the website, you indicate that you have read, understood, and accepted the terms of this agreement.

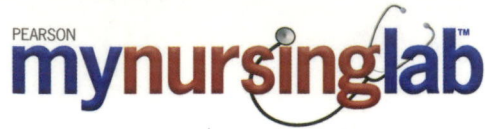
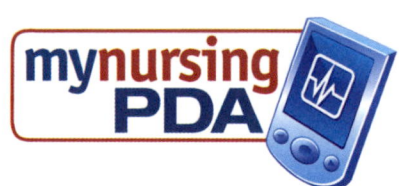

COMPREHENSIVE
Nursing Care

Second Edition

Roberta Pavy Ramont, RN, MS, EdD
Corporate Director of Nursing
International Education Corporation
Irvine, California

Dolores Maldonado Niedringhaus, RN, BSN
Instructional Administrator of Medical Programs
North Orange County Regional Occupational Program
Anaheim, California

Mary Ann Towle, RN, MEd, MSN
Senior Instructor, Department of Nursing
Boise State University
Boise, Idaho

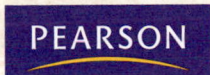

PEARSON

Upper Saddle River, New Jersey 07458

Library of Congress Cataloging-in-Publication Data

Ramont, Roberta Pavy.
  Comprehensive nursing care/Roberta Pavy Ramont, Dolores Maldonado
Niedringhaus, Mary Ann Towle. -- 2nd ed.
    p. ; cm.
  Includes bibliographical references and index.
  ISBN-13: 978-0-13-504099-7
  ISBN-10: 0-13-504099-X
  1. Practical nursing. I. Niedringhaus, Dolores Maldonado. II. Towle, Mary Ann. III. Title.
  [DNLM: 1. Nursing Care. 2. Nursing Process. 3. Nursing, Practical. WY 100 R175c 2010]
  RT62.R26 2010
  610.7306'93--dc22

                                                              2008049457

Publisher: Julie Levin Alexander
Executive Assistant: Regina Bruno
Editor-in-Chief: Maura Connor
Senior Acquisitions Editor: Kelly Trakalo
Development Editor: Rachel Bedard
Editorial Assistant: Lauren Sweeney
Managing Editor, Production: Patrick Walsh
Production Liaison: Yagnesh Jani
Production Editor: Carol Singer, GGS higher education resources
Manufacturing Manager: Ilene Sanford
Senior Design Coordinator: Maria Guglielmo-Walsh
Interior and Cover Design: Mary Siener
Media Product Manager: Travis Moses-Westphal
Media Project Manager: Lorena Cerisano
Senior Marketing Manager: Harper Coles
Marketing Specialist: Michael Sirinides
Marketing Assistant: Crystal Gonzalez
Manager, Rights and Permissions: Zina Arabia
Manager, Visual Research: Beth Brenzel
Manager, Cover Visual Research & Permissions: Karen Sanatar
Image Permission Coordinator: Craig A. Jones
Composition: GGS higher education resources
Cover Printer: Lehigh/Phoenix Color
Printer/Binder: Webcrafters

Pearson Education Ltd., London
Pearson Education Australia PTY, Limited
Pearson Education Singapore, Pte. Ltd.
Pearson Education North Asia Ltd., Singapore
Pearson Education, Canada, Inc.
Pearson Educación de Mexico, S.A. de C.V.
Pearson Education—Japan
Pearson Education Malaysia, Pte. Ltd
Pearson Education, Upper Saddle River, New Jersey

All photographs/illustrations not credited on page,
under or adjacent to the piece, were photographed/rendered
on assignment and are the property of
Pearson Education/Prentice Hall Health.

Golden wheat field cover image and background: Greg
Probst/Botanica/Jupiter Images. Dandelion photo on cover &
interior background: Grant V. Faint/Image Bank/Getty Images,
Inc. Waterfall photo on cover & interior: Digital Vision
Ltd./Royalty Free. Autumn leaves photo on cover & interior:
Digital Vision/Getty Images, Inc. Winter by the lake photo on
cover & interior: Brand X Pictures/Getty Images, Inc. Lily pad
with bloom photo on cover & interior: Eyewire Collection/Getty
Images, Inc. Fern bud photo on cover and interior: Eyewire
Collection/Getty Images, Inc. Fern leaves photo: Akita Keade/
Photodisc/Getty Images, Inc. Sunset behind clouds photo on cover &
interior: Getty Images, Inc. - Comstock Images Royalty Free.

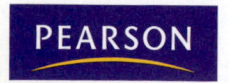

10 9 8 7 6 5 4 3 2 1
ISBN 13: 978-0-13-504099-7
ISBN 10:   0-13-504099-X

Preface

The LPN/LVN of today must be able to function as a bedside nurse, a team member, supervisor of unlicensed assistive personnel, and a client educator. It is not enough to be skilled in carrying out client care tasks. LVNs and LPNs must understand the meaning of signs and symptoms, and they must be able to distinguish between normal and abnormal laboratory results and diagnostics. They must be able to function in a variety of settings: in the acute hospital, sub-acute setting, long-term care facility, physicians' office, clinic, and home care.

We feel very strongly that the education of nurses at the LPN/LVN level is more important today than ever before. In many situations LPNs and LVNs are the nurses who will have direct contact with the healthcare consumer. They need to be competent, professional, and articulate, as well as compassionate. They must be able to gain the confidence of their clients.

Comprehensive Nursing Care addresses the LPN/LVN scope of practice, roles, and collaborative relationships with the registered nurse. It provides essential information in six core areas of the LPN/LVN curriculum (Fundamentals; Medical-Surgical/Adult Health; Maternal-Newborn; Pediatrics; Mental Health; and Leadership) and focuses on delivery of safe, professional care to clients.

Academic survival skills are provided in the opening chapters and woven through the text where appropriate. Many students entering LPN/LVN programs have not had the opportunity to develop their academic survival skills. They also have many outside responsibilities. We present them with solid information about study skills, tips on how to read a textbook, and strategies on test taking and time management that will help them to be successful as students and nurses.

Organization of subject manner within the textbook can be very important in making the book user friendly for students. Most LPN/LVN programs are taught from simple to complex, building on knowledge and skills already obtained. This book provides a building block approach:

- Units I through IV cover fundamental concepts
- Unit V covers medical-surgical/adult health
- Unit VI addresses the special needs of the older adult
- Unit VII addresses additional clients requiring specialized care
- Unit VIII covers mental health nursing
- Units IX and X cover maternal-newborn and pediatric nursing care
- Unit XI covers leadership and the transition from student to professional nurse

Comprehensive Nursing Care focuses on "need-to-know" information. Only skills and competencies that are within the LPN/LVN scope of practice have been included. Some of the current texts in LPN/LVN courses include skills and procedures that are beyond the LPN/LVN scope of practice. Others provide just a bare overview of LPN/LVN nursing actions. We have attempted to provide the skills and procedures the new nurse will need upon graduating and within the first six months of practice. Our goal has been to provide level-specific information and make this text truly an LPN/LVN-level book.

The role of the LPN or LVN differs from one area of practice to another, as well as from state to state. A nurse working in the acute setting has a much different role than one in a skilled nursing facility or in an ambulatory setting. We present information about these delineations in the unit on professional development.

Throughout the text, as appropriate, we include geriatric, pediatric/adolescent, and maternal and neonate considerations. Nursing process and theory are incorporated as appropriate.

Since much of client care is now delivered outside the acute hospital (in the home, skilled nursing facilities, physician's offices, and clinics), we address these concepts. Hospice and restorative nursing care are also discussed.

Critical thinking and problem solving situations are presented in each unit. "Real life" client scenarios allow students to demonstrate knowledge and capabilities and to develop higher-level skills in preparation for practice.

Methods for achieving and maintaining professionalism have been included in Unit XI and throughout the book. Changes in dress codes, demographics of LPNs/LVNs, and public relations require that professionalism be a focus of nursing education. Whereas once starched caps and white dresses identified the licensed nurse, now other indicators of the profession must be apparent in the healthcare setting to gain and sustain client confidence. Professional behavior, well-developed clinical reasoning, and conflict resolution skills are some of the hallmarks that define the professional LPN/LVN. Finally, *Comprehensive Nursing Care* text is in alignment with the NCLEX-PN® Test Plan. It is not our intention to "teach to the test," but rather to demonstrate in each chapter how the information relates to the broad categories of the Test Plan.

The second edition of *Comprehensive Nursing Care* provides greater depth and scope of information while maintaining the easy-to-access format. Sixteen new chapters include:

- Chapter 2: History of Nursing
- Chapter 8: Complementary and Alternative Therapies
- Chapter 18: Loss, Grief, and Death
- Chapter 22: Pain, the Fifth Vital Sign
- Chapter 24: Wound Care and Skin Integrity
- Chapter 25: Nutrition
- Chapter 28: IV Therapy
- Chapter 40: Clients with Reproductive Disorders

A new Gerontology Unit now includes one new chapter:

- Chapter 42: Health Promotion for Older Clients

A new Specialized Nursing Care Unit includes two new chapters:

- Chapter 46: Long-Term Care and Rehabilitation Nursing
- Chapter 48: Community Health Nursing

An expanded Maternal-Newborn Unit now includes normal and high-risk care of the pregnant woman and of the newborn child. New chapters include:

- Chapter 52: Care of Women During High-Risk Pregnancy
- Chapter 55: Care of High-Risk Postpartum Woman
- Chapter 57: Care of the High-Risk Neonate

An expanded Pediatric and Adolescent Unit contains two new chapters, including a transition chapter that highlights differences between care of children and adults.

- Chapter 58: Pediatric-Focused Nursing Care
- Chapter 60: Care and Illnesses of Preschool Children

In addition to new chapters, content has been given more depth is various ways:

- Expanded Unit Wrap-Ups encourage integrated review of unit content.
- A Pediatric Considerations thread runs through the Medical-Surgical section.
- Latest information on infection control, including Community Acquired MRSA
- Overview of National Medical Reserve Corps and Disaster Preparedness
- 2009 National Patient Safety Goals from the Joint Commission

Design and Features

Chapter Openers help focus students on what is important.

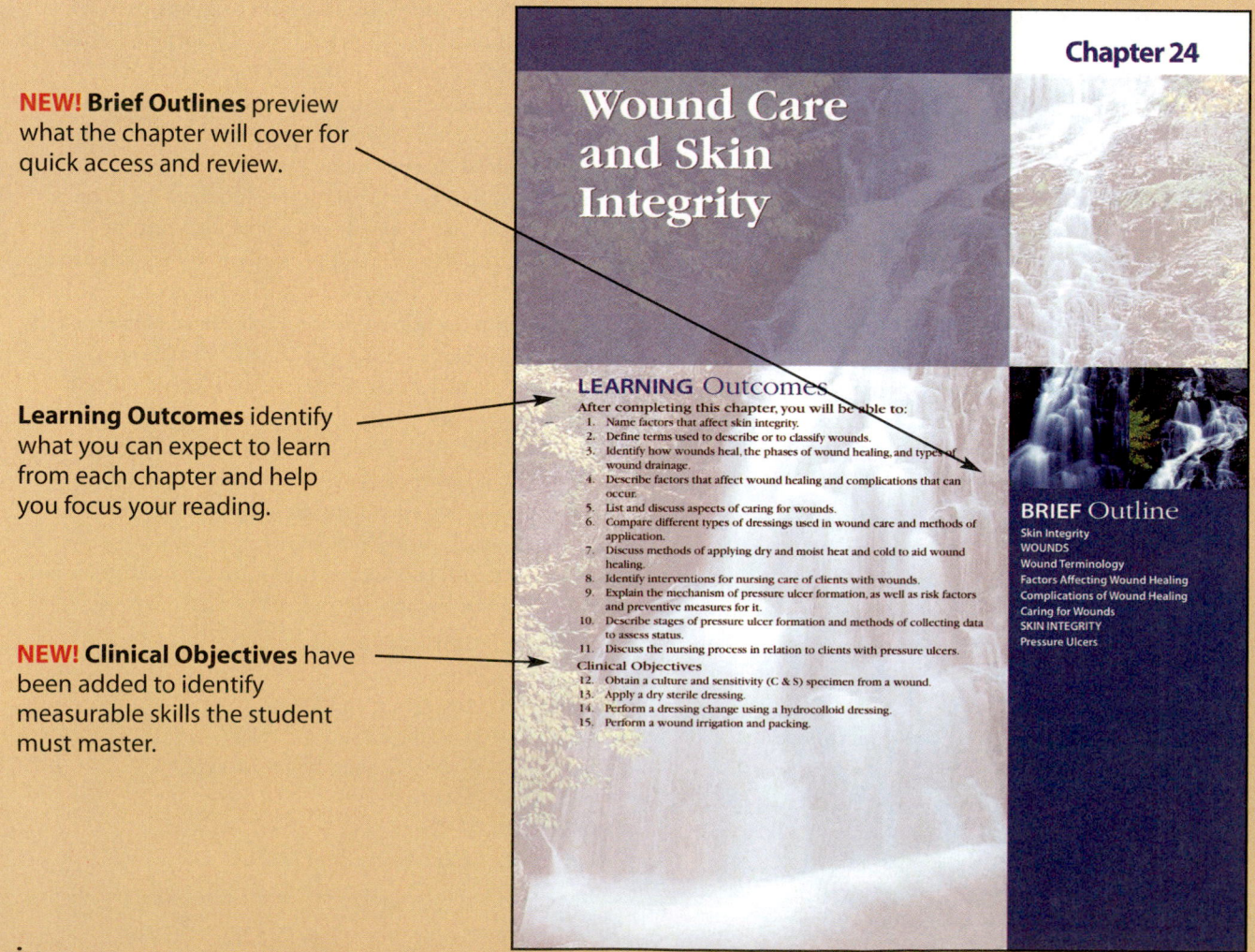

NEW! Brief Outlines preview what the chapter will cover for quick access and review.

Learning Outcomes identify what you can expect to learn from each chapter and help you focus your reading.

NEW! Clinical Objectives have been added to identify measurable skills the student must master.

Chapter 24

Wound Care and Skin Integrity

LEARNING Outcomes
After completing this chapter, you will be able to:
1. Name factors that affect skin integrity.
2. Define terms used to describe or to classify wounds.
3. Identify how wounds heal, the phases of wound healing, and types of wound drainage.
4. Describe factors that affect wound healing and complications that can occur.
5. List and discuss aspects of caring for wounds.
6. Compare different types of dressings used in wound care and methods of application.
7. Discuss methods of applying dry and moist heat and cold to aid wound healing.
8. Identify interventions for nursing care of clients with wounds.
9. Explain the mechanism of pressure ulcer formation, as well as risk factors and preventive measures for it.
10. Describe stages of pressure ulcer formation and methods of collecting data to assess status.
11. Discuss the nursing process in relation to clients with pressure ulcers.

Clinical Objectives
12. Obtain a culture and sensitivity (C & S) specimen from a wound.
13. Apply a dry sterile dressing.
14. Perform a dressing change using a hydrocolloid dressing.
15. Perform a wound irrigation and packing.

BRIEF Outline
Skin Integrity
WOUNDS
Wound Terminology
Factors Affecting Wound Healing
Complications of Wound Healing
Caring for Wounds
SKIN INTEGRITY
Pressure Ulcers

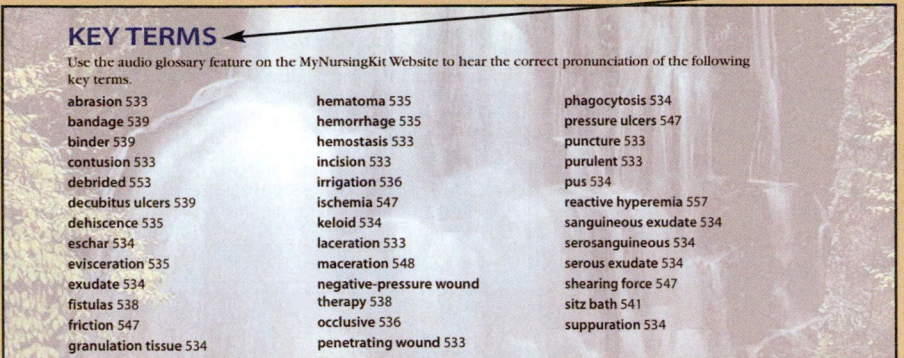

Key Terms are listed alphabetically, with page numbers, at the beginning of the chapter. They are also boldfaced and defined where they first appear in the text.

KEY TERMS

Use the audio glossary feature on the MyNursingKit Website to hear the correct pronunciation of the following key terms.

abrasion 533
bandage 539
binder 539
contusion 533
debrided 553
decubitus ulcers 539
dehiscence 535
eschar 534
evisceration 535
exudate 534
fistulas 538
friction 547
granulation tissue 534

hematoma 535
hemorrhage 535
hemostasis 533
incision 533
irrigation 536
ischemia 547
keloid 534
laceration 533
maceration 548
negative-pressure wound therapy 538
occlusive 536
penetrating wound 533

phagocytosis 534
pressure ulcers 547
puncture 533
purulent 533
pus 534
reactive hyperemia 557
sanguineous exudate 534
serosanguineous 534
serous exudate 534
shearing force 547
sitz bath 541
suppuration 534

Color-coded boxes and tables provide important information for students to remember.

Client Teaching and Population Focus boxes provide information on age-specific and other special needs of client groups, and help students prepare for client instruction.

BOX 24-1   POPULATION FOCUS

Factors That Inhibit Wound Healing in Older Adults
- Vascular changes associated with aging, such as atherosclerosis and atrophy of capillaries in the skin, can impair blood flow to the wound.
- Collagen tissue is less flexible.
- Changes in the immune system may reduce the formation of antibodies and monocytes necessary for wound healing.
- Nutritional deficiencies may reduce the numbers of red blood cells and leukocytes, thus impeding the delivery of oxygen and the inflammatory response essential for wound healing. Oxygen is needed for the synthesis of collagen and the formation of new epithelial cells.
- Scar tissue is less elastic than normal tissue. It is structurally different, being composed mostly of connective tissue made of collagen. Its density and composition can limit movement in badly damaged areas.

BOX 31-2   CULTURAL PULSE POINTS

Differences in Bone Structure and Density
There are many bicultural variations with the musculoskeletal system that you need to be aware of when performing an assessment. You will learn to distinguish between normal ethnic variation and abnormalities. Bone density varies greatly among different groups. African American males have the densest bone, which accounts for their very low incidence of osteoporosis. Most humans normally have 24 vertebrae. However, approximately 11% of African American females have 31, and 12% of Eskimo and Native American males have 25.

According to the National Osteoporosis Foundation (2008), it is estimated that 20% of Caucasian and Asian women over age 50 have osteoporosis, and 52% have low bone density (*osteopenia*). The risk for osteoporosis is rising most rapidly in Hispanic women over age 50.

Cultural Pulse Points boxes highlight transcultural nursing issues and prepare the student to deliver culturally proficient care .

BOX 24-7   NURSING CARE CHECKLIST

Treating Pressure Ulcers
- ☑ Minimize direct pressure on the ulcer. Reposition the client at least every 2 hours. Use a schedule, and record position changes on the client's chart.
- ☑ Clean the pressure ulcer daily. The method of cleaning depends on the stage of the ulcer and agency protocol. For example, a whirlpool bath may be indicated for a stage I ulcer and a wound irrigation for a stage IV ulcer (see Procedure 24-3).
- ☑ Clean and dress the ulcer using surgical asepsis.
- ☑ If the pressure ulcer is infected, obtain a sample of the drainage for culture and sensitivity to antiseptic agents (see Procedure 24-2).
- ☑ If the client cannot keep weight off the pressure ulcer, use pressure-relieving devices such as an egg-crate mattress.
- ☑ Teach the client to move, if only slightly, to relieve pressure.
- ☑ Provide range-of-motion (ROM) exercises as the client's condition permits.

Nursing Care Checklist boxes provide handy summaries of important nursing interventions.

BOX 44-1   PEDIATRIC CONSIDERATIONS

Care of the Child with a Chronic Illness
When caring for children with chronic illnesses, the nurse must be alert to developmental stages (see Erikson's developmental stages in Chapter 16 ⬤) and how a child's developmental stage may impact the plan of care. Children born with such chronic conditions as muscular dystrophy and cerebral palsy may never have known any other life. Still, they are often very aware of how they are different from their peers. Programs that focus on allowing "kids to be kids" within the level of their disability can be valuable in providing some degree of normalcy.

Chronically ill children pose many challenges to families. The challenges, both physically and financially, can be overwhelming, placing stress on relationships among family members. Knowledge of the support available through community services is essential. Appropriate referrals are needed so that families can manage care of their children and receive support when they are feeling overburdened.

Pediatric Considerations discuss content in context of the special needs of children.

Data Collection boxes summarize data collected and manifestations the nurse may observe .

clinical ALERT

Hemorrhage is an emergency that requires the application of extra sterile pressure dressings to the area, monitoring the client's vital signs, and notifying the physician. The risk of hemorrhage is greatest during the first 48 hours after surgery.

Clinical Alerts call attention to clinical roles and responsibilities for heightened awareness, monitoring, and/or reporting.

ASSESSING

Particular attention is paid to skin condition in areas most likely to break down: skinfolds (such as under the breasts), areas that are frequently moist (such as the perineum), and areas that receive extensive pressure (such as the coccyx and trochanters). Figure 24-16 ■ illustrates common sites of pressure ulcers. Box 24-6 ■ describes assessment of common pressure sites.

When a pressure ulcer is present, the nurse notes the following:

- Location of the lesion
- Size of lesion in centimeters (Measure length, width, and depth, beginning with length [head to toe] and then width [side to side]. To measure depth, gently insert a sterile swab at the deepest part of the wound, and then measure against a measuring guide.)
- Stage of the ulcer (see Figure 24-13)
- Color of the wound bed and location of necrosis or eschar
- Condition of the wound margins
- Integrity of surrounding skin
- Clinical signs of infection, such as redness, warmth, swelling, pain, odor, and exudate (note color of exudate)

DIAGNOSING, PLANNING, AND IMPLEMENTING

Nursing diagnoses that are common in clients with pressure ulcers are:

- *Impaired Skin Integrity* (commonly applies to stage I and II pressure ulcers)
- *Impaired Tissue Integrity* (applies to stage III and IV pressure ulcers)
- *Pain*

Nursing Care is presented in the five-step nursing process format and emphasizes the scope of practice for the LPN/LVN. Rationales after each nursing action explain why the action is important and support the evidence-based nursing process.

NURSING CARE
PRIORITIZING NURSING CARE

To maintain intact skin, the nurse attends to the client and checks pressure points regularly. The nurse adheres to turning and repositioning schedules and ensures that restraints are removed at frequent intervals, during which skin care is provided. When pressure breakdown has occurred, the nurse follows strict precautions to provide sterile care to the wound and assist healing. As of April 2008, Medicare and Medicaid will not reimburse costs associated with the acquisition of a pressure ulcer. It is the responsibility of the LPN/LVN to prevent skin breakdown. It is not enough to delegate to unlicensed assistive personnel. The nurse is responsible for following up and documenting that appropriate turning and skin care has been carried out. Once a client has been medicated, the sleep cycle is disturbed and the client will need to be turned and positioned. A turning clock can be placed on the door as a reminder to all staff.

Prioritizing Nursing Care helps the student transition from conceptual content about disorders to the LPN/LVN role of caring for clients.

Continuity of Care

Prior to discharge, the nurse must ensure that clients have an understanding of wound care. Clients should know how to change a dressing and how frequently to do so. They should understand what normal healing looks like. They should be given a list of signs that might indicate an infection or other complication and when to notify the physician.

The nurse reviews the client's self-care abilities, such as the ability to manage hygiene and other self-care, to perform wound care as needed, to manage tubes and stomas, and to manage prescribed medications. The nurse teaches about required supplies (dressings, hypoallergenic tape, etc.) or

Continuity of Care focuses on preparing clients for self-care and discharge.

Nursing Process Care Plans illustrate nursing care in a "real-life" scenario.

Critical Thinking Questions allow students to apply their new knowledge to a specific client.

NURSING PROCESS CARE PLAN
Client with Pressure (Decubitus) Ulcer

Jamie Lee, a 73-year-old female, was admitted to the hospital for a decubitus ulcer on her left hip. Jamie lives in a skilled nursing center and is being treated for diabetes. She takes insulin twice a day. Mrs. Lee is unhappy with the restrictions of her diabetic diet. The staff must remind her about the dangers of eating candy bars, which they frequently find in her bedside table. Her mobility is limited, and she complains when the staff encourages her to sit up. She favors her left side because she can watch the television from that angle easily.

Assessment
VS: T 99, apical P 76, R 22, BP 146/90. Blood sugar is 320; hemoglobin is 10; hematocrit is 36; and WBC count is 12,000. The decubitus ulcer is described as having full-thickness skin loss, measuring 2×2 across and 0.5 in. deep. No undermining noted.

Nursing Diagnosis
The following important nursing diagnoses (among others) are established for this client:

- *Impaired Skin Integrity*
- *Risk for Infection* related to decubitus ulcer
- *Activity Intolerance*
- *Powerlessness* related to illness-related regimen
- *Deficient Knowledge* related to diabetes

Critical Thinking in the Nursing Process
1. How will you reinforce Mrs. Lee's understanding of diabetes and wound healing?
2. Compare treatment for a stage III and stage IV decubitus ulcer.
3. Describe how nutrition can affect the healing process in pressure ulcers.

Note: Discussion of Critical Thinking questions appears on the MyNursingKit.

Procedures are located at the end of applicable chapters for easy access and provide step-by-step instructions and rationales for nursing actions. Special icons in the procedures reinforce essential preliminary steps in client care. "Live" documentation at the end of each procedure demonstrates samples of good record-keeping.

PROCEDURE 24-1 **Wound Dressings**

Purposes
- To provide a moist wound environment and promote wound healing
- To protect the wound from trauma and infectious agents
- To facilitate assessment of wound healing
- To prevent the entrance of microorganisms into the wound
- To minimize wound discomfort
- To promote autolysis of necrotic material by white blood cells
- To decrease the frequency of dressing changes

Equipment
- Disposable gloves
- Hair scissors or clippers
- Alcohol or acetone
- Moisture-proof bag
- Sterile gloves (optional)
- Sterile gauze and the wound-cleaning agents specified by the physician or agency (e.g., sterile saline)
- Wound barrier dressing
- Scissors
- Paper tape
- Dressing set
- Sterile normal saline or other cleaning agent used by the agency
- Hydrocolloid dressing at least 3 to 4 cm (1.5 in.) larger than wound on all four sides

MyNursingKit tabs located in page margins identify additional resources on the MyNursingKit website (www.mynursingkit.com). See the MyNursingKit page at the beginning of the book for information on how to access.

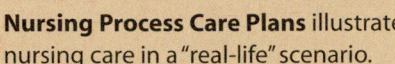
MyNursingKit | Collective bargaining

Comprehensive review
at the end of each chapter!

Key Points remind students of lifelong need-to-know items and ideas.

MyNursingKit (www.mynursingkit.com) provides interactive materials for online review, with video clips, websites, and learning exercises to explore. See the MyNursingKit page at the beginning of the book for instructions on how to access.

For Further Study identifies cross-references and draws together related content from other chapters in the book.

Chapter Review

KEY Points

- Skin integrity is the body's first line of defense.
- The wound healing process has three phases: inflammatory, proliferative, and maturation.
- Essential data for wounds include wound appearance, size, drainage, swelling, pain, and the presence of tubes and drains.
- Nurses are usually responsible for obtaining specimens of wound drainage for culture. Laboratory data support wound assessment.
- Nurses must wash hands before and after providing wound care to prevent infection and transmission of bloodborne pathogens.
- Major nursing responsibilities related to wound care include preventing infection, preventing further tissue damage, preventing hemorrhage, promoting healing, and preventing skin excoriation around draining wounds.
- Wound care may involve cleaning wounds, changing dressings, maintaining drains, irrigating, inserting packing, applying heat and cold, and applying bandages and binders.
- Nurses must use extra precautions when applying heat or cold to clients with neurosensory or circulatory impairment.
- Major types of wound exudate are serous, purulent, and sanguineous (hemorrhagic). The main complications of wound healing are hemorrhage, infection, dehiscence, and evisceration.
- A pressure ulcer is caused by unrelieved pressure resulting in damage to underlying tissues.
- Friction and shearing forces can also produce a pressure ulcer. Frequent change of position and care when moving a client can help prevent pressure ulcers.

- The nurse describes a pressure ulcer in terms of location, size, depth, stage, color, status of wound margins and surrounding skin, and specific signs of infection.
- Wound assessment continually requires visual inspection, palpation, and the sense of smell.

FOR FURTHER Study

For more information about infection control, see Chapter 10.
For further information about the body's normal responses to heat and cold, see Chapter 21.
See more on nutrition in Chapter 25.
Removal of sutures and staples is discussed in care of the client after surgery, in Chapter 29.
For more on the structure of normal skin and disorders that affect it see Chapter 30.
Chapter 31 addresses compartment syndrome.
See Procedure 47-1 for applying a sling.
Sitz baths are described in postpartum care, Chapter 54.

EXPLORE mynursingkit

MyNursingKit is your one stop for online chapter review materials and resources. Prepare for success with additional NCLEX®-style practice questions, interactive assignments and activities, web links, animations and videos, and more!

Register your access code from the front of your book at www.mynursingkit.com

560 Unit IV Promoting Physiological Health

An interactive **Critical Thinking Care Map** helps students to prioritize data and nursing interventions. Each map provides a case study, nursing diagnosis, and a list of data and interventions. The student selects which data and nursing interventions would relate to that client with that particular nursing diagnosis. Each map also sharpens reporting and charting skills by asking what should be documented and by providing examples of appropriate documentation.

Critical Thinking Care Map

Caring for a Debilitated Client
NCLEX-PN® Focus Area: Physiological Integrity

Case Study: Mr. Johns is an 84-year-old client being treated for a urinary tract disorder. Mr. Johns suffered a cerebrovascular accident (stroke) 6 months ago and has difficulty ambulating and attending to his own needs because of right-sided weakness. While assessing Mr. Johns, you note that he is thin for his 6-foot frame, weighs 135 lbs, is incontinent of foul-smelling urine, and has deeply reddened areas on his right hip, coccyx, and entire perineal area. He is alert and oriented to person, place, and time, but he has decreased sensation on his entire right side. He spends most of his time in bed or sitting at his bedside chair due to his difficulty with ambulation.

Nursing Diagnosis: *Risk for Impaired Skin Integrity*

COLLECT DATA

Subjective	Objective
_____	_____
_____	_____
_____	_____
_____	_____
_____	_____

Would you report this? Yes/No
If yes, report to: _____
What would you report? _____

Nursing Care

_____
_____
_____
_____
_____
_____
_____
_____

Would you report this? Yes/No
If yes, report to: _____
What would you report? _____
Compare your answers and documentation to those provided on the MyNursingKit Website.

Data Collected
(use only those that apply)

- Difficulty ambulating
- Height: 6 ft
- Weight: 135 lbs
- Client states,"I'm not hungry most of the time."
- Weakened
- BP 150/88
- Incontinent of urine
- General malaise
- Deeply reddened coccyx, right hip, and perineal area
- Alert and oriented
- Decreased sensation to his entire right side
- Right-sided weakness
- Negative for fecal blood
- TSH 5 mcgU/mL (microgram of international units/mL)

Nursing Interventions
(use only those that apply; list in priority order)

- Monitor urine output.
- Monitor reddened area.
- Check vital signs every 2 hours.
- Turn client every 2 hours.
- Refer to dietitian.
- Steadily increase ambulation.
- Weigh daily.
- Offer urinal frequently.

Chapter 24 Wound Care and Skin Integrity 561

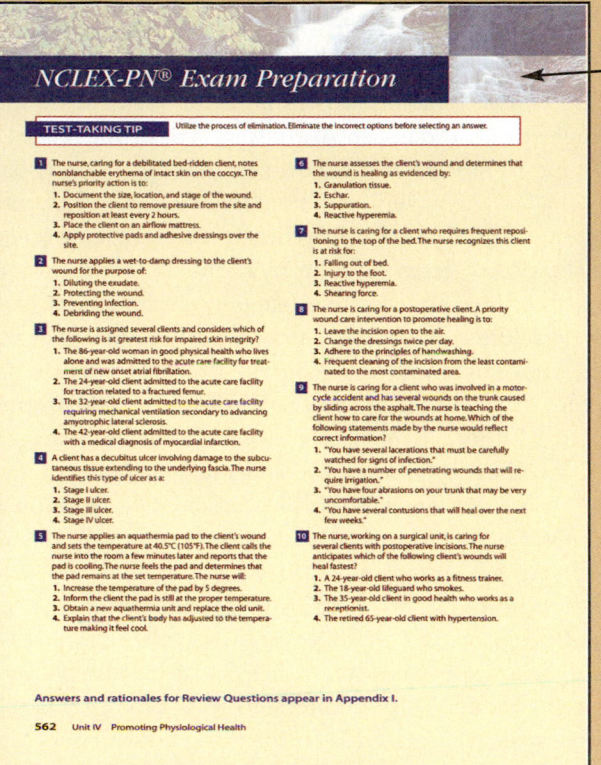

NCLEX-PN® Exam Preparation includes:
- Test-Taking Tip with a focused study hint
- NCLEX-PN® style questions for review and test practice, with both traditional and alternative formats. Answers are found in Appendix I.

After each unit in this book, use the **Thinking Strategically About...** pages as an opportunity to reflect on the important themes across the LPN/LVN curriculum. Short scenarios and project ideas spotlight the unit's content from a variety of angles. Review of concepts enables students to approach unit topics from a more integrated perspective.

Prioritizing Nursing Care questions give students practice in this essential nursing skill.

Critical Thinking questions highlight specific challenges new nurses will face as they strive to provide the best possible care.

Delegation scenarios provide opportunities to identify tasks that can be assigned to unlicensed assistive personnel.

Collaborative Care Strategies challenge students to think concretely about health care settings and to envision the many health care workers who may participate in a client's care.

Conflict Resolution issues help students think ahead about potentially difficult situations.

Culturally Competent Care strengthens the student's confidence by providing information and scenarios to familiarize them with cultural patterns and differences.

Time Management items offer hints for efficiency and organization.

Communication and Team Building presents ideas and activities for becoming a stronger communicator and a more effective professional.

Community Care Strategies discuss the nurse's role and responsibility in and beyond the workplace.

Compassionate Caring focuses on the caring and empathy that are at the core of the nursing profession.

Acknowledgments

Nursing is as exciting a profession today as it was 20, 30, 50, or even 100 years ago. Today people in the hospital require more care, have shorter stays, and are sent home to recover and be cared for by family members or home health nurses. Nurses need to be prepared to take on new care roles. Practical and vocational nurses must be more knowledgeable, and they must understand their scope of practice. The authors have much gratitude for specific LVNs or LPNs who influences their life paths. With this text we hope to express some of that gratitude by assisting today's practical and vocational students to become the nurses of the 21st century.

A project such as this could never have been accomplished without the contribution of many people. A teacher cannot teach without students. Our students have taught us much about persistence, motivation, culture, and life. You are our future and we are confident that you will be a credit to the profession.

Many nursing colleagues have provides us with encouragement. Our contributors provide their knowledge, skill, and time, writing selected chapters in the text. Reviewers provided quality assurance for the book as well as a nationwide perspective. They validated the content and provided objective opinions as this book came into being. Contributors and reviewers for *Comprehensive Nursing Care* are listed with their current affiliations following this preface. We especially want to thank Marti Burton, who provided a review of the entire book and who offered her skills as a nurse educator and writer to make this textbook complete, clear, and always geared directly to students.

The support, skills, and expertise of many people were involved in creating this text. Kelly Trakalo, our editor, has been with us throughout this revision. Her hands-on approach and knowledge of the field has guided us in such a way that this text will be current and competitive as it goes to press. Rachel Bedard, our developmental editor, skillfully turned a manuscript into a book. Our frequent conversations and e-mails have kept this project on track. We have worked and laughed and accomplished a dream. Thank you, Rachel, for keeping us focused on the goal even when the day-to-day details clouded the view. Teresa Himpsl assisted at every turn and kept the organization of materials intact. Lauren Sweeney, editorial assistant, attended to many critical details and coordinated all printed and electronic supplements. Yagnesh Jani, Production Editor, tracked and recorded all the pieces of the project, problem-solved, and monitored quality. Our special thanks are also due to many others. Patrick Walsh (Managing Production Editor), Ilene Sanford (Manufacturing Manager) guided scheduling, production, and manufacturing. Carol Singer, Trish Finley and the capable staff of GGS transformed the manuscript to printed page. Kathy Pruno did a superb copy-editing job, bringing consistency to more than 4000 manuscript pages. Mary Siener created a colorful, integrated design. Bridget Staton, research analyst, solicited information from educators and students, to help us shape the book to their needs. Harper Coles (Senior Marketing Manager) developed the marketing materials to show you this product and consistently offered input about new marketing ideas. Our thanks to all of you!

When this project was in the planning stage, we were asked what would make this book different from what is already available. We thought about all the things we have wished were in the texts we have used over the years. We also considered what students have asked for as support material to classroom lectures. We asked you what would encourage you to read and use a textbook. We have attempted to incorporate your ideas and to make this text "user friendly" for both student and teachers.

It is our hope that this text will enhance your knowledge and that it will make a difference in preparing you for success. We hope that as you enter the profession, you, too, will be a nurse who will make a difference.

About the Authors

Roberta Pavy Ramont, EdD, RN

Roberta Pavy Ramont is the Corporate Director of Nursing for International Education Corporation, where she oversees the nursing program. She is the owner of Educational Innovations, which provides curriculum and program development and assessment for schools offering career technical education. From 1991 to 2003 she was an Instructor of Vocational Nursing at the North Orange County Regional Occupational Program (ROP) in Anaheim, California. She received her initial nursing education at the Cooper Hospital School of Nursing in Camden, New Jersey. She received her baccalaureate degree from the University of Redlands and a masters in psychology–school counseling from the University of LaVerne. Dr. Ramont received her Ed.D. in Educational Leadership with an emphasis in training and development from Alliant International University.

Roberta served as curriculum chair for health careers education at the ROP. During that time she worked with the health occupations faculty to identify academic standards taught in the career technical classes. She has been involved in an extensive project to develop rubrics for alternate assessment of student work.

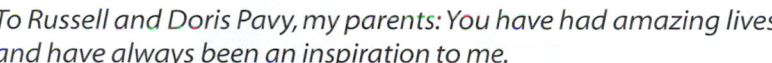

In addition to her teaching responsibilities, she has served as an advisor for Health Occupation Students of America, and as Cal-HOSA Inc. Board of Directors Chair. She served as President of the California Association of Health Careers Educators (CAHCE) during 2000–2001.

Over the years Roberta has had the privilege of serving on the NCLEX-PN® writing panel, and developing and presenting educational seminars on the adult learner and technology in the classroom. She has taught teacher credentialing classes for San Diego University and is serving on a task force with the California Department of Education of Teacher Credentialing for Health Occupation teachers.

Roberta has three children: twin daughters (Amy, an RN; and Alicia, a busy mom and a mortgage title processor); and Tom, a documentary filmmaker. She has three grandchildren: Haley, T.J., and Dylan Thomas. In addition, she has two special sons-in-law, Adam and Blaine, and an extra special daughter-in-law, Charlene. When time permits, she enjoys traveling and reading anything but textbooks. She credits her entrance into nursing to an LVN student who cared for her during an illness and saw something in her that she had not seen herself.

To Russell and Doris Pavy, my parents: You have had amazing lives and have always been an inspiration to me.

Roberta Ramont

Dee Maldonado Niedringhaus, RN, BSN

Dee Maldonado Niedringhaus is an Administrator of Instructional Programs for North Orange County Regional Occupational Programs (ROP). Dee's responsibility includes medical programs ranging from introductory medical care to our model vocational nursing program. Among the many health occupations courses taught are Medical Assistant Front and Back Office, Insurance Billing, Coding, and Emergency Medical Technician. In addition to her medical block, she directs two high schools with ROP classes.

Dee's nursing career began as a Nursing Assistant during her senior year in high school. She was accepted into the Nursing Program at USC/LACMC (Los Angeles County Medical Center) School of Nursing in California and graduated in 1973. She received her baccalaureate in nursing from Excelsior College, New York, in 2003. Dee worked as a Clinical Nurse III on the medical-surgical units at UCIMC (University

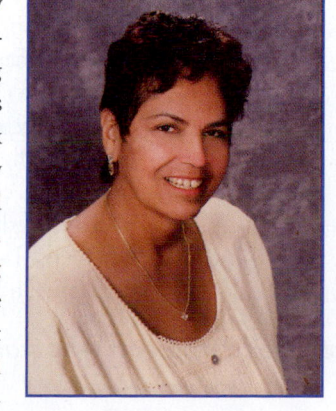

California at Irvine Medical Center) from 1973 to 1985. She taught a Nursing Assistant class during the summer of 1985 and found a new perspective of nursing as an instructor. She found that sharing her dedication to nursing with students was fulfilling and a way to give back to her profession. She then began teaching for the Vocational Nursing Program as a fulltime instructor from 1986 to 2001 at North Orange County ROP.

Dee worked as a Health Careers Consultant for the California Department of Education from 1991 to 2001. She was adjunct faculty to Cal Polytechnic University Pomona to teach and coordinate year III in the Health Careers Education Teacher Preparation Program. Dee developed and revised the curriculum. She was a writer for the Science for Health Care in 1991. She has participated on several committees that aligned the California health careers nursing standards with career performance standards.

California Superintendent Delaine Easton appointed her to the Reauthorization of the 1998 Perkins Advisory Council. Under Dee's administration, North Orange County ROP has added three new medical careers academies in Anaheim and Placentia-Yorba Linda school districts in the past 2 years.

Dee became involved in the California Health Occupations Students of America (Cal-HOSA) program in 1988. She initiated the NOCROP HOSA chapters with many successful levels of student recognition. She served as the Chairman of the Board of Directors, Inc for 1999–2000. She currently serves on the HOSA national Competitive Events Committee. Dee was named outstanding HOSA advisor in 1988 and 1998. In addition, Dee is a member of California Association of Health Careers Educators (CAHCE).

She has served as the Chairperson for the Ways and Means committee, and then as treasurer for the organization. Dee was CAHCE's Teacher of the Year in 1999. Dee was also honored by Orange County Department of Education, as a nominee for Teacher of the Year 2000.

Dee has been married for 35 years to her husband, Lee. They have two children, Josh and Jamie. Josh has completed his AA degree. Jamie has received a BA and teacher credential from Cal State Fullerton University; she is currently teaching third grade. Dee credits her family for her achievements because of their continuing support and encouragement. Dee enjoys traveling with family and friends. She has learned a new skill, scuba diving in tropical waters. Dee believes that nursing has always been at the core of everything she has done in her career.

To my husband, Lee, my children, Jamie and Josh, my father, Emmett Maldonado, and my mother, Dora. Your love and patience have always made the difference in my life.

Dee Maldonado Niedringhaus

Mary Ann Towle, RN, MSN

Mary Ann Towle "always wanted to be a nurse," but teaching science in high school also seemed appealing. After graduating from Idaho State University with a baccalaureate degree in nursing, she married and moved to Boise, Idaho, where she accepted a position at St. Luke's Medical Center. As a new nurse, Mary Ann felt confident with her entry-level knowledge, but was unsure of herself when it came to performing nursing procedures. Several LPNs helped her gain the needed skill and confidence. Within a few months she was working in the Coronary Intensive Care Unit as the evening charge nurse.

While Mary Ann enjoyed the direct client care of the CCU, she felt something was missing in her career. She taught a few in-service programs and workshops to nurses as well as respiratory therapy students from Boise State University. After 3 years, an opportunity became available to teach in the LPN program at Boise State University, and Mary Ann jumped at the chance to combine her love for nursing with her desire to teach.

All faculty in the Vocational-Technical Education programs were required to take education classes to improve their teaching performance. With a husband and two young children to care for and a fulltime teaching position, Mary Ann began attending classes two or three nights a week. In 1983, she completed a master of education degree with a specialty in vocational education. A proponent of life-long learning, Mary Ann again returned to school once her family was grown, and completed a master of science degree in nursing in 1998. Having taught the entire curriculum, Mary Ann sees herself as a generalist with experience in maternity, pediatrics, medical-surgical nursing, and geriatrics.

It has been 32 years since Mary Ann began her career as a nursing instructor at Boise State University. She has been recognized by the American Vocational Association as Vocational Teacher of the Year at the state and regional levels, and first runner-up at the national level. Mary Ann's students have received state and national recognition by Vocational Industrial Clubs of America (VICA).

Mary Ann is a strong advocate for LPNs, and works to advance their education and scope of practice within the healthcare community. Mary Ann feels that role modeling, positive feedback, and reducing the stress involved in learning can help all students develop into quality nurses who can think critically and function in any situation.

To Robert and Roma Messenger, my parents, who started my life's journey and believed in me.

Mary Ann Towle

Contributors

Cynthia Bartlau, MSN, RN, PHN
Long Beach City College
Long Beach, CA
Chapter 27

Michele Blash RN, MSN
Hagerstown Community College
Hagerstown, MD
Chapters 25, 31

Stephanie Bronsky, BSN, RN
TESST College of Technology
Alexandria, VA
Chapter 41

Janet McIlhenny Callaway, RN, BSHS
Everest College
Anaheim, CA
Chapters 33, 34

Peggy Denning, RN, MSN
Tri-State School of Practical Nursing
Erie, PA
Chapter 35

Karen Dietz, RN
North Orange County ROP
Anaheim, CA
Chapter 45

Jeanne Hately, RN, MSN, CNOR PhD
Professional Nurse Consultants, LLC
Aurora, CO
Chapter 8

Cherry A. Karl, RN, MSN, MA, PhD
Anne Arundel Community College
Arnold, MD
Chapter 19

Debra S. McKinney MSN, MBA/HCM, RN
University of Illinois Global Campus
Myrtle Beach, SC
End of chapter NCLEX® Questions
Chapters 13, 21, 32
Instructor and Student Supplements

Janet Tompkins McMahon, RN, MSN
Francis Marion University
Florence, SC
Chapter 47

Jill A. Scott, MS, RN, CNS
Tri-State Business Institute
Erie, PA
Chapter 44

Leann Thrapp-Fields
NewHaven Healing Center
Bolingbrook, IL
Chapter 18

Patricia C. Williams, MSN, RN
Hagerstown Community College
Hagerstown, MD
Chapters 9, 36

Reviewers

We would like to express our deep gratitude to more than 50 of our colleagues from schools across the country who have given their time generously over the last few years to help us create this learning package. These individuals helped us develop this textbook and supplements by reviewing chapters and media, and by answering a myriad of questions right up until time of publication. *Comprehensive Nursing Care* has benefited immeasurably from their efforts, insights, suggestions, objections, encouragement, and inspiration, as well as from their collective vast experience as teachers and nurses.

Donna Alt, RN, MSN
ATA Career Education
Louisville, KY

Sandy Barker, BSRN, MS
Tennessee Technology Center
Elizabethton, TN

LaVon Barrett, MSN, RN
Amarillo College
Amarillo, TX

Rebecca Michelle Barton, RN, BSN
Miami-Jacobs School of Nursing
Springboro, OH

Brenda Basile, RN, MSN
Okefenokee Technical College
Waycross, GA

Tracy Blanc, RN, BSN
Ivy Tech Community College
Terre Haute, IN

Connie J. Booth, RN, MSN
Des Moines Area Community College
Boone, IA

Victoria J. Brown, MSN, RN
Jefferson College
Hillsboro, MO

Brigette L. Casteel, RN, MSN
Mountain Empire Community College
Big Stone Gap, VA

Kerry Cave, RN, BSN
Indian River Community College
Fort Pierce, FL

Kim Cooper, RN, MSN
Ivy Tech Community College
Terre Haute, IN

Michelle D'Arcy-Evans, CN M, PhD
Lewis-Clark State College
Lewiston, ID

Peggy Denning, RN, MSN
Tri-State School of Practical Nursing
Erie, PA

Jodi Dobslaw, MSN, CRNP
Lancaster County Career and Technology Center
Willow Street, PA

Christy Dryer, MSN, RN-C
Cecil College
Northeast, MD

Lula J. English, RN, BSN, MSN
Reid State Technical College
Evergreen, AL

Sally Flesch, RN, PhD
Black Hawk College
Moline, IL

Judy S. Fuhrmann, MS, APRN, BC
Cecil College
MD

Dori Gilman, RN, MS
North Country College of Essex and Franklin County (NCCC)
Saranac Lake, NY

Catherine M. Griswold, RN, MSN, CLNC
Community College of Baltimore County
Baltimore, MD

Karen R. Hazzard, RN, BSN, MSN
Horry Georgetown Technical College
Georgetown, SC

Debra Hodge, RN, MSN
Academy of Careers and Technology
Mountain State University
Beckley, WV

Alice M. Hupp, BS, RN
North Central Texas College
Gainesville, TX

Margaret A. Johnson, RN, MSN
Indian River Community College
Fort Pierce, FL

Cherry A. Karl, RN, MSN, MA, PhD
Anne Arundel Community College
Arnold, MD

Misty Kershner, RN, MSN
Lehigh Carbon Community College
Schnecksville, PA

Thuy Lam, RN, MSN
J. F. Drake State Technical College
Huntsville, AL

Barbara Lee-Learned, MSN, RN
Technical College of the Lowcountry
Beaufort, SC

Carolyn Levi, RN, MSN
Grand Rapids Community College
Grand Rapids, MI

Barbara McGraw, MSN, RN, CNE
Central Community College
Grand Island, NE

Susie McGregor-Huyer, RN, MSN, CHPN, CLNC
University of Phoenix Online
Mahtomedi, IN

Laura M. Moskaluk, BSN, RN
Somerset County Technology Institute
Bridgewater, NJ

Cydney King Mullen, PhD, RN
Sandhills Community College
Pinehurst, NC

Anne Mulligan, BSN, MS
Olympic College
Bremerton, WA

Robbie L. Murphy, BSN, RN/BC-Gerontology
San Jacinto College North Campus
Houston, TX

Carolyn Neal, MSN, RN, CNE
Madisonville Community College
Madisonville, KY

Noel C. Piano, RN, MS
Lafayette School of Practical Nursing
Williamsburg, VA

Jennifer Ponto, RN, BSN
South Plains College
Levelland, TX

Alice Raymond, MSN, CRRN
J.F. Drake State Technical College
Huntsville, AL

Charlotte Riddle, RN, MSN
Tri-state Business Institute
Erie, PA

Elizabeth Rohan, AAS, RN
Wharton County Junior College
Wharton, TX

Terri Rudd, RN, MSN
Mount San Antonio College
Walnut, CA

Jill A. Scott, MS, RN, CNS
Tri-State Business Institute
Erie, PA

Brenda Shields, RN, BSN
Academy of Careers and Technology
Beckley, WV

Amanda Simmons, MSN, RN
Technical College of the Lowcountry
Beaufort, SC

Sue Ellen Smith, RN, MSN, Med
Iowa Western Community College
Council Bluffs, IA

JoAnne Sorci, RN, MS, ANP/BC
Trocaire College
Buffalo, NY

Russlyn St. John, RN, MSN
St. Charles Community College
Cottleville, MO

Martha M. Tingley, RN, MSN
Mercyhurst North East
North East, PA

Frances M. Warrick, MS, RN
El Centro/College
Dallas, TX

Kristi Wilkerson, RN, MSN
Southeastern Community College
West Burlington, IA

Lorraine White, RN, BSN, MA
North Country Community College
Malone, NY

Robyn Whitehair, RN, MSN, ARNP
Madisonville Community College
Madisonville, KY

Dian Wright, MSN, RN, Family Nurse Practitioner, MBA, CCM
Ivy Tech Community College
Sellersburg, IN

Kathleen Young, RN, MSN
Indiana County Technology Center
Indiana, PA

Contents

The Nature of Nursing

UNIT I

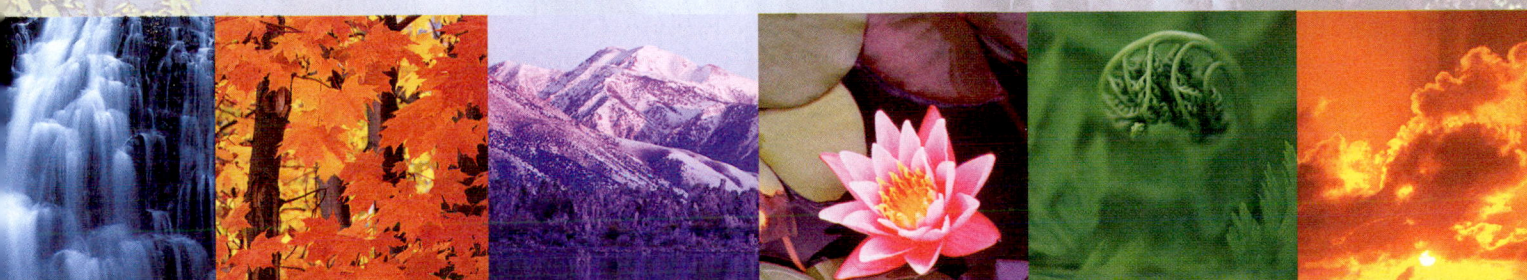

Chapter 1

Succeeding as a Nursing Student

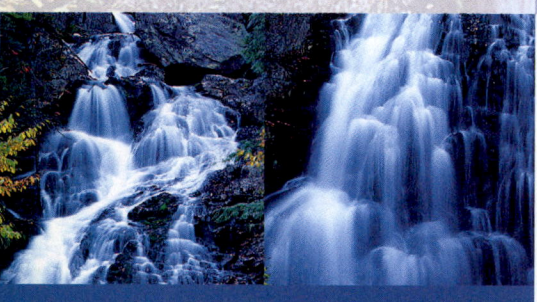

LEARNING Outcomes

After completing this chapter, you will be able to:

1. Relate essential nursing values to attitudes, personal qualities, and professional behaviors.
2. Explain ways to approach this textbook and plan your study time effectively.
3. Discuss the importance of time management for students in a nursing program.
4. Describe three important aspects of time management that support academic survival in nursing education.
5. Identify strategies to use when answering various types of test questions.
6. Discuss the responsibilities of the student nurse during clinical experiences.
7. Explain the importance of prioritizing in the clinical setting.

BRIEF Outline

Nursing Values and Characteristics
Reading This Textbook
Studying Effectively
Managing Time
Taking Tests
Participating in Clinical Experiences
Prioritizing in the Clinical Setting

KEY TERMS

Use the audio glossary feature on the MyNursingKit Website to hear the correct pronunciation of the following key terms.

analysis 6   comprehension 6
application 6   knowledge 6

Welcome to a career in nursing. You have made an excellent choice for a future helping others to regain or maintain health and function. Nursing is full of rewards and challenges that you will encounter while you are a student and also after you graduate. This text is designed to help you recognize and overcome those challenges as well as to appreciate the rewards.

LPN/LVN training programs for licensed practical nurses (LPNs) and licensed vocational nurses (LVNs) can be found in many different types of schools. In some states, they are part of high schools. In others, they are in community college settings, vocational training centers, or private schools.

The governing nursing board in each state dictates the length of the program. Some programs can be completed in about 9 months. Others take up to 2 years. Some are full-time day programs; others are part-time in the evening and/or on weekends.

People with a variety of backgrounds enter the nursing profession. Your classmates may represent a variety of life experiences, educational backgrounds, and ethnic/cultural influences. You can learn a great deal by collaborating with fellow students during your course of study. The ages of LPN/LVN students within a class may range from young adult to near retirement. Motives for attending nursing school may also vary. Students may be realizing a lifelong dream to become a nurse or making a career change.

Nursing Values and Characteristics

You have come to this profession for a variety of reasons, but to be successful, you will come to share certain values and behaviors that are hallmarks of professional nurses. Among these are caring, precision, timeliness, and hygiene. You may not have fully developed these values at this time, but all good nurses understand the importance of these values and strive to maintain them in practice.

Caring is perhaps the core characteristic of nursing. Nurses are guided by a philosophy of caring. By communication, manner, attire, and responsiveness, they show that they respect themselves and others. As a nurse, you care about and promote the health and well-being of the whole person—the physical, mental, emotional, and spiritual aspects that are all involved in a person's well-being.

Precision and timeliness are crucial in quality nursing. To be successful, nurses must value learning to do things accurately and within a given time frame. An example of this is administering medications. It not only would be unprofessional to be imprecise about how much, by what route, or when to give a medication, but also could be harmful or even life threatening to the client.

Good hygiene is another key value for nurses. It takes careful attention to assist clients in healing and to prevent the spread of infection. The importance of cleanliness and the environment was one of the foundations of nursing care first established by Florence Nightingale, and it remains a cornerstone of nursing today.

Besides these values, professional nurses develop characteristics that improve their quality of practice. These include confidentiality, accountability, teamwork, healthy communication, and critical thinking.

Following established guidelines, you will protect the confidentiality of your clients. You will take responsibility for your actions. On a daily basis, you will accept accountability for the safety of those assigned to your care.

As a healthcare team member, you will develop relationships that promote a positive work environment. This will mean broadening your viewpoint and learning to communicate with coworkers who are different from you. It will require you to move past your own biases and assumptions and learn to resolve conflicts that would interfere with quality nursing. In this course, you will learn communication tools and develop interpersonal skills so that you can better relate to clients and coworkers. After examining the elements of communication, you will have many new ways of expressing concern and asking for information.

Finally, you will demonstrate problem-solving skills and learn critical thinking. The elements of critical thinking that you learn here have potential for enriching all areas of your life. They can provide a path to lifelong learning as you enter your nursing career.

Reading This Textbook

It may have been a long time since you studied a subject that really mattered to you, or you may have recently been in school and studied with serious commitment. In either case, here are some academic survival skills to help you in your LPN/LVN course of study.

Begin by reading the preface and other material in the front of the book. Become familiar with how the book is organized and any special features that will make your reading and studying easier. Review the table of contents and look over the appendices. By spending a few minutes becoming familiar with the book, you will be ready to use your book when the first reading assignment is given. The textbook is a great stand-alone reference, as well as a source for clarifying lecture material.

Read through the textbook assignments before the class in which the material will be covered. Reading beforehand will help you organize your thoughts, and help you spell and define words that may be used in a lecture. Although many students use highlighter pens while reading, it is much better to save the highlighter for reviewing lecture notes or marking the location of answers to the chapter's study questions (Porter, n.d.).

Studying Effectively

It is easy to stare at a page of text and feel that you have spent time studying when, in fact, you may have understood very little. When you have a block of time set aside to study, make sure you use it wisely. For hints about what is most important in the text, look at the Learning Outcomes at the beginning of each chapter. These objectives guide you in discovering the information you need to obtain from the chapter as you read and study. For example, when an objective states, "Identify three strategies to use when . . . ," go to the text, find all three strategies, and write them down. As you study, review those three strategies and when you would use them.

Another technique to employ when studying is outlining. Some students find it helpful to outline the chapter after reading it. Under the main ideas, they organize the concepts and the information that supports those ideas. You can easily do this by using the main headings in the chapter as outline headings, then listing two or three main ideas from the paragraphs beneath those headings.

Study questions at the end of the chapter and/or in the student workbooks are another way to help you pull out the most important information in a chapter. First, try to answer the questions from what you have read and understood. If you are unable to answer them correctly or at all, look up the information within the chapter to find the correct answer. This will help you remember the information better than simply looking up each answer. Some students find it helpful to make up their own study questions. They try to anticipate what instructors might ask, using information from class notes.

Take advantage of all available tools. Use a computer at school or at home to access the Companion Website (www.prenhall.com/ramont) or the student CD for this text. These tools provide additional questions and case studies to bring the information to life and to prepare you for future practice. The website and CD also supply links to the Internet to help you with your school projects and research.

Studying with another person or a group of three or four people can be helpful in processing information and discussing ideas. To be successful, the groups must be well-organized. Study groups are discussed further in the next section.

Managing Time

The "average" LPN/LVN student is far from average. Proposing a one-time management template that would work for everyone is impossible. Still, being organized and having a plan will help you work within your time limits. Learning to manage your time is a skill that will benefit you during the nursing program and also in your career and in life.

Learning how to be a good student may be the most important lesson during the first few weeks of your nursing program. Study skills will support you throughout your student days and as you prepare for exams. The time taken to perfect these skills will be hours well spent. Figure 1-1 ■ illustrates a sample time management schedule.

PLANNING CALENDAR

To keep from feeling overwhelmed by your new role and its demands, start by using the following suggestions for time management:

- Obtain a blank calendar or planner for the entire year.
- Fill in holidays, vacations, medical or dental appointments, class times, and clinical days as soon as you know them.
- Add due dates, tests, homework, and projects as they are assigned.
- Schedule study time by writing it on your calendar or planner.
- Schedule personal time for relaxation and being with other people.

GROUP STUDY SESSIONS

Group study time can be very useful when you participate regularly. Learn to plan your group study time, just as you would plan other parts of your day. Stay focused on content, and resist the urge to talk about other things that are not study material. Bring four or five questions with you to discuss with the group. This can be especially helpful if you are having difficulty understanding certain concepts.

It is a good idea to break a study session down into segments. For example, a 2-hour session might include 30 minutes of lecture note review, 20 minutes of shared questions

	Monday	Tuesday	Wednesday	Thursday	Friday	Saturday	Sunday
0600	Sleep	Sleep	Sleep	Shower/dress	Shower/dress	Shower/dress	Sleep
0700	Shower/dress	Shower/dress	Shower/dress	Clinical	Clinical	Work	Sleep
0800	Class	Class	Class				Shower/dress
0900							Breakfast
1000							Church
1100							
1200	Lunch	Lunch	Lunch	Lunch	Lunch	Lunch	
1300	Class	Class					
1400		Library	Group project				Dinner with family
1500							
1600							
1700	Dinner	Dinner	Dinner	Dinner	Dinner	Dinner	
1800						Movie	
1900	Study group	Study	Study	Study			Laundry
2000							Study
2100			Personal time	Personal time			
2200	Personal time	Personal time	Sleep	Sleep	Personal time		Personal time
2300	Sleep	Sleep	Sleep	Sleep	Sleep		Sleep

Figure 1-1. ■ Sample time management schedule.

and answers, a 10-minute break, 30 minutes of quizzing, and 30 minutes of review of class objectives. This plan gives focus to the study time. The change in activities also helps to sustain people's interest and energy levels.

MAINTAINING CURRENT RESPONSIBILITIES

Another aspect of time management is the realization that involvement in a concentrated educational program such as an LPN/LVN program will impact your life as well as that of your family. Just because you are now a student, you cannot put the rest of your life on hold. You will still have family, financial, and personal responsibilities. It may be necessary to cut back on some of your extracurricular activities, but you should make every effort to maintain relationships with family and friends who support your goal of becoming an LPN/LVN. Unfortunately, there may be people in your life who are not supportive. If you have unsupportive people in your life, limit your contact with them, especially at times when you need encouragement.

A significant number of LPN/LVN students have children. Their needs cannot be ignored. Child care needs to be arranged, as well as backup, and it is also a good idea to have backup for your backup. Clinical days start early, so be sure that your day care accepts children early enough to meet your needs.

Previously we talked about study time. Trying to study when your children need attention takes skill and planning. Many students set a family study-time. Older children do their homework or read to younger children while mom or dad completes reading assignments, too. This can have a positive effect on children; as they observe a parent studying, they will imitate the behavior.

No matter how busy you are with school responsibilities, be sure to take time to show interest in what is going on in your family's day. On that wonderful day when you have finally reached your goal, your family will feel like this is something you have all accomplished together.

FINANCIAL PLANNING

Hopefully you have been able to plan financially for the next year. You will need to adjust your work schedule so that it does not conflict with your school or clinical schedule. It is most desirable to limit your work hours. If that is not possible, be sure you have talked in depth with your supervisor about your schedule. Most supervisors are willing to work with you as long as you give them sufficient notice. If you are working in the healthcare field, discuss your future with the organization when you complete your program. Some organizations offer reduced hours or financial assistance with the commitment of continued employment once you have graduated.

Your instructors will probably give you a calendar with test dates at the beginning of each course or module. When you have that information, arrange your work schedule with your supervisor so that you will not have to work a late shift the night before a final exam. This is a much better solution than to call in sick at work at the last minute.

Being a nursing student is a real balancing act. There may be times when you feel that everyone and everything is working against you. At these times, the effort you have put in to preplan will help you cope with the unexpected.

Taking Tests

ANSWERING MULTIPLE-CHOICE QUESTIONS

Most tests given in nursing programs will be objective, multiple-choice tests. These are the same types of questions used on the NCLEX-PN® exam. Multiple-choice questions can evaluate your knowledge of the facts, as well as your ability to apply that knowledge within a client care scenario. Each question will consist of a stem and answer choices. Read each question completely in order to understand what is being asked. Then read each of the choices. Try to eliminate one or more of the choices. Examine each choice to see if anything is incorrect within the answer itself. Watch out for choices that are correct and accurate on

their own, but that do not answer the question as it is written. See Box 1-1 ■ for an example.

Multiple-choice questions can test **knowledge, comprehension, application,** and **analysis** ability of the student. Table 1-1 ■ provides examples and comparisons of each type.

Questions that include choices such as "all of the above" or "none of the above" have been eliminated from the NCLEX-PN® examination. However, some textbooks have them as study questions, and some instructors may test

BOX 1-1	EXAMPLE OF A MULTIPLE-CHOICE QUESTION

Which of the following men was responsible for the reduction of maternal death related to infection transmitted by way of unwashed hands?

1. Joseph Lister
2. Louis Pasteur
3. Ignaz Semmelweis
4. Karl Crede

Although all four people were involved in prevention of infection and/or disease, the correct answer is 3. Ignaz Semmelweis was the person who discovered that puerperal fever was related to examination of mothers during the intra- and postpartum periods by doctors who had not washed their hands after performing autopsies.

TABLE 1-1	Test Questions and Levels of Learning		
LEVEL	**INFORMATION REQUIRED**	**EXAMPLE**	**RATIONALE**
Knowledge question	Requires recall of information. To answer a knowledge question, you need to commit facts to memory. Knowledge questions expect you to know terminology, specific facts, trends, sequences, classifications, categories, criteria, structures, principles, generalization, and/or theories.	What does the abbreviation BRP mean? a. Bathe daily b. Bed rest patient c. Blood pressure reading d. Bathroom privileges	To answer this question correctly, you have to know the meaning of the abbreviation BRP (bathroom privileges, answer d)
Comprehension question	Requires you to understand information. To answer a comprehension question, you must not only commit facts to memory, but also be able to translate, interpret, and determine the implications of information. You demonstrate understanding when you translate or paraphrase information, interpret or summarize information, or determine the implications of information. Comprehension questions expect you not only to know but also to understand the information being tested. You do not necessarily have to relate it to other material or see its fullest implications.	To evaluate the therapeutic effect of a cathartic, the nurse should assess the client for: a. Increased urinary output. b. A decrease in anxiety. c. A bowel movement. d. Pain relief.	To answer this question, you have to know not only that a cathartic is a potent laxative that stimulates the bowel, but also that the increase in peristalsis will result in a bowel movement (answer c).

TABLE 1-1	Test Questions and Levels of Learning (continued)		
LEVEL	**INFORMATION REQUIRED**	**EXAMPLE**	**RATIONALE**
Application question	Requires you to utilize knowledge. To answer an application question, you must take remembered and comprehended concepts and apply them to concrete situations. The abstractions may be theories, technical principles, rules of procedures, generalizations, or ideas that have to be applied in a scenario. Application questions test your ability to use information in a new situation.	An elderly client's skin looks dry, thin, and fragile. When providing back care, the nurse should: a. Apply a moisturizing body lotion. b. Wash back with soap and water. c. Massage back using short kneading strokes. d. Leave excess lubricant on the client's skin.	To answer this question, you must know that dry, thin, fragile skin is common in the elderly and that moisturizing lotion helps the skin to retain water and become more supple. When presented with this scenario, you have to apply your knowledge concerning developmental changes in the elderly and the benefits of using moisturizing lotion (answer a).
Analysis question	Requires you to interpret a variety of data and recognize the commonalities, differences, and interrelationships among present ideas. Analysis questions make assumptions that you know, understand, and can apply information. Now you must identify, examine, dissect, evaluate, or investigate the organization, systematic arrangement, or structure of the information presented in the question. This type of question tests your analytical ability.	A client who is undergoing cancer chemotherapy says to the nurse, "This is no way to live." Which of the following responses uses reflective technique? a. "Tell me more about what you are thinking." b. "You sound discouraged today." c. "This is all really hard to handle." d. "What are you saying?"	To answer this question, you must understand the communication techniques of reflection, clarification, and paraphrasing. You must also analyze the statements and identify which techniques are represented. This question requires you to understand, interpret, and differentiate information to know that the correct answer would be c.

with them. A choice of this type can be confirmed or eliminated easily. If you have identified one choice as being correct, then you can eliminate "none of the above." If you can identify one choice that is incorrect, then "all of the above" can also be eliminated. If you can identify at least two answers as correct, then the question qualifies as an "all of the above" answer.

If you are able to narrow your choice to two options, don't spend too much time deciding between them. More likely than not, your first impression is correct. Once you have identified your choice, do not go back and change it unless you later figure out the correct response with absolute certainty.

Most questions on the NCLEX-PN® exam are standard multiple choice, but some new types of questions are being added. Answering the study questions at the end of each chapter and in the student workbook will help you improve your ability to select correct answers in objective tests and prepare for the NCLEX-PN® exam. The NCLEX-PN® exam is discussed in more detail in Chapter 64 ⟨⟩.

Several techniques are useful in calling information to mind during a test (Figure 1-2 ■). For example, by using visualization, you may be able to "see" in your mind a poster or handout that was used during a class presentation. With some practice, you may be able to visualize a word or a passage that you read in the textbook.

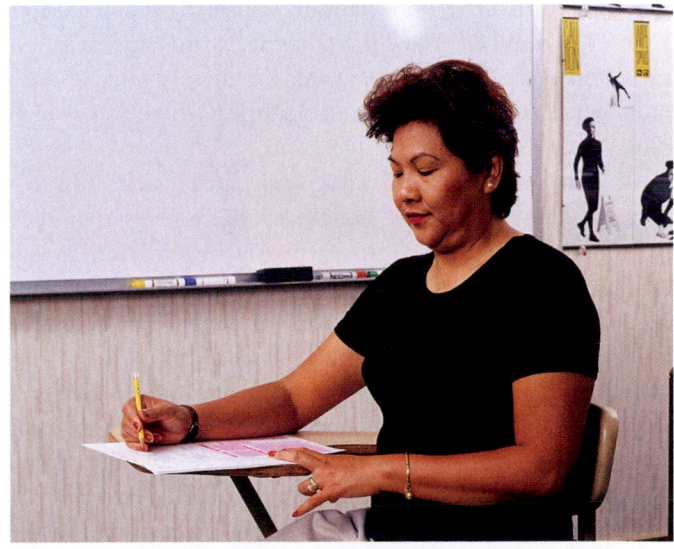

Figure 1-2. ■ Organize your thoughts prior to test taking, and pay attention to key words in questions. *Source:* Pearson Education/PH College.

ANSWERING ESSAY, SHORT-ANSWER, AND CALCULATION QUESTIONS

Answers to essay, short-answer, and calculation questions will require you to remember content and apply it as requested. Read the question carefully to determine what is being asked. Some students find it helpful to develop a brief

TABLE 1-2	Key Words in Essay Exams
KEY WORD	**EXPLANATION**
Compare	To point out similarities and differences
Contrast	To point out differences only
Define	Several connotations: (1) to give the meaning of, (2) to explain or describe essential qualities, (3) to place it in the class to which it belongs and set it off from other items in the same class
Describe	Enumerate (list) the special features of the topic
	Show how the topic is different from similar or related items
	Give an account of, tell about, or give a word picture of the topic
Discuss	Present various sides or points, talk over, consider the different sides; a discussion is usually longer than an explanation of the same subject
Explain	Make plain or clear, interpret, tell "how" to do
Identify	Show recognition
Illustrate	Describe in narrative form using "word pictures" to provide examples
Justify	Provide supporting data for opinions or actions
List or name	Present a group of names or items in a category
Outline	Give information systematically in headings and subheadings
Summarize	Present in condensed form; give main points briefly

outline before beginning an essay question. Check with the instructor to see if this can be written on the test paper or if you are permitted to use an additional sheet. The outline can help you organize your thoughts and can serve as a checkpoint that all important information was included. Usually, a number of key introductory words appear in essay questions (Table 1-2 ■). Look for these words, and do only what is required of you. Ignoring these key words causes many low grades.

Calculation questions are particularly troubling for many students who have convinced themselves that they cannot do math. Although math may be difficult, it is a necessary skill for a nurse. With extra practice, calculations are possible to learn. Several methods are used to do calculations (see Chapter 27 ⬭).

It is important that you show your work on calculations. If you are unable to arrive at the correct answer, your instructor can review your work and will be able to tell you where you went wrong. Memorizing formulas and frequently used conversions will make calculations on tests and in the clinical area much easier.

Participating in Clinical Experiences

A major part of your learning will occur during your clinical experiences. You will be assigned to assist with the care of one or more clients in a healthcare setting. This experience is extremely valuable in preparing you for the profession you have chosen. You will find that observing signs

and symptoms of an illness firsthand is far more impressive than reading about them.

At first you will care for just one client, with assistance from other healthcare workers as needed. As you progress through your course of study, you will be assigned more responsibility and more clients. The clients you care for will have more complex illnesses and needs. When you study and learn about performing skills and signs to watch for, you are learning what you need to know to be a safe healthcare practitioner.

As a student, your responsibilities in preparing for clinical experience include:

- Ensuring that you understand what you read and how to apply it to the care of real clients.
- Practicing skills repeatedly so that you know exactly what to do when called on to perform those skills quickly and efficiently in the clinical setting.
- Researching information about an assigned client's medical diagnosis, nursing diagnoses, problems, and needs so that you are prepared and can anticipate what could happen as you care for that client.
- Asking for help when you are not sure how to proceed, but proceeding when you are sure of what you need to do.
- Reporting any and all deviations from the baseline that you observe while caring for clients. (You may not realize the significance of your observation, especially early in the program, but other healthcare professionals will know what actions to take.)
- Taking advantage of all learning opportunities in the clinical setting. If a procedure is being done, ask if you

can observe, even though the client may not be assigned to you. Spend any "downtime" during your clinical experience observing, assisting, or listening to healthcare staff.

Prioritizing in the Clinical Setting

There are two major classifications of students who enter an LPN/LVN program: those with no previous healthcare experience, and those who have been trained and have worked as a nursing assistant, medical assistant, or other unlicensed healthcare worker. Nursing assistants are used to caring for a large number of clients, but their care has been limited to activities of daily living (ADL) and vital signs. Data collection, medications and treatments, and documentation must be added to the general care. It will no longer be sufficient just to deliver good care. You will also need to make observations and think critically about what those observations say about your client's condition.

The student who has worked as a medical assistant usually has good organizational skills, but he or she has not previously given complete client care such as bathing and bed making. These skills can be learned quickly. No matter what your background, you will need to learn how to prioritize in the clinical setting.

Prioritization begins before you walk onto the nursing unit at the beginning of your shift. Some schools will have the student go to the unit the evening before to review their assigned clients' medical records. Others have the

A

| Rm Number: _____ |
| Dr.: _____ |
| Code Status: Full DNR _____ |
| Allergies: _____ |
| _____ |
| Admitting Dx: _____ |
| _____ |
| DIET: _____ |
| _____ |

| Vitals: |
| 0800 B/P ____ AP ____ RR ____ Temp ____ |
| 1200 B/P ____ AP ____ RR ____ Temp ____ |

| Focus System: |
| Neuro Cardio Resp GI GU |
| Integ Psychosocial |

Nursing Dx: _____

Foley   IV: _____   Oxygen: _____

Other: _____

Neuro: _____

Cardio: _____

Resp: _____

PROCEDURES TO BE DONE:

ACCUCHECK   DRESSING time: _____

0700 _____   Loc: _____

1130 _____   Type: _____

Daily Weight _____   Size: _____

_____   Desc: _____

GI: _____

GU: _____

Integ: _____

Med Calculations:
On Hand   Ordered Give

	0700 _____ 1100 _____
	0800 _____ 1200 _____
	0900 _____ 1300 _____
	1000 _____ 1400 _____

	LABS	
4.3 – 10.8	WBC	_____
13 – 18	Hgb	_____
45 – 52	Hct	_____
150 – 450	Platelets	_____
70 – 110	Glucose	_____
3.5 – 5.5	K^+	_____
135 – 145	Na^+	_____
98 – 106	Cl^+	_____
7 – 18	BUN	_____
1 – 2	Creatinine	_____
35 – 45	CO_2	_____

PRE-OP	
LAB TESTS	_____
Informed consent signed?	_____
Check NPO	_____
GI prep	_____
Skin prep	_____
Resp prep	_____
Teach coughing	_____
Circulation	_____
Vital signs	_____
Catheter insertion	_____
Remove dentures (etc.)	_____

POST-OP	
Assess vitals	_____
Do assessment	_____
15 × 4	_____
30 × 4	_____
1hr × 4	_____
Pt on side or 45°	_____
Emesis basin present	_____
Blankets	_____
Check incision	_____
Check Foley	_____
TC DB q 2°	_____

Figure 1-3. ■ Student report sheets. **A.** Form where students hold information about a client.

B

Team Member				Break		Conference		Lunch			Date	
Team Leader			Special Assignment									
Room	Client	Bath	Activity	Diet	Fluids	To Be Checked		Treatments			Comments	
		Bed Self* Shower Tub Sitz	Bed Dangle BRP BRP help AMB. AMB. help Walker Crutches W.C.	Regular Soft Surg. liq. Full liq. Special NPO Tube feeding	Force NPO Limit Sips water Ice chips IV Dist. water	Blood pressure TPR Test urine ac & hs I & O Chest tube Foley Oxygen		Enema Harris Flush Douche Peri-care–Light Weigh Oral hygiene Special back care Prepare for surgery Prepare for x-ray O.T. P.T. E.C.T.				
		Bed Self* Shower Tub Sitz	Bed Dangle BRP BRP help AMB. AMB. help Walker Crutches W.C.	Regular Soft Surg. liq. Full liq. Special NPO Tube feeding	Force NPO Limit Sips water Ice chips IV Dist. water	Blood pressure TPR Test urine ac & hs I & O Chest tube Foley Oxygen		Enema Harris Flush Douche Peri-care–Light Weigh Oral hygiene Special back care Prepare for surgery Prepare for x-ray O.T. P.T. E.C.T.				
		Bed Self* Shower Tub Sitz	Bed Dangle BRP BRP help AMB. AMB. help Walker Crutches W.C.	Regular Soft Surg. liq. Full liq. Special NPO Tube feeding	Force NPO Limit Sips water Ice chips IV Dist. water	Blood pressure TPR Test urine ac & hs I & O Chest tube Foley Oxygen		Enema Harris Flush Douche Peri-care–Light Weigh Oral hygiene Special back care Prepare for surgery Prepare for x-ray O.T. P.T. E.C.T.				
		Bed Self* Shower Tub Sitz	Bed Dangle BRP BRP help AMB. AMB. help Walker Crutches W.C.	Regular Soft Surg. liq. Full liq. Special NPO Tube feeding	Force NPO Limit Sips water Ice chips IV Dist. water	Blood pressure TPR Test urine ac & hs I & O Chest tube Foley Oxygen		Enema Harris Flush Douche Peri-care–Light Weigh Oral hygiene Special back care Prepare for surgery Prepare for x-ray O.T. P.T. E.C.T.				
		Bed Self* Shower Tub Sitz	Bed Dangle BRP BRP help AMB. AMB. help Walker Crutches W.C.	Regular Soft Surg. liq. Full liq. Special NPO Tube feeding	Force NPO Limit Sips water Ice chips IV Dist. water	Blood pressure TPR Test urine ac & hs I & O Chest tube Foley Oxygen		Enema Harris Flush Douche Peri-care–Light Weigh Oral hygiene Special back care Prepare for surgery Prepare for x-ray O.T. P.T. E.C.T.				

Codes: *You wash back and legs
BRP Bathroom Privileges
AMB. Ambulatory
I & O Intake and Output

W.C. Wheelchair
BP Blood Pressure
NPO Nothing by Mouth
Dist. Distilled water

O.T. Occupational Therapy
P.T. Physical Therapy
E.C.T. Electroconvulsive Therapy

IV Intravenous
ac Before meals
hs At bedtime

Figure 1-3. ■ *Continued.* **B.** Form to use for several clients, including the tasks assigned to the student.

instructor make the assignment early on each clinical day and review the clients with the students during a pre-conference period. Both systems require that the student review the pertinent client information prior to delivering care. Many students make use of a report sheet to write down information about their clients that they will need during the shift. Figure 1-3 ■ illustrates an example of a student report sheet.

Once the shift report has been concluded, visit each of your clients and introduce yourself. Explain how each one fits into your plan for the day. You can say something like this: "Good morning, Mr. Torres, my name is Mary Jane Blaine and I am a practical nursing student at Vista College. I will be working with your nurse, Ms. Wheeler, today. I will be providing all your care, but feel free to call for Ms. Wheeler if you have any questions. My instructor is Ms. Saunders and she will be observing me as I provide some of your care. She may also ask you questions about the care I have provided. I have another assigned client I need to prepare for a procedure. Once I have completed that task, I will return and help you to get ready for breakfast. Is there

anything that you need immediately? If not, I will return in about 20 minutes." Your client now knows what to expect. As appropriate, you could add information about tests or procedures that are scheduled or ancillary services that the client will have during the day.

You will be able to collect data about your client's physical condition. This is done by a head-to-toe examination. The data collection needs to be accomplished prior to administering medication. Preparation of medications will take a good deal of time. If you are able to review your client's medical record the evening before, you will be able to research the medications and make a med card for each medication. Otherwise, gather the information you will need from your drug guide and make a card when you get home that night. In a few weeks, you will have a collection of drug cards for most of the drugs you will be giving. Prior to administering medications, review pertinent information from medication cards, and check for lab values that may be related to the drugs you will be giving. When it is time for your instructor to review your medications, you will be prepared and the process will go smoothly.

Advanced students or new graduates may tell you that they never have time to take a break. This is a bad habit to establish. First, many states require employees to take their designated breaks and lunch. Also, you need that time to regroup and nourish yourself so that you can work effectively. Having the time to take breaks and lunch is a matter of organization and time management. If you organize your day to include these two items, you will soon see that it is possible to complete your assignment and also take your breaks.

Flexibility is also a very important skill in prioritizing your clinical day. Nursing can be unpredictable: an emergency may occur, you may be assigned a newly admitted client, or a physician may decide to do a complicated procedure at the bedside. Do not let these things throw you. Make adjustments to your plan and move ahead.

Postconferences are an important part of the student's clinical day. This is an opportunity to discuss your day with your peers and your instructor. Sharing like this among students helps you to see where you could have been more efficient or allows you to pass on something that worked well for you. Once your organizational skills become well developed and your instructor is confident in your abilities and skills, you may be assigned as team leader. When you serve as team leader, you will be responsible for assisting several students and providing an extra pair of eyes and ears for the instructor. This is an opportunity where your organizational skills and your ability to prioritize can shine. Your clinical experience is a very important part of your nursing program. As you perfect your skills, practice your critical thinking, prioritization, and organizational skills. These will prepare you to be a competent and efficient nurse.

Although prioritizing and flexibility are important, the safety of the client, oneself, and one's coworkers must always be foremost in the nurse's mind. Safe practice includes personal safety as well as safety in administering medications. For specific guidelines for safety, see Chapter 9 ⚭. For the major discussion of infection control, see Chapter 10 ⚭.

Note: The references and resources for all chapters have been compiled at the back of the book.

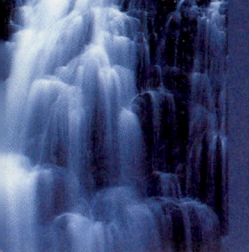

Chapter Review

KEY Points

- Learning good study skills now will serve you for the rest of your career.
- Knowing how to get an overview of a task, organize your time, and break large jobs into smaller tasks are all life skills that will help you both inside and outside of nursing.
- Spending a few minutes becoming familiar with the textbook will help you to be ready when the first reading assignment is given.
- The textbook is a great stand-alone reference, as well as a source for clarifying lecture material.
- Once you have identified your choice on a multiple-choice question, don't go back and change it unless you later figure out the correct response with absolute certainty.
- Comprehension questions expect you not only to know but also to understand the information being tested.
- Analysis questions make assumptions that you know, understand, and can apply information.
- It is important for you to review pertinent client information prior to delivering care. Once you know what needs to be done for your assigned client(s), you will be able to prioritize your day in order to accomplish all tasks in an appropriate and safe manner for your client and yourself.
- Prioritizing and being flexible is important, but the safety of the client, personal safety, and safety of coworkers must always be on the nurse's mind.

∞ FOR FURTHER Study

For specific safety guidelines, see the major discussion of safety in Chapter 9.

See Chapter 10 for a full discussion on infection control.

Math calculation methods and medication administration are described in Chapter 27.

The NCLEX-PN® exam is discussed in detail in Chapter 64.

PEARSON

EXPLORE **mynursingkit**™

MyNursingKit is your one stop for online chapter review materials and resources. Prepare for success with additional NCLEX®-style practice questions, interactive assignments and activities, web links, animations and videos, and more!

Register your access code from the front of your book at
www.mynursingkit.com

NCLEX-PN® Exam Preparation

1 A question that requires you to use knowledge, as well as take remembered and comprehended abstractions and apply them to concrete situations, is what type of question?
1. Knowledge
2. Comprehension
3. Application
4. Analysis

2 Which of the following indicates that the student needs more understanding of roles and responsibilities in the clinical setting?
1. The student has read about the clinical situation and understands how to apply the information to the care of individualized clients.
2. The student has practiced a skill repeatedly and can perform it quickly and efficiently in the clinical setting.
3. The student is not sure how to proceed but makes an educated guess and completes the procedure.
4. The student reports deviations from baseline to the team leader.

3 The new student nurse understands that which of the following situations demonstrate essential values of nursing? (Select all that apply.)
1. The student explains to the instructor that the appendectomy in room 208 is experiencing pain and has not had pain medication since 4 hours ago.
2. The student nurse requests a special diet for the client with religious beliefs forbidding meat products.
3. The student nurse takes notes to write a care plan but uses care not to include the client's name or any identifying information.
4. The student nurse makes a mistake while providing care to the client and immediately informs the instructor of the error.
5. The student nurse tells the client that the respiratory therapist does not know what he or she is doing but reassures the client that the nurse will supervise to make sure nothing is done wrong.

4 The student nurse has been given a textbook to be used in class. Which of the following should the student do before beginning to read the textbook? (Select all that apply.)
1. Read the preface.
2. Review the table of contents.
3. Look over appendices.
4. Highlight the first sentence in every paragraph.
5. Become familiar with the organization of the book.

5 When should the student nurse read for the first time the material that will be covered in class on Tuesday?
1. After the lecture so the information is familiar.
2. The weekend following the lecture so he or she can cover all the material for the week at the same time.
3. The night before the lecture.
4. There is no need to read the material if the lecture is thorough.

6 When studying for a quiz, the student nurse recognizes which of the following as an excellent hint to determine what will be in the test and what to study?
1. The biggest headings in the book
2. The boldest headings in the book
3. The things in the textbook that are italicized
4. The learning outcomes

7 Which of the following statements reflects a student nurse with good time management skills?
1. "Every student nurse should follow the same time management plan in order to succeed in nursing school."
2. "I got a calendar for the entire year and will fill in holidays, vacations, appointments, and school days as I learn about them."
3. "I plan to study whenever time allows throughout the day."
4. "I have filled every minute of the day with school, home, and family responsibilities and know that I won't have any personal time until I graduate."

8 The student nurse recognizes which of the following as important aspects of time management for academic survival? (Select all that apply.)
1. Maintain a planning calendar.
2. Maintain current responsibilities.
3. Plan his or her finances.
4. Ask the instructor to reduce homework assignments to prevent overload.
5. Reduce sleep time to no more than 4 hours per night.

9 The student nurse is taking the first quiz in the nursing program. Which of the following guidelines does the student follow when answering multiple-choice questions in order to improve a test score?
1. Read each question and all answer choices carefully and completely.
2. Try to choose the answer that includes terms like "always" or "never" because they are usually correct.
3. After completing the test, go back and change answers that seem wrong on second thought.
4. If there is a term in one of the answer choices that is unfamiliar, that is probably the correct answer.

10 What is the most important reason for the student nurse to prioritize in the clinical setting?
1. Each client has different needs and it is important to provide care in a logical manner that meets the most urgent needs first.
2. The student nurse will fail clinical if he or she is not able to prioritize.
3. Clients will get angry if the student nurse does not provide care in the correct order.
4. Good prioritizing skills will allow the student to be assigned more clients.

Answers and rationales for Review Questions appear in Appendix I.

Chapter 2

History of Nursing

LEARNING Outcomes

After completing this chapter, you will be able to:

1. Discuss historical and contemporary factors influencing the development of nursing.
2. Briefly discuss the key figures in nursing history.
3. Outline the contribution made to the profession by males.
4. Identify four major areas within the scope of LPN/LVN scope of practice.
5. Explain key contributions in practical/vocational nursing history.
6. Discuss the customers, purpose, standards, and work settings of LPNs/LVNs.
7. Identify professional organizations for the LPN/LVN and nursing students.

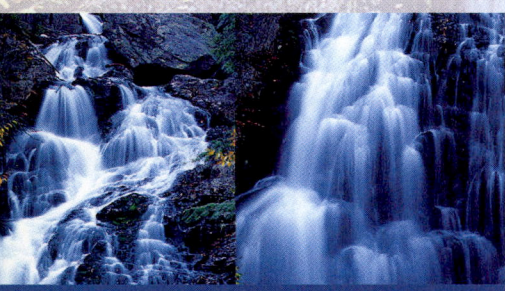

BRIEF Outline

Influences on the Development of Nursing

Leading Nurses of History

History of LPNs/LVNs

Practical and Vocational Nursing Today

Professional Organizations for LPN/LVN Students and Graduates

To fully appreciate your position as a contemporary LPN/LVN, you need to understand a bit about the history of nursing. Many women and men have been influential in developing nursing into the profession it is today.

Influences on the Development of Nursing

Nursing has undergone dramatic changes in response to societal needs and influences. A look at nursing's origins reveals its continuing struggle for autonomy and professionalization. In recent decades, a renewed interest in nursing history has produced a growing amount of related literature. This section highlights only selected aspects of events that have influenced nursing practice.

RELIGION

Although many of the world's religions encourage benevolence, Western nursing was strongly influenced by the Christian value of "love thy neighbor as thyself" and Christ's parable of the Good Samaritan. During the third and fourth centuries, several wealthy matrons of the Roman Empire, including Marcella, Fabiola (Figure 2-1 ■), and Paula, converted to Christianity and used their wealth to provide houses of care and healing (the forerunner of hospitals) for the poor, the sick, and the homeless.

These "deaconess groups" were suppressed during the Middle Ages by Western churches. However, groups of nursing providers resurfaced occasionally throughout the centuries. In 1836, Theodor Fliedner reinstituted the Order of Deaconesses and opened a small hospital and training school in Kaiserswerth, Germany. Florence Nightingale (Figure 2-2 ■) received her "training" in nursing at the Kaiserswerth School.

Early religious values, such as self-denial, spiritual calling, and devotion to duty and hard work, have dominated nursing throughout its history. Nurses' commitment to these values often resulted in exploitation and few monetary rewards. For some time, nurses themselves believed it was inappropriate to expect economic gain from their "calling."

WAR

Throughout history the need for nurses always increased during times of war. During the Crimean War (1854–1856), the inadequacy of care given to soldiers led to a public outcry in Great Britain. The role Florence Nightingale played in addressing this problem is well known. She was asked by Sir Sidney Herbert of the British War Department to recruit a group of female nurses to provide care to the sick and injured in Crimea. Nightingale and her nurses transformed the military hospitals by setting up kitchens, a laundry, recreation centers, and reading rooms and by organizing classes for orderlies. Nightingale is credited with performing miracles. The mortality rate in the Barrack Hospital in Turkey, for example, was reduced to 1 percent by the end of the war.

During the American Civil War (1861–1865), several nurses contributed greatly to a country torn by internal strife. Harriet Tubman and Sojourner Truth (Figure 2-3 ■) provided care and safety to slaves fleeing to the North on the "Underground Railroad." Mother Biekerdyke and Clara Barton searched the battlefields and gave care to injured and dying soldiers. Noted authors Walt Whitman and Louisa May Alcott volunteered as nurses to give care to injured soldiers in military hospitals.

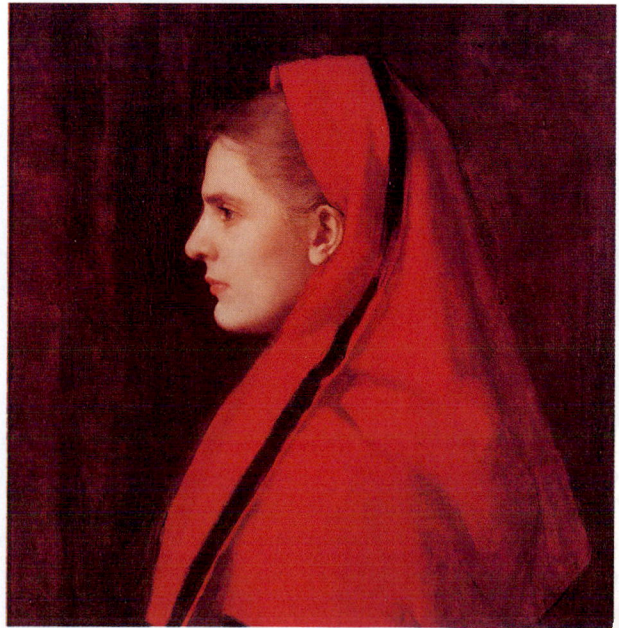

Figure 2-1. ■ Wealthy Roman matrons like Fabiola (circa A.D. 400)—viewed by some as the patron saint of early nursing—u position and wealth to establish hospitals for the sick. Fabiola Jean-Jacques Henner (1829–1905 French). (*Source:* Super Stoc

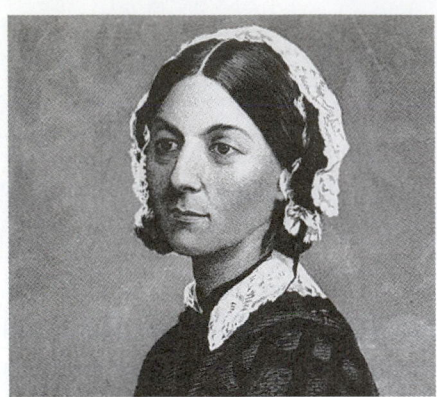

Figure 2-2. ■ Considered to be the founder of modern nursing, Florence Nightingale (1820–1910) was influential in developing nursing education, practice, and administration. Her 1859 publication *Notes on Nursing: What It Is, and What It Is Not* was intended for all women. (*Source:* © Bettmann/CORBIS. Reprinted with permission.)

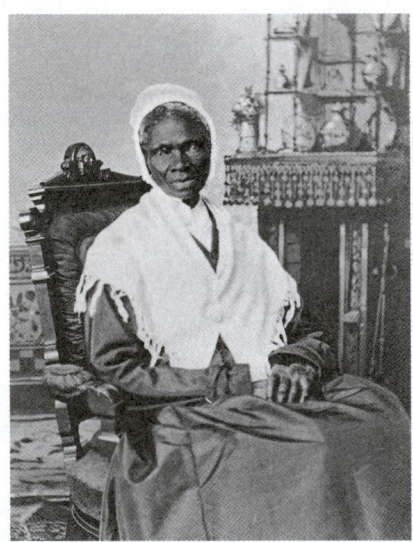

Figure 2-3. ■ Sojourner Truth (1797–1883), abolitionist, Underground Railroad agent, preacher, and women's rights advocate was a nurse for 4 years during the Civil War and worked as a nurse and counselor for the Freedom Relief Association after the war. (*Source:* Courtesy of the National Portrait Gallery, Smithsonian Institution.)

Nurses continued to provide care and assistance through [t]urn of the 20th century and World War I. However, [World] War II casualties created an acute shortage of care. It [was at] this time that auxiliary healthcare workers became [promin]ent. Practical nurses, aides, and technicians pro[vided m]uch of the actual nursing care under the instruction [and sup]ervision of registered nurses. At the same time, [many] specialties arose to meet the needs of hospitalized [patients. N]urse Ruby Bradley was the most decorated woman

ever to serve in the U.S. military. As a POW for 37 months in a Japanese prison camp, she slowly starved so that children could eat. She dropped to 86 pounds and was able to smuggle surgical supplies into POW camp under her ill-fitting uniform. Miss Bradley earned 34 medals and citations for bravery, including two Bronze Stars. Dr. Elizabeth Norman, in her book *We Band of Angels*, wrote about the sacrifice, terror, and contribution of nurses involved in the Bataan March in the Philippines. Military nurses experienced life, death, joy, and sorrow all within the time span of a duty shift.

It is estimated that between 4,000 and 15,000 nurses served during the Vietnam War. Very little has been written to document nurses' contributions during that time, but their work is commemorated near the Vietnam Memorial in Washington, D.C. (Figure 2-4 ■).

Nurses continue to provide care to military personnel as well as civilians. Nurses served with distinction during Desert Storm, treated victims of terrorist attacks in the United States, and provide nursing care in Afghanistan and Iraq. The combat nurse through the years has been on the cutting edge. Risk and ingenuity in the war zone have led to many accepted nursing practices used today.

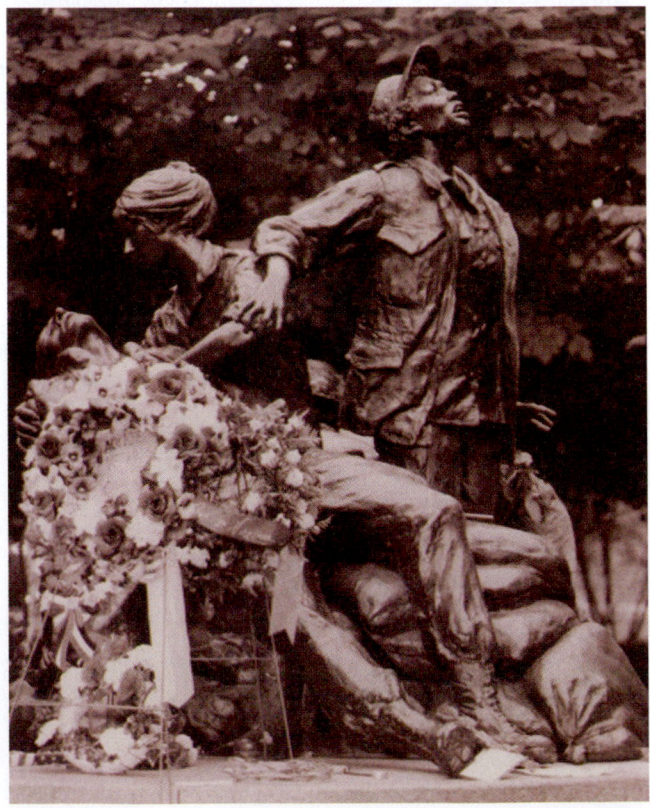

Figure 2-4. ■ Nurses served with distinction during the Vietnam War, but little has been written about them to date.

SOCIETAL ATTITUDES

Society's attitudes about nurses and nursing have significantly influenced professional nursing. Before the mid-1800s, nursing was without organization, education, or social status. The prevailing attitude was that a woman's place was in the home and that no respectable woman should have a career. The writings of Charles Dickens reflect societal attitudes about nursing during much of the 1800s. The character of Sairy Gamp (in his 1896 novel *Martin Chuzzlewit*, Figure 2-5 ■) epitomizes the nurse of the day. Sairy was a midwife who lived and worked in appalling environments. Dickens characterized nurse's work as a repugnant form of domestic service, for which little or no special training was required. This portrayal greatly influenced attitudes toward nurses and training.

The "Guardian Angel" or "Angel of Mercy" image arose in the latter part of the 19th century, largely because of the work of Florence Nightingale. After Nightingale brought respectability to the nursing profession, nurses were viewed as noble, compassionate, moral, religious, dedicated, and self-sacrificing. Another image that arose in the late 19th century was the nurse as doctor's handmaiden. This image developed when women did not yet have the right to vote, when family structures were largely paternalistic, and when the use of scientific knowledge was viewed as a male domain.

Leading Nurses of History

NIGHTINGALE (1820–1910)

Florence Nightingale's contributions to nursing are well documented. Her achievements in improving the standards for the care of war casualties in Crimea earned her the title "Lady with the Lamp." Her efforts in reforming hospitals and in producing and implementing public health policies also made her an accomplished political nurse. She was the first nurse to exert political pressure on government. She is also recognized as nursing's first scientist-theorist for her work *Notes on Nursing: What It Is, and What It Is Not*.

When she returned from Crimea, a grateful English public gave Nightingale an honorarium of £4,500. She used this money to establish the Nightingale Training School for Nurses in 1860. At St. Thomas Hospital in London, England, she taught her straightforward requirements.

Nightingale believed that nursing education should develop both the intellect and character of the nurse. She gave students a solid background in science to understand the theory behind their care. To develop character, by increasing their understanding of human ethics and morals, she assigned readings in the humanities. She believed that nurses should never stop learning. To her nurses she wrote, "[Nursing] is a field of which one may safely say: there is no end in what we may be learning everyday" (Schuyler, 1992). The school served as a model for other training schools. Its graduates traveled to other countries to manage hospitals and to institute training programs for nurses.

Nightingale's vision of nursing, which included public health and health promotion roles for nurses, was only partially addressed in the early days. The focus first was on developing the profession within hospitals. Although Miss Nightingale died in 1910, her influence continues in nursing today.

BARTON (1821–1912)

Clara Barton (Figure 2-6 ■) was a schoolteacher who volunteered as a nurse during the American Civil War. Her responsibility was to organize the nursing services. Barton is

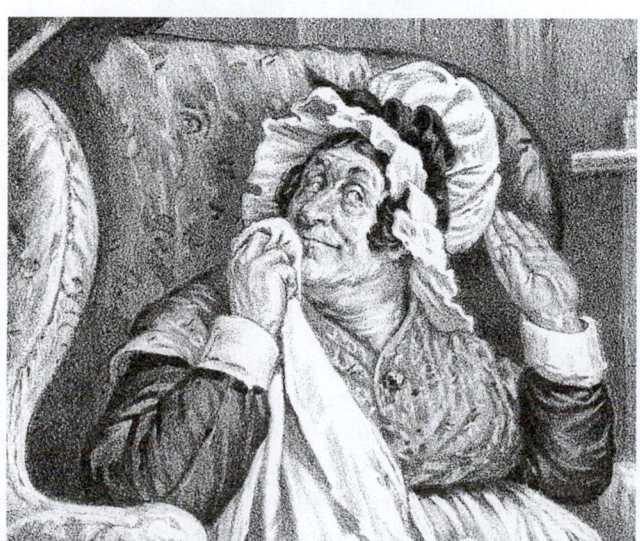

Figure 2-5. ■ Sairy Gamp, a character in Dickens' book *Martin Chuzzlewit*, epitomizes nurses of the early 1800s.

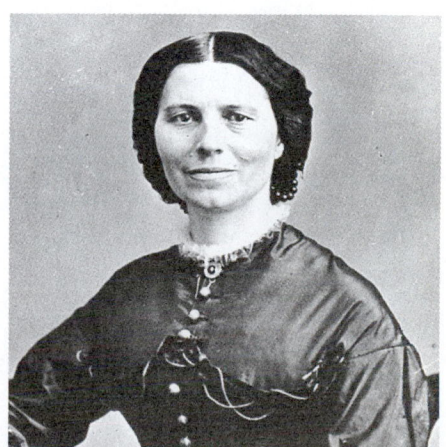

Figure 2-6. ■ Clara Barton (1821–1912) organized the American Red Cross, which linked with the International Red Cross when the U.S. Congress ratified the Geneva Convention in 1882. (*Source:* © Bettmann/CORBIS. Reprinted with permission.)

noted for her role in establishing the American Red Cross, which linked with the International Red Cross when the United States Congress ratified the Treaty of Geneva (Geneva Convention). In 1882, Barton persuaded Congress to ratify this treaty so that the Red Cross could perform humanitarian efforts in times of peace.

WALD (1867–1940)

Lillian Wald (Figure 2-7 ■) is considered the founder of public health nursing. Wald and Mary Brewster were the first to offer trained nursing services to the poor in the New York slums. They founded the Henry Street Settlement and Visiting Nurse Service, which provided nursing and social services, and also organized educational and cultural activities. Soon after the founding of the Henry Street Settlement, school nursing was established as an adjunct to visiting nursing.

DOCK (1858–1956)

Lavinia L. Dock (Figure 2-8 ■) was a feminist, as well as a prolific writer, political activist, suffragist, and friend of Wald. She participated in protest movements for women's rights that resulted in the 1920 passage of the 19th Amendment to the U.S. Constitution, which granted women the right to vote. In addition, Dock campaigned for legislation to allow nurses rather than physicians to control their profession. In 1893, Dock, Mary Adelaide Nutting, and Isabel Hampton Robb founded the American Society of Superintendents of Training Schools for Nurses of the United States and Canada. This was a precursor to the current National League for Nursing (NLN).

SANGER (1879–1966)

Margaret Higgins Sanger (Figure 2-9 ■), a public health nurse from New York, has had a lasting impact on women's health care. Imprisoned for opening the first birth control

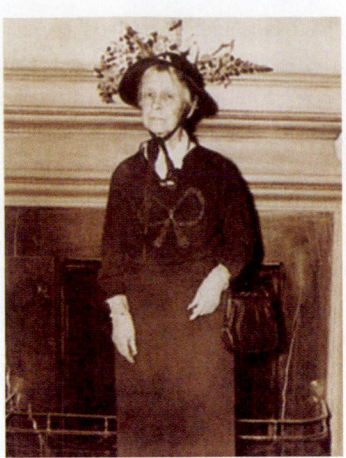

Figure 2-8. ■ Nursing leader and suffragist Lavinia L. Dock (1858–1956) was active in the protest movement for women's rights that resulted in the 1920 U.S. constitutional amendment allowing women to vote. (*Source:* Courtesy of Milbank Memorial Library, Teachers College, Columbia University. Reprinted with permission.)

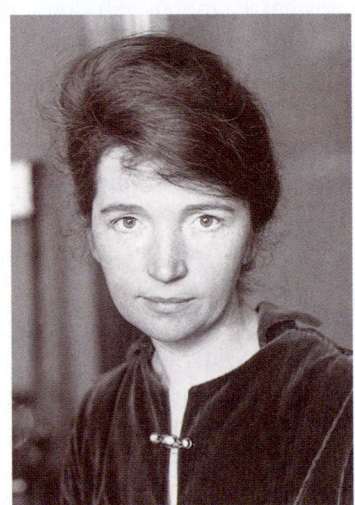

Figure 2-9. ■ Nurse activist Margaret Sanger, considered to be the founder of Planned Parenthood, was imprisoned for opening the first birth control information clinic in Baltimore in 1916. (*Source:* © Bettmann/CORBIS. Reprinted with permission.)

information clinic in America, she is considered the founder of Planned Parenthood.

BRECKINRIDGE (1881–1965)

After World War I, the Frontier Nursing Service (FNS) was established by a notable pioneer nurse, Mary Breckinridge (Figure 2-10 ■). In 1918 she worked with the American Committee for Devastated France distributing food, clothing, and supplies to rural villages and taking care of sick children. In 1921 Breckinridge returned to the United States with plans to provide health care to the people of rural America.

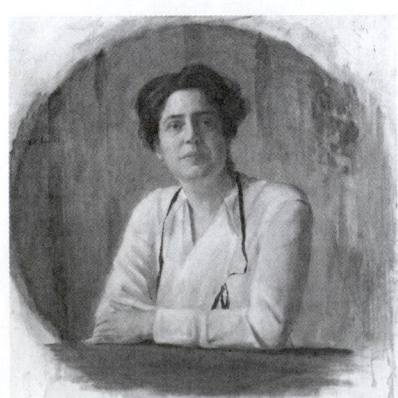

Figure 2-7. ■ Lillian Wald (1867–1940) founded the Henry Street Settlement and Visiting Nurse Service (circa 1893), which provided nursing and social services and organized educational and cultural activities. She is considered to be the founder of public health nursing. (*Source:* University of Iowa, College of Nursing, Iowa City, IA.)

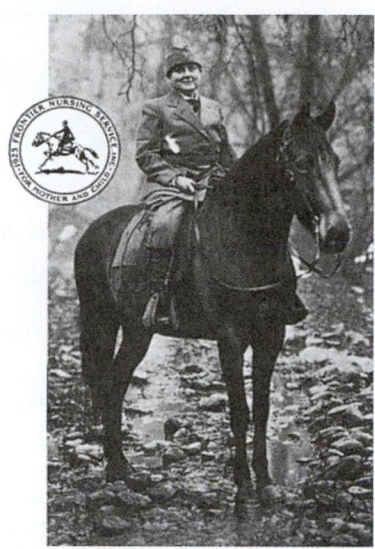

Figure 2-10. ■ Mary Breckinridge, a nurse who practiced midwifery in England, Australia, and New Zealand, founded the Frontier Nursing Services in Kentucky in 1925 to provide family-centered health care to rural populations. (*Source:* Reprinted with permission of Frontier Nursing Service.)

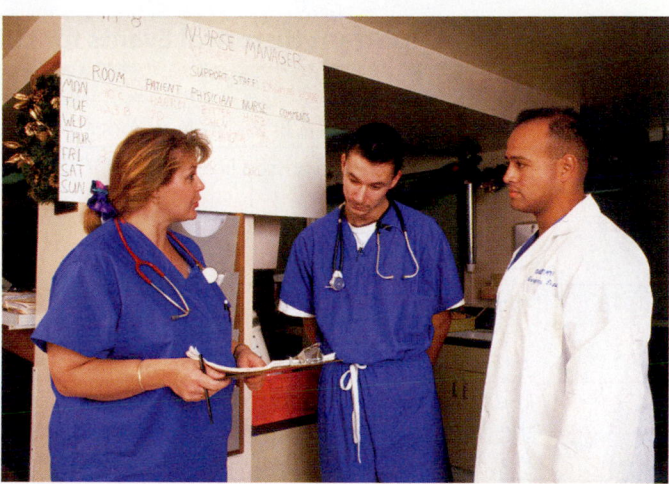

Figure 2-11. ■ Modern male nurses work side by side with their female colleagues to provide care to hospitalized clients.

In 1925 Breckinridge and two other nurses began the Frontier Nursing Service in Leslie County, Kentucky. Within this organization, Breckinridge started one of the first midwifery training schools in the United States.

KENNY (1880–1952)

Sister Elizabeth Kenny, an Australian nurse, is remembered for her efforts to fight poliomyelitis. She devised a method for treatment of poliomyelitis by stimulating and reeducating affected muscles. In the early 1940s she came to the United States. She gained the support of the American Medical Association, and in 1943 established the Elizabeth Kenny Institute in Minneapolis, Minnesota, to train nurses and physiotherapists in her methods. Sister Kenny's death in 1952 prevented her from seeing the introduction of the Salk vaccine program, which has virtually put an end to the disease she dedicated her life to treat.

MALE NURSES IN HISTORY

Women were not the sole providers of nursing services. The first nursing school in the world was started in India in about 250 B.C. Only men were considered to be "pure" enough to fulfill the role of a nurse at that time. In Jesus' parable in the New Testament, the Good Samaritan paid an innkeeper to provide care for the injured man. Paying a man to provide nursing care was fairly common. During the Crusades, several orders of knights provided nursing care to their sick and injured comrades and also built hospitals. The organization and management of their hospitals set a standard for the administration of hospitals throughout Europe at that time. St. Camillus de Lellis started out as a soldier and later turned to nursing. He started the sign of the Red Cross and developed the first ambulance service. Friar Juan de Mena was shipwrecked off the south Texas coast in 1554. He is the first identified nurse in what would become the United States. James Derham, a black slave who worked as a nurse in New Orleans in the late 1700s, saved the money he earned to purchase his freedom. Later, he studied medicine and became a well-respected physician in Philadelphia. During the Civil War, both sides had military men who cared for the sick and wounded.

In 1876, only 3 years after the first U.S. nurse received her diploma from New England Hospital for Women and Children, the Alexian Brothers opened their first hospital in the United States and a school to educate men in nursing.

During the years from the Civil War to the Korean War, men were not permitted to serve as nurses in the military. Today, men have resumed their historical place in the profession. As the history of nursing continues to be written, men and women will work side by side (Figure 2-11 ■).

History of LPNs/LVNs

The site for the first training for practical nurses was at the Young Women's Christian Association (YWCA) in New York City in 1862. However, it was not until 1893 that the first official school for the education of LPNs was established. This later became the Ballard School in New York. The program of study was 3 months long, and the participants studied special techniques for caring for the sick as well as a variety of homemaking techniques.

Much of the care during this time was done in the client's home, making the LPN a home health or visiting

TABLE 2-1	Important Historical Events for LPNs/LVNs	
DATE	**EVENT**	**IMPORTANCE**
1893	Ballard School at YWCA, Brooklyn, New York	First formal training for practical nurses.
1914	Mississippi legislature passed license laws for practical nurses	First laws passed to govern the practice of practical nurses.
1917	Smith-Hughes Act	Provided federal funding for vocationally oriented schools of practical nursing.
1918	Third school established	Even with new schools and federal assistance, the need for nurses could not be met because of the demand created by the war and epidemics.
1941	The Association of Practical Nurse Schools was founded; the name was changed to National Association for Practical Nurse Education and Service (NAPNES) in 1942	Standards for practical nurse education were established.
1944	U.S. Department of Education commissioned an intensive study differentiating tasks of the practical nurse	The outcome of the study differentiated tasks performed by the practical nurse from those performed by the registered nurse. State boards of nursing established tasks that could be performed by both groups.
1945	New York established mandatory licensure for practical nurses	The first state to require licensure; by 1955 all other states had followed suit.
1949	The National Federation of Licensed Practical Nurses (NFLPN) was founded by Lillian Kuster; the name was changed to the National Association for Licensed Practical Nurse Education and Services in 1959	The discipline now had an official organization with membership limited to LPNs/LVNs.
1955	All states passed licensing laws for practical/vocational nurses	Practice of nursing by licensed practical nursing was regulated in all states.
1961	The National League of Nursing established a Department of Practical Nursing	Through this department, schools of practical nursing could be accredited by the NLN.
1965	American Nurses Association published a position paper that influenced attitudes about practical and vocational nursing	The paper clearly defined the two levels of nursing: registered nursing and technical nursing. The exclusion of the term *practical/vocational nurse* necessitated that the LPN/LVN prove his or her worth to provide valuable nursing interventions under the direction of a registered nurse.
1994	Computerized NCLEX-PN® examination available to graduates of LPN/LVN programs in all states	Allowed for more availability of test dates and interstate endorsement of licensure.

nurse. Eleven years later a second school, the Thompson Practical Nursing School, was established.

In 1914, the state legislature in Mississippi passed the first laws governing the practice of practical nurses. Other states were slow to follow. By 1940, only six states had passed nurse practice acts relating to practical nurses. In 1955, the state board test pool of the NLN Education Committee established the procedures for testing graduates of approved practical/vocational education programs in all states. Graduates who passed the examination became licensed practical nurses (LPNs) or, in California and Texas, licensed vocational nurses (LVNs). Each state set its own passing score.

Today, a graduate of an approved LPN/LVN training program is eligible to take the national council licensure examination for practical nursing (**NCLEX-PN**®). The examination is computerized, with a "pass" score that is standardized throughout the United States. A nurse must successfully pass the licensure examination in order to practice nursing. All states have licensing laws. *Interstate endorsement* (reciprocity between states) exists. This means that an LPN/LVN from one state can apply for licensure in another state without retesting. It is the responsibility of the individual nurse to contact the board of nursing in the jurisdiction where he or she wishes to work. The nurse must apply for licensure and for information regarding the scope of practice within that state. Table 2-1 ■ lists important events in the history of practical/vocational nursing.

NURSE LICENSURE COMPACT

The mutual recognition model of nurse licensure allows a nurse to have one license (in his or her state of residency) and to practice in other states (both physically and electronically [via computer]), subject to each state's practice law and regulation. Under mutual recognition, a nurse may practice across state lines unless otherwise restricted.

On January 10, 2000, the Nurse Licensure Compact Administrators (NLCA) were organized to protect the public's health and safety by promoting compliance with the laws governing the practice of nursing in each party state through the mutual recognition of party state licenses. As of October 2007 there were 22 Nurse Licensure Compact (NLC) states. The National Council State Boards of Nursing's website is a good source for current NLC states.

To achieve mutual recognition, each state must enact legislation or regulation authorizing the NLC. States entering the compact also adopt administrative rules and regulations for implementation of the compact. Once the compact is enacted, each compact state designates a Nurse Licensure Compact Administrator to facilitate the exchange of information between the states relating to compact nurse licensure and regulation.

A nurse must legally reside in an NLC state to be eligible to have a multistate license. The board of nursing in your state of residence can answer questions related to multistate license or privilege to practice.

Practical and Vocational Nursing Today

OUR CUSTOMERS

The "customers" we serve in nursing today are sometimes called consumers, patients, or clients. A **consumer** is an individual, a group of people, or a community that uses a service or commodity. People who use healthcare products or services are consumers of health care. A **patient** is a person who is waiting for or undergoing medical treatment and care. The word *patient* comes from a Latin word meaning "to suffer" or "to bear." Traditionally, the person receiving health care has been called a patient. People become patients when they seek assistance because of illness. Some nurses believe that the word *patient* implies passive acceptance of the decisions and care of health professionals. Because nurses interact with family, friends, and healthy people as well as those who are ill, nurses increasingly refer to recipients of health care as *clients*.

A **client** is a person who engages the advice or services of someone who is qualified to provide the service. Therefore, a client is a collaborator, a person who is also responsible for his or her own health. The health status of a client is the responsibility of the individual in collaboration with health professionals. In this book, *client* is the preferred term, although *consumer* and *patient* may be used in some instances.

OUR PURPOSE

Nurses provide care for individuals, families, and communities. The scope of nursing practice involves four areas: promoting health and wellness, preventing illness, restoring health, and caring for the dying.

Promoting Health and Wellness

Wellness is a state of well-being. It means engaging in attitudes and behavior that enhance the quality of life and maximize personal potential. Nurses promote wellness in individuals and groups who are healthy or ill. Nurses may hold blood pressure clinics, teach about healthy lifestyles, give talks about drug and alcohol abuse, and instruct about safety in the home and workplace. Nurses who work in public health, community clinics, mental health facilities, and occupation health settings promote health and wellness.

Preventing Illness

Illness may be defined as the highly individualized response a person has to a disease. The goal of illness prevention programs is to maintain optimal health by preventing disease. Nurses in physicians' offices or health clinics administer immunizations, provide prenatal and infant care, and teach about the prevention of sexually transmitted infections.

Restoring Health

Restoring health means focusing on the ill client from early detection of disease through the recovery period. Nurses in acute care and rehabilitation facilities perform all of the following:

- Provide direct care to the client such as administering medications, assisting with activities of daily living, and performing specific procedures and treatments.
- Perform procedures that provide data for diagnosis and assessment, such as measuring blood pressure and examining feces for occult blood.
- Consult with other healthcare professionals about client problems.
- Teach clients about recovery activities, such as exercises that will hasten recovery after a stroke.
- Rehabilitate clients to their optimal functional level following physical or mental illness, injury, or chemical addiction.

Caring for the Dying

This area of nursing practice involves comforting and caring for people of all ages who are dying. It includes helping clients live as comfortably as possible until death and helping clients' support persons cope with death. Nurses carry out these activities in homes, hospitals, and extended care facilities. Some agencies, called hospices, are specifically designed for this purpose (see Chapter 44 ⚭).

OUR STANDARDS

Nurse practice acts, or legal acts for professional nursing practice, regulate the practice of nursing in the United States and Canada. Each state in the United States and each province in Canada has its own practice act.

Although practice acts may differ in various jurisdictions, they all have a common purpose: to protect the public. The title of *nurse* can legally be used *only* by an individual who is licensed as an RN or an LPN/LVN. For additional information, see Chapter 63 ⚭.

During your nursing education program, you will develop, clarify, and internalize professional values. The National Federation of Licensed Practical Nurses (NFLPN) Inc. has

identified specific standards (Box 2-1 ■). LPNs/LVNs in all areas of practice should adhere to these standards.

OUR WORK SETTINGS

In the past, the acute care hospital was the major practice setting open to most nurses. Today the LPN/LVN works in hospitals, clients' homes, community agencies, ambulatory clinics, health maintenance organizations, and skilled nursing facilities (see Chapter 7 ⚭). See also Chapter 65 ⚭ for a description of opportunities available to the LPN/LVN.

LPNs/LVNs work under their own license under direct supervision of a physician or a registered nurse. LPNs/LVNs may be involved in clinical planning meetings because of

---

BOX 2-1	NURSING PRACTICE STANDARDS FOR THE LICENSED PRACTICAL/VOCATIONAL NURSE

Education

The licensed practical/vocational nurse:

1. Shall complete a formal education program in practical nursing approved by the appropriate nursing authority in a state.
2. Shall successfully pass the National Council Licensure Examination for Practical Nurses.
3. Shall participate in initial orientation within the employing institution.

Legal/Ethical Status

The licensed practical/vocational nurse:

1. Shall hold a current license to practice nursing as an LPN/LVN in accordance with the law of the state wherein employed.
2. Shall know the scope of nursing practice authorized by the Nursing Practice Act in the state wherein employed.
3. Shall have a personal commitment to fulfill the legal responsibilities inherent in good nursing practice.
4. Shall take responsible actions in situations wherein there is unprofessional conduct by a peer or other healthcare provider.
5. Shall recognize and commit to meet the ethical and moral obligations of the practice of nursing.
6. Shall not accept or perform professional responsibilities that the individual knows he or she is not competent to perform.

Practice

The licensed practical/vocational nurse:

1. Shall accept accountability for assigned responsibilities as a member of the healthcare team.
2. Shall function within the limits of educational preparation and experience, as related to the assigned duties.
3. Shall function with other members of the healthcare team in promoting and maintaining health, preventing disease and disability, caring for and rehabilitating individuals who are

experiencing an altered health state, and contributing to the ultimate quality of life until death.
4. Shall know and utilize the nursing process in planning, implementing, and evaluating health services and nursing care for the individual patient or group.
   a. Planning: The planning of nursing includes:
      1. Assessment of health status of the individual patient, the family, and community groups
      2. Analysis of the information gained from assessment
      3. Identification of health goals
   b. Implementation: The plan for nursing care is put into practice to achieve the stated goals and includes:
      1. Observing, recording, and reporting significant changes that require intervention or different goals
      2. Applying nursing knowledge and skills to promote and maintain health, to prevent disease and disability, and to optimize functional capabilities of an individual patient
      3. Assisting the patient and family with activities of daily living and encouraging self-care as appropriate
      4. Carrying out therapeutic regimens and protocols prescribed by an RN, physician, or other persons authorized by state law
   c. Evaluation: The plan for nursing care and its implementations are evaluated to measure the progress toward the stated goals and will include appropriate persons and/or groups to determine:
      1. The relevancy of current goals in relation to the progress of the individual patient
      2. The involvement of the recipients of care in the evaluation process
      3. The quality of the nursing action in the implementation of the plan
      4. A reordering of priorities or new goal setting in the care plan

5. Shall participate in peer review and other evaluation processes.
6. Shall participate in the development of policies concerning the health and nursing needs of society and in the roles and functions of the LPN/LVN.

Continuing Education

The licensed practical/vocational nurse:

1. Shall be responsible for maintaining the highest possible level of professional competence at all times.
2. Shall periodically reassess career goals and select continuing education activities that will help to achieve these goals.
3. Shall take advantage of continuing education opportunities that will lead to personal growth and professional development.
4. Shall seek and participate in continuing education activities that are approved for credit by appropriate organizations, such as the NFLPN.

Specialized Nursing Practice

The licensed practical/vocational nurse:

1. Shall have had at least one year's experience in nursing at the staff level.
2. Shall present personal qualifications that are indicative of potential abilities for practice in the chosen specialized nursing area.
3. Shall present evidence of completion of a program or course that is approved by an appropriate agency to provide the knowledge and skills necessary for effective nursing services in the specialized field.
4. Shall meet all of the standards of practice as set forth in this document.

"Patient," not "client," is used here as quoted by NFLPN.
Source: National Federation of Licensed Practical Nurses, Inc. Copyright © 1991.

---

their expertise, but they are required to do this less than other licensed healthcare providers. Their primary duty is to deliver care to the client.

Professional Organizations for LPN/LVN Students and Graduates

When a professional organization is in place to oversee the operation of a group, it becomes a **profession** rather than an occupation. Several organizations oversee the profession of practical/vocational nursing.

Operation under the umbrella of a professional organization differentiates a profession from an occupation.

NATIONAL ASSOCIATION FOR PRACTICAL NURSE EDUCATION AND SERVICE

The National Association for Practical Nurse Education and Service (NAPNES) was established in 1941. This was the first national organization for the practical/vocational level of nursing. NAPNES was responsible for the accreditation of LPN/LVN education programs from 1945 until 1984.

NATIONAL FEDERATION OF LICENSED PRACTICAL NURSES

In 1949, Lillian Kuster founded the National Federation of Licensed Practical Nurses (NFLPN). This organization is considered to be the official membership organization for LPNs and LVNs. Only individuals with those licenses may join the organization. The National League for Nursing, formed in 1952, is an organization of both individuals and

agencies. In 1961 the NLN established the Council for Practical Nursing Programs. This arm of the organization assumed responsibility for promoting the interests of LPNs/LVNs in the NLN. All of these organizations provide continuing education opportunities and publish literature of interest to the LPN/LVN.

NFLPN welcomes LPN/LVN students as members. NFLPN provides leadership for nearly one million licensed LPNs and LVNs employed in the United States. It also fosters high standards of LPN/LVN education and practice so that the best nursing care will be available to every client. The NFLPN serves as the central source of information on what is new and changing in practical/vocational nursing education and practice on the local, state, and national level. The organization is a three-tiered concept of local, state, and national enrollment. By participating in local, state, and national meetings and conferences, the LPN/LVN student can learn firsthand how a professional organization works to maintain the professional status of the membership. NFLPN also encourages continuing education and publishes a quarterly magazine *Practical Nursing Today.* Through relationships with the National Council of State Boards of Nursing and the U.S. Congress, the NFLPN enables policy makers to better understand the role of practical/vocational nursing in the nation's healthcare delivery system (NFLPN, 2003).

HEALTH OCCUPATION STUDENTS OF AMERICA

Health Occupation Students of America (HOSA) is a nationally recognized career technical student organization, which was founded in 1976. HOSA provides a unique program of leadership and team building development, motivation, and recognition experience. HOSA is an instructional tool integrated into the health careers classroom by the instructor. It is an intracurricular activity, which reinforces technical skills and supports service to the community. HOSA helps to develop the "total person." The national organization is made up of health occupation students from the 40 affiliated states. HOSA's membership is made up of secondary, postsecondary, and collegiate students. Healthcare professionals, alumni, and business and industry members are also welcome. There is also an associate membership category for students who are interested in health careers but who are not enrolled in a program. Through participation, the LPN/LVN student can network with other health careers students. Involvement in a student organization demonstrates to students the benefits of participating in professional organizations once they have graduated.

Note: The references and resources for all chapters have been compiled at the back of the book.

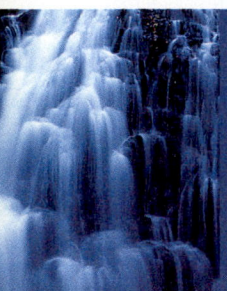

Chapter Review

KEY Points

- Nursing values have traditionally included compassion, devotion to duty, and hard work. Nurses today are regarded as a vital part of the healthcare team. All levels of staff work together to provide the best possible care for clients.

- Practical and vocational schools have existed since the late 1800s, but it was only in the 1950s that a procedure was established to test graduates of approved schools in all states. Individual states still govern many factors of LPN/LVN practice.

- The terms *consumer, patient,* and *client* all refer to the recipient of healthcare services. The term *client* indicates that the person is actively involved in all phases of decision making and planning care.

- The scope of nursing practice includes promoting wellness, preventing illness, restoring health, and caring for the dying.

- Nurse practice acts vary among states and provinces, and nurses are responsible for knowing the act that governs their practice.

- Standards of clinical nursing practice provide measurement criteria for the effectiveness of nursing care and for professional performance behaviors.

- Traditionally, the majority of nurses were employed in hospital settings. Today, more nurses are working in home health care, ambulatory care, and community health settings.

- Professional and student organizations help the nursing profession and individual nurses. Participation in nursing associations encourages individual growth and helps nurses influence policies that affect nursing practice.

⊂⊃ FOR FURTHER Study

Chapter 7 contains information about the variety of healthcare settings in which LPNs/LVNs work.

Some agencies, called hospices, are specifically designed for caring for the dying (see Chapter 44).

Licensure as an LPN/LVN is discussed further in Chapter 63.

See Chapter 65 for a description of employment opportunities available to the LPN/LVN.

NCLEX-PN® Exam Preparation

TEST-TAKING TIP Do not focus on memorizing dates. Focus on people, relationships, and what happened. Most tests use dates as a frame of reference, not as the most important thing to remember.

1 A male student nurse asks the instructor if there have ever been any men who made a significant contribution to nursing. The instructor's best response would be:
1. "Yes, male nurses played a critical role in the Korean War."
2. "Yes, the Alexian Brothers opened their first hospital in the United States and a school to educate men in nursing."
3. "No, the role of men in nursing is too recent to have led to any significant contributions to nursing yet."
4. "Men have not played a significant role in nursing since the Crusades."

2 The nurse recognizes that the role of nurses has been impacted in the past by all of the following factors *except*:
1. Religion.
2. War.
3. Societal attitudes.
4. Cost containment.

3 Nurses consider Florence Nightingale to be nursing's first scientist-theorist because:
1. She reformed hospitals and pressured government to implement public health policies.
2. She described the basic elements of the nursing profession in her work *Notes on Nursing: What It Is, and What It Is Not*.
3. She believed that nurses should never stop learning.
4. She taught that an understanding of human ethics and morals was essential to the development of nursing students.

4 The nurse recognizes which of the following as the founder of public health nursing?
1. Barton
2. Wald
3. Dock
4. Nightingale

5 What is the significance of the Smith-Hughes Act for LPNs/LVNs?
1. It required licensure for practical nurses.
2. It differentiated the practice of LPNs and LVNs from RNs.
3. It provided federal funds to support practical nurse education.
4. It established computerized testing centers for licensure exams.

6 The LPN/LVN recognizes which of the following as a major area within the LPN/LVN scope of practice? (Select all that apply.)
1. The LPN/LVN is accountable for the care delivered.
2. The LPN/LVN functions within the limits of educational preparation and experience.
3. The LPN/LVN functions as a member of the healthcare team.
4. The LPN/LVN creates the plan of care for the client.
5. The LPN/LVN determines medical needs of the client.

7 The nurse's customers include which of the following? (Select all that apply.)
1. An individual client
2. A group of people
3. A community
4. Peers
5. Physicians

8 The unlicensed assistive personnel (UAP) asks a group of nurses why they are considered professionals whereas the UAP's job is considered an occupation. The nurse would explain the difference between an occupation and a profession by explaining that a profession:
1. Requires licensure.
2. Has a longer educational program.
3. Has an overseeing organization.
4. Has nationally recognized testing.

9 In 1949, Lillian Kuster founded which of the following organizations?
1. Health Occupations Students of America (HOSA)
2. National Council of State Boards of Nursing
3. National Federation of Licensed Practical Nurses (NFLPN)
4. Henry Street Settlement House

10 The nurse practice act provides:
1. The NCLEX-PN® test plan.
2. The scope of practice for LPNs/LVNs in individual states.
3. Guidelines for the ethical practice of nursing.
4. Questions to prepare for the licensing exam.

Answers and rationales for Review Questions appear in Appendix I.

Chapter 3

Promoting Culturally Proficient Care

LEARNING Outcomes

After completing this chapter, you will be able to:

1. Develop an understanding of the history of transcultural nursing.
2. Define terminology of transcultural nursing.
3. Describe the 12 domains of culture.
4. Identify the effect of healthcare disparities among members of various cultural groups.
5. Discuss the role of communication in the delivery of culturally proficient care to hospitalized clients and their families.
6. List the components of a cultural assessment.
7. Discuss the subculture of health care, including cultural diversity among nurses.

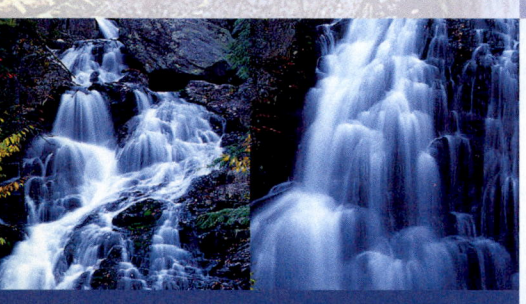

BRIEF Outline

Development of Transcultural Nursing

Theoretical Basis of Transcultural Nursing

Racial and Ethnic Disparities in Health Care

Culturally Based Communication

Transcultural Communication and Client Concerns

Conducting the Cultural Assessment

Subculture of Health Care

KEY TERMS

Use the audio glossary feature on the MyNursingKit Website to hear the correct pronunciation of the following key terms.

acculturation 33

biocultural ecology 34

cultural awareness 27

cultural competence 27

cultural empathy 35

cultural sensitivity 27

discrimination 31

domains 30

ethnocentrism 28

intercultural communication 32

prejudice 29

segregation 31

stereotypes 28

For more than 30 years, nursing has been concerned with the cultural differences among clients. In the early years, culture was equated with ethnicity. Ethnicity was identified by a code on the client's chart or on the addressograph plate. As the profession became aware of the need to provide for the client holistically, the term **cultural awareness** (knowing about the similarities and differences among cultures) crept into the professional vocabulary. The goal of cultural awareness was to end prejudice and discrimination. In fact, though, awareness often resulted in a focus on differences, without providing the nurse with the tools to meet the culturally related needs of the client.

To break down the barriers among cultures, there was a movement toward **cultural sensitivity** (being aware of the needs and feelings of your own culture and of other cultures). Since the 1990s, a new term has been added. The profession has been talking about **cultural competence**—a set of practice skills, knowledge, and attitudes that must encompass the following elements:

1. Awareness and acceptance of differences
2. Awareness of one's own cultural values
3. Understanding of the dynamics of difference
4. Development of cultural knowledge
5. Ability to adapt practice skills to fit the cultural context of the client

It is very difficult to separate cultural heritage from family traits. Studying the family gives insight to beliefs about roles, health practices, and religion. Box 3-1 ■ offers some insights into the family in the four major cultural groups. Refer to Chapter 18 🔗 for more information on beliefs about death and dying and Table 44-1 🔗 for mourning and after-death rites of major cultural groups.

BOX 3-1	CULTURAL PULSE POINTS

Major Cultural Groups and Traits

Rasa-Latina Group

Rasa-Latina families are those whose native language is Spanish and whose religion, most commonly, is Catholic. The family is led by a male head of the household, who is strong but distant, especially with father-son relationships. Mothers and daughters have a very close relationship. In the traditional family, the mother's role is to care for the home and children and to teach daughters to do the same. The Rasa-Latina family functions in the here and now. Customs, ethnic foods, and music are important and they are passed on, especially during celebrations. The family may follow native healthcare practices rather than seeking medical care. This is frequently related to lack of access to medical care. Healthcare professionals frequently become frustrated with Rasa-Latina mothers who are reluctant to make healthcare decisions, especially for their children. Before she can make a decision, the Rasa-Latina woman must often discuss it with the head of the household. (Note: Modern Rasa-Latina women are changing. Many are seeking education and job training. Attempts to increase their independence may cause resentment and family disruptions.)

Asian Pacific (or Pacific Rim) Group

The Asian Pacific or Pacific Rim group includes Japanese, Chinese, Vietnamese, Filipinos, Pacific Islanders, etc. These cultures do not have a common language or religion. The one common thread with this culture is the fact that they are not time limited. When Asian Pacific individuals speak of family, they are including many generations of ancestors. The family is a continuation of those who have gone before. An individual who brings shame upon him- or herself brings shame on the entire family. Many times a young Asian female who becomes pregnant prior to marriage may be reluctant to confide in her family because of the disgrace she perceives she has brought upon her family. When young people marry, they do not form a new family. Instead, the young wife is absorbed into the family of the new husband. Although the westernization of young Asian individuals has precipitated change, many families continue to arrange marriages. Health practices may involve Eastern medical treatment with the acceptance of some alternative medical practices in this country. Asians are more comfortable using Western medicine along with the native healthcare practices. In the Asian Pacific family, the father is the head of the household. His main responsibility is providing for the family. Traditionally, he leaves all household and childbearing responsibilities to the wife. An Asian Pacific mother would seek medical care for the children and herself, and make decisions in this area independently.

American Black Group

The American Black (or African American) family is traditionally a matriarchal family. This is a result of husbands and fathers being separated from the family during the slavery period in the United States. Today there continues to be an alarming number of fatherless Black American families. This is especially true in lower socioeconomic areas. Middle-class Black American families are frequently two-parent families. Many of them also are two-income families. Black American children often have the advantage of care by extended family members. Children contribute to the household early on by learning to do chores. They often seek employment as soon as they are of age. Family, as well as the church, is the center of the Black American family social support system. Health-seeking behaviors in the lower socioeconomic area continue to be a problem. Access is difficult,

and many Black American children are without a primary health-care provider. In many urban areas, hospital emergency rooms have become the primary provider for Black children. This fact is frightening when it is noted that the highest infant mortality rates in this country are in three of our largest urban areas (Philadelphia, Detroit, and Washington, DC).

Caucasian Group

The Caucasian family in the United States has changed dramatically since the mid-1970s. Once the middle-class family was provided for by the husband and father, and the mother was the homemaker and primary caregiver for the children. Now, a second income is often required, and child care is provided outside the home. Caucasian women are better educated than other groups and often seek a career. Women are no longer completely dependent on the status of their husbands. For Caucasians, the "American dream" includes not only a house and one or more cars, but also health care. Good health care is viewed as a right by middle-class White families. They also believe that health care should be paid for by their employer and that they should have a choice in who delivers the care. Caucasian workers may turn down a career opportunity because of benefits that do not equal those of the present job. The White American family differs from other family groups in that individual needs frequently take precedence over the needs of the family.

Now it is time to take the next step past competency to culturally proficient care. For culturally proficient nurses, the five components of cultural care will be second nature. Care for clients will include consideration of their physical, psychosocial, emotional, spiritual, and cultural components.

Development of Transcultural Nursing

The study of transcultural nursing began in the 1950s, when Dr. Madeleine Leininger noted differences in culture among clients and nurses. As she studied cultural differences, she realized that health and illness are influenced by culture. Dr. Leininger's work encouraged a broader awareness of cultural issues (Box 3-2 ■) and led to the study of culture within the nursing curriculum.

Although diversity of population can be one of a country's greatest assets, it also represents a range of health improvement challenges. Nurses need to be prepared to meet the holistic needs of their clients, including those affected by client culture.

One pitfall in communicating with a person from a different culture is ethnocentrism. **Ethnocentrism** means interpreting the beliefs and behavior of others in terms of one's own cultural values and traditions. It assumes that

one's own culture is superior. It is difficult to avoid the tendency toward ethnocentrism. Nurses, though, must be extra diligent to avoid **stereotypes** (oversimplified conceptions, opinions, or beliefs about some aspect of a group of people). Individuals vary greatly within any ethnic group, just as children vary within one family. The nurse must look for ways to care for each client as a unique person, regardless of category.

BOX 3-2	EVENTS IN THE HISTORY OF CULTURAL CARE
1974	Transcultural Nursing Society was established as the official organization of transcultural nursing.
1991	Dr. Leininger published theory of cultural care diversity and universality.
2000	The U.S. Department of Health and Human Services (USDHHS) stated, *"Healthy People 2010* is firmly dedicated to the principle that—regardless of age, gender, race or ethnicity, income, education, geographical location, disability and sexual orientation—every person in every community across the nation deserves equal access to comprehensive, culturally competent, community-based health care systems that are committed to serving the needs of the individual and promoting community health"* (USDHHS, 2000).

Providing cultural care for pediatric clients is a bit different than that for adults. Children are more tolerant than adults, although they can be very blunt and inquisitive. They may ask questions about the color of a nurse's skin or accent. They may be reluctant to share a room with another child who is different from them.

Theoretical Basis of Transcultural Nursing

Nursing theories base their views on four concepts: nursing, person/client, health, and environment. (See Chapter 5 ⬤⬤ for more information on nursing models and theories.) Leininger's cultural care diversity and universality theory (see Table 5-4 ⬤⬤) is still the only theory focused specifically on transcultural nursing with a cultural care focus. It is used world-wide today. Leininger's "Sunrise" model is probably the best known of all nursing theories related to culture. Figure 3-1 ■ provides a visual representation of Dr. Leininger's theory.

Leininger's theory can be used with individuals, families, groups, communities, and institutions. Her ideas are important to nursing care today not only because of the diversity of the healthcare clients, but also because travel and communication have made us a global society. A competent, effective nurse must be aware of his or her feelings and behaviors and must be able to view the client without **prejudice** (prejudgment or bias based on characteristics such as race, age, or gender).

Dorothea Orem's theory (see selected nursing theories in Table 5-4 ⬤⬤), which looks at self-care deficits and the client's level of performance of self-care, must be considered in light of a client's culture. Orem added several observations about cultural issues in nursing. She recognized that some ethnic or cultural groups tend not to seek Western-style health care. They may either try folk remedies or avoid care altogether. In many instances, this can result in a self-care deficit and worsening of the condition. Healthcare professionals and community health educators need to be aware of this resistance and work to provide clients with the skills they need to develop self-care. The lack of access can also be a problem. If individuals have been unable to obtain health care in the past, they may avoid seeking it in the future. This again compounds the health issues.

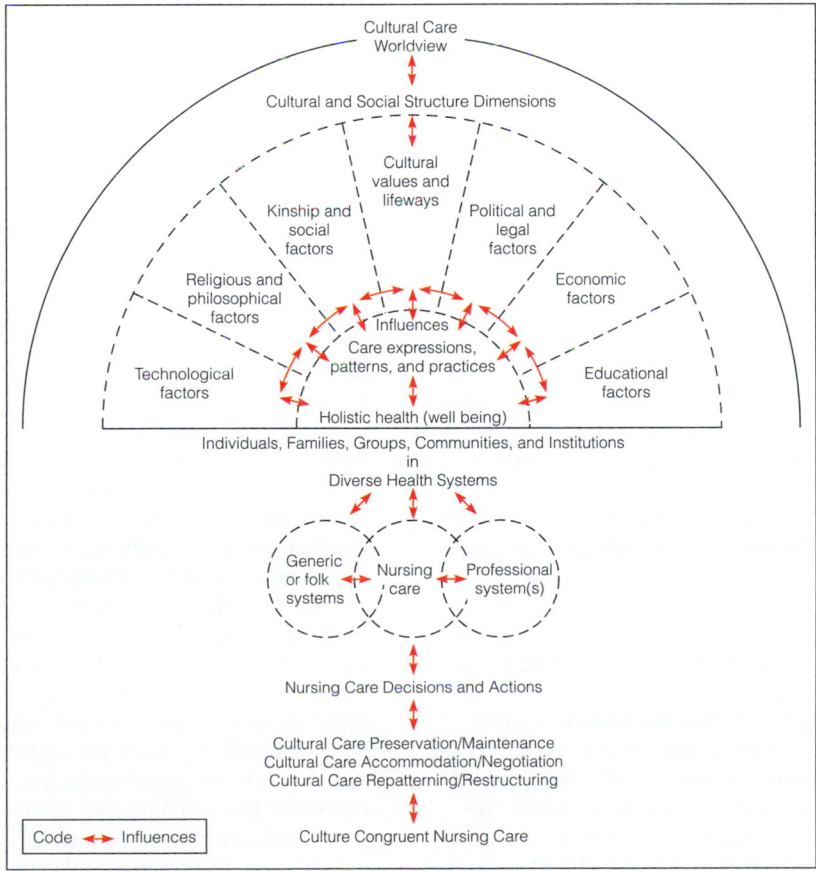

Figure 3-1. ■ Leininger's "Sunrise" model, depicting the cultural care diversity and universality theory. (*Source:* From *Cultural Care Diversity and Universality: A Theory of Nursing*, by M. M. Leininger, 1991, New York: National League for Nursing Press. Reprinted by permission.)

Larry Purnell and B. J. Paulanka (2008) developed a model for cultural competence that describes 12 **domains** (elements that describe a scientific variable) of culture. This assessment tool identifies ethnocultural attributes of an individual, family, or group. Box 3-3 ■ provides information about cultural domains.

In everyday practice as a practical or vocational nurse LPN/LVN, you will need to be aware of these domains. You will develop knowledge of different cultures, especially those in the area where you live and work. This should include becoming familiar with the part of the world where those cultures were established and the heritage of the people. It is also important for you to realize that individuals within a particular culture may have characteristics that don't "fit" their group. It is important not to generalize and stereotype a member of a group (Purnell & Paulanka, 2008).

BOX 3-3	TWELVE DOMAINS OF CULTURE

Overview, Inhabited Localities, and Topography—include concepts related to country of origin, the effects of topography of country of origin and present residence on health, economics, politics, reasons for migration, educational status, and occupations. An awareness of the geographic residence of an ethnocultural group increases opportunities for collaborating with healthcare providers in these areas; this is essential for disease prevention and treatment, health promotion and maintenance, and health teaching.

Communication—includes dominant language and dialects, cultural communication patterns, temporal relationships, and format of names. Healthcare professionals who need to communicate with non-English-speaking clients should be aware of the following:

Use an interpreter not just a translator; a translator merely restates the words in the other language, whereas the interpreter can decode the words and provide the meaning behind the language.

Use interpreters who have a healthcare background whenever possible.

Beware that interpreters may affect the reporting of symptoms, insert their own ideas, or omit information.

Avoid using family members, who may not be objective.

Maintain eye contact with both the client and interpreter to read nonverbal cues and encourage feedback.

Personal space is another issue in communication. Personal space needs to be respected. The European Americans, Canadians, and British tend to need at least 18 inches between them and another person, whereas Middle Eastern clients may stand very close during conversation.

Family Roles and Organization—are interrelated to all other domains; they include head of household and gender roles; prescribed, restricted, and taboo behaviors of children and adolescents; family goals and priorities; and alternate lifestyles. The nurse must be aware of these issues in order to not offend the client or become frustrated when the client or family members do not respond in an expected manner.

Workforce Issues—include culture in the workplace and issues of autonomy. By 2080, 51% of the workforce in this country will be made of various minorities. Today a significant number of technical, laboratory, and service workers in health care are foreign born and/or trained. The educational level of healthcare professionals in some countries may not compare to the education in the United States. Additional education and training may be needed prior to the foreign professional being licensed to practice in the United States.

Cultural differences related to assertiveness can have an influence on how healthcare professionals relate to one another. For example, Asian nurses may not be as assertive with physicians as an American nurse. Foreign nurses who do not have previous experience with autonomy at the same level as American nurses may accept being more assertive in their duties if they are placed in the context of legal and professional requirements.

Biocultural Ecology—includes physical, biologic, and physiologic variations of racial and ethnic origins, such as skin color, endemic conditions that tend to occur continuously in a specific racial or ethnic group, and variation in drug metabolism.

High-Risk Behavior—is shared across cultures, although some groups do not place value on avoiding high-risk behaviors such as tobacco, recreational drugs, alcohol, nonuse of safety measures (seat belts or helmet), high-calorie diets, and lack of physical activity. Healthcare practices, such as a lack of healthcare promotion and safety practices, can present a major threat to some groups. Control of risk factors through ethnic-specific interventions is aimed at health promotion and health risk prevention through educational programs.

Nutrition—includes meaning of food, common foods and food rituals, dietary practices for health promotion as well as nutritional deficiencies and food limitations. Food is a very important component of most cultures; it is not looked at merely as a means for maintaining life, but rather as a part of the social structure. The British have their afternoon tea, whereas Americans have their morning coffee. Special occasions and holidays are frequently associated with ethnic foods. Religion also plays a large part in this domain; Jews and Muslims have very strict dietary laws that need to be adhered to even when hospitalized or ill.

Pregnancy and Childbearing Practices—include fertility practices and views toward pregnancy as well as prescriptive, restrictive, and taboo practices in the childbearing family. Fertility control in most cultures is the responsibility of the woman, although in China it is a government issue. The one-child law has made abortion a method of birth control. What is not commonly known outside the country is the fact that more than one child is permissible if the family is willing or able to pay a tax or fine equivalent to 4,000 American dollars. Most cultural groups have prescribed, restricted, and taboo beliefs for maternal behavior and delivery of a healthy infant. These beliefs affect lifestyle and

(continued)

BOX 3-3   *(continued)*

sexual behavior during prenatal, intrapartum, and postpartum periods. These practices may be in conflict with nursing practices and hospital policy. In hospitals that are "breastfeeding friendly," the practice of Hispanic women not breastfeeding until they leave the hospital goes against the knowledge of the importance of colostrum to the infant and to milk production.

Death Rituals—involve how individuals and their society view death, preparation for death, grieving and bereavement, burial practices, and euthanasia.

Spirituality—includes more than the beliefs related to organized religion, faith and affiliation, and use of prayer. Spirituality is a component of health related to the essence of life. A client's religious beliefs may have a profound effect on health care. Some cultures promote the feeling that illness is a result of sin. Clients may express that they will not get well because of some wrongdoing in their lives. Others believe that wellness and spirituality go hand-in-hand. At a time of serious illness or impending death, many clients and their families turn to the religious practices of their origin. The nurse needs to be supportive and assist them in contacting the clergy of their choice as well as provide them with the privacy so that they may carry out religious rituals.

Healthcare Practices—are interrelated with all the other domains. They include health-seeking beliefs and behaviors, responsibility for health care, folk practices, barriers to health care, cultural responses to health and illness as well as blood transfusions and organ donations. Mental health issues in many Asian, Pacific Islander, and Latino cultures are considered a disgrace; the family may keep the individual at home and not seek needed care.

Healthcare Practitioners—include the status, use, and perception of the traditional, magicoreligious, and biomedical healthcare providers. Many cultures make use of traditional as well as folk healers and magicoreligious healers. They may seek out a practitioner of folk medicine prior to seeking care from a traditional practitioner. In some cultural groups, folk and magicoreligious healthcare providers may be more respected and superior to biomedically educated physicians and nurses. The family may be more comfortable with a folk healer who is known to the family, spends time with them, and engages in small talk unrelated to the health problems in order to accomplish their objectives. It is important that traditional healthcare practitioners establish a satisfactory interpersonal relationship in order to improve health care and education within these ethnic groups.

The American Nurses Association (ANA) has recognized the importance of understanding the concepts of transcultural nursing. Its *Position Statement on Cultural Diversity in Nursing Practice, 1991*, maintains that:

- Cultural assessment of the client is an expected nursing function.
- Sensitive nursing care and appropriate client advocacy cannot be accomplished without knowledge of cultural diversity.

SEGREGATION AND DISCRIMINATION

Segregation (physical separation of housing and services based on race) and **discrimination** (unfair and unequal treatment or access to services based on race, culture, or other bias) have permeated the global community. Although the United States has moved beyond segregation in many areas, there are still inequalities based on lack of access to equal health care. Discrimination, as it relates to health services, can involve more than just race or ethnicity. The nurse must also guard against unequal treatment related to an individual's gender, sexual orientation, or legal status. If a client feels that the nurse is being judgmental because of his or her differences, the therapeutic relationship is compromised.

Racial and Ethnic Disparities in Health Care

The Institute of Medicine's Committee on Understanding and Eliminating Racial and Ethnic Disparities in Health Care defined *disparities* in health care as racial or ethnic differences in the quality of health care that are not due to access-related factors or clinical needs, preferences, and appropriateness of interventions. In the context of disparities, discrimination refers to differences in care that result from bias, prejudices, stereotyping, and uncertainty in clinical communication and decision making.

This topic cannot be adequately covered within the confines of this chapter. Some studies have demonstrated that racial and ethnic minorities experience a lower quality of health services and are less likely to receive even routine medical procedures than are White Americans. African Americans and, in some cases, Hispanics are less likely to receive appropriate cardiac medication or to undergo coronary bypass surgery, are less likely to receive dialysis and kidney transplantation, and are likely to receive a lower quality of basic clinical services such as intensive care, even when variations in such factors as insurance status, income, age, comorbid conditions, and symptom expression are taken into account.

Racial and ethnic disparities are also found in a range of other health service categories, including diabetes care, pediatric care and maternal and child health, mental health, rehabilitative and nursing home services, and many surgical procedures.

The sources of disparities in care are a range of client-level, provider-level, and system-level factors.

Racial and ethnic disparities in care may emerge, at least in part, from a number of client-level attributes. For example, minority clients are more likely to refuse recommended services, adhere poorly to treatment regimens, and delay seeking care. These behaviors and attitudes develop as a result of a poor cultural match between the client and the care provider, mistrust, misunderstanding of provider instructions, poor prior interactions with healthcare systems, or simply a lack of knowledge of how best to use healthcare services.

Given that stereotypes, bias, and clinical uncertainty may influence diagnostic and treatment decisions, education may be one of the most important tools as part of an overall strategy to eliminate healthcare disparities. The nurse needs to become aware of racial and ethnic disparities in health care, and the fact that these disparities exist, often despite providers' best intentions. In addition, as a future healthcare provider, you can benefit from cross-cultural education. Through your classroom studies and clinical experience you will have the opportunity to develop an enhanced awareness of how cultural and social factors influence health care. Cross-cultural education can be divided into three conceptual approaches focusing on *attitudes* (cultural sensitivity/awareness approach), *knowledge* (multicultural/categorical approach), and *skills* (cross-cultural approach). Training will be effective in improving your knowledge of cultural and behavioral aspects of health care and building effective communication strategies.

Culturally Based Communication

Intercultural communication occurs when members of two or more cultures exchange messages in a manner that is influenced by their different cultural perceptions (Adler et al., 1998). Communication is interrelated with all other domains. It includes verbal communication (dialects, the context in which language is used, etc.) and nonverbal communication. Clients may communicate quite differently with family and close friends than with unfamiliar healthcare professionals.

VERBAL COMMUNICATION

One of the first questions that should be asked in any healthcare situation is "What language do you normally use to communicate?" Even though a client may understand English in a casual conversation, he or she may not be able to communicate on the technical level required during a health interview. Healthcare workers need to be aware of the dominant language of an area, as well as problems that may be caused by particular dialects. Clients from Mexico may speak 1 of more than 50 dialects. People from the Philippines may speak 1 of 87. The dialect may pose a communication barrier even if a nurse speaks the same language. Dialect differences increase the difficulty of obtaining accurate information.

NONVERBAL COMMUNICATION

Many times much more is learned from what is not said than from what is said. Nonverbal communication is vital to communicating with clients, but here cultural variations can have a big impact. For example, in Western cultures, people are expected to make eye contact during communication. In other cultures, Asian specifically, making eye contact is a demonstration of lack of respect.

Nurses can learn ways of identifying a particular client's normal behavior. For example, in any culture a client may be reluctant to make eye contact with the health professional when sensitive issues are being discussed. The nurse may wonder whether embarrassment about the topic or cultural behavior is the reason. To assess the situation, the nurse can move to a less sensitive topic and observe the client's response. If the client continues to avoid eye contact, the nurse who is culturally sensitive will be able to interpret such behavior accurately.

Touch can convey much, but again, cultures differ on what they permit and accept. It is important for the nurse to be aware of the client's reaction to touch. During the first contact with a client, the nurse should ask permission to touch the client. When performing a procedure that involves touch, the nurse should fully explain the procedure before touching the client.

Appropriate touch for children may vary by culture. Box 3-4 ■ describes some variations in ways of touching children.

Personal space must be respected, both when caring for multicultural clients and when interacting with coworkers. For example, European Americans usually keep a minimum of 18 inches between themselves and the person with whom they are communicating. Middle Easterners tend to stand very close and stare during conversation. A European American nurse who does not know about this difference may feel threatened during a conversation with a Middle Eastern physician. The nurse may feel the physician is invading his or her personal space. Information about cultural norms is important to staff education to preserve a comfortable work environment.

BOX 3-4	PEDIATRIC CONSIDERATIONS

Cultural Views on Touching Children

In the Latino culture as well as many in Asia, Africa, and some parts of Europe, patting a child on the head is considered a demeaning touch, as if you were touching a thing like a dog. Some groups even see touching the child's head as placing a curse on the child.

With mothers and infants of Hispanic descent, it is important to say something like "what a cute baby" when touching the infant (other than on the head). Touching the baby without complimenting him or her is thought to bring bad luck.

Facial expressions and hand gestures also have different meanings from one culture to another. For example, individuals of Jewish, Hispanic, and Italian heritage rarely smile because showing one's teeth can be viewed as a sign of aggression. A therapeutic relationship can be promoted or hampered by the nurse's understanding of transcultural communication.

Transcultural Communication and Client Concerns

PREVENTING ERRORS AND NONCOMPLIANCE

Transcultural communication is applicable in all healthcare situations. It can help to prevent errors and noncompliance during client teaching. For example, the nurse may tell a mother with limited English to give her child Tylenol (acetaminophen) elixir if the child develops a fever. Medication to lower a fever is the usual intervention in American culture. A mother from an Asian or Latin American culture, however, may view the fever as resulting from an upset of body balance. It is important for the nurse to teach the mother that a fever in a young child can spike very quickly and may even result in a seizure. For this reason, cooling measures and antipyretic medication (like acetaminophen) should be used when the fever reaches 38.3°C (101°F). Besides giving clear and specific instructions, nurses should also make sure instructions are understood before ending the communication.

ENSURING INFORMED CONSENT

Informed consent can also present enormous difficulties. Whenever possible, family members (especially children) should not be used to interpret medical information. Although they may have better English skills than the client, they may be too emotionally involved to give clear information. They may not have the language skills to ensure a clear understanding of the procedures to which the client is consenting. Also, including a family member in discussions can involve violations of confidentiality. Newly instituted Health Insurance Portability and Accountability Act (HIPAA) regulations prevent information from being given to a family member without specific permission from the client. The hospital or healthcare institution must make provisions for maintaining privacy. (See more about HIPAA in Chapter 14 ⬤⬤.)

Many healthcare facilities designate qualified employees to provide translation services. Each unit will have contact information for these individuals. Frequently these staff members are compensated for their skill. Nurses who have the ability to speak, write, or translate another language should provide that information to their facilities' human resources departments.

REDUCING CLIENT STRESS AND ANXIETY

Stress and anxiety are alleviated when there is adequate understanding and communication. Clients whose questions and concerns are addressed in a language with which they are comfortable will be more cooperative, less anxious, and more able to cope with hospitalization than clients who are having communication problems.

PROVIDING CUSTOMER SATISFACTION

Good communication is also important because customer service has become an important part of health care. Health care is a service industry, and clients are increasingly aware consumers. Clients frequently research their disease and the available treatments. When they come for a consultation, they expect to be given all the appropriate information. If information is not given to their satisfaction, they may look elsewhere for care. They may change doctors or refuse to allow a particular healthcare professional to administer treatment to them. Taking time to communicate effectively on first contact is not wasting time. In fact, it may save time, because corrections will not have to be made. Further, a well-informed client is likely to be more willing to participate in the treatment plan than one who is not well informed.

Conducting the Cultural Assessment

Nurses learn general concepts about transcultural nursing and specific facts about various cultures so that they can provide ethical and effective care to all their clients. They must understand how ideas from other cultures agree with or differ from their own. Nurses must be sensitive to issues of race, gender, sexual orientation, social class, and economic situation in their everyday work.

A cultural assessment has four basic elements. These elements are highlighted in Box 3-5 ■.

When performing the cultural assessment, the nurse needs to consider many of the cultural domains that were mentioned earlier (see Box 3-3).

Heritage and residence are important. Immigrants commonly relocate to an area where there is an established population of the same background. When individuals settle and work in ethnic communities, their primary social support is enhanced. However, **acculturation** (the modification of a group's or individual's culture as a result of contact with another group) may be hindered. The nurse can increase the opportunities for clients to cooperate in health promotion, health maintenance, and disease prevention by being aware of the geographic location of a cultural group. Communities with large cultural groups may have specific

BOX 3-5   DATA COLLECTION

Elements and Questions for a Cultural Assessment

There are four elements in a cultural assessment. Data for cultural assessment of a client can be collected by the LPN/LVN.

1. *The cultural identity of the client.*
   - How does the client identify himself or herself culturally?
   - Does the client feel closer to the native culture or to the host culture?
   - What is the client's language preference?
2. *The cultural factors related to the client's psychosocial environment.*
   - What stressors are there in the local environment?
   - What role does religion play in the individual's life?
   - What kind of support systems does the client have?
3. *The cultural elements of the relationship between the healthcare provider and the client.*
   - What kind of experiences has the client had with healthcare providers, either now or in the past? (The nurse should also consider what differences exist between the provider's and the client's culture and social status. These differences are important in communicating and in negotiating an appropriate relationship.)
4. *The cultural explanation of the client's illness.*
   - What is the client's cultural explanation of the illness?
   - What idioms does the client use to describe it? (For example, the client may say she is suffering from *ataque de nervios*—an attack of the nerves. This is a syndrome in Hispanic cultures that closely resembles anxiety and depressive disorders.)
   - Is there a name or category used by the client's family or community to identify the condition? For care to be client centered, no matter what culture the client is, the nurse has to elicit specific information from the client and use it to organize strategies for care.

services available to meet their population's healthcare needs while also considering their cultural practices.

Educational status must also be considered. Primary learning styles vary among individuals from different cultures. The nurse adjusts teaching strategies to fit the individual's educational values and modes of learning.

The client's occupation is also of importance. Knowledge about a client's current *work and work history* is essential for health screening. For example, individuals who worked in the mines in their home country may need to be evaluated for respiratory conditions.

Family roles and organization may need to be considered. Dominant family roles determine who will make healthcare decisions. Some cultures (such as Italian and Filipino families) are patriarchal. (No major health decisions would be made without consulting with the male head-of-the-house.) The African American family is primarily *matriarchal* (headed by the mother or grandmother). European American families

are more *egalitarian* (sharing the leadership role). Family roles also describe gender-related roles of men and women in the family system.

Biocultural ecology involves the assessment of skin color and biologic variations. Skin color may pose special problems or concerns for healthcare professionals. For example, to collect data about anemia in an African American client, the nurse needs to know to assess the oral mucosa. Nurses must also identify biologic variations in body structure. For example, many Asian children are small by American standards. This must be considered by the nurse when gathering data on a standard growth chart.

The nurse will need to identify *specific risk factors* related to topography or climate. Hereditary or genetic diseases or conditions, as well as endemic diseases specific to a cultural or ethnic group, must be identified. Some groups have an increased susceptibility to certain diseases or health conditions. This knowledge is important for health screening and prevention. Finally, variations in drug metabolism, interaction, and related side effects should be considered.

Assessment should take into consideration specific *high-risk behaviors* that are common among the client's culture of origin. The nurse should explore behaviors related to the use of tobacco, alcohol, and recreational drugs. Healthcare practices, or the client's reluctance to follow safety practices, may provide some essential information. The client should be assessed for the level of physical activity in his or her lifestyle. Clients should also be asked about the use of safety measures, such as seat belts or motorcycle or bike helmets.

Healthcare practices and the use of health practitioners are also part of the cultural assessment. Questions related to *lifespan issues*, specifically pregnancy and childbearing practices and death rituals, can provide vital information. For a complete cultural assessment, the nurse may explore the client's views and practices related to fertility control and pregnancy. Many cultures have prescriptive, restrictive, and taboo practices related to childbearing. These may interfere with instructions given by the healthcare provider. By identifying these issues, the client and the provider can address them while maintaining an open therapeutic relationship. During the cultural assessment, practices related to food, exercise, intercourse, and avoidance of weather-related conditions should also be addressed.

Many nurses find it uncomfortable to discuss the client's views on *death and dying*. However, this too is a key part of the cultural assessment. It is important for the nurse to understand the mourning practices of cultural groups, so that respect and privacy can be provided for the family. The nurse must also be aware of the client's individual desires. Some may want to talk about the meaning of death, dying, and the afterlife. Others may feel that this is private and not something to be discussed.

Subculture of Health Care

No matter how proficient the nurse is in understanding his or her own culture, there is an added barrier to communication. The healthcare profession itself is a kind of subculture, and all nurses are members of it. The subculture of nursing affects the nurse's views and actions, no matter what the culture of origin. A Hispanic nurse may have been raised in an environment where folk medicine, a variety of prayers, poultices, and herbs were used to treat illness. After training, the nurse may view certain health-seeking behaviors of clients as being primitive or even foolish, even when members of the nurse's own family practice those behaviors. The Hispanic client may treat the nurse as a member of the "establishment" and an oppressor rather than as someone who shares the same background and has experienced the same social treatment.

Nurses cannot prevent their education and training from affecting their thinking and perhaps even their cultural values. However, if they have insight into their own changes in thinking, their interactions with clients will be more positive. They will be able to interact with clients with more acceptance and empathy.

Healthcare facilities can provide training and policies to encourage culturally proficient care, but staff attitudes are another important consideration. Facilities must regularly assess staff attitudes and take steps to correct those that hamper the mission of delivering culturally proficient care. Box 3-6 ■ offers some questions for reviewing your own attitudes.

CULTURAL EMPATHY

Cultural empathy involves the ability to experience "as" the client experiences rather than "how" they experience themselves. It is the ability to express genuine interest in the struggles, challenges, and conflicts surrounding the client's health-related problems (Andrews & Boyle, 2007). The nurse has a responsibility to help the client explore his or her feelings, thoughts, and behaviors. It is important to validate the client's feelings and to demonstrate genuine concern. Without these positive actions, the client is not likely to perceive that the nurse cares.

CULTURAL DIVERSITY AMONG NURSES

At one time the profession of nursing was predominantly White women of European descent. That has changed dramatically, especially in large metropolitan coastal cities. The nursing population now closely resembles the population as a whole. It was once enough to teach nursing students about other predominant cultures that they might encounter with the client for whom they would be caring. Today nurses must also learn how to work with other nurses from different cultures (Figure 3-2 ■).

Nurses of different ethnic and racial backgrounds will be of two types: those who received their education locally, and

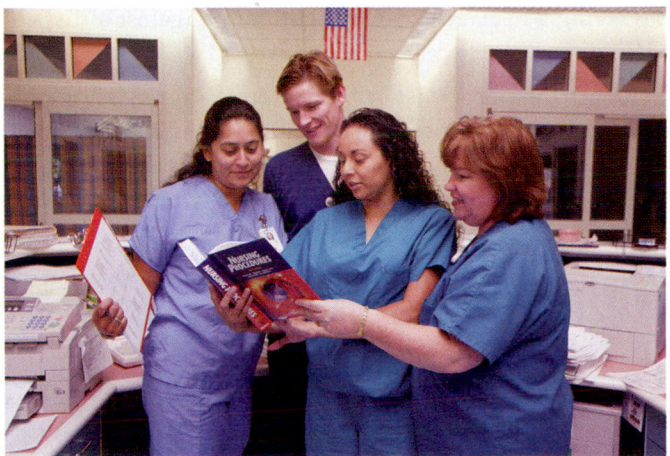

Figure 3-2. ■ Nurses today are of many backgrounds and cultures. It is important both for the needs of clients and for the success of institutions for nurses to make adaptations to account for the differences in culture. *Source:* Photoedit Inc.

BOX 3-6	REVIEWING YOUR ATTITUDES TOWARD CULTURAL DIVERSITY

The following are some reflective questions about attitudes toward other cultures. Rate yourself on the following scale:
1—Strongly agree; 2—Agree; 3—Neither agree nor disagree; 4—Disagree; 5—Strongly disagree.

I react negatively if the client has an accent.	1 2 3 4 5
I am open to differences among cultures and different ways of doing things.	1 2 3 4 5
I respect diverse practices and requests without judgment.	1 2 3 4 5
I recognize and actively accommodate clients' choices about their care.	1 2 3 4 5
I assume that I know how to determine what a client wants or needs.	1 2 3 4 5
I identify the need for resources to overcome barriers, such as poor or insufficient English proficiency or lack of support networks.	1 2 3 4 5
I identify the need for, and obtain knowledge of, sources of extra social support, such as community organizations.	1 2 3 4 5

those who were foreign trained. Of the second group, the LPN/LVN may come in contact with a fellow staff member or student who was trained as a physician or a registered nurse in another country but who is now working or training as an LPN/LVN. The American-trained, non-White nurse will share much of the philosophy of nursing as the traditionally trained White nurse, while having some very distinct ethnocentric views. Foreign-born and foreign-trained nurses may have a different philosophy of care, as well as very diverse cultural attitudes.

It is important that nurses of all backgrounds be able to work together for the good of the clients as well as the nursing unit.

When a significant number of staff on a unit are from one ethnic or racial group, a number of issues can arise that can cause tension among the staff. They include the following:

- Speaking a native language in front of other staff members
- Criticizing an entire group when one member of that group is not performing up to standards
- Having a manager who is biased for or against a particular group when granting requests

When tensions exist among groups in a class or on a nursing unit, care should be taken to discuss the real issues and to encourage individuals to broaden their knowledge and understanding of others' backgrounds.

NURSING CARE

PRIORITIZING NURSING CARE

Nurses at all levels have the responsibility to deliver culturally proficient care. Because LPNs/LVNs work so closely with clients and families, they carry a large share of this responsibility. Before nurses can provide proficient transcultural care, they must have an understanding of their own culture.

For example, if a nurse discovers that immigrants of his or her own culture (French) once competed heavily for jobs with Irish immigrants, the "instant dislike" the nurse feels for Irish clients may be seen in a new light. This awareness of bias in oneself may also help the nurse understand why some Irish clients react negatively toward him or her "for no reason." By recognizing such biases in one's own culture, the nurse will be able to identify those unhelpful reactions and learn to overcome them.

Both the nurse and the client are influenced by their cultural identity, ethnic history, values, kinship, and family. Illness and stress may cause these aspects of a person's life and cultural, religious, and spiritual beliefs to become more pronounced. Philosophic points of view and moral and ethical perspectives also influence the nurse–client relationship.

ASSESSING

To meet the holistic needs of clients, the nurse must complete a holistic assessment (described earlier in the chapter), not just a physical assessment. This includes information about the client's physical, psychosocial, emotional, and spiritual status, as well as cultural status. The cultural assessment may be done as discussed previously. Review Box 3-5 for questions that are part of a cultural assessment.

It may be necessary to work with an interpreter while completing the assessment. The team leader or RN usually obtains the full assessment, but ongoing assessment requires the same full awareness. Box 3-7 ■ provides guidelines for working with interpreters.

Pain Expression

Pain and pain expression are an important area of consideration in nursing. Pain is a universal occurrence. Pain is the most frequent reason for seeking health care, and chronic pain is now the leading cause of disability in the country.

It is difficult to define pain, partly because of its complex nature and partly because of the many different perspectives on pain that exist. The medical definition of pain, established in the late 1800s, is a sensation associated with real or potential tissue damage involving chemical disturbances

BOX 3-7	WORKING WITH INTERPRETERS

Obtain an interpreter from the facility's designated interpreters list (when available).*

Avoid using family members.

Confirm the issue of confidentiality with the interpreter and reassure the client of same.

Allow additional time for the assessment or interview.

Brief the interpreter and provide background information prior to the encounter with the client.

Use simple language and pause between sentences to allow the interpreter to translate every word.

Talk directly to the client, not the interpreter. The interpreter is just a voice.

If the client and the interpreter begin to talk to each other, ask for a translation. Do not be left out.

If possible, use the same interpreter for all such contacts with the client.

Validate the client's understanding by asking for brief summaries. Important ideas can be lost during translation.

Encourage the interpreter to inform the nurse of any cultural differences that may lead to misunderstanding or lack of compliance. (Interpreters are usually bicultural as well as bilingual; they can be a source of information about the culture, customs, and worldview of the client.)

Respect the interpreter's suggestions but do not allow him or her to take over.

*A list of interpreters is usually available through the human resources or social services department.

along neurologic pathways. However, we know that pain is much more. It is a very personal experience. Perception of pain is based on cultural learning, the meaning of the situation, and factors unique to each individual.

Culturally Specific Responses

Responses to pain culturally have been divided into two categories: *stoic* and *emotive*. Stoic clients are less expressive of their pain and tend to "grin and bear it." They tend to withdraw socially. Emotive clients are more likely to verbalize their expressions of pain. They desire people around to react to their pain and assist them with their suffering. Expressive clients often come from Hispanic, Middle Eastern, and Mediterranean backgrounds. Stoic clients often come from Northern European and Asian backgrounds. However, ethnicity alone does not predict accurately how a person will respond to pain. Some individuals tolerate even the most severe pain with little more than a clenched jaw and frequently refuse pain medication.

Pain has both personal and cultural meanings. It is a subjective and universal experience of human existence that affects individuals of every age and every culture. Pain has physical, emotional, social, and spiritual components. There are vast differences in the expression of pain, and culture plays a major role in these pain experiences. Culture significantly affects the assessment and management of people in pain.

Cultural diversity affects care of the client in pain. The influx of minorities from other countries is predicted to continue, along with the growth of the proportion of minorities within the United States. This changing population means that we as healthcare providers must learn how to respond to pain in a wide range of clients. Cultural background affects pain perception. Cultural background has long been recognized as having a major influence on how one perceives and reacts to painful situations. Pain has both personal and cultural meanings. Although clients from two different cultures may experience a similar condition or surgical procedure, their pain response may differ dramatically. An understanding of pain from a cultural perspective is vital if healthcare providers are to respond to clients in a helpful manner.

Caregivers must also be aware that people within cultural groups may differ biologically from those in other groups. This is true with medications affecting the central nervous system that may be used for pain or symptoms related to pain. Clients with a genetic alteration in a drug-metabolizing enzyme cannot metabolize codeine to morphine properly, so they do not experience an analgesic response. About 5% to 10% of the population does not receive an analgesic effect from codeine.

When treating a client from a different culture, the *client's concern for symptoms* must be treated with as much concern as the actual physical symptoms that are present. People often attribute meaning to their pain. Clients attempt to order the experience of their pain (what it means to them and those close to them) through personal narratives of their illness. These stories are not fixed, but constantly told and retold. In a sense, the narratives not only reflect the pain experience but create it.

Key metaphors and rhetorical devices appear to be chosen by the client as a way to make sense of the pain experience. A client might use a rhetorical device such as *amplification*, which involves repeating a word or expression while adding more detail to it in order to emphasize what might otherwise be passed over. An example of this would be, "I am in pain. My pain is so severe, it feels like bugs are crawling under my skin. It feels like they are biting me. My skin is on fire. I just can't stand this pain anymore." Metaphors are also used by clients. An example would be "the pain in my side is a hot poker piercing my skin."

Nurses' Views about Pain Response

Nursing, medical, and hospital cultures influence pain assessment, decision making, and care. An understanding of the impact of culture on the pain experience is crucial to providing effective care. Because cultural or religious reasons may keep a person from requesting pain medication even when it is medically necessary, it is often best to anticipate a client's pain needs.

DIAGNOSING, PLANNING, AND IMPLEMENTING

The nurse's number one responsibility is to establish an open nurse–client relationship. Nurses must always present themselves as supportive, effective, competent, and empathetic professionals. The nurse–client relationship should be one of respect, genuineness, and warmth. These behaviors constitute the essence of transcultural nursing. If the client gets the impression that the nurse is looking down on him or her, the relationship will be damaged.

The nurse must respect the client as an individual, whether the nurse is meeting the client's physical or psychosocial needs. When the professional loses sight of the individual, stereotyping based on culture can occur. Prejudging a client's needs can place the client in jeopardy. One example of this is related to protocols for breast cancer treatment. A client who has a mixed heritage of African American and Native American will usually be African American in appearance. However, African Americans and Native Americans may have quite different responses to chemotherapeutic drugs. The physician may prescribe treatment according to protocols developed through research with an African American group. The assumption that the client is genetically identical to the research group may lead to unexpected reactions. In this instance, cultural assessment could have provided the physician with valuable information. Collaboration with the RN or the physician on cultural information can be an important function of the LPN/LVN.

Partly as a result of the nursing subculture, nurses often expect people to be objective about a really subjective experience. In clinical practice, the nurse may expect clients to give a detailed description of their pain, and to give the description without displaying an emotional response. When a client complains, cries, or screams, he or she may be labeled as overreacting or having an excessive need for additional medication.

Extensive research has been done about nurses' reactions to clients in pain. Nurses bring their own attitudes about pain to each interaction. It is important for them to identify their beliefs and opinions about pain relief. They should also examine how they express and manage their own pain. Then, they must begin to understand that there is no right or wrong way to express pain. Only when nurses have dealt with their own attitudes about pain will they be able to help their clients who are in pain.

EVALUATING

Discharge planning is also a responsibility of the nurse. Depending on the type of healthcare facility, the LPN/LVN will participate to a greater or lesser degree. Cultural care should continue throughout the nursing process. Points that are considered especially important for clients from diverse cultural backgrounds are listed in Box 3-8 ■.

It is no longer acceptable to treat a client without considering his or her culture throughout the hospital stay. As you

BOX 3-8	DISCHARGE PLANNING

The nurse should consider the following questions when evaluating discharge planning:

Do you use an interpreter when necessary to facilitate communication about discharge planning?

Do you start discharge planning as early as possible in the hospitalization period?

Do you consider the client's medical and nonmedical needs?

Do you employ a multidisciplinary approach?

Do you allow clients and their families to be involved in planning their care?

Do you check that the clients, family/support people, and care providers fully understand the proposed plan?

Do you ensure that posthospital care involves cooperation and collaboration among the hospital, home care agencies, community services, or alternate care facilities?

work your way through this text, you will find cultural applications in every chapter called "Cultural Pulse Points." They will be found as a box for easy reference.

Technology and travel have expanded our community such that now we are part of a global community. As we develop a fuller understanding of the cultures of the people with whom we come in contact, we as nurses can become more accepting of differences. As we become more accepting, we will be able to provide culturally proficient nursing care.

Note: The references and resources for all chapters have been compiled at the back of the book.

Chapter Review

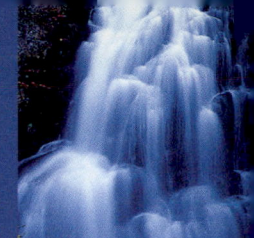

KEY Points

- The goal of cultural awareness is to end prejudice and discrimination.
- Theories of transcultural nursing, begun by Dr. Madeleine Leininger in the 1950s, are a vital part of nursing care in our diverse society.
- Ethnocentrism is a common tendency. Nurses must be extra careful not to stereotype their clients, because their work depends on their ability to see each client as unique.
- The LPN/LVN will need to develop knowledge of different cultures, especially those that relate to groups where the nurse lives and works.
- Nonverbal communication is vital to communicating with clients. Cultural variations have a big impact on nonverbal communication.
- Transcultural communication is applicable in all healthcare situations. It can help to prevent error and noncompliance during client teaching.
- Whenever possible, family members (especially children) should not be used to interpret medical information.
- A trained nurse may view the health-seeking behaviors of clients as being primitive or even foolish, even when members of the nurse's own family practice those behaviors.
- Healthcare practices and the use of health practitioners are part of the cultural assessment.

⊕ FOR FURTHER Study

For more information on nursing theories and models, see Chapter 5 and Table 5-4.

For the major discussion about HIPAA, see Chapter 14.

Refer to Chapter 18 for more information on beliefs about death and dying in major cultural groups.

See Table 44-1 for mourning and after-death rites of major cultural groups.

NCLEX-PN® Exam Preparation

TEST-TAKING TIP Questions related to cultural care are frequently subjective. When faced with a question concerning the client's culture, be on guard against using stereotypes from your own background.

1 During shift report, the night nurse states, "Maria Sanchez in Room 402 has been yelling all night 'delaude, delaude,' but she doesn't look like she is in pain. You know those people have a very low pain tolerance." The nurse is using:

1. Stereotypes.
2. Ethnocentrism.
3. Acculturation.
4. Cultural awareness.

2 The nursing theorist whose theory focused specifically on transcultural nursing with a culture care focus is:

1. Dorothea Orem.
2. Martha Rogers.
3. Madeleine Leininger.
4. Betty Neuman.

3 The nurse displays cultural competence by being aware of and accepting differences in others, understanding the dynamics of difference, being aware of his or her own cultural values, developing cultural knowledge, and the ability to:

1. Communicate in the client's native language.
2. Adapt practice skills to fit the cultural context of the client.
3. Ignore cultural differences while providing nursing care.
4. Provide complementary or alternative health care to culturally diverse clients.

4 The nurse, working in a culturally diverse facility, anticipates finding which of the following to be true? (Select all that apply.)

1. Some team members may not be as competent as others, depending on their cultural background.
2. The unit director will give preference to staff members who share the same cultural background as the director.
3. All staff members will be expected to meet minimum standards of competence for their designated job title.
4. Nurses from different cultures may have different approaches to client care.
5. Some nurses may be less dependable because they will need religious holidays off.

5 A Caucasian nurse raised in the American culture and viewing Western medicine as the only option can be said to be:

1. Prejudiced.
2. Culturally sensitive.
3. Ethnocentric.
4. Culturally competent.

6 When a nurse makes a statement based on ethnic stereotyping, the nurse assumes:

1. All members of an ethnic group are alike.
2. All members of a cultural group have the same health beliefs.

3. Commonalities occur among cultures.
4. Individuals of specific groups respond to medical treatment differently.

7 An Asian mother brings her child in for follow-up after an ear infection. The physician suggests surgery to place ear tubes. The mother becomes agitated when pushed to schedule surgery. With your knowledge of cultural responses, you determine that:

1. She does not understand why the procedure must be done.
2. It is important to consider who has the authority to make healthcare decisions in the family.
3. She is concerned that her health insurance may not pay for the procedure.
4. An interpreter should be provided when consent for surgery is obtained.

8 A Hispanic mother who had expressed a desire to breastfeed is giving her baby a bottle. She states, "I don't have any milk yet. I will breastfeed when I get home." From her statement the nurse would conclude:

1. She does not understand the importance of colostrum to provide immunity for the baby.
2. She does not understand the concept of supply and demand for milk production.
3. Some cultural groups are extremely modest and are only comfortable breastfeeding in private.
4. She really does not plan to breastfeed. She just feels pressured by the staff to agree to it.

9 A Jewish rabbi in traction refuses the nurse's help to eat roast pork, vegetables, roll, and butter and drink a carton of milk. Which statement made by the nurse would be appropriate?

1. "It is very important that you have a diet high in protein and calcium in order for your body to heal."
2. "If you don't like the meal they have sent, I can see what else is available."
3. "I know it is difficult to be dependent. Once you are out of traction you will be able to do it on your own."
4. "Do you follow kosher dietary laws? I will have the dietitian speak with you about a diet that will meet your needs."

10 The nurse, performing a cultural assessment, would assess which of the following? (Select all that apply.)

1. Religious beliefs
2. Cultural elements of the relationship with the healthcare provider
3. The client's race
4. Cultural identity
5. Heritage and residence

Answers and rationales for Review Questions appear in Appendix I.

Chapter 4

Legal and Ethical Issues of Nursing

LEARNING Outcomes

After completing this chapter, you will be able to:

1. Describe aspects of law that affect nursing practice, including the difference between crimes and torts, and give examples in nursing.
2. Define unprofessional conduct: negligence, assault/battery, false imprisonment, invasion of privacy, and defamation.
3. Describe regulation of nursing practice, standards of care, agency policies, and nurse practice acts that affect the scope of nursing practice.
4. Describe legal protection for nurses, including Good Samaritan and the Americans with Disabilities acts.
5. Explain the purpose of liability insurance.
6. Identify ways nurses and nursing students can minimize their chances of liability.
7. Discuss several legal aspects of nursing practice, including privileged communication in the nurse–client relationship.
8. List information that needs to be included in an incident report.
9. Explain the purposes and limitations of professional codes of ethics and how they relate to nursing practice.
10. Discuss the advocacy role of the nurse.
11. Discuss approaches to making ethical decisions.
12. Discuss common ethical issues currently facing healthcare professionals.

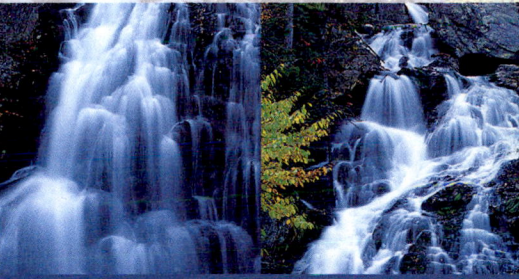

KEY TERMS

Use the audio glossary feature on the MyNursingKit Website to hear the correct pronunciation of the following key terms.

advocate 55	credentialing 45	libel 44
arbitration 47	crime 45	malpractice 43
assault 44	defamation 44	negligence 43
attitudes 54	ethics 54	scope of practice 46
autonomy 55	false imprisonment 44	sexual harassment 53
battery 44	impaired nurse 52	slander 45
beliefs 54	invasion of privacy 44	statute of limitations 43
bioethics 54	law 42	tort 43
code of ethics 56	liability 46	values 54

Nursing practice is governed by many legal concepts. It is important for nurses to know the basics of legal concepts because nurses are accountable for their professional judgments and actions. Nurses must know laws that regulate and affect nursing practice for two reasons:

1. To ensure that their decisions and actions are consistent with current legal principles.
2. To protect themselves from liability.

UNDERSTANDING LEGAL ISSUES

Law can be defined as "those rules made by humans which regulate social conduct in a formally prescribed and legally binding manner" (Bernzweig, 1996, p. 3).

The law serves a number of functions in nursing:

- It provides a framework for establishing which nursing actions in the care of clients are legal.
- It differentiates the nurse's responsibilities from those of other healthcare professionals.
- It helps establish the boundaries of independent nursing action.
- It assists in maintaining a standard of nursing practice by making nurses accountable under the law.

The regulation of nursing is a function of state law in the United States and of provincial law in Canada. State or provincial legislatures pass statutes that define and regulate nursing, that is, nurse practice acts. These acts, however, must be consistent with constitutional and federal provisions. See Table 4-1 ■ for selected categories of law affecting nurses.

Kinds of Legal Actions

There are two kinds of legal actions: civil or private actions and criminal actions. Civil actions deal with the relationships among individuals in society. For example, a man may file a suit against a person who he believes cheated him. Civil actions that are of concern to nurses include the contracts and torts listed in Table 4-1. Criminal actions deal

TABLE 4-1	Selected Categories of Laws Affecting Nurses
CATEGORY	**EXAMPLES**
Constitutional	Due process
	Equal protection
Statutory (legislative)	Nurse practice acts
	Good Samaritan acts
	Child and adult abuse laws
	Living wills
	Sexual harassment laws
	Americans with Disabilities Act
Criminal (public)	Homicide, manslaughter
	Theft
	Arson
	Active euthanasia
	Sexual assault
	Illegal possession of controlled drugs
Contracts (private/civil)	Nurse and client
	Nurse and employer
	Nurse and insurance
	Client and agency
Torts (private/civil)	Negligence
	Assault and battery
	False imprisonment
	Invasion of privacy
	Libel and slander

with disputes between an individual and the society as a whole. For example, if a man shoots a person, society brings him to trial. The major difference between criminal and civil law is the potential outcome for the defendant. If found guilty in a civil action, such as malpractice, the defendant will have to pay a sum of money. If found guilty in a criminal action, the defendant may lose money, be jailed, or be executed. Nurses could lose their license. The action of a lawsuit is called *litigation*, and lawyers who participate in lawsuits may be referred to as *litigators*.

CIVIL LAW

A **tort** is a civil wrong committed against a person or a person's property. Torts are usually litigated in court by civil action between individuals. In other words, the person or persons claimed to be responsible for the tort are sued for damages. Tort liability almost always is based on fault, that is, something was done incorrectly (an unreasonable act of commission) or something should have been done but was not (an act of omission).

Torts may be classified as unintentional or intentional.

Unintentional Torts

Negligence and malpractice are examples of unintentional torts that may occur in the healthcare setting. **Negligence** is misconduct or practice that is below the standard expected of an ordinary, reasonable, and prudent practitioner, which places another person at risk for harm. Gross negligence involves an extreme lack of knowledge, skill, or decision making. The person clearly should have known that such behavior would put clients at risk for harm. **Malpractice** is negligence that occurred while the person was performing as a professional. Malpractice applies to physicians, dentists, lawyers, and, in some cases, nurses. Four elements must be present for a case of nursing negligence or malpractice to be proven:

1. The nurse has a working relationship with the client (duty).
2. The nurse fails to uphold the appropriate standard of care (breach).
3. The client must have suffered harm, injury, or damage (harm).
4. The harm has to be a direct result of the nurse's failure to provide appropriate care (causation).

If a lawsuit is filed for a negligent act performed by a nurse, it will also name the nurse's employer. In addition, employers may be held liable for negligence if they fail to provide adequate human and material resources for nursing care, to properly educate nurses on the use of new equipment or procedures, or to orient nurses to the facility. Sometimes the harm cannot be traced to a specific healthcare provider or standard but does not normally occur unless there has been a negligent act. An example is harm that results when surgical instruments or sponges are accidentally left in a client during surgery.

To defend against a negligence suit, the nurse must prove that one or more of the required elements is not met. There is also a limit to the amount of time that can pass between recognition of harm and the bringing of a suit. This is referred to as the **statute of limitations.** In some cases, an additional defense is "contributory or comparative negligence" on the part of the injured client. In these situations, the client was at least partly responsible for his or her own injury. When clients choose not to follow healthcare advice, such as remaining in bed while recovering from a treatment, the court may reduce any verdict against the nurse by an amount considered to be the plaintiff's own contribution.

To avoid charges of malpractice, nurses need to recognize those nursing situations in which negligent actions are most likely to occur and to take measures to prevent them (Box 4-1 ■). The most common situation is the medication error. Because of the large number of medications on the market today and the variety of methods of administration, these errors may be on the increase. Nurses always need to check medications very carefully (see Chapter 27 ⚭). Even after checking, the nurse is wise to recheck the medication order and the medication before administering it if the client states, for example, "I did not have a green pill before."

A relatively frequent malpractice action attributed to nurses is causing a burn to a client. Elderly, comatose, and diabetic people are particularly vulnerable to burns because of their decreased sensitivity to pain and temperature. Hot objects can burn these people before they notice it.

BOX 4-1	BASIC NURSING CARE ERRORS RESULTING IN NEGLIGENCE

Assessment Errors

Failing to
- Gather and chart client information adequately.
- Recognize the significance of certain information (e.g., laboratory values, vital signs).

Planning Errors

Failing to
- Chart each identified problem.
- Use language in the care plan that other caregivers understand.
- Ensure continuity of care by ignoring the care plan.
- Give discharge instructions that the client understands.

Intervention Errors

Failing to
- Administer and document medications correctly.
- Interpret and carry out a doctor's orders.
- Perform nursing tasks correctly.
- Pursue the physician if the doctor doesn't respond to calls or notify the nurse-manager if the physician is unavailable.

Clients often fall accidentally, sometimes with resultant injury. Some falls can be prevented by elevating the side rails on the cribs, beds, and stretchers of babies and small children and, when necessary, of adults. A nurse who leaves the rails down or leaves a baby unattended on a bath table is guilty of malpractice if the client falls and is injured as a direct result. The nurse needs to follow facility policies regarding side rails and injury prevention. Information about providing a safe environment for the client can be found in Chapter 9 🔗.

In some instances, ignoring a client's complaints can constitute malpractice. This type of malpractice is termed *failure to observe and take appropriate action*. If a nurse does not report a client's complaint of acute abdominal pain and the client sustains a ruptured appendix, the nurse is negligent and may be found guilty of malpractice. If a nurse fails to check vital signs and the dressing of a client who has just had surgery, important assessments are omitted. If the client hemorrhages and dies, the nurse may be held responsible for the death as a result of this malpractice.

Incorrectly identifying clients is a problem, particularly in busy hospital units. Failure to check identification bands before administering medication can result in injury to the client if the medication is given to the wrong person. Checking the medication administration record (MAR) against the armband at the bedside every time can prevent cases of mistaken identity, which are costly to the client and render the nurse liable for malpractice.

Intentional Torts

In the United States, the terms *assault* and *battery* are often heard together, but each has its own meaning. **Assault** can be described as an attempt or threat to touch another person unjustifiably. Assault precedes battery; it is the act that causes the person to believe a battery is about to occur. For example, the person who threatens someone by making a menacing gesture with a club or a closed fist is guilty of assault. In nursing, a nurse who threatens a client with an injection after the client refuses to take the medication orally would be committing assault.

Battery is the willful touching of a person (or the person's clothes, or even something the person is carrying) that may or may not cause harm. To be illegal, however, the touching must be wrong in some way. For example, it must be done without permission, be embarrassing, or cause injury. In the previous example, if the nurse followed through on the threat and gave the injection without the client's consent, the nurse would be committing battery. Even though the physician ordered the medication and even if the client benefits from the administration of the medication, the nurse is still liable.

In Canada, the term *battery* is not used. Instead, there are three categories of assault: assault with intent to injure

(e.g., threatening someone with a knife), assault causing bodily injury, and sexual assault.

To perform procedures without consent is considered battery. (See discussion on informed consent later in this chapter.)

False imprisonment is the "unlawful restraint or detention of another person against his or her wishes." False imprisonment does not require force; the fear of force to restrain or detain the individual is sufficient (Bernzweig, 1996). False imprisonment accompanied by forceful restraint or threat of restraint is battery.

Nurses may suggest under certain circumstances that a client remain in the hospital room or in bed, but the client must not be detained against the client's will. The client has a right to insist on leaving, even though it may be detrimental to his or her health. The client can leave by signing an absence without authority (AWA) or against medical advice (AMA) form. As with assault or battery, client competency is a factor in determining whether there is a case of false imprisonment or a situation of protecting a client from injury. Agencies usually have clear policies about the application of restraints to guide nurses in such dilemmas. See Chapter 9 🔗 for information about restraints.

Invasion of privacy is a direct wrong of a personal nature that injures the feelings of the person and does not take into account the effect of revealed information on the standing of the person in the community. Privacy is the right of individuals to withhold themselves and their lives from public scrutiny, or the right to be left alone. Liability can result if the nurse breaches confidentiality by passing along confidential client information to others or by intruding into the client's private domain.

Necessary discussion about a client's medical condition is usually considered appropriate, but unnecessary discussions and gossip are considered a breach of confidentiality. Necessary discussion involves only those people engaged in the client's care. Four major categories of client information must be reported: (1) vital statistics, such as births and deaths; (2) infections and communicable diseases, such as syphilis; (3) child or elder abuse; and (4) violent incidents, such as knife wounds. As of April 14, 2003, healthcare agencies and providers must adhere to the Health Insurance Portability and Accountability Act of 1996 (HIPAA). See Chapter 14 🔗 for HIPAA guidelines.

False Communication

Defamation is communication that is false, or made with a careless disregard for the truth, and that results in injury to the reputation of a person. Both libel and slander are wrongful actions that come under the heading of defamation. **Libel** is defamation by means of print, writing, or pictures. Writing in the nurse's notes that a physician is incompetent because he did not respond immediately to a call is an example of libel. **Slander** is defamation by the spoken word, stating information or false words that can cause damage to a person's reputation. An example of slander would be for the nurse to tell a client that another nurse is incompetent.

If a comment that criticizes a person's competence is made to that person in private, it is not defamation because a third party did not hear it. It is slander only if the comment is communicated to a third party.

Nurses are allowed to make statements that could be considered defamatory, but only as a part of nursing practice and only to a physician or another healthcare team member caring directly for the client. For example, the nurse is allowed to say, "The client exhibits inappropriate sexual behavior."

Loss of Client Property

Client property, such as jewelry, money, eyeglasses, and dentures, is a constant concern to hospital personnel. Today, agencies are taking less responsibility for property and are generally requesting clients to sign a waiver on admission relieving the hospital and its employees of any responsibility for property. Situations arise, however, in which the client cannot sign a waiver and the nursing staff must follow prescribed policies for safeguarding the client's property (see Chapter 12 ⚭). Nurses are expected to take reasonable precautions to safeguard a client's property, and they can be held liable for its loss or damage if they do not exercise reasonable care.

CRIMINAL LAW

A **crime** is an act committed in violation of public (criminal) law and punishable by a fine or imprisonment. A crime does not have to be intended in order to be a crime. For example, a nurse may commit a crime by accidentally giving a client an additional and lethal dose of a narcotic to relieve discomfort.

Crimes are classified as either felonies (or in Canada, indictable offenses) or misdemeanors (or in Canada, summary conviction offenses). Crimes are punished through criminal action by the state or province against an individual. A *felony* is a crime of a serious nature, such as murder, punishable by a term in prison. In some areas, second-degree murder is called *manslaughter*. A nurse who accidentally gives an additional and lethal dose of a narcotic can be accused of manslaughter.

A *misdemeanor* is a less serious offense than a felony and is usually punishable by a fine, a short-term jail sentence, or both. A nurse who slaps a client's face could be charged with a misdemeanor.

Regulation of Nursing Practice

Credentialing is the process of determining and maintaining competence in nursing practice. The credentialing process is one way in which the nursing profession maintains standards of practice and accountability for the educational preparation of its members. Credentialing includes licensure, registration, certification, and accreditation.

LICENSURE AND REGISTRATION

There are two types of licensure and registration: mandatory and permissive. In the United States, nursing licensure is mandatory in all states. In Canada, permissive licensure and registration are allowed in some provinces, which means that people who are not licensed or registered can perform nursing duties. Note, however, that licensure and registration are mandatory in most Canadian provinces.

A nurse in any state or province can have his or her license revoked for just cause. These causes are defined in the nurse practice acts. They include incompetent nursing practice, professional misconduct, and conviction of a crime such as using illegal drugs or selling drugs illegally. In each situation, all of the facts are generally reviewed by a committee at a hearing. Nurses are entitled to be represented by legal counsel at such a hearing. If the nurse's license is revoked as a result of the hearing, either the nurse can appeal the decision to a court of law or, in some states, an agency is designated to review the decision before any court action is initiated.

CERTIFICATION

Most certifications are awarded to RNs and advanced practice nurses. However, an LPN/LVN can be certified in long-term care and IV therapy through the National Federation of Licensed Practical Nurses (NFLPN).

ACCREDITATION/APPROVAL OF BASIC NURSING EDUCATION PROGRAMS

Accreditation is a process by which a private organization, such as the National League for Nursing, or a governmental agency, such as the state board of nursing, appraises and grants accredited status to institutions, programs, or services that meet predetermined standards. Minimum standards for basic nursing education programs are established in each state of the United States and in each province in Canada. State accreditation or provincial approval is granted to schools of nursing that meet the minimum criteria.

NURSE PRACTICE ACTS

Each state in the United States has a nurse practice act, and each province in Canada has a nurse practice act or an act for professional nursing practice. Nurse practice acts legally define and describe the scope of nursing practice, which the law seeks to regulate, thereby protecting the public as well. See the website of the National Council of State Boards of Nursing for more information. State boards of nursing also have Internet websites that provide valuable information on the nurse practice acts and scope of practice for the LPN/LVN.

STANDARDS OF PRACTICE

Another way the nursing profession attempts to ensure that its practitioners are competent and safe to practice is through the establishment of standards of practice. These standards are often used to evaluate the quality of care nurses provide. Standards of practice for the LPN/LVN are outlined in the **scope of practice,** a document developed by the board of nursing that governs practice within each state. This document was seen earlier in Chapter 2, Box 2-1 ⚭.

Legal Roles of Nurses

Nurses have three separate, interdependent legal roles, each with rights and associated responsibilities: provider of service, employee or contractor for service, and citizen. As the nurse carries out these roles, the issue of liability must be considered. **Liability** means being legally responsible for one's acts and omissions. When a nurse carries out treatments ordered by the physician, the responsibility for the nursing activity is the nurse's. When a nurse is asked to carry out an activity that the nurse believes could injure the client, the nurse's legal responsibility is to refuse to carry out the order and report this to the nurse's supervisor. An example of this would be a medication that is ordered by a physician, but the dose far exceeds the normal adult dose. If the LPN/LVN would give the medication without questioning the dose and the client was harmed, he or she would be liable. The person administering the medication must be knowledgeable of the medication, the recommended doses, and side effects. Failure to use this knowledge violates the nurse's legal responsibility.

PROVIDER OF SERVICE

The nurse is expected to provide safe and competent care so that harm (physical, psychological, or material) to the recipient of the service is prevented.

EMPLOYEE OR CONTRACTOR FOR SERVICE

A nurse who is employed by an agency works as a representative of the agency. A nurse who is employed directly by a client, for example, a private nurse, may have a written contract with that client to provide professional services for a certain fee. If the nurse becomes ill or dies and cannot fulfill the contract, that is understood. But if a nurse does not fulfill the contract because his or her car broke down or because of personal problems, the nurse broke the contract.

A nurse employed by a hospital functions within an employer–employee relationship, in which the nurse represents and acts for the hospital and therefore must function within the policies of the employing agency. The employer assumes responsibility for the conduct of the employee and can also be held responsible for malpractice by the employee. The nurse's conduct, therefore, is the hospital's responsibility.

This does not mean that the nurse cannot be held liable as an individual. If the employee's actions are extraordinarily inappropriate, the employer might not be held liable. For example, if a nurse hits a client in the face, the employer would not be responsible because this behavior is inappropriate. Criminal acts, such as assisting with criminal abortions or taking drugs from a client's supply for personal use, would also be considered extraordinarily inappropriate behavior. Nurses can be held liable for failure to act as well. For example, a nurse who sees another nurse hitting a client and fails to do anything to protect the client may be considered negligent.

The nurse has obligations to the employer, the client, and other personnel. Nurses must give appropriate care and perform only those responsibilities that they are competent to perform.

The nurse is expected to respect the rights and responsibilities of other healthcare team members. For example, the nurse explains nursing activities to a client but does not have the right to comment on the client's medical care in a way that disturbs the client or criticizes the physician. The nurse also has the right to expect reasonable and prudent conduct from other healthcare professionals.

One area in which nurses and the employer are sometimes in conflict is the practice of "floating" nurses from their assigned unit to one where the level of care and type of client are different. An example of this would be a maternal-infant nurse being floated to a medical-surgical unit. The nurse has the responsibility to make sure he or she has the knowledge and experience to care for the assigned clients properly. The supervisor (the employer) also must evaluate the individual's ability to perform the skills necessary so as not to cause harm to the clients. Injury to the client could present liability issues for both the nurse and the employer. The nurse cannot refuse the assignment to float, but should request assistance with tasks that he or she does not feel capable of performing. The nurse could say something like this, "My assigned client has a newly inserted chest tube. I have not worked with chest tubes since I was a first-year graduate. Would you please assist me with the tube? I will be glad to help you with some of your clients to make up for the time you are spending with me."

Collective Bargaining

Collective bargaining is the formalized decision-making process between representatives of management and representatives of labor to negotiate wages and conditions of employment, including work hours, working environment, and fringe benefits of employment (e.g., vacation time, sick leave, and personal leave). Through a written agreement, both employer and employees legally commit themselves to observe the terms and conditions of employment.

When collective bargaining breaks down because an agreement cannot be reached, the employees usually call a strike. A *strike* is an organized work stoppage by a group of employees to express a grievance, enforce a demand for changes in conditions of employment, or solve a dispute with management.

Because nursing practice is a service to people (often ill people), striking presents a moral dilemma to many nurses. Actions taken by nurses can affect the safety of people. When faced with a strike, each nurse must make an individual decision to cross or not to cross a picket line.

Arbitration (an agreement negotiated by a designated impartial person) may be required to prevent a strike or to settle a strike.

CITIZEN

The rights and responsibilities of the nurse in the role of citizen are the same as those of any individual under the legal system. Nurses move in and out of these roles when carrying out professional and personal responsibilities.

Legal Protection for Nurses

GOOD SAMARITAN ACTS

Good Samaritan acts are laws designed to protect healthcare providers who provide assistance at the scene of an emergency against claims of malpractice, unless it can be shown that there was a gross departure from the normal standard of care or willful wrongdoing on their part. Gross negligence usually involves further injury or harm to the person. For example, a nurse who went to get help, leaving an injured child on the shoulder of the road might be charged with gross negligence if the child was then struck by a passing automobile.

In the United States, most state statutes do not require citizens to give aid to people in distress. Such assistance is considered more of an ethical than a legal duty. A few states and provinces, however, have enacted legislation that requires people to stop and help persons in danger (Fletcher, 1996). In Canada, some provinces specify that it is the responsibility of people to give aid at the scene of an emergency.

To encourage citizens to be "Good Samaritans," most states have now enacted legislation releasing a Good Samaritan from legal liability for injuries caused under such circumstances, even if the injuries resulted from negligence of the person offering emergency aid.

It is generally believed that a person who renders help in an emergency, at a level that would be provided by any reasonably prudent person under similar circumstances, cannot be held liable. The same reasoning applies to nurses, who are among the people best prepared to help at an emergency scene. If the level of care a nurse provides is of the caliber that would have been provided by any other nurse, then the nurse will not be held liable. Guidelines for nurses who choose to render emergency care are:

- Limit actions to those normally considered first aid if possible.
- Do not perform actions that you do not know how to do.
- Offer assistance, but do not insist.
- Do not leave the scene until the injured person leaves or another qualified person takes over.

AMERICANS WITH DISABILITIES ACT

The Americans with Disabilities Act (ADA), passed by the U.S. Congress in 1990 and fully implemented in 1994, prohibits discrimination on the basis of disability in employment, public services, and public accommodations. The purposes of the act are:

- To provide a clear and comprehensive national mandate for eliminating discrimination against individuals with disabilities.
- To provide clear, strong, consistent, enforceable standards addressing discrimination against individuals with disabilities.
- To ensure that the federal government plays a central role in enforcing standards established under the act.

An employer may not refuse to hire a nurse with disabilities if the nurse is able to fulfill the duties of the work role. The ADA also enables individuals of normal intelligence who have a physical or learning disability to pursue a nursing curriculum through alternative learning methods.

PROFESSIONAL LIABILITY INSURANCE

Because of the increase in the number of malpractice lawsuits against health professionals, nurses are advised in many areas to carry their own liability insurance. Most hospitals have liability insurance that covers all employees, including all nurses. However, some smaller facilities, such as "walk-in" clinics, may not. Thus the nurse should always check with the employer at the time of hiring to see what coverage the facility provides. A physician or a hospital can be sued because of the negligent conduct of a nurse, and the nurse can also be sued and held liable for negligence or malpractice. Because hospitals have been known to countersue nurses when they have been found negligent and the hospital was required to pay, nurses are advised to provide their own insurance coverage and not rely on hospital-provided insurance.

Additionally, nurses often provide nursing services outside of employment-related activities, such as being available for first aid at children's sport or social activities or providing health screening and education at health fairs. Neighbors or friends may seek advice about illnesses or treatment for themselves or family members. In such situations, the nurse may be tempted to give advice, but it is always advisable for the nurse to refer the friend or neighbor to the family physician. The nurse may be protected from liability under Good Samaritan acts when nursing service is volunteered. However, if the nurse receives any compensation or if there is a written or verbal agreement outlining the nurse's responsibility to the group, the nurse needs liability coverage to cover legal expenses in the event that the nurse is sued.

Students and teachers of nursing are unlikely to be covered by the insurance carried by hospitals and health agencies. It is advisable for them to check with their school about the coverage that applies to them. In some states, hospitals do not allow nursing students to provide nursing care without liability insurance.

MINIMIZING CHANCE OF LIABILITY

To protect themselves from legal action, nurses should always follow the policies and protocols of the facility where they work. Methods of legal protection for nurses are summarized in Box 4-2 ∎.

STUDENT NURSES

Nursing students are responsible for their own actions and liable for their own acts of negligence committed during the course of clinical experiences. When they perform duties that are within the scope of professional nursing, such as administering an injection, they are legally held to the same standard of skill and competence as a licensed nurse. Lower standards are not applied to the actions of nursing students.

Students in clinical situations must be assigned activity within their capabilities and be given reasonable guidance

---

BOX 4-2	NURSING CARE CHECKLIST

Legal Precautions for Nurses

☑ Function within the scope of your education, job description, and area nurse practice act. This enables you to function within the scope of the description and know what is and what is not expected.

☑ Follow the procedures and policies of the employing agency.

☑ Build and maintain good rapport with clients. Keeping clients informed about diagnostic and treatment plans, giving feedback on their progress, and showing concern for the outcome of their care prevent a sense of powerlessness and a buildup of hostility in the client.

☑ Always identify clients, particularly before initiating major interventions (e.g., surgical or other invasive procedures or when administering medications or blood transfusions).

☑ Observe and monitor the client accurately. Communicate and record significant changes in the client's condition to the physician.

☑ Promptly and accurately document all assessments and care given. Records must show that the nurse provided and supervised the client's care daily.

☑ Be alert when implementing nursing interventions and give each task your full attention and skill.

☑ Perform procedures appropriately. Negligent incidents during procedures generally relate to equipment failure, improper technique, and improper performance of the procedure. For instance, the nurse must know how to safeguard the client in the event that a respirator or other equipment fails.

☑ Make sure the correct medications are given in the correct dose, by the right route, at the scheduled time, and to the right client. See Chapter 27 ⬭ for more detailed information about the administration of medications.

☑ When delegating nursing responsibilities, make sure that the person who is delegated a task understands what to do and that the person has the required knowledge and skill. As the delegating nurse, you can be held liable for harm caused by the person to whom the care was delegated.

☑ Protect clients from injury. Inform clients of hazards and use appropriate safety devices and measures to prevent falls, burns, or other injuries.

☑ Report all incidents involving clients. Prompt reporting enables those responsible to attend to the client's well-being, to analyze why the incident occurred, and to prevent recurrences.

☑ Always check any order that a client questions and ensure that verbal orders are accurate and documented appropriately. Question and confirm standing orders if you are inexperienced in a particular area.

☑ Know your own strengths and weaknesses. Ask for assistance and supervision in situations for which you feel inadequately prepared.

☑ Maintain your clinical competence. For students, this demands study and practice before caring for clients. For graduate nurses, it means continued study, including maintaining and updating clinical knowledge and skills.

and supervision. Nursing instructors are responsible for assigning students to the care of clients and for providing reasonable supervision.

Although it is the responsibility of the clinical instructor to supervise the students, students have the responsibility for study, lab practice, and seeking extra assistance when they do not understand a concept. Taking personal responsibility is a necessary skill that needs to be learned early in the student's career.

To fulfill responsibilities to clients and to minimize chances for liability, nursing students need to:

- Make sure they are prepared to carry out the necessary care for assigned clients.
- Ask for additional help or supervision in situations for which they feel inadequately prepared.
- Comply with the policies of the agency in which they obtain their clinical experience.
- Comply with the policies and definitions of responsibility supplied by the school of nursing.

Students who work as part-time or temporary nursing assistants or aides must also remember that legally they can perform only those tasks that appear in the job description of a nurse's aide or assistant. Even though a student may have received instruction and acquired competence in administering injections or suctioning a tracheostomy tube, the student cannot legally perform these tasks while employed as an aide or assistant. While acting as a paid worker, the student is covered for negligent acts by the employer, not the school of nursing.

Selected Legal Aspects of Nursing Practice

PRIVILEGED COMMUNICATION

A *privileged communication* is information given to a professional person who is forbidden by law from disclosing the information in a court without the consent of the person who provided it. See the earlier discussion of invasion of privacy.

Legislation regarding privileged communications is highly complicated. Many states with statutes granting privileged communications among the client and various healthcare providers do not extend the privilege to nurse–client communication.

INFORMED CONSENT

Informed consent is an agreement by a client to accept a course of treatment or a procedure after complete information has been provided by a healthcare provider. Information includes the risks of the treatment and facts relating to it. Usually, the client signs a form provided by the agency. The form is a record of the informed consent, not the informed consent itself. Consent forms may be available in languages other than English. For example, in areas with large Hispanic populations, they are often available in Spanish.

Obtaining informed consent for specific medical and surgical treatments is the responsibility of the physician or the care provider who is performing the procedure (e.g., nurse practitioner, advance practice RN, physician's assistant). The task of obtaining the signature is delegated to nurses in some agencies, and no laws prohibit the nurse from being part of the information-giving process (repeating information). However, if the client did not understand when the procedure was explained, the physician or other practitioner must be notified. It is not appropriate for the LPN/LVN to explain the procedure or to have a client sign a consent form for a procedure that is not fully understood. The LPN/LVN should be a witness to the signature itself, not to whether the client understands what will occur.

Usually a consenting adult (the client or the client's parent) signs the consent form. Box 4-3 ■ describes situations of informed consent that involve children.

Witnessing Informed Consent

Often, the nurse's responsibility is to witness the giving of informed consent for medical procedures. This involves:

- Witnessing the exchange between the client and the physician.
- Establishing that the client really did understand, that is, was really informed.
- Witnessing the client's signature.

If a nurse witnesses only the client's signature and not the exchange between the client and the physician, the nurse

---

BOX 4-3	PEDIATRIC CONSIDERATIONS

Informed Consent for Children

- Informed consent—The parent or legal guardian is the person who must give consent for medical procedures for a minor child until the child reaches the age of 18. The exception is if the child becomes emancipated, marries, or has a child of his or her own. Emancipation requires a court proceeding.
- Refusal of treatment—A child is not legally allowed to refuse medical treatment until the age of 18 is reached or the child has become emancipated. Ethically, an adolescent should be consulted, but if the parent wants the care to continue, the physician legally must follow the parent's wishes.
- Refusal of treatment for the child by the parent—When a parent refuses treatment for a child, the physician or healthcare facility will need to obtain a court order making the child a ward of the state. Once this is done, an advocate will be appointed for the child and the advocate will be able to give consent.

should write "witnessing signature only" on the form. If the nurse finds that the client really does not understand the physician's explanation, then the physician must be notified.

Obtaining informed consent for nursing procedures is the responsibility of nurses when they perform direct care such as insertion of nasogastric tubes or medication administration.

It can be a challenge to determine the amount and type of information required for the client to make an informed decision. General guidelines include:

- The purposes of the treatment.
- What the client can expect to feel or experience.
- The intended benefits of the treatment.
- Possible risks or negative outcomes of the treatment.
- Advantages and disadvantages of possible alternatives to the treatment (including no treatment).

There are three major elements of informed consent:

1. The consent must be given voluntarily.
2. The client must have the capacity and competence to understand.
3. The client must be given enough information to be the ultimate decision maker.

To give informed consent voluntarily, the client must not feel coerced. Sometimes fear of disapproval by a health professional can be the reason the client gives consent. Such consent is not voluntarily given.

Technical words and language barriers can keep clients from understanding information about the procedure. If a client cannot read, the consent form must be read to the client before it is signed. If the client does not speak the same language as the health professional who is giving the information, an interpreter must be provided.

A client who is confused, disoriented, or sedated is not considered *functionally competent* (able to understand and give informed consent).

Ensuring informed consent is also important when providing nursing care in the home. Because home care often occurs over an extended period of time, the nurse has many opportunities to ensure that the plan of treatment is accepted.

Exceptions to Informed Consent

Three groups of people cannot provide consent. The first is a dependent child, under the age of 18 (minor). In most areas, a parent or guardian must give consent before minors can obtain treatment. Adults who have the mental capacity of a child and who have an appointed guardian also fall into this category. There are some exceptions. Some states allow minors to give consent for such procedures as blood donations, treatment for drug dependence and sexually transmitted infections, and procedures for obstetric care. Minors who are married, pregnant, parents, members of the military, or

emancipated (living on their own) may be legally allowed to give their own consent. These statutes may vary by state or province.

The second group includes persons who are unconscious or injured so that they are unable to give consent. In these situations, consent is usually obtained from the closest adult relative if existing statutes permit. In a life-threatening emergency, if consent cannot be obtained from the client or a relative, the law generally agrees that consent is implied (agreed to).

The third group consists of people with mental illnesses who have been judged by professionals to be incompetent. State and provincial mental health acts or similar statutes generally provide definitions of mental illness and specify the rights of the mentally ill under the law as well as the rights of the staff caring for such clients.

CARRYING OUT PHYSICIANS' ORDERS

Nurses are expected to analyze procedures and medications ordered by the physician. It is the nurse's responsibility to seek clarification of ambiguous or seemingly erroneous orders from the prescribing physician. Clarification from any other source is unacceptable and regarded as a departure from competent nursing practice.

There are several categories of orders that nurses must question to protect themselves legally:

- Question any order a client questions. For example, if a client who has been receiving an intramuscular injection tells the nurse that the doctor changed the order from an injectable to an oral medication, the nurse should recheck the order before giving the medication.
- Question any order if the client's condition has changed. The nurse is considered responsible for notifying the physician of any significant changes in the client's condition, whether the physician requests notification or not. For example, if a client who is receiving an intravenous infusion suddenly develops a rapid pulse, chest pain, and a cough, the nurse must notify the physician immediately and question continuance of the ordered rate of infusion.
- Question and record verbal orders to avoid miscommunications. In addition to recording the time, the date, the physician's name, and the orders, the nurse documents the circumstances that occasioned the call to the physician, reads the orders back to the physician, and documents that the physician confirmed the orders as the nurse read them back.
- Question any order that is illegible, unclear, or incomplete. Misinterpretations in the name of a drug or in dose, for example, can easily occur with handwritten orders. The nurse is responsible for ensuring that the order is interpreted the way it was intended and that it is a safe and appropriate order.

PROVIDING COMPETENT NURSING CARE

Competent practice is a major legal safeguard for nurses. Nurses need to provide care that is within the legal boundaries of their practice and within the boundaries of agency policies and procedures. Nurses, therefore, must be familiar with their various job descriptions, which may be different from agency to agency. All nurses are responsible for ensuring that their various education and experience are adequate to meet the responsibilities delineated in their job descriptions.

Competency also involves care that protects clients from harm. Nurses need to anticipate sources of client injury, educate clients about hazards, and implement measures to prevent injury.

Application of the nursing process is another essential aspect of providing safe and effective client care. Clients need to be assessed and monitored appropriately and involved in care decisions. All assessments and care must be documented accurately. Effective communication can also protect the nurse from negligence claims. Nurses need to approach every client with sincere concern and include the client in conversations. In addition, nurses should always acknowledge when they do not know the answer to a client's questions, tell the client they will find out the answer, and then follow through.

RECORD KEEPING

The client's medical record is a legal document and can be produced in court as evidence. Often, the record is used to remind a witness of events surrounding a lawsuit, because several months or years can elapse before a suit goes to trial. The effectiveness of a witness's testimony can depend on the accuracy of such records. Nurses, therefore, need to keep accurate and complete records of nursing care provided to clients. Failure to keep proper records can constitute negligence and be the basis for tort liability. Insufficient or inaccurate assessments and documentation can hinder proper diagnosis and treatment and result in injury to the client. See Chapter 13 🔗 for types of records and facts about recording.

THE INCIDENT REPORT

An incident report is an agency record of an accident or unusual occurrence. Incident reports are used to make all the facts available to agency personnel, to contribute to statistical data about injuries or incidents, and to help healthcare personnel prevent future incidents or injuries. All injuries are usually reported on incident forms. Some agencies also report other incidents, such as the occurrence of client infection or the loss of personal effects. Box 4-4 ■ lists the information to be included in an incident report. The report should be completed as soon as possible and filed according to agency policy. Because incident reports are not part of the

---

BOX 4-4	INFORMATION TO INCLUDE IN AN INCIDENT REPORT

- Identify the client by name, initials, and hospital or identification number.
- Give the date, time, and place of the incident.
- Describe the facts of the incident. Avoid any conclusions or blame. Describe the incident as you saw it even if your impressions differ from those of others.
- Identify all witnesses to the incident.
- Identify any equipment by number and any medication by name and number.
- Document any circumstance surrounding the incident, for example, that another client was experiencing cardiac arrest.

---

client's medical record, the facts of the incident should also be noted in the medical record. Do not record in the client record that an incident report has been completed.

The incident report should be completed by the person who identifies that the incident occurred. This may not be the same person actually involved with the incident. For example, the nurse who discovers that an incorrect medication has been administered completes the form even if it was another nurse who administered the medication. In addition, all witnesses to an incident, such as a client fall, are listed on the incident form even if they were not directly involved.

Incident reports are often reviewed by an agency risk management committee, which decides whether to investigate the incident further. Nurses may be required to answer questions such as what they believe precipitated the incident, how it could have been prevented, and whether any equipment should be adjusted. Incident reports are discussed further in Chapter 63 and a sample is shown in Figure 63-1 🔗.

HAVING BACKGROUND CHECKS AND FINGERPRINTING

In 2005 the Joint Commission established a policy that students and volunteers be considered the same as employees as far as requiring background checks and fingerprinting. If a hospital requires their employees to be fingerprinted, go through a background check, or be drug tested, then they will require the same of nursing students prior to clinical assignment. Normally these actions are done one time prior to the first clinical rotation. This is not a law or a requirement of the boards of nursing for nursing students. The state boards of nursing require fingerprints prior to sitting for the NCLEX®, not before. Students who are unable to pass the requirements for clinical assignment may not be able to continue in the program, since they will not be able to obtain the necessary clinical hours to complete the program.

REPORTING CRIMES, TORTS, AND UNSAFE PRACTICES

Nurses may need to report nursing colleagues or other health professionals for practices that endanger the health and safety of clients. For instance, alcohol and drug use, theft from a client or agency, and unsafe nursing practice should be reported. Reporting a colleague is not easy. The person reporting may feel disloyal, incur the disapproval of others, or perceive that chances for promotion are endangered. When reporting an incident or series of incidents, the nurse must be careful to describe observed behavior only and not make inferences as to what might be happening. Reporting these events is referred to as *whistle-blowing*. Many states have laws that prevent wrongful termination of whistle-blowers by employers. Reporting illegal, unethical, or incompetent performance is an expectation found in the code of ethics of the NFLPN.

Controlled Substances

Laws in the United States and Canada regulate the distribution and use of controlled substances such as narcotics, depressants, stimulants, and hallucinogens. Misuse of controlled substances leads to criminal penalties. See Chapter 27 ⟳ for the legal aspects of drug administration.

The Impaired Nurse

The term **impaired nurse** refers to a nurse whose practice has been negatively affected because of chemical abuse, specifically the use of alcohol and drugs. Chemical dependence in healthcare workers has become a problem because of the high levels of stress involved in many healthcare settings and the easy access to addictive drugs. Substance abuse is the most common reason for actions against nurses' licenses. Between 10% and 15% of nurses are estimated to be chemically impaired. This is about the same percentage as in the general population. Employers must have sound policies and procedures for identifying situations that involve a possibly impaired nurse. Intervention in such situations is important to protect clients and to get treatment for the impaired nurse quickly.

A variety of programs have been developed to assist impaired nurses to recover. In many states, impaired nurses who enter an intervention program for treatment (diversion program) are closely supervised and restricted in practice, but do not have to surrender their nursing license.

A nurse who works while impaired can place her clients and other staff members in jeopardy. It is important to recognize when a coworker is working in an unsafe condition. See Box 4-5 ■ for behaviors frequently seen in nurses who are impaired.

BOX 4-5	SIGNS OF AN IMPAIRED NURSE

Actual or potential impairment is identified through signs of deteriorating performance including, but not limited to, the following:
- Problems with lateness, missing work
- Increasing numbers of incidents and errors with nursing care
- Observed or reported incidence of interpersonal conflict
- Complaints of poor quality nursing care
- Decreased productivity
- Awkward, ineffective, inaccurate psychomotor skills
- Elaborate, implausible excuses for behavior
- Emotional lability
- Coming to work intoxicated or "hung over"
- Falling asleep at work
- Appearance of complaints of unrelieved pain from assigned clients when medications should have been given (nurse is "diverting drugs")
- Frequent requests to "waste" narcotic doses
- Need of peers and others to compensate for the imbalance of care (Note: Coworkers may overlook impaired performance, lateness, and absenteeism.)

Impaired Student Nurses

It is important that impaired students learn to self-identify their impairment and take steps to correct the problem, since such behavior can be cause for dismissal from the program or prevent them from being eligible to be licensed to practice nursing. Many schools have policies such as these:

- The use of psychoactive substances while performing or learning to perform nursing care is not acceptable.
- When a student's performance is impaired, safe, effective care is at risk whether it occurs in the classroom, the learning skills laboratory, or the clinical setting.
- Alcohol and drug abuse and addiction are primary illnesses as are psychiatric and physical illnesses; each can be successfully treated with rehabilitation resulting in return to optimal function.
- Students who are willing to cooperate with a program of assistance to them and who accept treatment, rehabilitation, and monitoring should be allowed to continue their nursing education, provided they cooperate fully and comply with requirements for treatment and monitoring of their continued well-being. This applies to any illness causing impairment.
- Habitual impairment is cause for disciplinary procedure. This applies to students identified as impaired or potentially impaired who are unwilling to be rehabilitated.
- Legal transgressions such as theft; falsification of records; diversion of drugs for sale or supply to another; or the substitution, alteration, or denial of prescribed medications to

clients will trigger the disciplinary process as well as the assistance process.

SEXUAL HARASSMENT

Sexual harassment is a violation of the individual's rights and a form of discrimination. In 1987, the law prohibiting sexual discrimination was clarified to apply to all educational and employing institutions receiving federal funding. The Equal Employment Opportunity Commission (EEOC) defines sexual harassment as "unwelcome sexual advances, requests for sexual favors, and other verbal or physical conduct of a sexual nature" occurring in the following circumstances (EEOC, 1980, sections 3950.10–3950.11):

- When submission to such conduct is considered, either explicitly or implicitly, a condition of an individual's employment
- When submission to or rejection of such conduct is used as the basis for employment decisions affecting the individual
- When such conduct interferes with an individual's work performance or creates an "intimidating, hostile, or offensive working environment"

In health care, both clients and healthcare professionals may experience sexual harassment. Because sexual harassment is generally related to a power imbalance, female nurses are more likely than male nurses to experience sexual harassment from male physicians or administrators. Nurses may be "sexually propositioned," "suggestively touched," or "sexually insulted" during their careers. Such behavior is considered sexual harassment and can negatively affect client care. For example, to avoid uncomfortable situations, a nurse may be reluctant to work with the clients of a particular offensive physician or work on a unit with an offensive administrator, or a nurse may avoid calling a physician to report changes in client status or to suggest changes to improve client care.

The victim or the harasser may be male or female. The victim does not have to be of the opposite sex. Furthermore, the victim does not have to be the person harassed. Anyone who is affected by the offensive conduct may be considered a victim. Nurses must develop skills of assertiveness to deter sexual harassment in the workplace. Box 4-6 ■ describes nursing strategies for dealing with inappropriate sexual behavior.

Nurses must be familiar with the sexual harassment policy and procedures that are in place in every institution. These will include information regarding the grievance policy, the person to whom incidents should be reported, and the resolution process.

NURSES AS WITNESSES

A nurse may be called to testify in a legal action for a variety of reasons (Figure 4-1 ■). The nurse may be a defendant in a malpractice or negligence action or may have been a member

BOX 4-6	NURSING STRATEGIES FOR DEALING WITH INAPPROPRIATE SEXUAL BEHAVIOR

- Identify the behavior you expect: "Please call me by my name, not 'honey'" or "I expect you to keep yourself covered when I am in the room. If you are feeling hot or something is uncomfortable, let me know, and I will try to make you more comfortable."
- Set firm limits: Take the client's hand and move it away, use direct eye contact, and say, "Don't do that!"
- Communicate that the behavior is not acceptable by saying, for example, "I really do not like the things you are saying" or "I see you are not dressed. I will be back in 10 minutes and will help you with breakfast when you have your clothes on."
- Tell the client how the behavior makes you feel: "When you act like that toward me, I don't want to come into your room. It embarrasses me and makes it hard for me to give you the kind of nursing care you need."
- Try to refocus clients from the inappropriate behavior to their real concerns and fears. Sometimes people talk inappropriately when they are concerned about the sexual part of their life and how their illness will affect them. Offer to discuss sexuality concerns: "All morning you have been making very personal sexual comments about yourself. Are there things that you have questions about or would like to talk about?"
- Clarify the consequences of continued inappropriate behavior (avoidance, withdrawal of services, no chance to help resolve underlying concerns of client).
- Report the incident to your nursing instructor, charge nurse, or clinical nurse specialist. Discuss the incident, your feelings, and possible interventions.
- If you feel you are not being successful in getting the client to change behavior, ask your supervisor to assign another nurse to the client.

of the healthcare team that provided care to the plaintiff. If a nurse is going to testify, he or she should consult an attorney first. If the action is against the nurse's employer, the same

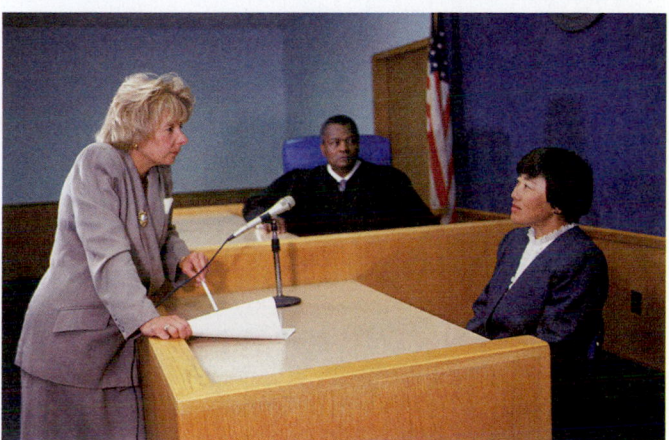

Figure 4-1. ■ Nurse testifying in court. *Source:* PhotoEdit Inc.

attorney will assist the nurse. If the action is against the nurse, he or she should retain a separate attorney.

A nurse may also be asked to provide testimony as an expert witness. An *expert witness* has special training, experience, or skill and offers an opinion on some issue within the nurse's area of expertise. Nurses usually are called to help a judge or jury understand evidence pertaining to the extent of damage or the standard of care.

UNDERSTANDING ETHICAL ISSUES

In the course of their daily work, nurses deal with such fundamental events as birth, suffering, and death. They must decide the morality of their own actions when they face these ethical issues. The present cost-driven environment of managed care tends to give highest priority to business values. This creates new moral problems and exaggerates old ones. It is more critical than ever for nurses to make sound moral decisions. Therefore, nurses need to develop an understanding of the ethical dimensions of nursing practice by examining their values. Early on in their practice, nurses must look ahead to the kinds of moral problems they are likely to face and begin to understand how values influence their decisions.

Ethical Concepts

Values are freely chosen, enduring beliefs or attitudes about the worth of a person, object, idea, or action. Values are important because they influence decisions and actions. Values are often taken for granted. In the same way that people are not aware of their breathing, they usually do not think about their values; they simply accept them and act on them. The word *values* usually brings to mind things such as honesty, fairness, friendship, safety, or family unity. Of course, not all values are moral values. For example, some people hold money, work, power, and politics as values in their lives.

Although values consist of freely chosen and enduring beliefs and attitudes, beliefs and attitudes are related, but not identical, to values.

Values are learned through observation and experience. They are transmitted to others through the influence of environment—that is, by family and peer groups, by cultural, ethnic, and religious groups. For example, if a parent consistently demonstrates honesty in dealing with others, the child will probably begin to value honesty. Nurses should keep in mind the influence of values on health. In some cultures, folk healers are valued over treatment by a physician.

Beliefs or opinions are interpretations or conclusions that people accept as being true; they do not necessarily involve values. For example, the statement "I believe if I study hard I will get a good grade" expresses a belief that does not involve a value. By contrast, the statement "Good grades are really important to me. I believe I must study hard to obtain good grades" involves both a belief and a value.

Attitudes are mental positions or feelings toward a person, object, or idea (e.g., acceptance, compassion, openness). Attitudes are often judged as good or bad, positive or negative, whereas beliefs are judged as correct or incorrect.

The term **ethics** has several meanings in common use. It refers to (1) a method of inquiry that helps people to understand the morality of human behavior (i.e., it is the study of morality), (2) the practices or beliefs of a certain group (e.g., medical ethics, nursing ethics), and (3) the expected standards of moral behavior of a particular group as described in the group's formal code of professional ethics. **Bioethics** is ethics as applied to life (e.g., decisions about abortion or euthanasia). Nursing ethics refers to ethical issues that occur in nursing practice. The NFLPN holds nurses accountable for their legal and ethical conduct in the *Nursing Practice Standards for the Licensed Practical/Vocational Nurse* (2003).

Moral Concepts

Morality (or morals) is similar to ethics, and many people use the terms interchangeably. *Morality* usually refers to private, personal standards of what is right and wrong in conduct, character, and attitude. Sometimes the first clue to the moral nature of a situation is an aroused conscience or an awareness of feelings such as guilt, hope, or shame. Another indicator is the tendency to respond to the situation with words such as *ought, should, right, wrong, good,* and *bad*. Moral issues are concerned with important social values and norms; they are not about trivial things.

Nurses should distinguish between morality and law. An action can be legal but not moral. For example, an order for full resuscitation of a dying client is legal, but one could still question whether the act is moral. On the other hand, an action can be moral but illegal. For example, if a child at home stops breathing, it is moral but not legal to exceed the speed limit when driving to the hospital.

Moral principles are statements about broad, general, philosophic concepts such as autonomy and justice. They provide the foundation for moral rules, which are specific prescriptions for actions. Principles are useful in ethical discussions because even if people disagree about which action is right in a situation, they may be able to agree on the principles that apply. Such an agreement can serve as the basis for a solution that is acceptable to all parties. Ethical issues are looked at differently among people of different cultures; the nurse must consider these differences when providing care. See Box 4-7 ■ for cultural pulse points related to legal and ethical considerations.

Autonomy refers to the right to make one's own decisions. Nurses who follow this principle recognize that each client is unique, has the right to be what that person is, and has the right to choose personal goals.

Honoring the principle of autonomy means that the nurse respects a client's right to make decisions even when those choices seem not to be in the client's best interest. It also means treating others with consideration. In a healthcare setting, this principle is violated, for example, when a nurse disregards a client's report of the severity of his or her pain.

Nonmaleficence is a duty to do no harm. Although this would seem to be a simple principle to follow, in reality it is complex. Harm can mean intentional harm, risk of harm, and unintentional harm. In nursing, intentional harm is never acceptable. However, the risk of harm is not always clear. A client may be at risk of harm during a nursing intervention that is intended to be helpful. For example, a client may react adversely to a medication, and caregivers may or may not always agree on the degree to which a risk is morally permissible.

Beneficence means "doing good." Nurses are obligated to do good, that is, to implement actions that benefit clients and their support persons. However, doing good can also pose a risk of doing harm. For example, a nurse may advise a client about a strenuous exercise program to improve general health, but should not do so if the client is at risk of a heart attack.

Justice is often referred to as fairness. Nurses often face decisions in which a sense of justice should prevail. For example, a nurse making home visits finds one client tearful and depressed, and knows she could help by staying for 30 more minutes to talk. However, that would take time from her next client, who is a diabetic who needs a great deal of teaching and observation. The nurse will need to weigh the facts of each situation carefully in order to divide her time justly among her clients.

Fidelity means to be faithful to agreements and promises. By virtue of their standing as professional caregivers, nurses have responsibilities to clients, employers, the government, and society, as well as to themselves. Nurses often make promises such as "I'll be right back with your pain medication," "You'll be all right," or "I'll find out for you." Clients take such promises seriously, and so should nurses.

Veracity refers to telling the truth. Although this seems straightforward, in practice, choices are not always clear. Should a nurse tell the truth when it is known that it will cause harm? Does a nurse tell a lie when it is known that the lie will relieve anxiety and fear? The loss of trust in the nurse and the anxiety caused by not knowing the truth, for example, usually outweigh any benefits derived from lying. Lying to sick or dying people is rarely justified.

Client Advocacy

An **advocate** is one who expresses and defends the cause of another. A client advocate is an advocate for clients' rights. The healthcare system is complex, and many clients are too ill to deal with it. If they are to keep from "falling through the cracks," clients need an advocate to cut through the

---

BOX 4-7	CULTURAL PULSE POINTS

Female Circumcision

Because of the increase in the number of immigrants now living in the United States, nurses working in a multicultural setting may encounter women who have had procedures such as *female circumcision* (removal of part or all of the clitoris and/or labia, sometimes with suturing that leaves only a small opening for menstruation and urination). Some may ask for it to be performed on their daughters. This presents an ethical issue for healthcare professionals in this country. Although female circumcision has been illegal in the United States since the Federal Prohibition of Female Genital Mutilation bill passed in 1996, the procedure is widely performed in 27 different countries. Members of societies where these procedures are widely practiced do not consider them to be mutilation, as do many healthcare professionals in the United States. Many immediate and long-term health effects are related to the procedures. The procedure creates a physical risk for hemorrhage, pain, and infection; painful or difficult intercourse; and impairment of vaginal childbirth. Psychologically it may be associated with frigidity, anxiety, or depression (Reichert, 1998).

Nursing intervention strategies for ethical problems of traditional cultural practices should be addressed honestly and with respect. Healthcare professionals need to listen and express respect for the perspective of the client and the family (Andrews & Boyle, 2008). All interactions must be conducted in such a way that the client is an equal partner with the professional.

While expressing respect for the practices of all cultures, there must be a recognition that traditional practices may need to be viewed differently. This can be done by collaborating with the client to:

- Identify and prioritize the current values.
- Identify the goals of the values.
- Identify alternative methods to achieve the same goal.

BOX 4-8	VALUES BASIC TO CLIENT ADVOCACY

- The client is a holistic, autonomous being who has the right to make choices and decisions.
- Clients have the right to expect a nurse–client relationship that is based on shared respect, trust, and collaboration in solving problems related to health and healthcare needs, and consideration of their thoughts and feelings.
- Clients are responsible for their own health.
- It is the nurse's responsibility to ensure that the client has access to healthcare services that meet health needs.

layers of bureaucracy and help them get what they require. Values basic to client advocacy are shown in Box 4-8 ■.

The overall goal of the client advocate is to protect clients' rights. Being an effective client advocate involves:

- Being assertive.
- Recognizing that the rights and values of clients and families must take precedence when they conflict with those of healthcare providers.
- Being aware that conflicts may arise over issues that require consultation, confrontation, or negotiation between the nurse and administrative personnel or between the nurse and physician.
- Working with unfamiliar community agencies and lay practitioners.
- Knowing that advocacy may require political action—communicating a client's healthcare needs to government and other officials who have the authority to do something about these needs.

Nursing Ethics

In the past, nurses looked on ethical decision making as the physician's responsibility. However, no one profession is responsible for ethical decisions, nor does expertise in one discipline such as medicine or nursing necessarily make a person an expert in ethics. As situations become more complex, input from all caregivers becomes increasingly important.

Most healthcare institutions have ethics committees. Ethical standards of the Joint Commission that grants accreditation to healthcare organizations support nurses' involvement on these committees. Ethics committees typically review cases, write guidelines and policies, and provide education and counseling. They ensure that relevant facts of a case are brought out, provide a forum in which diverse views can be expressed, provide support for caregivers, and can reduce legal risks.

A **code of ethics** is a formal statement of a group's ideals and values. It is a set of ethical principles that (1) is shared by members of the group, (2) reflects their moral judgments

over time, and (3) serves as a standard for their professional actions. Codes of ethics usually have higher requirements than legal standards, and they are never lower than the legal standards of the profession. Nurses are responsible for being familiar with the code that governs their practice.

International, national, state, and provincial nursing associations have established codes of ethics.

Nursing codes of ethics have the following purposes:

1. Inform the public about the minimum standards of the profession and help them understand professional nursing conduct.
2. Provide a sign of the profession's commitment to the public it serves.
3. Outline the major ethical considerations of the profession.
4. Provide general guidelines for professional behavior.
5. Guide the profession in self-regulation.
6. Remind nurses of the special responsibility they assume when caring for the sick.

ORIGINS OF ETHICAL PROBLEMS IN NURSING

Nurses' growing awareness of ethical problems has occurred largely because of (1) social and technologic changes and (2) nurses' conflicting loyalties and obligations.

Social and Technological Changes

Social changes, such as the women's movement and a growing consumerism, expose ethical problems. Presently, the large number of people without health insurance, the high cost of health care, and workplace redesign under managed care are all raising issues of fairness and allocation of resources.

Technology creates new issues that did not exist in earlier, simpler times. Before monitors, ventilators, and parenteral feedings, there was no question about whether to "allow" an 800-gram premature infant to die. Today, with treatments that can prolong biologic life almost indefinitely, the questions are: Should we do what we know we can? Who should be treated—everyone, only those who can pay, only those who have a chance to improve?

Conflicting Loyalties and Obligations

Because of their unique position in the healthcare system, nurses experience conflicts among their loyalties and obligations to clients, families, physicians, employing institutions, and licensing bodies. Client needs may conflict with institutional policies, physician preferences, needs of the client's family, or even laws of the state. According to the nursing code of ethics, the nurse's first loyalty is to the client. However, it is not always easy to determine which action best serves the client's needs. For instance, a nurse may think that a client needs to be told a truth that others have been withholding. But this might damage the client–physician relationship, in the long run causing harm to the client rather than the intended good.

MAKING ETHICAL DECISIONS

Responsible ethical reasoning is rational and systematic. It should be based on ethical principles and codes rather than on emotions, intuition, fixed policies, or precedent. (A *precedent* is an earlier similar occurrence.)

A good decision is one that is in the client's best interest and at the same time preserves the integrity of all involved. Nurses have ethical obligations to their clients, to the agency that employs them, and to physicians. Therefore, nurses must weigh competing factors when making ethical decisions (Box 4-9 ■). See also Chapter 5 ⬭, the section on critical thinking.

Although the nurse's input is important, in reality several people are usually involved in making an ethical decision. Therefore, collaboration, communication, and compromise are important skills for health professionals. When nurses do not have the autonomy to act on their moral or ethical choices, compromise becomes essential.

Integrity-preserving compromises are most likely to be produced by collaborative decision making. See Box 4-10 ■ for strategies to enhance ethical decisions and practice.

Specific Ethical Issues

The American Nurses Association (ANA) Center for Ethics and Human Rights conducted a survey at the 1994 ANA convention that indicated the following as some of the ethical problems nurses encounter most frequently: cost-containment issues that jeopardize client welfare and access to health care (resource allocation), end-of-life decisions, breaches of client confidentiality (e.g., computerized information management), use of advance directives, informed consent and procedures, and issues in the care of HIV/AIDS clients (Scanlon, 2003). These and other issues are discussed in this section.

BOX 4-9   EXAMPLES OF NURSES' OBLIGATIONS IN ETHICAL DECISIONS

- Maximize the client's well-being.
- Balance the client's need for autonomy with family members' responsibilities for the client's well-being.
- Support each family member and enhance the family support system.
- Carry out hospital policies.
- Protect clients' well-being.
- Protect the nurse's own standards of care.

BOX 4-10   STRATEGIES TO ENHANCE ETHICAL NURSING PRACTICE

- Become aware of your own values and the ethical aspects of nursing.
- Be familiar with nursing codes of ethics.
- Respect the values, opinions, and responsibilities of other healthcare professionals that may be different from your own.
- Participate in or establish ethics rounds. Ethics rounds using hypothetical cases based on real situations incorporate the traditional teaching approach for clinical rounds, but focus on the ethical dimensions of client care rather than the client's clinical diagnosis and treatment.
- Serve on institutional ethics committees.
- Strive for collaborative practice in which nurses function effectively in cooperation with other healthcare professionals.

HIV AND AIDS

Because of its association with sexual behavior, prostitution, illicit drug use, and inevitable physical decline and death, AIDS bears a social stigma. Nurses caring for AIDS clients frequently have conflicting feelings of anger, fear, sympathy, fatigue, helplessness, and self-enhancement.

According to an ANA (2001) position statement titled *HIV Infections and Nursing Students*, "Nursing Curriculum including current HIV information should be provided by faculty with expertise in HIV disease at the onset of the academic program and as applicable throughout their course. . . . Each school of nursing should demonstrate the availability of a post-exposure management program for students who sustain exposure to blood and certain body fluids in the clinical practice setting. . . . Nursing students should be assured workplace/clinical setting protections consistent with those of employees according to OSHA Standards. . . . Nursing students and applicants to nursing programs should not be deprived of access to schools of nursing nor dismissed based solely on HIV positive status. . . . There must be confidentiality of all HIV-related information to safeguard nursing students' right to privacy."

Other ethical issues center on testing for HIV status and for the presence of AIDS in health professionals and clients. Questions arise as to whether testing should be mandatory or voluntary and to whom test results should be given. The Centers for Disease Control and Prevention (CDC) provides recommendations as to which persons should be considered for HIV antibody counseling and testing. It also recommends that voluntary testing be made available to anyone, including all healthcare professionals. In addition, the CDC recommends that HIV-positive healthcare professionals avoid performing "exposure prone procedures" (CDC, 2001).

ABORTION

Abortion is a highly publicized issue about which many people, including nurses, feel very strongly. Debate continues, pitting the principle of sanctity of life against the principle of autonomy and the woman's right to control her own body. This is an especially volatile issue because no public consensus has yet been reached.

Most state and provincial laws have provisions known as conscience clauses that permit individual physicians and nurses, as well as institutions, to refuse to assist with an abortion if doing so violates their religious or moral principles. However, nurses have no right to impose their values on a client. Abortion laws provide specific guidelines for nurses about what is legally permissible, although the U.S. Supreme Court and state legislatures continue to struggle with the issue of abortion.

ORGAN TRANSPLANTATION

Organs for transplantation may come from living donors or from donors who have just died. Many living people choose to become donors by giving consent under the Uniform Anatomical Gift Act. Ethical issues related to organ transplantation include allocation of organs, selling of body parts, involvement of children as potential donors, consent, clear definition of death, and conflicts of interest between potential donors and recipients. In some situations, a person's religious beliefs may also present conflict. For example, certain religions forbid the mutilation of the body, even for the benefit of another person.

END-OF-LIFE ISSUES

Some of the most frequent disturbing ethical problems for nurses involve issues that arise around death and dying. These include euthanasia, assisted suicide, termination of life-sustaining treatment, and the withdrawing or withholding of food and fluids.

Many moral problems surrounding the end of life can be resolved if clients complete advance directives such as the power of attorney for health care (Figure 4-2 ■). Presently, all 50 of the United States have enacted advance directive legislation (Scanlon, 2003). Advance directives direct caregivers as to the client's wishes about treatments, providing an ongoing voice for clients when they have lost the capacity to make or communicate their decisions. See Chapter 18 🔗 for a full discussion of advance directives.

Euthanasia and Assisted Suicide

Euthanasia, a Greek word meaning "good death," is popularly known as "mercy killing." Active euthanasia involves actions to directly bring about the client's death, with or without client consent. An example of this would be the administration of a lethal medication to end the client's suffering. Regardless of the caregiver's intent, active euthanasia is forbidden by law and can result in criminal charges of murder.

Active euthanasia includes assisted suicide, or giving clients the means to kill themselves if they request it (e.g., providing pills or a weapon). Nurses should recall that legality and morality are not one and the same. Determining whether an action is legal is only one aspect of deciding whether it is ethical. The questions of suicide and assisted suicide are still controversial in our society. The ANA's (1995) position statement on assisted suicide states that active euthanasia and assisted suicide are in violation of the Code for Nurses.

Passive euthanasia involves the withdrawal of extraordinary means of life support, such as removing a ventilator or making a client a "no code (do not resuscitate). The legality of passive euthanasia is dependent on the laws of a particular jurisdiction and/or facility, even though not a violation of the ANA code" (ANA, 1995).

Termination of Life-Sustaining Treatment

Antibiotics, organ transplants, and technologic advances (e.g., ventilators) help to prolong life, but not necessarily to restore health. Clients may specify that they wish to have life-sustaining measures withdrawn, they may have advance directives on this matter, or they may appoint a surrogate decision maker. There is no ethical or legal distinction between the withholding or withdrawing of treatments. However, it is usually more troubling for healthcare professionals to withdraw a treatment than to decide initially not to begin it. Nurses must understand that a decision to withdraw treatment is not a decision to withdraw care. As the primary caregivers, nurses must ensure that sensitive care and comfort measures are given as the client's illness progresses.

Withdrawing or Withholding Food and Fluids

It is generally accepted that providing food and fluids is part of ordinary nursing practice and, therefore, a moral duty. However, when food and fluids are administered by tube to a dying client, or are given over a long period of time to an unconscious client who is not expected to improve, then some consider it to be an extraordinary, or heroic, measure. A nurse is morally obligated to withhold food and fluids when it is more harmful to administer them than to withhold them. In addition, "It is morally as well as legally permissible for nurses to honor the refusal of food and fluids by competent patients in their care" (ANA, 1998, p. 3). The ANA Code for Nurses supports this position

POWER OF ATTORNEY FOR HEALTH CARE

(1) **DESIGNATION OF AGENT:** I designate the following individual as my agent to make health care decisions for me: _____

_____
(Name of individual you choose as agent)

_____
(address) (city) (state) (zip code)

_____
(home phone) (work phone)

OPTIONAL: If I revoke my agent's authority or if my agent is not willing, able, or reasonably available to make a health care decision for me, I designate as my first alternate agent:

_____
(Name of individual you choose as first alternate agent)

_____
(address) (city) (state) (zip code)

_____
(home phone) (work phone)

OPTIONAL: If I revoke the authority of my agent and first alternate agent or if neither is willing, able, or reasonably available to make a health care decision for me, I designate as my second alternate agent:

_____
(Name of individual you choose as second alternate agent)

_____
(address) (city) (state) (zip code)

_____
(home phone) (work phone)

(2) **AGENT'S AUTHORITY:** My agent is authorized to make all health care decisions for me, including decisions to provide, withhold, or withdraw artificial nutrition and hydration, and all other forms of health care to keep me alive, **except** as I state here:

(3) **WHEN AGENT'S AUTHORITY BECOMES EFFECTIVE:** My agent's authority becomes effective when my primary physician determines that I am unable to make my own health care decisions unless I mark the following box. If I mark this box [ ], my agent's authority to make health care decisions for me takes effect immediately.

(4) **AGENT'S OBLIGATION:** My agent shall make health care decisions for me in accordance with this power of attorney for health care, any instructions I give below, and my other wishes to the extent known to my agent. To the extent my wishes are unknown, my agent shall make health care decisions for me in accordance with what my agent determines to be in my best interest. In determining my best interest, my agent shall consider my personal values to the extent known to my agent.

(5) **AGENT'S POSTDEATH AUTHORITY:** My agent is authorized to make anatomical gifts, authorize an autopsy, and direct disposition of my remains, except as I state here or elsewhere in this form:

INSTRUCTIONS FOR HEALTH CARE
Strike any wording you do not want.

(6) **END-OF-LIFE DECISIONS:** I direct that my health care providers and others involved in my care provide, withhold, or withdraw treatment in accordance with the choice I have marked below: **(Initial only one box)**
[ ] (a) **Choice NOT To Prolong Life**
I do not want my life to be prolonged if (1) I have an incurable and irreversible condition that will result in my death within a relatively short time, (2) I become unconscious and, to a reasonable degree of medical certainty, I will not regain consciousness, or (3) the likely risks and burdens of treatment would outweigh the expected benefits, **OR**
[ ] (b) **Choice To Prolong Life**
I want my life to be prolonged as long as possible within the limits of generally accepted health care standards.

(7) **RELIEF FROM PAIN:** Except as I state in the following space, I direct that treatment for alleviation of pain or discomfort should be provided at all times even if it hastens my death:

DONATION OF ORGANS AT DEATH
(8) Upon my death: (mark applicable box)
[ ] (a) I give any needed organs, tissues, or parts,
OR
[ ] (b) I give the following organs, tissues, or parts only: _____
[ ] (c) My gift is for the following purposes:
(strike any of the following you do not want)
(1) Transplant
(2) Therapy
(3) Research
(4) Education

(9) **EFFECT OF COPY:** A copy of this form has the same effect as the original.

(10) **SIGNATURE:** Sign and date the form here:

_____　_____
(date)　　　　　　　　　　　　　　(sign your name)

_____　_____
(address)　　　　　　　　　　　　　(print your name)

_____　_____
(city)　　　　　　　　　　　　　　(state)

(11) **WITNESSES:** This advance health care directive will not be valid for making health care decisions unless it is either: (1) signed by two (2) qualified adult witnesses who are personally known to you and who are present when you sign or acknowledge your signature; or (2) acknowledged before a notary public.

Figure 4-2. ■ Power of attorney for health care.

through the nurse's role as a client advocate and through the moral principle of autonomy.

ALLOCATION OF HEALTH RESOURCES

Allocation of healthcare goods and services, including organ transplants, artificial joints, and the services of specialists, has become an especially urgent issue as medical costs continue to rise and more stringent cost-containment measures are implemented.

Nursing care is also a health resource. Most institutions have been implementing "workplace redesign" in order to cut costs. As a result, nursing units are staffed with fewer nurses and more unlicensed caregivers. Nurses must continue to look for ways to balance economics and caring in the allocation of health resources.

MANAGEMENT OF COMPUTERIZED INFORMATION

In keeping with the principle of autonomy, nurses are obligated to respect clients' privacy and confidentiality. Clients must be able to trust that nurses will reveal details of their situations only as appropriate and will communicate only the information necessary to provide for their health care. Computerized client records make sensitive data accessible to more people and accent issues of confidentiality. Nurses should help develop and follow security measures and policies to ensure appropriate use of client data. For example, nurses should not give their system security codes to unauthorized persons.

Note: The references and resources for all chapters have been compiled at the back of the book.

Chapter Review

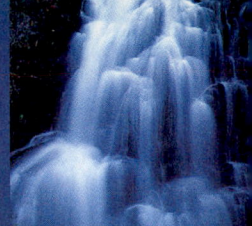

KEY Points

- Accountability is an essential concept of professional nursing practice under the law.
- Nurses need to understand laws that regulate and affect nursing practice to ensure that the nurses' actions are consistent with current legal principles and to protect the nurse from liability.
- Nurse practice acts legally define and describe the scope of nursing practice that the law seeks to regulate.
- Nurses can be held liable for intentional torts, such as invasion of privacy, defamation, assault and battery, and false imprisonment, and for unintentional torts, such as negligence and malpractice.
- Negligence or malpractice of nurses can be established when (1) the nurse (defendant) owed a duty to the client, (2) the nurse failed to carry out that duty according to standards, (3) the client (plaintiff) was injured, and (4) the client's injury was caused by the nurse's failure to follow the standard.
- Good Samaritan acts protect health professionals from claims of malpractice when they offer assistance at the scene of an emergency, provided that there is no willful wrongdoing or gross departure from normal standards of care.
- Chemical dependence in healthcare workers has become a problem because of the high levels of stress involved in many healthcare settings and the easy access to addictive drugs. The nurse needs to know the proper procedure for reporting nursing colleagues who are chemically impaired.
- Sexual harassment is a violation of the individual's rights and is a form of discrimination. Sexual harassment can happen to both nurses and clients. The nurse needs to be aware of strategies to deter harassing behavior.
- Nursing students need to make certain that they are prepared to provide the necessary care to assigned clients and to ask for help or supervision in situations for which they feel inadequately prepared.
- Moral issues and ethical problems are created as a result of advances in technology and nurses' conflicting loyalties and obligations.
- Client advocacy involves concern for an action on behalf of another person or organization in order to bring about change.

∞ FOR FURTHER Study

Chapter 2, Box 2-1 provides the standards of practice for the LPN/LVN.

Chapter 5 has the major discussion of critical thinking in nursing.

See Chapter 9 for more information about providing a safe client environment and the correct use of restraints.

See Chapter 12 for policies for safeguarding clients' property when they are being admitted to a facility.

See Chapter 13 for information about types of records and how to document care.

See Chapter 14 for more information on HIPAA.

See Chapter 18 for a full discussion about advance directives.

See Chapter 27 for information about administering medications and documenting their administration.

See Chapter 63 for more information about incident reports.

PEARSON

EXPLORE mynursingkit™

MyNursingKit is your one stop for online chapter review materials and resources. Prepare for success with additional NCLEX®-style practice questions, interactive assignments and activities, web links, animations and videos, and more!

Register your access code from the front of your book at
www.mynursingkit.com

NCLEX-PN® Exam Preparation

1 A client has signed the consent for surgery, which is scheduled for the morning. The nurse enters the room and finds the client crying. The client says, "I don't want to have surgery, but the doctor and my family tell me I must." The nurse should consider which of the following dilemmas? (Select all that apply.)

1. Has the client given informed consent?
2. Do the client and family disagree on treatment?
3. Has the client already signed the consent?
4. Has the treatment team followed the principle of beneficence?
5. What time is the client scheduled to go to surgery?

2 The nurse, caring for a client who has been placed in restraints, fails to follow the hospital policy on frequency of assessment and periodic release of restraints. This behavior could be considered which of the following?

1. Negligence
2. False imprisonment
3. Ethical misconduct
4. Defamation

3 The nurse recognizes that the major difference between civil and criminal law is:

1. If found guilty of a civil action, the defendant may lose money or be jailed.
2. If found guilty of a criminal action, the defendant will be jailed.
3. The potential outcome for the defendant if found guilty.
4. If found guilty of a criminal or civil action, the defendant will be jailed.

4 When an LPN/LVN obtains a license, it indicates to the public that the nurse:

1. Is a safe practitioner who can handle any client situation that may arise.
2. Has graduated from an approved school of nursing and has met the minimum standards for licensure.
3. Is competent to perform all nursing tasks.
4. Demonstrates competence in all areas of nursing practice.

5 The nurse understands that the Americans with Disabilities Act:

1. Enables a person with a learning disability, who is physically capable, to pursue a nursing curriculum through alternate methods.
2. Provides retraining for nurses who have been injured on the job.
3. Sets limits on lifting requirements for employers of nurses.
4. Has no significant impact on nursing practice.

6 Which of the following behaviors performed by the student nurse will minimize the chance of liability? (Select all that apply.)

1. The nurse builds rapport with clients by sharing personal information.
2. The nurse never documents an error so there is no proof of the mistake.
3. The nurse identifies clients by asking, "What is your name?" as opposed to "Are you Mr. Jones?"
4. The nurse is familiar with, and follows, policies and procedures.
5. The nurse functions within his or her scope of practice.

7 An incident report should be completed by:

1. The nurse involved in the incident.
2. The immediate supervisor of the nurse involved in the incident.
3. The nurse who discovers the incident.
4. The risk management department of the facility.

8 The nursing code of ethics is a formal statement of:

1. Directions for dealing with any ethical dilemma that may arise in nursing practice.
2. Legal standards for making ethical decisions.
3. Nursing's ideals and values.
4. The nurse's requirements for coping with ethical issues that arise in nursing.

9 The nurse's primary goal when making an ethical decision is:

1. A decision that is in the client's best interest and preserves the integrity of all involved.
2. A decision that meets the ethical obligations held to the employer and the physician.
3. A decision that allows for integrity-preserving compromises.
4. A decision that is based on ethical principles, ethical codes, intuition, and emotions.

10 Your supervisor has asked you to serve on the committee to develop guidelines for the new computerized client record system. Coworkers are concerned about confidentiality. The best response to their concerns would be:

1. "Medical records on the Internet are guaranteed to be secure."
2. "The best ways we can protect the client's information is by following security policies and keeping our security codes private."
3. "There is no way to protect confidentiality, but the benefits of the system outweigh the risks."
4. "As long as we save after each entry, the records are secure."

Answers and rationales for Review Questions appear in Appendix I.

Chapter 5

Critical Thinking and Nursing Theory/Models

LEARNING Outcomes

After completing this chapter, you will be able to:

1. Discuss the characteristics, skills, and attitudes of critical thinking.
2. Explain the importance of critical thinking to the nursing process.
3. Define nursing theory.
4. Compare selected theories of nursing in terms of client, environment, health, and nursing.
5. Identify areas in which LPN/LVNs can incorporate critical thinking into their nursing practice.
6. Explain the concept of evidence-based practice and describe ways in which the LPN/LVN can participate in evidence-based practice.

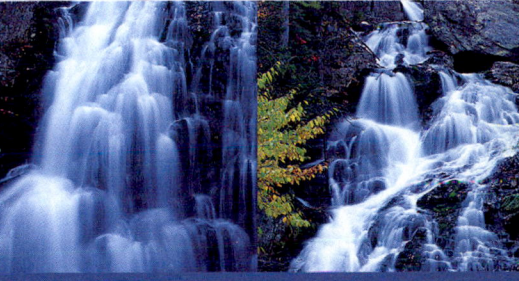

BRIEF Outline

Critical Thinking
Theories and Models
Evidence-Based Practice

KEY TERMS

Use the audio glossary feature on the MyNursingKit Website to hear the correct pronunciation of the following key terms.

critical thinking 64	**inductive reasoning** 65	**subjective data** 67
deductive reasoning 65	**objective data** 68	**theories** 68
environment 65		

Nursing instructors as well as staff nurses in the clinical setting continually challenge nursing students to become critical thinkers. You may ask a question about a client, only to be asked a question in return. Your instructor or staff nurse is trying to help you think like a nurse. For example, you may ask, "Can my client ambulate in the hall?" And your instructor may reply, "Think about your client's diagnosis and the results of the ultrasound of her leg this morning. What could happen if she ambulates?" Beginning LPN/LVN students certainly may be puzzled when confronted with such a situation. From the very beginning of the training program, the LPN/LVN student is challenged to begin to think like a nurse. Thinking like a nurse is different from thinking like a doctor or a teacher or a lawyer. Seeing the client as a whole person and dealing with problems that arise when providing care are what defines thinking for the nurse.

A nurse's thinking is not limited to problem solving or decision making. Nurses must also make reliable observations, draw sound conclusions, create new information and ideas, evaluate other people's ways of reasoning, and improve their own self-knowledge. Critical thinking goes hand in hand with the nursing process. As you work your way through this chapter and Chapter 6 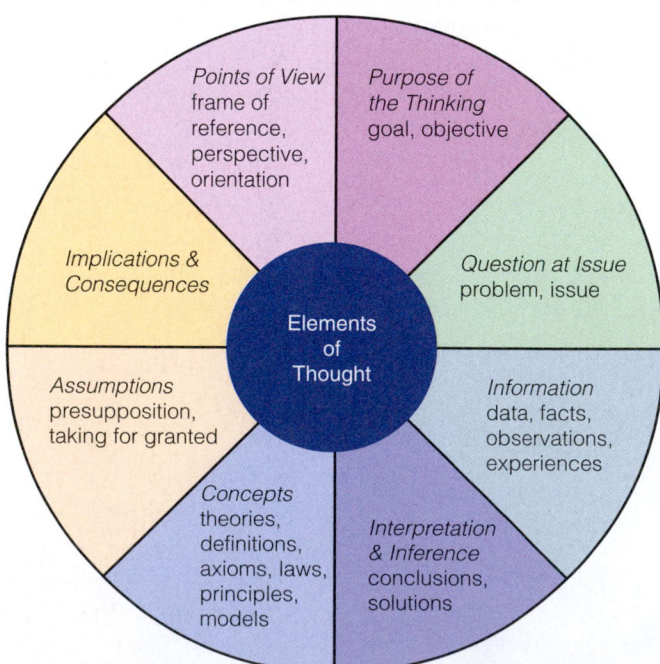, you will begin to see how the pieces fit together.

You will develop many critical-thinking skills and abilities, such as information gathering, focusing, remembering, organizing, analyzing, generating, integrating, and evaluating. As you progress through your program, you will encounter increasingly more complex situations. This is the challenge of nursing: *thoughtful, thorough nursing practice based on sound reasoning and committed to safe and effective client care.* To accomplish this goal, you will be required to reason about nursing by reading, writing, listening, and speaking critically. By thinking critically about nursing, you will gain in-depth knowledge about the practice of nursing as a professional.

Critical Thinking

The thinking process that guides nursing practice must be organized, logical, purposeful, and disciplined rather than random or undirected. Paul and Elder (2005) describe **critical thinking** as "the art of thinking about thinking." *Critical*, in this context, does not mean "eager to find fault," but instead "capable of judging carefully and accurately."

METHODS OF PROBLEM SOLVING

When solving problems, the nurse makes inferences, sorts out facts from opinions, evaluates the credibility of information sources, and uses a variety of other cognitive skills. The LPN/LVN employs questioning skills when listening to an end-of-shift report, reviewing a history or progress notes, planning care, or discussing a client's care with colleagues. For example, during the end-of-shift report about a client who has just been diagnosed with terminal cancer, the nurse coming on shift may ask, "What has the family been told about the client's prognosis?" This helps the staff understand the family's knowledge level and needs. Asking such questions gives the nurse additional information to use when applying inductive and deductive reasoning.

TYPES OF REASONING

The nurse learns to approach problems from several angles in order to apply reasoning skills. Figure 5-1 ■ highlights the different factors that go into the process of reasoning.

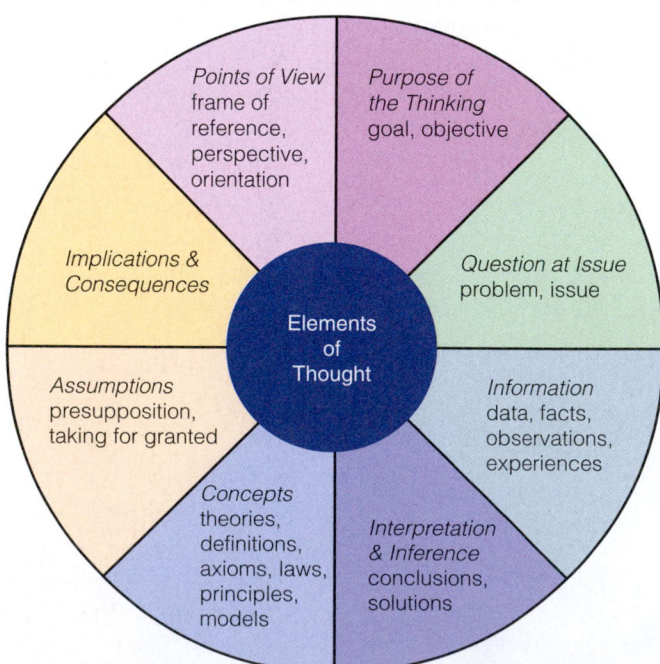

Figure 5-1. ■ The elements of reasoning that are employed in the process of critical thinking. (*Source:* Adapted from "Critical Thinking" by R. Paul and L. Elder, 2005, Dillon Beach, CA: Foundation for Critical Thinking. Reprinted with permission.)

Two other skills used in critical thinking are inductive and deductive reasoning.

- **Inductive reasoning** is a process of forming generalizations from individual pieces of data. Inductive reasoning is like looking at the pieces of a jigsaw puzzle and attempting to describe the whole (without seeing a picture of the completed puzzle). As the person puts more and more pieces together, the whole picture becomes clearer. For example, the nurse who observes that a client has dry skin, poor turgor, sunken eyes, and dark amber urine may make the generalization that the client appears dehydrated.

- **Deductive reasoning** is a process of moving logically from a general statement or concept to related specifics. In deductive reasoning, the thinker sees the whole picture (from the puzzle box cover) and puts the puzzle together by organizing the pieces into border pieces, or colors, or some other grouping. For example, nurses know that people who have experienced several days of vomiting and diarrhea are likely to be dehydrated. In a client who has had vomiting and diarrhea for 2 days, the nurse would confirm this generalization deductively by checking skin turgor, appearance of the client's eyes, and color and quantity of the client's urine.

By using critical thinking, the nurse will also separate facts, inferences, judgments, and opinions (Table 5-1 ■). Box 5-1 ■ lists the characteristics of a critical thinker.

APPLYING CRITICAL THINKING TO NURSING

LPNs/LVNs use their critical-thinking skills in a variety of ways. Nursing students must take knowledge from the classroom and apply it to real-life client situations. You will study lifespan development, nutrition, communication, and psychosocial issues in addition to nursing courses so that you can acquire a strong foundation on which to build your nursing knowledge and skill. You will use the knowledge from all of your courses when you care for your clients. For

---

BOX 5-1	CHARACTERISTICS OF CRITICAL THINKERS

As Critical Thinkers:
- We analyze our thinking.
- We subject the *egocentric* (self-centered) root of our thinking to close scrutiny.
- We expose inappropriate standards and replace them with sound ones.
- We learn how to raise our thinking to conscious examination, to free ourselves from traps of undisciplined, instinctive thought.
- We develop tools for analyzing and assessing our participation in logical systems in which we live.
- We take explicit intellectual and emotional command of who we are, what we are, and the ends to which our lives are tending.
- We learn how to govern the thoughts that govern us.

---

example, you may be assigned to care for a 17-year-old with Crohn's disease, a disorder of the small intestine. Your client will have needs in a variety of areas:

- She is a normal adolescent with the same needs as any 17-year-old.
- She has nutritional needs due to poor absorption of nutrients from her small intestine.
- She has communication needs regarding her feelings and issues about hospitalization and illness.
- She has psychological needs because she is away from her friends and family and her "normal life."

These needs are in addition to the technical aspects of her nursing care, which may include managing total parenteral nutrition, IV therapy, medications, and pain. You will pull together concepts from many different courses when you care for this client.

Nurses deal with change in a stressful **environment** (internal and external surroundings that affect the client). Treatments, medications, and technology change constantly, and a client's condition may change from minute to minute. When

---

TABLE 5-1	Differentiating Types of Statements	
STATEMENT	**DESCRIPTION**	**EXAMPLE**
Facts	Can be verified through investigation	Birth control pills do not protect against sexually transmitted infections (STIs).
Inferences	Conclusions drawn from the facts; going beyond facts to make a statement about something not currently known	A person in a sexual relationship with a client with an STI should not rely on birth control pills alone but should consider using a method that provides a physical barrier.
Judgments	Evaluation of facts or information that reflect values or other criteria; a type of opinion	Having multiple sexual partners can lead to serious health consequences.
Opinions	Beliefs formed over time that include judgments and may fit facts or be in error	It is wrong not to wait until marriage to have sex.

unexpected situations arise, critical thinking enables the nurse to recognize important cues, respond quickly, and adapt interventions to meet specific client needs. An example of this is the client about to be discharged who is stable when you arrive on shift, but over the next several hours has a drop in blood pressure, an increase in pulse, and develops an irregular heart rate. Although the plan was to discharge the client and admit another person into the room, the nurse must assess the situation and respond to changes that have occurred. In addition to responding to the changes in the client's vital signs and implementing care to stabilize him, the nurse must notify the physician, cancel the discharge, and let admitting know that a new person cannot be admitted to the room.

During the course of a workday, nurses make vital decisions of many kinds. These decisions may be made independently by the LPN/LVN or in collaboration with an RN or other team member. It is important that the decisions be sound. LPNs/LVNs use critical-thinking skills when collecting information. For example, consider a nurse who is caring for a client who states that he feels itchy on his back. The nurse must recognize that this itchy feeling could be a sign of a reaction to a medication. The nurse must decide if this problem is indeed a possible drug reaction and must notify the physician if that is the case. The nurse may decide to seek collaboration with the RN to determine whether a drug reaction is taking place. Or, the nurse may decide it is not a serious problem and take steps to make the client more comfortable, while still monitoring the situation for any changes.

Nurses do not always have to think critically and make critical decisions. Some things come naturally without too much thought, like selecting clothes or deciding what to eat for lunch. Nurses often do familiar tasks, such as taking vital signs, without thinking much about how to do the job. But the higher-order skills of critical thinking are put into play as soon as a new idea is encountered or a less-than-routine decision must be made. An example of this is the nurse who uses critical thinking when deciding which clients need to be cared for first, second, or third as the shift begins.

USING CRITICAL THINKING TO MAKE NURSING DECISIONS

The Nursing Process

One model for making decisions is the nursing process, which is a systematic method of assessing, planning, implementing, and evaluating nursing care (see Chapter 6 🔗). Critical thinking is used throughout the nursing process (Table 5-2 ■).

Nurses use critical thinking to resolve problems related to client care. The nurse obtains information that clarifies the problem and suggests possible solutions. The nurse then carefully evaluates the possible solutions and chooses the best one to implement. The nurse monitors the situation carefully over time to ensure its initial and continued effectiveness. The nurse does not discard the other solutions but keeps them in mind. They may be useful if the first solution is not effective, or if a different client with a similar problem prefers an alternative solution. For example, a nurse may be attempting to solve the problem of a client who refuses most of the food on his tray. The nurse considers possible solutions: asking for a consult with the dietician, talking with the client about his food likes and dislikes, checking to see if chewing or swallowing is difficult for him, and asking questions that might indicate if he is discouraged and therefore not eating. The nurse chooses the best solution to implement by checking to see if the client has difficulty chewing or swallowing and determines that no problem exists. The nurse next checks with the client about his food preferences and includes this information in his care plan. The nurse then evaluates how the client is eating for the next several days and, if needed, asks for a dietary consult. The next time the nurse encounters a similar client situation, this problem-solving experience will be remembered and used as a resource.

Nursing Decisions

Nurses make many types of decisions throughout the day. They make value decisions, such as ways to keep client information confidential, and time management decisions, such as taking clean linen to the client's room at the same time as the medication in order to save steps. They make scheduling decisions, such as the decision to bathe the client before scheduled physical therapy, and priority decisions, such as preparing a client for surgery before giving a bath to another client.

Decision making is a critical-thinking process for choosing the best actions to meet a desired goal. Nurses must make decisions and assist clients to make decisions. When two call lights are ringing, an IV pump is beeping, and a physician is calling, the nurse must decide which situation to handle first. When a client is faced with choices about chemotherapy and radiation therapy to treat cancer, the nurse may need to provide information or resources the client can use in making a decision. See Table 5-3 ■ for a description of a seven-step decision-making process.

PRACTICING CRITICAL THINKING

The day in and day out use of critical thinking and problem solving takes a great deal of practice. As a student, you may feel overwhelmed right now. That is why your instructors and other healthcare professionals will continue to challenge your thinking and decision making throughout your course of study. Every chapter in this text provides

TABLE 5-2	Questions about Critical Thinking Throughout the Nursing Process
NURSING PROCESS	**QUESTIONS TO ASK**
COLLECTING DATA FOR THE ASSESSMENT	
	Are the data complete?
	What other data do I need?
	What are the possible sources of the data?
	What assumptions and biases do I have about the situation?
	What is the client's point of view?
PLANNING FOR AND IMPLEMENTING THE NURSING DIAGNOSIS	
Diagnosing	What do these data mean?
	What else could be happening?
	Are there any gaps in the data?
	How are these data similar and how are they different?
	What assumptions or biases do I have in this situation?
	Have my assumptions affected my interpretation of the data?
Planning	What are the goals for the client?
	What do I want to accomplish?
	How are my goals related to what the client wants to accomplish?
	What are the expected outcomes for this client?
	What interventions are to be used?
	How much involvement can the client and family have at this time?
Implementing	What is the client's current status?
	What are the most critical steps in this intervention?
	How must I alter the interventions to best meet this client's needs and maintain the principles of safety?
	What is the client's response during and after the intervention?
	Is there a need to alter the intervention in any way? If so, how?
Evaluating	Were the interventions successful in helping the client to meet the desired goals?
	How could things have been done differently?
	What data do I need to make new decisions?
	Where will I get the data?
	Were there assumptions, biases, or points of view that I missed that affected the outcomes?

review questions to strengthen your thinking. Chapters 8 through 62 ⚭ also provide care plans and care maps to encourage you to apply your critical-thinking skills to nursing situations.

Critical Thinking Care Map

As LPNs/LVNs collect assessment data about a client, they use critical-thinking skills to organize data into **subjective data** (information apparent only to the person

TABLE 5-3	Seven-Step Decision-Making Process
STEP	**EXPLANATION**
Identify the purpose.	Identify the why and what.
Set the criteria.	Question what needs to be achieved, preserved, avoided.
Weigh the criteria.	Set priorities in order of importance.
Seek alternatives.	Identify all possibilities for meeting the criteria.
Test alternatives.	Study alternatives for objective rationales for choosing one alternative over another.
Troubleshoot.	Determine what might go wrong and develop a plan to prevent, minimize, or overcome problems.
Evaluate the action.	Determine how effective the actions were and if they achieved the purpose.

being affected) and **objective data** (information detectable by an observer). These data contribute to the development of nursing diagnoses (see Chapter 6 ⚭). For example, an LPN/LVN assesses a client who has not been taking his medication consistently. The blood pressure is elevated, and the nurse reports it to the physician. The physician orders an increase in the dose of blood pressure medication. The nurse knows the client is not compliant in taking the medication due to lack of understanding of its importance. The client is at risk for complications of elevated blood pressure and stroke. LPNs/LVNs also use critical thinking to determine which interventions would be appropriate for specific nursing diagnoses. They think critically when they frame their narrative notes for the client's chart.

A sample Critical Thinking Care Map is shown on page 69. The case studies supplied in Chapters 8 through 62 ⚭ will focus on one of the NCLEX-PN® focus areas, to help you think in terms of the broad categories of nursing you will master. An appropriate nursing diagnosis will be supplied, and you will select and sort objective and subjective data that apply to this nursing diagnosis. You will decide which of the data you would report immediately to a supervisor or physician. You will select appropriate interventions from the list provided. You will also practice documenting the important information. When you take time to complete these Critical Thinking Care Maps, you will practice and sharpen your critical-thinking skills.

Theories and Models

Besides thinking critically about a client's condition and care, nurses must also think critically about nursing itself. Starting with Florence Nightingale, nurses have been doing just that. Several have developed theories of nursing. **Theories** are ways of looking at a discipline, such as nursing, in clear, explicit terms that can be communicated to others.

INTRODUCTION TO NURSING THEORIES

Until 1859, when Florence Nightingale penned her *Notes on Nursing: What It Is, and What It Is Not*, nursing practice was based on borrowed theory from medicine. Nursing continues to draw on the medical communities for knowledge, but since the middle of the 20th century, nursing has begun to develop its unique theory. Theory development gained momentum in the 1960s and has progressed since then through the work of several nurse-theorists and nurses. Each theory bears the name of the person or group that developed it and reflects the beliefs of the developer.

ESSENTIAL ELEMENTS IN NURSING THEORY

Nursing theories address and specify relationships about four major ideas. These four concepts are central to nursing:

1. Nursing—the attributes, characteristics, and actions of the nurse providing care on behalf of, or in conjunction with, the client
2. Person or client—the recipient of nursing care (includes individuals, families, and communities)
3. Health—the degree of wellness or well-being that the client experiences
4. Environment—the internal and external surroundings that affect the client, including people in the physical environment, such as families, friends, and significant others.

Each nurse-theorist's definitions of the four major concepts vary in accordance with personal philosophy, scientific orientation, and experience in nursing. See Table 5-4 ■ for selected theorists' definitions and descriptions of nursing, person/client, health, and environment.

NON-NURSING MODELS

Models and theories of health and wellness are also used by nurses, even though they are not specifically about nursing.

Wellness Model

Nurses use wellness models to assist clients to identify health risks and to explore lifestyle habits and health behaviors, beliefs, values, and attitudes that influence levels of wellness. Such models generally include the following:

- Health history
- Physical fitness evaluation
- Nutritional assessment
- Life-stress analysis
- Lifestyle and health habits
- Health beliefs
- Sexual health
- Spiritual health
- Relationships
- Health risk appraisal

Non-nursing models are included in LPN/LVN training programs to assist the nurse in gathering data and processing it. Nurses usually will use more than one model at a time to obtain a complete history.

Body Systems Model

Closely related to the medical model, the body systems model focuses on abnormalities. The client is assessed and treated according to the body system that is affected by the primary or presenting diagnosis. The model does have one very significant downfall: It is not effective when treating a client with a disease process that has multisystem effects.

(Text continues on p. 74.)

This line provides an appropriate nursing diagnosis.

This line provides the appropriate NCLEX-PN® focus area.

This information is provided to give you basic information about the client.

Sample Critical Thinking Care Map

Caring for a Client with Hypertension

NCLEX-PN® Focus Area: Physiological Integrity

Case Study: Jose Salazar, a 45-year-old Latino male, complains of severe headache. He is 20 lb overweight and his blood pressure is 180/95 mm Hg. He states he has been taking high blood pressure pills only when he has a headache. He is a self-employed gardener; he lives with his wife, mother-in-law, and four children.

Nursing Diagnosis: Deficient Knowledge R/T Medication Regimen

COLLECT DATA

Subjective	Objective
_____	_____
_____	_____
_____	_____
_____	_____
_____	_____
_____	_____

Would you report this data? Yes/No

If yes, to: _____

What would you report? _____

Nursing Care

_____
_____
_____
_____
_____
_____
_____

How would you document this? _____
_____
_____

Data Collected
(use those that apply)

- Self-employed gardener
- Married
- Lives with wife, four children (16, 14, 10, and 4), and mother-in-law
- Wife works ½ day at the 10-year-old's school
- Mother-in-law cares for 4-year-old and cooks traditional meals
- VS: T 98.8, P 86, R 24, BP 180/95 mm Hg
- Weight: 206 lb
- Height: 5'9"
- Procardia XL 30 mg daily
- Admits to taking meds only when he has a headache
- History of Type II diabetes mellitus controlled with diet
- Diet: 2,000 cal ADA/NSA (no added salt)
- Mrs. Salazar stated, "Jose complains of dizzy spells when working out in the heat."
- Client states, "I can't follow the diet. My mother-in-law does the cooking and doesn't always follow the plan."

Nursing Interventions
(use all that apply; list in priority order)

- Discuss treatment options.
- Help client identify community resources.
- Acknowledge racial/ethnic differences at the onset of care.
- Determine client's previous knowledge related to diagnosis.
- Report noncompliance to the physician.
- Review medications with client and discuss indications for use.
- Teach client or family member procedure for taking blood pressure.
- Discuss with client reasons for not taking medications.
- Discuss food likes and dislikes with client.

Carefully consider the data. What statements and data collected would support this nursing diagnosis? What data are subjective and what data are objective? What data are not relevant?

Subjective data: Only takes blood pressure medication when he has a headache, severe headache, dizzy when working outside in heat, not following diet

Objective data: VS: T 98.8, P 86, R 24, BP 180/95 mm Hg, weight 206, height 5'9", 2,000 cal ADA diet (no salt added), Procardia XL 30 mg daily

Irrelevant data: Self-employed gardener; married; lives with wife, four children (16, 14, 10, and 4), and mother-in-law; wife works ½ day at the 10-year-old's school; mother-in-law cares for 4-year-old and cooks traditional meals.

Think about the data you have collected. Are any of the data abnormal? Would they indicate deficient knowledge that could have a negative impact on the client's health? Would it be important to report this information? If so, to which person? **Yes, report dizziness and blood pressure reading to physician.**

This question allows you to practice your documentation. It is not necessary to document all the data or interventions for this exercise. For example, the assessment documentation might be:

(date) Client admitted through ER following dizzy spell at work. BP 150/95, complaining of severe headache. Hx of hypertension, treated with Procardia KL 30 mg. q.d. Client admits to taking meds only when he has a headache. Marge Smith, LPN

Consider the client's deficient knowledge about the medication regimen. Make a decision about which interventions are relevant and which are not relevant.

Relevant interventions: Acknowledge racial/ethnic differences at the onset of care. Determine client's previous knowledge related to diagnosis. Review medications with client and discuss indications for use. Teach client or family member procedure for taking blood pressure. Discuss with client reasons for not taking medications. Report noncompliance to the physician.

Irrelevant interventions: Discuss treatment options. Help client identify community resources. Discuss food likes and dislikes with client.

TABLE 5-4 Selected Nursing Theories and the Nursing Process

THEORY	NURSING	PERSON/CLIENT	HEALTH	ENVIRONMENT	COLLECTING DATA FOR ASSESSMENT	PLANNING AND IMPLEMENTING THE DIAGNOSIS	EVALUATING
Florence Nightingale's environmental theory (1859)	Provision of optimal conditions to enhance the person's reparative processes and prevent the reparative process from being interrupted.	An individual with vital reparative processes to deal with disease and desirous of health but passive in terms of influencing the environment or nurse.	Being well and using one's powers to the fullest extent. Health is maintained through prevention of disease via environmental health factors. Disease is a reparative process nature institutes because of some want of attention.	The major concepts for health are ventilation, warmth, light, diet, cleanliness, and absence of noise. Although the environment has social, emotional, and physical aspects, Nightingale emphasized the physical aspects.	"The most important practical lesson that can be given to nurses is to teach them what to observe, how to observe, what symptoms indicate improvement, what the reverse indicates, which are of importance, which are not, which are the evidence of neglect, and what kind of neglect." In this statement Nightingale was teaching the first step.	**Diagnosing/planning:** The concept of nursing diagnoses came much later, but she did identify particular needs and problems presented by the client. Through observation she was able to title problems such as lack of appetite or difficulty breathing so that they could be addressed immediately. Nurses were able to plan care, basing it on the prioritizing of patients' needs. **Implementing:** The plan of care was directly related to Nightingale's theory of environment. Nurses were responsible not only for personal care of the client but also for washing the floors and walls and maintenance of the stove to provide warmth in the environment.	The client's progress was evaluated and reassessed by observation. She determined that the evaluation of the client's status was critical to the process of providing adequate care, and to determining if care should be continued or altered.
Dorothea Orem's general theory of nursing (1980)	A helping or assisting service to persons who are wholly or partly dependent—infants, children, and adults—when they, their parents, guardians, or other adults responsible for their care are no longer able to give or supervise their care. A creative effort of one human being to help another human being. Nursing is	An entity who can be viewed as functioning biologically, symbolically, and socially and who initiates and performs self-care activities on one's own behalf in maintaining life, health, and well-being. Self-care activities deal with	Health is a state that is characterized by soundness or wholeness of developed human structures and of bodily and mental functioning. It includes physical, psychological, interpersonal, and social aspects. Well-being is used	The environment is linked to the individual, forming an integrated and interactive system.	Involves collecting data about the client's capacities (knowledge, skills, and motivation) to perform universal, developmental, and health-deviation self-care requisites. Determines self-care deficits.	**Diagnosing:** Stated in terms of the client's limitations for maintaining self-care (a deficit in self-care agency). **Planning:** Involves considering and designing, with the client's participation, an appropriate nursing system (wholly compensatory, partially compensatory, supportive-educative, or a mix) that will help the	Determining the client's level of achievement in resolving self-care deficits and in performing self-care.

TABLE 5-4 Selected Nursing Theories and the Nursing Process (continued)

THEORY	NURSING	PERSON/CLIENT	HEALTH	ENVIRONMENT	COLLECTING DATA FOR ASSESSMENT	PLANNING AND IMPLEMENTING THE DIAGNOSIS	EVALUATING
	deliberate action, a function of the practical intelligence of nurses, and action to bring about humanely desirable conditions in persons and their environments. It is distinguished from other human services and other forms of care by its focus on human beings.	air, water, food, elimination, activity and rest, solitude and social interaction, prevention of hazards to life and well-being, and promotion of human functioning.	in the sense of individuals' perceived condition of existence. Well-being is a state characterized by experiences of contentment, pleasure, and certain kinds of happiness; by spiritual experiences; by movement toward fulfillment of one's self-ideal; and by continuing personalization. Well-being is associated with health, with success in personal endeavors, and with sufficiency of resources.			client achieve an optimal level of self-care (i.e., enhance the client's self-care agency). **Implementing:** Assisting the client by acting for or doing for, guiding, supporting, providing a developmental environment, and teaching.	
Betty Neuman's system model (1982)	A unique profession in that it is concerned with all of the variables affecting an individual's response to stressors, which are intra-, inter-, and extrapersonal in nature. The concern of nursing is to prevent stress invasion, or, following stress invasion, to protect the client's basic structure and obtain or maintain a maximum level of wellness. The nurse helps the client, through primary, secondary, and	Open system consisting of a basic structure or central core of survival factors surrounded by concentric rings that are bounded by lines of resistance, a normal line of defense, and a flexible line of defense. The total person is a composite of physiological, psychological, sociocultural,	Wellness is the condition in which all parts and subparts of an individual are in harmony with the whole system. Wholeness is based on interrelationships of variables that determine the resistance of an individual to any stressor. Illness indicates lack of harmony among	Both internal and external environments exist, and a person maintains varying degrees of harmony and balance between them. It is all factors affecting and affected by the system.	Proper assessment requires consideration of both the client's and the caregiver's perceptions of the basic structure, the lines of resistance and defense, and the internal and external environments.	**Diagnosing:** The nursing diagnosis must be a comprehensive statement that encompasses the client's general condition and circumstances, including actual and potential variances from wellness. **Planning:** The diagnostic statements are used to formulate and prioritize the client's needs and to identify interactions. **Implementing:** Nursing interventions focus on retaining or maintaining	The final stage of the nursing process according to Neuman occurs when the client's outcomes are evaluated to confirm their attainment or guide reformulation of the goals.

(continued)

	Nursing	Person	Environment	Health	Nursing process
			the parts and subparts of the system of the individual and developmental variables.	Health is viewed as a point along a continuum from wellness to illness; health is dynamic (i.e., constantly subject to change). Optimal wellness or stability indicates that all of a person's needs are being met. A reduced state of wellness is the result of unmet systemic needs. The individual is in a dynamic state of wellness–illness, in varying degrees, at any given time.	tertiary prevention modes, to adjust to environmental stressors and maintain client system stability. … system stability. Interventions are carried out on three preventive levels: primary, secondary, and tertiary.
Sister Callista Roy's adaptation model (1970)	Nursing involves the care and well-being of human persons; the value-based stance of the discipline is rooted in beliefs about the human person. As a science, nursing is a developing system of knowledge about persons used to serve, classify, and relate the processes by which persons positively affect their health status. As a practice discipline, nursing's scientific body of knowledge is used to provide an essential service to people, that is, to promote the ability to affect health positively.	A biopsychosocial being who is in constant interaction with the environment and who has four modes of adaptation, based on physiological needs, self-concept (physical self, moral-ethical self, self-consistency, self-ideal and expectancy, and self-esteem), role function, and interdependence relations. Persons are coextensive with their physical	All the conditions, circumstances, and influences surrounding and affecting the development and behavior of persons or groups; the input into the person as an adaptive system involving both internal and external factors.	A state and a process of being and becoming an integrated and whole person. Lack of integration represents lack of health.	Involves two levels. First-level assessment includes collecting data about output behaviors related to the four adaptive modes (physiological, self-concept, role function, and interdependence modes). Second-level assessment includes collecting data about internal and external stimuli (focal, contextual, or residual) that are influencing the identified behaviors. **Diagnosing:** Focuses on adaptation problems and uses one of three alternative methods: 1. Stating behaviors within one mode with their most relevant influencing stimuli. 2. Clustering behavioral information and labeling it according to indicators of positive adaptation and a typology of common adaptation problems related to each mode. Roy provides a typology of indicators of positive adaptation and a typology of commonly recurring adaptation problems … Determining the client's output behaviors with those identified in the goals.

THEORY	NURSING	PERSON/CLIENT	HEALTH	ENVIRONMENT	COLLECTING DATA FOR ASSESSMENT	PLANNING AND IMPLEMENTING THE DIAGNOSIS	EVALUATING
		and social environments. Persons and the earth are one; they are in god and of god.				according to each of the four modes. 3. Labeling a behavioral pattern when more than one mode is being affected by the same stimuli. **Planning**: Setting goals in terms of behaviors the client is to achieve and planning nursing interventions to promote the effectiveness of the client's coping mechanisms and adaptive behaviors. **Implementing**: Altering and manipulating the focal, contextual, and residual stimuli by increasing, decreasing, or maintaining them.	
Madeleine Leininger's cultural care diversity and universality theory (1991)	A learned humanistic art and science that focuses on personalized behaviors, functions, and processes to promote and maintain health or recovery from illness. It has physical, psychosocial, and cultural significance for those being assisted. It uses a problem-solving approach, as depicted in the sunrise model, (see Figure 3-1), and three models of action: culture care preservation, culture care accommodation, and culture care repatterning.	Human beings are caring and capable of feeling concern for others. Caring about human beings is universal, but ways of caring vary across cultures.	A state of well-being that is culturally defined, valued, and practiced. It is universal across cultures but is defined differently by each culture. It includes health systems, healthcare practices, health patterns, and health maintenance and promotion.	Not specifically defined, but concepts of worldview, social structure, and environmental context are closely related to the concept of culture.	Must take into account biocultural variations in health and illness (e.g., assessing cyanosis, jaundice, anemia, and related clinical manifestations of disease in darkly pigmented clients).	**Diagnosing**: Focuses on meeting healthcare needs in the context of clients' patterns. **Planning**: The nurse plans, negotiates, and accommodates the client's specific cultural wants and needs (e.g., food preferences, religious practices, and treatment practices). **Implementing**: Healthcare personnel should work toward an understanding of care and the values, health beliefs, and lifestyles of different cultures, which will form the basis for providing culture-specific care.	When the client chooses to follow only folk medicine/ treatment and refuses all prescribed medical or nursing interventions, nursing goals for the client need to be adjusted.

Body systems covered by this model include:

- Integumentary system
- Respiratory system
- Cardiovascular system
- Nervous system
- Musculoskeletal system
- Gastrointestinal system
- Genitourinary system
- Reproductive system

Maslow's Hierarchy of Needs

Maslow's hierarchy of needs theory assists the nurse in identifying needs and setting priorities. It clusters data pertaining to the following:

- Physiological needs (survival needs)
- Safety and security needs
- Love and belonging needs
- Self-esteem needs
- Self-actualization needs

See Figure 6-4 and Chapter 15 ☍ for more details about this theory.

Developmental Theories

Developmental theories assist the nurse in treating the client holistically. Several physical, psychosocial, cognitive, and moral developmental theories may be used by the nurse in specific situations. Examples include the following:

- Freud's five stages of development
- Erikson's eight stages of development
- Piaget's phases of cognitive development
- Kohlberg's stages of moral development

The theories and theorists are discussed in Chapter 15 ☍ as they relate to lifespan development.

SIGNIFICANCE OF MODELS AND THEORIES

Why is it important for an LPN/LVN to have an understanding of nursing theories? A theoretical understanding of nursing helps you view your clients as more than a medical diagnosis from which you will perform nursing tasks. This understanding will help you develop a personal nursing philosophy. It will help you to understand and participate in the nursing process and collaborate with registered nurses and other staff. It will also help you to discern the differences in scope among levels of nursing practice. It will help you provide culturally competent care (Box 5-2 ■). Most schools of nursing and healthcare agencies have developed their own structured assessment tools. Many of these are based on selected nursing theories.

Today the LPN/LVN has a great deal of responsibility and must think critically to make sound decisions. Understanding

BOX 5-2	CULTURAL PULSE POINTS

Thinking Clearly about Clients of Other Cultures

When culture is an issue in the delivery of client care, the nurse must make use of his or her critical-thinking ability. Cultural awareness does not take the process far enough. Cultural awareness can be used to categorize, rather than individualize, care. Focusing too heavily on race, culture, and ethnicity is one danger associated with transcultural nursing theories and models.

Nurses must not label people by culture and race. Do not assume that the characteristics of a certain cultural group are true for every client who belongs to that racial, ethnic, or cultural group. The information we learn about cultural groups is no more than an overview. To fill in the picture would take many books. Nurses must always be aware of what people may be thinking that may differ from our own thoughts, and that other sources outside the traditional medical community exist to help the client.

the four concepts that are central to nursing will help the LPN/LVN process information and make appropriate judgments. As nurses progress in formal education or lifelong learning, they will develop a personal theory of nursing. Understanding the basic principles will prepare the LPN/LVN for nursing of the future.

Evidence-Based Practice

Evidence-based practice (EBP) is a thoughtful integration of the best available evidence coupled with clinical expertise. As such, it enables the nurse as well as other health practitioners to address healthcare questions with an evaluative and qualitative approach. EBP allows practitioners to assess current and past research, clinical guidelines, and other information resources. Evidence-based practice includes five fundamental steps.

Step 1: Formulating a well-built question A well-built clinical question includes the following components:

- The client's disorder or disease
- The intervention or finding under review
- A comparison of interventions (if applicable—not always present)
- The outcome

The acronym *PICO* assists in remembering the steps (*P*, patient or problem; *I*, intervention; *C*, comparison intervention; *O*, outcomes).

Step 2: Identifying articles and other evidence-based resources that answer the question Applying PICO is a systematic way to identify important concepts in a case and to formulate a question for searching. There often is not a comparison intervention, and EBP resources may require different levels of specificity. Depending on the type of resource being used, all the PICO components might not be part of the search at first. However, no matter what type of resources are ultimately used to look for answers, the nurse should always start by applying PICO to the question so strategic thinking can be instituted.

Step 3: Critically appraising the evidence to assess its validity   After identifying an article or resource that seems appropriate to the question, the nurse appraises the information critically. If the study is from a primary source, its *validity* (closeness-to-truth) must be checked. To check for validity, the nurse will ask questions related to diagnosis, therapy, harm, and prognosis.

Step 4: Applying the evidence   Once it has been determined that a study is internally valid (Step 3), it must be decided how the study or other information applies to the question. To reach this conclusion, the nurse may consult questions related to diagnosis, therapy, harm, and prognosis. Information must be interpreted based on a number of criteria. Depending on the nurse's skill and experience, he or she may need to confer with a peer.

Step 5: Reevaluating the application of evidence and areas for improvement   In the process of executing evidence-based practice, a clinical question must be developed (Step 1); answers must be verified to support the clinical decision (Steps 2 and 3); and, ultimately, the findings must be applied to the client (Step 4). The final step in this process is to evaluate the effectiveness and efficacy of the decision in direct relationship to the client. This is done by asking questions such as the following:

Was the diagnosis and treatment successful?
Is there new information or data in the literature?
How can I improve or update my clinical decisions?

THE LPN/LVN ROLE IN EVIDENCE-BASED PRACTICE

Evidence-based practice is based in research, and research is usually done by the RN. However, just as care plans are used as learning activities in LPN/LVN courses, evidence-based practice can also be used to teach students better ways of providing client care. Evidence-based practice gives you the opportunity to read current literature (nursing journals). This is a very good habit to develop during your nursing program. Regularly updating your knowledge is an important activity that should be carried on throughout your career.

As a licensed nurse, you may have the opportunity to work on a unit that is involved in evidence-based practice. It will be your responsibility to collect data and collaborate with RNs and other healthcare professionals to evaluate whether the treatment has been successful, and if improvements and updating can be made in practice.

Note: The references and resources for all chapters have been compiled at the back of the book.

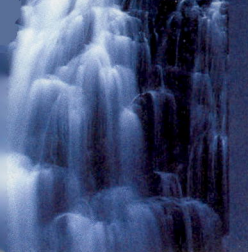

Chapter Review

KEY Points

- Critical thinking is a purposeful, organized, logical, and disciplined mental activity in which ideas are produced and evaluated and judgments made.

- Critical thinking is reasonable, rational, reflective, autonomous, creative, and fair; it inspires an attitude of inquiry that focuses on deciding what to believe or do.

- Critical thinkers have certain attributes: independence of thought, humility, courage, integrity, perseverance, empathy, and fair-mindedness.

- Everyone has at least some level of critical-thinking skill, and that skill can be developed with practice.

- Nursing theories help us view the client more completely or understand the goals of nursing better.

- Nursing theories explore the meaning of client environment, health, and nursing and add perspective to our own individual way of approaching our profession.

- Non-nursing theories help nurses as they gather and process data, particularly when completing a client history.

- Evidence-based practice is generally carried out by RNs, but participating in research and keeping up with current nursing literature can improve the quality of care provided by LPNs/LVNs as well.

⊕ FOR FURTHER Study

Figure 3-1 depicts the sunrise model.

Chapter 6 contains the main discussion about the nursing process; see Figure 6-4 for Maslow's hierarchy of needs.

Chapters 8 through 62 provide Critical Thinking Care Maps.

Chapter 15 provides details about theories as they relate to lifespan development.

PEARSON

EXPLORE **mynursingkit**™

MyNursingKit is your one stop for online chapter review materials and resources. Prepare for success with additional NCLEX®-style practice questions, interactive assignments and activities, web links, animations and videos, and more!

Register your access code from the front of your book at
www.mynursingkit.com

NCLEX-PN® Exam Preparation

TEST-TAKING TIP Identify the components of the question. The case situation gives you the information about the clinical health problem and the information you need to consider when answering the question. Always read all of the information and every word of the case situation.

1 The nurse who uses critical thinking:
1. Finds fault with statements of fact.
2. Thinks about thinking.
3. Makes decisions considering only one point of view.
4. Makes random and undirected decisions.

2 The nurse considers personal assumptions or biases about the situation during what phase of the nursing process?
1. Assessment/data collection
2. Diagnosing
3. Planning
4. Evaluation

3 The nurse applies critical thinking to the teaching process, aware of potential pitfalls and limitations, by:
1. Evaluating the cognitive ability of the client.
2. Giving the client written instructions and allowing time to read them.
3. Instructing the client to call the home health nurse if problems develop.
4. Arranging for a family member to be present during teaching.

4 The primary model used by nursing for making decisions using critical thinking is:
1. Nursing Code of Ethics.
2. Data collection.
3. Collaboration with peers.
4. The nursing process.

5 The nurse works at the community hospital. The nurse is a member of the union. The union has called for a strike. All of the nurses at the hospital will go on strike, therefore the nurse must strike. This sequence of thinking is called:
1. Inductive reasoning.
2. Deductive reasoning.
3. Opinion.
4. Belief.

6 Which of the following situations indicates that a nurse is using evidence-based practice?
1. The nurse who reads nursing research articles and uses the findings to change the way care is delivered, even if that differs from facility policy.

2. The nurse who joins the standards and practice committee to contribute research findings to improving current facility policies and procedures.
3. The nurse who changes his or her practice after reading one nursing research article.
4. The nurse who tells coworkers, "According to the article I read we're doing this all wrong."

7 Which of the following interventions is aimed at addressing the nursing theory concept of environment?
1. Teaching a community class on proper nutrition.
2. Actively listening to a client who expresses concerns about upcoming surgery.
3. Limiting external stimulation for a client who has increased intracranial pressure.
4. Instructing a client to do range-of-motion exercises in preparation for walking following a cerebrovascular accident.

8 The Neuman system model's unique focus is on:
1. Responses to a constantly changing environment.
2. Clients' reactions to stress.
3. Nurses' actions related to therapeutic self-care.
4. Culturally competent care.

9 The environment theory is attributed to which of the following nursing theorists?
1. Florence Nightingale
2. Sister Callista Roy
3. Betty Neuman
4. Madeleine Leininger

10 The dominant, distinctive, and unifying feature of nursing is human caring, which varies by culture. Which of the following theorists identified this feature of nursing?
1. Dorothea Orem
2. Sister Callista Roy
3. Betty Neuman
4. Madeleine Leininger

Answers and rationales for Review Questions appear in Appendix I.

Chapter 6

The LPN/LVN and the Nursing Process

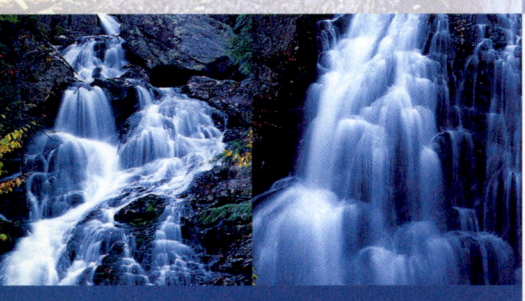

BRIEF Outline

The Nursing Process
Assessment
Diagnosis
Planning
Implementation
Evaluation

LEARNING Outcomes

After completing this chapter, you will be able to:

1. Identify essential characteristics of the nursing process.
2. Describe the components of the nursing process.
3. Describe the role of the LPN/LVN in the assessment process.
4. Define the purpose of collecting data and how the data will be used.
5. Differentiate objective and subjective data, and primary and secondary data.
6. Identify three methods of data collection and give examples of how each is useful.
7. Describe the importance and the elements of nursing diagnoses.
8. Discuss the planning step of the nursing process.
9. Discuss the activities of the implementing phase.
10. Explain the value of evaluating and how evaluating relates to other phases of the nursing process.

KEY TERMS

Use the audio glossary feature on the MyNursingKit Website to hear the correct pronunciation of the following key terms.

In 1961, the nursing process was defined at the Catholic University of America. It was developed as a template for thinking that was exclusively for nursing. The process was designed with the RN in mind, but use of the nursing process provides a common way of thinking for all licensed nurses. All licensed nurses collect data for assessment. They plan, implement, and evaluate. Although RNs are responsible for diagnosing, LPNs and LVNs contribute to the diagnosis through the data they collect and through their ongoing evaluation of the client.

The Nursing Process

The **nursing process** is a systematic, logical method of providing individualized nursing care. The purpose of the nursing process is to identify a client's health status and actual or potential healthcare problems or needs, to establish plans to meet the identified needs, and to deliver specific nursing interventions to meet those needs.

The components of the nursing process follow a logical sequence, but more than one component may be involved at any one time (Figure 6-1 ■). The nursing process consists of five steps: assessing, diagnosing, planning, implementing, and evaluating. Nursing theorists may use different terms to describe these steps. For example, nursing diagnosis may sometimes be called analysis. Implementation (implementing) may be called intervention or intervening. However, the activities of the nurse using the process are similar. An overview of the five-phase nursing process is shown in Table 6-1 ■.

The nursing process "provides the framework in which nurses use their knowledge and skills to express human caring" and to help clients with their actual and potential health problems (Wilkinson, 2009, p. 10). The nursing process has unique properties that enable it to respond to the changing health status of the client.

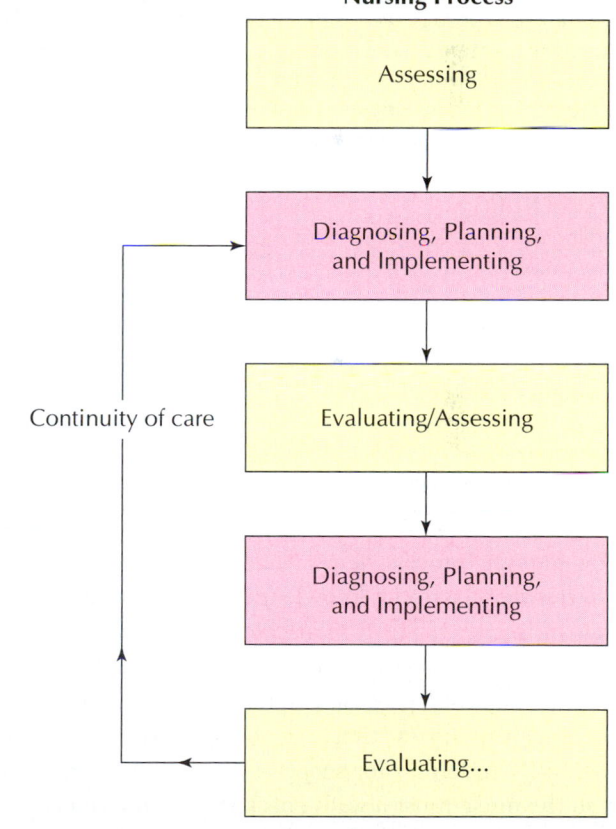

Nursing Process

Figure 6-1. ■ The nursing process in action.

ROLE OF THE LPN/LVN IN THE NURSING PROCESS

LPNs/LVNs, as important members of the healthcare team, should be educated to use all aspects of the nursing process that fall within their scope of practice. Each step includes functions delegated to the LPN/LVN, functions carried out in collaboration with or under the direction of the RN, and functions implemented by the RN. It is very important for the LPN/LVN to understand the entire nursing process.

TABLE 6-1	Overview of the Nursing Process		
COMPONENT AND DESCRIPTION	**PURPOSE**		**LPN/LVN ROLE**
ASSESSING Collecting, organizing, validating, and documenting client data	To establish a database about the client's response to health concerns or illness and the ability to manage healthcare needs		To collect data, to make observations of client status, to report changes in client condition or abnormal results of data collection to the RN or primary nurse
DIAGNOSING Analyzing and synthesizing data	To identify client strengths and health problems that can be prevented or resolved by collaborative and independent nursing interventions and to promote health maintenance To develop a list of nursing diagnoses and collaborative problems		To understand the nursing diagnoses identified by the RN as it relates to the client's condition
PLANNING Determining how to prevent, reduce, or resolve the identified client problems; how to support client strengths; and how to implement nursing interventions in an organized, individualized, and goal-directed manner	To develop an individualized care plan that specifies client goals/desired outcomes and related nursing interventions		To review and follow the care plan
IMPLEMENTING Carrying out the planned nursing interventions	To assist the client in taking steps to meet desired goals/outcomes, promote wellness, prevent illness and disease, restore health, and facilitate coping with altered functioning		To carry out nursing interventions as assigned
EVALUATING Measuring the degree to which goals/outcomes have been achieved and identifying factors that positively or negatively influence goal achievement	To determine whether to continue, modify, or terminate the plan or individual parts of the plan of care		To observe or measure client responses to nursing interventions and to report any responses or data that might require alteration in the care plan

The nursing process helps students to think critically and to transfer classroom knowledge to the clinical setting. (See also Chapter 5 👥 for critical thinking.) The nursing process provides both structure and guidance for LPNs/LVNs as they provide client care. This chapter will define specific duties that can be carried out by the LPN/LVN. Guidelines for scope of practice do vary, however, so the nurse must always check state regulations.

Assessment

Assessment is the systematic collection, organization, *validation* (proving or supporting), and documentation of data. All phases of the nursing process depend on accurate and complete collection of data (information). Nursing assessments focus on a client's responses to a health problem. The Joint Commission that gives accreditation to healthcare organizations (JCAHO, 2002) recommended that each client receive a documented assessment on admission to an agency. The initial assessment is done by or in collaboration with the RN.

In some situations, ongoing assessments are done only by RNs. This may be stated in the nurse practice act of the state or may be a management decision of a particular facility. The LPN/LVN is responsible for contributing by collecting data.

clinical ALERT

The LPN/LVN is responsible for reading the assessment *prior to* beginning care of assigned clients.

The assessment process involves four closely related activities: collecting data, organizing data, validating data, and documenting data.

COLLECTING DATA FOR ASSESSMENT

Data collection is the process of gathering information about a client. It must be both systematic and continuous, and it must reflect a client's changing health status. Approaches for collecting head-to-toe client data are discussed in Chapter 19 👥. Methods for gathering information through the interview process are described in Chapter 11 👥.

A client's **database** (baseline data) includes information from many sources: (1) the nursing health history (Box 6-1 ■), (2) the nurse's physical assessment (see Chapter 19 👥), (3) the physician's history and physical examination, (4) results

BOX 6-1	COMPONENTS OF A NURSING HEALTH HISTORY

Biographic Data

- Client's name, address, age, sex, marital status, occupation, religious preference, healthcare financing, and usual source of medical care

Chief Complaint or Reason for Visit

- The answer given to the question "Why did you come here today?"

History of Present Illness

- Provocation or palliation: what causes it, what relieves it
- Quality and quantity: type of pain and intensity
- Region or radiation: where it is, where it goes
- Scale of pain: 1 to 10
- Timing: when it began, how long it lasts, and how often it occurs

Past History

- Childhood illnesses
- Childhood immunizations
- Allergies
- Injuries
- Hospitalization for serious illnesses
- Medication: all currently used prescription and over-the-counter medication, such as aspirin, nasal spray, vitamins, laxatives, supplements, and complementary medications such as St. John's wort, ginseng, etc.

Family History of Illness

- Heart disease, cancer, genetic abnormalities

Lifestyle

- Personal habits: tobacco, alcohol, coffee, recreational drugs, etc.
- Diet
- Sleep/rest patterns
- Activities of daily living (ADLs): any difficulties in performing the basic activities
- Recreation/hobbies

Social Data

- Client's support system: family, friends, professional counseling
- Ethnic affiliation
- Highest level of education
- Occupation and employment: Has illness affected ability to work?
- Health insurance
- Home and neighborhood conditions (if applicable)

Psychological Data

- Major stressors
- Usual coping pattern
- Communication style

BOX 6-2	CULTURAL PULSE POINTS

Assessing across Cultural Differences

The assessment step of the nursing process is extremely important when clients and nurses have different ethnic backgrounds. To gather data about a client of a culture different from your own, you need to view the person in the context within which he or she exists. It is important to ask, not to assume, information. A helpful strategy is to repeat back information as a question, in order to validate what the client has said.

patterns. To collect data accurately, both the client and nurse must participate actively. The assessment should also consider the culture of each client (Box 6-2 ▪).

TYPES OF DATA

Data can be subjective or objective. **Subjective data,** also referred to as **symptoms,** are apparent only to the person affected. Itching, pain, and feelings of worry are examples of subjective data. Subjective data include the client's sensations, feelings, values, beliefs, attitudes, and perception of personal health status and life situation. Information supplied by family members and significant others is also considered subjective. The following statements are examples of subjective data:

- "I feel weak all over when I exert myself."
- "I'm short of breath."
- "He doesn't seem so sad today," wife states.
- Client states he has a cramping pain in his abdomen. States, "I feel sick to my stomach."
- "I would like to see the chaplain before surgery."

Objective data, also referred to as **signs,** are detectable by an observer or can be tested against an accepted standard. They can be seen, heard, felt, or smelled. The following data are examples of objective data:

- Blood pressure 90/50
- Apical pulse 104
- Skin pale and diaphoretic
- Vomited 100 mL green-tinged fluid
- Cried during interview
- Lung sounds clear bilaterally
- Holding open Bible

During the head-to-toe assessment, the nurse obtains the objective data needed to validate subjective data. A complete database of both subjective and objective data provides a baseline for comparing the client's responses to nursing and medical interventions. Together, subjective and objective data are called **manifestations.**

SOURCES OF DATA

The client is the *primary source* of data. All sources other than the client are considered *secondary sources.* The nurse should indicate on the nursing history when the data

of laboratory and diagnostic tests, and (5) information contributed by other health personnel.

Client data should include past history as well as current problems. For example, a history of an allergic reaction to penicillin is a vital piece of historical data. Current data relate to present circumstances, such as pain, nausea, or sleep are obtained from a secondary source (a parent, a cousin, a friend).

The nurse must always consider the information in client records in light of the current situation. For example, if the most recent medical record is 10 years old, it is likely that the client's health practices and coping behaviors have changed. The nurse should document any changes that have been reported.

DATA COLLECTION METHODS

The primary methods used to collect data are observing, interviewing, and examining.

Observing

Observation is gathering data by using the senses. Observation occurs whenever the nurse is in contact with the client or support persons. Although nurses observe mainly through sight, most of the senses are engaged during careful observations. Examples of client data observed through four of the five senses are shown in Table 6-2 ■.

Observation involves interpretation of data. The LPN/LVN and the RN work together (*collaborate*) to determine the meaning of the observation.

Interviewing

An **interview** is a planned communication or a conversation with a purpose. Interviewing is used mainly while taking the nursing health history. In interviews, the nurse gets or gives information, identifies problems of mutual concern, evaluates change, teaches, and provides support, counseling, or therapy. Interviewing is a process the nurse applies in most phases of the nursing process. During the assessment phase, however, the primary purpose of the interview is to gather data. (Note: See Chapter 11 ⚭ for the main discussion of interviewing and communication techniques.)

Examining

The physical **examination** or physical assessment is a systematic data collection method. To conduct the examination, the nurse uses techniques of inspection, auscultation, palpation, and percussion. These techniques are discussed in Chapter 19 ⚭.

DOCUMENTING DATA

To complete the assessment phase, the nurse records client data. Accurate documentation is essential and should include all data collected about the client's health status. Data are recorded in a factual manner and not interpreted by the nurse. For example, the nurse records the client's breakfast intake (objective data) as "coffee 240 mL, juice 120 mL, 1 egg, and 1 slice of toast," not as "appetite good" (a judgment). A judgment or conclusion such as "appetite good" or "normal appetite" may have different meanings for different people.

To increase accuracy, the nurse records subjective data in the client's own words. Rewording what someone says increases the chance of changing the original meaning. The main discussion about documenting data and interventions is discussed in Chapter 13 ⚭.

Diagnosis

Diagnosing is the second phase of the nursing process. In this phase, nurses use critical-thinking skills to interpret assessment data, identify client strengths, and describe health problems. As mentioned earlier, this phase is the responsibility of the RN. The LPN/LVN discusses the collected data with the RN. The RN identifies appropriate nursing diagnoses for the client and initiates the nursing care plan.

A **nursing diagnosis** is a statement about an alteration in the client's health status. It refers to a condition that nurses are licensed to treat. A *medical diagnosis* is one made by a physician and refers to a condition that only a physician can treat. Table 6-3 ■ compares nursing and medical diagnoses.

The identification and development of nursing diagnoses began formally in 1973, and international recognition came in 1977 with the First Canadian Conference. In 1982, the conference group accepted the name North American Nursing Diagnosis Association (NANDA, now NANDA International), recognizing the participation and contributions

TABLE 6-2	Observational Skills
SENSES	**EXAMPLES OF CLIENT DATA**
Vision	Overall appearance (body size, general weight, posture, grooming); signs of distress or discomfort; facial and body gestures; skin color and lesions; abnormalities of movement; nonverbal demeanor (e.g., signs of anger or anxiety); religious or cultural artifacts (e.g., books, icons, candles, beads)
Smell	Body or breath odors
Hearing	Breath and heart sounds; bowel sounds; ability to communicate; language spoken; ability to initiate conversation; ability to respond when spoken to; orientation to time, person, and place; thoughts and feelings about self, others, and health status
Touch	Skin temperature and moisture; muscle strength (e.g., hand grip); pulse rate, rhythm, and volume; palpatory lesions (e.g., lumps, masses, nodules)

TABLE 6-3	Comparison of Medical Diagnosis, Nursing Diagnosis, and Collaborative Problem		
CATEGORY	MEDICAL DIAGNOSIS	NURSING DIAGNOSIS	COLLABORATIVE PROBLEM
Description	Describes disease and pathology; does not consider other human response; usually consists of not more than three words	Describes human responses to disease process or health problems; consists of a one-, two-, or three-part statement, usually including problem and etiology	Involves human responses, mainly physiological complications of disease, test, or treatments; consists of a two-part statement of situation/ pathophysiology and the potential complication
Example	Myocardial infarction	*Activity Intolerance* related to decreased cardiac output	Potential complication of myocardial infarction: congestive heart failure
Duration	Remains the same while disease is present	Can change frequently	Present when disease or situation is present
Treatment orders	Physician orders primary interventions to prevent and treat	Nurse plans interventions to prevent and treat the nursing diagnosis	Nurse collaborates with physician and other healthcare professionals to prevent and treat
Nursing focus	Implement medical orders for treatment and monitor status of condition	Provide interventions for the nursing diagnosis	Prevent and monitor for onset or status of condition

of nurses in the United States and Canada. NANDA updates its list of nursing diagnoses every 2 years (see Appendix II on the Companion Website).

DEFINITIONS

In 1990, NANDA adopted an official working definition for the term *nursing diagnosis:* "Nursing diagnosis is a clinical judgment about individual, family, or community responses to actual and potential health problems/life processes. Nursing diagnoses provide the basis for selection of nursing interventions to achieve outcomes for which the nurse is accountable." They also defined the term *wellness diagnosis* as follows: "A wellness diagnosis is a clinical judgment about an individual, family, or community in transition from a specific level of wellness to a higher level of wellness." *Readiness for Enhanced Spiritual Well-Being* and *Readiness for Enhanced Nutrition* are examples of possible wellness diagnoses.

Linda Carpenito (2005b) provided a definition of nursing diagnosis that is perhaps easier to understand. According to her, nursing diagnoses are "actual or potential health problems which nurses, by virtue of their education and experience, are capable and licensed to treat" (p. 3).

Both of these definitions imply the following:

- Registered nurses are responsible for making nursing diagnoses, even though other nursing personnel may contribute data to the process of diagnosing and may implement specified nursing care.
- Nursing diagnoses describe a continuum of health states: deviations from health, presence of risk factors, and areas of enriched personal growth or areas of improved health.

- The domain of nursing diagnosis includes *only* those health states that nurses are educated and licensed to treat. For example, nurses are not educated to diagnose or treat diseases such as diabetes mellitus. This task is legally within the practice of medicine. Yet nurses can diagnose and treat *Deficient Knowledge, Ineffective Individual Resilience,* or *Imbalanced Nutrition,* all of which may accompany diabetes mellitus.
- A nursing diagnosis is a statement made only after thorough, systematic data collection.

COMPONENTS OF A NANDA NURSING DIAGNOSIS

A nursing diagnosis has three components: the problem, defining characteristics, and etiology. Each diagnostic label approved by NANDA carries a definition that clarifies its meaning. For example, the definition of the label *Activity Intolerance* is: A state in which an individual has insufficient physiological or psychological energy to endure or complete required or desired daily activities.

Problem (Diagnostic Label)

The problem statement, or *diagnostic label,* describes the client's health problem or response for which nursing theory is given in clear, concise terms. (See Appendix II on the Companion Website.) The purpose of the nursing diagnosis is to direct the formation of client goals and desired outcomes. It may also suggest some nursing interventions.

Defining Characteristics

Defining characteristics are the cluster of manifestations (signs and symptoms) that indicate the presence of a particular diagnostic statement. *Major and critical defining characteristics* are those that must be present for the diagnosis to be valid. For example, if the nursing diagnosis is *Activity Intolerance*, the client must have manifestations that include:

- Altered response to activity (such as dyspnea, tachypnea, shortness of breath)
- A weak, thready, or irregular pulse; tachycardia; increased pulse that does not return to resting heart rate after 3 minutes
- Blood pressure that does not increase with activity, hypotension, increased diastolic pressure of 15 mm Hg
- Weakness and fatigue

Minor characteristics may or may not be present. The client with *Activity Intolerance* might or might not have the following manifestations:

- Pallor
- Cyanosis
- Vertigo
- Diaphoresis
- Confusion

For *actual* nursing diagnoses, the defining characteristics are the client's signs and symptoms. For *risk* nursing diagnoses, characteristics are the factors that cause the client to be more than "normally" vulnerable to the problem.

Qualifiers

When a NANDA label is followed by the word (*specify*), the nurse states the area in which the problem occurs. For example, *Deficient Knowledge* (medications) and *Deficient Knowledge* (dietary adjustments) specify the particular area in which teaching is needed.

Qualifiers are added to some NANDA statements to give additional meaning to the diagnostic statement. For example, NANDA uses these qualifications:

- *Imbalanced* (a change from baseline)
- *Impaired* (made worse, weakened, damaged, reduced, deteriorated)
- *Decreased* (smaller in size, amount, or degree)
- *Ineffective* (not producing the desired effect)
- *Acute* (severe or of short duration)
- *Chronic* (lasting a long time, recurring, or constant)

Etiology

The **etiology** piece (related and risk factors) of the nursing diagnosis identifies probable causes of the health problem. It gives direction to the required nursing therapy, and enables nurses to individualize the client's care.

Take the example of a nursing diagnosis of *Constipation*. In one client, the etiology of constipation may be long-term laxative use. In another, it may be inactivity and insufficient fluid intake. In a third, it may be a diet that is very low in fiber and high in refined and processed foods.

TWO-PART AND THREE-PART NURSING DIAGNOSIS STATEMENTS

Most nursing diagnoses are written as two-part or three-part statements. Basic two-part statements are used for potential problems or "at risk for" statements. The basic two-part statement includes the following:

1. Problem (P): statement of the client's response (NANDA label)
2. Etiology (E): factors contributing to or probable causes of the response

The two parts are joined by the words *related to* to imply a relationship (such as *Ineffective Breastfeeding* related to breast engorgement).

Basic three-part statements are used for actual problems. The basic three-part nursing diagnosis statement is in the PES format and includes:

1. Problem (P): statement of the client's response (NANDA label)
2. Etiology (E): factors contributing to or probable causes of the response
3. Signs and symptoms (S): defining characteristics manifested by the client

Box 6-3 ■ provides an example of a three-part diagnostic statement.

Planning

Planning is the third step in the nursing process. **Planning** is the process of designing nursing activities required to prevent, reduce, or eliminate a client's health problems. It involves decision making and problem solving. In planning, the nurse refers to the client's assessment data and diagnostic statements for direction in formulating client goals. All planning is aimed at preventing, reducing, or eliminating the client's health problems. The product of the planning phase is a client **care plan.**

The input of the LPN/LVN and support persons is essential if a plan is to be effective. Nurses do not plan for the client, but encourage the client to participate as actively as

---

BOX 6-3	BASIC THREE-PART DIAGNOSTIC STATEMENT

Problem
Situational Low Self-Esteem related to (r/t)
Etiology
Rejection by husband as manifested by (a.m.b.)
Signs and Symptoms
Hypersensitivity to criticism; states, "I don't know if I can manage by myself" and rejects positive feedback

possible in making a plan together. In a home setting, the client's support people and caregivers are the ones who implement the plan of care. They should help create the care plan because its effectiveness depends largely on them.

According to the NCLEX-PN® test plan, the role of the LPN/LVN in the planning phase is to do the following:

1. Assist in the formation of the goals of care:
   - Participate in identifying nursing interventions required to achieve goals.
   - Communicate client needs that may require alteration of the goals of care.
2. Assist in developing the plan of care:
   - Involve the client and healthcare team members in the selection of nursing interventions.
   - Plan for the client's safety, comfort, and maintenance of optimum functioning.
   - Select nursing interventions for delivery of client's care. (Anderson, 2005, p. 234)

TYPES OF PLANNING

Planning is the process of mapping out a logical, prioritized sequence of actions for future use. Planning begins with the first client contact and continues until the nurse–client relationship ends, usually when the client is discharged from the healthcare agency.

The RN who performs the admission assessment usually develops the *initial comprehensive plan of care*. Planning should be initiated as soon as possible after the initial assessment, especially because of the trend toward shorter hospital stays. The LPN/LVN assists with data collection.

Ongoing planning is done by all nurses who work with the client. As nurses obtain new information and evaluate the client's responses to care, they can individualize the initial care plan further.

Discharge planning involves anticipating and planning for needs after discharge. It is a crucial part of comprehensive health care and should be addressed in each client's care plan. Although many clients are discharged to other agencies (e.g., nursing homes), follow-up care is increasingly being delivered in the home. Effective discharge planning begins at first client contact and involves comprehensive and ongoing assessment to obtain information about the client's ongoing needs. For details about discharge planning, see Chapter 14 🔗 .

NURSING CARE PLANS

The end product of the planning phase of the nursing process is a formal or informal plan of care. An informal plan is a plan of action that exists in the nurse's mind. For example, the nurse may think, "Mrs. Phan is very tired. I will need to reinforce her teaching after she is rested." A formal nursing care plan is a written guide that organizes information about the client's care. The most obvious benefit of a formal written care plan is that it provides continuity of care. When nurses use the client's nursing diagnoses to develop goals and nursing interventions, the result is a holistic, individualized plan of care that will best meet the client's unique needs.

Standardized care plans (Figure 6-2 ■) specify the nursing care for groups of clients with common needs (e.g., all clients with myocardial infarction). Individualized care plans are tailored to meet the unique needs of a specific client—needs that are not addressed by the standardized plans.

Kardex® Care Plans

Kardex® is a trade name for a system in which client information and instructions for some of the client's care are kept on a large card in a central file, making information quickly accessible. The Kardex® usually contains information about diet, activity levels, self-care/hygiene needs, treatments, and procedures (Figure 6-3 ■). Kardex® information may change frequently. It is usually recorded in pencil so that the Kardex® can be changed and kept up to date. For more information about documentation, see Chapter 13 🔗 .

Computerized Care Plans

Computers are increasingly being used to create and store nursing care plans. The computer can also generate both standardized and individualized care plans. Nurses access the client's stored care plan from a centrally located terminal at the nurses' station or from terminals in client rooms.

Regardless of whether care plans are handwritten, computerized, or standardized, nursing care must be individualized to fit the unique needs of each client. The nurse uses standardized care plans for predictable, commonly occurring problems. Individual plans are used for unusual problems or problems that need special attention.

Student Care Plans

Because student care plans are a learning activity as well as a plan of care, they may be more lengthy and detailed than care plans used by working nurses. To help students learn to write a care plan, educators generally require that it be individualized. They may also modify the care plan by adding a column for "Rationale" after the nursing orders column (Table 6-4 ■). A **rationale** is the scientific principle given as the reason for selecting a particular nursing intervention.

The student may find it helpful to follow these guidelines when writing nursing care plans:

1. Use these category headings: "Nursing Diagnoses," "Goals/Desired Outcomes," "Evaluation Statement," "Nursing Orders/Interventions," "Rationales," and include a date for the evaluation of each goal.

Standardized Care Plan for Nursing Diagnosis of DEFICIENT FLUID VOLUME

Etiology	Desired Outcomes	Nursing Order (Identify Frequency)
✓Decreased oral intake	✓Urinary output > 30 mL/hr	✓Monitor intake and output q _1_ h
✓Nausea	✓Urine specific gravity 1.005 ±1.025	✓Weigh daily
__Depression		✓Monitor serum electrolyte levels X 1 _or until normal_
✓Fatigue, weakness	✓Serum Na⁺ normal	✓Check skin turgor and mucus membranes q _8_ h
__Difficulty swallowing	✓Mucus membranes moist	✓Monitor temperature q _4_ h
__Other:_____	✓Skin turgor good	✓Administer prescribed IV therapy (Monitor according to protocol for Intravenous Therapy) _1000 mL D₅ LR_
✓Excess fluid loss	✓No weight loss	✓Offer oral liquids q _1_ h _at 100 mL/hr_
✓Fever or increased metabolic rate	✓8-hour intake =	Type _clear, cold_____
✓Diaphoresis	_400 mL oral_	✓Instruct client regarding amount, type, and schedule of fluid intake
✓Vomiting	Other:	✓Assess understanding of type of fluid loss; teach accordingly
__Diarrhea		✓Mouth care prn with _mouthwash_
__Burns		✓Institute measures to reduce fever (e.g., lower room temperature, remove bed covers, offer cold liquids)
__Other_____		Other Nursing Orders:_____

In the Nursing Order section after "Other Nursing Orders:":

Monitor urine specific gravity
q̄ shift

Defining Characteristics

✓Insufficient intake
✓Negative balance of intake and output
✓Dry mucus membranes
✓Poor skin turgor
__Concentrated urine
__Hypernatremia
✓Rapid, weak pulse
__Falling B/P
__Weight loss

Plan Initiated by: _M. Medina RN_____ Date _[date]_____

Plan/outcomes evaluated_____ Date_____

Plan/outcomes evaluated_____ Date_____

Client: _Amanda Aquilini_____

Figure 6-2. ■ A standardized care plan for the nursing diagnosis of *Deficient Fluid Volume*.

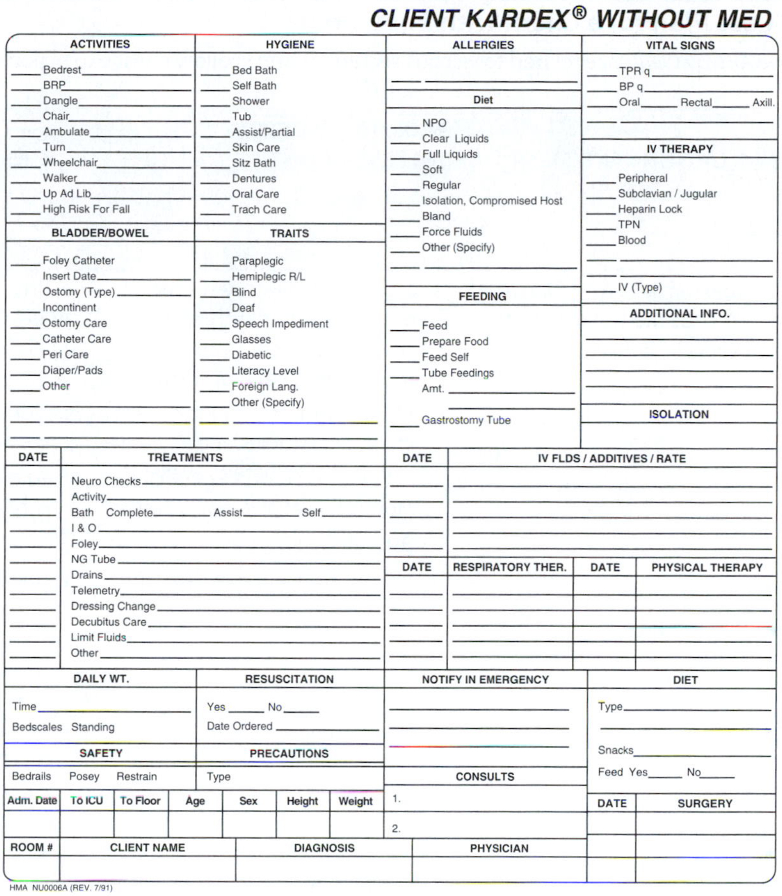

Figure 6-3. ■ Kardex®.

2. Use standardized medical or English abbreviations and key words, not complete sentences, to communicate your ideas. Be sure to use only acceptable abbreviations. See Table 13-1 ⚭ for a list of standard medical abbreviations.

3. Refer to procedure books or other sources of information rather than including all the steps on a written plan.

4. Tailor the plan to the unique characteristics of the client by ensuring that the client's choices, such as preferences about the times of care and the methods used, are included. This reinforces the client's individuality and sense of control. For example, the written nursing order "Provide prune juice at breakfast rather than regular juice" indicates that the client was given a choice of beverages. Adaptations to the plan of care are also important when working with children. Box 6-4 ■ describes a few adaptations that can make the nursing process more suited to care of children.

5. Ensure that the nursing plan incorporates preventive and health maintenance aspects as well as restorative ones. For example, carrying out the order "Provide active-assistance ROM (range-of-motion) exercises to affected limbs every 2 h" prevents joint contractures and maintains muscle strength and joint mobility.

6. Ensure that the plan contains orders for ongoing assessment of the client (e.g., "Inspect incision every 8 h").

7. Include collaborative and coordination activities in the plan. For example, the RN may write orders to ask a nutritionist or physical therapist about specific aspects of the client's care.

8. Include plans for the client's discharge and home care needs. It is often necessary to consult and make arrangements with the community health nurse, social worker, and specific agencies that supply client information and needed equipment.

9. Date and sign the plan. The date the plan is written is essential for evaluation, review, and future planning. The nurse's signature demonstrates accountability to the client and to the nursing profession, since the effectiveness of nursing actions can be evaluated.

Chapters 8 through 62 ⚭ provide Nursing Process Care Plans like the sample one given here. You will be asked to review the care plans and answer questions that call on your critical-thinking skills.

TABLE 6-4	Partial Care Plan for a Client with Pneumonia		
Nursing Diagnosis: *Ineffective Airway Clearance* related to viscous secretions and shallow chest expansion secondary to deficient fluid volume, pain, and fatigue.			
DESIRED/EXPECTED OUTCOMES	**EVALUATION STATEMENTS**	**NURSING ORDERS/ INTERVENTIONS**	**RATIONALE**
Demonstrates adequate air exchange, as evidenced by			
1. Absence of pallor and cyanosis (skin and mucous membranes)	1. Goal partially met. Skin and mucous membranes not cyanotic, but still pale.	a. Monitor respiratory status every 4 h; rate, depth, effort, skin color, mucous membranes, amount and color of sputum. b. Monitor results of blood gases, chest x-ray studies, and incentive spirometer volume as available. c. Monitor level of consciousness. d. Auscultate lungs every 4 h.	a, b, c, d. To identify progress toward or deviations from goal. *Ineffective Airway Clearance* leads to poor oxygenation, evidenced by pallor, cyanosis, lethargy, and drowsiness. *Retain nursing orders to continue to identify progress. Goal status indicates problem not resolved.*
2. Using correct breathing/coughing technique after instruction	2. Goal partially met. Uses correct technique when pain well controlled by narcotic analgesics.	e. Vital signs every 4 h (TPR, BP).	e. Inadequate oxygenation causes increased pulse rate. Respiratory rate may be decreased by narcotic analgesics or increased by dyspnea and anxiety.
3. Productive cough	3. Goal met. Cough productive of moderate amounts of thick, yellow, pink-tinged sputum.	f. Instruct in breathing and coughing techniques. Remind to perform and assist every 3 h. Support and encourage. g. Administer prescribed expectorant; schedule for maximum effectiveness.	f. Does not need to be reinstructed as client demonstrates correct techniques. May still need support and encouragement because of fatigue and pain. g. Helps loosen secretions so they can be coughed up and expelled.
4. Demonstrating symmetric chest excursion of at least 4 cm	4. Goal not met. Chest excursion = 3 cm.	h. Maintain Fowler's or semi-Fowler's position.	h. Gravity allows for fuller lung expansion by decreasing pressure of abdomen on diaphragm.

BOX 6-4	PEDIATRIC CONSIDERATIONS

Adapting the Nursing Process to the Care of Children

Some simple ways that the LPN/LVN can adapt the nursing process to pediatric clients are:

- Change the order of data collecting so that any painful or potentially frightening measurements in small children are taken last.
- Permit infants or toddlers with separation anxiety to be held by a parent whenever possible.
- With infants and small children, plan the timing of procedures as much as possible to allow the normal pattern of eating and sleeping.
- With preschoolers a procedure can be demonstrated on a doll or a teddy bear, or children can be allowed to manipulate equipment, so they will not be frightened.
- Evaluate the effectiveness of nursing actions by addressing the adolescent, not the parent. Communication with teens is improved by speaking as equals with them.

NURSING PROCESS CARE PLAN
Client with Pneumonia

Amanda Aquilini is a 28-year-old female attorney who lives with her husband and 3-year-old daughter; her husband is on a business trip and will return tomorrow. The child is staying with a neighbor until her husband returns. Amanda was admitted to an acute care facility with shortness of breath (S.O.B.) on exertion, chest pain on inspiration, and fever, following a chest cold of 2 weeks' duration.

Assessment

The client states, "The doctor says I have pneumonia"; anxious, "I can't breathe when lying down"; states "I feel weak"; experiencing chills; VS: T 103, P 92, R 28, BP 122/80 sitting, pulse ox 95% on room air; skin dry, cheeks are flushed; respirations shallow, productive cough—pale pink sputum, inspiratory crackles right upper and lower chest, diminished breath sounds on right side.

Nursing Diagnosis

The following important nursing diagnosis (among others) is established for this client:

- *Ineffective Airway Clearance*

Expected Outcomes

The expected outcomes specify that Ms. Aquilini will:

- Demonstrate adequate air exchange, as evidenced by (AEB) absence of pallor and cyanosis.
- Use correct breathing/coughing technique after instruction.
- Have a productive cough.
- Have symmetric chest excursion of at least 4 cm.
- Verbalize chest pain of less than 4 on a 1–10 scale within 30 minutes after receiving PO analgesic.

Planning and Implementation

The following nursing interventions are planned and implemented:

- Monitor respiratory status every 4 h: rate, depth, effort, skin color, mucous membranes, amount and color of sputum.
- Monitor results of blood gases, chest x-ray studies, and incentive spirometer volume as available.
- Monitor level of consciousness.
- Auscultate lungs every 4 h.
- Take vital signs every 4 h (TPR, BP).
- Instruct in breathing and coughing techniques.
- Administer prescribed expectorant.
- Administer prescribed analgesic.
- Administer oxygen by nasal cannula.
- Assist with postural drainage daily.
- Administer prescribed antibiotic to maintain blood level.

Evaluation

Skin and mucous membranes not cyanotic, but still pale. Uses correct technique when pain well controlled by narcotic analgesics. Cough productive of moderate amounts of thick, yellow, pink-tinged sputum. Chest excursion = 3 cm. Stated "Easier to breathe," rated pain at 3, and cough effective 30 minutes after oral analgesics. Scattered crackles throughout right anterior and posterior chest on auscultation. Respirations 26/min, pulse 96.

The physician orders:

- Chest x-ray
- Sputum culture and sensitivity
- Antibiotic therapy
- Expectorant
- Analgesics

Critical Thinking in the Nursing Process

1. Identify and prioritize your nursing activities at this time.

2. Why does the physician order culture and sensitivity? Why must this be done prior to beginning antibiotic therapy?
3. Ms. Aquilini states, "I can't breathe." What nursing activities can you perform to relieve her anxiety and ease her breathing?
4. What discharge teaching should be given to continue recovery and prevent another respiratory infection?

Note: Discussion of Critical Thinking questions appears on the MyNursingKit Website.

LPN/LVN LONG-TERM CARE PLANNING

The LPN/LVN working in long-term or home care may be assigned greater responsibilities related to care planning. (See Chapter 46 ⬭ for in-depth discussion about long-term care.) Once the initial assessment has been completed by the RN, the care plan will be developed as a collaborative process. The LPN/LVN will be responsible for implementing, evaluating, and reporting back to the RN on the achievement of the client's goals. Most long-term facilities and home care agencies have regularly scheduled client care conferences so that the healthcare team can interact and plan for the client's future needs.

SETTING PRIORITIES

Priority setting is the process of identifying nursing diagnoses and interventions in order from most important or critical to least important. Life-threatening problems, such as loss of respiratory or cardiac function, are given highest priority. Health-threatening problems, such as pain and decreased coping ability, are assigned medium priority because they may result in delayed development or cause destructive physical or emotional changes. A low-priority problem is one that arises from normal developmental needs or that requires only minimal nursing support.

Nurses frequently use Maslow's hierarchy of needs when setting priorities. In Maslow's hierarchy, physiologic needs that are basic to life (such as air, food, and water) are listed at the base of the pyramid (Figure 6-4 ■). They receive higher priority than the need for security or activity. Growth needs, such as self-esteem, are not perceived as "basic" in this framework. So, nursing diagnoses such as *Ineffective Airway Clearance* and *Impaired Gas Exchange* would take priority over nursing diagnoses such as *Anxiety* or *Ineffective Coping*. Table 6-5 ■ provides an example of high, medium, and low priorities for a client.

Establishing Client Goals/Expected Outcomes

After establishing priorities, the nurse and client set goals for each nursing diagnosis. (*Note:* The terms *goal* and *expected outcome* are used interchangeably in this text.) On a care plan, the **goals** or **desired/expected outcomes**

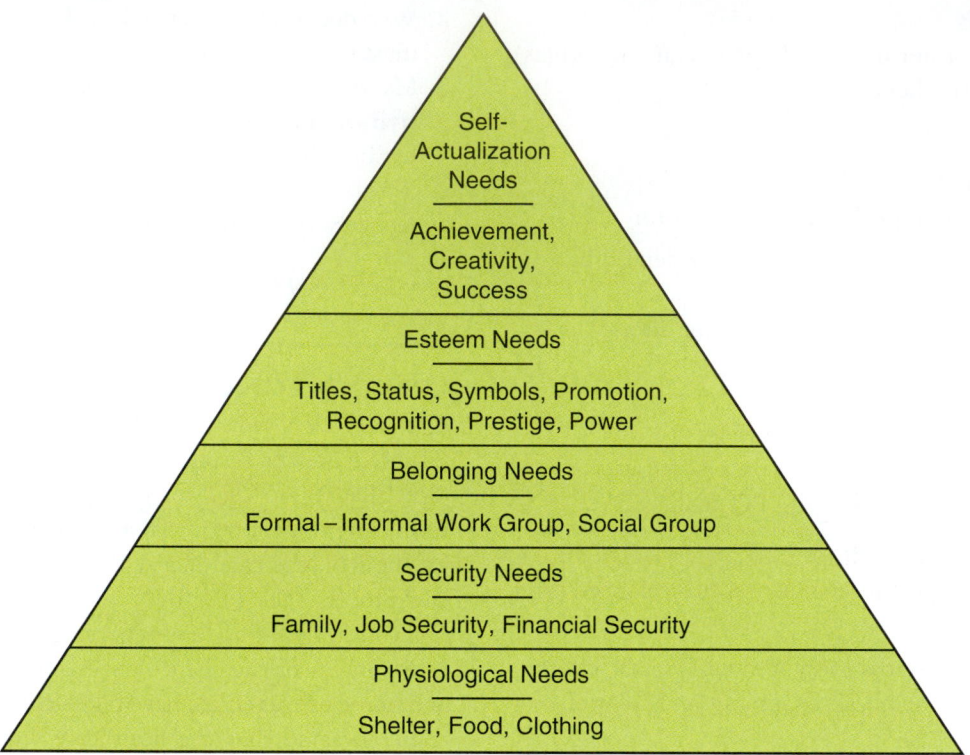

Figure 6-4. ■ Maslow's hierarchy of needs.

TABLE 6-5	**Prioritizing Nursing Diagnoses for a Client with Pneumonia**	
NURSING DIAGNOSIS	**PRIORITY**	**RATIONALE**
Ineffective Airway Clearance related to (1) viscous secretions secondary to deficient fluid volume and (2) shallow chest expansion secondary to pain and fatigue	High priority	Loss of respiratory functioning is a life-threatening problem. The nurse's primary concern must be to promote the client's oxygenation by addressing the etiologies of this problem.
Deficient Fluid Volume: intake insufficient to replace fluid loss related to fever and diaphoresis	High priority	Severe fluid volume deficit is life threatening. Although not that severe for this client, it is a high-priority problem because it is also a contributing factor for *Ineffective Airway Clearance.* Collaborative efforts to improve hydration have already begun (intravenous fluids). The nurse must immediately and continuously assess and promote hydration.
Anxiety related to (1) difficulty breathing and (2) concerns over work and parenting roles	Medium priority	Although the client is concerned about work and parenting roles, these are not a threat to life. Also, treatment of her high-priority problem, *Ineffective Airway Clearance,* will relieve one of the etiologies of this problem (dyspnea). Meanwhile, the nurse must provide symptomatic relief of the client's anxiety during periods of dyspnea because extreme anxiety could further compromise oxygenation by causing her to breathe ineffectively and increasing the rate at which she uses oxygen.
Imbalanced Nutrition: Less than Body Requirements related to decreased appetite, nausea, and increased metabolism secondary to disease process	Low priority	This problem is not currently health threatening, but it could be if it were to persist. It will almost certainly resolve in a day or two as the medical problem is treated. If the medical problem does not resolve quickly, this will change to a medium priority.
Interrupted Family Processes related to mother's illness and temporary unavailability of father to provide child care	Low priority	Client's child is currently being cared for. If the husband returns as planned, this potential problem will not develop into an actual problem. No interventions are needed at present, except for continued assessment and reassurance.

describe, in terms of observable client responses, what the nurse hopes the client will achieve by implementing the nursing orders.

LONG-TERM AND SHORT-TERM GOALS. Goals may be short term or long term. A short-term goal might be "Client will raise right arm to shoulder height by Friday." In the same context, a long-term goal might be "Client will regain full use of right arm in 6 weeks." Long-term goals are often used for clients who live at home and have chronic health problems and for clients in nursing homes, extended-care facilities, and rehabilitation centers.

DEVELOPING DESIRED OUTCOMES FROM NURSING DIAGNOSES. Goals are derived from and relate to the client's nursing diagnoses. For every nursing diagnosis, there will be at least one desired outcome that, when achieved, directly helps resolve the problem. When developing goals/desired outcomes, ask the following questions:

1. What is the problem statement?
2. What is the opposite, healthy response?
3. How will the client look or behave if the healthy response is achieved? (What will I be able to see, hear, palpate, smell, or otherwise observe with my senses?)
4. What must the client do and how well must the client do it to demonstrate problem resolution or to demonstrate the ability to resolve the problem?

For example, if the nursing diagnosis is *"Risk for Deficient Fluid Volume* related to diarrhea and inadequate intake secondary to nausea," the related goal statement might be "Maintain fluid balance, as evidenced by urinary output in balance with fluid intake, normal skin turgor, and moist mucous membranes." In this example, a general goal (fluid balance) is stated as the opposite of the problem (deficient fluid volume) and then followed by a list of observable desired outcomes. If achieved, the outcomes would be evidence that the problem, *Deficient Fluid Volume*, has been prevented. Table 6-6 ■ provides examples of establishing goals and desired outcomes from nursing diagnoses.

WRITING DESIRED OUTCOME STATEMENTS. Goals/desired outcome statements should usually have the following four elements:

1. *Subject.* The subject is the client, any part of the client, or some attribute of the client (such as the client's pulse or urinary output). You do not need to write "the client" or "the client's pulse" in each statement, although as you begin to write care plans, stating, "the client will," will make sure you are writing a client outcome. It is assumed that the subject is the client unless otherwise stated.
2. *Action verb.* The verb specifies an action the client is to perform, for example, what the client is to do, learn, or experience. Some action verbs that express directly observable behaviors are *apply, describe, explain, inject, move, sleep, turn,* and *verbalize.*
3. *Measurable modifiers.* Conditions or modifiers may be added to the verb to explain the circumstances under which the behavior is to be performed. They explain:
   - *How*—"Walks with the help of a walker."
   - *When*—"After attending two group diabetes classes, lists signs and symptoms of diabetes."
   - *Where*—"When at home, maintains weight at existing level."
   - *What*—"Discusses food pyramid and recommended daily servings."
4. *Criteria of desired performance.* The criteria indicate the standard by which a performance is evaluated, or the level at which the client will perform the behavior. These criteria may specify time or speed, accuracy, distance, and quality. Examples follow:
   - To establish a time-achievement criterion, the nurse asks *"How long?"*—"Weighs 75 kg by April."
   - To establish an accuracy criterion, the nurse asks *"How well?"*—"Lists five out of six signs of diabetes in 2 weeks."

TABLE 6-6	**Deriving Desired Outcomes from Nursing Diagnoses**	
NURSING DIAGNOSIS	**OPPOSITE HEALTHY RESPONSE (GOALS)**	**DESIRED OUTCOMES**
Impaired Physical Mobility: inability to bear weight on left leg, related to inflammation of knee joint	Improved mobility: ability to bear weight on left leg	Ambulate with crutches by end of the week. Be able to stand without assistance by end of the month.
Ineffective Airway Clearance related to poor cough effort, secondary to incision pain and fear of damaging sutures	Effective airway clearance	Lungs will be clear to auscultation during entire postoperative period. No skin pallor or cyanosis by 12 hours postoperation. Within 24 hours after surgery, will demonstrate good cough effort.

- To establish distance, the nurse asks *"How far?"*—"Walks one block per day."
- To establish quality, the nurse asks *"What is the expected standard?"*—"Administers insulin using aseptic technique in 3 days."

Students can use the guidelines listed in Box 6-5 ■ to help them develop useful outcome statements.

BOX 6-5 | NURSING CARE CHECKLIST

Student Guidelines for Writing Desired Outcomes

☑ Write goals/outcomes in terms of client responses, not nurse activities. Begin each goal statement with "The client will" to focus it on client behaviors and responses. Avoid statements that start with *enable, facilitate, allow, let, permit.* These indicate what the *nurse* hopes to accomplish, not what the *client* will do.
Correct: The client will drink 100 mL of water per hour. (*client behavior*)

Incorrect: Maintain client hydration. (*nursing action*)

☑ Be sure that desired outcomes are realistic for the client's capabilities, limitations, and designated time span, if it is indicated. Limitations include finances, equipment, family support, social services, physical and mental condition, and time. For example, the outcome "Measures insulin accurately" may be unrealistic for a client who has poor vision due to cataracts.

☑ Ensure that the desired outcomes are compatible with the therapies of other professionals. For example, the outcome "The client will increase the time spent out of bed by 15 minutes each day" is not compatible with a physician's prescribed therapy of bed rest.

☑ Make sure that each goal is derived from only one nursing diagnosis. For example, the goal "The client will increase the amount of nutrients ingested and show progress in the ability to feed self" is derived from two nursing diagnoses: *Feeding Self-Care Deficit* and *Imbalanced Nutrition: Less than Body Requirements.*

☑ Use observable, measurable terms for outcomes. Avoid words that are vague and require interpretation or judgment by the observer. Phrases such as "increase daily exercise" and "improve knowledge of nutrition" can mean different things to different people. They are not clear and specific enough to guide the nurse when evaluating client responses.

☑ Make sure the client considers the goals important and values them. The nurse must actively listen to the client to determine personal values, goals, and desired outcomes in relation to current health concerns. Clients are usually motivated to reach goals they consider important. They may resist goals they feel they are told they "should do."

Implementation

Implementation is the fourth step of the nursing process. It is the phase of the nursing process in which selected nursing interventions and activities occur. Nursing **interventions** are the actions that are initiated by the nurse to achieve client goals. The specific strategies should focus on eliminating or reducing the cause of the nursing diagnosis.

The process of implementing normally includes five steps: (1) reassessing the client, (2) determining the nurse's need for assistance, (3) implementing nursing orders, (4) delegating and supervising, and (5) documenting nursing actions.

REASSESSING THE CLIENT

Just before implementing an order, the nurse must reassess the client to make sure the intervention is still needed, because the client's condition may have changed. For example, Gayle Fischer has a nursing diagnosis of *Disturbed Sleep Pattern* related to anxiety and unfamiliar surroundings. During rounds, the nurse discovers that Gayle is sleeping and therefore does not perform the back rub that had been planned as a relaxation strategy.

New data may indicate a need to change the priorities of care or the nursing strategies. For example, a nurse begins to teach Ms. Eves, who has diabetes, how to give herself insulin injections. Shortly after beginning the teaching, the nurse realizes that Ms. Eves is not concentrating on the lesson. In discussion, the nurse learns that Ms. Eves is worried about her eyesight and fears she is going blind. Realizing that the client's level of stress is interfering with her learning, the nurse ends the lesson. She documents the client's response to the teaching and discusses Ms. Eves's concerns with the RN. The nurse continues to provide support to help the client cope with her stress.

DETERMINING THE NURSE'S NEED FOR ASSISTANCE

When implementing some nursing strategies, the nurse may require assistance for one of the following reasons:

- The nurse is unable to implement the nursing strategies safely alone (e.g., turning an obese client in bed).
- Assistance would reduce stress on the client (e.g., turning a person who experiences acute pain when moved).
- The nurse lacks the knowledge or skills to implement a particular nursing activity (e.g., a nurse who is not familiar with a particular model of oxygen mask needs assistance the first time it is applied).

IMPLEMENTING NURSING ORDERS (STRATEGIES)

It is important to explain to the client what will be done, what sensations to expect, and what the client is expected to do. For many nursing actions, it is also important to ensure the client's privacy, for example, by closing doors, pulling curtains, or draping the client.

DELEGATING AND SUPERVISING

The LPN/LVN may have the opportunity to delegate to nursing assistants or other unlicensed staff. It is the responsibility of the delegator to assess the abilities of the staff member being assigned the task. Delegating does not relieve the nurse of the ultimate responsibility for the task. When in doubt, the nurse and the unlicensed person should work together until the unlicensed person's understanding of the assigned task and ability to perform it are confirmed.

DOCUMENTING AND REPORTING NURSING ACTIONS

After carrying out the nursing orders, the nurse completes the implementing phase by recording the interventions and client responses in the nursing progress notes. These are a part of the agency's permanent record for the client. Nursing actions must not be recorded in advance because, on reassessment, the nurse may find that the action should not or cannot be implemented. For example, a nurse is authorized to inject 10 mg of morphine sulfate subcutaneously to a client, but the nurse finds that the client's respiratory rate is 4 breaths per minute. This finding contraindicates the administration of morphine (a respiratory depressant). The nurse withholds the morphine and reports the client's respiratory rate to the nurse in charge and/or physician.

The nurse may record routine or recurring activities (e.g., mouth care) at the end of a shift. In the meantime, the nurse maintains a personal record of these interventions. Many agencies have special forms for this type of recording.

clinical ALERT

In some instances, it is important to record a nursing action immediately after it is implemented. Recorded data about a client must be up to date, accurate, and available to other nurses and healthcare professionals. This is particularly true of the administration of medications and treatments. For example, immediate recording helps safeguard the client from receiving a second dose of medication.

Nursing actions are communicated verbally as well as in writing. When a client's health is changing rapidly, the charge nurse and/or the physician may want to be kept up to date with verbal reports.

Interdisciplinary documentation forms require the nurse to chart in a timely manner. When others are using the same form, delayed charting may find the nurse without a place to document, making it necessary to document a late entry.

Nurses also give verbal reports at a change of shift and on a client's discharge to another unit or health agency. For information on documenting and reporting, see Chapter 13 🔗.

TYPES OF NURSING INTERVENTIONS

Nursing interventions that were identified and written during the planning step of the nursing process are performed during the implementing step. McCloskey and Bulechek (2003) define a nursing intervention as "any treatment, based upon clinical judgment and knowledge, that a nurse performs to enhance patient/client outcomes" (p. 3). Nursing interventions include:

- *Direct care*—An intervention performed through interaction with the client, such as giving a back massage.
- *Indirect care*—An intervention performed away from but on behalf of the client, such as obtaining a referral for physical therapy.

Nursing interventions can also be independent, dependent, or collaborative:

- **Independent interventions**—Independent or nurse-initiated interventions are those activities that nurses are licensed to do on the basis of their knowledge and skills. An example of an independent action is planning and providing special mouth care for a client based on a nursing diagnosis of *Impaired Oral Mucous Membranes*.
- **Dependent interventions**—Dependent (physician-initiated) interventions are activities carried out under the physician's orders or supervision, or according to specified routines.
- **Collaborative interventions**—These are nursing activities that reflect the overlapping responsibilities among healthcare personnel. A collaborative problem is a type of potential problem that nurses manage using both independent and physician-prescribed interventions.

Independent nursing interventions for a collaborative problem focus mainly on monitoring the client's condition and preventing development of the potential complication. For example, the physician might order physical therapy to teach the client crutch-walking. The nurse would be responsible for informing the physical therapy department and for coordinating the client's care to include the physical therapy sessions. When the client returns to the nursing unit, the nurse would assist with crutch-walking and collaborate with the physical therapist to evaluate the client's progress.

The nurse is responsible for explaining, assessing the need for, and administering the medical orders. The RN may write nursing orders to individualize the medical order based on the client's status. For example, for a medical order of "Progressive ambulation, as tolerated," the nursing orders might be:

1. Dangle for 5 min, 12 h postop.
2. Stand at bedside 24 h postop; observe for pallor, dizziness, and weakness.
3. Check pulse before and after ambulating. Do not progress if pulse 110.

The nurse should consider the consequences of each strategy and develop an understanding of the rationale for performing each intervention. Usually several possible interventions can be identified for each nursing diagnosis. The nurse's task is to choose those that are most likely to achieve the desired client outcomes. An intervention may have more than one consequence. For example, the strategy "Provide accurate information" could result in the following client behaviors:

- Increased anxiety
- Decreased anxiety
- Wish to talk with the physician
- Desire to leave the hospital
- Relaxation

After considering the consequences of the alternative interventions, the nurse chooses one or more that are likely to be most effective. Although the nurse bases this decision on knowledge and experience, the client's input is important. The LPN/LVN must use judgment (or critical thinking) in implementing them.

The following criteria can help the nurse choose the best nursing strategy. The planned action must be:

- Safe and appropriate for the individual's age, health, and condition.
- Achievable with the resources available. For example, a home care nurse might wish to include a nursing order for an elderly client to "Check blood glucose daily," but if the client is legally blind, a daily visit by a capable support person or a home care nurse must be available and affordable.
- Compatible with the client's values, beliefs, and culture.
- Compatible with other therapies (e.g., if the client is not permitted food, the strategy of taking medication with an evening snack is not workable).
- Based on nursing knowledge and experience or on scientific knowledge (i.e., based on a rationale). For examples of rationales, refer to Table 6-5.
- Within established standards of care as determined by state laws and the policies of the institution.

IMPLEMENTATION SKILLS

Nurses employ a wide variety of skills in providing client care:

1. *Cognitive* (intellectual) skills include problem solving, decision making, critical thinking, and creative thinking. They are crucial to safe, intelligent nursing care.
2. *Interpersonal* skills are all the verbal and nonverbal activities people use when communicating directly with one another. The effectiveness of a nursing action often depends largely on the nurse's ability to communicate with others. Even when giving medication to a client, the nurse needs to understand the client and in turn be understood. A nurse who is delegating a nursing action also needs to be understood. Communication skills are discussed in detail in Chapter 11 🔗 .

   Interpersonal skills are necessary for all nursing activities. Caring, comforting, referring, counseling, and supporting are just a few. Interpersonal skills also include conveying knowledge, attitudes, feelings, interest, and appreciation of the client's cultural values and lifestyle.
3. *Technical* skills or **procedures** are "hands-on" skills such as manipulating equipment, giving injections, doing dressing changes, and moving, lifting, and repositioning clients. Procedures, also called psychomotor skills, always require communicating with the client. However, they also require knowledge and, frequently, manual dexterity. The number of technical skills expected of a nurse has greatly increased in recent years because of the increased use of technology, especially in acute care hospitals.

ESSENTIAL PROCEDURES IN IMPLEMENTING CARE

The procedures provided in this book give you some of the basic skills you will need to provide excellent client care. Procedures should always begin with an initial set of actions that ensure a safe, efficient, and caring environment. See Procedure 6-1 ■ for an example. These actions will become second nature to you as you continue your nursing training. Icons will be used to represent this initial set of actions at the start of each procedure. In some instances, an action may be optional. However, most are not. The icons (Figure 6-5 ■) are a reminder to do these basic, important interventions in nursing care:

1. Check the physician's order (Figure 6-5A).
2. Gather the necessary equipment (Figure 6-5B).
3. Introduce yourself to the client (Figure 6-5C).
4. Identify the client (check the client's wristband against the chart [Figure 6-5D]).
5. Provide privacy as needed (close the curtain [Figure 6-5E]).

PROCEDURE 6-1 — Basic Procedure Steps and Admission Information

Purpose

- To obtain all pertinent data on hospital admission.

Equipment

- Admission kit
- Thermometer
- Blood pressure cuff and stethoscope
- Appropriate scale of client's need
- Urine container (if UA needed)
- Kardex®, care plan
- Client's medical record

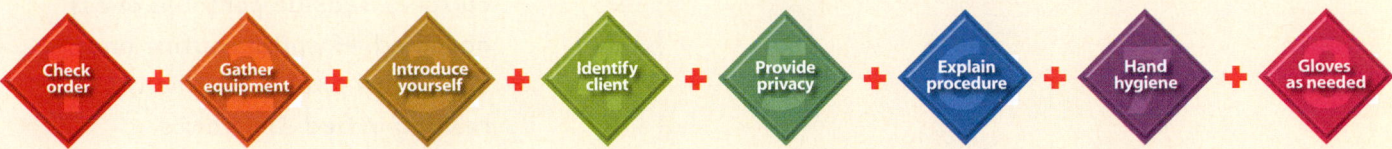

Check order + Gather equipment + Introduce yourself + Identify client + Provide privacy + Explain procedure + Hand hygiene + Gloves as needed

Interventions and Rationales

1. Perform preparatory steps (see icon bar above).

2. Check physician's orders. *All dependent nursing interventions require a physician's order.*

3. Gather the necessary equipment. *Collecting all necessary equipment prior to beginning procedure will save steps, time, and ensure that you will have what you need to complete procedure correctly.*

4. Introduce yourself. Address the client by Mr., Mrs., Ms., followed by first and last name.

5. Compare the wristband to the name and medical record number on the client's chart to make sure procedure is being done on the correct client.

6. Provide privacy. *By closing the door or pulling the bed curtain, you can assure the client that confidentiality will be maintained.*

7. Explain the procedure. *This will help relieve client anxiety and help establish rapport between you and the client.*

8. Wash hands. *Hand hygiene is the most important thing that the nurse can do to stop the spread of infectious disease. This should be done prior to any client contact.*

9. Put on gloves if necessary. Some facilities say, "If it's wet and you are not, put on gloves." Other facilities may require gloves for all client contact. *(Note: Throughout the text, steps 1–8 will be identified with icons only to remind you to complete the steps before starting the procedure.)* Rationales follow the procedure steps in italics.

10. Place a hospital gown on the client and assist him or her into bed. *Wearing a hospital gown will be necessary during the physical assessment, and the client will be more comfortable in bed during the assessment.*

11. Explain equipment and hospital routine. *To assist the client to adjust to hospital environment with minimal distress.*

12. Open and place admission kit on the bedside table. Fill and place water pitcher and cup on the overbed table unless the client is NPO (nothing by mouth). *Supplies and water will be easily accessible to the client.*

13. Record personal belongings on the admission form and encourage family to take valuables home. (Valuables can be placed in the hospital safe if no family available.) *This will serve as a checklist on discharge to be sure all belongings are sent home with the client. Valuables should not be kept at the bedside to prevent loss.*

14. Obtain client's height and weight using a bed or floor scale. *Height and weight need to be available for physician and pharmacy for proper dosage of medication, and as a baseline of client's nutritional status.*

15. Take vital signs. *This is a baseline to determine the client's status.*

16. Collect data for the client's health history. *A complete history provides a total picture of client's condition and present health problems.*

17. Complete the bedside assessment (if this is within the LPN's/LVN's scope in your area of practice). *To obtain as much data as possible about the client's chief complaint.*

18. Document the procedure. *"If it is not documented, it is not done." (Each procedure in the clinical chapters will provide a sample documentation.)*

19. Obtain a urine specimen, and notify laboratory, x-ray, and ECG of client's admission. *Client may need to have admission laboratory studies, ECG, and chest x-ray done as a baseline.*

20. Document all findings in the client's medical record on the admission form. *Complete, accurate, timely documentation is necessary to provide continuity of care.*

21. Collaborate with the RN to write and initiate the care plan. *Initiation of care plan will be the first step on client's road to recovery.*

22. Notify the physician that the client has been admitted and obtain orders if they are not on the floor. *It is important that the physician be notified in a timely manner so that treatment can begin as soon as possible.*

SAMPLE CHARTING (DOCUMENTATION)

(date)	Admission procedure completed
(time)	on a 28-year-old female, admitted with pneumonia. See admission form for vital signs and assessment. V.A. obtained and sent to lab. Blood sample drawn by lab for CBC and blood culture. Bedside portable chest obtained. Hospital routine and equipment explained. Client resting in bed. Dr. Katz's exchange notified. _____
	_____ M. Smith, LPN

6. Explain the procedure (Figure 6-5F).
7. Wash your hands. Hand hygiene is the single most effective way to prevent disease transmission (Figure 6-5G).
8. Don gloves as needed. (If the client is wet, wear gloves.) (Figure 6-5H)

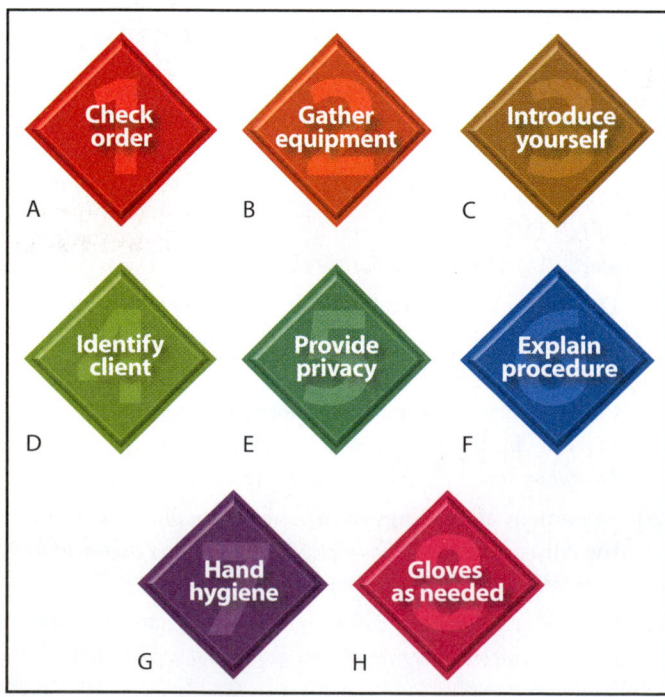

Figure 6-5. ■ Icons of initial nursing actions.

Evaluation

Evaluation is the fifth and last phase of the nursing process, but many times the evaluation phase is overlooked. **Evaluation** is a planned, ongoing, purposeful activity in which client and healthcare professionals determine the client's progress toward goal achievement and the effectiveness of the nursing care plan. Without evaluation, an intervention may be discarded as ineffective without taking time to discover why it did not work. One thing that sets the LPN/LVN apart from a certified nursing assistant (CNA) is the knowledge and ability to evaluate.

Clients need to be evaluated continuously through the day. The best way to evaluate an intervention is to determine if the objective from the written care plan has been met, and if not, why not. Through evaluating, nurses accept responsibility for their actions. They indicate interest in the results of the nursing actions. They also demonstrate a desire to replace ineffective actions with more effective ones. After determining whether a goal has been met, the nurse writes an evaluative statement (either on the care plan or in the nurse's notes). These notes help the RN to review and modify the nursing care plan so that individualized nursing care can continue. Once the care plan is modified, the nursing process cycle begins again.

Note: The references and resources for all chapters have been compiled at the back of the book.

Chapter Review

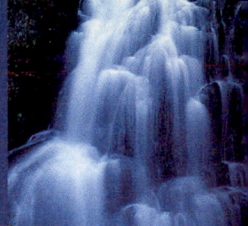

KEY Points

- The nursing process is a systematic, rational method of planning and providing individualized nursing care for individuals, families, groups, and communities.

- The nursing process can be used in all healthcare settings. It is client centered, interpersonal, and collaborative. It provides a framework for nurses' accountability and responsibility.

- The five phases of the nursing process—assessing, diagnosing, planning, implementing, and evaluating—are ongoing and interconnected. The primary functions of the LPN/LVN are gathering data for assessment, implementing, and evaluating.

- The nurse collects data for assessment (1) to help establish nursing diagnoses and care plans, (2) to ensure that the ordered intervention is appropriate, and (3) to evaluate whether nursing actions have been effective.

- Subjective data is information such as pain or worry that is apparent only to the person involved. Objective data is information that can be observed or measured from the outside.

- Nursing diagnoses define health conditions that nurses are legally qualified to treat. A nursing diagnosis has three components: the problem, the etiology (cause), and the defining characteristics (signs and symptoms). Professional standards require that RNs establish nursing diagnoses.

- Planning involves establishing goals and designing nursing activities to prevent, reduce, or eliminate a client's health problems. The client and family should be involved in establishing desired outcomes.

- Planning is generally done by registered nurses, but LPNs/LVNs in long-term care may be called on to identify problems and initiate the plan of care.

- Implementing is carrying out or delegating the nursing interventions. It incorporates all the activities performed to promote health, prevent complications, treat present problems, and facilitate the client's coping with chronic alterations in health status. Documenting is an important piece of this step of care.

- Evaluating is the process of comparing client responses to established goals/outcomes to determine whether goals have been met. It includes review and modification of the care plan.

- Goal statements and desired outcomes are written in terms of the client's behavior. They describe specific and measurable client responses and help the nurse evaluate the effectiveness of the nursing interventions.

- The desired outcomes determine the data that must be collected to evaluate the client's health status. The data are used to confirm or change the nursing diagnoses, maintain or alter the plan of care, and continue or change nursing interventions.

⚭ FOR FURTHER Study

For the main discussion about critical-thinking process, see Chapter 5.

Chapters 8 through 62 include a Nursing Process Care Plan.

See Chapter 11 for interviewing and communication techniques.

See Chapter 13 for more information on documenting and reporting, the Kardex® system, and Table 13-1, which lists common medical abbreviations.

For details about discharge planning, see Chapter 14.

For the full discussion on examination techniques see Chapter 19.

See Chapter 46 for in-depth discussion about long-term care.

PEARSON

EXPLORE **mynursingkit**™

MyNursingKit is your one stop for online chapter review materials and resources. Prepare for success with additional NCLEX®-style practice questions, interactive assignments and activities, web links, animations and videos, and more!

Register your access code from the front of your book at
www.mynursingkit.com

Critical Thinking Care Map

Caring for a Client with Alzheimer's

NCLEX-PN® Focus Area: Nursing Process

Case Study: Charles Weldon, a 78-year-old male, was diagnosed with Alzheimer's disease 3 years ago. His wife, Mary, has been his primary caregiver. They reside in their own retirement apartment in Lakeview Manor, a full-care retirement community. Mr. Weldon has been admitted to the skilled nursing area on a trial basis while Mrs. Weldon attends her granddaughter's college graduation out of state. She comes to visit to tell him good-bye before her trip. He says he doesn't know her and that they won't give him any food. She begins to cry and says, "It was a bad idea to plan this trip. I should stay and take Charles home with me."

Nursing Diagnosis: Compromised Family Coping

COLLECT DATA

Subjective	Objective
_____	_____
_____	_____
_____	_____
_____	_____
_____	_____
_____	_____
_____	_____

Would you report this? Yes/No

If yes, report to: _____

What would you report? _____

Nursing Care

_____
_____
_____
_____
_____
_____
_____
_____
_____
_____
_____
_____

How would you document this? _____
_____
_____

Compare your answers and documentation to those provided on the MyNursingKit Website.

Data Collected
(use only those that apply)

- Aricept
- Says they won't give him any food
- Coreg 6.125 mg every day (hold if SBP <110)
- Ativan 1 mg prn every 6 hours for anxiety
- Regular insulin per sliding scale ac and at bedtime
- "It was a bad idea to plan this trip. I should stay and take Charles home with me."
- NPH Humulin 30 units every am
- Diet: mechanical soft diet
- VS: T 98.2, P 68, R 16, BP 104/60
- He doesn't know her.

Nursing Interventions
(use only those that apply; list in priority order)

- Assist significant person with expanding repertoire of coping skills.
- Observe for any symptoms of elder abuse.
- Assess the client's awareness of deficits that may result from normal aging.
- Assess for dietary intake of essential nutrients.
- Help family members recognize the need for help and teach them how to ask for it.
- Encourage family members to verbalize feelings.
- Provide finger food and place in hands as needed to cue.
- Validate the family's feelings regarding the impact of client's illness on family lifestyle.

NCLEX-PN® Exam Preparation

TEST-TAKING TIP Remember you are taking a nursing exam and the answer to the question involves something that is included in the nursing care plan, rather than the medical plan.

1 Assessment can be distinguished from evaluation in which of the following ways?

1. Assessment is done throughout the nursing process; evaluation is done only when the client is ready for discharge.
2. Assessment is done by the LPN/LVN, evaluation is always done by the RN.
3. Assessment identifies the client's current status, whereas evaluation determines the client's progress toward a desired outcome.
4. Assessment is based on subjective data, whereas evaluation is based on objective data.

2 The second phase of the nursing process involves analyzing data and identifying health problems, risks, and strengths. This phase is known as:

1. Planning.
2. Evaluating.
3. Diagnosing.
4. Implementing.

3 During the assessment phase of the nursing process, which of the following are included in the LPN's/LVN's role? (Select all that apply.)

1. Collect data.
2. Respond to abnormal results of data collection.
3. Make observations of client status.
4. Report changes in client's condition.
5. Develop the plan of care.

4 The nurse collects data for the primary purpose of:

1. Determining the client's biographical data.
2. Gathering information about the client to contribute to the individualized plan of care needed to assist the client to regain optimal levels of health.
3. Learning about the client's past history.
4. Creating a database.

5 The LPN/LVN collects data on a newly admitted client. Which of the following data is objective data? (Select all that apply.)

1. Temperature is 98.2 degrees Fahrenheit.
2. Pain is rated as 8 on a 0–10 scale and is located in left lower quadrant of abdomen.

3. Client has history of drinking four beers per week for the past 2 years.
4. Breath sounds clear bilaterally in all lung fields.
5. Client complains of feeling short of breath with a respiratory rate of 14 breaths per minute.

6 The nurse collects objective data using which of the following data collection methods?

1. Observing
2. Interviewing
3. Examining
4. Observing and examining

7 The nursing care plan is put into action during which phase of the nursing process?

1. Planning
2. Implementing
3. Assessing
4. Evaluating

8 Delegating occurs in which stage of the nursing process?

1. Assessing
2. Diagnosing
3. Planning
4. Implementing

9 Evaluation statements consist of which two parts?

1. Effectiveness of plan of care and supporting data
2. Desired outcome and rationale
3. Problem status and client's response
4. Reassessment and data comparison

10 The nursing process can be described as a(n):

1. Strategy for implementing evidence-based nursing practice.
2. Holistic nursing assessment.
3. Organized framework for professional nursing practice.
4. Contributing factor for nursing diagnosis.

Answers and rationales for Review Questions appear in Appendix I.

Thinking Strategically About . . .

Carlos, an LVN with several years' experience, begins working in a long-term care facility. Within a few weeks, it becomes apparent that the night nurse is treating elderly clients unkindly, and there seems to be an increase in reported skin tears on the nights when she works. He speaks to this nurse about his concerns, but he sees no change in the situation. One morning, arriving at work early for a staff meeting, he overhears her verbally abusing a confused resident who will not take his medications. Carlos reports his observation to the director of nursing. When there is no improvement, Carlos returns to the director and says that he is considering speaking to the administrator or making a formal complaint to the state nursing board.

The alleged abuser is a long-time employee at the facility and popular with the nursing assistants and other staff. When the supervisor finally speaks to her about the complaint, the identity of the reporter becomes clear. Carlos is ostracized by most of the staff. He is criticized in front of residents and family members, and the night nurse continuously makes racial slurs when referring to him with other staff members. After several months Carlos feels he can no longer tolerate the working conditions and accepts a job at another facility.

CRITICAL THINKING

- Would you consider Carlos to be a "whistleblower"?
- Was Carlos's decision to report what he observed a legal or an ethical issue?
- Does Carlos have any legal recourse for his treatment?

COMMUNICATION

Consider the instances of communication that occurred in this case study: between the abusive nurse and the client, between the two nurses, between Carlos and the director of nursing, and between the staff and Carlos. In pairs or small groups, role-play these interactions as you think they probably occurred.

DELEGATING

How could the nurse who had become visibly frustrated with facility residents have used delegation to help her deal with the frustration that was the cause of her abusive behavior?

COMMUNITY

Why could this nurse's action or inaction be considered a community issue?

CONFLICT RESOLUTION

As a class or in an essay, review Carlos's decisions, using what you know about conflict resolution as a guide. What other alternatives might Carlos have had? How could Carlos have handled the situation differently?

CLIENT TEACHING

Develop a teaching plan to assist a client in not becoming a victim of mistreatment by others (e.g. staff or family members).

DOCUMENTING AND REPORTING

- Identify the form or forms that should be used to document mistreatment of a client by another staff member.
- What outside agencies should be involved when client mistreatment is suspected and facility administration fails to take action?

Introduction to Clinical Practice

UNIT II

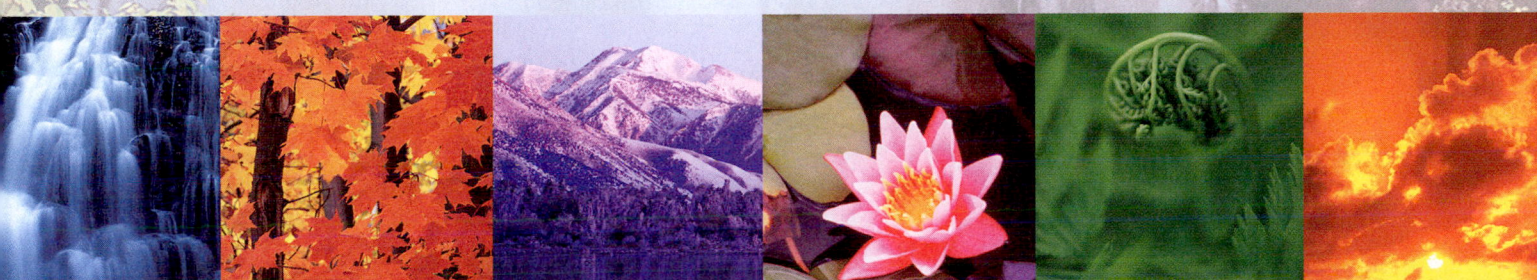

Healthcare Delivery Systems

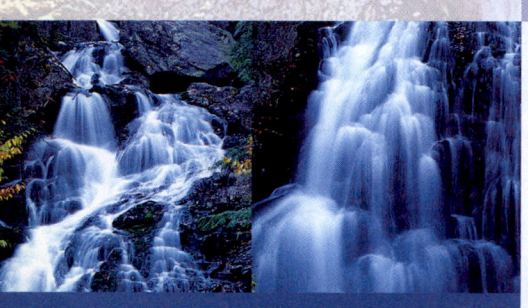

LEARNING Outcomes

After completing this chapter, you will be able to:

1. Differentiate primary, secondary, and tertiary healthcare delivery services.
2. Compare the characteristics of nursing in the outpatient setting to those of institutionalized nursing care.
3. Describe the functions and purposes of the healthcare agencies outlined in this chapter.
4. Discuss health care as a right and the essentials of the Patient's Bill of Rights.
5. Identify the roles of various healthcare professionals.
6. Describe factors that affect healthcare delivery.
7. Differentiate among the various models of care.
8. Compare various systems of payment for healthcare services.

KEY TERMS

A **healthcare system** is the totality of services offered by all health disciplines. Healthcare services are commonly categorized according to type and level.

Types of Health Care

Three types of services are often described: (1) health promotion and illness prevention, (2) diagnosis and treatment, and (3) rehabilitation and health restoration.

HEALTH PROMOTION AND ILLNESS PREVENTION

Based on the notion of maintaining an optimum level of wellness, the U.S. Department of Health and Human Services (DHHS) has developed a systematic approach to health improvement. A DHHS report, *Healthy People 2010* (2000), "focuses on improving health—the health of each individual, the health of the communities, and the health of the nation." However, the *Healthy People 2010* goals and objectives cannot by themselves improve the health status of the nation; instead, they need to be recognized as a part of a larger systemic approach to health improvement.

Since the 1980s, more and more people have recognized the advantages of staying healthy and avoiding illness. Health promotion programs address areas such as adequate and proper nutrition, weight control and exercise, and stress reduction. Health promotion activities emphasize the important role clients play in maintaining their own health and encourage them to maintain the highest level of wellness they can achieve. Recent transitions in health care also reflect a growing support for community-based nursing and health care that capitalizes on health promotion activities.

The healthcare delivery system also offers illness prevention programs. They may be directed at the client or the community and involve such practices as providing immunizations, identifying risk factors for illnesses (e.g., cardiovascular disease), and helping people take measures to prevent these illnesses from occurring.

DIAGNOSIS AND TREATMENT

Traditionally, the largest segment of the healthcare delivery system has been dedicated to the diagnosis and treatment of illness. Hospitals and physicians' offices were the major agencies offering these services. More recently, however, community-based agencies have been instrumental in providing these services (see Chapter 48). For example, clinics in some communities provide mammograms and education regarding the early detection of cancer of the breast. Voluntary HIV testing and counseling is another example of the shift in services from traditional healthcare settings to community-based agencies. Some shopping malls and shopping centers have walk-in clinics that provide diagnostic screening tests, such as screening for cholesterol and high blood pressure.

REHABILITATION AND HEALTH RESTORATION

Rehabilitation is a process of restoring ill or injured people to optimum and functional levels of wellness. Rehabilitative care emphasizes the importance of assisting clients to function adequately in the physical, mental, social, economic, and vocational areas of their lives. The goal of rehabilitation is to help people move to their previous level of health (i.e., to their previous capabilities) or to the highest level they are capable of given their current health status. Rehabilitation may begin in the hospital but will eventually lead clients back out into the community for further treatment and follow-up once health has been restored. The topic is discussed with long-term care in Chapter 46 .

Levels of Health Care

Healthcare delivery services can also be categorized according to the complexity or level of the services provided: primary, secondary, or tertiary. Table 7-1 ■ provides levels of care and the kinds of services provided at each level. Nurses play a key

TABLE 7-1	Types of Healthcare Services by Increasing Complexity
LEVEL	**NURSING SERVICES**
Primary (ambulatory care settings)	Health promotion (e.g., scoliosis screening, see Chapter 48)
	Preventive care (e.g., immunization; see Chapters 35 and 60)
	Health education (e.g., community education program about new vaccine against HPV)
	Environmental protection (e.g., distribution of iodine tablets to people living near nuclear power plants, to take in case of accidental emission of radioactivity)
Secondary (hospitals and ERs)	Emergency care (emergency departments)
	Diagnosis and treatment (complex illnesses)
	Acute care (hospitalization, surgery, etc.)
Tertiary (long-term care or rehabilitation facilities, hospices, or homes)	Long-term care
	Care of the dying (e.g., hospice)
	Rehabilitation (e.g., assisting return to highest possible level of functioning)

role in health promotion activities and in providing primary health care, whether in the hospital or in the community.

Types of Healthcare Settings

Healthcare agencies and settings are both varied and numerous. Some agencies provide a number of services; for example, a hospital may provide acute inpatient services, outpatient or ambulatory care services, and emergency services. In addition, the same services may be found in other community-based agencies. For example, hospice services may be provided in the hospital, in the home, or in another agency within the community.

A client may be categorized as an inpatient or an outpatient. An *inpatient* is a person who enters a setting such as a hospital and remains for at least 24 hours. An *outpatient* is a person who requires health care but does not need to stay in an institution such as a hospital.

Because the array of healthcare services and agencies is so great, nurses often need to help clients choose the service that best suits their needs. Clients may be seen in any number of these agencies, depending on their care and ability to pay for the services. Traditional nursing roles and responsibilities are also changing in response to the movement of client care from the hospital into the community. The LPN/LVN is currently being employed in almost every type of healthcare setting.

OUTPATIENT SETTINGS
Public Health

Health agencies at the state, county, or city level vary according to the needs of the area. Their funds, usually generated from taxes, are administered by elected or appointed officials. Local health departments (county, bicounty, or tricounty) traditionally have responsibility for developing programs to meet the health needs of the people, providing the necessary staff and facilities to carry out these programs, continually evaluating the effectiveness of the programs, and monitoring changing needs. State health organizations are responsible for assisting the local health departments. In some remote areas, state departments also provide direct services to people.

The Centers for Disease Control and Prevention (CDC) in Atlanta, Georgia, administers a broad program related to surveillance of diseases. By means of laboratory and epidemiologic investigations, data are made available to the appropriate authorities. The CDC also publishes recommendations about the prevention and control of infections and administers a national health program. The federal government also administers a number of Veterans Administration services in the United States.

Physicians' Offices

In North America, the physician's office is a traditional primary care setting. Most physicians either have their own offices or work with several other physicians in a group practice. Clients usually go to a physician's office for routine health screening, illness diagnosis, and treatment. People often seek consultation from physicians when they are experiencing symptoms of illness or when a significant other considers the person to be ill.

Nurses employed in physician's offices have a variety of roles and responsibilities. Some nurses carry out traditional functions including registering the client, preparing the client for an examination, obtaining health information, and providing information. Other functions may include obtaining specimens, assisting with procedures, and providing some treatments.

Ambulatory Care Centers

Ambulatory care centers are being used more frequently in many communities. Most ambulatory care centers have diagnostic and treatment facilities providing medical, nursing, laboratory, and radiologic services, and they may or may not be attached to or associated with an acute care hospital. Some ambulatory care centers provide services to people who require minor surgical procedures that can be performed outside the hospital. Nurses in ambulatory care centers may have specialized knowledge and skills to enable them to assist physicians with procedures. The term *ambulatory care center* has replaced the term *clinic* in many places.

General Clinics

The term *clinic* can refer to a department inside or outside the hospital, managed by a group of physicians or by nurses. Some may provide a specialized type of health service such as infant immunizations. Nurses in clinics perform many of the same functions as nurses employed in a physician's office.

Industrial Clinics

The industrial clinics are gaining importance as a setting for employee health care. Employee health has long been recognized as important to productivity. Nursing functions in industrial health care include work safety and health education, annual employee health screening for tuberculosis, and maintaining immunization information. Other functions may include screening for such health problems as hypertension and obesity, caring for employees following injury, and counseling.

Home Healthcare Agencies

The implementation of prospective payment (discussed later in this chapter) and the resulting earlier discharge of clients from hospitals have made home care an essential aspect of the healthcare delivery system. As concerns about the cost of health care have escalated, the use of the home as a care delivery site has increased. In addition, the scope of services offered in the home has broadened. Home healthcare agencies offer education to clients and families and also provide comprehensive care to acute, chronic, and terminally ill clients. Once the RN has opened the home care case, the LPN/LVN may be assigned to provide care and to supervise the home health aide or the individual providing homemaker services. Figure 7-1 ■ shows a documentation excerpt from home health care.

There are several different types of home health agencies:

- Official or public agencies are operated by state or local governments and financed primarily by tax funds.
- Voluntary or private not-for-profit agencies are supported by donations, endowments, charities such as the United Way, and third-party reimbursement. Because these agencies are not for profit, they are exempt from federal income tax.

- Private, proprietary agencies are for-profit organizations and are governed by either individual owners or national corporations. Some of these agencies participate in third-party reimbursement; others rely on "private-pay" sources.
- Institution-based agencies operate under a parent organization, such as a hospital.

Regardless of the type of agency, all home health agencies must meet specific standards for licensing, certification, and accreditation. See Box 7-1 ■ for the unique aspects of home care nursing.

Day Care Centers

Day care centers serve many functions and many age groups. A relatively new concept is centers that provide care for adults who cannot be left at home alone but do not need to be in an institution. Elder care centers often provide care involving socializing, exercise programs, and stimulation. Some centers provide counseling and physical therapy. Nurses who are employed in adult day care centers may provide medications, treatments, and counseling, thereby facilitating continuity between day care and home care. Adult day care is another work opportunity for the LPN/LVN.

INPATIENT SETTINGS

Hospitals

Hospitals traditionally have provided restorative care to the ill and injured. Although hospitals are chiefly viewed as institutions that provide care, they have other functions, such as providing sources for health-related research and teaching.

BOX 7-1	**UNIQUE ASPECTS OF HOME HEALTH NURSING**

The nurse:
- Functions independently.
- Must establish rapport with client and family.
- Provides care while family is present.

The family:
- May feel more free to question advice than when in the hospital setting.
- Will set their own schedule and priorities.
- Has more responsibility for care of client.

Positive Aspects
- Setting is more intimate and relaxed.
- Behaviors are more natural.
- Cultural beliefs and practices are more visible.
- Multigenerational interaction can take place.

Negative Aspects
- Caregiver demands may continue for months or years.
- Living conditions and support systems may be inadequate.
- There is risk of psychological or physical problems for caregiver.

na Nursing Associates

Triboro Office
555-5555

CLINICAL NOTES

CLIENT'S NAME _Eleanor Butler_

DATE & TIME	NARRATIVE
Thurs. (date)	0700 ~ cl. awake & states she is having arthritis pain. Rates her pain level @
7 AM - 10 AM	7 out of 10. Medicated c̄ oxycontin ṫ tab. po @ 0710. Assisted to sitting position
Ø BM	@ side of bed for breakfast. AM meds given c̄ meal. Cl. refused colace stating,
	"I want to talk to my doctor about that before I take it." 0800 ~ ate 1 egg,
	1 1/2 pc. toast, slice of watermelon & cup of hot tea. 0835 ~ Routine AM &
	oral care given. 0910 ~ cl. returned to bed. 0925 ~ Daughter-in-law called
	to check on her. Brief report given. Pain level ↓ to 2/10. Oxycontin
	appears to have been effective in pain relief. ———————————
	————————————————— Nancy Carpenter LPN
Fri. (date)	0700 ~ cl. incont. of lg. amt. urine. Routine AM care given.
7 AM - 9 AM	0735-0813. In w/c for breakfast. 0755-ate 1 egg, 1/2 pc. toast & cup of hot tea.
Ø BM	Having pain level @ 6/10. AM meds & oxycontin ṫ tab given c̄ H₂0.
	Ct. refused colace & MOM today. Oral care given. Fresh linens applied to
	bed, & cl. returned to bed @ 0850. ——————————
	————————————————— Nancy Carpenter LPN
Mon. (date)	0700 ~ cl. incont. of lg. amt. urine. Routine AM care given.
7 AM - 8:30 AM	Lotion applied to reddened areas on hips. Depends applied & out of
⊕ BM over W/E	bed to wheelchair for breakfast. Fresh linens applied to bed. All AM meds
	given c̄ breakfast including colace per ct's. request. Cl. ate 2 tsp Activia only
	for breakfast. Back to bed @ 0820. ——————————
	————————————————— Nancy Carpenter LPN

Figure 7-1. ■ Documentation sample from a home healthcare chart.

Hospitals are classified by the services they provide. General hospitals admit clients requiring a variety of services, such as medical, surgical, obstetric, pediatric, and psychiatric services. Other hospitals offer only specialty services, such as psychiatric or pediatric care. Hospitals can be further described as acute care or chronic (long-term) care. An acute care hospital provides assistance to clients who are acutely ill or whose illness and need for hospitalization are relatively short term. Long-term care hospitals provide services for longer periods, sometimes for years or the remainder of the client's life.

The variety of healthcare services hospitals provide usually depends on their size and location. The large urban hospitals usually have inpatient beds, emergency services, diagnostic facilities, ambulatory surgery centers, pharmacy services, intensive and coronary care services, and multiple outpatient services provided by clinics. Some large hospitals have other specialized services such as spinal cord injury and burn units, oncology services, and infusion and dialysis units. In addition, some hospitals have substance abuse treatment units and health promotion units. Small rural hospitals often are limited to inpatient beds, radiology and laboratory services, and basic emergency services. The number of services a rural hospital provides is usually directly related to its size and its distance from an urban center.

Hospitals in the United States have undergone massive changes. Many hospitals have merged with other hospitals or have been sold to large multihospital for-profit corporations.

Another change relates to the client population. Most clients in hospitals are seriously ill and require complex nursing care. With the increasing acuity (severity) of illness among clients, general hospitals have virtually become complex care centers. Because so many of the seriously ill are elderly, some general hospitals are becoming acute care hospitals solely for the elderly.

Nurses in hospitals have multiple responsibilities such as coordinating client care, assessing and monitoring client health, and providing direct care. The LPN/LVN works closely with the RN and provides much of the direct client care. While working in the acute care hospital, LPNs/LVNs have excellent opportunities to continue their education and then obtain RN positions.

Extended-Care (Long-Term Care) Facilities

Traditionally, all extended-care facilities were called nursing homes and provided care only for elderly clients. Today's facilities provide care to clients of all ages who require rehabilitation or custodial care. They can include skilled nursing facilities (intermediate care) and extended-care facilities (long-term care) that provide personal care for those who are chronically ill or are unable to care for themselves without

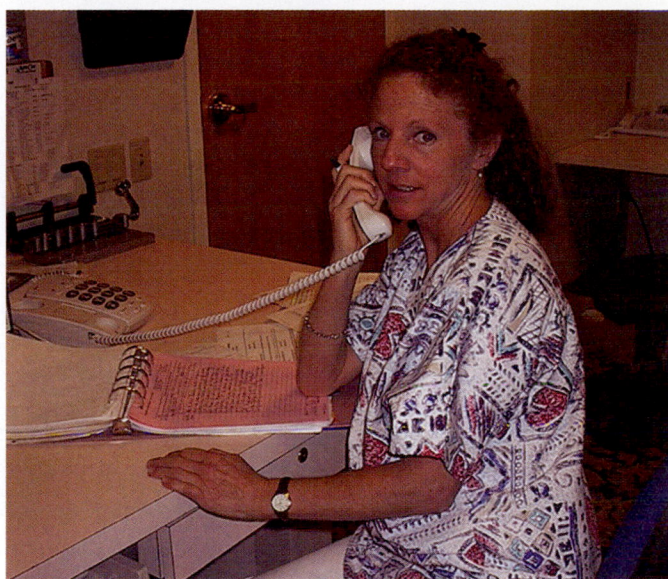

Figure 7-2. ■ The LPN/LVN charge nurse in the long-term setting serves as a liaison between resident, family, and physician.

assistance. LPNs/LVNs often have an increased level of responsibility in these settings (Figure 7-2 ■). The major discussion of long-term care is in Chapter 46 ⏩.

In 1987, as part of the **Omnibus Budget Reconciliation Act** (OBRA), the Congress of the United States passed legislation to bring a measure of quality improvement to the nursing home and extended-care facility industry. In response to a growing concern about whether minimal essential standards were being met in many facilities, OBRA instituted requirements for nurse's aide training. Requirements include a certification program for nurse's aides and competence evaluations of the aides.

Retirement and Assisted Living Centers

Retirement or assisted living centers consist of separate houses, condominiums, or apartments for residents. Residents live relatively independently. However, many of these facilities offer meals, laundry services, nursing care, transportation, and social activities. Some centers have a separate hospital to care for residents with short-term or long-term illness. Often, these centers also work collaboratively with other community services including case managers, social services, and a hospice to meet the needs of the residents who live there. The retirement or assisted living center is intended to meet the needs of people who are unable to remain at home but do not require hospital or nursing home care. Nurses in retirement and assisted living centers provide limited care to residents, usually related to the administration of medications and minor treatments. An LPN/LVN may be the only licensed nurse in an assisted living facility.

Rehabilitation Centers

Rehabilitation centers usually are independent community centers or special units. However, because rehabilitation ideally starts the moment the client enters the healthcare system, nurses who are employed on pediatric, psychiatric, or surgical units of hospitals also help to rehabilitate clients. Rehabilitation centers play an important role in assisting clients to restore their health and recuperate. Drug and alcohol rehabilitation centers, for example, help free clients of drug and alcohol dependence, and assist them in reentering the community. Physical rehabilitation centers help clients to regain purpose, function, and dignity. The focus is on assisting them to function at the maximum level possible and return to their community. Today, the concept of rehabilitation is applied to all illness (physical and mental), to injury, and to chemical addiction. Nurses in the rehabilitation setting coordinate client activities and ensure that clients are complying with their treatments. This type of nursing often requires specialized skills and knowledge. (Rehabilitation nursing is discussed in Chapter 46 ⚭ with long-term care.)

MIXED SETTINGS

Hospice Services

The hospice movement provides a variety of services to clients who are terminally ill, their families, and support persons. In the 1970s, the movement gained momentum, through the work of such people as Elisabeth Kübler-Ross, whose books challenged prevailing attitudes, and Cicely Saunders, founder of St. Christopher's Hospice in London, England. Saunders believed that the physical and social environments of dying people are as important as medical interventions on their behalf. The central concept of the hospice movement, as distinct from the acute care model, is not saving life but improving or maintaining the quality of life until death. The LPN/LVN works under the direction of an RN case manager to provide care for terminally ill clients in their home, long-term care facilities, or inpatient hospice centers. The main discussion of hospice is in Chapter 44; for some additional information about psychosocial aspects of care at hospice, see Chapter 18 ⚭ .

Crisis Centers

Crisis centers provide emergency services to clients experiencing life crises. These centers may operate out of a hospital or in the community, and most provide 24-hour telephone service. Some also provide direct counseling to people at the center or in their homes. The primary purpose of a crisis center is to help people cope with an immediate crisis and then provide guidance and support for long-term therapy. The LPN/LVN with specialized training may be employed and work with RNs, counselors, and psychologists in these settings.

Mutual Support and Self-Help Groups

Mutual support or self-help groups exist for nearly every major health problem or life crisis people experience. Alcoholics Anonymous, which formed in 1935, served as the model for many of these groups. The National Self-Help Clearinghouse provides information on current support groups and guidelines about how to start a self-help group. Many of these groups are facilitated by lay volunteers, although social workers or other healthcare professionals may carry out responsibilities for self-help groups.

Rights and Health Care

The movement for clients' rights in health care arose in the late 1960s. Today, clients are also seeking more self-determination and control over their own bodies when they are ill. Informed consent, confidentiality, and the right of the client to refuse treatment are all aspects of this self-determination. Today, the goals of health include the return of autonomy and independence to the client and the acceptance of good health as a responsibility of the client, the care providers, and society. These goals cannot be met unless clients accept active responsibility for their health and health care, and unless clients and care providers have mutual respect.

When people are ill, they are frequently unable to assert their rights as they would if they were healthy. Asserting rights requires energy and an underlying awareness of one's rights in the situation.

PATIENT'S BILL OF RIGHTS

In 1973, the American Hospital Association (AHA) published *A Patient's Bill of Rights* to promote the rights of hospitalized clients (Box 7-2 ■). The publication was revised in 1992. Included in this bill of rights are the right of clients to considerate and respectful care; consideration of privacy for clients, including confidentiality of all records and communications regarding their care; and the right to make decisions about their care, including the right to refuse a treatment or plan of care. In addition, clients have a right to make a statement such as a living will, which should be followed by the agency as permitted by law.

The AHA bill of rights states that clients have the right to review all of their medical records and have them explained; to receive requested care and services, provided these are reasonable; and to be informed of any business arrangements among institutions or people involved in their care. In addition, clients have the right to be informed of resources that can be used to resolve a dispute or grievance and of hospital policies and practices that relate to client care, treatment, and responsibilities, and to be informed of hospital charges and available payment methods.

BOX 7-2   PATIENT'S BILL OF RIGHTS

A patient's* bill of rights was first adopted by the American Hospital Association (AHA) in 1973. The bill of rights below incorporates the AHA update as well as bill of rights information from the American Academy of Pain Management and the National Institutes of Health.

Bill of Rights

These rights can be exercised on the client's behalf by a designated surrogate or proxy decision maker if the client* lacks decision-making capacity, is legally incompetent, or is a minor.

1. The client has the right to considerate and respectful care.
2. The client has the right to and is encouraged to obtain from physicians and other direct caregivers relevant, current, and understandable information about diagnosis, treatment, and prognosis.

   Except in emergencies when the client lacks decision-making capacity and the need for treatment is urgent, the client is entitled to the opportunity to discuss and request information related to specific procedures and treatments, the risks involved, the possible length of recuperation, and the medically reasonable alternatives and their accompanying risks and benefits.

   Clients have the right to know the identity of physicians, nurses, and others involved in their care, as well as when those involved are students, residents, or other trainees. The client also has the right to know the immediate and long-term financial implications of treatment choices insofar as they are known.
3. The client has the right to make decisions about the plan of care prior to and during the course of treatment and to refuse recommended treatment or plan of care to the extent permitted by law and hospital policy and to be informed of the medical consequences of this action. In case of such refusal, the client is entitled to other appropriate care and services that the hospital provides or transfer to another hospital. The hospital should notify clients of any policy that might affect client choice within the institution.
4. The client has the right to have an advance directive (such as a living will, health care proxy, or durable power of attorney for health care) concerning treatment or designating a surrogate decision maker with the expectation that the hospital will honor the intent of that directive to the extent permitted by law and hospital policy.

   Health care institutions must advise clients of their rights under state law and hospital policy to make informed medical choices, ask if the client has an advance directive, and include that information in client records. The client has the right to timely information about hospital policy that may limit its ability to implement fully a legally valid advance directive.
5. The client has the right to have every consideration of privacy. Case discussion, consultation, examination, and treatment should be conducted so as to protect each client's privacy.
6. The client has the right to expect that all communications and records pertaining to his/her care will be treated as confidential by the hospital, except in cases of suspected abuse or public health hazards when reporting is permitted or

required by law. The client has the right to expect that the hospital will emphasize the confidentiality of this information when it releases it to any other parties entitled to review information in these records.
7. The client has the right to review the records pertaining to his/her medical care and have information explained or interpreted as necessary, except when restricted by law.
8. The client has the right to expect that, within its capacity and policies, a hospital will make reasonable response to the request of a client for appropriate and medically indicated care and services. The hospital must provide evaluation, services, and/or referral, as indicated by the urgency of the case. When medically appropriate and legally permissible, or when a client has so requested, a client may be transferred to another facility. The institution to which the client is to be transferred must first have accepted the client for transfer. The client must also have the benefit of complete information and explanation concerning the need for, risks, benefits, and alternatives to such a transfer.
9. The client has the right to ask and be informed of the existence of business relationships among the hospital, educational institutions, other health care providers, or payers that may influence the client's treatment and care.
10. The client has the right to consent to or decline to participate in proposed research studies or human experimentation affecting care and treatment or requiring direct client involvement, and to have those studies fully explained prior to consent. A client who declines to participate in research or experimentation is entitled to the most effective care that the hospital can otherwise provide.
11. The client has the right to expect reasonable continuity of care when appropriate and to be informed by physicians and other caregivers of available and realistic client care options when hospital care is no longer appropriate.
12. The client has the right to be informed of hospital policies and practices that relate to client care, treatment, and responsibilities. The client has the right to be informed of available resources for resolving disputes, grievances, and conflicts such as ethics committees, client representatives, or other mechanisms available in the institution. The client has the right to be informed of the hospital's charges for services and available payment methods.
13. The client has the privilege to examine and receive an explanation of the bill.
14. The client has the right to expect that medical information about him or her discovered at the clinical center, as well as an account of his or her medical program here, will be communicated to the referring physician.
15. The client has the right, at any time during the medical program, to designate additional physicians or organizations to receive medical updates. The client should inform the outpatient department staff of these additions.

*Note: This book uses the word *client* instead of *patient* to indicate that the person is an active participant in the process of achieving or maintaining health.

Sources: American Hospital Association, Chicago, IL; American Academy of Pain Management, Sonora, CA; National Institutes of Health, Washington, DC.

Furthermore, the AHA bill states that clients have the right to refuse to participate in any research study, to expect reasonable continuity of care, and to have options explained when hospital care is no longer appropriate.

The Patient's Bill of Rights, by federal law, must be explained verbally and signed by the client before care can be provided. Verification of compliance is an important nursing function at the time of admission. The client should be asked about any advance directive (e.g., not to be resuscitated in the event of a cardiac arrest), and this information must be on the client's record. If the hospital's policy limits its ability to implement any advance directive, the client has a right to be informed of this before any problem arises. See details about advance directives in Chapter 18 .

If a client lacks decision-making capacity, is legally incompetent, or is a minor, these rights can be exercised on the client's behalf by a designated surrogate or proxy decision maker.

Other bills of rights have been proposed for healthcare recipients. See, for example, the Mourner's Bill of Rights in Chapter 18 .

Providers of Health Care

The providers of health care, also referred to as the healthcare team or health professionals, are health personnel from different disciplines who coordinate their skills to assist clients and perhaps their support persons. Their mutual goal is to restore a client's health and promote wellness. The choice of personnel for a particular client depends on the needs of the client. In the present system of health care in North America, health teams commonly include the personnel discussed in the following subsections.

NURSE

The role of the nurse varies with the needs of the client. As nursing roles have expanded, new dimensions for nursing practice have been established. See Chapter 1 for the roles of the nurse. Nurses can pursue a variety of practice specialties (e.g., critical care, mental health, oncology). An RN assesses a client's health status, identifies health problems, and develops and coordinates care. An LPN/LVN provides direct client care under the direction of a registered nurse.

NURSE PRACTITIONER

A nurse practitioner is a registered nurse who has advanced training and a master of science in nursing degree. These nurses are responsible for screening, diagnosis, and treatment of uncomplicated illnesses and injury. They have prescriptive authority and may order diagnostic tests. They often work directly with a physician in his or her office. In

some settings, the nurse practitioner may have a solo practice, but generally will work closely with a physician for referral if necessary.

PHYSICIAN

The physician is responsible for determining medical diagnoses and for determining the therapy required by a person who has a disease or injury. The physician's traditional role is the treatment of disease and trauma (injury); however, many physicians are now including health promotion and disease prevention in their practice. Some physicians specialize in specific areas such as surgery or oncology.

HOSPITALIST

The term *hospitalist* was first used in 1996 in an article in the *New England Journal of Medicine*. By the summer of 1998 it had become a very popular career choice. The demand for hospitalists exceeded the supply of doctors to fill the positions. The hospitalist focuses on inpatient care. In general, the duties of the hospitalist are to provide prompt, efficient, and competent care to hospitalized clients. The clients are usually referred by a primary care provider or an emergency room physician. The bulk of their workload involves acute admissions. Once the client has been discharged from the hospital, he or she will be referred back to the primary physician for follow-up care.

PHYSICIAN'S ASSISTANT

Physician's assistants (PAs) perform certain tasks under the direction of a physician. They diagnose and treat certain diseases and injuries. In most states, physician's assistants also have limited prescriptive authority.

UNLICENSED ASSISTIVE PERSONNEL

Unlicensed assistive personnel (UAPs) are healthcare staff such as certified nurse assistants, hospital attendants, nurse technicians, and orderlies who assume aspects of client care that do not require nursing judgment. These tasks include bathing, assisting with feeding, exercise, and range of motion. Individual facilities may provide training for unlicensed personnel to perform additional tasks.

DENTIST

Dentists diagnose and treat dental problems. Dentists are also actively involved in preventive measures to maintain healthy oral structures (e.g., teeth and gums). Many hospitals, especially long-term care facilities, have dentists on staff.

PHARMACIST

A pharmacist prepares and dispenses pharmaceuticals in hospital and community settings. The role of the pharmacist in monitoring and evaluating the actions and effects of medications on clients is becoming increasingly prominent.

A clinical pharmacist is a specialist who guides physicians in prescribing medications. A pharmacy technician/assistant is also recognized in some states. This person administers medications to clients or works in the pharmacy under the direction of the pharmacist.

DIETITIAN OR NUTRITIONIST

When dietary and nutritional services are required, the dietitian or nutritionist may be a member of a health team. A dietitian, often a registered dietitian (RD), has special knowledge about the diets required to maintain health and to treat disease. Dietitians in hospitals generally are concerned with therapeutic diets, may design special diets to meet the nutritional needs of individual clients, and supervise the preparation of the meals to ensure that clients receive the proper diet.

A nutritionist is a person who has special knowledge about nutrition and food. The nutritionist in a community setting recommends healthy diets and gives broad advisory services about the purchase and preparation of foods. Community nutritionists often function at the preventive level. They promote health and prevent disease, for example, by advising families about balanced diets for growing children and pregnant women.

PHYSICAL THERAPIST

The physical therapist (PT) assists clients with musculoskeletal problems. He or she provides physical therapy in response to a physician's order. The physiotherapist's functions include assessing clients' mobility and strength, providing therapeutic measures (e.g., exercises and heat applications to improve mobility and strength), and teaching new skills (e.g., how to walk with an artificial leg). Some physiotherapists provide their services in hospitals; often, however, independent practitioners establish offices in communities and serve clients either at the office or in the home.

RESPIRATORY THERAPIST

A respiratory therapist (RT) is skilled in therapeutic measures used in the care of clients with respiratory problems. These therapists are knowledgeable about oxygen therapy devices, intermittent positive-pressure breathing respirators, artificial mechanical ventilators, and accessory devices used in inhalation therapy.

OCCUPATIONAL THERAPIST

An occupational therapist (OT) assists clients with impaired function to gain the skills needed to perform activities of daily living. The therapist also teaches skills that are therapeutic and at the same time provide some satisfaction, such as crafts, puzzles, woodworking, and needlework.

PARAMEDICAL TECHNOLOGISTS

Paramedical means having some connection with medicine. Laboratory technologists examine specimens such as urine, feces, blood, and discharges from wounds to provide exact information that facilitates the medical diagnosis and the prescription of a therapeutic regimen. The radiologic technologist assists with a wide variety of x-ray film procedures, from simple chest radiography to more complex fluoroscopy. The nuclear medicine technologist uses radioactive substances to provide diagnostic information.

SOCIAL WORKER

A social worker counsels clients and support persons about social problems, such as finances, family interactions, parenting, and adoption. It is not unusual for health problems to produce problems in living and vice versa. Social workers usually make the placement arrangements for acute care hospital clients who require rehabilitation services in skilled nursing facilities or in the home. They also help families make choices when loved ones can no longer live at home.

SPIRITUAL SUPPORT PERSON

Chaplains, pastors, rabbis, priests, and so on serve as part of the healthcare team by attending to the spiritual needs of clients. In most facilities, local clergy volunteer their services on a regular or on-call basis. Hospitals affiliated with specific religions, as well as many large medical centers, have fulltime chaplains on staff. They usually offer regularly scheduled religious services. The nurse is often instrumental in identifying the client's desire for spiritual support and notifying the appropriate person. A relatively new nursing specialty is that of parish nurse. A parish nurse helps meet the health needs in the community while including spiritual aspects of care. They are affiliated with a church or group of churches and provide health screening and information for church members and the surrounding community.

CASE MANAGERS

The case manager's role is to ensure fiscally sound, appropriate care in the best setting. This role is often filled by the member of the healthcare team who is most involved in the client's care. Depending on the nature of the client's concerns, the case manager may be a nurse, a social worker, an OT, a PT, or any member of the healthcare team.

ALTERNATIVE CARE PROVIDERS

Chiropractors, herbalists, acupuncturists, and other nontraditional healthcare providers are playing increasing roles in the contemporary healthcare system. These providers may practice alongside traditional healthcare providers, or clients may use their services in conjunction with, or in lieu of, traditional therapies. Box 7-3 ■ lists types of alternative

BOX 7-3	ALTERNATIVE CARE PROVIDERS

- Chiropractor—provides care by manipulating spinal vertebrae to relieve interference with nerve function.
- Herbalist—provides information and consultation regarding the use of herbal remedies for various symptoms and illnesses.
- Acupuncturist—provides relief of pain and other symptoms by gently inserting long, hollow needles at various points in the body to stimulate the flow of energy along meridians.
- Homeopathist—provides treatment for certain illnesses by giving small doses of substances that help build up the body's natural defenses against the specific disease or illness.
- Massage therapist—provides relief of muscle pain, spasm, and tension by stroking and kneading soft tissue.

care providers. The main discussion of complementary and alternative medical care (CAM) appears in Chapter 8 ⚭ .

Factors Affecting Healthcare Delivery

Today's healthcare consumers have greater knowledge about their health than in previous years, and they are increasingly influencing healthcare delivery. Formerly, people expected a physician to make decisions about their care; today, however, consumers expect to be involved in making any decisions. Consumers have also become aware of how lifestyle affects health. As a result, they desire more information and services related to health promotion and illness prevention. A number of other factors affect the healthcare delivery system.

INCREASING NUMBER OF ELDERLY

By the year 2020, it is estimated that the number of adults over the age of 65 years will be nearly 56 million in the United States (Abrams et al., 2004). Long-term illnesses are prevalent among this group and frequently require special housing, treatment services, financial support, and social networks.

The frail elderly, considered to be people over age 85, are projected to be the fastest growing population in North America and will constitute 9.6 million by 2030 (Lee & Estes, 2003).

Because only 5 percent of older people with health problems are institutionalized, substantial home management and nursing support services are required to assist those in their homes and communities.

ADVANCES IN TECHNOLOGY

Scientific knowledge and technology related to health care are rapidly increasing. Improved diagnostic procedures and sophisticated equipment permit early recognition of diseases that might otherwise have remained undetected. New antibiotics and medications are continually being manufactured to treat infections and multiple-drug-resistant organisms. Surgical procedures that were nonexistent 20 years ago are common today. Laser and microscopic procedures streamline the treatment of diseases that required surgery in the past. Computers, bedside charting, and the ability to store and retrieve large volumes of information in databases are commonplace in healthcare organizations. All the technological advances and specialized treatments and procedures come, unfortunately, with a high price tag.

WOMEN'S HEALTH

The women's movement has been instrumental in changing healthcare practices. Examples are the provision of childbirth services in more relaxed settings such as birthing centers, and the provision of overnight facilities for parents in children's hospitals. Traditionally, women's health issues have focused on the reproductive aspects of health, disregarding many healthcare concerns that are unique to women. Today, research and treatment focuses on many areas of women's health care such as breast cancer, osteoporosis, abuse, treatment of sexually transmitted infections, and issues on aging. An expert panel on women's health of the American Academy of Nursing (AAN) recommends that "understanding women's health requires more than a biomedical view; it requires awareness of the context of women's lives" (AAN Panel on Women's Health, 1997, p. 7).

UNEVEN DISTRIBUTION OF SERVICES

Serious problems in the distribution of health services exist in the United States. In many remote and rural locations, insufficient services and healthcare professionals are available to meet the healthcare needs of individuals. Uneven distribution is evidenced by the relatively higher number of physicians and nurses per capita in the New England states than in the South, which has the lowest number per capita.

Because of the highly specialized techniques and new knowledge that have emerged during the past 30 years, an increasing number of healthcare personnel provide specialized services. This specialization leads to fragmentation of care and, often, increased cost of care. To clients, it may mean receiving care from 5 to 30 people during their hospital experience. This seemingly endless stream of personnel is often confusing and frightening.

ACCESS TO HEALTH CARE

Another problem plaguing individuals is access to health care. Low income has been associated with relatively higher rates of infectious diseases, problems with substance abuse, rape, violence, and chronic diseases. The use of healthcare services is also affected by unemployment and poverty. Even though some government assistance is available, eligibility for such assistance and type of benefits vary considerably from state to state.

HOMELESS POPULATIONS

The growing number of homeless individuals in towns and cities is a major health problem. The homeless differ from those who are poor. They are alone, lack some type of permanent residence, and are disaffiliated from family and friends. Limited access to healthcare services and compliance from the client contributes to the general poor health of the homeless in the United States. Box 7-4 ■ provides factors contributing to health problems among the homeless.

DEMOGRAPHIC CHANGES

The characteristics of the North American family have changed considerably in the last few decades. The number of single-parent families and alternative family structures has increased markedly. Most of the single-parent families are headed by women, many of whom work and require assistance with child care or when a child is sick at home.

BOX 7-4	POPULATION FOCUS

Risk Factors for Health Problems among the Homeless

- Poor physical environment resulting in increased susceptibility to infections
- Inadequate rest and privacy
- Improper nutrition
- Poor access to facilities for personal hygiene
- Exposure to the elements
- Lack of social support
- Few personal resources
- Questionable personal safety (physical assault is a constant threat)
- Inadequate health care
- Poor compliance with treatment plans

BOX 7-5	CULTURAL PULSE POINTS

Healthcare Delivery Systems

A number of elements can enhance a healthcare agency's ability to provide culturally proficient care. These include but are not limited to:

- Service delivery that reflects an understanding of cultural diversity (as evidenced by signs such as "Se habla espanol")
- Institutionalized knowledge of culture (a statistical database that can aid in diagnosis and care)
- Consciousness of dynamics that are inherent when cultures interact (as in workshops or seminars on areas of conflict)
- Valuing diversity (hiring people of varied cultural, racial, or ethnic backgrounds)
- Capacity for cultural self-assessment (awareness and review from the administrative level down to assess the facility's own functioning)

Recognition of cultural and ethnic diversity is also increasing. Healthcare professionals and agencies are aware of this diversity and are employing means to meet the challenges it presents (Box 7-5 ■).

Contemporary Frameworks for Care

Approaches to client care that support continuity of care and cost effectiveness include managed care and case management.

MANAGED CARE

Managed care describes a healthcare system whose goals are to provide cost-effective, quality care that focuses on improved outcomes for groups of clients. The care of a client is carefully planned from initial contact to the conclusion of the specific health problem. In managed care, healthcare providers and agencies collaborate so as to render the most appropriate, fiscally responsible care possible. Managed care emphasizes cost controls, customer satisfaction, health promotion, and preventive services. Health maintenance organizations and preferred provider organizations are examples of provider systems committed to managed care.

CASE MANAGEMENT

Case management describes a range of models for integrating healthcare services for individuals or groups. Various case management models strive to provide cost-effective care and ensure quality outcomes. Generally, case management involves nurse–physician teams that assume collaborative responsibility for planning, assessing needs, and coordinating, implementing, and evaluating care for groups of clients from preadmission to discharge or transfer and recuperation. A case manager, however, may be a social worker or other appropriate professional.

Case management may be used as a cost-containment strategy in managed care. Case management is usually the responsibility of the RN. Occasionally in a long-term care setting, an LPN/LVN may be specially trained to carry out these duties. Both case management and managed care systems often use clinical pathways to track the client's progress (Figure 7-3 ■). **Clinical pathways** provide an expected path of client needs, care, teaching, and progress for specific diagnoses. Case managers use them for planning care and anticipating potential problems in the progression of a client's recovery.

Models of Care

Contemporary configurations for the delivery of nursing include collaborative arrangements such as managed care, case management, and client-focused care. Other models

CRITICAL PATHWAY: TOTAL HIP REPLACEMENT

	DOS/Day 1	Days 2–3
Pain Management	Outcome: • Verbalizes comfort or tolerance of pain Circle: V NV Variance:	Outcome: • Verbalizes comfort with pain control measures Circle: V NV Variance:
Respiratory	Outcomes: • Breath sounds clear to auscultation • Achieves 50% of volume goal on incentive spirometer Circle: V NV Variance:	Outcomes: • Breath sounds clear to auscultation • Achieves 100% of volume goal on incentive spirometer Circle: V NV Variance:

Key: V = Variance NV = No Variance	
Signature:	Initials:
Signature:	Initials:

Figure 7-3. ■ Excerpt from a critical pathway documentation form.

specifically designed for the provision of nursing are the case method, the functional method, team nursing, and primary nursing.

CLIENT-FOCUSED CARE

Client-focused care is a delivery model that brings all services and care providers to the clients. The supposition is that if activities normally provided by auxiliary personnel (e.g., physical therapy, respiratory therapy, electrocardiographic [ECG] testing, and phlebotomy) are moved closer to the client, the number of personnel involved and the number of steps involved to get the work done are decreased. Proponents of this type of system believe that clients will perceive improved care and service and the agency will achieve cost savings.

Cross-training, development of multiskilled workers who can perform tasks or functions in more than one discipline, is an essential element of client-focused care. For example, a healthcare worker may be taught to obtain a 12-lead ECG and perform phlebotomy. Individuals who are already certified in one profession can take on a second certification such as medical laboratory and x-ray technology, nursing and respiratory therapy, physical therapy and occupational therapy. Cross-training will be integral to the managed care system in the future.

CASE METHOD

The **case method**, also referred to as total care, is one of the earliest nursing models developed. In this client-centered method, one nurse is assigned to and is responsible for the comprehensive care of a group of clients during an 8- or 12-hour shift. Facilities that function under the case method employ RNs only for bedside care. With the shortage of nursing personnel during World War II, the case method could no longer be the chief mode of care for clients. Many hospitals reinstituted a form of total care, called primary care, beginning in the mid-1970s and continuing for many years.

FUNCTIONAL METHOD

The **functional method** focuses on the jobs to be completed (e.g., bed making, temperature measurement). In this task-oriented approach, personnel with less preparation than the professional nurse perform less complex care requirements. It is based on a production and efficiency model that gives authority and responsibility to the person assigning the work, for example, the head nurse. Clearly defined job descriptions, procedures, policies, and lines of communication are required. The functional approach to nursing is economical and efficient and permits centralized direction and control. Its disadvantages are fragmentation of care and the possibility that nonquantifiable aspects of care, such as meeting the client's emotional needs, may be overlooked.

TEAM NURSING

In the early 1950s, Eleanor Lambertson and her colleagues proposed a system of team nursing to overcome the fragmentation of care resulting from the task-oriented functional approach and to meet increasing demands for professional nurses created by advances in technological aspects of care. **Team nursing** is the delivery of individualized nursing care to clients by a nursing team led by a professional nurse. A nursing team consists of RNs, LPNs/LVNs, and often nurse's aides. This team is responsible for providing coordinated nursing care to a group of clients during an 8- or 12-hour shift.

With the advent of managed care, team nursing is experiencing a resurgence. In this revisited form of team nursing, licensed nursing personnel (RNs and LPNs/LVNs) are frequently paired with UAPs. The licensed nurse retains responsibility and authority for client care but delegates appropriate tasks to the UAP. Contemporary proponents of this model believe the team approach increases the efficiency of the licensed nurse. Opponents state that inpatients' high acuity of illness leaves little to be delegated.

PRIMARY NURSING

Primary nursing, a system in which one nurse is responsible for total care of a number of clients 24 hours a day, 7 days a week, was introduced at the Loeb Center for Nursing and Rehabilitation, the Bronx, New York, in the early 1960s. It is a method of providing comprehensive, individualized, and consistent care.

Primary nursing uses the nurse's technical knowledge and management skills. The primary nurse assesses and prioritizes each client's needs, identifies nursing diagnoses, develops a plan of care with the client, and evaluates the effectiveness of care. Associates provide some care, but the primary nurse co-ordinates it and communicates information about the client's health to other nurses and other health professionals. Primary nursing encompasses all aspects of the professional role (RN), including teaching, advocacy, decision making, and continu-ity of care. The primary nurse is the first-line manager of the client's care with all of its inherent accountabilities and responsibilities. With today's nursing shortage and high cost of health care, this model of nursing care is being replaced.

Healthcare Economics

Although efforts have been made to control the costs of health care, these costs continue to increase. Employers, legislators, insurers, and healthcare providers continue to collaborate in efforts to resolve the issues surrounding how to best finance healthcare costs.

PAYMENT SOURCES

Medicare and Medicaid

In the United States, the 1965 Medicare amendments (Title 18) to the Social Security Act provided a national and state health insurance program for older adults. **Medicare** is divided into two parts: Part A is available to people with disabilities and people age 65 years and over. It provides in-surance toward hospitalization, home care, and hospice care. Part B is voluntary and provides partial coverage of physician services to people eligible for Part A. Clients pay a monthly premium for this coverage. Medicare does not cover dental care, dentures, eyeglasses, hearing aids, or examinations to prescribe and fit hearing aids. Most preventive care, includ-ing routine physical examinations and associated diagnostic tests, is also not included.

In 2006, Medicare prescription drug coverage was insti-tuted. Everyone with Medicare is eligible for the coverage regardless of income and resources, health status, or current prescription expense.

Participants must select a plan during the open enrollment period, normally November 15–December 31. Choosing an appropriate plan may be a daunting task for an older individ-ual. Family members and healthcare providers should become familiar with available plans in order to assist the client.

Medicaid was also established in 1965 under Title 19 of the Social Security Act. **Medicaid** is a federal public assistance program paid out of general taxes to people who require finan-cial assistance. Medicaid is paid by federal and state govern-ments. Each state program is distinct. Some states provide very limited coverage, whereas others pay for dental care, eye-glasses, and prescription drugs.

Supplemental Security Income

In addition, people who are blind or have a disability may be eligible for special payments called **Supplemental Security Income** (SSI) benefits. These benefits are also available to people not eligible for Social Security, and payments are not restricted to healthcare costs. Clients often use this money to purchase medicines or to cover costs of extended health care.

PROSPECTIVE PAYMENT SYSTEM

In 1983 the United States Congress passed legislation putting the **prospective payment system** (PPS) into effect. This legislation limits the amount paid to hospitals that are reimbursed by Medicare. Reimbursement is made according to a classification system known as **diagnostic-related groups** (DRGs). Prospective payment or billing is formu-lated before the client is even admitted to the hospital; thus, the record of admission, rather than the record of treatment, now governs payment. DRG rates are set in advance of the prospective year during which they apply and are considered fixed except for major, uncontrollable occurrences.

INSURANCE PLANS

A variety of plans have come into existence to finance health care in the United States. These include private insurance and group insurance. Each individual and group plan offers different options for consumers to consider when choosing a prepaid healthcare program.

Private Insurance

Commercial health insurance carriers offer a wide range of coverage plans. There are two types of private insurance: not-for-profit (e.g., Blue Shield) and for-profit companies (e.g., commercial companies such as Metropolitan Life, Travelers, and Aetna). Private health insurance is known as third-party reimbursement because the insurance company pays either the entire bill or, more often, 80 percent of the costs of healthcare services. With private health insurance plans, the insurance company reimburses the healthcare provider a fee for each service provided (fee-for-service).

These insurance plans may be purchased either as an indi-vidual plan or as part of a group plan through a person's em-ployer, union, student association, or similar organization.

Group Plans

Healthcare group plans provide blanket medical service in exchange for a predetermined monthly payment. Each group plan offers different options for consumers to con-sider when choosing a prepaid healthcare program.

HEALTH MAINTENANCE ORGANIZATIONS. A **health mainte-nance organization** (HMO) is a group healthcare agency that provides basic and supplemental health maintenance and treatment services to voluntary enrollees. A fee is set without regard to the amount or kind of services provided.

The HMO plan emphasizes client wellness; the better the health of the person, the fewer HMO services are needed and the greater the agency's profit. Members of HMOs choose a primary care provider (PCP), who evaluates their health status and coordinates their care. The PCP has two options: Treat the condition or refer the client to a specialist. To reduce costs, HMOs will pay for a specialty physician's services only if the PCP has made the referral. It is an expectation between the HMO and physicians being reimbursed under their plans that PCPs will treat clients and reduce costs whenever possible. Thus, under HMO plans, clients are limited in their ability to select healthcare providers and services. Because health promotion and illness prevention are highly emphasized in HMOs, nurses in HMOs focus on these aspects of care.

PREFERRED PROVIDER ORGANIZATIONS. The **preferred provider organization** (PPO) has emerged as another alternative in the healthcare delivery system. PPOs consist of a group of physicians and perhaps a healthcare agency (often a hospital) that provide an insurance company or employer with health services at a discounted rate. One advantage of the PPO is that it provides clients with a choice of healthcare providers and services. Physicians can belong to one or several PPOs, and the client can choose among the physicians belonging to the PPO. A disadvantage of PPOs is that they tend to be slightly more expensive than HMO plans, and if individuals wish to join a PPO, they might have to pay more for the additional choices. PPOs were first established in 1980 in the United States.

PREFERRED PROVIDER ARRANGEMENTS. **Preferred provider arrangements** (PPAs) are similar to PPOs. The main difference is that the PPAs can be contracted with individual healthcare providers, whereas PPOs involve an organization of healthcare providers.

INDEPENDENT PRACTICE ASSOCIATIONS. **Independent practice associations** (IPAs) are somewhat like HMOs and PPOs. The difference is that clients pay a fixed prospective payment to the IPA, and the IPA pays the provider. The provider receives a fixed fee for services given. At the end of the fiscal year, any surplus money is divided among the providers; any loss is assumed by the IPA.

PHYSICIAN/HOSPITAL ORGANIZATIONS. Physician/hospital organizations (PHOs) are joint ventures between a group of private practice physicians and a hospital. PHOs combine both resources and personnel to provide managed care alternatives and medical services. PHOs work with a variety of insurers to provide services. A typical PHO will include primary care providers and specialists.

A PHO may be part of an **integrated delivery system** (IDS). Such a system incorporates acute care services, home health care, extended and skilled care facilities, and outpatient services. Most integrated delivery systems provide care throughout the life span. An IDS enhances continuity of care and communication among professionals and various agencies providing managed care.

Other Payment Options

In rural communities and in some areas of the country, payment for services may not be mediated by any sort of private or governmental agency. Among the Amish in Ohio, Indiana, or Pennsylvania, for example, payment is generally made in cash, and no insurer is involved. Oftentimes for major medical events, the religious community works together to pay costs, and physicians and hospitals make private arrangements with them.

Individual care providers may make other private arrangements in the communities where they work.

A relatively new innovative healthcare delivery method is being used by some physicians in larger metropolitan areas. The physician charges a yearly fee to clients to cover provided services. The fee is quite substantial, but the physician limits the number of clients who are "members" in the plan. The physician does not accept any insurance. This method is appealing to affluent, self-employed individuals who would be paying very high premiums for health insurance coverage. The advantage of this method is personalized care from a personal physician. The disadvantage is the need to carry catastrophic or hospitalization insurance for surgery or hospital care.

Note: The references and resources for all chapters have been compiled at the back of the book.

Chapter Review

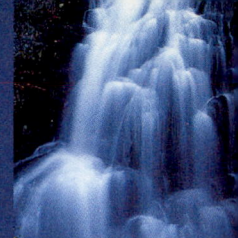

KEY Points

- Healthcare delivery services can be categorized as primary, secondary, or tertiary, and generally, they can also be grouped by the type of service: (1) health promotion and illness prevention, (2) diagnosis and treatment, and (3) rehabilitation.

- Health care can be considered a right of all people.

- Hospitals provide a wide variety of services on an inpatient and outpatient basis. Hospitals can be categorized as for-profit or not-for-profit, public or private, acute care or long-term care facilities. Many other settings, such as clinics, offices, and day care centers, also provide care.

- Various providers of health care coordinate their skills to assist a client. Their mutual goal is to restore a client's health and promote wellness.

- The many factors affecting healthcare delivery include increased participation in their own care by healthcare consumers, economic factors, increased costs, the increasing number of elderly people, advances in knowledge and technology, women's health, uneven distribution of health services, access to health care, health care of the homeless, and demographic changes.

- There are a number of frameworks for client health care, including managed care, case management, and client-focused care.

- In the United States, health care is financed largely through government agencies and private organizations that provide healthcare insurance, prepaid plans, and federally funded programs.

FOR FURTHER Study

To find out more about the roles of nurses, see Chapter 1.

Chapter 8 provides a discussion of CAM medicine.

For additional information about advance directives and the psychosocial aspects of care at hospice, see Chapter 18.

Hospice services are discussed in Chapter 44.

For complete discussion on long-term care and rehabilitation facilities, see Chapter 46.

For community-based and ambulatory settings that include various screenings, see Chapter 48.

For an immunization schedule for children, see Chapter 59.

PEARSON

EXPLORE **mynursingkit**™

MyNursingKit is your one stop for online chapter review materials and resources. Prepare for success with additional NCLEX®-style practice questions, interactive assignments and activities, web links, animations and videos, and more!

Register your access code from the front of your book at
www.mynursingkit.com

NCLEX-PN® Exam Preparation

1 Which is NOT a right of hospitalized clients according to the Patient's Bill of Rights?
1. The right to considerate and respectful care
2. The right to determine the schedule of care
3. The right to make decisions about care
4. The right to refuse treatment or care

2 The Omnibus Budget Reconciliation Act is important in health care because it:
1. Instituted specific training requirements for nurse's aides working long-term care.
2. Outlined guidelines for death with dignity.
3. Governs Medicare payments for individuals receiving Social Security.
4. Set the nurse–client ratio in acute care hospitals.

3 A homeless client is brought by a police officer to the emergency department for treatment. Which of the following would you recognize as a major contributing factor for his or her health problems?
1. Mistrust of the system and healthcare providers
2. Transportation for follow-up visits
3. Poor physical environment exacerbating chronic health problems
4. Lack of motivation to work and provide for self

4 Which model of nursing care is more favorable under managed care?
1. Primary care
2. Case method
3. Client-focused care
4. Team nursing

5 A person who is over age 65 may have national health insurance called:
1. Medicaid.
2. Medi-Cal.
3. Medi-Soft.
4. Medicare.

6 Diagnostic-related groups were developed to:
1. Create physician groups that specialize in diagnostic procedures.
2. Provide special insurance for persons with disabilities.
3. Limit amounts paid to hospitals by Medicare.
4. Provide medical care for groups of people with the same diagnoses.

7 Which of the following is not considered to be a paramedical technologist?
1. Occupational therapist
2. Physiotherapist
3. Laboratory technician
4. Spiritual support person

8 One of the benefits of managed care can be to:
1. Emphasize wellness through access to a primary care physician.
2. Offer insurance companies health services for a discounted rate.
3. Increase the amount of time nurses spend with each client.
4. Provide payment to physicians for each service provided.

9 The physician's office where you work is paid monthly by the insurance company by the number of enrollees, not the service provided. You understand that the office is part of a(n):
1. IPA—independent practice association.
2. HMO—health maintenance organization.
3. PPO—preferred provider organization.
4. PHO—physician/hospital organization.

10 Preventive care such as immunizations is classified as what type of healthcare service?
1. Primary
2. Secondary
3. Tertiary
4. Prospective

Answers and rationales for Review Questions appear in Appendix I.

Complementary and Alternative Medicine in Health Care

LEARNING Outcomes

After completing this chapter, you will be able to:

1. Describe the historical basis for complementary and alternative medical therapy.
2. Define terminology used in complementary and alternative therapy.
3. Identify some nontraditional complementary and alternative medical therapies that the client may already use or that may be helpful in addition to conventional therapy.
4. Identify complementary and alternative therapies that are performed only by a trained professional.
5. Explain the reasons for eliciting information about complementary and alternative medical therapies being used by clients.
6. Demonstrate the use of the nursing process when caring for a client who uses CAM.

Clinical Objectives

7. Collect data on complementary therapies that may interact with the client's medications or treatment.
8. Provide client teaching on the importance of informing the care provider of all complementary or alternative medical therapies being used.

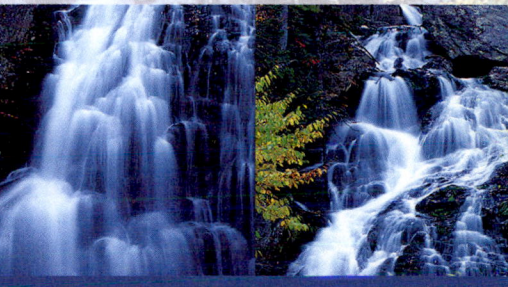

BRIEF Outline

Defining Terms Related to Complementary and Alternative Medicine
Use of CAM Therapies
CAM Therapies and Nursing Practice
Communicating with Clients about CAM Therapies

KEY TERMS

Use the audio glossary feature on the MyNursingKit Website to hear the correct pronunciation of the following key terms.

alternative medicine 121   **conventional medicine** 121   **naturopathic medicine** 121

complementary 121   **integrative medicine** 121

complementary and alternative medicine 121

More persons than ever are using complementary and alternative medicine (CAM) to self-medicate and treat various conditions. The practicing nurse needs to know about CAM therapies in order to provide safe nursing care to clients. Centuries ago many of the effective medications that were available were plant-based. Today, many popularly prescribed medications still originate from plant sources. Digitalis, from the foxglove plant, is very effective in treating some cardiac problems. Morphine, an effective pain reliever, is a derivative of the opium poppy plant. Quinidine and quinine, used to treat cardiac arrhythmias and malaria, are taken from the willow bark of certain South American trees. Ginkgo biloba, from the leaves of the ginkgo tree, is a very popular treatment for memory loss and also a potent anticoagulant. Discovery of these remedies, though made through primitive experimentation, has served the development of important modern pharmaceuticals used today.

Sometimes, medicinal properties were discovered through disaster. For example, the anticoagulant property of sweet clover was discovered while investigating deaths of cattle. In the early part of the 20th century, farmers in the northern prairie states of the United States and Canada began planting sweet clover plants brought from Europe. Although the sweet clover was nutritious when used as fodder for cattle, it also brought a fatal disease that decimated cattle herds and horrified farmers. Cattle with this disease, called *sweet clover disease*, developed uncontrolled, spontaneous bleeding. A veterinary pathologist in Alberta by the name of Schofield reported in 1921 that the disease was caused by consumption of spoiled sweet clover hay. The *fresh* clover plant, which contained the compound coumarin (a known anticoagulant), did not cause the cattle disease. The mystery of why spoiled hay caused the disease was solved by Karl Paul Link and his coworkers in 1940. They discovered that in moldy hay coumarin is oxidized to 4-hydroxycoumarin, which (coupled with formaldehyde and another coumarin component) forms dicoumarol, an anticoagulant. This chemical alteration was responsible for the disease. Dicoumarol was patented in 1941 and is still therapeutically used in humans for its anticoagulant properties.

In the United States the sale of herbal remedies to the public has been occurring for hundreds of years. In the 1800s and early 1900s traveling salesmen promoted so-called herbal-based miracle drugs. Some of these "miracle drugs" contained sugar water; others may have contained addictive substances such as opiates or alcohol.

Today many herbal remedies are marketed and sold as dietary supplements that are not subject to regulations by the U.S. Food and Drug Administration (FDA). Interestingly, until 1994 all dietary supplements were regulated as food and were evaluated for safety before being placed on the market for purchase by consumers. In 1994 Congress passed the Dietary Supplement Health and Education Act (DSHEA). This act established new regulatory guidelines for dietary supplements. As a result of this act, herbal remedies can now be sold without FDA approval.

Manufacturers of herbal remedies are not required by the FDA to submit proof of their product's safety and efficacy before the product is marketed to the public. Unlike prescription medications, which undergo clinical trials and years of testing, herbal remedies do not have to be regulated or tested for potency and purity. Also, an herbal remedy's recommended use (e.g., for allergies) may be on the label, but its side effects or potential interactions are not listed. Proof of product purity and accuracy of the amount of the herbs contained in the preparation are also not required by law on the label. In short, there are no established standards requiring information about the herbal remedy to be supplied on the product label.

Herbal remedies cannot be marketed to the public as being able to prevent, diagnose, treat, or cure disease. Nevertheless, the DSHEA permits manufacturers to label herbal remedies with statements explaining their usage and their perceived effect(s) on the human body. The FDA regulates herbal remedies in much the same way it regulates food and nutritional supplements, but herbal remedies do not have to undergo the same research protocols as prescription medications or over-the-counter medications prior to their release to the public.

Whole plants such as garlic cannot be patented, which means that no one manufacturer has exclusive rights to an herb. If the FDA has reason to suspect that an herb is unsafe, then the agency may require it to be removed from the market.

In 1998, the FDA put forth the "Regulations on Statements Made for Dietary Supplements Concerning the Effect of the Product on the Structure or Function of the Body." These regulations specifically state that "under the proposal, dietary supplements that expressly or implicitly claim to diagnose, treat, prevent, or cure a disease continue to be regarded as drugs and have to meet the safety and effectiveness standards for drugs under the Food, Drug and Cosmetic Act." Therefore, herbal remedy manufacturers can claim that the herb or product "promotes vascular health" but it cannot claim that the product "reduces blood pressure." It also cannot state what other actions the herb may have on the body (e.g., anticoagulation properties).

Many herbal product manufacturers add information to their product labeling or advertisements that includes the disclaimer that the product is not intended to diagnose, treat, cure, or prevent any disease. This disclaimer and ones similar to it keep the product from being subjected to FDA regulations. This marketing technique allows manufacturers to avoid regulations by using legally sound wording that avoids further scrutiny by the FDA.

Nurses and their clients need to be aware of the lack of regulation of herbal medications and make judgments accordingly. With this knowledge, the nurse can understand and counsel clients about the herbal medications they are taking.

Defining Terms Related to Complementary and Alternative Medicine

Conventional medicine is defined as medicine practiced by holders of a medical doctor (MD) or doctor of osteopathy (DO) degree and by other health professionals such as nurses, physical therapists, and psychologists. Some examples of areas of conventional medicine include internal medicine, cardiology, rheumatology, and oncology.

Healing philosophies, approaches, and therapies that exist largely outside the main frame of conventional treatment are known as **complementary and alternative medicine** (CAM). According to the National Center for Complementary and Alternative Medicine, a division of National Institutes of Health (NIH), CAM is a group of diverse medical and healthcare systems, practices, and products that are not considered by the Western medical model to be part of conventional medicine (National Institutes of Health, 2007). However, they often add to (*complement*) conventional medicine; hence, the name complementary. When a therapy is used together with conventional medicine, it is considered **complementary**. An example would be the use of massage to help a client who is anxious about an impending procedure to relax (Figure 8-1 ■).

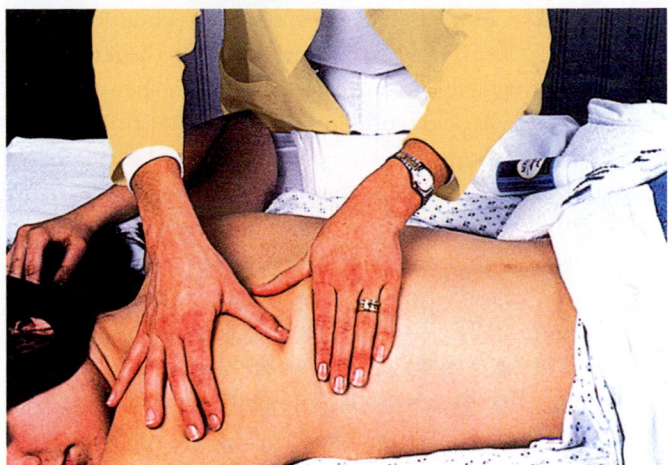

Figure 8-1. ■ Massage is a type of complementary therapy that is familiar to most people and is commonly used both inside and outside the healthcare setting.

Alternative medicine is a medical treatment used in place of conventional medicine. An example of alternative medicine would be use of a special diet as treatment for cancer. Radical dietary therapy would be used in place of the surgery, radiation, and chemotherapy that are conventional treatments recommended by physicians or surgeons.

Some healthcare providers have seen the benefits of both traditional and nontraditional medicine and have decided to practice both CAM and conventional medicine. For example, some physicians (MDs) have taken additional training as a Doctor of Naturopathic Medicine (ND). **Naturopathic medicine** is a complete alternative care system that uses a wide range of approaches to healing, such as nutrition, herbs, manipulation of the body, exercise, stress reduction, and acupuncture.

Integrative medicine is a practice that integrates treatments and therapies from conventional medicine with complementary and alternative medicines that have been deemed safe and effective. For example, the Consortium of Academic Health Centers for Integrative Medicine (2005) states that its mission is "to help transform medicine and healthcare through rigorous scientific studies, new models of clinical care, and innovative educational programs that integrate biomedicine, the complexity of human beings, the intrinsic nature of healing, and the rich diversity of therapeutic systems." This center offers alternative and complementary services in addition to conventional medicine and is physician managed. For example, the physician may prescribe massage or music therapy for clients who are undergoing chemotherapy to relax the client and release tense muscles and toxins.

Although there is scientific evidence demonstrating the benefits of some CAM therapies, for most some key questions are yet to be answered through well-designed scientific studies and research. Questions do exist about whether some CAM therapies are safe and whether they work for the diseases or medical conditions for which they are used.

Despite the lack of solid research about efficacy, there has been an upsurge in the use of herbal remedies and other products. Consider the number of herbal teas or enhanced water drinks available in most supermarkets today. There are also energy-enhancing drinks that offer a "natural energy boost." These products can cause damage in clients with preexisting conditions such as cardiac conditions (increased caffeine causes increased heart rate) and kidney disorders (possible adrenaline surge stressing the adrenal glands). Other so-called natural ingredients can be harmful to clients who have a sensitivity to those ingredients. It is important for the nurse to instruct the client to read the label and know what ingredients are being ingested.

New types of CAM are periodically introduced, so the list of what is considered to be CAM changes. The list of CAM therapies is updated as individual therapies are proved to be safe and effective and are adopted into conventional health care, and as new approaches to health care emerge. Table 8-1 ■ describes some accepted types of CAM therapy, who performs it, methods, and possible outcomes.

TABLE 8-1	Types of CAM Therapy, Providers, and Descriptions	
TYPE OF CAM	**PROVIDER OF CAM (PRACTITIONER OR CLIENT)**	**HOW IS IT DONE? WHAT DOES IT DO?**
Acupressure	Trained practitioner or self	The practitioner uses the fingers to press key points on the surface of the skin to stimulate the body's natural self-curative abilities. When these points are pressed, they release muscular tension and promote the circulation of blood and the body's life force to aid healing. Some nurses use acupressure in their practice. The client may also use these pressure points himself or herself.
Acupuncture	Trained practitioner	The practitioner uses the same points and premise as acupressure but needles are used instead of the hands to release the muscular tension and promote circulation.
Ayurveda	Trained practitioner	Ayurvedic medicine emphasizes reestablishing balance in the body through diet, lifestyle, exercise, and body cleansing, focusing on the health of the mind, body, and spirit.
Chiropractic medicine	Trained practitioner	The chiropractor uses the hands and/or devices to manipulate the spine or extremities to gain proper alignment, increased well-being, and health. Chiropractic medicine is one of the oldest healing practices.
Healing or essential oils	Trained practitioner or self	Healing or essential oils are subtle, volatile, aromatic liquids that are extracted from flowers, leaves, seeds, stems, bark, and roots of herbs, shrubs, bushes, and trees through the distillation process. They can be used for massage, diffusing, direct application (with caution), inhalation, in the bath or shower, and cleaning. Most oils come with a caution regarding use as they can cause damage to skin and mucous membranes if applied full-strength to the skin.
Herbalism or use of Chinese Medicine	Trained practitioner or self	Practice of using plant-derived preparations for therapeutic and prevention purpose.
Hypnosis	Trained practitioner or self	Carefully worded instructions are given with the goal of helping the client enter a state of deep relaxation. Some nurse anesthetists use hypnosis in the operating room either alone or as an adjunct to anesthesia.
Homeopathy	Trained practitioner or self	Treatment involves giving very small doses of substances that, according to practitioners, would produce the same or similar symptoms of illness in healthy people if they were given in larger doses. The small doses stimulate the body's immune system to effect a cure.
Magnet therapy	Usually self; can be recommended by others	Magnets can be worn, applied to the skin, or used in mattresses and shoe inserts. It is believed that magnets can increase endorphins, promote blood flow, relax muscles, improve circulation, and relieve pain.
Massage therapy	Trained practitioner, nurse, aides, or self	The therapist manipulates the muscles and other soft tissues of the body using varying pressures and movements. The intent is to relax the soft tissues, increase delivery of blood and oxygen to the massaged areas, warm them, and decrease pain. Some nurses use massage therapy in their practice.

TABLE 8-1	Types of CAM Therapy, Providers, and Descriptions (continued)	
TYPE OF CAM	**PROVIDER OF CAM (PRACTITIONER OR CLIENT)**	**HOW IS IT DONE? WHAT DOES IT DO?**
Meditation	Trained practitioner or self	Meditation is a group of techniques used by clients either for religious or cultural reasons or for health and wellness purposes. This practice is believed to result in a state of greater physical relaxation, mental calmness, and psychological balance.
Music therapy	Moderator or self	Music is played to enhance physical, mental, and emotional well-being to the listener. Some nurses use music therapy in their practice.
Naturopathy	Trained practitioner	The practitioner uses natural and least invasive methods of treatment such as hydrotherapy (water treatments), gentle exercise, herbal medications, wholesome dietary approaches, and exposure to sun and air.
Reiki	Trained practitioner or self	Reiki is a method of energy-based healing in which a practitioner lays his or her hands on the client to promote a deep sense of relaxation. Some nurses use Reiki in their practice.
Yoga, Pilates, Qigong, or Tai Chi	Trained practitioner or self	Mind-body exercises that use specific movements, breathing, and mindfulness to achieve the desired outcome, which in most cases is a disciplined mind and a toned body. Some nurses use any or all of these therapies in their practice.

Use of CAM Therapies

Approximately two-thirds of the world's population seek health care from sources other than conventional medicine. Most of them seek care from practitioners of traditional, indigenous systems of medicine, such as Ayurveda, Native American medicine, Traditional Chinese Medicine, and folk systems. Despite the diverse cultures, languages, geographic locations, and worldviews from which these medical systems originated, they have common characteristics and philosophies:

- They may use multiple botanical products in complex interventions.
- They individualize the diagnosis and treatment of clients.
- They emphasize disease prevention instead of disease treatment.
- They believe in maximizing the body's inherent healing ability.
- They treat the "whole" client (physical, mental, and spiritual) rather than a single pathology (i.e., provide *holistic care*).

The number of clients seeking CAM is growing exponentially. The reasons for this changing scenario are many (Pal, 2002). Clients want to take charge of their health and limit their costs as consumers. They do their own research or listen to family, friends, or the media to make their decisions about what therapies might work best for them and their specific conditions. Many people who believe in the value of CAM therapies self-medicate with herbs or herbal preparations. *Note:* CAM therapies are included as appropriate in Complementary Therapies boxes throughout this text (for example, Chapters 22, 29, 32, 33, and 40 ⟳).

Many healthcare facilities are offering CAM therapies to inpatients and outpatients as components of total client care. Approximately 15% of institutions are offering CAM therapies to clients as a part of their total care package or on a private-pay basis.

Many clients use CAM for daily stress management. Clients may practice meditation, controlled breathing, and massage to facilitate their healing process. Stress can contribute to illness and delay healing, and CAM can be very effective in decreasing the client's symptoms and improving the quality of life. In the healthcare environment, a common example of CAM is use of music therapy through earphones or as background to lessen client anxiety and promote relaxation.

CAM Therapies and Nursing Practice

Holistic nursing is based on some of the same philosophies and theories that underlie CAM therapies. Nurses often integrate complementary therapies (such as non-pharmacologic methods of pain relief) as part of nursing practice. Nurses care for the physical, emotional, and spiritual concerns of the client. Thus, the nurse addresses the needs of the whole client rather than an isolated part.

As more clients use a variety of CAM therapies, nurses need to become more knowledgeable about them. Approximately half of the state boards of nursing recognize that CAM therapies are a part of nursing practice and include provisions for the safe practice of these modalities by nurses (Sparber, 2001).

Nurses must have an understanding of CAM therapies. Clients may want to continue using their therapies while in the healthcare facility as their condition permits. The nurse may be asked to administer herbal medications, topical herbal preparations, or supplements to clients. Also, the nurse may be asked to assist clients in providing the setting for religious or ethnic healing practices within the healthcare facility or in the home. Box 8-1 ■ provides a few traditional herbal preparations from different cultures.

CAM practices can influence client signs and symptoms. They have the potential to interfere with prescription medications or medical regimens. They can also affect intra- or postoperative outcomes (Fessenden, 2001). The nurse who has knowledge of these therapies can look at the whole picture instead of just one piece of the puzzle.

Communicating with Clients about CAM Therapies

It is important for the nurse to establish a caring relationship with the client so that information can be shared openly. The nurse asks whether the client is using any CAM therapies on a regular basis. This must be done in a nonjudgmental manner so that the client feels free to share information.

In certain situations, knowledge of CAM therapy may be life saving. For example, if the client is scheduled for surgery (see Chapter 29 ⊙⊙), the nurse must establish which herbal medicines or supplements the client is taking. Many herbal preparations contain *anticoagulant* (blood-thinning) properties. If the client is being prepared for surgery and is taking ginkgo biloba daily for memory loss, the nurse needs to know that this herb has anticoagulant properties. The continued use of this herb until surgery can result in excessive bleeding intraoperatively.

It is recommended that the client stop taking all anticoagulant preparations at least 2 weeks before a scheduled surgery. In this situation, use of the herbal medication is a significant piece of information that could create complications during and after surgery (Cheng, 2002). Table 8-2 ■ provides information about common herbal remedies that have anticoagulant properties.

The nurse will also determine other CAM therapies the client practices. For example, if the client practices yoga, Qigong, Tai Chi, or Pilates on a regular basis and is scheduled for abdominal surgery, the client will need teaching to refrain from these exercises for a period of time postoperatively. Yoga (Figure 8-2 ■), Qigong, Tai Chi, and Pilates are all examples of mind-body methods of toning the body (NIH, 2006). They use specific body movements that may seriously injure a postoperative surgical client who has had major abdominal surgery.

BOX 8-1	CULTURAL PULSE POINTS

Selected CAM Therapies for Common Ailments

The following complementary therapies are used in other cultures for common ailments. Note that practices in other cultures may *complement* (add to) pharmaceutical methods to include cultural remedies, as in the Philippines below.

China

In China, a few slices of ginger and the roots of two to three green onions are diced and brought to a boil with two cups of water. The mixture is simmered for about 20 minutes; then the person drinks the broth. This remedy is recommended at the first sign of cold or fever.

Ginger is used to ease an upset stomach, including morning and motion sickness, and to aid in digestion. It is also used to relieve symptoms of irritable bowel syndrome and other intestinal afflictions.

Philippines

In the Philippines, besides using a fever reducer such as aspirin for a cold or fever, the juice of five squeezed calamansis (part of the citrus family) is prepared. It is mixed with half a cup of water. Sugar may be added to the preparation for children since it can be quite sour.

A washcloth soaked in warm water and vinegar or just vinegar may be placed on the forehead at night to "draw out" fever. In the northern Philippines (Ilocos), a folk remedy for fever was to harvest young leaves from a fruit tree (atis leaves), salt them, and apply them to the forehead.

For stomach problems such as diarrhea, there are several remedies:

- a mixture of one cup of sarsaparilla, one tablespoon of flour, and an egg
- the tea of boiled guava leaves
- the brew of the lining of chicken intestines, washed, dried, and ground into a texture similar to coffee grounds

For flatulence, an oil called *aceite de manzanilla* was rubbed on the stomach, and the stomach was tapped to relieve gas and bloating.

Russia

In Russia, a spoonful of honey in warm water is drunk before lying down to rest. Hot tea is a must, though cold drinks can also be drunk. Dressing warmly and staying indoors are necessary for prevention of and recovery from sickness.

Raspberry "varenie," a liquid jam, is used to prevent colds by taking a tablespoon a day.

TABLE 8-2 Common Herbs with Anticoagulant Properties

HERB NAME (COMMON AND *SCIENTIFIC*)	COMMON USES	SIDE EFFECTS	DRUG INTERACTIONS OR CONTRAINDICATIONS
Black cohosh (*Cimicifuga racemosa*)	Premenstrual discomfort, dysmenorrhea, menopausal symptoms	GI discomfort	Anticoagulants, antiplatelets
Butcher's broom (*Ruscus aculeatus*)	Circulatory disorders, leg cramps, inflammation, hemorrhoids, varicose veins	GI discomfort, nausea	Anticoagulants, antiplatelets, monoamine oxidase inhibitor (MAOI)
Catnip (*Nepeta cataria*)	Migraine, anxiety, colic, common cold, digestive disorders, influenza	Headache, GI discomfort	-May increase effects of sedatives and alcohol if used concurrently -Should not be used during pregnancy because of mild uterine stimulant action
Cat's claw (*Uncaria tomentosa*)	Birth control, cancer treatment, GI disorders, inflammation, HIV, AIDS	Diarrhea, lower blood pressure	Antihypertensives, anticoagulants, antiplatelets
Chamomile (*Matricaria chamomilla*)	Colic, GI disorders, spasms, infections, intestinal gas, inflammation, skin ulcers	Allergic reaction in people with sensitivity to ragweed; is known abortifacient—should not be used during pregnancy	Anticoagulants, antiplatelets, sedatives
Devil's claw (*Harpagophytum procumbens*)	Arteriosclerosis, arthritis, inflammation, muscle pain, osteoarthritis	Diarrhea, possible slow pulse rate	Antacids/H2 antagonist, beta-blockers, anticoagulants
Dong quai (*Angelica sinensis*)	Dysmenorrhea, PMS, menopausal symptoms	Photosensitivity	Anticoagulants
Fenugreek (*Trigonella foenum-graecum*)	GI complaints; topically: promotes wound healing	Bleeding, hypoglycemia	Anticoagulants, antidiabetic agents
Garlic (*Allium sativum*)	Decrease cholesterol, circulatory disorders, hypertension	Headache, fatigue, potential for bleeding, sweating, hypoglycemia	Insulin and hypoglycemic drugs, anticoagulant, antiplatelets
Ginger (*Zingiber officinale*)	Antioxidant, motion sickness, sore throat, nausea, vomiting, migraine headaches	Nausea, vomiting, skin hypersensitivity	-Anticoagulants, antiplatelets, may increase absorption of oral medications -Should not be used in pregnancy due to abortifacient effects
Ginko (*Ginkgo biloba*)	Asthma, bronchitis, heart disease, memory loss	Headache, dizziness, GI upset, subarachnoid hemorrhage, palpitations	Anticoagulants, antiplatelets, antipsychotics, MAOI
Ginseng, Asian (*Panax ginseng*)	Diabetes, health maintenance, cancer, clotting, strength, stamina	Headache, tachycardia, nausea, vomiting, diarrhea, insomnia	Anticoagulants, insulin, MAOI
Goldenseal (*Hydrastis canadensis*)	Digestive aid, expectorant, postpartum hemorrhage, improve bile secretion	GI distress, hallucinations, delirium	Antihypertensives, anticoagulants, antiplatelets, barbiturates
Horse chestnut (*Aesculus hippocastanum*)	Varicose veins, circulatory disorders, hemorrhoids, diarrhea, phlebitis	GI distress, muscle twitching, paralysis	Anticoagulants, antiplatelets
Pau d'arco (*Tabebuia impetiginosa*)	Ulcers, diarrhea, rheumatism, cancers, inflammation	GI distress, dizziness, anemia, bleeding	Anticoagulants, antiplatelets
Red clover (*Trifolium pratense*)	Respiratory congestion, spasms, cancers, menopausal symptoms	Breast tenderness, weight gain, allergic reactions (hives, swelling)	Anticoagulants, antiplatelets
Sweet clover (*Melilotus officinalis*)	Blunt injuries, hemorrhoids, venous conditions	Headache, stupor, possible liver damage	Anticoagulants
Turmeric (*Amomum curcuma*)	Dyspepsia, bloating, flatulence, headaches	GI distress	Anticoagulants, antiplatelets
Willow bark (*Salix alba*)	Migraines, fever, arthritis, inflammation, pain, influenza	GI distress, tinnitus, renal damage	Anticoagulants, antiplatelets, NSAIDs

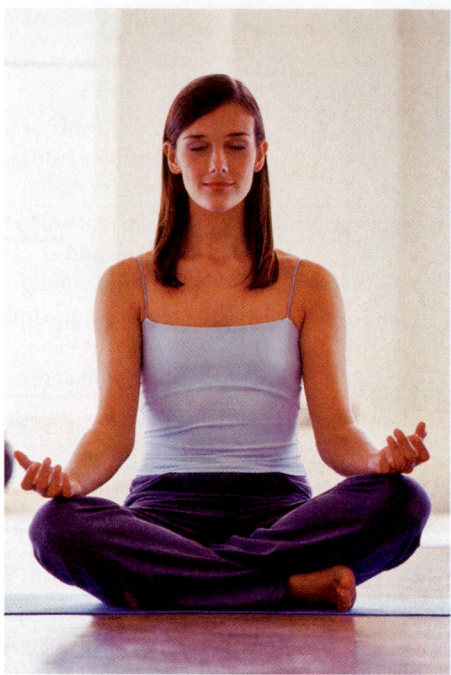

Figure 8-2. ■ Yoga can provide healing relaxation to an anxious client. However, caution would be required if a client had had recent abdominal surgery, because some yoga postures or deep breathing could strain an incision. *Source:* Getty Images Inc.—Stone Allstock.

NURSING CARE

PRIORITIZING NURSING CARE

The first priority in nursing care of the client who uses CAM therapies is to determine what type of treatment the client is using. Is the client using herbal medicines, and will their use affect or interact with the client's medical treatment? Knowing what CAM therapies the client is using will help the nurse determine whether there is potential for interactions or alterations in care or healing.

ASSESSING

When LPNs/LVNs are assigned the responsibility of collecting data about the client's use of CAM therapies, they must develop a method for gaining this information. This information is not necessarily on the client's chart and may not have been determined before the client's admission to the facility. The LPN/LVN must review the client's chart, including the medication history, to see if any notes were taken about CAM therapies. Often clients are reluctant to tell healthcare professionals about their use of herbs or other CAM therapies because they fear admonishment. Also, they may not realize the importance of providing this information to the nurse

Ginkgo Biloba and Asthma

Because herbal medications are advertised as "safe," parents seeking remedies for a child with asthma may give the child ginkgo biloba for relief of the asthma. Unfortunately, ginkgo biloba can cause headaches, dizziness, hemorrhage, and possible heart palpitations. Parents should be aware of potential side effects of herbal medications. They should always verify with the primary care provider that the herbal preparations are suitable for children.

or primary care provider. Review the communication skills in Chapter 11 ⚭ for ways to ask for information from clients.

Many healthcare professionals still consider herbal medications safe and do not see the need to ask the client. However, research has shown that CAM therapies can have a profound impact on concurrent medical care. Ignoring this information can be harmful or fatal to the client. Box 8-2 ■ illustrates a situation in which CAM therapy should not be used in children.

When asking the client questions about CAM usage, the nurse must use terminology that the client understands, and that is nonjudgmental.

DIAGNOSING, PLANNING, AND IMPLEMENTING

Nursing diagnoses for use of complementary and alternative medicine include the following:

- Deficient Knowledge
- Risk for Injury

Client outcomes for a client who uses CAM would include that the client will:

- Understand that procedures such as surgery can be affected by herbal medications, and will know possible side effects.
- Report use of CAM therapies to the registered nurse. *The LPN/LVN is responsible for reporting any CAM therapies the client is using if the CAM therapies may be detrimental to the client's well-being.*
- Make use of available resources to understand the CAM therapies they are using. As with the administration of any medication, the nurse checks for potential allergies, side effects, and interactions. If the client asks to keep taking herbal medications that are dangerous to the client's present condition, the LPN/LVN reports this desire to the supervising nurse. *Using resources to understand the effects of herbal preparations will*

increase the nurse's knowledge. Even though the medications are considered herbal and "safe," the nurse still must follow the standards of care regarding medication administration.

■ Reinforce client teaching (see Chapter 12 🔗) about the CAM therapies the client is using, and educate the client about potential risks related to their use while in the facility or during the postoperative period. *LPNs/LVNs have a responsibility to answer questions and reinforce teaching.*

■ If it is determined that the CAM therapy practiced by the client will not be harmful, the LPN/LVN documents continuation of the CAM. *Reporting and documenting provide continuity of care.*

EVALUATING

If the client is permitted to continue CAM herbal use, the nurse must observe the client for side effects of herbal medications. If the client is permitted to practice CAM therapy (e.g., yoga, Tai Chi), the nurse assesses the client for adverse reactions. If side effects or adverse reactions are noted, the nurse reports these to the RN and primary care provider. The administration of herbal medications or practice of any types of CAM in the clinical setting must be documented on the client's chart.

NURSING PROCESS CARE PLAN
CAM Therapy Use by Clients

Nancy Case is a 28-year-old runner who has just been admitted to the unit for preoperative assessment for repair of her torn right Achilles tendon tomorrow.

Assessment

Client is admitted with crutches to the unit. She has an elastic bandage on her right foot/ankle area. The bandage is dry and intact. She brings a bag of herbal medications with her and explains that she wants to continue taking them while in the hospital. She says she has been taking these medications up until yesterday. In the bag are the following: black cohosh, chamomile, ginkgo biloba, and sweet clover. She also has aspirin in the bag. When questioned about other medication intake, she states these medications are the only ones she takes. She explains the reasons she is using each herbal medication and states she "feels better" when she takes them.

Nursing Diagnosis

The following important nursing diagnoses (among others) are established for this client:

■ Risk for Bleeding during the perioperative period because of the herbal medications she is taking.

■ Deficient Knowledge regarding the side effects and potential for bleeding during surgery related to the continued herbal medication intake.

Expected Outcomes

■ Surgery may have to be postponed.

■ If surgery continues as scheduled, the anesthesia provider, surgeon, and members of the surgical team will have to be alerted to the potential for intra- and postoperative bleeding.

■ The client will remain free from adverse reactions.

Planning and Implementation

■ Notify the RN of the potential for complications related to herbal medication intake. *Ginkgo biloba is an anticoagulant and should have been stopped 2 weeks prior to surgery.*

■ Educate the client about the potential for bleeding from the herbal medications she is taking and explain why she should not take them while in the hospital or until her surgeon tells her she can resume. *Understanding improves compliance.*

Evaluation

Client verbalized understanding about the side effects of the herbal medications. Surgical team was prepared for potential bleeding risks during surgery. Bleeding was controlled during surgery. Discharge planning was initiated. Client teaching was reinforced about the risks of herbal medication intake until cleared by the surgeon.

Critical Thinking in the Nursing Process

1. What questions would the nurse ask of the client who reports using some form of CAM therapies in self-treatment?

2. What specific CAM therapies should the nurse be alerted to when caring for clients in the clinical setting, specifically preoperative and labor settings?

3. Why would the nurse report a client's continued use of ginkgo biloba?

Note: Discussion of Critical Thinking questions appears on the MyNursingKit Website.

Note: The references and resources for all chapters have been compiled at the back of the book.

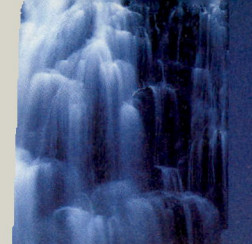

Chapter Review

KEY Points

- Conventional medicine is defined as medicine practiced by an MD, DO, nurses, physical therapists, psychologists, and other healthcare professionals.

- Massage therapy is an example of a nontraditional complementary therapy used to help relax a client who is anxious about a surgical procedure.

- Alternative medicine is a medical treatment used in place of conventional medicine such as use of a special diet as an adjunct treatment for cancer.

- Naturopathic medicine is a complete alternative care system that uses a wide range of approaches to healing, such as nutrition, herbs, manipulation of the body, exercise, stress reduction, and acupuncture.

- Nurses should elicit information about any complementary and alternative medical therapies used by clients to determine why the client is using the specific therapy, to determine possible underlying illnesses, and to make sure the client is not in danger of possible side effects or reactions from the therapies.

- Healthcare professionals who assist clients with their CAM therapies are listed in Table 8-1.

∞ FOR FURTHER Study

Review the communication skills in Chapter 11 for ways to ask for information from clients.

The main discussion of client teaching is in Chapter 12.

Care of the client who is having surgery is discussed in Chapter 29.

CAM therapies are included as appropriate in Complementary Therapies boxes throughout this text (for example, Chapters 22, 29, 32, 33, and 40).

PEARSON
EXPLORE mynursingkit™

MyNursingKit is your one stop for online chapter review materials and resources. Prepare for success with additional NCLEX®-style practice questions, interactive assignments and activities, web links, animations and videos, and more!

Register your access code from the front of your book at
www.mynursingkit.com

Critical Thinking Care Map

Caring for a Client Who Uses CAM Therapies

NCLEX-PN® Focus Area: Physiological Integrity

Case Study: Suzanne, a 28-year-old, gravida 4, para 0, has had several miscarriages in the past 5 years and tearfully confides her depression about whether she will ever have a child. When asked about herbal supplementation use, she tells the nurse that she drinks chamomile tea four times a day.

Nursing Diagnosis: Deficient Knowledge related to herbal medicine intake.

COLLECT DATA

Subjective	Objective
_____	_____
_____	_____
_____	_____
_____	_____
_____	_____
_____	_____
_____	_____

Would you report this? Yes/No

If yes, report to: _____

What would you report?_____

Nursing Care

_____
_____
_____
_____
_____
_____
_____
_____
_____

How would you document this? _____
_____
_____
_____

Compare your answers and documentation to those provided on the MyNursingKit Website.

Data Collected
(use only those that apply)

- Drinks 4 cups of chamomile tea per day
- Four miscarriages in 5 years
- Client is wanting to drink more water for hydration
- Client appears depressed, is crying
- Client's mother visits her twice a day
- Chamomile is a known abortifacient
- Client's husband is supportive of his wife

Nursing Interventions
(use only those that apply; list in priority order)

- Refer client to physician
- Educate client about side effects of chamomile
- Raise side rails when client is sleeping
- Document client's intake of chamomile
- Offer coffee instead of tea to the client
- Note client's statements about depression
- Provide pamphlet regarding common herbal medications and side effects
- Refer client to group therapy

NCLEX-PN® Exam Preparation

1 The nurse, teaching a community class on supplements, makes a correct statement when saying:

1. "Dietary supplements have never been regulated and are not regulated today."
2. "Dietary supplements are not regulated by the FDA but they are regulated as food and evaluated for safety."
3. "The Dietary Supplement Health and Education Act established regulatory guidelines for dietary supplements but are not regulated by the FDA."
4. "Dietary supplements do not need to be regulated because they are harmless."

2 The client with cancer chose nutrition, herbs, manipulation of the body, exercise, stress reduction, and acupuncture instead of conventional Western medical treatment. This client is using:

1. Integrative medicine.
2. Naturopathic medicine.
3. Complementary medicine.
4. Complementary and alternative medicine.

3 The client tells the nurse that she practices Ayurveda. This form of CAM, offered by a trained practitioner, involves:

1. The insertion of needles into specific pressure points to release muscular tension and promote circulation.
2. Subtle, volatile aromatic liquids extracted from flowers, leaves, seeds, and other plants used for massage, inhalation, direct application, and cleaning.
3. Manipulation of the spine or extremities to gain proper alignment and to increase well-being.
4. Reestablishing balance in the body through diet, lifestyle, exercise, and body cleansing focusing on the health of mind, body, and spirit.

4 In a physician's office, the nurse collecting admission history data asks if the client takes any medications. When the client responds, "No," the next question should be:

1. "Do you take any over-the-counter medications, dietary supplements, or herbal medicines?"
2. "Do you have any allergies?"
3. "You don't take any medications of any kind?"
4. "Can you tell me what brings you to the doctor today?"

5 Which of the following treatments require the use of a trained practitioner? (Select all that apply.)

1. Acupressure
2. Acupuncture
3. Chiropractic medicine
4. Naturopathy
5. Magnet therapy

6 The nurse in acute care discovers that a client did not disclose complementary therapy and supplements previously. Which of the following statements would be appropriate for the nurse to make at this time?

1. "Although supplements and complementary therapy can be very helpful, it is very important for you to inform us of them, because they can have an impact on your plan of care."
2. "Oh, I take St. John's wort as well. Does it work for you?"
3. "You should never take supplemental medication without your physician permission. It could be dangerous."
4. "When did you start taking these supplements?"

7 What is the nurse's primary role in complementary and alternative therapy?

1. Nurses are not involved. The client should seek complementary and alternative therapy from other providers.
2. Nurses should provide holistic care, integrating complementary therapies into their plan of care.
3. Nurses coordinate with alternative healthcare providers who work with the client.
4. Nurses should learn more about CAM so they can explain the dangers of these therapies to the client.

8 The LPN/LVN is caring for a newly admitted client with a medical diagnosis of GI bleeding. The client reports taking supplements including garlic, ginkgo biloba, and ginseng. The nurse's priority action would be to:

1. Inform the RN of the client's use of supplements because they may be contributing to the client's medical condition.
2. Instruct the client to stop taking these medications immediately and explain that the medical condition is caused by supplement use.
3. Continue gathering information from the client because there is nothing significant in this information.
4. Explain to the client that by taking these supplements she is poisoning herself.

9 The mother of a 3-year-old child diagnosed with asthma says, "I've read that ginkgo biloba can be helpful for children with asthma. What do you think?" The nurse's best response would be:

1. "I've heard that some children get great results from ginkgo, but I don't know for sure if it works."
2. "Don't use supplements. They are very dangerous."
3. "You can talk to the primary provider about that, but he's going to tell you not to take supplements."
4. "Some supplements can cause unexpected side effects. I suggest you discuss this supplement with the provider."

10 Which would be an appropriate nursing outcome for a client who uses complementary and alternative medicines?

1. The client stops using all complementary and alternative medications.
2. The client stops taking complementary and alternative medications 12 hours prior to surgery.
3. The client understands the potential side effects and uses of complementary and alternative medications he is using.
4. The client understands potential risks of complementary and alternative medications.

Answers and rationales for Review Questions appear in Appendix I.

Chapter 9

Safety

LEARNING Outcomes

After completing this chapter, you will be able to:

1. Discuss factors that affect safety and people's ability to protect themselves from injury.
2. List points for client teaching about safety across the life span.
3. Identify common preventable injuries in the home and in healthcare settings.
4. Name institutional strategies for maintaining safety.
5. List triage and emergency codes that are used in healthcare settings.
6. Describe the use and legal implications of restraints.
7. Name several alternatives to restraints.
8. Identify ways to prevent self-injury while delivering client care.
9. List strategies for self-protection in violent or potentially violent situations.

Clinical Objectives

10. Provide safety teaching for clients of various ages.
11. Demonstrate proper body mechanics for lifting and transferring clients.

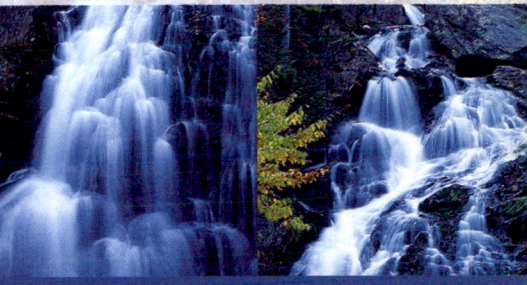

BRIEF Outline

Factors that Affect Safety
Preventing Specific Hazards
Hospital and Institutional Safety
Restraining Clients
Body Mechanics for Nurses
Protection from Violence in the Healthcare Setting

A fundamental concern of nurses, which extends from the bedside to the home and to the community, is prevention of injury, as well as assisting the injured. Motor vehicle crashes, falls, drowning, fire and burns, poisoning, inhalation and ingestion of foreign objects, and firearm use are major causes of injury and death.

Nurses need to be aware of what constitutes a safe environment for a particular person, or for a group of people, in a variety of healthcare settings. Injuries that are caused by human conduct, such as carelessness, impulsiveness, or poor judgment, can often be prevented.

Factors that Affect Safety

The ability of people to protect themselves from injury is affected by such factors as age and development, lifestyle, mobility and health status, sensory–perceptual alterations, cognitive awareness, emotional state, ability to communicate, safety awareness, and the environment. Nurses need to assess each of these factors when they plan care or teach clients to protect themselves.

AGE AND DEVELOPMENT

Through knowledge and accurate assessment of the environment, people learn to protect themselves from many injuries. Young children's curiosity often exceeds their judgment. However, through knowledge and experience, children do learn what is safe and what is potentially harmful. Elderly people can have difficulty with movement, thought processes, and diminished senses, which contribute to the likelihood of injury.

Measures to ensure the safety of people of all ages focus on two things:

1. Observation or prediction of potentially harmful situations so that injury can be avoided.
2. Client education that empowers clients to safeguard themselves and their families from injury.

Specific age-related potential hazards and preventive measures are discussed later in this chapter. See Box 9-1 ■ for safety measures for each age group. Box 9-2 ■ describes cultural issues related to safety.

LIFESTYLE

Lifestyle factors that place people at risk include unsafe work environments; residence in neighborhoods with high crime rates; access to guns and ammunition; insufficient income to buy safety equipment or make necessary repairs; and access to illicit drugs, which may also be contaminated by harmful additives. Risk-taking behavior is a factor in some accidents.

MOBILITY AND HEALTH STATUS

People who have impaired mobility due to paralysis, muscle weakness, and poor balance or coordination are obviously prone to injury. Clients with spinal cord injury and paralysis of both legs may be unable to move even when they perceive discomfort. Hemiplegic clients or clients with leg casts often have poor balance and fall easily. Clients weakened by illness or surgery are not always fully aware of their condition. Clients using any mind-altering medications, such as narcotics or antidepressants, are at risk for injury due to lack of coordination or impaired judgment.

SENSORY–PERCEPTUAL ALTERATIONS

Accurate sensory perception of environmental stimuli is vital to safety. People with impaired touch perception, hearing, taste, smell, and vision are highly susceptible to injury. A person who does not see well may trip over a toy or not see an electric cord. People with impaired hearing may not hear a siren in traffic, and people with impaired olfactory sense may not smell burning food or escaping gas. Elderly clients may elect to not have their cataracts removed and corrected; so their vision will be poor. Those with hearing aids may limit the purchase of the replacement batteries due to the cost or may not use them unless they go out to functions to conserve the battery source.

COGNITIVE AWARENESS

Awareness is the ability to perceive environmental stimuli and body reactions and to respond appropriately through thought and action. Clients with impaired awareness include people lacking in sleep, unconscious or semiconscious persons, disoriented people (i.e., those who may not understand

(Text continues on p.135.)

BOX 9-1   LIFESPAN CONSIDERATIONS

Safety Measures Throughout the Life Span

Newborns and Infants (Ages 0–12 months)

- Use a federally approved car seat at all times (including coming home from the hospital). Place children in the back seat when traveling in a car. (The middle of the back seat is recommended if the car seat can fit in the car.) If the child must ride in the front seat, ensure that the car seat is facing toward the rear of the car and the seat is positioned as far from the dashboard as possible. The air bag on the passenger side of the front seat should also be disengaged in this situation.
- Never leave the infant unattended in a vehicle.
- Never leave the infant unattended on a raised surface.
- Check the temperature of the infant's bathwater and formula by using the inside of your wrist.
- Hold the infant upright during feeding. Do not prop the bottle. Cut soft, easily swallowed, or dissolvable foods into small pieces, and do not feed the infant peanuts, raisins, or popcorn.
- Investigate the infant's crib for compliance with federal safety regulations: slats no more than $2\frac{3}{8}$ inches apart, lead-free paint, height of crib sides, and a tight fit of mattress to crib. Use crib sheets that are tight-fitting; avoid stuffed animals in cribs or bassinets.
- Use a playpen with sides made of small-sized netting. Never leave playpen sides down.
- Provide large, soft toys with no small detachable or sharp-edged parts. Read the labels on packages for age-appropriate toys.
- Use guard gates on stairs and screens on windows. Supervise the infant in the walker, swing, and highchair.
- Cover electric outlets. Coil cords out of reach.
- Place plants, household cleaners, and wastebaskets out of reach. Lock away potential poisons, such as medicines, paint, and gasoline.

Toddlers (Ages 1–3 years)

- Continue to use a federally approved car seat or seat belts at all times, and make sure they are properly inserted in the vehicles. In most communities, the police, fire, or rescue departments have personnel trained to inspect car seats and their insertion stability for safety of the children.
- Teach children not to put objects in the mouth, including pills (unless given by parent).
- Keep objects with sharp edges (such as furniture and knives) out of children's reach. Pad corners of fireplaces or other sharp items, such as coffee tables or end tables, in the home or simply remove them until the child is older.
- Place hot pots on back burners with handles turned inward.
- Teach toddlers to avoid the fireplace or other heating sources in the home, especially the floor grates and kerosene heaters.
- Keep cleaning solutions, insecticides, and medicines in locked cupboards.
- Keep windows and balconies screened. Keep cribs or beds away from windows that are screened to prevent a child from falling through the screen. Make sure the

balconies or decks are properly installed with proper width between the rails.
- Teach children to swim. Fence in pools with locks, and supervise at all times. Do not overfill the bathtub. Do not let toddlers play near ditches or wells.
- Teach children not to run or ride a tricycle, scooters, or roller blades into the street or on decks with stairs or without safety railings or gates.
- Obtain a low bed when the child begins to climb.
- Cover outlets with safety covers or plugs.

Preschoolers (Ages 3–5 years)

- Do not allow children to run with candy or other objects in the mouth.
- Teach children not to put small objects in the mouth, nose, and ears.
- Remove doors from unused equipment, such as refrigerators.
- Teach preschoolers to cross streets safely and obey traffic signals.
- Check Halloween treats before allowing children to eat them. Discard loose or open candy.
- Teach children to play in safe areas, not on streets and railroad tracks.
- Teach preschoolers the dangers of playing with matches and playing near barbeque grills, fire, and heating appliances.
- Teach children to keep parents informed of their whereabouts and to avoid strangers. Have child fingerprinted or videotaped for identification purposes. Ask that health fairs or police department community functions provide this service and teach children the importance of safety. Arrange with a neighbor (or someone in the community) to volunteer to be a safe place for the child to seek help in case of any fears or threats from strangers.
- Teach preschoolers not to walk in front of swings and not to push others off playground equipment.
- Teach parents to reinforce the importance of proper child restraints in vehicles.

School-Age Children (Ages 5–12 years)

- Teach children safety rules for recreational and sports activities: Never swim alone; always wear a life jacket when in a boat; and wear a protective helmet and knee and elbow pads when needed, especially with bicycles, scooters, roller blades, skateboards, and motorized equipment.
- Supervise contact sports and activities in which children aim at a target (e.g., archery or darts). Inspect playground equipment and sports equipment prior to participation. For example, children have been injured or died when soccer goals that were not anchored properly fell over onto children while playing.
- Teach children to obey all traffic and safety rules for bicycling, skateboarding, and roller-skating. Reinforce the importance of safety restraints in vehicles.
- Teach children to use a flashing light or reflective clothing when walking or cycling at night.
- Teach children safe ways to use the stove, garden tools, and other equipment.

MyNursingKit | Lead poisoning

- Supervise children when they use saws, electric appliances, tools, and other potentially dangerous equipment.
- Teach children not to play with fireworks, gunpowder, or firearms. Keep firearms unloaded, locked up, and out of reach. Keep ammunition locked up in a separate place from the firearms.
- Teach children to avoid excavations, quarries, vacant buildings, and playing around heavy machinery.
- Teach children the effects of drugs and alcohol on judgment and coordination.

Adolescents (Ages 13–18 years)
- Have adolescents complete a driver's education course, and take practice drives with them in various kinds of weather. For example, industrial parking lots (on weekends) or vacant parking lots are recommended as practice driving areas.
- Reinforce the importance of safety restraints in the vehicle while driving and the need to ensure that all passengers are properly restrained before moving the vehicle.
- Limit the passenger load of other teens, especially when the teen is inexperienced. Set firm limits on automobile use, namely, never to drive after drinking or using drugs, and never to ride with a driver who has done so. Encourage adolescents to call home for a ride if they have been drinking, assuring them they can do so without a reprimand.
- Teach the young adult the importance of not using tobacco products and the hazards of their use.
- Teach adolescents to avoid using the cell phone for calls and not to send text messages while driving. Many crashes are tied to cell phone use, CD players, and other distractions from the road.
- Teach adolescents to wear a safety helmet when riding motorcycles, scooters, and other sports vehicles. Teach safety rules for water sports.
- Encourage adolescents to use proper equipment when participating in sports. Schedule a physical examination before participation, and be certain there is medical supervision for all athletic activities.
- Encourage adolescents to swim, jog, and go boating in groups so they can obtain help in case of an emergency. Explain the reasons to avoid drinking alcohol while boating.
- Teach rules for hunting and the proper care, storage, and use of firearms. Avoid alcohol while using hunting equipment. Blaze orange vests or hats are a necessity when hunting.
- Inform the adolescent of the dangers of drugs, alcohol, and unprotected sex. Be alert to changes in the adolescent's mood and behavior. Listen to and maintain open communication with the adolescent. Open communication is a powerful preventive measure.
- Remember to set a good example of behavior that the adolescent can follow.

Young Adults (Ages 19–40 years)
- Reinforce motor vehicle safety: Drive defensively, use "designated drivers" if alcohol is consumed, routinely check brakes and tires, and use seat and shoulder belts or age-appropriate car seats for all passengers.

- Remind the young adult to repair potential fire hazards, such as faulty electric wiring and overuse of extension cords.
- Reinforce to the young adult the importance of not using tobacco products and the hazards of their use, especially around their children or those with health issues.
- Teach water safety: know the depth of a pool before diving; supervise backyard pools and other water activities.
- Discuss evaluating the potential for workplace injuries or death when making decisions about a career or occupation. Encourage the young adult to participate actively in programs that reduce occupational hazards.
- Discuss avoiding excessive sun radiation by limiting exposure, using sun-blocking agents, and wearing protective clothing. Explain the skin changes that may indicate a cancerous condition.
- Encourage young adults who are unable to cope with the pressures, responsibilities, and expectations of adulthood to seek counseling. Encourage counseling or treatment for any addiction problems.

Middle-Aged Adults (Ages 40–65 years)
- Reinforce motor vehicle safety: Use seat belts and drive within the speed limit. Test visual acuity periodically.
- Make certain stairways and walkways are well lighted and uncluttered.
- Equip bathrooms with grab bars and nonskid bath mats.
- Test smoke detectors and fire alarms and replace batteries regularly, such as every 3 to 6 months.
- Keep all machines and tools in good working condition at work and at home. Follow safety precautions when using machinery.
- Advocate regular exercise of the person's choice and healthful diet to maintain a strong body.

Older Adults (Ages 66+ years)
- Encourage the client to have regular vision and hearing tests.
- Assist the client with setting up a home hazard appraisal, such as limiting the use of rugs, lighting at night and on stairs, temperature control on hot water heaters, etc.
- Encourage the client to keep as active as possible.
- Teach clients to beware of phone or selling scamming, such as home repairs or paying money for a reward, etc. For example, remind the elderly to be alert of phone calls or home visits asking for money to do a particular job, such as paving or sealing the driveway or selling magazines. The elderly want to help people and are very vulnerable to these requests. Make suggestions to post a "No Solicitors" sign on their front doors or entrances to their neighborhoods.
- Teach the elderly to keep doors locked at all times and to not answer the door to someone they may not know or when not expecting someone to call, especially in the evenings and at night.
- Encourage those who live alone to subscribe to an alarm system for falls or illnesses, such as the "LifeLine" services; or to arrange to have a family member or neighbor check on the client regularly.

where they are or what to do to help themselves), people who perceive stimuli that do not exist, and people whose judgment is altered by disease or medications (such as narcotics, tranquilizers, hypnotics, and sedatives). Mildly confused clients may momentarily forget where they are, wander from their rooms, take an extra dose of medication, or misplace personal belongings.

EMOTIONAL STATE

Extreme emotional states can alter the ability to perceive environmental hazards. Stressful situations can reduce a person's level of concentration, cause errors of judgment, and decrease awareness of external stimuli. Depressed people may think and react to environmental stimuli more slowly than usual.

ABILITY TO COMMUNICATE

People with diminished ability to receive and convey information are also at risk for injury. Aphasic clients, people with language barriers, and those unable to read are among them. For example, a person who cannot interpret the sign "No smoking—Oxygen in use" may cause a fire.

SAFETY AWARENESS

Information is crucial to safety. Clients in unfamiliar environments frequently need specific safety information. Lack of knowledge about unfamiliar equipment, such as oxygen tanks, intravenous tubing, and hot pads/packs, is a potential hazard. Healthy clients need knowledge about

water safety, car safety, fire prevention, ways to prevent the ingestion of harmful substances, and preventive measures for age-related hazards.

ENVIRONMENT

The environment in which people live and work can increase their risk for injury. Nurses should assess the home environment for potential hazards such as living in an area where there are environmental contaminants from chemicals and other industrial wastes. Nurses should encourage parents to remove all mercury thermometers from the home and replace with a digital thermometer. In addition, parents should be instructed to avoid smoking due to the risks of secondhand smoke. In the employment setting, nurses should assess the environment for exposure to hazardous chemicals through inhalation or contact, dangerous equipment, and excessive noise.

Preventing Specific Hazards

Measures to prevent specific hazards or injuries (such as burns, fire, poisoning, falls, suffocation, excessive noise, electrocution, and radiation injury) are critical aspects of nursing care. Teaching clients about safety is another important aspect. Nurses usually have opportunities to teach while providing care.

SCALDS AND BURNS

A **scald** is a burn from a hot liquid or vapor, such as steam. A burn results from excessive exposure to thermal, chemical, electric, or radioactive agents. Burns can occur from hot liquids, vapors, acids, or alkaline chemicals. Burns are classified as superficial, partial thickness, or full thickness burns. Clients need to be assured that safety is top priority in the workplace and in the home. Employing agencies must be made aware of and follow OSHA guidelines for worker safety.

In healthcare agencies, the risk of scalds and burns is greater for clients whose skin sensitivity to temperature is impaired. Scalds can occur from overly hot bathwater, and burns can occur from therapeutic applications of heat (see Chapter 24). Nurses should assess their clients' skin at regular intervals to ensure that therapeutic appliances have not malfunctioned and resulted in injury. It is important for the nurse to assess how well clients can protect themselves and what special precautions, if any, need to be taken.

FIRES

Fires continue to be a constant risk in both healthcare settings and homes. Agency fires usually result from malfunctioning electric equipment or combustion of anesthetic gas. In the home, fires can result from cooking, heating appliances such as kerosene or natural gas heaters, and smoking. Children may also start fires in the home if they have access to matches or lighters.

Agency Fires

In healthcare agencies, fire is particularly hazardous when people are incapacitated and unable to leave the building without assistance. Smoking materials must be removed from the client's room and the client must be under close observation if allowed to smoke in the agency. This makes it extremely important for nurses to be aware of the fire safety regulations and fire prevention practices of the agency in which they work. When a fire occurs, the nurse follows four sequential priorities. Using the acronym RACE can help you remember the procedure (Figure 9-1 ■):

Rescue clients in immediate danger.
Alarm (pull alarm or call to report).
Contain the fire.
Extinguish the fire *or* **E**scape the fire.

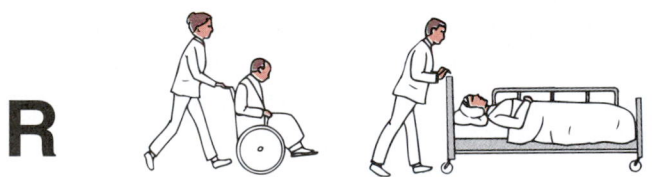

R

Remove all patients or personnel in the immediate vicinity of the fire.

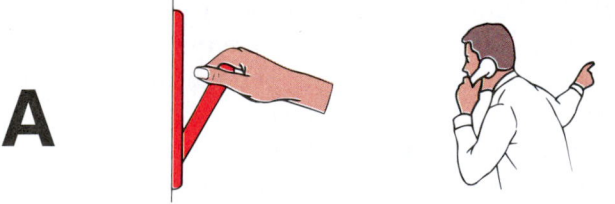

A

Activate the alarm and notify other staff members that a fire exists.

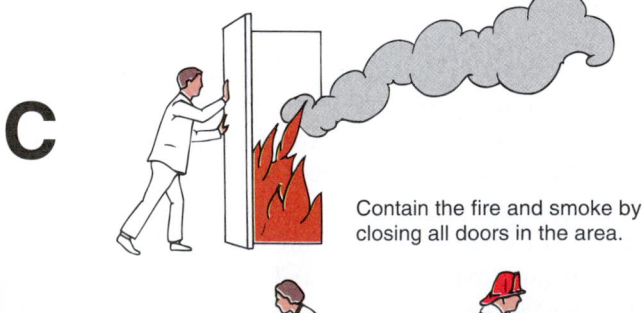

C

Contain the fire and smoke by closing all doors in the area.

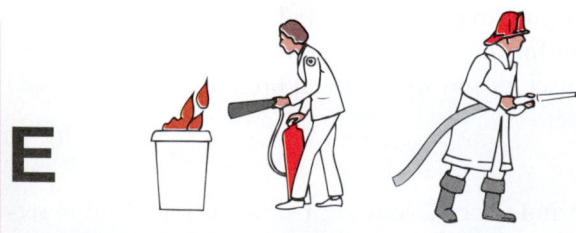

E

Extinguish the fire, if it is a very small fire, or allow the fire department to extinguish it.

Figure 9-1. ■ The RACE system for protecting clients in case of fire.

Extinguishing the fire requires knowledge of three categories of fire, classified according to the type of material that is burning:

Class A: Paper, wood, upholstery, rags, ordinary rubbish
Class B: Flammable liquids and gases
Class C: Electrical

The right type of extinguisher must be used to fight the fire. Each extinguisher has picture symbols showing the type of fire for which it is to be used. Directions for use are also attached. When using an extinguisher, remember PASS:

Pull (the pin on the extinguisher)
Aim (at the base of the fire)
Squeeze (the extinguisher trigger)
Sweep (the extinguisher from side to side).

Home Fires

In the home, adults should be educated about measures to reduce their risk of fires. If they use a kerosene or natural gas heater, they need to be certain to keep all combustible materials including paper and cloth products away from the heater. Educating adults to be vigilant when cooking with oils and to avoid cooking when they are very tired and likely to fall asleep can reduce the risk of fires from cooking. A fire extinguisher should also be kept close to cooking areas and heating sources, such as kerosene heaters, with all family members familiar with its operation. The nurse should encourage the family to maintain working smoke detectors near sleeping and cooking areas. The smoke detectors should be checked at least every 3 months and batteries changed every 6 months. Many community fire departments offer the homeowner a free fire risk assessment and will install smoke detectors in the home for free or a minimal fee. Children should also be educated to avoid playing with matches and how to respond in case of fire. The elderly need extra reminders to avoid nightclothes that are flammable and to keep clothing away from flames.

All families should develop a fire escape plan. In homes with bars or other protective coverings over the windows to prevent burglary, the family needs to have an escape route or a way to remove the covering to escape through a window. In an upstairs room, an escape plan is particularly important since people can become trapped if the fire starts in the downstairs living area. An outside stairwell or ladder that can be attached to the window and lowered to the ground can be effective measures to prevent trapping. Families should be encouraged to practice their fire escape plan so that all family members are familiar with it.

POISONING

Accidental poisoning can occur through swallowing or inhaling toxic substances, from bites and stings, or through contact with poisonous items such as poison ivy. Infants and children are prone to swallowing substances they may find as they explore. Adolescent and adult poisonings are usually related to the ingestion of recreational drugs or suicide attempts. Older adults are at risk for poisoning through overdoses of prescribed medications.

Prevent accidental poisonings by keeping toxic substances locked up and out of reach. Both young children and elders with dementia should have a "safe" environment with plants, flowers, medications, and small objects kept out of reach. Food poisoning can be prevented by properly washing and cooking foods. The Poison Control Center (800-222-1222) can provide current information about potential hazards and recommended treatments.

Clients and staff in healthcare facilities can be at risk for poisonings because of potentially toxic substances in the environment, such as cleaning solutions. Healthcare facilities will generally have posted instructions and alerts for accidental ingestion of poisonous substances. Medication errors can lead to drug interactions and overdoses, and medication administration procedures should always be followed to prevent errors from occurring (see Chapter 27 ⊕).

All clients and families that have furnaces or heaters should have them checked and cleaned on a regular basis to prevent the chance of carbon monoxide poisoning and death. Carbon monoxide (CO) detectors must also be checked on a regular basis. It is recommended that CO alarms be installed on every level of the home, including habitable portions of basements and attics in most residences. On levels with sleeping areas, CO alarms should be installed within 10 feet of bedroom doors. These detectors must be installed low to the floor surfaces following the manufacturer's recommendations.

FALLS

People of any age can fall, but infants and older adults are particularly prone to falling and serious injury. Falls are the leading cause of injury among older adults. They are also a major cause of hospital and nursing home admissions. Most falls occur in the home and are a major threat to the independence of older adults. Fear of falling is common in older adults, even in those who have not experienced a fall. This fear is of particular concern for those who live alone and who anticipate being helpless and unable to summon help after a fall. For these individuals the nurse can make the following recommendations:

- Encourage daily or more frequent contact with a friend or family member.
- Install a personal emergency response system.
- Maintain a physical environment that prevents falls.

Risk factors and associated preventive measures are shown in Table 9-1 ∎.

TABLE 9-1	**Risk Factors for Falls and Preventive Measures**
RISK FACTOR	**PREVENTIVE MEASURES**
Poor vision	Ensure eyeglasses are functional.
	Ensure appropriate lighting.
	Mark doorways and edges of steps as needed.
	Keep the environment tidy. Remove throw rugs and cords from walking paths.
Cognitive dysfunction (confusion, disorientation, impaired memory or judgment)	Set safe limits to activities (e.g., going for walks with a companion, not alone).
	Remove unsafe objects.
	Remove electrical equipment that could start a fire if left unattended *or* install safety switches.
	Enlist family or friends to check on client at regular intervals.
	Move client to a home or facility where supervision can be provided.
Impaired gait or balance and difficulty walking because of lower extremity dysfunction (e.g., arthritis)	Wear shoes or well-fitted slippers with nonskid soles.
	Use ambulatory devices as necessary (cane, crutches, walker, braces, and wheelchair).
	Provide assistance with ambulation as needed.
	Monitor gait and balance.
	Adapt living arrangements to one floor if necessary.
	Encourage exercise and activity as tolerated to maintain muscle strength, joint flexibility, and balance.
	Ensure uncluttered environment with securely fastened rugs.
	Adjust activity to time period when client has increased mobility.
	Provide portable or mobile telephones that are easy for the client to carry with them or to access.
	Use an intercom system at entry doors. (This can prevent falls caused by rushing to answer the door.)

TABLE 9-1	Risk Factors for Falls and Preventive Measures (continued)
RISK FACTOR	**PREVENTIVE MEASURES**
Difficulty getting in and out of chair or in and out of bed	Encourage the client to request assistance. Keep the bed in the low position. Install grab bars in the bathroom. Provide a raised toilet seat. Obtain a lift chair that can bring the client closer to a standing position.
Orthostatic hypotension	Instruct client to rise slowly from a lying to sitting to standing position, and to stand in place for several seconds before walking.
Urinary frequency or receiving diuretics	Provide a bedside commode. Assist with voiding on a frequent and scheduled basis.
Weakness from disease process or therapy	Encourage client to summon help. Monitor activity tolerance.
Current medication regimen that includes sedatives, hypnotics, tranquilizers, narcotic analgesics, diuretics	Attach side rails to the bed. Keep side rails in place when the bed is in the lowest position. Monitor orientation and alertness status. Encourage annual or more frequent review of all medications prescribed.

Prevention of falls in healthcare agencies is an ongoing concern. Healthcare environments are designed with many safety features. These include railings along corridors; call bells at each bedside; safety bars and emergency pull cords in toilet areas; locks on beds, wheelchairs, and stretchers; side rails on beds; and nightlights. In addition, nurses can implement measures to decrease the incidence of falls, as described in Box 9-3 ■.

Safety monitoring devices are also available to prevent falls. Some monitoring systems use a chair or bed sensor (Figure 9-2 ■); others use a leg band. These devices trigger an alarm when the client attempts to get out of bed or a chair unassisted. Procedure 9-1 ■ on page 155 describes how to use these devices.

SUFFOCATION OR CHOKING

Suffocation, or *asphyxiation*, is lack of oxygen due to interrupted breathing. Suffocation occurs when the air source is cut off for any reason. One common reason for choking is that food or a foreign object becomes lodged in the throat. The universal sign of distress in this case is observation of the victim's grasping and pointing to the neck and throat area without speaking. The emergency response is the Heimlich maneuver, or abdominal thrust, which can dislodge the foreign object and reestablish an airway (Figure 9-3 ■).

EXCESSIVE NOISE

Excessive noise is a health hazard that can cause hearing loss, depending on the overall level of noise, the frequency range of the noise, the duration of exposure, and individual susceptibility. When ill or injured, people are frequently sensitive to noises that normally would not disturb them. Loud voices, the clatter of dishes, and even a nearby television can disturb clients, some of whom react angrily. Physiological effects of noise include (1) increased heart and respiratory rates, (2) increased muscular activity, (3) nausea, and (4) hearing loss, if the noise is sufficiently loud.

BOX 9-3	NURSING CARE CHECKLIST

Preventing Falls in Healthcare Agencies

☑ Orient clients on admission to their surroundings, and explain the call system.

☑ Carefully assess each client's risk for falling.

☑ Alert all personnel to the client's risk for falling.

☑ Assign clients at risk for falls to rooms near the nursing station where they can be more closely supervised.

☑ Encourage the client and family to use the call bell to request assistance; ensure that the bell is within easy reach.

☑ Answer call bells promptly.

☑ Place bedside tables and over-the-bed tables near the bed or chair so that clients do not overreach and consequently lose their balance.

☑ Always keep hospital beds in the low position when not providing care so that clients can move in or out of bed easily. Use age-appropriate equipment (e.g., high-topped cribs for infants or toddlers).

☑ Keep side rails up and the bed in the low position for sedated and unconscious clients when they are unattended. (Or, keep the upper side rails in the raised position.) Be familiar with facility policies about side rails and their positioning.

☑ Lock wheels on beds, wheelchairs, client movers/lifters, and stretchers.

☑ Ensure that the client wears nonskid footwear.

☑ Use bed or chair safety monitoring devices as needed.

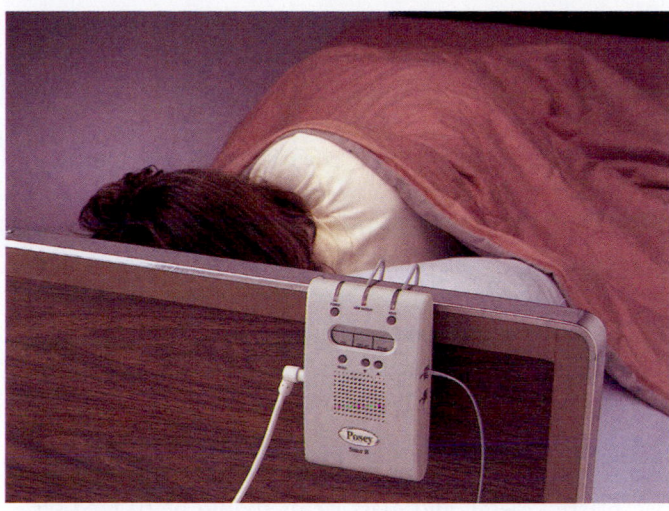

Figure 9-2. ■ Bed exit monitoring device; sounds an alarm if client exits bed. (*Source:* Courtesy of J. T. Posey Company. Reprinted with permission.)

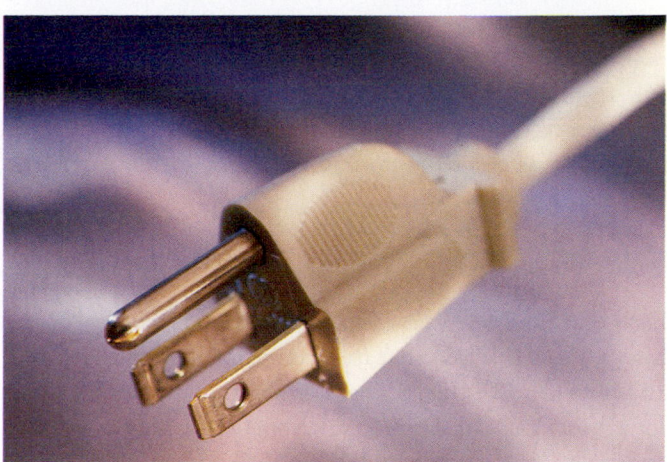

Figure 9-4. ■ Three-pronged grounded plug. (*Source:* Ambularm Co.) *Source:* Getty Images—Photodisc.

Faulty equipment (e.g., equipment with a frayed cord) presents a danger of electric shock or may start a fire. For example, an electric spark near certain anesthetic gases or a high concentration of oxygen can cause a serious fire. Electric shock occurs when a current travels through the body to the ground rather than through electric wiring, or from static electricity that builds up on the body. Using machines in good repair, wearing shoes with rubber soles, standing on a nonconductive floor, and using nonconductive gloves are all ways to prevent shock. If the nurse identifies faulty equipment, the nurse is responsible for removing this equipment from service and making a report to the appropriate person at the healthcare facility.

RADIATION

Radiation injury can occur from overexposure to radioactive materials used in diagnostic and therapeutic procedures. Clients being examined using radiography or fluoroscopy generally receive minimal exposure, and few precautions are necessary.

Nurses need to protect themselves from radiation when some clients are receiving radiation therapy. Exposure to radiation can be minimized by (1) limiting the time near the source, (2) providing as much distance as possible from the source, and (3) using shielding devices such as lead aprons or shields when near the source. Nurses need to become familiar with agency protocols related to radiation therapy.

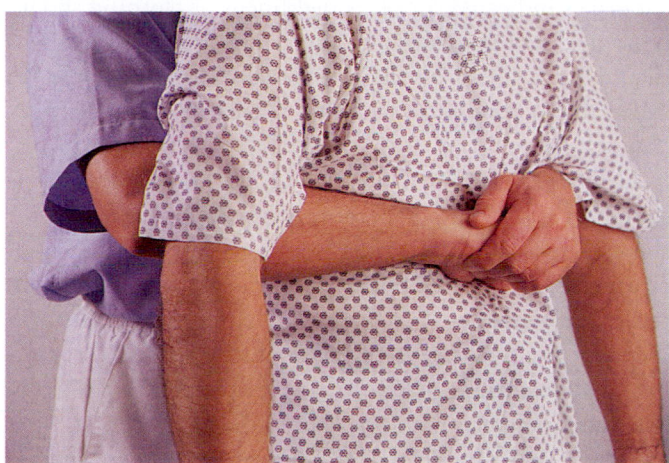

Figure 9-3. ■ Performing the Heimlich maneuver. (Photographer Elena Dorfman.)

Noise can be minimized in several ways. Acoustic tile on ceilings, walls, and floors as well as drapes and carpeting absorb sound. Background music can mask noise and have a calming effect on some people. During the change-of-shift reports, nurses should be careful to keep their voices low or to give reports in areas away from clients' rooms. It is important for nurses to minimize noise in any healthcare setting and to encourage clients to protect their hearing as much as possible.

ELECTRICAL HAZARDS

All electric equipment must be properly grounded. The electric plug of grounded equipment has three prongs. The two short prongs transmit the power to the equipment. The third, longer prong is the grounding device, which carries short circuits or stray electric current to the ground (Figure 9-4 ■). Grounding prongs offer a path of least resistance to stray electric currents.

PREVENTING PROCEDURE-RELATED AND EQUIPMENT-RELATED INJURY

Risk assessment in the healthcare setting must include risks related to procedures and equipment. Whether giving a medication or assisting a client out of bed, nurses need to follow safeguards to prevent errors or injuries. Most healthcare agencies establish protocols that are designed to prevent injuries. When in doubt about a course of action, the nurse should consult the appropriate written guidelines before proceeding.

When an injury or error does occur, most agencies require that the incident be reported. The nurse completes the report immediately after taking whatever action is required to safeguard the client and notifying the charge nurse. For additional information about incident reports, see Chapters 4 and 63 ⚭.

Hospital and Institutional Safety

Each year the Joint Commission publishes National Patient Safety Goals (NPSG) that focus on problems in health care and how to solve them. Their annual updates are based on input from the Commission's national accreditation surveys and a national advisory group. NPSG for 2009 appear in Chapter 63, Table 63-3. Healthcare professionals can keep current by accessing the Joint Commission's website.

The Department of Labor's Occupational Safety and Health Administration (OSHA) has supplied guidelines to ensure that every worker in the United States is employed in a safe environment. Employees are required to follow OSHA regulations; fines are imposed for violations. Although student nurses are not specifically addressed by OSHA regulations, they are expected to comply with healthcare policies and procedures.

SAFETY DEVICES

To protect healthcare workers' safety, OSHA has implemented several requirements for the use of safety devices in the healthcare setting. One example of these safety devices is the use of needleless systems and safeguards to prevent needlestick injury to healthcare workers. OSHA has also encouraged the use of assistive equipment to prevent musculoskeletal injuries. Musculoskeletal injuries, such as lower back and shoulder injuries are one of the most common injuries of healthcare workers today. These injuries can be so severe that the employee can no longer provide direct client care.

INFECTIOUS WASTE

OSHA has developed two standards dealing with infection control activities in the healthcare setting: the *Bloodborne Pathogens Standards* and the *Occupational Exposure to Tuberculosis Standard*. Healthcare facilities are required to develop exposure control plans. In addition, healthcare facilities must provide training to employees. When an employee is exposed to infectious agents, the facility must have a plan in place to provide appropriate intervention and follow-up. It is important that students and nurses be familiar with the requirements for controlling exposure.

Disposal of Used or Soiled Equipment from an Isolation Room

Most facilities have policies and procedures in place that state specifically how to dispose of equipment and supplies that have been contaminated. Be familiar with these policies! Materials may be disposed of, cleaned, disinfected, or sterilized. Some equipment and supplies are for single use only, whereas other materials are meant to be used many times.

Bagging is a technique recommended by the CDC for removal of materials from a client's room. The purpose is to prevent exposure from items contaminated with body secretions. The bag must be **impervious** (impenetrable) to microorganisms. The bags may come in specific colors (e.g., red) and have labels that indicate they contain infectious materials.

The CDC recommends placing contaminated disposable items in the plastic bags that line the waste containers. Nondisposable or reusable items should be put into a labeled bag before being removed from the client's room and sent to a central processing area for decontamination. Rubber, plastic, metal, and glass items should be bagged separately. (Metal and glass can be autoclaved, but rubber and plastic need to be exposed to gas sterilization.)

Special procedure trays should be disassembled and bagged as indicated above. Soiled linens or clothing should be bagged and sent to the facility laundry or home. Linens should be handled as little as possible. They should be rolled into a bundle before being placed in the bag (do *not* shake the linens).

Laboratory specimens should be put into a leak-proof container. If the container is contaminated on the outside, it should be put in a plastic bag before sending it to the laboratory. Dishes are often made of paper and are disposed of in the refuse container. Blood pressure equipment, if kept in the room, needs no special precautions. If it becomes contaminated, follow the agency's cleaning procedures. Nondisposable thermometers should be disinfected after use according to agency protocols. Needles, syringes, and other "sharps" should be placed in a puncture-resistant container kept in the room.

Clients' personal objects (such as toys) that are contaminated should be bagged and sent home for cleaning. For additional information on infection control, see Chapter 10 ⚭.

HAZARDOUS WASTE

Every work area is responsible for having Material Safety Data Sheets (MSDS) available for all chemicals used in that work area. Common substances considered to be hazardous include bleach and other disinfectants. Chemotherapeutic or antineoplastic agents are among the most hazardous substances for nurses. As an LPN/LVN, you will not be administering these drugs without special training.

Each person is responsible for knowing the chemical used and any potential risks to themselves and their clients. The containers must be labeled with the chemical name as well as the function. The labels must also tell any danger or hazard that may exist with that chemical or ingredients and the name, address, and phone number of the manufacturer.

BOX 9-4　MSDS REQUIRED INFORMATION

OSHA suggests that each MSDS shall be in English, and shall contain at least the following information:

1. The identity (product name) used on the label and the chemical and common name(s) of ingredients that have been determined to be health hazards and that comprise 1% or greater of the composition; carcinogens shall be listed if the concentrations are 0.1% or greater.
2. The chemical and common name(s) of all ingredients that have been determined to present a physical hazard when present in the mixture.
3. Relevant physical and chemical characteristics of the hazardous chemical (such as vapor pressure, flash point).
4. Relevant physical hazards, including the potential for fire, explosion, and reactivity.
5. Relevant health hazards, including signs and symptoms of exposure, and any medical conditions generally recognized as being aggravated by exposure to the chemical.
6. The primary route(s) of entry into the body.
7. The OSHA permissible exposure limit and the American Conference of Governmental Industrial Hygienists (ACGIH) threshold limit value. Additional applicable exposure limits may be listed.
8. Whether the hazardous chemical is listed in the National Toxicology Program (NTP) Annual Report on Carcinogens (latest edition) or has been found to be a potential carcinogen in the International Agency for Research on Cancer (IARC) Monographs (latest editions), or by OSHA.
9. Precautions for safe handling and use, including appropriate hygienic practices, protective measures during repair and maintenance of contaminated equipment, and procedures for cleanup of spills and leaks.
10. Appropriate control measures, such as engineering controls, work practices, or personal protective equipment.
11. Emergency and first aid procedures.
12. The date of preparation of the MSDS or the last change to it.
13. The name, address, and telephone number of the chemical manufacturer, importer, employer, or other responsible party preparing or distributing the MSDS, who can provide additional information on the hazardous chemical and appropriate emergency procedures, if necessary.

Always read the label before using. If labels become illegible, do not use the bottle and report it so the bottle or label can be replaced. Know where the MSDS are kept and how to access them. Extensive information about the chemical can be found on the sheets. Box 9-4 ■ lists the required information for MSDS.

DISASTER PLAN

Disasters can be external or internal or a combination of both for a healthcare facility. **External disasters** include events outside the hospital that produce a large number of victims (e.g., fires, plane or train crashes, earthquakes, or violent civil disturbances). **Internal disasters** are events within the hospital that interrupt services and produce victims (e.g., utility interruption or chemical spill). Disasters such as earthquakes with building damage, tornadoes, and floods can be both internal and external. The Department of Homeland Security has increased the awareness of preparing for and responding to emergencies resulting in loss of electricity, heat, water, food, and/or shelter. The events of Hurricane Katrina in the Gulf of Mexico region and wildfires in the West are reminders to all that nature's effects can be massive and destructive.

The Medical Reserve Corps (MRC), founded in 2002, is a partner program with Citizen Corps, a national network of volunteers dedicated to ensuring hometown security. The mission of the MRC is to improve the health and safety of communities across the country by organizing and utilizing public health, medical, and other volunteers. MRC volunteers supplement existing emergency and public health resources.

MRC volunteers include medical and public health professionals such as physicians, nurses, pharmacists, dentists, veterinarians, and epidemiologists. Interpreters, chaplains, office workers, legal advisors, and others—can also fill key support positions.

MRC volunteers can choose to support communities outside their local area. When the Southeast was battered by hurricanes in 2004, MRC volunteers helped communities by filling in at hospitals and shelters, and by providing first aid to those injured by the storms, assisting the American Red Cross (ARC) and the Federal Emergency Management Agency (FEMA). During the 2005 hurricane season, more than 1,500 MRC members were willing to deploy outside their local jurisdiction on optional missions to the disaster-affected areas with their state agencies, the ARC, and HHS. Of these, almost 200 volunteers from 25 MRC units were activated by HHS, and more than 400 volunteers from more than 80 local MRC units were activated to support ARC disaster operations in Gulf Coast areas.

Joining the community MRC is one way healthcare professionals can assist during a local or national disaster and give back to their communities.

Teaching about Disaster Planning

Nurses and members of the community need to be proactive and involved in community efforts to plan for the event of a disaster. The following list will guide nurses in teaching clients to plan ahead for disasters:

- Evacuation plans must be adhered to when mandated by government agencies.
- Discuss the options of staying in their own homes or seeking shelter in a community source or with relatives.
- Have at least 3 days of food and water and extra medications in their homes, as well as a list of all family members with ages, allergies, medications, and health histories.

- Have cell phones or battery-powered radios available to keep aware of situations, whether weather related or terrorist threats, etc.
- Refer clients to the Homeland Security website or to the local Red Cross offices for additional preparation suggestions.
- Include pets in the disaster plan.

Teamwork and cooperation are essential to any disaster plan. Many communities hold annual disaster drills in cooperation with hospitals, police and fire departments, and public works offices. Mock disasters can provide much valuable information for all involved agencies.

Triage is an important consideration during a disaster. Clients in the hospital will be assessed for possible discharge if necessary. Victims are prioritized according to their care needs, from most severe to least injured or ill. Victims are identified by universal emergency medical services (EMS) disaster triage codes:

- *Red:* The most severely injured—likely to need surgery or hospitalization in the intensive care unit (ICU)
- *Yellow:* Significant injuries—require quick attention to prevent worsening of condition; may require hospitalization after treatment
- *Green:* Persons who are "walking wounded" and have non-life-threatening injuries that must eventually be treated to restore client to normal functioning; may not require hospitalization
- *Black:* Deceased, DOA, code blue; transport to morgue

Not all victims arrive at the hospital with an EMS triage tag. The "walking wounded" may arrive by private car and will need to be assessed in the emergency department.

During a disaster, healthcare workers must be willing to perform tasks as assigned by the command center director or supervisor. During this time, personal communication should be put on hold in order not to tie up communication systems. It is important to observe client confidentiality and not perpetuate rumors. Each person should stay in his or her assigned area until directed to do otherwise. The facility will usually have a public information officer who will make statements to the media; it is imperative that all questions be referred to that person or office. Do not fall into the trap of giving unauthorized information.

EMERGENCY CODES

All healthcare facilities have emergency codes. Eleven codes have been identified. There is a real push to have all hospitals use a universal code system. Code Red and Code Blue are widely accepted, but much work is needed to bring other codes into line in all facilities. Box 9-5 ■ lists commonly used emergency codes. It is important that both students and nurses know the specific codes used in each facility where they work or are affiliated.

BOX 9-5	EMERGENCY CODES

- *Code Red:* Fire
- *Code Blue:* Medical emergency adult
- *Code White:* Medical emergency pediatric
- *Code Pink:* Infant abduction
- *Code Purple:* Child abduction
- *Code Yellow:* Bomb threat
- *Code Gray:* Combative person
- *Code Silver:* Person with a weapon and/or hostage situation
- *Code Orange:* Hazardous material spill/release
- *Code Triage Internal:* An internal disaster
- *Code Triage External:* An external disaster

Note: Regional or teaching hospitals may have code *stroke* or code *MI*, for example, to identify those who need immediate attention for these illnesses for rapid treatment to prevent further tissue damage or death.

Codes may vary by facility. Be sure to know the color coding of the facility in which you work!

EMERGENCY NURSING AND FIRST AID

You may be called on to deal with healthcare emergencies inside and outside of the healthcare facility. Nurses who give emergency care in the community should seek first aid training. Such training provides the individual with specific skills that can be used to serve and protect the community. It is important to administer first aid treatment and/or cardiopulmonary resuscitation (CPR) in the manner in which you have been trained (Figure 9-5 ■). *Note:* CPR for children must be done carefully to prevent broken ribs and injury. CPR for infants requires special certification (see Figure 47-4 ⚭).

Any nurse who volunteers his or her time at community activities to provide first aid should contact a local certifying agency (such as the Red Cross) to obtain a first aid certification. As long as you provide appropriate and safe care within the guidelines of your state practice act, most states offer you protection under Good Samaritan laws. (*Note:* First aid is also discussed in the chapter on emergency and urgent care centers, Chapter 47 ⚭ .)

Cardiopulmonary Resuscitation

CPR certification is required for healthcare professionals by most healthcare facilities (Box 9-6 ■). Several different agencies including the American Heart Association (AHA) and the Red Cross provide certification programs that meet these requirements. Many facilities and schools provide the classes for employees and students. It is important to maintain current certification as a nurse as well as a responsible citizen. In 2005, the AHA issued new guidelines for CPR. Those holding a CPR card should refer to the guidelines frequently and practice the skills on a regular basis. For more information, contact a local provider of

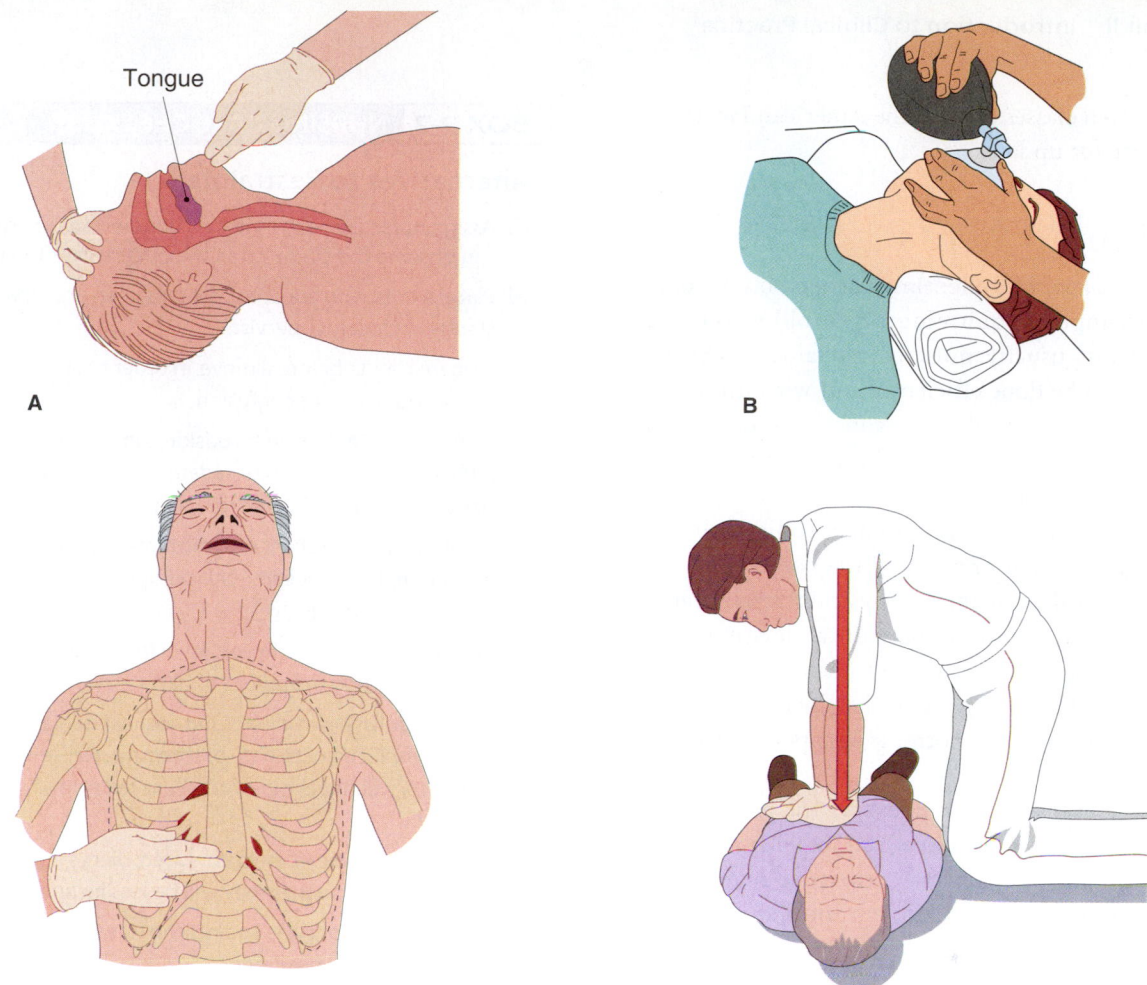

Figure 9-5. ■ CPR. **A.** Use the head tilt/chin lift method to open the airway. **B.** If not breathing, give two full breaths using a pocket mask, mouth shield, or bag-valve-mask device. Observe the chest rise and fall during ventilation. **C.** Locate the compression site by following the edge of the rib cage to the notch where the ribs join the sternum. **D.** Position your hands and begin chest compressions with your arms vertical over the victim.

BOX 9-6	CPR FOR ADULTS BY HEALTHCARE PROVIDER

If you find an unresponsive adult, place flat on back on a firm surface; move an injured adult only if necessary, and turn the head, neck, and body as a unit. If the rescuer suspects the collapse is the result of asphyxiation due to an obstructed airway, the rescuer should perform approximately 2 minutes of CPR and then call for help and retrieve the automated external defibrillator (AED).

1. Shout for help. If alone, phone the emergency response number or 911 and retrieve the AED and emergency equipment.
2. **A** Open the airway:
   Perform a head tilt/chin lift maneuver.
   If neck injury is suspected, use jaw thrust.
3. **B** Check for breathing (look, listen, and feel).
   If breathing is not adequate, provide 2 breaths at 1 second per breath. Take a normal breath (not a deep breath) with each rescue breath.
   Use bag-valve-mask device with oxygen or barrier device. Be sure chest rises with each breath.
   If chest does not rise, reopen the airway and try again.
4. **C** Check for signs of circulation (pulse, breathing, coughing, or movement).

Signs of circulation but no breathing:
- Provide rescue breathing (one breath every 5 to 6 seconds). Each breath is over 1 second.

No pulse, no signs of circulation present:
- *If AED is available:* Power on, attach electrodes, follow prompts.

One shock should be delivered followed immediately by CPR. Rhythm checks will be performed every 2 minutes.
- *If no AED available:* Perform chest compressions:
  —Compress lower half of sternum.
  —Rate approximately 100 times per minute.
  —30 compressions, then two breaths (repeat) for all victims.

5. CPR: Provide 30 compressions and two breaths (repeat) until client is intubated. If client is intubated, compressions are given continually, without pauses for breaths (8 to 10 breaths per minute are provided while compressions are being given).

If the nurse is working with infants or children, they should be familiar with the current emergency care guidelines.

Source: Adapted from guidelines of American Heart Association (2005).

CPR certification classes or view the American Heart Association website for updates.

Restraining Clients

Sometimes the safety of a client may depend on use of a restraint. For example, a squirming 2-year-old who needs to have a blood test usually must be restrained so that the venipuncture can be done efficiently and with minimal injury. Likewise, an older adult who cannot maintain a sitting position independently would need a restraint in order to leave the room in a wheelchair.

Restraints are protective devices used to limit the physical activity of the client or a part of the body. They can be classified as physical or chemical. Physical restraints are any manual method or physical or mechanical device, material, or equipment attached to the client's body. They cannot be removed easily, and they restrict the client's movement. Chemical restraints are psychotropic agents used to control disruptive behavior.

The purpose of restraints is to ensure the physical safety of the person who is being restrained, or of other persons whom the restrained person may otherwise harm. Nurses are encouraged to reduce the use of restraints and use safe alternatives whenever possible. Alternatives to restraints are listed in Box 9-7 ■.

To safeguard clients in long-term care facilities, the U.S. government regulated the use of mechanical restraints. The Omnibus Budget Reconciliation Act clearly states that restraints should be applied only as a last resort. Regulations also require that (1) restraints be applied only under a physician's written order, one that specifies why the restraint is being used and for how long it will be used; (2) the client or designated medical power of attorney (POA) agrees to be restrained; and (3) the client be free of physical restraints not required to treat the client's medical symptoms.

LEGAL IMPLICATIONS OF RESTRAINTS

Because restraints restrict a person's ability to move freely, their use has legal implications. Box 9-8 ■ lists guidelines about the legal implications of using restraints.

SELECTING A RESTRAINT

Before selecting a restraint, nurses need to understand clearly its purpose and measure it against the following five criteria:

1. It restricts the client's movement as little as possible. If a client needs to have one arm restrained, do not restrain the entire body.
2. It does not interfere with the client's treatment or health problem. If a client has poor blood circulation to the hands, apply a restraint that will not aggravate that circulatory problem.

BOX 9-7 NURSING CARE CHECKLIST

Alternatives to Restraints

☑ Assign nurses in pairs to act as "buddies" so that one nurse can observe the client when the other leaves the unit.

☑ Place clients who are at risk for falls in an area that is constantly or closely supervised.

☑ Prepare clients before a move, in order to limit relocation shock and resultant confusion.

☑ Stay with a client using a bedside commode or bathroom if the client is confused or sedated or has a gait disturbance or a high-risk score for falling.

☑ Monitor all of the client's medications and, if possible, attempt to lower or eliminate dosages of sedatives or psychotropic drugs.

☑ Position beds at their lowest level from the floor to facilitate getting in and out of bed.

☑ Report confusion in clients and request full-length side rails be replaced with half- or three-quarter-length rails, so clients will not climb over rails or fall from the end of the bed.

☑ Use rocking chairs to help confused clients expend some of their energy so that they will be less inclined to wander.

☑ Wedge pillows or pads against the sides of wheelchairs to keep clients well positioned.

☑ Place a removable lap tray on a wheelchair to provide support and help keep the client in place.

☑ To quiet agitated clients, try a warm beverage, soft lights, a back rub, or a walk.

☑ Use "environmental restraints," such as pieces of furniture or large plants as barriers, to keep clients from wandering beyond appropriate areas.

☑ Place a picture or other personal item on the door to clients' rooms to help them identify their room.

☑ Try to determine the causes of the client's *sundown syndrome* (nocturnal wandering and disorientation as darkness falls, associated with dementia). Possible causes include poor hearing, poor eyesight, or pain.

☑ Establish ongoing assessment to monitor changes in physical and cognitive functional abilities and risk factors.

---

3. It is readily changeable. Restraints need to be changed frequently, especially if they become soiled. Keeping other guidelines in mind, choose a restraint that can be changed with minimal disturbance to the client.
4. It is safe for the particular client. Choose a restraint with which the client cannot self-inflict injury. For example, a physically active child could incur injury trying to climb out of a crib if one wrist is tied to the side

BOX 9-8   LEGAL IMPLICATIONS FOR USE OF RESTRAINTS

To protect clients and to avoid legal problems, the nurse should follow these guidelines:

- Know the agency's restraint policies. Policies should cover all types of physical and chemical restraints and specify how and when to apply them and what procedures to follow.
- When determining the need for a restraint, always assess the underlying reason for a client's restlessness, agitation, or confusion.
- Apply restraints only when necessary for the client's health and safety, not for convenience or to cope with understaffing.
- Avoid being influenced by a family member's advice not to restrain the client, even when the person offers to sit with the client. Nurses cannot legally delegate responsibility to a family member.
- Obtain a physician's order before applying a restraint whenever possible. If the client needs to be restrained immediately, apply the restraint and then notify the physician directly afterward. In many agencies, standing orders allow the use of restraints under certain circumstances, provided that a written order is obtained from the physician within 24 hours.
- Recognize the competent adult's right to make decisions regarding personal care and treatment, and obtain appropriate consent. Check agency policies if necessary restraint is refused. An agency may require the client to sign a release of

liability should injury result; otherwise, the agency has the option of refusing to continue care. For clients who are declared legally incompetent, obtain consent from an appointed guardian or surrogate as permitted by law.
- Keep in mind the principle of least restriction; that is, restrain the client only to the extent necessary to accomplish the restraint's purpose.
- Make sure that a physical restraint fits properly.
- When a restraint is applied, document the following:
  a. The specific behavior that made it necessary and all the unsuccessful interventions used prior to restraining as proof of attempting to de-escalate the client's behavior
  b. The type of restraint used
  c. The substance of explanations given to the client and support persons
  d. The client's consent
  e. The exact times the restraint was applied and removed
  f. The client's behavior while the restraint was applied
  g. The frequency of care given while the restraint was applied and removed (e.g., assessment of circulation and range-of-motion exercises)
  h. Notification of the physician
- Periodically reevaluate the need for the restraint.
- Some facilities may have a policy requiring a one-on-one observation for certain types of restraints or behaviors.

of the crib. A jacket restraint would restrain the child more safely.

5. It is the least obvious to others. Both clients and visitors are often embarrassed by a restraint, even though they understand why it is being used. The less obvious the restraint, the more comfortable people feel.

KINDS OF RESTRAINTS

There are several kinds of restraints (Figure 9-6 ■ through 9-8 ■). Among the most common are the jacket or vest restraint, the belt restraint, the mitt or hand restraint, limb restraints, elbow restraints, mummy restraints, and crib nets. Geri chairs and wheelchairs used to confine client activity can also be considered restraints.

There are several types of vest restraints (see Figure 9-6A), but all are essentially sleeveless jackets (vests) with straps (tails) that can be tied to the bed frame under the mattress or to the legs of a chair. These body restraints are used to ensure the safety of confused or sedated clients in beds or wheelchairs. The Food and Drug Administration (FDA) advises that manufacturers place "front" and "back" labels on vest restraints. To put a restraining vest on a client, make sure the front or back opening is placed according to manufacturer's recommendations. Pull the tie on the end of the vest flap across the chest, and place it through the slit on

the opposite side of the chest. Repeat for the other tie. Use a half-bow knot to secure each tie. Do not tie the vest to the head of the bed. Fasten the ties together behind the chair using a square knot. Ensure that the client is positioned appropriately to enable maximum chest expansion for breathing.

Belt or safety strap body restraints (see Figure 9-6B) are used to ensure the safety of all clients who are being moved on stretchers or in wheelchairs. If the client is on a stretcher, one portion of the belt (the longer portion) is placed beneath the client, and the shorter portion is placed over the client's gown, with a finger width between the belt and the client. For clients in a wheelchair, attach the belt around the client's waist and fasten it at the back of the chair. Some wheelchairs have a soft padded safety bar that attaches to side brackets installed under the armrests. To prevent the person from slumping forward, the nurse attaches a shoulder "Y" strap to the bar and over the client's shoulders to the rear handles. Other safety belt models have a three-loop design. One loop surrounds the person's waist and attaches to the rear handles. If such restraints are unavailable, the nurse can place a folded towel or small sheet around the client's waist and fasten it at the back of the wheelchair. Belt restraints may also be used for certain clients confined to bed or to chairs.

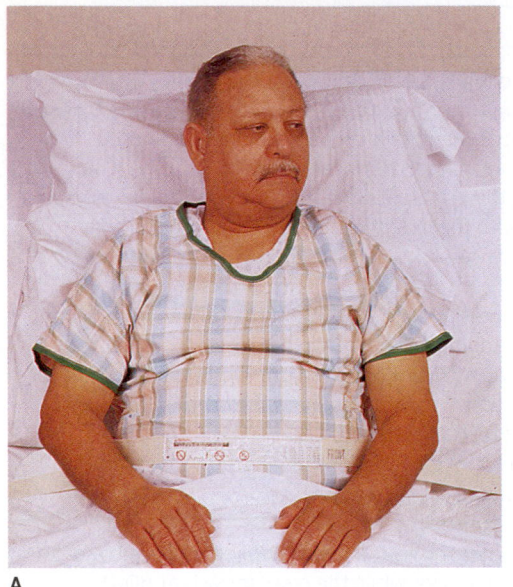 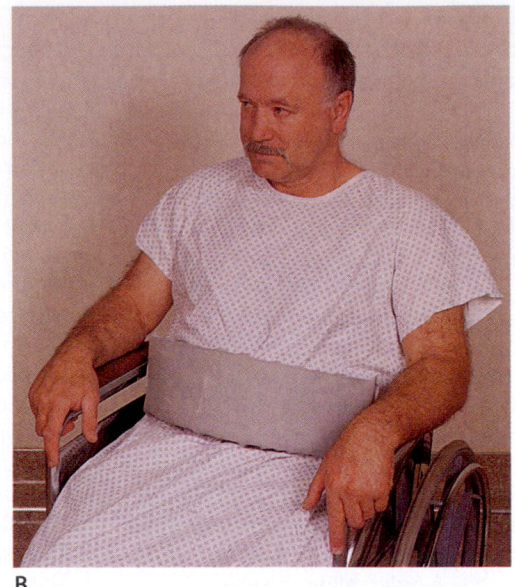 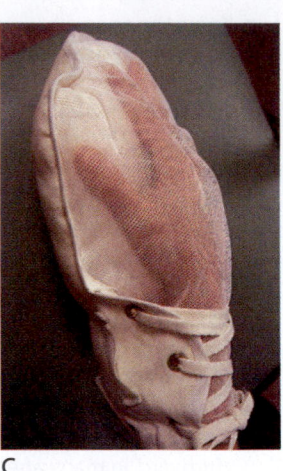

A   B   C

Figure 9-6. ■ **A.** Poncho-type vest restraint. **B.** Belt restraint (safety belt restraint). **C.** Mitt restraint. (*Source:* Jenny Thomas Photography, photos A and B.)

A mitt or hand restraint (see Figure 9-6C) is used to prevent confused clients from using their hands or fingers to scratch and injure themselves. For example, a confused client may need to be prevented from pulling at intravenous tubing or a bandage following surgery. Hand or mitt restraints allow the client to be ambulatory and/or to move the arm freely rather than be confined to a bed or a chair. Follow the manufacturer's directions for securing the mitt. When applying the mitt restraint, make sure the fingers can be slightly flexed and

are not caught under the hand. Be sure to remove at least every 2 to 4 hours for washing and exercising the client's hand. Assess the client's hand circulation shortly after the mitt is applied and at regular intervals. Monitor for feelings of numbness or discomfort or inability to move the fingers.

Limb restraints (see Figures 9-7A and B) are generally made of cloth. They may be used to immobilize a limb, primarily for therapeutic reasons (e.g., to maintain an intravenous infusion).

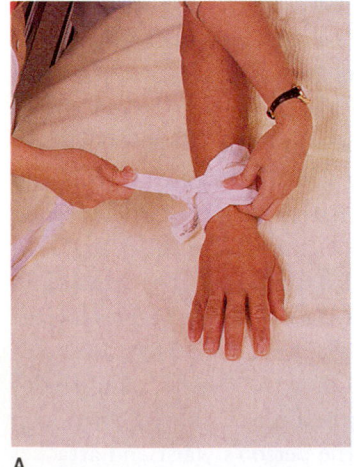 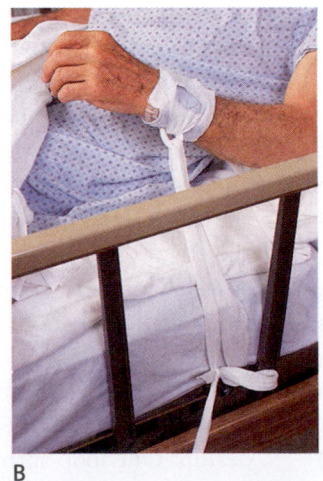 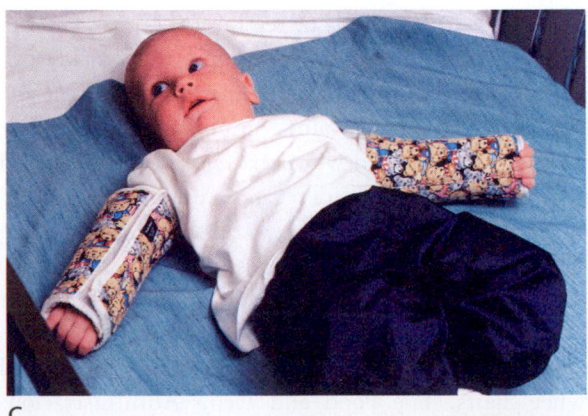

A   B   C

Figure 9-7. ■ **A, B.** Wrist or ankle restraint. Pad bony prominences to prevent skin breakdown. Pull the tie of the commercially made restraint through the slit or through the buckle, and secure the tie to the bed frame. **C.** Elbow restraint. Place the child's elbow in the center of the restraint. Make sure that the ends of the tongue depressors are covered by padded material to prevent irritation. Wrap the restraint smoothly around the arm and secure it with safety pins, ties, or tape. Pinning it to the child's shirt prevents it from sliding down the arm. Monitor for tightness and obstructed blood circulation. (*Source:* Jenny Thomas Photography, photo A.)

Elbow restraints (see Figure 9-7C) are used to prevent infants or small children from flexing their elbows to touch or scratch a skin lesion or to reach the head when a scalp vein infusion is in place. This restraint consists of a piece of material with pockets into which plastic or wooden tongue depressors are inserted to provide rigidity.

The mummy restraint is a special folding of a blanket or sheet around a child to prevent movement during a procedure such as gastric washing, eye irrigation, or collection of a blood specimen. See Figure 9-8 for folding instructions.

General guidelines for applying and monitoring restraints are presented in Box 9-9 ■.

Attaching restraints to a bed or chair requires the use of knots, which must be secure but easily untied by staff in an emergency situation. See Figure 9-9 ■ for instructions on tying a half-bow knot and Figure 9-10 ■ for a square knot.

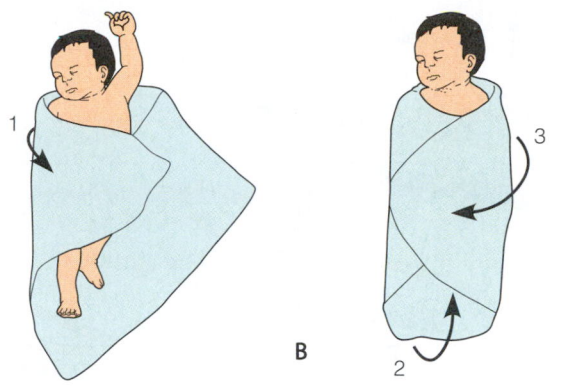

Figure 9-8. ■ Making a mummy restraint. **A.** Use a blanket about twice the length of the infant's body. Fold down one corner, and place the baby's shoulders on it in the supine position. Fold the right side of the blanket over the infant's body, leaving the left arm free (1). The right arm is in a natural position at the side. **B.** Fold the excess blanket at the bottom up under the infant (2). With the infant's left arm in a natural position beside the body, fold the left side of the blanket over the infant, including the arm, and tuck the blanket under the body (3).

BOX 9-9   NURSING CARE CHECKLIST

Applying and Monitoring Restraints

☑ Apply the selected restraint. Obtain consent from the client or guardian.

☑ Ensure that a physician's order has been provided, or in an emergency, obtain one within 24 hours after applying the restraint.

☑ Assure the client and the client's support people that the restraint is temporary and protective. A restraint must never be applied as punishment for any behavior or merely for the nurse's convenience.

☑ Apply the restraint in such a way that the client can move as freely as possible without defeating the purpose of the restraint.

☑ Ensure that limb restraints are applied securely but not so tightly that they impede blood circulation to any body area or extremity.

☑ Assess the restraint every 10 to 30 minutes. Some facilities have specific forms, policies, and procedures to be used to record ongoing assessment.

☑ Release all restraints at least every 2 to 4 hours, and provide range-of-motion (ROM) exercises (see Chapter 23 ⬤⬤) and skin care. This is the time to offer toileting and fluids or nourishment. Be sure to document that the physiological needs were offered to the client.

☑ If more than one limb is restrained, remove one restraint at a time. When a restraint is temporarily removed, do not leave the client unattended.

☑ Reassess the continued need for the restraint at least every 8 hours. Include an assessment of the underlying cause of the behavior necessitating use of the restraints.

☑ Immediately report to the nurse in charge and record on the client's chart any persistent reddened or broken skin areas under the restraint.

☑ At the first indication of cyanosis or pallor, coldness of a skin area, or a client's complaint of a tingling sensation, pain, or numbness, loosen the restraint and exercise the limb.

☑ Apply a restraint so that it can be released quickly in case of an emergency and with the body part in a normal anatomic position.

☑ Provide emotional support verbally and through touch.

☑ Determine that restraint is in good condition and is the appropriate size for the client.

☑ Explain to client and support people the purpose and procedure for using the restraint.

☑ Document relevant information for all types of restraints.

☑ Record on the client's chart the time the physician was notified, the type of restraint applied, the time it was applied, the reason for its application, the client's response to the restraint, and the times that the restraints are removed and skin care given.

☑ Record any other interventions, assessments, and explanations to client and significant others.

☑ Adjust the nursing care plan as required, for example, to include releasing the restraint every 2 h, assessing circulation, sensation, and motion of restrained extremities; and providing skin care, toileting, fluids, snacks or meals, and ROM exercises.

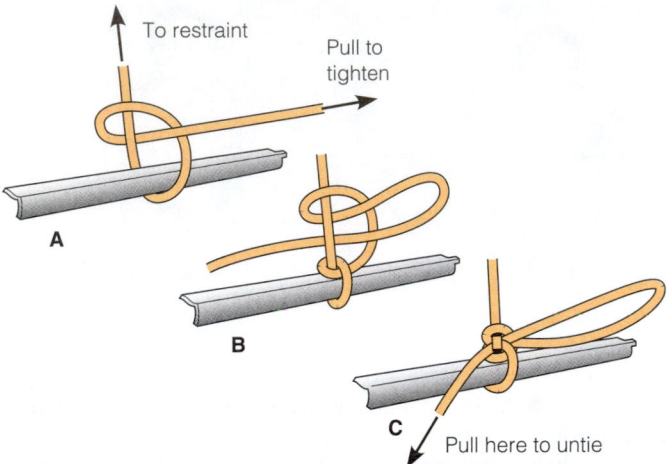

Figure 9-9. ■ To make a half-bow (quick-release) knot, first place the restraint tie under the side frame of the bed (or around a chair leg). **A.** Bring the free end up, around, under, and over the attached end of the tie and pull it tight. **B.** Again take the free end over and under the attached end of the tie, but this time make a half-bow loop. **C.** Tighten the free end of the tie and the bow until the knot is secure. To untie the knot, pull the end of the tie and then loosen the first cross over the tie.

NURSING CARE

PRIORITIZING NURSING CARE

The nurse's focus in relation to safety is to follow CDC and facility guidelines carefully. An important aspect of maintaining safety is to be fully aware of the potential risks when viewing a situation or beginning an intervention. Careful attention to basic handwashing technique is one of the best ways for the nurse to prevent the spread of microorganisms. Remember to follow safety guidelines even if you see others who do not.

ASSESSING

Assessing clients at risk for injury involves (1) noting risk indicators in the nursing history and physical examination, (2) using specifically developed risk assessment tools, and (3) evaluating the client's home environment.

The nursing history and physical examination can reveal considerable data about the client's safety practices and risks for injury. Data include age and developmental level; general health status; mobility status; presence or absence of physiologic or perceptual deficits such as olfactory, visual, tactile, taste, or other sensory impairments; altered thought processes or other impaired cognitive or emotional capabilities; substance abuse; any indications of abuse or neglect; and an injury history. A safety history also needs to include the client's awareness of hazards, knowledge of safety precautions both at home and work, and any perceived threats to safety.

Risk Assessment Tools

Risk assessment tools are available to determine clients at risk for both specific kinds of injury, such as falls, and skin impairment. In general, these tools direct the nurse to appraise the factors affecting safety as they have been outlined earlier. See Figure 24-15 ⬭ for one skin impairment assessment tool.

DIAGNOSING, PLANNING, AND IMPLEMENTING

An RN will identify nursing diagnoses and develop the care plan for each client. A primary NANDA diagnostic label that relates to safety issues is *Risk for Injury*, a state in which the individual is at risk for injury as a result of environmental conditions interacting with the individual's adaptive and defense resources. One of the subcategories of this diagnosis

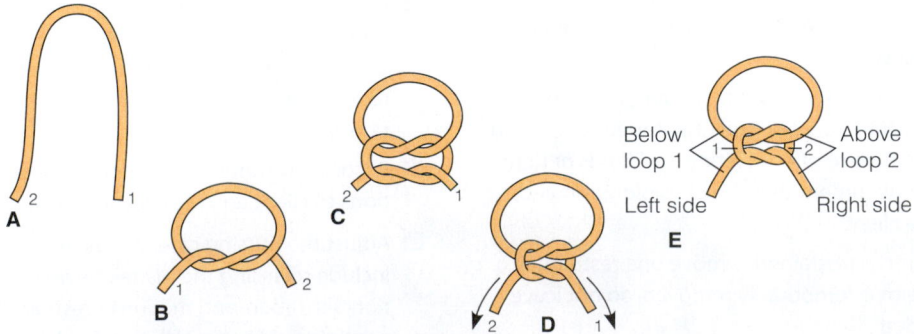

Figure 9-10. ■ To make a square (reef) knot: **A.** Form a "U" loop. **B.** Pass one end (1) over and under the other. **C.** Take the same end (1), and pass it over, under, and over the other. **D.** Pull knot tight. **E.** When the knot is tied correctly, the ties on each side are both either above or below the loop. Attach the other end of the commercial restraint to the movable portion of the bed frame, never to the side rails or to the nonmoving bed frame. If the ties are attached to the movable portion, the wrist or ankle will not be pulled when the bed position is changed.

may be preferred when the nurse wants to isolate suitable interventions. These subcategories are:

- Risk for Poisoning
- Risk for Suffocation
- Risk for Trauma
- Impaired Home Maintenance
- Ineffective Protection

(Refer to Appendix II on the Companion Website 🔗 for a complete list of nursing diagnoses related to safety.)

When planning care to prevent injury, the nurse considers all factors affecting the client's safety, specifies desired outcomes, and selects nursing activities to meet these outcomes. The major goal for clients with safety risks is to prevent injury. To meet this goal, clients often need to change their health behavior and may need to modify the environment.

Desired outcomes associated with preventing injury depend on the individual client. Examples of desired outcomes follow. The nurse needs to individualize these for clients. The client:

- Describes methods to prevent specific hazards (e.g., falls, suffocation, choking, fires, drowning, electric shock).
- Reports use of home safety measures (e.g., fire safety measures, smoke detector maintenance, fall prevention strategies, burn prevention measures, poison prevention measures, safe storage of hazardous materials, firearm safety precautions, electrocution prevention, water safety precautions, bicycle safety, motor vehicle safety).
- Alters home physical environment to reduce the risk of injury.
- Describes emergency procedures for poisoning and fire.
- Describes age-specific risks, work safety risks, or community safety risks.
- Demonstrates correct use of child safety seats.
- Demonstrates correct administration of cardiopulmonary resuscitation.

Nursing interventions to meet desired outcomes are largely directed toward helping the client and family to:

- Identify environmental hazards in home and community.
- Demonstrate safety practices appropriate to the home healthcare agency, community, and workplace.
- Demonstrate safe childrearing practices or lifestyle practices.

EVALUATING

In preventing client injury, the nurse's role is largely one of education. The nurse evaluates whether the client has learned about safety hazards, incorporated safety practice into behavior, and acquired skills to perform in the event of certain emergencies.

Continuity of Care

If clients require an alarm system when they return home, caregivers would need instruction in its setup and use.

Instruct them to test the monitoring device every 12 to 24 hours to ensure that it is working. Also, have them check the volume of the alarm to be sure they can hear it.

If a client is in danger of falling, remind caregivers to:

- Clear the floor of wires or loose rugs.
- Provide lighting at night between bedroom and bathroom.
- Encourage clients to rise in stages from lying to sitting to standing, and to get their balance before starting to walk.
- Provide assistive devices (e.g., cane, walker) as needed.

If the client has a visual impairment, instruct the family members that the client needs to be informed of any changes to the environment. Otherwise, the change in the client's environment may pose a risk because many clients with visual impairments will memorize the layout of their home.

NURSING PROCESS CARE PLAN
Client with Fractured Hip

Mr. Moore is a 72-year-old widower who is recovering from a fall in which he fractured his hip and underwent surgical repair 1 week ago. He is returning home after staying with his son for 2 weeks. Once he is home, his son will visit nightly after work. He will receive Meals-on-Wheels once a day, and a home healthcare attendant will visit weekly to assist him with hygienic care until he is more independent. Mr. Moore's wife died 3 years ago, but he has remained independent and continued his social functions. He lives in a small three-bedroom house with his dog and cat, and he enjoys gardening. Prior to fracturing his hip, he walked his dog daily. After the initial visit from the RN, you will be his home healthcare nurse.

Assessment

Home care nurse (LPN/LVN) visited on the second day in client's own home. The home health attendant assisted with shower and dressing. The client is doing well physically with no complaints of pain. VS stable: 98.2/74/18, BP 132/84. Surgical incision well healed with no redness or drainage, open to air. AAO ×3. Throw rugs and furniture in pathway from bed to bathroom. Safety devices installed in bathroom: grab bar and raised toilet seat. Family members' phone numbers are programmed on speed dial on phone. Client states, "It is so good to be home, I had the best night's sleep last night." Walked 20 feet from front door to car using a walker. Client reports he is looking forward to being able to walk his dog.

Nursing Diagnosis

The following important nursing diagnoses (among others) are established for this client:

- *Ineffective Health Maintenance*
- *Impaired Physical Mobility*
- *Risk for Injury*

Expected Outcomes

Mr. Moore will:

- Follow mutually agreed-on healthcare maintenance plan.
- Participate in activities of daily living at the maximum of functional ability.
- Demonstrate use of adaptive equipment (e.g., walker) to increase mobility.

Planning and Implementation

- Assess client's awareness of deficits that may result from normal aging.
- Give client information about community resources for the elderly (home visitors, emergency call systems, and transportation to appointments).
- Evaluate the client's knowledge of and compliance with hip precautions.
- Monitor client for physiological complaints, including pain and medication effects.
- Monitor the use of any assistive devices needed for activity in coordination with the physical therapist (PT).
- Initiate a walking program in coordination with the PT in which the client walks with or without help every day as part of his daily routine.
- Ensure the removal of the throw rugs and other obstacles in the client's path from the bed to the bathroom.

Evaluation

Two weeks after discharge, Mr. Moore is in his own home. You make your first home visit.

- Client and family have established regular schedule of caretakers' and family members' visits to allow independence.
- Meals-on-Wheels scheduled 6 days per week.
- Client spending one weekend day with family.
- Mr. Moore is able to shower and dress with assistance of home health attendant. Home safety evaluation reveals that nightlights have been installed and furniture has been rearranged for easy access from bedroom to bath.
- PT home visits 2× per week. Able to get in and out of bed. Using walker in house and outside when accompanied.
- Client demonstrates compliance with hip precautions.
- No complaints of pain or medication side effects.

Critical Thinking in the Nursing Process

1. While hospitalized, Mr. Moore tried to get out of bed without assistance and almost fell, but his nurses decided not to restrain him. What are the best reasons for avoiding the use of restraints for clients such as Mr. Moore? What are some alternatives to restraints that could be used in this situation?

2. What strengths do you note about Mr. Moore's case that may protect him from injury when he returns home?

3. What other safety issues are important to consider in this situation?

Note: Discussion of Critical Thinking questions appears on the MyNursingKit Website.

Body Mechanics for Nurses

Nurses routinely protect the safety of the client for whom they care. However, little thought is given to the nurse's personal safety until the nurse sustains an injury. A nurse cannot provide for clients effectively unless he or she is free from injury.

Body mechanics is the term used to describe safe, efficient use of the body to move objects and carry out activities of daily living. The purpose of body mechanics is to ensure safe and efficient use of appropriate muscle groups to maintain balance, reduce fatigue and energy expended, and prevent injury.

Body mechanics involves the concepts of alignment and posture. When a person moves, the center of gravity shifts continuously in the direction of moving body parts. The closer the line of gravity is to the center of the base of support, the greater the person's stability (Figure 9-11A ■). Conversely, the closer the line of gravity is to the edge of the base of support, the more precarious the balance (Figure 9-11B). If the line of gravity falls outside the base of support, the person falls (Figure 9-11C).

Body balance can be greatly enhanced by (1) widening the base of support and (2) lowering the center of gravity, bringing it closer to the base of support. The base of support may be easily widened by spreading the feet farther apart. The center of gravity is readily lowered by flexing the hips and knees until a squatting position is achieved. Use of these two techniques is vital to nurses to prevent work-related back injuries.

PREVENTING BACK INJURIES

Many factors increase the potential for lower back injury. Low back pain can be caused by a number of factors, from injuries to the effects of aging. The American Nurses Association has initiated a campaign called Handle with Care. This campaign is designed to reduce the risks for injury to nurses and other healthcare workers who provide direct client care. The focus of the campaign is to encourage facilities to purchase equipment to assist employees in moving clients and to implement safety committees to review policy and evaluate risks for injury as a result of lifting.

Undesirable **twisting** can be prevented by facing the direction of movement squarely, whether pushing, pulling, or sliding, and by moving the object directly toward or away from one's center of gravity (Figure 9-12 ■).

> **clinical ALERT**
>
> Twisting (rotation) of the thoracolumbar spine and stooping (acute flexion of the back with hips and knees straight) must always be avoided because of the potential for causing back injury.

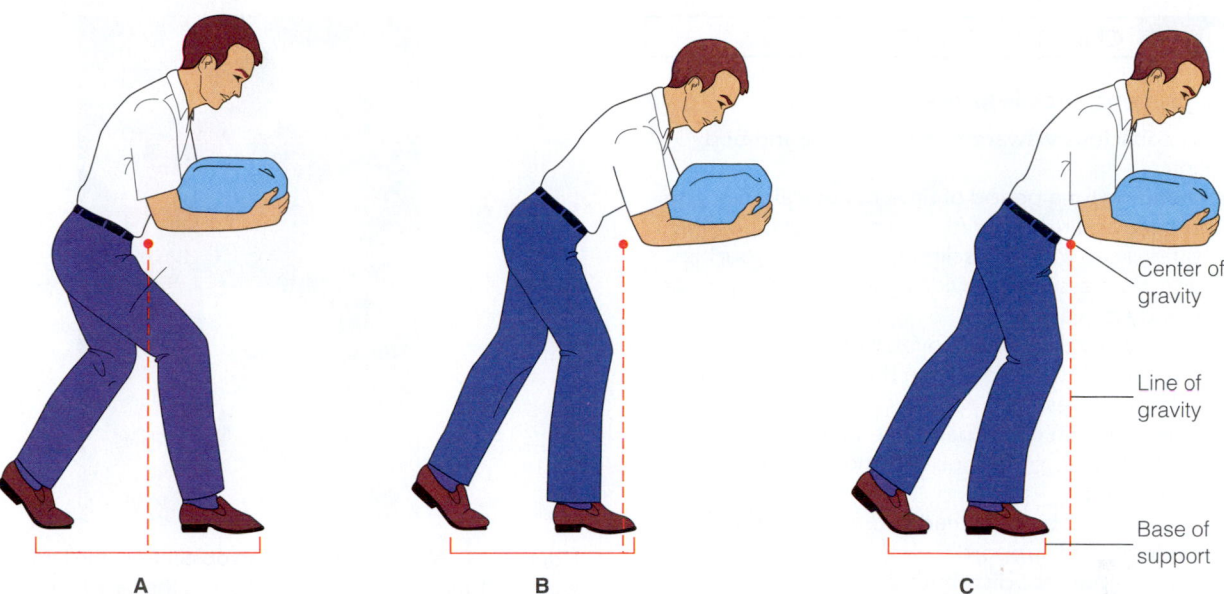

Center of gravity

Line of gravity

Base of support

A   B   C

Figure 9-11. ■ **A.** Balance is maintained when the line of gravity falls close to the base of support. **B.** Balance is precarious when the line of gravity falls at the edge of the base of support. **C.** Balance cannot be maintained when the line of gravity falls outside the base of support.

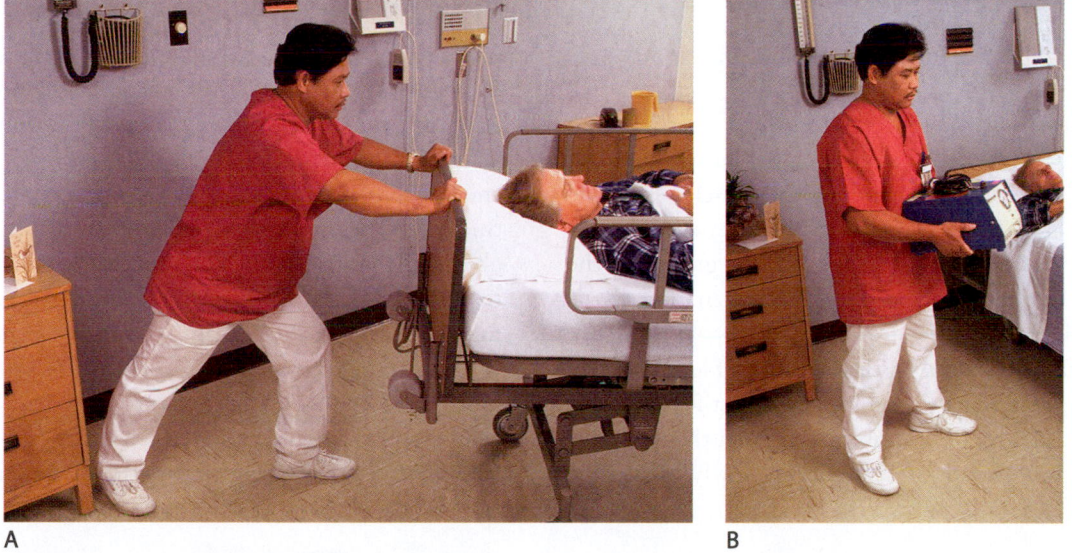

A   B

Figure 9-12. ■ Correct body mechanics for the proper method of carrying or moving an object. **A.** Face the object squarely before pushing or pulling. **B.** When turning with an object, turn the feet as well as the body; do not twist the spine while holding a heavy object. *Source: Pearson Education/PH College.*

Low Back Sprain and Strain

The muscles of the low back provide power and strength for activities such as standing, walking, and lifting. A strain of the muscle can occur when the muscle is poorly conditioned or overworked. The ligaments of the low back interconnect the five vertebral bones and provide support or stability for the low back. A sprain of the low back can occur when a sudden, forceful movement injures a ligament that has become stiff or weak through poor conditioning or overuse. These injuries, or sprain and strain, are the most common causes of low back pain. Although you cannot totally halt the progress of these effects, they can be slowed by regular exercise, knowing the proper way to lift and move objects,

proper nutrition, and good posture. Box 9-10 ■ lists guidelines for preventing back injury in nurses or in clients.

LIFTING

When a person lifts or carries an object, the object's weight becomes part of body weight. This weight change affects the center of gravity, which becomes displaced in the direction of the added weight. To counteract this potential imbalance, body parts (e.g., arm, trunk) move away from the weight, so the center of gravity is maintained at the same point in the base of support. By holding an object as close to the body as possible, the lifter avoids displacing the center of gravity and achieves greater stability.

BOX 9-10 CLIENT TEACHING

How to Prevent Back Injuries

- Become consciously aware of your posture and body mechanics.
- When standing for a period of time, periodically flex one hip and knee and rest your foot on an object if possible.
- When sitting, keep your knees slightly higher than your hips.
- Use a firm mattress that provides good body support at natural body curvatures.
- Exercise regularly to maintain overall physical condition; include exercises that strengthen the pelvic, abdominal, and lumbar muscles.
- Avoid exercises that cause pain or require spinal flexion with straight legs (e.g., toe-touching and sit-ups) or spinal rotation (twisting).
- When moving an object, spread your feet apart to provide a wide base of support.
- When lifting an object, distribute the weight between large muscles of the legs and arms.
- Wear clothing that allows you to use good body mechanics and comfortable low-heeled shoes that provide good foot support, such as an athletic or walking shoe, and will not cause you to slip, stumble, or turn your ankle.

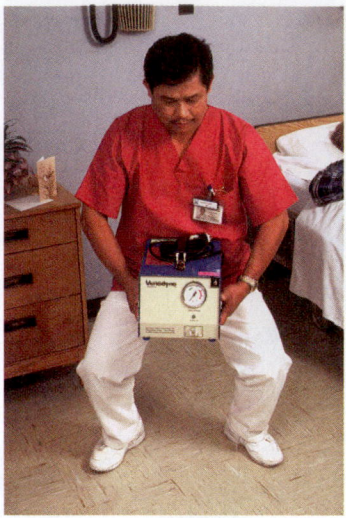

Figure 9-14. ■ Stages in lifting an object from the floor to the waist. First, move close to the object, flex the back and knees, and grasp the object. Then (see photo) start the lift by keeping the back flexed while the knees begin to straighten so that the leg muscles can exert an upward thrust. *Source:* Pearson Education/PH College.

People can lift more weight when using a lever. Human bones function as levers—the joint is the **fulcrum** (fixed point about which a lever moves) and the muscles exert the force (Figure 9-13 ■). Lifting involves movement against gravity, so the nurse must use major muscle groups of the thighs, knees, upper and lower arms, abdomen, and pelvis to prevent back strain.

Another technique based on the principle of leverage may be used when lifting objects from floor to waist level. In this technique, the back and knees are flexed until the load is at thigh level. Then the back straightens slowly while the knees remain flexed to provide thrust (Figure 9-14 ■). This maneuver provides for better balance and leverage. The muscles work together (in *synchronization*), which helps prevent injury. When an object is lifted to knee level, the abdominal and lumbar muscles contract for leverage and pull. The thigh and leg muscles exert the upward thrust to bring the object off the floor. When an object is lifted from mid-thigh to waist level, force is primarily exerted by leg and thigh muscles, while back and lumbar muscles remain contracted.

For all lifting positions, it is necessary to maintain a distance of 30 cm (12 inches) or more between the feet and to keep the load close to the body, especially when it is at knee level. Before attempting to lift, the nurse must ensure that

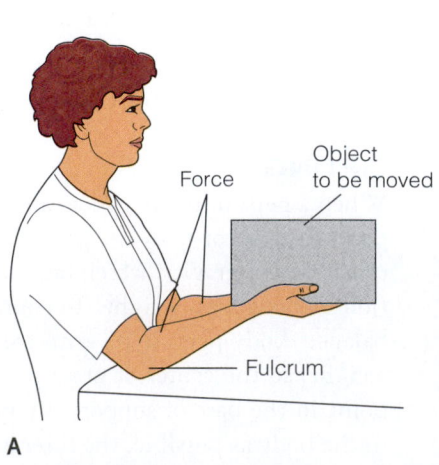

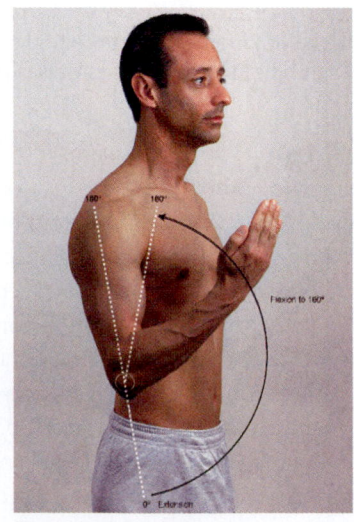

A   B

Figure 9-13. ■ **A.** Principles of using arm as a lever. **B.** Correct posture when using arm as a lever. *Source:* Pearson Education/PH College.

there are no hazards on the floor, there is a clear path for moving the object, and the nurse's base of support is secure.

PUSHING AND PULLING

When pushing or pulling an object, a person maintains balance with the least effort when the base of the support is enlarged in the direction in which the movement is to be produced or opposed. It is easier and safer to pull an object toward one's own center of gravity than to push it away, because the person can exert more control of the object's movement when pulling it.

PIVOTING

Pivoting is a technique in which the body is turned in such a way to avoid twisting of the spine. To pivot, place one foot ahead of the other, raise the heels very slightly, and put the weight on the balls of the feet. When the weight is off the heels, the frictional surface is decreased and the knees are not twisted when turning. Keeping the body aligned, turn (pivot) about 90 degrees in the desired direction. The foot that was forward will now be behind. A summary of principles and guidelines related to body mechanics is shown in Table 9-2 ■.

TABLE 9-2	Summary of Guidelines and Principles Related to Body Mechanics
GUIDELINES	**PRINCIPLES**
Plan the move or transfer carefully. Free the surrounding area of obstacles and move required equipment near the head or foot of the bed.	Appropriate preparation prevents potential falls and injury and safeguards the client and equipment.
Obtain the assistance of other people or use mechanical devices to move objects that are too heavy. Encourage clients to assist as much as possible by pushing or pulling themselves to reduce your muscular effort. Use arms as levers whenever possible to increase lifting power.	The heavier an object, the greater the force needed to move the object.
Adjust the working area to waist level, and keep the body close to the area. Elevate adjustable beds and over-the-bed tables or lower the side rails of beds to prevent stretching and reaching.	Objects that are close to the center of gravity are moved with the least effort.
Provide a firm, smooth, dry bed foundation before moving a client in bed or use a pull sheet.	Less energy is required when you reduce the friction between the object moved and the surface on which it is moved.
Always face the direction of the movement.	Ineffective use of major muscle groups occurs when the spine is rotated or twisted.
Start any body movement with proper alignment. Stand as close as possible to the object to be moved. Avoid stretching, reaching, and twisting, which may place the line of gravity outside the base of support.	Balance is maintained and muscle strain is avoided as long as the line of gravity passes through the base of support.
Before moving an object, increase your stability by widening your stance and flexing your knees, hips, and ankles.	The wider the base of support and the lower the center of gravity, the greater the stability.
Before moving an object, contract your gluteal, abdominal, leg, and arm muscles to prepare them for action.	The greater the preparatory isometric tensing, or contraction of muscles, before moving an object, the less energy required to move it, and the less likelihood of musculoskeletal strain and injury.
Avoid working against gravity. Pull, push, roll, or turn objects instead of lifting them. Lower the head of the client's bed before moving the client up in bed.	Moving an object along a level surface requires less energy than moving an object up an inclined surface or lifting it against the force of gravity. Pulling creates less friction than pushing.
Use your gluteal and leg muscles rather than the sacrospinal muscles of your back to exert an upward thrust when lifting. Distribute the workload between both arms and legs to prevent back strain. Balance is maintained with minimal effort when the base of support is enlarged in the direction in which the movement will occur.	The synchronized use of as many large muscle groups as possible during an activity increases overall strength and prevents muscle fatigue and injury.
When *pushing* an object, enlarge the base of support by moving the front foot forward. When *pulling* an object, enlarge the base of support by either moving the rear leg back if facing the object or moving the front foot forward if facing away from the object.	Balance is maintained with minimal effort when the base of support is enlarged in the direction in which the movement will occur.
When moving or carrying objects, hold them as close as possible to your center of gravity.	The closer the line of gravity to the center of the base of support, the greater the stability.
Use the weight of the body as a force for pulling or pushing by rocking on the feet or leaning forward or backward.	Body weight adds force to counteract the weight of the object and reduces the amount of strain on the arms and back.
Alternate rest periods with periods of muscle use to help prevent fatigue.	Continuous muscle exertion can result in muscle strain and injury.

Protection from Violence in the Healthcare Setting

Anyone in the healthcare setting, from the admitting clerk to the phlebotomist to the security guard, is potentially at risk for violence. Each healthcare facility must have a policy in place to protect employees, clients, and visitors.

clinical ALERT

Because of the risk of violent behavior, healthcare facilities must have policies stating that violence or potential violence is unacceptable in or on the facility property.

Clients whose behavior escalates toward violence are a danger to themselves, visitors, other clients, and staff. Early recognition of escalating behaviors and immediate intervention are keys to preventing violent outcomes. Training to de-escalate potentially violent behavior is necessary. This training allows healthcare workers to become aware of subtle hints that danger is possible. Box 9-11 ■ provides important concepts about self-protection and de-escalating potentially violent situations.

At times it is not a client but a visitor or someone seeking revenge on a staff member or client who may be the violent one. Units with the highest potential for violence are emergency departments, intensive care units, maternity units, pediatric units, and mental health units. Facilities generally have a code to alert staff to these situations via an overhead paging system. Security would secure doors to keep the person from exiting into other areas. For example, "Attention all staff . . . Code grey in west stairwell."

Dementia units in extended-care facilities are at high risk for violence because of clients' confusion and disorientation. Rarely, these clients may become violent, so it is important to learn and to avoid actions that have the potential

| BOX 9-11 | VIOLENT OR POTENTIALLY VIOLENT SITUATIONS |

The following are some suggestions for situations of potential or actual violence:

- Never allow the client/visitor to stand between you and the door. Prevent the potential for restraint and harm by keeping a clear path to safety.
- Stay attuned to visitor behavior. Observe for escalation of voices, tearfulness of the client, or anything that is suspicious in nature.
- Notice and report any unusual behavior in a coworker that might be the result of domestic abuse. Dark glasses, new and fading bruises, and withdrawal from coworkers may be manifestations of abuse that could escalate in the workplace.
- Never allow an audience to observe escalation in someone who is angry. Take the person to a quiet environment, such as an office or unoccupied waiting area, to allow the person to calm down or vent frustrations. Use a calm voice and direct eye contact, but be cautious with touch.
- Always call or have a coworker notify the security officer and/or supervisor to report escalating behaviors. Some facilities have client advocates who can intercede and who are trained to listen and offer empathy.
- Know your facility's code and the proper procedure to follow when it is used.
- Ask for an ID badge neck strap (lanyard) that breaks away when pulled. This prevents use of the strap as a strangling device.
- Be alert for everyday objects that could be used as weapons. Examples include ink pens, scissors, clamps, and pencils.

to trigger violent reactions. (*Note*: If a confused or violent client has an IV infusing, the IV tubing will not break, but will continue to stretch.)

Note: The references and resources for all chapters have been compiled at the back of the book.

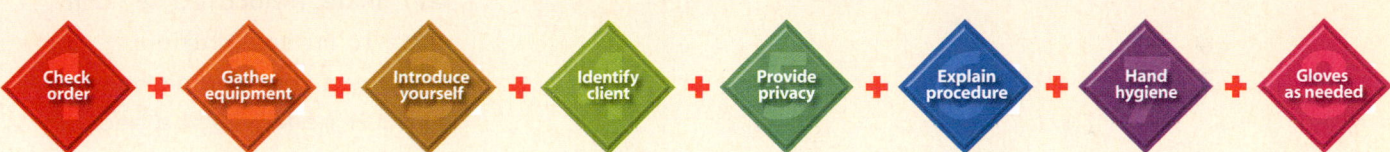

PROCEDURE 9-1   Using a Safety Monitoring Device for Bed or Chair

A bed or chair safety monitor (Figure 9-15 ■) is an electronic device with a position-sensitive switch that triggers an audio alarm when the client attempts to get out of the bed or chair unassisted. When activated, the alarm alerts the nurse and provides an opportunity for the nurse to intervene.

Purposes

■ To alert the nurse that the client is attempting to get out of bed

■ To help decrease the risk of client falls

Equipment

■ Alarm and control device
■ Connection to nurse call system (optional)
■ Sensor device

Check order + Gather equipment + Introduce yourself + Identify client + Provide privacy + Explain procedure + Hand hygiene + Gloves as needed

Interventions and Rationales

1. Perform preparatory steps (see icon bar above).

2. Explain to the client and support people the purpose and procedure for using safety monitoring.
   ■ Explain that the device does not limit mobility in any manner; rather, it alerts the staff when the client is about to get out of bed or a chair.
   ■ Explain that the nurse must be called when the client needs to get out of bed. *These measures reduce anxiety and protect the client from injury.*

3. Obtain the appropriate sensor device and control unit.

4. Test the battery device and alarm sound. *This ensures that the device is functioning properly prior to use. (Locate the extra batteries to ensure continuous functioning.)*

5. Apply the sensor pad or leg band.
   ■ Place the leg band according to the manufacturer's recommendations. The usual position for a bed or chair sensor is under the mattress (see Figure 9-15) or chair cushion directly beneath the client's buttocks. For clients at high risk of falling, the sensor may be placed under the shoulders. *Placement must be individualized to the client's needs.*
   ■ For a bed or chair device, set the time delay for determining the client's movement patterns from 1 to 12 seconds.
   ■ Connect the sensor pad to the control unit and the nurse call system. *The alarm device is position sensitive. For example, when a leg band approaches a near-vertical position (such as in walking, crawling, or kneeling as the*

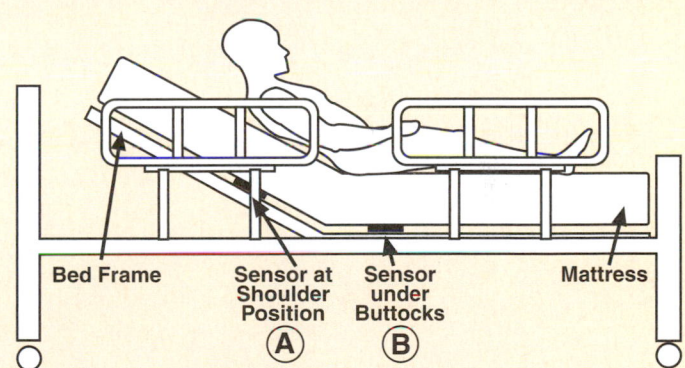

Bed Frame   **Sensor at Shoulder Position** Ⓐ   **Sensor under Buttocks** Ⓑ   **Mattress**

Figure 9-15. ■ Bed exit monitoring device; the sensor is usually placed under the client's buttocks. (*Source:* Courtesy of J. T. Posey Company. Reprinted with permission.)

client attempts to get out of bed), the audio alarm is triggered, causing a sharp, shrill sound.

6. Instruct the client to call the nurse when the client wants or needs to get up, and assist as required. *This reassures the client that he or she will not be confined indefinitely.*
   ■ Before assisting the client to rise, deactivate the alarm by unsnapping the alarm device from the elastic band. *This prevents the alarm from being triggered.*
   ■ Assist the client back to bed, and reattach the alarm device to the sensor. *The alarm provides a safeguard against client injury.*

7. Ensure client safety with additional safety precautions.
   ■ Place call light within client reach, lift all side rails, and lower the bed to its lowest position. *The alarm device is not a substitute for other precautionary measures.*

- Place monitoring device stickers on the client's door, chart, and Kardex. *This communicates use of the alarm to other personnel.*

8. Document relevant data. *An action that is not documented is not legally considered to be done.*
   - Record that monitoring device is intact when applied.
   - Record all assessments.
   - Record all safety precautions and interventions discussed and employed. *Documentation is crucial for client safety and to ensure quality of care.*

SAMPLE DOCUMENTATION

(date) Focus

0930   Safety D[Data] Attempting to climb out of bed over side rail. Confused. Stated "I need to go home and feed my dogs."
A[Action] Reoriented, placed call light within reach. Instructed to call before attempting to get out of bed. Wander-guard® attached to left ankle. Relocated to room close to nurses' station. Explained that the alarm will sound if he leaves the bed. Contacted family members to reassure client that the dogs are being cared for. Instruct nursing assistant to check every 15 min and respond immediately to alarm.

1030   R[Response] Alarm activated 3 times within one hour. Asked that alarm be removed. Offered reassurance, explained purpose of alarm. Alarm remains in place. Resting quietly after reorientation. _____
K. Adams, LPN

Chapter Review

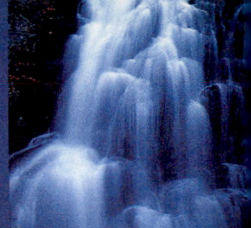

KEY Points

- Education is a major health protection strategy in preventing injuries.
- When planning to meet safety needs of clients, nurses need to consider physical factors in the environment and the psychological and physiological state of the individual.
- Injuries are a major cause of death among individuals of all ages in the United States and Canada.
- Hazards to safety occur at all ages and vary according to the age and development of the individual.
- To ensure safety, focus on (1) observing or predicting situations that are potentially harmful and (2) educating clients to safeguard themselves and their families. It is often necessary to modify the environment to make it safe.
- Nurses must be familiar with the fire procedures in the healthcare agency where they practice. In the event of a fire, the nurse must (1) protect clients from injury, (2) report, (3) contain, and (4) put out the fire.
- Use the RACE acronym in event of fire. **R**emove the client from the room; **A**ctivate the **A**larm system or dial the facility code for Code Red or 911; **C**onfine the area by closing the door to the room and if in a facility close all doors to the adjoining area or rooms; **E**xtinguish the blaze if a small fire, or **E**scape using the plans of the facility.
  - Please be sure to follow the plans of the facility for escape and notification of the proper authorities.
  - By all means do not reenter the smoke-filled room or a room with a blaze.
- To prevent falls, the nurse must provide constant surveillance for infants and young children and assess older clients' safety needs carefully.
- Prolonged exposure to excessive noise can produce hearing loss. Ill or injured people may be especially sensitive to noises.
- Electrical injuries can be prevented by using grounded outlets and plugs, putting protective covers over outlets, and making sure that electric wiring and circuits meet safety standards.
- In hospitals, radioactive substances are used for both diagnostic and treatment purposes. Follow agency policy to safeguard clients and staff from exposure.

- Side rails and handrails protect hospitalized clients from falls. Restraints keep clients from inflicting injuries on themselves and others.
- Because restraints restrict a client's basic freedom to move, they should be used as a last resort. Careful assessment and accurate, complete documentation are important when restraints are used.
- A nurse cannot provide for clients effectively unless he or she is free from injury.
- Planning moves or transfers will help prevent falls and injuries and safeguard the client and equipment.

FOR FURTHER Study

For additional information about incident reports, see Chapters 4 and 63.

For additional information on infection control, see Chapter 10.

For directions on passive ROM exercises, see Chapter 23.

See Chapter 24 for therapeutic applications of heat and cold, and Figure 24-14 for an example of a skin assessment tool.

Chapter 27 provides information about avoiding medication errors.

First aid is also discussed in Chapter 47.

Appendix II on the Companion Website lists nursing diagnoses related to safety.

Critical Thinking Care Map

Caring for a Client with Risk for Injury
NCLEX-PN® Focus Area: Safety

Case Study: George Whitman is a 75-year-old man with a history of Parkinson's disease. He was admitted to the hospital following a fall, which resulted in an intertrochanteric fracture of his right hip. The fracture was treated with an open reduction internal fixation (ORIF). For the past 7 days he has been in the transitional care unit receiving physical therapy and mobility training. He is currently able to ambulate with a walker.

Nursing Diagnosis: *Ineffective Protection*

COLLECT DATA

Subjective	Objective
_____	_____
_____	_____
_____	_____
_____	_____
_____	_____
_____	_____

Would you report this? Yes/No

If yes, report to:_____

What would you report?_____

Nursing Care

_____
_____
_____
_____
_____
_____
_____
_____
_____
_____
_____

How would you document this? _____
_____
_____

Compare your answers and documentation to those provided on the MyNursingKit Website.

Data Collected
(use only those that apply)

- Client's wife expressed concerns about his upcoming discharge
- Lives with wife in a two-story house
- Does yard work
- Socializes with the neighbors
- Daughter and three grandchildren live 75 miles away
- Mrs. Whitman and the daughter feel the couple should move to a retirement apartment
- Mr. Whitman expressed, "Selling the house would be a sign that I am just giving up."
- Rigidity due to the Parkinson's
- Soft diet—difficulty in swallowing
- Large bruise on his left leg and right forearm
- Routine medications: Sinemet 25/100 t.i.d., Tasmar 100 t.i.d., DSS capsule 100 mg daily, ferrous sulfate 325 mg daily, heparin 5,000 units SQ b.i.d.
- VS: T 98.2, P 76, R 20, BP 140/88
- Lab results: H&H 13.2 40.4, PT 13.5 sec, PTT 90 sec

Nursing Interventions
(use only those that apply; list in priority order)

- Monitor risk for bleeding.
- Assess pain severity on 1–10 scale.
- Help client perform prescribed exercises every 8 h.
- Refer family to appropriate community resources.
- Observe client for cause of impaired mobility.
- Evaluate client for signs of depression.
- Observe for causes of inability to feed self independently.
- Take temperature, pulse, and blood pressure every 4 h.
- Observe nutritional status.
- Teach client and family signs of bleeding, precautions to take to prevent bleeding.
- Work with dietitian to improve nutritional status.
- Teach caregiver feeding techniques that prevent choking.

NCLEX-PN® Exam Preparation

1 You are asked to teach a parenting class on safety at a community center. One of the parents asks why young children are so prone to injury. Of the following, which is the best answer?

1. Young children are uncoordinated, so they are more likely to fall.
2. Misbehavior results in many injuries to children.
3. Young children's curiosity exceeds their judgment.
4. Children are unable to remember safety instructions.

2 The nurse is preparing to restrain a client who has been pulling at the intravenous lines and surgical incision. The most appropriate restraint device in this situation would be:

1. A vest restraint.
2. Mitt restraints.
3. Bed alarm.
4. Arm restraints.

3 A nurse is working in a facility where she uses a variety of chemicals. Which is the most important safety consideration for this nurse?

1. The name of the chemical
2. The nurse's access to MSDS
3. The nurse's years of experience using these chemicals
4. The nurse's previous exposure to the chemicals

4 Your client is being discharged following a total hip replacement. You provide discharge instructions involving home safety in the presence of the son. Which of the following statements would demonstrate the need for more teaching?

1. "Dad will be staying with us until he is completely recovered."
2. "We have removed the throw rugs from the bedroom and bathroom."
3. "Dad will need to use the walker only when leaving the house."
4. "When Dad gets out of bed, we will have him get up slowly and gain his balance before walking."

5 The safe and efficient use of the body to move objects and carry out activities of daily living is:

1. Physical therapy.
2. Body mechanics.

3. A nursing intervention.
4. Occupational therapy.

6 The government agency responsible for a safe work environment is the:

1. CDC.
2. OSHA.
3. JCAHO.
4. Department of Labor.

7 You are assigned to care for a client in isolation. After you have changed the bed, you need to remove the soiled linen from the room. What is the procedure for dealing with soiled linen?

1. Linen remains in the room until the client is discharged.
2. Carry the rolled-up linen without touching your uniform.
3. Place the soiled linen in a bag, which is held by another person outside the isolation room.
4. Dispose of the linen in the refuse container.

8 The nurse is providing education regarding home fire prevention to a group of families. The nurse should include which instruction?

1. Avoid the use of electric heaters.
2. Keep paper and cloth away from heating appliances.
3. Use of bars over windows can increase fire safety.
4. Fire extinguishers should be stored close to sleeping areas.

9 The nurse is preparing to assist a client to transfer from the bed to a wheelchair. To safely transfer this client, the nurse would:

1. Keep the client at arm's length.
2. Have both feet close together.
3. Encourage the client to perform the transfer while the nurse is standing close to the client's side.
4. Hold the client close to the nurse's center of gravity with feet about hip-width apart.

10 When discovering a fire in a client's room, the nurse would take which of the following actions? (Select all that apply.)

1. Remove the client from the area.
2. Contact the client's physician.
3. Activate the alarm system.
4. Contain the fire by closing doors.

Answers and rationales for Review Questions appear in Appendix I.

Infection Control and Asepsis

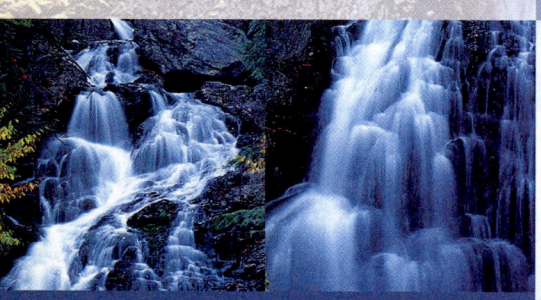

LEARNING Outcomes

After completing this chapter, you will be able to:

1. Define terms and name helpful and harmful actions of microorganisms.
2. Define infectious and communicable diseases and name agencies that try to control their spread.
3. Define types of infection, including nosocomial infection.
4. Name six links in the chain of infection.
5. Identify factors that increase client risk of infection.
6. Compare nonspecific and specific defense systems of the body.
7. Describe drug-resistant organisms, as well as nursing care and client teaching for them.
8. Identify important means of controlling microorganisms in the environment.
9. Describe Standard Precautions and Transmission-based Precautions as well as CDC Guidelines.
10. Name equipment used for infection control.
11. List relevant nursing diagnoses and interventions for clients with an infection or at risk of developing an infection.

Clinical Objectives

12. Demonstrate aseptic techniques including hand hygiene, donning and removing sterile and nonsterile gloves, and donning personal protective equipment.
13. Establish and maintain a sterile field.

KEY TERMS

Use the audio glossary feature on the MyNursingKit Website to hear the correct pronunciation of the following key terms.

Infection control is a primary concern in nursing care. Nurses play an important role in establishing a biologically safe environment for their clients.

Microorganisms

Microorganisms are tiny living bodies that are visible only with a microscope. The most common are classified as bacteria, viruses, fungi, and parasites. Microorganisms are present in the environment and on body surfaces (such as the skin), in the intestinal tract, mouth, upper respiratory tract, lower urinary tract, and vaginal tract. These are referred to as *normal flora*. Although we frequently refer to microorganisms as "germs," most are harmless and some are even helpful because they perform essential functions for the body. For example, normal flora is the body's first line of protection against infection for clients and care providers.

TYPES OF MICROORGANISMS

Bacteria are the most common type of disease-causing microorganisms. They can live in and be transported through the air, water, food, soil, inanimate objects, and body tissues or fluids. **Viruses** are the smallest known disease-causing agents. They must enter living cells to reproduce. Viruses cannot survive or maintain their infectiousness outside a living host. Viral infections are generally self-limiting (e.g., rhinovirus, which causes the common cold). Others can cause serious illness or death (hepatitis, herpes, and human immunodeficiency virus [HIV]). **Fungi** are either yeasts or molds. Examples are the fungi that cause athlete's foot and yeast infections. **Parasites** live on other living organisms.

Examples are protozoa (which cause malaria), helminths (worms), and arthropods (mites, ticks, and fleas).

HELPFUL ACTIONS OF MICROORGANISMS

Resident flora (normal flora) are harmless microorganisms. They can be found in and on the body. Many of them perform useful protective functions. For example, intestinal flora help to synthesize vitamin K, which is important to the body's blood-clotting mechanism. Various other microorganisms make antibiotic-like substances and toxic substances that slow or stop the growth of other organisms.

The process of *colonization* occurs when strains of microorganisms become resident flora. Resident flora can grow in or on the body and not cause disease. However, if a person's defenses are weak, flora may invade a part of the body they normally would not, and cause illness or infection. *Escherichia coli* (*E. coli*), a normal resident flora of the intestinal tract, causes illness if transmitted elsewhere. For example, if proper hygiene is not used after a bowel movement, *E. coli* may be moved to the urethra and cause a urinary tract infection. (Table 10-1 ■ provides some common resident organisms.)

HARMFUL ACTIONS OF MICROORGANISMS

An **infection** is defined as an invasion of the body by a disease-causing organism called the *infectious agent*. Microorganisms that cause disease are called **pathogens**. A "true" pathogen causes disease or infection in a healthy person. An **opportunistic pathogen** causes a disease only in a susceptible person, that is, someone whose immune system is not functioning as a defense system.

TABLE 10-1	Examples of Normal Flora
BODY AREA	**ORGANISMS**
Skin	*Staphylococcus epidermidis*
	Propionibacterium acnes
	Staphylococcus aureus
	Coagulase-negative staphylococcus
	Bacillus species
	Pityrosporum ovale (yeast)
Nasal passages	Coagulase-negative staphylococci
	Staphylococcus epidermidis
	Neisseria species
	Haemophilus species
Oropharynx	*Streptococcus pneumoniae*
Bronchi, lungs	None
Mouth	Coagulase-negative staphylococci
	Lactobacillus
	Bacteroides
	Actinomyces
Stomach	None
Esophagus	None
Intestine	*Bacteroides*
	Fusobacterium
	Eubacterium
	Lactobacillus
	Streptococcus
	Enterobacteriaceae
	Escherichia coli
	Klebsiella species
Urethral orifice	*Staphylococcus epidermidis*
Urethra (lower)	*Proteus*
Bladder, ureters, kidneys	None
Vagina	*Lactobacillus*
	Bacteroides
	Clostridium
	Candida albicans
Blood, lymph system	None

When an infection occurs, the signs and symptoms of the infection are distinctive, and the person's health is recognized as being different from the normal. **Disease** causes a detectable change in the way the body functions. In some cases, the microorganism will not cause any signs or symptoms of disease, and the infection is called *asymptomatic* or *subclinical*. For example, many cases of mumps are asymptomatic.

Various microorganisms are stronger than others and are called more *virulent*. **Virulence** refers to the organism's ability to produce disease and survive both inside and outside the body. Microorganisms also differ in their strength and their communicability (how easily they can be spread). The cold or the annual strain of influenza can be easily spread by hands and coughing or sneezing, whereas bloodborne pathogens such as hepatitis C and AIDS are not easily transmitted. They require blood-to-blood contact to pose a risk for transmission. A **communicable disease** is one that is spread or transmitted by direct or indirect contact. (*Note:* Communicable diseases often affect people during childhood and are discussed in the Pediatric section (see Chapter 59 of this text.)

The transmission of an organism can be caused by a **vector** or vehicle (an insect, or a used drinking glass, for instance). West Nile virus is the newest vector-borne disease. It has been in the United States only a short time but has been spread across the United States by migrating birds. Birds contract the disease and die. Mosquitoes then pick up the virus from dead birds and pass the disease on to humans. Microorganisms can also be airborne and carried by air currents. For example, an airborne disease such as tuberculosis (TB) can be transmitted from one person to another in a close living situation. Although not a highly communicable disease, the disease has been the cause of epidemics for centuries.

Microorganisms that develop resistance to various antibiotics can lead to outbreaks of infections in both the medical facility and community. One example is methicillin-resistant *Staphylococcus aureus* (MRSA), discussed later in this chapter under Drug-Resistant Organisms. This strain of staph has been responsible for deaths in hospitals and in the community setting. This infection has become an issue in gyms, prisons, and school locker rooms.

AGENCIES FOR CONTROLLING COMMUNICABLE DISEASES

Infectious and communicable diseases (see Chapters 60 and 61) are the major cause of death throughout the world. They account for a significant threat to public health and for many deaths annually in the United States. The World Health Organization works on the international level to protect people from communicable forms of disease. An **infectious disease** is primarily one that affects the client. It is not necessarily one that can be transmitted to another person. For example, most pneumonias are infectious. If caused by staphylococcus bacteria, they may be communicable. A communicable disease can be transmitted from one person to another under certain conditions.

In the United States, the Centers for Disease Control and Prevention (CDC), a division of the U.S. Public Health Service, is the main agency concerned with protecting the public from disease and controlling its spread on a national level.

The CDC also surveys for trends in all aspects of health and safety. Health departments in states, counties, and cities follow epidemics and illnesses when hospitals, physicians, and other healthcare providers make reports. These reports are required by law and are reported to the CDC each month and tabulated each year to assist with trend/need identification. The U.S. Public Health Service and the CDC are part of the Department of Health and Human Services. They are not part of the Department of Homeland Security.

Infection control is an ever-changing concern. It seems that every year there is a new infection to worry about. Too many people, including healthcare professionals, have taken the attitude that any new health concern can be taken care of with a course of medication. In reality, however, bacteria and viruses are arising faster than the ability to develop new treatments. Most adults under 40 years of age do not even remember most of the childhood illnesses. Medical science and research have provided immunizations that, when administered in a timely manner, have virtually eliminated polio, measles, mumps, rubella, diphtheria, tetanus, and whooping cough. They also have the ability to prevent hepatitis A and B, as well as *haemophilus influenza*. The unfortunate result of not experiencing the illness is that many have lost sight of the importance of keeping immunizations current, so we are seeing a rising incidence of childhood communicable diseases in the community.

Infection

TYPES OF INFECTION

Disease may be referred to as being infectious or communicable. Infectious disease presents as illness in the client but may not be transmissible to others. Communicable diseases are transmissible to others. Infection in a client may be either local or systemic. A **local infection** occurs when the microorganisms are in only a specific part of the body. A **systemic infection** is one that exists when the microorganisms spread to other body areas. The person has *bacteremia* if the microorganisms enter the bloodstream. When bacteremia spreads through all of the body's systems, the condition is called **septicemia.**

Acute infections occur suddenly or last a short time. *Chronic infections* happen slowly over a long period and may last months or years. For example, an ear infection may be described as an acute infection. Hepatitis C viral infection may be described as a chronic infection in some clients.

Infections that occur after hospital admission, and for which the client had no symptoms at the time of admission, are called **nosocomial infections** (hospital-acquired infections). By the end of 2006, the National Center for Preparedness, Detection, and Control of Infectious Diseases had identified 28 different hospital-acquired infections. The nurse as a client advocate has a responsibility to take every precaution to

prevent injury to the client from a hospital-acquired infection (HAI). Surgical site infections account for 30% of all HAIs, and clients who develop a surgical site infection are twice as likely to die as other surgical clients (Odom-Forren, 2006).

Many factors contribute to nosocomial infections. An example of this would be bacteremia caused by an infected or contaminated intravenous (IV) site. An infection directly caused by any diagnostic or therapeutic source (healthcare provider) is called an **iatrogenic infection**. For an example of an iatrogenic infection, see the historical perspective at the beginning of the chapter. Another example would be a urinary tract infection resulting from a break in sterile technique during catheterization.

A microorganism that comes from the client's own body and causes a nosocomial infection is referred to as being from an *endogenous* source. If the organism causing the infection comes from the healthcare environment or personnel, it is from an *exogenous* source. (*Exo* means outside, as in exoskeleton.) The three most common microorganisms causing exogenous infections are *E. coli*, *S. aureus*, and *Enterococcus* species (Table 10-2 ■).

TABLE 10-2	Nosocomial Infections
MOST COMMON ORGANISMS	**CAUSES**
URINARY TRACT	
Escherichia coli	Poor catheterization technique
Enterococcus species	Contamination of closed drainage system
Pseudomonas aeruginosa	Inadequate hand hygiene
SURGICAL SITES	
Staphylococcus aureus	Inadequate hand hygiene
Enterococcus species	Improper dressing change technique
Pseudomonas aeruginosa	Environmental contamination
BLOODSTREAM	
Coagulase-negative staphylococci	Inadequate hand hygiene
Staphylococcus aureus	Improper intravenous fluid, tubing, and site care technique, site prep prior to insertion
Enterococcus species	
PNEUMONIA	
Staphylococcus aureus	Inadequate hand hygiene
Pseudomonas aeruginosa	Improper suctioning technique, improper positioning, lack of respiratory care after anesthesia
Enterobacter species	

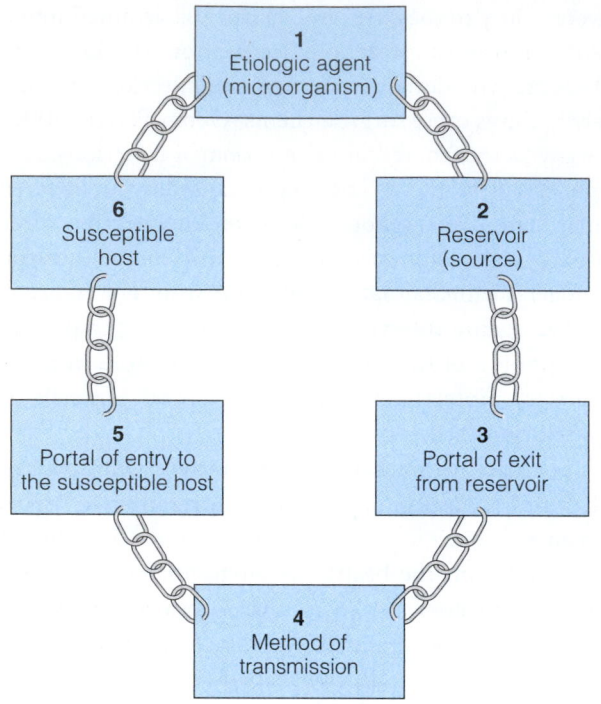

Figure 10-1. ■ The chain of infection.

Factors in the Chain of Infection

The chain of infection is made up of six factors (Figure 10-1 ■): agent, reservoir, portal of exit, method or mode of transmission, portal of entry, and susceptibility of the host.

AGENT/MICROORGANISM

The first link in the chain of infection is the **etiologic agent** (source of the infection). Several factors affect whether or not a microorganism invades the body and causes an infection. These factors include the number of organisms present (dose), how virulent or potent they are, and whether the organisms can live in the host's body. Some organisms, such as bacteria, survive well outside the body in the presence of nutrients and the proper temperature. Others, such as the viruses, do not. For example, HIV virus does not survive outside the body. Some organisms can be present in a person and not present with signs and symptoms. This person may be called a *carrier*. A **carrier** is a potential source of infection for others. For example, a person infected with hepatitis B may be a carrier and be able to transmit the disease to others through his or her blood or through sexual contact.

RESERVOIR

The second link in the chain of infection is the place where the microorganism naturally lives, its reservoir. The source, or **reservoir**, of the microorganism can be many different places: the individual, other humans, animals, plants, insects, birds, or the environment. Food, water, milk, or anything that can be ingested could also be considered a reservoir (Table 10-3 ■). The more a person's resistance is lowered, the more susceptible the person becomes and the more easily he or she will be infected from the reservoir of microorganisms.

TABLE 10-3	Human Reservoirs, Common Infectious Microorganisms, and Portals of Exit	
BODY AREA (SOURCE)	**COMMON INFECTIOUS ORGANISMS**	**PORTALS OF EXIT**
Respiratory tract	Parainfluenza virus *Mycobacterium tuberculosis* *Staphylococcus aureus*	Nose or mouth through sneezing, coughing, talking; endotracheal tubes or tracheostomies
Gastrointestinal tract	Hepatitis A virus *Salmonella* species	Mouth: saliva, vomitus; anus: feces; ostomies: drainage tubes (e.g., nasogastric or T-tubes)
Urinary tract	*Escherichia coli* enterococci *Pseudomonas aeruginosa*	Urethral meatus and urinary diversion ostomies
Reproductive tract (including genitals)	*Neisseria gonorrhoeae* *Treponema pallidum* Herpes simplex virus type 2 Hepatitis B virus	Vagina: vaginal discharge; urinary meatus: urine semen (hepatitis B virus, hepatitis C virus, HIV virus via sexual contact)
Blood	Hepatitis B virus (HBV) Hepatitis C (HCV) HIV *Staphylococcus aureus* *Staphylococcus epidermidis*	Open wound, needle puncture site, any disruption of intact skin or mucous membrane surfaces
Tissue	*Staphylococcus aureus* *Escherichia coli* *Proteus* species *Streptococcus* beta-hemolytic A or B	Drainage from cut or wound

PORTAL OF EXIT FROM THE RESERVOIR

The third link in the chain is the **portal of exit,** a way of leaving the reservoir. The microorganism must leave the reservoir in order to spread the infection. Any body fluid can provide an exit from the source. Wound drainage, blood, urine, feces, mucus, or any break in the skin or mucous membrane can all provide a portal of exit.

METHODS OR MODES OF TRANSMISSION

The fourth link in the chain of infection is a method, or mode, of **transmission**. It is the manner in which the microorganism gets to the host. There are three modes of transmission. The first is direct contact. This occurs differently for different diseases. For bloodborne diseases, blood-to-blood contact must occur.

The second method is indirect contact. An example would be that of a nurse who has an open cut on her hand and picks up a piece of equipment that has blood on it. Another example is *vector-borne transmission,* which could occur when an animal or insect bites or injects the microorganism through saliva into the host, or leaves feces or other material on the host's traumatized skin. An example is West Nile virus infection. Water, food, blood products, or contact with a **fomite** (an inanimate object such as a toy, cooking or eating utensil, or contaminated instrument) are all examples of *vehicle-borne transmission.* When a person eats poorly cooked chicken contaminated with the *Salmonella* species and becomes ill, the microorganism was transmitted by a vehicle.

The third method of transmission is droplet or airborne transmission. These modes usually involve droplet nuclei, the remains of droplets coming from an infected person, which are suspended in the air. An example of airborne transmission is when someone infected with untreated pulmonary tuberculosis coughs. The bacteria are expelled into the air, and another individual then inhales it into his or her lungs. An example of droplet transmission is influenza (flu). Dust particles can also carry infectious spores, viruses, and bacteria. Microorganisms can be inhaled into the lungs when dust is disturbed and becomes airborne. An example of this might be anthrax.

PORTAL OF ENTRY

The fifth link in the chain of infection is a **portal of entry** into the host. Intact skin is a barrier to pathogenic microorganisms. However, broken skin provides a portal of entry for a pathogen. Most microorganisms enter the body through the same routes they use to leave it. For example, an organism that was inhaled into the lungs can then be coughed out to infect someone else.

SUSCEPTIBLE HOST

The sixth link in the chain of infection is the **susceptibility of the host**. The body provides natural defenses to fight off infection. Immune response serves to protect from infection even if an exposure were to occur. An individual who has impaired immune response and is at risk for developing an infection is called a **susceptible host**. A *compromised host* is someone who has a higher risk for getting an infection, for one or more reasons. An example would be a geriatric client with emphysema; this person is at a higher risk for developing pneumonia than someone of the same age without emphysema.

It is important to recognize that these six factors must all come together for transmission to possibly result in infection. They cannot function independently and cause infection. And, even if they all come together, that does not mean infection will occur because the immune system may respond and protect the person. In the provision of health care, it is important to remember that exposure does not always mean infection.

Factors that Reduce Host Resistance

Some factors will impact and reduce the body's immune response. Age is a factor influencing the risk of infection. Both the very young and the elderly have reduced defenses. Newborns have immature immune systems and are protected for only the first 2 or 3 months by immunities they received from their mother. Immunizations against communicable diseases are started at about 2 months of age, when the infant's immune system can respond.

The immune system becomes weak in the elderly, and as they age they develop infections more easily or suffer from chronic disease. The CDC recommends annual immunizations for them against influenza and pneumonia, particularly if they have histories of cardiac, renal, respiratory, or metabolic diseases. Heredity may also influence the development of infections. People may have a genetic susceptibility to them.

Stressors in life can influence susceptibility to infection. Stressors can be physical, emotional, or both. The nature, number, and duration of the stressors may all influence whether or not the individual develops an infection. Stressors elevate blood cortisol. Cortisol is a hormone in the body that is secreted by the adrenal glands. This hormone is responsible for regulating blood pressure, immune function, and proper glucose metabolism. Small increases in cortisol can result in some very positive effects: (1) increased energy, (2) increased immunity, (3) lower sensitivity to pain, and (4) heightened memory. Prolonged elevation of cortisol decreases anti-inflammatory responses; drains energy stores, causing exhaustion; decreases resistance to infection; impairs cognitive performance; suppresses thyroid function; decreases bone density; and creates sugar imbalances.

Nutrition plays a role in resistance to infection. Good nutrition provides ample proteins, which allow the body to manufacture antibodies. Medical therapies may contribute to the development of infection. Radiation treatments for cancer and diagnostic procedures that penetrate the skin or sterile body cavities are examples of procedures that increase infection risk.

Some medications can increase the chance of infection by depressing bone marrow production of white blood cells (leukocytes). Also, corticosteroids (steroids) slow down the inflammatory response needed to fight infection. Antibiotics, however, may kill not only infectious organisms but also the resident flora. This would allow other strains, which would not normally grow, to multiply. Some microorganisms may become resistant to certain medications, making them more difficult to treat. Smoking has been clearly recognized as a factor that impacts or lowers immune response.

Chronic diseases (*pathologies*) that lessen the body's defense system increase the risk for infection. Some examples are pulmonary diseases (emphysema, asthma), burns, peripheral vascular diseases, diseases of the blood, and diabetes mellitus.

Defenses against Infection

NONSPECIFIC DEFENSES

The body has normal defenses to protect it against infection. **Nonspecific defenses** include anatomic and physiological barriers and the inflammatory response:

- Intact skin protects against pathogens. Organisms can live on the skin but cannot penetrate it. Resident flora (bacteria) on the skin stops other bacteria from growing. The skin's slight acidity also inhibits bacterial growth.
- Moist mucous membranes and cilia in the nose trap microorganisms, dust, and foreign materials.
- Special cells in the lungs (called macrophages or phagocytes) ingest microorganisms and foreign particles.
- Saliva in the mouth helps to prevent infection by its washing action. The presence of enzymes also serves as a protective measure.
- Tears (which have an enzyme in them) wash away organisms and protect the eyes. Tears also reduce the number load (dose) of organisms present.
- Stomach acids protect the stomach from infection. Resident flora in the large intestine stops the growth of other microorganisms.

- Vaginal secretions have a pH that stops the growth of many disease-producing bacteria.
- The flow of urine flushes the urethra and keeps bacteria from entering the bladder. Urine is a sterile body fluid.
- Gastric acids and bile serve to kill some organisms.
- Chemical agents in the immune system, such as interferon, kill viruses.

SPECIFIC OR IMMUNE DEFENSES

Specific defenses are also known as *immune defenses*. They work against identified foreign proteins such as bacteria, fungi, viruses, and other infectious agents, which are considered to be invading agents and are called **antigens**.

The resistance of the body to infection is known as **immunity** (Table 10-4 ■). In *active immunity,* the body produces its own antibodies to natural antigens (e.g., infection) or artificial antigens (e.g., vaccines). For example, if you acquire chickenpox, you will develop acquired immunity. The same is true if you receive the chickenpox vaccine. *Passive immunity* refers to receipt of natural antibodies (e.g., from a nursing mother). Two systems are working and overlapping during the immune response. See Box 10-1 ■ for specific cultural immunity issues.

Antibody-Mediated Defense

Immune response is made up of two separate but interrelated systems. These systems are mediated by B and T lymphocytes. B cells originate in the bone marrow from stem cells. T cells also originate in the bone marrow but in more primitive stem cells.

The *antibody-mediated defense* (also called circulating or *humoral immunity*) depends primarily on the B lymphocytes. They are mediated by antibodies produced from B cells, which flow through the bloodstream. These antibodies are also called immunoglobulins (Ig) and are part of the body's plasma proteins. The B cells are activated and attack when they recognize a foreign invader (antigens). B cells secrete antibodies to assist in the destruction of antigens. B cells bind to the antigens, which makes it easier for phagocytes to get to the antigens.

TABLE 10-4	Types of Acquired Immunity	
TYPE	**ANTIGEN OR ANTIBODY SOURCE**	**DURATION**
Active immunity	Antibodies are produced by the body in response to an antigen.	Long
a. Natural	Antibodies are formed in the presence of active infection in the body.	Lifelong
b. Artificial	Antigens (vaccines or toxoids) are administered to stimulate antibody production.	Many years: the immunity must be reinforced by booster inoculations
Passive immunity	Antibodies are produced by another source, animal or human.	Short
a. Natural	Antibodies are transferred naturally from an immune mother to her baby through the placenta or in colostrum.	6 months to 1 year
b. Artificial	Immune serum (antibody) from an animal or another human is injected.	2 to 3 weeks

Infection

Although susceptibility to infectious/communicable diseases is frequently linked to socioeconomic factors such as overcrowding and poor nutrition, there are some ethnic factors that should be considered:

■ Ethnicity appears to be a factor in the incidence of tuberculosis and hepatitis B viral infection. Native Americans living in the southwest, Vietnamese refugees, and Mexican Americans have a relatively high incidence of these diseases.

■ Africans possessing sickle cell trait are known to have increased immunity to malaria.

■ Childhood illnesses caused by viruses such as rubeola and varicella are considered to be benign in a majority of children. However, many countries do not have the vaccine and immunization programs in place that are standard here in the United States.

■ HIV infections continue to be a major health problem, with racial/ethnic minorities suffering a disproportionate share of the disease.

Cell-Mediated Defense

The *cell-mediated defense* acts through the T-cell system. When a person is exposed to an antigen, the lymphoid tissue produces and releases large numbers of T cells into the lymphatic fluid and system. If T-cell immunity is lost, people cannot defend themselves against most viral, bacterial, and fungal infections. An example of depressed T-cell function is HIV infection. This system serves as the first line of protection from illness and disease.

Inflammatory Response

The **inflammatory response** is a local nonspecific defense reaction of tissues when they are exposed to infection or injury. The inflammatory response destroys or dilutes microorganisms and prevents their spread. There are five primary signs of inflammation: pain, swelling, redness, heat, and (if there is severe injury) weakened function of a body part. Inflammation of a part is indicated by the suffix *-itis*. For example, appendicitis is inflammation of the appendix.

There are three stages to the inflammatory response:

■ *First stage: vascular and cellular response.* During the cellular and vascular response, blood vessels first constrict at the site of injury. This is quickly followed by dilation of small vessels in the area, which causes increased blood flow and redness (*hyperemia*) with increased warmth. Fluid enters the interstitial space, causing edema and irritation to the nerve endings and producing pain. Blood flow eventually slows down in the capillaries, and *leukocytes* (white blood cells) move out of them into the tissues to work against the microorganisms.

■ *Second stage: exudate production.* The exudate consists of dead phagocytic cells (cells that attacked the microorganism).

During this stage the microorganisms are killed. The exudate is removed when it drains into the lymphatic system channels or leaves the body as drainage. The major types of exudates are serous, purulent, and hemorrhagic (sanguineous). (See types of cultures in Chapters 23, 24, 27, and 28 ⚭ .)

■ *Third stage: reparative phase.* In the reparative phase, the tissues regenerate cells that are similar or identical in structure and function to the dead cells. Some tissues (such as skin) regenerate well; others (such as nerve tissue) regenerate little if at all. The sequence of repair of damaged tissue is discussed in detail in Chapter 24 ⚭ .

LABORATORY TESTS FOR INFECTION

Some abnormal values from laboratory tests indicate infection. Elevated white blood cell counts with changes in specific types of cells are seen on the differential count. Neutrophils increase with bacterial infections. Lymphocytes are elevated with viral infections. The erythrocyte sedimentation rate (ESR) increases with the inflammatory response. Cultures of body fluids and any drainage can identify specific organisms.

Drug-Resistant Organisms

During the past two decades, there has been rising concern regarding the increased incidence of nosocomial (hospital-acquired) infections involving drug-resistant organisms. The overuse and misuse of antibiotics, as well as the tendency of clients not to complete a prescribed course of treatment, have impacted the development of resistant organisms. In the 1980s, drug companies were not developing new antibiotics. There seemed to be a feeling that bacterial infections were a thing of the past. Bacteria can become resistant to antibiotics "naturally." This happens because when antibiotics are taken and bacteria are killed, the antibiotic will leave behind some bacteria that caused resistance to occur. Added to this is the fact that when new antibiotics are developed, physicians tend to prescribe them en masse, overlooking common and less expensive antibiotics. Resistance develops, and the number of antibiotics available to treat an infection is fewer. Clients often demand that their physicians give them antibiotics even when they are not needed. For example, clients may ask for antibiotics when they have the flu, but an antibiotic is not effective against the flu virus. Box 10-2 ■ provides teaching for clients about taking antibiotic medications.

Another factor that may lead to the development of resistance is failure to complete a full course of prescribed medication. For example, when clients with tuberculosis do not complete their full course of treatment, they may develop drug-resistant tuberculosis. Currently, the three most

BOX 10-2   CLIENT TEACHING

Taking Antibiotics

Client Teaching

Complete the full course of medication prescribed.
Do not take antibiotics for viral illnesses.
Older, more common antibiotics work well.

Rationale

Failure to complete the full course of treatment may result in prolonged illness and the development of drug resistance. Antibiotics are for the treatment of bacterial infections only. Overuse of new, more powerful antibiotics may lead to resistance.

prominent types of drug-resistant organisms are MRSA, vancomycin-resistant enterococci (VRE), and multi-drug-resistant TB. Hospitalized clients whose immune systems are already compromised are at the greatest risk.

Failure to perform appropriate hand hygiene is considered to be the leading cause of healthcare-associated infections and spread of multi-drug-resistant organisms and has been recognized as a substantial contributor to outbreaks (CDC, 2002).

METHICILLIN-RESISTANT STAPHYLOCOCCUS AUREUS

During the summer and fall of 2007, there was a public concern about MRSA (methicillin-resistant *Staphylococcus aureus*). Once thought to be a hospital-acquired infection (HAMRSA), it has been reported as community-acquired methicillin-resistant *Staphylococcus aureus* (CAMRSA) in medical literature for about 8 years. Reports emerged of a much higher estimated incidence of infection (32/100,000) and higher death rate than previously thought. The report of the death of a student in Virginia from MRSA resulted in public hysteria.

In reality, only 14% of invasive infections of MRSA are community acquired. News reports of a school-based epidemic were also exaggerated; since the incidence of infection rates in 5- to 17-year-olds is only 1.4/100,000. This is much lower than the incidence of infection in the 65 and older age group of 128/100,000. Although public health officers do not consider CAMRSA a superbug, healthcare professionals and the general population need to recognize and respect it.

Table 10-5 ■ provides a comparison of CAMRSA and HAMRSA.

Transmission

The MRSA organism is colonized in the nose. It inoculates a wound by hand transfer or is transferred by hand-to-hand contact and then is introduced to nasal mucosa from the hand (Figure 10-2 ■).

Risk factors for infection include:

■ Compromised skin
■ Contact skin-to-skin
■ Contaminated items or surfaces
■ Crowding
■ Poor hygiene

Staphylococcus aureus skin infection usually presents initially as a small lesion, which is frequently confused with a spider bite. Some of the confusion occurs because the initial lesion will itch or sting. Left untreated, the lesion will develop into furuncles (boils) (Figure 10-3A ■) and progress to cellulitis (Figure 10-3B).

Prevention and Control

The first line of defense is proper personal hygiene including frequent hand washing. (*Note:* It is important not to share towels used for drying.) Hygiene also includes regular bathing and not sharing personal care items. All cuts and scrapes need to be covered with a bandage to avoid infection. Youth need to be advised of the potential for infection when engaging in sports activities (Box 10-3 ■).

Treatment

Draining and packing wounds is the primary treatment in young healthy individuals. "Incision and drainage without antibiotic therapy is effective in management of CAMRSA skin and soft-tissue abscesses less than 5 cm in immunocompetent children" (Lee et al., 2004, p. 123).

Antibiotic therapy includes:

■ Trimethoprim—sulfamethoxazole
■ Clindamycin
■ Rifampin
■ Vancomycin
■ Linezolid (last resort; very expensive)

TABLE 10-5   Comparison of CAMRSA and HAMRSA

COMMUNITY-ACQUIRED METHICILLIN-RESISTANT *STAPHYLOCOCCUS AUREUS* (CAMRSA)	HOSPITAL-ACQUIRED METHICILLIN-RESISTANT *STAPHYLOCOCCUS AUREUS* (HAMRSA)
Causes skin and soft tissue infections; invasive infections rare	Invasive infections common (pneumonia, bacteremia)
Typically affects young healthy persons	Most common in hospitals and nursing homes
Resistant to penicillins and cephalosporins, but sensitive to several oral antibiotics (Bactrim, clindamycin, rifampin, and others)	Multi-drug-resistant organisms, usually sensitive only to IV antibiotics
Toxin production common	Usually no toxin production

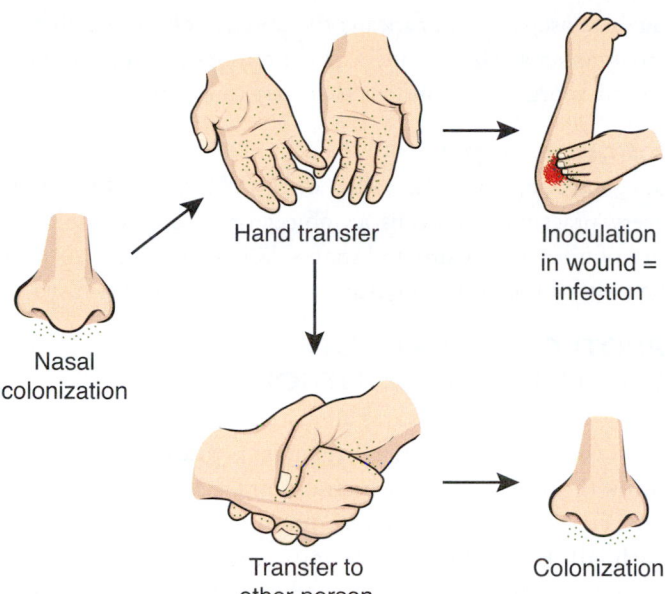

Figure 10-2. ■ Transmission of *Staphylococcus aureus*.

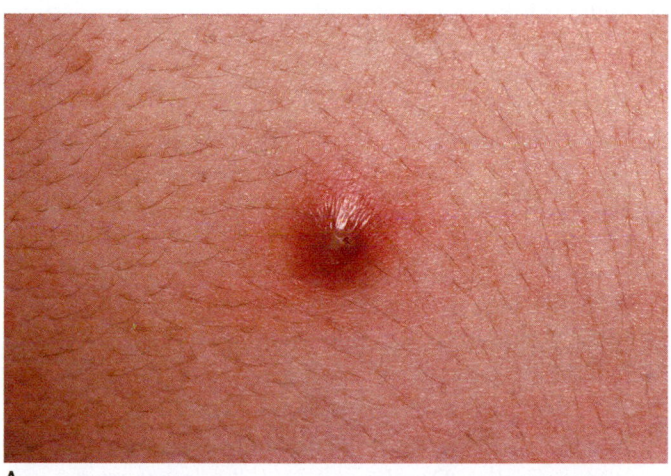

A

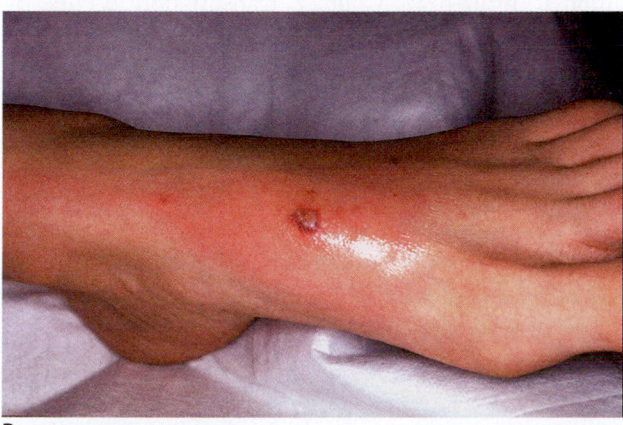

B

Figure 10-3. ■ **A.** Development of *S. aureus* infection into furunculosis (boils). *Source:* Phototake NYC. **B.** Cellulitis spreading out from the source of the infection. *Source:* Charles Stewart MD FACEP, FAAEM.

BOX 10-3	PEDIATRIC CONSIDERATIONS

Sports and the Potential for Infection

Shared sports equipment and contaminated surfaces are a significant source of infection. Laundering and disinfection must be done frequently and thoroughly. Items must be cleaned to remove any organic material prior to disinfection. Disinfectants used must be appropriate for the surface and must be effective against staph infection.

Students with infections must be adequately managed. Infected lesions must be covered with bandage material sufficient to contain any drainage for the entire school day.

Controlling Microorganisms in the Environment

CLINICAL GUIDELINES FOR HAND HYGIENE

Recommendations by the CDC for hand hygiene and hand antisepsis follow:

- When hands are visibly dirty or contaminated with proteinaceous material or are visibly soiled with blood or body fluids, wash hands with either a non-antimicrobial (microbe destroying) soap and water or an **antimicrobial** soap and water (waterless hand cleaner cannot remove organic material).
- If hands are not visibly soiled, use alcohol-based hand rub for routinely decontaminating hands in all other clinical situations.
- When decontaminating hands with an alcohol-based hand rub, apply product to palm of one hand and rub together, covering all surfaces of hands and fingers, until hands are dry.
- Hands should also be washed with soap and water after glove removal. (CDC, 2002)

See Procedure 10-1 ■ on page 178 for hand hygiene instructions.

AGENTS FOR CONTROLLING MICROORGANISMS

Maintaining a clean environment helps to inhibit the growth and multiplication of organisms. The very process of cleaning slows down the growth of microorganisms. **Antiseptics** (agents that inhibit the growth of some microorganisms) and **disinfectants** (agents that destroy pathogens other than spores) help to keep control of organisms in the environment.

Disinfection requires the use of a disinfectant solution that contains a chemical preparation, such as phenol, bleach, or other chemical compounds. These substances should not

---

BOX 10-4   NURSING CARE CHECKLIST

Using Bactericidal and Bacteriostatic Agents

When disinfecting, remember to:

☑ Use the recommended concentration of the solution and keep it on the area for the required amount of time.

☑ Know the type and number of infectious organisms. Make certain no soap is present on the item since some disinfectants will not work when soap is present.

☑ Keep the room temperature within a normal range because some disinfectants will not work otherwise.

☑ Be certain there is no organic material (e.g., blood, pus, excretions) present because the disinfectants may be inactivated.

☑ Treat all exposed surface areas and crevices.

---

be used on tissue because they are often caustic or toxic. Both antiseptics (which can be used on tissue) and disinfectants have bactericidal and/or bacteriostatic properties. A **bactericidal agent** destroys bacteria, whereas a **bacteriostatic agent** prevents growth and reproduction of only some bacteria. Important points to remember when disinfecting are listed in Box 10-4 ■. Using boiling water for a minimum of 15 minutes is a good method for the home setting.

Sterilization destroys all microorganisms, viruses, and spores. Moist heat (steam) can be used under pressure or as a free agent to sterilize. Autoclaves provide steam under pressure, with temperatures ranging from 121 to 123°C (250 to 254°F) and 15 to 17 lbs of pressure. Free steam at 100°C (212°F) must be used for at least 30 minutes for 3 consecutive days. Gas sterilization is effective for heat-sensitive items. An example is ethylene oxide gas. However, it is toxic, and staff working with this form of sterilization must wear badges to monitor exposure. Radiation can also be employed in sterilization. Ionizing radiation is often used for foods and drugs that are sensitive to heat, although it is a very costly process. This is not routinely used in the healthcare setting.

ASEPTIC TECHNIQUE

Asepsis is the absence of disease-causing microorganisms. **Sepsis** is the opposite, the presence of infection. It can take many forms in the human body. **Aseptic technique** is used to prevent the possibility of transferring microorganisms from one place or person to another.

Medical Asepsis

Medical asepsis includes all practices that are used to confine a specific microorganism to a specific area, or to limit the number of microorganisms, their growth, and their transmission. Objects are referred to as clean or dirty in medical asepsis. *Clean* means the absence of almost all microorganisms. *Dirty* (soiled or contaminated) means there are microorganisms present that may cause an infection.

Surgical Asepsis

Surgical asepsis is also called *sterile technique*, and it means every practice that keeps an object or an area completely free of microorganisms and spores. When dealing with sterile areas of the body, only surgical asepsis should be used.

PROTECTIVE PRECAUTIONS FOR INFECTION CONTROL

Infection control measures are used in institutions to prevent the spread of microorganisms. **Standard Precautions** (Figure 10-4 ■), which are practiced in all healthcare facilities, are guidelines for special care to be used with all body fluids, especially those associated with bloodborne pathogens (e.g., hepatitis B and C, and HIV infections). In 1996, the CDC presented new guidelines for isolation precautions that included two levels: Tier 1 or Standard Precautions, and Tier 2 or Transmission-based Precautions.

Standard Precautions

Standard Precautions are used in the care of all clients. They are applied to all body fluids, blood, secretions, excretions (except sweat), mucous membranes, and nonintact skin.

Transmission-based Precautions

Transmission-based Precautions are used in addition to Standard Precautions for any client with known or suspected infections that are spread by airborne or droplet transmission or by physical contact. Airborne nuclei are those agents smaller than 3 microns (e.g., tuberculosis, measles, varicella). Droplets are particles larger than 3 microns (e.g., diphtheria, streptococcal pharyngitis, mumps, pneumonia, influenza). Contact transmission occurs by touching items in the client's environment that are contaminated. Contact precautions would be appropriate for MRSA- and VRE-infected clients.

ISOLATION PRACTICES.   Isolation practices are initiated after assessing the client's condition. CDC guidelines, institutional policies, nursing assessment, and laboratory study results are used to make the decision to place an individual in an isolated environment. Other factors that must be considered are the status of the client's defense mechanisms, the source of the infection, and its mode of transmission.

TRANSPORTING CLIENTS WITH INFECTIONS.   Clients with infections are not transported outside of their own rooms unless it is necessary for testing or treatment. If they need to be moved to another area, the environment must be

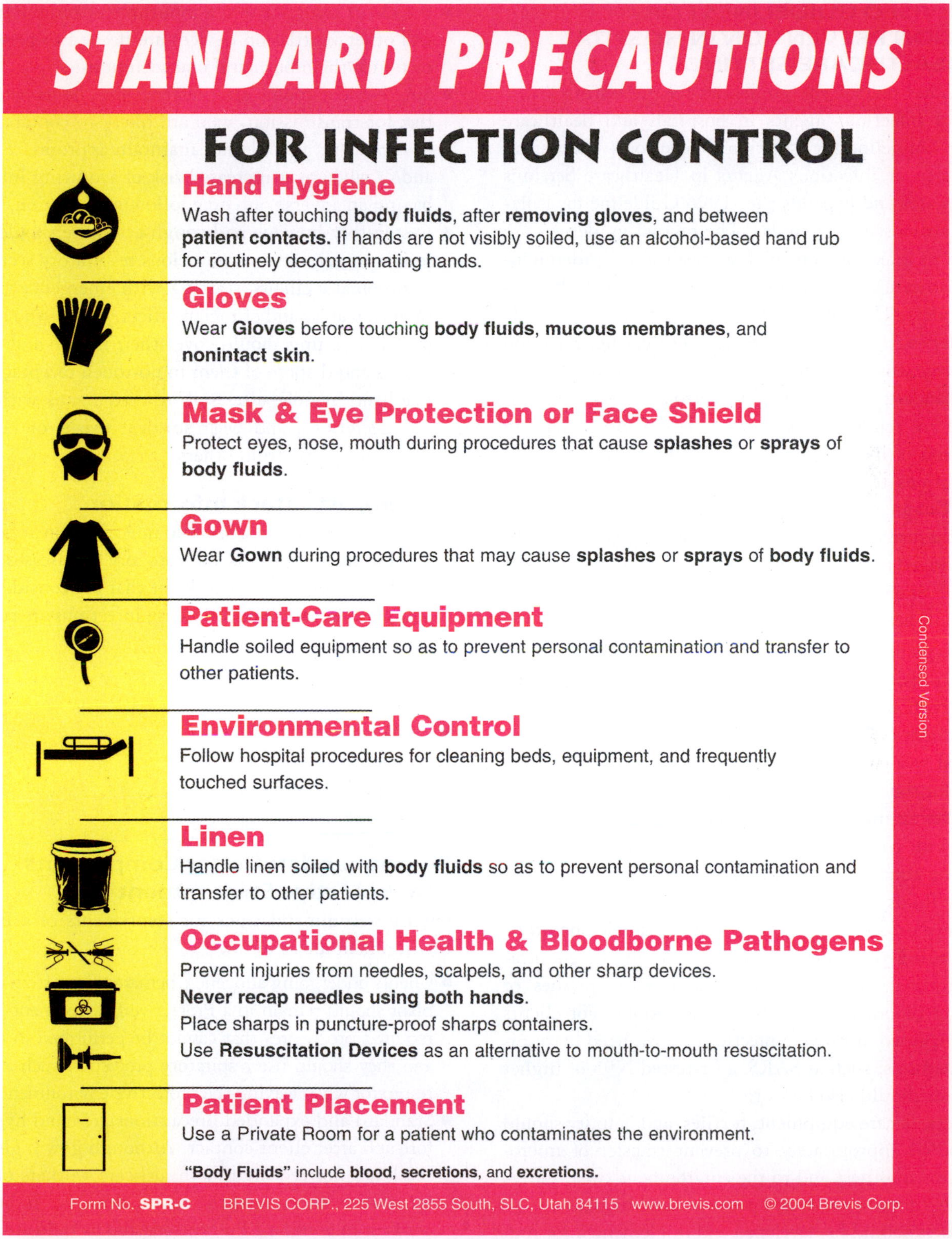

STANDARD PRECAUTIONS

FOR INFECTION CONTROL

Hand Hygiene
Wash after touching **body fluids**, after **removing gloves**, and between **patient contacts.** If hands are not visibly soiled, use an alcohol-based hand rub for routinely decontaminating hands.

Gloves
Wear **Gloves** before touching **body fluids**, **mucous membranes**, and **nonintact skin**.

Mask & Eye Protection or Face Shield
Protect eyes, nose, mouth during procedures that cause **splashes** or **sprays** of **body fluids**.

Gown
Wear **Gown** during procedures that may cause **splashes** or **sprays** of **body fluids**.

Patient-Care Equipment
Handle soiled equipment so as to prevent personal contamination and transfer to other patients.

Environmental Control
Follow hospital procedures for cleaning beds, equipment, and frequently touched surfaces.

Linen
Handle linen soiled with **body fluids** so as to prevent personal contamination and transfer to other patients.

Occupational Health & Bloodborne Pathogens
Prevent injuries from needles, scalpels, and other sharp devices.
Never recap needles using both hands.
Place sharps in puncture-proof sharps containers.
Use **Resuscitation Devices** as an alternative to mouth-to-mouth resuscitation.

Patient Placement
Use a Private Room for a patient who contaminates the environment.

"Body Fluids" include **blood**, **secretions**, and **excretions**.

Condensed Version

Form No. **SPR-C**   BREVIS CORP., 225 West 2855 South, SLC, Utah 84115   www.brevis.com   © 2004 Brevis Corp.

Figure 10-4. ■ Standard Precautions for infection control. (*Source:* Courtesy of BREVIS Corporation.)

protected to avoid contamination. The client should wear a surgical mask if the infection is airborne, and all draining wounds should be covered with dressings that will not leak. The area the client is going to should be advised of the isolation precautions ordered so that they can take precautions to maintain the environment. The client should wear clean clothing, so as not to contaminate wheelchairs or transportation carts.

CDC REVISED GUIDELINES FOR INFECTION PREVENTION IN HOSPITAL AND HEALTHCARE SETTINGS

The CDC has revised the guidelines for preventing transmission of infectious agents in hospitals and healthcare settings. "Guideline for Isolation Precautions: Preventing Transmission of Infectious Agents in Healthcare Settings 2007" updates and expands the "1996 Guideline for Isolation Precautions in Hospitals." The revised guidelines are addressed to infection control staff, healthcare epidemiologists, healthcare administrators, nurses, and other healthcare providers. They also address other persons responsible for developing, implementing, and evaluating infection control programs in a variety of healthcare settings.

The Standard Precautions first introduced in the 1996 guideline are reinforced as the foundation for preventing transmission of infectious agents in all healthcare settings. New additions to these recommendations are Respiratory Hygiene/Cough Etiquette and safe injection practices, including the use of a mask when performing certain high-risk, prolonged procedures involving spinal canal punctures.

Specific Standard Precautions recommendations for all clients in all healthcare settings are as follows:

- Hand hygiene should be performed after touching blood, body fluids, secretions, excretions, and contaminated items, both immediately after removing gloves and between client contacts.
- Personal protective equipment (PE) should include gloves for touching blood, body fluids, secretions, excretions, contaminated items, mucous membranes, and non-intact skin; gown during client procedures and activities involving contact of clothing or exposed skin with blood or body fluids, secretions, and excretions.
- Mask, eye protection (goggles), and face shield should be worn during procedures such as suctioning or endotracheal intubation that are associated with splashes or sprays of blood, body fluids, and secretions. For clients with suspected or proven infections transmitted by respiratory aerosols, such as SARS, a fit-tested N95 or higher respirator should also be worn.
- Soiled client-care equipment, textiles, and laundry should be handled appropriately to prevent transfer of microorganisms to others and to the environment (wear gloves if visibly contaminated, and perform hand hygiene).
- Procedures should be developed and implemented for routine care, cleaning, and disinfecting environmental surfaces, especially frequently touched surfaces in client care areas.
- Used needles should not be recapped, bent, broken, or manipulated by hand. A one-handed scoop technique only should be used when recapping is required. Safety features should be used when available and used "sharps" should be placed in a puncture-resistant container.

- For client resuscitation, a mouthpiece, resuscitation bag, and other ventilation devices are needed to prevent contact with the mouth and oral secretions.
- Single-client rooms are preferred for clients at increased risk for transmission, who are likely to contaminate the environment, who do not maintain appropriate hygiene, and/or who are at increased risk of acquiring infection or having an adverse outcome following infection.
- Respiratory hygiene and cough etiquette should include source containment of infectious respiratory secretions in symptomatic clients, starting with emergency triage and reception areas and clinician offices. Those who are sneezing or coughing should cover their mouth and nose, use tissues and dispose of them in no-touch receptacles, practice hand hygiene after soiling their hands with respiratory secretions, and wear surgical masks or keep more than 3 feet away from others.

Bioterrorist Attack Information

The guidelines describe specific infection control considerations for high-priority (CDC category A) diseases that may result from bioterrorist attacks or that are considered to be bioterrorist threats. The following infections are considered potential bioterrorist agents:

- Anthrax
- Botulism
- Ebola hemorrhagic fever
- Plague
- Smallpox
- Tularemia

Recommendations for Components of a Protective Environment

Specific recommendations for components of a Protective Environment are as follows:

- Clients undergoing allogeneic hematopoietic stem cell transplant should remain in a Protective Environment except for required procedures that cannot be performed in the room, and they should use respiratory protection such as an N95 respirator when leaving the protective environment.
- Standard and expanded precautions are hand hygiene before and after client contact. Although gown, gloves, and mask are not required for healthcare workers or visitors for routine entry into the room, these are indicated according to Standard Precautions and as indicated for suspected or proven infections for which Transmission-based Precautions are recommended.
- Engineering features should include central or point-of-use high-efficiency particulate air (HEPA; 99.97% efficiency) filters that can remove particles 0.3 μm in diameter for supply (incoming) air; well-sealed rooms; properly constructed windows, doors, and intake and exhaust ports;

smooth ceilings free of fissures, open joints, and crevices; walls sealed above and below the ceiling; repairs of any leakage detected; ventilation to maintain more than 12 air changes per hour; directed airflow with air supply and exhaust grills located so that clean, filtered air enters from one side of the room, flows across the client's bed, and exits on the opposite side of the room; positive room air pressure relative to the hallway; pressure differential of greater than 2.5 Pa (0.01-inch water gauge); daily visual monitoring of airflow patterns; self-closing door on all room exits; and back-up ventilation equipment.

- Clients needing both a protective environment and airborne infection isolation should have an anteroom to provide proper air balance relationships and independent exhaust of contaminated air to the outside, or a HEPA filter should be placed in the exhaust duct. In place of an anteroom, the client may be placed in an airborne infection isolation room with portable ventilation units and industrial-grade HEPA filters to enhance filtration of spores.

- Horizontal surfaces should be wet-dusted daily with cloths moistened with Environmental Protection Agency–registered hospital disinfectant and detergent. Methods that stir up dust should be avoided, as should carpeting in client rooms or hallways, upholstered furniture and furnishings, and fresh or dried flowers or potted plants in PE rooms or areas. When vacuum cleaning is needed, the vacuum should be equipped with HEPA filters.

See Box 10-5 ■ for a summary of the CDC recommendations.

clinical ALERT

The use of alcohol-based solutions is preferred to hand washing with soap and water in most situations following contact with a client or medical equipment.

According to the current guidelines, healthcare workers should wear masks when caring for clients with droplet precautions. However, masks are not necessary during client transport if the client is wearing a mask, and there were no recommendations made regarding eye protection for such clients.

EQUIPMENT FOR INFECTION CONTROL

Personal Protective Equipment

Particular items are used to protect the personnel, the client, and the environment when administering care. They include gloves, gowns, protective eyewear, and masks.

Gloves are used to protect the nurse's hands from coming in contact with body fluids and contaminated items. They also protect the client from the nurse's microorganisms. Gloves reduce the transmission of microorganisms from one client to another, or to any object (*fomite*) where microorganisms might grow. Hands are washed before and after wearing gloves. Gloves are not a primary protection measure.

BOX 10-5 NURSING CARE CHECKLIST

CDC Recommendations for Infection Control

When hands become visibly soiled or there is possible contact with spores (such as *C. difficile*) in a client care setting, they should be carefully washed with soap and water. Otherwise, alcohol-based hand gels are the preferred method for hand decontamination between clients. Decontamination should be performed after contact with a client as well as after contact with medical equipment.

Artificial fingernails should be avoided among healthcare providers.

In pediatric practices, toys provided to clients should be easy to clean and disinfect. Sharing of stuffed animals should be avoided.

Clients who are coughing or sneezing in the waiting area should ideally be separated by at least 3 feet from other clients.

Personal protective equipment, such as gloves and gowns, should be readily available at all times. Healthcare workers should put on such equipment prior to contact with a potential pathogen and remove and discard it in the client room.

Healthcare workers should wear an appropriate mask in caring for clients with droplet precautions in their hospital room, but masks are not necessary for workers transporting such clients as long as the client is wearing a mask. No recommendation was made regarding the use of eye protection when caring for clients with droplet precautions.

Clients with airborne infection precautions should be placed in an appropriate isolation room with at least six air changes per hour (for newer buildings, 12 or more air changes per hour) and a direct vent to outside the building for exhausted air.

Clients suspected of having illnesses such as tuberculosis or SARS in ambulatory settings should be placed in an examination room and should wear a surgical mask. This room should not be used for 1 hour after the client departs to ensure an adequate exchange of air.

It is not clear whether healthcare workers with a presumed immunity to measles or varicella zoster who are caring for clients with active measles or varicella should wear personal protective equipment. It also is unclear what the best type of equipment to wear to prevent transmission of infection from these clients is.

Dried and fresh flowers should be prohibited from client care areas, as should potted plants.

For injected medications, single-dose vials are preferred to multiple-dose vials.

For many activities, only clean gloves are worn, and no special technique is used to put them on. Removal of soiled gloves should be done in such a way that the hand does not touch the soiled surface. This can be accomplished by pulling the glove off the hand while turning the soiled side to the inside of the glove. Place the first glove in the palm of the second gloved hand and remove the glove in the same manner as the first. The soiled side is now encased and it can be dropped into a trash container.

Sterile gloves are worn if the nurse works with a wound or when the nurse's hands enter a body orifice. A specific technique is used to apply and remove sterile gloves (Procedure 10-2 ■ on page 179). If a gown is worn, the cuff of the glove is pulled over the gown's sleeve.

Gowns are used only once before being either discarded or laundered. Gowns should be water resistant and clean. Sterile gowns are used in surgery and in cases of reverse isolation (wherein the client is protected from organisms carried by the staff) or when the nurse is changing dressings on extensive wounds (e.g., burns). No special technique is used to put on a clean gown or to take it off if it is not visibly soiled. If there is a large amount of contamination, the nurse should avoid touching the contaminated area and roll the gown up with the soiled area inside. The gown is then disposed of in the proper container. Sterile gowns are grasped at the crease near the neck and held away from the body. They are allowed to unfold without touching anything. If the gown's outer surface does touch something, it is contaminated. The nurse's hands are put into the shoulders and sleeves without touching the outside of the gown. The hands can be put through the cuff using the open method of sterile gloving. A coworker will tie the gown at the neck and at the back without touching the outside surface (Procedure 10-3 ■ on page 181).

Face masks are worn to stop the spread of microorganism and airborne droplets from either the nurse to the client, or the client to the nurse. They also protect against splatters from body fluids. Many face masks now have transparent protective eye coverings. Otherwise, protective glasses or goggles should be worn if there is a possibility of body fluid splatters. The CDC recommends that people within 3 feet of the client should wear masks if the infection is transmitted by large particle droplets. If the infection is transmitted by small particle or droplet nuclei, all persons entering the room should wear masks. Masks should be disposable and worn only once. They should be replaced if they become wet or soiled. They are to be disposed of in the appropriate waste container.

Particulate respirators are also used to protect against droplet transmission. Many different types are available, and some are disposable. The CDC recommends those with a rating of N95, which means a category N respirator that has 95% efficiency and meets the tuberculosis control criteria. The use of this mask by the nurse requires a medical evaluation and fit testing to ensure a proper fit and the absence of health problems that would interfere with the nurse's ability to wear a respirator. The Occupational Safety and Health Administration (OSHA) has published a specific regulation, *Respiratory Standard 1910.134*, that addresses the use of respirators.

When removing soiled protective equipment:

1. Remove the gloves first (if the gown is tied in the front, undo the ties before removing the gloves).

2. After removing the gloves, remove the mask, holding it by the strings.
3. Remove the gown next.
4. Finally, remove any eyewear.
5. Wash the hands and wrists thoroughly.

Cleaning Reusable Equipment

Washing items to remove any organic material is important. Cold-water rinses should be done first, because hot water coagulates the protein of organic material and causes it to stick to items. Then wash items in hot water with soap to emulsify and dislodge dirt. Abrasive action with stiff-bristled brushes will help to remove material from crevices in equipment. Rinse articles with warm to hot water and dry thoroughly. Items are now considered clean. However, the process is not complete until the basin or sink and any brushes or tools used for cleaning the items are also cleaned with a disinfectant. This task is generally assigned to housekeeping or central service staff.

NURSING CARE

PRIORITIZING NURSING CARE

Standard Precautions, including hand hygiene, are the first line of defense against hospital-acquired infections. Prevention is so much better than treatment when dealing with the drug-resistant organisms that are currently widespread in the hospital environment. Healthcare professionals routinely need to wash hands with soap and water at the beginning of the shift, plus whenever hands are visibly soiled or have been contaminated with organic material. Waterless hand cleaner should be used between each client contact and after glove removal. Gloves should be worn whenever contamination is possible. A good rule of thumb is: "If it is wet and you are not, wear gloves." Gloves should not be worn outside the client unit (e.g., when going from room to room).

Be observant of any signs of infection. Examine the client's skin during bathing. Document any signs of infection. Be vigilant when performing sterile procedures such as dressing changes and catheterizations. A break in sterile procedure can cause long-term problems for the client. Infection control is everyone's responsibility.

ASSESSING

The client history is one of the most important parts of the assessment. It gives you specific information on the client's signs/symptoms and information on what the client has tried for treatment or relief of the problem. The nursing history allows the nurse to assess the client's degree of risk for developing an infection and symptoms that suggest the presence of an infection. Along with reviewing the chart, the nurse will interview the client to collect objective data that are significant. Such data would include anything that might influence the development of an infection, history of recurring infections, immunization history, nutritional status, emotional stressors, and current medications and/or therapeutic measures. In light of the potential for a pandemic, travel history is also an important part of assessment especially for a client with respiratory symptoms.

Subjective data can be obtained from clients when they are asked about any symptoms they have experienced that may indicate infection. These include headache, lethargy, nausea or vomiting, rash, and pain.

Along with data already collected, the nurse looks for signs and symptoms of infection associated with specific body systems. Sneezing or watery, discolored discharge from the nose suggests sinus infection. Cloudy urine may indicate bladder infection. Vital signs also show changes, such as increased temperature, pulse, and respirations. Other observations may include anorexia and lymph node enlargement or rash.

DIAGNOSING, PLANNING, AND IMPLEMENTING

The primary nursing diagnosis for the transmission of pathologic microorganisms is *Risk for Infection*. Some of the specific risk factors include traumatized or broken skin, stasis of body fluids, altered peristalsis, change in pH of secretions, decreased ciliary action, rash and wound contamination. Contributing factors to the nursing diagnosis include immunosuppression, anemia, and suppressed inflammatory response.

Other contributing nursing diagnoses that may result from the infection are:

- *Impaired Physical Mobility*
- *Imbalanced Nutrition*
- *Pain* related to tissue damage
- *Hyperthermia* related to infection
- *Risk for Imbalanced Fluid Volume*
- *Anxiety*
- *Situational Low Self-Esteem*
- *Impaired Social Interaction*

Nursing goals in the planning stage of the nursing process include:

- Restoring and maintaining body defenses against infection
- Preventing the spread of infection and its complications
- Maintaining hydration to prevent fluid and electrolyte imbalances.

To achieve these goals, nursing care must include thorough aseptic technique, supporting the host's defenses, client teaching that emphasizes protective measures to prevent infections and their spread, and appropriate hydration

measures. Some common nursing interventions for the client at risk for infection include:

- Help the client as necessary with routine hygiene (including oral hygiene) and skin care. *Practicing consistent and good hygiene reduces the number of microorganisms. Maintaining intact skin prevents the possibility of infection.*
- Appropriately dispose of, or change, any clothing or linens, bandages, or dressing whenever they become soiled or wet. *Microorganisms grow easily and live in soiled or wet cloth.*
- Dispose of feces and urine appropriately. *Human waste contains many microorganisms that can cause infection or transfer bacteria and viruses to others.*
- Cover all containers of fluid (e.g., water bottles) at the client's bedside. *Uncapped containers holding liquids increase the risk of contamination and microbial growth.*
- Empty all drainage containers (e.g., suction bottles, catheter bags) before they become full, and at the end of each nursing shift, or according to agency policy. Hold containers steady and level to prevent spillage. *Body fluids and drainage contain microorganisms that grow and increase in numbers and can potentially be transmitted to others.*
- When giving care, avoid reaching over, talking, sneezing, or coughing across open wounds. Also, cover the mouth and nose when coughing or sneezing. *This limits the number of microorganisms falling from the caregiver's skin or escaping from the respiratory tract and prevents contamination of the wound.*
- Start all client care using Standard Precautions. *Anyone may have infectious microorganisms that can potentially be transmitted to others.*
- Wash hands before and after any client contact. *Correct hand hygiene controls and prevents the spread and transmission of microorganisms.*
- Wear masks and eye protection when caring for clients who have infections transmitted by droplets from the respiratory tract, or when sprays of body fluid may occur (e.g., during wound irrigations). *Masks and eye protection reduce the spread of microorganisms from droplet secretion contamination.*
- Wear gloves (and gowns if there is a possibility of soiling clothing) when handling any secretions or excretions from the client. *Gloves and gowns prevent contamination with microorganisms by contact.*
- Provide every client with his or her own individual hygiene and personal care items. *This prevents cross contamination of microorganisms from others.*
- Use sterile technique for all invasive procedures (e.g., injections, catheterizations, suctioning) and for open wounds. *When the body's natural defense mechanisms (e.g., skin, body cavities) are penetrated, the barriers to microorganisms are broken.*

- Use only appropriate puncture-proof containers for all disposal of used needles, knife blades, and syringes. The use of needle safe or needleless systems are now required. *Infectious diseases can be transmitted to healthcare workers and others by puncture injuries from contaminated needles, blades, and syringes. The U.S. Congress passed the Needlestick Safety and Prevention Act in 2000, which requires that all sharps be needle safe or needleless. OSHA is also enforcing this mandate.*
- Provide a balanced diet for the client. *A well-balanced diet provides all the nutrients needed to maintain and build body tissues* (see Chapter 25 ⊚).

Practicing Sterile Technique

Many client care procedures require the use of sterile technique. Objects are only sterile when free of all microorganisms. When practicing sterile technique, the basic principles of surgical asepsis are used.

A **sterile field** is a microorganism-free area. Nurses use sterile drapes and the inside of sterile wrappers to create the sterile field (Procedure 10-4 ■ on page 183). Some general concepts to keep in mind when creating and working with a sterile field are listed in Box 10-6 ■.

EVALUATING

During the evaluation process, the nurse reviews both positive and negative outcomes of the care and instructions given to the client. Revisions in care are made as needed until the desired result is achieved. Examples of positive outcomes and obtaining stated goals in client care are:

- All dressings are kept dry and are changed when they are soiled or become wet.
- The client eats a well-balanced diet and has adequate fluid intake to maintain nutrition and hydration.
- Clients participate in self-care to the degree possible, and good hygiene is maintained.
- All contaminated equipment and linens are disposed of appropriately and according to agency standards.
- All containers holding human waste or drainage are disposed of appropriately.
- All materials used for invasive procedures (e.g., needles, syringes, catheters) are disposed of in a sharps container located at the site of use.

Continuity of Care

Education is an important aspect of the nurse's role in treating a client with an infection or potential for infection. Some appropriate points follow:

- Teach clients and their significant others why articles must be clean, disinfected, or sterilized. Teach how this is to be done.
- Teach clients and significant others to wash their hands before eating or handling food, after toileting, or after handling any infectious materials.
- Educate or remind clients and significant others about the importance of immunizations and booster shots.

Clients and support people must often provide home care of a person with an infectious disease or partially healed wound. The following instructions can be useful:

- Wash hands carefully before and after any hands-on care.
- Keep fingernails clean, short, and well trimmed.
- If there is no running water, use commercially available hand hygiene agents that require no water.
- Use soap and paper towels when washing hands.
- Teach young children hand hygiene as soon as they can participate.
- Keep pets out of the area when setting up for and performing sterile procedures.
- Clean and wipe dry a flat surface for the sterile field.
- Dispose of all soiled materials in a waterproof bag. Check with the home care nurse as to how to dispose of medical waste.

BOX 10-6   NURSING CARE CHECKLIST

Creating and Maintaining a Sterile Field

☑ Wear sterile gloves to work with the equipment on the field, or use sterile forceps to move items around on it.

☑ Never reach across a sterile field once it is established. (Microorganisms can be dropped on it and cause contamination.)

☑ If the field becomes wet, it is considered contaminated.

☑ If an unsterile object touches a sterile object, it is then contaminated.

☑ The edges of the sterile field are considered unsterile.

☑ If an object is below the nurse's waist level or is out of sight, it is considered unsterile.

☑ If objects must be left open to the air for a prolonged period of time, cover the sterile field with sterile drapes to prevent contamination by airborne microorganisms.

☑ Nursing qualities that are essential in maintaining a sterile field are alertness, honesty, and conscientiousness.

☑ Follow the old adage: "If there is any doubt about sterility, the object or field is unsterile."

NURSING PROCESS CARE PLAN
Client with Respiratory Infection

Mrs. Chase is a 76-year-old woman who has a 10-year history of emphysema. She has a history of smoking a pack a day for 25 years, and continues to do so. Recently, she began coughing much more frequently and expectorating larger volumes of yellow/green-colored mucus. She was admitted to the hospital with complaints of fatigue, coughing, a poor appetite, and a fever with chills. She is sitting on the edge of the bed, coughing, with her hand pressing against her chest. There are used tissues scattered all over the bed.

Assessment

VS: T 101.4, P 90, R 22 and shallow, BP 146/88. Pain 4/10 in the chest while coughing and less between episodes. Weight is 108 lbs, height 5' 9". The client's skin is hot, flushed, and dry. Skin turgor is fair. She is alert and oriented, but restless and anxious. She coughs frequently and expectorates moderate amounts of thick, yellow/green-tinged mucus. She has a barrel chest, and on auscultation slight wheezes are heard in both lungs. Nail beds show slight cyanosis. Specimens of blood and sputum have already been collected. The WBC count is elevated. The sputum specimen shows a streptococcal upper respiratory tract infection. The chest x-ray shows bilateral pneumonia. Mrs. Chase states she had been caring for her young grandchild who had a "strep throat."

Nursing Diagnosis

The following important nursing diagnoses (among others) are established for this client:

- *Risk for Infection* due to decreased ciliary action in lungs
- *Deficient Fluid Volume* related to high fever and poor appetite
- *Impaired Gas Exchange* related to rapid respirations, copious secretions, alveolar destruction, and air trapping
- *Ineffective Airway Clearance* related to increased secretions and a weak cough
- *Deficient Knowledge* related to infectious process and status of compromised host

Expected Outcomes

The expected outcomes for the plan of care are that Mrs. Chase will:

- Regain prior lung function.
- Maintain adequate hydration and circulating blood volume.
- Improve gas exchange as demonstrated by respirations within normal limits, normal pulse, and blood gases.
- Maintain a patent airway with decreased volume of secretions.
- Understand and be able to verbalize the process of contamination, susceptibility to infection, and how to prevent the spread of organisms.

Planning and Implementation

The following nursing interventions are implemented for Mrs. Chase. Ongoing assessments are done to monitor her condition.

- Monitor character of respirations including rate and rhythm, blood gases, and skin color every 2 to 4 hours.
- Auscultate breath sounds. Encourage deep breathing and coughing.
- Monitor vital signs every 4 h and intake and output every shift.
- Encourage fluids. Find out what liquids she likes and offer her 8 ounces of preferred fluid every hour.
- Have client deep breathe and cough every 2 h while awake. Position in semi-Fowler's or Fowler's position. Change client's position from back to sides often.
- Document volume of secretions as well as color and character. Request order for chest physiotherapy. Suction as necessary. See also Chapter 32 🔗.
- Administer medications (antibiotics, analgesics, expectorants, antitussives) on time.
- Follow orders from respiratory therapy.
- Teach Mrs. Chase to limit her exposure to others who are ill, because her history of emphysema and advanced age make her more susceptible to infection.
- Discuss hand hygiene techniques, and emphasize that she should wash her hands after coughing or sneezing into them and after handling objects used by other ill persons.
- Place waste container next to patient to decrease potential for contamination of other surfaces. Remind her to throw contaminated tissues into a waste container to maintain a clean environment.

Evaluation

At the end of the shift, Mrs. Chase's lung sounds were improved with less wheezing. Mucus was clear in color, thin, and "easier to cough out." The rate, rhythm, and character of her respirations were adequate. Her blood gases were within normal limits, and she showed no signs of cyanosis. Her temperature was 99.9°F and her pulse was 82. She was resting easily with her oxygen on. She was eating and taking fluids well with good urinary output.

Critical Thinking in the Nursing Process

1. Why was caring for her ill grandchild endangering Mrs. Chase's health?
2. What is the connection between the used tissues and the spread of infection?
3. Which of Mrs. Chase's assessment findings are consistent with a bacterial infection?

Note: Discussion of Critical Thinking questions appears on the MyNursingKit Website.

Note: The references and resources for all chapters have been compiled at the back of the book.

PROCEDURE 10-1 Hand Hygiene/Washing

Purposes

- To reduce the number of microorganisms on the hands
- To reduce the risk of transmission of microorganisms to clients
- To reduce the risk of cross-contamination among clients and equipment
- To reduce the risk of transmission of infectious organisms to oneself

Equipment

- Soap
- Warm running water
- Towels
- Alcohol-based foam or gel

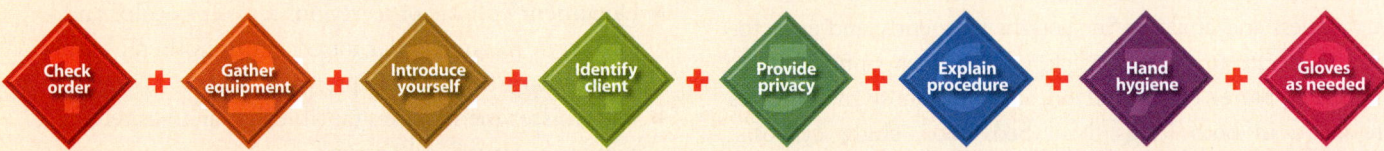

Check order + Gather equipment + Introduce yourself + Identify client + Provide privacy + Explain procedure + Hand hygiene + Gloves as needed

Interventions and Rationales

1. Perform preparatory steps (see icon bar above).

2. Prepare and assess the hands.
   - File the nails short. *Short nails are less likely to harbor microorganisms, scratch a client, or puncture gloves.* Do not wear artificial nails or extensions. *These can pass organisms on to clients. Note: The CDC recommends that nail enhancements not be worm by nurses working in areas such as the OR, L&D, or NICU. Many facilities have made this recommendation a policy for all employees who have contact with clients.*
   - Remove all jewelry. Some nurses prefer to slide their watches up above their elbows. Others pin the watch to the uniform. *Microorganisms can lodge in the settings of jewelry and under rings. Removal facilitates proper cleaning.*
   - Check hands for breaks in the skin, such as hangnails or cuts. Use lotions to prevent hangnails and cracked, dry skin. *A nurse who has broken skin areas may have to wear a dressing. If the area is too large to cover, then work reassignment is required.*

3. Turn on the water and adjust the flow.
   - There are five common types of faucet controls:
     a. Hand-operated handles.
     b. Knee levers. Move these with the knee to regulate flow and temperature.
     c. Foot pedals. Press these with the foot to regulate flow and temperature.
     d. Elbow controls. Move these with the elbows instead of the hands.
     e. Infrared controls. The water runs when motion is detected at a preset distance.
   - Adjust the flow so that the water is warm. Warm water removes less of the protective oil of the skin than hot water and is more effective than cold water for producing lather.

4. Wet the hands thoroughly by holding them under the running water, and apply soap to the hands.
   - Hold the hands lower than the elbows so that the water flows from the arms to the fingertips (Figure 10-5 ■). *The water should flow from the least contaminated to the most contaminated area; the hands are generally considered more contaminated than the lower arms.*
   - Apply 2 to 4 mL (1 tsp) of liquid soap; rub it firmly between the hands.

5. Thoroughly wash and rinse the hands.
   - Wash hands for a minimum of 10 to 15 seconds. For a more thorough washing, extend the time for wetting, washing, and rinsing.
   - Use firm rubbing and circular movements to wash the palm, back, and wrist of each hand. Interlace the fingers and thumbs and move the hands back and forth, continuing the motion for 10 seconds. *The circular action helps remove microorganisms mechanically.*

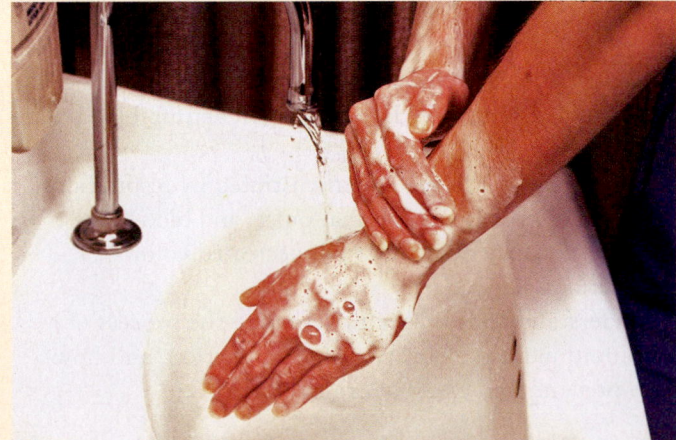

Figure 10-5. ■ The hands are held lower than the elbows to allow water to run down and off the hands. *Source:* Michael Heron Photography.

Interlacing the fingers and thumbs cleans between the fingers.
- Rinse the hands.
6. Thoroughly dry the hands and arms.
   - Dry hands and arms thoroughly with a paper towel. *Moist skin becomes chapped readily; chapping produces lesions.*
   - Discard the paper towel in the appropriate container.
7. Turn off the water.
   - Use a dry paper towel to grasp a hand-operated control (Figure 10-6 ■). *This prevents the nurse from picking up microorganisms from the faucet handles.*

Hand hygiene as described is to be done when hands are visibly soiled. When not visibly soiled, alcohol-based foams and gels are to be used. They are located outside the entrance to each client room.

Variation: Hand Hygiene Before Sterile Techniques

- Apply the soap and wash as described in step 4, but hold the hands higher than the elbows during this hand hygiene procedure. Wet the hands and forearms under the running water, letting it run from the fingertips to the elbows so that the hands become cleaner than the elbows. *In this way, the water runs from the area with the fewest microorganisms to areas with a relatively greater number.*
- After washing and rinsing, use a towel to dry one hand thoroughly in a rotating motion from the fingers to the elbow. Use a clean towel to dry the other hand and arm. *A clean towel prevents the transfer of microorganisms from one elbow (least clean area) to the other hand (cleanest area).*

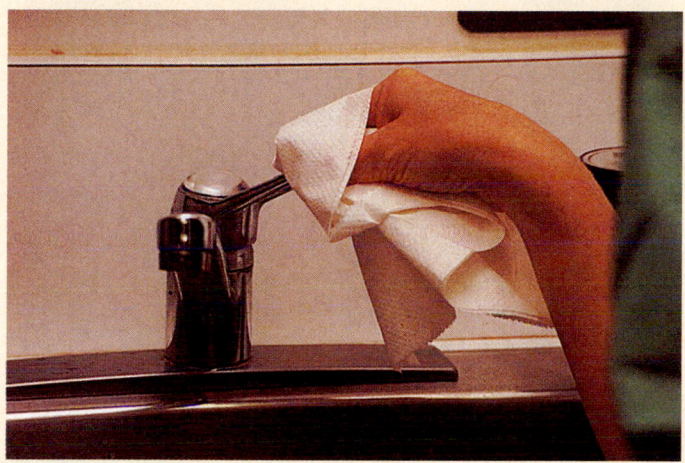

Figure 10-6. ■ Using a paper towel to grasp the hand-operated faucet. (Photographer: Elena Dorfman.)

SAMPLE DOCUMENTATION

[date] [time] Hand hygiene done for 3 minutes per hospital protocol prior to clean dressing change. _____

_____ A. Parsons, LVN

PROCEDURE 10-2   Donning and Removing Sterile Gloves (Open Method)

Purposes
- To enable the nurse to handle sterile objects freely
- To prevent clients at risk (e.g., those with open wounds) from becoming infected by microorganisms on the nurse's hands

Equipment
- Package of sterile gloves

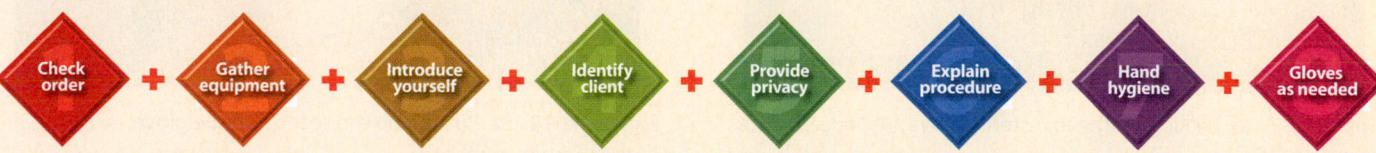

Check order + Gather equipment + Introduce yourself + Identify client + Provide privacy + Explain procedure + Hand hygiene + Gloves as needed

Interventions and Rationales

1. Perform preparatory steps (see icon bar).

2. Open the package of sterile gloves.
   - Place the package of gloves on a clean dry surface. *Any moisture on the surface could contaminate the gloves.*
   - Some gloves are packed in an inner as well as an outer package. Open the outer package without contaminating the gloves or the inner package.
   - Remove the inner package from the outer package.
   - Open the inner package as in step 2 of Procedure 10-3 or according to the manufacturer's directions. *Some manufacturers provide a numbered sequence for opening the flaps and folded tabs to grasp for opening the flaps.* If no tabs are provided, pluck the flap so that the fingers do not touch the inner surfaces. *The inner surfaces, which are next to the sterile gloves, will remain sterile.*

3. Put the first glove on the dominant hand.
   - If the gloves are packaged so that they lie side by side, grasp the glove for the dominant hand by its cuff (on the palmar side) with the thumb and first finger of the nondominant hand. Touch only the inside of the cuff (Figure 10-7 ■). *The hands are not sterile. By touching only the inside of the glove, the nurse avoids contaminating the outside.*
   or
   If the gloves are packaged one on top of the other, grasp the cuff of the top glove as above, using the opposite hand.
   - Insert the dominant hand into the glove and pull the glove on. Keep the thumb of the inserted hand against the palm of the hand during insertion (Figure 10-8 ■). *If the thumb is kept against the palm, it is less likely to contaminate the outside of the glove.*
   - Leave the cuff turned down.

4. Put the second glove on the nondominant hand.
   - Pick up the other glove with the sterile gloved hand, inserting the gloved fingers under the cuff and holding the gloved thumb close to the gloved palm (Figure 10-9 ■). *This helps prevent accidental contamination of the glove by the bare hand.*

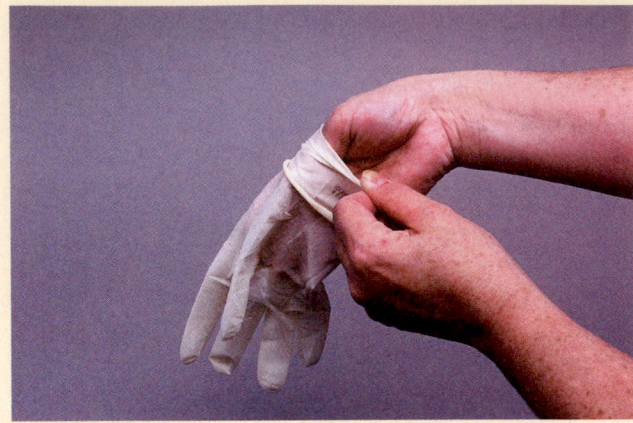

Figure 10-8. ■ Putting on the first sterile glove. (Al Dodge, Pearson Education/PH.)

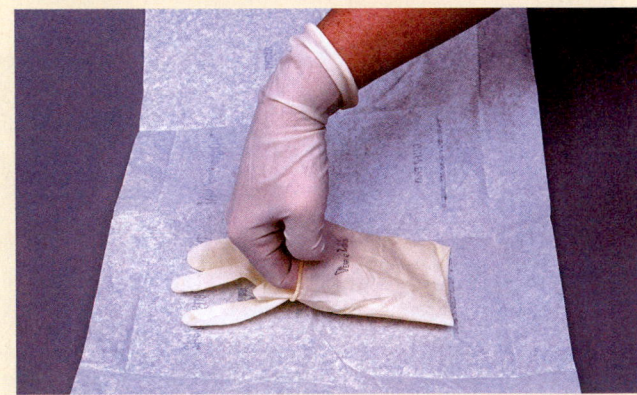

Figure 10-9. ■ Picking up the second sterile glove. (Al Dodge, Pearson Education/PH.)

   - Pull on the second glove carefully. Hold the thumb of the gloved first hand as far as possible from the palm (Figure 10-10 ■). *In this position, the thumb is less likely to touch the arm and become contaminated.*
   - Adjust each glove so that it fits smoothly, and carefully pull the cuffs up by sliding the fingers under the cuffs.

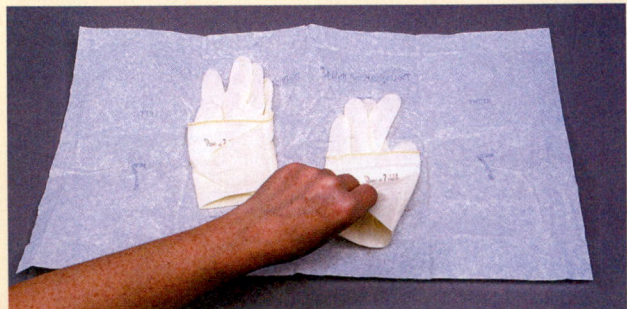

Figure 10-7. ■ Picking up the first sterile glove. (Al Dodge, Pearson Education/PH.)

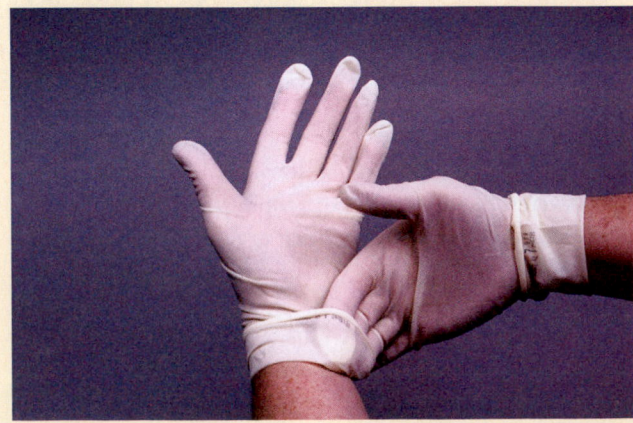

Figure 10-10. ■ Putting on the second sterile glove. (Al Dodge, Pearson Education/PH.)

5. Remove and dispose of used gloves.
   - To remove sterile gloves that are soiled with secretions, hold the palmar surface below the cuff and turn it inside out. Insert fingers into the second glove, and turn it inside out while removing it (Figure 10-11 ■).

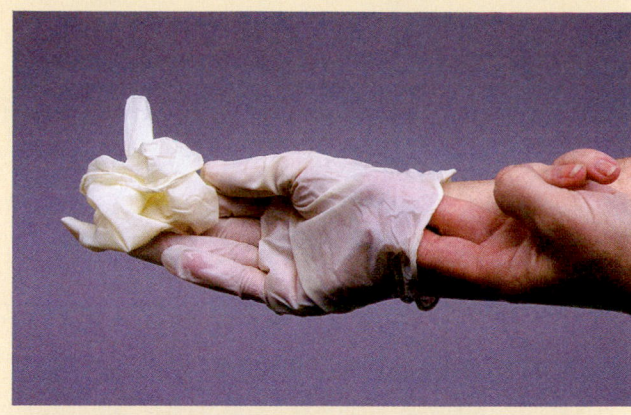

B

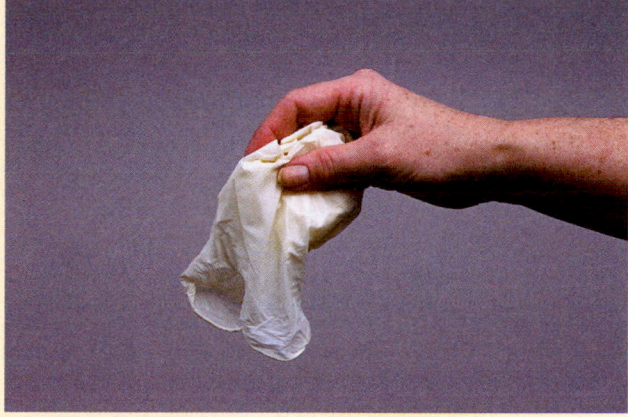

C

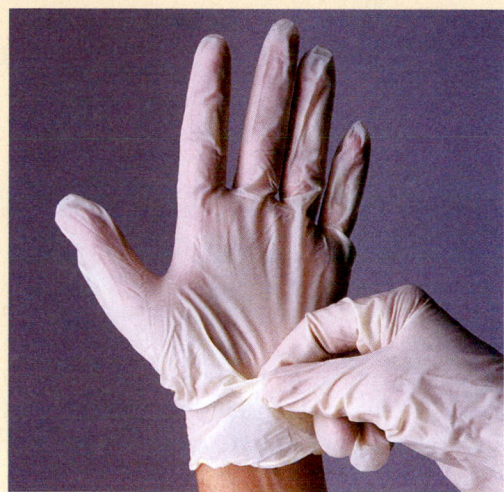

A

Figure 10-11. ■ **A.** Plucking the palmar surface below the cuff of a contaminated glove. **B.** Inserting fingers to remove the second contaminated glove. **C.** Holding contaminated gloves, which are inside out. (Al Dodge, Pearson Education/PH.)

SAMPLE DOCUMENTATION

[date] [time] Donned sterile gloves according to institutional protocol. Changed dressing. Wound pink, granulation tissue visible. _____

P. Morgan, LVN

| PROCEDURE 10-3 | Donning Personal Protective Equipment |

Purposes

- To enable the nurse to work close to a sterile field and handle sterile objects freely
- To protect clients from becoming contaminated with microorganisms on the nurse's hands, arms, and clothing

Equipment

- A sterile pack containing a sterile gown
- A package of sterile gloves

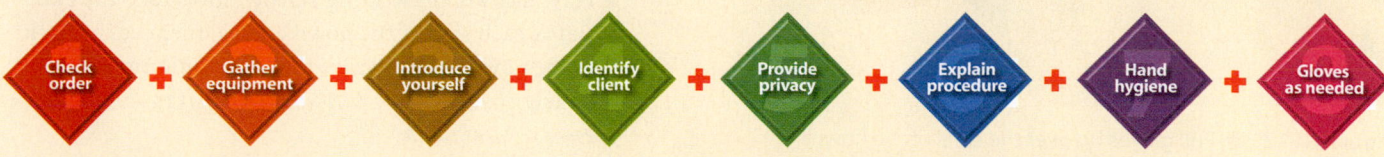

Check order + Gather equipment + Introduce yourself + Identify client + Provide privacy + Explain procedure + Hand hygiene + Gloves as needed

Interventions and Rationales

DONNING A STERILE GOWN

1. Perform preparatory steps (see icon bar above).

2. Open the package of sterile gloves.
   - Remove the outer wrap from the sterile gloves and leave the gloves in their inner sterile wrap on the sterile field. *If the inner wrapper is not touched, it will remain sterile.*

3. Unwrap the sterile gown pack.

4. Wash and dry hands carefully. See "Variation" at the end of Procedure 10-1 and review agency practice.

5. Put on the sterile gown (Figure 10-12 ■).
   - *Grasp the sterile gown at the crease near the neck, hold it away from you, and permit it to unfold freely without touching anything, including the uniform. The gown will be unsterile if its outer surface touches any unsterile objects.*
   - Put the hands inside the shoulders of the gown, and work the arms partway into the sleeves without touching the outside of the gown.
   - If donning sterile gloves by using the closed method (*see below*), work the hands down the sleeves only to the proximal edge of the cuffs.
   or

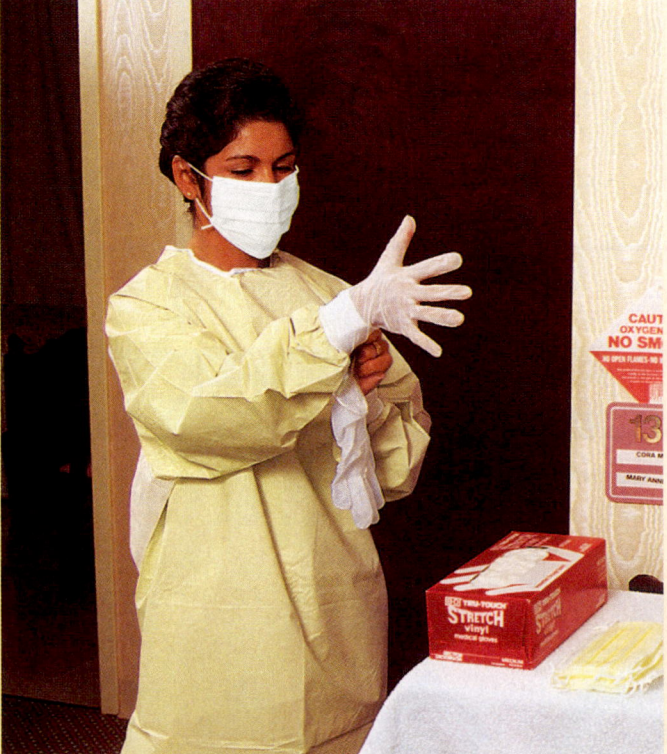

Figure 10-12. ■ Pull gloves up over the cuffs of the gown.

If donning sterile gloves by using the open method, work the hands down the sleeves and through the cuffs.
- Have a coworker wearing a hair cover and mask grasp the neck ties without touching the outside of the gown and pull the gown upward to cover the neckline of your uniform in front and back. The coworker ties the neck ties. Gowning continues at step 6.

DONNING STERILE GLOVES (CLOSED METHOD)

1. Open the sterile wrapper containing the sterile gloves.
   - Open the sterile glove wrapper while the hands are still covered by the sleeves.

2. Put the glove on the nondominant hand. The steps for a right-handed person follow.
   - With the dominant hand, pick up the opposite glove with the thumb and index finger, handling it through the sleeve.
   - Lay the glove on the opposite gown cuff, thumb side down, with the glove opening pointed toward the fingers. Position the dominant hand palm upward inside the sleeve.
   - Use the nondominant hand to grasp the cuff of the glove through the gown cuff, and firmly anchor it.
   - With the dominant hand working through its sleeve, grasp the upper side of the glove's cuff, and stretch it over the cuff of the gown. *This covers the nonsterile skin of the wrist and creates a solid sterile area from gloves to gown.*
   - Pull the sleeve up to draw the cuff over the wrist as you extend the fingers of the nondominant hand into the glove's fingers.

3. Put the glove on the dominant hand.
   - Place the fingers of the gloved hand under the cuff of the remaining glove.
   - Place the glove over the cuff of the second sleeve.
   - Extend the fingers into the glove as you pull the glove up over the cuff.

COMPLETION OF GOWNING

6. Complete gowning as follows:
   - Have a coworker wearing a hair cover and mask hold the waist tie of your gown, using sterile gloves or sterile forceps or a drape. *This approach keeps the ties sterile.*
   - Make a three-quarter turn, then take the tie and secure it in front of the gown.
   or
   - Have a coworker wearing sterile gloves take the two ties at each side of the gown and tie them at the back of the gown, making sure that your uniform is completely covered. *Both methods ensure that the back of the gown remains sterile.*

■ When worn, sterile gowns should be considered sterile in front from the waist to the shoulder. The sleeves should be considered sterile from 2 inches above the elbow to the cuff, since the arms of a scrubbed person must move across a sterile field. Moisture collection and friction areas such as the neckline, shoulders, underarms, back, and sleeve cuffs should be considered unsterile.

SAMPLE DOCUMENTATION

[date] [time] Prior to entering reverse isolation, sterile gown, gloves, and mask applied utilizing proper procedure, and according to institutional protocol. _____

P. Morgan, LVN

Special note: *This type of documentation will become more important as hospitals are required by law to report hospital-acquired (nosocomial) infection rates. These rates will be available to the public at large.*

PROCEDURE 10-4   Establishing and Maintaining a Sterile Field

Purpose

■ To maintain the sterility of supplies and equipment

Equipment

■ Package containing a sterile drape

■ Sterile equipment as needed (e.g., wrapped sterile gauze, wrapped sterile bowl, antiseptic solution, sterile forceps)

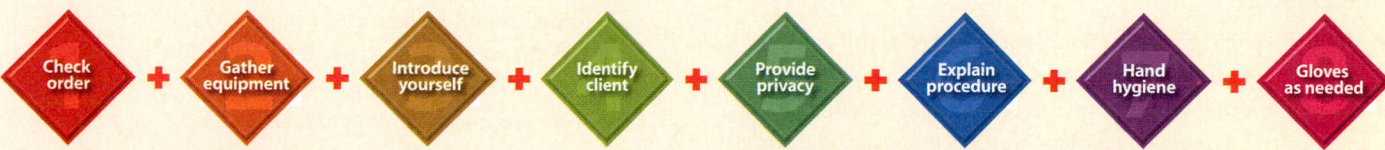

Check order + Gather equipment + Introduce yourself + Identify client + Provide privacy + Explain procedure + Hand hygiene + Gloves as needed

Interventions and Rationales

1. Perform preparatory steps (see icon bar above).
2. Confirm the sterility of the package.
   ■ Ensure that the package is clean and dry. *If moist, it is considered contaminated and must be discarded.*
   ■ Check the sterilization expiration dates on the package, and look for any indications that it has been previously opened.
3. Open the package.

TO OPEN A WRAPPED PACKAGE ON A SURFACE

■ Place the package in the center of the work area so that the top flap of the wrapper opens away from you. *This position prevents the nurse from subsequently reaching directly over the exposed sterile contents, which could contaminate them.*

■ Reaching around the package (not over it), pinch the first flap on the outside of the wrapper between the thumb and

index finger (Figure 10-13 ■). *Touching only the outside of the wrapper maintains the sterility of the inside of the wrapper.* Pull the flap open, laying it flat on the far surface.

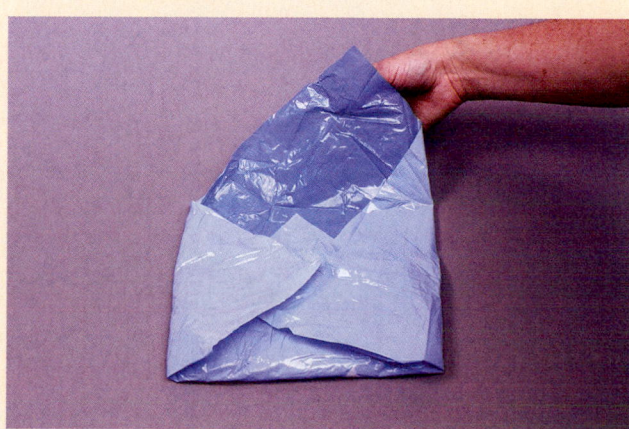

Figure 10-13. ■ Opening the first flap of a sterile, wrapped package. (Al Dodge, Pearson Education/PH.)

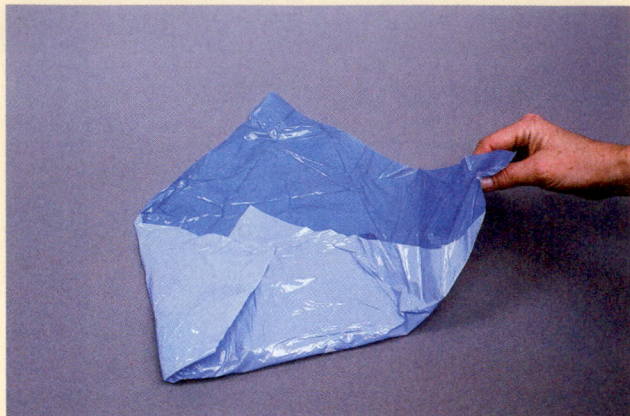

Figure 10-14. ■ Opening the second flap to the side. (Al Dodge, Pearson Education/PH.)

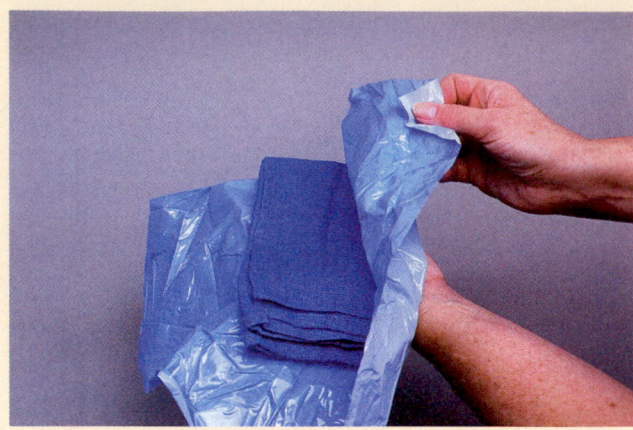

Figure 10-16. ■ Opening a wrapped package while holding it. (Al Dodge, Pearson Education/PH.)

- Repeat for the side flaps, opening the top one first. Use the right hand for the right flap, and the left hand for the left flap (Figure 10-14 ■). *By using both hands, the nurse avoids reaching over the sterile contents.*
- Pull the fourth flap toward you by grasping the corner that is turned down (Figure 10-15 ■). Make sure that the flap does not touch any object. *If the inner surface touches any unsterile article, it is contaminated. Note:* One inch along the edges of a sterile package is not considered to be sterile.

TO OPEN A WRAPPED PACKAGE WHILE HOLDING IT

- Hold the package in one hand with the top flap opening away from you.
- Using the other hand, open the package as described above, pulling the corners of the flaps well back and not reaching across the contents of the package (Figure 10-16 ■). *The hands are considered contaminated, and at no time should they touch the contents of the package.*

TO OPEN COMMERCIALLY PREPARED PACKAGES

Commercially prepared sterile packages and containers usually have manufacturer's directions for opening.

- If the flap of the package has an unsealed corner, hold the package in one hand and pull back on the flap with the other hand (Figure 10-17 ■).
- If the package has a partially sealed edge, grasp both sides of the edge, one with each hand, and pull apart gently.

4. Establish a sterile field by using a drape.
   - Open the package containing the drape as described in step 3.
   - With one hand, pluck the corner of the drape that is folded back on the top.
   - Lift the drape out of the cover and allow it to open freely without touching any objects (Figure 10-18 ■). *If the drape touches the outside of the package or any unsterile surface or object, it is considered contaminated.*
   - Discard the cover.
   - With the other hand, carefully pick up another corner of the drape, holding it well away from yourself.

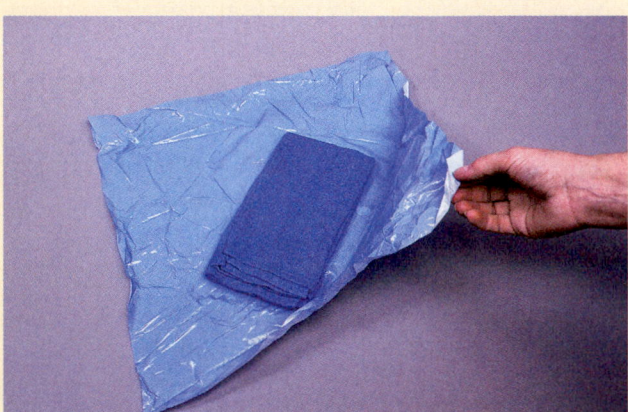

Figure 10-15. ■ Pulling the last flap toward oneself by grasping the corner. (Al Dodge, Pearson Education/PH.)

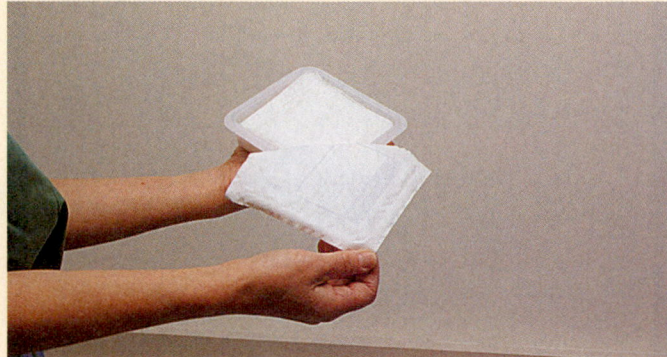

Figure 10-17. ■ Opening a sterile package that has an unsealed corner. (Photographer: Elena Dorfman.)

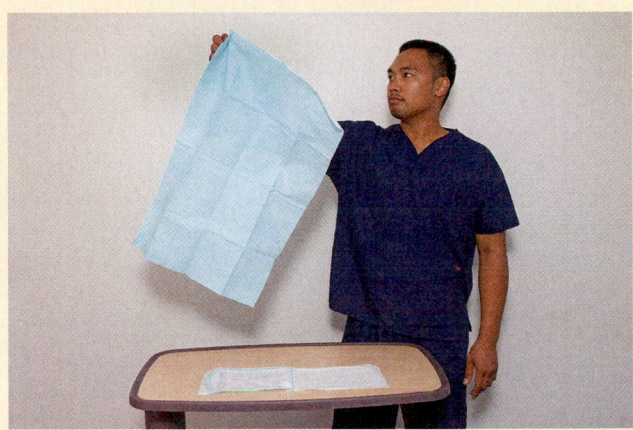

Figure 10-18. ■ Allowing a drape to open freely without touching any objects. (Patrick Watson.)

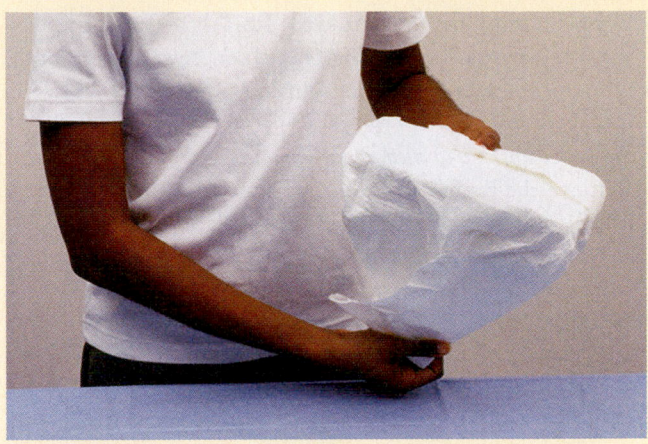

Figure 10-20. ■ Adding wrapped sterile supplies to a sterile field. (Patrick Watson.)

■ Lay the drape on a clean and dry surface, placing the bottom (i.e., the freely hanging side) farthest from you (Figure 10-19 ■). *By placing the lowermost side farthest away, the nurse avoids leaning over the sterile field and contaminating it.*

5. Add necessary sterile supplies.

TO ADD WRAPPED SUPPLIES TO A STERILE FIELD

■ Open each wrapped package as described in the preceding steps.
■ With the free hand, grasp the corners of the wrapper and hold them against the wrist of the other hand (Figure 10-20 ■). *The unsterile hand is now covered by the sterile wrapper.*
■ Place the sterile bowl, drape, or other supply on the sterile field by approaching from an angle rather than holding the arm over the field.
■ Discard the wrapper.

TO ADD COMMERCIALLY PACKAGED SUPPLIES TO A STERILE FIELD

■ Open each package as previously described.
■ Hold the package 15 cm (6 in.) above the field and allow the contents to drop on the field (Figure 10-21 ■). *Keep in mind that 2.5 cm (1 in.) around the edge of the field is considered contaminated. At a height of 15 cm (6 in.), the outside of the package is not likely to touch and contaminate the sterile field.*

TO ADD STERILE SOLUTION TO A STERILE BOWL

Sterile liquids (e.g., normal saline) frequently need to be poured into metal or nonabsorbent containers within a sterile field. *Unwrapped bottles or flasks that contain sterile solution are considered sterile on the inside and contaminated on the outside because the bottle may have been handled. Bottles used in an operating room may be sterilized on the outside as well as the inside, however, and these are handled with sterile gloves.*

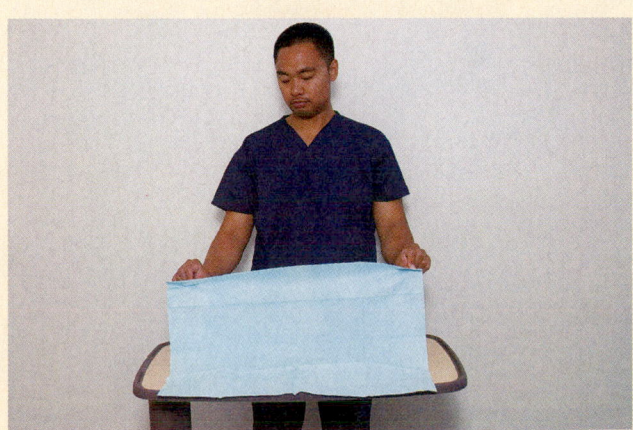

Figure 10-19. ■ Placing a drape on a surface. (Patrick Watson.)

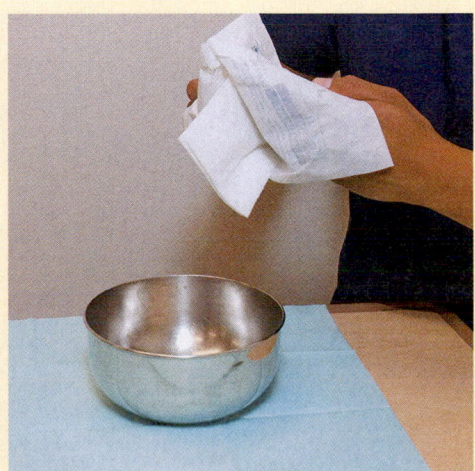

Figure 10-21. ■ Adding commercially packaged gauze to a sterile field. (Patrick Watson.)

- Before pouring any liquid, read the label three times to make sure you have the correct solution and concentration (strength).
- Obtain the exact amount of solution, if possible. *Once a sterile container has been opened, its sterility cannot be ensured for future use unless it is used again immediately.*
- Remove the lid or cap from the bottle and turn the lid upside down before placing it on a surface that is not sterile. *Inverting the lid keeps the inside surface sterile, because it is not allowed to touch an unsterile surface.*
- Hold the bottle at a slight angle so that the label is uppermost. *Any solution that flows down the outside of the bottle during pouring will not damage the label or make it unreadable.*
- Hold the bottle of fluid at a height of 10 to 15 cm (4 to 6 in.) over the bowl and to the side of the sterile field so that as little of the bottle as possible is over the field. *At this height, there is less likelihood of contaminating the sterile field by touching the field or by reaching an arm over it.*
- Pour the solution gently to avoid splashing the liquid. *If the sterile drape is on an unsterile surface, moisture will contaminate the field by allowing the movement of microorganisms through the sterile drape.*
- Replace the lid securely on the bottle if you plan to use it again, and provide the date and time of opening according to agency policy. *Replacing the lid immediately maintains the sterility of the inner aspect of the lid and the solution. In many agencies, a sterile container of solution that is opened is used only once and then discarded.*

6. Use sterile forceps to handle certain sterile supplies. Forceps are commonly used for such techniques as changing a sterile dressing and shortening a drain. Transfer forceps are usually used to move a sterile article from one place to another, for example, when transferring sterile gauze from its package to a sterile dressing tray. Forceps may be discarded or resterilized after use. Commonly used forceps include hemostats or artery forceps (Figure 10-22 ■) and tissue forceps (Figure 10-23 ■).

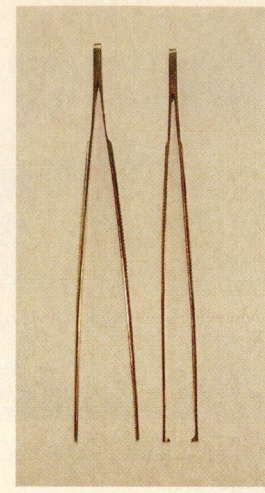

Figure 10-23. ■ Tissue forceps. (Alexandra Truitt & Terry Marshall.)

- Keep the tips of wet forceps lower than the wrist at all times, unless you are wearing sterile gloves (Figure 10-24 ■). *Gravity prevents liquids on the tips of the forceps from flowing to the handles and later back to the tips, thus making the forceps unsterile. The handles are unsterile once they are held by the bare hand.*
- Hold sterile forceps above waist level. *Items held below waist level are considered contaminated.*
- Hold sterile forceps within sight. *While out of sight, forceps may, unknown to the user, become unsterile. Any forceps that go out of sight should be considered unsterile.*
- When using forceps to lift sterile supplies out of a commercially prepared package, be sure that the forceps do not touch the edges or outside of the wrapper. *The edges and outside of the package are exposed to the air and handled and are thus unsterile.*
- When placing forceps whose handles were in contact with the bare hand, position the handles outside the

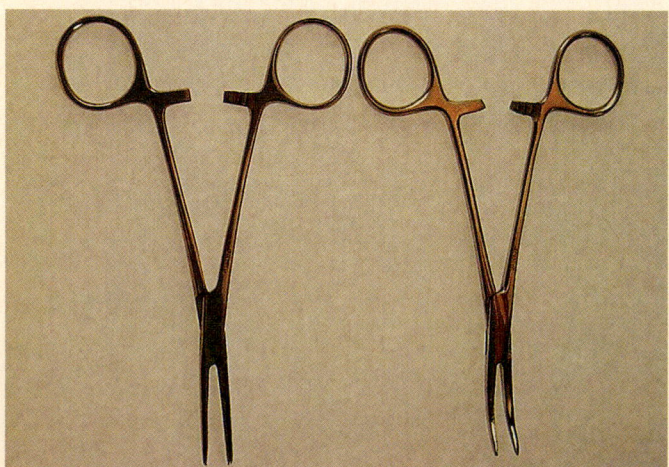

Figure 10-22. ■ Hemostats or artery forceps. (Alexandra Truitt & Terry Marshall.)

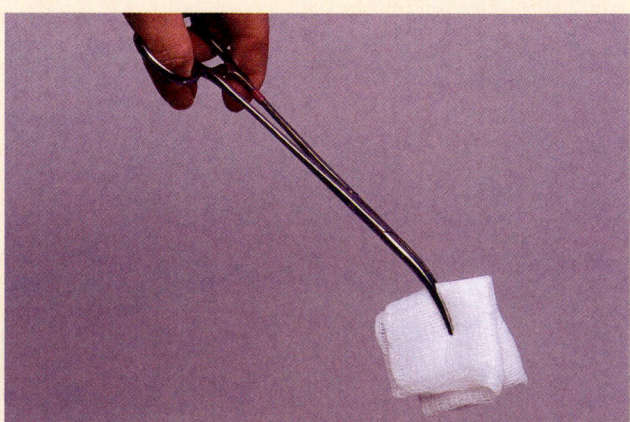

Figure 10-24. ■ Holding forceps with an ungloved hand, keeping the tips lower than the wrist. (Al Dodge, Pearson Education/PH.)

sterile area. *The handles of these forceps harbor microorganisms from the bare hand.*

- Deposit a sterile item on a sterile field without permitting moist forceps to touch the sterile field when the surface under the absorbent sterile field is unsterile and a barrier drape is not used. *A barrier drape is resistant to moisture (e.g., blood and antiseptics) and should be used whenever a procedure involves the use of liquids. Made of chemically treated cotton or synthetic materials, barrier drapes prevent a sterile field from becoming unsterile when the drape becomes wet. If the underlying surface is sterile (e.g., a plastic container), the field will not become unsterile when moist.*

SAMPLE DOCUMENTATION

[date] [time] A sterile field was set up according to hospital protocol using aseptic technique for abdominal wound irrigation and dressing change. _____
M. Stuart, LVN

Chapter Review

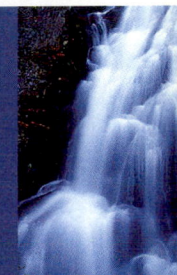

KEY Points

- Microorganisms are everywhere in our environment and in or on our body. Most of them are harmless and perform essential functions.
- Infections are invasions and growth of microorganisms in a body tissue or organ.
- Microorganisms are different in their strength and communicability.
- The medical and nursing communities use aseptic technique to prevent the transfer of microorganisms from one place or person to another.
- Nosocomial infections occur as a result of healthcare delivery in a healthcare setting.
- The chain of infection is composed of six links, all of which must be present to cause the infectious process.
- Specific defenses are immune defenses and work against identified foreign proteins and other infectious agents.
- Age is a factor that affects the risk of infection. Both the very young and the elderly have reduced defenses.
- Cleaning, disinfecting, and sterilizing are proven ways of inhibiting the growth and multiplication of microorganisms and of maintaining the environment.
- Isolation practices that protect the client, the healthcare provider, and others are initiated after assessing the client's condition. They are practiced according to institutional policies and the recommendations of the CDC.

- If there is any doubt about sterility, the object or field is unsterile.

FOR FURTHER Study

For more information on wound healing, see Chapter 24.

For more information on obtaining different types of cultures, see Chapters 23, 24, 27, and 28.

Chapter 32 provides information about oxygenation.

For further information about nutrition in healing, see Chapter 25.

For more about disposal of sharps, see Chapter 27.

Communicable diseases often affect people during childhood and are discussed in the Pediatric section, Chapters 59 to 62.

PEARSON
EXPLORE **mynursingkit**™

MyNursingKit is your one stop for online chapter review materials and resources. Prepare for success with additional NCLEX®-style practice questions, interactive assignments and activities, web links, animations and videos, and more!

Register your access code from the front of your book at
www.mynursingkit.com

Critical Thinking Care Map

Caring for a Client with a Stasis Ulcer

NCLEX-PN® Focus Area: Physiological Integrity

Case Study: George Gower has been admitted to the hospital with an open wound from an arterial stasis ulcer on his inner right lower leg. The wound has increased in size and is now draining small amounts of yellow/green secretions. There is a foul odor. The WBC count is elevated and he has an oral temperature of 101°F.

Nursing Diagnosis: Risk for Infection

COLLECT DATA

Subjective	Objective
_____	_____
_____	_____
_____	_____
_____	_____
_____	_____
_____	_____

Would you report this? Yes/No

If yes, report to:_____

What would you report?_____

Nursing Care

_____
_____
_____
_____
_____
_____
_____
_____
_____
_____
_____

How would you document this? _____
_____
_____

Compare your answers and documentation to those provided on the MyNursingKit Website.

Data Collected
(use only those that apply)

- Complains of burning pain in area of wound
- Yellow/green secretions
- Foul odor from wound and secretions
- Poor pedal pulses
- Says his foot is cold
- States elevating his foot hurts his hip
- Edema around wound, and feet are swollen
- Feet appear slightly cyanotic
- Says he has not washed right leg in several days
- States he left wound open because "air is good for it"

Nursing Interventions
(use only those that apply; list in priority order)

- Administer analgesics as ordered by physician.
- Report poor pedal pulses and edema.
- Look for hazards in the environment.
- Consult with physical therapist about positioning.
- Cleanse wound and apply wound dressings as ordered.
- Keep feet warm.
- Elevate feet.
- Keep the leg uncovered.
- Put feet in a dependent position.
- Teach client about airborne contamination.
- Consult with dietitian regarding diet.
- Keep the leg immobilized.

NCLEX-PN® Exam Preparation

1 A man has a history of a draining wound infection in his lower right leg. He was admitted with a wet, soiled dressing and the following vital signs: T 100.6, P 90, R 20, BP 136/70. A nursing priority would be:

1. Elevation of the right leg.
2. Placing the person in isolation.
3. Medicating the client for an elevated temperature.
4. Changing the wound dressing.

2 A client was admitted with active tuberculosis with moderate amounts of pink-tinged sputum. She was placed in isolation. The nurse knows that the type of isolation initiated would be:

1. Tier 1.
2. Tier 2.
3. The use of clean gowns.
4. The use of masks by the client while in their room.

3 When preparing a sterile field for the provider, the nurse would:

1. Use sterile forceps while reaching across the tray to place the contents in their proper location.
2. Wear clean gloves to handle the contents of the tray.
3. Prepare the tray 30 minutes in advance of the provider's arrival and cover it with a sterile towel while unattended.
4. Don sterile gloves while handling the contents of the tray.

4 The nurse, caring for a child admitted with pneumonia and placed in isolation, instructs the parents to take all clothing and toys home and:

1. Wash all the clothing and toys in very hot water before putting them away.
2. Throw all the clothes and toys away.
3. No other actions would be necessary.
4. Air the clothes and toys to destroy the organisms.

5 The nurse recognizes that microorganisms are:

1. Always dangerous and must be eliminated whenever they occur.
2. Tiny bacteria that are only visible with a microscope.
3. Are germs that invade and damage the body.
4. Are mostly harmless and may even be helpful.

6 The nurse is caring for a client who was admitted with a diagnosis of hiatal hernia. Following surgery the client develops a wound infection. The nurse recognizes this infection is a/an:

1. Nosocomial infection.
2. Systemic infection.

3. Septicemia.
4. Nosocomial or iatrogenic infection.

7 When leaving the room of a client diagnosed with HIV-related pneumonia, the nurse removes personal protective equipment in what order?

1. Gown, mask, and then gloves.
2. Mask, gloves, and then gown.
3. Gloves, mask, and then gown.
4. Gown first and then either the gloves or the mask.

8 An 82-year-old client with a history of emphysema was being seen for a possible upper respiratory tract infection (URI). Several family members had been ill with colds during the previous week. The nurse is aware that the client may be considered:

1. A susceptible host.
2. A compromised host.
3. To be in no special danger of the infection since the family was ill last week.
4. To have a chronic URI.

9 The nurse performs hand hygiene in order to reduce what link in the chain of infection?

1. Agent.
2. Reservoir.
3. Portal of exit.
4. Mode of transmission.

10 The student nurse asks the nurse how to reduce the risk of a client becoming infected with a drug-resistant organism. Which of the following would be the nurse's best response? (Select all that apply.)

1. "Teach clients to take all of the antibiotics that are prescribed and to not stop taking them when they feel better."
2. "Teach clients to avoid taking antibiotics when they aren't needed, such as when the symptoms are caused by a virus."
3. "Bacteria can become resistant to antibiotics when antibiotics don't work properly and leave some bacteria behind."
4. "Washing the hands is the best way of preventing the spread of drug-resistant organisms to the client."
5. "The most common drug-resistant organisms are MRSA, vancomycin-resistant enterococci, and multi-dose-resistant streptococcus."

Answers and rationales for Review Questions appear in Appendix I.

Chapter 11

Client Communication

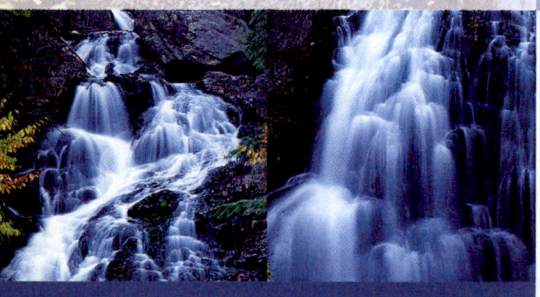

LEARNING Outcomes

After completing this chapter, you will be able to:

1. Describe essential aspects of communication and the communication process.
2. Name several factors that influence the communication process.
3. Differentiate between verbal and nonverbal modes of communication.
4. Explain therapeutic techniques the nurse can use to help the client express thoughts, feelings, and concerns.
5. List principles of communication in the clinical setting.
6. Identify barriers to the development of therapeutic communication.
7. Name two approaches to interviewing a client.
8. Identify nursing approaches for interviewing clients.
9. Discuss types of interview questions.
10. Describe factors that affect client interviews.
11. List the stages of an interview.

Clinical Objectives

12. Reflect on and write a journal entry about a conversation with a client that included therapeutic communication strategies.
13. Interview a client regarding health history.
14. Demonstrate ways nonverbal communication can affect client relationships.

The term **communication** has various meanings, depending on the context in which it is used. To some, communication is the exchange of information or thoughts between two or more people. The person who initiates the communication is the **sender.** The one who is the endpoint of the communication is the **receiver.** The information being passed from the sender to the receiver is the message and the response of the receiver is feedback. This kind of communication uses talking and listening, or writing and reading. Painting, dancing, and storytelling are other methods of communication. In addition, gestures and body actions convey thoughts to others, sometimes "speaking louder than words." Our self-presentation is a form of communication, whether we are aware of it or not.

The intent of any communication is to obtain a response. Communication has two main purposes: to influence others and to obtain information. **Helpful communication** encourages a sharing of information, thoughts, or feelings between two or more people. **Unhelpful communication** hinders or blocks the transfer of information and feelings. Communication techniques that help or hinder effective communication are discussed later in this chapter.

Factors Influencing Communication

Many factors influence the communication process in a therapeutic setting.

DEVELOPMENT

Language, psychosocial, and intellectual development move through stages across the life span. Knowledge of a client's developmental stage allows the nurse to modify the message to reach the listener. This is particularly true in a client teaching situation.

From an early age, females and males communicate differently. Girls tend to use language to seek confirmation, minimize differences, and establish intimacy. Boys use language to establish independence and negotiate status within a group. These differences can continue into adulthood so that a man and a woman may interpret the same communication differently. Many studies have found that men and women communicate differently in both content and process of communication. There is evidence to suggest that more effective communication occurs when the care provider and the client are of the same gender.

Because each person has unique personality traits, values, and life experiences, each will perceive and interpret messages and experiences differently. It is important for the nurse to be aware of a client's values and to validate or correct perceptions to avoid creating barriers in the nurse–client relationship. (**Validation** is a form of feedback that provides confirmation that both parties have the same basic understanding of the message and the feedback.)

PERSONAL SPACE

Personal space is the distance people prefer in interactions with others. In contrast to public space, which is often 6 feet or more, personal space may be inches to a few feet between one person and another. The amount of personal space varies with individuals and cultures.

It is a natural protective instinct for people to maintain a certain amount of space immediately around them. When someone who wants to communicate steps too close, the receiver automatically steps back a pace or two. As they provide nursing care, however, nurses may need to invade a client's personal space. It is important to be aware of this and to warn the client when this will occur.

Territoriality is a concept of the space and things that an individual considers as belonging to the self. For example, clients in a hospital often consider their territory as bounded by the curtains around the bed unit. If a visitor or nurse removes a chair to use at another bed, the client may feel upset or somewhat threatened. Nurses should obtain permission from clients to remove, rearrange, or borrow objects in their hospital area.

ROLES AND RELATIONSHIPS

Roles and relationships affect the communication process. Roles vary when communication occurs. Choices of words and tone of voice are different depending on the roles of the communicators. Nursing student and instructor, client and physician, or parent and child are examples of such roles. The specific relationship between communicators is also significant. The nurse who meets with a client for the first time needs to establish a relationship with that client.

ENVIRONMENT

Communication occurs best in a comfortable, private environment. Nurses should be careful to provide for both. Environmental distractions, such as loud noises or lack of privacy, can impair and distort communication.

GROUP COMMUNICATION

A **group** is more than two people who have shared needs and goals, who take each other into account in their actions, and who thus are held together and set apart from others because of their interactions. Examples of groups are families, peer groups, work groups, and religious groups. Communication within a group depends on each member of the group and his or her motivations (the reasons for participating in the group).

Self-help groups are composed of individuals who share a similar health, social, or daily living problem. The belief of self-help groups is that people who have experienced a similar problem understand better than those who have not experienced the problem. Examples of self-help groups include Alcoholics Anonymous (the first of this type) and groups for those who have experienced stillbirth, divorce, drug abuse, cancer, mental illness, and diabetes.

Nurses may spend time together outside of work to help relieve work-related stress. Nurses who understand work stress can help encourage and support others. They can share the joys of success and the frustration of failure.

Modes of Communication

Communication is generally carried out in two different modes: verbal and nonverbal. **Verbal communication** is exchange of ideas using the spoken or written word. Besides books, newspapers, magazines, and brochures, it also includes electronic forms of communication (television, movies, videos, Internet, text mail, and e-mail). **Nonverbal communication** uses other forms, such as gestures or facial expressions, and touch. Although both kinds of communication occur at the same time, as much as 80% to 90% of what is actually communicated is nonverbal. Learning about nonverbal communication is very important for nurses, so they can develop effective communication patterns and relationships with clients.

VERBAL COMMUNICATION

Verbal communication is largely conscious. People choose the words they use. Their choices are often guided by their culture, socioeconomic background, age, and education. As a result, countless possibilities exist for the way ideas are exchanged.

An important form of verbal communication is written communication. Today more and more messages are being conveyed in this manner. E-mail and text messaging have replaced much face-to-face talking. In addition, communication is done through memos, reports, written documents, and published materials such as this textbook. Written communication must be accurate and clear. It should also be polite and follow social conventions. There is more danger of legal repercussions with written communication, because there is a record of what was said.

Written communication in health care takes many forms, including all of those mentioned above plus documentation and charting. Chapter 13 ⊖⊖ provides the major discussion of documentation.

NONVERBAL COMMUNICATION

Nonverbal communication is sometimes called body language. It includes **gestures,** body movements, touch, and physical appearance (Figure 11-1 ■). Nonverbal behavior is controlled less consciously than verbal behavior. So, nonverbal communication often tells others more about what a person is feeling than what is actually said. Nonverbal communication either reinforces or contradicts what is said verbally. If a nurse says to a client, "I'd be happy to sit here and talk to you for a while," yet glances nervously at a watch every few seconds, the actions contradict the verbal message. The client is more likely to believe the nonverbal behavior, which implies "I am very busy and need to leave."

Observing and interpreting the client's nonverbal behavior is an essential skill for nurses to develop. To observe nonverbal behavior efficiently, the nurse must make a systematic assessment of the person's overall physical appearance, posture, gait, facial expressions, and gestures. The nurse should always exercise caution in interpreting, and always confirm any observation with the client.

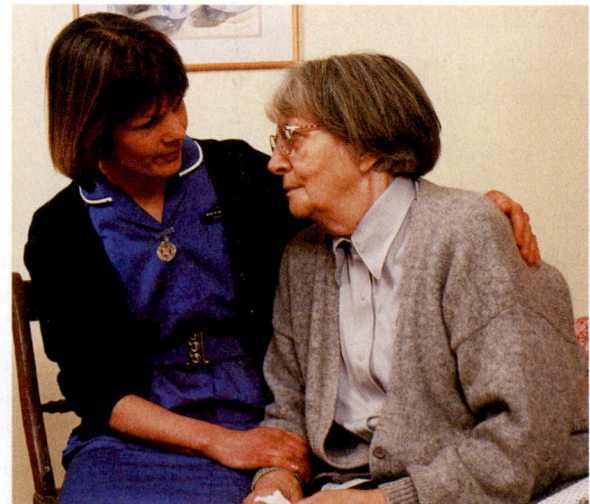

Figure 11-1. ■ Appropriate forms of touch can communicate caring. *Source:* Photo Researchers, Inc.

Nonverbal communication varies widely among cultures. Even behaviors such as smiling and handshaking can mean different things in different cultures.

Personal appearance, clothing, and adornments can say a lot about a person. Clothing may convey social and financial status, culture, religion, group association, and self-concept. Jewelry may be worn as a decoration or as a protection against harm. When the symbolic meaning of an object is unfamiliar, the nurse should ask about its significance. How a person dresses is often an indicator of how the person feels. When a person known for immaculate grooming becomes sloppy in appearance, the nurse may suspect a physical illness or a loss of self-esteem.

The ways people walk and carry themselves are often reliable indicators of self-concept, current mood, and health. The posture of people when they are sitting or lying can also indicate feelings or mood. The nurse can validate the interpretation of the behavior by asking, for example, "You look like it really hurts you to move. I'm wondering how your pain is and if you might need something to make you more comfortable?"

No part of the body is as expressive as the face. Facial expressions can convey surprise, fear, anger, disgust, happiness, and sadness. When the message is not clear, it is important to get feedback to be sure what the person intends.

Nurses need to be aware of their own facial expressions and what they are communicating to others (Figure 11-2 ■). Clients are quick to notice the nurse's expression, particularly when they feel unsure or uncomfortable. It is impossible to control all facial expression. However, the nurse should learn to control expressions such as fear or disgust.

Eye contact is another essential element of facial communication. In many cultures, mutual eye contact means you recognize the other person and are willing to maintain communication.

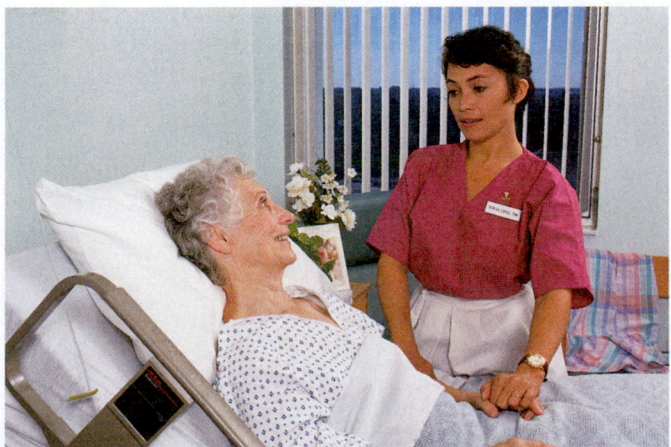

Figure 11-2. ■ The nurse's facial expression communicates warmth and caring. *Source:* Pearson Education/PH College.

Gestures

Hand and body gestures may emphasize and clarify the spoken word. They may occur without words to indicate a particular feeling or to give a sign. Some gestures, however, may have different meanings depending on one's culture. For example, the American gesture meaning "shoo" or "go away" means "come here" or "come back" in some Asian cultures.

For people with special communication problems, such as the deaf, the hands are invaluable in communication. Many deaf people learn sign language. Ill persons who are unable to reply verbally can similarly devise a communication system using the hands. (See also Chapter 12 ∞.)

Therapeutic Communication

Therapeutic communication is client-centered, goal-directed, and time-limited communication. Nurses use therapeutic communication to determine client concerns, problems, and feelings. It is important for the nurse to know how to help clients explore their own feelings and how to avoid shutting down communication by saying the wrong thing.

THERAPEUTIC TECHNIQUES

Nurses can use a variety of responses to client's comments to help them explore or expand on the client's thoughts and feelings. This is important if the nurse is to help the client achieve goals and overcome obstacles. Table 11-1 ■ lists therapeutic communication techniques with examples.

As you talk with clients, you will find you are most comfortable using certain techniques such as offering self, using touch, and providing general leads. However, it is good to try new techniques periodically, especially if the techniques you usually use do not seem to be working.

Communication techniques should be comfortable for you, so that the conversation flows and is not stilted. Be careful not to overuse any one technique, because it may seem to the client that you are being insincere or uncaring. Overuse of silence or reflecting, for example, may slow down communication.

Principles of Communication for the Clinical Setting

Effective communication in the clinical setting can be accomplished using the following communication principles:

- Use therapeutic communication techniques to communicate with clients.
- Think before you speak. Communicating with a client is different than speaking with a friend or another student. Share only what is appropriate, and always remember ethical principles and confidentiality.

TABLE 11-1	Therapeutic Communication Techniques	
TECHNIQUE	**DESCRIPTION**	**EXAMPLES**
VERBAL TECHNIQUES		
Using silence	Accepting pauses or silences that may extend for several seconds or minutes without interjecting any verbal response.	Sitting quietly (or walking with the client) and waiting attentively until the client is able to put thoughts and feelings into words.
Providing general leads	Using statements or questions that (1) encourage the client to verbalize; (2) choose a topic of conversation; and (3) facilitate continued verbalization.	"Perhaps you would like to talk about. . . ." "Would it help to discuss your feelings?" "Where would you like to begin?" "And then what?" "I follow what you are saying."
Being specific vs. tentative	Making statements that are specific rather than general, and tentative rather than absolute.	"You scratched my arm." (specific statement) "You are as clumsy as an ox." (general statement) "You seem unconcerned about Mary." (tentative statement) "You don't give a damn about Mary and you never will." (absolute statement)
Using open-ended questions	Asking broad questions that lead or invite the client to explore (elaborate, clarify, describe, compare, or illustrate) thoughts or feelings. Open-ended questions specify only the topic to be discussed and invite answers that are longer than one or two words.	"I'd like to hear more about that." "Tell me about. . . ." "How have you been feeling lately?" "What brought you to the hospital?" "What is your opinion?" "You said you were frightened yesterday. How do you feel now?"
Restating or paraphrasing	Actively listening for the client's basic message and then repeating those thoughts and/or feelings in similar words. This conveys that the nurse has listened and understood the client's basic message and also offers clients a clearer idea of what they have said.	*Client:* "I couldn't manage to eat any dinner last night—not even the dessert." *Nurse:* "You had difficulty eating yesterday." *Client:* "Yes, I was very upset after my family left." *Client:* "I have trouble talking to strangers." *Nurse:* "You find it difficult talking to people you do not know?"
Seeking clarification	A method of making the client's broad overall meaning of the message more understandable. It is used when paraphrasing is difficult or when the communication is rambling or garbled. To clarify the message, the nurse can restate the basic message or confess confusion and ask the client to repeat or restate the message. Nurses can also clarify their own message with statements.	"I'm puzzled." "I'm not sure I understand that." "Would you please say that again?" "Would you tell me more?" "I meant this rather than that." "I guess I didn't make that clear—I'll go over it again."
Checking perception or seeking consensual validation	A method similar to clarifying that verifies the meaning of specific words rather than the overall meaning of a message.	*Client:* "My husband never gives me any presents." *Nurse:* "You mean he has never given you a present for your birthday or Christmas?" *Client:* "Well—not never. He does get me something for my birthday and Christmas, but he never thinks of giving me anything at any other time."
Offering self	Suggesting one's presence, interest, or wish to understand the client without making any demands or attaching conditions that the client must comply with to receive the nurse's attention.	"I'll stay with you until your daughter arrives." "We can sit here quietly for a while; we don't need to talk unless you would like to." "I'll help you to dress to go home."
Giving information	Providing, in a simple and direct manner, specific factual information the client may or may not request. When information is not known, the nurse states this and indicates who has it or when the nurse will obtain it.	"Your surgery is scheduled for 11 A.M. tomorrow." "You will feel a pulling sensation when the tube is removed from your abdomen." "I do not know the answer to that, but I will find out from Mrs. King, the nurse in charge."

TABLE 11-1	Therapeutic Communication Techniques (continued)	
TECHNIQUE	**DESCRIPTION**	**EXAMPLES**
Acknowledging	Giving recognition, in a nonjudgmental way, of a change in behavior, an effort the client has made, or a contribution to a communication. Acknowledgment may be with or without understanding, verbal or nonverbal.	"You trimmed your beard and mustache and washed your hair." "I notice you keep squinting your eyes. Are you having difficulty seeing?" "You walked twice as far today with your walker."
Clarifying time or sequence	Helping the client clarify an event, situation, or happening in relationship to time.	*Client:* "I vomited this morning." *Nurse:* "Was that after breakfast?" *Client:* "I feel that I have been asleep for weeks." *Nurse:* "You had your operation Monday, and today is Tuesday."
Presenting reality	Helping the client to differentiate the real from the unreal.	"That telephone ring came from the program on television." "That's not a dead mouse in the corner; it is a discarded washcloth." "Your magazine is here in the drawer. It has not been stolen."
Focusing	Helping the client expand on and develop a topic of importance. It is important for the nurse to wait until the client finishes stating the main concerns before attempting to focus. The focus may be an idea or a feeling; however, the nurse often emphasizes a feeling to help the client recognize an emotion disguised behind words.	*Client:* "My wife says she will look after me, but I don't think she can, what with the children to take care of, and they're always after her about something—clothes, homework, what's for dinner that night." *Nurse:* "You are worried about how well she can manage."
Reflecting	Directing ideas, feelings, questions, or content back to clients to enable them to explore their own ideas and feelings about a situation.	*Client:* "What can I do?" *Nurse:* "What do you think would be helpful?" *Client:* "Do you think I should tell my husband?" *Nurse:* "You seem unsure about telling your husband."
Summarizing and planning	Stating the main points of a discussion to clarify the relevant points discussed. This technique is useful at the end of an interview or to review a health teaching session. It often acts as an introduction to future care planning.	"During the past half hour we have talked about. . . ." "Tomorrow afternoon we may explore this further." "In a few days I'll review what you have learned about the actions and effects of your insulin."
NONVERBAL TECHNIQUES		
Using touch	Providing appropriate forms of touch to reinforce caring feelings. Because tactile contacts vary considerably among individuals, families, and cultures, the nurse must be sensitive to the differences in attitudes and practices of clients and self.	Putting an arm over the client's shoulder. Placing your hand over the client's hand.
Using posture and position	Using body stance and direction to indicate interest and attention.	Facing the client, sitting at the same level as the client, leaning forward when listening to the client, keeping arms relaxed and not crossed.
Using facial expression	Presenting a calm and friendly expression.	Eye contact (as much as seems comfortable for the client), a relaxed face and occasional smile (as appropriate), openness of expression (indicating listening), appearing to be "in the present" (not preoccupied).
Using gestures	Moving the body, especially the hands and arms.	Clapping (to express praise or pleasure), making motions that help describe a procedure or process, demonstrating position of a needle for SC injection.

- Be quiet and gentle in your communication. Do not communicate in any way that could increase the stress or discomfort of clients, families, or staff.
- Ask appropriate questions. Questions are asked to obtain information needed to care for clients, not to satisfy your curiosity. You should not make it a habit to read charts or look up information on the computer about clients to whom you are not assigned. When information is needed for educational purposes, the client's name and personal information must be removed. Client

records should not be copied and removed from the hospital by a student.

- Keep information confidential. Do not talk about clients or their families in inappropriate places. Avoid discussing clients in the elevator, cafeteria, or anywhere visitors can overhear.
- Be respectful in your communication. Speak to physicians, nursing assistants, instructors, and visitors with equal respect.
- Find out what you don't know. Don't pretend that you know something if you don't. This could inadvertently harm a client. Do not expect your instructor to give you all the answers. Instead, take responsibility for your own learning.
- Give a clear concise report. Shift report is an important form of communication (see Chapter 23 ⬤⬤).

ATTENTIVE LISTENING

Attentive listening or active listening involves listening for key themes in communication with clients. The nurse should not interrupt the speaker, should take time to think about the message, and should ask questions to clarify or obtain additional information if needed. Attentive behaviors are a type of nonverbal communication. The nurse should lean slightly toward the client and have direct eye contact with the client. (Clients may have personal or cultural reasons for not returning eye contact. In these cases, the nurse would still make sure to make eye contact often.) The nurse should use open and expansive gestures as well as nonverbal cues such as nodding and smiling.

Attentive listening is a highly developed skill, but it can be learned with practice. A nurse can convey attentiveness in listening to clients in various ways (Figure 11-3 ■). Common responses are nodding the head, uttering "uh huh" or "mmm," repeating the words that the client has used, or

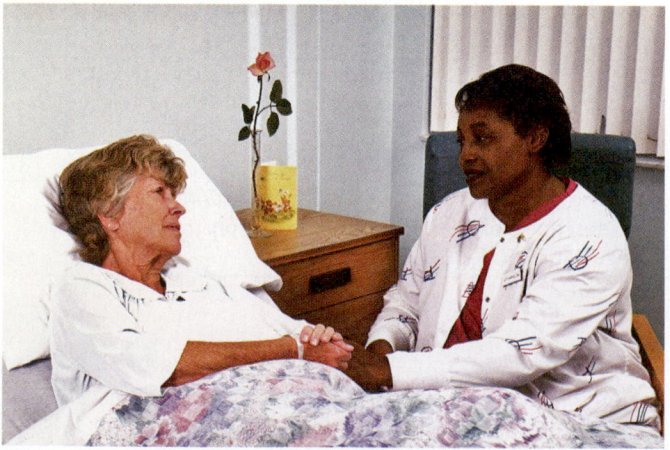

Figure 11-3. ■ The nurse conveys attentive listening through a posture of involvement. *Source:* Pearson Education/PH College.

saying "I see what you mean." Each nurse has characteristic ways of responding, and the nurse must take care not to sound insincere or phony.

CONFIDENTIALITY IN COMMUNICATION

Federal law as well as facility policy governs communication in health care. HIPAA (Health Insurance Portability and Accountability Act of 1996) makes violation of confidentiality of client information a punishable offense. See Chapters 4 and 14 ⬤⬤ for coverage of HIPAA information.

BARRIERS TO COMMUNICATION

Have you ever had a conversation with someone who responded in a way that made you feel it was useless to keep talking to that person? Chances are good that you experienced a barrier to communication. Everyone uses communication barriers from time to time, but nurses need to be especially careful to avoid them when speaking with clients. Communication barriers are described in Table 11-2 ■.

It is very important to recognize when a barrier to communication has been used. You may respond to a client and then realize that you have used a barrier. When this happens, it is perfectly acceptable to say, "Let me say that differently." Or, "I'm sorry, that did not come out the way I meant it." If you realize later that you have used a barrier and shut down communication with a client, you can speak with the client again. You can tell the client that you would like to talk about the subject again and that you did not mean to be abrupt earlier.

Interviewing

An **interview** is a planned communication or a conversation with a purpose, for example, to get or give information. Interviewing is used in most phases of the nursing process, and is especially important when obtaining the nursing health history.

There are two approaches to interviewing: directive and nondirective. The *directive interview* is structured and is used to discover specific information. The nurse explains the purpose of the interview and asks closed-ended questions (see the next section) that call for specific data. The client gives responses without discussion. Directive interviews are used to gather and to give information when time is limited, such as in an emergency situation.

A *nondirective interview* allows the client to control the situation. *Rapport*, an understanding between two or more people, is built in this type of interview. The nurse encourages communication by asking open-ended questions (see the next section) and by providing empathetic responses.

A combination of directive and nondirective approaches is usually appropriate during the information-gathering

TABLE 11-2	Barriers to Communication	
TECHNIQUE	**DESCRIPTION**	**EXAMPLES**
Stereotyping	Offering generalized and oversimplified beliefs about groups of people that are based on experiences too limited to be valid. These responses categorize clients and negate their uniqueness as individuals.	"Two-year-olds are brats." "Women are complainers." "Men don't cry." "Most people don't have any pain after this type of surgery."
Agreeing and disagreeing	Akin to judgmental responses, agreeing and disagreeing imply that the client is either right or wrong and that the nurse is in a position to judge this. These responses deter clients from thinking through their position and may cause them to become defensive.	*Client:* "I don't think Dr. Broad is a very good doctor. He doesn't seem interested in his patients." *Nurse:* "Dr. Broad is head of the Department of Surgery and is an excellent surgeon."
Being defensive	Attempting to protect a person or healthcare services from negative comments. These responses prevent the client from expressing true concerns. The nurse is saying, "You have no right to complain." Defensive responses protect the nurse from admitting weaknesses in the healthcare services, including personal weaknesses.	*Client:* "Those night nurses must just sit around and talk all night. They didn't answer my light for over an hour." *Nurse:* "I'll have you know we literally run around on nights. You're not the only client, you know."
Challenging	Giving a response that makes clients prove their statement or point of view. These responses indicate that the nurse is failing to consider the client's feelings, making the client feel it necessary to defend a position.	*Client:* "I felt nauseated after that red pill." *Nurse:* "Surely you don't think I gave you the wrong pill?" *Client:* "I feel as if I am dying." *Nurse:* "How can you feel that way when your pulse is 60?" *Client:* "I believe my husband doesn't love me." *Nurse:* "You can't say that; why, he visits you every day."
Probing	Asking for information chiefly out of curiosity rather than with the intent to assist the client. These responses are considered prying and violate the client's privacy. Asking "why" is often probing and places the client in a defensive position.	*Client:* "I was speeding along the street and didn't see the stop sign." *Nurse:* "Why were you speeding?" *Client:* "I didn't ask the doctor when he was here." *Nurse:* "Why didn't you?"
Testing	Asking questions that make the client admit to something. These responses permit the client only limited answers and often meet the nurse's need rather than the client's.	"Who do you think you are?" (forces people to admit their status is only that of client) "Do you think I am not busy?" (forces the client to admit that the nurse really is busy)
Rejecting	Refusing to discuss certain topics with the client. These responses often make clients feel that the nurse is rejecting not only their communication but also the clients themselves.	"I don't want to discuss that. Let's talk about. . . ." "Let's discuss other areas of interest to you rather than the two problems you keep mentioning." "I can't talk now. It's time for my coffee break."
Changing topics and subjects	Directing the communication into areas of self-interest rather than considering the client's concerns is often a self-protective response to a topic that causes anxiety. These responses imply that what the nurse considers important will be discussed and that clients should not discuss certain topics.	*Client:* "I'm separated from my wife. Do you think I should have sexual relations with another woman?" *Nurse:* "I see that you're 36 and that you like gardening. This sunshine is good for my roses. I have a beautiful rose garden."
Using unwarranted reassurance	Using clichés or comforting statements of advice as a means to reassure the client. These responses block the fears, feelings, and other thoughts of the client.	"You'll feel better soon." "I'm sure everything will turn out all right." "Don't worry."
Passing judgment	Giving opinions and approving or disapproving responses, moralizing, or implying one's own values. These responses imply that the client must think as the nurse thinks, fostering client dependence.	"That's good (bad)." "You shouldn't do that." "That's not good enough." "What you did was wrong (right)."
Giving common advice	Telling the client what to do. These responses deny the client's right to be an equal partner. Note that giving expert rather than common advice is therapeutic.	*Client:* "Should I move from my home to a nursing home?" *Nurse:* "If I were you, I'd go to a nursing home, where you'll get your meals cooked for you."

BOX 11-1 NURSING CARE CHECKLIST

Guidelines for Wording Verbal Communication

☑ Pay attention to your tone of voice, manner, and pace of speech. They can change the feeling and impact of the message. Your intonation can express enthusiasm, sadness, anger, or amusement. Your pace of speech may indicate interest, anxiety, boredom, or fear.

☑ Use simple terms and give complete information. Complex technical terms become natural to nurses, but laypeople often misunderstand them. Instead of saying to a client, "The nurses will be catheterizing you tomorrow for a urine analysis," it may be more understandable to say, "Tomorrow we need to get a sample of your urine, so we will collect it by putting a small tube into your bladder." Speak clearly and briefly. A message that is direct and simple is effective. Clarity is saying precisely what you mean, and brevity is using the fewest words necessary. The result is a message that is simple and clear.

☑ Use consistency in verbal and nonverbal communication. The nurse's behavior must match the words spoken. When the nurse tells the client, "I am interested in hearing what you have to say," the nonverbal behavior would include the nurse facing the client, making eye contact, and leaning forward.

☑ Keep communication relevant and well timed. The timing of any message needs to be appropriate to ensure that words are heard. Messages should address the person's interests and concerns, and be given when the client can hear and understand them. Nurses need to be aware of both relevance and timing when communicating with clients. Avoid asking several questions at once or asking questions without waiting for an answer. For example, a nurse might enter a client's room and say in one breath, "Good morning. How are you this morning? Did you sleep well last night? Your husband is coming to see you before your surgery, isn't he?" The client no doubt would wonder which question to answer first.

☑ Be adaptable when communicating. Spoken messages should be adapted to behavioral cues from the client. What the nurse says and how it is said must show sensitivity. For example, a nurse who is usually friendly and jovial may notice that a client seems very withdrawn and distressed. The nurse should modify his or her tone of speech with this client, and share observations about the client's expression and mood.

☑ Be credible (believable). Credibility may be the most important requirement for effective communication. Nurses foster credibility by being consistent, dependable, and honest. They should be knowledgeable about what is being discussed and have accurate information. Nurses should convey confidence and certainty in what they are saying. If they don't know the answer, they should say so: "I don't know the answer to that, but I will find someone who does."

☑ Use humor, but use it with care. Humor can be a positive and powerful tool in the nurse–client relationship. Humor can help clients adjust to difficult and painful situations by providing a different perspective and promoting a sense of well-being. The physical act of laughter can be both an emotional and physical release that reduces tension. Healthful humor must be distinguished from harmful humor. Healthful humor elicits laughter, it is appropriate to the situation, and it protects a person's dignity. Harmful humor ridicules other people by laughing at them. Humor is also harmful if used to avoid resolving problems.

---

interview. The nurse begins by asking open-ended questions to determine areas of concern for the client. If, for example, a client expresses worry about surgery, the nurse pauses to explore the client's worry and to provide support. Simply to note the worry, without dealing with it, can leave the impression that the nurse does not care about the client's concerns or dismisses them as unimportant. As the interview evolves, the nurse may use closed-ended questions to obtain more specific data and to complete the nursing health history. See the nursing care checklist in Box 11-1 ■ for guidelines for wording verbal communication.

KINDS OF INTERVIEW QUESTIONS

Questions are classified as closed or open ended, and as neutral or leading. **Closed-ended questions,** used in the directive interview, generally require only "yes" or "no" or short factual answers giving specific information. Thus the amount of information gained is generally limited. Closed questions often begin with "when," "where," "who," "what," "do (did, does)," "is (are, was)," and sometimes "how." Examples of closed questions are "What medication did you take?" "Are you having pain now? Show me where it is." "How old are you?" "When did you fall?" The highly stressed person and the person who has difficulty communicating will find closed-ended questions easier to answer than open-ended questions.

Open-ended questions, used in the nondirective interview, invite clients to discover and explore their thoughts or feelings. They allow clients the freedom to talk about what they wish. An open-ended question specifies only the broad topic to be discussed, and invites answers longer than one or two words. The open-ended question is useful at the beginning of an interview or to change topics and to elicit attitudes.

The type of question a nurse chooses depends on the situation. For example, the nurse asks closed-ended questions in an emergency when information must be obtained quickly. Nurses often find it necessary to use a combination of open- and closed-ended questions throughout an interview to obtain needed information. A comparison of open- and closed-ended questions appears in Box 11-2 ■.

A *neutral question* is a question the client can answer without direction or pressure from the nurse. Examples are "How do you feel about that?" and "Why do you think you had the operation?" A *leading question*, by contrast, directs the client's answer. The phrasing of the question suggests what answer is expected. Examples are "You're stressed about surgery tomorrow, aren't you?" and "You will take your medicine, won't you?" The leading question gives the client less opportunity to decide whether the answer is true or not. Leading questions create problems if the client gives inaccurate responses in order to please the nurse. This can result in inaccurate data.

FACTORS THAT INFLUENCE THE INTERVIEW

Before beginning an interview, the nurse reviews available information. The following factors can have a great effect on the success or failure of the client interview.

Time

Nurses need to schedule interviews with hospitalized clients for a time when the client is comfortable and when interruptions are unlikely. Nurses should schedule interviews with home care clients at a time selected by the client. In all instances, the client should be comfortable and unhurried.

Place

The place for an interview should be comfortable, well lit, private, and quiet. Most people are uncomfortable about answering personal questions or expressing strong feelings in the sight or hearing of others.

Seating Arrangement

When a client is in bed, the nurse can sit at a 45-degree angle to the bed. This position is less formal than sitting behind a table or standing at the foot of the bed. During an initial admission interview, a client may feel less confronted if there is an overbed table between the client and the nurse. Sitting on a client's bed may make the client uncomfortable.

Distance

People feel uncomfortable when talking to someone who is too close or too far away. Most people feel comfortable at a distance of 3 to 4 feet during an interview. Some clients require more or less personal space, depending on their cultural and personal needs (Box 11-3 ■).

Height also affects communication. When a nurse is standing and looking down at a client, the client may feel intimidated.

STAGES OF AN INTERVIEW

An interview has three major stages: the opening or introduction, the body or development, and the closing.

The Opening

The opening can be the most important part of the interview because what is said and done at that time sets the tone for the remainder of the interview. The purposes of the opening are to establish rapport and orient the interviewee.

Establishing rapport is a process of creating goodwill and trust. It can begin with a greeting ("Good morning, Mr. Johnson") or a self-introduction ("Good morning. I'm

Becky James, a nursing student") accompanied by nonverbal gestures such as a smile, a handshake, and a friendly manner. A brief amount of small talk about the person, the weather, sports, and families is appropriate to develop rapport, but too much superficial talk can cause anxiety. The nurse then orients the client by explaining the purpose and nature of the interview, what information is needed, how long it will take, and what is expected of the client. The nurse usually states that the client has the right not to provide data and tells the client how the information will be used.

The following is an example of an interview introduction:

STEP 1: ESTABLISH RAPPORT

Nurse: Hello, Ms. Goodwin. I'm Sharon Fellows, and I will be assisting with your care today. I am a nursing student at the technical center.

Client: It's nice to meet you. My sister-in-law teaches at the technical center. Do you know Dorothy Goodwin?

Nurse: No, I don't believe I have met her. What does she teach?

Client: Something in computers. I don't actually understand it! Will you be bringing me my medicine today?

STEP 2: PROVIDE ORIENTATION

Nurse: Yes, that will be part of my responsibilities. I also need to ask you a few questions about your health and illness. Do you need any pain medicine or other medicines before we talk for about 10 minutes?

Client: No, I am fine. Just wondered if you would be doing the medicines today.

Nurse: I will. Don't hesitate to ask for anything you need.

Client: What do you need to know?

Nurse: I need to ask you about what you might need after you leave the hospital. If you don't want to discuss something I bring up, just let me know. I will be making notes so we can arrange for you to have follow-up doctor visits and nursing care if you need it.

Client: I probably will. My husband cannot do much because he is nearly blind and has a heart condition. My daughter will be coming to stay for a few days, though.

The Body

In the body of the interview, the client communicates what he or she thinks, feels, knows, and perceives in response to questions from the nurse. The nurse can make the transition from the opening stage to this stage by asking an open-ended question that is related to the

---

BOX 11-4	NURSING CARE CHECKLIST

Communication during an Interview

☑ Listen attentively, using all your senses, and speak slowly and clearly.

☑ Use language the client understands. Clarify points that are not understood.

☑ Plan questions to follow a logical sequence.

☑ Ask only one question at a time. Double questions limit the client to one choice and may confuse both the nurse and the client.

☑ Allow the client the opportunity to look at things the way they appear to him or her and not the way they appear to the nurse or someone else.

☑ Do not impose your own values on the client.

☑ Avoid using personal examples, such as saying "If I were you. . . ."

☑ Nonverbally convey respect, concern, interest, and acceptance.

☑ Use and accept silence to help the client search for more thoughts or to organize them.

☑ Use eye contact and be calm, unhurried, and sympathetic.

---

stated purpose, such as "What brought you to the hospital today?"

The nurse must use communication techniques that make both parties feel comfortable and serve the purpose of the interview. Communication techniques are covered in Table 11-1. Brief guidelines for communicating during an interview are outlined in Box 11-4 ∎.

The Closing

The nurse usually terminates the interview when the needed information has been obtained. In some cases, however, a client terminates it, for example, when deciding not to give any more information or when unable to offer more information for some other reason—fatigue, for example. The closing is important in maintaining rapport. The following techniques are commonly used to close an interview (Stewart & Cash, 2006):

1. Signal that the interview is coming to an end by offering to answer questions: "Do you have any questions?" "I would be glad to answer any questions you have." Be sure to allow time for the person to answer, or the offer will be regarded as insincere.

2. Declare completion of the purpose or task by saying "Well, that's about all I need to know for now" or "Well, those are all the questions I have for now."

Preceding a remark with the word *well* generally signals that the end of the interaction is near.

3. State appreciation or satisfaction about what was accomplished: "I really enjoyed meeting you, and I think we accomplished a great deal." "Those are all the questions I have. Thank you for your time and help." "The questions you have answered will be helpful in planning your nursing care."

NURSING CARE

PRIORITIZING NURSING CARE

Good nursing requires an understanding of the many factors involved in communicating. A client may state that she is "all set" for the next day's gallbladder surgery. However, the nurse may observe that the client has a fearful expression and is trembling. If the nurse focuses on only the client's verbal communication, he or she is unlikely to provide good care or accurate documentation. The nurse must always be attuned to the verbal and nonverbal messages from the client.

ASSESSING

The nurse collects assessment data through closed- or open-ended questions, depending on the task at hand and the time available. When collecting data for a shift change, the nurse might focus on vital signs, status of IVs, and so on. When giving a client a sponge bath before sleep, the nurse might ask open-ended questions that would give the client the opportunity to reminisce and think of pleasant events.

The nurse will need to vary communication and interviewing techniques when caring for clients of different ages and those who have communication-related disabilities. Box 11-5 ■ provides specific communication and interviewing guidelines for clients of different ages.

DIAGNOSING, PLANNING, AND IMPLEMENTING

Certain nursing diagnoses (among others) that may affect communication with a client are:

- *Anxiety*
- *Ineffective Coping*
- *Ineffective Denial*
- *Hopelessness*
- *Disturbed Sensory Perception*

Be prepared to address the client's feelings, and to adapt the pace and style of your communication.

The following interventions are useful in interviewing clients:

- Before beginning an interview, know what information to collect. *This will ensure that the exchange with the client is*

| BOX 11-5 | LIFESPAN CONSIDERATIONS |

Interviews

Children

- Determine the words that a young child uses for "bathroom," "bottle," or an important comfort item so he or she does not become frustrated when trying to communicate wants.
- Talk to the child and ask questions of him or her even when parents are there and are providing most of the information. This will help the child feel that his or her needs are being considered.
- Ask adolescents if they want to have the parent present during the interview or care. (There may be a reluctance to give full information or to ask questions if the parent is present.)

Older Adults

- Assess hearing ability prior to beginning an interview. If the client has trouble hearing, conduct the interview in an area without a lot of background noise (e.g., turn off the TV, turn down air conditioners or fans).
- Older clients may be more reserved about discussing personal health issues. Delay asking personal or embarrassing questions until they feel more comfortable with you.
- Conduct the interview when the client is rested and during the time of day when he or she is most alert, if possible.
- If family members are present, ask the client if she or he wishes the interview to be in private or to have the family remain.

Clients with Communication Deficits

- Determine what deficit the client has.
- If the client is hearing impaired and wears a hearing aid, have the client put it on prior to the interview.
- If the client uses sign language, provide an interpreter.
- A client who has experienced a stroke may have intact receptive language but have difficulty expressing ideas. Allow extra time if needed. Give clients a choice of words if they are struggling for the right one.
- Provide a client who is nonverbal or unable to speak (e.g., following surgery) with paper and pencil to write answers or requests.
- Make use of available communication devices such as picture boards, signs, or cards.

---

smooth and efficient. It will also free you to observe the client more during the interaction.

- Schedule interviews at a time that is as convenient as possible for the client, and when interruptions are not likely to occur. Allow home care clients to select a time. *This will allow the interview to be relaxed and unhurried. Most people are uncomfortable about answering personal questions or expressing strong feelings in the sight or hearing of others.*
- If possible, sit at a 45-degree angle to the bed or chair where the client is, and about 3 to 4 feet from the client.

Sitting too close to, or standing over, the client can make the client feel threatened. Sitting far away may suggest lack of interest.

- Open the interview with a friendly greeting and introduce yourself. If appropriate, start with some general conversation. Then explain why you are there. *This approach expresses respect for the client and builds rapport. The client can be more relaxed about the interview once its purpose is stated.*

- Ask an open-ended question that is related to the stated purpose, is easy to answer, and does not embarrass or place stress on the person. *This helps make the transition into the main part of the interview.*

- Throughout the interview, use good communication techniques. If you feel you have put up a block to communication, apologize and restate the question in a better way. If a client appears suddenly embarrassed or concerned, look for the underlying reason (Box 11-6 ■). Pay attention to both verbal and nonverbal messages from the client. *When the nurse recognizes a communication block and attempts to correct it, communication can continue.*

- When the necessary information has been obtained, ask if the client has any questions. If the client decides to stop the interview, state what you have accomplished and, if needed, say what follow-up will be required. Suggest a follow-up time. *If all questions have been answered, the open-ended question signals that the interview is ending. If a client is too tired or refuses to give any more information, the restatement will help them to know what has been accomplished and what more they will be asked to do at another time.*

- Thank clients for their time and express hope for a positive outcome. *This again expresses your respect and concern for them.*

EVALUATING

In evaluating professional communications with a client, the nurse first looks at the client's verbal and nonverbal expressions of comfort. Does the client seem relaxed, or does he appear flushed and tense? Does the client express satisfaction at understanding better, or does he appear anxious and confused?

The nurse also mentally reviews the interaction to determine the success of the communication process. What communication techniques were effective in the situation? Which were not effective? Did any blocks to communication arise? Was a way found to move past them? If not, can the nurse think of a possible way past the block now that the interaction is over? Has the nurse experienced any similar communications that might provide insights?

NURSING PROCESS CARE PLAN
Client Affected by Nurse Communication Barriers

Lucy, an LPN, is assigned to care for Mr. Levowitz. He is currently in the recovery room after surgery to remove prostate cancer that had spread to his abdomen. His wife comes into the room crying. Lucy asks her what is wrong. Mrs. Levowitz continues to sob and is unable to answer. Lucy gets chairs for herself and Mrs. Levowitz and urges her to sit down. Lucy says, "Come on now. The news can't be that bad, can it?" Mrs. Levowitz responds by telling Lucy that the doctor has said the cancer is so bad that there is nothing they can do. Lucy then says, "I am so very sorry. That must be difficult news to hear." Mrs. Levowitz cries a bit longer, then says she doesn't know how she can live without him. Lucy tells her, "You should wait and see how the chemotherapy and radiation treatments go before you think about living without him. Things may still turn out all right." Mrs. Levowitz grasps at that hope and says, "Oh, do you really think those treatments could help him? That he doesn't really have cancer that bad?" Lucy says, "It's been known to happen. I really have to go see some other patients now. Everything will be okay for you. It will turn out just fine."

BOX 11-6	CULTURAL PULSE POINTS

Handling Miscommunications

Miscommunication is a frequent problem in hospitals. The most obvious miscommunication occurs when the client and hospital staff do not speak the same language. Language problems, however, can also occur among English-speaking people. In England, Australia, and South Africa, the word *fanny* is a derogatory term referring to a woman's vagina. Imagine the reaction of a British woman when asked to prepare for a shot in the fanny. But the more subtle problems are those that result from cultural differences in meaning of nonverbal behavior. Many Asians consider it disrespectful to look someone directly in the eye, especially if that person is a nurse. An Asian client may avoid eye contact out of respect for the superior status of the nurse. Many Middle Easterners see direct eye contact between a man and a woman as a sexual invitation. Knowing what the norm within the culture is will facilitate understanding and lessen miscommunication.

The nursing diagnosis "*Impaired Verbal Communication* related to cultural difference" is defined by NANDA as being relevant when "an individual experiences a decreased or absent ability to use or understand language in human interaction." This diagnosis implies that the client's verbal communication and ability to understand and utilize language is impaired in some way regardless of the cause. An individual who speaks a different language than that used by the healthcare provider may be capable of both use and comprehension of a familiar language when interacting with a person fluent in the language. In this situation if the client is verbally impaired, the nurse is equally impaired. It is clear that this NANDA diagnosis does not adequately address the issue of nonverbal communication, an essential assessment factor in transcultural nursing.

Assessment

The client and his wife live alone in a small cottage several miles outside the city. Mrs. Levowitz does not drive and has always been a stay-at-home wife. She also expresses concerns about caring for him at home and getting him to his treatment appointments. Mr. Levowitz is very controlled and sits quietly not joining in the conversation with the LPN and his wife.

Nursing Diagnosis

The following important nursing diagnoses (among others) are established for these clients:

- *Caregiver Role Strain* related to need for significant home care
- *Compromised Family Coping* related to inadequate resources available
- *Grieving* related to potential loss of significant others
- *Ineffective Role Performance* related to change in physical capacity to resume prior role

Expected Outcomes

The expected outcomes for the plan of care are:

- Caregiver identifies resources available to help in giving care.
- Identifies need for and seeks outside support.
- Plans for future one day at a time.
- Accepts physical limitation regarding role responsibility and considers ways to change lifestyle to accomplish goals associated with role performance.

Planning and Implementation

The following nursing interventions are implemented:

- Monitor caregiver for psychological distress and signs of depression.
- Assess health of the caregiver at intervals, especially if she has a chronic illness in addition to caregiver role.

- Help caregiver identify ways to equitably distribute workload among family.
- Assist in finding transportation for treatment and family visit.
- Refer family to appropriate resources for assistance as indicated.
- Involve client and family in planning care as much as possible.
- Use therapeutic communication with open-ended questions such as "What are your fears and thoughts?"
- Actively listen to client's/family's expression of grief; do not interrupt, do not tell own story, and do not offer meaningless platitudes such as "It will be better this way."
- Refer to family counseling if needed for adjustment of role change.
- Identify ways to compensate for physical disabilities.

Evaluation

Mrs. Levowitz spoke with a social worker, and arrangements were made for her and her husband to move temporarily to an assisted living arrangement during treatment. Mrs. Levowitz expressed that "I will keep an open mind, maybe we will consider moving permanently to the assisted living apartment." Both client and wife expressed a desire to discuss the future once a therapeutic communication dialogue was started. Mr. Levowitz expressed an understanding of his physical limitation, but stated, "They can't get rid of me that easy. I am going to fight this as long as my wife is by my side."

Critical Thinking in the Nursing Process

1. What communication techniques did Lucy use?
2. What barriers to communication did Lucy use?
3. What nonverbal communication did Lucy use?

Note: Discussion of Critical Thinking questions appears on the MyNursingKit Website.

Note: The references and resources for all chapters have been compiled at the back of the book.

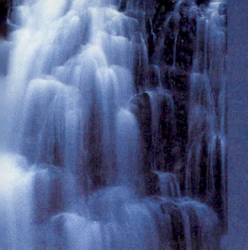

Chapter Review

KEY Points

- Communication is a critical nursing skill used to gather information, to teach and persuade, and to express caring and comfort.
- Communication is the exchange of information or thoughts between two or more people. Messages are both verbal and nonverbal.
- The effectiveness of verbal communication depends on many factors, including pace and intonation, simplicity, clarity and brevity, timing, relevance, adaptability, and credibility.
- Nonverbal communication includes personal appearance, posture and gait, facial expressions, and gestures. It often reveals more about a person's thoughts and feelings than words do. The "receiver" is more likely to believe a nonverbal message than a verbal one.
- When communication is effective, verbal and nonverbal expressions are consistent.
- When assessing verbal and nonverbal behaviors, nurses need to consider cultural influences. A single nonverbal expression can indicate a variety of feelings, and one word can have several meanings.
- Many techniques facilitate therapeutic communication: attentive listening; paraphrasing; clarifying; using open-ended questions and statements; focusing; being specific; using touch and silence; clarifying reality, time, or sequence; providing general leads; and summarizing.
- To communicate well, the nurse must be seen as trustworthy.
- Offering unwarranted reassurance, stating approval or disapproval, giving common (not expert) advice, stereotyping, and being defensive are barriers to communication that destroy trust.

⊕ FOR FURTHER Study

Chapters 4 and 14 provide information about legal aspects of nursing, including client confidentiality and HIPAA.

See Chapter 12 for more on communication techniques in relation to client teaching.

For more information on shift change reporting, see Chapter 13.

Chapter 13 provides the major discussion of communication for the purpose of documentation in the client's record.

Critical Thinking Care Map

Caring for a Client with Anorexia

NCLEX-PN® Focus Area: Coping and Adaptation

Case Study: Erlene Barnes, age 18, has been diagnosed with anorexia. She expresses that she feels she is fat although she admits to losing 15 pounds in the last 2 months. She is planning to leave home to go to college in about 3 months. She has come for her college physical. Her mother accompanied her and insists on being in the room during the exam, and attempts to answer all questions directed to Ms. Barnes.

Nursing Diagnosis: *Ineffective Family Therapeutic Regimen Management* related to family conflict

COLLECT DATA

Subjective	Objective
_____	_____
_____	_____
_____	_____
_____	_____
_____	_____
_____	_____

Would you report this? Yes/No

If yes, report to: _____

What would you report _____

Nursing Care

_____
_____
_____
_____
_____
_____
_____
_____
_____
_____

How would you document this? _____
_____
_____
_____

Compare your answers and documentation to those provided on the MyNursingKit Website.

Data Collected
(use only those that apply)

- Height 5'9"
- Weight 98 lbs, down from 117 lbs 2 months ago
- States feels fat
- LMP 3 months ago
- VS: T 96.8, P 100, R 18, BP 90/66
- Exercises 2 hours per day in addition to cheerleading practice.
- Mother states she is a straight A student and very popular; "We are so proud of Erlene. She has a full scholarship to my college; she is going to be an attorney just like her father."
- Erlene was asked what she eats on a normal day. Mother replied, "She is so busy she just grabs breakfast on the run. I am sure she eats lunch at school, 'cause she says she isn't hungry at dinner time."
- When Erlene is sent to restroom to collect a urine sample, her mother states, "She hasn't had a period in 3 months. Do you think she could be pregnant?"
- Takes no prescription medications; does admit to taking laxatives for "constipation."

Nursing Interventions
(use only those that apply; list in priority order)

- Review with family members the congruence and incongruence of family behaviors.
- Help family to mobilize social support.
- Encourage client to use "I" statements and to accept responsibility for and consequences of actions.
- Review client's current medication.
- Facilitate modeling and role-playing for family regarding healthy ways to communicate and interact.
- Establish open and trusting relationship within the family.
- Provide knowledge to support decisions regarding therapeutic regimens.
- Assess client's level of anxiety and physical reaction to anxiety.
- Model age and cognitively appropriate caregiver skills by communicating with the client at an appropriate cognitive level.

NCLEX-PN® Exam Preparation

TEST-TAKING TIP Unusual or highly technical language typically indicates that the option is not correct.

1. The nurse is providing preoperative teaching to a client who is frequently interrupted by cell phone calls. In between calls the client appears distracted and does not seem to be listening to the nurse. The aspect of communication that is missing in this situation is:
   1. The sender.
   2. The receiver.
   3. The message.
   4. The feedback.

2. The nurse is gathering data for a client history while sitting on the client's bed. The client seems to be answering questions reluctantly. A factor that may be creating a negative influence on this nurse–client communication is:
   1. The client's developmental level.
   2. The client's need for personal space.
   3. The relationship between the nurse and the client.
   4. The environment in which the communication is occurring.

3. The client asks the nurse if he can ask a few questions about an upcoming treatment he is about to receive. The nurse says yes, glances at the clock, and stands in the doorway, tapping a foot. What message will the client receive?
   1. The nurse is happy to answer the client's questions and is open to discussing anything the client wants to know.
   2. The nurse is overworked but wants to provide quality care to the client.
   3. The nurse is in a hurry and annoyed that the client wants to ask questions.
   4. The client's needs come first with the nurse.

4. The nurse is caring for a client who has just been diagnosed with a terminal illness. The client says, "I can't believe this. I feel . . ." and pauses. The most effective technique for the nurse to use at this time would be:
   1. Silence.
   2. Providing general leads.
   3. Seeking clarification.
   4. Restating or paraphrasing.

5. The nurse is teaching a class of unlicensed assistive personnel about principles of communication in a clinical setting. Which of the following statements, made by the nurse, would relay correct information?
   1. "If you aren't sure what the correct answer is for a question the client asks, give them the best answer you can."
   2. "It is best to call clients by their first name in order to make the relationship more intimate."
   3. "Sharing personal experiences will improve the relationship with the client."
   4. "Avoid questions that just satisfy your curiosity and only ask questions that are appropriate,"

6. The nurse has been developing rapport with a new client but then inadvertently creates a communication barrier. The nurse's best response would be to:
   1. Change the subject and continue talking with the client.
   2. Stop and make a statement such as, "I'm sorry; that didn't come out the way I meant it."
   3. Ignore the mistake; the client probably did not notice.
   4. End the session, and leave the room as quickly as possible.

7. While communicating with the client, the nurse demonstrates active listening when:
   1. Interrupting the client to clarify information being given.
   2. Leaning forward slightly, making eye contact, and giving nonverbal clues while listening.
   3. Making notes so as not to miss what the client is saying.
   4. Sitting quietly with hands folded in the lap.

8. The nurse is performing preoperative teaching and sees the client wringing her hands and displaying signs of anxiety. The nurse responds, "You are anxious about your surgery tomorrow, aren't you?" The nurse is using what type of question?
   1. Neutral.
   2. Open-ended.
   3. Leading.
   4. Directed interview.

9. The stage of the interview when the nurse is listening as clients communicate what they think, feel, know, and perceive is:
   1. Establishing rapport.
   2. The orientation.
   3. The opening.
   4. The body.

10. The nurse has completed an interview with the client and ends the interview by:
    1. Glancing at the clock, closing the chart, and standing.
    2. Saying, "I really enjoyed meeting with you. I think we have accomplished a great deal."
    3. Saying "I have other clients I need to see. I will stop back later on."
    4. Saying, "Time really flew. I have all the information I need."

Answers and rationales for Review Questions appear in Appendix I.

Chapter 12

Client Teaching

LEARNING Outcomes

After completing this chapter, you will be able to:

1. Identify key concepts about learning and list topics for client education.
2. Name and describe three main theories of human learning.
3. Identify the three domains of learning.
4. Describe factors that facilitate learning and factors that inhibit learning.
5. Contrast the nursing process and teaching process.
6. Identify the role of LPNs/LVNs in client teaching.
7. Identify effective teaching strategies.
8. Discuss the challenges of teaching clients of different cultures.
9. Identify methods to evaluate learning.

Clinical Objectives

10. Design and deliver client teaching in a clinical setting.
11. Demonstrate effective documentation of teaching–learning activities.
12. Implement teaching strategies used when working with children.

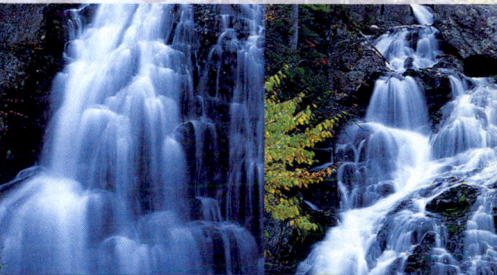

BRIEF Outline

LEARNING
Client Education
Learning Theories
Factors that Facilitate Learning
Factors that Inhibit Learning
TEACHING
Role of LPNs/LVNs in Teaching

KEY TERMS

Use the audio glossary feature on the MyNursingKit Website to hear the correct pronunciation of the following key terms.

affective domain 209

behaviorism 208

behavior modification 219

client education 208

cognitive domain 209

cognitivism 209

compliance 208

feedback 211

humanism 209

learning 208

motivation 209

psychomotor domain 209

readiness 210

relevance 210

retention 211

teaching 212

Client education is a major nursing responsibility—both legally and professionally. Legislation regarding nursing defines client teaching as an independent nursing function.

LEARNING

Client Education

Client education is a dynamic, integrated, and multifaceted teaching–learning process in which the nurse and client work together to change client behaviors. Participants exchange information, emotions, perceptions, and attitudes.

Learning is a lifelong process of acquiring knowledge or skills that cannot be solely accounted for by human growth. This process is demonstrated by changes in behavior (Box 12-1 ■). Each client has unique learning needs regarding intellectual knowledge, skills, or behaviors.

An important aspect of learning is an individual's desire to learn and to act on the learning (Box 12-2 ■). In health care, **compliance** is the extent to which a person's behavior aligns with medical or health advice. Compliance is best demonstrated when the client embraces learning and then follows through with appropriate and expected behaviors. For example, a client who has been newly diagnosed with diabetes would show compliance by willingly studying the special diet and then planning and eating meals accordingly. Areas for client education include health promotion, protection, and maintenance (Box 12-3 ■).

Nurses can use the following concepts about learners as a guide for teaching adult clients:

- As people mature, they move from dependence to independence (see Chapter 16 ⊙).
- An adult's previous experiences can be used as a resource for learning.
- An adult's readiness to learn is often related to a developmental task or social role.
- People are more oriented to learning when the material is useful immediately, not sometime in the future.

Learning Theories

The three main theories of human learning are behaviorism, cognitivism, and humanism.

BEHAVIORISM

Behaviorism is the belief that environment influences behavior, which is the essential factor determining human action. Edward Thorndike, who pioneered the 20th-century behaviorist movement, asserted that learning should be based on the learner's behavior. B. F. Skinner introduced the importance of positive reinforcement to

---

BOX 12-1	SAMPLE DOCUMENTATION: CHANGES IN BEHAVIOR

Instructed regarding dietary changes: increased fruit and vegetable intake, decreasing fats, especially saturated fats. Instructed on need for physical activity within parameters prescribed by physician. Discussed need to stop smoking and available aids for this. Verbalized understanding of teaching when questioned.

—A. Martin, LPN

BOX 12-2	ATTRIBUTES OF LEARNING

Learning is:
- An experience that occurs inside the learner.
- The discovery of the personal meaning and relevance of ideas.
- A consequence of experience.
- A collaborative and cooperative process.
- An evolutionary process.
- A process that is both intellectual and emotional.
- A change in behavior.

BOX 12-3	AREAS FOR CLIENT EDUCATION

Promotion of Health

- Increasing a person's level of wellness
- Growth and development topics
- Fertility control
- Hygiene
- Nutrition
- Exercise
- Stress management
- Lifestyle modification
- Resources within the community

Prevention of Illness/Injury

- Health screening (e.g., blood glucose levels, blood pressure, blood cholesterol, Pap test, mammograms, vision, hearing, routine physical examinations)
- Reducing health risk factors (e.g., lowering cholesterol level, cessation of smoking, etc.)
- Specific protective health measures (e.g., immunizations, use of condoms, use of sunscreen, use of medication, umbilical cord care, having regular exercise)
- First aid
- Safety (e.g., using seat belts, helmets, walkers)

Restoration of Health

- Information about tests, diagnosis, treatment, medications
- Self-care skills or skills needed to care for family member
- Resources within healthcare setting and community

Adapting to Altered Health and Function

- Adaptations in lifestyle
- Problem-solving skills
- Adaptation to changing health status
- Strategies to deal with current problems (e.g., home IV skills, medications, diet, activity limits, prostheses)
- Strategies to deal with future problems (e.g., fear of pain with terminal cancer, future surgeries, or treatments)
- Information about treatments and likely outcomes
- Referrals to other healthcare facilities or services
- Facilitation of strong self-image
- Grief and bereavement counseling

encourage a person to repeat a desired action. Alfred Bandura claimed that most learning comes from observation and instruction rather than personal trial and error, so most people imitate or model observed behavior. Imitation and modeling of healthy behaviors are key goals of client teaching.

COGNITIVISM

Cognitivism defines learning largely as a complex thinking process. The learner constantly structures and processes information from many sources. Cognitivists emphasize the importance of individual perception and motivation, as

well as the teacher–learner relationship and environment. Developmental readiness and individual readiness (called client *motivation*) are other key factors.

J. Piaget and B. Bloom are important cognitive theorists. Bloom (1956) identified three *domains* (or areas) of learning: cognitive, affective, and psychomotor. The **cognitive domain** includes knowing, comprehending, and applying. The **affective domain** includes feelings, emotions, interests, attitudes, and appreciations. The **psychomotor domain** includes motor skills (such as giving an injection). Nurses should address each domain in client teaching. For example, a three-point teaching session on colostomy care would include the following:

1. Demonstration of irrigation technique (*psychomotor domain*)
2. Discussion of safe fluid volume for irrigation (*cognitive domain*)
3. Discussion of the client's change in body image (*affective domain*)

HUMANISM

Humanism (humanistic learning theory) focuses on both cognitive and affective qualities of the learner. Leading humanists include Abraham Maslow and Carl Rogers. According to humanistic theory, each individual is a unique composite of biological, psychological, social, cultural, and spiritual factors. Learning focuses on self-development, achieving full potential, and learning what the person needs (i.e., what is relevant). Autonomy and self-determination are most important. Learning is self-motivated, self-initiated, and self-evaluated. So, the learner is an active participant in every phase of the teaching process.

APPLYING LEARNING THEORIES

Each mode of teaching has benefits and drawbacks. Behaviorism is useful but may be hard to apply to complex learning situations. It also may limit the learner's role in the teaching process. Cognitivism recognizes complex and multiple learning domains. However, it may not address external factors that are beyond the nurse's control. Humanism addresses the client's first interest (him- or herself), but this may inhibit the teacher's role in the process. Table 12-1 ■ lists sample nursing applications for each mode of teaching.

Factors that Facilitate Learning

MOTIVATION

Motivation to learn is the desire to do so. It greatly influences how quickly and how much a person learns. Motivation is generally greatest when the client recognizes a need and believes he or she can meet it by learning. It is not

TABLE 12-1	Application of Learning Theory
LEARNING THEORY	**NURSING ACTIONS**
Behaviorism	■ Encourage learner problem solving through trial and error. ■ Provide an environment conducive to learning. ■ Encourage repetitive practice and redemonstration. ■ Praise the learner and provide positive feedback. ■ Provide role models of desired behavior.
Cognitivism	■ Obtain data about the learner's developmental capacity and readiness to learn. ■ Adapt teaching strategies accordingly. ■ Recognize the role of personality in selecting teaching methods to target different learning styles. ■ Recognize the role of perception in learning by using multisensory teaching methods. ■ Provide an environment conducive to learning. ■ Encourage a positive teacher–learner relationship.
Humanism	■ Encourage self-directed and active learning by serving as a facilitator, resource, or mentor for the learner. ■ Encourage the learner to establish and evaluate goals. ■ Expose the learner to relevant new information and ask appropriate questions to encourage fact seeking.

enough for the need to be identified and verbalized by the nurse. The need must be experienced by the client. Often, the nurse's primary task in teaching is to help the client (or significant others) to recognize the need. For example, smokers with heart disease need to understand the effects of nicotine before they recognize the need to quit.

READINESS

Readiness to learn is the demonstration of behaviors or cues that reflect the learner's motivation to learn at a specific time. Readiness reflects not only desire or willingness, but also ability to learn at a given time. The nurse's role in teaching is to identify and develop client readiness. For example, a client may want to learn ostomy care, but postoperative pain or a change in body image may inhibit him or her. The nurse can provide pain medication and emotional support to enhance readiness.

ACTIVE INVOLVEMENT

Active involvement in the learning process makes learning faster and more meaningful (Figure 12-1 ■). It also improves retention (holding, keeping; in the case of learning, retention means active remembering). *Active learning* promotes critical thinking and strengthens problem-solving ability. *Passive learning* (listening to lectures or watching television, for example) is much less effective. For example, clients who are actively learning about their therapeutic diets may be more able to apply the principles being taught to their cultural food preferences and their usual eating habits.

RELEVANCE

Relevance is importance or applicability. The knowledge or skill to be learned must be personally relevant to the learner. The client can learn more easily if he can connect the new knowledge to what he already possesses. For example, a morbidly obese patient may be more motivated to lose weight if he remembers having more energy when he weighed less. The nurse should emphasize and validate the relevance of learning throughout the teaching process.

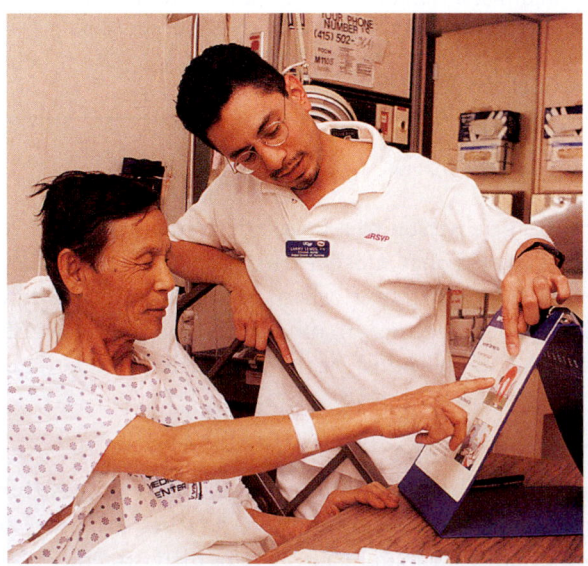

Figure 12-1. ■ Learning is facilitated when the client is interested and actively involved.

FEEDBACK

Feedback is shared information that relates a person's performance to the desired goal. Feedback must accompany the practice of psychomotor skills; it must be meaningful to help the person learn those skills. Praise, redirection, constructive criticism, and advice are ways of providing *positive feedback*. *Negative feedback*, such as ridicule, anger, or sarcasm, inhibits learning. Such feedback is viewed as a type of punishment and may cause clients to avoid the teacher.

NONJUDGMENTAL SUPPORT

People learn best when they believe they are accepted and will not be judged. Clients who expect to be judged (especially as "poor" students) will not learn as well as those who feel respected and accepted. Once learners have succeeded in accomplishing a task or understanding an idea, they gain self-confidence in their ability to learn. Self-confidence increases motivation and reduces anxiety and fear of failure.

SIMPLE TO COMPLEX METHOD

Material that is logically organized and proceeds from simple concept or task to the complex is easiest to learn. Such organization enables the learner to comprehend and assimilate knowledge to promote new understanding. Simple and complex are relative terms, however. What is simple for one client may be complex for another.

REPETITION

Repetitive practice of key facts and skills aids retention of newly introduced concepts. When combined with positive feedback from the nurse, repetition improves skill performance and the client's ability to apply this knowledge to other settings.

TIMING

People retain concepts best when the time between initial learning and active use is short. **Retention** (the ability to remember what is learned) decreases as the time between learning and practicing increases. For example, if an asthmatic is prescribed an inhaler for prn use and effectively demonstrates "practice" use one time, this does not mean that the client may remember how to use it 3 weeks later during an asthmatic episode.

ENVIRONMENT

Environmental factors affect learning. The optimal learning environment promotes physical and psychological comfort (see Chapter 11 ⌾). It is well lit (including glare-free lighting), well ventilated, neither too hot nor too cold, and with a minimum of noise and other distractions. Privacy is essential to some kinds of learning, such as when discussing confidential issues or demonstrating techniques such as perineal or ostomy care. Anxious or shy clients, however, may prefer to have a support person present. To ensure privacy, nurses should teach when visitors or other interruptions are unlikely.

Factors that Inhibit Learning

Many internal and external factors can create barriers to the learning process (Table 12-2 ■).

EMOTIONS

Emotions such as fear, anxiety, anger, and depression can impede learning. Clients experiencing intense emotions are preoccupied and unable to concentrate on incoming messages. Fear and anxiety may be minimized by providing factual information to counteract uncertainty or irrational thoughts. Severely depressed clients may require psychiatric and/or drug therapy to increase motivation and participation in the teaching process.

PHYSIOLOGICAL EVENTS

Learning can be inhibited by physiological events such as a critical illness, pain, or sensory deficits.

> **clinical ALERT**
>
> The nurse must identify and reduce physiological barriers to learning *before* teaching. When a client cannot concentrate and apply energy to learning, the learning itself becomes impaired.

CULTURAL BARRIERS

Cultural barriers to learning include language and values. Foreign language is a common barrier. Western medicine may conflict with clients' native healing beliefs and cultural practices. For example, a client who comes from a culture that does not value slimness may have difficulty learning about a reducing diet. To be effective, the nurse should directly address such conflict. Support persons such as translators should be involved whenever there is a language barrier.

PSYCHOMOTOR ABILITY

It is important that the LPN/LVN be aware of a client's psychomotor skills when collaborating with the RN to develop a teaching plan or in cooperation with other disciplines such as physical therapy. The following physical abilities are important for learning psychomotor skills:

1. *Muscle strength.* For example, an elderly client who cannot rise from a chair because of insufficient leg and muscle strength cannot be expected to learn to lift herself out of a bathtub.
2. *Motor coordination. Gross motor coordination* (coordination of large muscle groups) is necessary for walking. For example, a client who has advanced amyotrophic lateral

TABLE 12-2	Barriers to Learning	
BARRIER	**EXPLANATION**	**NURSING IMPLICATIONS**
Acute illness	Client requires all resources and energy to cope with illness.	Defer teaching until client is less ill.
Pain	Pain decreases ability to concentrate.	Deal with pain before teaching.
Prognosis	Client can be preoccupied with illness and unable to concentrate on new information.	Defer teaching to a better time.
Biorhythms	Mental and physical performances have a circadian (daily) rhythm.	Adapt time of teaching to suit client.
Emotion (e.g., anxiety, denial, depression, grief)	Emotions require energy and distract from learning.	Deal with emotions and possible misinformation first.
Language	Client may not be fluent in the nurse's language.	Obtain services of an interpreter or nurse with appropriate language skills.
Age—older adults	Vision, hearing, and motor control can be impaired.	Consider sensory and motor plan.
Age—children	Children have a shorter attention span.	Plan shorter, developmentally appropriate, and more active learning episodes.
Culture/religion	There may be cultural or religious restrictions on certain types of knowledge, for example, birth control information.	Collect data about the client's cultural/religious needs when planning learning activities.
Physical disability	Visual, hearing, sensory, or motor impairments may interfere with a client's ability to learn.	Plan teaching activities appropriate to learner's physical abilities. For example, provide audio learning tools for clients with visual impairments or who have trouble reading.
Mental disability	Impaired cognitive ability may affect the client's capacity for learning.	Determine the client's capacity for learning, and plan teaching activities to complement the client's ability while planning more complex learning for the client's caregivers.

sclerosis involving the lower limbs will probably be unable to use a walker. Likewise, fine motor coordination is needed when doing precise motions such as eating with a fork.

3. *Energy.* Learning psychomotor skills requires increased energy. The elderly and infirm often have limited energy resources, so practice sessions should be scheduled when the client's energy level is at its peak.

4. *Sensory acuity.* People depend on sight for most learning (e.g., walking with crutches, changing a dressing, drawing a medication into a syringe). Clients with visual impairments often need assistance as they learn to carry out such tasks.

TEACHING

Teaching is a system of activities intended to produce specific learning. Individualized teaching emphasizes reducing health risks and taking specific action to increase the client's level of personal wellness.

The teaching process and the nursing process are much alike. Table 12-3 ■ compares the two processes.

Role of LPNs/LVNs in Teaching

Nurses teach clients and their families in varied environments such as the home, a hospital, an assisted living center, or a long-term care facility. Clients may be instructed in groups or in one-on-one sessions (Figure 12-2 ■). For example, a nurse may teach about diabetic foot care to several clients at once, or the nurse may teach privately about wound care while changing a client's dressing. Nurses are often responsible for teaching clients' spouses and other caregivers.

Despite time constraints caused by short hospital stays, nurses are expected to provide education that will ensure the client's safe transition from one level of care to another. Nurses must make appropriate plans for follow-up education in the client's home. Discharge plans must include documentation of all teaching before discharge, and the

TABLE 12-3	Comparison of the Teaching Process and the Nursing Process	
STEP	**TEACHING PROCESS**	**NURSING PROCESS**
1	Collect data; analyze client's learning strengths and deficits.	Collect data; analyze client's strengths and deficits.
2	Make educational diagnoses.	Make nursing diagnoses.
3	Prepare teaching plan. ■ Write learning objectives. ■ Select content and time frame. ■ Select teaching strategies.	 ■ Write nursing goals. ■ Select measurable outcome criteria and time frame. ■ Select interventions.
4	Implement teaching plan.	Implement nursing strategies.
5	Evaluate client learning based on achievement of learning.	Evaluate client outcomes based on achievement of goal criteria.

learning goals yet to be achieved. See Chapters 13 and 14 ⚭, respectively, for more information about documentation and discharge.

TEACHING IN THE COMMUNITY

Nurses often participate in community health education programs. Teaching may be voluntary, such as for the Red Cross, or it may be compensated employment, such as for a government agency. Community teaching may be directed to large groups with a common interest in some aspect of health, such as nutrition, cardiopulmonary resuscitation (CPR), or bicycle and swimming safety. Community education programs can also be for small groups or individual learners, such as childbirth classes.

TEACHING HEALTH PERSONNEL

Nurses are responsible for supporting and maintaining the profession by teaching each other. In many facilities, nurses are required to present staff development sessions to colleagues. Experienced LPNs/LVNs may function as preceptors for new graduate LPNs/LVNs or for newly employed LPNs/LVNs. LPNs/LVNs reinforce teaching begun by the clinical nurse specialist and other members of the healthcare team. In some settings the LPN/LVN is responsible for all client teaching.

NURSING CARE

PRIORITIZING NURSING CARE

Recall that a key factor in communication is trust, and teaching is one way of communicating. To teach effectively, it will be important to have a therapeutic relationship with the client. The nurse will consider the different domains of learning and will provide teaching in as many domains and formats as possible. Teaching is individual, so the nurse must note what methods of teaching are most effective for each client. During and after teaching, the nurse will ask questions to determine whether teaching has been effective.

ASSESSING

Comprehensive assessment of learning needs incorporates data from the nursing history, physical assessment, and the client's support system. LPN/LVN observations are vital to the success of the overall assessment done by the RN. Data collection should include information regarding all aspects of learning, including readiness, motivation, reading ability, and comprehension level. The nurse also comes to know the common learning needs that groups of people with similar health problems have. The LPN/LVN must be constantly aware of changes in the client's health status and report these observations as learning needs and health status change.

Several elements in the nursing history provide clues to learning needs:

■ Age (and developmental status) dictates the choice of appropriate teaching strategies and health teaching content.

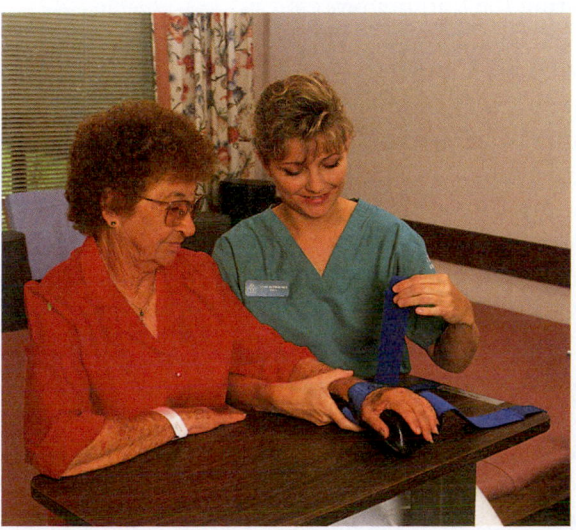

Figure 12-2. ■ Teaching activities may need to include hands-on client participation. (Photographer: Elena Dorfman.)

- Clients' perceptions of their current health problems and concerns may indicate knowledge deficits.
- A client's health beliefs and practices are always important to consider. Nurses must recognize that sometimes a client's health beliefs may interfere with healthful changes, and that it will not be possible to change that individual's core beliefs. Clients who do make changes usually believe they are personally at risk; they believe that the risk is serious; and they believe that changes in lifestyle will help to prevent the undesired outcome.
- The client's cultural group may have beliefs and practices related to diet, health, illness, and lifestyle. It is important to know how a client's practices and values affect their learning needs and their willingness to learn. Although clients may understand the healthcare information being taught, they may avoid it in the home where folk medicine practices prevail. It is important to know whether any advice or treatments given by the doctor conflict with their values or beliefs. If they seek the advice of traditional healers, or use herbs or folk treatments, it is important to verify whether their medical doctor knows about these. For additional information, see Chapter 3 ⭕, as well as the section on transcultural teaching later in this chapter.
- Economic factors can affect a client's learning. For example, elderly clients with diabetes may not have enough money to buy a large supply of sterile insulin syringes. The concern about cost may make it hard for them to focus on learning to administer the insulin.
- Learning styles vary. Some people are *visual learners* and learn best by watching or reading text. *Auditory learners* learn best by verbal explanations. Many learn best through touch and feel (*haptic learners*), such as by manipulating equipment to discover how it works. Some learn best in groups. For others, thinking about a skill and its logic promotes learning. The nurse should ask clients how they prefer to learn and have learned best in the past. The nurse can also discover a client's learning style by varying activities and techniques when teaching.
- The client's support system may include others who can assist the client's learning. Family members or close friends may help reinforce health teaching to maintain lifestyle changes at home.

The physical examination provides useful clues to the client's learning needs, such as mental status, energy level, and nutritional status. The exam provides data about the client's physical capacity (such as vision, hearing, and muscle strength) to learn and perform self-care. This information is vital in developing the teaching plan.

Readiness to Learn

A client who is ready to learn may seek information by asking questions and requesting reading materials. The client who is not yet ready is unlikely to demonstrate these behaviors and may even engage in avoidance behavior. For example, the nurse may ask, "When would you like me to show you how to inject insulin?" and the client might respond, "Oh, my wife will take care of everything."

The nurse collects data about the following:

- *Physical readiness.* Is the client in pain, fatigued, or immobile? If so, the client may not be ready.
- *Emotional readiness.* Is the client motivated toward self-care? Clients who are anxious, depressed, or grieving over their health status may not be ready.
- *Cognitive readiness.* What is the client's level of consciousness? Is disease (such as stroke) affecting the client's cognition? Are drugs affecting the client's judgment or concentration? If so, the client may not yet be ready to learn.

Nurses can promote learning readiness by providing physical and emotional support during the critical stage of recovery. As the client stabilizes physically and emotionally, the nurse can provide opportunities to learn.

Motivation

As discussed earlier, motivation is usually greatest when the client is ready, the learning need is recognized, and the information being offered is meaningful (relevant) to the client.

Nurses can increase a client's motivation by:

- Relating the learning to something the client values.
- Creating a welcoming, nonthreatening learning environment in which the client is likely to succeed.
- Encouraging autonomy and independence.
- Demonstrating a positive attitude about the client's ability to learn.
- Offering positive reinforcement and emotional support during the learning process.

Reading Level

The nurse should not assume that a client's reading level is equal to the level of formal education achieved. Nurses should ask clients about their reading proficiency. However, clients with literacy problems may be reluctant to discuss the issue. Reading materials for clients with low literacy should be at the eighth-grade level or lower.

To quickly determine the reading level of written materials, mark 10 sentences in a row at the beginning, middle, and end of the material. Then count every word within those 30 sentences with three or more syllables. If the same word appears more than once, count it each time it appears. Now total the number of words in all 30 sentences. For an eighth-grade reading level, you should have 21 to 30 multisyllable words.

DIAGNOSING, PLANNING, AND IMPLEMENTING

Three basic NANDA-approved diagnoses related to the learning process are *Deficient Knowledge, Readiness for Enhanced Self Health Management*, and *Noncompliance*. These diagnoses are used when a client's learning needs are the primary concern.

Whenever the diagnostic label *Deficient Knowledge* is used, either the client is seeking health information or the nurse has identified a learning need. An example of this would be *Deficient Knowledge: Low-Calorie Diet* related to inexperience with newly ordered therapy.

When *Readiness for Enhanced Self Health Management* is used, the client is seeking health-related information. This diagnosis is especially appropriate for clients attending community health education programs. A sample NANDA label would be *Readiness for Enhanced Self Health Management: Exercise and Activity* related to desire to improve health behaviors and decrease risk of heart disease.

Whenever the diagnostic label *Noncompliance* is used, factors are present that prevent the person from following advice given by health professionals.

clinical ALERT

The diagnosis *Noncompliance* must be used with caution, because failure to follow healthcare advice is not always the result of an unwilling attitude.

Noncompliance, as a nursing diagnosis, is associated with the desire to comply, but the inability to do so because of intervening factors (Carpenito, 2008). Intervening factors include communication barriers and financial limitations. A sample diagnosis is *Noncompliance: Hygienic Colostomy Care* related to insufficient funds to purchase necessary supplies.

A teaching plan is developed, using information collected during the nursing history and physical assessment, as well as observations from the LPN/LVN. Involving the client in this process is essential. This can be done by engaging them in conversation about their goals and by tailoring teaching to their goals. For example, the LPN/LVN would reinforce client teaching after a leg fracture. If the nurse learns that the person plans to walk his daughter down the aisle at her wedding this summer, the discussion about regaining normal gait, posture, and endurance can be framed in terms of those plans. Involved clients are more motivated and are more likely to achieve learning goals.

Determining Teaching Priorities

In the initial planning phase, the client and nurse collaborate to prioritize learning needs. For example, a client with heart disease may not be ready to learn about other lifestyle changes until she satisfies her need to learn how "to make food taste good without adding salt." Nurses can also use theoretical frameworks, such as Maslow's hierarchy of needs (see Figure 6-4 ⬭), to establish priorities.

Setting Learning Objectives

Learning objectives are equivalent to desired outcomes for other nursing diagnoses. They are written in the same way. Like client outcomes, learning objectives would do the following:

1. State the client (learner) behavior or performance, not nurse behavior. For example, "[Client] will identify personal risk factors for heart disease" (*client behavior*), not "Teach the client about cardiac risk factors" (*nurse behavior*).

2. Reflect an observable, measurable activity. The performance may be visible (e.g., walking) or invisible (e.g., adding a column of figures). The performance of an objective might be written: "Selects low-fat foods from a menu" (*observable*), not "understands low-fat diet" (*unobservable*). Verbs used for learning objectives would include *defines, describes, identifies, selects*, and so on. Outcomes would avoid such words as *knows, understands, believes*, and *appreciates*. They are neither observable nor measurable.

3. Use modifiers as required to clarify what, where, when, or how the behavior will be performed. For example, "Irrigates colostomy independently as taught" tells how the client does the task.

4. Specify the time by which learning should have occurred. For example, "The client will state three things that affect blood sugar level by end of second class on diabetes."

Learning objectives can reflect the learner's command of simple to complex concepts. For example, the learning objective "The client will list cardiac risk factors" simply requires the learner to identify all cardiac risk factors. In contrast, the learning objective "The client will list *personal* cardiac risk factors" requires that the learner learn how general cardiac risk factors apply to his or her own behaviors.

Nursing Outcomes Classifications

Many different outcomes will be appropriate depending on what is being taught (Moorehead, Johnson, & Maas, 2003). However, some general nursing outcomes classifications could include:

1802 Knowledge: Diet
1803 Knowledge: Disease process
1805 Knowledge: Health behavior
1823 Knowledge: Health promotion
1824 Knowledge: Illness care
1808 Knowledge: Medication
1811 Knowledge: Prescribed activity

1814 Knowledge: Treatment procedure
1813 Knowledge: Treatment regimen

Choosing Content

The content of teaching is determined by learning objectives. For instance, "Identify appropriate sites for insulin injection" means the nurse must include content about the body sites suitable for insulin injections. Nurses can select among many sources of information including books, nursing journals, and other nurses and physicians. Whatever sources the nurse chooses, content should be:

- Accurate.
- Current.
- Based on learning goals (outcomes).
- Adjusted for the learner's age, culture, and ability.
- Consistent with information the nurse is teaching.
- Selected with consideration of how much time and what resources are available for teaching.

Selecting Teaching Strategies

The method of teaching that the nurse chooses should be suited to the individual, to the material to be learned, and to the teacher (Figure 12-3 ■). For example, the person who cannot read needs to have material presented in other ways. The best strategy for teaching how to give an injection is not lecturing but demonstration. Teachers who lead group sessions should be poised, confident, and skilled at group facilitation. People who say they are visually oriented should be taught with visual aids. Table 12-4 ■ lists selected teaching strategies.

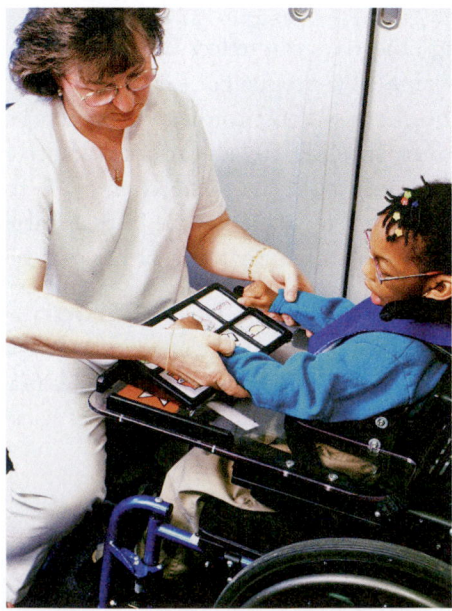

Figure 12-3. ■ Teaching materials and strategies should be suited to the client's age and learning abilities. *Source:* Creative Eye/MIRA.com.

Ordering Learning Experiences

To conserve nursing resources, some health agencies have developed their own teaching guides. These guides feature standardized content and teaching methods that all staff nurses are expected to use when teaching. Standardized teaching plans are convenient. These guides ensure consistent content for the learner, and they reduce the confusion that might occur when more than one teacher is involved. Consistency of content is key whether the nurse develops an original teaching plan or uses a standardized format. For example, when teaching multistep procedures (such as ostomy care), the nurse should repeat the steps in the same sequence, without altering the order. If possible, the nurse should use the same brands and types of equipment the client will be using at home. Topics for client teaching were provided in Box 12-3.

The nurse needs to be flexible in implementing any teaching plan because the plan may need revising. The client may tire sooner than anticipated or be faced with too much information too quickly.

clinical ALERT

Report
The LPN/LVN should report any changes in the client's physical or psychosocial condition that might require alteration in the teaching plan.

The client's needs may change. External factors may intervene. For example, the nurse and the client may have planned for the client to self-irrigate his colostomy at 10 A.M., but when the time comes, he wants more information before actually doing it himself. In this case, the nurse would discuss the desired information, provide written information, and defer teaching until the next day. The LPN/LVN would collaborate with the team leader and document accordingly. (See Table 12-2 for barriers to learning.)

Nursing Interventions Classifications

Many nursing interventions classifications (NICs) can be used when implementing client teaching (McCloskey & Bulechek, 2003). Some general classifications that apply include:

5602 Teaching: Disease process
5606 Teaching: Individual
5603 Teaching: Group
5612 Teaching: Prescribed activity/exercise
5614 Teaching: Prescribed diet
5616 Teaching: Medication
5618 Teaching: Procedure/treatment
5620 Teaching: Psychomotor skill

TABLE 12-4	Selected Teaching Strategies	
STRATEGY	**MAJOR TYPES OF LEARNING**	**CHARACTERISTICS**
Explanation or description (e.g., lecture)	Cognitive	Teacher controls content and pace. Learner is passive; therefore retains less information than when actively participating. Teacher determines feedback. Teacher may give explanation to individual or group.
One-to-one discussion	Affective, cognitive	Encourages participation by learner. Permits reinforcement and repetition at learner's level. Permits introduction of sensitive subjects.
Answering questions	Cognitive	Teacher must understand question and what it means to learner. Learner may need to overcome cultural perception that asking questions is impolite and may embarrass the teacher. Teacher can use with individuals and groups. Teacher should confirm personal responses by asking the learner, "Does that answer your question?" Teacher controls most of content and pace.
Demonstration	Psychomotor	Often used with explanation. Can be used with individuals, small or large groups. Does not permit use of equipment by learners; learner is passive.
Discovery	Cognitive, affective	Teacher guides problem-solving situation. Learner is active participant; retention of information is high.
Group discussions	Affective, cognitive	Group members assist and learn from each other. Teacher needs to keep the discussion focused and prevent monopolization by one or two learners.
Practice	Psychomotor	Allows repetition and immediate feedback. Permits hands-on experience.
Printed and audiovisual materials	Cognitive	Forms include books, pamphlets, films, programmed instruction, and computer learning. Learners can proceed at their own speed. Nurse can act as resource person; need not be present during learning. Potentially ineffective if reading level of materials is too high. Teacher needs to select language that meets learner needs if English is a second language.
Role-playing	Affective, cognitive	Permits expression of attitudes, values, and emotions. Can assist in development of communication skills. Involves active participation by learner. Teacher must create supportive, safe environment for learners to minimize anxiety.
Modeling	Affective, psychomotor	Nurse sets example by attitude, psychomotor skill.
Computer-assisted learning programs	All types of learning	Learner is active. Learner controls pace. Learning programs provide immediate reinforcement and review. Use with individuals or groups.

Implementing Client Education

When structuring client teaching sessions, the nurse should keep the following eight principles in mind:

1. *The optimal time for each session depends largely on the learner.* Whenever possible, ask the client for help to choose the best time, for example, when she feels most rested or when no other activities are scheduled.

2. *The pace of teaching affects learning.* A very rapid pace may confuse or frustrate the learner. When the pace is too slow, the client may become bored and distracted.

BOX 12-4 **PEDIATRIC CONSIDERATIONS**

Teaching Tools for Children

- *Visits.* Visiting the hospital and treatment rooms; seeing people dressed in uniforms, scrub suits, protective gear.
- *Dress-up.* Touching and dressing up in the clothing they will see and wear.
- *Coloring books.* Using coloring books to prepare for treatments, surgery, or hospitalization; shows what rooms, people, and equipment will look like.
- *Storybooks.* Storybooks describe how the child will feel, what will be done, and what the place will look like. Parents can read these stories to children several times before the experience. Younger children like this repetition.
- *Dolls.* Practicing procedures on dolls or teddy bears that they will later experience; gives a sense of mastery of the situation. For example, custom dolls are often available for inserting tubes and giving injections.
- *Puppet play.* Puppets can be used in role-play situations to provide information and show the child what the experience will be like; they help the child express emotions.
- *Health fairs.* Health fairs can educate children about their bodies and ways to stay healthy. Fairs can focus on high-risk problems children face, such as accident prevention, poison control, and other topics identified in the community as a concern.

(Loss of interest may also indicate that the client is fatigued.)

3. *Position and location affect learning.* Most people associate their bed with rest and sleep, not with learning. A client who is shown a videotape while in bed is more likely to become drowsy during instruction than a client who is sitting in a bedside chair.

4. *Teaching aids foster learning and attentiveness.* When selecting teaching aids, the nurse should choose identical products (such as ostomy pouches) to those the client will be using. When planning audiovisual presentations, the nurse should ensure that all equipment is functioning well before starting the session. Teaching aids should be appropriate to the client's developmental level (see Figure 12-3). For example, some anatomical models may contain tiny plastic parts that pose a choking hazard to young children. Box 12-4 ■ lists teaching tools that are specifically useful for children.

5. *Learning is more effective through self-directed activity.* The nurse can encourage independent learning by enabling the client to explore alternative sources of information. If the client chooses, the nurse may provide a list of related health topics to research.

6. *Repetition reinforces learning.* Summarizing content, rephrasing (using other words), and approaching the material from another point of view are ways of repeating and clarifying content. For instance, after discussing the kinds of foods that can be included in a diet, the nurse describes the foods again, but in the context of the three meals eaten during one day.

7. *Organize the material; connect new information to what the client has already learned.* For example, "You understand how urine flows down a catheter from the bladder. Now I will show you how to push fluid up the catheter to rinse the bladder."

8. *Always use simple language.* If possible, eliminate medical jargon. Even common terms such as *urine* and *feces* may be unfamiliar to clients. Avoid common abbreviations such as RR (recovery room) or CAD (coronary artery disease).

Teaching Strategies

Nurses can choose from a number of special teaching strategies. Any strategy the nurse selects must be appropriate for the learner and the learning goals.

Client Contracting

A learning contract with a client specifies certain objectives and when they are to be met. Here is an example of a self-contract:

> I, Amy Martin, will jog for 20 minutes three times per week for a period of 2 weeks and will then buy myself six yellow roses.
>
> Amy Martin
>
> [date]

The contract, drawn up and signed by the client and the nurse, should specify learning objectives, responsibilities of the client and the nurse, and the methods of follow-up and evaluation. The learning contract allows for freedom, mutual respect, and mutual responsibility. Contracts may be revised when the client chooses to set new goals.

Group Teaching

Group instruction is economical, and it provides members with an opportunity to share and learn from others. A small group allows for discussion in which everyone can participate. A large group often requires a lecture technique or use of films, videos, slides, or role-playing by teachers. All members involved in group instruction should have a common need (e.g., prenatal health or preoperative instruction). It is also important to consider sociocultural factors when forming a group (see Chapter 3 ⦾).

Computer-Assisted Instruction

Computer-assisted instruction is constantly advancing. Now, computers can be used to teach:

- Complex problem-solving skills.
- Application of information.
- Psychomotor skills.

"Virtual reality" programs and video clips can allow the client to "see" how the heart pumps blood or how nerves send messages to the brain. Learning is becoming increasingly visual.

Discovery/Problem Solving

In using the discovery/problem-solving technique, the nurse presents some initial information and then asks the learners a question or presents a situation related to the information. The learner applies the new information to the situation and decides what to do. Learners can work alone or in groups. This technique is well suited to family learning. The teacher guides the learners through the thinking process to reach the best solution or the best action to take in the situation. For example, the nurse-educator might present information on diabetes and glucose management. Then the nurse might ask the learners how they think their insulin and diet should be adjusted if their morning glucose reading was too low. In this way, clients learn what critical components they need to consider to reach the best solution to the problem.

Behavior Modification

Behaviorists believe that (1) human behaviors are learned and can be selectively strengthened, weakened, eliminated, or replaced and (2) a person's behavior is under conscious control. **Behavior modification** is a system of positive reinforcement in which desirable behavior is rewarded and undesirable behavior is ignored. For example, clients trying to quit smoking are not criticized when they smoke, but they are praised or rewarded when they go without a cigarette for a certain period of time. A client contract may increase the effectiveness of a behavior modification plan. The contract outlines the behavior modification plan and lists specific rewards.

Transcultural Teaching

When the nurse and client come from different ethnic or cultural backgrounds, natural communication barriers may exist. These barriers include language, differing concepts of time, or cultural beliefs and practices that may influence compliance with client teaching and health care. It is important to keep these differences in mind when you are teaching clients about their health care. Treat the client's cultural healing beliefs with respect and try to identify whether they are in agreement or in conflict with what is being taught. Then focus on the ones in agreement to promote the integration of new learning with familiar health practices. Explain why certain folk healing practices are harmful, and how the recommended health practices will improve health. See Chapter 3 ⟳ for more information on culturally proficient nursing. Guidelines for teaching clients from other ethnic or cultural groups are listed in Box 12-5 ■.

BOX 12-5 **CULTURAL PULSE POINTS**

Transcultural Teaching Guidelines

- **Enlist the aid of a translator when necessary.**
- **Obtain foreign language teaching materials.** The translator can assist by reading the materials to the nurse and can assist the nurse with adaptations of the material.
- **Use visual aids.** Many pictures, charts, and diagrams have universal meaning. Videos can allow the client to observe a skill or procedure, despite a language barrier. Audiovisual materials in which English is spoken slowly and clearly can benefit a client who may be learning English.
- **Use clear, simple language.** Avoid long sentences and big words. Use concrete rather than abstract terms. Avoid medical jargon.
- **Avoid slang or colloquialisms.** For example, if a nurse said that an amputee's new prosthesis was "hot" (meaning appealing), the client might misinterpret that to mean hot in terms of temperature.
- **Present only one idea at a time.**
- **Phrase questions positively.** For example, "Do you understand how far you may bend your hip after surgery?" is a much better question than "You don't know how far you may bend your hip, do you?"
- **Validate verbal communication in writing.** This is especially important if understanding the client's speech is a problem. For example, when collecting data, write down numbers or phrases and have the client read them to verify accuracy.

- **Use humor very cautiously.** Meaning can change in the translation process.
- **Specifically invite the client to ask questions or request help.** In some cultures, expressing a need is not appropriate. Expressing confusion or asking to be shown something again may be considered rude. Some clients may feel that asking questions or stating a lack of understanding may cause the nurse to "lose face."
- **Confirm nonverbal cues.** A client who nods, uses eye contact, or smiles may not really understand what is being taught. In some cultures these signals are merely indicators of respect.
- **Identify cultural gender issues.** When explaining procedures or functioning related to personal areas of the body, it may be appropriate to have a nurse of the same sex do the teaching. Because of modesty concerns, and cultural taboos about male–female interaction, it is wise to have a female nurse teach a female client about personal care, birth control, sexually transmitted infections, and other potentially sensitive areas. If a translator is needed during explanation of procedures or teaching, the translator should also be female.
- **Include the family in planning and teaching.** This promotes trust and mutual respect. Identify the authoritative family member and incorporate that person into the planning and teaching to promote compliance and support of health teaching. In some cultures, the male head of household is the critical family member to include in health teaching; in other cultures, it is the eldest female member.

(continued)

BOX 12-5 (continued)

■ **Consider the client's time orientation.**

■ The client may be oriented to the past, present, future, or a combination of these. Cultures with a predominant orientation to the present include the Mexican American, Navajo Native American, Appalachian, Eskimo, and Filipino American cultures. Preventing future problems may be less significant for these clients, so teaching prevention may be difficult. For example, teaching a client why and when to take medications may be more difficult if the client is oriented to the present. In such instances, the nurse can emphasize preventing short-term problems.

■ Schedules tend to be very flexible in present-oriented societies. Failure to keep clinic appointments or to arrive

on time is common in clients who have a present-time orientation. The nurse can help by arranging transportation and by accommodating these clients when they do come rather than rescheduling an appointment that they probably will not keep.

■ Teaching clients to take medications at bedtime or with a meal does not necessarily mean that these activities will occur at the same time each day. For this reason, the nurse should collect data about the client's daily routine before teaching the client to pair a treatment or medication with a daily event. When teaching a client when to take medication, the nurse should determine whether a clock or watch is available to the client and whether the client can tell time.

EVALUATING

Evaluating Learning

Evaluation is both an ongoing and a final process in which the client, the LPN/LVN in collaboration with the RN, and often the support people determine what has been learned. Learning is measured against the learning goals that were selected in the planning phase. For example, the objective "Selects foods that are low in carbohydrates" can be evaluated by asking the client to name such foods or to select low-carbohydrate foods from a list.

The best method for evaluating depends on the type of learning (cognitive, psychomotor, or affective). For cognitive learning, the client demonstrates the acquired knowledge. The client might:

■ Select the solution to a problem using the new knowledge.
■ Take written tests.
■ Respond to oral questioning (e.g., restate information or give correct responses to questions).
■ Self-report and self-monitor during follow-up phone calls, home visits, or computer-assisted instruction.
■ Verbally report, list, or describe the new knowledge.

For psychomotor skills, evaluation is best done by observing how well the client carries out a procedure such as changing a dressing.

Affective learning is more difficult to evaluate. The nurse may listen to the client's responses to questions, note how the client speaks about relevant subjects, and observe the client's behavior that expresses feelings and values. For example, have parents learned to value health enough to have their children immunized?

Following evaluation, teaching may have to be modified or repeated. Follow-up teaching in the home or by phone may be needed.

Behavior change does not always take place immediately. Often, individuals accept change intellectually first and then change their behavior only periodically (for example, a person who knows that he must lose weight may diet and exercise off and on). If the new behavior is to replace the old behavior, it must emerge gradually; otherwise, the old behavior may prevail. The nurse can support behavior change by anticipating client vacillation and by providing encouragement.

Evaluating Teaching

It is important for nurses to evaluate their own teaching and the content of the teaching program, just as they evaluate the effectiveness of nursing interventions for other nursing diagnoses. Evaluation should include all aspects of teaching, including timing, teaching strategies, content quality, and so on. The nurse may find, for example, that the client was excited about understanding how to control her diabetes and was motivated to learn more.

Both the client and the nurse should evaluate the learning experience. The client should be asked for detailed feedback. Feedback questionnaires and videotapes of the learning sessions can be helpful.

The nurse should not feel ineffective as a teacher if the client forgets some of what is taught. Forgetting is normal and should be anticipated. Having the client write down information, repeating it during teaching, giving handouts on the information, and having the client be active in the learning process all promote retention (Box 12-6 ■).

Documenting

Documentation of the teaching process is essential. Charting provides a legal record that the teaching occurred, and it communicates the teaching to other health professionals. If teaching is not documented, legally it did not occur.

Responses to teaching should always be documented. What did the client or support person say or do to indicate that learning occurred? Has the client demonstrated mastery of a skill or the acquisition of knowledge? Such documented responses provide evidence of learning. Many agencies have

BOX 12-6   NURSING CARE CHECKLIST

General Teaching and Client Teaching

General Teaching Guidelines

☑ **All teaching should be individualized.** If certain activities do not assist the learner, the nurse should make adaptations. For example, explanation alone may not be able to teach a client to handle a syringe. Actually handling the syringe may be more effective.

☑ **When the learner is involved in planning, the desire to learn is increased.**

☑ **Rapport between teacher and learner is essential.** The nurse should take time to establish rapport before teaching.

☑ **Teaching should build on the client's existing knowledge base.** For example, a person who already knows how to cook can use this knowledge when learning to prepare food for a special diet.

☑ **Communication must be clear, concise, and mutually understood.** For example, a client may understand the terms *damp* and *wet* to have very different meanings. So, when the nurse says, "Don't get the abdominal incision wet," the client may immediately understand that he may not shower or bathe, but may think that wiping the incision with a damp washcloth is allowed. The nurse should explain that no water or moisture should touch the incision.

☑ **Teaching that involves a number of the learner's senses often enhances learning.** For example, when teaching about changing a surgical dressing, the nurse can tell the client about the procedure (hearing), show how to change the dressing (sight), and show how to manipulate the equipment (touch).

☑ **Goal setting (determining learning objectives and outcomes) must be appropriate to the client's lifestyle and resources.** For example, it would be unreasonable to expect a woman to soak in a tub of hot water four times a day if she did not have a bathtub or hot running water.

Client Teaching Guidelines

☑ **Discover the client's knowledge or skill level.** Ask questions or have the client complete a written form, such as a pretest.

☑ **Identify fear, anxiety, or other barriers to learning. Address the source of anxieties before beginning to teach.** For example, a client's spouse may be reluctant to learn tracheostomy care due to fear of suffocating the client during suctioning.

☑ **Begin with relevant information in an area of client readiness.** For example, an adolescent may want to know how he may continue to play football before he can learn how to administer insulin to himself.

☑ **Teach the basics first.** Make sure the client demonstrates understanding of a procedure before you teach variations or give information on special circumstances or "troubleshooting." For example, when teaching a client to insert a retention catheter, explain the basic procedure in its entirety before discussing what to do if the catheter fails to drain properly.

☑ **Plan to review.** Schedule time to clarify content and to answer any questions the learner(s) may have.

---

multiple-copy client teaching forms that include the medical and nursing diagnoses, the treatment plan, and client education (see Figure 14-6 🔗). After the teaching session is completed, the client and the nurse sign the form and a copy of the form is given to the client to reinforce content and provide a record of the teaching. A second copy of the completed and signed form is placed in the client's chart.

Key aspects of the teaching process to be documented in the client record include:

- Diagnosed learning needs
- Learning objectives
- Topics taught
- Client outcomes
- Need for additional teaching
- Resources provided

The nurse's written teaching plan should include:

- Actual information and skills taught
- Teaching strategies used
- Time framework and content for each class
- Teaching outcomes and methods of evaluation

NURSING PROCESS CARE PLAN
Client with Laceration

Kevin Brewer is a 24-year-old male college student admitted to the emergency department (ED) with a 7-cm (2.5-in.) laceration on the left lower anterior leg, which occurred during a hockey game. The laceration was cleaned, sutured, and bandaged. The client was given an appointment to return to the health clinic in 10 days for suture removal. Client states that he lives in a college dormitory and is able to care for the wound if given instructions. Client states he is able to read and understand English.

Assessment
Mr. Brewer complains of a pain level of 5 related to the laceration to his left leg. Thirty-five minutes after administration of prn pain medication, stated pain at a level of 1. Client is able to ambulate with a slow, steady gait. His roommate is on his way to the ED to drive the client home.

Nursing Diagnosis

The following important nursing diagnosis (among others) is established for this client:

- *Deficient Knowledge* related to wound care

Expected Outcomes

The expected outcomes specify that Mr. Brewer will:

- Be able to describe signs and symptoms of wound infection.
- Respond to questions regarding wound care and perform return demonstration of wound cleansing and bandaging.
- Identify equipment needed for wound care.
- Describe appropriate action if complications arise.
- Identify date, time, and location of follow-up appointment for suture removal.

Planning and Implementation

The following nursing interventions are planned and implemented:

- Instruct client on what to look for regarding signs and symptoms of wound infection and appropriate action to take if complications arise.
- Demonstrate wound cleansing and bandaging, and allow time for a return demonstration by the client.

- Lay out equipment needed for wound care in front of client and encourage client to handle and become familiar with equipment.
- Provide written instructions for all implementations to client.
- Provide an appointment card for client with details for date, time, and location of suture removal appointment.

Evaluation

After teaching session, Mr. Brewer was able to fulfill all expected outcomes without difficulty.

Critical Thinking in the Nursing Process

1. Why is it necessary for Mr. Brewer to be able to identify the signs and symptoms of wound infection?
2. Why is it important for Mr. Brewer to be able to give a return demonstration of wound care?
3. Why should Mr. Brewer be allowed to handle the equipment needed for wound care?

Note: Discussion of Critical Thinking questions appears on the MyNursingKit Website.

Note: The references and resources for all chapters have been compiled at the back of the book.

Chapter Review

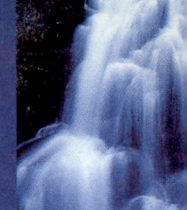

KEY Points

- Teaching clients and families about their health needs is a major role of the nurse.
- Learning is represented by a change in behavior.
- Three main theories of learning are behaviorism, cognitivism, and humanism.
- There are three learning domains: cognitive, affective, and psychomotor.
- Factors that facilitate learning include motivation, readiness, active involvement, relevance, feedback, nonjudgmental support, progression from simple to complex concepts, repetition, timing, and environment.
- Factors such as emotions (e.g., anxiety), certain physiological events (e.g., pain), cultural barriers, and psychomotor deficits may impede learning.
- Learning objectives guide the content of the teaching plan and are written in terms of client or learner behavior.
- Teaching strategies should be suited to the client, the material to be learned, and the teacher. They should be adjusted to the client's developmental level and health status.
- Teaching methods and materials must be adapted for clients who are illiterate, elderly, or from different cultural backgrounds.
- Documentation of client teaching is essential to communicate the teaching to other health professionals and to provide a record for legal and accreditation purposes.

ꝏ FOR FURTHER Study

Further steps to improve culturally proficient nursing are discussed in Chapter 3.

For Maslow's hierarchy of needs, see Figure 6-4.

For environmental considerations, see Chapter 11.

For documentation methods and guidelines, see Chapter 13.

For more about client teaching at discharge, see Chapter 14.

For growth and developmental issues as they affect clients, see Chapter 16.

PEARSON

EXPLORE mynursingkit™

MyNursingKit is your one stop for online chapter review materials and resources. Prepare for success with additional NCLEX®-style practice questions, interactive assignments and activities, web links, animations and videos, and more!

Register your access code from the front of your book at **www.mynursingkit.com**

Critical Thinking Care Map

Caring for a Client with Deficient Knowledge
NCLEX-PN® Focus Area: Physiological Integrity

Case Study: Mrs. Yorty, 59, is an African American bank vice president who is heavily relied on by her boss and coworkers. Three days ago she was admitted to the hospital with complaints of shortness of breath and mild chest pain. A diagnostic evaluation indicates that she has significant coronary artery disease but has not yet had a heart attack. Her physician indicated that Mrs. Yorty will need to make significant lifestyle changes to reduce her heart attack risk. Mrs. Yorty states that she rests a lot after work so she doesn't overwork her heart.

Nursing Diagnosis: *Deficient Knowledge* related to coronary artery disease

COLLECT DATA

Subjective	Objective
_____	_____
_____	_____
_____	_____
_____	_____
_____	_____
_____	_____

Would you report this? Yes/No

If yes, report to:_____

What would you report?_____

Nursing Care

_____
_____
_____
_____
_____
_____
_____
_____
_____
_____
_____

How would you document this? _____
_____
_____
_____

Data Collected
(use only those that apply)

- Weight: 180 lbs
- Height: 5'1"
- VS: T 98.5, P 80, BP 140/100
- Blood oxygen level 98%
- Lung sounds clear bilaterally
- Complains of shortness of breath on mild exertion
- Complains of occasional mild chest pain
- States she rests a lot after work so she doesn't overwork her heart
- States she has smoked one pack of cigarettes a day for 25 years

Nursing Interventions
(use only those that apply; list in priority order)

- Explain to client that physical activity can reduce her risk of heart attack. However, her doctor will prescribe how much activity she may do based on the severity of her coronary artery disease.
- Instruct client that she will die of a heart attack if she doesn't stop smoking.
- Encourage client to make dietary changes. Stress importance of cutting back on fat, especially saturated fats, which may help reduce cholesterol.
- Explain to client that smoking is a major risk factor and that by quitting she can significantly cut her risk of a heart attack.
- Obtain a physician's order for the client to meet with the hospital dietitian.
- Encourage client to eat a well-balanced diet with at least five servings of fruits and vegetables a day.

Compare your answers and documentation to those provided on the MyNursingKit Website.

NCLEX-PN® Exam Preparation

1. While teaching the diabetic client about diet management, the nurse gives praise and positive feedback each time the client makes an appropriate food choice. The nurse is applying what theory of learning?
   1. Behaviorism
   2. Cognitive
   3. Humanism
   4. Health promotion

2. The nurse provides information about tests, diagnosis, treatment, and medications in which area of client teaching?
   1. Promotion of health
   2. Prevention of illness/injury
   3. Restoration of heatlh
   4. Adapting to altered health and function

3. The client is scheduled for a first meeting with the physical therapist for mobility training following surgery. When the nurse administers pain medication prior to the session, the client's family asks why pain medication is being given at this time. The nurse's best response is:
   1. "The next dose is due during the time she is in physical therapy. I don't want to have to interrupt them."
   2. "The medication will allow her to rest following therapy."
   3. "I felt it would be best for her."
   4. "Pain decreases the ability to concentrate, so pain needs to be controlled before teaching begins."

4. You have just told your outpatient surgical client not to get the incision wet until after his follow-up visit. Which statement demonstrates a need for more instruction?
   1. "I will not take a shower until I see the doctor."
   2. "I will only wipe the area with a slightly damp washcloth daily."
   3. "I will be careful not to get the area wet while bathing."
   4. "The dressing should be kept clean and dry until I see the doctor."

5. You have been teaching your client self-administration of insulin. The first two times, she prepared the injection correctly. This morning she states, "I can't do it. How will I be able to take care of myself at home?" Which response is most appropriate?
   1. "You are right. I will arrange for a home health nurse to give you your insulin."
   2. "You did it just fine yesterday. What's wrong with you today?"
   3. "Many people feel overwhelmed at first. You did well yesterday and you will gain confidence with practice. Would you feel better if we had a family member sit with you?"
   4. "Maybe we should have your daughter learn to do this in case you aren't able to do it yourself."

6. An elderly Vietnamese client avoids eye contact during discharge instructions. The nurse recognizes this behavior means:
   1. The client does not understand the instructions but is ashamed to admit it.
   2. The client lacks interest.
   3. The client believes eye contact is a sign of disrespect.
   4. The client does not value the knowledge of the nurse and prefers to learn from the physician.

7. The nurse is using the nursing process as a guide to the teaching process. What activities would the nurse perform during the assessment phase of the teaching process? (Select all that apply.)
   1. Determine the client's education level.
   2. Determine the client's learning style.
   3. Select measurable outcomes for this client to obtain.
   4. Develop nursing strategies for teaching the client.
   5. Explore the client's motivation to learn.

8. The LPN/LVN's role in client teaching includes all of the following except:
   1. Collaborate with the RN to develop and carry out a teaching plan.
   2. Develop a plan of care including a teaching plan.
   3. Reinforce teaching begun by other members of the healthcare team.
   4. Assist the RN with data collection to determine client's needs.

9. The nurse avoids using negative feedback when teaching the adult client because negative feedback:
   1. Is viewed as a punishment and may cause clients to avoid or resent the teacher.
   2. Can only be applied to teaching psychomotor skills.
   3. Can only be used if presented in a joking manner.
   4. Only works when the nurse applies behavior modification theory.

10. The nurse is teaching a newly diagnosed diabetic client how to perform a fingerstick blood sugar using a glucometer. The nurse teaches the client how to troubleshoot the machine:
    1. Right after explaining how to use the glucometer, but before performing a fingerstick.
    2. At the very beginning of instruction, in case there are problems with the glucometer during the lesson.
    3. After the client performs one successful fingerstick blood sugar and glucometer reading.
    4. After the client is comfortable performing the fingerstick blood sugar and glucometer reading.

Answers and rationales for Review Questions appear in Appendix I.

Documentation

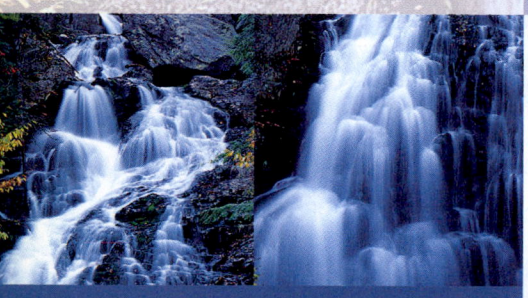

LEARNING Outcomes

After completing this chapter, you will be able to:

1. Define terms and discuss reasons for keeping client records.
2. Identify essential guidelines for reporting client data.
3. Identify abbreviations and symbols commonly used for charting.
4. Identify and discuss guidelines for effective recording that meet legal and ethical standards.
5. List the measures used to maintain the confidentiality of records, including computer records.
6. Compare and contrast different documentation systems, and explain how various forms in the client record are used to document steps of the nursing process.
7. Describe the nurse's role in reporting, conferring, and making referrals.
8. Compare and contrast the documentation needed for clients in acute care, home health care, and long-term care settings.

Clinical Objectives

9. Document client care performed, using a variety of documentation systems.
10. Give a change-of-shift report to the oncoming nurse using the client's Kardex®.
11. Listen to a taped report upon starting your shift.
12. Take a telephone order from the physician and transcribe the order.
13. Complete an incident report.
14. Graph vital signs.
15. Research and develop a nursing care plan for a client.
16. Complete the client flow sheet.

KEY TERMS

Use the audio glossary feature on the MyNursingKit Website to hear the correct pronunciation of the following key terms.

APIE 237

charting 227

charting by exception 238

clinical record 227

confer 243

CORE 238

DAR 238

database 235

discussion 227

documenting 227

FACT 238

flow sheets 245

focus charting 238

incident 244

Kardex® 244

medication administration records 245

nursing care conference 243

nursing rounds 243

objective data 236

PIE 237

problem-oriented medical record 234

record 227

report 227

SOAP 236

source-oriented record 234

subjective data 236

Effective communication among health professionals is vital to delivering high-quality client care. Generally, health personnel communicate through discussion, reports, and documentation in the medical records. A **discussion** is an informal conversation between two or more healthcare personnel to identify a problem or establish strategies to resolve a problem. Nurses frequently hold discussions about client care in order to seek another nurse's input before responding to a change in the client's status. A **report** is an oral, written, or computer-based communication intended to convey information to others. For example, nurses always report on clients at the end of a work shift. A **record** is a written or computer-based collection of data. The process of making an entry on a client record is called *recording*, **charting**, or **documenting.** A **clinical record,** also called a *chart* or *client record*, is the formal, legal document that provides evidence of a client's care. Although healthcare organizations use different systems and forms for documentation, all client records contain similar information.

Each healthcare organization has policies about recording and reporting client data, and each nurse is accountable for practicing in accordance with these standards. Agencies also indicate which nursing assessments and interventions must be recorded by a nurse and those items that may be delegated to unlicensed personnel. Nurse Practice Acts and Standards of Care vary slightly between locations, but all include requirements for documenting in the client's medical record. In addition, the Joint Commission that gives accreditation to healthcare organizations has policies on information management in the acute care setting specifying that record keeping should be timely, accurate, confidential, and client specific (JCAHO, 2000).

Purposes of Client Records

COMMUNICATION

The client record serves as the vehicle by which different health professionals who interact with a client communicate with each other. This prevents fragmentation, repetition, and delays in client care. The record also provides a central location for notifying health professionals of the client's needs, progress, and current health status. For example, when the nurse writes a progress note describing a change in the client's condition, this information will be used by the respiratory therapist, dietitian, social services, or the physician to amend the client's plan of care. Accurate and thorough communication among health team members improves the client's continuity of care.

PLANNING CLIENT CARE

Each health professional uses data from the client's record to plan care for that client. A physician, for example, may determine that laboratory tests reveal the presence of a certain microorganism and then orders an antibiotic. Nurses then use baseline and ongoing assessments to determine the effectiveness of interventions and the nursing care plan. The record also provides a base from which all healthcare disciplines may coordinate the client's care. Nurses may hold a nursing care conference to coordinate a comprehensive plan of care using the medical record to determine client needs, problems, and history.

LEGAL DOCUMENTATION

The client's record is a legal document and is admissible in court as evidence. In some jurisdictions, however, the record is considered inadmissible as evidence when the client objects, because information the client gives to the physician is confidential. It frequently takes many years for a court case to go to trial, so the medical record serves as a memory aid for those involved. If the care delivered is not documented, in the eyes of the court it did not occur, so thorough documentation of nursing care is very important. Legal aspects are discussed later in the chapter.

EDUCATION, RESEARCH, AND HEALTHCARE ANALYSIS

Students use client records as an essential educational tool. A record can frequently provide a comprehensive view of the client, the illness, treatment strategies, and factors that affect the outcome of the illness. The information contained in a record can be a valuable source of data for research. Review of treatment plans for clients with similar health problems can yield helpful information when treating new clients with the same problems.

Likewise, information from records may assist healthcare planners to identify agency needs. It can highlight overused and underused hospital services. It can identify services that cost the agency money and those that generate revenue.

AUDITING

An audit is a review of records. Client records are audited for quality improvement. Accrediting agencies such as the Joint Commission may review client records to determine if a particular health agency is meeting its stated standards. By carefully reviewing client records, outcomes can be examined to determine what actions are effective and what actions need to be amended or stopped.

REIMBURSEMENT

Documentation also helps a facility receive reimbursement from the federal government. For a facility to obtain payment through Medicare, the client's clinical record must contain the correct diagnosis-related group (DRG) codes and reveal that the appropriate care has been given. An insurance company may deny a claim if there is no documentation in the medical record to indicate that the procedure, medication, or problem occurred.

Guidelines for Recording

The client's record is a legal document and specific guidelines should be followed. Documenting not only is a legal obligation, but also carries an ethical obligation. The American Nurses Association Code of Ethics stresses the importance of respecting the human dignity in all encounters with every client by respecting client privacy and keeping the client's interests at the center of all nursing actions (ANA, 2003). Healthcare personnel must not only maintain the confidentiality of the client's record, but also meet legal standards in the process of recording.

DATE AND TIME

- Document the date and time you are writing the note with each entry.
- Make entries as soon as possible after performing a nursing action, whether assessment, intervention, or evaluation, in order to document thoroughly and accurately while the events are still memorable.
- Record the time using either conventional time, denoting A.M. or P.M., or using the 24-hour clock (military time) according to agency policy (Figure 13-1 ■).

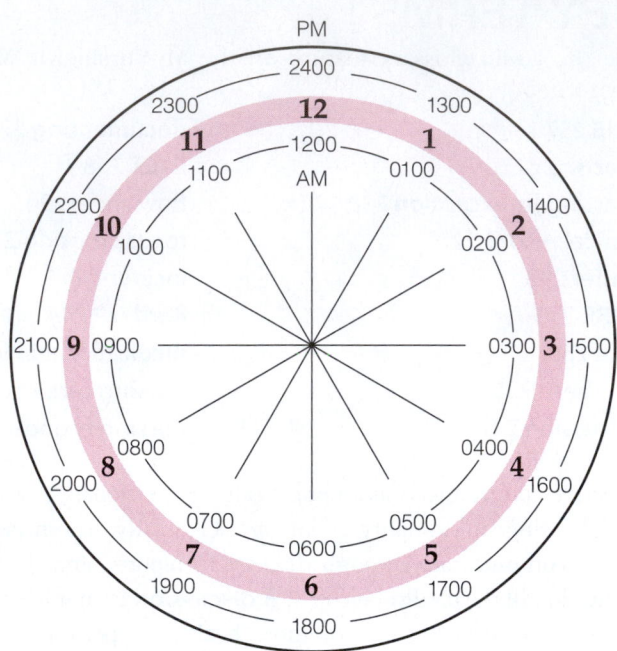

Figure 13-1. ■ The 24-hour clock.

- Some facilities avoid block-style charting in which an entire shift is documented under one date and time. Their reasoning is that block-style charting may lead to inaccurate notation, because something is bound to be forgotten or overlooked. Block-style charting may have less credibility should the record be used in court.

TIMING

- Follow agency policy regarding the minimum frequency of documenting, although more frequent documentation is acceptable if it is warranted.
- Adjust frequency of documentation as a client's condition indicates. An unstable client requires more frequent assessment and documentation than a stable client.
- Never record nursing care before it is provided. This is both unethical and illegal.

LEGIBILITY

- Make all entries legible and easy to read to prevent interpretation errors.
- Print your entries if your cursive writing is difficult to read.
- Follow agency policy regarding handwritten recording of nurses' notes.

PERMANENCE

- Make all entries on the client's record in permanent, non-erasable blue or black ink according to agency policy. This ensures that the record is permanent and that changes can be identified.
- Never use erasable ink or gel pens. Gel ink tends to fade with time and become illegible.

TABLE 13-1	Commonly Used Abbreviations		
ABBREVIATION	**TERM**	**ABBREVIATION**	**TERM**
abd	abdomen	meds	medications
ABO	the main blood group system	mL (ml)	milliliter
ac	before meals (ante cibum)	mod	moderate
ad lib	as desired (ad libitum)	neg	negative
ADLs	activities of daily living	nil	none
adm	admitted or admission	no. (#)	number
a.m.	morning (ante meridiem)	NPO (NBM)	nothing by mouth (per os)
amb	ambulatory	NS (N/S)	normal saline
amt	amount	O_2	oxygen
approx	approximately (about)	od	daily (omni die)
b.i.d.	twice daily (bis in die)	OD	overdose
BM (bm)	bowel movement	OOB	out of bed
BP	blood pressure	os	mouth or opening
BR	bed rest	pc	after meals (post cibum)
BRP	bathroom privileges	PE (PX)	physical examination
c̄	with	per	by or through
C	Celsius (centigrade)	p.m.	afternoon (post meridiem)
CBC	complete blood count	po	by mouth (per os)
CBR	complete bed rest	postop	postoperative (ly)
Cl	client	preop	preoperative (ly)
c/o	complains of	prep	preparation
DAT	diet as tolerated	prn	when necessary (pro re nata)
dc (disc)	discontinue	pt	patient
drsg	dressing	q2h, q3h, and so on	every 2 hours, 3 hours, and so on
Dx	diagnosis	req	requisition
ECG (EKG)	electrocardiogram	Rt (rt, R)	right
F	Fahrenheit	s̄	without (sine)
fld	fluid	SI	seriously ill
GI	gastrointestinal	spec	specimen
GP	general practitioner	stat	at once, immediately (statim)
gtt	drops (guttae)	t.i.d.	three times a day (ter in die)
h (hr)	hour (hora)	TL	team leader
H_2O	water	TLC	tender loving care
I&O	intake and output	TPR	temperature, pulse, respirations
IV	intravenous	Tr	tincture
lab	laboratory	VO	verbal order
liq	liquid	VS (vs)	vital signs
LMP	last menstrual period	WNL	within normal limits
lt (L)	left	wt	weight

ACCEPTED TERMINOLOGY

- Use only commonly accepted abbreviations and symbols. Many agencies have lists of acceptable and unacceptable abbreviations. Many client care errors can occur as the result of using improper abbreviations. See Table 13-1 ■ for common abbreviations and Table 13-2 ■ for common

symbols. See Chapter 27 🔗 for abbreviations related to medication administration. Access the Joint Commission website for a current list of unacceptable abbreviations.

- It is best to write a term out in full if doubt exists about whether an abbreviation is acceptable.

TABLE 13-2	**Commonly Used Symbols**		
SYMBOL	**TERM**	**SYMBOL**	**NUMBER**
>	greater than	ō	0
<	less than	ss̄	1/2
=	equal to	i	1
↑	increased	ii	2
↓	decreased	iii	3
♀	female	iv	4
♂	male	v̄	5
°	degree	vi	6
#	number; fracture	vii	7
ℨ	dram	viii	8
℥	ounce	ix	9
×	times	x̄	10
@	at		

CORRECT SPELLING

- Use correct spelling to ensure accuracy in documentation and gain credibility as a professional.
- Look words up in a dictionary or other resource book if unsure of the correct spelling. Most nursing units have medical dictionaries available.
- Spell similar medication names correctly to avoid medication errors. (For example, *Celebrex* and *Cerebyx* are two decidedly different medications.)

SIGNATURE

- Sign entries made in the nurses' notes at the time you make the entry.
- Use your name and title in the signature. For example, the signatures "Susan J. Green, LPN" or "S. Green, LPN" would be correct, depending on facility policy.
- Full signature should appear at least once on each page.
- Use correct title abbreviations: RN for registered nurse, LPN for licensed practical nurse, LVN for licensed vocational nurse, SN for student nurse in an RN program, and SVN/SPN for student vocational/practical nurse. (Some schools use VNS or PNS for vocational/practical nursing student.)
- Some facilities maintain a signature log. You sign your name to the signature log only once and follow it with your initials. Once your name appears on the log, you may use your initials to sign any future entries. Follow facility policy if a signature log is used.

ACCURACY

- Check that you have the correct chart by verifying the client's name and identification information stamped or written on each page before making any entry or filing a report.
- Make accurate notations—ones that consist of facts or observations rather than opinions or interpretations. Describe what you see and hear, not what you think or interpret for client actions.
- Quote the client directly in the client's exact words when documenting client's concerns. For example, "Stated: 'I'm worried about my leg.'" If you are quoting several client statements, there is no need to keep repeating "The client said." Separate client statements by a comma with each statement in complete quotes. For example: Client states, "I'm worried about my leg," "My leg really doesn't seem to be healing."
- Chart specific data rather than using general terms such as *large, good*, or *normal* that can be misinterpreted. For example, "2 cm by 3 cm bruise" is more accurate than "large bruise."
- Document a description of behavior you observed rather than using terms such as *anxiety* or *agitation*. For example, "Crying, pacing in room, talking on phone states, 'I'm so scared that surgery won't go well.'" is far more accurate than your interpretation of what the behavior means.
- Document objectively—what you see, or hear, feel, or smell. Avoid subjective statements, interpretations of actions, or suppositions.
- Correct an error in documentation by drawing a single line through the error and writing the word *error* above it, with your initials or name, depending on agency policy.
- Do not erase, overwrite, blot out, or use correction fluid. The original entry must remain visible.
- Write on every line but never between lines.
- Draw a line through any blank space and sign the notation. In this way, no additional information can be recorded at any other time or by any other person.
- Never leave blank lines above your entry or between your entries (Figure 13-2 ■).

SEQUENCE

- Document events in the order in which they occur: assessments, interventions, and client responses. Every intervention needs an evaluation in order to be considered complete.
- Make a late entry by clearly labeling your entry as late according to facility policy. For example, "Late entry [date] [time]" or "[date] [time] Late entry" could be correct. (See Figure 13-2.)
- Do not make a late entry more than 24 hours after the event. This is not usually permitted by facility policy.

Date	Time	Nursing Note
1/1/11	0015	BP 150/82, P 92 irregular/irregular ECG leads in place, Resp 22
		unlabored O_2 2L/min via N/C. NG tube placement verified via
		auscultation and litmus strip testing, low intermittent suction
		continues. C/O nausea, phenergan 25mg suppository given rectally.
		Color normal for race, skin warm and dry to touch. --------S. Oradei LPN
----------	--------	-- ----
1/1/11	0200	Wakeful watching TV states relief of nausea. ----------------S. Oradei LPN
1/1/11	0600	~~BP 152/90~~ error S.O. -- BP 152/80, P 90 irregular/irregular ECG leads
		in place. Resp 24 unlabored O_2 2L/min via NC occasional dry
		non-productive cough, lung sounds clear to auscultation. Denies
		nausea at this time. ---S. Oradei
1/1/11		LPN
	0400	Late entry – Telemetry unit reports irregular signal. Leads checked,
		lead left low chest loose, pad replaced and lead reattached. Verified
		signal with telemetry.-------------------------------------S. Oradei
1/1/11		LPN
	0700	Vomited approximately 100cc of dark green liquid, black flecks noted
		in emesis. Denies nausea prior to emesis---(Continued) --S. Oradei
		LPN
Jones, Adam (male - 51y/o) / 410A / Dr. A. Amsterdamm / Partial Gastrectomy , A.Fib, HTN / NKDA		

Date	Time	Nursing Notes
1/1/11	0700	(Continued) – and denies nausea at this time. BP 168/90, P 100
		irregular/irregular, Resp 26 O_2 2L/min via N/C, no cough noted at this
		time. Color pale, skin moist. .----------------------------------S. Oradei
		LPN
1/1/11	0715	Dr. Amsterdamm notified of client condition, no new orders noted.
		--S. Oradei
		LPN
1/1/11	0800	Dr. Amsterdamm to see client. New orders noted for IV Zantac BID, and
		labs to be drawn stat. Lab & Pharmacy notified.----------- *K. Hamrick LPN*

Figure 13-2. ■ Sample narrative notes with error correction, a skipped line, and a continued note.

CONTINUED NOTES

■ Continue entries to another page by indicating that the note continues and signing the entry. On the next page, enter the date/time of the note, which should contain the same date and time as the note on the previous page that you are continuing, and start it by indicating that it is a continuation (see Figure 13-2).

APPROPRIATENESS AND COMPLETENESS

■ Record only information that pertains to the client's health problems and care.

■ Record all assessments, dependent and independent nursing interventions, client problems, client comments and responses to interventions and tests, progress toward goals, and communication with other disciplines.

■ Document any care that was omitted and include why it was omitted and who was notified.

■ Use descriptions that are appropriate and accurate. Avoid stereotyping (Box 13-1 ■).

■ Avoid use of inflammatory or biased words such as *but, noncompliant*, or any judgmental terminology. For example, "Client complains of pain *but* he is watching TV and laughing." The simple word *but* says you don't believe he is in pain. When healthcare team members do not perform as you desire, avoid writing statements such as, "Paged Dr. Jones 4 times and he never responded." Instead write, "Dr. Jones paged. Consulted with supervisor and emergency room physician, Dr. Smith, informed of change in client's condition." It is far less inflammatory and more professional.

■ Avoid use of swear words when quoting clients unless absolutely essential.

■ When working with an infant or child, document the pediatric client and the family (Box 13-2 ■).

BOX 13-1	CULTURAL PULSE POINTS

Documentation

When documenting information in nurses' notes or on a cultural or psychosocial assessment, it is important to use terminology that is free of derogatory racial terms. Biological variations, as well as cultural beliefs and practices, do need to be recorded. They give the healthcare team essential information. However, take care to use exact and appropriate terms in all documentation.

Documentation with Pediatric Clients

When documenting the chart of pediatric clients, it will usually be necessary to provide documentation about the family of the client as well as the client. Document parenting skills and style, parental involvement in care, family concerns or questions, as well as any sibling visitation if it is pertinent to the child's care.

CONCISENESS

- Do not use the client's name when charting. In many facilities, the use of *client, resident*, or *patient* is common practice. However, some people feel that use of these words in charting is repetitive, because the whole chart is about the client. They suggest avoiding these terms when charting in order to keep notes brief and save time. Check policies and procedures for your facility.
- Use of the word *client* is essential when family members are also being quoted, such as, "client complains of pain, wife says he has been moaning."
- End each thought or sentence with a period. It is not necessary to use complete sentences.
- Write notes so that data that follows a comma is associated with the data that preceded it, such as "awake, alert, denies pain, sitting in chair, ate entire breakfast."

LEGAL PRUDENCE

- Document accurately and completely to protect the healthcare staff, facility, client, and yourself. The clinical record is a legal document that provides proof of the quality of care given to a client. Your documentation reflects your nursing care.
- Follow the general principle, "If it isn't charted, it wasn't done."
- Follow agency policy and procedures for intervention and documentation in all situations, especially high-risk situations.

ADDITIONAL TIPS FOR DOCUMENTATION

Special care is needed when caring for clients with the same last name to prevent documentation mistakes. Many agencies have a policy about flagging charts when name confusion could occur. Do not identify charts by room number only.

LEGAL AND ETHICAL ASPECTS OF DOCUMENTATION

As has already been stated, the client record is a legal document, admissible in a court of law. All information in the document is open to scrutiny by attorneys. However, a client may object to having the record admitted into court because of the confidential information it contains. It is very important that nurses remember that the chart could someday be read in court when they enter information in it.

The client's record is usually considered the property of the agency but the information contained within the record belongs to the client. The client generally has a right to a copy of the information, though the client will need to make a written request and may need to pay a copying fee. The client can also sign a release allowing access to the record by anyone the client designates in the release, including an attorney, insurance company, or family member (Figure 13-3 ■).

When you are charting, be sure to use objective, factual information rather than opinions or interpretations. It is more accurate, for example, to write that a client "refused medication" (fact) than to write that the client "was uncooperative" (opinion). To write that a client "was crying" (observation) is preferable to noting that the client "was depressed" (interpretation). Avoid using the word *seems* or *appears* regarding the client. Write that the client is "resting in bed with eyes closed" rather than the client "seems to be sleeping."

Not all data about a client should be recorded. Any personal information the client shares that does not pertain to the client's health problems and care is inappropriate for the record. Recording irrelevant information may be considered an invasion of the client's privacy and could be considered libelous.

For the best legal protection, the nurse should not only adhere to professional standards of nursing care, but also follow agency policy and procedures for intervention and documentation in all situations, especially high-risk situations. Below is an example of such documentation:

> 1100 hours—Complained of feeling dizzy. Side rails raised, instructed to stay in bed and ring call bell for assistance. K. Gandenberger, LVN
>
> 1130 hours—found beside bed on floor. Said, "I climbed over these rails all by myself." Denies pain when questioned, replies, "I feel fine but a little dizzy." BP 100/60 P 90 R 24. Assessed for injuries, no complaints of pain or discomfort, assisted back to bed. Dr. RJ Naden notified. R.S. Woo, LVN

Documentation is the determining factor in a great percentage of malpractice cases involving client care, so it is important that you document client care clearly, concisely, and accurately.

| clinical ALERT |

Always remember to chart the five W's: who, what, when, where, and what resulted. *Who* was involved, *what occurred, when* did it happen, *where* did it happen, and *what was the outcome?* If you cover all of these aspects when you document, you will reflect the same quality of care you delivered.

Chapter 13 Documentation **233**

CONDITIONS OF TREATMENT AND ADMISSION

CLIENT'S NAME _____ ATTENDING PHYSICIAN _____

ACCOUNT NO. _____ DATE & TIME OF ADMISSION _____

CONSENT TO HOSPITAL CARE AND TREATMENT

I AM PRESENTING MYSELF FOR EMERGENCY SERVICES OR ADMISSION TO THE HOSPITAL AND I VOLUNTARILY CONSENT TO THE RENDERING OF SUCH CARE, INCLUDING DIAGNOSTIC TESTS AND MEDICAL TREATMENT, BY AUTHORIZED AGENTS AND EMPLOYEES OF THE HOSPITAL, AND BY ITS MEDICAL STAFF, OR THEIR DESIGNEES, AS MAY IN THEIR PROFESSIONAL JUDGEMENT BE DEEMED NECESSARY OR BENEFICIAL TO MY WELL BEING.

I ACKNOWLEDGE AND UNDERSTAND THAT MANY OF THE PHYSICIANS ON THE STAFF OF THIS HOSPITAL, INCLUDING THE ATTENDING PHYSICIAN(S) NAMED ABOVE, AND RADIOLOGISTS, ANESTHESIOLOGISTS, PATHOLOGISTS AND EMERGENCY PHYSICIANS, ARE NOT EMPLOYEES OR AGENTS OF THE HOSPITAL, BUT RATHER ARE INDEPENDENT CONTRACTORS WHO HAVE BEEN GRANTED THE PRIVILEGE OF USING THE HOSPITAL FACILITIES FOR THE CARE AND TREATMENT OF THEIR PATIENTS. I AGREE TO ACCEPT THEIR CARE EVEN THOUGH THEY ARE NOT EMPLOYED BY THE HOSPITAL.

I UNDERSTAND THAT THE EXAMINATION AND TREATMENT THAT I RECEIVE ON AN EMERGENCY BASIS IS NOT INTENDED AS A SUBSTITUTION OR REPLACEMENT FOR COMPLETE MEDICAL CARE.

CONSENT TO RELEASE INFORMATION

I HEREBY AUTHORIZE THE HOSPITAL TO DISCLOSE TO INSURANCE COMPANIES, INCLUDING WORKERS COMPENSATION CARRIERS, OR OTHER PARTIES THAT MAY BE LIABLE FOR ALL OR PART OF THE HOSPITAL CHARGES, ALL OR PART OF MY HOSPITAL RECORDS AS MAY BE NECESSARY (INCLUDING ANY TREATMENT FOR ALCOHOL OR DRUG ABUSE OR DEPENDENCE), TO DETERMINE BENEFITS ENTITLEMENT AND PROCESS PAYMENT CLAIMS FOR HEALTH CARE SERVICES PROVIDED.

MEDICARE CERTIFICATION RELEASE

I CERTIFY THAT THE INFORMATION GIVEN BY ME IN APPLYING FOR PAYMENT UNDER THE TITLE XVIII AND TITLE XIX OF THE SOCIAL SECURITY ACT IS CORRECT. I AUTHORIZE ANY HOLDER OF MEDICAL OR OTHER INFORMATION ABOUT ME TO RELEASE TO THE SOCIAL SECURITY ADMINISTRATION OR ITS INTERMEDIARIES OR CARRIERS ANY INFORMATION NEEDED FOR THIS OR A RELATED MEDICARE CLAIM. I REQUEST THAT PAYMENT OF AUTHORIZED BENEFITS BE MADE ON MY BEHALF TO THE HOSPITAL OR TO THE PHYSICIAN WHO ACCEPTS ASSIGNMENT.

PERSONAL EFFECTS AND VALUABLES

I UNDERSTAND THAT THE HOSPITAL SHALL NOT BE LIABLE FOR THE LOSS OR DAMAGE OF ANY PERSONAL EFFECTS OR VALUABLES (MONEY, JEWELRY, GLASSES, DENTURES, DOCUMENTS, CLOTHING, ETC.) UNLESS SUCH ITEMS ARE DEPOSITED IN THE HOSPITAL SAFE. THE HOSPITAL WILL NOT BE LIABLE IN EXCESS OF $50 FOR THE LOSS OR DAMAGE OF ANY PERSONAL EFFECTS OR VALUABLES DEPOSITED WITHIN THE HOSPITAL SAFE.

ABOUT YOUR BILL

I UNDERSTAND THAT I WILL RECEIVE A BILL FROM THE HOSPITAL FOR PROVISION OF THE HOSPITAL SERVICES, INCLUDING STAFF AND EQUIPMENT, AND FOR ANY SUPPLIES OR MEDICINES UTILIZED. I WILL ALSO RECEIVE A BILL FROM ANY PHYSICIAN WHO PROVIDES PROFESSIONAL CARE TO ME, FOR EXAMPLE, I MAY RECEIVE A SEPARATE BILL FROM ONE OR MORE OF THE FOLLOWING TYPES OF PHYSICIANS WHO RENDER SERVICES TO ME: MY ATTENDING PHYSICIAN OR PERSONAL PHYSICIAN, EMERGENCY ROOM PHYSICIAN, RADIOLOGIST, ANESTHESIOLOGIST, PATHOLOGIST, OR ANY OTHER SPECIALIST.

INSURANCE ASSIGNMENT

I HEREBY ASSIGN TO AND AUTHORIZE THE HOSPITAL AND PHYSICIANS INVOLVED IN CARE DURING THIS PERIOD OF ILLNESS OR TREATMENT (HEREINAFTER "PHYSICIANS"), OR THEIR DULY AUTHORIZED ASSIGNS TO TAKE ALL NECESSARY STEPS, WITHOUT LIMITATIONS, TO ENSURE THAT ANY INSURANCE BENEFITS OTHERWISE PAYABLE TO ME OR MY ESTATE ARE PAID DIRECTLY TO THE HOSPITAL OR PHYSICIANS. THIS ASSIGNMENT OF INSURANCE BENEFITS INCLUDES BUT IS NOT LIMITED TO BILLING INSURANCE, FILING PETITIONS, FILING SUIT, IN MY NAME OR ON BEHALF OF THE HOSPITAL OR PHYSICIANS, FILING PROOFS OF CLAIM, FILING PROBATE CLAIMS AND FILING GRIEVANCES AND ALL OTHER SIMILAR PROCEDURES, AS MAY BE AMENDED FROM TIME TO TIME WITH THE STATE DEPARTMENT OF INSURANCE. I ALSO AGREE TO PROVIDE AND SIGN ANY OTHER DOCUMENTS THAT MAY BE REASONABLY NECESSARY TO ACCOMPLISH ANY OF THE OTHER PURPOSES.

STATEMENT OF FINANCIAL RESPONSIBILITY

I UNDERSTAND THAT I AM FINANCIALLY AND LEGALLY RESPONSIBLE FOR CHARGES NOT COVERED IN FULL BY ANY THIRD PARTY. I FURTHER AGREE THAT SHOULD I NOT PAY THE BALANCE WITHIN THIRTY (30) DAYS AFTER THE DATE OF DISCHARGE, MY ACCOUNT WILL BE CONSIDERED DELINQUENT. I AGREE TO PAY COSTS OF COLLECTION, INCLUDING REASONABLE ATTORNEY'S FEES AND COSTS, COLLECTION AGENCY FEES AND COSTS, AND INTEREST WHICH SHALL ACCRUE AT THE MAXIMUM RATE ALLOWED BY LAW.

FRAUD

ANY PERSON WHO KNOWINGLY AND WITH INTENT TO INJURE, DEFRAUD, OR DECEIVE ANY INSURANCE COMPANY, OR FILES A STATEMENT OF CLAIM CONTAINING FALSE, INCOMPLETE OR MISLEADING INFORMATION MAY BE SUBJECT TO PROSECUTION UNDER APPLICABLE LAW.

ADVANCE DIRECTIVE (FOR ADMISSION TO HOSPITAL ONLY)

IF I AM TO BE ADMITTED TO THE HOSPITAL, I HAVE BEEN GIVEN WRITTEN MATERIALS ABOUT MY RIGHT TO ACCEPT OR REFUSE MEDICAL TREATMENT. I HAVE BEEN INFORMED OF MY RIGHTS TO FORMULATE ADVANCE DIRECTIVES. I UNDERSTAND THAT I AM NOT REQUIRED TO HAVE AN ADVANCE DIRECTIVE IN ORDER TO RECEIVE MEDICAL TREATMENT AT THIS HOSPITAL. I UNDERSTAND THAT THE HOSPITAL AND MY CAREGIVERS WILL FOLLOW THE TERMS OF ANY ADVANCE DIRECTIVE THAT I HAVE EXECUTED TO THE EXTENT PERMITTED BY LAW.

(INITIAL THE FOLLOWING OPTION THAT APPLIES)

* I HAVE EXECUTED AN ADVANCE DIRECTIVE AND WILL PROVIDE A COPY OF THIS FOR MY MEDICAL RECORD WITHIN A REASONABLE AMOUNT OF TIME. _____ INIT.

* I HAVE NOT EXECUTED AN ADVANCE DIRECTIVE AND DO NOT WISH TO DO SO. _____ INIT.   (FOLLOW-UP DONE BY _____ DATE _____)

* I WISH TO COMPLETE AN ADVANCE DIRECTIVE DURING THIS HOSPITALIZATION. _____ INIT.

I CERTIFY THAT I HAVE READ (OR HAVE BEEN READ) THE ABOVE CONSENTS AND CERTIFICATIONS AND UNDERSTAND AND AGREE WITH THEM.

DATE: _____ _____ _____
      MONTH   DAY   YEAR

_____
SIGNATURE OF CLIENT OR LEGALLY AUTHORIZED REPRESENTATIVE

_____
WITNESS

_____
PRINT NAME OF PERSON ABOVE

Figure 13-3. ■ Medical release record.

Confidentiality of Client Records

The client's record is protected legally as a private record of the client's care. (See discussion of the nurse's legal responsibilities in Chapter 4 ⚭.) Access to the record is restricted to health professionals directly involved in giving care to the client. Insurance companies, for example, have no legal right to demand access to medical records, even though they may

be determining compensation to the client. Therefore, a client who is making a claim for compensation may ask to have the medical history used as evidence. In order for an agency to provide the requested information, the client must sign an authorization for review, copying, or release of information. This form must specifically indicate what information is to be released and to whom. A nurse should not allow access to a client's record by significant others or any person other than the healthcare providers who are directly involved in the care of the client, often referred to as a "need to know." If the person requesting access to the record does not need to know the information contained within the record, they should be denied access.

For purposes of education and research, most agencies allow student and graduate health professionals access to client records. The records are used in client conferences, clinics, rounds, and written papers or client studies. The student is bound by a strict ethical code to hold all information in confidence. It is the responsibility of the student and health professionals to protect the client's privacy by not using a name or any statements in the notations that would identify the client. *When writing care plans or papers on individual clients, coding such as initials should be used in place of the client's name.* Additionally, it is very important for staff and students to maintain confidentiality with worksheets and assignment sheets. Caution must be used to ensure that papers are not left where visitors and clients may see them, and they should never be removed from the facility if they contain the client's name or anything that would personally identify the client. Many facilities have special receptacles for discarding papers containing client identification. The papers in these special receptacles are shredded or burned before being thrown away. For additional information, see the discussion in Chapter 14 about the Health Insurance Portability and Accountability Act (HIPAA).

ENSURING CONFIDENTIALITY OF COMPUTER RECORDS

Because of the increased use of computerized client records, healthcare agencies have developed policies and procedures to ensure the privacy and confidentiality of client information stored in computers. Most facilities have tracking software that allows them to see what all computer users within the facility are viewing. Accessing information that you have no need to view can be grounds for termination in many facilities. The following are some suggestions for ensuring the confidentiality of computerized records:

1. Each healthcare worker needs a password to enter and sign off computer files. Do not share this password with anyone. Do not write down your password where others may find it.
2. After logging on, never leave a computer terminal unattended. If your agency provides handheld computers, ensure that you do not leave them unattended.
3. Do not leave client information displayed on the monitor where others may see it.
4. Position monitor screens so that visitors cannot see them when you are documenting or working with private medical information.

5. Follow agency procedures for documenting sensitive material. Conditions of confidentiality for computerized documents are the same as those for paper charts.
6. Never access medical information on clients for whom you are not specifically providing care.

Documentation Systems

A number of documentation systems are in current use: source-oriented record, problem-oriented record, PIE, focus charting, charting by exception, FACT, CORE, outcome documentation, computerized documentation, and case management are a few of the more common systems in use, but there are others that are less frequently seen. It is essential that nurses become familiar with the documentation system used by their facility and follow agency policies and procedures for documentation.

SOURCE-ORIENTED RECORD

The traditional client record is source oriented. The **source-oriented record** is segmented into sections such as physician's orders, nurse's notes, radiology, and lab, to name a few. Each person or department makes notations in a separate section or sections of the client's chart. As a result, information about a particular problem is distributed throughout the record. For example, the physician writes orders in the physician order section, the nurse documents in the nursing notes section, and lab work or radiology results will be in their individual section. To gather data about an individual client problem, all sections of the chart would need to be reviewed. See Table 13-3 ■ for the components of a source-oriented record.

Narrative charting is a traditional part of the source-oriented record. It consists of written notes, often written in block format, that include routine care, normal findings, and client problems. There is no right or wrong order to the information, although chronological order is most frequently used. Currently, narrative recording is being replaced by other systems, such as PIE, charting by exception, and focus charting. Narrative charting is expedient in emergency situations or when the space provided on a flow sheet is insufficient for the information that needs to be documented (see Figure 13-2 for an example of a narrative note).

Source-oriented records are convenient because care providers from each discipline can easily locate the forms on which to record data, and it is easy to trace the information specific to one's discipline. The disadvantage is that information about a specific problem is scattered throughout the chart, so it can be difficult to find chronological information on a client's problems and progress.

PROBLEM-ORIENTED MEDICAL RECORD

In the 1960s Lawrence Weed established the **problem-oriented medical record** (POMR), or *problem-oriented record*

TABLE 13-3	Components of the Source-Oriented Record
FORM	**INFORMATION**
Admission (face) sheet	Demographic data
	Emergency contact information or next of kin
	Admitting diagnosis
	Allergies
	Admitting (attending) physician
	Insurance information
	Any assigned DRG
Initial nursing assessment	Findings from the initial nursing history and physical health assessment
Graphic record	Body temperature, pulse rate, respiratory rate, blood pressure, daily weight, and special measurements, such as fluid intake and output
Daily care record	Activity, diet, bathing, and elimination records; may also include restraints, isolation precautions
Special flow sheets	Examples: 24-hour fluid balance record, frequent vital signs records, intensive care flow sheets, client education flow sheet
Medication record (see Chapter 27 ⚭)	Flow sheet containing medications administered with date, time, route, and initials of person administering
Narrative nurses' notes	Pertinent assessment of client-specific nursing care including teaching and client's responses, client's complaints, and how client is coping
Medical history and physical examination	Past and family medical history, present medical problems, differential or current diagnoses, findings of physical examination by the physician, social history
Physician's order sheet	Orders written by the physician for care of the client including medications, diet, and treatments
Physician's progress notes	This is the physician's narrative notes about assessments, plans for care or discharge, evaluation of treatment, and client concerns
Consultation records	Reports by medical and clinical specialists asked to assist with client care such as anesthesiologists, cardiologists, or dietitians
Diagnostic reports	Examples: laboratory reports, x-ray reports, CT scan reports; this section may be divided into one for laboratory reports and another for radiology reports
Consultation reports	Physical therapy, respiratory therapy
Client discharge plan and referral summary	Started on admission and completed upon discharge; includes nursing problems, general information, educational requirements log, and referral data

(POR). The data are arranged according to the individual problems the client has rather than the source of the information. All of the members of the healthcare team contribute to the same problem list, plan of care, and progress notes. Plans for each active or potential problem are drawn up, and progress notes are recorded for each problem.

The advantages of POMR are that it encourages collaboration and that the problem list in the front of the chart alerts caregivers to the client's needs, making it easier to track the status of each problem. It also works well for the nursing care plan because the medical problems are clearly stated. This allows the nurse to identify the nursing diagnosis based on the client's problems, and then to individualize the care based on client needs. Its disadvantages are that caregivers differ in their ability to use the required charting format, it takes constant vigilance to maintain an up-to-date problem list, and it is somewhat inefficient because assessments and interventions that apply to more than one problem must be repeated.

The POMR has four basic components: database, problem list, plan of care, and progress notes. In addition, flow sheets and discharge notes are added to the record as needed.

The **database** contains all information known about the client from the nursing assessment, physician's history, and the family. This database is updated as needed. The problem list (Figure 13-4 ■) is kept at the front of the chart and serves as an index for the numbered entries in the progress notes. As problems are resolved they are marked off. As new ones appear, they are identified and numbered. As the client's needs change, problems are redefined (see problems 1B and 1C in Figure 13-4). All caregivers may contribute to the problem list. The plan of care is based on the list of active problems and includes both physician's orders and nursing orders (generally written by RNs) aimed at resolving the problems. All healthcare professionals involved in the client's care make progress notes, numbered to correspond to the problems on the list. When you

No.	Date Entered	Date Inactive	Client Problem
#1	3/9/11		CVA resulting in Rt hemiplegia and left-sided weakness
#1A	3/9/11		Self-care deficit (hygiene, toileting, grooming, feeding)
#1B	3/9/11		Impaired physical mobility (unable to turn and position self) *Redefined 2/7/12*
#1C	3/9/11		Total urinary incontinence *Redefined 1/17/12*
#1D	3/9/11		Progressive dysphasia
#2	3/9/11		Constipation r/t immobility *Redefined 6/10/11*
#3	3/9/11		History of depression
#4	3/9/11		Essential hypertension
~~#5~~	~~6/6/11~~	~~7/11/11~~	~~Pruritus~~
#2	6/10/11		*Risk for constipation r/t insufficient fiber intake*
#1C	1/17/12		Nocturnal urinary incontinence
#1B	2/7/12		*Impaired physical mobility (needs major assistance to transfer and walk)*

Figure 13-4. ■ Client problem list in the POMR system.

want to read about care addressing a specific problem, you go through the notes to find all entries with that problem number.

Types of Documentation Methods

Several methods are available for documenting data in the progress notes: SOAP, which has evolved into SOAPIE and SOAPIER in some facilities; PIE or APIE; focus charting; FACT, CORE, or DAE format; charting by exception; outcome documentation; computerized documentation; and case management. Some methods are more adaptable to source-oriented record keeping, whereas others lend themselves better to problem-oriented methods.

SOAP

SOAP is an acronym for subjective data, objective data, assessment, and planning.

   S—**Subjective data** are information obtained from what the client says. They describe the client's perceptions and experience of a problem. When possible, the nurse quotes the client's words; otherwise, they are summarized.

Subjective data are included only when they are important and relevant to the problem. Refer to the section on accuracy for more information regarding quoting the client.

   O—**Objective data** consist of information that is measured or observed by use of the senses (e.g., vital signs, laboratory and x-ray results). Examples of subjective and objective data are provided in Chapter 6 ∞.

   A—Assessment is the interpretation or conclusions drawn about the subjective and objective data. During the initial assessment, the problem list is created from the database, so the initial "A" entry should be a statement of the problem, such as a nursing diagnosis. In all subsequent SOAP notes for that problem, the "A" should describe the client's condition and level of progress rather than merely restating the diagnosis or problem.

   P—The plan is the plan of care designed to resolve the stated problem. In other words, what are you planning to do about the problem? The person who entered the problem into the record writes the initial plan. All subsequent plans, including revisions, are entered into the progress notes.

Over the years, the SOAP format has been modified. The acronyms SOAPIE and SOAPIER refer to formats that add interventions, evaluation, and revision.

I—Intervention refers to the specific interventions that have actually been performed by the caregiver, or what was done to resolve the problem.

E—Evaluation includes client responses to nursing interventions and medical treatments. This is primarily reassessment data.

R—Revision reflects care plan modifications suggested by the evaluation. Changes may be made in desired outcomes, interventions, or target dates.

Figure 13-5 ■ illustrates an example of progress notes using the SOAP, SOAPIER, and PIE formats.

PIE /APIE CHARTING

PIE charting, which is similar to SOAPIE charting, stands for problem, intervention, and evaluation and is based on the nursing process. PIE charting consists mainly of assessment flow sheets and progress notes. On admission, the nurse, generally an RN, completes a thorough assessment and identifies and documents specific problems on the progress notes using NANDA diagnoses. If there is no NANDA diagnosis for the client's particular problem, then a problem statement is formulated based on the NANDA format (see Chapter 6 🔗). Each problem is numbered P1, P2, P3, and so on. As problems are revised, the numbers are changed to P1A, P1B, and so on. Interventions and evaluations are numbered similarly.

After the initial assessment, 24-hour flow sheets are used, which include specific assessment criteria in a structured format. Some PIE systems use **APIE,** in which "A" stands for assessment. The assessment data are included in your problem list to support the PIE portion of the documentation.

The PIE or APIE system eliminates the traditional care plan by incorporating an ongoing care plan into the progress notes. The major disadvantage is that the nurse must review all of the progress notes before giving care, to determine which problems are current and which interventions were effective. See Figure 13-5 to view a sample of the PIE system.

SOAP Format

[date]   #5   Generalized pruritus

[time]   S—"My skin is itchy on my back and arms, and it's been like this for a week."

O—Skin appears clear—no rash or irritations noted. Marks where client has scratched noted on left and right forearms. Allergic to elastoplast but has not been in contact. No previous history of pruritus.

A—Altered comfort (pruritus): cause unknown.

P—Instructed to not scratch skin.
  —Applied calamine lotion to back and arms at 1430 h.
  —Cut fingernails.
  —Assess further to determine whether recurrence associated with specific drugs or foods.
  —Refer to physician and pharmacist for assessment.

SOAPIER Format

[date]   #5   Generalized pruritus

[time]   S—"My skin is itchy on my back and arms, and it's been like this for a week."

O—Skin appears clear—no rash or irritation noted. Marks where client has scratched noted on left and right forearms. Allergic to elastoplast but has not been in contact. No previous history of pruritus.

A—Altered comfort.

P—Instruct to not scratch skin.
  —Apply calamine lotion as necessary.
  —Cut nails to avoid scratches.
  —Assess further to determine whether recurrence associated with specific drugs or foods.
  —Refer to physician and pharmacist for assessment.

I —Instructed not to scratch skin. Applied calamine lotion to back and arms at 1430 h. Assisted to cut fingernails. Notified physician and pharmacist of problem.

1600   E—States, "I'm still itchy. That lotion didn't help."

R—Remove calamine lotion and apply hydrocortisone ungt. as ordered.

PIE Format

[date]   #5   Generalized pruritus r/t unknown cause

[time]   P— Instruct not to scratch skin.
  —Apply calamine lotion as necessary.
  —Cut nails to avoid scratches.
  —Assess further to determine whether recurrence associated with specific drugs or foods.
  —Refer to doctor and pharmacist for assessment.

I —Instructed not to scratch skin. Applied calamine lotion to back and arms at 1430 h. Assisted to cut fingernails. Notified physician and pharmacist of problem.

E—States, "I'm still itchy. That lotion didn't help."

Figure 13-5. ■ SOAP, SOAPIER, and PIE charting examples.

FOCUS CHARTING

Focus charting is a type of record intended to make the client, along with client concerns and strengths, the focus of care. Three columns for recording are usually used: date and time, focus, and progress notes (see the example at the end of this section). The focus may be a condition, a nursing diagnosis, a behavior, a sign or symptom, an acute change in the client's condition, or a client's strength. The progress notes are organized into data (**D**), action (**A**), and response (**R**), referred to as **DAR.** The data category consists of observations of client status and behaviors, including data from flow sheets (e.g., vital signs, pupil reactivity). The nurse records both subjective and objective data in this section.

The action category includes immediate and future nursing actions. It may also include any changes to the plan of care. The response category describes the client's response to any nursing and medical care.

The focus charting system provides a holistic perspective of the client and the client's needs. It also provides a framework for the progress notes (DAR). The three components do not need to be recorded in order, and each note does not need to have all three categories. Flow sheets are frequently used on the client's chart to augment recording data.

DATE/HOUR	FOCUS	PROGRESS NOTES
[date] [time]	Neuro status	**D:** Unresponsive to verbal stimuli; responsive to painful stimuli. Pupils pinpoint and equal. Dr. Ward visited. **A:** Neuro assessment and VS every 2 h. **R:** See flow sheets. S. Myers, LVN

CORE

The **CORE** documentation system focuses on the nursing process. It consists of a database, plans of care, flow sheets, progress notes, and discharge summary. CORE documentation calls for assessing the client's functional and cognitive status within 8 hours of admission.

The progress notes use a DAE format:

Data

Action

Evaluation

This system has been found to be most useful in acute care and long-term care facilities.

CHARTING BY EXCEPTION

Charting by exception (CBE) is a documentation system in which only significant findings or exceptions to norms are recorded. CBE involves three distinct components:

1. Unique flow sheets that highlight significant findings and define assessment parameters and findings. The flow sheets include a sheet for the nursing and physician orders to perform assessments or interventions, the graphic record (Figure 13-6 ■), the client teaching record, and the client discharge note.

2. Documentation by reference to the agency's printed standards of nursing practice. This eliminates much of the repetitive charting of routine care. An agency using CBE must develop its own specific standards or definitions of nursing practice that identify the minimum criteria for client care or status regardless of clinical area. Some units may also have unit-specific standards unique to their type of client; for example, "The nurse must ensure that the unconscious client has oral care at least every 4 h." Documentation of care according to these specified standards involves only a check mark in the routine standards box on the graphic record. If all of the standards are not implemented, an asterisk or other mark is made on the flow sheet with reference to the nurses' notes. All exceptions to the standards are fully described in narrative form on the nurses' notes.

3. Documentation forms at the bedside. Flow sheets are kept at the client's bedside for immediate recording. This eliminates the need to transcribe data from the nurse's worksheet to the permanent record.

CBE lends itself well to computerized documentation systems. The advantage to CBE is that it makes charting quick and easy, eliminates lengthy repetitive narrative notes, and makes changes in the client's condition more obvious. Inherent in CBE is the presumption that the nurse performed the assessment and determined what responses were normal and abnormal. Disadvantages are that nurses frequently feel vulnerable because of the belief that if it isn't charted it wasn't done (Berman, Snyder, Kozier, & Erb, 2008). Sullivan (2004) suggests avoiding leaving any blank spaces and instead writing "N/A" on flow sheets where the items are not applicable. This prevents the possible misinterpretation that the assessment or intervention simply was not performed by the nurse.

FACT

The **FACT** system of documentation is named for its elements. It has many similarities to CBE and is designed to eliminate redundant and irrelevant data and inconsistencies in recording. The four main elements are:

Flow sheets that are individualized.

Assessment sheet that is standardized with baseline parameters.

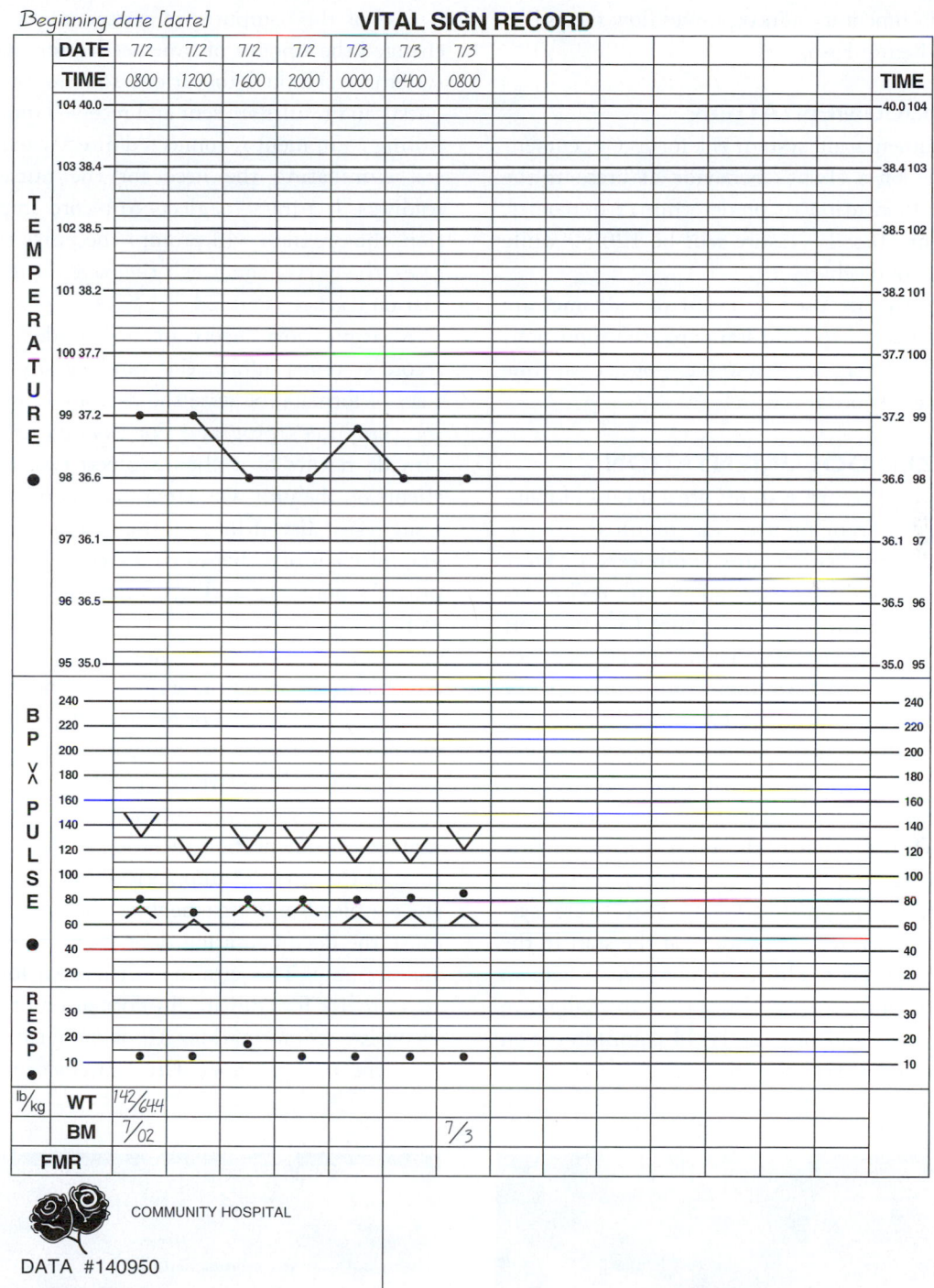

Figure 13-6. ■ Graphic flow sheet.

Concise integrated progress notes and flow sheets that are used to document the client's condition and response.

Timely entries that are recorded after care is given.

To use FACT documentation, the nurse must start with a complete database on each client. Only significant information and exceptions to the normal are recorded. The comprehensive assessment is recorded on an assessment action flow sheet. Another flow sheet is used for frequent assessments,

such as blood pressure or neurologic assessments. Progress notes are written in narrative style to document a client's clinical progress and any significant changes in health status.

FACT documentation is computer ready. It eliminates duplication and supports consistent language, making this system efficient and time saving. Inherent to this system is the complete initial assessment of the client, along with reassessment when the client's condition changes significantly. The

FACT system of documentation incorporates flow sheets like that illustrated in Figure 13-6.

OUTCOME DOCUMENTATION

The outcome documentation system is a form of documentation that focuses on a client's behavior. It presents the client's condition in relation to predetermined outcomes, such as "The client's blood pressure will be 120/80 while sitting by the time of discharge."

The standards that are used to evaluate outcomes are specific client behavior, a specific standard, the conditions under which the behaviors occur, and a target date or time by which the behaviors occur.

COMPUTERIZED DOCUMENTATION

Computerized clinical record systems are a means of managing the huge volume of information required in contemporary health care. Nurses use computers to store the client's database, add new data, create and revise care plans, and document client progress (Figure 13-7 ■). Some institutions have a computer terminal at each client's bedside, or nurses carry a small handheld unit, enabling the nurse to document care immediately after it is given. Many acute care facilities have already changed to computerized documentation; long-term care facilities are beginning to make the transition. One disadvantage of computerized documentation is the high cost of startup. When transitioning to computers, facilities must purchase the necessary equipment, create a software system that works for their facility, and train the staff in the use of the new equipment. However, computers help to reduce errors, allow for more rapid response to changes in a client's plan of care, and provide rapid communication within and between departments.

Use of the computer in documentation has drastically changed the amount of time needed for charting. Since the systems are linked to various sources of information, requests and results are sent and received quickly. Some monitoring equipment is connected directly to bedside computers, eliminating the need for the nurse to record the readings. If a nurse neglects to record important information, the program will prompt the nurse to do so. In some cases, the nurse cannot exit the page until all critical information has been entered.

Multiple flow sheets are not needed in computerized record systems. Information can be easily retrieved in a variety of formats, because the data are cross-indexed within the computer's program. For example, the computer can provide results of a client's blood test, a schedule of all clients on the unit who are to have surgery during the day, a suggested list of interventions for a nursing diagnosis, a graphic chart of a client's vital signs, or a printout of all the progress notes for a client. Many systems can generate a work list for the shift, with a list of all the treatments, procedures, and medications needed by the client. It is also possible to run a computer query to find out whether documentation was missed or medication is due. Some facilities use e-mail between departments so that questions about client care can be answered quickly.

Other advantages of computerized documentation over written documentation include the fact that the date and time of the entry is automatically recorded and all entries are legible. Reimbursement to the facility is quicker because the documentation done by a computer is complete and accurate. This eliminates the need for the third-party payer to ask for additional information or the correction of inconsistent information. All of these factors combined reduce the risk of errors. Drug interactions are flagged by

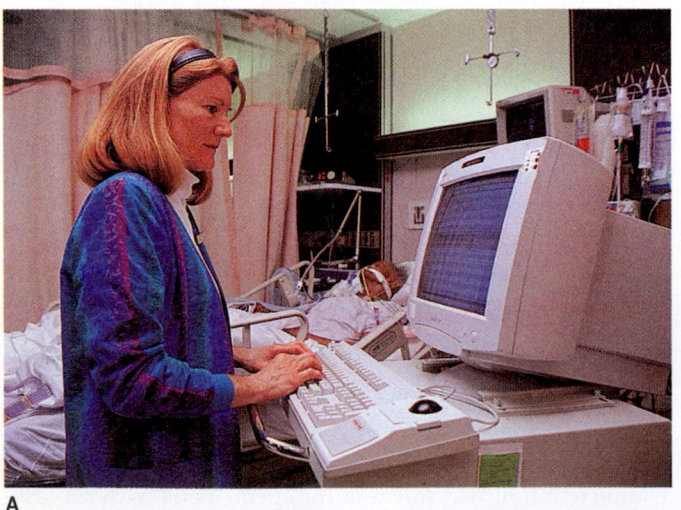

A

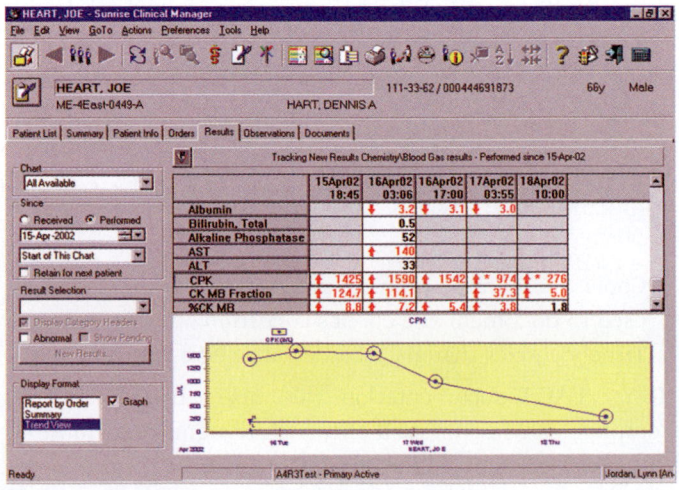

B

Figure 13-7. ■ **A.** The nurse using a bedside computer. (Photographer: Elena Dorfman.) **B.** Portion of a computer charting document.

computer software; physician's orders are relayed to the client's chart immediately with no need for a unit clerk to transcribe the orders; and nurses carrying small handheld PDAs can be notified of changes to the client's treatment plan immediately. Computerized documentation allows multiple users to access client data at the same time, eliminating the need to find out who has the client's chart when another member of the healthcare team needs it.

Computers make care planning and documentation relatively easy and efficient. In most facilities, nurses record nursing actions and client responses by choosing from standardized lists of care and interventions using a touch screen, much like the CBE method. The nurse can also type narrative information into the computer for further explanation or to note exceptions. Some computer programs produce a flow sheet with expected outcomes and nursing interventions. The nurse chooses the appropriate interventions for the specific client and initials them, indicating they were implemented. Others use the problem-oriented format, producing a problem list in priority order. The nurse then selects the appropriate nursing diagnoses, expected outcomes, and nursing interventions by using a light-pen on the screen. The nurse uses the keyboard to type in additional information.

In the future, automated speech-recognition technology may allow nurses to enter data by voice and have it converted to written documentation. Handwriting-recognition technology reduces the need for typing on the handheld units. As computers become less expensive and smaller, it is possible to give every member of the healthcare team his or her own handheld computer to carry at work.

As documentation on computers becomes more prevalent, the problems related to use of computers are being overcome. The issue that is most often cited is that system downtime makes information temporarily unavailable and documenting impossible. Client confidentiality is always of concern. Making systems secure and protecting information on computer screens both require constant vigilance. Adequate backup of computer information is essential.

CASE MANAGEMENT

The case management model emphasizes quality, cost-effective care delivered within an established length of stay. This model uses a multidisciplinary approach to planning and documenting client care using critical (or clinical) pathways; it is most effective when there is a predictable outcome. These forms identify the outcomes that certain groups of clients are expected to achieve on each day of care, along with the interventions necessary for each day. See Chapter 7 ⚭ for more information about critical pathways and case management. See the Unit Wrap Up ⚭ for a sample critical pathway.

Along with critical pathways, the case management model incorporates graphics and flow sheets. Progress notes typically use some type of CBE. For example, if goals are met, no further charting is required. Goals that are not met are called *variances*. Deviations or variances are unexpected occurrences that affect the planned care or the client's responses to care. When a variance occurs, the nurse writes a note documenting the unexpected event, the cause, and actions taken to correct it. Or, the note may justify the actions taken. See Table 13-4 ■ for an example of how a variance might be documented.

The case management model promotes collaboration and teamwork among caregivers, helps to decrease length of stay, and makes efficient use of time. Because care is goal focused, the quality may improve. However, critical pathways work best for clients with one or two diagnoses and few individualized needs. Clients with multiple diagnoses (e.g., a client with a hip fracture, pneumonia, diabetes, and pressure sore) or those with an unpredictable course of symptoms (e.g., a neurologic client with seizures) are difficult to document on a critical path.

TABLE 13-4	**Examples of Variance Documentation (Portion of a Critical Pathway)**

An elderly client has had a below-the-knee amputation. On the third postoperative day, he has a temperature of 38.8°C (102°F). Lung sounds are clear, and he is not coughing. The nurse notices redness and skin breakdown over the client's sacrum. The critical pathway outcomes specified for Day 3 are "Oral temperature less than 37.7°C (100°F)" and "Skin intact over bony prominences." The nurse should chart the following variances:

DATE/TIME	VARIATION	CAUSE	ACTION TAKEN/PLANS
[date] [time]	Elevated temperature	Possible sepsis	[date]—Blood cultures ×3 per order. Monitor temp. every 1 h. Monitor I&O, hydration, and mental status.
[date] [time]	*Impaired Skin Integrity:* pressure on sacrum	Client does not move about in bed unless reminded	[date]—Positioned on L side. Turn side-to-side every 2 h while awake. On every client contact, remind client to move about in bed. Apply DuoDERM daily after bath.

Reporting

Reports can be either oral or written. The purpose of reporting is to communicate specific information to a person or group of people. A report should be concise, including pertinent information, but should not include any extraneous detail.

CHANGE-OF-SHIFT REPORTS

Change-of-shift reports may be given to a group of nurses on the oncoming shift, or may be individualized to the nurse taking over care of a nurse's assigned clients. Its purpose is to provide continuity of care for clients by providing the new caregivers with a quick summary of client needs, changes in client condition, description of the prior day's events, and details of care to be given.

Change-of-shift reports may be written or given orally, either in a face-to-face exchange or by audiotape recording. The face-to-face report permits the listener to ask questions during the report. Written and tape-recorded reports are often briefer and less time-consuming. Reports are sometimes given at the bedside, and clients as well as nurses may participate in the exchange of information. See Box 13-3 ■ for key elements of a change-of-shift report. Also see information on reporting in Chapter 63 🔗.

TELEPHONE REPORTS

Health professionals frequently report about a client by telephone. Nurses inform physicians about a change in a client's condition; a radiologist reports the results of an x-ray study; a nurse may confer with a nurse on another unit about a transferred client, or the laboratory may call to report an abnormal result.

The nurse receiving a telephone report should document the date and time, the name of the person giving the information, and what information was received, and should sign the notation. It is essential that the nurse write down what is being relayed to prevent inaccuracies due to memory lapses. Many hospitals use the abbreviation VORB (verbal order received by) or TORB (telephone order received by). Follow your facility policy for writing verbal and telephone orders. An example of a telephone order might read:

> [date] [time] GL Messina, laboratory technician, reported by telephone that Mrs. Sara Ames's hematocrit was 39/100 mL. _____ Barbara Ireland, LPN

If there is any doubt about the information given over the telephone, the person receiving the information should repeat it back to the sender to ensure accuracy.

When giving a telephone report to a physician, it is important that the nurse be concise and accurate. Begin with your name, credentials, and relationship to the client (e.g., "This is Jana Gomez; I'm calling about your patient, Dorothy

Mendes. I'm the LPN/LVN caring for her on the 7 P.M. to 7 A.M. shift.")

Telephone reports usually include the client's name and medical diagnosis, changes in nursing assessment, vital signs related to baseline vital signs, significant laboratory data, and related nursing interventions. The nurse should have the client's chart ready to give the physician any further information.

BOX 13-3	KEY ELEMENTS OF A CHANGE-OF-SHIFT REPORT

- Follow a particular order (e.g., provide a head-to-toe review or a system-by-system review).
- Provide basic identifying information for each client (e.g., name, room number, bed designation).
- For new clients, provide the reason for admission or medical diagnosis (or diagnoses), pertinent medical history, surgery (date), diagnostic tests, and therapies in past 24 hours along with a concise list of the client's problems.
- Include significant changes in client's condition and present information in order (i.e., assessment, nursing diagnoses, interventions, outcomes, and evaluation). For example, "Mr. Ronald Oakes said he had an aching pain in his left calf at 1400 hours. Inspection revealed no other signs. Rest and elevation of his legs on a footstool for 30 minutes provided relief."
- Provide exact information, such as "Ms. Jessie Jones received Demerol 100 mg intramuscularly at 2000 hours," not "Ms. Jessie Jones received some Demerol during the evening."
- Report clients' need for special emotional support. For example, a client who has just learned that his biopsy results revealed malignancy and who is now scheduled for a laryngectomy needs time to discuss his feelings before preoperative teaching is begun.
- Include current nurse-prescribed and physician-prescribed orders.
- Provide a summary of newly admitted clients, including diagnosis, age, general condition, plan of therapy, and significant information about the client's support people.
- Report clients who have been transferred or discharged from the unit.
- Clearly state priorities of care and care that is due after the shift begins. For example, in a 7:00 A.M. report, the nurse might say, "Mr. Li's vital signs are due at 0730, and his IV bag will need to be replaced by 0800." Give this information at the end of that client's report, because memory is best for the first and last information given.
- Be concise. Don't elaborate on background data or routine care (e.g., do not report "Vital signs at 0800 and 1200" when that is the unit standard). Do not report coming and going of visitors unless there is a problem or concern, or visitors are involved in teaching and care. Social support and visits are the norm.

After reporting, the nurse should document the date, time, and content of the call. (See Table 63-1 ⚭ for guidelines for calling a physician.) For example:

[date] [time] 24-year-old Asian female admitted from ED to Room 301B with c/o burning and pain URQ. BP 120/80, P 100, R 22, T 99.8. Had received Demerol 100 mg IM in ED at 11:10. States pain "10" on a scale of 1 to 10. See Admission Sheet for admission assessment. _____K. Hamrick, LVN. [date] [time] states pain unchanged. Color pale and perspiring profusely. BP 100/60, P 105, R 24, T 100.4. Dr. Burns notified via telephone new order noted for stat MRI of abd. _____K. Hamrick, LVN

TELEPHONE ORDERS

Physicians often order a therapy (e.g., a medication) for a client by telephone. Most agencies have specific policies about telephone orders. Some agency policies require that only registered nurses take telephone orders. (See also Chapter 63 ⚭.) *Note:* The Joint Commission requires that any information given over the phone (lab results, doctors orders, etc.) be repeated to the caller and documented as "100% read back."

When the physician gives the order, write it down and repeat it back to the physician to ensure accuracy. Question the physician about any order that is ambiguous, unusual (e.g., an abnormally high dosage of a medication), or contraindicated by the client's condition. When preparing to receive verbal or telephone orders, you should have the client's chart with you so that you may verify allergies or review current medication orders while the physician is talking to you. These efforts will prevent you from having to contact the physician to clarify the order or provide omitted information. Then transcribe the order onto the physician's order sheet, indicating it as a verbal order or telephone order. Refer to Box 13-4 ■ for guidelines concerning telephone orders.

Once the order is transcribed on the physician's order sheet, the order must be countersigned by the physician within a time period described by agency policy. Many acute care hospitals require that this be done within 24 hours, whereas most long-term care facilities require physician signatures within 72 hours.

FAX AND E-MAIL COMMUNICATION

Faxing and e-mailing are convenient ways of sending large amounts of information, laboratory results, or copies of progress notes. These routes of communication should not be used in emergency situations as a primary method of communication. In the nurse's notes, document how the information was sent and the date and time of the fax or e-mail.

When faxing or e-mailing information, a follow-up phone call is needed to ensure that the information was received. You should also document the follow-up call.

| BOX 13-4 | NURSING CARE CHECKLIST |

Guidelines for Telephone Orders

☑ Do not accept an order from a prescriber you do not know.

☑ Ask the prescriber to speak slowly and clearly.

☑ Ask the prescriber to spell out the name of the medication.

☑ Question the drug, dosage, or changes if they seem inappropriate for this client.

☑ Read the order back to the prescriber before hanging up. Use words for abbreviations (i.e., three times a day for *t.i.d.*).

☑ When writing a dosage, always put a zero (0) before a decimal (i.e., 0.3 mL) but never after a decimal (i.e., 6 mg, not 6.0 mg).

☑ Write out units (i.e., 20 units of insulin, not 20 U of insulin).

☑ Follow agency protocol about the prescriber's signature on telephone orders (e.g., within 24 hours).

☑ Note that the Joint Commission requires 100% read back for all telephone orders.

Include the person's name who verified receipt of the fax or e-mail, as well as the date and time of your call. To maintain client confidentiality, it is important that fax machines transmitting personal health information be located in an area that will prevent viewing by visitors or those who should not have access to the material.

NURSING CARE CONFERENCE

A **nursing care conference** is a meeting of a group of nurses to discuss possible solutions to certain client problems, such as inability to cope with an event or lack of progress toward reaching goals. The goal of a nursing care conference is to work as a group to create a plan of care that is consistent and that addresses client needs in a way that will help the client move toward the desired outcomes.

To **confer** is to consult another person or persons for advice, information, ideas, or instructions. Nursing conferences are most effective when there is a climate of respect—that is, nonjudgmental acceptance of others even though their values, opinions, and beliefs may seem different. Nurses will gain the most information and insight about a client's situation by listening with an open mind to what others are saying, even when there is disagreement (see Chapter 5 ⚭).

NURSING ROUNDS

Nursing rounds are conducted by choosing a group of nurses who visit selected clients at each client's bedside to:

- Obtain information that will help plan nursing care.
- Provide clients the opportunity to discuss their care.
- Evaluate the nursing care the client has received.

To help clients participate in nursing rounds, nurses need to use terms that clients can understand and encourage the client to participate without fear of retaliation or judgment.

INTERDISCIPLINARY CARE PLAN MEETINGS

Skilled nursing units, rehabilitation facilities, and long-term care facilities have regularly scheduled meetings where care is coordinated for a common plan of care. Often nursing services or social workers are the primary coordinators for these meetings. They may include respiratory therapists, physical therapists, physicians, dietitians, and/or pharmacists.

INCIDENT REPORTS

An **incident** can be defined as any unexpected event, such as a medication error or a fall. Each agency defines what it considers an incident, which forms need to be completed, and which protocols are to be implemented. An incident event needs to be documented in the nurse's notes. However, the words "incident report completed" should never be included in the nurse's notes. Events should be written objectively, reporting only what is known to be true and never drawing conclusions or assumptions. Incident reports are for the agency's use. They are not generally part of the client's medical record. Incident reports are discussed in Chapter 63 ⚭.

NURSING CARE

PRIORITIZING NURSING CARE

The client record should describe the client's ongoing status and reflect the full range of the nursing process. Regardless of the records system used in an agency, nurses document the same types of evidence of the nursing process on a variety of forms throughout the clinical record (Table 13-5 ■).

ASSESSING

Admission Nursing Assessment

A comprehensive admission assessment, also referred to as an initial assessment, initial database, nursing history, or nursing assessment, is completed when the client is admitted to the nursing unit. The initial nursing assessment is a snapshot of the client's condition and needs upon admission. This comprehensive and accurate evaluation of the client guides care and interventions. See Figure 14-1 ⚭ for an example of an admission assessment document.

The LPN/LVN assists with the admission assessment by gathering data such as client vital signs, allergies, or current medications. Ongoing assessments are performed each time care is delivered and significant data should be recorded on the flow sheet, graphic record, or documented in a narrative form in the client's record.

DIAGNOSING, PLANNING, AND IMPLEMENTING

Nursing Care Plans

The Joint Commission's *Accreditation Manual for Hospitals* (2000) requires that the clinical record include evidence of client assessments, nursing diagnoses and/or client needs, nursing interventions, and client outcomes, but the standards no longer require a separate nursing care plan. Depending on the records system being used, the nursing care plan may be separate from the client's chart, recorded in progress notes and other forms in the client record, or incorporated into a multidisciplinary plan of care.

There are two types of nursing care plans: traditional and standardized. The traditional care plan is written for each client. The form varies from agency to agency according to the needs of the client and the department. Most forms have three columns: one for nursing diagnoses, a second for expected outcomes, and a third for nursing interventions.

Standardized care plans have been developed to save documentation time. See Chapter 6, Figure 6-2 ⚭, for additional information. These plans are based on an institution's standards of practice for specific medical diagnoses, nursing diagnoses, or client problems; they help maintain the quality of nursing care. However, the nurse must individualize standardized plans in order to address individual client needs properly. To do this, the nurse selects from a list of interventions relating to a specific nursing diagnosis, then fills in data specific to the client.

Kardex®

The **Kardex®** (see Figure 6-3 ⚭) is a widely used, concise method of organizing and recording data about a client, making information quickly accessible to all health professionals. The system consists of a single card or a series of cards kept in a portable index file or on computer-generated forms. The cards for a particular client can be quickly turned over to obtain specific data. The Kardex® may or may not become a part of the client's permanent record. In some organizations, it is a temporary worksheet written in pencil for ease in recording when frequent changes in

TABLE 13-5	Documenting the Nursing Process	
STEP*	**DOCUMENTATION FORMS**
Assessment	Initial assessment form, various flow sheets
Nursing diagnosis	Nursing care plan, Kardex®, critical path, progress notes, problem list
Planning	Nursing care plan, critical path
Intervention	Progress notes, flow sheets
Evaluation	Progress notes

*All steps are recorded on discharge/referral summaries.

details of a client's care must be made. The information on a Kardex® may be organized into sections, for example:

- Pertinent information about the client, such as name, room number, age, religion, marital status, admission date, physician's name, diagnosis, type of surgery and date, occupation, and next of kin
- List of intravenous fluids, with dates of infusions; medications may also be listed
- List of daily treatments and procedures, such as dressing changes, postural drainage, or measurement of vital signs
- List of diagnostic procedures ordered
- Allergies
- Specific data on how the client's physical needs are to be met, such as type of diet, assistance needed with feeding, elimination devices, activity, hygienic needs, and safety precautions (e.g., use of side rails)
- A problem list, stated goals, and a list of nursing approaches to meet the goals and relieve the problems

Although much of the information on the Kardex® may be recorded by the nurse in charge or a delegate (e.g., the ward clerk), any nurse who cares for the client plays a key role in initiating the record and keeping the data current. Students must avoid planning care based solely on information found on the Kardex®, because it is necessary to review the client's record in order to obtain the most up-to-date information. For the Kardex® to be useful, nurses must update it on every shift as the treatment plan and needs of the client change.

Flow Sheets

Flow sheets, also called abbreviated progress notes, enable nurses to record nursing data quickly and concisely and provide an easy-to-read record of the client's condition over time.

The time parameters for flow sheets can vary from minutes to months. In a hospital intensive care unit, a client's blood pressure may be monitored by the minute, whereas in an ambulatory clinic, a client's blood glucose level may be recorded once a month.

Flow sheets commonly used are the graphic (clinical) record, the fluid intake and output record, the medication record, and daily nursing care records.

Graphic (Clinical) Record

This record (see Figure 13-6) indicates body temperature, pulse, respiratory rate, blood pressure, weight, and, in some agencies, other significant clinical data such as admission or postoperative day, bowel movements, appetite, and activity.

24-Hour Fluid Balance Record

All routes of fluid intake and all routes of fluid loss or output are measured and recorded on this form. Information about ways to measure and record specific amounts of fluid

intake and output are described in Chapter 26 ∞. This record is often called an I&O sheet.

Medication Record

Medication flow sheets are also called **medication administration records** (MARs). They usually include designated areas for the date of the medication order, the expiration date, the medication name and dose, the frequency of administration and route, and the nurse's signature. Many records also include a place to document the client's allergies. A sample medication record is shown in Chapter 27 ∞. When changes are made to the MAR, the initials of the nurse making the changes and the date and time of the changes should be included. Frequently, facilities will use a colored highlighter to cross through medications that have been discontinued (dc), for easy identification.

Daily Nursing Care Record

Daily nursing care for activities of daily living (ADLs) are most frequently recorded on a flow sheet such as the one in Figure 13-8 ∎. These records may include categories related to diet, hygiene, activity, elimination, treatments, protective precautions, diagnostic studies, and so on. Depending on the agency, licensed nurses may delegate the completion of this flow sheet to unlicensed staff.

Progress Notes

Progress notes made by nurses provide information about the progress a client is making toward achieving the desired outcomes. Therefore, in addition to assessment and reassessment data, progress notes include information about client problems and nursing interventions. The format used depends on the documentation system in place in the institution. Various kinds of nursing progress notes were discussed earlier in this chapter.

Nursing Discharge/Referral Summaries

Discharge notes are completed when the client is being discharged, although discharge planning is an ongoing process that begins at the time of admission. See Figure 14-4 in the discharge planning section of Chapter 14 ∞ and the assessment parameters suggested when preparing clients to go home. Many discharge forms combine the discharge plan, including instructions for care, and the final progress note. Many forms are designed with checklists to facilitate data recording.

If the client is being transferred to another institution or to a home setting where a visit by a home health nurse is required, the discharge note takes the form of a referral summary. Regardless of format, the nurse includes some or all of the elements noted in Box 13-5 ∎ in discharge and referral summaries.

MED/SURG/TELE/ONC
DAILY CARE RECORD

PeaceHealth

Date: _____

12	13	14	15	16	17	18	19	20	21	22	23

Pain Intervention Key:
1. Medicated   4. Repositioned
2. Cold   5. Diversion
3. Heat   6. PCA/Epidural

Sedation Scale:
0 – None; alert
1 – Mild; occasionally drowsy, easy to arouse
2 – Moderate; frequently drowsy, easy to arouse
3 – Severe; somnolent, difficult to arouse

Diversion Therapies Key:
A - Audio   V - Visual   T - Tactile

Hygiene Key:
S–Self   A–Assist   D–Depend
CB – Complete bath
SH – Shower   PC – Peri Care
OC – Oral Care   HS – HS Care
FC – Foley Care

Toileting Key:
BRP – Bathroom Privileges
C – Commode   U – Urinal
BP – Bed Pan   I – Incontinent
FC – Foley Catheter

Activity Key:
S–Self   A–Assist   D–Depend
BR – Bed Rest   T – Turn
C – Chair   AMB – Ambulate

Positioning Key:
R – Right   L – Left   S – Supine

12	13	14	15	16	17	18	19	20	21	22	23

Pulmonary Toilet Key:
IS – Incentive Spirometer
C&DB – Cough & Deep Breathe
RT – Respiratory Therapy

Diet Function Key:
FS – Feeds Self
A – Setup Assist
CS – Constant Supervision
F – Total Feed
FF – Force Fluids
RF – Restrict Fluids

Dysphagia Eval Key:
CH – Choke   CO – Cough
V – Change in Voice   N – None

Oversight of Care: Initials Indicate RN Delegation and Oversight of Care:

Initials	Signature	Initials	Signature	Initials	Signature

Figure 13-8. ■ Daily record of care. (Courtesy of PeaceHealth St. John Medical Center, Longview, WA.)

BOX 13-5   NURSING CARE CHECKLIST

Discharge or Referral Summary

The nurse would include some or all of the following in the client summary for discharge or referral:

- ☑ Description of client's physical, mental, and emotional status at discharge or transfer
- ☑ Resolved health problems
- ☑ Unresolved continuing health problems and continuing care needs; may include a review-of-systems checklist (e.g., integumentary, respiratory, cardiovascular problems)
- ☑ Treatments that are to be continued (e.g., wound care, oxygen therapy)
- ☑ Current medications
- ☑ Restrictions that relate to:
  - ☑ Activities, such as lifting, stair climbing, walking, driving, working
  - ☑ Diet
  - ☑ Bathing, such as sponge bath, tub, or shower
- ☑ Functional/self-care abilities in terms of vision, hearing, speech, mobility with or without aids, meal preparation and eating, preparation and administration of medications, and so on
- ☑ Comfort level
- ☑ Support networks including family, significant others, religious adviser, community self-help groups, and home care and other community agencies available
- ☑ Client education provided in relation to disease process, activities and exercise, special diet, medications, specialized care or treatments, follow-up appointments, and so on
- ☑ Discharge destination (e.g., home, nursing home) and mode of discharge (e.g., walking, wheelchair, ambulance)
- ☑ Referral services (e.g., social worker, home health nurse)

Educational Records

Educational records are used to document learning needs of the client. Part of Figure 14-5 ⚭ shows one way of documenting an educational record. As teaching takes place, the nurse evaluates the client's learning as requiring more reinforcement, demonstrating understanding, or being able to provide self-care. For example, a diabetic client's educational record might include self-administration of insulin, foot care, nutritional needs, and dealing with illness. When the nurse teaches the client how to administer insulin, it would be documented on the educational record with a notation that further reinforcement is needed. When the client self-administers insulin for the first time, the nurse would document how the client performed the skill and any corrections that were needed. When the client is able to self-administer insulin without coaching, it would be documented that the client (or family member) is able to provide self-care for this skill.

Long-Term Care Documentation

Requirements for documentation in long-term care settings are based on professional standards, federal and state regulations, and the policies of the healthcare agency. The Health Care Financing Administration (HCFA), a branch of the Department of Health and Human Services, and the Omnibus Budget Reconciliation Act (OBRA) of 1987 determine the kind and frequency of documentation required. As stated in Chapter 7 ⚭, the OBRA law requires that (1) a comprehensive assessment (the Minimum Data Set [MDS] for Resident Assessment and Care Screening) be performed within 14 days of a client's admission to a long-term care facility, (2) a formulated plan of care be completed within 7 days of completion of the MDS, and (3) the comprehensive assessment and care screening process be reviewed every 90 days. (The major discussion of long-term care is in Chapter 46 ⚭.)

clinical ALERT

It is essential for the nurse to be aware of the clients' status in order to identify changes in the client's condition. In long-term care, a client's condition can change significantly in hours, and the nurse must be alert to these changes.

Report

The nurse must document and report changes in a client's condition within 24 hours to the physician and the client's family, and institute appropriate care measures.

Documentation also must comply with requirements set by Medicare and Medicaid. These requirements vary with the level of service provided and other factors. For example, Medicare provides little reimbursement for care provided in long-term care facilities except for services that require skilled care such as chemotherapy, tube feedings, and mechanical ventilation. For such clients, the nurse must provide daily documentation to verify the need for service and reimbursement.

Nurses need to familiarize themselves with regulations that influence the kind and frequency of documentation required in long-term care facilities. Usually, the nurse completes a nursing care summary at least once a week for clients requiring skilled care and every 2 to 4 weeks for those requiring intermediate care. Clients in a skilled nursing unit within a long-term care facility should be assessed daily or each shift, depending on the skilled services needed by the client. Summaries should address the following:

- Specific problems noted in the care plan
- Mental status
- ADLs
- Rehabilitative or restorative interventions, with comments about progress made
- Hydration and nutrition status
- Safety measures needed (e.g., bed rails)

- Medications and treatments
- Skin condition and wound treatments if applicable
- Preventive measures

Nurses should also keep a record of visits and phone calls to the client from family, friends, and other visitors.

Home Care Documentation

The HCFA mandated that home healthcare agencies standardize their documentation methods to meet requirements for Medicare and Medicaid and other third-party disbursements. Two records are required: (1) a home health certification and plan of treatment form and (2) a medical update and client information form. The nurse assigned to the home care client usually completes the forms, which must be signed by both the nurse and the attending physician. Box 13-6 ■ provides guidelines for home healthcare documentation.

Some home health agencies provide nurses with laptop or handheld computers to make records available in multiple locations. With the use of a modem, the nurse can add new client information to records at the agency without traveling to the office.

BOX 13-6	NURSING CARE CHECKLIST

Home Healthcare Documentation

☑ Complete a comprehensive nursing assessment and develop a plan of care to meet Medicare and other third-party payer requirements. Some agencies use the certification and plan of treatment form as the client's official plan of care.

☑ Write a progress note at each client visit, noting any changes in the client's condition; nursing interventions performed (including education and instructional brochures and materials provided to the client and home caregiver); client responses to nursing care; and vital signs as indicated.

☑ Provide a monthly progress nursing summary to the attending physician and to the reimburser to confirm the need to continue services.

☑ Keep a copy of the care plan in the client's home and update it as the client's condition changes.

☑ Report changes in the plan of care to the physician and document that these were reported. Medicare and Medicaid will reimburse only for the skilled services provided that are reported to the physician.

☑ Encourage the client or home caregiver to record data when appropriate.

☑ Write a discharge summary for the physician to approve the discharge and to notify the reimbursers that services have been discontinued. Include all services provided, the client's health status at discharge, outcomes achieved, and recommendations for further care.

EVALUATING

Evaluation of client status, goals, and outcomes is an ongoing part of the nursing process. Documentation of client changes is recorded on progress notes daily. Periodic evaluations are performed and documented at regular intervals, depending on client status and institutional policy. Anytime an intervention is performed, the nurse should evaluate how the client responded. This is true for any intervention, whether pain management, a procedure, or teaching.

NURSING PROCESS CARE PLAN
Client with Ineffective Protection

Amy is a 14-year-old girl who is popular in school. She has recently been diagnosed with leukemia. Amy lives with her mother, father, and two brothers who are also active in school activities. The physician has ordered Amy be started on chemotherapeutics and corticosteroids.

Assessment
VS: 99.2 oral-72-16, BP 124/68 in the left arm while sitting. Height: 5 ft, 2 inches. Weight: 105 lbs.
Client states:

"I have several of my friends coming to visit me tonight."
"I don't like to eat much. I have to keep my weight down."
"I have leukemia. I'm not sure what that means."
"I get tired easily."

Nursing Diagnosis
The following important nursing diagnoses (among others) are established for this client:

- *Ineffective Protection* related to chemotherapy and cortisone therapy
- *Imbalanced Nutrition: Less than body requirements*

Expected Outcomes
- Client will not have symptoms of infection.
- Client will demonstrate knowledge and understanding of asepsis.
- Client will demonstrate understanding of need for balanced diet.
- Client will demonstrate understanding of need for energy conservation.

Planning and Implementation
- Take VS every 4 hours. *Vital signs should be monitored at least every 4 hours to detect any change in condition.*
- Monitor WBC levels. *WBCs are the best indicator of response to treatment in a client with leukemia.*

- Administer medications per doctor's orders. *It is important the client receive the medications ordered by the physician.*
- Post signs regarding neutropenic precautions. *This client has a reduced immune response and care must be taken to prevent infection.*
- Provide client teaching regarding hand hygiene and need for asepsis. *Teaching the family the importance of hand hygiene and asepsis will reduce the client's risk for infection.*
- Observe return demonstration of proper hand hygiene. *Once the family is taught proper hand hygiene, observe their technique to ensure that they are performing the procedure properly.*
- Have client verbalize understanding of asepsis. *The client must understand how to reduce the risk for infection through the proper use of asepsis.*
- Provide client teaching regarding neutropenic precautions. *The client must understand how to reduce the risk of infection by following neutropenic precautions in order to keep safe after discharge until her white count returns to acceptable levels.*
- Have client verbalize understanding of precautions. *Having the client verbalize what she understands about precautions allows the nurse to evaluate the effectiveness of teaching and the need for review of specific topics.*
- Have client verbalize willingness to comply with precautions. *Asking the client "Is this something you will be able to do?" will help the nurse determine alterations or additional teaching regarding precautions for the client.*
- Provide age-appropriate education for visiting friends. *Providing age-appropriate information will increase the visiting friends' understanding of what is required of them.*
- Provide client education regarding proper nutrition. *Nutrition is particularly important in clients who are diagnosed with leukemia, particularly because of the potential for gastric distress related to the treatment regimen.*
- Have client verbalize understanding of need for balanced diet (without raw/uncooked foods). *Raw or uncooked foods can contain pathogens that the immunocompromised client would be particularly susceptible to.*
- Obtain dietitian consult regarding dietary needs. *A dietitian can sit with the client and plan a daily meal plan that will consider client preferences along with specific nutrient requirements related to the client's diagnosis and treatment.*
- Provide client teaching regarding energy conservation. *Leukemia, and the treatment regimen, may sap the client's energy, and it will be important that she avoid unnecessary calorie use.*
- Have client verbalize understanding regarding grouping activities and resting between activities. *Have the client explain how daily activities will be completed in order to allow for energy conservation.*
- Provide client teaching regarding signs and symptoms of infection. *It is important that both the client and family understand the signs and symptoms of infection, and whom to notify, because rapid intervention is needed.*
- Have client verbalize signs and symptoms of infection and verbalize understanding of the need to immediately report signs/symptoms if noted. *Evaluating the client's understanding of teaching is important to determine additional teaching that may be required.*

Evaluation

Two days after admission, Amy has met all of her educational needs. She verbalizes that she is unhappy about not being able to have plants in her room but is willing to comply. You note that she is washing her hands regularly and wears a mask when her friends come to visit. The dietitian reports that Amy is not eating a balanced diet and has scheduled further meetings with both Amy and her parents. She must be reminded to rest during the day, especially when friends are visiting. Amy's parents are supportive and cooperative with protocols. Amy is 48 hours into her chemotherapy and corticosteroids treatments, and is free of any signs of infection at this time.

Critical Thinking in the Nursing Process

1. What is Amy's priority need at this time?
2. Amy's friends do not understand why Amy wears a mask. They say that they thought you couldn't catch cancer. How will you explain this to them?
3. Four days into her treatment, Amy reports a sore throat. Her VS are T 101.4°F, P 92, R 18, BP 136/74. What is your next action and why?
4. Ten days into her treatment, Amy is upset about her "fat face" and wants to know what is causing it. When you tell her it is a side effect of the steroids, she wants to know why she's taking them. How will you answer her?

Note: Discussion of Critical Thinking questions appears on the MyNursingKit Website.

Note: The references and resources for all chapters have been compiled at the back of the book.

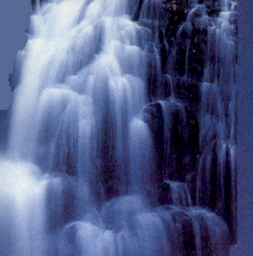

Chapter Review

KEY Points

- Nurses must accurately document each step of the nursing process in a timely manner, regardless of the documentation system used.

- Entries into the client's record must be legible, concise, sequential, complete, and signed by the healthcare provider making the entry.

- The client record is a legal document. All parts of the client's record are admissible into a court of law as evidence.

- The most common documentation systems are SOAP, PIE, focus charting, CORE, CBE, FACT, outcome documentation, and case management.

- Computers have increased the ease of documenting most nursing interventions. Most documentation systems can be adapted to computer use. Terminals at bedsides and handheld units permit immediate documentation of care.

- Case management uses critical pathways that incorporate the care plan into the documentation form.

- Long-term care documentation is essentially the same as documentation made in the acute care setting but has a different focus. Acute care charting focuses on progress toward a wellness goal. Long-term care charting focuses on daily functioning and maintenance of function with the use of restorative and preventive measures. Long-term care charting is also less frequent.

- Accuracy is important in the home care setting because there are fewer caregivers. Documentation in the home care setting is used to obtain reimbursement from third-party payers and to justify continued home care.

- Confidentiality must be maintained at all times, regardless of location of care, documentation method, or whether or not computers are used.

⊘ FOR FURTHER Study

The main discussion of the nurse's legal responsibilities is in Chapter 4.

For further discussion about listening with an open mind and other aspects of critical thinking, see Chapter 5.

For additional information about subjective and objective data, student nursing care plans (Figure 6-2), Kardex® (Figure 6-3), and formulating NANDA diagnoses, see Chapter 6.

For additional discussion about OBRA, critical pathways, and case management, see Chapter 7.

See Chapter 14 for the main discussion of HIPAA and for information about discharge planning; Figure 14-1 provides an admission document; Figure 14-5 shows an educational record as part of a discharge form.

For additional information about fluid monitoring of intake and output, see Chapter 26.

For information about abbreviations used for medication administration and a sample MAR, see Chapter 27.

The main discussion of long-term care is in Chapter 46.

For additional information on change-of-shift report, taking telephone orders, and reporting, including incident reporting and when to call a physician, see Chapter 63.

See the Unit Wrap Up for a sample critical pathway.

Critical Thinking Care Map

Caring for a Client with Complicated Grieving
NCLEX-PN® Focus Area: Coping and Adaptation

Case Study: Mrs. Estella Rodriguez is an 87-year-old female admitted 3 days ago for treatment of bilateral pneumonia. She has lost 1 kilogram (2.2 lbs) since admission, and her records note that she does not eat well at mealtimes. The dietitian reports that Mrs. Rodriguez does not fill out her menus and declines assistance. When her son visits later in the shift, you ask him about food preferences. Her son reports that she hasn't had much of an appetite since his father died 2 years ago, and has lost "quite a bit" of weight. He also reports that she used to be very active in church and hardly leaves the house anymore. The daughter-in-law comments that Mrs. Rodriguez cries frequently and occasionally talks as if her husband is still alive. The son tells you that they had been married 62 years.

Nursing Diagnosis: *Complicated Grieving* related to loss of spouse

COLLECT DATA

Subjective	Objective
_____	_____
_____	_____
_____	_____
_____	_____
_____	_____
_____	_____
_____	_____

Would you report this? Yes/No

If yes, report to: _____

What would you report? _____

Nursing Care

_____
_____
_____
_____
_____
_____
_____
_____
_____
_____

How would you document this? _____
_____
_____

Compare your answers and documentation to those provided on the MyNursingKit Website.

Data Collected
(use only those that apply)

- 87 years old
- Weight 36.63 kg (85 lbs)
- Weight loss since admission
- Height 152 cm (5'2")
- Crying
- Talks as if spouse is alive
- States "I don't know how to cook for one person."
- Not wearing makeup, hair not combed
- Decreased social activity
- Belongs to the Catholic Church
- VS: T 98.2°F, P 84, R 18, BP 150/82
- Complains of hunger
- Watches TV much of day
- Decreased interest in surroundings

Nursing Interventions
(use only those that apply; list in priority order)

- Obtain referral to grief counselor.
- Encourage family to choose an adult singles group for their mother.
- Obtain referral to appropriate grief support group.
- Dietitian consult for meal planning upon discharge.
- Suggest to family that the client's priest should visit regularly.
- Provide reality orientation.
- Suggest weight gain program and recommend a 6.5-kg weight gain by end of the month.
- Schedule follow-up visit in doctor's office, for 1 week from today.
- Schedule time during the shift where you can spend one-on-one time with client.
- Encourage client to talk about spouse.

NCLEX-PN® Exam Preparation

1 A client has told you that she wishes she were dead. When you ask her about her feelings, she tells you that since her husband died a year ago nothing has mattered to her. You would best document this as:

1. Client has suicidal tendencies.
2. Client is grieving for her spouse.
3. Client is expressing dysfunctional grieving and states that she wishes she was dead. Physician notified.
4. Referral for psychiatric evaluation made at this time.

2 The nurse would breach confidentiality in which of the following situations?

1. Notifying the pharmacist of the blood level of an antibiotic.
2. Discussing the progress of a rehabilitation client with the case manager.
3. Explaining to a visitor what the "contact isolation" notice on a family member's door means.
4. Telling a coworker about a client's attempted suicide on another unit.

3 The nurse is working in a facility that uses the source-oriented record system. The nurse would find notes written by nurses in what section?

1. In different sections depending on the client problem addressed in the note.
2. All of the notes written by care providers, including nurses, would be found in the notes section.
3. In the database.
4. In the section labeled "nursing."

4 A client tells you that he did not like his care and is going to sue. He is demanding a copy of his records. You would tell him that:

1. He will need to contact medical records and complete necessary paperwork before he may receive a copy.
2. Because he is going to sue, he cannot have a copy of his records for legal reasons.
3. The chart belongs to the facility and he has no right to it.
4. There is a $100 copy fee and it will take 6 to 8 weeks to receive it.

5 You are making an entry into the nurses' notes and discovered that you forgot to enter something that happened half an hour ago. You would best correct this omission by:

1. Crossing through the entry you are now making, writing *error*, initialing it, and then making the entry you forgot to enter earlier.
2. Making the entry now with the current time since that is when you are documenting it.
3. Making the entry with the time the event happened, and labeling it as a late entry.
4. Doing nothing—it is too late.

6 Dr. Jones calls and relays several telephone orders. Prior to hanging up with the physician it is important for the nurse to:

1. Write the orders down and sign them.
2. Read the written orders back to the physician and confirm they are correct.
3. Research each medication ordered to make sure the dosage ordered is correct.
4. Notify the charge nurse that orders have been obtained.

7 An unlicensed assistive personnel (UAP) says, "You nurses spend so much time charting. I don't know why you bother!" The nurse's best response would be:

1. "The client's medical record serves as a vital means of communicating the client's care and response to treatment, so it is essential that it be accurate and thorough."
2. "We do all this writing because the facility policies require it."
3. "It's important we do a thorough job of documenting in order to prevent lawsuits."
4. "Some nurses don't understand what needs to be written so they spend a lot more time documenting than would be required if they knew what they were doing."

8 The nurse discovers that a client has received the wrong medication on the previous shift. It would be important for the nurse to do which of the following: (Select all that apply.)

1. Complete an incident report.
2. Notify the client's primary care provider.
3. Notify the RN.
4. Call the risk management department.
5. Assess the client.

9 You are working at a long-term care facility and lab reports have just arrived. You plan to fax the lab results to the individual doctors. You should:

1. Not fax lab reports.
2. Follow up with a phone call to the physician's office to ensure receipt of the fax.
3. Fax the lab results and include a request for the office staff to call you if they don't get the fax.
4. Call the abnormal lab values in to the office.

10 You are doing walking rounds with the nurse coming on shift. You come to Room 402 and stand in the doorway to discuss the conditions and progress of the clients in bed A and bed B. You should be aware that:

1. This is normal procedure.
2. If you are not careful, you may create a breach of confidentiality.
3. Walking rounds are done only on critical care units.
4. Taped reports are a better form of shift-to-shift communication.

Answers and rationales for Review Questions appear in Appendix I.

Chapter 14

Admission, Transfer, and Discharge

LEARNING Outcomes

After completing this chapter, you will be able to:

1. Discuss the common reactions that a client might have on admission to a facility.
2. List steps in the admission procedure and important issues when admitting a client.
3. Discuss rules for distributing HIPAA information.
4. Name several interventions for orienting and caring for a newly admitted client.
5. List aspects of nursing care for admitting a client.
6. Identify reasons and guidelines for transferring a client.
7. Describe nursing care for a client who is being transferred.
8. Name important factors in discharging clients.
9. Explain the nurse's responsibility related to discharging a client.

Clinical Objectives

10. Complete selected portions of admission paperwork for an assigned client.
11. Orient a client upon admission to the hospital.
12. Transfer a client to another unit with appropriate documentation.
13. Provide discharge teaching for a client and family.

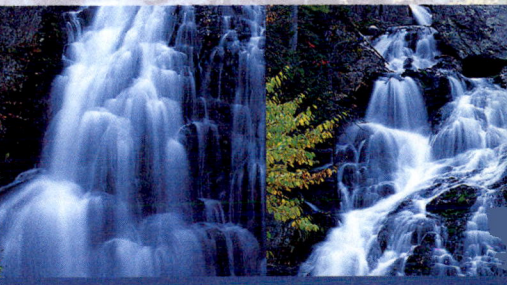

BRIEF Outline

Admitting a Client
Transferring a Client
Discharging a Client

Everyone, during the course of a lifetime, experiences changes in health status. At times, these changes will require medical treatment in a hospital or other healthcare facility. The person in need of such medical care, the client, will be admitted, possibly transferred, and eventually discharged from the hospital or other healthcare setting.

This chapter addresses the processes of admission, transfer, and discharge of clients in these settings. It also includes the responsibilities of the nurse in helping clients through these processes successfully, with caring attention to all clients' needs and concerns. Many research studies conducted in healthcare settings demonstrate that nursing care, and specifically the quality of the client–nurse interaction, is a part of medical treatment that affects clients' health status.

The goal of nursing care is to ensure the continuity of individualized client care during admission, transfer, and discharge. The nursing process (see Chapter 6 ⚭) is used as a framework for achieving these objectives. In this chapter, the nursing process is applied in the discussion of each section: admission, transfer, and discharge.

Admitting a Client

COMMON RESPONSES TO HOSPITAL ADMISSION

Hospital admission is entry into the hospital. It is usually a very stressful time for a client and his or her family or significant others. The nurses who initially provide assistance with admission and orientation will influence the client's reaction to hospitalization and treatment. Therefore, it is important to make a positive first impression. Each individual client deserves to be greeted in a caring manner that demonstrates concern and respect.

The **admission** process elicits many different responses from clients. Clients' responses, although unique, are influenced by their particular gender, age, culture, religion, and **coping behaviors** (behaviors such as crying, acting angry, sexual "acting out," overeating, or smoking, which people perform in times of crisis or stress in an attempt to deal with their feelings). The client's responses are also related to needs identified by Maslow (see Figure 6-4 ⚭ and discussed in Chapter 15 ⚭).

Two of the most common responses to hospital admission are anxiety and fear of the unknown. Clients already are vulnerable to these responses because of the medical need for which they are entering the hospital. Anxiety causes emotional discomfort. It may have physical effects as well, such as an increase in vital signs. Fear of the unknown causes a sense of insecurity. Clients can be helped to feel more secure by reassuring them that their needs will be met promptly and their questions answered thoroughly.

Unfortunately, the healthcare environment promotes **dehumanization** (removal of unique human qualities) by asking clients to surrender their belongings, privacy, and independence. A loss of self-identity occurs when individuals are referred to as a number, a diagnosis, or a nickname or when they are called by their first name without having given permission. Children have other anxieties and fears that may be expressed during the admission process. For example, they are likely to experience separation anxiety if their parents are not allowed to stay with them throughout the admission procedures.

It is the nurse's responsibility to help protect the client from feeling dehumanized by anticipating and avoiding situations that are likely to provoke these feelings. In addition, the nurse must strive to help reduce the specific fears and anxieties of each client. The client's integrity and personal dignity must always be maintained (see Chapter 44 ⚭).

CULTURAL CONSIDERATIONS

Culture is a set of learned attitudes and behaviors associated with particular values, ethnic traditions, and religious beliefs. Clients come from many different cultures, and so have a variety of attitudes and beliefs related to illness and medical treatment. Clients' views about health care and their behavior during hospitalization may be expressions of their cultural beliefs. Often, the client's views are different from the nurse's view. Regardless of the cultural differences between the nurse and the client, it is the nurse's obligation to provide culturally sensitive care (see Chapter 3 ⚭).

Suggestions for communicating with culturally diverse clients during admission, transfer, and discharge procedures include the following:

1. Address clients by their last name. In some cultures, the informal use of first names is offensive. It is best to ask clients how they wish to be addressed.
2. Respect the clients' values and beliefs about health care and illness.

3. Use culturally sensitive language (this may include the term *African American* instead of *black*, *gay* or *lesbian* instead of *homosexual*, etc.). Take your cues from the client.

4. Use clear, common English. The use of slang is usually not appropriate.

5. If a language barrier exists, find an interpreter. According to the Joint Commission (JCAHO) standards, the interpreter should be a medical professional to avoid miscommunication. Family members should not be relied on to interpret medical information.

6. Schedule teaching for periods after the client has rested, because translating or working through an interpreter can be tiring.

Further steps to improve cultural sensitivity are discussed in detail in Chapter 3 ⚭.

ADMISSION PROCEDURE GUIDELINES

Each healthcare facility has its own policies concerning admission procedures. Immediately upon entering the hospital, the client usually goes to the admitting office, where clerical personnel start the admission process. However, clients may also be admitted directly from the emergency department or physician's office.

The client's medical record is initiated in the admitting department (Figure 14-1 ■). It usually includes demographic data, such as age, gender, birthday, Social Security number, next of kin, and insurance information. At this time, clients are usually informed about their legal rights. Forms for durable power of attorney and do-not-resuscitate (DNR) orders are presented. The client may sign or waive them, but most facilities require that these forms be in the client's file. If the person does not sign the forms, a notation is made to document that the client waived the signature (see more about legal issues in Chapter 4 ⚭).

The admitting clerk places an identification bracelet on the client's arm. The bracelet is worn throughout the client's stay in the facility. Clients who have allergies will also need to have an additional armband. Some facilities have specific armbands, for example, to denote DNR status. Check with the facility to be sure that all necessary identification requirements have been met. When all appropriate information has been collected and the client is ready to be transferred to a room, the admitting personnel notify the nurse or unit clerk. The client is usually transported to the nursing unit by wheelchair.

The nurse should prepare the room before the client arrives on the unit. A room that is neat and clean, has good lighting, is the appropriate temperature, and is equipped with basic supplies makes a client feel welcome and safe. When the client arrives on the unit, he or she should be greeted warmly and with a smile. The greeting is a way to begin the client–nurse relationship on a positive note.

HIPAA

Hospitals and health systems are responsible for protecting the privacy and confidentiality of their clients and client information. The Health Insurance Portability and Accountability Act (HIPAA) of 1996 mandated regulations that govern privacy standards for healthcare information. HIPAA regulations specify the purposes for which information may and may not be released without authorization from the client. These regulations have been in effect since April 2003. Failure to comply with these regulations can result in fines being levied against the facility and in some cases against individuals. It is important that all hospital personnel, including nursing students, understand and adhere to these federal regulations. Refer to Table 14-1 ■ for a summary of client information that can be released.

Hospitals and other healthcare facilities usually have a staff member or department that handles the disbursement of information. All inquiries from nonfamily members for client information should be referred to that individual or department. The individual may have a title such as public information officer. Note that information also cannot be given to family or friends without the client's permission. This permission may be a formal document such as a durable power of attorney for health care or informally when a client gives permission for the individual during discussion of treatment or prognosis.

Exercise good judgment in situations where clients cannot express a preference for release of information. In some cases, clients will not have had the opportunity to state a preference related to the release of their information. For example, a client's medical condition may prevent hospital staff from asking about information preferences upon admission. In those circumstances, condition and location information should be released only if, *in the hospital's professional judgment*, releasing such information would be in the client's best interest. As soon as the client recovers sufficiently, the hospital must ask about information preferences. Each hospital should develop policies and procedures to guide staff in making these judgments.

When a client has opted out of the hospital directory (the information as to client's name and room number available through the hospital operator) by requesting information not be included, the hospital should not say that it has no information on the client or that it is unable to confirm the client's presence in the facility, since the media may then infer that the client is at the hospital. Under the HIPAA medical privacy rule, a hospital is permitted to release only directory information (i.e., the client's one-word condition [see Table 14-1] and location) to individuals who inquire about the client by name unless the client has requested that information be withheld. In response to a media inquiry about a client who has opted out of the directory, therefore, the

(Text continues on p. 259.)

ADMISSION DATA

Date _(date)_ Time _3:15 p.m._ Primary Language _English_

Arrived Via: ☐ Wheelchair ☐ Stretcher ☑ Ambulatory

From: ☐ Admitting ☐ ER ☑ Home ☐ Nursing Home ☐ Other

Admitting M.D. _R. Katz_ Time Notified _5 p.m._

ORIENTATION TO UNIT

	YES	NO		YES	NO
Arm Band Correct	☑	☐	Visiting Hours	☑	☐
Alllergy Band	☑	☐	Smoking Policy	☑	☐
Telephone	☑	☐	TV, Lights, Bed Controls,		
Electrical Policy	☑	☐	Call Lights, Side Rails	☑	☐
Educational Mat©	☑	☐	Nurses Station	☑	☐
(TV Brochure)	☑	☐			

Family M.D. _R. Katz_

Weight _125 lb._ Height _5ft. 2in._ BP:R — L _122 / 80_

Temp. _103F_ Pulse _92, weak_ Resp. _28, shallow_

Source Providing Information ☑ Patient ☐ Other_____

Unable to Obtain History ☐ _____

Reason for Admission (Onset, Duration, Pt. ⓒ Perception) _"Chest cold" X2 weeks S.O.B. on exertion. "Lung pain, fever." "Dr. says I have pneumonia."_

ALLERGIES & REACTIONS

Drugs _Penicillin_

Food/Other_____

Signs & symptoms _Rash, nausea_

Blood Reaction ☐ Yes ☑ No Dyes/Shellfish ☐ Yes ☑ No

MEDICATIONS

Current Meds	Dose/Freg.	Last Dose
Synthroid	0.1 mg. daily	4-16, 8 a.m.

Disposition of Meds: ☑ Home ☐ Pharmacy ☐ Safe *At Bedside

MEDICAL HISTORY

☑ No Major Problems ☐ Gastro_____
☐ Cardiac_____ ☐ Arthritis_____
☐ Hyper/Hypotension_____ ☐ Stroke_____
☐ Diabetes_____ ☐ Seizures_____
☐ Cancer_____ ☐ Glaucoma_____
☐ Respiratory_____ ☑ Other _Childbirth - (year)_

Surgery/Procedures	Date
Appendectomy	(year)
Partial thyroidectomy	(year)

SPECIAL ASSISTIVE DEVICES

☐ Wheelchair ☐ Contacts ☐ Venous ☐ Dentures
☐ Braces ☐ Hearing Aid Access ☐ Partial
☐ Cane/Crutches ☐ Prosthesis Device ☐ Upper
☐ Walker ☐ Glasses ☐ Epidural Catheter ☐ Lower
☐ Other_____ _None_

VALUABLES

Client informed Hospital not responsible for personal belongings.

Valuables Disposition: ☐ Client ☐ Safe ☐ Given to_____

Client/SO Signature _None_

PSYCHOSOCIAL HISTORY

Recent Stress _None_

Coping Mechanism _Not assessed because of fatigue_

Support System _Husband, coworkers, friends_

Calm: ☑ Yes ☐ No_____

Anxious: _Facial muscles tense; trembling_

Religion _Catholic, would want Last Rites_

Tobacco Use: ☐ Yes ☑ No_____

Alcohol Use: ☐ Yes ☑ No_____

Drug Use: ☐ Yes ☑ No_____

NEUROLOGICAL

Oriented: ☑ Person ☑ Place ☑ Time ☐ Confused ☐ Sedated
☐ Alert ☐ Restless ☑ Lethargic ☐ Comatose

Pupils: ☑ Equal ☐ Unequal ☑ Reactive ☐ Sluggish
☐ Other _3mm._

Extremity Strength: ☑ Equal ☐ Unequal

Speech: ☑ Clear ☐ Slurred ☐ Other_____

MUSCULO-SKELETAL

Normal ROM of Extremities ☑ Yes ☐ No

☑ Weakness ☐ Paralysis ☐ Contractures ☐ Joint swelling ☑ Pain
☐ Other _↓ related to fatigue_ _when coughing_

RESPIRATORY

Pattern: ☐ Even ☐ Uneven ☑ Shallow ☑ Dyspnea
☑ Other _diminished breath sounds_

Breathing Sounds: ☐ Clear ☑ Other _inspiratory crackles_

Secretions: ☐ None ☑ Other _pink, thick sputum_

Cough: ☐ None ☑ Productive ☐ Nonproductive

CARDIOVASCULAR

Pulses: Apical Rate _92-W_ ☑ Reg. ☐ Irregular ☐ Pacemaker
S = Strong W = Weak A = Absent D = Doppler

Radial R _92_ L _____ Pedal R _____ L _____

Edema: ☑ Absent ☐ Present Site_____

Perfusion: ☐ Warm ☐ Dry ☑ Diaphoretic ☐ Cool (Hot)

GASTROINTESTINAL

Oral Mucosa ☐ Normal ☑ Other _pale and dry_

Bowel Sounds: ☑ Normal ☐ Other _Abd. soft_

Wt. Change ☐ ☑ N/V Stool Frequency/Character _1/day soft_

Last B/M _(date)_ ☐ Ostomy (type)_____

Equip._____

GENITOURINARY

Urine: Last Voided _This morning_

☐ Normal ☐ Anuria ☐ Hematuria ☐ Dysuri ☐ Incontinent
☑ Other _↓ amount & frequency since ill_
☐ Catheter (type)_____ Other_____

LMP _(date)_ ☐ Vaginal/Penile Discharge

Other_____

SELF CARE

Need Assist with: ☐ Ambulating ☐ Elimination
☐ Meals ☑ Hygiene ☐ Dressing
while fatigued

Amanda Aquilini [F. age 28]
_#4637651_

⁂ **NORTH BROWARD HOSPITAL DISTRICT**
NURSING ADMINISTRATION ASSESSMENT

Figure 14-1. ■ Adult admission assessment. (Courtesy of North Broward Hospital District.)

NUTRITION

General Appearance: ☑ Well Nourished   ☐ Emaciated
☐ Other _____

Appetite: ☐ Good   ☐ Fair   ☑ Poor - *X2 days*
Diet _Liquid_   **Meal Pattern** _3/day_
☐ Feeds Self   ☐ Assist   ☐ Total Feed

SKIN ASSESSMENT

Color: ☐ Normal ☐ Flushed ☑ Pale ☐ Dusky ☐ Cyanotic
☐ Jaundiced ☑ Other _Cheeks flushed, hot_
General Description _Surgical scars;_
RLQ abdomen; anterior neck
_____
_____
_____
_____
Note Cultures Obtained _____
_____
_____

PRESSURE SORE™ AT RISKS SCREENING CRITERIA

OVERALL SKIN CONDITION

Grade
- ☐ 0 Turgor (elasticity adequate, skin warm and moist)
- ☑ 1 Poor turgor, skin cold & dry
- ☐ 2 Areas mottled, red or denuded
- ☐ 3 Existing skin ulcer/lesions

BOWEL AND BLADDER CONTROL

Grade
- ☑ 0 Always able to ask for bedpan
- ☐ 1 Incontinence of urine
- ☐ 2 Incontinence of feces
- ☐ 3 Totally incontinent Confined to bed

REHABILITATIVE STATE

Grade
- ☐ 0 Fully ambulatory
- ☑ 1 Ambulated with assistance
- ☐ 2 Chair to bed ambulation only
- ☐ 3 Confined to bed
- ☐ 4 Immobile in bed

NUTRITIONAL STATE

Grade
- ☐ 0 Eats all
- ☑ 1 Eats very little
- ☐ 2 Refuses food often
- ☐ 2 Tube feeding
- ☐ 4 Intravenous feeding

MENTAL STATE

Grade
- ☑ 0 Alert and clear
- ☐ 1 Confused
- ☐ 2 Disoriented/senile
- ☐ 3 Stuporous
- ☐ 4 Unconscious

CHRONIC DISEASE STATUS (i.e. COPD, ASCVD, Peripheral Vascular Disease, Diabetes, or Renal Disease, Cancer, Motor or Sensory Deficits, Elderly, Other)

Grade
- ☑ 0 Absent
- ☐ 1 One Present
- ☐ 2 Two Present
- ☐ 3 Three or more Present

TOTAL _____   Refer to Skin Care Protocol

FALLS SCREENING

If one or more of the following are checked institute fall precautions/plan of care
☐ History of Falls ☐ Unsteady Gait ☐ Confusion/Disorientation ☐ Dizziness

If two or more of the following are checked institute fall precautions/plan of care
☐ Age over 80   ☐ Utilizes cane, walker, w/c   ☐ Sleeplessness
☐ Impaired vision   ☐ Urgency/frequency in elimination
☐ Multiple Diagnoses   ☐ Impaired hearing
☐ Medication/Sedative /Diuretic etc.
☐ Inability to understand or follow directions

NURSE SIGNATURE/TITLE	DATE	TIME
Mary Medina, RN	(date)	3:30 p.m.
NURSE SIGNATURE/TITLE	**DATE**	**TIME**

EDUCATION/DISCHARGE PLANNING

1. **What do you know about your present illness?** _"Dr. says I have pneumonia." "I will have an I.V."_
2. **What information do you want or need about your illness?**
3. **Would you like family/SO involved in your care?** _Husband, Michael_
4. **How long do you expect to be in the hospital?** _"1-2 days_
5. **What concerns do you have about leaving the hospital?**—

CHECK APPROPRIATE BOX

Will client need post discharge assistance with ADLs/physical functioning?   ☐ Yes ☑ No ☐ Unknown

Does client have family capable of and willing to provide assistance post dishcarge?
☑ Yes ☐ No   ☐ Unknown   ☐ No family

Is assistance needed beyond that which family can provide?
☐ Yes ☑ No   ☐ Unknown

Previous admission in the last six months?
☐ Yes ☑ No   ☐ Unknown

Client lives with _Husband and child_
Planned discharge to _Home_
Comments _Fatigue and anxiety may have interfered with learning. Re-teach anything covered at admission later._
_____

Social Services Notified ☐ Yes ☑ No

ADVANCE DIRECTIVES:

Does client have a Living Will? ☑ Yes ☐ No   If Yes, please obtain a copy for the medical record. If unable to obtain a copy, document intent of Advace Directive in the medical record. Please refer to Interdisciplinary Patient/Family Education Record for documentation of Education regarding Advance Directives/Living Will.

Is the client an Organ Donor? ☑ Yes ☐ No   If no, explain in progress notes.

If "No", provided information on organ donation ☐ Yes ☐ No

NARRATIVE NOTES

S—c/o sharp chest pain when coughing and dyspnea on exertion. States unable to carry out regular daily exercise for past week. Coughing relieved "if I sit up and sit still." Nausea associated with coughing. Having occasional "chills." Occasionally becomes frightened stating, "I can't breathe." Well groomed but "too tired to put on make-up."

O—Chest expansion < 3cm, no nasal flaring or use of accessory muscles. Breath sounds and insp. crackles in ® upper and lower chest.

Assesses own supports as "good" (e.g., relationship ē husband). Is "worried" about daughter. States husband will be out of town until tomorrow. Left 3-year-old daughter with neighbor. Concerned too about her work (is attorney). "I'll never get caught up." Had water at noon—no food today. Informed of need to save urine for 24 hr. specimen. IV D5W LR 1000 mL started in ® arm, 100 mL/hr. Slow capillary refill. Keeping head of bed ↑ to facilitate breathing.

✿ **NORTH BROWARD HOSPITAL DISTRICT**
NURSING ADMINISTRATION ASSESSMENT

Figure 14-1. ■ Continued

TABLE 14-1	HIPAA Information Distribution Rules			
INFORMATION CATEGORY	INFORMATION THAT CAN BE RELEASED WITHOUT PERMISSION	TO WHOM INFORMATION CAN BE RELEASED	CONDITIONS FOR INFORMATION RELEASE	NO INFORMATION CAN BE GIVEN
Condition and location of clients	General condition; location such as inpatient, outpatient, or emergency department	Any inquirer including the press	Released only if inquirer identifies client *specifically* by name	If the client requests that the information not be released
Inquiry from clergy	Client's name and location; religion (names of all clients of a particular religious affiliation can be given to an affiliated clergy member)	HIPAA gives specific permission to clergy	Clergy do not have to identify client by name	Hospitals are not required to ask about clients' religious affiliations, and clients do not have to supply that information
One-word condition and location	One-word condition; use the terms *undetermined, good, fair, serious,* or *critical*	To an individual who identifies client by name or to clergy	N/A	Without obtaining prior client authorization
Death of a client	Information about the cause of death must come from the client's physician, and a legal representative of the deceased must approve its release	To the authorities by the hospital, as required by law	Public information about a death will be disclosed after efforts have been made to notify the next of kin	Hospitals cannot share information with the media on the specifics about sudden, violent, or accidental deaths, or deaths from natural causes without the permission of the decedent's next of kin or other legal representative
Obstetric client	Confirm that the client is in labor and delivery or has been released from labor and delivery	Information can be released to individual who identifies client by name	This is more information than general condition, so information cannot be released	Without individual authorization, unless the disclosure is to family members or friends involved in the client's care or payment for the client's care
Client treated and released	A hospital may disclose, to individuals who ask for the client by name, that a client was treated and released because this only provides the client's general condition (that they were treated at the hospital) and the client's location (that the client is no longer at the hospital)	No specific health information is provided	Information, however, can be released to the client's family members or friends involved in the client's care, as long as the client has not opted out of such disclosures and such information is relevant to the person's involvement in the client's care	Although a hospital may disclose that a client was treated and released (with regard to the client's location—or lack thereof—in the hospital), it may not release information regarding the date of release or where the client went upon release without client authorization
Media access to client	Drafting a detailed statement (i.e., anything beyond the one-word condition) for approval by the client or the client's legal representative ■ Taking photographs of clients ■ Interviewing clients	Press or broadcast media	Require written authorization from the client	If the client is a minor, permission for any of these activities must be obtained from a parent or legal guardian; under certain circumstances, minors can authorize disclosure of information without parental approval or notification; state laws may vary

TABLE 14-1	HIPAA Information Distribution Rules (continued)			
INFORMATION CATEGORY	**INFORMATION THAT CAN BE RELEASED WITHOUT PERMISSION**	**TO WHOM INFORMATION CAN BE RELEASED**	**CONDITIONS FOR INFORMATION RELEASE**	**NO INFORMATION CAN BE GIVEN**
Information that could embarrass or endanger clients	Situations where room location information could embarrass clients include (but are not limited to) admission to a psychiatric or substance abuse unit; admission to an obstetrics unit following a miscarriage, ectopic pregnancy, or other adverse outcome; or admission to an isolation room for treatment of an infectious disease	Any inquirer	Be aware that federal laws prohibit hospitals from releasing any information regarding a client undergoing treatment for alcohol or substance abuse	Knowledge of a client's location could potentially endanger that individual (i.e., the hospital has knowledge of a stalker or abusive partner); no information of any kind should be given, including confirmation of the client's presence at the facility

hospital should respond by stating that the federal medical privacy regulations allow the hospital to release to the media only the information in the hospital's directory and that the hospital does not have any information about the person in its directory.

Client privacy can be protected (1) by making sure discussions between healthcare professionals are not conducted in public areas, (2) by keeping medical records and forms such as flow sheets in the nurses' station, and (3) by not posting clients' names where they can be viewed by visitors (e.g., scheduling on assignment board). Facilities who use computerized medical records are required to have safeguards in place. Computer screens should be obscured from view. Passwords must be secure, and users should always log out before leaving the computer.

ORIENTATION

All new clients are oriented to the hospital unit. **Orientation** is the introduction of clients to the people and the facility into which they have been admitted. It starts with the nurse introducing himself or herself and explaining the roles of the staff who will care for the client. If the client is in a semiprivate room, the roommate is also introduced. Important elements to include in the orientation are listed in Box 14-1 ■.

CLIENT'S VALUABLES AND CLOTHING

Clients might bring jewelry, money, credit cards, prescription medications, and other valuables with them to the hospital. During the admission process they should be instructed to give those items to a family member to take home. If this is not possible, the valuables can usually be stored in the hospital safe. The hospital's policy for storing

BOX 14-1   NURSING CARE CHECKLIST

Orienting a Client on Admission

When admitting a person to a facility, the nurse should provide the following information and instructions:

- ☑ The location of the room in relation to the nurse's desk
- ☑ How to use the intercom system
- ☑ How to call the nurse's station from the bed and bathroom
- ☑ How to use the phone
- ☑ How to adjust the bed (The bed should always be in the low position when the client enters.)
- ☑ How to operate the television
- ☑ Location of the bathroom
- ☑ How to adjust the lights
- ☑ Times at which meals are served
- ☑ Location of personal care items
- ☑ Hospital policies that apply to the clients, such as visiting times
- ☑ A gown and instructions on how to wear it (if the client does not have a gown or pajamas); assist client to change if necessary
- ☑ Explanation of why an identification band is necessary
- ☑ Information about when laboratory or other diagnostic tests will be performed
- ☑ Information about when the physician usually visits

personal items should be explained carefully to the client and family. An inventory with a general description of each item (such as a "gold-colored ring with a clear stone," instead of "gold diamond ring") should be documented on the

Valuables		
Cash		
Currency	Coins	
Watch and Jewelry		
Wallet		
Keys		
Driver's License		
Insurance Cards		
Credit Cards		
Documents		
Admitting Date	Time	Received by
Dept Use		
Disposition of Valuables	Client/Designate Signature Date	
	Witness Signature Date	

Envelope No.
This facility assumes **NO RESPONSIBILITY** for the loss or damage of personal property not enclosed within the envelope
Client Identification

Client Valuables Record

Figure 14-2. ■ Excerpt from client's valuables record.

proper forms required by the hospital (Figure 14-2 ■). The client and a designated member of the hospital staff must sign these forms.

The client may keep personal items such as clothing, glasses, contact lenses, dentures, and hearing aids in the room. These items must also be listed on the inventory sheet. When forms are completed and signed, a copy is given to the client and a copy is placed in the client's medical record.

NURSING CARE

PRIORITIZING NURSING CARE

Although the priority for the RN will be to complete the initial assessment, the priority for the LPN/LVN will be to orient the client and accompanying family members to the hospital and the nursing unit. The LPN/LVN should:

- Assist the client to change into a gown so that he or she will be ready for the assessment.
- Record all belongings on the admission sheet, and send valuables home with family member if possible. Arrange for valuables that must remain to be taken to the safe.

- Make sure the client and family members are comfortable, and explain how to contact the nurse both from inside and outside the hospital. Explain the policy on visiting.
- Assist the RN in collecting data such as vital signs and specimens as ordered. Be sure to allow client and family members to ask questions and express concerns. Complete all documentation.

ASSESSING

The initial assessment should be started once the client is settled into the room. The Joint Commission requires that an RN perform the admission assessment. Subjective and objective data are collected throughout the interview, medical history, and physical assessment. However, the RN may delegate parts of the assessment to the LPN/LVN. This may include baseline information such as level of consciousness, vital signs, skin condition, height and weight, bowel sounds, lung sounds, specimen collection, and clarification of the client's questions and concerns. The collected data are then organized, prioritized, and reviewed. They are used to construct nursing diagnoses and to identify areas in which the client may need teaching before discharge. (See Chapter 19 ∞ for more on focused head-to-toe assessment, Chapter 21 ∞ for vital signs assessment, and Chapter 39 ∞ for obtaining urine specimens.)

When the client is admitted, the physician is notified, and orders are requested if they were not sent with the client from the admitting office.

DIAGNOSING, PLANNING, AND IMPLEMENTING

As mentioned, some common nursing diagnoses of clients at admission are *Anxiety, Fear, Powerlessness, Social Isolation*, and *Disturbed Personal Identity*. For example, the RN might write "*Anxiety* related to unfamiliar hospital environment" as an admission nursing diagnosis.

As part of the planning process, the nurse and the client set the client's short- and long-term goals. The client's choices and decisions about his or her health care are discussed and noted at this time. Nursing interventions are then planned to help the client reach these goals. Common interventions follow:

- Orient the client to the hospital staff and environment (see Box 14-1). It is important for the client to know who should receive what information and to become acquainted with various caregiver roles. For example: "You will be visited by a laboratory technician who will draw some blood for examination." It is equally important for the client to know where the nurse's station and lounge are in relation to the room. Familiarity increases comfort.

- Monitor client's level of understanding. Becoming familiar with the client's educational, cultural, and familial background makes communication easier. It also will make your choice of words more appropriate.
- Provide the opportunity for clients to place belongings in the room as they wish, and assist as needed. This simple courtesy helps the client avoid feeling a loss of control and encourages a sense of ownership of the environment.
- Provide the opportunity for the client to ask questions. Answer only what you know and obtain answers quickly to questions you do not have answers for. Do not appear hurried during the admission process. Appearing hurried will prevent the client from asking questions and will increase stress.

EVALUATING

The evaluation step is measured by assessing whether or not the goals have been met. For example, for a client with anxiety, an evaluation statement might be "Client states 'less anxious' after orientation." The plan of care is consistently reevaluated to determine if the client's changing needs are being met as treatment progresses.

NURSING PROCESS CARE PLAN
Admission of a Client from the Emergency Department

David Reynolds is a 42-year-old accounting executive with chest pain admitted from the emergency department. Janet, the admitting nurse, introduces herself and welcomes him to the cardiovascular unit. As Janet begins to obtain Mr. Reynolds's vital signs, he says: "I got this really sharp pain at work. Someone called the ambulance and also called my wife. She should have been here by now." He adds: "My father died of a heart attack at 47." While Mr. Reynolds was in the ED, he was examined by the cardiologist, who admitted him for observation and diagnostic tests. Mr. Reynolds is not receiving intravenous fluids. His right hand is on the left side of his neck. He says he is feeling his pulse.

Assessment
Mr. Reynolds' temperature is 100°F. Radial pulse is 120 and regular. Apical pulse is 118 and regular. Respirations are 28, audible and shallow. BP is 160/94.

Mr. Reynolds rates his pain as a 4 on a scale of 1 to 10. He says he is just a "little nauseated." His color is pink, and his skin is cool and dry. He is frowning, his face appears taut, and his hands are shaking. Janet is asking Mr. Reynolds about his pain—when it started, its character, and the location. She also asks him if this pain has ever been present before. He says he has never had pain this sharp or in his chest before but has had some pain in his stomach on occasion after eating a lot late at night. Mr. Reynolds interrupts Janet's questioning: "Where the heck is my wife? I could be biting the big one here! I wonder if she went to the wrong hospital."

Nursing Diagnosis
The following important nursing diagnoses (among others) are established for this client:

- *Acute Pain* (midline chest)
- *Nausea*
- *Fear*
- *Anxiety*

Expected Outcomes
The current expected outcomes specify that Mr. Reynolds will:

- Obtain relief from pain.
- Obtain relief from nausea.
- State his fears.
- Become less anxious.
- Regain and maintain vital signs within normal limits.

Planning and Implementation
The interventions indicated for Mr. Reynolds are:

- Orient to the unit.
- Explain the purpose of admission (observation and diagnosis).
- Position for greater comfort in breathing.
- Respond to need for information regarding wife.
- Encourage to talk about fears.
- Listen attentively to concerns.
- Welcome questions.
- Arrange room (client belongings) according to preferences.
- Monitor vital signs frequently as specified by physician's orders.
- Assess rate, rhythm, and character of pulse and respiration.
- Assess pain occurrence, including intensity, duration, and location.
- Assess skin color.
- Assess presence of nausea.
- Explain diagnostic procedures ordered (procedure and purpose).

Evaluation
By the third day of hospitalization, Mr. Reynolds has learned that he did not have a heart attack (myocardial infarction) but instead has a peptic ulcer. Treatment for the

ulcer is continuing. Discharge planning has begun. Stress management will be one of the teaching initiatives.

Critical Thinking in the Nursing Process

1. What nursing care problems did Mr. Reynolds present at the time of admission that would be reported to the nurse team leader?
2. What aspects of Mr. Reynolds' verbal and nonverbal communication were significant indicators of fear and anxiety?
3. What effect would arranging Mr. Reynolds' room according to his preferences have in reducing his anxiety?

Note: Discussion of Critical Thinking questions appears on the MyNursingKit Website.

Transferring a Client

COMMON RESPONSES TO TRANSFER

The client may require **transfer** (a move) to another unit in the hospital or to a different healthcare facility as a result of a client or physician request. The usual reasons for transfer are:

- The client may request another room (e.g., the client may need a quieter environment).
- The client's health condition may change and require more specialized nursing care (e.g., a severely elevated heart rate may require that the client be moved into intensive care).
- The client's condition may improve, permitting transfer from ICU to a medical/surgical or a transitional care unit.
- The client's condition may require a transfer to another facility (e.g., from an acute care setting to a rehab unit).
- The client may be disturbing others.

Transferring from one room, department, or facility to another is always somewhat stressful for the client and significant others. Clients may be concerned about people not being informed or about staff losing their belongings during the transfer. Anxieties tend to be lessened when the client is being transferred to a step-down or rehabilitation unit. However, when the physician orders the transfer for the purpose of having the client receive more specialized care (such as intensive care), the client's initial response is fear. Concerned that his or her condition has worsened, the client's fears may escalate into fear of death. Obviously, whatever the client's response, individualized nursing care is required.

Parents may be upset when a child needs to be transferred for whatever reason. Special high-topped cribs are available for transferring infants, toddlers, and small children (Figure 14-3 ■). Points the nurse needs to remember when transferring a child are provided in Box 14-2 ■.

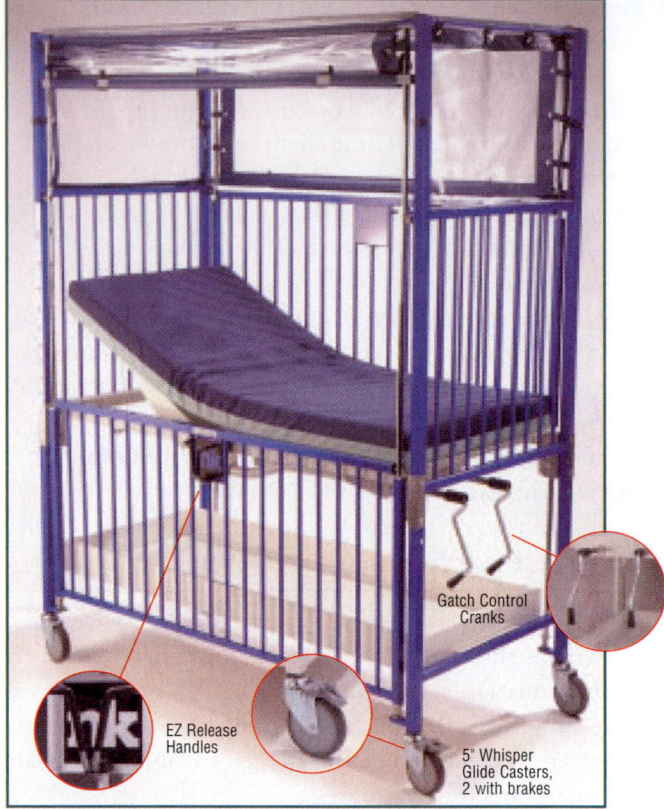

Figure 14-3. ■ Bubble-top crib for safe transfer of pediatric clients. (Courtesy of nk Medical Products.)

Labels in figure: Gatch Control Cranks; EZ Release Handles; 5" Whisper Glide Casters, 2 with brakes

---

BOX 14-2	Pediatric Considerations

Transferring a Child

If the child is to be transported to another area of the hospital for the diagnostic exam or treatment, safety is an issue.

- The child can be transported in:
  - A crib with high sides
  - A youth bed
  - A wheelchair with a safety harness
  - On a stretcher
- The child should be lying down with the side rails raised.
- A vinyl-top crib protects a climbing child from injury.
- A safety belt may be fastened across the child's abdomen to prevent the child from falling off the stretcher.
- Children should never be left unattended.

TRANSFER GUIDELINES

Each hospital has written policies for transferring a client. The procedure usually requires the following:

1. Receiving a physician's order
2. Informing the client and family about the reason for the transfer
3. Assisting the client to gather all belongings
4. Completing the required documentation

SKILLED NURSING FACILITY (SNF)
Transfer Record

Client's Name _____ DOB _____ Insurance No. _____

SNF Name _____

Hosp. Admission Date _____ Discharge Date _____ SNF Admission Date _____

Principal Diagnosis (es):

Surgical Procedures and Dates:

Client Allergies:

Diet:

Physician Transfer Orders: (Medicines, Therapy, Lab Work, etc.)

Physician's Signature _____

Nursing Evaluation:

Date of Foley Insertion _____ Date of Last BM _____

Decubitus size / condition _____

Nursing Assessment:

Nurse's Signature _____

**Community Hospital
of Lancaster**

Figure 14-4. ■ Skilled nursing facility transfer record.

Figure 14-4 ■ illustrates one type of transfer form.

NURSING CARE

PRIORITIZING NURSING CARE

When a client is being transferred from one room to another or to a different level of care, be sure that the client is informed prior to initiating the transfer procedure. If the client is a minor or elderly person, the family also needs to be informed. As a courtesy, the next of kin should be notified so that they do not arrive at the client's room and find an empty bed.

Call the new unit to determine the time they can accept the transferred client. Arrange for a transporter. Complete all documentation, and make sure all medications and treatment supplies are sent with the client unless facility policy prohibits it. Match client's belongings against the admission sheet. Be sure that nothing is left behind.

Accompany the client to the new room or unit and introduce him or her and any accompanying family members to a new staff member. Do not leave the client until report has been given to a nurse and all questions have been answered. Be sure the client is stable and comfortable before returning to your own unit.

ASSESSING

Although it is not the responsibility of the LPN/LVN to determine if, where, or when a client is transferred, he or she may participate in the process. The nurse may be involved in assessing and reporting client problems related to transfer. The LPN/LVN may also assist in implementing transfer procedures as directed by the registered nurse.

The following are common assessment issues related to transfer:

1. Client's health status. Physical and emotional support may be necessary throughout the process of transfer.
2. The client's and significant others' level of understanding about the reason for the transfer.
3. Safety precautions. Special equipment (such as wheelchair, stretcher, and portable IV apparatus) may be required to ensure client safety.

DIAGNOSING, PLANNING, AND IMPLEMENTING

Nursing diagnoses for clients who are being transferred are identified upon reviewing assessment issues. The following are examples:

- *Deficient Knowledge* related to need for transfer
- *Risk for Injury* related to the transfer procedure
- *Anxiety* related to a new environment

Implementation of the care plan or nursing actions addresses client issues directly related to the nursing diagnoses. All nursing actions related to transfer should be directed toward managing the transfer process in an efficient and calm manner. These nursing actions include:

- *Explaining the transfer process.* Sharing information with the client and significant others decreases anxiety. It also generally increases compliance.
- *Taking safety precautions.* There is risk for injury in transfer situations. Also, if the transfer is delayed, there is potential for client discomfort. (For example, the client may have to wait a long time on a transfer bed or in a wheelchair. Clients in hospital gowns may become chilled.)
- *Checking and recording vital signs.* It is important to document client status before transfer. This documentation can be used as a reference point should the client's condition change.

clinical ALERT

Report
It is important to report all aspects of the transfer process immediately upon completion. Reporting completion of a transfer will allow several steps to occur:

1. Details about room number and client status at the time of transfer will be communicated.
2. The physician will be notified, usually by the unit clerk, that the client has been transferred.
3. The empty room will be cleaned and prepared for the next client.

The nurse may be directed to accompany the client to the new environment. If so, it is the nurse's responsibility to ensure that the client is greeted by the staff member of the new unit or facility who will be caring for the client. When accompanying a client to a new environment, it is also necessary to inform the registered nurse manager that transfer has occurred. Any change in the client's health status during transfer, or any problem encountered during the process, is also reported to the registered nurse who will oversee the client's care.

EVALUATING

After transfer, the nurse evaluates whether the client's vital signs and general health status have remained stable, and determines whether the transfer was completed safely. The time of transfer and the client's reaction to transfer are also noted.

Discharging a Client

Discharge is the official procedure by which the client leaves the healthcare facility and returns home or to another setting. Written permission from the physician is required for discharge. A client's leaving the hospital or healthcare facility without the written permission of a primary care provider is **against medical advice** (AMA). It is reported to the registered nurse manager immediately. If the client is rational and a court order does not exist to detain the client, he or she cannot be forcibly detained. The nurse or designated supervisor is responsible for notifying the physician. The client and supervisor sign and complete the proper forms. If the client refuses to sign the forms, this is documented in the client's medical record.

Clients are generally discharged from the hospital and return home because their condition has improved or has become stable. Client discharge to another healthcare facility, however, may occur for various reasons. For example, the discharged client may be a resident of a nursing home or may require the type of care received in a rehabilitation center. Clients may be discharged by wheelchair to their personal vehicle or by wheelchair or stretcher to some other form of transport such as an ambulance. Depending on the condition of the client at the time of discharge and the type of facility receiving the client, a nurse may accompany the client. In many healthcare facilities, there is a particular time for discharge of clients (for example, 11 A.M.), which precedes a designated admission time. Regardless of the policies and procedures in a healthcare setting, it is the nurse's responsibility to manage discharge efficiently and in a manner that ensures the client's physical and emotional comfort.

DISCHARGE GUIDELINES

Each hospital has written guidelines about the discharge procedure. They generally consist of the following:

- Receiving written physician's order for discharge
- Completing discharge teaching documentation (Figure 14-5 ■)
- Sending notification of discharge to the business office
- Assisting the client to prepare for discharge
- Ensuring that all client belongings are assembled for discharge
- Explaining referral agencies and providing information about people or groups to contact (if this is not required prior to discharge)

Discharge Charting

Content Items marked with (✓) required on all Clients	Identified Client/Family Educational Needs		Date	Instruction Educator's Initials	Learner's Response	Date	Instruction Educator's Initials	Learner's Response
	Pre-op	Other						
Teaching/Miscellaneous:								
OR / PACU Routine								
Report Time to Hospital								
Waiting Area/visitors								
SCD's								
IV Therapy								
Incision / Wound Care								
NPO status								
Drain Tubes								
Other:								
Rehabilitation Needs:								
Cane/Crutch/Walker Training/Transfer Training								
Hip/Knees/Back/Ankle/Upper Extremity Exercise								
Sling/Splint/Corset/Braces								
TENS								
CPM								
Total Hip Precautions								
ADL Adaptive Equipment								
Energy Conservation / Joint Protection								
Body Mechanics								
Safety								
Other:								
Lifestyle Changes / Interventions								
Activity Level								
Other:								
Community Resources								
Specify								
Grief Counseling / Training								

Figure 14-5. ■ Discharge teaching from interdisciplinary client/family education record.

■ Completing the teaching process; this includes all discharge instructions related to medication, nutrition and diet, self-care, allowable activity, and future appointments. (Figure 14-6 ■ provides a sample of discharge instructions.)

■ Transporting the client to the discharge location

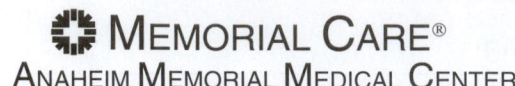

ADDRESSOGRAPH

MEMORIAL CARE®
ANAHEIM MEMORIAL MEDICAL CENTER

DISCHARGE INSTRUCTIONS

For medical questions, call your physician.
For medical emergencies, dial 9-1-1 immediately.

CLIENT NAME: _____

REASON FOR YOUR HOSPITAL STAY: _____

DATE ADMITTED: _____ DATE DISCHARGED: _____

DIET: REGULAR   SPECIAL (see "special instructions" below)

BATHING: AS DESIRED LIMITS (see "special instructions" below)

PAIN MANAGEMENT: MEDICATION TREATMENT OUTPATIENT FOLLOW-UP

ACTIVITY: NORMAL LIMITS (see "special instructions" below)

YOU CAN RESUME NORMAL ACTIVITIES WHEN: _____

_____

_____

_____

PRE-PRINTED INSTRUCTIONS PROVIDED & REVIEWED INCLUDING FOOD/DRUG AND

OTHER INTERACTIONS (LIST TITLE): _____

SPECIAL INSTRUCTIONS: _____

_____

_____

THINGS TO LET YOUR DOCTOR KNOW ABOUT: _____

_____

PHYSICIAN APPOINTMENTS / REFERRALS:

1. _____
   DATE   PHYSICIAN/SPECIALTY   PHONE

2. _____
   DATE   PHYSICIAN/SPECIALTY   PHONE

3. _____
   DATE   PHYSICIAN/SPECIALTY   PHONE

4. _____
   DATE   PHYSICIAN/SPECIALTY   PHONE

Home Health Services Ordered: _____

_____

_____

Co. _____ # _____

Medical Equipment Ordered: _____

_____

_____

Co. _____ # _____

Assisted Daily Living Needs: _____

_____

List of Homemaker Agencies Given? _____

Other Services Ordered/Resources Contacted?

_____

Co. _____ # _____

MEDICATION INSTRUCTIONS

NO.	DRUG / DOSE	ROUTE	TIME(S)	PURPOSE	DATE/TIME LAST GIVEN
1					/
2					/
3					/
4					/
5					/
6					/
7					/
8					/
9					/
10					/
11	Pain Medication: _____		CALL YOUR DOCTOR WITH QUESTIONS REGARDING PAIN.		

Prescription Given? ____ Yes ____ No   Medication Information Discussed? ____ Yes ____ No   Medication Side Effects Discussed? ____ Yes ____ No

Client requests additional information about medication ____ Yes ____ No   Pharmacy contacted ____ Yes ____ No   By whom: _____

Client verbalizes an understanding of above discharge instructions and states where to obtain medications.

Figure 14-6. ■ Discharge instruction sheet for client. (Courtesy of Anaheim Memorial Medical Center.)

Appointments such as those to physical therapy and referral to agencies such as home health are usually arranged by the social worker assigned to the client. Appointments and referrals are also sometimes scheduled by the nurse manager, discharge planner, or the unit clerk. The client or significant others may be instructed by the nurse or social worker in making the referral.

The physician orders referrals and appointments. An exception to a physician-ordered referral may occur when the client requests information regarding a particular problem or disease. The nurse may then refer the client to an organization by providing the name and number and perhaps some printed material. For example, a newly diagnosed diabetic client may ask where he or she can learn more about the disease and perhaps join a support group. In instances such as this, referral to community services is part of the nursing responsibility of promoting health education.

COMMON RESPONSES TO DISCHARGE

Most clients are excited and happy to be returning home. Others may be anxious about the support they will receive at home or about the consequences and nature of continued convalescence. Those who are going to an unfamiliar destination may feel uncomfortable. Clients generally feel concerned about how to care for themselves and how to follow the discharge instructions precisely.

NURSING CARE

PRIORITIZING NURSING CARE

Discharge planning begins the day the client is admitted to the hospital. The planning and teaching continue until clients are wheeled out the door and are safe in their transportation home. The first priority of discharge is that the client and family have been given the necessary information and training to continue the client's course of recovery. On the day of discharge, be sure that the client and family understand that they will need to remain until all discharge orders have been received. If the client has a Foley catheter that is to be removed and he or she must void prior to leaving, explain that to the client so that he/she will not become frustrated if the discharge is delayed. Gather all belongings, and retrieve any valuables from the safe. Inform all hospital departments of the pending discharge, and send a family member to the business office if necessary. If the client has a dressing, be sure it is clean, dry, and intact. If necessary, change it before helping the client to get dressed. Remove IV or other equipment.

Help the client dress. Ask the family member to bring the car to the door. Obtain a wheelchair to transport the client, and assist the client into the car. If the client is a child, be sure that an appropriate car seat is available. The parent should be responsible for installing it in the car and placing the child in it. Return to the unit and strip the room of any remaining supplies and equipment. This may be done by housekeeping or unlicensed assistive personnel, depending on facility policy and staffing. Complete all charting and give the chart to the ward secretary for proper disposition.

ASSESSING

The LPN/LVN may collect data about the following issues prior to discharge:

- *Client's physical and emotional readiness for discharge.* The nurse should provide the opportunity to listen to the client's feelings related to discharge. These concerns could be related to wondering how well the client will continue to progress at home or whether medical supplies or equipment will be accessible in the home.
- *Support system for client.* Significant others must become part of the discharge process. The nurse listens to their concerns about the client's return home or to a designated facility.
- *Understanding discharge instructions.* Assessing how the client interprets the instructions is essential. Confusion about diet, medication, special procedures, or exercise and activity may be present.
- *Progress expectations.* The client may not understand what to expect regarding convalescence. Clients may wonder how long they will need certain types of treatment or how long they will have certain symptoms.
- *Home environment and safety.* Clients may feel insecure about home safety. They may feel that their living space will not accommodate the medical supplies and equipment they need.

clinical ALERT

Report

LPNs/LVNs should inform the registered nurse of all concerns stated by the client that could potentially affect the client's continued progress toward wellness. Questions and concerns specifically related to discharge instructions and progress expectations should always be discussed with the registered nurse. In some instances, the registered nurse will refer questions to or obtain answers from the physician.

DIAGNOSING, PLANNING, AND IMPLEMENTING

Two of the most common nursing diagnoses that are identified when discharging clients are *Self-Care Deficit* and *Deficient Knowledge*. The planning and implementation of the nursing process related to discharge occur in response to these diagnoses.

Discharge planning actually begins with hospital admission. Teaching that was identified at admission and introduced during a client's stay is reinforced on the day of discharge. Written guidelines often are provided (see Figure 14-5). Underlying all care and treatment the client receives is the goal to restore the client, if possible, to the level of wellness that preceded hospitalization.

In collaboration with the RN, the LPN/LVN helps the client to clarify goals for discharge by assisting the client in anticipating and solving problems. For example, the client who lives alone may realize that he or she will need help to carry out activities of daily living (ADLs) and to follow discharge instructions. A goal would be set to obtain help and support from significant others, home health care, or other available agencies. The social worker may be notified and may provide special assistance in obtaining help and support.

Client outcomes and timelines are also developed to help the client and family during the transition. For example, for a very weak client, an initial goal might be to work gradually toward full participation in ADLs over a period of 2 weeks (if this is in keeping with physician's orders). The plan may include slowly increasing the time spent on each activity, or selecting one or two activities to complete and gradually increasing the number as strength permits.

The example of problem solving given above relates to planning (goal setting), but it is also an example of the implementation process associated with discharge. Perhaps the most important nursing actions at discharge are those directed toward giving the client the appropriate oral presentation and written resources related to discharge instructions. For example, if a particular diet is recommended, then the nutritionist can be contacted to discuss the diet with the client and provide helpful materials and menu ideas. Printed instructions are available on many topics and in almost every language (examples: insulin self-administration, dressing changes, and mobility devices). Large-print materials are also available.

However, the nurse must not simply give the client a pack of printed brochures or information sheets and consider the discharge process complete. Printed materials are intended as an information supplement and as a reference. Every discharge instruction should be explained verbally to the client. During oral instruction, the client should be encouraged to ask questions. The client should paraphrase the instructions, and the nurse should listen carefully to determine whether the client interprets the instructions accurately. Whenever possible, the nurse should ask the client to demonstrate procedures listed in the discharge instructions.

In addition to discharge instructions related to medical care, the client should also be informed about what to expect during convalescence, what symptoms to report and to whom, and what to regard as an emergency. Often, a number of physicians in different specialties have attended the client. The client may be confused about which one to call. Review physician names and phone numbers and scheduled appointments, or give directions for scheduling appointments.

The most important fact about discharge is not a set of discharge instructions but the client's departure. Saying good-bye and wishing the client well are aspects of nursing care that, in themselves, promote client well-being. An acknowledged departure provides closure for the client and for the nursing staff and can be personally satisfying to both.

EVALUATING

Evaluation of the discharge process involves reporting to the nurse manager that discharge is completed. A release form (obtained from the business office at the time of discharge) is usually returned to the nurse manager. Details about the discharge (time, who accompanied client, type of transportation) and the client's reaction are recorded on the client's medical record.

Either at the time of discharge or shortly after (through the mail), the client is given the opportunity to evaluate the nursing care and other aspects of hospitalization. Each facility has its own procedure for reviewing and disseminating the information. Generally, though, evaluations are shared with the nursing staff in the form of reports.

Note: The references and resources for all chapters have been compiled at the back of the book.

Chapter Review

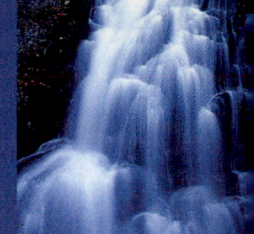

KEY Points

- Nurses can significantly affect how the client views and experiences the admission, transfer, and discharge processes.
- The client's feelings about admission help to determine the success of the hospital stay.
- The LPN/LVN participates in the baseline assessment of the new client.
- Common reactions of newly admitted clients include anxiety, feelings of loss of independence or loss of identity, and, in children, separation anxiety.
- Nurses are responsible for giving culturally sensitive care.
- The Health Insurance Portability and Accountability Act (HIPAA) provides strict guidelines for maintaining client privacy and confidentiality as well as providing for continuation of health insurance from one employer to another.
- The client's belongings and valuables must be properly identified and safely stored.
- Client transfer requires adherence to certain procedures designed to keep the client safe and comfortable during the process.
- Discharge planning and teaching actually begin during the admission process.
- The emphasis of nursing care during the discharge process is to assist the client in understanding the discharge instructions accurately and planning for any problems that may arise.

FOR FURTHER Study

Steps to improve cultural sensitivity are discussed in detail in Chapter 3.

For additional information about legal issues, see Chapter 4.

For more details on the nursing process, see Chapter 6.

For further information about needs as identified by Maslow, see Figure 6-4 and discussion in Chapter 15.

For further study on head-to-toe assessment, see Chapter 19; for vital signs assessment, Chapter 21; and for obtaining urine specimens, Chapter 39.

For more about maintaining the client's integrity and personal dignity, see Chapter 44.

EXPLORE PEARSON **mynursingkit**™

MyNursingKit is your one stop for online chapter review materials and resources. Prepare for success with additional NCLEX®-style practice questions, interactive assignments and activities, web links, animations and videos, and more!

Register your access code from the front of your book at **www.mynursingkit.com**

Critical Thinking Care Map

Caring for a Client Prior to Discharge

NCLEX-PN® Focus Area: Coping and Adaptation

Case Study: Amanda Carr is an 86-year-old client being discharged from the rehabilitation unit to an assisted living center. Two months ago, after a fall, she had a hip replacement. She has been in the medical center's rehab unit since that time. Before surgery, she lived with her two cats in a second-floor apartment with an outdoor metal staircase. Mrs. Carr is scheduled to leave the hospital in 1 week. She is resisting discharge planning and insists she is returning home. "My cats need me, and I can make do."

Nursing Diagnosis: *Ineffective Coping*

COLLECT DATA

Subjective	Objective
_____	_____
_____	_____
_____	_____
_____	_____
_____	_____

Would you report this? Yes/No

If yes, report to: _____

What would you report? _____

Nursing Care

_____
_____
_____
_____
_____
_____
_____
_____
_____

How would you document this? _____
_____
_____
_____

Compare your answers and documentation to those provided on the MyNursingKit Website.

Data Collected
(use only those that apply)

- "My cats need me, and I can make do."
- Daughter says client very independent
- Unsafe environment at home (outdoor entry and metal stairs)
- Chart indicates noncompliance with discharge plan to assisted living facility
- Height 5'9"
- Weight 100 lbs
- Reports "Nurses all mumble."

Nursing Interventions
(use only those that apply; list in priority order)

- Maintain a calm, quiet manner.
- Demonstrate firmness in seeking cooperation.
- Assess level of understanding regarding discharge and transfer.
- Explain purpose of transfer to assisted living.
- Encourage statement of concerns.
- Isolate from other clients.
- Allow time to answer questions about the assisted living facility.
- Inquire about family members who live in the area.

NCLEX-PN® Exam Preparation

1 The nurse is admitting a client to the acute care facility. Which of the following statements, made by the nurse, would help to reduce the two most common responses to hospitalization?

1. "I will explain everything I am going to do before I do it so you will always know what is coming."
2. "You don't have to wear the hospital gown if you're more comfortable in your own pajamas."
3. "Your wife can stay with you if you prefer."
4. "I respect you as an individual."

2 The nurse's understanding of culturally sensitive communication is best illustrated when the nurse:

1. Refers to a Native American as Indian.
2. Addresses clients by their first name.
3. Speaks in a loud but clear voice using simple words.
4. Arranges for an interpreter when the client does not speak English.

3 The nurse is transferring a client in acute respiratory distress to the intensive care unit. The priority nursing action is to:

1. Answer the client's and significant others' questions related to visiting hours in the ICU.
2. Account for all of the client's personal belongings.
3. Give report to the RN in the ICU.
4. Retrieve a portable oxygen tank, place it on the client's bed, and move the client's oxygen delivery system to the portable tank prior to transfer.

4 The nurse participates in admitting a client by:

1. Formulating the nursing diagnosis related to anxiety caused by the admission process.
2. Assessing the client's mental status and applying restraints if they are confused.
3. Collecting baseline subjective and objective data.
4. Developing a treatment plan to ensure the client meets optimal outcomes.

5 A newly admitted adult client in an acute care facility says to the nurse, "Please put my wallet, watch, and rings in the drawer for me." The nurse's best response would be:

1. "I'll put your things in the top drawer right here next to your bed."
2. "Is there a family member with you who could take these things home?"
3. "Valuables all need to be stored in the safe."
4. "I need to inventory and document your personal belongings and then I'll put them away."

6 When discharging a client to home the nurse's responsibility includes: (Select all that apply.)

1. Evaluate client's understanding of self-care at home.
2. Explain the physician's orders including medication teaching for any prescribed medications.
3. Assemble the client's belonging.
4. Assure discharge teaching documentation is completed.
5. Obtain approval from business office for client to be discharged.

7 Which of the following clients would the nurse understand is in particular need of advanced planning for discharge?

1. A 70-year-old male who is being discharged to the skilled unit for rehabilitation
2. A 24-year-old female, living with her husband, who broke her left tibia while skiing.
3. A 38-year-old Spanish speaking female, who is a newly diagnosed diabetic beginning insulin therapy
4. A 64-year-old African American male with a 20-year history of hypertension, controlled by medication

8 The nurse is called into the room of a newly admitted client by the unlicensed assistive personnel (UAP) who has arrived to take the client for diagnostic testing. The UAP reports the client does not have an identification bracelet. The priority nursing action would be to:

1. Call registration to replace the identification band before sending the client for the test.
2. Identify the client for the UAP.
3. Make a new ID band for the client after checking the client's identity using two separate methods.
4. Ask the client for her name, send her for the test so there is no delay in treatment, and replace the identification band when she returns.

9 The nurse is working in a pediatric unit and needs to move a child to another room. After transferring the child, the nurse's most important priority action will be to:

1. Call housekeeping to clean the child's old room.
2. Obtain a high-topped crib to move the child.
3. Obtain a physician's order for the transfer.
4. Notify the child's parents.

10 The nurse receives a phone call from a priest asking if any Catholic clients were admitted today. The nurse's best response would be:

1. "That is private information and I cannot answer your question."
2. "Mr. Jones in room 215 is Catholic and he was admitted this afternoon."
3. "Mr. Jones is a new admission who is Catholic. You should really try to visit him today because he's very anxious about his upcoming heart surgery."
4. "You'll have to call my nursing supervisor to request that information."

Answers and rationales for Review Questions appear in Appendix I.

Thinking Strategically About . . .

Deborah Mason, LPN, has been assigned to work with Laurene Carter, a triage nurse, in the emergency department (ED) of a large metropolitan hospital in the Southwest. Ms. Mason is responsible for conducting an "intake inquiry." This inquiry includes a brief history ("the chief complaint") and taking client vital signs. The information is charted and verbally communicated to Ms. Carter, who determines in which area of the ED clients will be treated and who will escort them there.

There are four clients who have been checked in and are ready to be seen by the triage nurses:

1. José Suarez, age 58, arrives at the ED accompanied by his wife, Mariela. Mr. Suarez is diaphoretic and visibly short of breath. Mr. Suarez reports that he feels like he has influenza, like he did a few years ago, except he does not have a sore throat. Petechiae are visible on his forearms. In broken English, he explains that he picks tomatoes at a small ranch and sells them to families living on the nearby military testing base, as well as to tourists. Mrs. Suarez interrupts him repeatedly in Spanish during the intake inquiry. He gestures impatiently and says, "She wants me to tell you I had to bury four dead sheep last week at the ranch." In recent weeks, there have been three reported cases of anthrax in the state.

2. Avery Johnson, a 17-year-old male, is brought in by his baseball coach. He was hit during a game, sustaining a laceration on his lip. He is bleeding from the lip. His parents are out of town, but his grandfather is on the way to the E.R. and has permission to sign for treatment in the parents' absence.

3. Helen Marlow, an 89-year-old woman, has a history of nausea and vomiting for 2 days. She is accompanied by her daughter and son-in-law. Mrs. Marlow uses a walker; she has low vision and is wearing a long robe and slip-on house shoes.

4. Sean Lee, 18 months, is accompanied by his mother, father, and 3-year-old sibling who wanders around the waiting room. Sean was playing on the bed with his brother when he fell and hit his head. He cried immediately, did not lose consciousness, and does not appear to be in distress.

CRITICAL THINKING

- What is the priority nursing concern for Mr. Suarez?
- What are the special safety concerns for each client?

PRIORITIZING NURSING CARE

The triage nurse asks you to decide the order in which the clients in the waiting room should be moved to an exam room. You have three open rooms. Two rooms are divided from others by a curtain, and the third is an enclosed room with a door. Considering safety and infection control, assign the clients rooms for treatment.

MANAGEMENT OF CARE

All of the clients have been placed in examination rooms. Mrs. Marlow and Mr. Suarez will be admitted. What tasks need to be accomplished for admission and transfer to an inpatient unit?

COLLABORATIVE CARE

Based on information gained from this scenario, what members of the healthcare team might need to be involved in assessment of Mr. Suarez?

CULTURAL CARE STRATEGIES

- What must be done to ensure that Mr. and Mrs. Suarez have the best possible communication with hospital staff?
- What cultural influences are apparent in their case study?

COMPASSIONATE CARE

What interventions might the nurse use to assist Mr. Suarez while he is in the ED?

DELEGATING

Are there any tasks that could be delegated to a UAP? If so, what are they and what follow-up will need to be carried out?

CLIENT TEACHING

Sean Lee and Avery Johnson are being discharged. What client teaching needs to be completed for each of these clients?

DOCUMENTING AND REPORTING

- What documentation needs to be completed on each client?
- Are there any external reporting requirements that need to be completed for any of these clients (e.g., public health, CDC, Child Protective Services)?

Promoting Psychosocial Health

UNIT III

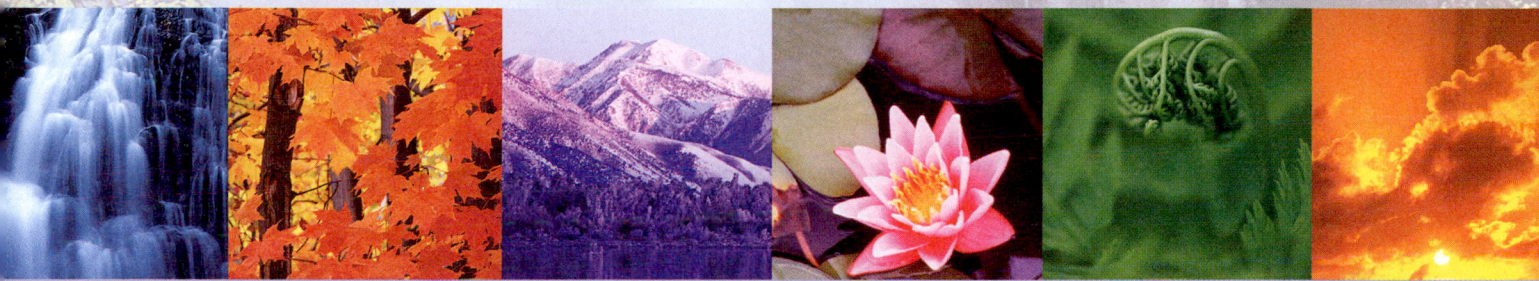

Theorists, Theories, and Therapies

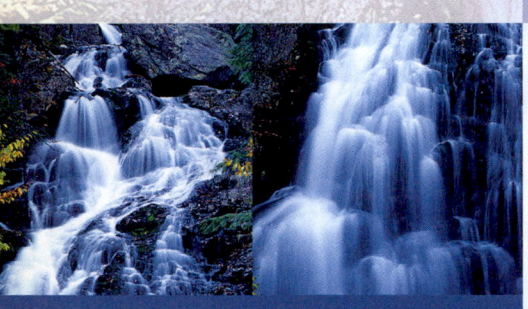

LEARNING Outcomes

After completing this chapter, you will be able to:

1. List Erikson's eight stages of psychosocial development and describe indicators of negative or positive resolution of each stage.
2. Compare and contrast theories of Freud and Erikson.
3. Identify Kohlberg's stages of moral development.
4. Explain Piaget's theory of cognitive development.
5. Describe Maslow's hierarchy of human needs.
6. Describe the key points of various developmental and psychological theories.
7. Identify and contrast several psychological therapies.

Clinical Objectives

8. Provide for clients' psychosocial needs following Maslow's hierarchy.

Individuals come into this world with a number of inborn personality characteristics, and each person's personality develops in stages. LPNs/LVNs provide care for clients at various stages of personality development. So, they need basic information about personality development to meet both **physiologic needs** (needs having to do with physical processes in the human body) and **psychosocial needs** (needs having to do with relationships within oneself and others). No one theorist or theory completely explains human psychic development throughout the life span. It is important to study a number of theorists to reach a clear understanding of why clients behave in certain ways.

THEORISTS AND THEIR THEORIES

Freud's Psychosexual Theory

The concepts of the conscious, subconscious, and unconscious were described by Sigmund Freud in 1924. Through his personal analysis and work, he discovered that an individual is unaware of psychologic processes. The mind, he said, is somewhat like an iceberg: Only a small portion is above the surface and visible. The greater part of an iceberg lies below the surface. Although it is huge, it may not be noticed until a ship unexpectedly collides with it. Then the result is traumatic. The same thing happens with the mind. The individual goes along undisturbed by what lies below the surface until the conscious and subconscious worlds collide.

The *conscious* is the awareness of what is happening at the present moment. It involves the internal environment (thoughts and feelings). It also involves awareness of the external environment. The *subconscious*, sometimes called *preconscious*, consists of an individual's memory. It can be accessed easily and can include things in the past as well as things made for a future date (such as an appointment). The *unconscious* cannot be controlled, and the individual is unaware of it. The unconscious is the core of the individual's psyche. According to Freud, it is made up of many layers of repressed memories and experiences. In addition to the conscious, subconscious, and unconscious, Freud described the psyche as being made of three parts: id, ego, and superego.

The **id** is part of the unconscious. It has been described as the biological and psychologic drives with which an individual enters this world. The id is self-centered and is concerned with immediate gratification. The **ego** connects the psyche with reality and promotes well-being and survival.

The **superego** is concerned with moral behavior. Many people refer to it as the *conscience*. The superego takes into account the rules of society and the individual's personal values. Figure 15-1 ■ illustrates the structures of Freud's theory. According to Freud, the interaction of these components determines human behavior and affects how goals are met. The ability to resolve conflict depends on the mental health status of the individual.

Freud defined personality development in five stages, which are characterized by the source of pleasure at each stage. He felt that personality development began at birth

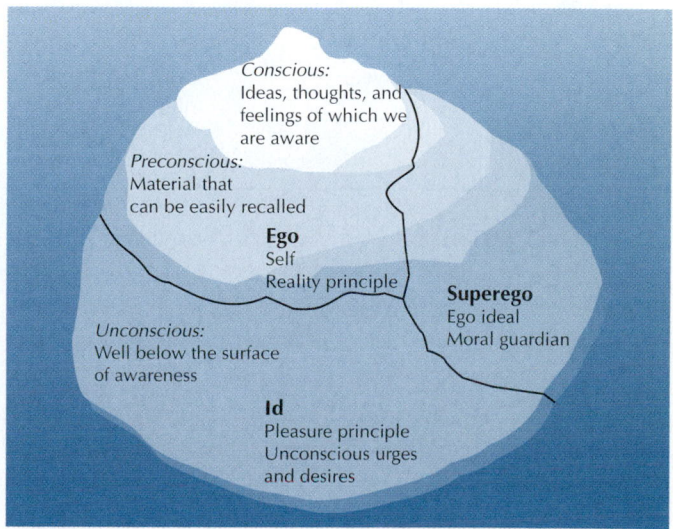

Figure 15-1. ■ The structural relationship formed by the id, ego, and superego. (*Source:* From *Understanding Psychology* [5th ed.], by C. G. Morris and A. A. Maisto, 2001, Upper Saddle River, NJ: Pearson/Prentice Hall. Used with permission.)

and was complete by the end of adolescence. His theory was titled *psychosexual development*. The stages are:

- *Oral stage.* Pleasure is focused on the mouth, lips, and tongue through behaviors such as sucking, tasting, and vocalizing.
- *Anal stage.* This stage coincides with control of urination and defecation. The expulsion of feces brings relief. The child learns to postpone gratification by controlling the sphincter muscles.
- *Phallic stage.* At approximately 3 years of age, the child develops an awareness of the genital area and learns about sexual identity. Masturbation is common during this stage.
- *Latency stage.* The fourth stage is latency. It begins with entrance into school. Freud felt that sexual development was dormant during this stage because psychic energy was devoted to acquiring knowledge.

- *Genital stage.* The final stage of psychosexual development occurs during adolescence. The goal of the genital stage is to develop satisfying relationships with the opposite sex. When the goal has been achieved, Freud felt that development was complete.

Erikson's Psychosocial Development Theory

Erikson described eight stages of development (Table 15-1 ■) spanning life from birth to old age. According to Erikson, the central crisis during infancy (stage 1) is *trust versus mistrust*. Infants depend on their primary caregivers for all physical and psychologic needs. The newborn reacts socially to caregivers by paying attention to the face or voice and by cuddling when held. The child interacts with the environment by responding to various stimuli such as touch and sound.

TABLE 15-1	**Erikson's Eight Stages of Development**			
STAGE	**AGE**	**CENTRAL TASK**	**INDICATORS OF POSITIVE RESOLUTION**	**INDICATORS OF NEGATIVE RESOLUTION**
Infancy	Birth to 18 months	Trust versus mistrust	Learning to trust others	Mistrust, withdrawal, estrangement
Early childhood	18 months to 3 years	Autonomy versus shame and doubt	Self-control without loss of self-esteem Ability to cooperate and to express oneself	Compulsive self-restraint or compliance Willfulness and defiance
Late childhood	3 to 5 years	Initiative versus guilt	Learning the degree to which assertiveness and purpose influence the environment Beginning ability to evaluate one's own behavior	Lack of self-confidence Pessimism, fear of wrong doing Overcontrol and overrestriction of own activity
School age	6 to 12 years	Industry versus inferiority	Beginning to create, develop, and manipulate Developing sense of competence and perseverance	Loss of hope, sense of being mediocre Withdrawal from school and peers
Adolescence	12 to 20 years	Identity versus role confusion	Coherent sense of self Plans to actualize one's abilities	Feelings of confusion, indecisiveness, and possible antisocial behavior
Young adulthood	18 to 25 years	Intimacy versus isolation	Intimate relationship with another person Commitment to work and relationships	Impersonal relationships Avoidance of relationship, career, or lifestyle commitments
Adulthood	25 to 65 years	Generativity versus stagnation	Creativity, productivity, concern for others	Self-indulgence, self-concern, lack of interests and commitments
Maturity	65 years to death	Integrity versus despair	Acceptance of worth and uniqueness of one's own life Acceptance of death	Sense of loss, contempt for others

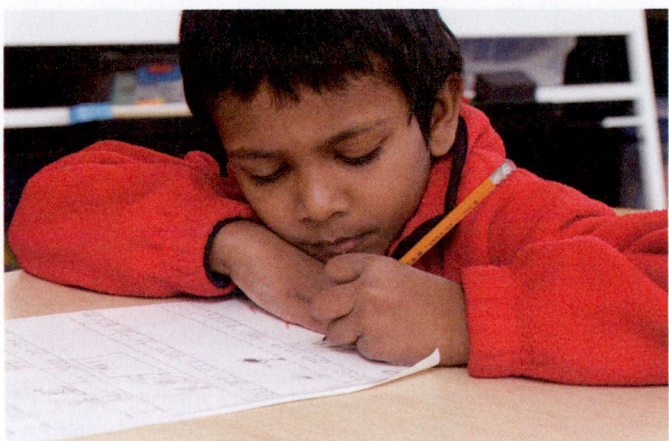

Figure 15-2. ■ School-age children use their increased cognitive skills to learn to accomplish tasks. *Source:* Ellen Senisi.

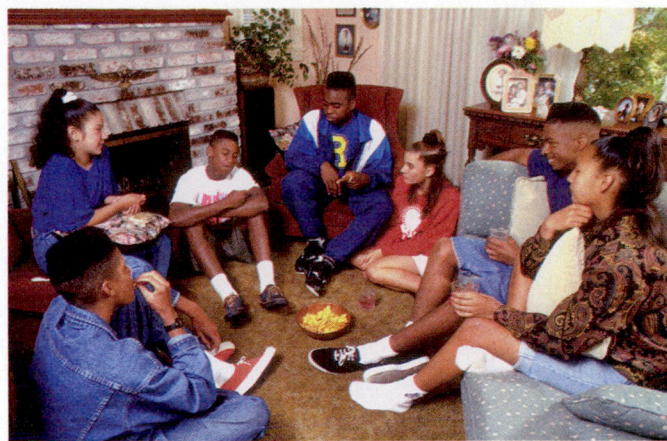

Figure 15-3. ■ Adolescents seem to focus entirely on their peer group but they still do need guidance from adults. *Source:* Lawrence Migdale/Pix.

Toddlers begin to develop their sense of *autonomy* by asserting themselves with frequent use of the word "no." Parents need to have a great deal of patience coupled with an understanding of the importance of this developmental milestone. A toddler whose development is frustrated during this period will develop *shame and doubt*. Erikson writes that the major developmental crisis of the preschooler is *initiative versus guilt*. Parents can enhance the self-concept of preschoolers by providing opportunities for new achievements that children can learn, repeat, and master. At this time children begin to create and develop a sense of competence and perseverance.

School-age children are motivated by activities that provide a sense of worth. They concentrate on mastering skills that will help them function in the adult world (Figure 15-2 ■; see also Table 15-1). Erikson identified this stage as *industry versus inferiority*. It is important for children of this age to feel that the work they have produced is worthwhile. Parents should be encouraged to reinforce or assist with school projects, but not to do projects for their children.

The psychosocial task of the adolescent is the establishment of *identity*. The danger of this stage is *role confusion*. Because of the adolescent's dramatic body changes, it is hard to develop a stable identity. Adolescents who are accepted, loved, and valued by family and peers generally tend to gain confidence and feel good about themselves. Adolescents who have difficulty forming relationships may develop poor self-image. Those who are perceived by peers as too different and who are not included in adolescent cliques may have low self-esteem. Adolescents still need guidance from their parents, although they appear to neither want nor need it. Their primary focus is on their peers (Figure 15-3 ■). The task of self-discovery is difficult for many young people. As they try out roles, it may also be a difficult time for their parents.

Young adults face a number of new experiences and changes in lifestyle as they progress toward maturity. Erikson called this stage *intimacy versus isolation*. Remaining single is becoming the lifestyle of more and more young adults. Many singles pursue an education and then take time to pursue their chosen vocations. Even so, it is important for the young adult to develop the ego strength of love. If the individual's development is not accomplished during this time period, he or she is in danger of becoming emotionally isolated.

Erikson views the developmental choice of the middle-aged adult as *generativity versus stagnation*. This is the time period when adults' development is focused on the transfer of skills, culture, and family heritage from their generation to the next. Failure to do so may result in stagnation of development.

According to Erikson, the developmental task during old age is *ego integrity versus despair* (see Table 15-1). People who attain ego integrity view life with a sense of wholeness. They derive satisfaction from past accomplishments. They view death as an acceptable completion of life. By contrast, people who despair often believe they have made poor choices during life and wish they could live life over.

In 1997 Joan Erikson (Erik Erikson's wife) published an expanded edition of her husband's theory and identified a ninth stage. This stage described the response of the older, more frail adult who has entered the eighth or ninth decade. Eyesight and hearing are not acute as they once were. Loss of capacities and disintegration may demand almost all of one's attention. "There is much sorrow to cope with plus a clear announcement that death's door is open and not so far away" (Erikson & Erikson, 1997, p. 105).

Kohlberg's Moral Development Theory

Lawrence Kohlberg began working on his theory of moral development during the 1970s (Table 15-2 ■). The theory looks at how individuals make decisions about **moral**

TABLE 15-2	Kohlberg's Stages of Moral Development	
LEVEL AND STAGE	**DEFINITION**	**EXAMPLE**
Level I: Preconventional Stage 1: Punishment and obedience orientation Stage 2: Instrumental-relativist orientation	The activity is wrong if one is punished, and the activity is right if one is not punished.	A nurse follows a physician's order so as not to be fired. A client in hospital agrees to stay in bed if the nurse will buy the client a newspaper.
Level II: Conventional Stage 3: Interpersonal concordance (good boy, nice girl) Stage 4: Law and order orientation	Action is taken to satisfy one's needs. Action is taken to please another and gain approval. Right behavior is obeying the law and following the rules.	A nurse gives elderly clients in hospital sedatives at bedtime because the night nurse wants all clients to sleep at night. A nurse does not permit a worried client to phone home because hospital rules stipulate no phone calls after 9:00 P.M.
Level III: Postconventional Stage 5: Social contract, legalistic orientation Stage 6: Universal-ethical principles	Standard of behavior is based on adhering to laws that protect the welfare and rights of others. Personal values and opinions are recognized, and violating the rights of others is avoided. Universal moral principles are internalized. Person respects other humans and believes that relationships are based on mutual trust.	A nurse arranges for an East Indian client to have privacy for prayer each evening. A nurse becomes an advocate for a hospitalized client by reporting to the nursing supervisor a conversation in which a physician threatened to withhold assistance unless the client agreed to surgery.

Source: Adapted from R. Duska and M. Whelan, *Moral Development: A Guide to Piaget and Kohlberg.* Copyright © 1975 by The Missionary Society of St. Paul the Apostle in the State of New York. Used by permission of Paulist Press.

conduct (conduct related to judgment of right and wrong). As individuals progress through the six stages, they develop ethical behavior. Kohlberg believed that the six identifiable stages could be more generally classified into three levels: preconventional, conventional, and postconventional.

Infants associate right and wrong with pleasure and pain. What gives them pleasure is right, since they are too young to reason otherwise. During the second year of life, children begin to know that some activities elicit affection and approval. Children can easily tell by changes in parental expression and voice tones whether their behavior is approved of or not. These early years are sometimes referred to as *premoral*.

The first level of moral thinking is found at the elementary school level. In the first stage of this level, children behave according to socially acceptable norms because they are told to do so. Authority figures (e.g., parent or teacher) compel obedience by threat of punishment. The second stage of this level is characterized by a view that right behavior means acting in one's own best interests.

The second level of moral thinking was named *conventional* by Kohlberg since this is the type of moral reasoning generally found in society. The first stage of the conventional level (stage 3) is characterized by an attitude that seeks to do what will gain the approval of others. The second stage is one oriented to abiding by the law and responding to the obligations of duty.

Kohlberg felt that a majority of adults never reach the postconventional stage, the third level of moral thinking

(see Table 15-2). Its first stage (stage 5) is an understanding of social mutuality and a genuine interest in the welfare of others. The last stage (stage 6) is based on respect for universal principles and the demands of individual conscience. While Kohlberg always believed in the existence of stage 6, the limited number of subjects who had achieved this level of reasoning made it virtually impossible to define or study over time. Kohlberg believed that individuals could only progress through these stages one stage at a time. They could not "jump" stages. They could only understand the moral rationale one stage above their own. Thus, according to Kohlberg, it was important to present them with moral dilemmas for discussion. These would help them to see the reasonableness of a "higher stage" morality and encourage their development in that direction. Kohlberg believed, as did Piaget, that most moral development occurs through social interaction.

Piaget's Cognitive Development Theory

Jean Piaget, a Swiss biologist and psychologist, constructed a model of child development and learning (Table 15-3 ■). It is based on the idea that the developing child builds cognitive structures, called *schemes*. These schemes are a mechanism for understanding and responding to physical experiences in one's environment. Piaget stated that a child's cognitive structure becomes more sophisticated at each

TABLE 15-3	Piaget's Phases of Cognitive Development	
PHASES	**AGE**	**SIGNIFICANT BEHAVIOR**
Sensorimotor phase	Birth to 2 years	At birth most action is reflexive. During the first 4 months, perception of events is centered on the body, and objects are an extension of self. From 4 to 8 months, the child acknowledges the external environment and actively makes changes in it. The infant gradually learns what goals are, how to obtain them, and how to find new goals. Rituals become important. Between 18 and 24 months, the child can interpret the environment and use make-believe and pretend play.
Preoperational phase (includes preconceptual phase—2 to 4 years, and intuitive thought phase—4 to 7 years)	2 to 7 years	The child uses an egocentric approach to the environment. Everything is significant as it relates to "me." The child explores the environment, develops language rapidly, and associates words first with objects, and then with thoughts. In the latter half of this phase, egocentric thinking decreases and the child begins to include others. The child thinks of one idea at a time.
Concrete operations phase	7 to 11 years	The child solves concrete problems and begins to understand relationships such as size and direction (right and left). The child can recognize different viewpoints.
Formal operations phase	11 to 15 years	The child uses rational thinking. Reasoning is deductive and futuristic.

Source: Adapted from *The Origin of Intelligence in Children,* by J. Piaget, 1966. International Universities Press, Inc. Copyright © 1966. Used by permission.

stage of growth and development. Individuals begin with a few inborn reflexes (crying and sucking), and progress to highly complex mental activities.

The theory of cognitive development is identified by four phases:

1. *Sensorimotor phase (birth to 2 years old).* Through physical interaction with the environment, the child develops concepts about reality and how it works. The child begins to learn that objects out of sight continue to exist (*object permanence*).

2. *Preoperational phase (ages 2 to 7).* The child thinks in concrete physical terms.

3. *Concrete operations phase (ages 7 to 11).* As physical experiences accumulate, the child starts to conceptualize, creating logical structures that explain the experiences. Abstract problem solving, such as arithmetic equations, can now be solved with numbers, not just with objects.

4. *Formal operations phase (beginning at ages 11 to 15).* By this point, the child's cognitive structures are like those of an adult and include conceptual reasoning.

During all developmental stages, the child experiences the environment using whatever mental maps and schemes he or she has constructed so far. Piaget outlined several principles for building cognitive structures. If the experience is repeated, it fits easily (*is assimilated*) into the cognitive structure so that the child maintains mental "equilibrium." If the experience is different or new, the child loses equilibrium and alters the cognitive structure to include the new conditions. In this way, the child gradually creates more complex cognitive structures. Cognitive structures are

completed during the formal operations period, from roughly 11 to 15 years (see Table 15-3).

Maslow's Hierarchy of Basic Human Needs

Abraham Maslow published his theory of human motivation in 1943. He believed that **actualization** (turning an idea into fact or action) was the driving force behind human personality. He established a hierarchy of human needs that has five levels (see Figure 6-4 ⭕):

1. *Physiologic:* hunger, thirst, shelter, sex, etc.
2. *Safety:* security, protection from physical and emotional harm
3. *Social:* affection, belonging, acceptance, friendship
4. **Esteem** *(also called ego):* Internal esteem includes self-respect, autonomy, and achievement; external esteem includes status, recognition, and attention
5. **Self-actualization:** doing things of one's choice, bringing ideas into action

Self-actualization is the highest drive. However, a person must first satisfy other, lower motivations such as hunger, safety, and belonging.

Maslow points out that the hierarchy is dynamic. In other words, the dominant need is always shifting. For example, a musician may be lost in the self-actualization of playing music. Eventually he or she becomes tired and hungry and so has to stop. Also, a single behavior may combine several levels. (Eating dinner can meet both physiologic and social needs.) The hierarchy does not exist by itself. It is affected by the situation and the general culture. Satisfaction is relative. An unsatisfied need is very important. In contrast, a satisfied need no longer motivates. For example, a hungry man feels desperate for food. Once he has had his fill, the promise of food no longer motivates him.

Maslow's hierarchy can be related to the life cycle. A newborn baby's needs are almost entirely physiologic. As the baby grows, it needs safety, then love. Toddlers are eager for social interaction. Teenagers are anxious about social needs. Young adults are concerned with esteem. Only more mature people transcend the first four levels to spend much time self-actualizing.

Other Theorists

FOWLER'S SPIRITUAL DEVELOPMENT THEORY

Fowler theorized six stages of **spiritual** development (development having to do with God or a higher power). Table 15-4 ■ lists a brief sketch of his theory. He called the toddler's stage of spiritual development *undifferentiated*. Toddlers may be aware of some religious practices. However, they are primarily involved in learning knowledge and emotional reactions. A toddler repeats prayers and conforms to a religious ritual because of the praise and affection that result.

In the *intuitive-projective* stage, many preschool children are enrolled in Sunday School or faith-oriented classes. The preschooler usually enjoys the social interaction of these classes (see Table 15-4). Faith at this stage is primarily a result of teaching by significant others, such as parents or teachers.

According to Fowler, the school-age child reaches stage 2 in spiritual development, the *mythic-literal* stage. Children learn to distinguish fantasy from fact. Spiritual facts are those beliefs that are accepted by a religious group. Parents and the minister, rabbi, or priest help the child distinguish fact from fantasy. They still influence the child more than peers in spiritual matters.

School-age children may ask many questions about God and religion in these years and will generally believe that God is good and always present to help. Just before puberty, children become aware that their prayers are not always answered and become disappointed.

The adolescent or young adult reaches Fowler's third stage of spiritual development: the *synthetic-conventional* stage. Adolescents become aware of differences among religions. Often, the adolescent believes that various religious beliefs and practices have more similarities than differences. The adolescent may reconcile differences in one of the following ways:

- Deciding any differences are wrong
- Compartmentalizing the differences (For example, a friend may not be able to go to dances on Friday evenings because of religious observances, but the friend can share activities on other days.)
- Obtaining advice from a significant other, such as a parent or a minister

According to Fowler, the individual enters the *individuating-reflexive* period sometime after 18 years of age (see Table 15-4). Not all adults progress through Fowler's stages to the fifth, called the *paradoxical-consolidative* stage. At this stage, the individual can view "truth" from a number of viewpoints. In middle age, people tend to be less dogmatic about religious beliefs. People in this age group often rely on spiritual beliefs to help them deal with illness, death, and tragedy.

TABLE 15-4	Fowler's Stages of Spiritual Development	
STAGE	**AGE**	**DESCRIPTION**
0. Undifferentiated	0 to 3 years	Infant unable to formulate concepts about self or the environment.
1. Intuitive-projective	4 to 6 years	A combination of images and beliefs given by trusted others, mixed with the child's own experience and imagination.
2. Mythic-literal	7 to 12 years	Private world of fantasy and wonder; symbols refer to something specific; dramatic stories and myths used to communicate spiritual meanings.
3. Synthetic-conventional	Adolescent or adult	World and ultimate environment structured by the expectations and judgments of others; interpersonal focus.
4. Individuating-reflexive	After 18 years	Constructing one's own explicit system; high degree of self-consciousness.
5. Paradoxical-consolidative	After 30 years	Awareness of truth from a variety of viewpoints.
6. Universalizing	Maybe never	Becoming an incarnation of the principles of love and justice.

Source: Data from *Life Maps: Conversations in the Journey of Faith*, by J. Fowler and S. Keen, 1985, Waco, TX: Word Books; *How to Help Your Child Have a Spiritual Life: A Parents' Guide to Inner Development*, by A. Hollander, 1980, New York: A and W Publishers; and A. M. Josephson and M. L. Dell (2004), Religion and spirituality in child and adolescent psychiatry: A new frontier, *Child Adolesc. Psychiatr. Clin. N. Am., 13*(1), 1–15.

BOX 15-1   CULTURAL PULSE POINTS

Adolescence in Different Cultures

Adolescence has a great significance in many cultures. Currently, in middle-class America, the term *vestibule adolescence* describes the period between age 18 and the mid-20s. This term refers to a delayed rite of passage from childhood to adult. The increased financial dependence on parents due to the costs of advanced education and the expense of living on their own are reasons for this delay. Other cultures view adolescence much differently. Here are a few examples:

- Young people from the Amish culture are encouraged to work away from home to gain experience, but wages are sent home. There is a period of tolerance for Amish young people to experiment with non-Amish dress and behavior. When this time is over, the Amish young adult is expected to be baptized, marry, and return to the discipline of the church.

- Arab adolescents are expected to remain within the family system. Family interests and opinions have great influence on marriage and choice of career. Adolescents strive to succeed in school because professional careers are closely connected to social status. Behavior that would bring dishonor to family is avoided.

- Mexican American children are highly valued. Adolescents and young adults are discouraged from leaving home. It is very difficult for a young woman to be independent from her family. Continuation of the family and culture is the ultimate goal.

- Navajo American females have an important ceremonial ritual that coincides with the onset of menarche. This is celebrated with special food and marks the entrance to adulthood. Men are excluded from this celebration. Other Native American tribes have rite of passage ceremonies for males, but the Navajos do not.

- Among Vietnamese Americans, respect for elders is a strong characteristic. The adolescent would avoid any activity that would bring dishonor to the family. Assimilation into the American educational system and society can cause conflict with Vietnamese parents.

Often, the older person's knowledge becomes wisdom, an inner resource for dealing with both positive and negative life experiences. Many older people have strong religious convictions and continue to attend religious meetings or services. Involvement in religion often helps the older adult to resolve issues related to the meaning of life, to adversity, or to good fortune. The "old-old" person who cannot attend formal services often continues religious participation in a more private manner. According to Fowler, some people enter the sixth stage of spiritual development, *universalizing*.

BOWLBY'S ATTACHMENT THEORY

John Bowlby served as a clinician, teacher, and researcher. He concentrated on child and family psychiatry, especially the effects of parents on children. Bowlby had a significant effect in the area of attachment relations and the social-emotional development of the young child. His 1952 report led to extensive changes in how children were treated in hospitals and institutions. He also emphasized the importance of the mother–child relationship.

Bowlby's theory describes the importance of healthy, secure, sustaining attachments in human development. According to Bowlby, when the caregiver nurtures attachment behaviors, the child develops a sense of security. With that security, the child can explore the world and develop a positive sense of self. The child who has rejecting or ambivalent caregivers is likely to develop insecurity.

When they are distressed or threatened, infants demonstrate attachment behaviors, such as seeking and clinging to the mother. With secure attachments, the mother can calm her infant and lessen the sense of external threat by her presence. As the child's relationship with the mother develops into a secure base, that child will be able to explore the environment, knowing that the mother will be available in case of danger.

CULTURAL ISSUES

The study of development must take culture into account. Cultural diversity can result in lifestyles and values that influence development. Box 15-1 ■ provides some cultural perspectives on adolescence.

THERAPIES

Psychoanalysis

Sigmund Freud developed psychoanalytic theory. Psychoanalysis is the classic form of psychotherapy. It involves the interpretation of thoughts and dreams. Freud was very interested in the effect of early childhood. He felt that all problems could be related to a person's early developmental years. With the introduction of psychotropic drugs in the 1950s, the practice of long-term analysis has declined. Although Freudian psychology has been joined by many other theories, some aspects of it are still used by many psychiatrists and counselors.

Behavior Modification

B. F. Skinner developed behavior modification or behavioral theory. He felt that behavior should be studied, that it was important to understand why a person behaves in certain ways. Skinner thought that a person's behavior could be controlled by rewards and punishments. He used the term *reinforcement* for rewards and *consequences* for punishments. Desired behaviors are reinforced so that they will continue. Undesirable behaviors are not rewarded, so they will not re-cur. Behavioral therapy is particularly useful in the field of education and in mental health nursing. Behavioral modifi-cation is frequently used with addictive disorders such as smoking. Behavioral theory helps the client and the nurse identify what is gained by continuing an inappropriate or harmful behavior. The theory is that individuals would not continue a behavior if there were no benefit associated with it. (This benefit is known as *secondary gain*.)

Cognitive Therapies

A number of theorists provided input into the development of cognitive theory and therapies. Piaget was mentioned earlier in the chapter. Aaron Beck added perspective about how individuals viewed themselves or their worlds.

Cognitive theory looks at distortion of thought as the cause of psychologic distress. For example, in the case of depression clients frequently have automatic negative thoughts. They respond negatively to stimuli that others might experience as positive. If a supervisor asks, "Why is this project running over budget?" a person with depression might think, "Nothing I do is right." A person who does not suffer from depression might think, "Let me go back through the records and find out what happened. Maybe I can set it up better next time."

The task of cognitive behavioral therapy (CBT) is partly to understand how emotions, behaviors, and thoughts in-terrelate. It also examines how these three components may be influenced by external stimuli, including early life events. CBT aims to help the client:

1. Become aware of thought distortions that are causing distress.
2. Become aware of behavioral patterns that reinforce the thought distortion.
3. Correct the thought distortion and the behavior. The objective is not to correct every distortion in a client's entire outlook, just those that may be at the root of distress.

Because of the interrelationship between thoughts, feelings, and behaviors, therapeutic interventions frequently involve the client's behavior. For instance, a client with a strong fear that a neighbor's dog might attack him if he walks past the neighbor's yard will go to great lengths to avoid that area of the street. This behavior prevents the client from learning whether the dog would actually attack or not. The therapist may help the client overcome this avoidance of the neigh-bor's yard. Walking past the yard is part of the process of correcting the distorted thought that doing so will result in injury. The goal of cognitive therapy is control of the nega-tive thoughts that trigger distress.

Person-Centered Therapies

Carl Rogers was the most influential psychologist in American history. He was the first to offer an alternative to psychiatry and psychoanalysis and the first to record and publish ther-apy sessions.

Rogers constantly reflected on his professional and personal life experiences, on the client–therapist relationship, and on the process of therapy. He felt that all individuals have the ability to guide their own lives in a manner that is personally satisfying and socially constructive. In the therapeutic help-ing relationship, individuals are free to find their inner wis-dom and confidence, which allows them to make increasingly healthier and more constructive choices. Rogers believed and trusted that human beings have within themselves vast resources for self-understanding and for altering their self-concepts, basic attitudes, and self-directed behavior. Rogers's goal for therapy was to move the individual toward matu-rity. Rogers believed that if a person were fully accepted for who he is, he could not help but change. The maturing process leads to positive choices and increased capacity for problem solving. Rogers believed that three characteristics were necessary to a supportive climate:

- Genuineness
- Unconditional positive regard
- Empathetic understanding

Rogers perfected the art of active listening. He made use of many therapeutic communication techniques. These included silences, minimal encouragement ("go on," "Ummm," "Uh-huh"), reflection, and *parroting* (repeating words exactly). These techniques can be used in therapeutic relationships between nurses and their clients (see Chapter 11 👓). With practice the nurse can use them proficiently and feel comfort-able with their use.

Nursing Responsibilities

Generally, LPNs/LVNs will work in nonpsychiatric set-tings. However, you may be called on to care for a client with a psychiatric disorder who is admitted to the hospi-tal with an acute physical illness. You will surely en-counter clients who exhibit stress or anxiety related to serious illness or hospitalization. It is the nurse's responsibility to establish a therapeutic relationship with clients and to provide interventions that treat the client holistically. The mind can have a significant effect on the body and response to illness. See Chapter 17 🔗 more information on psychosocial nursing issues and Chapter 49 🔗 for a discussion of caring for clients with mental disorders.

LPNs and LVNs use a variety of personality and psychologic theories. For example, they may implement Hildegard Peplau's theory, which described nursing as a therapeutic interpersonal process. Peplau identified communication growth and development and roles as major concepts of her theory. Following her theory, the nurse would identify the client's developmental stage in order to provide appropriate, holistic care. Also, the use of theories such as Maslow's hierarchy helps the nurse understand the importance of meeting basic physiologic needs. (A client who is unable to sleep will show little interest in attending a support group.)

NURSING CARE

PRIORITIZING NURSING CARE

Prioritizing nursing care involves consideration of the client's developmental level. The client's physical recovery may be dependent on the positive resolution of developmental tasks. Clients may regress to an earlier developmental level when experiencing a crisis such as illness or hospitalization. During the assessment process the nurse needs to be observant for behaviors that may indicate regression. Stages of development are not only important when caring for children. They are also important for clients continuing to move through the life span.

Meeting client needs is the most important consideration in nursing care. Maslow's hierarchy of human needs provides a template for delivery of nursing care. Clients must have their basic needs met before they can achieve the next level. For example, basic needs such as food and oxygen are necessary before the client can achieve safety and security.

ASSESSING

During the process of personality development, traits are established in the individual that permit interaction with the environment. Self-confidence, self-worth, and an ability to relate to others are a result of positive traits. If the individual is inflexible, manipulative, or hostile, these may be signs and symptoms of personality disorders. A psychosocial assessment (see Chapter 17 🔗) takes into account both the present condition of the client and the client's history (including family history; clients with mental health issues must be treated in the context of their family and their environment).

DIAGNOSING, PLANNING, AND IMPLEMENTING

The Diagnostic and Statistical Manual of Mental Disorders, 4th edition, text revision (2000), is used to group personality disorders into descriptive categories. (See discussion of mental disorders in Chapter 49 🔗.) In addition, some of the NANDA nursing diagnoses are specifically used for clients with mental health issues. Some of these are:

- *Acute Confusion*
- *Anxiety*
- *Decisional Conflict*
- *Disturbed Sleep Pattern*
- *Disturbed Body Image*
- *Ineffective Coping*
- *Impaired Social Interaction*
- *Ineffective Coping*
- *Noncompliance*

Planning involves identifying priorities. A threat to clients' self-esteem, dignity, or life is considered urgent. It is important for the nurse to identify whether problems affect normal development or an inability to meet Maslow's hierarchy of needs.

clinical ALERT

When treating clients with mental health or personality development issues, nursing implementations are much less physical than for clients with physical illness. Probably the most frequently used intervention is to establish or maintain a therapeutic environment. More discussion is provided in Chapter 11 🔗.

EVALUATING

Evaluation focuses on the client's present status and progress toward achievement of goals. A special consideration when evaluating clients with personality disorders is termination of the therapeutic relationship. This must be a gradual process. It can be compared to beginning discharge planning on admission for clients hospitalized with acute illnesses. In a similar way, termination of the therapeutic relationship must be introduced to the client early on. The client needs to know that once goals are accomplished, he or she will function within the environment without the nurse's intervention.

NURSING PROCESS CARE PLAN
Client with a Personality Disorder

James, a 70-year-old male, was admitted to the hospital complaining of heart palpitations. He has been employed by the Collins Company for 38 years. The company has just been acquired by another company. The rumor in the office is that some employees of the Collins Company will be forced into retirement.

Assessment

Personal strengths: Alert and oriented ×4; intact support system—family. No acute medical problems. Weaknesses: suspicious; angry; c/o work-related anxiety. Client states: "They are all talking about who is going to be forced to retire. I know it will be me, because they can replace me with someone who makes less money." "I heard them talking when they think no one is listening." Admits to waking frequently throughout the night, and experiences palpitations throughout the workday.

Nursing Diagnosis

The following important nursing diagnoses (among others) are established for this client:

- *Anxiety* r/t work uncertainties
- *Disturbed Personal Identity*
- *Disturbed Sleep Pattern*

Expected Outcomes

The expected outcomes are that James:

- Will demonstrate anxiety control as evidenced by a decrease in heart palpitations during workday.
- Will recognize that others do not see his beliefs as real.
- Will verbalize plan to implement bedtime routines.
- Will awaken refreshed and not be fatigued during the day.

Planning and Implementation

After ruling out physical causes of heart palpitations, the following interventions are planned and implemented for James:

- Determine current level of anxiety.
- Ask about client's sleep pattern and usual bedtime rituals.
- Note any changes in mental status.

- Observe for causes of altered thought processes.
- Focus discussion on the underlying feeling, rather than on the content of delusions.
- Encourage client to write feelings and conversations in a journal related to changes at work.

Evaluation

On a follow-up visit, physical manifestations of anxiety have decreased. James reports two episodes of heart palpitations during past week. One occurred during a meeting with the new owners, and one during lunch when coworkers were discussing the merger. James reports that he is relaxing and reading non-work-related material prior to bedtime. Regular bedtime has been maintained nightly ×1 week. Client recorded three conversations related to merger in his journal. He states that when he reread them, he was able to realize that they were not specific references to him.

Critical Thinking in the Nursing Process

1. Disturbed thought processes may be related to delusions or auditory hallucinations. Describe how you think the nurse should interact with a client experiencing delusions or hallucinations.
2. Why is it important to do a complete physical assessment in conjunction with a psychosocial assessment for a client who is experiencing physical symptoms related to a personality disorder?
3. Describe a therapeutic relationship that is appropriate for a client with a personality disorder.

Note: Discussion of Critical Thinking questions appears on the MyNursingKit Website.

Note: The references and resources for all chapters have been compiled at the back of the book.

Chapter Review

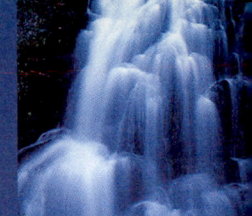

KEY Points

- Freud's psychosexual theory, which describes the oral, anal, phallic, latency, and genital stages of development, developed the idea that much of what we choose to do is governed by unconscious drives and impulses. Erikson's psychosocial theory does not have sexuality as a core motivator. He described eight stages of life and developmental tasks, with possible positive and negative outcomes for each stage.

- Kohlberg's stages of moral development are the preconventional, the conventional, and the postconventional.

- Piaget's theory of cognitive development describes mechanisms (schemes) for understanding and responding to experiences. These schemes become more sophisticated as a child goes through each phase of development, including sensorimotor, preoperational, concrete operations, and formal operations.

- Maslow's hierarchy of human needs identifies self-actualization as the driving force behind human personality. His hierarchy of human needs is illustrated as a pyramid with physiologic needs at the bottom and self-actualization at the top.

- Psychoanalysis, Freud's classic form of psychotherapy, centers on interpretation of thoughts and dreams, and the effects of early childhood. Skinner's behavior modification model is based on the idea that behavior can be controlled by rewards and punishments. Cognitive therapies identify distortion of thought as the cause of psychologic distress. Rogers' person-centered therapy relies on the client finding an inner wisdom and confidence to make better choices.

- Developmental theories provide information to help the healthcare professional understand what is taking place.

- Knowledge of developmental stages can help nurses plan appropriate interventions.

- Health promotion activities by the nurse assist the client to meet developmental milestones.

∞ FOR FURTHER Study

Maslow's hierarchy is illustrated as Figure 6-4.

For more on therapeutic relationships between nurses and their clients, see Chapter 11.

See Chapter 17 for more information on psychosocial nursing issues and psychosocial assessments.

See Chapter 49 for a discussion of caring for clients with mental disorders.

Critical Thinking Care Map

Caring for a Client with an Amputation
NCLEX-PN® Focus Area: Safety

Case Study: Craig is a 20-year-old male college student who was involved in an automobile accident 3 days ago, suffering a traumatic amputation of his left lower leg. Craig's mother has remained with him since the accident and is very supportive. His father is grief stricken and having difficulty dealing with Craig's condition, because Craig was captain of his college basketball team and had hopes of becoming a professional basketball player. Craig's condition is stable and he is being placed into a rehabilitation program immediately. Soon, he will be fitted for a leg prosthesis. Usually an outgoing individual, Craig is somber and untalkative. He does not look at his leg when dressings are being changed and he refuses to discuss his rehabilitation program.

Nursing Diagnosis: *Situational Low Self-Esteem*

COLLECT DATA

Subjective	Objective
_____	_____
_____	_____
_____	_____
_____	_____
_____	_____
_____	_____

Would you report this? Yes/No

If yes, report to: _____

What would you report? _____

Nursing Care

_____
_____
_____
_____
_____
_____
_____
_____

How would you document this? _____
_____
_____
_____

Compare your answers and documentation to those provided on the MyNursingKit Website.

Data Collected
(use only those that apply)

- Somber and untalkative
- 20-year-old male student
- Refuses to discuss rehabilitation
- Automobile accident 3 days ago
- Father is grief stricken and having difficulty dealing with Craig's condition because of traumatic amputation of his left lower leg
- Condition is stable
- Mother at bedside
- Captain of his college basketball team, shared aspirations of becoming a professional basketball player
- To be fitted for a leg prosthesis
- Usually an outgoing individual
- Does not look at his leg when dressings are being changed
- Rehabilitation program to begin immediately
- Mother very supportive

Nursing Interventions
(use only those that apply; list in priority order)

- Actively listen to, demonstrate respect for, and accept the client.
- Encourage client to get up and use crutches within 2 days.
- Assess for intergenerational family problems that can overwhelm coping abilities.
- Assess client for anger and identify previous outlets for anger.
- Have client list strengths.
- Encourage client to reminisce about basketball.
- Accept client's own pace in working through grief and crisis situation.
- Assess the strengths and deficiencies of the family system.
- Talk to family about the importance of sharing feelings and ways to do so.
- Note other stressors in the family.
- Assess for unhealthy coping mechanisms such as substance abuse.
- Provide information about support groups.
- Assess client's support system.

NCLEX-PN® Exam Preparation

1 The student nurse asks the instructor, "What is the difference between Freud's theory and Erikson's theory?" The instructor's best response would be:

1. "Freud looks at development from a psychosexual perspective while Erikson approaches development from a psychosocial perspective."
2. "Freud theorized that development occurred in a random and nonpredictable manner while Erikson theorized that development occurred in a prescribed sequence."
3. "Both Freud and Erikson believed that development occurred throughout childhood and ended in the late teens when the individual was fully developed."
4. "Freud's theory has 4 stages of development while Erikson's theory has 6 stages."

2 The nurse is caring for a 2-year-old child who requires the insertion of a nasogastric tube. In consideration of the child's development, a priority action for the nurse to perform before beginning the procedure is to:

1. Allow the child to examine and play with a similar tube.
2. Ask the child's permission to insert the tube.
3. Show the child a teddy bear or doll with the tube in place.
4. Tell the child she must hold still during insertion of the tube.

3 The nurse is caring for a 10-year-old boy with cystic fibrosis who has experienced numerous hospital admissions. The child wants to catch up on his homework and asks the nurse if he can call a classmate to drop off his assignments. The nurse agrees in order to help him achieve which of the following appropriate goals for his age?

1. Autonomy
2. Industry
3. Identity
4. Ego integrity

4 The nurse has been assigned to care for an elderly client who is scheduled for surgery in the morning. The client is anxious, cannot sleep, and wishes to phone a family member. Because the hospital rules stipulate no phone calls after 9 P.M., the nurse will not allow the client to make the call. These actions demonstrate which stage of moral development according to Kohlberg?

1. Stage 1: Punishment and obedience orientation
2. Stage 3: Interpersonal concordance
3. Stage 4: Law and order orientation
4. Stage 6: Universal-ethical principles

5 An adult who relies on spiritual beliefs to help her deal with illness, death, or tragedy is progressing to which stage of spiritual development according to Fowler?

1. Intuitive-projective
2. Mythical-literal
3. Synthetic-conventional
4. Paradoxical-consolidative

6 The nurse is caring for a retired 75-year-old woman who reports working daily on a book of poetry. The nurse identifies that this client is satisfying what level of need, according to Maslow?

1. Social level, because she can increase her friendships by giving poems as gifts
2. Ego integrity level, because she has always wanted to do this
3. Self-actualization level, because she has chosen this task and is making it happen
4. Esteem level, because she will be recognized for her achievement

7 The nurse, preparing to initiate IV therapy for a 4-year-old child, says, "Don't worry. I can get this started with one stick." How would this child interpret the nurse's statement using Piaget's theory of cognitive development?

1. The nurse will get the IV started using only one catheter so he or she will only be poked once.
2. The nurse is very skilled in initiating IV therapy.
3. The nurse is only going to require one branch from a tree but the child is not quite sure what the nurse is going to do with this stick.
4. The nurse is going to hurt him or her.

8 The nurse is using behavioral therapy to help a client. The nurse would avoid which of the following techniques?

1. Reinforcement of desired behavior.
2. Contracts about expectations for behavior.
3. Listing consequences for undesired behavior.
4. Negative reinforcement.

9 The nurse, creating a therapeutic environment according to Rogers, does which of the following?

1. Agrees with everything the client says.
2. Displays genuine concern for the client's needs.
3. Smiles and tells clients how well they are doing at every opportunity.
4. Nods and says "Yes?" or "Really?" to indicate they are listening even when their mind is on something else.

10 When providing care for clients with personality or mental disorders, the nurse should:

1. Use a direct and businesslike approach.
2. Collect physical data using a remote approach.
3. Apply restraints if the client appears agitated.
4. Play background music to distract and soothe the client.

Answers and rationales for Review Questions appear in Appendix I.

Chapter 16

Life Span, Health Promotion, and Family Systems

LEARNING Outcomes

After completing this chapter, you will be able to:

1. Define growth and development and describe how they progress.
2. List the components and principles of growth and development.
3. Describe normal development and some characteristic milestones for each age group.
4. Identify types of families and stages in the family life cycle.
5. Describe roles, functions, and parenting styles in families.
6. Describe nursing care as it relates to lifespan differences.

Clinical Objectives

7. Provide developmentally appropriate client/family teaching.
8. Conduct growth and development observations on clients of different developmental levels.

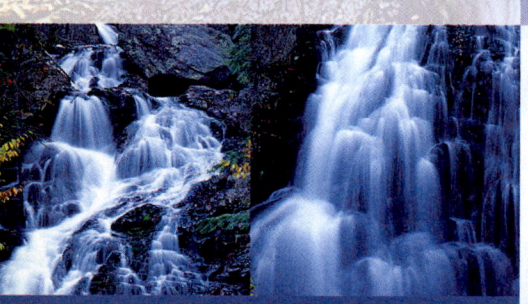

BRIEF Outline

Often used interchangeably, the terms *growth* and *development* have different meanings. **Growth** refers to physical change and increase in size. Indicators of growth include height, weight, bone size, and dentition. Although the pattern of physiological growth is similar for all people, growth rates vary during different stages of growth and development. For example, the growth rate is rapid during the prenatal, neonatal, infancy, and adolescent stages, but slows during childhood, and is minimal during adulthood.

Development is an increase in the complexity of function and skill progression. It refers to the person's capacity and skill to adapt to the environment. Development is the behavioral aspect of growth and includes the abilities to walk, to talk, and to run.

Growth and Development

Growth and development take place in an organized way, although they do not progress at the same rate with all individuals.

- *Cephalocaudally*—from the head down or literally from head (*cephalo*) to tail (*cauda*) (e.g., the infant gains head control before control of extremities). Figure 16-1 ■ illustrates the normal progression of growth and development.
- *Proximal to distal*—from the midline of the body to the extremities (e.g., the infant rolls over before grasp is perfected).
- *General to specific*—(e.g., walking is learned before running or skipping).

Growth and development are independent, interrelated processes. For example, an infant's muscles, bones, and nervous system must grow to a certain point before the infant can sit up or walk.

PRINCIPLES OF GROWTH AND DEVELOPMENT

Growth generally takes place during the first 20 years of life; development continues after that. Principles of growth and development follow:

- Growth and development are continuous, orderly, sequential processes influenced by maturational, environmental, and genetic factors.
- All humans follow the same pattern of growth and development.
- The sequence of each stage is predictable, although the time of onset, the length of the stage, and the effects of each stage vary with the person.
- Learning can either help or hinder the maturational process, depending on what is learned.
- Each developmental stage has its own characteristics.
- Growth and development occur in a cephalocaudal direction. They start at the head and move to the trunk, legs, and feet. This pattern is particularly obvious at birth, when the head of the infant is disproportionately large.
- Growth and development occur from the center of the body outward. For example, infants can roll over before they can grasp an object with the thumb and second finger.

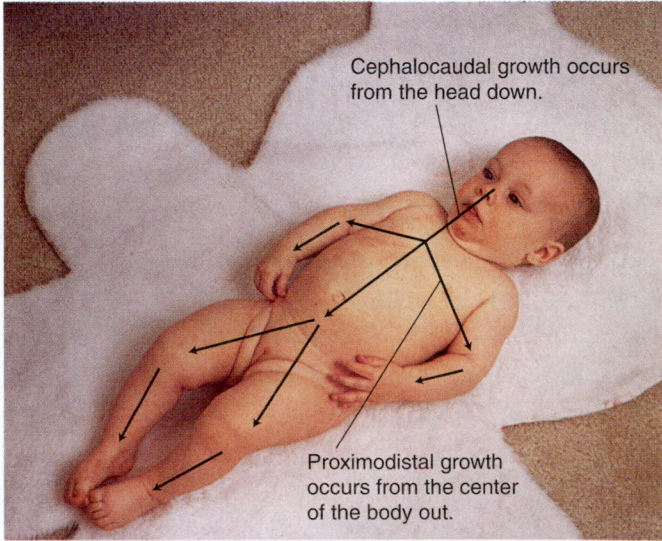

Figure 16-1. ■ Growth and development proceed from head to toe and from center to extremities.

- Development proceeds from simple to complex or from single acts to integrated acts. To drink and swallow from a cup, for example, the child must first learn eye–hand coordination, grasping, hand–mouth coordination, controlled tipping of the cup, and then mouth, lip, and tongue movements to drink and swallow.

- Development becomes increasingly differentiated. Differentiated development begins with a generalized response and progresses to a skilled specific response. For example, an infant's initial response to a stimulus involves the total body; a 5-year-old child can respond more specifically with laughter or fear.

- Certain stages of growth and development are more critical than others. It is known that the first 10 to 12 weeks after conception are critical. The incidence of congenital anomalies as a result of exposure to certain viruses, chemicals, or drugs is greater during this stage than others.

- The pace of growth and development is uneven. Asynchronous development is demonstrated by rapid growth of the head during infancy and of the extremities at puberty.

FACTORS THAT INFLUENCE GROWTH AND DEVELOPMENT

The factors that influence growth and development are genetic and environmental. The genetic inheritance of an individual is established at conception. It remains unchanged throughout life and determines such characteristics as sex, physical stature, and race. Environmental factors include family, religion, climate, culture, school, community, and nutrition. For example, poorly nourished children are more likely to have infections than are well-fed children, and they may not attain their full height potential. A cultural look at the stages of childhood is given in Box 16-1 ■.

Safety is an important topic as people grow and develop throughout the life span. Review Box 9-1 ⊙⊙ for lifespan safety considerations by age group.

COMPONENTS OF GROWTH AND DEVELOPMENT

The rate of a person's growth and development is highly individual. However, the sequence of growth and

BOX 16-1	CULTURAL PULSE POINTS

The Stages of Childhood

Five stages of human growth and development are common to *Homo sapiens*: infancy, childhood, juvenility, adolescence, and adulthood. Margaret Mead described lap children (infants, ages 0–1), knee children (toddlers, 2–3), yard children (preschool, 4–5), and community children (juveniles in middle childhood, 6–12). Anthropologists analyze the cultural meaning of the very idea of "stages," because stages are used to account for children's behavior ("He's crying but it's okay, because he's still a toddler") and to assure and define normal and appropriate development ("She is eight and old enough to start helping run our household").

Human cultures weave wonderful variations, meanings, and stories around panhuman maturational stages of childhood. The Beng of the Ivory Coast, for example, believe that young children are still partly in yet another stage, a cultural world called *wrugbe*, where ancestors share life with prebirth children who are ambivalent about leaving that world. This helps explain for Beng why infants cry or are sickly: They want to return to *wrugbe*.

development is predictable. Stages of growth usually correspond to certain developmental changes, as shown in Table 16-1 ■.

Growth and development are commonly thought of as having five major components:

- **Physiological**—relating to physical processes in the human body
- **Psychosocial**—pertaining to the relationship between oneself and others
- **Cognitive**—having to do with awareness of and interaction between oneself and the environment
- **Moral**—relating to judgments of right or wrong
- **Spiritual**—pertaining to relationship with God or a higher power

Knowledge of growth and development is essential for nurses if they are to identify developmental needs and problems and participate in health assessment and promotion. Growth and development encompass the prenatal period and the life span: from the neonate to older adult including the physiological, psychosocial, cognitive, moral, and spiritual aspects of each life stage.

TABLE 16-1	**Stages and Milestones of Growth and Development**			
STAGE AND SELECTED MILESTONES	**AGE**	**SIGNIFICANT CHARACTERISTICS**	**NURSING IMPLICATIONS**
Neonate Sample Milestones: Follows objects and closes hand reflexively around another's finger (Figure 16-2A 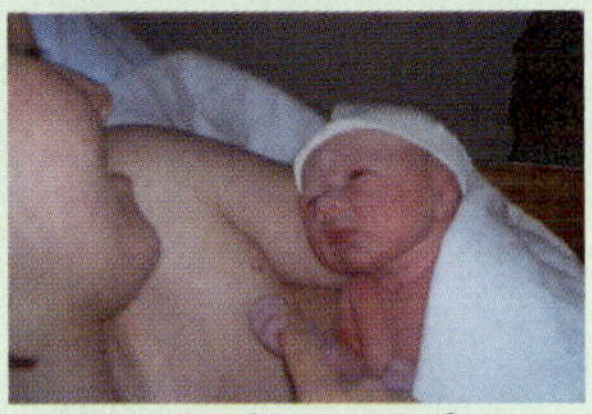 ■) **Figure 16-2.** ■ **A.** Grasps finger.	Birth–28 days	Behavior is largely reflexive and develops to more purposeful behavior.	Assist parents to identify and meet unmet needs.
Infant Sample Milestones: Sits, crawls, and stands (Figure 16-2B and C) 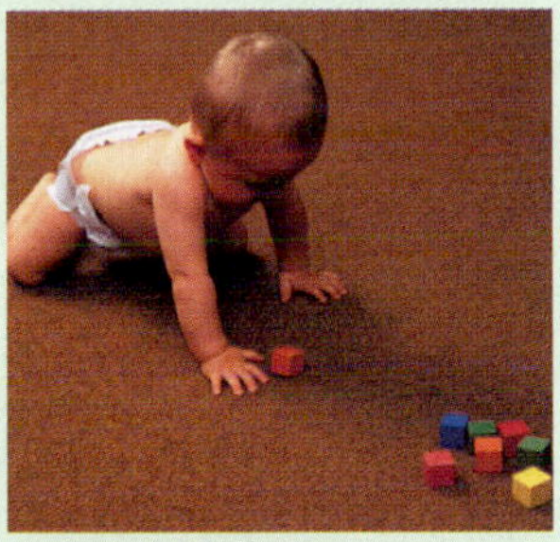 **Figure 16-2.** ■ **B.** Crawls or pulls the body up.	1 month–1 year	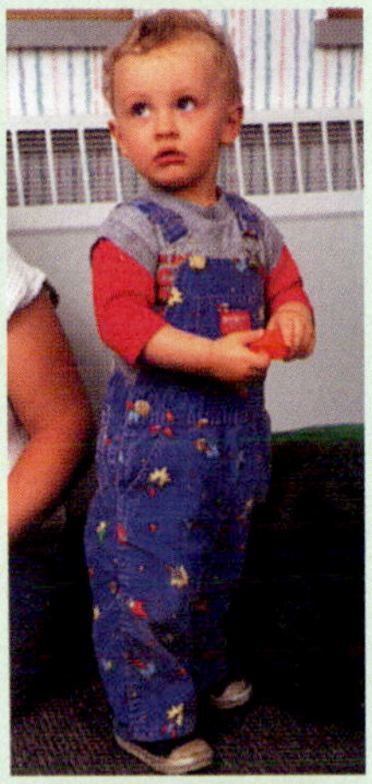 Physical growth is rapid.	Control the infant's environment so that physical and psychological needs are met.
Toddler Sample Milestones: Gains skill with spoon, begins to eat with fork (Figure 16-2D), goes up and down stairs, has daytime bowel and bladder control. 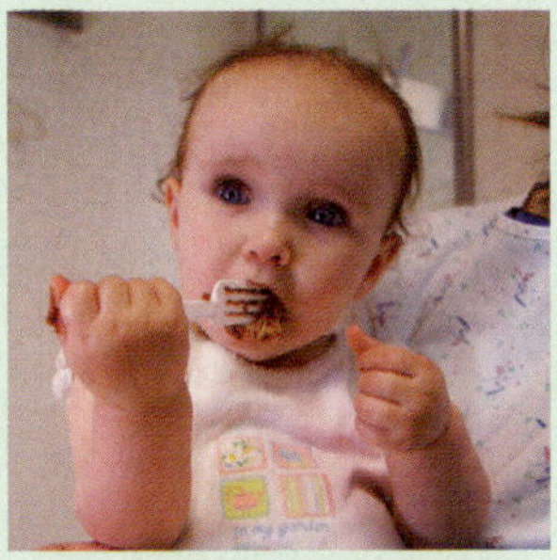 **Figure 16-2.** ■ **D.** Uses utensils.	1–3 years	Motor development permits increased physical autonomy. Psychosocial skills increase.	Safety and risk-taking strategies must be balanced to permit growth.

Figure 16-2. ■ **C.** Stands alone.

(continued)

TABLE 16-1	Stages and Milestones of Growth and Development (continued)		
STAGE AND SELECTED MILESTONES	AGE	SIGNIFICANT CHARACTERISTICS	NURSING IMPLICATIONS
Preschooler Sample Milestones: Climbs well, rides three-wheeler, and learns letters and numbers (Figure 16-2E); vocabulary increases to 1,000 or more words (has a direct relationship to the number of years the child attends preschool) 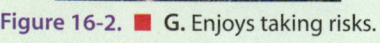 **Figure 16-2.** ■ E. Scribbles. *Source: Dorling Kindersley Media Library.*	3–6 years	The preschooler's world is expanding. New experiences and the preschooler's social role are tried during play. Physical growth is slower.	Provide opportunities for play and social activity.
School-age child Sample Milestones: May learn musical instrument; participates in group activities such as team and scouts; accomplishment of tasks important (Figure 16-2F) **Figure 16-2.** ■ F. Plays musical instruments.	6–12 years	Stage includes the preadolescent period (10 to 12 years). Peer group increasingly influences behavior. Physical, cognitive, and social development increases, and communication skills improve.	Allow time and energy for the school-age child to pursue hobbies and school activities. Recognize and support child's achievement.
Adolescent Sample Milestones: Puberty begins, peers and independence become central; risk taking behaviors may occur (Figure 16-2G) **Figure 16-2.** ■ G. Enjoys taking risks.	12–20 years	Self-concept changes with biologic development. Values are tested. Physical growth accelerates. Stress increases, especially in the face of conflicts.	Assist adolescents to develop coping behaviors. Help adolescents develop strategies for resolving conflicts.

TABLE 16-1 **Stages and Milestones of Growth and Development (continued)**

STAGE AND SELECTED MILESTONES	AGE	SIGNIFICANT CHARACTERISTICS	NURSING IMPLICATIONS
Young adult Sample Milestones: Begin to establish long-term relationships and find life path (Figure 16-2H) **Figure 16-2.** ■ **H.** Planning a future. *Source:* PhotoEdit Inc.	20–40 years	A personal lifestyle develops. Person establishes a relationship with a significant other and a commitment to something.	Accept adult's chosen lifestyle and assist with necessary adjustments relating to health. Recognize the person's commitments. Support change as necessary for health.
Middle adult Sample Milestones: Careers important; often continue pleasurable activities of youth (Figure 16-2I); may have commitments to children and aging parents **Figure 16-2.** ■ **I.** Sharing skill with grandchild.	40–65 years	Lifestyle changes due to other changes; for example, children leave home, occupational goals change.	Assist clients to plan for anticipated changes in life, to recognize the risk factors related to health, and to focus on strengths rather than weaknesses.
Older adult ("Young-old") Sample Milestones: (Figure 16-2J) Retirement or semiretirement; time for new activities or longtime hobbies **Figure 16-2.** ■ **J.** Having time to pursue pleasurable interests.	65–74 years	Adaptation to retirement and changing physical abilities is often necessary. Chronic illness may develop.	Assist clients to keep physically and socially active and to maintain peer group interactions.

(continued)

TABLE 16-1	Stages and Milestones of Growth and Development (continued)		
STAGE AND SELECTED MILESTONES	**AGE**	**SIGNIFICANT CHARACTERISTICS**	**NURSING IMPLICATIONS**
Middle-old adult Sample Milestones: Adaptations for physical and sensory changes; still active time (Figure 16-2K) **Figure 16-2.** ■ K. Adapting activities to support body changes. *Source:* Photo Researchers, Inc.	75–84 years	Adaptation to decline in speed of movement, reaction time, and sensory abilities and increasing dependence on others may be necessary.	Assist clients to cope with loss (e.g., hearing, eyesight, death of loved one). Provide necessary safety measures.
Old-old adult Sample Milestones: Assistive devices may be needed (Figure 16-2L); may need help with ADLs; adapting to loss **Figure 16-2.** ■ L. Using adaptive devices to maintain independence. *Source:* Geri Engberg Photography.	85 years and up	Increasing physical problems may develop.	Assist clients with self-care as required, and with maintaining as much independence as possible.

LIFE STAGES

Havighurst was one theorist who described developmental tasks associated with life stages. Box 16-2 ■ reviews Havighurst's approach to the tasks in each stage.

Conception and Prenatal Development

Prenatal or intrauterine development lasts approximately 38 to 40 weeks. *Note:* The major discussion of this period is in Unit IX ⚭, which discusses maternal and newborn care. Traditionally, pregnancy has been divided into three periods, called *trimesters*, each of which lasts about 3 months. Each trimester includes certain landmarks for developmental changes in the mother and the fetus. There are two phases of intrauterine life: embryonic and fetal.

The *embryonic phase* is the period during which the fertilized ovum develops into an organism with most of the features of the human. This period takes place during the first trimester of pregnancy. During the first 3 weeks:

1. The embryo is implanted.
2. Tissues differentiate into three layers. From these layers all of the body's complex organs and systems are formed.
3. Placental function starts. Its functions are to exchange nutrients and gases between the embryo or fetus and the mother.
4. The fetal membranes differentiate.

BOX 16-2   HAVIGHURST'S AGE PERIODS AND DEVELOPMENTAL TASKS

Infancy and Early Childhood

1. Learning to walk
2. Learning to take solid foods
3. Learning to talk
4. Learning to control the elimination of body wastes
5. Learning sex differences and sexual modesty
6. Achieving psychological stability
7. Forming simple concepts of social and physical reality
8. Learning to relate emotionally to parents, siblings, and other people
9. Learning to distinguish right from wrong and developing a conscience

Middle Childhood

1. Learning physical skills necessary for ordinary games
2. Building wholesome attitudes toward oneself as a growing organism
3. Learning to get along with age-mates
4. Learning an appropriate masculine or feminine social role
5. Developing fundamental skills in reading, writing, and calculating
6. Developing concepts necessary for everyday living
7. Developing conscience, morality, and a scale of values
8. Achieving personal independence
9. Developing attitudes toward social groups and institutions

Adolescence

1. Achieving new and more mature relations with age-mates of both sexes
2. Achieving a masculine or feminine social role
3. Accepting one's physique and using the body effectively
4. Achieving emotional independence from parents and other adults
5. Achieving assurance of economic independence
6. Selecting and preparing for an occupation
7. Preparing for marriage and family life
8. Developing intellectual skills and concepts necessary for civic competence

9. Desiring and achieving socially responsible behavior
10. Acquiring a set of values and an ethical system as a guide to behavior

Early Adulthood

1. Selecting a mate
2. Learning to live with a partner
3. Starting a family
4. Rearing children
5. Managing a home
6. Getting started in an occupation
7. Taking on civic responsibility
8. Finding a congenial social group

Middle Age

1. Achieving adult civic and social responsibility
2. Establishing and maintaining an economic standard of living
3. Assisting teenage children to become responsible and happy adults
4. Developing adult leisure-time activities
5. Relating oneself to one's spouse as a person
6. Accepting and adjusting to the physiological changes of middle age
7. Adjusting to aging parents

Later Maturity

1. Adjusting to decreasing physical strength and health
2. Adjusting to retirement and reduced income
3. Adjusting to death of a spouse
4. Establishing an explicit affiliation with one's age group
5. Meeting social and civil obligations
6. Establishing satisfactory physical living arrangements

Source: From Robert J. Havighurst, *Developmental Tasks and Education*, 3rd ed. Published by Allyn and Bacon, Boston, MA. Copyright © 1972 by Pearson Education.

The *fetal phase* of development is characterized by a period of rapid growth in the size of the fetus. Both genetic and environmental factors affect its growth.

At the end of the second trimester, the fetus resembles a small baby. The skin appears wrinkled, red, and transparent. A protective covering (called *vernix caseosa*) begins to develop over the skin. This is a white cheeselike substance that adheres to the skin. *Lanugo*, a fine downy hair, also covers the body. At about 5 months, the mother first perceives movement by the fetus, and the first fetal heartbeat may be heard.

At the end of the third trimester, the fetus has developed to approximately 20 inches and 7.0 to 7.5 pounds. The lanugo has disappeared, and the skin is a more normal color and appears less wrinkled. The last 2 months *in utero* are largely devoted to accumulating weight.

Neonates and Infants (Birth to 1 Year)

Babies are considered neonates from birth to the end of 1 month. Infants are babies from 1 month of age to 1 year. *Note:* See Unit X, the Pediatric unit, for in-depth discussion.

PHYSICAL DEVELOPMENT

An infant's basic task is survival, which requires breathing, sleeping, sucking, eating, swallowing, digesting, and eliminating. Infants undergo significant physiological change in these areas: weight, length, head growth, vision, and motor development.

Just after birth, most infants lose 5% to 10% of their birth weight because of fluid loss. This weight loss is normal, and infants usually regain that weight in about 1 week. Usual weight gain is 5 to 7 ounces weekly for 6 months. By 5 months of age infants usually reach twice their birth weight, and by age 12 months, three times their birth weight.

The average length of a newborn is about 20 inches. Two recumbent lengths are measured: the crown-to-rump length (the sitting length), which is approximately the same as the head circumference, and the head-to-heel length (from the top of the head to the base of the heels). By 12 months, the infant's length increases by approximately one-half of the birth length. The procedures for taking an infant's height, weight, and circumference are provided in Chapter 56 ⚭.

Assessment of head circumference is of particular importance in infants and children to determine the growth rate of the skull and the brain (Figure 16-3 ■). An infant's head should be measured at every visit to the physician or nurse until the child is 2 years old.

Normal head circumference (*normocephaly*) is often related to chest circumference. The chest circumference of the newborn is usually less than the head circumference. As the infant grows, the chest circumference becomes larger than the head circumference.

Head Molding

The heads of most newborn babies are misshapen because of the molding of the head that occurs during vaginal deliveries. Molding of the head is made possible by **fontanels** (unossified membranous gaps) in the bone structure of the skull and by overriding of the *sutures* (junction lines of the skull bones). Within a week of birth, a newborn's head usually regains its symmetry. The posterior fontanel closes from 4 to 8 weeks after birth. The larger anterior fontanel, which is diamond shaped, closes between 9 and 18 months. Figure 16-4 ■ shows fontanels and suture lines.

Sensory Abilities

VISION

- The newborn can follow large moving objects and blinks in response to bright light.
- The newborn eyes cannot focus on close objects.
- At 4 months, the infant can recognize familiar objects and follow moving ones.
- At 6 months, the infant can perceive colors.
- At 9 months, most can recognize facial characteristics and often smile in response to a familiar face.
- At 12 months, depth perception has developed.

HEARING

- Newborns with intact hearing will react with a startle to a loud noise. In many locales, newborn hearing screenings are now mandated prior to hospital discharge. Computerized equipment makes this possible. Within a few days infants can tell the difference between their mother's voice and that of another woman.
- At 5 months of age, the infant will pause while sucking in order to listen to the mother's voice.
- A 9-month-old infant is able to locate the source of sounds and recognizes familiar ones.
- At 1 year, the infant listens to sounds, begins to distinguish words, and responds to simple commands.

SMELL AND TASTE. The senses of smell and taste are functional shortly after birth. Newborns prefer sweet tastes and tend to decrease their sucking in response to liquids with a salty content. They are able to recognize the smell of their mother's milk and respond to this smell by turning toward the mother.

TOUCH. The sense of touch is well developed at birth. Skin-to-skin touching is important for an infant's development. The infant responds positively to the warmth, love, and security it perceives when touched, held, and cuddled. The newborn

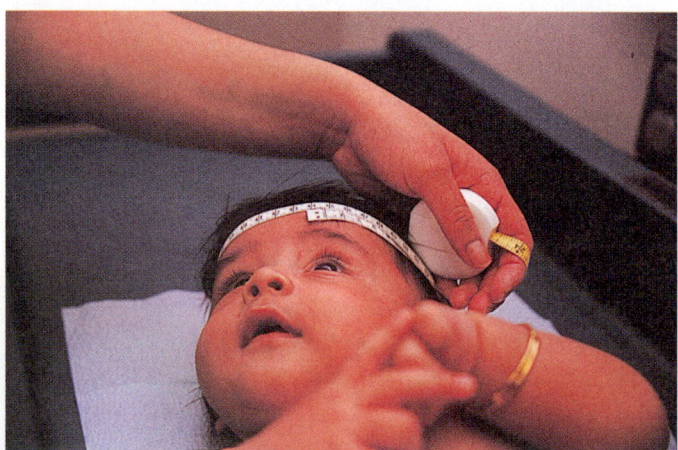

Figure 16-3. ■ Head circumference is an important indicator for newborns and children up to 36 months.

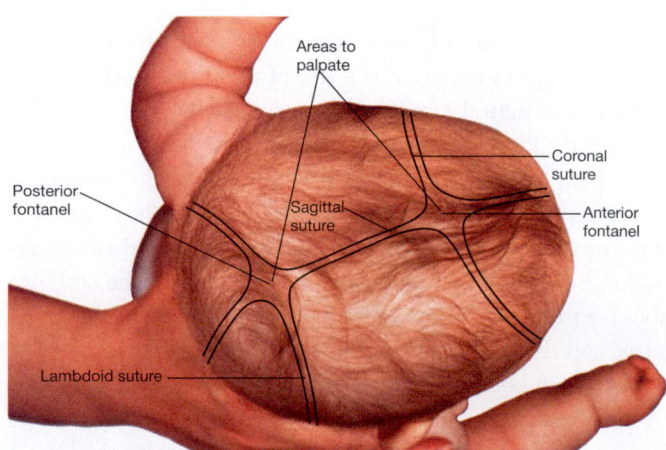

Figure 16-4. ■ The bones of the skull, showing the fontanels and the suture lines.

TABLE 16-2	Infant Reflexes
REFLEX	**DESCRIPTION**
Sucking reflex	A feeding reflex that occurs when the infant's lips are touched. The reflex persists throughout infancy.
Rooting reflex	A feeding reflex elicited by touching the baby's cheek, causing the baby's head to turn to the side that was touched. This reflex usually disappears after 4 months.
Palmar grasp reflex	Occurs when a small object is placed against the palm of the hand, causing the fingers to curl around it. This reflex disappears after 3 months.
Plantar reflex	Similar to the palmar grasp reflex; an object placed just beneath the toes causes them to curl around it. This reflex disappears after 8 months.
Stepping reflex (walking or dancing reflex)	Elicited by holding the baby upright so that the feet touch a flat surface. The legs then move up and down as if the baby were walking. This reflex usually disappears at about 2 months.
Tonic neck reflex or fencing reflex	A postural reflex. When a baby who is lying on its back turns its head to the right side, for example, the left side of the body shows a flexing of the left arm and the left leg. This reflex disappears after 4 months.
Moro reflex	Often assessed to estimate the maturity of the central nervous system. A loud noise, a sudden change in position, or an abrupt jarring of the crib elicits this reflex. The infant reacts by extending both arms and legs outward with the fingers spread, then suddenly retracting the limbs. Often, the infant cries at the same time. This reflex disappears after 4 months.
Babinski's reflex	When the sole of the foot is stroked, the big toe rises and the other toes fan out. A newborn baby has a positive Babinski. After age 1, the infant exhibits a negative Babinski; that is, the toes curl downward. A positive Babinski after age 1 indicates brain damage.

is also sensitive to temperature extremes and pain; however, babies react diffusely and cannot isolate the discomfort.

REFLEXES.   The **reflexes** of the newborn are unconscious, involuntary responses. They are neither learned nor consciously carried out; rather, they are nervous system responses to a number of stimuli. Table 16-2 ■ and Figure 16-5 ■ describe infant reflexes. For more in-depth content on newborn infants, see Chapter 56 ⊘⊘.

Motor Abilities

Motor development is the development of the baby's abilities to move and to control the body. Initially, the neonate turns the head from side to side when in a prone position and grasps by reflex when an object is placed in the palm of the hand. By 6 months, the normal infant can lift chest and shoulders off a surface when prone and can bear weight on the hands. The 6-month-old also manipulates small objects. By 9 months, infants can creep and crawl. They can hold something tight in a pincer grasp with the thumb and forefinger. At the age of 1 year, infants walk alone with help and have learned to use a spoon to feed themselves.

PSYCHOSOCIAL DEVELOPMENT

Erikson described eight stages of development in humans (see Table 15-1 ⊘⊘). According to Erikson, the central crisis at this stage is trust versus mistrust. Infants depend on the primary caregivers for all their physiological and psychological needs.

The newborn reacts socially to caregivers by paying attention to the face or voice and by cuddling when held. It is able to interact with the environment by responding to various stimuli such as touch and sound. It displays displeasure by crying and satisfaction by soft vocalizations.

By 6 months, the infant starts to imitate sounds and vocalizes one-syllable sounds such as "ma ma," "da da." At 9 months infants can comply with simple verbal commands such as "wave bye-bye." They may begin to display fear of being left alone (e.g., going to bed). By 1 year, infants have developed separation anxiety. They cling to their mother in unfamiliar situations. They are able to display emotions such as anger and affection.

COGNITIVE DEVELOPMENT

According to Piaget, **cognitive development** is a result of interaction between an individual and the environment. Piaget identified stages and significant behaviors for different age groups (see Table 15-3 ⊘⊘). Infants' initial period of cognitive development was named the sensorimotor phase.

MORAL DEVELOPMENT

Infants associate right and wrong with pleasure and pain. What gives them pleasure is right, since they are too young to reason otherwise. In later months and years, children can tell easily and quickly by changes in parental facial expressions and voice tones that their behavior is either approved or disapproved.

HEALTH ASSESSMENT AND PROMOTION

Nursing care of infants involves some specific tests. Newborn babies are assessed at birth and at 5 minutes by the Apgar scoring system. This provides a numeric indicator of the baby's physiological capacities to adapt to extrauterine

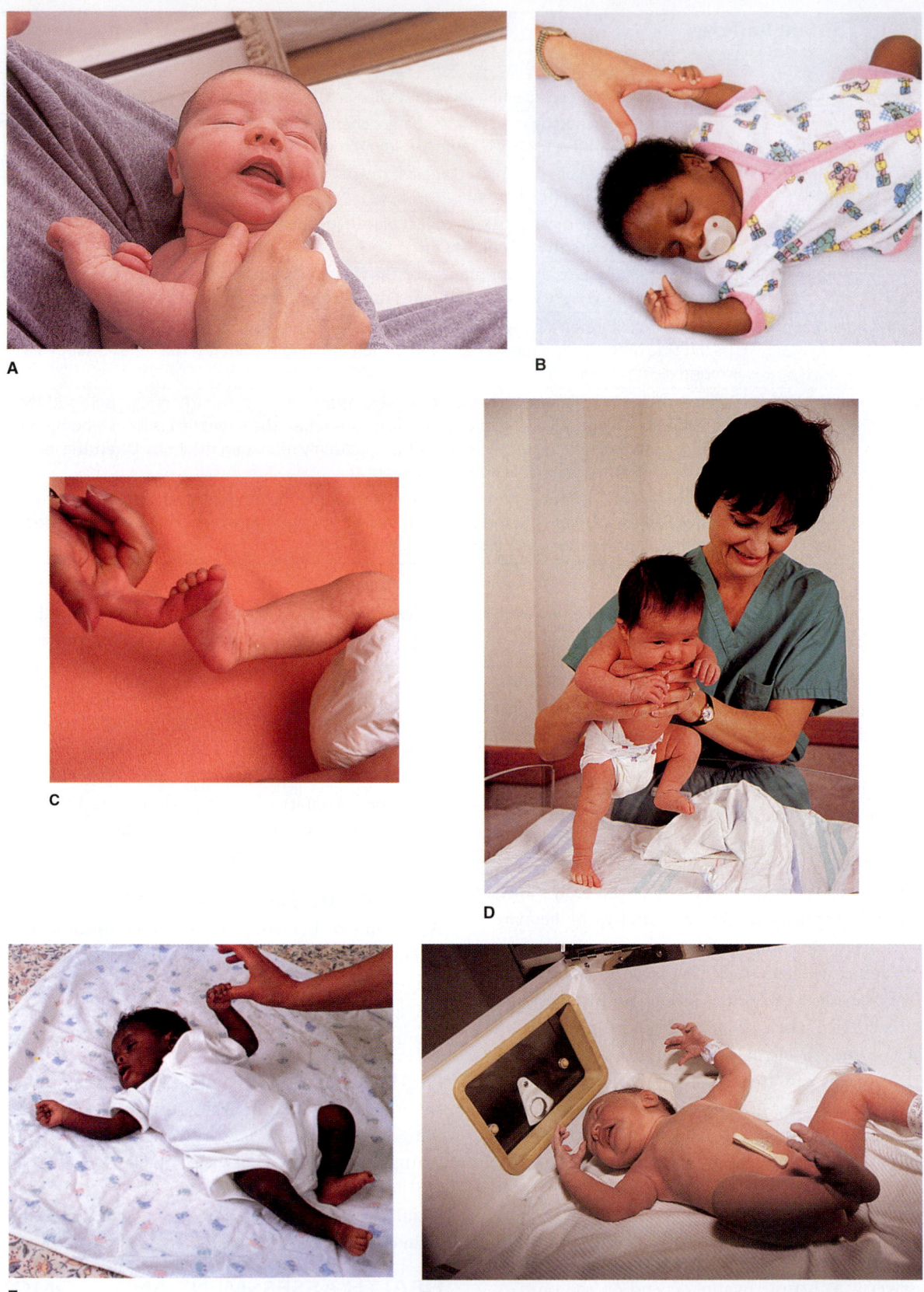

Figure 16-5. ■ Reflexes of the neonate reflect neurologic integrity: **A.** Rooting reflex. **B.** Palmar grasp reflex. **C.** Plantar grasp reflex. **D.** Stepping reflex. **E.** Tonic neck reflex. **F.** Moro (startle) reflex.

life. You can find the steps for performing the Apgar scoring system in Chapter 56 🔗.

During well-check visits, the nurse examines and observes the infant, noting normal progression and variations from the norm in developmental age and activity.

Health promotion is a crucial part of nursing care for parents of newborns and infants. Table 16-3 ■ provides health promotion and client teaching guidelines for infants, toddlers, and preschoolers. For additional information on health promotion, nursing, and health care, see Chapters 59 and 60 🔗.

Developmental Screening Tests

Development can be assessed by observing the infant's behavior and by using standardized tests such as the Denver Developmental Screening Test (DDST). The DDST (see Figure 58-15 🔗) is used to screen children from birth to 6 years of age. The test is intended to estimate the abilities of a child compared to those of an average group of children of the same age and ethnic group.

Toddlers (1 to 3 Years)

Toddlers develop from having no voluntary control to being able to walk and speak. They also learn to control their bladder and bowels, and they acquire all kinds of information about their environment.

TABLE 16-3	Health Promotion Guidelines for Infants, Toddlers, and Preschoolers		
GUIDELINES	**INFANTS**	**TODDLERS**	**PRESCHOOLERS**
Health examinations	At 2 weeks and at 2, 4, 6, and 12 months	At 15 and 18 months and then as recommended by the physician Dental visits starting at age 3 Hearing tests by 18 months or earlier	Every 1 to 2 years
Protective measures	Immunizations: diphtheria-pertussis-tetanus (DPT), oral poliovirus vaccine (OPV), measles-mumps-rubella (MMR), *Haemophilus influenzae* type B, and hepatitis B and varicella vaccines as recommended Fluoride supplements if there is inadequate water fluoridation (less than 0.7 parts per million [ppm]) Screening for tuberculosis Screening for phenylketonuria (PKU) Prompt attention for illnesses Appropriate skin hygiene and clothing	Immunizations: continuing DPT, OPV series, MMR, *Haemophilus influenzae* type B, and hepatitis B vaccines as recommended Screenings for tuberculosis and lead poisoning Fluoride supplements if there is inadequate water fluoridation (less than 0.7 ppm)	Immunizations: continuing DPT, OPV series, MMR vaccine; other immunizations as recommended Screening for tuberculosis Vision and hearing screening Regular dental screenings and fluoride treatment
Safety	Importance of supervision Car seat, crib, playpen, bath, and home environment safety measures Feeding measures (e.g., avoid propping bottle) Providing toys with no small parts or sharp edges	Importance of supervision and teaching child to obey commands Home environment safety measures (e.g., lock medicine cabinet) Outdoor safety measures (e.g., close supervision near water) Appropriate toys	Educating child about simple safety rules (e.g., crossing the street) Teaching child to play safely (e.g., bicycle and playground safety) Educating to prevent poisoning
Nutrition	Breastfeeding and bottle-feeding techniques Formula preparation Feeding schedule Introduction of solid foods Need for iron supplements at 4–6 months	Focus on soft foods and finger foods and those that do not present a choking hazard. Provide nutritious meals and snacks and do not force child to eat set foods or amounts of food Teach simple mealtime manners and allow toddler to participate in dental care	Give variety of foods; begin to teach importance of nutritious meals and snacks Have preschooler participate in daily oral care
Elimination	Characteristics and frequency of stool and urine elimination Diarrhea and its effects	Toilet training techniques	Teaching proper hygiene (e.g., washing hands after using bathroom)

(continued)

TABLE 16-3	Health Promotion Guidelines for Infants, Toddlers, and Preschoolers (continued)		
GUIDELINES	INFANTS	TODDLERS	PRESCHOOLERS
Rest/sleep	Usual sleep and rest patterns	Dealing with sleep disturbances	Dealing with sleep disturbances (e.g., nightmares)
Sensory stimulation/play	Touch: holding, cuddling, rocking Vision: colorful, moving toys Hearing: soothing voice tones, music, singing Play: toys appropriate for development	Providing adequate space and a variety of activities Toys that allow "acting on" behaviors and provide motor and sensory stimulation	Providing times for group play activities Teaching child simple games that require cooperation and interaction Providing toys and dress-ups for role-playing

PHYSICAL DEVELOPMENT

Toddlers are usually chubby, with relatively short legs and a large head (Figure 16-6 ■). The face appears small when compared to the skull. Toddlers have a pronounced lumbar lordosis and a protruding abdomen. The abdominal muscles develop gradually with growth, and the abdomen flattens.

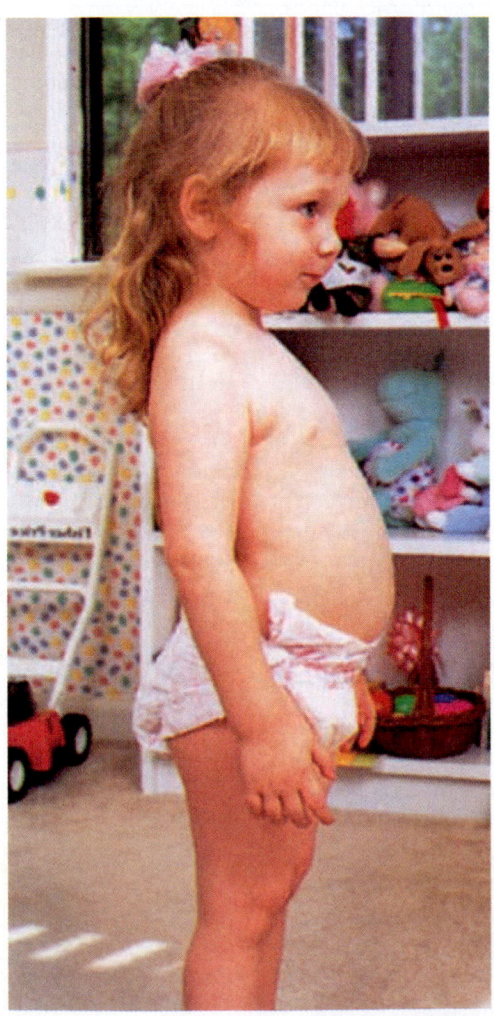

Figure 16-6. ■ The toddler appears chubby with relatively short legs and a large head. (Photographer: Michael Newman.)

Two-year-olds can be expected to weigh approximately four times their birth weight. The weight gain is about 5 lbs between 1 and 2 years and about 2 to 5 lbs between 2 and 3 years.

A toddler's height can be measured as height or length. Height is measured while the toddler stands, and length is measured while the toddler is in a recumbent position. Between ages 1 and 2 years, the average growth in height is 4 to 5 inches, and between 2 and 3 years it slows to 2.5 to 3.5 inches.

The head circumference of the toddler increases about 1 inch on average. By 24 months, the head is 80% of the average adult size and the brain is 70% of its adult size.

Sensory Abilities

Visual acuity is fairly well established at 1 year; average estimates of acuity for the toddler are 20/70 at 18 months and 20/40 at 2 years of age. Accommodation to near and far objects is fairly well developed by 18 months and continues to mature with age. Hearing in the 3-year-old is at adult levels. The taste buds of the toddler are sensitive to the natural flavors of food, and the 3-year-old prefers familiar odors and tastes. Touch is a very important sense, and a distressed toddler is often soothed by tactile sensations.

Motor Abilities

Fine muscle coordination and gross motor skills improve during toddlerhood. At 18 months, the child can:

- Pick up small beads and place them in a receptacle.
- Hold a spoon and a cup.
- Walk upstairs with assistance.
- Crawl down the stairs.

At 2 years, toddlers can:

- Hold a spoon and put it into the mouth correctly.
- Run (with steady gait).
- Balance on one foot.
- Ride a tricycle.

By 3 years most children are toilet trained, with occasional nighttime accidents or when playing.

PSYCHOSOCIAL DEVELOPMENT

Toddlers begin to develop their sense of autonomy by asserting themselves with the frequent use of the word *no.* Parents need to have a great deal of patience coupled with an understanding of the importance of this developmental milestone. See Table 15-1 ⚭ for Erikson's stage for toddlers.

Although toddlers like to explore the environment, they always need to have a significant person nearby. During the toddler stage, receptive and expressive language skills are developing quickly. Children can understand words and follow directions long before they can actually form them into sentences. By 1 year of age, toddlers can recognize their own names.

COGNITIVE DEVELOPMENT

According to Piaget, the toddler completes the fifth and sixth stages of the sensorimotor phase and starts the preconceptual phase at about 2 years of age.

MORAL DEVELOPMENT

Kohlberg established six stages of **moral development.** According to Kohlberg, the first level of moral development is the preconventional when children respond to punishment and reward. During the second year of life, children begin to know that some activities elicit affection and approval.

SPIRITUAL DEVELOPMENT

Fowler theorized six stages of **spiritual development.** According to Fowler, the toddler's stage of spiritual development is undifferentiated. Toddlers may be aware of some religious practices, but they are primarily involved in learning knowledge and emotional reactions rather than establishing spiritual beliefs. A toddler may repeat short prayers at bedtime, conforming to a ritual, because praise and affection result.

HEALTH ASSESSMENT AND PROMOTION

Assessment activities for the toddler are similar to those for the infant in terms of measuring weight, length (height), and vital signs. Promoting health and wellness includes such areas as injury prevention, toilet training, and good dental hygiene. See Table 16-3 for health promotion guidelines. See also the Nursing Care section later in the chapter.

Preschoolers (3 to 6 Years)

During the preschool period, physical growth slows, but control of the body and coordination increase greatly.

PHYSICAL DEVELOPMENT

By the time children are 4 or 5 years old, they appear taller and thinner than toddlers. The preschooler's brain reaches almost its adult size by 5 years. The extremities of the body grow more quickly than the body trunk, making the child's body appear somewhat out of proportion.

Weight gain in preschool children is generally slow. By 5 years, they have added only another 7 to 12 lbs to their 3-year-old weight. Preschool children grow about 2.0 to 2.5 inches each year.

Sensory Abilities

VISION. Preschool children are generally *hyperopic* (farsighted), that is, unable to focus on near objects. By the end of the preschool years, visual ability has improved to approximately 20/30.

HEARING AND TASTE.   The hearing of the preschool child has reached optimal levels, and the ability to listen (attending to and comprehending what is said) has matured since the toddler age. As for the sense of taste, preschoolers show their preferences by asking for something "yummy," and may refuse something they consider "yucky."

Motor Abilities

By 5 years of age, children are able to wash their hands and face and brush their teeth. They are self-conscious about exposing their bodies and go to the bathroom without telling others. Typically, preschool children run with increasing skill each year. By 5 years of age, they run skillfully and can jump three steps. Preschoolers can balance on their toes and dress themselves without assistance.

PSYCHOSOCIAL DEVELOPMENT

Erikson writes that the major developmental crisis of the preschooler is initiative versus guilt. Parents can enhance the self-concept of the preschooler by providing opportunities for new achievements where the child can learn, repeat, and master.

The self-concept of the preschooler is also based on gender identification. Preschoolers are aware of the two sexes and identify with the correct one. They may mimic the parent's behavior, attitudes, and appearance (Figure 16-7 ■).

Preschool children gradually emerge as social beings. At the age of 3 or 4, they learn to play with a small number of their peers. They gradually learn to play with more people as they grow older. Preschoolers also learn about their feelings; they know the words *cry, sad,* and *laugh,* and the feelings related to them. They also begin to learn how to control their feelings and behavior. The preschooler uses the same types of coping mechanisms in response to stress as the toddler does, although protest behavior (kicking, screaming) is less likely to occur in the older preschooler.

COGNITIVE, MORAL, AND SPIRITUAL DEVELOPMENT

The preschooler's cognitive development, according to Piaget, is the phase of intuitive thought. Reading skills also start to develop at this age.

MyNursingKit | Handling temper tantrums

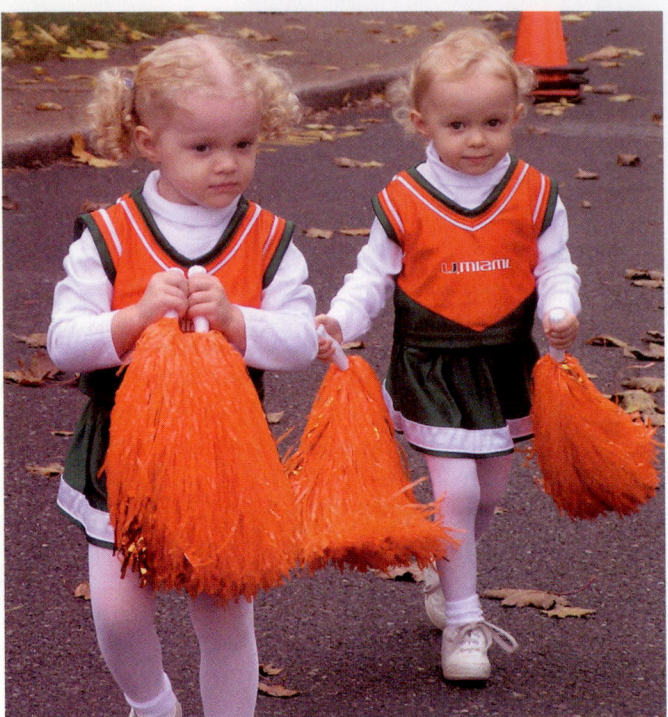

Figure 16-7. ■ Preschoolers often identify with the parent of the same sex and like to mimic behavior.

Preschoolers are capable of prosocial behavior, that is, any action that a person takes to benefit someone else. The term *prosocial* is synonymous with *kind* and connotes sharing, helping, protecting, giving aid, befriending, showing affection, and giving encouragement. Moral behavior to a preschooler may mean taking turns at play or sharing. It is important for parents to answer preschoolers' "why" questions and discuss values with them.

Many preschoolers enroll in Sunday school or faith-oriented classes. The preschooler usually enjoys the social interaction of these classes. Faith at this stage is primarily a result of the teaching of significant others, such as parents and teachers.

HEALTH ASSESSMENT AND PROMOTION

During assessment, the preschooler can often participate in answering questions with assistance from parents or caregivers. Health promotion guidelines for the preschooler were shown in Table 16-3. Further information on nursing care follows later in the chapter. For further discussion on preschoolers, child, see Chapter 60 ⬛⬛.

School-Age Children (6 to 12 Years)

The school-age period starts when children are about 6 years of age, when the deciduous teeth are shed. This period includes the preadolescent (*prepuberty*) period. It ends at about 12 years, with the onset of puberty. **Puberty** is the age when the reproductive organs become functional and secondary sex characteristics develop. See Chapter 62 ⬛⬛ for further discussion of sexuality and sexual development. In general, the period from 6 to 12 years is one of rapid and dramatic change.

PHYSICAL DEVELOPMENT

The school-age child gains weight rapidly and thus appears less thin than previously. At 6 years boys tend to weigh about 2 lbs more than girls. The weight gain of schoolchildren from 6 to 12 years of age averages 7 lbs per year, but the major weight gains occur from ages 10 to 12 for boys and from 9 to 12 for girls.

At 6 years both boys and girls are about the same height. Before puberty, children of both sexes have a growth spurt, girls between 10 and 12 years and boys between 12 and 14 years. Thus, girls may well be taller than boys at 12 years, but boys are usually stronger.

Little change takes place in the reproductive and endocrine systems until the prepuberty period. During prepuberty, at about ages 9 to 13, endocrine functions slowly increase. This change in endocrine function can result in increased perspiration and more active sebaceous glands.

Sensory Abilities

VISION. The depth and distance perception of children 6 to 8 years of age is accurate. By age 6, children have full binocular vision. The eye muscles are well developed and coordinated, and both eyes can focus on one object at the same time. A child's 20/20 vision is usually well established between 9 and 16 years of age.

HEARING AND TOUCH. Auditory perception is fully developed in school-age children, who are able to identify fine differences in voices, both in sound and in pitch. At this stage, children also have a well-developed sense of touch and are able to locate points of heat and cold on all body surfaces. They are also able to identify an unseen object, such as a pencil or a book, simply by touch. This ability is called *stereognosis*.

Motor Abilities

During the middle years (6 to 10), children perfect their muscular skills and coordination. By 9 years most children are becoming skilled in games of interest, such as football or baseball. These skills are often associated with school, and many of them are learned there. By 9 years most children have sufficient fine motor control for such activities as building models or sewing.

PSYCHOSOCIAL DEVELOPMENT

At this time children begin to create and develop a sense of competence and perseverance. School-age children are motivated by activities that provide a sense of worth. They

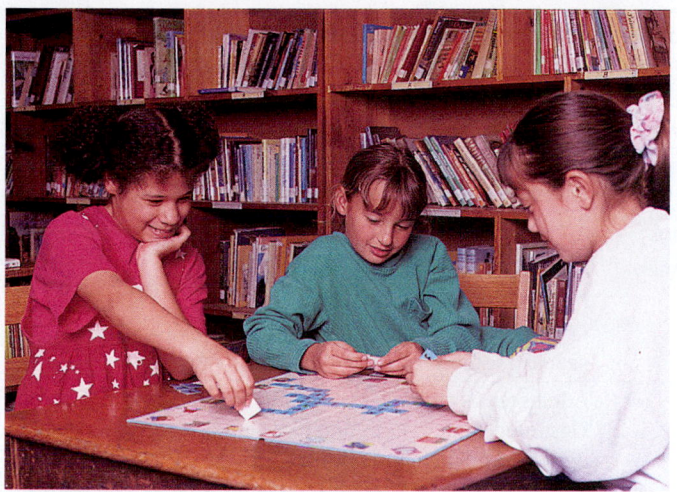

Figure 16-8. ■ Expanding cognitive skills enable school-age children to interact cooperatively in activities of an increasingly complex nature, as shown by the children playing this board game. (Photographer: Jane Wattenburg.)

concentrate on mastering skills that will help them function in the adult world (Figure 16-8 ■).

As they grow older, schoolchildren learn to play with more children at one time. Usually, the 6- or 7-year-old is a member of a peer group. This group can have a greater influence than the family in teaching attitudes.

The schoolchild's self-concept continues to mature. Children recognize similarities and differences between themselves and others. School-age children compare themselves with others and obtain feedback from teachers and peers.

COGNITIVE, MORAL, AND SPIRITUAL DEVELOPMENT

According to Piaget, the ages 7 to 11 years mark the phase of concrete operations. During this stage, the child changes from egocentric interactions to cooperative interactions.

Some school-age children are at Kohlberg's stage 1 of the preconventional level (punishment and obedience); that is, they act to avoid being punished. Some school-age children, however, are at stage 2 (instrumental-relativist orientation). These children do things to benefit themselves. Fairness (everyone getting a fair share or chance) becomes important.

According to Fowler, the school-age child is at stage 2 in spiritual development, the mythic-literal stage. Children learn to distinguish fantasy from fact. Spiritual facts are those beliefs that are accepted by a religious group. Parents and the minister, rabbi, or priest help the child distinguish fact from fantasy. These people still influence the child more than peers in spiritual matters.

School-age children may ask many questions about God and religion in these years and will generally believe that God is good and always present to help. Just before puberty, children become aware that their prayers are not always answered and become disappointed.

HEALTH ASSESSMENT AND PROMOTION

During the assessment interview, the nurse responds to questions from the parent or other caregiver, gives appropriate feedback, and lends encouragement and support. Promoting health and wellness includes dental hygiene and regular dental examinations, safety measures to prevent accidents, physical fitness, autonomy and self-esteem, and hygiene measures to prevent infections. See Table 16-4 ■ for health promotion guidelines for school-age children and adolescents.

Adolescents (12 to 20 Years)

Adolescence is the period during which the person becomes physically and psychologically mature and acquires a personal identity. At the end of this critical period in development, the person is ready to enter adulthood and assume its responsibilities. Puberty is the first stage of adolescence in which sexual organs begin to grow and mature.

PHYSICAL DEVELOPMENT

During puberty, growth is markedly accelerated compared to the slow, steady growth of the child. This period, marked by sudden and dramatic physical changes, is referred to as the adolescent growth spurt. In boys, the growth spurt usually begins between ages 12 and 16; in girls, it begins earlier, usually between ages 10 and 14. Because the growth spurt begins earlier in girls, many girls surpass boys in height at this time.

Physical growth continues throughout adolescence. Growth is fastest for boys at about 14 years, and the maximum height is often reached at about 18 or 19 years. Some men add another 1 or 2 cm to their height during their 20s as the vertebral column gradually continues to grow. During the period from 10 to 18 years of age, the average American male doubles his weight and grows about 16 inches.

Growth is noted first in the musculoskeletal system. This growth follows a sequential pattern: The head, hands, and feet are the first to grow to adult status. Next, the extremities reach their adult size. Because the extremities grow before the trunk, the adolescent looks leggy, awkward, and uncoordinated. After the trunk grows to full size, the shoulders, chest, and hips grow. Skull and facial bones also change proportions: The forehead becomes more prominent, and the jawbones develop.

Glandular Changes

The eccrine and apocrine glands increase their secretions and become fully functional during puberty.

Sexual Characteristics

During puberty, both primary and secondary sex characteristics develop. Primary sexual characteristics relate to the organs necessary for reproduction, such as the testes, penis, vagina, and uterus. Secondary sexual characteristics

TABLE 16-4	Health Promotion Guidelines for School-Age Children and Adolescents	
GUIDELINES	**SCHOOL-AGE CHILDREN**	**ADOLESCENTS**
Health examinations	Annual physical examination or as recommended	As recommended by the physician
Protective measures	Immunizations as recommended Screening for tuberculosis Periodic vision, speech, and hearing screenings Regular dental screenings and fluoride treatment Providing accurate information about sexual issues (e.g., reproduction, AIDS)	Immunizations as recommended, such as adult tetanus-diphtheria (Td) vaccine and hepatitis B vaccine Screening for tuberculosis Periodic vision and hearing screenings Regular dental assessments Obtaining and providing accurate information about sexual issues
Safety	Using proper equipment when participating in sports and other physical activities (e.g., helmets, pads) Encouraging child to take responsibility for own safety (e.g., participating in bicycle and water safety courses)	Adolescent's taking responsibility for using motor vehicles safely (e.g., completing a driver's education course, wearing seat belt and helmet) Making certain that proper precautions are taken during all athletic activities (e.g., medical supervision, proper equipment) Parents' keeping lines of communication open and being alert to signs of substance abuse and emotional disturbances in the adolescent
Nutrition, elimination, exercise	Importance of child not skipping meals and eating a balanced diet Experiences with food that may lead to obesity Utilizing positive approaches for elimination problems (e.g., enuresis)	Importance of healthy snacks and appropriate patterns of food intake and exercise Factors that may lead to nutritional problems (e.g., obesity, anorexia nervosa, bulimia) Balancing sedentary activities with regular exercise
Play and social interactions	Providing opportunities for a variety of organized group activities Accepting realistic expectations of child's abilities Acting as role models in acceptance of other persons who may be different Providing a home environment that limits TV viewing and video games and encourages completion of homework	Encouraging adolescent to establish relationships that promote discussion of feelings, concerns, and fears Parents' encouraging adolescent peer group activities that promote appropriate moral and spiritual values Parents' acting as role models for appropriate social interactions Parents' providing a comfortable home environment for appropriate adolescent peer group activities

differentiate the male from the female but do not relate directly to reproduction. See discussion in Nursing Care for Adolescents, Chapter 62 ⬤.

The first noticeable sign that puberty has begun in males is the appearance of pubic hair. Sexual maturity is achieved by age 18. Often, the first noticeable sign of puberty in females is the appearance of the breast bud, although the appearance of hair along the labia may precede this. The milestone of female puberty is the *menarche* (beginning of menstrual cycles), which occurs about 2 years after the breast bud appears. At first, menstrual periods are scanty and irregular and may occur without ovulation. Ovulation is usually established 1 to 2 years after menarche. Female internal reproductive organs reach adult size at about age 18 to 20.

PSYCHOSOCIAL DEVELOPMENT

The psychosocial task of the adolescent is the establishment of identity. The danger of this stage is role confusion. Because of the adolescent's dramatic body changes, the development of a stable identity is difficult. Adolescents who are accepted, loved, and valued by family and peers generally tend to gain confidence and feel good about themselves. Adolescents who have difficulty forming relationships or who are perceived by peers as too different and not included in adolescent cliques may develop less favorable self-images and have low self-esteem.

Adolescents still need guidance from their parents, although they appear to neither want it nor need it. However, adolescents need to know that their parents care about them and that their parents still want to help them. Restrictions and guidance need to be presented in a manner that makes adolescents feel loved. They need consistency in guidance and fewer restrictions than previously. They should have the independence they can handle yet know that their parents will assist them when they need help.

During adolescence, peer groups assume great importance (Figure 16-9 ■).

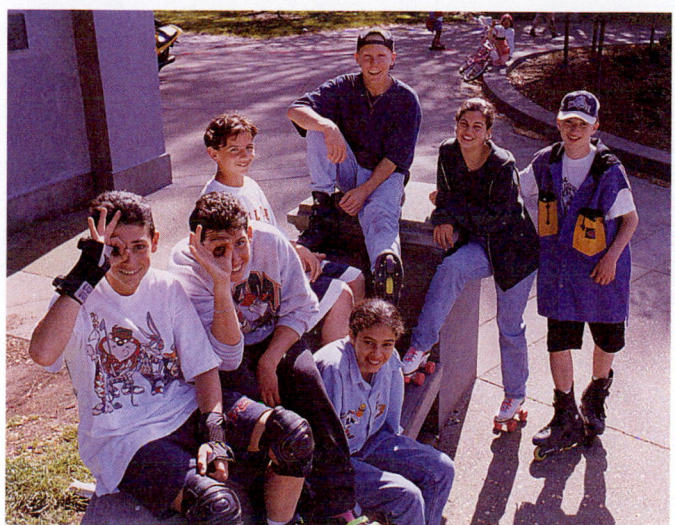

Figure 16-9. ■ Adolescent peer group relationships enhance a sense of belonging, self-esteem, and self-identity. (Photographer: Elena Dorfman.)

COGNITIVE DEVELOPMENT

Cognitive abilities mature during adolescence. Between the ages of 11 and 15, the adolescent begins the formal operations stage of cognitive development. The adolescent becomes more informed about the world and environment. Adolescents use new information to solve everyday problems and can communicate with adults on most subjects.

MORAL DEVELOPMENT

According to Kohlberg, the young adolescent is usually at the conventional level of moral development. Most still accept the Golden Rule and want to abide by social order and existing laws. Adolescents examine their values, standards, and morals. They may discard the values they have adopted from parents in favor of values they consider more suitable. See Kohlberg's stages of moral development in Table 15-2 .

SPIRITUAL DEVELOPMENT

According to Fowler, the adolescent or young adult reaches the synthetic-conventional stage of spiritual development. The adolescent may reconcile the differences in one of the following ways:

- Deciding any differences are wrong
- Compartmentalizing the differences (For example, a friend may not be able to go to dances on Friday evenings because of religious observances, but the friend can share activities on other days.)
- Obtaining advice from a significant other, such as a parent or a minister

Often, the adolescent believes that various religious beliefs and practices have more similarities than differences.

HEALTH ASSESSMENT AND PROMOTION

Adolescents are usually self-directed in meeting their health needs. Because of maturation changes, however, they need teaching and guidance in a number of healthcare areas.

Promoting health and wellness includes screening for tobacco, alcohol, and drug use and for sexual practices, and checking blood pressure, height, and weight. See Table 16-4 for health promotion guidelines for adolescents. For more information on the adolescent client, see Chapter 62 .

Young Adults (20 to 40 Years)

Legally, a person in the United States can vote at 18 years of age. Another criterion of adulthood is financial independence, which is also highly variable. Some adults are financially dependent on their families for many years during prolonged educational courses.

Moving away from home and establishing one's own living arrangements may also indicate adulthood. Many adults under age 30 continue to live with parents due to high housing costs and unemployment rates, as well as social issues such as high divorce rates, single parenting, and the problems resulting from substance abuse. Some young people who are employed fulltime receive only minimum wage and are unable to earn enough money to be totally self-supporting.

Young adults are typically busy people who face many challenges. They are expected to assume new roles at work, in the home, and in the community, and to develop interests, values, and attitudes related to these roles.

PHYSICAL DEVELOPMENT

People in their early 20s are in their prime years physically. The musculoskeletal system is well developed and coordinated. This is the period when athletic endeavors reach their peak.

Although physical changes are minimal during this stage, weight and muscle mass may change as a result of diet and exercise. In addition, extensive physical and psychosocial changes occur in pregnant and lactating women. These changes are discussed in maternal/child textbooks.

PSYCHOSOCIAL DEVELOPMENT

In contrast to the minimal physical changes, psychosocial development and stresses of the young adult are great. Young adults face a number of new experiences and changes in lifestyle as they progress toward maturity.

Remaining single is becoming the lifestyle choice of more and more young adults. Many people choose to remain single, perhaps to pursue an education and then to have the freedom to pursue their chosen vocation. Some

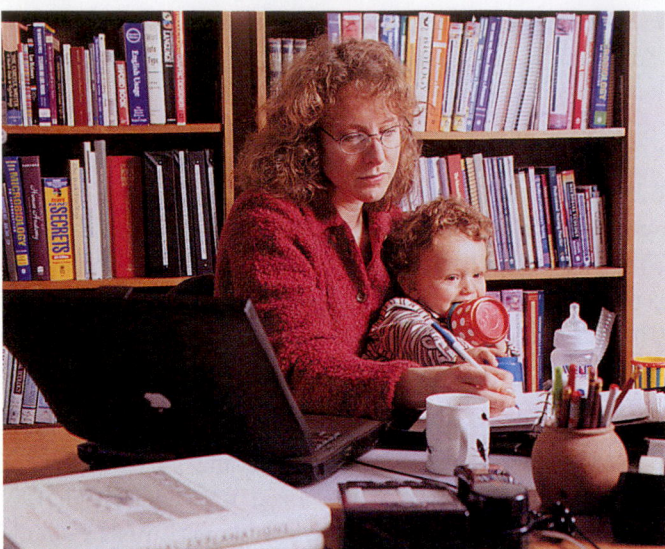

Figure 16-10. ■ Many young women combine active careers with motherhood. (Photographer: Elena Dorfman.)

unmarried individuals choose to live with another person of the opposite or same sex and share living arrangements and certain expenses. Some unmarried people are gay or lesbian and live with or are involved with a partner to whom they are committed.

The multiple roles of adulthood (citizen, worker, taxpayer, homeowner, wife/husband, daughter/son, brother/sister, parent, friend, etc.) may also create stress as a result of role conflict (Figure 16-10 ■).

COGNITIVE, MORAL, AND SPIRITUAL DEVELOPMENT

Cognitive structures were completed during the formal operations period, from roughly 11 to 15 years.

Young adults who have mastered the previous stages of Kohlberg's theory of moral development now enter the postconventional level. At this time, the person is able to separate self from the expectations and rules of others and to define morality in terms of personal principles.

According to Fowler, the individual enters the individuating-reflective period sometime after 18 years of age. You may review the theorists in Chapter 15 ⊙.

HEALTH ASSESSMENT AND PROMOTION

Young adults are usually interested in meeting their health needs. However, because of the many stresses and changes that occur throughout this 20-year period, the nurse needs to offer teaching and guidance in several healthcare areas. The nurse may wish to discuss some or all of the health promotion topics outlined for adults in Table 16-5 ■.

Middle-Age Adults (40 to 65 Years)

The middle years, from 40 to 65, have been called the years of stability and consolidation. For most people, it is a time when children have grown and moved away or are moving away from home. Thus, partners generally have more time for and with each other and time to pursue interests they may have deferred for years.

PHYSICAL DEVELOPMENT

A number of changes take place during the middle years. At age 40, most adults can function as effectively as they did in their 20s. However, during ages 40 to 65, many physical changes take place. Normal changes of aging, which become more pronounced among older adults, are described in Table 16-5.

PSYCHOSOCIAL DEVELOPMENT

Before the mid-1900s, the developmental tasks of middle-aged adults received little attention. Havighurst outlined seven tasks for this age group (see Box 16-2). Erikson views the developmental choice of the middle-aged adult as generativity versus stagnation. *Generativity* is defined as the concern for establishing and guiding the next generation. In other words, the concern about providing for the welfare of humankind is equal to the concern of providing for self.

The middle-aged person looks older and feels older. Although people of these ages are reaching their prime, they begin to recognize that time is at a premium and that life is finite. Youthfulness and physical strength can no longer be taken for granted.

Some researchers suggest that it is not the events themselves that make midlife a crisis, but an individual's response to these life events. Internal and external resources include physical health, family income, the social support system, intelligence, and personality. Thus, the crisis or transitions of midlife are not just within the individual, but also between the individual and the individual's world.

COGNITIVE, MORAL, AND SPIRITUAL DEVELOPMENT

The middle-aged adult's cognitive and intellectual abilities change very little. Cognitive processes include reaction time, memory, perception, learning, problem solving, and creativity. Learning continues and can be enhanced by increased motivation at this time in life.

Middle-aged adults are able to carry out all the strategies described in Piaget's phase of formal operations.

According to Kohlberg, the adult can move beyond the conventional level to the postconventional level.

TABLE 16-5	Health Promotion Guidelines for Young Adults, Middle-Aged Adults, and Older Adults		
GUIDELINES	**YOUNG ADULTS**	**MIDDLE-AGED ADULTS**	**OLDER ADULTS**
Health tests and screenings	Routine physical examination (every 1–3 years for females; every 5 years for males) Immunizations as recommended, such as Td boosters Regular dental assessments (e.g., annually) Periodic vision and hearing screenings Breast self-examination monthly, 1 week after onset of period Professional breast examination every 1–3 years Papanicolaou smear annually or at onset of sexual activity Testicular self-examination every month Screening for cardiovascular disease (e.g., cholesterol test every 5 years if results are normal; blood pressure to detect hypertension; baseline electrocardiogram at age 35 for males) Tuberculosis skin test every 2 years	Routine physical examination (annually for females; every 2–3 years or as directed by physician for males) Immunizations as recommended, such as a tetanus booster every 10–15 years and influenza and pneumococcal vaccinations Regular dental assessments (e.g., yearly) Tonometry for signs of glaucoma and other eye disease every 2–3 years or annually if indicated Breast self-examination as for young adults and first day of every month after menopause Testicular self-examination monthly Screenings for cardiovascular disease (e.g., blood pressure measurement; electrocardiogram and cholesterol test as directed by the physician) Screenings for colorectal, breast, cervical, uterine, and prostate cancer Screening for tuberculosis every 2 years	Same as middle-aged adults
Safety	Motor safety reinforcement (e.g., using designated drivers when drinking, maintaining brakes and tires) Sun protection measures Workplace safety measures Water safety reinforcement (e.g., no diving in shallow water)	Motor vehicle safety reinforcement, especially when driving at night Workplace safety measures Home safety measures: keeping hallways and stairways lighted and uncluttered, using smoke detectors, using nonskid mats and handrails in the bathrooms	Home safety measures to prevent falls, fire, burns, scalds, and electrocution Motor vehicle safety reinforcement, especially when driving at night Precautions to prevent pedestrian accidents
Nutrition, exercise, and elimination	Importance of adequate iron intake in diet Nutritional and exercise factors that may lead to cardiovascular disease (e.g., obesity, cholesterol and fat intake, lack of vigorous exercise)	Importance of adequate protein, calcium, and vitamin D in diet Nutritional and exercise factors that may lead to cardiovascular disease (e.g., obesity, cholesterol and fat intake, lack of vigorous exercise) An exercise program that emphasizes skill and coordination	Importance of a well-balanced diet with fewer calories to accommodate lower metabolic rate and decreased physical activity Importance of sufficient amounts of vitamin D and calcium to prevent osteoporosis Nutritional and exercise factors that may lead to cardiovascular disease (e.g., obesity, cholesterol and fat intake, lack of exercise) A regular program of moderate exercise to maintain joint mobility, muscle tone, and bone calcification Importance of adequate roughage in the diet, adequate exercise, and at least six 8-ounce glasses of fluid daily to prevent constipation

(continued)

TABLE 16-5	Health Promotion Guidelines for Young Adults, Middle-Aged Adults, and Older Adults (continued)		
GUIDELINES	YOUNG ADULTS	MIDDLE-AGED ADULTS	OLDER ADULTS
Social interactions	Encouraging personal relationships that promote discussion of feelings, concerns, and fears Setting short- and long-term goals for work and career choices	The possibility of a midlife crisis: encourage discussion of feelings, concerns, and fears Providing time to expand and review previous interests Retirement planning (financial and possible diversional activities), with partner if appropriate	Encouraging intellectual and recreational pursuits Encouraging personal relationships that promote discussion of feelings, concerns, and fears Availability of social community centers and programs for seniors

Not all adults progress through Fowler's stages to the fifth, called the paradoxical-consolidative stage. At this stage, the individual can view "truth" from a number of viewpoints. In middle age, people tend to be less dogmatic about religious beliefs. People in this age group often rely on spiritual beliefs to help them deal with illness, death, and tragedy.

HEALTH ASSESSMENT AND PROMOTION

Guidelines for health promotion for the middle-aged adult are shown in Table 16-5. Further discussion of nursing care is provided in the Nursing Care section of this chapter.

Older Adults (Over 65 Years)

In 2000, the number of Americans age 65 and older was about 14% of the population. By the year 2030, that percentage is projected to increase to more than 18% of the population. The group of older individuals who are 85 years and older is rapidly increasing (Figure 16-11 ■). Census projections estimate that the population over age 85 will almost triple by the year 2020 (U.S. Bureau of the Census, 2000).

Various systems are used to categorize the aging population. *Frail elderly*, a term used to describe the extremely aged, is more likely to be used to describe the elderly individual who has significant physiological and functional impairment, whatever the age.

PHYSICAL CHANGES

As the person ages, a number of physical changes occur; some are visible, some are not. Older adults will experience changes in every body system. For example, the skin will become drier and more fragile. The muscles will atrophy if not used, and reaction time will slow. Generally speaking, the body will experience the consequences of lifestyle choices and genetic inheritance.

An in-depth discussion of the healthy older adult is found in Chapter 42 . Discussion of the ill older adult is found in Chapter 43 .

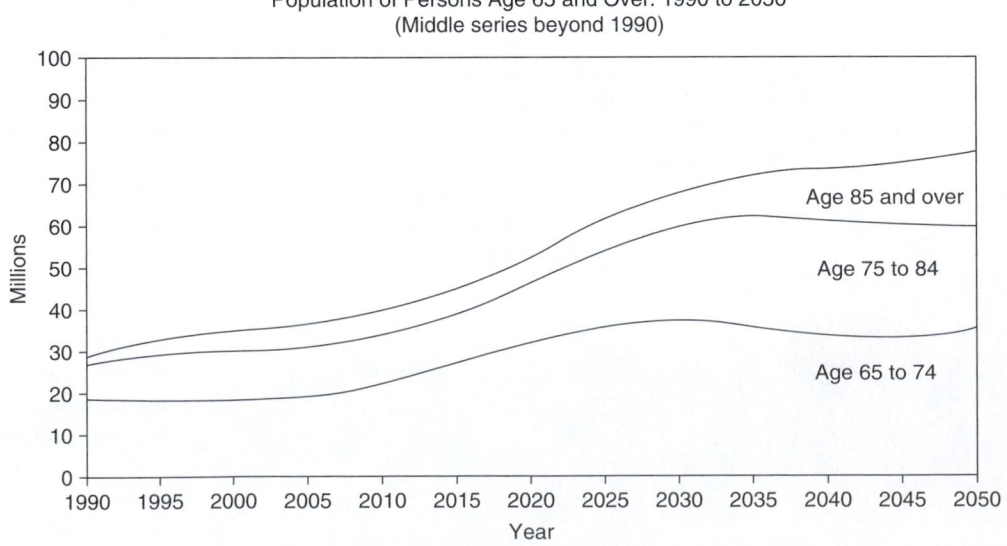

Population of Persons Age 65 and Over: 1990 to 2050
(Middle series beyond 1990)

Age 85 and over
Age 75 to 84
Age 65 to 74

Figure 16-11. ■ Census data show a tremendous increase in the older adult population.

PSYCHOSOCIAL DEVELOPMENT

According to Erikson, the developmental task at this time is ego integrity versus despair (see Table 15-1 ⚭). People who attain ego integrity view life with a sense of wholeness and derive satisfaction from past accomplishments. They view death as an acceptable completion of life. By contrast, people who despair often believe they have made poor choices during life and wish they could live life over.

Most elderly people thrive on independence (Figure 16-12 ■). Having to begin to depend on others is a difficult life transition. For full coverage of the effects of retirement, economic changes, relocation, and maintaining independence, refer to Chapters 42 and 43 ⚭ . Older adults, no matter what their current health status, realize that life cannot continue forever. As friends and perhaps even a spouse dies, they must face their own mortality. Refer to Chapter 18 ⚭ for discussion of death, dying, and grieving.

COGNITIVE DEVELOPMENT

Piaget's phases of cognitive development end with the formal operations phase. Intellectual capacity includes perception, cognitive agility, memory, and learning. If the aging person's senses are impaired, the ability to perceive the environment and react appropriately is diminished. Overall, the older adult maintains intelligence, problem solving, judgment, creativity, and other well-practiced cognitive skills. Intellectual loss generally reflects a disease process. Most older adults do not experience cognitive impairments.

In older adults, retrieval of information from long-term memory can be slower, especially if the information is not frequently used. Most age-related differences occur in short-term memory. Older adults tend to forget the recent past. This forgetfulness can be improved by the use of memory aids, making notes or lists, and placing objects in consistent locations. The older person should remain mentally active to maintain cognitive ability at the highest possible level.

MORAL DEVELOPMENT

According to Kohlberg, moral development is completed in the early adult years. Most older people stay at Kohlberg's conventional level of moral development. The value and belief patterns that are important to older adults are cultural background, life experiences, gender, religion, and socioeconomic status. The nurse must identify and consider the specific values of the older client when nursing care is planned.

SPIRITUAL DEVELOPMENT

Often, the older person's knowledge becomes wisdom, an inner resource for dealing with both positive and negative life experiences. Many older people have strong religious convictions and continue to attend religious meetings or services. Involvement in religion often helps the older adult to resolve issues related to the meaning of life, to adversity, or to good fortune. The "old-old" person who cannot attend formal services often continues religious participation in a more private manner. According to Fowler, some people enter the sixth stage of spiritual development, universalizing.

HEALTH ASSESSMENT AND PROMOTION

Assessment activities may include questions about the following:

- Usual dietary pattern
- Any problems with bowel or urinary elimination
- Activity/exercise and sleep/rest patterns
- Family and social activities and interests
- Any problems with reading, writing, or problem solving
- Adjustment to retirement or loss of partner

Healthcare professionals must also be alert for the following:

- Symptoms of depression
- Risk factors for suicide
- Signs of abnormal bereavement
- Changes in cognitive function

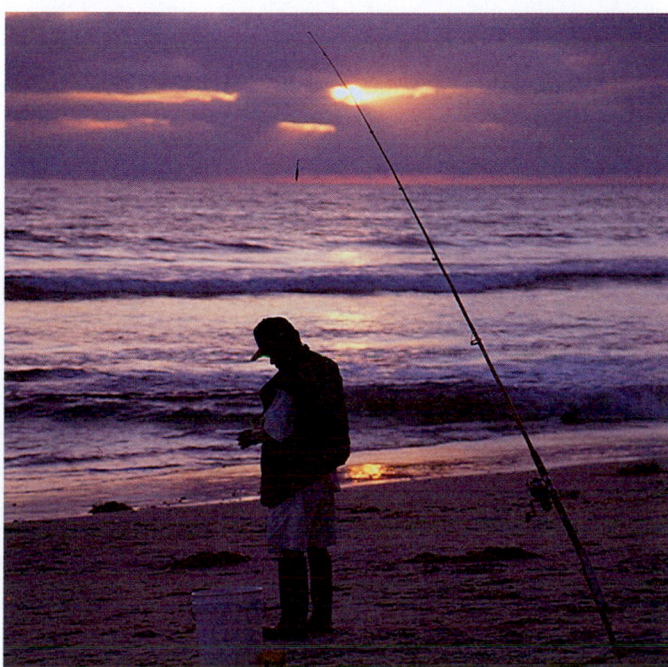

Figure 16-12. ■ Many elderly people find creative outlets during retirement. (Photographer: Elena Dorfman/AWL.)

- Medications that increase risk of falls
- Signs of physical abuse or neglect
- Skin lesions (malignant and peripheral)
- Tooth decay, gingivitis, loose teeth

Older persons are usually concerned about their health and are interested in information and behavioral strategies directed toward improving it. Refer to Box 9-1 and Chapter 42 ⚭ for health promotion topics.

FAMILY SYSTEMS

When planning care for the individual client, it is important to consider the needs of the family as well. This is most obvious in the areas of maternal-infant care, pediatrics, geriatrics, and mental health. **Family-centered care** is treatment to a designated client with recognition that the family system or unit may also need intervention. This is especially important in maternal-newborn, pediatric, and mental health nursing.

Like the individual, the family is a developing system (Carter, 1999). For the individual to have a healthy development, the family must progress through predictable

stages of a family life cycle. Table 16-6 ■ provides a snapshot of stages in the family life cycle.

What is a **family**? The classic definition of family is two or more people related by blood or marriage who reside together. In recent years the definition has been broadened to two or more individuals who come together for the purpose of nurturing. The structure of families traditionally is linked to the relationship between parent and child, between spouses, or both.

Traditionally family types are **nuclear family** (a family consisting of parents and biological offspring). This type of

TABLE 16-6	Stages in the Family Life Cycle	
STAGE	**FAMILY TASKS**	**FAMILY ROLES**
I Beginning family (*no children*)	■ Learning to live together ■ Relating harmoniously to three families (families of origin and newly established family) ■ Planning for family (whether or not to have children) ■ Making satisfactory sexual and marital role adjustment	Husband Wife Parents In-laws
II Early childbearing (*birth of first child until infant reaches 30 months of age*)	■ Developing a stable family unit with new parent role ■ Reconciling conflicting developmental tasks of family members ■ Facilitating development needs of family members to strengthen the family unit ■ Accepting new child's personality	Husband Wife Parents In-laws Grandparents
III Families with preschool children (*1st born 2 1/2 to age 5*)	■ Helping child explore environment ■ Establishing privacy, housing, and adequate space ■ Encouraging husband-father to be more involved in household responsibilities ■ Helping preschooler assume responsibilities of self-care ■ Enabling socialization of children ■ Integrating new family members ■ Dealing with separation from children as they enter school	Husband Wife Parents In-laws Grandparents Child Sibling
IV Families with school-age children (1st born 6 to 13 years)	■ Promoting school achievement of children ■ Maintaining satisfying marital relationships ■ Promoting open communication in family ■ Accepting adolescence	Husband Wife Parents In-laws Grandparents Child Sibling

TABLE 16-6	Stages in the Family Life Cycle (continued)	
STAGE	**FAMILY TASKS**	**FAMILY ROLES**
V Families with teenagers	■ Maintaining satisfying marital relationships while handling parental responsibilities ■ Maintaining open communication between generations ■ Maintaining family ethical and moral standards while teens are searching for their own beliefs and values ■ Allowing children to experiment with independence	Husband Wife Parents In-laws Grandparents Chlid Sibling Adolescent
VI Launching-center families (*first child through last child leaving home*)	■ Expanding the family circle to include new members by marriage ■ Accepting new couple's own lifestyle and values ■ Devoting time to other activities and relationships by parents ■ Reestablishing the wife and husband roles as children achieve independence ■ Assisting aging and ill parents of husband or wife	Husband Wife Parents In-laws Grandparents Child Sibling Young Adult
VII Families of middle years (*"empty nest" period through retirement*)	■ Maintaining a sense of well-being psychologically and physiologically by living in a healthy environment ■ Attaining and enjoying a career or other creative accomplishments by cultivating leisure-time activities and interests ■ Sustaining satisfying and meaningful relationships with aging parents and children ■ Strengthening the marital relationship	Husband Wife Parents In-laws Grandparents Child Sibling Young Adult Great-Grandparents
VIII Families in retirement and old age (*begins with retirement of one or both spouses, continues until loss of one spouse to death, and terminates with death of the other spouse*)	■ Maintaining satisfying living relationship ■ Maintaining marital relationship ■ Adjusting to reduced income ■ Adjusting to loss of spouse	Children Caring for Elderly, Frail Parents

family usually maintains relatively close ties with kin. **Extended family** refers to an egocentric network of relatives (e.g., grandparents, aunt, uncles, and cousins). Today we see many other types of families. In a single-parent family, either a mother or father raises children alone. Divorced parent families account for more than half of American families today. Many will find themselves in a stepfamily situation, or blended family. The term **blended family** describes a situation in which one or both spouses have had a previous marriage and children from that marriage. Guardians, foster care, and adoptions provide a family for almost 2 million children in this country. Interracial families are an ever-growing part of family groupings. (By 2000, nearly 7 million Americans of all ages were identified as more than one race.) Unmarried partners with or without children form a large number of families. In the 2000 census, the number of these families had increased 72% in the last decade (including same-sex and heterosexual

couples). The final family type is the **communal family**. This family includes adults and children who may or may not be related. In this type of family, family decisions and responsibilities are shared. A communal family should not be confused with a cult family, where a leader makes all decisions and controls the actions of all those who live there.

Roles and Functions

The functions of the family are to:

■ Provide economic support for other family members.
■ Satisfy emotional needs for love and security.
■ Provide a sense of place and position in society.

Roles play an important part in healthy family functioning. Clear family roles within a family are directly connected to the family's ability to deal with day-to-day life. Individual members occupy specific roles (child, sibling, grandchild). As family members mature, they take on new roles such as spouse, parent, or grandparent. A person's role is always expanding or changing, depending on age and family stage. Family expectations are closely connected to roles. Parents are expected to teach, discipline, and provide for their children. Children are expected to cooperate with and respect their parents.

Parenting Styles

Parenting styles play an important part in family expectations. Two important factors to consider when analyzing parenting styles are:

- **Demandingness**, which relates to the demands that parents make on the children, their expectations for mature behavior, the discipline and supervision they provide, and their willingness to confront behavioral problems.
- **Responsiveness**, which relates to how much they foster individuality, self-assertion, and self-regulation; and how responsive they are to special needs and demands.

Table 16-7 ■ lists types and descriptions of some parenting styles.

Culture is also an important consideration in family groups. In the United States, there are four main cultural groups: Rasa Latina, Asian Pacific, American Black, and Caucasian. Family roles, views, and expectations vary widely among these groups. Box 3-1 ⬭ provided some insight into these cultural groups.

NURSING CARE

PRIORITIZING NURSING CARE

The LPN/LVN must have a good basic understanding of lifespan development and family systems. With understanding of that information comes the ability to plan nursing care to promote continued development even in times of crisis. When caring for a young child, knowing whether a child has achieved bowel and bladder control or is not toilet trained will help the nurse decide if trips to the bathroom need to be scheduled.

Adolescents need to be given the choice of whether or not to have a parent present when being examined.

Middle adult clients frequently have stressful family and job concerns while hospitalized. A serious illness can have an effect on their ability to support the family. A mother may worry about who will carry out the home responsibilities during her recovery. The nurse needs to be supportive and encourage them to talk to their spouse or other family member or social worker about these concerns, so that they can concentrate on their health and recovery.

Development of older adults depends a lot on their life up to this point. If their life has been fulfilling, they may express that they are ready to die in a very comfortable, almost anticipatory manner. The nurse should encourage them to talk about their life and to talk with family and bring closure. Other older adults may become sullen and difficult to please. With these clients, the nurse will strive to make the client comfortable. Understanding the client stage of development is always a priority.

ASSESSING

Data for assessment should always take into consideration the normal growth and developmental level of the client. For example, normal assessment information for an infant would include head circumference as well as height and weight. Normal assessment data for a 14-year-old girl would include presence and frequency of menstrual cycles.

DIAGNOSING, PLANNING, AND IMPLEMENTING

Nursing diagnoses for clients with developmentally related concerns might include:

- *Risk for Impaired Parenting*
- *Relocation Stress Syndrome*
- *Situational Low Self-Esteem*

Some outcomes for clients with developmentally related concerns might include:

- Parents will state belief in positive outcomes for child demonstrated by effective coping behaviors as evidenced by holding and helping with infant care.

TABLE 16-7	**Parenting Styles**		
STYLE	CONTROL	WARMTH	DESCRIPTION
Authoritative	High	High	Parents allow give-and-take communication and have clear expectations for behavior. Children are mature, resilient, and achievement oriented. *"We can talk about it."*
Authoritarian	High	Low	Parents are highly directive and value obedience. Children show lower internalization of prosocial values and ego development. *"Because I said so."*
Permissive	Low	High	Parents make few demands, allow children to regulate themselves, and avoid confrontational behavior. A common phrase is, *"Do whatever you want."*
			Children who are encouraged to make decisions before they are mature enough to make them may feel confused, overwhelmed, or paralyzed at the thought of taking action in the world.

- Client will request information about new environment.
- Client will report a sense of control over life situations.

The nurse's role in providing support for these clients would include the following:

- *Encourage parents to hold and interact with the child during the pre- and postoperative periods to promote bonding.*
- *Reduce differences between old and new environment; promote continuity of care in new environment.*
- *Provide encouragement while a task or skill is being performed. Allow client to perform as independently as possible.*

Planning at all levels of nursing care should incorporate an understanding of the client's age, developmental level, and any particular issues that might affect the client's progress toward wellness.

Awareness of a client's developmental level is especially important in implementing nursing care. A young child will usually respond better if a parent or safe adult is present for nursing care. An adolescent may prefer to have the parent leave the room during physical examination (especially a parent of the opposite sex). An older adult with an age-related hearing impairment would benefit from having a family member or caregiver present to listen to discharge instructions. Sensitivity to developmental issues is a great aid to nurses both in listening and in providing teaching. (See also Chapter 12 🔗 for client teaching.)

EVALUATING

The nurse collects data to determine whether outcomes have been met. If goals have not been achieved, the nurse can consider the need to adapt interventions to address developmental needs more closely.

NURSING PROCESS CARE PLAN
Client with Involutional* Depression

Sandra Peterson is a 48-year-old woman experiencing perimenopause. She feels that she is "losing her mind." She constantly forgets things, and her mood is unpredictable. She often becomes irritable for no apparent reason and then feels guilty for being hypercritical. She has a tendency to overdramatize events. According to her family, she "always has to be right." Sandra accidentally burns herself every time she uses the oven, and refuses to recognize the limitations of her aging body. Her arms have burn scars that are obviously months old, and now she has

---

*Involutional depression—A major depressive episode associated with the end of the female productive cycle.

sustained a severe burn. Sandra lives with her husband, but the close family frequently interacts, although she reports, "My kids continually make excuses not to attend family gatherings."

Assessment

- C/o persistent physical symptoms that do not respond to treatment: headaches, digestive disorders, chronic pain.
- Weight 135 lbs, height 62", increase of 7 lbs over the last month
- VS: T 97.2, P 76, R 18, BP 110/78; c/o palpitations
- Lab test
- H&H 12.8, 33
- T_3, T_4 within normal
- Serum calcium low

Nursing Diagnosis

The following important nursing diagnoses (among others) are established for this client:

- *Chronic Low Self-Esteem* related to repeated unmet expectations
- *Energy Field Disturbance* related to disharmony
- *Self-Mutilation* related to inability to express tension verbally

Expected Outcomes

The expected outcomes for the plan of care are:

- Verbalizes increased self-acceptance through use of positive self-statements.
- States feeling of relaxation.
- States appropriate ways to cope with increased psychological or physiological tension.

Planning and Implementation

The following nursing interventions are implemented:

- Demonstrate and promote effective communication techniques.
- Encourage realistic and achievable goal setting; recognize the value of attempts and accomplishment.
- Assist client with evaluating the impact of family on feelings of self-worth.
- Administer therapeutic touch to induce relaxation.
- Validate the client's feelings and concerns related to sense of disharmony or energy disturbance.
- Provide medical treatment for injuries. Use careful aseptic technique when caring for burns.
- Assess for signs of depression, anxiety, and impulsivity.
- Establish trust.

Evaluation

On recheck, the client reports participating in yoga class 3× per week for relaxation. Reports that she has had no injuries this week. No digestive problems or headaches this week. Family reports she seems less stressed.

Critical Thinking in the Nursing Process

1. What might be some of the reasons for Mrs. Peterson's burns?

2. According to Erikson's developmental stages, Mrs. Peterson is in the generativity vs. stagnation stage. Her behavior demonstrates negative resolution (self-indulgence, self-concern, and lack of interest and commitments). What recommendations could you make as a nurse that would help produce positive resolution?

3. Mrs. Peterson's family is very concerned about her injuries and behavior. What can they do to help her through this difficult time?

Note: Discussion of Critical Thinking questions appears on the MyNursingKit Website.

Note: The references and resources for all chapters have been compiled at the back of the book.

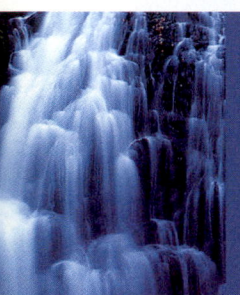

Chapter Review

KEY Points

- Growth and development are influenced by both genetics and environment. Development begins at conception and continues into old age.
- Growth and development happen individually but follow general predictable patterns.
- Growth and development have five major components: physiological, psychosocial, cognitive, moral, and spiritual.
- Health assessment and promotion activities by the nurse assist the client to meet developmental milestones.
- As the population grows older, growth and development needs of the elderly will affect health care to a greater extent.
- Parenting styles have a great impact on family dynamics.
- Families go through developmental stages just as individuals do.

FOR FURTHER Study

Box 3-1 provides some insight into the four main cultural groups.

See Box 9-1 for lifespan safety considerations.

See Chapter 12 for client teaching.

For a review of theorists and therapies related to see Chapter 15.

Refer to Chapter 18 for discussion of death, dying, and grieving.

For an in-depth discussion of the healthy older adult, see Chapter 42; discussion of the ill older adult is found in Chapter 43.

See Chapter 56 for the procedures for taking an infant's height, weight, and circumference and for more in-depth content on newborn infants.

For a sample of the Denver Developmental Screening Test, see Figure 58-15.

For additional information on health promotion, nursing, and health care for toddlers and preschoolers, see Chapters 59 and 60.

See Chapter 62 for a discussion of nursing care for adolescents.

PEARSON
EXPLORE mynursingkit™

MyNursingKit is your one stop for online chapter review materials and resources. Prepare for success with additional NCLEX®-style practice questions, interactive assignments and activities, web links, animations and videos, and more!

Register your access code from the front of your book at **www.mynursingkit.com**

Critical Thinking Care Map

Caring for a Toddler with Risk for Injury
NCLEX-PN® Focus Area: Safety

Case Study: Todd Underwood, a 2-year-old, is brought into the clinic by his mother, Kelly. He has been brought in for a recheck following an ear infection. When you enter the exam room to take his vital signs, you observe Kelly frantically chasing Todd around the room. He is climbing on the furniture, opening all the cupboards, and pulling the paper off the exam table. Kelly states, "I'm worn out from chasing him and worried about his safety. Over the weekend he got into the medicine cabinet and was able to open several bottles. He also has learned how to unlock the patio door, which leads to the backyard Jacuzzi." Todd lives with his parents. A 12-year-old half-sister visits on alternate weekends.

Nursing Diagnosis: *Risk for Injury/Trauma*

COLLECT DATA

Subjective	Objective
_____	_____
_____	_____
_____	_____
_____	_____
_____	_____
_____	_____

Would you report this? Yes/No

If yes, report to: _____

What would you report? _____

Nursing Care

_____
_____
_____
_____
_____
_____
_____
_____
_____
_____

How would you document this? _____
_____
_____

Compare your answers and documentation to those provided on the MyNursingKit Website.

Data Collected
(use only those that apply)

- 2-year-old male child
- Lives with parents
- Half-sister, child of father's previous marriage, visits alternate weekends
- Both parents work outside the home
- Is cared for by maternal grandmother during the week
- VS: T 98.8 (tympanic), P 80, R 18
- Weight 29 lbs
- Height 34"
- Amoxicillin 500 mg (10-day course completed 2 days ago)
- Diet: appetite fair; grandmother has trouble getting him to sit down for meals, usually resorts to finger food; takes a bottle at night
- Mother states opened medicine bottles from home medicine cabinet
- Able to open patio door near backyard Jacuzzi
- Mother states she is worn out from chasing Todd

Nursing Interventions
(use only those that apply; list in priority order)

- Explain individual differences in child temperaments and compare and contrast with the reality of parent expectations.
- Inform parents of available CPR and first aid training in the community.
- Assist parents in devising a plan to childproof the home.
- Advise parent to eliminate all sweets from the child's diet.
- Teach caregiver the need for close supervision of young children.
- Provide poison control number to mother.
- Initiate referrals to parent education opportunities and stress management training.
- Observe for cause of family problem.
- Help caregiver find personal time to meet own needs and learn stress management.
- Discuss sound disciplinary techniques (e.g., time out).

NCLEX-PN® Exam Preparation

1 You are assessing a 2-month-old infant. The mother tells you that he has been lifting his head and looking around but cannot roll over. She is expressing concerns about the baby's development. Your best response would be:

1. "Don't worry, he will roll over at about 4 months."
2. "Development is very individualized, but it does progress in an orderly manner."
3. "Babies who sleep on their backs don't try to roll over as soon as babies who sleep on their stomachs."
4. "Heavier babies are slower to roll over."

2 The nurse admits a child to the pediatric unit who graphs as falling into the 5th percentile for height, weight, and head circumference. The nurse recognizes this child:

1. Is developmentally delayed.
2. Is lagging behind in growth and development.
3. Requires further assessment to determine why he or she is not growing normally.
4. Has failure to thrive.

3 The nurse is providing care for a child who eats fairly well with a spoon, controls bladder and bowel during the day, and can climb stairs. The nurse recognizes this is normal development for a/an:

1. Toddler.
2. Preschooler.
3. School-aged child.
4. Infant.

4 The nurse is caring for a woman whose last child has recently moved out of the family home and into an apartment. The woman describes feeling a lack of purpose and no longer knows how to fill the hours when her husband is at work. The nurse recognizes this family is in what stage?

1. Beginning family – stage I
2. Launching – stage VI.
3. Middle years – stage VII.
4. Pre-retirement – stage VIII.

5 The nurse overhears two parents talking in the waiting room. Parent A says, "I tell my child what to do and if he questions me, I tell him to do what I said because I said so!" Parent B responds: "In our family we discuss rules and reach decisions together that we can all be happy with." What parenting styles are these parents displaying?

1. Parent A is demonstrating authoritative parenting while parent B is demonstrating authoritarian parenting style.
2. Parent A is demonstrating authoritarian parenting while parent B is demonstrating permissive parenting style.
3. Parent A is demonstrating authoritarian parenting while parent B is demonstrating authoritative parenting style.

4. Parent A is demonstrating permissive parenting while parent B is demonstrating authoritarian parenting style.

6 The nurse, working in a physician's office, calls an adolescent female to be seen. The teen's mother begins to follow along. Which of the following statements by the nurse would be appropriate and correct?

1. "We normally prefer to see clients without their family members. Would you feel better if your mother came with you?"
2. "Your mother is not allowed in the examination room."
3. "I'm so glad you're coming along. I prefer to have parents in the examination room with children."
4. "Do you need your mother to come with us?"

7 The nurse, working in the newborn nursery, enters the room of a new mother to take a newborn to the nursery for the pediatrician to examine. The mother says, "Oh, I'm so glad you're here. It's been crying for the last 30 minutes and all I want to do is sleep. Could you please take it to the nursery for a few hours?" The nurse recognizes that which of the following would be an appropriate nursing diagnosis for this family?

1. Altered sleep patterns.
2. Risk for impaired parenting.
3. Situational low self-esteem.
4. Altered family roles.

8 The nurse is contributing to a health promotion teaching plan for a middle-aged adult and recognizes which of the following is an important factor to include for this client?

1. Home safety measures such as keeping hallways and stairways clear of clutter.
2. Sun protection measures.
3. Home safety to prevent falls.
4. Water safety measures.

9 The nurse is caring for a 6-month-old infant and anticipates which of the following reflexes would still be present?

1. Rooting reflex.
2. Moro reflex.
3. Plantar reflex.
4. Tonic neck reflex.

10 The nurse teaches the young adult male the importance of which of the following? (Choose all that apply.)

1. Importance of adequate iron intake.
2. Actions to prevent or reduce the risk of sexually transmitted infections.
3. Reduction in calories to match reduced caloric needs.
4. Importance of adequate folic acid in the diet.

Answers and rationales for Review Questions appear in Appendix I.

Chapter 17

Psychosocial Nursing of the Physically Ill Client

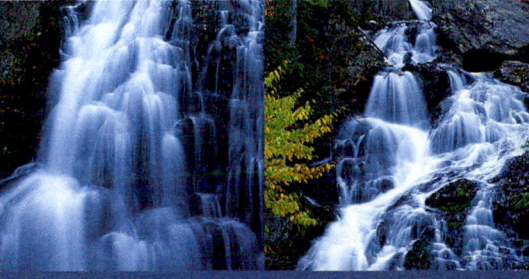

LEARNING Outcomes

After completing this chapter, you will be able to:

1. Explain the types of data collected for a psychosocial assessment.
2. List the components of a mental status exam.
3. Name common psychological responses to serious medical illness.
4. Identify types of depression, its manifestations at different ages, and therapies used to treat depression.
5. List conditions associated with increased risk of suicide and the emotional or behavioral changes that may be seen.
6. Contrast stress and anxiety, and describe ways clients can cope with these conditions.
7. Identify ways clients cope, including defense mechanisms.
8. Discuss psychosocial factors in medical illness.
9. Name ways the LPN/LVN can meet the psychosocial needs of the medically ill adult or child.
10. Discuss the nursing process in terms of meeting the psychosocial needs of the client.

Clinical Objectives

11. Perform a psychosocial evaluation on a physically ill client.
12. Provide for clients' psychosocial needs following Maslow's hierarchy.

BRIEF Outline

KEY TERMS

Use the audio glossary feature on the MyNursingKit Website to hear the correct pronunciation of the following key terms.

affect 320	dual diagnosis 333	posttraumatic stress disorder 331
anger 329	fight-or-flight response 328	projection 334
anxiety 329	general adaptation	psychiatrist 321
bipolar affective disorder 321	syndrome 327	psychologist 323
caregiver burden 332	ICU psychosis 335	psychosocial assessment 318
clinical depression 320	identification 335	rationalization 334
compensation 335	intellectualization 334	reaction formation 334
coping 332	introjection 335	regression 335
counseling 323	labile 319	repression 334
crisis 338	obsessive-compulsive	seasonal affective disorder 321
defense mechanisms 332	disorder 330	self-help 331
denial 334	panic attacks 330	stressors 326
depression 320	phobias 330	suicidal ideation 325
displacement 334	postnatal depression 331	undoing 334

The nurse should view every client as a total person. A *holistic* view incorporates the person's physical, mental, emotional, spiritual, behavioral, and social dimensions.

The connection between mind and body has been shown to affect a person's health and well-being. It is important for nurses to consider this connection when providing physical care. Failure to do so can have a negative effect on the client and may slow down physical recovery.

People who undergo a life-threatening disease or chronic illness must often deal with distressing physical side effects and changes in body image. Clients who have body-altering procedures (colostomies, mastectomies) frequently have psychosocial concerns that must be considered. Clients who have had a cardiac arrest or coronary bypass may experience severe psychosocial reactions. It is important for the nurse to know whether clients have coping strategies and social supports to help them deal with the consequences of illness.

Individuals diagnosed with mental illness may also experience health problems that require hospitalization in an acute care hospital. At times, a medical-surgical nurse may be called on to provide care for a client who also suffers from mental disorders. Delivery of care to these individuals increases the nurse's responsibility to address the psychosocial needs of clients along with their physical needs.

Components of holistic assessment include a physical assessment (see Procedure 19-1 ⚭), psychosocial assessment, assessment of usual coping strategies, and an overall quality-of-life assessment, including ability to attend to activities of daily living (ADLs), social activities, social supports, and client's perception of quality of life, feelings, and pain. Religious or spiritual assessment and assessment of cultural beliefs are covered as part of the inquiry into social supports.

Psychosocial Assessment

To meet the client's psychosocial needs, the nurse must conduct a psychosocial assessment as part of the admission process. The RN normally is responsible for the complete assessment. LVNs and LPNs may be in charge of certain aspects of data collection to assist with this process.

The **psychosocial assessment** can be defined as the gathering of data about the emotional, behavioral, mental, environmental, spiritual, and interactional processes of the client. Information is gathered in an effort to identify the client's past and current level of functioning. This is much more than the nurse asking a series of questions. Instead, it is an interactive process. The client is evaluated in different situations to determine his or her present level of functioning in all the areas listed above.

COMPONENTS OF THE PSYCHOSOCIAL ASSESSMENT

A psychosocial assessment, like a physical assessment, has prescribed areas for which the nurse elicits information. Box 17-1 ■ lists important components of a psychosocial assessment.

Problem Identification and Clarification

The information from the psychosocial assessment is used to identify problems. Both subjective and objective data are collected to determine what psychosocial problems might exist.

Once a problem has been identified, further data collection determines the "who, what, where, why, when, how, and how much" of the problem. The nurse will participate

BOX 17-1   DATA COLLECTION

Psychosocial Status

- Demographic information: name, birth date, age, gender, marital status, and religious preference; include also a mental health diagnosis if one has been given
- Family members or other support system
- Admission data
  - Length of admission
  - Type of admission: voluntary/involuntary (see Chapter 14 ⚭), crisis situation
- Presenting problem
  - Client's perception of reason for admission/clinic visit: describe using client's own words; this may or may not be the actual reason
  - Actual factors precipitating admission/clinic visit: identify actual facts leading to admission (e.g., family quarrels, bizarre public or private behaviors, violence to self or others, poor medication compliance, inability to care for self, confusion, disorientation, hearing voices, etc.)
- Previous medical history: inpatient/outpatient, treatment, effectiveness
- Previous psychiatric history: inpatient/outpatient, reasons for the types of treatment, and their effectiveness
- Drug and alcohol use/abuse: amount, frequency, duration of past or present use of legal/illegal substance, date and time of last use; include medications they are taking
- Disturbance in patterns of daily living: sleep, intake, elimination, sexual activity, work leisure, self-care, and hygiene
- Support systems: amount of contact, nature/quality of relationships, and availability of support
- General appearance: type and condition of clothing, cleanliness, physical condition, and posture
- Behavior during interview
  - Anger: overt, covert, verbal, or physical
  - Degree of cooperation, resistance, evasiveness

- Social skills: positive/unpleasant habits, shyness, withdrawal
- Motor activity: amount and type (e.g., psychomotor retardation, agitation, restlessness, tics, tremors, hypervigilance, lack of activity)
- Orientation to time, place, person, and level of consciousness
- Memory: recent/remote, amnesia, blackouts, confabulation
- Thought processes reflected in speech (e.g., blocking, *circumstantiality* [providing an excessive amount of unnecessary detail], loose associations, flight of ideas, *perseveration* [constant repetition of a meaningless word or phrase], tangential ideas, ambivalence, *neologisms* [made-up words or words used with a new meaning], or "word salad")
- Thought content (e.g., expressing helplessness, hopelessness, worthlessness, guilt, suicidal ideas/plans, homicidal ideas/plans, suspiciousness, phobias, obsessions, compulsions, preoccupations, antisocial attitudes, blaming others, poverty of comfort, denial)
- Hallucinations: visual, auditory, others
- Delusions (e.g., persecution ["they are after me"], grandeur ["I am king"], religious ["I am the Messiah"], or somatic ["My legs are solar-powered machines"])
- Intellectual functioning: use of language and knowledge, abstract vs. concrete thinking, proverbs, calculations
- Affect and mood refer to the client's emotions/feeling tone (e.g., anxiety level, blunted, or flat affect, volatile; quickly springing from one emotion to another [called **labile**]; elated; euphoric; depressed; tearful; motivated; caring; protective; open and receptive; closed and noncommunicative; suspicious; irritable; annoyed; angry; inappropriate)
- Insight: degree of awareness of problems and their causes
- Judgment: soundness of problem solving and decisions
- Motivation for treatment

---

in planning with the client. This includes setting goals, developing and implementing interventions, and evaluating the effectiveness of those interventions in relation to established goals. To set workable goals and create a care plan that is unique to the client, the nurse must gather historic information about the client. Exploration into the following areas is done:

- Social history (discussed in Box 17-1)
  - What is the client's religion/spirituality?
  - What is the client's occupation?
  - What other interests does the client have?
  - Does the client have the ability to socialize?
  - What is the pattern of communication with significant others?
  - What roles does the client play within family, community?
  - How is conflict handled within family?

- Usual coping patterns
  - How does client usually manage stressors?
  - What happened the last time the person was under severe stress?
  - How does client rate the current stress level?
- Understanding of current illness and need for hospitalization
- History of psychiatric disorders
- Major issues raised by the current illness (i.e., how is institutionalization affecting client and family?)
- *Neurovegetative changes* (physical problems related to psychosocial issues)
- Body image
  - Describe your appearance (draw a picture).
  - What are your feelings about your body?
  - What do you like about your body?
  - If you could change your body, what, if anything, would you change?

- Self-concept
  - How would you describe yourself to others? What are your strengths and weaknesses?
  - Who would you like to be?
  - Who or what has influenced your self-expectations?
  - What are your expectations in life? Are they realistic?
- Self-esteem (Do you like who you are?)
- Competence (How do you feel about your ability to do all the things your roles demand?)
- Goals (Where do you see yourself in 1 month? 1 year? 5 years?)
- Power (To what extent do you feel able to control your life?)
- Spirituality
  - Is there a spiritual belief system that is important to you? How is it important?
  - What gives meaning to your life or makes you want to live?
  - Does your spiritual system help when you are not feeling well?
  - Does your spiritual system influence healthcare decisions in any way? How?
  - Do you have any beliefs of a religious or spiritual nature about the cause or treatment of your problems?
- Interpersonal relations (family, school, work, community, dependence/independence)
- Sexuality (see Box 17-1)
  - Are you sexually active?
  - Are you satisfied with your sex life?
  - Has your desire for sex or interest in sex changed? If so, how?
  - How has the state of physical health affected you and your spouse or partner?
  - Is your significant other living? (If yes) Is your relationship satisfying? (If no) How do you cope with the loss of that relationship?
- Activities of daily living (ADLs)

Mental Status Exam

The mental status examination is part of a psychosocial assessment. However, when the client is in crisis, it is often done independently of the complete assessment (see also Procedure 19-1 and Chapter 49 ⬤⬤). The RN would perform this assessment initially, but LPNs/LVNs will also monitor the following in the course of daily care:

- General appearance
- Behavior (such as *catatonic* [rigid], agitated, compulsive; client's words and actions in agreement)
  - Speech (pressured, disconnected)
  - Thought content and thought processes

  - Whether the person's statements make sense and are logical
  - Themes in the client's thinking
  - Evidence of delusions
  - Sensation/perception
  - Evidence of hallucinations
  - Trust/mistrust
  - Actions/statements suggesting suspicion, mistrust of others (paranoia)
- **Affect**—outward appearance of emotional state (e.g., tense, angry, happy, flat, blunted, labile or changeable)
- Mood—client's subjective description of emotional state
- Memory—immediate, recent, and remote
- Orientation, attention, and judgment
- Abstract thinking
- Insight and general intelligence

Psychological Responses to Serious Medical Illness

Common responses to physical illness are depression, anxiety, stress, grief, denial, and fear of dependency.

DEPRESSION

Depression describes a range of moods, from the low spirits that we all experience to a severe problem that interferes with everyday life. *Major depressive disorder*, or **clinical depression,** is diagnosed when a person loses interest in life and displays signs of severe sadness that last more than 2 weeks. Major depressive disorder and bipolar disorder are complex and are discussed in depth in Chapter 49 ⬤⬤. Any degree of depression is a risk factor for medical noncompliance. The odds are three times greater that depressed clients will be noncompliant with medical treatment recommendations than will nondepressed clients.

Depression can affect anyone, of any culture, age, or background. About twice as many women as men seek help for depression, though this may reflect a greater readiness by women to discuss their problems. Clients who seek care for physical problems (such as headaches, lethargy, stomach upsets, or joint pain) may actually be suffering from depression. Because of the stigma attached to depression and other mental health disorders, they may find it easier to seek help for the physical symptoms of their emotional distress rather than to face that distress directly. Questions about the person's perceived quality of life (Box 17-2 ■) can help identify depression.

A client's depression may be the cause of physical ailments; physical illness may be the cause of depression; or the client may suffer from a physical problem and unrelated depression. Good listening skills are a crucial part of helping clients bring

BOX 17-2   DATA COLLECTION

Quality of Life

The following are examples of questions that can be addressed with the client to assess quality of life.

1. How would you describe your overall quality of life?

Symptom issues:

2. How would you rate your current control of your symptoms?
3. To what extent does your physical discomfort impact your ability to enjoy your day?

Functional issues:

4. How many times each week are you able to do many of the things you like to do?
5. What are your favorite activities?
6. Does your contentment with life depend on being active and being independent in your personal care?

Interpersonal issues:

7. Do you feel that you have been able to say important things to the people close to you?
8. At present, how much time do you spend with family and friends?
9. Is it important to you to have close personal relationships?

Well-being:

10. Do you feel that your affairs are in order and that you could die today with a clear mind?

Transcendent issues:

11. Do you have a better sense of meaning in your life now than you had in the past?
12. Is it important for you to feel that your life has meaning?

important information to light (see the discussion of therapeutic communication in Chapter 11 ⬭). Several types of depression (see Chapter 49 ⬭) may be present in physically ill clients for whom you are caring.

Bipolar Affective Disorder (Manic Depression)

Bipolar affective disorder is a condition characterized by both "high" and "low" swings of mood, along with changes in thoughts, emotions, and physical health. It is discussed in depth in Chapter 49 ⬭.

Postnatal Depression

Postnatal depression (PND or postpartum depression) is a condition experienced by about 1 in 10 women in the first year after having a baby. It involves an extended depressed state and sometimes psychotic behavior. PND is more serious than "baby blues," which frequently occur about 3 or 4 days following delivery and are related to changes in hormone levels.

Seasonal Affective Disorder

Seasonal affective disorder is depression related to decreased sunlight. People describe feeling depressed regularly at certain times of the year. Usually this kind of depression starts in the autumn or winter, when daylight is reduced.

Major Depressive Disorder

Clients with severe depression (major depressive disorder) may experience prolonged periods of low mood, loss of interest and pleasure, and feelings of worthlessness and guilt. These feelings may manifest themselves as tearfulness, poor concentration, reduced energy, reduced or increased appetite and weight, sleep problems, and anxiety. They may even feel that life is not worth living and plan or attempt suicide.

Not all people with depression will show all symptoms or have them to the same degree. People with four or more symptoms for more than 2 weeks should consult a medical doctor or psychiatrist. Major depression shares some characteristics with other disorders, including unipolar depression, bipolar illness, anxiety disorder, and attention deficit disorder with or without hyperactivity. Remember that only a medical doctor can diagnose depression.

Symptoms of major depression vary by age group. It is important to understand what constitutes "normal" development in infants, children, and adolescents. You may not see a drastic change in a child's or adolescent's behavior or mood if he or she was born with a depressive illness.

In children, depressive illnesses/anxiety may present as school phobia or school avoidance, social phobia or social avoidance, excessive separation anxiety, running away, obsessions, compulsions, or everyday rituals, such as having to go to bed at the exact time each night for fear something bad may happen. Chronic illnesses may be present also because depression weakens the immune system.

Among adolescents, depressive illness or anxiety may be disguised as eating disorders (see Chapter 50 ⬭), substance abuse, sexual promiscuity, or risk-taking behavior (reckless driving, unprotected sex, carelessness on bridges or cliffs). Other behaviors may include social isolation, running away, constant disobedience, getting into trouble with the law, physical or sexual assaults against others, obnoxious behavior, failure to care about appearance/hygiene, no sense of self or of values/morals, difficulty cultivating relationships, or inability to establish/stick with occupational/educational goals.

Many people feel that it is normal for elderly persons to be depressed. This is a dangerous misconception. If you suspect an older adult is suffering from a depressive illness, a thorough medical examination should be given as soon as possible. Symptoms may be the result of a reversible physical condition. Table 17-1 ■ lists age-related clinical manifestations of depression. (Chapter 43 ⬭ discusses depression in the elderly.)

Treatment

MENTAL HEALTH PROFESSIONALS.   A number of mental health professionals may collaborate with nursing staff when a client is experiencing psychosocial issues. A **psychiatrist** is a

TABLE 17-1	Age-Related Clinical Manifestations of Depression
AGE GROUP	**CLINICAL MANIFESTATIONS**
Infant	Unresponsive when talked to or touched, never smiles or cries, or may cry often, being difficult to soothe
	Failure to gain weight (not due to other medical illness)
	Unmotivated in play
	Restless, oversensitive to noise or touch
	Problems with eating or sleeping
	Digestive disorders (constipation/diarrhea)
Child	Persistent unhappiness, negativity, complaining, chronic boredom, no initiative
	Uncontrollable anger with aggressive or destructive behavior, possibly hitting themselves or others, kicking, self-biting, head banging, harming animals
	Continual disobedience
	Easily frustrated, frequently crying, low self-esteem, overly sensitive
	Inability to pay attention, remember, or make decisions; easily distracted; mind goes blank
	Energy fluctuations from lethargic to frenzied activity, with periods of normalcy
	Eating or sleeping problems
	Bedwetting, constipation, diarrhea, impulsiveness, accident-prone
	Chronic worry and fear, clingy, panic attacks
	Extreme self-consciousness
	Slowed speech and body movements
	Disorganized speech; hard to follow when telling you a story
	Physical symptoms such as dizziness, headaches, stomachaches, arms or legs hurt, nail-biting, pulling out hair or eyelashes (ruling out other medical causes)
	Suicidal talk or attempts
Adolescent	Physical symptoms such as dizziness, headaches, stomachaches, neck aches, arms or legs hurt due to muscle tension, digestive disorders (ruling out other medical causes)
	Persistent unhappiness, negativity, irritability
	Uncontrollable anger or outbursts of rage
	Excessive self-criticism, unwarranted guilt, low self-esteem (possibly expressed by such behaviors as having sex, using drugs or alcohol, or taking risks); inability to concentrate, think straight, remember, or make decisions, possibly resulting in refusal to study in school or an inability (due to depression or attention deficit disorder) to do schoolwork
	Slowed or hesitant speech or body movements, restlessness (anxiety)
	Loss of interest in once pleasurable activities
	Low energy, chronic fatigue, sluggishness
	Change in appetite, noticeable weight loss or weight gain, or abnormal eating patterns
	Chronic worry, excessive fear
	Preoccupation with death themes in literature, music, drawings; speaking of death repeatedly; fascination with guns/knives
	Suicidal thoughts, plans, or attempts
Adult	Persistent sad or "empty" mood
	Feeling hopeless, helpless, worthless, pessimistic, and/or guilty
	Substance abuse
	Fatigue or loss of interest in ordinary activities, including sex
	Disturbances in eating and sleeping patterns
	Irritability, increased crying, anxiety, or panic attacks
	Difficulty concentrating, remembering, or making decisions
	Thoughts of suicide; suicide plans or attempts
	Persistent physical symptoms or pains that do not respond to treatment

TABLE 17-1	Age-Related Clinical Manifestations of Depression (continued)
AGE GROUP	**CLINICAL MANIFESTATIONS**
Elderly	Unusual complaints of aches and pains (back, stomach, arms, legs, head, chest), fatigue, slowed movements and speech, loss of appetite, inability to sleep, weight increase or decrease, blurred vision, dizziness, heart racing, anxiety
	Inability to concentrate, remember, or think straight (sometimes mistaken for dementia); an overall sadness or apathy, withdrawal; inability to find pleasure in anything
	Irritability, mood swings, or constant complaining; nothing seems to make the person happy
	Talk of worthlessness, not being needed anymore, excessive and unwarranted guilt
	Frequent doctor visits without relief in symptoms; all tests come out negative
	Alcoholism, which can mask an underlying depression

physician who specializes in the branch of health science that deals with the study, treatment, and prevention of mental disorders. A client requiring treatment with psychotropic drugs will usually be followed by a psychiatrist. A clinical **psychologist** is a trained professional who provides counseling and testing for clients with mental health and/or developmental issues. A counseling professional may have been trained as a marriage and family counselor, a psychiatric social worker, or a clinical social worker; have graduate-level education; and provide counseling for individuals and groups. Some facilities will allow the LPN/LVN to participate in a group session. Occasionally an instructor may arrange for students to observe a group.

DRUG TREATMENT AND COGNITIVE BEHAVIORAL THERAPY.
Treatment for depression often includes medication and cognitive therapy. Antidepressant drugs act by increasing the activity of brain chemicals that affect the way we feel. Antidepressants are thought to help two out of three people with depression. Several types of antidepressants exist. Three to four weeks are normally required before the client experiences relief. New drugs seem to have fewer side effects, but some clients experience *idiosyncratic* (unpredictable) reactions, so they must be closely observed during the initial dosage. Clients must be taught the importance of following the medication regime exactly. They should be cautioned always to consult the doctor before discontinuing antidepressants, because the withdrawal effects may be severe.

Cognitive behavioral therapy and interpersonal therapy, which focuses on people's relationships and on problems such as trouble communicating or coping with bereavement, have in some instances been as effective as medication. **Counseling** is a form of therapy in which trained professionals help people think about the problems they are experiencing in their lives and find new ways of coping. Counselors give support and help people find their own solutions, rather than offering advice or treatment. Box 17-3 ■ provides some suggestions for reducing depression.

ELECTROCONVULSIVE THERAPY.
Electroconvulsive therapy (ECT) may be used for people with severe depression who have not responded well to medication or other treatments. In ECT, an electrical "shock" is applied to the brain through electrodes placed on the head. Some people say that ECT is very helpful in relieving their depression. Others have reported unpleasant experiences, including memory problems. (See further discussion in Chapter 49 ⬭ .)

BOX 17-3	CLIENT TEACHING

Suggestions for Reducing Depression

- Keep in touch with friends. If you are already depressed, you may find it very difficult to be sociable, and this can make you feel more depressed. So, it is important for you to keep in contact with friends and find someone to talk to when you are feeling low.
- Keep active. Being more active is associated with lower levels of depression. Outdoor activity seems to be particularly important in staving off depression in older men.
- Review your eating habits. Recent research has suggested that people who are depressed may have low levels of certain essential fatty acids, which are found in fish oils. It has therefore been suggested that people with depression should change their eating habits, for example, eating more oily fish such as sardines or taking fish oil supplements.
- Investigate self-help techniques. Some people have reported benefits from various self-help techniques such as meditation, listening to music, and acupuncture.
- Take control. Some people find it helps if they have some control over what happens. This helps to guard against the kind of "hopelessness" that is associated with depression. Activities that involve making a fresh start have been shown to help people recover from long-lasting depression. Similarly, learning to set small or manageable goals can give you a sense of achievement and make you feel better.
- Seek medical attention if you are unable to carry out normal daily functioning.

Suicide

Each year in the United States, 30,000 lives are lost to suicide. More people die from suicide than from homicide. Suicide is the 11th leading cause of death for all Americans. Males are four times more likely to die from suicide than are females. However, females are more likely to attempt suicide than are males (Centers for Disease Control and Prevention [CDC], 2001).

SUICIDE AMONG THE YOUNG. Persons under age 25 account for 14 percent of all suicides. The incidence of suicide among adolescents and young adults nearly tripled between 1952 and 1995. Suicide is the third leading cause of death for people 15 to 24 years old, following unintentional injury and homicide. More teenagers and young adults died from suicide than from cancer, heart disease, AIDS, birth defects, stroke, and chronic lung disease combined. There has also been a dramatic increase in the suicide rate among 10- to 14-year-olds. There is an urgent need to intensify prevention efforts among persons in this age group (CDC, 2001). Box 17-4 ■ gives some of the behaviors associated with suicide in young people.

SUICIDE AMONG THE ELDERLY. The elderly are also at risk for suicide. Suicide rates increase with age and are highest among Americans aged 65 years and older. Men account for 84 percent of suicides in this age group. Suicide rates among the elderly are highest for those who are divorced or widowed. Older persons have a higher prevalence of depression, have often visited a healthcare provider before their suicide, and have more physical illnesses. A suicidal person urgently needs to see a doctor or psychiatrist (CDC, 2001).

BOX 17-4	PEDIATRIC CONSIDERATIONS

Suicide among Youth

The Department of Health and Human Services—Center for Disease Control and Prevention's National Youth Risk Behavior Survey 1991–2005 monitored priority health risk behaviors that contributed to the leading causes of death, disabilities, and social problems among youth. The following behaviors were identified.

■ Rarely or never wore seatbelts
■ Rode with driver who had been drinking alcohol
■ Carried a weapon
■ Attempted suicide
■ Currently abused substances (alcohol, cocaine, marijuana, tobacco)
■ Had unprotected sexual activity

COMMON MISCONCEPTIONS ABOUT SUICIDE. Suicide is probably the most misunderstood mental health issue. There continues to be much stigma associated with it. Families who have experienced death of a family member by suicide are reluctant to talk of the cause, and many times feel ostracized by friends and associates. Table 17-2 ■ describes some of the common misconceptions associated with suicide.

CONDITIONS ASSOCIATED WITH INCREASED RISK OF SUICIDE. Increased risk of suicide is associated with the following conditions:

■ Death or terminal illness of relative or friend.
■ Divorce, separation, broken relationship, stress on family.
■ Loss of health (real or imaginary).
■ Overwhelming pain: pain that threatens to exceed the person's pain-coping capacity. Suicidal feelings are often

TABLE 17-2	Myths Associated with Suicide	
MYTH	**TRUTH**	
"People who talk about suicide won't really do it."	Almost everyone who commits or attempts suicide has given some clue or warning. Do not ignore suicide threats. Statements such as "You'll be sorry when I'm dead" or "I can't see any way out"—no matter how casually or jokingly said—may indicate serious suicidal feelings.	
"Anyone who tries to kill him/herself must be crazy."	Most suicidal people are not psychotic or insane. They must be upset, grief stricken, depressed, or despairing, but extreme distress and emotional pain are not necessarily signs of mental illness.	
"If a person is determined to kill him/herself, nothing is going to stop him/her."	Even the most severely depressed person has mixed feelings about death. Suicidal people are wavering until the very last moment between wanting to live and wanting to die. Most suicidal people do not want death; they want the pain to stop. The impulse to end it all, however overpowering, does not last forever.	
"People who commit suicide are people who were unwilling to seek help."	Studies of suicide victims have shown that more than half had sought medical help within 6 months before their deaths.	
"Talking with clients about suicide may give them the idea."	You don't give a suicidal person morbid ideas by talking about suicide. The opposite is true—bringing up the subject of suicide and discussing it openly is one of the most helpful things you can do.	

the result of long-standing problems that have been exacerbated by recent precipitating events. The precipitating factors may be new pain or the loss of pain-coping resources.

- Loss of job, home, money, status, self-esteem, personal security.
- Alcohol or drug abuse.
- Depression. In the young, depression may be masked by hyperactivity or acting-out behavior. In the elderly it may be incorrectly attributed to the natural effects of aging. Depression that seems to disappear quickly for no apparent reason is cause for concern. The early stages of recovery from depression can be a high-risk period. Recent studies have associated anxiety disorders with increased risk for attempted suicide.
- Difficult times: holidays, anniversaries, and the first week after discharge from a hospital; just before and after diagnosis of a major illness; just before and during disciplinary proceedings. Undocumented status adds to the stress of a crisis.

EMOTIONAL AND BEHAVIORAL CHANGES ASSOCIATED WITH SUICIDE.
Box 17-5 ■ lists some of the warning signs of suicide. In general, a person who is depressed is at risk for suicide. Some of the following indicators may exist:

- Hopelessness: the feeling that the pain will continue or get worse; things will never get better
- Powerlessness: the feeling that one's resources for reducing pain are exhausted
- Feelings of worthlessness, shame, guilt, self-hatred, "no one cares," fears of losing control, harming self or others
- Person becomes sad, withdrawn, tired, apathetic, anxious, irritable, or prone to angry outbursts
- Declining performance in school, work, or other activities (Occasionally the reverse may be true: People may volunteer for extra duties just to fill up their time and keep themselves from being alone.)
- Social isolation; or association with a group that has different moral standards than those of the family

---

BOX 17-5	WARNING SIGNS OF SUICIDE

- Talking about suicide
- Statements about hopelessness, helplessness, or worthlessness
- Preoccupation with death
- Suddenly happier, calmer manner after
- Loss of interest in things one cares about
- Visiting or calling people one cares about
- Making arrangements; setting one's affairs in order
- Giving things away

- Declining interest in sex, friends, or activities previously enjoyed
- Neglect of personal welfare and deteriorating physical appearance
- Alterations in sleeping or eating habits
- Self-starvation, dietary mismanagement, disobeying medical instructions (particularly in the elderly)

SUICIDAL BEHAVIOR

- Previous suicide attempts, "mini-attempts"
- Explicit statements of **suicidal ideation** (suicidal thinking) or feelings
- Development of suicidal plan, acquiring the means, "rehearsal" behavior, setting a time for the attempt
- Self-inflicted injuries, such as cuts, burns, or head banging
- Risky behavior
- Unexplained accidents among children and the elderly
- Making out a will or giving away favorite possessions
- Inappropriately saying goodbye
- Verbal behavior that is ambiguous or indirect: "I'm going away on a real long trip," "You won't have to worry about me anymore," "I want to go to sleep and never wake up," "I'm so depressed, I just can't go on," "Does God punish suicides?" "Voices are telling me to do bad things," requests for euthanasia information, inappropriate joking, stories or essays on morbid themes

NURSING CONSIDERATIONS.
If the nurse suspects that a client is contemplating suicide, it is crucial to respond in a nonjudgmental manner. Do not say, "Oh, you wouldn't want to do that" or suggest that they do not really mean what they say. Be careful not to minimize their concerns. If they say, "Everyone hates me," do not respond with a statement like, "No, I'm sure there are people who love you." Instead, empathize with their feelings and ask them to say more. Most people who consider suicide want help to overcome these feelings.

Report any suspicion of risk for suicide to the supervising nurse at once. The nurse may ask, "Are you thinking about hurting yourself?" If the client says yes and has a workable, lethal plan, immediate action is necessary. Counseling by a qualified professional should be arranged, and the person should not be left alone. The nurse may need to call a support person to meet and stay with the client.

STRESS

Stress is a condition that requires a response. Stress has numerous consequences (Figure 17-1 ■):

- *Physiological*—Can threaten a person's physiological homeostasis.

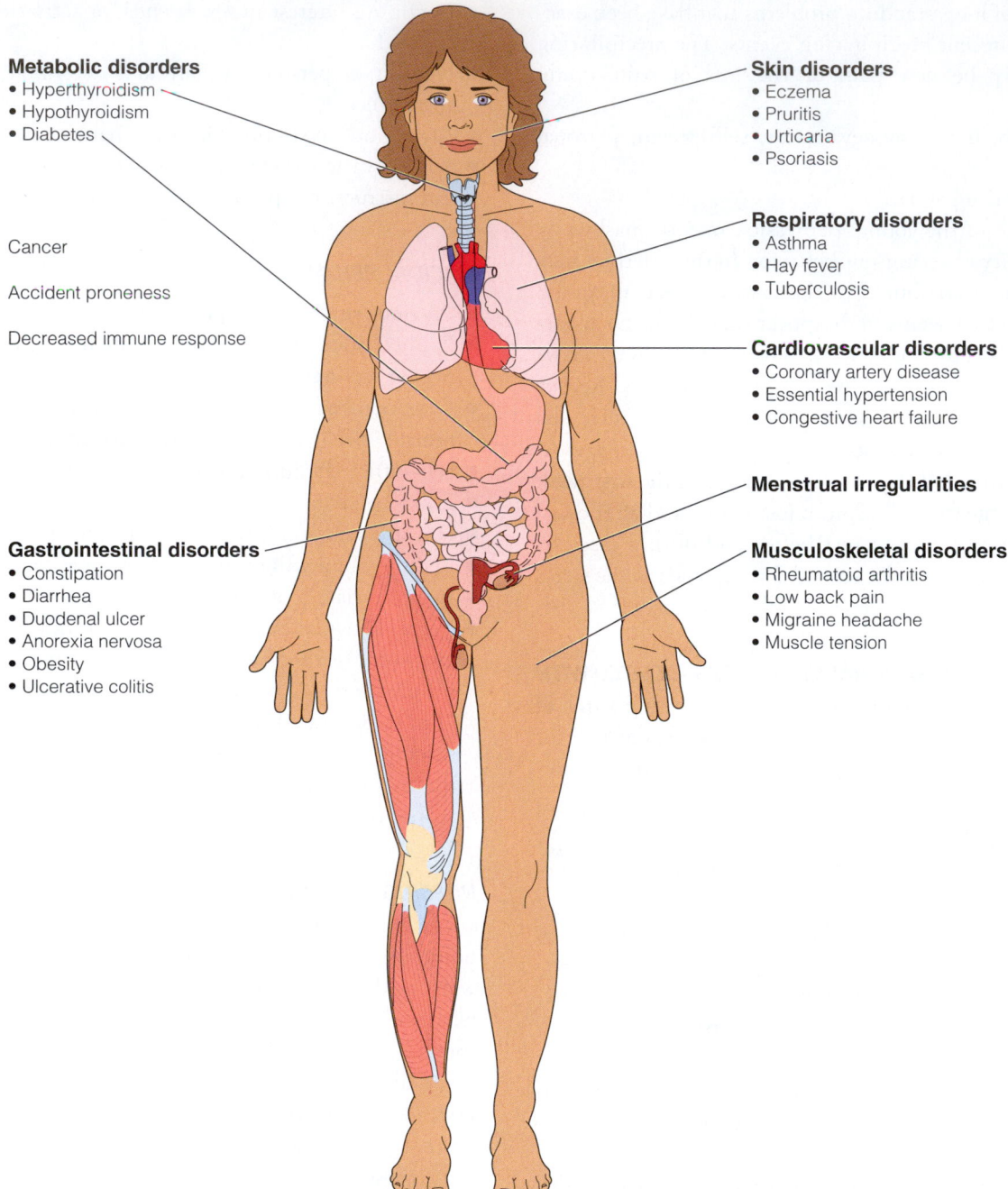

Metabolic disorders
- Hyperthyroidism
- Hypothyroidism
- Diabetes

Cancer

Accident proneness

Decreased immune response

Gastrointestinal disorders
- Constipation
- Diarrhea
- Duodenal ulcer
- Anorexia nervosa
- Obesity
- Ulcerative colitis

Skin disorders
- Eczema
- Pruritis
- Urticaria
- Psoriasis

Respiratory disorders
- Asthma
- Hay fever
- Tuberculosis

Cardiovascular disorders
- Coronary artery disease
- Essential hypertension
- Congestive heart failure

Menstrual irregularities

Musculoskeletal disorders
- Rheumatoid arthritis
- Low back pain
- Migraine headache
- Muscle tension

Figure 17-1. ■ Many physical disorders can be caused or aggravated by stress.

- *Emotional*—Can produce negative or unconstructive feelings about the self.
- *Intellectual*—Can influence a person's perceptual and problem-solving abilities.
- *Social*—Can alter a person's relationships with others.
- *Spiritual*—Can challenge one's beliefs and values.

An individual is considered to be mentally healthy if he or she is able to love (form relationships), work, and cope simultaneously. Coping with stress then becomes an important factor in maintaining mental homeostasis or emotional balance.

Sources of Stress

Sources of stress can be broadly classified as either internal or external **stressors**. They may also be developmental or situational stressors, or both. Internal stressors originate within a person. Examples are receiving a diagnosis of cancer or experiencing feelings of depression. External stressors originate outside the individual. Examples are moving to another city, experiencing a death in the family, or feeling pressure from peers. Developmental stressors occur at predictable times throughout an individual's life. Examples of these are shown in Table 17-3 ■. Within each developmental

TABLE 17-3	Selected Stressors Associated with Developmental Stages
DEVELOPMENTAL STAGE	**STRESSORS**
Child	Conflict between independence and dependence
	Beginning school
	Establishing peer relationships and adjustments
	Peer competition
Adolescent	Changing physique
	Developing relationships involving sexual attraction
	Achieving independence
	Choosing a career
Young adult	Getting married
	Having a home
	Managing a home
	Getting started in an occupation
	Continuing one's education
	Rearing children
Middle adult	Physical changes of aging
	Maintaining social status and standard of living
	Teenage children becoming independent
	Adjusting to aging parents
Older adult	Decreasing physical abilities and health
	Changes in residence
	Retirement and reduced income
	Death of spouse and friends

stage, certain tasks must be achieved to prevent or reduce stress. Situational stressors are unpredictable and may occur at any time during life. Situational stress may be positive or negative. Examples of this type of stress include:

- Death of a family member
- Marriage or divorce
- Birth of a child
- New job
- Illness

Models of Stress

The three main models used to explain the effects of stress are the stimulus-based, response-based, and transaction-based models. Nurses use knowledge of these models to help clients use healthy coping responses and change unhealthy, unproductive responses.

STIMULUS-BASED MODELS. In the stimulus-based model, stress is defined as a life event, or a set of circumstances that arouses physiological and/or psychological reactions that may increase the individual's vulnerability to illness. Holmes and Rahe (1967) created a scale that assigned a numerical value to 43 life changes or events. Similar scales have since been developed, but all such scales require

caution because the degree of stress an event presents can be highly individual.

The scale of stressful life events is used to document a person's relatively recent experiences, such as divorce, pregnancy, and retirement. In this view, both positive and negative events are considered stressful. Research has shown that people who have a high level of stress are often more prone to illness. They also have a lowered ability to cope with an illness and subsequent stress.

RESPONSE-BASED MODELS. Stress may also be considered as a response to illness. Hans Selye (1976), a recognized authority in the field of stress, observed:

> Whether a man suffers from severe blood loss, an infection or advanced cancer; he loses his appetite, strength, and ambition; usually he also loses weight and even his facial expression betrays his illness. I felt that the syndrome of "Just being sick," which is essentially the same no matter what disease we have, could be analyzed and expressed scientifically. (p. 12)

Selye realized that changes in the body occurred in the presence of stress (see Figure 17-1), and this became the basis of his identification of the **general adaptation syndrome** (GAS). He proposed three stages in this syndrome

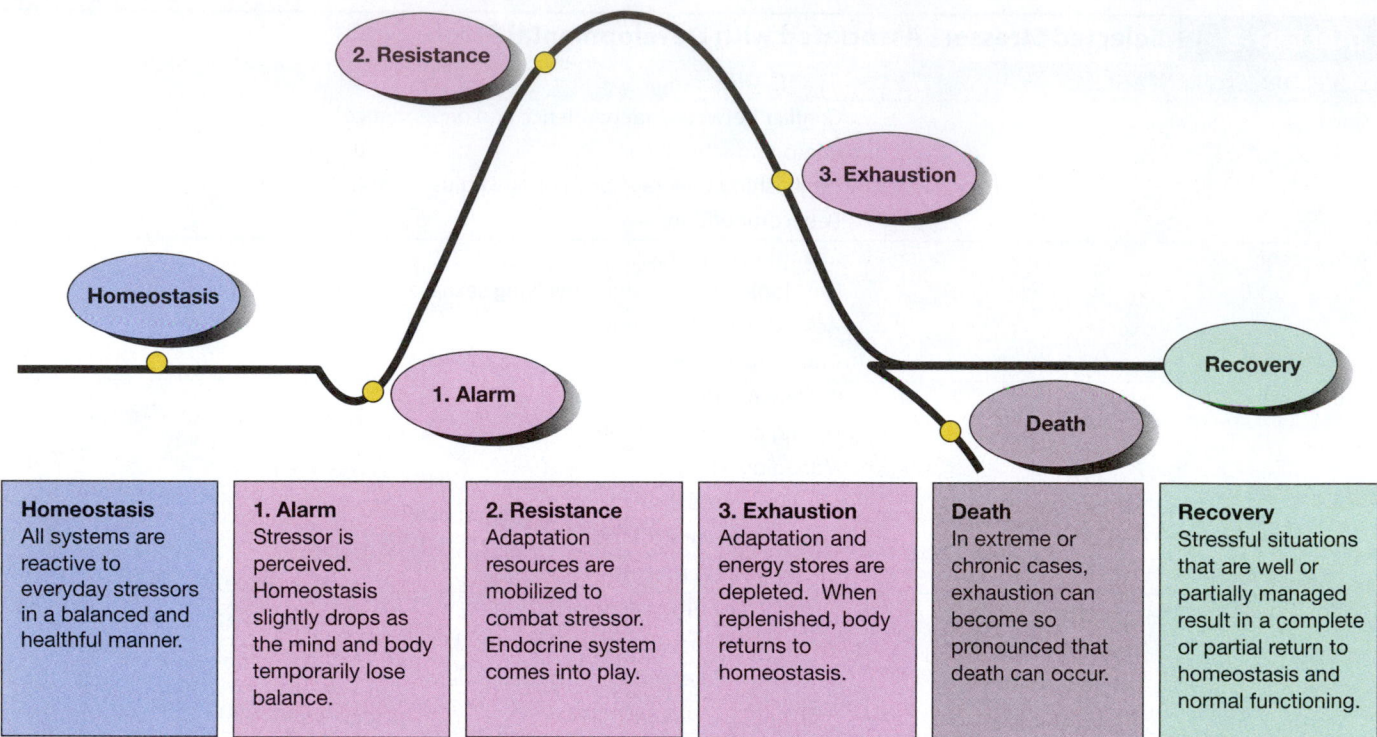

Homeostasis	1. Alarm	2. Resistance	3. Exhaustion	Death	Recovery
Homeostasis All systems are reactive to everyday stressors in a balanced and healthful manner.	**1. Alarm** Stressor is perceived. Homeostasis slightly drops as the mind and body temporarily lose balance.	**2. Resistance** Adaptation resources are mobilized to combat stressor. Endocrine system comes into play.	**3. Exhaustion** Adaptation and energy stores are depleted. When replenished, body returns to homeostasis.	**Death** In extreme or chronic cases, exhaustion can become so pronounced that death can occur.	**Recovery** Stressful situations that are well or partially managed result in a complete or partial return to homeostasis and normal functioning.

Figure 17-2. ■ Three stages of adaptation to stress: the alarm reaction, the stage of resistance, and the stage of exhaustion. (*Source*: From *Wellness: Concepts and Application*, 6th ed. (p. 298) by D. M. Anspaugh, M. Hamrick, and F. D. Rosato, 2005, New York: McGraw-Hill).

(Figure 17-2 ■): alarm reaction, resistance, and exhaustion. Box 17-6 ■ provides a description of these stages. Selye's general adaptation syndrome encompasses a range of physiological responses to stressors in the body as a whole.

TRANSACTION-BASED MODELS.   The transactional view was developed by Richard Lazarus (1965). It focuses on individual differences in response to stress, rather than to events or reactions. The transactional view attempts to answer the following: Which factors lead some persons and not others to respond effectively to stressful events? Why are some persons more sensitive and vulnerable to stressful

events? And why are some persons able to adapt better than others over longer periods to stressful events?

The Lazarus transactional stress theory includes cognitive, affective, and adaptive (coping) responses. This theory states that the person and the environment are inseparable; each affects and is affected by the other. Stress "refers to any event in which environmental demands, internal demands, or both tax or exceed the adaptive resources of an individual, social system, or tissue system" (Monat & Lazarus, 1991, p. 3). The individual responds to perceived environmental changes by adaptive (coping) responses. See the Coping section later in this chapter.

Indicators of Stress

Indicators of an individual's stress may be physiological or psychological.

Responses to stress vary depending on the individual's perception of events. The physiological signs and symptoms of stress result from the activation of the sympathetic and neuroendocrine systems of the body. The autonomic nervous system reacts to a perceived threat by releasing large amounts of epinephrine (adrenaline) and cortisone into the body. The person is then ready for "fight or flight." The **fight-or-flight response** of the sympathetic nervous system and the adrenal glands can be described as a generalized response to an emergency situation. The heart rate, respiratory rates, blood pressure, and blood flow to the muscles are increased. This response prepares the body to either

---

BOX 17-6   GENERAL ADAPTATION SYNDROME STAGES

Stage 1: Alarm reaction—This is the immediate reaction to stress or a stressor. A fight-or-flight response occurs. This response can diminish the effectiveness of the immune system, decreasing resistance.

Stage 2: Stage of resistance—As the stress continues, the body adapts to the stressors. The body changes at different levels in order to reduce the effects of stress.

Stage 3: Stage of exhaustion—The stress has been continuous; the body's resistance is lowered or can fail. People experiencing long-term stress may have severe physical manifestations such as a heart attack or severe immunodeficiencies.

BOX 17-7	PHYSIOLOGICAL INDICATORS OF STRESS

- Pupils dilate to increase visual perception when serious threats to the body arise.
- Sweat production (*diaphoresis*) increases to control elevated body heat due to increased metabolism.
- The heart rate increases, which leads to an increased pulse rate to transport nutrients and by-products of metabolism more efficiently.
- Skin is pallid because of constriction of peripheral blood vessels, an effect of norepinephrine.
- The rate and depth of respirations increase because of dilation of the bronchioles, promoting hyperventilation.
- Urinary output decreases.
- The mouth may be dry.
- Peristalsis of the intestines decreases, resulting in possible constipation and flatus.
- For serious threats, mental alertness improves.
- Muscle tension increases to prepare for rapid motor activity or defense.
- Blood sugar increases because of release of glucocorticoids and gluconeogenesis.

flee or fight (Jacobs, 2001). Box 17-7 ■ lists physiological indicators of stress.

ANXIETY. A common reaction to stress is anxiety. **Anxiety** can be described as a state of mental uneasiness, apprehension, dread, or foreboding. It can also be a feeling of helplessness related to an unidentified threat to self or significant relationships. Anxiety can be experienced at the conscious, subconscious, or unconscious levels. It differs from fear in four ways:

- The source of anxiety may not be identifiable; the source of fear is identifiable.
- Anxiety is related to the future, that is, to an anticipated event. Fear is related to the present.
- Anxiety is vague, whereas fear is definite.
- Anxiety is the result of psychological or emotional conflict; fear is the result of a physical or psychological reality.

All people experience anxiety to some degree most of the time. Mild or moderate anxiety helps people accomplish developmental tasks and meet goals. In this sense, anxiety is an effective coping strategy. For example, mild anxiety motivates students to study. Excessive anxiety, however, often has destructive effects. The overly anxious student may be unable to sleep or to eat, and may do poorly on a test as a result.

Anxiety may be manifested on four levels:

1. Mild anxiety produces a slight arousal state that enhances perception, learning, and productive abilities. Most healthy people experience mild anxiety, perhaps as a feeling of mild restlessness that prompts a person to seek information and ask questions.

2. Moderate anxiety increases the arousal state to a point where the person expresses feelings of tension, nervousness, or concern. Perceptual abilities are narrowed. Attention is focused on a particular aspect of a situation.

3. Severe anxiety consumes most of the person's energies and requires intervention. The person, unable to focus on what is really happening, focuses on only one specific detail of the situation causing the anxiety.

4. Panic is an overpowering, frightening level of anxiety that causes the person to lose control. It is less frequently experienced than other levels of anxiety. A panicked person may distort events as a result of altered perception.

Table 17-4 ■ provides indicators of these anxiety levels.

FEAR. Fear is an emotion or feeling of apprehension aroused by impending danger, pain, or other perceived threat. People may fear something that has already occurred, a current threat, or something they believe will happen. The fear may or may not be based in reality. For example, beginning nursing students may fear their first experience in a client care setting. They may be worried that clients will not want to be cared for by students or that they might inadvertently harm the clients. The nursing students' feelings of fear are real and will probably elicit a stress response. However, the instructor arranges the students' first client assignment so that the students' feared outcomes are unlikely to occur.

ANGER. **Anger** is an emotional state that includes feelings of animosity or strong displeasure. Many people feel guilty when they feel anger because they have been taught that to feel angry is wrong. When anger is expressed in a nonalienating verbal manner, it is considered a positive emotion. Anger can be a sign of emotional maturity when growth and positive interactions result from it.

A verbal expression of anger is a signal of internal psychological discomfort and a call for assistance to deal with perceived stress. Anger, hostility, violence, and aggression differ:

- *Anger* is an emotional state that includes feelings of animosity or strong displeasure.
- *Hostility* is usually marked by antagonism and harmful or destructive behavior.
- *Violence* is the exertion of physical force to injure or abuse.
- *Aggression* is an unprovoked attack or a hostile, injurious, or destructive action or outlook.

Verbally expressed anger is not the same as hostility, aggression, or violence. However, if anger persists unabated, it can lead to destructiveness and violence.

When an angry person tells another person about the anger and carefully identifies the source, this is constructive. Clear communication gets the anger out into the open

TABLE 17-4	Indicators of Levels of Anxiety			
	LEVEL OF ANXIETY			
CATEGORY	**MILD**	**MODERATE**	**SEVERE**	**PANIC**
Verbalization changes	Increased questioning	Voice tremors and pitch changes	Communication difficult to understand	Communication may not be understandable
Motor activity changes	Mild restlessness Sleeplessness	Tremors, facial twitches, and shakiness Increased muscle tension	Increased motor activity, inability to relax Fearful facial expression	Increased motor activity, agitation Unpredictable responses Trembling, poor motor coordination
Perception and attention changes	Feelings of increased arousal and alertness Uses learning to adapt	Narrowed focus of attention Able to focus but selectively inattentive Learning slightly impaired	Inability to focus or concentrate Easily distracted Learning severely impaired	Perception distorted or exaggerated Unable to learn or function
Respiratory and circulatory changes	None	Slightly increased respiratory and heart rates	Tachycardia, hyperventilation	Dyspnea, palpitations, choking, chest pain or pressure
Other changes	None	Mild gastric symptoms, e.g., "butterflies in the stomach"	Headache, dizziness, nausea	Feeling of impending doom Paresthesia, sweating

Data from Carpenito, L. J. (2007). *Nursing Diagnosis: Application to Clinical Practice* (12th ed.). Philadelphia: Lippincott; Fontaine, K. L. J. S. (2008). *Essentials of Mental Health Nursing* (6th ed.). Upper Saddle River, NJ: Prentice Hall; Wilkinson, J., Ahern, N. (2009). *Nursing Diagnosis Handbook* (9th ed.). Upper Saddle River, NJ: Prentice Hall.

so it can be dealt with appropriately. The angry person "gets it off the chest" and an emotional buildup is prevented.

DEPRESSION. Depression is a common reaction to overwhelming or negative events. The signs and symptoms of depression vary with the client. Emotional symptoms can include feelings of tiredness, sadness, emptiness, or numbness. Behavioral signs of depression include irritability, inability to concentrate, difficulty making decisions, loss of sexual desire, crying, sleep disturbance, and social withdrawal. Physical signs of depression may include loss of appetite, weight loss, constipation, headache, and dizziness. Most people experience short periods of depression in response to overwhelming stressful events, such as the death of a loved one or loss of a job. When depression is prolonged, it is a cause for concern and may require treatment.

The main types of anxiety are:

- **Phobias:** a specific type of anxiety, defined as out-of-proportion fears (Figure 17-3 ■). Examples include *zoophobia* (fear of animals), *arachnophobia* (fear of spiders), *acrophobia* (fear of heights), or *claustrophobia* (fear of small spaces), and many others.
- **Panic attacks:** a sudden and intense sensation of fear and impending doom.
- **Obsessive-compulsive disorder:** an anxiety disorder characterized by patterned behaviors that are focused on some topic of fixation (or obsession) and that are repeated

in order to relieve the anxiety. *Obsessions* are recurrent, persistent thoughts, images, or impulses that are unwanted or distressing that come involuntarily to mind despite attempts to ignore the thoughts. *Compulsions* are a recurrent, unwanted, and distressing urge to perform an act in order to stop obsessional thoughts.

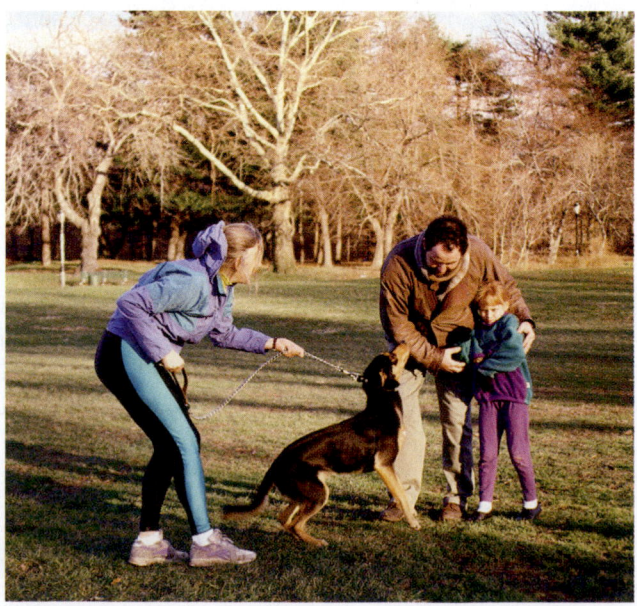

Figure 17-3. ■ People with specific phobias experience high levels of anxiety when confronted with the feared situation or object. (*Source:* Innervisions.)

Treatment

Today many individuals experience stress and anxiety. In fact, the phrase *worried well* describes the emotional situation in which day-to-day problems continue to increase stress and cause anxiety.

Since the mid-1980s the self-help movement has become popular. Many people have attempted to diagnosis and self-treat their emotional problems. **Self-help** is based on the idea that as you begin to understand your personal levels of stress and anxiety, you are able to develop more control over them and are, therefore, more likely to be able to cope with them in the future.

Healthcare professionals can do a number of things to help prevent or lessen the impact of anxiety, personally as well as with their clients, whatever its form. Box 17-8 ■ offers suggestions for helping clients to deal with anxiety. Drug treatments provide short-term help, but are not a cure for the underlying causes of anxiety. Drugs may be most useful when combined with other treatments or support.

Counseling allows the client to talk about anxieties. Cognitive behavioral therapy is called *cognitive* (related to thinking) because the way anxiety is experienced is shaped by how the client thinks about it. It is called *behavioral* because it stresses the importance of practicing new behaviors, particularly facing up to whatever we fear and learning

---

BOX 17-8	CLIENT TEACHING

Mechanisms for Coping with Anxiety

- *Awareness/education:* Try to learn more about your anxiety. The more you are able to understand your anxiety, the less you will fear it.
- *Positive thinking:* Try to have a positive outlook, taking one day at a time. Do not be too hard on yourself. No one is perfect.
- *Structure:* Try to find ways of motivating yourself, such as setting small and achievable goals. This may involve writing lists of things that may help in situations where you are likely to become anxious.
- *Relaxation:* Try to learn to relax by thinking about things that make you feel calm such as listening to music or reading. You could also use specific relaxation techniques.
- *Exercise:* Physical exercise can trigger brain chemicals that will improve your mood. Feeling fit can make you feel more positive about yourself.
- *Diet:* Eating a low-fat, high-fiber diet, with lots of fresh vegetables and fruit, will increase body energy. Also, try to avoid drinking too much tea and coffee because caffeine can increase anxiety levels. If your anxiety gets worse when you miss a meal, try avoiding "fast burn" sugar and refined starch, which can produce dips in your blood sugar.
- *Talking:* Share and discuss your worries and the tasks you have set for yourself with your friends and family.

---

that we are able to cope. In addition to one-on-one counseling, support groups with other people who have experienced anxiety have been shown to be helpful. People have reported benefits from a range of alternative or complementary therapies, including herbal remedies (e.g., valerian), homeopathy, and acupuncture. Some studies have also suggested benefits from massage and from aromatherapy; for example, lavender oil can help if you have problems sleeping.

Posttraumatic Stress Disorder

Posttraumatic stress disorder (PTSD) is an anxiety disorder that can develop after exposure to one or more terrifying events in which grave physical harm occurred or was threatened. It is a severe and ongoing emotional reaction to an extreme psychological trauma. The stressors may involve someone's actual death or a threat to the client's or someone else's life, serious physical injury, or threat to physical and/or psychological integrity, to a degree that usual coping strategies are not effective.

PTSD is believed to be caused by psychological trauma, such as experiencing or witnessing childhood physical, emotional, or sexual abuse; in addition, by experiencing or witnessing an event perceived as life-threatening such as physical assault, adult experiences of sexual assault, accidents, drug addiction, illnesses, medical complications, or the experience of, or employment in occupations exposed to war (such as soldiers) or disaster (such as emergency service workers).

DIAGNOSIS. The diagnostic criteria for PTSD, per the *Diagnostic and Statistical Manual of Mental Disorders IV (Text Revision) (DSM-IV-TR)*, may be summarized as:

A. Exposure to a traumatic event
B. Persistent reexperience (e.g., flashbacks, nightmares)
C. Persistent avoidance of stimuli associated with the trauma (e.g., inability to talk about things even related to the experience, avoidance of things and discussions that trigger flashbacks and reexperiencing symptoms, fear of losing control and harming another person)
D. Persistent symptoms of increased arousal (e.g., difficulty falling or staying asleep, anger, and hypervigilance)
E. Duration of symptoms more than 1 month
F. Significant impairment in social, occupational, or other important areas of functioning (e.g., problems with work and relationships)

TREATMENT. Basic counseling for PTSD includes education about the condition and provision of safety and support. Cognitive therapy shows good results, and group therapy may be helpful in reducing isolation and social stigma.

In recent history, catastrophes (by human means or not) such as the terrorist attack of September 11, 2001, and the devastation in New Orleans by Hurricane Katrina may have caused PTSD in many survivors and rescue workers. Relief workers from organizations such as the Red Cross and the Salvation Army provide counseling after major disasters as part of their standard procedures to curb severe cases of PTSD.

Reports of battle-associated stress appear as early as the 6th century B.C. Although PTSD-like symptoms have also been recognized in combat veterans of many military conflicts since then, the modern understanding of PTSD dates from the 1970s, largely as a result of the problems that were still being experienced by Vietnam veterans. Because United States Marines in combat in the wars in Iraq and Afghanistan have faced significant physical, emotional, and relational disruptions on returning home, the United States Marine Corps has instituted programs to assist them in readjusting to life, and in particular marriage, outside of the Marine Corps.

Propranolol, a beta-blocker that appears to inhibit the formation of traumatic memories by blocking adrenaline's effects, has been used in an attempt to reduce the impact of traumatic events. PTSD is commonly treated with a combination of psychotherapy and medications.

GRIEF AND LOSS

Feelings of grief and loss are normal reactions to any physical illness that creates a major permanent change. Dynamics involved in coping with these feelings are similar to those in people dealing with their or a loved one's imminent death. Grieving involves spiritual changes, as well as emotional changes, and as such requires client spiritual assessment. The main discussion of grief and loss is in Chapter 18 ⚭ .

DENIAL

Denial may cause clients to minimize symptoms such as pain, or may cause them to focus on the positive while ignoring negative information about an illness. Caregivers may unwittingly assist with the person's denial by not performing complete assessments or by accepting the person's subjective appraisals.

FEAR OF DEPENDENCY

People may respond to being dependent with anger, inability to accept nurturing, or refusal of treatment. Others may fear that dependency needs will go unmet, so they do not express any negative feelings to caregivers. Suppressed negative feelings may emerge as somatic symptoms (headaches, stomachaches, etc.).

Coping

Coping means dealing with problems and situations. A coping strategy (coping mechanism) is an inborn or learned way of responding to a changing environment, specific

---

BOX 17-9	FACTORS INFLUENCING THE EFFECTIVENESS OF COPING

- The number, duration, and intensity of the stressors
- Past experiences of the individual
- Support systems available to the individual
- Personal qualities of the person

---

problem, or situation. Several factors influence how well a person copes (Box 17-9 ■).

Two types of coping strategies are problem-focused and emotion-focused coping. *Problem-focused coping* involves taking action to improve a situation. *Emotion-focused coping* involves using thoughts and actions to relieve emotional distress. Emotion-focused coping does not improve the situation but may help alleviate anxiety.

Coping can also be adaptive or maladaptive. *Adaptive coping* helps the person to deal effectively with stressful events and minimizes distress associated with them. *Maladaptive coping* can result in unnecessary distress for the person. Effective coping results in adaptation; ineffective coping results in maladaptation. When clients exhibit appropriate behavior, nurses should remember that clients are attempting to cope through such behavior.

If a person is under stress beyond the ability to cope, he or she will become exhausted and be at risk for developing health problems. Family members who undertake the care of a person in the home for a long period develop long-term stress called **caregiver burden**. Responses such as chronic fatigue, sleeping difficulties, and high blood pressure are common in caregivers.

When coping strategies or defense mechanisms become ineffective, the individual may experience interpersonal problems, work difficulties, and inability to meet basic human needs (Table 17-5 ■). Sometimes, prolonged stress can result in mental illness.

DEFENSE MECHANISMS

Defense mechanisms are unconscious attempts to manage anxiety. They protect us from being consciously aware of a thought or feeling that we cannot tolerate. The defense only allows the unconscious thought or feeling to be expressed indirectly in a disguised form. Defense mechanisms are coping mechanisms and are generally healthy. However, if used to the extreme, they become unhealthy. Defense mechanisms help us cope with unpleasant aspects of reality, but overreliance on them can create serious problems.

Besides defense mechanisms, individuals also have a repertoire of coping behaviors. These are classified as effective and ineffective.

Effective coping behaviors include reviewing strengths and weaknesses; setting short- and long-range goals, and

TABLE 17-5	Examples of the Effects of Stress on Basic Human Needs	
NEEDS	**EXAMPLES**
Physiological	Altered elimination pattern
	Change in appetite
	Altered sleep pattern
Safety and security	Expresses nervousness and feelings of being threatened
	Focuses on stressors and inattention to safety measures
Love and belonging	Isolated and withdrawn
	Becomes overly dependent
	Blames others for own problems
Self-esteem	Fails to socialize with others
	Becomes a workaholic
	Draws attention to self
Self-actualization	Preoccupied with own problems
	Shows lack of control
	Unable to accept reality

formulating a plan of action to deal with anxiety-producing situations. Ineffective coping behaviors are things such as physical fights, substance abuse, social withdrawal, or addictive behaviors. (See more on these topics in Chapter 50 ⬭.) Table 17-6 ■ describes how various defenses might be used.

clinical ALERT

Healthcare professionals frequently have the same feelings of stress as their clients. Many people, especially professionals, are reluctant to seek help. They feel that it is an admission of failure. This is not the case! If stress becomes unmanageable, it is important to get help as soon as possible.

Other Psychosocial Factors in Medical Illness

Stress, depression, and loneliness can create an unhealthy psychosocial environment and increase the risk of disease. Stress reduction and support can bring about improvement in a number of physical illnesses. Anyone facing a serious medical condition needs a variety of supports and may benefit from learning new coping skills.

HUMAN RIGHTS ABUSES OF PERSONS WITH STIGMATIZING MEDICAL ILLNESSES

Persons with stigmatizing medical illnesses include those who are human immunodeficiency virus (HIV) positive and people who have had transgender surgery or treatment. Stigmatization can result in inadequate care, undue stress, worsening of physical illness, and even death. Examples of human rights abuse include neglect in fully investigating somatic complaints in the emergency department, avoiding contact with or refusing to care for such persons, labeling hastily with a psychiatric diagnosis, and inappropriate psychiatric admission. These situations occur more frequently among those who lack family support, are from lower socioeconomic classes, are newly arrived immigrants, or have an "unacceptable" alternative lifestyle. (See more on care of clients with HIV in Chapter 35 ⬭.)

Psychosocial issues associated with HIV infection are sometimes overwhelming to both nurses and clients. Counseling at the time of HIV testing requires great sensitivity. HIV encephalopathy and the central nervous system infections of cryptococcosis and toxoplasmosis have created a need for psychiatric instruction for caretakers. The fact that many HIV clients are young has given rise to special needs for support and respite. The middle-aged population has become caretakers for their ill children and for their aging parents as well.

DUAL DIAGNOSIS

Dual diagnosis is the presence of substance abuse along with a concurrent psychiatric disorder. The origin of a dual diagnosis is one of three things:

- Two independent disorders occurred together.
- Substance abuse caused the other mental disorder.
- The person with the mental disorder uses substances in an effort to self-medicate or to feel better (Fontaine, 2008).

Clients hospitalized for surgery have particular problems related to their substance abuse and the need for anesthesia and/or pain medication. It is very important for nurses to maintain their objectivity and not become judgmental when confronted with such clients. The convalescent period following surgery or other serious illness is not necessarily the time to initiate a treatment program for substance abuse.

Diagnostic Groupings

Mental disorders are classified in the *Diagnostic and Statistical Manual of Mental Disorders*, fourth edition, text revision (*DSM-IV-TR*, 2000). All members of the healthcare team use this manual for diagnosis or reference. *DSM-IV* has been designed for use across settings, inpatient, outpatient, partial hospital, consultation-liaison, clinic, private practice, and primary care, and with community populations and by psychiatrists, psychologists, social workers, nurses, occupational and rehabilitation therapists, counselors, and other health and mental health professionals. The diagnostic classification is the list of the mental disorders that are officially part of the *DSM* system. These diagnostic codes are derived from the coding system used by all healthcare professionals in the United States, known as the ICD-9-CM. The LPN/LVN should become familiar with the system and use

TABLE 17-6	Defense Mechanisms		
DEFENSE MECHANISMS	**DESCRIPTION**	**EXAMPLE**	**USE/PURPOSE**
Denial	An attempt to ignore unacceptable realities by refusing to acknowledge them.	A client has just been given a diagnosis of cancer and the need to start treatment has been explained. She tells the nurse that she is glad the doctor is discharging her because she is going on vacation to Europe next week.	Self-protection from unpleasant reality by refusal to face or accept the problems of a certain unpleasant reality, such as addiction problems. It is seen in codependency, physical abuse, domestic violence, and so forth.
Repression	Threatening thoughts, feelings, and desires are kept from becoming conscious; the repressed material is denied access into the conscious.	A woman witnesses a shooting during a bank robbery, but when the police question her she cannot remember any of the details of the incident.	Preventing painful/dangerous thoughts from entering our consciousness. Repression is unconscious. Suppression is conscious prevention of painful thoughts. When individuals stop themselves from thinking, they are suppressing their thoughts.
Rationalization	Justification of certain behaviors by faulty logic and ascription of motives that are socially acceptable but did not in fact inspire the behavior.	A woman cuts flowers from her neighbor's garden to take to a sick friend, saying she won't even miss them, she has so many.	Proving one's behavior is justifiable, rational, and thus worthy of self and social approval. The client is justifying the behavior.
Projection	A process in which blame is attached to others for unacceptable thoughts, desires, shortcomings, and mistakes.	A group of students were suspected of cheating on an exam; their explanation was that the test covered material that had not been fully explained, so if the teacher had done his job they would not have needed to cheat. Another example: A man may blame his partner for having an affair, when he is the one who is being unfaithful.	Individuals are projecting feelings onto someone else, placing blame onto others, or attributing their own unethical desires to others.
Reaction formation	A mechanism that causes people to act exactly opposite to the way they feel.	A student nurse is angry that she has been put on probation for excessive absences, but tells her clinical instructor that she appreciates the constructive criticism and knows she will be a better nurse because of it. Another example: "Gay bashing."	Preventing dangerous desires from being expressed by exaggerating opposed attitudes or types of behavior.
Displacement	The transferring of emotional reactions from one person to another.	A man is reprimanded at work by his boss. Rather than respond, when he returns home he yells at his wife. Or the boss yells at an employee and he goes home and kicks the cat.	Discharging pent-up feelings, usually of hostility, onto less threatening subjects.
Intellectualization	A mechanism by which an emotional response that normally would accompany an uncomfortable or painful incident is evaded by the use of rational explanation that removes from the incident any personal significance and feelings.	A young man loses his job because of cutbacks throughout the company. His response is that it is for the best because he does not want to work for a failing company.	Happens with bright, educated people; they use logic to cut off emotionally charged situations. By focusing on logic, they avoid connecting with their feelings.
Undoing	An action or words designed to cancel some disapproved thoughts, impulses, or acts in which the person relieves guilt by making reparation.	A father gets busy at work and misses his son's softball game. The next day he brings him an expensive new mitt.	Atoning for and thus counteracting immoral desires and acts.

TABLE 17-6	Defense Mechanisms (continued)		
DEFENSE MECHANISMS	**DESCRIPTION**	**EXAMPLE**	**USE/PURPOSE**
Regression	Resorting to an earlier, more comfortable level of functioning that is characterized by fewer demands and responsibilities.	A young adult male who is hospitalized is perfectly happy to have his mother stay with him and provide all his care.	Retreating to an earlier developmental level, involving a less mature response and usually a lower level of aspiration.
Identification	An attempt to manage anxiety by imitating the behavior of someone feared or respected.	A teenage girl, who is shy, begins to dress and act like the girls from the popular group in order to be accepted.	Increasing the feeling of worth by identifying self with a person or an institution of illustrious standing, losing person identity in the process and instead identifying with that person or entity.
Introjection	A form of identification that allows for acceptance of others' norms and values into oneself, even when contrary to one's previous assumptions.	The 8-year-old sister tells her little brother to put on his helmet before he rides his bike. She introjected the instructions of her parents. Or, a gang member reforms and becomes a police officer in order to legalize behaviors such as carrying a weapon and being the tough guy.	Incorporating external values and standards into the ego so that the individual is not at the mercy of external threat. (If individuals don't incorporate their values/standards into their ego structure, they are going to be at their mercy of the external threat.)
Compensation	Covering up weaknesses by emphasizing a more desirable trait or by overachievement in a more comfortable area.	Unable to become a star athlete, an individual becomes an author of books about athletes' achievements. Or, short men become muscle builders to compensate for their height.	Covering up weakness by emphasizing desirable traits or making up for frustrations in one area by overgratification in another area.

it as a reference when questions arise about a psychiatric diagnosis of an assigned client. For an explanation of the classifications, see Chapter 49 .

ICU PSYCHOSIS

A particularly severe psychosocial reaction to serious illness and hospitalization is ICU psychosis. **ICU psychosis** is a disorder in which clients in an intensive care unit (ICU) or a similar setting become temporarily psychotic and lose touch with reality. They may experience anxiety, hear voices, see things that are not there, and become paranoid, severely disoriented in time and place, very agitated, or even violent.

ICU psychosis is a form of *delirium*, or acute brain failure. Organic factors that contribute to or cause the disorder include dehydration, *hypoxia* (diminished oxygen availability to tissue), heart failure (inadequate cardiac output), infection, and drugs.

Causes

The causes of ICU psychosis are not fully known. Something about the ICU causes some people, who are already experiencing great infirmity, stress, and pain, to "lose their minds." Among the factors believed to contribute to ICU psychosis are:

- Sensory deprivation—being put in a room that often has no windows and is away from family, friends, and all that is familiar and comforting
- Sensory overload—being hooked up to noisy machines that run day and night
- Pain—which may not be adequately controlled in an ICU
- Sleep deprivation—hospital staff coming at all hours to check vital signs, give medications, etc.
- Disruption of the normal rhythm of day and night related to no natural light and room lighting continuously on
- Almost total loss of control over their lives while lying in intensive care

Treatment

The treatment of ICU psychosis depends on the cause(s). Family members, familiar objects, and calm words may help. Dehydration is remedied by administering fluids. Heart failure requires treatment with digitalis or other cardiac glycosides. See Chapter 33 for coverage of treatment of cardiac failure. Infections must be diagnosed and treated. Sedation with antipsychotic agents may help. ICU psychosis often vanishes magically with the coming of morning or the arrival of some sleep. Although it may linger through the day, severe agitation usually occurs only at night. (This phenomenon of increased confusion at dusk, called *sundowning*, is common in nursing homes.) Refer to Chapter 36 ⚭ for coverage of sundowner syndrome.

ICU psychosis usually resolves completely when the client leaves the ICU. Approximately one client in every three who spends more than 5 days in an ICU experiences some form of psychotic reaction. As the numbers of ICUs and the populations in them grow, the disorder is likely to increase.

Meeting Psychosocial Needs of the Seriously Ill or Dying Child

Children who are chronically or terminally ill must withstand the stress of strange hospital environments, procedures performed by strangers, time away from family and friends, and other stressors. They are actively developing, but development may be interrupted by the stress of illness. Regression to an earlier stage of development may occur. Chapter 58 ⚭ discusses the special concerns that occur with hospitalization of chronically or terminally ill children.

The child with a terminal illness has the same need for love, emotional support, and normal activities as any person facing death. Love, respect, and dignity are all important factors in caring for a dying child. Box 17-10 ■ provides guidelines about psychosocial needs of the dying child that should be considered.

NURSING CARE

PRIORITIZING NURSING CARE

The key to assisting clients with psychosocial needs is good communication and creation of a safe environment. Emotional aspects of care can be difficult for clients to express. The nurse needs to practice good listening skills in order to encourage the client to share what may feel like embarrassing, "silly," or frightening thoughts. It is important to take the client's concerns seriously and to avoid condescending responses. The client needs your empathy and support. Chapter 11 ⚭ discusses techniques a nurse can use to provide therapeutic communication.

ASSESSING

When assessing a client's psychosocial response to hospitalization, the nurse needs to be aware of signs and symptoms of stress, anxiety, or depression. Nurses must also be alert to the meaning of illness to their clients (Box 17-11 ■). A client with a dual diagnosis presents specific problems for

BOX 17-10	PEDIATRIC CONSIDERATIONS

Psychosocial Needs of Seriously Ill or Dying Children

- *Time to be a child*: Engage in activities such as age-appropriate play.
- *Communication/listening/expression of fears or anger*: Children should have someone they can talk to about their fears, joys, angers, or simply the weather. Listening to them is the most important way to help. Accepting that a seriously ill or dying child may not want to talk about dying is also important.
- *Depression and withdrawal*: Many physical changes that occur before death can make the child very dependent for even simple tasks. The older the child, the more stressful this dependence may be. Independence and control need to be given to the dying teenager whenever possible.
- *Spiritual and cultural needs*: The nurse should respect and provide for spiritual and cultural needs. Rituals that allow the child and his/her family to honor the transition from getting well to letting go or dying by:
  - Remembering
  - Giving thanks and expressing gratitude
  - Trusting God's presence in the experience for both the child who is dying and those who will be grieving
  - Saying goodbye
- *Wish fulfillment*: Some organizations provide funding for a "wish" for seriously and/or terminally ill children. If possible, help the child decide what he or she would most like to do before dying. These wishes often create wonderful memories for families of children with a terminal illness.
- *Permission from loved ones to die*: Some children seem to require "permission" to die. Many children fear their death will hurt their parents and make them very sad. It has been observed that children will cling to life through pain and suffering until they get "permission" from their parents to die.
- *Comfort in knowing they are not alone in the dying process*: The dying child most often wants reassurance that they will not die alone and that he/she will be missed. Parents and loved ones need to comfort the child and tell him/her that, when death occurs, they will be right at the bedside.
- *Limit setting*: Parents need to continue setting appropriate limits on a child's behavior and not let their guilt or grief inhibit their normal parenting, the consequence of which can be children becoming or feeling out of control.

the nurse who is collecting data for assessment. Clients may show signs of stress and fear. They may be experiencing withdrawal reactions. Because substance abusers are often also addicted to nicotine, they may object to being confined in an area where smoking is not allowed. Nurses should carry out all actions in a nonjudgmental manner. The nurse can ask the client about smoking habits early,

BOX 17-11	CULTURAL PULSE POINTS

Mental Illness and Minorities

- Minorities are just as likely as nonminorities to experience severe mental disorders such as anxiety, depression, bipolar disorder, and schizophrenia, but they are far less likely to receive treatment. Reasons include a lack of access to services, cultural and language barriers, and limited research concerning mental health and minorities.

- Lack of access to services is associated with one's level of income and access to medical insurance. Racial and ethnic minorities have higher rates of poverty and a much greater likelihood of being uninsured. The percentage of uninsured minorities is more than half that of Whites. Individuals experiencing symptoms of a mental disorder are most likely to seek help from their primary care physician; approximately 30 percent of Hispanics and 20 percent of African Americans do not have a primary healthcare provider.

- Language is a significant barrier to receiving appropriate mental health care. Diagnosis and treatment of mental disorders greatly depends on the ability of clients to explain their symptoms to their physician and understand steps for treatment. The language barrier often deters individuals from seeking treatment.

- Culture significantly influences the definition and treatment of mental illness, affecting the way individuals describe their symptoms and the symptoms they exhibit. For instance, African Americans may describe symptoms such as isolated sleep paralysis, or the inability to move while falling asleep or waking up. Some Hispanics experience symptoms of anxiety that include uncontrollable screaming, crying, trembling, and seizure-like fainting. Cultural beliefs about mental health strongly affect whether or not some people seek treatment, a person's coping styles and social supports, and the stigma they attach to mental illness.

- Many people from different cultures see mental illness as shameful and delay treatment until symptoms reach crisis proportions. The culture of physicians and mental health professionals influences how they interpret symptoms and interact with clients.

BOX 17-12	REMINDERS FOR CONDUCTING A THERAPEUTIC INTERVIEW

- The interview should be goal directed.
- Both participants must share actively in the process and each is influenced by the other.
- The relationship-building interaction of nurse and client determines the success or failure of the interview as an assessment tool.
- The nurse should have developed these interviewing skills:
  - Careful listening and attending
  - Demonstration of sincere interest in the importance of what the client has to say
  - Persistence in attempts to validate
  - Ability to pick up on/respond to cues from the client
- The client will have certain expectations of the interviewer:
  - Client expectations influence how the interview process will go.
  - At least initially, clients respond more positively to interviewers who meet their expectations/preferences.
  - The nurse will be the confident expert.
  - The professional will convey warmth and authentic concern while maintaining emotional objectivity (nonjudgmental).
  - The nurse will be competent at initiating and maintaining the flow of the interview.
  - The nurse will be knowledgeable about human behavior and able to interpret the client's behavior in proper context.

termination) are discussed in detail in Chapter 11 . Box 17-12 ■ lists several factors that help ensure that an interview is therapeutic. It is especially important with physically ill clients who have mental disorders to make clear from the start that your relationship will end when the client is discharged.

DIAGNOSING, PLANNING, AND IMPLEMENTING

Several NANDA diagnoses relate to psychosocial coping during physical illness. Examples of these are *Anxiety, Fear*, and *Social Isolation*. Examples of desired outcomes would be:

- Describes causes of anxiety as appropriate.
- Identifies personal strengths.
- Identifies reasons for feeling isolated.

Clients with varying levels of anxiety, stress, and depression are found in the acute hospital setting. Physical illness, coupled with the need to adjust to an unfamiliar environment, is stress producing. Stress can manifest itself in behaviors such as anger, agitation, fear, withdrawal, or inappropriate behavior. And, as mentioned, sensory overload and strange surroundings in the ICU can cause a severe reaction.

and then consult with the physician on the possibility of a nicotine patch.

Nursing diagnoses, as well as *DSM-IV-TR* diagnoses, begin with data collection. Collecting data for assessment is every nurse's responsibility and should be done at every client encounter as part of a comprehensive, ongoing assessment. The initial formal psychosocial assessment frequently is the responsibility of the RN. The LPN/LVN participates in ongoing evaluation of the client's psychosocial status. This is important, because significant changes can occur during the course of hospitalization or even in the course of a shift.

The interview is part of the therapeutic relationship that is formed between the client and the nurse. The three stages of the interview process (introductory, working, and

Encouraging Health Promotion Strategies

Useful intervention strategies for reducing stress and inducing relaxation include meditation, guided imagery, breathing exercises, progressive muscle relaxation, and biofeedback. Cognitive approaches such as journal keeping, restructuring, setting priorities and goals, cognitive reframing, and assertiveness training may be useful. Healthcare professionals at all levels should be role models for health promotion strategies. Physical exercise, optimal nutrition, adequate rest and sleep, and time management are all ways to promote health and reduce stress.

Exercise

Regular exercise promotes both physical and emotional health. Physiological benefits include improved muscle tone, increased cardiopulmonary function, and weight control. Psychological benefits include relief of tension, a feeling of well-being, and relaxation. In general, health guidelines recommend exercise at least three times a week for 60 to 90 minutes.

Nutrition

Optimal nutrition is essential for health and in increasing the body's resistance to stress. To minimize the effects of a stress response (e.g., irritability, hyperactivity, anxiety), people need to avoid excessive caffeine, salt, sugar, fat, and deficiencies in vitamins and minerals. Guidelines for a well-balanced, healthful diet are detailed in Chapter 25 ⚭.

Rest and Sleep

Rest and sleep restore the body's energy levels and are an essential aspect of stress management. To ensure adequate rest and sleep, clients may need comfort measures such as pain management. Nurses may need to teach techniques that promote peace of mind and relaxation. Rest and sleep are discussed further in Chapter 23 ⚭.

Relaxation Techniques

Several relaxation techniques can be used to quiet the mind, release tension, and counteract the fight-or-flight response of GAS, discussed earlier in this chapter. Nurses can teach these techniques to clients and encourage their use during and after hospitalization. Relaxation tapes can be purchased if desired. Some clients make their own recordings. Specific relaxation techniques that may be used are summarized in Box 17-13 ■. Review Table 8-1 ⚭ in the Complementary Therapies chapter for details.

Time Management

People who manage their time effectively usually experience less stress because they feel more in control of their circumstances. Feeling overwhelmed may indicate the need to prioritize tasks and make modifications in role demands. Responding appropriately to the demands of others is also

BOX 17-13	RELAXATION TECHNIQUES

- Breathing exercises
- Massage
- Progressive relaxation
- Imagery
- Biofeedback
- Yoga
- Meditation
- Therapeutic touch
- Music therapy
- Humor and laughter

an important aspect of effective time management. Since all requests made by others cannot always be met, individuals must decide which requests they can honor without undue stress, which ones can be negotiated, and which ones need to be declined. Another way to manage time effectively is to schedule daily or weekly times to do specific tasks. When people feel overwhelmed, they need to reexamine the "should, ought, and must" approach to their actions and develop more realistic self-expectations.

Minimizing Anxiety

Nurses have always carried out measures to minimize clients' anxiety and stress. For example, nurses encourage clients to take deep breaths before an injection, explain procedures before they are implemented including sensations likely to be experienced during the procedure, administer a back or neck rub to help the client relax, and offer support to clients and families during times of illness.

Mediating Anger

Often nurses find clients' anger difficult to handle. Caring for the client who is angry is difficult for two reasons:

- Clients rarely state, "I feel angry or frustrated," and rarely indicate the reason for their anger. Instead, they may refuse treatment, become verbally abusive or demanding, threaten violence, or become overly critical. Their complaints rarely reflect the cause of their anger.
- Anger from clients can elicit fear and anger in the nurse, who may respond in a manner that intensifies the client's anger, even to the point of violence. The majority of nurses respond in a way that reduces their own stress rather than the client's stress. Box 17-14 ■ lists some strategies for dealing with clients' anger.

Specific relaxation techniques that may be used were summarized in Box 17-13.

Intervening in Crisis Situations

A **crisis** is an acute, time-limited state of emotional imbalance resulting from sources of stress. It can be defined as a turning point in a person's life—a point at which usual resources and coping skills are no longer effective. A person in

---

BOX 17-14   STRATEGIES FOR DEALING WITH ANGER

Fontaine (2008) recommends the following strategies for dealing with clients' anger:

- Know and understand your own response to the feelings and expressions of anger.
- Accept the client's right to be angry; feelings are real and cannot be discounted or ignored.
- Ask the client in what way you may have contributed to the anger.
- Help the client "own" the anger—do not assume responsibility for her or his feelings.

---

crisis is temporarily unable to cope with or adapt to the stressor by using previous methods of problem solving. People in crisis generally see a stressor as overwhelming. They often do not have adequate situational support, and do not have adequate coping mechanisms.

Because a state of emotional imbalance is so uncomfortable, a crisis is self-limiting. However, a person experiencing a crisis alone has more difficulty handling the situation than a person working through a crisis with help.

Nurses in acute care or short-term care settings may not see the long-term effects of their crisis interventions. Typically, nurses in these settings will assess the crisis, and begin implementing a crisis intervention plan.

The nurse can help the client adjust in several ways:

- Provide compassionate, consistent care.
- Do not take client's reactions personally.
- Explain all care and procedures before beginning interventions.

EVALUATING

The desired outcomes developed during the planning stage are reviewed when collecting data about a client's current status. To determine if the outcomes have been achieved, the nurse will ask questions such as:

- How does the client perceive the problem?
- Is there an underlying problem that has not been identified?
- How does the client perceive the effectiveness of new coping strategies?
- Have family members and significant others provided effective support?

Although stress is part of everyday life, it is also highly individual. The addition of physical illness and hospitalization may require more intense intervention. Nurses need to be sensitive to clients' needs and reactions, and choose interventions that will be most effective for each individual. Establishing and maintaining an environment that will help the client to relax and to feel secure will help the client adjust to the situation at hand.

Continuity of Care

Clients with severe psychosocial reaction to physical illness or hospitalization may need ongoing support after discharge. Now is the time to discuss with the client the need to deal with substance abuse problems. During hospitalization, clients are sometimes able to face the need to deal with psychosocial issues. They may more readily accept the idea of getting treatment for their substance abuse. Inpatient care or a "12-step" program could be beneficial. Resources and referrals are crucial to enable clients and families ready access to ongoing sources of support.

NURSING PROCESS CARE PLAN
Physically Ill Client with Psychosocial Issues

Mr. Severs is a 54-year-old salesman who was hospitalized 3 days ago for treatment of aortic dissection. He was admitted to the CCU from the recovery room. He has been heavily medicated since the surgery. He has a closed chest drainage system. Mr. Severs has a history of alcohol (ETOH) addiction.

Assessment

VS: T 97.8, P 86, R 20, BP 128/88. Urinary output 60 mL/hr Foley catheter. IV D_5 in 0.45 NSS 100 mL/hr. Peripheral pulses strong and equal bilaterally. Drifting in and out of consciousness; moans in response to pain. Client attempting to pull out chest tube, IV, and Foley catheter.

Nursing Diagnosis

The following nursing diagnoses (among others) are identified for Mr. Severs:

- *Anxiety* r/t serious medical condition
- *Disturbed Sensory Perception* (visual and auditory)
- *Acute Confusion* r/t misinterpretation of environmental stimuli
- *Risk for Injury* r/t environmental conditions interacting with client's adaptive and defensive resources

Expected Outcomes

The expected outcomes of the plan of care specify that Mr. Severs will:

- Have posture, facial expression, gestures, and activity level that reflect decreased distress.
- Demonstrate relaxed body movements and facial expressions.
- Have cognitive status restored to baseline.
- Remain free of injury.

Planning and Implementation

The following interventions are planned and implemented:

- Monitor client's level of anxiety and physical reaction to anxiety (e.g., tachycardia, tachypnea, nonverbal expression of anxiety).
- Check client's behavior and cognition systematically throughout the day and night as appropriate.
- Explain care and interventions to client prior to initiation.
- Talk to client even if nonresponsive.
- Provide uninterrupted rest/sleep periods whenever possible.

Evaluation

Mr. Severs was discharged from the CCU on post-op day 4. Chest tube removed. Client calmer; no longer attempting to pull out tubes. Awake and oriented to name; still confused as to date and time; knows he has had surgery. Asks questions about last 3 days.

Critical Thinking in the Nursing Process

1. Speculate about the relationship of Mr. Severs' ETOH addiction and the severity of his psychosocial reactions during his stay in the CCU.
2. Explain how ICU psychosis can be prevented.
3. Discuss the progression and resolution of severe psychosocial reactions to hospitalization (ICU psychosis).

Note: Discussion of Critical Thinking questions appears on the MyNursingKit Website.

Note: The references and resources for all chapters have been compiled at the back of the book.

Chapter Review

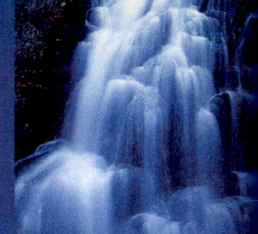

KEY Points

- Components of holistic assessment include a psychosocial assessment, assessment of usual coping strategies, and an overall quality-of-life assessment.

- Common responses to physical illness are depression, anxiety, substance use, denial, and anger.

- Verbalization is an effective outlet for anxiety, but ability to verbalize may be compromised by cultural expectations, disability, or lack of a listener.

- Anyone facing a serious medical condition needs a variety of supports and may benefit from learning new coping skills.

- Defense mechanisms protect us from being consciously aware of a thought or feeling that we cannot tolerate.

- A dual diagnosis indicates (1) two independent disorders occurring together, (2) substance abuse causing another mental disorder, or (3) a person with a mental disorder using substances in an effort to self-medicate or to feel better.

- Suicide is probably the most misunderstood mental health issue. A number of myths exist that must be recognized by healthcare professionals in order to better deal with this problem.

◑ FOR FURTHER Study

Table 8-1 provides information on various complementary therapies that can help clients with psychosocial disorders.

The three stages of the interview process, communication and listening techniques are discussed in Chapter 11.

See Chapter 14 for a discussion of types of admission.

The main discussion of grief and death is in Chapter 18.

Procedure 19-1 lists the steps in a focused physical assessment.

Rest and sleep are discussed further in Chapter 23.

Guidelines for a well-balanced, healthful diet are detailed in Chapter 25.

See Chapter 33 for coverage of treatment of cardiac failure.

Chapter 35 provides more information on care of clients with HIV and AIDS.

See Chapter 36 for a discussion of sundowning or sundowner syndrome.

Depression in ill older adults is discussed in Chapter 43.

Mental health disorders and their treatment are discussed in Chapter 49.

Substance abuse and eating disorders are discussed in Chapter 50.

Refer to Chapter 58 for information on chronically or terminally ill children.

Critical Thinking Care Map

Caring for a Client with Myocardial Infarction

NCLEX-PN® Focus Area: Psychosocial Integrity, Coping, and Adaptation

Case Study: Darryl Johnson, a 47-year-old accountant, was admitted to the emergency department with a heart attack. He says, "I'm scared about this. My dad died of a heart attack when he was 48 years old." He appears restless, questions everything that is going on, and is hyperventilating.

Nursing Diagnosis: *Anxiety*

COLLECT DATA

Subjective	Objective
_____	_____
_____	_____
_____	_____
_____	_____
_____	_____
_____	_____
_____	_____

Would you report this? Yes/No

If yes, report to: _____

What would you report? _____

Nursing Care

_____

_____

_____

_____

_____

_____

_____

_____

_____

_____

How would you document this? _____

_____

_____

_____

Compare your answers and documentation to those provided on the MyNursingKit Website.

Data Collected
(use only those that apply)

- Alert and oriented to time, place, and person.
- VS: 99.6/88/28 BP140/82
- Peripheral pulse strong and equal
- Cap refill less than 3 seconds
- Lungs clear
- Pale; skin cool and diaphoretic
- Nail bed pink
- ECG normal sinus rhythm
- Severe chest pain

Nursing Interventions
(use only those that apply; list in priority order)

- Assess client's level of anxiety and physical reaction to anxiety.
- Avoid confrontation.
- Assess for subtle signs of denial.
- Validate observations by asking client, "Are you feeling anxious now?"
- Assess source of fear with client.
- Allow and reinforce client's personal reaction to or expression of pain, discomfort, or threat to well-being.
- Explain all activities, procedures, and issues that involve the client; use nonmedical terms and calm, slow speech. Do this in advance of procedures when possible, and validate client's understanding.
- Encourage realistic and achievable goal setting.
- Explore coping skills previously used by the client to relieve anxiety; reinforce these skills and explore other outlets.
- Provide back rub to decrease anxiety.

NCLEX-PN® Exam Preparation

TEST-TAKING TIP Remember that this is a nursing examination and the answer to the question involves something that is included in the nursing care plan, rather than the medical plan.

1 The nurse, assisting with a psychosocial assessment, would gather information about all of the following processes except:

1. Emotional
2. Behavioral
3. Interactional
4. Physical

2 The client was diagnosed with a myocardial infarction 2 days ago and is on bed rest, allowed up to the chair only for meals. The client has followed the order until today, when the nurse enters the room and finds the client sitting on the floor doing sit-ups. The nurse recognizes the client is demonstrating what defense mechanism?

1. Repression
2. Sublimation
3. Identification
4. Denial

3 The nurse is contributing to a mental status examination of a client who has been alert, oriented, with clear speech, and normal thought content and thought processes. What other information would the nurse *observe*?

1. Sensation/perception
2. Trust/mistrust
3. Affect
4. Memory

4 The nurse explains to the client that anxiety can sometimes be helpful by producing a slight arousal state that enhances perception, learning, and productive abilities. What level of anxiety is the nurse describing?

1. Mild
2. Moderate
3. Severe
4. Panic

5 The nurse is caring for a client with prolonged periods of low mood, loss of interest, and feelings of worthlessness that manifest when the client sleeps most of the day, has no energy or appetite, and has been losing weight. The nurse recognizes the client is demonstrating what type of depression?

1. Seasonal affective disorder
2. Major depressive disorder
3. Bipolar affective disorder
4. Postnatal depression

6 The nurse is caring for a client with a medical diagnosis of asthma who becomes very anxious during acute attacks. The nurse's priority response is to:

1. Ignore the anxiety because the physiological needs are more acute
2. Notify the physician and request an order for a sedative

3. Tell the client not to be anxious because it makes the asthma attack more severe
4. Work with the client to reduce anxiety using antianxiety techniques

7 The nurse would anticipate feelings of loss in all of the following clients except:

1. The parents of a newborn infant born prematurely at 28 weeks who is stable and doing well
2. The client who was just diagnosed with rheumatoid arthritis
3. The client who was informed that her lab result was confused with another client's resulting in a misdiagnosis of Grave's disease
4. The client who has just been informed of a diagnosis of cancer with a good chance of recovery following chemotherapy

8 The nurse is caring for a 26-year-old client requiring cardiorespiratory monitoring secondary to sleep apnea. The client is placed on a noninvasive mechanical ventilator at night. The client's sleep is frequently disturbed by alarms from both the monitor and the ventilator. When the nurse enters the room the client reports hearing voices and seeing things that are not there. The nurse recognizes the client is experiencing:

1. Posttraumatic stress disorder
2. ICU psychosis
3. Onset of schizophrenia
4. Major depressive episode

9 The nurse is caring for a client with a nursing diagnosis of social isolation. Which of the following is a desired outcome for this client?

1. Able to list actions to reduce anxiety
2. No longer feels socially isolated
3. Able to list strategies for reducing feelings of isolation
4. Describes situations that cause anxiety

10 The nurse, caring for a client who required amputation of the left arm, recognizes that the stress of accepting changes in physique and developing intimate relationships with others will be particularly difficult for this client because he or she is in what stage of development?

1. School-aged child
2. Adolescent
3. Young adult
4. Middle adult

Answers and rationales for Review Questions appear in Appendix I.

Loss, Grief, and Death

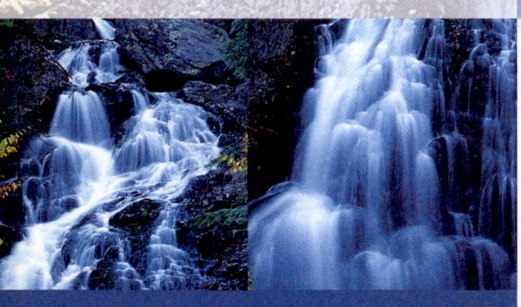

BRIEF Outline

LEARNING Outcomes

After completing this chapter, you will be able to:

1. Discuss the relationship between loss, grief, and death.
2. Identify factors that affect a loss or grief response.
3. Identify common myths about grief in relation to children.
4. Discuss different stages and manifestations of grieving.
5. Name the "four tasks" of William Worden's grief model.
6. Discuss the mourner's bill of rights and six reconciliation needs.
7. Name three legal issues that arise when a client is dying.
8. Identify strategies nurses can use when assisting clients and families at times of grief, loss, or death.
9. Describe the importance of self-care for the nurse working with dying clients.

Clinical Objective

10. Provide support for client and family during the grief process.

KEY TERMS

Loss, grief, and death are experienced by everyone at some time during life. People may suffer the loss of valued relationships through life changes, such as moving from one city to another, separation, divorce, or the death of a parent, spouse, or friend. People may grieve changing life roles as they watch grown children leave home or they retire from their lifelong work. The loss of valued pets or material objects can evoke feelings of grief and loss. When people's lives are affected by civil or national strife, they may grieve the loss of valued ideals such as safety, freedom, or democracy. Although the grieving process has certain similarities for all important losses in life, the most traumatic grieving is usually associated with the loss of one's own life (as you have known it), or that of a loved one.

Nurses will interact with those experiencing loss in a variety of settings, from a miscarriage, stillbirth, or neonatal death to an accidental death, dismemberment, or attempted suicide of a teen to the elderly client who finally succumbs to a chronic illness. Nurses must recognize the various aspects of a loss or death—legal, ethical, religious and spiritual, biologic, intellectual, personal—and be prepared to provide sensitive, skilled, and supportive care to all those affected. This section offers general guidelines that will assist the nurse in caring for people who are dying or experiencing a loss, and in helping family members who are sharing the experience.

Loss, Grief, and Dying

Loss describes a real or potential situation in which something that is valued is gone, is unavailable, or is changed. People can experience a loss in many different ways, and sometimes it helps to categorize loss. **Situational loss** is related to a specific occurrence such as loss of a job due to a job transfer. **Maturational loss** can be related to loss of endurance or an increase in dependence due to aging.

Accidental loss can be related to loss of a body part due to an accident or disease.

Grief is the whole range of feelings, thoughts, and behaviors related to loss and signifying emotional responses, especially overwhelming distress and sorrow. **Bereavement** is the normal grieving period experienced by the surviving loved ones. **Mourning** involves the process and rituals through which grief is eventually resolved. It is influenced by culture, beliefs, and customs. Normal ways of expressing grief include sorrow and a change in sleep patterns, eating habits, activity level, or communication patterns. This type of grieving is called **anticipatory grieving. Dysfunctional grieving** describes grief that is characterized by an extended period of denial, depression, severe physiological symptoms, or suicidal thoughts. **Disenfranchised grief** describes the grief that occurs when a mourner is judged by a social norm that does not recognize the validity of the loss. A mourner cannot publicly mourn because others do not validate the relationship to the person lost. (This kind of grief is not restricted to, but often affects, those with loss of a loved one to AIDS, addiction, or prostitution.)

Grief can have negative effects on health, and symptoms may not be recognized as relating to the grief process. Survivors may experience such manifestations as depression, anxiety, fatigue, headaches, chest pain, dyspnea, dizziness, palpitations, or menstrual irregularities. Unresolved grief can lead to continued physical and emotional problems. To achieve mental and physical health, survivors must work through and resolve their grief.

Factors Influencing Loss and Grief Responses

A number of factors affect a person's response to a loss or death. Nurses learn general concepts about the influence of these factors of the grieving experience, but it is important to remember that these factors and their significance vary from individual to individual.

Age

Age affects a person's understanding of and reaction to loss. With experience, people usually increase their understanding and acceptance of life, loss, and death.

Childhood

Children differ from adults not only in their understanding of loss and death but also in how they are affected by the loss of others. The child's patterns of growth and development progress rapidly; adult patterns are generally more stable. The loss of a parent or other significant person can threaten the child's ability to develop, and regression sometimes results. Assisting the child with the grief experience includes helping the child regain the normal continuity and pace of emotional development. Table 18-1 ■ describes some myths and realities that the Hospice Foundation of America has identified about children and grief. Further information can be found by visiting their website.

In situations of crisis and loss, children are sometimes pushed aside in an attempt to protect them from the pain. They can feel afraid, abandoned, and lonely. Careful work with bereaved children is especially necessary because experiencing a loss in childhood can have serious effects later in life.

Early and Middle Adulthood

As people grow, they come to experience loss as part of normal development. By middle age, for example, the loss of a parent through death seems a normal occurrence compared to the death of a younger person. Coping with the death of an aged parent has even been viewed as a necessary developmental task of the middle-aged adult.

The middle-aged adult will experience losses other than death. For example, losses resulting from impaired health or body function and losses of various role functions can be difficult for the middle-aged adult. How the middle-aged adult responds to such losses is influenced by previous experiences with loss, the person's sense of self-esteem, and the strength and availability of support.

Late Adulthood

Losses experienced by older adults include loss of health, loss of mobility, loss of independence, and loss of work role (see Chapter 16 ◯◯). Limited income and the need to change one's living accommodations can also lead to feelings of loss and grieving.

For older adults, the loss through death of a longtime mate is profound (Figure 18-1 ■). Although individuals differ in their ability to deal with such a loss, research suggests that health problems and mortality for widows and widowers increase in the period of bereavement following

TABLE 18-1	Myths and Realities about Children and Grief
MYTH	**REALITY**
Children do not grieve.	**Children of all ages grieve.** The child's development and experiences affect the grieving process.
The death of a loved one is the only major loss children and adolescents experience.	**Young people experience a variety of losses.** These include losses of pets, separations caused by divorce or relocations, losses of friends and relationships, as well as losses due to illness or death. All of these losses generate grief.
Children should be shielded from loss.	**It is impossible to protect children from loss.** Adults can teach ways of adapting to loss by including young people in the grieving process.
Children should not go to funerals.	**Allow young people to make their own choice.**
Children should always attend funerals.	They should decide how they wish to participate in funerals or other services. Adults must provide information, options, and support.
Children get over loss quickly.	**No one gets over significant loss.** Children, like adults, will learn to live with the loss. They may revisit that loss at different points in their lives and experience grief again.
Children are permanently scarred by loss.	**Children are resilient.** By providing solid support and strong consistent care, adults can help children cope with loss.
Talking with children and adolescents is the most effective approach in dealing with loss.	**Different approaches are helpful to young people.** It is important to talk openly with children and adolescents; it is also helpful to let young people use creative approaches. Play, art, dance, music, and ritual are all valuable modes of expression that allow them to say what words cannot.
Helping children and adolescents deal with loss is the family's responsibility.	**Other individuals and organizations can share this responsibility.**

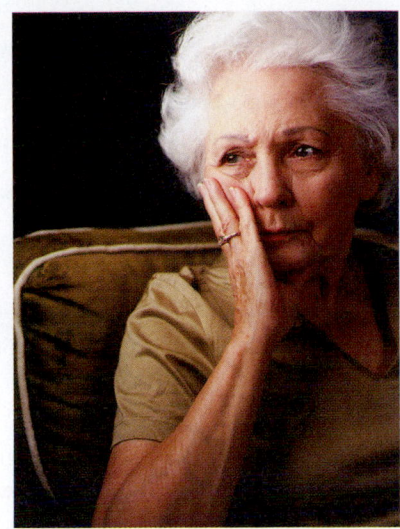

Figure 18-1. ■ The loss of a long-term partner can have a devastating effect on an older adult.

the death of the spouse (Hart et al., 2007). Because the majority of deaths occur among elderly people, and because the number of elderly people is increasing in North America, nurses will need to be especially alert to the potential problems of older grieving adults. **Bereavement overload** is a condition that can occur when older adults have to deal with a succession of losses in overlapping time frames, which can interfere with a normal grieving period.

SPIRITUAL BELIEFS

Spiritual beliefs and practices greatly influence both a person's reaction to loss and subsequent behavior. Most religious groups have practices related to dying, and these are often important to the client and support people. To provide support at a time of death, nurses need to understand the client's particular beliefs and practices. Ask the client and family if they have any spiritual beliefs and practices, so the healthcare team can accommodate their wishes at the time of death.

GENDER

The gender roles into which many people are socialized in the United States and Canada affect their reactions at times of loss. Men are frequently expected to "be strong" and show very little emotion during grief, whereas it is acceptable for women to show grief by crying. Often when a wife dies, the husband, who is the chief mourner, is expected to repress his own emotions and to comfort sons and daughters in their grieving.

SOCIOECONOMIC STATUS

The socioeconomic status of an individual often affects the support system available at the time of a loss. A pension plan or insurance, for example, can offer a widowed or disabled person a choice of ways to deal with a loss. A person who loses a hand and can no longer carry out work-related tasks may be able to pursue vocational reeducation. A wealthy person whose spouse has died may decide to take a cruise or visit relatives. On the other hand, a person who is confronted with both severe loss and economic hardship may not be able to cope with either.

SUPPORT SYSTEMS

The people closest to the grieving individual are often the first to recognize and provide needed emotional, physical, and functional assistance. However, because many people are uncomfortable or inexperienced in dealing with losses, the usual support people may instead withdraw from the grieving individual. Also, support may be available when the loss is first recognized, but as the support people return to their usual activities, the need for ongoing support may be unmet. Sometimes, the grieving individual is unable or unready to accept support when it is offered.

CULTURE

Culture influences an individual's reaction to loss. How grief is expressed is often determined by the customs of the culture. In the United States and Canada, unless an extended family structure exists, grief is usually handled by the nuclear family. The death of a family member in a typical nuclear European American family leaves a great void, because the same few individuals fill most of the roles. In cultures where several generations and extended family members either live in the same household or are physically close, the impact of a family member's death may be softened, because the roles of the deceased are quickly filled by other relatives.

Many Americans appear to have adopted the belief that grief is a private matter to be endured internally. Therefore, feelings tend to be repressed and may remain unidentified. People who have been socialized to "be strong" and "make the best of the situation" may not express deep feelings or personal concerns when they experience a serious loss.

Some cultural groups value social support and the expression of loss. In some groups, the expression of grief through wailing, crying, physical prostration, and other outward demonstrations are acceptable and encouraged. Other groups may frown on this demonstration as a loss of control, favoring a more quiet and stoic expression of grief. In cultural groups where strong kinship ties are maintained, physical and emotional support and assistance are provided by family members.

Supporting Death Rituals

Death rituals are as varied as the number of cultures and religions in any given locale. Differences in these rituals involve the client's beliefs and actions as well as the mourning rituals of the family. Throughout the dying process, the healthcare team should make every effort to provide the time and privacy necessary to carry out the rituals that will show respect for the client. Allow spiritual counselors private time with the client and family. If death is imminent, provide care as unobtrusively as possible so as to not interfere with death rituals. Some cultures use music, drums, and incense. If this is the case, it might be necessary to remove other clients from the area so as to allow the dying client to be cared for in a culturally sensitive way while not disturbing other clients.

DEATH-RELATED RELIGIOUS AND CULTURAL PRACTICES

Thanatology is the academic study of death and dying. It is an interdisciplinary study, researching into cultural practices, attitudes, sociology, and psychology of death among human beings.

Cultural and religious traditions and practices help people cope with death, dying, and the grieving process. They give crucial comfort to survivors. Nurses are often present through the dying process and at the moment of death. Knowledge of the client's religious and cultural beliefs helps nurses provide individualized care to clients and their families, even though they may not participate in the family's rituals.

Nurses also need to be knowledgeable about the client's death-related rituals, such as last rites, administration of Holy Communion, or chanting at the bedside (Box 18-1 ■). There may be ritual procedures for washing, dressing, positioning, and shrouding the dead. Certain ethnic groups may wish to retain their native customs, in which family members of the same sex wash and prepare the body for burial and cremation. Muslims also customarily turn the body toward Mecca. Nurses need to ask family members about their preferences and verify who will carry out these activities. The nurse must ensure that any ritual items that were brought to the institution be given to the family or to the funeral home at the time of death to prevent such items from being lost. Culturally diverse traditions about mourning and after-death rites will be seen later in this book, in Table 44-1 ⚭.

Stages and Manifestations of Grief

Many authors have described the process of grief. The most famous is Dr. Elisabeth Kübler-Ross, who set the foundation in the field of thanatology when she described five

Stages of Grief	
Shock	No! I don't believe it!
Anger	**It's not fair! I don't deserve this!**
Bargaining	If you just make me better, *I promise* I'll. . . .
Depression	*Leave me alone.*
Acceptance	I am ready now.

Figure 18-2. ■ Stages of grieving as identified by Kübler-Ross.

stages of grief. Nurses can observe clinical signs to determine a person's stage of grieving (Figure 18-2 ■).

1. **Denial.** The client refuses to believe that the loss is happening and is not ready to deal with practical problems, such as use of prosthesis after loss of a leg. The client may assume artificial cheerfulness to prolong denial. This stage is important and necessary and can assist to cushion the impact of the client's awareness.

2. **Anger.** The client resents the fact that others will remain healthy and alive while he or she must die. The client or family may direct anger at the nurse or staff about matters that normally would not bother them.

3. **Bargaining.** The client promises a change in behavior to avoid loss and may express feelings of guilt or fear of punishment for past sins, real or imagined. The client promises to be good in exchange for prolonged time.

4. **Depression.** The client grieves over what has happened and what cannot be. The client may talk freely (e.g., remembering past losses such as money or job) or may withdraw. The client then enters a state of "preparatory grief" getting ready for the arrival of death.

5. **Acceptance.** The client comes to terms with loss and may have decreased interest in physical surroundings and support people. The client may wish to begin making plans (e.g., will, prosthesis, altered living arrangements).

Note that not everyone goes through these stages of grief in the exact order listed. Also, individuals may move back and forth between stages. The amount of time one remains in each stage differs from person to person, and some individuals may never reach the acceptance stage. A study confirming the existence of five stages of grief (Maciejewski et al., 2007) suggested that people may need professional counseling if they do not experience the five stages within 6 months of a grief event.

Tasks, Rights, and Needs of the Grieving Person

Other theorists have since elaborated on Kübler-Ross's work. William Worden (2003) developed a model of four basic tasks confronting a person experiencing loss and grief. These include:

Task One: To accept the reality of the loss.
Task Two: To work through the pain of grief.
Task Three: To adjust to a different type of environment.
Task Four: To emotionally relocate the deceased and move on with life (Jeffers, 2001).

Alan Wolfelt (2003) has further defined the rights and needs of those who grieve. He has identified a mourner's "bill of rights" (Box 18-2 ■) that supports the grieving person's unique experience.

Besides **grieving** (the internal process of working through the effects of loss), Wolfelt (2003) suggested that people have a need for mourning (the outward expression of those who are grieving a loss). He encouraged mourners to take time to address certain basic needs as they are recovering from a loss. He encouraged those who mourn to reconcile themselves to the following six needs:

- The need to acknowledge the reality of the loved one's death.
- The need to be open to the pain of the loss, allowing oneself "doses" of grief (time) when one feels the grief completely and without distraction) followed by periods when one is not dwelling in the grief. At the beginning, the "doses" may be frequent. It takes patience to accept them and allow them to be expressed.
- The need to create a relationship with the deceased person as part of the past. This allows the mourner to maintain

---

BOX 18-2   THE MOURNER'S BILL OF RIGHTS

Though you should reach out to others as you do the work of mourning, you should not feel obligated to accept the unhelpful responses you may receive from some people. You are the one who is grieving, and as such, you have certain "rights" no one should try to take away from you.

The following list is intended both to empower you to heal and to decide how others can and cannot help. This is not to discourage you from reaching out to others for help, but rather to assist you in distinguishing useful responses from hurtful ones.

1. *You have the right to experience your own unique grief.* No one else will grieve in exactly the same way you do. So, when you turn to others for help, don't allow them to tell what you should or should not be feeling.

2. *You have the right to talk about your grief.* Talking about your grief will help you heal. Seek out others who will allow you to talk as much as you want, as often as you want, about your grief. If at times you don't feel like talking, you also have the right to be silent.

3. *You have the right to feel a multitude of emotions.* Confusion, disorientation, fear, guilt and relief are just a few of the emotions you might feel as part of your grief journey. Others may try to tell you that feeling angry, for example, is wrong. Don't take these judgmental responses to heart. Instead, find listeners who will accept your feelings without condition.

4. *You have the right to be tolerant of your physical and emotional limits.* Your feelings of loss and sadness will probably leave you feeling fatigued. Respect what your body and mind are telling you. Get daily rest. Eat balanced meals. And don't allow others to push you into doing things you don't feel ready to do.

5. *You have the right to experience "griefbursts."* Sometimes, out of nowhere, a powerful surge of grief may overcome you. This can be frightening, but is normal and natural. Find someone who understands and will let you talk it out.

6. *You have the right to make use of ritual.* The funeral ritual does more than acknowledge the death of someone loved. It helps provide you with the support of caring people. More importantly, the funeral is a way for you to mourn. If others tell you the funeral or other healing rituals such as these are silly or unnecessary, don't listen.

7. *You have the right to embrace your spirituality.* If faith is a part of your life, express it in ways that seem appropriate to you. Allow yourself to be around people who understand and support your religious beliefs. If you feel angry at God, find someone to talk with who won't be critical of your feelings of hurt and abandonment.

8. *You have the right to search for meaning.* You may find yourself asking, "Why did he or she die? Why this way? Why now?" Some of your questions may have answers, but some may not. And watch out for the clichéd responses some people may give you. Comments like, "It was God's will" or "Think of what you have to be thankful for" are not helpful and you do not have to accept them.

9. *You have the right to treasure your memories.* Memories are one of the best legacies that exist after the death of someone loved. You will always remember. Instead of ignoring your memories, find others with whom you can share them.

10. *You have the right to move toward your grief and heal.* Reconciling your grief will not happen quickly. Remember, grief is a process, not an event. Be patient and tolerant with yourself and avoid people who are impatient and intolerant with you. Neither you nor those around you must forget that the death of someone loved changes your life forever.

Source: Wolfelt, Alan. (2003) Used with permission.

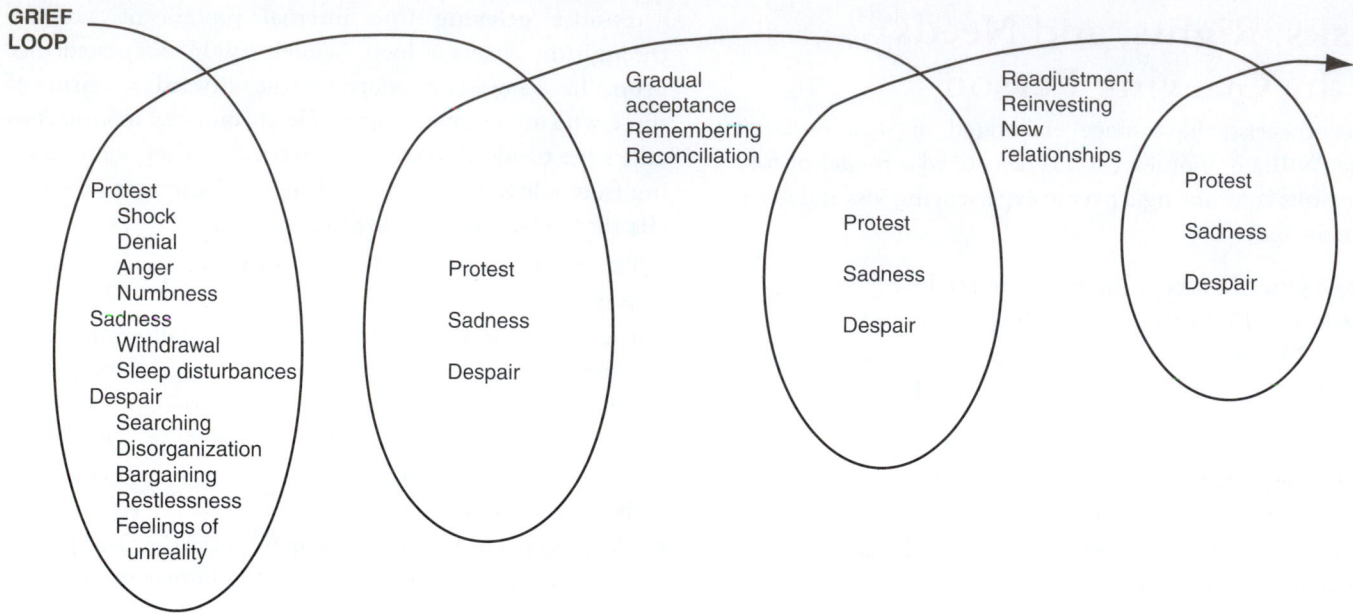

GRIEF LOOP

Protest
Shock
Denial
Anger
Numbness
Sadness
Withdrawal
Sleep disturbances
Despair
Searching
Disorganization
Bargaining
Restlessness
Feelings of
unreality

Protest
Sadness
Despair

Gradual
acceptance
Remembering
Reconciliation

Protest
Sadness
Despair

Readjustment
Reinvesting
New
relationships

Protest
Sadness
Despair

Figure 18-3. ■ The linear model of the stages of grieving has been modified to a more process-oriented model. This approach provides a more fluid view of how grief evolves over time.

the past relationship and to be open to new experiences in the future.

- The need to create a new self-identity, perhaps adopting roles that the loved one filled previously.
- The need to search for meaning. Whether one has a spiritual practice or not, the death of a loved one raises the question of "Why" and "What's it all about?" Doubts are natural, but the mourner will have to find reasons for going on with life.
- The need to have support from others. Support is a healthy human need, and the mourning person may require support periodically for many years. The approach of seeing mourning as something to "get over" quickly leads to repression, not resolution, of grief.

Worden, Wolfelt, and others differed from Kübler-Ross by describing grief not in stages but as a fluid process that evolves over time. Figure 18-3 ■ illustrates this idea.

Legal Issues

The nurse's roles in legal issues related to death are determined by the laws of the region and the policies of the healthcare institution. For example, in some states a nasogastric feeding tube cannot be removed from a person in a coma without a prior directive from the client. In other states, the removal is allowed at the family's request or on a physician's order. These legal issues raise strong ethical concerns. The nurse may need support from other team members in understanding issues and providing appropriate care to clients facing death.

ADVANCE DIRECTIVES

The Patient Self-Determination Act, implemented in 1991, requires all healthcare facilities receiving Medicare and Medicaid reimbursement to do the following:

- Recognize advance directives.
- Ask clients whether they have advance directives.
- Provide educational materials advising clients of their rights to declare their personal wishes regarding treatment decisions, including the right to refuse medical treatment.

There are two types of advance medical directives: the living will and the healthcare proxy or surrogate. The **living will** provides specific instructions about what medical treatment the client chooses to omit or refuse in the event that the client becomes unable to make those decisions. Treatments that are commonly included are cardiopulmonary resuscitation (CPR), intubation, ventilatory (breathing) support, and feeding (intravenously and/or via tube placement).

The healthcare proxy document (also called a **durable power of attorney for health care** or **medical power of attorney**) is a written statement appointing someone else to manage healthcare treatment decisions when the client is unable to do so (see Figure 4-2). The healthcare proxy is often a relative or trusted friend.

The proxy document is often used for specific clients who are in a coma, are having life-sustaining procedures, or are receiving artificial nutrition or hydration.

If a durable power of attorney for health care is not appointed and the client becomes unable to make healthcare decisions, the attending physician will appoint a healthcare surrogate. A **healthcare surrogate** is an adult who is appointed to make healthcare decisions in the event a client becomes incapacitated and has not executed a living will or medical power of attorney.

DO-NOT-RESUSCITATE ORDERS

Physicians may order "no code" or **do-not-resuscitate** (DNR) orders for clients who are in a stage of terminal, irreversible illness or expected death. A DNR order is generally written when the client or surrogate has asked for no CPR (cardiopulmonary resuscitation) to take place in the event the client's breathing stops or the heart stops beating. Medications will not be administered. A *comfort measures only* order is written to indicate that the goal of treatment is a comfortable, dignified death and that further life-sustaining measures are not indicated. Pain relief is an important element of comfort measures only.

ORGAN DONATION

The Uniform Anatomical Gift Act and the National Organ Transplant Act in the United States, and the Human Tissue Act in Canada, are acts governing organ donation. Under these acts, people who are 18 years of age or older and of sound mind may become organ donors. They make a gift of all or any part of their own bodies for the following purposes: medical or dental education, research, advancement of medical or dental science, therapy, or transplantation.

Nurses may serve as witnesses for people consenting to donate organs or revoking the organ donor designation. In many states, healthcare workers are required to ask survivors for consent to donate the deceased's organs. Organ donation can be an emotional issue for the bereaved.

NURSING CARE

PRIORITIZING NURSING CARE

Providing care in relation to loss can be a challenge for nurses. As a healthcare provider, do not presume to know what the client and family need. Instead, ask them directly. When caring for clients who are dying, focus your care on meeting physiological, spiritual, and psychological needs and on providing support to the family.

Sometimes nurses avoid caring for dying clients because they do not want to "bother" the client. Give personal care as you would to any client to keep them clean and comfortable. Educate and empower the family to participate in the care as much as possible. Teach the family simple skills such as mouth care or turning and positioning techniques. Other comfort measures should include dimmed lighting, soft music, and gentle touch. Helping with care may reduce their anxiety.

Clients near death are often able to communicate verbally or nonverbally, so ask them what they need. It is generally believed that hearing is the last sense to leave, so always speak to the client and explain what you are doing. Dying clients need to feel safe and secure, and communication is a very real way of providing for these needs. If the client is unconscious, consult the family because they will likely know the client's wishes.

It is important to give the family information about vital signs and other indicators of the client's status. Remember, family members may not understand the implications of these physiological changes, so be sure to explain the process in detail. Show kindness and empathy, even if the family seems angry or hostile. They may be angry because their loved one is leaving them or angry at the staff for being unable to save the client. Again, understand that the anger is not meant for you personally. Offer a private area for the family to grieve.

ASSESSING

Past Losses and Coping Techniques

During the health care of a client, the nurse poses questions about previous losses and coping techniques. If there is a current or recent loss, greater detail is needed.

Clients do not always associate physical ailments with emotional responses such as grief. The nurse may need to ask specific questions to help identify possible loss-related stresses. If the client reports significant losses, it is important to understand how the client usually copes with loss and what resources are available to assist the client to cope. This information is gathered to help determine a plan of care. Box 18-3 ■ lists interview questions nurses may ask about loss and grief.

In collecting data on the client's response to a current loss, the nurse may identify dysfunctional grief. This is best treated by a healthcare professional who is expert in assisting such clients. If the observation reveals severe physical or psychological signs and symptoms, the client should be referred to an appropriate care provider.

Awareness of Approaching Loss

When gathering data to assess a dying client, the nurse must pay attention to the level of awareness of the client

---

BOX 18-3   DATA COLLECTION

Interview for Loss and Grieving

Previous Losses

- Have you ever lost someone or something very important to you?
- Have you or your family ever moved your home?
- What was it like for you when you first started school? Moved away from home? Got a job? Retired?
- Are you physically able to do all the things you like to do? Used to do?
- Do you think there will be any losses in your life in the near future?

Previous Grieving

- Tell me about (the loss). What was losing _____ like for you?
- Did you have trouble sleeping? Eating? Concentrating?
- What kinds of things did you do to make yourself feel better when something like that happened?
- Are there spiritual or cultural practices you observed when you had a loss like that?
- Who was a person you could turn to if you were very upset about (the loss)?
- How long did it take you to feel more like yourself again and go back to your usual activities?

Current Loss

- What have you been told about (the loss)? Is there anything else you would like to know or don't understand?
- What changes do you think this (illness, surgery) will cause in your life? What do you think it will be like without (the lost object)?
- Have you ever experienced a loss like this before?
- Can you think of anything good that might come out of this?
- What kind of help do you think you will need? Who is going to be helping you with this loss?
- Are there any people or organizations in your community that might be able to help?

Current Grieving

- Are you having trouble sleeping? Eating? Concentrating? Breathing?
- Do you have any pain or other new physical problems?
- Are you taking any drugs or medications to help you cope with this loss?
- What are you doing to help you deal with this loss?
- Do you feel like you are suffering?

and the family. The type of awareness must be considered when planning care and communicating with caregivers. There are three basic types of awareness:

- *Closed awareness.* The client and family are unaware of impending death. They may not completely

understand why the client is ill. They believe the client will recover.
- *Mutual pretense.* The client, family, and health personnel know that the prognosis is terminal. However, they do not talk about it and they try not to raise the subject.
- *Open awareness.* Both client and others know about the impending death and feel comfortable discussing it, even though it is difficult.

Physical Signs of Impending Death

Nursing care includes collecting data to make accurate assessment of the signs of approaching death. In addition to signs related to the client's specific disease, the four main physical signs of impending death are:

- Loss of muscle tone.
- Slowing of the circulation.
- Changes in respirations.
- Impairment of senses.

See Box 44-3 🔗 for additional signs of approaching death.

Various consciousness levels can occur just before death. Some clients are alert. Others are drowsy, stuporous, or comatose. However, hearing is always thought to be the last of the five senses lost so speak slowly, softly, and clearly. Loved ones may be comforted by knowing that they can talk to the dying loved one and say all the things they want to tell them.

DIAGNOSING, PLANNING, AND IMPLEMENTING

Some of the most common priority nursing diagnoses related to loss and grieving are the following:

- *Grieving (Complicated)*
- *Fear*
- *Hopelessness*
- *Powerlessness*
- *Risk for Caregiver Role Strain*
- *Interrupted Family Processes*

When planning care with clients who are confronting a loss or death, the Dying Person's Bill of Rights can be a useful guide (Figure 18-4 ■).

The major nursing responsibility for clients who are dying is to assist the client to a peaceful death. Other specific responsibilities in relation to a dying person include the following:

- Maintain the client's comfort and dignity.
- Provide relief from loneliness, fear, and depression (Figure 18-5 ■). This can be achieved by active listening, therapeutic touch, or just your presence.

The Dying Person's Bill of Rights

As we face death, what are our rights as human beings? This bill of rights was created at a workshop on "The Terminally Ill Patient and the Helping Person," sponsored by the Southwestern Michigan Insurance Education Council and conducted by Amelia J. Barbus.

- I have the right to be treated as a living human being until I die.
- I have the right to maintain a sense of hopefulness, however changing its focus may be.
- I have the right to be cared for by those who can maintain a sense of hopefulness, however changing this might be.
- I have the right to express my feelings and emotions about my approaching death in my own way.
- I have the right to participate in decisions concerning my care.
- I have the right to expect continuing medical and nursing attention even though "cure" goals must be changed to "comfort" goals.
- I have the right not to die alone.
- I have the right to be free from pain.
- I have the right to have my questions answered honestly.
- I have the right not to be deceived.
- I have the right to have help from and for my family in accepting my death.
- I have the right to die in peace and dignity.
- I have the right to retain my individuality and not be judged for my decisions which may be contrary to beliefs of others.
- I have the right to discuss and enlarge my religious and/or spiritual experiences, whatever these may mean to others.
- I have the right to expect that the sanctity of the human body will be respected after death.
- I have the right to be cared for by caring, sensitive, knowledgeable people who will attempt to understand my needs and will be able to gain some satisfaction in helping me face my death.

Figure 18-4. ■ The Dying Person's Bill of Rights.

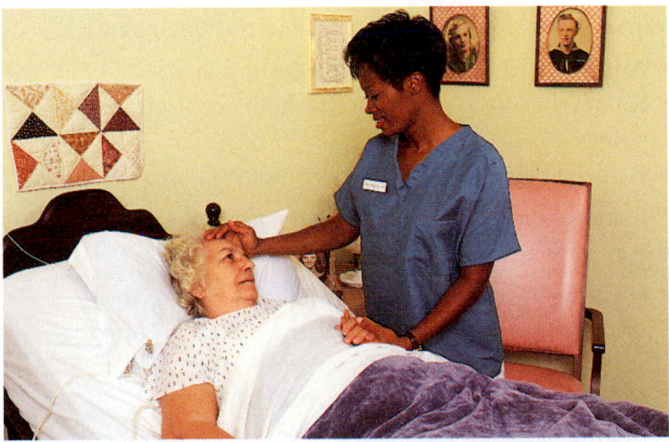

Figure 18-5. ■ The touch of your hand may be the dying person's last memory.

- Maintain the client's sense of security, self-confidence, dignity, and self-worth. *Allowing the client to make treatment decisions and to maintain self-care duties is a way of reinforcing self-worth.*
- Maintain hope. *Empower clients to make decisions about their care. When recovery is not possible, people can still make peace with their death.*

- Help the client accept losses. *Allowing grief to be expressed encourages healthy grieving.*
- Provide physical comfort or healing touch. (See Chapter 8 ⊂⊃ for other complementary and alternative therapies.) Box 18-4 ■ describes some forms of complementary therapy the nurse or family could employ (Linde et al., 2001). *Healing touch, a back rub, and a warm bath are physical ways to express your concern for the client's well-being.*
- Eliminate suffering. Suffering is different from physical pain. *Provide psychological support and open communication to the client.*
- Provide spiritual support. As desired, arrange access to individuals who can provide spiritual or cultural care. *Not all clients have a specific religious faith or belief. However, most people need a sense of meaning in their lives, especially when they know they have a terminal illness. The nurse's responsibilities include seeing that the client's spiritual needs are met.*

Meeting Physiological Needs of the Dying Client

Dying clients experience homeostatic imbalances and a slowing of body processes. Nursing interventions address the need to provide comfort and dignity to the dying

BOX 18-4	COMPLEMENTARY THERAPIES

Providing Comfort to Dying Clients

The Center for Complementary and Alternative Medicine groups complementary and alternative medicine (CAM) into four domains: mind-body medicine, biologically based practices, manipulative and body-based practices, and energy medicine. The two domains commonly used in hospice care are mind-body medicine and energy medicine.

Mind-body medicine is based on the belief that the mind can affect the body. Imagery and visualization are some examples:

- **Imagery** is a technique designed to replace unpleasant thoughts and feelings with positive ones that encourage a change in attitudes, behaviors, or physiologic reactions. The client imagines scenes or experiences that help the body heal and relax.
- **Visualization,** often used with imagery, refers to picturing something in the mind's eye and "seeing" healing, pain relief, relaxation, and so on.

Meditation, prayer, biofeedback, art, and music are also classified under mind-body medicine.

Energy medicine involves the belief that the body has energy fields that can be used for health and wellness. Energy medicine therapies include Reiki, therapeutic touch, and others:

- **Reiki** (RAY-key) is a form of healing touch therapy that directs energy through the hands of the provider to assist healing. Reiki is a gentle technique that uses 12 to 15 hand positions to direct energy through the hands of the provider to replenish and rebalance energy.
- **Therapeutic touch** is energy directed through the hands of the practitioner (usually held slightly away from the client's body) to activate the healing response of the recipient.
- Qigong and bioelectromagnetic therapies (see Chapter 8 ⚭) are other energy medicine therapies.

person. Physical care of the terminally ill client is discussed in detail in Chapter 44 ⚭ . Safeguarding respiratory status, helping to control pain, assisting with ADLs and position changes, supporting client's needs for nutrition and elimination, and monitoring for sensory overload or deficit are basic nursing interventions.

Encouraging Coping

The nurse can assist the person to work through grief. Possible interventions would include the following:

- Provide opportunities for the client to participate in decision making about daily activities. *Involvement in decision making is empowering and helps the client begin to organize the experience.*
- Encourage the client to share loss with significant others. *This will assist with acceptance of loss.*

- Encourage the client to get increasingly involved in usual activities. *This will help the client establish a routine and help with closure.*
- Encourage the client to get enough sleep and adequate nutrition. *This will help keep the client from getting ill.*
- Encourage the client to seek out support services and resources available to assist during difficult episodes. *This will help promote healthy grieving. An objective listener can sometimes help a person get past an emotional barrier.*
- Encourage the client to verbalize positive expectations for the future. *This will help promote a positive focus.*
- Practice active and attentive listening, open and closed questioning, paraphrasing, clarifying and reflecting feelings, and summarizing. *These communication techniques allow clients to explore their own feelings. It is less helpful to clients for the nurse to respond by giving advice and evaluating, by interpreting and analyzing, or by giving empty reassurance. (See also Chapter 11 ⚭ .)*

Communication with grieving clients needs to be appropriate to their stage of grief. For example, denial or depression can affect how a client hears a message or how the nurse interprets the client's comments. Box 18-5 ■ describes specific interventions nurses can perform as they relate to Kübler-Ross's five stages of grieving.

Supporting the Family

When clients lose a loved one, priority outcomes are:

- Adjusting to the actual or impending loss.
- Remembering that person without feeling intense pain.
- Redirecting emotional energy into one's own life.

The nurse can help the client find specific ways of reaching these outcomes.

- Learn to listen. No intervention can reverse the inevitable dying process, but the nurse can provide a caring presence. *Many times, the best intervention nurses can offer is their caring attention.* Refer to Chapter 11 ⚭ for a full discussion on therapeutic communication.
- Present a calm and patient demeanor and allow client and family to express their grief. When grieving family members have not absorbed some information, the nurse can reinforce what is happening or what the family can expect. Some clients or families may need to have information repeated several times.
- Encourage family members to participate in the physical care of the dying person if they want to and are able. The nurse can suggest they assist with bathing, speak or read to the client, or hold hands. *Assisting the*

BOX 18-5	NURSING CARE CHECKLIST

Assisting Clients in Different Stages of Grief

Denial Stage
- ☑ Verbally support client but do not reinforce denial.
- ☑ Examine your own behavior to ensure that you do not share in client's denial.

Anger Stage
- ☑ Help client understand that anger is a normal response to feelings of loss and powerlessness.
- ☑ Avoid withdrawal or retaliation; do not take anger personally.
- ☑ Deal with client's needs that underlie any angry reaction.
- ☑ Provide structure and continuity to promote feelings of security.
- ☑ Allow clients as much control as possible over their lives.

Bargaining Stage
- ☑ Listen attentively, and encourage client to talk to relieve guilt and irrational fear.
- ☑ If appropriate, offer spiritual support.

Depression Stage
- ☑ Allow client to express sadness.
- ☑ Communicate nonverbally by sitting quietly without expecting conversation.
- ☑ Convey caring by touch.

Acceptance Stage
- ☑ Help family and friends understand client's decreased need to socialize.
- ☑ Encourage client to participate as much as possible in the treatment program.

dying person may relieve anxiety and reduce the feeling of helplessness.

- Recognize that every family member's desire and ability to help may be different. Some may feel unable to be with the dying person. They also require support from the nurse and from other family members. They should be shown to a quiet waiting area if they just wish to stay nearby.
- Tell children exactly what to expect if they are going to visit the dying person. *It may be unsettling for a child to see an unresponsive person or a loved one attached to medical equipment. Having information ahead of time will make the situation less frightening.*
- Encourage support among family members. *Close contact among several generations may help the survivors cope with the loss.*

Teaching the Family about the Grieving Process

It is often helpful for clients to know more about the process of grieving. For example, nurses can inform clients of the grief stages they can expect to experience over time. They can prepare survivors for feelings of guilt that may arise as they recover from the initial impact of a loss. They can emphasize that holidays and other significant dates may be especially stressful for them. For some people, events and/or anniversaries will trigger painful feelings of loss long after the loss occurred (see Figure 18-2). These feelings can be alarming to someone who thought they had "gotten over it."

Whenever possible, nurses provide clients with resources to use in the future. They can teach clients that many people go back and forth through the stages of grief at different times. Preparing clients for these times and providing information about support groups and counseling are important aspects of teaching.

Children also should be included in nursing care and client teaching about grief. The Hospice Foundation of America (2008) identified myths about children and grief that require education and change (see Table 18-1).

Providing Care after Death

After death, avoid the temptation to rush the body to the morgue before the family arrives. Many families expect to be in control during the time of death and want to have time alone with their loved one. Allow the family the opportunity for remembrance and closure.

The main goal of care immediately following the death is personal care, such as bathing the deceased person, and advocating for the personal wishes of the deceased. Nurses may need to provide postmortem care to the dying. For this discussion and procedure, see Chapter 44 🔗 .

Documenting Care

Documentation should include the care and treatment provided; progress or lack of progress to care and treatment; skilled observations; vital signs; physical; emotional, and spiritual support provided; significant family and client interactions; and physician communications.

EVALUATING

The nurse evaluates care of the dying client by observing the client's relationship with significant others and by listening to the client directly. The client's feelings and thoughts are the focus. Is the client as physically comfortable as possible? Is pain sufficiently relieved? Does the client find the treatment plan acceptable? Is the client satisfied with visitation of family and support people?

NURSING PROCESS CARE PLAN
Client in Denial

Mrs. Smith is a 52-year-old smoker with a diagnosis of chronic obstructive pulmonary disease (COPD). She has been smoking a pack of cigarettes a day for 32 years. She was admitted to the hospital for shortness of breath. Her condition has worsened during the last 5 years. She has increased periods of shortness of breath and less quality of life. She needs continuous oxygen therapy. Her primary physician has begun speaking to her and her family about hospice care. Mrs. Smith explains to her physician that she does not want to go somewhere to die. She believes she will get better and she continues to go outside the hospital and smoke.

Assessment

She has several crisis episodes in which skin color is dusky and her nail beds are blue despite being on continuous oxygen therapy. Her physician speaks to her again about palliative care and hospice. This time Mrs. Smith agrees to hospice but she is very angry at her physician for "giving up." The physician writes the order for the social worker and discharge planning nurse to make the hospice referral.

Nursing Diagnosis

The following important nursing diagnoses (among others) are established for this client:

- *Powerlessness* related to terminal illness
- *Grieving* related to terminal illness

Expected Outcomes

The expected outcomes specify that Mrs. Smith will:

- Participate in self-care activities as much as she is able.
- Make choices related to care and treatment.
- Maintain physiological comfort.
- Share values and personal meaning of life.
- Gain acceptance of the terminal state of her illness.

Planning and Implementation

The following nursing interventions are planned and implemented:

- Teach client and family about hospice and its philosophy.
- Reinforce to the client and family that hospice care is not about "giving up."
- Reinforce to the client and family that hospice is no longer about treating the "disease" but managing the "symptoms" of the disease. *This information*

will help the client and family adapt to the reality of the situation.

- Allow the client to verbalize feelings. *The client must express feelings in order to move forward.*
- Identify support systems available to client and family. *Support will be needed to confront the upcoming loss.*
- Allow the client to participate in decision making about daily activities. *Self-determination is important throughout one's life.*
- Encourage client in self-care activities. *Doing self-care enhances a sense of well-being.*
- Teach the client and family about appropriate grieving responses. *Information about the process can reduce the stress the person feels and reinforce that it is okay to experience these emotions.*

Evaluation

After 3 months in home hospice, Mrs. Smith's symptoms are under control with medications and oxygen. Her appetite has significantly decreased and she sleeps most of the time. After the fourth month in home hospice, Mrs. Smith dies peacefully at home.

Critical Thinking in the Nursing Process

1. Why is it important to allow Mrs. Smith to participate in self-care activities and decision making?
2. Why has Mrs. Smith's appetite decreased?
3. To control Mrs. Smith's pain, a combination fast-acting and long-acting narcotic is used. Why is this combination of medications ordered for terminally ill clients?

Note: Discussion of Critical Thinking questions appears on the MyNursingKit Website.

Nurse's Self-Care in Relation to Death

Distancing is an unconscious response of professionals in which they hold back emotionally from clients, especially dying clients. Distancing is especially prevalent when the client is not aware of the truth. This behavior can enhance loneliness and fear in the client.

Although being a nurse of any kind has moments that are difficult, it takes a special person to care for the sick and dying. Care of the sick and dying requires discipline, dedication, and compassion. It can easily become a balancing act between being empathetic to the client and family and creating a healthy balance mentally, physically, emotionally, and spiritually. Proactively caring for oneself first will allow a healthy balance.

When working with clients who are chronically and terminally ill, it is natural for a nurse to form a bond with them. A nurse's personal views about death and dying and his or her personal coping techniques can affect how the nurse handles the death of a client. Nonetheless, it can still be hard to lose someone with whom you have become close. Some things you can do to promote your own healthy grieving are to recognize your grief and to cry if necessary. Some nurses attend memorial services or funeral services to provide the closure they need. Some units may hold their own special services or rituals to remember those who have died.

Note: The references and resources for all chapters have been compiled at the back of the book.

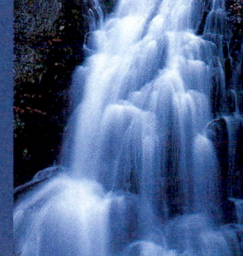

Chapter Review

KEY Points

- Nurses help clients deal with all kind of losses, such as loss of body image, loss of limbs, loss of function, and death.

- Grieving is a normal, subjective emotional response to loss. It is essential for mental and physical health.

- How an individual deals with loss is related to many factors, such as the individual's stage of development, personal resources, social support, and others.

- Nurses must recognize myths that exist surrounding children and death. It is important to ask questions and not to assume you know what the child is thinking.

- Thanatology is the academic study of death and dying.

- Knowledge of different stages of grieving can help the nurse understand the responses and needs of the client.

- The work of Kübler-Ross, Worden, Wolfelt, and other theorists provides help to nurses in working with dying clients and their families.

- Nurses must know their responsibilities with regard to legal and policy issues surrounding death.

- Dying is a normal process. Dying clients and their families require open communication, as well as physical, emotional, and spiritual support to achieve a peaceful and dignified death.

- Caring for the dying and bereaved is one of the nurse's most challenging responsibilities, but it can also be rewarding to give comfort and support at this difficult time.

- Nurses must make time to take care of themselves as they work with loss, grief, and death issues. Burnout can result if nurses ignore their own emotions or physical needs.

∞ FOR FURTHER Study

See Figure 4-2 for a durable power of attorney for health care.

See Chapter 8 for other complementary and alternative therapies.

Refer to Chapter 11 for a full discussion on therapeutic communication.

Losses experienced by older adults are discussed in Chapter 16.

Refer to Chapter 44 for care of the chronically or terminally ill clients, including Table 44-1 Cultural Traditions in Mourning and After-Death Rites.

PEARSON

EXPLORE mynursingkit™

MyNursingKit is your one stop for online chapter review materials and resources. Prepare for success with additional NCLEX®-style practice questions, interactive assignments and activities, web links, animations and videos, and more!

Register your access code from the front of your book at
www.mynursingkit.com

Critical Thinking Care Map

Caring for a Client Who Is Grieving

NCLEX-PN® Focus Area: Psychosocial Integrity

Case Study: Mr. Morris is at the end stages of advanced stage IV lung cancer. He has been admitted to an inpatient hospice setting because the family is having difficulty taking care of him at home.

Nursing Diagnosis: *Grieving*

COLLECT DATA

Subjective	Objective
_____	_____
_____	_____
_____	_____
_____	_____
_____	_____
_____	_____

Would you report this? Yes/No

If yes, report to: _____

What would you report? _____

Nursing Care

_____
_____
_____
_____
_____
_____
_____
_____
_____
_____

How would you document this? _____
_____
_____
_____

Compare your answers and documentation to those provided on the MyNursingKit Website.

Data Collected
(use only those that apply)

- Reports poor appetite
- Easily fatigued
- Skin color pink
- Skin color dusky
- Increased appetite
- Drowsy
- BP 90/40
- States pain is 9 on scale of 1 to 10

Nursing Interventions
(use only those that apply; list in priority order)

- Auscultate breath sounds with RN.
- Position client for comfort.
- Encourage client to take a shower.
- Encourage client to eat.
- Set up for a bed bath.
- Moisten client's lips as needed.
- Administer oxygen as needed.
- Use therapeutic touch and encourage family communication.
- Administer pain medications as ordered around the clock.
- Observe family responses to grieving and offer appropriate support.

NCLEX-PN® Exam Preparation

TEST-TAKING TIP   Try to get up early in the morning to study. It is better to study when you are refreshed from a night's sleep. If you are caring for children or working full time while attending school, you may feel too exhausted at the end of the day to remain awake and retain any information.

1   A client in end-stage renal failure and her family are aware of the signs of approaching death, but they do not talk about it. They are manifesting which state of awareness?

1. Closed awareness
2. Mutual pretense
3. Open awareness
4. Undisclosed pretense

2   A client diagnosed with inoperable lung cancer states, "Please get my discharge papers ready. We had vacation plans before I got this cold, and I feel well enough to go." The client is experiencing which stage of the grief process?

1. Denial
2. Anger
3. Bargaining
4. Acceptance

3   An unmarried adult is admitted following a motor vehicle crash. He is unresponsive and has been placed on life support. His mother and domestic partner arrive. His mother states, "I can't bear to take him off life support. I know he would want everything to be done." The domestic partner produces a notarized Durable Power of Attorney for Health Care that states no life support is to be used and that gives control to the partner. The physician must consider:

1. The mother's wishes.
2. The domestic partner's wishes.
3. The instructions outlined in the document.
4. The ER physician's assessment.

4   Following the death of a client, the nursing assistant leaves the room quickly and is found sobbing in the utility room. Which action would be the most supportive?

1. Sending the nursing assistant home for the rest of the shift
2. Reassigning the nursing assistant to an area where it is unlikely that a client may die
3. Sitting with her and allowing her to express how she feels
4. Insisting that she perform postmortem care for the client

5   The parents of a stillborn infant wish to see the body. The nurse should:

1. Show them the baby through the glass nursery window.
2. Allow the parents to hold the baby and give them a picture with a lock of hair.
3. Discourage them from seeing the infant because they will be distressed by its appearance.
4. Show them the baby but the nurse should hold it.

6   A widower reports headache, loss of appetite, and inability to sleep following his wife's death. He related that his symptoms increased on his wife's birthday. He states he would just like to die and be with her. The most appropriate nursing diagnosis is:

1. *Anticipatory Grief.*
2. *Compromised Family Coping.*

3. *Complicated Grieving.*
4. *Compromised Individual Coping.*

7   An 11-year-old child's grandfather has just died. Of the following statements, which is most developmentally appropriate?

1. "Grampa will get better and come home soon."
2. "I got mad because my grandfather would not buy me a video game. That is why he got sick."
3. "What happens after someone dies? Will Grampa's body go to heaven or just his heart?"
4. "When people die they go to live with God. I'm sad but Grampa isn't sick anymore, so that is good."

8   The nurse is caring for a client diagnosed with terminal breast cancer. The client's husband sits with the woman when she dies and says, "I just can't tell the children their mother has died. I think it would be better if I told them she'll be in the hospital for a while to help them adjust to being without her." The nurse's best response would be:

1. "Telling the children will be difficult, but you can teach them ways of adapting to loss by including them in the grieving process."
2. "Take some time to deal with your own emotions before informing the children."
3. "You must tell the children because they will know there is something wrong, and if you don't tell them they'll never trust you again."
4. "I'm sure you know what is best for your children."

9   The nurse is caring for an elderly client who lost her husband several years ago. The client says, "I've met a wonderful man and he wants to marry me. I know my husband would want me to be happy so I think I'm going to get remarried." The nurse recognizes this client is achieving which of Worden's basic tasks?

1. Task one: Acceptance
2. Task two: Grief work
3. Task three: Adjustment
4. Task four: Emotional relocation

10   The nurse is talking with a bereaved family about the mourner's bill of rights. Which of the following statements made by the nurse would be inaccurate?

1. "Everyone grieves differently and no one should tell you how to feel."
2. "Talking about your grief will help you heal so seek out those who will allow you to talk as much as you need to about your loss."
3. "Confusion, disorientation, fear, or guilt are signs of dysfunctional grieving."
4. "It is normal to have powerful surges of grief that overcome you."

Answers and rationales for Review Questions appear in Appendix I.

Thinking Strategically About...

You have been assigned your first case as an LPN/LVN working for a community hospice agency. The client is a 68-year-old Hispanic woman whose breast cancer has metastasized to her spine. The RN completed the intake interview with the family yesterday at the hospital. The client has been discharged to her home. You have reviewed her discharge plan and see that no additional treatment has been recommended because of her rapidly advancing disease.

When you arrive at home, the client's daughter meets you in the driveway and asks you to remove your name badge, which indicates you are from the hospice organization. She states, "Mother doesn't know how sick she is. We want her last days to be happy. We don't want her to think about dying." The daughter asks you to say that the doctor sent you to help with her bath and to see if all the equipment arrived.

You observe that the family relationship is very close and loving, but that there seems to be an underlying strain. You adhere to the daughter's request during that visit, but when you return to the agency you ask to have a conference with the RN and the social worker.

While bathing Mrs. Esparza you observe that she is having pain when moving side to side and lifting her legs. She has a reddened area on her back and around her surgical incision.

CRITICAL THINKING

Are you violating your nursing ethics and your ability to be a client advocate by complying with the family's request that you remove your name tag and hide the fact that you are from hospice?

PRIORITIZING NURSING CARE

- What are your priorities in nursing care for your first visit with Mrs. Esparza?
- Would your priorities be different in subsequent visits? If so, what would they be?

DELEGATING

You will continue to see Mrs. Esparza 3 times per week. A caregiver will be assigned to her 10 hours a day while her family is at work. A caregiver will also be available during the night or for respite 1 to 2 times per month if needed. What care should you delegate to the caregiver and what follow-up will be needed?

CULTURAL CARE STRATEGIES

- Do you think that the request to keep the terminal diagnosis from the client has any relationship to the client's culture?
- How can a nurse who adheres to values of honesty and individualism maintain integrity while honoring this client's culture?

PROBLEM SOLVING

- What legal and ethical issues occur when a client's "right-to-know" is not addressed?
- What are the implications of this for healthcare institutions and workers?

COMPASSIONATE CARING

- How can you help the client to obtain a sense of closure if the family refuses to talk about the impending death?
- What tools are available that do not violate the family's specific request?

COMMUNITY CARE STRATEGIES

Arrange a visit to a family support group for people in hospice. Observe how the facilitator works with families to draw them out. List communication strategies used in these settings to allow people to face the death of a loved one and to cope with their grief.

CLIENT TEACHING

What client and/or family teaching should be carried out? Are there other professionals who could be involved to assist the family through the transitions of the process of dying?

DOCUMENTING AND REPORTING

- What routine documentation should be done during each of your visits?
- What kind of documentation should you instruct the caregiver to do on a daily basis?
- What information needs to be reported immediately to the RN or the physician, and what can wait until the nurse's weekly visit?

Promoting Physiological Health

UNIT IV

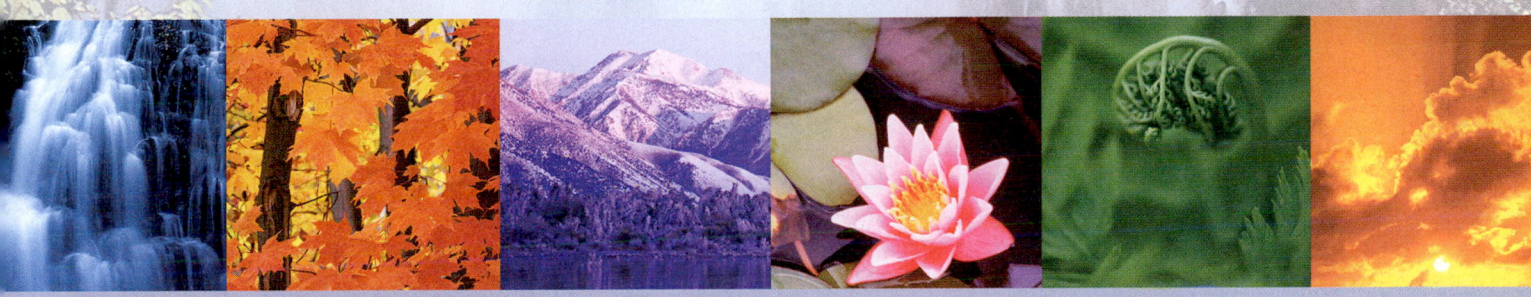

Chapter 19

Health Assessment/ Head-to-Toe Data Collection

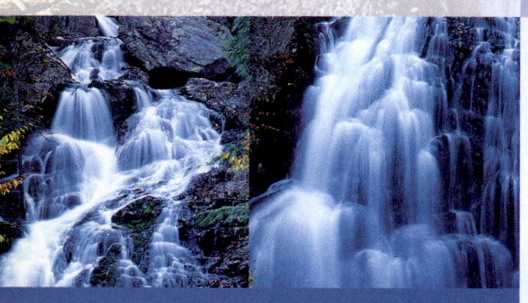

BRIEF Outline

Physical Health Assessment
Preparation for Assessment
Methods of Examination
Terminology for Documenting Data

LEARNING Outcomes

After completing this chapter, you will be able to:

1. Name three types of physical health assessment and discuss the role of the LPN/LVN in health assessment.
2. Identify elements to check by body system.
3. Discuss preparation of client and environment for examination.
4. Identify potential variables in data by age or condition.
5. Name four methods of examination and state which are commonly used by LPNs/LVNs.
6. List common terms for identifying body parts and locations during examination.
7. Describe nursing care of the client undergoing an assessment.
8. Identify terms used in physical health assessment of the lungs.
9. Describe suggested sequencing to conduct a physical health assessment in an orderly fashion.

Clinical Objectives

10. Perform head-to-toe data collection on several clients.
11. Demonstrate auscultation of the lungs, heart, and abdomen.
12. Measure height and weight and document findings.
13. Determine the level of consciousness and orientation of a variety of clients.
14. Evaluate and document pupil reaction.

KEY TERMS

Use the audio glossary feature on the MyNursingKit Website to hear the correct pronunciation of the following key terms.

Assessing a client's health status is a major component of nursing care. There are two aspects of assessment: the nursing health history and the physical examination. The physical examination or assessment is the focus of this chapter.

Physical Health Assessment

A **physical assessment** can be any of three types:

1. A complete assessment, normally an admission assessment
2. A focused assessment by body system (Figure 19-1 ■), normally a daily assessment
3. A focused assessment of a body part, normally done during the shift

Box 19-1 ■ provides some guidelines for assessment by body systems.

COMPLETE ASSESSMENT

An RN conducts a complete assessment when the client is admitted to the healthcare facility. The LPN/LVN may be asked to collect data for this. The complete assessment includes a full head-to-toe assessment as well as a complete health history, information that pertains to the client's level of functioning. Information collected may include allergies; client's level of ambulation; personal property brought to the facility by the client, and people with whom any valuables are sent home; chronic health conditions and any medications taken for these conditions; past medical history; fall risk assessment; dietary habits; and impairments and disabilities (see Figure 14-1 ⬭). This complete assessment

should remain in the client's chart so that all staff involved in the client's care may refer to it. This assessment also provides baseline information about the client to all staff members. The RN may delegate to LPNs/LVNs a variety of data-collecting tasks that become part of the full assessment. It is important to know and follow the scope of practice defined by the state board of nursing and facility policy.

FOCUSED ASSESSMENT

A focused assessment or shift assessment may be conducted by the LPN/LVN at the beginning and end of the shift. It may be conducted in several ways. One efficient method is to start at the head and proceed in a systematic manner downward to the toes. The procedure can vary according to the age of the individual, the severity of the illness, the method preferences of the nurse, the location of the examination, and the agency's priorities and required procedures. Regardless of what type of procedure is used, the client's energy and time need to be considered. The physical health assessment is always conducted in a systematic and efficient manner that requires the fewest position changes for the client.

The sequence of the assessment differs with children and adults. Box 19-2 ■ discusses age-related differences and considerations.

A focused assessment of a body part may occur when the nurse assesses a specific system's body part or area instead of the entire body. These specific (or focused) assessments are made in relation to client complaints, the nurse's own observation of problems, the client's presenting problem, the nursing interventions provided, and medical therapies.

(Text continues on p. 368.)

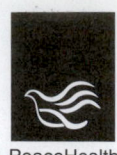

PeaceHealth

ST. JOHN MEDICAL CENTER
LONGVIEW, WASHINGTON

MED / SURG / TELE / ONC - DAILY CARE RECORD

Symbol Key
Empty box = Not assessed
✓ = Assessment matches normal parameters
X = Variation, describe in Comments
→ = Variations same as last assessment
* = See progress notes
Initial each assessment block on line
Use right box for reassessment or daily care (dc) assessment

Date:	NOC - Time: /	DAY - Time: /	EVE - Time: /
SYSTEMS ASSESSMENTS	Comments Reassess ☐ D/C ☐	Comments Reassess ☐ D/C ☐	Comments Reassess ☐ D/C ☐
Pain If other than 0-10 scale used, check appropriate box: ☐ APP ☐ Faces	Intensity _____ If > 0, see Focused Assessment section	Intensity _____ If > 0, see Focused Assessment section	Intensity _____ If > 0, see Focused Assessment section
Neurological LEVEL OF CONSCIOUSNESS: alert SPEECH: coherent, clearly understandable speech, symmetry of facial expression SWALLOWING: handles oral secretions ORIENTATION: aware of time, place, person; short-term memory intact BEHAVIOR: interactions appropriate to situation	☐ ____ ____ ☐	☐ ____ ____ ☐	☐ ____ ____ ☐
Cardiovascular VITAL SIGNS: HR reg, BP & temp WNL for pt. RADIAL PULSE: easily palpated and regular SKIN: warm, dry, natural color for patient CIRCULATION: no peripheral edema or calf pain	☐ ____ ____ ☐	☐ ____ ____ ☐	☐ ____ ____ ☐
Respiratory RATE: regular pattern, rate WNL for patient EFFORT: unlabored at rest on room air BREATH SOUNDS: no audible wheeze, stridor, rattles or other adventitious sounds COUGH: none reported or observed SPUTUM: absent or reported clear	☐ ____ ____ ☐	☐ ____ ____ ☐	☐ ____ ____ ☐
Gastrointestinal PALPATION: soft, non-tender AUSCULTATION: normally active bowel sounds INTAKE: tolerating at least half of prescribed diet without nausea/vomiting BM: continent of soft, formed stool within past 48°	☐ ____ ____ ☐	☐ ____ ____ ☐	☐ ____ ____ ☐
Genitourinary URINATION: observed/reported continent voiding of clear urine in sufficient quantity; no dysuria BLADDER DISTENTION: none visible GENITALIA: no observed/reported genital discharge or swelling	☐ ____ ____ ☐	☐ ____ ____ ☐	☐ ____ ____ ☐
Musculoskeletal EXTREMITIES: functional, non-painful ROM x4 MOVEMENT: independent gait, transfers and ambulates without use of assistive devices	☐ ____ ____ ☐	☐ ____ ____ ☐	☐ ____ ____ ☐
Integumentary/Wounds PRESSURE: no blanching or redness at boney prominences. No skin breakdown. HYDRATION: normal skin turgor; moist mucosa WOUND: well-approximated edges, no redness, swelling, drainage OR dressing clean, dry, intact	☐ ____ ____ ☐	☐ ____ ____ ☐	☐ ____ ____ ☐
Psych/Soc SUPPORT: fam/soc support sys evident/ reported AFFECT: calm, cooperative, normal eye contact (within cultural context) SLEEP PATTERNS: able to sleep at night if undisturbed; absence of unusual fatigue	☐ ____ ____ ☐	☐ ____ ____ ☐	☐ ____ ____ ☐
IV Site Assessment No redness Dressing CD&I No swelling Site < 72 hr old No pain	☐ Site #1 _____ ☐ Site #2 _____ ☐ Site #3 _____	☐ Site #1 _____ ☐ Site #2 _____ ☐ Site #3 _____	☐ Site #1 _____ ☐ Site #2 _____ ☐ Site #3 _____
If Site > 72 hr old, reason not DC'd			
Site care	☐ Site #1 _____	☐ Site #2 _____	☐ Site #3 _____

Figure 19-1. ■ Focused assessment by body system. (Courtesy of PeaceHealth St. John Medical Center, Longview, WA. Used with permission.)

BOX 19-1   NURSING CARE CHECKLIST

Assessment by Body Systems

(Terms here are defined in the pertinent body system chapter.)

Neurologic (see Chapter 36 ⚭)

☑ LOC (level of consciousness):
- Alert, lethargic, sedated, unconscious

☑ Orientation:
- O × 3 (oriented to name, time, and place)

☑ Verbal response:
- Clear
- Incoherent, rambling, slurred, stuttering
- Dysphasia, aphasia

☑ Motor response (less on one side, equal bilaterally, greater on one side):
- Grips (note strength)
- Obeys commands, localizes pain, withdrawal, flexion, extension, none
- Pain—sharp, burning, intense, sudden, agonizing, throbbing, stabbing
- Pain level 0–10 (0 = no pain); for children or other clients unable to verbally respond, the facial pain scale 1–5 is used

☑ Assess pupils:
- Note shape
- Pupils are equally round and reactive to light, and accommodation (PERRLA)
  - 1 mm after surgery
  - 2–3 mm normal
  - 6–9 mm "blown"; if permanent, possible herniation
  - Pupils should be equal

Integumentary (see Chapter 30 ⚭)

☑ General appearance:
- Pale, flushed, cyanotic, discolored, freckled
- Moist, diaphoretic, clammy
- Hot, warm, cold
- Dry, scaly, oily
- Rash, abrasion, laceration, incisions, broken, sores, lesions, scars, calloused, contusions
- Tanned, glossy, tattoos
- Swollen, coarse or fine texture

☑ Skin turgor:
- Normal
- Loose
- Tight
- Tenting

☑ Integrity:
- Intact
- Impaired

☑ Mucous membranes:
- Color
- Condition

Cardiovascular—normal pulse 60–100 (see Chapter 33 ⚭)

☑ Apical, B/P, radial (present; less than/greater than (on one side); = bilaterally):
- Rate/rhythm
  - Regular
  - Irregular
  - Strong
  - Rapid
  - Weak
  - Absent
  - Thready
- Intensity (force of blood flow felt at pulse site)
  - 1, 2 (hypo)
  - 4 (hyper or bounding)
- Doppler

☑ Skin—pale, flushed, cyanotic, discolored, moist, cold, clammy

☑ Edema—present or absent, pitting or nonpitting

☑ Capillary refilling time less than 3 seconds

☑ Positive or negative Homans' sign (this is controversial) *or* ask if there is any calf pain and assess for redness or swelling before proceeding to dorsiflex the foot (Avoid Homans' sign after orthopedic surgery because of the complication of deep vein thrombosis [DVT].)

Respiratory—10–20 normal respirations/minute (see Chapter 32 ⚭)

☑ Breathing:
- Tachypnea (greater than 24/minute)
- Bradypnea (less than 10/minute)
- Dyspnea
- Apnea
- Deep/shallow

☑ S.O.B. (shortness of breath):
- With which activities?

☑ Chest:
- Excursion symmetrical/asymmetrical (Respiratory sounds seem to move from usual course or location in chest to another area.)

☑ Lung sounds (audible all lobes):
- **Crackles/rales** (Sound created by air passing over airway secretions; crackles and rales are synonymous.)
- **Rhonchi** (A continuous musical sound heard with a stethoscope; it occurs in asthma, croup, hay fever, and can also result from tumor or obstruction.)
- Wheezes

☑ Sputum:
- Clear
- Thin/thick
- Tenacious
- Note color

☑ Measure O_2 saturation:
- Pulse oximeter

(continued)

BOX 19-1 · NURSING CARE CHECKLIST (continued)

Gastrointestinal (see Chapter 37 ⚭)

☑ Abdomen:
- Soft, firm, rigid, tender, sensitive to touch
- Enlarged, distended, flat, round
- Note any rebound tenderness

☑ Bowel sounds (listen all four quadrants—2 to 5 minutes):
- Normoactive, faint, hypoactive, absent, hyperactive

☑ BM size (sm, med, lg)

☑ N/V (nausea/vomiting)—amount/color/frequency:
- Milliliters; small, large
- Blood tinged, fecal
- Projectile

☑ Diarrhea (amt/color/freq)

☑ Appetite (tolerance to prescribed diet):
- Percentage

Genitourinary—30 mL/h normal output in adults (see Chapter 39 ⚭)

☑ Urination—independent, catheter, incontinent:
- Amount
- Color—yellow, amber, bloody, brown, dark red
- Appearance—clear, cloudy, sediment
- Odor—offensive, foul, musty, aromatic, ammonia-like, odorless

☑ I/O (intake/output)—all fluids should be balanced with output

☑ Bladder distention:
- Check, feel, palpate

Musculoskeletal (see Chapter 31 ⚭)

☑ ROM (range of motion)

☑ Gait

☑ Deformities

Psychosocial

☑ Mental and spiritual:
- Mood, affect, judgment, abilities, lifestyle, patterns, age

BOX 19-2 · LIFESPAN CONSIDERATIONS

Assessment Differences by Age or Condition

Infants and Children

Skin
- Jaundice (yellowish skin) possible in newborns for several weeks after birth.
- May have increased pigmentation in sacral area of infants and young children of dark-skinned races.
- Possible milia (whiteheads) over the nose and face, and vernix caseosa (white, greasy, protective material) on skin of newborns.

Head
- Shape altered by delivery for about 1 week in most newborns.
- Posterior *fontanel* (soft spot) generally closes by 8 weeks and anterior fontanel by 18 months.
- Voluntary head control by 6 months of age.

Eyes, Ears, Nose, and Mouth
- Horizontal line from eye to top of the ear is normal. Auricle should angle no more than 10 degrees from vertical. (*Note:* Variation may indicate developmental abnormality or renal abnormalities.)
- Infants may blink at a sharp sound. (*Note:* To assess gross hearing, ring a bell from behind the infant or have the parent call the child's name to check for a response. At 3 to 4 months, the infant will turn head and eyes toward the sound.)
- Tooth development should be appropriate for age; permanent teeth are darker than deciduous teeth.
- Inspect the palate for a cleft.

Chest, Heart, and Lungs
- Infants and children up to age 6 tend to breathe more from abdomen than from chest.
- Chest circumference measurements at delivery and up to 9 months rule out birth injuries, congenital anomalies, or other dysfunction.
- Auscultated sounds are louder and harsher because of thinner chest wall.
- A third heart sound, best heard at the apex, is present in about one-third of all children.
- Palpation of pulses in the lower extremities (particularly the femoral pulses) can be used to screen for certain heart abnormalities.

Gastrointestinal
- Abdomen of the newborn and infant is round. Characteristic "pot belly" appearance of toddlers persists until about age 5.
- Peristaltic waves usually more visible than in adults.
- Children may not be able to pinpoint areas of tenderness. Observe facial expressions to determine areas of maximum tenderness.
- Liver is relatively larger than in adults, and can be palpated 1 to 2 cm below the right costal margin.

Musculoskeletal
- Lordosis (swayback) is common in young children.
- Pronation (in-turning) of the feet is common between 12 and 30 months of age.
- *Genu varum* (bowleg) is normal for 1 year after beginning to walk.

- Asymmetric gluteal folds, asymmetric abduction of the legs, or apparent shortening of the femur suggest developmental dysplasia of the hip (congenital dislocation).

Pregnant Women
- Breast, areola, and nipple size increase.
- Areolae and nipples darken. Nipples may become more erect. Areolae contain small, scattered, elevated Montgomery's glands.
- Superficial veins become more prominent. Stretch marks may develop.
- Colostrum (thick yellow fluid) may be expressed from the nipples after the first trimester.

Older Adults
Skin, Hair, and Nails
- Skin loses elasticity, appears thin, translucent, more wrinkled.
- Skin often dry and flaky, when testing for skin turgor, the skin takes longer to return to its natural shape after being tented between the thumb and finger.
- Increased number of discolorations and skin lesions.
- Scalp and facial hair grays.
- Toenails grow more slowly and thicken.
- Longitudinal bands commonly develop on fingernails in older adults, and the nails tend to split.

Eyes, Ears, Nose, and Mouth
- Ears may appear dry, with increased coarse hair growth.
- Tympanic membrane is more translucent and less flexible.
- Earwax is drier.
- Hearing loss (presbycusis) occurs.
- Eyes may have a ring around the pupil area known as *arcus senilis*.
- Oral mucosa may be drier because of decreased salivary gland activity or dehydration.
- Gums recede, giving an appearance of increased toothiness.
- Taste sensations diminish due to atrophy of the taste buds and a decreased sense of smell.
- Tooth loss may occur as a result of gum disease.

Chest, Heart, and Lungs
- Anteroposterior diameter of the chest deepens, giving the person a barrel-chested appearance due to loss of skeletal muscle strength in the thorax and diaphragm and constant lung inflation (from excessive expiratory pressure on the alveoli).
- Breathing rate and rhythm are unchanged at rest; heart rate after activity may take longer to return to the resting rate.
- Inspiratory muscles become less powerful, and depth of respiration decreases.
- Expiration may require the use of accessory muscles. The amount of air remaining in the lungs at the end of a normal breath increases.
- Cilia in the airways become fewer and are less effective in removing mucus.
- Heart size remains the same (if no disease is present).
- Cardiac output and strength of contractions decrease, so activity tolerance is less.
- Sudden emotional and physical stresses may result in cardiac arrhythmias and heart failure.
- Overall effectiveness of blood vessels decreases; lower extremities are more likely to show signs of impairment.
- Systolic and diastolic blood pressures may increase.
- Peripheral edema is frequently observed.

clinical ALERT

Clients with a blood pressure reading above 140/90 should be referred for follow-up assessments. (*Note:* The American Heart Association has lowered the numbers to as low as 120/80 as a risk factor for heart disease, particularly in those with other risk factors.)

Gastrointestinal
- Abdomen may appear round due to increase in adipose (fatty) tissue and decreased muscle tone. Abdominal wall is slacker and thinner, so palpation is easier and more accurate.
- Side effects of drugs are often manifested by nausea, vomiting, and diarrhea.
- Pain threshold is often higher; major abdominal problems such as appendicitis or other acute emergencies may therefore go undetected.
- Gastrointestinal pain needs to be differentiated from cardiac pain. (*Note:* Gastrointestinal pain may be located in the chest or abdomen, whereas cardiac pain is usually located in the chest. Factors aggravating gastrointestinal pain are usually related to either ingestion or lack of food intake; antacids, food, or an upright position usually relieve gastrointestinal pain. Common factors that can aggravate cardiac pain are activity or anxiety; rest or nitroglycerin relieves cardiac pain.)
- Emptying time of the stomach is slower because gastric acid secretion is decreased, resulting in indigestion and intolerance of certain foods. Decreases in the production of pancreatic enzymes also contribute to complaints of indigestion and anorexia.
- Stool passes through the intestines at a slower rate, and the perception of stimuli that produce the urge to defecate often diminishes.
- Fecal incontinence may occur in older adults who are confused or neurologically impaired.
- Decreased absorption of oral medications.
- In the liver, impaired metabolism of certain drugs may occur.

clinical ALERT

Absence of a daily bowel movement does not signify constipation. When assessing for constipation, the nurse must consider the client's diet, activity, and medications; the characteristics of feces and ease or difficulty in defecating; and the frequency of bowel movements.

Musculoskeletal
- Muscle mass decreases progressively with age, but there are wide variations among individuals.
- Decreases in speed, strength, resistance to fatigue, reaction time, and coordination occur.
- Bones become more fragile. Osteoporosis leads to a loss of total bone mass, predisposition to fractures, and compressed vertebrae.
- Osteoarthritic changes in joints may be observed.
- Curvature in the spine may occur from osteoporosis causing a somewhat diminished stature.

TABLE 19-1	Selected Client Situations and Focused Assessments
SITUATION	**PHYSICAL ASSESSMENT**
Client complains of abdominal pain.	Inspect, auscultate, and palpate the abdomen; assess vital signs and levels of pain. Avoid palpation if the abdominal pain is acute.
Client is admitted with a head injury.	Assess level of consciousness using Glasgow Coma Scale (see Table 19-2); assess pupils for reaction to light and accommodation; assess vital signs.
The nurse prepares to administer a cardiotonic drug to a client.	Assess apical pulse and compare with baseline data.
The nurse administers postural drainage.	Auscultate lungs before and after the procedure.
The client has just had a cast applied to the lower leg.	Assess peripheral perfusion of toes, capillary blanch test, dorsalis pedis pulse if able, and vital signs.
The client's fluid intake is minimal.	Assess tissue (skin) turgor, fluid intake and output, and vital signs.

Examples of client situations and focused assessments are presented in Table 19-1 ■.

Preparation for Assessment

PREPARING THE CLIENT

Most clients need an explanation of the physical health assessment. Explain when and where it will take place, why it is important, and what will happen during the assessment. Assist the client as needed to undress and put on an examination gown.

Clients should be instructed to empty their bladders before the examination. Doing so helps them feel more relaxed and facilitates palpation of the abdomen and pubic area. If a urinalysis is required, the urine should be collected at this time. Often, clients are anxious about what the nurse will find. They can be reassured during the assessment by explanations at each step.

> **clinical ALERT**
>
> Health assessments are usually painless. However, it is important to determine, in advance, any positions that are contraindicated for a particular client.

Positioning

Frequently, several positions are required during the physical assessment. It is important to consider the client's ability to assume a position. The client's physical condition, energy level, and age should also be taken into consideration. The assessment is organized so that several body areas can be assessed in one position. The LPN/LVN most frequently assesses the client in (1) the prone or supine position in bed (Figure 19-2 ■) or (2) sitting in bed or in a chair.

Draping

Drapes, usually the client's bed linens, should be arranged so that the area to be assessed is exposed while other body areas are covered. Exposure of the body is frequently embarrassing to clients. Drapes provide not only privacy but also warmth.

PREPARING THE ENVIRONMENT

It is important to prepare the environment before starting the assessment. The time for the physical assessment should be convenient for both the client and the nurse. The environment should be well lit and the equipment organized for use.

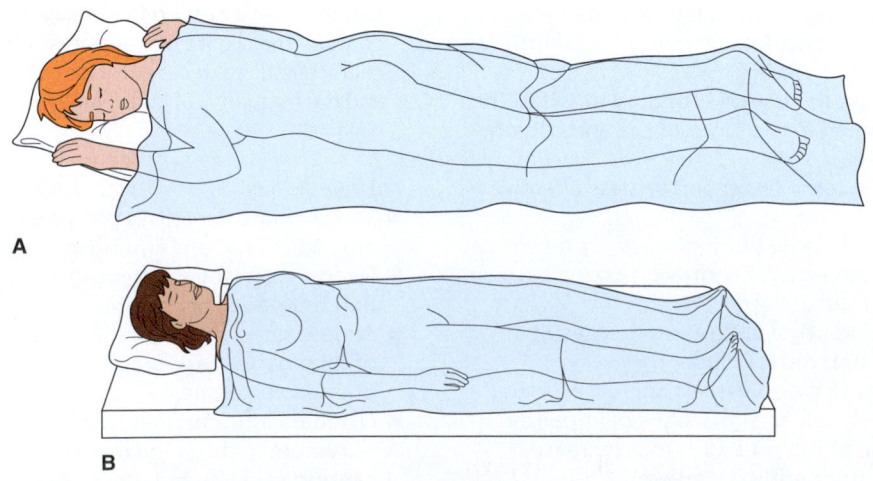

Figure 19-2. ■ Two most common client positions for assessment in bed: **A.** prone; **B.** supine.

Providing privacy is important. Curtains should be drawn. Most people are embarrassed if others can overhear or view them during the assessment. Family and friends should not be present during the examination unless the client specifically requests their presence.

The room temperature should be warm enough to be comfortable for the client. A well-prepared environment affects the client's response to the examination. The client who is physically relaxed usually experiences little discomfort.

Methods of Examination

Three primary techniques used by the LPN/LVN in the physical examination are inspection, auscultation, and palpation. A fourth technique, percussion, is learned in later training and is used in specific procedures. These techniques are defined and discussed throughout this chapter as they apply to each body system.

INSPECTION

Inspection is visual examination, that is, assessing by using the sense of sight. Inspection should be deliberate, purposeful, and systematic. In addition to visual observations, olfactory (smelling) and auditory (hearing) cues are noted. Nurses frequently use visual inspection to assess moisture, color, and texture of body surfaces, as well as shape, position, size, color, and symmetry of the body. Lighting must be sufficient for the nurse to see clearly; either natural or artificial light can be used. When using the auditory senses, it is important to have a quiet environment for accurate hearing. Inspection can be combined with the other assessment techniques.

AUSCULTATION

Auscultation is the process of listening to sounds produced within the body. Auscultation may be direct or indirect. Direct auscultation is the use of the unaided ear, for example, to listen to a respiratory wheeze or the grating of a moving joint. Indirect auscultation (shown in Procedure 19-1 ■ on page 379) is done with the use of a stethoscope. The stethoscope amplifies the sounds and conveys them to the nurse's ears. A stethoscope is used primarily to listen to sounds from within the body, such as bowel sounds in the abdomen or valve sounds of the heart.

PALPATION

Palpation is the examination of the body using the sense of touch. The pads of the fingers are used because their concentration of nerve endings makes them highly sensitive and able to detect small differences or changes. Palpation is used to determine (1) texture (e.g., of the hair); (2) temperature (e.g., of a skin area); (3) vibration (e.g., of a joint); (4) position, size, consistency, and mobility of organs or masses; (5) distention (e.g., of the urinary bladder); (6) pulsation; and (7) the presence of pain upon pressure.

There are two types of palpation: light and deep. The LPN/LVN is trained in light palpation. Deep palpation is not usually done by the LPN/LVN, because pressure can damage internal organs. It is usually avoided in clients who have acute abdominal pain or who have pain that is not yet diagnosed.

PERCUSSION

Percussion is the act of striking a body part with short, sharp blows (1) to help gather data about internal organs, (2) to assist in massage, or (3) to help a client to clear the respiratory tract.

Terminology for Documenting Data

ANATOMIC POSITIONS AND BODY PLANES

The starting position, when collecting data about the human body, is the **anatomic position.** In this position the body is upright with the face front, arms at the sides with palms facing forward, and feet parallel (Figure 19-3 ■). Basic anatomic terms for direction are provided in Box 19-3 ■.

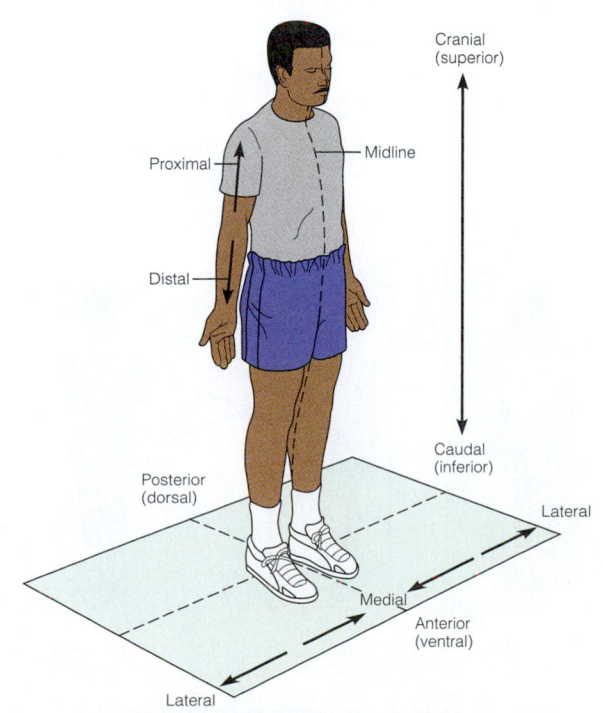

Figure 19-3. ■ Correct anatomic position.

BOX 19-3 **ANATOMIC TERMS FOR DIRECTION**

- **Anterior** or **ventral**—toward the front of the body or the belly
- **Posterior** or **dorsal**—toward the back of; the opposite of ventral
- **Superior**—above or in a higher position
- **Inferior**—a point lower than or below a reference point
- Superficial—situated near the surface of an object
- Deep—below the surface of an object
- **Medial**—closer to the middle of the body
- **Lateral**—toward the side; the opposite of medial
- **Proximal**—nearer the origin of a structure
- **Distal**—farther from the origin of a structure

In anatomy, the body is often pictured as being divided by an imaginary flat surface (**plane**) that divides it into two portions. There are three commonly designated types of planes (Figure 19-4 ■):

- **Sagittal plane,** a line running from front to back, separating the body into left and right. If the left and right divisions are equal, the plane is called midsagittal.
- **Frontal plane,** a line running from one side of the body to the other. The front plane separates the body into front and back portions.
- **Transverse plane,** a line running across the body horizontally, creates a *superior* (higher) and an *inferior* (lower) portion.

Body Cavities

It is also important to know terms to describe the body cavities for which data need to be collected. There are two large spaces or cavities that house various organs (Figure 19-5 ■):

- *Dorsal cavity* (including the cranial and the spinal cavities)

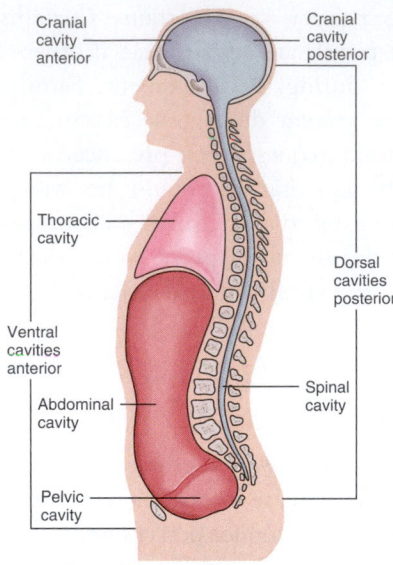

Figure 19-5. ■ Major body cavities.

- *Ventral cavity* (including the thoracic cavity and the abdominopelvic cavity)
  - The *thoracic cavity*, above the diaphragm, contains the heart, the major blood vessels, and the lungs.
  - The *abdominopelvic cavity*, below the diaphragm, contains the stomach, kidneys, liver, spleen, gallbladder, and most of the intestines (these are named *upper abdominal organs*). It also includes the urinary bladder, rectum, and internal parts of the male and female reproductive systems (called *pelvic organs*). Figure 19-6 ■ shows a common way of mapping the abdomen in order to document findings.

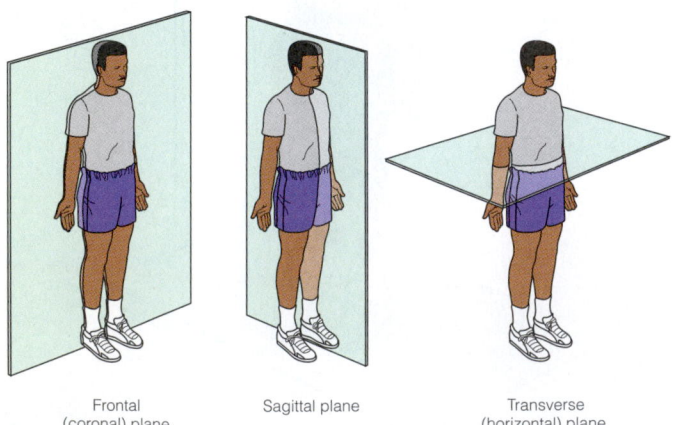

Frontal (coronal) plane | Sagittal plane | Transverse (horizontal) plane

Figure 19-4. ■ Body planes: frontal or coronal, sagittal, and transverse or horizontal.

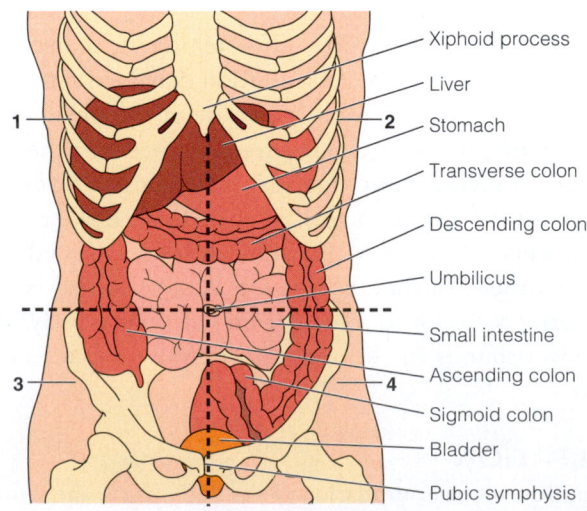

Figure 19-6. ■ The four abdominal quadrants and their underlying organs: 1, right upper quadrant (RUQ); 2, left upper quadrant (LUQ); 3, right lower quadrant (RLQ); 4, left lower quadrant (LLQ).

NURSING CARE

PRIORITIZING NURSING CARE

When preparing to collect data for assessment, the LPN/LVN focuses on having all necessary equipment and preparing a comfortable environment. The physical status and developmental level of the client are included as factors in determining the order of data collection. The LPN/LVN always keeps in mind scope of practice and facility policy when collecting data for assessment.

ASSESSING

General Survey

Physical assessment begins with a general survey that involves observation of the client's general appearance and behavior, and measurement of vital signs, height, and weight.

Many components of the general survey, to include psychosocial and cultural issues, are assessed when the RN takes the client's health history, such as the client's body build, posture, hygiene, and mental status. (See Chapter 17 for more inclusive information about psychosocial issues and Chapter 3 about cultural issues ⚭ .) Variations that relate to racial or ethnic background may occur (Box 19-4 ■). These data can be used by the LPN/LVN as a baseline with which to compare future assessment findings. Procedure 19-1 describes how to perform a focused physical assessment by body system.

The general appearance and behavior of an individual must be assessed in relationship to current circumstances. For example, an individual who has recently experienced a personal loss may appropriately appear depressed. Also, the client's age, sex, and race are useful factors in interpreting findings that suggest increased risk for known conditions.

BOX 19-4	CULTURAL PULSE POINTS

Data for Assessment

- Certain acquired and genetic disorders occur more frequently in specific cultural groups (e.g., hypertension, sickle cell anemia, Tay-Sachs disease, lactose intolerance).
- The client may have distinctive physical features that are characteristic of ethnic or cultural groups (e.g., hair texture or skin color). These are known as biocultural variations. The client may also have variations in anatomic characteristics such as body structure, height, weight, facial shape, and structure (e.g., nose, eye, facial contour) that can be identified with their ethnic heritage.
- Some cultural groups have a higher incidence of some socio-environmental conditions. These include HIV/AIDS, drug abuse, family violence, lead poisoning, alcoholism, and ear infections.

Neurologic Status

Level of Consciousness

Level of consciousness (LOC) can lie anywhere along a continuum from a state of alertness to coma. A fully alert client responds to questions spontaneously; a comatose client may not respond at all to verbal stimuli. The Glasgow Coma Scale (Table 19-2 ■) was originally developed to predict recovery from a head injury; however, many professionals use it to assess LOC. It is a practical and standardized system for assessing the degree of consciousness impairment. It tests in three major areas: eye response, motor response, and verbal response. An assessment totaling 15 points indicates the client is alert and completely oriented. A comatose client scores 7 or less.

clinical ALERT

CAUTION: Any score lower than a 10 on the Glasgow Coma Scale should be reported.

The Glasgow Coma Scale was developed in 1974 to provide a way for healthcare professionals to arrive at the same conclusion regarding clients' status. It saves time because the ratings are done numerically rather than with descriptions.

Orientation

The nurse determines the client's orientation to time, place, and person by tactful questioning. **Orientation** (as used when collecting data) is the client's ability to remember city

TABLE 19-2	Levels of Consciousness: Glasgow Coma Scale	
FACULTY MEASURED	**RESPONSE**	**SCORE**
Eye response	Spontaneous	4
	To verbal command	3
	To pain	2
	No response	1
Motor response	To verbal command	6
	To localized pain	5
	Flexes and withdraws	4
	Flexes abnormally	3
	Extends abnormally	2
	No response	1
Verbal response	Oriented, converses	5
	Disoriented, converses	4
	Uses inappropriate words	3
	Makes incomprehensible sounds	2
	No response	1

and state of residence, time of day, date, day of the week, duration of illness, and names of family members. More direct questioning may be necessary for some people; for example, "Where are you now?" "What day is it today?" Most people readily respond and accept these questions. The nurse listens for quantity of speech (amount and pace), quality (loudness, clarity, and inflection), and organization (coherent thought, connection to what was asked, overgeneralization, or vagueness). This is recorded as oriented times (×) 1, 2, or 3, depending on the response of the client. (A sample narrative note would be, "Client oriented ×3."

Pupil Reaction

Pupils are normally black, are equal in size (about 3 to 7 mm in diameter), and have round, smooth borders. Cloudy pupils often indicate cataracts. Unequal pupils (anisocoria) may result from a central nervous system disorder; however, slight variations may be normal. The reactions a nurse must check are discussed in Procedure 19-1. They include:

1. **Direct response**—In a semidarkened room, a pupil should constrict or close when a bright light is shone into the eye.
2. **Consensual response**—When the bright light is shone on the same pupil a second time, the pupil of the other eye should also constrict.
3. **Accommodation**—A person alternates looking from a near object (about 10 cm or 4 in from the bridge of the nose) to a distant object (such as a point on the far wall). Accommodation is the alternating change in pupil size (constricts when looking at the near object, dilates when looking at the distant one).

A normal assessment of the pupils is recorded using the abbreviation **PERRLA** (pupils equal round, reactive to light and accommodation).

Skull

The skull of an adult client is not usually directly assessed. However, if the client has had head trauma or a procedure involving this area, the skull is assessed.

Part A of Procedure 19-1 focuses on assessing general appearance and mental status.

Vital Signs

Vital signs are measurements of temperature, pulse, respirations, and blood pressure. Some agencies are identifying pain as the fifth vital sign and it belongs in that assessment category. They are measured (1) to establish baseline data against which to compare future measurements and (2) to detect actual and potential health problems. Normal adult vital signs are T 98.6°F (37°C); P 60 to 100 per minute, average 80 beats per minute; R 12 to 20 per minute, average 16 per minute; BP 120/80. See

Chapter 21 🔗 for full information and instructions related to taking vital signs.

Height and Weight

In adults, the ratio of weight to height provides a general measure of health. It is also important that the nurse and client be aware of any significant unintentional weight gain or loss. The height and weight are usually measured when a client is admitted to a healthcare agency. Measurement of height and weight is discussed in Chapter 25 🔗.

Weight may also be measured regularly, for example, each morning before breakfast. When accuracy is essential, the nurse should use the same scale each time (because every scale weighs differently). The weight should be measured at the same time each day, making sure the client wears the same kind of clothing and no shoes. The client usually stands on a platform, and the weight is read from a digital display panel or a balancing arm. Clients who cannot stand are weighed on bed or chair scales.

Integumentary System

The integumentary system includes the skin, hair, and nails. In most documentation paperwork, condition of hair would be documented as a narrative note only in the event of a problem. Examination begins with a generalized inspection using a good source of lighting, preferably indirect natural daylight.

Skin

Assessment of the skin involves inspection and palpation. The nurse may also need to use the nose (olfactory sense) to detect unusual skin odors. These odors are usually most evident in the skinfolds or in the axillae. Pungent body odor is frequently related to poor hygiene, *hyperhidrosis* (excessive perspiration), or *bromhidrosis* (foul-smelling perspiration). The entire skin surface may be assessed at one time or as each aspect of the body is assessed.

Pallor occurs when there is too little circulating blood or hemoglobin, which results in reduced amounts of oxygen being carried to body tissues. It is usually characterized by the absence of underlying red tones in the skin and may be most readily seen in the buccal mucosa. In brown-skinned clients, pallor may appear as a yellowish brown tinge; in black-skinned clients, the skin may appear ashen gray. When assessing clients with darker skin color, look for changes in skin color such as purple, brown, or bluish tones that are darker than surrounding skin. It is usually best to assess darker skin in natural or halogen light. Fluorescent light casts a blue color, making skin assessment more difficult and less accurate. Pallor in all people is usually most evident in areas with the least pigmentation such as the conjunctiva, oral mucous membranes, nail beds, palms of the hand, and soles of the feet. Pallor may be seen in clients with anemia and in decreased blood flow as in fainting or insufficient arterial blood flow.

The integument can also be characterized as cyanotic, erythematous, or edematous. **Cyanosis** (a bluish tinge) is most evident in the nail beds, lips, and buccal mucosa. Common causes of cyanosis include advanced lung disease, congenital heart disease, and abnormal hemoglobins. Bruised areas normally blanch when pressure is applied. Cyanotic skin does not blanch to the same degree as bruised skin.

Jaundice is a yellowish color of skin, sclera, palms of hands, and oral mucous membranes. Jaundice is usually indicative of liver disease, pancreatic disease, or common bile duct obstruction. In the dark-skinned client, jaundice usually presents as yellowish-green and is most obviously seen in the sclera of the eye. Do not confuse jaundice with yellow pigmentation in palms of hands and soles of feet, which is typical in the healthy dark-skinned client.

Erythema is a redness associated with a variety of rashes. **Edema** is the presence of excess interstitial fluid (see Procedure 19-1B). Elasticity or **turgor** (fullness) of the skin is also observed.

A skin **lesion** is an alteration in a client's normal skin appearance. Nurses are responsible for describing skin lesions accurately in terms of location (e.g., face), distribution (i.e., body regions involved), and configuration (the arrangement or position of several lesions). They also note the color, shape, size, firmness, texture, and characteristics of individual lesions.

Assessment of the feet is an important consideration. This is especially important for clients with diabetes or peripheral vascular disease, or for clients in traction from musculoskeletal injury or surgery (Table 19-3 ■).

Nails

Nails are inspected for nail plate shape, nail texture, nail bed color, the intactness of the tissues around the nails, and the angle between the nail and the nail bed (Figure 19-7 ■).

Nail texture is normally smooth. Excessively thick nails can appear in the elderly, in the presence of poor circulation, or in relation to a chronic fungal infection. A bluish or purplish tint to the nail bed may reflect cyanosis. Pallor in the nail bed may reflect poor arterial circulation.

A blanch test can be carried out to test the **capillary refill time** (the time the nail bed takes to return to its usual color after being pressed), to assess peripheral circulation. Normal nail bed capillaries blanch when pressed but quickly turn pink or their usual color when pressure is released. A capillary refill rate of more than 3 seconds may indicate circulatory problems.

Procedure 19-1, Part B, describes how to assess the skin and nails.

Cardiovascular System

Heart

In every physical assessment, it is important to listen to and count the apical **pulse** (heartbeat) for 1 full minute. Note pulse quality (bounding, normal, thready). Also note extra or skipped beats.

Associated with these sounds are systole and diastole. **Systole** is the period in which the ventricles contract. It begins with the first heart sound and ends at the second heart sound. Systole is normally shorter than diastole. **Diastole** is the period in which the ventricles relax. It starts with the second sound and ends at the following first sound. Both sounds are low in pitch and heard best at the apical site, with the bell of the stethoscope, and with the client lying on the left side. Palpation and/or auscultation of an irregular rhythm reliably indicate atrial fibrillation.

TABLE 19-3	Assessment of the Feet	
METHOD	**NORMAL FINDINGS**	**DEVIATIONS FROM NORMAL**
Inspect all skin surfaces, particularly between the toes, for cleanliness, odor, dryness, inflammation, swelling, abrasions, or other lesions.	Intact skin Absence of swelling or inflammation	Excessive dryness Areas of inflammation or swelling (e.g., corns, calluses) Fissures Scaling and cracking of skin (e.g., athlete's foot) Plantar warts
Palpate anterior and posterior surfaces of ankles and feet for edema.	No swelling	Swelling or pitting edema (see Procedure 19-1)
Palpate dorsalis pedis pulse on dorsal surface of foot.	Strong, regular pulses in both feet	Weak or absent pulses
Compare skin temperatures of the two feet.	Warm skin temperature	Cool skin temperature in one or both feet

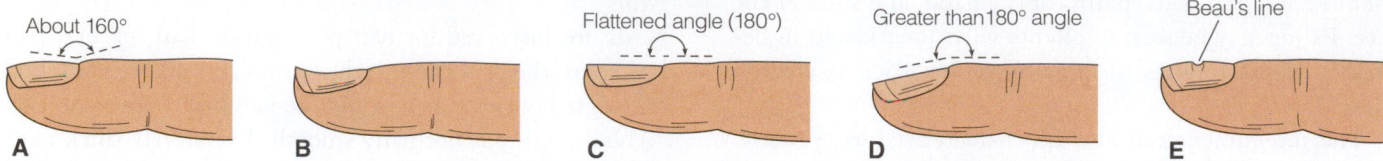

About 160° A

Flattened angle (180°) B

Greater than180° angle C

D

Beau's line E

Figure 19-7. ■ **A.** A normal nail, showing the convex shape and the plate angle of about 160 degrees. **B.** A spoon-shaped nail, which may be seen in clients with iron-deficiency anemia. **C.** Early clubbing. **D.** Late clubbing (may be caused by long-term oxygen lack). **E.** Beau's line on nail (may result from severe injury or illness).

To accurately determine all other irregular patterns, an electrocardiogram is needed to identify the arrhythmia (see pattern to auscultation in Procedure 19-1).

Peripheral Vascular System

The peripheral vascular system includes all of the blood vessels that carry oxygenated blood to body tissues and organs and return deoxygenated blood to the heart and lungs. When palpating peripheral pulses (Figure 19-8 ■), note quality of pulses; document as bounding (palpable, forceful), normal, weak (difficult to palpate and easily stopped by pressure), or absent (not palpable).

Assessing the peripheral vascular system also includes measuring the blood pressure; inspecting, palpating, and auscultating the carotid pulse; inspecting the jugular and peripheral veins; and inspecting the skin and tissues

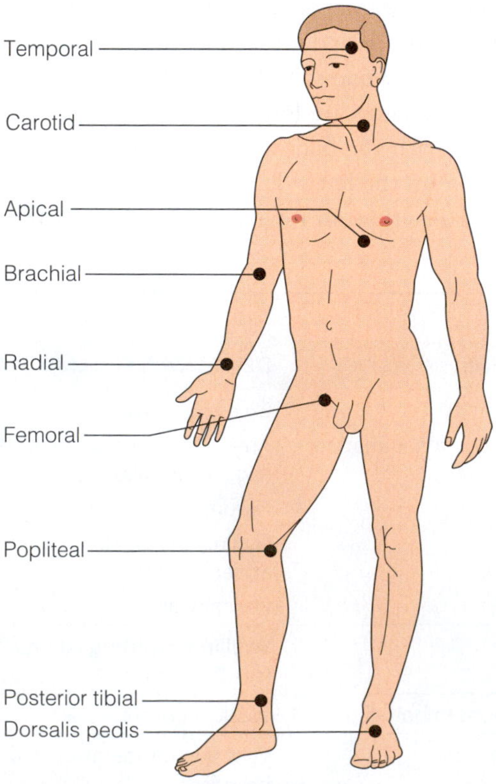

Temporal
Carotid
Apical
Brachial
Radial
Femoral
Popliteal
Posterior tibial
Dorsalis pedis

Figure 19-8. ■ Nine sites commonly used for assessing a pulse.

to determine **perfusion** (blood supply to an area) to the extremities.

The force of the pulse indicates the strength of the heart's stroke volume and is recorded using a three-point scale: 3+, full bounding; 2+, normal; and 1+, weak, thready. Certain aspects of peripheral vascular assessment are often incorporated into other parts of the assessment procedure. For example, blood pressure is usually measured at the beginning of the physical examination (see Chapter 21 ⚭, the section on pulse sites and Procedure 21-2 ⚭; see also Procedure 21-4 ⚭ on assessing blood pressure). Procedure 19-1, Part C, describes how to assess the cardiovascular and peripheral vascular systems.

Edema is also measured on examination of the cardiovascular or peripheral vascular assessment. Edema is described as present or absent, pitting or nonpitting. Pitting edema may be measured by depth or by counting the time that it takes to have the skin turgor return to normal. For example, the feet may have 1+, 2+, 3+, or 4+ pitting edema: 1+ = return to normal after blanching within 5 seconds, 2+ = 10 seconds, 3+ = 15 seconds, and 4+ = 20 seconds or longer to return to normal turgor. Other resources use 1+ as mild pitting edema, 2+ as moderate, 3+ as deep pitting, and 4+ as very deep pitting and indentation lasting a long time.

Respiratory System

Thorax and Lungs

Abnormal breath sounds, called adventitious breath sounds, occur when air passes through narrowed airways or airways filled with fluid or mucus, or when pleural linings are inflamed. **Adventitious breath sounds**—crackles (referred to as *rales* or crepitations), gurgles, pleural friction rub, and wheezes—are often superimposed over normal sounds. Table 19-4 ■ describes normal sounds and adventitious breath sounds. Absence of breath sounds over some lung areas is also a significant finding; it is associated with collapsed and surgically removed lobes. Oxygenation is discussed in depth in Chapter 32 ⚭.

Assessing the lungs is frequently critical to assessing the client's air exchange status. Changes in the respiratory system can come about slowly or quickly. In clients with

TABLE 19-4	**Normal and Adventitious Breath Sounds**		
TYPE/NAME	DESCRIPTION	CHARACTERISTICS/CAUSES	LOCATION
NORMAL BREATH SOUNDS			
Vesicular sound	Soft-intensity, low-pitched, "gentle sighing" sounds created by air moving through smaller airways (bronchioles and alveoli)	Best heard on inspiration, which is about 2.5 times longer than the expiratory phase (5:2 ratio)	Over peripheral lung; best heard at base of lungs
Bronchovesicular sound	Moderate-intensity and moderate-pitched "blowing" sounds created by air moving through larger airways (bronchi)	Equal inspiratory and expiratory phases (1:1 ratio)	Between the scapulae and lateral to the sternum at the first and second intercostal spaces
Bronchial (tubular) sound	High-pitched, loud, "harsh" sounds created by air moving through the trachea	Louder than vesicular sounds; have a short inspiratory phase and long expiratory phase (1:2 ratio)	Anteriorly over the trachea; not normally heard over lung tissue
ADVENTITIOUS BREATH SOUNDS			
Crackles (rales)	Fine, short, interrupted crackling sounds; alveolar rales are high-pitched. Sound can be simulated by rolling a lock of hair near the ear. Best heard on inspiration but can be heard on both inspiration and expiration. *May not be cleared by coughing.*	Air passing through fluid or mucus in any air passage	Most commonly heard in the bases of the lower lung lobes
Gurgles (rhonchi)	Continuous, low-pitched, coarse, gurgling, harsh, louder sounds with a moaning or snoring quality. Best heard on expiration but can be heard on both inspiration and expiration. *May be altered by coughing.*	Air passing through narrowed air passages as a result of secretions, swelling, tumors	Loud sounds can be heard over most lung areas but predominate over the trachea and bronchi
Friction rub	Superficial grating or creaking sounds heard during inspiration and expiration. *Not relieved by coughing.*	Rubbing together of inflamed pleural surfaces	Heard most often in areas of greatest thoracic expansion (e.g., lower anterior and lateral chest)
Wheezing	Continuous, high-pitched, squeaky musical sounds. Best heard on expiration. *Not usually altered by coughing.*	Air passing through constricted bronchi as a result of secretions, swelling, tumors	Heard over all lung fields

MyNursingKit | Normal lung sounds: 4 years old

chronic obstructive pulmonary disease (COPD), such as chronic bronchitis, emphysema, and asthma, changes often occur gradually as the body attempts to increase lung expansion.

Auscultation

To hear the breath sounds accurately, the nurse performs auscultation with the stethoscope on the skin, not through clothing. For efficiency, the nurse usually examines the posterior chest first, then the anterior chest. For posterior and lateral chest examinations, the client is uncovered to the waist and is in a sitting position. A sitting or lying position may be used for anterior chest examination. The sitting position is preferred because it maximizes chest expansion. However, if the client is unable to sit up, the examination can be performed with the client lying on his or her side.

Ask the client to take slow, deep breaths through the mouth while the exam is performed. This allows the client to move a greater amount of air through the lungs, which helps the nurse detect abnormal sounds. It can sometimes be helpful to have the client cough two or three times before the nurse begins auscultation. Coughing helps to clear the lung fields, which in turn clears airway secretions in the healthy lower respiratory track. If crackles, rhonchi, or wheezes can be heard following patient cough, then these adventitious lung sounds need further evaluation.

To auscultate the anterior chest, begin just above the clavicle starting on the client's right side. Move to the left side. Move to each lobe in a right-to-left pattern. When auscultating the anterior chest of a female client, it may be necessary to have her lie down so that her breasts fall to the side, allowing more accurate auscultation of the lung fields.

Respirations should also be counted at this time. Respirations normally range from 18 to 20 breaths per minute in an adult. Respirations should be described as present, absent, deep, shallow, and with or without difficulty. A procedure called pulse oximetry is frequently conducted on clients with respiratory impairment (see Procedure 32-1 ⚭ for an explanation of the use of an oximeter).

The nurse should also note any sputum, its appearance, and amount. See Box 19-1 for description of sputum. It is also important to note if the client is short of breath and which activity, if any, produces shortness of breath (also known as *dyspnea on exertion*). Procedure 19-1, Part D, describes how to assess the lungs.

Gastrointestinal System

Upper GI

When assessing the mouth and oropharynx, the nurse should observe for the following: inflammation of the tongue and oral mucosa; accumulation of food, microorganisms, and epithelial elements on the teeth and gums (referred to as *sordes*); or bleeding of the gums (which may be due to disease process or medication). Note that cancer of the lip and cancer of the tongue are the most common cancers of the mouth. Any persistent nodule or ulcer should be suspect and should be further evaluated.

The mouth is the beginning of the gastrointestinal system (digestive system) and should be assessed carefully. The Centers for Disease Control and Prevention (CDC) recommends that nurses wear gloves when in contact with the buccal mucosa (Figures 19-9A and B ■). A tongue blade can be used to aid inspection.

The nurse should note any difficulty swallowing and obtain further information about the cause. The nurse also notes any subjective indications of discomfort or nausea and records the client's statement of when these manifestations began and how long they have persisted. Frequent vomiting along with macerated knuckles, swollen salivary glands, and dental caries may indicate an eating disorder. Any abnormal findings or change in client condition should be reported to the team leader.

Abdomen

To assist in obtaining valid observations and to enhance client comfort, as mentioned previously, the nurse asks the client to urinate before beginning the assessment. If necessary, the nurse assists the client to a supine position, with arms placed comfortably at the sides. The nurse also places small pillows beneath the knees and the head. This position and an empty bladder prevent tension in the abdominal muscles. By contrast, the abdominal muscles tense when the client is sitting or when the client is supine with knees and arms extended and hands clasped behind the head.

The nurse exposes only the client's abdomen from chest line to the pubic area to avoid chilling and shivering, which can also tense the abdominal muscles.

The nurse locates and describes abdominal findings in a client by dividing the abdomen into quadrants, imagining a vertical line from the xiphoid process to the pubic symphysis, and a horizontal line across the umbilicus (see Figure 19-6). These quadrants are labeled (1) right upper quadrant (RUQ), (2) left upper quadrant (LUQ), (3) right lower quadrant (RLQ), and (4) left lower quadrant (LLQ). Assessment of the abdomen involves all four methods of examination (inspection, auscultation, palpation, and percussion). As mentioned already, inspection, auscultation, and light palpation are the skills first practiced by LPNs/LVNs.

The nurse performs inspection first, followed by auscultation, and palpation last. Auscultation is done before palpation because palpation causes movement or stimulation of the bowel. This can increase bowel motility and heighten bowel sounds, creating false results.

Thus, the order of abdominal assessment should be:

1. *Look.* While standing at the side of the supine client, inspect the abdomen for contour and symmetry. Is it flat, rounded, or concave? If rounded, is it distended (stretched out)? When distention is present, measure the abdominal girth by placing a tape around the abdomen at the level of the umbilicus (Figure 19-10 ■).

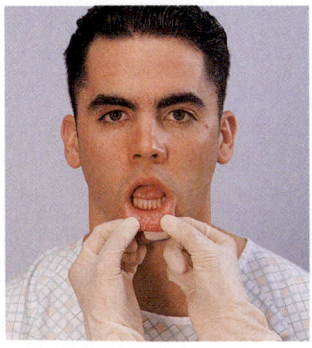 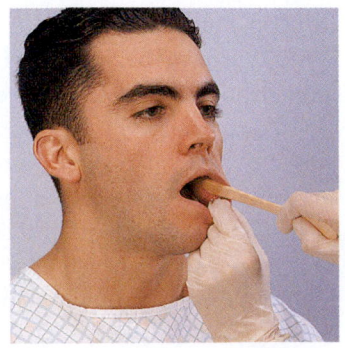

A B

Figure 19-9. ■ A. Inspecting the mucosa of the lower lip. B. Inspecting the buccal mucosa using a tongue blade.

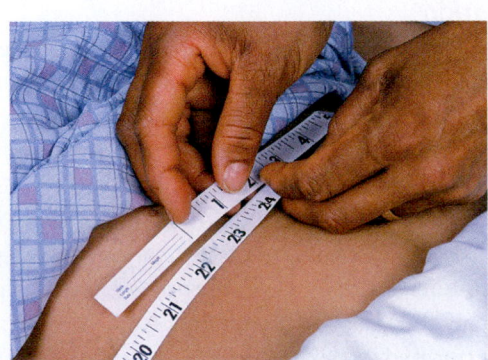

Figure 19-10. ■ Measuring abdominal girth at the level of the umbilicus. (Al Dodge, Pearson Education/PH.)

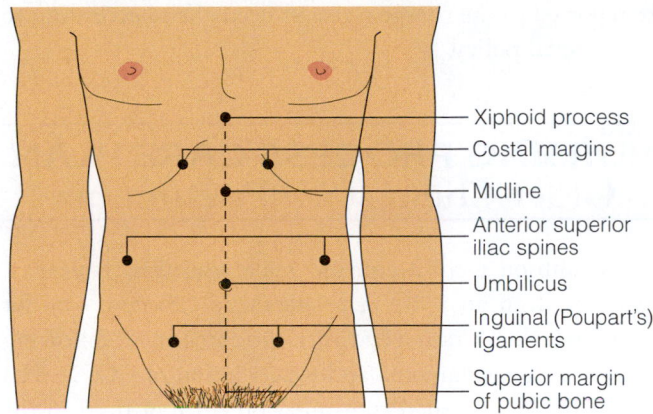

Figure 19-11. ■ Landmarks commonly used to identify abdominal areas.

Labels:
- Xiphoid process
- Costal margins
- Midline
- Anterior superior iliac spines
- Umbilicus
- Inguinal (Poupart's) ligaments
- Superior margin of pubic bone

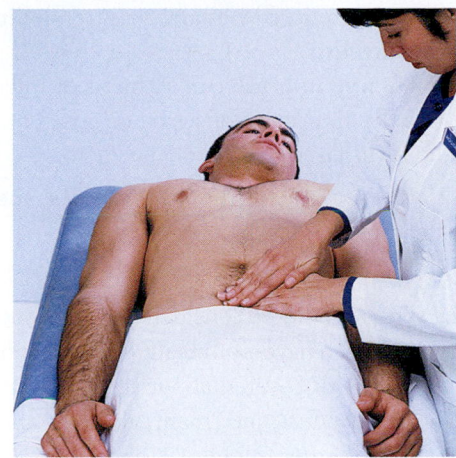

Figure 19-12. ■ Palpating the bladder.

Look for movement associated with peristalsis or pulsations.

2. *Listen.* Place the diaphragm of your stethoscope lightly on the client's abdomen and listen for bowel sounds in all four quadrants (see Figure 19-6). Landmarks for identifying abdominal areas are shown in Figure 19-11 ■. Are sounds normal, increased, decreased, or absent? If you suspect absent bowel sounds, listen for 5 minutes. Be sure that the client's bladder is empty before reporting absent bowel sounds. A full bladder may obscure sounds.

3. *Feel.* Light palpation is used mainly for determining areas of tenderness. Palpate in all four quadrants. The best indicator of tenderness is the client's facial expression. Pain with pressure, such as in palpation or percussion, in the costovertebral angle may suggest kidney infection or a musculoskeletal cause. In either case, further and more focused assessment should be conducted. Tenderness and rigidity 1 to 2 inches above the anterosuperior spine of the right ilium and the umbilicus (McBurney's point) are indicative of appendicitis. Caution should be used when palpating this area of the abdomen if there is complaint of pain. Voluntary or involuntary guarding may be present.

Procedure 19-1, Part E, describes how to assess the abdomen.

Genitourinary System

Note whether the client is continent or incontinent of urine or if an indwelling catheter is present. The amount, color, frequency, and odor of the urine should be described. This is a good opportunity to check the client's intake and output.

In some clients, it may be necessary to palpate the bladder to determine whether the client has emptied it completely (Figure 19-12 ■). Locate the edge of the bladder by pressing in the midline about 1 to 2 inches above the symphysis pubis. If the bladder is palpable, the nurse will feel a smooth, firm, slightly bouncy area. The client may indicate the urge to empty the bladder when it is palpated. During the postpartum period, the bladder can be easily palpated by first identifying the fundus of the uterus and then creeping the fingers down toward the symphysis pubis.

Procedure 19-1, Part F, describes how to assess the bladder and urine.

Musculoskeletal System

The musculoskeletal system encompasses the muscles, bones, and joints (see Chapter 31 ⬭).

Range of Motion

There are two types of range of motion (ROM): active and passive. In **active range of motion,** the extremities and joints are moved by the client through a systematic series of movements. The nurse asks the client to move each joint through a full range of motion. The nurse notes the degree and type of pain or weakness, or any limitation of movement. Each movement is compared with the same movement on the other side. The nurse proceeds to passive ROM if the client is unable to perform active ROM.

In **passive range of motion,** the client's extremities and joints are supported and moved by the nurse. The same series of movements are made as in active ROM. Any pain or increased limitation of movement is noted, and each movement is compared with the other side. If a client is able to stand or walk, observe his or her ability. Also describe any deformities. (See Procedure 23-1 ⬭ for passive ROM exercises.) The nurse should be especially alert to signs of inflammation and arthritis in joints.

■ *Swelling*: May indicate synovitis; swelling may involve the synovial membrane, effusion from excess synovial fluid within the joint space, or soft-tissue injury.

- *Warmth*: May be indicative of arthritis, tendonitis, bursitis, or osteomyelitis.
- *Tenderness*: Usually indicative of arthritis or infection.
- *Redness*: Usually indicative of septic or gouty arthritis or rheumatoid arthritis.

Procedure 19-1, Part G, describes how to assess the extremities, joints, and movement.

Psychosocial Status

Psychosocial status should be considered. The client's mental and spiritual status can have significant effects on physical recovery. Much can be discovered about the client through an assessment of mood, affect, judgment, abilities, and lifestyle patterns. Refer to Chapters 3, 11, 12, and 17 ⚭ for more about psychosocial aspects of care.

Variations in the Geriatric Assessment

The elderly client should be kept warm and comfortable during the physical assessment. Loss of subcutaneous fat in the elderly decreases their ability to stay warm. It may be necessary to adapt assessment and positioning to physical limitations. Perform as much of the assessment as possible in the position most comfortable for the client.

The elderly client's skin is fragile and care should be used when assessing the skin and or helping the client change positions. Use care when removing tape and bandages to prevent skin tears.

Sensory deficits (loss of hearing, sight, touch) can occur in the elderly. Provide a quiet environment with minimal distractions.

Avoid using vigorous assessment techniques such as hopping on one foot or doing deep knee bends when doing musculoskeletal assessments of the elderly. Elderly clients have limited range of motion and decreased balance.

DIAGNOSING, PLANNING, AND IMPLEMENTING

Data from focused assessments are used to shape the plan of care and provide appropriate interventions to suit the client's needs. The nurse learns to assess using all of the senses and is always alert to changes in the client's condition.

An accurate picture of the client's health can be achieved by thorough, organized assessment of all the body systems and by regular communication of all findings to the team leader. Assessment serves as a tool to all members of the healthcare team who care for the client.

EVALUATING

The LPN/LVN performs the focused assessment as ordered. A focused assessment is usually done at the beginning of a shift and throughout the shift. The results are then shared in an end-of-shift report. During a shift, changes in status are reported to the charge nurse as needed and according to institutional policy.

NURSING PROCESS CARE PLAN
Older Client with Pneumonia

James Johnson is a 72-year-old male who was transferred yesterday from an acute care agency to subacute care for continued rehabilitation and antibiotic treatment following a diagnosis of pneumonia and exacerbation of COPD. His chest x-ray has revealed continued presence of fluid in the right lower lobe, but he is no longer in the acute phase of pneumonia. He needs to regain his mobility and be prepared to return home. His intravenous antibiotics will continue to be infused in his PICC (peripherally inserted central catheter) line (see Chapter 28 ⚭).

Assessment

During the daily focused assessment, the LPN/LVN notes that Mr. Johnson is very dyspneic on exertion following his ambulation to the bathroom. The following data is collected: T 100.8 (F), P 112, B/P 118/88, R 32 and labored, Pulse Ox 88. He has coarse, gurgling lung sounds heard in the upper lobes. On auscultation, the right lower lobe has crackles. He has a cough with thick dark sputum and complains that he cannot catch his breath. His nail beds and oral mucosa are cyanotic. He is not currently on oxygen.

The following problems were reported to the RN:

- Dyspnea on exertion
- Unable to attend to normal activities of daily living
- Altered oxygen level as evidenced by low pulse oximetry level

Nursing Diagnoses

The following important nursing diagnoses (among others) were established for this client:

- *Ineffective Breathing Pattern* related to low oxygen level and increased respiratory rate
- *Activity Intolerance* related to dyspnea on exertion
- *Toileting Self-Care Deficit* related to impaired ability to help himself without exertion
- *Risk for Infection* related to pulmonary disease process

Expected Outcomes

Expected outcomes are that the client will:

- Have the breathing pattern return to baseline.
- Be able to complete activities of daily living without assistance.
- Be able to ambulate without increasing respiratory rate and pattern.
- Will be clear of infection following antibiotic therapy.

Planning and Implementation

- Apply oxygen via nasal cannula at 2 liters/min. *Low oxygen saturation in the blood indicates the need for supplemental oxygen.*
- Auscultate lungs and monitor respiratory status. *Condition may change suddenly.*
- Monitor vital signs for signs of increased temperature related to pneumonia. *Increase in temperature indicates infection.*
- Encourage fluids. *Fluids are needed to clear lung secretions.*
- Have the client use the incentive spirometer every hour. *The incentive spirometer exercises the lungs to prevent lung collapse (atelectasis).*

Evaluation

After 48 hours, Mr. Johnson stated he felt "less tired after walking than before." Heart rate and respirations at high end of normal range after ambulation. No crackles noted on auscultation of right lower lobes. Nail beds pink, capillary refill 3 seconds.

Critical Thinking in the Nursing Process

1. Describe why pneumonia makes it hard for a client to exercise without having difficulty breathing.
2. Explain why oxygen administration can lessen the blue-tinged color (cyanosis) of the client's nail beds.
3. If the client stated a preference to remain lying in one position through the night, what might the nurse respond?

Note: Discussion of Critical Thinking questions appears on the MyNursingKit Website.

Note: The references and resources for all chapters have been compiled at the back of the book.

PROCEDURE 19-1 # Focused Physical Assessment by Body Systems*

Purposes

- To obtain measurements to compare to baseline data
- To obtain information to assess effect of medications
- To determine health and comfort status of the client before or after a procedure or at the end of shift

Equipment

- Stethoscope or Doppler ultrasound (DUS)
- Penlight or flashlight
- Thermometer
- Sphygmomanometer and cuff

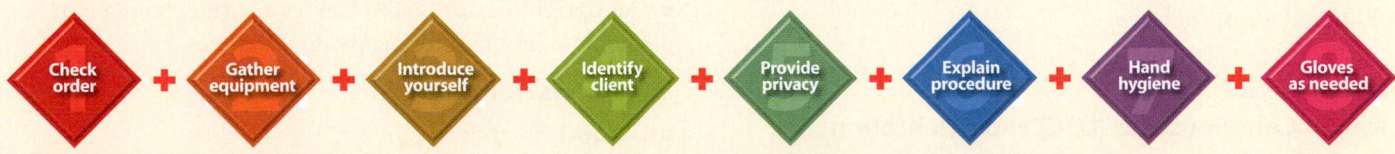

Check order + Gather equipment + Introduce yourself + Identify client + Provide privacy + Explain procedure + Hand hygiene + Gloves as needed

Part A: General Appearance and Mental Status

Interventions and Rationales

GENERAL APPEARANCE

Inspection

1. Observe body build, height, and weight in relation to the client's age, lifestyle, and health.
2. Observe the client's posture and gait, standing, sitting, and walking.
3. Observe the client's overall hygiene and grooming. Relate these to the person's activities prior to the assessment.
4. Note body and breath odor in relation to activity level.
5. Observe for signs of distress in posture (e.g., bending over because of abdominal pain) or facial expression (e.g., wincing or labored breathing).
6. Note obvious signs of health or illness (e.g., in skin color or breathing).

Behavior

1. Assess the client's attitude.
2. Note the client's affect/mood; assess the appropriateness of the client's response and level of orientation to time, place, and persons.

---

*This is an abbreviated assessment that can be conducted by the LPN/LVN at the beginning and/or end of the shift. A complete physical assessment is done by the RN on admission.

3. Listen for quantity of speech (amount and pace), quality (loudness, clarity, inflection), and organization (coherence of thought, overgeneralization, vagueness).

4. Listen for relevance and organization of thoughts.

Normal Findings

- Varies with lifestyle
- Relaxed, erect posture; coordinated movement
- Clean, neat
- No body odor or minor body odor relative to work or exercise; no breath odor
- Healthy appearance
- Cooperative
- Appropriate to situation
- Understandable, moderate pace
- Exhibits thought association
- Logical sequence
- Makes sense; has sense of reality

Deviations from Normal

- Excessively thin or obese
- Tense, slouched, bent posture; uncoordinated movement; tremors
- Dirty, unkempt
- Foul body odor; ammonia odor; acetone breath odor; foul breath
- Pallor; weakness; obvious illness
- Negative, hostile, withdrawn
- Inappropriate to situation
- Rapid or slow pace
- Uses generalizations; lacks association
- Illogical sequence
- Flight of ideas; confusion

NEUROLOGIC

Level of Consciousness (LOC) and Orientation

1. Ask client to give name, present location, and date or time of day.

Normal Findings

- Alert and oriented ×3: able to give correct name, location, and/or time of day or date

Deviations from Normal

- Inability to correctly name one or more items
- Lethargic or not responsive

Verbal Response

1. Assess how the client communicates rather than what is communicated, through normal conversation.

Normal Findings

- Clear
- Rate consistent with overall psychomotor status
- Volume audible, normal conversational tone

- Modulation and flow—fluid and expressive
- Production—able to produce words

Deviations from Normal

- Incoherent, rambling, slurred, stuttering
- Monotone
- Dysphasia, **aphasia** (impairment in understanding and producing verbal or written language)
- Pressured speech
- **Dysarthria,** difficulty articulating words, possibly resulting from medication or from neurologic damage

ASSESSING MOTOR RESPONSE

Grips

1. Ask the client to grasp your index and middle finger while you try to pull the fingers out.

Pushes/Pulls

1. Have the client hold arm up and resist while you try to push it down.

2. Have the client fully extend each arm and try to flex it while you attempt to hold arm in extension.

3. Have the client resist while you attempt to dorsiflex the foot and again while you attempt to flex the foot.

Walking Gait

1. Ask the client to walk across the room and back with eyesight focused ahead; assess the client's gait.

Normal Findings

- Bilateral/equal 100% normal strength; normal full movement; against gravity and against full resistance
- Has upright posture and steady gait with opposing arm swing; walks unaided, maintaining balance

Deviations from Normal

- Unequal strength
- 10% of normal strength; no movement, contraction of muscle is palpable or visible
- Has poor posture and unsteady, irregular, staggering gait with wide stance; bends legs only from hips; has rigid or no arm movements

ASSESSING PUPIL REACTIONS

Direct and Consensual Reaction to Light

1. Partially darken the room.

2. Ask the client to look straight ahead.

3. Using a penlight or flashlight and approaching from the side, shine a light on the pupil.

4. Observe the response of the illuminated pupil. It should constrict (direct response).

5. Shine the light on the pupil again, and observe the response of the other pupil. It should also constrict (consensual response).

Reaction to Accommodation

1. Hold an object (a penlight or pencil) about 10 cm (4 in.) from the bridge of the client's nose.

2. Ask the client to look first at the top of the object and then at a distant object (e.g., the far wall) behind the penlight. Alternate the gaze from the near to the far object.

3. Observe the pupil response. The pupils should constrict when looking at the near object and dilate when looking at the far object.

4. Next, move the penlight or pencil toward the client's nose. The pupils should converge.

5. To record normal assessment of the pupils, use the abbreviation PERRLA (pupils equally round and react to light and accommodation).

6. Assess each pupil's reaction to accommodation.

Normal Findings

- Pupils constrict when looking at near object; pupils dilate when looking at far object; pupils converge when near object is moved toward nose

Deviations from Normal

- One or both pupils fail to constrict, dilate, or converge

Part B: Integumentary Assessment
Interventions and Rationales
ASSESSING THE SKIN

1. Inspect skin color (best assessed under natural light and on areas not exposed to the sun).

2. Inspect uniformity of skin color.

3. Assess edema, if present (i.e., location, color, temperature, and the degree to which the skin remains indented or pitted when pressed by a finger). See Figure 19-13 ■.

4. Inspect and describe skin lesions.

clinical ALERT

Assess skin turgor over the sternum in older adults. Loss of subcutaneous tissue in aging makes the skin of the arms a less reliable indicator of fluid status.

5. Observe and palpate skin moisture.

6. Palpate skin temperature. Compare the two feet and the two hands, using the backs of your fingers.

Backs of fingers pick up temperature differences more readily.

7. Note skin turgor (fullness or elasticity) by lifting and pulling the skin on an extremity into a tent position.

Normal Findings

- Varies from light to deep brown; from ruddy pink to light pink; from yellow overtones to olive
- Generally uniform except in areas exposed to the sun; areas of lighter pigmentation (palms, lips, nail beds) in dark-skinned people

  One Scale for Describing Edema
  1 = Barely detectable
  2 = Indentation of less than 5 mm
  3 = Indentation of 5 to 10 mm
  4 = Indentation of more than 10 mm

  Alternate Scale for Describing Edema
  1+ = if the indentation of the fingers remains for more than 5 seconds
  2+ = if the indentation of the fingers remains for more than 10 seconds
  3+ = if the indentation of the fingers remains for more than 15 seconds
  4+ = if the indentation of the fingers remains for more than 20 seconds

- Freckles, some birthmarks, some flat and raised *nevi* (moles); no abrasions or other lesions
- Moisture in skinfolds and the axillae (varies with environmental temperature and humidity, body temperature, and activity)
- Uniform; within normal range
- When tented, skin springs back to previous state

Deviations from Normal

- Pallor, cyanosis, jaundice, erythema
- Areas of either hyperpigmentation or hypopigmentation (e.g., vitiligo, albinism, edema)
- Various interruptions in skin integrity

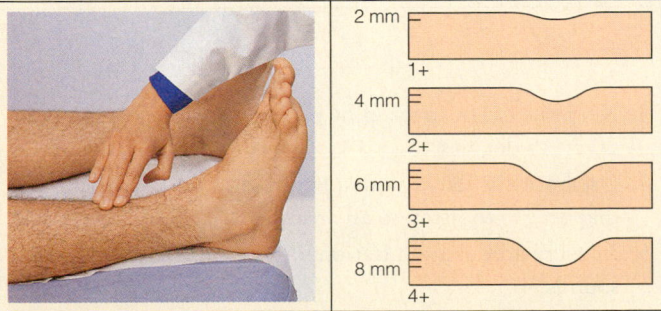

Figure 19-13. ■ Assess edema by pressing your finger firmly against client's skin for several seconds (especially in ankle area). After removing your finger, observe for lasting impression or indentation.

- Excessive moisture (e.g., in hyperthermia); excessive dryness (e.g., in dehydration)
- Generalized hyperthermia (e.g., in fever); generalized hypothermia (e.g., in shock); localized hyperthermia (e.g., in infection); localized hypothermia (e.g., in arteriosclerosis)
- Skin stays tented or moves back slowly (e.g., in dehydration)

ASSESSING MUCOUS MEMBRANES

1. Inspect and palpate the inner lips and buccal mucosa for color, moisture, texture, and the presence of lesions. Uniform pink color (darker, e.g., bluish hue, in dark-skinned clients).

Normal Findings

- Soft, moist, smooth texture
- Uniform pink color (freckled brown pigmentation in dark-skinned clients)
- Moist, smooth, soft, glistening, and elastic texture

Deviations from Normal

- Pallor; cyanosis
- Blisters; generalized or localized swelling; fissures, crusts, or scales (may result from excessive moisture, nutritional deficiency, or fluid deficit)
- Inability to purse lips (indicative of facial nerve damage)
- Pallor; white patches (leukoplakia)
- Excessive dryness

ASSESSING TEETH AND GUMS

1. Inspect the teeth and gums while examining the inner lips and buccal mucosa.

Normal Findings

- 32 adult teeth
- Smooth, white, shiny tooth enamel
- Pink gums (bluish or dark patches in dark-skinned clients)
- Moist, firm texture to gums
- No retraction of gums (pulling away from the crown of the tooth)

Deviations from Normal

- Missing teeth
- Ill-fitting dentures
- Brown or black discoloration of the enamel (may indicate staining or the presence of caries)
- Excessively red gums
- Spongy texture; bleeding; tenderness (may indicate periodontal disease)
- Receding, atrophied gums; swelling that partially covers the teeth
- Dry, furry tongue (associated with fluid deficit)
- Nodes, ulcerations, discolorations (white or red areas); areas of tenderness
- Restricted mobility
- Swelling, ulceration
- Swelling, nodules
- Inflammation (redness and swelling)
- Discoloration (e.g., jaundice or pallor)
- Palates the same color
- Irritations
- Bony growths (exostoses) growing from the hard palate
- Deviation to one side from tumor or trauma; immobility (may indicate damage to trigeminal [fifth cranial] nerve or vagus [tenth cranial] nerve)
- Reddened or edematous; presence of lesions, plaques, or exudate
- Inflamed
- Presence of discharge
- Swollen
- Sordes (accumulation of brown crusts on teeth and lips; may be related to mild elevated temperature)

ASSESSING THE NAILS

1. Note the color of the nail bed. Bluish nails suggest cyanosis.
2. Perform a capillary refill test if necessary. A capillary refill time of more than 3 seconds may indicate circulatory problems.
3. Abnormal clubbing can be noted with chronic respiratory disease.

Part C: Cardiovascular Assessment
Interventions and Rationales

ASSESSING HEART SOUNDS

1. Auscultate the heart in all four anatomic sites: aortic, pulmonic, tricuspid, and apical (mitral). Auscultation need not be limited to these areas. However, the nurse may need to move the stethoscope to find the most audible sounds for each client.
2. Eliminate all sources of room noise. *Heart sounds are of low intensity, and other noise hinders the nurse's ability to hear them.*
3. Keep the client in a supine position with head elevated 30 to 45 degrees.
4. Use both the flat-disk diaphragm and the bell-shaped diaphragm to listen to all areas.
5. In every area of auscultation, distinguish both S_1 and S_2 sounds.
6. When auscultating, concentrate on one particular sound at a time in each area: the first heart sound, followed by systole, then the second heart sound, then diastole. Systole and diastole are normally silent intervals.

7. Later, reexamine the heart while the client is in the upright sitting position. *Certain sounds are more audible in this position.*

Normal Findings

- S_1: usually heard at all sites; usually louder at the apical and tricuspid areas
- S_2: usually heard at all sites; usually louder at base of heart and aortic and pulmonic areas
- Systole: silent interval; slightly shorter duration than diastole at normal heart rate (60–90 bpm)
- Diastole: silent interval; slightly longer duration than systole at normal heart rates
- S_3 in children and young adults
- S_4 in many older adults

Deviations from Normal

- Increased or decreased intensity
- Varying intensity with different beats
- Increased intensity at aortic area
- Increased intensity at pulmonic area
- Sharp-sounding ejection clicks
- S_3 in older adults
- S_4 may be a sign of hypertension

ASSESSING THE PERIPHERAL VASCULAR SYSTEM

Peripheral Pulses

1. Palpate the peripheral pulses (except the carotid pulse) on both sides of the client's body simultaneously and systematically to determine the symmetry of pulse volume. *This method helps to determine the symmetry of pulse volume.*

2. Assess radial pulses and compare. Check capillary refill. Ask client to wiggle fingers. Ask client not to look at his or her feet. Touch the client's feet one at a time, asking the client if he or she is able to feel your touch. *This will determine level of touch perception.*

3. Assess pedal pulses and compare one side to the other. Note strength of pulse. If pedal pulses are not palpable, palpate posterior tibial pulse and compare one side to the other. Check capillary refill in toes. Ask client to wiggle toes. Ask the client if he or she experiences numbness or tingling in extremities or sensation of cold. *Tibial pulse should be more palpable because it is closer to the heart.*

4. Palpate skin temperature. Compare the two feet and the two hands, using the backs of your fingers. *Coolness may indicate lack of tissue perfusion.*

5. Note color of feet and toes and edema of the lower extremities.

6. Check for Homans' sign. To perform this test, the nurse supports the leg while flexing the foot in dorsiflexion. Ask the client if pain is felt as foot is flexed. Palpate muscles of calf for tender, hot areas. *A positive Homans' sign indicates venous thrombosis (blood clots). Some facilities prefer to have the nurse check for warmth and/or swelling, and to ask whether the client has any calf pain.*

Normal Findings

- Symmetric pulse volumes
- Full pulsations
- In dependent position, distention and nodular bulges at calves are present
- When limbs are elevated, veins collapse (veins may appear tortuous or distended in older people)
- Limbs not tender
- Symmetric in size

Deviations from Normal

- Asymmetric volumes (indicate impaired circulation)
- Absence of pulsation (indicates arterial spasm or occlusion)
- Decreased, weak, thready pulsations (indicate impaired cardiac output)
- Increased pulse volume (may indicate hypertension, high cardiac output, or circulatory overload)
- Distended veins in the anteromedial part of thigh and/or lower leg or on posterolateral part of calf from knee to ankle
- Tenderness on palpation
- Pain in calf muscles with passive dorsiflexion of the foot (Homans' sign)
- Warmth and redness over vein
- Swelling of one calf or leg

Peripheral Perfusion

1. Inspect the skin of the hands and feet for color, temperature, edema, and skin changes. These factors can identify poor blood perfusion.

clinical ALERT

Report

If signs of arterial insufficiency occur, report findings to charge nurse.

2. Assess the adequacy of arterial flow if arterial insufficiency is suspected.

Normal Findings

- Natural skin color
- Skin temperature not excessively warm or cold
- No edema
- Skin texture resilient and moist
- Buerger's test: original color returns in 10 seconds; veins in feet or hands fill in about 15 seconds
- Capillary refill test: Immediate return of color

Deviations from Normal

- Cyanosis, pallor
- Skin cool
- Marked edema
- Skin thin and shiny or thick, waxy, shiny, and fragile, reduced hair, ulceration

- Delayed color return or mottled appearance; delayed venous filling; marked redness of arms or legs (indicates arterial insufficiency)
- Delayed return of color (arterial insufficiency)

Part D: Respiratory Assessment

Interventions and Rationales

ASSESSING THE THORAX AND LUNGS

Posterior Thorax

1. Inspect the shape and symmetry of the thorax from posterior and lateral views.

2. Palpate the posterior thorax.

3. For clients who have no respiratory complaints, rapidly assess the temperature and integrity of all chest skin.

4. For clients who do have respiratory complaints, palpate all chest areas for bulges, tenderness, or abnormal movements. Do not perform deep palpation. Observe caution when palpating (lightly). *If rib is fractured, deep palpation could lead to displacement of the bone fragment against the lungs.*

Normal Finding

- Chest symmetric

Deviations from Normal

- Chest asymmetric
- Bulges, tenderness, or abnormal movements in chest area

Anterior Thorax

1. Auscultate the chest using the flat-disk diaphragm of the stethoscope. Use the systematic zigzag procedure used in percussion (Figure 19-14 ■). *The flat-disk side is best for transmitting the high-pitched breath sounds. This ensures that no areas are missed.*

2. Ask the client to take slow, deep breaths through the mouth. Listen at each point to the breath sounds during

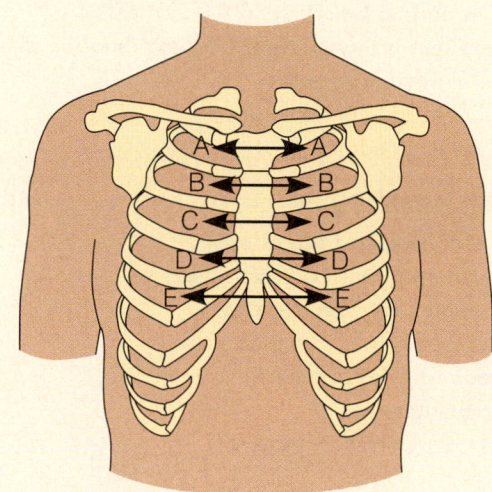

Figure 19-14. ■ Systematic zigzag pattern.

a complete inspiration and expiration. Compare findings at each point with the corresponding point on the opposite side of the chest. *Slow, deep breaths move more air and allow abnormalities to be heard.*

Normal Findings

- Quiet, rhythmic, and effortless respirations
- Full, symmetric respiratory effort

Deviations from Normal

- Adventitious breath sounds (e.g., crackles, rhonchi, wheezes, friction rub)
- Absence of breath sounds (associated with collapsed and surgically removed lung lobes)
- Asymmetric and/or decreased respiratory exchange

Part E: Abdominal Assessment

Interventions and Rationales

Inspection

1. Inspect the abdomen for skin integrity (refer to the discussion of skin assessment earlier in this chapter).

2. Inspect the abdomen for contour and symmetry.

3. Observe the abdominal contour (profile line from the rib margin to the pubic bone) while standing at the client's side when the client is supine.

4. Ask the client to take a deep breath and to hold it (makes any abnormality such as an enlarged liver or spleen more obvious).

5. Assess the symmetry of contour while standing at the foot of the bed.

6. If distention is present, measure the abdominal girth by placing a tape around the abdomen at the level of the umbilicus. *Distention may indicate hidden fluid imbalances.*

Normal Findings

- Unblemished skin
- Uniform color
- Silver-white striae or surgical scars
- Flat, rounded (convex), or scaphoid (concave or boat shaped)
- No evidence of enlargement of liver or spleen
- Symmetric contour

Deviations from Normal

- Presence of rash or other lesions
- Tense, glistening skin (may indicate ascites, edema)
- Purple striae (associated with Cushing's disease)
- Generalized distention (associated with gas retention, obesity, ascites, or tumors)
- Lower abdominal distention (may indicate bladder distention, pregnancy, or ovarian mass)
- Markedly *scaphoid* (concave or boat-shaped) abdomen (associated with malnutrition)
- Evidence of enlargement of liver or spleen
- Asymmetric contour, such as localized protrusions around umbilicus, inguinal ligaments, or scars (possible hernia or tumor)

AUSCULTATION

1. Auscultate the abdomen for bowel sounds and vascular sounds.

2. Warm the hands and the stethoscope diaphragms. *Cold hands and a cold stethoscope may cause the client to contract the abdominal muscles, and these contractions may be heard during auscultation.*

For Bowel Sounds

1. Use the flat-disk diaphragm. *Intestinal sounds are relatively high pitched and best accentuated by the flat-disk diaphragm. Light pressure with the stethoscope is adequate to detect sounds.*

2. Ask when the client last ate. *The frequency of sounds relates to the state of digestion or the presence of food in the gastrointestinal tract. Shortly after or long after eating, bowel sounds may normally increase. They are loudest when a meal is long overdue. Four to 7 hours after a meal, bowel sounds in the RLQ may be heard continuously over the ileocecal valve area while the digestive contents from the small intestine empty through the valve into the large intestine.*

3. Place the flat-disk diaphragm of the stethoscope in each of the four quadrants of the abdomen (Figure 19-15 ■). Many nurses begin in the lower right quadrant in the area of the cecum.

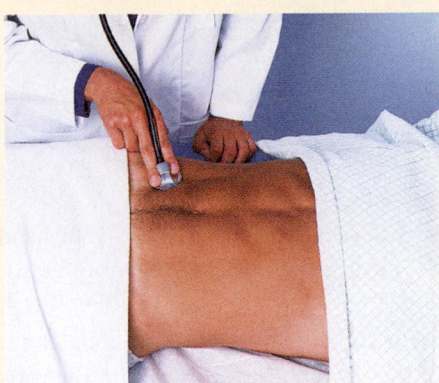

Figure 19-15. ■ Auscultating the abdomen for bowel sounds.

4. Listen for active bowel sounds—irregular gurgling noises occurring about every 5 to 20 seconds. *The duration of a single sound may range from less than a second to more than several seconds.*

5. Normal bowel sounds are described as audible. Alterations in sounds are described as absent or hypoactive, that is, extremely soft and infrequent (e.g., one per minute), and hyperactive or increased, that is, high-pitched, loud, rushing sounds that occur frequently (e.g., every 3 seconds) also known as borborygmi. *Absence of sounds indicates a cessation of intestinal motility. Hypoactive sounds indicate decreased motility and are usually associated with manipulation of the bowel during surgery, inflammation, paralytic ileus, or late bowel obstruction. Hyperactive sounds indicate increased intestinal motility and are usually associated with diarrhea, an early bowel obstruction, or the use of laxatives.*

For Absent, Hypoactive, or Hyperactive Bowel Sounds

1. If bowel sounds appear to be absent, listen for 3 to 5 minutes before concluding that they are absent. *Because bowel sounds are so irregular, a longer time and more sites are used to confirm absence of sounds.*

Normal Finding

- Audible bowel sounds

Deviations from Normal

- Limited movement due to pain or disease process
- Visible peristalsis in nonlean clients (with bowel obstruction)

Palpation

1. Perform light palpation first to detect areas of tenderness and/or muscle guarding. Systematically explore all four quadrants. *Palpation is used to detect tenderness, the presence of masses or distention, and the outline and position of abdominal organs (e.g., the liver, spleen, and kidneys). Two types of palpation are used: light and deep. In some practice settings,*

palpation is limited to light abdominal palpation to assess tenderness and bladder palpation to assess for distention.

2. Before palpation, ensure that the client's position is appropriate for relaxation of the abdominal muscles, and warm the hands. *Cold hands can cause muscle tension and thus impede palpatory evaluation.*

3. For light palpation, hold the palm of your hand slightly above the client's abdomen, with your fingers parallel to the abdomen.

4. Depress the abdominal wall lightly, about 1 cm or to the depth of the subcutaneous tissue, with the pads of your fingers (Figure 19-16 ■).

5. Move the finger pads in a slight circular motion.

6. Note areas of slight tenderness or superficial pain, large masses, and muscle guarding. To determine areas of tenderness, ask the client to tell you about them, watch for changes in the client's facial expressions, and note areas of muscle guarding.

Normal Findings

■ No tenderness; relaxed soft abdomen with smooth, consistent tension; pain free

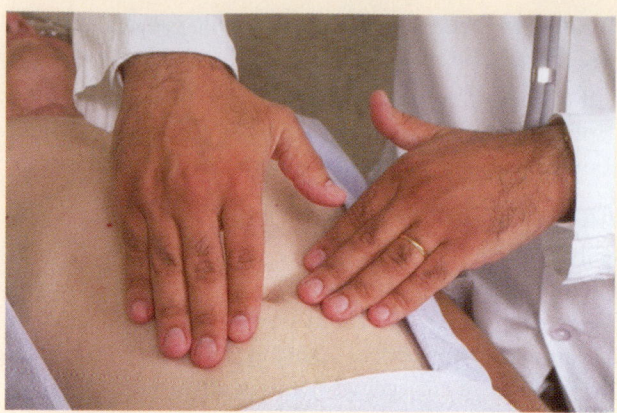

Figure 19-16. ■ For light palpation of the abdomen, depress the abdominal wall lightly, about 1 cm or to the depth of the subcutaneous tissue, with the pads of your fingers.

Deviations from Normal

■ Tenderness and hypersensitivity
■ Superficial masses
■ Localized areas of increased tension
■ Generalized or localized areas of tenderness

Part F: Genitourinary Assessment

Interventions and Rationales

URINATION

1. Assess client for continence and independent urination.

Normal Finding

■ Continent

Deviation from Normal

■ Incontinent

Indwelling Catheter

1. Assess amount, color, odor, clarity, sediment, and frequency.

Normal Findings/Deviations from Normal

■ Refer to Table 39-3 ⬭ for normal characteristics of urine.

Palpation of the Bladder

1. Palpate the area above the pubic symphysis if the client's history indicates possible urinary retention.

Normal Finding

■ Not palpable

Deviation from Normal

■ Distended and palpable as smooth, round, tense mass (indicates urinary retention)

Part G: Musculoskeletal System Assessment

Interventions and Rationales

MUSCLES

1. Inspect the muscles for size. Compare the muscles on one side of the body (e.g., of the arm, thigh, and calf) to the same muscle on the other side. For any discrepancies, measure the muscles with a tape.

2. Inspect the muscles and tendons for contractures (shortening).

3. Inspect the muscles for fasciculations and tremors. Inspect any tremors of the hands and arms by having the client hold the arms in front of the body.

BONES

1. Inspect the skeleton for normal structure and deformities.

2. Examine for scoliosis in persons over age 12. Client stands facing away from the nurse and bends over to touch the toes.

JOINTS

1. Inspect the joints for swelling.
2. Palpate each joint for tenderness, smoothness of movement, swelling, crepitation, or presence of nodules.
3. Assess joint range of motion.

Normal Findings

- Equal size on both sides of the body
- No contractures
- No fasciculations or tremors
- Normally firm
- Smooth coordinated movements
- Equal strength on each body side
- No deformities
- Straight spine
- No tenderness, swelling, crepitation, or nodules
- Joints move smoothly
- Varies to some degree in accordance with person's genetic makeup and degree of physical activity

Deviations from Normal

- Atrophy (a decrease in size) or hypertrophy (an increase in size)
- Malposition of body part (e.g., a foot fixed in dorsiflexion)
- Presence of fasciculation or tremor
- Atonic (lacking tone)
- Flaccidity (weakness or laxness) or spasticity (sudden involuntary muscle contraction)
- 25% or less of normal strength

- Bones misaligned
- A hump in the thoracic spine indicating a lateral curve
- Presence of tenderness or swelling (may indicate fractures, neoplasms, or osteoporosis)
- One or more swollen joints
- Presence of tenderness, swelling, crepitation, or nodules
- Limited range of motion in one or more joints

SAMPLE DOCUMENTATION

[date] [time] Client alert and oriented x3, eyes PERRLA, I&O 700 mL in 6 h; BP 130/80; R 16; P 80; breath sounds clear; bowel sounds present and active in all quadrants. Abdominal incision open to air, without redness or swelling, staples intact. Complained of incision pain with a stated pain level of 7. PRN Pain meds given 1100. Pain level 1 at 1145. _____

_____ Barbara Cook, LPN

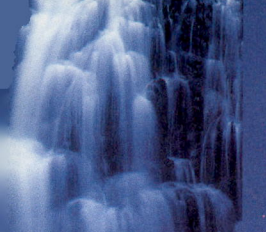

Chapter Review

KEY Points

- The health examination is conducted to assess the function and integrity of the client's body parts.
- The health examination may entail a complete head-to-toe assessment or focused assessment of one or more body systems, or focused assessment of a body part. If the head-to-toe assessment is performed during the admission process, the RN carries it out.
- Findings by the LPN/LVN during the focused assessment should be brought to the attention of the RN.
- Accurate terminology when documenting physical examination is important.
- LPNs/LVNs commonly use the techniques of inspection, auscultation, and light palpation.
- The health assessment is conducted in a systematic manner that requires the fewest position changes for the client.
- Adaptations should be made in the order of data collection if the person (for example, a child or an older adult) has attention or other issues that affect the exam.
- Aspects of the physical assessment procedures should be incorporated in the assessment, intervention, and evaluation phases of the nursing process.
- Data obtained in the physical health examination are reported to the team leader. They are used to help establish nursing diagnoses and are helpful to all nursing staff in planning the client's care and evaluating nursing care outcomes.
- Initial assessment findings provide baseline data about the client's functional abilities. Subsequent assessment findings are compared to them.

☜ FOR FURTHER Study

Refer to Chapters 3, 11, 12, and 17 for more about psychosocial aspects of care.

Chapter 14 provides more information about collecting health history data.

See Chapter 21, Procedures 21-1 through 21-4 for detailed instructions related to measuring vital signs (body temperature, pulse, respirations, and blood pressure).

See Procedure 23-1 for passive range-of-motion exercises.

Measurement of height and weight is also discussed in Chapter 25.

Chapter 28 discusses intravenous therapy.

Chapter 30 focuses on the integumentary system.

Chapter 31 illustrates and discusses the musculoskeletal system.

See Chapter 32 for more discussion of oxygenation and assessing respirations; see Procedure 32-1 for using a pulse oximeter.

Chapter 33 discusses the cardiovascular system in depth.

Chapter 36 focuses on the neurological system and special senses.

Chapter 37 provides an in-depth discussion of the gastrointestinal system.

Chapter 39 focuses on the genitourinary system; see Table 39-3 for characteristics of urine.

Critical Thinking Care Map

Caring for a Client with Activity Intolerance
NCLEX-PN® Focus Area: Physiological Integrity

Case Study: Theresa Harris, 88, was admitted from a long-term care facility yesterday to rule out pneumonia. Theresa states, "I get dizzy when I get out of bed." Theresa has a history of cerebrovascular accident with some residual weakness of the left hand.

Nursing Diagnosis: *Activity Intolerance*

COLLECT DATA

Subjective	Objective
_____	_____
_____	_____
_____	_____
_____	_____
_____	_____
_____	_____
_____	_____

Would you report this? Yes/No

If yes, report to: _____

What would you report? _____

Nursing Care

_____
_____
_____
_____
_____
_____
_____
_____
_____
_____

How would you document this? _____

_____
_____
_____

Compare your answers and documentation to those provided on the MyNursingKit Website.

Data Collected
(use only those that apply)

- Weight 135 lbs
- BP 128/80—110/72—90/50; lying/sitting/standing
- Pulse 89
- Respiratory rate at rest 18 and shallow; 26 and shallow on exertion
- Temp 99.0°F
- Skin is pale and client is diaphoretic
- Complains of dizziness on standing
- Skin dry and flaky
- Oral mucosa dry
- Taking oral antibiotics every 4 hours
- Pitcher of water is on the left side of the bed and is full
- Family not present, uninvolved in care of client
- Saline lock in place and patent
- Complains of loss of appetite over the past week
- Crackles noted in lower lobes of lungs, bilaterally
- Nonproductive cough
- Blood oxygen level 98%
- Client unmotivated to get better
- Pupils PERRLA

Nursing Interventions
(use only those that apply; list in priority order)

- Place water pitcher on client's right side, within reach.
- Determine cause of activity intolerance: physical, psychological, motivational.
- State, "You need to eat your meals to get better."
- Encourage client to change positions slowly.
- Instruct client to sit up in bed for a few minutes before standing.
- Put a bed alarm in place according to agency policy.
- Slow pace of care, allowing client extra time.
- Check orders for IV fluid administration and discuss with RN.
- When mobilizing client, monitor for orthostatic hypotension accompanied by dizziness/fainting.
- Encourage client to deep breathe and cough.
- Encourage client to increase clear fluid intake.
- Instruct client to call for assistance before ambulating.
- Use a walking belt when ambulating client.

NCLEX-PN® Exam Preparation

1. The nurse is admitting a new client to the unit. What type of assessment will be performed by the nurse on this client?
   1. Complete assessment
   2. Health history
   3. Focused assessment
   4. Focused assessment on body part causing admission

2. The nurse has performed percussion and postural drainage on a client diagnosed with pneumonia. After performing this procedure, the priority assessment would be:
   1. Level of consciousness using the Glasgow Coma Scale.
   2. Inspect, auscultate, and palpate the abdomen.
   3. Heart rate and blood pressure.
   4. Auscultation of breath sounds.

3. Assessing skin turgor, intake and output, and vital signs would be the priority assessment for which of the following clients?
   1. The client with a medical diagnosis of closed head injury.
   2. The client with a medical diagnosis of myocardial infarction.
   3. The client with a medical diagnosis of hypovolemia.
   4. The client with a medical diagnosis of right tibia fracture with a newly applied cast.

4. The nurse notes longitudinal bands on the client's fingernails, the tympanic membrane is more translucent and less flexible, and the heart rate takes longer to return to baseline after exercise. The nurse recognizes these are normal findings for a/an:
   1. Infant.
   2. School-aged child.
   3. Middle-aged adult.
   4. Elderly adult.

5. The nurse, working in a physician's office, admits a client requiring a complete annual physical examination. The client says, "I'm scared. I've never had a complete physical exam before." The nurse recognizes a priority action for preparing this client would be:
   1. Explaining what the client will experience during the examination.
   2. Measuring vital signs.
   3. Having the client undress and put on an examination gown.
   4. Inviting a family member or friend to stay with the client.

6. The nurse, working in a physician's office, admits a client who cut the palm of the right hand while using a power saw. The priority method the nurse will use to examine this client will be:
   1. Auscultation.
   2. Percussion.
   3. Palpation.
   4. Inspection.

7. The nurse examines the client's wound on the thigh close to the knee and documents the wound's location as:
   1. Superior to the knee.
   2. Medial to the knee.
   3. Distal to the knee.
   4. Proximal to the knee.

8. You are assigned to assist with the admission assessment of a client who has been living alone and is unable to provide for his own hygiene needs. As you examine the integumentary system, you notice numerous red lesions, which appear as "red tracks" under the skin. Which of the following would be an appropriate nursing action?
   1. Don gloves prior to continuing your assessment.
   2. Postpone your assessment until the nursing assistant has bathed the client.
   3. Place the client in isolation.
   4. Proceed with the assessment but do not touch the client.

9. The nurse examines the client's breath sounds and hears continuous low-pitched coarse, harsh sounds that are best heard on expiration but can also be heard on inspiration. The nurse documents these lung sounds, specifically, as:
   1. Adventitious breath sounds.
   2. Rhonchi.
   3. Rales.
   4. Wheeze.

10. Which of the following considerations would direct the order in which the nurse performs an assessment on a young child?
   1. Perform a head-to-toe assessment in order to avoid missing something.
   2. Perform a system-by-system examination in order to assess every organ system.
   3. Perform a focused assessment only on the area causing problems.
   4. Leave painful or uncomfortable examinations for last.

Answers and rationales for Review Questions appear in Appendix I.

Chapter 20

Hygiene

LEARNING Outcomes

After completing this chapter, you will be able to:

1. Describe the kinds of hygienic care provided to clients.
2. Identify factors influencing personal hygiene.
3. Identify normal and abnormal findings and interventions for nursing care of the skin, feet, and nails.
4. List and describe different kinds of baths and purposes of baths.
5. Name several points for teaching clients about foot care.
6. Identify normal and abnormal findings and interventions for nursing care of the hair.
7. Identify normal and abnormal findings and interventions for nursing care of the mouth, eyes, ears, and nose.
8. Describe ways to support a hygienic environment.
9. Describe methods of making an unoccupied and an occupied bed.
10. Identify infection control measures that are part of bed-making procedures.

Clinical Objectives

11. Provide a bed bath for an adult or pediatric client.
12. Demonstrate hair care for female and male clients.
13. Provide oral care for the unconscious client.
14. Demonstrate care of hearing aids.
15. Demonstrate bed-making procedures for occupied, unoccupied, and surgical beds.

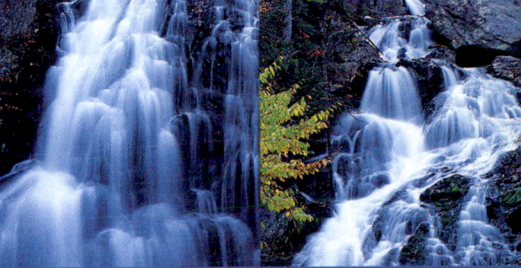

BRIEF Outline

Skin, Foot, and Nail Care

Hair Care

Mouth Care

Eye Care

Ear Care

Nose Care

Supporting a Hygienic Environment

KEY TERMS

Use the audio glossary feature on the MyNursingKit Website to hear the correct pronunciation of the following key terms.

afternoon care 393	**dandruff** 400	**hygiene** 392
alopecia 400	**dentures** 405	**lanugo** 400
as-needed (prn) care 393	**early morning care** 392	**morning care** 393
bed cradle 411	**gingiva** 403	**pediculosis** 400
caries 403	**halitosis** 404	**scabies** 401
cerumen 409	**hearing aid** 409	**sebum** 393
cleaning baths 393	**hirsutism** 401	**therapeutic baths** 393
contact lenses 407	**hour of sleep (HS) care** 393	**ticks** 400

Hygiene is the science of health and its maintenance. Personal hygiene is the self-care by which people attend to such functions as bathing, toileting, general body hygiene, and grooming. Hygiene is a highly personal matter determined by individual values and practices. Culture plays a role in how often a person bathes and how much privacy a person needs when bathing (Box 20-1 ■). Economics also plays a role, because access to warm water, soap, shampoo, and so on may be limited.

Hygiene involves care of the skin (including perineal and genital areas), hair, nails, teeth, oral and nasal cavities, eyes, and ears. Nursing assistance with hygiene also includes bed making and changing clients' clothes.

It is important for the LPN/LVN to know exactly how much assistance a client needs for hygienic care. Clients may require help after urinating or defecating, after vomiting, and whenever they become soiled, such as from wound drainage or profuse perspiration. Box 20-2 ■ lists factors that influence hygiene practices.

BOX 20-1   CULTURAL PULSE POINTS

Bathing and Body Odor

Personal hygiene is a cultural issue. The dominant North American culture seems to have an obsession with minimizing natural body odors. Daily bathing and use of deodorant, mouthwash, and perfumes is the norm. However, a client may have been raised in an area where water was limited and bathing was restricted. Or, the client may follow religious or cultural practices that prohibit bathing during the menstrual cycle or following childbirth. You may be called on to care for clients from cultures that are not bothered by body odor and do not cover up natural smells. It is important not to prejudge the person because of different values.

Another cultural issue related to bathing is gender separation. For example, in traditional Muslim families there is a strict separation of men and women socially. There are many rules for behavior and dress. The nurse will need to be sensitive to client concerns about not being bathed by a person of another gender, as well as about not having body parts uncovered.

BOX 20-2   FACTORS INFLUENCING INDIVIDUAL HYGIENIC PRACTICES

Culture: As mentioned in Box 20-1, North American culture places a high value on cleanliness. Many North Americans bathe or shower once or twice a day, whereas people from some other cultures bathe once a week. Some cultures consider privacy essential for bathing, whereas others practice communal bathing. Body odor is offensive in some cultures and accepted as normal in others.

Religion: Ceremonial washings are practiced by some religions.

Environment: Finances may affect the availability of facilities for bathing. For example, homeless people may not have warm water available; soap, shampoo, shaving lotion, and deodorants may be too expensive for people who have limited resources.

Developmental level: Children learn hygiene in the home. Practices vary according to the individual's age; for example, preschoolers can carry out most tasks independently with encouragement.

Health and energy: Ill people may not have the motivation or energy to attend to hygiene. Some clients who have neuromuscular impairments may be unable to perform hygienic care.

Personal preferences: Some people prefer a shower to a tub bath.

An important consideration when providing personal care is protection of the client's modesty. Some cultures may prohibit personal care being provided by someone of the opposite sex. Other individuals may just feel uncomfortable. If an objection is made, nursing staff should make arrangements to honor the client's request. Making sure privacy is protected and taking care to keep the client covered will alleviate the client's discomfort. A client's cultural and religious beliefs should be adhered to at all times.

The following terms are commonly used to describe types of hygienic care. **Early morning care** is provided to clients as they awaken in the morning. This care consists of providing a urinal or bedpan to the client confined to bed, washing the face and hands, and giving oral care.

Morning care is provided after clients have breakfast. It usually includes the provision of a urinal or bedpan (to clients who are not ambulatory), a bath or shower, perineal care, back massages, and oral, nail, and hair care. It also includes making the client's bed. **Afternoon care** often includes providing a bedpan or urinal, washing the hands and face, and assisting with oral care to refresh clients' mouths. **Hour of sleep (HS) care** is provided to clients before they retire for the night. It usually involves providing for elimination needs, washing face and hands, giving oral care, and giving a back massage. **As-needed (prn) care** is provided as required by the client. For example, a client who is *diaphoretic* (sweating profusely) may need frequent bathing and changes of clothes and linen.

Skin, Foot, and Nail Care

The skin is the largest organ of the body. As described in Chapter 24 ⧉, the skin protects underlying tissues from injury. It regulates body temperature. (See Chapter 21 ⧉ for a detailed discussion of body heat losses and gains.) Skin secretes an oily substance called **sebum** that softens and lubricates the hair and skin. Sebum decreases water loss from the skin when the external humidity is low. Fat is a poor conductor of heat, so sebum lessens the amount of heat lost from the skin. Sebum also has a *bactericidal* (bacteria-killing) action. Skin transmits sensations through nerve receptors, which are sensitive to pain, temperature, touch, and pressure. It also produces and absorbs vitamin D in conjunction with ultraviolet rays from the sun. The normal skin of a healthy person has transient and resident microorganisms that are not usually harmful. (See Table 10-1 ⧉.) Elderly clients exhibit skin changes that need to be considered when bathing. Their skin loses its elasticity, vascular changes occur, and many times nutritional deficiencies are present. See Box 24-1 ⧉ for factors that inhibit wound healing in older adults.

TYPES OF BATHS

Two categories of baths are given to clients: cleaning and therapeutic. **Cleaning baths** are given chiefly for hygiene purposes and include these types:

- *Complete bed bath.* The LPN/LVN washes the entire body of a dependent client in bed.
- *Self-assist bed bath.* Clients confined to bed are able to bathe themselves with assistance for the back and perhaps the feet.
- *Partial bath.* Only the parts of the client's body that might cause discomfort or odor, if neglected, are washed: the face, hands, axillae, perineal area, and back. Omitted are the arms, chest, abdomen, legs, and feet. The LPN/LVN provides this care for dependent clients and assists self-sufficient clients confined to bed by washing

their backs. Some ambulatory clients prefer to take a partial bath at the sink. The client can be assisted with washing the back.

- *Bag bath.* Required equipment consists of a plastic bag, 10 to 12 washcloths, and a cleanser and water mixture that does not require rinsing. The solution and washcloths are placed in a warmer. Each area of the body is cleaned with a different cloth and then air dried. Because the body is not rubbed dry, the emollient in the solution remains on the skin. Some agencies may provide commercially prepared, disposable bag baths. Each pack usually contains enough wipes to bathe the entire body. These are warmed in the warmer according to directions on the packaging.
- *Tub bath.* Tub baths are preferred to bed baths because it is easier to wash and rinse in a tub. Tubs are also used for therapeutic baths. The amount of assistance offered depends on the abilities of the client. Specially designed tubs are available for dependent clients. These tubs greatly reduce the work and potential for injury in lifting clients in and out of the tub and offer greater benefits than a sponge bath in bed.
- *Shower.* Many ambulatory clients are able to use shower facilities and require only minimal assistance.

Therapeutic baths are given for physical effects, such as to soothe irritated skin or to treat an area (e.g., the perineum). Medications may be placed in the water. A therapeutic bath is generally taken in a tub one-third or one-half full, about 114 L (30 gal). The client remains in the bath for a designated time, often 20 to 30 minutes. If the client's back, chest, and arms are to be treated, these areas need to be immersed in the solution. The bath temperature is generally included in the order; 37.7° to 46°C (100° to 115°F) may be ordered for adults, and 40.5°C (105°F) is usually ordered for infants. Procedure 20-1 ▪ on page 413 provides guidelines for bathing clients.

Purposes of Baths

Bathing removes accumulated oil, perspiration, dead skin cells, and some bacteria. The uppermost layer of the epidermis is composed of dead cells that are continuously being shed by the millions and replaced.

Excessive bathing, however, can interfere with the intended lubricating effect of the sebum, causing dryness of the skin. This is an important consideration, especially for older adults, who produce less sebum.

In addition to cleaning the skin, bathing stimulates circulation. A warm or hot bath dilates superficial arterioles, bringing more blood and nourishment to the skin. Vigorous rubbing has the same effect. Rubbing with long smooth strokes from the distal to proximal parts of extremities (from the point farthest from the body to the point closest) is particularly effective in facilitating venous blood flow.

Bathing also produces a sense of well-being. It is refreshing and relaxing and frequently improves morale, appearance, and self-respect. Some people take a morning shower for its refreshing, stimulating effect. Others prefer an evening bath because it is relaxing. These effects are more evident when a person is ill. For example, it is not uncommon for clients who have had a restless or sleepless night to feel relaxed, comfortable, and sleepy after a morning bath.

Bathing offers an excellent opportunity for the LPN/LVN to assess ill clients. During the bath, it is easy to observe the condition of the client's skin and physical conditions such as sacral edema or rashes. While assisting a client with a bath, the LPN/LVN can also assess the client's psychosocial needs, such as orientation to time and ability to cope with the illness. Learning needs, such as a diabetic client's need to learn foot care, can also be assessed.

Toileting before Baths

To feel most relaxed, people generally use toileting facilities before taking a bath. Clients who are restricted to bed may need assistance in using a bedpan. There are two main types of bedpans: the regular high-back pan and the fracture pan.

The fracture pan has a low back and is used for clients who cannot raise their buttocks. Nursing guidelines for placing and removing a bedpan are presented in Box 20-3 ■ and Figures 20-1 and 20-2 ■. Female clients use a bedpan for both urine and feces. Male clients use a urinal for urine.

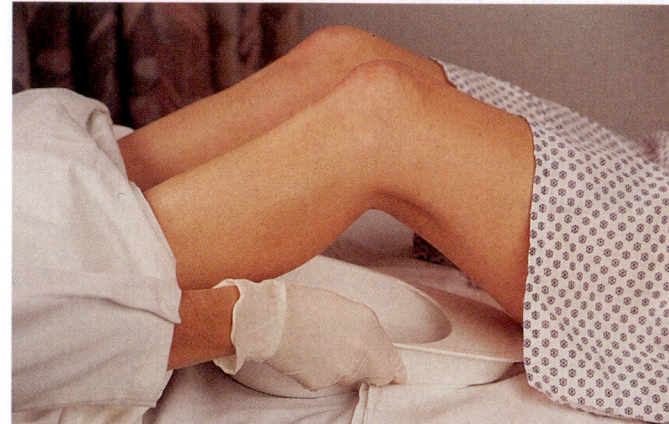

Figure 20-1. ■ Placing a slipper (fracture) pan under the buttocks of a client. (*Source:* © Elena Dorfman.)

BOX 20-3　NURSING CARE CHECKLIST

Giving and Removing a Bedpan

- ☑ Provide privacy.
- ☑ Wear disposable gloves.
- ☑ If the bedpan is metal, warm it by rinsing it with warm water.
- ☑ Adjust the bed to a height appropriate to prevent back strain.
- ☑ Elevate the side rail on the opposite side to prevent the client from falling out of bed.
- ☑ Ask the client to assist by flexing the knees, resting the weight on the back and heels, and raising the buttocks, or by using a trapeze bar, if present.
- ☑ Help lift the client as needed by placing one hand under the lower back, resting your elbow on the mattress, and using your forearm as a lever.
- ☑ Place a regular bedpan so that the client's buttocks rest on the smooth, rounded rim. Place a fracture pan with the flat, low end under the client's buttocks (Figure 20-1).
- ☑ For the client who cannot assist, obtain the assistance of another nurse to help lift the client onto the bedpan. Or, place the client on his or her side, place the bedpan against the buttocks (Figure 20-2), and roll the client back onto the bedpan.
- ☑ To provide a more normal position for the client's lower back, elevate the client's bed to a semi-Fowler's position, if permitted. If elevation is contraindicated, support the client's back with pillows as needed to prevent hyperextension of the back.

- ☑ Cover the client with bed linen to maintain comfort and self-dignity.
- ☑ Provide toilet tissue, place the call light within reach, lower the bed to the low position, elevate the side rail if indicated, and leave the client alone.
- ☑ Answer the call bell promptly.
- ☑ When removing the bedpan, return the bed to the position used when giving the bedpan. Hold the bedpan steady to prevent spillage of its contents. Cover the bedpan, and place it on the bedside chair.
- ☑ If the client needs assistance with cleaning, don gloves and wipe the client's perineal area with several layers of toilet tissue. If a specimen is to be collected, discard the soiled tissue into a moisture-proof receptacle other than the bedpan. For female clients, clean from the urethra toward the anus to prevent the transfer of rectal microorganisms into the urinary meatus.
- ☑ Wash the perineal area of dependent clients with soap and water as indicated, and dry the area thoroughly.
- ☑ For all clients, offer warm water, soap, a washcloth, and a towel to wash the hands.
- ☑ Assist the client to a comfortable position, empty and clean the bedpan, and return it to the bedside.
- ☑ Remove and discard your gloves and wash your hands.
- ☑ Document color, odor, amount, and consistency of urine and feces, and the condition of the perineal area.

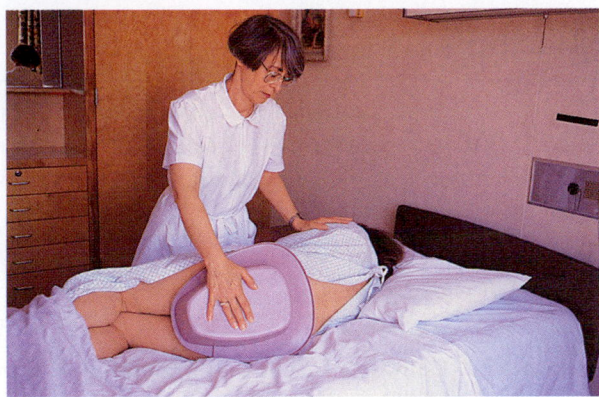

Figure 20-2. ■ Placing a bedpan against a client's buttocks.

Most male clients can use a urinal independently either in bed or when standing at the bedside. If the client needs support to stand, the nurse remains with him. If the client cannot stand at the bedside, the urinal can be placed between the client's legs with the handle uppermost so that urine will flow into it.

FEET

The feet are essential for ambulation. They need attention even when people are confined to bed. Children's feet are easily damaged by tight, binding stockings and ill-fitting shoes. They should be well supported, and the bony structure and the feet should grow without restrictions. Feet are not fully grown until about age 20. Healthy feet remain relatively unchanged during life. However, the elderly often require special attention for their feet. Reduced blood supply and accompanying arteriosclerosis can make a foot prone to infection following trauma. Common foot problems include calluses, corns, unpleasant odors, plantar warts, fissures between the toes, and fungal infections such as athlete's foot.

NAILS

Nails are normally present at birth. They continue to grow throughout life and change very little until people are elderly. At that time, the nails tend to be tougher, more brittle, and in some cases thicker. The nails of an older person normally grow less quickly than those of a younger person and may be ridged and grooved.

NURSING CARE

PRIORITIZING NURSING CARE

Bathing and skin care are frequently delegated to unlicensed assistive personnel (UAP) because of time constraints on the licensed nurse. These tasks should be made a priority since bathing, hair, nail, and foot care provide an opportunity to collect a large amount of data. It is the one time when the nurse can observe the client's whole body. Although the UAP can make general observations of the condition of the skin, feet, hair, and nails, they do not have the knowledge to interpret minute changes that may be significant and may signal future problems.

Bathing also gives the nurse the opportunity to complete a general psychosocial assessment and to provide emotional support by communicating with the client during the procedure. Hygiene and the cleanliness of the environment were at the center of Nightingale's nursing theory and practice; they should still be a priority for nurses today.

ASSESSING

The LPN/LVN checks the nursing history for the client's skin care practices, self-care abilities, and past or current skin problems. Data about the client's skin care practices enable the LPN/LVN to incorporate the client's needs and preferences as much as possible in the plan of care and to determine necessary learning needs. Clients may have difficulty performing bathing activities. They may not be able to wash the body or certain body parts, to obtain or get to a water source, or to regulate water temperature or flow. Clients may also have difficulties in dressing and grooming. They may not be able to obtain, put on, take off, fasten, or replace articles of clothing; and to maintain appearance at a satisfactory level. They may have difficulties with toileting, such as getting to the toilet or commode, or sitting on and rising from it. Also, clients may have trouble manipulating their clothes for toileting, cleaning themselves after using the toilet, flushing the toilet, or emptying the *commode* (portable toilet, often used at the bedside by people who have limited mobility).

The client's self-care abilities determine the amount of nursing assistance and the kind of bath (bed, tub, or shower) the client requires. The client's balance, coordination, and strength are important factors. The confused or very ill client will lack the motivation and energy to provide self-care. It is important to determine the client's functional level, so the nurse can maintain and promote as much client independence as possible. This also enables the LPN/LVN to identify the client's potential for growth and rehabilitation.

A physical assessment of the skin is performed, and clients who are at risk for developing skin impairment are identified (Box 20-4 ■). The presence of past or current skin problems alerts the LPN/LVN to specific nursing interventions or referrals the client may require. Common skin problems and implications for nursing interventions are shown in Table 20-1 ■. Refer to Chapter 30 ∞ for types and descriptions of skin lesions.

Physical assessment of the skin, feet, and nails, which involves inspection and palpation, is discussed in Chapter 19 ∞ (see Table 19-3 and Figures 19-4 and 19-13) and described further in Integumentary Disorders, Chapter 30 ∞.

BOX 20-4	RISK FACTORS FOR SELF-CARE DEFICIT

- Visual impairment
- Activity intolerance or weakness
- Pain or discomfort
- Mental impairment
- Neuromuscular or skeletal impairment
- Psychological or motivation impairment
- Medically prescribed restriction
- Therapeutic procedure restraining mobility (e.g., intravenous infusion, cast)
- Environmental barriers

A systematic head-to-toe assessment includes collection of data about skin color, uniformity of color, texture, turgor, temperature, intactness, and lesions.

Attention is paid to risk factors for foot problems (such as diabetes) and foot discomfort. The feet are assessed at the beginning and end of each shift, unless otherwise ordered. Changes are reported to the RN.

DIAGNOSING, PLANNING, AND IMPLEMENTING

For clients who have problems performing hygiene care, *Self-Care Deficit* diagnoses are used in collaboration with the LPN/LVN. Three *Self-Care Deficit* diagnoses are discussed in this chapter:

- *Bathing Self-Care Deficit*
- *Dressing Self-Care Deficit*
- *Toileting Self-Care Deficit*

Associated diagnoses commonly include *Deficient Knowledge* (e.g., related to lack of experience with skin condition and treatment) and *Risk for Situational Low Self-Esteem* (e.g., related to body odor). The diagnoses *Risk for Impaired Skin Integrity* and *Impaired Skin Integrity* are discussed in Chapter 24 ⬭.

In planning care, the LPN/LVN identifies nursing interventions that will assist the client to maintain or improve skin cleanliness, maintain circulation to the skin, and improve or maintain a sense of well-being. Nursing activities for hygiene include assisting dependent clients with bathing,

TABLE 20-1	Common Skin Problems and Nursing Implications
PROBLEM AND APPEARANCE	**NURSING IMPLICATIONS**
ABRASION Superficial layers of the skin are scraped or rubbed away. Area is reddened and may have localized bleeding or serous weeping.	1. Prone to infection; therefore, wound should be kept clean and dry. 2. Do not wear rings or jewelry when providing care to avoid causing abrasions to clients. 3. Lift, do not pull, a client across a bed. See Chapter 23 ⬭ .
EXCESSIVE DRYNESS Skin can appear flaky and rough.	1. Prone to infection if the skin cracks; therefore, provide alcohol-free lotions to moisturize the skin and prevent cracking. 2. Bathe client less frequently; use no soap, or limit use of nonirritating soap. Rinse skin thoroughly because soap can be irritating and drying. 3. Encourage increased fluid intake if health permits to prevent dehydration.
AMMONIA DERMATITIS (DIAPER RASH) Caused by skin bacteria reacting with urea in the urine. The skin becomes reddened and is sore.	1. Keep skin dry and clean by applying protective ointments containing zinc oxide to areas at risk. (Ointments may require a physician's order.)
ACNE Inflammatory condition with papules and pustules.	1. Keep the skin clean to prevent secondary infection. 2. Treatment varies widely.
ERYTHEMA Redness associated with a variety of conditions, such as rashes, exposure to sun, elevated body temperature.	1. Wash area carefully to remove excess microorganisms. 2. Apply antiseptic spray or lotion to prevent itching, promote healing, and prevent skin breakdown.
HIRSUTISM Excessive hair on a person's body and face, particularly in women.	1. Remove unwanted hair by using depilatories, shaving, electrolysis, or tweezing. 2. Enhance client's self-concept. See Chapter 17 ⬭ .

skin and nail care, and perineal care; providing back massages to promote circulation (discussed in Chapter 23 ⚭); and providing instruction to clients about ways to promote good hygiene and prevent skin lesions.

When planning to assist a client with personal hygiene, the nurse considers the client's personal preferences, health, and limitations; the best time to give the care; and the equipment, facilities, and personnel available. A client's personal preferences about when and how to bathe should be followed as long as they are compatible with the client's health and the equipment available. The LPN/LVN provides whatever assistance the client requires, either directly or by delegating this task to other nursing personnel.

Examples of desired outcomes for clients with self-care deficits might be:

- Client bathes in tub twice weekly with assistance.
- Client participates in self-care (foot hygiene) to optimal level of capacity (specify).
- Client reports satisfaction with appearance.
- Client demonstrates nail care as instructed.

Nursing guidelines for providing skin care to clients are listed in Box 20-5 ■.

Bathing

Sponge baths are suggested for the newborn to prevent hypothermia. An infant's ability to regulate body temperature has not yet fully developed. Body surface area is very large in relation to body mass, contributing to heat loss. Infants perspire minimally, and shivering starts at a lower temperature. Therefore, significant heat loss occurs before shivering begins. After the bath, the infant should be immediately dried and wrapped (swaddled) for warmth.

Caution is needed when bathing clients who are receiving intravenous therapy. Easy-to-remove gowns that have Velcro or snap fasteners along the sleeves may be used. If a special gown is not available, the LPN/LVN must pay special attention when changing the client's gown after the bath (or whenever the gown becomes soiled). Guidelines for changing a hospital gown are provided in Box 20-6 ■. These guidelines do not apply if the client has an IV pump or controller. In this situation, use a special gown or do not put the sleeve of a gown over the client's involved arm.

The water for a bath should feel comfortably warm to the client. People vary in their sensitivity to heat; generally, the temperature should be 43° to 46°C (110° to 115°F). Most clients can verify a comfortable temperature. The water for a bed bath should be changed at least once.

Perineal-Genital Care

Perineal-genital care is also referred to as perineal care or peri-care. Perineal care as part of the bed bath is embarrassing for many clients. LPNs/LVNs also may find it embarrassing

| BOX 20-5 | NURSING CARE CHECKLIST |

Skin Care Guidelines
Dry Skin
- ☑ Use cleansing creams to clean the skin rather than soap or detergent, which cause drying and, in some cases, allergic reactions.
- ☑ Use bath oils, but take precautions to prevent falls caused by slippery tub surfaces.
- ☑ Thoroughly rinse soap or detergent (if used) from the skin.
- ☑ Bathe less frequently when environmental temperature and humidity are low.
- ☑ Increase fluid intake.
- ☑ Humidify the air with a humidifier.
- ☑ Use moisturizing or emollient creams that contain lanolin, petroleum jelly, or cocoa butter to retain skin moisture.

Skin Rashes
- ☑ Keep the area clean by washing it with a mild soap. Rinse the skin well, and pat it dry.
- ☑ To relieve itching, try a tepid bath or soak. Some over-the-counter preparations, such as Caladryl lotion, may help but should be used with full knowledge of the product.
- ☑ Avoid scratching the rash to prevent inflammation, infection, and further skin lesions.
- ☑ Choose clothing carefully. Too much can cause perspiration and aggravate a rash.

Acne
- ☑ Wash the face frequently with mild soap or detergent and water to remove oil and dirt.
- ☑ Avoid using oily creams, which aggravate the condition.
- ☑ Avoid using cosmetics that block the ducts of the sebaceous glands and the hair follicles.
- ☑ Never squeeze or pick at the lesions. This increases the potential for infection and scarring.

initially, particularly with clients of the opposite sex. Most clients who require a bed bath are able to clean their own genital areas with minimal assistance. The LPN/LVN may need to hand a moistened washcloth and soap to the client, rinse the washcloth, and provide a towel.

Because some clients are unfamiliar with terminology for the genitals and perineum, it may be difficult to explain what is expected. Most clients, however, understand what is meant if the LPN/LVN simply says, "I'll give you a washcloth to finish your bath." Older clients may be familiar with the term "private parts." Whatever expression is used, it needs to be one that the client understands and one that is comfortable for the LPN/LVN to use.

BOX 20-6   NURSING CARE CHECKLIST

Changing a Hospital Gown for a Client with an IV Infusion

☑ Slip the gown completely off the arm without the infusion and onto the tubing connected to the arm with the infusion.

☑ Holding the container above the client's arm, slide the sleeve up over the container to remove the used gown.

☑ Place the clean gown sleeve for the arm with the infusion over the container as if it were an extension of the client's arm, from the inside of the gown to the sleeve cuff.

☑ Rehang the container. Slide the gown carefully over the tubing toward the client's hand.

☑ Guide the client's arm and tubing into the sleeve, taking care not to pull on the tubing.

☑ Assist the client to put the other arm into the second sleeve of the gown, and fasten as usual.

☑ Count the rate of flow of the infusion to make sure it is correct before leaving the bedside. Immediately report an incorrect rate of flow to the RN.

The LPN/LVN needs to provide perineal care efficiently and matter-of-factly. Nurses wear gloves while providing this care, both for the comfort of the client and to protect themselves from infection. Part B of Procedure 20-1 explains how to provide perineal-genital care.

Foot

Interventions may include teaching the client about correct nail and foot care, proper footwear, and ways to prevent potential foot problems (e.g., infection, injury, and decreased circulation). For clients with self-care difficulties, the LPN/LVN plans a schedule for soaking the client's feet and assisting with regular cleaning and trimming of nails (if not contraindicated and within agency policy). Foot and nail care is often provided during the client's bath but may be provided at any time in the day to accommodate the client's preference or schedule. The LPN/LVN and client determine the frequency of foot care. It is based on objective assessment data and the client's specific problems. For some clients, the feet need to be bathed daily; for those whose feet perspire excessively, bathing more than once a day may be necessary.

Part C of Procedure 20-1 describes how to provide foot care. (See also discussion of nails.) During these procedures, the LPN/LVN has the opportunity to teach the client appropriate methods for foot care (see Continuity of Care in next column). Clients with reduced peripheral circulation to the feet, such as clients with diabetes or peripheral vascular disease, may require specialized care by a physician or podiatrist. These clients should be discouraged from attempting

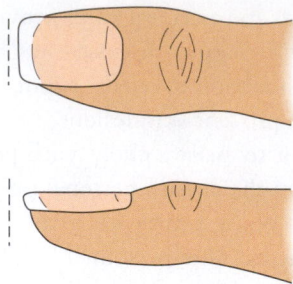

Figure 20-3. ■ Fingernails are trimmed straight across.

some aspects of personal foot care and cautioned about "commercial" pedicures, such as at salons or spas.

Nails

One hand or foot is soaked, if needed, and dried. Then the nail is cut or filed straight across beyond the end of the finger or toe (Figure 20-3 ■). Avoid trimming or digging into nails at the lateral corners. (This predisposes the client to ingrown toenails.) File rather than cut the nails of clients who have diabetes or circulatory problems. Inadvertent injury to tissues can occur if scissors are used. After the initial cut or filing, file the nail to round the corners, and clean under the nail. Push the cuticle back gently, taking care not to injure it. Care for the next finger or toe in the same manner. Record and report any abnormality, such as inflammation of the tissue around the nail, to the RN.

EVALUATING

Using data collected during care, the LPN/LVN judges whether desired outcomes have been achieved, and documents changes in self-care. The nurse determines whether the client maintains skin cleanliness, reports satisfaction with appearance, states that feet are not as sore, and so on. If the outcomes are not achieved, the LPN/LVN explores reasons why. For example:

■ Did the LPN/LVN overestimate the client's functional abilities (physical, mental, emotional) for self-care?

■ Were provided instructions not clear?

■ Were appropriate assistive devices or supplies not available to the client?

■ Did the client's condition change?

■ Were required analgesics provided before hygienic care?

■ What currently prescribed medications and therapies could affect the client's abilities or tissue integrity?

■ Is the client's fluid and food intake adequate or appropriate to maintain skin and mucous membrane moisture and integrity?

Continuity of Care

To provide for continuity of care when a client is to be discharged, the nurse assesses the client's and family's abilities for care. Referrals and home health services may be required.

BOX 20-7   CLIENT TEACHING

Teaching for Discharge: Foot Care

- Wash the feet daily, and dry them well, especially between the toes.
- When washing, inspect the skin of the feet for breaks or red or swollen areas. Use a mirror if needed to visualize all areas.
- To prevent burns, check the water temperature before immersing the feet.
- Use creams or lotions to moisten the skin, or soak the feet in warm water with Epsom salts to avoid excessive drying of the skin of the feet. Lotion will also soften calluses. A lotion that reduces dryness effectively is a mixture of lanolin and mineral oil.
- To prevent or control an unpleasant odor due to excessive foot perspiration, wash the feet frequently and change socks and shoes at least daily. Special deodorant sprays or absorbent foot powders are also helpful.
- File the toenails rather than cutting them to avoid skin injury. File the nails straight across the ends of the toes. If the nails are too thick or misshapen to file, consult a podiatrist.
- Wear clean stockings or socks daily. Avoid socks with holes or darns that can cause pressure areas.
- Wear correctly fitting shoes that neither restrict the foot nor rub on any area; rubbing can cause corns and calluses. Check worn shoes for rough spots in the lining. Break in new shoes gradually by increasing the wearing time 30 to 60 minutes each day.
- Avoid walking barefoot, because injury and infection may result. Wear slippers in public showers and in change areas to avoid contracting athlete's foot or other infections.
- Several times each day exercise the feet to promote circulation. Point the feet upward, point them downward, and move them in circles.
- Avoid wearing constricting garments such as knee-high elastic stockings and avoid sitting with the legs crossed at the knees, which may decrease circulation.
- When the feet are cold, use extra blankets and wear warm socks rather than using heating pads or hot water bottles, which may cause burns. Test bathwater before stepping into it.
- Wash any cut on the foot thoroughly, apply a mild antiseptic, and notify the physician.
- Avoid self-treatment for corns or calluses. Pumice stones and some callus and corn applications are injurious to the skin. Consult a podiatrist or physician first.
- Notify the physician if you notice abnormal sores or drainage, pain, or changes in temperature, color, and sensation of the foot.

Also, the nurse determines the client's learning needs and provides written or verbal instructions as needed. Use the guidelines listed in Box 20-5 to provide client teaching on general skin care. Clients with impaired circulation or diabetes are especially in need of teaching about foot care (Box 20-7 ■).

NURSING PROCESS CARE PLAN
Client with Diabetes

Gerard Bucholz is a 52-year-old, divorced man who was admitted to the hospital with a nonhealing cut on his left, great toe. The cut occurred when Mr. Bucholz trimmed his toenails a month ago. He is an insulin-dependent diabetic and was diagnosed 6 years ago. It has taken him most of the 6 years to begin managing his diabetes well and to comply with his prescribed diet. Although his blood sugars have been in good control over the last 1.5 years, the high blood sugar in the past has resulted in poor peripheral circulation. His lower extremities are mainly affected, but he does complain of decreased sensation in his fingertips. Mr. Bucholz states, "Nobody ever told me I shouldn't cut my nails."

Assessment
T 98.6, P 72, R 18, BP 130/72. Pedal pulses weak, bilaterally, radial pulses palpable. Feet cold to touch; client denies feeling in toes when touched. Hands cool; client states he has feeling in the tips when touched. Ulcerated area on left, great toe, approximately 2 cm by 2 cm. Skin around and inside ulcer is black; client denies pain. The bone is visible.

Nursing Diagnosis
The following important nursing diagnoses (among others) are established for this client:

- *Impaired Skin Integrity* related to nonhealing skin injury
- *Deficient Knowledge* (diabetic nail care) related to possible lack of exposure to information

Expected Outcomes
The expected outcomes for the plan of care are that Mr. Bucholz will:

- Demonstrate proper nail care.
- Have no further injuries to the extremities as a result of improper nail care.

Planning and Implementation
The following nursing interventions are implemented for Mr. Bucholz:

- Discuss with client the relationship between diabetes and decreased peripheral circulation.
- Discuss with client other activities that may cause impaired skin integrity, for example, possible burn related to use of a heating pad on areas with impaired circulation, going without proper footwear outside.

- Demonstrate proper nail care techniques to client.
- Supply client with handouts explaining proper nail care techniques and encourage him to keep them in an accessible area at home.

Evaluation

Mr. Bucholz is able to repeat information given to him regarding proper nail care. He has made a monthly appointment with a podiatrist near his home.

Critical Thinking in the Nursing Process

1. What might have helped Mr. Bucholz to avoid cutting himself in the first place?

2. Why is it important to note in the evaluation that Mr. Bucholz has contacted a podiatrist and has a standing appointment?

3. What is the possible consequence of untreated foot injuries for clients with poor peripheral circulation?

Note: Discussion of Critical Thinking questions appears on the MyNursingKit Website.

Hair Care

The appearance of the hair often reflects a person's feelings or general state of health. A person who feels ill may neglect grooming. Changes in hair texture and volume can result from disease or medication. For example, hypothyroidism may cause excessively thin, dry, or brittle hair. Chemotherapy or radiation to treat cancer often causes hair loss (**alopecia**).

Newborns may have **lanugo** (the fine hair on the body of the fetus, also referred to as down or woolly hair) over their shoulders, back, and sacrum. This generally disappears, and the hair distribution on the eyebrows, head, and eyelashes of young children becomes noticeable. Some newborns have hair on their scalps. Others grow hair over the scalp during the first year.

Pubic hair usually appears in early puberty followed in about 6 months by the growth of axillary hair. Boys develop facial hair in later puberty. In adolescence, sebaceous glands activity increases. Hair follicle openings enlarge to accommodate increased sebum, which can make the adolescent's hair more oily.

In older adults, the hair is generally thinner, grows more slowly, and loses its color as a result of aging tissues and diminishing circulation. Men often lose their scalp hair and may become completely bald. Male baldness is influenced by genetics; it may occur even when a man is relatively young. The older person's hair also tends to become drier. Axillary and pubic hair becomes finer and scanter, but eyebrows become bristly and coarse. Many women develop some facial hair.

NURSING CARE

PRIORITIZING NURSING CARE

Hair care needs to be provided on a daily basis. Clean and groomed hair can help the client to feel better. Long hair should be braided to keep it contained and prevent it from getting matted. Hair that has been soiled by vomitus, blood, or perspiration should be shampooed. If the client is unable to shower, a waterless shampoo or "bag shampoo" may be used. The nurse should be observant of any conditions of the scalp that require medical treatment.

ASSESSING

During the nursing history, data about usual hair care, self-care abilities, history of hair or scalp problems, and conditions (such as hypothyroidism) that affect the hair are obtained. Questions about medications, hair dyes, and curling or straightening preparations can provide more information to assess dry and brittle hair. Common hair problems follow.

Often accompanied by itching, **dandruff** appears as a diffuse scaling of the scalp. In severe cases, it involves the auditory canals and the eyebrows. Dandruff can usually be treated effectively with a commercial shampoo. In severe or persistent cases, the client may need the advice of a physician.

Hair loss and growth are continual processes. By middle age, some permanent thinning of hair normally occurs. Baldness, common in men, is thought to be a hereditary problem. Hairpieces, surgical hair transplantation, and various medications address the issue of baldness.

Ticks are small, gray-brown parasites that bite into tissue and suck blood. Ticks transmit several diseases to people, including Rocky Mountain spotted fever, Lyme disease, babesiosis, and tularemia. Ticks should never be forcibly pulled from the skin because the sucking apparatus remains and may become infected. To ease removal, cover the tick with mineral oil or a lubricating jelly such as petroleum jelly. This deprives the tick of oxygen, and allows it to be removed more easily.

Lice are parasitic insects that infest mammals. They are very small, grayish white, and difficult to see. The crab louse in the pubic area has red legs. Lice may be contracted from infested clothes and direct contact with an infested person. Infestation with lice is called **pediculosis.** Hundreds of varieties of lice infest humans. Three common kinds are *Pediculus capitis* (the head louse), *Pediculus corporis* (the body louse), and *Pediculus pubis* (the crab louse).

Pediculus capitis tends to stay hidden in scalp hair; similarly, *Pediculus pubis* stays in pubic hair. Head and pubic lice lay their eggs on the hairs. The eggs are oval, similar to dandruff, and they cling to the hair. Bites and pustular eruptions may be noticed at the hairline and behind the ears. *Pediculus corporis* tends to cling to clothing, so when a client undresses, the lice may not be seen on the body. These lice suck blood from the person and lay their eggs on the clothing. The nurse can suspect their presence in the clothing if (1) the person habitually scratches, (2) there are scratches on the skin, and (3) there are hemorrhagic spots on the skin where the lice have sucked blood.

Gamma benzene hexachloride (Kwell) was widely used for treatment of pediculosis, but serious side effects and parasite resistance with its use were reported. It is more common now to use an over-the-counter preparation such as pyrethrin shampoo. If the client has head lice, the hair is washed with the shampoo and the bed linens are changed. This treatment is repeated 12 to 24 hours later if needed. A client with pubic or body lice takes a bath or shower, dries, and applies the lotion or cream—to the entire body surface for body lice, and to the pubic area and adjacent areas for pubic lice. After 12 to 24 hours the lotion is washed off, and clean clothing and linens are supplied.

Scabies is a contagious skin infestation by the itch mite. The characteristic lesion is the burrow produced by the female mite as it penetrates into the upper layers of the skin. Burrows are short, wavy, brown or black threadlike lesions, usually seen between the webs of the fingers and the folds of the wrists and elbows. The mites cause intense itching. Itching is more pronounced at night, because the increased warmth of the skin stimulates the parasites. Secondary lesions caused by scratching include vesicles, papules, pustules, excoriations, and crusts. Treatment involves thorough cleansing of the body with soap and water to remove scales and debris from crusts, and then an application of a scabicide lotion. All bed linens and clothing are washed in very hot or boiling water.

clinical ALERT

Because some conditions of the scalp are highly contagious, the nurse should always don gloves for the initial physical assessment of the scalp and hair.

The growth of excessive body hair is called **hirsutism.** The acceptance of body hair in the axillae and on the legs is largely dictated by culture. In North America media, well-groomed women are depicted with no hair on the legs or under axillae. In many other cultures, it is customary for women not to remove this hair. Excessive facial hair on a woman is thought unattractive in most Western and Asian cultures.

The cause of excessive body hair is not always known. Older women may have some on their faces, and women in menopause may also experience the growth of facial hair. These conditions may be due to hormonal changes. Heredity also influences the pattern of hair distribution and the production of androgens by the adrenal glands.

Inflammation, flaking, and itching may also be produced by a fungal infection of the skin. When it appears on the upper body, it is sometimes called *ringworm*. When it appears in the groin, it is commonly called *jock itch*. A fungal infection of the feet produces redness, peeling, and cracking of the skin and is commonly known as *athlete's foot*.

DIAGNOSING, PLANNING, AND IMPLEMENTING

Nursing diagnoses related to hair hygiene and hair and scalp problems include:

- *Dressing Self-Care Deficit*
- *Impaired Skin Integrity*
- *Risk for Infection*
- *Disturbed Body Image*

Factors such as imposed immobility (bed rest), pain in upper extremities, and insect bite can contribute to these diagnoses.

Examples of desired outcomes might be:

- Client performs hair grooming with assistance (specify).
- Client has reduced or absent scalp lesions or infestations.
- Client takes preventive measures for specific hair problem (e.g., dandruff).

Plans for assisting the client should take into account the client's personal preferences, health, and energy resources as well as the time, equipment, and personnel available. Often, clients like to receive hair care after a bath, before receiving visitors, and before retiring. At some agencies, shampoos can be given to clients only after a physician's order.

Shampooing the Hair

Hair should be washed as often as needed to keep it clean. There are several ways to shampoo clients' hair, depending on their health, strength, and age. The client who is well enough to take a shower can shampoo there. The client who is unable to shower may be given a shampoo while sitting on a chair in front of a sink. The client who must remain in bed can be given a shampoo with water brought to the bedside. Shampoo basins to catch the water and direct it to the washbasin or other receptacle are usually made of plastic or metal. A pail or large washbasin can be used to catch the shampoo water. If possible, the receptacle should be large enough to hold all of the shampoo water so that it does not have to be emptied during the shampoo.

Water used for the shampoo should be 40.5°C (105°F) for an adult or child to be comfortable and not injure the scalp. Usually the client will supply a liquid or cream shampoo. If the shampoo is being given to destroy lice, a medicated shampoo should be used. Dry shampoos are also available. They will remove some of the dirt, odor, and oil. Their main disadvantage is that they dry the hair and scalp.

How often a person needs a shampoo is highly individual, depending largely on the person's activities and the amount of sebum secreted by the scalp. Oily hair tends to look stringy and dirty, and it feels unclean to the person.

Another option available for shampoo for bed rest clients is commercial "bag shampoo." The shampoo solution is in a shower cap that can be warmed in the microwave or a warming device and then used in the same manner as the "bag bath" discussed earlier. After warming, the cap is placed on the client's head for 20 minutes. The nurse massages the client's head through the cap prior to removing. The hair is towel dried and styled. Part A of Procedure 20-2 ■ on page 418 explains how to provide a shampoo for a client confined to bed.

Brushing and Combing Hair

To be healthy, hair needs to be brushed daily. Brushing stimulates the circulation of blood in the scalp, distributes the oil along the hair shaft, and helps to arrange the hair.

For clients confined to bed, hair should be combed and brushed at least once a day to prevent matting. A brush with stiff bristles provides the best stimulation to the scalp, but bristles should not be sharp enough to injure the client's scalp. A comb with dull, even teeth is advisable. Some clients are pleased to have their hair tied neatly in the back or braided until other assistance is available or until they feel better and can look after it themselves.

African American people often have thicker, drier, curlier hair than many Caucasian people. Spiraled or very curly hair may stand out from the scalp and has less strength than straight hair. If straightened, it tends to tangle and mat easily, especially at the back and the sides if the client is confined to bed. Some African Americans style their hair in small braids (Figure 20-4 ■). These braids do not have to be unbraided for shampooing and washing. The LPN/LVN should obtain the client's permission before any such unbraiding. Some people with spiraled hair need to oil their hair daily to prevent hair strands from breaking and the scalp from becoming too dry.

Procedure 20-2, Part B, describes how to provide hair care for African American clients.

Beard and Mustache Care

Beards and mustaches also require daily care. The most important aspect of the care is to keep them clean. Food particles tend to collect in beards and mustaches, and they need

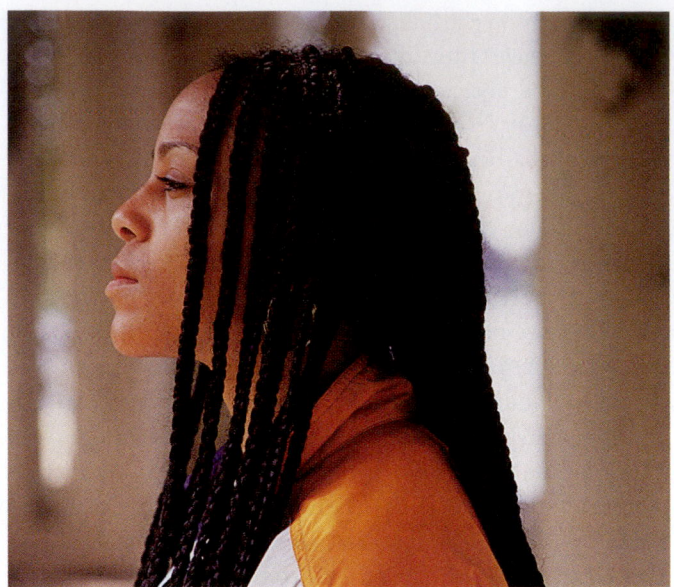

Figure 20-4. ■ An African American's hair styled with braids. (Photographer: Elena Dorfman.)

washing and combing periodically. Clients may also wish a beard or mustache trim to maintain a well-groomed appearance. A beard or mustache should not be shaved off without the client's consent.

Male clients often shave or are shaved after a bath. Frequently clients supply their own electric or safety razors. Box 20-8 ■ lists the steps involved in shaving facial hair with a safety razor.

BOX 20-8   NURSING CARE CHECKLIST

Using a Safety Razor to Shave Facial Hair

☑ Don gloves in case there are facial nicks and contact with blood.

☑ Check client's medication record for drugs in which shaving with a blade is contraindicated (i.e., anticoagulants).

☑ Apply shaving cream or soap and water to soften the bristles and make the skin more pliable.

☑ Hold the skin taut, particularly around creases, to prevent cutting the skin.

☑ Hold the razor so that the blade is at a 45-degree angle to the skin, and shave in short, firm strokes in the direction of hair growth.

☑ After shaving the entire area, wipe the client's face with a wet washcloth to remove any remaining shaving cream and hair.

☑ Dry the face well, then apply aftershave lotion or powder as the client prefers.

☑ To prevent irritating the skin, pat on the lotion with the fingers and avoid rubbing the face.

EVALUATING

The nurse collects data to determine whether desired outcomes have been reached.

Mouth Care

Teeth begin to appear 5 to 8 months after birth, and by age 2 years, children usually have all 20 temporary teeth (Figure 20-5A ■). These are gradually replaced by the 32 permanent teeth (Figure 20-5B) by age 25.

The incidence of periodontal disease increases during pregnancy. Many pregnant women experience more bleeding during brushing and increased redness and swelling of the **gingiva** (the gums).

Older adults may lose permanent teeth; some have dentures. Loss of permanent teeth is usually due to periodontal disease (gum disease) rather than dental **caries** (cavities). However, caries are also common in middle-aged adults.

Some receding of the gums and a brownish pigmentation of the gums occur with age. Saliva production decreases with age, so dryness of the oral mucosa is a common finding in older people.

Poor oral hygiene, dry mouth, and poor nutrition are common causes of oral problems. Poor oral hygiene may be the result of a lack of knowledge or illness. Confused, depressed, physically weak, or comatose clients generally have poor oral hygiene. Clients who have nasogastric tubes, are on oxygen, or breathe through their mouths experience increased oral dryness. Dry mouth is also caused by aging and medication. Older adults experience decreased saliva production and thinning of the oral mucosa. Medications that cause dry mouth include diuretics, laxatives (if used excessively), tranquilizers such as chlorpromazine (Thorazine) and diazepam (Valium), and chemotherapeutic agents to treat cancer. Dry mouth is aggravated by anxiety, poor fluid intake (dehydration), high salt intake, and smoking. Current medications being used to stimulate saliva production include Salagen (pilocarpine HCl) and Evoxac (cevimeline). Poor eating habits, such as excessive intake of salt and refined sugars, can erode tooth enamel, increasing risk. Recent mouth injury or surgery increases the risk of infection. Clients with impaired immune systems (such as those on chemotherapy or with HIV) and those who wear dental appliances (such as retainers) are at increased risk of developing mouth lesions.

NURSING CARE

PRIORITIZING NURSING CARE

Mouth care should be offered to the client prior to all meals, and at other times as necessary. A toothbrush, refreshing swabs, or mouthwash can be offered. Clients on oxygen

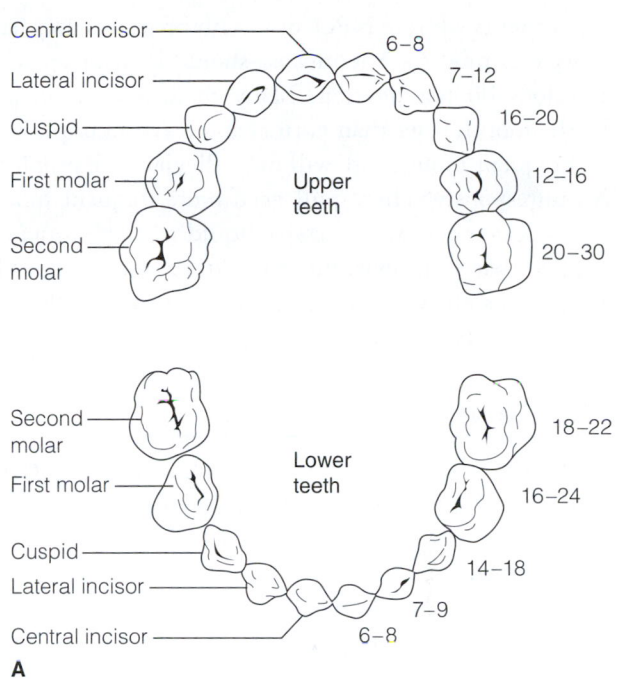

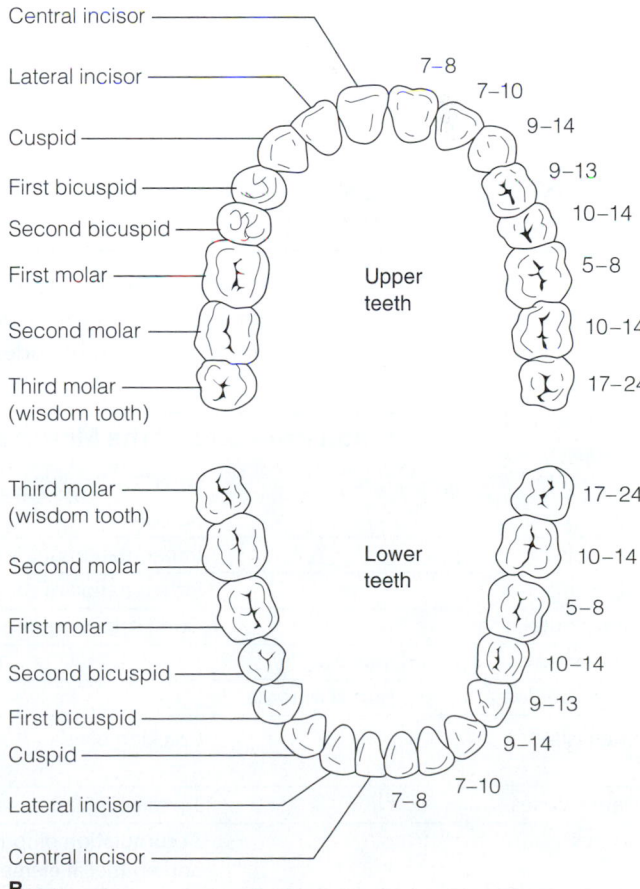

Figure 20-5. ■ **A.** Temporary teeth and their times of eruption (stated in months). **B.** Permanent teeth and their times of eruption (stated in years).

therapy, clients who are NPO, or mouth breathers may have very dry oral mucosa. The mucosa should be kept moist so that lesions do not develop. Many medications can also make the mouth drier than normal and leave an unpleasant taste. Frequent mouth care will help alleviate the problem.

An unresponsive client will need more frequent mouth care. Take care not to use excessive liquid when cleaning the mouth, so that secretions, mouthwash, or water cannot be aspirated. The client should be positioned to the side with the head slightly forward.

ASSESSING

Assessment of the client's mouth and hygiene practices includes (1) a nursing history, (2) physical assessment of the mouth, and (3) identification of clients at risk for developing oral problems.

During the nursing history, data are obtained about the client's oral hygiene practices, including dental visits, self-care abilities, and past or current mouth problems. Learning needs and client preferences are also determined. Clients whose hand coordination is impaired, whose cognitive function is impaired, whose illness alters energy levels and motivation, or whose therapy imposes restrictions on activities will need assistance.

Common problems of the mouth and nursing implications are detailed in Table 20-2 ■. For more information about mouth assessment, see also Chapter 19 ⊂⊃ .

DIAGNOSING, PLANNING, AND IMPLEMENTING

Three nursing diagnoses related to problems with oral hygiene and the oral cavity are *Self-Care Deficit, Impaired Oral Mucous Membrane,* and *Deficient Knowledge.* NANDA includes oral hygiene in the diagnostic label *Bathing Self-Care Deficit.* In this book, the diagnosis *Bathing Self-Care Deficit: Oral Hygiene* is used for clients who cannot perform oral care independently. This includes the inability to brush or floss teeth or clean dentures.

The diagnosis *Impaired Oral Mucous Membrane* refers to the state in which an individual experiences disruptions in the tissue layers of the oral cavity. Manifestations include a coated tongue; dry mouth; dental caries; **halitosis** (bad breath); gingivitis; oral plaque, pain, discomfort, erythema, lesions, or ulcers; and lack of or decreased salivation. These may be the result of inadequate oral hygiene; physical injury or drying effect (e.g., mouth breathing, oxygen therapy); mechanical trauma (e.g., surgery, injury from oral tube, broken teeth, or ill-fitting dentures); chemical trauma (e.g., side effects of medications); or radiation injury. The diagnosis *Deficient Knowledge* is discussed in detail in Chapter 12 ⊂⊃ .

A major goal for clients with oral hygiene or oral problems is to maintain or restore the integrity of the oral tissues and to prevent associated risks. Examples of desired outcomes include:

- Gums are firm, well hydrated, uniform in color, and do not bleed.
- Client brushes and flosses teeth after meals and at bedtime.
- Mucosa, tongue, and lips are pink, moist, and intact.

Good oral hygiene includes daily stimulation of the gums, mechanical brushing and flossing of the teeth, and flushing of the mouth. The LPN/LVN is often in a position to help people maintain oral hygiene by helping or teaching them to clean the teeth and oral cavity, and by inspecting whether clients (especially children) have done so. They can provide special oral hygiene for clients who are debilitated, unconscious, or have lesions of the mucous membranes or other oral tissues. (See Procedure 20-3 ■.) The LPN/LVN

TABLE 20-2	Common Problems of the Mouth and Nursing Implications	
PROBLEM	**DESCRIPTION**	**NURSING IMPLICATIONS**
Halitosis	Bad breath	Teach or provide regular oral hygiene.
Glossitis	Inflammation of the tongue	As above.
Gingivitis	Inflammation of the gums	As above.
Periodontal disease	Gums appear spongy and bleeding	As above; advise client to see a dentist.
Reddened or excoriated mucosa		Check for ill-fitting dentures.
Excessive dryness of the buccal mucosa		Increase fluid intake as health permits.
Cheilosis	Cracking of lips	Lubricate lips; use antimicrobial ointment to prevent infection.
Dental caries	Teeth have darkened areas, may be painful	Advise client to see a dentist.
Sordes	Accumulation of foul matter (food, microorganisms, and epithelial elements) in the mouth	Teach or provide regular cleaning.
Stomatitis	Inflammation of the oral mucosa	Teach or provide regular cleaning.
Parotitis	Inflammation of the parotid salivary glands	Teach or provide regular oral hygiene.

can also be instrumental in identifying problems that require the intervention of a dentist or oral surgeon and in arranging a referral. These problems should be discussed with the RN before conferring with the physician.

Promoting Oral Health through the Life Span

A major role of the LPN/LVN in promoting oral health is to teach clients about specific oral hygiene measures. Most dentists recommend that dental hygiene should begin when the first tooth erupts and be practiced after each feeding. Cleaning can be accomplished by using a wet washcloth or a cotton ball or small gauze moistened with water.

Dental caries (cavities) occur frequently during the toddler period, often as a result of the excessive intake of sweets or a prolonged use of the bottle during naps and at bedtime. The LPN/LVN should give parents the following instructions to promote and maintain dental health:

- Beginning at about 18 months of age, brush the child's teeth with a soft toothbrush. Use only a toothbrush moistened with water. Introduce toothpaste later; use one that contains fluoride.
- Give a fluoride supplement daily or as recommended by the physician or dentist, unless the drinking water is fluoridated.
- Schedule an initial dental visit for the child at about 2 or 3 years of age, as soon as all 20 primary teeth have erupted.
- Some dentists recommend an inspection type of visit when the child is about 18 months old to provide an early pleasant introduction to the dental examination.
- Seek professional dental attention for any problems such as discoloring of the teeth, chipping, or signs of infection such as redness and swelling.

Because deciduous teeth guide the entrance of permanent teeth, dental care for preschoolers and school-age children is essential to keep these teeth in good repair. Abnormally placed or lost deciduous teeth can cause misalignment of permanent teeth. Fluoride helps prevent dental caries. Preschoolers need to be taught to brush their teeth after eating, and parents should limit the child's intake of refined sugars. Regular dental checkups are required during these years when permanent teeth appear.

Proper diet and mouth care should be taught to adolescents and adults.

Care of Teeth

Brushing and Flossing the Teeth

Thorough brushing of the teeth is important in preventing tooth decay. The mechanical action of brushing removes food particles that can harbor and incubate bacteria. It also stimulates circulation in the gums, maintaining their healthy firmness. Fluoride toothpaste is often recommended

because of its antibacterial protection. An effective toothpaste can also be made by combining two parts table salt to one part baking soda. (However, this paste is not to be used by clients on sodium-restricted diets.) Part A of Procedure 20-3 on page 420 provides instruction in brushing and flossing the client's teeth.

Caring for Dentures

Dentures (a "plate" of artificial teeth for one jaw) may be worn to replace upper or lower teeth or both. When only a few artificial teeth are needed, a "bridge" may be worn. Bridges may be fixed or removable. Clients should always be encouraged to wear their dentures (or other oral prostheses) to prevent gum shrinkage and further tooth loss.

Like natural teeth, dentures collect microorganisms and food. They need to be cleaned at least once a day. Dentures may be removed, scrubbed with a toothbrush, rinsed, and reinserted. Some people use toothpaste; others use commercial cleaning compounds or soaking solutions for plates. Always rinse dentures thoroughly before inserting into the mouth, especially after soaking. Procedure 20-3, Part B, describes how to clean dentures.

Assisting Clients with Oral Care

When providing mouth care for partially or totally dependent clients, the LPN/LVN should wear gloves. Required equipment includes a curved basin that fits snugly under the client's chin (e.g., a kidney basin) to receive the rinse water and a towel to protect the client and the bedclothes (see Part A of Procedure 20-3). Foam swabs are often used in healthcare agencies to clean the mouths of dependent clients. These swabs are convenient and effective in removing excess debris from the teeth and mouth but should be used infrequently and for short periods (i.e., less than 3 days); foam swabs are not as effective as a toothbrush in removing plaque from "sheltered" areas of the teeth and gingival crevices.

Most people prefer privacy when they take their artificial teeth out to clean them. Many do not like to be seen without their teeth. One of the first requests of many postoperative clients is "May I have my teeth in, please?"

For the client who is debilitated or unconscious or who has excessive dryness, sores, or irritations of the mouth, it may be necessary to clean the oral mucosa and tongue in addition to the teeth. Agency practices differ in regard to special mouth care and the frequency with which it is provided. Depending on the health of the client's mouth, special care may be needed every 2 to 8 hours. Mouth care for unconscious or debilitated people is important because their mouths tend to become dry and consequently predisposed to infections. Dryness occurs because the client cannot take fluids by mouth, is often breathing through the mouth, or may be receiving oxygen, which tends to dry the mucous membranes. The nurse can request an order for humidified oxygen to decrease dryness for the client.

The LPN/LVN can use commercially prepared applicators of lemon oil juice and oil glycerin to clean the mucous membranes. If these are unavailable, a gauze square wrapped around a tongue blade and dipped into lemon juice and oil or into mouthwash usually suffices. Note, however, that most commercial mouthwashes contain alcohol, which can lead to further dryness of the mucosa. An alcohol-free mouthwash is usually available from agency pharmacies or central supply units. Mineral oil is contraindicated because aspiration could cause an infection. Hydrogen peroxide is not recommended for use in oral care, because if not diluted properly, it can irritate healthy oral mucosa and may alter the microflora of the mouth (Grap et al., 2003). Normal saline solution is recommended for oral hygiene for the dependent client.

Procedure 20-3, Part C, focuses on oral care for the unconscious client but may be adapted for conscious clients who are seriously ill or have mouth problems.

EVALUATING

To evaluate care of the mouth, data are collected on the status of oral mucosa, lips, tongue, and teeth. The nursing team determines whether desired outcomes have been achieved. If they are not achieved, the RN, LPN/LVN, and client explore the reasons. The care plan may be modified.

Eye Care

Normally eyes require no special hygiene, because *lacrimal fluid* (tears) continually washes the eyes, and because the eyelids and lashes prevent the entrance of foreign particles. However, special interventions are needed for unconscious clients and for clients recovering from eye surgery or having eye injuries, irritations, or infections. In unconscious clients, the blink reflex may be absent, and excessive drainage may accumulate along eyelid margins. In clients with eye trauma or eye infections, excessive discharge or drainage is common. Excessive secretions on the lashes need to be removed before they dry on the lashes as crusts. Clients who wear eyeglasses, contact lenses, or an artificial eye also may require instruction and care by the LPN/LVN.

NURSING CARE

PRIORITIZING NURSING CARE

Loss of vision can be very traumatic to a client. The nurse should always be observant for possible problems, so that injury or infection can be prevented or treated in a timely manner. Clients who wear contacts need to have them removed prior to surgery. An unresponsive client may not have blink reflex, so the nurse needs to be sure the eyes are protected. When caring for an elderly or confused client, be sure to protect eyeglasses from loss or damage. Glasses frequently end up in the laundry or in dietary when they are lost in the linen or left on the food tray. Placing them on a crowded bedside table at night can result in them being knocked on the floor and stepped on, or damaged on equipment that is moved in the darkened room.

ASSESSING

During the nursing history, the RN obtains data about the client's eyeglasses or contact lenses, recent examination by an ophthalmologist, and any history of eye problems and related treatments. In the physical assessment, all external eye structures are inspected for signs of inflammation, excessive drainage, encrustations, or other obvious abnormalities. Inspection of the external eye structures is detailed in Chapter 19 ⚭ .

DIAGNOSING, PLANNING, AND IMPLEMENTING

Nursing diagnoses related to eye problems may include:

- *Dressing Self-Care Deficit* (such as contact lens insertion, removal, and cleaning)
- *Risk for Infection* (as with accumulation of secretions on eyelids)
- *Risk for Injury* (for example, related to absence of the blink reflex associated with unconsciousness)

Nursing activities are identified that will assist the client in maintaining the integrity of the eye structures or a prosthesis and in preventing eye injury and infection. Nursing activities may include teaching clients about how to insert, clean, and remove contact lenses or a prosthesis, and ways to protect the eyes from injury and strain. Examples of desired outcomes to evaluate the effectiveness of nursing interventions follow:

- Eyelids free of secretions
- No eye discomfort
- Demonstrates appropriate methods of caring for contact lenses

Eye Care

When giving eye care, always wear clean gloves. Dried secretions that have accumulated on the lashes need to be softened and wiped away. Soften dried secretions by placing a sterile cotton ball moistened with sterile water or normal saline over the lid margins. Wipe the loosened secretions from the inner canthus of the eye to the outer canthus to prevent the particles and fluid from draining into the lacrimal sac and nasolacrimal duct.

If the client is unconscious and lacks a blink reflex or cannot close the eyelids completely, drying and irritation of the cornea must be prevented. Lubricating eye drops may be ordered. See Box 20-9 ■ for eye care for the comatose client.

BOX 20-9 NURSING CARE CHECKLIST

Eye Care for the Comatose Client

When a comatose client's corneal reflex is impaired, eye care is essential to keep moist the areas of the cornea that are exposed to air.

☑ Administer moist compresses to cover the eyes every 2 to 4 hours.

☑ Clean the eyes with saline solution and cotton balls. Wipe from the inner to outer canthus. This prevents debris from being washed into the nasolacrimal duct.

☑ Use a new cotton ball for each wipe. This prevents extending infection in one eye or to the other eye.

☑ Instill ophthalmic ointment or artificial tears into the lower lids as ordered. This keeps the eyes moist.

☑ If the client's corneal reflex is absent, keep the eyes moist with artificial tears and protect the eye with a protective shield. These should be ordered by a physician.

☑ Monitor the eyes for redness, exudate, or ulceration.

Eyeglass Care

It is essential to exercise caution when cleaning eyeglasses to prevent breaking or scratching the lenses. Glass lenses can be cleaned with warm water and dried with a soft tissue that will not scratch the lenses. Plastic lenses are more easily scratched; they may require special cleaning solutions and drying tissues. When not being worn, all glasses should be placed in a case that is labeled appropriately. They should be stored in the client's bedside table drawer.

Contact Lens Care

Contact lenses, thin curved disks of hard or soft plastic, fit on the cornea of the eye directly over the pupil. They float on the tear layer of the eye. For some people, contact lenses offer several advantages over eyeglasses. They cannot be seen and thus have cosmetic value. They are highly effective in correcting some astigmatisms. They are safer than glasses for some physical activities. They do not fog, as eyeglasses do. They provide better vision in many cases.

Contact lenses may be either hard or soft or a compromise between the two types—gas-permeable (GP) lenses. Hard contact lenses are made of a rigid, unwettable, airtight plastic that does not absorb water or saline solutions. They usually cannot be worn for more than 12 to 14 hours and are rarely recommended for first-time wearers.

Soft contact lenses cover the entire cornea. Because they are more pliable and soft, they mold to the eye for a firmer fit. The duration of extended wear varies by brand from 1 to 30 days or more. Eye specialists recommend that long-wear brands be removed and cleaned at least once a week. These lenses require very careful care and handling.

GP lenses are rigid enough to provide clear vision but are more flexible than the traditional hard lens. They permit oxygen to reach the cornea, thus providing greater comfort, and will not cause serious damage to the eye if left in place for several days.

Most clients normally care for their own contact lenses. In general, each lens manufacturer provides detailed cleaning instructions. Depending on the type of lens and cleaning method, warm tap water, normal saline, or special rinsing or soaking solutions may be used.

clinical ALERT

Never substitute saline marked "for injection" as a wetting or cleansing solution. Injectable saline may harm soft lenses or the client's eye.

All users should have a special container for their lenses. Each lens container has a slot with a label indicating whether it is for the right or left lens. Lenses must be stored in the appropriate slot so that they are placed in the correct eye.

Removing Contact Lenses

Hard contact lenses must be positioned directly over the cornea for proper removal. If the lens is displaced, the LPN/LVN asks the client to look straight ahead, and gently exerts pressure on the upper and lower lids to move the lens back onto the cornea. Figures 20-6A–C ■ show the steps needed to remove a hard lens. To avoid lens mix-ups, always place the first lens in its designated storage cup before removing the second lens.

Soft lenses can be removed in two ways. First, after separating the eyelids with the nondominant hand, move the lens down to the inferior part of the sclera using the pad of the dominant index finger (Figure 20-7A ■). This reduces the risk of damage to the cornea. Second, remove the lens by gently pinching it between the pads of the thumb and index finger of your dominant hand (Figure 20-7B). Pinching causes the lens to double up, so that air entering under the lens overcomes the suction and allows removal. Use the pads of the fingers to prevent scratching the eye or the lens with the fingernails.

Inserting Contact Lenses

Seriously ill clients whose contact lenses have been removed do not need them reinserted until they become more active in their care and require the lenses to see properly. Contact lenses need to be lubricated in a sterile, nonirritating wetting solution (usually a saline solution) before they are inserted. The wetting solution helps the lens glide over the cornea and reduces the risk of injury. Most clients, when well, will reinsert the lenses independently.

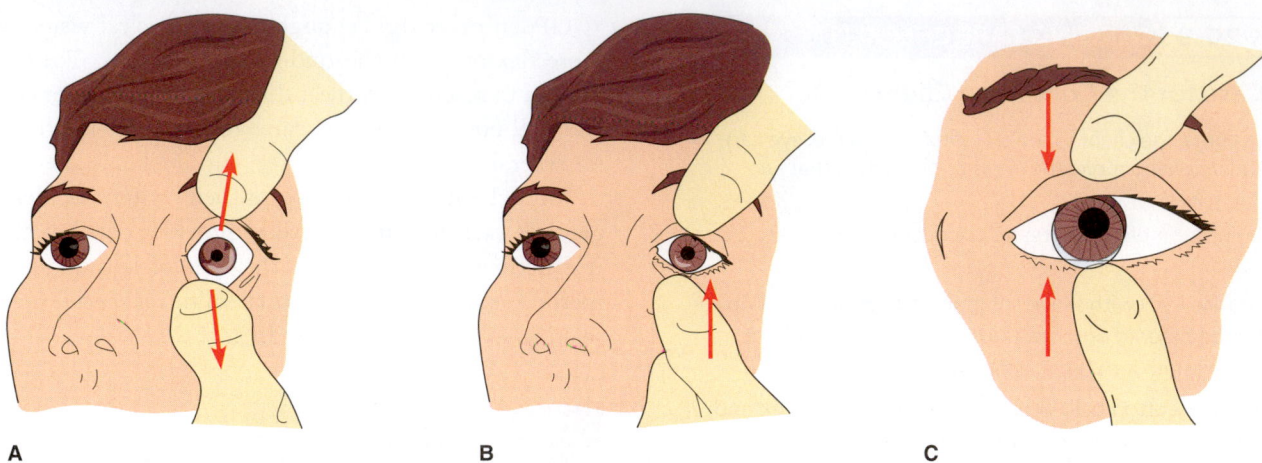

A   **B**   **C**

Figure 20-6. ■ Removing hard contact lenses: **A.** Separate the eyelids until they are beyond the edge of the lens. **B.** Hold the top eyelid stationary at the edge to the lens, and lift the bottom edge of the contact lens by pressing the lower lid at its margin. **C.** After the lens is slightly tipped, slide the lens out of the eye by moving both eyelids toward each other.

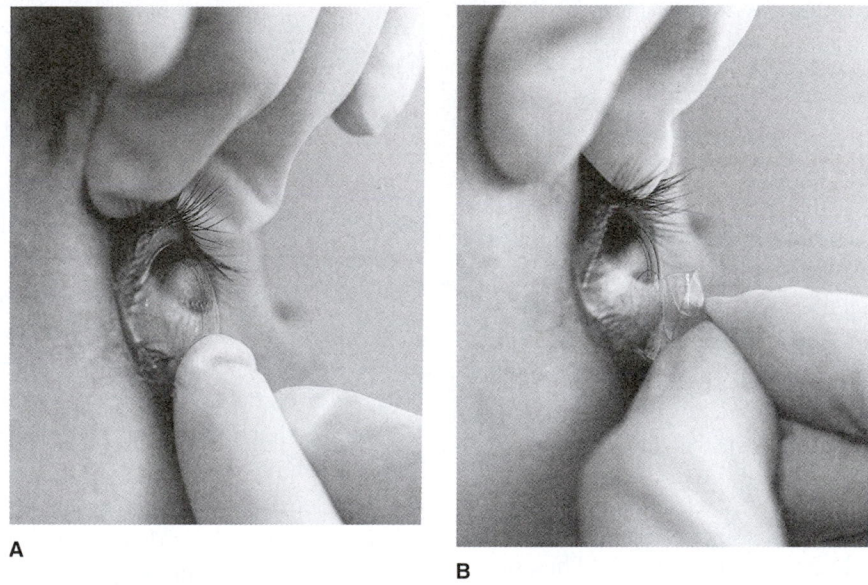

A   **B**

Figure 20-7. ■ **A.** Moving a soft lens down to the inferior part of the sclera. **B.** Removing a soft lens by pinching it between the pads of the thumb and index finger. (Photographer: William Thompson.)

Artificial Eyes

Artificial eyes are usually made of glass or plastic. Some are permanently implanted; others are removed regularly for cleaning. Most clients who wear a removable artificial eye follow their own care regimen. Even for an unconscious client, daily removal and cleaning are not necessary.

To remove an artificial eye, the LPN/LVN dons clean gloves and uses the dominant thumb to pull the client's lower eyelid down over the infraorbital bone, exerting slight pressure below the eyelid to overcome the suction in the eye socket (Figure 20-8A ■). An alternate method is to compress a small rubber bulb and apply the tip directly to the eye. As the pressure on the bulb is gradually released, the suction of the bulb counteracts the suction to draw the eye out of the socket.

The eye is cleaned with warm normal saline and placed in a container filled with water or saline solution. The socket and tissues around the eye are usually cleaned with cotton wipes and normal saline. To reinsert the eye, the thumb and index finger of one hand are used to retract the eyelids, exerting pressure on the supraorbital and infraorbital bones. The nurse holds the eye between the thumb and index finger of the other hand and slips the eye gently into the socket (Figure 20-8B).

EVALUATING

Evaluation of the eyes is part of a regular head-to-toe or body systems assessment. Any unusual redness, discharge, or pain should be documented and reported to the team leader. Changes in vision or unusual dryness should be noted.

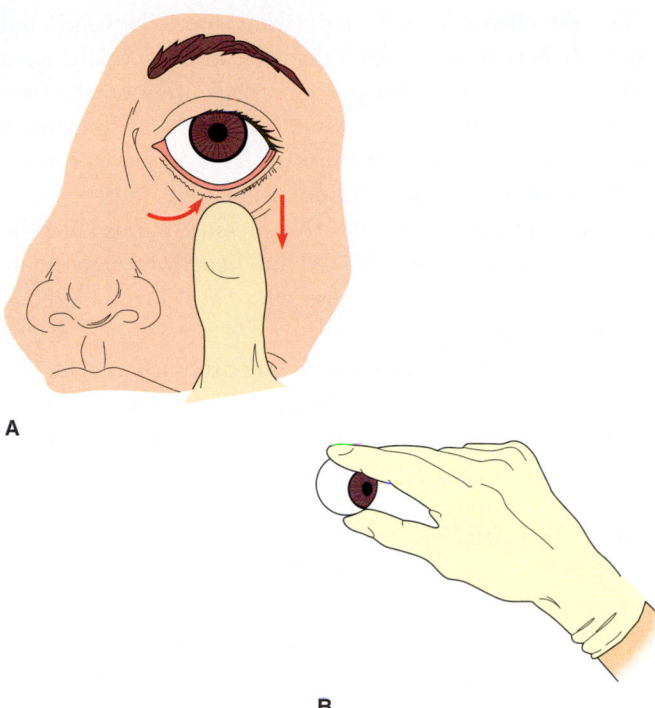

A

B

Figure 20-8. ■ **A.** Remove an artificial eye by retracting the lower eyelid and exerting slight pressure below the eyelid. **B.** Hold an artificial eye between the thumb and index finger for insertion.

Continuity of Care

Many clients may need to learn specific information about care of the eyes. The nurse can provide these general guidelines:

- Avoid home remedies for eye problems. Eye irritations or injuries at any age should be treated medically and immediately.
- If dirt or dust gets into the eyes, clean them copiously with clean, tepid water as an emergency treatment.

- Take measures to guard against eyestrain and to protect vision, such as maintaining adequate lighting for reading and obtaining shatterproof lenses for glasses.
- Schedule regular eye examinations, particularly after age 40, to detect problems such as cataracts and glaucoma.

Ear Care

Normal ears require minimal hygiene. Clients who have excessive **cerumen** (earwax) and dependent clients who have hearing aids may require assistance with hygiene tasks. Hearing aids are usually removed before surgery.

CLEANING THE EARS

The auricles of the ear are cleaned during the bed bath. The LPN/LVN or client removes excessive cerumen that is visible or that causes discomfort or hearing difficulty. Visible cerumen may be loosened and removed by retracting the auricle downward. If this measure is ineffective, irrigation is necessary (see the procedure on otic irrigation in Chapter 60 ⚭). Clients should be advised never to use bobby pins, toothpicks, or cotton-tipped applicators to remove cerumen. Bobby pins and toothpicks can injure the ear canal and rupture the tympanic membrane. Cotton-tipped applicators can cause wax to become impacted within the canal.

CARE OF HEARING AIDS

A **hearing aid** is a battery-powered, sound-amplifying device used by people with hearing impairments (Figures 20-9A and B ■). It consists of a microphone that picks up sound and converts it to electric energy, an amplifier that magnifies the electric energy electronically, a receiver that converts the amplified energy back to sound energy,

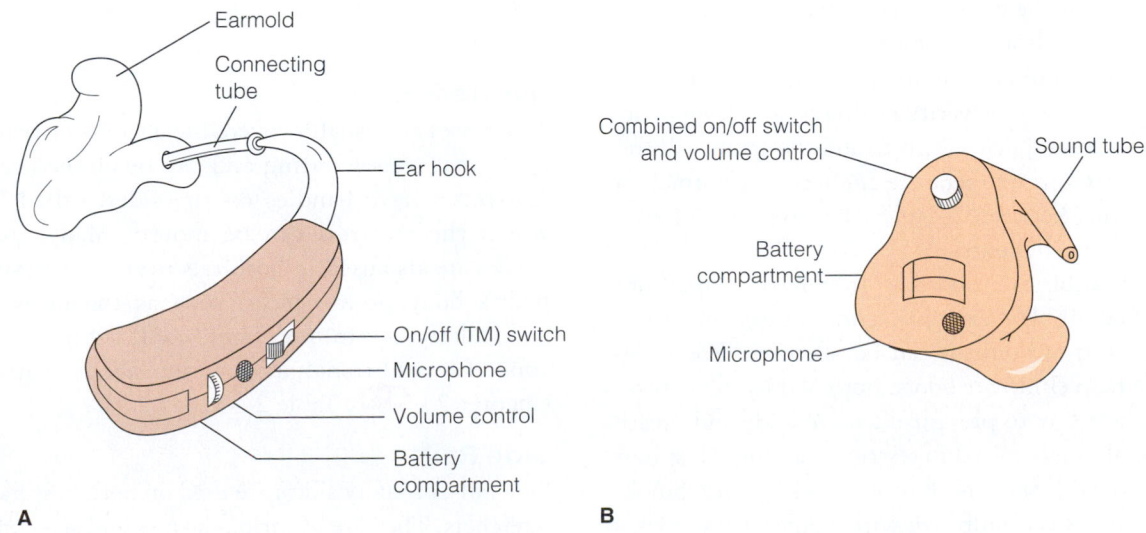

A

B

Figure 20-9. ■ **A.** A behind-the-ear hearing aid. **B.** An in-the-ear hearing aid.

and an earmold that directs the sound into the ear. There are several types of hearing aids. They may be positioned in or behind the ear or on the body.

Procedure 20-4 ■ on page 424 describes how to remove, clean, and insert a hearing aid.

Nose Care

The LPN/LVN usually does not need to provide special care for the nose. Clients can ordinarily clear nasal secretions by blowing gently into a soft tissue. When the external nares are encrusted with dried secretions, they should be cleaned with a cotton-tipped applicator or moistened with saline or water. The applicator should not be inserted beyond the length of the cotton tip; inserting it further may cause injury to the mucosa.

Supporting a Hygienic Environment

Because ill people are usually confined to bed, often for long periods, the bed becomes an important element in the client's life. A place that is clean, safe, and comfortable contributes to the client's ability to rest and sleep and to a sense of well-being. Basic furniture in a healthcare facility includes the bed, bedside table, overbed table, one or more chairs, and a storage space for clothing. Most bed units also have a call light, light fixtures, electric outlets, and hygienic equipment in the bedside table. Three types of equipment that are often installed in an acute care facility are a suction outlet for several kinds of suction, an oxygen outlet for most oxygen equipment, and a sphygmomanometer (blood pressure cuff and gauge) to measure the client's blood pressure. Some long-term care agencies also permit clients to have personal furniture, such as a television, a chair, and lamps, at the bedside. In the home, a client often has personal and medical equipment.

To provide a comfortable environment, it is important to consider the client's age, severity of illness, and level of activity. The very young, the very old, and the acutely ill frequently need a room temperature higher than normal. A room temperature between 20° and 23°C (68° and 74°F) is comfortable for most clients.

Good ventilation is important to remove unpleasant odors and stale air. For example, odors caused by urine, draining wounds, or vomitus can be offensive. Room deodorizers can help eliminate odors, but good hygienic practices are the best way to prevent offensive body and breath odors. Hospitals are required to restrict smoking. Hospitals often have an outside staff and visitors' smoking area. Smoking in client rooms is prohibited; with a physician's order, a client may be taken outside to smoke.

Certain clients may benefit from specially ventilated rooms. Infection can be contained by using special rooms with different types of air pressure, depending on the type of infection. A negative-pressure room is used for clients with a highly communicable disease. This negative pressure filters the contamination without allowing it to pass out of the room into other areas. Positive-pressure rooms keep the contamination out; they are used for clients who are vulnerable to infection, such as those who have just undergone transplant surgery.

Ill persons are usually sensitive to noise such as clanging of metal equipment, loud talking, and laughter. The nursing staff always tries to control noise in healthcare settings. (See Chapter 23 ⚭ .)

HOSPITAL BEDS

The frame of a hospital bed is divided into three sections. This permits the head and the foot to be elevated separately. Most hospital beds have electric motors to operate the movable joints. The motor is activated by pressing a button or by moving a small lever, located either at the side of the bed, in the side rail, or on a small panel separate from the bed but attached to it by a cable, which the client can readily use. Common bed positions are described in Table 20-3 ■.

Hospital beds are usually narrower than the usual bed, so that the nursing staff can reach the client from either side of the bed without undue stretching. The length is usually 1.9 m (6.5 ft). Some beds can be extended in length to accommodate very tall clients. Long-term care facilities for ambulatory clients usually have low beds to facilitate movement in and out of bed. Most hospital beds have "high" and "low" positions that can be adjusted either mechanically or electrically by a button or lever. The high position permits the nursing staff to reach the client without undue stretching or stooping. The low position allows the client to step easily to the floor.

Mattresses

Mattresses are usually covered with a water-repellent material that resists soiling and can be cleaned easily. Most mattresses have handles on the sides, called "lugs," by which the mattress can be moved. Many special mattresses are also used in hospitals to relieve pressure on the body's bony prominences, such as the heels. They are particularly helpful for clients confined to bed for a long time. For additional information about mattresses, see Chapter 24 ⚭ , Table 24-5.

Side Rails

Side rails, or safety sides, are used on both hospital beds and stretchers. They are of various shapes and sizes and are usually made of metal. Devices to raise and lower them differ.

TABLE 20-3	Commonly Used Bed Positions	
POSITION	**DESCRIPTION**	**INDICATIONS FOR USE**
Flat	Mattress is completely horizontal.	Client sleeping in a variety of bed positions, such as back-lying, side-lying, and prone (face down) To maintain spinal alignment for clients with spinal injuries To assist clients to move and turn in bed Bed making by LPN/LVN
Fowler's position	Semisitting position in which head of bed is raised to angle of at least 45°. Knees may be flexed or horizontal.	Convenient for eating, reading, visiting, watching TV Relief from lying positions To promote lung expansion for client with respiratory problem To assist a client to a sitting position on the edge of the bed
Semi-Fowler's position	Head of bed is raised only to 30° angle.	Relief from lying position To promote lung expansion
Trendelenburg's position	Head of bed is lowered and the foot raised in a straight incline.	To promote venous circulation in certain clients To provide postural drainage of basal lung lobes.
Reverse Trendelenburg's position	Head of bed raised and the foot lowered. Straight tilt in direction opposite to Trendelenburg's position.	To promote stomach emptying and prevent esophageal reflex in client with hiatal hernia.

When side rails are being used, it is crucial that the client's bedside is never elevated while the rail is lowered. Some agencies have a release form that the client can sign if the use of side rails is refused.

Footboard or Footboot

Footboards are used to support the immobilized client's foot in a normal right angle to the legs to prevent plantar flexion contractures.

Bed Cradles

A **bed cradle,** sometimes called an Anderson frame, is a device designed to keep the top bedclothes off the feet, legs, and even abdomen of a client (e.g., a client with a skin condition in which contact with covers could cause pain or irritation). The bedclothes are arranged over the device and may be pinned in place. There are several types of bed cradles. One of the most common is a curved metal rod that fits over the bed. Part of the cradle fits under the mattress, and small metal brackets press down on each side of the mattress to keep the cradle in place. The frame of some cradles extends over half of the width of the bed, above one leg.

INTRAVENOUS RODS

Intravenous (IV) rods (poles, stands, standards), usually made of metal, support IV infusion containers while fluid is being administered to a client. These rods were traditionally freestanding on the floor beside the bed. Now, intravenous rods are often attached to the hospital beds.

Some special care units have overhead hanging rods on a track for IVs.

MAKING BEDS

The LPN/LVN needs to be able to prepare hospital beds in different ways for specific purposes. In most instances, beds are made after the client receives certain care and when beds are unoccupied. However, at times it may be necessary to make an occupied bed or prepare a bed for a client who is having surgery (an anesthetic, postoperative, or surgical bed). No matter what type of bed equipment is available, whether the bed is occupied or unoccupied, or why the bed is being prepared, certain guidelines apply. The guidelines for bed making are summarized in Box 20-10 ■.

An unoccupied bed can be either closed or open. Generally the top covers of an *open bed* are folded back (thus the term open bed) to make it easier for a client to get in. Open and closed beds are made the same way, except that the top sheet, blanket, and bedspread of a *closed bed* are drawn up to the top of the bed and under the pillows.

A surgical or postoperative bed is similar to an open bed. The purpose is to be able to transfer the postoperative client into the bed easily. The top sheet is not tucked or mitered at the bottom of the bed. The top sheets can be folded low at the bottom to be pulled up over the client or folded lengthwise to be pulled across the client.

Beds are often changed after bed baths, although the linen is not usually changed unless it is soiled. Check the policy at each clinical agency. Unfitted sheets, blankets, and

BOX 20-10 NURSING CARE CHECKLIST

Bed Making and Infection Control Issues

☑ Wash hands thoroughly after handling a client's bed linen. Linens and equipment that have been soiled with secretions and excretions harbor microorganisms that can be transmitted to others directly or by the LPN's/LVN's hands or uniform.

☑ Hold soiled linen away from uniform.

☑ Linen for one client is never (even momentarily) placed on another client's bed.

☑ Place soiled linen directly in a portable linen hamper or tucked into a pillowcase at the end of the bed before it is gathered up for disposal.

☑ Do not shake soiled linen in the air because shaking can disseminate secretions and excretions and the microorganisms they contain.

☑ When stripping and making a bed, conserve time and energy by stripping and making up one side as much as possible before working on the other side.

☑ To avoid unnecessary trips to the linen supply area, gather all linen before starting to strip a bed.

bedspreads are *mitered* at the corners of the bed. The purpose of mitering is to secure the bedclothes while the bed is occupied. Figure 20-10 ■ shows how to miter the corner of a bed.

Part A of Procedure 20-5 ■ on page 426 explains how to change an unoccupied bed.

Changing an Occupied Bed

Some clients may be too weak to get out of bed because of the nature of their illness. Others may be restricted in bed by the presence of traction or other therapies. When changing an occupied bed, the LPN/LVN works quickly and disturbs the client as little as possible. To conserve the client's energy, use the following guidelines:

■ Maintain the client in good body alignment. Never move or position a client in a manner that is contraindicated by the client's health. Obtain help if necessary to ensure safety.

■ Move the client gently and smoothly. Rough handling can cause the client discomfort and abrade the skin.

■ Throughout the procedure, explain what you plan to do before you do it. Use terms that the client can understand.

■ Use the bed-making time, like the bed bath time, to assess and meet the client's needs.

Part B of Procedure 20-5 describes how to change an occupied bed.

Note: The references and resources for all chapters have been compiled at the back of the book.

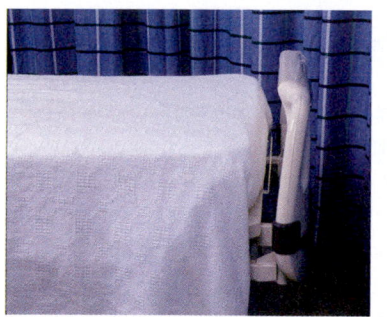
A

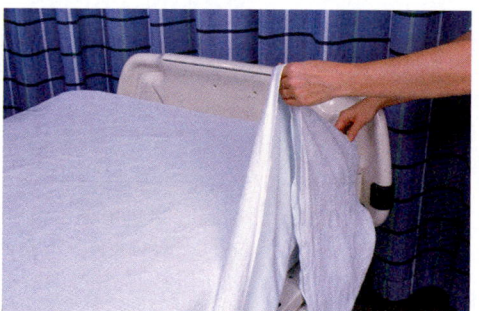
B

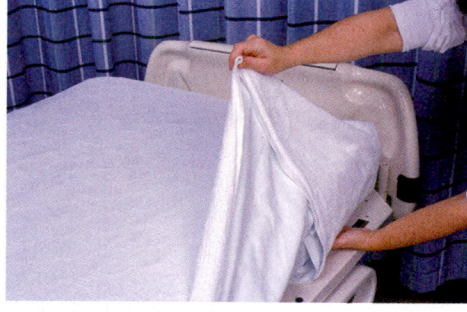
C

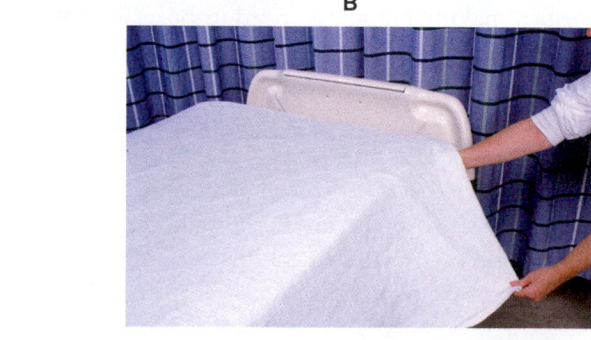
D

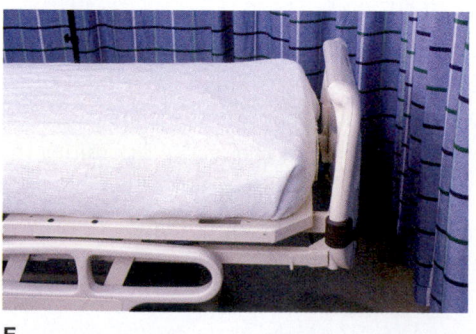
E

Figure 20-10. ■ Mitering the corner of a bed: **A.** Tuck in the bedcover (sheet, blanket, and/or spread) firmly under the mattress at the bottom or top of the bed. **B.** Lift the bedcover at point 1 so that it forms a triangle with the side edge of the bed and the edge of the bedcover is parallel to the end of the bed. **C.** Tuck the part of the cover that hangs below the mattress under the mattress while holding the cover against the side of the mattress. **D.** Bring point 1 down toward the floor while the other hand holds the fold of the cover against the side of the mattress. **E.** Remove the hand and tuck the remainder of the cover under the mattress, if appropriate. The side of the top sheet, blanket, and bedspread may be left hanging freely rather than tucked in. The bedspread is mitered separately and left hanging freely if the top sheet and blanket are tucked in.

PROCEDURE 20-1   Bathing Clients

Purposes

- To remove transient microorganisms, body secretions and excretions, dead skin cells, and normal secretions and odors
- To stimulate circulation to the skin
- To produce a sense of well-being
- To promote relaxation and comfort
- To prevent or eliminate unpleasant body odors
- To maintain skin integrity

Equipment

- Bedpan or urinal
- Changing table
- Bath blanket
- Gloves (if giving perineal care)
- Washcloth

- Soap
- Washbasin
- Water between 43° and 46°C (110° and 115°F) for adults, 38° and 40°C (100° and 105°F) for children
- Two bath towels
- Additional bed linen and towels, if required
- Hygiene supplies such as lotion and deodorant
- Clean gown or pajamas as needed
- Cotton balls or swabs
- Solution bottle, pitcher, or container filled with warm water or a prescribed solution
- Bedpan to receive rinse water
- Moisture-resistant bag or receptacle for used cotton swabs
- Moisture-resistant disposable pad
- Pillow (optional)

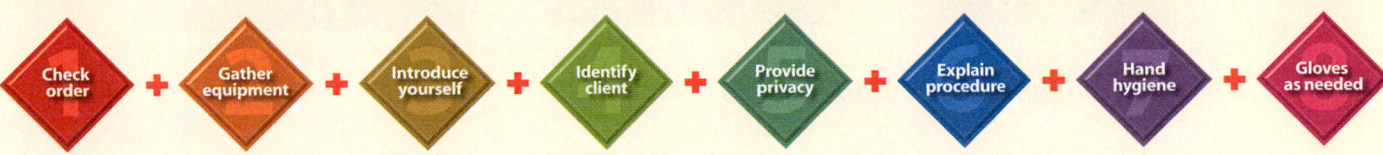

Part A: Bathing an Adult or Pediatric Client

Interventions and Rationales

1. Perform preparatory steps (see icon bar above).
   - Invite a parent or family member to participate if desired.
   - Close the windows and doors to make sure that the room is free from drafts. *Air currents increase loss of heat from the body by convection.*
   - Provide privacy by drawing the curtains or closing the door. *Hygiene is a personal matter. Some agencies provide signs indicating the need for privacy.*
   - Offer the client a bedpan or urinal or ask whether the client wishes to use the toilet or commode. *The client will be more comfortable after voiding, and voiding before cleaning the perineum is advisable.*
   - During the bath, assess each area of the skin carefully.

For a Bed Bath

2. Prepare the bed, and position the client appropriately.
   - Place the bed in the high position. Place an infant or small child on a changing table or elevated crib. *This avoids undue strain on the LPN's/LVN's back.*
   - Remove the top bed linen and replace it with the bath blanket. If the bed linen is to be reused, place it over the bedside chair. If it is to be changed, place it in the linen hamper.
   - Assist the client to move near you. *This helps prevent undue reaching and straining.*
   - Remove the client's gown.

3. Make a bath mitt with the washcloth (Figure 20-11 ■).
   A bath mitt retains water and heat better than a loosely held cloth.
   - Triangular method: (1) Lay your hand on the washcloth; (2) fold the top corner over your hand; (3, 4) fold the side corners over your hand; and (5) tuck the second corner under the cloth on the palmar side to secure the mitt.
   - Rectangular method: (1) Lay your hand on the washcloth and fold one side over your hand; (2) fold the second side over your hand; (3) fold the top of the cloth down; and (4) tuck it under the folded side against your palm to secure the mitt.

4. Wash the face.
   - Place one towel across the client's chest.
   - Wash the client's eyes with water only and dry them well. Use a separate corner of the washcloth for each eye. *Using separate corners prevents transmitting microorganisms from one eye to the other.* Wipe from the inner to the outer canthus. *Cleaning from the inner to the outer canthus prevents secretions from entering the nasolacrimal ducts.*
   - Ask whether the client wants soap used on the face. *Soap has a drying effect, and the face, which is exposed to the air more than other body parts, tends to be drier.*
   - Wash, rinse, and dry the client's face, neck, and ears.

5. Wash the arms and hands. (Omit the arms for a partial bath.)
   - Place the bath towel lengthwise under the arm. *It protects the bed from becoming wet.*

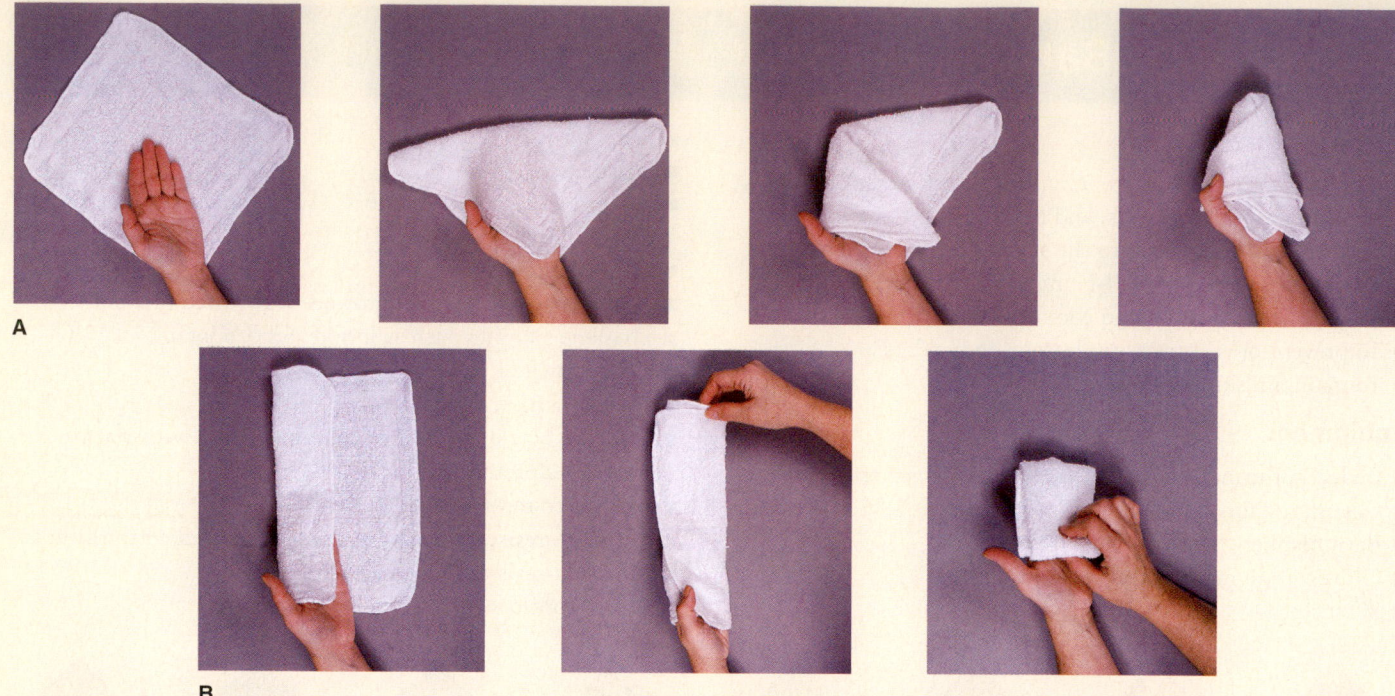

Figure 20-11. ■ Making a bath mitt: **A.** triangular method; **B.** rectangular method.

■ Wash, rinse, and dry the arm, using long, firm strokes from distal to proximal areas (from the point farthest from the body to the point closest). *Firm strokes from distal to proximal areas increase venous blood return.*

■ Wash the axilla well. Repeat for the other arm. Exercise caution if an intravenous infusion is present, and check its flow after moving the arm. Immediately report any problems with the IV to the RN.

■ Place a towel directly on the bed and put the basin on it. Place the client's hands in the basin. *Many clients enjoy immersing their hands in the basin and washing themselves. Assist the client as needed to wash, rinse, and dry the hands, paying particular attention to the spaces between the fingers.*

6. Wash the chest and abdomen. (Omit the chest and abdomen for a partial bath. However, the areas under a woman's breast may require bathing if they are irritated.)

■ Fold the bath blanket down to the client's pubic area, and place the towel alongside the chest and abdomen.

■ Wash, rinse, and dry the chest and abdomen, giving special attention to the skinfold under the breasts. Keep the chest and abdomen covered with the towel between the wash and the rinse.

■ Replace the bath blanket when the areas have been dried. Avoid undue exposure when washing the chest and abdomen. For some clients, it may be preferable to wash the chest and the abdomen separately. In that case, place the bath towel horizontally across the abdomen first and then across the chest.

7. Wash the legs and feet. (Omit legs and feet for a partial bath.)

■ Wrap one of the client's legs and feet with the bath blanket, ensuring that the pubic area is well covered.

■ Place the bath towel lengthwise under the other leg, and wash that leg. Use long, smooth, firm strokes, washing from the ankle to the knee to the thigh. *Washing from distal to proximal areas stimulates venous blood flow.*

■ Rinse and dry that leg, reverse the coverings, and repeat for the other leg.

■ Wash the feet by placing them in the basin of water.

■ Dry each foot. Pay particular attention to the spaces between the toes. If you prefer, wash one foot after that leg, before washing the other leg.

■ Obtain fresh, warm bathwater now or when necessary. *Water may become dirty or cold. Because surface skin cells are removed with washing, the bathwater from dark-skinned clients may be dark; however, this does not mean the client is dirty.*

8. Wash the back and then the perineum.

■ Assist the client to turn to a prone position or side-lying position facing away from you, and place the bath towel lengthwise alongside the back and buttocks.

■ Wash and dry the back, buttocks, and upper thighs, paying particular attention to the gluteal folds. Avoid undue exposure of the client, as for the abdomen and chest in step 6.

■ Assist the client to the supine position, and determine whether the client can wash the perineal-genital area independently. If the client cannot do so, drape the

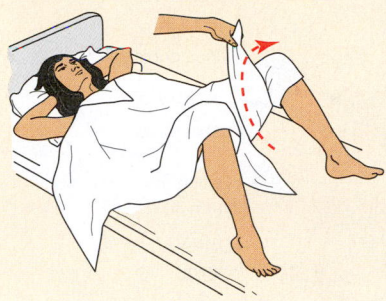

Figure 20-12. ■ Draping the client for perineal-genital care.

client as shown in Figure 20-12 ■ and wash the area. See also Procedure 20-1, Part B.

9. Assist the client with grooming aids such as lotion or deodorant.
   - Help the client to put on a clean gown or pajamas.
   - Assist the client to care for hair, mouth, and nails. *Some people prefer or need mouth care prior to the bath.*

10. Document pertinent data.
    - Record assessments, such as excoriation in the folds beneath the breasts or reddened areas over bony prominences and report changes to the RN.
    - Record the type of bath given (i.e., complete, partial, or self-help). *This is usually recorded on a flow sheet.*

For a Tub Bath or Shower

11. Prepare the client and the tub.
    - Fill the tub about one-third to one-half full of water at 43° to 46°C (110° to 115°F). *Sufficient water is needed to cover the perineal area.*
    - Cover all intravenous catheters or wound dressings with plastic coverings, and instruct client to prevent wetting these areas if possible.
    - Obtain assistance with holding a pediatric client as indicated. *Holding minimizes contamination of open skin areas.*
    - Apply a rubber bath mat or towel to the floor of the tub if safety strips are not on tub floor. *These prevent the client from slipping during the bath or shower.*

- Use a small basin or large sink for a small child. *Smaller containers decrease the danger of slipping and possible drowning.*

12. Assist the client into the shower or tub.
    - Assist the client taking a standing shower with the initial adjustment of the water temperature and water flow pressure, as needed. *Some clients need a chair to sit in the shower because of weakness. Elderly people often feel faint under hot water.*
    - If the client requires considerable assistance with a tub bath, additional staff may be needed. To provide support as the client sits down in the tub, fold a towel lengthwise and place it around the chest under both axillae; then hold the ends securely at the back as the client sits. It may be helpful to seat the client on the edge of the tub or on a chair beside the tub before transferring the client into the tub.
    - Explain how the client can signal for help, leave the client for 2 to 5 minutes, and place an "occupied" sign on the door.
    - Never leave an infant or small pediatric client unattended in a tub. *Slippage and drowning can occur in a matter of seconds and in very little water.*

13. Assist the client with washing and getting out of the tub.
    - Wash the client's back, lower legs, and feet, if necessary.
    - Assist the client out of the tub. If the client is unsteady, place a bath towel over the client's shoulders and drain the tub of water before the client attempts to get out of it. *Draining the water first lessens the likelihood of a fall. The towel prevents chilling.*

14. Dry the client, and assist with follow-up care.
    - Follow step 9.
    - Assist the client back to the room.
    - Clean the tub or shower in accordance with agency practice, discard used linen in the laundry dry hamper, and place the "unoccupied" sign on the door.

15. Document pertinent data.
    - Follow step 10.

Part B: Providing Perineal-Genital Care

Interventions and Rationales

1. Prepare the client.
   - Offer the client an appropriate explanation, being particularly sensitive to any embarrassment felt by the client.
   - Determine whether the client is experiencing any discomfort in the perineal-genital area.
   - Fold the top bed linen to the foot of the bed, and fold the gown up to expose the genital area.
   - Place a bath towel under the client's hips. *The bath towel prevents the bed from becoming soiled.*

2. Position and drape the client, and clean the upper inner thighs.

For Females
   - Position the female in a back-lying position, with the knees flexed and spread well apart (abducted).
   - Cover her body and legs with the bath blanket. Drape the legs by tucking the bottom corners of the bath

blanket under the inner sides of the legs (see Figure 20-12). *Minimum exposure lessens embarrassment and helps to provide warmth.* Bring the middle portion of the base of the blanket up over the pubic area.

- Don gloves, and wash and dry the upper inner thighs.

For Males

- Position the male client in a supine position with knees slightly flexed and hips slightly externally rotated.
- Don gloves, and wash and dry the upper inner thighs.

3. Inspect the perineal area.
   - Note particular areas of inflammation, excoriation, or swelling, especially between the labia in females and the scrotal folds in males.
   - Also note excessive discharge or secretions from the orifices and the presence of odors.

4. Wash and dry the perineal-genital area.

For Females

- Clean the labia majora. Then spread the labia to wash the folds between the labia majora and the labia minora (Figure 20-13A ■). *Secretions that tend to collect around the labia minora facilitate bacterial growth.*
- Use separate quarters of the washcloth for each stroke, and wipe from the pubis to the rectum. For menstruating women and clients with indwelling catheters, use disposable wipes, cotton balls, or gauze. Use a clean ball for each stroke. *Using separate quarters of the washcloth or new cotton balls or gauzes prevents the transmission of microorganisms from one area to the other.* Wipe from the area of least contamination (the pubis) to that of greatest (the rectum).
- Rinse the area well. You may place the client on a bedpan and use a periwash or solution bottle to pour warm water over the area. Dry the perineum thoroughly, paying particular attention to the folds between the labia. *Moisture supports the growth of many microorganisms.*

For Males

- Wash and dry the penis, using firm strokes. *Handling the penis firmly may prevent an erection.*
- If the client is uncircumcised, retract the prepuce (foreskin) to expose the glans penis (the tip of the penis) for cleaning. Replace the foreskin after cleaning

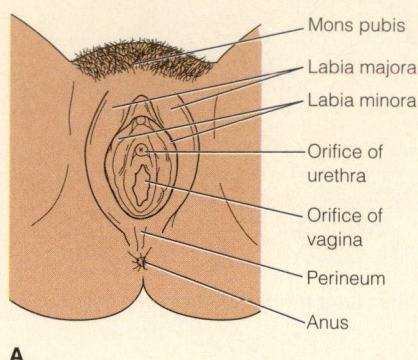

A

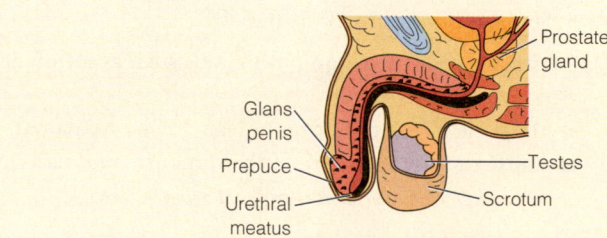

B

Figure 20-13. ■ **A.** Female genitals; **B.** male genitals.

the glans penis (Figure 20-13B). *Retracting the foreskin is necessary to remove the smegma that collects under the foreskin and facilitates bacterial growth.*

- Wash and dry the scrotum. The posterior folds of the scrotum may need to be cleaned in step 6 with the buttocks. *The scrotum tends to be more soiled than the penis because of its proximity to the rectum; thus it is usually cleaned after the penis.*

5. Inspect perineal orifices for intactness.
   - Inspect particularly around the urethra in clients with indwelling catheters. *A catheter may cause excoriation around the urethra.*

6. Clean between the buttocks.
   - Assist the client to turn onto the side facing away from you.
   - Pay particular attention to the anal area and posterior folds of the scrotum in males. Clean the anus with toilet tissue before washing it, if necessary.
   - Dry the area well.
   - For postdelivery or menstruating females, apply a perineal pad as needed from front to back. *This prevents contamination of the vagina and urethra from the anal area.*

7. Document any assessments (redness, swelling, discharge) and report findings to RN.

Part C: Providing Foot Care
Interventions and Rationales

1. Prepare the equipment and the client.
   - Fill the washbasin with warm water at about 40° to 43°C (105° to 110°F). *Warm water promotes circulation, comforts, and refreshes.*
   - Assist the ambulatory client to a sitting position in a chair, or the bed client to a supine or semi-Fowler's position.
   - Place a pillow under the bed client's knees. *This provides support and prevents muscle fatigue.*
   - Place the washbasin on the moisture-resistant pad at the foot of the bed for a bed client or on the floor in front of the chair for an ambulatory client.
   - For a bed client, pad the rim of the washbasin with a towel. *The towel prevents undue pressure on the skin.*

2. Wash the foot and soak it as required (Figure 20-14 ■).
   - Place one of the client's feet in the basin, and wash it with soap, paying particular attention to the interdigital areas. *Prolonged soaking is generally not recommended for diabetic clients or individuals with peripheral vascular disease. Prolonged soaking may remove natural skin oils, thus drying the skin and making it more susceptible to cracking and injury.*

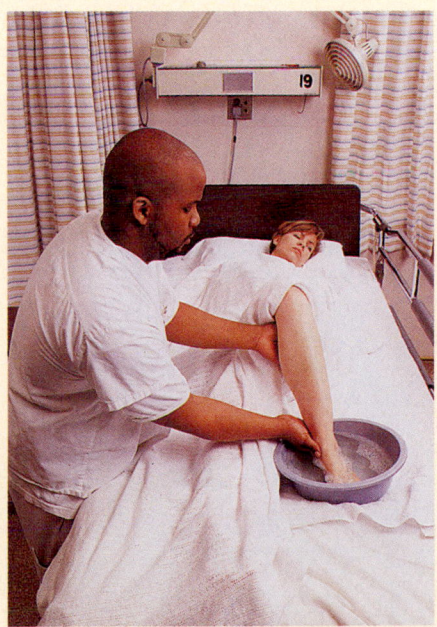

Figure 20-14. ■ Soaking a foot in a basin.
(Photographer: Jenny Thomas.)

   - Rinse the foot well to remove soap. *Soap irritates the skin if not properly removed.*
   - Rub callused areas of the foot with the washcloth. *This helps remove dead skin layers.*

   - If the nails are brittle or thick and require trimming, replace the water and allow the foot to soak for 10 to 20 minutes. *Soaking softens the nails and loosens debris under them.* Clean the nails as required with an orange stick or the blunt end of a toothpick. *This removes excess debris that harbors microorganisms.*
   - Remove the foot from the basin and place it on the towel.

3. Dry the foot thoroughly and apply lotion or foot powder.
   - Blot the foot gently with the towel to dry it thoroughly, particularly between the toes. *Harsh rubbing can damage the skin. Thorough drying reduces the risk of infection.*
   - Apply lotion or lanolin cream. Gently massage the feet until the lotion is absorbed. *This lubricates dry skin and increases circulation. (See Chapter 38 ⊙⊙ for specialized foot care for diabetic clients.)*

4. *If agency policy permits,* trim the nails of the first foot while the second foot is soaking.
   - See the discussion on nails for the appropriate method to trim nails. Note that in many agencies, toenail trimming requires a physician's order or is contraindicated for clients with diabetes mellitus, toe infections, and peripheral vascular disease, unless performed by a podiatrist or general practice physician.

5. Document any foot problems observed and report them to the RN.
   - Foot care is not generally recorded unless problems are noted.
   - Record any signs of inflammation, infection, breaks in the skin, corns, troublesome calluses, bunions, and pressure areas. *This is of particular importance for clients with peripheral vascular disease and diabetes.*

SAMPLE DOCUMENTATION

[date] [time] Self-help, bed bath given. Client tolerated bath without complaint. Client able to complete bath with assistance only for back. Skin intact, no redness or inflammation noted.

_____ Lisa Patel, LPN

Providing Hair Care

Purposes

- To stimulate blood circulation to the scalp through massage
- To clean the hair and increase the client's sense of well-being
- To distribute hair oils and provide a healthy sheen
- To assess or monitor hair or scalp problems (e.g., matted hair or dandruff)

Equipment

- Comb and brush
- Plastic sheet or pad
- Two bath towels
- Shampoo basin
- Washcloth or pad
- Bath blanket
- Receptacle for the shampoo water
- Cotton balls (optional)
- Pitcher of water
- Bath thermometer
- Liquid or cream shampoo
- Hair dryer
- Large, open-toothed or long-toothed comb (a pick)
- Lubricant (optional)

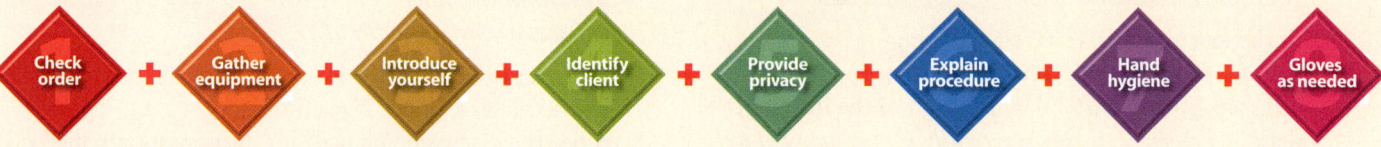

Check order ✚ Gather equipment ✚ Introduce yourself ✚ Identify client ✚ Provide privacy ✚ Explain procedure ✚ Hand hygiene ✚ Gloves as needed

Part A: Shampooing the Hair

Interventions and Rationales

1. Perform preparatory steps (see icon bar above).
   - Verify agency policy and the physician's order.
   - Determine whether a physician's order is needed before a shampoo can be given. *Some agencies require an order.*
   - Determine the type of shampoo to be used (e.g., medicated shampoo).

2. Prepare the client.
   - Determine the best time of day for the shampoo. Discuss this with the client. *A person who must remain in bed may find the shampoo tiring.* Choose a time when the client is rested and can rest after the procedure.
   - Assist the client to the side of the bed from which you will work.
   - Remove pins and ribbons from the hair, and brush and comb it to remove any tangles.

3. Arrange the equipment.
   - Put the plastic sheet or pad on the bed under the head. *The plastic keeps the bedding dry.*
   - Remove the pillow from under the client's head, and place it under the shoulders. *This hyperextends the neck.*
   - Tuck a bath towel around the client's shoulders. *This keeps the shoulders dry.*
   - Place the shampoo basin under the head (Figure 20-15 ■), putting a folded washcloth or pad where the client's neck rests on the edge of the basin. *If the client is on a stretcher, the neck can rest on the edge of the sink with the washcloth as padding. Padding supports the muscles of the neck and prevents undue strain and discomfort.*

   - Fanfold the top bedding down to the waist, and cover the upper part of the client with the bath blanket. *The folded bedding will stay dry, and the bath blanket, which can be discarded after the shampoo, will keep the client warm.*
   - Place the receiving receptacle on a table or chair at the bedside. Put the spout of the shampoo basin over the receptacle.

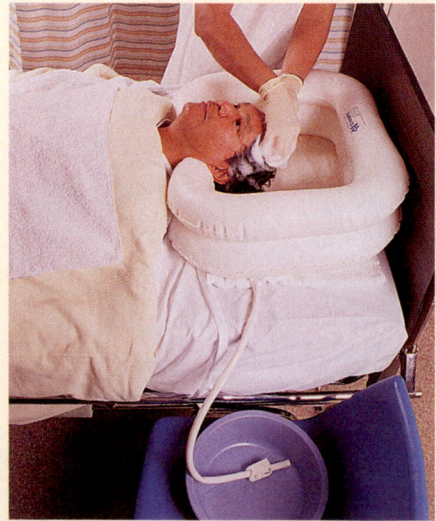

Figure 20-15. ■ Shampooing the hair of a client confined to bed. Note the shampoo basin and the receptacle below. (Photographer: Jenny Thomas.)

4. Protect the client's eyes and ears.
   - A damp washcloth may be placed over the client's eyes. *The washcloth protects the eyes from soapy water. A damp washcloth will not slip.*
   - Place cotton balls in the client's ears if indicated. *These keep water from collecting in the ear canals.*

5. Shampoo the hair.
   - Wet the hair thoroughly with the water.
   - Apply shampoo to the scalp. Make a good lather with the shampoo while massaging the scalp with the pads of your fingertips. Massage all areas of the scalp systematically, for example, starting at the front and working toward the back of the head. *Massaging stimulates the blood circulation in the scalp. The pads of the fingers are used so that the fingernails will not scratch the scalp.*
   - Rinse the hair briefly, and apply shampoo again.
   - Make a good lather and massage the scalp as before.
   - Rinse the hair thoroughly this time to remove all the shampoo. *Shampoo remaining in the hair may dry and irritate the hair and scalp.*
   - Squeeze as much water as possible out of the hair with your hands.

6. Dry the hair thoroughly.
   - Rub the client's hair with a heavy towel.
   - Dry the hair with the dryer. Set the temperature at "warm."
   - Continually move the dryer to prevent burning the client's scalp.

7. Ensure client comfort.
   - Assist the person confined to bed to a comfortable position.
   - Arrange the hair using a clean brush and comb.

8. Document the shampoo and any assessments.
   - Report any problems noted to the RN.

Part B: Providing Hair Care for African American Clients

Interventions and Rationales

1. Position and prepare the client appropriately.
   - Assist the client who can sit to move to a chair. *Hair is more easily brushed and combed when the client is in a sitting position.* If health permits, assist a client confined to a bed to a sitting position by raising the head of the bed. Otherwise, assist the client to alternate sidelying positions, and do one side of the head at a time.
   - If the client remains in bed, place a clean towel over the pillow and the client's shoulders. Place it over the sitting client's shoulders. *The towel collects any removed hair, dirt, and scaly material.*
   - Remove any pins or ribbons in the hair.

2. Comb the hair.
   - Apply a lubricant as the client indicates or as needed.
   - Using a large and open-toothed comb, start at the neckline and lift and fluff the hair outward, moving upward toward the forehead (Figure 20-16 ■).
   - Continue fluffing the hair outward and upward until all of the hair is combed on half of the head. Repeat the procedure for the other half.

3. Remove tangles gradually.
   - After the hair has been lubricated, weave and lift your opened fingers through the hair to ease the tangles free.
   or
   Support the hair securely at the base of the scalp, if possible, to prevent pulling and discomfort. Insert a long-toothed comb into the ends of the hair and carefully comb out the ends of the tangles (Figure 20-16A).

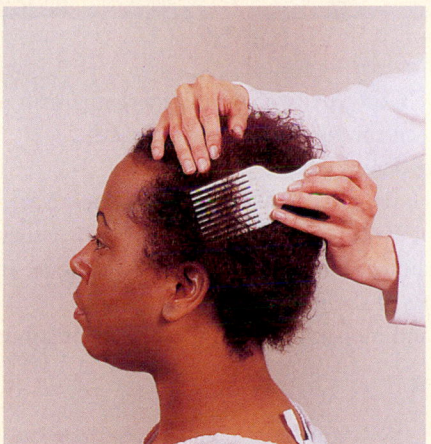

A

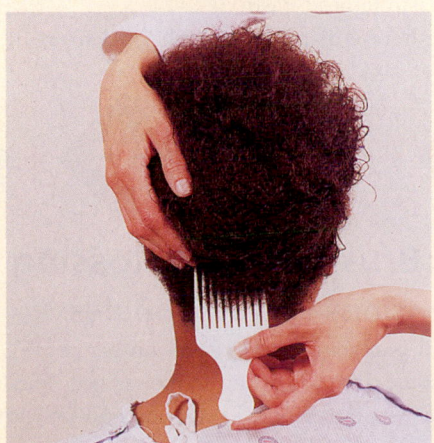

B

Figure 20-16. ■ **A.** Removing tangles with a long open-toothed comb. **B.** Using a long open-toothed comb to comb an African American client's hair from the neckline upward toward the forehead. (Photographer: Jenny Thomas.)

- Repeat this step, each time working the comb farther up the hair shaft toward the scalp, until the hair is untangled.

4. Document assessments and special nursing interventions.
   - Daily combing and brushing of hair are not normally recorded.
   - Record problems such as excessive dandruff, very dry or very oily hair, or the presence of lice.

PROCEDURE 20-3 Providing Oral Care

Purposes

- To remove food particles and microorganisms from around and between the teeth and artificial teeth
- To remove dental plaque
- To enhance the client's feelings of well-being
- To prevent sordes and infection of the oral tissues
- To maintain the continuity of the lips, tongue, and mucous membranes of the mouth
- To clean and moisten the membranes of the mouth and lips

Equipment

- Towel
- Disposable gloves
- Curved basin (emesis basin)
- Toothbrush (or stiff-bristled brush for dentures)
- Cup of tepid water
- Toothpaste or denture cleaner
- Mouthwash
- Dental floss, at least two pieces 20 cm (8 in.) in length
- Floss holder (optional)
- Tissue or piece of gauze
- Denture container
- Clean washcloth
- Bite-block to hold the mouth open and teeth apart
- Rubber-tipped bulb syringe
- Suction catheter with suction apparatus (optional)
- Applicators and cleaning solution for cleaning the mucous membranes
- Petroleum jelly (Vaseline)

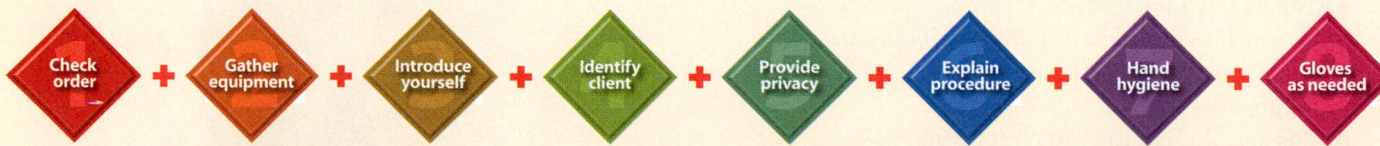

Check order + Gather equipment + Introduce yourself + Identify client + Provide privacy + Explain procedure + Hand hygiene + Gloves as needed

Part A: Brushing and Flossing the Teeth
Interventions and Rationales

1. Perform preparatory steps (see icon bar above).
   - Assist the client to a sitting position in bed, if health permits. If not, assist the client to a side-lying position with the head on a pillow so that the client can spit out the rinse water.

2. Prepare the equipment.
   - Place the towel under the client's chin.
   - Don gloves. *Wearing gloves while providing mouth care prevents the LPN/LVN from acquiring infections.*

Gloves also prevent transmission of microorganisms to the client.
   - Moisten the bristles of the toothbrush with tepid water, and apply the toothpaste to the toothbrush.
   - Use a soft toothbrush (a small one for a child) and the client's choice of toothpaste. For the person who does not have toothpaste, use a mixture of salt and baking soda.
   - For the client who must remain in bed, place or hold the curved basin under the client's chin, fitting the small curve around the chin or neck.

■ Inspect the mouth and teeth.
3. Brush the teeth.
   ■ Hand the toothbrush to the client, or brush the client's teeth as follows:
   a. Hold the brush against the teeth with the bristles at a 45-degree angle (Figure 20-17 ■). The tips of the

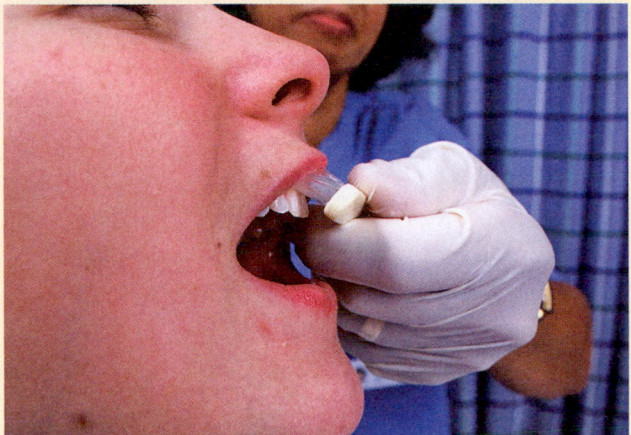

A

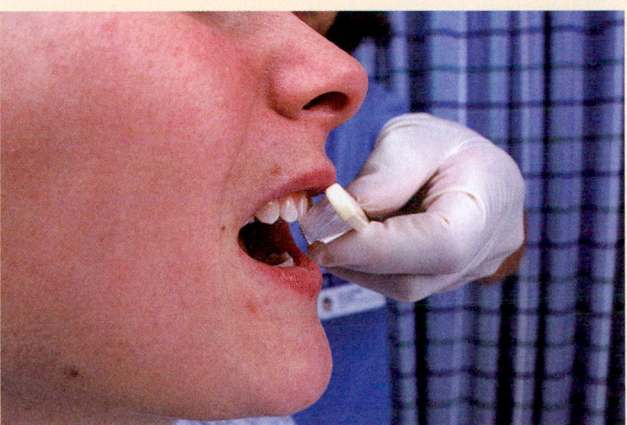

B

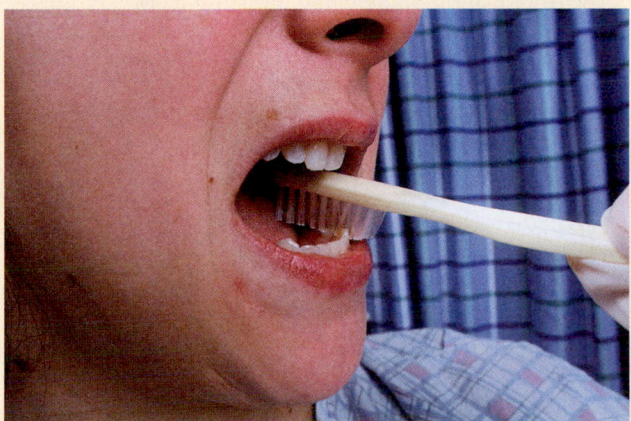

C

Figure 20-17. ■ **A.** The sulcular technique: placing the bristles at a 45-degree angle against the teeth. **B.** Brushing from the sulcus to the crown of the teeth. **C.** Brushing the biting surfaces. (Al Dodge, Pearson Education/PH.)

outer bristles should rest against and penetrate under the gingival sulcus (Figure 20-17B). *The brush will clean under the sulcus of two or three teeth at one time. This sulcular technique removes plaque and cleans under the gingival margin.*
   b. Move the bristles back and forth using a vibrating or jiggling motion, from the sulcus to the crowns of the teeth.
   c. Repeat until all outer and inner surfaces of the teeth and sulci of the gums are cleaned.
   d. Clean the biting surfaces by moving the brush back and forth over them in short strokes (Figure 20-17C).
   e. If the tongue is coated, brush it gently with the toothbrush. *Brushing removes accumulated materials and coatings. A coated tongue may be caused by poor oral hygiene and low fluid intake. Brushing gently and carefully helps prevent gagging or vomiting.*
   ■ Hand the client the water cup or mouthwash to rinse the mouth vigorously. Then ask the client to spit the water and excess toothpaste into the basin. Some agencies supply a standard mouthwash. Alternatively, a mouth rinse of normal saline can be an effective cleaner and moisturizer. *Vigorous rinsing loosens food particles and washes out already loosened particles.*
   ■ Repeat the preceding steps until the mouth is free of toothpaste and food particles.
   ■ Remove the curved basin, and help the client wipe the mouth.
4. Floss the teeth.
   ■ Assist the client to floss independently, or floss the teeth as follows. Waxed floss is less likely to fray than unwaxed floss; particles between the teeth attach more readily to unwaxed floss than to waxed floss. Some believe that waxed floss leaves a residue on the teeth and that plaque then adheres to the wax.
   a. Wrap one end of the floss around the third finger of each hand (Figure 20-18 ■).
   b. To floss the upper teeth, use your thumb and index finger to stretch the floss (Figure 20-18B). Move the floss up and down between the teeth from the tops of the crowns to the gum and along the gum lines as far as possible. Make a "C" with the floss around the tooth edge being flossed. Start at the back on the right side and work around to the back of the left side, or work from the center teeth to the back of the jaw on either side.
   c. To floss the lower teeth, use your index fingers to stretch the floss (Figure 20-18C).
   ■ Give the client tepid water or mouthwash to rinse the mouth and a curved basin in which to spit the water.
   ■ Assist the client in wiping the mouth.

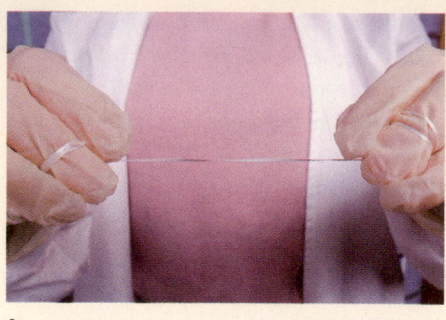

A

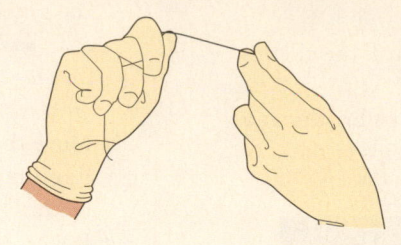

B

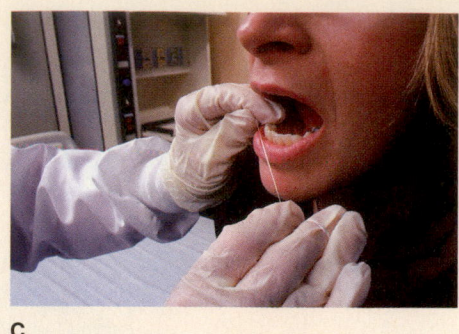

C

Figure 20-18. ■ **A.** Stretching the floss between the third finger of each hand. **B.** Flossing the upper teeth by using the thumbs and index fingers to stretch the floss. **C.** Flossing the lower teeth by using the index finger to stretch the floss.

5. Remove and dispose of equipment appropriately.
   - Remove and clean the curved basin.
   - Remove and discard the gloves.
6. Document assessment of the teeth, tongue, gums, and oral mucosa. Include any problems such as sores or

inflammation and swelling of the gums and report findings to RN. *Brushing and flossing teeth are not usually recorded.*

Part B: Cleaning Dentures

Before beginning to clean dentures, determine (1) areas in the mouth that require ongoing assessment and (2) whether the client has upper and lower dentures.

Interventions and Rationales

1. Place denture solution in denture container according to directions.
2. Prepare the client.
   - Assist the client to a sitting or side-lying position.
3. Remove the dentures.
   - Don gloves. *Wearing gloves protects the LPN/LVN and client from infection.*
   - If the client cannot remove the dentures, take the tissue or gauze, grasp the upper plate at the front teeth with your thumb and second finger, and move the denture up and down slightly (Figure 20-19 ■). The slight movement breaks the suction that holds the plate on the roof of the mouth.
   - Lower the upper plate, move it out of the mouth, and place it in the denture container.
   - Lift the lower plate, turning it so that the left side, for example, is slightly lower than the right, to remove the plate from the mouth without stretching the lips. Place the lower plate in the denture container.
4. Inspect the dentures and the mouth.
   - Observe the dentures for any rough, sharp, or worn areas that could irritate the tongue or mucous membranes of the mouth, lips, and gums.

- Inspect the mouth for any redness, irritated areas, or indications of infection.
- Assess the fit of the dentures. People who have them should see a dentist at least once a year to check the fit and the presence of any irritation to the soft tissues of the mouth. *Clients who need repairs to their dentures or new dentures may need a referral for financial assistance.*

5. Return the dentures to the mouth.
   - Offer some mouthwash and a curved basin to rinse the mouth. If the client cannot insert the dentures independently, insert the plates one at a time. Hold each plate at a slight angle while inserting it, to avoid injuring the lips (Figure 20-20 ■).

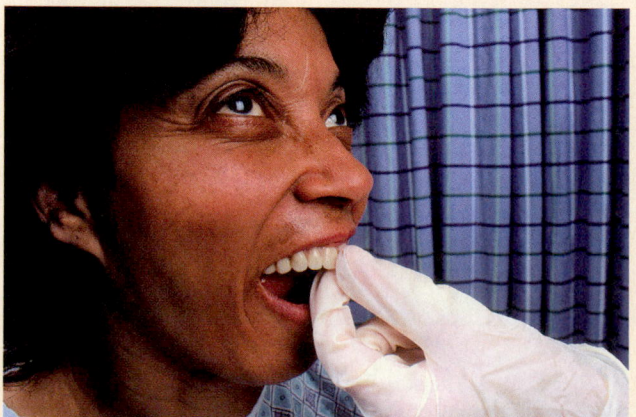

Figure 20-19. ■ Removing the top dentures by first breaking the suction.

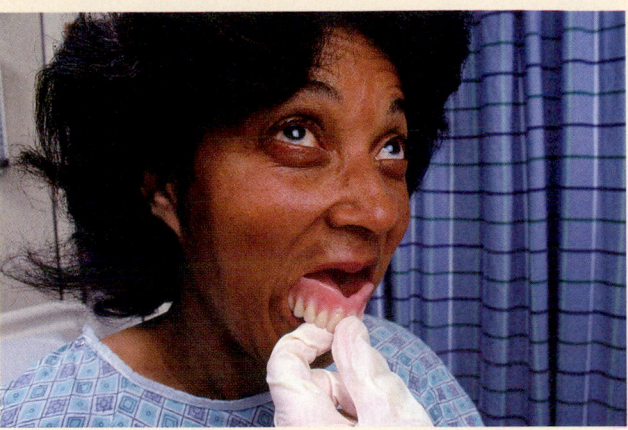

Figure 20-20. ■ Inserting the denture at a slight angle.

6. Assist the client as needed.
   - Wipe the client's hands and mouth with the towel.
   - If the client does not want to or cannot wear the dentures, store them in a denture container with water. Label the cup with the client's name and identification number.

7. Remove and discard gloves.

8. Document all relevant information.
   - Document all assessments, and include any problems, such as an irritated area on the mucous membrane and report findings to the RN.
   - Once dentures are clean, replace them in client's mouth unless client prefers them to be left out.

Part C: Providing Special Oral Care

Interventions and Rationales

1. Prepare the client.
   - Position the unconscious client in a side-lying position, with the head of the bed lowered. *In this position, the saliva automatically runs out by gravity rather than being aspirated into the lungs. This position is the one of choice for the unconscious client receiving mouth care.* If the client's head cannot be lowered, turn it to one side. *The fluid will readily run out of the mouth or pool in the side of the mouth, where it can be suctioned.*
   - Place the towel under the client's chin.
   - Place the curved basin against the client's chin and lower cheek to receive the fluid from the mouth (Figure 20-21 ■).
   - Don gloves.

2. Clean the teeth and rinse the mouth.
   - If the client has natural teeth, brush the teeth as described in Procedure 20-3, Part A. Brush gently and carefully to avoid injuring the gums. If the client has artificial teeth, clean them as described in Procedure 20-3, Part B.
   - Rinse the client's mouth by drawing about 10 mL of water or mouthwash into the syringe and injecting it gently into each side of the mouth. *If the solution is injected with force, some of it may flow down the client's throat and be aspirated into the lungs.*
   - Watch carefully to make sure that all the rinsing solution has run out of the mouth into the basin. If not, suction the fluid from the mouth. See the section on oropharyngeal suctioning in Chapter 32 ⊙⊙. *Fluid remaining in the mouth may be aspirated into the lungs.*
   - Repeat rinsing until the mouth is free of toothpaste, if used.

3. Inspect and clean the oral tissues.
   - If the tissues appear dry or unclean, clean them with the applicators or gauze and cleaning solution following agency policy.
   - Picking up one applicator, wipe the mucous membrane of one cheek. If no commercially prepared applicators are available, wrap a small gauze square around a tongue blade and moisten it. Discard the applicator or tongue blade in a waste container, and with a fresh one clean the next area. *Using separate applicators for each area of the mouth prevents the transfer of microorganisms from one area to another.*
   - Clean all the mouth tissues in an orderly progression, using separate applicators: the cheeks, roof of the mouth, base of the mouth, and tongue.
   - Observe the tissues closely for inflammation and dryness.
   - Rinse the client's mouth as described in step 2.
   - Remove and discard gloves.

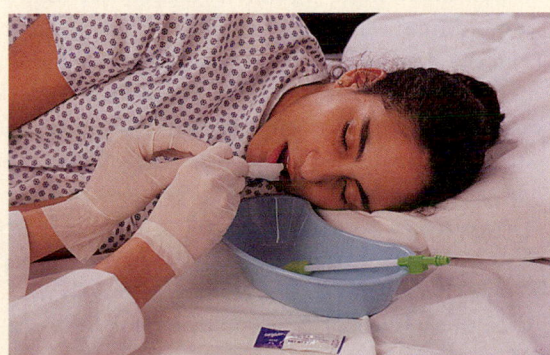

Figure 20-21. ■ Position of the client and placement of curved basin when providing special mouth care. (Photographer: Elena Dorfman.)

4. Ensure client comfort.
   - Remove the basin, and dry around the client's mouth with the towel. Replace artificial dentures, if indicated.
   - Lubricate the client's lips with petroleum jelly. *Lubrication prevents cracking and subsequent infection.*
5. Document pertinent data.
   - Record special oral hygiene and pertinent observations.
   - Report problems to the RN in charge.

SAMPLE DOCUMENTATION

[date] [time] Assisted client with oral care. Client able to brush and floss teeth. Partial denture soaked and replaced in client's mouth. Oral mucosa intact without signs and symptoms of irritation or infection. Client states dentures fit comfortably without slipping. _____
_____ Daniel Fortune, LPN

PROCEDURE 20-4   Removing, Cleaning, and Inserting a Hearing Aid

Purpose

- To maintain proper hearing aid function

Equipment

- Client's hearing aid
- Soap, water, and towels or a damp cloth
- Pipe cleaner or toothpick (optional)
- New battery (if needed)

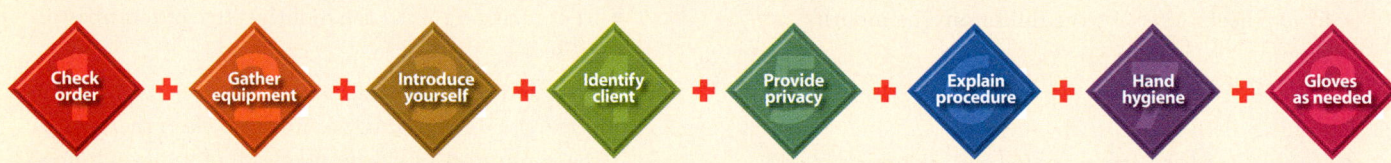

Interventions and Rationales

1. Perform preparatory steps (see icon bar above).

2. Remove the hearing aid.
   - Turn the hearing aid off and lower the volume. The on/off switch may be labeled "O" (off), "M" (microphone), "T" (telephone), or "TM" (telephone/microphone). *The batteries continue to run if the aid is not turned off.*
   - Remove the earmold by rotating it slightly forward and pulling it outward.
   - If the aid is not to be used for several days, remove the battery. *Removal prevents corrosion of the aid from battery leakage.*
   - Store the hearing aid in a safe place. Avoid exposure to heat and moisture. *Proper storage prevents loss or damage.*

3. Clean the earmold.
   - Detach the earmold if possible. Disconnect the earmold from the receiver of a body hearing aid or from the hearing aid case of behind-the-ear and eyeglasses aids where the tubing meets the hook of the case. Do not remove the earmold if it is glued or secured by a small metal ring. *Removal facilitates cleaning and prevents inadvertent damage to the other parts.*
   - If the earmold is detachable, soak it in a mild soapy solution. Rinse and dry it well. Do not use isopropyl alcohol. *Alcohol can damage the hearing aid.*
   - If the earmold is not detachable or is for an in-the-ear aid, wipe the earmold with a damp cloth.
   - Check that the earmold opening is patent. Blow any excess moisture through the opening or remove debris (e.g., earwax) with a pipe cleaner or toothpick.

■ Reattach the earmold if it was detached from the rest of the hearing aid.

4. Insert the hearing aid.
   ■ Determine from the client if the earmold is for the left or the right ear.
   ■ Check that the battery is inserted in the hearing aid. Turn off the hearing aid, and make sure the volume is turned all the way down. *A volume that is too loud is distressing*.
   ■ Inspect the earmold to identify the ear canal portion. Some earmolds are fitted for only the ear canal and concha; others are fitted for all the contours of the ear. *The canal portion, common to all, can be used as a guide for correct insertion.*
   ■ Line up the parts of the earmold with the corresponding parts of the client's ear.
   ■ Rotate the earmold slightly forward, and insert the ear canal portion.
   ■ Gently press the earmold into the ear while rotating it backward.
   ■ Check that the earmold fits snugly by asking the client if it feels secure and comfortable.
   ■ Adjust the other components of a behind-the-ear or body hearing aid.
   ■ Turn the hearing aid on, and adjust the volume according to the client's needs.

5. Correct problems associated with improper functioning.
   ■ If the sound is weak or there is no sound:
   a. Ensure that the volume is turned high enough.
   b. Ensure that the earmold opening is not clogged.
   c. Check the battery by turning the aid on, turning up the volume, cupping your hand over the

earmold, and listening. A constant whistling sound indicates the battery is functioning. If necessary, replace the battery. Be sure that the negative ($-$) and positive ($+$) signs on the battery match those on the aid.
   d. Ensure that the ear canal is not blocked with wax. *Wax can obstruct sound waves.*
   ■ If the client reports a whistling sound or squeal after insertion:
   a Turn the volume down.
   b. Ensure that the earmold is properly attached to the receiver.
   c. Reinsert the earmold.

6. Document pertinent data.
   ■ The removal and the insertion of a hearing aid are not normally recorded.
   ■ Record any problems the client has with the hearing aid and report findings to the RN.

SAMPLE DOCUMENTATION

[date] [time] No wax buildup in external ear canal noted. Client denies ear discomfort. Hearing aid inserted and volume adjusted by client. Client denies discomfort upon insertion and states adequacy of hearing acuity.
_____ Alfred Donofrio, LPN

PROCEDURE 20-5 | **Changing a Bed**

Purposes

■ To promote the client's comfort
■ To provide a clean, neat environment for the client
■ To provide a smooth, wrinkle-free bed foundation, thus minimizing sources of skin irritation
■ To conserve the client's energy and maintain current health status

Equipment

■ Two large sheets (some agencies may use fitted bottom sheets)
■ Cloth draw sheet (optional)
■ One blanket
■ One bedspread (some agencies do not use bedspreads)
■ Waterproof draw sheet or waterproof pads (optional)
■ Pillowcase(s) for the head pillow(s)
■ Portable linen hamper, if available

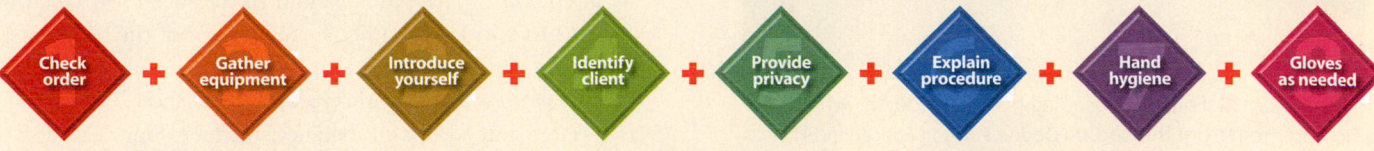

Check order + Gather equipment + Introduce yourself + Identify client + Provide privacy + Explain procedure + Hand hygiene + Gloves as needed

Part A: Changing an Unoccupied Bed
Interventions and Rationales

1. Perform preparatory steps (see icon bar above).

2. Place the fresh linen on the client's chair or overbed table; do not use another client's bed. *This prevents cross contamination (the movement of microorganisms from one client to another) via soiled linen.*

3. Assess and assist the client out of bed.
   - Make sure that this is an appropriate and convenient time for the client to be out of bed.
   - Assess the client's health status to determine that the person can safely get out of bed. *In some hospitals, it is necessary to have a written order if the client has been in bed continuously.*
   - Assess the client's pulse and respirations if indicated.
   - Assist the client to a comfortable chair.

4. Strip the bed.
   - Check bed linens for any items belonging to the client, and detach the call bell or any drainage tubes from the bed linen.
   - Loosen all bedding systematically, starting at the head of the bed on the far side and moving around the bed up to the head of the bed on the near side. *Moving around the bed systematically prevents stretching and reaching and possible muscle strain.*
   - Remove the pillowcases, if soiled, and place the pillows on the bedside chair near the foot of the bed.
   - Fold reusable linens, such as the bedspread and top sheet on the bed, into fourths. First, fold the linen in half by bringing the top edge even with the bottom edge, and then grasp it at the center of the middle fold and bottom edges (Figure 20-22 ■). *Folding linens saves time and energy when reapplying the linens on the bed.*
   - Remove the waterproof pad and discard it if soiled.
   - Roll all soiled linen inside the bottom sheet, hold it away from your uniform, and place it directly in the linen hamper. These actions are essential to prevent the transmission of microorganisms to the LPN/LVN and others.
   - Grasp the mattress securely, using the lugs if present, and move the mattress up to the head of the bed.

5. Apply the bottom sheet and draw sheet.
   - Place the folded bottom sheet with its center fold on the center of the bed. Make sure the sheet is hemside down for a smooth foundation. Spread the sheet out over the mattress, and allow a sufficient amount of sheet at the top to tuck under the mattress. The top of the sheet needs to be well tucked under to remain securely in place, especially when the head of the bed is elevated. Place the sheet along the edge of the mattress at the foot of the bed and do not tuck it in (unless it is a contour sheet).
   - If the bottom sheet is not fitted, miter the sheet at the top corner on the near side (see Figure 20-10) and tuck the sheet under the mattress, working from the head of the bed to the foot.
   - If a waterproof draw sheet is used, place it over the bottom sheet so that the center fold is at the center line of the bed and the top and bottom edges will extend from the middle of the client's back to the area of the mid thigh or knee. Fanfold the uppermost half of the folded draw sheet at the center or far edge of the bed and tuck in the near edge.
   - Lay the cloth draw sheet over the waterproof sheet in the same manner.
   - *Optional*: Before moving to the other side of the bed, place the top linens on the bed hemside up, unfold them, tuck them in, and miter the bottom corners. *Completing the entire side of the bed saves time and energy.*

6. Move to the other side and secure the bottom linens.
   - Tuck the bottom sheet in under the head of the mattress, pull the sheet firmly, and miter the corner of the sheet if a fitted sheet is not being used.
   - Pull the remainder of the sheet firmly so that there are no wrinkles. *Wrinkles can cause discomfort for the client. Tuck the sheet in at the side.*
   - Complete this same process for the draw sheet(s).

7. Apply or complete the top sheet, blanket, and spread.
   - Place the top sheet, hemside up, on the bed so that its center fold is at the center of the bed and the top edge is even with the top edge of the mattress.
   - Unfold the sheet over the bed.
   - *Optional*: Make a vertical or a horizontal toe pleat in the sheet to provide additional room for the client's feet.
   a. *Vertical toe pleat:* Make a fold in the sheet 5 to 10 cm (2 to 4 in.) perpendicular to the foot of the bed (Figure 20-23A ■).
   b. *Horizontal toe pleat:* Make a fold in the sheet 5 to 10 cm (2 to 4 in.) across the bed near the foot (Figure 20-23B).

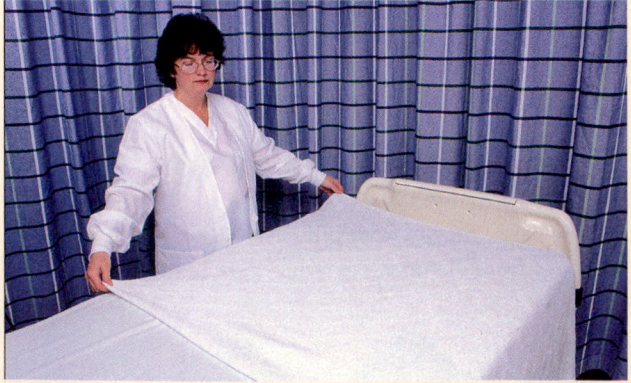

Figure 20-22. ■ Folding reusable linens into fourths when removing them from the bed. (Al Dodge, Pearson Education/PH.)

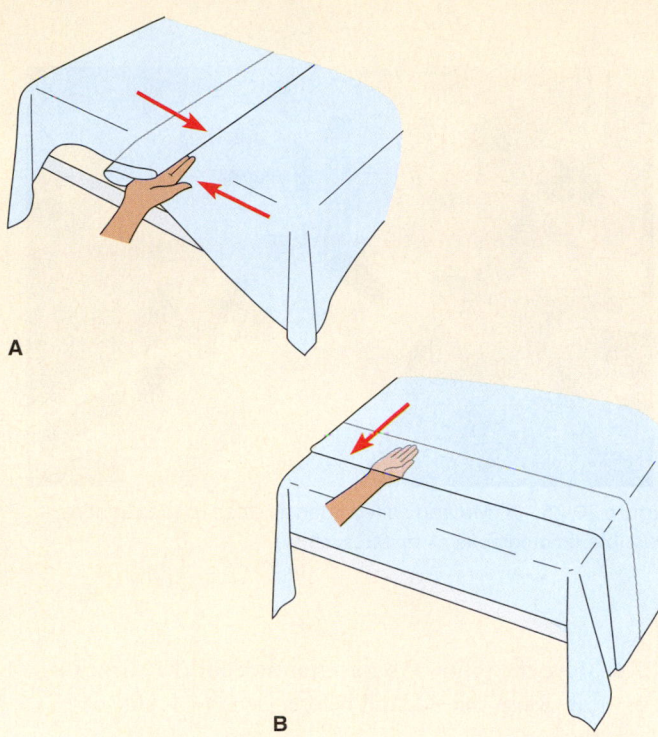

A

B

Figure 20-23. ■ **A.** A vertical toe pleat; **B.** a horizontal toe pleat.

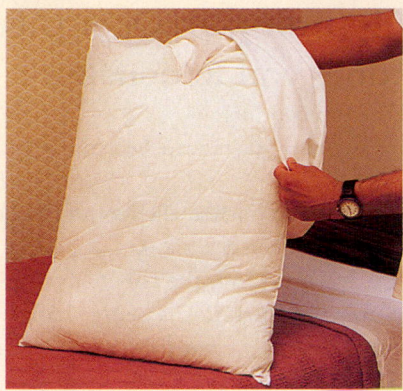

Figure 20-24. ■ Method for putting a clean pillowcase on a pillow.

Loosening the top covers around the feet after the client is in bed is another way to provide additional space.

■ Follow the same procedure for the blanket and the spread, but place the top edges about 15 cm (6 in.) from the head of the bed to allow a cuff of sheet to be folded over them.

■ Tuck in the sheet, blanket, and spread at the foot of the bed, and miter the corner, using all three layers of linen. Leave the sides of the top sheet, blanket, and spread hanging freely unless toe pleats were provided.

■ Fold the top of the top sheet down over the spread, providing a cuff. *The cuff of sheet makes it easier for the client to pull the covers up.*

■ Move to the other side of the bed and secure the top bedding in the same manner.

■ *Postsurgical*: When preparing a bed for a client returning from surgery, handle the top sheet and spread in one of the following ways.

a. Leave them untucked.

b. Fanfold the sheet and spread it to the side of the bed away from the door. Or create a triangle by folding the top sheet and bedspread sides to the middle of the bed. Then narrowly fanfold the triangle to the bottom of the bed. *When the client returns to the room, the gurney is placed alongside the bed. The client can be transferred without being encumbered by the sheets and can quickly and easily be covered once in bed.*

c. Do not place the pillow on the bed at this time. *The pillow can be placed under the client's head if permitted once the client is properly positioned.*

d. Incontinence pads can be placed under the draw sheet. An additional draw sheet can be placed at the head of the bed. *This will prevent the need to change the bed completely in case of emesis or drainage.*

8. Put clean pillowcases on the pillows as required.

■ Grasp the closed end of the pillowcase at the center with one hand.

■ Gather up the sides of the pillowcase and place them over the hand grasping the case. Then grasp the center of one short side of the pillow through the pillowcase (Figure 20-24 ■).

■ With the free hand, pull the pillowcase over the pillow.

■ Adjust the pillowcase so that the pillow fits into the corners of the case and the seams are straight. *A smoothly fitting pillowcase is more comfortable than a wrinkled one.*

■ Place the pillows appropriately at the head of the bed.

9. Provide for client comfort and safety.

■ Attach the signal cord so that the client can conveniently use it. Some cords have clamps that attach to the sheet or pillowcase. Others are attached by a safety pin.

■ If the bed is currently being used by a client, either fold back the top covers at one side or fanfold them down to the center of the bed. *This makes it easier for the client to get into the bed.*

■ Place the bedside table and the overbed table so that they are available to the client.

■ Leave the bed in the high position if the client is returning by stretcher, or place in the low position if the client is returning to bed after being up.

10. Document and report pertinent data.

■ Bed making is not normally recorded.

■ Record any nursing assessments, such as the client's physical status and pulse and respiratory rates before and after being out of bed, as indicated. Report any changes in client's status to the RN.

Part B: Changing an Occupied Bed
Interventions and Rationales

1. Remove the top bedding.
   - Remove any equipment attached to the bed linen, such as a signal light.
   - Loosen all the top linen at the foot of the bed, and remove the spread and the blanket.
   - Leave the top sheet over the client (the top sheet can remain over the client if it is being changed and if it will provide sufficient warmth), or replace it with a bath blanket as follows:
   a. Spread the bath blanket over the top sheet.
   b. Ask the client to hold the top edge of the blanket.
   c. Reaching under the blanket from the side, grasp the top edge of the sheet and draw it down to the foot of the bed, leaving the blanket in place.
   d. Remove the sheet from the bed and place it in the soiled linen hamper.

2. Move the mattress up on the bed.
   - Place the bed in the flat position, if the client's health permits.
   - Grasp the mattress lugs and, using good body mechanics, move the mattress up to the head of the bed. Ask the client to assist, if permitted, by grasping the head of the bed and pulling as you push. If the client is heavy, you may need help from another staff member.

3. Change the bottom sheet and draw sheet.
   - Assist the client to turn on the side facing away from the side where the clean linen is.
   - Raise the side rail nearest the client. This protects the client from falling. If there is no side rail, have another staff member support the client at the edge of the bed.
   - Loosen the foundation of the linen on the side of the bed near the linen supply.
   - Fanfold the draw sheet and the bottom sheet at the center of the bed (Figure 20-25 ■), as close to the client as possible. *Doing this leaves the near half of the bed free to be changed.*
   - Place the new bottom sheet on the bed, and vertically fanfold the half to be used on the far side of the bed as close to the client as possible. Tuck the sheet under the near half of the bed and miter the corner if a fitted sheet is not being used.
   - Place the clean draw sheet on the bed with the center fold at the center of the bed. Fanfold the uppermost half vertically at the center of the bed and tuck the near side edge under the side of the mattress.
   - Assist the client to roll over toward you onto the clean side of the bed. The client rolls over the fanfolded linen at the center of the bed.

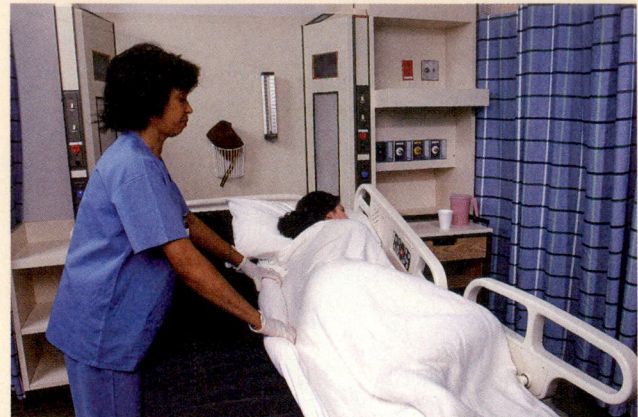

Figure 20-25. ■ Moving soiled linen as close to the client as possible. (Photographer: Alain McLaughlin.)

   - Move the pillows to the clean side for the client's use. Raise the side rail before leaving the side of the bed.
   - Move to the other side of the bed and lower the side rail.
   - Remove the used linen and place it in the portable hamper.
   - Unfold the fanfolded bottom sheet from the center of the bed.
   - Facing the side of the bed, use both hands to pull the bottom sheet so that it is smooth and tuck the excess under the side of the mattress.
   - Unfold the draw sheet fanfolded at the center of the bed and pull it tightly with both hands. Pull the sheet in three sections: (a) face the side of the bed to pull the middle section; (b) face the far top corner to pull the bottom section; and (c) face the far bottom corner to pull the top section.
   - Tuck the excess draw sheet under the side of the mattress.

4. Reposition the client in the center of the bed.
   - Reposition the pillows at the center of the bed.
   - Assist the client to the center of the bed. Determine what position the client requires or prefers and assist the client to that position. If the client needs to be moved up in bed, follow Procedure 23-2 ⬭ on page 523.

5. Apply or complete the top bedding.
   - Spread the top sheet over the client and either ask the client to hold the top edge of the sheet or tuck it under the shoulders. *The sheet should remain over the client when the bath blanket or used sheet is removed.*
   - Complete the top of the bed.

6. Ensure continued safety of the client.
   - Raise the side rails. Place the bed in the low position before leaving the bedside.
   - Attach the signal cord to the bed linen within the client's reach.
   - Put items used by the client within easy reach.

Chapter Review

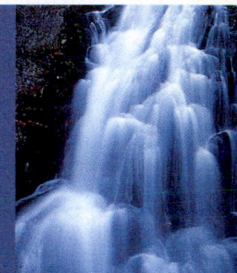

KEY Points

- Clients' hygienic practices are influenced to a large degree by their sociocultural background.
- When clients cannot meet their own hygiene needs, the LPN/LVN assists them.
- The major functions of the skin are to help regulate body temperature, to protect underlying tissues, to secrete sebum, and to contain nerve receptors that act in sensory perception.
- When planning hygiene care, the LPN/LVN must consider client preferences.
- The LPN/LVN provides perineal-genital care for clients who are unable to do so for themselves.
- The LPN/LVN can often teach clients how to prevent foot problems.
- Oral hygiene should include daily dental flossing and mechanical brushing of the teeth.
- Regular dental checkups and fluoride supplements are recommended to maintain healthy teeth.
- The LPN/LVN provides special oral care to clients who are helpless (e.g., unconscious) and who have oral problems.
- Hair care includes daily combing and brushing and regular shampooing.
- African American clients' hair may require special care.
- The LPN/LVN may need to assist clients with their artificial eyes, eyeglasses, and contact lenses.
- Clients with a hearing aid may require nursing assistance with the device.
- Changing bed linens is a part of maintaining hygiene.
- It is important to keep beds clean and comfortable for clients.

FOR FURTHER Study

Table 10-1 lists examples of normal flora found on the skin.

The diagnosis *Deficient Knowledge* is discussed in detail in Chapter 12.

For more about enhancing a client's self-concept, see Chapter 17.

For detailed information about physical assessment, see Chapter 19.

Assessment of skin, feet, and nails is discussed in Chapter 19.

For a detailed discussion of body heat losses and gains, see Chapter 21.

For information on controlling noise in healthcare settings and providing back massages, see Chapter 23.

For discussion of skin integrity, skin impairment, and heat and cold applications, see Chapter 24; Table 24-5 provides additional information about mattresses.

See Chapter 32 for more information on oropharyngeal suctioning.

For additional information on otic irrigation, see Chapter 60.

Critical Thinking Care Map

Caring for a Client with Oral Cavity Problems

NCLEX-PN® Focus Area: Health Promotion and Maintenance: Prevention and Early Detection of Disease

Case Study: Joe Kwan, 46 years old, was admitted with a fractured femur. On bed rest and in Buck's traction; scheduled for an ORIF at 11:00 A.M. Maureen Stiffel, LVN, has been assigned to assist him with his bath and oral hygiene. NPO; Foley catheter in place. Intravenous 5% D/W in NSS in place and infusing at 100 mL/h. VS: T 99.2, P 78, R 20, BP 134/82; pulse ox 98% on room air.

Nursing Diagnosis: *Impaired Oral Mucous Membrane*

COLLECT DATA

Subjective	Objective
_____	_____
_____	_____
_____	_____
_____	_____
_____	_____
_____	_____

Would you report this? Yes/No

If yes, report to: _____

What would you report? _____

Nursing Care

_____
_____
_____
_____
_____
_____
_____
_____
_____
_____

How would you document this? _____
_____
_____
_____

Compare your answers and documentation to those provided on the MyNursingKit Website.

Data Collected
(use only those that apply)

- Teeth stained from heavy smoking
- One large cavity evident in second lower left molar
- Tartar buildup along gum margins
- Pronounced halitosis
- Gums are reddened in some areas and bleed when flossed
- States, "I can't remember when I last saw a dentist."

Nursing Interventions
(use only those that apply; list in priority order)

- Thoroughly orient the client to environment. Place call light within reach and show how to call for assistance. Answer call light promptly.
- Use tap water or normal saline to provide oral care; do not use commercial mouthwash containing alcohol or hydrogen peroxide.
- Plan care activities around periods of greatest comfort whenever possible.
- Use foam sticks to moisten the oral mucous membrane, clean out debris, and swab while client is NPO.
- Keep lips well lubricated using petroleum jelly or a similar product.
- Encourage client to take deep breaths and cough at intervals.
- Inspect oral cavity at least once daily and note any discoloration, lesions, edema, bleeding, exudate, or dryness.
- Determine client's usual method of oral care and address any concerns related to oral care.
- Identify reasons client has not seen a dentist regularly.

NCLEX-PN® Exam Preparation

1 When providing A.M. care to the client the nurse performs which of the following?

1. Take the client's vital signs.
2. Complete the initial assessment.
3. Help the client with oral care and face and hand hygiene.
4. Give the client a shower or bath and ambulate the client.

2 The nurse prepares to assist a client with personal hygiene. The client has a number of personal preferences for how and when hygiene should be performed. The nurse's best action would be to:

1. Follow the client's preferences whenever possible.
2. Explain to the client that as a professional nurse you will provide personal hygiene in an effective and efficient manner.
3. Delegate care of this client to an unlicensed assistive personnel who has more time to deliver care as the client wishes.
4. Smile and agree with the client, but provide hygiene care as usual because this is the correct method.

3 While caring for a client with impaired circulation of the lower extremities, the nurse assesses the client's feet and finds that the skin is very dry and the heels have reddened areas. The nurse's priority action is to:

1. Ensure that the bottom sheet is taut and free of wrinkles.
2. Massage the feet and allow them to air dry.
3. Bathe the feet and dry briskly.
4. Apply extra blankets over the leg and feet to keep them warm.

4 The nurse is meeting the client's hygienic needs, which include all of the following *except*:

1. Skin, hair, nail, and oral care.
2. Care of the nasal cavities, eyes, and ears.
3. Bed making.
4. Changing and washing the client's clothes.

5 The nurse is providing oral hygiene for an unconscious client and places the client in what position?

1. High Fowler's
2. Side-lying
3. Prone
4. Supine

6 The nurse notes that the client is scratching her head frequently, especially behind the ears. Upon assessing the scalp, the nurse finds small grayish white spots moving on the scalp. When providing care to this client, the nurse should:

1. Stand back at least 2 to 3 feet.
2. Wash the client's hair as normal using an over-the-counter pyrethrin shampoo.
3. Wear mask, gloves, gown, and goggles when washing the client's hair with pyrethrin shampoo.
4. Wear head cover while assisting the client to shampoo the hair with pyrethrin shampoo.

7 The nurse is teaching the client about foot care and instructs the client to:

1. Use the hottest water tolerable.
2. Allow the feet to air dry to avoid injury.
3. Soak the foot for 3 to 5 minutes prior to trimming the toenails.
4. Rub callused areas of the foot with a washcloth to remove dead skin layers.

8 The nurse is changing the client's bed linens and begins by removing the old linen. The nurse takes the soiled linen and:

1. Places it on the floor at the foot of the bed and slightly under the bed until the new linen is applied.
2. Places it on the chair in the client's room until the new linen is placed.
3. Carries it to a proper linen bag by holding it close to the uniform to avoid dropping it.
4. Carries the soiled linen to the linen bag placed just outside the client's room, taking care not to touch the uniform.

9 The nurse is providing eye care for an unconscious client. A priority nursing action is:

1. Wiping from the outer to the inner canthus.
2. Using a different cotton ball for each wipe.
3. Covering the eyes with an eye shield.
4. Using fresh water to cleanse each eye.

10 The nurse is changing linen on an occupied bed and begins by:

1. Removing the top bedding.
2. Moving the mattress up on the bed.
3. Turning the client toward the side where the linen will be changed.
4. Loosening the foundation of the bottom linen on the side of the bed nearest the linen supply.

Answers and rationales for Review Questions appear in Appendix I.

Chapter 21

Vital Signs

LEARNING Outcomes

After completing this chapter, you will be able to:

1. Identify times when vital signs should be measured.
2. Identify normal ranges for each vital sign by age.
3. Describe factors that affect temperature and its accurate measurement.
4. Describe factors that affect pulse rate and its accurate measurement.
5. Point to the nine sites commonly used to assess the pulse and state the reasons each site might be used.
6. Identify normal ranges for pulse rate and quality when assessing a client's pulse.
7. Describe factors that affect respiration and its accurate measurement.
8. Describe the mechanics of breathing and identify the components of a respiratory assessment.
9. Describe factors that affect blood pressure and its accurate measurement.
10. Differentiate systolic from diastolic blood pressure and describe five phases of Korotkoff's sounds.

Clinical Objectives

11. Demonstrate the procedure for assessing body temperature, pulse, and respirations.
12. Demonstrate techniques for obtaining blood pressure.
13. Demonstrate the proper response to abnormal vital sign measurements.

KEY TERMS

Use the audio glossary feature on the MyNursingKit Website to hear the correct pronunciation of the following key terms.

afebrile 436
antipyretic 436
apical pulse 441
apical–radial pulse 444
apnea 447
arrhythmia 443
arteriosclerosis 448
auscultatory gap 453
basal metabolic rate 435
bladder 450
blood pressure 448
blood volume 448
body temperature 434
bradycardia 443
bradypnea 447
bubbling 447
cardiac output 441
Celsius 440
Cheyne-Stokes respirations 447
circadian rhythm 435
compliance 441
conduction 435
constant fever 436
convection 435
core temperature 434
costal breathing 445
crackles 447
crisis 437
diaphragmatic breathing 445
diastolic pressure 448
diurnal variations 435
dyspnea 447

dysrhythmia 443
eupnea 447
evaporation 435
exhalation 445
expiration 445
external respiration 445
Fahrenheit 440
febrile 436
fever 436
flail chest 447
hematocrit 449
hemoptysis 447
hyperpyrexia 436
hypertension 441
hyperthermia 436
hyperventilation 445
hypotension 449
hypothermia 437
hypoventilation 445
inhalation 445
insensible water loss 435
inspiration 445
intercostal retractions 447
intermittent fever 436
internal respiration 445
Korotkoff's sounds 451
labored breathing 448
lumen 448
nonproductive cough 447
orthopnea 447
orthostatic hypotension 449
parallax 450

peripheral pulse 441
peripheral vascular resistance 448
point of maximal impulse 442
polycythemia 449
productive cough 447
pulse 441
pulse deficit 444
pulse oximeter 448
pulse pressure 448
pulse volume 443
pyrexia 436
radiation 435
rales 447
relapsing fever 436
remittent fever 436
respiration 445
secondary hypertension 449
sphygmomanometer 450
stertor 447
stridor 447
substernal retractions 447
suprasternal retractions 447
systolic pressure 448
tachycardia 443
tachypnea 447
thermoregulation 440
tidal volume 447
vaporization 435
viscosity 448
vital signs 443
wheeze 447

Vital signs include body temperature, pulse rate, respiratory rate, and blood pressure. They are called *vital* signs because they monitor vital function and are an excellent means of assessing the client's status. Recently, many agencies have designated pain as a fifth vital sign to be monitored at the same time as the other four. Pain assessment is covered in Chapter 22 ⬭. (Pulse oximetry is also commonly measured at the same time as traditional vital signs. Measurement of oxygen saturation is discussed in Chapter 32 ⬭.) Monitoring a client's vital signs should be a thoughtful, scientific assessment evaluated in total and never performed casually or automatically without thought or consideration. Vital signs must be evaluated with reference

to the client's present and prior health status and be compared to accepted normal standards (Table 21-1 ▪).

Frequency of vital sign collection is chiefly a nursing judgment, depending on the client's health status. Some medical facilities have policies about how often to take the clients' vital signs. Physicians may also order vital signs (e.g., "blood pressure every 2 hours") to be taken at specific times. Ordered assessments, however, should be considered the minimum. A nurse should measure vital signs more often if the client's health status requires it and should always measure vital signs before calling the doctor to report a change in the client's condition. Vital signs are routinely assessed in the following order: temperature first; pulse and

TABLE 21-1	Variations in Normal Vital Signs by Age			
AGE	TEMPERATURE IN DEGREES CELSIUS	AVERAGE PULSE (RANGES)	AVERAGE RESPIRATIONS (RANGES)	BLOOD PRESSURE (MM HG)
Newborns	36.8 (axillary)	130 (80–180)	35 (30–80)	73/55
1–3 years	37.7 (rectal)	120 (80–140)	30 (20–40)	90/55
6–8 years	37 (oral)	100 (75–120)	20 (15–25)	95/57
10 years	37 (oral)	70 (50–90)	19 (15–25)	102/62
Teen years	37 (oral)	70 (50–90)	18 (15–20)	120/80
Adult	37 (oral)	80 (60–100)	16 (12–20)	120/80
Older adult (>70 years)	36 (oral)	80 (60–100)	16 (15–20)	Possible increased diastolic

BOX 21-1 NURSING CARE CHECKLIST

When to Measure Vital Signs

- ☑ On admission to a facility
- ☑ Prior to transfer to a new unit
- ☑ Upon arrival at the new unit
- ☑ Prior to discharge
- ☑ Any change in the client's status
- ☑ Prior to calling the physician
- ☑ Before and after any procedure that could impact vital signs
- ☑ Thirty minutes after a client ceases shivering
- ☑ Before and after administration of a medication that can impact vital signs (antihypertensives, antipyretics, etc.)
- ☑ Every 15 minutes for 1 hour, then every 30 minutes for 2 hours, then every hour for 4 hours, then every 4 hours following surgery
- ☑ As often as every 1 to 2 minutes if the client is unstable or has a deteriorating condition
- ☑ At least every 4 hours if the client had an elevated temperature within the last 24 hours

respirations are taken while the thermometer is in place, if possible. Respirations should be assessed while your fingers are still touching the pulse point, so that the client will be unaware and not alter the breathing pattern. The blood pressure should be performed following the other vital signs. Examples of times to assess vital signs are listed in Box 21-1 ■.

Body Temperature

Body temperature reflects the balance between the heat produced and the heat lost from the body, measured in heat units called degrees. The normal body temperature (temperature of deep tissues of the body) is actually a range of temperatures and depends on the site used for measurement.

When measured orally, the average body temperature of an adult is between 36.7°C (98°F) and 37°C (98.6°F) (Figure 21-1 ■). Measurement of temperature rectally will measure one degree higher, 37.5°C (99.6°F), because it is an enclosed space and does not have air movement over the thermometer like the oral cavity has. Axillary temperatures measure one degree lower than oral, 35.4°C (97.6°F), and a normal tympanic temperature measures 37.6°C (99.7°F). The most accurate means of measuring temperature is rectally because this is a measurement of the **core temperature** (the temperature of deep tissues of the body). In contrast, an axillary temperature measures surface temperature (the temperature of the skin, subcutaneous tissue, and fat cells) (Moran & Mendal, 2002). Surface temperature can be influenced by changes in environmental temperature.

The body continually produces heat as a by-product of metabolism. When the amount of heat produced by the body exactly equals the amount of heat lost, the person is in

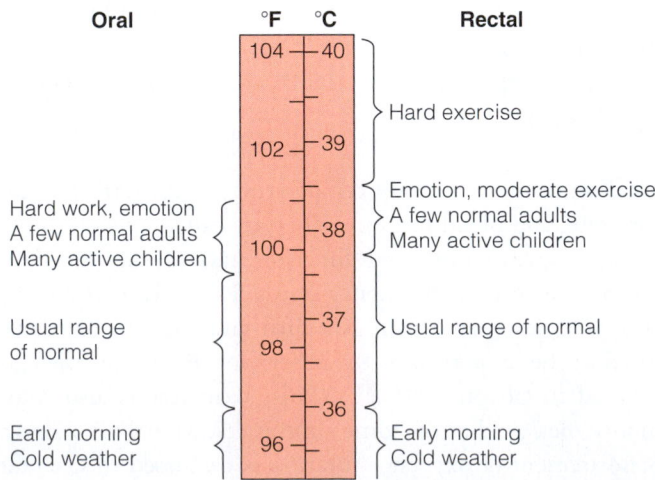

Figure 21-1. ■ Estimated ranges of body temperatures in normal persons. (*Source:* E. F. DuBois, *Fever and the regulation of body temperature,* Springfield, IL: Charles C. Thomas, 1948. Courtesy of Charles C. Thomas, Publisher.)

heat balance. A number of factors affect the body's heat production. The most important are these five:

1. *Basal metabolic rate.* The **basal metabolic rate** (BMR) is the rate of energy utilization in the body required to maintain essential activities such as breathing. Metabolic rates decrease with age. In general, the younger the person, the higher the BMR.
2. *Muscle activity.* Muscle activity, including shivering, increases the metabolic rate.
3. *Thyroxine output.* Increased thyroxine output increases the rate of cellular metabolism throughout the body and increases heat.
4. *Epinephrine, norepinephrine, and sympathetic stimulation.* These hormones immediately increase the rate of cellular metabolism in many body tissues.
5. *Fever.* Fever increases the cellular metabolic rate and thus increases the body's temperature further.

Heat loss occurs through radiation, conduction, convection, and vaporization. **Radiation** is the transfer of heat from one object to another without the two objects touching. An example would be the effects of walking outside on a sunny day and having the skin warmed by the sun, or the application of a heat lamp to the skin of a client. **Conduction** is the transfer of heat from one molecule to another of lower temperature. An example of conduction would be jumping into a swimming pool filled with cold water. The body will quickly lose heat to the water in the pool. **Convection** is the dispersion of heat by air currents, which explains why it feels colder on a windy day than a still day. **Vaporization** (or **evaporation**) is a continuous change into vapor of moisture from the respiratory tract, mucosa of the mouth, and perspiration on the skin. The result of vaporization is **insensible water loss,** a continuous and unnoticed loss of water from the body.

REGULATION OF BODY TEMPERATURE

The hypothalamus in the brain is the primary regulator of body temperature. When the skin becomes chilled over the entire body or when cold sensors in the brain are stimulated, three physiological processes take place to increase the body temperature:

1. *Shivering* increases heat production.
2. *Sweating* is inhibited to decrease heat loss.
3. *Vasoconstriction* pulls circulating blood volume away from the skin to decrease heat loss through conduction.

When the sensors in the hypothalamus of the brain detect heat, they send out signals intended to reduce the temperature. The body decreases heat production and increases heat loss by:

1. Sweating, which increases vaporization and cooling.
2. Peripheral vasodilation, which facilitates cooling.

Also, when sensors are stimulated, the person consciously makes appropriate adjustments, such as putting on additional

---

BOX 21-2	PEDIATRIC CONSIDERATIONS

Brown Fat

Newborns do not have the normal temperature regulators found in the older child or adult and depend on a substance called brown fat located around the kidneys and spinal cord. When the newborn becomes cold, the brown fat is burned to raise temperature. Rapid burning of brown fat can cause damage to the kidney and spinal cord, so temperature regulation is an important component when caring for a newborn.

clothing in response to cold or turning on a fan in response to heat.

Factors Affecting Body Temperature

Nurses should be aware of the factors that can affect a client's body temperature. They should recognize normal temperature variations and understand the significance of body temperature measurements that deviate from normal. Among factors affecting body temperature are:

- *Age.* The infant is greatly influenced by the temperature of the environment and must be protected from extreme changes (Box 21-2 ■). Children's temperatures continue to fluctuate more than those of adults until puberty. Older people, particularly those over 75 years of age, are sensitive to extremes in temperature, and are at risk of hypothermia (temperatures below 36°C [96.8°F]). Some of the reasons for this include inadequate diet, loss of subcutaneous fat, lack of activity, and reduced efficiency of the temperature-regulating system (see Table 21-1).
- **Diurnal variations (circadian rhythm).** Body temperatures normally change throughout the day, varying as much as 1.0°C (1.8°F) between the early morning and the late afternoon. The point of highest body temperature is usually reached between 1600 and 2000 hours (4:00 P.M. and 8 P.M.), and the lowest point is reached during sleep between 0400 and 0600 hours (4:00 A.M. and 6:00 A.M.) (Figure 21-2 ■).
- *Exercise.* Hard work or strenuous exercise can increase body temperature to as high as 38.3° to 40°C (101° to 104°F) measured rectally because of the increased heat produced by working muscles.

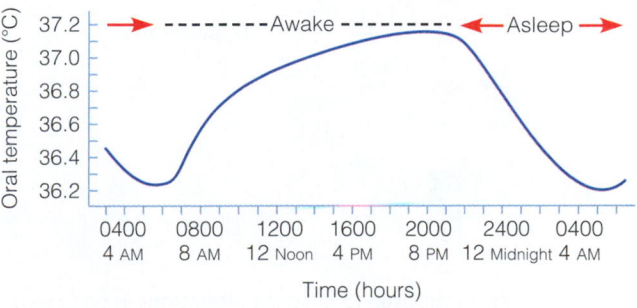

Figure 21-2. ■ Range of oral temperatures during 24 hours for a healthy young adult.

- *Hormones.* Women usually experience more hormonal fluctuations than men. In women, progesterone secretion at the time of ovulation raises body temperature by about 0.3° to 0.6°C (0.5° to 1.0°F) above basal temperature. This is best recognized by measuring body temperature upon waking, before getting out of bed.
- *Stress.* Stimulation of the sympathetic nervous system can increase the production of epinephrine and norepinephrine, thereby increasing metabolic activity and heat production. Nurses may anticipate that a highly stressed or anxious client could have an elevated body temperature for that reason.
- *Environment.* Extremes in environmental temperatures can affect a person's temperature-regulating systems. If the temperature is assessed in a very warm room, the temperature may be falsely elevated. Similarly, if the client has been outside in extremely cold weather without suitable clothing, the body temperature may be low. Core temperature is less affected than surface temperature by the environment.

ALTERATIONS IN BODY TEMPERATURE

Pyrexia

A body temperature above the usual range is called **pyrexia, hyperthermia,** or **fever.** A very high fever, such as 41°C (105.8°F), is called **hyperpyrexia** (Figure 21-3 ■). The client who has a fever is referred to as **febrile;** one who does not have a fever is referred to as **afebrile.**

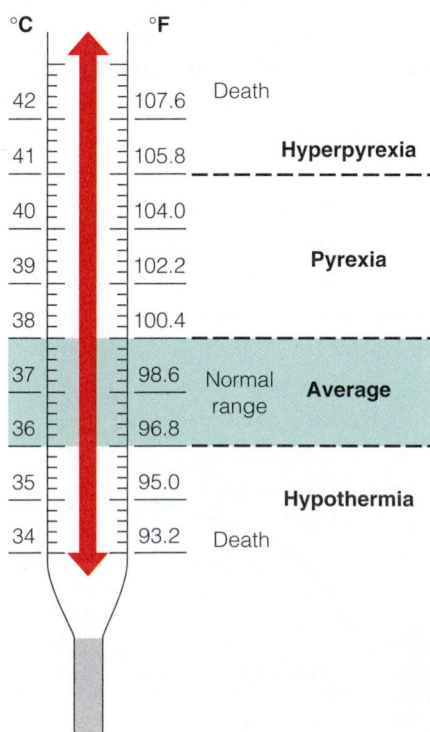

Figure 21-3. ■ Terms used to describe alterations in body temperature (oral measurements) and ranges in Celsius (centigrade) and Fahrenheit scales.

Four common types of fevers are intermittent, remittent, relapsing, and constant. During an **intermittent fever,** the body temperature alternates at regular intervals between periods of fever and periods of normal or subnormal temperatures without the use of **antipyretics** (medications that help to reduce an elevated temperature). During a **remittent fever,** the temperature remains elevated but fluctuates widely (more than 2°C [3.6°F]) over a 24-hour period. In a **relapsing fever,** the client will have a fever for a few days, then be afebrile for a few days before the fever returns again. With a **constant fever,** the body temperature fluctuates minimally but always remains above normal. The manifestations of fever vary with the onset, cause, course, and abatement stages of the fever (Box 21-3 ■).

Very high temperatures, such as 41° to 42°C (106° to 108°F), damage cells throughout the body, particularly in the brain where destruction of neuronal cells is irreversible. Damage to the liver, kidneys, and other body organs can also be great enough to disrupt functioning and eventually cause death.

When the cause of the high temperature is suddenly removed, the body's thermostat is reset to a lower value, perhaps even back to the original normal level. In this instance, the hypothalamus now attempts to lower the temperature to 37°C (98.6°F). Heat loss responses cause a reduction of the body temperature to occur; manifestations are excessive sweating

BOX 21-3	MANIFESTATIONS OF FEVER

Onset (Cold or Chill Stage)

- Increased heart rate
- Increased respiratory rate and depth
- Shivering
- Pallid, cold skin
- Complaints of feeling cold
- Cyanotic nail beds
- "Gooseflesh" appearance of the skin
- Cessation of sweating

Course

- Absence of chills
- Skin that feels warm
- Photosensitivity
- Glassy-eyed appearance
- Increased pulse and respiratory rates
- Increased thirst

Mild to Severe Dehydration

- Drowsiness, restlessness, delirium, or convulsions
- Herpetic lesions of the mouth
- Loss of appetite (if the fever is prolonged)
- Malaise, weakness, and aching muscles

Defervescence (Fever Abatement)

- Skin that appears flushed and feels warm
- Sweating
- Decreased shivering
- Possible dehydration

and a hot, flushed skin due to sudden vasodilation. This sudden change of events is known as the **crisis** of a pyrexic condition. A more gradual return of the body temperature to normal is referred to as a *resolution by lysis*. Nursing interventions for a client who has a fever are designed to support the body's normal physiological processes, provide comfort, and prevent complications. During the course of fever, the nurse needs to monitor the client's vital signs closely (Box 21-4 ■).

Nursing measures during the chill phase are designed to help the client decrease heat loss and raise the core body temperature. During flushing or the crisis phase, body processes are attempting to lower the core temperature to normal. At this time, the nurse takes measures to increase heat loss and decrease heat production.

The nurse may provide a cooling sponge bath to reduce a client's fever (see use of cold and heat in Chapter 24 ⚭). The bath consists of water or a combination of alcohol and water that is below body temperature. Alcohol evaporates at a low temperature and therefore removes body heat rapidly. However, alcohol-and-water sponge baths are less frequently used than in the past because alcohol has a drying effect on the skin. The temperatures for cooling sponge baths range from 18° to 32°C (65° to 90°F).

clinical ALERT

Alcohol sponge baths are of particular danger to children because the alcohol can be absorbed through the skin (Boggan, 2003).

A tepid sponge bath generally refers to one in which the water temperature is 32°C (90°F) throughout the bath. The decision to give a tepid sponge bath is generally made only when a marked fever or a temperature increase is noted. Some agencies require a physician's order; others permit a decision by a nurse.

Hypothermia

Hypothermia is core body temperature below the lower limit of normal. The three physiological mechanisms of hypothermia are (1) excessive heat loss, (2) inadequate heat production to counteract the heat loss, and (3) impaired hypothalamic temperature regulation. The manifestations of hypothermia are given in Box 21-5 ■.

Hypothermia may be accidental or induced. Accidental hypothermia can occur as a result of (1) exposure to a cold environment (i.e., below 16°C [60.8°F]), (2) immersion in cold water, and (3) lack of adequate clothing, shelter, or heat. In older people the problem can be compounded by a decreased metabolic rate and the use of sedatives, which depress the metabolic rate further. Alcohol and drug abuse can also increase the risk of hypothermia.

Managing the hypothermia involves removing the client from the cold and rewarming the client's body gradually. For the client with mild hypothermia, the body is rewarmed by applying blankets. For the client with severe hypothermia, a hyperthermia blanket (an electronically controlled warming blanket that provides a specified temperature) is applied, warm saline stomach lavage, and warm intravenous fluids are given. In the most extreme cases a dialysis machine with warming coils may be used to warm

---

BOX 21-4	NURSING CARE CHECKLIST

Clients with Fever

- ☑ Monitor vital signs.
- ☑ Assess skin color and temperature.
- ☑ Monitor white blood cell count, hematocrit value, and other pertinent laboratory reports for indications of infection or dehydration.
- ☑ Remove excess blankets when the client feels warm, but provide extra warmth when the client feels chilled, especially if the client is shivering, which raises body temperature through excess muscle work.
- ☑ Provide adequate nutrition and fluids (e.g., 2500 to 3000 mL per day) to meet the increased metabolic demands and prevent dehydration. Clients who sweat profusely can become dehydrated and fever increases insensible water loss. Dehydration can increase temperature.
- ☑ Measure intake and output.
- ☑ Reduce physical activity to limit heat production, especially during the flush stage.
- ☑ Administer antipyretics as ordered.
- ☑ Provide oral hygiene to keep the mucous membranes moist. They can become dry and cracked as a result of excessive fluid loss.
- ☑ Provide a tepid sponge bath to increase heat loss through conduction, but stop the bath immediately if shivering occurs.
- ☑ Provide dry clothing and bed linens if they become wet from diaphoresis.

BOX 21-5	MANIFESTATIONS OF HYPOTHERMIA

- Decreased body temperature, pulse, and respirations
- Severe shivering (initially)
- Feelings of cold and chills
- Pale, cool, waxy skin
- Hypotension
- Decreased urinary output
- Lack of muscle coordination
- Disorientation
- Drowsiness progressing to coma
- In the most extreme cases of hypothermia, physical stimulation of the body can lead to ventricular fibrillation

BOX 21-6   NURSING CARE CHECKLIST

Clients with Hypothermia

☑ Provide a warm environment (room temperature).

☑ Provide dry clothing.

☑ Apply warm blankets.

☑ Keep limbs close to body.

☑ Cover the client's scalp with a cap or turban.

☑ Supply warm oral or intravenous fluids.

☑ Apply warming pads.

clinical ALERT

The client who is hypothermic should never be declared dead if cardiac function stops. A client cannot be declared dead until he or she is warmed and still does not respond to resuscitation efforts.

the circulating blood volume. Wet clothing, which increases heat loss because of the high conductivity of water, should be replaced with dry clothing. See Box 21-6 ■ for nursing interventions for clients who have hypothermia.

Induced hypothermia is the deliberate lowering of the body temperature to decrease the need for oxygen by the body tissues. Induced hypothermia can involve the whole body or a body part. It is sometimes indicated prior to surgery (e.g., cardiac and brain surgery).

TEMPERATURE ASSESSMENT METHODS

The four most common sites for measuring body temperature are oral, rectal, axillary, and the tympanic membrane. Each of the sites has advantages and disadvantages (Table 21-2 ■). Products exist on the market to measure skin temperature by applying a sensor to the skin, such as the forehead, but these methods should not be used for anything other than screening purposes owing to the unreliability of the reading.

The tympanic membrane thermometer (Figure 21-4 ■) is becoming the preferred method for taking body temperature. Tympanic membrane temperature readings average 1.1 to 1.5°F higher than oral temperature readings. Like the sublingual oral site, the tympanic membrane has an abundant arterial blood supply. The tympanic infrared method is quickly

TABLE 21-2   Comparison of Four Sites for Measuring Body Temperature

SITE	ADVANTAGES	DISADVANTAGES
Oral	Most accessible and convenient	Mercury-in-glass thermometers can break if bitten; therefore they are contraindicated for children under 6 years and clients who are confused or who have convulsive disorders.
		Inaccurate if client has just ingested hot or cold food or fluid or smoked.
		Could injure the mouth following oral surgery.
		Contraindicated in children who are unable to cooperate with the procedure.
Rectal	Most reliable measurement	Inconvenient, invasive, and more unpleasant for clients; difficult for client who cannot turn to the side.
		Could injure the rectum following rectal surgery or if inserted improperly.
		Placement of the thermometer at different sites within the rectum yields different temperatures, yet placement at the same site each time is difficult.
		A rectal glass thermometer does not respond to changes in arterial temperatures as quickly as an oral thermometer, a fact that may be potentially dangerous for febrile clients because misleading information may be acquired.
		Presence of stool may interfere with thermometer placement. If the stool is soft, the thermometer may be embedded in stool rather than pressed against the wall of the rectum. If the stool is impacted, the depth of the thermometer insertion may be insufficient.
		In newborns and infants, insertion of the rectal thermometer has resulted in ulcerations and rectal perforations. Many agencies advise against using rectal thermometers on neonates. Movement of the child during measurement can result in puncture of the bowel.
Axillary	Safest and most noninvasive	The thermometer must be left in place a long time to obtain an accurate measurement.
		Measures surface body temperature instead of core temperature and can be affected by environmental temperature.
Tympanic membrane	Readily accessible; reflects the core temperature; very fast	Can be uncomfortable and involves risk of injuring the membrane if the probe is inserted too far.
		Repeated measurements may vary.
		Right and left measurements can differ.
		Presence of cerumen can affect the reading.
		Inaccurate in children younger than 2 years of age due to the small circumference of the ear canal.

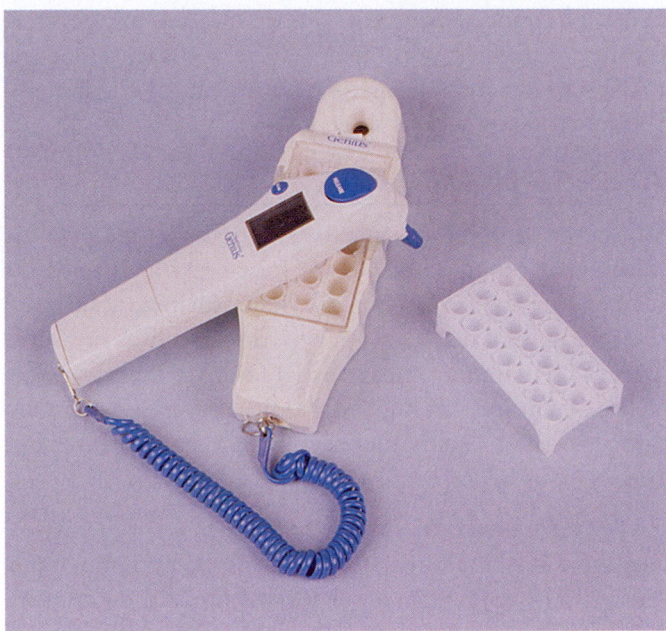

Figure 21-4. ■ A tympanic thermometer.

becoming the method of choice in clients over 2 years of age. The oral site is an equally preferred site. This method reflects changing body temperature more quickly than the rectal method. Rectal temperature readings are considered to be the most accurate. The axilla is the preferred site for measuring temperature in newborns because it is accessible and offers no possibility of rectal perforation. Nursing students should check facility protocol when taking the temperature of newborns, infants, toddlers, and children. Clients for whom the axillary method of temperature assessment is appropriate include adult clients with oral inflammation or wired jaws, clients recovering from oral surgery, clients who are breathing through their mouths (e.g., following nasal surgery), irrational clients, and clients for whom other temperature sites are contraindicated.

In addition to the four common sites for measuring temperature, the forehead may also be used. Body temperature is measured by using a chemical thermometer. Forehead temperature measurements are most useful for screening infants and children where a more invasive measurement is not necessary. If the forehead indicates a temperature elevation, a glass or electronic thermometer should be used to obtain a more accurate measurement.

Types of Thermometers

Traditionally, body temperatures have been measured using mercury-in-glass thermometers. Due to the risk of mercury poisoning from broken thermometers, many facilities have discontinued using mercury-in-glass thermometers and instead use mercury-free glass thermometers (Figure 21-5 ■). Oral thermometers may have long, slender tips or short, rounded tips. The rounded thermometer can be used at the rectal as well as other sites. In some medical facilities, thermometers may be

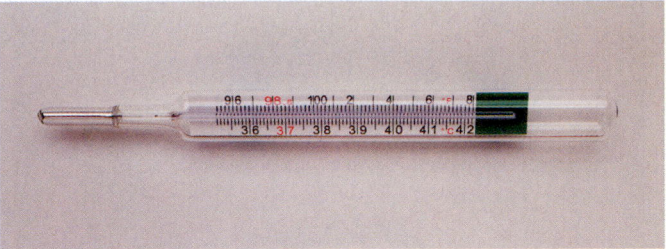

Figure 21-5. ■ Nonmercury glass thermometer. *Source:* Pearson Learning Photo Studio.

color coded (red thermometers for rectal temperatures, silver or blue for oral and axillary temperatures).

Electronic thermometers offer another method of assessing body temperatures. They can provide a reading in only 2 to 60 seconds, depending on the model. The equipment consists of a battery-operated portable electronic unit, a probe that the nurse attaches to the unit, and a probe cover, which is usually disposable (Figure 21-6 ■).

Chemical disposable thermometers are also used to measure body temperatures. Chemical thermometers using liquid crystal dots, bars, or heat-sensitive tape or patches applied to the forehead change color to indicate temperature. Some of these are single use and others may be reused several times. To read the temperature, the nurse notes the highest reading among the dots or bars that have changed color (Figure 21-7 ■).

Temperature-sensitive tape is used to obtain a general indication of body surface temperature. When applied to dry skin, usually of the forehead or abdomen, the temperature digits on the tape respond by changing color after the length of time specified by the manufacturer (e.g., 15 seconds). The

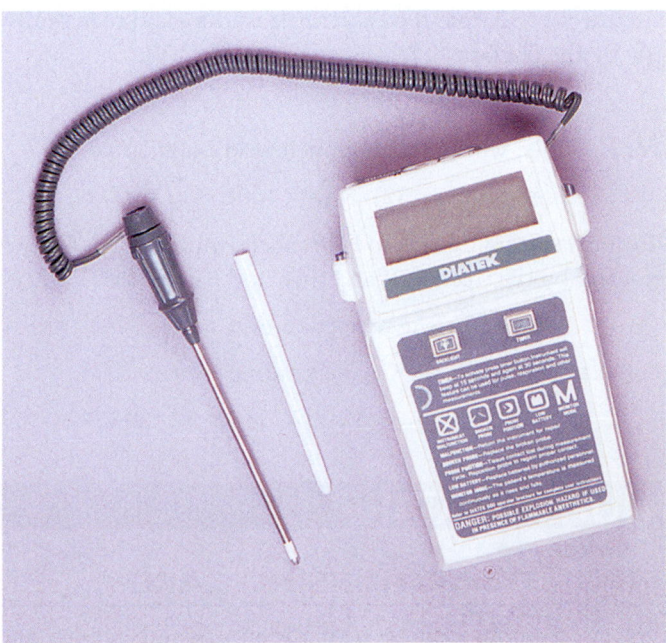

Figure 21-6. ■ An electronic thermometer. Note the probe and probe cover. (© Elena Dorfman.)

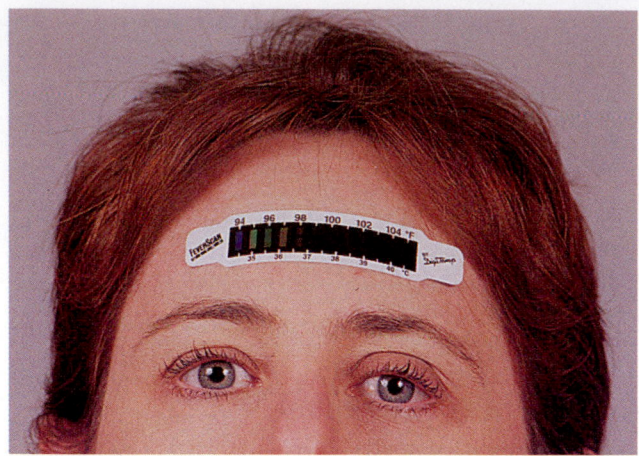

Figure 21-7. ■ A temperature-sensitive skin tape. (© Jenny Thomas.)

tape is removed and discarded after the color has been compared to the scale provided by the manufacturer. This method is particularly useful at home and for infants whose temperatures are to be monitored for any reason, but it should be used for screening purposes only. If the tape indicates the presence of a fever, an oral, axillary, rectal, or tympanic temperature should be obtained.

Temperature Scales

The body temperature is measured in degrees on two scales: Celsius (centigrade) and Fahrenheit. On a glass thermometer, the **Celsius** scale normally extends from 34.0° to 42.0°C. The **Fahrenheit** scale usually extends from 94° to 108°F. Body temperatures rarely extend beyond these scales (see Figure 21-3).

Sometimes a nurse needs to convert a Celsius reading to Fahrenheit, or vice versa. To convert from Fahrenheit to Celsius, deduct 32 from the Fahrenheit reading and then multiply by the fraction $\frac{5}{9}$, that is:

$$C = (\text{Fahrenheit temperature} - 32) \times \tfrac{5}{9}$$

For example, when the Fahrenheit reading is 100:

$$C = (100 - 32) \times \tfrac{5}{9} = (68) \times \tfrac{5}{9} = 37.7$$

To convert from Celsius to Fahrenheit, multiply the Celsius reading by the fraction $\frac{9}{5}$ and then add 32; that is:

$$F = (\text{Celsius temperature} \times \tfrac{9}{5}) + 32$$

For example, when the Celsius reading is 40:

$$F = (40 \times \tfrac{9}{5}) + 32 = (72) + 32 = 104$$

NURSING CARE

PRIORITIZING NURSING CARE

When caring for a client with a fever, the nurse must take measures to reduce the fever, prevent complications of hyperthermia, and contribute to determining the cause. Assess hydration status, encourage fluids, measure temperature reading frequently until temperature approaches and remains within normal limits, and document the client's temperature and any actions taken.

ASSESSING

Whenever a fever is assessed, follow-up temperature measurements should be done at least every hour until the temperature approaches normal. Many antipyretics control fever for up to 4 hours, so temperature should be measured every 4 hours in any client with a fever until they remain afebrile for at least 24 hours. In addition to measuring temperature, assess clients for other symptoms of a fever (see Box 21-3) or hypothermia (see Box 21-5).

Safety Precautions

Safety is a major consideration when assessing temperature due to the disadvantages of the various sites and equipment. Never force any type of thermometer into place. If it does not enter easily, reassess the site and consider using a different location or type of thermometer.

The oral site should not be used if the client cannot cooperate or there is a risk that he or she may bite a glass thermometer. The rectal thermometer should always be held in place and never be left unattended. Severe injury could occur if the client rolled onto the thermometer or sits up on the thermometer. Glass thermometers must be handled carefully since they pose a safety hazard if broken. If a glass thermometer does not shake down easily or has any signs of cracks, it should be disposed of according to facility policy. (The nurse who frequently shakes down a thermometer is at increased risk for carpal tunnel syndrome.)

Electronic thermometers and other electrical equipment should not be used if damaged, since malfunctioning equipment can present a shock hazard to both the client and the nurse.

DIAGNOSING, PLANNING, AND IMPLEMENTING

The most common nursing diagnosis for clients with alterations of temperature beyond normal limits is *Ineffective Thermoregulation*. **Thermoregulation** is the control of temperature to maintain a normal, or near-normal, reading. Refer to Table 21-2 for selecting an appropriate site for measuring body temperature. Procedure 21-1 ■ on page [455] explains how to measure body temperature. Box 21-4 provides nursing implementations for clients with a fever.

EVALUATING

The temperature measurement is compared to baseline data and normal range. Client's age, time of day, site used for measurement, and any other influencing factors are considered. Temperature readings are reviewed in relation to other vital signs. Always monitor the febrile client's temperature at least every 4 hours until the client remains afebrile for at least 24 hours.

Continuity of Care

- Teach the client accurate use and reading of the type of thermometer to be used. Reinforce the importance of reporting the site and type of thermometer used and the value of using one type of thermometer consistently. Provide a recording chart or table if indicated.
- Discuss means of keeping the thermometer clean, such as warm water and soap, and avoiding cross-contamination.
- Ensure that the client has water-soluble lubricant if using a rectal thermometer.
- Have the client or family member demonstrate use of the thermometer so proper technique can be reinforced.
- Instruct the client or family member to notify the healthcare provider if the temperature is 37.7°C (100°F) or higher. A temperature of 37.7°C (100°F) or higher in an infant less than 6 months of age requires immediate medical intervention to screen for sepsis.

Pulse

The **pulse** is a wave of blood flowing through the artery created by contraction of the left ventricle of the heart. The heart is a pulsating pump, and the blood enters the arteries with each contraction, causing pressure pulses or pulse waves. These pulse waves can be palpated in areas where the artery passes over a bone. Generally, the pulse wave represents the **cardiac output** (stroke volume × pulse rate) and the amount of blood that enters the arteries with each ventricular contraction. When an adult is resting, normal cardiac output is approximately 5 liters of blood each minute. **Compliance** of the arteries is their ability to contract and expand. When a person's arteries lose their ability to expand, as can happen in old age, greater pressure is required to pump the blood into the arteries because the rigid arterial walls offer resistance resulting in elevated blood pressure or **hypertension.**

In a healthy person, the pulse reflects the heartbeat. In other words, the pulse rate is the same as the rate of the ventricular contractions of the heart. However, in some types of cardiovascular disease, the heartbeat and pulse rates can differ. For example, a client's heart may produce very weak or small pulse waves that are not detectable in a peripheral pulse far from the heart. In these instances, the nurse should assess the apical and peripheral pulse at the same time. See the section on assessing the apical pulse later in this chapter. A **peripheral pulse** is a pulse taken away from the heart, for example, in the foot, hand, or neck. The **apical pulse,** in contrast, is a central pulse; that is, it is a pulse taken directly at the heart.

FACTORS AFFECTING PULSE RATE

The rate of the pulse is expressed in beats per minute (bpm). A pulse rate varies according to a number of factors. The nurse should consider each of the following factors when assessing a client's pulse:

- *Age.* As age increases, the pulse rate gradually decreases. See Table 21-1 for specific variations in pulse rates from birth to adulthood.
- *Sex.* After puberty, the average male's pulse rate is slightly lower than the female's.
- *Exercise.* The pulse rate normally increases with activity. The rate of increase in the professional athlete is often less than in the average person because of greater cardiac size, strength, and efficiency. The athlete will normally have a slower resting heart rate than the average person; it could be normal when it measures as low as 45 to 55 bpm.
- *Fever.* The pulse rate increases (1) in response to the lowered blood pressure that results from peripheral vasodilation associated with elevated body temperature and (2) because of the increased metabolic rate.
- *Medications.* Some medications decrease the pulse rate, and others increase it. For example, cardiotonics (e.g., digitalis preparations) decrease the heart rate, whereas epinephrine causes an increase.
- *Hemorrhage.* Loss of blood from the vascular system (hemorrhage) normally increases pulse rate. In adults, the loss of a small amount of blood (e.g., 500 mL, the amount lost after a blood donation) results in a temporary adjustment of the heart rate as the body compensates for the lost blood volume. An adult has about 5 liters of blood circulating in the vascular system and can usually lose up to 10% without adverse effects.
- *Stress.* In response to stress, sympathetic nervous stimulation increases the overall activity of the heart. Stress increases the rate as well as the force of the heartbeat. Fear and anxiety, as well as the perception of severe pain, stimulate the sympathetic system. Box 21-7 ■ describes effects of stress in the pediatric client.
- *Position changes.* When a person assumes a sitting or standing position, blood usually pools in dependent vessels of the venous system. Pooling results in a transient decrease in the venous blood return to the heart and a subsequent reduction in blood pressure and increase in heart rate.

BOX 21-7 PEDIATRIC CONSIDERATIONS

Crying and Pulse Rate

Crying can increase pediatric pulse rates. Every attempt should be made to measure children's heart rates while they are calm or sleeping. It is normal for pediatric pulse rhythm to be slightly irregular, with pauses between beats if the child holds his or her breath while crying, or more rapid pulsations if the child hyperventilates.

PULSE SITES

A pulse is commonly taken in any of nine sites (see Figure 19-8 🔗):

1. *Temporal*, where the temporal artery passes over the temporal bone of the head. The site is superior (above) and lateral to (away from the midline of) the eye.
2. *Carotid*, at the side of the neck where the carotid artery runs between the trachea and the sternocleidomastoid muscle. Never press both carotids at the same time because this can cause a reflex drop in blood pressure or pulse rate and reduce blood flow to the brain.
3. *Apical* pulse is heard at the apex of the heart using a stethoscope. In an adult, this is located on the left side of the chest, no more than 8 cm (3 in.) to the left of the sternum (breastbone) and at the fourth, fifth, or sixth intercostal space (area between the ribs). For a child 7 to 9 years of age, the apical pulse is located at the fourth or fifth intercostal spaces. Before 4 years of age, it is left of the midclavicular line (MCL); between 4 and 6 years, it is at the MCL (Figure 21-8 ■). The area where the pulse is heard the loudest and strongest is called the **point of maximal impulse** (PMI).
4. *Brachial*, at the inner aspect of the biceps muscle of the arm (especially in infants) or medially in the antecubital space (elbow crease). This pulse spot will be discussed in more detail later in the chapter as it is used for measuring blood pressure.
5. *Radial*, where the radial artery runs along the radial bone, on the thumb side of the inner aspect of the wrist.
6. *Femoral*, where the femoral artery passes alongside the inguinal ligament, palpated in the medial crease where the femur meets the pelvis.
7. *Popliteal*, where the popliteal artery passes behind the knee. This point is difficult to find, but it can be best palpated if the client flexes the knee slightly (see Figure 19-8 🔗).

TABLE 21-3	Reasons for Using Specific Pulse Sites
PULSE SITE	**REASONS FOR USE**
Radial	Readily accessible
Temporal	Used when radial pulse is not accessible
Carotid	Used for infants
	Used in cases of cardiac arrest
	Used to determine circulation to the brain
Apical	Routinely used for infants and children up to 3 years of age
	Used to determine discrepancies with radial pulse
	Used in conjunction with some medications
Brachial	Used to measure blood pressure
	Used during cardiac arrest for infants
Femoral	Used in cases of cardiac arrest
	Used for infants and children
	Used to determine circulation to a leg
Popliteal	Used to determine circulation to the lower leg
Posterior tibial	Used to determine circulation to the foot
Pedal	Used to determine circulation to the foot

8. *Posterior tibial*, on the medial surface of the ankle where the posterior tibial artery passes behind the medial malleolus.
9. *Pedal (dorsalis pedis)*, where the dorsalis pedis artery passes over the bones of the foot. This artery can be palpated by feeling the *dorsum* (upper surface) of the foot on an imaginary line drawn from the middle of the ankle to the space between the big and second toes. This pulse may be difficult to palpate in clients with peripheral vascular disease and may require the use of a Doppler ultrasound.

The radial site is most commonly used. It is easily found in most people and is readily accessible. The reasons for use of each site are given in Table 21-3 ■.

NURSING CARE

PRIORITIZING NURSING CARE

Changes in heart rate can impact other organ systems because of reduced blood perfusion resulting in decreased oxygen supply. The nurse should measure and document pulse rate, rhythm, and strength of pulsation. If the pulse rate is outside the normal limits, it should be reported to the nursing supervisor and/or physician along with assessment of how the change in pulse rate is affecting the client's mental status, respiratory status, and peripheral perfusion. It is important for an abnormal pulse rate to be verified by obtaining an apical pulse to determine if it is a peripheral perfusion problem versus an abnormal heart rate.

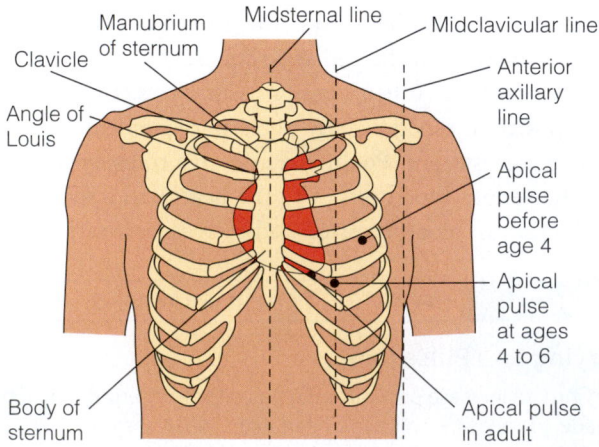

Figure 21-8. ■ Location of the apical pulse for a child under 4 years, a child 4 to 6 years, and an adult. The dots show the *point of maximal impulse* for different ages.

ASSESSING

A pulse is commonly assessed by palpation (feeling) or auscultation (hearing). The middle three fingertips are used for palpating all pulse sites except the apex of the heart. A stethoscope is used for assessing apical pulses and fetal heart tones. A Doppler ultrasound stethoscope (DUS; Figure 21-9 ▪) is used for pulses that are difficult to assess. The DUS headset has earpieces similar to standard stethoscope earpieces, but it has a long cord attached to a volume-controlled audio unit and an ultrasound transducer. The DUS detects movement of red blood cells through a blood vessel. In contrast to the conventional stethoscope, it excludes environmental sounds. It cannot detect blood flow in deep vessels or in blood vessels underlying bone, such as the vessels in the abdomen, thorax, or skull.

A pulse is normally palpated by applying moderate pressure with the three middle fingers of the hand. The pads on the most distal aspects of the finger are the most sensitive areas for detecting a pulse. The thumb should not be used for palpation because the pulsation in the thumb may cause the nurse to count his or her own pulse instead of the pulse of the client. With excessive pressure the nurse can obliterate the pulse, whereas with too little pressure, the nurse may

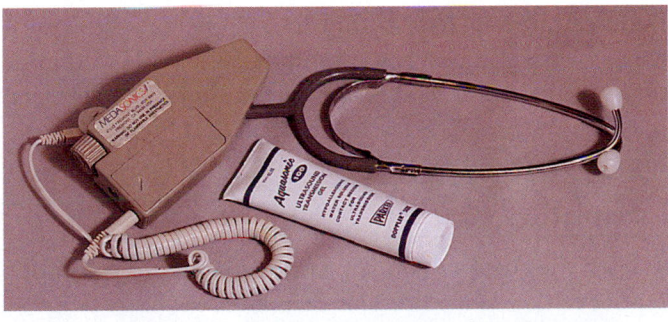

Figure 21-9. ▪ An ultrasound (Doppler or DUS) stethoscope.
(© Elena Dorfman.)

not be able to detect it. Before the nurse assesses the resting pulse, the client should assume a comfortable position. The nurse should also be aware of the following:

- Whether the client has taken any medication that could affect the heart rate.
- Whether the client has been physically active. If so, wait 10 to 15 minutes until the client has rested and the pulse has slowed to its usual rate.
- Whether any baseline data exist about the normal heart rate for the client. For example, a physically fit athlete may have a heart rate below 60 bpm.
- Whether the client should assume a particular position (e.g., sitting). In some clients, the rate changes with the position because of changes in blood flow volume and autonomic nervous system activity.

When assessing the pulse, the nurse collects the following data: the rate, rhythm, volume, arterial wall elasticity, and presence or absence of bilateral equality. The normal pulse rates are shown in Table 21-1. An excessively fast heart rate (e.g., more than 100 bpm in an adult) is referred to as **tachycardia.** A heart rate in an adult of 60 bpm or less is called **bradycardia.** If a client has either tachycardia or bradycardia, the apical pulse should be assessed.

The pulse rhythm is the pattern of the beats and the intervals between the beats (Table 21-4 ▪). Normal pulsations are regular, with equal time elapsing between beats. A pulse with an irregular rhythm is referred to as a **dysrhythmia** or **arrhythmia.** It may consist of random, irregular beats or a predictable pattern of irregular beats. When a dysrhythmia is detected, the apical pulse should be assessed for one full minute. An electrocardiogram (ECG or EKG) is necessary to define the dysrhythmia further.

Pulse volume, also called the pulse strength or amplitude, refers to the force of the blood in the artery with each heartbeat. Usually, the pulse volume is the same with each

TABLE 21-4	Basic Heart Sounds	
HEART SOUNDS	**NORMAL FINDINGS**	**ABNORMAL FINDINGS**
S_1	Usually heard at all sites Usually louder at apical and tricuspid areas	Increased intensity at aortic area Increased intensity at pulmonic area Sharp-sounding ejection clicks
S_2	Usually heard at all sites Usually louder at the base of the heart and aortic and pulmonic areas	Increased or decreased intensity Varying intensity with different beats Sharp-sounding ejection clicks
SYSTOLE	Silent interval Slightly shorter duration than diastole at normal heart rate (60–90 bpm)	
DIASTOLE	Silent interval Slightly longer duration than systole at normal heart rate	
S_3	Normal to hear in children and young adults	S_3 in older adults
S_4	Normal to auscultate in many older adults	S_4 may be a sign of hypertension

TABLE 21-5	Scale for Measuring Pulse Volume
SCALE	DESCRIPTION OF PULSE
0	Absent, not discernible
1	Thready or weak, difficult to feel, easily obliterated
2	Normal, detected readily, obliterated by strong pressure
3	Bounding, difficult to obliterate, can sometimes be visualized

beat. It can range from absent to bounding. A normal pulse can be felt with moderate pressure of the fingers and can be obliterated (unable to be felt) with greater pressure. A forceful or full blood volume that is obliterated only with difficulty is called a *full* or *bounding pulse*. A pulse that is readily obliterated with pressure from the fingers is referred to as weak, feeble, or *thready*. A pulse volume is usually measured on a scale of 0 to 3 (Table 21-5 ■).

The elasticity of the arterial wall reflects its ability to expand or respond to increased pressures. A healthy, normal artery feels straight, smooth, soft, and pliable. Older people often have inelastic arteries that feel twisted (*tortuous*) and irregular on palpation.

When assessing a peripheral pulse to determine the adequacy of blood flow to a particular area of the body, the nurse should compare the corresponding pulse on the other side of the body. The second assessment gives the nurse data with which to compare the pulses. For example, when assessing the blood flow to the right foot, the nurse assesses the right dorsalis pedis pulse and then the left dorsalis pedis pulse. If the client's right and left pulses are the same, the client's dorsalis pedis pulses are said to be *bilaterally equal*. If a pulse is absent, or cannot be palpated, use of the Doppler ultrasound can reveal the pulsations. The nurse should assess circulatory competence to the extremity with the missing pulse. Pale, cool skin that differs from the other extremity can indicate inadequate blood flow to the extremity and requires immediate medical intervention to prevent loss of the limb.

Peripheral Pulse

A peripheral pulse, usually the radial pulse, is assessed by palpation in all individuals except:

- Newborns and children up to 2 or 3 years. Apical pulses are assessed in these clients.
- Very obese or elderly clients, whose radial pulse may be difficult to palpate. Doppler equipment may be used for these clients, or the apical pulse is assessed.
- Individuals with a heart disease, who require apical pulse assessment.
- Individuals in whom the circulation to a specific body part must be assessed; for example, following leg surgery, the pedal (dorsalis pedis) pulse is assessed.

Apical–Radial Pulse

An **apical–radial pulse** may need to be assessed for clients with certain cardiovascular disorders. Normally, the apical and radial rates are identical. An apical pulse rate greater than a radial pulse rate can indicate that the thrust of the blood from the heart is too feeble for the wave to be felt at the peripheral pulse site, or it can indicate that vascular disease is preventing impulses from being transmitted. Any differences between the two pulse rates (called a **pulse deficit**) need to be reported promptly. In no instance is the radial pulse greater than the apical pulse.

An apical–radial pulse can be taken by two nurses or one nurse, although the two-nurse technique may be more accurate. It takes practice for one nurse to perform apical–radial assessment competently.

DIAGNOSING, PLANNING, AND IMPLEMENTING

A possible nursing diagnosis would be *Decreased Cardiac Output*. Refer to Table 21-3 for selection of an appropriate site. Procedure 21-2 ■ on page 457 provides guidelines for various methods of assessing pulse.

EVALUATING

Evaluate pulse in relationship to baseline data or normal range for age of client, relationship of pulse rate and volume to other vital signs, and health status. Compare peripheral pulses by assessing equality, rate, and volume in corresponding extremities.

Continuity of Care

- Teach the client or family member to monitor the pulse prior to taking medications that affect the heart rate.
- Tell the client to report any notable changes in heart rate or rhythm (regularity) to the healthcare provider.
- Ensure that the client or family member is aware of which pulse findings should be reported and to whom.

NURSING PROCESS CARE PLAN
Client with Left-Sided Heart Failure

Marie McGhee, an 81-year-old female, has been a resident at Knight's Bridge Road Retirement Center since her husband died 6 months ago. She was admitted through the ED for left-sided heart failure. Mrs. McGhee expresses a dislike for her low-sodium diet. She admits to taking no medication except "natural" therapy prescribed by her herbalist.

She is presently taking multivitamins and dried English hawthorn to decrease her blood pressure and decrease her oxygen needs. She states, "I don't want to take drugs because they gave them to my husband and he died anyway."

Assessment

VS: T 97.4, apical pulse 102 and irregular, respirations 28 and labored, BP 148/90, pulse ox 94%; orthopnea; inspiratory crackles and wheezes at the base of the lungs; nonproductive cough; states "I have to sleep sitting up in a chair." 3+ bilateral ankle edema, abdomen distended. ECG reflects atrial fibrillation. Chest x-ray reveals cardiomegaly.

Nursing Diagnosis

The following important nursing diagnoses (among others) are established for this client:

- *Excess Fluid Volume* related to impaired excretion of sodium and water
- *Activity Intolerance* related to weakness, fatigue
- *Powerlessness* related to illness-related regimen

Expected Outcomes

The expected outcomes specify that Mrs. Munson will:

- Maintain clear lung sounds, with no evidence of dyspnea or orthopnea.
- Express an understanding of need to balance rest and activity.
- Participate in planning care; make decision regarding care and treatments when possible.

Planning and Implementation

The following nursing interventions are planned and implemented:

- Monitor location and extent of edema; using a measuring tape, record ankle and abdominal circumference in millimeters in the same area at the same time each day to reflect any changes in the amount of edema in the extremities and abdomen.
- Monitor lung sounds for crackles; monitor respirations for effort and determine the presence and severity of orthopnea.
- Recognize that the presence of risk factors for excessive fluid volume is particularly serious in the elderly.
- Slow the pace of care. Allow client extra time to carry out activities and provide with rest periods.
- Encourage family and/or caretaker to help while allowing the client to be as independent in whatever activities as possible.
- Refer client to physical therapy to help increase activity tolerance and strength.
- Establish therapeutic relationship by listening; give the client choices and accept her statement of limitations.

- Help client identify factors not under her control.
- Validate client's feelings regarding the impact of health status on current lifestyle.

Evaluation

Mrs. Munson is being discharged to the skilled nursing center in her retirement community, after 4 days of hospitalization. Her respirations are unlabored at rest and edema in ankles reduced to +2. Lungs clear, able to sleep in low Fowler's position. Mrs. Munson referred to dietitian at the care facility to develop an eating plan that she can live with; stated "I will take my meals in the dining room after I return to my own apartment so that I can follow my prescribed diet." Participating in PT 3 days per week, can ambulate 25 feet without difficulty or shortness of breath. Taking Lasix 20 mg every day and still refusing other medications. BP 140/80. Mrs. Munson expresses fear of having a stroke.

Critical Thinking in the Nursing Process

1. Mrs. Munson expressed a wish to return to her own apartment as soon as possible. Design an activity program that will help her regain her strength and mobility.
2. Mrs. Munson wants to continue her natural medicine. What would be your response to her desire?
3. Mrs. Munson is fearful that she may have a stroke. What warning signs should she be aware of, and what actions should she take if they occur?

Note: Discussion of Critical Thinking questions appears on the MyNursingKit Website.

Respirations

Respiration is the act of breathing. **External respiration** refers to the interchange of oxygen and carbon dioxide between the alveoli of the lungs and the pulmonary blood. **Internal respiration** is the interchange of these same gases between the circulating blood and the cells of the body tissues.

Inhalation, or **inspiration,** refers to the intake of air into the lungs. **Exhalation,** or **expiration,** refers to breathing out or the movement of gases from the lungs to the atmosphere. *Ventilation* is also used to refer to the movement of air in and out of the lungs. **Hyperventilation** refers to very deep, rapid respirations; **hypoventilation** refers to very shallow inadequate respirations.

There are two types of breathing. **Costal** (thoracic) **breathing** involves external intercostal and accessory muscles. It can be observed by the movement of the chest upward and outward. **Diaphragmatic** (abdominal) **breathing** involves contraction and relaxation of the diaphragm. The abdomen moves with the diaphragm's contraction and downward movement. *Note: In infants and young children, the main muscle for breathing is the diaphragm.*

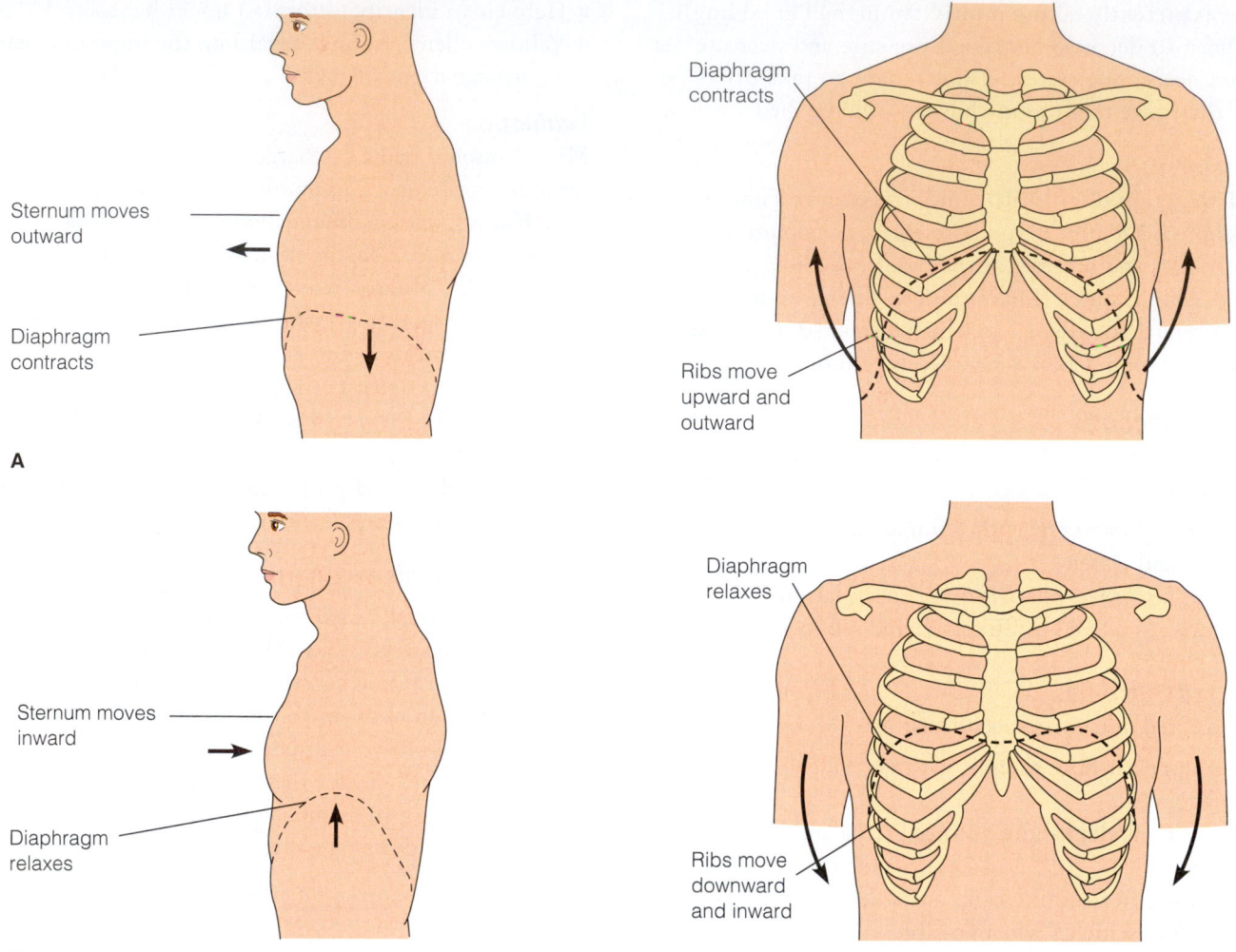

Figure 21-10. ■ **A.** Respiratory inhalation: *left:* lateral view; *right:* anterior view. **B.** Respiratory exhalation: *left:* lateral view; *right:* anterior view.

MECHANICS AND REGULATION

During inhalation, the diaphragm contracts, the ribs move upward and outward, and the sternum moves outward (Figure 21-10 ■). During exhalation, the diaphragm relaxes, the ribs move downward and inward, and the sternum moves inward, decreasing the size of the thorax as the lungs are compressed. Inspiration requires the use of energy, whereas exhalation is passive and results from relaxation of the diaphragm. Normal breathing is automatic and effortless. Inspiration lasts 1 to 1.5 seconds, and expiration lasts 2 to 3 seconds.

Respiration is controlled by (1) respiratory centers in the medulla oblongata and the pons of the brain and (2) chemoreceptors located centrally in the medulla and peripherally in the carotid and aortic bodies. These centers and receptors respond to changes in the concentrations of oxygen (O_2), carbon dioxide (CO_2), and hydrogen (H) in the arterial blood. See Chapter 32 ⬭ for further details.

NURSING CARE

PRIORITIZING NURSING CARE

The client's respiratory status affects all of the body's other organ systems, and alteration in oxygenation is an emergency situation. When measuring respirations the nurse should assess rate, effort, and rhythm. The nurse should never leave a client in respiratory distress alone. Stay with the client and seek help to notify the nursing supervisor or physician. Assessment of oxygen saturation, vital signs, perfusion, and mental status should be performed prior to notifying the primary provider.

ASSESSING

Resting respirations should be assessed when the client is relaxed. Both exercise and anxiety increase respiratory rate and depth. Respirations may also need to be assessed after

BOX 21-8 ALTERED BREATHING PATTERNS AND SOUNDS

Breathing Patterns

Rate

- **Tachypnea**—rapid respiration marked by quick, shallow breaths
- **Bradypnea**—abnormally slow breathing
- **Apnea**—cessation of breathing
- **Eupnea**—normal respirations

Volume

- Hyperventilation—an increase in the amount of air in the lungs characterized by prolonged and deep breaths; may be associated with anxiety
- Hypoventilation—a reduction in the amount of air in the lungs, characterized by shallow respirations

Rhythm

- **Cheyne-Stokes respirations**—rhythmic waxing and waning of respirations, from very deep to very shallow breathing and temporary apnea; often associated with cardiac failure, increased intracranial pressure, or brain damage

Ease or Effort

- **Dyspnea**—difficult and labored breathing during which the individual has a persistent, unsatisfied need for air and feels distressed
- **Orthopnea**—ability to breathe only in upright sitting or standing positions

Breath Sounds

Audible without Amplification

- **Stridor**—a shrill, harsh sound heard during inspiration with laryngeal obstruction

- **Stertor**—snoring or sonorous respiration, usually due to a partial obstruction of the upper airway
- **Wheeze**—continuous, high-pitched musical squeak or whistling sound occurring on expiration and sometimes on inspiration when air moves through a narrowed or partially obstructed airway
- **Bubbling**—gurgling sounds heard as air passes through moist secretions in the respiratory tract
- **Rales** (also referred to as **crackles**)—fine, short, interrupted crackling sounds (like sound of lock of hair being rubbed between thumb and finger), best heard on inspiration but can also be heard on expiration; may not be cleared by coughing

Chest Movements

- **Intercostal retraction**—indrawing between the ribs
- **Substernal retraction**—indrawing beneath the breastbone
- **Suprasternal retraction**—indrawing above the clavicles
- **Flail chest**—the ballooning out of the chest wall through injured rib spaces; results in paradoxical breathing, during which the chest wall balloons on expiration but is depressed or sucked inward on inspiration

Secretions and Coughing

- **Hemoptysis**—the presence of blood in the sputum
- **Productive cough**—a cough accompanied by expectorated secretions
- **Nonproductive cough**—a dry, harsh cough without secretions

---

exercise to identify the client's tolerance to activity. Before assessing a client's respirations, a nurse should be aware of:

- The client's normal breathing pattern.
- The influence of health problems on respirations.
- Any medications or therapies that might affect the client's respirations.
- The relationship of respirations to cardiovascular function.

The rate, depth, rhythm, and special characteristics of respirations should always be assessed. Box 21-8 ■ provides terms for breathing patterns, sounds, and movements. For the respiratory rates for different age groups, see Table 21-1. Several factors influence respiratory rate; major factors are listed in Table 21-6 ■.

The depth of a person's respirations can be established by watching the movement of the chest. Respiratory depth is generally described as normal, deep, or shallow. During a normal inspiration and expiration, an adult takes in about 500 mL of air. The normal quantity of air exchanged with each breath is called **tidal volume.** Body position also affects the amount of air that can be inhaled. People in a

supine position experience two physiological processes that suppress respiration: an increase in the volume of blood inside the thoracic cavity and compression of the chest. So, clients lying on their back have poorer lung aeration. This predisposes them to the stasis of fluids and subsequent infection. Certain medications also affect the respiratory depth. For example, barbiturates in large doses depress the respiratory centers in the brain, thereby depressing the respiratory rate and depth.

TABLE 21-6	Major Factors Influencing Respiratory Rate	
FACTOR	**EFFECT**
Exercise: increases metabolism	Increase
Stress: readies the body for "fight or flight"	Increase
Environment: increased temperature	Increase
Environment: decreased temperature	Decrease
Increased altitude: lower oxygen concentration	Increase
Certain medications (e.g., narcotic, analgesic)	Decrease
Increased intracranial pressure	Decrease

Respiratory rhythm or pattern refers to the regularity of expirations and inspirations. Normally, respirations are evenly spaced. Respiratory rhythm can be described as regular or irregular. An infant's respiratory rhythm may be less regular than an adult's.

Respiratory quality or character refers to those aspects of breathing that are different from normal, effortless breathing. Two of these are the amount of effort a client must exert to breathe and the sound of breathing. Usually, breathing does not require noticeable effort; some clients, however, breathe only with decided effort, referred to as **labored breathing.**

The sound of breathing is also significant. Normal breathing is silent. Many sounds occur as a result of the presence of fluid in the lungs, and are most clearly heard with a stethoscope (see Box 21-8).

The effectiveness of respirations is measured in part by the uptake of oxygen from the air into the blood and the release of carbon dioxide from the blood into expired air. The amount of hemoglobin in arterial blood that is saturated with oxygen can be measured indirectly through a **pulse oximeter.** (See Chapter 32 🔗 for an illustration of a pulse oximeter.)

DIAGNOSING, PLANNING, AND IMPLEMENTING

A common nursing diagnosis for clients with respiratory difficulty is *Ineffective Breathing Pattern.* Procedure 21-3 ■ on page 461 provides guidelines for assessing respirations.

Implementations to improve respiration might include repositioning, administration of oxygen, or postural drainage. Chapter 32 🔗 discusses respiratory care.

EVALUATING

Respirations are evaluated in relationship to the client's baseline data or normal range for age. The nurse documents the rate, volume, rhythm, and effort of respirations and notifies the primary care provider and nursing supervisor if significant changes occur in the client's normal pattern of respirations.

Blood Pressure

Arterial **blood pressure** is a measure of the force exerted by the blood as it flows through the arteries. Because the blood moves in waves, there are two blood pressure measurements. The **systolic pressure** is the pressure of the blood as a result of contraction of the ventricles (the pressure at the height of the blood wave). The **diastolic pressure** is the pressure when the ventricles are at rest; it is the lower pressure that is present at all times within the arteries. The difference between the diastolic and the systolic pressures is called the **pulse pressure.**

Blood pressure is measured in millimeters of mercury (mm Hg) and recorded as a fraction. The systolic pressure is written over the diastolic pressure. The average blood pressure

of a healthy adult is a range of 90–140 systolic and 60–90 diastolic. A number of factors influence blood pressure, and a change in blood pressure can indicate several different conditions. Blood pressure is not static and normally changes from minute to minute.

DETERMINANTS OF BLOOD PRESSURE

Arterial blood pressure is the result of several factors: the pumping action of the heart, the **peripheral vascular resistance** (the resistance supplied by the blood vessels as a result of compliance), and the **blood volume** (quantity of circulating fluid in the blood vessels) and **viscosity** (thickness of the blood).

Cardiac output is the volume of blood pumped into the arteries by the heart. When the pumping action of the heart is weak, less blood is pumped into the arteries, and the blood pressure decreases. When the heart's pumping action is strong, and the volume of blood pumped into the circulation increases, the blood pressure increases.

Peripheral vascular resistance is the amount of pressure applied by the arteries in the peripheral circulation. Increased peripheral vascular resistance can increase blood pressure. The diastolic pressure is especially affected by peripheral vascular resistance. Some factors that create resistance in the arterial system are the size of the arterioles and capillaries, the *compliance* of the arteries (ability to expand and contract), and the viscosity of the blood.

The size of the arterioles and the capillaries determines, in great part, the peripheral resistance. A **lumen** is a channel within a tube. The smaller the lumen of a vessel, the greater the resistance. Normally, the arterioles are in a state of partial constriction. Increased vasoconstriction raises the blood pressure, whereas decreased vasoconstriction lowers the blood pressure.

The arteries account for most of the peripheral resistance. The major factor reducing arterial compliance is pathologic change affecting the arterial walls. When elastic and muscular tissues of the arteries are replaced with fibrous tissue, the arteries lose much of their compliance. This condition, most common in middle-aged and elderly adults, is known as **arteriosclerosis.**

When the blood volume decreases (e.g., from hemorrhage or dehydration), the blood pressure decreases because of decreased circulating fluid in the arteries. When the volume increases (e.g., with an intravenous infusion or inadequate kidney function), the blood pressure increases because of the greater fluid volume within the circulatory system.

Blood *viscosity* is a physical property that results from friction of molecules in a fluid. In viscous (or "thick") fluid, there is a great deal of friction among the molecules as they slide by each other. The blood pressure is higher when the blood is highly viscous, that is, when the proportion of red blood cells to the blood plasma is high. This proportion is referred to as the **hematocrit.** The viscosity increases markedly when the hematocrit is more than 60% to 65%. One example would be the condition called **polycythemia,** which is an increased red blood cell count.

FACTORS AFFECTING BLOOD PRESSURE

Among the factors influencing blood pressure are:

- *Age.* Newborns have a mean systolic pressure of about 75 mm Hg. The pressure rises with age, reaching a peak at the onset of puberty, and then tends to decline somewhat. One quick way to determine the normal systolic blood pressure of a child is to use the following formula:

Normal systolic BP $= 80 + (2 \times$ child's age in years)

In older people, elasticity of the arteries is decreased—the arteries are more rigid and less yielding to the pressure of the blood. This produces an elevated systolic pressure. Because the walls no longer retract as flexibly with decreased pressure, the diastolic pressure is also higher. (See Table 21-1.)

- *Exercise.* Physical activity increases the cardiac output and the blood pressure. So, 20 to 30 minutes of rest following exercise is indicated before the resting blood pressure can be reliably assessed.

- *Stress.* Stimulation of the sympathetic nervous system increases cardiac output and vasoconstriction of the arterioles, increasing the blood pressure reading. However, severe pain can decrease blood pressure greatly and cause shock by inhibiting the vasomotor center and producing vasodilation. *White coat syndrome* describes the situation in which clients' blood pressure elevates when they visit the doctor because they feel stress. To rule out an element of white coat syndrome, the client with chronic hypertension can make a log of daily blood pressures measured at home.

- *Race.* African American males over 35 years of age have higher blood pressures than European American males of the same age (Box 21-9 ■).

- *Obesity.* Pressure is generally higher in some overweight and obese people than in people of normal weight.

- *Sex.* After puberty, females usually have lower blood pressures than males of the same age; this difference is thought to be due to hormonal variations. Women generally have higher blood pressures after menopause than during child-bearing years.

- *Medications.* Many medications may increase or decrease the blood pressure. Nurses should be aware of the specific medications a client is receiving and consider their possible impact when interpreting blood pressure readings.

- *Diurnal variations.* Blood pressure is usually lowest early in the morning, when the metabolic rate is lowest, then rises throughout the day and peaks in the late afternoon or early evening.

- *Disease process.* Any condition affecting the cardiac output, blood volume, blood viscosity, or compliance of the arteries has a direct effect on blood pressure.

HYPERTENSION

A blood pressure that is persistently above normal is called *hypertension.* It is usually asymptomatic and is often a contributing factor to myocardial infarctions (heart attacks) and cerebral vascular accidents (strokes). An elevated blood pressure of unknown cause is called *primary hypertension.* An elevated blood pressure as a result of a known problem, such as kidney damage, is called **secondary hypertension.** Hypertension is a widespread health problem. The diagnosis is made when the average of two or more diastolic readings on two visits following the initial assessment is 90 mm Hg or higher, or when the average of multiple systolic blood pressure readings is higher than 140 mm Hg. Categories of hypertension have been identified and are described in Table 21-7 ■. Factors associated with hypertension include thickening of the arterial walls, which reduces the size of the arterial lumen; inelasticity of the arteries (may result from *arteriosclerosis*—a buildup of plaque on the arterial lumen); and lifestyle factors such as cigarette smoking, obesity, heavy alcohol consumption, lack of physical exercise, high blood cholesterol levels, and continued exposure to stress. Follow-up care should include lifestyle changes conducive to lowering the blood pressure as well as monitoring the pressure itself.

HYPOTENSION

Hypotension is a blood pressure that is below normal (a systolic reading consistently below 90 mm Hg in an adult). **Orthostatic hypotension** is a blood pressure that drops when the client sits or stands. It is usually the result of peripheral vasodilation in which the blood flow leaves the central body organs, especially the brain, and moves to the periphery, often causing the person to feel faint or dizzy. Hypotension can also be caused by narcotic analgesics such as meperidine hydrochloride (Demerol), bleeding, severe burns, and prolonged diarrhea and vomiting. It is important to monitor hypotensive clients carefully to prevent falls. Box 21-10 ■ provides instructions for measuring blood pressure for clients with orthostatic hypotension.

BOX 21-9	CULTURAL PULSE POINTS

African Americans and Hypertension

African Americans are at increased risk of high blood pressure in proportion to Caucasian Americans. They also suffer disproportionately more adverse health effects as a result of hypertension.

Research (Sundquist, Winkleby, Pudaric, 2001) is attempting to determine if African Americans are more prone to die from heart disease because the disease follows a different and more severe course than it does in Caucasians, because they are exposed to more risk factors, or because they have reduced access to medical care.

TABLE 21-7	Follow-up Recommendations for Blood Pressure Measurement for Adults Older Than 18 Years	
INITIAL SCREENING BLOOD PRESSURE (mm Hg)[a]		
SYSTOLIC	**DIASTOLIC**	**FOLLOW-UP RECOMMENDED[b]**
Less than 130	Less than 85	Recheck in 2 years.
130–139	85–89	Recheck in 1 year.[c]
140–159	90–99	Confirm within 2 months.
160–179	100–109	Evaluate or refer to source of care within 1 month.
180–209	110–119	Evaluate or refer to source of care within 1 week.
210 or higher	120 or higher	Evaluate or refer to source of care immediately.

[a]If the systolic and diastolic categories are different, follow recommendation for the shorter time to follow up (e.g., 160/85 mm Hg should be evaluated or referred to source of care within 1 month).

[b]The scheduling of follow-up should be modified by reliable information about past blood pressure measurements, other cardiovascular risk factors, or target-organ disease.

[c]Consider providing advice about lifestyle modifications.

Source: From the fifth report of the Joint National Committee for the Detection, Evaluation, and Treatment of High Blood Pressure, National Heart, Lung, and Blood Institute, National Institutes of Health, 1993, *Archives of Internal Medicine, 329,* 1912; and USDHHS (2005). NIH Publication No. 05–5267.

BOX 21-10 MEASURING BLOOD PRESSURE FOR ORTHOSTATIC HYPOTENSION

When measuring the blood pressure of a client who has orthostatic hypotension:

- Place the client in a supine position for 2 to 3 minutes. This allows the blood pressure and pulse to stabilize in this position.
- Record the client's pulse and blood pressure.
- Assist the client to sit or stand slowly leaving the blood pressure cuff in place. Support the client to prevent a fall in case of faintness.
- After 1 minute in the upright position, recheck the client's pulse and blood pressure in the same sites as previously measured.

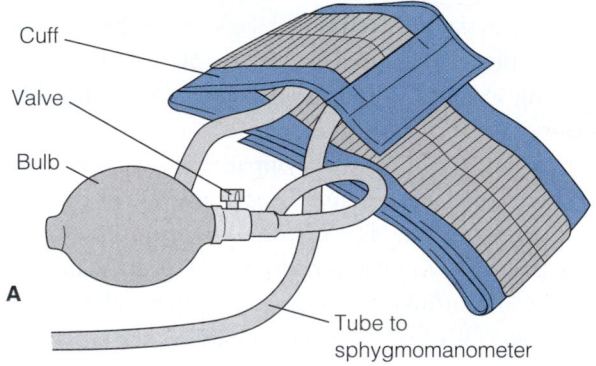

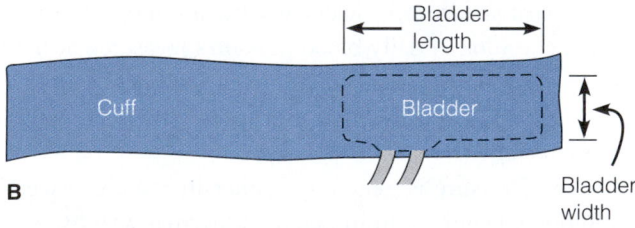

Figure 21-11. ■ **A.** Blood pressure cuff and bulb; **B.** bladder inside the cuff.

BLOOD PRESSURE EQUIPMENT

Blood pressure is measured with a blood pressure cuff, called a **sphygmomanometer,** and a stethoscope. The blood pressure cuff consists of a rubber bag, called a **bladder,** that can be inflated with air (Figure 21-11 ■). It is covered with cloth and has two tubes attached to it. One tube connects to a rubber bulb that inflates the bladder. A small valve on the side of this bulb releases the air in the bladder. When the valve is closed, air pumped into the bladder remains trapped inside. The other tube is attached to a sphygmomanometer that measures the amount of pressure being exerted against the skin as a result of the inflated bladder.

There are two types of sphygmomanometers: aneroid and mercury (Figure 21-12 ■). The aneroid sphygmomanometer is a calibrated dial with a needle that points to the number representing the pressure exerted by the bladder against the skin. The mercury sphygmomanometer is a calibrated cylinder filled with mercury. The pressure is indicated at the point to which the rounded curve (the base) of the meniscus

(the curved top of a column of liquid in a small tube) rises (Figure 21-13 ■). The blood pressure reading should be made with the eye at the level of the rounded curve in order to be accurate. If the eye is looking up or down, a distortion in the reading can occur. A distortion that occurs as a result of the angle of view is called **parallax.** Like mercury thermometers, mercury sphygmomanometers are being replaced with aneroid sphygmomanometers due to the risk created by potential mercury spills.

Some medical facilities use electronic sphygmomanometers (Figure 21-14 ■), which inflate automatically and determine the client's blood pressure, eliminating the need to

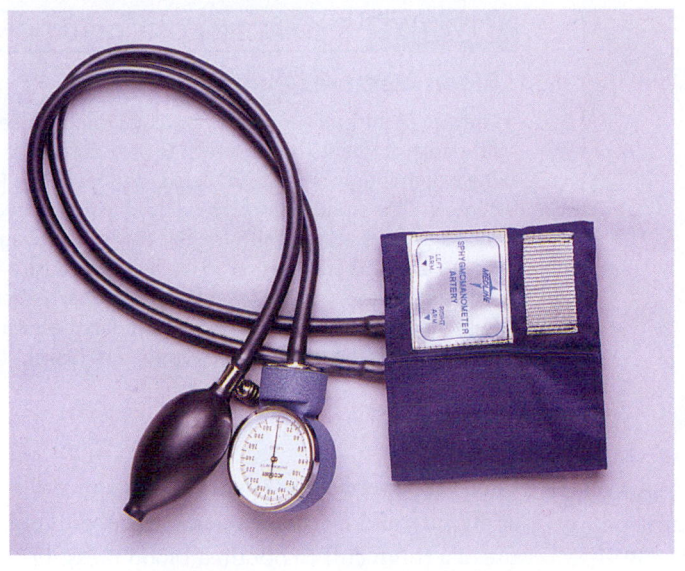

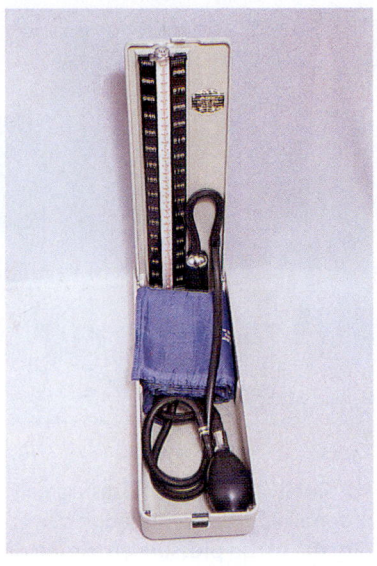

A   **B**

Figure 21-12. ■ Blood pressure equipment: **A.** aneroid manometer and cuff; **B.** mercury manometer and cuff.

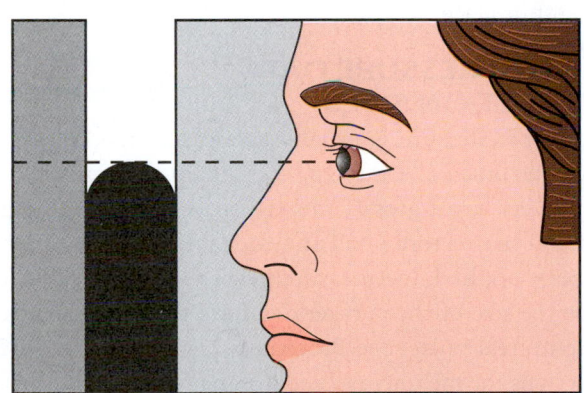

Figure 21-13. ■ To obtain an accurate reading from a mercury manometer, position the meniscus at eye level.

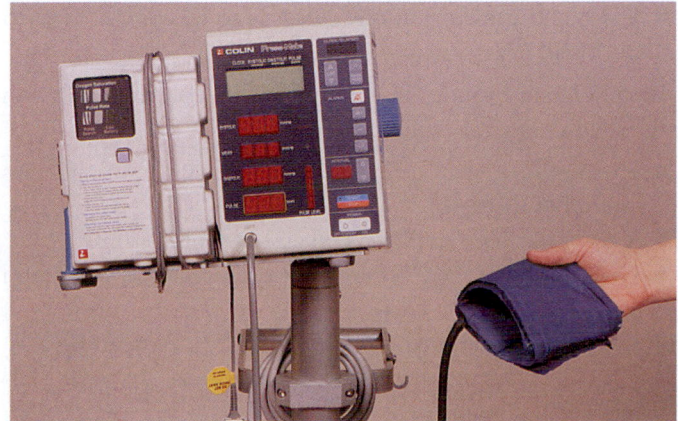

Figure 21-14. ■ Electronic blood pressure monitors automatically register systolic, diastolic, and mean blood pressures. (© Jenny Thomas.)

listen to the sounds of the client's systolic and diastolic blood pressures using a stethoscope. Electronic blood pressure devices should be calibrated against a mercury sphygmomanometer to check that they are accurate. Research indicates that automated electronic devices produce higher values than manual readings. Abnormal results obtained from an electronic sphygmomanometer should always be checked using a manual sphygmomanometer and stethoscope to avoid treating the client for an incorrect reading.

Korotkoff's sounds are the sounds heard through the stethoscope when measuring blood pressure. Doppler ultrasound stethoscopes can be used to assess blood pressure when Korotkoff's sounds are difficult to hear, such as in infants, obese clients, and clients in shock (see Figure 21-9). A systolic blood pressure assessed with a DUS is recorded with a large D, for example, 85D. Systolic pressure may be the only blood pressure obtainable with some ultrasound models.

Blood pressure cuffs come in various sizes because the bladder must be the correct width and length for the client's arm (Figure 21-15 ■). If the bladder is too narrow, the blood pressure reading will be erroneously elevated; if it is too wide, the reading will be erroneously low. The arm circumference, not the age of the client, should always be used to determine bladder size (Figure 21-16 ■). Box 21-11 ■ describes pediatric adaptations for taking blood pressure.

Blood pressure cuffs that are too small, whether too short or too narrow, will result in abnormally high readings. Blood pressure cuffs that are too big, either too long or too wide, will result in abnormally low blood pressure readings. To prevent treating a client for an abnormal blood pressure reading that is not accurate, proper choice of blood pressure cuffs is

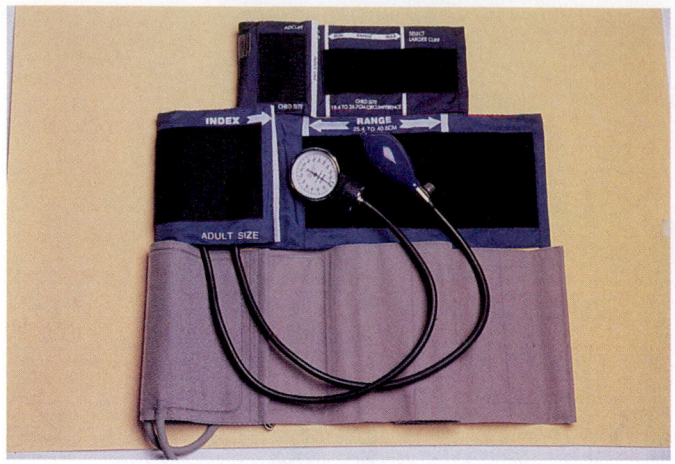

Figure 21-15. ■ Three standard cuff sizes: a small cuff for an infant, small child, or frail adult; a normal adult-size cuff; and a large cuff for measuring the blood pressure on the leg or on the arm of an obese adult. (© Elena Dorfman.)

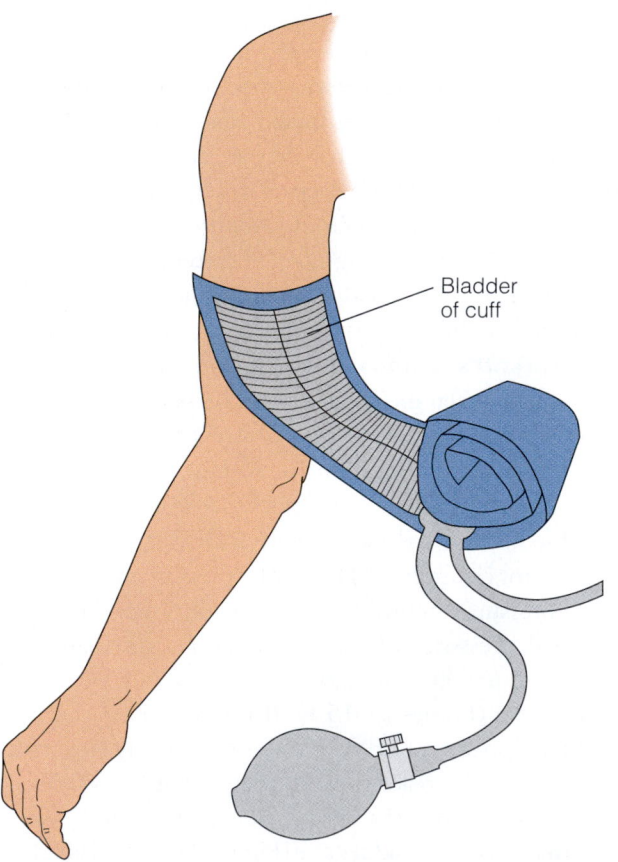

Bladder of cuff

Figure 21-16. ■ To ensure an accurate reading, the nurse must determine that the bladder of a blood pressure cuff is 40% of the arm circumference or 20% wider than the diameter of the midpoint of the limb. To do this, the nurse lays the cuff lengthwise at the midpoint of the upper arm, holding the outermost side of the bladder edge laterally on the arm. With the other hand, the nurse wraps the width of the cuff around the arm to ensure that it covers 40% of the arm's circumference.

BOX 21-11	PEDIATRIC CONSIDERATIONS

Blood Pressure Readings

The size of the cuff used is of particular importance when caring for pediatric clients because of the vast difference in the size of the extremities in a newborn versus an older child. Pediatric cuffs come in sizes small enough to be used in a premature infant and range to sizes appropriate for the older school-aged child (see Figure 21-15). A cuff that is too small could cause a false increase in blood pressure of 25–35 mm Hg. A properly sized cuff should fully encircle the arm, with room to overlap the Velcro, and should be two-thirds the length of the upper arm (Baker, 2000).

essential. Overweight clients may require the use of a large adult cuff, and clients who are very obese might require the use of a thigh cuff to obtain a blood pressure in the arm.

Blood pressure cuffs are made of nondistensible material so that an even pressure is exerted around the limb. Most cuffs are held in place by hooks, snaps, or Velcro. Of these, Velcro is by far the most commonly used material to hold the cuff in place.

BLOOD PRESSURE DATA COLLECTION SITES

The blood pressure is usually assessed in the client's arm using the brachial artery and a standard stethoscope. If the arm is very large, grossly misshapen, or the client has had a bilateral mastectomy and the conventional cuff cannot be properly applied, leg measurements can be taken to determine the size of the cuff needed for a thigh pressure using the popliteal pulse. See Procedure 21-4 ■ on page 462 for directions for measuring blood pressure on the thigh.

Assessing the blood pressure on a client's thigh is usually indicated in these situations:

- The blood pressure cannot be measured on either arm (e.g., because of burns, bilateral mastectomy, or other trauma).
- The blood pressure in one thigh is to be compared with the blood pressure in the other thigh.

Blood pressure is not measured on a client's arm or thigh in the following situations:

- The shoulder, arm, or hand (or the hip, knee, or ankle) is injured or diseased.
- A cast or bulky bandage is on any part of the limb.
- The client has had removal of axillary (or hip) lymph nodes on that side, such as following a mastectomy.
- The client has an intravenous infusion in that limb.
- The client has an arteriovenous fistula (e.g., for renal dialysis) in that limb.

To obtain a forearm blood pressure, apply an appropriate-sized cuff to the forearm 14 cm (5 in.) below the elbow. Blood pressure sounds can then be heard from the radial artery.

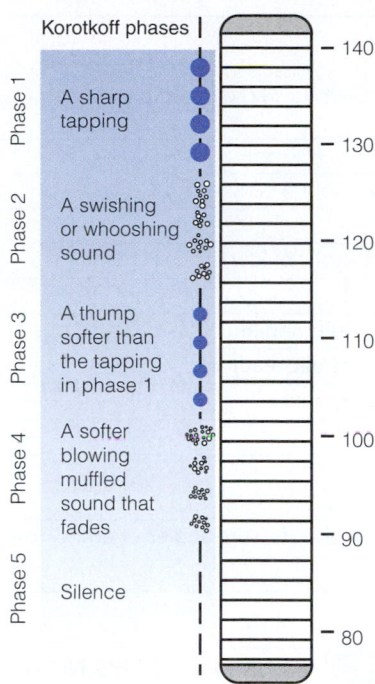

Figure 21-17. ■ Korotkoff's sounds can be differentiated into five phases. In the illustration, the blood pressure is 138/90 or 138/102/90.

Labels within figure:
Korotkoff phases

- Phase 1: A sharp tapping
- Phase 2: A swishing or whooshing sound
- Phase 3: A thump softer than the tapping in phase 1
- Phase 4: A softer blowing muffled sound that fades
- Phase 5: Silence

Scale values: 140, 130, 120, 110, 100, 90, 80

BLOOD PRESSURE DATA COLLECTION METHODS

Blood pressure can be assessed directly or indirectly. Direct (invasive monitoring) measurement involves the insertion of a catheter into the brachial, radial, or femoral artery. Arterial pressure is represented as wavelike forms displayed on an oscilloscope. With correct placement and calibration of the transducer, this pressure reading is highly accurate and allows a constant reading of blood pressure to be seen on the bedside monitor.

Two noninvasive indirect methods of measuring blood pressure are the auscultatory and palpatory methods. The auscultatory method is most commonly used in hospitals, clinics, and homes. When carried out correctly, the auscultatory method is relatively accurate.

When taking a blood pressure using a stethoscope, the nurse identifies five phases in the series of sounds called Korotkoff's sounds (Figure 21-17 ■). Box 21-12 ■ describes Korotkoff's phases.

NURSING CARE

PRIORITIZING NURSING CARE

The client's blood pressure is an indication of perfusion and should be accurately measured and recorded. Blood pressure readings outside the range of normal should be checked in both arms to determine any differences. If the unlicensed

---

BOX 21-12 KOROTKOFF'S SOUNDS

- **Phase 1:** The pressure level at which the first faint, clear tapping or thumping sounds are heard. These sounds gradually become more intense. To ensure that they are not extraneous sounds, the nurse should identify at least two consecutive tapping sounds. The first tapping sound heard during deflation of the cuff is the systolic blood pressure.
- **Phase 2:** The period during deflation when the sounds have a muffled, whooshing, or swishing quality.
- **Phase 3:** The period during which the blood flows freely through an increasingly open artery and the sounds become crisper and more intense and again assume a thumping quality but softer than in phase 1.
- **Phase 4:** The time when the sounds become muffled and have a soft, blowing quality.
- **Phase 5:** The pressure level when the last sound is heard. This is followed by a period of silence. The pressure at which the last sound is heard is the diastolic blood pressure in adults.[a]

[a]For children, the USDHHS (2005) recommends that if phase 5 (disappearance of sounds) can be heard down to zero, the measurement be repeated with less pressure on the head of the stethoscope. Then, if Korotkoff's sounds are still heard to zero, the onset of phase 4 (muffling of sounds) would be considered the diastolic pressure. In agencies in which the fourth phase is considered the diastolic pressure of adults, three measures are recommended (systolic pressure, diastolic pressure, and phase 5). These may be referred to as systolic, first diastolic, and second diastolic pressures. The phase 5 (second diastolic pressure) reading may be zero; that is, the muffled sounds are heard even when there is no air pressure in the blood pressure cuff. In some instances, muffled sounds are never heard, in which case a dash is inserted where the reading would normally be recorded (e.g., 190/–/110).

---

assistive personnel reports abnormal blood pressure readings, the nurse should verify the accuracy of the reading before notifying the physician. Hypotension can impact the client's mental status and should be assessed if blood pressure falls below normal limits. Hypertension requires rapid intervention by the nurse to prevent complications. Any client reporting lightheadedness, dizziness, or a severe headache should have blood pressure assessed.

ASSESSING

The palpatory method is sometimes used when Korotkoff's sounds cannot be heard and electronic equipment to amplify the sounds is not available, or when an auscultatory gap occurs. An **auscultatory gap,** which occurs particularly in hypertensive clients, is the temporary disappearance of sounds normally heard over the brachial artery when the cuff pressure is high followed by the reappearance of the sounds at a lower level. This temporary disappearance of sounds occurs in the latter part of phase 1 and phase 2 and may cover a range of 40 mm Hg. Instead of listening for the blood flow sounds, the nurse palpates the pulsations of the artery as the pressure in the cuff is released. The systolic pressure is read from the sphygmomanometer when the first pulsation is

TABLE 21-8	Blood Pressure Data Collection Errors
ERROR	**EFFECT**
Bladder cuff too narrow	Erroneously high
Bladder cuff too wide	Erroneously low
Arm unsupported	Erroneously high
Insufficient rest before the assessment	Erroneously high
Repeating assessment too quickly	Erroneously high systolic or low diastolic readings
Cuff wrapped too loosely or unevenly	Erroneously high
Deflating cuff too quickly	Erroneously low systolic and high diastolic readings
Deflating cuff too slowly	Erroneously high diastolic reading
Failure to use the same arm consistently	Inconsistent measurements
Arm above level of the heart	Erroneously low
Assessing immediately after a meal or while client smokes or has pain	Erroneously high
Failure to identify auscultatory gap	Erroneously low systolic pressure and erroneously low diastolic pressure

felt. A single whiplike vibration, felt in addition to the pulsations, identifies the point at which the pressure in the cuff nears the diastolic pressure. This vibration is no longer felt when the cuff pressure is below the diastolic pressure. To palpate the diastolic pressure, the nurse applies light to moderate pressure over the pulse point.

Common Errors in Collecting Data for Blood Pressure

The importance of the accuracy of blood pressure assessments cannot be overemphasized. Many judgments about a client's health are made on the basis of blood pressure. It is an important indicator of the client's condition and is used extensively as a basis for nursing interventions. Some reasons for erroneous blood pressure readings are given in Table 21-8 ■.

clinical ALERT

Because BP varies among individuals, the nurse must know a client's baseline BP. If a client's usual BP is 180/100 mm Hg, but after surgery is 120/80 mm Hg, report this drop in pressure to the physician. Similarly, if the client's baseline blood pressure is 92/64 and is currently reading 140/90, this is a significant increase in blood pressure and should also be reported to the physician or nurse supervisor.

DIAGNOSING, PLANNING, AND IMPLEMENTING

A frequent nursing diagnosis for clients with problems of blood pressure is *Ineffective Family Therapeutic Regimen Management*. Procedure 21-4 gives guidelines for assessing blood pressure.

Vital signs are documented in a flow sheet (see Figure 13-6 ⦾) or in graphic form in most facilities. This type of documentation provides easy access for the physician and

BOX 21-13	SAMPLE NURSE'S NOTES CONTAINING VITAL SIGNS

Focus			
CVS	D	0835	VS 99.8/100/24 158/90 c/o chest pain 5/10. Sitting in chair.
	A		PRN ms given as prescribed. Assisted to return to bed. K. Turner LVN
	R	0915	Client resting comfortably; chest pain resolved. 0/10. VS 98.8/86/20 140/88. K. Turner LVN

other members of the healthcare team. Occasionally, a nurse will insert vital signs in a nurse's note. Box 21-13 ■ illustrates an example of this.

EVALUATING

Each vital sign, as well as vital signs assessed as a group, tell the nurse what is happening with the client. The nurse knows that a low blood pressure (hypotension) in the presence of a rapid pulse (tachycardia) can be signs of hemorrhage and impending shock. Widening pulse pressure—a separation of more than 40 mm Hg between the systolic and diastolic blood pressure readings—should alert the nurse to possible increased intracranial pressure. In the presence of pain, vital signs may be elevated. It is important to consider not only the vital sign readings, but also the picture created by performing a complete assessment. The data obtained from vital signs measurement, in combination with your assessment, will aid you in making sound judgments regarding the client's care and needs.

Note: The references and resources for all chapters have been compiled at the back of the book.

PROCEDURE 21-1   Measuring Body Temperature

Purposes

- To establish baseline data for follow-up evaluation
- To identify whether the core temperature is within normal range
- To monitor clients at risk for change in temperature (e.g., clients at risk for infection or diagnosis of infection; those who have been exposed to temperature extremes; those with a leukocyte count below 5,000 or above 12,000)

- To identify clients requiring treatment for abnormal temperature readings

Equipment

- Oral, rectal, or axillary thermometer
- Towel, if the axillary site is used
- Lubricant and tissue, if the rectal site is used
- Disposable gloves, if the rectal site is used

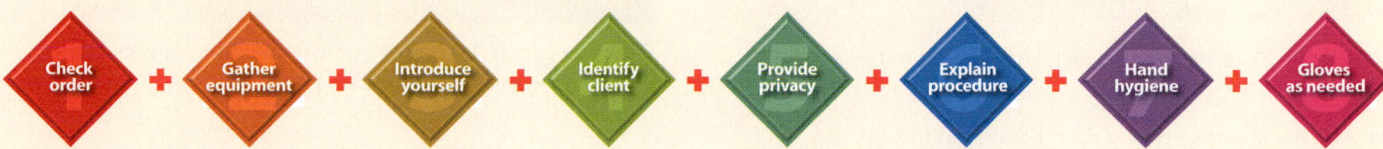

Check order ✚ Gather equipment ✚ Introduce yourself ✚ Identify client ✚ Provide privacy ✚ Explain procedure ✚ Hand hygiene ✚ Gloves as needed

Interventions and Rationales

1. Perform preparatory steps (see icon bar above).
2. Prepare client.

FOR AN ORAL TEMPERATURE

- Determine the time the client last took hot or cold food or fluids or smoked. *To obtain an accurate oral temperature reading, allow 15 to 30 minutes to elapse between a client's intake or smoking and obtaining a measurement.*

FOR A RECTAL TEMPERATURE

- Assist the client to assume a lateral position. Place newborn in a lateral or prone position. Place a young child in a lateral position with knees flexed, or prone across the lap.

FOR COMFORT AND SAFETY

- Provide privacy before folding the bedclothes back to expose the buttocks. *Privacy is essential because exposure of the buttocks embarrasses most people.*

FOR AN AXILLARY TEMPERATURE

- Expose the client's axilla. If the axilla is moist, dry it with the towel, using a patting motion. *Friction created by rubbing can raise the temperature of the axilla.*

3. Prepare the equipment.
   - Remove the thermometer from its storage container, and check the temperature reading on the thermometer.
   - Shake down the mercury (if necessary) by holding the thermometer between the thumb and forefinger at the end farthest from the bulb. Snap the wrist downward. Repeat until the mercury is below 35°C (95°F).
   - Place the thermometer in a plastic sheath according to agency policy. *Disposable sheaths prevent spread of infections.*
4. Take the temperature.

FOR AN ORAL TEMPERATURE

- Place the thermometer or probe at the base of the tongue to the right or left of the frenulum, in the posterior sublingual pocket (Figure 21-18 ■). *The thermometer needs to reflect the core temperature of the blood in the larger blood vessels of the posterior pocket.*
- Ask the client to close the lips, not the teeth, around the thermometer and refrain from speaking. *A client who bites a glass thermometer can break it and injure the mouth. When the client speaks, air is passed over the thermometer and can result in an abnormally lower temperature.*
- Leave the thermometer in place a sufficient time for the temperature to register or for the length of time recommended by the agency. *The recommended time is generally 2 minutes.*

FOR A RECTAL TEMPERATURE

- Place some lubricant on a piece of tissue. Then apply lubricant to the thermometer. *The lubricant facilitates insertion of the thermometer without irritating the mucous membrane.*
- Put on disposable gloves. With the nondominant hand, raise the client's upper buttock to expose the anus.

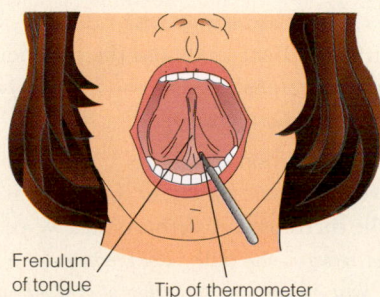

Frenulum of tongue   Tip of thermometer

Figure 21-18. ■ The tip of the oral thermometer is placed beside the frenulum below the tongue.

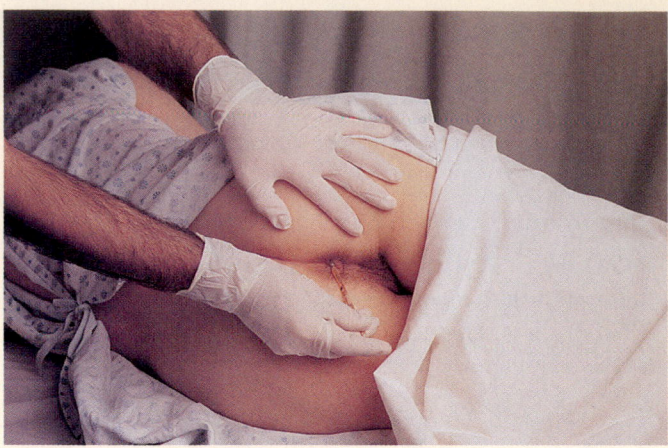

Figure 21-19. ■ Inserting a rectal thermometer. (Patrick Watson.)

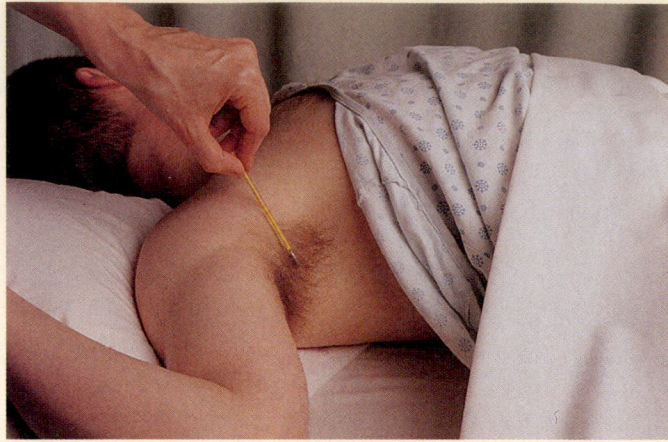

Figure 21-20. ■ Placing the bulb of the thermometer in the center of the axilla. (Patrick Watson.)

■ Ask the client to take a deep breath, and insert the thermometer into the anus anywhere from 1.5 to 4 cm (0.5 to 1.5 in.), depending on the age and size of the client (for example, 1.5 cm [0.5 in.] for an infant, 2.5 cm [0.9 in.] for a child, and 3.7 cm [1.5 in.] for an adult) (Figure 21-19 ■). *Taking a deep breath often relaxes the external sphincter muscle, thus easing insertion.*

■ Do not force insertion of the thermometer. *Inability to insert the thermometer into a newborn could indicate the rectum is not patent.*

■ Hold the thermometer in place for 3 minutes or for the length of time recommended by the agency in adults and children. For neonates, hold the thermometer in place for 5 minutes or according to agency protocol. Hold the young child firmly while the probe is in the rectum. *The thermometer may become displaced inside or outside the anus if not held in place.*

FOR AN AXILLARY TEMPERATURE

■ Place the thermometer in the center of the client's axilla (Figure 21-20 ■). *This allows the thermometer to come in contact with the axillary blood supply.*

■ Assist the client to place the arm tightly across the chest to keep the thermometer in place. *This maintains the proper position.*

■ Leave the thermometer in place for 9 minutes or according to agency protocol. For infants and children, leave the thermometer in place 5 minutes. *Device must stay in position long enough to ensure an accurate temperature.*

■ Remain with the client, and hold the thermometer in place if the client is irrational or very young. *This provides safety for the client and prevents breakage.*

5. Remove the thermometer.

■ Remove the plastic sheath, or if a sheath is not used, wipe the thermometer with a tissue. Wipe in a rotating manner toward the bulb. *The thermometer is wiped from the area of least contamination to that of greatest contamination.*

■ Discard the tissue or sheath in a receptacle used for contaminated items. *This prevents spread of infection.*

6. Read the temperature.

■ Hold the thermometer at eye level and rotate it until the mercury column is clearly visible. The upper end of the mercury column registers the client's body temperature. On the Fahrenheit thermometer, each long line reflects 1 degree, and each short line 0.2 degree. On the Celsius (centigrade) thermometer, each long line reflects 0.5 degree, and each short line 0.1 degree.

7. Clean and shake down the thermometer.

■ Wash the thermometer in tepid, soapy water. Rinse the thermometer in cold water, dry it, and store it dry. *Organic material, such as mucus, must be removed before the thermometer can be stored. Organic materials on the thermometer can harbor microorganisms. Hot water expands the mercury and may break the thermometer.*

■ Shake down the thermometer and return it to its container or discard it. *Some agencies also have special equipment for spinning down the mercury levels.*

■ If the thermometer is to be disinfected before storage, follow agency policy.

8. Document the temperature.

■ Record the temperature to the nearest indicated tenth (for example, 37.1°C, 98.4°F) on a designated flow sheet. See Figure 13-6 ⬭. *Recording the temperature immediately ensures it is not forgotten.*

VARIATION: USING AN ELECTRONIC THERMOMETER

■ Remove the electronic unit from the battery charging area.

■ Remove the temperature probe. If the probe is not attached, attach it to the appropriate circuit (oral, rectal, or axillary) in models that have separate circuits for each.

■ Place a disposable cover securely on the probe.

■ Warm up the machine by switching it on if removal of the probe does not automatically prepare the machine for functioning.

■ Take the temperature as indicated in step 3.

- Listen for a sound indicating that the maximum measurement has been reached, and read the temperature on the dial or readout.
- Remove the thermometer.
- Record the temperature.
- Remove and discard the probe cover.
- Return the unit to the charging base.

VARIATION: USING A TYMPANIC (INFRARED) THERMOMETER

- Apply a disposable sheath to the probe. Different sheaths fit adults and infants. They can be applied without being touched.
- Select the ear opposite the side on which the client may have been lying. *The ear against a surface can be much warmer.*
- Use your right hand to hold the thermometer when using the client's right ear, left hand for the left ear. This helps achieve the proper angle for a good seal.
- Gently pull the pinna upward and back for children over age 3 and adults (Figure 21-21 ■), straight back for children under age 3. *This straightens the ear canal so the thermometer is properly pointed toward the tympanic membrane.*
- Place the probe tip into the outer position of the ear canal just at the opening pointing toward the opposite eyebrow. The probe tip seals the opening of the canal.
- Press the button on the electronic thermometer. Do not wait too long to do this. The presence of the probe can "draw down" the temperature reading.
- Remove the thermometer when it beeps or indicates the reading is complete.
- Read the temperature on the screen. *Within 1 to 2 seconds, the temperature is displayed on the screen.*

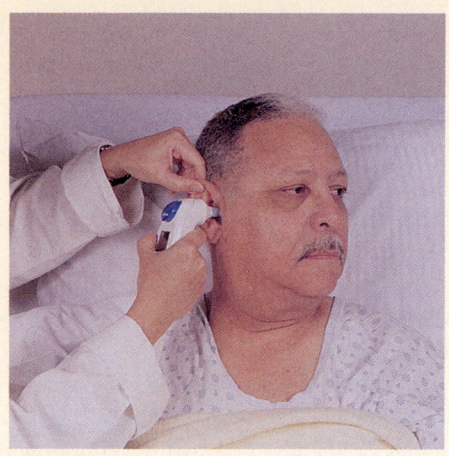

Figure 21-21. ■ Pull the pinna of the ear up and back while inserting the tympanic thermometer.

- Remove and discard the probe cover. Covers can be ejected without being touched.
- Return the unit to the charging base.

SAMPLE DOCUMENTATION

[date] [time] [*temperature portion only*]
Temp 102.4 ax. Skin hot and dry, cheeks flushed, client complains of feeling warm. Dr. Siebels notified and orders received.
_____ C. Marx, LVN

PROCEDURE 21-2 Measuring a Pulse

Purposes

- To establish baseline data for subsequent evaluation
- To identify whether the pulse rate is within normal range
- To determine whether the pulse rhythm is regular and the pulse volume is appropriate
- To compare the equality of corresponding peripheral pulses on each side of the body
- To monitor and assess changes in the client's health status
- To monitor clients at risk for pulse alterations (e.g., those with a history of heart disease or experiencing cardiac arrhythmias, hemorrhage, acute pain, infusion of large volumes of fluids, fever)
- To obtain the heart rate of newborns, infants, and children 2 to 3 years old or of an adult with an irregular peripheral pulse
- To determine whether the cardiac rate is within normal range and the rhythm is regular
- To monitor clients with cardiac disease and those receiving medications to improve heart action
- To determine adequacy of peripheral circulation or presence of pulse deficit

Equipment

- Watch with a second hand or indicator
- If using Doppler ultrasound stethoscope, the transducer in the DUS probe, a stethoscope headset, and transmission gel
- Antiseptic wipes
- Stethoscope with a bell-shaped or flat disk (Figure 21-22 ■)
- Stethoscope

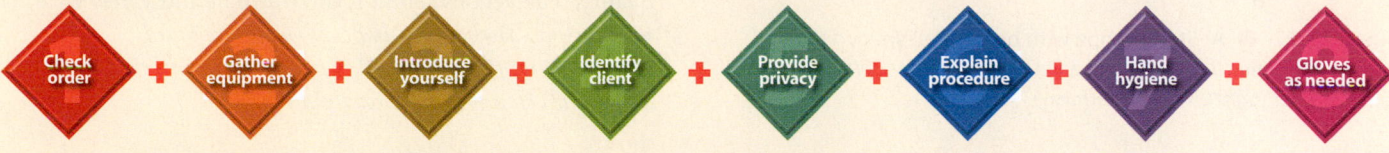

Part A: Peripheral Pulse
Interventions and Rationales

1. Perform preparatory steps (see icon bar above).

2. Prepare the client.
   - Select the pulse point. *Normally, the radial pulse is taken unless it cannot be exposed or circulation to another body area is to be assessed.*
   - Assist the client to a comfortable resting position. When the radial pulse is assessed, the client's arm can rest alongside the body, the palm facing downward. Or the forearm can rest at a 90-degree angle across the chest with the palm downward. For the client who can sit, the forearm can rest across the thigh, with the palm of the hand facing downward or medially. Position a child comfortably in the parent's arms, or have the parent remain close by. *Having the parent close or holding the child may decrease anxiety and yield more accurate results.*

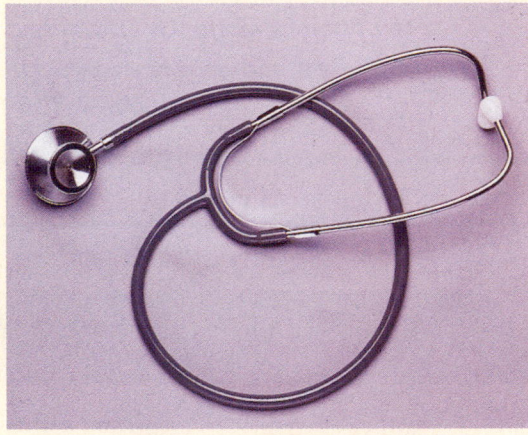

A

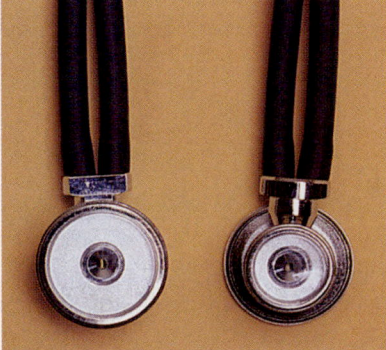

B

Figure 21-22. ■ **A.** Stethoscope with both a bell-shaped and flat-disk amplifier. **B.** Close-up of a flat-disk amplifier (*left*) and a bell amplifier (*right*). (© Elena Dorfman.)

3. Palpate and count the pulse (Figure 21-23 ■).
   - Place two or three middle fingertips lightly and squarely over the pulse point (Figure 21-23B). *Using the thumb is contraindicated because the thumb has a pulse that the nurse could mistake for the client's pulse.*
   - If the pulse is regular, count for 30 seconds and multiply by 2. If it is irregular, count for 1 minute. When taking a client's pulse for the first time, or obtaining baseline data, count the pulse for a full minute. *An irregular pulse requires a full minute's count for a correct assessment and indicates the need to take the apical pulse.*

4. Assess the pulse rhythm and volume.
   - Assess the pulse rhythm by noting the pattern of the intervals between the beats. *A normal pulse has equal time periods between beats.* If this is an initial assessment, assess for 1 minute.
   - Assess the pulse volume. *A normal pulse can be felt with moderate pressure, and the pressure is equal with each beat. A forceful pulse volume is full; an easily obliterated pulse is weak.*

5. Document and report to the nurse in charge pertinent assessment data.
   - Record the pulse rate, rhythm, and volume on the appropriate records.
   - Report to the nurse in charge pertinent data such as (1) pale skin color and cool skin temperature; (2) a pulse rate faster or slower than normal for the client; (3) a full, bounding, or weak pulse volume; and (4) an irregular pulse rhythm.

VARIATION: USING A DUS

- Plug the stethoscope headset into one of the two output jacks located next to the volume control. DUS units may have two jacks so that a second person can listen to the signals (see Figure 21-9).
- Apply transmission gel either to the probe at the narrow end of the plastic case housing the transducer or to the client's skin. Ultrasound beams do not travel well through air. *The gel makes an airtight seal, which then promotes optimal ultrasound wave transmission.*
- Press the "on" button.
- Hold the probe against the skin over the pulse site. Use light pressure, and keep the probe in contact with the skin. *Too much pressure can stop the blood flow and obliterate the signal.*
- Distinguish artery sounds from vein sounds. The artery sound (signal) is distinctively pulsating and has a pumping quality. The venous sound is intermittent and varies with respirations. *Both artery and vein sounds are heard simultaneously through the DUS because major arteries and veins are situated close together throughout the body.*

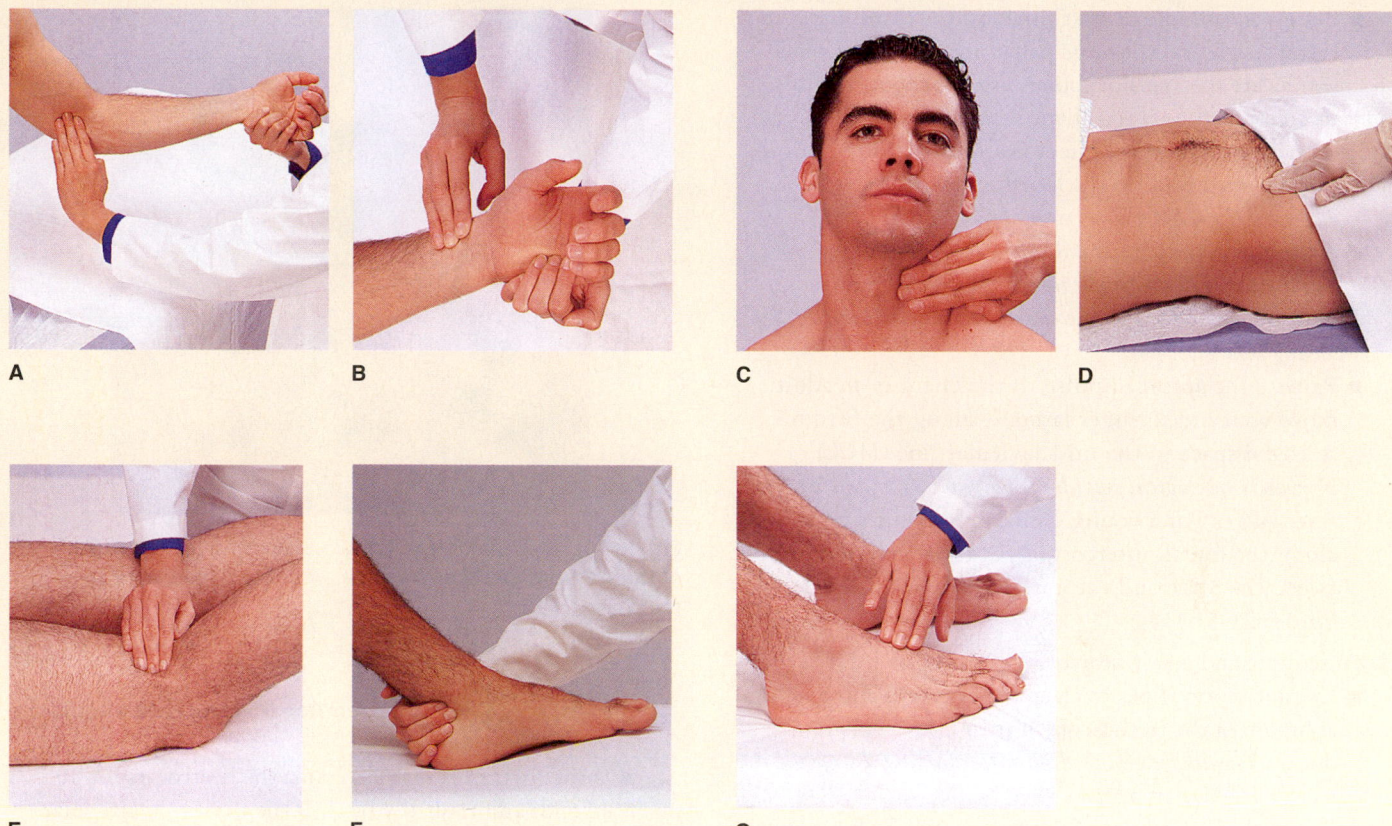

Figure 21-23. ■ Assessing the pulses: **A.** Brachial; **B.** radial; **C.** carotid; **D.** femoral; **E.** popliteal; **F.** posterior tibial; **G.** pedal (dorsalis pedis).

■ If arterial sounds cannot be easily heard, reposition the probe.

■ After assessing the pulse, remove all gel from the probe to prevent damage to its surface. Clean the transducer with

aqueous solutions. *Alcohol or other disinfectants may damage the face of the transducer.* Remove all gel from the client using a tissue or damp washcloth.

Part B: Apical Pulse
Interventions and Rationales

1. Prepare client. Position the client appropriately.
   ■ Assist an adult or young child to a comfortable supine position or to a sitting position.
   ■ Place a baby in a supine position, and offer a pacifier if the baby is crying or restless. *Crying and physical activity will increase the pulse rate.* Take the apical pulse rate of infants and small children before assessing body temperatures or performing any distressing assessments.
   ■ Demonstrate the procedure to the child using a stuffed animal or doll, and allow the child to handle the stethoscope before beginning the procedure. If the child is particularly anxious, allow them to listen to your apical pulse. *This will decrease anxiety and promote cooperation.*

■ Expose the area of the chest over the apex of the heart. *Clothing may interfere with ability to assess heartbeat.*

2. Locate the apical impulse.
   ■ This is the point over the apex of the heart where the apical pulse can be most clearly heard. It is referred to as the point of maximal impulse (PMI).
   ■ Palpate the angle of Louis (the angle between the manubrium, the top of the sternum, and the body of the sternum). It is palpated just below the suprasternal notch and is felt as a prominence (see Figure 21-8).
   ■ Slide your index finger just to the left of the client's sternum, and palpate the second intercostal space.

■ Place your middle or next finger in the third intercostal space, and continue palpating downward until you locate the apical impulse, usually about the fifth intercostal space if the client is an adult or a child 7 years or older. If the client is a young child, palpate downward to the fourth intercostal space. *The apex of the heart is normally located in the fifth intercostal space in individuals who are 7 years of age and over; it is in the fourth intercostal space in young children, and one or two spaces above the adult apex during infancy.*

■ Palpate the apical impulse. If the client is an adult, move your index finger laterally along the fifth intercostal space to the midclavicular line (MCL). *Normally, the apical impulse is palpable at or just medial to the MCL.* For a young child, move your finger along the fourth intercostal space to a position between the MCL and the anterior axillary line (see Figure 21-8).

3. Auscultate and count heartbeats.

■ Use antiseptic wipes to clean the earpieces and diaphragm of the stethoscope if their cleanliness is in doubt. *The diaphragm needs to be cleaned and disinfected if soiled with body substances.*

■ Warm the diaphragm of the stethoscope by holding it in the palm of the hand for a moment. *The metal of the diaphragm is usually cold and can startle the client when placed immediately on the chest.*

■ Insert the earpieces of the stethoscope into your ears in the direction of the ear canals, or slightly forward. *This facilitates hearing.*

■ Tap your finger lightly on the diaphragm to be sure it is the active side of the head. If necessary, rotate the head to select the diaphragm side.

■ Place the diaphragm of the stethoscope over the apical impulse (Figure 21-24 ■) and listen for the normal S_1 and S_2 heart sounds, which are heard as "lub-dub." Each lub-dub is counted as one heartbeat. The heartbeat is normally loudest over the apex of the heart. The two heart sounds are produced by closure of the valves of the heart. The S_1 heart sound (lub) occurs when the atrioventricular valves close after the ventricles have been sufficiently filled. The S_2 heart sound

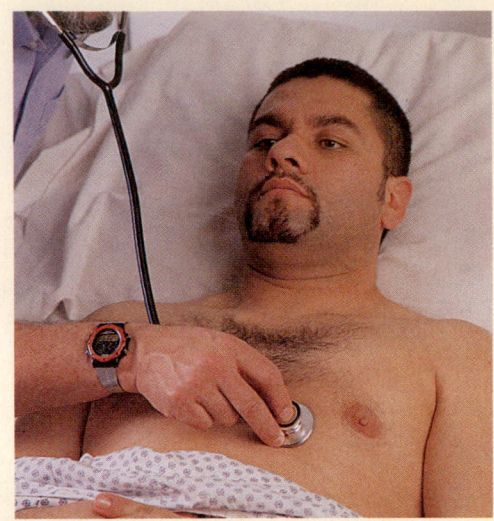

Figure 21-24. ■ Taking an apical pulse using the flat disk of the stethoscope. Note how the amplifier is held against the chest.

(dub) occurs when the semilunar valves close after the ventricles empty.

■ If the rhythm is regular, count the heartbeats for 30 seconds and multiply by 2. If the rhythm is irregular or if the apical impulse is being taken on an infant or child, count the beats for 60 seconds. *A 60-second count provides a more accurate assessment of an irregular pulse than a 30-second count.*

4. Assess the rhythm and the strength of the heartbeat.

■ Assess the rhythm of the heartbeat by noting the pattern of intervals between the beats. *A normal pulse has equal time periods between beats.*

■ Assess the strength (volume) of the heartbeat. *Normally, the heartbeats are equal in strength and can be described as strong or weak.*

5. Document and report pertinent assessment data.

■ Record the pulse site and rate, rhythm, and volume on the appropriate records.

■ Report to the nurse in charge any pertinent data such as pallor, cyanosis, dyspnea, tachycardia, bradycardia, irregular rhythm, and reduced strength of the heartbeat.

Part C: Apical–Radial Pulse

Interventions and Rationales

1. Position the client appropriately.

■ Assist the client to assume the position described for taking the apical pulse (on page 466).

■ If previous measurements were taken, determine what position the client assumed and use the same position. *This ensures an accurate comparative measurement.*

2. Locate the apical and radial pulse sites.

3. Count the apical and radial pulse rates.

TWO-NURSE TECHNIQUE

■ In the two-nurse technique, one nurse locates the apical impulse by palpation or with the stethoscope while the other nurse palpates the radial pulse site.

- Place the watch where both nurses can see it. The nurse who is taking the radial pulse may hold the watch.
- Decide on a time to begin counting. *A time when the second hand is on 12, 3, 6, or 9 is usually selected to help in obtaining an accurate reading.* The nurse taking the radial pulse says "Start" at the designated time. *This ensures that simultaneous counts are taken.*
- Each nurse counts the pulse rate for 60 seconds. Both nurses end the count when the nurse taking the radial pulse says "Stop." *A full 60-second count is necessary for accurate assessment of any differences between the two pulse sites.*
- The nurse who assesses the apical rate also assesses the apical pulse rhythm and volume (i.e., whether the heartbeat is strong or weak). If the pulse is irregular, note whether the irregular beats come at random or predictable times.
- The nurse assessing the radial pulse rate also assesses the radial pulse rhythm and volume.

ONE-NURSE TECHNIQUE (NOT RECOMMENDED FOR CLIENTS WITH IRREGULAR HEARTBEAT OR NURSES LACKING EXPERIENCE)

- Assess the apical pulse for 60 seconds.
- Assess the radial pulse for 60 seconds.

4. Document and report pertinent assessment data.
   - Promptly report any notable changes from previous measurements or any difference between the two pulses.
   - Document the apical and radial (AR) pulse rates, rhythm, volume, and any pulse deficit.
   - Record any other pertinent observations, such as pallor, cyanosis, or dyspnea.
   - Check the physician's orders for any directions related to a difference in the AR pulse rates.

SAMPLE DOCUMENTATION

[date] [time] Apical–radial pulse taken: 80 apical strong and regular, 65 radial at left wrist and weak. Edema left arm +3.
_____ S. Markham, LPN

PROCEDURE 21-3   Measuring Respirations

Purposes

- To acquire baseline data against which future measurements can be compared
- To monitor abnormal respirations and respiratory patterns and identify changes
- To assess respirations before the administration of a medication such as morphine (an abnormally slow respiratory rate may warrant withholding the medication)
- To monitor respirations following the administration of a general anesthetic or any medication that influences respirations
- To monitor clients at risk for respiratory alterations (e.g., those with fever, pain, acute anxiety, chronic obstructive pulmonary disease, respiratory infection, pulmonary edema or emboli, chest trauma or constriction, brainstem injury)

Equipment

- Watch with a second hand or indicator

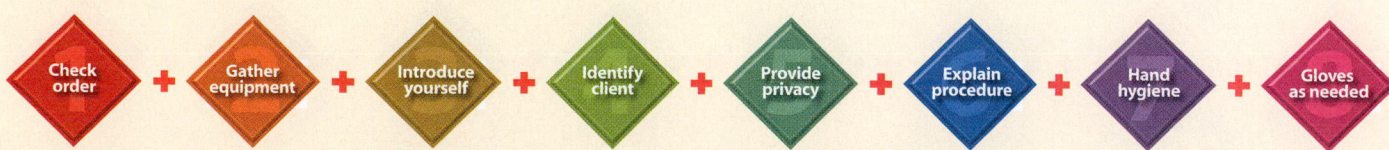

Check order + Gather equipment + Introduce yourself + Identify client + Provide privacy + Explain procedure + Hand hygiene + Gloves as needed

Interventions and Rationales

1. Perform preparatory steps (see icon bar above).
2. Determine the client's activity schedule.
   - Choose a suitable time to monitor the respirations. *A client who has been exercising will need to rest for a few minutes to permit the accelerated respiratory rate to return to normal. An infant or child who is crying will have an abnormal respiratory rate and will need time to calm down before respirations can be accurately assessed.*
3. Observe or palpate and count the respiratory rate.

- Place a hand against the client's chest to feel the client's chest movements, or place the client's arm across the chest and observe the chest movements while appearing to take the radial pulse. Because young children are diaphragmatic breathers, observe the rise and fall of the abdomen. *Awareness of respiratory rate assessment could cause the client to voluntarily alter the respiratory pattern.*
- Count the respiratory rate for 30 seconds and multiply by 2 if the respirations are regular. Count for 60 seconds if they are irregular. An inhalation and an exhalation count as one respiration.

4. Observe the depth, rhythm, and character of respirations.
- Observe the respirations for depth by watching the movement of the chest. *During deep respirations, a large volume of air is exchanged causing greater chest expansion; during shallow respirations, a small volume is exchanged and respirations may be difficult to assess due to poor chest excursion.*
- Observe the respirations for regular or irregular rhythm. *Normally, respirations are evenly spaced.*
- Observe the character of respirations—the sound they produce and the effort they require. *Normally, respirations are silent and effortless. Presence of abnormal breath sounds, retractions, grunting, or nasal flaring should be reported to the charge nurse or physician.*

5. Document and report pertinent assessment data.
- Document the respiratory rate, depth, rhythm, and character on the appropriate records.
- Report:
  a. Respiratory rate significantly above or below the normal range and any notable change in respirations from previous assessments.
  b. Irregular respiratory rhythm.
  c. Inadequate respiratory depth.
  d. Abnormal character of breathing—orthopnea, wheezing, stridor, or bubbling.
  e. Any complaints of dyspnea, retractions, nasal flaring, grunting, or posturing.

SAMPLE DOCUMENTATION

[date] [time] Client c/o difficulty breathing.
R 26. Wheezing noted.
Encouraged huff coughing.
Expelled thick yellow sputum.
R 20. Resting in semi-Fowler.
_____ Erin McClellan, LVN

PROCEDURE 21-4 Measuring Blood Pressure

Purposes

- To obtain a baseline measure of arterial blood pressure for subsequent evaluation
- To determine the client's hemodynamic status (e.g., stroke volume of the heart and blood vessel resistance)
- To identify and monitor changes in blood pressure resulting from a disease process and medical therapy (e.g., presence or history of cardiovascular disease, renal disease, circulatory shock, or acute pain; rapid infusion of fluids or blood products)

Equipment

- Stethoscope or DUS
- Blood pressure cuff of the appropriate size (newborn, infant, child, small adult, adult, large adult, thigh)
- Sphygmomanometer

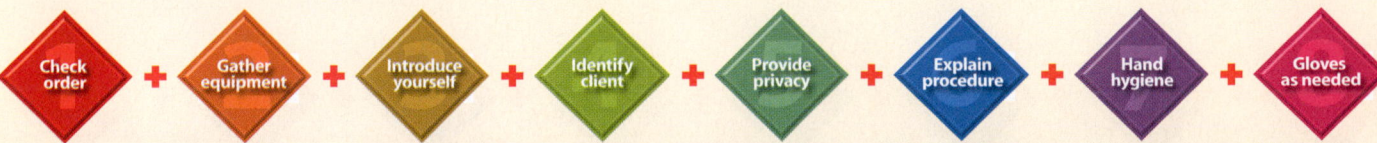

Check order + Gather equipment + Introduce yourself + Identify client + Provide privacy + Explain procedure + Hand hygiene + Gloves as needed

Interventions and Rationales

1. Perform preparatory steps (see icon bar above).
2. Prepare and position the client appropriately.
   - Make sure that the client has not smoked or ingested caffeine within 30 minutes prior to measurement. *Nicotine and caffeine can elevate BP.*
   - Make sure that the bladder of the cuff covers at least two-thirds of the arm and that the length of the cuff is appropriate (see Figure 21-16). *Inappropriate size can result in altered readings.*
   - Position the client in a sitting position unless otherwise specified. The elbow should be slightly flexed with the

palm of the hand facing up and the forearm supported at heart level. *Readings in any other position should be specified. The blood pressure is normally similar in sitting, standing, and lying positions, but it can vary significantly by position in certain people. The blood pressure increases when the arm is below heart level and decreases when the arm is above heart level.*

■ Expose the upper arm.

3. Wrap the deflated cuff evenly around the upper arm.
   ■ Locate the brachial artery (Figure 21-25 ■).
   ■ Apply the center of the bladder directly over the artery. *The bladder inside the cuff must be directly over the artery to be compressed if the reading is to be accurate.*
   ■ For an adult, place the lower border of the cuff approximately 2.5 cm (1 in.) above the antecubital space. The lower edge can be closer to the antecubital space of an infant. The thigh may be a more appropriate site for measuring blood pressure in neonates or young infants.
   ■ If this is the client's initial examination, perform a preliminary palpatory determination of systolic pressure. *The initial estimate tells the nurse the maximal pressure to which the manometer needs to be elevated in subsequent determinations. It also prevents underestimation of the systolic pressure or overestimation of the diastolic pressure should an auscultatory gap occur.*
   ■ Palpate the brachial artery with the fingertips.

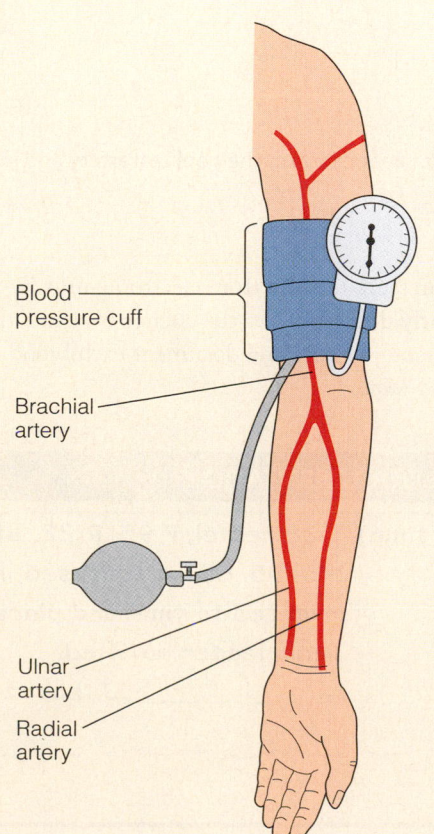

Blood pressure cuff

Brachial artery

Ulnar artery

Radial artery

Figure 21-25. ■ Location of the brachial artery and application of the cuff.

■ Close the valve on the pump by turning the knob clockwise.
■ Pump up the cuff until you no longer feel the brachial pulse. *At that pressure the blood cannot flow through the artery.*
■ Note the pressure on the sphygmomanometer at which the pulse is no longer felt. *This gives an estimate of the maximum pressure required to measure the systolic pressure.*
■ Release the pressure completely in the cuff, and wait 1 to 2 minutes before making further measurements. *A waiting period gives the blood trapped in the veins time to be released.*

4. Position the stethoscope appropriately.
   ■ Clean the earpieces with alcohol or recommended disinfectant. *Infection control measures are necessary unless a nurse is using a personal stethoscope.*
   ■ Insert the ear attachments of the stethoscope in your ears so that they tilt slightly forward. *Sounds are heard more clearly when the ear attachments follow the direction of the ear canal.*
   ■ Ensure that the stethoscope hangs freely from the ears to the diaphragm. *Rubbing the stethoscope against an object can obliterate the sounds of the blood within an artery.*
   ■ Place the bell side of the stethoscope (see Figure 21-22) over the brachial pulse. *Because the blood pressure is a low-frequency sound, it is best heard with the bell-shaped diaphragm.* Hold the diaphragm snugly against the skin with the thumb and index finger. *Holding the diaphragm snugly against the skin prevents noise in the room from entering the stethoscope, making it easier to hear Korotkoff's sounds.*

5. Auscultate the client's blood pressure.
   ■ Pump up the cuff until the sphygmomanometer registers about 30 mm Hg above the point where the brachial pulse disappeared.
   ■ Release the valve on the cuff carefully so that the pressure decreases at the rate of 2 to 3 mm Hg per second. *If the rate is faster or slower an inaccurate reading may be obtained.*
   ■ As the pressure falls, identify the manometer reading at each of the five phases.
   ■ Deflate the cuff rapidly and completely.
   ■ Wait 1 to 2 minutes before making further measurements. *This permits blood trapped in the veins to be released.*
   ■ Repeat the preceding steps once or twice as necessary to confirm the accuracy of the reading. Use the opposite extremity if the reading is done more than twice.

6. Remove the cuff.
   ■ Wipe the cuff with an approved disinfectant. *Cuffs can become significantly contaminated.*
   ■ If this is the client's initial examination, repeat the procedure on the client's other arm.
   ■ There should be a difference of no more than 5 to 10 mm Hg between the arms.

■ The arm found to have the higher pressure should be used for subsequent examinations.

7. Document and report pertinent assessment data.

■ Document the blood pressure according to agency policy. Record the systolic and diastolic pressures in the format of "130/80" where "130" is the systolic (phase 1) and "80" is the diastolic (phase 5) pressure. Record three pressures in the form "130/110/90," where "130" is the systolic, "110" is the first diastolic (phase 4), and "90" is the second diastolic (phase 5) pressure. Use the abbreviations RA for right arm and LA for left arm. Record a difference of greater than 10 mm Hg in the arms.

■ Report any significant change in the client's blood pressure. Also report these findings:
  a. Systolic blood pressure (of an adult) above 140 mm Hg
  b. Diastolic blood pressure (of an adult) above 90 mm Hg
  c. Systolic blood pressure (of an adult) below 100 mm Hg

VARIATION: TAKING A THIGH BLOOD PRESSURE

■ Help the client to assume a prone position. If the client cannot assume this position, measure the blood pressure while the client is in a supine position with the knee slightly flexed. *Slight flexing of the knee will facilitate placing the stethoscope on the popliteal space.*

■ Expose the thigh, taking care not to expose the client unduly.

■ Locate the popliteal artery (Figure 21-26 ■).

■ Wrap the cuff evenly around the mid thigh with the compression bladder over the posterior aspect of the thigh and the bottom edge above the knee. The bladder must be directly over the posterior popliteal artery if the reading is to be accurate.

■ If this is the client's initial examination, perform a preliminary palpatory determination of systolic pressure by palpating the popliteal artery. The systolic pressure in the popliteal artery is usually 20 to 30 mm Hg higher than that in the brachial artery because of use of a larger bladder; the diastolic pressure is usually the same.

■ Auscultate the pressure as for the arm.

VARIATION: USING AN ELECTRONIC INDIRECT BLOOD PRESSURE MONITORING DEVICE

■ Unplug the electronic unit from the electrical outlet.
■ Place the blood pressure cuff on the extremity according to the manufacturer's guidelines.
■ Turn on the blood pressure switch.
■ When the device has determined the blood pressure reading, note the digital results.
■ Record the blood pressure according to agency policy.

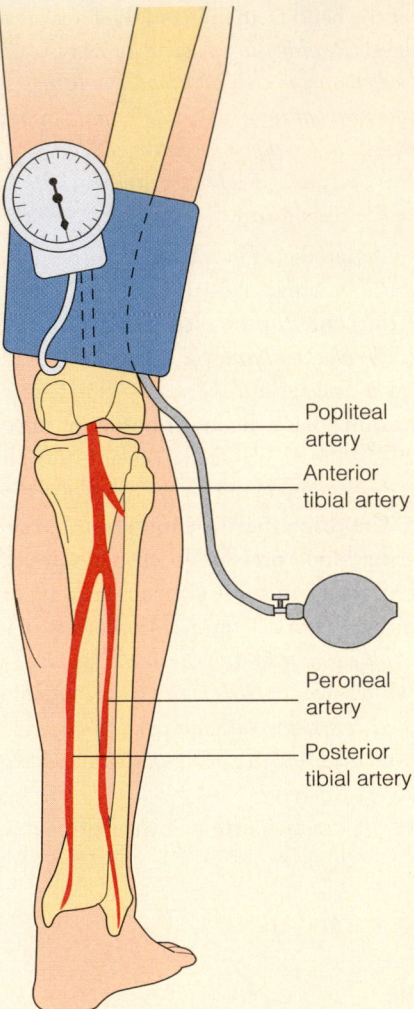

Popliteal artery

Anterior tibial artery

Peroneal artery

Posterior tibial artery

Figure 21-26. ■ Location of the popliteal artery and application of the cuff.

■ If blood pressure reading from electronic unit is significantly different than the client's baseline, take a manual blood pressure and document each blood pressure as *auto* and *manual*.

SAMPLE DOCUMENTATION

[date] [time] T 38 rectal, P 95, R 22, BP 145/95. Client confused, not oriented to time and place. Team leader notified. _____
_____ J. Lopez, LPN

Chapter Review

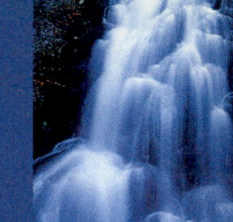

KEY Points

- Vital signs reflect changes in body function that otherwise might not be observed.
- Various sites and methods can be used to assess vital signs. The nurse selects the site and method that is safe for the client and that will provide the most accurate measurement possible.
- The most accurate values are obtained when the client is at rest and comfortable.
- Changes in one vital sign can trigger changes in other vital signs.
- Vital signs are assessed when a client is admitted to a healthcare agency to establish baseline data and when there is a change or possibility of a change in the client's condition.
- Data obtained from measurements of vital signs are used to plan and implement appropriate nursing interventions and to evaluate a client's response to these interventions or prescribed medical therapy.
- Body temperature is the balance between heat produced by the body and heat lost from the body.
- Knowledge of factors affecting heat production and heat loss helps the nurse to implement appropriate interventions when the client has a fever or hypothermia.
- Factors affecting body temperature include age, diurnal variations, exercise, hormones, stress, and environmental temperatures.
- Pyrexia (fever) is a common sign of disease. Four common types of fever are intermittent, remittent, relapsing, and constant. Clinical signs of fever vary during the onset, course, and abatement stages.
- Hypothermia involves three mechanisms: excessive heat loss, inadequate heat production by body cells, and increasing impairment of hypothalamic temperature regulation.
- Body temperature can be measured orally, tympanically, rectally, or by axilla. The nurse selects the most appropriate site according to the client's age and condition.

- Normally a peripheral pulse reflects the client's heartbeat, but it may differ from the heartbeat in clients with certain cardiovascular diseases; in these instances, the nurse takes an apical pulse and compares it to the peripheral pulse.
- Many factors affect a person's pulse rate: age, sex, exercise, presence of fever, certain medications, hemorrhage, stress, and (in some situations) position changes.
- Respirations are normally quiet, effortless, and automatic and are assessed by observing respiratory rate, depth, rhythm, and sound.
- Blood pressure reflects cardiac output, peripheral vascular resistance, blood volume, and blood viscosity. Peripheral vascular resistance varies according to the size of the arterioles and capillaries, and the elasticity of the arteries.

⊙ FOR FURTHER Study

See Figure 13-6 for a graphic flow sheet documenting vitals signs.

See Figure 19-8 for nine sites for obtaining a pulse and for overall information about collecting data for assessment.

See Chapter 22 for an in-depth discussion of pain.

Use of cold and heat is described in Chapter 24.

See Chapter 32 for more information about regulation of breathing and about pulse oximetry.

Critical Thinking Care Map

Caring for a Client after a Heart Attack

NCLEX–PN® Focus Area: Physiological Adaptation

Case Study: Edgar Wilson, a 50-year-old African American, was brought to the ED after chest pain of 1 hour's duration. He was admitted to rule out myocardial infarction (MI). The pain radiating to his back and down his left arm is 9/10. After receiving morphine sulfate 4 mg IV, his pain is now 5/10. He has a history of hypertension (treated with Verapamil) and a family history of cardiovascular disease. His father died of a heart attack at 56. His mother had a disabling stroke at age 60.

Vital signs: T 99.8 oral, P 100, R 24 BP 158/90. Height 5'10", weight 295 lbs. Cardiac monitoring showed sinus tachycardia with occasional PVC. Twelve-lead ECG and cardiac enzymes obtained in ED.

Mr. Wilson was in a motor vehicle crash 1 week ago in which he sustained a head injury. He lives with his wife; a son lives nearby. He is a history teacher at a local community college. Mr. Wilson states, "I probably won't live to an old age. I have bad genes for heart attack and stroke."

Nursing Diagnosis: *Acute Pain*

COLLECT DATA

Subjective	Objective
_____	_____
_____	_____
_____	_____
_____	_____
_____	_____
_____	_____
_____	_____

Would you report this? Yes/No

If yes, report to: _____

What would you report? _____

Nursing Care

_____
_____
_____
_____
_____
_____
_____
_____
_____
_____

How would you document this? _____
_____
_____

Compare your answers and documentation to those provided on the MyNursingKit Website.

Data Collected
(use only those that apply)

- 50-year-old African American male
- Chest pain, radiating to back and left arm 9/10. Morphine sulfate 4 mg IV × 3; pain now 5/10
- Verapamil ED. 180 mg bid for hypertension
- Father died of a heart attack age 56
- Mother stroke at 60; now 69, disabled
- VS: T 99.8, P 100, R 24 BP 158/90
- Height 5'10", weight 295 lbs
- Diet: "I normally eat fast food for lunch. My wife does make healthy dinners."
- Sinus tachycardia with occasional PVC
- 12-lead ECG and cardiac enzymes obtained in ED (no report)
- MVC 1 week ago sustained a head injury
- Lives with wife; one son nearby
- History teacher at local college
- "I probably won't live to an old age. I have bad genes for heart attack and stroke."

Nursing Interventions
(use those that apply; list in priority order)

- Assess client's feelings, values, and reasons for not following prescribed plan of care.
- Discuss client's beliefs about health and his ability to maintain health.
- Identify barriers and benefits to being healthy.
- Help client to choose healthy lifestyle and to have appropriate diagnostic tests.
- Compare client's height and weight to standards for age and height.
- Encourage client to eat a diet with fresh foods, low saturated fat, and no added salt.
- Teach stress-relieving techniques.
- Assess for the influences of culture and values on the client's beliefs about health.
- Identify support groups related to the disease process.

NCLEX-PN® Exam Preparation

TEST-TAKING TIP   If there are words in the stem that are unfamiliar, try to figure out the meaning in terms of the context, or break down the words using your medical terminology skills.

1 The nurse is assigned to take morning vital signs on several clients on a medical surgical unit. Of the following vital signs, which would the nurse immediately report to the RN?

   1. 99.6 (R), 86, 24, 140/88
   2. 97.2 (O), 110, 18, 110/78
   3. 101.8 (A), 72, 18, 90/60
   4. 98 (O), 100, 26, 148/80

2 The nurse's assigned client has a history of mastectomy of the right breast, 1 year ago. She has been admitted with a fracture of her left humerus. The nurse would measure blood pressure by:

   1. Applying the cuff to the right arm, being careful not to pump it up above 150 mm.
   2. Obtaining a large cuff and assessing her blood pressure using her thigh.
   3. Placing the cuff below her left elbow and palpating her radial pulse.
   4. Take her other vital signs and chart that you were unable to assess the blood pressure.

3 The nurse observes an unlicensed assistive personnel measure blood pressure using a cuff that is too small for the client. The nurse anticipates the blood pressure reading will be:

   1. Erroneously high
   2. Erroneously low
   3. Erroneously low diastolic
   4. Erroneously high systolic

4 The nurse recognizes phase 5 of Korotkoff's sounds when which of the following is heard?

   1. The systolic blood pressure
   2. The diastolic blood pressure in an adult
   3. The diastolic blood pressure in a child
   4. The period of silence at the end of the blood pressure

5 The nurse receives an order to administer Tylenol (acetaminophen) for a temperature over 101°F . When measuring the temperature, the nurse gets a reading of 38.6°C and converts this temperature to what on the Fahrenheit scale?

   1. 100.6
   2. 104

   3. 103.2
   4. 101.5

6 The nurse admits a 30-month old toddler to the pediatric care unit and measures pulse rate using what site?

   1. Radial
   2. Carotid
   3. Brachial
   4. Apical

7 The nurse, caring for a 6-year-old child, recognizes which of the following blood pressures as falling within normal range?

   1. Systolic blood pressure of 92
   2. 100/70
   3. Diastolic blood pressure of 80
   4. 72/40

8 The nurse measures blood pressure while the client is lying, sitting, and standing and records these measurements as:

   1. Orthostatic blood pressure readings.
   2. Orthostatic hypotension.
   3. Pulse deficit.
   4. Auscultatory gap.

9 The client has a physician's order for digoxin. Prior to administering the medication the nurse should:

   1. Assess the blood pressure and give medication if systolic pressure is greater than 140.
   2. Assess the radial pulse and hold if it is greater than 100.
   3. Assess the apical pulse and hold if less than 60.
   4. Assess the apical pulse and give if less than 60.

10 The client is being discharged home. The physician has ordered MS Contin for pain control. The nurse would teach the client and support people to do which of the following prior to administering the medication?

   1. Measure blood pressure prior to administration.
   2. Measure blood pressure 20 minutes after administration.
   3. Assess respirations following administration.
   4. Assess apical pulse prior to administration.

Answers and rationales for Review Questions appear in Appendix I.

Pain: The Fifth Vital Sign

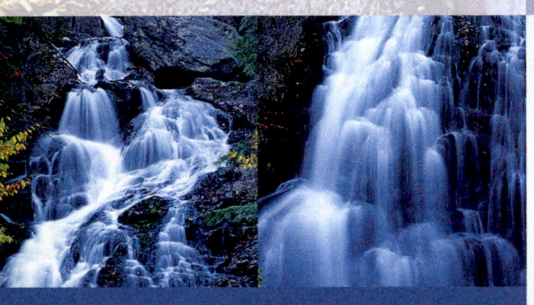

BRIEF Outline

LEARNING Outcomes

After completing this chapter, you will be able to:

1. Identify types and categories of pain according to location, etiology, and duration.
2. Define and contrast pain threshold, pain tolerance, and other concepts associated with pain.
3. Discuss the physiology of pain and three types of pain stimuli.
4. Explain the gate control theory and its application to nursing care.
5. Identify factors that affect the experience of pain.
6. Describe the World Health Organization's three-step ladder approach to cancer pain.
7. List pharmacologic interventions for pain and nursing implications.
8. Describe nonpharmacologic pain control interventions.
9. Discuss key factors in providing effective pain management.
10. State rationales for using various analgesic delivery routes.
11. Identify barriers to effective pain management.
12. Describe nursing care for the client in pain, including data to collect and important interventions.
13. Identify adaptations by developmental level in the care of clients with pain.
14. State criteria by which to evaluate a client's response to interventions for pain.

Clinical Objectives

15. Make use of various pain scales to evaluate a client's pain.
16. Provide nonpharmacologic interventions for a client experiencing pain.

KEY TERMS

Pain is a highly unpleasant and very personal sensation. Pain can consume a person's thoughts and take over daily activities. Yet pain is a difficult concept for a client to communicate. A nurse can neither feel nor see a client's pain.

No two people experience pain in exactly the same way. Because of the differences in how individuals perceive and react to pain, as well as the many causes of pain, the nurse is faced with a complex situation when developing a plan to relieve pain and provide comfort. Effective pain management is an important aspect of care.

As we have learned more about pain, we have seen a shift in focus toward pain control and pain management independent of the cause of the pain. Severe pain is now being viewed as an emergency situation deserving anticipation and prompt treatment. Pain is more than a symptom of a problem; it is a high-priority problem in itself. Pain presents both physiological and psychological dangers to health and recovery. Pain increases morbidity and mortality. Unresolved pain has been shown to prolong hospital stays, delay the healing process, and contribute to depression.

Types of Pain

Although pain is a universal experience, its exact nature remains a mystery. There are a number of definitions of pain. Pain is sensation that is highly subjective and individual; it is one of the body's defense mechanisms indicating that a problem exists.

McCaffery (1979), in a classic work, defined pain as "whatever the experiencing person says it is, existing whenever he (or she) says it does" (p. 11). The most vital part of this definition is the care provider's willingness to believe that the client is experiencing pain and that the client is the real authority on that pain.

Pain may be described in terms of its duration, location, or etiology. When pain lasts only through the expected recovery period, it is described as **acute pain,** whether it has a sudden or slow onset and regardless of the intensity. **Chronic pain** lasts beyond the typical healing time period. Pain lasting longer than 3 to 6 months is generally labeled chronic. Chronic pain can be further classified as chronic malignant pain, when associated with cancer or other life-threatening conditions, or as chronic nonmalignant pain when the etiology is a nonprogressive disorder, such as damage from trauma. Chronic pain that persists despite therapeutic interventions is classified as **intractable pain.** Acute and chronic pain result in different physiological and behavioral responses, shown in Table 22-1 ■.

Pain can be categorized according to its origin as cutaneous, deep somatic, or visceral. **Cutaneous pain** originates in the skin or subcutaneous tissue. A paper cut causing a sharp pain with some burning is an example of cutaneous pain. **Somatic pain** arises from ligaments, tendons, bones, blood vessels, and nerves. It is diffuse and tends to last longer than cutaneous pain. An ankle sprain is an example of deep somatic pain. **Visceral pain** results from stimulation of pain receptors in the abdominal cavity, cranium, and thorax. Visceral pain tends to appear diffuse and often feels like deep somatic pain, that is, burning, aching, or creating a feeling of pressure. Visceral pain is frequently caused by stretching of the tissues, ischemia, or muscle spasms. For example, an obstructed bowel will result in visceral pain.

Pain may also be described according to where it is experienced in the body. **Radiating pain** is perceived at the source of the pain and extends to nearby tissues. For example, cardiac pain may be felt not only in the chest but also along the left shoulder and down the arm. **Referred pain** is pain felt in a part of the body that is considerably removed from the tissues causing the pain. The pain is felt along the nerve pathways for the tissue of origin. For example, pain from one part of the abdominal viscera may be perceived in an area of the skin remote from the organ causing the pain (Figure 22-1 ■).

Intractable pain is pain that is highly resistant to relief. One example is the pain from an advanced malignancy. Often, nurses are challenged to use a number of methods, such as imagery and patient-controlled **analgesia** (pain relief), to provide a client with pain relief.

Neuropathic pain is the result of a disturbance of the nerve pathways either from past or continuing tissue damage that results in pain. Neuropathic pain is described as

TABLE 22-1	Comparison of Acute and Chronic Pain
ACUTE PAIN	**CHRONIC PAIN**
Mild to severe	Mild to severe
Lasts expected amount of time; generally less than 3 to 6 months' duration	Does not resolve in expected time; lasts longer than 6 months

Sympathetic nervous system responses:
   Increased pulse rate
   Increased respiratory rate
   Elevated blood pressure
   Diaphoresis
   Dilated pupils
	Parasympathetic nervous system responses:
	   Vital signs normal
	   Dry, warm skin
	   Pupils normal or dilated

Related to tissue injury; resolves with healing	Continues beyond healing
Client appears restless and anxious	Client appears depressed and withdrawn
Client reports pain	Client often does not mention pain unless asked
Client exhibits behavior indicative of pain: crying, rubbing area, holding area	Pain behavior often absent

shooting or stabbing and is often severe. Clients with conditions such as AIDS and diabetes often suffer from neuropathic pain.

Phantom pain, which is a painful sensation perceived in a body part that is missing (e.g., an amputated leg) or paralyzed by a spinal cord injury, is also an example of neuropathic pain. This can be distinguished from phantom sensation, that is, the feeling that the missing body part is still present.

Concepts Associated with Pain

When an individual perceives pain from injured tissue, the pain threshold is reached. An individual's **pain threshold** is the amount of pain stimulation a person requires in order to feel pain. People's pain threshold is generally fairly uniform; however, it can change. For example, the same stimuli that once produced mild pain can at another time produce intense pain.

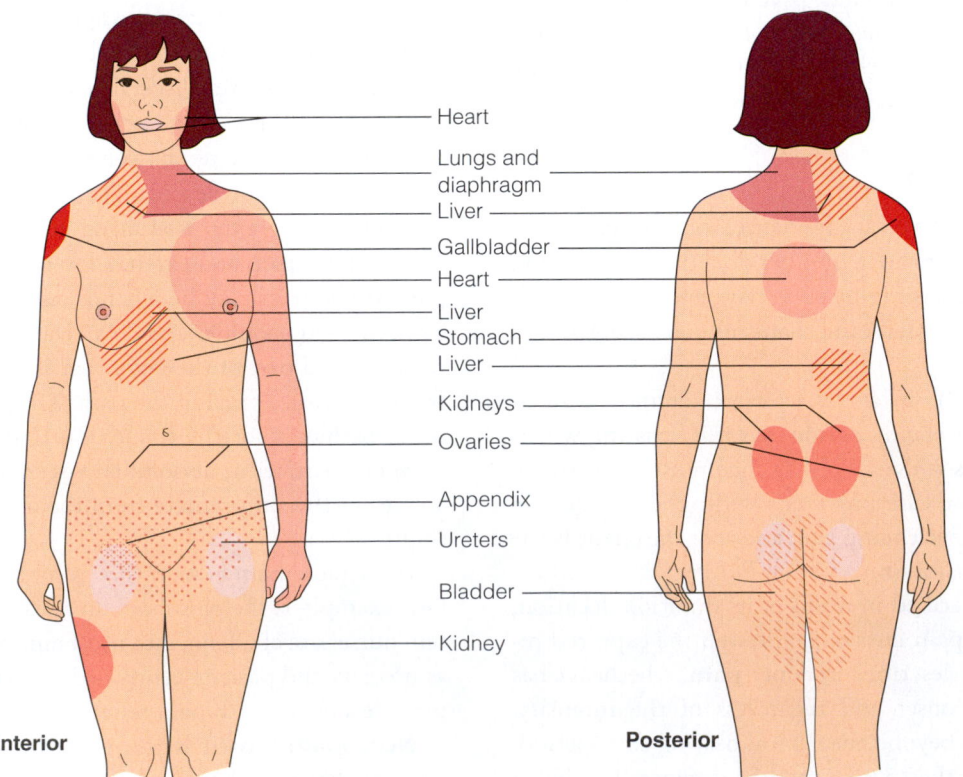

Heart
Lungs and diaphragm
Liver
Gallbladder
Heart
Liver
Stomach
Liver
Kidneys
Ovaries
Appendix
Ureters
Bladder
Kidney

Anterior   **Posterior**

Figure 22-1. ■ Common sites of referred pain from various body organs.

Two additional terms used in the context of pain are pain reaction and tolerance. **Pain reaction** includes the autonomic nervous system and behavioral responses to pain. The *autonomic nervous system response* is the automatic reaction of the body that often protects the individual from further harm, such as the automatic withdrawal of the hand from a hot stove. The *behavioral response* is a learned response used as a method of coping with the pain. Behavioral responses can be related to the anticipation of pain, the sensation of pain, or the aftermath of pain. For example, explaining to a client what he or she will feel prior to administering an injection may reduce the behavioral reaction to the injection.

Pain tolerance is the maximum amount and duration of pain that an individual is willing to endure. Some clients are unable to tolerate even the slightest pain, whereas others are willing to endure severe pain rather than be treated for it. Thus, pain tolerance varies greatly among people and is widely influenced by psychological and sociocultural factors. Pain tolerance may increase with age.

Physiology of Pain

How pain is transmitted and perceived is still incompletely understood. Whether pain is perceived and to what degree depend on the interaction between the body's analgesia system and the nervous system's transmission and interpretation of stimuli.

TRANSMISSION AND PERCEPTION

The peripheral nervous system includes primary sensory neurons specialized to detect tissue damage and to evoke the sensation of touch, heat, cold, pain, and pressure. **Nociceptor** is related to a pain receptor, whereas proprioceptor is a response to stimuli within the body of pressure, position, or stretch, including pacinian corpuscles, which includes sensory nerve endings (Figure 22-2 ■). These pain receptors or nociceptors can be excited by mechanical, thermal, or chemical stimuli (Table 22-2 ■). When there are sufficient noxious stimuli, biochemical mediators are released that sensitize or activate the nociceptors. These chemicals cause the cardinal signs and symptoms we see when tissue damage has occurred. The release of inflammatory chemicals causes vasodilation (redness) and increased capillary permeability (swelling); it also contributes to the conduction of nociception. (See also Chapter 24 ⬭.)

Pain impulses are transmitted via two types of fibers. The A-delta (large-diameter) fibers are *myelinated* (they conduct electrical impulses rapidly). These fibers are associated with the sensation of sharp, pricking pain. The C fibers (small-diameter, unmyelinated fibers) transmit the impulse more slowly and mediate long-lasting, burning pain. The fast A fibers primarily conduct impulses from mechanical

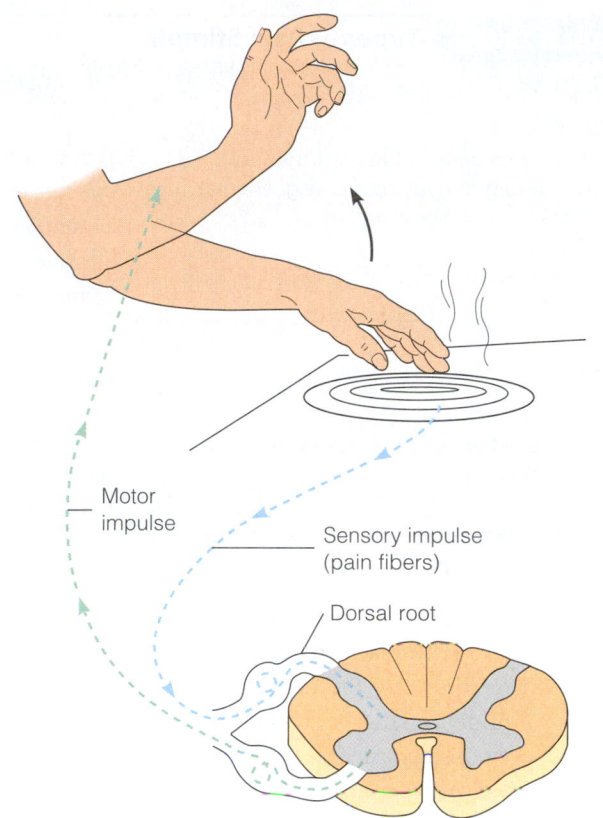

Figure 22-2. ■ Proprioceptive reflex to a pain stimulus.

and thermal pain. The slow, type C fibers conduct impulses from mechanical, thermal, and chemical stimuli.

As pain impulses stimulate the brain, nerve fibers conduct impulses from the brain to the spinal cord, where the pain impulses are inhibited in the spinal cord by the release of endogenous opioids. The three classes of **endogenous opioids** are enkephalins, dynorphins, and beta-endorphins. These substances bind to opiate receptor sites in the central and peripheral nervous system, decreasing or blocking any pain impulse. The opiate binding sites are the same sites where **exogenous opioid analgesics** (e.g., morphine) bind to provide pain relief.

GATE CONTROL THEORY

In 1965, Melzack and Wall proposed the **gate control theory.** According to this theory, peripheral nerve fibers carrying pain to the spinal cord can have their message modified at the spinal cord level before transmission to the brain. Synapses in the spinal cord act as gates that close to keep messages from reaching the brain or open to permit messages to ascend to the brain.

According to the gate control theory, small-diameter nerve fibers carry pain stimuli through a gate, but large-diameter nerve fibers going through the same gate can inhibit the transmission of those pain messages—that is, close

TABLE 22-2	Types of Pain Stimuli
STIMULUS TYPE	**PHYSIOLOGICAL BASIS OF PAIN**
MECHANICAL	
1. Trauma to body tissues (e.g., surgery)	Tissue damage; direct irritation of the pain receptors; inflammation
2. Alterations in body tissues (e.g., edema)	Pressure on pain receptors
3. Blockage of a body duct	Distention of the lumen of the duct
4. Tumor	Pressure on pain receptors; irritation of nerve endings
5. Muscle spasm	Stimulation of pain receptors (also see chemical stimuli)
THERMAL	
Extreme heat or cold (e.g., burns)	Tissue destruction; stimulation of thermosensitive pain receptors
CHEMICAL	
1. Tissue ischemia (e.g., blocked coronary artery)	Stimulation of pain receptors because of accumulated lactic acid (and other chemicals, such as bradykinin and enzymes) in tissues
2. Muscle spasm	Tissue ischemia secondary to mechanical stimulation (see above)

the gate (Figure 22-3 ■). Because a limited amount of sensory information can reach the brain at any given time, certain cells can interrupt the pain messages. The brain also appears to influence whether the gate is open or closed. For example, previous experiences with pain are known to affect how an individual responds to pain. The involvement of the brain helps explain why people interpret painful stimuli differently. Although the gate control theory is not unanimously accepted, it does help explain why electrical and mechanical interventions as well as heat and pressure can relieve pain. The gate control theory, simply put, suggests that a nerve pathway can only carry a few messages at a time. To inhibit the pain message, we must send another message on the nerve pathway for the brain to interpret. For

example, a back massage may stimulate impulses in large nerves, which in turn close the gate to back pain allowing only the message of tactile stimulation to reach the brain, not the message of pain.

RESPONSE TO PAIN

The body's response to pain is a complex process rather than a specific action. It involves physiological and psychosocial aspects. Initially the sympathetic nervous system responds, resulting in the fight-or-flight response. As pain continues, the body adapts; the parasympathetic nervous system takes over, reversing many of the initial physiological responses. This adaptation to the pain occurs after several hours or days of pain. The actual pain receptors adapt very little and continue to transmit the pain message. This keeps the person continually aware of the damaging stimuli causing the pain (Guyton & Hall, 2006). The person may learn to cope with the pain through cognitive and behavioral activities, such as diversions, imagery, and excessive sleeping. The individual may respond to pain by seeking out physical interventions to manage the pain, such as analgesics, massage, and exercise.

FACTORS AFFECTING THE PAIN EXPERIENCE

Numerous factors can affect a person's perception of and reaction to pain. These include the person's ethnic and cultural values, developmental stage, environment and support people, previous pain experiences, and the meaning of the current pain, as well as anxiety and stress (Box 22-1 ■).

Management of Pain

PHARMACOLOGIC MANAGEMENT

Pharmacologic pain management involves the use of opioids (narcotics), nonpioids or nonsteroidal anti-inflammatory drugs (NSAIDs), and adjuvants, or coanalgesic drugs.

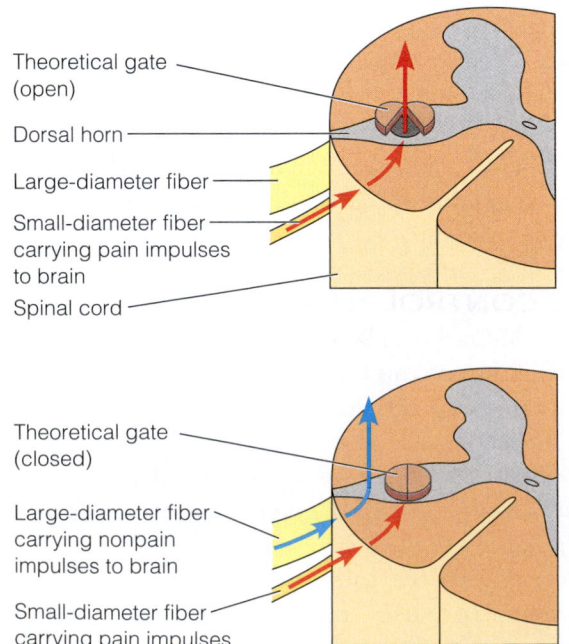

Theoretical gate (open)
Dorsal horn
Large-diameter fiber
Small-diameter fiber carrying pain impulses to brain
Spinal cord

Theoretical gate (closed)
Large-diameter fiber carrying nonpain impulses to brain
Small-diameter fiber carrying pain impulses

Figure 22-3. ■ A schematic illustration of the gate control theory.

BOX 22-1   FACTORS AFFECTING THE PAIN EXPERIENCE

Ethnic and Cultural Values

- Ethnic background and cultural heritage influence the experience of pain. Behavior related to pain is a part of the socialization process.
- There appears to be little variation in pain threshold, but cultural background can affect the level of pain that an individual is willing to tolerate. In some Middle Eastern and African cultures, self-infliction of pain is a sign of mourning or grief. In other groups, pain may be anticipated as part of the ritualistic practices, and therefore tolerance of pain signifies strength and endurance. Additionally, studies have shown that individuals of northern European descent tend to be more stoic and less expressive of their pain than people from southern European backgrounds. For more discussion of cultural considerations, refer to Chapter 3 ⚭ .

Developmental Stage

- Behavioral observation is recommended for pain assessment in infants since physiological responses vary greatly.
- Children are less able to articulate their experience or needs related to pain; therefore, their pain is often undertreated.
- The prevalence of pain in the older population is generally higher due to both acute and chronic disease conditions.
- Pain threshold does not appear to change with aging, although the effect of analgesics may increase due to physiological changes related to drug metabolism.

Environment and Support People

- A strange environment such as a hospital, with its noises, lights, and activity, can compound pain.
- A person who is without a support network may perceive pain as severe, whereas the person who has supportive people around may perceive less pain.
- Some people prefer to withdraw when they are in pain, whereas others prefer the distraction of people and activity around them.
- Family caregivers can be a significant support for a person in pain. With the increase in outpatient and home care, families are assuming an increased responsibility for the management of pain.
- Education related to the assessment and management of pain can positively affect the perceived quality of life for both clients and their caregivers.
- Expectations of significant others can affect a person's perceptions of and responses to pain (e.g., girls may be permitted to express pain more openly than boys).
- Family role can also affect how a person perceives or responds to pain (e.g., a single mother supporting three children may ignore pain because of her need to stay on the job).

- The presence of support people often changes a client's reaction to pain (e.g., toddlers often tolerate pain more readily when supportive parents or nurses are nearby).

Past Pain Experiences

- Previous pain experiences alter a client's sensitivity to pain. People who have personally experienced pain or who have been exposed to the suffering of someone close are often more threatened by anticipated pain than people without a pain experience.
- The success or lack of success of pain relief measures influences a person's expectations for relief (e.g., a person who has tried several pain relief measures without success may have little hope about the helpfulness of nursing interventions).

Meaning of Pain

- Some clients may accept pain more readily than others, depending on the circumstances and the client's interpretation of its significance.
- A client who associates the pain with a positive outcome may withstand the pain amazingly well (e.g., a woman giving birth to a child or an athlete undergoing knee surgery to prolong his career may tolerate pain better because of the benefit associated with it).
- Clients with unrelenting chronic pain may suffer more intensely. They may respond with despair, anxiety, and depression because they cannot attach a positive significance or purpose to the pain. In this situation, the pain may be looked upon as a threat to body image or lifestyle and as a sign of possible impending death.

Anxiety and Stress

- Anxiety often accompanies pain. Threat of the unknown and the inability to control the pain or the events surrounding it often augment the pain perception. See Chapter 17 ⚭ for more on effects of stress.
- Fatigue also reduces a person's ability to cope, thereby increasing pain perception. When pain interferes with sleep, it often leads to fatigue and muscle tension. Tiredness and tension increase the pain, and a cycle of pain, fatigue, and more pain develops.
- People in pain who believe that they have control of their pain have decreased fear and anxiety, which decreases their pain perception.
- A perception of lacking control or a sense of helplessness tends to increase pain perception.
- The expression of pain to an attentive listener and the participation in pain management decisions can increase the sense of control.

WHO Three-Step Ladder Approach

The World Health Organization (WHO) recommends a sequential or three-step ladder approach to manage cancer pain (Figure 22-4 ■). This approach may also apply to pain resulting from causes other than cancer. Therapy begins with a nonopioid/NSAID (step 1). If the client receives the maximum recommended dose of nonopioids and continues

to experience pain, a weak opioid is given (step 2). The dose of the weak opioid is increased until the ceiling dose is reached. If the client continues to experience pain, a stronger opioid is given (step 3). Adjuvant drugs may also be given at any stage of therapy.

A complete review of drugs for pain relief is beyond the scope of this chapter. However, LPNs/LVNs should

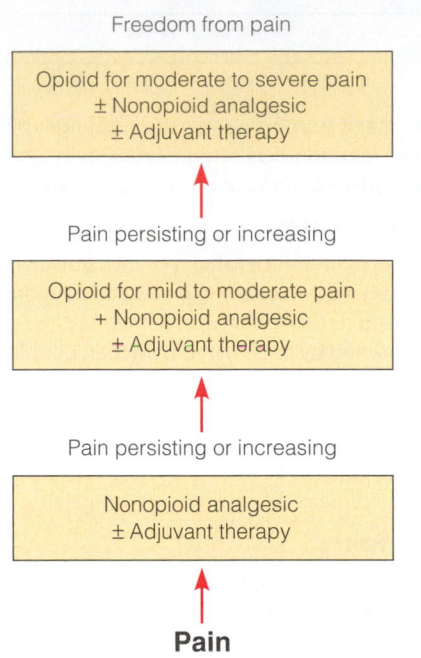

Freedom from pain

Opioid for moderate to severe pain
± Nonopioid analgesic
± Adjuvant therapy

Pain persisting or increasing

Opioid for mild to moderate pain
+ Nonopioid analgesic
± Adjuvant therapy

Pain persisting or increasing

Nonopioid analgesic
± Adjuvant therapy

Pain

Figure 22-4. ■ The WHO three-step analgesic ladder. (*Source:* World Health Organization.)

become familiar with commonly used pain medications and the nursing implications for their use. Table 22-3 ■ provides a brief overview of selected drugs used for relief of pain.

Opioid Analgesics

Opioid (narcotic) analgesics include opium derivatives, such as morphine and codeine. Narcotics relieve pain and provide a sense of euphoria largely by binding to opiate receptors and activating endogenous pain suppression in the central nervous system.

When administering any analgesic, the nurse must review side effects. All opioids result in some initial drowsiness when first administered, but with regular administration, this side effect tends to decrease. Opioids also may cause nausea, vomiting, constipation, and respiratory depression. The most common and most troubling side effect of opioids is constipation. If a client requires long-term opioid therapy, a laxative should be prescribed along with the opioid.

clinical ALERT

Before administering narcotics, the nurse needs to assess a client's level of alertness and respiratory rate for baseline data. An increased sedation level can be an early warning sign of impending respiratory depression.

Opioids must be used cautiously in clients with respiratory problems. If the client experiences significant respiratory depression (e.g., a drop from 18 to 12) or is overly sedated, the dosage is excessive. See the sedation rating scale

TABLE 22-3	Selected Drugs Used for Pain Management	
CLASS	**REASON FOR USE**	**SELECTED GENERIC DRUGS AND BRAND NAMES**
Opioids	Severe pain	*Opioid agonists:*
		codeine, morphine sulfate (Duramorph, etc.), oxycodone (OxyContin), propoxyphene hydrochloride (Darvon), meperidine hydrochloride (Demerol)
		Opioid antagonist:
		naloxone hydrochloride (Narcan)
		Opioids with mixed agonist-antagonist effects:
		butorphanol tartrate (Stadol), nalbuphine hydrochloride (Nubain)
Nonopioid analgesics	Mild to moderate pain, fever Inflammation	*Acetaminophen* (Tylenol); has no anti-inflammatory effect
		Nonsteroidal anti-inflammatory drugs (NSAIDs):
		Selective COX-2 inhibitors:
		Celecoxib (Celebrex)
		Nonsalicylates:
		Naproxen (Naprosyn), naproxen sodium (Aleve, Anaprox), ibuprofen (Advil, Motrin), tolmetin (Tolectin)
		Salicylates:
		aspirin (acetylsalicylic acid, ASA), salsalate (Disalcid)
		Centrally acting agents:
		clonidine (Catapres), tramadol (Ultram)

TABLE 22-3	Selected Drugs Used for Pain Management (continued)	
CLASS	**REASON FOR USE**	**SELECTED GENERIC DRUGS AND BRAND NAMES**
Antimigraine drugs	Relief or prevention of migraine headaches	*For relieving migraine:* *Ergotamine alkaloids:* dihydroergotamine mesylate (Migranal) or ergotamine tartrate (Ergostat) *Triptans:* sumatriptan (Imitrex), almotriptan (Axert), eletriptan (Relpax), frovatriptan (Frova), naratriptan (Amerge), rizatriptan (Maxalt) *For preventing migraines:* *Triptans:* almotriptan, eletriptan, frovatriptan *Beta-adrenergic blockers:* atenolol (Tenormin), metoprolol (Lopressor), propranolol hydrochloride (Inderal), timolol (Blocadren) *Calcium channel blockers:* verapamil hydrochloride (Calan), nifedipine (Procardia), nimodipine (Nimotop) *Tricyclic antidepressants:* amitriptyline (Elavil), imipramine (Tofranil) *Miscellaneous agents:* valproic acid (Depakene, Depakote), methysergide (Sansert), riboflavin (vitamin B_2)

in Box 22-2 ■. Often clients will manifest an increase in sedation before they manifest a decrease in respiratory rate and depth. The nurse should assess and document the client's level of sedation at the same time that respiratory status is checked. Early recognition of an increasing level of sedation or respiratory depression will enable the nurse to implement appropriate measures promptly (e.g., obtaining an order to decrease the opioid dosage). Healthcare providers should never allow the fear of respiratory depression to inhibit adequate pain control. Box 22-3 ■ provides common side effects of, and preventive measures for, opioid analgesics.

Older clients are particularly sensitive to the analgesic properties of opioids and often require less medication than younger clients. This sensitivity may be related to reduced excretion of the drug in elderly clients.

Nonopioids/NSAIDs

Nonopioids (nonnarcotic analgesics) include NSAIDs such as aspirin and ibuprofen. These analgesics have anti-inflammatory, analgesic, and antipyretic effects. (Acetaminophen has only analgesic and antipyretic effects.) They relieve pain by acting on peripheral nerve endings at the injury site and decreasing the level of inflammatory mediators generated at the site of injury.

Individual drugs in this category vary widely in their analgesic properties, metabolism, excretion, and side effects. In addition, the analgesic activity of these drugs has a ceiling effect—the level at which increasing the dose results in no further increase in analgesia.

The most common side effect of nonopioid analgesics is indigestion, which can be prevented by taking the medication with antacid or food. Stomach ulcers and gastric bleeding have also been reported. NSAIDs reduce the dose of opioids needed when the drugs are given together and provide better pain relief than use of either type separately. These drugs must be ordered by the physician; they all have a maximum daily dose limit.

Pharmacologic management of mild to moderate pain should begin with NSAIDs, unless there is a specific contraindication (Holland and Adams, 2007). NSAIDs are contraindicated, for example, in clients with impaired blood clotting, gastrointestinal bleeding or ulcer risk, renal disease, thrombocytopenia, and possibly infection (because NSAIDs will obscure fever).

Adjuvant Analgesics

Adjuvant analgesics are medications that were developed for uses other than analgesia but have been found to reduce certain types of chronic pain in addition to their primary action. For example, mild sedatives or tranquilizers, such as diazepam (Valium), may help reduce painful muscle spasms as well as anxiety, stress, and tension so that the client can obtain a good night's sleep. Antidepressants, such as amitriptyline hydrochloride (Elavil), are used to treat underlying depression or mood disorders but may also enhance other pain

BOX 22-2	SEDATION RATING SCALE

S = sleeping, easily aroused; requires no action
1 = awake and alert; requires no action
2 = occasionally drowsy, easy to arouse; requires no action
3 = frequently drowsy, arousable, drifts off to sleep during conversation; decrease the opioid dose
4 = somnolent, minimal or no response to stimuli; discontinue opioid and consider use of naloxone (Narcan)

Source: McCaffery, M., & Pasero, C. (1999). *Pain: Clinical manual,* p. 267. (2nd ed.). St. Louis, MO: Mosby. Reprinted by permission.

BOX 22-3 COMMON OPIOID SIDE EFFECTS AND PREVENTIVE MEASURES

Constipation

- Increase fluid intake (e.g., to 8 glasses daily).
- Increase fiber and bulk-forming agents in the diet (e.g., fresh fruits and vegetables).
- Increase exercise regimen.
- Administer stool softeners and provide a mild laxative if necessary.

Nausea and Vomiting

- Inform client that tolerance to this emetic effect generally develops after several days of opiate therapy.
- Provide an antiemetic as required.
- Change the analgesic as indicated.

Sedation

- Inform client that tolerance usually develops over 3 to 5 days.
- Administer a stimulant, such as dextroamphetamine sulfate (Dexedrine) or methylphenidate hydrochloride (Ritalin) each morning to clients who receive opiate therapy for chronic pain and do not develop tolerance.

Respiratory Depression

- Administer an opioid antagonist, such as naloxone hydrochloride (Narcan), until respirations return to an acceptable rate. Administer the medication slowly by intravenous route with 10 mL of saline. Monitor the client, and repeat the procedure as required.
- If the client is receiving intravenous patient-controlled analgesia (PCA), stop or slow the infusion.

Pruritus

- Apply cool packs, lotion, and diversional activity.
- Administer an antihistamine (e.g., diphenhydramine hydrochloride [Benadryl]).
- Inform the client that tolerance also develops to pruritus.

Urinary Retention

- May need to catheterize client.
- Administer narcotic antagonist (naloxone hydrochloride [Narcan]).

strategies. Anticonvulsants, such as carbamazepine (Tegretol) and clonazepam (Klonopin), usually prescribed to treat seizures, can be useful in controlling painful neuropathies such as herpes zoster (shingles) and diabetic neuropathies.

NONPHARMACOLOGIC PAIN MANAGEMENT

Nonpharmacologic pain management consists of a variety of physical and cognitive-behavioral pain management strategies. Physical interventions include cutaneous stimulation, immobilization, transcutaneous electrical nerve stimulation (TENS), and acupuncture. Mind-body (cognitive-behavioral) interventions include distraction activities,

relaxation techniques, imagery, meditation, biofeedback, hypnosis, and therapeutic touch. Box 22-4 ■ provides a detailed description of these interventions.

BOX 22-4 NONPHARMACOLOGIC PAIN INTERVENTIONS

Cutaneous Stimulation

Cutaneous stimulation can provide effective temporary pain relief. It distracts the client and focuses attention on the tactile stimuli, away from the painful sensations, thus reducing pain perception. Cutaneous stimulation can be applied directly to the painful area, proximal to the pain, distal to the pain, and contralateral (opposite side) to the pain. Cutaneous stimulation techniques include the following:

- *Massage.* Massage is a comfort measure that can aid relaxation, decrease muscle tension, and may ease anxiety. Massage can also decrease pain intensity by increasing superficial circulation to the area. Massage can involve the back and neck, hands and arms, or feet. The use of ointments or liniments may provide localized pain relief with joint or muscle pain.
- *Heat and Cold Applications.* A warm bath, heating pads, ice bags, ice massage, hot or cold compresses, and warm or cold sitz baths in general relieve pain and promote healing of injured tissues.
- *Acupressure.* Acupressure developed from the ancient Chinese healing system of acupuncture. The therapist applies finger pressure to points that correspond to many of the points used in acupuncture.
- *Contralateral Stimulation.* Contralateral stimulation can be accomplished by stimulating the skin in an area opposite to the painful area (e.g., stimulating the left knee if the pain is in the right knee). The contralateral area may be scratched for itching, massaged for cramps, or treated with cold packs or analgesic ointments. This method is particularly useful when the painful area cannot be touched because it is hypersensitive, inaccessible by a cast or bandages, or when the pain is felt in a missing part (phantom pain).

Transcutaneous Electrical Nerve Stimulation

TENS is a method of applying low-voltage electrical stimulation directly over identified pain areas, at an acupressure point, along peripheral nerve areas that innervate the pain area, or along the spinal column. The TENS unit consists of a portable, battery-operated device with lead wire and electrode pads that are applied to the chosen area of skin. Cutaneous stimulation from the TENS unit is thought to activate large-diameter fibers that modulate the transmission of the nociceptive impulse in the peripheral and central nervous system (closing the pain "gate"), resulting in pain relief. This stimulation may also cause a release of endorphins from the central nervous system centers.

Distraction

Distraction draws the person's attention away from the pain and lessens the perception of pain. In some instances, distraction can make a client completely unaware of pain. For example, a client recovering from surgery may feel no pain while

(continued)

BOX 22-4   *Continued*

watching a football game on television, yet feel pain again when the game is over.

Visual Distraction
- Reading or watching TV
- Watching a baseball game
- Guided imagery

Auditory Distraction
- Humor
- Listening to music

Tactile Distraction
- Slow, rhythmic breathing
- Massage
- Holding or stroking a pet or toy

Intellectual Distraction
- Crossword puzzles
- Card games (e.g., bridge)
- Hobbies (e.g., stamp collecting, writing a story)

Nonpharmacologic Invasive Therapies

A nerve block is a chemical interruption of a nerve pathway, affected by injecting a local anesthetic into the nerve. Nerve blocks are widely used during dental work. The injected drug blocks nerve pathways from the painful tooth, thus stopping the transmission of pain impulses to the brain. Nerve blocks are often used to relieve the pain of whiplash injury, lower back disorders, bursitis, and cancer.

Surgery

Pain conduction pathways can be interrupted surgically. Because this disruption is permanent, surgery is performed only as a last resort, generally for intractable pain. Several surgical procedures may be performed and depend on area of pain origin.

Key Factors in Effective Pain Management

ACKNOWLEDGING AND ACCEPTING

Basic to all strategies for reducing pain is that nurses convey to clients that they believe the client is having pain. Four ways of communicating this belief follow:

1. Verbally acknowledge the presence of the pain: "I understand your leg is very painful. How do you feel about the pain?"
2. Listen attentively to what the client says about the pain.
3. Convey that you are assessing the client's pain to understand it better, not to determine whether the pain is real, for example, "How does your pain feel now?" or "Tell me how it feels compared to an hour ago."
4. Attend to the client's needs promptly.

ASSISTING SUPPORT PERSONS

Support persons often need assistance to respond positively to the client experiencing pain. Enlisting the aid of support persons in the provision of pain relief to the client, such as massaging the client's back, may diminish his or her feelings of helplessness and foster a more positive attitude toward the client's pain experience. Support persons also may need the nurse's verbal recognition of their concern and participation in the client's care.

REDUCING MISCONCEPTIONS ABOUT PAIN

Reducing a client's misconceptions about the pain and its treatment will often avoid intensifying the pain. The nurse should explain to the client that pain is a highly individual experience and that it is only the client who really experiences the pain, although others can understand and empathize. Misconceptions are also dealt with when nurse and client discuss why the pain has increased or decreased at certain times. For example, a client whose pain increases in the evening may mistakenly think this is the result of eating dinner rather than the result of fatigue.

REDUCING FEAR AND ANXIETY

It is important to help relieve the emotional component, that is, anxiety or fear, associated with the pain. When clients have no opportunity to talk about their pain and associated fears, their perceptions and reactions to the pain can be intensified. The client may become angry or complain about the nurse's care when the problem really is a belief that the pain is not being attended to. If the nurse is honest and sincere and promptly attends to the client's needs, the client is much more likely to know that the nurse does believe the client is in pain.

By providing accurate information, the nurse can also reduce many of the client's fears, such as a fear of addiction or a fear that the pain will always be present. It also helps many clients to have privacy when they are experiencing pain.

PREVENTING PAIN

A preventive approach to pain management involves the provision of measures to treat the pain before it occurs or before it becomes severe. **Preemptive analgesia** is the administration of analgesics prior to an invasive or operative procedure. Nurses can also use a preemptive approach by providing analgesic around-the-clock (ATC), rather than as needed (prn). For clients who routinely feel pain, for example, with diseases such as cancer, administering pain medication at scheduled intervals maintains the level of analgesia without allowing the peaks and valleys associated with metabolism of the medication given on a prn basis. PCA pumps allow clients to self-administer medication to lessen breakthrough pain (Figure 22-5 ■).

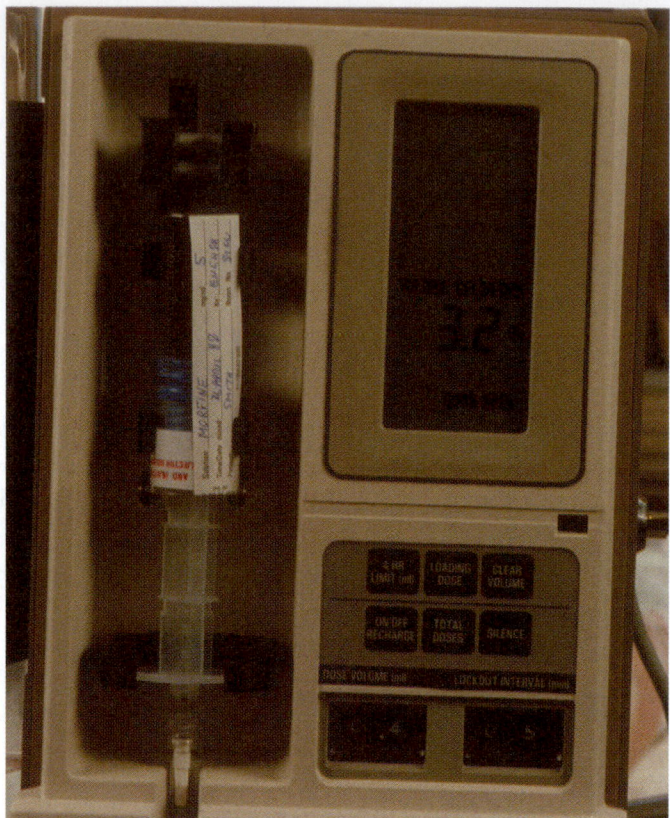

Figure 22-5. ■ A continuous, subcutaneous PCA infusion device.

Administering Pain Medication

ROUTES FOR OPIATE DELIVERY

Opioids have traditionally been administered by oral, subcutaneous, intramuscular, and intravenous routes. In addition, newer methods of delivering opiates have been developed to circumvent potential obstacles that occur with these traditional routes. Examples are transnasal and transdermal drug therapy, continuous subcutaneous infusions, and intraspinal infusion. Table 22-4 ■ lists routes and their benefits.

Barriers to Pain Management

Misconceptions and biases can affect pain management. Some of these involve attitudes of the nurse or the client as well as knowledge deficits. Clients respond to pain experiences based on their culture (Box 22-5 ■), personal experiences, and the meaning the pain has for them. For many people, pain is expected and accepted as a normal aspect of illness. Clients and families may lack knowledge of the adverse effects of pain and may have misinformation regarding the use of analgesics. Clients may not report pain because they expect nothing can be done, they think it is not severe enough, or they feel it would distract or prejudice the healthcare provider. Other common misconceptions are shown in Table 22-5 ■.

NURSING CARE

PRIORITIZING NURSING CARE

Pain control is the number one priority for the nurse. When clients are as pain free as possible, they are more likely to participate fully in their recovery. A pain assessment should be conducted when vital signs are taken and as necessary. Anticipate your clients' need for pain medication and arrange your schedule so that you do not have to delay medicating them. A delay of even 20 or 30 minutes can cause the pain level to be unmanageable to clients.

Make use of nonpharmacologic comfort techniques in tandem with medication. A back massage, linen change, or quiet, restful environment can assist with pain management. It is extremely important to remember that pain tolerance is very personal. The pain level is the client's perception and not that of the nurse. The nurse should not deny the client medication because the pain does not appear to be as severe as a client is reporting.

ASSESSING

Accurate pain assessment is essential for effective pain management. Because pain is subjective and experienced uniquely by each individual, nurses need to assess all factors affecting the pain experience—physiological, psychological, behavioral, emotional, and sociocultural.

Pain is considered the fifth vital sign, and should be assessed at least every 4 hours. Pain is also assessed following pain management interventions. Pain intensity should be reassessed at an interval appropriate for the intervention. For example, following the intravenous administration of morphine, the severity of pain should be reassessed in 20 to 30 minutes.

clinical ALERT

A quick pain assessment rubric is PQRST:

P—Precipitation/Palliation: What causes (*precipitates*) your pain? What relieves (or palliates) your pain?
Q—Quality: What does your pain feel like (sharp, dull, shooting, etc.)?
R—Region/Radiation: Where did the pain start? Does it radiate (travel to another location)?
S—Severity: How bad is the pain on a pain scale with zero meaning no pain and ten meaning the worst pain imaginable?
T—Timing: When did the pain start? How long does it last?

Because many people will not voice their pain unless asked about it, pain assessments *must* be initiated by the nurse. Some of the many reasons clients may be reluctant

TABLE 22-4	Routes of Administration for Pain Medications and Their Benefits
ROUTE OF ADMINISTRATION	BENEFITS
Oral route	Oral administration of opiates remains the preferred route of delivery because of ease of administration. Because the duration of action of most opiates is approximately 4 hours, people with chronic pain have had to awaken several times during the night to be medicated for pain. To circumvent this problem, long-acting forms of morphine with a duration of 8 or more hours have been developed. Two examples of long-acting morphine are MS Contin and Oramorph SR. Clients receiving long-acting morphine also may need prn rescue doses of immediate-release analgesics (e.g., short-acting morphine) for acute breakthrough pain. Another new method of oral opiate delivery is high-concentration liquid morphine. This formulation enables clients who can swallow only small amounts to continue taking the drug orally.
Nasal route	Transnasal administration has the advantage of rapid action of the medication because of direct absorption through the vascular nasal mucosa. A commonly used agent is butorphanol (Stadol) for acute headaches.
Transdermal route	Transdermal drug therapy is advantageous in that it delivers a relatively stable plasma drug level and is noninvasive. Fentanyl (Duragesic) is an opioid currently available as a skin patch with various dosages. It provides drug delivery for up to 72 hours.
Rectal route	Several opiates are now available in suppository form. The rectal route is particularly useful for clients who have dysphagia (difficulty swallowing) or nausea and vomiting. Oral analgesics, with the exception of sustained-release analgesics, may be crushed, dissolved in water, and given rectally (McCaffery & Pasero, 1999).
Subcutaneous route	Although the subcutaneous (SC) route has been used extensively to deliver opioids, a new technique uses subcutaneous catheters and infusion pumps to provide continuous subcutaneous infusion (CSCI) of narcotics. CSCI is particularly helpful for clients (1) whose pain is poorly controlled by oral medications, (2) who are experiencing dysphagia or gastrointestinal obstruction, or (3) who have a need for prolonged use of parenteral narcotics. CSCI involves the use of a small, light, battery-operated pump that administers the drug through a 23- or 25-gauge butterfly needle. The needle can be inserted into the anterior chest, the subclavicular region, the abdominal wall, the outer aspects of the upper arms, or the thighs. Client mobility is maintained with the application of a shoulder bag or holster to hold the pump. The frequency of site change ranges from 3 to 7 days.
Intramuscular route	The intramuscular (IM) route is the least desirable route for opioid administration because of variable absorption, pain involved with administration, and the need to repeat administration every 3 to 4 hours.
Intravenous route	The intravenous (IV) route provides rapid and effective pain relief with few side effects. The analgesic can be administered by IV bolus or by continuous infusion controlled by the client using a PCA machine at the bedside.
Intraspinal route	Another recent method of delivery is the infusion of opiates into the epidural or intrathecal (subarachnoid) space. Intraspinal analgesics act directly on opiate receptors in the spinal cord. Two commonly used medications are preservative-free morphine sulfate and fentanyl. The major benefit of intraspinal drug therapy is that it exerts a lesser sedative effect than do systemic opiates. The epidural space is most commonly used because the dura mater acts as a protective barrier against infection, including meningitis.
Patient-controlled analgesia	PCA is the self-administration of an analgesic by a client who has been instructed about the process. The physician prescribes the analgesic dose, route, and frequency, with the client administering the medication. With parenteral routes, an infusion pump is used to deliver the medication. Whether in an acute hospital setting, an ambulatory clinic, or with home care, the nurse is responsible for the initial instruction regarding use of the PCA and for the ongoing monitoring of the therapy. The client's pain must be assessed at regular intervals and analgesic use is documented in the client's record. PCA can be effectively used for clients with acute pain related to a surgical incision, traumatic injury, or labor and delivery, and for chronic pain, as with cancer. In some settings, PCAs are used even if the client is unable to initiate a dose by pushing the button, as long as a caregiver is willing to accept the responsibility, for example, when the client is an infant or toddler or is physically or cognitively impaired (Pasero & McCaffery, 1996). The benefits of this mode of administration include: ■ Self-control over pain relief. ■ More stable analgesic blood level for sustained pain relief. ■ Tendency for the client to need less medication for pain relief. PCA pumps usually have a chamber or cartridge that contains the analgesic, a mechanism for setting the ordered dose, and a control for client activation (see Figure 22-5). When clients want a dose of analgesic, they can push a button attached to the infusion pump and the preset dose is delivered. A programmable lockout interval (usually 10 to 15 minutes) follows the dose, when an additional dose cannot be given even if the client activates the button. It is also possible to program the maximum dose that can be delivered over a period of hours (usually 4). Many pumps are capable of delivering a low continuous infusion, or basal rate, to provide sustained analgesia during times of rest and sleep.

BOX 22-5   **CULTURAL PULSE POINTS**

Pain Experiences and Culture

The meaning and expression of pain are influenced by people's cultural backgrounds. Pain is not just a physiological response to tissue damage. Not everyone in a culture conforms to a set of expected behaviors or beliefs, so cultural stereotyping can lead to inadequate assessment and treatment of pain. Healthcare professionals need to be aware of their own values and perceptions because they affect how they evaluate the client's response to pain and ultimately how pain is treated. Even subtle cultural and individual differences, particularly in nonverbal, spoken, and written language, between healthcare providers and client can impact care.

---

to report pain are listed in Box 22-6 ■. Nurses must listen to and rely on the client's perceptions of pain. Believing the person experiencing and conveying the perceptions is crucial in establishing a sense of trust. (See Chapter 11 ⚭.)

Pain assessments consist of a pain history to obtain facts from the client and direct observation of behavioral and physiological responses of the client. The goal of assessment is to gain an objective understanding of a subjective experience.

While taking pain histories, the nurse must provide an opportunity for clients to express in their own words how they view the pain and the situation. This will help the nurse understand what the pain means to the client and how the client is coping with it. Remember that each person's pain experience is unique and that the client is the best interpreter of the pain experience. The initial pain assessment for someone in severe acute pain may consist of only a few questions before intervention occurs, such as location, intensity, and quality. For the person with chronic pain, the nurse may focus on the client's coping mechanisms, effectiveness of current pain management, and ways in which the pain has affected activities of daily living (ADLs).

Location

To identify the specific location of the pain, ask the individual to point to the site of the discomfort. A chart consisting of drawings of the body can assist in identifying pain locations. The client marks the location of pain on the chart. This tool can be especially effective with clients who have more than one source of pain.

When assessing the location of a child's pain, the nurse needs to understand the child's vocabulary. For example, "tummy" might mean the abdomen or part of the chest. Asking the child to point to the pain helps clarify the child's word usage to identify location. Again, the use of figure drawings can assist in identifying pain locations (Figure 22-6 ■.) Parents can also be helpful in interpreting the meaning of a child's words.

Intensity

The single most important indicator of the intensity of pain is the client's report of pain. Studies have shown that healthcare providers may underrate or overrate the pain

---

BOX 22-6   **WHY CLIENTS MAY BE RELUCTANT TO REPORT PAIN**

- Unwillingness to trouble staff who are perceived as busy
- Fear of the injectable route of analgesic administration (children in particular)
- Belief that pain is to be expected as part of the recovery process
- Belief that pain is a normal part of aging or a necessary part of life (older adults in particular)
- Belief that expressions of pain reveal weakness
- Difficulty expressing personal discomfort
- Concern about risks associated with opioid drugs (e.g., addiction)
- Fear about the cause of pain or that reporting pain will lead to further tests and expenses
- Concern about unwanted side effects, especially of opioid drugs
- Concern that use of drugs now will render the drug inefficient if or when the pain becomes worse

---

TABLE 22-5	Common Misconceptions about Pain
MISCONCEPTION	**CORRECTION**
Clients experience severe pain only when they have had major surgery.	Even after minor surgery, clients can experience intense pain.
The nurse and other healthcare professionals are the authorities on a client's pain.	The person who experiences the pain is the only authority on its existence and nature.
Administering analgesics regularly for pain will lead to addiction.	Clients are unlikely to become addicted to an analgesic provided to treat pain.
The amount of tissue damage is directly related to the amount of pain.	Pain is a subjective experience, and the intensity and duration of pain vary considerably among individuals.
Visible physiological or behavioral signs accompany pain and can be used to verify its existence.	Even with severe pain, periods of physiological and behavioral adaptation can occur.

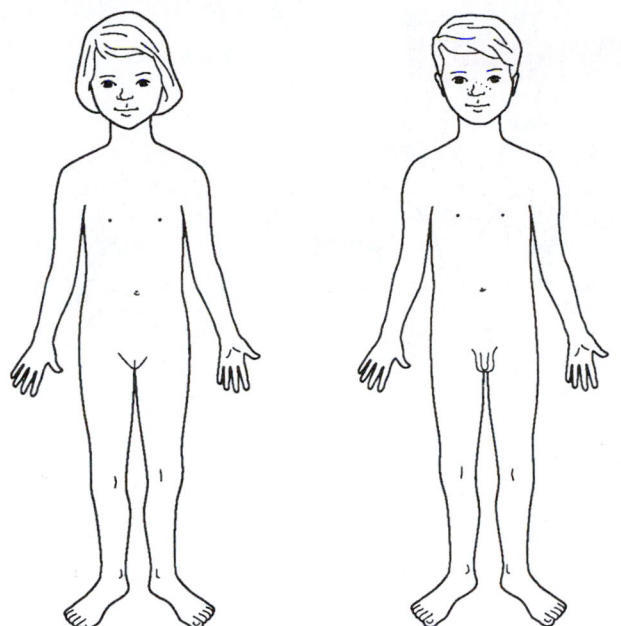

Figure 22-6. ■ The nurse can use a simple gender-specific drawing of a child's body to help the child pinpoint the location of the pain.

intensity. The use of pain intensity scales is an easy and reliable method of determining pain intensity. Such scales provide consistency for nurses to communicate with the client and other healthcare providers. Most scales use either a 0-to-5 or 0-to-10 range with 0 indicating "no pain" and the highest number indicating the "worst pain possible" for that individual. A 10-point rating scale is shown in Figure 22-7A ■. It is important for the nurse to understand that the pain scale is intended to compare the client to himself or herself, not to other individuals. A nurse should never compare one client's rating of pain with another client's rating of pain. The scale is intended to gauge the amount of relief or distress the client is in at any given time. It should not be used to compare levels of pain perception.

When noting pain intensity, it is important to determine any related factors that may be affecting the pain. When the intensity changes, the nurse needs to consider the possible cause. For example, the abrupt cessation of acute abdominal pain may indicate a ruptured appendix. Several factors affect the perception of intensity: (1) the amount of distraction, or the client's concentration on another event; (2) the client's state of consciousness; (3) the level of activity; and (4) the client's expectations.

Not all clients can understand or relate to numerical pain intensity scales. These include children who are unable to communicate discomfort verbally, elderly clients with impairments in cognition or communication, and people who do not speak English. For these clients, the Wong/Baker Faces Rating Scale (Figure 22-7B) may be easier to use

(Pasero, 1997). The face scale includes a number scale in relation to each expression so that the pain intensity can be documented. When it is not possible to use any kind of rating scale with a client, the nurse must rely on observation of behavior and the physiological cues discussed later in this section. The input of the client's significant others, such as parents or caregivers, can assist the nurse in interpreting the observations. An objective description of the behavior and the physiological data are then documented.

For effective use of pain rating scales, clients need to not only understand the use of the scale but also be educated about how the information will be used to determine changes in their condition and the effectiveness of pain management interventions. Clients should also be asked to indicate what level of comfort is acceptable so that they can perform specific activities. This will ensure that adequate pain management is achieved.

Quality

Descriptive adjectives help people communicate the quality of pain. A headache may be described as "hammer-like" or an abdominal pain as "piercing like a knife." Sometimes clients have difficulty describing pain because they have never experienced any sensation like it. Terms commonly used to describe pain can be classified as sensory words and affective words. Examples of sensory words are *searing, scalding, sharp, piercing, drilling, wrenching, shooting, splitting, crushing, penetrating, numb, radiating, dull, aching,* and *cramping.* Examples of affective words are *unbearable, killing, intense, torturing, agonizing, terrifying, grueling, suffocating, frightful, punishing, miserable, annoying, nagging, tiring,* and *troublesome.*

Nurses need to record the exact words clients use to describe pain. A client's words are more accurate and descriptive than an interpretation in the nurse's words. Exact information can be significant in both the diagnosis of the pain etiology and in the treatment choices made. For example, pain described as hot, electrical, and sharp tends to be neuropathic in origin and will be more responsive to anticonvulsants (e.g., Tegretol) than to an opioid (e.g., morphine).

Pattern

The pattern of pain includes time of onset, duration, and recurrence or intervals without pain. The nurse therefore determines when the pain began; how long the pain lasts; whether it recurs and, if so, the length of the interval without pain; and when the pain last occurred.

Precipitating Factors

Certain activities sometimes precede pain; for example, physical exertion may precede chest pain, or abdominal pain may occur after eating. These observations can help prevent pain and determine its cause.

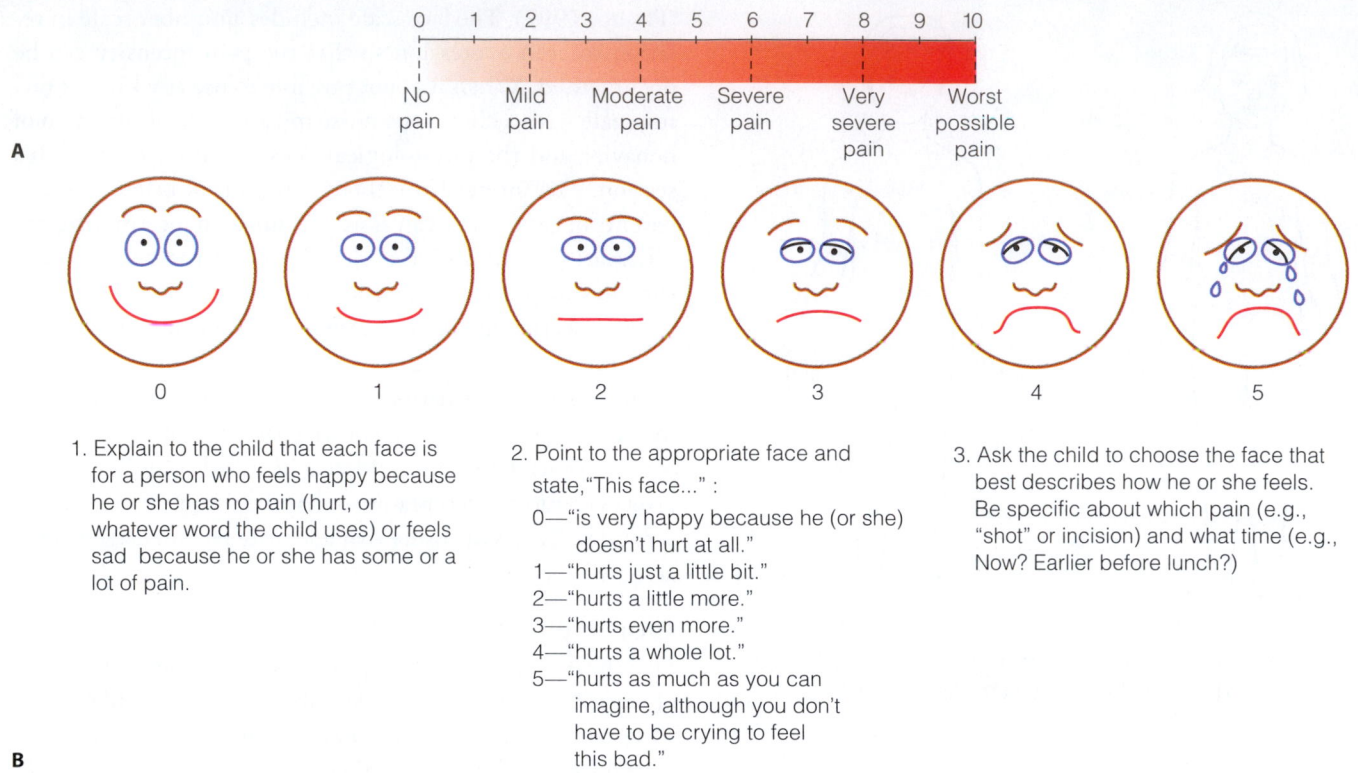

Figure 22-7. ■ **A.** A 10-point pain intensity scale with word modifiers. **B.** The Wong/Baker Faces Rating Scale. (*Source:* Wong, D. L. (2001). *Wong's Essentials of Pediatric Nursing* (6th ed.). St. Louis, MO: Mosby. Reprinted with permission.)

Environmental factors such as extreme cold or heat and extremes of humidity can affect some types of pain. For example, sudden exercise on a hot day can cause muscle spasm.

Physical and emotional stressors can also precipitate pain. Emotional tension frequently brings on a migraine headache. Intense fear or physical exertion can cause angina.

Alleviating Factors

Nurses must ask clients to describe anything that they have done to help alleviate the pain (e.g., home remedies such as herbal teas, or medications, rest, applications of heat or cold, prayer, or distractions such as watching TV). It is important to explore the effect any of these measures had on the pain, whether or not relief was obtained, or whether the pain became worse.

Associated Symptoms

Also included in the clinical appraisal of pain are other associated symptoms, such as nausea, vomiting, dizziness, and diarrhea. These symptoms may relate to the onset of the pain or they may result from the presence of the pain.

Effect on Activities of Daily Living

When caring for clients with chronic pain, knowing how ADLs are affected helps the nurse understand the client's perspective on the pain's severity. The nurse asks the client to describe how the pain has affected the following aspects of life:

- Sleep
- Appetite
- Concentration
- Work/school
- Interpersonal relationships
- Marital relations/sex
- Home activities
- Driving/walking
- Leisure activities
- Emotional status (mood, irritability, depression, anxiety)

A rating scale of none, a little, or a great deal or another range can be used to determine the degree of alteration.

Coping Resources

Each individual will exhibit personal ways of coping with pain. Strategies may relate to past pain experiences or the specific meaning of the pain; some may reflect religious or cultural influences. Nurses can encourage and support the client's use of methods known to have helped in modifying pain. Strategies may include withdrawal, use of distraction, prayer or other religious practices, and support from significant others.

Affective Responses

Affective responses vary according to the situation, the degree and duration of pain, the interpretation of it, and many other factors. The nurse needs to explore the client's feelings—for example, anxiety, fear, exhaustion, depression, or a sense of failure. Because many people with chronic pain become depressed and potentially suicidal, it may also be necessary to assess the client's suicide risk. In such situations, the nurse needs to ask the client, "Do you ever feel so bad that you want to die? Do you feel that way now?"

Observation of Behavioral and Physiological Responses

There are wide variations in nonverbal responses to pain. For clients who are very young, aphasic, confused, or disoriented, nonverbal expressions may be the only means of communicating pain. Facial expression is often the first indication of pain, and it may be the only one. Clenched teeth, tightly shut eyes, open somber eyes, biting of the lower lip, and other facial grimaces may be indicative of pain. Vocalizations such as moaning and groaning or crying and screaming are also associated with pain.

Immobilization of the body or a part of the body may also indicate pain. The client with chest pain often holds the left arm across the chest. A person with abdominal pain may assume the position of greatest comfort, often with the knees and hips flexed, and move reluctantly.

Purposeless body movements can also indicate pain—for example, tossing and turning in bed or flinging the arms about. Involuntary movements such as a reflexive jerking away from a needle inserted through the skin indicate pain. An adult may be able to control this reflex; however, a child may be unable or unwilling to do so.

Rhythmic body movements or rubbing may indicate pain. An adult or child may assume a fetal position and rock back and forth when experiencing abdominal pain. During labor a woman may massage her abdomen rhythmically with her hands.

It is important to note that behavioral responses can be controlled and so may not be very revealing. When pain is chronic, there are rarely overt behavioral responses because the individual develops personal coping styles for dealing with pain, discomfort, or suffering. Therefore, it is imperative that nurses believe clients when they report they are in pain. It is unacceptable for the nurse to doubt a client who reports pain because "he did not look like he was hurting."

Physiological responses vary with the origin and duration of the pain. Early in the onset of acute pain, the sympathetic nervous system is stimulated, resulting in increased blood pressure, pulse rate, respiratory rate, pallor, diaphoresis, and pupil dilation. However, in clients with chronic pain, the sympathetic nervous system adapts to the stimulus, making the physiological responses less evident or even absent. When people experience visceral pain, signs of parasympathetic stimulation may be observed, such as decreased blood pressure and pulse rate, pupil constriction, and warm, dry skin.

Daily Pain Diary

For clients who experience chronic pain, a daily diary may help the client and nurse identify pain patterns and factors that exacerbate or mediate the pain experience. In home care, the family or other caregiver can be taught to complete the diary.

The record can include time or onset of pain, activity before pain, pain-related positions or behaviors, pain intensity level, use of analgesics or other relief measures, duration of pain, and time spent in relief activities. Recorded data can provide the basis for developing or modifying the plan for care. The client can use the mnemonic HILDA as a reminder for including data:

How does your pain feel?
Intensity (0–10)
Location
Duration
Aggravating or alleviating factors

For a pain diary to be effective, it is important that the nurse educate the client and family about the value and use of the diary in achieving effective pain control. Determining the client's abilities to use the diary is essential.

DIAGNOSING, PLANNING, AND IMPLEMENTING

The North American Nursing Diagnosis Association (NANDA) includes the following diagnostic labels for clients experiencing pain or discomfort:

- *Acute Pain*
- *Chronic Pain*

Goals and interventions for clients should be individualized for the client, the particular pain process, and developmental level (Box 22-7 ■).

Because the presence of pain can affect so many areas of a person's functioning, pain may be the etiology of other nursing diagnoses. Examples of such nursing diagnoses follow:

- *Ineffective Airway Clearance* related to postoperative incisional chest pain
- *Powerlessness* related to past experiences of poor control of pain (See also Chapter 17 ⊂⊃ .)
- *Ineffective Coping* related to prolonged continuous back pain, ineffective pain management, and inadequate support systems
- *Impaired Physical Mobility* related to arthritic pain in knee and ankle joints
- *Disturbed Sleep Pattern* related to increased pain perception at night

Preventing Pain

Review the section Key Factors in Effective Pain Management on page 477. As mentioned, the nurse provides measures to treat the pain before it occurs or before it

---

BOX 22-7 | **LIFESPAN CONSIDERATIONS**

Selected Nursing Interventions for Pain by Developmental Level

Infant
- Give a glucose pacifier.
- Use tactile stimulation. Play music or tapes of a heartbeat.

Toddler/preschooler
- Distract the child with toys, books, pictures.
- Involve the child in blowing bubbles as a way of "blowing away the pain."
- Appeal to the child's belief in magic by using a "magic" blanket or glove to take away pain.
- Hold the child to provide comfort.
- Explore misconceptions about pain.

School-age child
- Use imagery to turn off "pain switches."
- Provide a behavioral rehearsal of what to expect and how it will look and feel.
- Provide support and nurturing.

Adolescent
- Provide opportunities to discuss pain.
- Provide privacy.
- Present choices for dealing with pain.
- Encourage music or TV for distraction.

Adult
- Deal with any misconceptions about pain.
- Focus on the client's control in dealing with the pain.
- Allay fears and anxiety when possible.

Older adult
- Spend time with the client, and listen carefully.
- Clarify misconceptions.
- Encourage independence whenever possible.

---

becomes severe. Preemptive analgesia is appropriate before an invasive or operative procedure. It is often appropriate for clients with chronic pain. Administering pain medication at scheduled intervals maintains the level of analgesia without allowing the peaks and valleys in pain relief. Box 22-8 ■ lists guidelines for individualizing care for clients with pain.

BOX 22-8 | **NURSING CARE CHECKLIST**

Individualizing Care for Clients with Pain

- ☑ Establish a trusting relationship. Convey your concern, and acknowledge that you believe that the client is experiencing pain. A trusting relationship promotes expression of the client's thoughts and feelings and enhances effectiveness of planned pain therapies.

- ☑ Consider the client's ability and willingness to participate actively in pain relief measures. Some clients who are excessively fatigued, are sedated, or have altered levels of consciousness (LOC) are less able to participate actively. For example, a client with an altered LOC or altered thought processes may not be able to deal with PCA. In contrast, a fatigued client may express a willingness to use pain relief measures that require little effort, such as listening to music or performing relaxation techniques.

- ☑ Use a variety of pain relief measures. It is thought that using more than one measure has an additive effect in relieving pain. Two measures that should always be part of any pain relief plan are (1) establishing a client–nurse relationship and (2) client teaching. Because a client's pain may vary throughout a 24-hour period, different types of pain relief are often indicated during that time.

- ☑ Provide measures to relieve pain before it becomes severe. For example, providing an analgesic before the onset of pain is preferable to waiting for the client to complain of pain, when a larger dose may be required.

- ☑ Use pain relief measures that the client believes are effective. It has been recognized that clients are usually the authorities on their own pain. Thus, incorporating the client's measures into a pain relief plan is sensible unless they are harmful.

- ☑ Base the choice of pain relief measure on the client's report of the severity of the pain. If a client reports mild pain, an analgesic such as aspirin may be indicated, whereas a client who reports severe pain often requires a more potent relief measure.

- ☑ If a pain relief measure is ineffective, encourage the client to try it once or twice more before abandoning it. Anxiety may diminish the effects of a pain measure, and some approaches, such as distraction strategies, require practice before they are effective.

- ☑ Maintain an unbiased attitude (open mind) about what may relieve the pain. New ways to relieve pain are continually being developed. It is not always possible to explain pain relief measures; however, measures should be supported unless they are harmful.

- ☑ Keep trying. Do not ignore a client because pain persists in spite of measures. In these circumstances, reassess the pain, and consider other relief measures.

- ☑ Prevent harm to the client. Pain therapy should not increase discomfort or harm the client. Some pain relief measures may have adverse untoward effects, such as fatigue, but they should not disable the client.

- ☑ Educate the client and support people about pain. Clients and support people need to be informed about possible causes of pain, precipitating and alleviating factors, and alternatives to drug therapy. Misconceptions also need to be corrected.

Supporting the Client and Significant Others

Nurses assist the client who is in pain by assessing pain regularly. Open-ended questions that allow the client to describe the type, location, or level of pain are much more useful than closed questions. For example, "How is your side feeling now?" encourages the client to answer more fully than "Did that medication work?" An attentive attitude and prompt attention to the client's needs help to build trust and reduce the anxiety that often accompanies severe or unremitting pain. The nurse can also help the client analyze when and why the pain worsens. Understanding more about the pain can sometimes help the client feel more in control.

The nurse's attitude of respect for the client in pain is important. Nurses can help family members by giving them accurate information about medications and about expected resolution of pain (e.g., period of recovery after surgery). Explaining when pain is likely to be the worst, when pain medication begins to take effect, and when the effect of medication wears off will enable support persons to organize their time and efforts to help the client. Providing accurate information about possible side effects, as well as reassurance that medications used appropriately will not cause addiction, is also a part of client teaching. The nurse can encourage family members to participate in client care and to provide distractions they know the client would enjoy.

Chronic pain is debilitating and frustrating. When chronic pain exists, the nurse can serve an important role in reminding support people that only the client really knows the pain. The client is the source about the client's pain. However, family and significant others can provide caring, encouragement, distraction, and empathy, all of which support the client.

EVALUATING

The nurse reviews client goals and outcomes to determine whether they have been achieved. Both subjective data (physical stance and facial expression) and objective data (heart rate and respirations) are collected to evaluate client comfort.

To assist in the evaluation process, flow sheet records or a client diary may be helpful. A weekly log or diary can be structured in a similar fashion for the individual client. For example, columns including day, time, onset of pain, activity before pain, pain relief measure, and duration of pain can be devised to help the client and nurse determine the effectiveness of pain relief strategies.

If outcomes are not achieved, the nurse and client might consider the following:

- Would the client benefit from a change in dose or in the time interval between doses?

- Did the client understate the pain experience for some reason?
- Did the client and support people understand the instructions about pain management techniques?
- Is the client receiving adequate support from significant others?
- Has the client's physical condition changed?

NURSING PROCESS CARE PLAN
Client with Pain

Mrs. Lundahl underwent abdominal surgery approximately 6 hours ago. She has a 21-cm midline incision that is covered with a dry and intact surgical dressing.

Assessment

Mrs. Lundahl is perspiring, lying in a rigid position, holding her abdomen, and grimacing. Her blood pressure is 150/90, heart rate 100, and respiratory rate 32. When asked to rate her pain on a scale of 1 to 10, Mrs. Lundahl rates her pain as 5.

Nursing Diagnosis

The following important nursing diagnosis (among others) is established for this client:

- *Acute Pain* related to surgical incision

Expected Outcomes

The expected outcomes specify that Mrs. Lundahl will:

- State postoperative discomfort is relieved "to a pain level of (whatever level client has identified as acceptable)" within 20 to 30 minutes of verbalized pain.
- Practice one relaxation technique for relief of pain by end of second postop day.
- Turn, cough, and deep breathe with minimum of discomfort by second postop day.

Planning and Implementation

The following interventions are planned and implemented for Mrs. Lundahl:

- Teach Mrs. Lundahl about her medications, as well as side effects and how to treat them.
- Encourage Mrs. Lundahl to request prn analgesics before pain becomes unmanageable.
- Teach Mrs. Lundahl relaxation and distraction techniques.

Evaluation

Mrs. Lundahl c/o dizziness following 2 tabs Vicodin ES; 1 tab adequately relieved pain without noticeable side effects in 30 minutes. Able to space prn pain meds to 5 to 6 hours by using relaxation technique (deep breathing and muscle group relaxation). Mrs. Lundahl using pillow to splint during coughing, able to change position and transfer to chair from bed without discomfort.

Critical Thinking in the Nursing Process

1. Can any conclusions be drawn about Mrs. Lundahl's pain status? Does Mrs. Lundahl's rating her pain as 5 mean that she is not experiencing pain severe enough to warrant intervention?
2. What type of pain is Mrs. Lundahl experiencing?

3. What interventions, in addition to pain medication, may be useful in reducing Mrs. Lundahl's pain? How will you know if your interventions have been effective?

Note: Discussion of Critical Thinking questions appears on the MyNursingKit Website.

> **Note:** The references and resources for all chapters have been compiled at the back of the book.

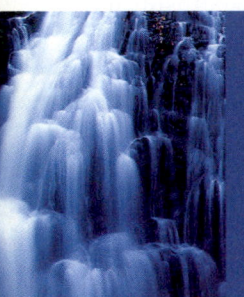

Chapter Review

KEY Points

- Pain is a subjective sensation. Pain can directly impair health and prolong recovery from surgery, disease, and trauma.
- Ethnic and cultural values, age, environment and support people, anxiety, and stress all influence a person's perception and reaction to pain.
- The overall client goal is to increase a client's functional capacity by preventing, modifying, or eliminating pain.
- The most reliable indicator of the presence or intensity of pain is the client's self-report.
- Nurses must acknowledge and convey belief in the client's report of pain and reduce fear and anxiety associated with the pain. Nurses should also assist support people and reduce misconceptions about pain.
- Do not allow fear of potential side effects to inhibit full and aggressive treatment of a client's pain.
- The nurse's evaluation of the client's pain therapy is multifaceted and should include the response of the client, changes in the pain, and the client's perceptions of the effectiveness of therapy.

FOR FURTHER Study

For more discussion of cultural considerations, refer to Chapter 3.

For more information about communicating effectively with clients, see Chapter 11.

For further discussion of listening skills, see Chapters 11 and 12.

For effects of anxiety and stress, as well as powerlessness in relation to pain, see Chapter 17.

For more information on incisional or wound pain, see Chapter 24.

Critical Thinking Care Map

Caring for a Client with Postoperative Pain

NCLEX-PN® Focus Area: Physiological Adaptation

Case Study: Mr. Lee Chin is a 57-year-old Chinese businessman who was admitted to the surgical unit for treatment of a possible strangulated inguinal hernia. Two days ago he had a partial bowel resection.

Nursing Diagnosis: *Acute Pain* related to surgical incision

COLLECT DATA

Subjective	Objective
_____	_____
_____	_____
_____	_____
_____	_____
_____	_____
_____	_____

Would you report this? Yes/No

If yes, report to:_____

What would you report?_____

Nursing Care

_____
_____
_____
_____
_____
_____
_____
_____
_____

How would you document this? _____

_____
_____
_____

Compare your answers and documentation to those provided on the MyNursingKit Website.

Data Collected
(use only those that apply)

- Height: 188 cm (6′3″)
- Weight: 90.0 kg (200 lbs)
- Temperature: 37°C (98.6°F)
- Pulse: 90 bpm
- Respirations: 24/min
- Blood pressure: 158/82 mm Hg
- Lying in dorsal recumbent position with legs drawn up
- Skin pale and moist, pupils dilated
- NPO, intravenous infusion of D_5 ½ NS at 125 mL/h left arm, nasogastric tube to low intermittent suction
- Restless
- Complaint of pain (7 on a scale of 1–10)
- "I am cold and tired, I wish I could sleep."
- Complaint of being thirsty
- Midline abdominal incision, sutures dry and intact
- Chest x-ray and urinalysis negative
- WBC 12,000
- Complaint of nausea but no vomiting

Nursing Interventions
(use only those that apply; list in priority order)

- Medicate before an activity to increase participation.
- Teach client to use incentive spirometer.
- Evaluate the effectiveness of the pain control measures used through ongoing assessment.
- Assess wound drainage at each dressing change.
- Provide extra blanket for warmth.
- Determine analgesic selections (narcotic, nonnarcotic, or NSAID) based on type and severity of pain.
- Institute safety precautions as appropriate if receiving narcotic analgesics.
- Encourage coughing and deep breathing.
- Instruct client to request prn pain medication before the pain is severe.
- Create a quiet, nondisruptive environment with dim lights and comfortable temperature when possible.

NCLEX-PN® Exam Preparation

1 A client with angina secondary to a 70% blockage of a coronary artery complains of chest pain. The nurse recognizes this is what type of pain?

1. Mechanical pain
2. Thermal pain
3. Chemical pain
4. A-delta fiber pain

2 Which of the following statements, made by the nurse, would elicit the most useful information for determining what the client is feeling?

1. "On a scale of 0 to 10 where 0 is no pain and 10 is the kind of pain you felt just before you delivered your son, how you would rank the pain you are feeling right now?"
2. "Where is the pain, when did it start, what have you done for it, and how much does it hurt?"
3. "On a scale of 0 to 10 with 10 being the worst imaginable pain, how would you rate the pain you are currently feeling and where is the pain located?"
4. "Would you describe your pain as mild, moderate, or severe?"

3 The nurse administers a narcotic analgesic to a client complaining of pain rating 10 on the 0–10 scale and the client denies relief. The nurse administers a nonnarcotic analgesic, and the client still gets no relief from pain. The client reports that nothing has worked for this pain since it started 8 months ago. This client is experiencing what type of pain? (Select all that apply.)

1. Chronic pain
2. Intractable pain
3. Referred pain
4. Visceral pain

4 The nurse is caring for a client with severe cancer pain whose current dosage of narcotic analgesics is no longer controlling the client's pain. The nurse receives a physician's order to increase the dose to improve pain control. After administering the new dosage IM, the priority nursing action would be to:

1. Evaluate the effectiveness of pain control.
2. Assess the client's respiratory status over the next 10 to 30 minutes.
3. Darken the room and ask visitors to allow the client to sleep.
4. Measure the client's vital signs every 15 minutes for the next 2 hours.

5 The nurse is caring for a client complaining of severe pain. After administering a narcotic analgesic, the nurse provides a back massage based on the:

1. Need to relax the client so the pain medication can work.
2. Pain response.
3. Pain tolerance.
4. Gate control theory.

6 The unlicensed assistive personnel tells the nurse, "That client is a complainer. Other people go through the same procedure and they don't complain but this client says she has pain that is 8 out of 10. I think she's overreacting, don't you?" The nurse's best response would be:

1. "Pain reaction is an automatic reaction that helps to protect the body from harm. I'll give the client medication."
2. "Pain tolerance is highly individualized and every client responds to, and feels, pain differently. I'll go talk to her."
3. "Some people use medical problems as a means of obtaining attention. Please document the client's complaint of pain and try providing a back massage to calm her."
4. "Everyone is different."

7 A 4-month-old infant had cardiac surgery this morning and has an incision from the top of the sternum to the xiphoid process. Which of the following symptoms would suggest the infant is in pain? (Select all that apply.)

1. Restlessness with rapid heart rate
2. Awake and quiet with decreased blood pressure
3. Crying vigorously with increased heart rate, respiratory rate, and blood pressure
4. Sleeping quietly with stable vital signs and quiet respirations
5. Grimacing, crying softly, with decreased heart rate

8 The nurse follows the World Health Organization's recommendations for managing cancer pain by administering which of the following until relief of pain is obtained? (Select all that apply.)

1. First give the largest safe dose of a strong opioid to reduce the pain quickly.
2. Increase the dosage of the weak opioid until the ceiling dose is achieved.
3. Second, give a nonsteroidal anti-inflammatory medication to work in conjunction with the opioid.
4. Second, administer a weak opioid.
5. First, administer a nonsteroidal anti-inflammatory medication.

9 The nurse recognizes that which of the following barriers to pain management is not impacting the client's comfort level?

1. The client fears addiction to narcotics.
2. The client's culture teaches that voicing pain is considered weak and that pain should be handled stoically.
3. The client declines specific medications to avoid the side effect of constipation.
4. The dosage schedule is every 12 hours, but the physician has said to call if the pain medication is not effective.

10 A client with chronic pain requires regular dosages of oral narcotic analgesics. The client complains that his sleep is disturbed because the medication stops working after 4 hours in the middle of the night. He has trouble getting back to sleep until the next dose takes effect. The nurse would suggest:

1. Taking the medication parenterally for faster effects.
2. Increasing the dosage before bedtime to increase the length of effect and reduce nighttime waking.
3. Recommending the client take naps during the day.
4. Requesting an order from the physician for a longer-lasting medication.

Answers and rationales for Review Questions appear in Appendix I.

Chapter 23

Activity, Rest, and Sleep

LEARNING Outcomes

After completing this chapter, you will be able to:

1. Describe basic elements of normal movement.
2. Name factors affecting body alignment and mobility.
3. Identify effects of immobility on body systems.
4. Describe assistive devices used to support mobility.
5. Explain how the nursing process relates to clients with immobility.
6. List and compare different body positions.
7. Name and describe actions the nurse performs to support client mobility.
8. Describe proper procedures for assisting a client with mobility issues.
9. Describe the stages and functions of sleep.
10. Identify factors that affect sleep, and variables related to age or stage of development.
11. Name common sleep disorders and interventions to promote normal sleep.
12. Identify tests used to diagnose sleep disorders.

Clinical Objectives

13. Provide nursing care for clients with sleep disorders.
14. Use proper body mechanics when positioning, moving, lifting, and ambulating clients.
15. Provide passive range-of-motion exercise for a client.
16. Instruct a client in proper techniques of active range-of-motion exercise.

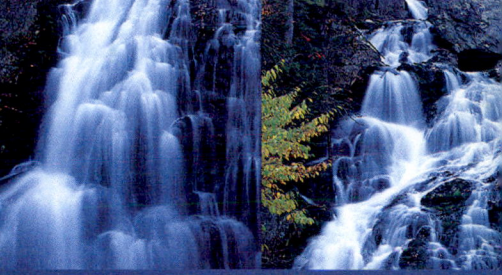

BRIEF Outline

ambulation 503	**infarction** 493	**postural tonus** 490
ankylosed 492	**insomnia** 507	**range of motion (ROM)** 491
atelectasis 494	**labyrinth** 491	**REM sleep** 506
atrophy 492	**line of gravity** 490	**sleep apnea** 508
center of gravity 490	**narcolepsy** 508	**thrombophlebitis** 493
effleurage 527	**NREM sleep** 505	**thrombus** 493
emboli 493	**osteoporosis** 492	**urinary stasis** 494
equilibrium 491	**parasomnia** 508	**vertigo** 491
hypersomnia 508	**pétrissage** 527	**vital capacity** 493

Balanced activity, rest, and sleep are essential to health. Most people equate physical well-being with freedom of mobility. Mobility is vital to independence. Inability to perform routine activities of daily living (ADLs) such as bathing, cooking, shopping, and engaging in recreational sports or work can adversely effect a client's self-esteem and mental health.

ACTIVITY

Normal Movement

Body movement is dependent on the integrated and interdependent activity of the musculoskeletal, nervous, and *vestibular* (inner ear) systems. Normal movement involves four bodily aspects: *alignment* (posture), joint mobility, *balance* (stability), and coordination. Alignment and joint mobility are discussed briefly here.

ALIGNMENT AND POSTURE

When the body is aligned, organs are properly supported. This allows them to function at their best, while also maintaining balance.

The **line of gravity** is an imaginary vertical line drawn through the body's center of gravity (Figure 23-1 ■). The **center of gravity** is the point at which all of the body's mass is centered and the base of support (the foundation on which the body rests) achieves balance. In humans, the usual line of gravity is drawn from the top of the head, down between the shoulders, through the trunk slightly anterior to the sacrum, and between the weightbearing joints (hips, knees) and base of support (feet). In the upright position, the center of gravity occurs in the pelvis approximately midway between the umbilicus and the symphysis pubis. When standing, an adult must center body weight symmetrically along the line of gravity to maintain stability. Greater stability and balance are achieved in the sitting or supine position because a chair or bed provides a wider base of support with a lower center of gravity. When the body is well aligned, there is little strain on the joints, muscles, tendons, or ligaments.

The musculoskeletal system continuously works to maintain erect posture and to offset the constant pull of gravity. The sustained muscle contraction required to maintain the upright position is called **postural tonus.** Posture

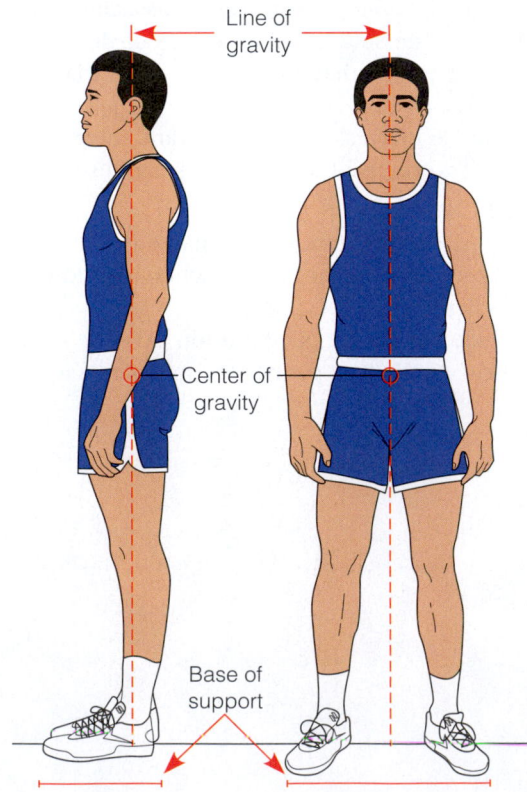

Figure 23-1. ■ Center of gravity and the line of gravity influence standing alignment.

TABLE 23-1	Synovial Joint Movements and Their Actions		
MOVEMENT	**ACTION**	**MOVEMENT**	**ACTION**
Flexion	Decreasing the angle of the joint (e.g., bending the elbow)	Eversion	Turning the sole of the foot outward by moving the ankle joint
Extension	Increasing the angle of the joint (e.g., straightening the arm at the elbow)	Inversion	Turning the sole of the foot inward by moving the ankle joint
Hyperextension	Further extension or straightening of a joint (e.g., bending the head backward)	Pronation	Moving the bones of the forearm so that the palm of the hand faces downward when held in front of the body
Abduction	Movement of the bone away from the midline of the body	Supination	Moving the bones of the forearm so that the palm of the hand faces upward when held in front of the body
Adduction	Movement of the bone toward the midline of the body	Protraction	Moving a part of the body forward in the same plane parallel to the ground
Rotation	Movement of the bone around its central axis	Retraction	Moving a part of the body backward in the same plane parallel to the ground
Circumduction	Movement of the distal part of the bone in a circle while the proximal end remains fixed		

is one criterion for assessing general health, physical fitness, and beauty. Posture reflects the mood, self-esteem, and personality of an individual.

JOINT MOBILITY

Most skeletal muscles are attached to two bones at the joint. These muscles are defined by the movement they produce and are therefore called flexors, extensors, internal rotators, and so on. Types of synovial joint movement are shown in Table 23-1 ■.

Flexors are stronger than extensors, so when a person is inactive, joints become pulled into the *flexed* (bent) position. Constant immobility causes muscles to shorten permanently and become fixed in the "flexed" position (see later section on immobility). The **range of motion (ROM)** of a joint is the maximum movement possible for that joint. Range of motion varies by individual and is determined by heredity, age, injury or disease, and level of physical activity. Many mechanisms are responsible for maintaining human balance.

Equilibrium (the sense of balance) depends on the integration of stimuli from several organs: the muscles and tendons of the head and neck (vestibulospinal input), the eyes (vestibulo-ocular input), and the inner ear. The inner ear or **labyrinth** consists of the cochlea, vestibule, and semicircular canals. The semicircular canals and vestibule govern equilibrium.

Factors Affecting Body Alignment and Activity

Numerous factors affect an individual's body alignment, mobility, and daily activity level. These include growth and development, physical health, mental health, nutrition, personal values and attitudes, and other external factors.

GROWTH AND DEVELOPMENT

A person's age and musculoskeletal and nervous system development affect posture, body proportions, body mass, body movements, and reflexes. Refer to Chapter 16 🔗 for age-related considerations.

PHYSICAL HEALTH

Mobility is directly affected by any disorder of the musculoskeletal or nervous systems, or by any vestibular (inner ear) disorders. Congenital anomalies, such as hip dysplasia and spina bifida, affect motor function. Musculoskeletal trauma limiting mobility includes strains, sprains, fractures, joint dislocations, amputations, and joint replacement. Nervous system disorders such as cerebral palsy, Parkinson's disease, multiple sclerosis, tumors, infections (e.g., meningitis), and injuries to the spinal cord or brain such as cerebrovascular accidents (strokes) may leave muscles weakened, paralyzed, spastic (with too much muscle tone), or flaccid (without muscle tone). Disorders of the vestibular apparatus, such as an ear infection or Ménière's disease, cause **vertigo,** a strong sensation of spinning around in space, which impairs balance.

Illnesses that limit the supply of oxygen to vital organs affect activity tolerance. Examples include chronic obstructive pulmonary disease (COPD), emphysema, anemia, angina, and congestive heart failure (CHF).

MENTAL HEALTH

Mental or *affective* (emotional) disorders affect personal motivation. Anxiety may produce an increase in physical activity. Chronic stress, however, depletes the body's energy reserves, producing fatigue. Slumped posture may indicate lassitude or depression. A depressed client may lack the physical energy required for daily hygiene. Exercise is necessary to mental health. Movement energizes the client and facilitates coping.

NUTRITION

Undernutrition and overnutrition influence body alignment and mobility. Obesity distorts posture and balance, causing strain on muscles and joints. More energy is expended on movement, which produces fatigue.

Effects of Immobility

A sedentary lifestyle or history of inactivity due to injury or illness increases the risk of major disease. The level of risk depends on the duration of inactivity, the client's general health, and sensory awareness. Nurses must understand these risks and encourage client mobility. Early ambulation after illness or surgery is an essential preventive measure.

MUSCULOSKELETAL SYSTEM

Signs of prolonged immobility are most often manifested in the musculoskeletal system. Muscular strength decreases in the absence of physical activity. Common musculoskeletal problems resulting from prolonged immobility include:

- *Disuse osteoporosis*. Without the stress of weightbearing activity, bones demineralize. Ninety-nine percent of body calcium is located in the bones. Calcium, which gives bones density and strength, becomes depleted when the body is immobile. Despite adequate calcium in the diet, this demineralization process, known as **osteoporosis,** continues during immobility. Bones become spongy and deformed, and they fracture easily. Intake of calcium matters little. What does matter is the output or, more importantly, the final balance. This explains why active people who take in small amounts of calcium may have healthy bones, whereas immobile people who take in large amounts of calcium may be osteoporotic and have hip fractures.

  Protein in excess of daily needs can cause severe calcium wasting. On a high-protein diet, more calcium is lost in the urine than can be deposited in the bones. On an extremely high-protein diet, even extremely high calcium intake can result in a negative balance. When dietary protein is sharply increased, urinary excretion of calcium increases also, and the person goes into a negative balance for calcium. Most Americans eat 2 to 5 times more protein than they need for maintenance, ingesting as much as 125 grams daily, when 35 to 50 grams is the minimum requirement. As little as 75 grams of protein a day can be enough to trigger negative calcium balance.

- *Disuse atrophy*. Unused muscles **atrophy** (decrease in size), losing most of their normal strength and function.

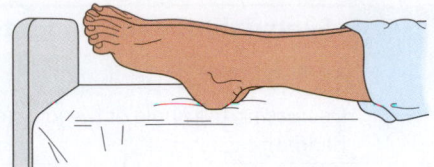

Figure 23-2. ■ Plantar flexion contracture (foot drop).

- *Contractures*. When muscle fibers are not able to shorten and lengthen for a prolonged time, a contracture (permanent shortening of the muscle) develops. This process involves the tendons, ligaments, and joint capsules, causing permanent fixation of the joint—irreversible except by surgical intervention. Joint deformities such as foot drop (Figure 23-2 ■) and external hip rotation occur when a stronger muscle dominates the opposite muscle.

- *Joint pain and stiffness*. Without movement, *collagen* (connective tissue) at the joint becomes **ankylosed** (permanently immobile). In addition, as the bones demineralize, excess calcium may deposit in the joints, contributing to stiffness and pain.

CARDIOVASCULAR SYSTEM
Diminished Cardiac Reserve

Decreased mobility creates an imbalance in the autonomic nervous system, resulting in increased heart rate. During immobility a rapid heart rate reduces diastolic pressure, coronary blood flow, and heart capacity available to respond to metabolic demands. Because of this diminished reserve, an immobilized person may experience tachycardia and angina with minimal exertion.

Increased Use of the Valsalva Maneuver

The Valsalva maneuver occurs when forceful exhalation against the closed glottis increases intrathoracic pressure, which in turn reduces venous blood return to the heart. This is the kind of breath holding that is done when straining to make a bowel movement or attempting to move up in bed. As the glottis opens and breath is released, blood suddenly surges to the heart. Tachycardia or cardiac arrhythmia may result.

Orthostatic Hypotension

Orthostatic hypotension (postural hypotension) is common with prolonged bed rest. It is marked by a sudden drop in blood pressure when a client stands and blood pools in the lower extremities. Cerebral perfusion is compromised, creating dizziness or fainting. This sequence is usually accompanied by a sudden and marked increase in heart rate, the body's effort to protect the brain from an inadequate blood supply.

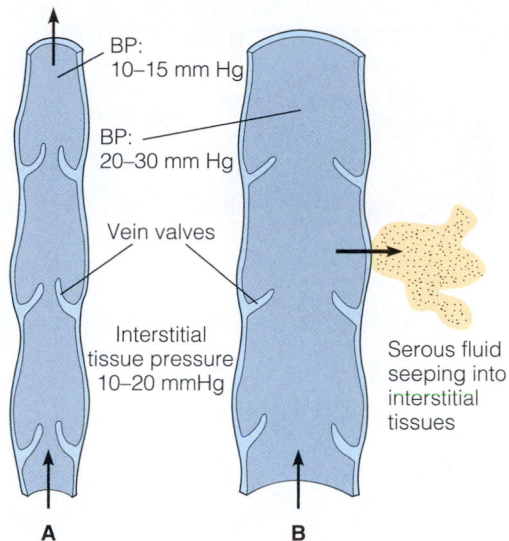

Figure 23-3. ■ Leg veins: **A.** in a mobile person; **B.** in an immobile person.

Venous Vasodilation and Stasis

The skeletal muscles of an active person contract with each movement. They compress the blood vessels to pump the blood back to the heart against gravity. Valves in the leg veins, which remain constricted, aid in venous return to the heart by preventing backflow. Atrophied muscles cannot assist in pumping blood back to the heart against gravity. Blood pools in the leg veins, causing vasodilation and engorgement (Figure 23-3 ■).

Dependent Edema

When venous pressure is great, serum is forced from the blood vessels into the surrounding interstitial space, causing *edema* (swelling). Edema occurs most commonly in the lower body, below the level of the heart. Prolonged bed rest is likely to cause edema at the sacrum. Prolonged sitting generally causes edema in the lower legs.

Thrombophlebitis and Emboli

Venous vasodilation and stasis predispose the client to **thrombus** (blood clot) formation. Impaired venous return to the heart, blood hypercoagulability, and injury to a vessel wall may result in **thrombophlebitis** (one or more clots loosely attached to an inflamed vessel wall). Thrombi become very dangerous when they break loose. **Emboli** (clots moved from their place of origin, causing circulatory obstruction elsewhere) may lodge in vessels supplying vital organs. Large *pulmonary* (lung) emboli may cause **infarction** (death of tissue) and sudden death. Emboli in the coronary or cerebral vessels are equally life threatening.

RESPIRATORY SYSTEM

Decreased Respiratory Movement

In a recumbent, immobile client, ventilation of the lungs is passively altered. The rigid bed presses against the body and curtails chest movement. Abdominal organs push against the diaphragm, further restricting chest movement and lung expansion. An immobile recumbent person rarely sighs, because muscle atrophy affects the respiratory muscles. Without periodic stretching movements, the cartilaginous intercostal joints become fixed in an *expiratory* (sunken chest) position, further restricting the potential for maximum ventilation. These changes produce shallow respirations and reduced **vital capacity** (the maximum volume of air that can be exhaled after maximum inhalation). Up to 25% to 50% of normal vital capacity may be compromised in an immobile, paralyzed client. For more information about oxygenation, see Chapter 32 ⚭ .

Pooling of Respiratory Secretions

Secretions are normally expelled by coughing and posture changes. Inactivity allows respiratory secretions to pool by gravity (Figure 23-4 ■), interfering with the normal exchange of oxygen and carbon dioxide in the alveoli. Cough may be diminished due to loss of respiratory muscle tone, dehydration (which thickens mucus), or sedatives, which depress the cough reflex. Poor oxygenation and buildup of

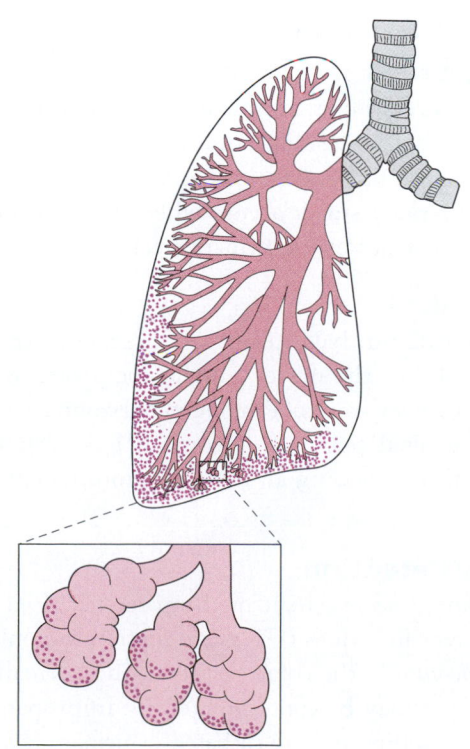

Figure 23-4. ■ Pooling of secretions in the lungs of an immobile person.

carbon dioxide in the blood can result in respiratory acidosis, a potentially lethal imbalance of body pH.

Atelectasis

As a result of changes in pulmonary blood flow, bed rest decreases surfactant production. *Surfactant* enables the alveoli to remain open. Decreased surfactant combined with mucous blockage of a bronchiole may cause **atelectasis** (the collapse of a lobe or of an entire lung) distal to the blockage. Immobile, elderly, and postoperative clients are at greatest risk of atelectasis.

Hypostatic Pneumonia

Pneumonia (inflammation of the lung) caused by static secretions in the alveoli is a common cause of death among weakened immobile persons, especially heavy smokers.

METABOLIC SYSTEM

Loss of Appetite

Loss of appetite occurs as a result of decreased metabolic rate and increased catabolism. Reduced caloric intake is usually a response to decreased energy requirements. Reduced dietary protein intake increases the risk of negative nitrogen balance and malnutrition.

Negative Calcium Balance

Negative calcium balance occurs as a result of calcium loss from bone.

URINARY SYSTEM

Urinary Stasis

Gravity plays an important role in the emptying of the kidneys and bladder. The client in a supine (back-lying) position must push upward against gravity (Figure 23-5 ■) to urinate. **Urinary stasis** occurs when urine *stagnates* in (does not move out of) the urinary tract.

Renal Calculi

Negative calcium balance causes increased excretion of calcium salts in the urine, which precipitate as crystals or calculi (kidney stones). Prolonged horizontal positioning causes the renal pelvis to become filled with stagnant alkaline urine, creating an ideal environment for calculi formation.

Urinary Retention

Static urine is an excellent medium for bacterial growth. Urinary tract infections (UTIs) are most commonly caused by *Escherichia coli*, the colon bacillus. The normally sterile urinary tract may be contaminated by improper perineal care, an indwelling urinary catheter, or urinary *reflux* (backward flow). See Chapter 39 ⚭ for conditions related to the urinary tract.

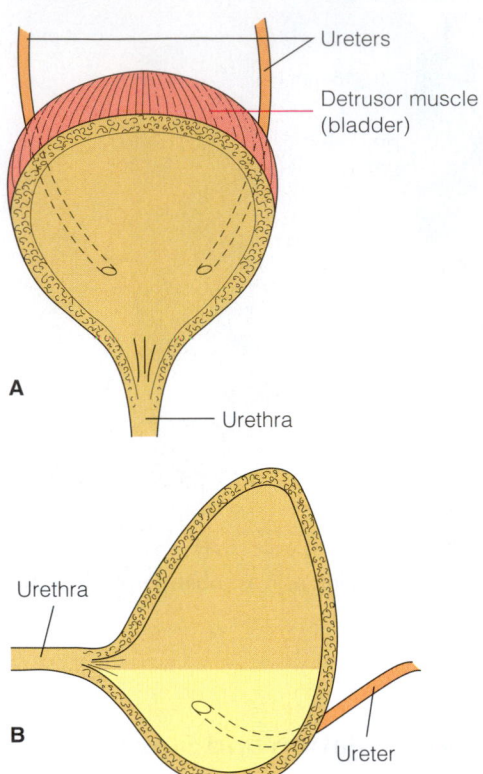

Figure 23-5. ■ Pooling of urine in the urinary bladder: **A.** The client is in an upright position. **B.** The client is in a back-lying position.

GASTROINTESTINAL SYSTEM

Decreased peristalsis, colon motility, and strength of the abdominal and perineal muscles used in defecation cause constipation. Disruption of normal bowel habits, caused by the embarrassment or discomfort of using a bedpan, may cause the client to postpone or ignore the urge for elimination. Repeated postponement suppresses the urge and weakens the defecation reflex. A bedfast person may lack the strength required to expel hardened stool. See Chapter 37 ⚭ for discussion of concerns related to bowel elimination.

INTEGUMENTARY SYSTEM

Reduced Skin Turgor

Skin can atrophy as a result of prolonged immobility. Shifts in body fluids between fluid compartments can affect the consistency and health of the dermis and subcutaneous tissues, eventually causing a gradual loss in skin *turgor* (elasticity). See Chapter 30 ⚭ for a full discussion of the skin.

Skin Breakdown

Normal blood circulation relies on muscle activity. Immobility impedes circulation and diminishes the supply of nutrients. As a result, skin breakdown and formation of pressure ulcers can occur (see Chapter 24 ⬭).

PSYCHONEUROLOGICAL SYSTEM

People who are unable to carry out usual activities related to their roles (e.g., breadwinner, spouse, parent, or athlete) become dependent on others. Loss of independence damages self-esteem, and may in turn provoke exaggerated emotional response. Reactions vary considerably. Some individuals become apathetic or withdrawn; others become angry or aggressive.

Assistive Devices

Hospitalized clients with limited mobility due to surgery, trauma, or a disease process may need assistive devices in order to regain mobility (Figure 23-6 ■). In most facilities, selection, fitting, and training in use of these devices is the responsibility of the physical therapy department. It is the LPN's or LVN's responsibility to reinforce the teaching and ensure that the client can use them safely both in the hospital and at home after discharge. See Box 23-1 ■ for teaching clients to use walking aids.

CANES

Three types of canes are used today: the standard straight-legged cane; the tripod or crab cane, which has three feet; and the quad cane, which has four feet and provides the most support.

WALKERS

Walkers are mechanical devices for ambulatory clients who need more support than a cane provides. Walkers come in many shapes and sizes, with devices suited to individual needs. The standard type of walker is made of polished aluminum. It has four legs with rubber tips and plastic hand grips (Figure 23-6B). Many walkers have adjustable legs.

Two- or four-wheeled walkers do not need to be picked up to be moved. However, they are less stable than the standard walkers. Clients who are too weak or unstable to pick up and move the walker with each step use wheeled walkers.

CRUTCHES

Crutches may be a temporary need for some people and a permanent one for others. Crutches should enable a person to ambulate independently, so it is important to learn to use them properly. There are several kinds of crutches (Figure 23-6C). The most frequently used are the underarm crutch or axillary crutch with hand bars, and the Lofstrand or forearm crutch, which extends to the forearm. The Lofstrand crutch is a single adjustable tube of aluminum to which a curved piece of steel, a rubber-covered hand bar, and a metal forearm cuff are attached. The Canadian or elbow extensor crutch, like the Lofstrand, is made of a single tube of aluminum with lateral attachments, a hand bar, and a cuff for the forearm, but it also has a cuff for the upper arm. This crutch is usually used by clients who require support for weak extensor muscles of the arm (e.g., weak triceps brachii).

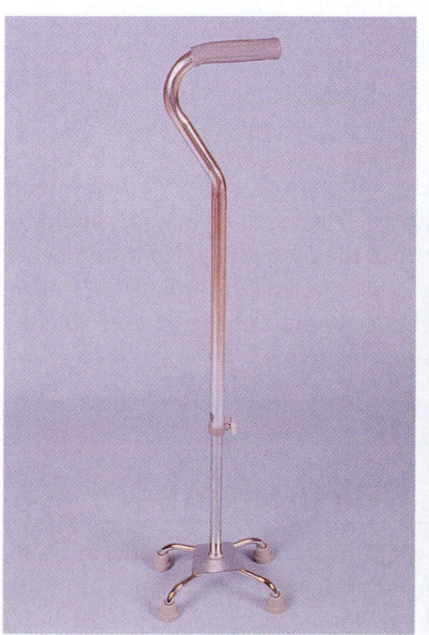
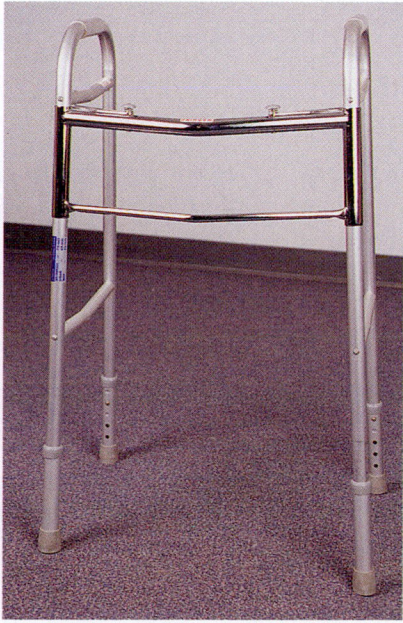
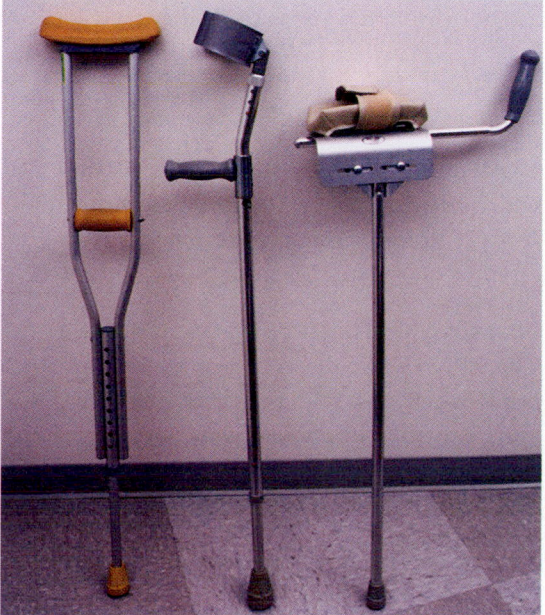

A   B   C

Figure 23-6. ■ Walking aids: **A.** Quad cane. (Photographer: Jenny Thomas.) **B.** Standard walker. (Photographer: Elena Dorfman.) **C.** Three types of crutches: C1, axillary crutch; C2, Lofstrand crutch; C3, Canadian, or elbow extensor, crutch.

BOX 23-1   CLIENT TEACHING

Using Walking Aids

Canes

- Hold the cane with the hand on the stronger side of the body to provide maximum support and appropriate body alignment when walking.
- Position the tip of a standard cane (and the nearest tip of other canes) about 15 cm (6 in.) to the side and 15 cm (6 in.) in front of the near foot, so that the elbow is slightly flexed.

When Maximum Support Is Required

- Move the cane forward about 30 cm (1 ft), or a distance that is comfortable while the body weight is borne by both legs.
- Then move the affected (weak) leg forward to the cane while the weight is borne by the cane and stronger leg.
- Next, move the unaffected (stronger) leg forward ahead of the cane and weak leg while the weight is borne by the cane and weak leg.
- Repeat the steps. This pattern of moving provides at least two points of support on the floor at all times.

As You Become Stronger and Require Less Support

- Move the cane and weak leg forward at the same time, while the weight is borne by the stronger leg.
- Move the stronger leg forward, while the weight is borne by the cane and the weak leg.

Walkers

When Maximum Support Is Required

- Move the walker ahead about 15 cm (6 in.) while your body weight is borne by both legs.
- Then move the right foot up to the walker while your body weight is borne by the left leg and both arms.
- Next, move the left foot up to the right foot while your body weight is borne by the right leg and both arms.

If One Leg Is Weaker than the Other

- Move the walker and the weak leg ahead together about 15 cm (6 in.) while your weight is borne by the stronger leg.
- Then move the stronger leg ahead while your weight is borne by the affected leg and both arms.

Crutches

- Follow the plan of exercises developed for you to strengthen your arm muscles before beginning crutch walking.
- Have a healthcare professional establish the correct length for your crutches and the correct placement of the handpieces. Crutches that are too long force your shoulders upward and make it difficult for you to push your body off the ground. Crutches that are too short will make you hunch over and develop an improper body stance.
- The weight of your body should be borne by the arms rather than the axillae (armpits). Continual pressure on the axillae can injure the radial nerve and eventually cause crutch palsy, a weakness of the muscles of the forearm, wrist, and hand.
- Maintain an erect posture as much as possible to prevent strain on muscles and joints and to maintain balance.
- Each step taken with crutches should be a comfortable distance for you. It is wise to start with a small rather than large step.
- Inspect the crutch tips regularly, and replace them if worn.
- Keep the crutch tips dry and clean to maintain their surface friction. If the tips become wet, dry them well before use.
- Wear a tie shoe with a low heel that grips the floor.

All crutches require suction tips, usually made of rubber, which help to prevent the crutches from slipping on a floor surface. Proper measurement for and fitting of crutches is essential to ensure client safety.

Nursing Considerations

The LPN/LVN collects information from the client, from other nurses, and from the client's records. The examination and history are important sources of information about disabilities affecting the client's mobility and activity status, such as contractures, edema, pain in the extremities, or generalized fatigue.

An activity and exercise history is usually part of the comprehensive nursing history form and includes daily activity level, activity tolerance, type and frequency of exercise, and factors affecting mobility. If the client indicates a recent pattern change or difficulties with mobility, a more detailed history is required. This detailed history should include the specific nature of the problem; when it first began and its frequency; its causes, if known; how the problem affects daily living; client coping strategies; and whether these methods have been effective.

NURSING CARE

PRIORITIZING NURSING CARE

In working with a client with mobility issues, the nurse focuses first on providing or ensuring safety to prevent injury. Then, the nurse works to support and encourage mobility through teaching, therapeutic communication, and providing a good role model.

ASSESSING

Body Alignment

Assessment of body alignment includes an inspection of the client while the client stands. To assess alignment the nurse views the client from lateral, anterior, and posterior perspectives.

The "slumped" posture (Figure 23-7 ■) is the most common problem that occurs when people stand. The neck is flexed far forward, the abdomen protrudes, the pelvis is thrust forward to create *lordosis* (an exaggerated curvature of the lumbar spine), and the knees are markedly hyperextended. Lower back pain and fatigue occur quickly in people with poor posture. Refer to Figure 23-1 for correct posture.

Gait

The characteristic pattern of a person's *gait* (walk) is assessed to determine the client's mobility and risk for injury due to falling. The nurse assesses gait as the client walks into the room or asks the client to walk a distance of 10 feet down a hallway and observes for the following:

- Head is erect, gaze is straight ahead, and vertebral column is upright.
- Heel strikes the ground before the toe.
- Feet are dorsiflexed in the swing phase.
- Arm opposite the swing-through foot moves forward at the same time.
- Gait is smooth, coordinated, and rhythmic, with even weight borne on each foot; it produces minimal body swing from side to side and directs movement straight ahead; and it starts and stops with ease.

The nurse should also note the client's need for a prosthesis or assistive device, such as a cane or walker. For a client

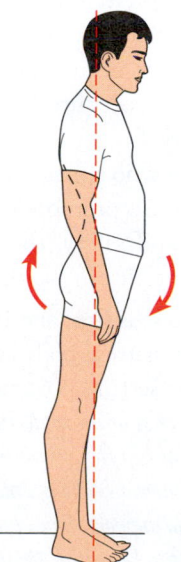

Figure 23-7. ■ Poor trunk alignment. The arrows indicate the direction in which the pelvis is tilted.

who uses assistive aids, the nurse assesses gait without the device and compares the assisted and unassisted gaits.

Appearance and Movement of Joints

Physical examination of the joints involves inspection; palpation; assessment of range of active motion; and, if active motion is not possible, assessment of range of passive motion. The following joints may be given special attention: neck, shoulder, elbow, wrist, hip, knee, and ankle. Box 23-2 ■ gives points for the nurse to remember in teaching clients to do active ROM exercises. Assessment of range of motion should not be unduly fatiguing, and the joint movements need to be performed smoothly, slowly, and rhythmically. No joint should be forced. Uneven, jerky movement and forcing can injure the joint and its surrounding muscles and ligaments.

The nurse also assesses the amount of assistance the client requires for the following:

- Moving in the bed. In particular, observe for the amount of assistance the client requires for turning:
  - From a supine position to a lateral position.
  - From a lateral position on one side to a lateral position on the other.
  - From a supine position to a sitting position in bed.
- Rising from a lying position to a sitting position on the edge of the bed. Healthy people can normally rise without support from the arms.
- Rising from a chair to a standing position. Normally this can be done without pushing with the arms.
- Range of motion of joints needed to complete transfer movements (see previous section).
- Coordination and balance. Determine the client's abilities to hold the body erect, to bear weight and keep balance in a standing position on both legs or only one, to take steps, and to push off from a chair or bed.

BOX 23-2   **NURSING CARE CHECKLIST**

Active ROM Exercises

☑ Perform each ROM exercise as taught to the point of slight resistance, but not beyond, and never to the point of discomfort.

☑ Perform the movements systematically, using the same sequence during each session.

☑ Perform each exercise three times.

☑ Perform each series of exercises twice daily.

For Older Adults

☑ For older adults, it is not essential to achieve full range of motion in all joints. Instead, emphasize achieving a sufficient range of motion to carry out activities of daily living (ADLs), such as walking, dressing, combing hair, showering, and preparing a meal.

MyNursingKit | ROM exercise

See Procedure 23-1 ■ on page 511 for instruction in providing passive ROM exercises.

Activity Tolerance

By observation of certain activities, the nurse can predict whether the client has the strength and endurance to participate in activities that require similar expenditures of energy. The most useful measures in predicting activity tolerance are heart rate, strength, and rhythm; respiratory rate, depth, and rhythm; and blood pressure. If the client tolerates an activity well, and if the client's heart rate returns to baseline within 5 minutes after activity, the activity is considered safe. This activity, then, can serve as a standard for predicting the client's tolerance for similar activities.

When collecting data pertaining to the problems of immobility, the nurse uses inspection, palpation, and auscultation; monitors results of laboratory tests; and takes measurements, including body weight, fluid intake, and fluid output.

DIAGNOSING, PLANNING, AND IMPLEMENTING

The LPN/LVN in collaboration with the RN develops a nursing care plan using a NANDA list. Examples of NANDA diagnoses that relate to activity are:

- *Activity Intolerance*
- *Impaired Physical Mobility*
- *Risk for Injury*

See Appendix II ⬤⬤ on the MyNursingKit website for a complete NANDA list.

Positioning, transferring, and ambulating clients are almost always independent nursing functions. The physician usually orders specific body positions only after surgery, anesthesia, or trauma involving the nervous and musculoskeletal systems. All clients should have an activity order written by a physician on admission.

As part of planning, the nurse is responsible for identifying clients who need assistance with body alignment and determining the degree of assistance required. The nurse must be sensitive to the client's need for independence, yet must provide assistance when warranted.

Most clients require specific knowledge to achieve and maintain proper body mechanics. The nurse is responsible for teaching such skills. For example, a client with a back injury must learn how to get out of bed safely and comfortably; a client with an injured leg needs to know how to transfer from bed to wheelchair safely; and a client with a newly acquired walker needs to learn how to use it safely. Nurses often teach family members or caregivers safe moving, lifting, and transfer techniques in the home setting.

The goals established for clients vary according to the nursing diagnosis and anticipated outcome for each individual. Examples of overall goals for clients with actual or potential problems related to mobility or activity follow:

- Increase tolerance for physical activity.
- Avoid injury from falling or improper use of body mechanics.
- Avoid any complications associated with immobility.

Nursing strategies to maintain or promote body alignment and mobility involve positioning clients appropriately, moving and turning clients in bed, transferring clients, providing ROM exercises, ambulating clients with or without mechanical aids, and preventing the complications of immobility. Whenever positioning, moving, lifting, and ambulating clients, nurses must use proper body mechanics to avoid personal injury. Refer to Chapter 9 ⬤⬤ for more information related to body mechanics and the nurse.

Positioning Clients

Positioning a client in good body alignment and changing position regularly and systematically are essential aspects of nursing practice. Clients who move easily automatically reposition for comfort. These people generally require minimal assistance from nurses, other than guidance about ways to maintain body alignment and exercise their joints. However, those who are weak, frail, in pain, paralyzed, or unconscious rely on nurses to provide or assist with position changes. For all clients, it is important to assess the skin and provide skin care before and after a position change.

Any position, if unchanged for a prolonged period, becomes detrimental. Frequent changes of position prevent muscle discomfort, pressure damage to superficial nerves and blood vessels, decubiti, and contractures. Position changes maintain muscle tone and stimulate postural reflexes.

When the client is not able to move independently or assist with moving, the preferred method is to have two or more people move or turn the client. Appropriate assistance reduces the risk of muscle strain and body injury to both the client and nurse. See Procedure 23-2 ■ on page 515 for moving a client in bed.

Sometimes a person who appears well aligned may be experiencing discomfort. To promote the client's proper body alignment, comfort, and safety, the nurse should perform the following interventions:

- Make sure the mattress is firm and level yet yields enough to fill in and support natural body curvatures. Mattress inspection in the home setting is particularly important. *A sagging or too soft mattress or an underfilled waterbed may contribute to development of hip flexion contractures or low back strain and pain. A plywood bedboard may be placed beneath a sagging mattress to add support. Some bedboards are hinged to allow the head of the bed to be raised. Bedboards are strongly recommended for clients who are at risk for back problems.*
- Ensure that the bed is clean and dry. Make sure extremities can move freely whenever possible. For example, top

BOX 23-3 SUPPORT DEVICES

- *Pillows.* Different sizes are available. Used for support or elevation of a body part (e.g., an arm). Specially designed dense pillows can be used to elevate the upper body.
- *Mattresses.* There are two types of mattresses: ones that fit on the bed frame (e.g., standard bed mattress) and mattresses that fit on the standard bed mattress (e.g., egg-crate mattress). Mattresses should be evenly supportive. See Chapter 24 🔗 for additional information and Table 24-5 🔗 for devices that reduce pressure on body parts.
- *Bedboards.* Bedboards are usually made of wood and are placed under the mattress to provide support.
- *Chair beds.* These beds can be placed into the position of a chair for clients who cannot move from the bed but require a sitting position.
- *Foot boot.* These are made of a variety of substances. They usually have a firm exterior and padding of foam to protect the skin. They provide support to the feet in a natural position and keep the weight of covers off the toes. Without support, an immobilized client's feet assume a plantar flexion position (foot drop). Prolonged assumption of this position results in permanent contracture of the gastrocnemius muscle and tendon.
- *Footboard.* A flat panel often made of plastic or wood. It keeps the feet in dorsiflexion to prevent plantar flexion.

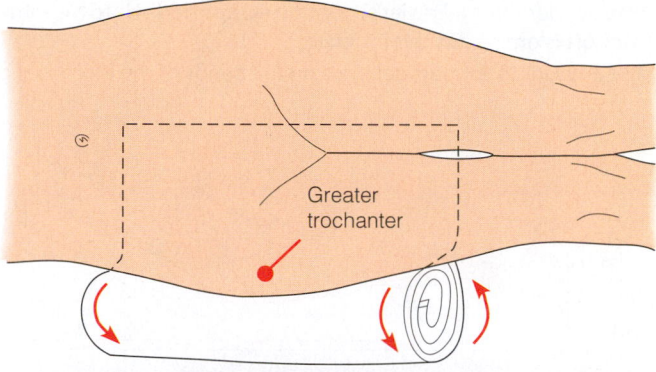

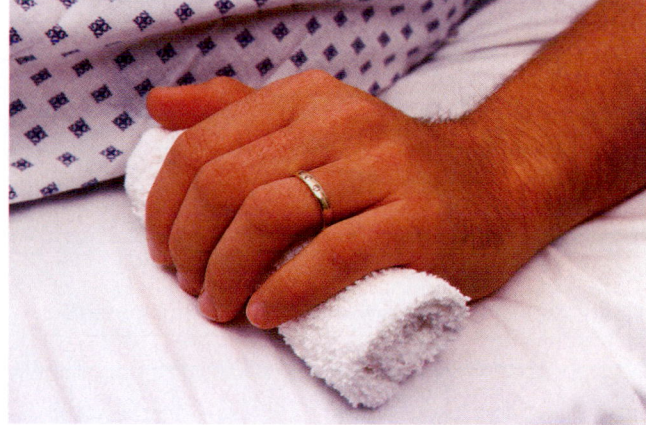

Figure 23-8. ■ Making a trochanter or hand roll: (1) Fold the towel in half lengthwise. (2) Roll the towel tightly, starting at one narrow edge and rolling within approximately 30 cm (1 ft.) of the other edge. (3) Invert the roll. Then palpate the greater trochanter of the femur and place the roll with the center at the level of the greater trochanter; place the flat part of the towel under the client; then roll the towel snugly against the hip (*top*); or place into the palm (*bottom*).

sheets need to be loose for the client to move the feet. *Wrinkled or damp sheets increase the risk of pressure ulcer formation (see Chapter 24 🔗).*

- Place support devices in specified areas according to the client's position. Box 23-3 ■ lists commonly used support devices. Use only those devices needed to maintain alignment (a trochanter or hand roll, Figure 23-8 ■) and prevent stress on muscles and joints. *If the person is mobile, too many devices limit movement and increase the potential for injury.*
- Avoid placing one body part, particularly one with bony prominences, directly on top of another body part. *Excessive pressure can damage veins and predispose the client to thrombus formation. Pressure against the popliteal space can damage nerves and blood vessels in this area.*
- Plan a systematic 24-hour schedule for position changes. See Chapter 24 🔗 .

Positioning the Bed
Fowler's Position

Fowler's position, or a semisitting position, is a bed position in which the head and trunk are raised 45 to 60 degrees. In low-Fowler's or semi-Fowler's position, the head and trunk are raised 15 to 45 degrees. In high-Fowler's position, the head and trunk are raised 60 to 90 degrees. See illustrations of positions in Table 23-2 ■ (Figures 23-9A–E ■). In this position, the knees may or may not be flexed.

Nurses need to clarify the meaning of the term *Fowler's position* in a particular agency. Fowler's position may refer to

elevation of the upper part of the body without knee flexion, and the term *semi-Fowler's* may refer to the sitting position with knee flexion.

Fowler's position is the position of choice for people who have difficulty breathing and for clients with heart problems. When the client is in this position, gravity pulls the diaphragm downward, allowing greater chest expansion and lung ventilation.

A common error nurses make when aligning clients in Fowler's position involves pillow usage. Overly plump or multiple pillows placed behind the client's head promote the development of neck flexion contractures. The nurse should encourage the client to rest without a pillow for several hours each day to extend the neck fully and counteract the effects of poor neck alignment.

Orthopneic Position

The orthopneic position is an adaptation of high-Fowler's position in which the client sits in bed or at bedside with an overbed table across the lap (Figure 23-10 ■). This position allows maximum chest expansion, eases breathing, and is

(*Text continues on pg. 502.*)

| TABLE 23-2 | Positions |

POSITIONS	UNSUPPORTED POSITION

Low-Fowler's (semi-Fowler's) position (supported). Note that arm support is omitted in this instance.

The amount of support depends on the needs of the individual client.

Bed-sitting position with upper part of body elevated 15–90° commencing at hips

Head rests on bed surface

Arms fall at sides

Legs lie flat and straight on lower bed surface

Legs are externally rotated

Heels rest on bed surface

Feet are in plantar flexion

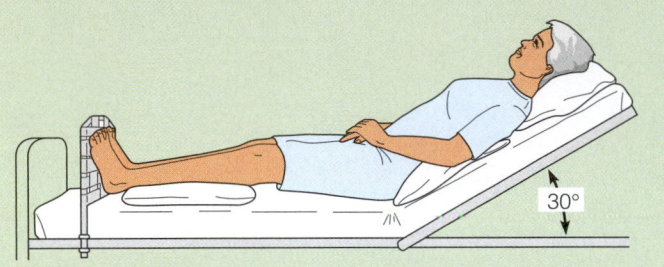

30°

Figure 23-9A. ■ Low-Fowler's (semi-Fowler's) position (supported).

Head and shoulders are slightly elevated on a small pillow

Lumbar curvature of spine is apparent

Legs may be externally rotated

Legs are extended

Feet assume plantar flexion position

Heels are on bed surface

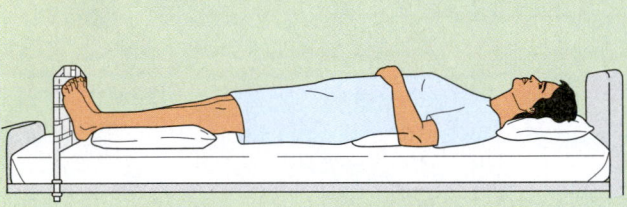

Figure 23-9B. ■ Dorsal recumbent position (supported).

Head is turned to side and neck is slightly flexed

Body lies flat on abdomen accentuating lumbar curvature

Toes rest on bed surface; feet are in plantar flexion

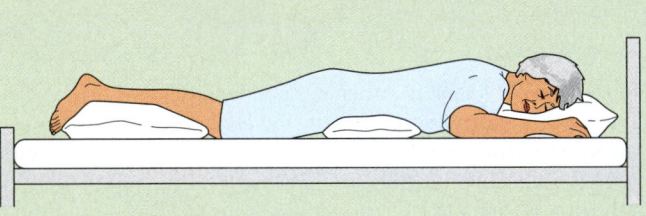

Figure 23-9C. ■ Prone position (supported).

Body is turned to side, both arms in front of body, weight resting primarily on lateral aspects of scapula and ilium

Upper arm and shoulder are rotated internally and adducted

Upper thigh and leg are rotated internally and adducted

Internal rotation and adduction of femur; twisting of the spine

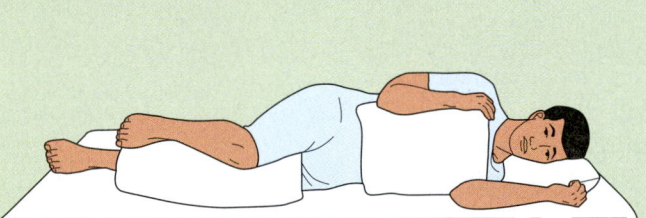

Figure 23-9D. ■ Lateral (supported).

Head rests on pillow; weight is borne by lateral aspects of cranial and facial bones

Upper shoulder and arm are internally rotated

Upper leg and thigh are adducted and internally rotated

Feet assume plantar flexion

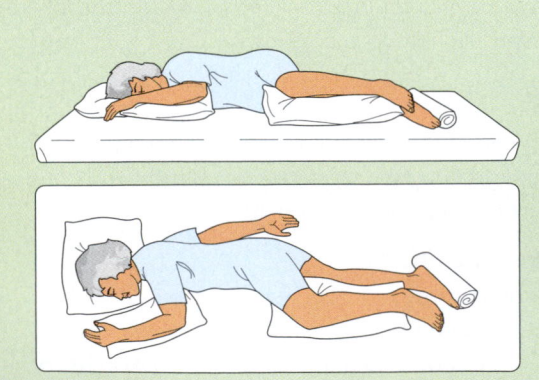

Figure 23-9E. ■ Sims' position (unsupported and supported).

PROBLEM TO BE PREVENTED	CORRECTIVE MEASURE
Posterior flexion of lumbar curvature	Pillow at lower back (lumbar region) to support lumbar region
Hyperextension of neck	Pillows to support head, neck, and upper back
Shoulder muscle strain, possible dislocation of shoulders, edema of hands and arms with flaccid paralysis, flexion contracture of the wrist	Pillow under forearms to eliminate pull on shoulder and assist venous blood flow from hands and lower arms
Hyperextension of knees	Small pillow under thighs to flex knees
External rotation of hips	Trochanter roll lateral to femur (Figure 23-8)
Pressure on heels	Pillow under lower legs
Plantar flexion of feet (foot drop)	Footboard to provide support for dorsal flexion
Hyperextension of neck in thick-chested person	Pillow of suitable thickness under head and shoulders if necessary for alignment
Posterior flexion of lumbar curvature	Roll or small pillow under lumbar curvature
External rotation of legs	Roll or sandbag placed laterally to trochanter of femur (optional)
Hyperextension of knees	Small pillow under thigh to flex knee slightly
Plantar flexion (foot drop)	Footboard or rolled pillow to support feet in dorsal flexion
Pressure on heels	Pillow under lower legs
Flexion or hyperextension of neck	Small pillow under head unless contraindicated because of promotion of mucous drainage from mouth
Hyperextension of lumbar curvature; difficulty breathing; pressure on breasts (women); pressure on genitals (men)	Small pillow or roll under abdomen just below diaphragm
Plantar flexion of feet (foot drop)	Allow feet to fall naturally over end of mattress, or support lower legs on a pillow so that toes do not touch the bed
Lateral flexion and fatigue of sternocleidomastoid muscles	Pillow under head and neck to provide good alignment
Internal rotation and adduction of shoulder and subsequent limited function; impaired chest expansion	Pillow under upper arm to place it in good alignment; lower arm should be flexed comfortably
Internal rotation and adduction of femur; twisting of the spine	Pillow under leg and thigh to place them in good alignment; shoulders and hips should be aligned
Lateral flexion of neck	Pillow supports head, maintaining it in good alignment unless drainage from the mouth is required
Internal rotation of shoulder and arm; pressure on chest, restricting expansion during breathing	Pillow under upper arm to prevent internal rotation
Internal rotation and adduction of hip and leg	Pillow under upper leg to support it in alignment
Foot drop	Sandbags to support feet in dorsal flexion

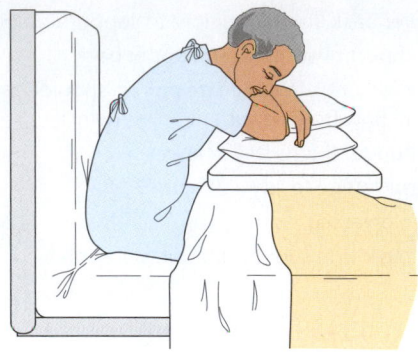

Figure 23-10. ■ Orthopneic position.

especially helpful to clients with COPD. In this position, the client can press the lower chest against the edge of the overbed table to assist with exhalation.

Dorsal Recumbent Position

In the *dorsal recumbent* (back-lying) position, the client's head and shoulders are slightly elevated on a small pillow. In some agencies, the terms *dorsal recumbent* and *supine* are used interchangeably. However, in the supine or dorsal position, the head and shoulders are not elevated (see Figure 23-9B). In both positions, the client's forearms may be elevated on pillows or placed at the client's sides. Supports are similar in both positions, except for the head pillow (see Table 23-2). The dorsal recumbent position is used to provide comfort and to facilitate healing after certain surgeries or anesthetics (e.g., spinal).

Prone Position

In the *prone* position (see Figure 23-9C), the client lies on the abdomen with the head turned to one side. The hips are not flexed. Both children and adults often sleep in this position, at times with one or both arms flexed over their heads. This position has several advantages. Prone is the only bed position that allows full extension of the hip and knee joints. When used periodically, the prone position helps to prevent flexion contractures of the hips and knees, thereby counteracting a problem caused by all other bed positions. Prone position promotes drainage from the mouth and is especially useful for unconscious clients or those clients recovering from surgery of the mouth or throat.

The prone position also has distinct disadvantages. The pull of gravity on the trunk produces a marked lordosis in most people, so that the neck is rotated laterally to a significant degree. For this reason, the prone position must be avoided by clients with spinal abnormalities and employed only when the client's back is properly aligned and maintained only for a brief time. This position also causes plantar flexion. Clients with cardiac or respiratory problems can find the prone position confining or suffocating because chest expansion is inhibited. Infants should not be placed in the prone position to sleep; sleeping prone is considered a risk for the occurrence of sudden infant death syndrome (SIDS).

Lateral Position

In the *lateral* (side-lying) position, the person lies on one side of the body (Figure 23-9D). Flexing the top hip and knee and placing this leg in front of the body creates a wide, triangular base of support that achieves greater stability. The greater the flexion of the top hip and knee, the greater the stability and balance. This flexion reduces lordosis and promotes good spinal alignment, making the lateral position optimal for resting and sleeping. The lateral position helps to relieve pressure on the sacrum and heels in people who sit much of the day or are confined to bed in Fowler's or dorsal recumbent positions. In the lateral position, most of the body's weight is borne by the lateral aspect of the lower scapula, the lateral aspect of the ilium, and the greater trochanter of the femur. People who have sensory or motor deficits on one side of the body usually find that lying on the uninvolved side is more comfortable.

Sims' Position

In *Sims'* (semiprone) position, the client assumes a posture halfway between the lateral and prone positions (see Figure 23-9E). The lower arm is positioned behind the client, and the upper arm is flexed at the shoulder and the elbow. Both legs are flexed in front of the client. The upper leg is more acutely flexed at both the hip and the knee than the lower one is.

Sims' position is occasionally used for unconscious clients because it facilitates drainage from the mouth and prevents aspiration of fluids. It is also used for paralyzed clients because it reduces pressure over the sacrum and greater trochanter of the hip. The Sims' position is often used for clients receiving enemas and occasionally for clients undergoing examinations or treatments of the perineal area. Many people, especially pregnant women, find Sims' position comfortable for sleeping. People with sensory or motor deficits on one side of the body usually find that lying on the uninvolved side is more comfortable.

Moving and Turning Clients in Bed

The level of assistance required for moving clients depends on client mobility and health status. Nurses must be empathetic regarding the client's need for independence while assisting with movement (see Procedure 23-2).

When a nurse assists, correct body mechanics must be employed so the nurse is not injured. Correct client body alignment must be maintained to avoid excessive stress on the musculoskeletal system. Strategies for preventing strains and sprains in nurses are provided in Chapter 9 🔗.

Transferring Clients

Many clients require assistance in transferring between bed and chair, wheelchair, toilet, or stretcher. The nurse must determine the client's capacity to participate and plan the maneuver before initiating a transfer. Methods of client transfer are given in Procedure 23-3 ■ on page 520.

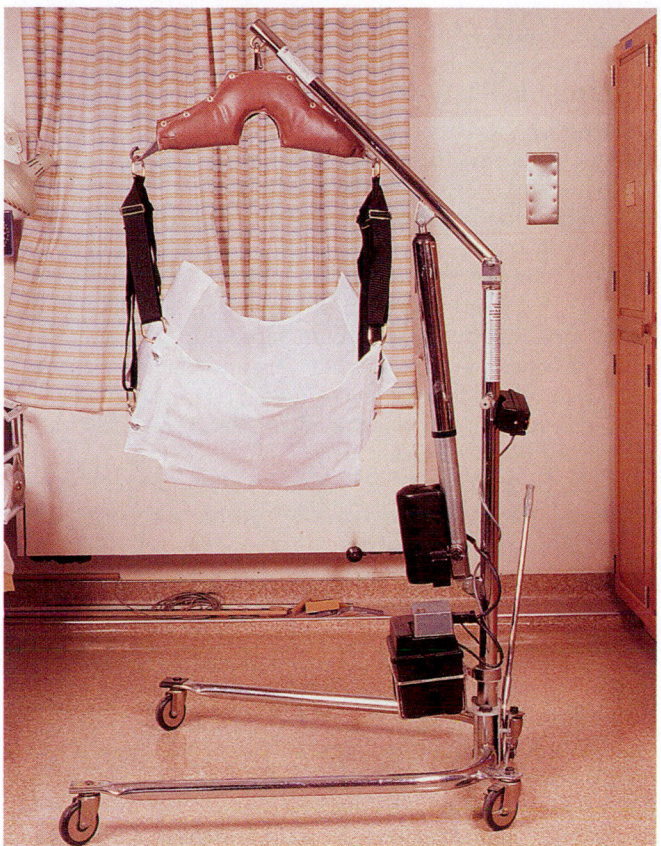

Figure 23-11. ■ A one-piece seat hydraulic lift. (Photographer: Jenny Thomas.)

Using a Hydraulic Lift

Hydraulic lifts, such as the Hoyer lift, are used primarily for clients who cannot assist or are too heavy for others to lift safely. The lift can be used in transferring the client between bed and wheelchair, bathtub, or stretcher. The *Hoyer lift* consists of a base on casters, a hydraulic mechanical pump, a mast boom, and a sling (Figure 23-11 ■). The sling may consist of a one-piece or two-piece canvas seat. The one-piece seat stretches from the client's head to the knees. The two-piece seat has one canvas strap to support the client's buttocks and thighs and a second strap extending up to the axillae to support the back. It is important to be familiar with the model used and the practices to accompany use. Before using the lift, the nurse ensures that it is in working order and that the hooks, chains, straps, and canvas seat are in good repair. Most agencies recommend that two nurses operate a lift. See Procedure 23-4 ■ on pages 523–524 for instructions for using a Hoyer lift.

Providing ROM Exercises

When people are ill, they often need ROM exercises until they regain normal activity. *Active ROM exercise* is isotonic exercise in which the client moves each joint in the body through its complete range of movement, stretching all muscle groups as far as possible within each plane over the joint (see illustrations in Procedure 23-1 for muscle groups).

They help to maintain cardiorespiratory function in an immobilized client and prevent deterioration of joint capsules, ankylosis, and contractures. See Box 23-2 for reminders about instructing clients to perform active ROM exercises.

The nurse may need to conduct passive ROM exercises until the client can accomplish these independently (see Procedure 23-1). During *passive ROM exercises*, the nurse (or an assistant) moves each of the client's joints through its complete range of movement, gently yet fully stretching all muscle groups over each joint. Passive ROM exercises are useful in maintaining joint flexibility. Passive exercises should be administered only when the client is unable to accomplish the movements independently.

Passive ROM exercises should be performed in a series, including each movement of the arms, legs, and neck that the client is unable to achieve. As with active ROM exercises, passive ROM should progress to the point of slight resistance, but never to the point of discomfort. Each exercise should consist of three repetitions, and the entire series is performed twice daily. One series should be performed during bath time.

During *active-assistive ROM exercises*, the client moves the immobile limb as far as possible, using the stronger arm or leg to move it. The nurse then continues the ROM to its maximal degree. Clients who begin with passive ROM exercises after disability generally progress to active-assistive ROM exercises and, finally, to active exercises.

Ambulating Clients

Ambulation (the act of walking) is a function most people take for granted. Prolonged bed rest (even 1 or 2 days) can make a person feel weak, unsteady, and shaky when first getting out of bed. Weakness is more pronounced in elderly and postoperative clients. Early ambulation greatly reduces the risks associated with immobility. Nurses should encourage clients to perform ADLs, maintain good body alignment, and carry out active ROM exercises to the maximum degree possible while on bed rest to prepare for ambulation.

Preambulatory Exercises

Clients on prolonged bed rest need exercises to strengthen the muscles used for walking before attempting to walk. One of the most important muscle groups is the quadriceps femoris, which extends the knee and flexes the thigh, enabling leg lifting, for example, to walk upstairs. To strengthen these muscles, the client consciously tenses them, drawing the kneecap upward and inward. The client pushes the popliteal space of the knee against the bed surface, relaxing the heels on the bed surface (Figure 23-12 ■). On the count of 1, the muscles are tensed; they are held during the counts of 2, 3, 4; and they are relaxed at the count of 5. These exercises are called *quadriceps drills* or sets and should be performed within the client's tolerance, that is, without fatiguing the muscles. This simple exercise builds muscle

Crutch instruction

MyNursingKit

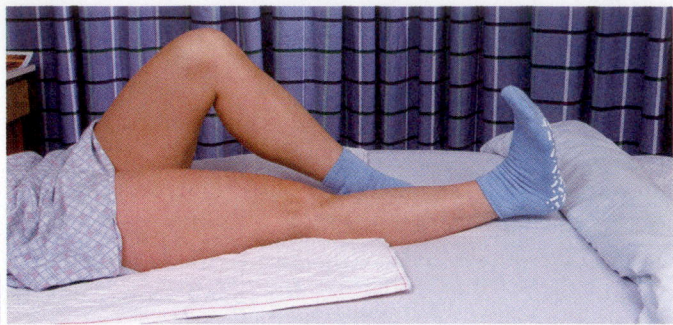

Figure 23-12. ■ Tensing the quadriceps femoris muscles before ambulation.

strength when carried out several times an hour while the client is awake.

Assisting Clients to Ambulate

Clients who have been immobilized for even a few days may require assistance to ambulate. The level required depends on the client's condition, including age, health status, and length of inactivity. Assistance may mean walking alongside the client while providing physical support (see Procedure 23-5 ■ on page 525) or providing instruction regarding the use of assistive devices such as a cane, walker, or crutches.

Clients may experience postural (*orthostatic*) hypotension and may exhibit the following symptoms: pallor, diaphoresis, nausea, tachycardia, and dizziness. If any of these are present, the client should be assisted to the supine position in bed and closely monitored. Box 23-4 ■ provides client teaching for ways to manage postural hypotension.

EVALUATING

The goals established during the planning phase are evaluated according to specific desired outcomes, also established in that phase. If outcomes are not achieved, the nurse, client, and support person (if appropriate) need to explore the reasons before modifying the care plan.

NURSING PROCESS CARE PLAN
Client in Traction

Kevin Andrews, a 17-year-old high school gymnast, fell from the parallel bars and fractured his left femur. Kevin has been on bed rest in skeletal traction since the injury. He is depressed and bored with the hospital routine of care. Because of painful muscle spasms, he often refuses to be turned or to move voluntarily. His appetite is poor, and he often refuses his hospital meals. He needs encouragement from the nursing staff to cough and deep breathe.

Assessment
- Height 175.3 cm (5′ 8″)
- Weight 70 kg (154 lbs) on admission

BOX 23-4 | **CLIENT TEACHING**

Controlling Postural Hypotension

- Sleep with the head of the bed elevated 8 to 12 inches (20.3–30.5 cm). This position makes the position change on rising less severe.
- Avoid sudden changes in position. Arise from bed in three stages:
  1. Sit up in bed for 1 minute.
  2. Sit on the side of the bed with legs dangling for 1 minute.
  3. Stand with care, holding onto the edge of the bed or another nonmovable object for 1 minute. Gradual changes in position stimulate *renin* (a kidney enzyme that has a role in regulating blood pressure), which prevents a dramatic drop in pressure.
- Never bend down all the way to the floor or stand up too quickly after stooping. *Baroreceptors* (sensory nerve endings in the walls of blood vessels) cannot accommodate rapid change.
- Postpone activities such as shaving and hair grooming for at least 1 hour after rising. Baroreceptor reflexes are slow to respond after a night of recumbency during sleep.
- Wear elastic stockings at night to inhibit venous pooling in the legs.
- Be aware that the symptoms of hypotension are most severe at the following times:
  - 30 to 60 minutes after a heavy meal
  - 1 to 2 hours after taking an antihypertension medication
- Get out of a hot bath very slowly, because high temperatures can lead to venous pooling.
- Use a rocking chair to improve circulation in the lower extremities. Even mild leg conditioning can strengthen muscle tone and enhance circulation.
- Refrain from any strenuous activity that results in holding the breath and bearing down. This Valsalva maneuver slows the heart rate, leading to subsequent lowering of blood pressure.

- 37°C (98.6°F)
- 80 bpm
- 16/minute
- BP 114/70 mm Hg
- Diagnostic data: chest x-ray negative, urinalysis negative, Hgb 13.3 g/dL, Hct 37%

Nursing Diagnosis
The following important nursing diagnosis (among others) is established for this client:

- *Risk for Disuse Syndrome* related to depression and reluctance to move secondary to painful muscle spasms

Expected Outcomes
The expected outcomes specify that:

- The client will perform ADLs within limitation of skeletal traction.
- The client will perform ROM exercises of upper limbs and unaffected lower limb tid.

- The client will use overhead trapeze every 3 h to strengthen muscles in upper limbs by day 3.
- The traction site remains free of drainage and odor.
- Homans' sign remains negative.

Planning and Implementation

The following nursing interventions are implemented for Kevin:

Traction/Immobilization Care
- Maintain proper position in bed to enhance traction.
- Ensure that the pull of ropes and weights remains along the axis of the fractured bone.
- Monitor pin insertion sites.
- Perform pin insertion site care.
- Monitor circulation, movement, and sensation of affected extremity.
- Monitor for complications of immobility.
- Administer appropriate skin care at friction points.
- Provide trapeze for movement in bed.
- Instruct Kevin on the importance of adequate nutrition for bone healing.

Exercise Therapy: Joint Mobility
- Determine Kevin's motivation level for maintaining or restoring joint movement.
- Explain to Kevin and his family the purpose and plan for joint exercises.

- Initiate pain control measures before beginning joint exercise.
- Assist Kevin to the optimal body position for each passive or active joint movement.
- Encourage active ROM exercises according to a regular schedule.
- Collaborate with a physical therapist in developing and executing an exercise program.

Evaluation

Goals partially met. Kevin performs active ROM exercises only once a day and refuses the other two sessions. He uses the overhead trapeze when repositioning frequently throughout the day but is reluctant to bathe and states "Just leave me alone for a while." His appetite has not improved and he eats approximately 40% to 50% of each meal. The skin surrounding the pin site remains odorless, dry, and intact. Homans' sign is negative; pulses are strong bilaterally.

Critical Thinking in the Nursing Process

1. What nursing intervention can be done for Kevin to relieve muscle spasms?
2. Kevin is refusing hospital meals. What can you do to improve Kevin's nutritional status needs to promote healing?
3. Describe diversion activities appropriate for a 17-year-old in traction.

Note: Discussion of Critical Thinking questions appears on the MyNursingKit Website.

REST AND SLEEP

Rest and sleep are essential to health. Normal sleep is characterized by minimal physical activity, variable levels of consciousness, changes in the body's physiologic processes, and decreased responsiveness to external stimuli. Some environmental stimuli, such as a smoke detector alarm, will awaken the sleeper, whereas other noises will not. Individuals respond to meaningful stimuli while sleeping and selectively disregard unmeaningful stimuli. Clients often complain that rest and sleep are difficult to achieve in the hospital environment. When deprived of sleep, clients become fatigued, depressed, or irritable. Nurses are responsible for providing an environment conducive to rest and sleep.

Physiology of Sleep

Sleep is a complex biologic rhythm. When a person's biologic clock coincides with sleep–wake patterns, the person is awake when the physiological and psychological rhythms are most active and is asleep when the physiological and psychological rhythms are most inactive. Infants are awake most often in the early morning and the late afternoon. After 4 months of age, infants enter a 24-hour cycle in which they sleep mostly

during the night. By the end of the fifth or sixth month, infants' sleep–wake patterns are almost like those of adults.

Two types of sleep have been identified: non–rapid eye movement (NREM or non-REM) sleep and REM (rapid eye movement) sleep.

NREM SLEEP

Most sleep during a night is **NREM sleep.** It is a deep, restful sleep with some decreased physiological functions. NREM sleep is divided into four stages:

- Stage I is very light sleep. The person feels drowsy and relaxed. The sleeper can be readily awakened. This stage lasts only a few minutes.
- Stage II is light sleep during which body processes continue to slow down. The eyes are generally still, the heart and respiratory rates decrease slightly, and body temperature falls. Stage II lasts about 10 to 15 minutes.
- Stage III occurs when the heart and respiratory rates, as well as other body processes, slow further because of the domination of the parasympathetic nervous system. The sleeper becomes more difficult to arouse.

BOX 23-5   CHARACTERISTICS OF SLEEP

NREM Sleep

- Arterial blood pressure falls.
- Pulse rate decreases.
- Peripheral blood vessels dilate.
- Activity of the gastrointestinal tract occasionally increases.
- Skeletal muscles relax.
- Basal metabolic rate decreases 10% to 30%.

REM Sleep

- Active dreaming occurs, and dreams are remembered.
- The sleeper may be difficult to arouse or may wake spontaneously.
- Muscle tone is depressed.
- Heart rate and respiratory rate often are irregular.
- A few irregular muscle movements occur—in particular, rapid eye movements.
- The brain is very active.

Source: Adapted from A. C. Guyton and J. E. Hall, *Textbook of Medical Physiology*, 9th ed. Philadelphia: Saunders, 1996, pp. 762–763. Reprinted with permission.

■ Stage IV signals deep sleep, called delta sleep. The sleeper's heart and respiratory rates are 20% to 30% below waking rates. The sleeper is very relaxed, rarely moves, and is difficult to arouse. Stage IV is thought to restore the body physically. During this stage, the eyes usually roll, and some dreaming occurs.

REM SLEEP

REM sleep constitutes about 25% of the sleep of a young adult. It usually recurs about every 90 minutes and lasts 5 to 30 minutes. REM sleep is not as restful as NREM sleep. Most dreams take place during REM sleep. Box 23-5 ■ lists characteristics of sleep.

Functions of Sleep

Sleep exerts physiological effects on body systems and restores normal levels of activity and balance within the nervous system. The effects of sleep on the body are not fully understood. However, it is known that the activity of the sympathetic nervous system is greater while the person is awake, as are impulses to the body's muscles, which increase muscle tone. During sleep, the activity of the parasympathetic nervous system increases, causing the physiological changes. Sleep is necessary for protein synthesis and cellular repair.

Research suggests that maintaining a regular sleep–wake rhythm (sleep hygiene) is more important than the actual number of hours slept. Some people, for example, can function well on as little as 5 hours' sleep each night. Reestablishing the sleep–wake cycle (e.g., after the disruption of surgery) is an important aspect of nursing.

Factors Affecting Sleep

Both the quality and the quantity of sleep are affected by a number of factors. Sleep quality refers to an individual's ability to stay asleep and to get appropriate amounts of REM and NREM sleep. Quantity of sleep is the total time the individual sleeps and it varies with age (Box 23-6 ■).

ILLNESS

Illness increases the need for sleep, but disease often disrupts normal sleep rhythms. Respiratory conditions affect sleep. Shortness of breath, nasal congestion, or sinus drainage and coughing disrupt sleep by causing frequent arousal.

People who have gastric or duodenal ulcers may find their sleep disturbed due to pain, the result of increased gastric secretions occurring during REM sleep. Endocrine disorders affect sleep. Hyperthyroidism lengthens presleep time, making it difficult to fall asleep. Hypothyroidism, conversely, decreases stage IV sleep. Elevated body temperatures can cause some reduction in stages III and IV NREM sleep and REM sleep.

The need to urinate during the night (*enuresis*) also disrupts sleep. People who awaken at night to urinate sometimes have difficulty getting back to sleep.

BOX 23-6   LIFESPAN CONSIDERATIONS

Age-Related Sleep Habits

Newborns: Sleep on and off throughout the day and night—2 to 4 hours at a time—usually related to their feeding cycle.

Infants: By 4 months of age will sleep 6 to 8 hours at night; by 6 months, 10 to 12 hours. Most babies still wake up at least once a night until 9 months of age.

Toddlers and preschoolers: Continue to need one to two daytime naps and sleep 11 to 14 hours at night.

School-age children: Still need between 9 and 12 hours of sleep at night. This is the age when children become more sleep deprived. They can fall asleep and wake up easily, and should be awake and alert all day.

Adolescents: Should have 9.5 hours sleep from ages 13 to 15. About 40% of adolescents report some kind of sleep problems. Most teenagers get an insufficient amount of sleep, usually 7.5 hours or less.

Adults: Should have a minimum of 7 hours nightly, although everyone is different. Adults who consistently do not get enough sleep do not perform at their highest potential.

Seniors: Need to keep a regular sleep schedule. Napping may interfere with nighttime sleeping. Lack of exercise can cause the client not to feel sleepy or to be sleepy all the time. Seniors tend to take more medications, and side effects or a combination of drugs can affect sleep. Tips for senior clients are to limit caffeine late in the day, avoid alcohol before bedtime, satisfy hunger prior to bed, avoid big meals or spicy foods just before bedtime, and minimize liquid intake before sleep.

ENVIRONMENT

Environment can promote or hinder sleep. Changes in the level of sound, light, and room temperatures adversely affect sleep. Unfamiliar surroundings may contribute to anxiety, which disturbs sleep. Over time, however, most individuals adjust to these changes.

LIFESTYLE

Moderate exercise is conducive to sleep, but excessive exercise can delay sleep. The ability to relax before retiring is an important factor affecting the ability to fall asleep. Shift work affects the quality of rest and sleep. Night shift workers may experience effects of lack of synchronicity between the body's internal clock and waking/working hours. Moving shifts forward (day to evening; evening to night; night to day) can be helpful in preventing fatigue, illness, or work error.

EMOTIONAL STRESS

Anxiety and depression frequently disturb sleep. Anxiety increases the norepinephrine blood levels through stimulation of the sympathetic nervous system.

CULTURE

The hospital environment is strange to anyone who is newly admitted. However, cultural or ethnic customs may have an added impact on a client's ability to achieve rest and sleep (Box 23-7 ■).

ALCOHOL AND STIMULANTS

Excessive alcohol intake disrupts REM sleep, although it may hasten the onset of sleep. While making up for lost REM sleep after some of the effects of the alcohol have worn off, people often experience nightmares. Caffeine-containing beverages act as stimulants of the central nervous system, thus interfering with sleep.

SMOKING

Nicotine is a stimulant. Therefore, smokers generally suffer from poor sleep. Smokers have difficulty falling asleep and maintaining sleep. Avoiding tobacco after the evening meal improves sleep.

DIET

Weight change may affect sleep. Weight loss is associated with reduced total sleep time and early awakening. Weight gain is associated with fewer arousals, later awakening, and an increase in total sleep time.

The amino acid L-tryptophan is believed to enhance sleep. Milk and cheese are rich dietary sources of L-tryptophan, which may explain why warm milk helps some people fall asleep.

MOTIVATION

A strong desire to stay awake can counteract fatigue. An individual will find it easier to stay awake when engaged in an interesting activity, whereas boredom invites sleep.

MEDICATIONS

Medications affect the quality of sleep. Sedative-hypnotics (e.g., secobarbital) interfere with stages III and IV NREM sleep and suppress REM sleep. Beta-blockers can cause insomnia and nightmares. Narcotics such as meperidine hydrochloride (Demerol) and morphine and tranquilizers suppress REM sleep and cause frequent awakenings and drowsiness. The following drugs may cause such sleep problems as disrupted REM sleep, delayed onset of sleep, decreased sleep time, nightmares, and increased daytime drowsiness:

- Amphetamines
- Antidepressants
- Beta-blockers
- Bronchodilators
- Caffeine
- Decongestants
- Narcotics
- Steroids

BOX 23-7	CULTURAL PULSE POINTS

Effect of Culture on Rest and Sleep

Inability to rest or sleep in the hospital is one of the most frequent complaints from clients. Hospital noise, lights, and timing of procedures make it difficult to meet rest needs. Getting quality rest becomes more difficult when cultural issues are a factor. Some clients may be more comfortable resting or sleeping on a mat on the floor, or sleeping with others in the same room or in the same bed. Others may be used to sleeping alone or in separate rooms. They may find it uncomfortable to share a room with one or more "strangers."

Women from Middle Eastern cultures may be uncomfortable leaving their rooms because of male clients who may be walking the hall in nightclothes. They may have difficulty sleeping, knowing that strange men are sleeping nearby.

Common Sleep Disorders

INSOMNIA

Insomnia, the inability to obtain an adequate amount or quality of sleep, is the most common sleep disorder. People suffering from insomnia do not feel refreshed on arising.

Insomnia is most commonly caused by mental overstimulation due to anxiety, but may result from physical discomfort. Clients may become anxious because they think they might not be able to sleep. Drug and alcohol abusers generally suffer from insomnia.

Treatment for insomnia routinely includes a behavior modification plan in which the client learns new habits to foster sleep. The therapeutic value of sleep-inducing drugs is considered debatable because these drugs treat only the symptom and not the root cause of sleeplessness. Furthermore, prolonged usage creates drug dependency.

HYPERSOMNIA

Hypersomnia, or excessive daytime sleep (EDS), can result from many diseases. Central nervous system, kidney, liver, or metabolic disorders, such as diabetic acidosis and hypothyroidism, cause sleepiness. Hypersomnia can be linked to mental disorders; depressed persons may use sleep as an escape mechanism.

NARCOLEPSY

Narcolepsy is an underrecognized and poorly understood disorder believed to be genetic or autoimmune. Narcolepsy sufferers experience regular REM-onset sleep attacks lasting from a few seconds to several hours. Nighttime sleep may be fragmented by vivid dreams or nightmares. Central nervous system stimulants such as methylphenidate (Ritalin) or amphetamine may be prescribed to control excessive daytime sleepiness. Tricyclic antidepressants may be given to suppress REM sleep.

SLEEP APNEA

Sleep apnea is the periodic cessation of breathing during sleep. Apnea occurs most often in men over age 50 and postmenopausal women. Sufferers may experience up to 600 episodes per night during NREM sleep, each lasting from 10 seconds to 2 minutes. These multiple arousals cause fatigue and EDS.

An apneic episode begins with snoring. Breathing ceases, followed by gasping or snorting as breathing resumes. Breathlessness causes increased carbon dioxide levels in the blood, which trigger awakening.

Treatment is aimed at the cause of the apnea; for example, enlarged tonsils may be removed. The use of a nasal continuous positive airway pressure (CPAP) device at night is often effective.

Sleep apnea profoundly affects a person's work or school performance. In addition, prolonged sleep apnea can cause a sharp rise in blood pressure and may lead to cardiac arrest. Over time, apneic episodes can cause cardiac arrhythmias, pulmonary hypertension, and left-sided heart failure.

PARASOMNIAS

A **parasomnia** is behavior that may interfere with sleep. Examples of this are sleepwalking (*somnambulism*), sleep talking, bedwetting (*nocturnal enuresis*), nocturnal erection, and teeth grinding and clenching (*bruxism*).

SLEEP DEPRIVATION

Sleep deprivation is the reduction in the amount, quality, or consistency of sleep. This syndrome produces both physiological and behavioral symptoms whose severity depends on the degree and type of deprivation (i.e., REM or NREM sleep). Combined REM/NREM deprivation increases the severity of symptoms. Table 23-3 ■ provides types, causes, and manifestations of sleep deprivation.

Diagnostic Studies for Sleep Disorders

Sleep may be measured objectively in a sleep laboratory by an electroencephalogram (EEG), electromyogram (EMG), and electro-oculogram (EOG) recorded simultaneously. This

TABLE 23-3	Types, Causes, and Signs of Sleep Deprivation	
TYPE	**CAUSES**	**CLINICAL SIGNS**
REM deprivation	Alcohol, barbiturates, shift work, jet lag, extended ICU hospitalization, morphine, meperidine hydrochloride (Demerol)	Excitability, restlessness, irritability, and increased sensitivity to pain Confusion and suspiciousness Emotional lability
NREM deprivation	All the above plus diazepam (Valium), flurazepam hydrochloride (Dalmane), hypothyroidism, depression, respiratory distress disorders, sleep apnea, and age (common in the elderly)	Withdrawal, apathy, hyporesponsiveness Feeling physically uncomfortable Lack of facial expression Speech deterioration Excessive sleepiness
Both REM and NREM deprivation	As above	Decreased reasoning ability (judgment) and ability to concentrate Inattentiveness Marked fatigue manifested by blurred vision, itchy eyes, nausea, headache Difficulty performing ADLs Lack of memory, mental confusion, visual or auditory hallucinations, and illusions

recording divides sleep into REM and NREM phases. Electrodes are placed on the scalp to record brain waves (EEG), at the outer canthus of each eye to record movement (EOG), and on the chin to record muscle contractions (EMG). Respiratory effort and airflow, ECG, leg movements, and oxygen saturation of arterial blood by pulse oximeter may also be monitored. Pulse oximetry and ECG recordings are of particular significance if sleep apnea is suspected. Video cameras may also be used to record the client's activity (movements, struggling, noisy respirations) during sleep.

NURSING CARE

PRIORITIZING NURSING CARE

The nurse's focus in relation to sleep issues is to help individual clients understand the factors that promote or interfere with normal sleep patterns. When providing interventions, the nurse attempts to schedule procedures and medications to limit interruptions and to encourage a restful environment.

ASSESSING

Sleep assessment includes a sleep history (sleep diary), physical examination, and review of diagnostic studies.

A brief general sleep history is obtained for all clients entering a healthcare facility. This enables the nurse to incorporate the client's needs and preferences in the plan of care.

Sleep Diary

A sleep diary may include all of the following information or selected aspects that pertain to the client's specific problem:

- Total number of sleep hours per day
- Activities performed 2 to 3 hours before bedtime (type, duration, and time)
- Bedtime rituals (e.g., ingestion of food, fluid, or medication, or ADLs such as prayer or bathing)
- Time of (1) going to bed, (2) trying to fall asleep, (3) falling asleep (approximate), (4) any instances of waking up and duration of these waking periods, and (5) waking up in the morning
- Any worries that the client believes may affect sleep
- Factors the client believes have a positive or negative effect on sleep

Physical Examination

Examination includes observation of the client's physical appearance, behavior, and energy level. Evidence of a deviated nasal septum, enlarged neck, obesity, and snoring may indicate obstructive sleep apnea. Irritability, restlessness, inattentiveness, slowed speech, yawning, rubbing the eyes,

confusion, incoordination, and physical weakness or lethargy also suggest sleep problems.

DIAGNOSING, PLANNING, AND IMPLEMENTING

Sleep Deprivation and *Disturbed Sleep Pattern* are NANDA nursing diagnoses that may be assigned to clients by the RN following assessment. See Appendix II 🔗 on the MyNursingKit Website for a complete NANDA list. These diagnoses may include further descriptions such as "difficulty falling asleep."

Nursing interventions to enhance clients' sleep primarily involve nonpharmacologic measures. These include teaching sleep hygiene, supporting bedtime rituals, providing a restful environment, and providing comfort measures to promote relaxation and reduce anxiety.

Promoting client sleep during hospitalization is challenging to the nurse and requires organization, caring, and creativity to control the many external factors affecting sleep. Assistive techniques to promote rest are described in Box 23-8 ■.

Supporting Bedtime Rituals

Most people have developed presleep routines to help them relax. Altering or eliminating these routines can affect sleep. Common adult bedtime rituals include an evening stroll, listening to music, watching television, taking a bath, and praying. Children's rituals may include a bedtime

---

| **BOX 23-8** | **NURSING CARE CHECKLIST** |

Reducing Environmental Distractions in Hospitals

- ☑ Close window curtains if street lights shine through.
- ☑ Close curtains between clients in semiprivate and larger rooms.
- ☑ Reduce or eliminate overhead lighting; provide a night-light at the bedside or in the bathroom.
- ☑ Close the door of the client's room.
- ☑ Adhere to agency policy about times to turn off communal televisions or radios.
- ☑ Lower the ring tone of nearby telephones.
- ☑ Discontinue use of the paging system after a certain hour (e.g., 2100 hours), or reduce its volume.
- ☑ Keep required staff conversations at low levels; conduct nursing reports or other discussions in a separate area away from client rooms.
- ☑ Wear rubber-soled shoes.
- ☑ Ensure that all cart wheels are well oiled.
- ☑ Perform only essential nursing tasks during sleeping hours.

story, hugging a favorite toy or blanket, and kissing everyone goodnight. Sleep is generally preceded by hygienic routines, such as washing the face and hands (or bathing), brushing the teeth, and voiding.

In institutional settings, nurses can provide similar bedtime rituals. Talking about events such as a visit from friends or the weather can help clients relax.

Creating a Restful Environment

To create a restful environment, the nurse needs to ensure safety, reduce sleep interruptions and environmental distractions, and provide room temperature satisfactory to the client. Interventions to reduce environmental distractions, especially noise, are listed in Box 23-8.

Clients must also feel safe in order to rest comfortably. People who are not accustomed to narrow hospital beds may feel more secure with side rails.

Additional safety measures include:

- Placing beds in low positions.
- Using night-lights.
- Placing call bells within easy reach.

Promoting Comfort and Relaxation

Comfort measures are essential to help the client fall asleep and stay asleep, especially when disease interferes with sleep. A concerned, caring attitude, along with the following interventions, can significantly promote client comfort, relaxation, and sleep:

- Provide loose-fitting nightwear.
- Assist clients with hygienic routines and other bedtime rituals.
- Make sure the bed linen is smooth, clean, and dry.
- Assist or encourage the client to void before bedtime.
- Provide a back massage before sleep (see Procedure 23-6 ■ on page 527).
- Position dependent clients appropriately to aid muscle relaxation.
- Provide supportive devices to protect pressure areas.
- Schedule medications, especially diuretics, to prevent nocturnal awakenings.
- Manage pain by administering analgesics 30 minutes before sleep; change dressings and/or apply warm or cool compresses or splints to painful areas.
- Facilitate effective breathing by administering prescribed medications such as bronchodilators before bedtime and position clients appropriately (e.g., semi-Fowler's position).
- Encourage slow deep breathing followed by tonic muscle exercises (rhythmic contraction and relaxation) to promote relaxation.
- Encourage the client to share concerns; actively listen and address problems as they arise.

| BOX 23-9 | NURSING CARE CHECKLIST |

Helping Older Clients Keep Warm in Bed

☑ Before the client goes to bed, warm the bed with hot water bottles or prewarmed bath blankets. Remove the hot water bottle before the client gets into bed to avoid the risk of a burn.

☑ Use 100% cotton flannel sheets, if possible, for warmth. Alternatively, apply thermal blankets between the sheet and bedspread.

☑ Encourage the client to wear own clothing, such as flannel nightgown or pajamas, loose-fitting jogging suit, thermal socks, leg warmers, long underwear, sleeping cap (if scalp hair is sparse), sweater, or a favorite quilt or blanket.

People, especially older adults, are unable to sleep well if they feel cold. Changes in circulation, metabolism, and body tissue density reduce the older person's ability to generate and conserve heat. Interventions to keep elderly clients warm during sleep are listed in Box 23-9 ■.

Enhancing Sleep with Medications

Sleep medications (most often prescribed on a prn or as-needed basis) include sedative-hypnotics to induce sleep and tranquilizers (benzodiazepines) to decrease anxiety and tension. In institutional settings, the nurse shares responsibility with the client regarding when to administer them. Both nurses and clients must be aware of the actions, effects, and risks of medication prescribed. Medication should be administered only when indicated and once the client has demonstrated understanding of the drug's action and effects. Whenever possible, nonpharmacologic interventions (discussed earlier) are the preferred interventions.

EVALUATING

If the desired outcomes are not achieved, the nurse, client, and support people, if appropriate, should explore the reasons. In many facilities, a client care conference may be convened to discuss client progress and analyze collected data. The desired outcome can be continued or revised at that time. If the goal is to be continued, a new timeline will be set.

Continuity of Care

Nurses can play a key role in teaching clients how to improve patterns of rest and sleep. This can speed recovery and add to quality of life. Box 23-10 ■ provides discharge teaching about promoting rest and sleep.

Note: The references and resources for all chapters have been compiled at the back of the book.

BOX 23-10   CLIENT TEACHING

Promoting Rest and Sleep

Sleep Pattern

- Establish a regular bedtime and wake-up time for all days of the week to prevent disruptions in your biologic rhythm. Eliminate lengthy naps, or if a daytime nap is necessary, take it at the same time each day and limit the time to 30 minutes, preferably once a day.
- Get adequate exercise during the day to reduce stress, but avoid excessive physical exertion 2 hours before bedtime.
- Avoid dealing with office work or family problems before bedtime.
- Establish a regular routine before sleep such as reading, listening to soft music, taking a warm bath, or doing some other quiet activity you enjoy.
- When you are unable to sleep, pursue some relaxing activity until you feel drowsy.
- If you have trouble falling asleep, get up and pursue nonstrenuous activity until you feel sleepy.
- Use the bed mainly for sleep, so that you associate it with sleep.

Environment

- Ensure appropriate lighting, temperature, and ventilation.
- Keep noise to a minimum; block out extraneous noise as necessary with soft music.

Diet

- Avoid heavy meals 3 hours before bedtime.
- Avoid alcohol and caffeine-containing foods and beverages (coffee, tea, chocolate) at least 4 hours before bedtime. These act as diuretics, creating the need to void during sleep time.
- Decrease fluid intake 2 to 4 hours before sleep if necessary to avoid the need to use the bathroom during sleeping hours.
- If a bedtime snack is necessary, consume only light carbohydrates or a milk drink. Heavy or spicy foods can cause gastrointestinal upsets that disturb sleep.

Medications

- Use sleeping medications only as a last resort. Take them judiciously (e.g., three times a week). Use over-the-counter medications sparingly because many contain antihistamines that cause daytime drowsiness.
- Take analgesics 30 minutes before bedtime to relieve aches and pains.
- Consult with your healthcare provider about adjusting other medications that may cause insomnia.

PROCEDURE 23-1   # Providing Passive Range-of-Motion Exercises

Purposes

- To maintain joint flexibility
- To provide exercise when the client is unable to accomplish movement actively

Equipment

- No special equipment is needed except a bed or exercise mat or table.

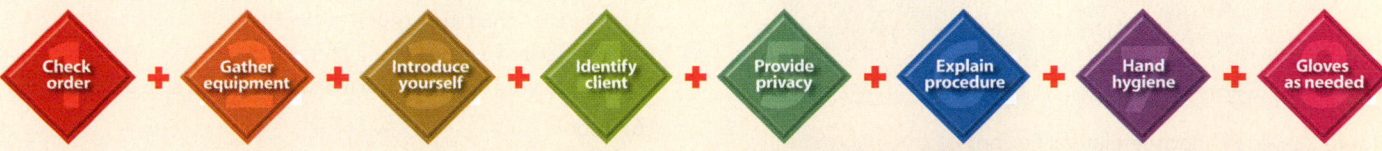
Check order + Gather equipment + Introduce yourself + Identify client + Provide privacy + Explain procedure + Hand hygiene + Gloves as needed

Interventions and Rationales

1. Perform preparatory steps (see icon bar above).

2. Perform exercises in an organized format from head to toe. Repeat each movement three times, supporting the joint. *This allows the muscles to stretch and warm.*

3. Observe the client for nonverbal clues of pain. *This can reduce discomfort and prevent further injury.*

4. Neck
   - Remove pillow.
   - Flex and extend the neck (Figure 23-13 ■):
     a. Place palm of one hand under client's head and the other on the chin.

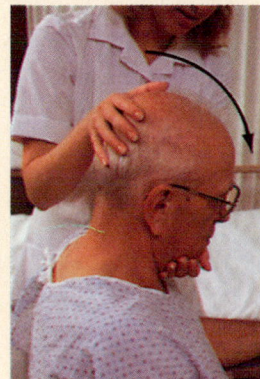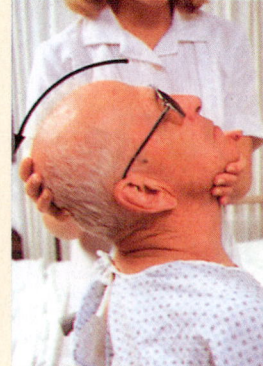

Figure 23-13. ■ Head flexion and extension.

b. Move head forward from an upright position until the chin rests on the chest.

c. Move the head back to the resting supine position.

■ Lateral flexion of neck (Figure 23-14 ■):

a. Place heels of the hands on each side of client's cheeks.

b. Move head laterally toward the right and left shoulders.

■ Rotation (Figure 23-15 ■):

a. Place heels of the hands on client's cheeks.

b. Turn face as far as possible to the right and left.

5. Shoulder

■ Flexion/extension (Figure 23-16 ■):

a. With client's arms at the side, grasp the arm beneath the elbow with one hand and beneath the wrist with the other hand.

b. Raise the arm forward and upward to a position beside the head.

c. Move the arm from a vertical position beside the head forward and down to a resting position at the side of the body.

■ Abduction/adduction (Figure 23-17 ■):

a. Move arm laterally from the resting position at the side to a side position above the head, palm of the hand away from the head.

b. Move the arm laterally from beside the head downward laterally and across the front on the body as far as possible.

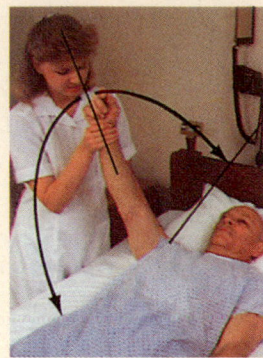

Figure 23-16. ■ Shoulder flexion and extension.

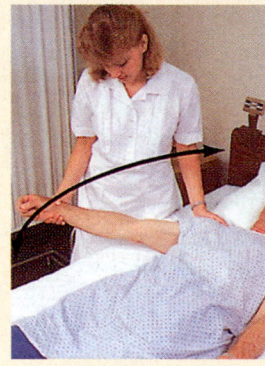

Figure 23-17. ■ Shoulder abduction and adduction.

■ External/internal rotation:

a. With arm held out to the side at shoulder level and elbow at a right angle and fingers pointing downward, move the arm upward so that the fingers are pointing up and the back of the hand touches the bed or mat.

b. With arm held out to the side at the level of the shoulder and the elbow bent at a right angle, fingers pointing up, bring the arm forward and down so that the palm touches the mat.

■ Circumduction:

a. Move the arm forward and backward in a full circle.

6. Elbow

■ Flexion/extension (Figure 23-18 ■):

a. Bring lower arm forward and upward so that hand is at shoulder level.

b. Bring lower arm forward and downward, straightening the arm.

■ Rotation for supination/pronation (Figure 23-19 ■):

a. Grasp the client's hand with a handshaking motion and turn the palm upward. Make sure only the forearm and not the shoulder moves.

b. Turn the palm downward, moving only the forearm.

7. Wrist

■ Flexion/extension (Figure 23-20 ■):

a. Flex client's arm at the elbow until the forearm is at a right angle to the bed or mat. Support the wrist

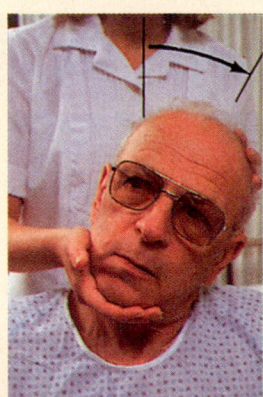
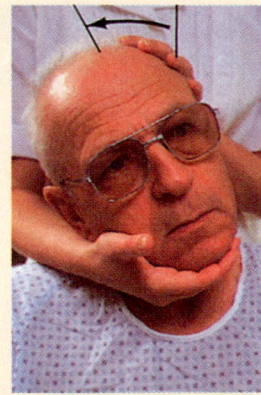

Figure 23-14. ■ Right/left lateral flexion.

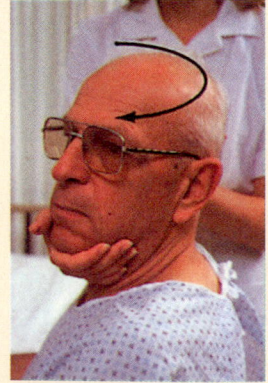
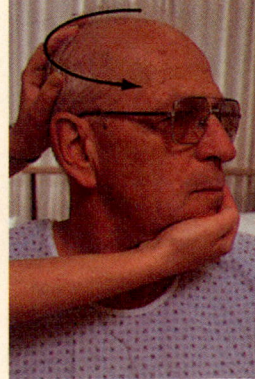

Figure 23-15. ■ Right/left rotation.

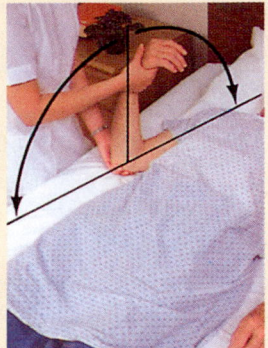

Figure 23-18. ■ Elbow flexion and extension.

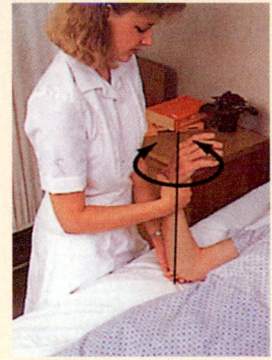

Figure 23-19. ■ Forearm pronation and supination.

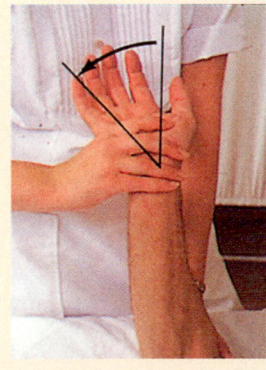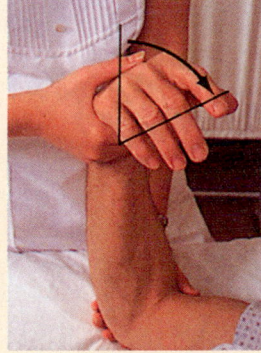

Figure 23-20. ■ Wrist flexion and extension.

joint with one hand while manipulating the joint with your other hand.
   b. Bring the fingers of the hand toward the inner aspect of the arm.
   c. Straighten the hand to the same plane as the arm.
■ Hyperflexion:
   a. Bend fingers of the hand back as far as possible.
■ Radial flexion (abduction)/ulnar flexion (adduction) (Figure 23-21 ■):
   a. Bend wrist laterally toward the thumb side.
   b. Bend the wrist laterally toward the fifth finger.

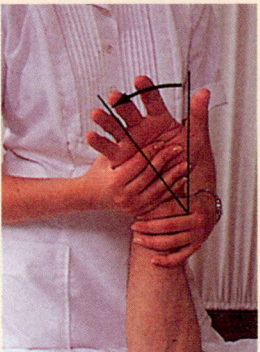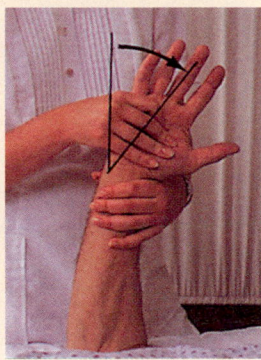

Figure 23-21. ■ Ulnar and radial deviation.

8. Hand and fingers
   ■ Flexion/extension (Figure 23-22 ■):
      a. Make client's hand into a fist.
      b. Straighten the fingers.
   ■ Hyperextension:
      a. Gently bend fingers back.
   ■ Adduction/abduction (Figure 23-23 ■):
      a. Bring fingers together.
      b. Spread fingers of the hand apart.
9. Thumb
   ■ Flexion/extension:
      a. Move thumb across the palmar surface toward the fifth finger.
      b. Move the thumb away from the hand.

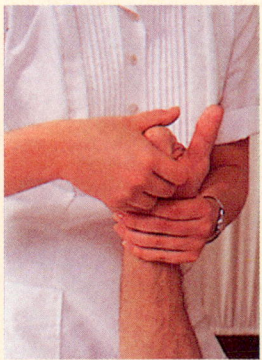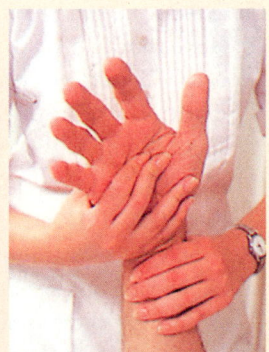

Figure 23-22. ■ Finger flexion and extension.

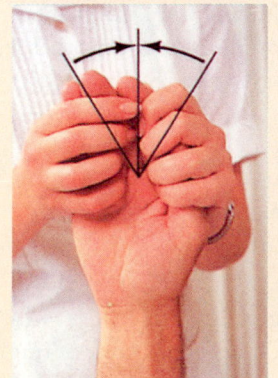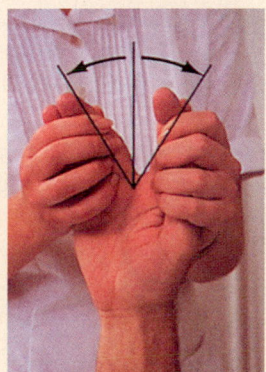

Figure 23-23. ■ Finger adduction and abduction.

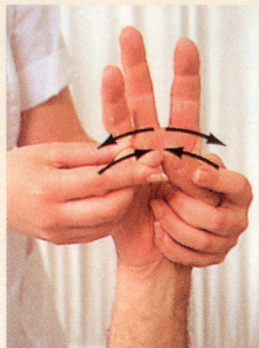

Figure 23-24. ■ Finger–thumb opposition.

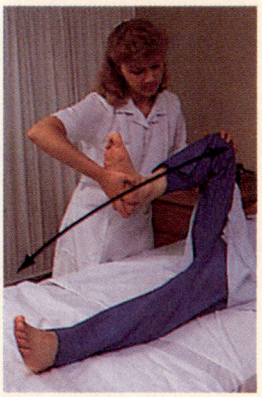

Figure 23-25. ■ Hip/knee flexion and extension.

- ■ Abduction/adduction:
  a. Extend the thumb laterally.
  b. Move thumb back to the hand. *Note: Can be done when abducting and adducting fingers.*
- ■ Opposition (Figure 23-24 ■):
  a. Touch thumb to the top of each finger of the same hand.

10. Hip: To exercise hip and leg, place one hand under the client's knee and the other under the ankle.
  - ■ Flexion/extension (Figure 23-25 ■):
    a. Lift the leg and bend the knee, moving the knee up toward the chest as far as possible.
    b. Bring leg down, straighten the knee, and lower the leg to the bed.
  - ■ Abduction/adduction (Figure 23-26 ■):
    a. Move the leg to the side away from the client.
    b. Move leg back across and in front of the other leg.
  - ■ Slowly raise and lower leg (Figure 23-27 ■):
  - ■ Circumduction:
    a. Move the leg in a circle.
  - ■ Internal/external rotation:
    a. Roll the foot and leg inward.
    b. Roll foot and leg outward.

11. Knee
  - ■ Flexion/extension (see Figure 23-25):
    a. Bend leg, bringing the heel toward back of thigh. *Note: Can be done with hip flexion.*
    b. Straighten the leg and return the foot to the bed.

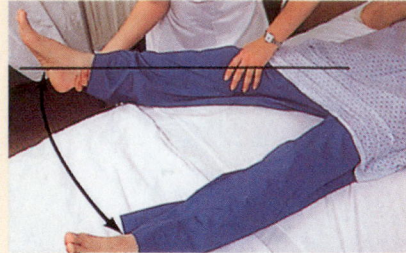

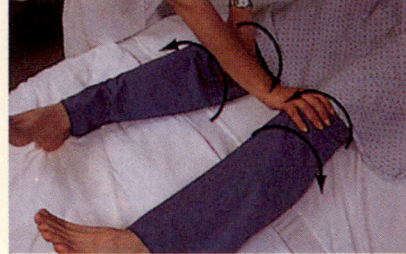

Figure 23-26. ■ Hip abduction and adduction.

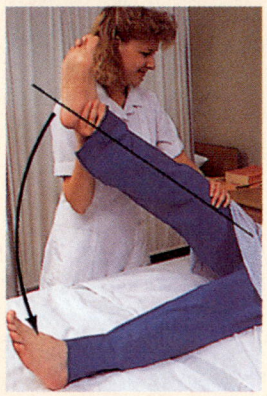

Figure 23-27. ■ Straight leg raising.

12. Ankle
  - ■ Extension/flexion (Figure 23-28 ■):
    a. Plantar flexion: Move the foot so that the toes are pointed downward.
    b. Dorsiflexion: Move foot so toes are pointed upward.

13. Foot
  - ■ Eversion/inversion:
    a. Place one hand under the client's ankle and the other over the arch.
    b. Turn the whole foot outward.
    c. Turn the whole foot inward.

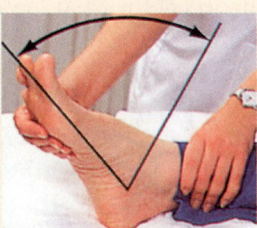

Figure 23-28. ■ Ankle dorsiflexion and plantar flexion.

14. Toes
    - Flexion/extension (Figure 23-29 ■):
      a. Place one hand over arch.
      b. Place the fingers of the other hand over toes and curl downward.
      c. Place fingers under the toes and bend toes upward.

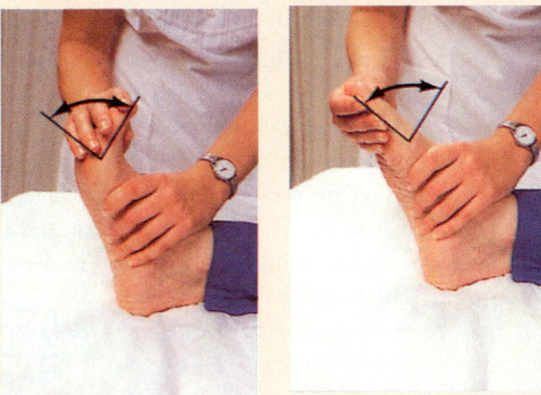

Figure 23-29. ■ Toe flexion and extension.

- Abduction/adduction:
  a. Spread toes apart.
  b. Bring toes together.

PROCEDURE 23-2   Moving a Client in Bed

Purpose

- To reposition clients who have slid down in bed from the Fowler's position or been pulled down by traction

Equipment

- None needed
- Second person may be needed to assist with some clients

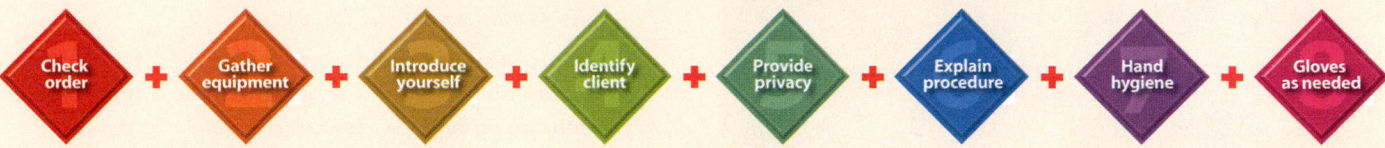

Check order + Gather equipment + Introduce yourself + Identify client + Provide privacy + Explain procedure + Hand hygiene + Gloves as needed

Part A: Moving a Client in Bed
Interventions and Rationales

1. Perform preparatory steps (see icon bar above).
2. Adjust the bed and the client's position.
   - Adjust the head of the bed to a flat position or as low as the client can tolerate. *Moving the client upward against gravity requires more force and can cause back strain.*
   - Raise the bed to the height of your center of gravity.
   - Lock the wheels on the bed and raise the rail on the side of the bed opposite you.
   - Remove all pillows, then place one against the head of the bed. *This pillow protects the client's head from inadvertent injury against the top of the bed during the upward move.*

3. Ask for the client's help in lessening your workload.
   - Ask the client to flex the hips and knees and position the feet so that they can be used effectively for pushing. *Flexing the hips and knees keeps the entire lower leg off the bed surface, preventing friction during movement, and ensures use of the large muscle groups in the client's legs when pushing, thus increasing the force of movement.*
   - Ask the client to:
     a. Grasp the head of the bed with both hands and pull during the move.
     or
     b. Raise the upper part of the body on the elbows and push with the hands and forearms during the move
     or

c. Grasp the overhead trapeze with both hands and lift and pull during the move. *Client assistance provides additional power to overcome inertia and friction during the move. These actions also keep the client's arms partially off the bed surface, reducing friction during movement, and make use of the large muscle groups of the client's arms to increase the force during movement.*

4. Position yourself appropriately, and move the client.
   - Face the direction of the movement, and then assume a broad stance, with the foot nearest the bed behind the forward foot and weight on the forward foot. Incline your trunk forward from the hips. Flex hips, knees, and ankles.
   - Place your near arm under the client's thighs (Figure 23-30 ■). *This supports the heaviest part of the body (the buttocks).* Push down on the mattress with the far arm. *The far arm acts as a lever during the move.*
   - Tighten your gluteal, abdominal, leg, and arm muscles, and rock from the back leg to the front leg and back again. Then shift your weight to the front leg as the client pushes with the heels and pulls with the arms, so that the client moves toward the head of the bed. *Tightening your muscles helps to prevent strain. Moving the client as you shift your weight adds momentum.*

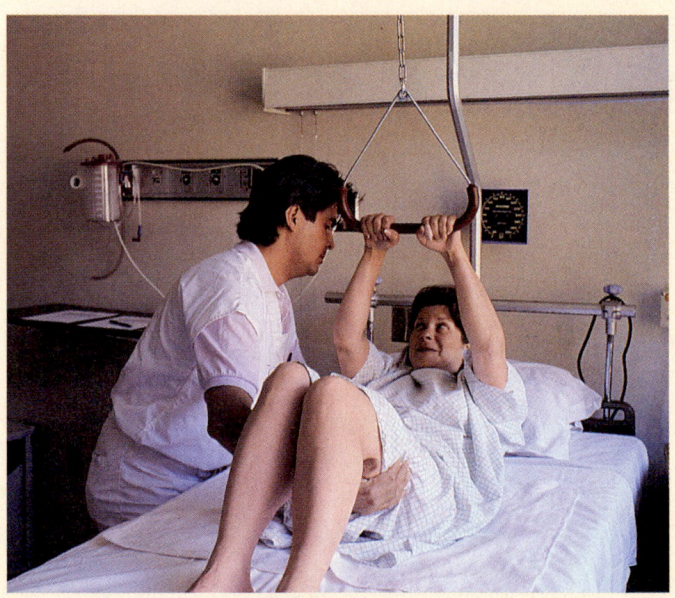

Figure 23-30. ■ Moving a client up in bed.

5. Ensure client comfort.
   - Elevate the head of the bed and provide appropriate support devices for the client's new position.
   - See the sections on positioning clients earlier in this chapter.

VARIATION: A CLIENT WHO HAS LIMITED STRENGTH OF THE UPPER EXTREMITIES

- Assist the client to flex the hips and knees as in step 2 previously. Place the client's arms across the chest. *This keeps them off the bed surface and minimizes friction during movement.* Ask the client to flex the neck during the move and keep the head off the bed surface.
- Position yourself as in step 3, and place one arm under the client's back and shoulders and the other arm under the client's thighs. *This placement of the arms distributes the client's weight and supports the heaviest part of the body (the buttocks).* Shift your weight as in step 3.

VARIATION: TWO NURSES USING A HAND–FOREARM INTERLOCK

Two people are required to move clients who are unable to assist because of their condition or weight. Using the technique described in step 3, with the second staff member on the opposite side of the bed, both of you interlock your forearms under the client's thighs and shoulders and lift the client up in bed.

VARIATION: TWO NURSES USING A TURN SHEET

Two nurses can use a turn sheet to move a client up in bed. *A turn sheet distributes the client's weight more evenly, decreases friction, and exerts a more even force on the client during the move. In addition, it prevents injury of the client's skin, because the friction created between two sheets when one is moved is less than that created by the client's body moving over the sheet.*

- Place a draw sheet or a full sheet folded in half under the client, extending from the shoulders to the thighs. Each of you rolls up or fanfolds the turn sheet close to the client's body on either side.
- Both of you then grasp the sheet close to the shoulders and buttocks of the client. *This draws the weight closer to the nurses' center of gravity and increases the nurses' balance and stability, permitting a smoother movement.* Then follow the method of moving clients with limited upper extremity strength, described earlier.

Part B: Turning a Client to a Lateral or Prone Position in Bed

Movement to a lateral (side-lying) position may be necessary when placing a bedpan beneath the client, when changing the client's bed linen, or when repositioning the client.

Interventions and Rationales

1. Position yourself and the client appropriately before performing the move.

- Move the client closer to the side of the bed opposite the side the client will face when turned. *This ensures that the client will be positioned safely in the center of the bed after turning.* Use a pull sheet beneath the client's trunk and thighs to pull the client to the side of the bed. Roll up the sheet as close as possible to the client's body and pull the client to the side of the bed. Adjust the client's head and reposition the legs appropriately.

- While standing on the side of the bed nearest the client, place the client's near arm across the chest. Abduct the client's far shoulder slightly from the side of the body. *Pulling the one arm forward facilitates the turning motion. Pulling the other arm away from the body prevents that arm from being caught beneath the client's body during the roll.*
- Place the client's near ankle and foot across the far ankle and foot. *This facilitates the turning motion. Making these preparations on the side of the bed closest to the client helps prevent unnecessary reaching.*
- Raise the side rail next to the client before going to the other side of the bed. *This ensures that the client, who is close to the edge of the mattress, will not fall.*
- Position yourself on the side of the bed toward which the client will turn, directly in line with the client's waistline and as close to the bed as possible.
- Incline your trunk forward from the hips. Flex your hips, knees, and ankles. Assume a broad stance with one foot forward and the weight placed on this forward foot.

2. Pull or roll the client to a lateral position.
   - Place one hand on the client's far hip and the other hand on the client's far shoulder (Figure 23-31 ■). *This position of the hands supports the client at the two heaviest parts of the body, providing greater control in movement during the roll.*
   - Tighten your gluteal, abdominal, leg, and arm muscles; rock backward, shifting your weight from the forward to the backward foot; and roll the client onto the side of the body to face you (see Figure 23-31B).

VARIATION: TURNING THE CLIENT TO A PRONE POSITION

To turn a client to the prone position, follow the preceding steps, with two exceptions:

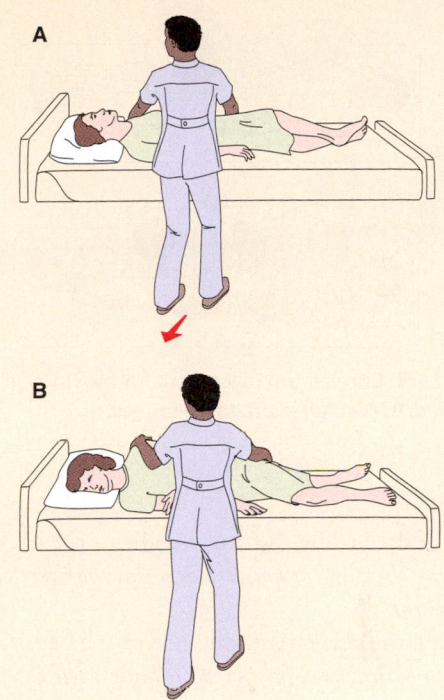

Figure 23-31. ■ **A, B.** Moving a client to a lateral position.

- Instead of abducting the far arm, keep the client's arm alongside the body for the client to roll over. *Keeping the arm alongside the body prevents it from being pinned under the client when the client is rolled.*
- Roll the client completely onto the abdomen. It is essential to move the client as close as possible to the edge of the bed before the turn so that the client will be lying on the center of the bed after rolling. Never pull a client across the bed while the client is in the prone position. Doing so can injure a woman's breasts or a man's genitals.

Part C: Logrolling a Client

Logrolling is a technique used to turn a client whose body must at all times be kept in straight alignment (like a log). *An example is the client with a spinal injury. Considerable care must be taken to prevent additional injury.* This technique requires two nurses or, if the client is large, three nurses. For the client who has a cervical injury, one nurse must maintain the client's head and neck alignment throughout the procedure.

Interventions and Rationales

1. Position yourselves and the client appropriately before the move.
   - Stand on the same side of the bed, and assume a broad stance with one foot ahead of the other.

- Place the client's arms across the chest. *Doing so ensures that they will not be injured or become trapped under the body when the body is turned.*
- Incline your trunk, and flex your hips, knees, and ankles.
- Place your arms under the client as shown in Figure 23-32A ■ or B, depending on the client's size. *Each staff member then has a major weight area of the client centered between the arms.*
- Tighten your gluteal, abdominal, leg, and arm muscles. *This provides support to your back muscles to prevent strain.*

2. Pull the client to the side of the bed.
   - One nurse counts, "One, two, three, go." Then at the same time, all staff members pull the client to the

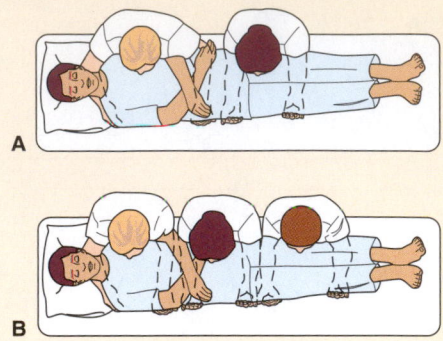

Figure 23-32. ■ Correct arm placement for moving a client to the side of the bed: **A.** two nurses; **B.** three nurses.

side of the bed by shifting weight to the back foot. *Moving the client in unison maintains the client's body alignment.*

■ Elevate the side rail on this side of the bed. *This prevents the client from falling while lying so close to the edge of the bed.*

3. Move to the other side of the bed, and place supportive devices for the client when turned.

■ Place a pillow where it will support the client's head after the turn. *The pillow prevents lateral flexion of the neck and ensures alignment of the cervical spine.*

■ Place one or two pillows between the client's legs to support the upper leg when the client is turned. *This pillow prevents adduction of the upper leg and keeps the legs parallel and aligned.*

4. Roll and position the client in proper alignment.

■ All nurses flex the hips, knees, and ankles and assume a broad stance with one foot forward.

■ All nurses reach over the client and place hands as shown in Figure 23-33 ■. *Doing so centers a major weight area of the client between each nurse's arms.*

■ One nurse counts, "One, two, three, go." Then at the same time, all nurses roll the client to a lateral position.

■ Place pillows to maintain the client's lateral position. See the discussion of the lateral position.

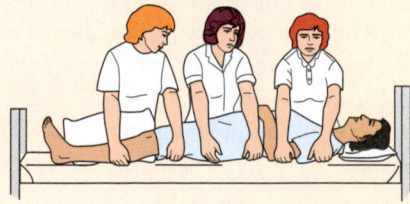

Figure 23-33. ■ Correct hand placement for logrolling a client.

VARIATION: USING A TURN OR LIFT SHEET

■ Use a turn sheet to facilitate logrolling. First, stand with another nurse on the same side of the bed. Assume a broad stance with one foot forward, and grasp half of the fanfolded or rolled edge of the turn sheet. On a signal, pull the client toward both of you (Figure 23-34 ■).

■ Before turning the client, place pillow supports for the head and legs, as described in step 3 previously. *This helps maintain the client's alignment when turning.* Then go

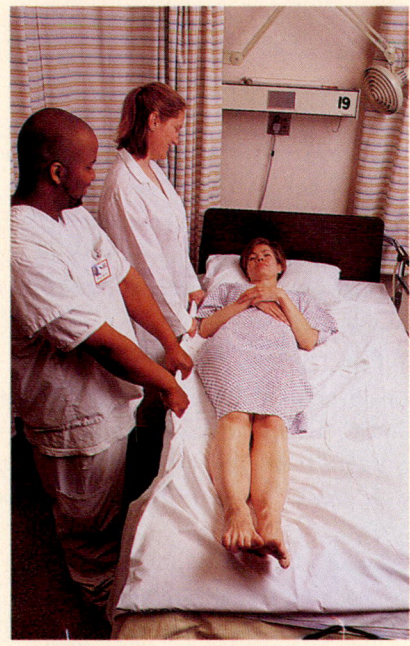

Figure 23-34. ■ Using the turn sheet, the nurses pull the sheet with the client on it to the edge of the bed. (Photographer: Jenny Thomas.)

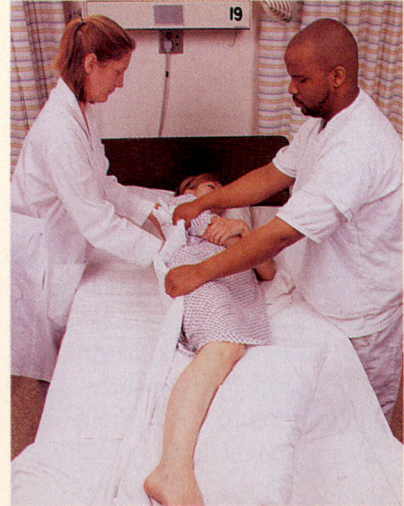

Figure 23-35. ■ The nurse on the right uses the far edge of the sheet to roll the client toward him; the nurse on the left remains behind the client and assists with turning. (Photographer: Jenny Thomas.)

to the other side of the bed (farthest from the client), and assume a stable stance. Reaching over the client, grasp the far edges of the turn sheet, and roll the client toward you (Figure 23-35 ■). The second nurse (behind the client) helps turn the client and provides pillow supports to ensure good alignment in the lateral position.

Part D: Moving a Client to a Sitting Position on the Edge of the Bed

The client assumes a sitting position on the edge of the bed before walking, moving to a chair or wheelchair, eating, or performing other activities.

Interventions and Rationales

1. Position yourself and the client appropriately before performing the move.
   - Assist the client to a lateral position facing you.
   - Raise the head of the bed slowly as high as it will go. *This decreases the distance that the client needs to move to sit up on the side of the bed.*
   - Position the client's feet and lower legs at the edge of the bed. *This enables the client's feet to move easily off the bed during the movement, and the client is aided by gravity into a sitting position.*
   - Stand beside the client's hips and face the far corner of the bottom of the bed (the angle in which movement will occur). Assume a broad stance, placing the foot nearest the client forward. Incline your trunk forward from the hips. Flex your hips, knees, and ankles (Figures 23-36A ■ and B).

2. Move the client to a sitting position.
   - Place one arm around the client's shoulders and the other arm beneath both of the client's thighs near the knees (see Figure 23-36A). *Supporting the client's shoulders prevents the client from falling backward during the movement. Supporting the client's thighs reduces friction of the thighs against the bed surface during the move and increases the force of the movement.*
   - Tighten your gluteal, abdominal, leg, and arm muscles. *This protects your own muscles from strain.*
   - Lift the client's thighs slightly. *This reduces the friction of the client's thighs and the nurse's arm against the bed surface.*
   - Pivot on the balls of your feet in the desired direction facing the foot of the bed while pulling the client's feet and legs off the bed (see Figure 23-36B). *Pivoting prevents twisting of the nurse's spine. The weight of the client's legs swinging downward increases downward movement of the lower body and helps make the client's upper body vertical.*
   - Keep supporting the client until the client is well balanced and comfortable. *This movement may cause some clients to faint.*
   - Assess vital signs (e.g., pulse, respirations, and blood pressure) as indicated by the client's health status.

VARIATION: TEACHING A CLIENT HOW TO SIT ON THE SIDE OF THE BED INDEPENDENTLY

A client who has had recent abdominal surgery or who is weak may have too much abdominal pain or too little strength to sit straight up in bed. This person can be taught to assume a "dangle" position without assistance. Instruct the client to:

- Roll to the side and lift the far leg over the near leg (Figure 23-37A ■).
- Grasp the mattress edge with the lower arm and push the fist of the upper arm into the mattress (Figure 23-37B).
- Push up with the arms as the heels and legs slide over the mattress edge (Figure 23-37B).
- Maintain the sitting position by pushing both fists into the mattress behind and to the sides of the buttocks.

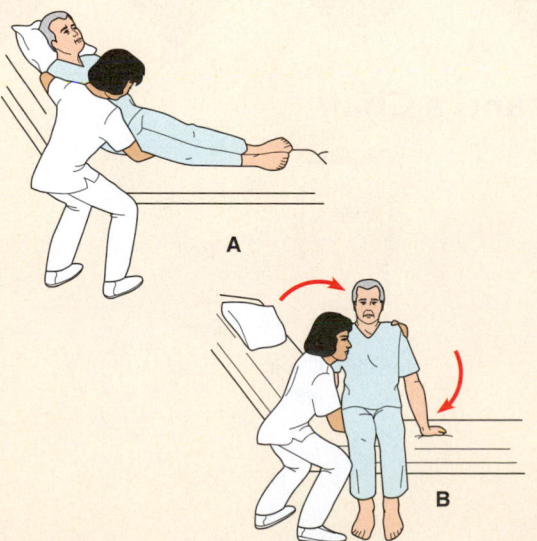

Figure 23-36. ■ A, B. Assisting a client to a sitting position on the edge of the bed.

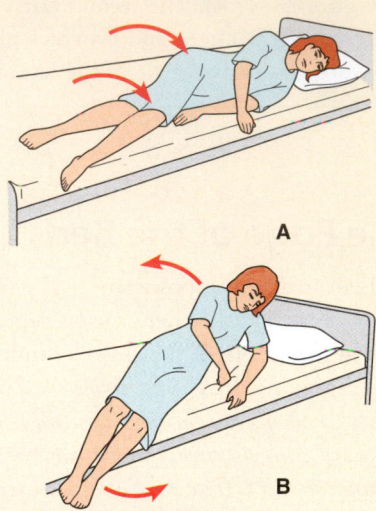

Figure 23-37. ■ **A, B.** Moving to a sitting position independently.

PROCEDURE 23-3   # Transferring a Client

Purpose

■ To safely move a client from bed to chair, wheelchair, or stretcher

Equipment

■ Transfer (walking) belt
■ Stretcher (if transferring to stretcher)
■ *Optional:* roller bar or long board (sliding board)

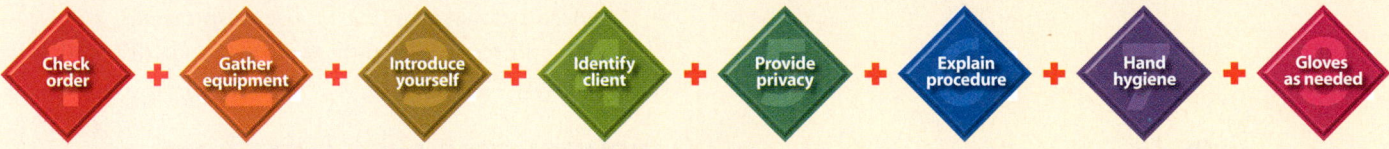

Check order + Gather equipment + Introduce yourself + Identify client + Provide privacy + Explain procedure + Hand hygiene + Gloves as needed

Part A: Transferring a Client between a Bed and a Chair

Interventions and Rationales

1. Perform preparatory steps (see icon bar above).

2. Position the equipment appropriately.
   ■ Lower the bed to its lowest position so that the client's feet will rest flat on the floor. Lock the wheels of the bed. *This helps to prevent risk of fall due to sudden movement.*
   ■ Place the wheelchair parallel to the bed as close to the bed as possible (Figure 23-38 ■). Lock the wheels of the wheelchair, and raise the footplate.

3. Prepare and assess the client.
   ■ Assist the client to a sitting position on the side of the bed. See Procedure 23-2, Part D.
   ■ Assess the client for orthostatic hypotension before moving the client from the bed. *Changes in posture could result in fainting.*

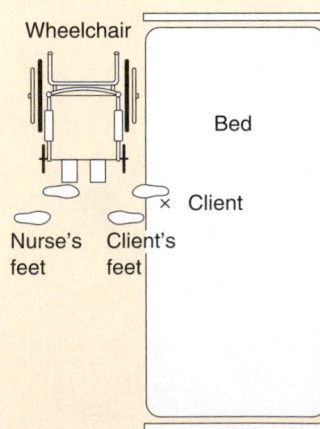

Figure 23-38. ■ The wheelchair is placed parallel to the bed as close to the bed as possible. Note that placement of the nurse's feet mirrors that of the client's feet.

- Assist the client in putting on a bathrobe and nonskid slippers or shoes. *These provide comfort and safety when walking.*
- Place a transfer belt snugly around the client's waist. Check to be certain that the belt is securely fastened.

4. Give explicit instructions to the client. Ask the client to:
   - Move forward and sit on the edge of the bed. *This brings the client's center of gravity closer to the nurse's.*
   - Lean forward slightly from the hips. *This brings the client's center of gravity more directly over the base of support and positions the head and trunk in the direction of the movement.*
   - Place the foot of the stronger leg beneath the edge of the bed and put the other foot forward. *In this way, the client can use the stronger leg muscles to stand and power the movement. A broader base of support makes the client more stable during the transfer.*
   - Place the client's hands on the bed surface or on your shoulders so that the client can push while standing. *This provides additional force for the movement and reduces the potential for strain on the nurse's back. The client should not grasp the nurse's neck for support. Doing so can injure the nurse.*

5. Position yourself correctly.
   - Stand directly in front of the client. Incline the trunk forward from the hips. Flex the hips, knees, and ankles. Assume a broad stance, placing one foot forward and one back. Mirror the placement of the client's feet, if possible. *This helps prevent loss of balance during the transfer.*
   - Encircle the client's waist with your arms, and grasp the transfer belt at the client's back (Figure 23-39 ■) with thumbs pointing downward. *The belt provides a secure handle for holding onto the client and controlling the*

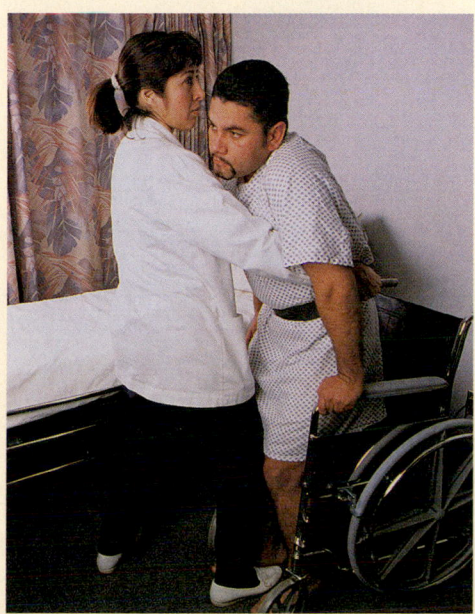

Figure 23-39. ■ Using a transfer (walking) belt. (Photographer: Elena Dorfman.)

movement. Downward placement of the thumbs prevents potential wrist injury as the nurse lifts. By supporting the client in this manner, you keep the client from tilting backward during the transfer.
   - Tighten your gluteal, abdominal, leg, and arm muscles.

6. Assist the client to stand, and then move together toward the wheelchair.
   - On the count of three:
     a. Ask the client to push with the back foot, rock to the forward foot, extend (straighten) the joints of the lower extremities, and push or pull up with the hands, while
     b. You push with the forward foot, rock to the back foot, extend the joints of the lower extremities, and pull the client (directly toward your center of gravity) into a standing position.
   - Support the client in an upright standing position for a few moments. *This allows the nurse and the client to extend the joints and provides the nurse with an opportunity to ensure that the client is all right before moving away from the bed.*
   - Together, pivot or take a few steps toward the wheelchair.

7. Assist the client to sit.
   - Ask the client to:
     a. Back up to the wheelchair and place the legs against the seat. *Having the client place the legs against the wheelchair seat minimizes the risk of the client's falling when sitting down.*
     b. Place the foot of the stronger leg slightly behind the other. *This supports body weight during the movement.*
     c. Keep the other foot forward. *This provides a broad base of support.*
     d. Place both hands on the wheelchair arms or on your shoulders. *This increases stability and lessens the strain on the nurse.*
   - Stand directly in front of the client. Place one foot forward and one back.
   - Tighten your grasp on the transfer belt, and tighten your gluteal, abdominal, leg, and arm muscles.
   - On the count of three:
     a. Have the client shift the body weight by rocking to the back foot, lower the body onto the edge of the wheelchair seat by flexing the joints of the legs and arms, and place some body weight on the arms, while
     b. You shift your body weight by stepping back with the forward foot and pivoting toward the chair while lowering the client onto the wheelchair seat.

8. Ensure client safety.
   - Ask the client to push back into the wheelchair seat. *Sitting well back on the seat provides a broader base of support and greater stability and minimizes the risk of falling from the wheelchair. A wheelchair can topple forward when the client sits on the edge of the seat and leans far forward.*
   - Lower the footplates, and place the client's feet on them.
   - Apply a seat belt as required.

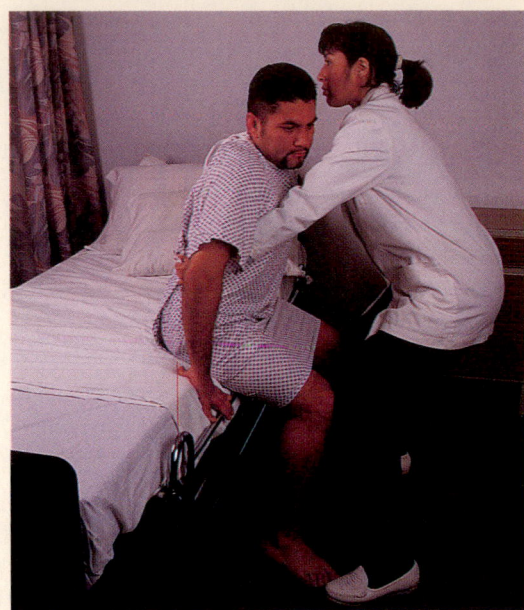

Figure 23-40. ■ Transferring without a belt. (Photographer: Elena Dorfman.)

VARIATION: ANGLING THE WHEELCHAIR

For clients who have difficulty walking, place the wheelchair at a 45-degree angle to the bed. *This enables the client to pivot into the chair and lessens the amount of body rotation required.*

VARIATION: TRANSFERRING WITHOUT A BELT

- For clients who need minimal assistance, place the hands against the sides of the client's chest (not at the axillae) during the transfer (Figure 23-40 ■). For clients who require more assistance, reach through the client's axillae and place the hands on the client's scapulae during the transfer. Avoid placing hands or pressure on the axillae, especially for clients who have upper extremity paralysis or paresis.
- Follow the steps described previously.

VARIATION: TRANSFERRING WITH A BELT AND TWO NURSES

- When the client is able to stand, position yourselves on both sides of the client, facing the same direction as the client. Flex your hips, knees, and ankles; grasp the client's

transfer belt with the hand closest to the client; and with the other hand support the client's elbows.
- Coordinating your efforts, all three of you stand simultaneously, pivot, and move to the wheelchair. Reverse the process to lower the client onto the wheelchair seat.

VARIATION: TRANSFERRING A CLIENT WITH AN INJURED LOWER EXTREMITY

When the client has an injured lower extremity, movement should always occur toward the client's unaffected (strong) side. For example, if the client's right leg is injured and the client is sitting on the edge of the bed preparing to transfer to a wheelchair, position the wheelchair on the client's left side. In this way, the client can use the unaffected leg most effectively and safely.

VARIATION: USING A SLIDING BOARD

Have a client who cannot stand use a sliding board to move without nursing assistance. *This method not only promotes the client's sense of independence but preserves your energy* (Figure 23-41 ■).

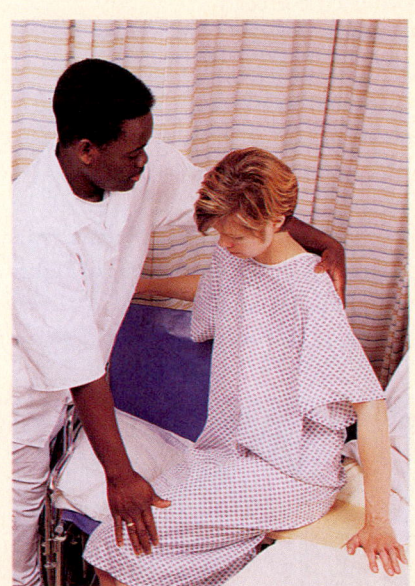

Figure 23-41. ■ Using a sliding board. (Photographer: Jenny Thomas.)

Part B: Transferring a Client between a Bed and a Stretcher

The stretcher, or gurney, is used to transfer supine clients from one location to another. Whenever the client is capable of accomplishing the transfer from bed to stretcher independently, either by lifting onto it or by rolling onto it, the client should be encouraged to do so. If the client cannot move onto the stretcher independently, at least two nurses are needed to assist with the transfer. More are needed if the client is totally helpless or is heavy.

Interventions and Rationales

1. Adjust the client's bed in preparation for the transfer.
   - Lower the head of the bed until it is flat or as low as the client can tolerate.
   - Raise the bed so that it is slightly higher than the surface of the stretcher. *It is easier for the client to move down an incline.*
   - Ensure that the wheels on the bed are locked.
   - Pull the draw sheet out from both sides of the bed.

2. Move the client to the edge of the bed, and position the stretcher.
   - Roll the draw sheet as close to the client's side as possible.
   - Pull the client to the edge of the bed, and cover the client with a sheet or bath blanket to maintain comfort.
   - Place the stretcher parallel to the bed, next to the client, and lock its wheels.
   - Fill the gap that exists between the bed and the stretcher loosely with the bath blankets (optional).

3. Transfer the client securely to the stretcher.
   - In unison with the other staff members, press your body tightly against the stretcher. *This prevents the stretcher from moving.*
   - Roll the pull sheet tightly against the client. *This achieves better control over client movement.*
   - Flex your hips, and pull the client on the pull sheet in unison directly toward you and onto the stretcher. *Pulling downward requires less force than pulling along a flat surface.*
   - Ask the client to flex the neck during the move, if possible, and place arms across the chest. *This prevents injury to these body parts.*

4. Ensure client comfort and safety.
   - Make the client comfortable, unlock the stretcher wheels, and move the stretcher away from the bed.
   - Immediately raise the stretcher side rails and/or fasten the safety straps across the client. *Because the stretcher is high and narrow, the client is in danger of falling unless these safety precautions are taken.*

VARIATION: USING A ROLLER BAR DURING THE TRANSFER

A roller bar is a metal frame covered with longitudinal rollers. Place the bar over the gap between the bed and the stretcher. Using a pull sheet, pull the client onto the roller bar, and roll the client easily onto the stretcher.

VARIATION: USING A LONG BOARD

The long board, which may be referred to as the Smooth Mover or Easyglide, is a lacquered or smooth polyethylene board measuring 45 to 55 cm (18 to 22 in.) by 182 cm (72 in.) with handholds along its edges. This device may be used by one nurse alone or up to four nurses together. Turn the client to a lateral position away from you, position the board close to the client's back, and roll the client onto the board. Pull the client and board across the bed to the stretcher. Safety belts may be placed over the chest, abdomen, and legs.

VARIATION: USING A DRAW SHEET

Position the client on the edge of the bed with the draw sheet or blanket supporting the client's head, torso, and upper thighs. Two or three people reach over the stretcher to lift and slide the client toward them. One person stands at the foot of the bed and transfers the client's feet. Two people reach across the bed as the client moves, assisting with the lift and transfer. The transfer is done in a coordinated motion or motions to provide smooth transfer.

This lift is not commonly used because of the risk for injury to those doing the transfer.

SAMPLE DOCUMENTATION

[date] [time] Found client sitting on edge of bed. Stated "waiting too long to get help." Assisted with transfer to chair. Reminded ct. wait for assistance to prevent a fall. Son visited 1/2 hour. _____

_____ R. Marino, LVN

PROCEDURE 23-4 # Hoyer (Sling) Transfer Lift

Purpose
- To lift and transfer client from bed to chair and back

Equipment
- Hoyer lift base
- Canvas pieces: 1 large, 1 small
- Canvas straps

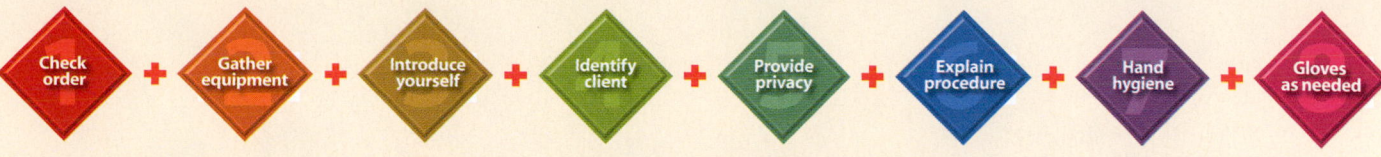

Check order ✛ Gather equipment ✛ Introduce yourself ✛ Identify client ✛ Provide privacy ✛ Explain procedure ✛ Hand hygiene ✛ Gloves as needed

Interventions and Rationales

1. Perform preparatory steps (see icon bar above).
2. Check orders and client care plan. Determine that lift can safely move the weight of the client.
3. Explain the procedure. *Client may be frightened by use of a mechanical device.*
4. Bring lift to bedside (Figure 23-42 ■). *Ensures safe elevation of client off bed.*
5. Lock wheels of bed. *Ensures that the bed will not move during transfer.*
6. Place client chair by the bedside. Allow adequate space to maneuver the lift.
7. Raise bed to high position with mattress flat. Lower side rail on the side closest to you. *Maintains nurses' alignment during transfer.*
8. Keep bed side rail up on the opposite side. *Maintains client safety.*
9. Roll client on side away from you.
10. Place hammock or canvas strips under client to form sling. Place two canvas pieces so that lower edge fits under client's knees (wide piece), and upper edge fits under client's shoulder (narrow piece). *Two different types of seats are supplied. Hammocks are better for clients who are flaccid, weak, and need support; canvas can be used for clients with normal muscle tone. Hooks should face away from client's skin. Place sling under client's center of gravity and greatest portion of body weight.*
11. Raise bed rail. *Maintains safety.*
12. Go to opposite side and lower side rail. *Maintains safety.*
13. Roll client to opposite side and pull Hammock (strip) through. *Completes positioning of client on lift sling.*
14. Roll client supine onto canvas seat. *Sling should extend from shoulder to knees to support client's body weight equally.*

15. Remove client's glasses, if appropriate. *Swivel bar can break eyeglasses.*
16. Place lift's horseshoe bar under side of bed (on side with chair). *Positions lift efficiently and promotes smooth transfer.*
17. Lower horizontal bar to sling level by releasing hydraulic valve. Lock the valve. *Position hydraulic lift close to client. Locking valve prevents injury to client.*
18. Attach hooks to strap (chain) to holes in sling. Short chains or straps hook to top holes of sling; long chains hook to bottom of sling. *Secures hydraulic lift to sling.*
19. Elevate head of bed. *Puts the client in a sitting position.*
20. Fold client's arms over chest. *Prevents injury to paralyzed arms.*
21. Pump hydraulic handle using long, slow, even strokes until client is raised off of the bed.
22. Use steering handle to pull lift from bed and maneuver to chair. *Moves client from bed to chair.*
23. Roll base around chair. *Positions lift in front of chair to which client is to be transferred.*
24. Release valve slowly (turn to lift) and lower client into chair. *Safely guides client back as chair descends.*
25. Close valve as soon as client *is* on the chair or stretcher and straps can be released. *If valve is left open, boom may continue to lower and injure the client.*
26. Remove straps and lift. *Prevents damage to skin and underlying tissues from canvas or hooks.*
27. Check client's sitting alignment and correct if necessary. *Prevents injury from poor posture.*
28. Perform hand hygiene. *Reduces transmission of microorganisms.*
29. Evaluate client's tolerance and level of fatigue and comfort. *These clients may find transfer very fatiguing and will need posttransfer interventions to restore a level of comfort.*
30. Return client to bed using reverse method.

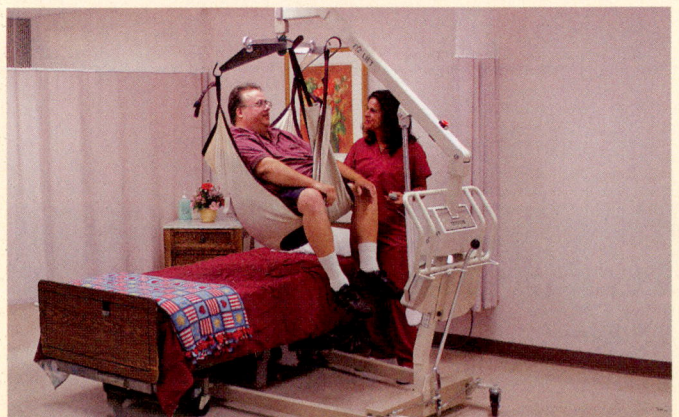

Figure 23-42. ■ Client in lift. Courtesy of EZ Way, Inc.

SAMPLE DOCUMENTATION

[date] [time] Assisted client with transfer from bed to chair with Hoyer. Ct. stated chilly outside of bed. Provided warm blanket. _____

_____ T. Tobias, LVN

PROCEDURE 23-5   # Assisting a Client to Walk

Purpose

- To provide safety for the client who is weak

Equipment

- Walking belt (optional)

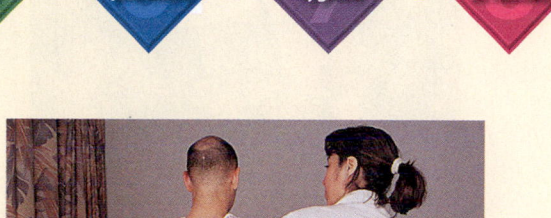

Check order + Gather equipment + Introduce yourself + Identify client + Provide privacy + Explain procedure + Hand hygiene + Gloves as needed

Interventions and Rationales

1. Perform preparatory steps (see icon bar above).

2. Prepare the client for ambulation.
   - Apply elastic (antiemboli) stockings as required. See Procedure 29-3 ⬭.
   - Assist the client to sit on the edge of the bed.
   - Assess the client carefully for signs and symptoms of orthostatic hypotension (dizziness, light-headedness, pallor, or a sudden increase in heart rate) prior to leaving the bedside.
   - Ensure that the client is appropriately dressed to walk and wears shoes or slippers with nonskid soles. *Proper attire and footwear prevent chilling and falling.*
   - Assist the client to stand by the side of the bed until the client feels secure.
   - Plan the length of the walk with the client, in light of the nursing or physician's orders. Be prepared to shorten the walk according to the person's activity tolerance.

ONE NURSE

3. Ensure client safety while assisting the client to ambulate.
   - Encourage the client to ambulate independently if the client is able, but walk beside the client.
   - Remain physically close to the client. *This gives you time to react in case assistance is needed at any point.*
   - Use a transfer or walking belt if the client is slightly weak and unstable. Make sure the belt is pulled snugly around the client's waist and fastened securely. Grasp the belt at the client's back, and walk behind and slightly to one side of the client (Figure 23-43 ■).
   - If it is the client's first time out of bed following surgery, injury, or an extended period of immobility, or if the client is quite weak or unstable, have an assistant follow you and the client with a wheelchair in case it is needed quickly.
   - If the client is moderately weak and unstable, interlock your forearm with the client's closest forearm, and walk on the client's weaker side. Encourage the client to press the forearm against your hip or waist for stability if desired. In addition, have the client wear a transfer or walking belt so that you can quickly grab the belt and prevent a fall if the client feels faint.

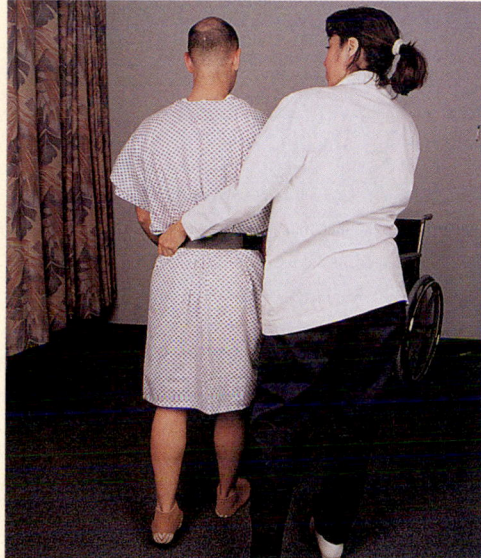

Figure 23-43. ■ Using a transfer (walking) belt to support the client. (Photographer: Elena Dorfman.)

   - If the client is very weak and unstable, place your near arm around the client's waist, and with your other arm support the client's near arm at the elbow. Walk on the client's stronger side. Again, have the client wear a transfer or walking belt in case of an emergency.
   - Encourage the client to assume a normal walking stance and gait as much as possible.

4. Protect the client who begins to fall while ambulating.
   - If a client begins to experience the signs and symptoms of orthostatic hypotension or extreme weakness, quickly assist the client into a nearby wheelchair or other chair, and help the client to lower the head between the knees. *Lowering the head facilitates blood flow to the brain.*
   - Stay with the client. *A client who faints while in this position could fall, head first, out of the chair.*
   - When the weakness subsides, assist the client back to bed.
   - If a chair is not close by, assist the client to a horizontal position on the floor before fainting occurs (Figure 23-44 ■). *A vertical position may increase feelings of faintness.*
     a. Assume a broad stance with one foot in front of the other. *A broad stance widens the nurse's base of support for*

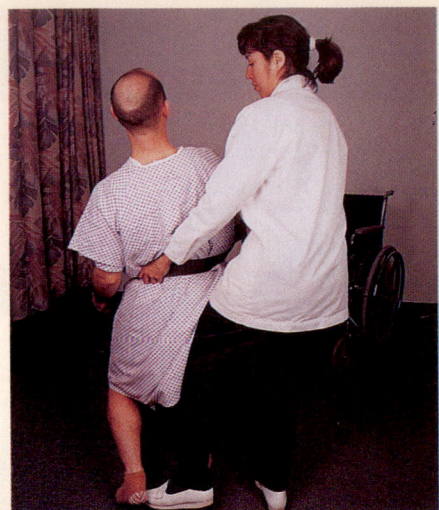

Figure 23-44. ■ Lowering a fainting client to the floor.
(Photographer: Elena Dorfman.)

stability. Placing one foot behind the other allows the nurse to rock backward and use the femoral muscles when supporting the client's weight and lowering the center of gravity (see step b), thus preventing back strain.

b. Bring the client backward so that your body supports the person. *Clients who do faint or start to fall and cannot regain their strength or balance usually drop straight downward or pitch slightly forward because of the momentum of ambulating; thus their head, hips, and knees are most vulnerable to injury. Bringing the client's weight backward against the nurse's body allows gradual movement to the floor without injury to the client.*

c. Allow the client to slide down your leg, and lower the person gently to the floor, making sure the client's head does not hit any objects.

TWO NURSES

5. Prepare the client.
   ■ See step 1 above.

6. Ensure client safety.
   ■ After the client stands, assume a position with one nurse at either side. Grasp the inferior aspect of the client's upper arm with your nearest hand and the client's lower arm or hand with your other hand (Figure 23-45 ■). *This provides a secure grip for each nurse.*
   ■ *Optional:* Place a walking belt around the client's waist. Each nurse grasps the side handle with the near hand and the lower aspect of the client's upper arm with the other hand.
   ■ Walk in unison with the client, using a smooth, even gait, at the same speed and with steps the same size as the client's. *This gives the client a greater feeling of security.*
   ■ If the client starts to fall and cannot regain strength or balance, each nurse slips an arm under the client's axillae and grasps the client's hands, and together the nurses lower the person gently to the floor or to a nearby chair

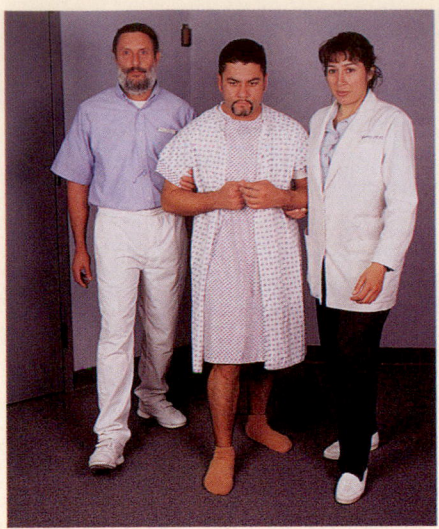

Figure 23-45. ■ Two nurses supporting an ambulatory client.
(Photographer: Elena Dorfman.)

(Figure 23-46 ■). *Placing the nurses' arms under the client's axillae evenly balances the client's weight between the two nurses, preventing injury to both the nurses and the client.*

7. Document all relevant information.
   ■ Document the time of the walk, the distance walked or time taken, and all nursing assessments.

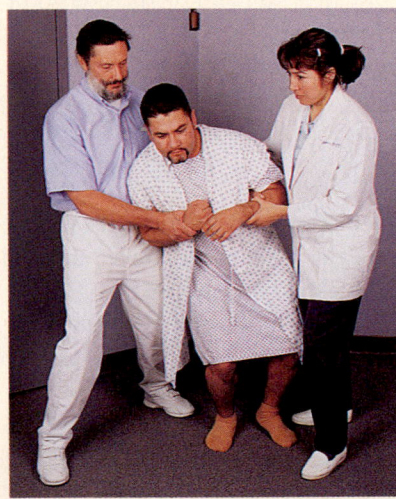

Figure 23-46. ■ Two nurses lowering a fainting client to the floor.
(Photographer: Elena Dorfman.)

SAMPLE DOCUMENTATION

[date] [time] Ambulated client from bed to nurse's station and returned. Client steady, no c/o dizziness. "Let's do more tomorrow!"

_____ E. Ketterer, LPN

PROCEDURE 23-6   Providing a Back Massage

Purposes
- To relieve muscle tension
- To promote physical and mental relaxation
- To relieve insomnia

Equipment
- Lotion or oil

Check order + Gather equipment + Introduce yourself + Identify client + Provide privacy + Explain procedure + Hand hygiene + Gloves as needed

Interventions and Rationales

1. Perform preparatory steps (see icon bar above).

2. Select an appropriate time free of interruptions and distractions.
   - Provide massage following the bath, before sleeping, and at other times as necessary to achieve relaxation and comfort for the client.
   - Assist the client to a prone or lateral position in bed. Remove the client's gown, or open the back of the gown.

3. Warm the massage lotion or oil before use. *This prevents the muscles from stiffening when it is used.*
   - Warm the lotion or oil by pouring and holding it in your hands or placing the container in warm water before applying it to the client's back. *Cold lotion may startle the client and increase discomfort.*

4. Massage the entire back. Two common types of massage strokes are **effleurage** (stroking the body; pronounced eh-flu-RAJ) and **pétrissage** (kneading or making large quick pinches of the skin, subcutaneous tissue, and muscle; pronounced PET-ri-saj).
   - Place your hands on either side of the lower spine. Using your palms and fingers, slowly massage using a circular motion and moving upward to the neck, gradually decreasing pressure as you get close to the neck. Use the circular motion over the shoulder blades and then slowly move down the lateral surface of the back (Figure 23-47 ■). *Effleurage has a relaxing, sedative effect if slow movement and light pressure are used.*
   - Repeat this massage pattern for 3 to 4 minutes.
   - Maintain contact with the skin during the massage.
   - Use your thumbs to apply friction strokes (strong circular motions).

5. Optional: Pétrissage the back and shoulders of the client.
   - Pétrissage first up the vertebral column and then over the entire back. *Pétrissage is stimulating, especially if done quickly and with firm pressure.*
   - Observe the client carefully to ensure that pétrissage does not cause pain or discomfort. *If the client grimaces or withdraws from the touch, ease the kneading pressure.*

- End the massage with long movements and tell the client you are finishing.

6. *Optional:* Effleurage and pétrissage the upper back and shoulders. *This area often experiences the most tension.*

7. Assist the client to a position of comfort.

8. Document the massage and your observations.

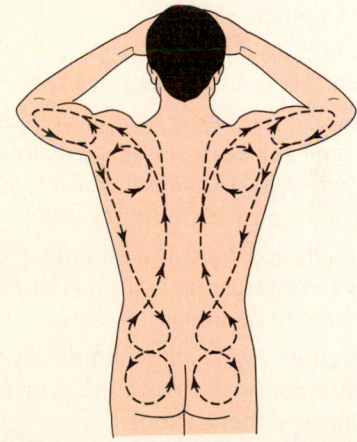

Figure 23-47. ■ A back rub pattern.

SAMPLE DOCUMENTATION

[date] [time] Client turned left laterally and placed in Sims' position w/foam wedges. Back care including effleurage to lower lumbar and sacral area. "Very relaxing." Skin intact and pink. _____

_____ J. Fontaine, LPN

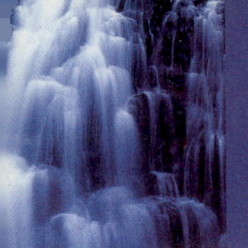

Chapter Review

KEY Points

- The ability to move freely, easily, and purposefully in the environment is essential for people to meet their basic needs.

- Purposeful coordinated movement relies on the integrated functioning of the musculoskeletal system, the nervous system, and the vestibular apparatus of the inner ear.

- Body alignment and activity are influenced by growth and development, physical health, and prescribed limitations to movement. They are also influenced by mental health, personal values, and attitudes.

- Immobility adversely affects almost every body organ and system. It also can cause psychosocial problems.

- The nurse must (1) prevent the complications of immobility and reduce the severity of any problems resulting from immobility and (2) design exercise programs for clients to promote wellness.

- Positioning a client in good body alignment and changing the position regularly and systematically are essential aspects of nursing practice.

- Safety measures must always be employed when the nurse uses a wheelchair or stretcher to move and transfer clients.

- The nurse should prepare clients for ambulation by helping them become as independent as possible while in bed. Techniques that facilitate normal walking yet provide required physical support are most effective.

- Sleep is a naturally occurring altered state of consciousness in which a person's perceptions of and reactions to the environment are decreased.

- Many factors affect sleep, including illness, age, environment, lifestyle, emotional stress, culture, alcohol, smoking, diet, motivation, and medications.

- Nursing responsibilities to help clients sleep include (1) teaching sleep hygiene, (2) supporting bedtime rituals, (3) creating a restful environment, (4) promoting comfort and relaxation, and (5) enhancing sleep with prescribed medications.

- Nonpharmacologic measures to induce and maintain sleep are always the preferred interventions.

◐ FOR FURTHER Study

Strategies for preventing strains and sprains in nurses are provided in Chapter 9.

See Chapter 16 for age-related considerations in regard to mobility.

See Chapter 24 for information on preventing and treating pressure ulcers.

See Procedure 29-3 for instructions on applying elastic (antiemboli) stockings.

See Chapter 30 for further discussion of the effects of immobility on the skin and risk for decubitus ulcer formation.

See Chapter 32 for information about oxygenation.

See Chapter 37 for more about the effects of immobility on bowel elimination.

See Chapter 39 for bladder considerations.

PEARSON

EXPLORE mynursingkit™

MyNursingKit is your one stop for online chapter review materials and resources. Prepare for success with additional NCLEX®-style practice questions, interactive assignments and activities, web links, animations and videos, and more!

Register your access code from the front of your book at
www.mynursingkit.com

Critical Thinking Care Map

Caring for a Client with Sleep Problems
NCLEX-PN® Focus Area: Physiological Integrity: Basic Care and Comfort

Case Study: Gillian Marks, 51, states she has had a problem falling asleep since her mastectomy 2 months ago. She says fears of prognosis become prominent when she is not active and busy. She has tried reading or watching TV, but neither makes her sleepy or relaxed. She appears agitated and restless. She is receiving her last radiation treatment. A decision has not been made as to the need for chemotherapy.

Nursing Diagnosis: *Disturbed Sleep Pattern: Insomnia*

COLLECT DATA

Subjective	Objective
_____	_____
_____	_____
_____	_____
_____	_____
_____	_____

Would you report this? Yes/No

If yes, report to: _____

What would you report?_____

Nursing Care

_____

_____

_____

_____

_____

_____

_____

_____

How would you document this? _____

_____

_____

_____

Compare your answers and documentation to those provided on the MyNursingKit Website.

Data Collected
(use only those that apply)

- Weight 126 lbs, 10-lb weight loss since surgery
- BP 128/86
- HR 84 and regular
- RR 16
- WBC 7,000
- H&H 12.8/36
- Skin pale; dark circles around eyes
- Surgical incision clean and healed well
- Radiation site irritated and red

Nursing Interventions
(use only those that apply; list in priority order)

- Assess client's sleep patterns and usual bedtime rituals and incorporate these into the plan of care.
- Encourage client to express feelings to others.
- Monitor client's defense mechanisms and support healthy defenses.
- Assess for signs of new onset of depression, depressed mood state, statement of hopelessness, and poor appetite.
- Expect client to meet responsibilities; give positive reinforcement.
- Observe client's medication, diet, and caffeine intake. Look for hidden sources of caffeine.
- Identify causes for and observe client's expression of sorrow.
- Advise client to avoid use of alcohol or hypnotics to induce sleep.
- Assist to resolve ambivalent feelings about illness and management of therapeutic regimen.

NCLEX-PN® Exam Preparation

TEST-TAKING TIP Data collection is the first step of the nursing process. When asked a question regarding your first or initial nursing action, select the response that deals with data collection.

1 The client tells the nurse that in physical therapy this morning the therapist kept referring to the center of gravity and asks what that means. The nurse's best response would be:

1. "The center of gravity is the point where the body's mass is centered and the base of support achieves balance."
2. "When you're standing upright, the center of gravity is just below your umbilicus, and balance is required to keep you from falling."
3. "It's an invisible line drawn from your head to your toes."
4. "It is an imaginary line drawn from left to right across your umbilicus."

2 The nurse, caring for a client confined to bed, recognizes which of the following conditions as the priority concern?

1. Contractures
2. Orthostatic hypotension
3. Osteoporosis
4. Disuse atrophy

3 The nurse, caring for a client with a sleep disorder, would not anticipate which of the following orders?

1. Electroencephalogram (EEG)
2. Electromyelogram (EMG)
3. Electro-oculogram (EOG)
4. Arterial blood gas (ABG)

4 The nurse teaches the client how to use an assistive mobility device and evaluates that further teaching is required when the client makes which of the following statements?

1. "My crutches are adjusted to the proper length if the pads are touching my underarms."
2. "I should be able to stand erect when using the crutches."
3. "I should start with small steps initially until I get comfortable with the crutches."
4. "I should replace the tips of the crutches if they become worn."

5 The nurse is caring for a client in respiratory distress and must position the client. What is the best position for reducing the client's respiratory effort?

1. Dorsal recumbent
2. Semi-Fowler's
3. Orthopneic
4. Sims

6 The nurse, working in the sleep apnea clinic, explains to a student nurse that body processes are dominated by the parasympathetic nervous system during which stage of NREM sleep?

1. Stage I
2. Stage II
3. Stage III
4. Stage IV

7 The nurse recognizes the client's stage IV sleep is decreased by which of the following conditions?

1. Hyperthyroidism
2. Respiratory conditions
3. Hypothyroidism
4. Enuresis

8 The nurse, working in a physician's office, admits a client complaining of insomnia. The nurse anticipates the first treatment will be:

1. Long-term use of sleep-inducing drugs.
2. Behavior modification.
3. Antidepressants.
4. Beta-blockers.

9 The nurse is working on a long-term care unit of an acute care facility. A priority action performed by the nurse to promote sleep and rest is:

1. Assess the client for depth of sleep during the night.
2. Schedule procedures and medications to reduce or limit interruptions.
3. Administer a sedative every night before sleep.
4. Turn off the overhead paging system.

10 A home care client has postural hypotension. The RN has recommended that the client sit in a rocking chair when out of bed. A family member questions why this is helpful. The nurse's best response would be:

1. "Using a rocking chair can strengthen leg muscle tone and enhance circulation."
2. "The rocking motion increases the blood flow to the upper body."
3. "Because she needs help to stand when in the rocking chair, there will be less danger of her falling."
4. "Sitting in the rocking chair will take her mind off her health problems and reduce her anxiety."

Answers and rationales for Review Questions appear in Appendix I.

Chapter 24

Wound Care and Skin Integrity

LEARNING Outcomes

After completing this chapter, you will be able to:

1. Name factors that affect skin integrity.
2. Define terms used to describe or to classify wounds.
3. Identify how wounds heal, the phases of wound healing, and types of wound drainage.
4. Describe factors that affect wound healing and complications that can occur.
5. List and discuss aspects of caring for wounds.
6. Compare different types of dressings used in wound care and methods of application.
7. Discuss methods of applying dry and moist heat and cold to aid wound healing.
8. Identify interventions for nursing care of clients with wounds.
9. Explain the mechanism of pressure ulcer formation, as well as risk factors and preventive measures for it.
10. Describe stages of pressure ulcer formation and methods of collecting data to assess status.
11. Discuss the nursing process in relation to clients with pressure ulcers.

Clinical Objectives

12. Obtain a culture and sensitivity (C & S) specimen from a wound.
13. Apply a dry sterile dressing.
14. Perform a dressing change using a hydrocolloid dressing.
15. Perform a wound irrigation and packing.

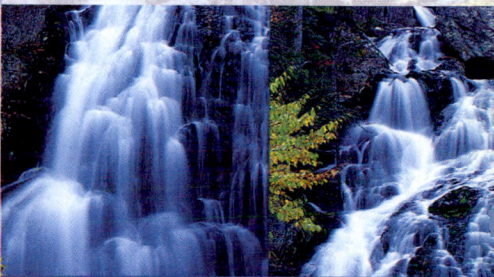

BRIEF Outline

Skin Integrity
WOUNDS
Wound Terminology
Wound Healing
Factors Affecting Wound Healing
Complications of Wound Healing
Caring for Wounds
SKIN INTEGRITY
Pressure Ulcers

The skin is the largest organ in the body. It protects the body and helps to maintain health. Nursing care of the skin includes promoting wound healing and maintaining skin integrity. Nurses must understand the physiology of wound healing. They must also be aware of risk factors of skin breakdown and specific measures to promote optimal skin conditions. Wounds and skin integrity (especially prevention and care of pressure ulcers) are two fundamental topics of nursing care.

Skin Integrity

Skin is referred to as *intact skin* when it is uninterrupted by wounds or lesions and has all normal layers. (See Chapter 30 ⚭ for a full description of skin and skin disorders.) Skin characteristics that can affect integrity (such as sensitivity to light or allergens) are governed largely by genetics.

Factors that increase risk for impaired skin integrity are aging, restricted mobility, chronic illnesses, trauma, and invasive healthcare procedures. Damage to skin can result from environmental exposure to light, heat, or cold. Age also influences skin integrity in both young and elder populations. Skin of infants and older adults is more fragile and susceptible to injury. However, wounds tend to heal much more rapidly in infants and children because of the rapid cell division that is associated with growth.

Skin integrity may be impaired in people with chronic illness, either because of the disease or because of treatment. For example, if peripheral arterial circulation is impaired, a client may have skin on the legs that lacks hair, that appears shiny and taut, and that damages easily. Clients who use steroids may develop thinning of the skin, which allows it to be damaged more easily. Certain antibiotics increase sensitivity to sunlight and can predispose a person to severe sunburns. Poor nutrition, associated with chronic illness, can interfere with the appearance and function of normal skin, as well as with healing.

WOUNDS

Wound Terminology

The nurse must be familiar with different ways of describing wounds. For example, body wounds are called *intentional traumas* if they occur during therapy. Operations and venipunctures are examples of intentional traumas that break skin integrity. Wounds may also be *unintentional* or accidental, such as broken bones from an automobile crash. Tissue that is damaged but has no break in the skin is a *closed wound*. When the skin or mucous membrane surface is broken, the wound is an *open wound*.

Wounds can be described according to the likelihood and degree of wound contamination:

- *Clean wounds* are uninfected wounds in which minimal inflammation is encountered. Clean wounds are primarily closed wounds.
- *Contaminated wounds* include open, fresh, accidental wounds and surgical wounds involving a major break in sterile technique. Contaminated wounds show evidence of inflammation.
- *Dirty* or *infected wounds* include old, accidental wounds contaminated with dead tissue and wounds with evidence

TABLE 24-1	Types of Wounds	
TYPE	**CAUSE**	**DESCRIPTION AND CHARACTERISTICS**
Incision	Sharp instrument (e.g., knife or scalpel)	Open wound; painful; deep or shallow
Contusion	Blow from a blunt instrument	Closed wound, skin appears ecchymotic (bruised) because of damaged blood vessels
Abrasion	Surface scrape, either unintentional (e.g., scraped knee from a fall) or intentional (e.g., dermal abrasion to remove pockmarks)	Open wound involving the skin; painful
Puncture	Penetration of the skin and often the underlying tissues by a sharp instrument, either intentional or unintentional	Open wound
Laceration	Tissues torn apart, often from accidents (e.g., with machinery)	Open wound; edges are often jagged
Penetrating wound	Penetration of the skin and the underlying tissues, usually unintentional (e.g., from a bullet or metal fragments)	Open wound

of a clinical infection, such as **purulent** (pus-filled) drainage.

Wounds are frequently described according to how they are acquired (Table 24-1 ■).

Wounds may be classified by depth, that is, the tissue layers involved in the wound. *Partial-thickness wounds* are confined to the skin (dermis and epidermis). *Full-thickness wounds* involve the dermis, epidermis, subcutaneous tissue, and possibly muscle and bone.

Pressure ulcers are a type of wound (usually preventable) that progresses from closed to open. They are a great concern in hospitals, in long-term care facilities, and in work with any client with impaired mobility. Pressure ulcers are discussed separately later in this chapter.

Wound Healing

Wound healing is the regeneration (renewal) of tissues. The two types of healing are distinguished by the amount of tissue loss. *Primary intention healing* (or first intention healing) occurs where the tissue surfaces have been *approximated* (closed) and there is minimal or no tissue loss. It characteristically has minimal granulation tissue and scarring. A closed surgical incision is an example of primary intention healing (Figure 24-1 ■).

A wound that is extensive and involves considerable tissue loss, and in which the edges cannot or should not be approximated, heals by *secondary intention healing*. A pressure ulcer is an example of a wound that heals by secondary intention. Secondary intention healing differs from primary intention healing in three ways: (1) The repair time is longer, (2) the scarring is greater, and (3) the risk of infection is greater.

PHASES OF WOUND HEALING

The phases of healing are the steps in the body's natural processes of tissue repair. The rate of healing varies depending on factors such as the type of healing, wound location

and size, and the health of the client. Wound healing can be broken down into three phases: inflammatory, proliferative, and maturation.

Inflammatory Phase

The inflammatory phase starts immediately after injury and lasts 3 to 6 days. Two major processes (hemostasis and phagocytosis) occur during this phase.

Hemostasis (the arrest or cessation of bleeding) results from vasoconstriction, *retraction* (drawing back) of injured blood vessels, the deposition of fibrin (connective tissue),

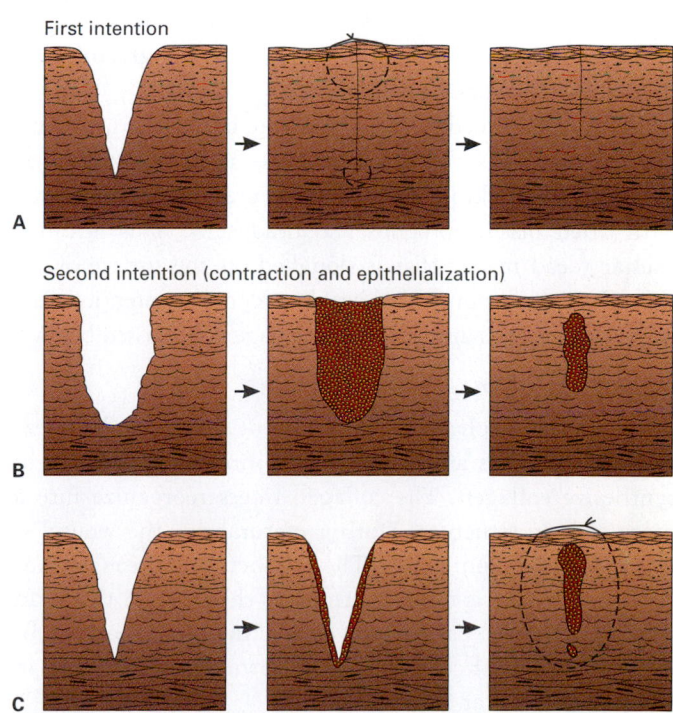

Figure 24-1. ■ Classification of wound healing: **A.** First intention: A clean incision is made with primary closure; there is minimal scarring. **B, C.** Second intention: The wound is left open so that granulation can result (B), or the wound is intentionally left open and later closed when there is no further evidence of infection (C).

and blood clot formation. The blood clots become the framework for cell repair. A scab, made of clots and dead or dying tissue, also forms on the surface of the wound. This scab aids hemostasis and helps prevent contamination of the wound by microorganisms.

During the inflammatory phase, vascular and cellular responses promote removal of foreign substances and dead or dying tissue. The blood supply to the wound increases, bringing with it substances and nutrients needed in the healing process. The area appears reddened and edematous as a result.

Macrophages (certain white blood cells) engulf microorganisms and cellular debris by a process known as **phagocytosis.** This inflammatory response is essential to healing. Measures that impair inflammation, such as use of steroid medications, can slow or prevent the healing process.

Proliferative Phase

The proliferative phase, the second phase in healing, extends from day 3 to about day 21 postinjury. *Fibroblasts* (connective tissue cells) migrate into the wound about 24 hours after injury. There they begin to synthesize collagen, a whitish protein substance that adds strength to the wound and gradually decreases the wound's chance of reopening.

Capillaries grow across the wound, increasing the blood supply, which brings oxygen and nutrients. Fibroblasts move from the bloodstream into the wound, depositing fibrin. As the capillary network develops, the tissue becomes a translucent red color. This tissue, called **granulation tissue,** is fragile and bleeds easily.

When the skin edges of a wound are not sutured, the area fills in with granulation tissue. If the wound does not close by *epithelialization* (skin formation), the area becomes covered with dried plasma proteins and dead cells. This is called **eschar** (dead matter that is sloughed off the surface of the skin). Initially, wounds that heal by secondary intention seep blood-tinged drainage. (Wound drainage is discussed below.)

Maturation Phase

The maturation phase begins on about day 21 and can extend 1 or 2 years after the injury. Fibroblasts continue to synthesize collagen. The collagen fibers reorganize into a more orderly structure. During maturation, the wound is remodeled and contracted. The scar becomes stronger, but the repaired area is never as strong as the original tissue. In some individuals, particularly dark-skinned persons, an abnormal amount of collagen is laid down. This can result in a hypertrophic scar (or **keloid**).

KINDS OF WOUND DRAINAGE

Exudate is material, such as fluid and cells, that has escaped from blood vessels during the inflammatory process and is deposited in tissue or on tissue surfaces. The nature and amount of exudate vary according to the tissue involved, the intensity and duration of the inflammation, and the presence of microorganisms.

There are three major types of exudate: serous, purulent, and sanguineous (hemorrhagic). A **serous exudate** consists chiefly of serum (the clear portion of the blood) derived from blood. It looks watery and has few cells.

A purulent exudate is thicker than serous exudate because it contains pus. **Pus** consists of leukocytes, liquefied dead tissue debris, and dead and living bacteria. The process of pus formation is referred to as **suppuration.** Purulent exudates may have tinges of blue, green, or yellow. The color may depend on the causative organism. However, not all microorganisms are *pyogenic* (pus producing).

A **sanguineous exudate** (also called *hemorrhagic*) consists of large amounts of red blood cells. This type of exudate indicates damage to capillaries that allows escape of red blood cells from the plasma. It is frequently seen in open wounds. Nurses often need to distinguish whether the sanguineous exudate is dark or bright. A bright sanguineous exudate indicates fresh bleeding. Dark sanguineous exudate denotes older bleeding. Mixed types of exudates are often observed.

When exudate is a combination of two types, the name used describes the combination. For example, wounds that heal by secondary intention initially release a watery, blood-tinged drainage called **serosanguineous** drainage.

Factors Affecting Wound Healing

AGE AND LIFESTYLE

Healthy children and adults often heal more quickly than older people. See Box 24-1 ■ for factors that inhibit wound healing in older adults.

People who exercise regularly tend to have good circulation. Because blood brings oxygen and nourishment to the wound, people who exercise are more likely to heal quickly. Smoking reduces the amount of functional hemoglobin in the blood, thus limiting the oxygen-carrying capacity of the blood.

NUTRITION

Wound healing requires a diet rich in protein, carbohydrates, lipids, vitamins A and C, and minerals, such as iron, zinc, and copper. Malnourished clients may require time to improve their nutritional status before surgery. Obese clients are at increased risk of wound infection and slower healing because *adipose* (fatty) tissue usually has a minimal blood supply.

Protein depletion can affect the rate and quality of wound healing. Protein is required as part of the inflammatory process, the immune response, and the development of

Factors That Inhibit Wound Healing in Older Adults

- Vascular changes associated with aging, such as atherosclerosis and atrophy of capillaries in the skin, can impair blood flow to the wound.
- Collagen tissue is less flexible.
- Changes in the immune system may reduce the formation of antibodies and monocytes necessary for wound healing.
- Nutritional deficiencies may reduce the numbers of red blood cells and leukocytes, thus impeding the delivery of oxygen and the inflammatory response essential for wound healing. Oxygen is needed for the synthesis of collagen and the formation of new epithelial cells.
- Scar tissue is less elastic than normal tissue. It is structurally different, being composed mostly of connective tissue made of collagen. Its density and composition can limit movement in badly damaged areas.

granulation tissue. The main protein synthesized during the healing process is collagen, and the strength of the collagen determines wound strength. Even short periods of low protein intake can significantly delay wound healing. Protein inadequacy has also been shown to affect remodeling of the wound. In extreme cases of protein deficiency, edema may develop.

During the healing process the body enters a hypermetabolic phase, requiring increased carbohydrate. When carbohydrate is insufficient, the body breaks down protein to provide glucose for cellular activity.

Vitamin C has an important role in collagen synthesis, helping in the formation of bonds between strands of collagen fiber. These bonds provide extra strength and stability to scar tissue.

Zinc is required for protein synthesis and is also a cofactor in enzymatic reactions. There is an increased demand for zinc during cell proliferation and protein secretion. Zinc also inhibits bacterial growth and is involved in the immune response.

Iron is a cofactor in collagen synthesis. Deficiency in iron delays wound healing. The major discussion of nutrition is in Chapter 25 ⬭ .

MEDICATIONS

Anti-inflammatory drugs (e.g., steroids and aspirin), heparin, and antineoplastic agents interfere with healing. Prolonged use of antibiotics may make a person susceptible to wound infection by resistant organisms.

CONTAMINATION AND INFECTION

Contamination of a wound surface with pathogenic microorganisms usually results in infection. These organisms compete with new cells for oxygen and nutrition and can impair wound healing. When the microorganisms multiply, infection occurs. Clients who are immunosuppressed (such as those with HIV or AIDS, cancer clients receiving chemotherapy, or organ recipients on immunosuppressive drugs) are especially susceptible to wound infections. Very old clients and children under age 2 years also have lesser immune function than others.

Complications of Wound Healing

HEMORRHAGE

Some escape of blood from a wound is normal. However, **hemorrhage** (persistent bleeding) is abnormal. It may be caused by a dislodged clot, a slipped suture, or erosion of a blood vessel.

- Internal hemorrhage may often be detected by swelling or distention in the area of the wound and or sanguineous drainage from a surgical drain. Some clients have a **hematoma,** a localized collection of blood underneath the skin that may appear as a reddish blue swelling.
- External hemorrhage often either appears under a dressing or escapes from the dressing and pools under the client due to gravity.

clinical ALERT

Hemorrhage is an emergency that requires the application of extra sterile pressure dressings to the area, monitoring the client's vital signs, and notifying the physician. The risk of hemorrhage is greatest during the first 48 hours after surgery.

INFECTION

A wound can be infected with microorganisms at the time of injury, during surgery, or postoperatively during open wound healing (see Chapter 10 ⬭). Wounds that occur as a result of injury (bullet and knife wounds) are most likely to be contaminated at the time of injury. Surgery involving the intestines can also result in infection from the microorganisms inside the intestine. Surgical infection is most likely to become apparent 2 to 11 days postoperatively.

DEHISCENCE WITH POSSIBLE EVISCERATION

Dehiscence is the partial or total rupturing of a sutured wound. Dehiscence usually involves an abdominal wound in which the layers below the skin also separate. **Evisceration** is the protrusion of the internal viscera through an incision. A number of factors, including obesity, poor nutrition, multiple trauma, failure of suturing, excessive coughing, vomiting, dehydration, and infection heighten a client's risk of wound dehiscence.

Caring for Wounds

LABORATORY DATA

Laboratory data often support the data the nurse collects about the wound's progress in healing. For example, if there is a decreased *leukocyte count*, healing may be delayed and the possibility of infection is increased. *Blood coagulation studies* are also significant. Prolonged coagulation times can result in excessive blood loss and prolonged clot absorption. *Serum protein analysis* provides an indication of the body's nutritional reserves for rebuilding cells. *Wound cultures* can either confirm or rule out the presence of infection. *Sensitivity studies* are helpful in selecting appropriate antibiotic therapy.

WOUND CLEANING

Wound cleaning has traditionally involved the removal of *debris* (e.g., foreign materials, excess slough, necrotic tissue, bacteria, and other microorganisms). Formerly, antimicrobial solutions such as povidone-iodine (Betadine), 3% hydrogen peroxide, 70% alcohol, and Dakin's solution were commonly used. However, these solutions have caustic effects on granulation tissue and the skin. The choices of cleaning agent and method now depend largely on agency protocol and the physician's preference.

WOUND IRRIGATION AND PACKING

An **irrigation** (also called *lavage*) is the washing or flushing out of an area. Sterile technique is required for wound irrigation, because there is a break in the skin integrity.

Using piston syringes instead of bulb syringes to irrigate a wound reduces the risk of aspirating drainage and provides safe, effective pressure. For deep wounds with small openings, a sterile straight catheter may also be necessary. Frequently used irrigation solutions are sterile normal saline, lactated Ringer's solution, and antibiotic solutions.

Gauze packing is placed in wounds to facilitate the formation of granulation tissue and healing by secondary intention. Generally, moistened 4×4 non-cotton-filled gauze dressings are used. Cotton fibers are contraindicated because they can pull loose and remain in the wound, encouraging bacterial growth and contamination.

The wet-to-damp technique is generally used to pack wounds. In this technique, moist gauzes are packed in the wound to absorb exudate, but they are not allowed to dry before removal.

WOUND DRESSINGS

Dressings are applied to wounds for the following purposes:

- To protect the wound from mechanical injury
- To protect the wound from microbial contamination
- To provide or maintain high humidity of the wound
- To provide thermal insulation
- To absorb drainage or debride a wound or both
- To prevent hemorrhage (when applied as a pressure dressing or with elastic bandages)
- To splint or immobilize the wound site and thereby facilitate healing and prevent injury
- To provide psychological comfort

Various dressing materials are available to cover wounds. The type of dressing used depends on several factors:

- The location, size, and type of the wound
- The amount of exudate
- Whether the wound requires debridement, is infected, or has sinus tracts
- Such considerations as frequency of dressing change, ease or difficulty of dressing application, and cost

Table 24-2 ■ describes materials for dressing wounds. Common gauze dressings (Figure 24-2 ■) may be applied in several ways to achieve different goals. Other dressing materials are used for specific types and conditions of wounds. Methods of applying gauze dressings are described in Table 24-3 ■.

Transparent Wound Barriers

Transparent dressings are often applied to wounds, including ulcerated or burned skin areas (Figure 24-3 ■). These dressings offer several advantages:

- They act as temporary skin.
- They are nonporous, self-adhesive dressings that do not require daily changing as other dressings do.
- They allow assessment of the wound without removal, because they are transparent.
- They are **occlusive** (closing off from the air), so the wound remains moist and retains the serous exudate, which promotes epithelial growth, hastens healing, and reduces the risk of infection.
- They are elastic, so they can be placed over a joint without disrupting the client's mobility.
- They adhere only to the skin area around the wound and not to the wound itself.
- They keep the wound moist.

TABLE 24-2	Selected Types of Wound Dressings		
DRESSING	**DESCRIPTION**	**PURPOSE**	**EXAMPLES**
Transparent adhesive films/wound barriers	Adhesive plastic, semipermeable, nonabsorbent dressings that allow exchange of oxygen between the atmosphere and wound bed. They are impermeable to bacteria and water.	To provide protection against contamination and friction; to maintain a clean moist surface that facilitates cellular migration; to provide insulation by preventing fluid evaporation; and to facilitate wound assessment.	Op-Site, Tegaderm, Bio-occlusive, ACU-derm
Impregnated nonadherent dressings	Woven or nonwoven cotton or synthetic materials that are impregnated with petrolatum, saline, zinc-saline, antimicrobials, or other agents. They require secondary dressings to secure them in place, retain moisture, and provide wound protection.	To cover, soothe, and protect partial- and full-thickness wounds without exudate.	Vaseline gauze, CarraGauze, Dermagran Wet Dressing, Xeroform
Hydrocolloids	Waterproof adhesive wafers, pastes, or powders. Wafers, designed to be worn for up to 7 days, consist of two layers. The inner adhesive layer has particles that absorb exudate and form a hydrated gel over the wound; the outer film provides a seal.	To absorb exudate; to produce a moist environment that facilitates healing but does not cause maceration of surrounding skin; to protect the wound from bacterial contamination, foreign debris, and urine or feces; and to prevent shearing.	DuoDERM, Comfeel, Tegasorb, Restore, RepliCare
Hydrogels	Glycerin or water-based, nonadhesive, jelly-like sheets, granules, or gels that are oxygen permeable, unless covered by a plastic film. They may require secondary occlusive dressing.	To liquefy necrotic tissue or slough, rehydrate the wound bed, and fill in dead space.	Aquasorb, Clear-Site, Elasto-Gel, Intra-Site, Vigilon
Polyurethane foams	Nonadherent hydrocolloid dressings that need to have their edges taped down or sealed. They require secondary dressings to obtain an occlusive environment. Surrounding skin must be protected to prevent maceration.	To absorb light to moderate amounts of exudate; to debride wounds.	LYOfoam, Allevyn, Nu-Derm, Flexzan
Exudate absorbers	Nonadherent dressings of powder, beads or granules, or paste that conform to the wound surface and absorb up to 20 times their weight in exudate. They require a secondary dressing.	To provide a moist wound surface by interacting with exudate; to form a gelatinous mass; to absorb exudate; to eliminate dead space or pack wounds; and to support debridement.	Debrisan, Triad paste, Sorbsan

- They allow the client to shower or bathe without removing the dressing.
- They can be removed without damaging wound tissue.

Part A of Procedure 24-1 ■ describes how to apply a moist transparent wound barrier.

Hydrocolloid Dressings

Hydrocolloid dressings (see Table 24-2) are frequently used over venous stasis leg ulcers and pressure ulcers. These dressings offer several advantages:

- They can last 5 to 7 days.
- They do not need a "cover" dressing and are water resistant.

- They can be molded to uneven body surfaces.
- They act as temporary skin and provide an effective bacterial barrier.
- They decrease pain and thus reduce the need for analgesics.
- They absorb some drainage and therefore can be used on draining wounds.
- They contain wound odor.

These dressings have certain limitations, however. Some of their disadvantages include the following:

- They are opaque and obscure wound visibility.
- They have a limited absorption.

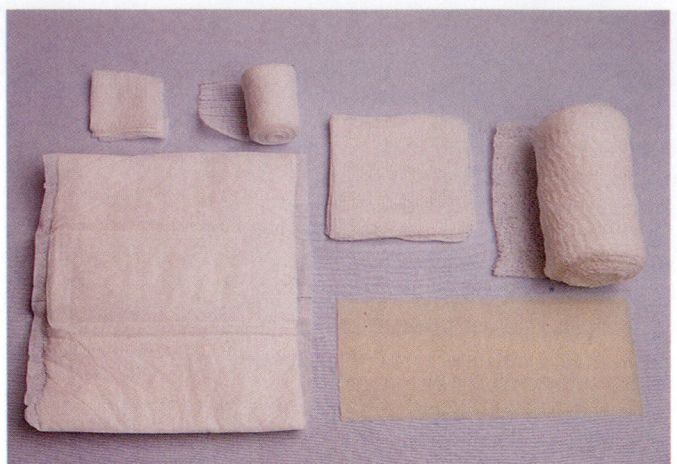

Figure 24-2. ■ Some frequently used dressing materials (clockwise from bottom left): Surgipad or abdominal pad, 2 × 2 gauze, 2-in. roller gauze, 4 × 4 gauze, 4-in. roller. (Photographer: Elena Dorfman.)

- They can facilitate anaerobic bacterial growth.
- They can soften and wrinkle at the edges with wear and movement.
- They can be difficult to remove and may leave a residue on the skin.

Hydrocolloid dressings should not be used for infected wounds or those with deep tracts or **fistulas** (abnormal passage that develops between a hollow organ and the skin or between two hollow organs). Part B of Procedure 24-1 describes how to apply hydrocolloid dressings.

Negative-Pressure Wound Therapy

Negative-pressure wound therapy (NPWT) is an advanced wound care method and treatment for chronic and acute wound types. Challenging cases of pressure ulcers, diabetic wounds, abdominal wounds, partial-thickness burns, trauma wounds, flaps, and grafts are being treated with NPWT (also called *wound vacuum* or *wound vac*). This therapy removes fluids and infectious materials; it helps promote perfusion, provides a moist healing environment, and aids in wound approximation. **Negative-pressure wound therapy** (also called *hyperbaric therapy*) is a treatment modality that provides a controlled application of subatmospheric pressure. The mechanized unit intermittently or continuously conveys negative pressure to a specialized wound dressing to promote wound healing. The resilient and foam-like dressing assists in tissue granulation and is sealed with an adhesive drape that contains the subatmospheric pressure at the wound site. The technology used regulates pressure at the wound site. The system directs drainage to a designated receptacle, reducing exposure to exudate and infectious materials. It decreases the number of dressing changes and diminishes the risk of

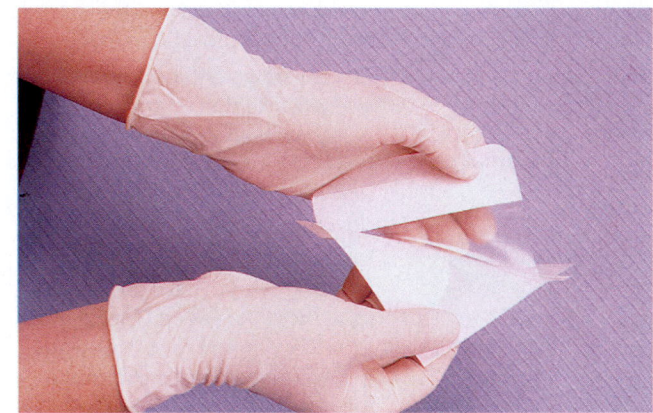

Figure 24-3. ■ A transparent wound dressing. (Photographer: Jenny Thomas.)

TABLE 24-3	Methods of Applying Gauze Dressings	
DRESSING	**DESCRIPTION**	**PURPOSE**
Dry-to-dry	A layer of wide-mesh cotton gauze lies next to the wound surface. A second layer of dry absorbent cotton or Dacron is on top.	Protect the wound. If the wound is open or draining, necrotic debris and exudates are trapped in the interstices of the gauze layer and are removed when the dressing is removed.
Wet-to-dry	Next to the wound surface is a layer of wide-mesh cotton gauze saturated with saline or an antimicrobial solution. This layer is covered by a moist absorbent material that is moistened with the same solution.	Debride the wound. Necrotic debris is softened by the solution and then adheres to the mesh gauze as it dries. It is removed when the dressing is removed. Also, moisture helps dilute viscous exudates.
Wet-to-damp	A variation of the wet-to-dry dressing, this dressing is removed before it is completely dry.	The wound is debrided when the gauze is removed.
Wet-to-wet	A layer of wide-mesh gauze saturated with antibacterial solution lies next to the wound surface. Above is a second layer of absorbent material saturated with the same solution. The entire dressing is kept moist with a wetting agent.	The wound surface is continually bathed. Moisture dilutes viscous exudate.

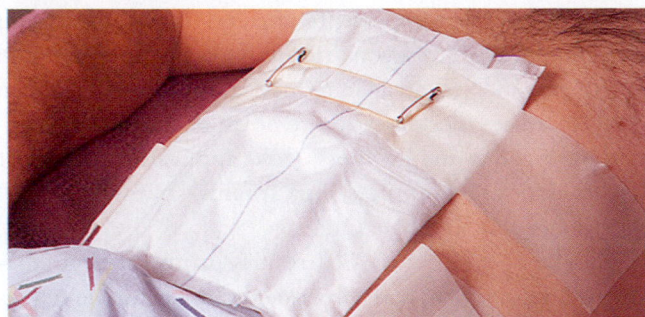

Figure 24-4. ■ Montgomery straps, or tie tapes, are used to secure large dressings that require frequent changing.

cross-contamination. Negative-pressure wound therapy is an expensive cutting edge procedure and thus is only used in the most involved cases.

Means of Securing Dressings

Dressings over wounds must cover the entire wound in order to protect it. They must also be secured so that they do not become dislodged, exposing the healing wound. The correct type of tape must be selected. For example, elastic tape can provide pressure; nonallergenic tape can be used when a client is allergic to other tape.

Montgomery straps (tie tapes) are commonly used for wounds that require frequent dressing changes (Figure 24-4 ■). These straps prevent skin irritation and discomfort caused by removing the adhesive each time the dressing is changed. The nurse can protect the skin by applying tincture of benzoin or other skin prep to the site where the adhesive is to be placed.

SUPPORTING AND IMMOBILIZING WOUNDS

Bandages and binders serve various purposes:

■ Supporting a wound (e.g., a fractured bone)
■ Immobilizing a wound (e.g., a strained shoulder)
■ Applying pressure (e.g., elastic bandages on the lower extremities to improve venous blood flow)
■ Securing a dressing (e.g., for an extensive abdominal surgical wound)
■ Retaining warmth (e.g., a flannel bandage on a rheumatoid joint)

Several types of bandages and binders are available, and they are applied in various ways. When correctly applied, they promote healing, provide comfort, and can prevent injury. Clinical guidelines for bandaging are discussed in the Nursing Care section starting on page 542.

Bandages

A **bandage** is a strip of cloth used to wrap some part of the body. Bandages are available in various widths, most commonly 1.5 to 7.5 cm (0.5 to 3 in.), and are usually supplied in rolls for easy application to a body part.

Many types of materials are used for bandages. Gauze is one of the most commonly used; it is light and porous and readily molds to the body. It is also relatively inexpensive, so it is generally discarded when soiled. Gauze is frequently used to retain dressings on wounds and to bandage the fingers, hands, toes, and feet. It supports dressings and at the same time permits air to circulate. It can also be saturated with petroleum jelly or other medications for application to wounds.

Many kinds of elasticized bandages are applied to provide pressure to an area. They are commonly used as tensor bandages or as partial stockings (TEDS). They provide support and improve the venous circulation in the legs.

The width of the bandage used depends on the size of the body part to be bandaged. The greater the circumference of a part, the wider the bandage should be. Padding (e.g., abdominal pads and gauze squares) is frequently used to cover bony prominences (e.g., the elbow) or to separate skin surfaces (e.g., the fingers).

Before applying a bandage, the nurse needs to know its purpose and to assess the area requiring support. Box 24-2 ■ lists assessment guidelines. When bandages are used to secure dressings, the nurse wears gloves to prevent contact with body fluids.

Binders

A **binder** is a type of bandage designed for a specific body part; for example, the triangular binder (sling) fits the arm. Binders are used to support large areas of the body, such as the abdomen, arm, or chest.

A triangular arm binder or *sling* is usually applied as a full triangle to support the arm, elbow, and forearm of the

---

BOX 24-2	ASSESSING CLIENTS BEFORE APPLYING BANDAGES OR BINDERS

■ Inspect and palpate the area for swelling.
■ Inspect for the presence of and status of wounds (open wounds will require a dressing before a bandage or binder is applied).
■ Note the presence of drainage (amount, color, odor, viscosity).
■ Inspect and palpate for adequacy of circulation (skin temperature, color, and sensation). Pale or cyanotic skin, cool temperature, tingling, and numbness can indicate impaired circulation.
■ Ask the client about any pain experienced (location, intensity, onset, quality).
■ Observe the ability of the client to reapply the bandage or binder when needed.
■ Note the capabilities of the client regarding activities of daily living (e.g., to eat, dress, comb hair, bathe) and assess the assistance required during the convalescence period.

client or to reduce or prevent swelling of a hand. Most agencies use commercial strap slings.

Straight abdominal binders are used to support the abdomen. A straight binder is also used to support the chest. Chest binders often have shoulder straps.

Heat and Cold Applications

Heat and cold can be useful in the healing process for closed wounds. They are applied to the body for local and systemic effects.

EFFECTS OF HEAT AND COLD. Heat causes vasodilation and increases blood flow to the affected area, bringing oxygen, nutrients, antibodies, and leukocytes. Table 24-4 ■ describes the physiological effects of heat and cold. Application of heat promotes soft tissue healing and increases suppuration. Heat is often used for clients with musculoskeletal problems such as joint stiffness from arthritis, contractures, and low back pain. Heat and cold therapies are also discussed in Chapter 31 ⚭ with musculoskeletal disorders.

A possible disadvantage of heat is that it increases capillary permeability, allowing extracellular fluid and substances such as plasma proteins to pass through the capillary walls. This may result in edema. Also, when heat is applied to a large body area, it may cause excessive peripheral vasodilation and a drop in blood pressure. A significant drop in blood pressure can cause fainting.

Cold lowers the temperature of the skin and underlying tissues and causes vasoconstriction, which reduces blood flow to the affected area. It reduces the supply of oxygen and metabolites, decreases the removal of wastes, and produces skin pallor and coolness. Cold applications are most often used for sports injuries (e.g., sprains, strains, fractures) to limit swelling and bleeding.

Prolonged exposure to cold results in impaired circulation, cell deprivation, and subsequent damage to the tissues from lack of oxygen and nourishment. The signs of tissue damage due to cold are a bluish purple mottled appearance of the skin, numbness, and sometimes blisters and pain.

Shivering is an initial, normal response to systemic cold, as the body attempts to warm itself (see also Chapter 21 ⚭). With extensive cold applications, a client's blood pressure can increase because vasoconstriction causes blood to be shunted from the cutaneous circulation to the internal blood vessels.

THERMAL TOLERANCE. Variables such as extremes of age, length of exposure, and intactness of the skin affect tolerance to heat and cold. Some body parts (such as the back of the hand and the foot) are not very temperature sensitive. Others (the neck, the inside of the wrist, the perineal area) are very sensitive to temperature. Certain conditions require added caution in the use of hot or cold applications:

- *Neurosensory impairment.* People who cannot perceive heat or cold normally are at risk for burns or tissue injury.
- *Impaired mental status.* People who are confused or have an altered level of consciousness need monitoring during applications to ensure safe therapy.
- *Impaired circulation.* People with peripheral vascular disease, diabetes, or congestive heart failure lack the normal ability to dissipate heat via the blood circulation. This puts them at risk for tissue damage with heat and cold applications.
- *Recent injury or surgery.* Immediately after injury or surgery, heat increases bleeding and swelling.

TABLE 24-4	Physiological Effects of Heat and Cold	
HEAT	**COLD**	
Vasodilation	Vasoconstriction	
Increases capillary permeability	Decreases capillary permeability	
Increases cellular metabolism	Decreases cellular metabolism	
Relaxes muscles	Relaxes muscles	
Increases inflammation; increases blood flow to an area	Slows bacterial growth; decreases inflammation	
Decreases pain by relaxing muscles	Decreases pain by numbing the area, by slowing the flow of pain impulses, and by increasing the pain threshold	
Sedative effect	Local anesthetic effect	
Reduces joint stiffness by decreasing viscosity of synovial fluids	Decreases bleeding	

■ *Open wounds.* Cold can decrease blood flow to the wound, thereby inhibiting healing.

METHODS FOR APPLYING HEAT AND COLD.   Heat can be applied to the body in both dry and moist forms. Dry heat is applied locally by means of a hot water bottle, electric pad, aquathermia pad, or disposable heat pack. Moist heat can be provided by compress, hot pack, soak, or sitz bath. (Sitz baths are described in postpartum care, Chapter 54 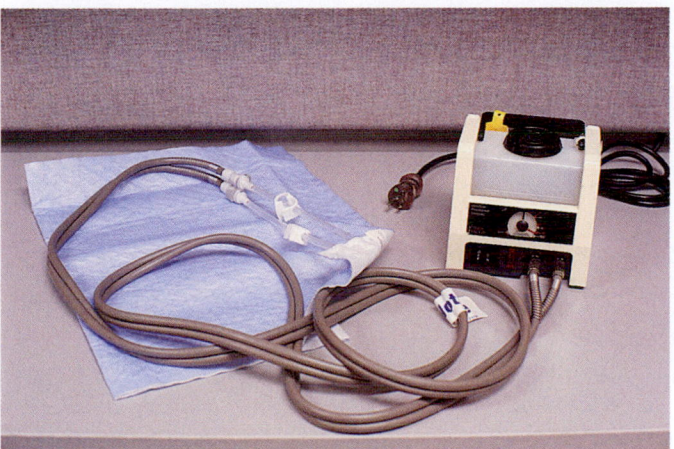.) Guidelines for nurses to follow for local applications of heat or cold are discussed in the following Nursing Care section. *Note:* A common reason for a charge of negligence is inadequate supervision of applications of heat and cold.

Aquathermia Pad.   The aquathermia or Aquamatic pad (also referred to as a K-pad) is a pad constructed with tubes containing water. The pad is attached by tubing to an electrically powered control unit that has an opening for water and a temperature gauge (Figure 24-5 ■). Some aquathermia pads have an absorbent surface through which moist heat can be applied. The other surface of the pad is waterproof. These pads are disposable.

Hot and Cold Packs.   Commercially prepared packs provide heat or cold for a designated time. Directions on the package tell how to initiate the heating or cooling process, such as by striking, squeezing, or kneading the pack.

Ice Bags, Ice Gloves, and Ice Collars.   Ice bags, ice gloves, and ice collars are filled either with ice chips or with an alcohol-based solution. They are applied to the body to provide cold to a localized area (e.g., a collar is often applied to the throat following a tonsillectomy).

Compresses.   Compresses can be either warm or cold. A *compress* is a moist gauze dressing applied to a wound. When hot compresses are ordered, the solution is heated to the temperature indicated by the order or according to agency protocol, for example, 40.5°C (105°F). When there is a break in the skin or when the body part (e.g., an eye) is vulnerable to microbial invasion, sterile technique is necessary. Sterile gloves are needed to apply the compress, and all materials must be sterile.

Soaks.   A *soak* refers to immersing a body part (e.g., an arm) in a solution or to wrapping a part in gauze dressings and then saturating the dressing with a solution. Sterile technique is generally indicated for open wounds, such as a burn or an unhealed surgical incision. Determine agency protocol regarding the temperature of the solution. Hot soaks are frequently done to soften and remove encrusted secretions and dead tissue.

Sitz Bath.   A **sitz bath** is used to soak a client's pelvic area. The client sits in a special tub or chair and is usually immersed from the mid thighs to the iliac crests or umbilicus. Special tubs or chairs are preferred because then the legs are also immersed and because a regular bathtub decreases blood circulation to the perineum or pelvic area. Disposable sitz baths are also available.

The temperature of the water should be from 40° to 43°C (105° to 110°F), unless the client is unable to tolerate the heat. Determine agency protocol. Some sitz tubs have temperature indicators attached to the water taps. The duration of the bath is generally 15 to 20 minutes, depending on the client's health. Clients with surgery in the perineal may benefit from sitz baths. The procedure for sitz baths is in the postpartum chapter, Chapter 54 .

Cooling Sponge Bath.   The purpose of a cooling sponge bath is to reduce a client's fever (see Chapter 21) by promoting heat loss through conduction and vaporization. A physician's order may be required, depending on the facility. A tepid bath uses water temperature of 32°C (90°F). An alcohol-and-water sponge bath is less commonly used than in the past because of alcohol's tendency to dry the skin. The temperatures for cooling sponge baths range from 18° to 32°C (65° to 90°F).

Hyperthermia and Hypothermia Blankets.   Hyperthermia and hypothermia blankets are used to increase or decrease a client's body temperature. The blanket has an associated control panel on which the desired temperature is set and the client's core temperature is registered. Follow institutional policy for further details.

Figure 24-5. ■ An aquathermia heating unit.

NURSING CARE

PRIORITIZING NURSING CARE

In caring for clients with wounds, the nurse must observe for characteristics of the wound and for changes (better or worse) in the wound size and overall condition (erythema, exudates, etc.). Precise documentation of wound appearance is crucial. The client's temperature should be monitored carefully as an early indicator of infection.

ASSESSING

The nurse examines the integument as part of a routine observation and assessment during regular care. During the review of systems as part of the nursing history, the nurse collects information about skin diseases, previous bruising, general skin condition, skin lesions, and usual healing of sores. Inspection and palpation of the skin focus on skin color distribution, skin turgor, presence of edema, pressure points, and characteristics of any lesions.

Untreated Wounds

Untreated wounds usually are seen shortly after an injury (e.g., at the scene of an emergency or in an emergency center). The following steps are important when assessing an untreated wound:

- Note size and severity of wound and check for associated injuries. Call for help to treat severe wounds.
- Inspect the wound for foreign bodies (soil, glass, etc.).
- If wound is contaminated with foreign material, assess need for tetanus immunization or booster.

Treated Wounds

Treated wounds, or sutured wounds, are usually assessed to determine the progress of healing. These wounds may be inspected during a dressing change unless a transparent dressing has been applied. If the wound itself cannot be inspected directly, the dressing is inspected and other data regarding the wound (e.g., the presence of pain) are assessed. Many treated wounds are covered with a transparent occlusive dressing that permits observation of the wound without exposure to the air.

Assessment of a treated wound includes observation of its appearance, size, and drainage; the presence of swelling or pain; and status of drains or tubes.

DIAGNOSING, PLANNING, AND IMPLEMENTING

Nursing diagnoses that relate to clients who have skin wounds or who are at risk for skin breakdown are:

- *Risk for Impaired Skin Integrity*
- *Impaired Skin Integrity* (commonly applies to superficial wounds extending through the epidermis but not through the dermis)
- *Impaired Tissue Integrity* (applies to wounds extending into subcutaneous tissue, muscle, or bone)
- *Risk for Infection*
- *Acute Pain* related to nerve involvement
- *Disturbed Body Image*

In planning nursing care, the primary goals are maintaining skin integrity and avoiding potential risks. For clients with *Impaired Skin Integrity* or *Impaired Tissue Integrity,* the goal is to achieve progressive wound healing and regain intact skin.

Nursing interventions for providing wound care involve supporting and immobilizing wounds, cleaning and dressing wounds, applying heat and cold, and supporting wound healing.

Maintaining Intact Skin

Besides attention to the wound area, clients with wounds need help in maintaining intact skin. Examples of nursing interventions follow:

- Inspect skin at regular intervals. *Changes in skin may indicate the beginning of breakdown or infection.*
- Keep skin clean, dry, and moisturized. *Clean, dry skin is less likely to break down; emollients provide moisture to prevent cracking.*
- Provide appropriate pressure-relieving devices and measures (Table 24-5 ■). *Prevention of pressure ulcers is a constant concern when clients are immobilized.*

Caring for Untreated Wounds

For clients with untreated wounds, the nurse performs the following interventions:

- Control severe bleeding, apply direct pressure to the wound, and elevate the extremity. *After a patent airway, bleeding is the top priority.*
- Prevent infection by cleansing or flushing abrasions or lacerations with water. Box 24-3 ■ provides guidelines for cleaning wounds. *Infection control and prevention are a major focus of nursing care.*
- If bleeding is severe or if internal bleeding is suspected, assess the client and report any signs of shock (rapid thready pulse, cold clammy skin, pallor, lowered blood pressure). *Any severe bleeding or signs of shock must be reported promptly to the supervising nurse or the physician.*
- Cover the wound with a clean dressing (a sterile dressing is preferred). If the first layer of dressing becomes saturated with blood, apply a second layer. *Removing the first layer of dressing might disturb blood clots, resulting in more bleeding.*

Supporting Wound Healing

To support wound healing, the following interventions can be performed:

- Encourage adequate fluid intake (2500 mL or more a day unless contraindicated). Provide a diet high in

TABLE 24-5	Mechanical Devices for Reducing Pressure on Body Parts
DEVICE	**DESCRIPTION/COMMENTS**
Gel flotation pads	Polyvinyl, silicone, or Silastic pads are filled with a gelatinous substance similar to fat.
Sheepskins (natural and artificial)	Some manufacturers produce mixed natural and synthetic pads; artificial pads are less likely to be damaged by washing but are more likely to make the client hot than natural skins.
Pillows and wedges (foam, gel and air, foam and fluid)	Can raise a body part (e.g., heels) off the bed surface.
Heel protectors (sheepskin boots, padded splints, foam wedges)	Limit pressure on heels when the client is in bed.
Egg-crate mattress	Polyurethane foam mattress resembling an egg crate; some types are flammable.
Foam mattress	Foam molds to the body.
Alternating pressure mattress	Composed of a number of cells in which the pressure alternately increases and decreases; uses a pump.
Water bed	Special mattress filled with water; controls temperature of water.
Air-fluidized (AF) bed (static high-air-loss bed)	Forced temperature-controlled air is circulated around millions of tiny silicone-coated beads, producing a fluid-like movement. Provides uniform support to body contours. Decreases skin maceration by its drying effect. Moisture from the client penetrates the bed sheet and soaks the beads. Airflow forces the beads away from the client and rapidly dries the sheet. A major disadvantage is that the head of the bed cannot be elevated.
Static low-air-loss (LAL) bed	Consists of many air-filled cushions divided into four or five sections. Separate controls permit each section to be inflated to a different level of firmness; thus pressure can be reduced on bony prominences but increased under other body areas for support.
Active or second-generation LAL bed	Like the static LAL, but in addition gently pulsates or rotates from side to side, thus stimulating capillary blood flow and facilitating movement of pulmonary secretions.

protein and with recommended daily vitamin content. *It is important to prevent dehydration. Adequate amounts of protein speed healing. Minimum daily amounts of vitamins should be ensured, but there is no evidence that megadoses of vitamins or minerals enhance healing.*

- Maintain infection control. *Clients need protection from microorganisms entering a wound. Clients and staff need protection from bloodborne pathogens.* (See Chapter 10 ∞ for more information about infection control.)
- Take wound cultures as needed. *A wound culture should be obtained whenever an infection is suspected.* Procedure 24-2 ■ provides guidelines for obtaining a specimen of wound drainage.
- Position clients to keep pressure off the wound. Move clients carefully to prevent shear or friction damage. *Clients with wounds may have impaired mobility, increasing the likelihood of skin breakdown.*
- Encourage the client to be as mobile as possible. *Activity enhances circulation.*
- If the client cannot move independently, implement range-of-motion exercises and a turning schedule. *These measures help to prevent skin breakdown.*

Cleaning, Irrigating, and Dressing Wounds

- Wear gloves and follow standard precautions to prevent transmission of bloodborne pathogens.
- Wash hands before and after caring for wounds. *Handwashing is the single action that is most effective against disease transmission.*
- Follow recommended guidelines for cleaning wounds (see Box 24-3). A major principle of cleaning wounds is always to clean from "clean to dirty." *Working from clean to dirty prevents the nurse from carrying microorganisms from contaminated tissue into healthy areas of the body.*
- Touch an open or fresh surgical wound only when wearing sterile gloves or using sterile forceps. Irrigate (flush out) the wound using sterile technique. *Sterile technique is required because of the break in skin integrity.* See Procedure 24-3 ■ on page 558 for the steps involved in irrigating a wound.
  - Pack the wound as ordered. Clinical guidelines for applying wet-to-damp dressings are described in Box 24-4 ■.
- Wash hands after removing gloves. *Bacteria increase in the moist environment inside a glove.*

BOX 24-3 | **NURSING CARE CHECKLIST**

Cleaning Wounds

☑ Use physiological solutions, such as isotonic saline or lactated Ringer's solution, to clean or irrigate wounds. If the physician orders antimicrobial solutions (such as Betadine), make sure they are diluted according to the physician's prescribed concentration. Ensure that saline bottles are dated when opened and that they are replaced according to facility policy, usually every 24 hours. (*Note:* Antimicrobial and antiseptic solutions are discussed in Chapter 10 ⚭.)

☑ When possible, warm the solution to body temperature before use. This prevents lowering of the wound temperature, which slows the healing process.

☑ If a wound is grossly contaminated by foreign material, bacteria, slough, or necrotic tissue, clean the wound at every dressing change. Foreign bodies and devitalized tissue act as a focus for infection and can delay healing.

☑ If a wound is clean, has little exudate, and reveals healthy granulation tissue, avoid repeated cleaning. Unnecessary cleaning can delay wound healing by traumatizing newly produced, delicate tissues, reducing the surface temperature of the wound, and removing exudate, which itself may have bactericidal properties.

☑ Use gauze squares for cleaning. Avoid using cotton balls and other products that shed fibers onto the wound surface. The fibers become embedded in granulation tissue and can act as foci for infection. They may also stimulate "foreign body" reactions, prolonging the inflammatory phase of healing and delaying the healing process.

☑ Clean superficial noninfected wounds by irrigating them with normal saline. The hydraulic pressure of an irrigating stream of fluid dislodges contaminating debris and reduces bacterial colonization.

☑ To retain wound moisture, avoid drying a wound after cleaning it.

■ *Note:* Removal of sutures and staples is discussed in care of the client after surgery, in Chapter 29 ⚭.

Securing Dressings

■ Ensure that the dressing covers the entire wound and select the appropriate tape to secure it. *Microorganisms can be introduced into wounds that are not completely covered.*

■ Place the tape so that the dressing cannot be folded back to expose the wound. Place strips at the ends of the dressing, and space tapes evenly in the middle (Figure 24-6 ■). *This placement prevents the wound from being exposed to airborne microorganisms.*

■ Ensure that the tape is long and wide enough to adhere to several inches of skin on each side of the dressing, but

BOX 24-4 | **NURSING CARE CHECKLIST**

Applying Wet-to-Damp Dressings

☑ Open the packages of the sterile dressing set, fine-mesh gauze, and sterile solution container.

☑ Pour the ordered solution into the solution container.

☑ Place the fine-mesh gauze dressings into the solution container, and thoroughly saturate them with solution. *The entire gauze must be moistened to enhance its absorptive abilities.*

☑ If agency protocol indicates, clean the wound.

☑ Wring out the packing material so that it is slightly moist. Avoid packing that is too wet. *An excessively wet wound bed creates an environment for bacterial growth and may macerate the surrounding skin.*

☑ Pack the moistened dressings into all depressions and grooves of the wound, ensuring that all exposed surfaces are covered. If necessary, use forceps to feed the gauze gradually into deep depressed areas. *Necrotic tissue is usually more prevalent in depressed wound areas and needs to be covered with gauze.*

☑ Avoid applying packing too tightly. *A tight application inhibits wound edges from contracting and compresses capillaries.*

☑ Pack only to the edge of the wound and do not overlap intact skin. *This prevents maceration of the surrounding skin.*

☑ If necessary, protect surrounding skin with a skin barrier (e.g., hydrocolloid dressing). *Sensitive skin may require extra protection.*

☑ Apply a secondary dressing (e.g., 4 × 4 gauze) over the wet dressings. *The secondary dressing will absorb excess exudate.*

☑ Cover all the dressings with a Surgipad or abdominal pad. *The pad protects the wound from external contaminants.*

☑ Remove gloves inside out and discard them. *This is proper procedure to prevent spread of pathogens.*

☑ To remove dressings, wear disposable gloves. If packing material adheres to any tissue during removal, soak it with normal saline. *Soaking facilitates removal and prevents tearing of new granulation tissue.*

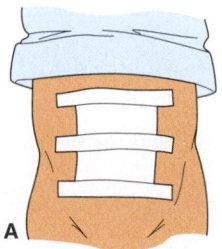 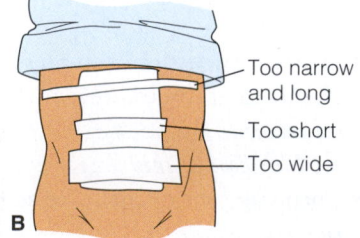

Figure 24-6. ■ The strips of tape should be placed at the ends of the dressing and must be sufficiently long and wide to secure the dressing. The tape should adhere to intact skin.

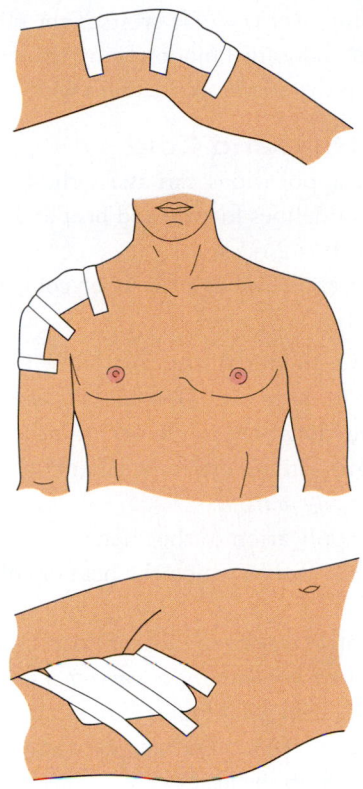

Figure 24-7. ■ Dressings over moving parts must remain secure in spite of the movement. Place the tape over a joint at a right angle to the direction the joint moves.

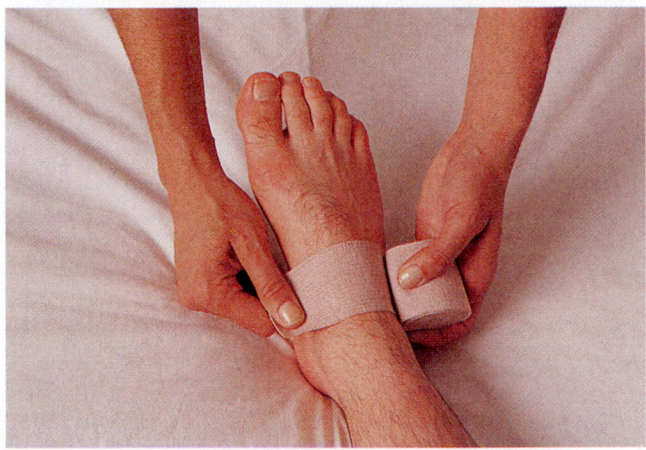

Figure 24-8. ■ Starting a bandage with two circular turns.

not so long or wide that the tape loosens with activity. *Firm coverage ensures protection.*

- Place the tape in the opposite direction from expected body action (Figure 24-7 ■). *This will prevent the tape from loosening or falling off.*

Applying Bandages and Binders

General guidelines for bandaging include the following interventions:

- Bandage the part in its normal position, with the joint flexed slightly. *This avoids putting strain on the ligaments and muscles of the joint.*
- Pad between skin surfaces and over bony areas. *This prevents friction and abrasion of the skin.*
- Bandage body parts from the distal to the proximal end. *This aids the return of venous blood.*
- If possible, leave the end of the body part (e.g., a toe) exposed. *This allows visual assessment of blood circulation to the extremity.*
- Cover the dressings with bandages at least 5 cm (2 in.) beyond the edges of the dressing. *This prevents the dressing and wound from becoming contaminated.*
- Face the client when applying the bandage. *This maintains uniform tension and alignment of the bandage.*

Circular turns are used chiefly to anchor bandages or to bandage certain areas, such as the proximal aspect of a finger or a wrist. Circular turns for roller bandages are done as follows:

- Apply the end of the bandage to the part of the body to be bandaged.
- Wrap the bandage around the body part a few times or as often as needed, each turn directly covering the previous turn (Figure 24-8 ■). This provides even support to the area. It is important not to wrap the bandage tightly, since that might impede circulation.
- Secure the end of the bandage with tape, metal clips, or a safety pin over an uninjured area. Clips and pins can be uncomfortable when situated over an injured area. When securing with tape, do not encircle the limb; in doing so, the circulation could be impaired.

Figure-eight turns are used to bandage an elbow, knee, or ankle, because they permit some movement after application. To apply a figure-eight turn with a roller bandage, follow these steps:

- Anchor the bandage with two circular turns.
- Carry the bandage above the joint, around it, and then below it, making a figure eight (Figure 24-9 ■).
- Continue above and below the joint, overlapping the previous turn by two-thirds the width of the bandage.
- End the bandage above the joint with two circular turns, and secure the end appropriately.

Binders are also sometimes called slings. To apply a large arm sling:

- Place one end of the unfolded triangular binder over the shoulder of the uninjured side so that the binder falls

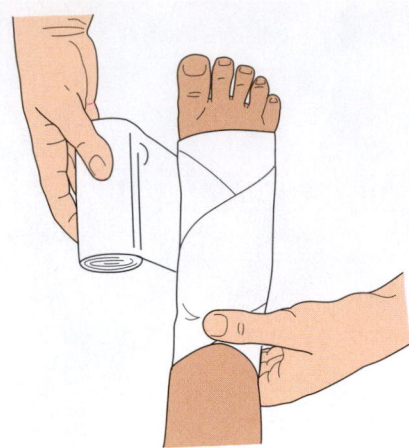

Figure 24-9. ■ Applying a figure-eight bandage.

down the front of the chest of the client with the point of the triangle (apex) under the elbow of the injured side.

- Take the upper corner, and carry it around the neck until it hangs over the shoulder on the injured side (Figure 24-10 ■). See also Procedure 47-1 for applying a sling.
- Bring the lower corner of the binder up over the arm to the shoulder of the injured side. Using a square knot, secure this corner to the upper corner at the side of the neck on the involved side.
- Fold the sling neatly at the elbow, and secure it with safety pins or tape. It may be folded and fastened at the front.

Straight abdominal binders are also useful. To apply straight abdominal binders, follow these steps:

- With the client in a supine position, place the abdominal binder smoothly under the client, with the upper border of the binder at the waist and the lower border at the level of the gluteal fold. *A binder placed above the waist can interfere with respiration. One placed too low can interfere with elimination and walking.*

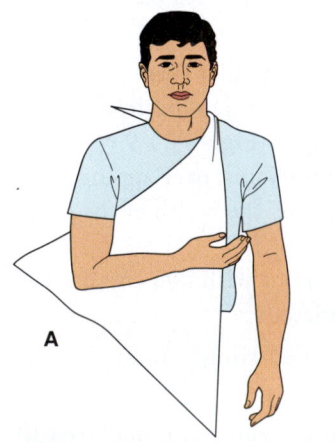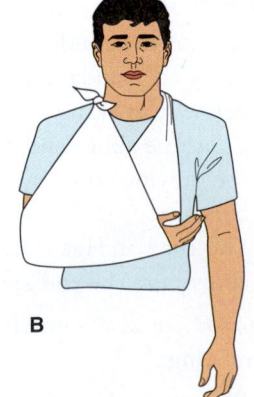

A   **B**

Figure 24-10. ■ Large arm sling.

- Apply padding over the iliac crests if the client is thin.
- For a straight abdominal binder, bring the ends around the client, overlap them, and secure them with pins or Velcro.

Applying Heat and Cold

Heat and cold applications can assist the healing process. Nursing care guidelines for selected heat and cold therapies are provided in Box 24-5 ■.

For all local applications of heat or cold, the following guidelines apply:

- Determine the client's ability to tolerate the therapy. *Some clients have an increased sensitivity to heat or cold.*
- Identify conditions that might contraindicate treatment (e.g., bleeding, circulatory impairment). *This protects the client from damage to tissue.*
- Explain the application to the client.
- Assess the skin area to which the heat or cold will be applied.
- Ask the client to report any discomfort. *Feedback will allow adjustments in placement or amount of heat or cold.*
- Return to the client 15 minutes after starting the heat or cold, and observe the local skin area for any untoward signs (e.g., redness). Stop the heat or cold if any problems occur.
- Remove the equipment at the designated time, and dispose of it appropriately. *Excess heat or cold can damage skin tissue.*
- Examine the area to which the heat or cold was applied, and record the client's response. *This contributes to ongoing, quality care.*

EVALUATING

To judge whether client outcomes have been achieved, the nurse uses data collected during care, such as skin status over bony prominences and perineal area, nutritional and fluid intake, mental status, and signs of healing if an ulcer is present. If outcomes are not achieved, the nurse should explore the reasons why:

- Has the client's physical condition changed?
- Were risk factors correctly identified?
- Were appropriate lifting devices and techniques used?
- Was the repositioning schedule adhered to?
- Are the client's nutritional and fluid intake adequate?

Continuity of Care

Before discharging the client, the nurse reviews the process of wound care and makes sure the client or family understands how to change a dressing and how frequently. The client should know what normal healing looks like. The nurse provides written instructions with a list of signs that might indicate infection or complication. The nurse ensures that the client understands when to notify the physician of a potential problem.

BOX 24-5	NURSING CARE CHECKLIST

Selected Heat and Cold Applications

Aquathermia Pad

☑ Fill the reservoir of the unit two-thirds full of distilled water.

☑ Set the desired temperature. Check the manufacturer's instructions. Most units are set at 40.5°C (105°F) for adults.

☑ Cover the pad and plug in the unit. Some manufacturers suggest warming the pad before applying it.

☑ Apply the pad to the body part. The treatment is usually continued for 10 to 15 minutes. Check orders and agency protocol.

Ice Bag, Glove, or Collar

☑ Always wrap the container in a cloth or towel before applying.

Sitz Bath

☑ Assist the client into the tub. Provide support for the client's feet; a footstool can prevent pressure on the backs of the thighs.

☑ Provide a bath blanket for the client's shoulders, and eliminate drafts to prevent chilling.

☑ Observe the client closely during the bath for signs of faintness, dizziness, weakness, accelerated pulse rate, and pallor.

☑ Maintain the water temperature.

☑ Following the sitz bath, assist the client out of the tub. Help the client to dry.

Cooling Sponge Bath

☑ Determine the client's vital signs (i.e., TPR).

☑ Protect the client's bed with moisture-proof material.

☑ Sponge the face, arms, legs, back, and buttocks. The chest and abdomen are not usually sponged. Each area is sponged slowly and gently. Rubbing may increase heat production.

☑ Leave each area wet, and cover with a damp towel.

☑ Place ice bags and cold packs, if used, or a cool cloth on the forehead for comfort and in each axilla and at the groin. These areas contain large superficial blood vessels that help the transfer of heat.

☑ Sponge one body part and then another. The sponge bath should take about 30 minutes. A bath given more quickly tends to increase the body's heat production by causing shivering.

☑ Discontinue the bath if the client becomes pale or cyanotic or shivers, or if the pulse becomes rapid or irregular.

☑ Pat each area dry.

☑ Reassess the vital signs at 15 minutes and after completing the sponge bath.

SKIN INTEGRITY

The structure of normal skin and disorders that affect it are discussed in depth in Chapter 30 🔗. Because they constitute a wound with serious consequences to the client's overall health, pressure ulcers are discussed here.

Pressure Ulcers

Decubitus ulcers, *pressure sores*, or *bed sores* are **pressure ulcers,** lesions caused by unrelieved pressure that results in damage to underlying tissue. Pressure ulcers are a significant problem whenever clients are immobilized (acute care, long-term care, and home settings).

Pressure ulcers are caused by localized **ischemia,** a deficiency in the blood supply to the tissue. The tissue is caught between two hard surfaces, usually the surface of the bed and the bony skeleton. When blood cannot reach the tissue, the cells are deprived of oxygen and nutrients, and waste products accumulate in the cells. Prolonged, unrelieved pressure damages the small blood vessels, and the tissue eventually dies.

Pressure ulcers usually occur over bony prominences. After the skin has been compressed, it appears pale. When pressure is relieved, the skin takes on a bright red flush, called **reactive hyperemia.** The flush is due to vasodilation; extra blood floods to the area to compensate for the impeded blood flow. If the redness disappears, no tissue damage can be anticipated. If the redness does not disappear, then tissue damage has occurred.

Besides pressure, two other factors often produce pressure ulcers: friction and shearing force. **Friction** is a force acting parallel to the skin surface. For example, sheets rubbing against skin create friction. Friction can remove the superficial layers, making the skin more prone to breakdown.

Shearing force is a combination of friction and pressure (Figure 24-11 ■). It occurs commonly when a client assumes a Fowler's position in bed. The body slides down toward the foot of the bed, but the skin over the sacrum tends not to move. The skin and superficial tissues are held by the bed surface, but the deeper tissues attached to the skeleton move downward. The shearing force occurs where the

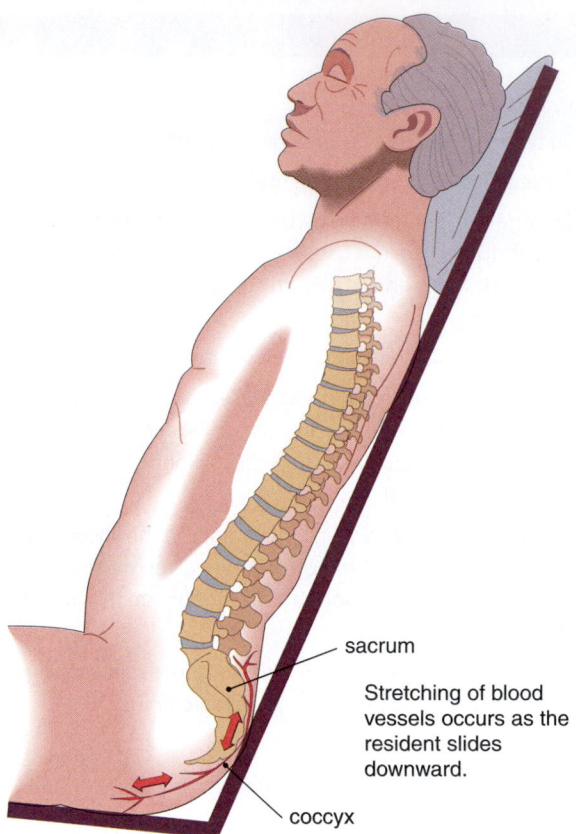

sacrum

Stretching of blood vessels occurs as the resident slides downward.

coccyx

Figure 24-11. ■ Shearing force can pull blood vessels at an angle, leading to impaired skin integrity.

deeper tissues and the superficial tissues meet. The force damages blood vessels and tissues in this area.

RISK FACTORS FOR FORMATION OF PRESSURE ULCERS

Several factors contribute to the formation of pressure ulcers:

■ *Immobility*. Immobility and inactivity are important risk factors for pressure ulcers. Immobility refers to a reduction in the amount of movement a person has. Paralysis, extreme weakness, or any cause of decreased activity can hinder a person's ability to change positions independently and relieve the pressure.

■ *Inadequate nutrition*. Nutritional factors are crucial in the development of pressure ulcers. Generally, prolonged inadequate nutrition causes weight loss, anemia, muscle atrophy, and the loss of subcutaneous tissue. Reduction in padding between the skin and the bones increases the risk of pressure sore development. Inadequate intake of protein, carbohydrates, fluids, and vitamin C specifically contributes to pressure ulcer formation.

■ *Edema*. The presence of excess fluid in the tissues, or edema, makes skin more prone to injury by decreasing its elasticity and resilience.

■ *Fecal and urinary incontinence*. Moisture from incontinence promotes skin **maceration** (softening of tissue by prolonged wetting) and makes the epidermis susceptible to injury. Digestive enzymes in feces also contribute to skin excoriation. Any accumulation of secretions or excretions is irritating to the skin, harbors microorganisms, and makes an individual prone to skin breakdown and infection.

■ *Decreased mental status*. Individuals with a reduced level of awareness and those who are unconscious or heavily sedated are at risk for pressure ulcers. They are less able to recognize and respond to pain associated with prolonged pressure.

■ *Diminished sensation*. Paralysis, or other neurologic disease causing loss of sensation, reduces a person's ability to respond to damaging levels of heat and cold and to feel the tingling ("pins and needles") that signals loss of circulation.

■ *Excessive body heat*. Body heat is another factor in the development of pressure sores. An elevated body temperature increases the body's metabolic rate, increasing the need for cellular oxygen. This increased need is severe in the cells of an area under pressure, which are already oxygen deficient. Severe infections with accompanying elevated body temperatures may affect the body's ability to deal with the effects of tissue compression.

■ *Advanced age*. The aging process can make older people more prone to impaired skin integrity. Older adults may be prone to loss of lean body mass, generalized thinning and dryness of the epidermis, and decreased strength and elasticity of the skin. They may have diminished pain perception due to decreased sensation of pressure and light touch. (See also Box 24-1.)

■ *Other factors*. Poor lifting techniques, incorrect positioning, repeated injections in the same area, hard support surfaces, and incorrect application of pressure-relieving devices also contribute to the formation of pressure sores.

PREVENTION OF PRESSURE ULCERS

The Center for Medicare and Medicaid is working with public health and infectious disease experts from the CDC to identify a list of hospital-acquired conditions. Pressure or decubitus ulcers were one of eight preventable events identified (others include falls and catheter-associated infections) as top priority for change.

Every year approximately 60,000 deaths result from pressure sores that developed during hospitalizations. In addition, pressure ulcers interfere with recovery, lengthen hospital stays, cause extreme pain and discomfort, and can increase the risk of infection. In acute-care hospitals, where clients stay for much shorter periods, prevention has been sporadic compared to the strides by long-term-care facilities.

The National Pressure Advisory Panel has updated its definition of the original four "stages" used to diagnose pressure ulcers, and added two new stages on deep-tissue injury and unstageable pressure ulcers. Hospitals are now required to track pressure ulcers present on admission and those that are facility acquired. As of October 1, 2008, in order to get the higher DRG payment, the presence of a PU on admission must be documented by a physician within 24 to 48 hours. Medicare and Medicaid Services will no longer reimburse hospitals for hospital-acquired pressure ulcers (Black et al., 2007).

Supportive Devices to Prevent Pressure Ulcers

For clients confined to bed, special support surfaces and positioning devices can be used to protect bony prominences. Three types of support surfaces can be used to relieve pressure.

- The *overlay mattress* or egg-crate mattress is a molded foam piece applied on top of the standard bed mattress.
- A *replacement mattress* is a mattress, usually made of foam and gel combinations, that replaces the standard mattress.
- A *specialty bed* is a replacement for hospital beds. Specialty beds, such as the alternating pressure mattress or active low-air-loss beds shown in Figure 24-12 ■, can provide pressure relief, eliminate shearing and friction, and decrease moisture. (See Table 24-5 for selected mechanical devices for reducing pressure on body parts.)

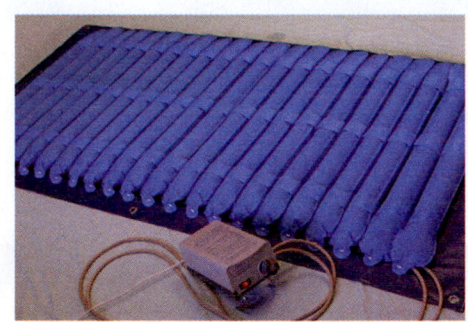

A

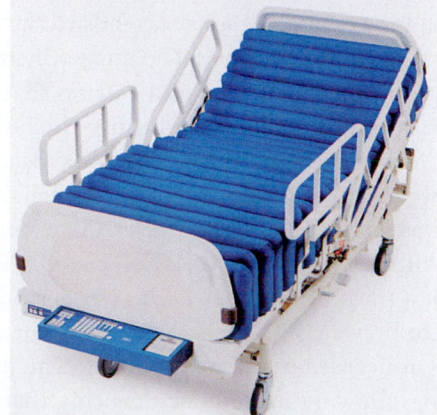

B

Figure 24-12. ■ A. An alternating pressure mattress provides comfort and helps distribute body weight evenly. (Courtesy of Ease.) **B.** Active low-air-loss beds pulsate or rotate from side to side. *Note:* KinAir MedSurg® courtesy of KCL Licensing, Inc., San Antonio, TX.

When a client is confined to bed or to a chair, pressure-reducing devices, such as pillows made of foam, gel, air, or a combination of these, can be used. When the client is sitting, weight should be distributed over the entire seating surface so that pressure does not center on just one area. To protect a client's heels in bed, supports such as wedges or pillows can be used to raise the heels completely off the bed. Doughnut-type devices should not be used (Panel for the Prediction and Prevention of Pressure Ulcers in Adults [PPPPUA], 1994).

STAGES OF PRESSURE ULCER FORMATION

The four stages in pressure ulcer formation relate to observable tissue damage (Figure 24-13 ■ and Figure 24-14 ■):

- *Stage I:* Nonblanchable erythema of intact skin.
- *Stage II:* Partial-thickness skin loss involving epidermis, dermis, or both. The ulcer is superficial and presents as an abrasion, blister, or shallow crater.
- *Stage III:* Full-thickness skin loss involving damage or necrosis of subcutaneous tissue that may extend down to, but not through, underlying fascia. The ulcer presents as a deep crater with or without undermining of adjacent tissue.
- *Stage IV:* Full-thickness skin loss with extensive destruction, tissue necrosis, or damage to muscle, bone, or supporting structures, such as a tendon or joint capsule. Undermining and sinus tracts may also be associated with stage IV pressure ulcers.

The National Pressure Ulcer Advisory Panel has recommended that two new stages be added to the current four. The first would precede Stage 1 and the other will follow stage 4. The are described in the following manner:

- *(Suspected) Deep Tissue Injury:* Purple or maroon localized area of discolored intact skin or blood-filled blister due to

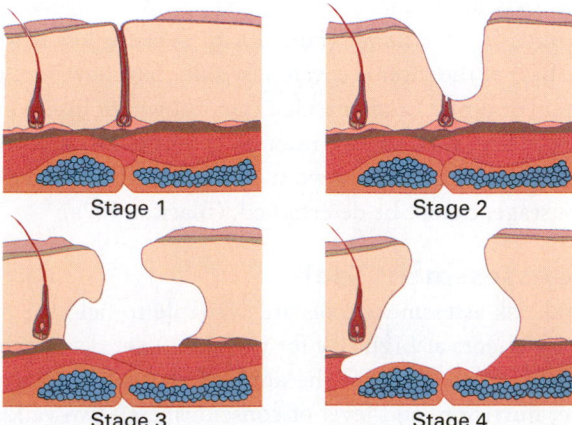

Stage 1

Stage 2

Stage 3

Stage 4

Figure 24-13. ■ Four stages of pressure ulcers. (*Source:* U.S. Department of Health and Human Services, PPPPUA, *Clinical Practice Guideline, Pressure Ulcers in Adults: Prediction and Prevention* AHCPR, Publication No. 92-0047, Rockville, MD: Public Health Service, 1992, p. 8.)

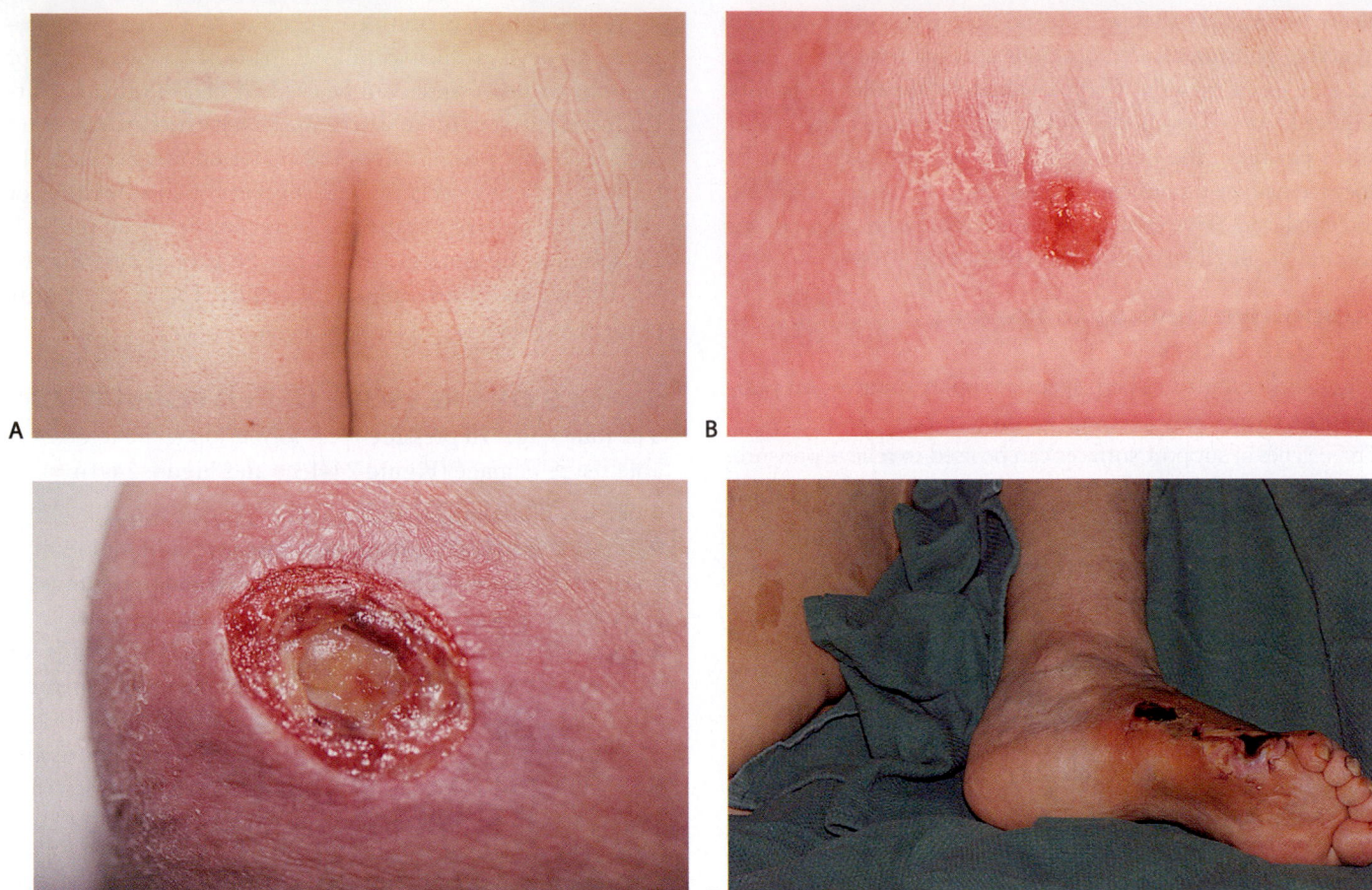

Figure 24-14. ■ The four stages of a decubitus ulcer: **A.** stage I—nonblanchable erythema signaling potential ulceration; **B.** stage II—abrasion, blister, or shallow crater involving the epidermis and possibly the dermis; **C.** stage III—deep ulcer exhibiting necrotic tissue and extending through the subcutaneous layer; **D.** stage IV—tissue necrosis and damage involving muscle, bone, or supporting structures. (**D.** © Caliendo/Custom Medical Stock Photo, Inc.)

damage of underlying soft tissue from pressure and/or shear. The change may be preceded by tissue that is painful, firm, mushy, boggy, or warmer or cooler than adjacent tissue.

■ *Unstageable Tissue Injury:* Full-thickness tissue loss in which the base of the ulcer is covered by slough (tallow, tan, gray, green, or brown) and/or eschar (tan, brown, or black) in the wound bed. Until enough slough and/or eschar is removed to expose the base of the wound, the true depth, and therefore stage, cannot be determined. (Black, 2007a)

Risk Assessment Tools

Several risk assessment tools are available to help the nurse identify clients at high risk for pressure ulcer development. Data collection includes the areas of immobility, incontinence, nutrition, and level of consciousness. Two validated assessment tools are the Braden scale (Figure 24-15 ■) and the Norton scale (Table 24-6 ■). These scales include subscales and categories that are assigned points. Scores of 16 or lower may be indicators of potential risk.

NURSING CARE

PRIORITIZING NURSING CARE

To maintain intact skin, the nurse attends to the client and checks pressure points regularly. The nurse adheres to turning and repositioning schedules and ensures that restraints are removed at frequent intervals, during which skin care is provided. When pressure breakdown has occurred, the nurse follows strict precautions to provide sterile care to the wound and assist healing. As of April 2008, Medicare and Medicaid will not reimburse costs associated with the acquisition of a pressure ulcer. It is the responsibility of the LPN/LVN to prevent skin breakdown. It is not enough to delegate to unlicensed assistive personnel. The nurse is responsible for following up and documenting that appropriate turning and skin care has been carried out. Once a client has been medicated, the sleep cycle is disturbed and the client will need to be turned and positioned. A turning clock can be placed on the door as a reminder to all staff.

BRADEN SCALE FOR PREDICTING PRESSURE SORE RISK

Client's Name _____   Evaluator's Name _____   Date of Assessment

SENSORY PERCEPTION — Ability to respond meaningfully to pressure-related discomfort	**1. Completely Limited:** Unresponsive (does not moan, flinch, or grasp) to painful stimuli, due to diminished level of consciousness or sedation, OR limited ability to feel pain over most of body surface.	**2. Very Limited:** Responds only to painful stimuli. Cannot communicate discomfort except by moaning or restlessness, OR has a sensory impairment which limits the ability to feel pain or discomfort over 1/2 of body.	**3. Slightly Limited:** Responds to verbal commands but cannot always communicate discomfort or need to be turned, OR has some sensory impairment which limits ability to feel pain or discomfort in 1 or 2 extremities.	**4. No Impairment:** Responds to verbal commands. Has no sensory deficit which would limit ability to feel or voice pain or discomfort.
MOISTURE — Degree to which skin is exposed to moisture	**1. Constantly Moist:** Skin is kept moist almost constantly by perspiration, urine, etc. Dampness is detected every time patient is moved or turned.	**2. Moist:** Skin is often but not always moist. Linen must be changed at least once a shift.	**3. Occasionally Moist:** Skin is occasionally moist, requiring an extra linen change approximately once a day.	**4. Rarely Moist:** Skin is usually dry; linen requires changing only at routine intervals.
ACTIVITY — Degree of physical activity	**1. Bedfast:** Confined to bed.	**2. Chairfast:** Ability to walk severely limited or nonexistent. Cannot bear own weight and/or must be assisted into chair or wheelchair.	**3. Walks Occasionally:** Walks occasionally during day but for very short distances, with or without assistance. Spends majority of each shift in bed or chair.	**4. Walks Frequently:** Walks outside the room at least twice a day and inside room at least once every 2 hours during waking hours.
MOBILITY — Ability to change and control body position	**1. Completely Immobile:** Does not make even slight changes in body or extremity position without assistance.	**2. Very Limited:** Makes occasional slight changes in body or extremity position but unable to make frequent or significant changes independently.	**3. Slightly Limited:** Makes frequent though slight changes in body or extremity position independently.	**4. No Limitations:** Makes major and frequent changes in position without assistance.
NUTRITION — Usual food intake pattern	**1. Very Poor:** Never eats a complete meal. Rarely eats more than 1/3 of any food offered. Eats 2 servings or less of protein (meat or dairy products) per day. Takes fluids poorly. Does not take a liquid dietary supplement, OR is NPO and/or maintained on clear liquids or IV's for more than 5 days.	**2. Probably Inadequate:** Rarely eats a complete meal and generally eats only about 1/2 of any food offered. Protein intake includes only 3 servings of meat or dairy products per day. Occasionally will take a dietary supplement, OR receives less than optimum amount of liquid diet or tube feeding.	**3. Adequate:** Eats over half of most meals. Eats a total of 4 servings of protein (meat, dairy products) each day. Occasionally will refuse a meal, but will usually take a supplement if offered, OR is on a tube feeding or TPN regimen, which probably meets most of nutritional needs.	**4. Excellent:** Eats most of every meal. Never refuses a meal. Usually eats a total of 4 or more servings of meat and dairy products. Occasionally eats between meals. Does not require supplementation.
FRICTION AND SHEAR	**1. Problem:** Requires moderate to maximum assistance in moving. Complete lifting without sliding against sheets is impossible. Frequently slides down in bed or chair, requiring frequent repositioning with maximum assistance. Spasticity, contractures, or agitation leads to almost constant friction.	**2. Potential Problem:** Moves feebly or requires minimum assistance. During a move skin probably slides to some extent against sheets, chair, restraints, or other devices. Maintains relatively good position in chair or bed most of the time but occasionally slides down.	**3. No Apparent Problem:** Moves in bed and in chair independently and has sufficient muscle strength to lift up completely during move. Maintains good position in bed or chair at all times.	

Total Score

Figure 24-15. ■ Braden Scale for Predicting Pressure Sore Risk. (*Source:* U.S. Department of Health and Human Services, *Clinical Practice Guideline, Pressure Ulcers in Adults: Prediction and Prevention,* Publication No. 92-0047, Rockville, MD: Public Health Service, 1992, pp. 16–17. Copyright © Barbara Braden and Nancy Bergstrom, 1988. Reprinted with permission.)

TABLE 24-6		Norton's Pressure Area Risk Assessment Form (Scoring System)							
GENERAL PHYSICAL CONDITION		**MENTAL STATE**		**ACTIVITY**		**MOBILITY**		**INCONTINENCE**	
Good	4	Alert	4	Ambulatory	4	Full	4	Absent	4
Fair	3	Apathetic	3	Walks with help	3	Slightly limited	3	Occasional	3
Poor	2	Confused	2	Chairbound	2	Very limited	2	Usually urinary	2
Very bad	1	Stuporous	1	Bedfast	1	Immobile	1	Double	1

Source: D. Norton, R. McLaren, and A.N. Exton-Smith, *An Investigation of Geriatric Nursing Problems in Hospital* (Edinburgh: Churchill Livingstone, 1962). Reissued 1975. Used by permission.

ASSESSING

Particular attention is paid to skin condition in areas most likely to break down: skinfolds (such as under the breasts), areas that are frequently moist (such as the perineum), and areas that receive extensive pressure (such as the coccyx and trochanters). Figure 24-16 ■ illustrates common sites of pressure ulcers. Box 24-6 ■ describes assessment of common pressure sites.

When a pressure ulcer is present, the nurse notes the following:

- Location of the lesion
- Size of lesion in centimeters (Measure length, width, and depth, beginning with length [head to toe] and then width [side to side]. To measure depth, gently insert a sterile swab at the deepest part of the wound, and then measure against a measuring guide.)
- Stage of the ulcer (see Figure 24-13)
- Color of the wound bed and location of necrosis or eschar
- Condition of the wound margins
- Integrity of surrounding skin
- Clinical signs of infection, such as redness, warmth, swelling, pain, odor, and exudate (note color of exudate)

DIAGNOSING, PLANNING, AND IMPLEMENTING

Nursing diagnoses that are common in clients with pressure ulcers are:

- *Impaired Skin Integrity* (commonly applies to stage I and II pressure ulcers)
- *Impaired Tissue Integrity* (applies to stage III and IV pressure ulcers)
- *Acute Pain*

Preventing Pressure Ulcers

To prevent pressure ulcers, the LPN/LVN, in collaboration with the RN, implements meticulous skin care as described earlier in the chapter:

- Provide nutritional supplements for nutritionally compromised clients. *An inadequate intake of calories,*

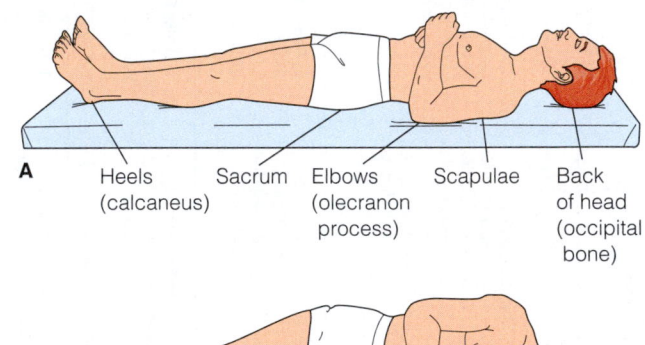

A   Heels (calcaneus)   Sacrum   Elbows (olecranon process)   Scapulae   Back of head (occipital bone)

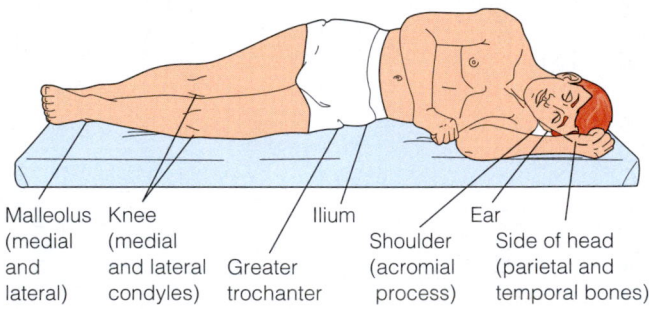

Malleolus (medial and lateral)   Knee (medial and lateral condyles)   Greater trochanter   Ilium   Shoulder (acromial process)   Ear   Side of head (parietal and temporal bones)

B

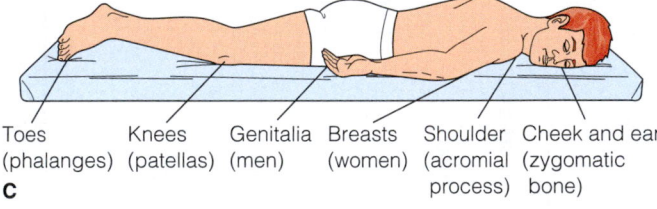

Toes (phalanges)   Knees (patellas)   Genitalia (men)   Breasts (women)   Shoulder (acromial process)   Cheek and ear (zygomatic bone)

C

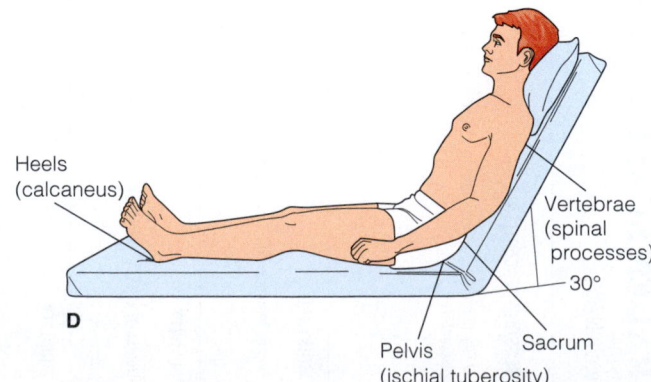

Heels (calcaneus)   Vertebrae (spinal processes)   30°   Pelvis (ischial tuberosity)   Sacrum

D

Figure 24-16. ■ Body pressure areas: **A.** supine position; **B.** lateral position; **C.** prone position; **D.** Fowler's position.

BOX 24-6 ASSESSING COMMON PRESSURE SITES

- Be sure there is good lighting, preferably natural or fluorescent.
- Regulate the environment before beginning the assessment so that the room is neither too hot nor too cold. Heat can cause the skin to flush; cold can cause the skin to blanch or become cyanotic.
- Inspect pressure areas for any whitish or reddened spots; discoloration can be caused by impaired blood circulation to the area. It should disappear in a few minutes when circulation is restored.
- Inspect pressure areas for abrasions and excoriations. An abrasion (wearing away of the skin) can occur when skin rubs against a sheet (e.g., when the client is pulled). Excoriations (loss of superficial layers of the skin) can occur when the skin has prolonged contact with body secretions or excretions or with dampness in skinfolds.
- Palpate the surface temperature of the skin over the pressure areas. Normally, the temperature is the same as that of the surrounding skin. Increased temperature is abnormal and may be due to inflammation or blood trapped in the area.
- Palpate over bony prominences and dependent body areas for the presence of edema, which feels spongy.

protein, and iron is believed to be a risk factor for pressure ulcer development.

- Keep the client's skin clean, dry, and free of irritation from urine, feces, and sweat. When bathing the client, avoid using hot water and apply minimal force and friction. Use mild cleansing agents that do not disrupt the skin's "natural barriers," and apply moisturizing lotions as needed. Also, minimize dryness by not exposing clients to cold and low humidity.
- Avoid massaging over bony prominences. *Nurses have used massage to stimulate blood circulation, with the intention of preventing pressure sores. Scientific evidence does not support this belief; in fact, massage may lead to deep tissue trauma.*
- Provide the client with a smooth, firm, and wrinkle-free foundation on which to sit or lie down. Position, transfer, and turn clients correctly. For bedridden clients, reduce shearing force by elevating the head of the bed to no more than 30 degrees, if this position is not contraindicated by the client's condition.
- Encourage or assist the client to shift weight every 15 to 30 minutes and, whenever possible, exercise or ambulate to stimulate blood circulation. *Frequent shifts in position, even if only slight, effectively change pressure points.*
- When lifting a client to change position, use a lifting device such as a trapeze rather than dragging the client across or up in bed. *The friction that results from dragging the skin against a sheet can cause blisters and abrasions, which may contribute to more extensive tissue damage.*

- At least every 2 hours, reposition any at-risk client who is confined to bed—even when a special support mattress is used. Establish a written schedule for turning and repositioning. This allows another body surface to bear the weight. Six body positions can be used: prone, supine, right and left lateral (side-lying), and right and left Sims' positions.

Treating Pressure Ulcers

To treat clients with pressure ulcers, the following interventions are performed:

- Follow the agency protocols and the physician's orders, if any.
- Protect wounds (such as those developing granulation tissue). Clean them gently, apply a topical antimicrobial agent, cover with a transparent film or hydrocolloid dressing, and disturb the dressing as infrequently as possible. *This will allow the healing process to continue uninterrupted.* Box 24-7 ■ provides guidelines for treating pressure ulcers.
- Clean wounds to remove drainage and nonviable tissue (see Procedure 24-3).
- Report any signs of infection and obtain a wound specimen with a physician's order (see Procedure 24-2).
- Provide supportive care of the client during removal of black (nonviable) tissue. Once the necrotic tissue has been removed (**debrided**), dress wound per physician orders.

EVALUATING

Pressure sores are a challenge for nurses because of the number of variables involved (e.g., risk factors, types

BOX 24-7 NURSING CARE CHECKLIST

Treating Pressure Ulcers

- ☑ Minimize direct pressure on the ulcer. Reposition the client at least every 2 hours. Use a schedule, and record position changes on the client's chart.
- ☑ Clean the pressure ulcer daily. The method of cleaning depends on the stage of the ulcer and agency protocol. For example, a whirlpool bath may be indicated for a stage I ulcer and a wound irrigation for a stage IV ulcer (see Procedure 24-3).
- ☑ Clean and dress the ulcer using surgical asepsis.
- ☑ If the pressure ulcer is infected, obtain a sample of the drainage for culture and sensitivity to antiseptic agents (see Procedure 24-2).
- ☑ If the client cannot keep weight off the pressure ulcer, use pressure-relieving devices such as an egg-crate mattress.
- ☑ Teach the client to move, if only slightly, to relieve pressure.
- ☑ Provide range-of-motion (ROM) exercises as the client's condition permits.

of ulcers, and degrees of impairment) and the many treatment measures that are advocated. Existing and potential infections are the most serious complications of pressure sores.

Evaluation of a client with pressure ulcers includes documentation of location, size, depth, stage, color, status of wound margins and surrounding skin, and specific signs of infection. Include care provided and client response to treatment.

Continuity of Care

Clients and their support people often need teaching in order to carry out measures to prevent pressure ulcers. The following information should be provided:

- Causes of pressure ulcers
- Skin care plan to keep the skin clean, lubricated, and protected from secretions and excretions
- Importance of maintaining or increasing correct activity level
- Avoidance of massage, doughnuts, and heat lamps
- Need to contact the physician when there is skin reddening, blister formation, or breakdown

NURSING PROCESS CARE PLAN
Client with Pressure (Decubitus) Ulcer

Jamie Lee, a 73-year-old female, was admitted to the hospital for a decubitus ulcer on her left hip. Jamie lives in a skilled nursing center and is being treated for diabetes. She takes insulin twice a day. Mrs. Lee is unhappy with the restrictions of her diabetic diet. The staff must remind her about the dangers of eating candy bars, which they frequently find in her bedside table. Her mobility is limited, and she complains when the staff encourages her to sit up. She favors her left side because she can watch the television from that angle easily.

Assessment
VS: T 99, apical P 76, R 22, BP 146/90. Blood sugar is 320; hemoglobin is 10; hematocrit is 36; and WBC count is 12,000. The decubitus ulcer is described as having full-thickness skin loss, measuring 2 × 2 across and 0.5 in. deep. No undermining noted.

Nursing Diagnosis
The following important nursing diagnoses (among others) are established for this client:

- *Impaired Skin Integrity*
- *Risk for Infection* related to decubitus ulcer
- *Activity Intolerance*
- *Powerlessness* related to illness-related regimen
- *Deficient Knowledge* related to diabetes

Expected Outcomes
The expected outcomes for the plan of care are:

- Skin integrity effectively managed.
- Wound is maintained without evidence of infection.
- Client expresses an understanding of need to balance rest and activity.
- Client participates in planning care; makes decisions regarding care and treatments when possible.
- Client expresses a basic understanding of the principles in diabetes care and treatment.

Planning and Implementation
The following nursing interventions are implemented:

- Monitor wound healing; measurements and documentation taken when dressing is changed.
- Maintain glucose levels with insulin adjustments.
- Observe for signs and symptoms of infection.
- Encourage the client to be independent in activities when possible.
- Determine the client's perception of activity level and strength.
  - Refer to physical therapy to help increase activity level and strength.
  - If possible, move TV so it can be viewed from another position.
- Reinforce diabetes teaching and understanding to family and client.

Evaluation
Mrs. Lee returns to her skilled nursing center after 5 days of hospitalization. Her vital signs are stable and glucose level has steadily dropped to 150. Wound cultures are negative for infection. Granulation tissue is apparent as evidence of healing progresses. Dressing changes will continue with nursing supervision. The client expresses understanding about mobility and position changes. She has been sitting up three times for meals and extends the time with each sitting. The client and family members understand the diabetic diet calorie restriction and the need to control blood sugars. She states she has a better understanding of diabetes and how it affects healing. She wants to take a more active role in her care and management.

Critical Thinking in the Nursing Process

1. How will you reinforce Mrs. Lee's understanding of diabetes and wound healing?
2. Compare treatment for a stage III and stage IV decubitus ulcer.
3. Describe how nutrition can affect the healing process in pressure ulcers.

Note: Discussion of Critical Thinking questions appears on the MyNursingKit Website.

Note: The references and resources for all chapters have been compiled at the back of the book.

Wound Dressings

Purposes

- To provide a moist wound environment and promote wound healing
- To protect the wound from trauma and infectious agents
- To facilitate assessment of wound healing
- To prevent the entrance of microorganisms into the wound
- To minimize wound discomfort
- To promote autolysis of necrotic material by white blood cells
- To decrease the frequency of dressing changes

Equipment

- Disposable gloves
- Hair scissors or clippers
- Alcohol or acetone
- Moisture-proof bag
- Sterile gloves (optional)
- Sterile gauze and the wound-cleaning agents specified by the physician or agency (e.g., sterile saline)
- Wound barrier dressing
- Scissors
- Paper tape
- Dressing set
- Sterile normal saline or other cleaning agent used by the agency
- Hydrocolloid dressing at least 3 to 4 cm (1.5 in.) larger than wound on all four sides

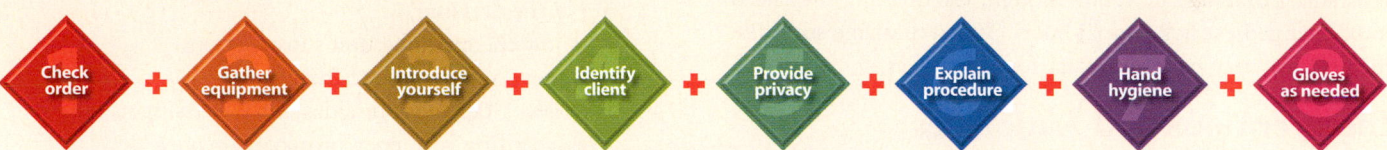

Check order + Gather equipment + Introduce yourself + Identify client + Provide privacy + Explain procedure + Hand hygiene + Gloves as needed

Part A: Moist Transparent Barrier Dressing

Before applying or changing a moist transparent wound barrier, (1) verify the physician's order regarding frequency and type of dressing change, and (2) determine agency protocol about solutions used to clean the wound and whether clean or sterile technique is to be used. Many agencies recommend clean rather than sterile technique for chronic wounds such as a decubitus ulcer.

ASSESSMENT FOCUS

Appearance and size of the wound; the amount and character of exudate; complaints of discomfort; signs of systemic infection (e.g., elevated body temperature, diaphoresis, malaise; leukocytosis).

Interventions and Rationales

1. Perform preparatory steps (see icon bar above).

2. Obtain assistance as needed.
   - If the size of the wound requires it, acquire the assistance of a coworker to help apply the dressing.

3. Thoroughly clean the skin area around the wound.
   - Put on disposable gloves.
   - Clean the skin well with normal saline or a mild cleansing agent. Always rinse the adjacent skin well prior to applying a dressing.
   - Clip the hair about 5 cm (2 in.) around the wound area if indicated.

- If adherence of the dressing is a concern, clean the area adjacent to the wound with alcohol or acetone, and allow it to dry. *Alcohol or acetone defats the skin. Defatted, clean, dry skin ensures better adhesion of the dressing.*
- Remove gloves, and dispose of them in the moisture-proof bag.

4. Clean the wound if indicated.
   - Put on clean disposable or sterile gloves in accordance with agency practice.
   - Clean the wound with the prescribed solution. Either (a) pour the sterile solution directly on the wound and collect drainage with an emesis basin, or (b) use a moist, sterile gauze and hold it so that the area that touches the wound remains sterile.
   - Dry the surrounding skin with a dry gauze.

5. Assess the wound.

6. Apply the wound barrier.
   - Remove part of the paper backing on the dressing. If you have an assistant, remove all of the paper backing; the two of you should hold the colored tabs attached to the dressing.
   - Apply the dressing at one edge of the wound site, allowing at least 2.5-cm (1-in.) coverage of the skin surrounding the wound.

- Gently lay or press the barrier over the wound. Keep it free of wrinkles, but avoid stretching it too tightly. *A stretched dressing restricts mobility*.
- Cut off the colored tabs after the wound is completely covered.
- Remove and dispose of gloves appropriately.

7. Reinforce the dressing only if absolutely needed.
   - Apply paper or other porous tape to the edges of the dressing.

8. Assess the wound at least daily.
   - Determine the extent of serous fluid accumulation under the dressing, wound healing, and the need to repair the dressing.

- If excessive serum has accumulated, consider replacing the transparent wound barrier with a more absorbent type of dressing, such as hydrocolloid.
- If the dressing is leaking, remove it and apply another dressing.

9. Document the procedure and all nursing assessments.

Part B: Hydrocolloid Dressing

A hydrocolloid dressing should be changed whenever it becomes dislodged, leaks, or develops an odor. If the wound has substantial drainage or yellow slough, the dressing may need to be changed every 24 to 72 hours. When drainage subsides, the dressing may be left in place for 3 to 7 days.

Interventions and Rationales

1. Remove the old dressing.
   - Put on disposable gloves.
   - Pull the dressing off gradually in the direction of hair growth. *This minimizes skin irritation*.
   - Dispose of the soiled dressing in the moisture-proof bag.

2. Clean the skin area around the wound.
   - Gently wash the skin surrounding the wound with a mild cleansing agent or with normal saline and dry it thoroughly with gauze squares.
   - Leave the residue that is difficult to remove on the skin. *This prevents unnecessary stretching of skin*.
   - Remove gloves and dispose of them in the moisture-proof bag.

3. Clean the wound if indicated.
   - Open the sterile dressing supplies.
   - Pour saline or other cleaning agent into the sterile container.
   - Put on disposable or sterile gloves in accordance with agency protocol.
   - Clean the wound with the prescribed solution.

4. Assess the wound.
   - Observe the appearance and the size of the wound and the amount and character of exudate.

- Determine presence of pain. *Subjective data is an important part of data collection*.

5. Apply the dressing.
   - Follow the manufacturer's instructions.
   - Remove and dispose of the gloves.
   - *Optional*: Tape all four sides of the dressing as required or according to agency protocol. *Taping prevents the dressing from sticking to bed linens and keeps the edges from lifting*.

6. Assess and change the dressing as indicated.
   - Inspect the dressing at least daily for leakage, dislodgement, odor, and wrinkling.
   - Change the dressing if any of these signs are present.

7. Document the technique and all nursing assessments.

SAMPLE DOCUMENTATION

[date] [time] Stage II superficial reddened wound 2 × 2 to coccyx cleansed with saline, hydrocolloid wafer applied and windowed with tape. Client complained of 3/10 on pain scale, medicated prior to procedure. _____

_____ D. Haus, LVN

| PROCEDURE 24-2 | **Obtaining a Specimen of Wound Drainage** |

Purposes

- To identify the microorganisms potentially causing an infection and the antibiotics to which they are sensitive
- To evaluate the effectiveness of antibiotic therapy

Equipment

- Disposable gloves
- Sterile gloves
- Moisture-resistant bag
- Sterile dressing set
- Normal saline and irrigating syringe
- Culture tube with swab and culture medium (aerobic and anaerobic tubes are available) and/or sterile syringe with needle for anaerobic culture
- Completed labels for each container
- Completed requisition to accompany the specimens to the laboratory

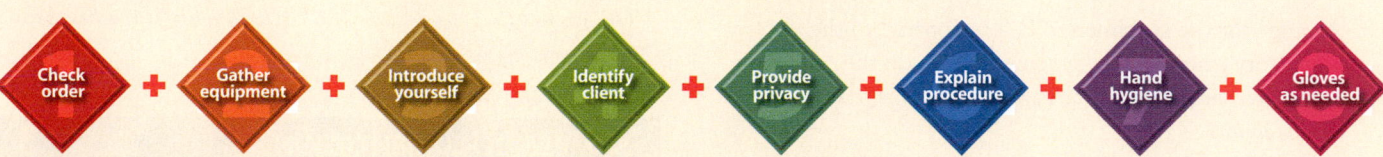

Check order + Gather equipment + Introduce yourself + Identify client + Provide privacy + Explain procedure + Hand hygiene + Gloves as needed

Interventions and Rationales

1. Perform preparatory steps (see icon bar above).
2. Remove any dressings that cover the wound.
   - Put on disposable gloves.
   - Remove the dressing, and observe any drainage on it. Hold the dressing so that the client does not see the drainage. *The appearance of the drainage could upset the client.*
   - Determine the amount of the drainage, for example, one 2 × 2 gauze saturated with pale yellow drainage.
   - Discard the dressing in the moisture-resistant bag. Handle it carefully so that the dressing does not touch the outside of the bag. *Touching the outside of the bag will contaminate it.*
   - Remove gloves and dispose of them properly.
3. Open the sterile dressing set using sterile technique.
4. Assess the wound.
   - Put on sterile gloves.
   - Assess the appearance of the tissues in and around the wound and the drainage. *Infection can cause reddened tissues with a thick discharge, which may be foul smelling, whitish, or colored.*
5. Clean the wound.
   - Irrigate the wound with normal saline until all visible exudate has been washed away. See Procedure 23-3.
   - After irrigating, apply a sterile gauze pad to the wound. *This absorbs excess saline.*
   - If a topical antimicrobial ointment or cream is being used to treat the wound, use a swab to remove it. *Residual antiseptic must be removed prior to culture.*
   - Remove and discard sterile gloves.

6. Obtain the culture.
   - Open a specimen culture tube and place the cap upside down on a firm, dry surface so that the inside will not become contaminated, or if the swab is attached to the lid, twist the cap to loosen the swab. Hold the tube in one hand, and take out the swab in the other (Figure 24-17 ■).
   - Rotate the swab back and forth over clean areas of granulation tissue from the sides or base of the wound. *Microorganisms most likely to be responsible for a wound infection reside in viable tissue.*
   - Do not use pus or pooled exudate to culture. *These secretions contain a mixture of contaminants that are not the same as those causing the infection.*
   - Avoid touching the swab to intact skin at the wound edges. *This prevents the introduction of superficial skin organisms into the culture.*
   - Return the swab to the culture tube, taking care not to touch the top or the outside of the tube.
   - Crush the inner ampule containing the medium for organism growth at the bottom of the tube. *This ensures*

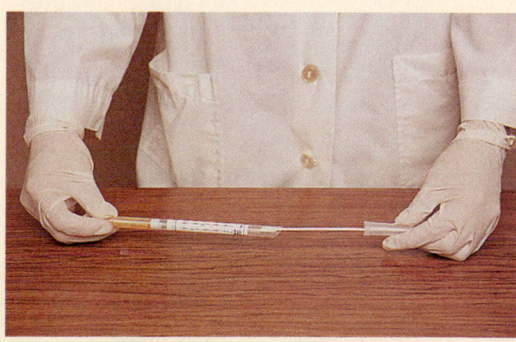

Figure 24-17. ■ A culture tube for a wound specimen.

that the swab with the specimen is surrounded by culture medium.

- Twist the cap to secure it.
- If a specimen is required from another site, repeat the preceding steps. Specify the exact site (e.g., inferior drain site or lower aspect of incision) on the label of each container. Be sure to put each swab in the appropriately labeled tube. *This ensures that tests can be carried out as intended.*

7. Dress the wound.
   - Apply any ordered medication to the wound.
   - Cover the wound with a sterile moist transparent wound dressing. See Procedure 24-1A.

8. Arrange for the specimen to be transported to the laboratory immediately. Be sure to include the completed requisition. *This prevents specimen from being lost or mislabeled.*

9. Document all relevant information.
   - Record on the client's chart the taking of the specimen and source.
   - Include the date and time; the examination requested; the appearance of the wound; the color, consistency, amount, and odor of any drainage; and any discomfort experienced by the client. *Complete documentation supports continuity of care.*

VARIATION: OBTAINING A SPECIMEN FOR ANAEROBIC CULTURE, USING A STERILE SYRINGE AND NEEDLE

- Insert a sterile 10-mL syringe (without needle) into the wound, and aspirate 1 to 5 mL of drainage into the syringe.
- Attach the #21 gauge needle to the syringe, and expel all air from the syringe and needle.
- Immediately inject the drainage into the anaerobic culture tube.
  or
  If a rubber stopper or cork is available, insert the needle into the rubber stopper or cork to prevent the entry of air.
- Label the tube or syringe appropriately.
- Send the syringe of drainage to the laboratory immediately. *This ensures that the specimen will be fresh when it reaches the laboratory.*

SAMPLE DOCUMENTATION

[date] [time] Anaerobic culture of lt. hip wound obtained and sent to the lab. _____

_____ D. Haus, LVN

PROCEDURE 24-3 ## Irrigating a Wound

Before irrigating a wound, determine (a) the type of irrigating solution to be used, (b) the frequency of irrigations, and (c) the temperature of the solution.

Purposes

- To clean the area
- To apply heat and hasten the healing process
- To apply an antimicrobial solution

Equipment

- Sterile dressing equipment and dressing materials
- Sterile irrigating syringes (e.g., a 30- to 50-mL piston syringe) with a catheter of an appropriate size (e.g., #18 or

#19) attached or a 250-mL squeezable bottle with irrigating tip
- Sterile basin for the irrigating solution
- Moisture-proof bag
- Sterile basin to receive the irrigation returns
- Irrigating solution, usually 200 mL (6.5 oz.) of solution warmed to body temperature, according to the agency's or physician's choice
- Clean disposable gloves
- Sterile gloves
- Moisture-proof sterile drape
- Sterile straight catheter or irrigating tip, if needed

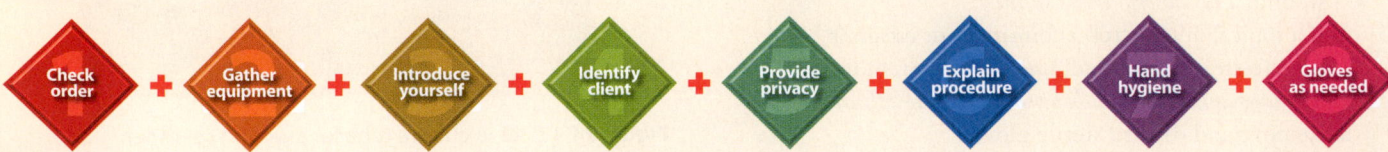

Check order + Gather equipment + Introduce yourself + Identify client + Provide privacy + Explain procedure + Hand hygiene + Gloves as needed

Interventions and Rationales

1. Perform preparatory steps (see icon bar above).

2. Verify the physician's order.
   - Confirm the type and strength of the solution.

3. Prepare the client.
   - Assist the client to a position in which the irrigating solution will flow by gravity from the upper end of the wound to the lower end and then into the basin.
   - Place the moisture-proof drape over the client and the bed.
   - Put on disposable gloves and remove and discard the old dressing.
   - Clean from the center of the wound outward, using circular strokes.
   - Use a separate swab for each stroke, and discard each swab after use. *This prevents the introduction of microorganisms to other wound areas.*
   - Assess the wound and drainage.
   - Remove and discard disposable gloves.

4. Prepare the equipment.
   - Open the sterile dressing set and supplies.
   - Pour the ordered solution into the solution container.
   - Put on sterile gloves.
   - Position the sterile basin below the wound to receive the irrigating fluid.

5. Irrigate the wound.
   - Instill a steady stream of irrigating solution into the wound. Make sure all areas of the wound are irrigated (Figure 24-18 ■).
   - Use either a syringe with a catheter attached or a 250-mL squeezable bottle with irrigating tip to flush the wound. *Effective irrigation requires 4 to 15 pounds per square inch of pressure. These devices provide this pressure; bulb syringes do not.*
   - If you are using a catheter, insert the catheter into the wound until resistance is met. Do not force the catheter. *Forcing the catheter can cause tissue damage.*
   - Continue irrigating until the solution becomes clear (no exudate is present). *The irrigation washes away tissue debris and drainage so that later returns are clearer.*
   - Dry the area around the wound. *Moisture left on the skin promotes the growth of microorganisms and can cause skin irritation and breakdown.*

6. Assess and dress the wound.
   - Assess the appearance of the wound, noting in particular the type and amount of exudate and the presence and extent of granulation tissue.
   - Pack the wound if ordered.
   - Apply a sterile dressing to the wound as described in Procedure 24-1.

7. Document all relevant information.
   - Document the irrigation, the solution used, the appearance of the irrigation returns, and nursing assessments. Note the presence of any exudate and sloughing tissue.

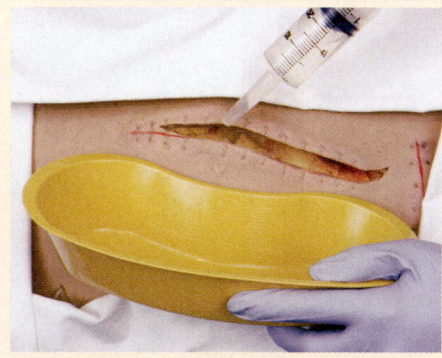

Figure 24-18. ■ Irrigating a wound.

SAMPLE DOCUMENTATION

[date] [time] Lt. hip wound, stage IV measured 2 inch × 4 inch, 1/2 inch (5 cm × 10 cm, 1 cm) depth. Drainage consists of yellow purulent material, no necrosis noted. Wound irrigated with saline solution and packed with 0.5-in. gauze, covered with gauze dressing. No sinus tract detected. Client complained of minimal pain, 4/10 on pain scale. Client medicated prior to procedure. _____

_____ D. Haus, LVN

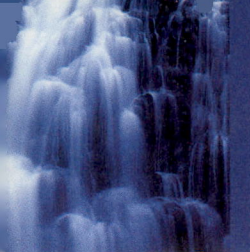

Chapter Review

KEY Points

- Skin integrity is the body's first line of defense.
- The wound healing process has three phases: inflammatory, proliferative, and maturation.
- Essential data for wounds include wound appearance, size, drainage, swelling, pain, and the presence of tubes and drains.
- Nurses are usually responsible for obtaining specimens of wound drainage for culture. Laboratory data support wound assessment.
- Nurses must wash hands before and after providing wound care to prevent infection and transmission of bloodborne pathogens.
- Major nursing responsibilities related to wound care include preventing infection, preventing further tissue damage, preventing hemorrhage, promoting healing, and preventing skin excoriation around draining wounds.
- Wound care may involve cleaning wounds, changing dressings, maintaining drains, irrigating, inserting packing, applying heat and cold, and applying bandages and binders.
- Nurses must use extra precautions when applying heat or cold to clients with neurosensory or circulatory impairment.
- Major types of wound exudate are serous, purulent, and sanguineous (hemorrhagic). The main complications of wound healing are hemorrhage, infection, dehiscence, and evisceration.
- A pressure ulcer is caused by unrelieved pressure resulting in damage to underlying tissues.
- Friction and shearing forces can also produce a pressure ulcer. Frequent change of position and care when moving a client can help prevent pressure ulcers.

- The nurse describes a pressure ulcer in terms of location, size, depth, stage, color, status of wound margins and surrounding skin, and specific signs of infection.
- Wound assessment continually requires visual inspection, palpation, and the sense of smell.

FOR FURTHER Study

For more information about infection control, see Chapter 10.

For further information about the body's normal responses to heat and cold, see Chapter 21.

See more on nutrition in Chapter 25.

Removal of sutures and staples is discussed in care of the client after surgery, in Chapter 29.

For more on the structure of normal skin and disorders that affect it see Chapter 30.

Chapter 31 addresses compartment syndrome.

See Procedure 47-1 for applying a sling.

Sitz baths are described in postpartum care, Chapter 54.

Critical Thinking Care Map

Caring for a Debilitated Client

NCLEX-PN® Focus Area: Physiological Integrity

Case Study: Mr. Johns is an 84-year-old client being treated for a urinary tract disorder. Mr. Johns suffered a cerebrovascular accident (stroke) 6 months ago and has difficulty ambulating and attending to his own needs because of right-sided weakness. While assessing Mr. Johns, you note that he is thin for his 6-foot frame, weighs 135 lbs, is incontinent of foul-smelling urine, and has deeply reddened areas on his right hip, coccyx, and entire perineal area. He is alert and oriented to person, place, and time, but he has decreased sensation on his entire right side. He spends most of his time in bed or sitting at his bedside chair due to his difficulty with ambulation.

Nursing Diagnosis: *Risk for Impaired Skin Integrity*

COLLECT DATA

Subjective	Objective
_____	_____
_____	_____
_____	_____
_____	_____
_____	_____
_____	_____
_____	_____

Would you report this? Yes/No

If yes, report to: _____

What would you report? _____

Nursing Care

_____
_____
_____
_____
_____
_____
_____
_____
_____
_____
_____

How would you document this? _____
_____
_____
_____

Compare your answers and documentation to those provided on the MyNursingKit Website.

Data Collected
(use only those that apply)

- Difficulty ambulating
- Height: 6 ft
- Weight: 135 lbs
- Client states, "I'm not hungry most of the time."
- Weakened
- BP 150/88
- Incontinent of urine
- General malaise
- Deeply reddened coccyx, right hip, and perineal area
- Alert and oriented
- Decreased sensation to his entire right side
- Right-sided weakness
- Negative for fecal blood
- TSH 5 mcgIU/mL (microgram of international units/mL)

Nursing Interventions
(use only those that apply; list in priority order)

- Monitor urine output.
- Monitor reddened area.
- Check vital signs every 2 hours.
- Turn client every 2 hours.
- Refer to dietitian.
- Steadily increase ambulation.
- Weigh daily.
- Offer urinal frequently.

NCLEX-PN® Exam Preparation

TEST-TAKING TIP Utilize the process of elimination. Eliminate the incorrect options before selecting an answer.

1 The nurse, caring for a debilitated bed-ridden client, notes nonblanchable erythema of intact skin on the coccyx. The nurse's priority action is to:

1. Document the size, location, and stage of the wound.
2. Position the client to remove pressure from the site and reposition at least every 2 hours.
3. Place the client on an airflow mattress.
4. Apply protective pads and adhesive dressings over the site.

2 The nurse applies a wet-to-damp dressing to the client's wound for the purpose of:

1. Diluting the exudate.
2. Protecting the wound.
3. Preventing infection.
4. Debriding the wound.

3 The nurse is assigned several clients and considers which of the following is at greatest risk for impaired skin integrity?

1. The 86-year-old woman in good physical health who lives alone and was admitted to the acute care facility for treatment of new onset atrial fibrillation.
2. The 24-year-old client admitted to the acute care facility for traction related to a fractured femur.
3. The 32-year-old client admitted to the acute care facility requiring mechanical ventilation secondary to advancing amyotrophic lateral sclerosis.
4. The 42-year-old client admitted to the acute care facility with a medical diagnosis of myocardial infarction.

4 A client has a decubitus ulcer involving damage to the subcutaneous tissue extending to the underlying fascia. The nurse identifies this type of ulcer as a:

1. Stage I ulcer.
2. Stage II ulcer.
3. Stage III ulcer.
4. Stage IV ulcer.

5 The nurse applies an aquathermia pad to the client's wound and sets the temperature at 40.5°C (105°F). The client calls the nurse into the room a few minutes later and reports that the pad is cooling. The nurse feels the pad and determines that the pad remains at the set temperature. The nurse will:

1. Increase the temperature of the pad by 5 degrees.
2. Inform the client the pad is still at the proper temperature.
3. Obtain a new aquathermia unit and replace the old unit.
4. Explain that the client's body has adjusted to the temperature making it feel cool.

6 The nurse assesses the client's wound and determines that the wound is healing as evidenced by:

1. Granulation tissue.
2. Eschar.
3. Suppuration.
4. Reactive hyperemia.

7 The nurse is caring for a client who requires frequent repositioning to the top of the bed. The nurse recognizes this client is at risk for:

1. Falling out of bed.
2. Injury to the foot.
3. Reactive hyperemia.
4. Shearing force.

8 The nurse is caring for a postoperative client. A priority wound care intervention to promote healing is to:

1. Leave the incision open to the air.
2. Change the dressings twice per day.
3. Adhere to the principles of handwashing.
4. Frequent cleaning of the incision from the least contaminated to the most contaminated area.

9 The nurse is caring for a client who was involved in a motorcycle accident and has several wounds on the trunk caused by sliding across the asphalt. The nurse is teaching the client how to care for the wounds at home. Which of the following statements made by the nurse would reflect correct information?

1. "You have several lacerations that must be carefully watched for signs of infection."
2. "You have a number of penetrating wounds that will require irrigation."
3. "You have four abrasions on your trunk that may be very uncomfortable."
4. "You have several contusions that will heal over the next few weeks."

10 The nurse, working on a surgical unit, is caring for several clients with postoperative incisions. The nurse anticipates which of the following client's wounds will heal fastest?

1. A 24-year-old client who works as a fitness trainer.
2. The 18-year-old lifeguard who smokes.
3. The 35-year-old client in good health who works as a receptionist.
4. The retired 65-year-old client with hypertension.

Answers and rationales for Review Questions appear in Appendix I.

Nutrition and Diet Therapy

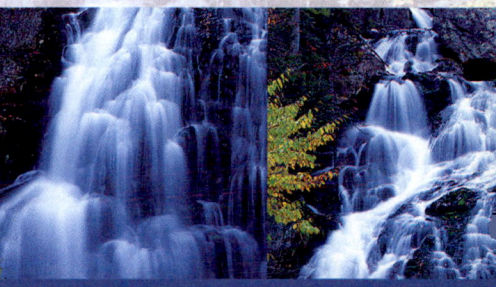

As healthcare providers, we work toward the goal that all people want to feel well, to enjoy good health. An essential part of this feeling of good health is to obtain the best available nutrient supply for the body. This chapter will introduce you to principles of nutrition and diet therapy, so that you can assist others in experiencing adequate nutrition.

Nutrients

Nutrients are the organic, inorganic, and energy-producing substances found in foods. These nutrients are required for body functioning. The result of this interaction between nutrients and the human body is **nutrition.** Specific nutrients in food allow growth, maintenance of all body tissues, and normal functioning of all body processes.

Nutrients have three major functions. They provide energy for body processes and movement. They provide structural material for body tissues. They regulate body processes. When a person's food intake is adequate, there is a balance of these essential nutrients:

- Water
- Macronutrients: carbohydrates, proteins, and fats (lipids)
- Micronutrients: vitamins and minerals

WATER

The body's most basic nutrient need is water. Water is vital to health and normal cellular function, serving as:

- A medium for metabolic reactions within cells
- A transporter for nutrients, waste products, and other substances
- A lubricant
- An insulator and shock absorber
- A means of regulating and maintaining body temperature

Age, body fat, and gender affect total body water. Infants have 70% to 80% of their body weight in water. The proportion of body water decreases with aging; in people over age 60, it is less than half of body weight. Fat tissue is essentially free of water; lean tissue contains a significant amount of water. So, water makes up a greater percentage of

a lean person's body weight than an obese person's. Women have proportionally more body fat than men, and so have a lower percentage of body water (Figure 25-1 ■).

MACRONUTRIENTS

Macronutrients provide fuel that converts to energy. These nutrients are found in carbohydrates, proteins, and fats (lipids).

Carbohydrates

Carbohydrates are composed of the elements carbon (C), hydrogen (H), and oxygen (O). There are two basic kinds: simple carbohydrates (sugars) and complex carbohydrates (starches and fiber).

Simple carbohydrates are made up of the monosaccharides and the disaccharides. Monosaccharides are single sugars, whereas disaccharides are composed of pairs of monosaccharides. Complex carbohydrates or polysaccharides are composed of many monosaccharides joined together.

Sugars, the simplest of all carbohydrates, are water soluble. Both plants and animals produce sugars. (Lactose is a sugar formed by combining glucose and galactose and is found in milk.) However, sugars are mostly produced naturally by plants, especially fruits, sugar cane, and sugar beets. Processed or refined sugars (e.g., table sugar, molasses, and corn syrup) are those that have been extracted and concentrated from natural sources. Processed sugars are added to foods such as soft drinks, cookies, candy, ice cream, and some cereals.

Starches are *insoluble* (they do not dissolve in water). Starches are nonsweet forms of carbohydrate. Like sugars, nearly all starches exist naturally in plants, such as grains, legumes, and potatoes. Starches are in foods such as cereals, breads, flour, and puddings.

Fiber is a complex carbohydrate derived from plants (whole grains, raw vegetables, etc.). It cannot be digested by humans but supplies roughage, or bulk, to the diet. This bulk satisfies the appetite and also helps the digestive tract to eliminate wastes. Fiber plays an important role in improving the function of various body systems. Fiber assists in

MyNursingKit | Carbohydrates

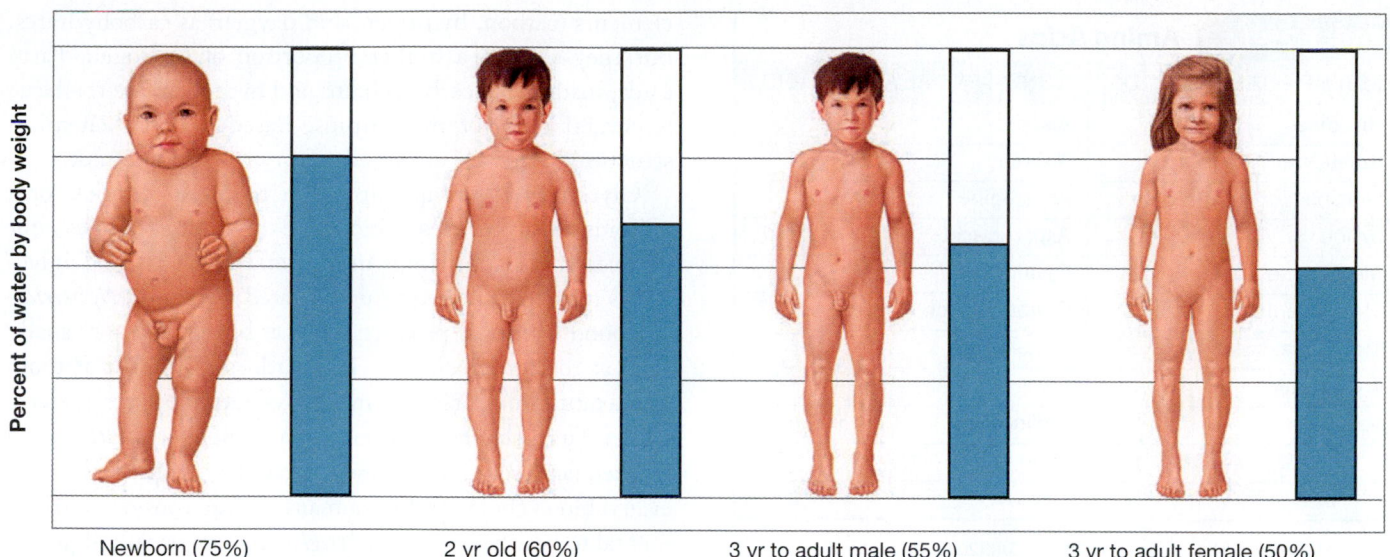

Newborn (75%)   2 yr old (60%)   3 yr to adult male (55%)   3 yr to adult female (50%)

Figure 25-1. ■ Percentage of body water by age group.

weight control by making us feel fuller so we consume less food. Fiber is important in the treatment of constipation and diverticular disease as well as potentially reducing colon cancer risk. Clients with heart disease benefit from fiber intake because fiber helps to lower blood cholesterol lipid levels.

Diabetics can use fiber to help stabilize blood glucose levels. The daily recommendation for fiber intake is based on age. Generally the recommended intake is between 20 to 38 grams per day. The average American diet is deficient in fiber.

It is important that carbohydrate intake include natural foods, not just processed foods. Natural sources of carbohydrates supply protein, vitamins, minerals, and dietary fiber; these are often missing in processed foods. Because processed carbohydrate foods are relatively low in nutrients and high in calories, they are often referred to as "empty calories."

The end products of carbohydrate digestion are monosaccharides (glucose, fructose, and galactose). Some simple sugars require no digestion. Examples of simple sugars include glucose, fructose, sucrose, and lactose. After the body breaks carbohydrates down into glucose, some glucose continues to circulate in the blood to maintain blood glucose levels and to provide a readily available source of energy. The unused glucose is converted to glycogen and then stored to be used at a later time, in a process called glycogenesis. In healthy persons, essentially all digested carbohydrate is absorbed by the small intestine (see Figure 37-4 ⬤⬤).

Insulin, a hormone secreted by the pancreas, is needed for glucose to be transported into the cells. So, the body's use of glucose is controlled by the pancreas's ability to produce insulin. When the pancreas is unable to produce insulin, or to produce enough insulin, the resulting condition is diabetes mellitus. Diabetes can negatively affect almost every body system.

Digested carbohydrates are maintained in the body either as **glycogen** (the stored form of glucose) or as fat. All body cells are capable of storing glycogen; however, most glycogen is stored in the liver and skeletal muscles. The process of glycogen formation is called **glycogenesis.** Glycogen can be converted back to glucose when needed to maintain blood levels or to provide energy by a process called **glycogenolysis.** Glucose that cannot be stored as glycogen is converted to fat.

Proteins

Proteins are organic substances composed of amino acids. Like carbohydrates, proteins contain carbon, hydrogen, and oxygen, but proteins also contain nitrogen. **Amino acids,** the building blocks of proteins, are categorized as essential or nonessential. *Essential amino acids* are those that cannot be manufactured in the body and must be supplied by ingesting protein. *Nonessential amino acids* are those that the body can manufacture. There are also *conditionally essential amino acids*. These are amino acids that in certain conditions (such as heavy exercise) cannot be produced in sufficient quantities from other amino acids. The amino acid l-glutamine is considered conditionally essential.

Table 25-1 ■ lists essential and nonessential amino acids. The body takes apart amino acids from food and reconstructs new ones from their basic elements (carbohydrates and nitrogen).

Proteins may be complete or incomplete. *Complete proteins* contain all nine essential amino acids plus many nonessential ones. Most animal proteins, including meats, poultry, fish, dairy products, and eggs, are complete proteins. Soybeans are the only plant source of complete proteins. *Incomplete proteins* lack one or more essential amino acids and are usually derived from vegetables.

TABLE 25-1	Amino Acids
ESSENTIAL AMINO ACIDS	**NONESSENTIAL AMINO ACIDS**
Histidine	Alanine
Isoleucine	Arginine
Leucine	Asparagine
Lysine	Aspartic acid
Methionine	Cysteine
Phenylalanine	Glutamic acid
Threonine	Glutamine
Tryptophan	Glycine
Valine	Proline
	Serine
	Tyrosine

Source: Whitney, E. N., Cataldo, C. B., & Rolfes, S. R. (2002). *Understanding normal and clinical nutrition.* Belmont, CA: Wadsworth/Thomson Learning.

When an appropriate mixture of plant proteins is provided in the diet, a balance of essential amino acids can be achieved. When foods containing some essential amino acids are combined with others so that together they contain all nine essential amino acids, the foods are called **complementary proteins.** For example, a combination of corn and beans is a complete protein. *Since complementary proteins are plant based they are less expensive and contain less fat then complete proteins.* Most protein is digested in the small intestine, where enzymes break it down into the end products of protein digestion, amino acids.

Amino acids are transported to the liver, where some are used to synthesize specific proteins such as albumin, globulin, and fibrinogen. Amino acids are also used to make protein for cell structures. In a sense, protein is "stored" as body tissue. The body cannot actually store excess amino acids for future use. However, a limited amount is available in the "metabolic pool" that exists as a result of the constant breakdown and buildup of the protein in body tissues.

Protein metabolism includes three activities: **anabolism** (building tissue), **catabolism** (breaking down tissue), and nitrogen balance. Because nitrogen is the element that distinguishes protein from lipids and carbohydrates, nitrogen balance reflects the status of protein nutrition in the body. **Nitrogen balance** is a measure of the intake and loss of nitrogen. When nitrogen intake equals nitrogen output, a state of nitrogen balance exists.

Lipids

Lipids are organic substances that are greasy and insoluble in water but soluble in alcohol or ether. *Fats* are lipids that are solid at room temperature; *oils* are lipids that are liquid at room temperature. In common use, the terms *fats* and *lipids* are used interchangeably. Lipids have the same elements (carbon, hydrogen, and oxygen) as carbohydrates, but they contain a higher proportion of hydrogen. Fatty acids, made up of carbon chains and hydrogen, are the basic structural units of most lipids. Based on their chemical structure, lipids are classified as simple or compound.

Glycerides, the simple lipids, are the most common form of lipids. **Triglycerides** (which have three fatty acids) account for over 90% of the lipids in food and in the body. Triglycerides may be saturated or unsaturated. *Saturated triglycerides* are found in animal products, such as butter, and are usually solid at room temperature. The hardness of the fat at room temperature indicates the amount of saturated fats present; harder fats such as beef tallow are more saturated than chicken fat, a softer fat. These saturated fats contribute to elevated blood cholesterol in humans and are considered detrimental to health. *Unsaturated triglycerides* are usually liquid at room temperature and are found in plant products, such as olive oil and corn oil. The unsaturated fats do not elevate but lower the blood cholesterol. Fish and low-fat foods would be included in selecting a diet with unsaturated fats. Knowing how to select fats that are less saturated can reduce the risk of heart disease.

Cholesterol is a fatlike substance that is both produced by the body and found in foods of animal origin. Most of the body's cholesterol is synthesized in the liver. However, some is absorbed from animal fats in the diet (e.g., from milk, egg yolk, and organ meats). Cholesterol is needed by the body to form bile acids and for the synthesis of steroid hormones. Cholesterol is also the primary lipid connected to heart disease. Testing for cholesterol levels is done to identify people at risk for developing coronary vessel disease. Table 25-2 ■ lists normal levels for cholesterol. Lipids are digested mainly in the small intestine, where they are broken down to glycerol, fatty acids, and cholesterol. These are immediately reassembled inside the intestinal cells into triglycerides and cholesterol esters (cholesterol with a fatty acid attached to it), which are not water soluble. For these reassembled products to be transported and used, the small intestine and the liver must convert them into soluble compounds called lipoproteins. Lipoproteins are made up of various lipids and a protein. One of the roles of lipoproteins is to carry the cholesterol throughout the body. Cholesterol testing is ordered through

TABLE 25-2	Normal Ranges for Cholesterol
CHOLESTEROL	**NORMAL LEVEL**
Total cholesterol	140–200 mg/dL
Triglycerides	40–190 mg/dL
HDL Men	37–70 mg/dL
HDL Women	40–88 mg/dL
LDL	Less than 130 mg/dL

lipid profiles, which test for lipoproteins and triglycerides. It is desirable to have a higher HDL (high-density lipoprotein) level and a lower LDL (low-density lipoprotein) level, because the risk of heart disease is greater when LDL is elevated. The LDL can be increased by the amount of saturated fats a person consumes.

The recommended daily cholesterol intake is 300 mg per day or less.

MICRONUTRIENTS

Vitamins

A **vitamin** is an organic compound that cannot be manufactured by the body and is needed in small quantities to *catalyze* (or trigger) metabolic processes. Thus, when vitamins are lacking in the diet, metabolic deficits result. Vitamins are generally classified as fat soluble or water soluble. *Water-soluble vitamins* include C (ascorbic acid) and the B-complex vitamins: B_1 (thiamine), B_2 (riboflavin), B_3 (niacin or nicotinic acid), B_6 (pyridoxine), B_9 (folic acid), B_{12}

(cobalamin), pantothenic acid, and biotin. The body cannot store water-soluble vitamins, so people must get a daily supply in the diet. Water-soluble vitamins can be affected by food processing, storage, and preparation. Vitamin content is highest in fresh foods that are consumed as soon as possible after harvest.

Fat-soluble vitamins include A, D, E, and K. The body can store these vitamins, though vitamins E and K can be stored only in limited amounts. Therefore, a daily supply of fat-soluble vitamins is not absolutely necessary.

Minerals

There are two categories of minerals. *Macrominerals* are those that people require daily in amounts over 100 mg. They include calcium, phosphorus, sodium, potassium, magnesium, chloride, and sulfur. *Microminerals* are those that people require daily in amounts less than 100 mg. They include iron, zinc, manganese, iodine, fluoride, copper, cobalt, chromium, and selenium. Both microminerals and macrominerals are found in vegetables, fruits, whole grains, and meats. Table 25-3 ■ describes vitamins and minerals

TABLE 25-3	Functions, Results of Deficiency or Toxicity, and Food Sources of Vitamins and Minerals			
VITAMIN OR MINERAL	**FUNCTION**	**RESULTS OF DEFICIENCY**	**RESULTS OF TOXICITY**	**FOOD SOURCES**
Vitamin C	Antioxidant; coenzyme; collagen formation; wound healing; iron absorption; hormone synthesis	Scurvy	Cramps, nausea, diarrhea	Citrus fruits, tomatoes, peppers, strawberries, broccoli
Thiamine (B_1)	Coenzyme energy metabolism; muscle, nerve action	Beriberi (wet or dry); Wernicke-Korsakoff syndrome	None	Lean pork, whole and enriched grains, legumes, nuts, seeds
Riboflavin (B_2)	Coenzyme energy metabolism	Ariboflavinosis with cheilosis, glossitis; may affect use of niacin and pyridoxine	None	Milk and dairy products, fish, poultry, eggs, dark, leafy greens, enriched breads/cereals
Niacin (B_3)	Cofactor to enzymes involved in energy metabolism; glycolysis	Pellagra (3Ds = diarrhea, dermatitis, dementia)	Vasodilation, liver damage, gout	Meat, poultry, fish, legumes, whole and enriched cereal, milk
Pyridoxine (B_6)	Coenzyme in metabolism of amino acids and protein; hemoglobin synthesis	Dermatitis, altered nerve function, weakness, microcytic anemia	Ataxia, sensory neuropathy	Whole grains and cereal, legumes, poultry, fish, pork, eggs
Folic acid (folate)	Coenzyme metabolism; fetal neural tube formation	Megaloblastic anemia; neural tube defects	Can mask presence of pernicious anemia	Leafy green vegetables, legumes
Cobalamin (B_{12})	Metabolism fatty acids; transport/storage of folate; develop and maintain myelin sheaths	Pernicious anemia, CNS damage	None	Animal protein
Vitamin A	Bone growth; maintain epithelial cells; vision; reproduction	Xerophthalmia; night blindness; keratomalacia; degeneration epithelial tissue	Blistered skin, weakness, anorexia, enlarged spleen and liver	Deep green, yellow, and orange fruits and vegetables; animal fat; whole milk and fortified low-fat and skim milk; butter; liver; egg yolks; fatty fish

(continued)

TABLE 25-3	Functions, Results of Deficiency or Toxicity, and Food Sources of Vitamins and Minerals (continued)			
VITAMIN OR MINERAL	**FUNCTION**	**RESULTS OF DEFICIENCY**	**RESULTS OF TOXICITY**	**FOOD SOURCES**
Vitamin D	Bone mineralization; calcium and phosphorus absorption	Rickets; osteomalacia	Hypercalcemia; hypercalciuria	Animal fat, butter, egg yolks, fatty fish, liver, fortified milk
Vitamin E	Antioxidant	Seen in disorders of fat absorption	None; can interfere with vitamin K activity	Vegetable oil, whole grains, seeds, nuts, leafy green vegetables
Vitamin K	Cofactor synthesis of blood clotting factors; protein formation	Blood coagulation inhibited; hemorrhagic disease in newborn	None	Green leafy vegetables, synthesized in intestines
Calcium	Bone and tooth formation; blood clotting; muscle contraction and relaxation; blood pressure	Decreased bone density; osteoporosis	Constipation, urinary stones, reduced iron and zinc absorption	Milk and milk products, green leafy vegetables, legumes
Phosphorus	Bone and tooth formation; energy metabolism; acid-base balance	Rare	Increased calcium excretion	Dairy products, eggs, meat, fish, poultry
Sodium	Fluid regulation; acid-base balance; nerve impulse and contraction; blood pressure	Headache, muscle cramps, weakness, mental status changes	Edema, hypertension, confusion, seizures	Table salt, processed food
Potassium	Fluid regulation; muscle function	Muscle weakness, confusion, cardiac dysrhythmias	Muscle weakness, vomiting, cardiac arrest	Fruits, vegetables, dairy products, meats, legumes
Magnesium	Bone structure; nerve and muscle function; blood clotting	Muscle twitching, weakness, mental status changes	Not related to dietary sources	Whole grains, legumes, green leafy vegetables, hard water
Chloride	Acid-base balance	Loss from the GI tract (emesis, NG output)	Results from dehydration	Table salt
Sulfur	Protein structure	None	None	Protein food sources
Iron	Role in hemoglobin formation	Microcytic anemia	Hemosiderosis, hemochromatosis	Meat, fish, poultry, egg yolks, vegetables, legumes, whole and enriched grains
Zinc	Carbohydrate metabolism; cofactor for enzymes	Decreased wound healing, decreased taste and smell, immune disorders	Vomiting, diarrhea, fever	Meat, fish, poultry, whole grains, legumes, eggs
Iodine	Thyroxine synthesis; regulate growth and development; regulation of basal metabolic rate	Decreased amount of thyroxine production, sluggishness, weight gain, goiter	Thyrotoxicosis	Iodized salt, saltwater fish and shellfish
Fluoride	Bone and tooth formation; protect against decay	Tooth decay and dental caries	Fluorosis (mottled teeth), headache, and gastric distress	Fluoridated water, tea, seafood, seaweed

used in the body, along with effects of deficiency or toxicity and food sources for them.

Nutritional needs are greatly affected by a person's age. Specific needs for macro- and micronutrients vary throughout the life span. Calorie requirements also rise and fall depending on the stage of life.

Standards for a Healthy Diet

Various daily food guides have been developed to help healthy people meet the daily requirements of essential nutrients and to facilitate meal planning. Food group plans emphasize the general types or groups of foods rather than

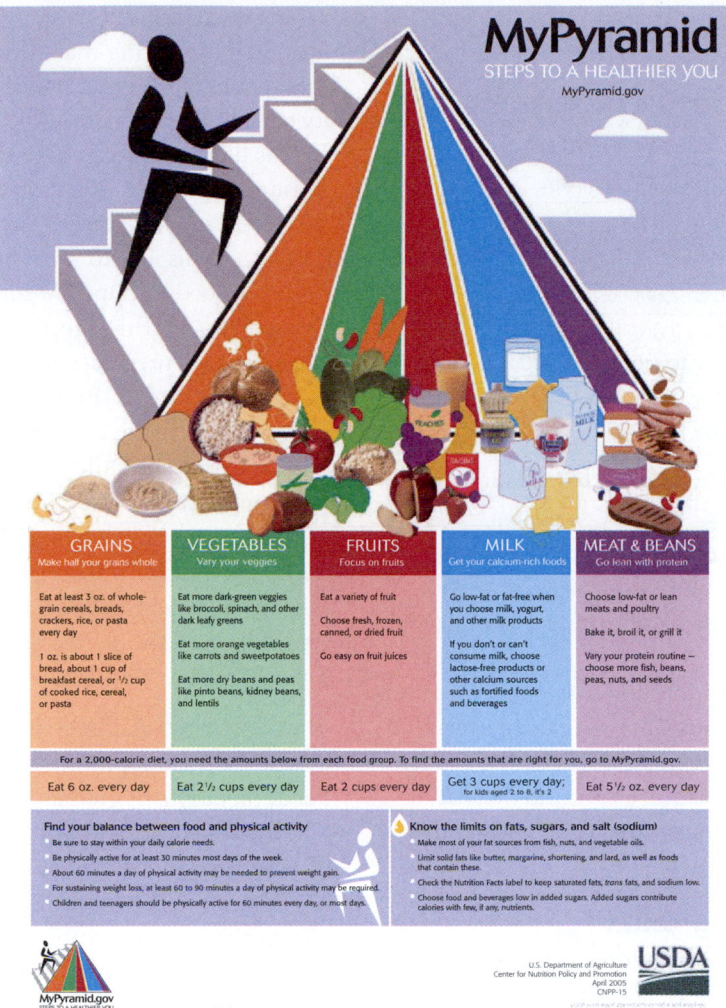

Figure 25-2. ■ The MyPyramid food guide. (*Source:* U.S. Department of Agriculture.)

the specific foods, because related foods are similar in composition and often have similar nutrient values. For example, all grains, whether wheat or oats, are significant sources of carbohydrates, iron, and the B vitamin thiamine.

The MyPyramid food guide has replaced the Food Guide Pyramid (Figure 25-2 ■). This is a web-based interactive tool that determines dietary recommendations based on an individual's age, sex, and activity level. It divides food into five groups: grains, vegetables, fruits, milk and dairy products, and meat and beans. Other daily food group guides include the 5-a-Day Program, which focuses on fruit and vegetable consumption, or Exchange Lists, which focus on the number of servings.

The USDA suggests that people eat a variety of whole foods to obtain the nutrients they need.

ENERGY BALANCE

Energy balance is the relationship between the energy obtained from food and the energy used by the body. The body gets energy in the form of **calories** (units of heat energy)

from carbohydrates, protein, fat, and alcohol. The body uses energy for voluntary activities (such as walking) and involuntary activities (such as breathing and growing). A person's energy balance is determined by comparing energy intake with energy output.

Metabolism is the term for all the biochemical and physiological processes by which the body grows and maintains itself. The **basal metabolic rate** (BMR) is the rate at which the body metabolizes food to maintain the energy requirements of a person who is awake and at rest. Lean, active people have a higher BMR than overweight and inactive people. In other words, lean people burn calories faster, even when at rest.

NUTRITIONAL REQUIREMENTS THROUGH THE LIFE SPAN

Nutritional considerations generally involve a diet that includes a proper distribution of intake from the major food groups, and that balances food intake with energy expenditure. Actual calories required at different stages of the life

TABLE 25-4	Calories Recommended by Life Stage	
AGE OF PERSON	**CALORIES RECOMMENDED**
Infant	100 to 200 kcal/kg/day
Toddler	1,100 to 1,300 kcal/day
Preschooler	1,300 to 1,600 kcal/day
School-age child	1,600 to 2,200 kcal/day*
Adolescent	2,200 to 2,800 kcal/day*
Adult female	1,300 to 2,000 kcal/day* change to 1,600 to 2,400 kcal/day
Adult male	2,200 to 2,600 kcal/day* change to 2,000 to 3,000 kcal/day

*Calories needed depend on many variables and should be individualized to the client.

span vary greatly. This chapter is not intended as a full course on nutrition. However, more information about nutrition can be found in the pediatric unit, Chapters 58 through 62 ⚭.

Infants have very special needs for the first year; these are addressed in Chapter 59 ⚭. Box 25-1 ■ gives an overview of infant nutrition. Throughout a person's life, one's gender, age, genetic makeup, and lifestyle affect nutritional requirements. Table 25-4 ■ lists recommended caloric intake by life stages.

Nutrition in the Growing Years

The nutritional needs of toddlers, children, and adolescents vary enormously and are affected by periods of growth. Toddlers may seem to eat practically nothing, and teens may appear to have an endless need for food. Neither state is

BOX 25-1	PEDIATRIC CONSIDERATIONS

Infant Nutrition

Nutrition for an infant during the first 12 months of life has an impact not only on growth and development, but also on the health of the infant in later life. Nurses play a key role in teaching parents about feeding infants.

For the first 4 to 6 months of life, formula or breast milk should be the sole source of nutrition for the infant. Sometime between 4 and 6 months, parents may start to introduce solid foods. Typically cereals, often iron fortified, are introduced first. Rice cereal is often the recommended first cereal because it is easy for most infants to digest. After cereal, fruits and vegetables are introduced next. The order of fruits or vegetables may be guided by the practitioner's recommendation. Meat is introduced last. New foods should be introduced one at a time about every 4 to 7 days to assess for food allergies. Cow's milk is not introduced before a year to prevent the development of iron-deficiency anemia. Raw honey should never be fed to an infant because of the risk of botulism. Parents also need to avoid any foods that may be choking hazards, such as popcorn, whole grapes, and hot dogs.

necessarily unhealthy; the body needs less when it is not growing and more during major "growth spurts." Overall, it is not the amount of food that provides for good health but the quality of food and the relationship of food intake to energy output.

It is best for parents of toddlers to look at the overall food consumption for several days versus intake at a single meal as their food intake patterns vary from meal to meal. It is important at this age to offer toddlers a wide variety of foods from all food groups. Mealtime is a social time for the preschooler. At this age the child may also wish to be involved in food preparation and can be given simple tasks such as setting the table. Providing preschoolers with a balanced diet, while limiting foods high in saturated fats, is the goal.

The school-age child begins to eat meals away from home. It is important that the child is given a nutritious breakfast to provide energy for learning. The child may wish to assist in packing a lunch. Teaching children healthy food choices at this age will help to influence food choices throughout life. At the end of the school-age period the child may begin a growth spurt as they enter into adolescence.

Nutrition in Adulthood

When the major physical growth processes stop in adulthood, metabolism gradually slows. To maintain (or achieve) a healthy weight, adults must pay attention to the volume of food they ingest and make necessary adjustments. Usually the most successful approach is to make incremental changes in eating habits (such as changing from whole to 2% milk, from 1% to skim) to reduce calories. It is also sensible to reduce fats ingested to 30% of the total calories consumed in a day. Table 25-5 ■ lists recommendations from the U.S. Department of Health and Human Services (2007) for daily consumption of food.

Nutrition for Older Adults

Changes in sensation and taste occur in older adults and can affect food intake. Clients may add salt to food to improve taste. They may need to be reminded of the dangers of high sodium intake. Encouraging them to add spices to food or try salt substitutes is an option. However, salt substitutes can be high in potassium. Often these clients do not consume enough calcium, which increases calcium loss from bones. Teach them that increasing calcium intake through food, supplements, or both is important. Vitamin D intake is important for the absorption of calcium. Pernicious anemia can develop as the production of intrinsic factor responsible for the absorption of vitamin B_{12} is reduced.

Finances may limit the types of foods the older adults can purchase. They may purchase more processed foods than fresh fruits and vegetables due to cost. The availability of transportation to purchase food can also influence food choices. Mobility problems may hinder the adults' ability to shop for food as well. Mobility can also play a role in the

TABLE 25-5	Recommended Amounts of Foods for Adults			
	AMOUNT RECOMMENDED		AVERAGE AMOUNT CONSUMED	
FOOD GROUP	MALES 31–50	FEMALES 31–50	MALES 31–50	FEMALES 31–50
Fruits	2 cups	1.5 cups	0.8 cups	0.8 cups
Vegetables	3 cups	2.5 cups	2.1 cups	1.6 cups
Grains	7 oz. eq.	6 oz. eq.	8.0 oz. eq.	5.9 oz. eq.
Meat and beans	6 oz. eq.	5 oz. eq.	7.4 oz. eq.	4.6 oz. eq.
Milk	3 cups	3 cups	1.8 cups	1.4 cups

individuals' ability to cook food. Eating alone or cooking for only one person may also influence the types of food purchased.

Issues for older adults are discussed in depth in Chapters 42, 43, and 46 ⬭. Special nursing concerns about dementia and Alzheimer's in older adults are discussed in Chapter 43 ⬭.

Specialized Diets

THERAPEUTIC DIETS

Alterations in the client's diet are often needed to treat a disease process such as diabetes mellitus, to prepare for a special examination or surgery, to increase or decrease weight, to restore nutritional deficits, or to allow an organ to rest and promote healing. Diets may be modified in texture, calories, specific nutrients, seasonings, or consistency (Box 25-2 ■).

Clients who do not have special needs eat the *regular* (*standard* or *house*) diet. The house diet is a balanced diet that supplies the metabolic requirements of a sedentary person (about 2,000 kcal). Most agencies offer clients a daily menu from which to select their meals for the next day. Others provide standard meals to each client on the general diet. A variation of the regular diet is the *light diet*, designed for postoperative and other clients who are not ready for the

regular diet. Foods in the light diet are plainly cooked; fat, bran, and high-fiber foods are usually omitted. Not all agencies provide a light diet.

Diets that are modified in consistency are often given to clients before and after surgery or to promote healing in clients with gastrointestinal distress. These diets include nothing by mouth (NPO, from the Latin *nil per os*), clear liquid, full liquid, soft, and diet as tolerated.

NPO or Nothing by Mouth

On an NPO diet, food and fluid are prohibited. This may be ordered before anesthesia or after surgery until bowel sounds return. IV fluids are often provided while a client is NPO to prevent dehydration. If a prolonged NPO diet is required, IV nutrition is usually ordered. *Note*: Enteral and parenteral feedings are discussed in Nursing Care and the procedures in this chapter.

Clear Liquid Diet

This diet is limited to water, tea, coffee, clear broths, ginger ale or other carbonated beverages, strained and clear juices, and plain gelatin. This diet provides the client with fluid and carbohydrate (in the form of sugar) but does not supply adequate protein, fat, vitamins, minerals, or calories (no more than 600 kcal/day). It is a short-term diet (24 to 36 hours) provided for clients after certain types of surgery or when infection occurs in the gastrointestinal system. The major objectives of this diet are to relieve thirst, prevent dehydration, and minimize stimulation of the gastrointestinal tract.

Full Liquid Diet

This diet contains only liquids or foods that turn to liquid at body temperature, such as ice cream. Full liquid diets are often eaten by clients who have gastrointestinal disturbances or are otherwise unable to tolerate solid or semisolid foods. This diet is not recommended for long-term use because it is low in iron, protein, and calories. In addition, its cholesterol content is high because of the amount of milk offered. If a client is on this diet for long periods, a nutritionally balanced oral supplement, such as Ensure, is usually ordered. Six or more feedings per day may work best for the client who must stay on this diet for a long period.

BOX 25-2	CULTURAL PULSE POINTS

Culture and Food Choices

Individual cultural practices often play a large role in the choice of food and diets. One's ethnic, national, and religious backgrounds have strong influences on food choices and eating patterns. Immigrants from another country may show preferences for their native foods. For example, Southeast Asians enjoy a diet high in fish, duck, chicken, eggs, pork, soybean products, rice, noodles, and tea, and they prepare foods by stir frying and steaming. It is helpful to be aware of cultural food preferences and demonstrate appreciation and respect for clients' choices. It is also helpful to incorporate these dietary preferences when helping a client to adjust to a dietary restriction.

Soft Diet

The soft diet is easily chewed and digested. It is often ordered for clients who have difficulty chewing and swallowing. It is a *low-residue* (low-fiber) diet with very few uncooked foods. The pureed diet is a modification of the soft diet. Liquid may be added to the food, which is then blended to a semisolid consistency.

Diet as Tolerated

Diet as tolerated is ordered when the client's appetite, ability to eat, and tolerance for certain foods change. For example, on the first postoperative day, a client may be given a clear liquid diet. If no nausea occurs, normal intestinal motility has returned, and the client feels like eating, the diet may be advanced to a full liquid, light, or regular diet.

DIET MODIFICATIONS FOR DISEASE

Many special diets may be prescribed to meet requirements for disease processes or altered metabolism. For example, a client with diabetes mellitus may need a diabetic diet recommended by the National Diabetic Association. An obese client may need a calorie-restricted diet. A cardiac client may need sodium and cholesterol restrictions. A client with allergies would need a nonallergenic diet. Some clients must follow certain diets (e.g., the diabetic diet) for a lifetime. If the diet is long term, the client must not only understand the diet, but also develop a healthy, positive attitude toward it. All dietary instructions must be individually designed to meet the client's intellectual ability, motivation level, lifestyle, culture, and economic status. Table 25-6 ■ provides specific information on dietary management of specific disorders.

TABLE 25-6	Dietary Management of Specific Disorders
FOR GASTROINTESTINAL DISORDERS	**DIETARY MANAGEMENT**
Low fiber	May be used with acute stages of diverticulosis, ulcerative colitis, and Crohn's disease Includes foods such as: ■ Milk products ■ Fruits without pulp or skins (need to be cooked or canned, not raw) ■ Vegetables without seeds or skins (need to be cooked or canned, not raw) ■ Refined bread and cereal products such as white bread, white rice, pasta, Cream of Wheat ■ Avoid products made with whole grains ■ Avoid products with nuts and seeds
High fiber	May be used for diverticular disease, constipation (prevention and treatment), and irritable bowel syndrome ■ Fiber intake goal for adults I 25 to 38 grams/day Includes foods such as: ■ Whole wheat bread, bran cereal, brown rice, and whole wheat pasta ■ Fruits with the skin on such as apples, pears, strawberries ■ Dried fruits ■ Beans ■ Vegetables such as broccoli, carrots, and peas ■ Popcorn, seeds (sunflower), and nuts
Gastroesophageal reflux disease (GERD)	Avoid or limit foods that relax the lower esophageal sphincter ■ Alcohol ■ Peppermint or spearmint oil ■ Chocolate ■ High-fat foods Avoid or limit foods that can irritate damaged intestinal mucosa ■ Carbonated beverages ■ Citrus fruits and juices ■ Coffee ■ Pepper ■ Spices ■ Tomatoes Food to encourage include: ■ Low-fat protein foods ■ Low-fat carbohydrate foods

TABLE 25-6	Dietary Management of Specific Disorders
FOR CARDIOVASCULAR DISORDERS	**DIETARY MANAGEMENT**
Low saturated fat, low cholesterol	Foods include: ■ Lean meats, skinless chicken, and fish ■ Low-fat or nonfat milk, cheese, and yogurt ■ Oils such as canola and olive ■ Limit trans fat intake (stick margarine, shortening, and processed foods made with hydrogenated fats) ■ High-fiber foods ■ Monounsaturated foods such as nuts, seeds, and avocado ■ Cholesterol intake of less than 300 mg/day ■ Avoid fried foods ■ Foods high in complex carbohydrates such as grains, fruits, and vegetables ■ Fish such as tuna and salmon (rich in omega-3 fatty acids)
Low-sodium diet	■ Can range from 250 mg to 3000 mg of sodium per day ■ Teach clients to read nutrition labels ■ Fresh foods contain less sodium than canned or processed foods ■ Fresh or frozen vegetables contain less sodium than canned vegetables ■ Snack foods are often high in sodium ■ Check sodium content of condiments such as catsup, pickles, soy sauce, and salad dressing ■ Avoid processed meat products such as lunch meat, bacon, and hot dogs ■ Cook with herbs or spices to flavor foods
Diabetes mellitus	■ Diet therapy individualized for each patient ■ < 10% saturated fat ■ Minimal intake of trans fat ■ < 300 mg cholesterol/day ■ Carbohydrate needs based on client's eating habits and blood glucose levels 　■ Choose complex carbohydrates ■ Limit foods high in sugar ■ High-fiber diet aids in lowering blood sugar

Sources: Data from Dudek, S. G. (2007). *Nutrition essentials for nursing practice* (5th ed.). Philadelphia, PA: Lippincott, Williams & Wilkins; Grodner, M., Long, S., & Walkingshaw, B. C. (2007). *Foundations & clinical applications of nutrition. A nursing approach* (4th ed.). St. Louis, MO: Mosby-Elsevier; and Hogan, M. A., Gingrich, M. M., Ricci, M. J., & Overby, P. (2006). *Fluids, electrolytes, and acid-base balance* (2nd ed.). Upper Saddle River, NJ: Prentice Hall.

VEGETARIAN AND OTHER ELECTIVE DIETS

The vegetarian diet presents special challenges to the nurse. For some people a vegetarian diet is a choice they make for the health benefits. For others, it may be cultural or religious. Diets for vegetarians fall into one of three categories.

Vegan diet: Diet consists of plant foods only.
Lacto vegetarian diet: Diet consists of plant foods along with dairy products.
Ovo-lacto vegetarian diet: Diet consists of plant foods, dairy products, and eggs.

The benefits of the vegetarian diet include decreased risk of obesity, heart disease, type 2 diabetes mellitus, and certain cancers. It takes careful diet planning to ensure that the individual who is following a vegetarian diet is consuming adequate amounts of certain nutrients, such as protein, iron, zinc, calcium, vitamin B_{12}, and vitamin D. (See previous discussion in this chapter regarding proteins and using plant protein in combination to make complete proteins.)

Calcium and vitamin D deficiencies can be seen in individuals who do not include dairy products in their diet. Iron, zinc, and vitamin B_{12} are all found in meat sources. Individuals need to find alternative sources for these nutrients or use supplements. Vitamin B_{12} is found only in food sources that are animal based. Deficiencies in this vitamin can take years to manifest and can cause permanent central nervous system damage. The client will need to take Vitamin B_{12} supplements or consume foods enriched with B_{12}. The nurse needs to educate clients choosing to follow a vegetarian diet on how to plan meals that will meet their individual dietary needs. The nurse may need to refer the client to a dietitian. The MyPyramid website also provides information on vegetarian diets.

As the U.S. population becomes more diverse, the nutrition and health needs of ethnic groups are being considered. Box 25-3 ■ offers variations to adapt the MyPyramid to ethnic diets.

FOOD ALLERGIES

It is important for the nurse to include food allergies when discussing allergies with a client. Food allergies occur when the immune system reacts to the ingestion of certain food proteins or molecules (see Chapter 35 ⬯ for more details on the immune response). The reaction can be immediate or delayed. The individual may experience nausea, vomiting, or itching. A severe reaction may lead to anaphylaxis (see Chapter 35 ⬯). In many cases food allergies develop during childhood, a time when new foods are being introduced. Again, this is why new foods should be introduced one at a time every 4 to 7 days during infancy. Allergy to foods presents a challenge to the child, parents, and caregivers, as well as teachers. Some of the common allergens are milk, nuts, wheat, and seafood.

Treating the allergy involves eliminating the food from the diet. Since most of the common allergens are found in many foods or are used in foods as fillers or stabilizers, clients need to become aware of what foods or food products may contain the allergen. Often a dietitian is needed to assist with meal planning and to ensure that nutritional needs are being met. The family needs to learn to read labels to determine whether allergens are in specific foods. They also need to know whether a machine that produces an allergen-free food is also used to produce foods that contain the allergen.

BOX 25-3	CULTURAL PULSE POINTS

Alternate Food Guides

Several variations have been made to adapt the food guide pyramid to ethnic diets.

Asian Diet Pyramid

A wide base of rice, rice products, noodles, breads, and grains; whole grains; and minimally processed foods
A second level of fruits; vegetables; and legumes, nuts, and seeds
Daily small amounts of vegetable oils; physical activity; and plant-based beverages (tea, sake, beer, or wine)
Optional daily fish, shellfish, or dairy
Weekly eggs or poultry and sweets
Monthly meats

Mediterranean Diet Pyramid

Abundance of food from plant sources, including fruits and vegetables, potatoes, breads and grains, beans, nuts, and seeds
Emphasis on a variety of minimally processed and seasonally fresh, locally grown foods
Olive oil as the principal fat
Daily consumption of low to moderate amounts of cheese and yogurt
Weekly low to moderate amounts of fish and zero to four eggs per week
Fresh fruit and typical daily dessert; sweets and saturated fat not more than a few times per week
Red meat a few times per week
Moderate consumption of wine, normally with meals
Regular physical activity

Native American Food Pyramid

Grain group divided into bread/cereal and rice/pasta—6 to 11 a day
Vegetables, 3 to 5 servings including corn, squash, and cactus
Fruits, 2 to 4 servings fresh whole fruits
Dairy, 2 to 3 servings including cheese, yogurt, and milk
Meat, poultry, fish, dried beans, eggs, and nuts, 2 to 3 servings
Fats and oils sparingly

NURSING CARE

PRIORITIZING NURSING CARE

The first priority in nursing care when performing a nutritional assessment is to obtain a height and weight. The nurse must know how to obtain the height and weight accurately using the appropriate equipment. The nurse will use the data from this assessment to assist the primary nurse in developing a plan of care for the client. Accurate height and weight measurement is also crucial in calculating medication doses.

ASSESSING

Size and weight are factors we notice almost without thinking. If a client is very thin or very heavy, this will be one of the first things the nurse observes. The nurse collects data about the client's height and weight. The nurse selects the appropriate type of scale to be used (Figures 25-3 ■ and 25-4 ■). Box 25-4 ■ provides guidelines about how to obtain a client's weight.

Ideal body weight (IBW) is the weight recommended for optimal health. A person is said to be overweight when body weight exceeds IBW by up to 20%. A person whose body weight exceeds IBW by more than 20% is said to have

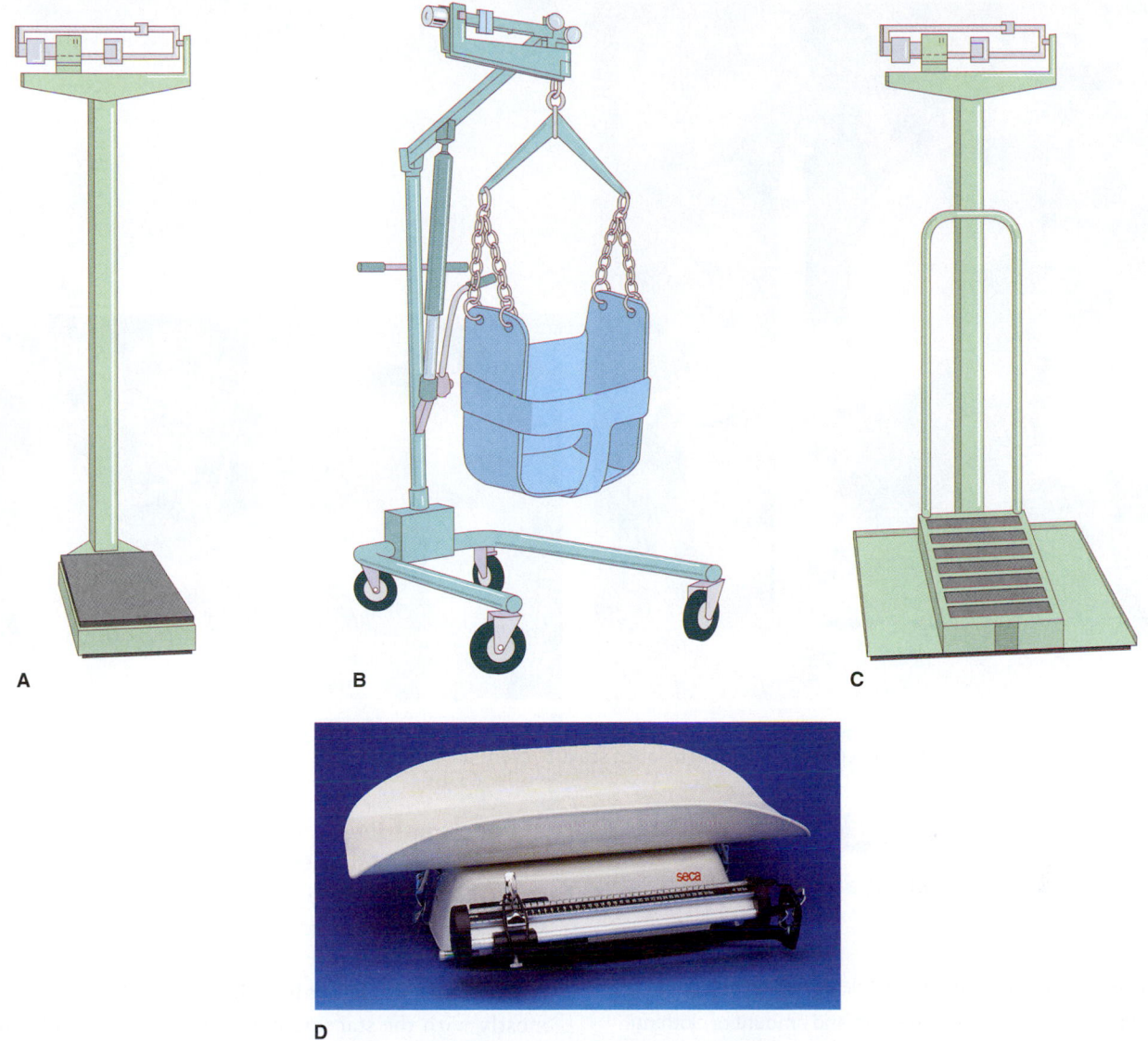

Figure 25-3. ■ Types of scales: **A.** standing balance scale; **B.** mechanical lift scale; **C.** wheelchair platform scale; **D.** neonate balance scale.

obesity. Standardized tables can provide approximate ideal weights, but they are not precise.

For people over 18 years old, the body mass index (BMI) may be a better indicator of whether a person's weight is appropriate for height. The BMI also may provide a useful estimate of malnutrition. However, the results must be used with caution in people who have fluid retention (e.g., ascites or edema). BMI results may be high in people who are athletes, since muscle tissue is heavy.

To calculate an individual's BMI, use this formula:

1. Measure the person's height in meters (1 meter = 3.3 ft, or 39 in.). Divide number of inches by 39 to find height in meters.
2. Measure the weight in kilograms (1 kg = 2.2 pounds). Divide number of pounds by 2.2 to find the weight in kilograms.

3. Calculate the BMI using the following formula:

$$\text{BMI} = \frac{\text{Weight in kilograms}}{(\text{Height in meters})^2}$$

4. Use the BMI number as follows: below 16, malnourished; 16–19, underweight; 20–25, normal; 26–30, overweight; 31–40, moderately to severely obese; and over 40, morbidly obese.

Problems of weight are among the most common health problems of adults. Excess body weight causes stress on body organs and contributes to chronic health problems such as hypertension and diabetes mellitus. Morbid obesity is obesity that interferes with mobility or breathing. Obese people may lack important nutrients even though they are eating excess calories.

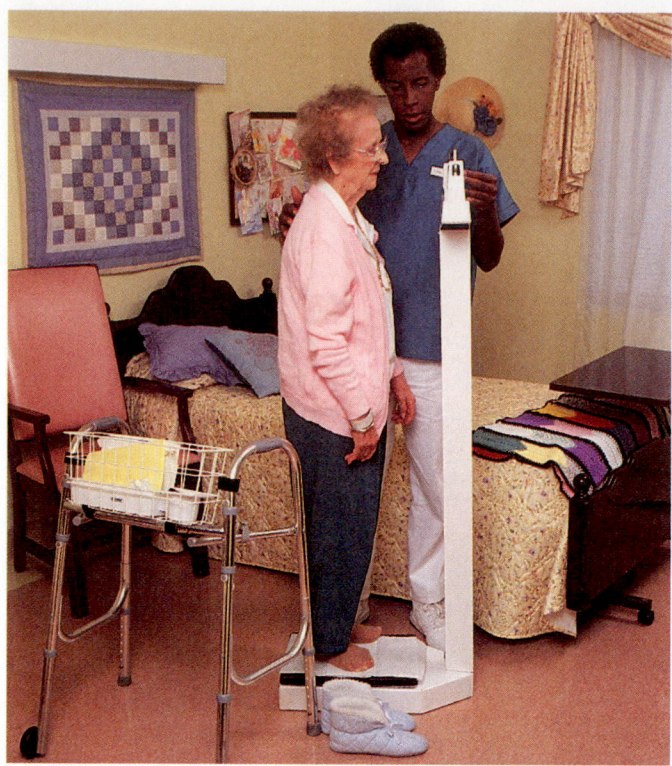

A

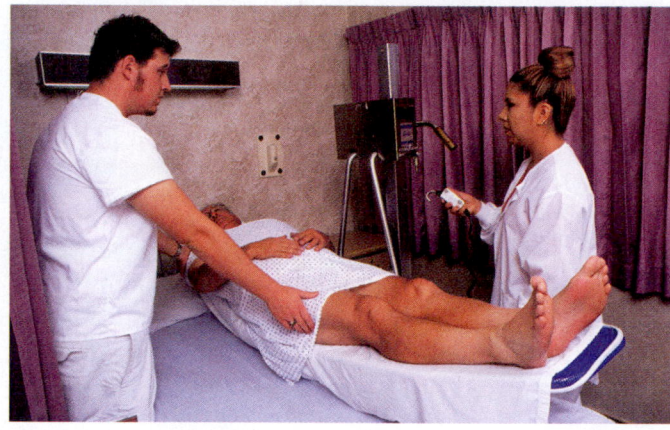

B

Figure 25-4. ■ Weighing the client: **A.** client on standing balance scale; **B.** client on bed scale.

BOX 25-4	NURSING CARE CHECKLIST

Obtaining a Client's Weight and Height

Adult Client
If client is able to stand:

☑ Take measurement at the same time each day.

☑ Have the client wear the same kind and amount of clothing each day, and no shoes.

☑ Have client stand on the weighing platform while the nurse reads and records the weight (see Figure 25-4A).

☑ For height obtain at the same time as weight with shoes off.

If client cannot stand:

☑ Weigh the client on a chair scale, *or*

☑ Weigh the client with a bed scale (canvas straps lift the client, and weight is recorded on a digital display or balance arm [see Figure 25-4B]).

☑ Some bed models also have a scale built in.

☑ For height have client lay flat on bed, measure from heel to top of head.

Pediatric Client

☑ Lay neonates flat on the balance (see Figure 25-3D).

☑ Weigh infants without any clothing.

☑ Weigh young children in their underwear.

☑ For height have infant lay flat on bed, measure from heel to top of head.

Undernutrition means that nutrient intake is insufficient to meet daily energy requirements. It can occur because the person does not eat enough food, or because he or she cannot digest or absorb food. Risk factors for undernutrition are listed in Box 25-5 ■.

Protein–calorie malnutrition (PCM), once associated mostly with the starving children of third world countries, is now recognized as a significant problem of clients with cancer and chronic disease. Characteristics of PCM are weight loss and visible muscle and fat wasting.

BOX 25-5	RISK FACTORS FOR UNDERNUTRITION

- Too few calories consumed
- Inability to digest or absorb food
- Inadequate production of hormones or enzymes
- Medical condition resulting in inflammation or obstruction of the gastrointestinal tract
- Inability to acquire and prepare food
- Lack of knowledge about essential nutrients and a balanced diet
- Discomfort during or after eating
- Dysphagia (difficulty swallowing)
- Nausea or vomiting
- Anorexia or bulimia
- Severe depression
- Elderly living alone and/or on fixed incomes

DIAGNOSING, PLANNING, AND IMPLEMENTING

The most frequent nursing diagnoses related to nutrition are *Imbalanced Nutrition: More than Body Requirements, Imbalanced Nutrition: Less than Body Requirements*, and *Risk for Imbalanced Nutrition* (as above). Nursing care of clients with imbalanced nutrition includes assisting with changes in diet, monitoring blood glucose, stimulating appetite, assisting with meals, and providing enteral nutrition.

Providing Therapeutic Diet

Nurses provide therapeutic diets as ordered, monitor food intake, and provide client teaching to reinforce the need for the diet. The nurse follows facility guidelines for progressing a diet after surgery or other procedures for which the client has been NPO.

Monitoring Blood Glucose

Clients who have diabetes may need to monitor random blood glucose levels throughout the day. This can be accomplished in the home setting by the client or family member, as well as by persons formally trained in medical care. By testing a single drop of blood, the client can receive a reading of the blood glucose present at the moment. Clients who understand the significance of this reading will be more likely to comply with their therapeutic diet for optimal management of their diabetes. Procedure 25-1 ■ on page 580 describes blood glucose monitoring. See main discussion in Chapter 38.

Stimulating the Appetite

Physical illness, unfamiliar or unpalatable food, environmental and psychological factors, and physical discomfort or pain may depress a client's appetite. A short-term decrease in food intake usually is not a problem for adults. However, over time, it leads to weight loss, decreased strength and stamina, and other nutritional problems. A decreased food intake is often accompanied by a decrease in fluid intake, which may cause dehydration. The nurse must determine the reason for a client's lack of appetite and then take steps to intervene. Reducing unpleasant odors, positioning the client comfortably, and sometimes cooling the room slightly are interventions that may help stimulate appetite.

Assisting Clients with Meals

Certain groups of people frequently require help with their meals. These groups include older adults who are infirm; people with physical impairments, such as clients who are blind; those who must remain in a back-lying position; and those who cannot use their hands. *Note:* The major discussion of this topic is found in Chapter 46 ∞, Nursing in Long-Term Care.

When feeding a client, ask in which order the client would like to eat the food. If the client cannot see, tell the client which food is being given. Always allow ample time for the client to chew and swallow the food before offering more. Also, provide fluids as requested. When the client is unable to communicate, offer fluids after every three or four mouthfuls of solid food. It is important to make the time a pleasant one, choosing topics of conversation that are of interest to clients who want to talk.

Although normal utensils should be used whenever possible, special utensils may be needed to assist a client to eat (see Figure 46-4 ∞). Many adaptive feeding aids are available to help clients maintain independence. A standard eating utensil with a built-up or widened handle helps clients who cannot grasp objects easily. Plates with rims and plastic or metal plate guards enable the client to pick up the food by first pushing it against this raised edge. A suction cup or damp sponge or cloth may be placed under the dish to keep it from moving while the client is eating. No-spill mugs and two-handled drinking cups are especially useful for persons with impaired hand coordination. Stretch terry cloth and knitted or crocheted glass covers enable the client to keep a secure grasp on a glass. Lidded tip-proof glasses are also available. Clients are more likely to participate in mealtime if their meal is set up for them as needed. The nursing staff may need to open packages and cartons to make the food accessible. Meat may need to be cut, a sugar packet opened, or tea bags placed in the hot water. These simple preparations encourage the client to begin eating. They also give a few moments for the nurse and client to engage in pleasant conversation, another stimulant for eating.

Providing Enteral Nutrition

Two types of alternative feeding methods are **enteral nutrition** (through the gastrointestinal system) and parenteral (intravenous) nutrition. **Parenteral nutrition,** also referred to as total parenteral nutrition (TPN), is provided when the client is unable to ingest or absorb foods.

Enteral Access Devices

Enteral access is achieved by nasogastric or nasointestinal tubes, or gastrostomy or jejunostomy tubes.

A nasogastric tube is inserted through one of the nostrils, down the nasopharynx, and into the stomach or small intestine. Traditional *nasogastric tubes* are firm and larger than 12 Fr in diameter. They are passed through the nose and pharynx to the stomach. An example is the Levin tube, a flexible rubber or plastic, single-lumen tube with holes near the tip. The commonly used Salem sump tube has two lumens, the smaller of the two for air entry to reduce the risk of a vacuum forming should the tube affix itself to the mucosal lining of the stomach. Softer tubes that are

MyNursingKit | NG tube

more flexible and smaller than 12 Fr in diameter are frequently used for total enteral nutrition (TEN).

Nasogastric tubes are used for clients who have intact gag and cough reflexes, who have adequate gastric emptying, and who require short-term feedings. Procedure 25-2 ■ on page 581 provides guidelines for inserting and removing a nasogastric tube.

Nasogastric tubes may be inserted for reasons other than providing a route for feeding the client. These include:

- To prevent nausea, vomiting, and gastric distention following surgery. In this case, the tube is attached to a suction source.
- To remove stomach contents for laboratory analysis.
- To *lavage* (wash) the stomach in cases of poisoning or overdose of medications.

A *nasoenteric tube* is a longer tube than the nasogastric tube (at least 40 inches for an adult). It is inserted into one nostril and through the pharynx, esophagus, and stomach into the upper small intestine. Some agencies may require that specially trained nurses or physicians do this procedure. Nasoenteric tubes are used when risk for aspiration is high. Clients are at risk for aspiration if any of the following exist:

- Decreased level of consciousness
- Poor cough or gag reflexes
- Endotracheal intubation
- Recent extubation
- Inability to cooperate with the procedure
- Restlessness or agitation

Gastrostomy and *jejunostomy devices* are used for long-term nutritional support, generally more than 6 to 8 weeks. Conventional tubes may be placed surgically or by laparoscopy through the abdominal wall into the stomach (**gastrostomy**) or into the jejunum (**jejunostomy**). More commonly, though, the percutaneous endoscopic gastrostomy (PEG) is used.

Testing Feeding Tube Placement

Before feedings are introduced, tube placement is confirmed by radiography, particularly when a small-bore tube has been inserted or when the client is at risk for aspiration. After placement is confirmed, the nurse marks the tube with indelible ink or tape at its exit point from the nose and documents the length of visible tubing for baseline data. Box 25-6 ■ lists items for the nurse to check prior to tube feeding.

Enteral Feedings and Medication

The frequency of feedings and amounts to be administered are ordered by the physician. Liquid feeding mixtures are available commercially, for example, Ensure, Osmolite, or Jevity. Enteral feedings may be ordered as intermittent or continuous. An **intermittent feeding** is the administration of 300 to 500 mL of enteral formula several times per day. These feedings are

| BOX 25-6 | NURSING CARE CHECKLIST |

Verifying Tube Placement for Enteral Feedings

- ☑ Aspirate 20 to 30 mL of gastrointestinal secretions. *Note:* Small-bore tubes offer more resistance during aspirations than large-bore tubes and are more likely to collapse when negative pressure is applied.
- ☑ Measure the pH of aspirated fluid. This is the recommended method to determine tube placement. The pH of gastric fluid is normally 6 or lower, different from the pH of respiratory or intestinal fluids.
- ☑ Auscultate the epigastrium while injecting 5 to 20 mL of air. Air injected into the stomach produces whooshing, gurgling, or bubbling sounds over the epigastrium and the upper left quadrant. This method is less reliable than pH testing.
- ☑ Ensure initial radiographic verification of small-bore tubes.
- ☑ Closely observe the client for signs of obvious distress, and suspect tube dislodgment after episodes of coughing, sneezing, and vomiting.

usually administered through the tube into the stomach over at least 30 minutes. **Continuous feedings** are generally administered over a 24-hour period using an infusion pump that guarantees a constant flow. Continuous feedings are essential when feedings are administered in the small bowel. *Cyclic feedings* are continuous feedings that are administered in less than 24 hours (e.g., 12 to 16 hours). These feedings, often administered at night and referred to as nocturnal feedings, allow the client to attempt to eat regular meals through the day. Because nocturnal feedings may use higher nutrient densities and higher infusion rates than the standard continuous feeding, the client should be assessed for fluid volume excess.

clinical ALERT

If a feeding tube accidentally becomes dislodged, formula could go into the lungs, causing aspiration or even death. Therefore, the nurse must verify that the tube is in the stomach before each intermittent feeding. In the case of continuous feedings, the nurse checks placement at least once per shift and before administering any medications through the tube.

Procedure 25-3 ■ on page 585 provides the essential steps for administering a tube feeding and for administering and evaluating a gastrostomy or jejunostomy tube feeding. Procedure 25-4 ■ describes how to administer medications through an enteral tube.

Before administering a tube feeding, the nurse must check for any food allergies and assess tolerance to previous feedings. The nurse must also check the expiration date on a commercially prepared formula or the preparation date and time of agency-prepared solution. Any formula that has passed the expiration date or solution that has been at room temperature for more than 8 hours must be discarded.

Providing Parenteral Nutrition

Feedings must sometimes be given intravenously when a client is unable to tolerate foods or formula through the gastrointestinal tract. Feeding is indicated when the client has a need for intensive nutritional support, as seen with burns, sepsis, and multiple trauma, or at times when the intestinal tract and/or accessory organs are not functioning or need to be rested, as occurs with inflammatory bowel disorders such as Crohn's disease and pancreatitis. There are two forms of parenteral nutrition:

- *Peripheral vein infusions.* Various solutions containing dextrose, amino acids, vitamins, and minerals can be infused into peripheral veins. However, hypertonic solutions are irritating to peripheral veins and the concentrations of such solutions must be less than 10% dextrose. This limits the concentrations and amount of fluids and nutrients that can be safely administered. This method of feeding is only used when the need for nutritional support is short term, usually less than 2 weeks.
- *Central vein infusions.* When the nutritional needs are great, the use of a large central vein is desirable. TPN is infused through a catheter that is surgically inserted into a central vein, such as the subclavian or femoral vein, or through a peripherally inserted central catheter, which is inserted into a peripheral vein and is threaded forward into a large central vein. The central catheter allows for infusion of larger volumes of nutrients and for longer periods of time. They carry an added risk of infection and must be closely monitored.

EVALUATING

To evaluate the client with imbalanced nutrition, the nurse would compare baseline weight with current data and determine the client's compliance with the recommended diet. Goals for activity would be assessed. The client's support system and sense of satisfaction with changes in weight would be reviewed. If necessary, plans and goals would be adjusted.

Continuity of Care

The nurse must be an educator in helping clients with nutritional imbalances. Positive effects of changes in diet must be emphasized. Negative effects of continued imbalances must also be addressed. Every effort must be made to have the client participate in the planned changes, because food choice is a central part of people's lifestyles. Discuss with the client what goals they have in mind, and point out how their therapeutic diet will help them reach those goals. If clients are involved and empowered, believing that they can make a difference, their chances for success are much improved. It is important to assess the support of family and friends available to the client.

NURSING PROCESS CARE PLAN
Client with Altered Nutrition

Andrea Brown is a 20-year-old single woman who has been diagnosed as having anorexia. She is underweight, weighs 22% less than IBW, and is weak. Despite her declining weight, she continues to make comments about being overweight such as "I am still too fat for my body build. I have no control over my life no matter what I do." Her hair appears to be thinning, and there are dark circles under her eyes. Upon collecting the meal tray one afternoon, the nurse notices that no food has been touched, and the client has requested soda crackers to go with her diet soda. Upon questioning, Ms. Brown states that she has had plenty to eat and is not hungry.

Assessment

VS: T 98, P 110, R 16, BP 110/74. Documentation of meals shows a poor intake, less than 25% at each meal since admission. Skin turgor is poor and mucous membranes dry. Lab tests indicate protein is below normal levels.

Nursing Diagnosis

The following important nursing diagnoses (among others) are established for this client:

- *Imbalanced Nutrition: Less than Body Requirements* related to anorexia
- *Adult Failure to Thrive* related to inadequate nutritive intake
- *Risk for Impaired Skin Integrity* related to alterations in nutritional state

Expected Outcomes

The expected outcomes for the plan of care are that Ms. Brown will:

- Establish and maintain protein lab levels of normal value.
- Participate in psychiatric counseling program on a regular basis.
- Demonstrate stable weight without further losses in immediate future.

Planning and Implementation

The following nursing interventions are implemented for Ms. Brown. Assessments are done frequently to monitor her condition.

- Monitor weight daily.
- Record oral intake each meal.
- Dietitian consult to identify daily caloric intake necessary to stabilize weight loss and reach target weight.
- If client refuses to eat, notify physician.

- Work with healthcare team members and client to establish goals for weight gain and increased food intake.
- Establish an atmosphere of trust with the client.
- Request psychiatric consult order. Follow recommendations offered by mental health practitioner.
- Monitor skin for redness and breakdown daily during bath.

Evaluation

Although the client agrees to participate in the plan recommended by the healthcare team, progress is made slowly. Her weight loss is slowed, but continued monitoring and support of the healthcare team are necessary.

Critical Thinking in the Nursing Process

1. What possible interventions may need to be implemented to address a nutritional and fluid balance for Ms. Brown?
2. What would be the role of the psychiatric clinician when anorexia is demonstrated with physical characteristics?
3. Why would the diagnosis *Disturbed Body Image* be appropriate for Ms. Brown?

Note: Discussion of Critical Thinking questions appears on the MyNursingKit Website.

> **Note:** The references and resources for all chapters have been compiled at the back of the book.

PROCEDURE 25-1 Monitoring Blood Glucose

Purposes

- To determine the client's blood glucose level
- To provide data for administering insulin in clients with diabetes mellitus or clients with disease processes requiring insulin

Equipment

- Chemical strips for reading glucose measurement
- Glucose monitor
- Lancet mechanism for obtaining blood
- Antiseptic agent (if required by agency)
- Cotton swabs
- Gloves
- Insulin sliding scale

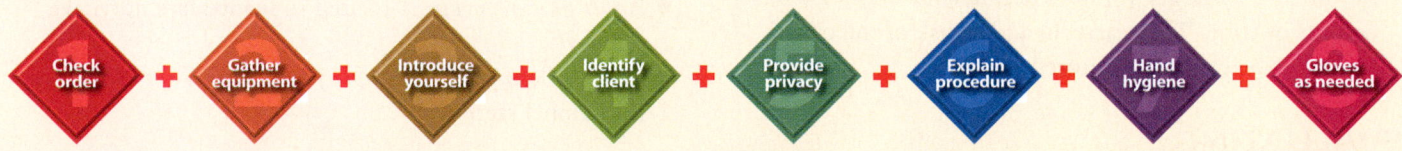

Check order + Gather equipment + Introduce yourself + Identify client + Provide privacy + Explain procedure + Hand hygiene + Gloves as needed

Interventions and Rationales

1. Perform preparatory steps (see icon bar above).
2. Prepare the client. Explain that a drop of blood is needed to determine the client's blood glucose level. *This promotes cooperation.*
3. Confirm the correct chemical strips with the machine code. *Matching the codes prevents a misreading.*
4. Remove chemical strip from container and place it in the machine.
5. Prepare the lancet for puncture.
6. Don gloves. *This supports infection control.*
7. Hold chosen finger downward and squeeze gently from base to fingertip. *This helps bring blood to the puncture site.*
8. Wipe intended puncture site (lateral pads of fingers) per hospital protocol.
9. Place lancet against side of finger and release spring or stick finger with darting motion. *Lateral side is less sensitive.*
10. Allow drop of blood to accumulate onto chemical strip.
11. Activate timing device if monitor is not equipped with automatic timer.
12. Apply pressure to puncture site.
13. Allow the appropriate time for a digital readout.
14. Obtain results from the digital reading.
15. Discard soiled materials and gloves in proper containers.
16. Position client for comfort with the call bell within reach.
17. Document appropriate dose of regular insulin from sliding scale if provided.

SAMPLE DOCUMENTATION

[date] [time] Blood Glucose: 250; Reg. Insulin
5 units given

SC per sliding scale in right
upper arm. _____
_____ N. Agarwal, LPN

Inserting and Removing Nasogastric Tubes

Purposes

- To administer tube feedings and medications directly into the GI tract for clients unable to eat by mouth or swallow a sufficient diet
- To establish a means for suctioning stomach contents to prevent gastric distention, nausea, and vomiting
- To remove stomach contents for laboratory analysis
- To *lavage* (wash) the stomach in case of poisoning, overdose of medications, or gastric bleeding

Equipment

- Nasogastric tube—Levin (single-lumen) or Salem sump (double-lumen)
- Towels, tissue, and an emesis basis
- Nonallergenic adhesive tape, 4 inches long and 1 inch wide or a NG tube clip
- Disposable gloves
- Water-soluble lubricant
- Glass of water and drinking straw
- Irrigating set with 20-mL syringe or 30-mL syringe with catheter tip
- pH test strip
- Stethoscope
- Clamp or plug for tubing
- Suction equipment if required
- Tincture of benzoin
- Tongue blade and penlight
- Rubber band and safety pin
- Plastic disposable bag
- Oral care supplies

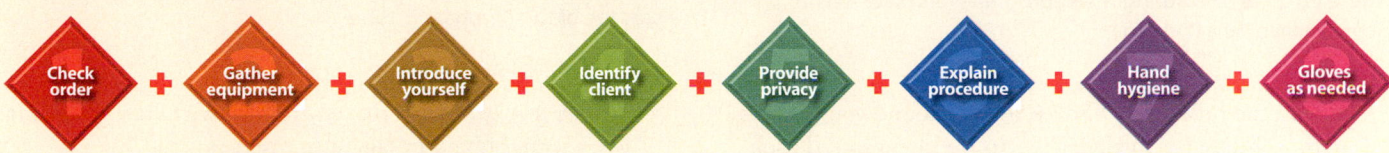

Part A: Inserting a Nasogastric Tube
Interventions and Rationales

1. Perform preparatory steps (see icon bar above).
2. Prepare the client.
   - Explain to the client what you plan to do. *The passage of a gastric tube is not painful, but it is unpleasant because the gag reflex is activated during insertion.* Tell the client how to breathe and swallow upon your direction to facilitate insertion of the tube. Establish with the client what sign he or she could use (such as raising hand) to indicate for you to pause due to discomfort or gagging. *This form of communication gives client reassurance.*
   - Assist the client to a high-Fowler's position if health condition permits, and support the head on a pillow. *This facilitates passage of the tube into the esophagus.* Place a towel across the chest.
      - Remove the client's dentures so they do not become loose and interfere with insertion of the tube. Place tissues and emesis basin near client.
3. Assess the client's nares.
   - Ask the client if he or she has had nasal surgery, trauma, or a bleeding disorder. *An NG may be contraindicated in clients with such a history.*
   - Examine the nares for any obstructions or deformities by asking the client to breathe through one nostril while occluding the other.
   - Select the nostril that has the greater airflow.
   - Have client blow nose to clear.
4. Prepare the tube.
   - If needed, chill the tube for less flexibility, or warm the tube for increased flexibility. *A tube that is firm but not rigid will pass most easily and with the least amount of trauma.*
5. Determine how far to insert the tube.
   - Use the tube to mark off the distance from the tip of the client's nose to the tip of the earlobe and then from the tip of the earlobe to the tip of the sternum (Figure 25-5 ■). This length approximates the distance from the nares to the stomach and may vary among individuals. Measuring the tube in this manner is more reliable than relying on tube markings and customizes the placement for this client. Mark the measured length with adhesive tape.
6. Insert the tube.
   - Lubricate the tip of the tube well with water-soluble lubricant or water to ease insertion, avoiding covering the holes on the tube with lubricant. *The lubricant reduces friction, thus reducing trauma. A water-soluble lubricant dissolves if the tube accidentally enters the lungs. An oil-based lubricant, such as petroleum jelly, will not dissolve and could cause respiratory complications if it enters the lungs.*

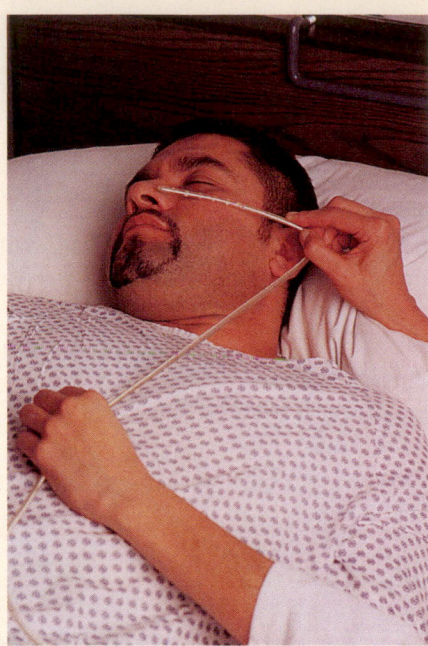

Figure 25-5. ■ Measuring the appropriate length of NG tube. (Photographer: Elena Dorfman.)

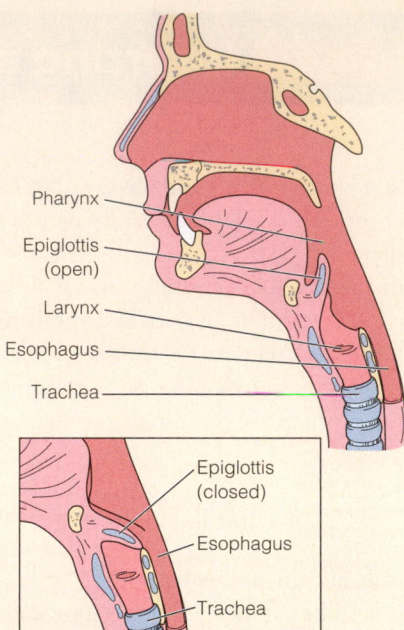

Figure 25-6. ■ Swallowing closes the epiglottis and allows passage of the nasogastric tube.

- Coil the tube's first 7 to 10 inches around your fingers to facilitate passage. Gently tip the client's head back and insert the tube, with its natural curve toward the client, into the selected nostril. Slowly advance the tube toward the nasopharynx by directing the tube toward the ear.
- If the tube meets resistance, withdraw it, relubricate it, and insert it in the other nostril. *The tube should never be forced against resistance, because of the possibility of trauma.*
- Once the tube reaches the pharynx the client will feel the tube in the throat and may gag and retch. You may need to pause and have the client rest for a few moments. Have the client take sips of water to calm the gag reflex.
- Ask the client to tilt the head forward, and encourage the client to drink sips of water and swallow (if not contraindicated). *Tilting the head forward facilitates passage of the tube into the posterior pharynx and esophagus rather than into the larynx; swallowing moves the epiglottis over the opening to the larynx* (Figure 25-6 ■).
- In cooperation with the client, pass the tube 5 to 10 cm (2 to 4 in.) with each swallow, until the indicated length is inserted.
- Stop the procedure and immediately remove tube if the client shows signs of coughing or cyanosis. *This could indicate that the tube has slipped into the trachea.*
- If the client continues to gag and the tube does not advance with each swallow, withdraw it slightly, and inspect the throat by looking through the mouth. *The*

tube may be coiled in the throat. If so, withdraw it until it is straight, and try again to insert it.

7. Ascertain correct placement of the tube. (This will vary based on institutional policy.)
   - Ask the client to speak or hum. *If unable to do so, the tube may have passed through the vocal cords or coiled in the back of the throat.*
   - Auscultate air insufflation. This is done by attaching a syringe with 10 to 20 mL of air in it to the end of the tube. Place your stethoscope over the left upper quadrant of the abdomen, and listen while the air is injected. *You will hear the movement of air if the placement is in the stomach. If the client belches, the tube may be in the esophagus.*
   - With the syringe in place, withdraw stomach contents to determine placement of the tube in the stomach. If unable to withdraw contents, turn client on left side, advance the tube 1 to 2 inches, and attempt again.
   - Check the pH of the stomach contents. *Gastric content normal pH is 6 or below.*
   - If the signs do not indicate placement in the stomach, advance the tube 5 cm (2 in.), and repeat the tests.
   - Placement may be verified by x-ray. *It is unsafe to place the end of the tube in water to check placement, because it places the client at risk for aspiration.*

8. Connect the tube to suction or plug the tube end.

9. Apply tincture of benzoin to the bridge of the nose where tape will be placed. *Taping will improve the security of the tube.*

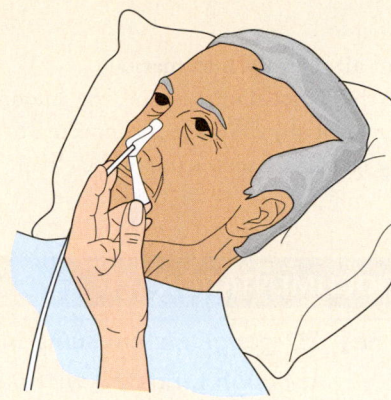

Figure 25-7. ■ Taping an NG tube to the bridge of the nose.

10. Prepare the tape by tearing it lengthwise halfway. Tape the unsplit end of tape to the nose and cross the split ends around the tubing (Figure 25-7 ■). *Do not tape tube to forehead because this may cause trauma to the nostril.*

11. To allow for client movement, make a slipknot with a rubber band around the tube. Secure the tube by pinning the rubber band to the client's gown.

12. To connect to suction, attach the larger lumen of the Salem sump. This begins intermittent or continuous suction (as ordered).

13. Document the insertion of the tube, including time, type of tube, size of tube, confirmation of placement, and client response.

14. Ensure the client's comfort.

15. Irrigate the tube every 2 hours or as ordered.

16. Specific care of the Salem sump:
    ■ Inject 10 to 20 mL of air into the smaller lumen, the blue port. *This will clear the air vent, preventing gastric mucosal trauma if the tube adheres to the stomach lining. You can test for proper functioning of the air vent by putting the port near your ear. You will hear a hissing sound if patency exists.* Do not let the port hang downward or stomach contents may drain from it.

17. Clean the nares and provide oral care every shift and as needed to prevent infection and promote comfort. Assess nares for skin irritation.
    ■ Apply water-soluble lubricant to the nostril if it appears dry or encrusted.
    ■ Change the adhesive tape as required.
    ■ Position client in semi-Fowler's position. *Head of bed must be elevated at least 30 degrees to minimize gastric reflux.*

18. Document placement checks and drainage amount, consistency, and color.

19. If suction is applied, ensure that the patency of both the nasogastric and suction tubes is maintained.
    ■ Irrigations of the tube with 30 mL of normal saline may be required at regular intervals. In some agencies, irrigations must be ordered by the physician.
    ■ Keep accurate records of the client's fluid intake and output, and record the amount and characteristics of the drainage. *This supports continuity of care.*

VARIATION: SMALL-BORE FEEDING TUBE

1. Prepare the tube for insertion.

2. Do not ice the tube or it will be too stiff.

3. Insert the stylet (guidewire) into the tube. Lubricate tube with water to activate lubricant.

4. After tube is in the stomach, have the client lean forward or to the right to help in advancing the tube. Leave the stylet in.

5. X-ray must confirm proper placement before any feeding is introduced. The stylet is removed after placement is confirmed.

PEDIATRIC CONSIDERATIONS

■ For infants and young children, restraints may be necessary during tube insertion and throughout therapy. Restraints will prevent accidental dislodging of the tube.

■ Place the infant in an infant seat, or position the infant with a rolled towel or pillow under the head and shoulders.

■ When assessing the nares, obstruct one of the infant's nares, and feel for air passage from the other. If the nasal passageway is very small or is obstructed, an orogastric tube may be more appropriate.

■ For infants and young children, measure appropriate NG tube length from the nose to the tip of the earlobe and then to the point midway between the umbilicus and the xiphoid process.

■ If an orogastric tube is used, measure from the tip of the earlobe to the corner of the mouth to the xiphoid process.

■ Do not hyperextend or hyperflex an infant's neck. *Hyperextension or hyperflexion of the neck could occlude the airway.*

■ For infants or small children, tape the tube to the area between the end of the nares and the upper lip, as well as to the cheek.

Part B: Removing a Nasogastric Tube
Interventions and Rationales

1. Confirm the physician's order to remove the tube.

2. Prepare the client.
   - Assist the client to a sitting position if health permits.
   - Place the towel or disposable pad across the client's chest to collect any spillage of mucous and gastric secretions from the tube.
   - Provide tissues to the client to wipe the nose and mouth after tube removal.

3. Discontinue suction. Disconnect the NG tube from the suction and plug the end of the tube.
   - Unpin the tube from the client's gown.
   - Remove the adhesive tape securing the tube to the nose.

4. Wash your hands and don disposable gloves to protect yourself from body fluids.

5. Remove the tube.
   - Ask the client to take a deep breath and to hold it. *This closes the glottis, thereby preventing accidental aspiration of any gastric contents.*
   - Pinch the tube with the gloved hand. *Pinching the tube prevents any contents inside the tube from draining into the client's throat.*
   - Slowly withdraw the tube for the first few inches, then quickly and smoothly withdraw the tube.
   - Place the tube in the plastic bag. *Placing the tube immediately into the bag prevents the transference of microorganisms from the tube to other articles or people.*

6. Ensure client comfort.
   - Provide oral care.
   - Assist the client as required to blow the nose. *Excessive secretions may have accumulated in the nasal passages.*

7. Dispose of the equipment appropriately.
   - Place the pad, bag with tube, and gloves in the receptacle designated by the agency. *Correct disposal prevents the transmission of microorganisms.*

8. Assess the nasogastric drainage if suction was used.
   - Measure the amount of gastric drainage, and record it on the client's fluid output record.
   - Inspect the drainage for appearance and consistency.

9. Document all relevant information.
   - Record the removal of the tube, the amount and appearance of any drainage if connected to suction, and any relevant assessments of the client.

SAMPLE DOCUMENTATION

[date][time]   20-gauge Salem sump inserted through L nostril without difficulty. Low intermittent suction attached with immediate return of 200 mL green viscous fluid. Client tolerated procedure with minor discomfort. Tube secured with tape to nose.
_____ J. Norris, LPN

[date][time]   NG tube, Salem sump, draining 50 mL of clear fluid during past 4 hours. Patency verified through irrigation with 20 mL NS. Placement confirmed by aspiration of gastric contents with a pH of 4. Oral care every 2 hours and upon request. Nares are free from irritation, with KY jelly applied. _____
_____ J. Norris, LPN

[date][time]   Bowel sounds present in all 4 quadrants, passed flatus. NG tube removed without difficulty. Client tolerated procedure well. Stated "relieved to have tube removed." No n/v or abdominal discomfort present. _____
_____ D. Hernandez, LPN

Administering a Tube Feeding

Purpose

- To restore or maintain nutritional status

Equipment

- Tube feeding formula
- 20- to 50-mL syringe with an adapter
- Emesis basin
- Stethoscope
- Large catheter-tip syringe with plunger

or

- Calibrated plastic feeding bag with tubing that can be attached to the feeding tube

or

- Prefilled bottle with a drip chamber, tubing, and a flow-regulator clamp

- pH test strip
- Measuring container from which to pour the feeding (if using open system)
- Water (60 mL unless otherwise specified) at room temperature
- Feeding pump as required
- Correct amount of feeding solution
- Graduated container to hold the feeding
- Graduated container with 60 mL of water to flush the tubing
- Graduated container to measure residual formula
- Four 3- × 4-in. gauze squares to cover the end of the tube
- Elastic band
- Mild soap and water

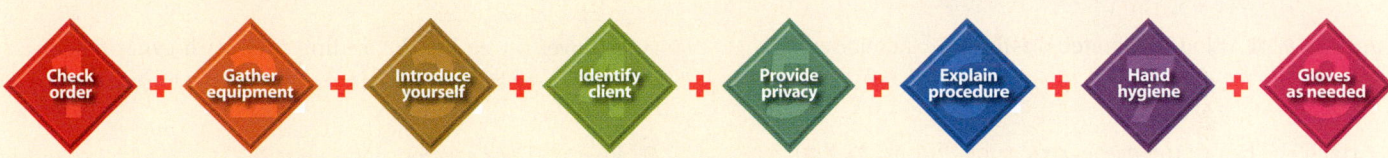

Part A: Nasogastric or Orogastric Feeding

Interventions and Rationales

1. Perform preparatory steps (see icon bar above).

2. Confirm physician order for specific type and amount of feeding.

3. Prepare the client.
   - Assist the client to a Fowler's position in bed or a sitting position in a chair, the normal position for eating. If a sitting position is contraindicated, a slightly elevated right side-lying position is acceptable. The head of the bed should be raised 30 to 45 degrees. *These positions enhance the gravitational flow of the solution and prevent aspiration of fluid into the lungs.*

4. Assess tube placement.
   - Auscultate placement of 20 to 30 mL of air into the tube with your stethoscope positioned over the epigastric area.
   - Attach the syringe to the open end of the tube; aspirate alimentary secretions. Check the pH at least an hour after medications have been given. *Gastric content normal pH is 6 or below.*

5. Assess residual feeding contents.
   - Aspirate all the stomach contents, and measure the residual amount prior to administering the feeding. *This is done to evaluate whether undigested formula from a previous feeding remains or the stomach is emptying properly.*
   - If 75 to 150 mL (or more than half the last feeding) is withdrawn, check with the nurse in charge or refer to agency policy before proceeding. The precise amount to infuse is usually determined by the physician's order or by agency policy. *At some agencies, a feeding is withheld when the specified amount or more of formula remains in the*

   stomach. In other agencies, the amount withdrawn is subtracted from the total feeding and that volume (less the undigested portion) is administered slowly.
   or
   - Reinstill the gastric contents into the stomach (to reduce fluid and electrolyte imbalance). Remove the syringe plunger, and pour the gastric contents via the syringe into the nasogastric tube. *Removal of the contents could disturb the client's electrolyte balance.*
   - If the client is on a continuous feeding, check the gastric residual every 4 hours or according to agency protocol. Agency protocol may dictate stopping a continuous feeding for a period of time prior to checking a residual. *The interval allows the stomach time to empty.*

6. Administer the feeding.
   - Before administering feeding:
     a. Check the expiration date of the feeding.
     b. Warm the feeding to room temperature. *An excessively cold feeding may cause cramps.*
   - When an open system is used, clean the top of the feeding container before opening it. *This minimizes the risk of contaminants entering the feeding syringe or feeding bag.*

FEEDING BAG (OPEN SYSTEM)

- Hang the bag from an infusion pole about 30 cm (12 in.) above the tube's point of insertion into the client.
- Clamp the tubing, and add the formula to the bag.
- Open the clamp, run the formula through the tubing, and reclamp the tube. *The formula will displace the air in the tubing, thus preventing the instillation of excess air into the client's stomach or intestine.*

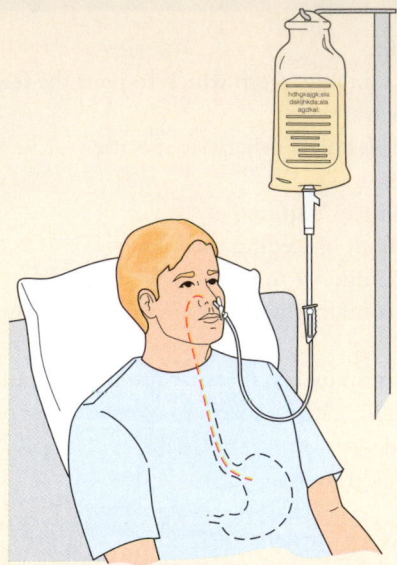

Figure 25-8. ■ Using a calibrated plastic bag to administer tube feeding.

■ Attach the bag to the nasogastric tube (Figure 25-8 ■). Regulate the drip by adjusting the clamp, or secure the tubing in the feeding pump for regulated administration.

SYRINGE (OPEN SYSTEM)

■ Remove the plunger from the syringe, and connect the syringe to a pinched or clamped nasogastric tube. *Pinching or clamping the tube prevents excess air from entering the stomach and causing distention.*

■ Pour a small amount of feeding into the syringe barrel.

■ Permit the feeding to flow in slowly at the prescribed rate. Raise or lower the syringe to adjust the flow as needed. Pinch or clamp the tubing to stop the flow for a minute if the client experiences discomfort. *If feeding is administered too quickly, flatus, crampy pain, and/or vomiting can occur.*

PREFILLED BOTTLE WITH DRIP CHAMBER (CLOSED SYSTEM)

■ Remove the screw-on cap from the container, and attach the administration set with the drip chamber and tubing.

■ Close the clamp on the tubing.

■ Hang the container on an intravenous pole about 30 cm (12 in.) above the tube's insertion point into the client. *At this height the formula should run at a safe rate into the stomach or intestine.*

■ Squeeze the drip chamber to fill it to one-third to one-half of its capacity.

■ Open the tubing clamp, run the formula through the tubing, and reclamp the tube. *The formula will displace the air in the tubing, thus preventing the instillation of excess air.*

■ Attach the feeding set tubing to the feeding tube, and regulate the drip rate to deliver the feeding over the desired length of time. *Prefilled tube-feeding sets can be attached to a feeding pump to regulate the flow.*

7. Rinse the feeding tube immediately before all of the formula has run through the tubing.
   ■ Instill 50 to 100 mL of water through the feeding tube. *Water flushes the lumen of the tube, preventing future blockage by sticky formula.*
   ■ Be sure to add the water before the feeding solution has drained from the neck of a syringe or from the tubing of an administration set. Before adding water to a feeding bag or prefilled tubing set, first clamp and disconnect both feeding and administration tubes. *Adding the water before the syringe or tubing is empty prevents the instillation of air into the stomach or intestine and thus prevents unnecessary distention.*

8. Clamp and cover the feeding tube.
   ■ Clamp the feeding tube before all of the water is instilled. *Clamping prevents leakage of feeding or air from entering the tube.*
   ■ Cover the end of the feeding tube with gauze held by an elastic band. *Covering the tube end prevents leakage from it.*

9. Ensure client comfort and safety.
   ■ Pin the tubing to the client's gown by slip knotting a rubber band over the tube. *This minimizes pulling of the tube, thus preventing discomfort and dislodgment.*
   ■ Ask the client to remain sitting upright in Fowler's position or in a slightly elevated right lateral position for at least 30 minutes. *These positions facilitate digestion and movement of the feeding from the stomach along the alimentary tract, and prevent potential aspiration of the feeding into the lungs. The head of the bed must remain elevated 30 to 45 degrees when a continuous feeding is taking place.*

10. Dispose of equipment appropriately.
    ■ If the open system bag and connected tube are to be reused, wash them thoroughly with soap and water so that they are ready for reuse. Hang to air dry.
    ■ Change the open system bag and connected tube every 24 hours or according to agency policy, as well as any syringes or irrigation fluid/set being used.

11. Monitor the client for possible problems.
    ■ Carefully assess clients receiving tube feedings for problems, particularly changes in lung sounds.
    ■ To prevent dehydration, give the client supplemental water in addition to the prescribed tube feeding as ordered.

12. Document all relevant information.
    ■ Document the feeding, including amount and kind of solution, duration of the feeding, and assessments of the client.
    ■ Document verification of placement of the feeding tube and the amount of residual obtained.
    ■ Record the volume of the feeding and water administered on the client's intake and output record.

VARIATION: CONTINUOUS-DRIP FEEDING

- If the feeding is a continuous-drip tube feeding, place a label on the container. *The label should indicate when the new feeding bag was hung.*
- Check residual as ordered or indicated by agency protocol. Then flush the tubing with 30 to 50 mL of water. *This verifies correct placement of the tube. If placement of a small-bore tube is questionable, a repeat x-ray should be done.*
- Determine agency protocol regarding withholding a feeding based on residual obtained. *Many agencies withhold the feeding for more than 75 to 150 mL of residual feeding.*
- To prevent spoilage or bacterial contamination, do not allow the feeding solution to hang longer than 8 hours. Check agency policy or manufacturer's recommendations regarding time limits.

- Follow agency policy regarding how frequently to change the feeding bag and tubing. *Changing the feeding bag and tubing every 24 hours reduces the risk of contamination.*

PEDIATRIC CONSIDERATIONS

- Feeding tubes may be reinserted at each feeding to prevent irritation of the mucous membrane, nasal airway obstruction, and stomach perforation that may occur if the tube is left in place continuously. Check agency practice.
- Position a small child or infant in your lap, provide a pacifier, and hold and cuddle the child during feedings. *This promotes comfort, supports the normal sucking reflex of the infant, and facilitates digestion.*
- Check agency policy or physician's orders for acceptable amounts of stomach aspirates and reinstillation of residual feedings.

Part B: Gastrostomy or Jejunostomy Feeding

Interventions and Rationales

1. Follow steps for NG feeding, including the following: Check placement, pour 15 to 30 mL of water into the syringe, remove the tube clamp, and allow the water to flow into the tube. *This determines the patency of the tube. If water flows freely, the tube is patent.* If the water does not flow freely, notify the nurse in charge and/or physician.

2. Administer the feeding.
   - Hold the syringe 7 to 15 cm (3 to 6 in.) above the ostomy opening.
   - Slowly pour the solution into the syringe and allow it to flow through the tube by gravity.
   - Just before all the formula has run through and the syringe is empty, add 30 mL of water. *Water flushes the tube and preserves its patency.*
   - If the tube is sutured in place, hold it upright, remove the syringe, and then clamp or plug the tube to prevent leakage. Cover the end of the tube with a 4 × 4 gauze, and secure the gauze with a rubber band.

3. Ensure client comfort and safety.
   - Assess status of peristomal skin. *Gastric or jejunal drainage contains digestive enzymes that can irritate the skin.* Document any redness and broken skin areas. Check orders about cleaning the peristomal skin, applying a skin protectant, and applying appropriate dressings. *Generally, the peristomal skin is washed with mild soap and water every shift and as needed.* Skin protectant may be applied around the stoma.
   - Observe for common complications of enteral feedings: aspiration, hyperglycemia, abdominal distention, diarrhea, and fecal impaction. Report findings to

physician. *Often, a change in formula or rate of administration can correct problems.*

VARIATION: PERCUTANEOUS ENDOSCOPIC GASTROSTOMY

- A percutaneous endoscopic gastrostomy (PEG) is kept in place with a short crosspiece or bolster near the skin level at the stoma.
- Clean the stoma daily with soap and water using a cotton swab or small piece of gauze in a circular motion.
- Rotate the bolster and clean the skin under it. Rotate the tube in a full circle between the thumb and forefinger daily.
- After cleaning, allow the skin to air dry.
- Report any signs of redness, pain, soreness, swelling, or drainage to the healthcare provider.
- Do not apply a dressing over the PEG. *A dressing and tape may result in skin excoriation and breakdown.*

4. Document all assessments and interventions.

SAMPLE DOCUMENTATION

[date][time] PEG-tube site assessed and cleaned with soap and water.

Client denies pain or soreness. No skin irritation present. Skin barrier cream applied. _____

_____ R. Diaz, LPN

PROCEDURE 25-4   Administering Medications via an Enteral Tube

Purpose

- To administer oral medications safely

Equipment

- 50- to 60-mL syringe
- Graduated container
- Medications to be administered
- Warm tap water (if needed to dissolve medications)
- Water for flushing tube
- Tongue blade or spoon to stir dissolved medications
- Disposable gloves
- pH test strip

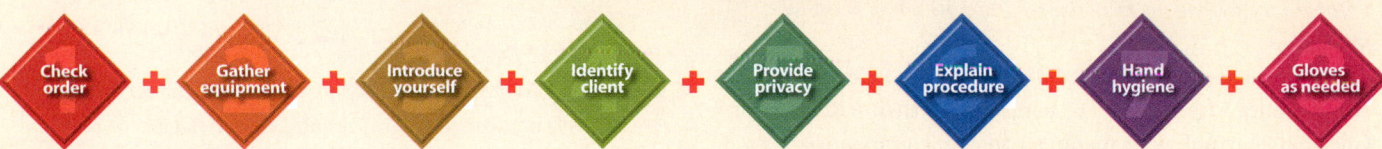

Check order + Gather equipment + Introduce yourself + Identify client + Provide privacy + Explain procedure + Hand hygiene + Gloves as needed

Interventions and Rationales

1. Perform preparatory steps (see icon bar above).

2. Prepare the medications.
   - Determine if client is allergic to any of the prescribed medications.
   - Obtain any necessary client data, such as pulse, blood pressure, and lab values.
   - Determine if the medication can be safely given through a tube. Liquid medications are the best choice. If only a pill form is available, it helps to dissolve the pill in a small amount of warm water before administering, so as not to clog the tube. Some pills will need to be crushed and then dissolved. *Note:* Enteric-coated and time-release pills should *NEVER* be crushed; if in a capsule form, do not open them. Crushing the pills or capsules alters their absorption and metabolism, resulting in unpredictable drug effects and sometimes producing a bolus dosing of the drug. When unsure if a drug can be crushed, consult a drug guide or check with the pharmacy.

3. Administer the medications.
   - Don clean gloves.
   - Ensure proper placement of tube.
   - Check for residual when indicated. This is usually done when client is receiving a continuous feeding and per agency policy. Feedings may need to be held before or after certain medications (see step 4).
   - Attach 50- to 60-mL syringe to feeding tube. An adaptor may be necessary for small-bore tubes.
   - Holding syringe upright at a 90-degree angle, administer 30 to 60 mL of tap water by pouring into syringe and allowing fluid to flow by gravity.
   - Administer medications, being sure to add sufficient water.
   - Flush between each individual medication. *This will allow identification if medication is spilled and prevents incompatible medications from clogging the tube.*

   - Administer another 30 to 60 mL of tap water after the medications have been administered. This helps to maintain tube patency.

4. Document medications.
   - Document fluid intake, being sure to include amount of fluid added to the medication.

5. Avoid drug–feeding interactions.
   - Never mix medications with the enteral feeding. The protein and mineral content of the feeding sometimes binds with the drug, thereby reducing drug absorption and availability.
   - Some medications that are known to interact with enteral feedings include:
     - *Antibiotics:* The mineral content reduces absorption of tetracycline, penicillin, and fluoroquinolones.
     - *Anticoagulants and antiepileptics:* The protein reduces absorption of warfarin (Coumadin) and phenytoin (Dilantin). Always check for specific interactions.
   - The interactions can be minimized by holding feedings for 1 hour before or for 2 hours after administration of meds.

SAMPLE DOCUMENTATION

[date][time] G tube client. 2.5 mL of residual noted.

Medications administered with 15 mL of H_2O. See MAR.

G tube flushed with 30 mL of H_2O to maintain patency.

Feeding continued, no c/o abdominal discomfort noted.
_____ J. Norris, LPN

Chapter Review

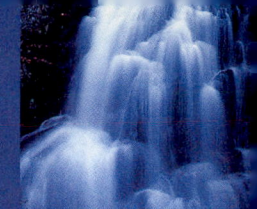

KEY Points

- For the body to grow, maintain body tissue, and perform all body functions normally, specific nutrients must be supplied. When a person is undernourished, carbohydrate reserves (stored as liver and muscle glycogen) meet energy requirements for a short time; then body protein is used. Over time, this may result in protein–calorie malnutrition.

- Homeostasis depends on many physiological processes. These processes regulate fluid intake and output. They also regulate the movement of water and dissolved substances between the body compartments.

- If diet therapy is long term, a client must not only understand the diet but also develop a healthy, positive attitude toward it. The client's belief that the diet will make a change is key to its success.

- Assessment of the vegetarian diet is important to prevent deficiencies in certain nutrients such as protein, calcium, vitamin D, vitamin B_{12}, zinc, and iron.

- After a feeding tube is inserted, and before feedings are introduced, tube placement is confirmed by radiography. Tube placement must be confirmed whenever possible dislodgment may have occurred, before administering medication or feeding through the tube, and at least daily for continuous feedings.

⊙ FOR FURTHER Study

See Chapter 35 for more details on the immune response and anaphylaxis.

To visualize the digestive tract, see Figure 37-4.

Issues for older adults are discussed in depth in Chapters 42, 43, and 46. Special nursing concerns about dementia and Alzheimer's in older adults are discussed in Chapter 43.

The major discussion on assisting clients with meals is found in Chapter 46. To see special utensils used to assist a client to eat, see Figure 46-4.

More information about nutrition can be found in the pediatric unit, Chapters 58 through 62.

PEARSON mynursingkit™

EXPLORE

MyNursingKit is your one stop for online chapter review materials and resources. Prepare for success with additional NCLEX®-style practice questions, interactive assignments and activities, web links, animations and videos, and more!

Register your access code from the front of your book at
www.mynursingkit.com

Critical Thinking Care Map

Caring for a Client with Nasogastric Tube Feeding
NCLEX-PN® Focus Area: Physiological Adaptation

Case Study: Angelica Del Monico, an 86-year-old female, was admitted from long-term care last evening for possible aspiration pneumonia. She has a history of cerebrovascular accidents (CVAs), with dysphagia, left side weakness. She has macular degeneration, which has severely compromised her vision; her hearing is assisted with bilateral hearing aids. Mrs. Del Monico is diabetic.

Nursing Diagnosis: *Imbalanced Nutrition: Less than Body Requirements*

COLLECT DATA

Subjective	Objective
_____	_____
_____	_____
_____	_____
_____	_____
_____	_____
_____	_____
_____	_____

Would you report this? Yes/No

If yes, report to: _____

What would you report? _____

Nursing Care

_____
_____
_____
_____
_____
_____
_____
_____
_____
_____

How would you document this?_____
_____
_____
_____

Compare your answers and documentation to those provided on the MyNursingKit Website.

Data Collected
(use only those that apply)

- Height: 150 cm (4'11")
- Weight: 39.55 kg (87 lbs)
- Temperature: 39°C (102.6°F)
- Pulse: 86 bpm
- Respirations: 30/min labored
- Blood Pressure: 130/82 mm Hg
- Skin pale and moist
- NPO, nasogastric tube 150 mL/hour Glucerna
- Blood glucose 236 at 7 A.M.
- Foley catheter in place draining dark amber urine
- Complaint of being thirsty
- Chest x-ray and urinalysis done—result pending
- WBC 28,000
- Client states "My chest hurts when I breathe"

Nursing Interventions
(use only those that apply; list in priority order)

- VS q 4 hr. Tylenol 650 mg PO q 4 hours prn for temp over 101.6°F.
- Cooling measures for temp over 102°F.
- Teach client to use incentive spirometer.
- Blood glucose monitoring a.c. and h.s.
- Insulin per sliding scale.
- Check tube placement and residual each shift and PRN.
- Flush tube with 100 mL following medication administration.
- Hold tube feeding for residual greater than 150 mL.
- Encourage coughing and deep breathing.
- Instruct client to request prn pain medication before the pain is severe.
- Create a quiet, nondisruptive environment with dim lights and comfortable temperature when possible.
- Offer oral fluids to increase urinary output.
- Encourage self-feeding.
- Encourage ambulation.
- Elevate head of bed 30 degrees.

TEST-TAKING TIP When considering a question that addresses priorities, remember that subjective and objective data should be gathered (assessment) before nursing interventions take place. In selecting the answer, ask yourself, "Does this client need further assessment before nursing interventions are performed?"

1 A client who follows a vegetarian diet asks the nurse why protein is necessary in the diet. The nurse's best response would be to explain that protein is needed to provide:
1. Adequate structural material for body tissues.
2. Adequate lubrication for the body's tissues.
3. Adequate calories for energy.
4. Adequate calcium for bone density.

2 The nurse is teaching the client about the low-fat diet to help the client reduce triglyceride and cholesterol levels when the client says, "I love to eat. Low-fat foods are so tasteless." The nurse's best response would be:
1. "If you don't reduce your fat intake, you won't live very long because your arteries will clog and you will end up with heart disease."
2. "There are ways to make all of your favorite foods with lower fat content without noticing a change in taste. Try a bite of each of these and tell me which one is low fat."
3. "The doctor says you have to lower your fat content but you could take pleasure in exercise and seeing your health improve instead of eating."
4. "Sometimes doing what is best for your health is not what is best for your taste buds."

3 A newly admitted client tells the nurse she has no appetite, hasn't been eating very well for the last few months, and has lost 15 pounds. The client is malnourished in appearance and very thin. The nurse's priority intervention is to:
1. Order a tray with many food options that are high in calories for the client.
2. Instruct the client on the importance of eating adequate quantities of nutrients for good health.
3. Document the client's lack of appetite and inform the physician.
4. Question the client about why she thinks she lost her appetite.

4 The spouse of a client diagnosed with coronary vessel disease asks the nurse how to prepare healthy meals. The nurse would instruct the spouse to:
1. Use cream sauces to enhance flavor whenever possible.
2. Replace red meat with fish and poultry as the entrée 4 to 5 days per week.
3. Buy food from health food stores whenever possible.
4. Substitute onion salt or celery salt for table salt to reduce sodium intake.

5 The client asks the nurse how to know if she is obese. The nurse's best response would include which of the following information?
1. Anyone who is 10% or more above ideal body weight is considered obese.
2. Anyone who is 20% or more than ideal body weight is considered to be obese.

3. Anyone who is 30% or more above ideal body weight is considered to be obese.
4. Anyone who is 20% to 30% above ideal body weight is overweight but is not obese if they are physically active.

6 After replacing a feeding tube accidentally removed by the client, the nurse's next action before restarting the feeding would be to:
1. Weigh the client.
2. Check tube placement.
3. Hang new fresh formula.
4. Apply restraints to prevent the client from removing this tube.

7 The nurse, caring for a newly diagnosed diabetic client, explains the primary function of carbohydrates is to:
1. Meet the body's energy needs.
2. Prevent heat loss.
3. Provide building blocks to repair new tissue.
4. Meet the body's fiber needs.

8 The nurse is assisting with passing meal trays. Which of the following foods would the nurse expect to find on the tray of a client on a clear liquid diet?
1. Milkshake.
2. Cranberry juice.
3. Apricot nectar.
4. Creamed soups.

9 The nurse is preparing to administer several different medications to the client via a nasogastric tube. The best procedure would be to:
1. Crush all of the medications together and dilute them with a small amount of water, then administer into the tube and flush with water.
2. Crush each tablet separately and then combine in a small amount of water, administer them together, and flush the nasogastric tube with water.
3. Crush and dilute each medication in its own cup, administer each medication one at a time, then flush the tube with water.
4. Crush and dilute each medication in its own cup, administer one medication, flush the tube with water, and then administer the next medication, flushing the tube after each medication is administered.

10 The nurse is feeding a client who requires assistance with eating. The nurse's best action would be to:
1. Encourage the client to perform independently as much as possible.
2. Feed all of the solid foods first, and then offer liquids.
3. Feed all of one food before moving to the next food.
4. Sit on the edge of the client's bed while feeding.

Answers and rationales for Review Questions appear in Appendix I.

Chapter 26

Fluids, Electrolytes, and Acid-Base Balance

BRIEF Outline

Body Fluids and Electrolyte Balance
Acid-Base Balance
Acid-Base Imbalances

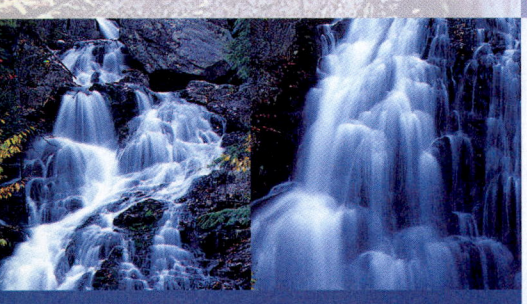

LEARNING Outcomes

After completing this chapter, you will be able to:

1. Discuss the definitions, composition, and distribution of fluids in the body.
2. Identify mechanisms for regulation of body fluids and electrolytes.
3. Identify the normal range of acid-base balance and name three important regulators of pH in the blood.
4. List important electrolytes, their normal ranges, and manifestations of imbalances.
5. Name four acid-base imbalances and state how they are treated.
6. List seven types of substances that are considered part of fluid intake.
7. Discuss nursing care for clients with fluid or acid-base disorders.

Clinical Objectives

8. Teach clients measures for maintaining fluid and electrolyte balances.
9. Demonstrate the procedure for collecting accurate intake and output.

KEY TERMS

Homeostasis (the processes by which body equilibrium is maintained) is essential to maintaining good health. To maintain homeostasis, the body must constantly receive feedback from the various regulatory mechanisms. One of the most delicate balances required for homeostasis is the balance between fluid, electrolytes, and pH. Almost every illness has the potential to threaten this balance. Even in normal daily living, high temperatures, vigorous exercise without adequate water and salt intake, or lack of adequate intake can disturb homeostasis. Many medical interventions such as diuretics, nasogastric suction, or intravenous fluid administration can cause fluid, electrolyte, or pH (acid-base) imbalances.

Body Fluids and Electrolyte Balance

The body's **fluid** (the liquid components of the body) is divided into two major compartments, intracellular and extracellular. Body water found within cells is referred to as **intracellular fluid** (ICF). It accounts for approximately two-thirds of the total body fluid in adults and is vital to normal cell functioning. ICF contains oxygen, electrolytes, and glucose.

Fluid found outside the cells is known as **extracellular fluid** (ECF). Extracellular fluid accounts for about one-third of total body fluid. ECF is the transport system that carries nutrients to, and waste products from, the cells. The ECF is subdivided into three compartments: intravascular, interstitial, and transcellular (Figure 26-1 ■). **Interstitial fluid** (three-quarters of the ECF) surrounds the cells and includes lymph. Interstitial fluid transports wastes from the cells by way of the lymph system, as well as directly in the blood plasma through capillaries. **Intravascular fluid** (or *plasma*) describes only that fluid which is found within the blood. **Transcellular fluid,** which some consider to be distinct from intracellular and extracellular fluids, includes cerebrospinal, pleural, peritoneal, and synovial fluids found in the body's cavities.

COMPOSITION OF BODY FLUIDS

Extracellular and intracellular fluids contain oxygen, nutrients, carbon dioxide, and salts that break up into electrically charged particles when dissolved in water (*ions* or *electrolytes*). These charged ions are called **electrolytes** because they are capable of conducting electricity. Ions that carry a positive charge are called **cations,** and ions carrying

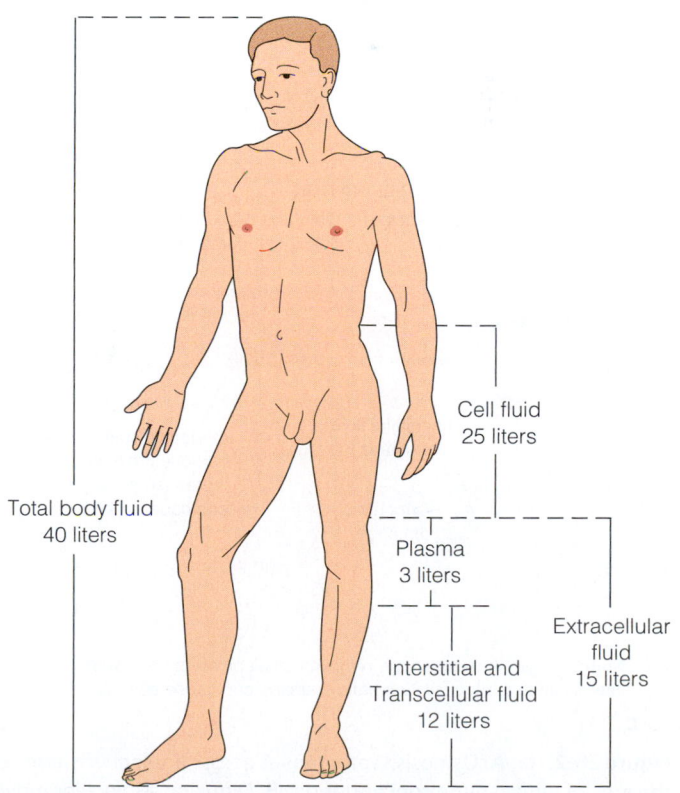

Total body fluid
40 liters

Cell fluid
25 liters

Plasma
3 liters

Interstitial and
Transcellular fluid
12 liters

Extracellular
fluid
15 liters

Figure 26-1. ■ Total body fluid represents 40 L in adult males weighing 70 kg. Fluid amounts are indicated for different body compartments.

a negative charge are called **anions.** Examples of cations are sodium, potassium, calcium, and magnesium. Anions include chloride, bicarbonate, phosphate, and sulfate. The composition of fluids varies from one body compartment to another.

In extracellular fluid, the principal electrolytes are sodium, chloride, and bicarbonate. Other electrolytes such as potassium, calcium, and magnesium are present, but in much smaller quantities. Plasma and interstitial fluid, the two primary components of ECF, contain essentially the same electrolytes and solutes, except for protein. Plasma is rich in protein, containing large amounts of albumin. Interstitial fluid, in contrast, contains little or no protein.

Intracellular fluid has a very different composition from ECF. Potassium and magnesium are the primary cations present in ICF; phosphate and sulfate are the major anions. Other electrolytes are present, but in much smaller concentrations.

A balance of fluid volumes and electrolyte compositions in the fluid compartments of the body is essential to health. Normal and unusual fluid and electrolyte losses must be replaced if homeostasis is to be maintained.

Other body fluids, such as gastric and intestinal secretions, also contain electrolytes. When these fluids are lost from the body during severe vomiting, diarrhea, or gastric suctioning, electrolyte imbalance can result. (See Figure 25-1 ⚭, which illustrates the relative proportions of fluid in infants, toddlers, children, and adults.)

FLUID TRANSPORT

Movement of particles occurs through transport mechanisms (Figure 26-2 ■). Mechanisms may be passive or active.

Passive transport is the movement of solutes through membranes without energy expenditure. Osmosis, passive diffusion, and filtration are types of passive transport. **Osmosis** is

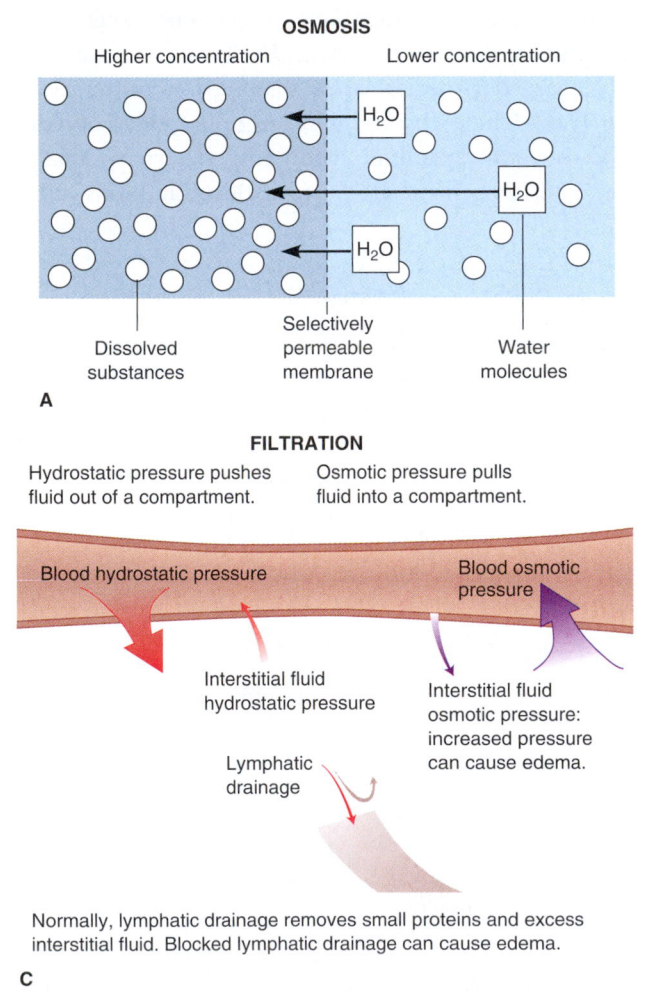

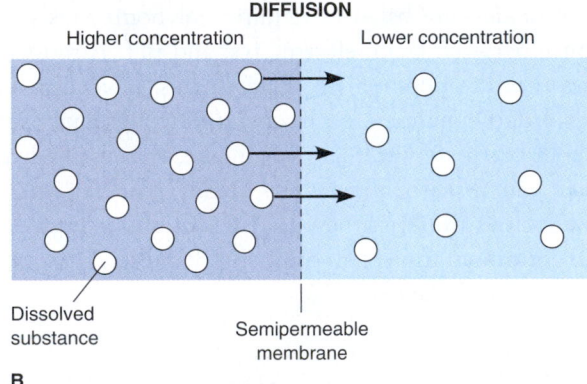

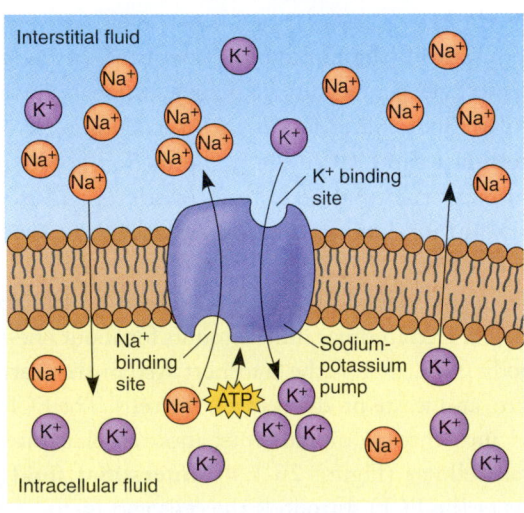

Figure 26-2. ■ **A.** Osmosis. Water moves across a selective permeable membrane into an area of higher solute concentration and out of the area of lower solute concentration. **B.** Diffusion. Molecules move across a semipermeable membrane from an area of higher solute concentration to an area of lower solute concentration. **C.** Filtration is the process by which water and solutes move across capillary membranes driven by fluid pressure. The pumping action of the heart and gravity push water and solutes into the interstitial space. Note that water is returned into the vascular space by osmosis. **D.** Active transport. ATP enables the movement of sodium and potassium ions across cell membranes against their concentration gradients.

BOX 26-1   MANIFESTATIONS OF FLUID IMBALANCES

Fluid Deficit

Low body temperature
Weight loss
Pulse rate can be increased or decreased
Low blood pressure
Sunken eyes
Poor skin turgor
Dry, cracked lips
Cool extremities
Diminished urine output
Increased hematocrit
Elevated electrolytes and bun levels
Increased serum osmolarity

Fluid Excess

Weight gain
High blood pressure
Bounding pulse
Jugular vein distention
Increased respiratory rate
Dyspnea
Moist crackles or rhonchi
Edema
Puffy eyelids
Periorbital edema
Low hematocrit
Decreased serum electrolytes and bun levels
Low serum osmolarity

---

the passage of water from an area of lower particle concentration toward an area of higher concentration of particles. An example is what happens to a hot dog when boiled in water; "it plumps when you cook it." **Osmotic pressure** is the force that develops as solute particles collide against each other. The concentration of solution with increased solute particles increases the collisions and creates increased osmotic pressure, causing the movement of fluid. The term **osmolarity** is the total number of osmotically active particles; it refers to the concentration of a solute in a volume of solution. The terms *osmolarity* and *osmotic pressure* are similar and are used interchangeably, although there are subtle differences. **Passive diffusion** is the movement of molecules randomly in all directions from a region of high concentration to an area of low concentration. There is no force to stop diffusion, and particles distribute themselves evenly. An example is how ink spreads in water. **Filtration** is the transfer of water and dissolved substances from a region of high pressure to a region of low pressure. Filtration moves in one particular direction due to hydrostatic pressure. Filtration causes water and electrolytes to move from capillaries into interstitial fluid. An example would be that of pouring a solution through a strainer in which the size of the opening determines the size of particles to be filtered.

Active transport occurs when it is necessary for electrolytes to move from an area of low concentration to an area of high concentration. For movement to occur against a concentration gradient, energy must be expended. Energy, released from the cell in the form of adenosine triphosphate (ATP), enables substances to pass through the cell membrane.

REGULATING BODY FLUIDS

In a healthy person, the volumes and chemical composition of the fluid compartments stay within narrow safe limits. Normally, fluid intake and fluid loss are balanced. Illness can upset this balance so that the body has too little or too much fluid (Box 26-1 ■). Many fluid and electrolyte imbalances are corrected with IV solutions. Solutions used to correct imbalances are isotonic, hypertonic, or hypotonic. **Isotonic** solutions are solutions that have the same concentration of solutes as blood plasma, so they cause cells neither to swell nor to shrink. **Hypertonic** solutions have a greater concentration of solutes than plasma; these move water out of cells. **Hypotonic** solutions have a lesser concentration of solutes; these move water into cells. IV solutions are discussed in detail in Chapter 28 and in Table 28-1 ⌾.

An exchange of fluid occurs continuously between the ICF and ECF. These changes occur as a result of changes in the volume or concentration of the plasma. Homeostasis of the internal environment occurs with intake and output that is relatively equal as in healthy adults.

Fluid Intake

During periods of moderate activity at moderate temperature, the average adult drinks about 1,500 mL per day but needs 2,500 mL per day. The difference, an additional 1,000 mL, is needed to replace *insensible water loss*, fluid lost by respirations and through the skin. This added volume is acquired as a by-product of food metabolism.

Fluid Output

Fluid losses from the body counterbalance the average daily intake of fluid. Fluid output occurs through several routes: urine, insensible losses, and feces. In children, fluid losses can have serious effects more quickly than fluid loss in adults (Box 26-2 ■).

Urine formed by the kidneys and excreted from the urinary bladder is the major avenue of fluid output. Normal urine output for an adult is 1,400 to 1,500 mL per 24 hours, or at least 30 to 50 mL per hour for adults. In healthy people, urine output may vary noticeably from day to day. Urine volume automatically increases as fluid

BOX 26-2 PEDIATRIC CONSIDERATIONS

Fluid Loss in Children

Children have a higher percentage of body water than adults and are subject to more severe responses to fluid losses than adults. Children must be seen and treated sooner than an adult if excessive fluid loss occurs from vomiting, diarrhea, or exposure to extreme heat.

intake increases. If fluid loss through perspiration is large, however, urine volume decreases to maintain fluid balance in the body.

As mentioned, insensible losses occur through the skin and through the lungs. They are usually not noticeable and cannot be measured. Insensible fluid loss through the skin occurs in two ways: through diffusion and through perspiration. Water losses through diffusion are not noticeable but normally account for 350 to 400 mL per day. This loss can be significantly increased if the protective layer of the skin is damaged, as with burns or large abrasions. Perspiration varies depending on factors such as environmental temperature and metabolic activity. Fever and exercise increase metabolic activity and heat production, thereby increasing fluid losses through the skin.

Insensible loss of water in exhaled air is normally 350 to 400 mL per day in an adult. When respiratory rate accelerates (as with exercise or an elevated body temperature), water loss can increase.

Loss through the intestines in feces usually amounts to 100 to 200 mL per day. The digested food that passes from the small intestine into the large intestine contains water and electrolytes. However, most fluid is reabsorbed in the proximal half of the large intestine.

REGULATING ELECTROLYTES

Electrolytes are present in all body fluids and fluid compartments. Just as maintaining the fluid balance is vital to normal body function, so is maintaining electrolyte balance (Box 26-3 ■). The concentration of specific electrolytes differs between fluid compartments, but a balance of *cations* (positively charged ions) and *anions* (negatively charged ions) should exist. Electrolytes are important for:

- Maintaining fluid balance.
- Contributing to acid-base regulation.
- Facilitating enzyme reactions.
- Assisting neuromuscular reactions.

Cations and anions are expressed in mEq (milliequivalents) per liter—mEq/L—rather than in mg (milligrams). Milliequivalents measure chemical activity rather than weight. The total cations and anions in a given compartment must be equal to have balance. Table 26-1 ■ describes the location, sources, and functions of electrolytes, as well as manifestations of imbalances.

BOX 26-3 CULTURAL PULSE POINTS

Electrolyte Imbalances in Ethnic Diets

Cultural food preferences and practices can play a large role in contributing to adequate and inadequate intake of electrolytes. A preference for certain foods can also contribute to the development of illness. African Americans often eat diets high in sodium content, which contributes to hypertension and heart disease. People of Southeast Asian background are often lactose intolerant and are at risk for osteoporosis and dental caries as a result of insufficient calcium intake. The nurse needs to be aware of cultural differences, help clients achieve a balanced diet based on preferences, and provide teaching when indicated.

TABLE 26-1 Location, Sources, and Function of Selected Electrolytes and Manifestations of Imbalances

ELECTROLYTE	LOCATION	SOURCES	FUNCTION	MANIFESTATIONS OF IMBALANCES
Sodium (Na^+) ■ Major cation in ECF ■ Normal serum level: 135–147 mEq/L	Extracellular fluid (most abundant cation)	Bacon, ham, processed cheese, table salt, most processed foods	Controls and regulates water balance	*Hyponatremia:* muscle weakness, decreased skin turgor, headache, tremor, seizures *Hypernatremia:* thirst, fever, flushed skin, oliguria, and dry, sticky membranes
Potassium (K^+) ■ Major cation in ICF ■ Normal serum level: 3.5–5.0 mEq/L	Intracellular fluid (most abundant cation)	Dark yellow and orange fruits, dark green leafy vegetables, meat, fish, and avocados	Helps maintain ECF and ICF water balance and acid-base balance; vital for skeletal, cardiac, and smooth muscle activity; supports ICF enzyme reactions	*Hypokalemia:* decreased GI, skeletal muscle, and cardiac muscle function; decreased reflexes, rapid, weak, irregular pulse, muscle weakness, or irritability; decreased blood pressure; nausea and vomiting, ileus *Hyperkalemia:* muscle weakness, nausea, diarrhea, oliguria

TABLE 26-1	Location, Sources, and Function of Selected Electrolytes and Manifestations of Imbalances *(continued)*			
ELECTROLYTE	**LOCATION**	**SOURCES**	**FUNCTION**	**MANIFESTATIONS OF IMBALANCES**
Calcium (Ca^{2+}) ■ Major cation in teeth and bones ■ Normal serum level: 8.5–10.5 mg/dL	Mostly in skeletal system, small amount in ECF	Milk and milk products; dark green leafy vegetables, canned salmon	Most found in bones and teeth, remaining 1% of total calcium found in serum; regulates muscle contraction/relaxation and neuromuscular and cardiac function. With aging, less calcium is absorbed in intestines and more is excreted via kidneys; weight-bearing exercise and vitamin D protect against osteoporosis and fractures	*Hypocalcemia:* muscle tremor, muscle cramps, tetany, tonic-clonic seizures, paresthesia, bleeding, arrhythmias, hypotension *Hypercalcemia:* lethargy, headache, muscle flaccidity, nausea, vomiting, anorexia, constipation, polydipsia, hypertension, polyuria
Magnesium (Mg^{2+}) ■ Major cation in ICF ■ Normal serum level: 1.3–2.1 mEq/L	Primarily in skeleton and ICF; only about 1% in ECF	Cereal grains, nuts, dried fruit, legumes, green leafy vegetables, dairy products, meat, and fish	Aids intracellular metabolism, especially adenosine triphosphate (ATP) production; necessary for protein and DNA synthesis within cells. In ECF, helps regulate neuromuscular and cardiac function	*Hypomagnesemia:* dizziness, confusion, convulsions, tremor, leg and foot cramps, hyperirritability, arrhythmias, vasomotor changes, anorexia, nausea *Hypermagnesemia:* drowsiness, lethargy, coma, arrhythmias, hypotension, vague neuromuscular changes (tremor), vague GI symptoms (nausea), slow weak pulse
Chloride (Cl^-) ■ Major anion in ECF ■ Normal serum level: 95–105 mEq/L	Major anion of ECF; major component of gastric fluid such as hydrochloric acid (HCl)	Found in the same foods as sodium	Functions with sodium to regulate serum osmolality and blood volume; concentration in ECF is regulated by sodium; is usually reabsorbed with sodium in the kidney; helps regulate acid-base balance; acts as buffer in the exchange of oxygen and carbon dioxide in red blood cells	*Hypochloremia:* increased muscle excitability, tetany, decreased respirations *Hyperchloremia:* stupor, rapid deep breathing, muscle weakness
Phosphorus (P^{2-}) ■ Major anion in ICF ■ Normal serum level: 3.5–4.5 mEq/dL	Major anion of ICF; also is found in ECF, bone, skeletal muscle, and nerve tissue; much higher levels in children, probably due to higher growth hormone	Found in many foods such as meat, fish, poultry, milk products, and legumes	Involved in many chemical actions of the cell; essential for functioning of muscles, nerves, and red blood cells; also involved in protein, fat, and carbohydrate metabolism; absorbed from the intestine	*Hypophosphatemia:* paresthesia (circumoral and peripheral), numbness, tingling, heightened sensitivity, lethargy, speech defects (such as stuttering or stammering) *Hyperphosphatemia:* renal failure, vague neuroexcitability ranging from tetany to convulsions, arrhythmias, and muscle twitching with sudden rise in phosphate levels
Bicarbonate (combination of hydrogen, oxygen, and carbon—HCO_3)	ICF and ECF; excreted and reabsorbed by kidneys	Produced in metabolic process, so dietary source unnecessary	Major body buffer involved in acid-base regulation	Acidosis or alkalosis

Most electrolytes enter the body through dietary intake and are excreted in the urine. Some electrolytes, such as sodium and chloride, are not stored and must be consumed daily to maintain normal levels.

Acid-Base Balance

There is a very narrow range of acceptable pH in the human body. The **pH** of fluid refers to the hydrogen ion concentration of that fluid. The normal pH of arterial blood is

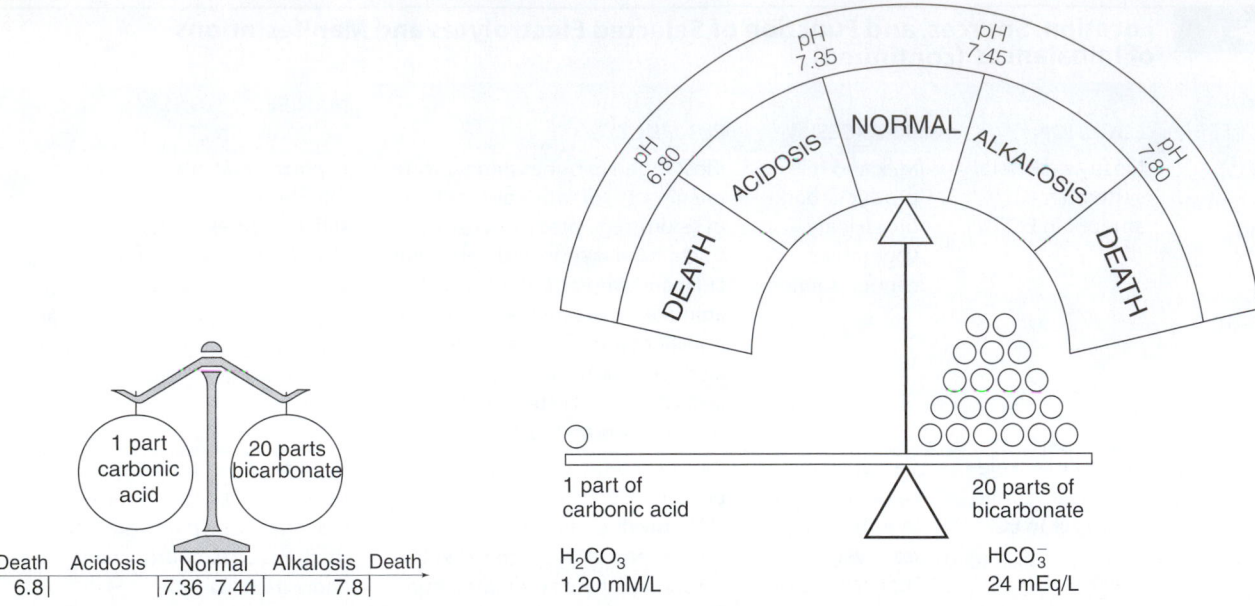

Figure 26-3. ■ The normal pH range is between 7.35 and 7.45 in adults (a ratio of 1 part carbonic acid to 20 parts bicarbonate). As little as 2 parts carbonic acid to 20 parts bicarbonate puts a client into respiratory acidosis (0.6 carbonic acid: 20 bicarbonate would be respiratory alkalosis). A reduction in bicarbonate (1 carbonic acid: 18 bicarbonate) results in metabolic acidosis. An increase in bicarbonate (1 carbonic acid: 22 bicarbonate) results in metabolic alkalosis. Movement past these ranges leads to death.

between 7.35 and 7.45. Body fluids are maintained at a slightly **alkaline** level (pH above 7 on a scale of 0 to 14). A pH of less than 7.35 reflects an increase of hydrogen ions, which can send the client into *acidosis*. A pH greater than 7.45 reflects a decrease in hydrogen ions, which can send the client into *alkalosis*. A variation of 0.4 above or below normal range can prove to be fatal (Alexander et al., 2006). Figure 26-3 ■ illustrates pH balance.

Acids are continually produced during metabolism. The body has many self-regulating mechanisms that help to keep the pH stable. Buffers in the digestive tract, the respiratory system, and the renal system work constantly to maintain the narrow pH range necessary for optimal function.

Three main regulators maintain the pH of the blood:

1. *Chemical buffer systems.* Chemical buffer systems act like sponges and combine with acid or alkali to prevent excessive changes in the hydrogen ion concentration.
2. *Respiratory system.* The lungs effectively regulate the blood levels of CO_2. CO_2 combines with H_2O to form carbonic acid. Increased levels of CO_2 decrease the pH level. Receptors in the brain identify pH changes and vary the rate and depth of breathing to compensate. Faster, deeper respirations reduce the CO_2 level in the lungs. The decrease in CO_2 increases the pH level. Respiratory response is rapid but short lived.
3. *Renal system.* The kidneys reabsorb or excrete acids and bases into the urine. They can produce bicarbonate to refill lost stores. The kidneys have a slower response, but long-term effects result.

BUFFER REGULATION

The body has a strong tendency toward acidity because acids are continually produced during metabolism. To maintain a safe pH, the body has a buffering system that is more base than acid.

Buffers neutralize excess acids or bases, preventing marked changes in hydrogen ion concentration. They are the body's first line of defense against acid-base balance changes in the body. The major buffer systems in extracellular fluids are bicarbonate and carbonic acid. The main buffer pair is sodium bicarbonate ($NaHCO_3$) and carbonic acid (H_2CO_3); they are responsible for 45% of hydrogen ion buffering. As long as a ratio of 20 parts of bicarbonate to 1 part of carbonic acid is maintained (Figure 26-3), the pH remains within its normal range of 7.35 to 7.45.

If bicarbonate is depleted while neutralizing a strong acid, the pH may drop below 7.35, resulting in a condition called *acidosis*. Likewise, if a strong base is added to ECF and depletes carbonic acid, the pH may rise over 7.45, resulting in a condition called *alkalosis*.

Bicarbonate is present in both intracellular and extracellular fluids. Extracellular bicarbonate levels are regulated by the kidneys. The kidneys excrete bicarbonate when too much is present. They regenerate and reabsorb bicarbonate ions if more is needed. Unlike other electrolytes that must be consumed in the diet, adequate amounts of bicarbonate are produced by the body to meet the body's needs.

In addition to the bicarbonate–carbonic acid buffer system, plasma proteins, hemoglobin, and phosphates also function as buffers in body fluids. Phosphate buffers are particularly effective in the renal tubules. Protein buffers are abundant in the body. Composed of hemoglobin and other proteins, they bind with acids and bases to cause neutralization.

RESPIRATORY SYSTEM REGULATION

The lungs help regulate acid-base balance by eliminating or retaining carbon dioxide, a potential acid. When carbon dioxide combines with water, it forms carbonic acid. This chemical reaction is reversible; carbonic acid can break down into carbon dioxide and water. Working together with the buffer system, the lungs regulate acid-base balance and pH by altering the rate and depth of respirations. The response of the respiratory system to changes in pH is rapid, occurring within minutes.

Carbon dioxide is a powerful stimulator of the respiratory center. When blood levels of carbonic acid and carbon dioxide rise, respiratory center stimulation causes the rate and depth of respirations to increase. By contrast, when bicarbonate levels are excessive, the rate and depth of respirations are reduced in order to retain carbon dioxide.

RENAL SYSTEM REGULATION

Although buffers and the respiratory system can compensate for changes in pH, it is the kidneys that provide the primary long-term regulation of acid-base balance. The kidneys cannot correct a pH imbalance as rapidly as the lungs. However, their response is more permanent and selective than that of the other systems. The kidneys maintain acid-base balance by selectively excreting or conserving bicarbonate and hydrogen ions. When excess hydrogen ions are present and the pH falls (*acidosis*), the kidneys reabsorb and regenerate bicarbonate and excrete hydrogen ions, helping to raise pH and reduce the amount of available acid. When there is excess bicarbonate and a high pH (*alkalosis*), the kidneys excrete bicarbonate and retain hydrogen ions in order to lower pH and make more acid available to offset the bicarbonate.

Acid-Base Imbalances

The key to acid-base balance is the regulation of hydrogen ion concentration of body fluids. There are two types of acid-base imbalances:

- Respiratory (carbonic acid deficit and excess) acidosis and alkalosis
- Metabolic (base bicarbonate deficit and excess) acidosis and alkalosis (Table 26-2 ■)

TABLE 26-2	Acid-Base Imbalances		
IMBALANCE	**ETIOLOGY**	**MANIFESTATIONS**	**TREATMENT**
Metabolic acidosis	Diarrhea Diabetic ketoacidosis Renal failure Acid ingestion Fistulas	Nausea and vomiting Kussmaul breathing Headache Drowsiness Increased breathing	Reverse underlying cause. Administer sodium bicarbonate per physician order.
Metabolic alkalosis	Gastric suctioning Vomiting Hypokalemia Potassium-losing diuretics Excessive alkali ingestion	Dizziness Tingling of the fingers Carpopedal spasm Depressed respirations Circumoral paresthesia	Reverse underlying cause. Administer chloride for the kidneys to excrete bicarbonate. Restore normal fluid volume.
Respiratory acidosis	Aspiration Cardiac arrest Severe pneumonia Emphysema Pulmonary edema Pneumothorax	Dizziness Palpitations Convulsions Weakness Mental changes Ventricular fibrillation	Improve ventilation. Use bronchodilators. Administer oxygen and fluids.
Respiratory alkalosis	Hyperventilation Anxiety Hypoxemia High fever Pulmonary emboli	Light-headedness Numbness and tingling of extremities Tinnitus Palpitations Blurred vision Chest tightness	Treat source of anxiety. Ask client to breathe slowly into a paper bag. Administer sedatives as ordered.

TABLE 26-3	Interpretation of ABG Test Results		
1. Look at pH	$\Uparrow$ = alkalosis		
	Normal (7.35 – 7.45)		
	$\Downarrow$ = acidosis		
2. Look at Pa_{CO_2} (normal 35–45 mm Hg)	= respiratory parameter		
3. Look at HCO_3 (normal 22–26 mEq/L)	= metabolic parameter		

DISORDER	pH	Pa_{CO_2}	HCO_3
Respiratory acidosis	$\Downarrow$	$\Uparrow$	—
Respiratory alkalosis	$\Uparrow$	$\Downarrow$	—
Metabolic acidosis	$\Downarrow$	—	$\Downarrow$
Metabolic alkalosis	$\Uparrow$	—	$\Uparrow$
pH normal with abnormal CO_2 and HCO_2 = fully compensated			
All values abnormal = partially compensated			
Two abnormal values and one normal value = uncompensated			

To determine acid-base balance in a client, blood work is obtained, called arterial blood gases (ABG). Normal arterial blood gases are as follows:

- pH = 7.35–7.45
- $PaCO_2$ = 35–45 mm Hg
- HCO_3 = 22–26 mEq/L

The ranges listed above are average values. Table 26-3 ■ illustrates interpretation of ABG test results. The mnemonic ROME can be used to help associate changes accurately:

RO–In respiratory imbalances (R), the arrows for pH and $PaCO_2$ in Table 26-3 go in opposite (O) directions.

ME–In metabolic imbalances (M), the arrows for pH and HCO_3 are "equal" (meaning they go in the same direction).

RESPIRATORY ACIDOSIS

When a deficiency occurs in the respiratory process, the acid-base balance is disturbed: The alveoli of the lungs are unable to reduce the carbon dioxide levels. Such a condition can be acute, as in excessive sedation, or chronic, as in chronic pulmonary disease.

As carbon dioxide is retained, it creates carbonic acid that builds up in the blood; the pH drops, creating **respiratory acidosis.** The changes in pH can be confirmed by an arterial blood gas (ABG) test showing a **$PaCO_2$** (carbon dioxide measured in arterial blood) level above 45 mm Hg and a pH below 7.35 (see Table 26-3). When the pH falls, hemoglobin is altered to make it give up its oxygen. This altered hemoglobin is alkaline and begins mopping up the excess carbonic acid. Oxygen saturation will drop. The increase in carbonic acid also causes changes in the respiratory center of the brain. Respirations become shallow and rapid in an attempt to blow off excess carbon dioxide. However, as pH continues to fall, respirations may become ineffective. The client may exhibit headache, nausea and vomiting, and a change in mental status.

If respiratory efforts fail to correct the imbalance, the $PaCO_2$ continues to rise. This triggers the kidneys to hold onto bicarbonate and sodium, which combine to form sodium bicarbonate, another buffer to mop up carbonic acid. However, it will take the kidney several days to compensate for respiratory acidosis. If these compensatory mechanisms fail to right the imbalance, hydrogen ions move into the cells and force the potassium out. With the potassium now unchecked, the client develops resultant hyperkalemia, heart arrhythmias, and a decreasing level of consciousness. The heart may experience such insult as to result in shock and even cardiac arrest. Treatment for respiratory acidosis is aimed at improving respiratory effort, including administration of oxygen or placing the client on a mechanical ventilator to provide adequate ventilation. If the cycle of increasing carbon dioxide and dropping pH is not reversed, it can result in death.

RESPIRATORY ALKALOSIS

Respiratory alkalosis may develop when the opposite situation, hyperventilation, occurs. By breathing too rapidly, CO_2 (an acid) is blown off, causing a decrease in $PaCO_2$ and an elevated pH. This can occur when pain, anxiety reactions, or fever cause a client to hyperventilate. Arterial blood gases confirm this situation by showing a pH above 7.45 and $PaCO_2$ below 35 mm Hg.

As the body defends itself, hydrogen ions leave the cells in exchange for potassium with resulting hypokalemia. The hydrogen ions join with the bicarbonate ions to lower the pH. As the $PaCO_2$ falls, the carotid and aortic bodies in the medulla are stimulated so the heart rate increases, but no change in the blood pressure occurs. There may be electrocardiographic (ECG) changes or chest pain, or the client may become restless and anxious. The blood vessels in the brain respond to the dropping $PaCO_2$ by constricting, reducing blood flow to the brain. The autonomic nervous system becomes overstimulated, and the client may exhibit dizziness and numbness or tingling in the fingers or toes. Eventually the client may lose consciousness, which often helps to regulate respirations if the hyperventilation is caused by stress or anxiety. If conscious, the client could be encouraged to breathe into a paper bag, which results in rebreathing CO_2 and increasing the level of CO_2 in the blood.

After about 6 hours of uncompensated alkalosis, the kidneys pour off the bicarbonate and hold back hydrogen ions. The client may show a decreased respiratory rate and hypoventilation. Eventually, the central nervous system (CNS) and the heart are overcome by the alkalosis, resulting in a change in level of consciousness, hyperreflexia, tetany, heart arrhythmias, seizures, and coma.

METABOLIC ACIDOSIS

Metabolic acidosis occurs when bicarbonate is lost or acid is increased within the plasma. When fatty acids change to ketone bodies (as perhaps from diabetes mellitus, starvation, or severe infection), metabolic acidosis may occur. Excessive loss of GI fluids, renal insufficiency, or renal failure may also cause metabolic acidosis. Arterial blood gases will confirm the imbalance with a pH below 7.35, a low bicarbonate level, and a low $PaCO_2$ level.

The first clue is hyperventilation as the respiratory system tries to blow off the acid. Although this will correct the imbalance initially, it will not be enough compensation to correct the metabolic imbalance. Deep and rapid respirations (*Kussmaul respirations*) may eventually develop. The CNS and the heart become depressed. Decreased cardiac function and hypotension may develop. The client develops weakness and headache as the blood vessels in the brain dilate. The client will show a change in the level of consciousness. Diminished muscle tone and deep tendon reflexes may be present. Nausea and vomiting are likely to occur. The kidneys try to correct the imbalance by secreting hydrogen, which combines with ammonia or phosphate and is excreted in the urine. Sodium and bicarbonate are held back by the kidneys to correct the acidosis. Hydrogen goes into the blood, forcing potassium out.

Signs of hyperkalemia may be seen, such as diarrhea, numbness and tingling of fingers or toes, weak or flaccid extremities, slowed heart rate, and ECG changes. The excess hydrogen ions cause further imbalance in the electrolytes, thereby reducing nervous system responses, resulting in CNS depression, lethargy, headache, confusion or stupor, and coma. To treat the acidosis, the underlying cause must be found. Insulin needs to be given for the diabetic client.

Insulin forces the potassium back into the cells, treating the hyperkalemia. A patent IV is necessary for effective reversal of this condition. Position the client to promote ventilation. Record intake and output and check oxygen saturation. Assess the level of consciousness frequently and make adaptations in the environment to promote the client's safety should confusion occur. In clients who fail to respond, the nurse should anticipate ventilatory support and possibly dialysis.

METABOLIC ALKALOSIS

Metabolic alkalosis occurs when the plasma loses hydrogen ions (acid) and gains bicarbonate. Arterial blood gases confirm this condition with a $PaCO_2$ less than 45 mm Hg and an elevated bicarbonate level. The metabolic alkalosis often occurs from diuretics that fail to conserve potassium. Loss of gastric fluids, as in vomiting or NG tube suction, is another primary cause for alkalosis. The excessive bicarbonate ions that do not bind with the chemical buffers depress the vital sign center of the brain, and the client develops a decreased respiratory rate with slow and shallow respirations, thus increasing the $PaCO_2$ in an attempt to compensate for the high bicarbonate level.

The kidneys let go of excess bicarbonate over time and hold on to the hydrogen ions to correct the imbalance. Sodium is thrown out by the kidneys, and the client displays polyuria followed by hypovolemia and thirst. To compensate for the hydrogen being excreted by the kidneys, the potassium moves into the cells and the client shows signs of hypokalemia such as anorexia, weakness, and diminished reflexes. Also in response to hydrogen being thrown out, sodium moves into the nerve cells and overstimulates them. The client may show tetany, irritability, disorientation, and seizures.

The underlying condition must be treated to reverse the imbalance. Untreated, the client may develop arrhythmias, and death may occur. A patent IV is required to treat this condition. Supplemental oxygen needs to be given when respiratory effort changes or oxygen saturations drop. NG suctioning should be discontinued, and nausea and vomiting treated with antiemetics. Seizure precautions need to be taken for client protection. As a precaution against metabolic alkalosis, NG tubes should be irrigated with normal saline instead of tap water and supplemental electrolytes may need to be administered to counter lost electrolytes from the gastric secretion removal.

NURSING CARE

PRIORITIZING NURSING CARE

Important factors to consider when assessing a client's fluid status are urine output, weight changes, and general condition. Fluid and electrolyte homeostasis is required for the normal function of all body systems, so alterations can impact each system differently. For example, dehydration can increase heart rate, reduce urine output, decrease thermoregulation by inhibiting sweating, cause alterations in electrolyte levels, and cause dry skin. As a result, a thorough assessment of the client's vital signs and general condition is required in order to put the whole picture together.

ASSESSING

In assessing the client's fluid balance, it is important to consider unusual factors that may affect intake and output. If a client is extremely diaphoretic or has rapid, deep respirations, fluid loss is occurring even if it cannot be measured.

clinical ALERT

Report
When there is a significant discrepancy between intake and output or when fluid intake or output is inadequate, report this information to the charge nurse, physician, or other care provider. The nurse may initiate intake and output without a physician's order.

Fluid imbalances may be difficult to detect. Poor skin turgor, or a rapid weak pulse with low blood pressure, may indicate dehydration. Noisy, wet respirations and edema may indicate fluid excess.

Acid-base imbalances may be detected initially by changes in respiratory effort, depth, or rate. Other vital signs may also change. The client may demonstrate a change in level of consciousness such as irritability/restlessness or lethargy, a change in muscle movement or reflexes, headache, nausea and/or vomiting, and a change in intake and output.

DIAGNOSING, PLANNING, AND IMPLEMENTING

Some common nursing diagnoses for clients with fluid and electrolyte or acid-base problems are *Deficient Fluid Volume*, *Excess Fluid Volume*, and *Impaired Gas Exchange* (see Chapter 32 ⭕ for information on monitoring oxygenation status). Nursing interventions center on helping the client achieve and maintain homeostasis. Nurses assist clients by monitoring intake and output, monitoring intravenous infusions (see Chapter 28 ⭕), administering supplemental electrolytes, and careful monitoring of drainage from tubes, drains, and wounds.

Monitoring Intake and Output

Intake and output (I&O) is the measurement and recording of all fluid taken in and excreted during a 24-hour period. It provides important data about the client's fluid and electrolyte balance. Generally, I&O is measured for hospitalized at-risk clients. The decision to place a client on intake and output can be an independent nursing measure.

Most agencies have a form for recording I&O; usually this is a bedside record on which the nurse lists all items measured and their quantities per shift (Figure 26-4 ■). It is important to inform clients, family members, and all caregivers that accurate measurements of the client's fluid intake and output are required. Nursing staff should explain why I&O is necessary and should emphasize the need to use a bedpan, urinal, commode, or in-toilet collection device. Clients who wish to be involved in recording fluid intake measurements need to be taught how to compute the values and what foods are considered fluids.

To measure fluid intake, the nurse records each item of fluid intake, specifying the time and type of fluid (Box 26-4 ■). All of the following fluids need to be recorded:

- *Oral fluids*. Include water, milk, juice, soft drinks, coffee, tea, cream, soup, and any other beverages. Include water taken with medications. To assess the amount of water taken from a water pitcher, measure what remains and subtract this amount from the volume of the full pitcher. Then refill the pitcher.

			CLIENT LABEL
	Intake and Output Record		
INTAKE	0600-1800	1800-0600	TOTAL
Oral			
Tube feeding			
IV (primary)			
IV Meds			
TPN			
Blood			
TOTAL			24-Hour Total
OUTPUT	0600-1800	1800-0600	TOTAL
Urine			
Emesis			
G.I. Suction			
Stool			
TOTAL			24-Hour Total

Figure 26-4. ■ Sample intake and output record. (Courtesy of El Camino Hospital, Mountain View, California.)

BOX 26-4   NURSING CARE CHECKLIST

Documenting Urine Output

☑ Wear clean gloves to prevent contact with body fluids.

☑ Ask client to void in a clean urinal, bedpan, commode, or toilet collection device.

☑ Instruct client to keep urine separate from feces and to avoid putting toilet paper in the urine collection container.

☑ Pour the voided urine into a calibrated container.

☑ Hold the container at eye level and read the amount in the container.

☑ If a specimen is required, pour some urine into the specimen container and discard the remainder, unless all urine is to be saved.

☑ Record the amount on the fluid I&O sheet.

☑ Rinse the urine collection and measuring containers with cool water and store.

☑ Remove gloves and wash hands.

☑ Calculate and document the total output at the end of each shift and at the end of 24 hours on the client's chart.

■ *Ice chips.* Measure ice chips and record the amount of fluid intake as one-half the amount of the ice chips.

■ *Foods that are or become liquid at room temperature.* These include ice cream, sherbet, broth, custard, and gelatin. Do not measure foods that are pureed, because purees are simply solid foods prepared in a different form.

■ *Tube feedings.* Record the amount of formula infused during the shift. Remember to include the 30- to 60-mL water rinse at the end of intermittent feedings or during continuous feedings.

■ *Parenteral fluids.* The exact amount of intravenous fluid administered is to be recorded, since some fluid containers may be overfilled. Blood transfusions are included.

■ *Intravenous medications.* Intravenous medications that are prepared with solutions such as normal saline (NS) and are administered as an intermittent or continuous infusion must also be included. These may infuse at a different rate than the primary IV and must be calculated and added to the I&O.

■ *Catheter or tube irrigants.* Fluid used to irrigate urinary catheters, NG tubes, and intestinal tubes must be measured and recorded if not immediately withdrawn.

To measure fluid output, measure the following fluids (remember to observe appropriate infection control precautions):

■ *Urinary output.* After the client voids, pour the urine into a measuring container. Measure the amount, then record the time and amount on the I&O form. For clients with retention catheters, empty the drainage bag into a measuring container at the end of the shift (or at prescribed times if output is to be measured more often). Note and record the amount of urine output. In intensive care areas, urine output is often measured hourly.

■ *Vomitus and liquid feces.* Measure in a graduated cylinder. Record the amount and type of fluid and the time. While solid feces are not measured, the frequency should be noted on the I&O form.

■ *Tube drainage.* Record the amount of drainage from gastric or intestinal drainage tubes.

■ *Wound drainage and draining fistulas.* Wound drainage may be documented by the type and number of dressings saturated with drainage or by measuring the exact amount of drainage collected in a vacuum drainage or gravity drainage system. To determine amount of fluid on the dressing, the nurse may weigh the dressing, then weigh a clean dry dressing of the same type, and subtract the dry dressing weight from the total weight.

When the nurse compares total intake and total output for a 24-hour period, fluid imbalance may be evident. Due to insensible water loss, a small difference in intake and output may be normal. However, if intake is significantly greater than output, the client has fluid volume excess. If intake is significantly less than output, fluid volume deficit may be a problem.

Assisting with IV Therapy

When a client is unable to drink fluids, IV therapy is ordered to prevent fluid volume deficit and to provide necessary electrolytes. State nursing practice acts govern the role of LPNs and LVNs in relation to IV therapy. Whatever the role, the LPN/LVN must be knowledgeable about care of clients receiving IV therapy. See Chapter 28 🔗 for the major discussion about IV therapy.

Monitoring for Acid-Base Disorders

It may be impossible to determine the exact imbalance through signs and symptoms. Nurses work in collaboration with the primary care provider, respiratory therapist, and laboratory personnel to identify the problem. Laboratory results—ABGs—determine the client's acid-base status. The LPN/LVN needs to be aware of normal values and should routinely check lab results to confirm clinical signs. Box 26-5 ■ provides reminders for review of lab results. The client should be monitored for changes in vital signs, especially in respiratory effort or rate. Lung sounds may be diminished or absent. The pulse oximeter recordings should be monitored for decreasing oxygen levels. (See Chapter 32 🔗 for more information about supporting oxygenation.) Level of consciousness and presence of seizures or changes in reflexes need to be followed to determine the extent and effects of the imbalance. Reflexes may be hyperreflexive or absent, depending on the particular imbalance. The client may complain of numbness or tingling in fingers or toes, lethargy, or headache. A change

---

BOX 26-5 | NURSING CARE CHECKLIST

Determining Acid-Base Imbalance

☑ Verify the pH level. A high level leads to alkalosis; a low one to acidosis.

☑ Establish the primary cause of the disturbance. Ascertain the $Paco_2$ and HCO_3 in relationship to the pH.

a. pH greater than 7.45, $Paco_2$ less than 35 mm Hg: The major imbalance is respiratory alkalosis. *$Paco_2$ is usually opposite of the pH. If the pH is low and $Paco_2$ is high or if pH is high with low $Paco_2$, then it is respiratory in origin.*

b. pH greater than 7.45, HCO_3 greater than 26 mEq/L: The major imbalance is metabolic alkalosis. *HCO_3 levels usually follow the pH level. If the pH is high and HCO_3 is high or if the pH is low with low HCO_3, then it is metabolic in origin.*

c. pH less than 7.35, $Paco_2$ greater than 45 mm Hg: The primary imbalance is metabolic acidosis.

d. pH less than 7.35, HCO_3 less than 22 mEq/L: The primary imbalance is metabolic acidosis.

☑ The next step is to decide if compensation has started. Monitor the value other than the major source of the imbalance. The other value shows the body's attempt to compensate. Compensation involves opposites. *If the major imbalance is metabolic acidosis, compensation will be accomplished by respiratory alkalosis.*

☑ Partial compensation occurs when the pH remains outside of the normal range.

---

in urinary output or NG output would be significant to report. (See Chapter 39, Box 39-1 ⚭, for measuring urine output.) The nurse performs regular assessment of mental status and vital signs. Any client who has an intake and output imbalance is at risk for acid-base imbalance, and should be monitored closely until homeostasis is achieved.

EVALUATING

The client with fluid and electrolyte or acid-base disorders must be monitored regularly and carefully. Data on vital signs and I&O should be collected. IV and respiratory therapy must be monitored as ordered. Changes in level of consciousness, abnormal or worsening vital signs, and fluid imbalances should be reported to the charge nurse or physician. Treatments aimed at correcting fluid, electrolyte, or acid-base imbalances require careful evaluation of the client to determine their response to treatment. It is possible to overcorrect, or undercorrect, an imbalance as the body tries to compensate and regain homeostasis.

Continuity of Care

Teaching needs to take place addressing the underlying cause of imbalances. How the client should take his or her medications, especially new prescriptions, should be reviewed, and the client's questions should be answered.

The client needs to know what signs might indicate that a respiratory compensation is beginning and what to report. Therapeutic dietary changes need to be reviewed and client should be helped to identify proper food choices.

NURSING PROCESS CARE PLAN
Client with Electrolyte Imbalance

Marcus Smith is a 69-year-old male who has been diagnosed with intrarenal renal failure. He has experienced damage to his nephrons and kidney tissue, resulting from an allergic reaction to contrasts dye administered during an intravenous pyelogram (IVP) to rule out renal calculi. He has been on a sodium-restricted diet in an attempt to regulate fluid balance. His weight has increased 11 lbs. in one week's time, due to fluid retention. He has expressed concern that he will need to begin dialysis if his condition does not improve.

Assessment
VS: T 99, P 110, R 28, BP 188/94. Weight today 196 pounds, c/o nausea, and lack of appetite. Urine output was 200 mL in the past 24 hours. Lab tests indicate elevated BUN and serum creatinine levels. Mr. Smith's daughter is concerned because he seems to be confused.

Nursing Diagnosis
The following important nursing diagnoses (among others) are established for Mr. Smith:

- *Impaired Urinary Elimination*
- *Risk for Ineffective Renal Tissue Perfusion*
- *Fluid Volume Excess*
- *Acute Confusion*

Expected Outcomes
The expected outcomes for the plan of care are that Mr. Smith will:

- Decrease weight 1–2 lb per day until normal weight obtained.
- Participate in psychiatric counseling program on a regular basis.
- Demonstrate stable weight without further losses in immediate future.
- Keep serum electrolytes within normal limits.

Planning and Implementation
The following nursing interventions are implemented for Mr. Smith. Assessments are done frequently to monitor his condition.

- Monitor weight daily.
- Monitor for electrolyte imbalance.

- Monitor fluid intake and urine output.
- Administer antihypertensives and diuretics per physician's orders.
- Offer several small meals of sodium-restricted, low protein diet.
- Administer vitamin supplements as ordered.
- Reorient client as needed.
- Provide opportunity for client and family to express feelings concerning possibility of dialysis treatment.

Evaluation

Appetite improved, able to eat small amounts without nausea. Weight decreased to 190 lbs. Sodium, calcium, and potassium levels within normal limits. Urinary output 800 mL/24 hours. Mr. Smith and his daughter are asking questions about dialysis.

Critical Thinking in the Nursing Process

1. Why would Mr. Smith be placed on a sodium-restricted diet when his sodium levels appear normal?
2. What is the probable cause of Mr. Smith's confusion and disorientation?
3. Mr. Smith's daughter asks how long he will need dialysis. What would be an appropriate answer to her question?

Note: Discussion of Critical Thinking questions appears on the MyNursingKit Website.

Note: The references and resources for all chapters have been compiled at the back of the book.

Chapter Review

KEY Points

- Water is the largest component of the body. Its functions include maintenance of blood volume, transportation of nutrients to and from cells, regulation of body temperature, and assistance with digestion.
- Homeostasis depends on many physiological processes. These processes regulate fluid intake and output. They also regulate the movement of water and dissolved substances between the body compartments.
- Fluid imbalances may signal the development of disease. Imbalances between fluid intake and fluid output need to be addressed without delay.
- The kidneys and lungs are the major organs in regulating acid-base imbalances.
- The key to acid-base balance is the regulation of hydrogen ion concentration of body fluids.
- Most electrolytes enter the body through dietary intake and are excreted in the urine. Some electrolytes, such as sodium and chloride, are not stored by the body and must be consumed daily to maintain normal levels.
- Changes in electrolyte levels and in acid-base balance can be life threatening. Clients with electrolyte or acid-base imbalances must be monitored often.
- If the flow of IV fluids is incorrect, problems such as hypervolemia, hypovolemia, or inadequate medication administration can result. The role of the LPN/LVN includes monitoring intake and output and effects of fluid administration. The LPN/LVN must consult a baseline assessment of the client's fluid status in order to evaluate fluid balance.

 FOR FURTHER Study

Figure 25-1 illustrates the percentage of fluid in clients of different ages.

See Chapter 28 for more information on IV therapy.

See Chapter 32 for information on monitoring oxygenation status.

Chapter 39 contains information on urinary system functioning and Box 39-1 describes how to measure urine output.

Critical Thinking Care Map

Caring for a Client with Risk for Deficient Fluid Volume

NCLEX-PN® Focus Area: Physiological Integrity

Case Study: Patti Glove, a 40-year-old female, was admitted to an acute care hospital for treatment of intractable nausea/vomiting and diarrhea. Patti states that she has been experiencing the nausea and vomiting for the past 3 days, with diarrhea beginning yesterday. She has not taken any medications at home for this condition. No fluids have been "kept down" for 3 days. Patti states that she has been very weak and feels faint when she stands up.

Nursing Diagnosis: *Deficient Fluid Volume*

COLLECT DATA

Subjective	Objective
_____	_____
_____	_____
_____	_____
_____	_____
_____	_____
_____	_____

Would you report this? Yes/No

If yes, report to: _____

What would you report? _____

Nursing Care

_____
_____
_____
_____
_____
_____
_____
_____
_____
_____
_____

How would you document this?_____
_____
_____
_____

Compare your answers and documentation to those provided on the MyNursingKit Website.

Data Collected
(use only those that apply)

- Weight: 145 lbs
- Blood pressure: 98/62
- Pulse: 110, regular
- Respirations: 16
- Mood: irritable, anxious
- States she is very thirsty
- Oxygen saturation: 93% on room air
- Nausea and vomiting present
- Mucous membranes dry
- Skin turgor poor
- Urine dark amber, 50 mL in last voiding

Nursing Interventions
(use only those that apply; list in priority order)

- Monitor and report abnormal lab results.
- Monitor and document intake and output.
- Encourage fluid intake.
- Regularly monitor abdominal girth.
- Teach client to stand slowly.
- Monitor color, amount, and frequency of fluid loss.
- Assess for vertigo and hypotension.
- Take daily weights.
- Give and monitor effectiveness of antinausea medication as ordered.
- Give and monitor effectiveness of antidiarrheal medications as ordered.
- Monitor orthostatic blood pressure every 4 hours.
- Administer IV therapy as ordered.
- Provide frequent oral care.
- Teach client about intake/output measurement.

NCLEX-PN® Exam Preparation

TEST-TAKING TIP   Read all the choices for answers and eliminate those that you know are incorrect. If you narrow your choices down to two options, reread the stem (question) and decide which of the two choices *BEST* answers the question.

1 A client is in a lot of pain and breathing rapidly. The nurse recognizes this will cause CO_2 (carbon dioxide) to be exhaled and the client may develop which acid-base imbalance?

_____

_____.

2 The nurse is calculating the intake and output on a client. Which of the following client conditions would be considered an insensible fluid loss? The client:

1. Has been perspiring heavily.
2. Had a large emesis.
3. Has a temperature of 36.8°C.
4. Had a blood pressure reading of 92/50.

3 You are totaling the intake and output record for your shift. The client's IV fluid intake for the shift is 1,200 mL, and the output is 2,200 mL from a Foley catheter drainage bag. The client received 1,000 mL PO, and had an emesis of 75 mL. What was the client's total output for your shift?

1. 3,125 mL
2. 2,275 mL
3. 2,200 mL
4. 2,125 mL

4 The nurse is teaching the client with hypertension about dietary factors to reduce blood pressure. The nurse would instruct the client to limit the intake of what electrolyte?

1. Potassium
2. Sodium
3. Calcium
4. Phosphorous

5 The nurse is calculating the fluid intake of a client. Which of the following would not be included in the calculation?

1. Ice chips
2. Gelatin dessert
3. Intravenous medications
4. Nasogastric tube secretions collected from continuous suctioning

6 When an isotonic solution is administered, fluid moves from an area of low concentration to an area of high concentration to achieve fluid balance. This occurs because the administered fluid:

1. Has a lower concentration than the blood.
2. Has a higher concentration than the blood.
3. Will cause a shift in fluids to expand intravascular compartments.
4. Has the same concentration as blood.

7 A client is admitted with diabetic ketoacidosis (DKA). Due to the ketone bodies formed, the client is most likely experiencing which of the following acid-base imbalances?

1. Metabolic acidosis
2. Metabolic alkalosis
3. Respiratory acidosis
4. Respiratory alkalosis

8 A client is experiencing a potassium deficiency secondary to diuretic therapy. The nurse recognizes this electrolyte deficiency could lead to:

1. Osteoporosis.
2. Abnormal cardiac function.
3. Stress fractures.
4. Excessive mucus production.

9 The nurse is caring for a client with a nursing diagnosis of *Fluid Volume Excess* who has been placed on a diet that restricts salt. The nurse explains to the client that the primary reason for limiting salt is that:

1. Increased sodium intake results in fluid retention.
2. Increased chloride intake results in fluid retention.
3. Increased sodium chloride intake results in potassium imbalances.
4. Salt contains a chemical that damages the kidneys and reduces urine output.

10 Which of the following signs and symptoms would indicate metabolic alkalosis (bicarbonate excess)?

1. Kussmaul respirations, breathing, confusion, increased respiratory rate
2. Tetany, soft tissue calcification, low pH
3. Poor skin turgor, sunken eyeballs, rapid pulse
4. Dizziness, tingling of fingers and toes, decreased respirations, and cardiac dysrhythmias

Answers and rationales for Review Questions appear in Appendix I.

Medications

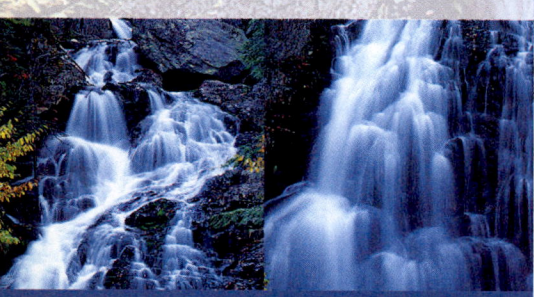

LEARNING Outcomes

After completing this chapter, you will be able to:

1. Define selected terms related to the administration of medication.
2. Describe drug standards and legal aspects of administering drugs.
3. Identify physiologic actions and effects of drugs, as well as factors affecting medication action.
4. Identify essential parts of medication orders, how to communicate about them, and how to avoid common errors.
5. Utilize systems of measurement and formulas commonly used in medication orders.
6. Identify equipment required for administering parenteral medications.
7. Describe various routes of medication administration and drug dispensing systems.
8. Explain important nursing interventions in relation to oral medication administration.
9. Outline steps required for administering nasogastric and gastrostomy tube medication.
10. Describe how to mix selected drugs from vials and ampules.
11. Describe essential steps for safely administering parenteral medications by intradermal, subcutaneous, and intramuscular routes.
12. Describe essential steps in safely administering topical medications.

Clinical Objectives

13. Demonstrate proper procedures for preparing medications for administration by the oral route, injection, ophthalmic instillation, otic instillation, vaginal instillation, and rectal instillation.
14. Demonstrate proper documentation of routine and prn medication administration.

KEY TERMS

Use the audio glossary feature on the MyNursingKit Website to hear the correct pronunciation of the following key terms.

absorption 614	generic 609	paste 610
adverse effects 612	half-life 613	pill 610
aerosol 610	household system 620	polypharmacy 616
ampule 628	hub 623	powder 610
anaphylaxis 613	iatrogenic disease 613	prescription 609
apothecaries' system 620	idiosyncratic effect 613	prn order 614
bevel 623	intradermal 624	side effects 612
buccal 624	intramuscular 624	single order 614
cannula 623	intravenous 624	solution 610
caplet 610	liniment 610	standing order 614
capsule 610	lotion 610	stat order 614
cream 610	lozenge 610	subcutaneous 624
cumulative effect 612	medication 609	sublingual 624
distribution 614	meniscus 638	suppository 610
drug allergy 613	metabolism 614	suspension 610
drug interaction 613	metric system 619	syringes 622
drug tolerance 613	nomogram 621	syrup 610
drug toxicity 612	NPO 624	tablet 610
elixir 610	ointment 610	therapeutic effect 612
excretion 614	ophthalmics 633	tincture 610
extract 610	otics 633	transdermal patch 610
gel 610	parenteral 624	vial 628

A **medication** is a substance administered for the diagnosis, cure, treatment, relief, or prevention of disease. In the healthcare context, the words *medication* and *drug* are used interchangeably.

In the United States and Canada, medications are usually dispensed by the order of physicians, nurse practitioners, and physician's assistants in some states, and dentists. The written direction for the preparation and administration of a drug is called a **prescription.**

A drug may have four different names:

1. The **generic** (family) name, given before a drug becomes official. The generic name is not capitalized (e.g., acetaminophen).
2. The *official* name, the name under which it is listed in one of the official publications (e.g., the *United States Pharmacopeia*).
3. The *chemical* name, which describes the drug constituents precisely. The chemical name is usually not used by the healthcare provider (e.g., -N-[4-hydroxyphenyl] acetamide).
4. The *trademark*, or *brand name*, which is the name used by the drug manufacturer. Because a drug may be manufactured by several companies, it can have several trade names. The trademark name should begin with a capital letter (e.g., Tylenol).

Medications are often available in a variety of forms. The drug form depends on the type of drug prescribed. Some drugs are only available in limited types of preparations. Some drugs may be delivered in several preparations (e.g., pills and suppositories), and some are only available in one type of preparation (e.g., aqueous solution for injection). The preparation may depend on the route ordered (e.g., oral vs. parenteral). Examples are given in Table 27-1 ■.

Drug Standards

Drugs may be made from natural (e.g., plant, mineral, and animal) sources, or they may be synthesized in the laboratory. For example, digitalis is plant derived, sodium chloride is a mineral, insulin has animal or human sources, and propoxyphene hydrochloride (the analgesic Darvon) is synthesized in a laboratory.

Drugs vary in strength and activity. Drugs must be pure and of uniform strength if drug dosages are to be predictable in their effect. Therefore, drug standards have been developed to ensure uniform quality. In the United States, official drugs are those designated by the Federal Food, Drug, and Cosmetic Act. These drugs are officially listed in the *United States Pharmacopeia (USP)* and described according to their source, physical and chemical properties, tests

TABLE 27-1	Types of Drug Preparations
TYPE	**DESCRIPTION**
Aerosol spray or foam	A liquid, powder, or foam deposited in a thin layer on the skin emitted by air pressure from the container
Aqueous **solution**	One or more drugs dissolved in water
Aqueous **suspension**	One or more drugs mixed with, but not dissolved in, water
Caplet	A solid form, shaped like a capsule, coated and easily swallowed
Capsule	A gelatinous container that holds a drug in powder, liquid, or oil form
Cream	A nongreasy, semisolid preparation used on the skin
Elixir	A sweetened and aromatic solution of alcohol used as a vehicle for medicinal agents
Extract	A concentrated form of a drug made from vegetables or animals
Gel or jelly	A clear or translucent semisolid that liquefies when applied to the skin
Liniment	A medication mixed with alcohol, oil, or soapy emollient and applied to the skin
Lotion	A medication in a liquid suspension applied to the skin
Lozenge (*troche*)	A flat, round, or oval preparation that dissolves and releases a drug when held in the mouth
Ointment (*salve, unction*)	A semisolid preparation of one or more drugs used for application to the skin and mucous membrane
Paste	A preparation like an ointment, but thicker and stiff, that penetrates the skin less than an ointment
Pill	One or more drugs mixed with a cohesive material, in oval, round, or flattened shapes
Powder	A finely ground drug or drugs; some are used internally, others externally
Suppository	One or several drugs mixed with a firm base such as gelatin and shaped for insertion into the body (e.g., the rectum); the base dissolves gradually at body temperature, releasing the drug
Syrup	An aqueous solution of sugar often used to disguise unpleasant-tasting drugs
Tablet	A powdered drug compressed into a hard, small disk; some are readily broken along a scored line; others are enteric coated to prevent them from dissolving in the stomach
Tincture	An alcohol or water-and-alcohol solution prepared from drugs derived from plants
Transdermal patch	A semipermeable membrane shaped in the form of a disk or patch that contains a drug to be absorbed through the skin over a long period of time

for purity and identity, method of storage, assay, category, and normal dosages. In Canada, the *British Pharmacopoeia* is used for the same purpose, although some drugs used in Canada conform to the *USP* because they are obtained from the United States.

LEGAL ASPECTS OF DRUG ADMINISTRATION

The administration, manufacture, distribution, and safety of drugs are controlled by law. Table 27-2 ■ summarizes drug legislation for the United States and Canada.

Nurses must:

1. Know how nursing practice acts in their areas define and limit their functions, since nurse practice acts vary from state to state. *Note:* The LPN/LVN must never function outside his or her scope of practice. He or she should be in constant communication with the RN. Knowing one's scope and reporting to the RN whenever necessary will ensure that the LPN/LVN is operating within the legal limits of the license as it relates to drug administration.

2. Be able to recognize the limits of their own knowledge and skill.

Under the law, nurses are responsible for their own actions whether or not a written order exists. Nurses administer thousands of medications and are responsible for assessing drug effects, including recognizing unfavorable reactions. Since it is impossible to memorize pertinent information about every drug, nurses must rely on references, such as the *Physician's Desk Reference (PDR)* or *Nurse's Drug Guide*. If a physician writes an incorrect order (e.g., Demerol 500 mg instead of Demerol 50 mg), the nurse who administers the incorrect dosage is responsible for the error. Therefore, nurses should question any order that appears unreasonable and refuse to give the medication until the order is clarified.

Another aspect of nursing practice governed by law is the use of controlled substances. Box 27-1 ■ provides the Drug Enforcement Agency's Schedules of Controlled Substances.

In hospitals (as in all healthcare facilities), controlled substances are kept in a locked drawer, cupboard, medication cart, or computer-controlled dispensing system. Agencies have special forms for recording the use of controlled substances. The information required usually includes the name of the client, drug name, the date and time of administration, the dosage, and the signature of the person

TABLE 27-2	**Important Drug Legislation for United States and Canada**
LEGISLATION	**CONTENT**
Pure Food and Drug Act (U.S. 1906)	First government intervention that established consumer protection in the manufacture of drugs and foods. It requires all drugs to meet minimal standards of strength, purity, and quality. Drug preparations containing morphine must be labeled as such. Established written resources for officially approved drugs, which became the *United States Pharmacopeia*/National Formulary (*USP*/NF).
Proprietary or Patent Medicine Act (Can. 1908)	Protects the public against unsafe and ineffective over-the-counter drugs.
Food, Drug, and Cosmetic Act (U.S. 1938)	Implemented by Food and Drug Administration (FDA); requires that labels be accurate and that all drugs be tested for harmful effects.
Durham-Humphrey Amendment (U.S. 1952)	Clearly differentiates drugs that can be sold only with a prescription, those that can be sold without a prescription, and those that should not be refilled without a new prescription.
Canada Food and Drugs Act (Can. 1953)	Prohibits advertising any food, drug, cosmetic, or device as a cure for certain specified diseases. Sets standards for manufacture, distribution, and sale of all drugs, with the exception of narcotics.
Canadian Narcotic Control Act (Can. 1961)	Allows only authorized people to possess narcotics. Specifies records about narcotics that must be kept.
Kefauver-Harris Amendment (U.S. 1962)	Requires proof of safety and efficacy of a drug for approval.
Comprehensive Drug Abuse Prevention and Control Act (U.S. 1970) (Controlled Substances Act)	Categorizes controlled substances and limits how often a prescription can be filled; established government-funded programs to prevent and treat drug dependence. (The Drug Enforcement Administration [DEA] was established as a bureau of the Department of Justice to enforce provisions of the act. This act also established five schedules of drugs based on their degree of danger for abuse or addiction, beginning with C-I for most abuse potential to C-V for low abuse potential [Woodrow, 2002].)

BOX 27-1 DEA SCHEDULES OF CONTROLLED SUBSTANCES

1. Schedule I
   A. The drug or other substance has a high potential for abuse.
   B. The drug or other substance has no currently accepted medical use in treatment in the United States.
   C. There is a lack of accepted safety for use of the drug or other substance under medical supervision.

2. Schedule II
   A. The drug or other substance has a high potential for abuse.
   B. The drug or other substance has a currently accepted medical use in treatment in the United States or a currently accepted medical use with severe restrictions.
   C. Abuse of the drug or other substances may lead to severe psychological or physical dependence.

3. Schedule III
   A. The drug or other substance has a potential for abuse less than the drugs or other substances in Schedules I and II.
   B. The drug or other substance has a currently accepted medical use in treatment in the United States.
   C. Abuse of the drug or other substance may lead to moderate or low physical dependence or high psychological dependence.

4. Schedule IV
   A. The drug or other substance has a low potential for abuse relative to the drugs or other substances in Schedule III.
   B. The drug or other substance has a currently accepted medical use in treatment in the United States.
   C. Abuse of the drug or other substance may lead to limited physical dependence or psychological dependence relative to the drugs or other substances in Schedule III.

5. Schedule V
   A. The drug or other substance has a low potential for abuse relative to the drugs or other substances in schedule IV.
   B. The drug or other substance has a currently accepted medical use in treatment in the United States.
   C. Abuse of the drug or other substance may lead to limited physical dependence or psychological dependence relative to the drugs or other substances in schedule IV.
   D. Initial schedules of controlled substances Schedules I, II, III, IV, and V shall, unless and until amended pursuant to section 811 of this title, consist of the following drugs or other substances, by whatever official name, common or usual name, chemical name, or brand name designated.

Food and Drug Administration Pregnancy Categories may also be included. The current categories for drug use in pregnancy follow (USFDA, 2001):

A - Adequate, well-controlled studies in pregnant women have not shown an increased risk of fetal abnormalities.

(continued)

BOX 27-1 (continued)

B - Animal studies have revealed no evidence of harm to the fetus, however, there are no adequate and well-controlled studies in pregnant women.

or

Animal studies have shown an adverse effect, but adequate and well-controlled studies in pregnant women have failed to demonstrate a risk to the fetus.

C - Animal studies have shown an adverse effect and there are no adequate and well-controlled studies in pregnant women.

or

No animal studies have been conducted and there are no adequate and well-controlled studies in pregnant women.

D - Studies, adequate well-controlled or observational, in pregnant women have demonstrated a risk to the fetus. However, the benefits of therapy may outweigh the potential risk.

X - Studies, adequate well-controlled or observational, in animals or pregnant women have demonstrated positive evidence of fetal abnormalities. The use of the product is contraindicated in women who are or may become pregnant.

Revised schedules are published in the Code of Federal Regulations, Part 1308 of Title 21, Food and Drugs.

who prepared and gave the drug. The name of the physician who ordered the drug may also be part of the record.

Included on this record are the controlled substances wasted during preparation. When a dose or portion of a dose is not used, it must be disposed of according to facility procedure. (Check facility protocol for wasting of any drug. It is no longer acceptable to flush drugs down the toilet, into a drain, or into a trash receptacle.) A second licensed nurse must witness and sign that the drug was wasted and disposed of properly. In most agencies, counts of controlled substances are taken at the end of each shift. The count total should tally with the total at the end of the last shift minus the number used. Discrepancies must be reported immediately.

Effects of Drugs

The **therapeutic effect** of a drug, also referred to as the *desired effect*, is the reason the drug is prescribed (the drug did what it was supposed [prescribed] to do). See Table 27-3 ■ for kinds of therapeutic actions.

Therapeutic drug level tests are usually performed to look for the presence and the amount of specific drugs in the blood. With most medications, a certain level of drug in the bloodstream is needed to obtain the desired effect. Some medications are toxic if the level rises too high and are ineffective if the levels are too low. Monitoring serum drug levels enables your healthcare provider to ensure that your drug levels are within an effective range.

A drug side effect is an unintended drug action. Unfavorable **side effects** are also called *untoward effects*. Untoward effects (such as slight stomach discomfort) may be tolerated for the sake of therapeutic effect. More severe side effects, also called **adverse effects** or *drug reactions* (such as a severe allergic reaction), may justify discontinuing the drug.

Drug toxicity (deleterious effects of a drug on an organism or tissue) results from overdosage, ingestion of a drug intended for external use, and **cumulative effect** (buildup of the drug in the blood because of impaired metabolism or excretion). Some toxic effects become apparent immediately; some are not apparent for weeks or months. Drug toxicity may be avoided by close monitoring of the drug dose

TABLE 27-3	**Therapeutic Actions of Drugs**	
DRUG TYPE	**DESCRIPTION**	**EXAMPLES**
Palliative	Relieves the symptoms of a disease but does not affect the disease itself.	Morphine sulfate, aspirin for pain
Curative	Cures a disease or condition.	Penicillin for infection
Supportive	Supports body function until other treatments or the body's response can take over.	Norepinephrine bitartrate for low blood pressure; aspirin for high body temperature
Substitutive	Replaces body fluids or substances.	Thyroxine for hypothyroidism, insulin for diabetes mellitus
Chemotherapeutic	Destroys malignant cells.	Busulfan for leukemia
Restorative	Returns the body to health.	Vitamin, mineral supplements, B_{12} injections for pernicious anemia

and client response. The elderly are most at risk for drug toxicity because of decreased kidney and liver function. Children are at risk for drug toxicity related to immature systems for handling drugs (Karch, 2008). In 2007, children's cold medications were pulled from the shelves of drug stores due to possible side effects, adverse reactions, and possible toxicity.

A **drug allergy** is an immunologic reaction to a drug. When a person is first exposed to a foreign substance (antigen), such as a drug, the body may react by producing antibodies, triggering an allergic reaction called anaphylaxis. Localized anaphylactic reactions include hay fever, hives, and gastroenteritis. Systemic **anaphylaxis** is a potentially life-threatening reaction to an allergen, with peripheral vasodilatation, bronchospasm, and laryngeal edema. Check for allergies before giving medications. Table 27-4 ■ describes common mild allergic responses.

Drug tolerance occurs when a person requires increases in dosage to maintain the therapeutic effect. Habituating drugs such as opiates, barbiturates, ethyl alcohol, and nicotine produce tolerance. A cumulative effect is the increasing response to repeated doses of a drug, which occurs when the rate of administration exceeds the rate of metabolism or excretion. As a result, the drug builds up in the client's body unless the dosage is adjusted.

An **idiosyncratic effect** (unexpected unique bodily response) causes unpredictable abnormal symptoms in clients, including opposite drug actions and over- and underresponse to medications (e.g., diphenhydramine [Benadryl] occasionally causes agitation instead of sedation in some clients).

A **drug interaction** occurs when the administration of one drug alters the effect of another drug. The effect of each drug may increase (*potentiating* or *synergistic effect*) or decrease (*inhibiting effect*). Drug interactions may be beneficial or harmful. For example, tetracycline should not be given with milk or milk products because it decreases the effectiveness of the medication. Foods and other natural substances, such as herbal supplements, may interact adversely with a medication; therefore, it is important for the nurse to assess the client for use of supplements of any kind (see Chapter 8).

Iatrogenic disease (an unintentional disease caused by medical therapy) can be due to drug administration.

ACTIONS OF DRUGS IN THE BODY

The action of a drug in the body can be described in terms of its half-life. **Half-life** is the time interval required for the body's elimination processes to reduce the concentration of the drug in the body by one-half. For example, if a drug's half-life is 8 hours, then the amount of drug in the body from one dose is as follows:

Initially: 100%
After 8 hours: 50%
After 16 hours: 25%
After 24 hours: 12.5%
After 32 hours: 6.25%

Because the purpose of most drug therapy is to maintain a constant drug level in the body, repeated doses are required to maintain that level. Figure 27-1 ■ illustrates drug half-life and maintenance of a therapeutic drug level in the blood.

Many variables affect the body's response to a drug. These may include age, weight (drug dosages are generally based on the weight of a 150-pound male), gender, environment, and physiological, psychological, pathological, and genetic factors (Karch, 2008). It is important to understand the four processes involved in drug actions. Box 27-2 ■ includes an explanation of the four processes of drug actions (absorption, distribution, metabolism, and excretion).

TABLE 27-4	Common Mild Allergic Responses
SYMPTOM	**DESCRIPTION/RATIONALE**
Skin rash (urticaria)	Either an intraepidermal vesicle rash or a rash typified by an urticarial wheal (hives) or macular eruption; rash is usually generalized over the body
Pruritus	Itching of the skin with or without a rash
Angioedema	Edema due to increased permeability of the blood capillaries
Rhinitis	Excessive watery discharge from the nose
Lacrimal tearing	Excessive watering of the eyes
Nausea, vomiting	Stimulation of centers in the brain causing stomach queasiness and possible loss of stomach contents
Wheezing and dyspnea	Labored respirations and high-pitched breathing noises upon inhalation and exhalation due to accumulated fluids and swelling of the respiratory tissues
Diarrhea	Irritation of the mucosa of the large intestine with resultant watery, loose stool

MyNursingKit | Drug metabolism

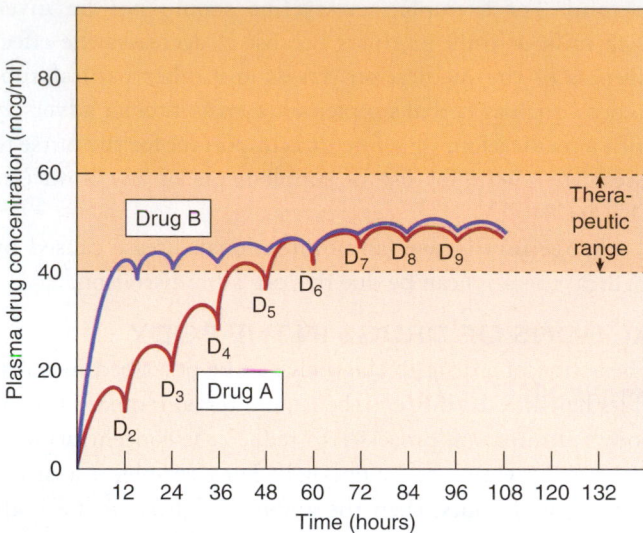

Figure 27-1. ■ Mechanism of drug half-life and maintenance of a therapeutic drug level in the blood.

| BOX 27-2 | KEY TERMS RELATED TO DRUG ACTION |

- **Onset of action:** The time after administration when the body initially responds to the drug
- **Peak plasma level:** The highest plasma level achieved by a single dose when the elimination rate of a drug equals the absorption rate
- **Drug half-life** (*elimination half-life*): The time required for the elimination process to reduce the concentration of the drug to one-half what it was at initial administration
- **Plateau:** A maintained concentration of a drug in the plasma during a series of scheduled doses

Processes of Drug Action

- **Absorption:** The process by which a drug passes into the bloodstream
- **Distribution:** The process by which the drug is sent to various body tissues
- **Metabolism:** The process by which some drugs are converted in the liver to inactive compounds
- **Excretion:** The process by which drugs are eliminated from the body, which most often occurs via the renal system

---

FACTORS AFFECTING MEDICATION ACTION

Medication action may be based on whether or not there are any changes in drug viability with exposure to light, air, heat, or moisture. Medications such as nitroglycerin lose potency in the presence of light, air, and moisture.

Various factors affect the action of a medication, and they vary based on the individual. For instance, an *idiosyncratic effect* is an unexpected and individual response to a drug. The drug may have a completely different effect from the normal one or cause unpredictable and unexplained symptoms in a particular client.

Ethnicity and culture may contribute to differences in responses to medications. It is thought that a toxic reaction may be due to a genetic defect that causes a person to be unable to eliminate a drug or to metabolize a drug too quickly.

Cultural practices can also affect a drug's actions. Herbal remedies may counteract prescribed medications. Age and development may also have an effect on medication. Box 27-3 ■ lists age-related considerations for medication administration.

The route of administration is another factor that affects medication action. Pharmaceutical preparations are generally designed for one or more specific routes of administration. Table 27-5 ■ lists the advantages and disadvantages of various routes of administration. The route of administration should always be indicated by the physician when the drug is ordered. When administering a drug, the nurse needs to ensure that the pharmaceutical preparation is appropriate for the route specified.

Medication Orders

A physician determines the client's medication needs and orders medications. Usually, the order is written, although telephone and verbal orders are acceptable in a number of agencies. Nursing students need to know the agency policies about medication orders. In most hospitals, for example, only licensed nurses are permitted to accept telephone and verbal orders.

Four common medication orders are the stat order, the single order, the standing order, and the prn order.

1. A **stat order** indicates that the medication is to be given immediately and only once unless subsequent doses are ordered to follow the immediate dose.
2. The **single order** or *one-time order* is for medication to be given once at a specified time.
3. The **standing order,** sometimes referred to as a *routine order,* may or may not have a termination date. A standing order may be carried out indefinitely (e.g., multiple vitamins daily) until an order is written to cancel it, or it may be carried out for a specified number of days.
4. A **prn order,** or *as-needed order,* permits the nurse to give a medication when, in the nurse's judgment, the client requires it. The nurse must use good judgment about when the medication is needed within the parameters provided by the physician (e.g., every 4 to 6 hours prn) and when it can be safely administered.

ESSENTIAL PARTS OF A MEDICATION ORDER

The drug order has seven essential parts, as listed in Box 27-4 ■. Unless it is a standing, or routine order, the order should state the number of doses or the number of days the

BOX 27-3	LIFESPAN CONSIDERATIONS

Medications for Infants and Children

- Knowledge of human growth and development is essential for the nurse. Oral medications for children are usually prepared in sweetened liquid form to make them more palatable. Never disguise with a necessary food (such as formula, milk, or juice), because the child may refuse that food in the future. Parents may provide suggestions.
- Infants usually require small dosages because of their body size and the immaturity of their organs, especially the liver and kidneys. They often do not have all of the enzymes required for drug metabolism and therefore may require different medications than adults. In adolescence or adulthood, allergic reactions may occur with drugs formerly tolerated.
- Children tend to fear any unfamiliar procedures, especially those in which needles are used. The nurse must acknowledge that the child will experience pain; denying this fact only fosters distrust. After an injection, the nurse (or parent) should cuddle and speak softly to the infant and/or give a toy to dispel the child's association of the nurse with pain.

Variation: Giving Oral Medications to Infants and Children

- Select an appropriate vehicle to measure and administer the medication, for example, a plastic disposable cup or an oral medication syringe. A plastic syringe without a needle is sometimes used but is not recommended because of increased likelihood of error. Whenever possible, give children a choice about use of a spoon, dropper, or oral medication syringe.
- Dilute the oral medication, if indicated, with a small amount of water. Many oral medications are readily swallowed if they are diluted with a small amount of water. If large quantities of water are used, the child may refuse to drink the entire amount and would receive only a portion of the medication.
- Unless contraindicated, crush medications that are not supplied in liquid form and mix them with substances available on most pediatric units, such as honey, flavored syrup, jam, or a fruit puree. *Note:* When selecting a substance to mix with a medication, avoid *essential* food items such as milk, cereal, and orange juice. If these foods are used, the child may refuse them in the future.
- Disguise disagreeable-tasting medications with sweet-tasting substances mentioned previously. However, present any altered medication to the child honestly and not as a food or treat.
- To prevent nausea, pour a carbonated beverage over finely crushed ice and give it before or immediately after the medication is administered.
- To prevent aspiration and choking, position infants in a semi-reclining position, and administer the medication slowly in divided doses by spoon or a plastic syringe.
- If using a spoon, retrieve and refeed medication that is thrust outward by the infant's tongue.
- If using a syringe, place it along the side of the infant's tongue. This position prevents gagging and expulsion of the medication.
- A child's parents or guardians may be able to provide valuable information on how best to give the child medications. However, a nurse may need to partially restrain a child who refuses to cooperate or consistently resists despite explanation, encouragement, and attempts to determine the reason for the behavior.
  - a. Place the child in your lap with the right arm behind you.
  - b. Grasp the child's left hand firmly with your left hand.
  - c. Secure the head between your arm and body.
- Follow all medication with a drink of water or juice, a soft drink, or a Popsicle or frozen juice bar. This removes any unpleasant aftertaste.
- For children who take sweetened medications on a long-term basis, follow the medication administration with oral hygiene. These children are at high risk for dental caries.
- For a young child, use a doll to demonstrate the procedure. This facilitates cooperation and decreases anxiety.
- For a young child or infant, enlist assistance to immobilize the arms and head. The parent may hold the infant or young child. This prevents accidental injury during medication administration.

Adults

- Maternal health considerations: During pregnancy, women must be very careful about taking medications. Most drugs are contraindicated because of the possible adverse effects on the fetus.
- Older adult physiological changes that affect responses to medications include the following:
  - Decreases in liver and renal function can affect the metabolism and excretion of drugs leading to an accumulation of the drug in the body, thereby increasing the risk for drug toxicity.
  - Decreased gastric motility and decreased gastric acid production and blood flow can impair drug absorption.
  - Increased adipose tissue and decreased total body fluid proportionate to the body mass can increase the possibility of drug toxicity.
  - Decreased number of protein-binding sites and changes in the blood–brain barrier can occur. The latter permits fat-soluble drugs to move readily to the brain, often resulting in dizziness and confusion. This is particularly evident with beta-blockers.
  - Impaired circulation delays the action of medications given intramuscularly or subcutaneously. Digitalis, which is frequently taken by older people, can accumulate to toxic levels and be lethal.
  - Older adults usually require smaller dosages of drugs, especially CNS depressants. Their reactions to medications, particularly sedatives, are unpredictable and often bizarre. Reactions to sedatives include irritability, confusion, disorientation, restlessness, and incontinence. Nurses therefore need to observe clients carefully for untoward (idiosyncratic) reactions.
  - Because memory and visual acuity of older adults may be impaired, the nurse needs to develop simple, realistic plans for clients to follow at home. For example, clients are more likely to remember to take medications if they are scheduled to be taken with meals or at bedtime. If they are likely to forget whether they have taken their medications, a special container for medications can be employed. An empty

(continued)

BOX 27-3 (continued)

container indicates that the person has already taken the pills. If the person has poor visual acuity, the nurse or a family member can write out the plan in block letters large enough to be read.

- Taking several different medications daily is called **polypharmacy.** The possibility of error increases with the number of medications taken.
- The greater number of medications also compounds the problem of drug interactions and side effects. A general rule to follow is to take as few medications as possible.

■ Older adult psychosocial problems (related to physiological changes, past experiences, and established attitudes toward medications) may affect how they view the use of medications.

- Attitudes of older people toward medical care and medications vary. Older people tend to believe in the wisdom of the physician more readily than younger people. Some

older people are bewildered by the prescription of several medications and may passively accept their medications and "cheek" them, spitting out tablets or capsules after the nurse leaves the room. For this reason, the nurse is advised to stay with clients until they have swallowed the medications. Others may be suspicious of medications and actively refuse them.

■ Older people are mature adults capable of reasoning. Therefore, the nurse needs to explain the reasons for and the effects of medications. This education can prevent clients from continuing to take a medication long after there is a need for it or discontinuing a drug too quickly. For example, clients should know that diuretics will cause them to urinate more frequently and may reduce ankle edema. Instructions about medications need to be given to all clients. These instructions should include when to take the drugs, what effects to expect, and when to consult a physician.

TABLE 27-5 Routes of Administration

ROUTE	ADVANTAGES	DISADVANTAGES
Oral	Most convenient Usually least expensive Safe, does not break skin barrier Administration usually does not cause stress	Inappropriate for clients with nausea or vomiting Drug may have unpleasant taste or odor Inappropriate when gastrointestinal tract has reduced motility Inappropriate if client cannot swallow or is unconscious Cannot be used before certain diagnostic tests or surgical procedures Drug may discolor teeth or harm tooth enamel Drug may irritate gastric mucosa Drug can be aspirated by seriously ill clients
Sublingual	Same as for oral, *plus* Drug can be administered for local effect Drug is rapidly absorbed into the bloodstream More potent than oral route because drug directly enters the blood and bypasses the liver	If swallowed, drug may be inactivated by gastric juice Drug must remain under tongue until dissolved and absorbed
Buccal	Same as for sublingual	Same as for sublingual
Rectal	Can be used when drug has objectionable taste or odor Drug released at slow, steady rate	Dose absorbed is unpredictable May be embarrassing to client
Vaginal	Provides local therapeutic effect	Limited use
Topical	Provides a local effect Few side effects	May be messy and may soil clothes Drug can enter body through abrasions and cause systemic effects
Transdermal	Prolonged systemic effect Few side effects Avoids gastrointestinal absorption problems	Leaves residue on the skin that may soil clothes May cause skin irritation
Subcutaneous	Onset of drug action faster than oral	Must involve aseptic technique because breaks skin barrier Risk for infection More expensive than oral

TABLE 27-5	Routes of Administration (continued)	
ROUTE	**ADVANTAGES**	**DISADVANTAGES**
Subcutaneous		Can administer only small volume Slower onset of action than intramuscular administration Some drugs can irritate tissues and cause pain Can be anxiety producing
Intramuscular	Pain from irritating drugs is minimized Can administer larger volume than subcutaneous Drug is rapidly absorbed	Must involve aseptic technique because breaks skin barrier Risk for infection Some drugs can irritate tissues and cause pain Can be anxiety producing
Intradermal	Absorption is slow (this is an advantage in testing for allergies)	Amount of drug administered must be small Limited use Must involve aseptic technique because breaks skin barrier Risk for infection
Intravenous	Rapid effect	Limited to highly soluble drugs Anxiety producing and causes pain Must involve aseptic technique because breaks skin barrier Risk for infection Only certain healthcare providers are allowed to administer IV medications Usually RN administers
Inhalation	Introduces drug through respiratory tract Rapid localized relief Drug can be administered to unconscious client	Drug intended for localized effect can have systemic effect

---

BOX 27-4	ESSENTIAL PARTS OF A DRUG ORDER

- Full name of the client
- Date and time the order is written
- Name of the drug to be administered
- Dosage of the drug
- Route of administration
- Frequency of administration
- Signature of the person writing the order

drug is to be administered. *Note:* Schedule II or opioid drugs, such as morphine, are only allowed by law to be prescribed for up to a 72-hour period. After that time, the doctor must write a new prescription to continue administering the drug.

COMMUNICATING A MEDICATION ORDER

A drug order is written on the client's chart by a physician or by a nurse who receives a telephone or verbal order from a physician. The medication order is then copied by a nurse or clerk to a medication administration record (MAR) and often a Kardex. Increasingly, nurses are provided with daily computer-generated MARs. This method saves time and reduces errors caused by hand copying of the physician's order.

Medication administration records (Figure 27-2 ■) vary in form, but all include the client's name, room, and bed number; drug name and dose; and times and method of administration. In most agencies, the date the order was prescribed and the date the order expires are also included.

The nurse should always question the physician about any order that is *ambiguous* (unclear or difficult to read), *unusual* (e.g., an abnormally high dosage of a medication), or contraindicated by the client's condition. When the LPN/LVN determines that a physician-ordered medication is inappropriate, the following actions are required:

1. Discuss the order with the RN and/or the nursing supervisor.
2. Contact the physician and discuss the rationale for believing the medication or dosage to be inappropriate.
3. Document in notes the following: time the physician was notified, by whom, information conveyed to the physician, and the physician's response (using the physician's words, if possible).

MEDICATION ADMINISTRATION RECORD

Seton Medical Center
100 Spurway Ave • Daly City
Seton Medical Center Coastside
100 Marine Blvd • Moss Beach

PAGE 1 OF 1
5 0507-02

VERIFIED BY: _____ DATE: _____

PRN#:
MRN#:   AGE:
ADM: 08-04-01   SEX:
DOB: HT:
DR.   HT:

DIAGNOSIS: *#ALOC
              *#PNEUMONIA

ALLERGIES: NO KNOWN DRUG ALLERGIES

GENERATED: 08-07-12   07:32am
FOR PERIOD: 08-07-12   08:00
THROUGH: 08-08-12   07:59

START	STOP	MEDICATION/I.V./IVPB/IRRIGATION		0800-1559	1600-2359	0000-0759
08-06 17	09-05 16	FERROUS SULFATE 300MG=5ML TWICE A DAY PO (FES04)	(973539)	09	17	
08-06 17	09-05 16	DOCUSATE SODIUM 100MG=1UDCUP TWICE A DAY PO (COLACE) 100MG/30ML UD HOLD FOR LOOSE STOOL	(973532)	09	17	
08-05 09	09-04 08	ASCORBIC ACID 500MG=1TAB TWICE A DAY PO (VITAMIN C) 500MG TAB	(972096)	09	17	
08-05 09	09-04 08	LEVOTHYROXINE 0.05MG=1TABDAILY PO (SYNTHROID) 0.05MG TAB	(972095)	09		
08-05 09	09-04 08	ASPIRIN 325MG=1 TAB DAILY PO (ASPIRIN) 325MG TAB *W/FOOD TO AVOID GI UPSET	(972094)	09		
08-04 23	08-14 22	CEFUROXIME ADDV. 1.500GM=1VIAL EVERY 8 HOUS IV (KEFUROX) 1.5GM ADDV *ATTACH TO D5W 50ML ADDV BAG *ACTIVATE BEFORE UNFUSION* * INFUSE OVER 30 MINS*	(971776)	14	22	06
		——— PRN ORDERS ———				
08-04 23	09-03 22	ACETAMINOPHEN 650MG=1SUPP EVERY 4 HOURS AS NEEDED PR (TYLENOL) 650MG SUPP	(971779)			

INITIALS	SIGNATURE	SHIFT	INITIALS	SIGNATURE	SHIFT	INITIALS	SIGNATURE	SHIFT

SITE CODES:
A. Right Upper Outer Gluteus
B. Left Upper Outer Quadrant Gluteus
C. Right Outer Aspect Arm
D. Left Outer Aspect Arm
E. Right Ventrogluteal
F. Left Ventrogluteal
G. Abdomen
H. Right Thigh
J. Left Thigh

Figure 27-2. ■ Medication administration record. (Courtesy of Seton Medical Center.)

4. If the physician cannot be reached, document all attempts to contact the physician and the reason for withholding the medication.

5. If someone else gives the medication that person must document that the drug was given, however the LPN/LVN may document data about the client's condition before and after the medication.

6. If an incident report is indicated, clearly document factual information.

COMMON STUDENT MEDICATION ERRORS

The Institute for Safe Medication Practices (2007) reported on an analysis of conditions that lead to student errors in medication administration. The following situations are most commonly involved in errors:

- *Dual assignment.* The nature of student environments in which both licensed and student nurses are caring for the same individuals is one element that can lead to over- or undermedication. In one case, the student and the licensed nurse may administer medication without realizing the other has done so. In the opposite case, both may think the other has administered the medication, so the client may miss a prescribed dose.

- *Documentation.* In the type of error just noted, lack of prompt, accurate documentation is a major factor.

- *Insulin errors.* Insulin is one of the most frequent drugs involved in errors, both among students and among staff. Errors include omitting doses, using the wrong type of insulin, administering the wrong amount (sliding-scale errors), and administering to the wrong client. Insulin and other high-alert drugs need special attention to avoid errors, including independent double-checking of all insulin doses by staff before administration.

- *Nonstandard dosage times.* Many omissions occur when a medication is to be administered at an unusual time, such as early in the morning.

- *Unavailability or ignoring of MAR.* The safest procedure is to bring the MAR to the client's bedside to check before administering medication. Duplicates should not be used, and student worksheets should never take the place of the MAR as the student's guide for drug administration.

- *Restrictions on routes of administration.* Errors have occurred when students assigned to clients were not certified to administer medications by IV, and staff were unaware of their lack of certification. Students sometimes think others will administer a medication and do not verify this. This results in delayed or missed medication.

- *Holding or discontinuing medication.* Staff and students must have clear communication about ways of signifying held or discontinued drugs. Otherwise, students may administer them.

- *Changes in lab values.* Students must learn to access the most recent lab results and understand how changing lab values will affect medication administration. Many medications are meant to be discontinued when lab values reach normal ranges.

- *Packaging.* Errors can occur when a medication is dispensed in a larger tablet or container than is needed. Students may assume that the entire amount provided is to be given in one dose.

- *Parenteral syringes.* Oral or enteral medications prepared in parenteral syringes have sometimes mistakenly been given by the IV route. This error can be avoided by always preparing oral medications in oral syringes.

- *Drugs for multiple clients.* When preparing more than one client's medications at a time, it is possible to group the medications incorrectly and give a medication to the wrong client.

Systems of Measurement

Three systems of measurement are used for the administration of medication: the metric system, the apothecaries' system, and the household system.

METRIC SYSTEM

The **metric system** is a decimal system based on units of 10. Units can be multiplied or divided by 10 to form secondary units. Multiples are calculated by moving the decimal point to the right, and division is accomplished by moving the decimal point to the left.

Basic units of measurement are the meter, the liter, and the gram. Prefixes (from Latin) indicate subdivision of the basic unit: *deci-* (1/10 or 0.1), *centi-* (1/100 or 0.01), and *milli-* (1/1,000 or 0.001). Multiples of the basic units (from Greek) are *deka-* (10), *hecto-* (100), and *kilo-* (1,000). See Figure 27-3 ■ for examples of how these numbers relate to one another.

In nursing practice, the kilogram (kg) is the only multiple of the gram used, and the milligram (mg) and microgram

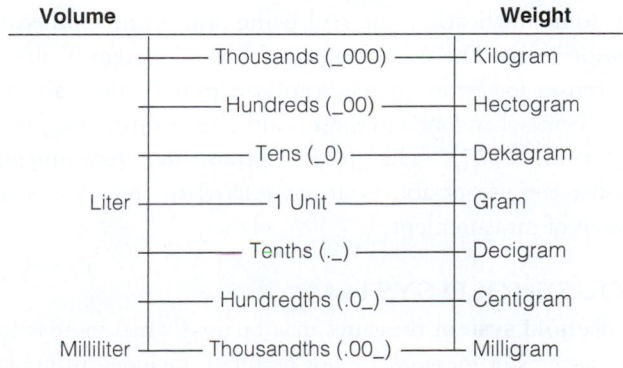

Figure 27-3. ■ Basic metric measurements of volume and weight.

TABLE 27-6	Approximate Equivalents: Metric, Apothecaries', and Household Systems	
METRIC	**APOTHECARIES'**	**HOUSEHOLD**
Volume		
1 mL	15 minims (min or m)	15 drops (gtt)
5 mL	75 min	1 measuring teaspoon
Generally not used		
15 mL	4 fluid drams	1 tablespoon (Tbsp)
30 mL	1 fluid ounce (oz)	1 fluid ounce
240 mL	8 oz	1 cup
500 mL	1 pint (pt)	1 pint
1,000 mL	1 quart (qt)	1 quart
4,000 mL	1 gallon (gal)	1 gallon
Weight		
1 milligram (mg)	1/60 grain	—
60 mg	1 grain (gr)	—
1 gram (g)	15 grains	—
		—
30 g	1 ounce	—
		—
1,000 g (1 kilogram [kg])	2.2 lbs	—

(mcg) are subdivisions. Fractional parts of the liter are usually expressed in milliliters (mL).

APOTHECARIES' SYSTEM

The **apothecaries' system** predates the metric system. The basic unit of weight in the apothecaries' system is the grain (gr), likened to a grain of wheat, and the basic unit of volume is the minim, a volume of water equal in weight to a grain of wheat. The word *minim* means "the least." Other units of weight are the dram, the ounce, and the pound. The units of volume are the fluid dram, the fluid ounce, the pint, the quart, and the gallon.

Quantities in the apothecaries' system are often expressed by lowercase Roman numerals (ii, iv, ix, etc.), particularly when the unit of measure is abbreviated. The Roman numeral follows the unit of measure. Although rarely used today, some medications are still being ordered in apothecary measurement. The use of the apothecaries' system is one of the causes for errors in medication administration, and its use is being abandoned in most healthcare facilities (Deglin & Vallerand, 2007). The Joint Commission recommends against the use of abbreviations related to the apothecary system of measurement.

HOUSEHOLD SYSTEM

Household system measures may be used when more accurate systems of measure are not required. Included in household measures are drops, teaspoons, tablespoons, cups, and

glasses. Although pints and quarts are often found in the home, they are defined as apothecaries' measures. Table 27-6 ■ lists measurement equivalents for the metric, apothecaries', and household systems.

clinical ALERT

A household teaspoon may hold 7.5 mL, which is one and a half times the amount in a measuring teaspoon. This caution should be included in discharge instructions. It is advisable to use a medication cup, oral syringe, or spoon with milliliter markings to prevent overdose of a drug.

CONVERTING UNITS OF WEIGHT AND MEASURE

Sometimes drugs are dispensed from the pharmacy in grams when the order specifies milligrams, or they are dispensed in milligrams though ordered in grains. For example, a physician orders morphine gr 1/4. The medication is available only in milligrams. The nurse knows that 1 mg equals 1/60 gr or 60 mg equals 1 grain. To convert the ordered dose to milligrams, the nurse calculates as follows:

$$\text{If } 60 \text{ mg} = 1 \text{gr}$$
$$\text{Then } x \text{ mg} = 1/4 \text{ gr } (or \ 0.25 \text{ gr})$$
$$x = \frac{(60 \times 0.25)}{1}$$
$$x = 15 \text{ mg}$$

Converting Weights within the Metric System

It is quite simple to find equivalent units of weight within the metric system, because the system is based on units of 10. Only three metric units of weight are used for drug dosages: the gram (g), milligram (mg), and microgram (mcg); 1,000 mg or 1,000,000 mcg equals 1 g. Equivalents are computed by dividing or multiplying. For example, to change milligrams to grams, the nurse divides the number of milligrams by 1,000. The simplest way to divide by 1,000 is to move the decimal point three places to the left: The gram is a *Larger* unit of measurement than milligram, so move the decimal point to the *Left*.

$$500 \text{ mg} = ? \text{ g}$$

Move the decimal point three places to the left:

$$\text{Answer} = 0.5 \text{ g}$$

Conversely, to convert grams to milligrams, multiply the number of grams by 1,000, or move the decimal point three places to the right: Milligram is a smaller unit of measurement than the gram, so the decimal point is moved toward the right.

$$0.006 \text{ g} = ? \text{ mg}$$

Move the decimal point three places to the right:

$$\text{Answer} = 6 \text{ mg}$$

Converting Weights and Measures between Systems

When preparing client medications, a nurse may need to convert weights or volumes from one system to another.

The units of weight most commonly used in nursing practice are the gram, milligram, and kilogram; and the grain and the pound. Household units of weight are generally not applicable (see Table 27-6). Learning these equivalents helps the nurse make weight conversions easily. For instance, if the nurse must give a medication based on the client's weight in kilograms, the amount of pounds the client weighs must be divided by 2.2.

$$150 \text{ lbs} \div 2.2 = 68.2 \text{ or } 68 \text{ kg}$$

CALCULATING DOSAGES

Several formulas can be used to calculate drug dosages. Nurses tend to choose the formula with which they are most comfortable; that the correct dosage is calculated is of most importance. One formula uses ratios:

$$\frac{\text{Dose on hand}}{\text{Quantity on hand}} = \frac{\text{Desired dose}}{\text{Quantity desired } (n)}$$

For example, erythromycin 500 mg is ordered. It is supplied in a liquid form containing 250 mg in 5 mL. To calculate the dosage, the nurse uses the formula

$$\frac{\text{Dose on hand (250 mg)}}{\text{Quantity on hand (5 mL)}} = \frac{\text{Desired dose (500 mg)}}{\text{Quantity desired } (n)}$$

Then the nurse cross-multiplies:

$$250 \times n = 5 \times 500$$
$$250 \times n = 2,500$$
$$n = \frac{2,500}{250}$$
$$n = 10 \text{ mL}$$

Therefore, the dose ordered is 10 mL. The nurse may also choose to use the following formula method to calculate dosages:

$$\frac{\text{Desired dose}}{\text{Dose on hand}} \times \text{Quantity on hand}$$

For example, heparin is often distributed in large vials in prepared dilutions of 10,000 units per mL. If the order calls for 5,000 units, the nurse can use the formula above to calculate:

$$n = \frac{5,000 \text{ units}}{10,000 \text{ units}} \times 1 \text{ mL}$$
$$n = 1/2 \text{ mL} = 0.5 \text{ mL}$$

Because the dosage is measured in mL, which is a liquid measure, the answer will be in decimal form—not a fraction. If the quantity on hand is a tablet, the answer would be written as a fraction rather than as a decimal.

Therefore, the nurse injects 0.5 mL for a 5,000-unit dose.

Dosages for Children

Although dosage is stated in the medication order, nurses must understand something about the safe dosage for children. Unlike adult dosages, children's dosages are not always standard. Body size significantly affects dosage. Following is the method for measuring pediatric doses based on body surface area.

BODY SURFACE AREA. Body surface area is determined by using a **nomogram** (a graph used to prescribe medications based on client size) and the child's height and weight. This is considered to be the most accurate method of calculating a child's dose. Standard nomograms give a child's body surface area according to weight and height (Figure 27-4 ■). The formula is the ratio of the child's body surface

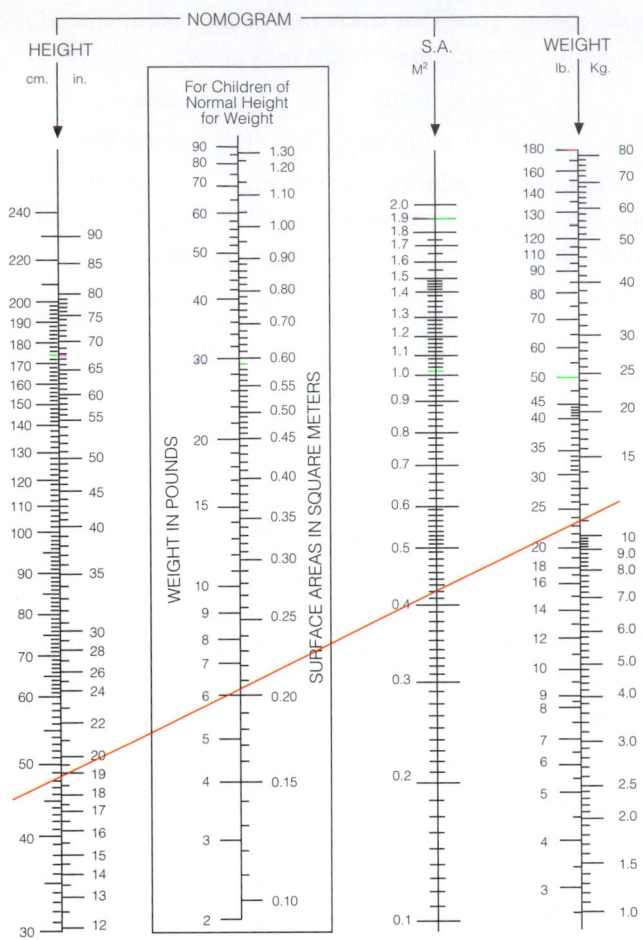

Figure 27-4. ■ Nomogram with estimated body surface area. A straight line is drawn between the child's height (on the left) and the child's weight (on the right). The point at which the line intersects the surface area column is the estimated body surface area.

area to the surface area of an average adult (1.7 square meters, or 1.7 m²), multiplied by the normal adult dose of the drug:

$$\text{Child's dose} = \frac{\text{Surface area of child (m}^2)}{1.7 \text{ m}^2} \times \text{Normal adult dose}$$

For example, a child who weighs 10 kg and is 50 cm tall has a body surface area of 0.4 m². Therefore, the child's dose of tetracycline corresponding to an adult dose of 250 mg would be as follows:

$$\text{Child's dose} = \frac{0.4 \text{ m}^2}{1.7 \text{ m}^2} \times 250 \text{ mg}$$

$$= 0.23 \times 250$$

$$= 58.82 \text{ mg}$$

Equipment

SYRINGES

To administer parenteral medications, nurses use special equipment. **Syringes** have three parts: the *tip*, which connects with the needle; the *barrel*, or fluid chamber, on which the scales are printed; and the *plunger*, which fits inside the barrel (Figure 27-5 ■).

To handle a syringe aseptically, the nurse may only touch the outside of the barrel and the plunger handle. The nurse must avoid letting any unsterile object contact the tip or inside of the barrel, the shaft of the plunger, or any part of the needle.

Syringes differ in size, shape, and material. The three most commonly used types are the standard hypodermic syringe, the insulin syringe, and the tuberculin syringe (Figure 27-6 ■). Standard hypodermic syringes generally come in 3-mL size (2-mL and 2.5-mL sizes are also possible). They usually have two scales marked on them: the minim and the milliliter. The milliliter scale is the one

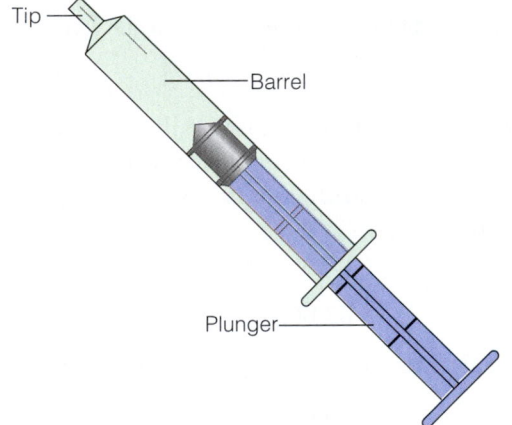

Figure 27-5. ■ The three parts of a syringe.

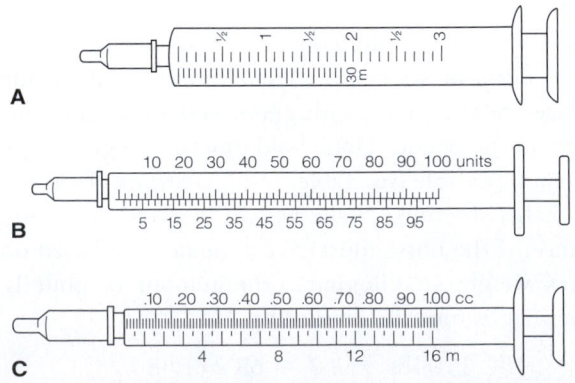

Figure 27-6. ■ Three kinds of syringes: **A.** hypodermic syringe marked in tenths (0.1) of milliliters and in minims; **B.** insulin syringe marked in 100 units; **C.** tuberculin syringe marked in tenths (0.1) and hundredths (0.01) of cubic millimeters and in minims.

normally used. Using the milliliter scale, the medication may be measured to the nearest tenth (e.g., 2.3 mL).

Insulin syringes are similar to hypodermic syringes, but they have a specially calibrated scale for use with U-100 insulin. In North America, all insulin syringes are calibrated this way. Most insulin syringes are disposable and have a nonremovable needle. Low-dose insulin syringes are also available. Low-dose insulin syringes only measure up to 50 units and are easier to read for small doses of insulin; the correct choice of syringe is based on the insulin dose. Although the U-100 syringe holds 1 mL of solution, the insulin syringe is not to be used for any medication other than insulin. Conversely the 1-mL or tuberculin syringe is not to be used for administering insulin.

The tuberculin syringe is a narrow-barrel syringe, calibrated in tenths and hundredths of a milliliter (up to 1 mL) on one scale and in sixteenths of a minim (up to 1 minim) on the other scale. (The minim scale is generally not in use.) Originally designed to administer tuberculin, this syringe is useful for administering other drugs, particularly when a small, precise measurement is necessary, such as 0.25 mL for pediatric doses.

Other syringes are manufactured in several sizes such as 5, 10, 20, and 50 mL (which are not used for intradermal, intramuscular, or subcutaneous injections). Most syringes used today are made of plastic and are individually packaged for sterility in a paper wrapper or a rigid plastic container (Figure 27-7 ■). The syringe and needle may be packaged together or separately.

Some injectable medications are supplied in disposable, prefilled unit-dose systems such as (1) ready-to-use syringes or (2) prefilled sterile cartridges and needles that require the attachment of a reusable holder (injection system) before use (Figure 27-8 ■). Examples of the latter system are the Tubex and Carpuject injection systems. The manufacturers provide specific directions for use.

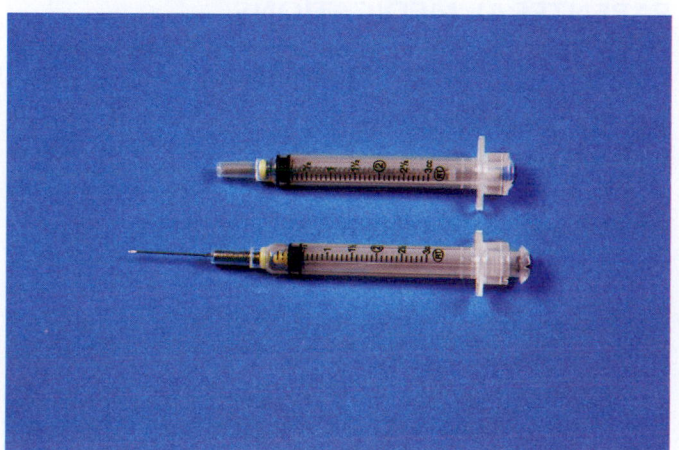

Figure 27-7. ■ Safety syringes. *Source:* Pearson Education/PH.

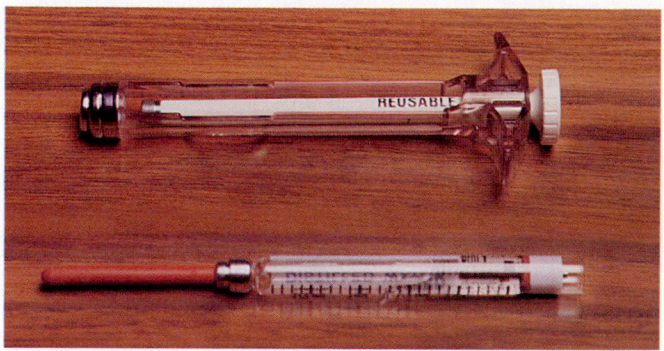

A

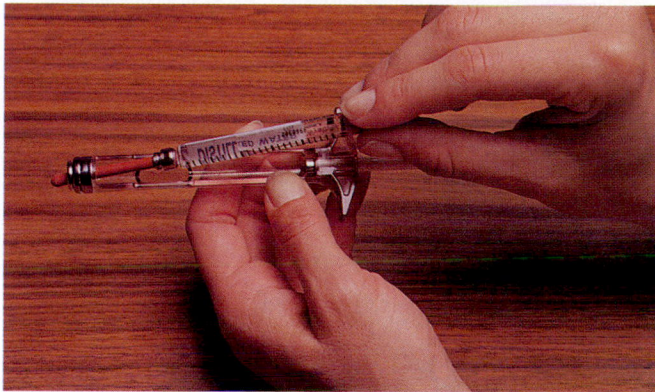

B

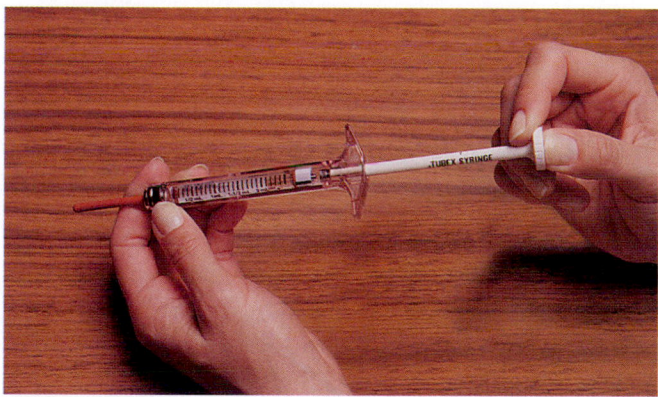

C

Figure 27-8. ■ **A.** Syringe and prefilled sterile cartridge with needle. **B.** Assembling the device. **C.** The cartridge slides into the syringe barrel, turns, and locks at the needle end. The plunger then screws into the cartridge end. (Photographer: Elena Dorfman.)

NEEDLES

Needles are made of stainless steel, and are disposable. A needle has three parts: the **hub,** which fits onto the syringe; the **cannula,** or *shaft,* which is attached to the hub; and the **bevel,** which is the slanted part of the tip (Figure 27-9 ■).

Needles have variable characteristics:

1. *Slant or length of the bevel.* Bevel length varies. Long-bevel needles are sharpest. They are best for intradermal,

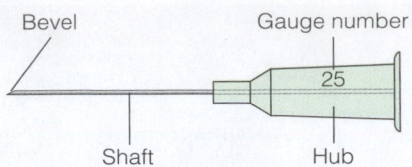

Figure 27-9. ■ The parts of a needle.

subcutaneous, and intramuscular injections because they cause the least discomfort.

2. *Length of the shaft.* The shaft length of commonly used needles varies from 1.25 to 5 cm (1/2 to 2 in.). The appropriate needle length is chosen according to the client's muscle development, the client's weight, and the type of injection.

3. *Gauge (or diameter) of the shaft.* The gauge varies from 16 to or 28. The larger the gauge number, the smaller the diameter of the shaft. Smaller gauges produce less tissue trauma, but larger gauges are necessary for viscous (thick) medications, such as penicillin.

Additional equipment is needed for intravenous administration.

Routes of Administration

ORAL MEDICATIONS

The oral route is the most common medication route. As long as a client can swallow effectively and retain the drug in the stomach, this is the route of choice. Procedure 27-1 ■ on page 637 describes how to give oral medications. Oral medications are contraindicated when a client is vomiting, has gastric or intestinal suction, is unconscious, or has swallowing difficulty, such as after a stroke. Such clients in the hospital are usually on orders for "nothing by mouth" (**NPO**).

There are two variations on the oral medication transmucosal route: sublingual and buccal. In **sublingual** administration, the drug is placed under the tongue (Figure 27-10 ■). The drug is absorbed into the blood vessels on the underside of the tongue. Nitroglycerin is one example of a drug commonly given in this manner.

Buccal means "pertaining to the cheek." In buccal administration, the tablet is held in the mouth next to the mucous membranes of the cheek until it dissolves (Figure 27-11 ■). The medication acts locally on the mucous membrane or systemically when the drug is absorbed into the blood vessels of the cheek (the same as the sublingual medication route).

NASOGASTRIC AND GASTROSTOMY MEDICATIONS

For the client who is NPO and has a nasogastric (NG) or gastrostomy (G) tube in place, medication may be administered via the tube. Medication is absorbed enterally because the

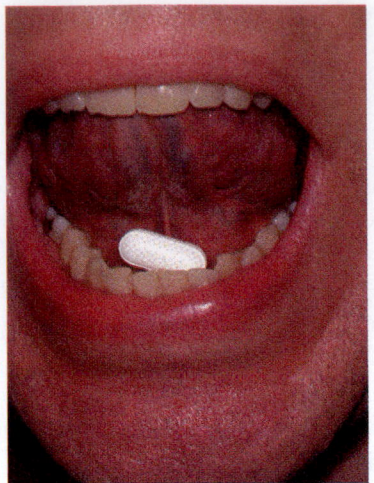

Figure 27-10. ■ Sublingual administration of a tablet.

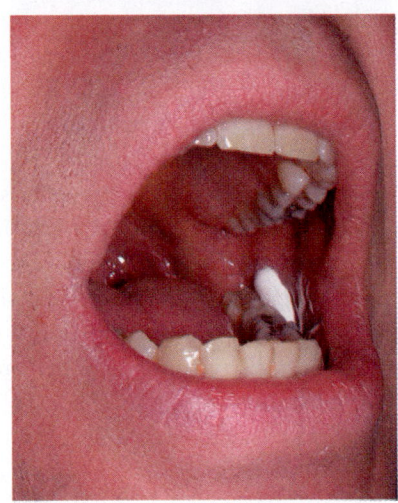

Figure 27-11. ■ Buccal administration of a tablet.

medication is delivered directly into the stomach or small intestine. See also Procedures 25-2 and 25-3 ∞.

PARENTERAL MEDICATIONS

LPNs/LVNs administer **parenteral** (injectable) medications. The routes are **intradermal** (ID or into the dermis or skin), **subcutaneous** (Sub-Q, subQ, or subcutaneously [per Joint Commission standards], below the skin), **intramuscular** (IM or into the muscle), and, in some states, **intravenous** (IV or into the vein). Figure 27-12 ■ illustrates the different angles of these injections and different ways of holding the syringe to administer them. Administration of medications via the parenteral route is discussed in the Nursing Care section of this chapter.

Because parenteral medications are absorbed rapidly and are irretrievable once injected, the nurse must prepare and administer them carefully and accurately. Administering parenteral drugs requires the same nursing knowledge as

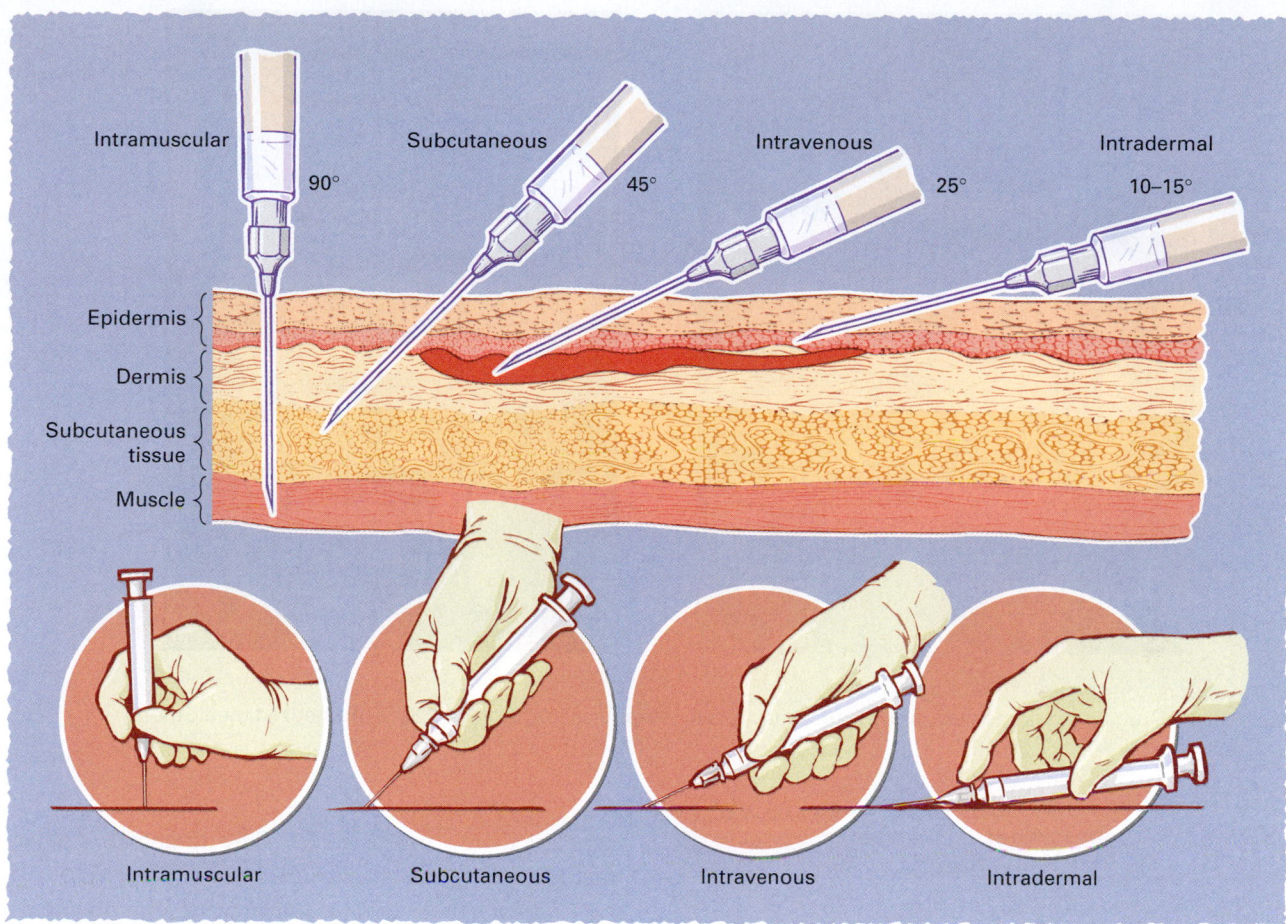

Figure 27-12. ■ Angles of needle insertion for four types of injection.

for oral and topical drugs. However, because injections are invasive procedures, aseptic technique must be used to minimize the risk of infection.

TOPICAL MEDICATIONS

Topical medications are those that are applied locally to the skin or to mucous membranes in areas such as the eye, external ear canal, nose, vagina, and rectum. Traditionally, topical application to the skin was limited to medications intended to produce a local effect at the administration site. However, several medications (e.g., nitroglycerin and estrogen) have been "packaged" in special transdermal delivery systems that gradually release a predictable amount of active substance into the bloodstream for as long as a week.

Drug Dispensing and Supply Systems

Medications are distributed to the nurse in various ways (Figure 27-13 ■). Facilities may use stock supply, unit-dose systems, and automated drug dispensary systems (such as the Omni-cell® machine). Many facilities use a medication cart. Carts may contain unit-dose supplies, bubble packs, or bulk. Unit doses are individually labeled drug packages consisting of one dose only. Bubble packs may be individually separated cards with an entire month's supply (e.g., routine meds) or with a supply for term of dosage (as with a course of antibiotics). Some drugs in the cart are in stock (bulk) supply (e.g., Tylenol and vitamins). Stock or bulk drugs may be stored in a manufacturer's labeled bottle in a separate drawer to be poured separately into a medication cup. Medication carts typically have separate drawers labeled for each client. However, in some facilities such as long-term care facilities, a large drawer may contain bubble packs separated by a divider for each resident. Medication cabinets may be located in the client's room in a locked cupboard for use by the nurse. Medication rooms typically contain storage for the medication cart, stock medications, refrigeration for medications, and a double-locked cabinet for controlled drugs.

Automated dispensing systems are computerized systems that allow the nurse access to a client's medications by using a password. The computerized system manages and controls the distribution of drugs.

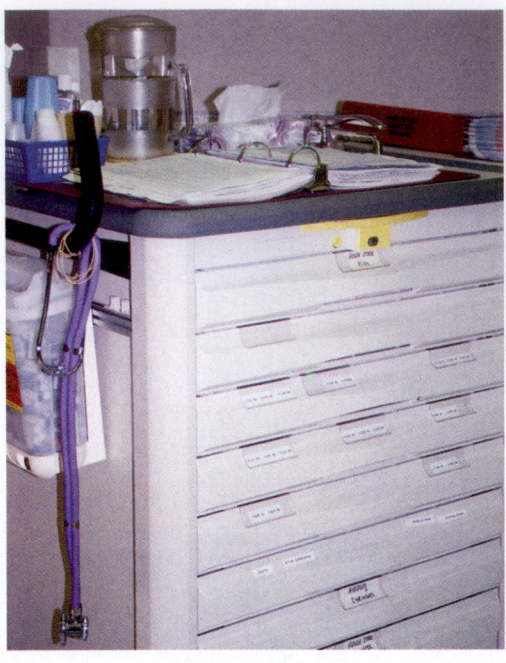

A

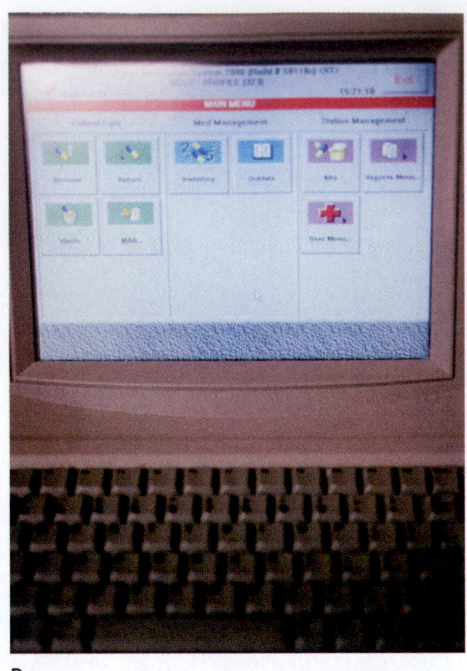

B

Figure 27-13. ■ Drug distributions systems the nurse may use. **A.** Portable medication cart. **B.** Computerized medication access system.

NURSING CARE

PRIORITIZING NURSING CARE

Priorities in the administration of drugs include identification of allergies; asepsis; six rights of medication administration; knowledge of each drug's usage, action, effects, and side effects; nursing assessments to be completed before and after drug administration; identification of side effects, adverse reactions, and allergies; safety; client education; and communication.

ASSESSING

When LPNs/LVNs are assigned the responsibility of administering medication, they must review the client's chart, including the medication history and nursing notes for assessment data, and discuss any concerns with the RN or physician.

DIAGNOSING, PLANNING, AND IMPLEMENTING

Providing Safety in Medication Administration

When administering any drug, regardless of the route of administration, the nurse must follow certain procedures. For a description of these procedures, see Table 27-7 ■. Box 27-5 ■ lists the six "rights" and the three "checks" for

accurate drug administration. The nurse who prepares the medication must also administer it to the client. Medications must never be left unattended on the medication cart or at the client's bedside.

Clients may take cultural remedies when they are ill, or they may have prohibitions against certain medications based on cultural and religious beliefs (Box 27-6 ■). These practices must be considered in the care of and planning for the client (see Chapter 8).

Observing Client's Response to the Drug

The kinds of behavior that reflect the action or lack of action of a drug and its untoward effects (both minor and major) are as variable as the purposes of the drugs themselves. For example, the effectiveness of a sedative-hypnotic may be directly observed by how well the client sleeps. The effectiveness of an antispasmodic must be based on the client's report of pain relief. It is essential to chart the client's drug response, but written notes are only one facet of communication needed for continuity of care. The LPN/LVN should also verbally report the client's response to the team leader or physician.

Administering Oral Medications

The nurse provides oral medications and water or other liquid as appropriate for the client. Some medications require the client to drink a full glass of water or to take the medication with food. This information is available in any

TABLE 27-7	Rules for Medication Administration
THE NURSE MUST ALWAYS	**DESCRIPTION**
Identify the client	In hospitals, most clients wear some sort of identification (ID), such as a wristband with name and hospital ID number. Before giving the client any drug, check the ID band against the MAR. As a double check, ask the client to state his or her name and birth date. The Joint Commission requires the use of two identifiers—neither of which can be the client's room number.
Inform the client	If the client is unfamiliar with the medication, the nurse should explain the intended action as well as any side effects or adverse effects that might occur.
Administer the drug	Read medication orders and records carefully; check both the client and drug name against the names on the drug packaging. If the client's medication is kept in a medication cart or computerized dispensary, check against this also.
Provide adjunctive interventions as indicated	Clients may need physical assistance, such as positioning for an injection. They may need teaching about measures to enhance drug effectiveness, such as changes in diet and fluid intake. Clients may express fear of medication. The LPN/LVN can allay fear through active listening and by offering factual information and emotional support.
Record the drug	Documentation must be completed immediately following the administration of a medication; never prechart medications. The name of the drug, dosage, method of administration, site of injection for parenteral medications, specific relevant data such as pulse rate, and any other pertinent information (e.g., date to be discontinued) are recorded in the chart in ink or by computer printout after being transcribed from the physician's order sheet. The record should also include the exact time of administration and the signature of the nurse providing the medication. Many medication records are designed in flowchart style so that the nurse signs once on the page and initials each medication administered. Any prn or stat medications, as well as the client's response to the drug, are recorded separately and should be documented in the nursing/progress notes. Nurses must be aware of all the medications a client is taking, and be alert for drug–drug or drug–food interactions.
Evaluate the client's response to the drug	In all nursing activities, nurses need to be aware of the medications that a client is taking and record their effectiveness as assessed by the client and the nurse on the client's chart. The nurse may also report the client's response to the RN or the physician.

BOX 27-5   SIX "RIGHTS" AND THREE "CHECKS" OF DRUG ADMINISTRATION

Right Client: Compare MAR to client name band and/or ask client for two identifiers.

Right Drug: Triple check the drug and watch for name discrepancies between generic and trade names.

Right Dose: Compute dosage. The drug dosage dispensed may not be the same as the order. Some drugs, such as insulin, must be double-checked with another licensed nurse.

Right Route: Is the drug to be given enterally or parenterally?

Right Time: Most facilities now use military time to decrease the risk of misinterpretation between AM and PM.

Right Documentation: Be certain to complete all pertinent information and write clearly, making sure you have the correct chart. Bring the MAR to the bedside and document as soon as the dose is taken (Institute for Safe Medication Practices, 2007).

Compare drug to MAR when removed from drawer.

Compare drug to MAR when pouring into cup.

Compare drug to MAR when returning container to the drawer.

nursing drug guide. The nurse remains with the client while the client swallows the medicine and assists if necessary. (*Note:* The nurse should be aware that some clients "pouch" medications in the cheek instead of swallowing them.)

Sublingual and buccal medications are placed under the tongue or between the cheek and the gum. They are not

BOX 27-6   CULTURAL PULSE POINTS

Cultural Remedies and Prohibitions

Cultural practices may affect which medications are acceptable to clients. For example, clients who follow strict Jewish dietary laws are not permitted to use pork insulin to treat diabetes. Muslims also do not consume pork products, but they are allowed to use medications made from pork. Many cultures prescribe herbal remedies based on cultural views of the nature of the illness. Many Native Americans, Hispanics, and Asians employ native health treatments before, or along with, Western medicine. These groups may consult an herbalist or medicine man. There is much more acceptance of alternative remedies in society now than in the past, but there still is need for caution. The client's record should always include herbs, remedies, or alternate medical practices as an important part of the client's database.

swallowed but allowed to dissolve in the mouth. No fluids are to be given until after the medication has fully dissolved.

Administering Nasogastric and Gastrostomy Medications

Clients may be NPO because of swallowing difficulties, illness, surgery, or another procedure. Medication may then be administered via nasogastric or gastrostomy tube. Nasogastric and gastric tubes are considered to be an enteral route because the medication is delivered to the gastrointestinal system. Guidelines for administering medications by NG or G tubes (American Journal of Nursing, 2005) are shown in Box 27-7 ■.

Assisting with IV Medication Administration

LPNs/LVNs, once licensed and certified in IV therapy, may be responsible for starting and hanging IVs. Until then, the LPN/LVN is responsible for assessing the site and may be responsible for removing the delivery system, once an

---

BOX 27-7 NURSING CARE CHECKLIST

Administering Medications by Nasogastric or Gastrostomy Tube

- ☑ Always check with the pharmacist to see if the client's medications come in liquid form, because liquids are less likely to cause tube obstruction.
- ☑ If not available, determine if the drug may be safely crushed. Enteric-coated, sustained-action, buccal, and sublingual medications should never be crushed.
- ☑ Dissolve crushed tablets in warm water. Cold liquids may congeal or cause client discomfort.
- ☑ Read medication labels carefully before opening a capsule.
- ☑ Open capsules and mix the contents with water only with the pharmacist's advice.
- ☑ Do not administer whole or undissolved medications.
- ☑ If the tube is connected to suction, disconnect the suction and keep the tube clamped for 20 to 30 minutes after giving the medication to enhance absorption. Positioning the patient toward the right side may facilitate gastric emptying.
- ☑ Always check and confirm NG tube placement before administering medications by checking gastric pH or by auscultating air.
- ☑ Flush the tube with at least 30 mL (5 to 10 mL for children) of water before administering medications.
- ☑ If you are giving several medications, administer each one separately and flush with at least 5 mL (3 mL for children) of water between each.
- ☑ When you have finished administering all medications, flush with another 30 mL of water to clear the tube.

BOX 27-8 NURSING CARE CHECKLIST

Discontinuing an Intravenous Device

- ☑ Check physician's order.
- ☑ Gather appropriate equipment.
- ☑ Identify the client and explain the procedure.
- ☑ Wash hands and don gloves.
- ☑ Stabilize needle or catheter while removing tape.
- ☑ Remove needle or catheter carefully and smoothly, keeping it almost flush with skin.
- ☑ Do not press down on top of needle point while it is in the vein.
- ☑ Once the catheter is removed, quickly press sterile pad over venipuncture site, and hold firmly until bleeding stops.
- ☑ Hold pressure for several minutes if client's drug therapy prolongs bleeding.
- ☑ Apply clean pad and tape in place.
- ☑ Elevate arm to reduce venous pressure and help facilitate clot formation.
- ☑ Observe venipuncture site for redness, swelling, or hematoma.
- ☑ Dispose of equipment.
- ☑ Wash hands.
- ☑ Check site again in 15 minutes.
- ☑ Record volume infused on intake and output (I&O) sheet.
- ☑ Document.

---

order has been given to discontinue. Box 27-8 ■ provides instructions for discontinuing an intravenous infusion. See also Procedure 28-11 ◯◯ .

Preparing Injectable Medications

Injectable medications can be prepared by withdrawing the medication from an ampule or vial into a sterile syringe, using prefilled syringes, or via a needleless injection system.

Ampules and Vials

Ampules and vials (Figure 27-14 ■) are frequently used to package sterile parenteral medications. An **ampule** is a clear glass container with a distinctive shape usually designed to hold a single dose of a drug. Ampule capacity ranges from 1 mL to 10 mL or more. Most ampules have colored score markings for opening. Refer to Procedure 27-2 ■ on page 640 for steps in preparing medications from ampules and vials.

A **vial** is a small glass bottle with a sealed rubber cap. Vials come in different sizes, from single to multidose, and have a metal or plastic cap that protects the rubber seal.

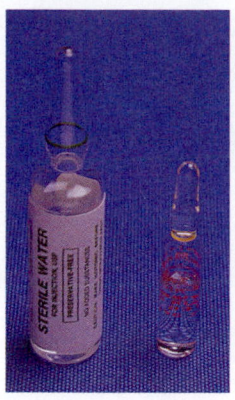 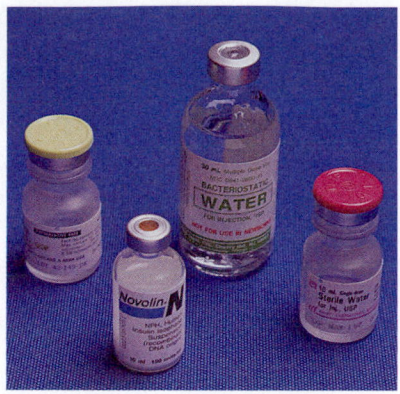

A   B

Figure 27-14. ■ **A.** Ampules; **B.** Vials.

Mixing Medications in One Syringe

Frequently, clients need more than one drug injected at the same time. To spare the client the experience of being injected twice, two drugs (if compatible) can be mixed together in one syringe. (See Procedure 27-2, Part C, for how to mix medications in one syringe.)

Preventing Needle-Stick Injuries

One of the most potentially hazardous procedures that healthcare personnel face is the use and disposal of needles and sharp instruments.

clinical ALERT

Needle-stick injuries present a major risk for infection with hepatitis B virus, human immunodeficiency virus (HIV), and many other pathogens. Standards have been set by the Occupational Safety and Health Administration to prevent such injuries.

To prevent needle-stick injury, the nurse must follow these guidelines carefully and consistently:

- Always use the designated puncture-proof disposal container provided (Figure 27-15 ■). Never throw sharps in wastebaskets. Never leave sharps unattended in public or client care areas.
- Handle all sharps with care, including any items that can cut or puncture skin, such as needles, surgical blades, lancets, razors, broken glass (including capillary pipettes and open ampules), exposed dental wires, reusable items (e.g., large-bore needles, hooks, rasps, drill points), or ANY SHARP INSTRUMENT!
- Never bend or break needles before disposal.
- When uncapping a needle, pull the needle and cap away from each other to minimize the risk of puncturing the fingers from reflexive action of the hands to come back together.

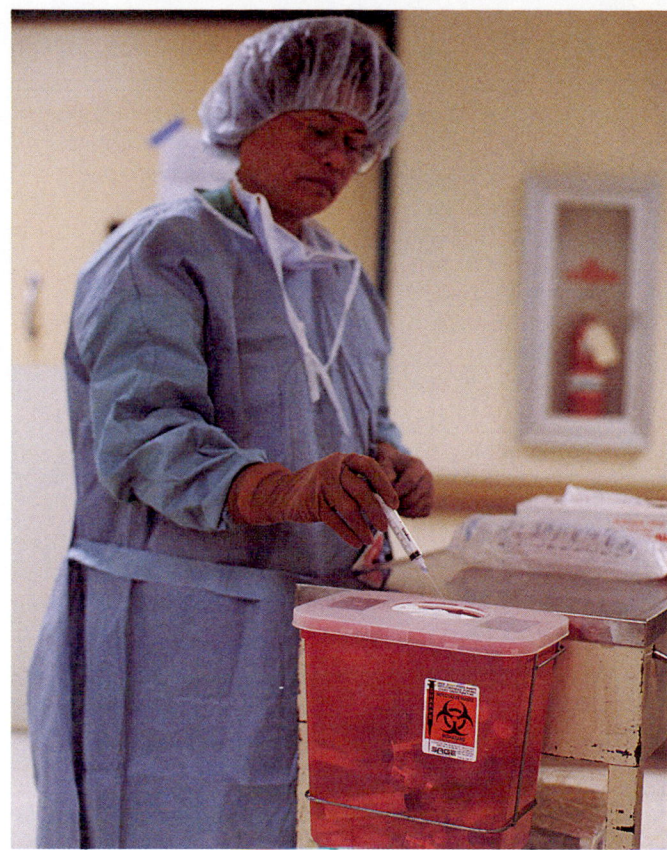

Figure 27-15. ■ Disposal container for contaminated needles and other sharps. (Photographer: Elena Dorfman.)

- Never recap used needles except under specified circumstances (e.g., when transporting a syringe to the laboratory for an arterial blood gas or blood culture).
- If you must recap a needle, use the one-handed "scoop" method. Set the needle cap and syringe horizontally on a flat surface. Insert the needle into the cap, using one hand (Figure 27-16 ■). Use your other hand to pick up the cap at its base (to avoid the risk of puncturing the fingers from the needle going through the cap) and tighten it to the needle hub.

If an accidental needle-stick injury occurs, follow specific steps outlined by the agency. A summary of these steps is provided in Box 27-9 ■. Safety syringes are now available to protect healthcare workers.

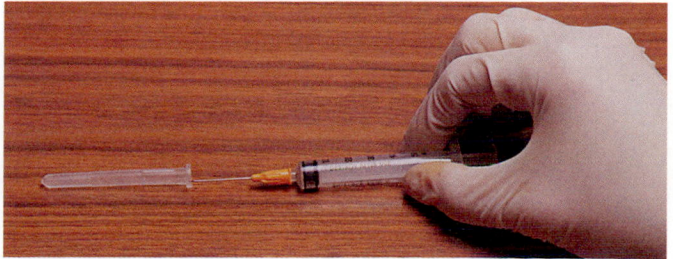

Figure 27-16. ■ Recapping a used needle using the scoop method. (Photographer: Elena Dorfman.)

Administering Intradermal Injections

An intradermal injection is the administration of a drug into the dermal layer of the skin just beneath the epidermis (see Figure 27-12). Intradermal injections generally use only a small amount of liquid, such as 0.1 mL. This method of administration is frequently indicated for allergy and tuberculin tests. Common sites for intradermal injections are the inner lower arm, the upper chest, and the back beneath the scapula (Figure 27-17 ■). Typically, the left arm is used for tuberculin tests and the right arm is used for all other tests.

The equipment normally used is a 1-mL syringe calibrated into hundredths of a milliliter. The needle is short and fine. After the site is cleaned, the skin is held tautly, and the syringe is held at about a 15-degree angle to the

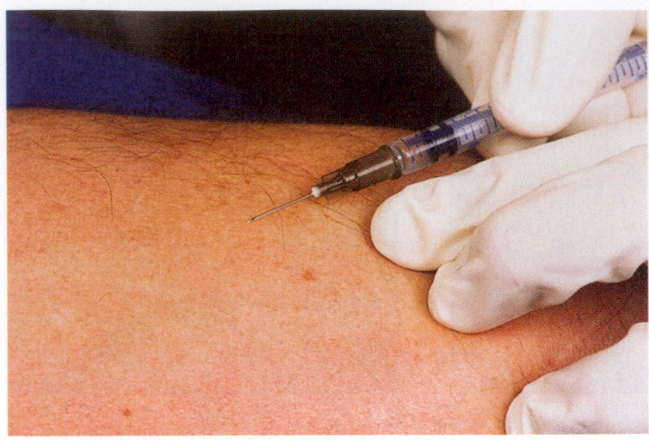

A

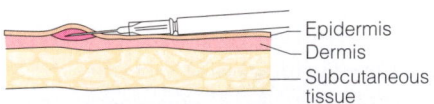

Epidermis
Dermis
Subcutaneous tissue

B

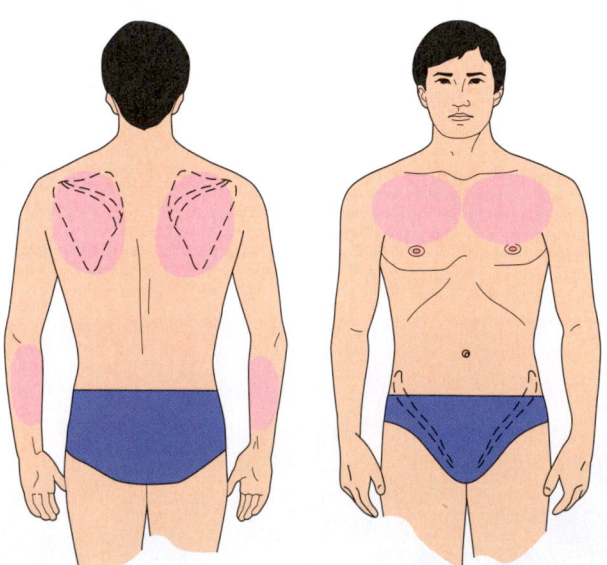

C

Figure 27-18. ■ For an intradermal injection: **A.** the needle enters the skin at a 15-degree angle; **B, C.** the medication forms a bleb under the epidermis.

skin, with the bevel of the needle upward. The needle is then inserted through the epidermis into the dermis, and the fluid is injected. The drug produces a small bleb or wheal just under the skin (Figure 27-18 ■). The needle is then withdrawn quickly, and the site is very lightly wiped with an antiseptic swab. The area is not massaged because the medication may disperse into the tissue or out through the needle insertion site. Intradermal injections are absorbed slowly through blood capillaries in the area.

Administering Subcutaneous Injections

Many kinds of drugs (such as insulin and heparin) are administered *subcutaneously* (just beneath the skin). Common sites for subcutaneous injections are the outer aspect of the upper arms and the anterior aspect of the thighs. These areas are convenient and normally have good blood circulation.

Figure 27-17. ■ Body sites commonly used for intradermal injections.

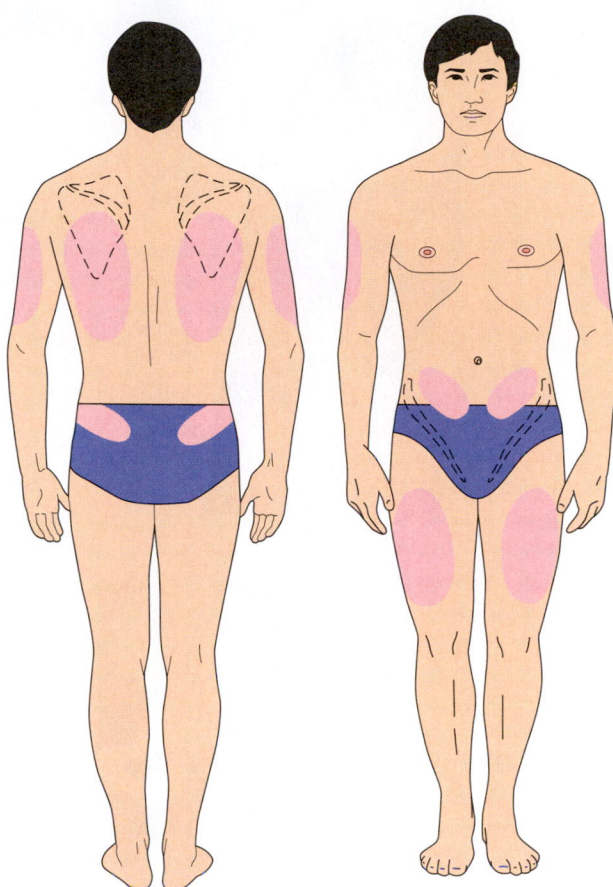

Figure 27-19. ■ Body sites commonly used for subcutaneous injections.

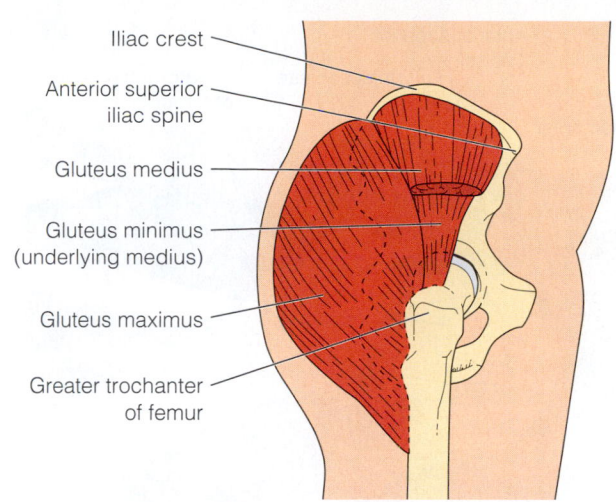

Figure 27-20. ■ Lateral view of the right buttock showing the three gluteal muscles used for intramuscular injections.

Other areas that can be used are the abdomen, the scapular areas of the upper back, and the upper ventrogluteal and dorsogluteal areas (Figure 27-19 ■). Only small doses (0.5 to 1 mL) of medication are usually injected via the subcutaneous route. Refer to Procedure 27-3 ■ on page 644 for instructions about subcutaneous injections.

Administering Intramuscular Injections

Injections into muscle tissue (IM injections) are absorbed more quickly than subcutaneous injections because of the greater blood supply to the body muscles. Muscles can also take a larger volume of fluid without discomfort than subcutaneous tissues can, although the amount varies somewhat, depending on muscle size, muscle condition, and the site used. An adult with well-developed muscles can usually safely tolerate up to 3 mL of medication in the gluteus medius and gluteus maximus muscles (Berman, Snyder, Kozier, & Erb, 2008).

A major consideration in the administration of IM injections is the selection of a safe site located away from large blood vessels, nerves, and bone. Several body sites can be used for IM injections. See Procedure 27-3, Part A, for administering IM injections.

Ventrogluteal Site

The ventrogluteal site is in the gluteus medius muscle, which lies over the gluteus minimus (Figure 27-20 ■). The ventrogluteal site is the preferred site for IM injections because the area (1) contains no large nerves or blood vessels, (2) provides the greatest thickness of gluteal muscle consisting of both the gluteus medius and gluteus minimus, (3) is sealed off by bone, and (4) contains consistently less fat than the buttock area, thus eliminating the need to determine the depth of subcutaneous fat.

The client position for the injection can be a supine, prone, or side-lying position. To establish the exact site, the nurse places the heel of the hand on the client's greater trochanter, with the fingers pointing toward the client's head. The right hand is used for the left hip, and the left hand for the right hip. With the index finger on the client's anterior superior iliac spine, the nurse stretches the middle finger dorsally, palpating the crest of the ilium and then pressing below it. The triangle formed by the index finger, the third finger, and the crest of the ilium is the injection site (Figure 27-21 ■).

Dorsogluteal Site

The dorsogluteal site is composed of the thick gluteal muscles of the buttocks (Figure 27-22 ■). The dorsogluteal site can be used for adults and for children with well-developed gluteal muscles. Because these muscles are developed by walking, this site should not be used for children under 3 years unless the child has been walking for at least 1 year. The nurse must choose the injection site carefully to avoid striking the sciatic nerve, major blood vessels, or bone.

The nurse palpates the posterior superior iliac spine, and then draws an imaginary line to the greater trochanter of the femur. This line is lateral to and parallel to the sciatic

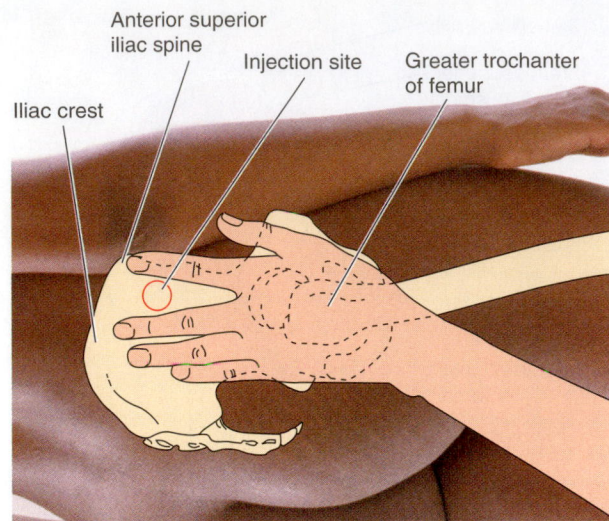

Figure 27-21. ■ The ventrogluteal site for an intramuscular injection.

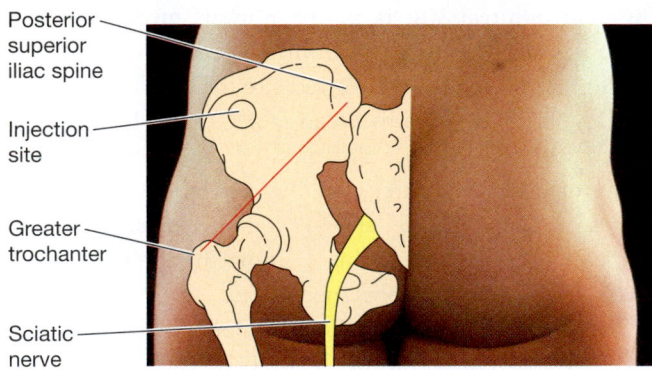

Figure 27-22. ■ The dorsogluteal site for an intramuscular injection. (*Source:* Custom Medical Stock Photo, Inc.)

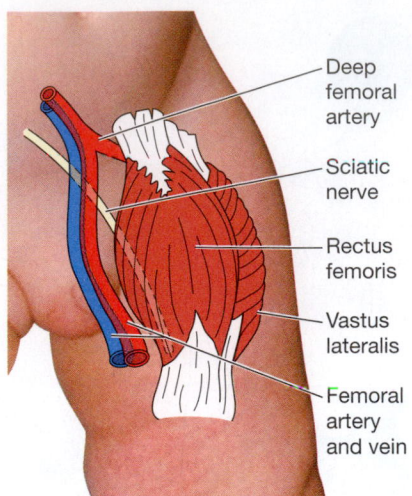

A

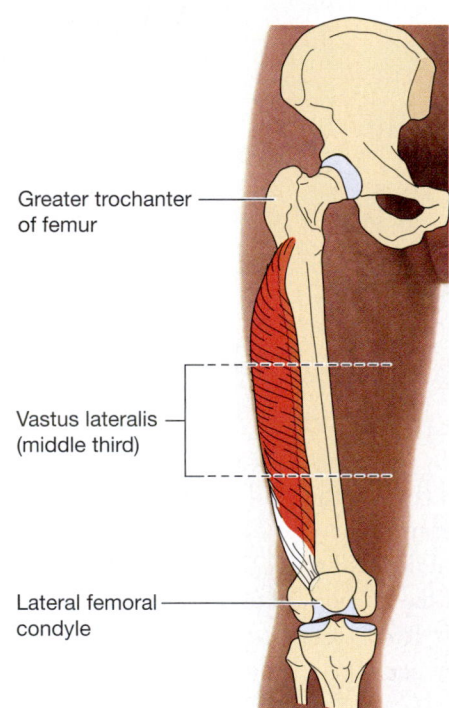

B

Figure 27-23. ■ **A.** The vastus lateralis muscle of the upper thigh, used for intramuscular injections. **B.** The vastus lateralis site of the right thigh, used for an intramuscular injection. (*Source:* Custom Medical Stock Photo, Inc.)

nerve. The injection site is lateral and superior to this line. Palpating the ilium and the trochanter is important. Visual calculations alone can result in an injection that is too low and that injures other structures.

It is best for the client to assume a prone position with the toes pointed inward, or a side-lying position with the upper knee flexed and in front of the lower leg. These positions promote muscle relaxation and minimize discomfort from the injection.

Vastus Lateralis Site

The vastus lateralis muscle is usually thick and well developed in both adults and children. It is recommended as the site of choice for IM injections for infants. Because there are no major blood vessels or nerves in the area, it is desirable for infants whose gluteal muscles are poorly developed. It is located on the anterior lateral aspect of the thigh (Figure 27-23 ■). The middle third of the muscle is suggested as the

site. This is established by dividing the area between the greater trochanter of the femur and the lateral femoral condyle into thirds and selecting the middle third (Figure 27-23B). The client can assume a back-lying or a sitting position for an injection into this site.

Deltoid Site

The deltoid muscle is found on the lateral aspect of the upper arm. It is not used often for IM injections, because it is a relatively small muscle and is very close to the radial nerve and radial artery. It is sometimes considered for use in adults because of rapid absorption from the deltoid area, but no more than 1 mL of solution can be administered. This site is recommended for the administration of hepatitis B vaccine in adults.

To locate the densest part of the muscle, the nurse palpates the lower edge of the acromion and the midpoint on the lateral aspect of the arm that is in line with the axilla. A triangle within these boundaries indicates the deltoid muscle about 5 cm (2 in.) below the acromion process (Figure 27-24 ■). Another method of establishing the deltoid site is to place four fingers across the deltoid muscle, with the first finger on the acromion process. The site is three finger-breadths below the acromion process (see Figure 27-24B).

Procedure 27-3, Part A, describes how to administer an IM injection using the *Z-track technique*. This technique is recommended for many IM injections. Medications that may irritate the tissue such as Vistaril (hydroxyzine hydrochloride solution) or drugs that may stain the tissue such as iron are examples of medications that require Z-track injection technique.

Although it is common practice to add 0.2 mL of air following the drawing up of medication, research has shown that use of an air bubble in the syringe is unnecessary with modern disposable syringes and can be potentially dangerous, causing overdoses (Beyea & Nicoll, 1996). Syringes are now calibrated to deliver correct dosages without the use of an air bubble. Some sources still advise the addition of 0.2 to 0.5 mL of air when administering medication by Z-track to clear the needle in order to prevent tracking of medication when the needle is withdrawn.

Administering Topical Applications

Skin Applications

Topical skin or dermatologic preparations include ointments, pastes, creams, lotions, powders, sprays, and patches (see Table 27-1 earlier in this chapter). Before applying a dermatologic preparation, remove any previously placed topical agent (e.g., skin patches) and clean off any remaining medication. Then thoroughly clean the area with mild soap and water and pat it dry. Medication absorption is affected by the buildup of skin secretions and previous topical medication. Human skin harbors microorganisms, so nurses should wear gloves when administering skin applications and always use surgical asepsis when an open wound is present.

Ophthalmic Instillations

Preparations for the eye (**ophthalmics**) come as liquids or ointments. Aseptic technique must be used to avoid contamination. Procedure 27-4 ■ on page 649 illustrates how to administer ophthalmic medications.

Otic Instillations

Medical aseptic technique is used to instill **otics** (ear preparations) unless the tympanic membrane is damaged,

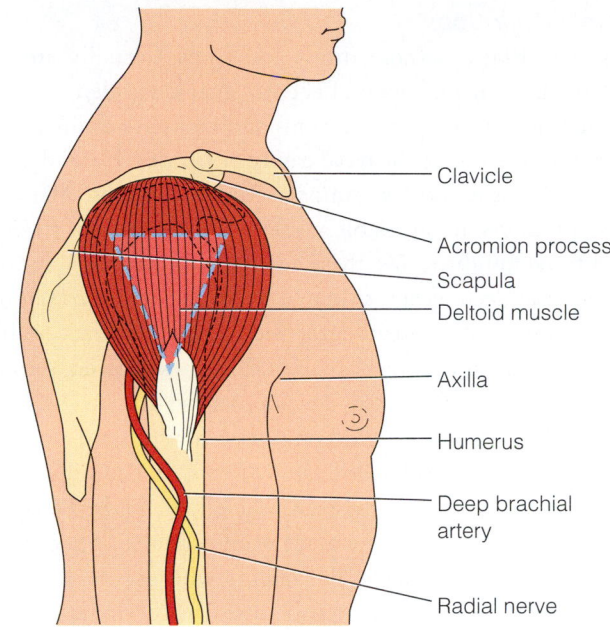

A

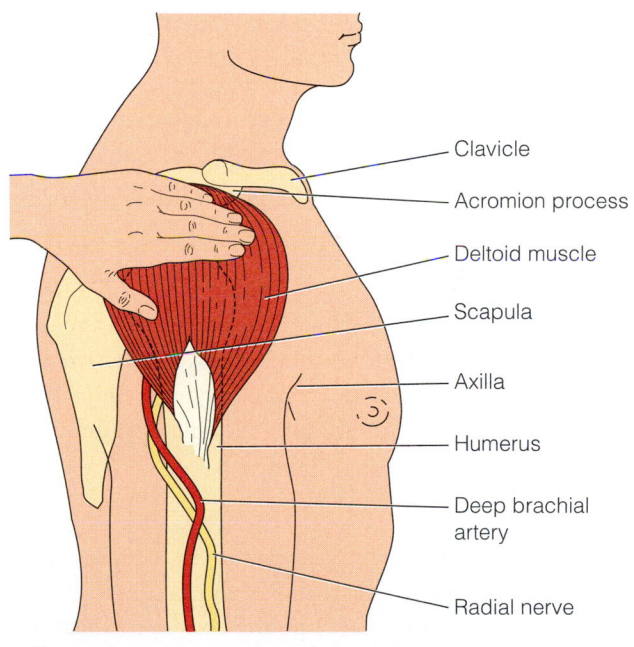

B

Figure 27-24. ■ **A.** The deltoid muscle of the upper arm, used for intramuscular injections. **B.** A method of establishing the deltoid muscle site for an intramuscular injection.

in which case sterile technique is required. The position of the external auditory canal varies with age. In the child under 3 years of age, the pinna (outer ear) is pulled down and back. In the adult, the pinna is pulled up and back in order to straighten the auditory canal. In the adult, the external auditory canal is a short tube about 2.5 cm (1 in.) long. Procedure 27-5 ■ on page 651 explains how to administer otic instillations.

Nasal Instillations

Nasal instillations (nose drops and sprays) usually are instilled for their *astringent* effect (to shrink swollen mucous membranes), to loosen secretions and facilitate drainage, or to treat infections of the nasal cavity or sinuses. Nasal decongestants are the most common nasal instillations. Many of these products are available without a prescription. Clients need to be taught to use these agents with caution. Chronic use of nasal decongestants may lead to a *rebound effect* (an increase in nasal congestion after the decongestant action has ended). If excess decongestant solution is swallowed, serious systemic effects may also develop, especially in children. Saline drops are safer as a decongestant for children.

Usually, clients self-administer sprays. In the supine position with the head tilted back, the client holds the tip of the container just inside the nares and inhales as the spray enters the nasal passages. For clients who use nasal sprays repeatedly, the nares need to be assessed for irritation. In children, nasal sprays are given with the head in an upright position to prevent excess spray from being swallowed.

The client should also be instructed to (1) blow the nose prior to nasal instillation, (2) breathe through the mouth to prevent aspiration of medication into the trachea and bronchi, (3) remain in a back-lying position for at least a minute so that the solution will come into contact with all of the nasal surface, and (4) avoid blowing the nose for several minutes.

Vaginal Instillations

Vaginal medications, or instillations, are inserted as creams, jellies, foams, or suppositories to treat infection or to relieve vaginal discomfort, such as itching, dryness, or pain. See Procedure 27-6 ■ on page 652 for guidelines on administering vaginal instillations.

Rectal Instillations

Insertion of medications into the rectum in the form of suppositories is a frequent practice. Rectal administration is a convenient and safe method of giving certain medications.

When rectal medication is to be given for constipation, the nurse should check the chart for the last bowel movement (BM) recorded. If no BM is recorded, then a digital exam should be done before giving a suppository. Procedure 27-7 ■ gives steps for administration of rectal medication.

Medication is occasionally given by enema. An example of this would be Kayexalate (sodium polystyrene sulfonate) to treat hyperkalemia (excessive potassium). See enema administration procedure in Chapter 37 ⬤⬤ .

Respiratory Inhalation Drugs

Medications administered by inhalation, such as bronchodilators, are frequently prescribed for clients with chronic respiratory disease such as asthma, emphysema, or bronchitis. Medications by inhalation are often administered by a respiratory therapist via a *nebulizer* (an inhaler machine that aerosolizes liquid as a fine mist delivered by mouthpiece or facial mask). This is done through a mask or mouthpiece, using oxygen, air under pressure, or an ultrasonic machine. An ultrasonic machine is often used by persons who cannot use a metered-dose inhaler, such as infants and young children, confused adults who cannot follow directions to inhale, and persons with severe asthma or other respiratory conditions requiring this type of medication administration method. The nebulizer is connected to a machine via plastic tubing to deliver the medication. A *metered-dose inhaler* (MDI) can be used by clients to self-administer measured doses of an aerosol medication. See Chapter 32 ⬤⬤ for more information.

To ensure correct delivery of the prescribed medication, nurses need to instruct clients on correct MDI use. To release medication through the mouthpiece, the client compresses the canister by hand while inhaling, and medication is released (Figure 27-25 ■). An extender or spacer may be attached to the mouthpiece to facilitate medication absorption for better results. *Spacers* are holding chambers into which the medication is fired and from which the client inhales, so that the dose is not lost by exhalation. Box 27-10 ■ provides instructions for clients about using an MDI. Newer, breath-activated MDIs are being produced in which inhalation triggers the release of a premeasured dose of medication.

Irrigations

An irrigation (or *lavage*) is the washing out of a body cavity by a stream of water or other fluid, which may contain medication. Stomach lavage may be used to remove medications

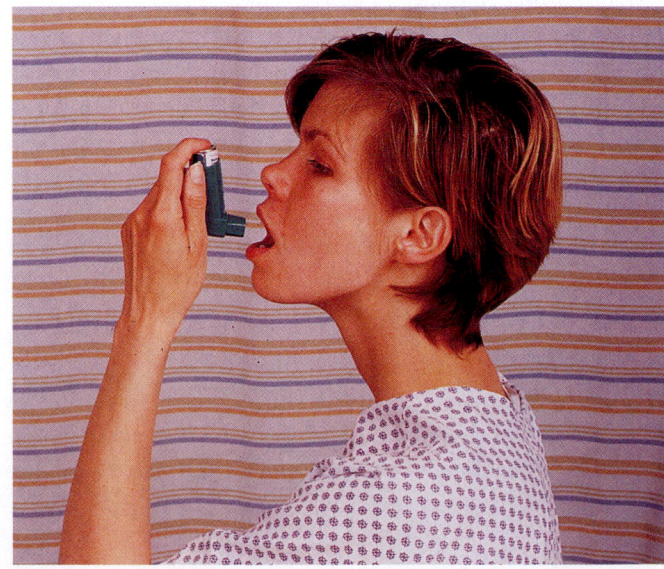

Figure 27-25. ■ The inhaler positioned away from the open mouth. (Photographer: Jenny Thomas.)

BOX 27-10 CLIENT TEACHING

Using a Metered-Dose Inhaler

- Make sure the canister is firmly and fully inserted into the inhaler.
- Remove the mouthpiece cap and, holding the inhaler upright; shake the inhaler for 3 to 5 seconds to mix the medication evenly.
- Tilt the head back slightly.
- Hold the canister upside down.
  a. Hold the MDI 1 to 2 cm (0.5 to 1 in.) from the open mouth (see Figure 27-25).
  b. If using a spacer, put the mouthpiece far enough into the mouth so that it extends beyond the teeth. Close the lips tightly around the mouthpiece. An MDI with a spacer or extender is always placed in the mouth.

Administering the Medication

- Inhale and exhale for several breaths, inhaling slowly and deeply through the nose.
- Then inhale slowly and deeply through the mouth while at the same time pressing down once on the medication canister. Continue to inhale for 2 to 3 seconds.
- Hold your breath for 5 to 10 seconds or longer, if possible.
- Remove the inhaler from or away from the mouth.
- Exhale slowly through pursed lips.
- If another puff is prescribed, wait for 1 to 3 minutes before the next inhalation. Remember to reshake the inhaler.
- After the inhalation is completed, rinse mouth with tap water and blow the nose to remove any remaining medication and reduce irritation and risk of infection.
- Remove the canister and clean the MDI mouthpiece after each use. Use mild soap and warm water, rinse it, and let it air dry before replacing it on the device.
- Disinfect the mouthpiece three times a week and air dry.
- Store the canister at room temperature. Avoid extremes of temperature.
- Follow the physician's orders about frequency of use.
- Report adverse reactions such as restlessness, palpitations, nervousness, or rash to your physician.

taken accidentally, or on purpose, that may be poisonous or toxic. In this case, a suction machine is attached to the catheter (NG tube) to remove or suck out any medications washed by the lavage. Guidelines for administering eye and ear irrigations are shown in Box 27-11 ■ (see also Procedure 60-1).

EVALUATING

After administering medication, the nurse observes the client to determine the effectiveness of the medication. The nurse also monitors the client for possible adverse effects and reports these to the team leader and physician. The nurse must promptly document administration of medications to provide client safety and prevent accidental overdose

of medications. Evaluation requires keen assessment skills by the nurse.

NURSING PROCESS CARE PLAN
Client with an Emergency Appendectomy

Kevin Ketron is a 20-year-old client who has just returned to the nursing unit from surgery after undergoing an emergency appendectomy.

Assessment

Client is awake and complaining of incisional pain at a level of 8/10. Dressing is dry and intact. Intravenous infusion of lactated Ringer's solution is running at 125 mL/h. Following surgery he received Kefzol (a cephalosporin antibiotic) 1 g intravenously every 4 hours until he was able to tolerate fluids. He now has been placed on oral Suprax (cefixime) 200 mg twice daily until discharged and for 1 week after returning home. He also has an order for morphine sulfate 10 mg to be given every 3 hours IM as necessary for pain.

Nursing Diagnosis

The following important nursing diagnoses (among others) are established for this client:

- *Risk for Deficient Fluid Volume* related to fluid restriction (although in the assessment it is stated that the client is receiving IV fluid until able to tolerate fluids)
- *Impaired Home Maintenance* related to deficient knowledge regarding self-care following appendectomy
- *Acute Pain* related to surgical incision
- *Risk for Infection* related to surgical incision

Expected Outcomes

The expected outcomes for the plan of care are:

- Maintains fluid volume balance.
- Maintains normal blood pressure, pulse, and body temperature.
- Follows mutually agreed-on healthcare home maintenance plan.
- Uses pain rating scale to identify current level of pain intensity and determine a comfort level.
- Remains free from symptoms of infection.

Planning and Implementation

- Monitor intake and output, skin turgor, and vital signs every 4 hours; observe for decreased pulse volume and increase in body temperature. *Intake and output measurements should be relatively equal. Intake and output measurements provide objective assessment of imbalances. Tenting of the skin, when assessing skin turgor, may indicate dehydration.*

BOX 27-11 NURSING CARE CHECKLIST

Administering Eye and Ear Irrigations

☑ Assess the site and surrounding structures for exudate, erythema, swelling, discharge, or other lesions before the irrigation. Determine the client's chief complaints (burning, pain, itching, etc.).

☑ Assemble required equipment: irrigating solution; appropriate irrigating syringe; receptacle to receive irrigation returns (e.g., kidney-shaped basin); moisture-proof drape; and cotton swabs as needed.

☑ Position the client appropriately in a sitting or lying position with the head tilted toward the affected eye or ear.

☑ Place the fluid-receiving receptacle below the affected area and a moisture-resistant pad beneath the receptacle.

☑ Put on disposable gloves and other PPE (personal protective equipment) as needed.

☑ Clean the eyelids or ear meatus before the irrigation as necessary, using moistened cotton swabs.

Administering the Irrigation

Eye Irrigation

☑ Expose the lower conjunctival sac by separating the lids with the thumb and forefinger to prevent reflex blinking. Or, to irrigate in stages, first hold the lower lid down, then hold the upper lid up. Exert pressure on the bony prominences of the cheekbone and beneath the eyebrow when holding the eyelids to minimize the possibility of pressing the eyeball and causing discomfort.

☑ Fill and hold the eye irrigator about 2.5 cm (1 in.) above the eye to ensure an even, safe pressure of the solution.

☑ Irrigate the eye, directing the solution on the lower conjunctival sac and from the inner canthus to the outer canthus. Directing the solution in this way prevents possible injury to the cornea and prevents fluid and contaminants from flowing down the nasolacrimal duct.

☑ Irrigate until the solution leaving the eye is clear (no discharge is present) or until all the solution has been used.

☑ Dry around the eye with tissue or gauze.

Ear Irrigation (see Procedure 60-1)

☑ Straighten the ear canal up and back in the adult and down and back in the child under 3 years of age.

☑ Insert a rubber-tipped syringe into the auditory meatus, and direct the solution gently upward against the top of the canal. The solution is instilled gently because strong pressure from the fluid can cause discomfort and damage the tympanic membrane.

☑ Dry the outside of the ear with absorbent cotton balls. Place a cotton fluff in the auditory meatus to absorb the excess fluid.

☑ Assist the client to a side-lying position on the affected side. Lying with the affected side down helps drain the excess fluid by gravity.

For All Irrigations

☑ Assess the client for any discomfort and the appearance and odor of the fluid returns.

☑ Document all relevant information, including all nursing assessments and interventions relative to the procedure; the type, concentration, amount, and temperature of the solution used; the appearance of the returns; and the presence of any discomfort.

- Provide fresh water and oral fluids preferred by the client; provide prescribed diet and snacks. *Clients will be more apt to comply with directions to increase fluid intake when the fluids are fresh and of client's preference.*
- Ensure that follow-up appointment is scheduled before discharge. *The physician needs to monitor the client's progress after discharge from the medical facility.*
- Provide detailed instruction for self-care, medications, and wound care; evaluate understanding of discharge instructions. *Client discharge education must be completed and documented prior to discharge.*
- Tell client to report location, intensity (using pain scale), and quality when experiencing pain. *The pain scale helps to objectify a subjective experience (pain) and allows the nurse to assess effectiveness of treatment.*
- Describe adverse effects of unrelieved pain. *Unrelieved pain can lead to muscle tension and fatigue which can lead to more pain and may cause depression.*

- Discuss client's fear of undertreated pain, overdose, and addiction. *By addressing client's fears, the nurse is better able to provide client education.*
- When opioids are administered, assess pain intensity, sedation, and respiratory status. *Opioids are used to relieve pain, but they can also cause drowsiness and a decrease in, or cessation of, respirations.*
- Use proper hand hygiene techniques before and after giving care to the client. *Prevention of the spread of pathogens is of primary importance for the healthcare worker.*
- Follow Standard Precautions and wear gloves during any contact with blood and body fluids. *Standard precautions are required for all clients regardless of infectious status.*
- Perform dressing changes using sterile technique. *A goal in wound care is to maintain asepsis in order to prevent infection.*
- Ensure client's appropriate hygienic care with correct hand hygiene; bathing; and hair, nails, and perineal care

performed by the nurse or client. *Reduction of pathogens on the client aids in the prevention of infection.*

Evaluation

Vital signs on second postoperative day are T 98.8, P 76, R 18, BP 128/78. He is taking a clear liquid diet, tolerated well with no complaints of nausea or vomiting, passing gas with a small amount of brown formed BM this morning. Discharge planning was initiated. The client will check with his roommate on ability to drive him to his follow-up appointment. Mr. Ketron was able to identify signs and symptoms of infection and describe when a physician should be notified. He understands the need to request pain medication while pain is still manageable. His pain is being maintained at a 2 to 3 level with prn M/S every 4 hours. The incision site is clean and dry with no drainage. Edges are well approximated, staples removed and Steri-Strips applied. Client has taken a shower.

Critical Thinking in the Nursing Process

1. It is always possible that a person receiving antibiotic drugs may experience side effects or an allergic reaction to the drug. How does an allergic reaction differ from a drug side effect?
2. Mr. Ketron is complaining of pain, and you have prepared his IM injection of morphine. How will you select the best site to give the morphine injection?
3. Mr. Ketron has been placed on oral antibiotics now that he is able to tolerate food and oral fluids. What difference, if any, does it make if this drug is given before or after meals?

Note: Discussion of Critical Thinking questions appears on the MyNursingKit Website.

Note: The references and resources for all chapters have been compiled at the back of the book.

PROCEDURE 27-1   Administering Oral Medications

Purpose

- To provide a medication that has systemic effects or local effects on the gastrointestinal tract or both (see specific drug action for each medication administered)

Equipment

- Medication tray or cart
- Disposable medication cups: small paper (souffle) or plastic cups for tablets and capsules, waxed or plastic calibrated medication cups for liquids
- Medication administration record (MAR) or computer printout
- Pill crusher
  or
- Syringe of appropriate size for child's mouth and medication amount
- Straws to administer medications that may discolor the teeth or to facilitate the ingestion of liquid medication for certain clients
- Water and water cups
- Applesauce or pudding may be needed to facilitate medication administration when pills must be crushed and for patients with swallowing difficulties

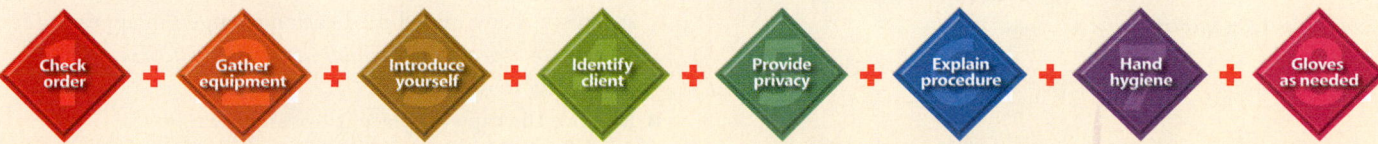

Check order + Gather equipment + Introduce yourself + Identify client + Provide privacy + Explain procedure + Hand hygiene + Gloves as needed

Interventions and Rationales

1. Perform preparatory steps (see icon bar above).
2. Verify the client's ability to take medication orally.
   - Determine whether the client can swallow well, is NPO, is nauseated or vomiting, has gastric suction, or has diminished or absent bowel sounds. Also, check for medication allergies.
3. Verify the order for accuracy.
   - Check the accuracy of the MAR or of the printout with the physician's written order. *It should contain the following information: client's name, drug name and dosage, time for administration, and route of administration.*
   - Check the expiration date for the order (e.g., opioid medications must be renewed every 72 hours).

■ Report any discrepancies in the order to the nurse in charge or the physician, as agency policy dictates.

4. Obtain appropriate medication.

■ Read the MAR and take the appropriate medication from the shelf, drawer, or refrigerator. The medication may be dispensed from the bottle, box, or unit-dose package.

■ Compare the label of the medication container or unit-dose package against the order on the MAR. If these are not identical, recheck the client's chart. If there is still a discrepancy, check with the nurse in charge or the pharmacist. *These checks are essential in providing the correct medication.*

5. Prepare the medication.

■ Prepare the correct amount of medication for the required dose, using aseptic technique.

■ While preparing the medication, recheck the MAR with each prepared drug and container. *This second check reduces the chance of error.*

TABLETS OR CAPSULES

■ Pour the required number into the bottle cap, and then transfer the medication to the disposable cup without touching the tablets (Figure 27-26 ■). Usually, all tablets or capsules to be given to the client are placed in the same cup.

■ Keep narcotics and medications that require specific assessments, such as pulse measurements, respiratory rate or depth, or blood pressure, separate from the others. *This enables the nurse to withhold the medication if indicated.*

■ Break scored tablets as needed to obtain the correct dosage. Use a file or cutting device if necessary (Figure 27-27 ■). Discard unused tablet pieces according to agency policy.

■ If the client has difficulty swallowing, crush the tablets to a fine powder with a pill crusher or between two medication cups or spoons. Mix the powder with a small amount of soft food (e.g., custard, applesauce). *Note:* Check with pharmacy before crushing tablets. *Sustained-action, enteric-coated, buccal, or sublingual tablets should not be crushed.*

■ Place packaged unit-dose capsules or tablets (Figure 27-28 ■) directly into the medicine cup. Do not remove the wrapper until at the bedside. *The wrapper keeps the medication clean and facilitates identification.*

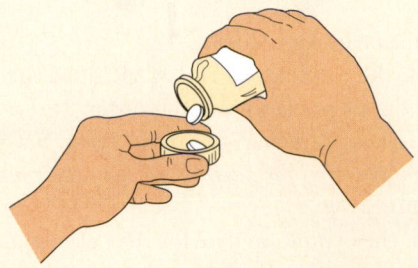

Figure 27-26. ■ Pouring a tablet into the container cap.

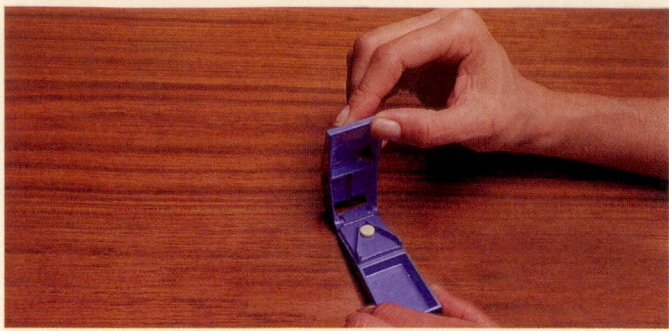

Figure 27-27. ■ A cutting device can be used to divide tablets. (Photographer: Elena Dorfman.)

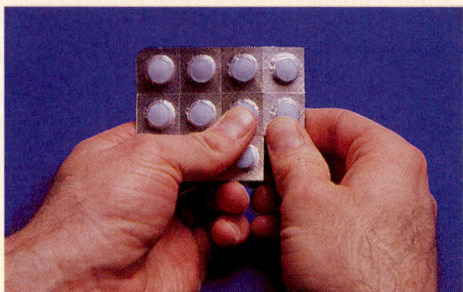

A

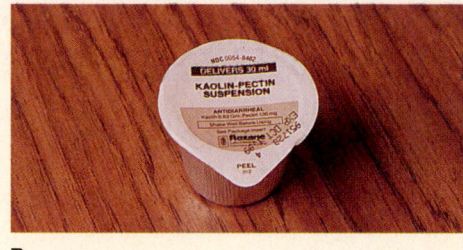

B

Figure 27-28. ■ Unit-dose packages: **A.** tablets; **B.** liquid medications. (Photographer: Elena Dorfman.)

LIQUID MEDICATION

■ Thoroughly mix the medication following label directions before pouring. Check expiration date for the medication and discard any mixed medication changed in appearance. *Changes in appearance may indicate contamination or expiration of the medication.*

■ Remove the cap and place it upside down on the countertop. *This helps to avoid contaminating its inside.*

■ Hold the bottle so the label is next to your palm, and pour the medication away from the label (Figure 27-29 ■). *This prevents the label from becoming soiled and illegible as a result of spilled liquids.*

■ Hold the medication cup at eye level and fill it to the desired level, using the bottom of the **meniscus** (crescent-shaped upper surface of a column of liquid) to align with the container scale (Figure 27-30 ■). (Marking the level

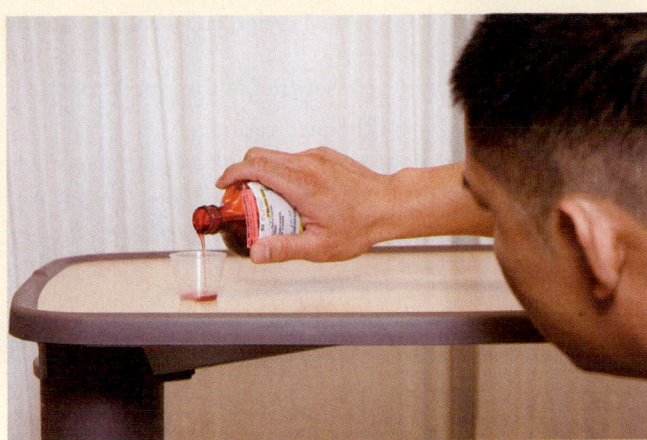

Figure 27-29. ■ Pouring a liquid medication from a bottle.

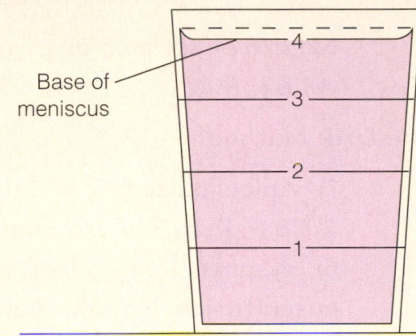

Base of meniscus

Figure 27-30. ■ The bottom of the meniscus is the measuring guide.

with an indelible marker or with one's finger helps to prevent overpouring of medication.) *This method ensures accuracy of measurement. Overage amounts may not be poured back into the bottle.*

■ Before capping the bottle, wipe the lip with a paper towel. *This prevents the cap from sticking.*

■ When giving small amounts of liquids (e.g., less than 5 mL), prepare the medication in a sterile syringe without the needle. *The use of a syringe allows for more precise measurement to the nearest milliliter.*

■ Keep unit-dose liquids in their package and open them at the bedside. *This practice helps to maintain asepsis and reduces wastage of drugs.*

ORAL NARCOTICS

■ If an agency uses a manual recording system for controlled substances, check the narcotic record for the previous drug count and compare it with the current supply available. *Some medications, including narcotics, are kept in plastic containers that are sectioned and numbered. This allows the drugs to be controlled securely.*

■ Remove the next available tablet using aseptic technique and drop it in the medicine cup.

■ After removing a tablet, record the necessary information on the appropriate narcotic control record and sign it. *Note:*

Computer-controlled dispensing systems allow access only to the selected drug and automatically records use.

■ Any time a narcotic must be wasted, it should be disposed of per agency protocol. A second licensed nurse must observe the wastage and both nurses must sign on the appropriate space on the narcotic record.

ALL MEDICATIONS

■ Place the prepared medication and MAR together on the tray or cart.

■ Return the bottle, box, or envelope to its storage place and recheck the label on the container. *This third check further reduces the risk of error.*

■ Avoid leaving prepared medications unattended. *This precaution prevents potential mishandling errors.*

■ For any medication, check the name of the drug, expiration date, dosage, frequency of administration, appropriateness of order, allergies, doctor's signature, and route suitability.

6. Administer the medication at the correct time. *Note:* Be aware of the difference between military time and Greenwich time notations to prevent timing errors.

■ Identify the client by comparing the name and hospital number on the medication record or list with the name and number on the client's identification bracelet and by asking the client's name. *Accurate identification is essential to prevent error. Remember, The Joint Commission requires the use of two identifiers.*

■ Explain the purpose of the medication and how it will help, using language the client can understand. Include relevant information about effects; for example, tell the client receiving a diuretic to expect an increase in urine. *Information facilitates acceptance of and compliance with the therapy.*

■ Assist the client to a sitting position or, if not possible, to a side-lying position. *These positions facilitate swallowing and prevent aspiration.*

■ Take the required assessment measures, such as pulse and respiratory rates or blood pressure. Take the apical pulse rate before administering digitalis preparations. Take blood pressure before giving hypotensive drugs. Take the respiratory rate prior to administering narcotics. *Narcotics depress the respiratory center.* If any of the findings are above or below the predetermined parameters, consult the physician before administering the medication.

■ Give the client sufficient water or preferred juice to swallow the medication. Before using juice, check for any food and medication incompatibilities. *(Grapefruit juice is contraindicated when administering most antihypertensive drugs.) Fluids ease swallowing and facilitate absorption from the gastrointestinal tract.*

■ If the client is unable to hold the pill cup, use the pill cup to introduce the medication into the client's mouth, and give only one tablet or capsule at a time. *Putting the cup to the client's mouth maintains the cleanliness of the nurse's hands. Giving one medication at a time eases swallowing.*

- If an older child or adult has difficulty swallowing, ask the client to place the medication on the back of the tongue before taking the water. *Stimulation of the back of the tongue produces the swallowing reflex.*
- If the medication has an objectionable taste, ask the client to suck a few ice chips beforehand, or give the medication with juice, applesauce, or bread if there are no contraindications. *The cold will desensitize the taste buds, and juices or bread can mask the taste of the medication.*
- If the client says that the medication you are about to give is different from what the client has been receiving, do not give the medication without checking the original order. *Most clients are familiar with the appearance of medications taken previously. Unfamiliar medications may signal a possible error.*
- Stay with the client until all medications have been swallowed. *The nurse must see the client swallow the medication before the drug administration can be recorded. This practice additionally allows the nurse to monitor the client for choking.* A physician's order or agency policy is required for medications left at the bedside.

7. Document each medication given.
   - Record the medication given, dosage, time, any complaints or assessments of the client, and your signature.
   - If medication was refused or omitted, record this fact on the appropriate record; document the reason, when possible, and the nurse's actions according to agency policy. *Recording the fact and the reason communicates the greatest amount of information, so that the charge nurse or physician can follow up.*

8. Dispose of all supplies appropriately.
   - Return the medication records to the appropriate file for the next administration time.

- Replenish stock (e.g., medication cups) and return cart to medicine room.
- Discard used disposable supplies in the proper container.

9. Evaluate the effects of the medication.
   - Return to the client when the medication is expected to take effect (usually 30 minutes). *This allows you to evaluate the effects of the medication on the client.*

SAMPLE DOCUMENTATION

[date]	Digoxin 0.5 mg held. AP 54.
[time]	Will reassess in 1 hour. (VS, i.e., BP 110/76, T 98.6, R 16). _____ M. Wirthwood, LVN
[time]	No c/o chest pain or dyspnea. AP 62. MW

Or use the DAR method:

[time]	D: Apical pulse 54, BP 110/76, T 98.6, R 16. No c/o chest pain or dyspnea. Lungs clear to auscultation. No s/s of digoxin toxicity.
	A: Digoxin 0.5 mg held. Physician notified. Order for digoxin level received. Will reassess apical pulse in 1 hour. _____ M. Wirthwood, LVN
[time]	R: Apical pulse 62. MW

PROCEDURE 27-2 ## Preparing Medications

Purpose

- To prepare medication for administration to client using safety and infection control rules

Equipment

- MAR or computer printout
- Ampule of sterile medication, or two vials of medication, or one vial and one ampule, or two ampules, or one vial or ampule and one cartridge

- File (if ampule is not scored) and small gauze square, or ampule opener
- Antiseptic swabs
- Sterile needle and syringe
- Filter needle (optional) (now mandated by The Joint Commission for use with ampule)
- Additional sterile subcutaneous or intramuscular needle (optional)
- Sterile water or normal saline, if drug is in powdered form

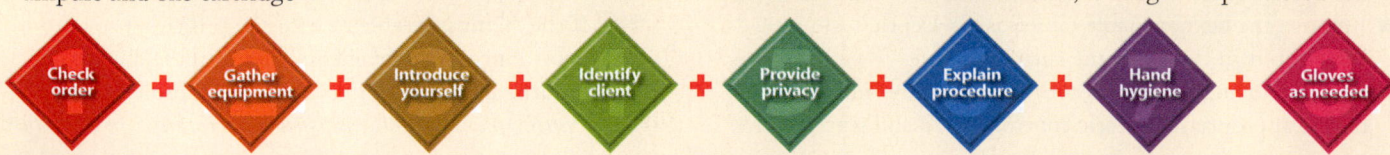

Check order + Gather equipment + Introduce yourself + Identify client + Provide privacy + Explain procedure + Hand hygiene + Gloves as needed

Part A: Preparing Medications from Ampules

Interventions and Rationales

1. Perform preparatory steps (see icon bar above).
2. Check the medication order, including drug administration. *This ensures accuracy.*
   - Check the label on the ampule carefully against the MAR or client's chart to make sure that the correct medication is being prepared.
   - Follow the three checks for administering medications. Read the label on the medication (1) before it is taken off the shelf, (2) before withdrawing the medication, and (3) after placing it back on the shelf.
3. Prepare the medication ampule for drug withdrawal.
   - Flick the upper stem of the ampule several times with a fingernail or, holding the upper stem of the ampule, make a large circle with the arm extended. *This will bring all the medication down to the main portion of the ampule.*
   - Partially file the neck of the ampule, if necessary, to start a clean break.
   - Place a piece of sterile gauze between your thumb and the ampule neck or around the ampule neck, and break off the top by bending it toward you (Figure 27-31 ■). *The sterile gauze protects the fingers from the broken glass and any glass fragments will spray away from the nurse.*
   or
   - Place the antiseptic wipe packet over the top of the ampule before breaking off the top. *This method ensures that all the glass fragments fall into the packet and reduces the risk of cuts.*
   - Dispose of the top of the ampule in the sharps container.
4. Withdraw the medication.
   - Place the ampule on a flat surface.
   - Obtain a filter needle to withdraw the medication. Disconnect the existing needle with cap on; attach the filter needle to the syringe. *Filter needles prevent glass particles from being drawn up with the medication.*
   - Remove the cap from the filter needle and insert the needle into the center of the ampule. Do not touch the rim of the ampule with the needle to keep it sterile. Withdraw the required dosage.
   - If necessary, tilt the ampule slightly to access all the medication (Figure 27-32 ■).
   - If a filter needle was used to withdraw the medication, replace it with a regular needle; tighten the cap at the hub before injecting the client.
   - If a filter needle was not used, recap the needle using the scoop method (carefully scooping the needle into the cap, which is placed on a flat surface, without contamination of the needle). *This prevents needle-stick injury while transporting medication to client's room.*

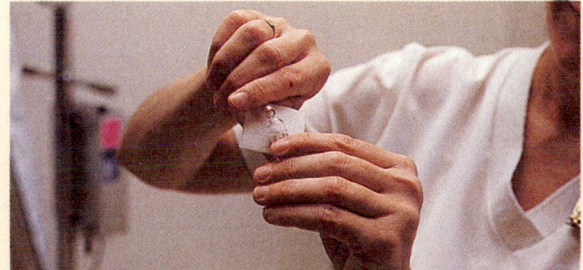

Figure 27-31. ■ Breaking the neck of an ampule. (Photographer: Jenny Thomas.)

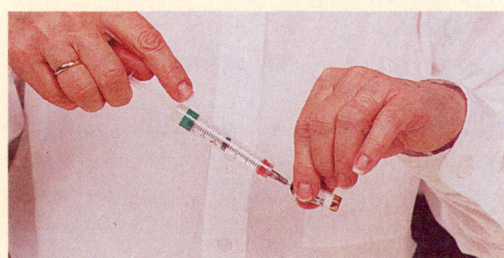

Figure 27-32. ■ Withdrawing a medication from an ampule. (Photographer: Jenny Thomas.)

Part B: Preparing Medications from Vials

Interventions and Rationales

1. Check the medication order, including drug administration, to ensure accuracy.
   - Check the label on the vial carefully against the MAR or client's chart to make sure that the correct medication is being prepared.
   - Follow the three checks for administering medications. Read the label on the medication (1) before it is taken off the shelf, (2) before withdrawing the medication, and (3) after placing it back on the shelf.
2. Prepare the medication vial for drug withdrawal.
   - Mix the solution, if necessary, by rotating the vial between the palms of the hands, not by shaking. *Some vials contain aqueous suspensions, which settle when they stand. In some instances, shaking is contraindicated because it may cause the mixture to foam.*
   - Remove the protective metal or plastic cap, and clean the rubber cap of a previously opened vial with an antiseptic wipe by rubbing in a circular motion and allow it to air dry. *The antiseptic cleans the cap of dust or grease and reduces the number of microorganisms.*

3. Withdraw the medication.

- Attach a filter needle as agency practice dictates to draw up premixed liquid medications from multidose vials. *The filter prevents any solid particles from being drawn up through the needle.*
- Ensure that the needle is firmly attached to the syringe.
- Remove the cap from the needle; then draw up into the syringe the amount of air equal to the volume of the medication to be withdrawn. *This practice will help to equalize pressure within the closed system of the vial.*
- Carefully insert the needle into the upright vial through the center of the rubber cap, maintaining the sterility of the needle.
- Inject the air into the vial, keeping the bevel of the needle above the surface of the medication (Figure 27-33 ■). *The air will allow the medication to be drawn out easily because negative pressure will not be created inside the vial. The bevel is kept above the medication to avoid creating bubbles in the medication.*
- Withdraw the prescribed amount of medication using either of the following methods:

  a. Hold the vial down (i.e., with the base lower than the top); move the needle tip so that it is below the fluid level; and withdraw the medication (Figure 27-34 ■). Avoid drawing up the last drops of the vial. *Proponents of this method say that keeping the vial in the upright position while withdrawing the medication allows particulate matter to precipitate to the bottom of the solution. Leaving the last few drops reduces the chance of withdrawing foreign particles.*

  or

  b. Invert the vial; ensure the needle tip is below the fluid level; and gradually withdraw the medication (Figure 27-34B). *Keeping the tip of the needle below the fluid level prevents air from being drawn into the syringe.*

- Hold the syringe and vial at eye level to determine that the correct dosage of drug is drawn into the syringe. Eject air remaining at the top of the syringe into the vial.

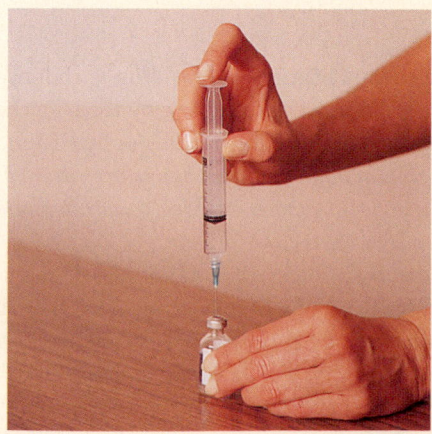

Figure 27-33. ■ Injecting air into a vial. (Photographer: Jenny Thomas.)

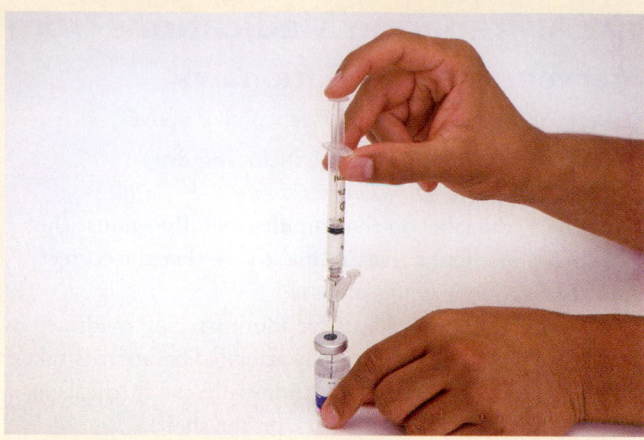

A

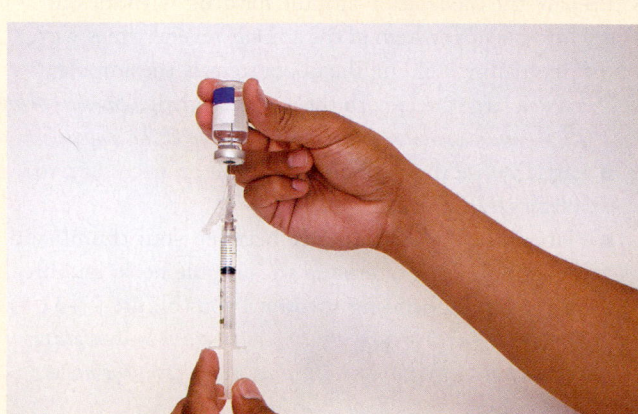

B

Figure 27-34. ■ **A.** Withdrawing a medication from a vial that is held with the base down. **B.** Withdrawing a medication from an inverted vial. (Photographer: Elena Dorfman.)

- When the correct volume of medication is obtained, withdraw the needle from the vial, and replace the cap over the needle (using the scoop method), thus maintaining its sterility.
- If air displacement changes the quantity, tap the syringe barrel to dislodge any air bubbles present in the syringe while the needle is still in the vial. (This decreases the need to reinsert the needle into the vial, which may dull the sharpness of the needle.) *The tapping motion will cause the air bubbles to rise to the top of the syringe where they can be ejected out of the syringe.*
- Replace the filter needle, if used, with a regular needle of the correct gauge and length before injecting the client.

VARIATION: PREPARING AND USING VIALS FOR RECONSTITUTION

- Read the manufacturer's directions to determine the amount and type of solution to be used for reconstitution. *Some solutions are unstable in solution and must be distributed in powder or crystalline form to be reconstituted at the time dosage is due.*

■ Add the amount of sterile water or saline indicated in the directions. An equivalent amount of air as the amount of solvent must be removed from the vial in order to equalize air pressure within the vial.

■ If a multidose vial is reconstituted, label the vial with the date and time it was prepared, the amount of drug contained in each milliliter of solution, and your initials. *Time is an important factor to consider in the expiration of these medications*.

■ Once the medication has been reconstituted, store it in a refrigerator or as recommended by the manufacturer.

Part C: Mixing Medications Using One Syringe

Interventions and Rationales

1. Check the medication order for accuracy.
   ■ Check the label on the ampule or vial carefully against the MAR or client's chart. *This makes sure that the correct medication is being prepared*.
   ■ Follow the three checks for administering medications. Read the label on the medication (1) before it is taken off the shelf, (2) before withdrawing the medication, and (3) after placing it back on the shelf.
   ■ Before preparing and combining the medications, ensure that the total volume of the injection is appropriate for the injection site.

2. Prepare the medication ampule or vial for drug withdrawal.
   ■ See Part A of this procedure for an ampule and Part B for a vial.
   ■ Inspect the appearance of the medication for clarity. *Some medications are always cloudy. Preparations that have changed in appearance should be discarded*.
   ■ If using insulin, thoroughly mix the solution in each vial prior to administration. Rotate the vials between the palms of the hands and invert the vials. Do not shake the vials. *Mixing ensures an adequate concentration and thus an accurate dose. Shaking insulin vials can make the medication frothy, making precise measurement difficult*.
   ■ Clean the tops of the vials with antiseptic swabs.

3. Withdraw the medications.

MIXING MEDICATIONS FROM TWO VIALS

■ Withdraw a volume of air equal to the total volume of medications to be withdrawn from vials A and B.

■ Inject a volume of air equal to the volume of medication to be withdrawn into vial A.

■ Withdraw the needle from vial A and inject the remaining air into vial B.

or

■ Draw up the volume of air equal to the amount of solution to be drawn from vial A and inject into vial A. Next, draw up the volume of air equal to the amount of solution to be drawn from vial B and inject into vial B. Leaving the needle in the vial, invert vial B and withdraw the prescribed amount of medication.

■ Withdraw the required amount of medication from vial B. The same needle is used to inject air into and withdraw medication from the second vial. *It must not be contaminated with the medication in vial A*.

■ Using a newly attached sterile needle, withdraw the required amount of medication from vial A. If using a syringe with a fused needle, withdraw the medication from vial A. The syringe now contains a mixture of medications from vials A and B. *With this method, neither vial is contaminated by microorganisms or by medication from the other vial*.

■ See also the variation on mixing insulins later in this procedure.

MIXING MEDICATIONS FROM ONE VIAL AND ONE AMPULE

■ First prepare and withdraw the medication from the vial. Ampules do not require the addition of air prior to withdrawal of the drug.

■ Then withdraw the required amount of medication from the ampule and discard the ampule. *Since ampules are single dose vehicles, the ampule must be discarded into the sharp's container after medication is drawn*.

MIXING MEDICATIONS FROM ONE CARTRIDGE AND ONE VIAL OR AMPULE

■ First, ensure that the correct dose of the medication is in the cartridge. Discard any excess medication and air. *Note*: If the medication is a narcotic, wastage must be witnessed and cosigned by a second licensed nurse.

■ Draw up the required medication from a vial or ampule into the cartridge. Note that when withdrawing medication from a vial, an equal amount of air must first be injected into the vial.

■ If the total volume to be injected exceeds the capacity of the cartridge, use a syringe with sufficient capacity to withdraw the desired amount of medication from the vial or ampule, and transfer the required amount from the cartridge to the syringe. When withdrawing medication from a cartridge, the nurse must first withdraw medication from the vial or ampule. Then the nurse

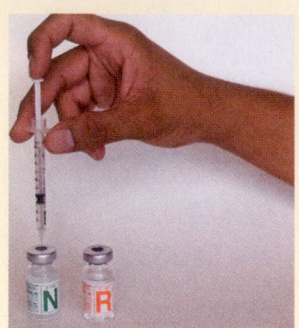

Step 1

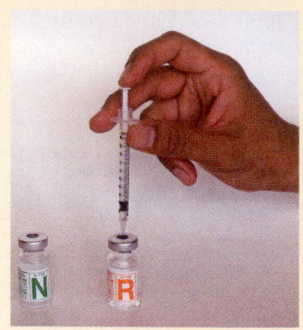

Step 2

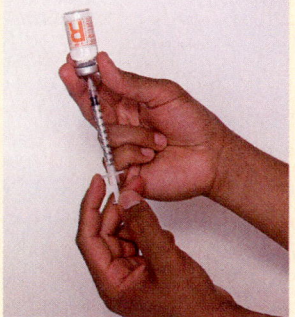

Step 3

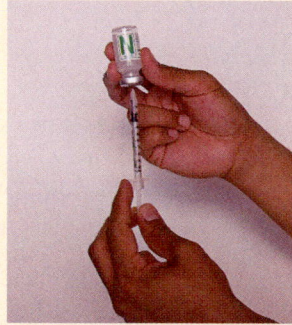

Step 4

Figure 27-35. ■ Mixing two types of insulin together. (Step 1) Inject 30 units of air into NPH vial without touching insulin. (Step 2) Inject 10 units of air into regular insulin vial. (Step 3) Immediately withdraw 10 units of regular insulin. (Step 4) Withdraw 30 units of NPH insulin.

removes the needle from the cartridge and pierces the rubber stopper with the needle of the syringe in order to extract the contents. It is not necessary to first instill air into a cartridge.

VARIATION: MIXING INSULINS

The following is an example of mixing 10 units of regular insulin and 30 units of NPH insulin. *Regular, or clear insulin, must be drawn first and NPH, or cloudy insulin, is drawn second.*

■ Inject 30 units of air into the NPH vial and withdraw the needle. (There should be no insulin in the needle.) The needle should not touch the insulin (Figure 27-35 ■, step 1).
■ Inject 10 units of air into the regular insulin vial and immediately withdraw 10 units of regular insulin (Figure 27-35, steps 2 and 3).
■ Reinsert the needle into the NPH insulin vial and withdraw 30 units of NPH insulin (Figure 27-35, step 4). (The air was previously injected into the vial.)

By using this method, you avoid adding NPH insulin to the regular insulin.

SAMPLE DOCUMENTATION

[date]	Focus pain
[time]	D—c/o incisional pain 7/10. Incision free of drainage and redness. Edges well approximated. A—Vistaril 50 mg, Demerol 75 mg IM
[time]	R—pain 2/10 resting comfortably _____ _____ A. Johnson, LVN

Administering Injections

Purposes

■ To provide a medication the client requires via the parenteral route (see specific drug action)
■ To provide a medication that is only available via the parenteral route (e.g., heparin may be administered subcutaneously or intravenously, but not orally or intramuscularly)
■ To allow slower absorption of a medication via the subcutaneous route as compared with either the intramuscular or intravenous route

Equipment

■ Client's MAR or computer printout
■ Sterile medication (usually provided in an ampule, cartridge, or vial)
■ Syringe and needle of a size appropriate for the amount of solution to be administered and for the site of administration
■ Antiseptic swabs
■ Dry sterile gauze for opening an ampule (optional)
■ Disposable gloves

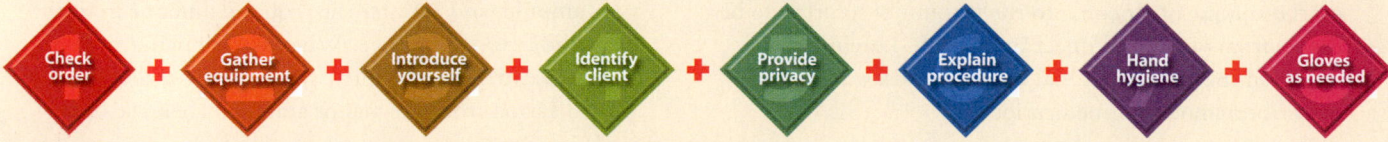

Part A: Intramuscular Injection

Interventions and Rationales

1. Perform preparatory steps (see icon bar above).

2. Check the medication order for accuracy.
   - See Procedure 27-1, step 3.

3. Prepare the medication from the vial or ampule.
   - See Procedure 27-2 (ampule or vial).
   - Whenever feasible, change the needle on the syringe before the injection. *Because the outside of a new needle is free of medication, it does not irritate subcutaneous tissues as it passes into the muscle.*
   - Invert the syringe needle uppermost and expel all excess air. (Some institutions subscribe to the practice of drawing up 0.2 to 0.3 mL of air to expel contents of syringe to prevent tracking through tissue layers and/or to seal medication into the site of injection.)

4. Identify the client, and assist the client to a comfortable position.
   - Check the client's identification band, and ask the client to tell you his or her name and date of birth. *The Joint Commission requires the use of two identifiers.*
   - Assist the client to a supine, lateral, prone, or sitting position, depending on the chosen site. If the target muscle is the gluteus medius (ventrogluteal site), have the client in the supine position flex the knee(s); in the lateral position, flex the upper leg; and in the prone position, "toe in." The preferred position for the dorsogluteal site is also the prone position with the toes pointed inward. *Appropriate positioning promotes relaxation of the target muscle.*
   - Obtain assistance to immobilize an infant or young child. The parent may hold the infant or young child, but provide clear instructions before beginning the injection. *This prevents accidental injury during the procedure.*

5. Select, locate, and clean the site.
   - Perform hand hygiene.
   - Select a site free of skin lesions, tenderness, swelling, hardness, or localized inflammation and one that has not been used frequently.
   - If injections are to be frequent, alternate sites. If necessary, discuss with the prescribing physician an alternative method of providing the medication.
   - Determine whether the size of the muscle is appropriate to the amount of medication to be injected. *An average adult's deltoid muscle can usually absorb 0.5 mL of medication, although some authorities believe 1 mL can be absorbed by a well-developed deltoid muscle. The gluteus medius muscle can often absorb 1 to 4 mL, although 4 mL may be very painful.*
   - Locate the exact site for the injection. (See the discussion of sites earlier in this chapter.)
   - Don gloves.

   - Clean the site with an antiseptic swab. Using a circular motion, start at the center and move outward about 5 cm (2 in.).
   - Transfer and hold the swab between the third and fourth fingers of your nondominant hand in readiness for needle withdrawal, or position the swab on the client's skin above the intended site. Allow skin to dry prior to injecting medication.

6. Prepare the syringe for injection.
   - Remove the needle cover without contaminating the needle.
   - Confirm that the medication and the dose are both correct.
   - If using a prefilled unit-dose medication, be careful to avoid dripping medication on the needle prior to injection. If this does occur, wipe the medication off the needle with a sterile gauze. *Medication left on the needle can cause pain when it is tracked through the subcutaneous tissue.*

7. Inject the medication.
   - After locating the proper site, use the nondominant hand to either pull the skin taut or pinch the skin and underlying tissue. *Pulling the skin and subcutaneous tissue or pinching the muscle makes it firmer and facilitates needle insertion.*
   - Holding the syringe between the thumb and forefinger (as if holding a pencil), pierce the skin quickly at a 90-degree angle (Figure 27-36 ■), and insert the needle into the muscle. *Using a quick motion lessens the client's discomfort.*
   - Aspirate by holding the barrel of the syringe steady with your nondominant hand and by pulling back on the plunger with your dominant hand. If blood appears in the syringe, withdraw the needle, discard the syringe, document the occurrence, and prepare a new injection. *This step determines whether the needle has been inserted into a blood vessel.*

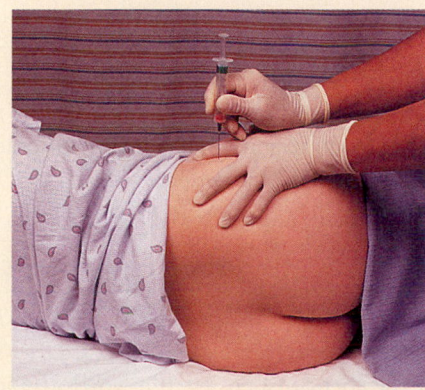

Figure 27-36. ■ Position for holding the syringe while administering an intramuscular injection into the ventrogluteal site.

- If blood does not appear, inject the medication steadily and slowly, holding the syringe steady. *Injecting medication slowly permits it to disperse into the muscle tissue, thus decreasing the client's discomfort. Holding the syringe steady minimizes discomfort.*

OR

8. If indicated, inject the medication using a Z-track technique.
   - Use the nondominant hand to pull the skin laterally and downward approximately 2.5 cm (1 in.) at the site (Figure 27-37 ■). Under some circumstances, such as for an emaciated client or an infant, the muscle may be pinched. *Pulling the skin and subcutaneous tissues laterally cause displacement of these tissues preventing return tracking of medication that may be painful or may stain the skin.*
   - Continue as for step 7.

9. Withdraw the needle and then release hand that has been holding skin laterally.
   - Withdraw the needle slowly and steadily in the same line as it was inserted. *This minimizes tissue injury.*

- Apply gentle pressure at the site with a dry sponge. If contraindicated, do not massage the site. *Massaging the site can result in tissue irritation.*
- If bleeding occurs, apply pressure with a dry sterile gauze until it stops.

10. Dispose of supplies appropriately.
   - Discard the uncapped needle and attached syringe into designated receptacles (e.g., sharps container). *Proper disposal protects the nurse and others from injury and contamination. The CDC recommends not capping the needle before disposal to reduce the risk of needle-stick injuries.*
   - Remove gloves. Perform hand hygiene.

11. Document all relevant information.
   - Include the time of administration, drug name, dose, route, site, and the client's reactions.

12. Assess effectiveness of the medication at the time it is expected to act.

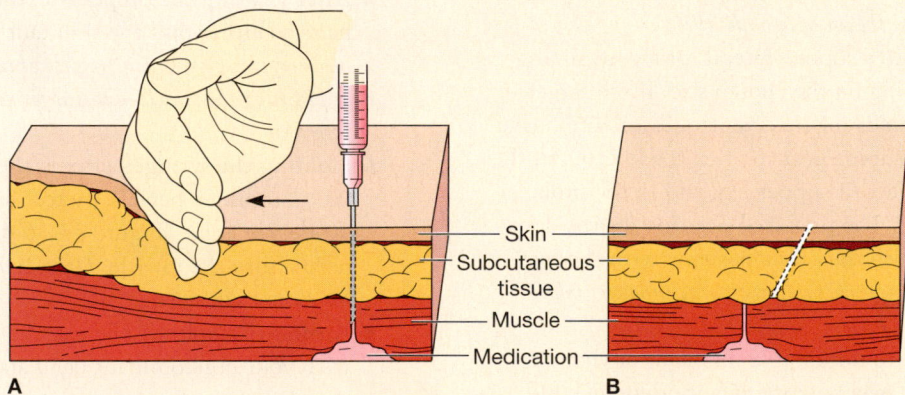

A **B**

Figure 27-37. ■ Inserting an intramuscular needle at a 90-degree angle using the Z-track method: **A.** Skin pulled to the side; **B.** skin released. *Note:* When the skin returns to its normal position after the needle is withdrawn, a seal is formed over the intramuscular site. This prevents seepage of the medication into the subcutaneous tissues and subsequent discomfort.

Labels in figure: Skin / Subcutaneous tissue / Muscle / Medication

Part B: Subcutaneous Injection

Interventions and Rationales

1. Check the medication order for accuracy.
   - See Procedure 27-1, step 3.

2. Prepare the medication from the vial or ampule.
   - See Procedure 27-2 (ampule or vial).

3. Identify the client, and assist the client to a comfortable position.
   - Check the client's identification band, and ask the client to tell you his or her name and date of birth. *The Joint Commission requires the use of two identifiers.*
   - Assist the client to a position in which the arm, leg, or abdomen can be relaxed, depending on the site to be used. *A relaxed position of the site minimizes discomfort.*

- Obtain assistance in holding an uncooperative client or small child. *This prevents injury due to sudden movement after needle insertion.*

4. Select and clean the site.
   - Select a site free of tenderness, hardness, swelling, scarring, itching, burning, or localized inflammation. Select a site that has not been used frequently. Save convenient sites (e.g., abdomen and legs) for self-administration of medications such as insulin. *These conditions could hinder the absorption of the medication and also increase the likelihood of injury and discomfort at the injection site.*
   - Don gloves.

■ Cleanse the skin with antiseptic per agency protocol. Swab the center of the site in a widening circle to about 5 cm (2 in.). Let the skin dry completely. *The mechanical action of swabbing removes skin secretions, which contain microorganisms.*

■ Hold the swab between the third and fourth fingers of the nondominant hand, or position the swab on the client's skin above the intended site. *This keeps the swab accessible when the needle is withdrawn.*

5. Prepare the syringe for injection.

■ Remove the needle cap while waiting for the antiseptic to dry. Pull the cap straight off to avoid contaminating the needle by the outside edge of the cap. *The needle will become contaminated if it touches anything but the inside of the cap, which is sterile.*

■ Confirm that the medication and the dosage are both correct. *This prevents medication error.*

6. Inject the medication.

■ Grasp the syringe in your dominant hand by holding it between your thumb and fingers. With palm facing to the side or upward for a 45-degree-angle insertion, or with the palm downward for a 90-degree-angle insertion, prepare to inject (Figure 27-38 ■; see also Figure 27-12).

■ Using the nondominant hand, pinch or spread the skin at the site, and insert the needle using the dominant hand and a firm steady push. *The nondominant hand can be used to immobilize the extremity of an infant or a young child as the needle is inserted.* Recommendations vary about whether to pinch or spread the skin and at what angle to administer subcutaneous injections. The most important consideration is the depth of the subcutaneous tissue in the area to be injected. *If the client has more than 1/2 inch of adipose tissue in the injection site, it would be safe to administer the injection at a 90-degree angle*

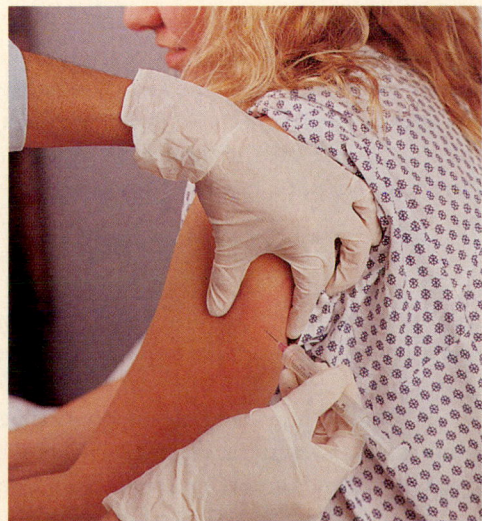

Figure 27-38. ■ Administering a subcutaneous injection into pinched tissue. (Photographer: Elena Dorfman.)

with the skin spread. If the client is thin or lean and lacks adipose tissue, the subcutaneous injection should be given with the skin pinched and at a 45- to 60-degree angle.

■ When the needle is inserted, move your nondominant hand to the end of the plunger. Some nurses find it easier to move the nondominant hand to the barrel of the syringe and the dominant hand to the end of the plunger. If the nondominant hand is holding the extremity of an infant or small child, use the dominant hand to aspirate and inject the medication.

■ Aspirate by pulling back on the plunger. If blood appears, withdraw the needle, discard the syringe, document the occurrence, and prepare a new injection. If no blood appears, inject the medication. *Subcutaneous medications can be very dangerous if injected directly into the bloodstream since these drugs require slow absorption.* See variation for administering a heparin injection.

■ Inject the medication by holding the syringe steady and depressing the plunger with a slow, even pressure. *Holding the syringe steady and injecting the medication at an even pressure minimizes discomfort for the client.*

7. Remove the needle.

■ Remove slowly and smoothly, pulling along the line of insertion while depressing the skin with your nondominant hand. *Depressing the skin places countertraction on it and minimizes the client's discomfort when the needle is withdrawn.*

■ If bleeding occurs, apply pressure to the site with dry sterile gauze until it stops. *Bleeding rarely occurs after subcutaneous injection.*

8. Dispose of supplies appropriately.

■ Discard the uncapped needle and attached syringe into designated receptacles. *Proper disposal protects the nurse and others from injury and contamination. The CDC recommends not capping the needle before disposal to reduce the risk of needle-stick injuries.*

■ Remove gloves. Perform hand hygiene.

9. Document all relevant information.

■ Document the medication given, dosage, time, route, injection site, any assessments, and add your signature.

■ Many agencies prefer that medication administration be recorded on the medication record. *The nurse's notes are used when prn medications are given or when there is a special problem.*

10. Assess the effectiveness of the medication at the time it is expected to act.

VARIATION: ADMINISTERING A BLOOD THINNER INJECTION (E.G., HEPARIN, LOVENOX)

The subcutaneous administration of blood thinners requires special precautions because of the drug's anticoagulant properties.

■ Select a site on the abdomen away from the umbilicus and above the level of the iliac crests. *Some agencies support the practice of subcutaneous injection of blood thinners in the thighs or arms as alternate sites to the abdomen.*

- Use a 5/8-in., 25- or 26-gauge needle, and insert it at a 90-degree angle. If a client is very lean or wasted, insert it at a 45-degree angle.
- Do not aspirate when giving heparin by subcutaneous injection. *Aspiration can possibly damage the surrounding tissue and cause bleeding as well as bruising.*

- Do not massage the site after the injection. *Massaging could cause bleeding and ecchymosis and hasten drug absorption.*
- Alternate the sites of subsequent injections.

Part C: Intradermal Injection
Interventions and Rationales

1. Check the medication order for accuracy.
   - See Procedure 27-1, step 3.

2. Prepare the medication from the vial or ampule.
   - See Procedure 27-2 (ampule or vial).

3. Identify the client, and assist the client to a comfortable position.
   - Check the client's identification band, and ask the client to tell you his or her name and date of birth. *The Joint Commission requires the use of two identifiers.*
   - Assist the client to a position in which the arm (or sometimes back) can be relaxed and easily available. *A relaxed position of the site minimizes discomfort.*

4. Select and clean the site.
   - Select a site on the forearm or upper back free of tenderness, hardness, swelling, scarring, itching, burning, or localized inflammation. *These conditions could hinder the absorption of the medication and increase the likelihood of injury and discomfort at the injection site. Since most intradermal injections are used to test for allergic reactions, any blemish may conceal a response.*
   - Don gloves.
   - Cleanse the skin with antiseptic per agency protocol. Swab the center of the site in a widening circle to about 5 cm (2 in.). Let the skin dry completely. *If you inject the skin before it dries, you might introduce antiseptic into the skin causing discomfort or an interference with test results.*

5. Prepare the syringe for injection. *Use a TB syringe or a 0.5- to 1-mL syringe, 26- or 27-gauge, 3/8-in. needle and do not draw up more than 0.1 mL of solution for injection for the intradermal route.*
   - Confirm that the medication and the dosage are both correct. *This prevents medication error.*
   - Remove the needle cap while waiting for the antiseptic to dry. Pull the cap straight off to avoid contaminating the needle by the outside edge of the cap. *The needle will become contaminated if it touches anything but the inside of the cap, which is sterile.*
   - Hold the client's arm in your nondominant hand and stretch the skin taut. *Stretching the skin tightly allows for ease of needle insertion.*

6. Inject the medication.
   - Hold the needle with the bevel side up at a 10- to 15-degree angle from the skin (almost parallel to the skin surface).
   - Slowly insert the needle into the first layer of skin so that the bevel is completely covered by the skin. The point of the needle should be slightly visible through the skin.
   - Inject the medication very slowly until a bleb or wheal (small white bubble) is formed just under the skin surface. *If no bubble forms, withdraw the needle slightly as it may be too deep. If solution leaks out as you inject, the needle is not deep enough. Do not aspirate when administering an intradermal injection because there are only small capillaries and no large vessels in the dermal layer of skin.*

7. Remove the needle.
   - Withdraw needle at same angle as insertion and lightly pat area with a sterile gauze pad. *Do not massage because this action may interfere with test results.*

8. Dispose of supplies appropriately.
   - Discard the uncapped needle and attached syringe into designated receptacles. *Proper disposal protects the nurse and others from injury and contamination. The CDC recommends not capping the needle before disposal to reduce the risk of needle-stick injuries.*
   - Remove gloves. Perform hand hygiene.

9. Document all relevant information.
   - Document the medication given, dosage, time, route, any assessments, injection site, and your signature.
   - Many agencies prefer that medication administration be recorded on the medication record. *The nurse's notes are used when prn medications are given or when there is a special problem.*
   - Clients undergoing allergy testing must be observed for a minimum of 30 minutes after the test for possible anaphylactic reaction. Emergency equipment and medication must be available before administering allergy testing.
   - Clients should be provided written instructions regarding when to return for reading. Clients should be instructed to avoid scrubbing, scratching, or rubbing the area of the injection and to report to an emergency facility if dyspnea, hives, or rash develops.

10. Assess the effectiveness of the medication at the time it is expected to act.
    - Since many intradermal injections are given for purposes of allergy sensitivity or tuberculosis testing, follow-up documentation may be required. *Tuberculosis testing, sometimes called a Mantoux or PPD skin test, must be read 48 to 72 hours after the test has been administered. Each agency has a policy on how the patient reaction is to be evaluated and recorded.*

PROCEDURE 27-4   Administering Ophthalmic Instillations

Purpose

- To provide an eye medication the client requires (e.g., an antibiotic) to treat an infection or for other reasons (see specific drug action)

Equipment

- Disposable gloves
- Sterile absorbent sponges soaked in sterile normal saline
- Medication
- Dry sterile absorbent sponges
- Sterile eye dressing (pad) as needed and paper tape to secure it

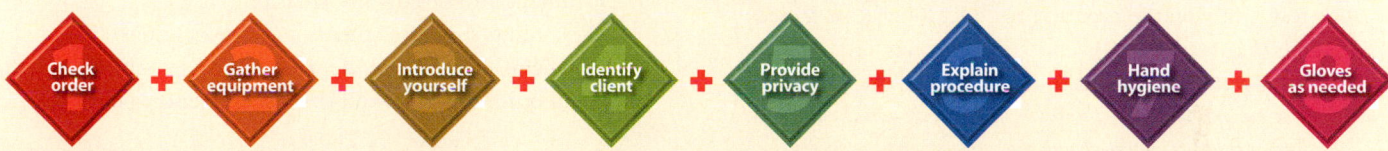

Check order + Gather equipment + Introduce yourself + Identify client + Provide privacy + Explain procedure + Hand hygiene + Gloves as needed

Interventions and Rationales

1. Perform preparatory steps (see icon bar above).

2. Check the medication order and the medication.
    - Carefully check the physician's order for the preparation, strength, and number of drops. Also, confirm the prescribed frequency of the instillation and which eye is to be treated. Abbreviations are frequently used to identify the eye: OD (right eye), OS (left eye), and OU (both eyes).

3. Prepare the client.
    - Check the client's identification band, and ask the client to tell you his or her name and date of birth. *The Joint Commission requires the use of two identifiers.*
    - Explain the technique to the client or to the parents of an infant or child. *The administration of an ophthalmic medication is not usually painful. Ointments are often soothing to the eye, but some liquid preparations may sting initially.*
    - Assist the client to a comfortable position, either sitting or lying.

4. Clean the eyelid and the eyelashes.
    - Don sterile gloves.
    - Use sterile cotton balls moistened with sterile irrigating solution or sterile normal saline, and wipe from the inner canthus to the outer canthus. *If not removed, material on the eyelid and lashes can be washed into the eye. Cleaning toward the outer canthus prevents contamination of the other eye and the lacrimal duct.*

5. Administer the eye medication.
    - Check the ophthalmic preparation for the name, strength, and number of drops if a liquid is used. Draw the correct number of drops into the shaft of the dropper if a dropper is used. If ointment is used, discard the first bead. *Checking medication data is essential to prevent a medication error. The first bead of ointment from a tube is considered to be contaminated.*
    - Instruct the client to look up to the ceiling. Give the client a dry sterile absorbent sponge. *The client is less likely to blink if looking up. While the client looks up, the cornea is partially protected by the top eyelid. A sponge is needed to press on the nasolacrimal duct after a liquid instillation or to wipe excess ointment from the eyelashes after an ointment is instilled.*
    - Expose the lower conjunctival sac by placing the thumb or fingers of your nondominant hand on the

client's cheekbone just below the eye and gently drawing down the skin on the cheek. If the tissues are edematous, handle the tissues carefully to avoid damaging them. *Placing the fingers on the cheekbone minimizes the possibility of touching the cornea, avoids putting any pressure on the eyeball, and prevents the person from blinking or squinting.*

■ Approach the eye from the side and instill the correct number of drops onto the outer third of the lower conjunctival sac. Hold the dropper 1 to 2 cm (0.4 to 0.8 in.) above the sac (Figure 27-39 ■). *The client is less likely to blink if a side approach is used. When instilled into the conjunctival sac, drops will not harm the cornea as they might if dropped directly on it.* The dropper must not touch the sac or the cornea.

or

■ Holding the tube above the lower conjunctival sac, squeeze 2 cm (0.8 in.) (or amount prescribed) of ointment from the tube into the lower conjunctival sac from the inner canthus outward.

■ Instruct the client to close the eyelids but not to squeeze them shut. *Closing the eye spreads the medication over the eyeball. Squeezing can injure the eye and push out the medication.*

■ For liquid medications, press firmly or have the client press firmly on the nasolacrimal duct for at least 30 seconds (Figure 27-40 ■). Check agency practice. *Pressing on the nasolacrimal duct prevents the medication from running out of the eye and down the lacrimal duct into the nasal mucosa where it could be absorbed into the systemic circulation..*

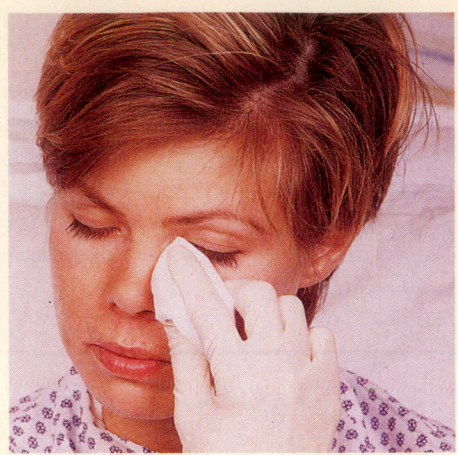

Figure 27-40. ■ Pressing on the nasolacrimal duct.
(Photographer: Jenny Thomas.)

6. Clean the eyelids as needed. Wipe the eyelids gently from the inner to the outer canthus to collect excess medication.

7. Apply an eye pad if needed, and secure it with paper tape.

8. Assess the client's response.
   ■ Assess responses immediately after the instillation and again after the medication should have acted.

9. Document all relevant information.
   ■ Record nursing assessments and interventions. Include the name of the drug, the strength, the number of drops if a liquid, the time, and the response of the client.

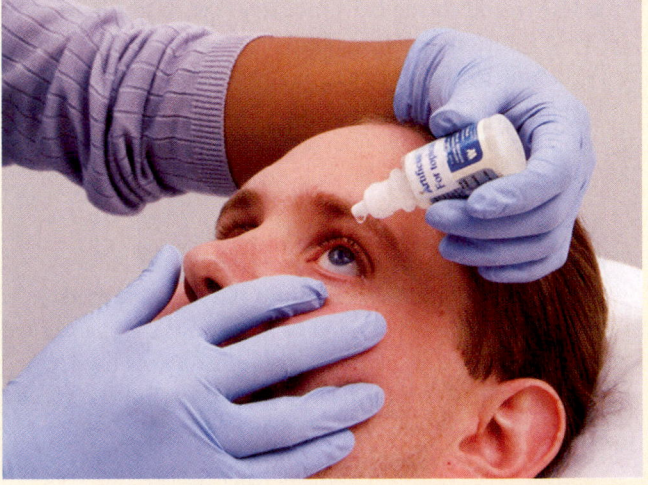

Figure 27-39. ■ Instilling an eye drop into the lower conjunctival sac. (Photographer: Elena Dorfman.)

SAMPLE DOCUMENTATION

[date] [time] Presented at ER following work-related injury. Experienced severe pain in rt. eye while using grinding wheel. Fluorescein NA 2 gtts instilled OD. Seen by Dr. Wilson 0.5-mm metal sliver removed. Eye irrigated with 25 mL NSS. Eye patch applied. _____
_____ R. Nelson, LVN

PROCEDURE 27-5 ## Administering Otic Instillations

Purposes

- To soften earwax so that it can be readily removed at a later time
- To provide local therapy to reduce inflammation, destroy infective organisms in the external ear canal, or both
- To relieve pain

Equipment

- Disposable gloves (optional)
- Cotton-tipped applicator
- Correct medication bottle with a dropper
- Flexible rubber tip (optional) for the end of the dropper, which prevents injury from sudden motion, for example, by a child or disoriented client
- Cotton fluff

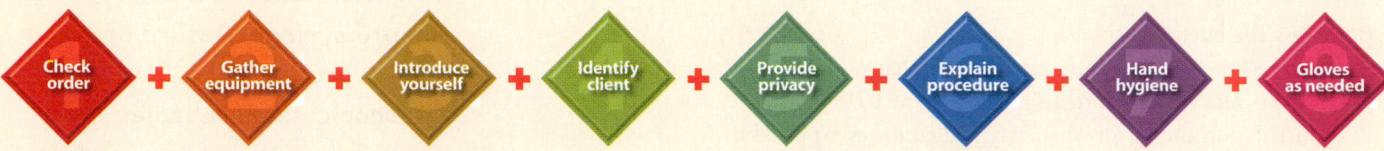

Check order ✛ Gather equipment ✛ Introduce yourself ✛ Identify client ✛ Provide privacy ✛ Explain procedure ✛ Hand hygiene ✛ Gloves as needed

Interventions and Rationales

1. Perform preparatory steps (see icon bar above).

2. Check the medication order.
   - Carefully check the physician's order for the kind of medication; the time, amount, and dosage; and which ear is to be treated. According to The Joint Commission guidelines, abbreviations for the ear (AU, AD, AS) are no longer acceptable.

3. Prepare the client.
   - Check the client's identification band, and ask the client to tell you his or her name and date of birth. *The Joint Commission requires the use of two identifiers.*
   - Explain the procedure to the client or to the parents of an infant or child. Client will need to remain in a side-lying position during and following the procedure so that the medication will remain in ear canal.
   - Obtain assistance to immobilize an infant or young child. *This prevents accidental injury due to sudden movement during the procedure.*
   - Assist the client to a side-lying position with the ear being treated uppermost.

4. Clean the pinna of the ear and the meatus of the ear canal.
   - Don gloves if infection is suspected.
   - Use cotton-tipped applicators and solution to wipe the pinna and auditory meatus. Remove any visible discharge before the instillation so that it won't be washed into the ear canal.

5. Administer the ear medication.
   - Warm the medication container in your hand, or place it in warm water for a short time. *This promotes client comfort and decreases the risk of causing the patient dizziness.*
   - Partially fill the ear dropper with medication.

- Straighten the auditory canal. For an infant, gently pull the pinna down and back (Figure 27-41 ■). For an adult or a child older than 3 years of age, pull the pinna upward and backward (see Figure 58-11 ⚭). *The auditory canal is straightened so that the solution can flow the entire length of the canal.*
- Instill the correct number of drops along the side of the ear canal (Figure 27-42 ■).

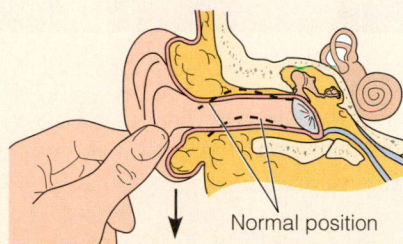

Normal position

Figure 27-41. ■ Straightening the ear canal of a child by pulling the pinna down and back.

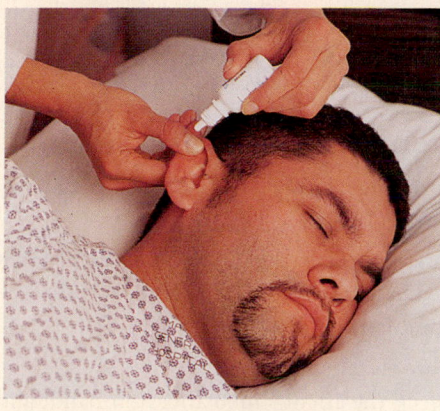

Figure 27-42. ■ Instilling eardrops, pulling up and back.

- Press gently but firmly a few times on the tragus of the ear. Pressing on the tragus assists the flow of medication into the ear canal.
- Ask the client to remain in the side-lying position for about 5 minutes. *This prevents the drops from escaping and allows the medication to reach all sides of the canal cavity.*
- Insert a small piece of cotton fluff loosely at the meatus of the auditory canal for 15 to 20 minutes. Do not press it into the canal. *The cotton helps retain the medication when the client is up. If pressed tightly into the canal, the cotton would interfere with the action of the drug and the outward movement of normal secretions.*

6. Assess the client's response.
   - Assess the character and amount of discharge, appearance of the canal, discomfort, and so on, immediately after the instillation and again when the medication is expected to act. Inspect the cotton ball for any drainage.

7. Document all relevant information.
   - Document all nursing assessments and interventions relative to the procedure.

- Include the time, the dose, and any complaints of pain. *Many agencies use flow sheets; others may require that a notation be made on the nurse's notes.*

SAMPLE DOCUMENTATION

[date] [time] Impacted cerumen ×2 weeks. Debrox gtts ii each ear daily ×5 days. Prepared for ear irrigation. 100 mL warm H_2O via Asepto syringe. Return of large amt of orange/yellow cerumen. Otoscopic exam revealed clear ear canal. Tolerated procedure well. _____

_____ O. Pearson, LVN

PROCEDURE 27-6 Administering Vaginal Instillations

Purposes

- To treat or prevent infection
- To reduce inflammation
- To relieve vaginal discomfort

Equipment

- Drape
- Correct vaginal suppository, foam, or cream
- Applicator for vaginal cream, foam, or suppository
- Disposable gloves
- Lubricant for suppository or applicator
- Disposable towel
- Clean perineal pad

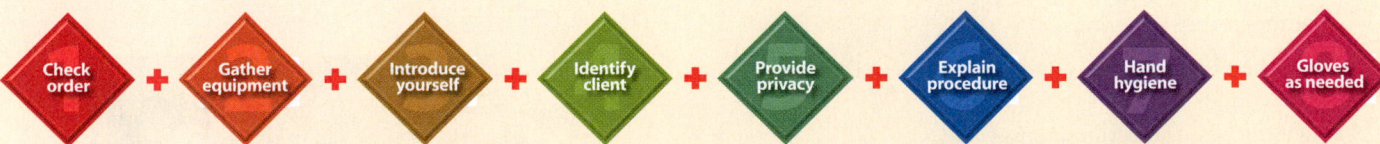

Check order + Gather equipment + Introduce yourself + Identify client + Provide privacy + Explain procedure + Hand hygiene + Gloves as needed

Interventions and Rationales

1. Perform preparatory steps (see icon bar above).
2. Check the medication order.
   - Carefully check the physician's order for the specific medication ordered, its dosage, and the time of administration.
3. Prepare the client.
   - Check the client's identification band, and ask the client to tell you his or her name and date of birth. *The Joint Commission requires the use of two identifiers.*
   - Explain to the client that a vaginal instillation is normally a painless procedure, and in fact may bring relief from itching and burning if an infection is present. *Many clients feel embarrassed about this procedure, and some may prefer to perform the procedure themselves if instruction is provided.*
   - Provide privacy, and ask the client to void. *If the bladder is empty, the client will have less discomfort during the*

treatment, and the possibility of injuring the vaginal lining is decreased.

4. Position and drape the client appropriately.
   - Assist the client to a back-lying position with the knees flexed and the hips rotated laterally.
   - Drape the client appropriately so that only the perineal area is exposed.

5. Prepare the equipment.
   - Unwrap the suppository, and put it on the opened wrapper.
   or
   - Fill the applicator with the prescribed cream, jelly, or foam. Directions are provided with the manufacturer's applicator.

6. Assess and clean the perineal area.
   - Don gloves. *Gloves prevent contamination of the nurse's hands from vaginal and perineal microorganisms.*
   - Inspect the vaginal orifice; note any redness, edema, odor, or discharge from the vagina; and ask about any vaginal discomfort.
   - Provide perineal care to remove secretions. *This decreases the chance of moving microorganisms into the vagina.*

7. Administer the vaginal suppository, cream, foam, or jelly.

VAGINAL SUPPOSITORY

- Lubricate with a water-soluble lubricant, such as KY jelly, the rounded (smooth) end of the suppository, which is inserted first. *Lubrication facilitates insertion.*
- Lubricate your gloved index finger.
- Expose the vaginal orifice by separating the labia with your nondominant hand.

- Insert the suppository about 8 to 10 cm (3 to 4 in.) along the posterior wall of the vagina, or as far as it will go (Figure 27-43 ■). The posterior wall of the vagina is about 2.5 cm (1 in.) longer than the anterior wall because the cervix protrudes into the uppermost portion of the anterior wall. The anterior wall is usually about 6 to 7.5 cm (2.5 to 3 in.).
- Withdraw the finger, and remove the gloves, turning them inside out. Discard appropriately. *Turning the gloves inside out prevents the spread of microorganisms.*
- Ask the client to remain lying in the supine position for 5 to 10 minutes following insertion. The hips may also be elevated on a pillow. *This position allows the medication to flow into the posterior fornix after it has melted.*

VAGINAL CREAM, JELLY, OR FOAM

- Lubricate applicator with water-soluble lubricant. Expose the vaginal orifice by gently separating labia with nondominant hand.
- Gently insert the applicator about 5 cm (2 in.).
- Slowly push the plunger until the applicator is empty (Figure 27-44 ■).
- Remove the applicator and place it on the towel. *The applicator is put on the towel to prevent the spread of microorganisms.*
- Discard the applicator if disposable or clean it according to the manufacturer's directions.
- Remove the gloves, turning them inside out. Discard appropriately.
- Ask the client to remain lying in the supine position for 5 to 10 minutes following the insertion.

8. Ensure client comfort.
   - Dry the perineum with tissues as required.

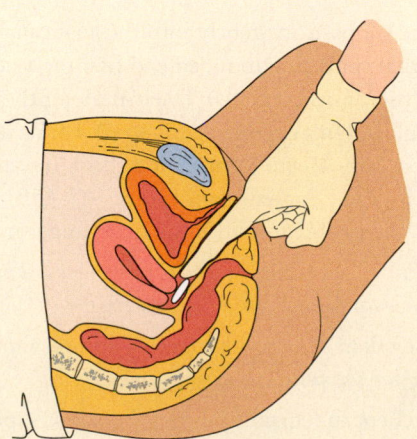

Figure 27-43. ■ Instilling a vaginal suppository.

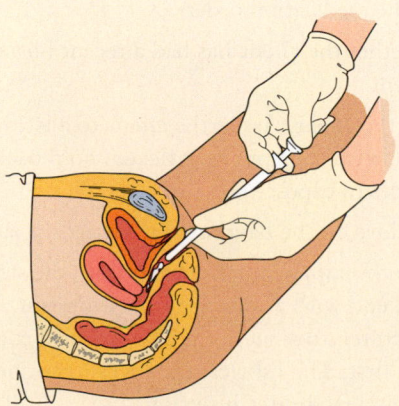

Figure 27-44. ■ Using an applicator to instill a vaginal cream.

- Apply a clean perineal pad and a T-binder if there is excessive drainage.

9. Document all relevant information.
   - Record the instillation and assessments as for other medications and instillations.

10. Assess and document the client's response.

PROCEDURE 27-7   # Administering Rectal Medication

Purpose

- To administer prescribed medication safely by the rectal route

Equipment

- Drape
- Correct rectal suppository
- Disposable gloves
- Lubricant for suppository
- Disposable towel
- Clean perineal pad

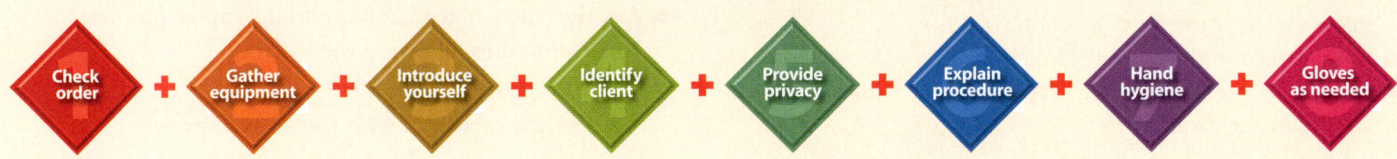

Check order + Gather equipment + Introduce yourself + Identify client + Provide privacy + Explain procedure + Hand hygiene + Gloves as needed

Interventions and Rationales

1. Perform preparatory steps (see icon bar above).

2. Check the medication order.

3. Ask whether the client has had a recent bowel movement.

4. Prepare the client. Assist the client to a left lateral position, with the upper leg flexed. Fold back the top bedclothes to expose the buttocks.

5. Don a glove on the hand used to insert the suppository.

6. Unwrap the suppository and lubricate the smooth rounded end with a water-soluble lubricant, or see manufacturer's instructions. The rounded end is usually inserted first. The lubricant reduces irritation of the mucosa and facilitates insertion.

7. Lubricate the gloved index finger. *This will allow for easier insertion.*

8. Encourage the client to relax by breathing through the mouth.

9. Insert the suppository gently into the anal canal beyond the internal sphincter, rounded end first (or according to manufacturer's instructions). Insert it along the rectal wall using a gloved finger (Figure 27-45 ■). For an adult, insert the suppository 10 cm (4 in.); for a child, insert it 2.5 to 5 cm (1 to 2 in.); for an infant (Figure 27-45B, insert it 1.25 to 2.5 cm (1/2 to 1 in.); the little finger may be used.

10. Avoid embedding the suppository in feces. *This would prevent the medication from being absorbed.*

11. Press the client's buttocks together for a few minutes. *This prevents the medication from being expelled.*

12. Ask the client to remain in the left lateral or supine position for at least 5 minutes to help retain the suppository. The suppository should be retained for at least 30 to 40 minutes or according to manufacturer's instructions.

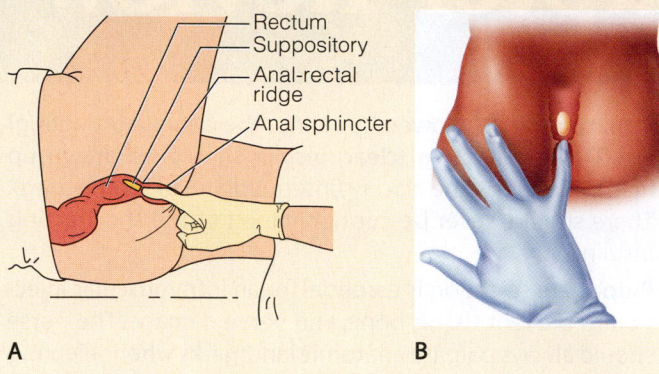

Rectum
Suppository
Anal-rectal ridge
Anal sphincter

A   B

Figure 27-45. ■ Inserting a rectal suppository beyond the internal sphincter and along the rectal wall. **A.** Inserting a suppository in an adult. **B.** Inserting a suppository in an infant.

SAMPLE DOCUMENTATION

[date]	T 101.8 F; 325 mg acetaminophen given rectally. _____ J. Sous, LVN
[time]	%100.1 F. Linens changed. Client states wants to nap. J. Sous, LVN (*Note:* This is only a piece of a full narrative note.)

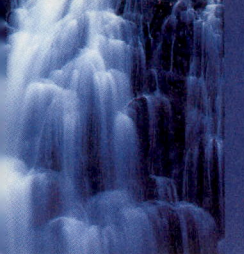

Chapter Review

KEY Points

- Nursing practice acts define limits on the nurse's responsibilities regarding medications.

- Medications have several names. Nurses need to know the generic and trade names of a medication and be aware of both its therapeutic and side effects.

- Adverse effects of medications include drug toxicity, drug allergy, drug tolerance, idiosyncratic effect, and drug interactions.

- Various routes are used to administer medications. The enteral (pertaining to the intestine) routes include oral, sublingual, buccal, rectal, or via a nasogastric (NG) or gastrostomy (G) tube. The parenteral routes include intravenous (IV), intramuscular (IM), subcutaneous (SubQ), intradermal (ID), vaginal, topical, transdermal, and inhalation.

- Medication orders must include the client name, date and time the order is written, name of the medication, dosage, route, frequency of administration, and signature of the person writing the order. Nurses must question any unclear orders before implementing the order.

- Three systems of measurement are used: the metric system, the apothecaries' system, and the household system. Weights and measures may need to be converted by the nurse within these three systems.

- When administering medications, the nurse observes the six "rights" to ensure accurate administration. When preparing medications, the nurse checks the medication container label against the medication card form or printout three times.

- The nurse who prepares the medication administers it and must never leave a prepared medication unattended.

- The nurse always identifies the client appropriately before administering a medication and stays with the client until the medication is taken.

- Medications, once given, are documented as soon as possible after administration.

- When mixing insulins in the same syringe, air should be injected into the cloudy (intermediate- or long-acting) insulin vial first, followed by air into the clear (short-acting) vial. The short-acting (clear) insulin should be drawn up first, followed by the cloudy (intermediate- or long-acting). There should never be contamination of the short-acting insulin.

- Proper site selection is essential for an intramuscular injection to prevent tissue, bone, and nerve damage. The nurse should always palpate anatomic landmarks when selecting a site.

- Clients receiving a series of injections should have the injection sites rotated.

- After use, needles should not be recapped but must be placed in puncture-resistant containers.

FOR FURTHER Study

For information on assessing the client for use of supplements, see Chapter 8.

For further information about inserting a nasogastric tube and tube feeding, see Procedures 25-2 and 25-3.

For information about discontinuing an intravenous device, see Procedure 28-11.

For more details about respiratory therapy, see Chapter 32.

For information about administering tube feedings or giving an enema, see Chapter 37.

For information on straightening the ear canal in young children, see Figure 58-12.

Critical Thinking Care Map

Caring for a Client with Insulin-Dependent Diabetes Mellitus

NCLEX-PN® Focus Area: Health Promotion and Maintenance

Case Study: Marissa Gonsalves is a 27-year-old elementary schoolteacher newly diagnosed with type 1 diabetes mellitus. She also attends school at night with plans to complete her master's degree in the spring. She lives with three roommates who have shared a house since their college days. She expresses concern over her diagnosis. "It will be hard to follow the diet at home. I don't eat on a regular schedule on my school nights and my roommates are big snackers."

Nursing Diagnosis: *Ineffective Therapeutic Regimen Management*

COLLECT DATA

Subjective	Objective
_____	_____
_____	_____
_____	_____
_____	_____
_____	_____
_____	_____

Would you report this? Yes/No

If yes, report to: _____

What would you report? _____

Nursing Care

_____
_____
_____
_____
_____
_____
_____
_____
_____
_____
_____

How would you document this? _____
_____
_____

Compare your answers and documentation to those provided on the MyNursingKit Website.

Data Collected
(use only those that apply)

- Weight: 156 lbs
- Fasting blood sugar 164 mg/mL
- Urine shows presence of ketones
- VS: T 99, P 132, R 28, BP 100/54
- Complains of excessive thirst and frequent urination
- States, "I have been so tired, but it is probably because I am working and going to school."
- Started on insulin injection and blood glucose monitoring; client hesitant to perform monitoring and injections herself
- 1,800-calorie ADA diet

Nursing Interventions
(use only those that apply, list in priority order)

- Review daily actions that are not therapeutic.
- Pay meticulous attention to foot care.
- Monitor skin condition at least once a day; determine whether client is experiencing loss of sensation.
- Demonstrate and allow client to perform monitoring and self-injection under supervision.
- Observe and report signs of infection such as redness, warmth, discharge, and increased body temperature.
- Provide information about the therapeutic regimen in various formats (video, brochures, written instructions).
- Deliberate with the client on changes that are possible to meet therapeutic goals.
- Assess client's locus of control related to her health.

NCLEX-PN® Exam Preparation

1 The physician wishes to give a medication by the fastest possible route. The nurse anticipates the medication will be ordered via what route?

1. Oral.
2. Rectal.
3. Topical.
4. Parenteral.

2 The physician has written an order that is illegible. It appears to be 5 mg of Ativan and the nurse gives the medication. The order in fact was 0.5 mg. Who is responsible for the error?

1. The nurse who administers the incorrect dosage is responsible for the error.
2. The physician who wrote the illegible order is responsible.
3. The unit secretary who transcribed the order is responsible.
4. The charge nurse who verified the order is responsible.

3 The nurse administers medications for what effect?

1. Side effect
2. Idiosyncratic effect
3. Therapeutic effect
4. Adverse effect

4 The nurse is caring for an elderly client with reduced hepatic and renal function. When transcribing medication orders, the nurse anticipates the dosage of medication will be:

1. Increased
2. Decreased
3. The same
4. Varying according to the medication

5 The physician has ordered Valium 5 mg "stat" for agitation. The nurse understands the order to mean:

1. The drug is to be given as needed.
2. The medication is to be given immediately and only once.
3. The order may be carried out indefinitely until an order is written to cancel it.
4. The drug is to be given on a regular schedule.

6 A preoperative order is given for atropine 0.4 mg. On hand is a multidose vial containing 1 mg/mL. What volume of the drug would the nurse give?

1. 2.5 mL
2. 0.2 mL
3. 0.4 mL
4. 4 mL

7 The nurse is providing discharge instructions for a mother of a 2-year-old. The physician has written a prescription for 1 teaspoon amoxicillin every 6 hours × 10 days. Which of the following statements would indicate that the mother understands the instructions provided?

1. "I will use a regular spoon to measure his medication."
2. "I will disguise the medicine in his milk to be sure he will take it."
3. "I will give him the medication with meals and his last dose before he goes to bed."
4. "I will use this medication cup to measure the correct dose."

8 The nurse is preparing a subcutaneous injection of heparin. Four thousand units have been ordered and 5,000 unit/mL is on hand. The nurse would prepare the medication using what syringe?

1. An insulin syringe
2. A tuberculin syringe
3. A 2-mL syringe with a 22-gauge 2.5-cm (1-in.) needle
4. A 3-mL syringe with a 23-gauge 3-cm (1.5-in.) needle

9 The primary reason nurses wear gloves when administering topical medications is:

1. To act as a barrier to prevent the nurse from absorbing some of the medication.
2. To prevent topical medication from irritating the nurse's skin.
3. To prevent transfer of the topical medication from one client to another on the nurse's hands.
4. To follow sterile technique.

10 The nurse is preparing to administer an intramuscular injection into a pediatric client when the mother requests the medication be given in the buttocks. The nurse explains that this site is not used for infants because:

1. It is difficult to restrain a child in the proper position to use this site.
2. This muscle is developed by walking so it should not be used until the child has been walking for 1 year.
3. Medication is absorbed slowly from this location.
4. The area is very vascular so there is a tendency for extensive bruising.

Answers and rationales for Review Questions appear in Appendix I.

Chapter 28

IV Therapy

LEARNING Outcomes

After completing this chapter, you will be able to:

1. Identify nursing responsibilities and concerns in IV therapy.
2. Discuss the purpose of IV therapy and the various solutions used.
3. Identify the equipment involved in providing parenteral therapy.
4. Describe how to calculate IV rates accurately.
5. Identify peripheral veins appropriate for use in IV therapy.
6. Describe factors that influence IV site and needle selection.
7. Explain venipuncture techniques and LPN/LVN responsibilities in monitoring IV drip rate.
8. Identify complications associated with infusion therapy.
9. Discuss the procedure for administering blood products and nursing measures for potential complications.

Clinical Objectives

10. Demonstrate proper venipuncture procedure.
11. Demonstrate accurate calculations for determining IV rates.
12. Demonstrate how to change a sterile central line dressing.
13. Prepare to administer blood/blood products.

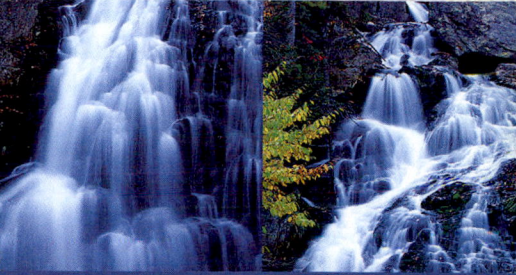

BRIEF Outline

Legal Implications and Safety Issues with IV Therapy

Purpose of Intravenous Therapy

IV Solutions

Equipment Overview

IV Rate Calculations

Preparing the Client for IV Therapy

Anatomy of Peripheral Veins

Factors Affecting IV Site Selection

Venipuncture Procedure

Peripheral IV Therapy Complications

Blood Transfusions

air embolism 676	homologous 675	septicemia 676
autologous 675	hypertonic 662	speed shock 677
bacteremia 676	hypotonic 662	stylet 664
circulatory overload 676	infiltration 673	thrombophlebitis 674
controller 665	infusate 667	thrombosis 674
designated 677	infusion pump 665	vasovagal response 674
drip factors 667	isotonic 662	venospasm 674
extravasation 675	osmolarity 662	
hematoma 673	phlebitis 673	

The LPN/LVN must be knowledgeable and skillful when delivering IV therapy. Rules and regulations regarding the role of LPNs/LVNs in IV therapy vary and are available from each state's Board of Nursing. LPNs/LVNs must know what is legal for them to do and must *always* perform duties within the scope of practice. Each state's nurse practice act defines scope of practice, including whether the nurse must complete boards and nurse's training before taking the IV course. The nurse must be trained and certified in IV therapy and must be fully aware of the standards of practice involved in providing it. Besides following state regulations, the LPN/LVN must also know and follow the policies and procedures of the employing agency. (The term *IV Certified* will usually be added to the license of the LPN/LVN upon first renewal, if the state requires certification only after the nurse has taken nursing boards.)

The LPN/LVN who provides IV therapy must advocate for the client in two important ways. First, the nurse must prepare and educate the client about IV therapy to ensure cooperation and a therapeutic relationship. Second, the nurse must observe the client closely for potential complications and provide early intervention if they should occur. Managing IV therapy is one of the most important roles that an LPN/LVN undertakes, whether the nurse is simply assisting and monitoring or providing fuller IV care.

Legal Implications and Safety Issues with IV Therapy

Laws about IV therapy differ widely from state to state, so you must be knowledgeable about the laws in your state. This section provides an overview of significant issues. There are three classifications of law that must be considered when administering IV therapy. *Common law* is court-made law and is most commonly found in the area of malpractice. *Criminal law* relates to a wrong against the public for which the government authority can prosecute criminal acts with imprisonment or fines. If carried out in an unlawful manner, IV therapy administration can be a criminal offense.

Civil law applies to the legal rights of private persons/ corporations. A private wrong or act of omission can result in a civil tort. Intentional torts that could be related to IV therapy are negligence, assault and battery, false imprisonment, slander, libel, and invasion of privacy. For example, forcing a rational adult client to allow placement of an IV cannula could constitute assault and battery charges.

Negligence is the failure to do something that a reasonable prudent person would do and is an unintentional tort (see Chapter 4). Malpractice, another type of unintentional tort, is acting in a manner that departs from the accepted standards of practice that the average qualified healthcare provider would deliver. *Note*: If an act of malpractice does not create harm, legal action cannot be initiated.

The rule of personal liability states that every person is liable for his or her own *tortuous conduct* (actions that could result in a tort). Therefore, nurses are liable for their own wrongdoings in carrying out physician orders. If, in his or her professional judgment, an LPN/LVN does not feel confident performing a particular IV task, then he or she can properly refuse to do so.

BREACH OF DUTY

Breaches of duty are certain events that may foreseeably cause a specific harm, for example, delay in medication administration, unfamiliarity with the drug, inappropriate route of administration, failure to qualify orders, and negligence in client teaching. More specific litigation for nurses can result from infiltration and phlebitis, extravasations, broken central venous catheters, nerve injury, and poor or inaccurate documentation.

STANDARDS OF CARE

The client is the focus of standards of care in healthcare organizations. The Joint Commission, which grants accreditation to healthcare organizations, has indicated that standards of care must be developed within organizations to measure quality based on expectations of service. Sources of standards of care include federal regulators, the Occupational Safety and

Health Administration (OSHA), the Food and Drug Administration (FDA), and the Centers for Disease Control and Prevention (CDC). State regulators include departments of health and human services, which enforce Health Insurance Portability and Accountability Act (HIPAA) regulations. Professional standards of care include those published by the American Nurses Association (ANA), the Infusion Nurses Society (INS), the Joint Commission, the American Association of Blood Banking (AABB), and the Environmental Protection Agency (EPA). Standards of care address nursing process, accountability, currency in practice, and outcomes of care and focus for the client.

OCCURRENCE/INCIDENT REPORT

A report should be filed every time something unusual or a deviation from the standard of care occurs. These reports are used for internal quality assurance purposes and as a record of the event. Incidents should be reported to the charge nurse/supervisor and objectively charted but not referenced in the client legal record. See Figure 63-3 ⊙⊙ for an example of an Occurrence/Incident Report.

CDC/OSHA GUIDELINES

All nursing personnel must follow Standard Precautions. All body fluids (not including sweat) are treated as if known to be infectious with HIV, hepatitis B and C, and other bloodborne pathogens. The main barriers include gloves (in combination with hand hygiene practices), eye protection, and mucous membrane protection (face shield or goggles and mask).

The Needlestick Safety and Prevention Act of November 2000 reinforced the need to use safe needles in order to reduce needle-stick injuries. Needleless systems and needle safety devices are being used to protect the safety of healthcare personnel. Built-in safety features such as syringes with a sliding sheath that shields the attached needle after use, needles that retract into a syringe after use, shielded or retracting catheters, and intravenous medical delivery systems that use a catheter port with a needle housed in a protective covering are currently being used.

---

clinical ALERT

If you are stuck by a needle or other sharp instrument, or get blood or other potentially infectious materials in your eyes, nose, mouth, or on broken skin:

- Immediately flood the exposed area with water and clean any wound with soap and water or a skin disinfectant if available.
- Report this immediately to your employer.
- Seek immediate medical attention.

POSTEXPOSURE PROPHYLAXIS

Healthcare agencies are required to have a plan in place prior to an exposure occurring. The treating agency will evaluate the risk of exposure, evaluate the source client, evaluate the exposed person, and decide on postexposure prophylaxis (PEP) or therapy and follow-up care.

Contaminated sharps have to be placed in a puncture-resistant, leak-proof, and labeled container. The container must be easily accessed, maintained upright, and replaced routinely. Hepatitis B vaccine must be offered at no charge to an employee "at a reasonable time and place" and "within ten days of initial assignment."

PHYSICAL HAZARDS

It is important to note abrasions, contusions, chemical exposure, and latex allergy. Small or undetected skin abrasions/contusions can be potential portals for microorganisms. Hand hygiene helps to prevent the invasion of microorganisms. The handling of cytotoxic drugs can be hazardous and is associated with human cancers. Latex allergies develop with an exposure to natural rubber latex. Reactions range from asthma to anaphylaxis. There is no treatment for latex allergy other than avoidance of latex. Nonlatex personal protective equipment is provided to personnel with a latex sensitivity.

Purpose of Intravenous Therapy

IV therapy is used to maintain blood volume, to deliver medications quickly, to provide nutrition, or to reestablish homeostasis when acid-base imbalance has occurred.

As discussed in Chapter 26 ⊙⊙, water is the largest component of the body. The functions of body fluids are to:

- Maintain blood volume.
- Transport nutrients to and from cells.
- Regulate body temperature.
- Assist in digestion.

When the body is dehydrated through injury, disease, or other mechanisms, rehydration by IV route may be required.

Electrolytes are either negatively or positively charged ions. As discussed in Chapter 26 ⊙⊙, these ions are expressed in mEq (milliequivalents) per liter, measuring chemical activity, rather than in mg (milligrams) that measure weight. Remember that the body needs a balance of cations and anions in any given compartment to maintain homeostasis. Review Box 26-1 and Table 26-1 ⊙⊙ for information about fluids and electrolytes. Imbalances in electrolytes can be life threatening. IV therapy is often used to correct electrolyte imbalances.

IV Solutions

Intravenous solutions can be classified as isotonic, hypotonic, or hypertonic (Table 28-1 ■). IV solutions that are **isotonic**, such as 0.9% sodium chloride (called normal saline or NS), have the same concentration of solutes as blood plasma. Isotonic solutions are often used to restore vascular volume. **Hypertonic** solutions, such as 0.9% sodium chloride with 5% dextrose, have a greater concentration of solutes than plasma. **Hypotonic** solutions, such as 0.45% sodium chloride, have a lesser concentration of solutes.

IV solutions can also be categorized according to their purpose: providing nutrition, replacing electrolytes, or expanding blood volume.

- *Nutrient solutions* contain carbohydrate in the form of dextrose. IV dextrose solutions provide 3.4 calories per gram. For example, 1 L of 5% dextrose provides 170 calories. The calories and fluid help to prevent dehydration and ketosis, but do not provide enough nutrients for body functions such as wound healing.

- *Electrolyte solutions* contain varying amounts of cations and anions. Commonly used solutions are normal saline (0.9% sodium chloride solution), Ringer's solution (which contains sodium, chloride, potassium, and calcium), and lactated Ringer's solution (which contains sodium, chloride, potassium, calcium, and lactate). Saline and balanced electrolyte solutions are commonly used to restore vascular volume, particularly after trauma or surgery. They also may be used to replace fluid and electrolytes for clients with continuous losses, such as gastric suction or wound drainage.

- *Volume expanders* are used to increase the blood volume following severe loss of blood (e.g., from hemorrhage) or loss of plasma (e.g., from severe burns, which draw large amounts of plasma from the bloodstream to the burn site). Common volume expanders are dextran, plasma, and human serum albumin. LPNs/LVNs who are allowed to administer IV fluids by their nurse practice act may or may not be allowed to administer volume expanders, so it is important to read your nurse practice act in the state where you are working.

The type of IV solution ordered depends on the need to change or maintain the client's body fluid status. The effect an IV solution has on the fluid compartments depends on how the solution's **osmolarity** (the concentration of a solute in a volume of solution) compares with the client's serum osmolarity. Normally, serum has the same osmolarity as other body fluids. A lower serum osmolarity suggests fluid overload (there is more water, so solute is less concentrated). A higher osmolarity suggests hemoconcentration and dehydration (more particles in less water).

TABLE 28-1	IV Solutions	
SOLUTION	**IV EXAMPLE**	**NURSING IMPLICATIONS**
Isotonic	Lactated Ringer's (LR) 0.9% NS D$_5$W	■ These solutions expand the intravascular compartment. Monitor client for signs of fluid overload particularly if the client has hypertension or congestive heart failure (CHF). ■ Don't give LR if the client has liver disease because of the inability to metabolize lactate. ■ Avoid giving D$_5$W to a client at risk for increased intracranial pressure (ICP). It acts like a hypotonic solution after administration. D$_5$W is quickly metabolized, leaving only water—a hypotonic solution.
Hypotonic	0.45% NS (½ NS) 0.33% NS D$_{2.5}$W	■ These solutions contain less sodium than ICF. They move water into cells, causing cells to swell and possibly burst. ■ These solutions can cause a sudden fluid shift from blood vessels into cells. This can cause cardiovascular collapse from intravascular fluid depletion and increased ICP from fluid shift into brain cells. ■ Avoid hypotonic solutions to clients at risk for ICP, CVA, stroke, head trauma, or neurosurgery. ■ Avoid hypotonic solutions for clients at risk for third spacing fluid shifts such as burns, trauma, or low serum protein levels.
Hypertonic	D 5% 0.45% NS (D$_5$½ NS) D 5% 0.9% NS (D$_5$NS) D 5% LR (D$_5$LR)	■ These solutions greatly expand the intravascular compartment. Monitor your client for circulatory overload. ■ Hypertonic solutions pull fluid from the ICF compartment. Avoid these solutions in clients with a condition that causes cellular dehydration such as diabetic ketoacidosis. ■ Avoid these solutions in clients with impaired heart or kidney function because this client is unable to manage extra fluid.

Equipment Overview

The LPN's/LVN's knowledge about IV equipment is essential in the safe delivery of IV therapy. Identification of the appropriate equipment and understanding the purpose of IV therapy for the client will assist the nurse in the selection of the necessary equipment. Typically IV containers are changed every 24 hours or per facility policy; this is usually performed with tubing changes. An IV container that is at a "keep-open" or slow rate could conceivably run as long as 24 hours and would need to be replaced in that time frame. (In that case, the IV tubing would be clamped briefly below the drip chamber. The old bag would be brought down and disconnected, and the new bag [and new tubing if due for tubing change] would be respiked or rehung. If the tubing was not changed, the clamp would be opened and the infusion would continue. If tubing was changed, the old tubing would be disconnected at the hub of the IV site and replaced with the new tubing before opening the clamp to continue infusing.)

Two types of infusion systems are used: glass or plastic systems. Glass bottles have a partial vacuum and require air vents. The glass system has the advantages of the glass being inert and being very clear, so the fluid level is more accurately read. The disadvantages are breakage, storage difficulties, rigidity, and difficult disposal. Glass construction is made with mixed materials that could cause incompatibilities with fluids or additives. Additionally, the potential for coring exists due to the rubber bung (stopper) when the administration set is inserted. In an open glass system, air enters through a plastic tube in the container and collects in the air space in the bottle allowing for displacement of the solution. In a closed glass system, air is filtered into the container via vented tubing to allow air into the container.

Plastic containers are used 90% to 95% of the time. They create no vacuum and they are flexible and collapsible. Plastic IV bags do not need air to replace fluid flowing from the container. Plastic containers are completely closed systems, lightweight, easy to store, and are made of polyvinyl chloride (PVC). Bags can be spiked with either a vented or nonvented administration set (Figure 28-1 ■). Disadvantages of plastic bags are that determining fluid level is more difficult and the bag can puncture easily. Plastic containers are made up of plasticizers and are not completely inert, so never use markers to write on the bag because the ink could be absorbed into the plastic.

All containers require some type of administration set to deliver fluid to the client. The most commonly used ones are the primary, or *macrodrip*, set and the pediatric, or *microdrip*, set. In the pediatric setting, buretrols and burettes are used to deliver a precise amount of fluid and prevent fluid overload. The primary sets are the basic administration

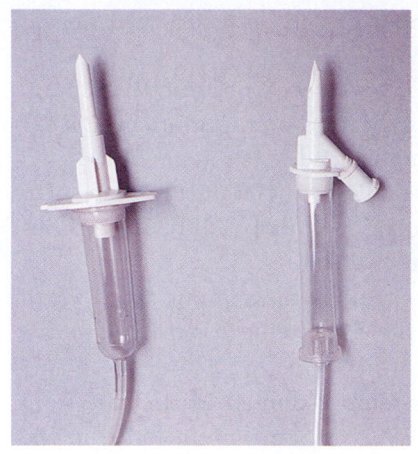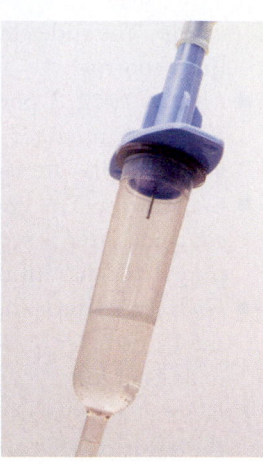

Figure 28-1. ■ Infusion spikes and drip chambers.

sets used for infusion of primary parenteral fluids. The drop factors of these commercial sets vary according to the manufacturer. Usually a macrodrip set ranges from 10 to 20 gtt/mL and the microdrip set is 60 gtt/mL. (*Note*: The macrodrips sets are larger, so the drops are fewer in number but bigger in size. The microdrips are smaller sets with smaller drips, so more drips are needed to release an equivalent amount.) A secondary administration set, called a *piggyback* set or a volume (meter or burette) controlled set, can be added to the primary line. (See Procedure 28-1 ■ on page 681.)

Primary and secondary continuous administration sets must be changed every 72 hours and immediately upon suspected contamination or compromise of product or system. When an increased rate of cannula-related infections occurs, the organization should revert to a 48-hour administration set change. Many hospitals adopt a 48-hour change rather than 72 hours; check your facility policy.

ADMINISTRATION SET COMPONENTS

- *Spike/piercing pin*: Sharp plastic end designed to be inserted into the IV fluid container. Connected to the flange, drop orifice, and drip chamber.
- *Flange*: Plastic guard that assists in protecting against contamination upon insertion of the spike.
- *Drop orifice*: The size and shape of the opening that determines the drop factor.
- *Drip chamber*: A flexible clear plastic tube that encloses the drop orifice and is connected to the tubing.
- *Tubing*: It is long (66–100 in.) for primary and shorter (28–42 in.) for secondary tubing.

A mixture of clamps, ports, connectors, or filters may be built in to the system.

- *Clamp*: A control device that compresses the tubing wall. The most common are a slide, roller, or screw clamp. The slide clamp is less precise when determining fluid control.

- *Injection ports*: A port is an access point into the tubing. Ports are used for medication administration; smaller gauge needles are recommended to ensure resealing.
- *Check valve*: This valve allows the main IV solution to continue after a secondary solution (IVPB, intravenous piggyback) has infused.
- *Hub*: An adaptor that connects the administration set to the IV catheter or needleless system. It is referred to as a male Luer lock.
- *Filter*: The final filter removes foreign particulate from the solution (Figure 28-2 ■). Some are included in the administration set or can be added. A 0.22-micron filter is considered adequate for bacterial/particulate reduction.

Extension tubing may be used to allow the IV tubing to be changed away from the insertion site, decreasing the risk of contamination. An IV loop also enables the tubing to be changed away from the device and promotes stabilization of the device. A T-connector is useful for simultaneous administration of fluids and drugs. It eliminates the need for insertion of a second venipuncture device. (See Procedures 28-2, 28-3, and 28-4 ■.)

Blood administration sets come in a Y-shaped or straight single tubing. The Y tubing allows for infusion of 0.9% normal saline before and after each blood product infusion. Blood administration sets come with an inline filter; the minimum pore size is 170 to 260 microns. Microaggregate blood filters can be added or may be inline. These filters are recommended for blood that has been stored longer than 5 days and when administering multiple units; refer to your facility's policy on adding these filters.

PERIPHERAL INFUSION DEVICES

Several types of peripheral infusion devices are available. Scalp vein needles (butterfly needles) and over-the-needle catheters (ONCs) are commonly used. When selecting a cannula it should be of the smallest gauge and shortest length possible to accommodate the necessary therapy. Cannulas have radiopaque material in them so that they are visible to x-rays.

Scalp Vein (Butterfly) Needles

Scalp vein (butterfly) needles are used for short-term therapy (Figure 28-3 ■). Gauges range from 17, 19, 21, and 23 to 25 at the smallest; their length is 0.5 to 1.0 in.; and the plastic tubing that extends from the wings is 3 to 12 in. long. A butterfly needle would be a good choice for single-dose therapy, blood withdrawal, or clients who are allergic to nylon or Teflon. Butterfly needles are also used for infants, children, the elderly, and adults with small veins. The wings assist with easy insertion and securing of the device. Butterfly needles, however, are stainless steel and inflexible, which may lead to easy needle displacement. There is also an increased risk of contamination with a stainless steel needle.

Over-the-Needle Catheter

An over-the-needle catheter or ONC is used for long-term peripheral infusion therapy for the delivery of viscous fluids (i.e., blood) (Figure 28-4 ■). Gauges range from 14, 16, 18, 20, and 22 to 24 at the smallest. Catheter length varies from 0.5 to 2.0 inches. The point of the needle (also known as the **stylet**) extends beyond the tip of the catheter, so that after the venipuncture, the needle is withdrawn and discarded, leaving the flexible catheter in the vein. These catheters are easy to insert and are patent longer than a steel needle. In

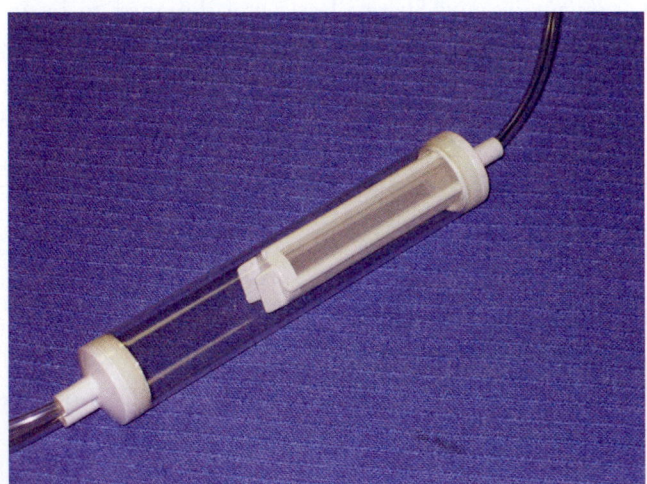

Figure 28-2. ■ Filter.

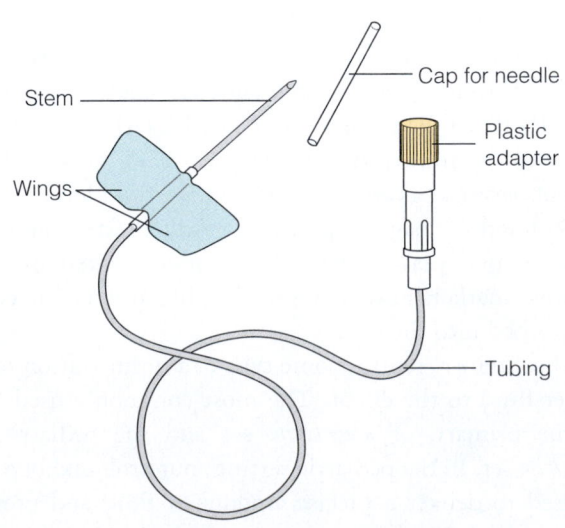

Figure 28-3. ■ Butterfly needle.

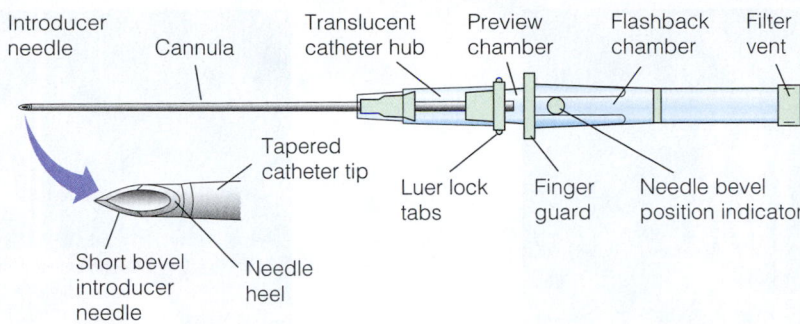

Figure 28-4. ■ Over-the-needle catheter (ONC).

addition, infiltration rate is lower, and they are radiopaque. Catheters with wings are easily taped. Some disadvantages are an increased risk of phlebitis; risk of puncture because the stylet (used when the skin is first punctured) is long and inflexible, and difficulty of taping some hubs. Box 28-1 ■ describes some uses for ONCs.

CENTRAL LINE DEVICES

Central line devices were developed for long-term IV therapy access. These devices are designed to increase client comfort and to decrease complications associated with numerous IV therapy needs. A central venous catheter is inserted into the subclavian vein or the internal jugular vein. The catheter tip end may be positioned in the superior vena cava or in the right atrium.

The LPN/LVN needs to be aware of the various types of central line devices (also known as centrally placed percutaneous catheters and are commonly referred to by site: subclavian, femoral, or jugular), central venous tunneled catheters (Groshong, Hickman, and Broviac), and implanted ports (Medi-Port, Port-A-Cath, Infuse-A-Port), all of which must be inserted by a physician. A fourth type of catheter is a peripherally inserted central catheter (PICC). This type can be inserted by a trained RN and is often used for acute, long-term, and home care settings.

Central catheters typically have double or triple *lumens* (openings for access), but can have a single lumen or as many as four. The LPN/LVN who is certified in IV therapy can change the site dressing on a central line, PICC line, or midline catheter. Check for the LPN/LVN scope of practice with regard to IV therapy in your state. (See Procedure 28-5 ■ on page 687.)

ELECTRONIC INFUSION DEVICES

The two basic groups of electronic infusion devices are controllers and pumps. These devices provide better control of the infusion flow rate than gravity or free flow. They are designed with alarms to signal a change in the normal flow of the IV solution. Electronic equipment has improved the accuracy of IV infusions, but the responsibility and accuracy remain with the nurse who monitors the IV. Machines are not infallible and must be checked for accuracy of the IV rates. The nurse using these machines must understand their use, their mechanical operation, and how to troubleshoot problems.

Controllers

A **controller** is a mechanism to regulate IV flow rate by gravity rather than by exertion or pressure (Figure 28-5 ■). A controller is appropriate for many infusions that do not require the accuracy of the volumetric pump. The drop size may vary among administration sets. If rate needs to be accurate, then an infusion pump should be used. Disadvantages of the controller are that they are unable to detect an infiltration and that the flow rate is affected by the height of the IV bag in relation to the IV site. The LPN/LVN should visually monitor the IV site often for signs of infiltration.

Infusion Pumps

An **infusion pump** is a positive-pressure pump (Figure 28-6 ■). These pumps are programmed to provide fluid more accurately than the controller. There are several types

BOX 28-1	GUIDE TO OVER-THE-NEEDLE CATHETER USE

Gauge	Use
14–16	Multiple trauma, heart surgery, and transplants
18	Major surgery or trauma and blood administration
20	Minor surgery or trauma and blood administration
22–24	Pediatric clients, clients with small veins, for platelets and plasma (Avoid this small gauge with packed RBCs, whole blood, and antibiotics.)

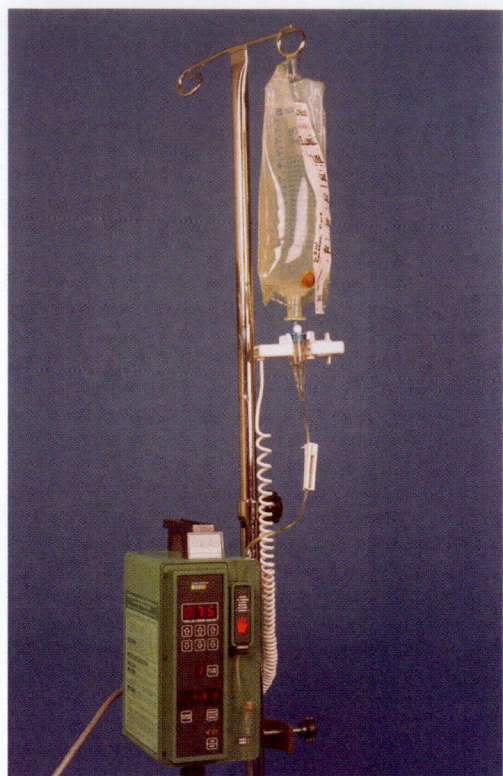

Figure 28-5. ■ Controller device.

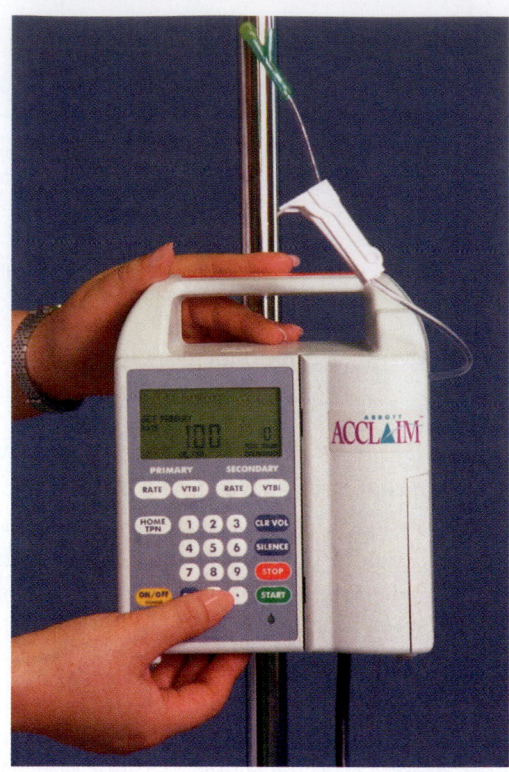

Figure 28-6. ■ Positive-pressure pump.

of pumps, with features such as more sensitive alarms and the ability to track the fluid volume infused.

- *Volumetric pumps* may require a type of cassette or cartridge to be used with the machine. The volumetric pump measures the volume of fluid that needs to be given at a specific rate, indicates the time period that said amount will take to infuse, and keeps track of the total amount of fluid infused over a period of time.
- *Peristaltic pumps* are used primarily to deliver enteral feedings. They use a rotary disk or rollers to compress the tubing, which propels the fluid forward. (See Procedure 28-6 ■ on page 690.)
- *Syringe pumps* provide precise infusion, controlling the rate by means of the drive speed and syringe size. They are valuable for critical infusions and small doses of high-potency drugs. Syringe pumps are used with patient-controlled analgesia (PCA).
- Other advanced systems are also in use, such as multichannel and *dual-channel pumps* that are computer controlled and deliver several medications concurrently or intermittently with the infusion solution (Figure 28-7 ■).
- Portable or *ambulatory pumps* are compact and lightweight. However, the life of the battery system is limited and requires frequent recharging.

As caregiver, you must be aware of the functional characteristics of the selected device prior to its use. Always read the manufacturer's directions before using any infusion pump. Typically the facility that employs you will provide you with in-service training on the electronic devices used.

NURSING CONSIDERATIONS FOR INFUSION DEVICES

- Peristaltic regulators are not appropriate for administration of blood due to their squeezing action.
- The administration set's drip chamber must be only half full to allow the sensor to monitor the drip rate; most sensors are placed at the top of the chamber.
- Tubing cassettes should be inverted for priming.
- Rate regulation devices do not take the place of nursing assessment; accurate function of the machine should be verified at regular intervals.
- All solutions should be labeled with flow strip tubing.
- Piggyback administration sets increase the risk of introducing air bubbles. Place them above the air detector device.
- Always check the package instructions to determine if a filter is compatible with a pump or controller.

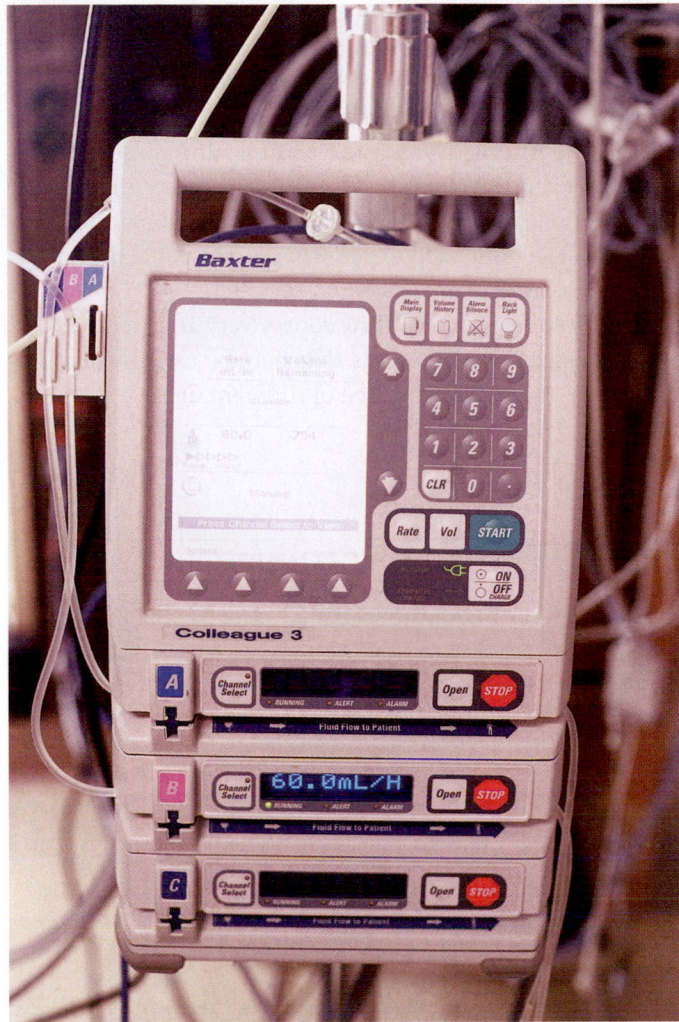

Figure 28-7. ■ Multichannel or dual-channel infusion pump.

- If the electronic device's alarm is going off, check for the most obvious problems in a systematic way: Follow the IV tubing from the insertion site to the IV bag. Look for kinked tubing; for instance, the client may be sitting on it. Check that roller/slide clamps are released. If the problem is the result of an infiltrate, remove and restart the IV in another location, either above the previous site or in the other arm.

ACCESSORY EQUIPMENT

Most transfusions do not need to be warmed. However, fluid/blood warmers are available and may be indicated for a rapid or massive transfusion, a neonatal transfusion exchange, or a client with potent cold agglutinins.

INTERMITTENT INFUSION DEVICE (PERIPHERAL SALINE LOCK/HEPARIN LOCK, PRN DEVICE)

An intermittent infusion device maintains venous access in the client who must receive IV medications regularly or intermittently but who does not require a continuous flow of fluids. The advantages of this device are that it:

- Minimizes the risk of fluid overload and electrolyte imbalance.
- Reduces cost.
- Increases client comfort and mobility.
- Reduces client anxiety.
- Allows for collection of blood samples.
- Allows access for emergency administration of medication.

Routine flushing is necessary to ensure and maintain patency of the cannula. It also prevents mixing of medications and solutions that are incompatible. LPNs/LVNs who hold an IV therapy certificate can instill a minute amount of heparin or normal saline into an intermittent infusion lock for the purpose of patency. Licensees must demonstrate competency prior to performing this procedure. (See Procedure 28-7 ■ on page 692.) Flushing is documented on the medication record/sheet and by the same LPN in the nurse's notes. Documentation includes date and time, amount given, patency of site, condition of site, client's tolerance of procedure, and LPN/LVN initials.

The CDC recommends that heparin be used only when intermittent infusion devices are being used for blood sampling. Studies indicate that 0.9% sodium chloride (normal saline) is just as effective as heparin in maintaining catheter patency and reducing phlebitis at the IV site.

IV Rate Calculations

IV rates can be calculated in a variety of ways. The infusion rate of the IV solution passes through and is regulated by the drip chamber. **Drip factors** (the rates at which IV solution passes through the drip chamber and into the tubing) vary by manufacturer and are found on the administration set box (Box 28-2 ■). When the physician writes an IV therapy order, it includes type of solution, quantity of **infusate** (the solution being administered by IV route), the time frame for administration, and, depending on the facility, the milliliters per hour. The nurse regulates the flow rate manually or by an electronic infusion device.

BOX 28-2	DRIP FACTORS
Infusion Administration Sets	**gtt/mL**
Standard sets (macrodrip)	10
	15
	20
Minidrip (microdrip; pediatric drip)	60
Buretrol set	60
Blood administration set	10
	6

The nurse is responsible for the regulation of flow rates by determining the infusion time or the total hours to be infused, calculating milliliters per hour and drops per minute. The nurse adjusts the rate by using the roller clamp on the tubing and counting the drops per minute. Hold the watch up to the drip chamber at eye level to count the drops manually for 1 minute. The nurse may also set the infusion rate on an electronic infusion device; see the following standard formula:

$$\frac{\text{Amount of fluid (in mL)} \times \text{drop factor}}{\text{Time to infuse in minutes}} = \text{drops per minute}$$

Problem: 1,000 mL of D_5W is to run over 8 hours with a drip factor of 10. What are the drops per minute?

$$\frac{\text{Amount of fluid (1,000 mL)} \times \text{drop factor (10)}}{\text{Time to infuse in minutes (8 hours)}} = \text{drops per minute}$$

Determine the fluid per hour: **1,000 mL** divided by **8 hours** = **125 mL**. Time to infuse is now 60 minutes or 1 hour.

$$\frac{\text{Amount of fluid (125 mL)} \times \text{drop factor (10)}}{\text{Time to infuse in minutes (60 min)}} = \text{drops per minute}$$

$$\frac{125 \times 10}{60} = \text{gtt/mL}$$

$$\frac{125 \times 1}{6} = 21 \text{ gtt/mL}$$

Here is a shorter, more practical method:

$$\frac{60 \text{ (minutes)}}{\text{Drop factor}}$$

The drop factor divided into 60 will give a number to be divided into the milliliters per hour. If the milliliters per hour rate are known, it is easy to find the drops per minute. The infusion time in hours divided into the amount to be infused gives milliliters per hour.

Problem: IV infusion of D_5LR 1,000 mL to run at 125 mL/h. The drop factor is 20 gtt/mL. What is the rate in gtt/min?

$$60 \div 20 = 3$$

$$125 \div 3 = 41.6 \text{ or } 42 \text{ gtt/minute (round off to the nearest whole number)}$$

Intravenous medications are not typically given by the LPN/LVN by secondary lines, push, or bolus. Check your state's nurse practice act for scope of practice.

Preparing the Client for IV Therapy

Client fear and anxiety about IV therapy are minimized through teaching. The LPN/LVN should instruct the client on the purpose of the IV, the mechanics of the insertion process, and the degree of discomfort expected. If the client is agitated or in pain, it might be advisable to delay the procedure. Distraction techniques are encouraged. Taking deep breaths and releasing them slowly during insertion is one technique. Alternately, tensing and relaxing muscle groups tends to focus the client on these actions rather than on the IV insertion. If the client has been prescribed pain medication, it is recommended to perform the procedure during the drug's peak effectiveness.

Children may find IV procedures very frightening. Box 28-3 ■ describes adaptations that may be useful when providing IV therapy to children of different ages.

| BOX 28-3 | PEDIATRIC CONSIDERATIONS |

Adapting IV Procedures for Children

All children. EMLA cream is often used with pediatric clients to reduce or eliminate pain from IV insertion. It can be used on infants as well as older children, and is especially useful if repeat IVs are indicated. (EMLA must have 15 to 20 minutes to provide effective pain relief, so it probably will not be used in an emergency situation.)

Infants. An infant's response to IV therapy is reflexive, with crying, body movements, and pulling back the extremities. Use distractions such as shaking a rattle, singing a song, or providing a toy. After the procedure, cuddle and rock the baby using soothing tones. (Suckling is allowed and is a great comfort.)

Toddlers. The toddler response is physical—hitting, biting, kicking, and screaming. The child may use the entire body to resist the nurse. Compliance may be improved by allowing the toddler to explore equipment such as the armboard, or to hold the tape. Use a treatment room to insert the IV, so that the child's room remains a "safe" place.

Preschoolers. The child 3 to 6 years old should be prepared for IV therapy just before the procedure is performed. Allow the child as much control as possible. Tell the child that crying is permitted but that it is important to hold still. An assistant should help manage the child. Suggest the child take a deep breath and blow air as if blowing bubbles. Another technique is to have the child push his or her hands together, thereby concentrating on the motion rather than the IV injection.

School-aged children. Children of school age like to try to be "grown up." Procedures should be explained shortly before they are to be performed. Generally, children of this age can be guided to use distraction. Remind them that it is all right to say "ow!" If possible, allow them some control in the situation.

Adolescents. Teens generally are as accepting of IV therapy as adults. They should be informed fully about what to expect. Because of body image issues, they may be concerned about the appearance of a continuous IV infusion line or infusion port.

Anatomy of Peripheral Veins

To perform IV therapy, LPNs/LVNs need an accurate understanding of the integumentary and venous systems. It is important to develop the ability to assess veins and determine suitability for venous access. Sites in children are more difficult to access. Figure 28-8 ■ illustrates venous access sites in adults and in children. Review the major veins in Figure 33-7 ⊕.

Veins are thin walled and less muscular than arteries (Table 28-2 ■). They can be distended easily under minimal pressure. Vein walls have three layers: The outermost layer, the *tunica adventitia*, surrounds and supports the vessel. It is made up of connective tissue and its appearance is likened to that of tree bark. This is the layer of the vein that allows movement with the skin. Movement of the vein under the skin is referred to as a *rolling vein*. When the vein is accessed with a venous catheter, the nurse can feel a pop upon penetrating the tunica adventitia.

The middle layer is the *tunica media*. This layer is composed of the muscle and elastic tissues that constrict and distend the vein. This venous layer can go into *venospasm*, causing pain and partially occluding the vessel. This layer is less rigid than the outermost layer and can have a tendency to collapse, resulting in what is referred to as *disappearing veins*.

The innermost layer is the *tunica intima*, or endothelial lining. This layer is thin and supports the valves pointing toward the heart, which prevent blood backflow. When a tourniquet is applied, the valves can be identified as visible bulges along the distended vein. Inaccurate venipuncture may traumatize the tunica intima, producing roughened endothelial edges. Platelets can adhere to the roughened area and lead to clot formation. (See Procedure 28-8 ■ on page 693.)

The most common sites for venipuncture are the veins of the hands and arms. When assessing suitability of a vein, the nurse palpates for a round, stable, elastic vein (Table 28-3 ■).

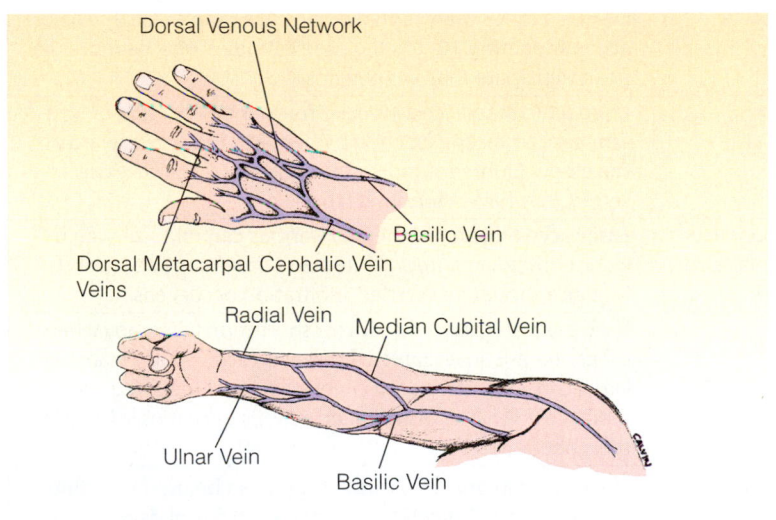

A

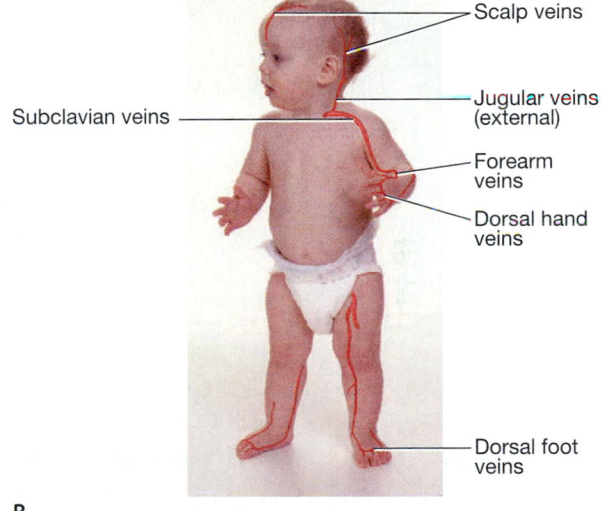

B

Figure 28-8. ■ Sites for venipuncture.

TABLE 28-2	Differences between Veins and Arteries	
	VEINS	**ARTERIES**
Blood color	Dark red, unoxygenated blood	Bright red, oxygenated blood
Pulse	No pulse	Pulsation with ventricular contraction
Valves	Seen as bulges along the vein Keep the blood flowing toward the heart	Do not occur in arteries where blood flows away from the heart
Location	Superficial veins are found just under the skin. They are the veins normally used for IV access.	Arteries are found deeper in the skin and surrounded by muscle, which protects them One in 10 are superficially located and identified as aberrant arteries
Tissue supplied	Multiple, and appear in a network formation. An injury to one usually is not serious because another will perform its function.	Supplies one area. An injury or occlusion can endanger the tissue supplied.

TABLE 28-3	Superficial Veins of the Arm and Suitability for IV Therapy	
VEINS	**LOCATION**	**IV SUITABILITY**
Digital vein	Found along lateral and dorsal areas of the fingers	Used when other sites are unavailable, for short-term therapy. Isotonic solutions and small-gauge (22-gauge) needles are appropriate for these veins. Use armboard or tongue blade to hold securely in place.
Metacarpal vein	Found on the dorsum of the hand, and formed by union of the digital veins between the knuckles	The hand veins are the best place to begin IV therapy because they are the most distal, allowing the veins above to be used as they are needed. Venous cannulas of 22 to 20 gauge with a short needle are easily inserted. Wrist mobility limited.
Cephalic vein	Formed by the metacarpal veins and function in the radial part of the forearm and upper arm	These can handle large-gauge needles from 22 to 16 gauge. Veins may have a tendency to roll. Larger veins can be used for rapid fluid infusion. Hypertonic fluids and fluids that irritate the veins can be infused more easily.
Antecubital cephalic vein	Found in the antecubital fossa, in front of the elbow	Antecubital site should be avoided unless warranted by an emergency. This area is difficult to splint and may be uncomfortable. Change site within 24 hours.
Accessory cephalic vein	Found along the radial bone following the metacarpal veins of the thumb	May be shorter than cephalic veins. Medium to large veins accommodating 18- to 20-gauge cannulas. May be more difficult to palpate than other veins.
Basilic vein	Follows along the ulnar side of the forearm	More difficult to access than veins on the radial side of forearm but can be approached by bending the arm upward at the elbow. Eighteen- to 22-gauge cannulas can be easily inserted. May have a tendency to roll.
Median vein	Forms from veins on the palm of the hand and extends up the front of the forearm on the ulnar side	Easily accessible for IV therapy. Various cannula sizes can be inserted. Median antebrachial areas have many nerve endings and should be avoided. Infiltration occurs easily.
Great saphenous vein	Found at the internal malleolus of the foot	Used as a last resort. Excellent for short-term IV therapy when other sites are unavailable. Large veins can accommodate larger cannulas. Can impair circulation of the lower leg and there is an increased risk of deep venous thrombosis. Avoid in the diabetic client.
Dorsal venous network	Found on the dorsal area of the foot	Suitable for infants and toddlers and can be used for adults as a last resort. Difficult to see. Increased risk of deep venous thrombosis. Avoid in the diabetic client.

The vein should feel bouncy, spongy, rubbery—similar to the feel of a water balloon.

Factors Affecting IV Site Selection

When selecting an IV site, these factors must first be considered:

- *Duration of IV therapy:* Select a vein that can support IV therapy for at least 72 hours. Begin therapy at the most distal area for long-term therapy, avoiding fingers. Follow routine site rotation, and alternate arms.
- *Cannula size:* Hemodilution is important to prevent vein irritation. The gauge of the cannula should be as small as possible to allow dilution as the infusate enters the vein.

The appropriate size for most situations is a 20- to 22-gauge cannula.

- *Type of solution:* Hypertonic solutions, potassium chloride, and antibiotics are irritating to the vein walls. Select a large vein to accommodate these solutions.
- *Condition of the vein:* Choose a soft, straight vein for venipuncture. Avoid veins that are bruised, red, swollen, or found near a previously infected site. Restart an IV infusion above a previous site. Palpate the vein and move your finger down the vein, observing how it refills.

clinical ALERT

A sluggish refill indicates that the vein is prone to collapsing.

- *Client's level of consciousness:* A combative client may make it difficult to secure the IV site. Use an armboard to protect the site. Avoid the wrist area if restraints are being used.
- *Client activity:* If the client is using crutches or a walker or uses the hands to steady movement and to get up and around, avoid the wrist and hands.
- *Client's age:* Veins in the elderly are more fragile; approach their veins cautiously and gently. Determine the need for a tourniquet. Infants have fewer available IV sites. Children under age 4 have increased body fat, so veins in the hands and feet may be the only accessible sites (see Figure 28-8).
- *Dominant hand:* The dominant hand usually has the most identifiable veins; avoid if possible. Active movement of the extremity can displace the cannula. Take into account the preference of the client.
- *Presence of preexisting disease:* Clients with dehydration or vascular disease can have limited available veins. Avoid sites affected by cerebrovascular accident, mastectomy, amputation, and orthopedic surgery or plastic surgery of the hand or arm. Clients on chemotherapy may have poor venous access. An extremity that has a shunt or graft access for dialysis should not be used for IV insertion. Clients on anticoagulants have a tendency to bleed.

The nurse is responsible for taking necessary precautions when choosing an IV site. Some guidelines include limiting tourniquet pressure for venous distention and use of the smallest cannula necessary to accomplish the necessary infusion.

Venipuncture Procedure

Prior to inserting an IV catheter, the LPN/LVN will check the physician's order, perform hand hygiene, collect and prepare the equipment, prepare and assess the client, and select the appropriate site. (See Procedure 28-2 on page 683.) In preparing the IV site, the nurse may need to remove excess hair to facilitate catheter insertion, taping, and dressing adherence. Infusion Nurse Society (INS) suggests the use of scissors for this because a razor can cause impairment of skin integrity. Ensure that the client does not have an iodine allergy prior to prepping the skin. Prep with alcohol, using a circular motion from the inside out, and allow the area to dry for 1 minute. Alcohol is an antimicrobial agent. It removes oils from the skin, and can be used alone if the client has an allergy to iodine (Betadine). If the client is not allergic, prep the area with Betadine, which is a germicidal solution. After drying for 1 minute, Betadine is effective for up to 6 hours.

Successful first sticks depend on proper preparation. Feeling rushed or nervous may lead to failure of the insertion. Put the client at ease by engaging in conversation. When the client is extremely nervous and has a needle phobia, a vasovagal response can ensue. The client can present with tachycardia and hypertension prior to insertion. Postcannulation, the client can experience bradycardia, pallor, diaphoresis, syncope, and a drop in blood pressure. These usually occur immediately. Keep the needle out of sight until the last minute, as this may decrease the severity of anxiety.

Here are some options for tourniquets (Figure 28-9 ■):

- A *flat rubberized band* can be used, but be careful not to pull hair. Avoid twisting the band, and keep the tails of the band away from the insertion site.
- A *Velcro-closure band* is more comfortable and easier to handle than the traditional rubberized band.
- A *blood pressure cuff* at 30 mm/Hg is preferred by some clinicians, especially with elderly clients or those with fragile veins. This prevents excessive engorgement.

(See Procedure 28-8 on page 693.)

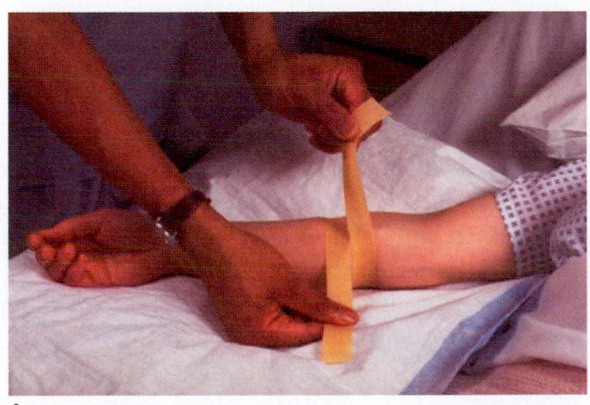

A

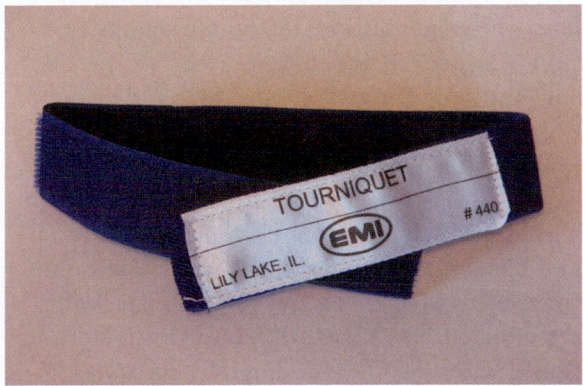

B

Figure 28-9. ■ **A.** Rubber tourniquet; **B.** Velcro tourniquet.

LOCAL ANESTHETIC

Lidocaine 1% without epinephrine can be used to numb the skin prior to a needle stick. However, there is controversy about this practice. The INS has stated that local anesthesia, including lidocaine, should not be used routinely for the insertion of a cannula.

Before using lidocaine, the IV nurse must receive instruction in the proper procedure and demonstrate knowledge, skill, and ability. Also, the nurse should have a physician's order. Check for history of allergies. Lidocaine may expose the client to complications, including:

- Allergic reaction
- Anaphylaxis
- Inadvertent injection of drug into the vascular system
- Obliteration of the vein

When lidocaine is used, the client feels touch and pressure and will have muscle control, but will not experience pain. The dose used is 0.1 mL of 1% lidocaine. The effect is felt within 15 to 30 seconds and lasts 30 to 45 minutes.

TECHNIQUES IN VENIPUNCTURE

Gloves should be applied before venipuncture is initiated. Two methods are used for vein entry.

- *Direct method* or one-step entry. The cannula enters the skin and the vein in one quick motion.
- *Indirect method* or two-step entry. The cannula is inserted through the skin; then the vein is relocated and entered.

Approaching the vein with the bevel up and to the side of the vein allows the nurse to feel the pop upon entering the vein. The vein will be easier to penetrate if the skin is held taut and the vein is pulled down slightly.

Several methods are used to advance the cannula. Smooth cannula insertion and advancement of the catheter prevent the cannula from being displaced. Four methods are described here.

1. The one-step technique is used by the more experienced nurse. In a one-step insertion, the cannula enters the skin and is advanced in one step.
2. "Floating" the cannula into the vein, advance the cannula one-third to one-half its length into the vein or until you see a backflow of blood. Attach the tubing and start the IV solution at a slow rate. Use one hand to maintain vein stretch while advancing the cannula with one hand.
3. For a two-handed method, insert the cannula into the vein half the length of the cannula or until you see a backflow of blood. With one hand, hold the hub of the cannula; with the other hand, retract the stylet. Maintain the vein stretch and advance the cannula until it is inserted completely.

4. When using catheters with a raised lip on the hub, push the cannula off the stylet, advancing the cannula halfway into the vein. Pressing your forefinger or thumb against the hub's lip, slide the cannula forward. It will move off the stylet and into the vein.

If you are not immediately successful in inserting the cannula, gently feel for the tip of the cannula. This gives you an idea of whether it is above, below, to the right or left of the vein. Do not spend too much time probing for a vein. If you are unable to locate the vein, remove the cannula and attempt venipuncture in another site.

Stabilize the catheter by one of three methods (see Chapter 24 ⚭):

- U method
- H method
- Chevron method

Determine whether an armboard is necessary to stabilize the catheter. Implement dressing management, with either a gauze dressing or a transparent semipermeable membrane (TSM). (See also Procedures 28-9 and 28-10 ■ starting on page 695.)

Documentation of IV therapy includes date of insertion, location, gauge and length of cannula, type of solution administered, client's response, and signature of the nurse inserting the IV.

PLACING IV CANNULAS IN INFANTS

Placing IV cannulas in infants requires expertise and specialized training. Scalp veins in infants are suitable for use until about 12 to 18 months of age. When scalp veins are used, always point the cannula downward in the direction of the infant's heart. Lower extremity veins are suitable for infants and toddlers, but are used as a last resort in adults. EMLA cream can help to prevent pain and anxiety in infants.

Peripheral IV Therapy Complications

Complications of IV therapy may be either localized or systemic. The nurse must take contributing factors into consideration. The following factors help the nurse determine the technique needed to start the IV, the need for restraints, the size of needle, the importance of timing (STAT or as needed), the client's level of understanding of the procedure, and so on:

- Age of the client
- Client's medical condition
- Skin integrity

- Site of infusion
- Duration of infusion
- Method of infusion
- Site and line maintenance
- Client activity
- Insertion technique

LOCALIZED COMPLICATIONS

Careful and frequent observation of the IV site will lead to early intervention for localized complications. Table 28-4 ■ lists localized IV complications, causes, nursing interventions, and preventive measures. Table 28-5 ■ provides the phlebitis scale for one of the most serious localized complications. (See also Procedure 28-11 ■ on page 700.)

SYSTEMIC COMPLICATIONS

Systemic complications of IV therapy can develop quickly or insidiously. They can be life threatening and must be recognized early to initiate prompt treatment. Table 28-6 ■ lists systemic IV complications of IV therapy, with causes, nursing interventions, and preventive measures.

Blood Transfusions

To provide safe therapeutic transfusion therapy, the nurse must be knowledgeable about the circulatory system and the management of blood products. The LPN/LVN is responsible for understanding and carrying out the facility criteria, policies, and procedures in transfusion therapy. Careful observation of the client for signs and symptoms of

TABLE 28-4	Local IV Complications		
COMPLICATION AND MANIFESTATIONS	**CAUSES**	**NURSING INTERVENTIONS**	**PREVENTIVE MEASURES**

Phlebitis (inflammation of the vein)
Tenderness at the tip of the catheter
Redness at the tip of the catheter and along the vein
Edema
Febrile
Vein is hardened on palpation
Types of phlebitis
   Mechanical
   Chemical
   Bacterial
	Friction related to cannula movement
	Cannula left in the vein for an extended period of time
	Clotting at the tip of the catheter
	High pH, low pH, or high osmolarity solutions causing vein irritation
	Rapid infusion
	Infection
	Increased risk with total parenteral nutrition (TPN), burns, multiple sticks, and immunosuppression
		Remove cannula.
		Apply warm compress to site.
		Notify physician.
		Document signs and symptoms, phlebitis scale (Table 28-5), and interventions.
			Tape cannula securely.
			Use filter.
			Review insertion technique.

Infiltration (passage of the IV solution out of the vein and into the surrounding tissue) Edema above the IV site Uncomfortable, painful burning Coolness at the site No backflow when IV bag lowered Tightness and blanching at the site IV rate decreased	Cannula dislodged or has perforated through the vein	Discontinue cannula. Apply cold pack and then warm compress. Elevate extremity. Assess circulation and capillary refill. Reinsert cannula above infiltration site or use other extremity. Document.	Observe site frequently. Avoid obscuring the site. Teach client to observe and report changes. Do not use tape that encircles the arm, causing constriction and obscuring the site.
Hematoma (pooling of blood in the tissue) Tenderness at IV site Bruising around the site Inability to advance or flush IV site	Vein has perforated through other vein wall at the time of insertion Leakage of blood from needle displacement	Remove venipuncture device. Apply pressure and warm compresses. Check for continued bleeding. Document.	Select a vein that accommodates the catheter needing to be inserted. Use a blood pressure cuff for a tourniquet. Release tourniquet once insertion is achieved.

(continued)

TABLE 28-4	Local IV Complications (continued)		
COMPLICATION AND MANIFESTATIONS	**CAUSES**	**NURSING INTERVENTIONS**	**PREVENTIVE MEASURES**
Venospasm (constriction of the inner lining of the vein) First symptom is pain along the vein Slow flow rate Blanched skin over the site	Common with blood transfusion or cold fluids Severe vein irritation from drugs or fluids Rapid IV flow rate	Apply warm compress over the vein. Slow the IV flow rate.	Use a blood warmer device. Use fluids at room temperature when possible.
Vasovagal response (a response characterized by tachycardia and hypertension prior to IV needle insertion, and by bradycardia, pallor, diaphoresis, syncope, and a drop in blood pressure after needle insertion) Vein collapse during venipuncture Pallor Sweating, faintness, dizziness, and nausea Low blood pressure	Anxiety or pain	Lower the head of the bed. Ask client to take deep breaths. Check vital signs.	Prepare and reassure the client. Use a local anesthetic if nurse has been authorized to do so. Remove venipuncture device.
Thrombosis (clot formation in the vein) Painful, reddened, and edematous vein Sluggish IV rate Febrile Malaise Unable to flush medication lock	Injury to the endothelial cells of the vein; platelets adhere and development of thrombus ensues Multiple sticks Through and through perforations of the vein	Reinsert IV in other extremity. Apply warm compresses. Be observant of potential infection process. Document.	Review venipuncture techniques. Use infusion devices to avoid blood from backing up. Use filters.
Thrombophlebitis (condition with inflammation and clot formation in a vein) Severe pain Reddened; edema; and vein is hardened Visible red line above the insertion site	Thrombosis and inflammation Use of lower extremity for infusion High pH, low pH, or high osmolarity solutions, causing vein irritation Insertion technique Client's condition	Remove venipuncture device. Reinsert IV in other extremity. Apply warm compresses. Document.	Observe site frequently. Secure catheter to prevent movement. Use proper IV insertion technique.
Nerve, Tendon, or Ligament Damage Severe pain similar to an electrical shock Numbness Muscle contraction May suffer delayed reaction Paralysis Deformity	Venipuncture technique Improper splinting or taping is too tight	Stop procedure. Document.	Review venipuncture technique. Avoid repeated attempts to insert venipuncture device into the same tissues. Tape securely without being too constricting. Pad armboards.

TABLE 28-4	Local IV Complications (continued)		
COMPLICATION AND MANIFESTATIONS	**CAUSES**	**NURSING INTERVENTIONS**	**PREVENTIVE MEASURES**
Extravasation (severe infiltration of a vesicant solution into the surrounding tissue) Severe pain or burning Skin sloughing Tissue necrosis Edema Skin tightness Coolness over the site Blanching Slow infusion rate Dressing may be moist	Venipuncture device dislodged Perforation of the vein wall Mechanical friction	Stop infusion and aspirate any fluid. Administer antidote per facility policy immediately. Apply cold packs unless vinca alkaloids are being infused, in which case cold application would be contraindicated. Photograph site per facility policy. Elevate arm per facility policy. Notify physician. Document.	Be skilled at IV insertion technique. Have knowledge of vesicant solutions. Access blood return of IV prior to infusion. Assess the condition of client's vein. Assess visibility of IV site.

TABLE 28-5	Phlebitis Scale	
STAGE	**INDICATORS**	**NURSING INTERVENTIONS**
0	No pain, redness, or edema at site	None
1+	Redness may extend above the IV site up to 1½ in.; may or may not be painful	Remove cannula.
2+	Redness may extend above the IV site up to 1½ in.; painful, edema	Remove cannula. Elevate extremity. Apply cool pack first and then warm compresses.
3+	Redness, edema, painful, and palpable cord less than 3 in. above the IV site	Remove cannula. Elevate extremity. Apply cool pack first and then warm compresses. Notify physician.
4+	Redness, edema, painful, induration, palpable cord less than 3 in. above the IV site	Remove cannula and culture tip. Elevate extremity. Apply cool pack first and then warm compresses. Notify physician.
5+	Purulent drainage, redness, edema, painful, induration, palpable cord less than 3 in. above the IV site	Remove cannula. Culture drainage, tip of the cannula. Elevate extremity. Apply cool pack first and then warm compresses. Notify physician.

transfusion reactions and condition changes can avert potential life-threatening problems. The use of 0.9% sodium chloride (NS) is common with transfusion therapy and is established in policies and procedures. (Box 28-4 ■ discusses cultural considerations surrounding blood transfusions.)

Clients receiving transfusions are tested for ABO and Rh grouping. Antibody screening and compatibility testing are performed prior to infusion of blood or blood products.

The purpose is to prevent antigen–antibody reactions and identify antibodies the recipient may have.

There are three types of blood donor collection methods. **Homologous** collection is a blood donation by someone other than the person receiving the blood. Strict guidelines have been in place to make sure the blood is safe for use. **Autologous** blood donation is when the client provides his or her own blood. This option is for a person who is likely

TABLE 28-6	Systemic Complications of IV Therapy		
COMPLICATIONS AND MANIFESTATIONS	**CAUSES**	**NURSING INTERVENTIONS**	**PREVENTIVE MEASURES**
Circulatory overload (excess fluid in the vasculature) Discomfort Neck vein engorgement Respiratory distress (pulmonary edema) Crackles Changes in I&O	Flow rate too rapid Error in fluid requirements Client with renal or cardiac condition	Raise the head of bed. Administer oxygen. Notify physician. Administer medications per physician order. Document.	Use infusion devices appropriately. Monitor infusions frequently. Make accurate fluid calculations.
Septicemia, Bacteremia (virulent microorganisms in the bloodstream from a localized source of infection; bacteria in the bloodstream; *blood poisoning*) Fluctuating febrile state Chills Elevated WBC Malaise IV site contaminated; no signs of infection at site Hypotension Tachycardia and tachypnea Mental status changes Diarrhea Vascular collapse, shock, and death	Nosocomial infection Primarily staphylococci and enterococci infections Lack of consistent hand hygiene Client risk factors: age, immunity, other infections Infusion factors: catheter, solutions, insertion site, length of infusion Inadequately maintained insertion site	Notify physician. Check vital signs. Monitor condition changes. Start antimicrobial therapy per physician order. Reinsert IV catheter in opposite extremity. Obtain cultures of equipment and client's blood. Document.	Practice consistent hand hygiene. Inspect equipment and solutions for malfunctions. Use Betadine for antimicrobial action. Ensure sterile dressing to insertion site. Monitor insertion site routinely. Change site per facility/INS protocol.
Air embolism (or venous air embolism, VAE, the entry of gas into the peripheral or central vasculature) Respiratory distress (dyspnea, cyanosis, tachypnea, wheezes, cough, and pulmonary edema) Inconsistent breath sounds Weakened pulse Palpitations, chest pain, and tachycardia Confusion, anxiousness, seizures Mental status changes Hemiplegia, aphasia, coma, and death	Solution runs dry Hanging a new IV bag and not clearing the line of air from a bag that ran dry Air in administration tubing cassettes Improper technique for tubing changes Loose connections	Place in Trendelenburg position. Call for assistance. Administer oxygen. Check vital signs. Notify physician. Keep emergency equipment on hand. Document.	Remove air from administration sets. Vent air from ports using a syringe. Use filters. Follow routine changes for tubing and dressings. Hang IV solutions prior to the bag running dry. Use infusion devices to monitor fluid infusion.
Allergic Reactions Itching Runny nose Bronchospasm Wheezing Rash Edema at site Anaphylactic reaction (within minutes up to an hour after exposure) Flushing, chills, anxiety, itching, agitation, ear throbbing, wheezing, coughing, convulsions, and death	Allergens, medications	Stop infusion immediately. Ensure patent airway. Notify physician. Administer antihistamine, steroid, anti-inflammatory, and antipyretic per physician order. Epinephrine is usually administered and can be repeated. Document.	Check client's allergy history. Test dose of medication, e.g., antibiotics. Monitor clients in the first 15 minutes of the infusion of a new drug.

TABLE 28-6	Systemic Complications of IV Therapy (continued)		
COMPLICATIONS AND MANIFESTATIONS	**CAUSES**	**NURSING INTERVENTIONS**	**PREVENTIVE MEASURES**
Speed shock (reaction to rapid induction of foreign substance or medication into the vascular system) Dizziness Headache Chest tightness Hypotension Irregular pulse Shock	IV administration of medications or fluids at a rapid rate	Ask for assistance. Notify the physician. Administer antidote. Administer emergency medications. Document.	Use microdrip administration sets (60 gtt/mL). Use infusion control flow devices. Avoid movement of the catheter. Monitor piggyback infusion.

> **BOX 28-4**   **CULTURAL PULSE POINTS**
>
> **Blood Transfusions**
> There are several religious or ethnic groups that set limitations on blood transfusion or prohibit them altogether. Jehovah's Witnesses, for example, believe that the Bible prohibits the consumption, storage, and transfusion of blood even in cases of emergency. In the last 20 years there has been a strong interest in bloodless surgery. This surgery may involve the use of techniques such as cell salvage, in which a device recycles and cleans blood from a client during an operation and redirects it back to the client's body. Other options include the use of blood substitutes that expand blood volume to prevent shock. Laser or sonic scalpels can be used to minimize bleeding during an operation.

to need blood for an elective surgery and donates prior to the operation. **Designated** blood is blood that is donated by friends and relatives of the client.

The main functions of the cardiovascular system are to deliver oxygenated blood and nutrients to the tissues. This transport system then removes waste substances from the tissues. Objectives for administering a blood transfusion are to:

- Restore and maintain blood volume.
- Improve the oxygen-carrying capacity of the circulatory system.
- Restore and maintain coagulation factors.
- Treat blood deficiencies such as anemia and other hematologic disorders.
- Permit neonatal blood exchange.

Various types of blood or blood components may be transfused (Table 28-7 ■). The client's condition and lab values determine the type of blood required. (See Procedure 28-12 ■.)

TRANSFUSION REACTIONS

Blood transfusions create a significant risk to clients for transfusion reactions (Table 28-8 ■). The nurse infusing blood products is charged with recognizing adverse signs and symptoms of a transfusion reaction. Implementing immediate action to stop or reverse the effects of transfusion

reaction can be lifesaving. Treat all reactions seriously until proven otherwise.

Monitor vital signs and remain with the client. Notify the blood bank and laboratory because urine and blood samples

clinical ALERT

Upon suspicion of a transfusion reaction, stop the transfusion, change the IV tubing, and start a saline solution infusion at a keep-open rate. Do not discard the blood container or administration set; they will be returned to the blood bank. Notify the physician.

will need to be obtained. Verify labels on blood containers with corresponding client identifications. Document time of the reaction, date, nursing interventions, including vital signs, specimens sent, treatment, and the client's response. Many facilities require a transfusion reaction report form.

Complications from blood transfusions can occur when blood is contaminated or the recipient's body reacts to donor lymphocytes. Table 28-9 ■ describes potential complications, manifestations, causes, and nursing interventions.

NURSING CARE

PRIORITIZING NURSING CARE

Priorities for the LPN/LVN in IV therapy include assessing the IV site for pain, swelling, phlebitis, or infection, and monitoring the infusion rate. It is important to review related lab values (especially sodium, potassium, glucose, and hematocrit). Important measurements include daily weights, intake and output, and body temperature.

ASSESSING

The nurse caring for a client with an IV observes the catheter site for signs of infection or infiltration (redness, warmth, dampness). The LPN/LVN assesses the condition of the site and the client's tolerance of IV therapy, and provides dressing changes as indicated.

TABLE 28-7	Blood/Blood Components		
COMPONENT	**INDICATOR**		**NURSING INTERVENTIONS**
Whole blood (500 mL) Composed of RBCs, plasma, WBCs, and platelets	To restore blood volume (most whole blood is broken down into three components)		Rarely transfused today. Use 20-gauge catheter or larger for infusion. Rate is 2–4 hours. Whole blood requires type and crossmatching and must be ABO identical.
Red blood cells (250–300 mL)	Improve oxygen-carrying capacity in symptomatic anemia Increase RBC mass Hemoglobin/hematocrit (H/H) values Client symptoms Blood loss Surgical procedures with blood loss of more than 1,200 mL		Determine severity of anemia and whether diet or vitamins could be an alternative. Assess client's age, presence of cardiopulmonary or vascular problems. Administer over 1–3 hours; never exceed 4 hours. Use 16- to 20-gauge catheter. Check vital signs.
Leukocyte-reduced RBCs (poor RBCs) (200 mL)	Prevention of febrile, nonhemolytic transfusion reactions Client with multiple transfusions (e.g., with leukemia or hemophilia)		Use Pall filter. Infuse over $1\frac{1}{2}$ to 4 hours. Administer same as whole blood and PRBCs. Watch for hypotension.
Platelets (50–500 mL) Responsible for hemostasis Live up to 12 days in blood Fragmented cells without nuclei or, hemoglobin and are unable to reproduce Normal platelet value: 150,000–300,000/μL	Prevent or control bleeding from platelet deficiencies Platelet counts <10,000/μL Thrombocytopenia Acute leukemia Control active bleeding with platelet counts of less than 50,000 μL Prophylactic with massive blood transfusions Prophylactic with cardiopulmonary bypass		Transfusions can be repeated every 1–3 days. Rapid transfusion. Usual rate is 5–10 min. Effectiveness can be altered if fever, infection, or active bleeding present. Use filter. Pooled platelets should be transfused within 4 hours.
Plasma and fresh frozen plasma (FFP) (200–250 mL)	*Plasma:* Replace plasma proteins *FFP:* Provide replacement coagulation factors (V, XI) Client with multiple coagulation factor deficiencies secondary to liver disease, disseminated intravascular coagulation (DIC) Coumarin drug reversal Thrombotic thrombocytopenia purpura		*Plasma:* Infusion rate is 220 mL/h. Medications/diluents are never added to plasma. *FFP:* Infusion rate is 1–2 hours. PT greater than 19 or PTT greater than 53. Must be thawed prior to infusion, about 30 min. ABO compatibility.
Cryoprecipitate (5–20 mL/unit volumes) Factor VIII Made from insoluble portion of plasma	Factor I, VIII, XIII, and von Willebrand factor deficiency Hypofibrinogenemia Uremic clients to control bleeding		Rate is 1–2 mL/min. ABO compatible. Use 170 micron filter. Rapid transfusion. Must be thawed prior to transfusion. Units are usually pooled.
Recombinant Factor VIII Recombinant DNA technology	Hemophilia Factor VIII or IX deficiency		Use bolus infusion. Store in refrigerator. Watch for allergic reactions.
Albumin 5%–25% (50–250 mL) Colloid volume expander Heat treated to prevent viral activation and hepatitis free Equal volume to plasma	Increase plasma volume Hypovolemic shock from trauma or surgery Support blood pressure Induce diuresis		Supplied in glass bottles. Use within 4 hours of opening. No filters are required. Rapid infusion. Watch for fluid overload.

TABLE 28-8	Transfusion Reactions, Manifestations, Causes, and Nursing Interventions	
REACTIONS AND MANIFESTATIONS	**CAUSES**	**NURSING INTERVENTIONS**
Acute hemolytic transfusion reaction Tachycardia, tachypnea, burning sensations along the vein, flushing, bleeding, low back, flank pain, vascular collapse, shock, death	Hemolysis occurs when antibodies in plasma attach to antigens on the donor's RBCs.	Stop transfusion. Treat shock. Maintain blood pressure. Administer diuretics as ordered. Monitor urine output. Prepare for potential dialysis. Obtain urine/blood samples required with a transfusion reaction. Document.
Delayed hemolytic reaction Lowered H/H, low-grade fever, jaundice, malaise	Occurs as a consequence to RBC destruction by alloantibodies, immunogenicity, or previous immunization through pregnancy.	Treatment is nonspecific. Monitor H/H. Monitor renal function.
Allergic reaction Rash, hives, itching, facial flushing, runny eyes and nose, anxiety, dyspnea, and wheezing	Recipient has sensitivity to donor's plasma proteins.	Stop transfusion. Treat with antihistamine per order. Restart transfusion slowly if a mild reaction. Monitor vital signs. Mild reactions can precede major allergic reactions.
Circulatory overload Cough, dyspnea, hypertension, pulmonary congestion/edema, hypervolemia, neck vein distention, and chest constriction	Rapid blood administration; the body is unable to make adjustment to fluid load.	Stop transfusion. Elevate head of bed. Administer diuretics. Administer oxygen. Notify physician. Collect blood and urine specimens.
Febrile nonhemolytic reaction Fever, chills, headache, nausea and vomiting, chest pain, cough, and malaise	Client has sensitivities to leukocyte, platelet, or protein antigens; bacterial contamination.	Stop transfusion. Monitor vital signs. Administer antipyretic per order. Notify physician. Restart transfusion slowly.
Anaphylactic transfusion reaction Anxiety, urticaria, wheezing, hypotension, shock, cardiac arrest, or death	Occurs when donor blood with IgA proteins is transfused into an IgA-deficient recipient who has developed an IgA antibody.	Stop transfusion. Resuscitate with CPR. Maintain blood pressure. Monitor vital signs. Administer steroids per order. Administer IV fluids.

DIAGNOSING, PLANNING, AND IMPLEMENTING

Nursing diagnoses common to IV therapy are:

- *Deficient Fluid Volume*
- *Risk for Deficient Fluid Volume*
- *Excess Fluid Volume*
- *Risk for Imbalanced Fluid Volume*
- *Imbalanced Nutrition: Less than Body Requirements*
- *Deficient Knowledge*
- *Risk for Infection*

Desired outcomes for clients with IV therapy might include:

- Client will maintain fluid volume balance.
- Client's electrolytes will be maintained within normal limits.
- Client will maintain a balanced nutrition status.
- Client will understand the purpose and medical treatment plan for IV therapy.
- Client will remain free from infection related to IV therapy.

In caring for a client with an IV, the nurse performs the following interventions:

- Monitor IV infusion sites often. Assess for redness, pain, or edema at the infusion site. *Visual observation of the infusion site helps to prevent (or identify and correct) complications.*

TABLE 28-9	**Transfusion Complications, Causes, and Nursing Interventions**	
COMPLICATIONS AND MANIFESTATIONS	**CAUSES**	**NURSING INTERVENTIONS**
Hepatitis B/C Anorexia, dark urine, increased liver enzymes, jaundice, pharyngitis	Viral infection; is spread by blood and serum. Incubation is 90 days.	Treat symptomatically. Encourage client to rest. Prevent transmission to others.
Graft versus host disease Fever, diarrhea, rash, and hepatitis	Recipient reacts to donor lymphocytes; T lymphocytes are activated and proliferate, attacking the host tissue cells. Client is immunocompromised.	Treat symptomatically. Realize that morbidity is high. Use leukocyte-reducing filter. Use irradiated blood.
HIV-1 Flulike symptoms, six stages of Walter Reed classification system, chronic fungal and viral infections	Viral infection is transmitted by bodily secretions from HIV-positive individual.	Realize there is no cure. Treat symptomatically. Follow CDC Standard Precautions.
Hyperkalemia (potassium toxicity) ECG changes, bradycardia, muscle twitching, asystole, diarrhea, oliguria to anuria to renal failure	Occurs most often in multiple transfusions. Potassium is released into blood during RBC destruction.	Stop or slow transfusion. Notify physician. Monitor EKG and potassium levels. Remove excess potassium.
Sepsis Febrile, chills, nausea and vomiting, diarrhea, hypotension, shock	Occurs when blood is contaminated.	Stop transfusion. Return blood container and tubing to the blood bank. Obtain blood culture. Administer antibiotics, fluid, steroids, and vasopressors as ordered.

■ Make sure bedding is not crushing the tubing or slowing flow and that solution or blood is not backing up in the tubing. Notify the team leader if problems are noted. *Planning is based on optimal flow. Changes in this could affect client outcomes.*

■ Be aware of IV bags that are near empty. Report them to the team leader so that trained personnel can change them. *Alerting the nurse supervisor about the near-empty bag ensures that air will not be allowed in the tubing line, resulting in an air embolism.*

■ If the pump alarm sounds, troubleshoot it or notify the team leader. Do not just turn it off and walk away. Do not resume flow until the reason for the alarm has been resolved. *If IV administration is within the responsibility of the LPN/LVN in your state, it is your responsibility to troubleshoot the alarm and determine why it was triggered. Resuming flow without knowing the cause of the alarm could result in severe complications for the client. If it is not within your scope of practice, the RN must determine the cause of the alarm.*

■ If an IV has been converted to a saline or heparin lock to provide a route for medication administration, monitor the converted site regularly. *These sites can clot off and then not be good for IV administration.*

■ If you suspect a transfusion reaction, stop the transfusion, change the IV tubing, and start a saline solution infusion at a keep-open rate. Do not discard the blood container or administration set. Notify the primary care provider. *Prompt response to a transfusion reaction can be life-saving. The tubing is changed to prevent more blood product from reaching the client. Saline helps to dilute the blood that has infused. The blood container will be returned to the blood bank to be examined for contamination. The physician is notified so that the treatment plan can be altered.*

EVALUATING

The client would have a patent, healthy IV site without signs or symptoms of infiltration or phlebitis. The client's intake and output would be adequate, and laboratory values would be within normal limits or returning to normal.

NURSING PROCESS CARE PLAN
Client with Dehydration

Margaret Greene is an 80-year-old woman living in an assisted living facility, but being for the most part self-sufficient. Her nurse's aide found her in her apartment very confused, still in her pajamas at 2:00 P.M. She told the aide that she had been throwing up and not able to keep anything down since last night. The aide tried to get some fluids down her but she refused. When the aide attempted to get some vital signs she became combative, which was unusual for this very gentle woman.

Assessment

VS: T 100.6, P 58 weak, R 24, BP 88/50. Client's skin is dry, skin turgor is tented. UA and C&S specimen were obtained and sent to the lab; urine was dark and concentrated. A serum blood BUN and H/H were also obtained. Ms. Greene continues to be confused but is taking sips of water. IV of D_5W at 100 mL/h placed per paramedics on transfer to the hospital.

Nursing Diagnosis

The following important nursing diagnoses (among others) are established for this client:

- *Deficient Fluid Volume* related to fluid loss related to vomiting
- *Acute Confusion* related to dehydration

Expected Outcomes

The expected outcomes for the plan of care are:

- Adequate hydration will be achieved.
- Confusion will dissipate with adequate hydration.
- Skin turgor will be improved.
- Electrolytes will return to balanced state.

Planning and Implementation

The following nursing interventions are implemented:

- Orient client to time, place, and surroundings.
- Monitor IV fluids and oral intake.
- Monitor electrolyte, BUN, and hematocrit lab values.
- Avoid fluid overload.
- Keep accurate intake and output records.

- Weigh client every day.
- Assess for skin turgor in the elderly over the sternum or forehead. (Skin elasticity is retained in this area in the elderly.)
- Monitor temperature. (Temperature may not appear elevated as the elderly client's normal body temperature is often a few degrees lower than that of a younger person.)

Evaluation

Ms. Greene is less disoriented and confused. IV infusion replaced lost fluids; I&O is balanced. Client is taking clear liquids at least 50%. Urine is yellow, straw colored.

Critical Thinking in the Nursing Process

1. Describe the difference between isotonic solutions and hypotonic solutions. Which solutions are used in the treatment of dehydration?
2. What symptoms might Ms. Greene exhibit if she is becoming overhydrated? What nursing implications are indicated?
3. Calculate drops per minute for an IV of D_5W to run at 100 mL/h with a drop factor of 15.

Note: Discussion of Critical Thinking questions appears on the MyNursingKit Website.

Note: The references and resources for all chapters have been compiled at the back of the book.

PROCEDURE 28-1 Using a Volume Control Set

Purposes

- To deliver limited amounts of medications or solution
- To monitor fluids for pediatric and critically ill clients
- To deliver intermittent administration of measured volumes of fluid with a calibrated chamber

Equipment

- IV solution
- Volume control administration set
- Extension tubing if desired
- Medication syringe (for RN's use)
- Antimicrobial swab
- Label

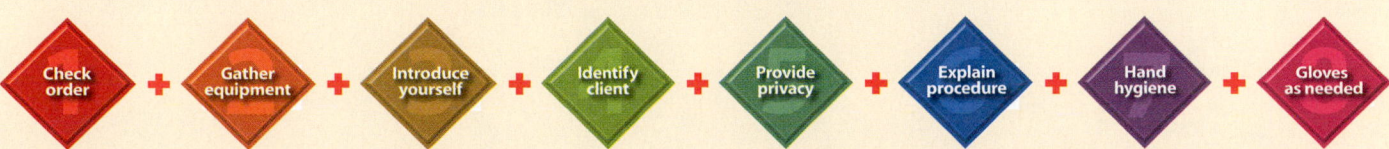

Check order + Gather equipment + Introduce yourself + Identify client + Provide privacy + Explain procedure + Hand hygiene + Gloves as needed

Interventions and Rationales

1. Perform preparatory steps (see icon bar above).
2. Add extension tubing to the volume control unit if necessary.
3. Close slide/roller clamps.
4. Open the air vent located on the top of the volume chamber.
5. Hang the IV solution and remove the plastic cap for insertion.

6. Remove the plastic covering from the spike. *Keep fingers below the flange to avoid contamination of the spike.*

7. Insert the spike into the IV bag.

8. Open the upper roller clamp that is between the IV bag and volume control set. Fill the chamber to about one-third full (Figure 28-10 ■).

9. Close the upper roller clamp.

10. Open the lower clamp and squeeze the drip chamber under the volume control set to about one-half full.

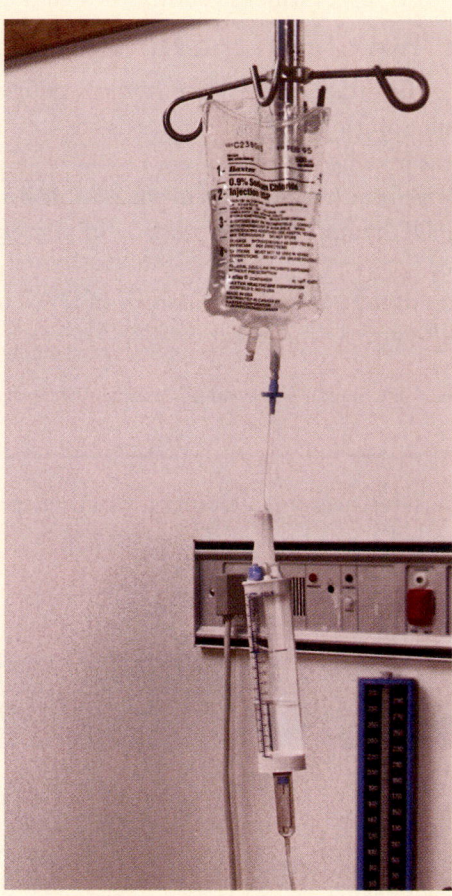

Figure 28-10. ■ Buretrol.

11. Prime the rest of the tubing and close the clamp.

12. Attach the tubing to the IV catheter site and begin infusion.

13. For a medication infusion:
   a. Swab injection port located on top of the volume control chamber with an antimicrobial solution. *The applicable INS standard indicates that injection access ports should be aseptically cleansed with an approved antimicrobial solution immediately before use.*
   b. Instill previously prepared medication into chamber and gently mix medication with IV solution.
   c. If further dilution is needed, add more IV solution to the chamber.
   d. Open the clamp below the IV chamber and adjust the prescribed drip rate.
   e. Label the volume control chamber and include the client's name, medication, dose, and the time the medication was started.

Note: A volume control set may also be referred to as a metered-volume chamber or buretrol.

SAMPLE DOCUMENTATION

[date]	Initiated first dose Kefzol 1 g in
[time]	50 mL of D_5 NS per physician order. Client tolerated well; no complaints noted. _____
	_____ M. Dedio, LVN

Note: This may be documented in the medication administration record (MAR) or IV therapy record rather than in the nurse narrative note.

PROCEDURE 28-2   # Preparing an Intravenous Solution

Purposes

- To maintain fluid and electrolyte balance
- To maintain daily nutritional requirements
- To restore and replace fluid losses

Equipment

- Infusate/IV solution in a bag (*Some glass bottles are used today for infusing certain medications.*)
- Primary administration tubing set
- Add-on particulate filter (*used according to facility policy*)
- Electronic infusion device or freestanding IV pole for gravity infusion
- Needleless Luer lock cannula
- Tubing date sticker
- Time strip

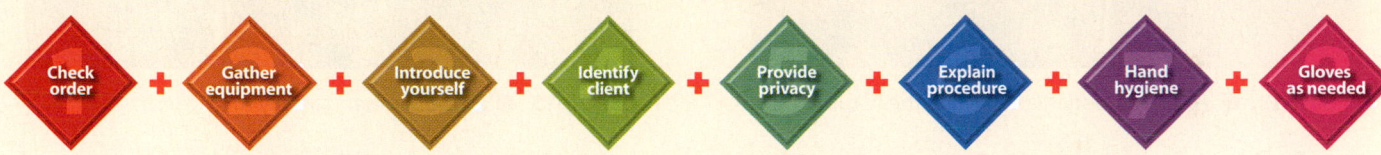

Check order + Gather equipment + Introduce yourself + Identify client + Provide privacy + Explain procedure + Hand hygiene + Gloves as needed

Interventions and Rationales

1. Perform preparatory steps (see icon bar above).

2. Remove outer plastic wrap by tearing at the precut tab. *There may be condensation on the bag and it may be wet.*

3. Examine bag carefully for any tears or leaks. Inspect the bag for discoloration, cloudiness, or particulate matter. *Evidence of change may indicate contamination. If contaminated, the bag must be discarded per facility policy.*

4. Hang the bag on the IV pole and affix the time strip (Figure 28-11 ■). *Avoid using a felt pen to write on the IV bag, the ink may leak through to the solution.*

5. Close the roller/slider clamp on the administration set (Figure 28-12 ■).

6. Remove the plastic cover on the tubing spike and the plastic protector on the bag port (Figure 28-13 ■).

7. While squeezing the drip chamber, insert the spike into the bag port (Figure 28-14 ■). *Squeezing the drip chamber prevents air from entering the bag. Keep fingers below the flange to avoid contamination of the spike.*

8. Release pressure to the drip chamber until it is half full of fluid (Figure 28-15 ■). *The drip chamber allows the monitoring of solution delivery.*

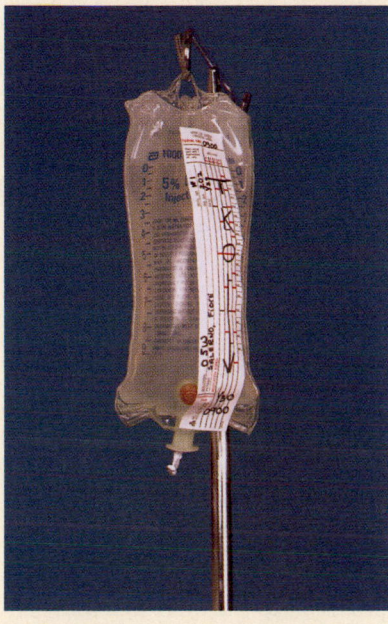

Figure 28-11. ■ IV time strip/bag suspended.

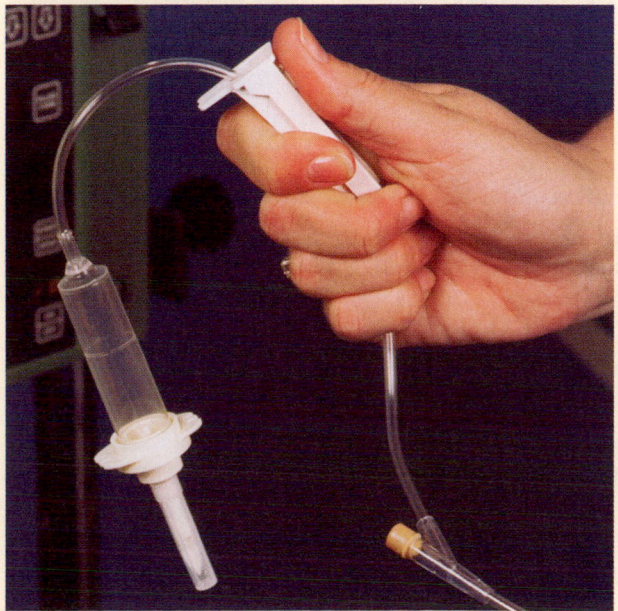

Figure 28-12. ■ Close to clamp.

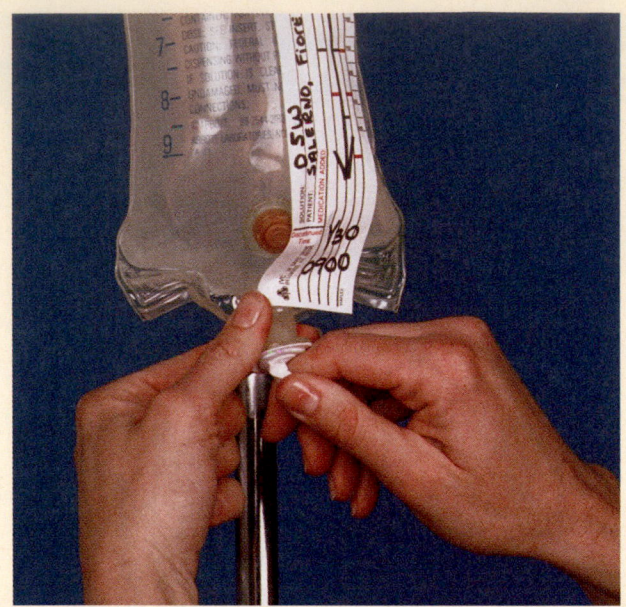

Figure 28-13. ■ Remove plastic protector on the IV tubing spike.

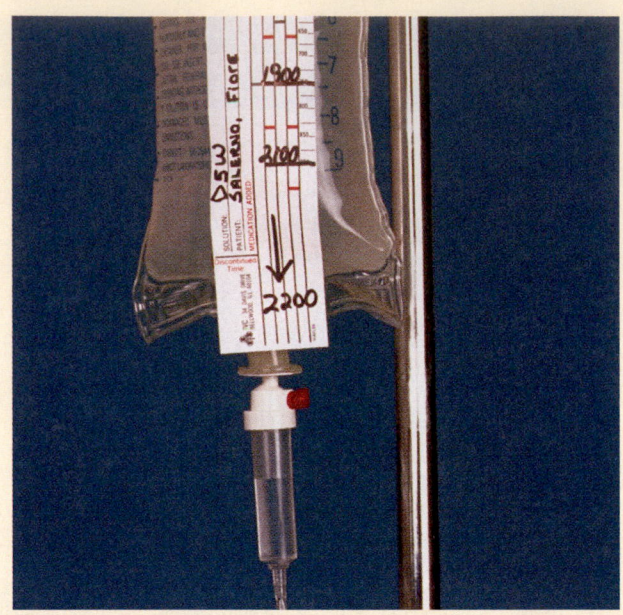

Figure 28-15. ■ Drip chamber partially full.

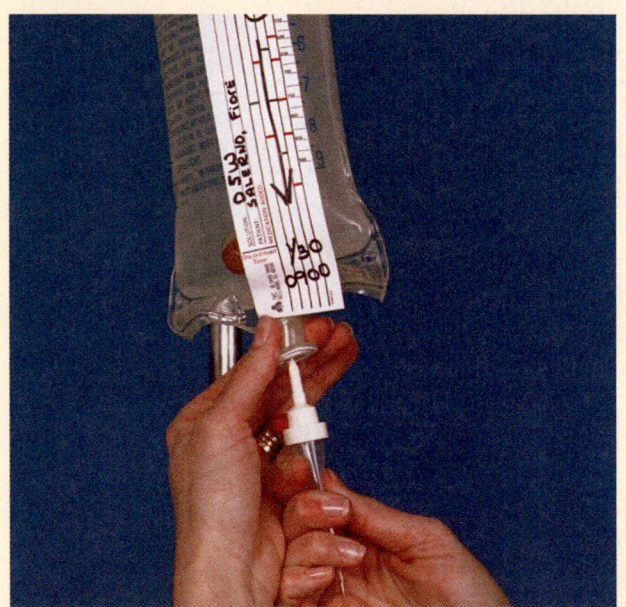

Figure 28-14. ■ Insert tubing spike while squeezing the drip chamber.

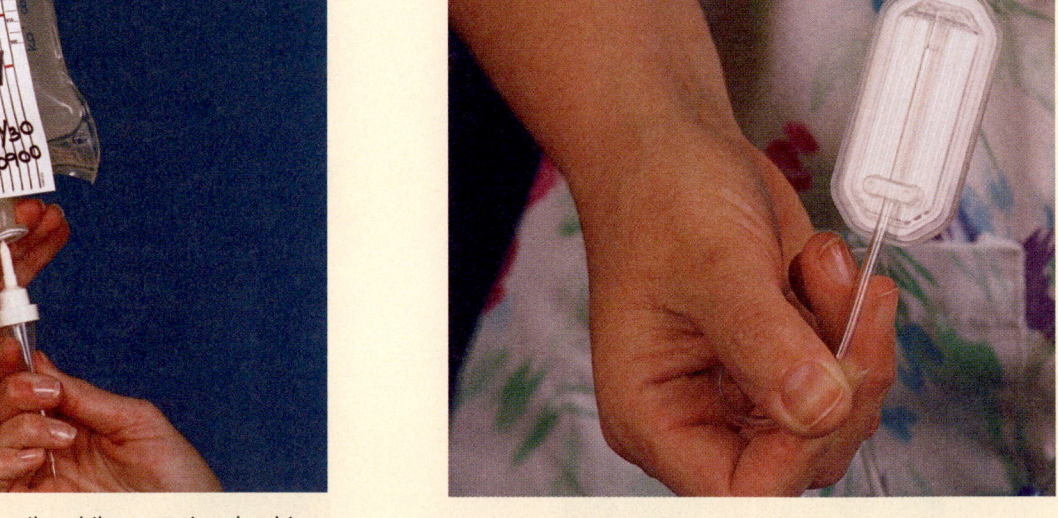

Figure 28-16. ■ Filter.

9. Attach add-on terminal filter when indicated (Figure 28-16 ■). *Filters reduce risk of infection or particulate contamination.*

10. Remove the protective cover at the end of tubing. Open the roller/slider clamp and prime/purge the tubing and filter of air. Hold the tubing tip at a higher level than the tubing loop while priming (Figure 28-17 ■). *Air rises and will pass out of the tubing as the fluid purges the tubing.*

11. Invert and tap Y injection ports to remove air bubbles as the tubing is primed. *Follow directions included in the administration set for priming pump cassettes. Careful air removal from the tubing prevents air embolism and supports administration set function.*

12. Hold filter (if attached) downward, allowing it to fill halfway and then invert the filter to complete the priming process. Tap the filter to remove air out of the filter as it primes.

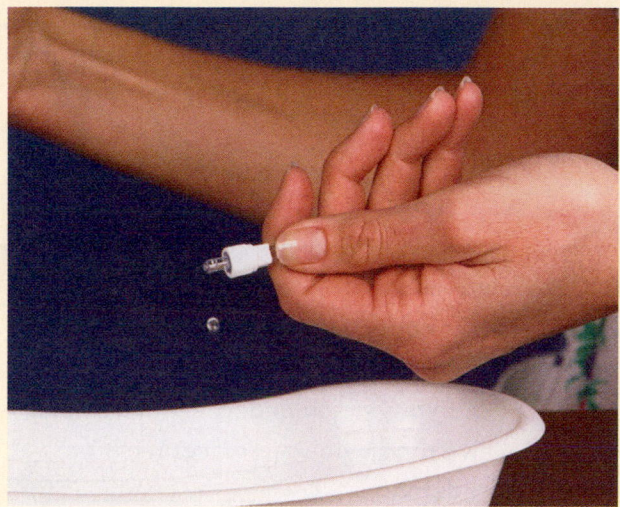

Figure 28-17. ■ Priming tubing.

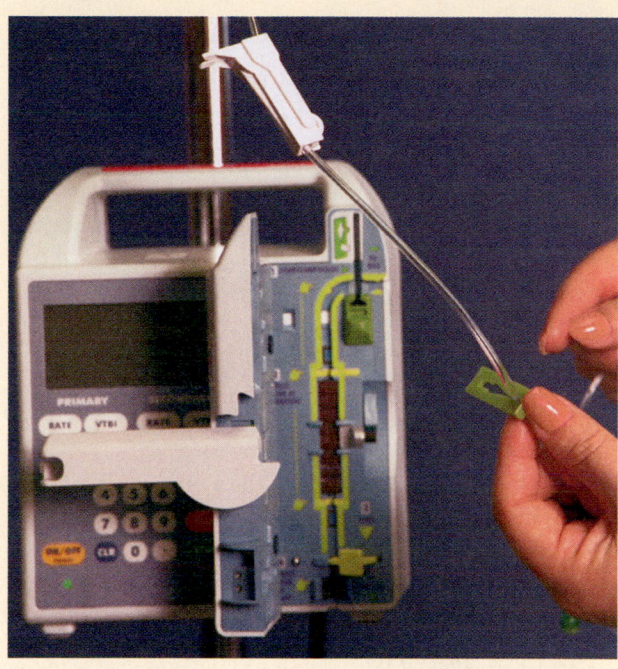

Figure 28-18. ■ Close tubing clamp when priming complete.

13. Close the roller clamp when priming is complete. Attach the needleless cannula on the end of the tubing (Figure 28-18 ■). *This maintains sterility before infusion is initiated. Needleless connections protect against needle sticks.*

14. Attach sticker with date of tubing use. *This helps to maintain consistency of tubing changes according to the facility's policy. INS standards recommend that primary tubing be changed every 72 hours or upon suspicion of contamination or compromise.*

15. Load administration set into the electronic device according to the manufacturer's directions. *Most devices require their tubing be used with detailed loading instructions.*

SAMPLE DOCUMENTATION

[date] [time]	IV infusion of D_5W 1,000 mL at 125 mL per hour initiated with #22 ONC to the left hand. IV site is clean and dry without evidence of erythema or edema. Client tolerated procedure well; no complaints of pain at the site.
	_____ C. Porter, LVN

PROCEDURE 28-3   Changing IV Solution Containers

Purposes

■ To follow physician orders for a change in IV solution
■ To continue the prescribed regimen for IV therapy with the next solution

Equipment

■ IV solution

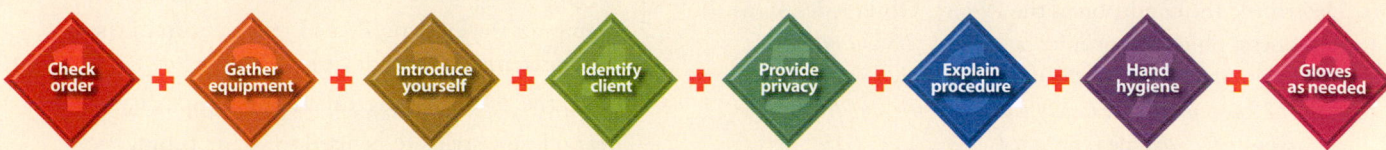

Check order + Gather equipment + Introduce yourself + Identify client + Provide privacy + Explain procedure + Hand hygiene + Gloves as needed

Interventions and Rationales

1. Perform preparatory steps (see icon bar above).

2. Remove outer plastic wrap by tearing at the precut tab. *There may be condensation on the bag and it may be wet.*

3. Examine bag carefully for any tears or leaks. Inspect the bag for discoloration, cloudiness, or particulate matter. *Evidence of change may indicate contamination. If contaminated, the bag must be discarded per facility policy.*

4. Hang the new IV container on the IV pole.

5. Remove the protective cap or tear the tab from the tubing insertion port. *Follow the manufacturer's direction to expose the insertion site of the IV bag.*

6. Slide the flow clamp closed on the administration set or close the roller clamp proximal to the IV bag.

7. Remove the current IV solution from the IV pole.

8. With one hand on the bag and one hand on the spike under the flange, loosen the spike from the IV solution. *Keep fingers below the flange to avoid contamination of the spike.*

9. While squeezing the drip chamber, insert the spike into the new bag port. *Squeezing the drip chamber prevents air from entering the bag. Release pressure to the drip chamber until it is half full of fluid. The drip chamber allows the monitoring of solution delivery.*

10. Open the slide/roller clamp and regulate the fluid rate as prescribed by physician order.

SAMPLE DOCUMENTATION

[date] [time]	IV container changed from D_5W to LR 1,000 mL at 125 mL per hour per physician order. IV is infusing with no evidence of redness or edema. _____ _____ K. James, LVN

Note: This may be recorded on the IV therapy flow sheet or I&O form in the client's chart rather than in narrative form in the nurse's notes.

PROCEDURE 28-4 — Changing IV Tubing

Purposes

- To change IV tubing every 72 hours as recommended by INS
- To maintain asepsis and Standard Precautions at all times

Equipment

- Gloves
- Administration set
- 2 × 2 sterile gauze
- Time strip
- IV tubing label
- Infusate/IV solution in a bag

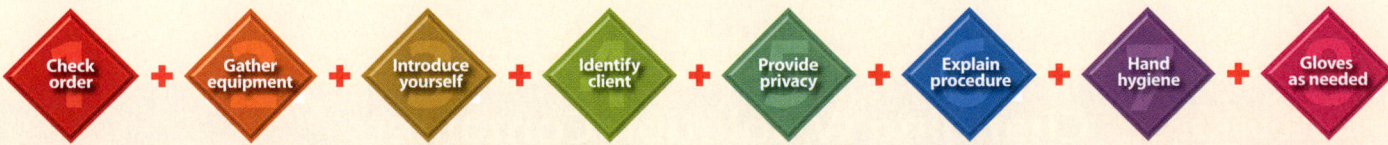

Check order + Gather equipment + Introduce yourself + Identify client + Provide privacy + Explain procedure + Hand hygiene + Gloves as needed

Interventions and Rationales

1. Perform preparatory steps (see icon bar).

2. Follow directions in Procedure 28-2, steps 1 through 13. *Changing IV tubing is normally done when the next IV solution is due.*

3. Determine the condition of the IV site. Observe for signs of redness, phlebitis, or infiltration. *The INS standard indicates that a peripheral short catheter should be removed every 72 hours and immediately when phlebitis, infiltration, or contamination to the site is suspected.*

4. Explain to the client the reason for changing the IV tubing. *Explaining the procedure to the client gives him or her information to enlist compliance and cooperation.*

5. Apply clean gloves.

6. Loosen tape that is securing the existing tubing to the catheter.

7. Clamp off the existing IV and remove it from the electronic monitoring device.

8. Open the 2 × 2 package, maintaining sterility.

9. Tear off tape strips to be used to secure tubing.

10. Detach the IV tubing. *Make sure the IV catheter is stabilized by gently twisting the tubing to loosen it. Put the 2 × 2 gauze under the IV site to contain any drops from the IV disconnection.*

11. Attach the new IV tubing to the catheter. *Twist the end of the new IV tubing into the catheter to lock into place.*

12. Retape the tubing securely.

13. Attach sticker with date of tubing change (Figure 28-19 ■). *To maintain consistency of tubing changes according to the facility's policy. INS standards recommend that primary tubing*

be changed every 72 hours or upon suspicion of contamination or compromise.

14. Load administration set into the electronic device according to the manufacturer's directions. *Most devices require their tubing be used with detailed loading instructions.*

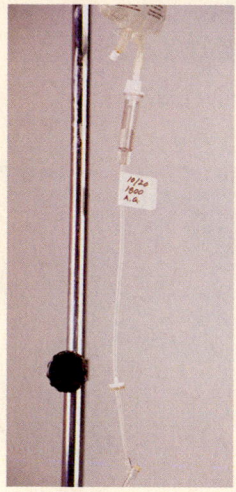

Figure 28-19. ■ IV bag with label.

SAMPLE DOCUMENTATION

[date]	IV tubing changed with #3 bag of
[time]	D_5 1/2NS at 100 mL per hour.
	IV site is clean and dry, no
	evidence of redness or edema.
	_____ B. Jones, LVN

Note: Tubing change can be noted on the IV therapy flow sheet or I&O form in the client's chart rather than in narrative form in the nurse's notes.

PROCEDURE 28-5 Changing a Central Line Dressing

Purposes

- To protect the central line catheter from contamination
- To prevent the central line catheter from becoming displaced
- To provide a visual means to observe the central line site

Equipment

- Betadine (povidone-iodine) swabs (3)
- Alcohol swabs (3)
- Central line dressing kit (optional)

- Transparent semipermeable dressing
- Precut sterile drain gauze (optional)
- Tape
- Receptacle for soiled dressing
- Clean gloves
- Sterile gloves
- Face mask (2)
- Sterile long-sleeved gown (check facility policy)
- Skin preparation/tincture of benzoin (check facility policy)

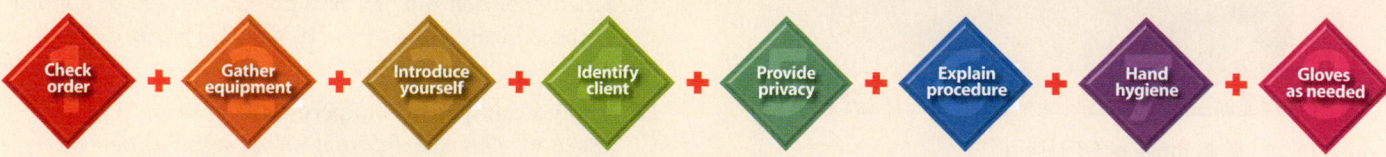

Interventions and Rationales

1. Perform preparatory steps (see icon bar above).

2. Explain the procedure to the client. *Giving instructions to the client prior to the procedure will prepare the client and encourage his or her cooperation during the procedure.*

3. Assist the client to a comfortable position while providing the client with privacy.

4. Expose the central line site. Apply a face mask. Assist the client to apply a mask if tolerated or ask the client to turn the head away from the central line dressing site. *This decreases the airborne risk of infection.*

5. Prepare the equipment needed. Open sterile supplies (Figure 28-20 ■).

6. Apply clean gloves and gently remove the soiled dressing and adhesive from the skin (Figure 28-21 ■). Start at the edges of the dressing and work toward the insertion site. Do not touch catheter insertion site. *Careful removal will prevent the central line catheter from being tugged or displaced.*

7. Discard the soiled dressing in the proper disposal receptacle. Remove gloves (Figure 28-22 ■).

8. Observe the site for signs and symptoms of infection, inflammation, and infiltration (Figure 28-23 ■).

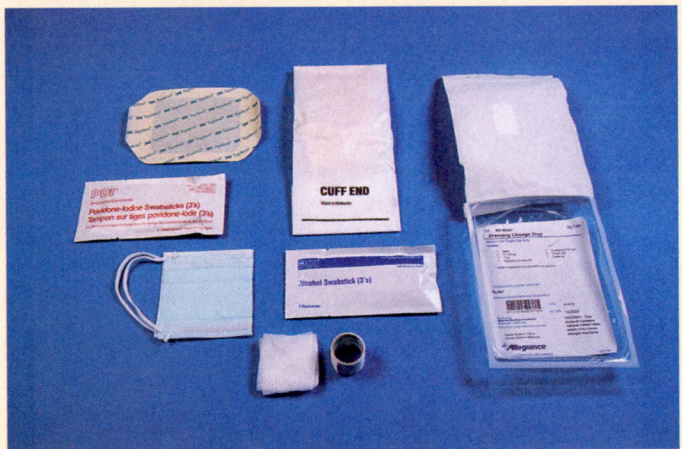

Figure 28-20. ■ Central dressing equipment.

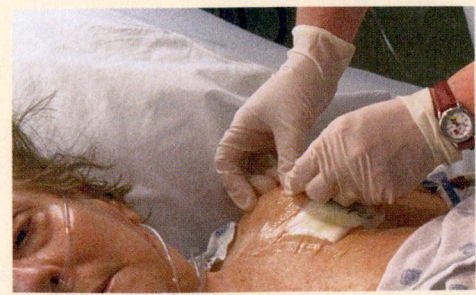

Figure 28-21. ■ Remove old dressing.

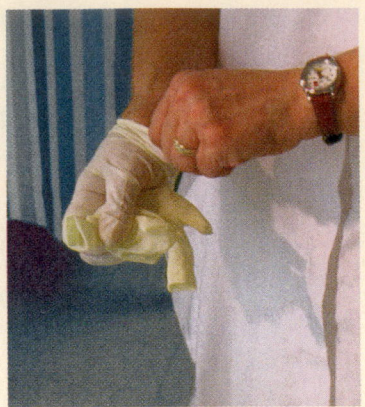

Figure 28-22. ■ Remove gloves.

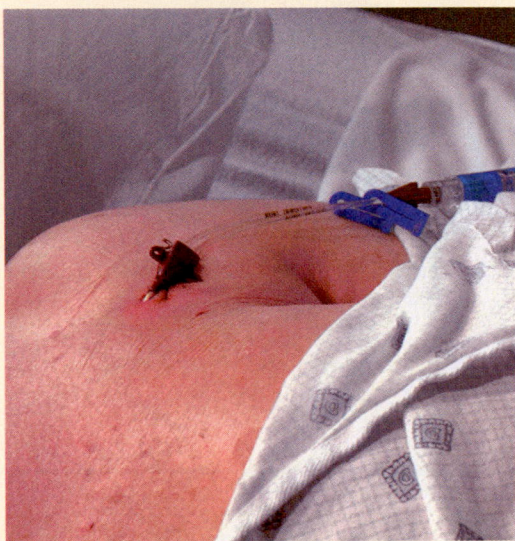

Figure 28-23. ■ Inspect insertion site.

Examine the site for loose sutures, drainage, and odor. Inspect the skin for changes and assess the length of the catheter. *Abnormal findings must be documented and the physician notified. A culture of the drainage may be necessary.*

9. Apply sterile gloves (Figure 28-24 ■). Cleanse the insertion site with three alcohol swabs in a circular motion working from the catheter insertion site outward 4 to 6 in. and allow the skin to dry (Figure 28-25 ■). Discard the swabs after each wipe. Repeat this same procedure with the three Betadine (povidone-iodine) swabs and allow the skin to dry. *Cleaning from the insertion site outward prevents contamination.*

10. Apply the precut sterile gauze dressing around the catheter. *The gauze is used to absorb exudate in the first 24 hours following the insertion of the catheter. Check facility policy with regard to using gauze dressing.*

11. Tincture of Benzoin or a skin preparation can be applied to the skin and allowed to dry. *The skin preparation protects the skin and promotes adhesion of the dressing.*

12. Apply a transparent semipermeable dressing (Figure 28-26 ■). *This type of dressing allows easy visualization of the*

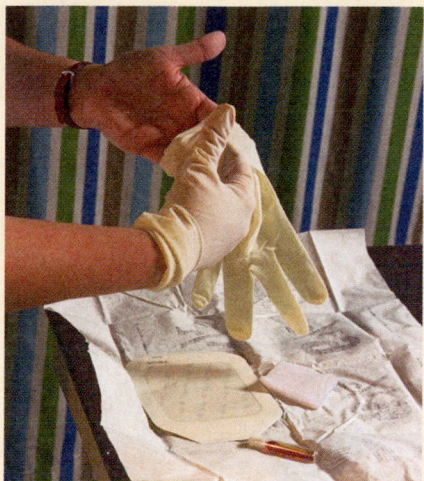

Figure 28-24. ■ Apply sterile gloves.

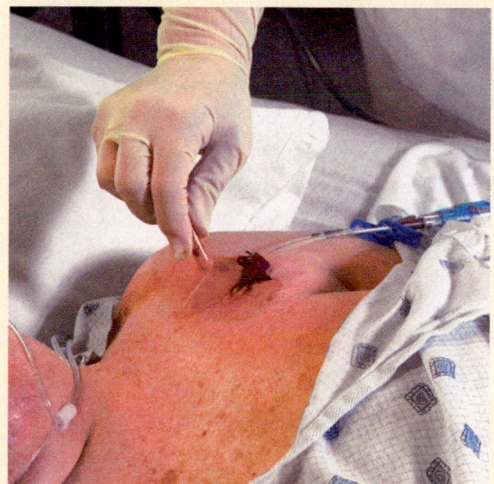

Figure 28-25. ■ Cleanse insertion site.

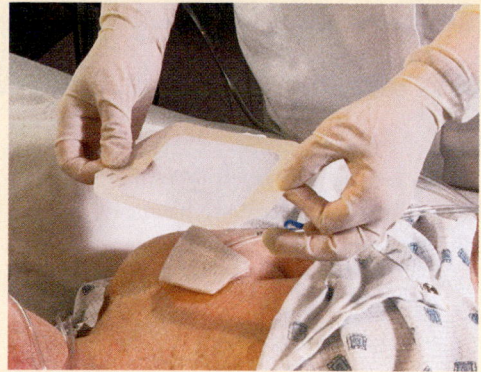

Figure 28-26. ■ Sterile transparent dressing.

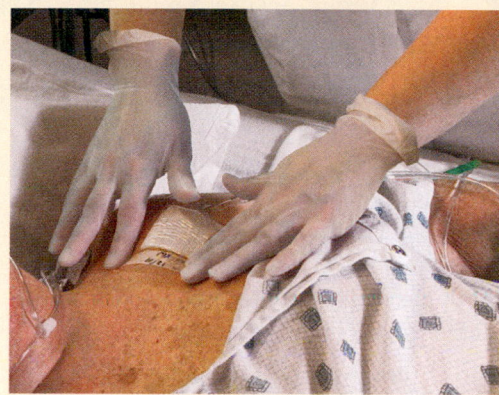

Figure 28-27. ■ Label dressing with date and initial.

site and skin. It allows gas exchange but is impermeable to fluids and microorganisms. Dressing changes may vary according to the facility. The INS recommends dressing changes at routine intervals. Most facilities require central line changes every 72 to 96 hours and immediately if the dressing becomes wet or is leaking.

13. Secure the catheter tubing. *Looping the tubing and taping it securely prevents pulling on the catheter and potential dislodgement of the catheter.*

14. Label the dressing with the date, time, and the initials of the nurse performing the dressing change (Figure 28-27 ■).

SAMPLE DOCUMENTATION

[date]	The central line dressing to the
[time]	left upper chest area was changed using sterile technique. The insertion site is reddened at the suture area. Nursing will monitor for increased redness to the suture site. No drainage, edema, or odor noted. TSM applied and secured in place. The client tolerated the procedure without pain or complaints.
	_____ Nellie Nguyen, LVN

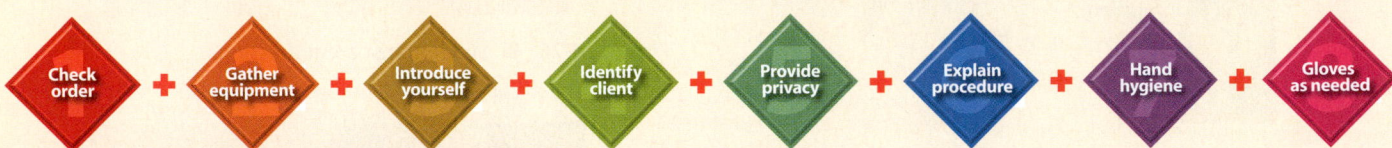

PROCEDURE 28-6   Setting the IV Flow Rate

Purposes

- To accurately set the prescribed IV rate
- To maintain fluid and electrolyte balance
- To maintain and restore fluid losses

Equipment

- Infusion device or pump
- IV administration set (compatible with device)
- Gloves
- Needleless cannula
- Tubing label

Check order + Gather equipment + Introduce yourself + Identify client + Provide privacy + Explain procedure + Hand hygiene + Gloves as needed

Interventions and Rationales

1. Perform preparatory steps (see icon bar above).

2. Follow the steps found in Procedure 28-2 for preparing intravenous solution. *Use the correct administrative set for the infusion device being utilized. Most pumps have dedicated tubing and require a specific method to load the machine. If using tubing with a cassette, follow the manufacturer's instructions for priming the line.*

3. Explain to the client about the purpose of the infusion controller/pump, the various sounds, and the sensitivity of the machine. Include when to notify the nurse if the alarm sounds. Inform the client that it runs on batteries when unplugged allowing for the client to be mobile. *Providing instruction regarding the equipment will promote client cooperation.*

Continue for controller infusion. For pump infusion, go to page 691 and continue at #4.

CONTROLLER INFUSION

4. Affix the controller to the IV pole and connect to the electrical outlet. *This device is less commonly used today. The function depends on gravity flow.*

5. Attach the eye sensor to the drip chamber above the level of fluid but below the drop opening. Make sure the photoelectric eye sensor is connected firmly into the controller. *The eye must be able to sense the fluid drop in order to give an accurate rate.*

6. Open the door of the device and insert the IV tubing into the controller. *Follow the manufacturer's instruction.* Close the door to the device and latch the handle.

7. Perform venipuncture or affix tubing to the existing IV catheter. (Follow the steps found in Procedure 28-9 for performing a venipuncture.)

8. Open all slide/roller clamps and turn on the power to the controller to initiate infusion.

9. Set the controls on the front of the controller to the appropriate infusion rate and volume. *Setting the volume to 50 to 100 mL less than the total volume gives the nurse time to attach a new bag before the previous bag is depleted.*

10. Count the drops for 15 seconds and multiply by 4 (Figure 28-28 ■). *Verifying the drops per minute ensures that the device is working correctly.*

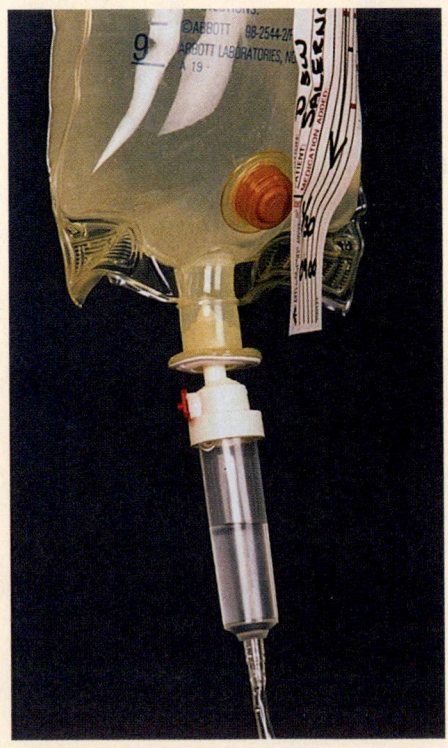

Figure 28-28. ■ Count drips per minute.

11. Ensure that the volume on the alarm is turned on. *The purpose of the alarm is to alert the nurse that the infusion is not proceeding as scheduled.*

12. Monitor the infusion every hour. Assess the volume that has been infused and compare to the time label on the bag. *This intervention will verify that the machine is functioning properly and the client is receiving the correct amount of fluid per hour.*

13. Troubleshoot if the machine alarms. Check:
    a. For kinks in the line.
    b. The fluid level in the drip chamber; ensure that it is half full, allowing the electronic eye to sense the drop.
    c. The placement of the electronic eye on the drip chamber.
    d. The position of the extremity with IV site, which can cause the machine to alarm.
    e. The rate and volume; verify accuracy.
    f. That the IV site is patent and free flowing.
    g. That IV tubing slide/roller clamps are open.
    h. The fluid in the IV container.

PUMP INFUSION

4. Affix the pump to the IV pole at eye level and connect to the electrical outlet. *This is a positive-pressure infusion, so the solution is delivered by applying pressure to the infusion to maintain the prescribed flow rate. It is extremely beneficial when administering viscous solutions, when the client's activity increases venous back pressure, or when the venipuncture catheter is a small gauge. The device can be placed at any level because it does not rely on gravity to function.*

5. Open the door of the device and insert the IV tubing into the controller. *Follow the manufacturer's instruction. If the tubing has a cassette attached, make sure that the cassette has been completely filled with fluid. It may need to be tilted and tapped to eliminate air bubbles. If air bubbles remain, it may cause the alarm to sound.* Close the door to the device and latch the handle.

6. Perform venipuncture or affix tubing to the existing IV catheter. Follow the steps found in Procedure 28-9 for performing a venipuncture.

7. Open all slide/roller clamps and turn on the power to the controller to initiate infusion.

8. Press the number pad for the prescribed drops per minute or milliliters per hour and push the start button.

9. Ensure that the volume on the alarm is turned on. *The purpose of the alarm is to alert the nurse that the infusion is not proceeding as scheduled.*

10. Monitor the infusion every hour. Assess the volume that has been infused and compare to the time label on the bag. *This intervention will verify that the machine is functioning properly and the client is receiving the correct amount of fluid per hour.*

11. Troubleshoot if the machine alarms. Check:
    a. For kinks in the line.
    b. The fluid level in the drip chamber; ensure that it is half full, allowing the electronic eye to sense the drop.
    c. The placement of the electronic eye on the drip chamber.
    d. The position of the extremity with IV site, which can cause the machine to alarm.
    e. The rate and volume; verify accuracy.
    f. That the IV site is patent and free flowing.
    g. That IV tubing slide/roller clamps are open.
    h. The fluid in the IV container.

SAMPLE DOCUMENTATION

[date]
[time]
IV initiated with D$_5$W infusing at 125 mL per hour using infusion pump. Venipuncture performed to the right hand with 20-gauge ONC. IV site is clean and dry. Client tolerated procedure well without complaints. _____
_____ Y. Yanez, LVN

Inserting a Medication Lock

Purposes

- To maintain a venous access for intermittent IV medication infusion
- To increase client's mobility and comfort
- To allow blood collection without repeated venipunctures
- To provide venous access for emergency medication delivery

Equipment

- Medication lock, prn device, or intermittent IV lock
- Needleless syringe
- Normal saline solution vial
- 2 × 2 sterile gauze
- Clean gloves

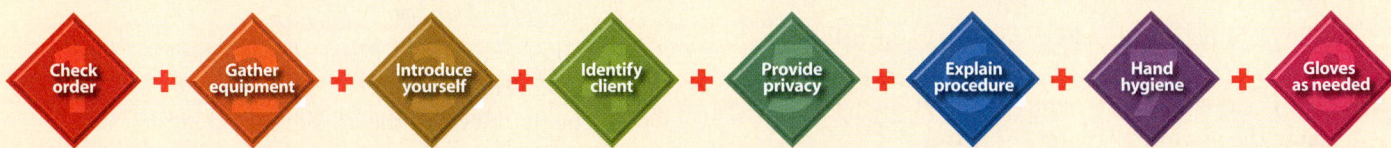

Check order + Gather equipment + Introduce yourself + Identify client + Provide privacy + Explain procedure + Hand hygiene + Gloves as needed

Interventions and Rationales

1. Perform preparatory steps (see icon bar above).

2. Determine the patency of the IV. Observe for signs of redness, phlebitis, or infiltration. *The INS standard indicates that a peripheral short catheter should be removed every 72 hours and immediately when phlebitis, infiltration, or contamination to the site is suspected.* Establish a new line (following the steps in Procedure 28-9 for performing a venipuncture using the ONC procedure) or use the existing line if patent.

3. Explain to the client the reason for an intermittent IV lock.

4. Apply clean gloves.

5. Loosen tape that may be obstructing the insertion of the intermittent device.

6. Clamp off the IV. It may be necessary to disconnect the IV from the electronic monitoring device when converting the existing IV line to an intermittent lock.

7. Open the 2 × 2 gauze package maintaining sterility.

8. Open the intermittent lock package and maintain sterility (Figure 28-29 ■).

9. Detach the IV tubing. Make sure to stabilize the IV catheter: gently twist the tubing to loosen it. Put the 2 × 2 gauze under the IV site to contain any drops from the IV disconnection.

10. Attach the lock to the hub of the cannula. Remove the protective cap. Twist the intermittent lock into place.

11. Clean the needleless injection port (Figure 28-30 ■) with an antimicrobial swab. *The INS standard indicates that injection access ports should be aseptically cleansed with an approved antimicrobial solution immediately before use.*

12. Infuse the saline solution as directed in the facility's procedures.

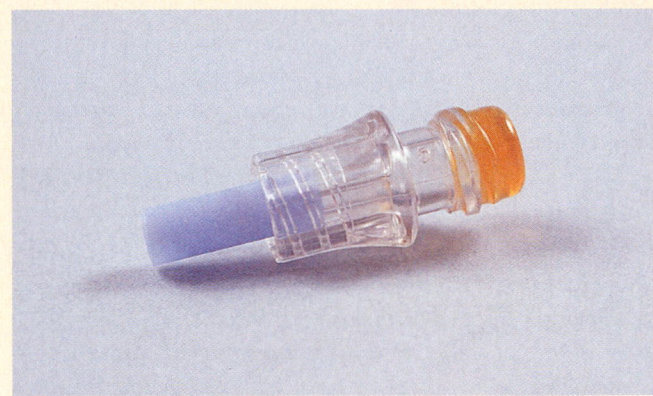

Figure 28-29. ■ Intermittent lock.

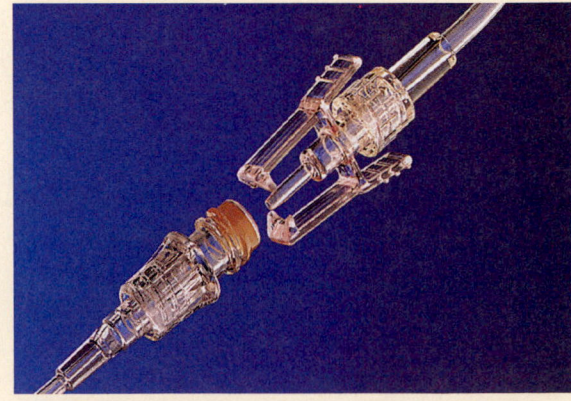

Figure 28-30. ■ Needle-free device. (Photograph reprinted courtesy of (BD) Becton, Dickinson and Company and courtesy of Baxter Healthcare Corporation. All rights reserved.)

13. Retape the catheter and intermittent device into place. The chevron or U method is recommended. A protective gauze bandage can be applied such as a stretch netting or a Kerlix dressing.

PROCEDURE 28-8   Applying a Tourniquet

Purposes

- To dilate a vein
- To perform intravenous venipuncture
- To perform phlebotomy

Equipment

- Alcohol swabs
- Blood pressure cuff (optional)
- Clean gloves when inserting IV needle/cannula
- IV insertion kit (optional)
- Tourniquet (flat, soft, 5 cm [2 in.] wide)
- Towel or disposable waterproof pad
- Velcro tourniquet (optional)
- Warm moist towel

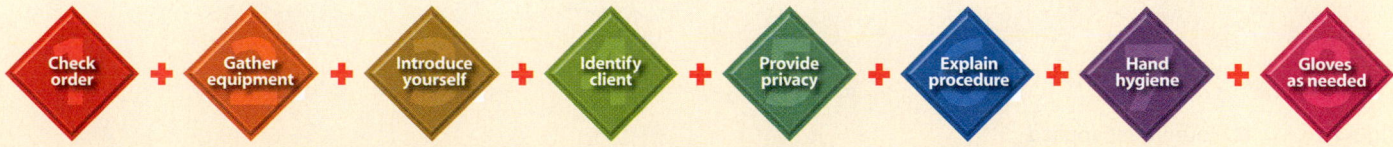

Check order + Gather equipment + Introduce yourself + Identify client + Provide privacy + Explain procedure + Hand hygiene + Gloves as needed

Interventions and Rationales

1. Perform preparatory steps (see icon bar above).
2. Assess the condition of the veins. Use a straight, soft, bouncy vein. Avoid previously used veins or area that has been infected or is reddened (graft, fistula, mastectomy, IV site, paralysis). Avoid valves in the veins. *A straight, soft, bouncy vein is easiest to access. Previously used veins and areas of potential infection or compromise all could be difficult to access and may lead to complications. Entering the vein at a valve could cause injury to the valve.*
3. Check that the cannula gauge is appropriate for the client's age and size. *A gauge that is too large may cause unnecessary discomfort and possible damage.*
4. Check the length of therapy and the client's activities. *The length and type of therapy may determine the type of gauge used as well as the client's extremity use.* Determine whether the client is using antithrombotics or anticoagulants. *Clotting time will be delayed in clients using these drugs.*
5. Select the nondominant hand first, unless one of the diseases/conditions listed in step 2 is present. Client preference is accommodated if possible. The most used veins are cephalic and basilic veins. The least used are feet and leg veins. *Use of the nondominant hand usually means the extremity is used less often than the dominant extremity when performing routine ADLs, diminishing movement and pressure to the extremity.*

6. Apply the tourniquet. Avoid rolling of the tourniquet. If it becomes twisted, reapply the tourniquet. Place the tourniquet flat 15 cm (6 in.) above the planned puncture site. Apply the two ends together; put one end on top of the other. Lift and stretch the tourniquet, then tuck the end on top underneath the tourniquet (Figure 28-31 ■). The tails should be out of the way of the planned site insertion or above the tourniquet (Figure 28-32 ■). Avoid pinching hair or skin. *This distends the vein.*

7. The tourniquet should be snug but avoid occluding the radial pulse. Leave the tourniquet in place for approximately 2 minutes. Observe for color changes or client complaints of a tingling sensation. *Marked darkening of the skin and complaints by the client can signal that tissue is not adequately perfused. Check the radial pulse. If it is absent, reapply the tourniquet.*

8. Have the client open and close his or her fist four to six times. *Opening and closing the fist dilates the vein.*

9. You can gently flick/tap the site or rub alcohol swabs on the skin. Avoid slapping the site. *Alcohol swabs and*

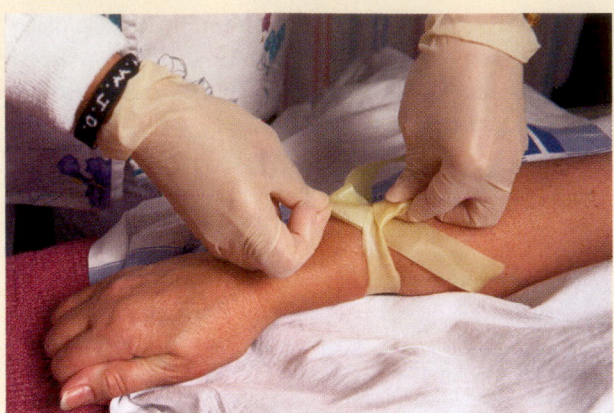

Figure 28-32. ■ Overlap with ends away from the site.

tapping distend the vein. Slapping will redden the skin and cause discomfort but will not increase the likelihood of finding a vein.

10. Use your index finger to feel for an insertion site. *The index finger is the most sensitive for palpation.*

11. If you are unable to find an adequate site for insertion, you can place the hand in a dependent position and/or use a warm compress then reapply the tourniquet. *These measures increase blood to the extremity.*

12. Repeat steps 7 through 10.

SAMPLE DOCUMENTATION

See Procedure 28-9.

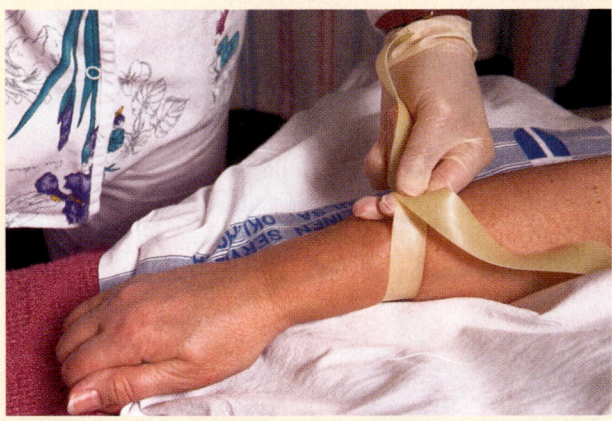

Figure 28-31. ■ Tourniquet applied.

Performing Venipuncture

Purposes

- To initiate vascular access for intravenous therapy
- To administer fluids and electrolytes
- To maintain parenteral nutrition
- To administer blood or blood components
- To provide vascular access for intravenous medications

Equipment

- Alcohol swabs
- Blood pressure cuff (optional)
- Clean gloves when inserting IV needle/cannula
- IV insertion kit (optional)
- Tourniquet (flat, soft, 5 cm [2 in.] wide)
- Towel or disposable waterproof pad
- Velcro tourniquet (optional)
- Warm moist towel
- Povidone-iodine wipes
- Scalp vein (butterfly or winged) needle *or* over-the-needle catheter (ONC)
- Prepared IV administration setup (see Procedure 28-2)
- Transparent semipermeable dressing
- Tape
- Armboard (optional)

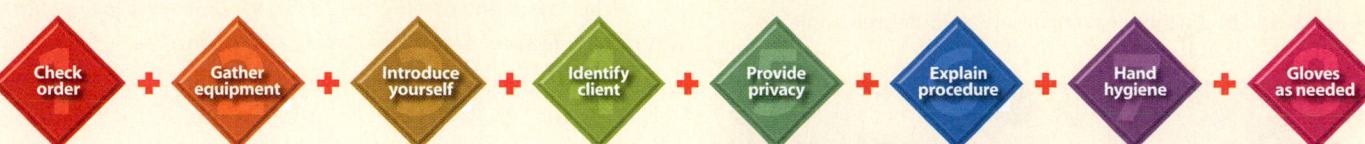

Check order + Gather equipment + Introduce yourself + Identify client + Provide privacy + Explain procedure + Hand hygiene + Gloves as needed

Interventions and Rationales

1. Perform preparatory steps (see icon bar above).

2. See applying a tourniquet (Procedure 28-8).

3. Prepare the site with povidone-iodine wipe. Use an alcohol prep (70%) if the client is allergic to iodine. Allow the preparation to dry completely. *Germicidal action occurs when the skin preparation dries. An antibacterial barrier can decrease risk for infection at the puncture site.*

4. Select appropriate scalp vein/butterfly/winged needle or an ONC device. *A winged needle is used primarily for short-term therapy, usually less than 24 hours. The butterfly needle has low rates of inflammation and phlebitis. The steel needle is not flexible and therefore has a tendency to dislodge or puncture the vein, increasing the risk of infiltration. The ONC is easy to insert and floats in the vein. It is used for long-term therapy; the material used in its manufacture is designed to minimize local reactions.*

Continue for scalp vein/butterfly/winged needle. For over-the-needle catheter, go to page 697 and continue at #5.

SCALP VEIN/BUTTERFLY/WINGED NEEDLE

5. Attach the end of the IV tubing to end of the scalp vein/butterfly/winged needle tubing.

6. Remove the plastic cover from the butterfly/winged needle and prime the fluid through the needle (Figure 28-33 ■). Clamp the tubing and replace the needle protector.

7. Anchor the vein by pulling the skin taut with the thumb of the nondominant hand beneath the selected site. *Controlling the vein prevents rolling and facilitates needle insertion.*

8. Holding the butterfly/winged needle by the wings with the bevel up, enter the client's skin at a 30-degree angle

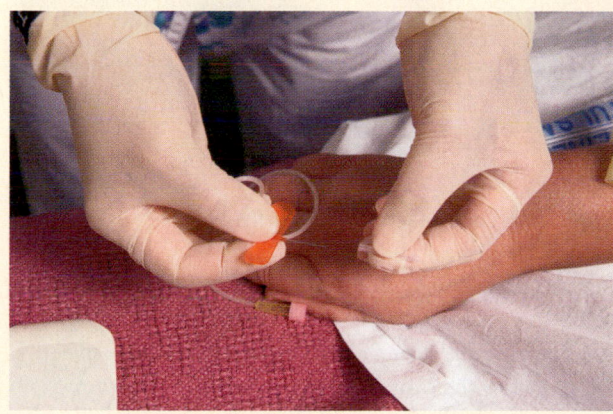

Figure 28-33. ■ Remove winged needle cap.

(Figure 28-34 ■). Two methods used to enter the vein:
   a. Enter the skin next to or along the vein. Drop the needle to a 15-degree angle and when the needle is under the skin enter the vein.
   b. Insert the needle into the skin below the intended site and directly into the vein. *Using the one-thrust method can result in hematoma formation.*

9. A pop is felt when the vein is entered. Observe for a flashback of blood in the tubing. Follow the course of the vein and advance the needle to the wings.

10. Release the tourniquet.

11. Attach sterile resealable injection cap (Figure 28-35 ■). Inject normal saline for peripheral saline lock (PSL) or connect to IV tubing. *The injection cap is used to flush the lock or when connecting to the infusion.* Open the roller clamp and monitor the drip chamber. *The fluid should be free flowing; observe for swelling at the insertion site.*

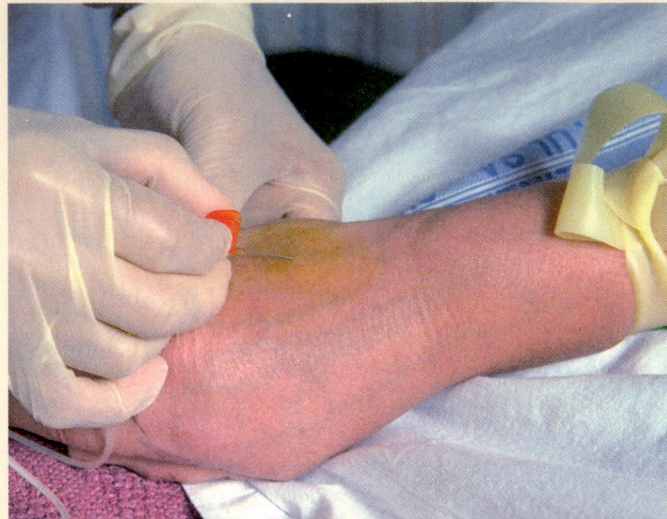

Figure 28-34. ■ Anchor vein and insert at 30-degree angle.

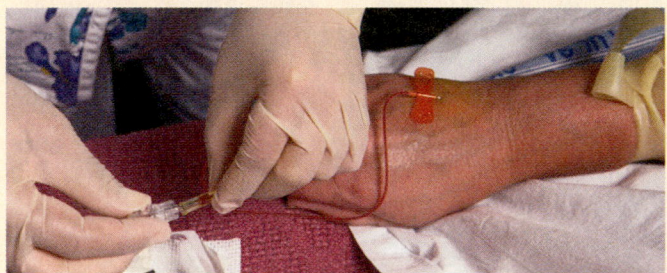

Figure 28-35. ■ Lock attached to butterfly.

12. Slow the infusion to a keep-open rate, and secure the needle and tubing to avoid the needle from becoming dislodged. Using ½-inch-wide tape with the adhesive side up under the tubing, cross the tape over the wings (Chevron method) (Figure 28-36 ■). Another taping method is to fold the tape end over the wings, making a U shape securing the needle (Figure 28-37 ■). Place another piece of tape across the wings of the chevron. Avoid adhering tape over the insertion site. *This allows for assessment and access.* Gloves can be removed here or after all taping is completed. *Wash hands if gloves have been removed.*

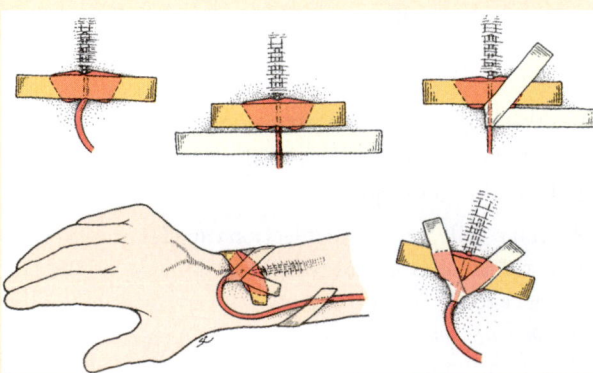

Figure 28-36. ■ Chevron method.

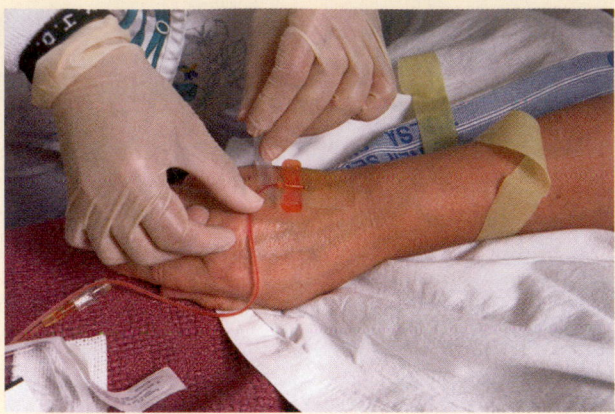

Figure 28-37. ■ Using U shape to tape.

13. Loop the butterfly/winged needle tubing to the side of the insertion site (Figure 28-38 ■). *Leave enough of a loop so as to avoid kinking the tubing at the wings.*

14. Apply the occlusive semipermeable transparent dressing (Figure 28-39 ■) over the insertion site. A 2 × 2 gauze square, taped occlusively, can also be used.

15. Label the dressing with date, time, and initials; include the size of needle used.

16. Regulate the infusion rate by pump or calculate the drip rate by gravity flow per minute.

17. Affix armboard to immobilize the hand in a flexion position. *This reduces risk of cannula displacement.*

18. Change IV every 48 to 72 hours. *INS recommends that a peripheral catheter be removed every 72 hours or immediately with suspected contamination or complications. An increased risk of phlebitis and bacteria colonization occurring after 72 hours has been documented.*

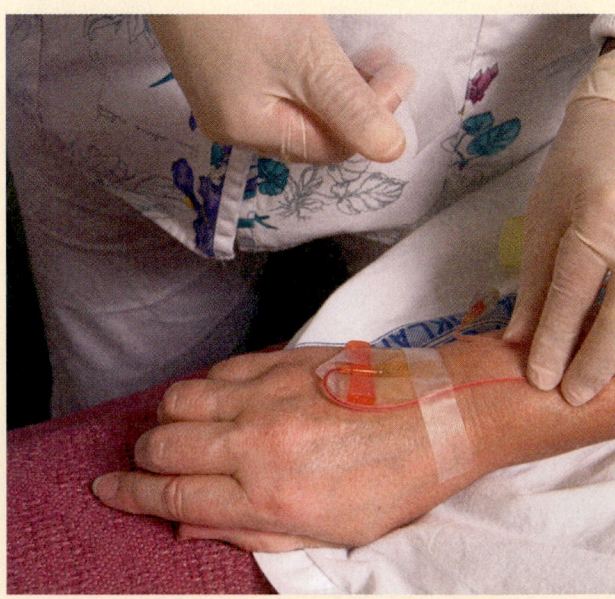

Figure 28-38. ■ Loop tubing and secure.

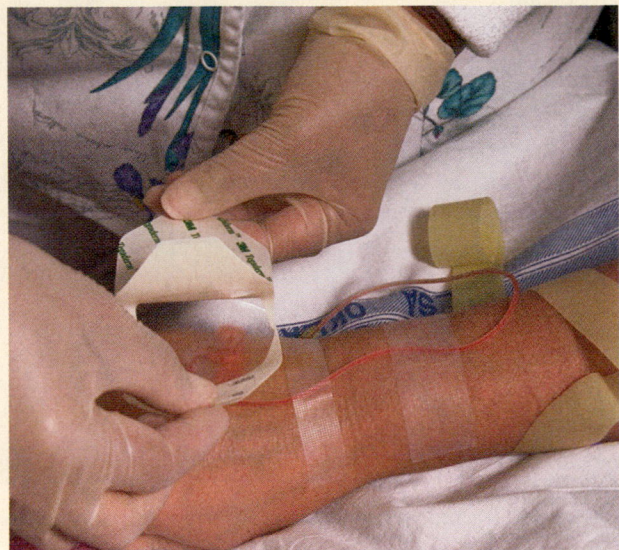

Figure 28-39. ■ Occlusive transparent dressing.

OVER-THE-NEEDLE CATHETER

5. Position the client's arm or hand. Select the appropriate size ONC for the purpose of the infusion. Open the catheter package and inspect for any product compromise.

6. Anchor the vein by pulling the skin taut with the nondominant thumb.

7. Stabilize the catheter with the needle bevel up and insert into the skin at a 45-degree angle (Figure 28-40 ■). As with the winged needle, the catheter can be inserted along the vein or distal to the site and directly into the vein.

8. Lower the cannula angle to 30 degrees and enter the vein. A pop sensation is usually felt. A backflash of blood will be seen in the plastic hub (Figure 28-41 ■). *A backflash of blood indicates the cannula is in the vein. If no blood is seen and you did not feel the catheter enter the vein, assess the vein's position. You can pull back slightly without exiting the vein and reattempt venipuncture. After*

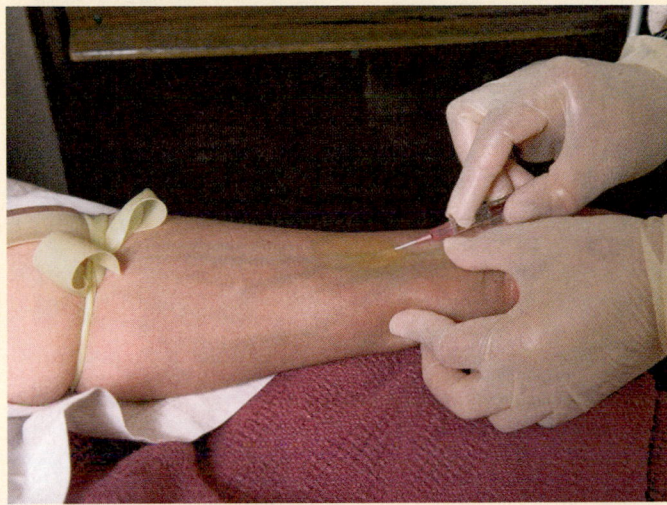

Figure 28-41. ■ Bevel up, blood flash.

two attempts at venipuncture without success, the nurse should notify the charge nurse or team leader for assistance.

9. Holding onto the needle/stylet, advance only the catheter into the lumen of the vein (Figure 28-42 ■). *By holding onto the needle/stylet there is a decreased risk of puncturing the vein. The catheter slides over the needle/stylet.*

10. Release the tourniquet. Leave the needle/stylet in place while taping the catheter in place. Tape the catheter wings in place and across the body of the catheter. Avoid touching the insertion site and the hub catheter junction to maintain aseptic technique.

11. Apply pressure to the distal end of the catheter and then remove the needle/stylet. *This action prevents blood loss.* If using a needleless catheter, use the button to retract the needle (Figure 28-43 ■).

12. Connect the end of the catheter to the primed administration set or needleless cap.

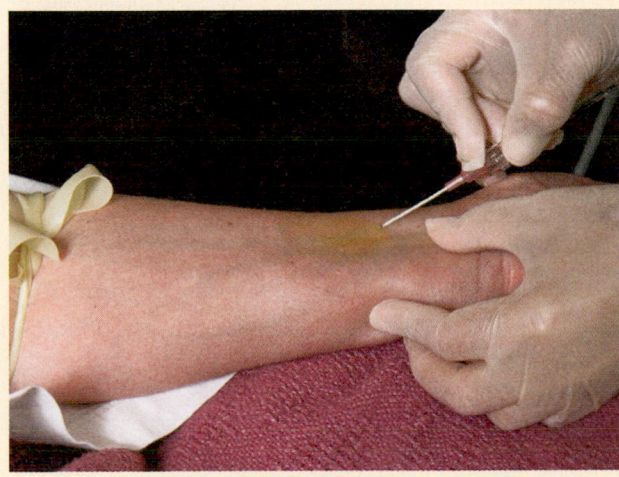

Figure 28-40. ■ Over the ONC, stabilize device.

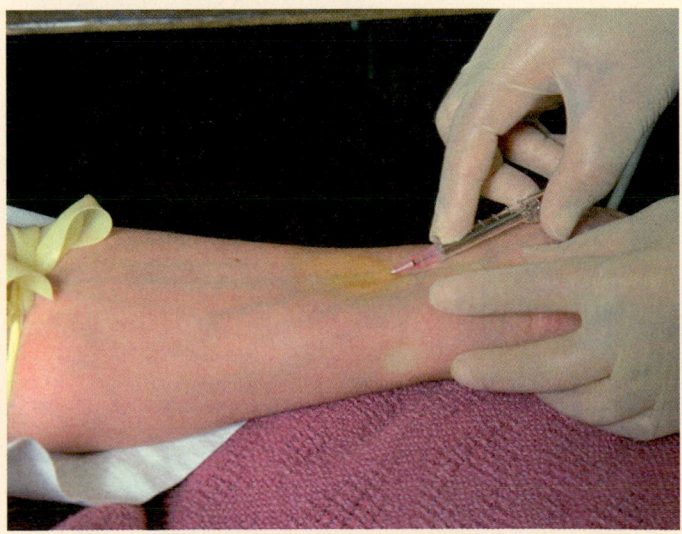

Figure 28-42. ■ After skin insertion, reduce angle and advance.

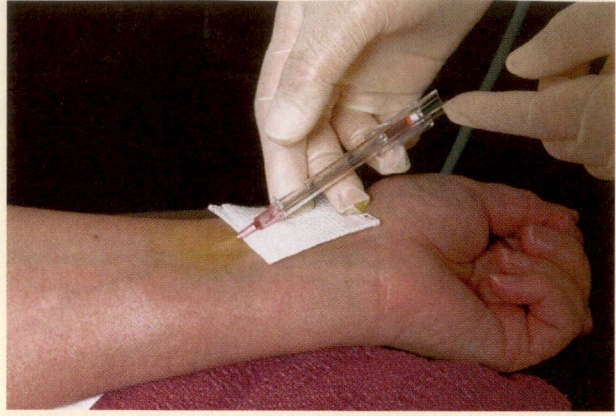

Figure 28-43. ■ Release tourniquet, gauze pad under hub, withdraw stylet, leaving catheter in place.

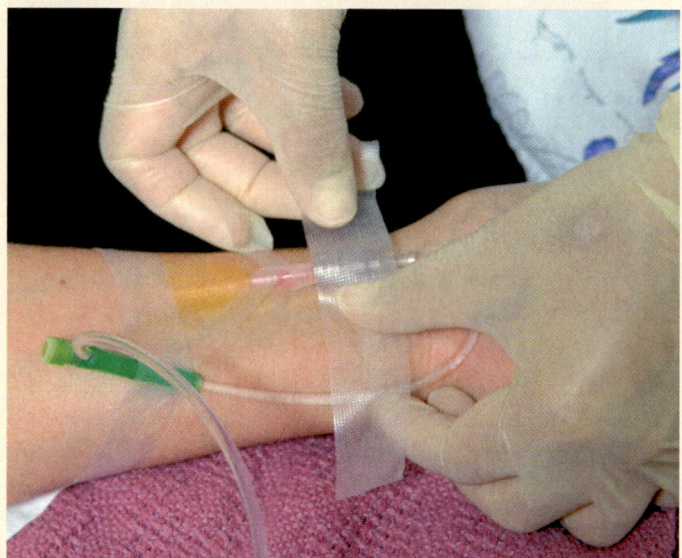

Figure 28-44. ■ Secure cannula with tape using the chevron method.

13. Open the roller clamp and observe the fluid flow in the drip chamber. Monitor the insertion site for signs of infiltration.

14. Decrease fluid flow and continue taping the catheter using the chevron method (Figure 28-44 ■).

15. Apply the occlusive semipermeable transparent dressing over the insertion site (Figure 28-45 ■). A 2 × 2 gauze square, taped occlusively, can also be used.

16. Loop the administration set tubing to the side of the insertion site and secure by taping.

17. Label the dressing with date, time, and initials (Figure 28-46 ■); include the size of needle used.

18. Regulate the infusion rate by pump or calculate the drip rate by gravity flow per minute.

19. Remove gloves and wash hands.

20. Change IV every 48 to 72 hours. *INS recommends that a peripheral catheter be removed every 72 hours or immediately with suspected contamination or complications. An increased risk of phlebitis and bacteria colonization occurring after 72 hours has been documented.*

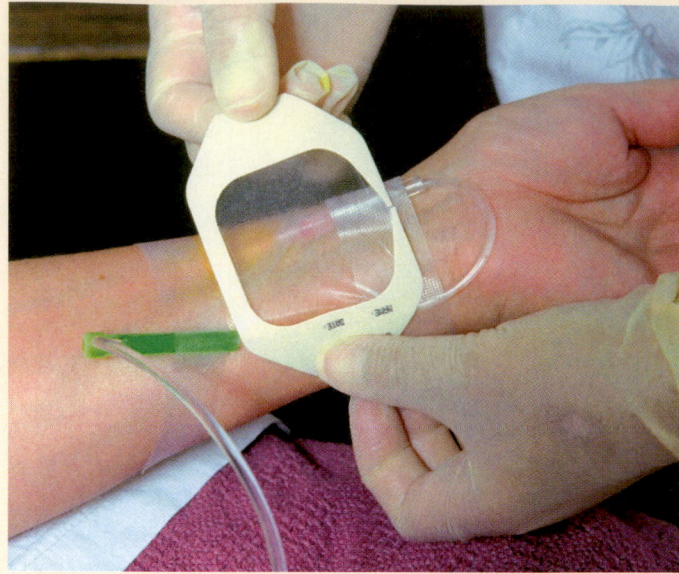

Figure 28-45. ■ Apply transparent dressing over site.

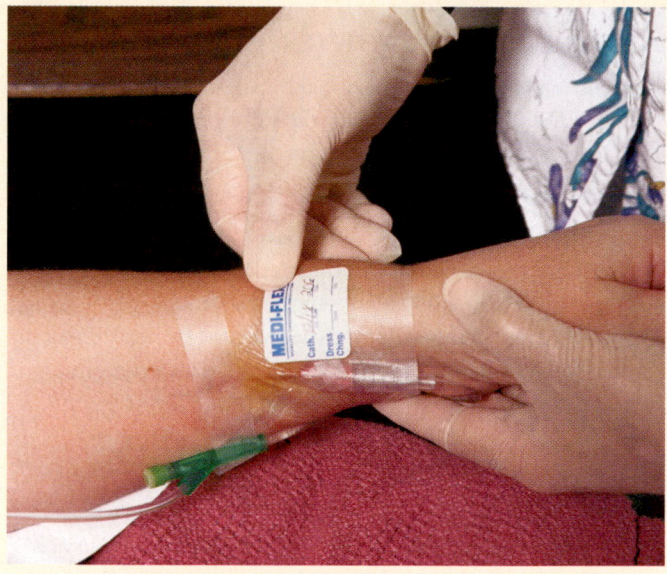

Figure 28-46. ■ Label with initials and date.

SAMPLE DOCUMENTATION

[date] [time]	IV infusion of D_5W 1,000 mL at 125 mL per hour initiated with #22 ONC to the left hand. IV site is clean and dry without evidence of erythema or edema. Client tolerated procedure well; no complaints of pain at the site. _____
	_____ C. Porter, LVN

PROCEDURE 28-10 # Assessing and Maintaining an IV Insertion Site

Purposes

- To assess the IV site regularly
- To evaluate for changes in the patency of the system
- To maintain the prescribed infusion rate
- To assess for complications and report to the physician

Equipment

- Clean gloves
- Tape

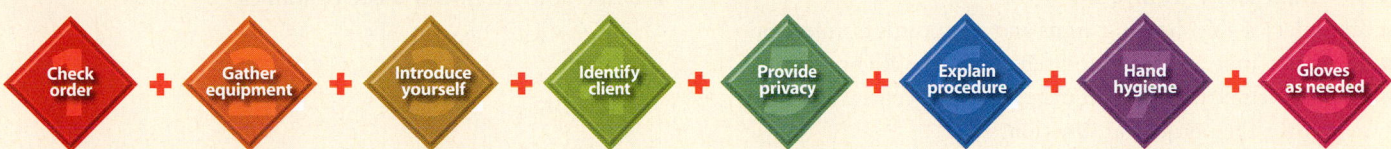

Check order + Gather equipment + Introduce yourself + Identify client + Provide privacy + Explain procedure + Hand hygiene + Gloves as needed

Interventions and Rationales

1. Perform preparatory steps (see icon bar above).

2. Explain the procedure to the client and enlist his or her cooperation. *The IV site should be evaluated every 8 hours for complications or more frequently if the client's condition warrants it.*

3. Provide the client with privacy.

4. Check the physician order and the sequence of the IV bags. Compare the IV label name and the client's identification band. *This confirms that the infusion is being given to the right client. If the IV bag and the ID band do not match, slow the IV container to a keep-open rate until corrective action can be implemented. Follow agency policy requiring incident reporting.*

5. Monitor the rate of flow and the volume infused hourly. Check the time strip as to the fluid remaining in the IV bag. *Although electronic devices used to monitor the volume and rate have improved IV therapy, they are not infallible and sometime need adjustment. Ultimately the responsibility lies with the nurse caring for the client. To read the volume remaining in the bag stretch the upper edges of the bag. If the rate is too slow, make adjustments to the predetermined rate. If the rate is too fast, the physician may need to be notified; follow agency policy. Infusing fluid too quickly can lead to fluid overload.*

6. Observe for the patency of the IV tubing and catheter. Check that the drip chamber is half full and make adjustments if needed. Examine the tubing for kinks and obstructions. *The client lying on the tubing can be an impediment to the flow. If the flow is less than prescribed, lower the IV bag and look for a blood return at the IV site. A blood return indicates that the needle is intact and properly placed in the vein. Venous pressure is stronger than the fluid pressure in the IV tubing giving a blood return. If no blood is returned, it may indicate that the catheter is no longer placed in the vein or is partially obstructed. Be aware that a soft catheter may not demonstrate a blood return and still be placed properly.*

7. Apply gloves. Palpate the site gently through the transparent dressing. *Note any redness or infiltration at the site. Observe for leakage and determine the cause. It could be a loosening at the catheter hub, in which case, tighten the connection. If that does not stop the leakage, change the tubing. If the flow continues to be less than ordered, adjust the level of the catheter bevel slowly. If by raising the catheter the fluid flow improves, place a 2 × 2 gauze under the hub and tape securely. The catheter bevel can be up against the wall of the vein, causing a partial obstruction of the infusate solution or a tendency to be positional.*

8. Check the date on the peripheral IV label. Change the IV to a new proximal site every 72 hours according to facility policy. *INS standards indicate that a peripheral short catheter should be removed every 72 hours and immediately upon suspected contamination.* See Procedure 28-9.

9. Check the date on the administration set and extension tubing. Change every 72 hours according to facility policy. This preventive measure can be routinely done with a new IV bag infusion. *INS standards indicate that primary and secondary administration sets should be changed every 72 hours and immediately upon suspected contamination.*

SAMPLE DOCUMENTATION

[date]
[time]   IV of D5LR #2 bag infusing at 80 mL per hour. IV seems to be positional, will monitor for changes. IV site to the right hand is clean and dry; there is no evidence of pain, redness, or edema. _____
_____ A. Parra, LVN

PROCEDURE 28-11   # Discontinuing or Terminating IV Therapy

Purposes

- To replace a compromised cannula
- To change an IV site after 72 to 96 hours (following hospital policy)
- To discontinue or terminate an IV per physician order
- To change an IV infiltration site
- To replace a site showing signs and symptoms of infection
- To discontinue an IV upon discharge of the client
- To discontinue an IV upon placement of a central line that takes over the peripheral function

Equipment

- Clean gloves
- Sterile (2 × 2 or 4 × 4) gauze pads (Avoid use of an alcohol wipe, it promotes stinging and bleeding.)
- Tape or adhesive bandage
- Disposable hazardous waste container

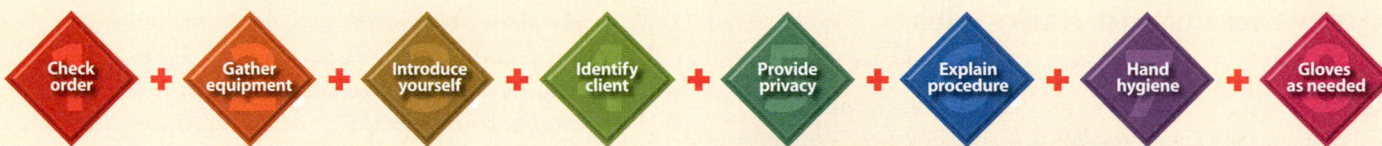

Check order ✚ Gather equipment ✚ Introduce yourself ✚ Identify client ✚ Provide privacy ✚ Explain procedure ✚ Hand hygiene ✚ Gloves as needed

Interventions and Rationales

1. Perform preparatory steps (see icon bar above).

2. Turn off the infusate with the slide/roller clamp (Figure 28-47 ■). Gloves optional. *This prevents the fluid from flowing out of the catheter onto the bed or client.*

3. Apply clean gloves. Loosen tape and dressing toward the cannula, while holding the needle or cannula firmly in place (Figure 28-48 ■). Apply countertraction to the skin. Adhesive remover can be used for the client who is particularly sensitive. *Movement of the catheter or cannula can injure the vein and cause the client discomfort. Countertraction prevents pulling the skin and causing discomfort or trauma.*

4. Stabilize the cannula. *Stabilizing the cannula avoids movement that can traumatize the site, causing increased bleeding and pain.*

5. Hold folded gauze over site while removing cannula/needle. Avoid pressure to site until cannula/needle is removed smoothly (Figure 28-49 ■). *Pressure applied prior to cannula removal causes the client discomfort.*

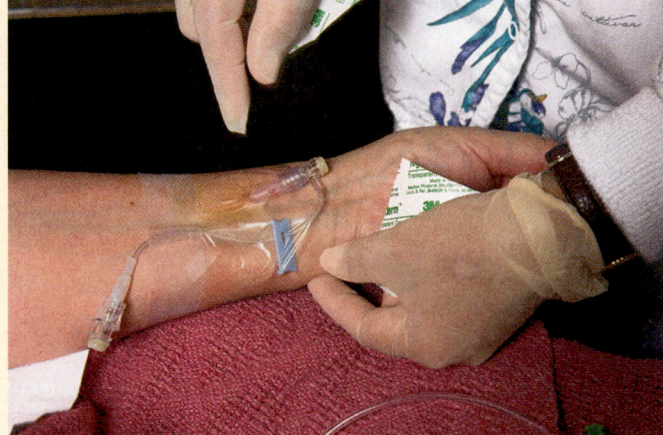

Figure 28-48. ■ Loosen dressing and tape.

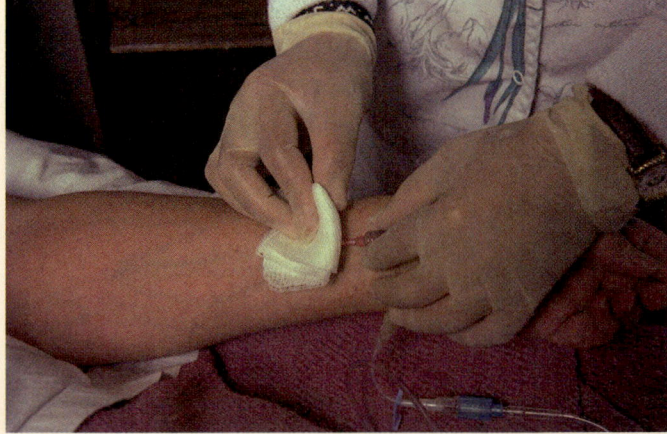

Figure 28-49. ■ Remove needle carefully and smoothly.

6. Apply gauze pressure to insertion site (Figure 28-50 ■). *Pressure stops bleeding. Avoid the use of an alcohol wipe, it promotes bleeding and causes stinging to the site.* Hold

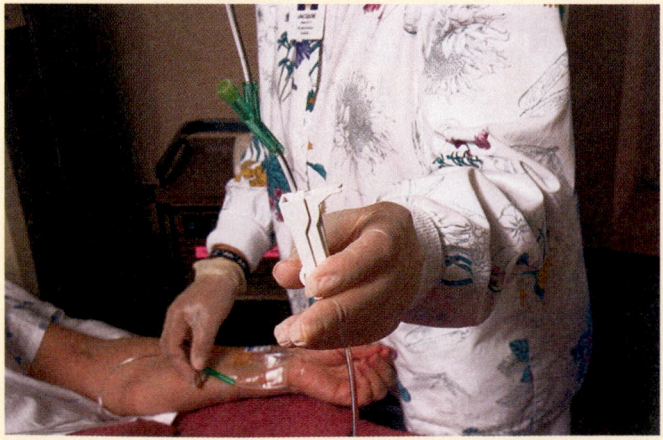

Figure 28-47. ■ Turn off infusion, discontinue IV.

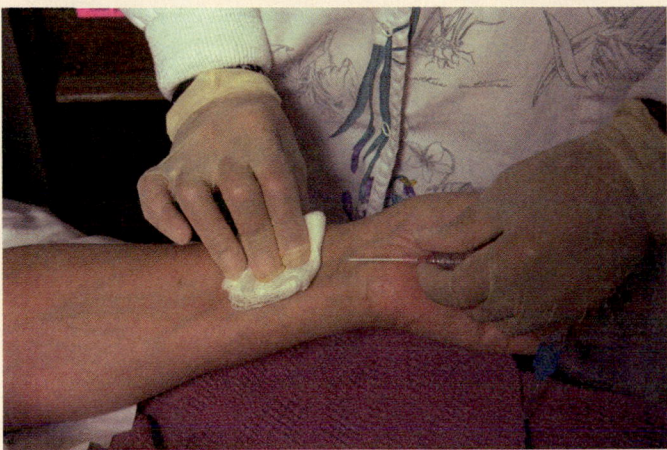

Figure 28-50. ■ Apply pressure to puncture site.

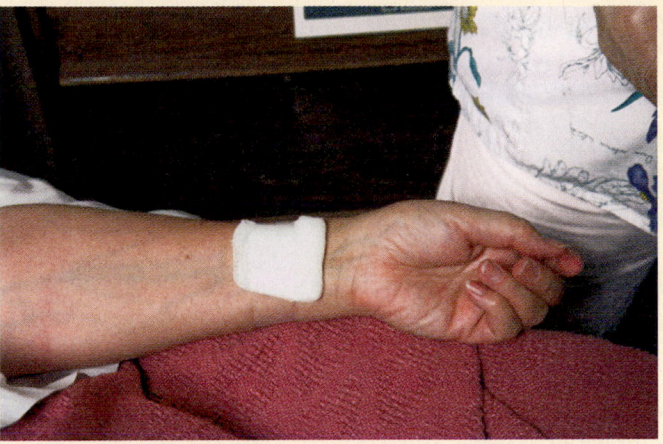

Figure 28-51. ■ Tape gauze into place.

pressure for a few minutes, longer if client is taking antithrombotics/anticoagulants. Do not walk away until bleeding has ceased. *Clotting time will be prolonged in clients using these drugs.* Hold the client's limb above the level of the heart if bleeding persists. *Raising the limb decreases blood flow to the area.*

7. Observe for signs of hematoma, redness, or swelling. Examine the catheter to make certain that it is intact. *These signs are potential complications of IV insertion. If a piece of the catheter or tubing remains in the client's vein, it could move toward the heart or lungs, causing serious problems. Immediately apply a tourniquet above the insertion site and report it to the physician and charge nurse.*

8. Tape gauze into place or use adhesive bandage (Figure 28-51 ■). *The dressing inhibits microorganisms from entering the open site.*

9. Dispose of equipment and gloves in the appropriate container. *Proper disposal inhibits transmission of microorganisms.*

10. Document pertinent information. Record the cannula size that was removed and document the fluid infused on the intake and output form according to the agency practice. Include the container number, type of solution, time of the IV discontinuance, and the client's response.

SAMPLE DOCUMENTATION

[date]   NS bag #2 and IV discontinued as
[time]   per physician order, cannula
         22 gauge fully intact. Site clean
         and dry; no evidence of further
         bleeding. Pressure dressing
         applied. Client tolerated the
         procedure well; no complaints of
         pain, edema, or ecchymosis at the
         site. _____

         _____ J. Ian, LVN

PROCEDURE 28-12 Transfusing Blood or Blood Components

Purposes

- To restore or expand blood volume
- To treat blood deficiencies such as anemia and other hematologic disorders
- To improve the oxygen-carrying capacity of the circulatory system

Equipment

- Normal saline solution (NSS), 500 mL
- Blood or component unit
- Y-set blood tubing with filter (170- to 240-micron filter)
- Venipuncture set (if site not established)
- Over-the-needle cannula (ONC), recommended 18–20 gauge or larger (22 gauge for limited transfusions)
- Needleless cannula
- Antimicrobial swabs
- Tape
- Electronic monitoring device designed for blood administration or freestanding IV pole
- Blood warming device (not required for routine transfusions)

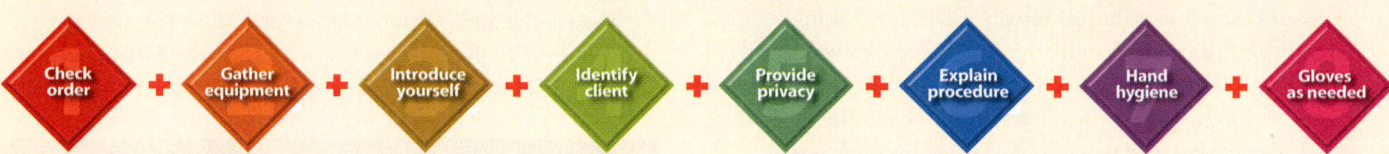

Interventions and Rationales

1. Perform preparatory steps (see icon bar above).

2. Verify physician's order. *The physician's order should be specific to the blood/blood components and the duration of transfusion.* Follow the facility's policies and procedures for transfusion therapy.

3. Check client's identification band, and ask client to state his or her name. *INS standards indicate that nurses are responsible for verification of client identification.*

4. Obtain or check the client's signed transfusion consent form. *INS standards indicate that the nurse is responsible for confirmation of an informed client consent.*

5. Assess the client's understanding of the purpose of blood transfusion and associated risks. *INS standards specify that nurses are responsible for client education.* Gather information regarding the client's previous blood transfusion response or allergic reactions.

6. Determine that the type and crossmatch has been processed and the blood/blood component is available in the blood bank.

7. Assess the patency of the client's current intravenous therapy. Initiate infusion with NSS 0.9%, using the Y-set blood tubing with filter (Figure 28-52 ■). *Normal saline is an isotonic solution that has an osmolarity equal to that of serum. Hypotonic solutions cause blood cells to burst, resulting in hemolysis, and hypertonic solutions cause blood cells to dilute and shrink. Blood and blood components should be filtered; the minimum pore size of a blood filter is between 170 and 260 microns.* Establish an intravenous line for the transfusion if IV is not available. Follow the steps in Procedure 28-9 for performing a venipuncture using the

ONC procedure with a cannula gauge of 18 to 20. *A cannula size of 18 to 20 gauge is necessary to provide adequate transfusion flow. A 22 gauge can be used for plasma products.*

8. Check the client's pretransfusion vital signs for baseline information. *An existing temperature elevation must be reported to the physician before proceeding.*

9. Obtain the blood or blood component from the blood bank (Figure 28-53 ■). The nurse verifies the blood/blood component bag with the laboratory technician, by checking component type, ABO and Rh, unit number, expiration date, and client identification number. The nurse's and laboratory technician's signatures/initials are required to validate and document that proper procedure has been followed. *Blood/blood component cannot be returned to the blood bank after it has been checked out for 20 minutes. Blood transfusion should be initiated within 30 minutes after being checked out of the blood bank. Blood is refrigerated at 33.6 to 42.8°F (1–6°C) in the blood bank; do not refrigerate blood on the nursing unit. Blood bank refrigerators are carefully monitored for constant control.* Check the blood unit for bubbles, cloudiness, color, and sediment. *These signs indicate bacterial contamination. If these signs are present, return the blood unit immediately and document your observations.*

10. The nurse returns to the unit and will again double check the blood/blood component with another licensed nurse before proceeding (Figure 28-54 ■). The nurse verifies the blood/blood component bag by checking component type, ABO and Rh, unit number, expiration date, and client identification number.

11. Record and document VS 5 minutes prior to initiating blood/blood component bag transfusion. The nurse verifies the client's name, identification number,

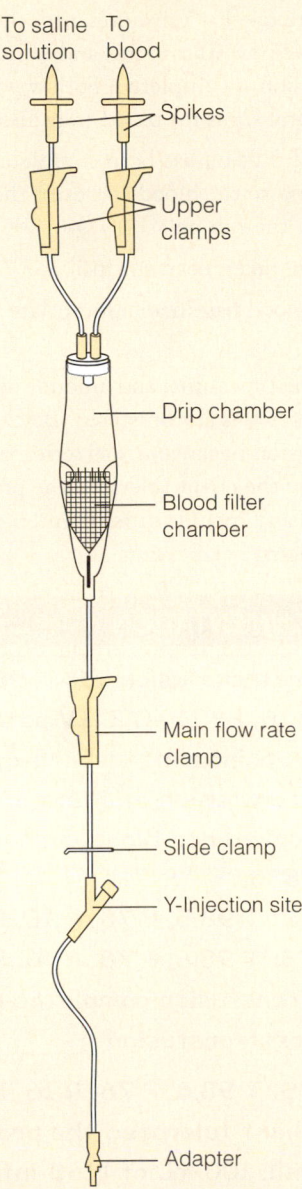

To saline solution — To blood

Spikes

Upper clamps

Drip chamber

Blood filter chamber

Main flow rate clamp

Slide clamp

Y-Injection site

Adapter

Figure 28-52. ■ Blood tubing.

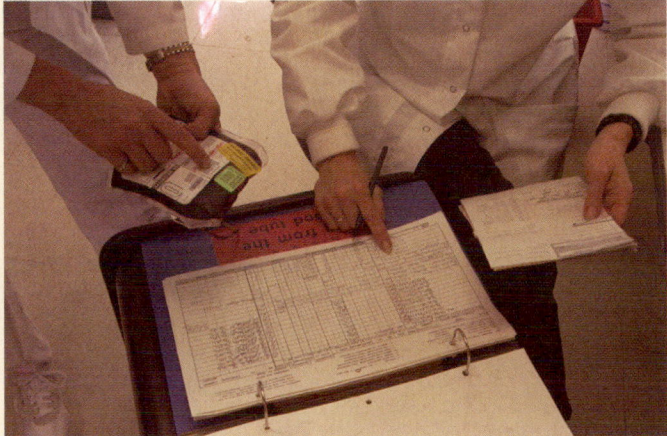

Figure 28-53. ■ Obtain ordered typed and matched blood or blood component bag from blood bank.

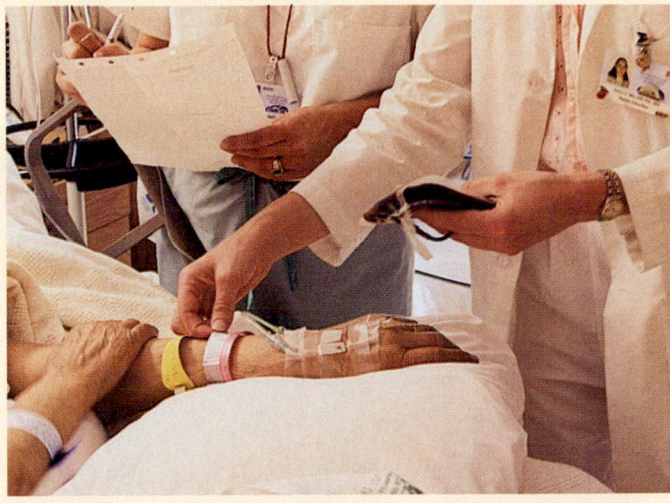

Figure 28-54. ■ Blood transfusion, verify label.

checking component type, ABO and Rh, unit number, and expiration date at the bedside.

12. Perform hand hygiene and apply clean gloves.

13. Prime tubing with NSS then close all clamps on the Y-set tubing (Figure 28-55 ■). Once the tubing has been primed attach the needleless cannula.

14. Remove the protective covering on the bag port and spike the blood bag with the Y-set. Open the clamps to the blood. Prime the tubing with blood/blood component. Agitate the blood/blood component bag. *This facilitates the mixing of blood with the anticoagulant additive in the bag.*

15. Initiate the blood transfusion slowly, it is recommended to start with 5 mL/min for the first 15 minutes of the transfusion. *Slowing the administration allows the nurse time to observe for adverse blood transfusion reactions* (Figure 28-56 ■). Blood/blood component should be infused within 4 hours. *Packed cells are routinely infused within 1 1/2 to 2 hours. Do not mix medications with blood/blood components. Stop the infusion immediately if an adverse transfusion reaction is apparent and notify the physician. Keep the vein open with a NSS. Follow agency policy for transfusion reactions, which may include sending the first voided urine specimen to the laboratory, documenting vital signs, and returning the blood container and tubing to the laboratory for further testing.*

16. Ensure that the electronic monitoring device being used is designed for use with blood/blood components. *Other types of infusion devices can cause hemolysis. Infusion devices control and regulate transfusion rate.*

17. Blood warming devices are not used for most transfusions but may be indicated for rapid transfusions or neonatal transfusion exchanges and clients receiving cold agglutinins. Follow manufacturer's instructions. *Do not attempt to warm blood in a microwave or hot water.*

18. Vital signs are taken 15 minutes after the transfusion begins followed by 30 minutes and 60 minutes thereafter until transfusion is completed. Follow your agency policy for routine vital signs for blood transfusions.

19. When the transfusion has been completed, close the clamps leading to the blood and open the clamp from the NSS flushing the tubing.

20. Vital signs are taken posttransfusion.

21. Discard the blood bag in an appropriate biohazard waste container.

22. Document the type, unit, and amount of blood/blood component that was administered. Be clear about the time the infusion began and was terminated. Note vital signs and how the client tolerated the procedure. Detail any reactions and include nursing interventions initiated. Record physician notification.

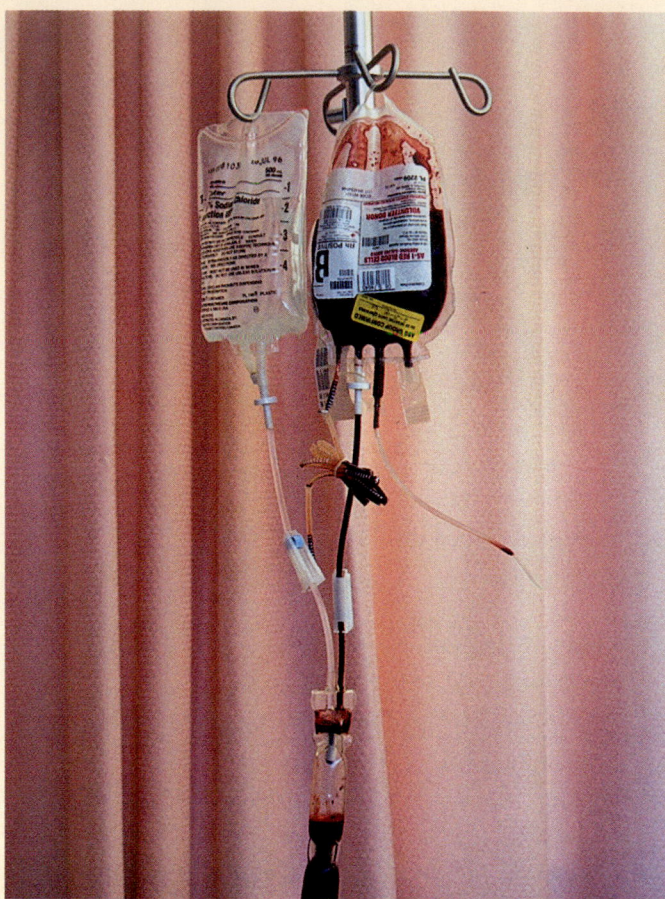

Figure 28-55. ■ Prime blood administration with normal saline before starting infusion with Y-set tubing.

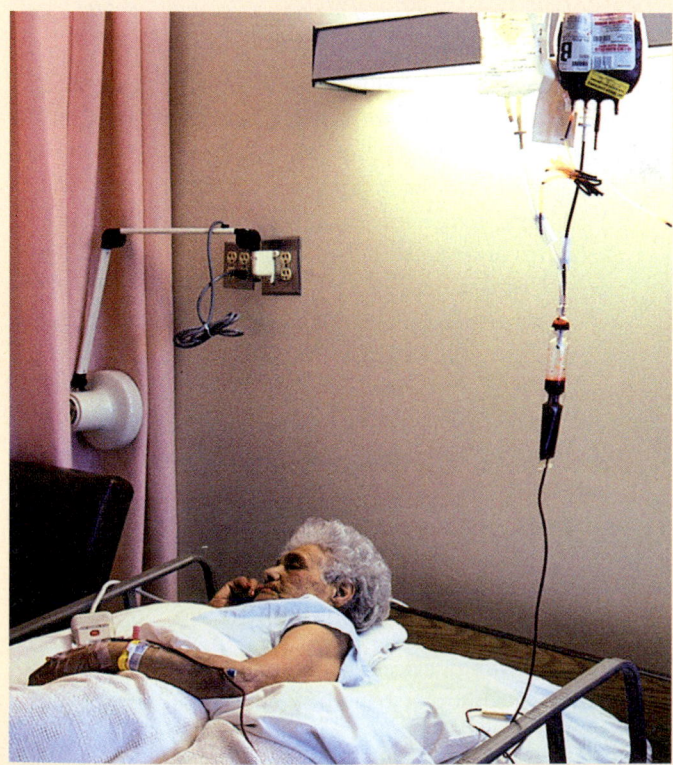

Figure 28-56. ■ Observe client for adverse signs.

SAMPLE DOCUMENTATION

[date]	Pretransfusion VS: T 98.7, P 76, R 16, BP 110/72. IV patent with
0825	NSS infusing at keep-open rate. Transfusion of 1 unit of 250 mL of packed red blood cells initiated at 0830.
0845	VS: T 98.5, P 78, R 18, BP 108/70.
0915	VS: T 98.6, P 78, R 16, BP 110/78. Transfusion completed at 1,000. Posttransfusion
	VS: T 98.6, P 76, R 16, BP 112/78. Client tolerated the procedure well. 100 mL of NSS infused. No adverse reactions noted. IV site is clean and dry. _____
	_____ J. French, LVN

Chapter Review

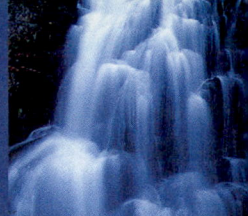

KEY Points

- The LPN/LVN must be knowledgeable and skillful when delivering IV therapy.
- A departure from the accepted standards of practice related to IV therapy is considered malpractice.
- IV therapy is used to maintain blood volume, to deliver medications quickly, to provide nutrition, or to reestablish homeostasis when acid-base imbalance has occurred.
- Standards of care must be developed within organizations to measure quality based on expectations of service. Organizations involved in IV therapy are OSHA, FDA, CDC, DHS, HIPAA, ANA, INS, the Joint Commission, AABB, and EPA.
- Identification of the appropriate equipment and understanding the purpose of IV therapy for the client will assist the nurse in the selection of the necessary equipment.
- Intravenous solutions can be classified as isotonic, hypotonic, or hypertonic. IV solutions can also be categorized according to their purpose: providing nutrition, replacing electrolytes, or expanding blood volume.
- The nurse is responsible for the regulation of flow rates by determining the infusion time or the total hours to be infused, calculating milliliters per hour and drops per minute.
- Knowledge of the integumentary and venous systems assists the nurse to determine vein suitability for IV therapy.
- A cannula should be of the smallest gauge and shortest length possible to accommodate the necessary therapy.
- Complications of IV therapy may be either localized or systemic. The nurse must take contributing factors into consideration.
- The LPN/LVN is responsible for monitoring the drip rate of an IV; even if the IV is on a pump, the nurse is still responsible for monitoring the amount infused.
- Three types of blood donation collection methods include homologous, autologous, and designated.
- Blood products are always infused using a "Y" infusion set; a saline infusion is hung on the nonfiltered chamber.

⊙⊙ FOR FURTHER Study

For more information on negligence in nursing, see Chapter 4.

For more information on stabilizing catheters, see Chapter 24.

See Chapter 26 for a discussion of fluids and electrolytes.

For a review of the major veins, see Figure 33-7.

See Figure 63-3 for an example of an Occurrence/Incident Report.

EXPLORE PEARSON **mynursingkit**™

MyNursingKit is your one stop for online chapter review materials and resources. Prepare for success with additional NCLEX®-style practice questions, interactive assignments and activities, web links, animations and videos, and more!

Register your access code from the front of your book at **www.mynursingkit.com**

Critical Thinking Care Map

Caring for a Client Requiring a Blood Transfusion
NCLEX-PN® Focus Area: Physiological Adaptation

Case Study: Margaret Woods is a 50-year-old woman who underwent a surgical procedure for a right hip replacement. Prior to admission for her surgery she participated in an autologous blood donation for two units of blood. Postoperatively, she returned to the hospital unit with a dressing to the right hip with some drainage and a Hemovac drain to suction that drained 150 mL of serosanguineous drainage.

Nursing Diagnosis: *Deficient Fluid Volume*

COLLECT DATA

Subjective	Objective
_____	_____
_____	_____
_____	_____
_____	_____
_____	_____
_____	_____
_____	_____

Would you report this? Yes/No

If yes, report to: _____

What would you report? _____

Nursing Care

_____
_____
_____
_____
_____
_____
_____
_____
_____
_____

How would you document this? _____
_____
_____

Compare your answers and documentation to those provided on the MyNursingKit Website.

Data Collected
(use only those that apply)

- 50-year-old female
- Surgery: right hip replacement
- Height: 5 ft 4 in.
- Weight: 200 lbs
- VS: T 99, P 110, R 22, BP 90/55
- Hemoglobin 6 g/dL, hematocrit 22%
- Hemovac 150 mL, serosanguineous drainage
- CXR clear
- Blood sugar 120
- Abductor pillow placed
- Pain level 8
- Ferrous sulfate 325 mg
- Demerol 75 mg every 4 hours prn for pain
- D_5W at 125 mL
- Soft diet
- Lethargic

Nursing Interventions
(use only those that apply; list in priority order)

- Arrange PT consult.
- Reinforce surgical dressing.
- Monitor I&O.
- Drain Hemovac and record drainage.
- Increase diet to Reg.
- Monitor H/H.
- Transfuse client with 1 unit PRBCs if H/H is less than 7 g/dL or 22%.
- Monitor VS every 4 hours.
- Elevate legs.

NCLEX-PN® Exam Preparation

1 The nurse is initiating IV therapy for the purpose of blood administration. The best catheter for the nurse to choose is:
1. 18 gauge.
2. 10 gauge.
3. 25 gauge.
4. 22 gauge.

2 The nurse is preparing to administer blood and selects Y tubing. What type of IV solution will the nurse hang with the infusing blood?
1. D5W
2. D51/2NS
3. LR
4. NS

3 The nurse is caring for a client with an intermittent infusion device and recognizes that the purpose of this device is to:
1. Prevent phlebitis.
2. Provide vascular access.
3. Prevent infiltration.
4. Administer solutions at a prescribed rate.

4 The physician orders 1,000 mL of IV fluid to be administered over 6 hours. The nurse chooses an administration set that delivers 10 drops per minute. There are no IV infusion devices available, and the nurse must adjust the rate of infusion by hand. How many drops per minute will the nurse deliver in order to properly carry out the physician's order?
1. 28 drops per minute
2. 17 drops per minute
3. 100 drops per minute
4. 167 drops per minute

5 The nurse is initiating IV therapy to administer antibiotics and blood. The nurse's best choice of an IV site is:
1. Cephalic.
2. Dorsal metacarpal vein.
3. Digital vein.
4. Median antecubital vein.

6 The experienced nurse is observing a nursing student initiate IV therapy. Which of the following would demonstrate correct technique?
1. The student inserts the IV catheter at a 45-degree angle with the bevel up.
2. When the student sees a blood return in the catheter, the IV tubing is connected to the catheter and the catheter is advanced while the fluid is flowing at a wide-open rate.
3. When blood backflow is seen in the catheter the student releases the vein stretch and advances the catheter into the vein.
4. The student nurse approaches the vein with the bevel up and to the side of the vein while holding the skin taut.

7 The nurse is caring for a normally healthy 15-year-old who has experienced acute vomiting and diarrhea over the past 2 days. The nurse notes dry mucous membranes and poor skin turgor; the client reports she has not voided in more than 12 hours. The nurse anticipates administration of what type of fluid?
1. Lactated Ringer's
2. 0.45% normal saline
3. D5LR
4. D5 0.9% NS

8 The nurse moves from one state to another state and begins work at the local hospital. The nurse determines the legalities of providing IV therapy by:
1. The facility policy.
2. The nurse practice act for that state.
3. Previous experience with IV therapy.
4. Both facility policy and the nurse practice act.

9 The nurse employs minidrip administration sets primarily when working with:
1. Pediatric clients.
2. Diabetic clients.
3. Any client admitted to an acute care facility.
4. Pregnant clients.

10 A client receiving IV therapy via a central line is exhibiting fluctuating temperature, profuse sweating, nausea, and a blood pressure that is lower than normal. The nurse suspects:
1. A local infection.
2. Septicemia.
3. Venous spasm.
4. Circulatory overload.

Answers and rationales for Review Questions appear in Appendix I.

Thinking Strategically About...

You are a newly graduated LPN/LVN assigned to a medical-surgical unit. You have been assigned to three clients.

Mr. Ramos is a 58-year-old male who was admitted for a prostatectomy (TURP) this morning. He is predominantly Spanish speaking, though he knows a few words of English and understands a little if he is spoken to slowly. He has returned from surgery. Initially he was sedated but begins to be more alert. He appears agitated and is yelling loudly at his roommate, who puts on his call light to summon the nurse. The roommate states, "Mr. Ramos is trying to climb out of bed and he is frightening me."

Mr. Drew is a 53-year-old male who was admitted directly from his physician's office with chest pain. His BP is 168/90 with tachycardia (heart rate 102). He is diaphoretic and is complaining of nausea.

Mr. Melezack is a 64-year-old male who had a colon resection 3 days ago. His NG tube has been clamped and he has been started on clear liquids. It was reported that he tolerated them well. The doctor has ordered that the tube can be removed if there is no nausea or vomiting.

CRITICAL THINKING

Mr. Ramos is frightening his roommate and trying to climb out of bed. He has an IV line and a three-way catheter that is draining dark red urine with clots. Outline the steps you would take to protect Mr. Ramos from himself and to relieve the concerns of the roommate.

PRIORITIZING NURSING CARE

You have received report. Using your knowledge of the three clients' diagnoses and present needs, prioritize your care for the shift.

MANAGEMENT OF CARE

- How frequently should you monitor Mr. Drew?
- Identify what care needs to be provided to each client and the time you will provide that care.

DELEGATING

What tasks can be delegated to a nursing assistant? What follow-up will need to be done?

CLIENT TEACHING

Mr. Drew's lab work has come back. You observe that his CPK values are within normal limits and that his chest pain is relieved with sublingual nitroglycerin spray. He will be discharged in the morning and you are to begin his discharge planning. In your teaching plan, state what activities would decrease the chance of recurrent angina and the risk factors that need to be controlled to decrease heart disease.

DOCUMENTING AND REPORTING

The client care assistant reports to you that Mr. Melezack is complaining of abdominal pain. He has vomited and asks to see you right away. After you go to his room to assess his present status, you will need to document and report your finding to the appropriate individuals. Write a medical record entry, using the Focus Charting method.

Medical Surgical Nursing Care

UNIT V

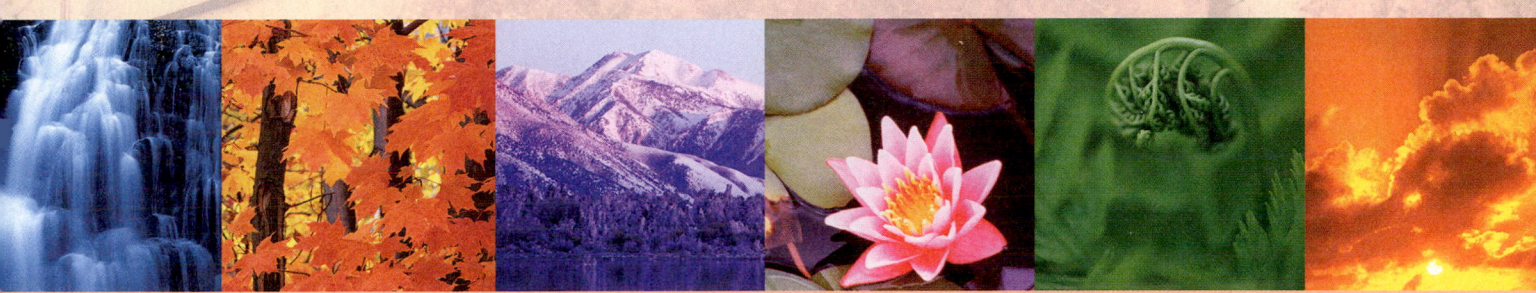

Chapter 29

Nursing Care of Clients Having Surgery

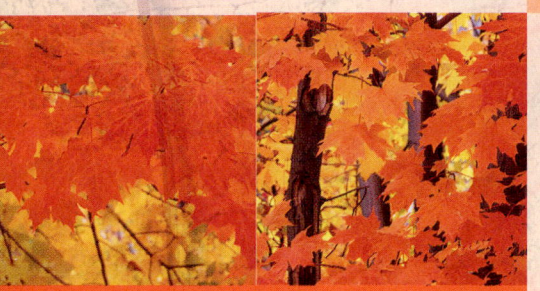

BRIEF Outline

LEARNING Outcomes

After completing this chapter, you will be able to:

1. Describe the phases of the perioperative period.
2. Discuss various types of surgery according to the purpose, degree of urgency, and degree of risk.
3. List the types of wounds and their potential complications.
4. Identify tests that may occur and overall nursing responsibilities in the perioperative period.
5. Describe essential preoperative teaching.
6. Name essential aspects of nursing care when preparing a client for surgery.
7. Describe the types of anesthesia that may be used intraoperatively.
8. Discuss the nurse's role in the care of the postoperative client.
9. Identify potential postoperative problems and preventive measures.
10. Describe ongoing care of the surgical client, including suture and staple removal and discharge considerations.
11. Explain ways that LPNs/LVNs can provide wound care and support healing.

Clinical Objectives

12. Demonstrate the procedure for preparing clients for surgery.
13. Perform a surgical prep (scrub and shave).
14. Provide preoperative teaching, including turning, coughing, and deep breathing.
15. Observe a client's postoperative vital signs and status.
16. Set up equipment for suctioning.

KEY TERMS

ablative 711

anesthesia 718

antiemboli stockings 717

aspiration pneumonia 720

atelectasis 720

closed wound drainage system 725

conscious sedation 718

dehiscence 721

diagnostic 711

elective surgery 711

embolus 721

emergency surgery 711

evisceration 721

general anesthesia 718

palliative 711

paralytic ileus 721

perioperative period 711

prostheses 716

pulmonary embolism 720

reconstructive 711

regional anesthesia 718

sequential compression device 717

surgery 711

sutures 725

thrombophlebitis 720

thrombus 721

tissue perfusion 719

transplant 711

tympanites 721

Surgery is a unique experience of a planned physical alteration by manual or operative methods. It encompasses three phases: preoperative, intraoperative, and postoperative. The *preoperative phase* occurs prior to surgery, the *intraoperative phase* occurs during surgery, and the *postoperative phase* occurs following surgery. These three phases are together referred to as the **perioperative period.** The LPN's and LVN's responsibilities are usually confined to client care in the postoperative period, although preoperative preparation is within the scope of the practical/vocational nurse.

Surgery

Surgical procedures are commonly grouped in one of three ways:

1. *Purpose.* Surgical procedures may be categorized according to their purpose (Box 29-1 ■).
2. *Degree of urgency.* Surgery is classified by its urgency and necessity to preserve the client's life, body part, or body function. **Emergency surgery** is performed immediately to preserve function or the life of the client. **Elective surgery** is performed when a condition is not immediately life threatening or to improve the client's life.
3. *Degree of risk.* Surgery is also classified as major or minor according to the degree of risk to the client.

> ### BOX 29-1 PURPOSE OF SURGICAL PROCEDURES
>
> **Diagnostic** Confirms or establishes a diagnosis (e.g., biopsy of a mass in a breast).
> **Palliative** Relieves or reduces pain or symptoms of a disease; does not cure (e.g., resection of nerve roots).
> **Ablative** Removes a diseased body part (e.g., removal of a gallbladder [cholecystectomy], removal of cancer tissue).
> **Reconstructive** Restores function or appearance that has been lost or reduced (e.g., breast implant).
> **Transplant** Replaces malfunctioning structures (e.g., hip replacement).

Major surgery involves a high degree of risk. In contrast, *minor surgery* normally involves little risk, produces few complications, and is often performed on an outpatient basis as "day surgery." The degree of risk involved in a surgical procedure is affected by the client's age, general health, nutritional status, use of medications, and mental status. Box 29-2 ■ lists health problems that increase surgical risk.

TYPES OF WOUNDS

As discussed in Chapter 24 ∞ , body wounds may be categorized in various ways. These include the following:

- intentional or unintentional trauma
- closed wound or open wound (see more about wounds and injury to the skin in Chapters 24 and 30 ∞)
- incision, contusion, abrasion, puncture, laceration, penetrating wound (see Table 24-1 ∞)
- contaminated or uncontaminated

Surgical wounds, of course, are a type of intentional trauma.

Wound care for postsurgical clients must be carried out with tremendous care, because skin integrity has been compromised. Poor wound care technique would lead to infection and perhaps other complications. Procedure 29-1 ■ provides steps in doing wound care for surgical dressings.

Complications of wound healing include hemorrhage, infection, dehiscence, and evisceration. Factors that can improve or impair wound healing are age and lifestyle, nutrition, medications, and contamination. These are described in detail in Chapter 24 ∞ .

Preoperative Phase

PREOPERATIVE CONSENT

Prior to any surgical procedure, clients must sign a consent form, which is generally supplied by the agency. This requirement protects clients from having any surgical procedure they do not want or do not understand. It also protects

BOX 29-2 RISK FACTORS FOR CLIENTS NEEDING SURGERY

- Malnutrition can lead to delayed wound healing, infection, and reduced energy. Protein and vitamins are needed for wound healing; vitamin K is essential for blood clotting.
- Obesity leads to hypertension, impaired cardiac function, and impaired respiratory ventilation. Obese clients are also more likely to have delayed wound healing and wound infection because adipose tissue impedes blood circulation and its delivery of nutrients, antibodies, and enzymes required for wound healing.
- Cardiac conditions such as angina pectoris, recent myocardial infarction, hypertension, and congestive heart failure weaken the heart. Well-controlled cardiac problems generally pose minimal operative risk.
- Blood coagulation disorders may lead to severe bleeding, hemorrhage, and subsequent shock. (Lab values of clients with hematologic disorders are monitored carefully preoperatively and postoperatively.)
- Upper respiratory tract infections or chronic obstructive pulmonary diseases (COPD) such as emphysema adversely affect pulmonary function, especially when exacerbated by the effects of general anesthesia. They also predispose the client to postoperative lung infections.
- Renal disease or insufficiency impairs regulation of the body's fluids and electrolytes and excretion of drugs and other toxins.

- Diabetes mellitus predisposes the client to wound infection and delayed healing.
- Liver disease (e.g., cirrhosis) impairs the liver's abilities to detoxify medications used during surgery, produce the prothrombin necessary for blood clotting, and metabolize nutrients essential for healing.
- Uncontrolled neurologic disease such as epilepsy may result in seizures during surgery or recovery.
- Aspirin increases blood coagulation time and risk of hemorrhage; it needs to be discontinued several days prior to surgery.
- Steroid therapy can delay or slow wound healing. Steroid medication needs to be withdrawn gradually.
- Many other medications can have adverse effects on the client during and following a surgical procedure. Inform the surgeon of all prescription and over-the-counter drugs, including vitamins, minerals, and herbal preparations, so that a decision can be made as to when they need to be discontinued if necessary.
- Older adults' body systems are less resilient, and recovery time is longer than in the young or middle-aged adults. Chronic conditions such as COPD may make general anesthesia a very high risk. See also Box 29-3 about cultural considerations.

the hospital and the health personnel from a claim by the client or family that permission was not granted. The consent form becomes a part of the client's record and goes to the operating room with the client. The surgical consent is transcribed from the physician's order sheet exactly as stated. Take care to ensure that the procedure is spelled correctly prior to having the consent signed.

Information about the procedure requiring consent is provided by the person performing the surgery. The consent form is signed by the client and may be witnessed by the LPN/LVN. For a complete discussion about informed consent, see Chapter 4 🔗. Box 29-3 ■ describes cultural considerations in consenting to surgery.

SCREENING TESTS

The physician orders preoperative diagnostic tests or screening tests and examinations to determine abnormalities. Check to be sure tests are ordered exactly as stated on the physician's orders. They need to be completed and results

placed in the medical record before the client is prepared for surgery. The surgeon or anesthesiologist should be informed of any abnormal results before the client is sent to the surgical on-call area. Abnormalities may warrant treatment prior to surgery. Table 29-1 ■ lists routine preoperative screening tests.

PREOPERATIVE TEACHING

Preoperative teaching is a vital part of nursing care. Studies have shown that preoperative teaching reduces clients' anxiety and postoperative complications. It also increases their satisfaction with the surgical experience. Thorough preoperative teaching aids the client's return to work and other activities of daily living.

Preoperative instructions for all clients are summarized in Box 29-4 ■. Prior to surgery, clients must learn exercises that will help them to maintain good oxygenation and circulation in the postoperative period. Procedure 29-2 ■ at the end of this chapter provides guidelines for teaching clients about moving, leg exercises, deep breathing, and coughing.

BOX 29-3 CULTURAL PULSE POINTS

Cultural Considerations in Having Surgery

Surgical procedures are acceptable in most cultures as a life-saving measure or a way to alleviate pain and disease. However, there are cultural and religious sanctions against the use of blood products, mainly among Jehovah's Witnesses and Christian Scientists. Some groups also require that amputated body parts be buried rather than discarded as medical waste.

clinical ALERT

Teaching for certain surgeries (nasal surgery, eye surgery, and cranial surgeries) has special requirements. For these surgeries, the client should be instructed to deep breathe but not to cough, because coughing can increase intracranial pressure and heighten the risk of bleeding.

TABLE 29-1	Routine Preoperative Screening Tests
TEST	**RATIONALE**
Complete blood count (CBC)	RBCs, hemoglobin (Hgb), and hematocrit (Hct) are important to the oxygen-carrying capacity of the blood; WBCs are an indicator of immune function
Blood grouping and cross-matching	Determined in case blood transfusion is required during or after surgery
Serum electrolytes (Na, K, Ca^2, Mg^2, Cl^2 HCO$_3$)	To evaluate fluid and electrolyte status
Fasting blood glucose	High levels may indicate undiagnosed diabetes mellitus
Blood urea nitrogen (BUN) and creatinine	To evaluate renal function
ALT, AST, LDH, and bilirubin	To evaluate liver function
Serum albumin and total protein	To evaluate nutritional status
Urinalysis	To determine urine composition and possible abnormal components (e.g., protein or glucose) or infection
Urine culture and sensitivity	To assess for the presence and type of infection
Chest x-ray	To evaluate respiratory status and heart size
Electrocardiogram (ECG)	To identify preexisting cardiac problems or disease

BOX 29-4 CLIENT TEACHING

Preoperative Instructions

- Explain the need for preoperative tests (e.g., laboratory, x-ray, ECG).
- Discuss bowel preparation, if required.
- Discuss skin preparation, including operative area and preoperative bath or shower.
- Discuss preoperative medications, if ordered.
- Explain individual therapies ordered by the physician, such as intravenous therapy, the insertion of a urinary catheter or nasogastric tube, the use of a spirometer, or antiemboli stockings.
- Discuss the visit by the anesthetist.
- Explain the need to restrict food and oral fluids at least 8 hours before surgery and to follow the written instructions about intake *precisely*. *Note:* If the client eats too much or too soon before surgery, the procedure will be canceled (because of the danger of aspiration) and will have to be rescheduled.

- Provide a general timetable for perioperative events, including the time of surgery.
- Discuss the need to remove jewelry, makeup, and all prostheses (e.g., eyeglasses, hearing aids, complete or partial dentures, wig) and all clothing immediately before surgery.
- Inform client about the preoperative holding area, and give the location of the waiting room for support people.
- Teach deep-breathing and coughing exercises (unless the type of surgery contraindicates coughing), leg exercises, ways to turn and move (see Procedure 29-2), and splinting techniques.
- Explain the method of analgesia that will be used postoperatively and explain that the client will need to ask for pain medication, usually every 3 to 4 hours.

PROVIDING PHYSICAL PREPARATION

Preoperative physical preparation includes the following areas: nutrition and fluids, elimination, hygiene, medications, rest, care of valuables (see Figure 14-2 ⬤) and prostheses, special orders, and surgical skin preparation. In many agencies a preoperative checklist (Figure 29-1 ■) is used on the day of surgery. The nurse checks the agency's forms and follows appropriate recording procedures (see Chapter 13 ⬤). Two things are essential:

1. All pertinent records (laboratory records, x-ray films, consents) must be assembled and completed so that operating and recovery room personnel can refer to them.
2. All physical preparation must be completed to ensure client safety.

NUTRITION AND FLUIDS

Adequate hydration and nutrition promote healing. Nurses need to record any signs of malnutrition or fluid imbalance. (See discussion of nutrition in Chapter 25 ⬤ and of fluids and acid-base balance in Chapter 26 ⬤ .)

Many preoperative clients are listed as NPO (nothing by mouth). Because anesthetics depress gastrointestinal functioning and create a danger that the client may vomit and aspirate vomitus during administration of a general anesthetic, the client usually fasts at least 6 to 8 hours before surgery.

Some recent research, however, no longer supports preoperative fasting. The typical order of "NPO after midnight" (or no liquid or food after 12 A.M. on the day of surgery) has been challenged in recent years. Studies have shown that

SURGERY/PROCEDURE CHECKLIST

PREPROCEDURE

Isolation Type:	❑ NA	❑ Advance Directive	❑ Conservator

NPO Since: (if less than 8 hours, notify Anesthesiologist)
Oral Meds Given @:

❑ NKA   ❑ Allergies (list):

Family Location: Pager #:

Invasive Procedure - Procedures involving puncture or incision of the skin or insertion of an instrument or foreign material into the body, including, but not limited to, percutaneous aspiration and biopsies, cardiac and vascular cauterizations, endoscopies, angioplasties and implantations and excluding venipuncture and intravenous therapy.

PRE-PROCEDURE AREA   **PROCEDURE AREA**

YES	NO	NA		YES	NO	NA
			History & physical (H&P) within 30 days prior to admission Date: _____ *If No notify O.R. or procedure area*	H & P Update within 24 hrs: Date: Time:		
			Informed Consent/Risks & Benefits documented check where found: ❑ H&P ❑ Consent ❑ Progress Notes *If No notify O.R. or procedure area*			
			❑ Appropriate Consent/s (i.e., general consent + sterilization as applicable) signed by client or appropriate surrogate ❑ Emergency procedure-consent unobtainable			
			Compare two (2) identifiers - name and D.O.B. with medical record, consent + have client state name if able			
			Procedure/Site verified: ❑ medical record ❑ consent ❑ surgery schedule ❑ client if able			
			MAR and Meditech Current Medication List on chart			
			Anesthesia Consent documented			
			Blood Consent documented Blood Products avail: ❑ Auto ❑ D.D. ❑ T&C ❑ T&H			
			Current Labs on chart/Pregnancy Test			
			X-ray available			
			EKG Date: _____			
			Prosthesis/Metal Implants Location: _____			
			Hearing Aid Disposition: _____			
			Dentures: ❑ Upper ❑ Lower ❑ Partial			
			Jewelry/Piercings left on: _____			
			Contact Lenses/Eyeglasses Disposition: _____			

	SIGNATURES	**ID #**	**DATE/TIME**
Pre Procedure Nurse			
Procedural Nurse			

***REVERSE SIDE COMPLETED IN PROCEDURAL AREA* Addendum A**   Client Label

Figure 29-1. ■ Preoperative checklist.

\multicolumn{3}{c}{**TO BE COMPLETED PRIOR TO PROCEDURE IN THE PROCEDURAL ROOM**}		
YES	**NA**	**CHECK**
		Review all documents (including consent) and studies referring to the client, procedure, site, laterality and position prior to beginning the procedure to verify accuracy of the procedure and site
		Verify the identity of the client by using two distinct client identifiers
		Surgical/Invasive site marked over or adjacent to proposed incision
		X-rays or imaging studies in room confirms client identity and surgical site
		Implants available
		Special equipment available
		"TIME OUT" immediately prior to start of procedure (*CORRECT client, procedure, site, positioning, implant & special equipment*)
	\multicolumn{2}{l}{Document members present for "TIME OUT": (O.R. staff document in Meditech)}
	\multicolumn{2}{l}{_____}
	\multicolumn{2}{l}{_____}
	\multicolumn{2}{l}{In case of discrepancy, procedural physician notified:}
	\multicolumn{2}{l}{Date: _____ Time: _____}
		Procedural physician final site and side verified and communicated with team

SIGNATURE	**ID #**	**DATE/TIME**
Procedure Nurse		

Figure 29-1. ■ Preoperative checklist (*continued*).   Client Label

pulmonary aspiration occurs only rarely as a complication of modern anesthesia (Winslow and Crenshaw, 2002).

In 1999 the American Society of Anesthesiology (ASA) revised its practice guidelines for preoperative fasting in healthy clients undergoing elective procedures. The newer, more liberal recommendations allow consumption of clear liquids up to 2 hours before elective surgery, a light breakfast (like tea and toast) 6 hours before the procedure, and a heavier meal 8 hours beforehand. Children typically are NPO for a shorter period of time. (See Chapter 58 for discussion about children and surgery.) A surgical client who is insulin dependent needs to have food intake and insulin balanced very carefully pre- and postoperatively. Facility policy should be followed.

ELIMINATION

Enemas before surgery are no longer routine, but cleansing enemas may be ordered if bowel surgery is planned (see procedure in Chapter 37). After surgery involving the intestines, peristalsis often does not return for 24 to 48 hours.

Prior to surgery, a retention catheter may be ordered to ensure that the bladder remains empty. This helps prevent inadvertent injury to the bladder, particularly during pelvic surgery. If the client does not have a catheter, it is important to empty the bladder prior to receiving preoperative medications. (See catheterization procedures in Chapter 39 .)

HYGIENE

In some settings, clients are asked to bathe or shower the evening or morning of surgery (or both). In some situations, they will wash the surgical site immediately before applying the antimicrobial agent in the practice setting. The purpose of hygienic measures is to reduce the risk of wound infection. The bath includes a shampoo whenever possible (see Chapter 20).

In most agencies, skin preparation is carried out during the intraoperative phase. The purpose of surgical skin prep/scrub is to reduce the risk of postoperative wound infection. Skin preparation and scrub remove soil and transient microorganisms from the skin. They reduce the resident microbial count quickly and with the least amount of tissue irritation. They also retard the rebound growth of microorganisms at the surgical site.

Hair removal at the surgical site should be performed according to physicians' orders or policies and procedures of the practice setting. Hair is best left at the surgical site, but the amount of hair, the location of the incision, or the type of surgical procedure to be performed may require removal. Hair should be removed as close to the time of surgery as possible and in a manner that preserves skin integrity (generally by electric clipper or depilatory cream rather than a razor). These actions will help prevent recolonization prior to surgery. Hair should not be removed in the vicinity of the sterile field because loose hair has the potential to contaminate the surgical site and sterile field.

The surgical site and surrounding area should be prepared with an antimicrobial agent. Preparation of surgical areas should include consideration of the length of the incision and all potential requirements for the surgical procedure. Potential requirements include extension of the incision, need for additional incisions, and all potential drain sites. It also includes area enough to avoid wound contamination by movement of drapes during the procedure.

Skin preparation is performed by progressing from the incision site to the periphery (Figure 29-2 ■). Each sponge is discarded when the periphery has been reached. A fresh sponge is used as the preparation continues. A sterile skin preparation set is contaminated when any part of it touches the skin, because the skin is not sterile. Removing soil and transient microbes, reducing resident microbial counts, and inhibiting rebound growth of microorganisms is accomplished through friction and antimicrobial agents, *not* through the use of sterile supplies.

Documentation of client skin preparation, according to the Association of periOperative Registered Nurses (AORN) recommended practices, includes condition of the skin, hair removal (if done), skin preparation, the name of the person or persons performing skin preparation, and development of any hypersensitivity reactions.

The client's nails should be trimmed and free of polish. All cosmetics should be removed so that the nail beds, skin, and lips are visible to observe circulation during and after surgery.

In some hospitals, clients may wear surgical caps the day of surgery. The surgical caps contain the client's hair and trap microorganisms on the hair and scalp.

Immediately before surgery, the nurse removes, or asks the client to remove, all hairpins and clips. Clips could cause pressure or accidental damage to the scalp when the client is unconscious. The client also removes personal clothing and puts on an operating room gown.

VALUABLES

Valuables such as jewelry and money should be sent home with support people. If this is impossible, they are labeled and placed in safekeeping (see Figure 14-2 and discussion in Chapter 14 ⬭). If a client wishes not to remove a wedding band, the nurse can usually tape it in place. However, wedding bands must be removed if there is danger of the fingers swelling after surgery. Situations requiring removal of rings are cast application to an arm and mastectomy with removal of the lymph nodes, because they may cause edema of the arm and hand.

PROSTHESES

All **prostheses** (artificial body parts, such as partial or complete dentures, contact lenses, artificial eyes, and artificial limbs), as well as eyeglasses, wigs, and false eyelashes, must be removed before surgery.

clinical ALERT

The Joint Commission recommends marking of the surgical site before the client is sedated. The nurse will ask the client which side is being operated on (e.g., left hip), and then will mark the area with a waterproof marking pen. In some facilities the procedure is that the client does the marking. In others, the nurse will label the surgical site with "yes" and the opposite site with "no."

MEDICATIONS

Preoperative medications may be given on the hospital unit or after the client goes to the operating room. Commonly used preoperative medications include:

- Sedatives and tranquilizers to reduce anxiety and ease anesthetic induction.
- Narcotic analgesics (opiates or opioids) to provide client sedation and reduce the required amount of anesthetic.
- Anticholinergics to reduce oral and pulmonary secretions and prevent laryngospasm.
- Histamine-receptor antihistamines to reduce gastric fluid volume and gastric acidity.
- Neuroleptic analgesic agents to induce general calmness and sleepiness.

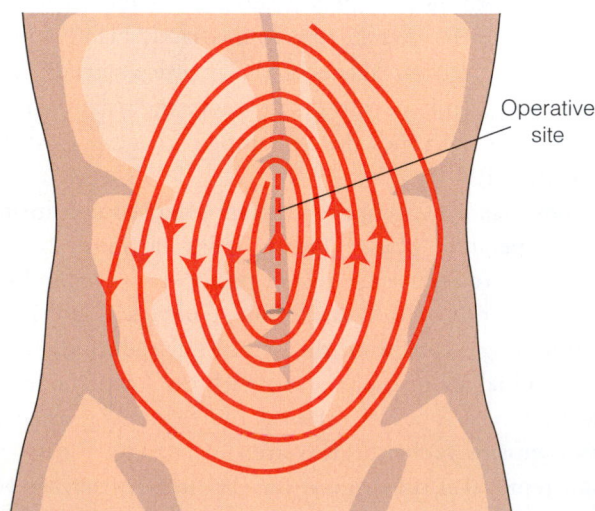

Operative site

Figure 29-2. ■ Surgical skin scrub.

Preoperative medications are given at a scheduled time or "on call," that is, when the operating room notifies the nurse to give the medication.

VITAL SIGNS

The nurse takes and records physical measurements or vital signs for baseline data. Abnormal findings, such as elevated blood pressure or elevated temperature, must be reported.

ANTIEMBOLI STOCKINGS

Antiemboli stockings are firm elastic hose that compress the veins of the legs and facilitate the return of venous blood to the heart. They are intended to prevent the formation of blood clots in the legs and edema of the legs and feet. These stockings are frequently applied both preoperatively and postoperatively. See Procedure 29-3 ■ for steps in applying antiemboli stockings.

SEQUENTIAL COMPRESSION DEVICES

Clients who are undergoing surgery may benefit from a **sequential compression device** (SCD)—also known as *pneumatic compression boots* or PCBs—to promote venous return from the legs. SCDs inflate and deflate plastic sleeves wrapped around the legs to promote venous flow. See Procedure 29-4 ■ for steps in applying a sequential compression device.

NURSING CARE

PRIORITIZING NURSING CARE

When you are caring for a client who is being prepared for surgery, give priority to the client's emotional needs and to thorough preparation. Clients are understandably nervous about an approaching surgery. Be careful not to belittle clients' concerns in this situation. Although nurses care for many clients with similar illnesses, the person undergoing the surgery is experiencing it as an individual. Listen to the client and allow concerns to be voiced. Avoid giving empty reassurances such as "Everything is going to be fine." Instead, be calm and reassuring, explaining what will be done and why. Instruct clients about how they can participate after surgery to decrease the possibility of complications. Have them practice coughing and deep breathing. Be vigilant in preparing the client for surgery by completing the surgery checklist carefully and following all preoperative orders exactly. Be prepared for delays in surgery times, but also anticipate that a case may cancel and your client may be called earlier than planned.

ASSESSING

Preoperative assessment includes collecting and reviewing specific client data to determine the client's needs both pre- and postoperatively. Physical, psychologic, and social needs are determined during data collection.

Anxiety is often a factor in preoperative nursing care. The nurse can help to reduce clients' anxiety by presenting a calm, confident presence and by asking about client concerns. People often have specific fears related to surgery, including:

- Fear of the procedure itself (e.g., general anesthesia, being "under the knife").
- Fear of the results of surgery (e.g., helplessness in early stages of recovery, potential for findings such as malignancies).
- Fear of pain.
- Uncertainty about what will happen after the surgery.
- Fear of the unknown.

Preoperatively, the nurse performs a brief but complete physical assessment, paying particular attention to systems that could affect the client's response to anesthesia or surgery. Respiratory and cardiovascular observations provide baseline data for evaluating the client's postoperative status. Preoperative screening test results (see Table 29-1) are reviewed. Abnormal test results are reported to the physician. If the LPN/LVN is assigned to prepare the client for surgery, he or she should check that the results of preoperative lab and diagnostic tests are on the chart. Discuss abnormal levels with the RN. Depending on facility policy, the LPN/LVN or RN will notify the physician. They also may alert care providers to a problem (e.g., a respiratory infection or irregular pulse rate) that may affect the client's response to surgery and anesthesia (see Box 29-2). The nurse checks that informed consent has been obtained. Although the nurse may witness the signing, it is not the nurse's responsibility to explain the procedure. Consents are usually the responsibility of the RN, although hospital policy may allow delegation of consents to the LPN/LVN. Check the date and time the consent was signed, noting the last time pain medication was administered.

DIAGNOSING, PLANNING, AND IMPLEMENTING

A number of NANDA nursing diagnoses may be appropriate for the preoperative client. The LPN/LVN will help implement many of the interventions. Two common nursing diagnoses for perioperative clients are:

- *Anxiety* related to threat of health status
- *Deficient Knowledge* r/t preoperative teaching

Goals for preoperative clients are to be physically, mentally, and emotionally prepared for surgery.

Outcomes for clients may include the following:

- Client will continue necessary activities even though anxiety persists.
- Client or family demonstrates ability to focus on new knowledge and skills.

Interventions the nurse performs for perioperative clients include:

- Assess and document client's level of anxiety, including physical reaction. *This will allow the nurse to recognize the client's coping skills and provide support and treatment to alleviate physical symptoms.*
- Explore with client techniques that have, and have not, reduced anxiety in the past. *This process helps the client identify personal coping skills.*
- Assist the client in setting realistic goals. *Realistic goals that are set by the client are more likely to be achieved than those set by a healthcare professional.*
- Relate new content to previous knowledge and experience. *Relating information taught to previous knowledge will help the client remember and apply the teaching.*

EVALUATING

The nurse evaluates specific desired outcomes. For example, the nurse would check whether vital signs are stable, the client understands and is ready for the upcoming surgery, and the client has learned how to do postoperative exercises. Client or family will identify the need for additional information about health promotion behavior (e.g., postsurgical prescribed diet).

Intraoperative Phase

RNs work intraoperatively as members of the surgical team, advocating for the client, maintaining safety, and continually assessing the needs of the client and the team. An LPN/LVN can also work in this specialized area with additional training.

While the client is in the operating room, the client's bed and room are prepared for the postoperative phase. The nurse must obtain and set up any special equipment, such as an intravenous pole, suction, oxygen equipment, and orthopedic appliances (e.g., traction). If these are not requested on the client's record, the nurse should consult with the perioperative nurse or surgeon. A report is usually called to the floor nurse by the postanesthesia care unit (PACU) nurse before the client is transferred to the floor.

TYPES OF ANESTHESIA

Anesthesia, the alteration in the level of sensation and consciousness, is classified as *general* (comprehensive) or *regional* (specific). Moderate sedation (**conscious sedation**), in which a client is able to respond to questions and has an increased pain threshold during surgery, is a minimal form of anesthesia. Anesthetic agents usually are administered by an anesthesiologist or nurse-anesthetist. Box 29-5 ■ provides a detailed explanation of the types of anesthesia.

| BOX 29-5 | TYPES OF ANESTHESIA |

General anesthesia is sedation that causes the loss of all sensation and consciousness.
- Protective reflexes such as cough and gag reflexes are lost.
- Blocks awareness centers in the brain so that amnesia (loss of memory), analgesia (insensibility to pain), hypnosis (artificial sleep), and relaxation (rendering a part of the body less tense) occur.
- Administered by intravenous infusion or by inhalation of gases through a mask or an endotracheal tube.

Regional anesthesia is the temporary interruption of the transmission of nerve impulses to and from a specific area or region of the body.
- *Topical* (surface) *anesthesia* is applied directly to the skin and mucous membranes, open skin surfaces, wounds, and burns.
- *Local anesthesia* (infiltration) is injected into a specific area and is used for minor surgical procedures such as suturing a small wound or performing a biopsy. *Nerve block* is a technique in which the anesthetic agent is injected into and around a nerve or small nerve group that supplies sensation to a small area of the body.
- *Spinal anesthesia* is injected, by way of a lumbar puncture, into the subarachnoid space surrounding the spinal cord. Spinal anesthesia is often categorized as a low, mid, or high spinal.
- *Epidural* (peridural) *anesthesia* is an injection of an anesthetic agent into the epidural space, the area inside the spinal column but outside the dura mater.

Moderate (conscious) sedation is anesthesia that produces minimal depression of the level of consciousness.
- It is used alone or in conjunction with regional anesthesia for diagnostic tests and surgical procedures.
- Client retains ability to consciously maintain a patent airway and respond verbally and physically.
- Increases the client's pain threshold.
- Induces a degree of amnesia but allows for prompt reversal of its effects.
- Rapid return to normal activities of daily living.

Postoperative Phase

Nursing during the postoperative phase is especially important for the client's recovery. Anesthesia impairs the ability of clients to respond to environmental stimuli and to help themselves, although the degree of consciousness of clients will vary. Moreover, surgery itself traumatizes the body by disrupting protective mechanisms and homeostasis.

IMMEDIATE POSTANESTHETIC PHASE

In the recovery room (postanesthesia care unit or PACU), the unconscious client is usually cared for by an RN. After the client has stabilized, he or she will be transferred to a nursing unit where an LPN/LVN may be assigned to continue postoperative care.

NURSING CARE

PRIORITIZING NURSING CARE

When you are notified that a client is returning from surgery to your unit, make that client your priority. Prepare for the client by determining that the room is ready and all anticipated equipment is at the bedside. Assist the surgery staff in moving the client from the stretcher to the bed. Do an immediate head-to-toe assessment of the client. This is a time when IV lines may loosen and leak, or catheters can be kinked. The client may be very drowsy and unable to give much information. Family members are anxious and ready to see their loved one. It takes skill to take care of all the technical needs of the client and the emotional needs of the family postoperatively. As the client becomes more responsive, pain management will be your next priority. Give pain medication as ordered and use other techniques such as distraction to help the client cope with postoperative pain. Another priority is detecting complications after surgery. Be vigilant in taking vital signs frequently as ordered to detect any changes in the client's condition. Observe for bleeding frequently by inspecting the dressing and checking beneath the client for pooling blood.

ASSESSING

As soon as the client returns to the nursing unit, the RN conducts an initial assessment. The sequence of these activities varies with the situation. The surgeon's postoperative orders will be consulted to learn the following:

- Food and fluids permitted by mouth
- Intravenous solutions and intravenous medications
- Position in bed
- Medications ordered (e.g., analgesics, antibiotics)
- Laboratory tests
- Intake and output, which in some agencies are monitored for all postoperative clients (e.g., 30 mL output is needed from the GU system after surgery)
- Activity permitted, including ambulation

The nurse also checks the PACU record for the following data:

- Operation performed
- Presence and location of any drains
- Anesthetic used
- Postoperative diagnosis
- Estimated blood loss
- Medications administered in the recovery room

Postoperative vital signs are usually taken every 15 minutes until stable, every hour for the next 4 hours, then every 4 hours for the next 2 days. *Note:* Assessments *must* be made

as often as the client's condition requires. The nurse collects data for the assessments described below.

Level of Consciousness

Check for orientation to time, place, and person. Most clients are fully conscious but drowsy when returned to their unit. Observe reaction to verbal stimuli and ability to move extremities.

Vital Signs and Pain

Take the client's vital signs (pulse, respiration, blood pressure, and oxygen saturation level) every 15 minutes until stable or in accordance with agency protocol. Compare initial findings with PACU data. In addition, assess the client's lung sounds and monitor for signs of common circulatory problems, such as postoperative hypotension, hemorrhage, or shock. (See the procedures in Chapter 32 🔗 for more about oxygenation.) Ask about pain level, which will normally increase after effects of anesthesia are gone and which may remain at a high level for up to 3 days after surgery. Potential postoperative problems with related manifestations and preventive measures are listed in Table 29-2 ■.

Skin Color, Temperature, and Wound Status

Skin color and temperature, particularly that of the lips and nail beds, are indicators of **tissue perfusion** (passage of blood through the vessels). Pale, cyanotic, cool, and moist skin may indicate circulatory problems.

The integument is examined regularly during routine nursing care. Treated wounds, or sutured wounds, are usually inspected during a dressing change unless a transparent dressing has been applied. If the wound itself cannot be inspected directly, the dressing is inspected and other data regarding the wound (e.g., the presence of pain) are collected. Many treated wounds are covered with a transparent occlusive dressing that permits observation of the wound without exposure.

Documentation of the wound status provides the physician and nursing staff with essential information for effective treatment and/or medication needs. Points to include in documentation are wound appearance, size, and drainage; the presence of swelling or pain; and status of drains or tubes.

Drains and Tubes

Determine color, consistency, and amount of drainage from all tubes and drains. All tubes should be *patent* (open), and tubes and suction equipment should be functioning. Drainage bags must be hanging properly.

Comfort

Ask about comfort when obtaining the client's vital signs and as needed between vital sign measurements. Determine the location and intensity of the pain. Do not assume that reported pain is incisional. Other causes may include muscle

(*Text continues on p. 722.*)

TABLE 29-2   **Potential Postoperative Problems**

PROBLEM/DESCRIPTION	CONTRIBUTING FACTORS	CLINICAL SIGNS	PREVENTIVE INTERVENTIONS
RESPIRATORY			
Pneumonia—inflammation of the alveoli	Infection, toxins, or irritants causing inflammatory process	Elevated temperature, cough, expectoration of blood-tinged or purulent sputum, dyspnea, chest pain	Turning and positioning until the client can move independently, coughing and deep-breathing exercises, moving in bed, early ambulation, incentive spirometer use
Infectious pneumonia—be limited to one or more lobes (*lobar*) or occur as scattered patches throughout the lungs (*bronchial*); also involve interstitial tissues of lungs	Common organisms include *Streptococcus pneumoniae*, *Haemophilus influenzae*, and *Staphylococcus aureus*		
Hypostatic pneumonia	Immobility and impaired ventilation result in atelectasis and promote growth of pathogens		Deep-breathing exercises and coughing, moving in bed, early ambulation, use of spirometer
Aspiration pneumonia—inflammatory process caused by irritation of lung tissue by aspirated material, particularly hydrochloric acid (HCl) from the stomach	Aspiration of gastric contents, food, or other substances; often related to loss of gag reflex		Elevate the head of the bed, evaluate for return of gag reflex prior to introducing oral fluid or food
Atelectasis—a condition in which alveoli collapse and are not ventilated	Mucous plugs blocking bronchial passageways, inadequate lung expansion, analgesics, immobility	Dyspnea, tachypnea, tachycardia; diaphoresis, anxiety; pleural pain, decreased chest wall movement; dull or absent breath sounds; decreased oxygen saturation (SaO_2)	Deep-breathing exercises and coughing, moving in bed, early ambulation
Pulmonary embolism (PE)—blood clot that has moved to the lungs blocks a pulmonary artery, thus obstructing blood flow to a portion of the lung	Stasis of venous blood from immobility, venous injury from fractures or during surgery, use of oral contraceptives high in estrogen, preexisting coagulation or circulatory disorder; childbirth is also a contributing factor to PE	Sudden chest pain, shortness of breath, cyanosis, shock (tachycardia, low blood pressure)	Turning, ambulation, antiemboli stockings, sequential compression devices (SCDs)
CIRCULATORY Hypovolemia—inadequate circulating blood volume	Fluid deficit, hemorrhage, nausea, and vomiting	Tachycardia, decreased urine output, decreased blood pressure	Early detection of signs; fluid and/or blood replacement; nausea and vomiting need to be managed because of their effect on fluid volume
Hemorrhage—internal or external bleeding	Disruption of sutures, insecure ligation of blood vessels	Overt bleeding (dressings saturated with bright blood; bright, free-flowing blood in drains or chest tubes), increased pain, increasing abdominal girth, swelling or bruising around incision	Early detection of signs
Hypovolemic shock—inadequate tissue perfusion resulting from markedly reduced circulating blood volume	Severe hypovolemia from fluid deficit or hemorrhage	Rapid weak pulse, dyspnea, tachypnea; restlessness and anxiety; urine output less than 30 mL/hr; decreased blood pressure; cool, clammy skin, thirst, pallor	Maintain blood volume through adequate fluid replacement, prevent hemorrhage; early detection of signs
Thrombophlebitis—inflammation of the veins, usually of the legs and associated with a blood clot	Slowed venous blood flow related to immobility or prolonged sitting; trauma to vein, resulting in inflammation and increased blood coagulability	Aching, cramping pain; affected area is swollen, red, and hot to touch; vein feels hard; discomfort in calf when foot is dorsiflexed or when client walks (Homans' sign)	Early ambulation, leg exercises, antiemboli stockings, sequential compression devices (SCDs), adequate fluid intake

PROBLEM/DESCRIPTION	CONTRIBUTING FACTORS	CLINICAL SIGNS	PREVENTIVE INTERVENTIONS
Thrombus—blood clot attached to wall of vein or artery (most commonly the leg veins)	As for thrombophlebitis for venous thrombi; disruption or inflammation of arterial wall for arterial thrombi	*Venous:* same as thrombophlebitis *Arterial:* pain and pallor of affected extremity; decreased or absent peripheral pulses	*Venous:* same as thrombophlebitis *Arterial:* maintaining prescribed position; early detection of signs
Embolus—foreign body or clot that has moved from its site of formation to another area of the body (e.g., lungs, heart, or brain)	Venous or arterial thrombus; broken intravenous catheter, fat, or amniotic fluid	In venous system, usually becomes a pulmonary embolus (see pulmonary embolism); signs of arterial emboli may depend on the location	As for thrombophlebitis or thrombus; careful maintenance of IV catheters
URINARY Urinary retention—inability to empty the bladder, with excessive accumulation of urine in the bladder	Depressed bladder muscle tone from narcotics and anesthetics; handling of tissues during surgery on adjacent organs (rectum, vagina)	Fluid intake larger than output; inability to void or frequent voiding of small amounts, bladder distention, suprapubic discomfort, restlessness	Monitoring of fluid intake and output, interventions to facilitate voiding, urinary catheterization as needed
Urinary tract infection (UTI)—inflammation of the bladder, ureters, or urethra	Immobilization and limited fluid intake, instrumentation of the urinary tract	Burning sensation when voiding, urgency, cloudy urine, lower abdominal pain	Adequate fluid intake, early ambulation, aseptic straight catheterization only as necessary, good perineal hygiene
GASTROINTESTINAL Nausea and vomiting	Pain, abdominal distention, ingesting food or fluids before return of peristalsis, certain medications, anxiety	Complaints of feeling sick to the stomach, retching or gagging	IV fluids until peristalsis returns; then clear fluids, full fluids, and regular diet; antiemetic drugs if ordered; analgesics for pain
Constipation—infrequent or no stool passage for abnormal length of time (e.g., within 48 hours after solid diet started)	Lack of dietary roughage, analgesics (decreased intestinal motility), immobility	Absence of stool elimination, abdominal distention, and discomfort	Adequate fluid intake, high-fiber diet, early ambulation
Tympanites—swelling of the abdomen from retention of gases within the intestines	Slowed motility of the intestines due to handling of the bowel during surgery and the effects of anesthesia	Obvious abdominal distention, abdominal discomfort (gas pains), absence of bowel sounds	Early ambulation; avoid using a straw, provide ice chips or water at room temperature
Paralytic ileus—intestinal obstruction characterized by lack of peristaltic activity	Handling the bowel during surgery, anesthesia, electrolyte imbalance, wound infection	Abdominal pain and distention; constipation; absent bowel sounds; vomiting	IV fluids until peristalsis returns, gradual reintroduction of oral feeding, early ambulation, measure abdominal girth
WOUND Wound infection—inflammation and infection of incision or drain site	Poor aseptic technique; laboratory analysis of wound swab identifies causative microorganism	Purulent exudate, redness, tenderness, elevated body temperature, wound odor	Keeping wound clean and dry, surgical aseptic technique when changing dressings
Wound **dehiscence**—separation of a suture line before the incision heals	Malnutrition (emaciation, obesity), poor circulation, excessive strain on suture line	Increased incision drainage, tissues underlying skin become visible along parts of the incision	Adequate nutrition, appropriate incisional support, and avoidance of strain
Wound **evisceration**—extrusion of internal organs and tissues through the incision	Same as for wound dehiscence	Opening of incision and visible protrusion of organs	Same as for wound dehiscence
PSYCHOLOGIC Postoperative depression—mental disorder characterized by altered mood	Weakness, surprise nature of emergency surgery, news of malignancy, severely altered body image, or other personal matter; may be a physiologic response to some surgeries	Anorexia, tearfulness, loss of ambition, withdrawal, rejection of others, feelings of dejection, sleep disturbances (insomnia, excessive sleeping)	Adequate rest, physical activity, opportunity to express anger and other negative feelings

strains, flatus, and angina. Ask the client to rate pain on a scale of 0 to 10, with 0 being no pain and 10 the worst pain imaginable. Evaluate the client for objective indicators of pain: pallor, perspiration, muscle tension, and reluctance to cough, move, or ambulate. Determine when and what analgesics were last administered, and assess the client for any side effects of medication such as nausea and vomiting. (See Chapter 22 🔗 for an in-depth discussion of pain.)

Fluid Balance

Note the type and amount of intravenous fluids, flow rate, and infusion site. LPN/LVN responsibilities related to IV therapy are defined in the scope of practice in each individual state. Monitor the client's fluid intake and output. In addition to watching for shock, monitor the client for signs of circulatory overload and for status of serum electrolytes.

Dressing and Bedclothes

Inspect the client's dressings and bedclothes underneath the client. Excessive bloody drainage on dressings or on bedclothes, often appearing underneath the client, can indicate hemorrhage. Record amount of drainage on dressings by describing the diameter of the stains or by noting the number and type of dressings saturated with drainage.

Document the client's time of arrival and all assessments. Many agencies have progress flow records for this purpose. Alter the frequency, parameters, and priorities to meet the individual needs of the client.

DIAGNOSING, PLANNING, AND IMPLEMENTING

Surgery can involve many body systems both directly and indirectly and is a complex experience for the client. So, nursing diagnoses focus on a wide variety of actual, potential, and collaborative problems. Appendix II 🔗 on the MyNursingKit Website lists NANDA diagnoses for the postoperative client. Nursing diagnoses that relate to clients who have skin wounds or who are at risk for skin breakdown are:

- *Risk for Impaired Skin Integrity*
- *Impaired Skin Integrity* (commonly applies to superficial wounds extending through the epidermis but not through the dermis)
- *Impaired Tissue Integrity* (applies to wounds extending into subcutaneous tissue, muscle, or bone)
- *Risk for Infection*
- *Acute Pain* related to nerve involvement
- *Disturbed Body Image*

In planning nursing care, the primary goals are maintaining skin integrity and avoiding potential risks. For clients with *Impaired Skin Integrity* or *Impaired Tissue Integrity*, the goal is to achieve progressive wound healing and regain intact skin.

Remember, postoperative care planning and discharge planning begin in the preoperative phase when preoperative teaching is implemented.

Some major client outcomes after surgery include maintaining comfort, healing, achieving wellness, and avoiding complications of surgery.

Pain Management

Pain is usually greatest 12 to 36 hours after surgery, decreasing after the second or third postoperative day. (See Chapter 22 🔗 for a more in-depth discussion of pain and pain management.) During the initial postoperative period, the physician may prescribe one of the following:

1. Patient-controlled analgesia (PCA) is self-administration of opioid medication by means of a programmed infusion pump (see Figure 22-5 🔗).
2. Continuous analgesic administration through an intravenous or epidural catheter. PRN parenteral or oral analgesics should be administered on a routine basis (every 2 to 6 hours, depending on the drug, route, and dose) for the first 24 to 36 hours. When routine analgesic administration is no longer necessary, the prescribed analgesic is generally given before scheduled activities and rest periods. *Clients need to be reminded that analgesics are most effective when taken on a regular basis or before pain becomes severe. An anti-inflammatory agent is often administered in conjunction with a narcotic analgesic to enhance pain relief.*
3. PRN parenteral or oral medication.

Provide nonpharmacologic measures in addition to prescribed analgesia. *Ensuring that the client is warm, and providing back rubs, position changes, diversional activities, and adjunctive measures such as use of imagery are all ways of reducing client anxiety and discomfort and providing holistic care.*

Positioning

- Position the client as ordered. Responsive clients who have had spinal anesthetics usually lie flat for 8 to 12 hours. A client who is not fully responsive is placed on one side with the head slightly elevated, if possible, or in a position that allows fluids to drain from the mouth. Unless contraindicated, elevate the affected extremities (e.g., following foot surgery) with the distal extremity higher than the heart. *Proper positioning can promote venous drainage, reduce swelling, and prevent choking in an unresponsive client.*

Deep-Breathing and Coughing Exercises

- Encourage deep-breathing exercises. *Exercises help remove mucus, which can form and remain in the lungs due to the effects of general anesthetic and analgesics. These drugs depress the action of both the cilia of the mucous membranes lining the respiratory tract and the respiratory center in the brain. Deep breathing increases lung expansion and prevents the accumulation of secretions. It helps prevent pneumonia and atelectasis (collapse of the alveoli), which may result from stagnation of fluid in the lungs* (see Procedure 29-2).

- An incentive spirometer is often ordered for the postoperative client to encourage deep breathing. This device measures the flow of air inhaled through a mouthpiece. See Chapter 32 🔗 for information about how to use an incentive spirometer. Instruct the client to breathe in through the mouthpiece until a certain level is achieved (usually measured by a ball within an enclosed chamber). *Inhalation and ventilation are enhanced using the incentive spirometer.*

- Encourage the client to do deep-breathing and coughing exercises hourly, or at least every 2 hours, during waking hours for the first few days. *Deep breathing frequently initiates the coughing reflex. Voluntary coughing in conjunction with deep breathing helps the client move and expel respiratory tract secretions* (see Procedure 29-2).

- Assist the client to a sitting position in bed or on the side of the bed. The client can splint the incision with a pillow when coughing, or the nurse can splint the incision for the client. *Splinting supports the wound area and reduces discomfort.*

Leg Exercises

- Encourage the client to do leg exercises taught in the preoperative period every 1 to 2 hours during waking hours. (See more about thrombus and embolus formation in Chapter 34 🔗.) *Muscle contractions compress the veins, preventing the stasis of blood in the veins, a cause of thrombus formation and subsequent thrombophlebitis and emboli. Contractions also promote arterial blood flow* (see Procedure 29-2).

Moving and Ambulating

- Encourage the client to turn from side to side at least every 2 hours. Clients who practice turning before surgery usually find it easier to do after surgery. *Turning allows alternate lungs to expand fully (the uppermost lung will have full expansion).*

- Avoid placing pillows or rolls under the client's knees. *Pressure on the popliteal blood vessels can reduce blood circulation to and from the lower extremities.*

- Encourage the client to ambulate as soon as possible after surgery in accordance with the surgeon's orders. Generally, clients begin ambulation the evening of the day of surgery or the first day after surgery, unless contraindicated. Schedule ambulation for periods after the client has taken an analgesic or when the client is comfortable. Ambulation should be gradual, starting with the client sitting on the bed and dangling the feet over the side. Safety must be a priority when ambulating a client. The nurse should stay with the client during the first time the client walks after surgery. *Early ambulation prevents respiratory, circulatory, urinary, and gastrointestinal complications. It also prevents general muscle weakness.*

- Periodically assist a client who cannot ambulate to a sitting position in bed, if allowed. Turn client frequently. *The sitting position permits the greatest lung expansion.* (See more about mobility in Chapter 23 🔗.)

Hydration

Intravenous infusions replace body fluids lost either before or during surgery.

- When oral intake is permitted, initially offer only small sips of water. Prior to the introduction of oral fluids, the nurse should assess whether the reflex has returned. This can be done by touching the back of the client's throat with a tongue depressor. *General anesthesia interrupts the gag reflex.*

- Provide ice chips instead of liquids. The client who cannot take fluids by mouth may be allowed by the surgeon's orders to suck ice chips. *Large amounts of water can induce vomiting because of the effects of anesthetics and narcotic analgesics on stomach motility.*

- Provide mouth care and place a mouthwash at the client's bedside. *Postoperative clients often complain of thirst and a dry, sticky mouth. These discomforts are a result of the preoperative fasting period, preoperative medications (such as atropine), and loss of body fluid.*

- Measure the client's fluid intake and output (see Figure 26-4 🔗) for at least 2 days or until fluid balance is stable without an intravenous infusion. Ensuring adequate fluid balance is important. *Fluids keep the respiratory mucous membranes and secretions moist. They help the client expectorate mucus while coughing. Also, fluid balance is important to maintain renal and cardiovascular function.*

Diet

- When "diet as tolerated" is ordered, offer clear liquids first. Assist very weak clients to eat. *The surgeon orders the client's postoperative diet. Depending on the extent of surgery and the organs involved, the client may be allowed nothing by mouth (NPO) for several days or may be able to resume oral intake when nausea is no longer present. If the client tolerates clear liquids with no nausea, the diet can often progress to full liquids and then to a regular diet, provided gastrointestinal functioning is normal.*

- Auscultate the abdomen for return of peristalsis (see Chapter 19 🔗). Bowel sounds should be carefully assessed every 4 to 6 hours. *Oral fluids and food are usually started after the return of peristalsis. Gurgling and rumbling sounds indicate peristalsis.*

- Observe the client's tolerance of the food and fluids ingested. Note and report the passage of flatus or abdominal distention. *These may be indicators of bowel activity or blockage.*

Urinary Elimination

- Provide measures that promote urinary elimination. For example, help male clients stand at the bedside, or help female clients to a bedside commode if allowed. Ensure that fluid intake is adequate. Report to the surgeon if a client does not void within 8 hours following surgery, unless another time frame is specified. *Lack of functioning could indicate a serious complication.*

- Generally, keep intake and output records (see Figure 26-4 ⊙⊙) for at least 2 days or until the client reestablishes fluid balance without an IV or catheter in place. *These provide documentation of client status.*

Suction

Some clients return from surgery with a gastric or intestinal tube in place and orders to connect the tube to suction. (For more information about gastrointestinal tubes, see Chapter 26 ⊙⊙ .) The suction ordered can be continuous or intermittent.

- Apply intermittent suction when a single-lumen gastric tube is used. *Intermittent suction reduces the risk of damaging the mucous membrane near the distal port of the tube.*

- Apply continuous suction if a double-lumen tube is in place. Fluids and electrolytes must be replaced intravenously when gastric suction or continuous drainage is ordered. *Replacement of suctioned fluid is necessary to maintain fluid balance.*

- Irrigate nasogastric tubes if the lumen becomes clogged. Nasogastric irrigation may require a physician's order, particularly following gastrointestinal surgery. *Tubes are generally irrigated before and after tube feedings or the instillation of medications.* Procedure 29-5 ■ describes the management of gastrointestinal suction.

- Monitor suction equipment. Check the receptacle frequently. Empty or change the receptacle according to agency policy. *Excess drainage can interfere with the suction apparatus.*

- Suction may be applied to other drainage tubes such as chest tubes or a wound drain. The type and amount of suction is ordered by the physician. A suction regulator with a drainage receptacle connects to a wall outlet that provides negative pressure. Portable electric suction units or pumps (e.g., the Gomco pump) may be used in the home or when wall suction is not available.

Wound Care

Most clients return from surgery with a sutured wound covered by a dressing, although in some cases the wound may be left unsutured.

BOX 29-6	**OBSERVING SURGICAL WOUNDS**

- *Appearance.* Inspect color of wound and surrounding area and approximation of wound edges.
- *Size.* Note size and location of suture lines as well as dehiscence (partial or total rupturing of a sutured wound), if present. If internal organs are visible (evisceration), notify physician immediately!
- *Drainage.* Observe location, color, consistency, odor, and degree of saturation of dressings. Note number of gauzes saturated or diameter of drainage on gauze.
- *Swelling.* Observe the amount of swelling; minimal to moderate swelling is normal in early stages of wound healing.
- *Pain.* Expect severe to moderate postoperative pain for 3 to 5 days; persistent severe pain or sudden onset of severe pain may indicate internal hemorrhaging or infection.
- *Drains or tubes.* Inspect drain security and placement, amount and character of drainage, and functioning of collecting apparatus, if present.

- Inspect dressings regularly to ensure that they are clean, dry, and intact. *Excessive drainage may indicate hemorrhage, infection, or an open wound.*

- When changing dressings, assess the wound for appearance, size, drainage, swelling, pain, and the status of a drain or tubes. Details about these observations are outlined in Box 29-6 ■. *These measures ensure continuity of care.*

Supporting Wound Healing

There are three major areas in which nurses can support wound healing: obtaining sufficient nutrition and fluids, preventing wound infections, and positioning the client properly.

- Assist the client to take in at least 2,500 mL of fluids a day unless conditions contraindicate this amount. Ensure that clients receive sufficient protein; vitamins C, A, B_1, and B_5, and zinc. *Although there is no evidence that excessive doses of vitamins or minerals enhance wound healing, adequate amounts are extremely important.*

- Provide excellent infection control. *Good nursing care can (1) prevent microorganisms from entering the wound and (2) prevent transmission of bloodborne pathogens to or from the client to others.* (See Chapter 10 ⊙⊙ for more information about infection control.)

- With physician's order, obtain a wound culture whenever an infection is suspected. See Chapter 24 ⊙⊙ for obtaining a specimen of wound drainage. *Prompt attention to a suspected infection promotes healing.*

- Position clients to keep pressure off the wound. *Changes of position and transfers must be accomplished without shear or friction damage.* (See Chapter 23 ⊙⊙ .)

- Encourage the client to be as mobile as possible. If the client cannot move independently, implement range-of-motion exercises and a turning schedule. *Activity enhances circulation.*

Cleaning, Irrigating, and Dressing Wounds

Chapter 24 ⚭ discusses wound cleaning, irrigating, and dressings. Not all surgical dressings require changing. Sometimes surgeons in the operating room apply a dressing that remains in place until the sutures are removed, and no further dressings are required. In many situations, however, surgical dressings are changed regularly to prevent the growth of microorganisms.

In some instances, a client may have a Penrose drain inserted directly into the incision. In this situation, the main surgical incision is considered cleaner than the surgical stab wound made for the drain insertion, because there is usually considerable drainage. The main incision is therefore cleaned first.

Cleaning a sutured wound and applying a sterile dressing are detailed in Procedure 29-1.

Wound Drains and Suction

Surgical drains, such as a Penrose drain, are inserted to permit the drainage of excess serosanguineous fluid and purulent material and to promote healing of underlying tissues. These drains may be inserted and sutured through the incision line, but they are most commonly inserted through stab wounds a few centimeters away from the incision line so that the incision itself may be kept dry. Without a drain, some wounds would heal on the surface and trap the discharge inside, and an abscess might form.

A **closed wound drainage system** consists of a drain connected to either an electric suction or a portable drainage suction, such as a Hemovac (Figure 29-3A ■). The closed system reduces the possible entry of microorganisms into the wound through the drain. The drainage tubes are sutured in place and connected to a reservoir. These portable wound suctions also provide for accurate measurement of the drainage. Generally, the suction is discontinued from 3 to 5 days postoperatively or when the drainage is minimal. Nurses are responsible for maintaining the wound suction, which hastens the healing process by draining excess exudate that might otherwise interfere with the formation of granulation tissue.

When emptying the container, the nurse should wear gloves and avoid touching the drainage port (see Figure 29-3B).

clinical ALERT

Materials that were used to clean a stab wound are never used again to clean the main incision. The main incision must be kept free of the microorganisms around the stab wound.

Sutures and Staples

Sutures are threads used to sew body tissues together. Sutures used to attach tissues beneath the skin are often made of an absorbable material that disappears in several days. Skin sutures, by contrast, are made of a variety of nonabsorbable materials.

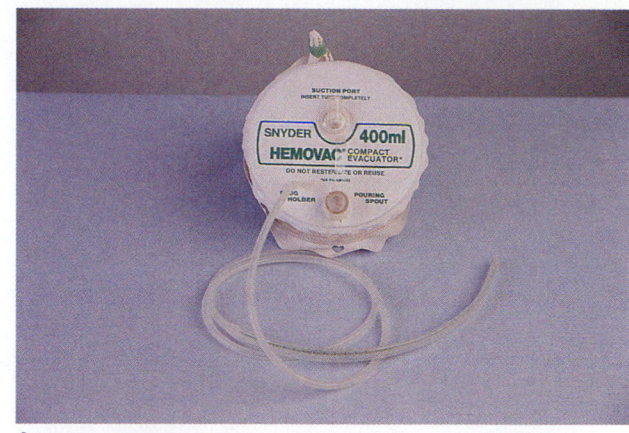

A

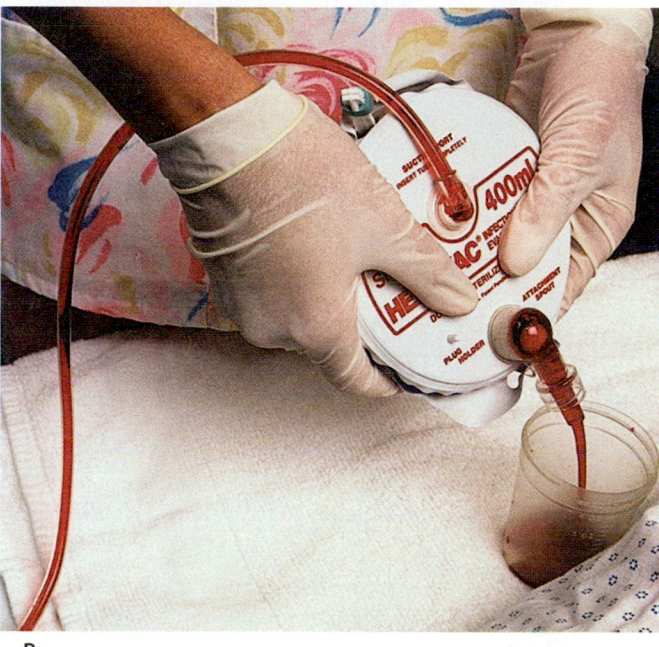

B

Figure 29-3. ■ Closed wound drainage system. **A.** Hemovac. **B.** Emptying drainage from Hemovac drainage system.

The physician orders the removal of sutures. In some agencies, only physicians remove sutures; in others, registered nurses and nursing students with appropriate supervision may do so. The LPN/LVN should review the LPN/LVN scope of practice regarding suture removal. Many states permit the removal of these on well-approximated, uncomplicated surgical wounds. Usually, skin sutures are removed 7 to 10 days after surgery. Nursing care guidelines for removing sutures are provided in Box 29-7 ■.

Sterile technique and special suture scissors are used in suture removal. The scissors have a short, curved cutting tip that readily slides under the suture (Figure 29-4A ■).

Silver wire clips or staples are also used to close surgical wounds. Wire clips or staples are removed with a special instrument that squeezes the center of the clip to remove it from the skin (Figure 29-4B). Nursing care guidelines for removal of staples can be found in Box 29-7.

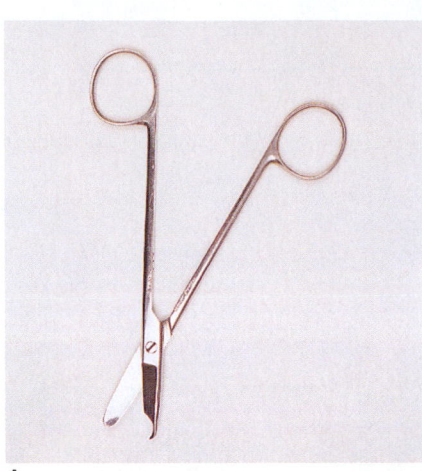

A

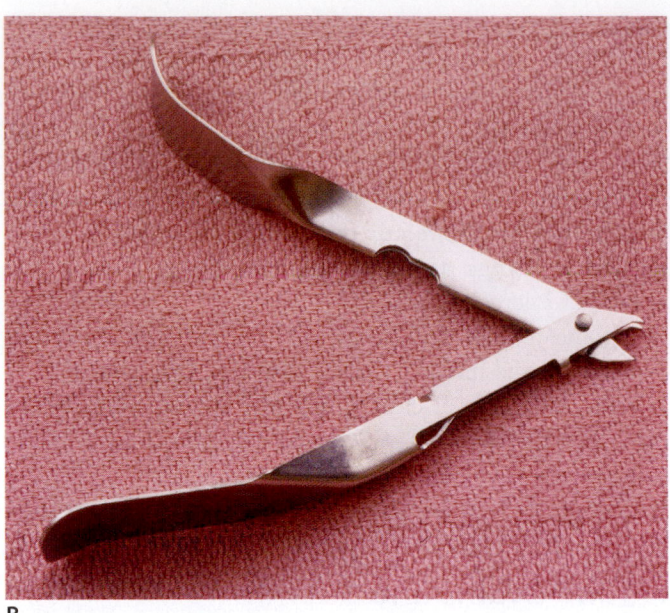

B

Figure 29-4. ■ **A.** Suture scissors. **B.** Staple removal device.

BOX 29-7 **NURSING CARE CHECKLIST**

Removing Skin Sutures and Staples

Part A: Plain Interrupted Sutures

☑ Before removing skin sutures, verify the orders for suture removal and whether a dressing is to be applied following suture removal.

☑ Inform the client that suture removal may produce slight discomfort, such as a pulling or stinging sensation, but should not be painful.

☑ Remove dressings and clean the incision in accordance with agency protocol.

☑ Put on sterile gloves.

☑ Grasp the suture at the knot with a pair of forceps.

☑ Place the curved tip of the suture scissors under the suture as close to the skin as possible, either on the side opposite the knot (Figure 29-5 ■) or directly under the knot. Cut the suture. *Sutures are cut as close to the skin as possible on one side of the visible part because the suture material that is visible to the eye is in contact with resident bacteria of the skin and must not be pulled beneath the skin during removal. Suture material that is beneath the skin is considered free from bacteria.*

☑ With the forceps, pull the suture out in one piece (Figure 29-5B). Inspect the suture carefully to make sure that all suture material is removed. *Suture material left beneath the skin acts as a foreign body and causes inflammation.*

☑ Discard the suture onto a piece of sterile gauze or into a moisture-proof bag. Be careful not to contaminate the forceps tips.

☑ Remove alternate sutures so that remaining sutures keep the skin edges in close approximation and prevent dehiscence. If no dehiscence occurs, remove the remaining sutures. If dehiscence does occur, do not remove the remaining sutures and report the dehiscence to the nurse in charge.

☑ If the physician orders Steri-Strips®, apply them to the wound after removing the sutures or clips. Reapply a dressing, if indicated.

☑ Instruct the client about follow-up wound care, such as contacting the physician if wound discharge appears.

Part B: Staples

☑ Before removing skin staples, verify the orders for removal and whether a dressing is to be applied following staple removal.

☑ Inform the client that suture removal may produce slight discomfort but should not be painful.

☑ Remove dressings and clean the incision in accordance with agency protocol.

☑ Put on sterile gloves.

☑ Place the two prongs of the staple remover under the first staple and clamp down completely (Figure 29-5C). *The single prong will bend the staple in the middle causing the "legs" of the staple to straighten out.*

☑ Gently rock the staple from side to side to remove it taking care not to pull at the incision site.

☑ Place the removed staple on a gauze pad.

BOX 29-7   **NURSING CARE CHECKLIST (continued)**

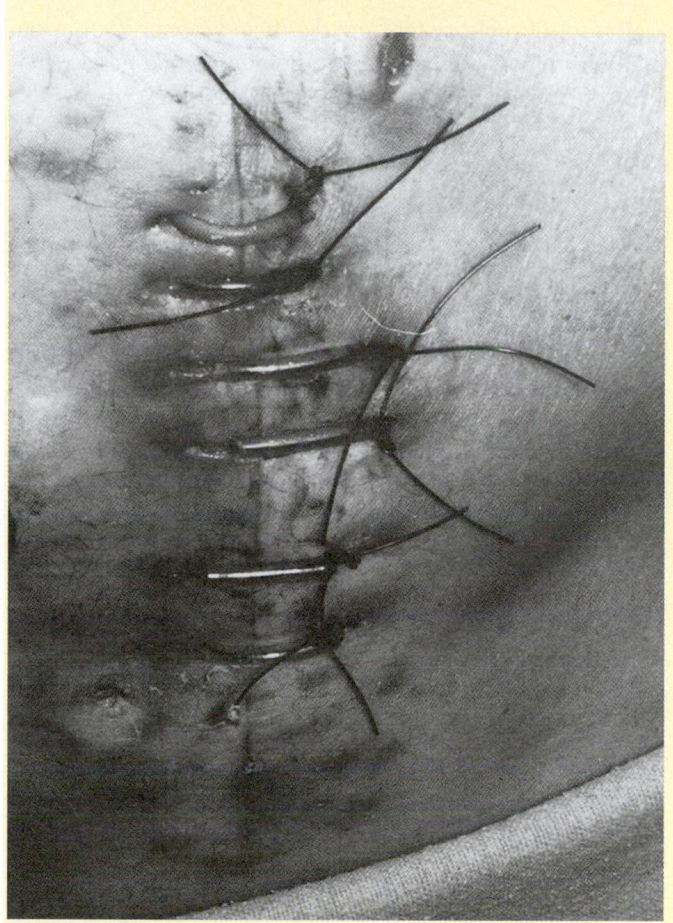
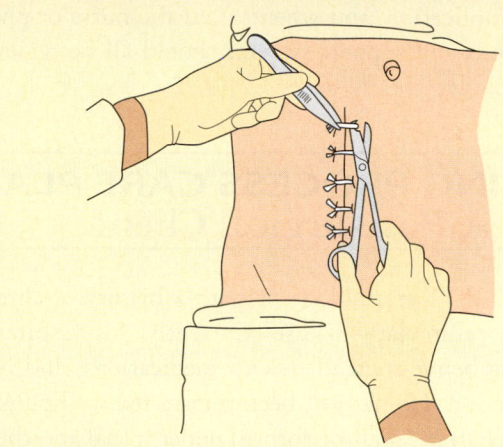
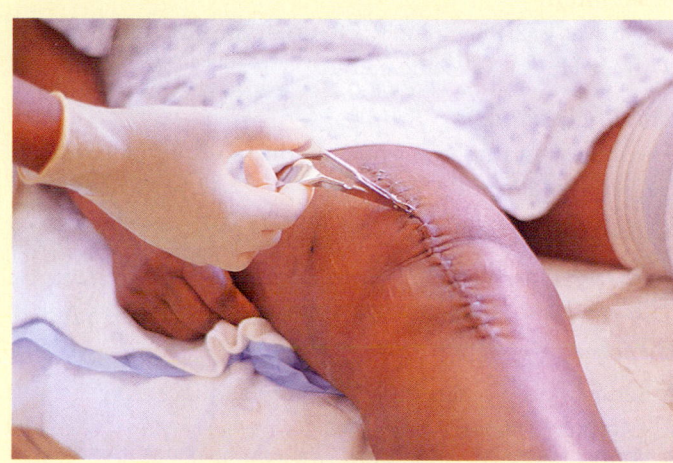

Figure 29-5. ■ **A.** Plain interrupted skin suture. **B.** Removing a plain interrupted skin suture. **C.** Removing surgical clips.

☑ Remove alternate staples along the incision, watching for any sign that the line is not staying closed.

☑ If Steri-Strips® are ordered, place them after the staples have been removed.

☑ When all staples have been removed, cover with a dressing, if ordered.

☑ Document the location, size, and condition of the incision. Record your intervention and client's tolerance.

☑ If at anytime during procedure the incision appears to be opening, do not remove any additional staples until the RN or physician has assessed the surgical site.

Following removal of sutures or staples, the physician may order the application of Steri-Strips® to support the surgical incision line until it is completely healed.

EVALUATING

The nurse collects vital signs measurements and data about client comfort, healing, restoring wellness, and preventing risks associated with surgery. Careful documentation always includes appearance and size of wound and type and amount of exudate. Using the goals developed during the planning stage, the nurse collects data to evaluate whether the identified goals and desired outcomes have been achieved.

Continuity of Care

Prior to discharge, the nurse must ensure that clients have an understanding of wound care. Clients should know how to change a dressing and how frequently to do so. They should understand what normal healing looks like. They should be given a list of signs that might indicate an infection or other complication and when to notify the physician.

The nurse reviews the client's self-care abilities, such as the ability to manage hygiene and other self-care, to perform wound care as needed, to manage tubes and stomas, and to manage prescribed medications. The nurse teaches about required supplies (dressings, hypoallergenic tape, etc.) or assistive devices (cane, raised toilet seat, grab bars in the shower). The client must know what occurrences might indicate a complication, and when to call the nurse or physician. Referrals and support systems should all be reviewed before discharge.

NURSING PROCESS CARE PLAN
A Postsurgical Client

Mr. Teng is a 77-year-old client with a history of chronic obstructive pulmonary disease. Currently, his respiratory condition is being controlled with medications, and he is free of infection. He has just been transferred to the PACU following a hernia repair performed under spinal anesthesia.

Assessment
His BP is 132/88, P 84, R 28, and tympanic temperature 97.8° F. He is awake and stable.

Nursing Diagnosis
The following important nursing diagnosis (among others) is established for this condition:

- Ineffective Breathing Pattern

Expected Outcomes
The expected outcomes for Mr. Teng's plan of care are that client will:

- Perform deep breathing, coughing, and incentive spirometry as instructed.
- Exhibit clear auscultated breath sounds.
- Have adequate respiratory excursion (depth).

Planning and Implementation
The following nursing interventions are planned and implemented for Mr. Teng:

- Monitor respiratory rate and depth and ease of respiration.
- Monitor client's oxygen saturation and blood gases.
- Encourage client to take deep breaths at prescribed intervals and do controlled coughing.
- Assist client to sit on side of bed and splint abdomen with pillow while coughing.
- Teach client to use incentive spirometer.

Evaluation
Client demonstrates ability to use incentive spirometer, cough, and deep breathe every 2 hours while awake. Splints abdomen while coughing to decrease discomfort. Lungs clear, no signs and symptoms of respiratory infection.

Critical Thinking in the Nursing Process

1. What factors place Mr. Teng at increased risk for the development of complications during and after surgery?
2. Speculate about why Mr. Teng's surgeon and anesthesiologist decided to perform Mr. Teng's surgery under regional anesthesia as opposed to general anesthesia.
3. What postoperative precautions are especially important to Mr. Teng in view of his chronic lung condition?

Note: Discussion of Critical Thinking questions appears on the MyNursingKit Website.

Note: The references and resources for all chapters have been compiled at the back of the book.

PROCEDURE 29-1 Cleaning Surgical Wounds and Applying Dressings

Purposes
- To promote wound healing
- To prevent infection
- To assess the healing process
- To protect the wound from mechanical trauma

Equipment
- Disposable gloves
- Hair scissors or clippers
- Acetone or another solution (if necessary to loosen adhesive)
- Moisture-proof bag
- Mask (optional)
- Sterile gloves
- Sterile gauze and the wound-cleaning agents specified by the physician or agency (e.g., sterile saline)
- Drape or towel
- Container for the cleaning solution
- Tape, tie tapes, or binder
- Two pairs of forceps (thumb or artery)

Equipment *continued*

- Gauze dressings and Surgipads/wound barrier dressing/ hydrocolloid dressing at least 3 to 4 cm (1.5 in.) larger than wound on all four sides/wet-to-damp dressing (as ordered)

- Applicators or tongue blades to apply ointments
- Additional supplies required for the particular dressing (e.g., extra gauze dressings and ointment, if ordered)

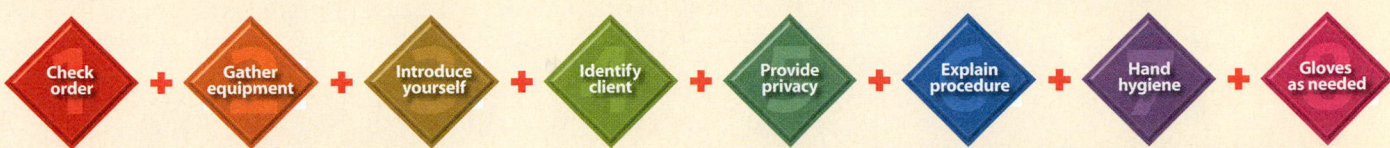

Interventions and Rationales

1. Perform preparatory steps (see icon bar above).

2. Prepare the client and assemble the equipment.
   - Acquire assistance for changing a dressing on a restless or confused adult. *The person might move and contaminate the sterile field or the wound.*
   - Assist the client to a comfortable position in which the wound can be readily exposed. Expose only the wound area, using a bath blanket to cover the client, if necessary. *Unnecessary exposure is physically and psychologically distressing to most people.*
   - Make a cuff on the moisture-proof bag for disposal of the soiled dressings, and place the bag within reach. It can be taped to the bedclothes or bedside table. *Making a cuff helps keep the outside of the bag free from contamination by the soiled dressings and prevents subsequent contamination of the nurse's hands or of sterile instrument tips when discarding dressing or sponges. Placement of the bag within reach prevents the nurse from reaching across the sterile field and the wound and potentially contaminating these areas.*
   - Put on a face mask, if required. *Some agencies require that a mask be worn for surgical dressing changes to prevent contamination of the wound by droplet spray from the nurse's respiratory tract.*

3. Remove binders and tape.
   - Remove binders, if used, and place them aside. Untie tie tapes, if used. (Discussion of wound dressings and binders is in Chapter 24 ⚭.)
   - If adhesive tape was used, remove it by holding down the skin and pulling the tape gently but firmly toward the wound. *Pressing down on the skin provides countertraction against the pulling motion. Tape is pulled toward the incision to prevent strain on the sutures or wound.*
   - Use a solvent to loosen tape, if required. *Moistening the tape with acetone or a similar solvent lessens the discomfort of removal, particularly from hairy surfaces.*

4. Remove and dispose of soiled dressings appropriately.
   - Put on clean disposable gloves, and remove the outer abdominal dressing or Surgipad.
   - Lift the outer dressing so that the underside is away from the client's face. *The appearance and odor of the drainage may be upsetting to the client.*

- Place the soiled dressing in the moisture-proof bag without touching the outside of the bag. *Contamination of the outside of the bag is avoided to prevent the spread of microorganisms to the nurse and others.*
- Remove the underdressings, taking care not to dislodge any drains. If the gauze sticks to the drain, support the drain with one hand and remove the gauze with the other.
- Note the location, type (color, consistency), and odor of wound drainage, and the number of gauzes saturated or the diameter of drainage collected on the dressings.
- Discard the soiled dressings in the bag as before.
- Remove gloves, dispose of them in the moisture-proof bag, and wash hands.

5. Set up the sterile supplies.
   - Open the sterile dressing set, using surgical aseptic technique.
   - Place the sterile drape beside the wound.
   - Open the sterile cleaning solution, and pour it over the gauze sponges in the plastic container.
   - Put on sterile gloves.

6. Clean the wound, if indicated.
   - Clean the wound, using your gloved hands or forceps and gauze swabs moistened with cleaning solution.
   - If using forceps, keep the forceps tips lower than the handles at all times. *This prevents their contamination by fluid traveling up to the handle and nurse's wrist and back to the tips.*
   - Use the cleaning methods illustrated and described in Figure 29-6 ■ or one recommended by agency protocol.
   - Use a separate swab for each stroke, and discard each swab after use. *This prevents the introduction of microorganisms to other wound areas.*
   - If a drain is present, clean it next, taking care to avoid reaching across the cleaned incision. Clean the skin around the drain site by swabbing in half or full circles from around the drain site outward, using separate swabs for each wipe. *This ensures that clean areas are not contaminated.*
   - Support and hold the drain erect while cleaning around it. Clean as many times as necessary to remove the drainage, taking care not to rub or irritate the skin.
   - Dry the surrounding skin with dry gauze swabs as required. Do not dry the incision or wound itself. *Moisture facilitates wound healing.*

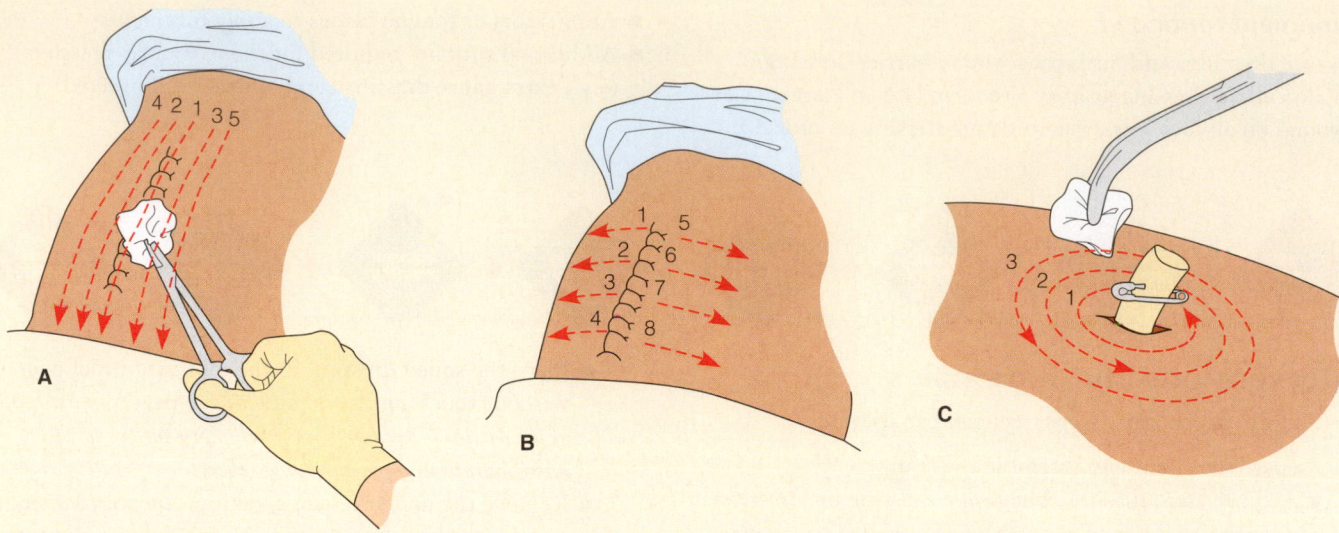

Figure 29-6. ■ Methods of cleaning surgical wounds: **A.** Cleaning the wound from top to bottom, starting at the center. **B.** Cleaning a wound outward from the incision. **C.** Cleaning around a drain site. For all methods, a clean sterile swab is used for each stroke.

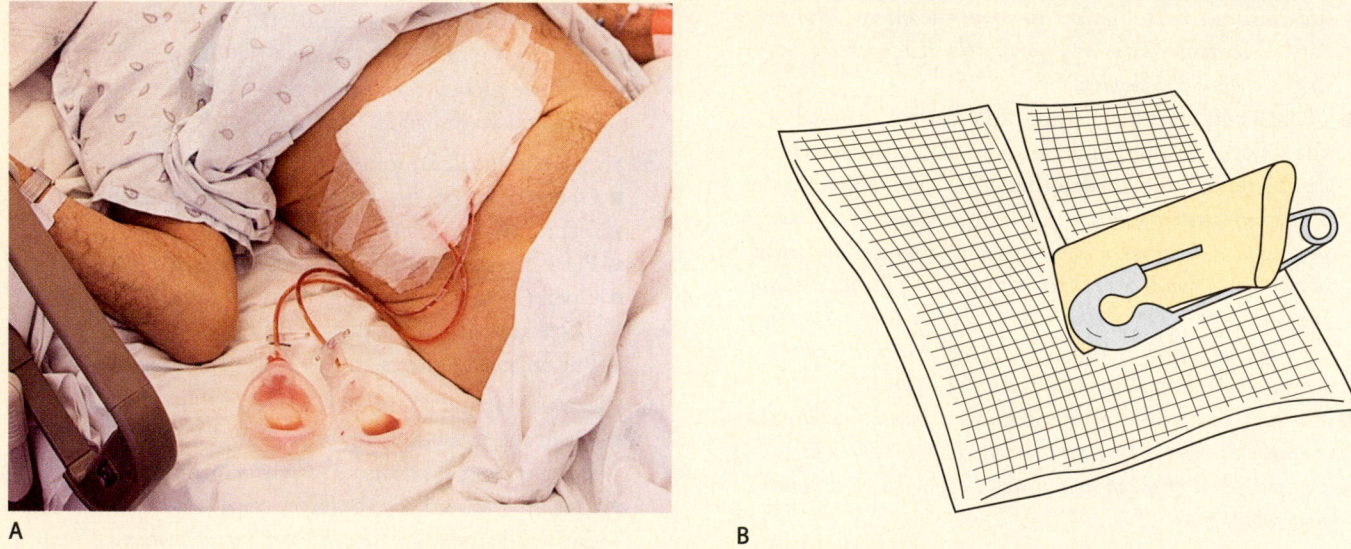

Figure 29-7. ■ **A.** Use drainage pouches for wounds with Jackson-Pratt drains. **B.** Precut gauze in place around a drain.

7. Apply dressings to the drain site and the incision (Figure 29-7 ■).

■ Place a precut 4×4 gauze snugly around the drain, or open a 4×4 gauze to 4×8, fold it lengthwise to 2×8, and place the 2×8 around the drain so that the ends overlap. *This dressing absorbs the drainage and helps prevent it from excoriating the skin. Using precut gauze or folding it as described, instead of cutting the gauze, prevents any threads from coming loose and getting into the wound, where they could cause inflammation and provide a site for infection.*

■ Apply the sterile dressings one at a time over the drain and the incision. Place the bulk of the dressings over the drain area and below the drain, depending on the client's usual position. *Layers of dressings are placed for best absorption of drainage, which flows by gravity.*

■ Apply the final Surgipad, remove gloves, and dispose of them. Secure the dressing with tape or ties.

8. Document the procedure and all data collected.

SAMPLE DOCUMENTATION

[date] [time] Transverse abdominal well approximated incision 4 cm in length, cleansed with saline. No drainage or signs of infection. Dressing reapplied. Tolerated the procedure well. _____

_____ D. Haus, LVN

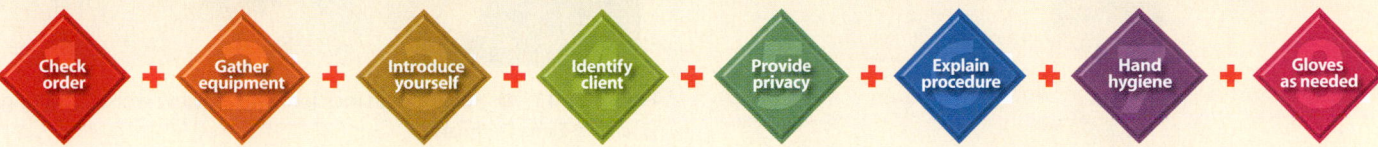

PROCEDURE 29-2   # Teaching Preoperative Exercises

Purposes

- To maintain blood circulation
- To stimulate respiratory function and lung aeration, preventing atelectasis and pneumonia
- To decrease stasis of gas in the intestines
- To facilitate early ambulation

- To stimulate blood circulation, thereby preventing thrombophlebitis and thrombus formation

Equipment

- Pillow

Check order + Gather equipment + Introduce yourself + Identify client + Provide privacy + Explain procedure + Hand hygiene + Gloves as needed

Interventions and Rationales

1. Perform preparatory steps (see icon bar above).

2. Show the client ways to turn in bed and to get out of bed.
   - Instruct a client who will have a right abdominal incision or a right-sided chest incision to turn to the left side of the bed and sit up as follows:
     a. Flex the knees.
     b. Splint the wound by holding the left arm and hand or a small pillow against the incision. *This minimizes pressure against the incision and reduces pain.*
     c. Turn to the left while pushing with the right foot and grasping a partial side rail on the left side of the bed with the right hand. *This puts least pressure on the side with the incision.*
     d. Come to a sitting position on the side of the bed by using the right arm and hand to push down against the mattress and swinging the feet over the edge of the bed.
   - Teach a client with left abdominal or left-sided chest incision to perform the same procedure but splint with the right arm and turn to the right.
   - For clients with orthopedic surgery (e.g., hip surgery), use special aids, such as a trapeze, to assist with movement.

3. Teach the client the following three leg exercises.
   - Alternate dorsiflexion and plantar flexion of the feet (Figure 29-8 ■). This exercise is sometimes referred to as calf pumping, because it alternately contracts and relaxes the calf muscles, including the gastrocnemius muscles (see also Figures 23-12 and 23-28 in Chapter 23 ⚭).
   - Flex and extend the knees, and press the backs of the knees into the bed while dorsiflexing the feet. Instruct clients who cannot raise their legs to do isometric exercises that contract and relax the muscles.
   - Raise and lower the legs alternately from the surface of the bed. Flex the knee of the stable leg and extend the

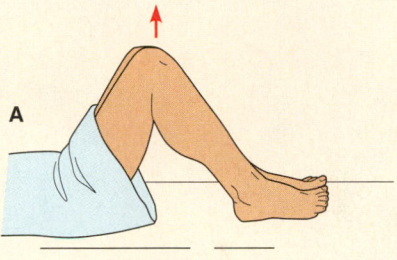
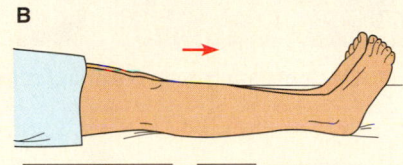
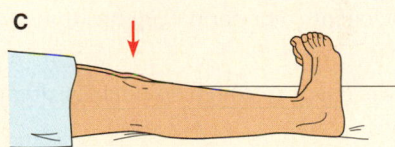

Figure 29-8. ■ Flexing and extending the knees; flexing and extending the ankles.

knee of the moving leg (Figure 29-9 ■). This exercise contracts and relaxes the quadriceps muscles.

4. Demonstrate deep-breathing (diaphragmatic) exercises as follows.
   - Place your hands palms down on the border of your rib cage, and inhale slowly and evenly through the nose until the greatest chest expansion is achieved (Figure 29-10 ■).
   - Hold your breath for 2 to 3 seconds.
   - Then exhale slowly through the mouth.
   - Continue exhalation until maximum chest contraction has been achieved.

5. Help the client perform deep-breathing exercises.
   - Ask the client to assume a sitting position.

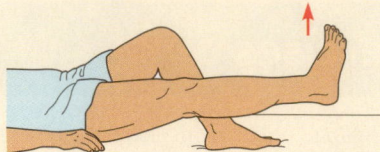

Figure 29-9. ■ Raising and lowering the legs.

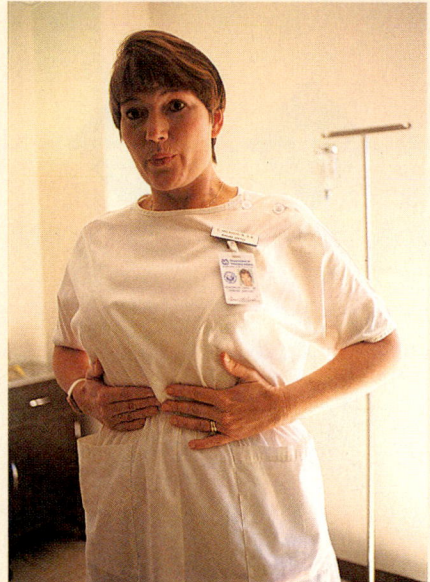

Figure 29-10. ■ Demonstrating deep breathing. (*Source*: © Elena Dorfman.)

- Place the palms of your hands on the border of the client's rib cage to assess respiratory depth.
- Ask the client to perform deep breathing, as described in step 4.

6. Instruct the client to cough voluntarily after a few deep inhalations.
   - Ask the client to inhale deeply, hold the breath for a few seconds, and then cough once or twice.
   - Ensure that the client coughs deeply and does not just clear the throat.

7. Demonstrate ways to splint the abdomen when coughing, if the incision will be painful when the client coughs.
   - Show the client how to support the incision by placing the palms of the hands on either side of the incision site or directly over the incision site, holding the palm of one hand over the other. *Coughing uses the abdominal and other accessory respiratory muscles. Splinting the incision may reduce pain while coughing if the incision is near any of these muscles. Note: Clients who have undergone nasal surgery, eye surgery, or cranial surgeries should not cough, since it could increase intracranial pressure and cause bleeding.*
   - Show the client how to splint the abdomen with clasped hands and a firmly rolled pillow held against the client's abdomen (Figure 29-11 ■).

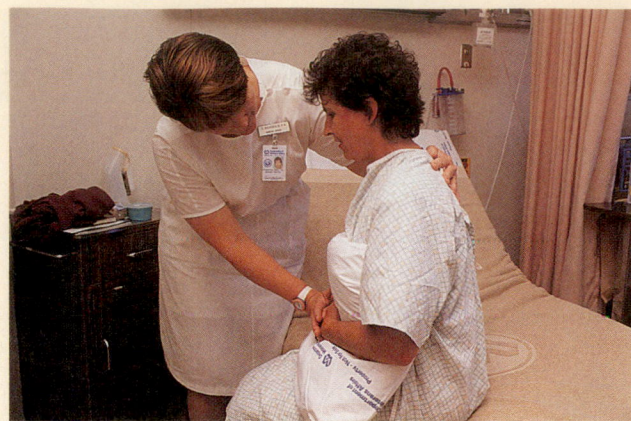

Figure 29-11. ■ Splinting an incision with a pillow while coughing. (*Source:* © Elena Dorfman.)

8. Inform the client about the expected frequency of these exercises. *This prepares the client mentally to perform them in the recovery period.*
   - Instruct the client to start the exercises as soon after surgery as possible. This promotes good oxygenation.
   - Encourage clients with abdominal or chest surgery to carry out deep-breathing and coughing exercises at least every 2 hours, taking a minimum of five breaths at each session. Note, however, that the number of breaths and frequency of deep breathing vary with the client's condition. *People who are susceptible to pulmonary problems may need deep-breathing exercises every hour. People with chronic respiratory disease may need special breathing exercises (e.g., pursed-lip breathing, abdominal breathing, exercises using various kinds of incentive spirometers).* See Chapter 32 ∞ .

9. Document the teaching and all assessments.

Continuous Passive Motion Machine for Postoperative Clients

The continuous passive motion (CPM) machine (Figure 29-12 ■) is a postoperative treatment method that is designed to assist in recovery after joint surgery. In most clients, after extensive joint

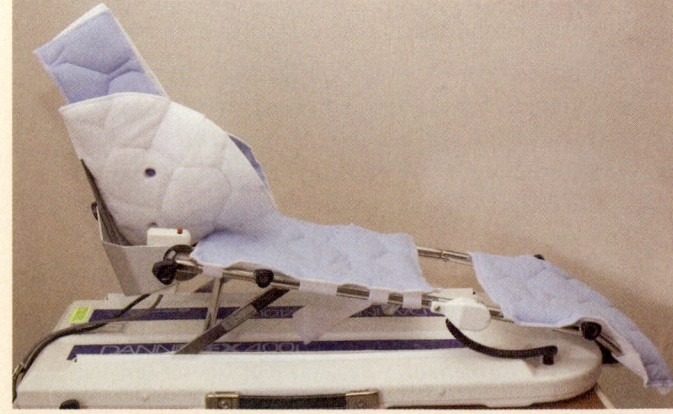

Figure 29-12. ■ Continuous passive motion machine for postoperative clients.

surgery, attempts at joint motion cause pain, so the client guards against joint movement. When this happens, the tissue around the joint becomes stiff and scar tissue forms, resulting in a joint that has limited range of motion.

Passive range of motion means that the joint is moved without the client's muscles being used (see Procedure 23-1 ⚭ for the full range of PROM exercises). Applied postoperatively, often in the PACU, a CPM machine may be used on an inpatient or outpatient basis. By using a motorized device to gradually move the joint, it is possible to accelerate recovery time significantly. Use of the CPM machine increases range of motion, decreases soft tissue stiffness, promotes healing of joint surfaces and soft tissue, and prevents the development of motion-limiting adhesions (scar tissue).

CPM devices are available for the knee, ankle, shoulder, elbow, wrist, and hand. The surgeon prescribes how the CPM unit should be used by the client (speed, duration of usage, amount of motion, rate of increase of motion, etc.).

SAMPLE DOCUMENTATION

[date] [time] Client coughing and deep breathing every 2 hours. Splinting abdomen while coughing. Lungs clear. _____

_____T. Thompson, LPN

PROCEDURE 29-3   Applying Antiemboli Stockings

Purposes

- To facilitate venous return from the lower extremities
- To prevent venous stasis and venous thrombosis
- To reduce peripheral edema

Equipment

- Tape measure
- Clean antiemboli stockings of appropriate size and of the type ordered
- Talcum powder

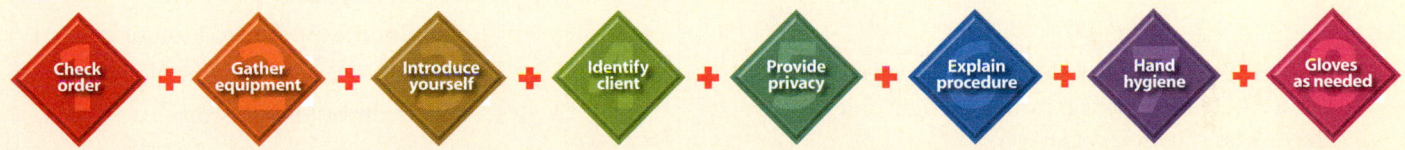

Check order + Gather equipment + Introduce yourself + Identify client + Provide privacy + Explain procedure + Hand hygiene + Gloves as needed

Interventions and Rationales

1. Perform preparatory steps (see icon bar above).
2. Take measurements as needed to obtain the appropriate size stockings.
   - Measure the length of both legs from the heel to the gluteal fold (for thigh-length stockings) or from the heel to the popliteal space (for knee-length stockings).
   - Measure the circumference of each calf and each thigh at the widest point.
   - Compare the measurements to the size chart to obtain stockings of correct size. Obtain two sizes if there is a significant difference. *Stockings that are too large for the client do not place adequate pressure on the legs to facilitate venous return and may bunch, increasing the risk of pressure and skin irritation. Stockings that are too small may impede blood flow to the feet and cause discomfort.*
3. Select an appropriate time to apply the stockings.
   - Apply stockings in the morning, if possible, before the client arises. *In sitting and standing positions, the veins can*

   become distended so that edema occurs; the stockings should be applied before this happens.
   - Assist the client who has been ambulating to lie down and elevate the legs for 15 to 30 minutes before applying the stockings. *This facilitates venous return and reduces swelling.*
4. Prepare the client.
   - Assist the client to a lying position in bed.
   - Wash and dry the legs as needed.
   - Dust the ankles with talcum powder. *This eases application.*
5. Apply the stockings.
   - Reach inside the stocking from the top, and grasping the heel, turn the upper portion of the stocking inside out over the foot portion. *Firm elastic stockings are easier to fit over the foot and calf when inverted in this manner rather than bunching the stocking up.*
   - Ask the client to point the toes, and position the stocking on the client's foot, taking care to place the toe and heel portions of the stocking appropriately (Figure 29-13 ■). *Pointing the toes makes application easier.*

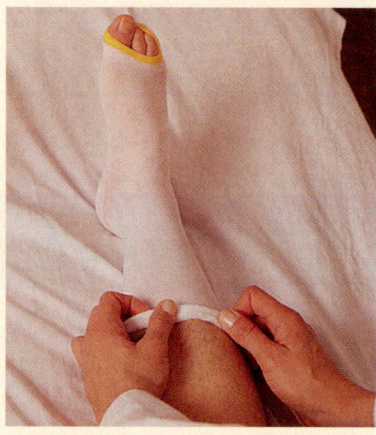

A

B

Figure 29-13. ■ **A.** Applying the inverted stocking over the toes. **B.** Pulling the stocking snugly over the leg. (*Source:* © Elena Dorfman.)

- Grasp the upper edge of the stocking and gently pull the stocking over the leg, turning it right side out in the process (Figure 29-13B).
- Inspect the client's leg and stocking, smoothing any folds or creases. Ensure that the stocking is not rolled down or bunched at the top or ankle. *Folds and creases*

can cause skin irritation under the stocking; bunching of the stocking can further impair venous return.

- Remove the stockings for 30 minutes every 8 hours, inspecting the legs and skin while the hose are off. *This allows early detection of problems.*
- Soiled stockings may be laundered by hand with warm water and mild soap. Hang to dry.

6. Document the procedure.
- Record the procedure, your assessment data, and when the stockings are removed and reapplied.

clinical ALERT

If you are having trouble adjusting stockings over a client's foot, this technique may help. Place the foot in a small plastic bag. (A clean bedside trash bag works well.) Adjust the stocking over the bag-covered foot and up the leg. Once the stocking has been adjusted, pull the plastic bag out through the open toe of the stocking. The elastic stocking will be smooth and wrinkle free without discomfort to the client.

SAMPLE DOCUMENTATION

[date] [time] Antiemboli stockings removed for bathing. Bilateral pedal pulses strong and regular. Skin warm, dry, and pink. No evidence of edema. Homans' sign negative. Stockings replaced, client ambulated from bed to chair. _____

_____ K. Turner, LVN

PROCEDURE 29-4 Applying Sequential Compression Devices

Purposes
- To facilitate venous return in immobilized clients
- To prevent thrombus formation

Equipment
- Measuring tape
- Antiembolism stockings
- Sequential compression device (SCD) including disposable sleeves, air pump, and tubing

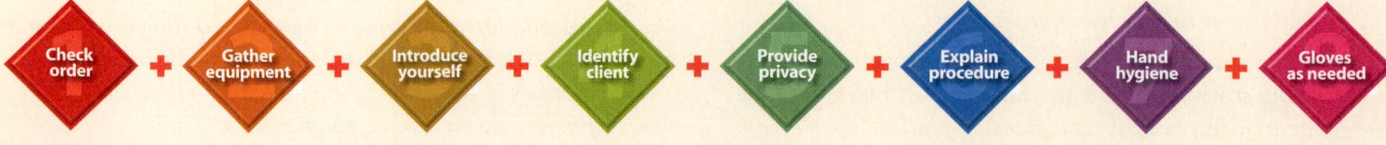

Check order + Gather equipment + Introduce yourself + Identify client + Provide privacy + Explain procedure + Hand hygiene + Gloves as needed

Interventions and Rationales

1. Perform preparatory steps (see icon bar).
2. Prepare the client.
   - Place the client in a dorsal recumbent or semi-Fowler's position. Provide for privacy and drape the client appropriately.
   - Measure the client's legs as recommended by the manufacturer if a thigh-length sleeve is required. *Knee-length sleeves come in just one size; the thigh circumference determines the size needed for a thigh-length sleeve.*
   - Apply antiembolism stockings. *Antiembolism stockings provide added support and reduce skin irritation from the compression sleeve.*
3. Apply the sequential compression sleeves.
   - Place a sleeve under each leg with the opening at the knee.
   - Wrap the sleeve securely around the leg, securing the Velcro tabs (Figure 29-14 ■). Allow two fingers to fit between the leg and the sleeve. *This amount of space ensures that the sleeve does not impair circulation when inflated.*
4. Connect the sleeves to the control unit and adjust the pressure as needed.
   - Connect the tubing to the sleeves and control unit, ensuring that arrows on the plug and the connector are in alignment and that the tubing is not kinked or twisted. *Improper alignment or obstruction of the tubing by kinks or twists will interfere with operation of the SCD.*

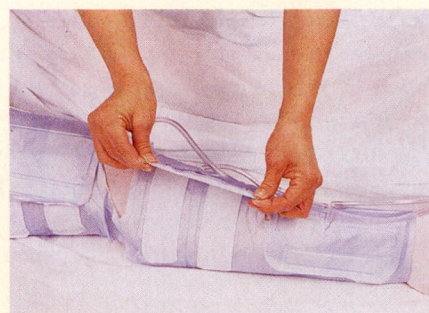

Figure 29-14. ■ Applying a sequential compression device to the leg. (*Source: © Jenny Thomas.*)

- Turn on the control unit and adjust the alarms and pressures as needed. The sleeve cooling control and alarm should be "on"; ankle pressure is usually set at 35 to 55 mm Hg. *It is important to have the sleeve cooling control on for comfort and to reduce the risk of skin irritation from moisture under the sleeve. Alarms warn of possible control unit malfunctions.*
5. Document the procedure.
   - Record baseline assessment data and application of the SCD. Note control unit settings.
   - Assess and document skin integrity and neurovascular status at least every 8 hours while the SCD is in place. Remove the unit and notify the physician if the client complains of numbness and tingling or leg pain. *These may be symptoms of nerve compression.*

SAMPLE DOCUMENTATION: FOCUS CHARTING

[date] [time] Data Action Response

[date] [time] **D**: Client is 1 day post Rt. THR. Antiembolism stockings & SCDs removed for bath.

A: Assessed pedal and popliteal pulses. Assessed CMS status. Assessed skin integrity before replacing thigh-high antiembolism stockings and SCDs. Instructed client to report any numbness, tingling, or leg pain.

R: CMS intact. The sleeve cooling control & alarm are "on" with sleeve pressure at 45 mm Hg. _____

_____ N. Nurse, LPN

PROCEDURE 29-5 Managing Nasogastric Suctioning

Purposes

- To relieve abdominal distention
- To maintain gastric decompression after surgery
- To remove blood and secretions from the gastrointestinal tract
- To relieve discomfort (e.g., when a client has a bowel obstruction)
- To maintain the patency of the nasogastric tube

Equipment

- Gastrointestinal tube in place in the client
- Basin
- 50-mL syringe with an adapter
- Stethoscope
- Suction device for either continuous or intermittent suction
- Connector and connecting tubing
- Disposable gloves

- Graduated container as required to measure gastric drainage
- Cotton-tipped applicators
- Ointment or lubricant
- Disposable irrigating set containing a sterile 50-mL syringe, moisture-resistant pad, basin, and graduated container
- Sterile normal saline (500 mL) or the ordered solution

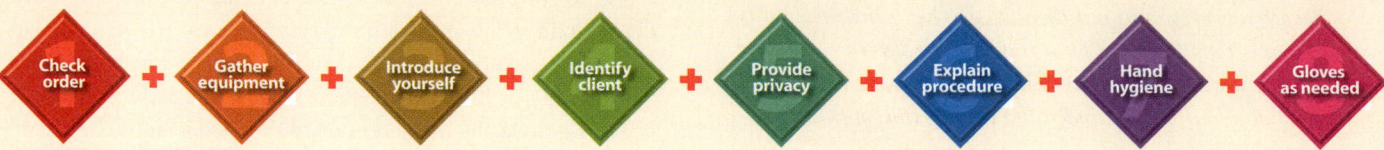

Check order + Gather equipment + Introduce yourself + Identify client + Provide privacy + Explain procedure + Hand hygiene + Gloves as needed

Interventions and Rationales

INITIATING SUCTION

1. Perform preparatory steps (see icon bar above).

2. Position the client appropriately.
   - Assist the client to a semi-Fowler's position if it is not contraindicated. *In semi-Fowler's position the tube is not as likely to lie against the wall of the stomach and will therefore suction most efficiently. Semi-Fowler's position also prevents reflux of gastric contents, which could lead to aspiration.*

3. Confirm that the tube is in the stomach.
   - Aspirate stomach contents and check their acidity using a pH test strip.
   - Insert air into the tube with the syringe and listen with a stethoscope over the stomach (just below the xiphoid process) for a swish of air.
   - Use other methods in accordance with agency protocol.

4. Set and check the suction (Figure 29-15 ■).
   - Connect the appropriate suction regulator to the wall suction outlet and the collection device to the regulator. Intermittent suction regulators generally are used with single-lumen tubes and apply suction for a set interval (15 to 60 seconds), followed by an interval of no suction. Intermittent low suction is set at 40 mm Hg or as ordered by the physician. Check the suction level by occluding the drainage tube and observing the regulator dial during a suction cycle. Continuous suction regulators are used with double-lumen (e.g., Salem sump) nasogastric tubes. Set continuous suction as ordered by the physician, or at 30 to 40 mm Hg. Intermittent high suction is set at 120 mm Hg or as ordered by the physician (Smith et al., 2008). *Note*: The air vent tube of a Salem sump must *always* remain open while the tube is connected to suction. This tube is not to be used for suction.
   - If using a portable suction machine, turn on the machine and regulate the suction as above. The Gomco pump has two settings: low intermittent for single-lumen tubes, and high for double-lumen tubes.
   - Test for proper suctioning by holding the open end of the suction tube to the ear and listening for a sucking noise or by occluding the end of the tube with a thumb.

5. Establish gastric suction.
   - Connect the gastrointestinal tube to the tubing from the suction by using the connector.
   - If a Salem sump tube is in place, connect the larger lumen to the suction equipment (see Figure 29-15B). This double-lumen tube has a smaller tube running inside the primary suction tube. *The smaller tube provides a continuous flow of atmospheric air through the drainage tube at its distal end and prevents excessive suction force on the gastric mucosa at the drainage outlets. This avoids damage to the gastric mucosa.*
   - Always keep the air vent tube of a Salem sump tube open and above the level of the stomach when suction is applied. *Closing the vent would stop the sump action and cause mucosal damage. Keeping the end of the air vent tube higher than the stomach prevents reflux of gastric contents into the air lumen of the tube.*
   - After suction is applied, watch the tubing for a few minutes until the gastric contents appear to be running through the tubing into the receptacle. A Salem sump tube makes a soft, hissing sound when it is functioning correctly.
   - If the suction is not working properly, check that all connections are tight and that the tubing is not kinked.
   - Coil and pin the tubing on the bed so that it does not loop below the suction bottle. *If the tubing falls below the suction bottle, the suction may be obstructed because of the pressure required to push the fluid against gravity.*

6. Assess the drainage.
   - Observe the amount, color, odor, and consistency of the drainage. *Normal gastric drainage has a mucoid consistency and is either colorless or yellow-green because of the presence of bile. A coffee-grounds color and consistency may indicate bleeding.*

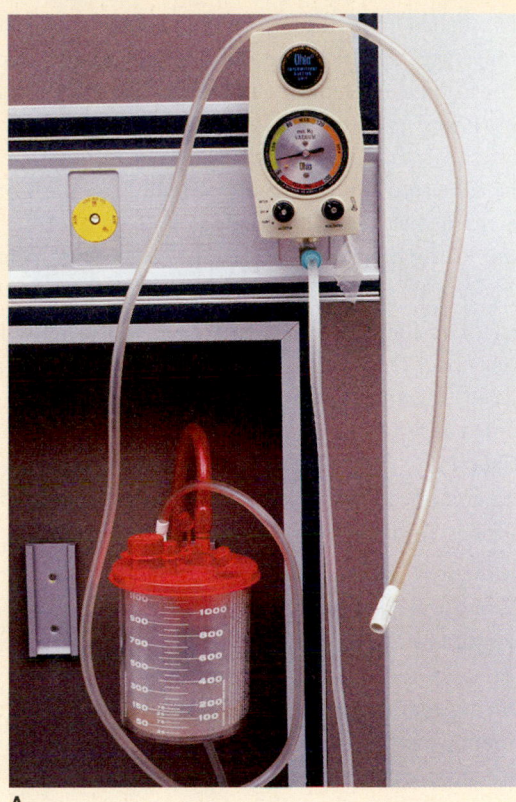

A

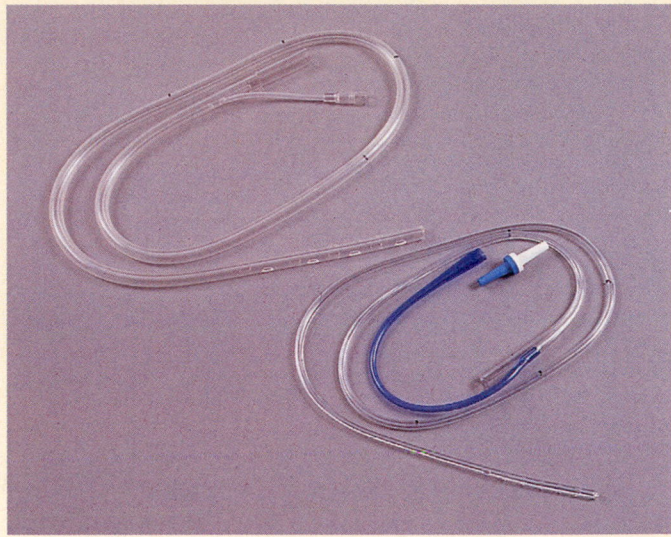

B

Figure 29-15. ■ **A.** Connect suction to suction source. **B.** Insert tapered adapter to connect the NG tube to the suction tubing. *Top:* Levin single-lumen tube; *bottom:* Salem double-lumen with antireflux valve. Insert blue side of antireflux valve into the Salem sump tube blue pigtail.

- Test the gastric drainage for pH and blood (by using Hematest) when indicated. *A person who has had gastrointestinal surgery can be expected to have some blood in the drainage.*

MAINTAINING SUCTION

7. Assess the client and the suction system regularly.
   - Assess the client every 30 minutes until the system is running effectively and then every 2 hours, or as the client's health indicates, to ensure that the suction is functioning properly. *If the client complains of fullness, nausea, or epigastric pain or if the flow of gastric secretions is absent in the tubing or in the collection bottle, ineffective suctioning or blockage of the nasogastric tube is likely.*
   - Inspect the suction system for patency of the system (e.g., kinks or blockages in the tubing) and tightness of the connections. *Loose connections can permit air to enter and thus decrease the effectiveness of the suction by decreasing the negative pressure.*

8. Relieve blockages if present.
   - Don gloves.
   - Check the suction equipment. To do this, disconnect the nasogastric tube from the suction over a collecting basin (to collect gastric drainage), and then, with the suction on, place the end of the suction tubing in a basin of water. *If water is drawn into the drainage bottle, the suction equipment is functioning properly,*

but the nasogastric tube is either blocked or positioned incorrectly.

- Reposition the client (e.g., to the other side) if permitted. *This may facilitate drainage.*
- Rotate the nasogastric tube, and reposition it. This step is contraindicated for clients with gastric surgery. *Moving the tube may interfere with gastric sutures.*
- Irrigate the nasogastric tube as agency protocol states or on the order of the physician. See steps 12 to 14.

9. Prevent reflux into the vent lumen of a Salem sump tube. *Reflux of gastric contents into the vent lumen may occur when stomach pressure exceeds atmospheric pressure. In this situation, gastric contents follow the path of least resistance and flow out the vent lumen rather than the drainage lumen.* To prevent reflux:
   - Place the vent tubing higher than the client's stomach.
   - Keep the drainage collection container below the level of the client's stomach and do not allow it to become overfull. *A collection device placed above the level of fluid in the stomach or that is too full may interfere with drainage, allowing reflux of gastric contents into the air lumen.*
   - Keep the drainage lumen free of particulate matter that may obstruct the lumen. See steps 12 to 14 for irrigating a nasogastric tube.

10. Ensure client comfort.

- Clean the client's nostrils as needed, using the cotton-tipped applicators and water. Apply a water-soluble lubricant or ointment.
- Provide mouth care every 2 to 4 hours and as needed. *Some postoperative clients are permitted to suck ice chips or a moist cloth to maintain the moisture of the oral mucous membranes.*

11. Empty the drainage receptacle according to agency policy or physician's order.
    - Clamp the nasogastric tube, and turn off the suction.
    - Don gloves.
    - If the receptacle is graduated, determine the amount of drainage.
    - Disconnect the receptacle.
    - If the receptacle is not graduated, empty the contents into a graduated container and measure.
    - Inspect the drainage carefully for color, consistency, and presence of substances (e.g., blood clots).
    - Discard and replace a full receptacle or rinse the receptacle with warm water and reattach it to the suction. Check agency policy.
    - Turn on the suction and unclamp the nasogastric tube.
    - Observe the system for several minutes to make sure function is reestablished.
    - Go to Step 15.

IRRIGATING A GASTROINTESTINAL TUBE

12. Prepare the client and the equipment.
    - Place the moisture-resistant pad under the end of the gastrointestinal tube.
    - Turn off the suction.
    - Don gloves.
    - Disconnect the gastrointestinal tube from the connector.
    - Determine that the tube is in the stomach. See step 3 above and in Procedure 25-3 ⦾. *This ensures that the irrigating solution enters the client's stomach.*

13. Irrigate the tube.
    - Draw up the ordered volume of irrigating solution in the syringe; 30 mL of solution per instillation is usual, but up to 60 mL may be given per instillation if ordered.
    - Attach the syringe to the nasogastric tube, and slowly inject the solution.
    - Gently aspirate the solution. *Forceful withdrawal could damage the gastric mucosa.*

- If you encounter difficulty in withdrawing the solution, inject 20 mL of air and aspirate again, and/or reposition the client or the nasogastric tube. *Air and repositioning may move the end of the tube away from the stomach wall.* If aspirating difficulty continues, reattach the tube to intermittent low suction, and notify the nurse in charge or physician.
- Repeat the preceding steps until the ordered amount of solution is used.

14. Reestablish suction.
    - Reconnect the nasogastric tube to suction.
    - If a Salem sump tube is used, inject the air vent lumen with 10 mL of air after reconnecting the tube to suction.
    - Observe the system for several minutes to make sure it is functioning.

15. Document all relevant information.
    - Record the time suction was started. Also record the pressure established, the color and consistency of the drainage, and nursing assessments.
    - During maintenance, record assessments, supportive nursing measures, and data about the suction system.
    - When irrigating the tube, record verification of tube placement; the time of the irrigation; the amount and type of irrigating solution used; the amount, color and consistency of the returns; the patency of the system following the irrigation; and nursing assessments. *Remember the saying, "If it isn't documented, it wasn't done."*

SAMPLE DOCUMENTATION

[date] [time] Abdominal distention decreased; bowel sounds present in all 4 quadrants; 450 mL of dark coffee-grounds gastric drainage; oral mucous pink and moist. _____

_____ D. Wilson, LPN

Chapter Review

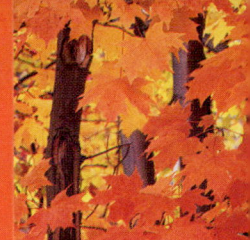

KEY Points

- The *preoperative phase* occurs prior to surgery, the *intraoperative phase* occurs during surgery, and the *postoperative phase* occurs following surgery. These three phases are together referred to as the perioperative period.

- Surgical procedures are commonly grouped in one of three ways: purpose, degree of urgency, and degree of risk.

- Surgery is a unique experience that creates stress and necessitates physical and psychologic changes.

- Factors such as age, general health, nutritional status, medication use, and mental status affect a client's risk during surgery.

- Clients must agree to surgery and sign an informed consent.

- Preoperative teaching should include moving, leg exercises, and coughing and deep-breathing exercises. Good preoperative teaching helps prevent postoperative complications.

- Physical preparation includes the following areas: nutrition and fluids, elimination, hygiene, rest, medications, care of valuables and prostheses, special orders, and surgical skin preparation.

- A preoperative checklist provides a guide to and documentation of a client's preparation before surgery.

- Initial and ongoing assessment of the postoperative client includes level of consciousness, vital signs, oxygen saturation, skin color and temperature, comfort, fluid balance, dressings, drains, and tubes.

- The overall goals of nursing care during the postoperative period are to promote comfort and healing, restore the highest possible level of wellness, and prevent associated risks such as infection or respiratory and cardiovascular complications.

- Surgical aseptic technique (sterile technique) is used when changing dressings on surgical wounds to promote healing and reduce the risk of infection. Sutures, wire clips, or staples are generally removed 7 to 10 days after surgery.

FOR FURTHER Study

For a complete discussion about informed consent, see Chapter 4.

See more about infections and resistant organisms in Chapter 10.

Recording and documenting procedures are discussed in depth in Chapter 13.

For handling of client valuables prior to surgery, see discussion in Chapter 14 and Figure 14-2.

For information about assessing the return of peristalsis by auscultating the abdomen, see Chapter 19.

For more information about hygiene, see Chapter 20.

For a more in-depth discussion of pain and pain management, see Chapter 22.

Chapter 23 provides information about mobility and exercises for clients.

For a discussion of wounds and wound care, see Chapter 24.

For more information on nutrition and nasogastric tubes, see Chapter 25.

For more information on fluids and acid-base balance, see Chapter 26.

For an illustration of an intake and output record, see Figure 26-4.

See more about disorders of the skin in Chapter 30.

Oxygenation and incentive spirometers are discussed in Chapter 32.

See more about thrombus and embolus formation in Chapter 34.

Chapter 37 covers the gastrointestinal system.

See catheterization procedures in Chapter 39.

See Chapter 58 for discussion about children and surgery.

Appendix II on the MyNursingKit Website lists the NANDA diagnoses.

PEARSON

EXPLORE mynursingkit™

MyNursingKit is your one stop for online chapter review materials and resources. Prepare for success with additional NCLEX®-style practice questions, interactive assignments and activities, web links, animations and videos, and more!

Register your access code from the front of your book at
www.mynursingkit.com

Critical Thinking Care Map

Caring for a Client with an Amputated Arm

NCLEX-PN® Focus Area: Psychosocial Integrity: Coping and Adaptation

Case Study: Tim Broughton is an 18-year-old college student. Six days ago, he was involved in a motorcycle accident. After every attempt to save his right arm, amputation below the shoulder was performed 2 days ago.

Nursing Diagnosis: *Disturbed Body Image*

COLLECT DATA

Subjective	Objective
_____	_____
_____	_____
_____	_____
_____	_____
_____	_____
_____	_____
_____	_____

Would you report this? Yes/No

If yes, report to: _____

What would you report?_____

Nursing Care

_____
_____
_____
_____
_____
_____
_____
_____
_____
_____

How would you document this? _____
_____
_____
_____

Compare your answers and documentation to those provided on the MyNursingKit Website.

Data Collected
(use only those that apply)

- Vital signs stable.
- Complains of pain.
- Refuses to respond to nurse's questions about pain level.
- Will not look at limb during dressing change.
- "I wish I had died in the accident; life will never be the same."
- Dressing dry and intact.
- Wound healing without signs of infection.

Nursing Interventions
(use only those that apply; list in priority order)

- Contact physician for social worker or psychologist referral.
- Acknowledge denial, anger, or depression as normal.
- Teach the importance of range-of-motion exercises.
- Ask client to describe past experiences with pain and effectiveness of methods used to manage pain.
- Encourage client to make own decisions, participate in plan of care, and accept both inadequacies and strengths.
- Obtain assistive devices needed for activity.
- Allow client gradual exposure to body change.
- Help client to accept help from others.
- Teach family appropriate care of surgical site.

NCLEX-PN® Exam Preparation

TEST-TAKING TIP   Remember the order of priority of AIRWAY, BREATHING, and CIRCULATION!

1 The client asks when the preoperative period ends. The nurse's best response would be:

1. "Why do you want to know that? You should just concentrate on getting prepared for surgery."
2. "The preoperative period ends when you are wheeled out of surgery."
3. "The preoperative period ends when you are wheeled into the holding area prior to surgery."
4. "The preoperative period ends when you are wheeled into the operating room."

2 The nurse, working on a surgical unit, is preparing several clients for the operating room this morning. The following clients request to keep their wedding rings on and the nurse tapes the ring in place except for which client who must remove the ring?

1. A 65-year-old male scheduled for a TURP (transurethral prostatectomy)
2. A 31-year-old female having a repeat C-section
3. A 72-year-old female having a total hip replacement
4. A 49-year-old female scheduled for a left modified radical mastectomy

3 After performing vital signs every 15 minutes for an hour, the nurse concludes that which of the following clients is not yet stable enough for vital sign measurements every 4 hours?

1. Vital signs have measured 98.2 oral, 88, 14, 112/68 for the past hour.
2. Vital signs have measured 96.8 axillary, 96, 20, 138/88 for the past hour.
3. Vital signs 98.4 oral, 60, 10, 92/58 when last checked.
4. Vital signs 99.2 oral, 104, 18, 138/84 when last checked.

4 After the client returns to the unit following surgery requiring spinal anesthesia, the nurse instructs the unlicensed assistive personnel to position the unresponsive client in the:

1. Prone position for 8 to 12 hours.
2. Side-lying position with slight elevation of the head.
3. Supine position for 8 to 12 hours.
4. Semi-Fowler's position.

5 The nurse teaches deep breathing and coughing to the client who is scheduled for surgery and recognizes the need for further teaching when the client makes which of the following statements?

1. "I will lie flat while coughing in order to control my pain."
2. "I will hold a pillow tightly against my abdomen when I cough."
3. "After taking a deep breath, I will cough forcefully."
4. "I will take a deep breath in through my nose prior to coughing."

6 The nurse is caring for a client who is scheduled for an appendectomy. The nurse recognizes this is what type of surgical procedure?

1. Diagnostic
2. Palliative
3. Ablative
4. Reconstructive

7 The nurse is preparing to ambulate the client the day after surgery when the client asks, "Why can't I just stay in bed? It hurts when I move." The nurse's best response would be:

1. "Your doctor has written an order for you to walk, and I must follow the doctor's orders."
2. "If you walk to the chair, it will be easier to change the bed while you are up."
3. "Walking is one of the best ways to prevent respiratory and circulatory complications."
4. "You need to move around to get better."

8 While preparing the client for surgery, the nurse recognizes the need to notify the physician immediately for which of the following data?

1. Vital signs 98.8–84–20, BP 132/80.
2. The client reports he took his pills with sips of water before coming to the hospital.
3. The client tells you he is having second thoughts about the need for surgery.
4. The client describes an acute systematic allergy to morphine sulfate.

9 The nurse is caring for a client with a Salem nasogastric tube and does which of the following to avoid reflux of gastric secretions into the vent?

1. Clamp the vent tube and turn up the suction.
2. Place the vent tubing higher than the client's stomach.
3. Place the vent tube lower than the stomach.
4. Irrigate the vent with normal saline.

10 While removing sutures from the client's postoperative wound, the edges of the incision separate and a portion of the intestine protrudes from the opening. The nurse notifies the physician of the:

1. Secondary intention.
2. Dehiscence.
3. Evisceration.
4. Granulation.

Answers and rationales for Review Questions appear in Appendix I.

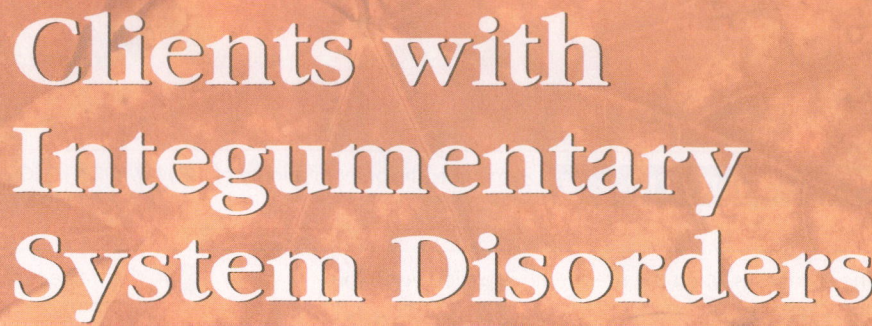

Clients with Integumentary System Disorders

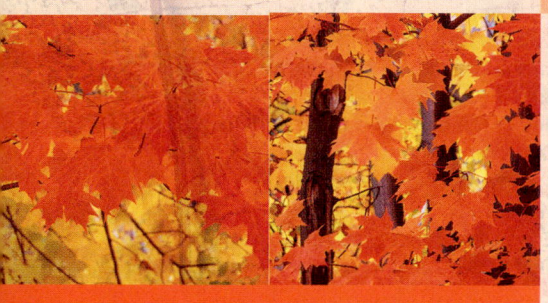

LEARNING Outcomes

After completing this chapter, you will be able to:

1. Explain the general structure and function of the integumentary system.
2. Define common terms to describe skin lesions.
3. List key points in preventing skin breakdown and preventing the spread of skin infection.
4. Discuss the symptoms, treatment, and nursing care for clients with infectious skin disorders.
5. Describe manifestations, treatment, and nursing care of clients with fungal skin disorders.
6. Identify types of parasitic skin disorders, treatment, and nursing considerations.
7. Discuss the nursing care of the client with a chronic skin condition.
8. List basic information about recognition and prevention of skin cancer.
9. Describe common types of plastic or reconstructive skin.

Clinical Objectives

10. Administer topical treatment for a skin disorder.
11. Demonstrate nursing interventions to prevent skin breakdown.
12. Care for a client with an infectious skin disease using the procedure for contact isolation.

KEY TERMS

Use the audio glossary feature on the MyNursingKit Website to hear the correct pronunciation of the following key terms.

albinism 745
alopecia 745
atrophy 746
bulla 746
capillary hemangioma 747
carbuncle 750
cerumen 745
crust 746
cyst 746
dermabrasion 759
dermis 743
ecchymosis 747
epidermis 743
erosion 746
fissure 746

furuncle 750
hematoma 747
herpes zoster 751
hirsutism 745
jaundice 745
keloid 746
lichenification 746
liposuction 759
macule 746
nodule 746
opportunistic 757
papule 746
petechiae 747
plaque 746

port-wine stain 747
postherpetic neuralgia 752
prodrome 751
purpura 747
pustule 746
pyemia 750
scale 746
scar 746
sebum 745
spider angioma 747
ulcer 746
venous star 747
vesicle 746
wheal 746

Nurses see many different skin integrity issues in daily practice. These lesions may be caused by abrupt injury (such as a motorcycle accident) or by immobility (as in a person in a coma). Whenever injury to the skin occurs, the client runs a high risk of infection. A review of the skin's anatomy will show why this is true.

Structure and Function of the Integumentary System

The skin, the largest organ, protects the body and helps to maintain health. It is often called the first line of defense against infection. The primary functions of the skin are:

- To protect the body from infection by preventing pathogens from entering.
- To prevent fluid loss and protect against dehydration.
- To regulate body temperature. This involves perspiration, as well as dilatation and constriction of vessels.
- To collect sensory information (pain, touch, pressure, temperature).

The skin and its associated structures (including the hair, nails, oil and sweat glands, blood vessels, nerves, and sensory organs) make up the integumentary system (*integumentary* means "covering"). Figure 30-1 ■ provides an illustration of skin structure. *Skin integrity* refers to the state in which the skin is not broken or open, and since that is the case, there is less chance for infection to enter the body. Common nursing diagnoses for clients with integumentary disorders are *Impaired Skin Integrity* or *Risk for Impaired Skin Integrity*. Clients have increased risk for impaired skin integrity when they are elderly, are immobile, have experienced trauma, have a chronic illness, or have undergone invasive procedures. Nursing care of clients with impaired skin integrity includes careful assessment and taking actions to promote wound healing. Nurses must understand the normal anatomy and physiology of the skin in order to identify skin disorders. They must also be aware of risk factors and specific measures for maintaining or restoring skin integrity. See Chapter 24 ◯◯ for more information on wounds and skin integrity.

The skin contains epithelial, connective, and nerve tissues. Adults have 17 to 20 square feet of skin on their bodies to protect them from mechanical, chemical, and microbial invasion. The skin also helps keep body temperature stable by evaporating sweat for cooling and by decreasing blood flow to maintain heat within the body. Included in the skin are multiple receptors for heat, cold, touch, pressure, and pain (Figure 30-2 ■). The skin manufactures vitamin D, which is needed for gastrointestinal absorption of calcium. It excretes fluids and electrolytes, and it stores fat.

EPIDERMIS

The **epidermis** is the tough outer external layer of the skin. It is only 1 millimeter thick and is made of stratified squamous and epithelial tissues. The epidermis sheds old cells as new cells in the dermis are pushed up. This layer replaces itself approximately every 4 weeks (about the length of time it takes to lose a tan).

DERMIS

The **dermis** consists of the inner thicker layer of skin, called the *true skin*. This layer contains most of the skin appendages (such as hair and nails), blood vessels, and nerve endings. Fibrous connective and collagen tissue is found in this layer.

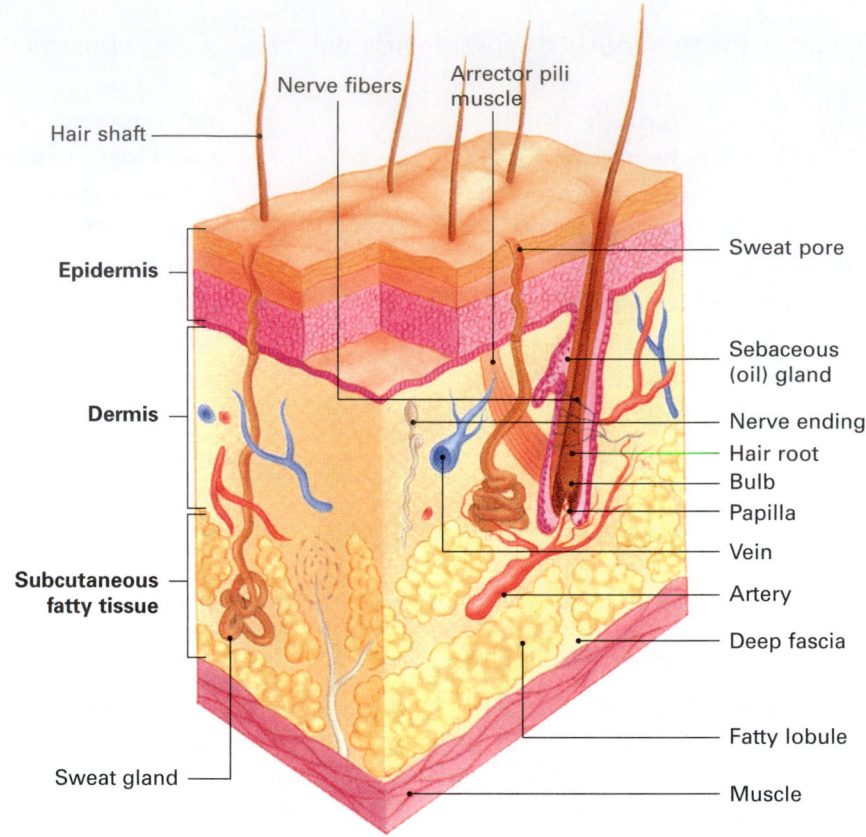

Figure 30-1. ■ Cross section of the skin.

The two layers are the papillary and reticular layers. The *papillary layer* is arranged in ridges with nipple-like projections. It contains capillaries that provide the nourishment for the *stratum germinativum* in the epidermis where new cells are made. The unchanging ridges and grooves found in the skin form an individual pattern that gives us our fingerprints. The *reticular layer* provides the rebound or elasticity in skin. When the skin is stretched it bounces back, but if it is stretched beyond its limits, *stretch marks* (uneven scarring) occur.

APPENDAGES

Hair covers all parts of the body except for the palms of the hands and the soles of the feet. The hair shaft is found in the stratum germinativum of the epidermis; the hair *follicle* (or

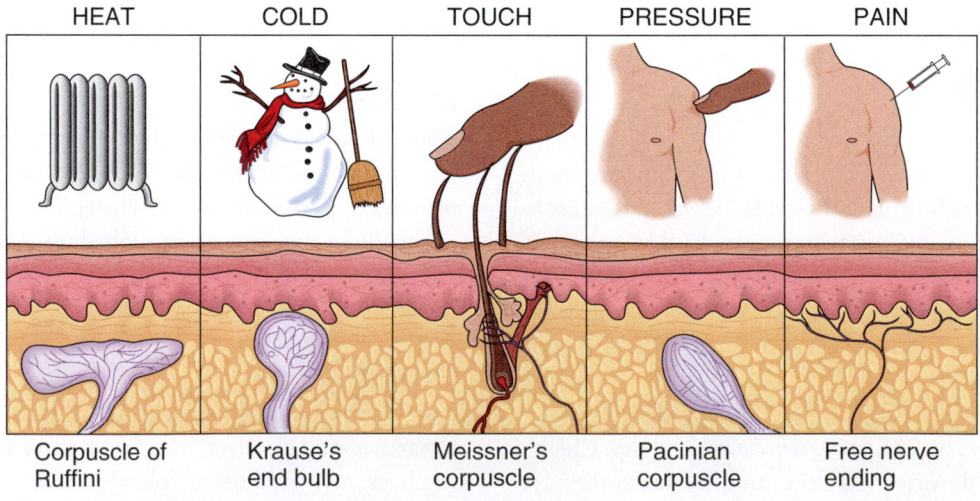

Figure 30-2. ■ The skin contains sensors for heat, cold, touch, pressure, and pain.

root) is located in the dermis. The shaft is the visible part of the hair, the medulla is the inner core of the hair, and the cortex is the outer portion around the medulla made up of keratinized cells. The *arrector pili muscle* is an involuntary muscle that pulls the hair upright when contracted, as in when you are cold or frightened (see Figure 30-1). When the hair is pulled, the skin forms a bump (called *goose bumps*). Hair color is determined by the amount of melanin in the cells. Darker hair contains more melanin than lighter hair.

The shape of the shaft determines hair type. When the shape is round and cylindrical, the hair shaft creates straight hair. A flat shaft produces wavy hair. The eyelashes, eyebrows, nose hair, and ear hair keep dust and insects from entering the body. People with excessive body hair have a condition known as **hirsutism.** The absence of hair on the head and/or body is called **alopecia.**

Sebaceous glands, small sacs in the dermis, secrete **sebum** (oil), and channel it into the hair follicles or directly onto the skin. The number of these glands increases during puberty. The sebum keeps the skin soft and hair supple. It acts as a lubricant and inhibits the growth of bacteria. The ceruminous gland, a modified sebaceous gland, is found in the auditory meatus of the ear. It secretes **cerumen** (earwax). The cerumen guards the sensitive tympanic membrane and protects the ear from microorganisms, dust, and insects.

Sudoriferous glands, or *sweat glands*, are exocrine glands that secrete fluid to the skin surface through a pore. There are approximately 3,000 per square inch of body surface. The two types of sudoriferous glands are the *eccrine glands,* which are small, and the *apocrine glands,* which are the larger glands found in the axillae and genital areas. When the fluid they secrete combines with bacteria on the skin, the result is body odor.

Nails are also skin appendages and are composed of keratinized epidermal cells. The portion of the nail you see is the nail body; beneath it is the nail bed, which is rich in blood vessels. The fold of skin around the nail is the cuticle. Beneath the cuticle is the nail root (Figure 30-3 ■). Nails grow approximately 0.5 mm per week, although fingernails grow at a quicker rate than toenails. Nails help us pick up small objects and protect the fingers and toes.

Blood vessels provide nourishment to the tissues. They also assist with heat regulation. When blood vessels open (*vasodilatation*), blood is brought closer to the body's surface, and heat loss is facilitated. When superficial blood vessels tighten (*vasoconstriction*), they help the body to conserve heat. In times of severe stress, the blood is routed to the major organs and the dermis temporarily manages with less blood flow.

Sensory receptors allow the skin to perceive sensations from the environment. Pain is transmitted through the nerve endings. Specific receptors are identified for pressure, heat, cold, and touch.

SUBCUTANEOUS LAYER

The subcutaneous layer of the skin is located beneath the dermis (see Figure 30-1). It contains elastic, fibrous, and *adipose* (fatty) tissue. Portions of the sudoriferous (sweat) and sebaceous (oil) glands are located here. The subcutaneous layer, also called the *superficial fascia,* insulates the body, cushions internal organs, stores energy, supports structures, and connects skin to surface muscles.

SKIN COLOR

Skin color is determined by the amount of melanin in the epidermis. Numerous factors, such as heredity, sunlight exposure, and hormone secretions (adrenocorticotropic hormone and melanocyte-stimulating hormone) affect skin color. Freckles (*lentigo*) are caused by irregular patches of melanin. When melanin is absent or unable to function, **albinism** occurs. **Jaundice** is a condition caused by excess bilirubin in the blood (see Chapter 37 ⬥). Racial differences make a difference in determining skin color changes (Box 30-1 ■).

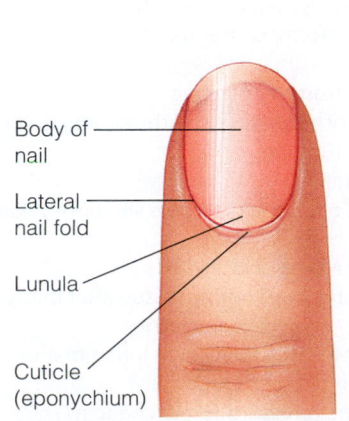

Figure 30-3. ■ Structure of the nail.

BOX 30-1 **CULTURAL PULSE POINTS**

Collecting Data on Changes in Skin Color

Numerous biocultural variations occur in the integumentary system. The range of normal skin color varies widely. It is important to establish a baseline color in order to be able to assess pertinent changes in a client.

The following skin assessment terms have different meanings for biocultural variations:

■ *Cyanosis* is a difficult clinical sign to observe in clients with dark skin. In light-skinned individuals, it appears as a yellowish skin discoloration. In dark-skinned individuals, it may appear as a grayish tone. Because cyanosis can signal decreased oxygenation to the brain, other clinical signs rather than skin color should be assessed.

■ *Jaundice* in both dark- and light-skinned clients can best be observed in the sclera, rather than the skin.

An abnormal condition known as *cyanosis* (from the color cyan, or blue) occurs when the blood does not contain enough oxygen, and the skin "turns blue." *Pallor* (paleness) is a temporary change in skin color caused by vasoconstriction. *Blushing* occurs as a response to vasodilatation.

Skin Integrity

Skin integrity is affected by many chronic illnesses and their treatments. When people have impaired peripheral circulation, they lose leg hair. The skin on the legs appears shiny and damages easily. Medications such as steroids can cause the skin to be fragile and easily torn. Some antibiotics, such as tetracyclines, cause sensitivity to sunlight and can predispose a person to severe sunburns. Skin does not heal well or have a normal appearance when a person has poor nutritional intake.

Changes in skin integrity are called *lesions*. It is important to be able to identify the different common lesions of the skin. Box 30-2 ■ provides terms and definitions of skin lesions. Figure 30-4 ■ illustrates primary skin lesions. Figure 30-5 ■ illustrates *secondary skin lesions* (those arising from a different disease process), and Figure 30-6 ■ depicts vascular lesions of the skin.

Now that you have reviewed the anatomy and physiology of the skin, you understand the importance of the skin in protecting clients with skin injury from infection. When a large part of the skin is affected, the risks for complications increase. When a client also has impaired mobility, the risk is high for a specific skin condition—pressure ulcers.

BOX 30-2 **COMMON SKIN LESIONS**

Primary Lesions (see Figure 30-4)

Cyst—a fluid-filled or semisolid sac originating in the subcutaneous tissue or dermis.
Examples: epidermoid (skin) cyst or sebaceous cyst seen in acne
Macule, patch—a discolored spot that is even with the skin's surface; macules are <1 cm, patches are >1 cm.
Examples: (of macule) freckles, petechiae; (of patch) port-wine stains, Mongolian spots
Nodule, tumor—a circumscribed, elevated mass of tissue extending deeper into the dermis than a papule; nodules are 0.5–2 cm; tumors are 2 cm or more and may have irregular borders.
Examples: (of nodule) squamous cell carcinoma or small lipoma (fatty growth); (of tumor) hemangioma, carcinoma
Papule, plaque—a circumscribed, solid elevation of the skin.
Examples: (of papule) elevated mole, warts; (of plaque) psoriasis, actinic keratosis
Pustule—a small, circumscribed elevation of the skin containing purulent matter.
Examples: infection from rose thorn
Vesicle, bulla—a small, circumscribed elevation of the skin containing fluid; vesicles are <0.5 cm; bullae are >0.5 cm.
Examples: (of vesicle) herpes simplex or cold sore; (of bulla) contact dermatitis or large burn blisters
Wheal—a circumscribed, slightly reddened, papule or irregular plaque of edema of the skin, usually accompanied by intense itching.
Examples: insect bites, hives

Secondary Lesions (see Figure 30-5)

Atrophy—a semitransparent, paper-like, sometimes wrinkled skin surface; a wasting of the skin.
Examples: aged or sun-damaged skin, striae ("stretch marks")
Crust—blood, pus, or serum that has dried on the surface of the skin after injury.
Examples: scab (after abrasion injury), eczema
Erosion—a wearing away of the superficial epidermis by friction or pressure.
Examples: scratches, ruptured vesicles
Fissure—a deep furrow or slit extending into the dermis.
Examples: athlete's foot lesions, cracks at the sides of the mouth with dehydration
Keloid—excess scar tissue; hyperplastic scar tissue with irregular bands of collagen, usually formed after trauma, surgery, burn or severe skin disease.
Examples: enlarged scars from ear piercing
Lichenification—leathery hardening and thickening of the skin, caused by scratching or rubbing.
Examples: chronic dermatitis
Scale—a small thin plate of epidermis that is shed from skin tissue.
Examples: dandruff, eczema, dry skin
Scar—fibrous tissue that replaces normal tissue after injury.
Examples: healed surgical wound, healed acne
Ulcer—superficial loss of tissue, usually with inflammation, on the surface of the skin or mucous membrane.
Examples: decubitus ulcers (pressure sores), chancres

BOX 30-2	COMMON SKIN LESIONS (continued)

Vascular Lesions (see Figure 30-6)

Ecchymosis—purplish patch caused by extravasation (leaking) of blood into the skin; like petechiae but >3 mm diameter.

Hematoma—localized mass of extravasated blood that is confined within an organ or tissue.

Petechiae—tiny hemorrhagic spots, from pinpoint to pinhead size.

Port-wine stain—a large, congenital vascular nevus with a purplish color; usually found on the head and neck.

Purpura—condition characterized by hemorrhaging into the skin.

Spider angioma—dilated arteriole in the skin with radiating capillary branches that look like the legs of a spider.

Capillary hemangioma or strawberry mark—an overgrowth of capillary blood vessels that resembles a strawberry in size, shape, and color; usually disappears in early childhood.

Venous star—a small varicose vein that occurs secondary to prolonged venous pressure.

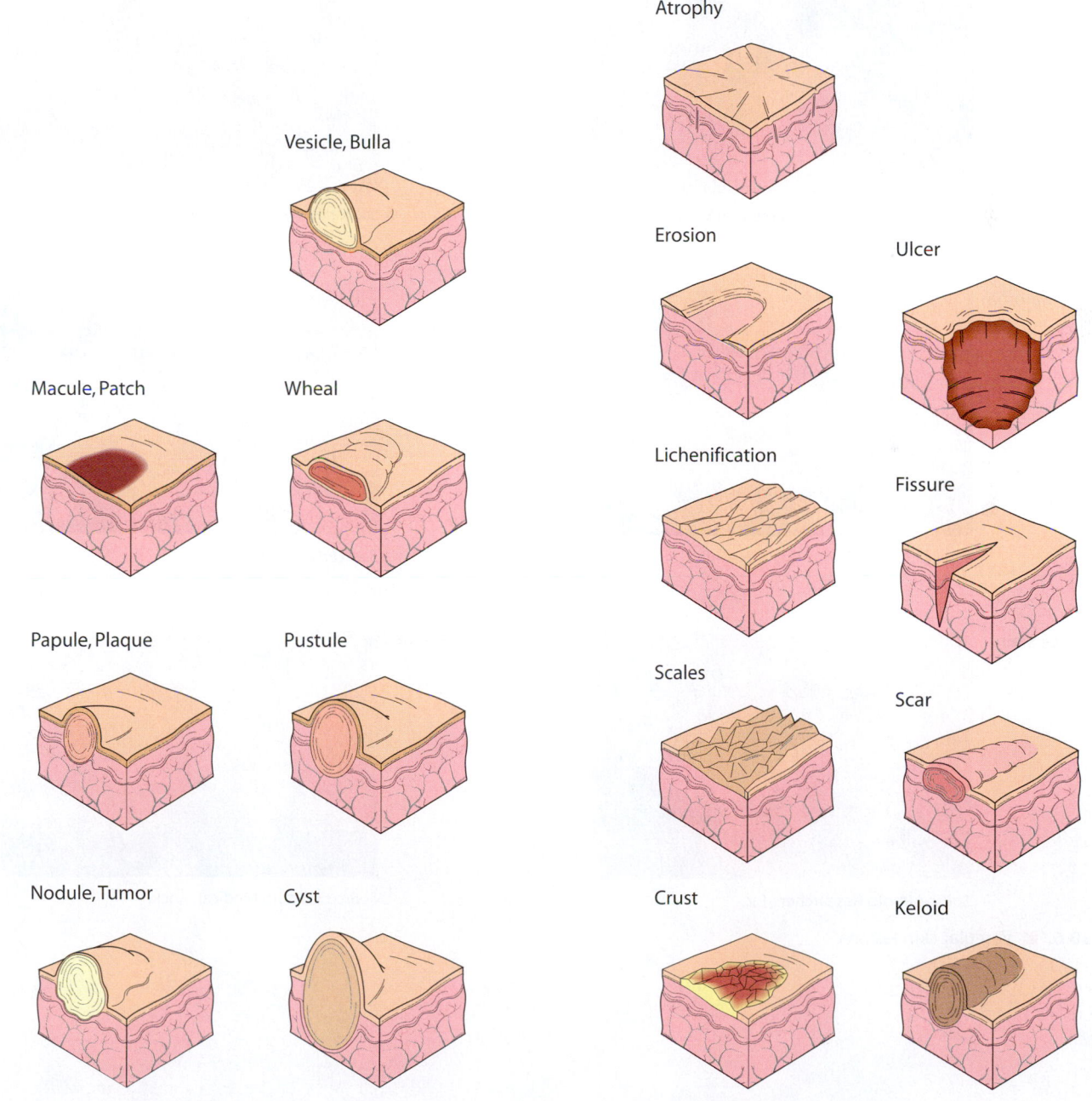

Figure 30-4. ■ Primary skin lesions.

Figure 30-5. ■ Secondary skin lesions.

Purpura

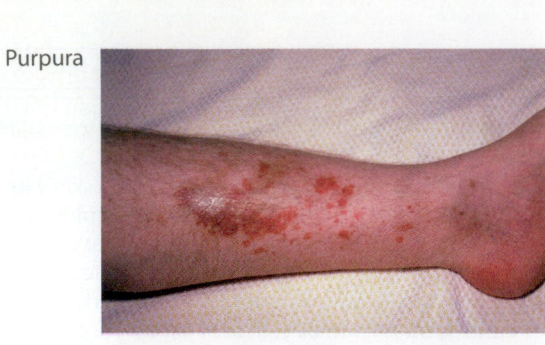

Source: Medical-On-Line Ltd.

Strawberry Mark

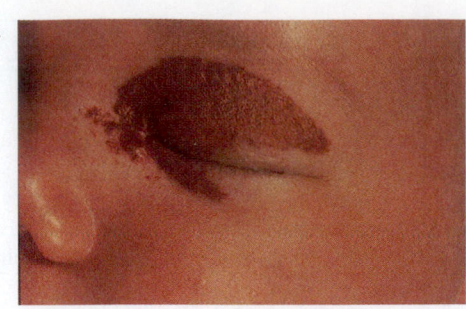

Source: NMSB/Custom Medical Stock Photo.

Ecchymosis

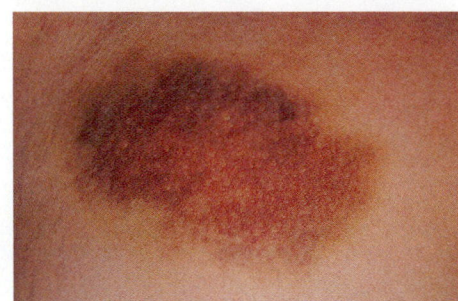

Source: DeGrazia/Custom Medical Stock Photo.

Spider Angioma

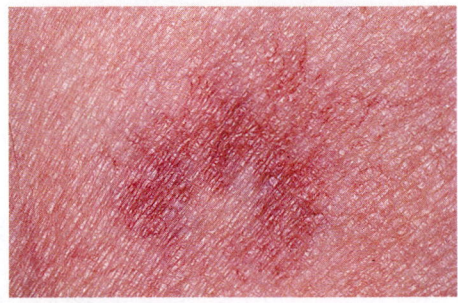

Source: Photo Researchers, Inc.

Hematoma

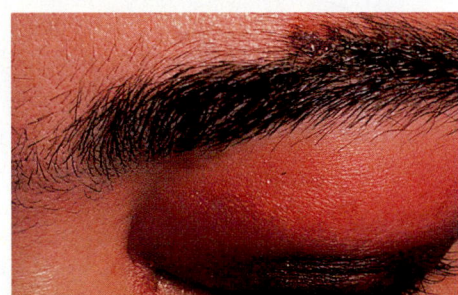

Source: Science Photo/Custom Medical Stock.

Venous Star

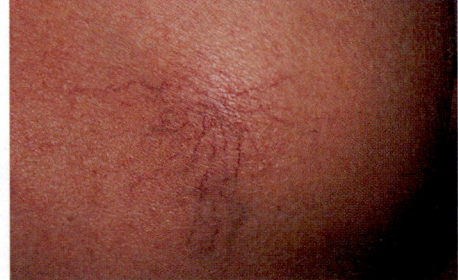

Source: Medichrome.

Port-Wine Stain

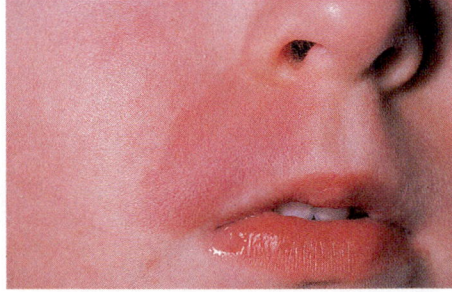

Source: Photo Researchers, Inc.

Petechiae

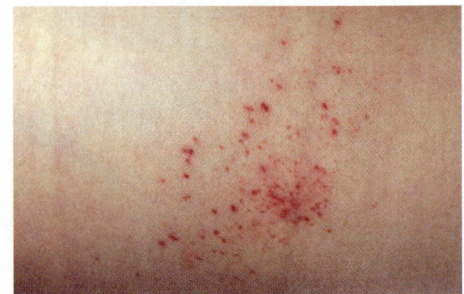

Source: Custom Medical Stock.

Figure 30-6. ■ Vascular skin lesions.

DIAGNOSING LESIONS

Much of the diagnosis of skin disorders is done by inspection and study of symptoms. If laboratory tests are ordered, they usually are limited to a complete blood count to indicate the presence of bacterial infection. Cultures may be done of certain skin conditions having pus or exudates.

PRESSURE ULCERS

Pressure ulcers are also called *decubitus ulcers, pressure sores,* or *bedsores.* They are lesions caused by unrelieved pressure that results in damage to underlying tissue. Pressure ulcers occur in all settings: acute care, long-term care, and home care. They are generally preventable, and prevention is a key nursing responsibility. The main discussion of pressure ulcers appears in Chapter 24 ⬤. Box 30-3 ■ provides suggestions for preventing skin breakdown.

Bacterial Infections

Many bacterial, viral, and fungal skin infections are very contagious. It is extremely important to prevent spread from client to client or client to staff when an individual with a skin infection is hospitalized. See Box 30-4 ■ for information on contact isolation.

BOX 30-3   PREVENTION OF SKIN BREAKDOWN

Education. Frequent, repeat educational efforts for staff, client, and family are needed. *The client and the medical staff must be made to realize that pressure ulcers can be prevented. However, no device or treatment measure, regardless of its cost or design, will effectively substitute for conscientious skin care.*

Identification of the high-risk client. People with impaired mobility, especially in combination with decreased sensation or alteration in the level of mental awareness, are obvious candidates for skin breakdown if they are neglected. These people must be identified at the time of admission in order to institute preventive measures.

Recognition of impending skin breakdown. All personnel must know how to recognize early skin changes that indicate impending breakdown of the skin. The earliest clinical evidence of damage, inflammation of the skin that blanches on application of digital pressure, is usually a completely reversible process. The appropriate response to this condition is immediate, complete elimination of pressure to the involved area.

Specific preventive measures for elimination or reduction of pressure. Pressure in excess of capillary pressure is the chief cause of pressure ulcers. So, primary preventive efforts are directed toward reducing or eliminating pressure over susceptible areas. Intermittent relief of pressure must be provided for all clients. Position changes must be made around the clock, but not less frequently than every 2 hours. Complete relief of pressure for each resting surface must be provided at regular intervals.

BOX 30-4   CONTACT ISOLATION

Personal Protective Equipment

- Use personal protective equipment (PPE).
  - Don gloves when entering the room or cubicle. Always wear gloves when touching the client's intact skin or surfaces *and* articles close to the client (e.g., medical equipment, bed rails).
  - Don a gown when entering the room or cubicle. Remove the gown and observe hand hygiene before leaving the client-care environment.
  - After gown removal, ensure that clothing and skin do not contact potentially contaminated surfaces.

Environment

- Use a single client room if available.
- If a single client room is impossible:
  - Avoid placing client with other clients who are immunocompromised, have open wounds, or have anticipated prolonged lengths of stay.
  - Ensure that clients are more than 3 feet apart from each other. Draw the privacy curtain between beds to minimize opportunities for direct contact.
  - Change protective attire and perform hand hygiene between contact with clients in the same room, regardless of whether one or both are on Contact Precautions.
- Prioritize rooms of clients on Contact Precautions for frequent cleaning and disinfection (e.g., at least daily) with a focus on

frequently touched surfaces (e.g., bed rails, overbed table, bedside commode, lavatory surfaces in bathrooms, doorknobs) and equipment in the immediate vicinity of the client.
- Discontinue Contact Precautions after signs and symptoms of the infection have been resolved.

Transport

- Limit transport and movement outside the room to medically necessary purposes.
- When transport is necessary, ensure that infected or colonized areas of the body are contained and covered.
- Remove and dispose of contaminated PPE and perform hand hygiene prior to transporting clients on Contact Precautions.
- Don clean PPE to handle the client at the transport destination.

Client-Care Equipment

- Handle client-care equipment according to Standard Precautions.
- Use disposable equipment (e.g., blood pressure cuffs) or dedicated equipment for the infected client. If common use of equipment for multiple clients is unavoidable, clean and disinfect such equipment before use on another client.

Source: U.S. Department of Health and Human Services CDC – Contact Precautions. [2007] *Guideline for Isolation Precautions: Preventing Transmission of Infectious Agents in Healthcare Settings 2007.* Atlanta, GA: Author.

IMPETIGO

Impetigo is a superficial infection of the skin and is caused by streptococci or staphylococci. It is highly contagious. While typically transferred between children, it can also affect adults. The lesions are most frequently found on the face, hands, neck, and extremities.

Manifestations

It begins with a small red macule that develops into a thin-walled vesicle (see Figure 30-4). The vesicle ruptures and the lesion is covered with a loosely adherent honey-yellow crust. The crust is removed easily but another crust quickly forms.

Treatment

Treatment of impetigo includes washing with a mild soap to remove the crusts, then applying a topical antibiotic medication such as neomycin or bacitracin. Remind family members to avoid touching the lesion directly to decrease the spread of infection. Oral antibiotics may also be used in more difficult cases.

FURUNCLES/CARBUNCLES

A **furuncle** (commonly known as a boil) is an acute inflammation caused by *Staphylococcus*. It starts deep in one or more hair follicles and spreads into the surrounding dermis. It begins as a *papule* (painful pimple). The area then enlarges and comes to a yellow point. A **carbuncle** is an extension of a furuncle. The infection is present in several follicles and an abscess develops in the dermis and subcutaneous tissue.

Manifestations

The client complains of a high fever and localized pain. The infection can occur anywhere on the body, but common sites are the axilla, the back of the neck, and buttocks.

Treatment

Treatment includes cleansing the area with an antibacterial soap and applying warm moist compresses. It is important to remind the client to avoid squeezing the boil. The physician will incise the boil to release the contents and dress the wound to absorb the drainage. Antibiotics are ordered to treat the infection. Special precautions are taken for boils found on the face. The infection from facial boils can spread to the cranial sinuses and cause **pyemia** (pus in the blood). If boils are in the anal or perineal area, bed rest is recommended. Clients should be instructed to keep the skin clean, maintain a healthy diet, and take antibiotics for the prescribed length of time.

CELLULITIS

Cellulitis (Figure 30-7 ■) is an infection of the dermis and epidermis. The causative organism produces a substance

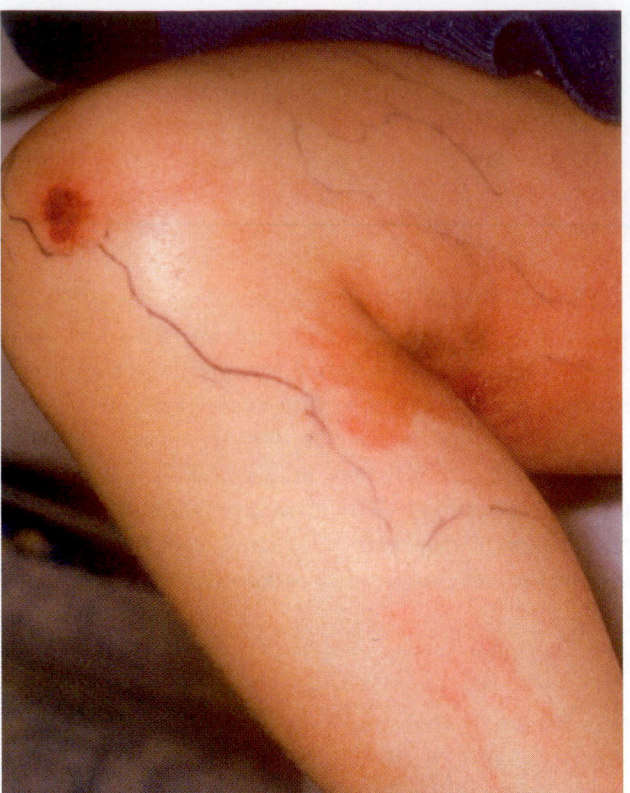

Figure 30-7. ■ The area with cellulitis is inflamed and painful. (*Source:* Medical-On-Line Ltd.)

called *hyaluronidase*. Hyaluronidase breaks down the barriers that normally keep infections localized. It causes an area of redness with edema that is often tender. Red streaking from the area of a localized infection may be seen. Without treatment, the area of affected tissue will spread and may lead to sepsis. Cellulitis is treated with antibiotics.

NURSING CONSIDERATIONS FOR BACTERIAL INFECTIONS

When caring for clients with skin infections, focus your care on preventing spread of the infection. When clients are contagious, such as those with impetigo, instruct them to avoid touching the lesions or allowing others to touch them, because the infection is spread by contact. Urge clients with boils (furuncles and carbuncles) to refrain from expressing pus or treating it with home remedies. Instead, encourage them to see a physician for incision and drainage of the area. Reinforce the need to comply with ordered oral antibiotics. When a client has cellulitis, monitor the condition closely to detect any spread of the reddened, edematous area, which indicates spreading of the infection beneath the skin. Notify the healthcare provider of any spread to prevent the possibility of sepsis from the cellulitis.

Viral Infections

HERPES SIMPLEX

Herpes simplex is a viral infection caused by herpes simplex virus type I (HSV-I) and type II (HSV-II). Type I is usually found above the waist. (Type II, usually found below the waist, is commonly called genital herpes and is discussed in Chapter 41 ⚭.) This chapter discusses type I, also known as a *fever blister, cold sore,* or *canker sore.* The herpes virus usually remains latent, perhaps since childhood. It can be activated by fever, emotional upsets, menses, cold, or sun. The virus is believed to be more contagious when blisters are present but can be transmitted without open lesions.

Manifestations

The appearance of the lesion may be preceded by a tingling sensation (**prodrome**—a warning sign). A single vesicle or cluster of vesicles appears on reddened inflamed skin. Pain and burning usually accompany the blister. Type I herpes simplex lesions are usually found near the mouth (Figure 30-8 ■) but can be inside the buccal cavity. Oral lesion occurrences can range from monthly to one or twice a year.

Treatment

Normally, blisters will subside without treatment in 2 to 10 days. Herpes simplex is usually treated with the antiviral medication acyclovir (Zovirax), valacyclovir (Valtrex), or famciclovir (Famvir). Therapy should be initiated as early as possible. Though the medication does not cure herpes or prevent recurrences, it does make outbreaks shorter, decreases viral shedding, and is less painful. Analgesics may be prescribed to help manage pain.

Complications

The herpes virus can infect the eye and lead to herpes keratitis resulting in severe eye pain. Other symptoms may include the feeling that something is in the eye, photosensitivity, and discharge. Treatment is aimed at prevention and avoidance of corneal scarring.

HERPES ZOSTER

Herpes zoster, also known as *shingles*, is caused by the varicella zoster virus, which is very similar to the chickenpox virus. After a person has varicella (chickenpox), the virus remains dormant in the nerve endings. When the virus becomes reactivated it travels through the nerves to the skin (Figure 30-9 ■). Approximately one-fifth of people who have had chickenpox will develop shingles during their life. It is more common in clients over the age of 50, those with weakened immune systems, in stressful situations, or in conjunction with another illness. Studies have shown that healthy children and adults who receive the chickenpox vaccine (Zostavax or VZV) are less likely to experience shingles than those who have experienced natural chickenpox.

Manifestations

Shingles begins with an itching, tingling, burning pain. The visible rash, which may not appear for a few days, is usually found on the trunk of the body. Headache and fever may accompany the vesicle formation. The vesicles are fluid filled and become *purulent* (pus-filled). The pain is felt along the region supplied by the affected nerves (see Figure 36-10 ⚭). The vesicles remain for 7 to 21 days and are typically found on one side of the body. Then the area crusts over and heals. The pain may continue even after the vesicles disappear. If a person has not already had the chickenpox and comes in

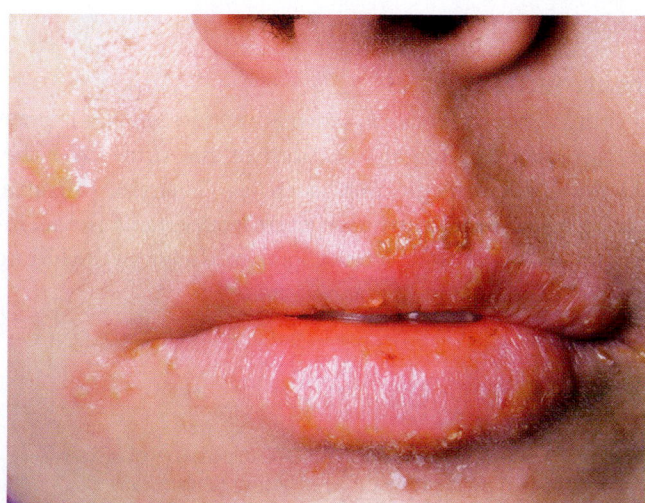

Figure 30-8. ■ Herpes simplex (cold sore). (*Source:* Medical-On-Line Ltd.)

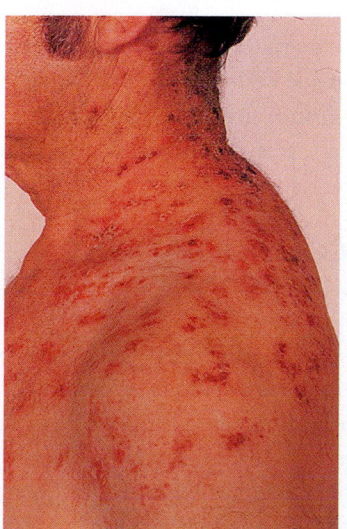

Figure 30-9. ■ Herpes zoster, also known as shingles. (*Source:* Custom Medical Stock, Inc.)

contact with the fluid of the vesicles during the initial 3 days of the infection, the person may develop chickenpox. Ophthalmic herpes zoster can result in corneal damage and blindness; an ophthalmologist may need to be called in as a consultant. The presence of constant pain, even after the blisters have healed, is referred to as **postherpetic neuralgia.**

Treatment

Treatment is usually aimed at relieving symptoms and preventing complications. Medications include analgesics for pain, antihistamines for the itching, and corticosteroids to decrease inflammation. Antiviral medications (acyclovir/Zovirax) inhibit viral shedding and lessen the extent of the lesions. Cool moist compresses help dry the vesicles. Capsaicin ointment can be applied to the lesions to help diminish the pain.

WARTS

Warts (*verrucae*) are caused by the human papillomavirus.

Manifestations

Most commonly they appear as round, raised thickened areas of skin. However, they may also be flat or tapered. Transmission is by skin contact. Common warts are most often seen on the hands or fingers, but they may appear anywhere on the skin or mucous membranes. *Plantar warts* are warts on the contact areas of the soles of the feet. Because of their location, they grow in, not out, and can become very painful. Nongenital warts are benign. *Condyloma acuminata* (genital warts) are transmitted through sexual contact and may be precancerous. They appear as cauliflower-like lesions on the vulva, the glans penis, or around the anus (see Chapter 41 ⬭).

Treatment

Topical treatments may be used to remove warts. Cryotherapy is common for resistant warts. Warts resolve spontaneously when immunity develops (up to 5 years). (*Note:* Genital warts are treated with sexually transmitted infections in Chapter 41 ⬭.)

NURSING CONSIDERATIONS FOR VIRAL INFECTIONS

Clients with viral skin infections need nursing care focused on alleviating pain for shingles and postherpetic neuralgia. Encourage clients to take pain medication as ordered and not to try to go without it when the pain begins. Nerve pain is very intense and clients need emotional support as well as pain medication. Clients with cold sores (herpes virus type I) are treated with similar medications, but the lesion is not as painful as herpes zoster. They should be encouraged to take the medication and keep the lips moisturized to prevent

cracking. Plantar warts can be painful and require surgical removal. Warts on the skin usually are not painful, but they may cause embarrassment to some clients.

Fungal Infections

TINEA

Dermatophytes are tiny organisms of the plant kingdom (fungi). Fungal skin infections that affect the surface of the skin are often referred to as *ringworm* or *tinea*.

Classifications and Manifestations

There are many types of tinea. Some forms are illustrated in Figure 30-10 ■. *Tinea pedis*, known as athlete's foot, is the most common of the fungal infections. The skin between the toes and on the soles of the feet becomes red, itchy, and scaly with painful skin cracks. It is highly contagious and can be spread by walking barefoot on common shower and locker room floors. *Tinea capitis* is a scalp fungus, often called ringworm. It is most common in children ages 3 to 10. It is the most frequent cause of hair loss in children, but the condition is temporary. The hair becomes brittle and breaks off when the fungus invades the scalp. Pustules may form around the edges of the ring of redness. The infection can be spread from kittens and puppies to humans, and from human to human by sharing combs, hairbrushes, or hats. *Tinea corporis* creates large, circumscribed lesions on the skin. *Tinea cruris* is a groin fungus, commonly called jock itch. It causes reddened, itching skin in the groin and can extend to the inner thighs and buttocks. It occurs most often in males and is frequently found in joggers. Perspiration in skin folds sets up an environment favorable to infection. *Tinea unguium* or *onychomycosis* is a nail fungus. This disorder causes thick, yellowed nails and has usually been associated with toenails.

Treatment

Antifungal topical lotions, ointments, powders, and sprays are used to treat fungal infections of the skin. Over-the-counter (OTC) medication such as Tinactin, Micatin, Lotrimin, and Lamisil are used to treat superficial fungal infections. For deeper infections, oral medications including Diflucan, Lamisil, and Sporanox are used.

clinical ALERT

Ask clients about prescription and OTC drugs. Use of antacids with these oral medications may interfere with the medication's absorption. Antifungals may also alter the effectiveness of warfarin.

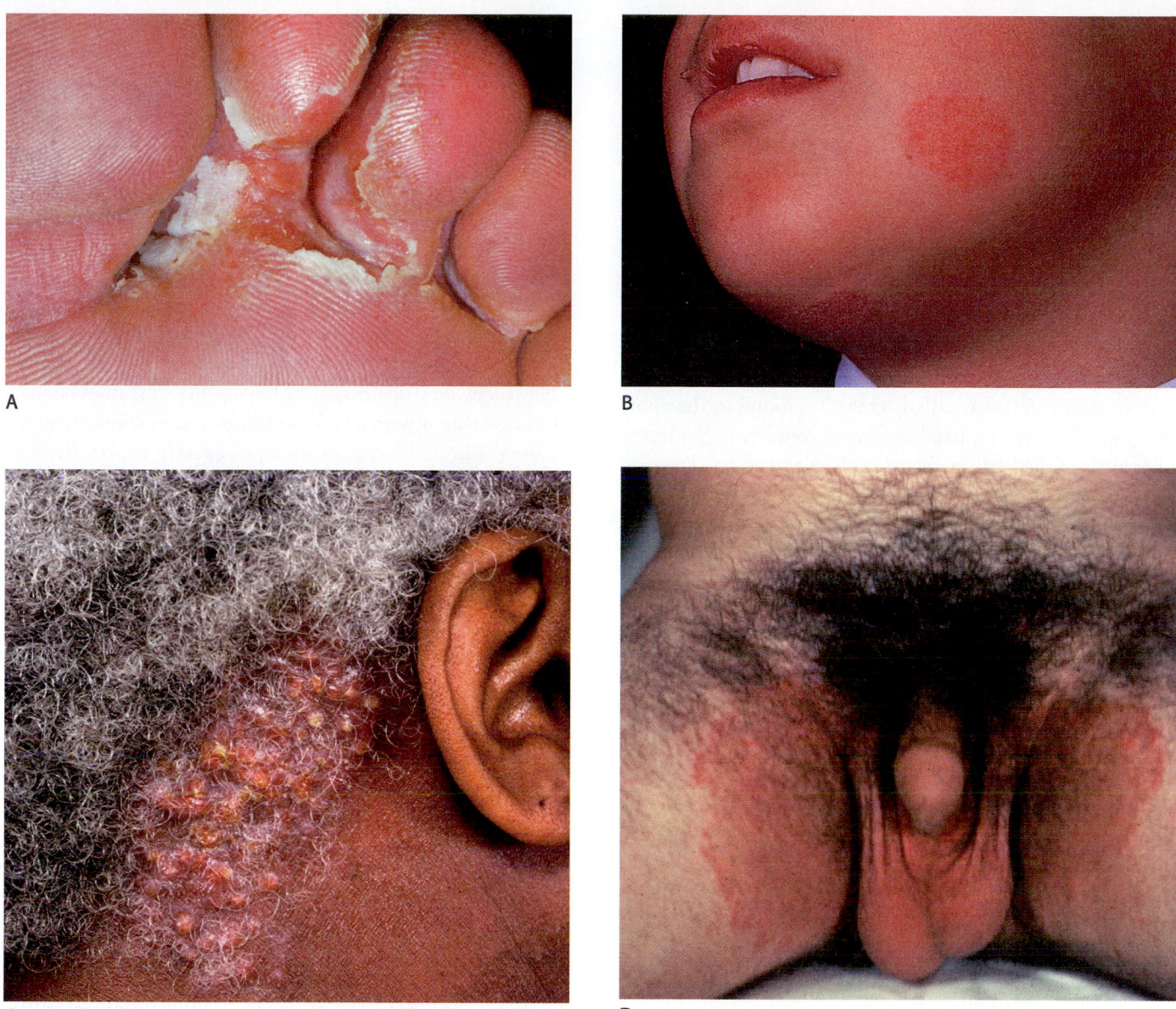

Figure 30-10. ■ **A.** Tinea pedis. **B.** Tinea corporis. **C.** Tinea capitis. **D.** Tinea cruris.   (*Source:* A, C, D: Medical-On-Line Ltd.; B: Custom Medical Stock, Inc.)

Griseofulvin is used when there is an allergy to the other antifungals. It is effective. However, it takes longer to clear the infection. Toenails grow slowly and treatment can take up to a year to be effective.

Nursing Considerations for Fungal Infections

Clients with tinea infections need care focused on preventing spread of the infection from person to person. Tinea corporis (ringworm) can be spread from animals to humans and from humans to humans. Encourage clients to follow instructions for over-the-counter antifungals and to consult their healthcare provider for prescription medications if those are not effective.

Parasitic Infestations

PEDICULOSIS

Pediculosis (lice infestation) is caused by a parasite that lives on the outside of the human host. It feeds on human blood about five times a day. Lice cause intense itching because they inject digestive juices and excrement into the skin.

Classifications and Manifestations

There are three forms of lice: *pediculosis capitis, corporis,* and *pubis. Pediculosis capitis* is the infestation of the scalp. The female tiny grayish brown louse lays nits (silvery oval eggs) close to the scalp. The nits cling to the hair shaft and the eggs hatch in about 10 days. The lice reach maturity in 2 weeks. The parasites are typically found on the back of the head and behind the ears. Their bites cause severe itching. Scratching can lead to infections and pustule formation. Impetigo or furunculosis can occur as a secondary infection. Head lice commonly affect children but can appear in persons of all ages. Children with lice are sent home from school to be treated. Students who have come in contact with those affected should be examined by the school nurse for the presence of lice or nits.

Pediculosis corporis (body lice) live in the seams of underwear and clothing. The bites cause a minute hemorrhagic point on the body. Secondary infections are usually due to scratching. Eczema may develop, causing the skin to become thickened, dry, and scaly.

Pediculosis pubis (also called "crabs") is found in the genital region. It is transmitted by sexual contact. It can infect other areas of the body such as the chest and axilla. The bite has a blue-gray, macular appearance and causes intense itching. The insect's excrement may appear as a reddish dust in the underwear.

Treatment

The treatment for pediculosis capitis is to wash the hair with an OTC shampoo such as Rid. Use as prescribed, then comb with a fine-toothed comb dipped in vinegar. The vinegar dissolves the substance that secures the nit to the hair shaft. Some of the nits may have to be picked off the hair shaft (hence the term *nitpicking*). It is important to remove the nits before they hatch. For pediculosis corporis and pubis, the treatment is to use Kwell (a pediculicide) lotion or cream after showering. The client should be instructed to shower, and to wash clothing and all bedding. Reinfestation will occur if the same clothing is used without proper washing.

Sexual partners of the client with pubic lice must be examined as well. Other medications used to treat all forms of pediculosis include antipruritics to alleviate itching, steroids to decrease inflammation, and possibly systemic antibiotics to fight infection.

SCABIES

The *Sarcoptes scabiei (scabies)* infestation is also referred to as *itch mite*. The mites are transferred by sexual or person-to-person contact. The adult female burrows into the skin to lay her eggs daily for 2 months. This leaves a dark line in the skin. The larva hatch in 6 days and then migrate to the skin surface. They reach maturity in 2 to 3 weeks. Symptoms appear in 4 weeks from contact. The itching occurs from the excrement left in the burrow. The itching and scratching intensify at night.

clinical ALERT

In recent years, the incidence of scabies has increased in skilled nursing facilities and convalescent homes.

Mites infect the fingers, forearms, axilla, waistline umbilical area, lower back, nipple area, and genitals. The client should shower, dry thoroughly, and apply Kwell lotion or cream. The cream is left on the skin for 8 to 12 hours. Then the client showers again. Bedding and clothing must be laundered. Itching may continue for several days following treatment. Close contacts must also be examined.

NURSING CONSIDERATIONS FOR PARASITIC INFESTATIONS

When you care for clients with parasitic skin infections, the focus of your care should be on killing the parasite and alleviating itching. It is also important to realize that many clients may be embarrassed by having lice or scabies because they associate it with a lack of cleanliness. Encourage clients to use medicated lotion or shampoo exactly as prescribed to eliminate the parasite. It is also very important for clients to comply with additional measures such as laundering bedding and clothing to prevent reinfestation. Be very sensitive to possible embarrassment in this situation. Be factual and nonjudgmental when giving instructions to clients.

Chronic Skin Conditions

ACNE

Acne is a disorder of the sebaceous glands. Sebum production responds to direct hormonal stimulation by androgens (testicular, adrenal, and ovarian). Therefore, acne typically appears in adolescents and young adults. Most acne lesions are *comedones* (pimples, whiteheads, and blackheads) that block the oil gland, leading to pimples or whiteheads. Inflammatory lesions also include pustules and cysts (see Figure 62-9). *Acne vulgaris* is common among teenagers and young adults. *Acne rosacea* (chronic facial acne) occurs more often in middle and older adults. Treatment is often by self-care with OTC preparations. Tetracycline is prescribed in severe and resistant cases. Isotretinoin (Accutane) is prescribed to treat cystic acne. See the discussion of this disorder in Chapter 62 .

clinical ALERT

Clients taking Accutane should not become pregnant because it can cause defects in the fetus. Birth control should be used 1 month before starting therapy, during therapy, and for 1 month after therapy is completed.

PSORIASIS

Psoriasis (Figure 30-11 ■) is chronic genetic inflammatory, noninfectious, noncontagious dermatosis. Researchers today conclude that psoriasis is an immune-mediated disease. Of the more than 4.5 million adults affected with psoriasis

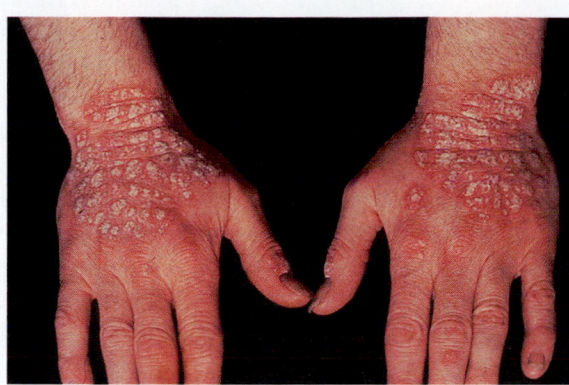

Figure 30-11. ■ Psoriasis often appears in matching patches on opposite sides of the body. (*Source:* NMSB/Custom Medical Stock Photo.)

in the United States, 10 to 30 percent also develop psoriatic arthritis (National Psoriasis Foundation, 2003). The pathology that occurs is called *epidermal proliferation*. This means that epidermal cells turn over at six to nine times the normal rate. It is believed that a signal sent out by the immune system speeds up the cell growth cycle. In normal skin the cells grow and move to the surface at a steady rate occurring once a month. In psoriasis this cycle is speeded up to 3 to 4 days.

Manifestations

Psoriasis lesions have bilateral symmetry. They appear as circular patches of varying size. The epidermis layer thickens and is raised with heaped up cells and inflammation. The blood vessels dilate and increase the nourishment to the cells. The dead surface cells are dry, silvery scales. When the scales are scraped away there is easy bleeding due to the increase in blood supply. The patches may cause itching and burning. Several factors may work together to cause an outbreak of the lesions (emotional stress, skin injury, infection, reaction to medication). Psoriasis commonly affects the scalp, elbows, knees, and lower back. Nail involvement is associated with psoriatic arthritis.

Diagnosis and Treatment

Psoriasis is diagnosed by clinical and physical manifestations. Diagnostic testing may be performed to determine secondary infections or other disease processes. There is no known cure, but research is learning more about the immune system and the cause of psoriasis. Treatment is varied, time-consuming, at times messy, and expensive for the client. The objective of care is to control the rapid growth of cells.

Some medications and treatments prescribed to treat psoriasis include steroids, anthralin, tazarotene, and phototherapy. Steroids are given either orally or topically to decrease inflammation and slow skin cell growth. Anthralin is

applied in cream or solution form. It decreases inflammation slowly and has longer lasting effects than steroids. Tazarotene (Tazorac) is a retinoid and vitamin derivative, prescribed as a gel or cream. It suppresses inflammation and blocks proliferation of the epidermis. Phototherapy may be prescribed to expose the skin to ultraviolet light to clear the lesions and maintain the skin.

ECZEMA (ATOPIC DERMATITIS)

Eczema is a skin disorder that has been linked to allergies and heredity. It is often seen in infants with food allergies.

Manifestations

Eczema causes patchy lesions on the skin. They contain papules and vesicles that rupture, leaving a yellow, crusty exudate. The areas of eczema are reddened and dry, with tiny cracks that cause further dryness as moisture leaves the skin. The lesions often itch and may be sensitive to touch.

Treatment

Treatment is aimed at removing the allergen if it can be identified and keeping the area moisturized with ointments or petroleum jelly. Steroid ointments are prescribed to relieve the itching and decrease inflammation. Infection is always a concern because of the breaks in skin integrity.

NURSING CONSIDERATIONS FOR CHRONIC SKIN CONDITIONS

One of the most important aspects of nursing care for clients with chronic skin conditions is to provide positive support for clients who are self-conscious or embarrassed by their condition. Acne may be devastating to a teen who is already struggling with self-esteem issues. Avoid blaming the client for causing the condition by diet or lack of good skin hygiene. Instead, be supportive and encouraging as the teen complies with OTC treatment regimens. Be alert to any indications of possible pregnancy when a client is taking Accutane. Psoriasis and eczema can be very noticeable to others, causing self-consciousness in clients with these disorders. Encourage compliance with treatment regimens and evaluate the effectiveness of treatments often.

NURSING CARE

PRIORITIZING NURSING CARE

Skin is the largest organ of the body and thus can provide much information about the client's overall health. The nurse should make frequent and complete observations of all skin surfaces. Blanching of the skin may be the first sign of potential breakdown. Recognition and quick action can prevent further injury. Serious problems such as pulmonary embolism can have skin signs (mediastinal petechiae), which can be a red flag that emergency action needs to be taken. Always make the skin the focus of your observation.

ASSESSING

As part of the client's initial assessment and history, information was gathered about skin diseases, previous bruising, general skin condition, skin lesions, and usual healing of sores. After this, nurses examine the integument as part of routine care. Inspection and palpation of the skin focus on skin color distribution, skin turgor, presence of edema, and characteristics of any lesions. *Note:* In dark-skinned clients, be aware that *erythema* (redness) may appear as a purple-gray cast. Palpate for warmth and signs of edema. Cyanosis (blue tint) assumes a gray tone. Inspect the area around the mouth, lips, earlobes, and cheekbones for color changes.

To determine skin turgor, the nurse lightly pinches the skin and then releases it. The skin should immediately rebound. If the skin *tents* (holds the pinched position), the client may be dehydrated. Edema is measured by a quantifying scale. (See Figure 19-13 ⬤⬤ for edema assessment.) Press your finger over the area of edema. A depression that does not resume its original form is an indication of pitting edema.

When a client has a skin disorder, the LPN/LVN collaborates with the RN to inspect the skin, and identify the general characteristics, the size of the area involved, the color and type of lesion, and to determine whether it is a primary or secondary lesion. Palpate the region (using clean gloves when appropriate) to determine texture and assess for edema, skin turgor, dryness or oiliness, and moistness of the skin. During this inspection, the nurse interviews the client to obtain more information about the outbreak. Document the information in concise medical terminology to assist the physician in treatment. This provides the baseline for changes in the condition.

DIAGNOSING, PLANNING, AND IMPLEMENTING

Nursing diagnoses that are common in clients with dermatologic disorders are:

- *Impaired Skin Integrity*
- *Impaired Tissue Integrity*
- *Acute Pain*
- *Latex Allergy Response*
- *Disturbed Body Image*
- *Risk for Infection*
- *Deficient Knowledge* related to changes in integument

To treat clients with dermatologic disorders, the following nursing interventions are performed:

- Follow agency protocols and the physician orders, if any. Keep the wounds clean and dry. *This ensures quality care and helps prevent infection.*

- Dress the wound as ordered. *Some skin disorders are covered to decrease the risk of infection or irritation. The physician may order a dry sterile dressing to cover lesions.*
- Medicate as ordered. *The physician generally orders medications to relieve itching, pain, and to prevent or treat infection. Analgesics and antihistamines are often prn orders. The nurse needs to determine the need for medication and provide it in a timely manner.*
- Implement comfort measures such as keeping the skin lubricated with lotion or medicated ointments if ordered. Keep the room cool and humidified. *These measures reduce itching.*
- Offer encouragement and allow the client to talk about his or her feelings. *Examine your feelings so that you can promote a sense of security and trust for the client. Skin problems can lead to psychosocial aspects for the client. Some skin conditions can be disfiguring, causing social isolation. Visible skin lesions, whether they are contagious or not, can cause depression, self-consciousness, and rejection. Treatment can last for weeks, months, or a lifetime. The client needs the support of the nursing staff to provide understanding and acceptance.*
- Report any evidence of secondary infection. The nurse should monitor the white blood cell count for elevation and check vital signs for changes. *Changes might indicate infection.*
- Provide educational resources for the client. *Support groups and foundations exist to assist people with chronic skin disorders such as psoriasis. Proper teaching about skin infections and infestations can help prevent recurrences.*
- Document care and the healing process. When noting information on the client's chart, be sure to include the location, size, color, and exudates of the lesions. *When lesions decrease in size and number, the effectiveness of the treatment can be validated. If lesions do not respond to treatment, documentation helps the physician.*

EVALUATING

The client will be able to verbalize diminished pain and increased comfort. The lesions will be controlled. The client is able to demonstrate self-care treatments. The client and family demonstrate effective appropriate coping mechanisms. The client has an understanding of the disease process. Documentation of the healing process; location, size, and depth of wound; color; exudates; and surrounding skin will provide a clear picture of the current condition of the wound.

Continuity of Care

Clients and their support people often need teaching in order to carry out measures to prevent further skin damage. The following information should be provided:

- A review of skin hygiene procedures
- A demonstration of dressing changes and medication application

- A list of the signs and symptoms of secondary infection that would require the client to notify the physician
- Timing for follow-up care and appointments
- A discussion of disease pathology
- A discussion of medication compliance measures and side effects

NURSING PROCESS CARE PLAN
Client with Herpes Zoster

William Barnard is a 78-year-old male client who has been transferred from assisted living to the skilled nursing unit at the Oakgrove Retirement Community. He was diagnosed with herpes zoster (shingles). He recently was involved in a traffic accident, which resulted in his son taking his car from the facility. The whole episode was quite stressful for Mr. Barnard. He also has a history of a weak immune system.

Assessment
Client complains of skin pain, sensitivity, and slight itching. There is a defused red rash with fluid-filled blisters on the left scapula of the back. There is one lesion under the left eye. Client has fever 101.4 F since this morning, complains of headache and upset stomach. The client states "I just feel sick." He has a history of progressive macular degeneration and hearing loss.

Nursing Diagnosis
The following important nursing diagnoses (among others) are established for this client:

- *Impaired Skin Integrity*
- *Acute Pain*
- *Decisional Conflict* related to loss of independence

Expected Outcomes
The expected outcomes for this client will include, but are not limited to, the following:

- Maintains skin integrity.
- Reports pain controlled consistently between 1 and 5 level on a scale of 0 to 10.
- Expresses understanding of son's concerns about driving.

Planning and Implementation
- Administer medication topically and oral antiviral drug as ordered.
- Apply cool moist compress to lesions prn.
- Apply capsaicin ointment for pain reduction.
- Encourage communication between client and son.
- Encourage client to find ways to maintain independence without having to drive.

Evaluation
Temperature 99.8 F at 12 noon and 4 pm; pain scale between 1 and 4 throughout the day. Son visited, client continues to be very angry that his car was taken away. States, "My vision isn't that bad. The sun was just in my eyes when I had the accident." Refuses to go on bus outing with other residents.

Critical Thinking in the Nursing Process

1. Why is it important for staff members who have not had chickenpox to avoid contact with the herpes lesions during the initial 3 days of the infection?
2. Identify some contributing factors that may have precipitated Mr. Barnard's herpes zoster outbreak.
3. Mr. Barnard's son asks you when the pain will go away. What is your best response?

Note: Discussion of Critical Thinking questions appears on the MyNursingKit Website.

Burns

Burns can destroy the epidermis, dermis, subcutaneous tissue, and bone. The degree of the burn (first through third) is determined by the depth of tissue destruction. Nursing care of clients with burns is a very specialized process because of the many complications that can occur. For discussion of burns, see Chapter 47 ∞.

Skin Cancer

Skin cancer is the most common and most preventable type of cancer. The three most common types are basal cell, squamous cell, and malignant melanoma, each named for the type of cell from which they arise (Figure 30-12A–C ■). *Mycosis fungoides* is another type of cancer affecting the skin. It is most often an **opportunistic** condition, meaning that it affects those with impaired immune function.

A major risk factor for the development of skin cancer and precancerous conditions is prolonged sun exposure, especially during childhood. Precancerous lesions of the skin are called *actinic keratosis* (see Figure 30-12D). A change in a mole or other skin lesion indicates increased risk of skin cancer. Exposure to ultraviolet light in tanning booths, certain chemicals containing hydrocarbons, and radiation are all factors that increase the incidence of skin cancer. When skin has been burned or traumatized, the risk of skin cancer in the area increases.

BASAL CELL CARCINOMA
Basal cell cancer (see Figure 30-12A) arises from the basal cells in the epidermis and is the most frequently seen skin cancer. The affected area appears as a pearly papule with a waxy border. It may develop a central crater. It is slow growing. Although it does not often spread, it can lead to tissue destruction. Basal cell cancer is easily detected. It most often appears

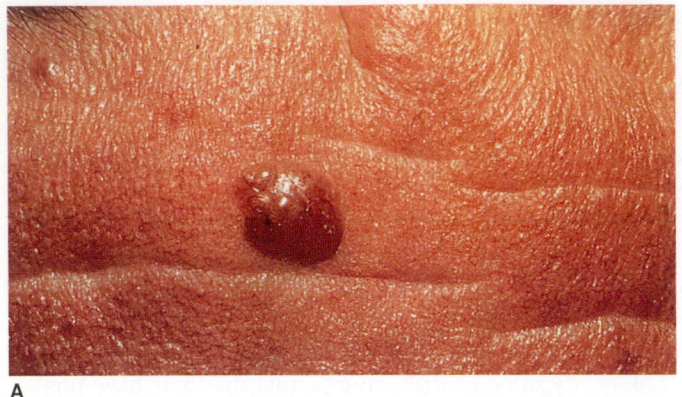

A

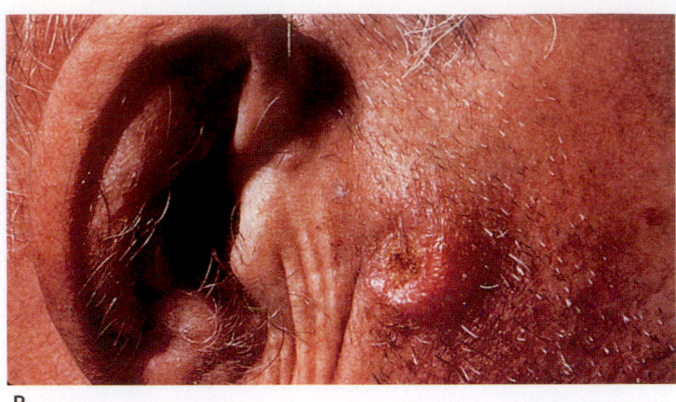

B

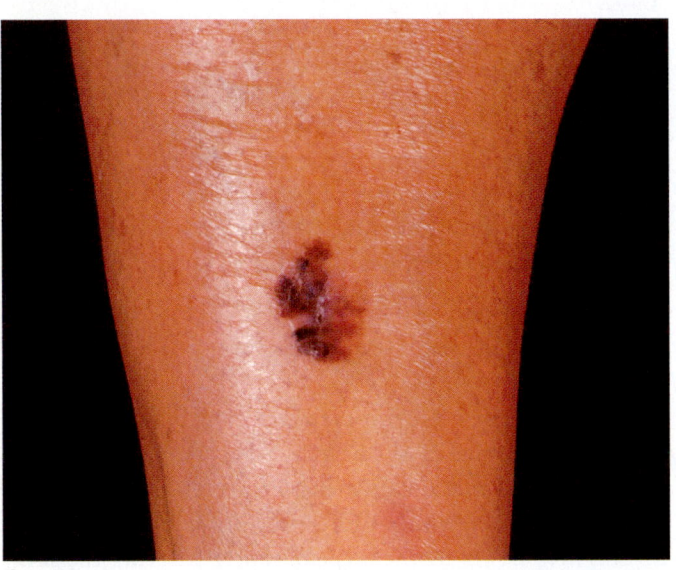

C

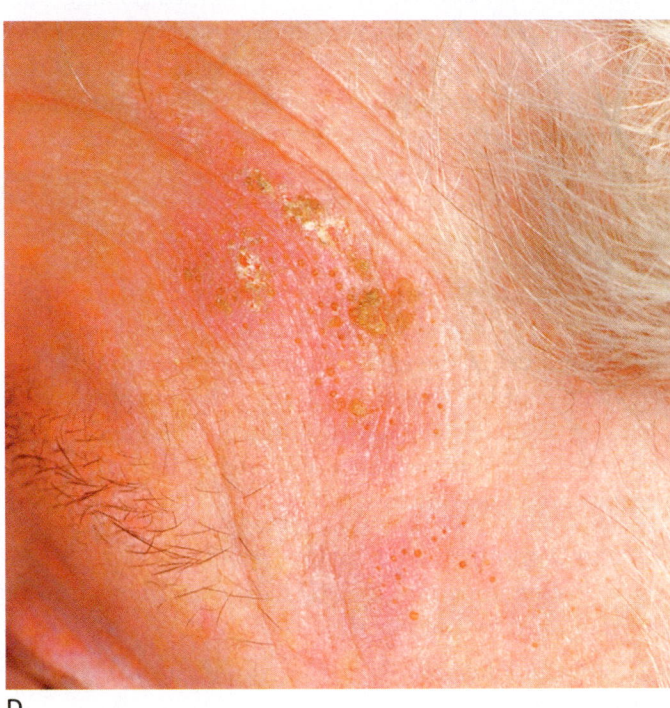

D

Figure 30-12. ■ **A.** Basal cell cancer. **B.** Squamous cell cancer. **C.** Malignant melanoma. **D.** Actinic keratosis. (*Source*: A, B: American Academy of Dermatology. Reprinted with permission. All rights reserved; C. Caliendo/Custom Medical Stock Photo; D. Medical-On-Line Ltd.)

on the face and upper trunk in areas frequently exposed to the sun. The treatment for this type of skin cancer is generally surgical removal of the lesion. It tends to recur. This type of cancer has recurred in 40% to 50% of the people affected.

SQUAMOUS CELL CARCINOMA

This type of skin cancer arises from the squamous cells in the epidermis. It appears as a firm nodule with a crust or central ulceration. The margins are hard. It may bleed and become painful as it grows. Squamous cell cancer (see Figure 30-12B) can spread quickly through the lymph system. Larger lesions spread most quickly. If this type of cancer is not treated, it can lead to death. It may be found on skin that has been burned or traumatized or on skin with chronic inflammation. The usual treatment for squamous

cell carcinoma is surgical or chemosurgical removal of the lesion.

MALIGNANT MELANOMA

Malignant melanoma (see Figure 30-12C) arises from the melanocytes in the dermis and epidermis. It is the most serious of all skin cancers. If the lesion is in the epidermis only, it is more easily removed. If it is also in the dermis, it easily spreads through the blood and lymph vessels to the body. The lesion may be at the site of an existing mole or in an area previously unaffected. The lesion may develop a raised appearance with smaller lesions (satellites) around the edges. The incidence of malignant melanoma is increasing. Peak incidence occurs between the ages of 21 and 45. This type of cancer can spread to all organs of the body through the blood and lymph.

The treatment for malignant melanoma is a wide surgical excision of the lesion and surrounding tissues. It may require skin grafts to close. Chemotherapy may also be used, especially to treat metastasis to other organs. Radiation therapy may be used to treat sites where the melanoma has spread, but is not used to treat the melanoma itself.

MYCOSIS FUNGOIDES

This type of cancer is also called *cutaneous T-cell lymphoma*. In early stages, the lesions look somewhat similar to psoriasis or seborrheic dermatitis. As the illness progresses, severe pruritus occurs. The skin develops ulcers and fissures, which become infected easily. In addition to skin symptoms, this cancer also affects multiple organs in the body. Even if the skin lesions respond to chemotherapy, the disease eventually causes death due to multiple-organ involvement. *Mycosis fungoides* is an opportunistic illness seen in clients with depressed immune systems, such as those with AIDS. It is not curable, but is treated with phototherapy to slow progression. Nursing care of clients with skin cancer focuses on wound care, teaching, and client support. See full discussion of care for clients with cancer in Chapter 45 ⚭.

Plastic and Reconstructive Surgery

Clients with skin disorders may require plastic or reconstructive surgery. Some types of plastic surgery are considered *cosmetic* surgery (desired by the client for alterations in appearance but not medically necessary). Some types of cosmetic surgeries are rhytidoplasty (face lifts), mammoplasty (breast reduction or augmentation), and rhinoplasty (repair of the nose). Many cosmetic surgeries are performed on an outpatient basis with the client going home to recover.

Plastic and reconstructive surgery is a combination of art and medicine to produce a natural appearance. Realistic expectations of the outcome should be discussed prior to the surgery. This type of surgery is done to repair cleft palates; trauma from burns, automobile accidents, and diseases; or after radical mastectomy.

Rhytidoplasty is cosmetic surgery done to tighten the normal crease lines in the face. The incisions are hidden in the hairline. Postoperatively, the face is quite edematous and the eyes are ecchymotic. The swelling diminishes and the appearance improves within 2 weeks.

Rhinoplasty may be performed for cosmetic reasons or to repair the nose allowing for better breathing. It helps improve the sense of smell and taste, as well as increase self-esteem.

Mammoplasty is defined as a change in the size and shape of the breast. A reduction mammoplasty may be performed when the breasts are so large that the client complains of poor posture, backache, pain due to the bra strap digging into the shoulder, and respiratory difficulties. A breast augmentation is done to increase the size of the breast. A saline-filled implant is placed between the chest wall and the breast to increase size without altering the normal breast function.

Dermabrasion is used to treat acne scars and gives a smooth appearance to the face. A recent advancement in acne treatment is called photodynamic therapy. This treatment starts with *microdermabrasion (scouring of the skin surface)*. Then a medication (aminolevulinic acid) is applied topically. This treatment is combined with laser or light therapy to enhance appearance.

SKIN GRAFTS

Skin grafts are used to close large open areas due to a severe burn, trauma to the body, or a wound that does not heal properly. Skin grafts are needed when the stratum germinativum has been destroyed and cannot grow new skin. For a graft to grow in the new location, it must have sufficient blood supply and be infection free. Excess fluid under the graft can separate the graft from the intended site. Skin grafts and burns are discussed in Chapter 47 ⚭.

LIPOSUCTION

Liposuction is a technique used to remove subcutaneous tissue. The purpose is to improve facial and body contours. It is not considered a replacement for dieting. The advantage of liposuction is that a significant amount of fat can be removed through a tiny incision. A firm scar forms between the layers of skin and fat to hold the body's contour. Ridges, dimpling, and irregular wrinkles can develop as the site heals. Postoperative complications include bleeding, serum accumulation in the liposuctioned area, and bruising. Deaths have been reported due to the removal of excessive amounts of fat coupled with extensive blood loss.

Note: The references and resources for all chapters have been compiled at the back of the book.

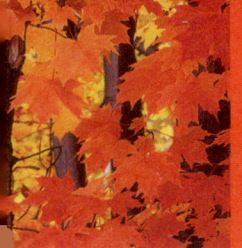

Chapter Review

KEY Points

- Skin integrity is the body's first line of defense.
- Assessment of the skin requires visual inspection, palpation, and the sense of smell. Essential data about skin lesions include appearance, size, drainage, swelling, and pain.
- Nursing care for clients with skin disorders involves attention both to physical and to psychosocial concerns. Disorders of the integument can be socially isolating and affect client self-esteem.

⊗ FOR FURTHER Study

See Figure 19-13 for edema assessment.

Refer to Chapter 24, including procedures, for a complete discussion on wound care and pressure ulcers.

For a full discussion on the nervous system see Chapter 36.

Jaundice is discussed further in Chapter 37.

Genital herpes and genital warts are discussed with sexually transmitted infections in Chapter 41.

Chapter 45 provides an in-depth discussion of caring for clients with cancer.

See Chapter 47 for a full discussion of burns.

Additional information on acne is located in Chapter 62.

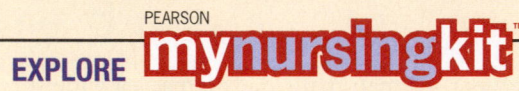

EXPLORE PEARSON **mynursingkit™**

MyNursingKit is your one stop for online chapter review materials and resources. Prepare for success with additional NCLEX®-style practice questions, interactive assignments and activities, web links, animations and videos, and more!

Register your access code from the front of your book at
www.mynursingkit.com

Critical Thinking Care Map

Caring for a Client with Secondary Infection

NCLEX-PN® Focus Area: Physiologic Integrity

Case Study: Mr. Wells is a 65-year-old client being treated for a secondary infection related to herpes zoster. Mr. Wells has a history of an autoimmune disorder and presents in a weakened and emaciated state. He is lethargic and unable to treat the lesions found on his left torso. He is having difficulty maintaining his weight and complains of not being hungry. He is 6 foot 2 inches tall and weighs 120 lb. While observing the lesions you note that there is a cluster of purulent vesicles on his left side that is oozing fluid that is draining down his abdomen. The dressing is odorous and appears to have been in place for several days. Mr. Wells is complaining of a 9 out of 10 on the pain scale. Mr. Wells is bent over on his left side with very little movement in the bed.

Nursing Diagnosis: *Impaired Skin Integrity*

COLLECT DATA

Subjective

_____
_____
_____
_____
_____
_____
_____

Objective

_____
_____
_____
_____
_____
_____
_____

Would you report this? Yes/No

If yes, report to: _____

What would you report? _____

Nursing Care

_____
_____
_____
_____
_____
_____
_____
_____
_____
_____
_____
_____

How would you document this? _____
_____
_____
_____

Compare your answers and documentation to those provided on the MyNursingKit Website.

Data Collected
(use only those that apply)

- Poor mobility
- Height 6' 2"
- Weight 120 lbs
- Client states, "I'm not hungry."
- Weakened
- Pulse is 110
- 9 out of 10 pain level
- Purulent cluster of vesicles
- Temperature 102.6°F
- WBC 12,500
- Eating 25% of diet
- Grimaces with movement

Nursing Interventions
(use only those that apply; list in priority order)

- Monitor urine output.
- Turn client every 2 hours.
- Change dressing every 4 hours.
- Monitor WBC.
- Monitor TSH.
- Refer to dietitian.
- Daily weights.
- Vital signs every 2 hours.

NCLEX-PN® Exam Preparation

1 The nurse is teaching staff members about anatomy and physiology of the skin and explains that what layer of the dermis is responsible for providing the elasticity of the skin?

1. Papillary layer
2. Appendage layer
3. Reticular layer
4. Stratum germinativum

2 The client is found to have a discolored spot that is not raised and less than a centimeter in size. The nurse documents this lesion as a:

1. Papule.
2. Nodule.
3. Macule.
4. Cyst.

3 The primary nursing action when treating a child with an impetigo lesion would be to:

1. Remove crusts and apply neomycin antibiotic ointment.
2. Administer oral analgesics.
3. Apply a dry sterile dressing.
4. Remove the crust and apply an antifungal ointment.

4 When providing education on antiviral medication for the client with herpes simplex, the nurse will emphasize that:

1. Therapy is best initiated early.
2. Analgesics are not necessary.
3. Medication will cure herpes simplex.
4. Viral shedding is increased.

5 A client has herpes zoster on the right side of his face and scalp. Which would concern the nurse most?

1. Complaints of pain on the right side of the scalp
2. Complaints of burning pain on the right side of the face
3. Presence of fluid-filled vesicles on the right side of the face
4. Complaints of pain in the right eye

6 A client is diagnosed with a severe nail fungus and is given a prescription for an oral antifungal medication. When looking over the client's daily meds, which one would cause concern?

1. Oral antidiabetic
2. Antihypertensive
3. Warfarin
4. Estrogen

7 A client is given a prescription for Kwell lotion. The nurse knows the client will need instruction about treating:

1. Lice or scabies.
2. Scabies or herpes zoster.
3. Lice or psoriasis.
4. Scabies or eczema.

8 The nurse knows that a client has the most serious type of skin cancer when the diagnosis is:

1. Basal cell carcinoma.
2. Squamous cell carcinoma.
3. Malignant melanoma.
4. Multiple myeloma.

9 A client with AIDS develops severe itching with skin lesions that ulcerate and become infected. The physician diagnoses *Mycosis fungoides*, which is a(n):

1. Skin cancer similar to basal cell carcinoma.
2. Opportunistic illness, also called T-cell lymphoma.
3. Fungal skin infection that leads to skin cancer.
4. Indication that the AIDS virus is now attacking the skin.

10 The nurse is caring for a postop client who has had a skin graft. Which of the following are possible reasons for a skin graft? (Select all that apply.)

1. A large area of skin was missing due to a burn.
2. A wound would not heal and had to be grafted closed.
3. Trauma to the skin destroyed the stratum germinativum layer.
4. The client had scabies, ringworm, and impetigo.
5. The client had wrinkles, freckles, or any skin discoloration the client wants repaired.

Answers and rationales for Review Questions appear in Appendix I.

Chapter 31

Clients with Musculoskeletal System Disorders

LEARNING Outcomes

After completing this chapter, you will be able to:

1. Discuss the anatomy and physiology of the musculoskeletal system.
2. List diagnostic tests for disorders of the musculoskeletal system.
3. Identify types of skeletal trauma, treatment, potential complications, and nursing care.
4. Define osteoporosis and describe prevention, treatment, and nursing care for a client with osteoporosis.
5. Identify disorders of bone tissue and describe proper nursing care for them.
6. Explain nursing care for a client in a cast or traction.
7. Distinguish among four inflammatory disorders of the musculoskeletal system and nursing care for them.
8. List the common nursing interventions in joint replacement surgery.
9. Describe the care of the client with spinal disorders.
10. Identify the most common joint and muscle disorders and nursing interventions for them.
11. Discuss advantages and disadvantages of heat and cold therapy for clients with musculoskeletal disorders.
12. Describe nursing care for clients with SLE or fibromyalgia.

Clinical Objectives

13. Teach clients ways to prevent or minimize osteoporosis.
14. Demonstrate application of moist and dry heat and cold to injured tissue.
15. Demonstrate nursing interventions for the client with a fracture.
16. Demonstrate necessary actions to deal with common complications of fracture.
17. Plan care for the client in a cast or traction. Include cast care, skin care, client safety, and psychological needs.
18. Develop a plan of care that promotes optimal healing for a client with an amputation.
19. Provide common nursing interventions for the client having joint replacement therapy.
20. Demonstrate common nursing interventions for sprains and strains.

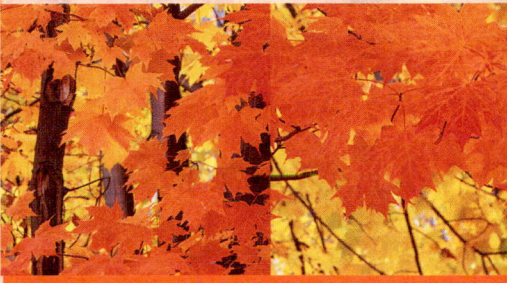

BRIEF Outline

Structure and Function of the Musculoskeletal System
Collaborative Care
Traumatic Bone Disorders
Inflammatory Disorders
Spinal Disorders
Joint and Muscle Disorders
Other Disorders

The musculoskeletal system of the body has three major functions: movement, support, and protection. There are two major parts to the musculoskeletal system: the skeletal muscles, which allow the bones to move, and the bones, which make up the skeleton of the body (Figures 31-1 ■ and 31-2 ■).

Structure and Function of the Musculoskeletal System

MUSCULAR SYSTEM

Movement of material in the body and of the body itself is generally due to the contraction of muscle tissue. There are three types of muscle tissue: skeletal, smooth, and cardiac. Each serves very different purposes.

Skeletal muscle is attached to the bones by tendons. It moves the bones and thus the body. It is sometimes called *voluntary muscle*, because it can be made to contract by conscious thought. At the cellular level, skeletal muscle has large, cylinder-shaped cells with striations (lines) and multiple nuclei.

Smooth (or *visceral*) *muscle* is found in the walls of the digestive organs, tubular structures such as blood vessels, and at the base of each body hair. Because this type of muscle contracts without conscious thought, it is said to be *involuntary*. Some functions include moving food and waste through the digestive tract and regulating blood pressure by contracting and relaxing blood vessels. The cells of smooth muscle are small and tapered, have no striations, and contain a single nucleus for each cell.

Cardiac muscle, as the name implies, forms the walls of the chambers of the heart and is also known as myocardium. It is another type of involuntary muscle.

The muscles of the body are responsible for producing movement. Skeletal movement occurs when muscles that are attached to bones contract. Food moves along when smooth muscle contracts in the digestive tract. Blood moves through the body when the heart muscle contracts. The contraction of skeletal muscle produces heat, helping to keep the body warm.

Skeletal muscles have four basic properties:

1. **Excitability** is the property that allows the muscle to receive a stimulus and act on that stimulus.
2. **Contractibility** is the property that causes the shortening of the muscle in response to a stimulus.
3. **Extensibility** is property that enables the muscle to lengthen or "extend" in response to a stimulus.
4. **Elasticity** is the property that causes the muscle to return to its normal shape and form after contracting or extending. Skeletal muscle must be used to retain its proper abilities. Muscles that are not used will undergo atrophy (a weakening and shortening of the muscle).

SKELETAL SYSTEM

There are 206 bones in the human body. Together, they form the skeletal system. The skeleton has five major functions:

1. Serves as the body's framework.
2. Protects delicate structures such as the brain and spinal cord.
3. Works with muscles as levers to produce movement.
4. Acts as a storehouse for calcium that can be used if calcium levels in the blood drop too low. Calcium is a very important component in muscle contractions and blood clotting.
5. Bones produce the blood cells in the red bone marrow. The cells produced are red blood cells, white blood cells, and platelets.

Bones are classified according to shape (Figure 31-3 ■). Long bones such as the femur are used for weight bearing. Short bones such as the phalanges of the finger are small and do not bear weight. Flat bones are thin and flat and are found in the skull, the ribs, and the sternum. Certain bones are unique in nature and are called irregular bones. One of these bones is the carpal bone in the wrist. The sesamoid bone develops within a tendon. An example of this bone is the patella.

Bone resorption and bone deposit are continually occurring in the body. These functions are regulated jointly by the action of hormones and by stress placed on the bone. If an extremity is not used, the bone will become weak from inactivity. Long bones are composed of an epiphysis at

MyNursingKit | Muscles

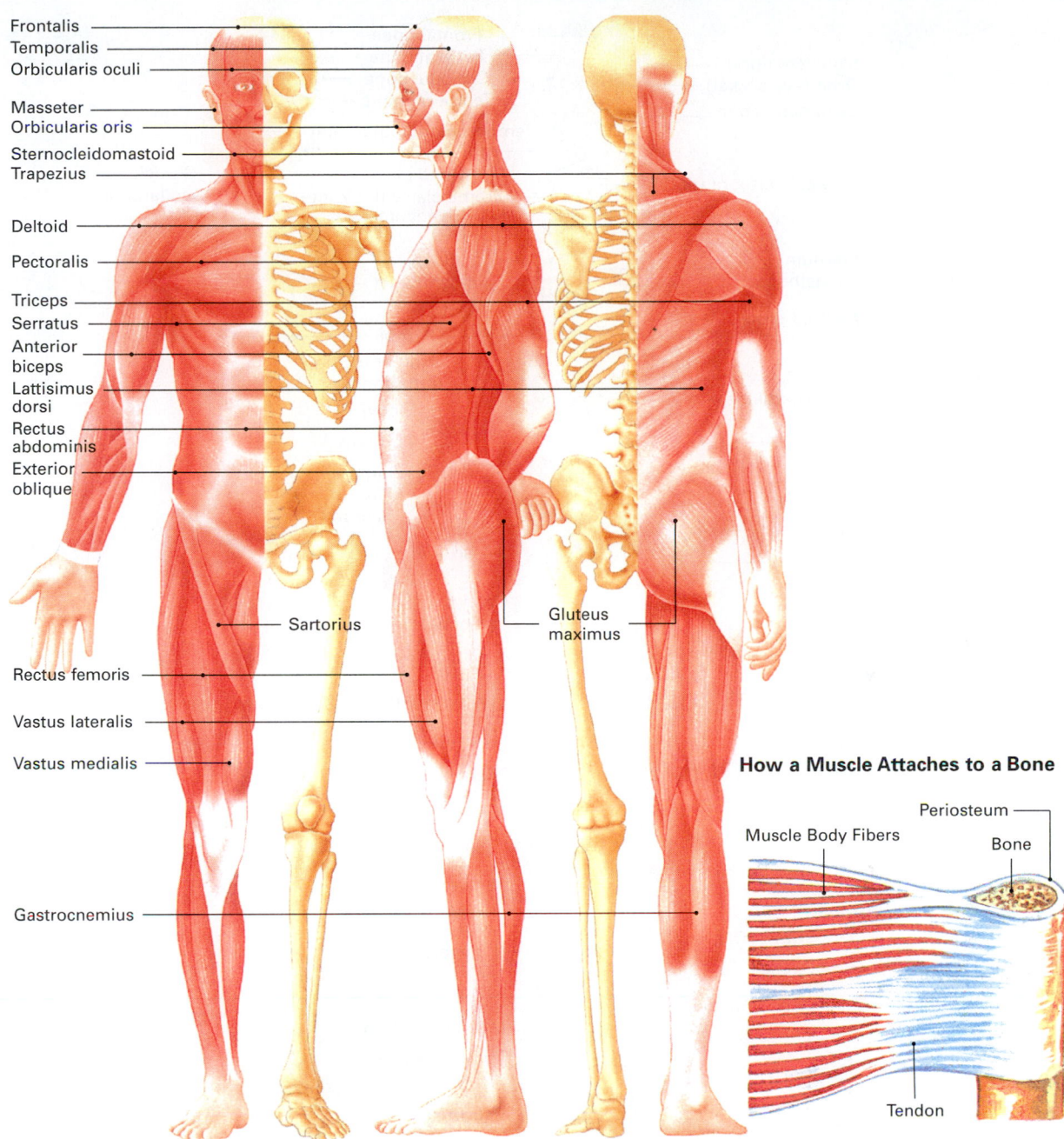

Frontalis
Temporalis
Orbicularis oculi
Masseter
Orbicularis oris
Sternocleidomastoid
Trapezius
Deltoid
Pectoralis
Triceps
Serratus
Anterior biceps
Lattisimus dorsi
Rectus abdominis
Exterior oblique
Sartorius
Gluteus maximus
Rectus femoris
Vastus lateralis
Vastus medialis
Gastrocnemius

How a Muscle Attaches to a Bone

Periosteum
Bone
Muscle Body Fibers
Tendon

Figure 31-1. ■ The musculature of the body. The skeletal muscles support the body and allow the bones to move.

either end with the diaphysis in the middle. The epiphysis is also known as the *growth plate*. Prior to puberty, the epiphysis remains open to allow for bone growth to occur. After puberty, the epiphysis solidifies and there is no further increase in the length of the bone.

Joints

The space where two bones meet is called a joint. Some joints allow for movement, whereas others are immovable. A joint that is immovable, such as the sutures

between the cranial bones, is classified as a synarthrosis joint. The joint spaces between the vertebrae are slightly moveable and are classified as amphiarthrosis. The largest category of joints is the diathrosis joints or the freely moveable joints. These include the joints of the limbs, shoulders, and hips. Various names are given to the moveable joints including ball and socket, hinge, condyloid, pivot, gliding, and saddle joints. Synovial fluid is secreted in the joint cavity to reduce friction and lubricate the joint (Figure 31-4 ■).

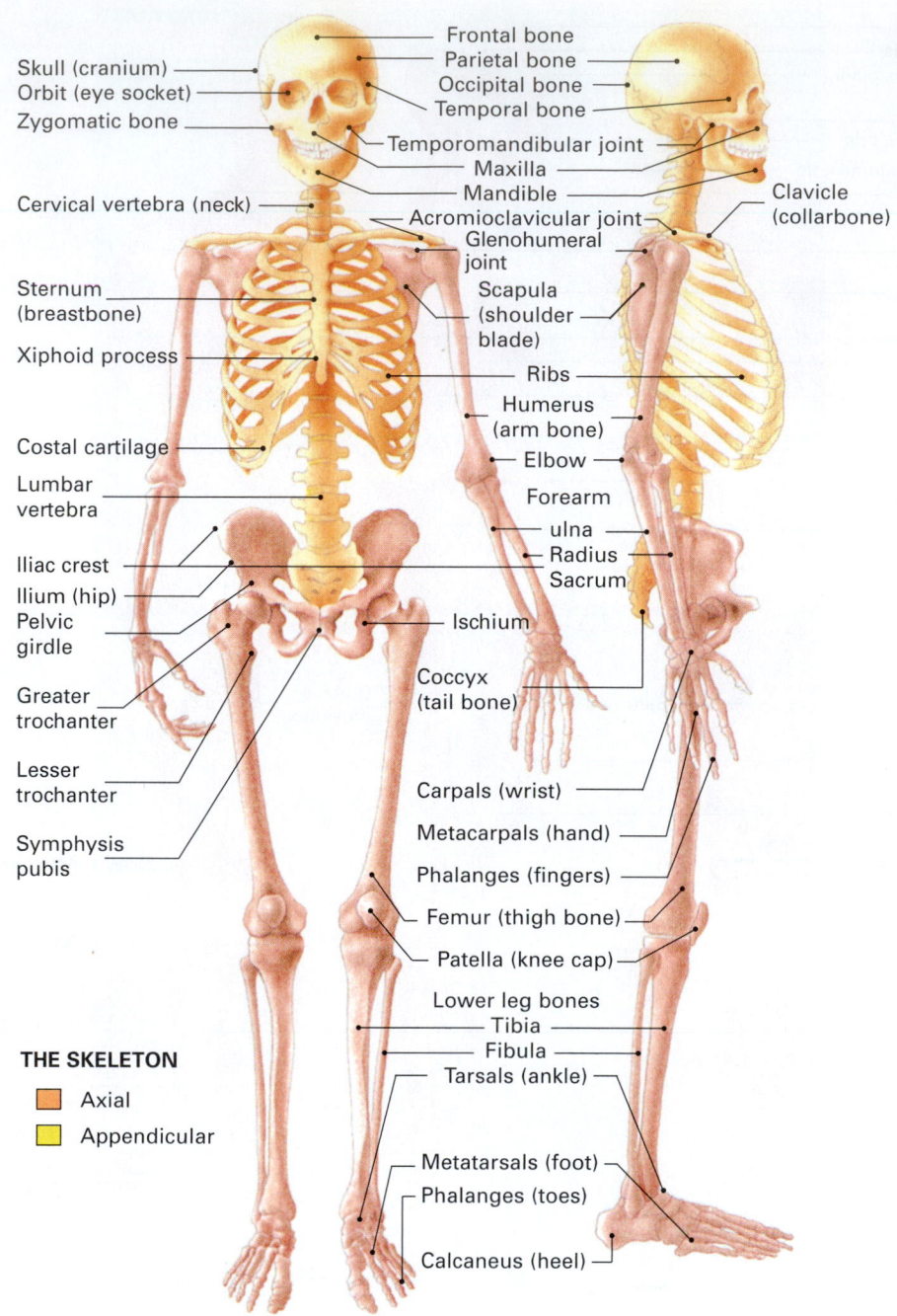

Frontal bone
Parietal bone
Occipital bone
Temporal bone
Skull (cranium)
Orbit (eye socket)
Zygomatic bone
Temporomandibular joint
Maxilla
Mandible
Clavicle (collarbone)
Cervical vertebra (neck)
Acromioclavicular joint
Glenohumeral joint
Sternum (breastbone)
Scapula (shoulder blade)
Xiphoid process
Ribs
Humerus (arm bone)
Costal cartilage
Elbow
Forearm
Lumbar vertebra
ulna
Radius
Sacrum
Iliac crest
Ilium (hip)
Ischium
Pelvic girdle
Coccyx (tail bone)
Greater trochanter
Carpals (wrist)
Lesser trochanter
Metacarpals (hand)
Phalanges (fingers)
Symphysis pubis
Femur (thigh bone)
Patella (knee cap)
Lower leg bones
Tibia
Fibula
Tarsals (ankle)

THE SKELETON
- Axial
- Appendicular

Metatarsals (foot)
Phalanges (toes)
Calcaneus (heel)

Figure 31-2. ■ The skeleton of the body.

Hard Connective Tissue

The skeleton consists of hard connective tissue, including cartilage and bone. (Other connective tissues include blood and lymph, loose connective tissue and fat, and fibrous connective tissue such as tendons.)

Three types of cartilage are found in the body. The most prevalent is *hyaline cartilage*. It is used by the body to reduce friction between moving parts such as bones, to attach the ribs to the sternum (breastbone), and to form the structure of the larynx.

The other two types of cartilage are *fibrocartilage* and *elastic cartilage*. Fibrocartilage, due to its highly compressible nature, is used by the body as a shock absorber and is found in the disks between the vertebrae of the spinal column. Elastic cartilage is more flexible than the other two types of cartilage and is found in the external ear.

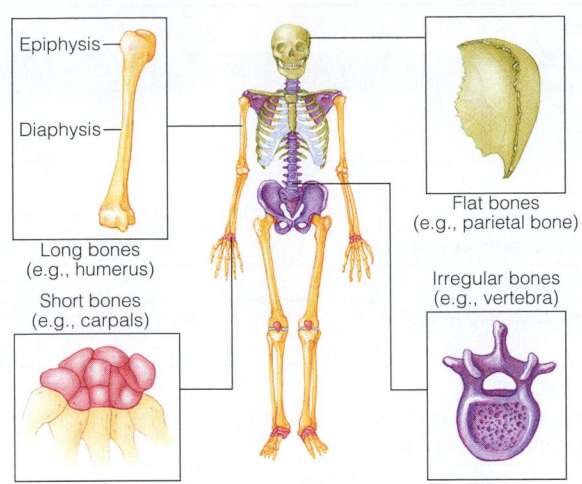

Figure 31-3. ■ Classification of long bones according to shape.

Cartilage has no blood vessels of its own, which means repair by the body takes a long time if it is damaged. In some cases, repair may not take place at all.

Bone or *osseous* tissue is similar to cartilage in its cellular structure, but it is harder and not flexible. The matrix consists of collagen fibers impregnated with calcium and phosphorous salts, which give bone its characteristic hardness.

As mentioned earlier, bones provide the framework of the body and are also the site of blood cell production.

Collaborative Care

DIAGNOSTIC TESTS

The most common tests used to confirm musculoskeletal disorders are x-rays. X-rays are most efficient at determining injuries of hard structures. Magnetic resonance imaging

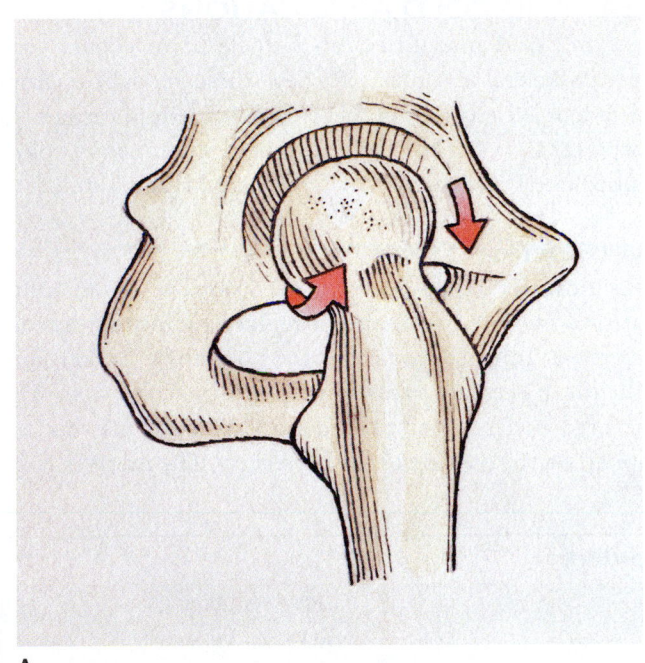

A

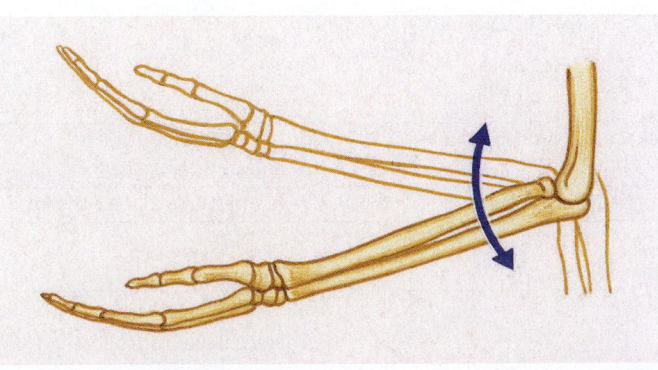

B

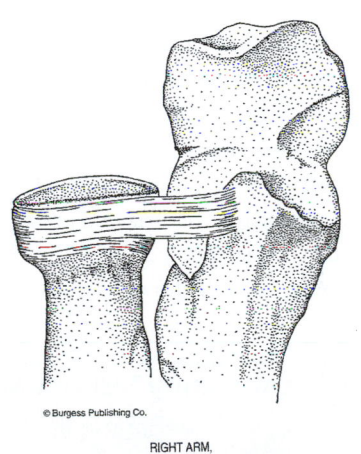

RIGHT ARM,
PROXIMAL ENDS OF RADIUS AND ULNA

C

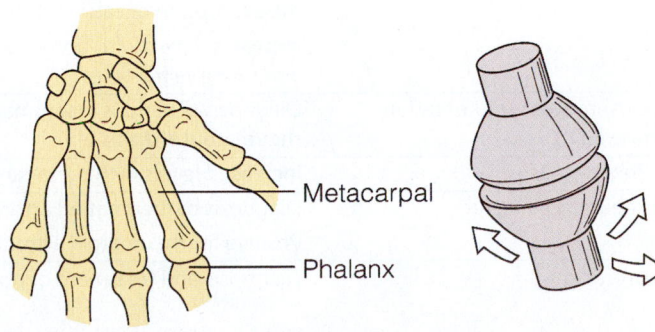

D

Figure 31-4. ■ Types of joint motion. **A.** Ball-and-socket joint. **B.** Hinge joint. **C.** Pivot joint (radioulnar articulation). **D.** Condyloid (wrist) and saddle joint (thumb). *Source:* A and B from Darling Kindersley Media Library; C from Pearson Education Custom Publishing; D from Pearson Education/PH College.

TABLE 31-1	Diagnostic Tests for Musculoskeletal Injuries
TEST	PURPOSE/USE
X-ray	Detect problems such as fractures Monitor treatment
CT scan	Evaluate bone trauma and bone abnormalities
MRI	Evaluate for conditions such as avascular necrosis, infection, tumors, disk disease, ligament or cartilage tears
Bone scan	Diagnose osteoporosis, osteomyelitis, bone cancer, and possible fractures
Bone density	Diagnose osteoporosis and monitor effectiveness of treatment
Electromyogram or myogram	Measure electrical activity of muscles during contraction and at rest
Myelogram	Diagnose herniated disk
Arthroscopy	Examine the inside of a joint (surgical procedure using an arthroscope); used for degenerative joint disease, rheumatoid arthritis, joint injuries such as ligament and meniscus tears
Arthrogram	Examine joint space after air or contrast medium injected into area; joint is moved as x-rays are taken
Arthrocentesis	Aspirate fluid from joint space Obtain fluid for diagnostic purposes and to remove excess fluid

(MRI) can determine the extent of soft tissue injury. Bone scans and computerized tomography (CT) scans are used for more detailed assessments. X-rays will be used at regular intervals to evaluate the progress of healing of the injury.

Arthroscopy and arthrograms can be used to evaluate joints. Table 31-1 ■ lists diagnostic tests for musculoskeletal injuries and their use.

Blood work may be ordered to evaluate the hemoglobin and hematocrit of the client. Fractures of the femur and the pelvis may cause significant bleeding. An erythrocyte sedimentation rate test may be ordered to evaluate the amount of inflammation present if rheumatoid arthritis or systemic lupus erythematosus is suspected. Table 31-2 ■ shows laboratory tests that may be done for musculoskeletal disorders.

HEAT AND COLD APPLICATIONS

Heat and cold modalities can be helpful to clients with musculoskeletal disorders. Review these modalities from the major discussion of heat and cold applications in Chapter 24 . The client may need a temporary splint applied (see Procedure 47-1 for splinting procedure).

SURGERY

Musculoskeletal disorders may need surgical treatment to realign a fractured bone and/or replace a joint that has deteriorated. Injuries that cause the bone to be broken into multiple pieces are treated with external fixation. The fractured bones are stabilized by rods and pins that are applied on the outside of the extremity. The frame is large

TABLE 31-2	Laboratory Tests for Musculoskeletal Disorders	
TEST	PURPOSE	NORMAL VALUES
Alkaline phosphatase (ALP)	Identify presence of bone disorder Elevated with bone cancer, healing fractures, rheumatoid arthritis	ALP1 42–136 unit/L ALP2 20–130 unit/L
Calcium	Decreased levels with lack of calcium and vitamin D intake and malabsorption of calcium from the GI tract Increased levels with bone neoplasms, immobilization, and multiple fractures	Serum 4.5–5.5 mEq/L or 9–11 mg/dL
Erythrocyte sedimentation rate (ESR)	Diagnosis of various inflammatory diseases including rheumatoid arthritis	Normal values vary with age and gender
Phosphorus	Increased levels with bone tumors and healing fractures	1.7–2.6 mEq/L or 2.5–4.5 mg/dL
Rheumatoid factor	Diagnosis of rheumatoid arthritis Positive for rheumatoid arthritis > 1:80	< 1:20 titer
Uric acid	Diagnosis and treatment of gout	Male: 3.5–8.0 mg/dL Female: 2.8–6.8 mg/dL Panic value > 12 mg/dL

Source: Adapted from Lemone, P., & Burke, K. (2008). *Medical surgical nursing: Critical thinking in client care* (4th ed.). Upper Saddle River, NJ: Prentice Hall.

and bulky and must be monitored frequently for any signs of infection. Surgery is discussed further under particular disorders.

Traumatic Bone Disorders

FRACTURES

(*Note:* Fractures as they relate to children are covered in Chapter 60 ⬭.) A **fracture** of a bone is defined as any disruption in the bone itself. It is classified as either open or closed (Figure 31-5 ■). An open fracture is also known as a *compound fracture*, meaning that the broken bone breaks the skin. A closed or *simple fracture* refers to a fracture that has not caused skin to be disrupted. A complete fracture refers to a break that goes through the entire bone. An incomplete fracture is one in which the break does not go completely through the bone. A *comminuted fracture* is one in which parts of the bone are broken into small pieces. A *displaced fracture* occurs when the broken sections of the bone are not in alignment with one another. A *spiral fracture* usually occurs when the extremity is twisted as in a sports injury. A spiral fracture that occurs in a child under the age of 2 should always be investigated as possible child abuse. A *greenstick fracture* occurs most commonly in children. Because the bones in a child are still flexible, the periosteum does not fracture easily. Greenstick fractures appear similar to a young branch of a

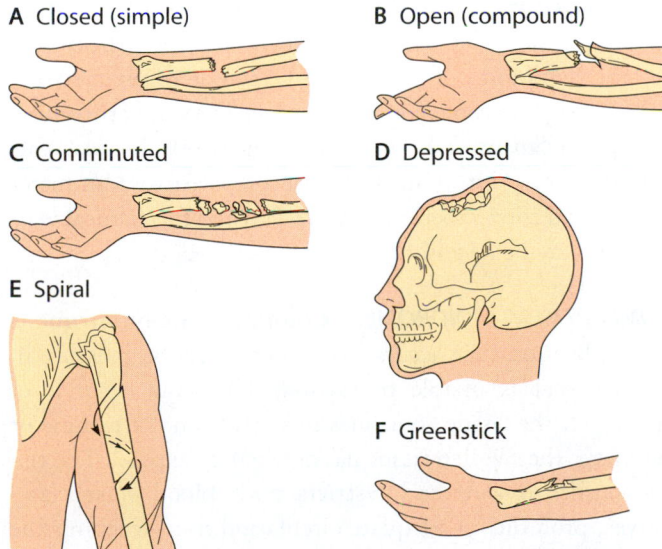

A Closed (simple) **B** Open (compound)

C Comminuted **D** Depressed

E Spiral

F Greenstick

Figure 31-5. ■ A fracture of a bone is defined as any disruption in the bone itself. It is classified as open or closed. **A.** Closed (simple)—skin over fracture remains intact. **B.** Open (compound)—broken bone protrudes through skin. **C.** Comminuted—bone fragments into many pieces. **D.** Depressed—broken bone is pressed inward (e.g., the skull). **E.** Spiral—jagged break due to twisting force. **F.** Greenstick—incomplete break along the length of the bone.

BOX 31-1	PEDIATRIC CONSIDERATIONS

Signs of Child Abuse

Musculoskeletal evidence of child abuse could include:
- Broken bones or black eyes
- Bruises, fading bruises, or other marks
- Unexplained burns or bites

The LPN/LVN must report any suspicion of child abuse.

Source: Child Welfare Information Gateway, Children's Bureau, Administration for Children and Families, U.S. Department of Health and Human Services.

---

tree when it is bent. The bone is too supple to break completely. A *pathological fracture* occurs as a result of a disease process that has weakened the bone resulting in a fracture. With a *compression fracture* the bone is crushed. An *impacted fracture* occurs when the ends of the fracture are forced into each other.

Manifestations

A fractured extremity will be swollen and extremely painful. The client may not be able to move the affected extremity. However, the ability to move an extremity does not indicate the absence of a fracture. There may be a visible deformity to the area. Crepitus may occur with movement. Bruising may or may not be present.

Fractures can be an indication of child abuse. Box 31-1 ■ lists other possible signs of child abuse.

Diagnosis

Fractures are diagnosed with the use of x-rays.

Treatment

A fractured bone must be placed in proper alignment to allow for healing and to maintain proper function of the bone and muscle involved. A fracture may be aligned externally by manipulation and casting to hold the bone in place while healing occurs (Figure 31-6 ■).

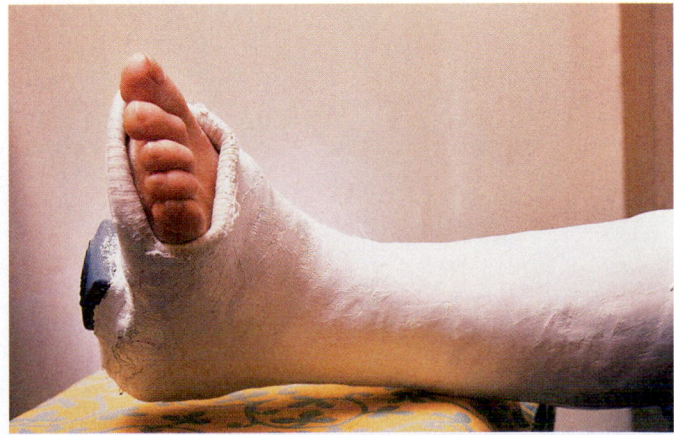

Figure 31-6. ■ A cast providing external fixation for a leg fracture. *Source:* Phototake NYC.

CASTS. A **cast** is a nonflexible encasement of a fractured extremity. Casts are traditionally applied to the joint above and below the fracture site to provide stability of the fractured bone. For example, to treat a fracture of the forearm, a cast would often be applied below the wrist to above the elbow. The client would not be able to twist or turn the forearm and the bone would be allowed to heal undisturbed. A cast is made of plaster of Paris or fiberglass. A plaster of Paris cast is inexpensive and is thicker, heavier, and bulkier than a fiberglass cast. A plaster of Paris cast may take up to 48 hours to dry completely. A fiberglass cast is much more expensive than a plaster of Paris cast. If waterproof material is used under the cast, the fiberglass cast can get wet. A fiberglass cast will dry very quickly, usually within a few hours.

Sometimes a cast is a combination of both materials. The plaster of Paris material is placed first and the fiberglass is added to the top of the cast. Fiberglass casts are popular with children because they are available in multiple colors and designs.

FIXATION OF FRACTURES. Fractures may also be treated by external or internal fixation (Figure 31-7 ■), with pins, plates, or screws securing the fracture area. With internal fixation, a surgical incision is made and the bone or bones are held together with wires, pins, plates, and screws completely within the body. This surgical procedure is known as an open reduction and internal fixation (ORIF). After internal fixation, a cast may or may not be used. With external fixation, pins are placed into the bones, above and below the fracture, that connect with an external fixation apparatus. Since the pins are placed into the bone, the area must be monitored for infection and pin care performed per agency policy.

Traction may also be used to treat a fracture for several reasons. Traction maintains the bone in good alignment until the fracture can be cast or the client can undergo a surgical repair of the fracture. Traction is used to fatigue the muscles that surround the fractured bone. These muscles often spasm and attempt to pull the fractured bone further out of alignment. **Traction** is a method of providing a steady and continuous pull that maintains the fractured bone in good alignment. There are several types of traction (Figure 31-8 ■):

- Buck's traction (straight traction) (Figure 31-8A): The extremity is pulled straight with a weight that is hung near the bottom of the bed frame. The weight is attached to an apparatus that adheres to the skin.
- Balanced suspended traction (Figure 31-8B): The client's fractured extremity is raised off the bed and the traction is applied in more than one way. The traction apparatus is usually applied to the skin.
- Skeletal traction (Figure 31-8C): The traction apparatus is applied directly to the bone through a pin inserted through the bone.

Procedure 31-1 ■ describes steps in applying traction.

Complications of a Fracture

FAT EMBOLISM. After the fracture of a long bone, fat globules may escape from the bone marrow and enter the bloodstream. Symptoms of fat embolism include respiratory distress, chest pain, confusion, and the development of petechiae. The physician must be notified immediately because this condition may result in death. Be prepared to administer oxygen and corticosteroids. Intubation and mechanical ventilation may be necessary.

COMPARTMENT SYNDROME. **Compartment syndrome** is a complication that occurs when there is excess pressure in a space that is unable to expand. This may occur after casting. If the tissue continues to swell from the trauma or bleeding, the swollen tissue has nowhere to expand. The tissue pushes inward and restricts both blood vessels and nerves, prohibiting adequate circulation from reaching the tissues distal to the swelling. This could result in death of those tissues.

Signs of compartment syndrome include severe pain that is not relieved by the prescribed pain medication. There may be decreased pulses in the extremity and the client will have extreme pain if asked to move the fingers or toes of the extremity. Other signs include pallor of the extremity, paresthesia, and paralysis.

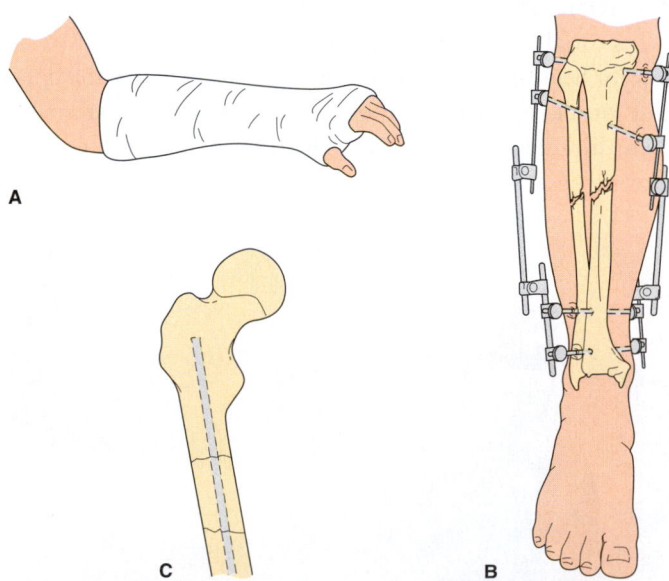

Figure 31-7. ■ **A.** Short arm cast. **B.** An external fixation device used to stabilize a fractured tibia and fibula. **C.** In internal fixation, the hardware is completely within the body. Plates, screws, or medullary nails (positioned lengthwise within the bone) can be used.

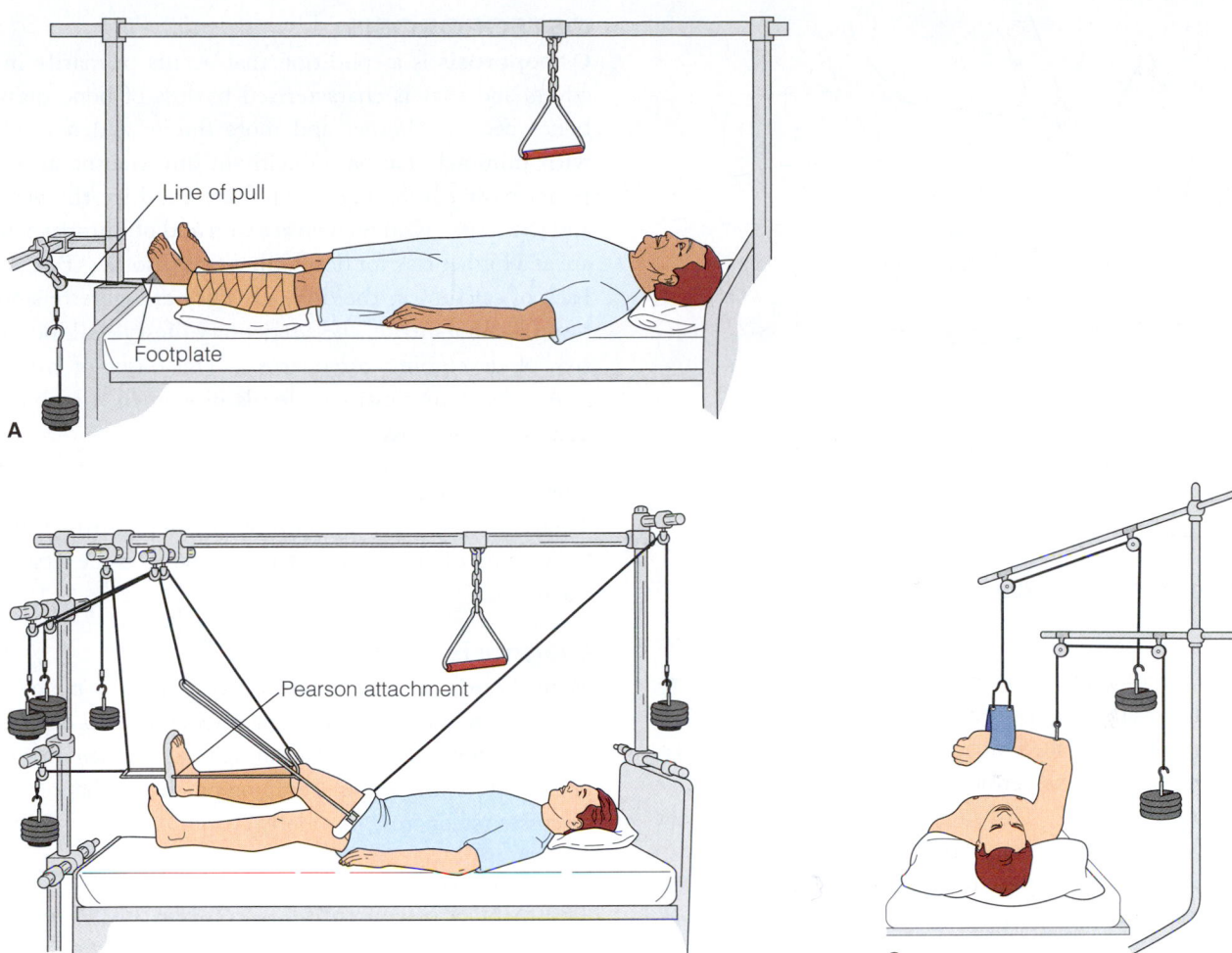

Figure 31-8. ■ Examples of traction: **A.** Buck's traction (straight skin traction). **B.** Balanced suspended traction for a femur fracture. **C.** Skeletal traction to stabilize a fractured humerus.

---

clinical ALERT

To prevent complications of compartment syndrome, look for and *report:*

- Pain
- Pallor
- Pulselessness
- Paralysis
- Paresthesia

If compartment syndrome is suspected, the cast must be bivalved and removed to prevent neurovascular complications (Figure 31-9 ■). In some severe cases, an incision will be made in the skin to relieve the pressure on the tissues. This procedure is called a **fasciotomy.** Compartment syndrome may also result from a crush injury.

DEEP VEIN THROMBOSIS.   Immobility and damage to the blood vessels in a fractured extremity leads to venous stasis and clot formation. If this clot dislodges it may travel to the brain, heart, or lungs and cause great damage to those tissues.

To prevent deep vein thrombosis (DVT), the client should be encouraged to ambulate as soon as possible. Anticoagulant therapy and compression stockings will often be ordered for clients who are unable to ambulate or who are on total bed rest. The client on enforced bed rest will usually receive some type of anticoagulant therapy to prevent the formation of blood clots during this period of inactivity. The nurse must assess for any signs of deep vein thrombosis every shift. Signs include swelling, warmth, redness, and tenderness at the site of the clot.

clinical ALERT

If a DVT is suspected, the nurse should elevate the extremity and notify the charge nurse immediately. Do not massage or rub the extremity with a suspected blood clot.

AMPUTATION.   An extremity or a portion of it may need to be amputated because of trauma or disease. Crushing injuries, trauma (e.g., gunshot wounds), or diseases such as diabetes or

MyNursingKit | Traction

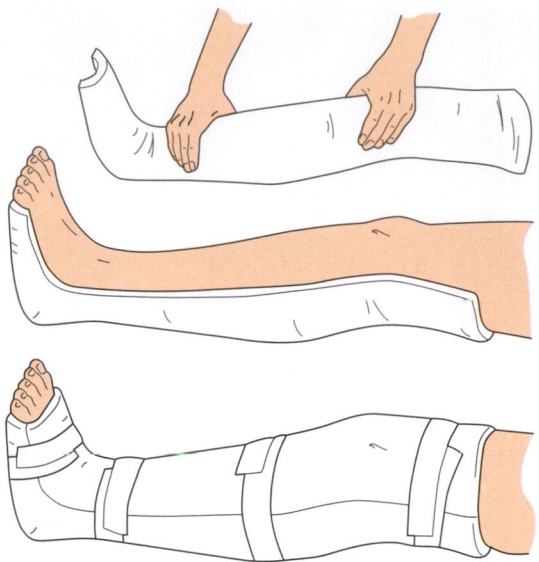

Figure 31-9. ■ Bivalving a cast.

peripheral vascular disease (PVD) can lead to the need for amputation. For example, **gangrene** (necrosis or tissue death) can result from the diminished blood supply of PVD or diabetes. Amputation may also be performed as a treatment for malignant tumors of the bone. This surgery will be used to prevent the spread of the tumor to other parts of the body.

Prior to amputation, the nurse will note a lack of circulation to the affected extremity. In the case of trauma, there may be obvious separation of tissues such as the foot from the leg or the hand from the arm. In other trauma situations, the nurse will note lack of pulses to the extremity and there will be coolness and lack of color to the extremity.

clinical ALERT

When the amputation occurs in the field, the nurse should instruct emergency workers or family members to wrap the amputated extremity in a towel and then place it in a plastic bag. The plastic bag should then be placed on ice and brought to the hospital.

When disease causes a lack of circulation, the nurse may note a darkening of the tissues or even a breakdown of the involved tissues.

The goal of care after an amputation is to ensure adequate healing of the stump to allow for placement of a prosthesis. Many clients will experience sensation in the absent extremity. This is called **phantom pain** (phantom limb sensation), and it is a normal phenomenon. Assure the client that this will go away over time. Phantom pain may occur because the brain remembers the nerve fibers. It can take some time for the brain to accommodate the loss of all of the tissue and nerves involved.

OSTEOPOROSIS

Osteoporosis is a condition that occurs primarily in older adults and that is characterized by loss of bone mass. The bones become thinner and more fragile and may fracture with minimal trauma, or without any trauma at all. The joints most commonly affected are the hip, the vertebrae, and the wrist. Women who are thin and of European descent are at a higher risk for developing this disorder (Box 31-2 ■). Lack of calcium in the diet, a history of cigarette smoking, heavy alcohol intake, and a sedentary lifestyle all increase the risk of developing osteoporosis. The onset of menopause causes decreasing estrogen levels in women, which also can accelerate bone loss.

Manifestations

There are few if any symptoms of osteoporosis. Often the fracture of a bone, such as the hip, will be the first sign of the disease.

Diagnosis

Many healthcare practitioners recommend a bone density x-ray for individuals at risk for osteoporosis to determine if this condition is present. Screening of all women over the age of 50 is becoming a more common practice. (Chapter 42 ⬭ discusses osteoporosis in elderly clients.)

Treatment

Treatment of osteoporosis is a combination of medication (Table 31-3 ■) and moderate exercise (Wilson et al., 2008). The medications used are bisphosphonates and/or hormone replacement therapy (HRT). The bisphosphonates such as alendronate (Fosamax) and risedronate (Actonel) inhibit the breakdown of bone, resulting in an increase in bone mass. HRT has been used to replace estrogen lost at menopause, thereby limiting the loss of bone mass. (Recent studies that indicate negative effects of HRT have made this practice

BOX 31-2	CULTURAL PULSE POINTS

Differences in Bone Structure and Density
There are many bicultural variations with the musculoskeletal system that you need to be aware of when performing an assessment. You will learn to distinguish between normal ethnic variation and abnormalities. Bone density varies greatly among different groups. African American males have the densest bone, which accounts for their very low incidence of osteoporosis. Most humans normally have 24 vertebrae. However, approximately 11% of African American females have 31, and 12% of Eskimo and Native American males have 25.

According to the National Osteoporosis Foundation (2008), it is estimated that 20% of Caucasian and Asian women over age 50 have osteoporosis, and 52% have low bone density (*osteopenia*). The risk for osteoporosis is rising most rapidly in Hispanic women over age 50.

less routine.) Another class of drugs being used is selective estrogen receptor modulators such as raloxifene (Evista), which mimics the effects of estrogen while reducing the risks associated with estrogen replacement. Treatment options may also include the use of calcitonin (Miacalcin), which increases bone formation. All women are encouraged to get adequate amounts of calcium in their diets with the help of dietary supplements. Calcium requirements range from 1,000 to 1,500 mg/day depending on age. Regular, moderate exercise, such as a walking program, has been proven to limit the loss of bone mass.

HIP FRACTURES.   Fractures of the hip in the elderly frequently result from osteoporosis. The neck of the femur is the most common site of a hip fracture. It is difficult to determine if the hip broke before the fall and caused the fall or if the individual fell and caused the fracture. The fracture must be surgically corrected to attain satisfactory healing of the bone. The surgeon will either place pins or plates and screws to stabilize the fracture site or replace the head and neck of the femur with a prosthesis. Occasionally the surgeon will perform a total hip replacement instead of repairing the fracture. Postoperatively, hip replacement clients need to be reminded (1) to keep the flexion of the affected hip at an angle of greater than 90 degrees and (2) to maintain abduction of

that joint. Bending the hip too far or crossing the legs can dislocate the hip.

OSTEOMALACIA

Osteomalacia is a reversible demineralization of the bone caused by a vitamin D deficiency. It is usually caused by a lack of dietary intake of vitamin D, such as not drinking milk, or a lack of exposure to sunlight. Clients with malabsorption disorders such as Crohn's disease or liver disorders may also develop osteomalacia because of an inability to absorb or store enough vitamin D.

Manifestations

Clients with osteomalacia complain of muscle weakness and stiffness that is similar to arthritis.

Diagnosis

X-rays will show demineralization of the bones. Pain will be greater at night or after activity. Osteomalacia is diagnosed with the use of x-rays and client symptoms.

Treatment

Treatment involves increasing the client's dietary intake of vitamin D as well as an increase in sun exposure. Vitamin D supplements may also be prescribed. The goal for the client

TABLE 31-3	**Medications for Osteoporosis**			
DRUG	**USUAL ROUTE/DOSE**	**CLASSIFICATION**	**SELECTED SIDE EFFECTS**	**NURSING CONSIDERATIONS**
Calcium	Calcium 1,000 mg to 1,500 mg daily	Calcium salt	Constipation, nausea	Administer after meals if GI upset occurs
Vitamin D	400 to 800 international units daily	Vitamin supplement		Food sources include fish, fortified milk
Fosamax (alendronate sodium)	10 mg once daily or 70 mg once a week	Bisphosphonates	Esophageal ulceration, nausea, vomiting, abdominal pain, dyspepsia	Administer in morning 30 minutes before food or beverage intake Client must remain upright for 30 minutes after taking medication
Actonel (risedronate sodium)	5 mg once daily or 35 mg once a week	Bisphosphonates	Diarrhea, headache, nausea, abdominal pain, arthralgia	Administer on an empty stomach with 6 to 8 ounces of water Client must remain upright for 30 minutes after taking medication
Evista (raloxifene hydrochloride)	60 mg daily	Selective estrogen receptor modulator (SERM)	Hot flashes, arthralgia,	Monitor for S/S of deep vein thrombosis Avoid other estrogen-containing medications
Miacalcin (calcitonin)	Intranasal 200 international units daily, alternating nostrils	Polypeptide hormone	Rhinitis, nausea, facial flushing, nasal congestion	Monitor patient for nasal irritation

Source : Data from Wilson, B.A., Shannon, M.T., Shields, K.M., & Stang, C.L. (2008). *Prentice Hall nurse's drug guide 2008.* Upper Saddle River, NJ: Prentice Hall.

with osteomalacia is that pain and weakness are resolved and bone mineralization is returned to normal.

OSTEOMYELITIS

Osteomyelitis is an infection of the bone (Figure 31-10 ■). It commonly follows some type of trauma though it can occur from any break in the skin. *Staphylococcus aureus* is the most common organism that causes infection of the bone.

Manifestations

The client will complain of fever and extreme tenderness at the site of the infection. The area will be red, swollen, and warm.

Treatment

Treatment consists of intravenous antibiotics for 10 days. The physician may also debride the infected portion of the bone. The client will be on bed rest until the physician determines that the infection is decreasing.

BONE CANCER

Tumors of the musculoskeletal system may be either primary or secondary. Primary tumors originate in the specific tissue such as the bone or the muscle. Secondary tumors are metastases of another primary tumor such as one in the breast or lung or colon. Primary bone tumors occur most commonly in adolescents who are experiencing a period of rapid bone growth. The most common primary bone tumors are osteosarcoma and Ewing's sarcoma.

Manifestations

The client will complain of pain at the site of the tumor. There will be swelling and impairment in the function of the extremity.

Diagnosis

Diagnosis is made by x-ray and a biopsy of the lesion.

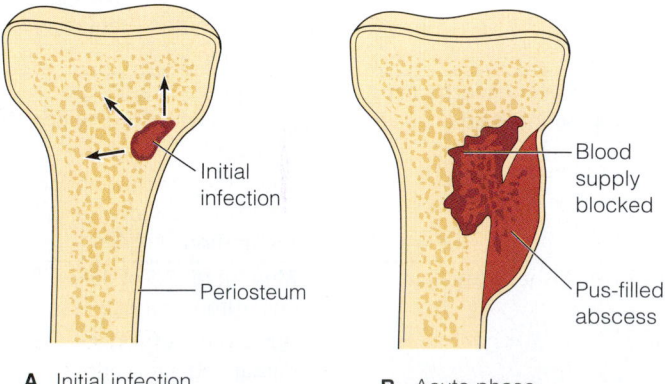

A Initial infection   **B** Acute phase

Figure 31-10. ■ Osteomyelitis. **A.** Bacteria enter and multiply in the bone. **B.** The infection spreads to other parts of the bone. If the infection reaches the outer part of the bone, the periosteum separates from the surface of the bone.

Treatment

The type of tumor and the location of the tumor determine treatment. Traditionally, the affected extremity was amputated. In recent years, surgeons have attempted to salvage the extremity if the tumor is small enough. The surgeon removes the entire tumor and inserts a metal rod and bone harvested from another site. Limb salvage surgery requires a longer recovery period but the client retains his or her own limb. Surgery is followed by chemotherapy and radiation therapy. Note: There are many psychosocial issues involved in loss of a limb. See Chapter 17 ⟲ for psychosocial issues and Chapter 18 ⟲ for discussion of loss and grief.

NURSING CARE

PRIORITIZING NURSING CARE

When you care for clients with bone disorders, focus your care on maintaining correct body alignment and managing pain. If the client has a cast applied, monitor the cast until it is dry to prevent indentations from forming that could cause pressure. Perform neurovascular checks every 2 hours to detect any circulatory compromise due to the cast. Instruct the client on cast care after discharge. Tell clients to report any complaints of numbness, tingling, or increased pain in the extremity. If the client is in traction or is waiting for surgery on a fracture, keep the affected extremity in correct body alignment. Monitor the traction equipment to be certain that the weights are hanging freely and the ropes are straight. After hip replacement surgery, keep the legs abducted to prevent dislocation of the prosthesis. An abduction pillow helps keep the legs in correct alignment. Always replace the pillow after you care for the client. When caring for clients with bone infections or tumors, make pain management your major priority. Give medication as ordered and anticipate the need for medication before procedures are performed.

ASSESSING

All clients who present with symptoms of bone disorders must have a careful history taken. The history should include the events preceding the pain and reports of any stiffness or limitation of motion. The nurse should also obtain a complete medication history from the client because some medications may have contributed to the client's complaint. For example, diuretics may cause a client to become dizzy upon arising, which could then cause the client to fall. It is also important to know if the client uses alcohol and, specifically, how much alcohol the client uses on a regular basis. Ask the client if he or she has any chronic diseases such as cancer or osteoporosis, which may signal a pathologic fracture. Include a nutritional assessment in the history because this may indicate a pattern of nutritional deficiencies.

DIAGNOSING, PLANNING, AND IMPLEMENTING

Possible nursing diagnoses for clients with bone disorders include:

- *Acute Pain*
- *Impaired Physical Mobility*
- *Risk for Peripheral Neurovascular Dysfunction*
- *Risk for Infection*
- *Disturbed Body Image*

Outcomes for these clients might be:

- Client states pain is relieved by medication.
- Client completes activities of daily living (ADLs) with use of assistive devices (see Figure 46-4 🔗).
- Neurovascular function is stable (or improved with medication and range-of-motion exercises).
- Client is free of infection.
- Client discusses ways to cope with changing physical abilities.
- When caring for clients with bone disorders, evaluate pain using a pain scale. *The pain scale helps provide an objective assessment.*
- Administer pain medication as ordered, carefully evaluating the client's response to the pain medication. *This evaluation helps the physician order the most effective pain management for the individual client.*
- Instruct clients with patient-controlled analgesia (PCA) units on how to use them and encourage their use. *PCA units allow the client to obtain effective pain management.*
- Monitor the client's pain. As the client improves after surgery or illness, the need for pain medication should decrease. If that is not the case, notify the physician. *Continued pain can indicate a complication.*
- Monitor clients with casts or in traction closely. The first thing to note is whether there is adequate circulation to the affected extremity. After surgical fixation of a fracture, it is very important to determine if there is any neurovascular compromise. The nurse will be responsible for checking capillary refill and asking the client to move fingers or toes. The nurse will determine if the client has feeling in the extremity and will check whether there is warmth in the extremity. Box 31-3 ■ provides a list for neurovascular assessment. *Careful attention can prevent complications due to impaired circulation to the extremity. Any negative findings could indicate impaired circulation, which can lead to tissue death.*

Cast Care

- If a plaster cast is applied, use the palms of the hands to handle the cast for the first 48 hours. *If the fingertips are used, the pressure of the fingertips may create pressure points on the underlying tissue.*

<table>
<tr><td>**BOX 31-3**</td><td>**COLLECTING DATA ABOUT CLIENTS FOR NEUROVASCULAR DISORDERS**</td></tr>
</table>

In clients with neurovascular disorders, the following data may be collected:

- Skin color distal to the injury is pale.
- Skin temperature distal to the injury is cool to the touch.
- Pulses distal to the injury are weak or absent.
- Client is unable to move the area distal to the injury.
- Client reports tingling or numbness distal to the injury.
- Capillary refill is greater than 3 seconds distal to the injury.
- Client reports pain increasing or not responding to pain medication.

- Turn the client frequently while the cast is drying. A hair dryer set on "cool" or a fan directed at the cast may also be used to assist with the drying process. *This allows all parts of the cast to be exposed to the air.*
- Report immediately any foul odor from a cast or oozing through the cast. Any symptoms of deep vein thrombosis, specifically chest pain or shortness of breath, should be reported to the physician immediately. Anticoagulants may be administered intravenously. *Odor could be an indication of infection beneath the cast. Chest pain or shortness of breath could signal a medical emergency. Anticoagulants are used to prevent further clot formation.*

Traction Care

Nursing care of the client in traction focuses on maintaining the traction and preventing complications from the traction.

- As in the case of all fractures, check the neurovascular status of the affected extremity frequently. *This determines if any circulatory compromise exists.*
- Always make sure that the weights are hanging freely. *This means the traction is operating correctly.*
- Never pick the weight up off the floor and reposition the client in bed. Using assistance, pull the client back up into position in the bed and allow the weight to hang freely. Use bolstering devices such as pillows. The client who is small or thin will have difficulty staying in good position. *Weight will tend to pull the individual down in the bed. Readjustments help the client stay in good position.*
- If the client has a pin placed in the bone for skeletal traction, follow the institutional policy for pin care. The pins are usually cleaned every shift with hydrogen peroxide and Betadine and wrapped with a sterile dressing. *Good care helps prevent the entrance of microorganisms through the skin into the bone.*
- Assess the skin every shift for breakdown. Change the client's position often. Keep sheets free of wrinkles. If the traction device is applied directly to the skin, assess this skin frequently for any signs of breakdown. *The client is unable to move very much while in traction. Frequent attention can prevent the chance of infection.*

- Provide diversionary activities for immobile clients. *Clients who are immobilized need distraction from the discomfort and boredom of confinement.*

Assisting Clients with Amputation

- When the client returns from surgery, a pressure dressing is usually in place on the stump. In some cases, a temporary prosthesis will also be in place. *This molds the stump to fit into the prosthesis after it heals.*
- Elevate the extremity and check the dressing frequently for any signs of bleeding. *Excessive edema or bleeding can indicate poor healing or a wound infection.*
- Use sterile technique when changing dressings. *This prevents infection.*
- While the skin is healing, wrap the stump with elastic bandages. *This helps compress the tissues and prepare them for fitting with a prosthesis (Figure 31-11 ■).*

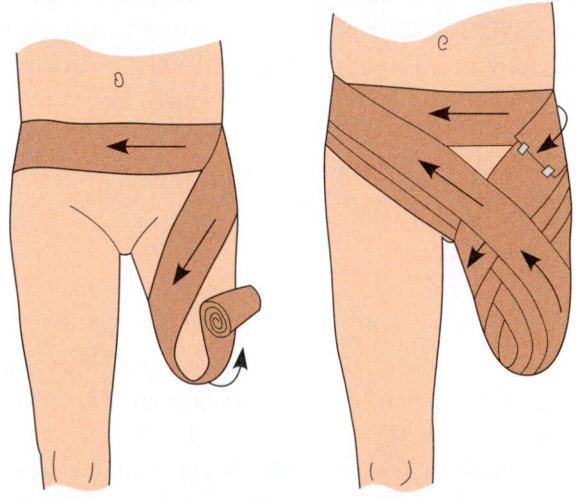

A

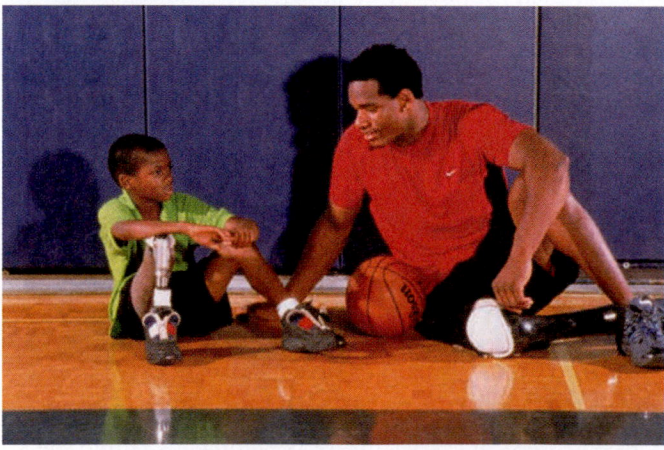

B

Figure 31-11. ■ A. With an above-the-knee amputation, a figure-eight bandage is wrapped around the waist, then brought down over the stump and back up around the hip. **B.** A role model can provide support and encouragement to a child learning to adapt to life with a prosthetic limb. (*Source: B: Photo Researchers, Inc.*)

- Allow clients to verbalize fears and frustration. Provide emotional support as the client works through stages of grieving over the lost limb. Help the client to begin to explore ways to function with the prosthetic limb. *Clients with bone cancer and amputation face particularly difficult recoveries due to change in body image.*

EVALUATING

The goal of care for clients with bone disorders involves evaluation of pain medication effectiveness, healing of fractures or infections, and assessing risk for further illness or injury.

NURSING PROCESS CARE PLAN
Client in Skeletal Traction

Jason McAllister is a 25-year-old man who broke his left femur in a motorcycle accident. The orthopedic surgeon placed him in skeletal traction. The surgeon told Jason that he expects him to remain in traction for approximately 2 weeks. Jason states, "I can't lie here for the next 2 weeks." He also expressed concern that he may lose his job while he is recovering from this injury.

Assessment

VS: T 97.8°F, P 84, R 16, BP 128/72. Client reports pain as a "4" on a scale of 1 to 10. Left leg is in skeletal traction with 6 pounds of weight at the end of the traction apparatus. Steinman pin inserted in left femur. Skin around pin, no sign of redness or edema.

Nursing Diagnosis

The following important nursing diagnoses (among others) are established for this condition:

- *Acute Pain* related to left femur fracture
- *Risk for Infection* related to pin in left femur
- *Risk for Impaired Skin Integrity* related to immobility
- *Ineffective Coping* related to fear of job loss

Expected Outcomes

The expected outcomes for the plan of care are that Mr. McAllister will:

- Rate pain as a "0 to 2" on a 0 to 10 scale.
- Remain free of infection.
- Remain free of any skin breakdown.
- Discuss financial needs with social worker.

Planning and Implementation

The following nursing interventions are implemented for Mr. McAllister:

- Monitor temperature every 4 hours.
- Instruct client to ask for pain medication before pain increases.

- Instruct client in the use of PCA if ordered.
- Administer pain medication as ordered.
- Assess pin site every 4 hours. Report any abnormalities to the physician.
- Perform pin care as ordered.
- Assess client's skin, especially back and sacral area, every shift.
- Keep linens free of wrinkles.
- Maintain client's body in good alignment to allow weight to hang freely.
- Provide client with activities such as books, magazines, TV, movies, and puzzle books.
- Ask social worker to discuss with client his employment status and financial needs.

Evaluation

The client's pain is slowly reduced to "0" on a scale of 0 to 10. Traction is removed after 10 days and a long leg cast is applied. The skin remained free of breakdown. The client applied for and received temporary disability while in the cast.

Critical Thinking in the Nursing Process

1. What possible nonpharmacologic techniques could be implemented to help Mr. McAllister with pain control?
2. What would be the most appropriate responses to Mr. McAllister's comments about his employment status?
3. Discuss the teaching regarding cast care that will need to be done with Mr. McAllister prior to discharge.

Note: Discussion of Critical Thinking questions appears on the MyNursingKit Website.

Inflammatory Disorders

RHEUMATOID ARTHRITIS

Rheumatoid arthritis (RA) is a chronic, systemic inflammatory disease of the connective tissue. It is thought to be autoimmune in origin. It is more common in women. Rheumatoid arthritis as it relates to children is covered in Chapter 61 .

Manifestations

The client complains of joint stiffness that is usually worse in the morning. This is often accompanied by fatigue, anorexia, weight loss, and possibly fever. Multiple joints may be involved. Joints may become red, warm, and swollen, with limited range of motion (ROM). The affected joints become deformed as the inflammatory process continues. The goal of treatment for the client with rheumatoid arthritis is to preserve function and limit deformity.

Diagnosis

Rheumatoid arthritis is diagnosed by symptoms and laboratory tests. Blood work is drawn for the presence of the rheumatoid factor (RF), erythrocyte sedimentation rate, and a complete blood count. Individuals with RA will usually have a *positive RF* (an antibody present with RA), an *elevated sedimentation rate* (an indication of inflammation), and the presence of *anemia*. X-rays of the affected joints will demonstrate *swelling of the soft tissue*.

Treatment

Treatment involves medication, application of heat and cold (described in Chapter 24), rest, and stress reduction. Stress reduction is necessary because stress (physiologic and psychologic) may increase the symptoms of rheumatoid arthritis. Various medications are used to control the disease. These medications include aspirin, other nonsteroidal, anti-inflammatory drugs (NSAIDs), corticosteroids, chemotherapeutic agents, and immune system modifiers. It is important that the client receiving chemotherapeutic agents understand that these drugs will damage a developing fetus. Therefore, good birth control should be practiced while taking these medications. The immune system modifiers have been found to dramatically limit the symptoms of rheumatoid arthritis, but they are very expensive and require the client to self-inject these medications on a regular basis. The client must be taught the importance of adequate rest. This should include rest periods during the day and uninterrupted sleep during the night. The client also needs regular exercise that has been approved by the physician.

Treatment for rheumatoid arthritis includes heat and cold applications. The client may use warm, moist heat around stiff joints to help combat stiffness. Warm paraffin treatments have been shown to lengthen the time without stiffness. The client places the hands or feet in liquid, warm paraffin (liquid wax). The paraffin is allowed to harden and is then removed. The use of cold applications during acute episodes of RA has been shown to relieve pain. The client may use frozen bags of vegetables that can form around the joint. It is important to teach the client that the source of cold must never be placed directly next to the skin. It must be wrapped in a towel or washcloth. Application of cold should be limited to 20 minutes every hour. The goal of treatment is to help the client retain function and mobility and be able to manage the pain and stiffness within the client's usual lifestyle.

DEGENERATIVE JOINT DISEASE (OSTEOARTHRITIS)

Degenerative joint disease (DJD), also known as **osteoarthritis,** is the most common form of arthritis. It is a "wear-and-tear" disease caused by overuse and/or injury to the joint. It is more common in older overweight adults. The hips and knees are the joints most commonly affected. Differences between rheumatoid arthritis and osteoarthritis are listed in Table 31-4 .

TABLE 31-4	Comparison of Rheumatoid Arthritis and Osteoarthritis	
RHEUMATOID ARTHRITIS	**OSTEOARTHRITIS (DEGENERATIVE JOINT DISEASE)**	
Chronic, systemic inflammatory disorder of connective tissue	Most common type of arthritis	
Autoimmune disorder of unknown cause	Caused by loss of cartilage in synovial joints (repetitive use, trauma, obesity, heredity, congenital or acquired defects)	
Typically involves multiple joints and occurs symmetrically		
Seen in joints of the fingers, wrists, knees, ankles, and toes	Most commonly seen in the weightbearing joints	
Affects more women than men	Affects men and women equally	
Usual onset from 30 to 50 years, may be abrupt; periods of exacerbation and remission (comes and goes)	Usual onset 50 or older; usually gradual with slow progression	
Fatigue, anorexia, weight loss, nonspecific aching and stiffness may appear before joint manifestations; anemia, low-grade fever	Deep aching pain in joints aggravated by use, relieved by rest, fatigue, Heberden's nodes, Bouchard's nodes, crepitation	
Joints are swollen, red, warm, tender, and painful; several joints involved; limited ROM	One or several joints; enlarged, cool, and hard on palpation; limited ROM	
Morning stiffness lasting more than 1 hour; pain and stiffness after prolonged immobility	Stiffness following immobility, subsides with activity	
Aspirin, NSAID, corticosteroids, immunosuppressive drugs, and disease modifying drugs, rest, exercise, hot, cold, assistive devices, joint arthroplasty	Analgesics such as aspirin, acetaminophen, NSAID, exercise, hot or cold, joint arthroplasty	

Manifestations

The client will complain of stiffness and pain in the affected joint. The pain is often described as a "deep ache." The joint may become enlarged over time but there is no swelling, warmth, or redness.

Diagnosis

Diagnosis is based on history and physical examination and x-ray.

Treatment

Treatment consists of weight loss if the client is overweight, rest of the joint followed by a return to moderate activity. Medications are used to reduce pain and inflammation. Traditionally the medication of choice has been an NSAID. The newest NSAID, celecoxib (Celebrex), has been proven effective in managing the pain and stiffness of osteoarthritis. This drug appears to have fewer gastrointestinal side effects, though it may increase the risk of heart attack or stroke. Oxycodone hydrochloride (OxyContin) is also used for this condition; it is a controlled drug that carries the risk of addiction. It must be monitored closely, especially in older adults because of reduced liver clearance.

Recent research has shown that the supplement glucosamine will repair the damaged joint tissue if begun before significant damage has occurred. The only other effective treatment is joint replacement surgery. This is used when the pain can no longer be managed with medication and/or the joint is no longer functional. Joint replacement surgery is also used in clients with rheumatoid arthritis.

TOTAL HIP REPLACEMENT. In total hip replacement surgery, the entire head of the femur and the surface of the acetabulum are replaced with a metal prosthesis (Figure 31-12 ■).

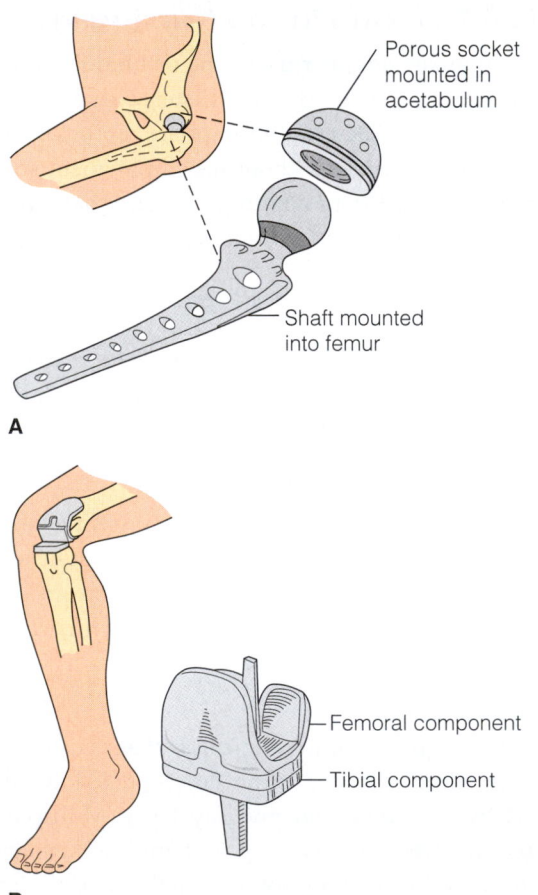

Figure 31-12. ■ **A.** Total hip replacement. **B.** Total knee replacement.

The surgeon makes an incision that is approximately 9 to 12 inches long. After the surgery, the client will have a drainage device such as a Hemovac. These are usually emptied once every shift and the drainage recorded. Newer surgical techniques use two to three smaller incisions. The surgeon uses a laparoscopic device to perform the hip replacement. The client has less blood loss and a quicker recovery time than with open procedures.

TOTAL KNEE REPLACEMENT.   In a total knee replacement, the knee joint is removed and replaced with a prosthesis attached to both the femur and the tibia (Figure 31-12B). The surgeon will make a long incision that extends from 2 inches above the knee to 2 inches below the knee. There will be a drainage device that must be emptied every shift if ordered by the physician. After surgery most clients will be placed in a continuous passive motion machine. This device moves the knee while the client is unable to do so. The movement helps to decrease swelling in the affected knee and also contributes to normal function of the knee joint.

The shoulder, elbow, and the joints of the fingers and toes may also be replaced. The goal after joint replacement surgery is to improve the client's mobility.

GOUT

Gout is an inflammatory disorder that causes uric acid crystals to form in a joint. The most common joint affected is the distal joint of the great toe. Gout may occur because the client does not excrete uric acid properly. It also may be caused by chronic renal disease, malignancies, starvation, and certain medications such as diuretics. Clients who abuse alcohol are at higher risk for gout because alcohol impairs the ability of the body to excrete uric acid. Gout occurs more often in men than in women. The first attack usually occurs after age 40.

Manifestations

The client will report sudden pain in the joint often occurring suddenly at night. The joint will be red, swollen, hot to the touch, and very painful.

Diagnosis

A number of diagnostic tests are used to establish a diagnosis of gout. Blood is drawn for a complete blood count (CBC), a uric acid level, and an eosinophil sedimentation rate (sed rate). The CBC is evaluated because the WBCs will be elevated above $20,000/mm^3$ during an attack of gout. Both the uric acid level and the sedimentation rate will also be elevated.

Treatment

Medication is the primary treatment for gout. NSAIDs are used to decrease the inflammation. Corticosteroids may also be used. Medications that decrease uric acid levels are used to prevent the occurrence of further attacks. Clients are also encouraged to follow a low-purine diet. Foods that are high in purines include meats and seafood. Other high-purine foods are beans and vegetables such as broccoli and mushrooms.

The treatment goal for the client with gout is a reduction in symptoms and the prevention of further attacks.

ANKYLOSING SPONDYLITIS

Ankylosing spondylitis is a type of arthritis that primarily affects the spine. It is an inflammatory disorder that causes the spine to stiffen and possibly fuse. There is no known cause for this disorder. It is more common in men than in women. It usually begins in early adulthood.

Manifestations

The client presents with symptoms of back pain accompanied by loss of mobility in the spine. The client complains of pain that is worse at night and may also occur in the hips and legs. The client may also have symptoms similar to the client with rheumatoid arthritis such as fatigue, weight loss, and fever.

Diagnosis

Ankylosing spondylitis is diagnosed by x-rays and blood work. The x-rays will show changes in the spine, and the blood work will show an elevated sed rate.

Treatment

Treatment includes the use of NSAIDs to combat the inflammatory process. The client is encouraged to participate in regular, prescribed exercise to help maintain spinal mobility. The treatment goal for this disorder is decreased spinal pain and stiffness and no loss of spinal mobility.

LYME DISEASE

Lyme disease is a musculoskeletal disorder that is caused by the bite of a deer tick. The deer tick infects the client with a bacterium that causes joint problems and systemic problems such as weight loss, fever, and fatigue.

Manifestations

The client will report symptoms that resemble the flu such as fever and generalized muscular discomfort. The client may or may not report a tick bite. A rash resembling a bull's-eye forms around the tick bite. Symptoms of Lyme disease begin anywhere from 1 to 3 weeks after the tick bite. After the flulike symptoms and the rash disappear, the client will complain of joint pain similar to arthritis.

Diagnosis and Treatment

When Lyme disease is suspected, blood is drawn and tested for the presence of antibodies to the bacterium from the deer tick. Lyme disease is treated with antibiotics such as tetracycline or amoxicillin. It is important to start treatment as quickly as possible to prevent the development of chronic joint symptoms. The client may need to take antibiotics for 1 month or longer. The treatment goal for the client with Lyme disease is no recurrence of symptoms.

NURSING CARE

PRIORITIZING NURSING CARE

When caring for clients with inflammatory joint disorders, make pain relief and preserving joint mobility your priorities. Give medication for pain as needed and help clients find other methods of pain relief such as warm, moist compresses or warm baths. Clients with arthritis tend to have some days when they feel less pain than other days. Encourage them to be more active on days when the pain is less intense, and allow themselves to rest during periods of exacerbation. Encourage clients to participate as much as possible in activities of daily living, but be prepared to assist if they are unable to complete them. Range of motion will be limited, so assist with areas they are unable to reach. Keep joints as mobile as possible. Perform passive range-of-motion exercises if active exercise is not feasible.

ASSESSING

Clients with inflammatory disorders must be carefully assessed to gather complete data about the problem. It is important to determine the time of day when the discomfort is the worst, as well as what types of activity, if any, bring on discomfort. A complete nursing history is taken with particular emphasis on exposure to ticks that could indicate Lyme disease. Information about diet and lifestyle are important clues to conditions such as gout.

DIAGNOSING, PLANNING, AND IMPLEMENTING

Possible nursing diagnoses for clients with inflammatory disorders of the joints include:

- *Acute Pain*
- *Activity Intolerance*
- *Risk for Injury*
- *Impaired Physical Mobility*
- *Disturbed Body Image*

When caring for clients with inflammatory disorders, it is important to evaluate pain management techniques for effectiveness. Some clients will be on pain medications of some type most of their remaining years.

- Discuss the pain management measures currently in use and determine their effectiveness. *This helps determine the most effective pain management regimen for the client.*
- Give pain medications as prescribed and check back frequently. Use other techniques such as distraction. *It is important to see if the medications are effective against the pain. Distraction helps decrease the client's focus on the pain.*

- Assist clients with ADLs as necessary. Provide frequent rest periods during activities. *These measures allow clients to be more comfortable.*
- Ensure safety for clients with mobility problems by clearing pathways of clutter and electrical cords. Make sure that clients who use walkers or canes have them fitted properly and use them correctly. *These interventions help prevent possible falls or injuries.*
- Allow clients to express their feelings about the chronic illness and the effect it has on their bodies. Be supportive and nonjudgmental, allowing clients to verbalize feelings of being a victim of the disease. *Clients with deforming disorders, such as rheumatoid arthritis, may have body image issues. Because this disorder often starts in young adulthood, this may be a life-long concern.*

Heat and Cold Applications

For many inflammatory disorders, heat and cold applications help relieve stiffness and pain. Heat and cold applications can assist the healing process. (See the main discussion of heat and cold applications in Chapter 24 ⃝.) Nursing care guidelines for selected heat and cold therapies are provided in Box 24-5 ⃝.

Assisting Clients with Joint Replacements

Postoperative care for clients with joint replacements is focused on detecting signs of infection or impaired circulation, as well as preventing postoperative complications.

- Take vital signs every 4 hours. Be especially alert for increased temperature. *Fever may indicate infection of the replaced joint, which would require removal of the prosthesis.*
- Check neurovascular status every 4 hours. Monitor dressing and drainage devices for excessive bleeding. *Early attention can prevent complications.*
- Encourage turning, coughing, and deep breathing and the use of an incentive spirometer (see Procedure 29-2 and Box 32-6 ⃝). Ambulate the client as soon as allowed by the physician. *These measures help prevent pneumonia that might result from inactivity of alveoli in the lungs, secondary to immobility and surgery.*
- Monitor intake and output. Clients will have a Foley catheter for 1 to 2 days. *Changes from normal urine output might signal hemorrhage or other complication.*
- Administer pain medication as needed. Encourage client to use PCA if ordered by physician. *These measures provide comfort and assist healing.*

Assisting Clients with Total Hip Replacement

A major focus of postoperative care for clients with total hip replacement is to prevent dislocation of the hip prosthesis. All hip replacement clients will return from surgery with a triangular-shaped pillow between the legs. This is called an *abduction pillow*. It prevents the client from crossing the legs, which could cause the hip prosthesis to become dislocated.

- Instruct the client that crossing of the legs is not allowed. Teach the client not to flex the hip more than 90 degrees. Ensure that the client's bathroom is equipped with an elevated toilet seat. *Crossing the legs or flexing the hips too far can dislocate the hip prosthesis.*

Assisting Clients with Lyme Disease

- Instruct clients to prevent tick bites by wearing long-sleeved shirts and pants and using tick repellent. Advise clients to avoid tick-infested areas such as the woods to prevent being bitten by a tick. *These measures help decrease the chances of contracting Lyme disease.*
- Stress the importance of continuing to take all prescribed medication, even if all symptoms are gone. *Antibiotic therapy must be completed to be totally effective.*

EVALUATING

In evaluating the progress of treatment of the client with Lyme disease, the client should report an absence of rash and of joint pain and stiffness. The client should verbalize understanding of the importance of completing treatment as well as the need to inspect the body each day for ticks and also to inspect the family pet for the presence of any ticks.

Spinal Disorders

KYPHOSIS, LORDOSIS, AND SCOLIOSIS

The screening for scoliosis is generally done in a community setting (see Chapter 48 ⚭). Scoliosis as it relates to children is discussed in Chapter 61 ⚭.

Manifestations

Scoliosis is a lateral curve of the spine (Figure 31-13A ■). It occurs most commonly in adolescents. Treatment is discussed in Chapter 61 ⚭. The curve may be either C or S shaped. The most serious complication of scoliosis is a decrease in the size of the thoracic cavity. This decreased space limits the ability of the lungs to expand and can cause serious problems if not corrected. **Kyphosis** is a forward rounding of the thoracic spine (Figure 31-13B). It can be caused by poor posture or by disorders such as severe osteoporosis. **Lordosis** is an exaggeration of the lumbar curve of the spine. It is often seen in obesity and during pregnancy. It is also seen in individuals with weak muscles who take this stance to improve balance.

Diagnosis

X-rays of the spine will demonstrate the presence of scoliosis and the type and degree of the curvature. The client with scoliosis may complain that clothes do not fit properly. Back pain may also be reported. Kyphosis and lordosis are diagnosed by visual inspection and may be confirmed by x-ray.

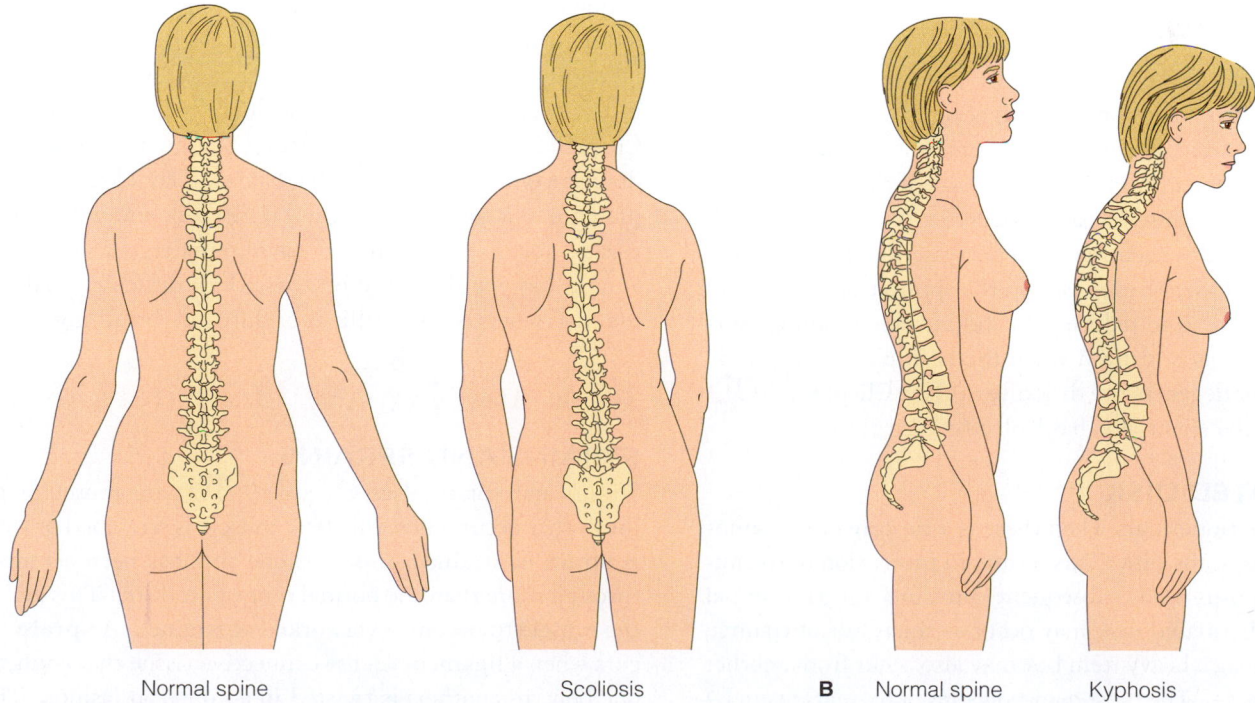

| A | Normal spine | Scoliosis | B | Normal spine | Kyphosis |

Figure 31-13. ■ **A.** Scoliosis, a lateral curvature of the spine. **B.** Kyphosis, exaggerated posterior curvature of the thoracic spine.

Treatment

Clients with kyphosis are instructed in the importance of proper posture. Medications for conditions such as osteoporosis will be prescribed. Clients with lordosis are advised to lose weight. Scoliosis may be treated conservatively with the use of exercise and bracing. Surgical treatment is recommended if the curve is significant. The most common surgical intervention is to fuse the spine and insert metal rods on either side of the fused spine to stabilize it.

LOW BACK PAIN

Low back pain is often muscular in nature, caused by twisting or straining of the muscles and tendons of the lower back. It may also be caused by a degenerative or herniated disk.

Manifestations

The client reports pain in the lumbar, lumbosacral, or the sacroiliac region of the back. The pain may be described as severe and sharp or dull and achy. It may be constant or intermittent. The client may report the pain as localized to a specific portion of the back or radiating down either leg. The pain may occur when changing positions, be brought on by specific positions, or be never ending. It is important to take a careful history of the client with special attention to events that preceded the pain and those events that aggravate the pain.

Diagnosis

It may be difficult to determine the exact cause of low back pain. An x-ray will be taken to determine if there is a skeletal cause for the pain. An MRI may be used to locate specific soft tissue abnormalities. Often, no specific cause for the pain can be determined.

Treatment

Treatment involves a combination of interventions. NSAIDs are used to decrease pain and inflammation. Muscle relaxants are used for a limited period of time if the pain is determined to be a muscle spasm. Bed rest is contraindicated. This has actually been found to decrease mobility over the long term. Moderate exercise and the application of heat and cold are also used to reduce pain and increase mobility. Surgical correction is utilized when the back pain is caused by herniated or degenerative disk disease. (See Chapter 29 ⚭ for care of the client who has had surgery.)

HERNIATED DISK

Disk herniation occurs when there is a rupture of the annulus fibrosus of the disk. This results in protrusion of the nucleus pulposus and subsequent pressure on the spinal nerves. A herniated disk may occur as the result of trauma, such as lifting a heavy item but may also occur from another disease process. The most common sites of herniation are L4 or L5 to S1 and C6 to C7.

Manifestations

The client reports pain often described as excruciating. With a lumbar disk herniation, the client may experience pain in the lower back that may radiate from the hip down the leg, muscle spasms, numbness and tingling of the leg, and possible decreased or absent knee and ankle reflexes. A client experiencing a cervical herniation may report pain in the neck and shoulder radiating down the arm, numbness and tingling in the shoulder and arm, and decreased arm strength.

Diagnosis

Diagnosis consists of x-ray, CT scan, and MRI of the area. A myelogram may also be done.

Treatment

Initial treatment involves pain management with NSAID and muscle relaxants. Conservative treatment includes heat applications and physical therapy. Epidural steroid injections can also be used. If the client does not obtain relief with conservative treatment, then surgery may be indicated. Surgery is also indicated in clients experiencing severe neurological deficits. Surgical options include laminectomy and spinal fusion.

A laminectomy is the removal of a portion of the vertebral lamina. A diskectomy may also be done to remove the nucleus pulposus, alone or in combination with a laminectomy. Spinal fusion is the insertion of a piece of bone between the vertebrae. Spinal fusion is done to stabilize the vertebrae.

Nursing Considerations

Following spinal surgery the client will need to be monitored for neurovascular complications. Along with monitoring vital signs, the nurse will also perform neurovascular checks. The client is turned using the logrolling technique (see Chapter 23, Procedure 23-2, Part C ⚭). The presence of drainage on the dressing with a halo sign could indicate the presence of a cerebrospinal fluid (CSF) leak and will require testing for glucose. Client's having undergone a cervical laminectomy will need to be assessed for difficulty swallowing, hoarseness, neck swelling, or difficulty breathing.

Joint and Muscle Disorders

STRAINS AND SPRAINS

Strains and sprains (see Chapter 9 ⚭) are muscular injuries that occur when a skeletal muscle is stretched or torn. A **strain** or strained muscle is one that has been extended through more than the normal range of motion. This allows the muscle to become overworked or strained. A **sprain** occurs when a ligament (dense connective tissue that connects one bone to another) is twisted in an unusual fashion. This causes tearing of the ligament involved. If the tear is extensive, the joint may become unstable. Repetitive motion injuries (such as *carpal tunnel syndrome*) are this type of injury.

Manifestations

The client complains of pain at the site of the injury. For both strains and sprains, swelling and lack of motion of the affected joint will be present.

Diagnosis and Treatment

X-rays may be taken to rule out fracture. Treatment of strains and sprains is known as RICE:

R   Rest
I   Ice
C   Compression
E   Elevation

Additionally, the sprained joint may be immobilized. If the sprain is in a weightbearing joint, the client may be advised to use crutches for 2 or 3 weeks to facilitate healing.

CARPAL TUNNEL SYNDROME

Carpal tunnel syndrome is a repetitive use injury that compresses the median nerve. This compression occurs as the result of inflammation and swelling of the tendons.

Manifestations

The client presents with numbness and tingling of the index finger, thumb, and middle finger. The pain may disrupt the client's sleep. Symptoms can progress to affecting the client's ability to perform activities that require precise movements.

Diagnosis

Diagnosis is confirmed by physical examination and history of a job that involves repetitive motion such as computer work.

Treatment

Pharmacologic treatment may include the use of NSAIDs or corticosteroid injections. Immobilization of the joint along with ice and then heat applications may also be used. Surgical intervention to enlarge the tunnel is also an option.

TEMPOROMANDIBULAR JOINT DISORDER

Temporomandibular joint disorder or TMJ disorder is common in adults. The TMJ provides the movements for chewing, swallowing, and speaking.

Manifestations

A client with TMJ disorder may experience any of the following symptoms: jaw pain, limited or painful jaw movement, headache, neck pain or stiffness, clicking or grating sound with movement, and a possible inability to open the mouth without pain. Often clients do not seek medical treatment for these symptoms.

Diagnosis

Diagnosis is based on physical assessment.

Treatment

Treatment is conservative. Acetaminophen or NSAID may be used for pain. Injections of local anesthetics or corticosteroids into the TMJ may be used.

DISLOCATIONS

A **dislocation** is an event that occurs when the end of the bone is no longer articulated in the joint capsule. Dislocations can occur as the result of trauma, such as a fall or during contact sports such as football. A dislocation can also occur following joint replacement surgery if positioning and movement precautions are not adhered to. This is seen most often with total hip replacements. A disease in the joint can cause a spontaneous dislocation. Although a dislocation can occur in any joint, the shoulder and hip are the two most common locations.

Manifestations

Client presents with pain, limited movement of the joint, and visible deformity. With a dislocated hip the affected leg will he shortened and internally rotated.

Diagnosis

Diagnosis is confirmed by physical examination and x-ray.

Treatment

Treatment consists of reducing the dislocation by manual reduction in the ER or operating room. Pain medication, muscle relaxants, and conscious sedation may be used to provide comfort for the client prior to a closed reduction.

NURSING CARE

PRIORITIZING NURSING CARE

Clients with strains and sprains need nursing care that is focused on decreasing pain and immobilizing the affected joint. Initially cold applications are applied and the limb is elevated to reduce swelling. Encourage the client to keep the extremity elevated and to avoid using it for a few days to several weeks, depending on the extent of the injury. Some healthcare providers recommend the use of heat after 48 hours, increasing circulation to the area to promote healing of soft tissue.

ASSESSING

One of the biggest concerns clients have when they suffer a sprain is whether or not the bone is broken. No one can tell simply by looking whether a joint is "only" sprained or whether a bone is broken. X-rays are the only way to determine this. Assess the joint for mobility, swelling, and pain. Note bruising and positioning. Clients may position the limb or joint in the most comfortable position, such as cradling a sprained wrist with the other hand.

DIAGNOSING, PLANNING, AND IMPLEMENTING

Possible nursing diagnoses for the client with a sprain or strain include:

- *Acute Pain*
- *Impaired Physical Mobility*

Heat and cold applications are used to treat the swelling and pain of strains and sprains. See Table 24-4 ⊙⊙ for the physiologic effects of heat and cold. Application of heat promotes soft tissue healing and increases **suppuration** (production of pus). Heat is often used for clients with musculoskeletal problems such as joint stiffness from arthritis, contractures, and low back pain. Advantages and disadvantages of heat and cold are reviewed in Table 31-5 ■.

Individuals vary in their tolerance of heat and cold. People with certain conditions require added caution in the use of heat or cold applications (Box 31-4 ■).

EVALUATING

The client should report decreased swelling and pain as well as improved mobility of the joint. The client should be instructed to resume normal activities slowly to prevent reinjuring the area.

Other Disorders

SYSTEMIC LUPUS ERYTHEMATOSUS

Systemic lupus erythematosus (SLE) is a chronic connective tissue disease that is inflammatory and is caused by an autoimmune disorder. Clients with SLE will present with

BOX 31-4	CLIENTS WITH RISK FACTORS FOR HEAT AND COLD APPLICATIONS

- People who cannot feel heat or cold normally
- People with altered level of consciousness
- People with mental confusion

Risks for Heat

- People with peripheral vascular disease, diabetes, or congestive heart failure (circulation is unable to dissipate heat)
- People who have recently been injured or had surgery (heat increases bleeding and swelling)

Risk for Cold

- People with open wounds (cold can decrease blood flow to the wound, thereby inhibiting healing)

complaints of fatigue, joint pain, fever, anorexia, and weight loss. Many clients with SLE will manifest a butterfly-shaped rash on the face (see Figure 35-13 ⊙⊙). SLE affects more women than men, and the first symptoms usually appear during the childbearing years. It is characterized by periods of outbreaks followed by periods of remission. As in RA, stress may cause an outbreak to occur. See Chapter 35 ⊙⊙ for the major discussion of this disorder.

FIBROMYALGIA

Fibromyalgia is a disorder that causes muscular pain, especially in the trunk and extremities. Some individuals report facial pain. It is believed that fibromyalgia is caused by a sleep disorder.

Manifestations

The client with fibromyalgia reports great fatigue, muscle stiffness, and pain. Most clients report that the pain and exhaustion prevent normal, daily activities. (*Note:* Clients with fibromyalgia or chronic fatigue syndrome have a manifestation of ongoing fatigue. Chronic fatigue syndrome is discussed in Chapter 36 ⊙⊙.)

TABLE 31-5	Advantages and Disadvantages of Heat and Cold Therapy	
TYPE OF THERAPY	**ADVANTAGES**	**DISADVANTAGES**
Heat applications	Increases blood flow that carries oxygen, nutrients, antibodies, and leukocytes to the affected area Promotes soft tissue healing	Increases suppuration Increases capillary permeability, which may lead to edema If used over large body area, may cause drop in blood pressure, increasing risk for falls
Cold applications	Limits postinjury swelling and bleeding May reduce pain by numbing the area	Causes vasoconstriction, which reduces blood flow (oxygen, nutrients, leukocytes) to the area, decreases removal of waste May increase pain (for example, in some clients with arthritis) Impairs circulation May cause increase in blood pressure as peripheral circulation is redirected to internal blood vessels and vital organs

Diagnosis

Fibromyalgia is diagnosed by the client's symptoms. There is no specific laboratory assessment that will demonstrate the presence of fibromyalgia. Most physicians will diagnose fibromyalgia if pain can be caused by palpating specific trigger points that usually cause pain in clients with fibromyalgia.

Treatment

Treating the sleep disorder is of primary importance. Medication is used to return the client to a normal sleep pattern. NSAIDs are used to ease the pain and stiffness of this disorder. The client is encouraged to get regular exercise to maintain muscle strength and mobility. The treatment goal for fibromyalgia is a normal sleep pattern and a decrease in fatigue, pain, and stiffness.

NURSING CARE

PRIORITIZING NURSING CARE

When caring for clients with SLE and/or fibromyalgia, focus your care on alleviating pain and stress. Stress increases symptoms of both disorders and clients frequently need to verbalize the stresses in their lives as they sort out ways to cope with them. Help clients identify medications and treatments that are most effective in relieving their pain. Promoting sleep is also a nursing priority. Keep the environment quiet and conducive to rest, with lights low. Do not interrupt sleep for routine procedures unless absolutely necessary.

ASSESSING

It is important to assess these clients for patterns in their symptom cycles, as well as any activities or stresses that tend to bring on symptoms. Sleep patterns and factors that interrupt sleep are also important.

DIAGNOSING, PLANNING, AND IMPLEMENTING

Possible nursing diagnoses for these clients include:

- *Risk for Infection* related to impaired immune system
- *Risk for Impaired Skin Integrity* related to facial skin changes
- *Acute Pain* related to joint involvement

SLE is a disease with many manifestations. The following interventions may assist clients in promoting health and preventing exacerbations of the disease:

- Encourage clients to decrease stress in their lives. Assist them in identifying stressors and positive coping strategies for dealing with them. *Stress causes exacerbations of these illnesses.*
- Teach and evaluate pain management techniques. *Pain medications must be evaluated so the most effective ones can be used to treat the pain.*
- Teach clients with SLE to limit the time they are in direct sunlight, to wear protective clothing such as a wide brim hat and long sleeves when in the sun, and to wear sunscreen. *Sun exposure can exacerbate the butterfly rash of SLE and other symptoms.*
- Teach clients with SLE to recognize fever, rash, cough, and increased joint pain as signs of an exacerbation. Also, instruct these clients in signs and symptoms of infection and monitor for signs of infection. *Because their white cell count is often low, these clients are at risk for developing infections. They should contact their physician quickly if these symptoms occur.*
- Advise clients with SLE to see their physician regularly. *This helps the physician detect any major organ involvement early so it can be treated quickly.*
- If clients are taking Plaquenil, they should be instructed to see an eye care professional on a regular basis. *The side effects of Plaquenil include retinopathy (see Chapter 42 ⚭).*
- Allow clients to verbalize distress and frustration. Offer your support. Refer them to the Lupus Foundation of America. *Clients with SLE have been diagnosed with a chronic and incurable disease. They need assistance and encouragement in order to cope.*

EVALUATING

To evaluate the client with systemic lupus erythematosus, the nurse would compare the client's perception of symptoms before and after treatment. The nurse would help the client to recognize anything that causes an increase in symptoms.

Note: The references and resources for all chapters have been compiled at the back of the book.

PROCEDURE 31-1 | Applying Traction

Purposes

- To ensure appropriate traction is applied
- To ensure proper body alignment is maintained
- To maintain safety and prevent further injury

Equipment

- Poles, pulleys, rope, weight, pads as ordered
- Elastic wrap for external traction

Check order **+** Gather equipment **+** Introduce yourself **+** Identify client **+** Provide privacy **+** Explain procedure **+** Hand hygiene **+** Gloves as needed

Interventions and Rationales

1. Perform preparatory steps (see icon bar above).

2. Place weights as ordered.

3. Apply traction as ordered to affected extremity. *Proper weights and placement will ensure correct treatment.*

4. Make the following assessments every 30 minutes initially, and then every 1 to 2 hours when stable:
   - Proper position of traction
   - Proper body alignment

clinical ALERT

When assessing neurovascular status in a pediatric client with musculoskeletal injury, the nurse looks for CMS:

- **c**irculation
- **m**ovement
- **s**ensation

Observe and document the five Ps: **P**aresthesia, **P**ain/pressure, **P**allor, **P**aralysis, **P**ulselessness.

- Neurovascular status of extremity; report any of the following: decreased or absent pulses, change in color of skin above or below sight of traction, warmth of the extremity, decreased sensation, decreased capillary refill, increased edema, limited movement of extremity, or pain, burning or tingling
- Condition of skin under and around traction application

- Skin over bony prominences
- Vital signs
- Pain
- Emotional state

These assessments will ensure quality of care.

5. Perform sterile pin care according to agency policy for internal traction or as ordered by physician. *Sterile cleansing is necessary to prevent introduction of microorganisms to compromised skin.*

6. Provide teaching and evaluation of technique if the family will maintain traction at home. *Client teaching and return demonstration will provide the family with the knowledge and skills they need to support the healing process.*

SAMPLE DOCUMENTATION

[date] [time] Traction to left lower extremity applied per order. Toes warm, pink, with appropriate ROM. Client is without complaint at present. Verbalized understanding of plan of care. Video provided for distraction. Call bell within reach. _____

_____ L. Atchley LPN

Source: Adams, E.D., & Towle, M. (2009). *Pediatric nursing care.* Upper Saddle River, NJ: Pearson Prentice Hall.

Chapter Review

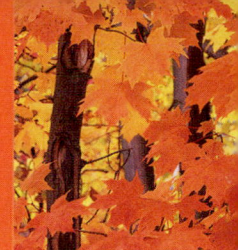

KEY Points

- Always immobilize an injured extremity until the type of injury is confirmed.
- Anaphylactic reaction is a life-threatening condition that must be reported and handled immediately.
- Injuries to the musculoskeletal system may result in complications related to immobility.
- Trauma to the tissues must be cared for carefully to prevent infection from occurring.
- Compartment syndrome can cause loss of limb; watch for pain, pallor, pulselessness, paralysis, and paresthesia.
- Clients with factures must be monitored carefully for complications such as fat emboli, compartment syndrome, deep vein thrombosis, and infection.
- All women should be given information related to prevention and treatment of osteoporosis.
- Heat and cold applications must be used carefully to prevent further injury to the tissues.
- Encourage the client with an amputation to be as independent as possible.
- Help the client with rheumatoid arthritis to understand the need for adequate rest to help prevent recurrent outbreaks of the disease.
- Prevention is an important component in the treatment of Lyme disease.

FOR FURTHER Study

For more discussion of strains and sprains, see Chapter 9.

See Chapter 17 for psychosocial issues and Chapter 18 for discussion of loss and grief.

Review the logrolling technique in Chapter 23, Procedure 23-2, Part C.

Review the major discussion of heat and cold applications in Chapter 24.

See Chapter 29 for care of the client who has had surgery.

For instructions on client use of an incentive spirometer, see Box 32-6.

See Chapter 35 for the major discussion of systemic lupus erythematosus.

Chronic fatigue syndrome is discussed in Chapter 36.

Retinopathy and osteoporosis in older adults are discussed in Chapter 42.

Figure 46-4 shows assistive devices used by clients to complete ADLs.

See Procedure 47-1 for splinting procedure.

The screening for scoliosis is provided in Chapter 48.

Fractures as they relate to children are covered in Chapter 60.

Chapter 61 discusses care of the child with scoliosis and care of the child with rheumatoid arthritis.

Critical Thinking Care Map

Caring for a Client with Rheumatoid Arthritis

NCLEX-PN® Focus Area: Physiologic Integrity

Case Study: Sharon Emelez, age 32, is the mother of four children. She has a 10-year-old girl and twin girls who are 22 months old. She also has a 5-year-old boy.

She comes to the physician's office with complaints of fever and swollen knee joints. She states she is fatigued and has lost weight recently. The physician diagnosed Ms. Emelez with rheumatoid arthritis.

Nursing Diagnosis: *Activity Intolerance*

COLLECT DATA

Subjective	Objective
_____	_____
_____	_____
_____	_____
_____	_____
_____	_____
_____	_____
_____	_____

Would you report this? Yes/No

If yes, report to: _____

What would you report? _____

Nursing Care

_____
_____
_____
_____
_____
_____
_____
_____
_____
_____
_____

How would you document this? _____
_____
_____
_____

Compare your answers and documentation to those provided on the MyNursingKit Website.

Data Collected
(use only those that apply)

- Fatigued
- Temperature 100.8°F
- Pulse 102, regular
- B/P 110/75
- Wt 112 (loss of 7 lbs)
- Awakens 2×/night
- Pain is 6 on a 0 to 10 scale
- Works part time
- Both knees swollen
- Both knees red
- Divorced
- Mother/2 hours away
- Receives WIC

Nursing Interventions
(use only those that apply; list in priority order)

- Instruct client in prescribed medication regime.
- Determine client's understanding of diagnosis of RA.
- Explore avenues of child care assistance.
- Discuss financial needs.
- Instruct client in relationship between adequate rest and acute episodes of disease.
- Review the use of heat and cold applications to assist with pain control.
- Explain need for well-balanced diet.

NCLEX-PN® Exam Preparation

1. The nurse, while teaching the staff about anatomy and physiology of the musculoskeletal system, explains that which of the following regulates bone resorption and bone deposit?
   1. Hormone activity and stress on the bones
   2. Biological modifiers
   3. Calcium intake
   4. Adequate supply of protein in the diet

2. When teaching the client how to provide self-care, the nurse explains the acronym RICE as useful for remembering how to:
   1. Determine if an injury is a strain or sprain.
   2. Locate the site of a fracture.
   3. Treat sprains and strains.
   4. Determine the time the injury should remain immobile.

3. When handling a damp plaster of Paris cast, the nurse should:
   1. Dry it with a handheld hair dryer set on high heat.
   2. Use the tips of the fingers to move the cast.
   3. Keep the client in one position until the cast has completely dried.
   4. Use the palms of the hands to manipulate the cast.

4. The nurse is preparing a client for arthroscopy when the client asks what the test is for. The nurse's best response would be:
   1. "Arthroscopy is done to evaluate the mass of the bone."
   2. "Arthroscopy is performed to look for torn or damaged ligaments."
   3. "Arthroscopy is done to evaluate the functioning of the joint."
   4. "I'll call the doctor because he should have explained that to you."

5. The client sustained a femur fracture of the right leg 2 days ago and is currently in skeletal traction. The client calls the nurse to the room to report severe pain at the site of the pin insertion. In assessing the leg the nurse notes the site is warm, edematous, and tender to touch. The nurse's priority action is to:
   1. Assist the client out of bed to help alleviate the pain.
   2. Notify the charge nurse.
   3. Massage the leg until it begins to feel better.
   4. Administer analgesia and reevaluate in 1 hour.

6. The nurse, working as a school nurse, examines a child found to have an exaggerated curve of the lumbar spine. The nurse instructs the parents to have the child evaluated by a physician for the possibility of:
   1. Scoliosis.
   2. Kyphosis.
   3. Lordosis.
   4. Ankylosing spondylitis.

7. The client, diagnosed with rheumatoid arthritis, asks the nurse why rest is so important. The nurse's best explanation would be that rest:
   1. Helps prevent acute episodes of rheumatoid arthritis.
   2. Makes the affected joints less stiff.
   3. Reduces the amount of medications needed for treatment.
   4. Prevents pain and deformity of the joints.

8. The nurse correctly instructs the client who has had hip replacement surgery to:
   1. Vigorously exercise the hip to prevent the formation of scar tissue.
   2. Cross the legs at the ankles instead of at the knees.
   3. Minimize use of the hip for 6 weeks until healing is complete.
   4. Never flex the hip greater than 90 degrees.

9. The nurse recognizes that which of the following clients is most at risk for developing osteoporosis?
   1. A 66-year-old African American woman
   2. A 57-year-old woman of European descent who smokes heavily
   3. A 51-year-old Caucasian man
   4. A 42-year-old Asian woman who drinks milk

10. The nurse instructs the client diagnosed with systemic lupus erythematous to do which of the following to reduce the recurrence of acute episodes?
    1. Dress warmly.
    2. Drink extra fluids.
    3. Exercise vigorously.
    4. Avoid exposure to direct sunlight.

Answers and rationales for Review Questions appear in Appendix I.

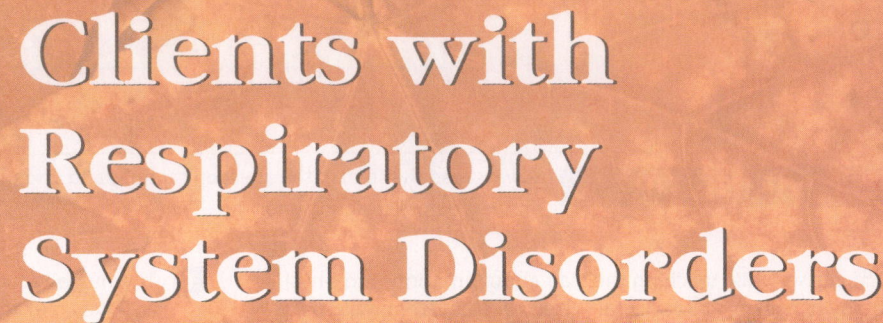

Clients with Respiratory System Disorders

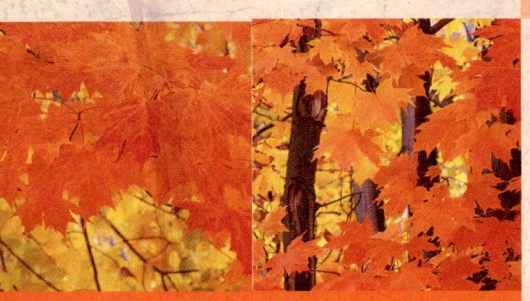

LEARNING Outcomes

After completing this chapter, you will be able to:

1. Outline the structure and function of the respiratory system.
2. Describe the processes of breathing (ventilation) and gas exchange (respiration).
3. Identify factors influencing respiratory function and oxygenation.
4. Name three major alterations in respiratory function and their manifestations.
5. List tests that are commonly done to diagnose respiratory disorders.
6. Name therapeutic measures used to promote respiratory function.
7. Identify nursing measures to promote oxygenation.
8. Name common disorders, manifestations, diagnostic measures, treatment, and nursing care for infections and inflammation of the upper respiratory system.
9. List common disorders, manifestations, diagnostic measures, treatment, and nursing care for trauma, obstruction, and tumors of the upper respiratory system.
10. Identify common disorders, manifestations, diagnostic measures, treatment, and nursing care for pulmonary embolism, pulmonary hypertension, chest trauma, inhalation injury, and near-drowning of the lower respiratory system.
11. Name common infections and inflammations of the lower respiratory system, including manifestations, diagnostic measures, treatment, and nursing care.
12. List obstructive disorders of the lower respiratory system, including manifestations, diagnostic measures, treatment, and nursing care.
13. Describe manifestations, diagnostic measures, treatment, and nursing care for clients with lung cancer and interstitial disorders.

Clinical Objectives

14. Obtain a throat and/or sputum culture from an assigned client.
15. Demonstrate competency in the use of pulse oximetry.
16. Demonstrate procedures for administering oxygen therapy.
17. Provide tracheostomy care and cleaning.
18. Demonstrate competency in oropharynx and nasopharyngeal suctioning techniques.
19. Demonstrate knowledge of normal hemoglobin and hematocrit, and the effects on the respiratory system.
20. Demonstrate competency in listening to and identifying lung sounds and breathing patterns.
21. Develop a plan of care for clients with chronic respiratory dysfunction.

KEY TERMS

Use the audio glossary feature on the MyNursingKit Website to hear the correct pronunciation of the following key terms.

asphyxiation 820
atelectasis 827
bronchitis 821
chronic obstructive pulmonary disease 824
clubbing 827
cor pulmonale 819
diffusion 793
emphysema 825
expiration 793
hematocrit 794
hemoglobin 794

hemothorax 809
hypercapnia 795
hypercarbia 795
hyperventilation 796
hypoxemia 795
hypoxia 795
induration 822
inspiration 793
Kussmaul respiration 796
lung abscess 822
mesothelioma 828
pleural effusion 822

pneumoconioses 828
pneumothorax 829
pulmonary function tests 797
retractions 793
shortness of breath 796
sputum 797
status asthmaticus 824
suctioning 804
tracheostomy 801
tubercle 822
ventilation 791

Oxygen, a clear, odorless gas that constitutes about 21 percent of the air we breathe, is necessary for all living cells. The absence of oxygen leads to death. Although the delivery of oxygen to body tissues is affected, at least indirectly, by all body systems, the respiratory system is central to this process. Impaired function of the respiratory system can significantly affect our ability to breathe and participate in everyday activities.

Respiration is the process of gas exchange between the individual and the environment. The process of respiration involves several components:

1. Pulmonary **ventilation** (breathing)—the movement of air between the atmosphere and the alveoli of the lungs
2. Diffusion of oxygen and carbon dioxide between the alveoli and pulmonary capillaries
3. Transport of oxygen and carbon dioxide in the blood to and from tissues
4. Diffusion of oxygen and carbon dioxide between the capillaries and the cells of body tissues

Structure and Function of the Respiratory System

Structures of the respiratory system function to move air, eliminate waste products, maintain acid-base balance, and protect the airway from infection. The primary function of the respiratory system is respiration, also known as gas exchange. The respiratory system consists of the lungs and the passages that lead to them. This system brings oxygen into the body where it enters the blood and is transported to all tissues of the body. Additionally, the respiratory system removes carbon dioxide, a waste product of cellular metabolism, from the body.

The respiratory system is structurally divided into the upper respiratory tract and the lower respiratory tract. The mouth, nose, pharynx, and larynx compose the upper respiratory tract (Figure 32-1 ■). The lower respiratory tract includes the trachea and lungs, with the bronchi, bronchioles, alveoli, pulmonary capillary network, and pleural membranes (Figure 32-2 ■).

Air enters through the nose, where it is warmed, humidified, and filtered. Large particles in the air are trapped by the hairs at the entrance of the *nares* (nostrils), and smaller particles are filtered and trapped by the *nasal turbinates* and septum inside the nose (see Figure 32-1). The sneeze reflex is initiated by irritants in nasal passages. During a sneeze, a large volume of air exits rapidly through the nose and mouth, helping to clear nasal passages.

Inspired air passes from the nose through the *pharynx*, commonly known as the throat. The pharynx is a shared pathway for air and food, divided into the nasopharynx, the oropharynx, and the laryngopharynx. It is richly supplied with lymphoid tissue that traps and destroys pathogens entering with the air.

The *larynx* can be identified externally, especially in men, and is known as the Adam's apple. In addition to its role in speech, the larynx is important for maintaining airway patency and protecting the lower airways from swallowed food and fluids. During swallowing, the inlet to the larynx (the epiglottis) closes, routing food to the esophagus. The epiglottis is open during breathing, allowing air to move freely into the lower airways.

Below the larynx, the trachea leads to the right and left main bronchi (primary bronchi) and the airways of the lungs. Within the lungs, the primary bronchi divide repeatedly into smaller and smaller bronchi, ending with the terminal bronchioles. Together these airways are

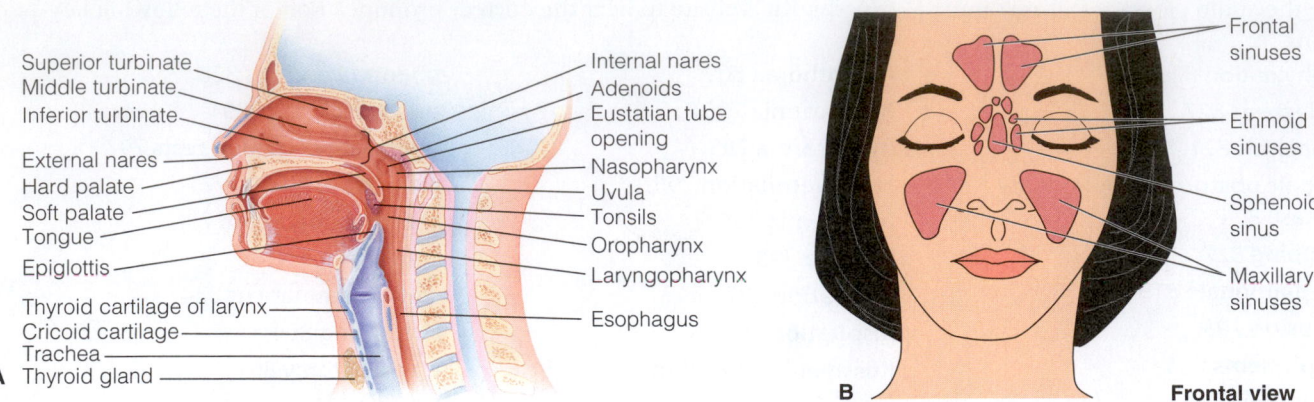

Figure 32-1. ■ **A.** Upper respiratory system. **B.** The sinuses.

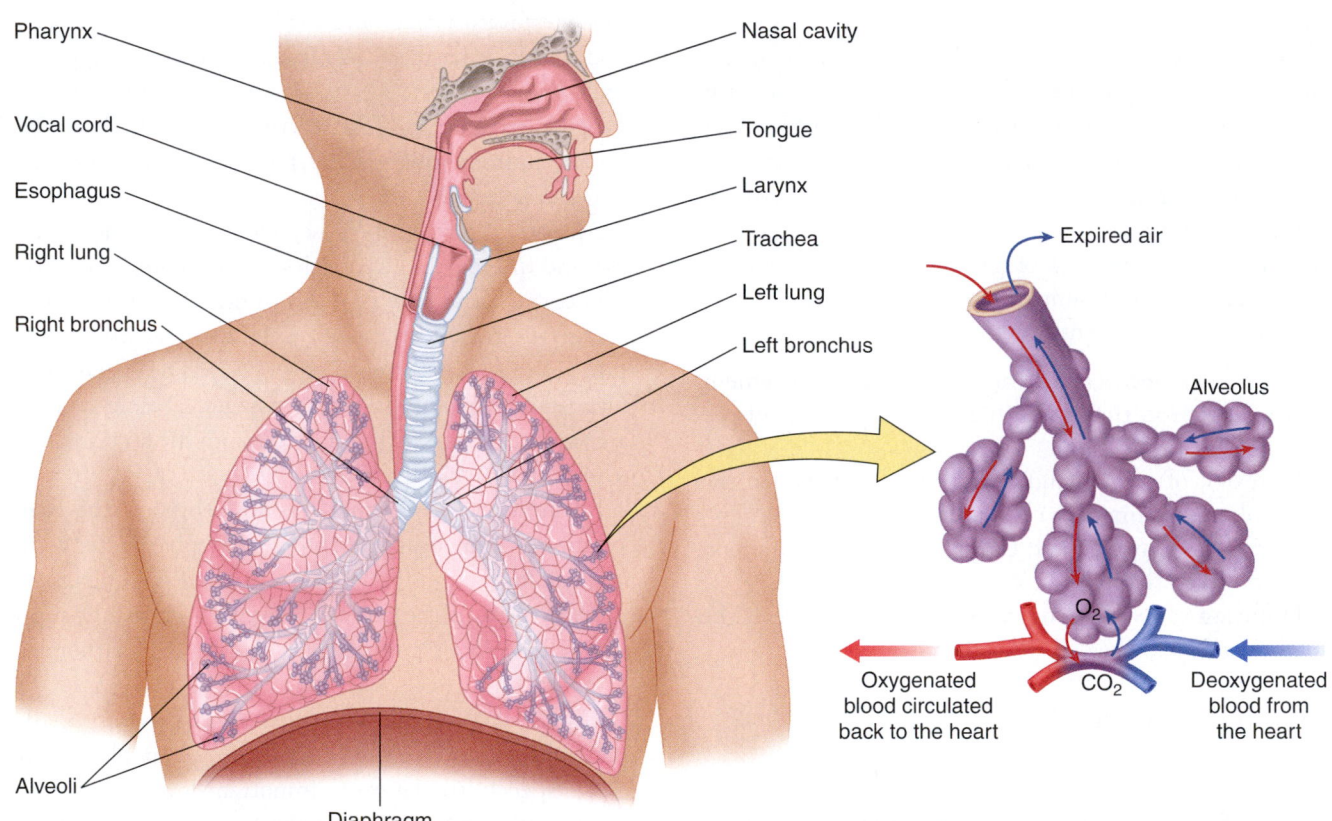

Figure 32-2. ■ Respiratory system. *Inset:* Exchange of oxygenated and deoxygenated air at the alveolar level.

known as the *bronchial tree*. The trachea and bronchi are lined with cells that produce a thin layer of mucus to trap pathogens and microscopic matter. These foreign particles are then swept upward toward the larynx and throat by *cilia*, tiny hairlike projections on the epithelial cells. The cough reflex is triggered by irritants in the larynx, trachea, or bronchi.

The respiratory zone of the lungs includes the respiratory bronchioles, the alveolar ducts, and the alveoli (see Figure 32-2). Until air enters the respiratory bronchioles and alveoli, no gas exchange occurs. Alveoli have very thin walls, composed of a single layer of epithelial cells covered by a thick mesh of pulmonary capillaries. The alveolar and capillary walls form the membrane where gas exchange occurs.

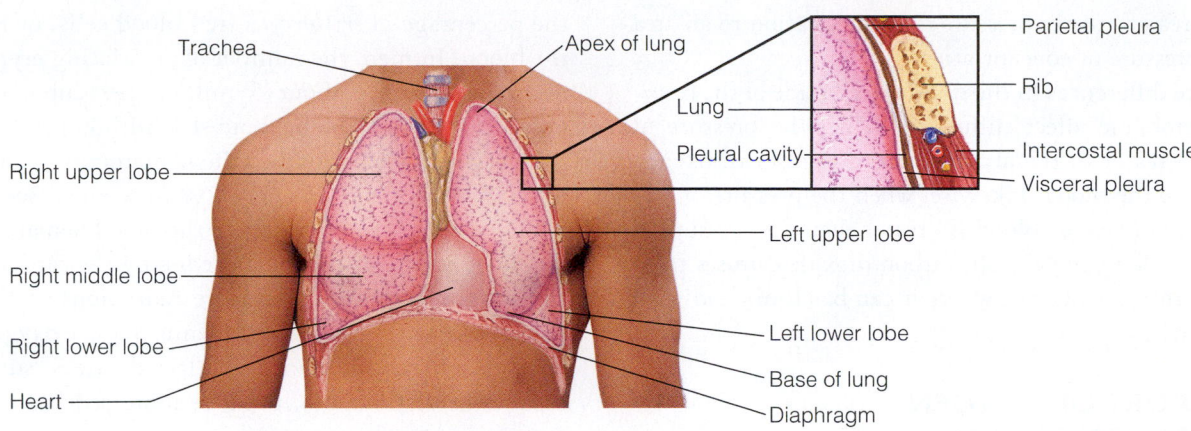

Figure 32-3. ■ The lower respiratory system, showing the layers of visceral and parietal pleura.

The outer surface of the lungs is covered by a thin, double layer of tissue known as the *pleura* (Figure 32-3 ■). The pleura has two parts:

1. The parietal pleura lines the thorax and surface of the diaphragm.
2. The visceral pleura (see Figure 32-3 *inset*) covers the external surface of the lungs.

Between these pleural layers is a space that contains a small amount of pleural fluid, a serous lubricating solution. This fluid prevents friction during the movements of breathing and keeps the layers adherent, much as a film of water can cause two glass slides to cling to each other.

PULMONARY VENTILATION

Ventilation (breathing) is accomplished through **inspiration** (inhalation), when air flows into the lungs, and **expiration** (exhalation), when air moves out of the lungs. If inflammation, edema, and/or excessive mucus production occur, small airways become clogged with these materials and block the walls of the airway, preventing gas exchange, which impairs ventilation. The more airways that are blocked in this manner, the greater the symptoms of respiratory distress that will be seen.

The respiratory centers of the medulla and pons in the brainstem control breathing. Severe head injury or drugs that depress the central nervous system (e.g., opiates or barbiturates) can affect the respiratory centers, impairing the drive to breathe.

The degree of chest expansion during normal breathing is minimal and requires little energy. However, when disease, trauma, or obstruction exists, the client must use accessory muscles of respiration, including the anterior neck muscles, intercostal muscles, and muscles of the abdomen (Figure 32-4 ■), to move air into and out of the chest. This use of accessory muscles for respiration is called **retractions.**

ALVEOLAR GAS EXCHANGE

The second phase of the respiratory process is the diffusion of oxygen from the alveoli into the pulmonary blood vessels. **Diffusion** is the movement of gases or other particles

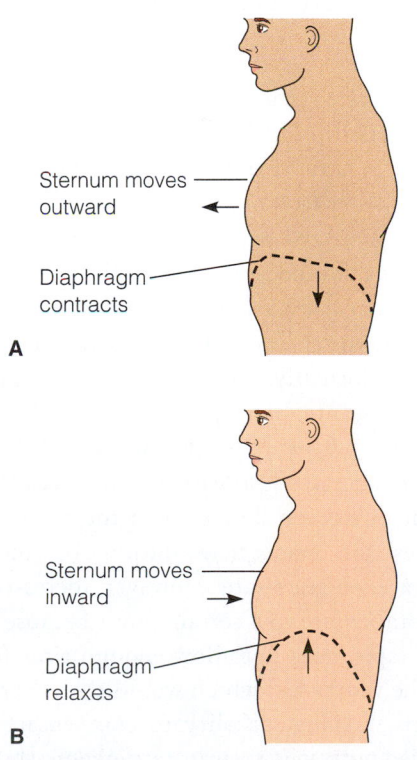

Figure 32-4. ■ **A.** During inspiration, the diaphragm contracts and flattens, and the intercostal muscles contract, moving the chest wall upward and outward. This increases the volume of the chest cavity. **B.** During expiration, the muscles relax, the diaphragm rises, and the lungs recoil.

from an area of greater pressure or concentration to an area of lower pressure or concentration.

Pressure differences in the gases on each side of the respiratory membrane affect diffusion. When the pressure of oxygen is greater in the alveoli than in the blood, oxygen diffuses into the blood. Likewise, when the pressure of carbon dioxide in venous blood is greater than the pressure of carbon dioxide in the alveoli, carbon dioxide diffuses from the blood into the alveoli, where it can be eliminated with expired air.

TRANSPORT OF OXYGEN AND CARBON DIOXIDE

The third part of the respiratory process involves the transport of respiratory gases. Oxygen needs to be transported from the lungs to the tissues, and carbon dioxide must be transported from the tissues back to the lungs. Normally, 97% of the oxygen combines loosely with **hemoglobin** (an oxygen-carrying red pigment) in the red blood cells. It is carried to the tissues as *oxyhemoglobin* (the compound of oxygen and hemoglobin). The remaining oxygen is dissolved and transported in the fluid of the plasma and cells.

Factors that Influence Respiratory Function

Several factors affect the rate of oxygen transport from the lungs to the tissues: cardiac output, number of *erythrocytes* (red blood cells), and exercise. When one of these factors changes, the other factors attempt to compensate to maintain a steady supply of oxygen to the tissues.

The amount of blood pumped by the heart is called cardiac output. Cardiac output is a product of heart rate and stroke volume, or the amount of blood ejected with each contraction. Normally, cardiac output is approximately 5 liters per minute. Any pathologic condition that decreases cardiac output (e.g., damage to the heart muscle, blood loss, or increased pressure in the arteries) diminishes the amount of oxygen delivered to the tissues. The heart compensates for inadequate output by increasing its pumping rate, or heart rate. However, increased heart rate can only compensate to a certain point because a heart rate that is too rapid does not allow enough time for adequate filling of the ventricles, which would then decrease cardiac output further. This inability to compensate for diminished cardiac output is seen in cardiogenic shock, congestive heart failure, or significant heart damage as might be seen in myocardial infarctions.

Another factor influencing oxygen transport is the number of erythrocytes. **Hematocrit** is a measurement of the percentage of *erythrocytes* (red blood cells, or RBCs) in the blood. In men, the number of circulating erythrocytes normally averages about 5 million per cubic milliliter of blood, and in women, about 4.5 million per cubic milliliter. The normal range of the hematocrit is about 40% to 54% in men and 37% to 47% in women (see Chapter 34 ⬤⬤). Excessive increases in the blood hematocrit raise the blood *viscosity* (thickness), reducing the cardiac output and oxygen transport. Excessive reductions in the blood hematocrit, such as occurs in anemia, reduce oxygen transport. People who live in high altitude areas, such as the mountains of Colorado, produce more red blood cells to compensate for the decrease in oxygen percentage found in the air at higher altitudes.

Exercise also has a direct influence on oxygen transport. Every muscle movement uses extra oxygen, so exercise increases the need for oxygen. In well-trained athletes, oxygen transport can be increased up to 20 times the normal rate, due in part to an increased cardiac output and to efficient use of oxygen by the cells. However, in clients whose ability to supply adequate oxygen to the tissues is compromised at rest, even minimal activity can push them beyond their ability to oxygenate the tissues.

RESPIRATORY REGULATION

Respiratory rate and depth are controlled by nerves and the concentration of certain gases in the blood. The brain regulates respirations to maintain correct concentrations of oxygen, carbon dioxide, and hydrogen ions in the body fluids.

An area in the medulla of the brain is highly responsive to increases in blood carbon dioxide (CO_2). When CO_2 or hydrogen ion concentration increases, the brain increases the rate and depth of respirations. In addition, special nerve receptors are sensitive to decreases in oxygen (O_2) concentration in the blood. When they sense decreases in the amount of oxygen in the arteries, they stimulate the respiratory center to increase respirations.

Of the three blood gases (hydrogen, oxygen, and carbon dioxide), increased carbon dioxide concentration normally stimulates respiration most strongly. (See also the discussion of acid-base balance in Chapter 26 ⬤⬤.)

ALTERATIONS IN RESPIRATORY FUNCTION

Respiratory function can be altered by conditions that affect:

- The movement of air into or out of the lungs.
- The diffusion of oxygen and carbon dioxide between the alveoli and the pulmonary capillaries.
- The transport of oxygen and carbon dioxide through the blood to and from the tissue cells.

Three major alterations in respiration are hypoxia, altered breathing patterns, and an obstructed or partially obstructed airway.

Hypoxia

Hypoxia is a condition of insufficient oxygen anywhere in the body. The inhaled air may lack enough oxygen, or an insufficient amount of oxygen may be delivered to the tissues. It can be related to ventilation, diffusion of gases, or transport of gases by the blood. It can be caused by any condition that alters one or more parts of the respiratory process.

Hypoventilation, or inadequate exchange of gases through the alveoli, can lead to hypoxia. Hypoventilation may be due to respiratory diseases, drugs, or anesthesia. It often causes **hypercarbia** or **hypercapnia.** Shallow or slow respirations would result in hypoventilation.

Hypoxia can also develop when oxygen does not diffuse effectively into the arterial blood (as in pulmonary edema). (The term **hypoxemia** refers to reduced oxygen in the blood only.) Hypoxia can also result from problems in the delivery of oxygen to the tissues. This occurs with anemia,

---

BOX 32-1   POPULATION FOCUS

Clients with COPD

Low-flow oxygen systems are essential for clients with COPD. People with COPD may have a chronically high carbon dioxide level. Their stimulus to breathe is not high levels of carbon dioxide but low levels of oxygen (*hypoxemia*). High flows of oxygen can potentially relieve this hypoxemia, but may also remove the stimulus to breathe. Low flows maintain a slightly hypoxemic state, thus maintaining the respiratory drive. Clients who have COPD and are receiving oxygen therapy should be observed carefully (especially when therapy is first initiated) for respiratory depression or arrest.

BOX 32-2   MANIFESTATIONS OF HYPOXIA

- Rapid pulse
- Rapid, shallow respirations and dyspnea
- Increased restlessness or light-headedness
- Flaring of the nares
- Substernal or intercostal retractions
- Cyanosis

---

heart failure, and pulmonary embolism. Box 32-2 ■ lists manifestations of hypoxia.

Cyanosis (bluish discoloration of the skin, nail beds, and mucous membranes due to reduced hemoglobin–oxygen saturation) may be present with hypoxia. The brain can tolerate hypoxia for only 4 to 6 minutes before permanent damage occurs. The face of the acutely hypoxic person usually appears anxious, tired, and drawn. The person usually assumes a sitting position, often leaning forward slightly to permit greater expansion of the thoracic cavity. Note that cyanosis in children is more serious a manifestation than cyanosis in an adult (Box 32-3 ■).

With chronic hypoxia, the client often appears fatigued and is lethargic. The client's fingers and toes may be clubbed as a result of long-term lack of oxygen. With *clubbing*, the base of the nail becomes swollen and the ends of the fingers and toes increase in size. The angle between the nail and the base of the nail increases to more than 180 degrees (see Figure 19-7D ○○).

Altered Breathing Patterns

Breathing patterns refer to the rate, volume, rhythm, and relative ease or effort of respiration. (See Chapter 21 ○○, the vital signs chapter, for an in-depth description of breathing patterns, chest movements, types of cough, and lung sounds.) Normal respiration (*eupnea*) is quiet, rhythmic, and effortless. Respirations are evenly spaced and vary little in depth. *Tachypnea* (rapid breathing rate) is seen with fevers, metabolic acidosis, pain, hypercapnia, respiratory distress, or hypoxemia. *Bradypnea* is an abnormally slow respiratory rate, which may be seen in clients who have taken narcotics, who have metabolic alkalosis, or who have increased intracranial pressure (e.g., from brain injuries). *Apnea* is defined as periods of no breathing. *Cheyne-Stokes* breathing is characterized by an increase and decrease in rate and depth of respirations followed by periods of apnea.

BOX 32-3   PEDIATRIC CONSIDERATIONS

Cyanosis in Children

Cyanosis is a *late* sign of hypoxia in young children. By the time cyanosis is seen, the child's oxygen saturation may be very low, and immediate intervention is required.

Hyperventilation is an increased rate and depth of respirations. In this situation, more CO_2 is eliminated than is produced. One particular type of hyperventilation that accompanies metabolic acidosis is called **Kussmaul respiration.** The body attempts to rid itself of excess body acids by blowing off the carbon dioxide through deep and rapid breathing. Hyperventilation also often occurs as a response to stress.

Abnormal respiratory rhythms create an irregular breathing pattern. With difficult or labored breathing (*dyspnea*), the client often appears anxious and may have **shortness of breath** (S.O.B). When a person is dyspneic, the nostrils may be flared because of the increased effort of inspiration, the skin may appear dusky, and there may be substernal (below the xiphoid process), suprasternal (above the clavicle and sternum), supraclavicular (above the clavicle), or intercostal (between the ribs) retractions assessed. Heart rate is increased.

Obstructed Airway

A completely or partially obstructed airway can occur anywhere along the upper or lower respiratory tract. An obstruction of the nose, pharynx, or larynx is an *upper airway obstruction*. It can be caused by a foreign object such as food, by the tongue blocking the oropharynx when a person is unconscious, or by secretions collecting in the passageways. In the last instance, the respirations sound gurgly or bubbly as the air attempts to pass through the secretions. (Review Box 21-8 🔗 for terminology.) *Lower airway obstruction* involves partial or complete blockage of the passageways in the bronchi and lungs. This can be caused by bronchospasm; increased production of secretions; thick, sticky secretions; or bronchial inflammation.

Maintaining an open (*patent*) airway is a primary nursing responsibility that takes priority over other nursing interventions. A low-pitched snoring sound during inhalation indicates partial obstruction of the upper airways. Complete obstruction is indicated by extreme inspiratory effort that produces no chest movement and prevents the client from coughing or making any sound. *Intercostal retractions* (the drawing of skin and muscle against the ribs) indicate this extreme effort. Lower airway obstruction is not always as easy to observe. *Stridor* (a harsh, high-pitched sound) may be heard during inspiration. The client may have altered arterial blood gas levels, restlessness, dyspnea, and *adventitious* (abnormal) breath sounds. (See Table 19-4 and Box 21-8 🔗 for information about lung sounds.)

Factors that Affect Oxygenation

In the healthy person, the cardiovascular and respiratory systems can provide sufficient oxygen to meet the body's needs. However, certain factors can affect respirations and/or ventilation:

- Diseases of the cardiovascular and/or respiratory systems (e.g., anemia, congestive heart failure, COPD, pneumonia).
- Medications. Narcotics such as morphine and meperidine (Demerol) depress the respiratory center in the medulla, causing decreased respiratory depth and rate.
- Stress. When stressed, some people hyperventilate. Oxygen levels in arterial blood rise and carbon dioxide levels fall. This causes symptoms of dizziness, numbness of fingers and toes, and numbness around the mouth.
- Gender may affect cardiopulmonary function. Through middle adulthood (until menopause), estrogen has a protective effect in women, slowing the progress of atherosclerosis and reducing the risk of cardiovascular disease. Among people in their 40s and 50s, men have a higher incidence of hypertension than women.
- Race may affect cardiopulmonary function. African Americans are at increased risk for asthma and hypertension, which can interfere with oxygen perfusion.

Tests for Respiratory Disorders

A variety of tests provide important information for clients with respiratory disorders.

PULSE OXIMETRY

A pulse oximeter is a noninvasive device that measures oxygen saturation (SaO_2, or O_2 Sat). The pulse oximeter is connected to a sensor attached to the client's finger (Figure 32-5 ■), toe, nose, earlobe, or forehead (or around the hand or foot of a neonate). The sensor detects hypoxemia before clinical signs and symptoms develop.

The pulse oximeter uses infrared light and a process known as spectrophotometry to measure the amount of oxygenated hemoglobin in arterial blood. Normal SaO_2 is 95%

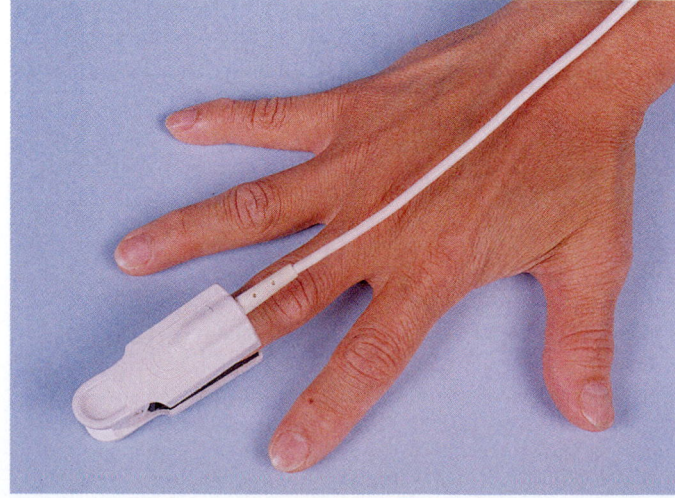

Figure 32-5. ■ A finger clip sensor for a pulse oximeter. (*Source:* © Jenny Thomas.)

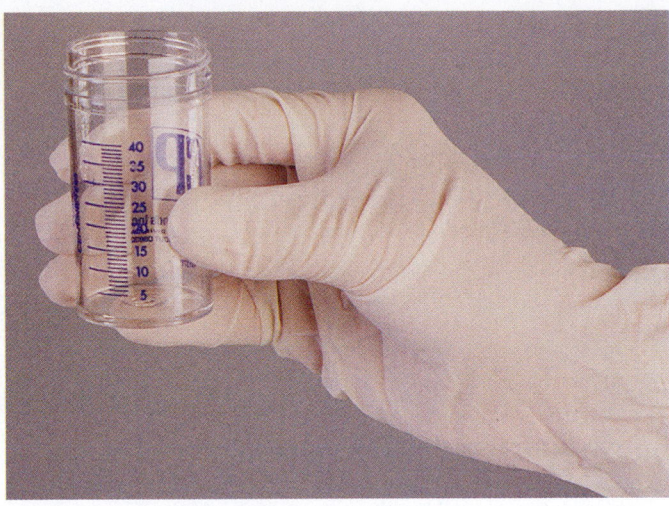

A

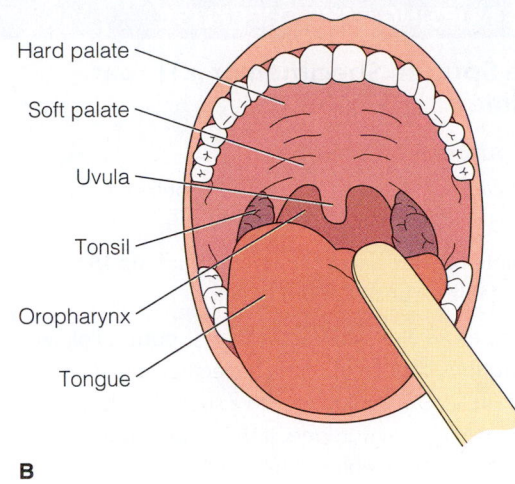

Hard palate

Soft palate

Uvula

Tonsil

Oropharynx

Tongue

B

Figure 32-6. ■ **A.** Sputum container. (*Source:* © Elena Dorfman.) **B.** Taking a throat culture.

to 100%. An SaO_2 below 70% is life threatening. Measurement of SaO_2 may be taken intermittently, often as an aspect of vital sign measurement, but it can also be continuously monitored. The procedure for using a pulse oximeter is described in Procedure 32-1 ■ at the end of the chapter. To obtain an accurate oxygen saturation reading, the probe must be placed on an area that is warm, well perfused, and still. Excess movement, reduced perfusion, or a cold area will all negatively impact the ability of the probe to assess oxygen saturation.

clinical ALERT

Pulse oximetry measures only the amount of oxygen that is bound with hemoglobin. Results can be misleading if the client's hemoglobin is bound to another substance, such as carbon monoxide.

DIAGNOSTIC STUDIES

The physician may order various diagnostic tests to assess respiratory status, function, and oxygenation. These tests include sputum specimens, throat cultures, skin testing for allergies, pulmonary function tests, and visualization procedures. Check the facility's policy for specimens that the LPN/LVN is responsible for collecting.

Specimens

Sputum is the mucus secreted by the lungs, bronchi, and trachea. It is important to differentiate it from saliva, the clear liquid secreted by the salivary glands in the mouth, sometimes referred to as "spit."

Healthy individuals produce smaller amounts of sputum than those with diseased lungs and would be unlikely to be able to produce enough for a specimen. Clients need to cough to bring sputum up from the lungs, bronchi, and trachea into the mouth in order to *expectorate* it (spit it out) into a collecting container (Figure 32-6A ■). The best time to collect a sputum specimen is first thing in the morning when there has been pooling of secretions secondary to the client's relatively fixed position during sleep.

A throat culture is collected from the mucosa of the oropharynx and tonsillar regions using a culture swab (Figure 32-6B). The sample is then cultured and examined for the presence of disease-producing microorganisms such as streptococci or staphylococci to name a few. Guidelines for obtaining a client sputum sample and a throat culture are provided in Box 32-4 ■.

Pulmonary Function Tests

Pulmonary function tests (PFTs) measure lung volume and capacity. Clients undergoing pulmonary function tests, which are usually carried out by a respiratory therapist, do not require an anesthetic. The client breathes into a tube attached to a machine and a computer. The tests are painless but often tiring, especially for clients with pulmonary or cardiac conditions. The test requires the client's full cooperation. Normal total lung capacity is 6,000 mL and vital capacity is 4,800 mL. PFTs also measure inspiratory reserve volume (3,100 mL), expiratory reserve volume (1,200 mL), and residual volume (1,200 mL). Figure 32-7 ■ illustrates lung volumes and capacities.

Visualization Procedures

A number of visualization procedures can be done to examine the respiratory tract and cardiovascular system. Roentgenography (x-ray), lung scan, *endoscopy* (in which a tube is threaded into the bronchus [bronchoscopy] or the larynx [laryngoscopy] for direct visualization), angiography, and echocar-

BOX 32-4 NURSING CARE CHECKLIST

Collecting a Sputum Specimen or a Throat Swab Specimen

Collecting a Sputum Specimen

☑ Offer mouth care so that the specimen will not be contaminated with microorganisms from the mouth.

☑ Ask the client to breathe deeply and then cough up 15 to 30 mL (1 or 2 tablespoons) of sputum.

☑ Wear gloves to avoid direct contact with the sputum. Follow special precautions if tuberculosis is suspected, obtaining the specimen in a room equipped with a special airflow system or ultraviolet light, or outdoors. If these options are not available, wear a mask capable of filtering droplet nuclei.

☑ Ask the client to *expectorate* (spit out) the sputum into the specimen container. Make sure the sputum does not contact the outside of the container (see Figure 32-6A). If the outside of the container does become contaminated, wash it with a disinfectant.

☑ Following sputum collection, offer mouthwash to remove any unpleasant taste.

☑ Document the amount of sputum collected, color, odor, consistency (thick, tenacious, watery), and presence of hemoptysis (blood in sputum).

Collecting a Throat Culture Specimen

☑ Don clean gloves.

☑ Insert the swab into the oropharynx, and run the swab along the tonsils and areas on the pharynx that are reddened or contain exudate. (The gag reflex is active in some clients. It may be decreased by having the client sit upright if health permits, open the mouth, extend the tongue, and say "ah," and by taking the specimen quickly.)

☑ If the posterior pharynx cannot be seen, use a light and depress the tongue with a tongue blade (see Figure 32-6B).

☑ Carefully place the swab into the culture container, being sure not to contaminate the outside of the container or the swab.

---

diography are a few visualization procedures. Bronchoscopy and laryngoscopy require numbing of the gag reflex and the client is usually sedated or anesthetized. Clients must be kept NPO until their gag reflex returns and should be assessed for any abnormal bleeding or airway obstruction.

Respiratory Therapies

OXYGEN THERAPY

Clients who have difficulty ventilating all areas of their lungs, have impaired gas exchange, or have perfusion problems (e.g., heart failure) may require oxygen therapy to prevent hypoxia. Oxygen can be administered via many different methods and concentrations.

Oxygen is classified as a medication and is prescribed by the physician, who specifies the concentration, method of delivery, and liter flow per minute. The nurse may initiate oxygen therapy in an emergency situation without an order, but an order should be obtained from the physician as soon as the situation allows. As mentioned earlier, a low-flow oxygen system is essential for clients who have chronic obstructive pulmonary disease (COPD). Safety precautions are essential during oxygen therapy. Box 32-5 ■ provides instructions for oxygen safety.

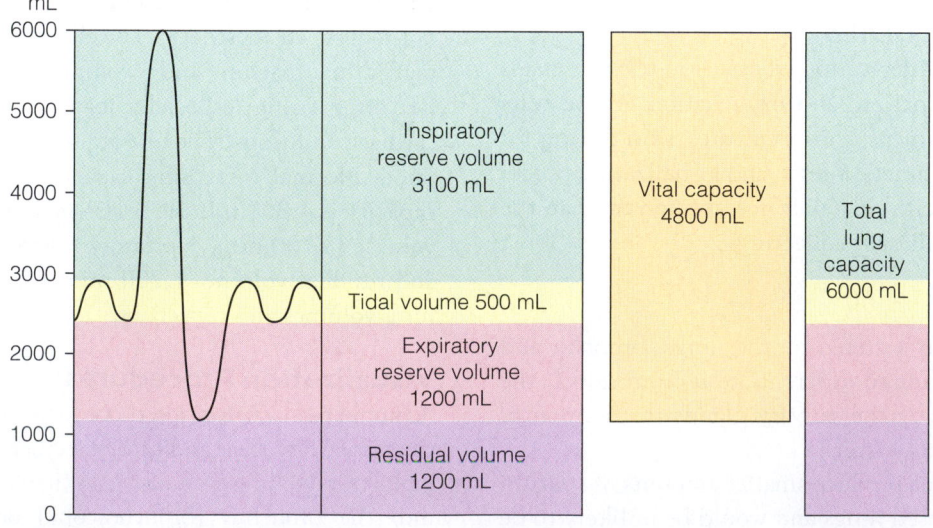

Figure 32-7. ■ The relationship of lung volumes and capacities. Volumes shown are for an average adult male.

BOX 32-5 NURSING CARE CHECKLIST

Oxygen Therapy Safety Precautions

- ☑ Place cautionary signs reading "No Smoking: Oxygen in Use" on the client's door, at the foot or head of the bed, and on the oxygen equipment.

- ☑ Handle and store oxygen cylinders with caution, and strap them securely in wheeled transport devices or stands to prevent possible falls and outlet breakages. Place them away from traffic areas and heaters.

- ☑ Instruct the client and visitors about the hazard of smoking with oxygen in use. Teach family members and roommates to smoke only outside or in provided smoking rooms away from the client.

- ☑ Make sure that electric devices (e.g., razors, hearing aids, radios, televisions, and heating pads) are in good working order to prevent the occurrence of short-circuit sparks.

- ☑ Avoid materials that generate static electricity, such as woolen blankets and synthetic fabrics. Advise clients and caregivers to wear cotton fabrics and use cotton blankets.

- ☑ Avoid the use of volatile, flammable materials, such as oils, greases, alcohol, ether, and acetone (e.g., nail polish remover), near clients receiving oxygen.

Because oxygen is colorless, odorless, and tasteless, people are often unaware of its presence. Although oxygen by itself will not burn or explode, it does facilitate combustion and burning. For example, a bed sheet ordinarily burns slowly when ignited in the atmosphere. However, if the sheet is saturated with oxygen and ignited by a spark, it will burn rapidly. The greater the concentration of the oxygen, the more rapidly fires start and burn, and the harder they are to extinguish.

Oxygen is supplied in several different ways. In hospitals and some long-term care facilities, it is usually piped into wall outlets at the client's bedside, making it readily available for use at all times (Figure 32-8 ■). Tanks or cylinders of oxygen under pressure are also frequently available for use when wall oxygen either is unavailable or impractical.

Oxygen administered from a cylinder or wall-outlet system is dry. Dry gases dehydrate the respiratory mucous membranes. Humidifying devices that add water vapor to inspired air are thus an essential component of oxygen therapy, particularly for liter flows over 2 liters per minute (see Figure 32-8B). These devices provide 20% to 40% humidity. The oxygen passes through distilled water and then along a line to the device through which the moistened

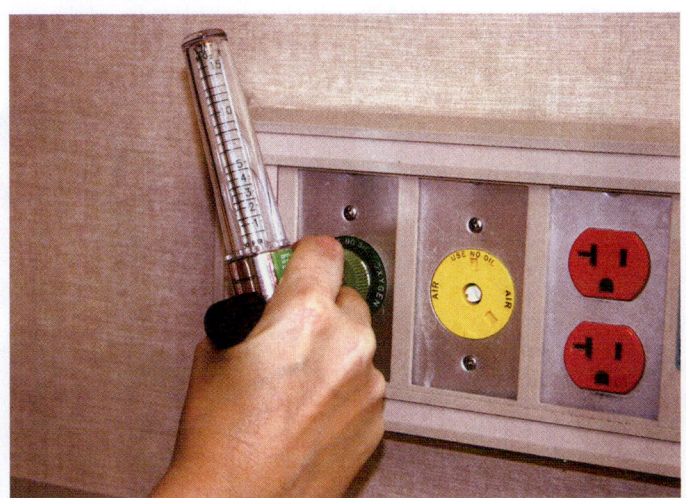
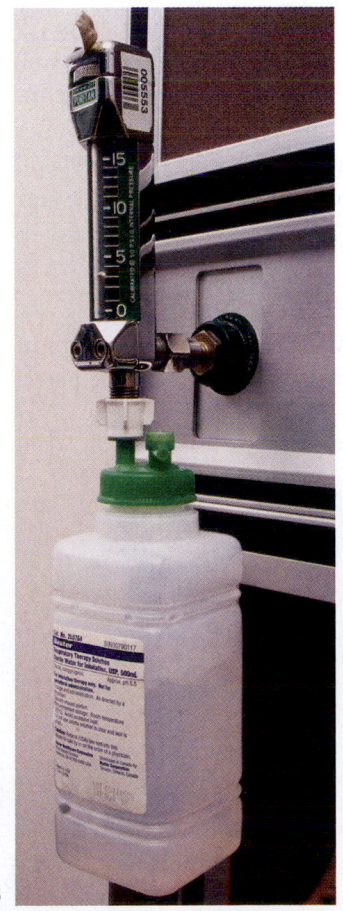

Figure 32-8. ■ **A.** An oxygen flowmeter attached to a wall outlet. (*Source:* © Jenny Thomas.) **B.** An oxygen humidifier. (*Source:* © Elena Dorfman.)

BOX 32-6 PEDIATRIC CONSIDERATIONS

Administering Oxygen to Infants

When administering oxygen to infants and young children, oxygen should be heated to prevent hypothermia. Oxygen is cold and can cause children's temperatures to drop. There are numerous forms of heaters that can be used, many that heat the humidifier, which then warms the oxygen as it bubbles through the water.

oxygen is inhaled (e.g., a nasal cannula or oxygen mask). Liter flows of 2 liters per minute or less by nasal cannula do not require humidification. Special consideration needs to be taken when administering oxygen to infants and young children (Box 32-6 ■).

clinical ALERT

There is a potential for bacterial growth in stagnant water. Hospitals may implement policies for frequent water changes or conduct cultures of the water in humidifiers. Follow your facility's policy for changing humidifier water to avoid risk of infection.

Clients who require oxygen therapy in the home, or in facilities without piped-in oxygen, may use small cylinders of oxygen, oxygen in liquid form, or an oxygen concentrator. Portable oxygen delivery systems are available to increase the client's independence (Figure 32-9 ■). Home oxygen therapy services are readily available in most communities. These services generally supply the oxygen and delivery devices, training for the client and family, equipment maintenance, and emergency services should a problem occur.

Oxygen Delivery Systems

Oxygen is most often delivered via cannula or face mask. When it is important to regulate the percentage of oxygen received by the client more precisely, a Venturi mask may

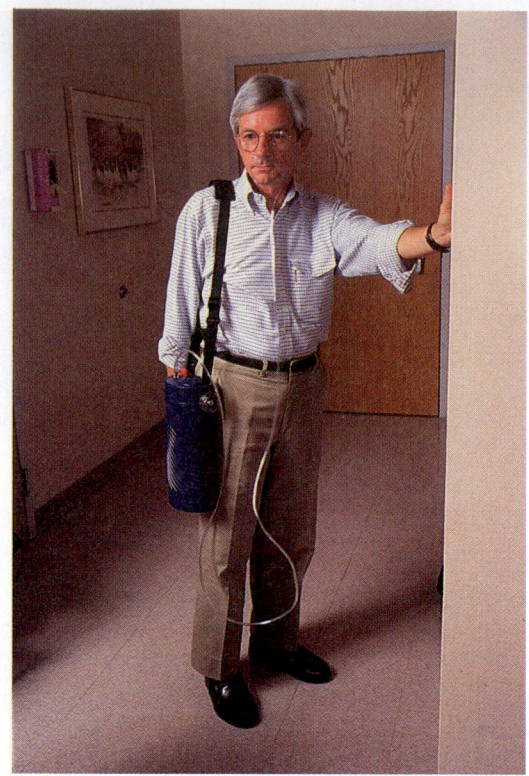

Figure 32-9. ■ Portable liquid oxygen supply gives the client more freedom.

be used. Refer to Procedure 32-2 ■ at the end of this chapter for steps in providing oxygen, descriptions of equipment, and illustrations.

Artificial Airways

Artificial airways are inserted to maintain a patent air passage for a client whose airway has become, or may become, obstructed such as postoperative clients who may be heavily sedated to keep their tongue from obstructing their airway. Three of the more common types of artificial airways are:

1. Oropharyngeal and nasopharyngeal airways (Figures 32-10A and B ■) are used to keep the upper air passages

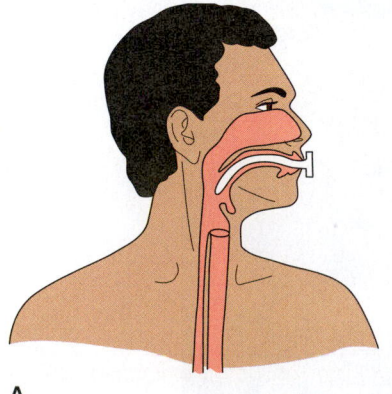
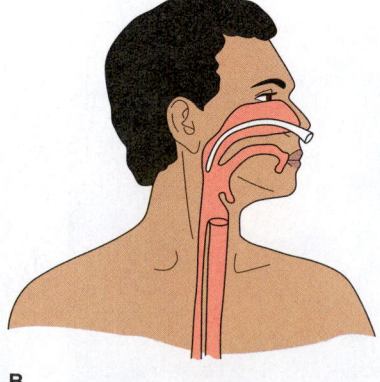
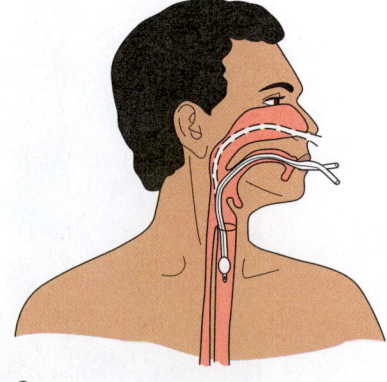

A **B** **C**

Figure 32-10. ■ **A.** An oropharyngeal airway. **B.** A nasopharyngeal airway. **C.** An endotracheal tube.

open when they may become obstructed by secretions or the tongue. These airways are easy to insert and have a low risk of complications.

2. Endotracheal tubes (Figure 32-10C) are most commonly inserted for clients who have had general anesthetics or for those in emergency situations where mechanical ventilation is required. An endotracheal tube is inserted by the physician or RN with specialized education through the mouth or nose and into the trachea. Because an endotracheal tube passes through the epiglottis and glottis, the client is unable to speak while it is in place.

3. Clients who need long-term airway support may have a **tracheostomy** (Figure 32-11 ■), a surgical incision in the trachea just below the larynx through which a tracheostomy tube is inserted.

Tracheostomy tubes may be either plastic or metal and are available in different sizes because the size of the trachea varies by both age and gender. Tracheostomy tubes (Figure 32-12 ■) usually have an inner and outer *cannula*. The outer cannula stays in place, and the inner cannula locks in place inside the outer cannula. The inner cannula can be removed for cleaning while still maintaining an open airway via the outer cannula. At the end of the inner cannula is a *flange* that rests against the neck and allows the tube to be secured in place with tape or ties. All tubes also have an *obturator*, which is used to stiffen the tracheostomy tube for insertion. The obturator must be removed once the tracheostomy tube is in place because it keeps air from moving into the airway. The obturator is kept at the client's bedside in case the tube becomes dislodged and needs to be reinserted. The obturator should be placed in a sealed container to keep pathogens and dust from collecting. Some tracheostomy tubes do not have an inner cannula.

Tracheostomy and endotracheal tubes may be cuffed (Figure 32-13 ■). Cuffed tubes are surrounded by an inflatable cuff that produces an airtight seal between the tube

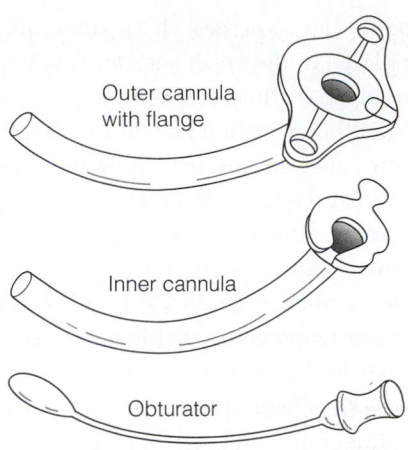

Figure 32-12. ■ Components of a tracheostomy tube.

and the trachea. This allows the client to move without concern that the tube will dislocate, but pressure must be carefully monitored to prevent excessive pressure on the trachea that could cause tissue necrosis. The air is instilled via a pigtail, or small tube, beside the flange. If the client with a cuffed tracheostomy tube complains of *air hunger* (a feeling of having insufficient air to breathe), the cuff should be checked to ensure that it is still inflated. Procedure 32-3 ■ at the end of this chapter describes tracheostomy care.

CHEST TUBES AND DRAINAGE SYSTEMS

Chest tubes may be inserted into the pleural cavity to correct a collapsed lung by restoring negative pressure. The negative pressure in the pleural cavity allows the lungs to easily inflate and deflate with inspiration and expiration. When the pleural cavity is exposed to the outside environment through even the smallest hole, the lung collapses and respiratory distress occurs. Insertion of the chest tube allows the lung to reinflate and provides a means to drain collected

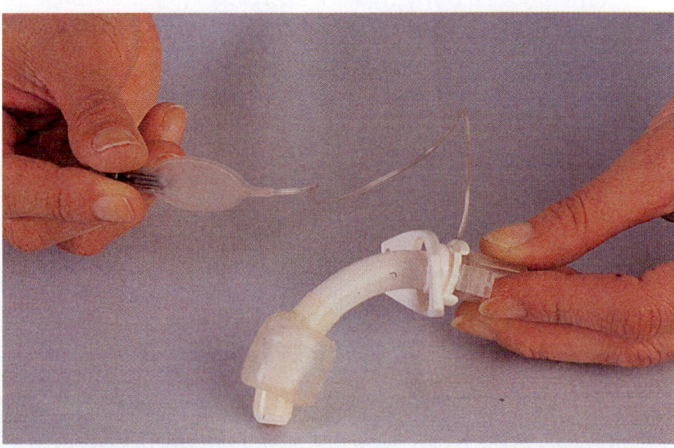

Figure 32-13. ■ A tracheostomy tube with a low-pressure cuff.
(*Source:* © Elena Dorfman.)

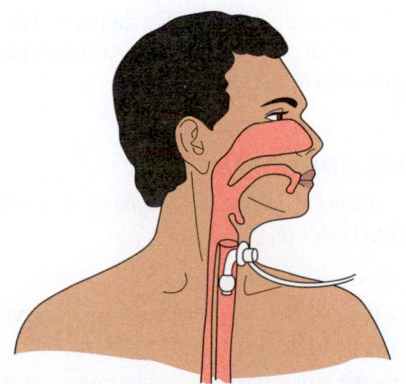

Figure 32-11. ■ A tracheostomy tube in place.

fluid or blood. Because air rises, chest tubes for pneumothorax are often placed in the upper anterior thorax. Chest tubes used to drain blood or fluid are usually placed in the lower lateral chest wall because fluid falls to the dependent area.

When chest tubes are inserted, they must be connected to a sealed drainage system or a one-way valve that allows air and fluid to be removed from the chest cavity but prevents air from entering from the outside. (See more on drainage systems in Chapter 29 ⚭.) Water-seal drainage systems are used to prevent outside air from entering the chest tube. Sterile disposable systems are commonly used (Figure 32-14 ■). These systems typically have a closed collection chamber for drainage that is connected to the water-seal chamber and allow for accurate measurement of drainage. When the client inhales, the water prevents air from entering the system from the atmosphere. During exhalation, however, air can exit the chest cavity, bubbling up through the water. Suction can be added to the system to help remove air and secretions from the chest cavity. Commonly used water-seal devices provide directions for how to set them up for use and should be followed exactly.

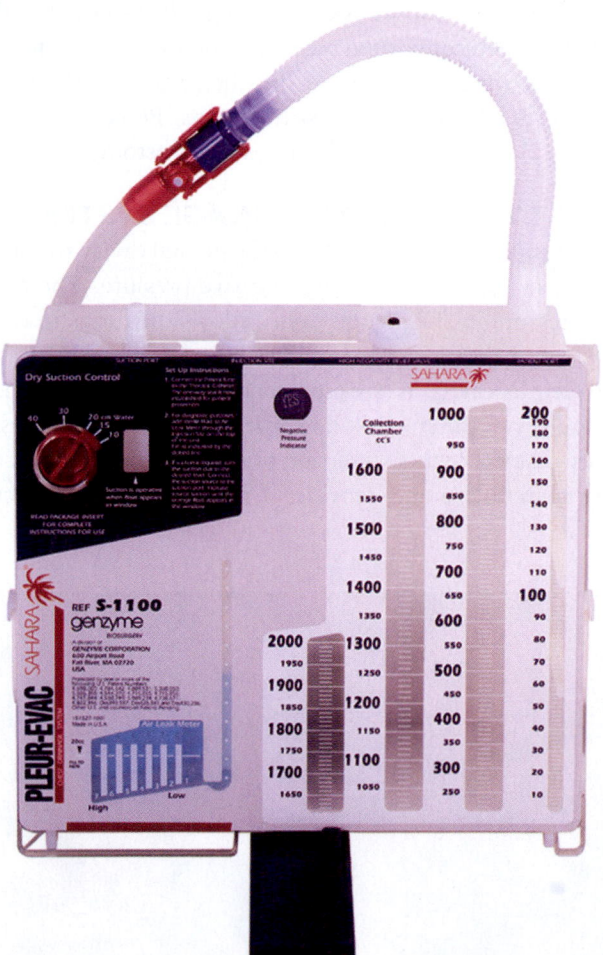

Figure 32-14. ■ A disposable chest drainage system. Fluid and blood collect in the white calibrated chambers. The red chamber provides the water seal, and the blue chamber is a suction-control chamber. (Courtesy of Teleflex Medical.)

clinical ALERT

Chest tube drainage systems should always be placed lower than the level of chest tube insertion to prevent backflow of drainage into the chest. Bubbling in the water-seal chamber indicates an air leak, or that air is being evacuated from the pleural space. Rapid or hard bubbling may be seen when the chest tube is first inserted if the client has a large pneumothorax or it could indicate a hole, leak, or disconnection in the tubing and must be carefully examined. It is normal for the water level in the water-seal chamber to rise with respirations and fall with expiration (the opposite will be seen if the client is receiving pressure generated mechanical ventilation).

BREATHING AND COUGHING EXERCISES

Breathing exercises are frequently indicated for clients with restricted chest expansion, such as people with COPD or clients recovering from surgery. Commonly employed breathing exercises are abdominal (diaphragmatic) breathing and pursed-lip breathing. Abdominal (diaphragmatic) breathing permits deep full breaths with little effort. Pursed-lip breathing helps the client develop control over breathing. The pursed lips create a resistance to the air flowing out of the lungs, prolonging exhalation, and preventing airway collapse by maintaining positive airway pressure. Box 32-7 ■ provides instructions for performing abdominal (diaphragmatic) and pursed-lip breathing. See also Procedure 29-2 ⚭ for preoperative exercises.

Clients can benefit from learning controlled coughing techniques, such as huff coughing. Instructions for coughing techniques are also included in Box 32-7. Coughing and deep-breathing exercises are taught to clients preoperatively to help reduce the risk of pneumonia and atelectasis.

clinical ALERT

Coughing may be contraindicated for clients at risk of increased intercranial pressure, because coughing increases pressure within the cranial space.

INCENTIVE SPIROMETRY

Incentive spirometers, also referred to as sustained maximal inspiration (SMI) devices, are used to:

- Improve pulmonary ventilation.
- Counteract the effects of anesthesia or hypoventilation.
- Loosen respiratory secretions.
- Facilitate respiratory gaseous exchange.
- Expand collapsed alveoli.

BOX 32-7 CLIENT TEACHING

Breathing and Coughing Techniques

Abdominal (Diaphragmatic) and Pursed-Lip Breathing

Teach client to:

- Assume a comfortable semi-sitting position in bed or a chair or a lying position in bed with one pillow.
- Flex the knees to relax the muscles of the abdomen.
- Place one or both hands on the abdomen, just below the ribs.
- Breathe in deeply through the nose, keeping the mouth closed.
- Concentrate on feeling the abdomen rise as far as possible; stay relaxed, and avoid arching the back. If it is difficult to raise the abdomen, take a quick, forceful breath through the nose.
- Then purse lips as if about to whistle, and breathe out slowly and gently, making a slow whooshing sound without puffing out the cheeks. This pursed-lip breathing creates a resistance to air flowing out of the lungs, increases pressure within the bronchi (main air passages), and minimizes collapse of smaller airways, a common problem for people with chronic obstructive pulmonary disease.
- Concentrate on feeling the abdomen fall or sink, and tighten (contract) the abdominal muscles while breathing out to enhance effective exhalation. Count to 7 during exhalation.
- Use this exercise whenever feeling short of breath, and increase gradually to 5 to 10 minutes four times a day. Regular practice will help you do this type of breathing without conscious effort. The exercise, once learned, can be performed when sitting upright, standing, and walking.

Controlled and Huff Coughing

- After using a bronchodilator treatment (if prescribed), inhale deeply and hold your breath for a few seconds.
- Cough twice. The first cough loosens the mucus; the second expels secretions.
- For huff coughing, lean forward and exhale sharply with a huff sound. This technique helps keep airways open while moving secretions up and out of the lungs.
- Inhale by taking rapid short breaths in succession (sniffing) to prevent mucus from moving back into smaller airways.
- Rest.
- Try to avoid prolonged episodes of coughing because it may cause fatigue and hypoxia.

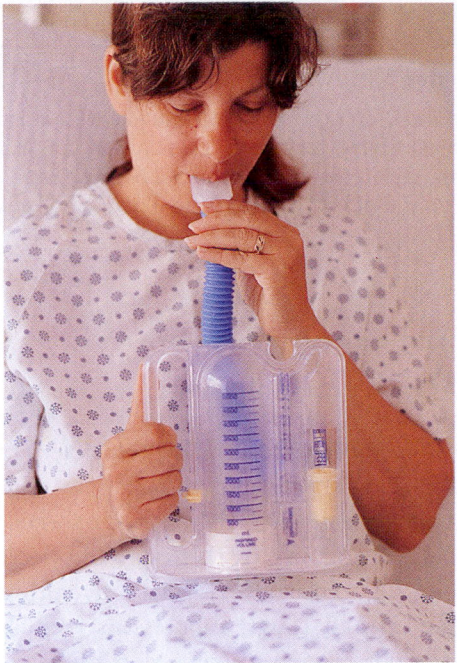

Figure 32-15. ■ Client using a plastic disposable volume-oriented incentive spirometer, or SMI.

BOX 32-8 CLIENT TEACHING

Using an Incentive Spirometer

- Hold or place the spirometer in an upright position. A tilted flow-oriented device requires less effort to raise the ball or disk; a volume-oriented device will not function correctly unless upright.
- Exhale normally.
- Seal the lips tightly around the mouthpiece.
- Take in a slow, deep breath to elevate the ball or cylinder, and then hold the breath for 2 seconds initially, increasing to 6 seconds (optimum), to keep the ball or cylinder elevated if possible.
- For a flow-oriented device, avoid brisk, low-volume breaths that snap the ball to the top of the chamber. Greater lung expansion is achieved with a very slow inspiration than with a brisk, shallow breath, even though it may not elevate the ball or keep it elevated while you hold your breath. Sustained elevation of the ball or cylinder ensures adequate ventilation of the alveoli (lung air sacs).
- If the client has difficulty breathing only through the mouth, a nose clip can be used.
- Remove the mouthpiece, and exhale normally.
- Cough after the incentive effort. Deep ventilation may loosen secretions, and coughing can facilitate their removal.
- Relax, and take several normal breaths before using the spirometer again.
- Do 5 to 10 repetitions. Practice increases inspiratory volume, maintains alveolar ventilation, and prevents atelectasis (collapse of the air sacs).
- Clean the mouthpiece with water and shake it dry. Change disposable mouthpieces every 24 hours.

Incentive spirometers measure the flow of air inhaled through the mouthpiece. They therefore offer an incentive to improve tidal volume, or the air taken in with each inhalation (Figure 32-15 ■). The client should be assisted to a fully upright position before using the incentive spirometer to allow the fullest possible lung expansion. Box 32-8 ■ lists instructions for clients in the use of incentive spirometers.

CLEARING SECRETIONS WITH HYDRATION

Adequate hydration maintains the moisture of the respiratory mucous membranes. Normally, respiratory tract secretions are thin and therefore moved readily by ciliary action. However, when the client is dehydrated or when the environment has a low humidity, the respiratory secretions can become thick and tenacious. Adequate hydration provides one the best natural cough suppressant because it helps to thin secretions enough to make a cough more effective, thereby clearing the lungs of the irritants causing the cough. This is far more effective than antitussive medications, which have only questionable effects especially in children (Box 32-9 ■). Fluid intake should be as great as the client can tolerate.

Humidifiers are devices that add water vapor to inspired air. Room humidifiers provide cool mist to room air. *Nebulizers* (atomizers, devices for throwing spray) are used to deliver humidity and medications. They also are used with oxygen delivery systems to provide moistened air directly to the client (Figure 32-16 ■).

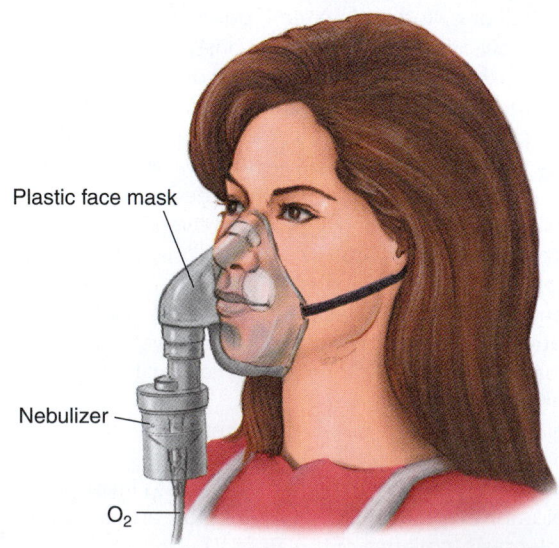

Plastic face mask

Nebulizer

O_2

Figure 32-16. ■ Nebulizer with attached face mask delivers humidity and medication at the same time. (*Source:* Pearson Education/PH College.)

PULMONARY TOILET

Percussion, vibration, and drainage (PVD) are dependent nursing functions performed according to a physician's order to assist clients in clearing pulmonary secretions. These procedures help loosen thick, tenacious secretions. The positions in postural drainage assist removal of secretions (Figure 32-17 ■). Nurses who work in areas where they are expected to assist with these procedures will receive additional training in PVD functions. Care must be taken when performing these procedures not to harm the client.

SUCTIONING

Suctioning means aspirating secretions, usually through a catheter connected to a suction machine or wall suction outlet. Suction catheters may be either open tipped or whistle tipped (Figure 32-18 ■). The whistle-tipped catheter is less irritating to respiratory tissues, although the open-tipped catheter may be more effective for removing thick mucous plugs. Most suction catheters have a thumb port on the side to control the suction. The catheter is connected to suction tubing, which in turn is connected to a collection chamber and suction control gauge (Figure 32-19 ■). Suctioning of the secretions in the mouth can be performed using clean technique. However, suctioning of tracheostomy or endotracheal tubes, because they involve entry into the lower respiratory tract, should be performed using sterile technique.

MECHANICAL VENTILATION

When a client is unable to provide adequate ventilation, it may be necessary to provide mechanical ventilation. Mechanical ventilation can be provided via continuous positive airway pressure (CPAP), also called noninvasive ventilation, or via a mechanical ventilator connected to an endotracheal or tracheostomy tube.

CPAP was developed as a treatment for clients with sleep apnea or other sleep-related respiratory disorders (discussed later in this chapter). The client places a mask snugly over the nose, or nose and mouth, connected to a machine that delivers continuous airway pressure to maintain an open airway and ease the work of breathing (Figure 32-20 ■). Side effects of this treatment can include abdominal bloating, gastroesophageal reflux, and other GI symptoms caused by excessive swallowing of air. Other side effects can include claustrophobia, increased nasal secretions, edema of the nasal mucous membranes, dry eyes, and facial or nasal pain. These complications can be reduced by ensuring proper fit of the CPAP mask, adequate humidification of the air, and gradual increases in pressure. Clients may find the treatment uncomfortable and compliance may drop. Client compliance improves if cognitive behavioral therapy accompanies the initiation of treatment (Aloia, Arnedt, Riggs, Heckt, & Borelli, 2004). In addition to sleep apnea, CPAP is also used to ease the

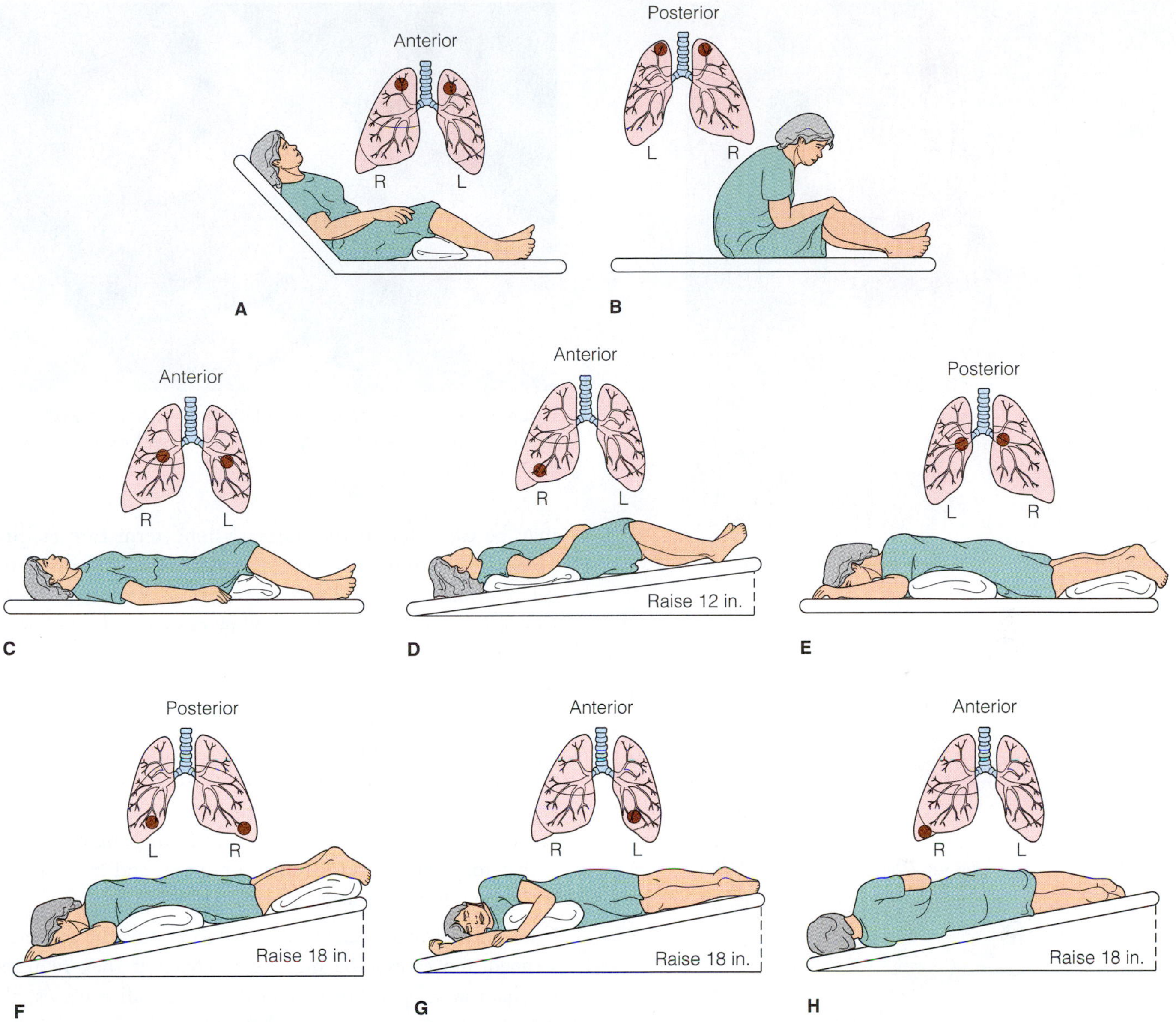

Anterior

Posterior

A

B

Anterior

Anterior

Posterior

Raise 12 in.

C

D

E

Posterior

Anterior

Anterior

Raise 18 in.

Raise 18 in.

Raise 18 in.

F

G

H

Figure 32-17. ■ Positions for postural drainage.

work of breathing in clients with reduced respiratory muscle function, such as those diagnosed with muscular dystrophy, prematurity of the newborn, and multiple sclerosis.

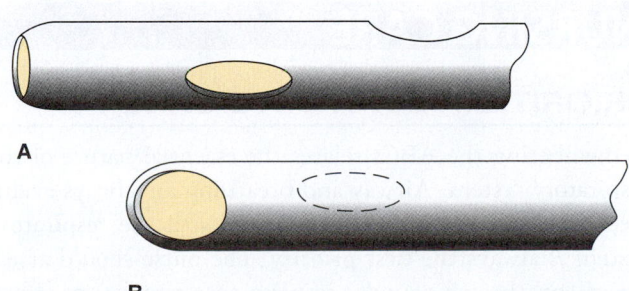

A

B

Figure 32-18. ■ Types of suction catheters. **A.** Open tipped. **B.** Whistle tipped.

Invasive mechanical ventilation requires the placement of an endotracheal or tracheostomy tube (Figure 32-21 ■). This is far more invasive than CPAP but provides greater ventilatory support. It also places the client at risk for introduction of pathogens into the lower respiratory tract and resulting respiratory infections. Mechanical ventilation can be provided using a pressure ventilator or a volume ventilator. Pressure ventilators deliver air at a preset pressure ordered by the physician and adjusted based on arterial blood gas analysis. Volume ventilators deliver a preset volume of air and must be carefully set to avoid causing trauma to the alveoli and airways. Table 32-1 ■ discusses types of pressures or volumes set on the ventilator.

Clients with degenerative muscle or respiratory disorders may require long-term mechanical ventilator support and

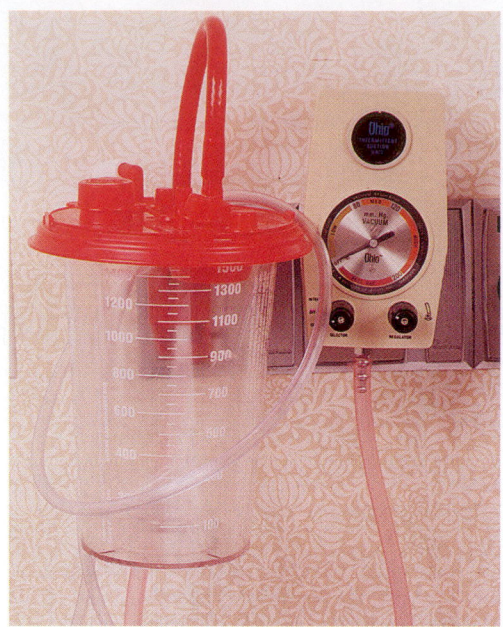

Figure 32-19. ■ A wall suction unit. (*Source:* © Jenny Thomas.)

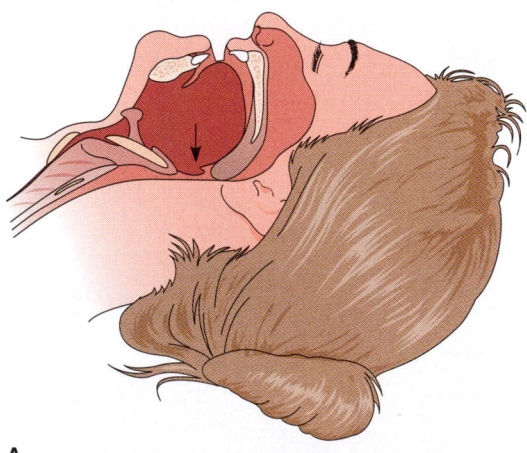

A

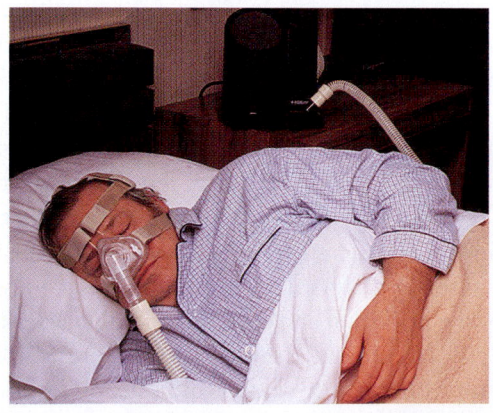

B

Figure 32-20. ■ **A.** In obstructive sleep apnea, the pharynx is obstructed by the soft palate and tongue. **B.** A client using a nasal mask and a CPAP machine to treat sleep apnea.

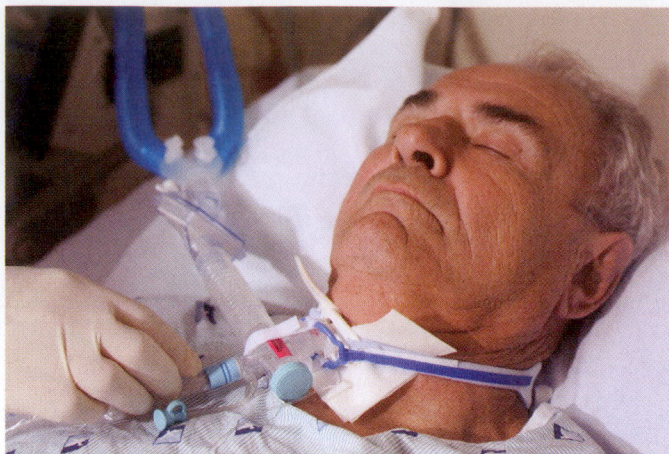

Figure 32-21. ■ Mechanical ventilation takes over the work of breathing for clients with long-term pulmonary disorder. *Source:* Phototake NYC.

may be cared for in the home or long-term care facility. LPNs/LVNs commonly care for clients requiring mechanical ventilation and will receive additional training. Priorities of care for the client receiving mechanical ventilation include:

- Maintaining a patent airway.
- Reducing client anxiety.
- Preventing infection.
- Maintaining proper mechanical ventilator settings.
- Client safety such as keeping ventilator alarms set, preventing undue pressure on the airway from hanging tubing that may collect fluid from humidifier, and maintaining adequate humidification of air.

Clients requiring mechanical ventilation must be gradually weaned and cannot be quickly removed if they required mechanical support for several days. Like all muscles, the muscles of respiration are weakened by lack of use. Gradual responsibility for respirations must be provided to the client to allow time for the respiratory muscles to strengthen in order for the client to provide adequate respiratory effort, without tiring, when the artificial airway is removed.

NURSING CARE

PRIORITIZING NURSING CARE

Remembering the ABCs relates the essential nature of the respiratory system. Airway and breathing are always evaluated first, and correcting a problem with the respiratory system is always the first priority. The nurse should assess the client's breath sounds, respirations, respiratory effort, and oxygenation at the beginning of every shift and then as often as indicated by the client's condition.

TABLE 32-1	**Ventilation Types and Settings**				
PRESSURE VENTILATOR SETTINGS			**VOLUME VENTILATOR SETTINGS**		
SETTINGS	DESCRIPTION	EFFECT ON VENTILATION	SETTINGS	DESCRIPTION	EFFECT ON VENTILATION
PIP (positive inspiratory pressure)	This is the maximum amount of pressure delivered on inhalation	Increases oxygenation	Tidal volume	Volume of air delivered with each inspiration	Increases in tidal volume improve PaO_2 and help to reduce $PaCO_2$ High volumes risk overinflation, too low risks atelectasis
PEEP (positive end expiratory pressure)	This is the amount of continuous pressure provided, even between inspirations	Increased PEEP pressures reduce $PaCO_2$ but can also reduce perfusion of blood through the pulmonary vessels	Sensitivity	May be set on some ventilators to recognize client's own attempt to breathe; helps clients who will be weaned from the ventilator take increasing responsibility for taking independent breaths	
Rate	This is the number of breaths to be delivered by the machine per minute	Faster rates reduce $PaCO_2$ levels	Rate	This is the number of breaths to be delivered by the machine per minute	Faster rates reduce $PaCO_2$ levels
Oxygen percentage	Sets the amount of oxygen delivered from room air to 100%	Effects PaO^2 levels	Oxygen percentage	Sets the amount of oxygen delivered from room air to 100%	Effects PaO_2 levels

ASSESSING

A nursing history and physical exam give valuable information about past health problems and current oxygenation status. During the physical exam, it is very important to evaluate the blood pressure in both arms to detect deficits (see Chapter 19 ⚭). There should be no more than 10 mm Hg difference between the arms.

Variations in the shape of the thorax may indicate adaptation to chronic respiratory conditions. For example, clients with emphysema frequently develop a barrel chest.

The nursing assessment specific to oxygenation includes pulse oximetry, cardiac monitoring, and the review of results of diagnostic tests. Nurses obtain sputum or throat swab cultures for culturing (see Box 32-4).

DIAGNOSING, PLANNING, AND IMPLEMENTING

Some of the NANDA diagnoses that may be appropriate for clients with oxygenation problems are:

- *Impaired Gas Exchange*
- *Ineffective Breathing Pattern*
- *Ineffective Peripheral Tissue Perfusion*

It is important to be familiar with the NANDA diagnoses; a complete list can be found in Appendix II ⚭ on the MyNursingKit Website.

Promoting Oxygenation

Most people in good health give little thought to their respiratory and cardiovascular function. Changing position frequently, ambulating, and exercising usually maintain adequate ventilation, gas exchange, and cardiovascular function in healthy people.

When people become ill, however, pain and immobility may cause shallow respirations or inadequate chest expansion. Respiratory secretions may pool in the lungs and promote infection. This situation is often compounded when clients are given narcotics for pain.

Nursing interventions to maintain the normal respirations of clients include:

- Position the client in semi-Fowler's or high-Fowler's if tolerated. *This position allows for maximum chest expansion.*

Some clients may oxygenate best in a tripod, or three-point, position to facilitate respirations (Figure 32-22 ■). They may experience hypoxia-related anxiety if required to sit back. Allow these clients to maintain the position that optimizes oxygenation.

- Encourage or provide frequent changes in position, especially from side to side. *This promotes lung expansion and mobilization of pulmonary secretions. The orthopneic position helps relieve pressure from abdominal organs on the diaphragm.*
- Encourage ambulation. *Ambulation promotes oxygenation, allows deep breathing, and helps prevent pooling of secretions.*
- Implement measures that promote comfort, such as giving pain medications. *The client who is comfortable will be able to rest and to heal.*
- Teach and encourage deep-breathing exercises and coughing (see Procedure 29-2 ⦿). *These exercises help remove secretions from the lungs.*
- Teach and reinforce coughing techniques, especially controlled or huff coughing. *Forceful coughing often is less effective than using controlled or huff coughing techniques (see Box 32-7).*
- Encourage use of an incentive spirometer and reinforce teaching as necessary. Assist client to an upright sitting position in bed or a chair. *With this device, the client can see how well the lungs are expanding and can see improvement with practice. The upright position facilitates maximum ventilation.*
- Ensure that humidifiers or nebulizers are working properly. *Oxygen can dry mucous membranes. Humidifiers and nebulizers prevent mucous membranes from drying and becoming irritated. They help loosen secretions for easier expectoration.*
- If trained, provide percussion to client as ordered. *Percussion loosens secretions for expectoration.*
- Provide suctioning as ordered, using sterile technique (Figure 32-23 ■). Introduce the suction catheter before

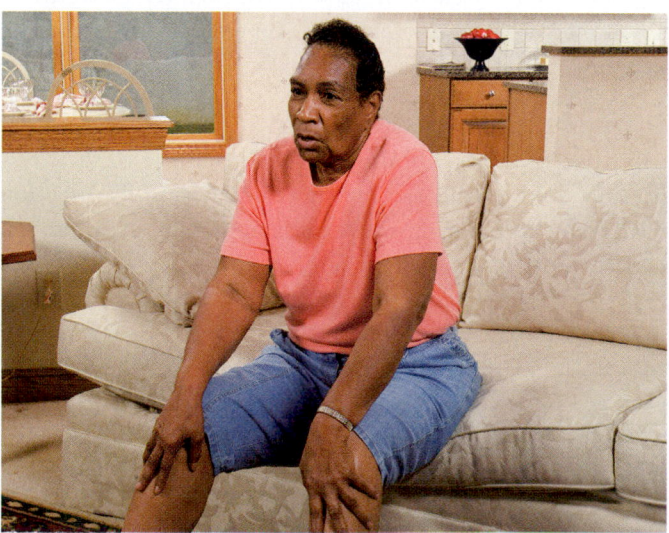

Figure 32-22. ■ Clients who have difficulty breathing often assume a tripod position as this person is doing. This posture allows greater lung expansion. *Source:* Pearson Education/PH College.

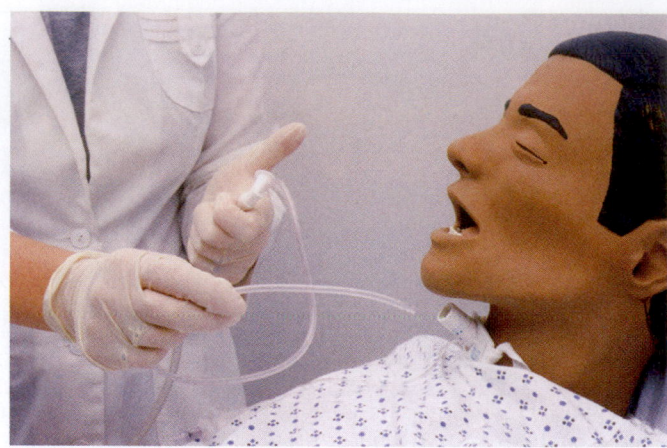

Figure 32-23. ■ Inserting the catheter into the trachea through the tracheostomy tube. *Note:* Suction is not applied until the catheter has been inserted.

applying suction. Steps in suctioning are described in Procedure 32-4 ■ at the end of this chapter. *When clients have difficulty expectorating their secretions or when an airway is in place, suctioning may be necessary to clear air passages. Even though the upper airways (the oropharynx and nasopharynx) are not sterile, sterile technique is recommended for all suctioning to avoid introducing pathogens into the airways.*

Monitoring Chest Tubes and Drainage Systems

Nurses are responsible for the care of clients with chest tubes and drainage systems in the pleural cavity. Nursing responsibilities regarding drainage systems are discussed with perioperative care in Chapter 29 ⦿ . They include the following:

- Assist with the insertion and removal of chest tubes. (See perioperative nursing in Chapter 29 ⦿ .)
- Maintain the water seal and patency of the drainage system. *A sealed suctioning unit provides the best drainage to the wound and promotes healing. A clogged unit will not drain the wound and could allow growth of microorganisms.*
- Assess the client's vital signs, cardiovascular status, and respiratory status. *These are baseline markers for nursing care and for prevention of complications.*
- Monitor the patency and integrity of the drainage system. *These are a nurse's responsibility.*
- Always keep the drainage system below the level of the client's chest. *This prevents fluid and drainage from being drawn back into the chest cavity.*
- Keep rubber-tipped clamps and a sterile occlusive dressing near the client. *The chest tube will need to be clamped quickly, close to the insertion site, if connections are broken or an air leak develops in the drainage system. If the chest tube is inadvertently pulled out, the wound should be immediately covered with a sterile occlusive dressing to protect against microorganisms.*

- Monitor the dressing around the chest tube insertion site and report excessive drainage, foul odor, and bubbling or air leakage.

Emergency Preparation

- Be prepared to perform cardiopulmonary resuscitation (CPR). *A respiratory arrest (pulmonary arrest) is the cessation of breathing. It often occurs as a result of a blocked airway, but it can occur following a cardiac arrest and for other reasons. A respiratory arrest may occur abruptly or be preceded by short, shallow breathing that becomes increasingly labored. If breathing stops for 4 to 6 minutes, the lack of oxygen supply to the brain can cause permanent and extensive damage. It is vital that all nurses be trained to perform CPR so that resuscitation measures can be initiated immediately when a cardiac or respiratory arrest occurs. Nurses can also be instrumental in increasing community awareness of the need for CPR training and ensuring its availability. Most healthcare agencies have established practices and policies governing CPR. See Chapter 47 ⚮ for more information on CPR.*

EVALUATING

Using the goals and desired outcomes identified in the planning stage of the nursing process, the nurse collects data to evaluate the effectiveness of interventions. If outcomes are not achieved, the nurse, client, and support person, if appropriate, need to explore the reasons before modifying the care plan. Outcomes for clients with alterations in oxygenation might include:

- Maintaining a patent airway with breath sounds clear/clearing and absence of dyspnea.
- Demonstrating behaviors to improve airway clearance (e.g., cough effectively and expectorate secretions).
- Demonstrating improved ventilation and adequate oxygenation of tissues by arterial blood gases within client's normal range and being free of symptoms of respiratory distress.
- Establishing a normal/effective respiratory pattern within client's normal range.
- Being free of cyanosis and other signs/symptoms of hypoxia.

Continuity of Care

The nurse provides client education about:

- Behaviors and lifestyle changes to regain and/or maintain appropriate weight.
- Interventions to prevent/reduce risk of infection.
- The condition or disease process and its treatment.
- Relationship of current signs and symptoms to the disease process and its causes.

NURSING PROCESS CARE PLAN
Client with Hemothorax

Jerry Markert, age 21, was admitted to the acute care facility following a biking accident in which he received multiple injuries, including a **hemothorax** (an accumulation of blood in the pleural space that causes partial or complete collapse of the lung on the affected side). He is receiving 6 L of oxygen by nasal cannula and has a chest tube connected to a closed drainage system.

Assessment

The client is alert, stable, and progressing well. Pulse oximeter indicates an oxygen saturation level of 89 percent, BP 110/60; pulse 120. C/o difficulty breathing. Multiple bruises noted on left side of torso, breath sounds absent in the left chest. Lacerations noted on forehead and legs, no evidence of extremity fracture. Chest x-ray revealed hemothorax.

Nursing Diagnosis

The following important nursing diagnoses (among others) are established for this condition:

- *Impaired Gas Exchange*
- *Risk for Injury*

Expected Outcomes

The expected outcomes specify that Mr. Markert will:

- Demonstrate improved ventilation and adequate oxygenation as evidenced by blood gases within client's normal parameters.
- Maintain clear lung fields and remain free of signs of respiratory distress.
- Remain free of injury as evidenced by chest tube in place and closed drainage system functioning properly.

Planning and Implementation

The following interventions are planned and implemented:

- Document vital signs, oxygen saturation, and respiratory status every 4 hours.
- Notify physician if vital signs outside the normal range (heart rate 60–100, respirations 12–20, systolic blood pressure 90–140, diastolic blood pressure 60–90) or oxygen saturation decreases below 90% to 92% depending on facility policy.
- Place in Fowler's position.
- Administer oxygen as ordered.
- Provide rest.
- Secure chest tube to chest wall and bedding to prevent tension during care.

- Prevent kinking of occlusion of chest tube to promote drainage.
- Keep drainage system below chest at all times.
- Observe for redness, swelling, drainage, or pain at insertion site.
- Assess chest tube and drainage system at least every 2 hours.
- Measure and record output from chest tube at least every 4 hours.
- Notify physician if drainage from chest tube exceeds predetermined amount (determined by physician's order or facility policy).
- If tube is inadvertently dislodged/removed, promptly seal with sterile occlusion dressing.
- Keep two padded clamps and petroleum dressings at bedside at all times.

Evaluation

Chest tube in place connected to closed drainage, secured to chest wall, 200 mL of bloody drainage. O₂ sat 98% on 2 L. Diminished breath sounds on left. R 20, HR 86, and BP 120/78.

Critical Thinking in the Nursing Process

1. If Mr. Markert is stable and progressing well, why is his oxygen saturation being monitored?
2. What precautions need to be taken when caring for Mr. Markert while his chest tube is in place?
3. Offer suggestions that would help Mr. Markert, or any person with a respiratory problem, to establish healthy breathing after his chest tube is removed.

Note: Discussion of Critical Thinking questions appears on the MyNursingKit Website.

UPPER RESPIRATORY DISORDERS

Disorders of the upper respiratory system may include diseases or structural disorders of the nose, sinuses, tonsils, adenoids, larynx, and pharynx. These structures are essential for effective breathing and communication. Although many of the disorders described in this section could be considered minor, they have the potential to cause serious medical emergencies. Diagnostic measures and treatment of upper respiratory disorders are outlined in Table 32-2 ■.

Infections and Inflammations

RHINITIS

Rhinitis is an inflammation of the nasal mucous membrane. It may be acute or chronic and may be caused by viruses, bacteria, or allergens. Acute rhinitis is also known as the common cold. Viral and bacterial rhinitis may be contagious. They are spread by droplet and direct contact. Allergic rhinitis, also called hay fever, is caused by reactions to allergens such as pollens. Allergic rhinitis may be seasonal or perennial. Excessive nasal dryness, exposure to damp and cool environmental temperatures, inhalation of large amounts of dust, stress or fatigue, a compromised immune system, and nasal injury may precipitate rhinitis.

Clinical manifestations of rhinitis include nasal congestion and drainage, which may affect breathing and alter the sense of smell. Congestion may also cause coughing, sinus headaches, and snoring. Fever, muscle aches, fatigue, sneezing, and watery, itchy eyes may occur.

See Table 32-2 for diagnosis and treatment of rhinitis.

SINUSITIS

Sinusitis is an inflammation of one or more of the sinus cavities creating narrowed or blocked passages. It is often seen as a complication of an upper respiratory tract infection, tooth infection or abscess, allergies, pneumonia, or the measles. Sinusitis may also be related to air pollution, diving, swimming, nasal structural defects, or prolonged nasotracheal intubation.

Chronic sinusitis typically results from repeated bouts of acute sinusitis. These bouts of acute sinusitis cause damage to the cilia lining the sinus cavity. Clients who smoke or frequently use nasal sprays are more susceptible to chronic sinusitis.

Headache, sinus tenderness, and nasal drainage or congestion are usually associated with sinusitis. Clients may also experience fever (not typical of chronic sinusitis), malaise, nausea, and dizziness. Visualization of the sinuses of a client with sinusitis may reveal erythema and inflammation of the nasal mucosa and enlarged turbinates.

For diagnosis and collaborative care of sinusitis, see Table 32-2.

INFLUENZA

An acute respiratory tract infection caused by a virus is called the flu or influenza. Influenza is easily transmitted by airborne droplet or direct contact. The incubation period following contact may be as short as 18 to 72 hours. Elderly clients, especially those with cardiac or lung disorders, are most susceptible to the disorder and the complications that can occur. Influenza may be caused by one of three viruses named A, B, or C.

Symptoms of influenza have a rapid onset due to the rapid replication of the virus within the respiratory

TABLE 32-2	Diagnostic Measures and Collaborative Care of Disorders of the Upper Respiratory Tract	
DISORDER	**DIAGNOSTIC MEASURES**	**COLLABORATIVE CARE**
Rhinitis	■ History and physical examination ■ White blood cell (WBC) count ■ Rhinorrhea culture	■ Comfort measures ■ Decongestants ■ Antihistamines ■ Analgesics
Sinusitis	■ X-rays, CT scans, or MRI of the sinuses ■ WBC count	■ Antibiotic therapy ■ Decongestants ■ Antihistamines ■ Mucolytic agents ■ Analgesics ■ Endoscopic sinus surgery ■ Antral irrigation ■ Caldwell-Luc procedure creating a nasal "window" ■ External sphenoethmoidectomy to remove diseased tissue and nasal polyps
Influenza	■ History and physical examination ■ WBC count	■ Prevention is accomplished through the yearly administration of the influenza vaccine ■ To reduce transmission following exposure: rimantadine (Flumadine) or amantadine (Symmetrel) ■ To reduce severity of symptoms: zanamivir (Relenza) or oseltamivir (Tamiflu) ■ Analgesics ■ Antitussives
Pharyngitis	■ Throat swab ■ Complete blood count (CBC)	■ Analgesics ■ Antipyretics ■ Penicillin
Tonsillitis	■ Throat swab ■ CBC	■ Analgesics ■ Antipyretics ■ Penicillin ■ For peritonsillar abscess: needle aspiration ■ For chronic tonsillitis: tonsillectomy usually including adenoidectomy
Laryngitis	■ History and physical examination	■ Vocal rest ■ Avoidance of other irritants ■ Analgesics
Epiglottitis	■ History and physical examination, although use of tongue blade is avoided due to risk of laryngospasm	■ Nasotracheal intubation ■ Antibiotic therapy ■ Corticosteroid to reduce inflammation

TABLE 32-2	Diagnostic Measures and Collaborative Care of Disorders of the Upper Respiratory Tract (continued)	
DISORDER	**DIAGNOSTIC MEASURES**	**COLLABORATIVE CARE**
Nasal trauma	■ Head and facial x-rays	■ Simple reduction ■ Applied external splints ■ Analgesics ■ Nasal packing ■ Rhinoplasty may be necessary to ensure adequate airway or for cosmetic reasons
Epistaxis	■ History and physical examination	■ Pressure applied to nasal septum for 5 to 10 minutes along with ice to the nose and forehead ■ Have client sit and lean forward ■ Topical vasoconstrictors ■ Chemical or surgical cauterization ■ Nasal packing
Deviated septum	■ Head and facial x-rays	■ Septoplasty ■ Nasal packing
Obstructive sleep apnea	■ Nocturnal sleep test with oximetry (portable or at a sleep testing lab)	■ Weight loss or smoking cessation ■ Removal of cause (e.g., enlarged tonsils) or treatment of associated medical problems ■ Oral appliance to maintain airway during sleep (Mayo Clinic, 2008) ■ CPAP machine during sleep ■ BiPAP ventilator during sleep
Tumors	■ Fiber-optic visualization ■ Biopsy ■ CT scans or MRIs	■ Vocal rest ■ Smoking cessation ■ Steroid inhalation ■ *Polypectomy* (removal of polyps) ■ External radiation or implanted iridium seeds ■ Chemotherapy ■ Partial or total laryngectomy ■ Speech restoration

epithelium. Respiratory symptoms of influenza include rhinorrhea or profuse nasal drainage, cough, and sore throat. Systemic symptoms are caused by the release of proteins in response to the inflammation. Systemic manifestations include fever, chills, gastrointestinal disturbances, and neuralgia.

The diagnosis and treatment of influenza are provided in Table 32-2.

PHARYNGITIS

Inflammation of the pharynx or pharyngitis may be viral (rhinovirus, influenza, or Epstein-Barr), bacterial (most commonly Group A beta-hemolytic streptococci or strep throat), or fungal (such as candidiasis) in nature. Environmental irritants such as smoking, dust, or smog may also bring about chronic pharyngitis. Pharyngitis, whether bacterial or viral, is spread by airborne droplet and may be transmitted for several days during the disease process.

Clinical manifestations of acute bacterial pharyngitis include a sudden onset of a sore throat, which may be scratchy or may produce difficulty swallowing, fatigue, fever, and muscle aches. On visualization of the pharynx, pus may be noted. Anterior lymph nodes may be tender and enlarged. Acute pharyngitis may be complicated by scarlet fever, rheumatic fever, toxic shock syndrome, and acute glomerulonephritis. Viral pharyngitis has a more gradual onset of symptoms including sore throat, low-grade fever, headache, and rhinorrhea. Fungal infections may produce white patches on the pharynx.

See Table 32-2 for diagnosis and treatment of pharyngitis.

TONSILLITIS

Inflammation of the palatine tonsils is called tonsillitis. The adenoids may also be inflamed as a result of tonsillitis. It may occur as a viral infection but is most commonly related to a streptococcal infection.

Tonsillitis is characterized by an extremely sore throat producing difficulty swallowing, high fever, tachycardia, otalgia, and malaise. On examination, the cervical lymph nodes may be found to be tender and enlarged. The tonsils appear bright red and edematous and are covered with white exudate. The uvula may also be enlarged. Tonsillitis may be complicated by otitis media, spontaneous rupture of the eardrum, or quinsy. Quinsy or peritonsillar abscess may result in increased swelling of the tonsil, deviation of the uvula, difficulty speaking, drooling, and tonic contractions of the jaw muscles.

Diagnosis and treatment of tonsillitis are discussed in Table 32-2.

LARYNGITIS

Laryngitis is an inflammation of the mucous membrane of the larynx associated with edematous vocal cords. Laryngitis may be acute or chronic. Acute laryngitis may be the result of either a viral or bacterial infection and is often associated with other upper respiratory infections. Overuse of the voice, exposure to allergens such as dust or smoke, or injury to the larynx due to hot or corrosive liquids may also cause acute laryngitis. Chronic laryngitis results following numerous episodes of acute laryngitis. Clients with chronic laryngitis have a granulation of the larynx that thickens and hardens over time and may cause a permanent change in the quality of the voice or chronic hypertrophic laryngitis.

Symptoms for laryngitis include a mild hoarseness, inability to speak or aphonia, sore or scratchy throat, decreased appetite, and a dry cough. Excessive inflammation of the larynx may produce impaired breathing.

See Table 32-2 for diagnosis and treatment of laryngitis.

EPIGLOTTITIS

Epiglottitis or supraglottis is a potentially life-threatening inflammation of the epiglottis. It is most commonly caused by *Haemophilus influenzae* type B but can also be caused by other bacteria, viruses, fungi, or trauma.

As the epiglottis swells, a sore throat and painful swallowing may occur. If the tissues adjacent to the epiglottis become inflamed, the epiglottis may be pushed into a posterior position causing dyspnea, drooling, and stridor.

See Table 32-2 for diagnosis and treatment of epiglottitis. Epiglottitis is a special danger to infants and young children (Box 32-10 ■). Epiglottitis is also discussed in the pediatric section, in Chapter 59 ◯◯.

BOX 32-10	PEDIATRIC CONSIDERATIONS

Epiglottitis in Infants and Young Children

Children, especially young children and newborns, have smaller airways and are at greater risk for airway obstruction. Diseases such as croup, bronchiectasis, epiglottitis, and pharyngitis are all diseases that risk obstruction of the pediatric airway. Monitor for stridor, increasing respiratory rate, and retractions which are much more common in children. Children who expend a great deal of effort attempting to breathe will tire easily, resulting in possible apnea. Pediatric clients must be closely monitored and all symptoms of respiratory distress must be reported immediately.

Trauma and Obstruction

AIRWAY OBSTRUCTION

Obstruction of the airway may be either partial or complete resulting in a medical emergency. Aspiration, trauma, anaphylaxis, or laryngospasm may cause airway obstruction. Laryngospasm is the spasmodic obstruction of the larynx caused by endotracheal intubation, aspiration, chemical irritation, or hypocalcemia. For more information, refer to Chapter 47 ◯◯, Emergency Room and Urgent Care Nursing.

NASAL TRAUMA

Fracture of the nose may occur as a result of trauma or sports injury. Nasal fracture is classified as bilateral, unilateral, or complex involving additional facial bones.

Tears in the mucous membrane may cause epistaxis or nosebleeds, ecchymosis of the eyes, bony crepitus, and septal hematomas. Septal deviation may also occur, putting the client at risk for airway obstruction.

Diagnosis and treatment of nasal trauma are provided in Table 32-2.

EPISTAXIS

Epistaxis results from a rupture of small blood vessels of the nasal septum. Nosebleeds are associated with trauma, deviated septum, introduction of a foreign body, nasal irritation due to allergies or the common cold, substance abuse (illicit drugs or nasal sprays), or nasal polyps or tumors. Epistaxis may be related to menstruation, hypertension, leukemia, thrombocytopenia, arteriosclerosis, and liver disease. It is also seen in clients receiving anti-inflammatories, anticoagulants, or antiplatelet drugs.

Diagnosis and treatment of epistaxis are provided in Table 32-2.

DEVIATED SEPTUM

Normally the nasal septum is straight. Deviated septum may be due to trauma or may have been present since birth. The deviated septum alters the passage of air through the nose and may significantly hinder breathing.

Epistaxis is more common with this condition. Clients with deviated septum may also snore loudly at night. Surgery is often needed to correct the problem.

Diagnosis and treatment of deviated septum are provided in Table 32-2.

OBSTRUCTIVE SLEEP APNEA

In obstructive sleep apnea, the client experiences periods of apnea and hypopnea during the transition phase from NREM to REM sleep. It is thought to be caused by obstruction of the airway due to a decrease in skeletal muscle tone causing pharyngeal collapse (Figure 32-20A).

For clients with sleep apnea, therapy including use of a continuous positive airway pressure (CPAP) machine is often prescribed (see Figure 32-20B). (For more information about care of clients with apnea and hypoxia, refer to Chapter 23 ⌒, Activity, Rest, and Sleep.) A BiPAP ventilator, which maintains high pressure during inspiration and lower pressure during expiration, is a newer alternative to the CPAP machine. See Table 32-2 for diagnosis and treatment.

Tumors

BENIGN LARYNGEAL TUMORS

Polyps and nodules of the larynx may develop in clients who are frequently exposed to cigarette smoke or environmental pollutants. Individuals who frequently have voice strain such as teachers, speakers, singers, or auctioneers may also be at risk for developing benign laryngeal tumors. Papillomas of the larynx are a result of viral infection.

These clients may speak with a hoarse tone or have a breathy quality to their voice. If the benign tumor is large, it could cause dyspnea or stridor.

Clinical management may include vocal rest, smoking cessation, steroid inhalation, or surgical removal. Diagnosis and treatment of tumors are provided in Table 32-2.

MALIGNANT TUMORS

The American Cancer Society estimates that, in 2004, about 10,270 people in the United States will have laryngeal cancer and 3,830 cases will be fatal. Fortunately, laryngeal cancer is easily cured if detected early. Risk factors for laryngeal cancer include male gender, compromised immune system, cigarette smoking, intake of alcohol, poor nutrition, particularly lack of vitamins A and B, history of human papillomavirus (HPV) infection, and exposure to asbestos and other pollutants. African Americans have a higher incidence of the disease.

Clinical manifestations of laryngeal cancer are related to the site of the tumor. The client may experience a change in the voice quality such as hoarseness, halitosis, difficulty swallowing accompanied by unilateral pain, dyspnea, otalgia,

and a palpable nodule in the neck. On examination, the practitioner may visualize leukoplakia or erythroplakia of the larynx. Leukoplakia is seen as thick, white patches, whereas erythroplakia is seen as a red, velvet patch.

Fiber-optic visualization, biopsy, and CT scans or MRIs are used to diagnose laryngeal cancer. Clinical management of laryngeal cancer is determined according to the stage of the cancer. External radiation or implanted iridium seeds can be used effectively. Chemotherapy may be used in addition to radiation.

Surgery may be necessary to optimize the client's chance for cure. If the tumor is limited to one part of the larynx, a partial laryngectomy may be performed. During this surgery at least 50% of the larynx is removed. Speech is often preserved with this type of surgery but the quality of the voice is at risk of being altered.

If the cancer is extensive, a total laryngectomy may be necessary. Along with the larynx, the epiglottis, thyroid cartilage, several tracheal rings, and the hyoid bone are removed. Speech is lost following the total laryngectomy. A permanent tracheostomy remains following this surgery. See Procedure 32-3, Providing Tracheostomy Care, at the end of this chapter.

Speech restoration may be accomplished through esophageal speech, with an artificial, battery-operated larynx or tracheoesophageal puncture (TEP). TEP (Figure 32-24 ■) places a prosthesis in the tracheal stoma allowing diversion of air from the trachea to the esophagus and oropharynx.

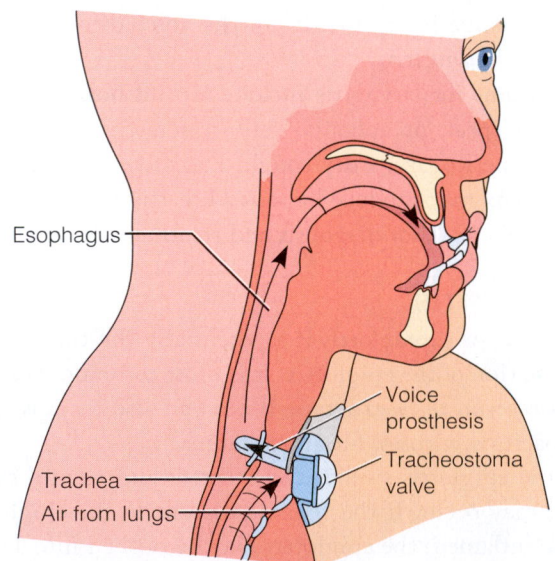

Figure 32-24. ■ Tracheoesophageal puncture (TEP) allows air from the trachea to be diverted through the prosthesis into the esophagus and oropharynx, producing speech when the tracheostomy stoma is occluded. A one-way valve prevents food from entering the trachea.

Speech is possible by occluding the stoma. For more information, refer to Chapter 45 ⚭, Caring for Clients with Cancer.

NURSING CARE

PRIORITIZING NURSING CARE

When caring for clients with disorders of the upper respiratory tract, focus your care on maintaining an open airway and monitoring for complications. When severe edema is present in the pharynx and larynx, the possibility of airway obstruction exists. Assess the client's respiratory status at least every 4 hours (more often if the risk for obstruction is high), checking for stridor, wheezes, or dyspnea. Count the respiratory rate. If it is above 26, the client is experiencing dyspnea. Assess the nail beds for cyanosis. Apply supplemental oxygen as ordered to help decrease the respiratory rate and effort. Keep the head of the bed elevated 30 degrees or more to help the client expand the chest with each breath and to decrease edema associated with trauma. In cases of severe dyspnea, high-Fowler's or the orthopneic position may be most effective. Assess the client's temperature every 4 hours to determine response to antibiotics. If the client's temperature remains elevated after 24 to 48 hours on antibiotics, report this to the healthcare provider since it could indicate that the antibiotics are not effectively treating the infection. Assess the client for evidence of spreading infection. For example, pharyngitis may spread to the middle ear. Assess for other complications. For example, spread of laryngeal tumors may cause loss of voice or airway obstruction.

ASSESSING

The nurse is responsible for obtaining a health history related to the upper respiratory system including symptoms, current medications, immunization history, and past medical and surgical history. Objective data and documentation obtained from a physical examination should include overall appearance, vital signs, lung sounds, characteristics of drainage, and skin color.

DIAGNOSING, PLANNING, AND IMPLEMENTING

Some common nursing diagnoses for clients with upper respiratory disorders are:

- *Ineffective Breathing Pattern*
- *Ineffective Airway Clearance*
- *Anxiety*
- *Acute Pain*

Typical outcomes for these clients might include:

- Client will maintain adequate ventilation as evidenced by respirations within normal limits and without effort.
- Client will have improved airway clearance as evidenced by clear lung sounds and productive cough.
- Client will express improved emotional status as evidenced by resolution of symptoms of anxiety.
- Client will remain pain free as evidenced by report of decreased pain level.

Upper respiratory infections are generally self-limiting. The nurse's role would include the following:

- Teach client the importance of covering mouth and nose when coughing or sneezing. Teach about proper disposal of tissues. *Most upper respiratory disorders are spread by droplet or by contact with secretions. Clients can limit the spread of the disease by covering mouth and nose completely. Teach them to dispose of tissues immediately in a trash receptacle and never to leave them on common surfaces.*
- Discuss the importance of hand washing. *Frequent hand washing can help to break the cycle of infection.*
- Provide for periods of rest. *Altered breathing patterns produce fatigue, which could further compromise ventilation.*
- Teach the client how to cough effectively and to keep nasal passages clear. *Opening airway passages by clearing the airway of secretions is essential to improved ventilation.*
- Encourage the client to maintain hydration. *Adequate fluid acts to decrease the viscosity of secretions. Thinner secretions are easier to expectorate.*
- Encourage slow, deep mouth breathing. *Ventilation is improved and anxiety is reduced when the client practices slow mouth breathing.*
- Discuss causes of anxiety with the client. *Exploring the client's reasons for anxiety gives them an opportunity to express feelings and concerns and then to explore options for coping.*
- Encourage the client to maintain an upright position. *Elevation of the head encourages drainage of nasal passages and sinuses and improves ventilation.*
- Encourage the use of nonpharmacologic pain methods and pharmacologic pain medications as necessary. *Prompt control of pain is essential in its management.*

Refer to Table 32-2 for diagnosis and treatment.

EVALUATING

The nurse revises care until expected outcomes are achieved. The expected outcomes for a client with an upper respiratory disorder include:

- Client maintains adequate ventilation.
- Client has improved airway clearance.
- Client reports anxiety decreased.
- Client reports reduction in pain level.

LOWER RESPIRATORY DISORDERS

Disorders of the lower respiratory system may include diseases or structural disorders of the trachea, lungs, pleura, bronchi, alveoli, rib cage, and intercostal muscles. These structures are essential for effective breathing and proper gas exchange. The lower respiratory system is also dependent on adequate function of the central nervous system, the heart, and the musculoskeletal system. Because many systems may be affected by lower respiratory disorders, clinical manifestations of these conditions may be local or systemic. Diagnostic and treatment measures for disorders of the lower respiratory tract are outlined in Table 32-3 ■.

Pulmonary Embolism

Pulmonary embolism is an obstruction of the pulmonary artery caused by an embolus. These *emboli* or blood clots usually originate from the legs or the pelvis. Pulmonary embolism is considered a medical emergency requiring prompt medical attention (see also Chapter 47 ⬤⬤).

Several risk factors predispose a client to pulmonary embolism: prolonged immobilization, obesity, older age, trauma to the legs and pelvis, surgery (of the lower abdomen, pelvis, or lower extremities), cancer, cardiovascular

TABLE 32-3	Diagnostic Measures and Collaborative Care of Disorders of the Lower Respiratory Tract	
DISORDER	**DIAGNOSTIC MEASURES**	**COLLABORATIVE CARE**
Pulmonary embolism	■ History and physical examination ■ Elevated plasma D-dimer levels ■ Perfusion and ventilation lung scans ■ Pulmonary angiography ■ ECG ■ Arterial blood gas (ABG) measurements ■ Coagulation studies	■ Anticoagulant therapy ■ Thrombolytic agents ■ Insertion of inferior vena cava filter ■ Oxygen therapy ■ Bed rest
Pulmonary hypertension	■ History and physical examination ■ CBC ■ Chest x-ray ■ ECG or echocardiogram ■ CT scan or MRI	■ Diuretic therapy ■ Anticoagulant therapy ■ Vasodilator therapy such as calcium channel blocker ■ Prostacyclin agents ■ Oxygen therapy ■ Lung or heart/lung transplant
Chest trauma	■ History and physical examination ■ Chest x-ray	■ Analgesics, possibly epidural ■ Intercostal nerve blocks ■ Immobilization devices such as belts, binders, and taping ■ For flail chest: fixation may be necessary; intubation, mechanical ventilation
Inhalation injuries	■ ABG measurements ■ Chest x-rays ■ Bronchoscopy	■ Endotracheal intubation ■ Mechanical ventilation ■ Oxygen therapy ■ Bronchodilator therapy ■ Chest physiotherapy
Near-drowning	■ ABG measurements ■ Chest x-rays ■ Serum electrolytes	■ Induced coma ■ Corticosteroid therapy ■ Osmotic diuretic therapy

TABLE 32-3	Diagnostic Measures and Collaborative Care of Disorders of the Lower Respiratory Tract (continued)	
DISORDER	**DIAGNOSTIC MEASURES**	**COLLABORATIVE CARE**
Bronchitis	■ History and physical examination ■ Chest x-ray	■ Antibiotic therapy ■ Expectorant in the day and cough suppression at night ■ Analgesics
Pneumonia	■ History and physical examination ■ Chest x-ray ■ Sputum culture and sensitivity ■ ABG measurements ■ Fiber-optic bronchoscopy	■ Prevention: pneumococcal vaccine ■ Antibiotic therapy ■ Bronchodilator therapy ■ Mucolytic agents ■ Incentive spirometry ■ Endotracheal suctioning prn ■ Oxygen therapy ■ Chest physiotherapy ■ Analgesics
Acute Respiratory Distress Syndrome (ARDS)	■ Chest x-rays ■ ABG measurements ■ Pulmonary function tests ■ Monitoring of pulmonary arterial pressure	■ Medication therapy including nitric oxide inhalants, surfactant, NSAIDs, corticosteroids, vasopressors, diuretics ■ Prone position or lateral rotation therapy ■ Careful fluid replacement ■ Oxygen administration ■ Mechanical ventilation
Pleuritis	■ Chest x-rays ■ ECG	■ Analgesics ■ For pleural effusion: thoracentesis
Lung abscess	■ History and physical examination ■ CBC ■ Sputum culture ■ Chest x-ray	■ Antibiotic therapy ■ Postural drainage ■ Bronchoscopy ■ Tube thoracostomy (chest tubes)
Tuberculosis	■ Sputum smear ■ Chest x-ray ■ Nucleic acid amplification (NAA)	■ Antituberculosis therapy such as isoniazid (INH), rifampin (Rifamate), pyrazinamide, streptomycin, and ethambutol (Myambutol)
Asthma	■ History and physical examination ■ Pulmonary function tests ■ Peak expiratory flow rate monitoring ■ WBC count ■ ABG measurements	■ Identification of triggers ■ Bronchodilator therapy ■ Anti-inflammatory therapy to include corticosteroids
Chronic obstructive pulmonary disease	■ History and physical examination ■ Chest x-ray ■ Pulmonary function tests ■ ABG measurements	■ Smoking cessation ■ Bronchodilator therapy ■ Annual immunization against pneumonia and influenza ■ Prompt treatment of infections with antibiotics ■ Corticosteroid therapy ■ Oxygen therapy ■ Exercise: aerobic and breathing ■ Lung transplantation

MyNursingKit | ARDS

TABLE 32-3	Diagnostic Measures and Collaborative Care of Disorders of the Lower Respiratory Tract (continued)	
DISORDER	**DIAGNOSTIC MEASURES**	**COLLABORATIVE CARE**
Bronchiectasis	■ Chest x-ray ■ CT scan ■ Bronchoscopy ■ Sputum studies	■ Antibiotic therapy ■ Inhaled bronchodilators such as Serevent Discus ■ Chest physiotherapy ■ Oxygen therapy ■ Percussion and postural drainage ■ Bronchoscopy ■ Surgical lung resection
Emphysema	■ Pulmonary function tests ■ Pulse oximetry ■ ABG measurements ■ Chest x-rays	■ Smoking cessation ■ Medication therapy including antibiotics, bronchodilators, corticosteroids, alpha-antitrypsin replacement therapy ■ Pulmonary hygiene measures such as hydration, effective coughing, percussion, postural drainage ■ Regular exercise ■ Breathing exercises ■ Oxygen therapy
Cystic fibrosis	■ Pilocarpine iontophoresis sweat chloride test ■ Chest x-ray ■ Fat analysis of stool ■ Pulmonary function studies	■ Annual immunization against pneumonia and influenza ■ Bronchodilator inhalers ■ Prompt treatment of infections with antibiotics ■ Anti-inflammatory agents ■ Oxygen therapy ■ Lung or heart/lung transplantation ■ Pancreatic enzyme replacement ■ High-calorie, high-protein diet
Atelectasis	■ Chest x-ray ■ CT scans	■ Suctioning ■ Coughing; position on unaffected side ■ Bronchoscopy ■ Vigorous chest physiotherapy ■ Antibiotic therapy ■ Possible surgical removal of affected segment

disease, diabetes mellitus, chronic lung disease, and use of oral contraceptives.

Manifestations

Clinical manifestations of pulmonary embolism depend on the size of the embolus and where it lodges. Onset of the symptoms is typically sudden. Most commonly the client will complain of dyspnea and intense chest pain. Tachypnea, tachycardia, hypotension, diaphoresis, hemoptysis, and cyanosis may develop. The client usually expresses anxiety and apprehension. Auscultation of the chest may reveal crackles and S_3/S_4 gallop (see Chapter 33 ⬭⬭).

Diagnosis and Treatment

See Table 32-3 for diagnosis and treatment of pulmonary embolism.

Nursing Considerations

Prevention and prompt attention to presenting symptoms are the key to managing pulmonary embolism effectively. Dorsiflexion, pulmonary exercises following surgery, early ambulation, removal of items such as pillows under the legs that could contribute to venous stasis, and external pneumatic compression devices can help the client to avoid this condition. The nurse is responsible for teaching the client to recognize and report symptoms of pulmonary embolism.

Pulmonary Hypertension

Pulmonary hypertension can be defined as an elevation in the pulmonary arterial pressure. It occurs when the arteries and capillaries in the lungs become narrow or are blocked or destroyed, making it harder for blood to flow through the lungs. It includes a pulmonary artery systolic pressure greater than 30 mm Hg or a pulmonary artery mean pressure greater than 20 mm Hg.

Classification and Manifestations

Primary pulmonary hypertension is rare and only occurs in 1 to 2 cases per 1 million persons yearly. The cause is unknown, but a familial association exists in some cases. In other instances, use of cocaine may contribute to pulmonary hypertension. The appetite suppressant fenfluramine was withdrawn from the market in 1997 because of a link to this disorder. A higher incidence of primary pulmonary hypertension occurs in females than in males. Clinical manifestations of primary pulmonary hypertension include dyspnea and chest pain on exertion and fatigue. Dizziness may also be present.

Secondary pulmonary hypertension occurs when a medical condition reduces the size of the pulmonary arteries and capillaries. Conditions related to secondary pulmonary hypertension include chronic obstructive lung diseases, sleep apnea, pulmonary embolism, left ventricular heart failure, AIDS, connective tissue disorders, lupus, chronic liver disease, and congenital heart disease. Symptoms are similar to primary pulmonary hypertension and include symptoms of the causative factor (Mayo Clinic, 2008).

Cor pulmonale, a complication of pulmonary hypertension, is right ventricular heart failure due to prolonged pulmonary hypertension. It may be acute, arising from pulmonary embolism, or chronic. Chronic cor pulmonale is typically associated with chronic obstructive pulmonary disease. In COPD, impaired pulmonary circulation creates altered blood flow through the pulmonary artery, reducing blood flow from the right ventricle and causing hypertrophy and dilatation. Symptoms resemble those of congestive heart failure including chronic productive cough, dependent edema, neck vein distention, and enlargement of the liver. (See disorders of the heart in Chapter 33 ⬭.) Other complications of pulmonary hypertension include pulmonary embolism, arrhythmias, and bleeding into the lungs.

Diagnosis and Treatment

Although pulmonary hypertension cannot be reversed, treatment can slow the process. Refer to Table 32-3 for diagnosis and treatment of pulmonary hypertension.

Chest Trauma

Injuries to the chest may be minor or life threatening, causing partial or complete disruption of respiratory or cardiac function. These traumatic events can be divided into two categories:

- *Blunt traumas* include injuries from a direct blow to the thoracic region, such as that from a steering wheel, seat belt, or heavy equipment. Blunt trauma may be associated with severe internal injuries.
- In a *penetrating trauma*, an object enters body tissues. Penetrating traumas include gunshot wounds, stabbings, and other objects that impale the thoracic region.

Manifestations

Pulmonary contusions are a kind of blunt trauma. They occur when the chest wall is abruptly compressed, such as in a crushing injury. Following compression, the chest wall is suddenly decompressed. Alveoli and pulmonary arterioles rupture. Inflammation and edema follow, impairing surfactant production and significantly affecting the client's ability to breathe. Oftentimes symptoms do not occur until 12 to 24 hours following the injury. Initial symptoms may include chest pain, difficulty breathing, hemoptysis, and anxiety. Ultimately the client may exhibit tachycardia, tachypnea, and cyanosis.

Fractures of the ribs may result from blunt traumas. This injury may also become a penetrating injury if the rib punctures underlying organs. Elderly clients with fractured ribs are at risk for pneumonia, atelectasis, and possible respiratory distress and failure. The primary symptom exhibited with fractured ribs is inspiratory pain. In an effort to reduce the pain, the client splints the injured site, stifles coughs, and reduces the depth of respirations. This decreased lung movement places the client at greater risk for developing pneumonia. The site of injury is often bruised. Crepitus may be palpated. Auscultation of breath sounds reveals diminished sounds in the bases of the lungs.

FLAIL CHEST.   When several ribs are fractured, a condition known as *flail chest* may occur. Lack of structural support hampers chest wall movement. The client's respiratory effort causes the chest wall to expand unequally. The affected side is depressed on inspiration and expands on expiration (Figure 32-25 ■).

Diagnosis and Treatment

See Table 32-3 for diagnosis and treatment of chest trauma and flail chest.

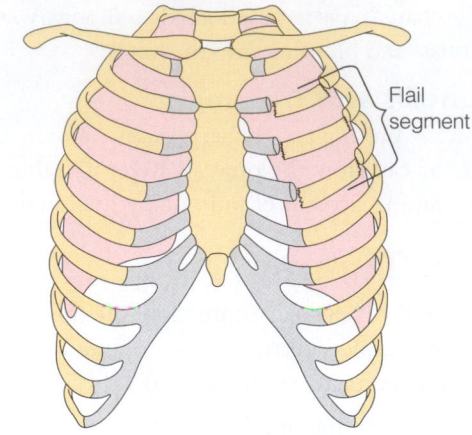

A Fracture pattern of flail chest

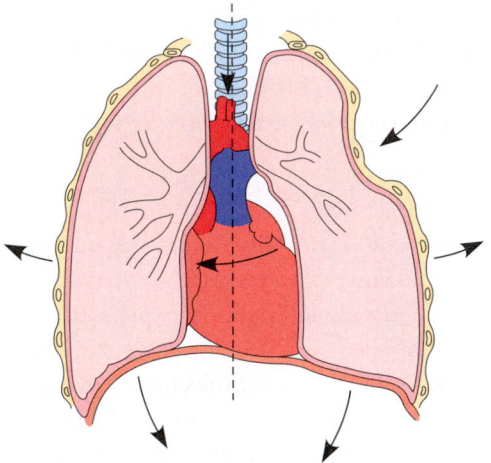

B Inspiration

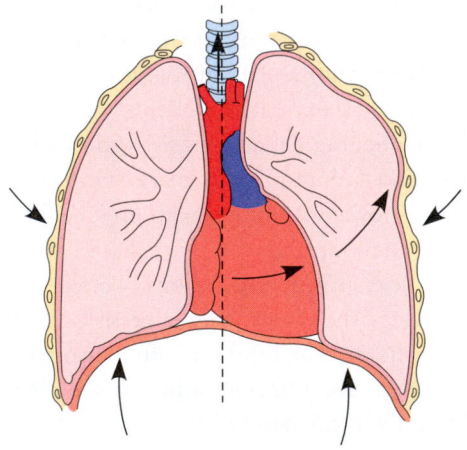

C Expiration

Figure 32-25. ■ Flail chest with paradoxic chest movement.

Inhalation Injuries

Pulmonary function can be severely compromised following inhalation of smoke, gases, fumes, toxins, and even hot air. Thermal damage, pulmonary irritation, or even asphyxiation may occur. Thermal damage may be a result of inhalation of steam, volatile gases, explosive gases, or the aspiration of hot liquids. **Asphyxiation** (oxygen deprivation or suffocation) can occur due to carbon monoxide poisoning or cyanide poisoning from the combustion of plastics, polyurethane, wool, silk, nylon, rubber, or paper products. Sulfur dioxide, ammonia, and chloride may be responsible for pulmonary irritation.

Manifestations

Clinical manifestations of inhalation injuries depend on the type of substance that was inhaled. Symptoms may include respiratory difficulties, cardiovascular changes, and neurologic symptoms.

Diagnosis and Treatment

Diagnosis and treatment of inhalation injuries are listed in Table 32-3.

Near-Drowning

In the United States, an average of 12 people per day will drown. It is the second leading cause of injury-related death for children ages 1 to 14. Drowning deaths are more common among men and occur more frequently when alcohol ingestion is involved. Drowning is also related to boating, particularly when individuals do not use personal flotation devices.

Manifestations

Individuals lose consciousness within 3 to 5 minutes following immersion in the water. Neurologic and circulatory impairment occurs after 5 to 10 minutes under water. Asphyxia and aspiration are the physical conditions most often associated with drowning or near-drowning. Figure 60-8 ∞ provides information on differences between fresh water and saltwater near-drowning.

The client who experiences near-drowning may be restless, lose consciousness at various levels, vomit, be cyanotic, experience tachypnea and tachycardia, or have hypotension and hypothermia. There is a difference in the clinical manifestations depending on the type of water the client aspirates:

■ Fresh water is hypotonic. It causes hypervolemia, hemodilution, hemolysis, electrolyte imbalances, and possible renal or respiratory failure.
■ Saltwater is hypertonic. It causes hypovolemia and hemoconcentration.

Either type of water puts a client at risk for pneumonia due to ingested bacteria and debris.

Diagnosis and Treatment

See Table 32-3 for diagnosis and treatment of near-drowning.

Nursing Considerations

When caring for clients with lower respiratory compromise or trauma, it is important to focus care on supporting the client and instituting emergency measures. Clients with pulmonary embolism, chest trauma, inhalation injuries, and near-drowning all need emergency treatment to prevent death. Place clients in the appropriate position to decrease respiratory effort and apply supplemental oxygen as ordered. Be ready to assist with intubation as necessary. Resuscitation bags should be at the client's bedside, connected to oxygen and ready to use. Intubation equipment should be nearby and checked to insure functionality. Clients with pulmonary hypertension must be monitored closely for signs of increasing heart failure such as dependent edema, neck vein distention, and moist lung sounds. Hypoxia causes anxiety. Clients who have difficulty breathing are often in a near-panic state, feeling they are going to die. Be very supportive of the client. Speak in calm, soothing tones, and remind clients to slow their breathing to increase the effectiveness of each breath. Reassure clients that the healthcare staff will not leave them alone.

Infections and Inflammations

BRONCHITIS

Bronchitis is the inflammation of one or more bronchi and may include the trachea. It may occur secondary to an upper respiratory tract infection. Bacteria and viral agents are the most common causes of bronchitis. However, it may also be caused by inhalation of physical and chemical irritants, such as tobacco smoke, dust, or automobile exhaust. Bronchitis may be either acute or chronic. Acute bronchitis is common in small children, the elderly, and the infirm client.

Rhinitis and pharyngitis may cause a persistent cough. Gradually this cough worsens and moves into the chest. The client may experience chest pain, fever, and purulent sputum. Wheezing or rhonchi may be heard on auscultation. Chronic bronchitis is associated with COPD, which is discussed in the next section. See Table 32-3 for diagnosis and treatment of bronchitis.

PNEUMONIA

Pneumonia is an inflammation of the lung that causes consolidation and exudation. In 2001 there were 61,777 deaths in the United States resulting from pneumonia. Clients considered at high risk for pneumonia include the elderly, infants, immobilized clients, and those with chronic conditions such as COPD, diabetes mellitus, congestive heart failure, and sickle cell anemia.

Pneumonia may be classified as either infectious or noninfectious. *Infectious pneumonia* may be caused by bacteria, viruses, fungi, or protozoa. Normal flora found in the respiratory tract may also cause pneumonia when the client is immunocompromised (see Chapter 35 ⬭). *Noninfectious pneumonia* results from aspiration and inhalation. Pneumonia may also be classified as community acquired, hospital acquired, or opportunistic. In pneumonia an inflammatory and immune response is initiated when the infecting agent is colonized in the alveoli. The substances released in these responses damage the mucous membranes. Ventilation and gas exchange are thus impaired.

The client may present with a variety of symptoms depending on the type and site of the pneumonia. An acute onset of fever, chills, cough with purulent or rust-colored sputum, and chest pain may occur. This pain is similar to pleuritis (discussed later in this chapter). Less common symptoms of pneumonia include nausea, vomiting, diarrhea, headache, sore throat, muscle aches, and fatigue. Due to resulting hypoxia, the elderly client may appear confused. On auscultation, the practitioner may hear diminished breath sounds, crackles, rales (see Box 21-8 ⬭), or pleural friction rub. See Table 32-3 for diagnosis and treatment of pneumonia.

ACUTE RESPIRATORY DISTRESS SYNDROME

Acute respiratory distress syndrome (ARDS) is a complication that results from other conditions, which may or may not involve the respiratory system. ARDS may result from head injury, shock, infection, drug overdosage, or trauma to the chest or pulmonary system. ARDS is a serious and potentially life-threatening complication that can result in death if rapid support and interventions are not supplied. In ARDS, the client's alveolar capillary membrane allows fluid to leak into the interstitial spaces and alveoli, causing the alveoli to become less elastic and collapse. Loss of alveoli results in impaired oxygenation, possible pulmonary hemorrhage, and pulmonary hypertension (increased pressure in the pulmonary artery and arterioles that reduces oxygenation still further). Clients with ARDS are at great risk for respiratory failure.

Manifestations

Clinical manifestations include dyspnea, tachypnea, tachycardia, cyanosis, and hypoxemia. For further information, see Chapter 47 ⬭, Emergency Room and Urgent Care Nursing.

Diagnosis and Treatment

It is important for the nurse to collect a thorough history when the client presents to the facility and assess the client's vital signs, respiratory effort, chest excursion, oxygenation, and breath sounds. Pulmonary function tests, arterial blood gases, and chest x-ray can be anticipated orders. ABG will reflect decreased PaO_2, increased $PaCO_2$, and respiratory acidosis. Chest x-ray may show thickened bronchial margins and/or infiltrates resulting from the changes in alveoli. See Table 32-3 for diagnosis and treatment of acute respiratory distress syndrome.

Nursing Considerations

The goal of nursing care is to optimize oxygenation and to treat the cause of ARDS. This client will often require mechanical ventilation and transfer to the critical care unit. This client will benefit from frequent repositioning and may be placed on a specialized bed that will rotate the client from side to side continuously to prevent further alveolar collapse. Frequent vital sign measurement and constant observation of this client is indicated.

PLEURITIS

Pleuritis or *pleurisy* is an inflammation of the pleura (see Figure 32-3 inset). Pleurisy may be related to pneumonia, tuberculosis, lung abscess, influenza, neoplasms, or injuries of the ribs. There are two types of pleuritis: dry or fibrinous and wet or pleural effusion. Dry pleurisy develops when the two layers of the pleura become inflamed and rub together causing unilateral pain. **Pleural effusion** develops when excess fluid accumulates in the pleural space. This fluid may be serous fluid, pus (empyema), blood (hemothorax), or blood and serous fluid (hemorrhagic pleural effusion). If this fluid is excessive, the lungs may collapse, causing a mediastinal shift. (See illustration and discussion of pneumothorax later in this chapter.)

Clinical manifestations of pleuritis include cough, fever, chills, pain worsening on inhalation, and rapid, shallow breaths. The nurse may observe limited chest excursion as the client guards against the pain. Auscultation may reveal diminished breath sounds and pleural friction rub. See Table 32-3 for diagnosis and treatment of pleuritis.

LUNG ABSCESS

A **lung abscess** is a necrotic area in the lung that forms as a result of consolidation. The area contains pus and is at risk for rupturing, spreading the infection into other parts of the respiratory system. Lung abscesses may occur as a result of pneumonia, tuberculosis, excessive ingestion of alcohol or illicit drugs, lung cancer, and general anesthesia.

Symptoms related to lung abscess may develop slowly over a period of 2 weeks. The client may experience a dry cough, chest pain, fever, chills, headache, dyspnea, odorous sputum, hemoptysis, and malaise. Breath sounds may be decreased or crackles heard when the practitioner listens to the chest cavity. See Table 32-3 for diagnosis and treatment of lung abscess.

TUBERCULOSIS

Tuberculosis (TB) is a chronic, infectious lung disease. TB is reportable to the Centers for Disease Control and Prevention. Each year, approximately 8 million people worldwide develop active TB and 3 million will die from the disease. In the United States 10 to 15 million people are infected and 1 in 10 of these will develop the active disease. Clients at greatest risk for developing TB include minorities, the elderly, intravenous drug abusers, the homeless and those living in poverty, immunocompromised clients, cancer clients, those with diabetes mellitus, those in long-term care facilities, and those in prisons.

The infecting agent for TB is *Mycobacterium tuberculosis*. It is spread via airborne droplets. Because TB is not highly contagious, repeated exposure usually transmits the organism. In the primary stage of the disease, a lesion called a **tubercle** develops (Figure 32-26 ■). This tubercle has a cheeselike (or *caseous*) center. Scar tissue then develops around the tubercle and calcification occurs. Those clients with effective immune systems will not develop the disease. However, the infection remains latent and may be reactivated if the client's immune system becomes compromised. At this time secondary TB develops and clinical symptoms may appear.

Manifestations

Clinical manifestations of secondary TB are fatigue, anorexia, weight loss, fever, night sweats, and a dry cough, which eventually produces purulent or blood-tinged sputum. Rupture of the tubercle may produce contamination of the pleural space, called *pleuritis*, or produce air in the pleural space, called *pneumothorax*.

Diagnosis and Treatment

TB may develop outside of the respiratory system. Areas of infestation include the blood, bone marrow, the urinary tract, the genitourinary tract, the subarachnoid space, and the bones and joints. Because of the risk of spread of this disease, the nurse is involved in selective screening for the TB infection. This is accomplished via two methods. The multiple-puncture tine test injects into the client's forearm a small amount of purified protein derivative (PPD) through a small multipronged device. The Mantoux test uses 0.1 mL of PPD injected intradermally also into the client's forearm. Results can be read 48 to 72 hours following the test. The nurse assesses for an area of **induration**, a raised, reddened area that may become hard (Figure 32-27 ■). This finding is considered positive and further diagnostic tests such as repeated PPD, chest x-rays, and sputum smears and cultures may be necessary.

See Table 32-3 for diagnosis and treatment of tuberculosis.

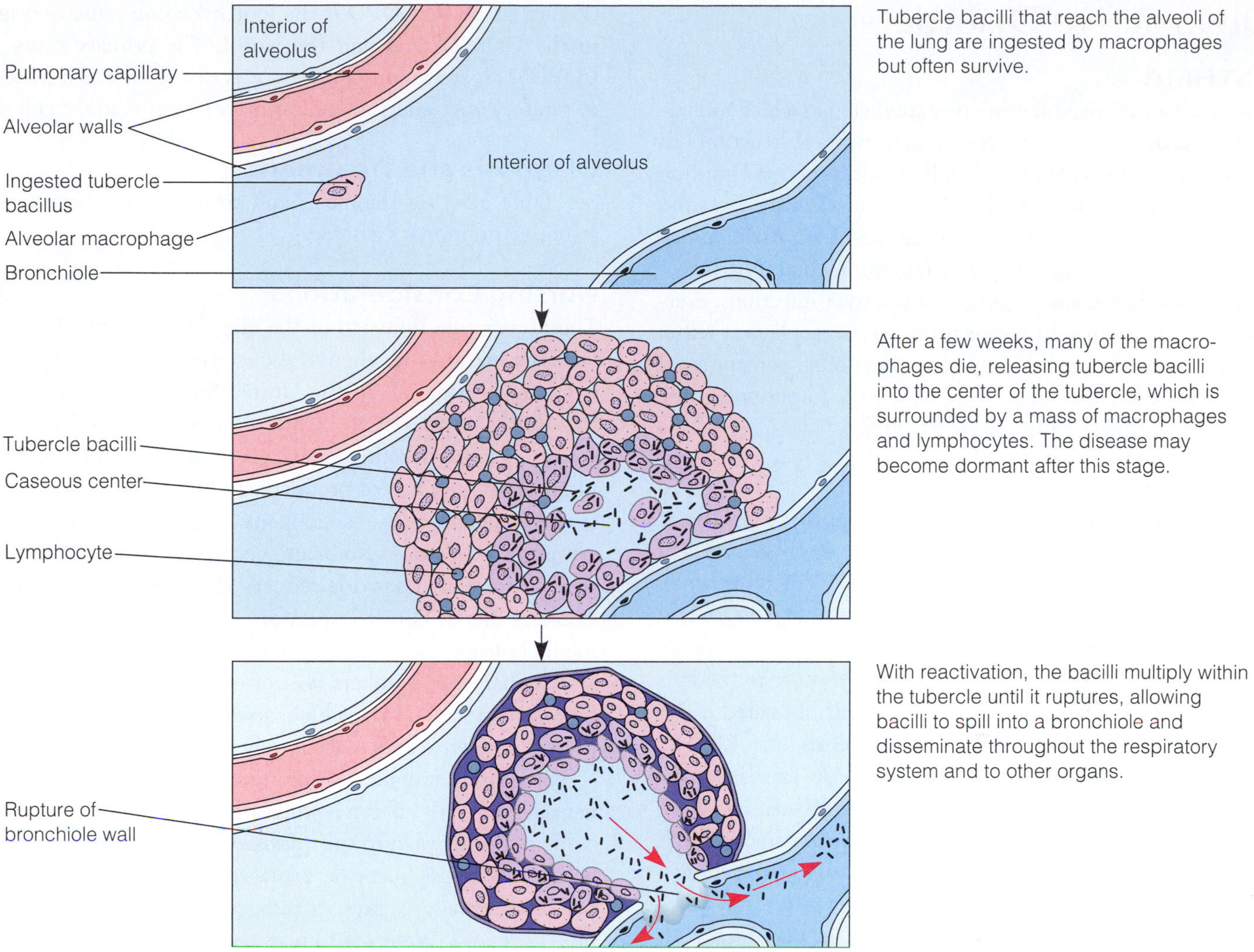

Interior of alveolus

Pulmonary capillary

Alveolar walls

Ingested tubercle bacillus

Alveolar macrophage

Bronchiole

Interior of alveolus

Tubercle bacilli that reach the alveoli of the lung are ingested by macrophages but often survive.

Tubercle bacilli

Caseous center

Lymphocyte

After a few weeks, many of the macrophages die, releasing tubercle bacilli into the center of the tubercle, which is surrounded by a mass of macrophages and lymphocytes. The disease may become dormant after this stage.

Rupture of bronchiole wall

With reactivation, the bacilli multiply within the tubercle until it ruptures, allowing bacilli to spill into a bronchiole and disseminate throughout the respiratory system and to other organs.

Figure 32-26. ■ The pathogenesis of tuberculosis. Tubercle bacilli multiply in macrophages and attract additional macrophages into the alveoli, forming a tubercle. The tubercle bacilli are surrounded by a mass of macrophages and lymphocytes. In a mature tubercle, a firm outer layer exists until reactivation and rupture.

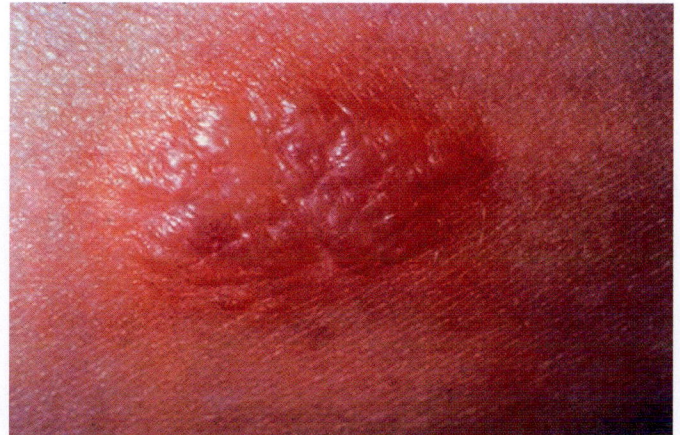

Figure 32-27. ■ Positive tuberculin skin test (Mantoux test), showing previous exposure to TB.

Nursing Considerations

When caring for clients with lower respiratory infections, make your priorities of care effective airway clearance, improved gas exchange, pain management, and prevention of complications. Maintain airborne or droplet precautions for clients with contagious illnesses, such as TB. Chest pain is a common symptom of lower respiratory infections. Ask clients about the location and intensity of the pain. Medicate as ordered, remembering that some pain medications can cause shallow respiratory effort. Keep the head of the bed elevated to increase lung expansion. Encourage deep breathing and coughing every 2 hours, using an incentive spirometer if ordered. Monitor vital signs every 4 hours, especially temperature and respirations, to evaluate the effectiveness of treatment. Instruct clients with TB to comply with their treatment regimen, which lasts for a year.

Obstructive Disorders

ASTHMA

Asthma is a chronic, inflammatory condition in which inflammation causes temporary, recurrent airway obstruction. In 2001 in the United States 14 million adults and 6.3 million children were diagnosed with asthma. It affects some races and ethnic groups more than others (Box 32-11 ■). Asthma may be caused by an allergic response (environmental, pharmacologic, or food), secondary to respiratory tract infections, exercise particularly in cold temperature, gastroesophageal reflux disease, and emotional responses. Asthma often is manifested in childhood and is discussed in Chapter 61. Common asthma triggers are illustrated in Figure 61-2 ⚭ .

Manifestations

Asthma occurs in two phases. The early-phase response is characterized by bronchospasm (see Figure 61-3 ⚭ , which provides a clear illustration of the mechanisms of asthma). The bronchospasm causes the client to wheeze, cough, and experience dyspnea and tightness of the chest. The late-phase response occurs 4 to 12 hours following exposure to the irritant. It is characterized by inflammation. If untreated it can lead to hypoxemia and respiratory alkalosis (see Chapter 26 ⚭). The client with asthma may also experience fatigue, anxiety, cyanosis of the lips and nail beds, and have pale, moist skin. A severe, prolonged asthma attack that is unresponsive to treatment is called **status asthmaticus.** Without resolution, status asthmaticus may result in respiratory failure. (See discussion of asthma in Chapter 61 ⚭ .)

Diagnosis and Treatment

Refer to Table 32-3 for diagnosis and treatment of asthma.

CHRONIC OBSTRUCTIVE PULMONARY DISEASE

Chronic obstructive pulmonary disease (COPD) is a pulmonary disorder characterized by airway obstruction caused by chronic bronchitis, bronchiectasis, or emphysema

---

(Figure 32-28 ■). COPD is the fourth leading cause of death in the United States and the world. The primary cause of COPD is cigarette smoking, but it is also related to recurrent respiratory tract infections and is more common in the elderly.

Diagnosis and Treatment

See Table 32-3 for diagnosis and treatment of chronic obstructive pulmonary disease.

Nursing Considerations

The nurse's role in assisting the client to prevent COPD is valuable. Educating clients about the effects of cigarette smoking is essential. In the United States one out of every five deaths is related to cigarette smoking. Besides being costly, cigarette smoking leads to periods of debilitation, hospitalization, and loss of productivity before death. Cigarette smoke contains many carcinogens. Nicotine stimulates the sympathetic nervous system and negatively affects the cardiac system. Carbon monoxide reduces the oxygen content of a smoker's blood. Direct respiratory effects of cigarette smoking include increased mucus production and narrowing of the airway diameter. Smokers will often have elevated levels of carbon monoxide in their bloodstream, which will cause the pulse oximeter to read inaccurately high.

Fortunately, stopping smoking can reverse many of these negative effects. Effective smoking cessation strategies include a specific plan to quit, including a date. Many clients will need to use nicotine replacement systems such as a patch, gum, nasal sprays, or inhalers. The substance bupropion (Zyban or Wellbutrin) may also be effective by increasing dopamine and epinephrine levels in the brain. Replacement activities such as exercise and creative activities should be encouraged. Support systems for quitting smoking can be helpful.

CHRONIC BRONCHITIS

Chronic bronchitis is defined as inflammation of the lining of the bronchial tubes with a mucus-producing cough that is present for 3 or more months (usually winter months) in 2 consecutive years. The inflammatory process causes vasodilation, congestion, and edema of the bronchial mucosa. The lengthy irritation of the bronchial tubes results in constant mucus production, and the bronchi become a breeding ground for infection. Incidence is higher in those over 45 years, and women are more than twice as likely to be diagnosed with this disorder as men.

Symptoms usually develop over a prolonged period of time, with recovery from colds taking longer with each event. There is a productive cough with thick sputum, cyanosis, right-sided heart failure, and loud rhonchi and wheezing on auscultation. Coughing is generally worse in the morning and in cold, damp weather (American Lung Association, 2007).

> ### BOX 32-11 · CULTURAL PULSE POINTS
>
> #### Frequency of Asthma
> Among adults, women of all races have higher rates of illness and death from asthma than do men. Death from asthma is two to six times more likely to occur among African Americans and Hispanics than among Whites. Rates for African Americans hospitalized for asthma are almost triple those for Whites. African Americans were four times more likely than Whites to visit an emergency department because of asthma. Asthma clients in general, and high-risk inner-city clients in particular, need to be able to recognize the signs and symptoms of uncontrolled asthma and know how to respond appropriately (U.S. Department of Health and Human Services, 2000).

MyNursingKit | Asthma

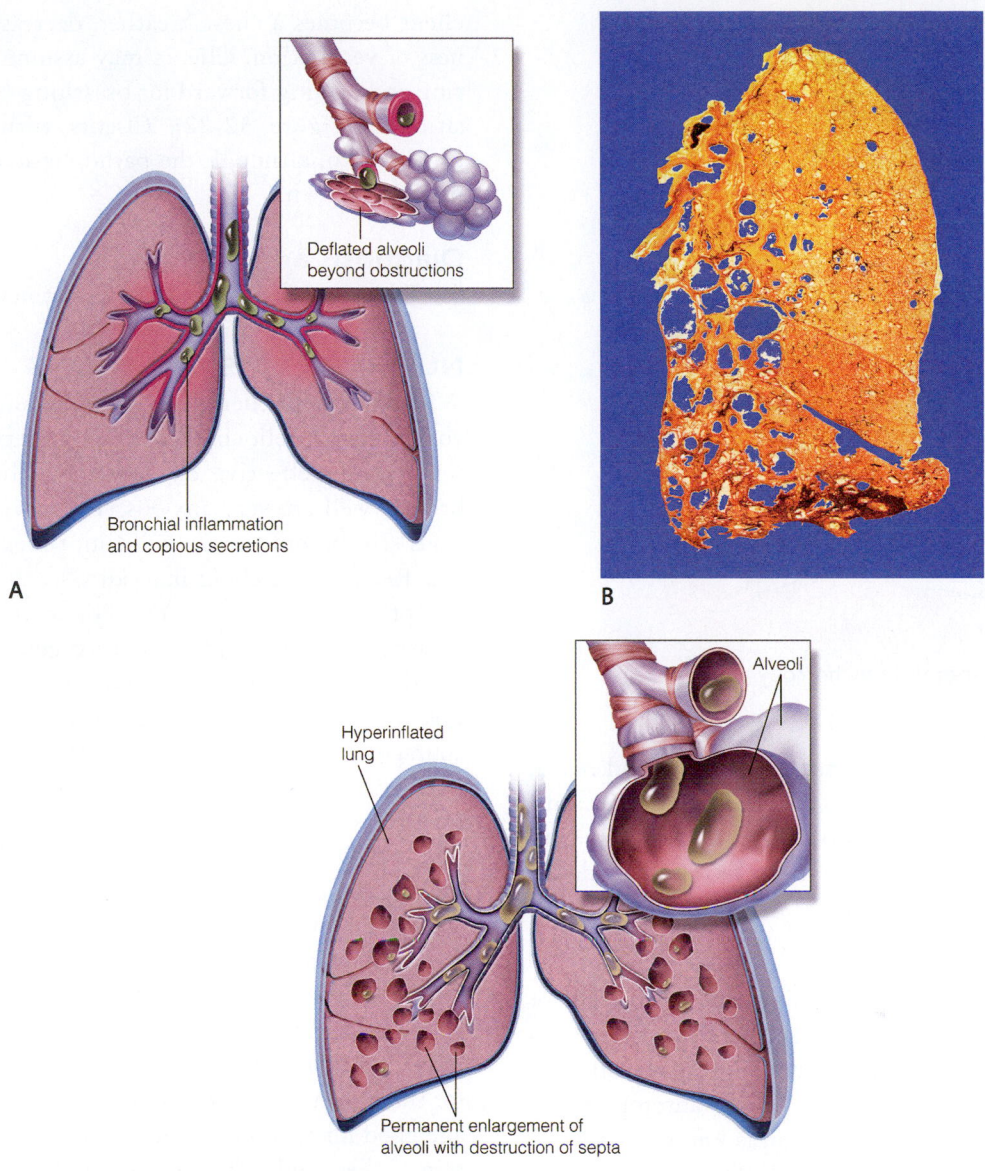

Figure 32-28. ■ COPD. **A.** Chronic bronchitis. With chronic bronchitis, sputum partially blocks the airway. The inset shows deflated clusters of alveoli past obstructed airways. **B.** Bronchiectasis. Gross anatomy of the lung showing abnormal dilation of the bronchi (bronchiectasis) of the lower lobe. *Source:* © Alain Pol. Phototake NYC. **C.** Emphysema. In emphysema permanent damage to the alveoli and pockets of air in the septa occur. The inset shows the interior of the alveoli.

BRONCHIECTASIS

Less common than chronic bronchitis, bronchiectasis is a chronic lung condition that obstructs pulmonary function. In bronchiectasis, there is an abnormal stretching and enlargement of the large airways (Figure 32-28B). With mucus accumulation and inflammation, the airways sometimes develop pockets in which infection can accumulate. The cycle of blocked airways and infection weakens the elasticity and musculature of the bronchial walls.

Manifestations

Clinical manifestations include copious sputum production, hemoptysis, foul-smelling breath, anorexia, anemia,

fever, pneumonia, wheezing, shortness of breath, and right-sided heart failure.

Diagnosis and Treatment

Diagnosis of bronchiectasis can be made through chest x-ray, CT scan, bronchoscopy (Figure 32-29 ■), and sputum studies. Clinical management is similar to that of atelectasis. Table 32-3 provides information about diagnosis and treatment of bronchiectasis.

EMPHYSEMA

Emphysema (Figure 32-28C) is a pulmonary condition characterized by overinflation and destruction of the alveolar walls. Lung elasticity and gas exchange are decreased, so

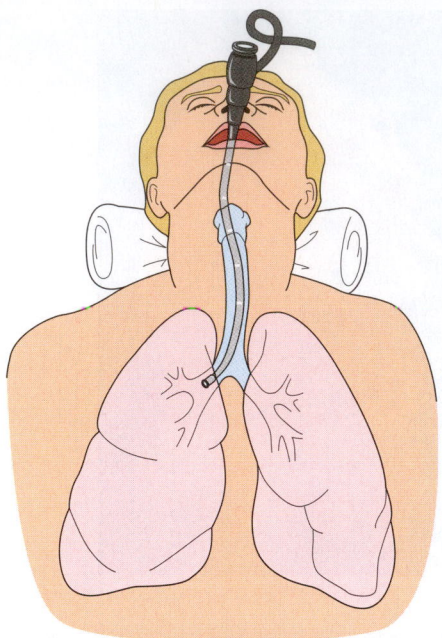

Figure 32-29. ■ Fiber-optic bronchoscopy.

air sacs within the lungs are unable to stretch and recoil, creating dead space where gas exchange should occur. Emphysema may accompany or follow chronic bronchitis. Cigarette smoking is implicated as a major factor in the development of this condition.

Manifestations

Dyspnea presents initially. Coughing may be present or not, productive or not. With worsening of the disease, increased amounts of air become trapped in the alveoli, flattening the diaphragm and increasing the anteroposterior diameter of the chest. This condition is known as a *barrel chest* (Figure 32-30 ■). Once barrel chest develops, the

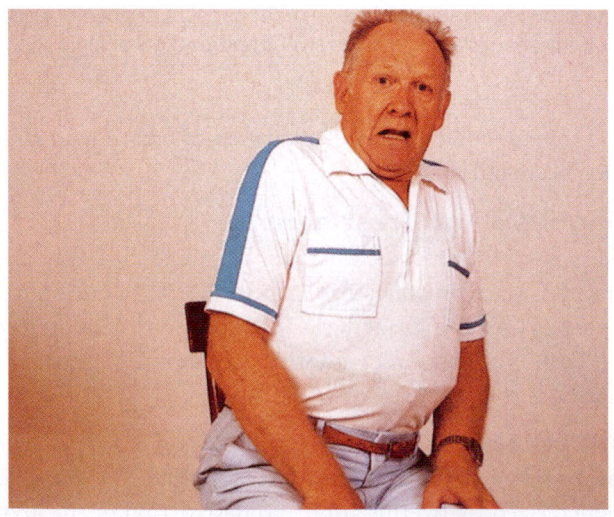

Figure 32-30. ■ Typical appearance of a client with emphysema.

client becomes a chest breather, decreasing the effectiveness of ventilation. Clients may assume a position of sitting and leaning forward for breathing (see the tripod position in Figure 32-22). Clients with emphysema are usually thin, although the pathophysiology for this finding is unknown.

Diagnosis and Treatment
See Table 32-3 for diagnosis and treatment of emphysema.

NURSING CONSIDERATIONS
When caring for clients with chronic lung disorders, focus your care on relieving anxiety, conserving energy, and maintaining effective oxygenation. Clients who cannot breathe well are very anxious. Those with chronic conditions still become anxious during times of extreme dyspnea. Reassure the client in a calm, soothing voice that you are present. Encourage the client to take slow deep breaths. Provide supplemental oxygen as ordered and assist the client to the most comfortable position for breathing, usually high-Fowler's or the orthopneic position. Encourage increased fluid intake to help thin secretions, making them easier to cough out. Provide a humidifier at the bedside, if ordered, to help moisten inspired air. Assess the client's respiratory rate every 2 to 4 hours, depending on the severity of the condition. Auscultate lung sounds for increases in wheezing or crackles. Check nail beds and mucous membranes for cyanosis. Encourage conservation of energy by helping clients plan their activities with rest periods. Because these clients use the neck and upper chest muscles to breathe, it is sometimes difficult for them to eat since it causes shortness of breath. Encourage good nutrition by offering frequent small meals, protein shakes, and other supplements as ordered. If ADLs cause extreme fatigue, encourage the client to step out of the shower and put on a terrycloth robe rather than trying to towel off. The client can then sit down and rest while getting dry.

CYSTIC FIBROSIS
Cystic fibrosis is an inherited recessive disorder affecting the epithelial cells of the respiratory, gastrointestinal, and reproductive tracts. The disorder causes dysfunction of the exocrine glands, leading to:

- Accumulation of excessively thick, adhesive, persistent mucus.
- Abnormal secretion of sweat and saliva.

About 30,000 American adults and children are living with cystic fibrosis. It is more common in Caucasians than African Americans. (Cystic fibrosis is diagnosed in infants or young children and is discussed in Chapter 59 ⬤⬤.)

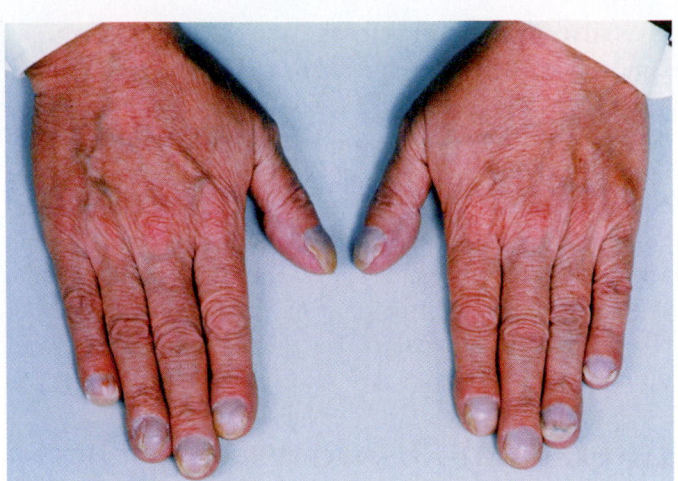

Figure 32-31. ■ Clubbing of fingers caused by chronic hypoxemia. (*Source:* John Radcliffe Hospital/Science Photo Library/Photo Researchers, Inc.)

Manifestations

The thick, sticky mucus that develops in the lungs causes dyspnea and increased susceptibility to infections, particularly infections of *Staphylococcus aureus*. Hypoxemia leads to **clubbing** (an increase in the angle between the base of the nail and the fingernail usually accompanied by increased depth, bulk, and sponginess of the end of the finger; Figure 32-31 ■) and barrel chest. The client may experience a productive cough with green-colored sputum. Pancreatic enzymes are prevented from reaching the duodenum by the thick, sticky mucus and this impairs digestion. Although appetite is not affected, weight gain and development often are. The client has abdominal pain and *steatorrhea*, excessive fat in the stool, causing stools to be frequent, bulky, and foul smelling. Reproductive effects include sterility in men and delayed menarche and infertility in women.

Diagnosis and Treatment

See Table 32-3 for diagnosis and treatment of cystic fibrosis.

ATELECTASIS

Atelectasis is a condition characterized by collapsed and airless lungs. This may occur partially, totally, acutely, or chronically. It is commonly caused by airway obstruction. Congenital atelectasis of the newborn often accompanies hyaline membrane disease. In the elderly client, airway obstruction may be due to secretions or a tumor. Postoperatively the client may fail to have the initiative to expand the lungs.

Manifestations

In acute atelectasis the client may experience dyspnea, cyanosis, fever, hypotension, or shock. Breath sounds may be diminished or absent. Chest excursion may be reduced.

Diagnosis and Treatment

See Table 32-3 for diagnosis and treatment of atelectasis.

Nursing Considerations

The client with atelectasis will need to have the airway obstruction removed. This can be accomplished through suctioning, coughing, bronchoscopy, and vigorous chest physiotherapy. Antibiotics may be necessary to treat infections. The nurse should promote drainage by placing the client on the unaffected side, helping the client make frequent position changes, and encouraging ambulation and deep breathing. Oral fluids may assist in liquefying secretions. In chronic atelectasis, surgery may be required to remove the affected section of the lung.

Lung Cancer

Lung and bronchus cancer is the second most common cancer among both men and women and is the leading cause of cancer death in both sexes. Men are more likely to have lung cancer, with African American males having the highest rate and American Indian males the lowest rate. More than 68,000 lung cancer deaths occur in women yearly. This is more than those who die from breast cancer. More women are diagnosed with breast cancer, but it is more treatable than lung cancer. Most women diagnosed with lung cancer will not live beyond 12 to 24 months.

The greatest risk of developing lung cancer is directly related to cigarette smoking. The more cigarettes smoked, and the more years a client smokes, the greater the risk. People who do not smoke but are exposed to second hand smoke, such as waitresses, family members of smokers, and those with frequent exposure to smokers, are also at risk for lung cancer. Lung cancer is also related to other inhaled carcinogens such as asbestos, radon, and arsenic.

Lung cancer is typically aggressive, invasive, and metastatic. The primary lesion is usually a mucosal lesion of the airway epithelium. The tumors are categorized as small-cell carcinoma (Figure 32-32A ■) and non-small-cell carcinoma. Twenty-five percent of lung cancers are small-cell and 75% are non-small-cell. Non-small-cell carcinomas are further classified as adenocarcinoma, squamous cell carcinoma, and large-cell carcinoma (see Figures 32-32B, C, and D).

Manifestations

Clinical manifestations may be absent or extremely vague. This fact means that at the time of diagnosis, most lung cancers are well advanced and the prognosis for these advanced cancers is poor. The earliest symptom may be a dry cough. Hemoptysis may be present. The client may experience wheezing, dyspnea, chest pain, and dysphagia. Anorexia, weight loss, weakness, and fatigue may occur. If the cancer

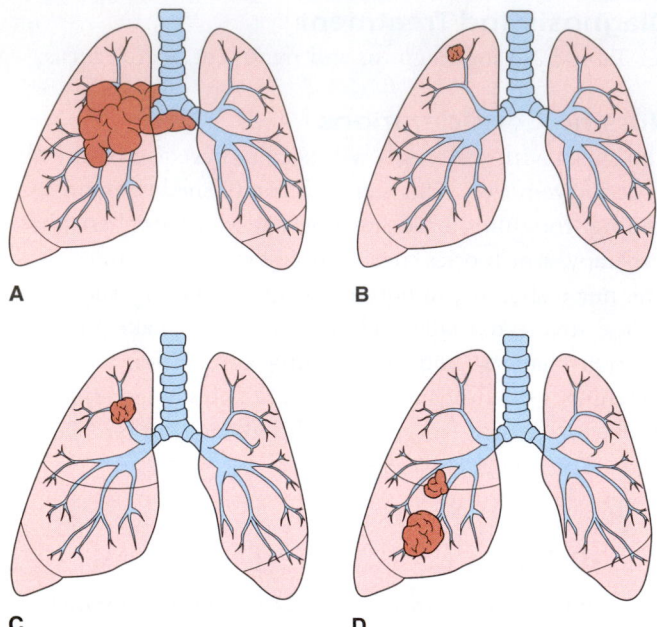

Figure 32-32. ■ Lung cancer: **A.** Small-cell (oat cell) carcinoma. **B.** Adenocarcinoma. **C.** Squamous cell carcinoma. **D.** Large-cell carcinoma.

metastasizes to the brain, confusion, impaired ambulation, headache, and personality changes may occur. With metastasis to the bone, pain, pathologic fractures, and spinal cord compression may occur. Liver metastasis results in jaundice and upper right quadrant pain. Cardiovascular symptoms include dizziness, vision disturbances, edema, flushing, and cyanosis. Respirations may be affected if laryngeal edema occurs.

Diagnosis and Treatment

The practitioner uses chest x-ray, sputum cytology, bronchoscopy, CT scan, tumor biopsy, CBC, liver function studies, and serum electrolytes to diagnose lung cancer. Clinical management of lung cancer will depend on the type of cancer diagnosed and the stage of disease. Chemotherapy, radiation, and surgery may be used alone or in conjunction with each other. Several chemotherapeutic agents are used together to attack the rapid growth of the cancer cells. Bronchodilators and analgesics may assist in combating side effects. Radiation goals include shrinking the size of the tumor and relieving clinical manifestations of lung cancer to make the client more comfortable. Intraluminal radiation or brachytherapy may be used. Several surgical procedures may be used to remove the tumor and surrounding cancerous tissue while leaving the lung in working order. The procedures used include laser bronchoscopy, mediastinoscopy, thoracotomy, wedge resection, segmental resection, sleeve resection, lobectomy, or pneumonectomy. *Note:* Chapter 45 🔗 discusses cancer and its treatment.

Nursing Considerations

Lung cancer is often interpreted by clients and loved ones as a death sentence because of its poor prognosis and aggressive nature. A primary nursing consideration is emotional support for both the client and support people. Encouraging the client to discuss fears and concerns while sharing in the decision making regarding treatment are important nursing actions. The nurse should support the client and loved ones as they work through the grieving process, but should not take away hope for recovery. For the main discussion about caring for clients with cancer, see Chapter 45 🔗.

Interstitial Disorders

OCCUPATIONAL LUNG DISEASES

Occupational lung diseases are caused by inhalation of hazardous substances in the work environment. Over time these inhaled substances cause an inflammatory response to the damaged alveolar epithelium. Lung scar tissue develops, causing the lungs to become stiff. Breathing now becomes difficult, lung volume decreases, and hypoxemia develops.

Classification and Manifestations

There are two types of these diseases. **Pneumoconioses** are chronic lung diseases caused when the client has long-term exposure to inorganic dusts such as asbestos or coal (black lung disease). Clients may be exposed to asbestos during mining, milling, manufacturing, or installation of products containing asbestos. Symptoms of dyspnea, exercise intolerance, and inspiratory crackles may not develop until 20 years following exposure.

Mesothelioma is a rare tumor of the pleura or peritoneum membranes that may develop as a result of asbestos exposure or other inhaled irritants. It carries a poor prognosis.

Hypersensitivity pneumonitis is an allergic lung disease that develops following exposure to organic dusts such as byssinosis (cotton), bagassosis (sugar cane), and moldy hay. This disease may be acute with symptoms of chills, fever, malaise, dyspnea, cough, and nausea occurring within 4 to 8 hours of exposure. It may also be chronic with symptoms of dyspnea, cough, anorexia, and weight loss occurring progressively.

Treatment

The nurse should be involved in protecting clients from occupational hazards by encouraging the use of masks to avoid inhalation of dangerous substances. Clinical management of these diseases is typically supportive in nature because no curative therapy is available.

SARCOIDOSIS

Sarcoidosis is a chronic condition in which granulomas form in response to an accelerated immune response. These granulomas are found most commonly in the lungs but may also be found in the lymph nodes, liver, eyes, skin, spleen, heart, and joints.

Manifestations

Clinical manifestations are related to the body system affected. In fact, it may be asymptomatic. Dyspnea, arthralgias, myalgias, fatigue, weight loss, fever, and skin lesions may develop.

Diagnosis and Treatment

To diagnose sarcoidosis, the practitioner may order blood work to review leukopenia, eosinophilia, and erythrocyte sedimentation rate. Chest x-rays, biopsies of the granuloma, and pulmonary function tests may also be ordered. Steroid and antibiotic therapy may be used to treat sarcoidosis.

PNEUMOTHORAX

Pneumothorax is an accumulation of air or gas in the pleural space that causes partial or complete collapse of the lung on the affected side. Pulmonary disease may cause a spontaneous pneumothorax. Air-filled blebs rupture and allow passage of air into the pleural space. The cause may be unknown or may be the result of conditions such as COPD, asthma, cystic fibrosis, ARDS, or TB.

A traumatic pneumothorax (Figure 32-33 ■) is a result of blunt or penetrating trauma of the chest wall and pleura. In an open pneumothorax, air from the environment enters the pleural space. *Hemothorax* or blood in the pleural space can occur as a result of an injury. Hemothorax may also be caused by TB, tumors, surgery, and infections. A closed pneumothorax occurs when air from the lung enters the pleural space. The iatrogenic pneumothorax occurs as a result of a medical procedure such as bronchoscopy, lung biopsy, or thoracentesis.

Manifestations

The client with spontaneous pneumothorax may experience chest pain, shortness of breath, tachypnea, tachycardia, hypotension, and asymmetrical chest wall movement.

Clinical manifestations of these types of pneumothorax are similar to a spontaneous pneumothorax. However, they may be difficult to discern from the symptoms resulting from the injury.

Tension pneumothorax (see Figure 32-33C) is a dangerous emergency situation that occurs when air flows into the pleural cavity from a bronchus but cannot escape. The pressure builds and places tension on the heart and opposite lung. Ventilation and cardiac output are affected. Shock may result. Prompt attention is necessary to correct the situation.

Diagnosis and Treatment

To diagnose pneumothorax, the practitioner uses oxygen saturation, arterial blood gas studies, and chest x-rays. Chest tubes may be inserted into the pleural cavity to restore negative pressure and drain collected fluid or blood. Because air rises, chest tubes for pneumothorax often are placed in the upper anterior thorax. Chest tubes used to drain blood or fluid are usually placed in the lower lateral chest wall.

When chest tubes are inserted, they must be connected to a sealed drainage system or a one-way valve that allows air and fluid to be removed from the chest cavity but prevents air from entering from the outside. Water-seal drainage systems (see Figure 32-14) are used to prevent outside air from entering the chest tube. Sterile disposable systems commonly are used. These systems typically have a closed collection chamber for drainage that is connected to the water-seal chamber. When the client inhales, the water prevents air from entering the system from the atmosphere. During exhalation, however, air can exit the chest cavity, bubbling up through the water. Suction can be added to the system to facilitate removal of air and secretions from the chest cavity.

The nurse must assess the system frequently, keep the collection chamber below chest level, ensure that the tubes are not kinked, measure drainage, and assist the client with frequent position changes as necessary.

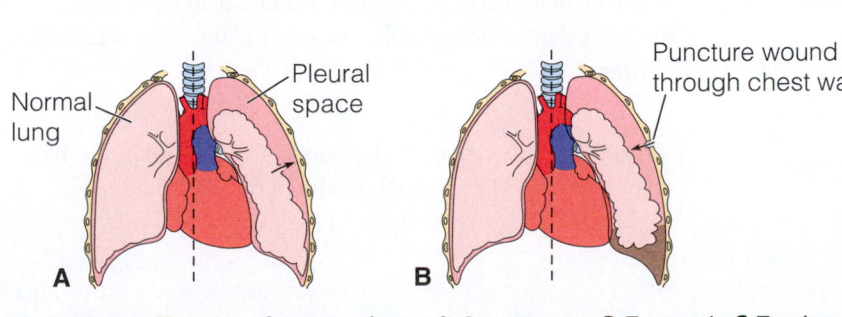

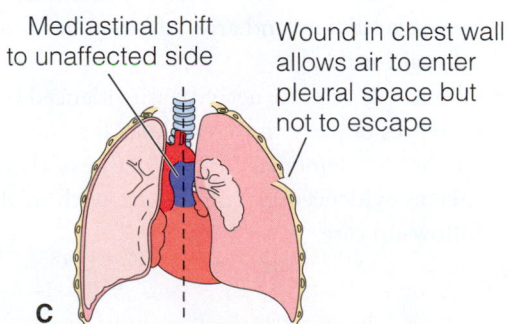

Figure 32-33. ■ Types of pneumothorax: **A.** Spontaneous. **B.** Traumatic. **C.** Tension.

NURSING CARE

PRIORITIZING NURSING CARE

The client experiencing respiratory distress will often demonstrate anxiety and requires the nurse to use therapeutic communication skills in addition to intervening to improve oxygenation. Reassure the client and attempt to reduce anxiety, which can increase respiratory distress. Position the client to optimize oxygenation. The health history may need to be delayed, except for most pertinent information, until the client is able to breathe comfortably enough to allow them to speak. Vital sign and pulse oximetry monitoring should be performed frequently until the client's condition stabilizes, and the nurse should seek help from the registered nurse and/or physician if the client's condition destabilizes. Rapid response teams are available for the client in acute distress to prevent further hypoxia and resulting complications.

ASSESSING

The nurse is responsible for obtaining a health history related to the lower and interstitial respiratory disorders including symptoms (especially dyspnea, cough, and chest pain), current medications, immunization history, smoking history, and past medical and surgical history. Objective data obtained from a physical examination should include overall appearance and level of distress, vital signs, lung sounds, respiratory *excursion* (rib and diaphragm movement), known allergies, and skin color.

DIAGNOSING, PLANNING, AND IMPLEMENTING

Some common nursing diagnoses for clients with lower respiratory and interstitial disorders are:

- *Ineffective Airway Clearance*
- *Activity Intolerance*
- *Ineffective Therapeutic Regimen Management*
- *Compromised Family Coping*

Typical outcomes for these clients might include:

- Client will have effective airway clearance as evidenced by patent airway and arterial blood gas levels within normal limits.
- Client will tolerate activity as evidenced by performing activities of daily living without fatigue.
- Client will demonstrate knowledge of therapeutic regimen as evidenced by compliance with medications and follow-up care.

- Client will express effective family coping as evidenced by the family's participation in the client's care.

Disorders of the lower respiratory system and interstitial disorders may be acute or chronic for the client and family. The nurse's role in providing support to these clients would include the following:

- Position the client in Fowler's or high-Fowler's position. *While in these positions the client may expand his or her chest more effectively; therefore, breathing will be facilitated.*
- Teach the client how to cough effectively and to breathe deeply. Provide suctioning prn. *These techniques assist the client to move secretions and clear the airway.*
- Collaborate with the client to plan activities of daily living to reduce drain on the client's energy. *Involving the client in these decisions will facilitate compliance with the medical regime. Combining activities will reduce the client's fatigue.*
- Provide range-of-motion exercises. *Keeping the muscles active and the joints mobile will assist the client to return to normal activity levels.*
- Involve the client's family in the medical regimen, particularly in assisting with stress reduction. *Enlisting the help of the client's support system will help to ensure compliance. Stress reduction is necessary to assist the client with avoiding fatigue.*
- When teaching the client and family about the therapeutic regimen, provide verbal and written instructions. *Written instructions allow the client and family to review the actions necessary for treatment of the disorder.*
- Provide an opportunity for the client's family to express their feelings regarding the client's disorder. *Expression of feelings is therapeutic to family members. It also allows the nurse to assess the level of support for the client and to plan interventions appropriately.*

EVALUATING

The nurse revises care until expected outcomes are achieved. The expected outcomes for a client with lower respiratory and interstitial disorders include:

- Client has improved airway clearance.
- Client demonstrates improved tolerance for activities of daily living.
- Client demonstrates effective therapeutic regimen.
- Client demonstrates effective coping and support for the client.

Note: The references and resources for all chapters have been compiled at the back of the book.

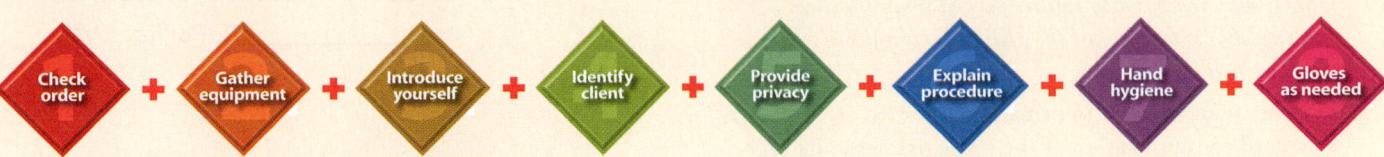

PROCEDURE 32-1 | # Measuring Pulse Oximetry

Purposes

- To measure the arterial blood oxygen saturation (SaO_2)
- To detect the presence of hypoxemia before visible signs develop

Equipment

- Pulse oximeter (Figure 32-34 ■)
- Nail polish remover as needed
- Sheet or towel

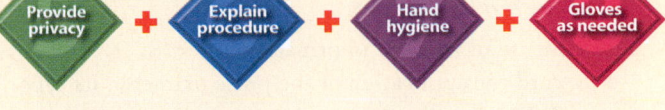

Check order ✚ Gather equipment ✚ Introduce yourself ✚ Identify client ✚ Provide privacy ✚ Explain procedure ✚ Hand hygiene ✚ Gloves as needed

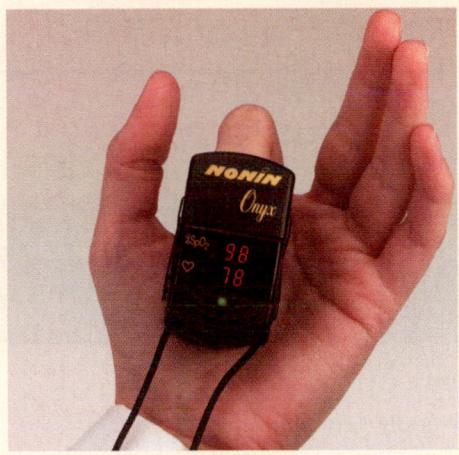

Figure 32-34. ■ Pulse oximeter with sensor reading. (Courtesy of Nonin Medical Inc.)

Interventions and Rationales

1. Perform preparatory steps (see icon bar above).

2. Select an appropriate sensor.
   - Choose a sensor appropriate for the client's weight and size. *Because weight limits of infant, pediatric, and adult sensors overlap, a neonatal sensor could be used for an infant or a pediatric sensor for a small adult.* See the manufacturer's directions for weight limits.
   - If the client is allergic to adhesive, use a clip or reflectance sensor without adhesive.

3. Select an appropriate site.
   - Use a location appropriate for the type of sensor.
   - If using an extremity, assess the proximal pulse and capillary refill at the point closest to the site. *Decreased circulation can alter the SaO_2 measurements.*
   - If the client has low tissue perfusion due to peripheral vascular disease or therapy using vasoconstrictive medications, use a nasal sensor or a reflectance sensor on the forehead.
   - Avoid using lower extremities that have compromised circulation and extremities that are used for infusions or other invasive monitoring.

4. Prepare the site.
   - Remove a female client's nail polish or acrylic nails. *These items can interfere with accurate measurements.*

5. Apply the sensor, and connect it to the pulse oximeter.
   - Make sure the LED and photodetector are accurately aligned, that is, opposite each other on either side of the finger, toe, nose, or earlobe. Many sensors have markings to facilitate correct alignment of the LED and photodetector. *Correct alignment is essential for accurate SaO_2 measurement.*
   - Attach the sensor cable to the connection outlet on the oximeter. Appropriate connection will be confirmed by an audible beep indicating each arterial pulsation. Turn on the machine according to the manufacturer's directions. Some devices have a wheel that can be turned clockwise to increase the signal volume and counterclockwise to decrease it.
   - Ensure that the bar of light or waveform on the face of the oximeter fluctuates with each pulsation and reflects the pulse volume or strength. *A signal that is too weak will not produce an accurate SaO_2 measurement.*

6. Set and turn on the alarm.
   - Check the preset alarm limits for high and low oxygen saturation and high and low pulse rates.
   - Change these alarm limits according to the manufacturer's directions as indicated.
   - Ensure that the audio and visual alarms are on before you leave the client. A tone will be heard and a number will blink on the faceplate.

7. Ensure client safety.
   - Inspect the location of an adhesive toe or finger sensor every 4 hours and a spring-tension sensor every 2 hours. Move it slightly or change the location as needed. *Movement prevents tissue necrosis due to prolonged pressure.*
   - Inspect the sensor site tissues for irritation from adhesive sensors.

8. Ensure the accuracy of measurement.
   - Minimize motion artifacts by using an adhesive sensor or immobilize the client's monitoring site. *Movement of*

the client's finger or toe may be misinterpreted by the oximeter as arterial pulsations.

- Cover a sensor with a sheet or towel to block large amounts of light from external sources (e.g., sunlight, procedure lamps, or bilirubin lights in the nursery). *Large amounts of outside light may be sensed by the photodetector and alter the SaO_2 value.*
- Verify that the client's hemoglobin level is normal. *An SaO_2 measurement may register normal when the client's hemoglobin is low because the available hemoglobin to carry oxygen is fully saturated.*

9. Document all relevant information.
   - Record the application of the pulse oximeter, its type and size, and all nursing assessments.

SAMPLE DOCUMENTATION

[date]
[time]

Oxygen saturation 91. Client c/o discomfort on rt second finger. Moved tester to rt third finger. Expressed comfort. T 36°C, P 62, R 15, BP 128/85.
_____ R. Parks, LVN

PROCEDURE 32-2

Administering Oxygen by Nasal Cannula or Face Mask

Purposes

- Nasal cannula: To deliver a relatively low concentration of oxygen when only minimal O_2 support is required
- To allow uninterrupted delivery of oxygen while the client ingests food or fluids
- Face mask: To provide moderate O_2 support and a higher concentration of oxygen and/or humidity than is provided by cannula

Equipment

- Oxygen supply with a flowmeter
- Humidifier with sterile, distilled, or tap water according to agency protocol
- Nasal cannula or prescribed face mask and tubing
- Gauze pads as needed

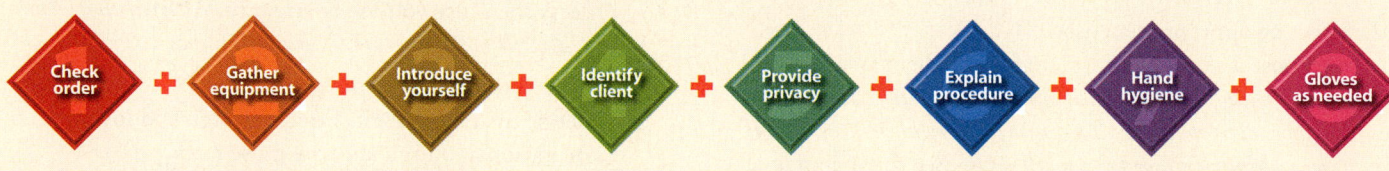

Check order + Gather equipment + Introduce yourself + Identify client + Provide privacy + Explain procedure + Hand hygiene + Gloves as needed

Interventions and Rationales

1. Perform preparatory steps (see icon bar above).
2. Determine the need for oxygen therapy, and verify the order for the therapy.
   - Perform a respiratory assessment. *This determines the need for O_2 therapy and develops baseline data if not already available.*
3. Prepare the client and support people.
   - Assist the client to a semi-Fowler's position if possible. *This position permits easier chest expansion and breathing.*
   - Explain that oxygen is not dangerous when safety precautions are observed and that it will ease the discomfort of dyspnea. Inform the client and support people about the safety precautions connected with oxygen use.

4. Set up the oxygen equipment and the humidifier.
5. Turn on the oxygen at the prescribed rate, and ensure proper functioning.
   - Check that the oxygen is flowing freely through the tubing. *There should be no kinks in the tubing, and the connections should be airtight. There should be bubbles in the humidifier as the oxygen flows through the water. You should feel the oxygen at the outlets of the cannula or mask.*
   - Set the oxygen at the flow rate ordered, for example, 2 to 6 L/min.
6. Apply the appropriate oxygen delivery device.

CANNULA

- Put the cannula over the client's face, with the outlet prongs fitting into the nares and the elastic band around the head (Figure 32-35 ■). Some models have a strap that adjusts under the chin.

■ If the cannula will not stay in place, tape it at the sides of the face.

■ Pad the tubing and band over the ears and cheekbones as needed. *This helps prevent skin breakdown.*

FACE MASKS

■ Guide the mask (Figures 32-36A–D ■) toward the client's face, and apply it from the nose downward.

■ Fit the mask to the contours of the client's face. *The mask should mold to the face, so that very little oxygen escapes into the eyes or around the cheeks and chin.*

■ Secure the elastic band around the client's head so that the mask is comfortable but snug.

■ Pad the band behind the ears and over bony prominences. *Padding will prevent irritation from the mask.*

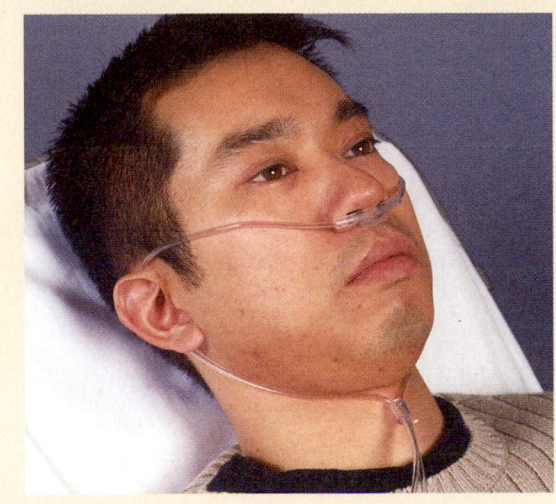

Figure 32-35. ■ Nasal cannula in place.

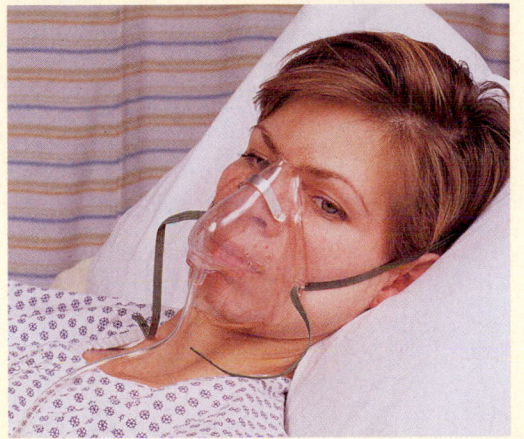

A

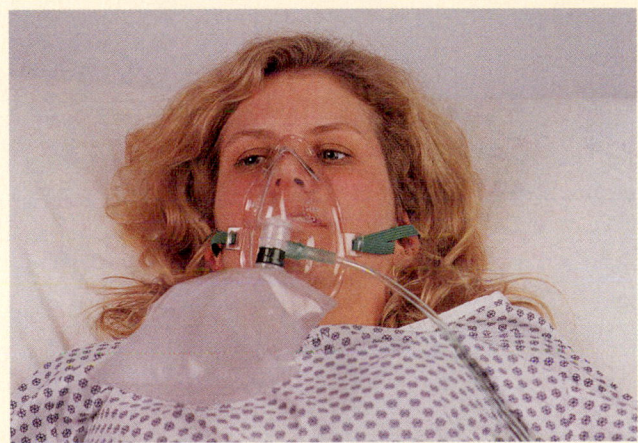

B

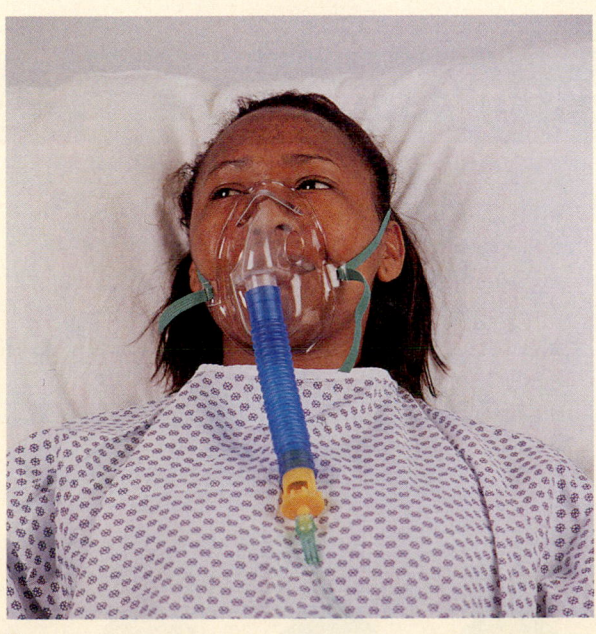

C

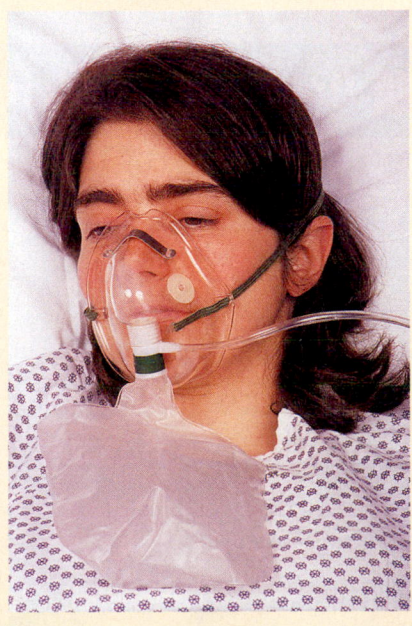

D

Figure 32-36. ■ **A.** A simple oxygen mask. (*Source:* © Jenny Thomas.) **B.** A partial rebreather mask. (*Source:* © Elena Dorfman.) **C.** A Venturi oxygen mask. (*Source:* © Elena Dorfman.) **D.** A nonrebreather mask. (*Source:* © Jenny Thomas.)

7. Assess the client regularly. *This allows early response to any changes or problems.*
   - Assess the client's level of anxiety, color, ease of respirations, and pulse oximeter reading (if available). Provide support while the client adjusts to the device.
   - Assess the client in 15 to 30 minutes, depending on the client's condition, and regularly thereafter. Assess vital signs, color, breathing patterns, and chest movements.
   - Assess the client regularly for clinical signs of hypoxia, tachycardia, confusion, dyspnea, restlessness, and cyanosis. Obtain arterial blood gas results if they are available.

NASAL CANNULA

- Assess the client's nares for encrustations and irritation. Apply a water-soluble lubricant as required. *Lubricants soothe the mucous membranes.*

FACE MASK

- Inspect the facial skin frequently for dampness or chafing, and dry and treat it as needed.

8. Inspect the equipment on a regular basis.
   - Check the liter flow and the level of water in the humidifier in 30 minutes and whenever providing care to the client.
   - Maintain the level of water in the humidifier.
   - Make sure that safety precautions are being followed.
9. Document relevant data.
   - Record the initiation of the therapy and all nursing assessments.

PROCEDURE 32-3 · Providing Tracheostomy Care

Purposes

- To maintain airway patency
- To maintain cleanliness and prevent infection at the tracheostomy site
- To facilitate healing and prevent skin excoriation around the tracheostomy incision
- To promote comfort

Equipment

- Sterile disposable tracheostomy cleaning kit or supplies including sterile containers, sterile nylon brush and/or pipe cleaners, sterile applicators, gauze squares
- Towel or drape to protect bed linens
- Hydrogen peroxide and sterile normal saline
- Sterile gloves (1 pair)
- Clean gloves
- Moisture-proof bag
- Commercially prepared sterile tracheostomy dressing or sterile 4×4 gauze dressing
- Cotton twill ties or commercially prepared self-closing ties
- Clean scissors

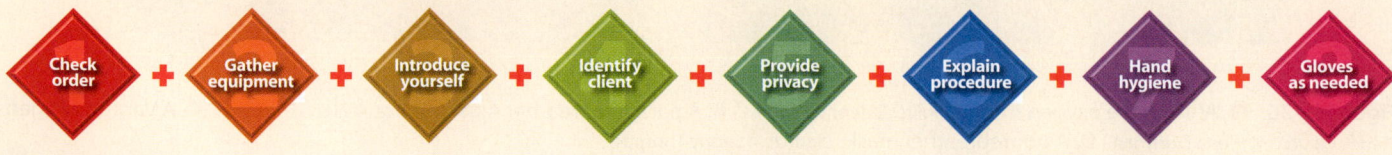

Check order + Gather equipment + Introduce yourself + Identify client + Provide privacy + Explain procedure + Hand hygiene + Gloves as needed

Interventions and Rationales

1. Perform preparatory steps (see icon bar).
   - Assist the client to a semi-Fowler's or Fowler's position. *This promotes lung expansion.*
   - Explain the procedure to the client and provide for a means of communication, such as eye blinking or raising a finger to indicate pain or distress. *This reduces client anxiety.*
   - Don clean gloves, remove the soiled tracheostomy dressing, and discard the glove and the dressing.
   - Open the tracheostomy kit or sterile basins. Pour sterile normal saline into both basins. Pour hydrogen peroxide into one basin only.
   - Establish a sterile field.
   - Don sterile gloves; place sterile towel on client's chest and under tracheostomy area.
   - Open other sterile supplies as needed including sterile applicators, and tracheostomy dressing.

2. Remove inner cannula.
   - Using one part of a fully opened 4 × 4 gauze, stabilize the flange with one hand. With the other end of the 4 × 4, use the other gloved hand to unlock the inner cannula (if present) and remove it by gently pulling it out toward you in line with its curvature. Place the inner cannula in the hydrogen peroxide solution to soak. *This moistens and loosens dried secretions.*

3. Clean the incision site and tube flange.
   - Using sterile applicators or gauze dressings moistened with normal saline, clean the stoma site (Figure 32-37 ■). Use each applicator or gauze dressing only once, then discard. *This avoids contaminating a clean area with a soiled gauze dressing or applicator.*
   - The hydrogen peroxide/saline solution may be used to remove encrustations. Thoroughly rinse the cleaned area, using gauze squares moistened with sterile normal saline. *Hydrogen peroxide can be irritating to the skin and inhibit healing if not thoroughly removed.*

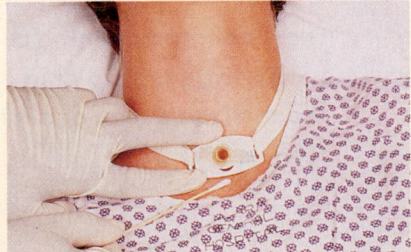

Figure 32-37. ■ Using an applicator stick to clean the tracheostomy site. (*Source:* © Jenny Thomas.)

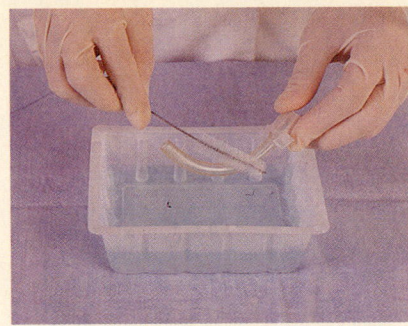

Figure 32-38. ■ Cleaning the inner cannula with a brush. (*Source:* © Elena Dorfman.)

   - Clean the flange of the tube in the same manner.
   - Thoroughly dry the client's skin and tube flanges with dry gauze squares.

4. Clean the inner cannula.
   - Remove the inner cannula from the soaking solution.
   - Clean the lumen and entire inner cannula thoroughly, using the brush or pipe cleaners moistened with sterile normal saline (Figure 32-38 ■). Inspect the cannula for cleanliness by holding it at eye level and looking through it into the light.
   - Rinse the inner cannula thoroughly in sterile normal saline. *Thorough rinsing is important to remove the hydrogen peroxide from the inner cannula.*
   - After rinsing, use a pipe cleaner folded in half to dry only the inside of the cannula; do not dry the outside. *This removes excess liquid from the cannula and prevents possible aspiration by the client, while leaving a film of moisture on the outer surface to lubricate the cannula for reinsertion.*

5. Replace the inner cannula, securing it in place.
   - Insert the inner cannula by grasping the outer flange and inserting the cannula in the direction of its curvature.
   - Lock the cannula in place by turning the lock (if present) into position to secure the flange of the inner cannula to the outer cannula.

6. Apply a sterile dressing.
   - Use a commercially prepared tracheostomy dressing of nonraveling material, or open and refold a 4 × 4 gauze dressing into a V shape as shown in Figure 32-39 ■. Avoid using cotton-filled gauze squares or cutting the 4 × 4 gauze. *Cotton lint or gauze fibers can be aspirated by the client, potentially creating a tracheal abscess.*
   - Place the dressing under the flange of the tracheostomy tube.
   - While applying the dressing, ensure that the tracheostomy tube is securely supported. *Excessive movement of the tracheostomy tube irritates the trachea.*

7. Change the tracheostomy ties.

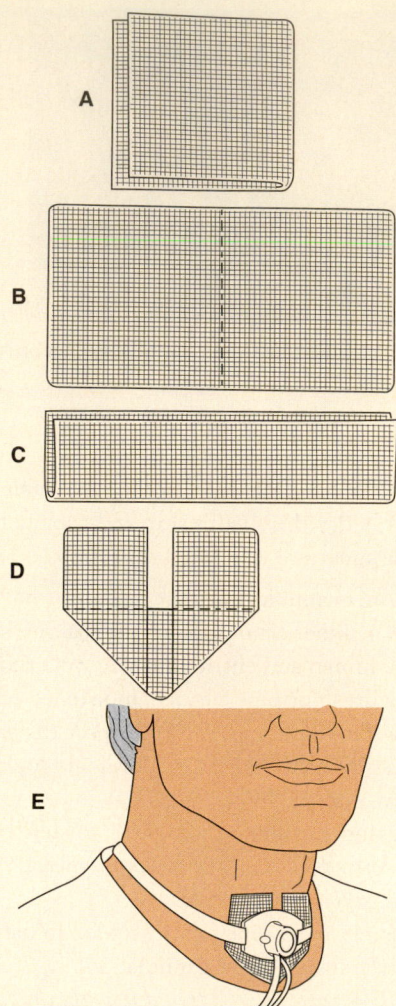

Figure 32-39. ■ Folding a 4 × 4 gauze to make a tracheostomy dressing.

ONE-STRIP METHOD

■ Cut a length of twill tape 2.5 times the length needed to go around the client's neck from one tube flange to the other.

■ Thread one end of the tape into the slot on one side of the flange.

■ Bring both ends of the tape together, and take them around the client's neck, keeping them flat and untwisted.

■ Thread the end of the tape next to the client's neck through the slot from the back to the front.

■ Have the client flex the neck. Tie the loose ends with a square knot at the side of the client's neck, allowing for slack by placing one finger under the ties as shown in Figure 32-40 ■. Cut off long ends.

8. Check the tightness of the ties.

■ Frequently check the tightness of the tracheostomy ties. *Neck movement may cause the ties to become too taut, interfering with coughing and circulation. Ties can loosen*

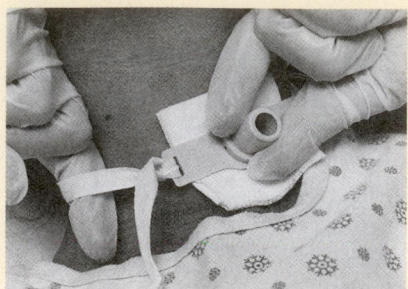

Figure 32-40. ■ Placing a finger underneath the tie tape before tying it. (*Source:* © Jenny Thomas.)

in restless clients, allowing the tracheostomy tube to extrude from the stoma.

9. Document all relevant information.

■ Record tracheostomy care and the dressing change, noting your assessments.

SAMPLE DOCUMENTATION: FOCUS CHARTING

Date	Time	Data Action Response
[date]	[time]	**D:** Encrustations noted around stoma; due for routine trach care. Breath sounds clear; no distress noted.

A: Using aseptic technique, removed soiled trach dressing. Set up sterile field per P&P and removed inner cannula for cleaning. Cleansed stoma site & flange. Reinserted inner cannula & locked into place. Applied clean ties using the one-strip method; 2 fingers fit tightly under ties. Applied around stoma and under flange. _____

R: Client tolerated procedure without S.O.B. or distress noted. Tracheal stoma pink, free of encrustations, and skin dry. Trach ties secure and inner cannula locked. _____

_____ N. Nurse, LVN

<table>
<tr><td>**PROCEDURE 32-4**</td><td># Suctioning</td></tr>
</table>

Purposes

- To remove secretions that obstruct the airway
- To facilitate ventilation
- To obtain secretions for diagnostic purposes
- To prevent infection that may result from accumulated secretions

Equipment

- Towel or moisture-resistant pad (sterile towel for tracheal or endotracheal suctioning)
- Portable or wall suction machine with tubing and collection receptacle
- Sterile disposable container for fluids
- Sterile normal saline or water

- Sterile gloves
- Sterile suction catheter kit (12 to 18 Fr for adults, 8 to 10 Fr for children, and 5 to 8 Fr for infants); if both the oropharynx and the nasopharynx are to be suctioned, one sterile catheter is required for each
- Water-soluble lubricant (for nasopharyngeal suctioning)
- Y-connector
- Sterile gauzes
- Moisture-resistant disposal bag
- Sputum trap, if specimen is to be collected
- Resuscitation bag (Ambu bag) connected to 100% oxygen for tracheal or endotracheal care
- Goggles and mask if necessary
- Gown (if necessary)

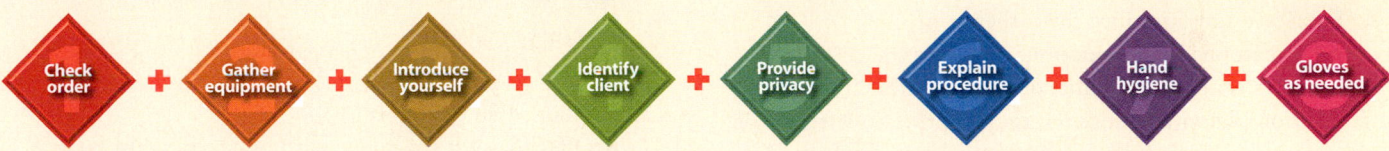

Check order + Gather equipment + Introduce yourself + Identify client + Provide privacy + Explain procedure + Hand hygiene + Gloves as needed

Part A: Oropharyngeal and Nasopharyngeal Cavities

Interventions and Rationales

1. Perform preparatory steps (see icon bar above).
   - Explain to the client that suctioning will relieve breathing difficulty and that the procedure is painless but may be uncomfortable and stimulate the cough, gag, or sneeze reflex. *Knowing that the procedure will relieve breathing problems is often reassuring and enlists the client's cooperation.*
   - Position a conscious person who has a functional gag reflex in the semi-Fowler's position with the head turned to one side for oral suctioning or with the neck hyperextended for nasal suctioning. *These positions facilitate the insertion of the catheter and help prevent aspiration of secretions.*
   - Position an unconscious client in the lateral position, facing you. *This position allows the tongue to fall forward, so that it will not obstruct the catheter on insertion. Lateral position also facilitates drainage of secretions from the pharynx and prevents the possibility of aspiration.*
   - Place the towel or moisture-resistant pad over the pillow or under the chin.

2. Prepare the equipment.
   - Set the pressure on the suction gauge, and turn on the suction. Many suction devices are calibrated to three pressure ranges:

   Wall unit:
   Adult: 100 to 120 mm Hg

   Child: 95 to 110 mm Hg
   Infant: 50 to 95 mm Hg

   Portable unit:
   Adult: 10 to 15 mm Hg
   Child: 5 to 10 mm Hg
   Infant: 2 to 5 mm Hg
   - Open the lubricant if performing nasopharyngeal suctioning.
   - Open the sterile suction package.
     a. Set up the cup or container, touching only its outside.
     b. Pour sterile water or saline into the container.
     c. Don sterile gloves and attach the catheter to the suction unit with the nondominant hand (Figure 32-41 ■). This hand will no longer be sterile. *The dominant hand maintains the sterility of the suction catheter, while the gloved nondominant hand prevents the transmission of the microorganisms to the nurse.*

3. Make an approximate measure of the depth for the insertion of the catheter and test the equipment.
   - Measure the distance between the tip of the client's nose and the earlobe, or about 13 cm (5 in.) for an adult.
   - Mark the position on the tube with the fingers of the sterile gloved hand.
   - Test the pressure of the suction and the patency of the catheter by applying your nonsterile gloved thumb to

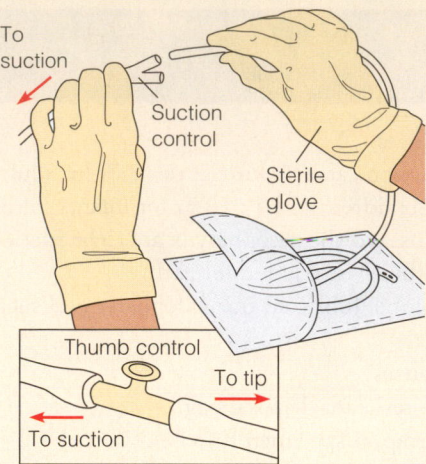

Figure 32-41. ■ Attaching the catheter to the suction unit.

the port or open branch of the Y-connector (the suction control) to create suction.

4. Lubricate and introduce the catheter.
   - For nasopharyngeal suction, lubricate the catheter tip with sterile water, saline, or water-soluble lubricant; for oropharyngeal suction, moisten the tip with sterile water or saline. *This reduces friction and eases insertion.*

FOR AN OROPHARYNGEAL SUCTION

- Pull the tongue forward, if necessary, using gauze.
- Do not apply suction (i.e., leave your thumb off the port) during insertion. *Applying suction during insertion causes trauma to the mucous membrane.*
- Advance the catheter about 10 to 15 cm (4 to 6 in.) along one side of the mouth into the oropharynx. *Directing the catheter along the side prevents gagging.*

FOR A NASOPHARYNGEAL SUCTION

- Without applying suction, insert the catheter the premeasured or recommended distance into either nares, and advance it along the floor of the nasal cavity. *This avoids the nasal turbinates.*
- Never force the catheter against an obstruction. If one nostril is obstructed, try the other.

5. Perform suctioning.
   - Apply your thumb to the suction control port to start suction, and gently rotate the catheter. *Gentle rotation of the catheter ensures that all surfaces are reached and prevents trauma to any one area of the respiratory mucosa due to prolonged suction.*
   - Apply suction for 5 to 10 seconds while slowly withdrawing the catheter, then remove your finger from the control, and remove the catheter.
   - A suction attempt should last only 10 to 15 seconds. During this time, the catheter is inserted, the suction is applied and discontinued, and the catheter removed. (Keep in mind that the client is deprived of oxygen during the suction procedure.)

- It may be necessary during oropharyngeal suctioning to apply suction to secretions that collect in the vestibule of the mouth and beneath the tongue.

6. Clean the catheter, and repeat suctioning as above.
   - Wipe off the catheter with sterile gauze if it is thickly coated with secretions. Dispose of the used gauze in a moisture-resistant bag.
   - Flush the catheter with sterile water or saline.
   - Relubricate the catheter, and repeat suctioning until the air passage is clear.
   - Allow 20- to 30-second intervals between each suction, and limit suction to 5 minutes in total. *Applying suction for too long may cause secretion to increase or decrease the client's oxygen supply.*
   - Alternate nares for repeat suctionings. *This will decrease irritation to mucosal lining.*

7. Encourage the client to breathe deeply and to cough between suctionings. *Coughing and deep breathing help carry secretions from the trachea and bronchi into the pharynx, where they can be reached with the suction catheter.*

8. Promote client comfort.
   - Offer to assist the client with oral or nasal hygiene.
   - Assist the client to a position that facilitates breathing.

9. Dispose of equipment and ensure availability for the next suction.
   - Dispose of the catheter, gloves, water, and waste container. Wrap the catheter around your sterile gloved hand, holding it as the glove is removed over it for disposal.
   - Rinse the suction tubing as needed by inserting the end of the tubing into the used water container. Empty and rinse the suction collection container as needed or indicated by protocol. Change the suction tubing and container daily. *This provides good infection control.*
   - Ensure that supplies are available for the next suctioning (suction kit, gloves, water or normal saline).

10. Assess the effectiveness of suctioning.
    - Auscultate the client's breath sounds to ensure they are clear of secretions. Observe skin color, dyspnea, and level of anxiety.

11. Document relevant data.
    - Record the procedure: the amount, consistency, color, and odor of sputum (e.g., foamy, white mucus; thick, green-tinged mucus; or blood-flecked mucus) and the client's breathing status before and after the procedure.
    - If the technique is carried out frequently, for example, every hour, it may be appropriate to record only once, at the end of the shift; however, the frequency of the suctioning must be recorded.

Part B: Tracheostomy or Endotracheal Tube
Interventions and Rationales

1. Prepare the client.
   - Inform the client that suctioning usually causes some intermittent coughing and that this assists in removing the secretions.
   - If not contraindicated because of health, place the client in semi-Fowler's position to promote deep breathing, maximum lung expansion, and productive coughing. *Deep breathing oxygenates the lungs, counteracts the hypoxic effects of suctioning, and may induce coughing. Coughing helps to loosen and move secretions.*
   - If necessary, provide analgesia prior to suctioning. *Endotracheal suctioning stimulates the cough reflex, which can cause pain for clients who have had thoracic or abdominal surgery or who have experienced traumatic injury. Premedication can increase the client's comfort during the suctioning procedure.*

2. Prepare the equipment.
   - Open the sterile supplies in readiness for use.
   - Place the sterile towel, if used, across the client's chest below the tracheostomy.
   - Turn on the suction, and set the pressure in accordance with agency policy. For a wall unit, pressure of about 100 to 120 mm Hg is normally used for adults, 50 to 95 mm Hg for infants and children.
   - Put on goggles, mask, and gown if necessary.
   - Put on sterile gloves. Some agencies recommend putting a sterile glove on the dominant hand and a nonsterile glove on the nondominant hand to protect the nurse.
   - Holding the catheter in the dominant hand and the connector in the nondominant hand, attach the suction catheter to the suction tubing (see Figure 32-41).

3. Flush and lubricate the catheter.
   - Using the dominant hand, place the catheter tip in the sterile saline solution.
   - Using the thumb of the nondominant hand, occlude the thumb control, and suction a small amount of the sterile solution through the catheter. *This determines that the suction equipment is working properly and lubricates the outside and the lumen of the catheter. Lubrication eases insertion and reduces tissue trauma during insertion. Lubricating the lumen also helps prevent secretions from sticking to the inside of the catheter.*

4. Quickly but gently insert the catheter without applying any suction.
   - With your nondominant thumb off the suction port, quickly but gently insert the catheter into the trachea through the tracheostomy tube (Figure 32-42 ■). *To prevent tissue trauma and oxygen loss, suction is not applied during insertion of the catheter.*
   - Insert the catheter about 12.5 cm (5 in.) for adults, less for children, or until the client coughs or you feel

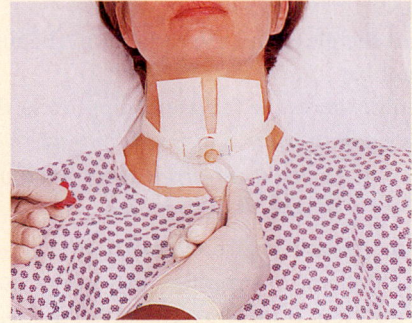

Figure 32-42. ■ Inserting the catheter into the trachea through the tracheostomy tube. (*Source:* © Jenny Thomas.)

resistance. *Resistance usually means that the catheter tip has reached the carina (bifurcation of the trachea into the main bronchi).* To prevent damaging the mucous membranes at the bifurcation, withdraw the catheter about 1 to 2 cm (0.4 to 0.8 in.) before applying suction.

5. Perform suctioning.
   - Apply intermittent suction for 5 to 10 seconds by placing the nondominant thumb over the thumb port. *Suction time is restricted to 10 seconds or less to minimize oxygen loss.*
   - Rotate the catheter by rolling it between your thumb and forefinger while slowly withdrawing it. *This prevents tissue trauma by minimizing the suction time against any part of the trachea.*
   - Withdraw the catheter completely, and release the suction.
   - Ventilate the client.
   - Then suction again.

6. Reassess the client's oxygenation status, and repeat suctioning.
   - Observe the client's respirations and skin color. Check the client's pulse if necessary, using your nondominant hand.
   - Encourage the client to breathe deeply and to cough between suctions.
   - Allow 2 to 3 minutes between suctions when possible. *This provides an opportunity for reoxygenation of the lungs.*
   - Flush the catheter, and repeat suctioning until the air passage is clear and the breathing is relatively effortless and quiet.
   - After each suction, pick up the resuscitation bag with your nondominant hand and ventilate the client with five breaths.

7. Dispose of equipment and ensure availability for the next suction.
   - Flush the catheter and suction tubing.
   - Turn off the suction, and disconnect the catheter from the suction tubing.

- Wrap the catheter around your sterile hand, and peel the glove off so that it turns inside out over the catheter.
- Discard the glove and the catheter in the moisture-resistant bag.
- Replenish the sterile fluid and supplies so that the suction is ready to be used again. *Clients who require suctioning often require it quickly, so it is essential to leave the equipment at the bedside ready for use.*

8. Provide for client comfort and safety.
   - Assist the client to a comfortable, safe position that aids breathing. *If the person is conscious, a semi-Fowler's position is frequently indicated. If the person is unconscious, Sims' position aids in the drainage of secretions from the mouth.*

9. Document relevant data.
   - Record the suctioning, including the amount and description of suction returns, the amount of sterile saline instilled, and any other relevant assessments.

SAMPLE DOCUMENTATION: FOCUS CHARTING

Date Time Data Action Response

[date] [time] **D:** Client w/audibly moist breath sounds; RR 30 and labored. Weak, ineffective cough. Rhonchi and coarse crackles auscultated A&P.

A: Positioned client in semi-Fowler's position. Maintaining sterile technique & following P&P, performed nasopharyngeal suctioning.

R: Copious amounts of thick, yellow secretions removed. RR 26 and less labored. Breath sounds with minimal coarse crackles @ bases bilaterally.

_____ N. Nurse, LVN.

Chapter Review

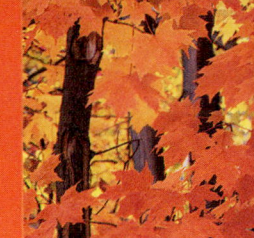

KEY Points

- The respiratory system includes pulmonary ventilation (the movement of air between the atmosphere and the lungs) and the diffusion of oxygen and carbon dioxide across the pulmonary membrane.
- The cardiovascular system transports these gases in the blood to the tissues, facilitates the diffusion of gases between the capillaries and body tissues, and carries away waste products from the tissues.
- Ninety-seven percent of oxygen is carried to the tissues loosely combined with hemoglobin in red blood cells (RBCs). Anemia, which is too few RBCs or low hemoglobin levels, impairs oxygen transportation.
- In most people, respirations are triggered by high carbon dioxide levels. However, people with COPD often have chronically high carbon dioxide levels, and their respirations are triggered by low oxygen (hypoxia). If they are given high levels of oxygen, they may stop breathing.
- Normal respirations are quiet and unlabored; altered respiratory patterns include tachypnea, bradypnea, hyperventilation, hypoventilation, and dyspnea. Shortness of breath is a subjective sensation of not getting enough air.
- A low-pitched snoring sound, stridor, and abnormal breath sounds may accompany partial airway obstruction.
- Managing disorders of the respiratory system require the nurse to fully understand the pathophysiology of the disorders and understand the multisystem effects caused by these disorders. Rapid intervention is required for the client experiencing hypoxia to prevent complications or death.
- Clients who are unable to meet body tissue oxygenation needs may require mechanical ventilation. The client with an artificial airway connected to a mechanical ventilator must be monitored closely and should have continuous cardiorespiratory and pulse oximetry monitoring. Ventilator alarms should be properly set and the nurse should respond to these alarms promptly when they ring to avoid life-threatening complications.

FOR FURTHER Study

See Chapter 19 for a full discussion on body assessment. For more information about respiratory patterns, see Table 19-4. For an illustration of clubbing, see Figure 19-7D.

For an in-depth discussion of steps in taking vital signs and lung sounds, see Chapter 21 and Box 21-8.

For more information about apnea and hypoxia, refer to Chapter 23.

For more information on respiratory and acid-base balance, refer to Chapter 26.

See Chapter 29 for nursing care of perioperative clients and Procedure 29-2 for steps in teaching postoperative exercises.

Pulmonary embolism and other cardiovascular disorders are discussed in more detail in Chapter 33.

For information about hematocrit and blood values, see Chapter 34.

Immunocompromised clients are discussed further in Chapter 35.

For more information on caring for the client with cancer, refer to Chapter 45.

See Chapter 47 for additional information on performing CPR and on the care of clients in emergency or urgent care facilities.

See Chapter 59 for more information on care of clients with upper respiratory infections and cystic fibrosis.

Figure 60-8 provides information on differences between fresh water and saltwater near-drowning.

See Chapter 61 for a discussion of asthma. Common asthma triggers are illustrated in Figure 61-2; Figure 61-3 provides a clear illustration of the mechanisms of asthma.

Critical Thinking Care Map

Caring for a Client with Pneumonia
NCLEX-PN® Focus Area: Physiologic Adaptation

Case Study: Betty Burt is a 39-year-old secretary who was admitted to the hospital with an elevated temperature, fatigue, and rapid labored respirations. Nursing history reveals that Ms. Burt has had a "bad cold" for several weeks that will not go away. She has been dieting for several months and skipping meals. In addition to her full-time job, she is attending college. She has smoked one pack of cigarettes per day since she was 18 years old. Chest x-ray confirms pneumonia.

Nursing Diagnosis: *Ineffective Airway Clearance*

COLLECT DATA

Subjective	Objective
_____	_____
_____	_____
_____	_____
_____	_____
_____	_____
_____	_____
_____	_____

Would you report this? Yes/No

If yes, report to: _____

What would you report? _____

Nursing Care

_____
_____
_____
_____
_____
_____
_____
_____
_____
_____
_____

How would you document this? _____
_____
_____
_____

Compare your answers and documentation to those provided on the MyNursingKit Website.

Data Collected
(use only those that apply)

- Height 5'6"
- Weight 120 lbs
- VS: T 103, P 82, R 24, BP 118/70
- Skin pale; cheeks flushed; chills; nasal flaring; use of accessory muscles; inspiratory crackles with diminished breath sounds right base; thick, yellow sputum
- Chest x-ray: right lobar infiltration
- WBC 14,000
- pH 7.48
- $PaCO_2$: 33 mm Hg
- HCO_3: 20 mEq/L
- $PaCO_2$: 80 mm Hg

Nursing Interventions
(use only those that apply; list in priority order)

- Assist Ms. Burt to a sitting position with head slightly flexed.
- Determine healthy body weight for age and height.
- Administer antipyretic medication for client comfort.
- Encourage client to relax the shoulders and flex the knees.
- Assess pain at least every 2 to 3 hours and administer analgesics as ordered.
- Provide written information as requested.
- Monitor intake, output, and daily weight.
- Arrange for dietary consult to determine calorie needs.
- Encourage her to take several deep breaths.
- Encourage her to take a deep breath, hold for 2 seconds, and cough two or three times in succession.
- Encourage use of incentive spirometry, as appropriate.
- Monitor rate, rhythm, depth, and effort of respirations.
- Auscultate breath sounds, noting area of decreased or absent ventilations and presence of adventitious sounds.
- Monitor respiratory secretions.
- Monitor increased restlessness, anxiety, and air hunger.

NCLEX-PN® Exam Preparation

1. The nurse helps the client to optimize oxygenation by placing the client in what position?
   1. Trendelenburg
   2. low-Fowler's
   3. Sims'
   4. high-Fowler's

2. The nurse notes the client's respirations increase and decrease in rate and depth with periods of apnea and documents:
   1. Kussmaul respirations.
   2. Tachypnea.
   3. Cheyne-Stokes respirations.
   4. Eupnea.

3. The nurse, caring for a 33-year-old client with a medical diagnosis of pneumonia, recognizes which of the following data as the highest priority?
   1. Size of pupils, presence of sneezing, oxygen saturation of 92%
   2. Presence of hiccups, amount of sweating, heart rate
   3. Capillary refill, amount of sputum, trembling, temperature
   4. Restlessness, chest wall movement, color of fingernails

4. The nurse is caring for a client experiencing an asthma attack and places the highest priority on which of the following outcomes?
   1. The client will report a decrease in anxiety level.
   2. The client will maintain an open airway with adequate gas exchange.
   3. The client will be afebrile.
   4. The client will maintain adequate fluid balance.

5. The nurse is caring for a client with dyspnea and recognizes that the client is experiencing orthopnea when the client demonstrates which of the following?
   1. Blood pressure decreases when standing upright.
   2. Blood gases indicate respiratory acidosis.
   3. Periods of apnea.
   4. Difficulty breathing unless sitting upright.

6. The nurse anticipates placement of a tracheostomy for which of the following clients?
   1. The postoperative client who will require mechanical ventilation for 2 to 3 days.
   2. The pediatric client who is unable to meet oxygenation requirements due to excess secretions caused by a respiratory infection.
   3. The client who is admitted with a fractured second cervical vertebrae and has no respiratory drive.
   4. The client with infection of the nasal sinuses and rhinorrhea.

7. An 87-year-old client is brought to the emergency room after being rescued from a house fire. Which of the following assessment findings would be of greatest concern to the nurse?
   1. Rapid, irregular respiration of 32/min
   2. Heart rate 124 beats per minute
   3. Partial and full thickness burns to the feet and legs
   4. Dry, nonproductive cough

8. The nurse, caring for an elderly client with a diagnosis of arterial insufficiency, is measuring oxygen saturation by placing the probe on the client's finger, which is pale and cool to touch. The oxygen saturation reads 74% and the client is alert, oriented, and breathing quietly at 14 breaths per minute. The nurse's priority action would be to:
   1. Call for assistance from the nursing supervisor, physician, or rapid response team.
   2. Apply oxygen at 2 liters per minute via nasal cannula and summon help.
   3. Document the reading and ask whether the client needs anything before leaving the room.
   4. Move the probe to the ear and obtain a new reading.

9. The nurse is caring for a client with a medical diagnosis of chronic obstructive pulmonary disease who requires the initiation of oxygen via nasal cannula. Which of the following orders would the nurse question before implementing?
   1. Apply oxygen via nasal cannula at 2 L/minute.
   2. Apply oxygen via nasal cannula at 3 L/minute.
   3. Apply oxygen via nasal cannula to maintain oxygen saturation greater than 95%.
   4. Apply oxygen via nasal cannula at 1 to 3 L/minute.

10. The nurse is performing tracheostomy care. Which of the following relates the steps to be followed in the proper order?
    1. Remove the old tracheostomy dressing; remove, clean and replace the inner cannula; change the tracheostomy ties; and apply a clean dressing.
    2. Remove, clean, and replace the inner cannula; remove the old tracheostomy dressing and replace with a clean one; and change the tracheostomy ties.
    3. Remove the old tracheostomy dressing; remove, clean, and replace the inner cannula; apply a clean dressing; and change the tracheostomy ties.
    4. Remove and replace the old tracheostomy dressing; remove, clean, and replace the inner cannula; and change the tracheostomy ties.

Answers and rationales for Review Questions appear in Appendix I.

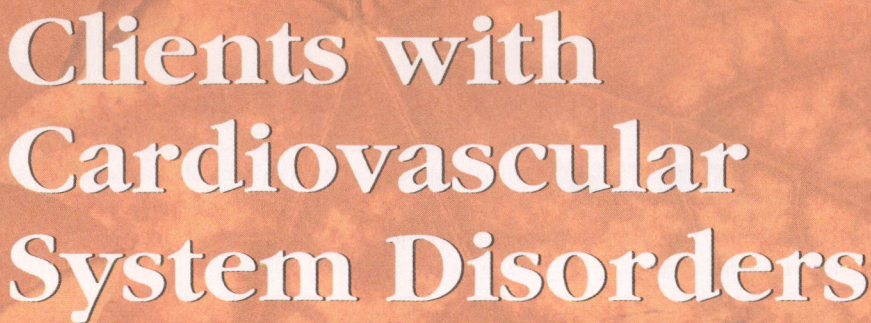

Chapter 33

Clients with Cardiovascular System Disorders

LEARNING Outcomes

After completing this chapter, you will be able to:

1. Review the structure and function of the cardiovascular system.
2. List factors that affect cardiovascular system function.
3. Describe tests for cardiovascular disorders.
4. Identify major heart disorders and nursing care for them.
5. Discuss normal and abnormal heart sounds.
6. Identify disorders that affect the heart and lungs and nursing care for them.
7. Describe valvular and inflammatory heart disorders and nursing care for them.
8. Identify conduction disorders and nursing care for them.
9. Discuss disorders affecting central circulation and nursing interventions for them.
10. Describe disorders affecting peripheral circulation and nursing care for them.

Clinical Objectives

11. Collect subjective and objective assessment data for clients with cardiovascular or peripheral vascular disorders.
12. Provide nursing care for clients undergoing diagnostic testing and monitoring for cardiovascular disorders.
13. Identify and correctly administer medications, with appropriate supervision, to clients with cardiovascular disorders, dysrhythmias, or peripheral vascular disorders.
14. Assist in the nursing care of clients undergoing invasive procedures or surgery of the heart.
15. Contribute to the care planning, and provide individualized nursing care, for clients with coronary heart disease and dysrhythmias.
16. Function as a member of the interdisciplinary team in providing appropriate care for cardiovascular clients, as allowed by state and local guidelines for an LPN/LVN.

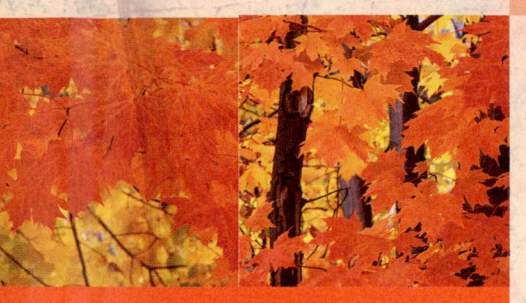

The respiratory and cardiovascular systems are closely linked and depend on each other to deliver oxygen to the tissues of the body. Alterations in function of either system can affect the other and lead to hypoxia, or lack of oxygen.

Two basic functions of the cardiovascular system are delivering oxygenated blood to the tissues and removing waste substances from the tissues.

The heart, blood vessels, and blood form the major transport system of the body, bringing oxygen and nutrients to the cells and removing wastes for disposal. The heart serves as the system pump, moving blood through the vessels to the tissues. The entire conduction system of the heart coordinates the contraction and relaxation (*cardiac cycle*) of the heart. Oxygen is continuously supplied to the cardiac muscle through the coronary arteries and a network of blood vessels.

Structure and Function of the Cardiovascular System

HEART

The heart is about the size of a fist. It lies against the diaphragm to the left of the sternum in the thoracic cavity (Figure 33-1 ■). The heart is anchored and protected by the **pericardium** (sac surrounding the heart). The pericardium has an inner and an outer layer. The outer fibrous pericardium attaches to the diaphragm and great vessels of the heart and the inner serous pericardium consisting of a

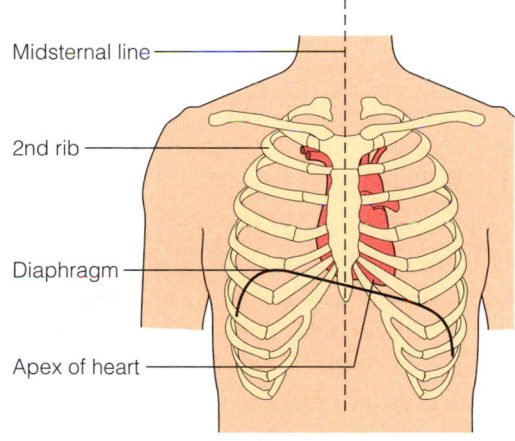

Figure 33-1. ■ Location of the heart within the chest cavity.

Midsternal line

2nd rib

Diaphragm

Apex of heart

double membrane (*outer parietal* and *inner viscera*). The space between these layers (*pericardial space*) is filled with serous fluid that provides cushioning for the heart as it beats.

In learning about the disease and disorders of the heart, it is helpful to have a mental picture of the heart's internal structure (Figure 33-2 ■). The wall of the heart has three layers: The outer layer is called the *epicardium*, the middle muscular layer the *myocardium* (the pumping force of the heart), and the inner lining the *endocardium*, which is in direct contact with the blood that passes through the heart.

The heart contains four chambers: two upper chambers and two lower chambers. A **septum** (wall) divides the left

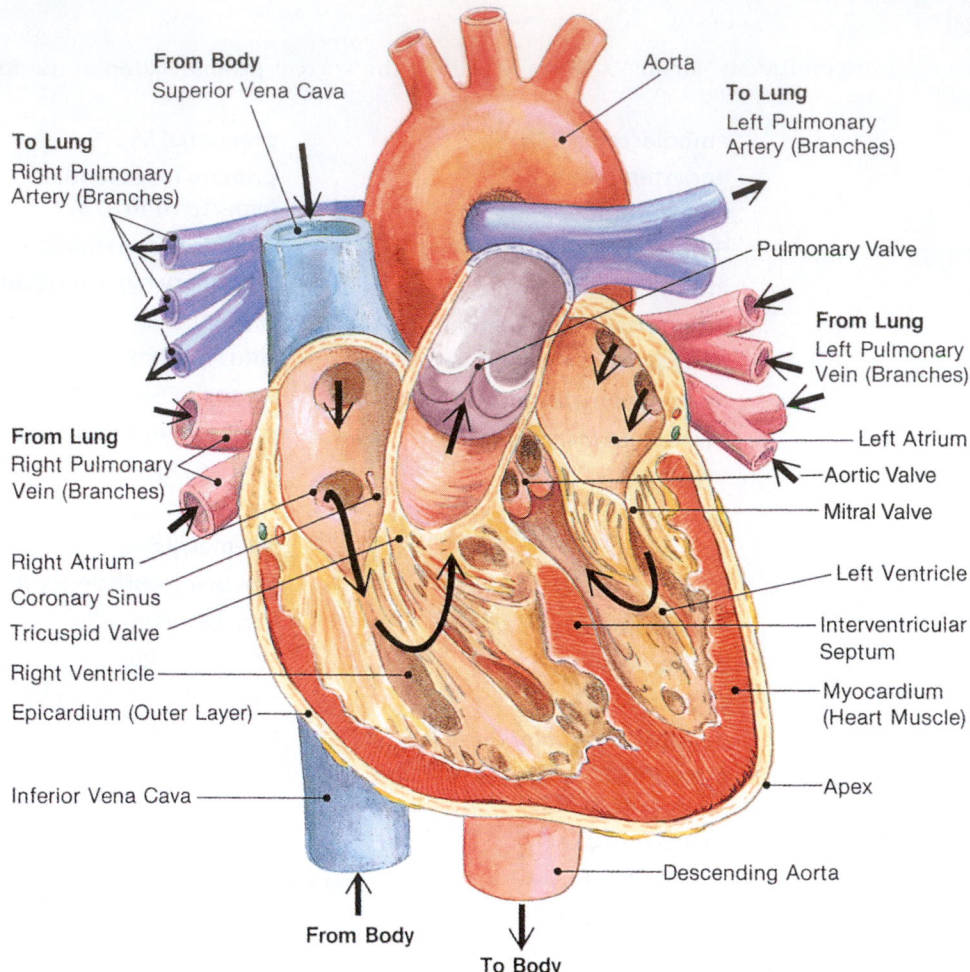

Figure 33-2. ■ The internal anatomy of the heart.

and right sides of the heart. The upper chambers are the right and left **atrium** (plural: *atria*). The lower chambers are the right and left **ventricle.** The atria and ventricles are separated by the *atrioventricular valves*. The flaps of these valves attach to the muscles of the ventricles, acting as one-way doors to prevent backflow when the ventricles contract.

The valve names reflect their shapes. The valve separating the right atrium from the right ventricle is the *tricuspid (three-leaf) valve*. The left atrium and ventricle are separated by the *bicuspid (two-leaf) valve*. The bicuspid valve is often called the *mitral valve* because its shape is similar to a bishop's hat, or miter.

Each ventricle connects to major blood vessels. The valves separating them from those vessels are the *semilunar (half-moon) valves*. As the blood travels through the heart, it enters the right atrium from the largest vein in the body, the vena cava. From the right atrium, it passes through the tricuspid valve and enters the right ventricle. When the ventricle contracts, the deoxygenated blood passes through the pulmonary valve into the large pulmonary artery which divides, taking the blood to the lungs for oxygenation

(Figure 33-3 ■). Blood is supplied to the heart muscle itself through *coronary circulation*. The left and right coronary arteries originate from the aorta and bring oxygenated blood to the heart muscle itself (Figure 33-4 ■).

The left atrium (see Figure 33-3) receives oxygenated blood from the lungs through the left and right pulmonary veins. The oxygenated blood in the left atrium then flows through the bicuspid (mitral) valve into the left ventricle. When the ventricle contracts, the blood passes through the aortic valve, into the aorta (the largest artery), which takes oxygenated blood throughout the body (systemic circulation). Facts about the heart in children are provided in Box 33-1 ■.

Conduction System

The heart beats because the specialized cells within the myocardium cause muscle contractions (about 60 to 100 times per minute). These specialized cells are the conduction system of the heart (Figure 33-5 ■). This entire sequence (contraction and relaxation of the heart) is called the **cardiac cycle** (Figure 33-6 ■).

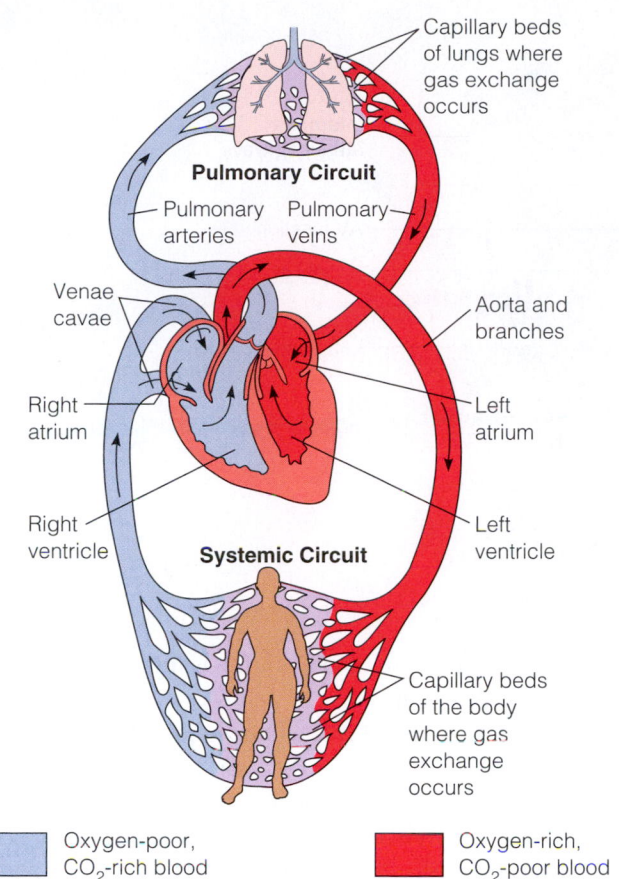

Figure 33-3. ■ Pulmonary and systemic circulation.

The initial electrical stimulation of the conduction system that starts the heartbeat takes place in the sinoatrial (SA) node in the right atrium. This is also called the *pacemaker* of the heart. The electrical stimulus then passes through internodal

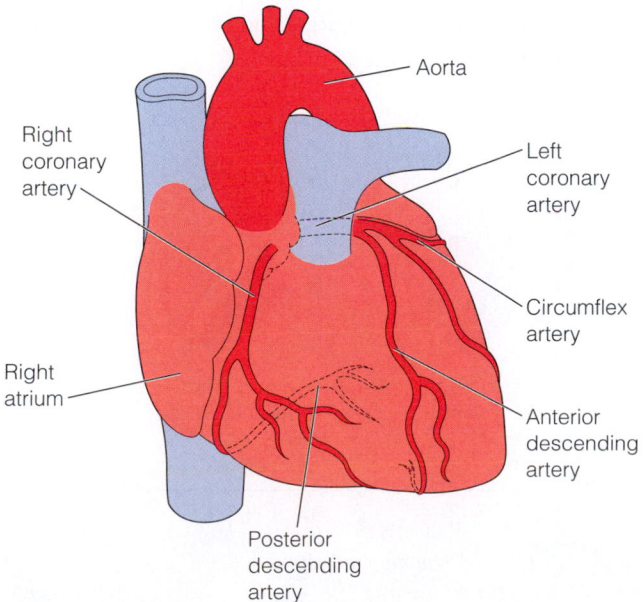

Figure 33-4. ■ Coronary arteries supply the heart muscle with oxygen.

BOX 33-1   PEDIATRIC CONSIDERATIONS

Pointers about the Heart

- In intrauterine life, the cardiovascular system is the first system to function.
- Newborns have high oxygen consumption and require a high cardiac output in the first few months of life.
- The normal range of blood pressure in neonates is between 65 and 95 mm Hg systolic over 30 to 60 mm Hg diastolic.
- Most heart defects in children are the result of imperfections in embryonic structure.
- Weighing the infant/child helps to determine the effectiveness of diuresis. Diapers must also be weighed to determine the output of urine.
- Every child should have blood pressure checked as part of the physical examination during childhood. Children whose parents have hypertension are more likely to develop hypertension.

---

pathways in the atria to the atrioventricular (AV) node located near the junction of the atria and ventricles. It then passes through the septum between the ventricles through tissue groups called the *bundle of His* (named for the German scientist who discovered it). As the stimulus passes through the right and left branches of the bundle and the Purkinje fibers in the ventricular walls, it causes the ventricles to contract.

The heart has an "all-or-nothing" response to electrical stimulation, meaning it always contracts as much as it is able. Between beats it briefly resists response (called the *refractory period*). The refractory period protects the heart from continuous contraction (*tetany*) or spasm.

The electrical impulse does not travel instantly to all parts of the heart. It slows slightly as it moves from the right atrium to the ventricles. On electrocardiogram (ECG or EKG), the movement of electricity through the heart can be seen as waveforms on the ECG strips.

One cardiac cycle equals one heartbeat. The ventricle fills during *diastole*, when the ventricles are relaxed. Toward the end of diastole, the atria contract, pumping 20% to 30% more blood into the ventricles (this is called *atrial kick*). Then the ventricles contract (*ventricular systole*), ejecting blood into the pulmonary and systemic circulation (see Figure 33-6). The amount of blood ejected from the heart in one contraction is called **stroke volume** (SV). In adults this is usually about 70 mL. **Cardiac output** (CO) is the amount of blood pumped by the ventricles in 1 minute (normally 4 to 8 liters per minute). The heart can adapt its function (i.e., pump slower or faster) to respond to the body's demands. *Heart rate* (the number of beats per minute) changes as we walk up a hill or sit in a chair. Cardiac output provides information on how well the heart is functioning. The cardiac output (CO) is determined by multiplying the heart rate (HR) by the stroke volume (SV). The average adult

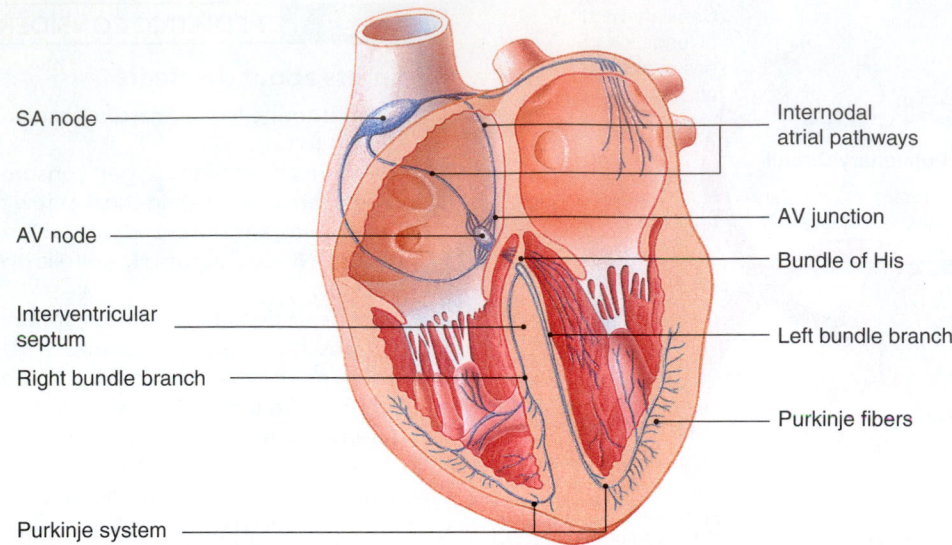

Figure 33-5. ■ Normal conduction pathways in the heart. (*Source:* Pearson Education/PH College.)

cardiac output ranges from 4 to 8 liters per minute. *Cardiac reserve* is the ability of the heart to increase output and blood pressure to meet demand.

Cardiac output is determined by four major factors: heart rate, preload, afterload, and contractility:

1. *Heart rate*—When the heart rate increases, it causes more blood to be pushed from the heart (cardiac output). We experience this when we run and our heart beats faster. However, if the rate of the heartbeat gets too rapid, the ventricles do not have time to fill completely, and cardiac output actually falls. If the heart rate is slow (below 60 bpm), cardiac output is low because the heart contracts less often.

2. *Preload*—Preload is the amount of blood in the ventricles before they contract. When the ventricles are full, they stretch and then contract more forcefully. Preload

decreases when the blood volume is low, as from hemorrhage or dehydration.

3. *Afterload*—Afterload is the force required for the ventricles to push blood out of the heart and into circulation. The right ventricle pushes blood to the lungs. The left ventricle has to work harder, because it pushes blood to circulate the blood through the whole body.

4. *Contractility*—Contractility refers to the natural ability of the cardiac muscle fibers to shorten (like an elastic band) during contraction, moving the blood into circulation. When the heart loses elasticity, the result is poor contractility, decreased stroke volume, and reduced ability of the ventricle to eject blood.

The percentage of blood in the ventricle (**ejection fraction**) that is ejected with each contraction is affected by preload, afterload, and contractility.

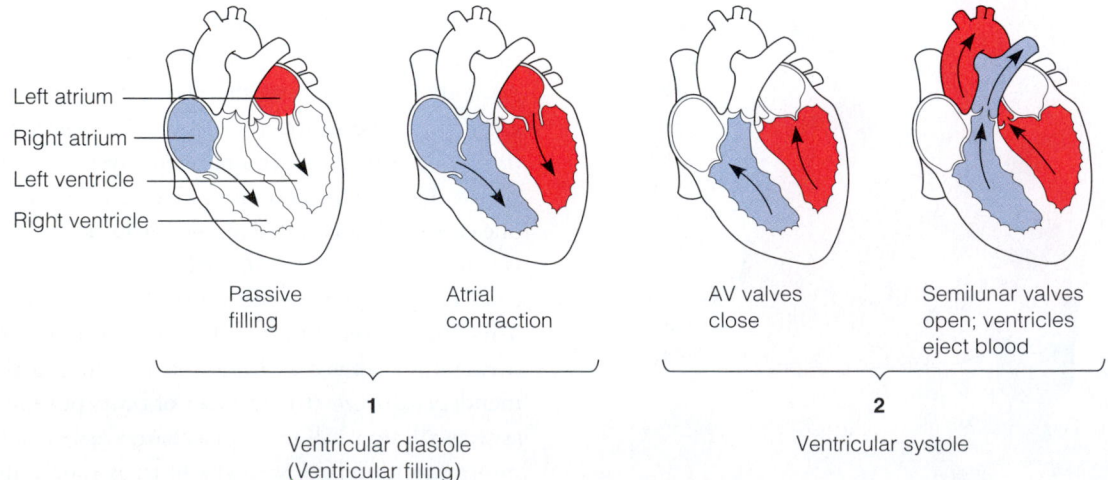

Figure 33-6. ■ Cardiac cycle: **1.** Ventricular filling occurs during diastole. **2.** Blood is pumped out of the heart to the pulmonary and systemic circulation during ventricular systole.

PERIPHERAL VASCULAR SYSTEM

The network of blood vessels that carry blood to the peripheral tissues and then back to the heart is called the peripheral vascular system. This network consists of arteries, veins, and capillaries (Figure 33-7 ■).

Arteries carry oxygenated blood away from the heart. The major artery, the *aorta*, branches into smaller arteries. These arteries then divide into smaller arteries called *arterioles*, which lead into hairlike arteries called *capillaries*. The capillaries lie within the organs and tissues and exchange the oxygen and nutrients for the metabolic waste. This waste, or deoxygenated blood, is then carried back to the heart through the *venules*, to the veins, and then to larger veins that empty the waste into the *inferior* and *superior venae cavae*. These large veins then empty into the right atrium of the heart. Blood vessel walls (except capillaries) have three layers (Figure 33-8 ■):

1. *Tunica intima, or endothelium*—innermost slick surface to assist blood flow
2. *Tunica media*—middle layer containing smooth muscle for expanding and contracting
3. *Tunica adventitia*—outermost layer of connective tissue that protects the vessel

The expanding (*dilation*) and contracting (*constriction*) of the arterioles maintain blood flow to the capillaries. This is a major factor in controlling blood pressure.

Veins have lower pressure, thinner walls, larger *lumen* (diameter), and a greater capacity than arteries. Veins have valves that assist in moving the blood back to the heart against gravity. The capillary beds contain both arterioles and venules and have one thin layer of tunica intima. This thin layer allows nutrients and gases to escape into the cells. It also allows metabolic waste products to enter the capillaries.

Arterial circulation is a balance of blood flow, peripheral vascular resistance, and blood pressure:

- *Blood flow* is the amount of blood in the body to be transported.
- *Peripheral vascular resistance (PVR)* is the force of blood that resists pushing by the heart. The amount of resistance is determined by how thick the blood is, how long the blood vessel is, and how large or small the blood vessel is:

  Blood viscosity (thickness)—thicker blood = greater resistance

  Vessel length—longer vessel = greater resistance

  Vessel diameter—smaller diameter = greater resistance

- *Blood pressure (BP)* is the force exerted by blood against the walls of the arteries:

  Systolic pressure—force exerted as the heart contracts (systole)

Diastolic pressure—force exerted when the heart is filling (diastole)

Example: $\dfrac{\text{Systolic} \rightarrow}{\text{Diastolic} \rightarrow} = \dfrac{120}{80}$

The average adult blood pressure is 120/80 mm Hg and is regulated by cardiac output and peripheral vascular resistance (PVR).

Additional factors can affect cardiac output, PVR, and blood pressure. These include diet, race, gender, age, weight, exercise, and emotional state. Note that several of these factors are controllable (diet, weight, exercise, and, generally speaking, emotional state).

Factors that Affect Cardiovascular System Function

In the healthy person, the cardiovascular and respiratory systems can provide sufficient oxygen to meet the body's needs. However, certain factors can affect the amount of oxygen entering the bloodstream and the function of the heart:

- Diseases of the cardiovascular or respiratory systems (e.g., anemia; see Chapter 34 ∞).
- Medications. Narcotics such as morphine and meperidine (Demerol) depress the respiratory center in the medulla, causing decreased respiratory depth and rate (see Chapter 27 ∞).
- Stress. When stressed, some people hyperventilate. Oxygen levels in arterial blood rise and carbon dioxide levels fall. This causes symptoms of dizziness, numbness of fingers and toes, and numbness around the mouth. (See hyperventilation in Chapter 26 and discussion of stress in Chapter 17 ∞ .)
- Anger may be connected to heart disease. Recent studies indicate that people who repress their anger or become hostile appear to have a higher incidence of heart disease.
- Gender may affect cardiopulmonary function. Through middle adulthood (until menopause), estrogen has a protective effect in women, slowing the progress of atherosclerosis and reducing the risk of cardiovascular disease. This effect is lost at menopause. (Hormone replacement therapy was considered to be beneficial in reducing this risk later in life. However, recent studies have raised doubts about its ability to protect the heart.) Among people in their 40s and 50s, men have a higher incidence of hypertension than women.

Cardiovascular disease (CVD) affects the ability of the heart and blood vessels to function normally. Cardiac functioning can be affected by obstruction, arrhythmias, inflammation or infection, and structural (valve and congenital) abnormalities.

The most common cause of heart disease is blockage or narrowing of the blood supply to the heart by the coronary

MAJOR ARTERIES

MAJOR VEINS

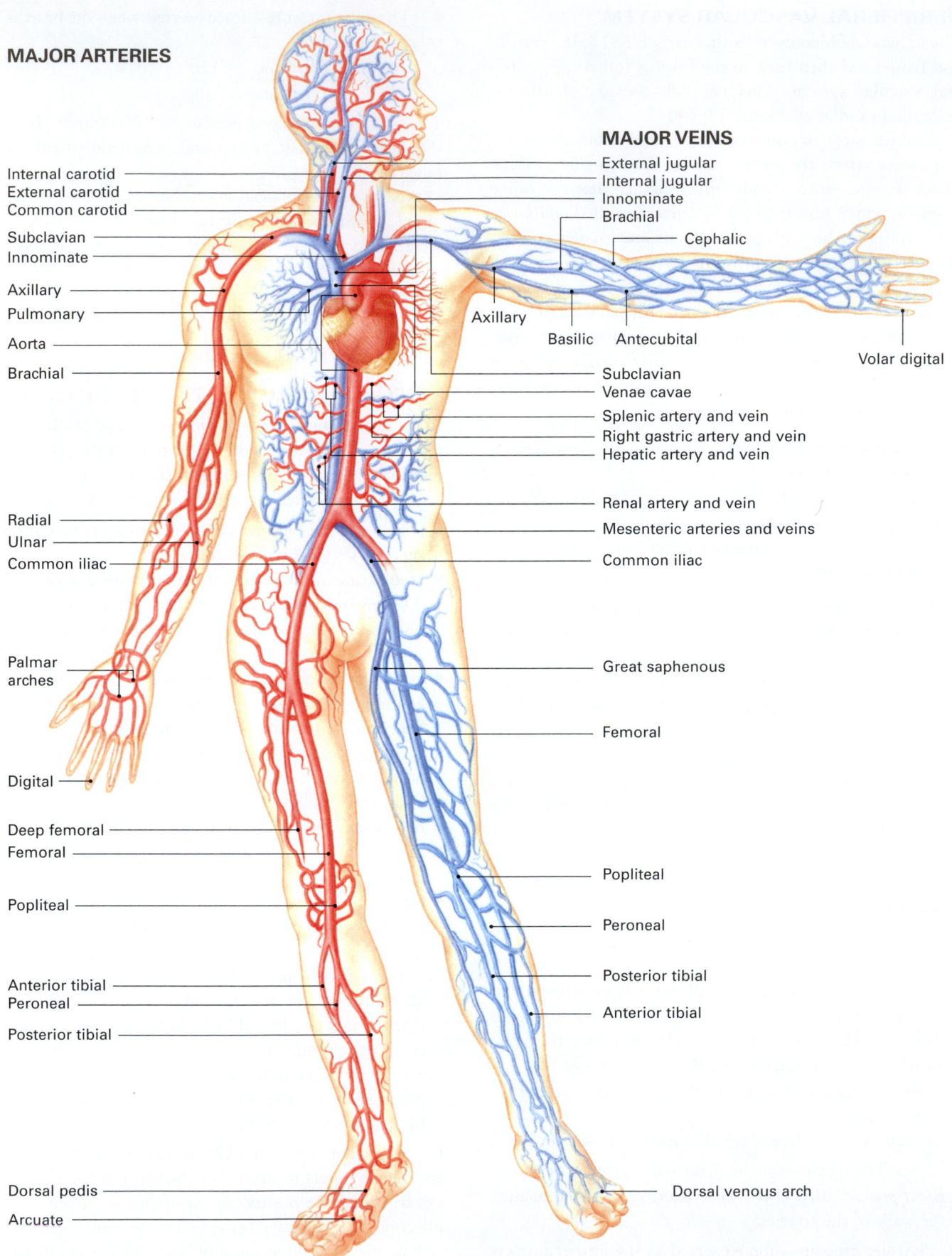

Figure 33-7. ■ Peripheral circulatory system.

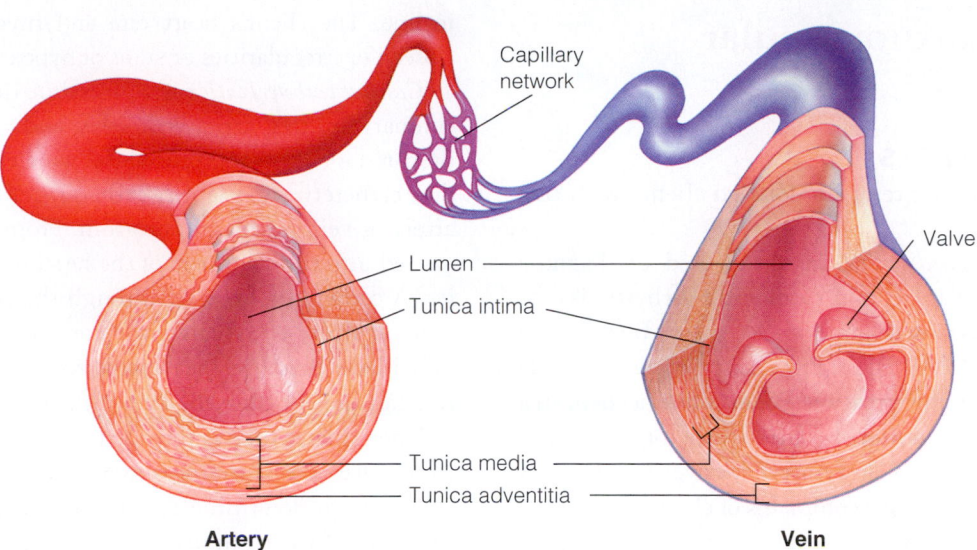

Figure 33-8. ■ Structure of arteries, veins, and capillaries.

arteries. This is associated with the elderly and those with diabetes. In **arteriosclerosis** the arteries lose elasticity and become hard and narrow. Blood supply decreases, leading to cardiac ischemia. Dead cells in the myocardium are replaced by scar tissue, which interferes with the heart's ability to pump and results in heart failure.

The World Health Organization (WHO, 2007) reports about 1.75 million people die annually due to CVD. The greater number of these deaths is from heart attacks and strokes. A considerable number of these deaths are preventable. Factors that lead to heart attacks and strokes include:

- Smoking
- Physical inactivity
- Hyperlipidemia
- Hypertension
- Diabetes mellitus
- Stress
- Oral contraceptives
- Heredity
- Obesity
- Family history
- Age
- Gender
- Race

Of these factors, heredity, family history, age (those over 65), gender (men more than women), and race are factors that cannot be changed. Other factors can be controlled or eliminated, such as smoking.

The heart and circulatory system are subject to many and varied disorders. Cardiac rhythm disorders are called *dysrhythmias* or *arrhythmias*. The heartbeats become irregular and may become abnormally fast (**tachycardia**) or abnormally slow (**bradycardia**).

PROGNOSIS

Most deaths related to heart disease are caused by coronary artery disease (CAD) and hypertension. Many CVDs can be treated or prevented. The most common CVDs are:

- **Angina pectoris** (chest pain caused by reduced oxygen supply to the heart)
- **Myocardial infarction** (MI or heart attack; death of heart tissue that results when an area of the heart does not receive oxygen or becomes *ischemic*)
- Congestive heart failure (CHF)
- Cardiac arrest
- Hypertension
- Peripheral vascular disease or PVD (emboli, arteriosclerosis, atherosclerosis, aneurysms, thrombophlebitis, varicose veins)

Other cardiovascular diseases include rheumatic fever, inflammation of the cardiac structure, pericarditis, myocarditis, endocarditis, or Raynaud's disease. Presenting signs and symptoms of cardiovascular disease are listed in Box 33-2 ■.

BOX 33-2	COMMON MANIFESTATIONS OF CARDIOVASCULAR DISEASE

- Chest pain
- Difficulty breathing with exertion (*dyspnea*)
- Rapid breathing (*tachypnea*)
- Rapid fluttering of the heart (*palpitations*)
- Blue coloration of lips, extremities (*cyanosis*)
- Pallor (paleness)
- Edema
- Fainting (*syncope*)
- Fatigue
- Anxiety

Tests for Cardiovascular Disorders

DIAGNOSTIC TESTS

A number of diagnostic tests are done on clients with cardiovascular disease.

Twelve-lead electrocardiograms are often used to diagnose heart rhythm irregularities and to monitor arrhythmias for response to medications (Figure 33-9A ■ and Box 33-3 ■ with Figure 33-10 ■). A 12-lead ECG can be done as a single test or can be an ongoing situation. For example, a client in a coronary care unit is monitored continuously for changes in rhythm. A client in a med-surg unit may have an order for a 12-lead ECG stat if he or she complains of chest pain.

A chest x-ray can look at the heart, lungs, and vessels. The x-ray will show the size and outline of the heart and whether the heart is enlarged. Changes or abnormalities of the lungs or fluid around the lungs that stem from heart problems can also be seen. If there is pulmonary congestion, it will show up as cloudy areas on the x-ray.

A *Holter monitor* (see Figure 33-9B) is used to obtain a 24-hour ECG tracing while the client is performing his or her daily routine. Some monitors record ECG tracings up to 72 hours continuously or intermittently. The monitor is small and portable, and is attached to the client's chest using one to four electrodes. It is carried on the belt or with a shoulder strap. The monitor is triggered to record heart activity on an ECG every time an irregularity is detected. The client is asked to keep a diary of activities and symptoms during the 24-hour period (or 72-hour period). The use of the Holter monitor is especially helpful in diagnosing clients who complain of heart irregularities that are not found on a resting 12-lead ECG.

A *treadmill* or *stress test* is done in a laboratory setting. The client is connected to an ECG monitor while performing specific exercises, such as walking on a treadmill at a 30-degree incline. The client's heart rate and rhythm are monitored closely for irregularities or signs of hypoxia during exercise.

Cardiac catheterization is a procedure done to visualize the coronary arteries, atria, ventricles, and valves. The client is prepared for a surgical procedure, which takes place in a cardiac catheterization lab. A catheter can be inserted into an artery or vein in the arm or groin. From there it can be advanced into the chambers of the heart or the coronary arteries. A catheter is inserted through the right groin into the femoral artery to visualize the coronary arteries and to obtain blood pressure measurements within the heart. The test can also measure the amount of oxygen in the blood.

The catheter then is threaded through the arterial system to the heart. Pressure measurements are taken within heart chambers to determine ejection fraction and contractility. Pressures of the right atrium and ventricle are obtained by inserting the catheter into the venous system. Radiopaque dye is injected through the catheter into the coronary arteries to detect blockages or narrowing of the lumen of the arteries. The process of visualizing blood vessels with injected dye is known as *angiography*. The client must lie flat for several hours after the procedure and the groin area is checked frequently for arterial bleeding or hematoma formation. During this procedure, the physician is able to detect valve malfunction and abnormalities of the heart.

A *thallium scan* is done to detect areas of the heart that are not receiving enough oxygen, or an area of infarction. Thallium is an intracellular ion that is transported easily into normal cells but does not enter abnormal cells. A "cold spot," or darkened area on the scan, indicates poor oxygenation in that area.

An *echocardiogram* is done to detect abnormalities in cardiac structures. High-frequency ultrasound waves outline heart tissue, showing the size, shape, and position of heart structures. It can also detect fluid in the pericardial sac, the size and thickness of the ventricular wall, size of the heart chambers, valve movement, and cardiac output.

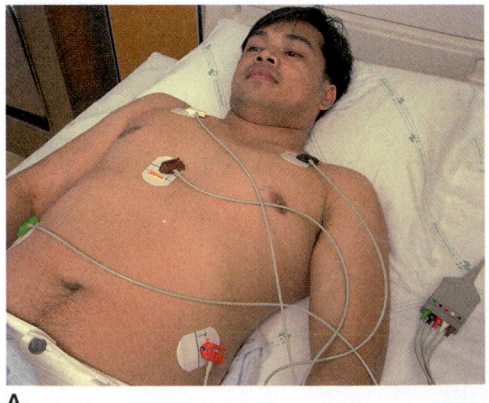
A

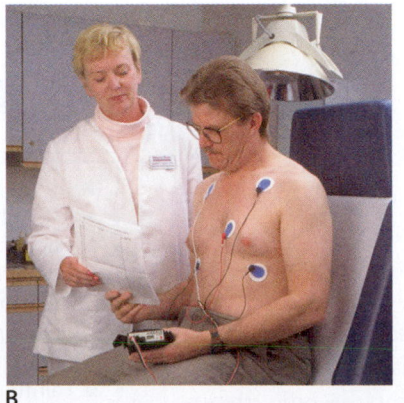
B

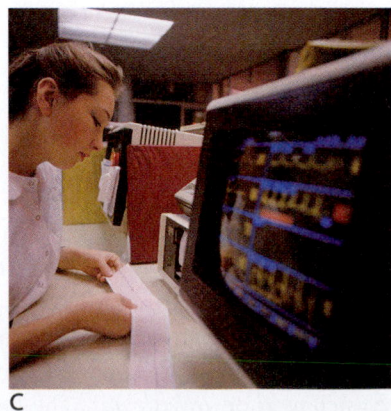
C

Figure 33-9. ■ **A.** Client with leads attached for electrocardiogram. **B.** A Holter monitor is portable and is used to follow a client during the client's normal routine. **C.** Nurse views ECG strip in front of ECG monitor. *Source:* Phototake NYC.

BOX 33-3   READING WAVEFORMS ON AN ELECTROCARDIOGRAM

An electrocardiogram (ECG) is a "picture" of the heart's electrical activity. Electrodes, coated with conductive gel, are placed directly onto the skin on different parts of the body. A standard 12-lead ECG includes recordings of six leads on the limbs and six leads that are **precordial** (relating to the area over the heart and lower thorax). The *limb leads* provide a view of the inferior and lateral walls of the heart. The *precordial leads* (chest or V leads) provide a view of the anterior, septal, lateral, and posterior walls of the heart.

Just as a camera captures more details of a scene by taking photos from different angles, the electrodes allow different views of the heart's electrical activity. The 12-lead ECG can reveal certain myocardial injury or damage.

ECG waveforms show the direction of electrical flow. Current moving toward the positive electrode causes an upward (positive) waveform; current moving away from it produces a downward (negative) waveform. When no electrical activity is occurring, a straight line, called the *isoelectric line*, is seen.

ECG waveforms are recorded on paper marked at intervals that represent time and voltage or amplitude (Figure 33-10A).

Each small box represents 0.04 second. Five small boxes make one large box, equivalent to 0.20 second. Five large boxes represent 1 full second.

The P, Q, R, S, and T waves represent the cardiac cycle (Figure 33-10B). The *P wave* shows the SA node impulse and atrial depolarization. It precedes the QRS complex and is normally smooth, round, and upright. The *PR interval* is the time required for the impulse to travel to the AV node and the bundle branches. It is measured from the beginning of the P wave to the beginning of the QRS complex. The PR interval is normally 0.12 to 0.20 second.

The *QRS complex* indicates ventricular depolarization. It occurs rapidly, lasting from 0.06 to 0.10 second. The *ST segment*, the period from the end of the QRS complex to the beginning of the T wave, is normally isoelectric. The *T wave* represents ventricular repolarization (or recovery of the ventricle). The T wave is smooth and rounded, and points in the same direction as the QRS complex. The *QT interval*, measured from the beginning of the QRS to the end of the T wave, indicates the total time for ventricular depolarization and repolarization.

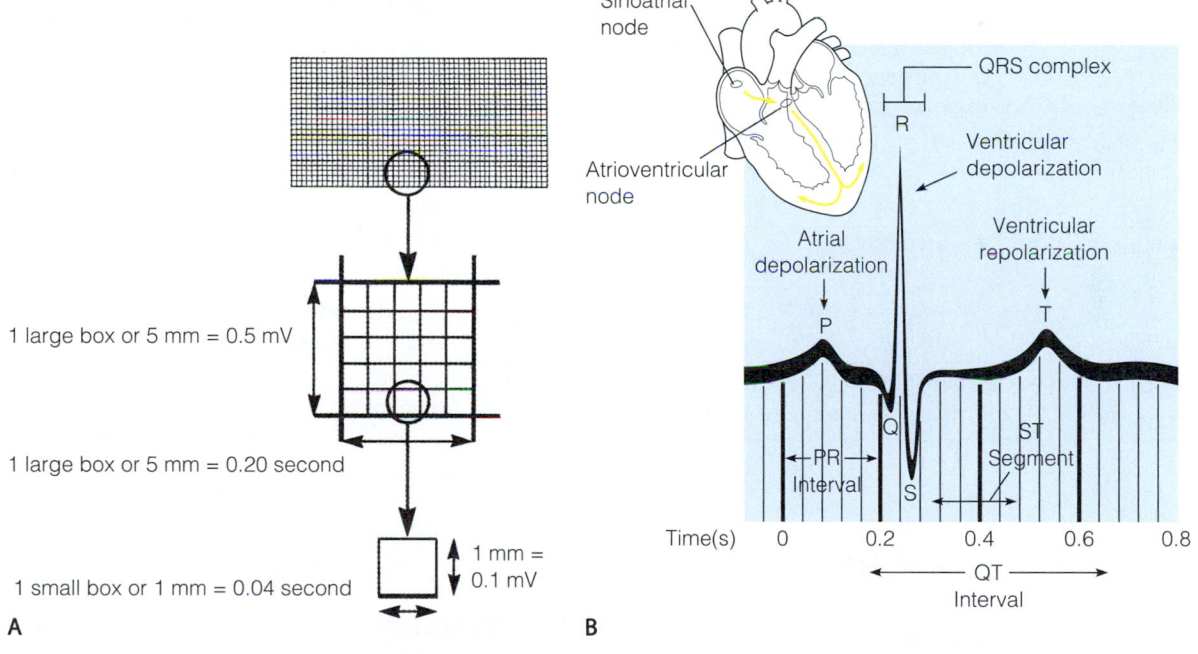

Figure 33-10. ■

Source: From *Medical Surgical Nursing Care* (2nd ed.), by K. M. Burke, P. LeMone, and E. L. Mohn-Brown, 2007, Upper Saddle River, NJ: Prentice Hall, Box 25-2, p. 600.

Positron-emission tomography (PET) scans are used to detect coronary artery disease without using a catheter to inject dye into the heart, so the risk to the client is greatly reduced. Radioactive substances used in the PET scan help physicians determine the function of the heart, showing which areas of the heart are contracting well and which areas are not. Physicians can then more easily determine which clients are the most appropriate candidates for angioplasty and surgery.

LABORATORY TESTS

Several laboratory tests are used to help diagnose cardiovascular disorders. See Table 33-1 ■ for some of the most common laboratory tests.

TABLE 33-1	Laboratory Tests for Cardiovascular Disorders	
LABORATORY TEST	**POTENTIAL ABNORMALITIES**	**SIGNIFICANCE**
Complete blood count	Low hemoglobin	Anemia, decreased oxygen-carrying capacity in the blood
	Elevated WBC	Infection or inflammation
	Elevated RBC	Compensation for chronic hypoxia
Coagulation studies	Elevated PT or PTT	Indication that client is receiving anticoagulation therapy
		Note: Monitor carefully to be sure levels do not rise above therapeutic levels.
Erythrocyte sedimentation rate (sed rate)	Elevated	May indicate rheumatic fever, MI, or endocarditis
Serum electrolytes	Low or elevated potassium	Either can cause life-threatening EKG changes
	Low or elevated sodium, calcium, magnesium	Any electrolyte imbalances can affect the ability of the cardiac muscle to contract
Serum lipids	Elevated cholesterol, especially LDL	Indicate risk for presence of or development of coronary artery disease
	Elevated triglycerides	
Arterial blood gases	Elevated pH	Systemic alkalosis
	Decreased pH	Systemic acidosis
	Decreased pO_2 and increased pCO_2	Indicates hypoxemia and lack of oxygen to tissues
Cardiac enzyme studies	Elevated creatinine phosphokinase, cardiac muscle (CPK-MB), lactic dehydrogenase (LDH), hydroxy-butyric dehydrogenase (HBD), serum glutamic-oxaloacetic transaminase (SGOT)	When elevated, all can indicate heart damage, and can determine if the client has had an MI, and whether thrombolytic therapy is appropriate
Serum cardiac markers, such as cardiac troponin I	Presence of dead cardiac cells in bloodstream	Indicates myocardial injury due to lack of oxygen
		Note: These levels are ordered on admission and again in 3 days
B type natriuretic peptide (BNP)	Elevated BNP indicates an increase in fluid pressure in the heart	A cardiac neurohormone
		Is cardioprotective
	It is secreted from the ventricle in response to heart failure	Important in differentiating the cause of dyspnea and response to diuretic therapy
International normalized ratio (INR)	Evaluates the ability of the blood to clot properly	Can be used to assess both bleeding and clotting tendencies
	Increased levels indicate prolonged bleeding times	

HEART DISORDERS

Coronary Artery Disease

Coronary heart disease (also *coronary artery disease* or *CAD*) is usually due to blockage (**occlusion**) of the arteries of the heart by a fibrous, fatty material called **plaque.** Plaque consists of cholesterol, lipids, collagen, and cellular debris. This occlusion or blockage is **atherosclerosis.** The plaque narrows the opening of the affected artery and restricts blood flow (Figure 33-11 ■). The reduced blood flow results in less oxygen reaching the heart muscle. CAD can lead to thrombus (blood clot), angina pectoris, or myocardial infarction.

ANGINA PECTORIS

Angina (Figure 33-12 ■) is pain that is the direct result of inadequate flow of oxygen to the myocardium (*myocardial ischemia*).

Manifestations

Angina pectoris is generally described as a squeezing, burning, crushing tightness in the chest beneath the sternum that radiates to the left arm, neck, jaw, or shoulder blade. It may also be described as originating in the epigastric area and radiating to the back, between the shoulder blades. An episode of angina may follow physical exertion, emotional excitement, exposure to cold, or a heavy meal. Angina has two major forms (stable and unstable) and an atypical form:

1. *Stable.* Pain is predictable in duration and frequency and is relieved with nitrates and rest.

2. *Unstable.* Pain increases in duration and frequency and can be easily induced. It occurs at rest or is worse than previous episodes.

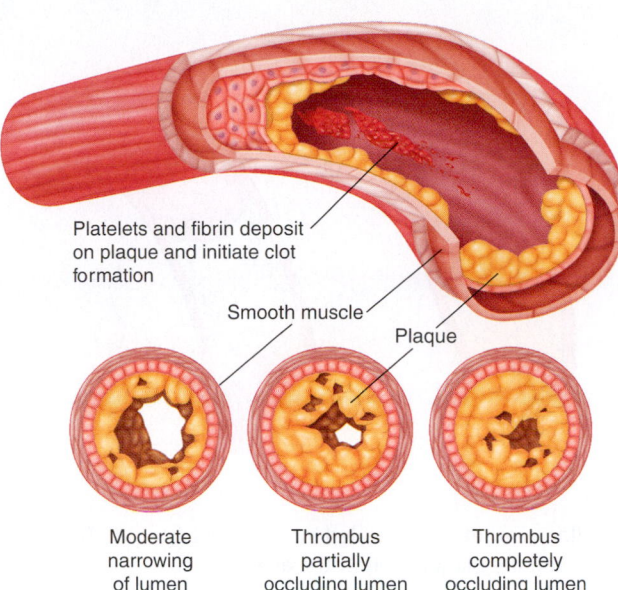

Figure 33-11. ■ Plaque and thrombus formation in the coronary artery. (*Source:* Pearson Education/PH College.)

3. *Prinzmetal's.* An atypical angina occurring when there are no precipitating causes, usually at the same time of day. It is generally caused by coronary artery spasm.

Severe, prolonged anginal pain suggests MI. (Myocardial infarction is discussed in the following pages.) With CAD,

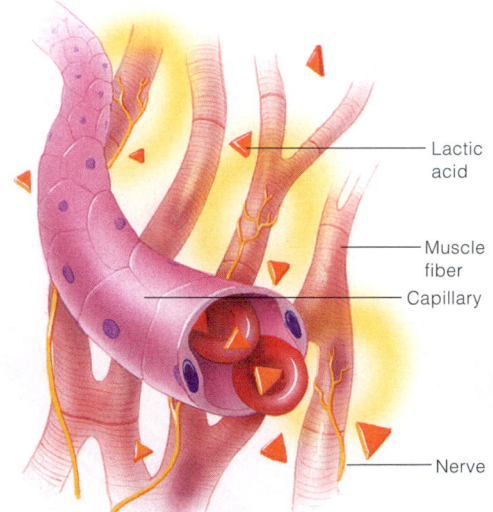

Figure 33-12. ■ Angina pectoris is characterized by episodes of chest pain, usually precipitated by exercise and relieved by rest. When myocardial oxygen needs are greater than partially occluded vessels can supply, myocardial cells become ischemic and shift to anaerobic metabolism. Anaerobic metabolism produces lactic acid, which stimulates nerve endings in the muscle, causing pain. The pain subsides when the oxygen supply again meets myocardial demand.

BOX 33-4	**MANIFESTATIONS OF CORONARY ARTERY DISEASE**

- Burning, pressure, or tight feeling in the chest
- Pain that may radiate (spread) to the left arm, neck, jaw, or shoulder blade
- Nausea, vomiting
- Fainting
- Sweating with cool extremities
- Occurrence of symptoms following physical exertion

the potential exists for fatal dysrhythmias and mechanical failure. Manifestations of CAD are listed in Box 33-4 ■.

Diagnosis and Treatment

The diagnosis of angina pectoris usually involves a careful assessment and history of signs and symptoms. The physician will order blood work, a resting ECG, echocardiogram, and exercise stress testing. Arteriograms are necessary if surgery is indicated.

Treatment for angina pectoris or MI consists of medications or surgery. Nitroglycerin is usually given sublingually or via oral spray for an angina attack. It generally relieves the pain of angina, but not the pain of an MI. Common pharmacologic treatments include nitrates, beta-adrenergic blockers, or calcium channel blockers. If medications are unsuccessful or blockage is advanced, coronary artery bypass surgery or angioplasty may be performed.

Coronary artery bypass grafting (CABG) is a surgical procedure in which a segment of a vein is grafted above and below the coronary artery blockage (Figure 33-13 ■). The vein

MyNursingKit | Angina

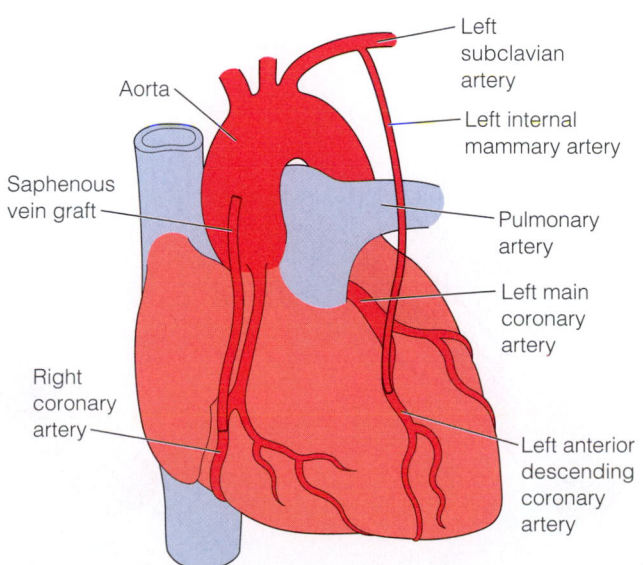

Figure 33-13. ■ Coronary artery bypass grafting using the internal mammary artery and a saphenous vein graft.

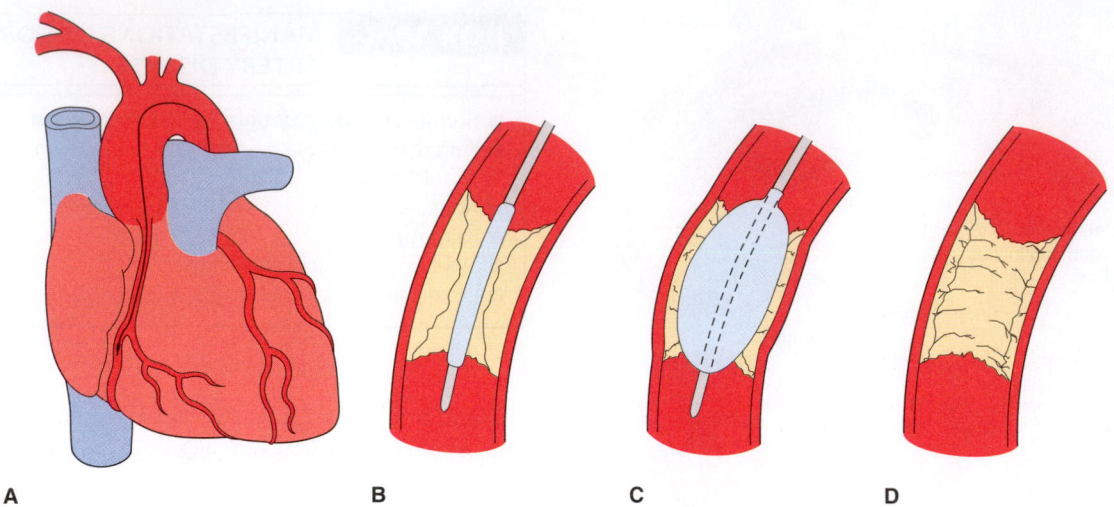

A   B   C   D

Figure 33-14. ■ **A.** Percutaneous transluminal coronary angioplasty. **B.** The balloon catheter is threaded into affected artery. **C.** The balloon is positioned across the area of obstruction. **D.** The balloon is then inflated, flattening the plaque against the arterial wall.

is usually harvested from the patient's calf (saphenous segment) and is placed in the opened chest with one end joined to the ascending aorta and the other end to a coronary artery distal to the blockage. The successful surgery restores blood flow to the myocardium, relieves pain, and improves the performance of the myocardium.

Percutaneous transluminal coronary angioplasty (PTCA) is a technique that is used to dilate an obstructed coronary artery without opening the chest catheter (Figure 33-14 ■). This involves passing a tiny catheter into the narrowed section of the artery and inflating the catheter's balloon tip. The inflated balloon causes the obstruction to be pressed against the walls of the artery so blood flow increases through the now unobstructed area. PTCA requires the use of three catheters: an introducer catheter, a guiding catheter, and a balloon. Often, a stent is inserted to provide

a permanent opening within the coronary artery. These procedures can be done in a catheterization lab.

Stent placement often follows angioplasty to prop open the artery (Figure 33-15 ■) and allow an increase in blood flow. In stent placement a stainless steel wire mesh tube is inserted through a balloon catheter to strengthen the wall of the blood vessel. Stents reduce the renarrowing that may occur after angioplasty and offer the client a noninvasive option.

Intracoronary streptokinase therapy (also referred to as *thrombolytic therapy*) consists of cardiac catheterization prior to infusion to pinpoint the obstructed artery. The infusion is directed into the occluded artery as close as possible to the blockage. The progress of the infusion is monitored by coronary angiography and ECG. Streptokinase disrupts the normal clotting process so there is a risk of hemorrhage. It is also a foreign protein that may trigger an allergic reaction.

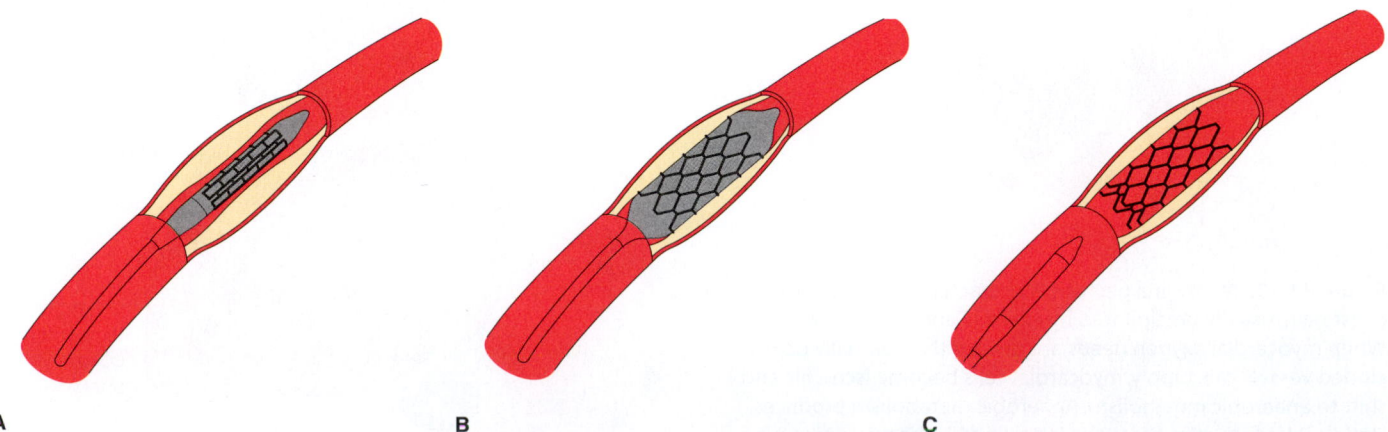

A   B   C

Figure 33-15. ■ Placement of an intracoronary stent: **A.** The stent is fitted over the balloon-tipped catheter. **B.** The stent is positioned in the area of narrowing and expanded with balloon inflation. **C.** The balloon is deflated and removed, leaving the stent in place.

The client should be monitored closely for color and temperature change at the site as indicators of bleeding. Symptoms of an allergic reaction may include nausea, itching, flushing, shortness of breath, and edema.

MYOCARDIAL INFARCTION

A myocardial infarction or heart attack occurs when blood flow through one of the coronary arteries is completely blocked, causing **ischemia** (decreased oxygenation) and **necrosis** (death) of an area of the cardiac muscle (Figure 33-16 ■). It differs from an angina attack because the coronary artery is completely blocked and damage to the heart is permanent. If circulation to the affected cardiac muscle is restored quickly, then the result is:

- Reduction in the amount of loss of functional muscle.
- Increased ability of the heart to maintain effective cardiac output.
- Decreased threat of cardiogenic shock (see also Chapter 47 ⬤⬤) and death.

The MI is a life-threatening condition. Most deaths occur within the first hour following the onset of symptoms. MI generally occurs in clients with preexisting coronary artery disease, although there is no identified specific cause. The coronary artery becomes blocked and the blood flow is reduced or stopped to a portion of the cardiac muscle. Cells deprived of oxygen and nutrients for an extended period of time (20 to 45 minutes) are irreversibly damaged. This results in cell death and tissue necrosis (*infarct*). The infarcted area no longer conducts electrical energy and therefore no longer contracts. This decreases cardiac output. *Collateral (supportive) vessels* in the coronary system dilate and enlarge to provide the blood flow needed to the cardiac muscle. If this collateral circulation is sufficient, it can help to reduce the size of an infarction. MI generally affects the left side (ventricle) of the heart, because of its greater size and oxygen demands.

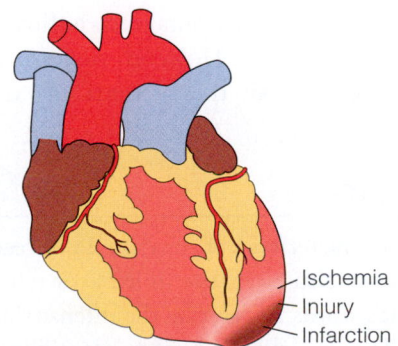

Ischemia
Injury
Infarction

Figure 33-16. ■ Myocardial infarction occurs when complete obstruction of the coronary artery interrupts blood flow to an area of heart muscle. Affected tissue becomes ischemic and eventually dies (infarcts) if the blood supply is not restored. Surrounding the area of an infarction is an area of tissue injury. Surrounding the injured tissue is an area of ischemic but undamaged tissue.

BOX 33-5	RISK FACTORS FOR MYOCARDIAL INFARCTION

- Positive family history
- Hypertension
- Smoking
- Elevated serum triglycerides, cholesterol, lipoprotein levels
- Diabetes mellitus
- Obesity
- Sedentary lifestyle
- Stress

Classification and Risk Factors

MIs are described by the area of the heart that is damaged:

Left anterior descending (LAD). Damages anterior portion of the left ventricle.
Left circumflex artery (LCA). Damages lateral portion.
Right ventricular, inferior, posterior (RCA). Occludes right coronary artery.
Posterior descending artery (PDA).
Transmural infarction. Involves all layers of heart.
Subendocardial infarction. Only involves inner layer of the heart.

The risk factors for MI are listed in Box 33-5 ■.

Manifestations

Signs and symptoms of MI include many of those listed for CAD (see Box 33-2). Pain in the chest is generally more persistent and may be described as crushing or viselike ("An elephant sitting on my chest") or severe pain ("The worst pain I have ever had in my life"). The pain may radiate to the arm, neck, jaw, and teeth. Weakness is a common symptom, and nausea and vomiting are common. Clients often experience shortness of breath, anxiety, and restlessness. When clients having an MI are assessed, common findings are pallor, hypotension, signs of shock, irregular heart rate, fever, diaphoresis, and erratic behavior. Table 33-2 ■ lists manifestations of heart attack in women.

TABLE 33-2	Manifestations of Heart Attack in Women
AREA OF BODY	**COMPLAINT**
Brain	Anxiety, trouble sleeping, dizziness
Chest	Chest pain, squeezing; throbbing ache in chest; feeling of fullness; arm, back, or shoulder pain
Skin	Pallor, diaphoresis
Lungs	Trouble breathing; or inability to catch one's breath when waking up
Stomach	Upset stomach, urge to vomit; vomiting

Diagnosis and Treatment

ECG and lab tests are ordered to confirm the diagnosis. The primary goals of treatment are to:

- Relieve chest pain by administering potent narcotics such as morphine (intravenously) and antianxiety agents such as Valium (orally or intravenously). Oxygen is generally administered immediately to improve hypoxemia.
- MONA is an acronym to remember for treating all chest pain. It stands for **M**orphine sulfate, **O**xygen, **N**itroglycerin, and **A**spirin (4–81 mg).
- Stabilize the heart rhythm by administering antiarrhythmics. Insertion of a pacemaker may be necessary.
- Reduce cardiac workload by minimizing exertion and keeping blood pressure within normal range.
- *Revascularize* (open up) the blocked coronary artery using fibrinolytic therapy or PTCA.

Fibrinolytics (also called thrombolytics) are medications that dissolve blood clots. One common medication used to dissolve clots that are blocking coronary arteries is streptokinase. Once the clot is dissolved, blood flow is once again established to the heart muscle. This helps decrease the size of the infarction and helps increase heart function.

PTCA is a procedure done by inserting a balloon-tipped catheter into the coronary artery containing the obstruction. Once positioned, the balloon is slowly inflated intermittently, to push the plaque against the walls of the artery and open the lumen so blood can flow through it.

Several serious and life-threatening complications can result from an MI. Box 33-6 ■ lists complications of MI.

NURSING CARE

PRIORITIZING NURSING CARE

When you care for clients with angina, you should keep a number of important things in mind. First and foremost, an angina attack can quickly lead to an MI. Never disregard a client's complaint of chest pain.

Clients with chest pain are understandably frightened. Some may be afraid of any exertion, even when they are stable. Patiently educate those clients about the benefits of mobility and the hazards of immobility. Other clients with chest

BOX 33-6	COMPLICATIONS OF MYOCARDIAL INFARCTION

- *Embolism.* A clot may originate in the heart and travel through the circulation to the lungs or brain; or the clot may form in the peripheral circulation and travel to the coronary arteries of the heart.
- *Ventricular aneurysm.* When an MI damages the ventricle, the wall of the ventricle may thin and balloon out; if it ruptures, death is imminent.
- *Pericarditis.* An inflammation of the sac that surrounds the heart; after an MI damages the ventricle, inflammation may set in.
- *Ventricular fibrillation.* A life-threatening arrhythmia that causes the ventricles to quiver rather than pump blood through the body; this occurs when the conduction system of the heart is interrupted by an MI and will result in death unless the heart is shocked into a life-sustaining rhythm (defibrillation).
- *Cardiogenic shock.* Loss of blood pressure with other symptoms of shock; this occurs because the heart is unable to pump blood to the vital organs effectively after damage from an MI.

pain tend to deny the seriousness of their situation and want to be too active, trying to prove that they have no heart disease. For those clients, it is important to explain the reasons for activity restrictions and the importance of gradually increasing activity so the heart can adjust to the exertion. Sometimes it is difficult to walk that fine line between encouraging activity and encouraging caution when caring for clients with chest pain. However, with patience, understanding, and education, these clients can do well after discharge.

ASSESSING

Location and characteristics of pain should be recorded, along with activities or situations that initiate or relieve the pain. Use the client's words to describe the intensity and character of the pain. Take the client's history, identifying any family history of heart disease, diabetes, hypertension, tobacco or alcohol use, stress, and other risk factors. It is important to note the frequency and duration of chest pain and the effectiveness of treatment measures (oxygen, rest, nitroglycerin). Monitor results of laboratory tests (complete blood count [CBC], cardiac enzymes, blood gases, and electrolytes). A physical assessment would include vital signs, heart and lung sounds, skin signs, urine output, and level of consciousness. The nurse would also monitor ECG rhythm and oxygen levels. Assess for subjective signs such as a feeling of impending death, factors that may have brought on the pain, changes in frequency or worsening of symptoms, and whether anything relieves the pain. Assess for objective signs such as behavior related to pain (grimacing, positioning, groaning, etc.), vital sign changes, diaphoresis, and anxious behavior.

When auscultating the heart, eliminate all sources of room noise. The heart is auscultated in all four anatomic sites (aortic, pulmonic, tricuspid, and apical). Find the most audible sounds for the client, using both sides of the stethoscope. Concentrate on one particular sound at a time in each area: the first heart sound, followed by systole, then the second heart sound, then diastole. Systole and diastole are normally silent intervals. Place the client supine with the head elevated 30 to 45 degrees, unless contraindicated. Table 33-3 ■ provides descriptions of normal and a few of the many abnormal heart sounds. See also Table 21-4 ⚭ .

DIAGNOSING, PLANNING, AND IMPLEMENTING

Clients with coronary artery disease often have the following nursing diagnoses:

- *Acute Pain* related to decreased myocardial oxygenation
- *Risk for Decreased Cardiac Tissue Perfusion* related to interruption in coronary arterial blood flow to myocardium
- *Activity Intolerance* related to chest pain with exertion
- *Anxiety* related to the threat of death (heart attack), change in health status causing inability to control pain and to cope with uncertainty about future
- *Deficient Knowledge* regarding disease and treatment

Expected outcomes are:

- Episodes of pain will be reduced and controlled as evidenced by verbalization that the pain is reduced, decreased frequency of need for medication, and ability to participate in moderate activity.
- Client will experience reduced anxiety and express an understanding of treatment or procedures.
- Client will maintain adequate cardiac output and tissue perfusion. These will be monitored by normal baseline ranges of vital signs (P, BP, R) and hemodynamic measurements of cardiac output, central venous pressure, and pulmonary artery pressure (CO, CVP, PAP, respectively), level of consciousness, urine output, and ECG rhythm.
- Dysrhythmias will be controlled or eliminated.

For Clients with Angina

- The primary nursing care focus is *education* of the client with angina in the causes of angina (atherosclerosis), the options for management of the disease, and pain control. *Clients can learn to manage the symptoms of their disease to increase their quality of life.*
- During angina episodes, monitor blood pressure and heart rate; record duration of pain and the amount of medication needed to relieve it. Keep nitroglycerin available for use and instruct the client to report pain in the chest, arm, or neck. (If a client is taking nitroglycerin, monitor the effectiveness of the medication by recording not only a change in anginal pain, but also the severity of the headache—if the client does not get a headache, it is a sign that the nitroglycerin may not be "good" anymore.) *These measures provide important data for treatment and support the client.*
- Answer questions about treatments that are planned, or arrange for someone to answer the client's questions.

TABLE 33-3	**Heart Sounds and Abnormalities**	
SOUND	**USUAL DETECTION SITE**	**FINDINGS ON EXAMINATION**
NORMAL S_1 (first)	Over the apex	Usually heard as one sound; is the "lub" of lub-dub. Indicates closure of mitral and tricuspid valves
S_2 (second)	Over the apex	Is the "dub" of lub-dub; indicates closure of aortic and pulmonic valves
ABNORMAL S_3 ventricular gallop	Over the apex; while client is supine or lt. lateral	Early diastolic low-pitched extra heart sound; increases with inspiration, exercise, elevation of legs, and with increased venous return
		Sound that follows S_1, S_2; heard as "Ken-tuck-y"; normal sound for children; may indicate heart failure in adults
S_4 atrial gallop	Over apex; client supine or lt. semilateral	Low pitch at late diastole or early systole. Increases with forceful inspiration, exercise, elevation of legs and with increased venous return
		Sound heard before S_1; sound resembles "Ten-nes-see"; sound may be associated with hypertensive heart disease

Clients will want to know the purpose of the procedure, what they will experience, any risks involved, and possible outcomes of the procedure. Providing information helps to reduce client anxiety.

- After procedures, monitor the catheter site for bleeding, check distal pulses, and offer fluids. *Bleeding or reduced distal pulses could signal a complication. Fluids are offered to counteract the effect of the dye.*

- After surgery, monitor and record chest pain, blood pressure, fluid intake and output, breath sounds, ECG, signs of ischemia, or dysrhythmias. Monitor, describe, and record vital signs and characteristics every 2 to 4 hours. *This information is crucial in determining the client's progress. Increases in pain, anxiety, and stress will increase client's blood pressure and pulse.*

- If vasodilator and nitroglycerin are ordered, keep them at the bedside for onset of pain. *Immediate treatment reduces the intensity and duration of the pain by relaxing the smooth muscle of coronary and peripheral vessels.*

- Start oxygen per nasal cannula as indicated. *This improves oxygenation to the myocardial tissue.*

- Teach client to modify or reduce activities that initiate angina attack. *Exertion increases oxygen consumption.* Once the client is stable, explain that a regular exercise program such as walking helps condition the heart so the demand for oxygen during exertion is decreased.

- Position client in semi- or high-Fowler's during angina attack. *This decreases oxygen requirement.*

- Determine the level of knowledge and understanding of angina. *Teaching effectiveness will be increased if the intervention is specific to meet the client needs.*

- Teach the client about the signs and symptoms of angina. *Teaching helps the client understand the pain as a warning necessitating immediate action.*

- Provide written instructions on medications and signs and symptoms of angina. *Written instructions are available to the client for future reference and reinforce the teaching.*

For Clients with MI

People who have suffered an MI often are seen in emergency settings (see Chapter 47 🔗) or are transferred to the ICU. Nursing care for these clients is intensive.

- Monitor, describe, and record vital signs and characteristics continuously. Immediate hourly assessments must be done until the client's condition is stable, and then every 2 to 4 hours. *Increases in pain, anxiety, and stress increase blood pressure/pulse.*

- Monitor level of consciousness and urine output. *Indicates decreased tissue perfusion and altered cerebral function due to decreased oxygenation.*

- Monitor ECG for any changes in heart rate or rhythm, and administer oxygen as ordered. *Abrupt change must be reported promptly. Oxygen supports the client and reduces cardiac workload.*

- Administer analgesic, vasodilator, antianxiety agent, sedative as ordered. Administer MONA. Aspirin is essential. *Pain medication inhibits pain pathways in the central nervous system; vasodilators increase blood flow to the myocardium thus reducing pain; and reducing anxiety provides for calm and increased rest.*

- Provide calm, quiet environment. *Increased periods of uninterrupted rest are essential. Nursing care is focused on preventing further myocardial damage by assessing for complications and promoting comfort and rest. Minimal stimuli reduce pain and anxiety.*

- Place in comfort position—semi-Fowler's. *Promoting comfort reduces pain and decreases respiratory effort.*

- Monitor and record severity of pain and its duration, blood pressure, ECG, fluid intake and output, and breath sounds. Encourage reports of any pain at onset. *Recurrence can indicate extension of the infarction with decreasing ventricular function and increased workload on the heart.*

- Assist with range of motion. *Range-of-motion exercises help prevent venous stasis and provide emotional support to reduce anxiety.*

EVALUATING

Client expresses acceptance of diagnosis, participation in plan of care, and involvement in restoration of optimal health and reduction in risk for additional cardiac events. Evaluate the effectiveness of the nursing care measures. Continue to monitor for any changes in condition to prevent sudden death and complications. Assess the willingness of the client to comply with physician's orders and to reduce or manage risk factors.

Continuity of Care

Emphasize the importance of maintaining and complying with the medication regimen. Explain dosages and therapy to promote compliance with drug regimen, and warn of any side effects and signs of toxicity. Some of the signs are nausea, vomiting, and anorexia. Digitalis patients may report yellow or double vision. Encourage moderate, regular exercise and dietary restrictions if warranted. Educate and give information about cessation of smoking. Review any diet or sexual activity restrictions and provide suggestions for compliance. Teach the client the importance of responding immediately to the signs and symptoms of an episode of angina and of reporting new or recurrent symptoms.

NURSING PROCESS CARE PLAN
Caring for a Client with Angina

Ms. Levitt is a 44-year-old divorced mother of three, ages 8, 11, and 14. In addition to her full-time job, she transports her children to numerous activities. She attends school part time in order to obtain a better paying job. She was recently divorced. Her ex-husband left the state and does not provide child support. Ms. Levitt was brought to the emergency room to rule out a heart attack, after experiencing a "crushing pain" in her chest that radiated to her arm. Health history unremarkable except for total abdominal hysterectomy 4 years ago.

Assessment
VS 98.6/102/30. BP 162/98. Pale, trembling. Complains of chest pain, "better now," rated as 8/10; holding chest and rubbing arm. Wt 189 (admits to a 20 lb weight gain over last year). Began smoking again 4 months ago (1–2 packs a day). C/o dyspnea on exertion and a sensation of choking during the past week when she is feeling rushed. ECG normal. Client states, "I thought I was having a heart attack, but I am okay now." It is determined that Ms. Levitt has experienced an angina attack.

Nursing Diagnosis
The following important nursing diagnoses (among others) are established for this condition:

- *Acute Pain* related to decreased myocardial oxygenation
- *Deficient Knowledge* related to causes of angina attacks and treatment
- *Anxiety* related to situational crisis
- *Ineffective Coping* related to recent life events and lack of personal support from ex-husband and others

Expected Outcomes
The expected outcomes of the plan of care specify that Ms. Levitt will:

- Experience few episodes of angina and that pain will be reduced and controlled by medication.
- Identify factors that may contribute to episodes of angina.
- Name factors in her life that she can control and change to help prevent further episodes.
- Verbalize ability to cope and to ask for help when needed.

Planning and Implementation
The following interventions are planned and implemented:

- Assess and document manifestations (e.g., dyspnea, pain, anxiety) and responses to treatment. *Accurate data gathering and evaluation of responses allows for appropriate measures to alleviate the client's symptoms.*

- Administer medication as ordered. Keep nitroglycerin available and instruct client to report pain in the chest, arm, or neck. *An understanding of the purpose of nitroglycerin as a vasodilator delivering more blood and more oxygen to heart muscle helps reduce pain and discomfort.*
- During an attack, place client in semi- or high-Fowler's position to aid breathing; monitor heart rate and blood pressure. *This position decreases the workload of the heart and the work of breathing.*
- Start oxygen by nasal cannula as ordered. *Supplemental oxygen increases oxygenation to myocardial tissue and therefore reduces pain.*
- Teach the client about signs and symptoms of angina. *An understanding of angina will enable the client to manage the disease better.*
- Teach client to identify activities that could induce an angina attack. Encourage client to modify or cut back on those activities. *A thorough understanding of activities that cause angina will promote adherence to medical regimen.*
- Explore coping skills previously used by the client to relieve anxiety; reinforce these skills, and explore other outlets. *An understanding and use of coping skills will decrease the sense of helplessness and powerlessness.*
- Encourage use of appropriate community resources. *Seeking assistance with a sudden change in lifestyle will enable clients to cope with the disease and realize they are not alone.*
- Provide client and family members with written information about manifestations of angina and medications used to treat it. *Information allows the family members to assist in care and lessen the feeling of helplessness.*

Evaluation
Ms. Levitt returns to the clinic in one week. VS are within normal limits. She reports one additional episode during the last week, relieved by one dose of nitroglycerin. She has arranged carpooling for some of her children's events. She reports reducing cigarettes to five a day and "taking a few minutes to slow down" during her lunch hour.

Critical Thinking in the Nursing Process

1. Speculate about the relationship between Ms. Levitt's health history and her cardiovascular symptoms.
2. Ms. Levitt's weight, hypertension, and smoking need to be addressed. How would you approach her on these issues?
3. What cues would alert you that Ms. Levitt is adapting to necessary lifestyle changes in a positive and healthy manner?

Note: Discussion of Critical Thinking questions appears on the MyNursingKit Website.

Disorders Affecting the Heart and Lungs

CONGESTIVE HEART FAILURE

Congestive heart failure (CHF) is the inability of the heart to pump enough blood throughout the body (decreased cardiac output) to maintain well-being. Blood that pools in the systemic venous circulation results in peripheral edema. Congestion of pulmonary circulation causes pulmonary edema. Pulmonary edema is an acute life-threatening emergency. CHF may be acute, a direct result of myocardial infarction. However, it is often a chronic disorder related to retention of salt and water by the kidneys.

Manifestations

The client experiences increasing *dyspnea* (shortness of breath). Cardiac and respiratory rates also increase. This results in greater stress and anxiety. The neck veins can become distended, and edema is usually found in the ankles. Box 33-7 ■ lists manifestations of CHF. Box 33-8 ■ lists risk factors associated with this disease.

BOX 33-7	MANIFESTATIONS OF CONGESTIVE HEART FAILURE

- Fatigue
- Shortness of breath (*dyspnea*)
- Distended neck veins
- Persistent cold
- Dry cough with wheezing
- Rapid breathing (*tachypnea*)
- Dependent edema
- Weight gain
- Nausea
- Chest tightness or angina
- Sweating (*diaphoresis*)
- Hypotension
- Pallor
- Anxiety
- Oliguria

BOX 33-8	RISK FACTORS FOR CONGESTIVE HEART FAILURE

Cardiovascular Causes

- Arteriosclerotic heart disease
- Myocardial infarction
- Prolonged hypertension
- Rheumatic heart disease
- Ischemic heart disease
- Cardiomyopathy
- Valvular disease
- Dysrhythmias
- Noncompliance with treatment for heart disease

Noncardiovascular Causes

- Pregnancy and childbirth
- Increased environmental temperature or humidity
- Severe physical or mental stress
- Thyrotoxicosis (see Chapter 38 ⚭)
- Diabetes mellitus
- Fluid replacement therapy
- Pulmonary embolism
- Severe infection
- Chronic obstructive pulmonary disease

Either side of the heart can fail, or both can fail (Table 33-4 ■). Left ventricular failure (also called *left-sided heart failure*) is the result of ventricular muscle damage or an overloading, in which the left side of the heart cannot pump enough blood to meet the body's needs. Blood backs up from the left ventricle into the lungs, and fluid leaks from the blood into the air spaces of the lungs. The hallmark symptom of left ventricular failure is shortness of breath. Additional symptoms include dyspnea (especially at night), pulmonary crackles, orthopnea, hemoptysis, and cough (Figure 33-17 ■).

Right ventricular failure (or *right-sided heart failure*) occurs when the right ventricle is not able to pump blood effectively to the lungs. This can be due to a backup in the lungs from left ventricular failure or it may be due to lung

TABLE 33-4	Left-Sided versus Right-Sided Heart Failure	
LEFT-SIDED HEART FAILURE	**RIGHT-SIDED HEART FAILURE**	
Blood becomes congested in the left ventricle, left atrium, and then pulmonary vasculature	Blood becomes congested and accumulates in the right ventricle, right atrium, the superior and inferior vena cava, and the venous vasculature	
Activity intolerance; fatigue	Activity intolerance; fatigue	
Weakness	Jugular vein distention	
Dizziness	Peripheral edema; weight gain	
Shortness of breath, cough, paroxysmal nocturnal dyspnea, orthopnea	Anorexia, nausea, abdominal distention	
Crackles in lung bases	Liver and spleen enlargement	

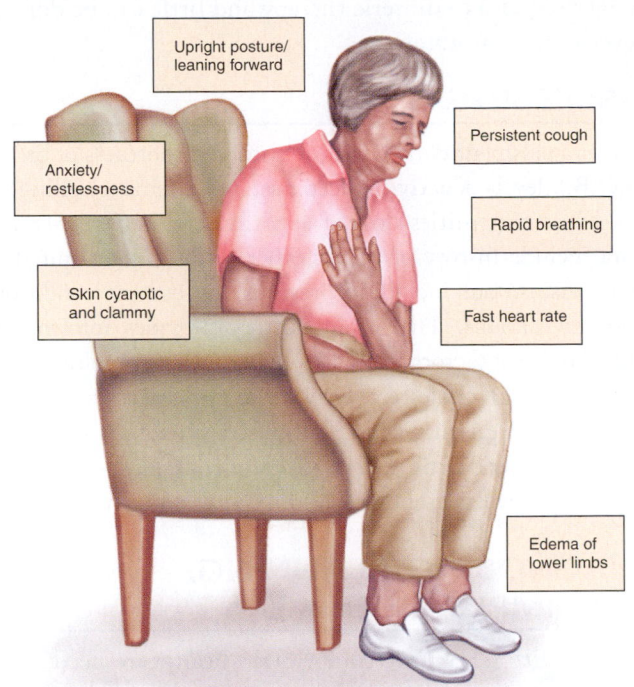

Upright posture/
leaning forward

Persistent cough

Anxiety/
restlessness

Rapid breathing

Skin cyanotic
and clammy

Fast heart rate

Edema of
lower limbs

Figure 33-17. ■ Signs and symptoms of the client with heart failure. (*Source:* Holland, N., and M. P. Adams. *Core Concepts in Pharmacology.* (2003). Upper Saddle River, NJ: Prentice Hall.)

disease. When this backup occurs, blood cannot leave the systemic circulation to enter the right side of the heart. The hallmark symptom of right ventricular failure is peripheral edema. Additional symptoms include jugular vein distention (JVD), abdominal distention, liver enlargement, ascites, and pronounced edema of the feet and ankles that may progress up to the knees.

The outlook for CHF clients depends on the cause of the syndrome and the response to treatment.

Reduced cardiac output triggers compensatory mechanisms:

- *Ventricular dilatation.* May lead to right ventricular failure.
- *Hypertrophy.* May require increased oxygen.
- *Increased sympathetic activity.* May restrict blood flow to the kidneys.

Diagnosis and Treatment

For CHF, an ECG, chest x-ray, and lab tests such as the BNP are commonly used tests. X-ray can show pulmonary vascular congestion and if the heart is enlarged. Pulmonary artery monitoring may also be used.

The treatment of CHF targets reduction of the workload of the heart in order to increase its efficiency. Digitalis strengthens and slows the heartbeat, whereas beta-blockers and angiotensin-converting enzyme (ACE) inhibitors increase blood flow. Vasodilators reduce the vascular pressure,

and diuretics reduce the volume of fluid being retained by the body. A diuretic is given to promote fluid and salt loss (*diuresis*) and to reduce blood volume and circulatory congestion. Treatment includes bed rest, antiembolism stockings to prevent fluid pooling in the legs, and medication to assist the heart. Medications are given to strengthen myocardial contractility and to increase cardiac output. Common diuretics are Lasix, HydroDIURIL, and Bumex. Common medications to assist in strengthening the heart rate are Lanoxin and Crystodigin.

clinical ALERT

Congestive heart failure in a child is evidenced by tachycardia, fatigue during feedings, and perspiration around the forehead. For congestive heart failure, Lanoxin is the preferred drug in children because of its rapid action and short half-life.

An herbal remedy is sometimes used to assist clients with early manifestations of heart failure. Box 33-9 ■ describes the use of hawthorn.

PULMONARY EDEMA

Pulmonary edema is a life-threatening complication of left-sided congestive heart failure. When fluids and blood accumulate in the lungs in large amounts, the alveoli fill up and air exchange is nonexistent.

Manifestations

The hallmark sign of pulmonary edema is pink, frothy sputum. This is caused by air, fluid, and red blood cells mixing in the alveoli. Additional symptoms include severe shortness of breath, productive cough of large amounts of pink frothy sputum, tachycardia, rapid respirations, restlessness, disorientation, and cool, clammy skin. The client may be

BOX 33-9   COMPLEMENTARY THERAPIES

Heart Failure

The client with heart failure may receive some benefit from the dried fruit of the hawthorn (also known as English hawthorn, maybush, or whitethorn) or a tincture or liquid extract of the hawthorn fruit or leaf. Hawthorn increases coronary blood flow and has positive inotropic effects. It increases cardiac output and decreases the blood pressure, cardiac workload, and oxygen consumption. It acts like an ACE inhibitor.

Clients should never begin herbal therapy without consulting a physician. Advise clients to consult their primary care provider before taking hawthorn or using it in conjunction with prescribed drugs.

Source: Adapted from Burke, K. M., LeMone, P., Mohn-Brown, E. L. *Medical-surgical nursing care.* (2nd ed.). (2007). Upper Saddle River, NJ: Prentice Hall, Table 27-4, p. 646. Used with permission.

pale or cyanotic. When lungs are auscultated, audible crackles and wheezes are noted.

Diagnosis and Treatment

Physical history may suggest pulmonary edema, and examination may detect a third heart sound (S_3). Blood tests to check for electrolytes, renal failure, liver enzymes, CBC, and coagulation will be ordered. Echocardiography will strengthen the diagnosis.

The client with pulmonary edema should be placed in the high-Fowler's position to facilitate lung expansion. Diuretics, such as furosemide (Lasix) intravenously (IV), are ordered to remove excess fluid from the lungs. Vasodilators and **inotropics** (drugs that increase force of contraction) are prescribed to decrease the workload of the heart, and nitroglycerin is given to increase blood supply to the heart muscle. Morphine sulfate or other analgesics may be prescribed to relieve pain and anxiety and to reduce the respiratory rate and oxygen demand.

COR PULMONALE

Cor pulmonale is an older name for pulmonary hypertension. This is an abnormal condition of the heart in which the right ventricle is enlarged due to hypertension in the pulmonary circulation. Usual causes of pulmonary hypertension are right-sided CHF and chronic obstructive pulmonary disease.

NURSING CARE

PRIORITIZING NURSING CARE

When you care for clients with cardiopulmonary disorders, it is important that you focus on maintaining effective circulation and oxygenation. The client with severe CHF or pulmonary edema is seriously ill. Focus your care on positioning the client in the high-Fowler's or the orthopneic position to increase respiratory capacity. Be vigilant about keeping the oxygen mask on the client and the oxygen at the ordered rate. If edema is a problem, be sure to elevate the client's feet when sitting to help decrease dependent edema. Clients with severe CHF and with pulmonary edema may be on a fluid restriction. They are generally placed on a restricted sodium diet to minimize sodium and water retention. (See Chapter 25 🔗 for low-sodium diet.) Be sure you follow the ordered amount of fluid for your shift and do not exceed it. Give frequent oral care and keep the lips moist when clients are on fluid restrictions.

Remember that clients who struggle to breathe may be frightened and confused. Always be calm and reassuring when you approach the client. In some cases, the client may be in end-stage CHF, which means that the kidneys no longer respond to diuretic therapy and little can be done to reverse the symptoms.

ASSESSING

Client assessment data include a history of shortness of breath (S.O.B.), levels of activity, sleep patterns, edema (swelling) of the lower extremities, loss of appetite, and nausea. Medical data include history of MI or other diseases not limited to heart disease but including previous and current conditions and medications. The family history provides information about the risk factors related to hypertension, smoking, diabetes, and high cholesterol levels. The physical assessment includes vital signs at rest and with activity, oxygen saturation levels, heart and lung sounds, level of consciousness, edema, skin turgor, weight, and daily fluid intake and output.

DIAGNOSING, PLANNING, AND IMPLEMENTING

Clients with CHF have complicated healthcare needs. The following nursing diagnoses commonly apply:

- *Anxiety* related to change in health status
- *Decreased Cardiac Output* related to changes in the heart
- *Excess Fluid Volume* related to inability of the heart to pump effectively

Outcomes for these clients would include the following:

- The client will be able to perform activities of daily living (ADLs) and participate in cardiac rehabilitation and manage medications.
- The client will tolerate increased activity levels and changes in dietary requirements.
- The client will verbalize understanding of the disease and its limitations and the medications necessary to manage the symptoms.

Nursing care for clients with CHF is supportive.

- Weigh the client at the same time daily. Monitor urinary intake and output and check daily for peripheral edema. *Daily monitoring of fluid intake and output indicates the status of fluid retention and evaluates the effect of the treatment with diuretics.*
- Take vital signs frequently. Auscultate the heart and lungs for abnormal sounds such as rales (crackles) and rhonchi. *Problems may be signaled by increases in respiratory rate, heart rate, and narrowing pulse pressure.*
- Check mental status. *Changes could indicate increased intracranial pressure and decreased tissue perfusion to the brain.*
- Perform range-of-motion (ROM) exercises. *This helps to prevent deep vein thrombosis (DVT).*
- Apply antiembolism stockings or compression stockings (see Procedures 29-3 and 29-4 🔗). Check for calf pain

and tenderness. Record and report any changes. *Calf pain and tenderness can signal the presence of a thrombus or clot that could dislodge and become an embolus. Emboli can be life threatening.*

- Administer antianxiety/sedative agent as directed. *Reduces anxiety to help provide calmness to increase potential for rest.*
- Monitor, describe, and record vital signs and hemodynamic status. *Provides indicators to cardiac function status and potential for failure.*
- Administer diuretics as ordered. *Diuretics increase sodium and water excretion.*
- Monitor intake and output (I&O) every hour, or as appropriate, and weigh daily. *To determine effectiveness of diuretic therapy.*
- Administer oxygen as needed. *Increases the blood oxygenation to decrease potential for ischemia.*
- Check heart and breath sounds regularly. *Increasing crackles, S.O.B. may indicate worsening condition.*
- Monitor mental status, urine output, skin, diminished pulses, pallor or cyanosis, and dysrhythmias. *These are indications of a decrease in tissue perfusion.*
- Encourage bed rest and a quiet environment. *Reduces anxiety, oxygen consumption, and cardiac workload.*

EVALUATING

Anxiety will be within manageable levels with coping and problem-solving skills evidenced by statements that the anxiety is reduced, and the client will participate in care activities and the development of a plan for managing the disease. The client will exhibit adequate cardiac output and tissue perfusion as evidenced by vital signs within normal baseline ranges, absence of dysrhythmias, pulmonary edema, and fluid volume excess. Hemodynamic monitoring may be used to assess cardiac function, assess circulatory status, and evaluate the client's response to treatment. The monitoring requires a multilumen catheter inserted by the physician through the central vein to the right side of the heart.

Continuity of Care

The primary goal is compliance with the treatment plan. Explain to the client that the medication taken may provide immediate improvement but controlling the episodes requires continued medication, dietary, and activity compliance. Explain the purpose for restricting the intake of sodium and fluid. Instruct the client to report if pulse is irregular or slow and if the client experiences dizziness, blurred vision, S.O.B., a persistent dry cough, palpitations, increased fatigue, swollen ankles, decreased urinary output, or a weight increase of 3 to 5 pounds in a week. These changes indicate decreased cardiac output caused by heart failure.

Other Heart Disorders

VALVULAR DISEASE

Valvular heart disease can be acquired or congenital and may involve any of the four valves in the heart. The most common cause of valvular heart disease is rheumatic fever, which can lead to mitral and aortic valve disorders.

Rheumatic Fever

Rheumatic fever is a disease that usually follows untreated strep throat and upper respiratory infections in childhood. If treatment is not sought, or the treatment is inadequate, the strep infection can progress to inflammatory disease of rheumatic fever. This condition can affect heart valves, although it may take 10 to 40 years for it to happen. It causes vegetative growth on the leaflets of the valves, called **Aschoff's nodules.** The valve then thickens and hardens so that it is unable to open and close correctly. This condition is sometimes referred to as *rheumatic heart disease* (RHD).

The condition may take two forms: insufficiency or stenosis.

Valvular Insufficiency

Valvular insufficiency is the failure of the valves to close completely, so blood is forced back into the previous chamber when the heart contracts. The mitral valve fails to close completely and blood flows from the left ventricle back into the left atrium. The signs and symptoms of mitral insufficiency are dyspnea, fatigue, and a murmur. The diagnosis is based on the patient history, physical examination revealing a murmur, and an ECG. Treatment includes bed rest, oxygen therapy, antibiotics if infection is detected, and fluid restrictions and diuretic therapy if other complications exist such as CHF.

Valvular Stenosis

Stenosis is a hardening of the cusps of the valves that prevents the valves from opening completely and slows blood flow into the next chamber. The mitral valve is the most commonly affected valve. The valve lies between the left atrium and the left ventricle. The signs and symptoms are dyspnea on exertion, fatigue, cough, palpitations, and in severe cases cyanosis. Mitral stenosis (Figure 33-18 ■) is diagnosed by the presence of a cardiac murmur, including a diastolic murmur, and is confirmed by an ECG. Treatment includes limiting salt intake and administration of diuretics and anticoagulants to prevent formation of clots. The treatment is to reduce the workload on the heart. Surgical intervention may be necessary to free the valve to provide adequate blood flow.

Clients with suspected valvular disease may have complaints of fatigue or weakness, chest pain with exertion,

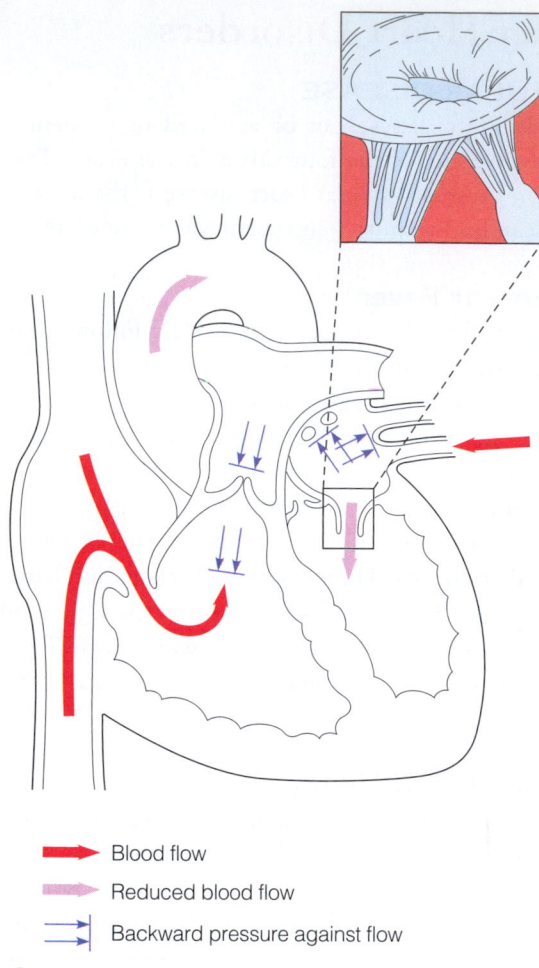

- ➡ (red) Blood flow
- ➡ (pink) Reduced blood flow
- ⇉ Backward pressure against flow

Figure 33-18. ■ Mitral stenosis.

dizziness, and fainting. On assessment of lung sounds, the nurse may hear a heart murmur and wheezes or crackles in the lungs. The client may also have edema of the lower legs and feet.

INFLAMMATORY HEART DISORDERS

Each of the three layers of the heart can become inflamed. When this happens, the heart is unable to pump effectively. In addition to inflammation of these layers, the heart muscle itself can become impaired, resulting in cardiomyopathy.

Pericarditis

Pericarditis is an inflammation, acute or chronic, of the sac (pericardium) that encloses and protects the heart. Causative agents are viruses, bacteria, trauma, rheumatic fever, or inflammation or infection elsewhere in the body. Friction and irritation result when there is blood or exudate between the pericardium and the epicardium.

Clients with pericarditis and cardiac arrest are at risk for cardiac tamponade. In **cardiac tamponade,** fluid accumulation in the pericardial sac impairs the diastolic filling of the heart. This can compress the heart and not allow the

pericardial sac to stretch. Rapid accumulation of fluid is potentially fatal and requires immediate lifesaving measures.

MANIFESTATIONS. Signs and symptoms of cardiac tamponade include neck vein distention, reduced arterial blood pressure, muffled heart sounds, and an abnormal drop in systemic blood pressure greater than 15 mm Hg. If this occurs, a **pericardiocentesis** (surgical drainage of the pericardium) is performed to remove the fluid from the pericardial sac and relieve restriction of heart movement (Figure 33-19 ■). Signs and symptoms include fever, chest pain, "pounding heart," dyspnea, chills, malaise, and often tachycardia. Auscultation may reveal friction rub or a grating sound.

DIAGNOSIS AND TREATMENT. Diagnosis is made through blood studies, cardiac enzyme levels and ECG.

Treatment requires antibiotic drugs, possibly surgical drainage, aspiration, bed rest, analgesics, antipyretics, and nonsteroidal anti-inflammatory drugs (NSAIDs).

Myocarditis

Myocarditis is the inflammation of the heart muscle. The condition may be acute or chronic and can occur at any age. The causative agent may be a viral, bacterial, fungal, or protozoal infection; it may be a complication of another disease, associated with an MI, or due to certain toxic agents (chronic cocaine use, alcoholism, radiation).

DIAGNOSIS AND TREATMENT. Diagnosis is made through labs, radiographic chest film, and ECG.

Treatment includes rest, medications (quinidine, procainamide), analgesics, oxygen, and anti-inflammatory medication.

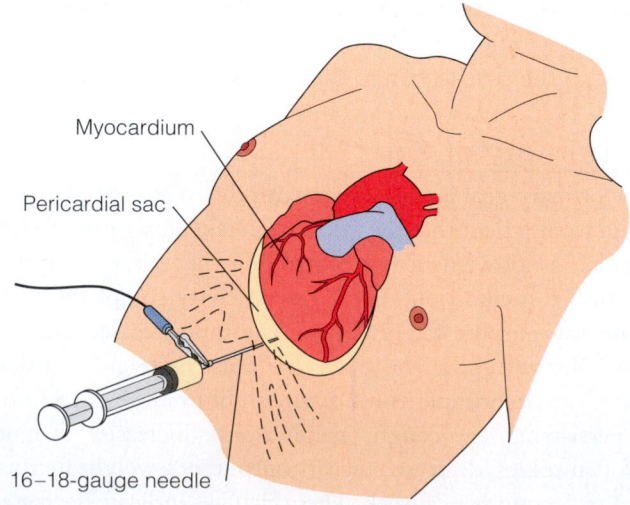

Myocardium

Pericardial sac

16–18-gauge needle

Figure 33-19. ■ Pericardiocentesis removes fluid from the pericardial sac.

Endocarditis

Endocarditis is the inflammation of the valves and lining of the heart. It can indicate infection elsewhere in the body. Because the infective organisms are embedded in the heart lining and valve tissue, vegetative growths on the valves may be released into the blood as emboli that can lodge and cause ischemia. They may also cause infection or abscesses in organs where they lodge. Infective endocarditis is seen most often in clients who have RHD or congestive heart failure and in IV drug users. To help prevent the development of endocarditis in high-risk clients, prophylactic antibiotics are given prior to any invasive procedure if the client has valvular disease. For example, a client with mitral stenosis should inform the dentist before having invasive dental work done. Antibiotics are usually ordered prior to and after the dental work to help prevent the development of endocarditis.

Signs and symptoms of infection may include fever, chills, night sweats, anorexia, fatigue, and weakness.

DIAGNOSIS AND TREATMENT.   Diagnosis includes a cardiac murmur on auscultation, CBC, blood cultures to identify the causative agent, and ECG.

Treatment includes IV antibiotics, antipyretics, anticoagulants, bed rest, and surgical repair if cardiac valves are damaged.

CARDIOMYOPATHY

Cardiomyopathy is a term given to a group of diseases that affect the heart muscle. The muscle of the ventricles becomes flaccid and is unable to pump effectively. Congestive heart failure is common as cardiac output falls. Clients older than 55 years have a poor prognosis, with death usually occurring within 2 years of symptoms.

NURSING CARE

PRIORITIZING NURSING CARE

Clients with valvular disease may have had the condition since childhood or may have a new diagnosis. Focus your care on managing discomfort and increasing heart and lung function. Explain to clients the reason for remaining on bed rest: to decrease the workload on the heart. Keep the feet elevated when the client is sitting up in a chair to prevent dependent edema. Encourage compliance with medications, especially diuretics and anticoagulants. For clients with inflammatory heart disorders, focus your care on managing chest pain and maintaining rest so the heart can heal. Be vigilant for any signs of emboli. For example, any changes in the level of consciousness or respiratory status could indicate an embolus to the brain or lungs.

ASSESSING

Clients with valvular and inflammatory heart disorders need to have a thorough history taken and a physical exam. It is important to determine when the symptoms began and how severe they have become. Auscultate the heart for murmurs and friction rubs and the lungs for crackles. Monitor lab work for signs of infection and inflammation. Assess for edema of the lower extremities. Assess vital signs, oxygen saturation, and balance of intake and output.

DIAGNOSING, PLANNING, AND IMPLEMENTING

Because the end result of valvular disease is usually congestive heart failure, the outcomes, nursing diagnoses, and nursing interventions are the same as those for CHF. Possible nursing diagnoses for clients with inflammatory heart disease include:

- *Acute Pain*
- *Activity Intolerance* related to fatigue, shortness of breath, and chest pain
- *Risk for Infection*

Outcomes for these clients would include the following:

- The client will be able to perform ADLs.
- The client will tolerate increased activity levels.
- The client will verbalize understanding of the disease and the medications necessary to manage the symptoms.

Nursing care for clients with valvular and inflammatory diseases includes:

- Weigh the client at the same time daily. Monitor urinary intake and output and check daily for peripheral edema. *Daily monitoring of fluid intake and output indicates the status of fluid retention and evaluates the effect of the treatment with diuretics.*
- Take vital signs frequently. *Problems may be signaled by increases in respiratory rate, heart rate, and narrowing pulse pressure. Narrowing pulse pressure can indicate impending cardiac tamponade.*
- Auscultate the heart and lungs for abnormal sounds every shift. *Presence of rales and rhonchi can indicate worsening heart failure in severe cases. Murmurs and friction rubs help diagnose valve disorders and pericarditis.*
- Apply antiembolism stockings. Check for calf pain and tenderness. Record and report any changes. *Calf pain and tenderness can signal the presence of a thrombus or clot that could dislodge and become an embolus. Emboli can be life threatening.*
- Administer antibiotics and anti-inflammatory medication as ordered. *Antibiotics help resolve the infections present or prevent infections in clients with valvular and inflammatory heart disease. Anti-inflammatory drugs decrease symptoms and effusion in pericarditis and endocarditis.*

- Administer diuretics as ordered. *Diuretics increase sodium and water excretion.*
- Monitor I&O every hour, or as appropriate, and weigh daily. *This helps in the determination of the effectiveness of diuretic therapy.*
- Administer oxygen as needed. *Increases blood oxygenation and decreases the potential for ischemia.*
- Monitor mental status, urine output, skin, diminished pulses, pallor or cyanosis, and dysrhythmias. *These are indications of a decrease in tissue perfusion.*
- Encourage bed rest and a quiet environment. *Reduces anxiety, oxygen consumption, and cardiac workload.*

EVALUATING

Assess the client for participation in care activities and the development of a plan for managing life with a heart valve problem. Inflammatory heart disorders usually resolve with treatment, but the client can be at risk for recurring problems. Data are gathered to assess for adequate cardiac output and tissue perfusion as evidenced by vital signs and hemodynamic measurements within normal baseline ranges and absence of dysrhythmias.

Continuity of Care

The primary goal is to reduce the workload of the heart for clients with valvular disease. Explain the need to pace oneself in exertion and activities. Discuss the possible need for valve replacement surgery or **commissurotomy** (surgical separation of valve leaflets). Explain the purpose for restricting the intake of sodium and fluid. Instruct the patient to report increased fatigue, swollen ankles, decreased urinary output, or a weight increase of 3 to 5 pounds in a week. These changes indicate decreased cardiac output caused by heart failure.

Conduction Disorders (Dysrhythmias)

Clients with heart disease are at risk for developing cardiac dysrhythmias (sometimes called *arrhythmias*). Cardiac **dysrhythmias** are deviations from the normal heartbeat (normal sinus rhythm) and are also called irregular heartbeats. Some dysrhythmias may develop without any underlying heart disease. Clients are often on **telemetry** (remote monitoring) for constant observation of the heart rhythm.

Sinus rhythm is the name for a regular heartbeat that originates in the sinoatrial node, or pacemaker, of the heart. Sinus tachycardia describes a regular heartbeat with a rate of more than 100 beats per minute. Sinus bradycardia describes a regular heart rhythm at a rate below 60 beats per minute.

Manifestations

The most common manifestations of dysrhythmias are palpitations. Chest pain, paleness, sweating, lowered blood pressure, dizziness, and fainting may also occur.

Diagnosis and Treatment

The primary care provider will order an ECG, ambulatory cardiac monitoring, or echocardiogram. Electrophysiology study (EPS) or coronary angiography may be performed.

The major dysrhythmias are atrial fibrillation, ventricular fibrillation, ventricular tachycardia, and atrioventricular block. Table 33-5 ■ shows ECG tracings, manifestations, and management for each of these dysrhythmias.

Treatment for serious incidents of dysrhythmia includes intravenous medications, defibrillation, or implantation of a pacemaker.

PACEMAKERS

An invasive therapy to restore an effective heart rate when the heart's natural pacemakers fail is an artificial **pacemaker.** The pacemaker sends an electrical impulse through the electrode catheter to the heart and then back to the pacemaker (Figure 33-21 ■). Pacemakers can be temporary or permanent.

There are three types of pacemakers: single-chamber, dual-chamber, and biventricular-chamber (using 3 leads). The single-chamber pacemaker has one lead either in the upper chamber (right atrium) or lower chamber (right ventricle). The dual-chamber pacemaker has one lead in the upper chamber and one lead in the lower chamber. The biventricular-chamber pacemaker has one lead in the upper chamber (right atrium), one lead in the lower chamber (right ventricle), and one lead in the left ventricle. The physician determines which pacemaker would be beneficial for the client's condition.

The electrode catheter is placed into a peripheral vein and the battery-powered generator of the temporary pacemaker is worn on the chest, waist, or arm. A permanent pacemaker is self-contained and may operate for up to 20 years. It is implanted in a pocket beneath the skin and operates on demand (senses the heart rate and fires accordingly).

Candidates for permanent pacemakers are some heart attack victims, clients with complete heart block, or people with slow ventricular rates from congenital or degenerative heart disease.

CARDIOVERSION

Cardioversion is a noninvasive therapy that attempts to restore the heart's natural pacemaker, the sinoatrial node. It is used to convert to normal sinus rhythm by using an electric current to slow down the heart rate. The procedure uses anterior/posterior (A/P) paddle electrodes or right-upper-chest and left-lower-chest electrodes. It requires announcement of

(Text continues on p. 873.)

TABLE 33-5   Selected Cardiac Rhythms, Manifestations, and Management

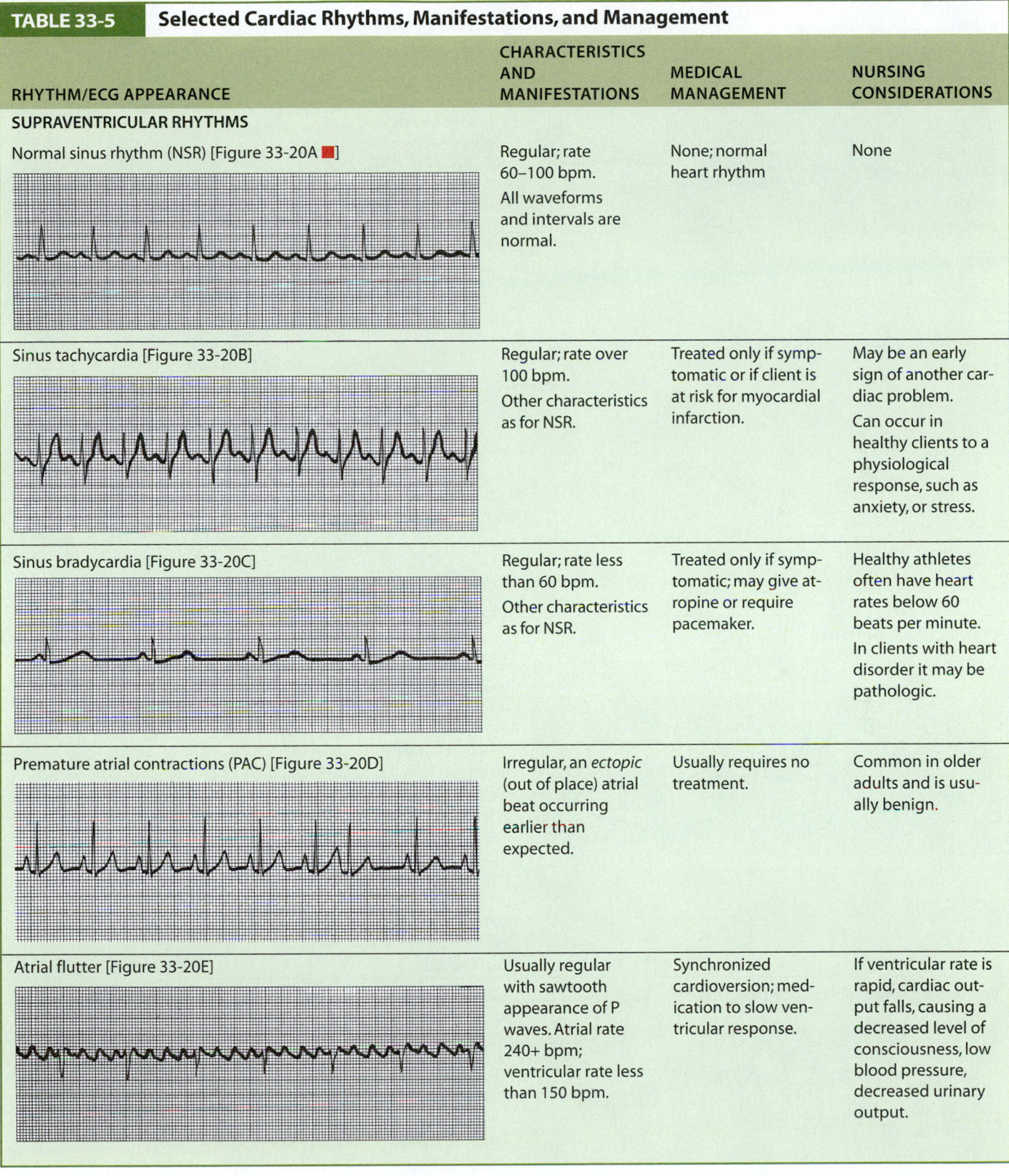

RHYTHM/ECG APPEARANCE	CHARACTERISTICS AND MANIFESTATIONS	MEDICAL MANAGEMENT	NURSING CONSIDERATIONS
SUPRAVENTRICULAR RHYTHMS			
Normal sinus rhythm (NSR) [Figure 33-20A ▪]	Regular; rate 60–100 bpm. All waveforms and intervals are normal.	None; normal heart rhythm	None
Sinus tachycardia [Figure 33-20B]	Regular; rate over 100 bpm. Other characteristics as for NSR.	Treated only if symptomatic or if client is at risk for myocardial infarction.	May be an early sign of another cardiac problem. Can occur in healthy clients to a physiological response, such as anxiety, or stress.
Sinus bradycardia [Figure 33-20C]	Regular; rate less than 60 bpm. Other characteristics as for NSR.	Treated only if symptomatic; may give atropine or require pacemaker.	Healthy athletes often have heart rates below 60 beats per minute. In clients with heart disorder it may be pathologic.
Premature atrial contractions (PAC) [Figure 33-20D]	Irregular, an *ectopic* (out of place) atrial beat occurring earlier than expected.	Usually requires no treatment.	Common in older adults and is usually benign.
Atrial flutter [Figure 33-20E]	Usually regular with sawtooth appearance of P waves. Atrial rate 240+ bpm; ventricular rate less than 150 bpm.	Synchronized cardioversion; medication to slow ventricular response.	If ventricular rate is rapid, cardiac output falls, causing a decreased level of consciousness, low blood pressure, decreased urinary output.

RHYTHM/ECG APPEARANCE	CHARACTERISTICS AND MANIFESTATIONS	MEDICAL MANAGEMENT	NURSING CONSIDERATIONS
Atrial fibrillation [Figure 33-20F] 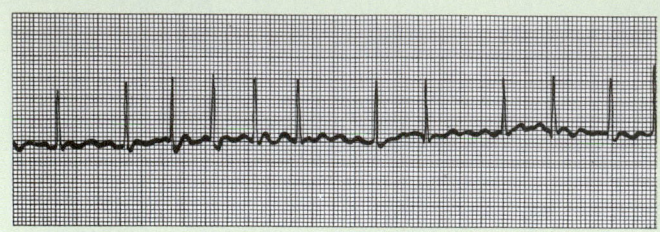	Irregular, no identifiable P waves; the atria are quivering, not pumping blood; when ventricles respond to the stimulus, may have rate as high as 180 bpm.	Cardioversion medications: ■ Digoxin to slow and strengthen heartbeat ■ Calcium channel blockers to relax the coronary artery walls so they can carry more blood to heart muscle ■ Anticoagulants to prevent emboli from forming in quivering atria and to reduce the risk of stroke A surgical procedure can be done if the client does not respond to cardioversion; called Maze procedure; a new conduction pathway is created in the heart.	Increased risk for thromboemboli.
VENTRICULAR RHYTHMS			
Premature ventricular contractions (PVC) [Figure 33-20G] 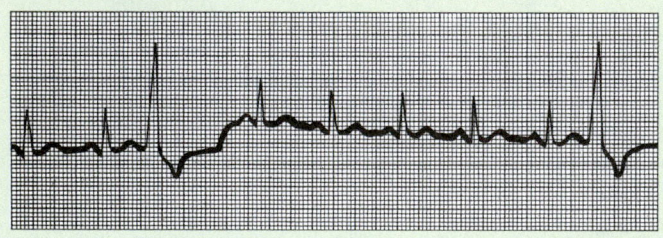	Client feels like heart is skipping a beat or flip-flopping; tracing on ECG shows early beat that is wide and bizarre because beat originates in the ventricle, not the SA node (ectopic QRS wide and bizarre). When PVCs occur in pairs or runs, they can cause ventricular tachycardia and lead to death.	Antidysrhythmics such as lidocaine (IV), procainamide, bretylium. Tell client to abstain from nicotine, caffeine.	Can be triggered by anxiety, stress, tobacco, alcohol, or caffeine.
Ventricular tachycardia (VT or v-tach) [Figure 33-20H] 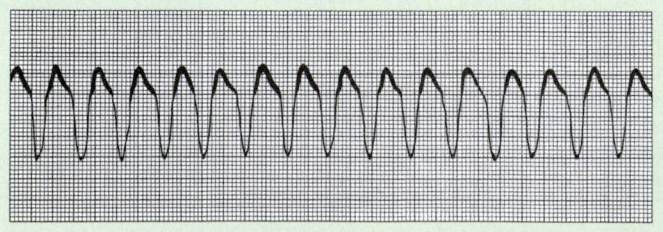	Wide, bizarre, PVC pattern with no sinus beats; rate is regular and rapid at 140–240 bpm; no identifiable P waves, QRS wide and bizarre. Generally caused by hypoxemia, digitalis toxicity, electrolyte imbalance, pronounced bradycardia.	Procainamide (Pronestyl) is given to depress the ventricular response to electrical stimulation. Lidocaine is used only if an MI or cardiac ischemia is the cause of the v-tach. Cardioversion or defibrillation if unconscious or unstable.	If dysrhythmia continues, client will become unconscious and pulseless, requiring defibrillation.

(continued)

TABLE 33-5	Selected Cardiac Rhythms, Manifestations, and Management (continued)

RHYTHM/ECG APPEARANCE	CHARACTERISTICS AND MANIFESTATIONS	MEDICAL MANAGEMENT	NURSING CONSIDERATIONS
Ventricular fibrillation (v-fib) [Figure 33-20I] 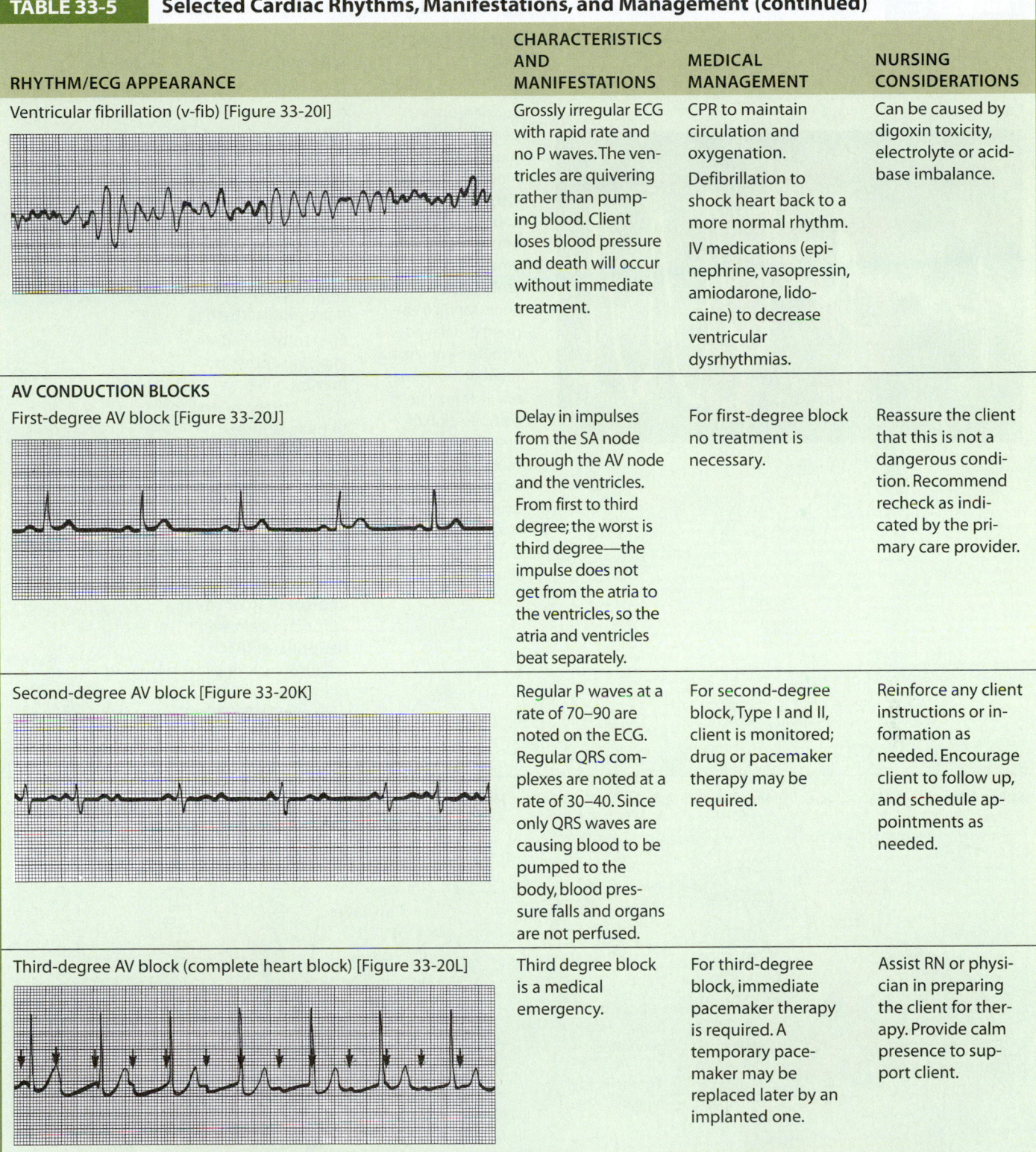	Grossly irregular ECG with rapid rate and no P waves. The ventricles are quivering rather than pumping blood. Client loses blood pressure and death will occur without immediate treatment.	CPR to maintain circulation and oxygenation. Defibrillation to shock heart back to a more normal rhythm. IV medications (epinephrine, vasopressin, amiodarone, lidocaine) to decrease ventricular dysrhythmias.	Can be caused by digoxin toxicity, electrolyte or acid-base imbalance.
AV CONDUCTION BLOCKS First-degree AV block [Figure 33-20J]	Delay in impulses from the SA node through the AV node and the ventricles. From first to third degree; the worst is third degree—the impulse does not get from the atria to the ventricles, so the atria and ventricles beat separately.	For first-degree block no treatment is necessary.	Reassure the client that this is not a dangerous condition. Recommend recheck as indicated by the primary care provider.
Second-degree AV block [Figure 33-20K]	Regular P waves at a rate of 70–90 are noted on the ECG. Regular QRS complexes are noted at a rate of 30–40. Since only QRS waves are causing blood to be pumped to the body, blood pressure falls and organs are not perfused.	For second-degree block, Type I and II, client is monitored; drug or pacemaker therapy may be required.	Reinforce any client instructions or information as needed. Encourage client to follow up, and schedule appointments as needed.
Third-degree AV block (complete heart block) [Figure 33-20L]	Third degree block is a medical emergency.	For third-degree block, immediate pacemaker therapy is required. A temporary pacemaker may be replaced later by an implanted one.	Assist RN or physician in preparing the client for therapy. Provide calm presence to support client.

TABLE 33-5	Selected Cardiac Rhythms, Manifestations, and Management (continued)

RHYTHM/ECG APPEARANCE	CHARACTERISTICS AND MANIFESTATIONS	MEDICAL MANAGEMENT	NURSING CONSIDERATIONS
Cardiac arrest 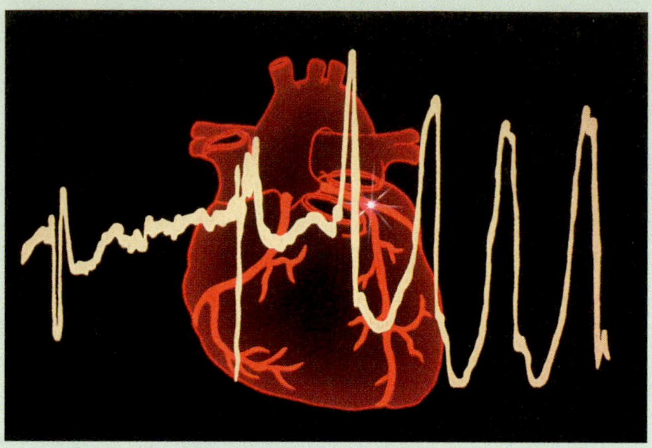	Sudden, unexpected cessation of the heart's pumping function; the client loses consciousness and stops breathing. This is a medical emergency and rapid treatment is necessary. If treatment is delayed 3–5 minutes, irreversible brain damage may result. It may be a complication of heart disease or be due to respiratory arrest, electrocution, drowning, severe trauma, massive hemorrhage, and drug overdose.	Call Code Blue immediately and begin CPR. CPR must be started within 3–5 minutes of the arrest. Defibrillation will be done during code to shock heart into a more regular rhythm. Epinephrine (Adrenalin), vasopressin may be given to stimulate the heart to beat, isoproterenol (Isuprel) and dobutamine to maintain blood pressure, lidocaine and bretylium to decrease cardiac arrhythmias. Implantation of an automated external defibrillator (AED) or an automatic implantable cardioverter defibrillator (AICD) or a pacemaker.	

Source: Adapted from *Medical Surgical Nursing Care,* by K. M. Burke, P. LeMone, and E. L. Mohn-Brown, 2003, Upper Saddle River, NJ: Prentice Hall, Table 22-1, pp. 543–545.

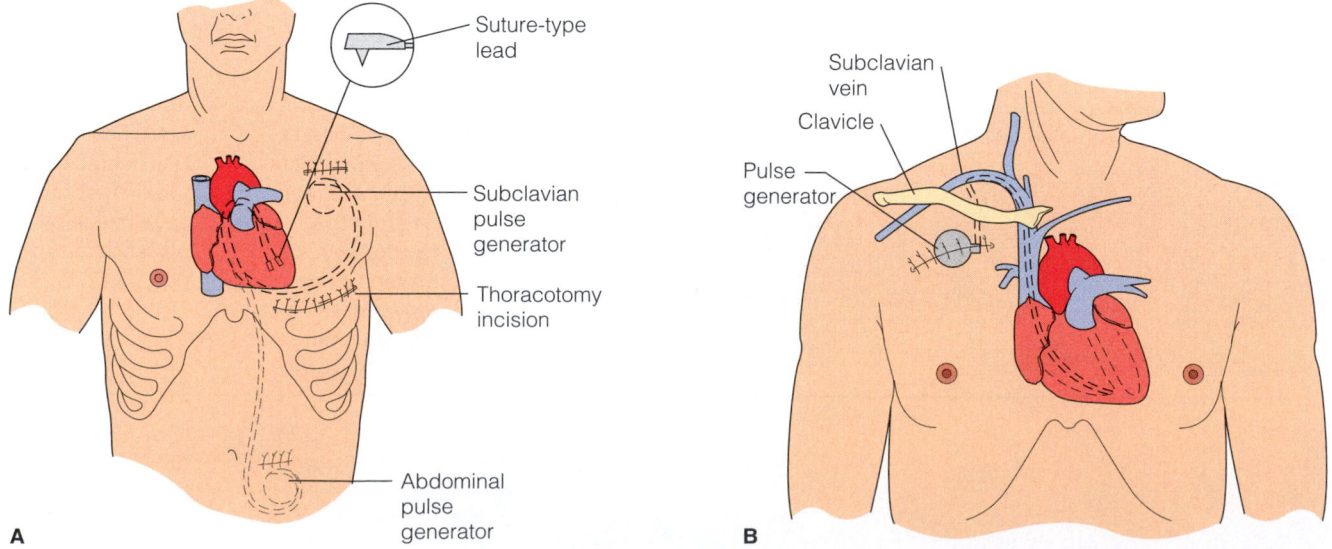

Figure 33-21. ■ **A.** A permanent epicardial pacemaker. The pulse generator may be placed in subcutaneous pockets in the subclavian or abdominal regions. **B.** A permanent transvenous (endocardial) pacemaker with the lead placed in the right ventricle via the subclavian vein.

"ready, stand back, all clear" to make sure all present are away from the client to decrease the potential for grounding and shocks (see Figure 47-5 ⚭).

Nursing Considerations

When caring for clients with cardiac dysrhythmias, focus on maintaining the telemetry unit at all times and the client's response to exertion and activity. If you need to remove the telemetry unit to assist the client to the shower, for example, be sure to call the monitor station first and notify them of your intent. Monitor the client's pulse before, during, and after activity, such as walking in the hallway. Stop the activity if the client's pulse goes above 100 or the client complains of dizziness, faintness, shortness of breath, or chest pain. Whenever the client complains of any of these symptoms, call the monitor room and ask about the client's rhythm during the episode. Be constantly aware that the client could go from having frequent PVCs to ventricular tachycardia to ventricular fibrillation to cardiac arrest in a matter of a moment or two.

Congenital Heart Defects

Congenital heart disease is a heart-related problem that is present at birth and often forms even before birth. Congenital heart defects are more common when a child has been exposed to rubella, alcohol, or drugs during intrauterine development. Other factors that increase the risk of congenital heart defects include other congenital or genetic defects, advanced maternal age, maternal disorders such as lupus and diabetes, and siblings or parents with congenital defects. The more common types of congenital heart defects include openings between chambers of the heart (atrial-septal defect, ventricular-septal defect, and patent ductus arteriosus) and defects of blood vessels (tetralogy of Fallot, coarctation of the aorta, and transposition of the great vessels). Most of these defects require surgical correction, although some may resolve without surgery as the child grows. For in-depth information about congenital heart defects, see Chapter 59 ⚭ .

Central Circulatory Disorders

HYPERTENSION

Primary (or **essential**) **hypertension** is a condition of abnormally high blood pressure in the arterial system. A blood pressure of 120/80 mm Hg is the most desirable per the American Heart Association. Prehypertension is a blood pressure of 120–139/80–89. Systolic blood pressure of 140/90 is considered high and should be evaluated by a physician. If either number is elevated, the finding is considered hypertension. The cause of essential hypertension is not known. However, the condition of the heart and blood vessels will have the most profound outcome on the blood pressure.

Manifestations and Risk Factors

The client exhibits few signs or symptoms following an insidious onset until damage has occurred. Hypertensive heart disease is the most prevalent cardiovascular disorder in the United States. Certain groups have a markedly higher incidence of this disease (Box 33-10 ■). Hypertensive heart disease is the result of chronically elevated pressure in the vascular system, causing the heart to work

---

| **BOX 33-10** | **CULTURAL PULSE POINTS** |

Clients with Cardiovascular System Disorders

Race has been a recognized risk factor in hypertension and cardiovascular disease. This has been particularly true with African American males. Recent research funded by the American Heart Association has found an increased risk of cardiovascular disease in African American and Mexican women. African American women living in the United States have a higher incidence of hypertension (HTN) than any other race-sex groups. African American women irrespective of age are much more susceptible to high blood pressure than Caucasian women, and it is the leading cause of death among African American women.

High blood pressure usually has no symptoms. It is referred to as the "silent killer" because the client may not have any evidence of the disease. Possible manifestations of hypertension include headaches, blurred vision, *epistaxis* (nose bleeds), and light-headedness or fainting (**syncope**).

Individuals with HTN may also experience a variety of secondary symptoms, including fatigue, reduced activity tolerance, dizziness, palpitations, angina, and dyspnea. Although symptoms for African Americans may be the same, descriptive verbal expressions of symptoms may have cultural differences. (For example, when an African American woman responds only with an affirmative nod to a question, a nurse of a different culture may conclude that she does not understand, when indeed she does.) Risk factors for HTN in African American women include a high prevalence of obesity, particularly central abdominal obesity; weight gain; cigarette smoking; excessive sodium diet; high cholesterol; alcohol intake; drug abuse; and propensity for other diseases such as diabetes. These behaviors increase the individual's risk for HTN; however, these risk factors can be reduced with lifestyle changes.

Education is the most effective way of preventing HTN. Understanding the racial difference in risk factors may lead to better health outcomes in African American women. Therefore, it is imperative that nurses, in a culturally sensitive manner, educate and support clients and their families in their efforts to lead healthier lives. In addition, education focusing on access to services in local communities and community health agencies should be an integral part of the treatment and prevention of HTN for African American women.

harder to pump against the resistance. Conditions that cause the heart to pump harder are:

- *Atherosclerosis*. A buildup of fatty plaque on the inside of the arteries causes narrowing of the lumen to the point of blockage.
- *Arteriosclerosis*. The walls of the arteries become thick and stiff, losing elasticity, and the walls calcify.
- *Renal disease*. Kidneys are no longer able to remove excess fluid from the blood, leading to fluid overload and increased workload on the heart.

Additional factors that can contribute to hypertension are stress, age (more frequent in older adults), heredity, smoking, obesity, and a *type A* (focused, driven) personality. Risk factors for hypertension are listed in Box 33-11 ■.

Secondary hypertension is elevated blood pressure due to another medical diagnosis. Examples of those diagnoses would include hormonal imbalances, especially involving cortisol; kidney disease; pregnancy; and brain trauma. Hypertension occurs as a complication of the underlying diagnosis.

Malignant hypertension, which is not cancer, is a medical emergency. The blood pressure elevates rapidly and progressively until the diastolic pressure is greater than 120 mm Hg. Malignant hypertension can cause irreversible damage to the arterioles of organs throughout the body. It is often difficult to determine the cause of malignant hypertension.

When hypertension is untreated for a long period of time, it can cause damage to many organs in the body. The heart may be damaged due to coronary artery disease, left ventricular hypertrophy, heart failure, and possible dysrhythmias. Hypertension may cause renal insufficiency or renal failure. The brain may be affected by stroke or cerebral edema, and sustained hypertension can cause peripheral vascular disorders.

Diagnosis and Treatment

Hypertension is diagnosed by frequent checks of the blood pressure. When the blood pressure remains at or above 140/90, the diagnosis is made. In addition, a history and physical are performed, with laboratory tests to determine if any organ damage has occurred.

Hypertension can be treated with a variety of medications and combinations of medications. *Diuretics* are given to reduce circulating blood volume and are often combined with *vasodilators* to dilate blood vessels and reduce blood pressure in two ways. *Beta-adrenergic blockers* and calcium channel blockers work to reduce blood pressure by slowing the heartbeat. Beta-blockers also dilate blood vessels. *ACE inhibitors* produce vasodilation to increase renal blood flow.

In addition to medications, clients should be advised to limit sodium intake, lose weight if they are overweight, stop smoking, exercise regularly, and take measures to reduce or manage stress.

ANEURYSMS

An **aneurysm** is a weakening and dilation in the wall of a blood vessel. Most aneurysms occur in the aorta and the arteries due to high pressure within these vessels. Aneurysms are caused by atherosclerosis, arteriosclerosis, trauma, or congenital weakness in the vessel wall. Aneurysms are classified by their location and shape (Figure 33-22 ■). The most common locations are in either the thoracic or the abdominal aorta. Three common shapes of aneurysms include:

- Fusiform, in which the walls of the artery dilate about equally, causing a tubular pouching.
- Saccular, in which one side of the wall of the artery pouches out.
- Dissecting, in which the lining of the artery pulls away from the pouch itself, allowing blood to flow between the artery layers.

If not treated immediately, the tearing of the dissecting aneurysm continues until the client goes into shock from blood loss. Dissecting aneurysms often result in death.

Manifestations

Fusiform or saccular aneurysms may be asymptomatic until they are found on a CAT scan, x-ray, ultrasound, or MRI. Abdominal aortic aneurysms are sometimes detected by observation of a pulsing in the abdominal area that matches the heart rate. Thoracic aneurysms may cause chest, back, or neck pain, with edema of the face and neck, distended neck veins, dyspnea, cough, and hoarseness. Abdominal aneurysms may cause abdominal or lower back pain, a pulsating abdominal mass, and cool, cyanotic, or pale extremities.

When the aneurysm dissects or ruptures, the client will have symptoms of shock such as hypotension, tachycardia, diaphoresis, pallor, and weakness. The client may complain of sudden severe chest pain, back pain, or abdominal pain as well. Blood pressure in the upper extremities will fall, and radial pulses may be absent.

BOX 33-11	RISK FACTORS FOR HYPERTENSION

- *Smoking.* Nicotine constricts blood vessels, elevating blood pressure.
- *High cholesterol.* Causes atherosclerosis, which narrows the lumen of the arteries.
- *Alcohol.* Increases chemicals (epinephrine and norepinephrine) in the blood that constrict blood vessels, which increases blood pressure.
- *Emotional stress.* Causes constricted peripheral blood vessels due to sympathetic nervous system stimulation.
- *Obesity and sedentary lifestyle.* Increase blood volume and cardiac demand; regular, consistent, mild exercise, such as walking, can help reduce blood pressure.

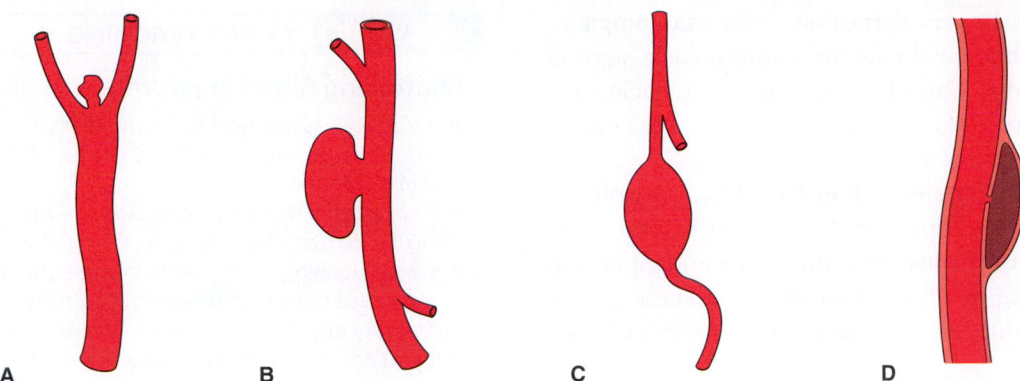

Figure 33-22. ■ Types of aneurysms. **A.** A berry aneurysm is a small sac on a stem or stalk. **B.** A saccular aneurysm is formed from a distended small portion of the vessel wall. **C.** A fusiform aneurysm is an enlarged area of the entire blood vessel. **D.** A dissecting aneurysm is formed when blood fills the area between the tunica media and the tunica intima.

Diagnosis and Treatment

Aneurysms are often noticed by chest or abdominal x-ray, or by ultrasound if an abdominal aneurysm is suspected. An MRI or CT can also be used for detection and estimation of the size of an aneurysm.

Dissected or ruptured aneurysms are often fatal. Prompt surgical intervention is needed if the client is to survive.

EMBOLI

Emboli are clots of aggregated material (usually blood but they can be air bubbles, fat globules, bacterial clumps, or pieces of tissue) that travel through a vessel, lodge in a blood vessel, and block the flow of blood. The most common is a venous thrombosis that forms in the deep veins of the legs. Part of the clot can break off and become lodged in another area of the venous system, often in the lungs. Clots can form in the heart and travel to the carotid and cerebral arteries, resulting in CVAs (*cerebrovascular accidents* or *strokes;* see Chapter 36 ◯◯ for full discussion).

Arterial emboli can also occur, in which a blood clot travels through the arterial circulation, then lodges in a small arteriole, destroying blood flow to the area. When this occurs, the client experiences sudden severe pain in the area.

Manifestations

Signs and symptoms of emboli include sudden or insidious pain in an affected area and numbness or tingling of the extremity. The affected area, often an extremity, is pale and cold to the touch. The pulses are absent distal to an arterial blockage. The client may also experience nausea and vomiting, fainting, and signs of shock.

Diagnosis and Treatment

Emboli are usually diagnosed using Doppler ultrasound studies to evaluate blood flow. A venogram may be done, injecting dye into the veins to look for a blockage.

Treatment for emboli depends on the area of involvement and the resulting urgency. Pulmonary embolism, MI, and CVA require immediate and aggressive treatment. Arterial embolism also requires immediate treatment to decrease the potential for tissue death. Blood flow is restored to the affected area by lowering the limb, maintaining warmth to the area, and treating the constriction. Medications that deter further clot formation are *heparin* or *enoxaparin (Lovenox)*. *Urokinase,* a *fibrinolytic* (clot-dissolving) drug, can be administered to a coronary embolism to break it down.

Surgery, or **embolectomy,** may be necessary to remove the obstruction and restore blood flow to the area. When a client has had surgery to remove an arterial embolus, observe for indications of complications such as further clot formation, infection, impaired circulation, and arterial hemorrhage.

NURSING CARE

PRIORITIZING NURSING CARE

When caring for clients with circulatory disorders such as hypertension, aneurysms, and emboli, it is important to focus your care on maintaining effective circulation. Clients with hypertension are at risk for developing many complications. Because they may not feel symptoms of their elevated blood pressure, they may not seek medical care or take antihypertensive medications continuously. It is very important to educate these clients frequently about signs and symptoms to report, how to monitor their own blood pressure daily, and the necessity of taking medications as prescribed.

Clients with aneurysms who also have hypertension are at risk for rupture or dissection of the aneurysm. Again, many people do not know they have an aneurysm until it is a critical problem. Be very alert to any client who complains of back pain or abdominal pain and exhibits early signs of shock or blood loss. This client may be experiencing the dissection or rupture of an aneurysm, and will need immediate surgery to prevent death.

Always be alert for signs of an embolus, especially in your clients with hypertension. Changes in mental alertness and level of consciousness can indicate an embolus to the brain resulting in a CVA. Complaints of chest pain or difficulty breathing can indicate an embolus to the heart or lungs.

ASSESSING

When assessing clients with known hypertension, inquire about whether the client has been taking antihypertensive medication as directed. Take the client's blood pressure in both arms in lying, sitting, and standing positions to establish a baseline (see Procedure 21-4 ⬭). It is not uncommon for blood pressure readings to vary with different positions. Clients on certain antihypertensive medications may have a drop in pressure when they change from lying to sitting or standing (*orthostatic hypotension;* see Chapter 21 ⬭). Auscultate heart sounds for murmurs or extra sounds. Monitor vital signs and assess for pain; check peripheral pulses for equality and strength, color, temperature, and capillary refill to detect emboli.

Assess clients with hypertension for complaints of headache, blurred vision, dizziness, and fatigue. Determine the client's level of knowledge about the disease and its management.

DIAGNOSING, PLANNING, AND IMPLEMENTING

Some common nursing diagnoses for clients with circulatory disorders include the following:

- *Anxiety*
- *Impaired Physical Mobility*
- *Acute Pain*
- *Deficient Knowledge* regarding the importance of controlling blood pressure and risk factors for high blood pressure
- *Ineffective Therapeutic Regimen Management*
- *Ineffective Health Maintenance* related to lifestyle behaviors

Desired outcomes for these clients would include the following:

- The client will understand the disease and the medication recommended for management of the disease.
- The client will develop a plan for a realistic, regular exercise program.
- The client will explore coping mechanisms to reduce stress.

| BOX 33-12 | CLIENT TEACHING |

Controlling Blood Pressure

- Avoid excess salt and fat in the diet to decrease the workload on the heart. See Chapter 25 ⬭ for nutrition guidelines.
- If symptoms decrease, it means the medication is working, so do not stop taking it.
- If you suddenly stop taking some antihypertensives, it can cause your blood pressure to suddenly increase dramatically and can lead to severe complications.
- If you are having undesirable side effects from the medication, talk with your healthcare provider about them rather than discontinuing the medication yourself.
- Set up a system so you know that you have taken the medication at the same time each day.

For Clients with Hypertension

Education is a very important aspect of managing this chronic health problem.

- Teach the client how and when to monitor blood pressure. *Understanding the significance and effect of hypertension on the body may result in compliance with medication therapy and changes in lifestyle behaviors.*
- Discuss ways to modify risk factors and how they contribute to hypertension (see Box 33-11). *Knowledge and understanding that lifestyle changes decrease the risk for hypertension helps the client take control and manage the disease.*
- Instruct the client about controlling blood pressure (Box 33-12 ■). *Understanding the importance of diet and medications will increase the likelihood of compliance with prescribed treatment and lifestyle changes.*
- Teach the client the importance of stopping smoking. *The client who understands the link between smoking and hypertension may be motivated to make positive lifestyle changes.*

For Clients with Thrombus and Embolus

- Instruct the client to avoid crossing the legs, to keep the extremities in a dependent position, and to change position frequently. *These measures will help prevent further formation of thrombi and emboli.*
- Encourage clients to report any edema, pain, warmth, or redness in the legs to their healthcare provider immediately. *Fibrinolytic (thrombolytic) therapy should be initiated immediately to dissolve the clot.*

For Clients with Aneurysm

Clients present both pre- and postoperatively for repair or treatment of an expanding or ruptured aneurysm with high levels of anxiety. Nurses caring for these clients need to manage these elevated anxiety levels, which result from the urgent nature of the disorder.

- Open communication and active listening by the nurse help establish trust and acknowledge the concerns of the client. *The stress level of the client will decrease as a result of the calm and reassuring demeanor of the nurse.*

EVALUATING

Collect data to determine client knowledge and understanding of hypertension, its signs and symptoms and treatment. Review with the client the lifestyle changes such as diet, exercise, and cessation of smoking that may positively impact control of the disease. Advise client that stroke and heart attack are a result of uncontrolled hypertension.

Continuity of Care

Teach the client that there is no cure for hypertension but that compliance with drug therapy can control it. Provide suggestions on altering contributing factors such as stress, salt intake, obesity, and smoking. Encourage the client to examine dietary and lifestyle habits and make appropriate changes. Additional types of therapy include dietary management, reduction of sodium, weight loss, exercise, and stress reduction. Teach the significance of the blood pressure reading and the indicators associated with an elevation in the numbers. Refer client to community-based programs that support the efforts to control contributing factors.

PERIPHERAL VASCULAR DISORDERS

The term **peripheral vascular disease** (PVD) refers to conditions of the arteries, veins, and lymph vessels outside the heart. Some diseases only affect arteries, whereas others affect veins.

Normal aging affects blood vessels by causing them to become less elastic and the walls to thicken. This inflexibility causes increasing peripheral vascular resistance and leads to increased blood pressure. Smoking increases the risks for development of peripheral arterial disease because the nicotine in tobacco causes constriction of both arteries and veins. As these vessels constrict, the blood pressure increases and circulation to the extremities decreases. The carbon monoxide in the smoke affects the amount of oxygen the blood can carry to the body.

Disorders of the Arteries

Whenever an artery is blocked or diseased and cannot deliver oxygenated blood to the tissues (ischemia), the first symptom the client experiences will be pain. The most common chronic disorder affecting the arteries is arteriosclerosis. **Intermittent claudication** is a symptom of ischemia that causes cramping pains and weakness in the calves of the legs while walking. It is relieved with rest. As the arterial disease worsens, so does the pain, to the point that it is not even relieved at rest. The client may experience burning, tingling, and numbness of the legs at night.

ARTERIOSCLEROSIS OBLITERANS

Arteriosclerosis obliterans is simply atherosclerosis of the peripheral arteries, often seen in the femoral and/or popliteal arteries. The lumen of the artery narrows due to plaque deposits, until the artery is partially or completely blocked and the tissue supplied by the artery becomes severely ischemic.

Manifestations

When an artery completely occludes, the client will exhibit signs and symptoms known as the "five Ps":

- Pain
- Pallor
- Pulselessness
- Paresthesia
- Paralysis

Diagnosis and Treatment

Arterial blockage in the legs is diagnosed using a variety of tests. The client may be placed on a treadmill to walk until the pain begins. Doppler ultrasounds, MRI, and angiography are also used to diagnose arteriosclerosis obliterans.

Treatment for this disorder includes medical management if the occlusion is not complete. Anticoagulants and possibly vasodilators are given, although studies show that vasodilators may not be effective for this condition. Fibrolytics, such as urokinase, may be instilled into the artery. Surgical treatment includes embolectomy to remove the blockage itself, **endarterectomy** (removal of the lining of the artery), angioplasty, and bypass of the occluded artery (femoral-popliteal or femoral posterior tibial bypass grafts). In the worst-case scenario, the extremity would be amputated.

BUERGER'S DISEASE

Buerger's disease is the inflammation of the peripheral arteries and veins with clot formation. The primary cause of the disease is long-term tobacco smoking. The upper or lower extremities can be affected but most often the leg or foot is affected. It is seen most often in men between the ages of 20 and 40.

Manifestations

Signs and symptoms include intense pain in the affected area (legs, instep) that is relieved by rest. The extremity involved may be pale, and cool or cold to touch. Circulation restoration will prevent atrophy, ulcers, and gangrene.

Diagnosis and Treatment

Diagnosis is based on reported pain, arteriogram, and ultrasonogram. Treatment is complete cessation of smoking, exercises to improve circulation (Buerger-Allen), rest, surgical intervention, or amputation if the limb is gangrenous.

RAYNAUD'S DISEASE

Raynaud's disease is a condition causing arterial spasm of the fingers, hands, or feet that causes pain, numbness, and discoloration. Usually the cause is unknown. It is seen most frequently in women between the ages of 20 and 40. Cold precipitates this condition. Signs and symptoms include a whiteness, or blanching, followed by a blue color due to the venous flow remaining, and then red/purple when the circulation is restored to areas. Treatment includes slowly warming the area, avoidance of cold, cessation of smoking, and reduction of stress.

Disorders of the Veins

THROMBOPHLEBITIS

Thrombophlebitis is an inflammation of a vein with the formation of a thrombus on the vessel wall. The cause may be *venous stasis* (blood pooling), increased blood *coagulability* (clotting), trauma to the vessel wall, or surgery. A common site for thrombophlebitis to occur is the calf of the leg. People who travel a great deal and are unable to get up and move about, such as those on long airplane flights, are at risk for developing thrombophlebitis. Blood flow back to the heart can be partially or completely blocked.

Manifestations

Manifestations include pain, swelling, heaviness and warmth in the area, chills, fever, and positive Homans' sign.

Diagnosis and Treatment

Thrombophlebitis is diagnosed by visible edema of the area, measurable circumference difference, tenderness to palpation, radiographic venography, and ultrasonography.

Immediate treatment is needed. Superficial clots can be treated with rest, leg elevation, and moist heat applications. NSAIDs are given to decrease pain as well as to slightly anticoagulate the blood. If the clot is in a deep vein (DVT), hospitalization is required. Immobilizing the affected part prevents the thrombus from dislodging and spreading. Anticoagulants are administered to reduce the possibility of pulmonary embolism. Warm, moist compresses are applied over area to relieve symptoms.

Prevention of thrombophlebitis is an important aspect of client teaching. Encourage clients to avoid sitting and standing for long periods. Tight stockings or knee-high stockings should be avoided. Encourage clients to elevate feet on a footstool when sitting to decrease dependent edema. Clients with possible thrombophlebitis should avoid massaging the extremities to prevent dislodging a clot.

VARICOSE VEINS

Varicose veins are swollen, knotted, and tortuous veins with poorly functioning valves (Figure 33-23 ■). The valves may be congenitally defective, absent, or can no longer close correctly.

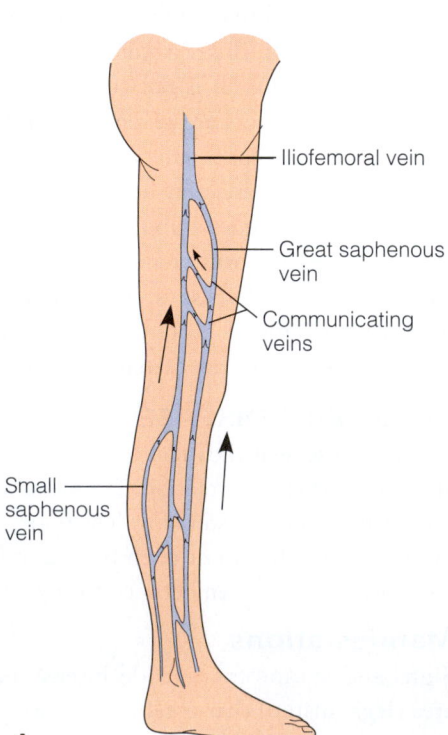

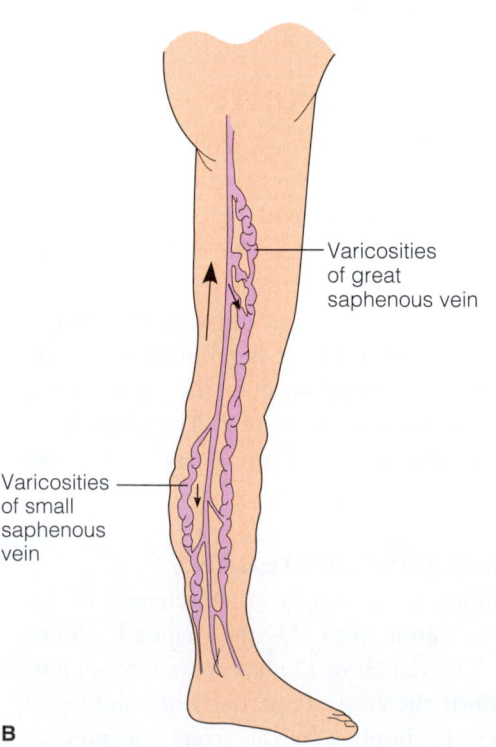

A — Iliofemoral vein — Great saphenous vein — Communicating veins — Small saphenous vein

B — Varicosities of great saphenous vein — Varicosities of small saphenous vein

Figure 33-23. ■ **A.** Normal leg vein. **B.** Varicose veins.

Varicose veins may develop in veins anywhere in the body. These veins usually develop gradually in the lower legs. Increased pressure stretching the vessel wall from prolonged standing, obesity, venous thrombosis, and pressure in the abdomen due to pregnancy can lead to varicose veins. The action of the leg muscles contracting and relaxing with normal movement causes the blood to be pushed upward. Extended periods of sitting or standing allow gravity to push the blood downward, resulting in increased pressure in the vein. The increased pressure decreases the blood return to the heart, the veins stretch, and the valves cannot close properly (*incompetence*). Varicose veins can result in venous insufficiency, which leads to stasis dermatitis and stasis ulcers.

Manifestations

Signs and symptoms of varicose veins include twisted, swollen, knotted veins in the lower legs, fatigue in the legs, dull aching, leg cramps, and swollen ankles. The veins feel hard when palpated.

Diagnosis and Treatment

Varicose veins are diagnosed using visual inspection, Doppler ultrasonic flow tests, and angiography.

Conservative treatment for varicose veins includes antiembolism (compression) stockings to help the blood flow back to the heart, daily walking, elevating and resting legs periodically through the day, and avoiding prolonged standing or sitting. Surgery may be required to treat varicose veins. The surgical procedures include **compression sclerotherapy,** which obliterates the vein by injecting a hardening agent into it. A compression dressing is then applied. Another surgery, **vein stripping,** is the surgical removal of the varicose veins.

clinical ALERT

After a vein stripping, check the client closely and often for bleeding. If bleeding occurs, apply pressure immediately and elevate the leg. Notify the physician stat.

Elastic bandages are applied to the legs and kept in place with a snug fit and no wrinkles. Early ambulation is important to help increase venous return to the heart.

VENOUS STASIS ULCERS

Venous stasis ulcers are open sores that appear on the lower legs due to poor circulation to the legs. Tissue cells die due to lack of oxygenated blood and slough off, causing open sores. These are different than decubitus ulcers (pressure sores) that occur over bony prominences and are due to pressure preventing blood circulation.

Manifestations

The client with venous stasis ulcers often complains of pain and burning in the area.

BOX 33-13 | CLIENT TEACHING

Foot Care with Peripheral Vascular Disease

- Keep legs and feet clean, dry, and comfortable.
- Wear shoes that fit well and do not rub or pinch the feet.
- Wear protective footwear at all times and avoid going barefoot to help prevent accidents and injuries to the feet.
- Observe any scratch or minor injury to the feet or lower legs for redness, swelling, or drainage. Report these signs immediately because infection sets in very quickly when circulation is compromised.
- Sit with legs elevated to improve circulatory return from the feet and legs to the heart.

Diagnosis and Treatment

Venous stasis ulcers are diagnosed by visual inspection. Dietary considerations are important in the treatment of stasis ulcers. Vitamins A and C and zinc help promote tissue healing, and protein lost through the ulcers must be replaced. Treatment of the ulcers themselves involves debridement of the necrotic tissue with chemical agents, wet-to-dry dressings, or surgical debridement. Dressing changes are ordered frequently to keep the ulcer clean and dry. It is easy for these ulcers to become infected, so it is important to keep them clean and watch for signs of infection.

Box 33-13 ■ provides client teaching about foot and ankle care for clients with PVD.

NURSING CARE

PRIORITIZING NURSING CARE

When caring for clients with peripheral vascular diseases, your focus needs to be on maintaining circulation to the area, decreasing edema, and managing pain. Overbed cradles (Figure 33-24 ■) can be used to keep sheets off tender extremities. Assess pain rating frequently and evaluate the effectiveness of pain management techniques. Assess circulation to extremities every shift by palpating pedal pulses and post tibial pulses. If these pulses are difficult to find, mark the client's foot with an X using a pen or marker. That way all nursing staff will be able to detect pulses in the same place. Compare right and left pulses for strength. Note any differences in strength. Inspect lower extremities for evidence of impaired circulation such as paleness or cyanosis. Check capillary refill in the toes and compare right and left feet. Feel the feet for coolness. Keep legs and feet elevated when the client is sitting to decrease dependent edema.

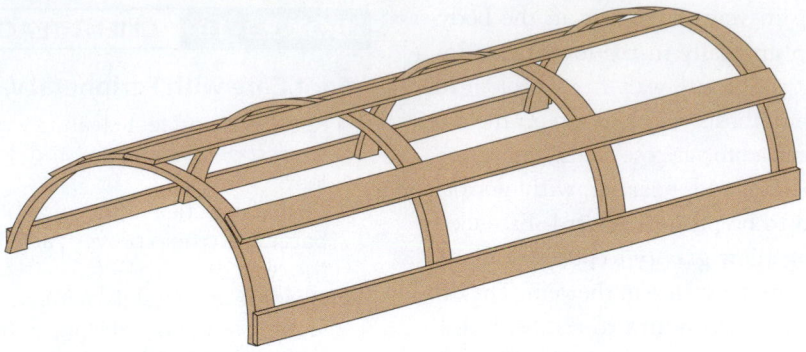

Figure 33-24. ■ Bed cradles are used to keep bed linens off a part of the client's body.

ASSESSING

Review Procedure 19-1, Part C ⊂⊃, for steps in collecting data about the peripheral vascular system. See Box 33-14 ■ for abnormal findings when assessing the peripheral vascular system. Refer to Chapter 19 ⊂⊃ for further guidelines for assessing this system.

Collect subjective data on pain and its onset, characteristics, severity, and relationship to activities. Note any additional manifestations such as burning, numbness, leg fatigue or cramps, swelling of the ankles, and the effects of positioning. The client medical and family history should include disorders and diseases, previous surgeries, and current medications. The dietary history should be included as well as any history of smoking and exercise habits. The objective data include vital signs, peripheral pulses, capillary refill, presence of edema, and skin color, turgor, and integrity.

DIAGNOSING, PLANNING, AND IMPLEMENTING

Possible nursing diagnoses for clients with peripheral vascular disease include:

- *Ineffective Peripheral Tissue Perfusion* peripherally related to alteration in blood flow
- *Acute Pain* related to physical factors or reduced blood flow
- *Risk for Impaired Skin Integrity* related to internal factor of altered circulation
- *Risk for Infection* in open areas such as stasis ulcers

Nursing interventions include:

- Assess for pain, peripheral pulse, capillary refill, color, and coldness. *Pain, weak or absent peripheral pulse, increased capillary refill time, sudden coldness, and pallor indicate reduction of blood flow to the extremities.*
- Assess skin for intactness, ulcerations, or breakdown. *Diminished blood flow can result in tissue damage and poor healing when tissue does not receive oxygen and nutrients.*
- Position extremities in dependent position and provide warm environmental temperature unless edema is a problem. *Gravity and warmth promote blood flow to the extremities.*
- Assess pain level and report acute or severe pain accompanied by a pale, cold extremity. *The effectiveness of pain medication can be determined and the immediate treatment for acute pain may save an extremity.*
- Provide gentle ROM exercises as ordered. (See Procedure 23-1 ⊂⊃, Providing Passive Range-of-Motion Exercises.) *ROM exercises promote circulation to the affected extremities.*

For Clients with Thrombophlebitis

- Maintain bed rest and elevate legs, assessing regularly for pain. Administer medication as ordered. Report

---

BOX 33-14   ABNORMAL FINDINGS FOR PERIPHERAL VASCULAR FUNCTION

Deviations from Normal—Pulses

- Asymmetric volumes (indicate impaired circulation)
- Absence of pulsation (indicates arterial spasm or occlusion)
- Decreased, weak, thready pulsations (indicate impaired cardiac output)
- Increased pulse volume (may indicate hypertension, high cardiac output, or circulatory overload)
- Distended veins in the anteromedial part of thigh and/or lower leg or on posterolateral part of calf from knee to ankle
- Tenderness on palpation
- Pain in calf muscles with passive dorsiflexion of the foot (Homans' sign)
- Warmth and redness over vein
- Swelling of one calf or leg

Deviations from Normal—Perfusion

- Cyanosis, pallor of extremity
- Skin on extremity cool to touch
- Marked edema of extremity
- Skin thin and shiny or thick, waxy, shiny, and fragile; reduced hair, ulceration
- Delayed color return or mottled appearance; delayed venous filling; marked redness of arms or legs (indicates arterial insufficiency)
- Delayed return of color (arterial insufficiency)

increased pain. *Using leg muscles increases inflammation and pain. Elevation of legs promotes venous return, decreases peripheral edema, and reduces pain. Increased pain may indicate extension of the inflammation and the clot.*

- Monitor the color of the extremity for skin integrity and capillary refill. Assess peripheral pulses and measure the extremity affected to monitor any increase in swelling. *Swelling indicates further inflammation and increased impaired circulation to the tissue.*

- Assess skin of the affected leg and foot frequently. *Careful assessment can lead to early detection of skin breakdown, which allows for early intervention to prevent continued breakdown.*

- Encourage frequent position change and active ROM exercises. *Position changes and ROM exercises increase circulation and prevent skin breakdown due to venous stasis and immobility.*

For Postoperative Clients after Vascular Surgery

Immediately report signs of graft leakage such as:

- Bruising of scrotum, perineum, or penis; hematoma at incision
- Increased abdominal girth
- Weak or absent peripheral pulses; impaired movement or sensation of extremities
- Decreased blood pressure, increased pulse; low urine output (less than 30 mL/hr)
- Increased abdominal, back, or groin pain
- Drop in hematocrit, hemoglobin, and red blood cell levels

Maintain intravenous fluids and administer blood as ordered. Report evidence of complications:

- *Lower extremity embolism:* pain and numbness, diminished pulses, and pale, cool, or cyanotic skin
- *Bowel ischemia:* blood in stools, diarrhea, severe abdominal pain, and abdominal distention
- *Impaired renal function:* output less than 30 mL/h, fixed specific gravity, increasing blood urea nitrogen and serum creatinine levels
- *Spinal cord ischemia:* lower extremity weakness and paraplegia

If ordered, apply a sequential compression device (SCD). See Procedure 29-4 ⟲ to review steps in applying SCDs.

EVALUATING

Collect subjective and objective data on pain, color, numbness, coldness, family history, and diet. Determine the strength and equality of the peripheral pulses and capillary refill. Provide teaching about managing PVD through exercise, stress reduction, and medications.

Continuity of Care

Self-care instruction to the client should include cessation of smoking, daily walking, elevating of the legs, exercises to tighten and relax the leg muscles, and application techniques for antiembolism stockings. (Review Procedure 29-3 ⟲ for instructions on applying antiembolism stockings.)

Note: The references and resources for all chapters have been compiled at the back of the book.

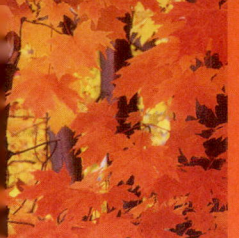

Chapter Review

KEY Points

- Arteries carry oxygen-rich blood to the body. Veins carry deoxygenated blood back to the heart and lungs.

- The pediatric client's anatomical and physiological immaturity, and vital signs (pulse, respirations, and blood pressure) vary with age and from the adult.

- There are many forms of cardiovascular disease such as atherosclerosis (hardening of the arteries), coronary artery disease, angina, stroke, high blood pressure (hypertension), and heart failure.

- The three biggest risk factors for cardiovascular disease are smoking, high blood pressure, and high blood cholesterol.

- Coronary artery disease occurs when the coronary vessels are narrowed due to the buildup of plaque.

- Angina pain is often relieved by rest, and no permanent damage results.

- In myocardial infarction, a portion of the heart muscle dies, causing permanent damage.

- Clients with complaints of chest pain unrelieved by nitroglycerin given three times, 5 minutes apart, should be treated as though an MI is impending. Immediate medical care is required.

- Signs of a heart attack include chest discomfort/pressure spreading pain to arms, back, jaw, or stomach, cold sweats, and nausea.

- In congestive heart failure, the heart muscle contracts poorly, leaving fluid in the peripheral tissues and lungs. Nursing care focuses on improving gas exchange and decreasing edema.

- Valvular diseases cause poor opening or closing of heart valves. When the problem is severe, symptoms similar to those of CHF result.

- Inflammatory heart diseases affect the heart's ability to pump well. Supplemental oxygen, pain medication, positioning, rest, and reduction of the heart workload are all key nursing interventions.

- Conduction disorders range from mild problems to medical emergencies. Pacemakers, cardioversion, defibrillation, and implantable defibrillators are all used to treat conduction disorders.

- With hypertension, one major focus of nursing care is educating the client about medications, lifestyle, diet, and exercise to decrease blood pressure.

- Peripheral vascular disease can affect veins or arteries. Nursing care includes careful assessment, meticulous foot and skin care, decreasing edema, and managing pain.

- Arterial disorders are characterized by cool, pale skin, diminished pulses, and pain. Venous disorders are characterized by reddish brown leathery skin and edema.

FOR FURTHER Study

For information about stress, see Chapter 17.

Review Procedure 19-1, Part C, for steps in collecting data about the peripheral vascular system.

For further information on heart and blood pressure measurements, see Chapter 21.

See Procedure 23-1 for passive range-of-motion exercises.

See Chapter 25 for low-sodium and other medically prescribed diets.

Hyperventilation is discussed in Chapter 26.

See Chapter 27 for administering medications.

Review Procedure 29-3 for application of antiemboli stockings, and Procedure 29-4 for steps in applying a sequential compression device.

For a more in-depth discussion of anemia, see Chapter 34.

See Chapter 36 for cerebrovascular accidents or strokes.

Thyrotoxicosis is discussed in Chapter 38.

See Figure 47-5 for cardioversion equipment.

For information about congenital heart defects, see Chapter 59.

PEARSON

EXPLORE **mynursingkit**™

MyNursingKit is your one stop for online chapter review materials and resources. Prepare for success with additional NCLEX®-style practice questions, interactive assignments and activities, web links, animations and videos, and more!

Register your access code from the front of your book at
www.mynursingkit.com

Critical Thinking Care Map

Caring for a Client with Congestive Heart Failure (CHF)
NCLEX-PN® Focus Area: Physiological Adaptation

Case Study: Mary Hart, a 75-year-old female of African-American descent, has been hospitalized for the fourth time in 6 months. She has a history of type II diabetes (NIDDM). Family brought her to the ED last night because she was experiencing shortness of breath.

Nursing Diagnosis: *Imbalanced Nutrition: Less than Body Requirements*

COLLECT DATA

Subjective	Objective
_____	_____
_____	_____
_____	_____
_____	_____
_____	_____
_____	_____
_____	_____

Would you report this? Yes/No

If yes, report to: _____

What would you report? _____

Nursing Care

_____
_____
_____
_____
_____
_____
_____
_____
_____

How would you document this? _____
_____
_____
_____

Compare your answers and documentation to those provided on the MyNursingKit Website.

Data Collected
(use only those that apply)

- Vital signs T 98.2, P 100, R 21, BP 168/92
- C/O weakness, fatigue
- Son-in-law is concerned because she is showing signs of confusion
- +4 edema lower extremities
- Persistent cough
- Restlessness/Anxiety
- Skin cyanotic and clammy
- Blood glucose 180
- Urine output 200 mL in 8 hours
- Weight 146
- Lives with daughter and son-in-law and 3 teenage grandchildren
- Hemoglobin 12.9 and hematocrit 34
- Potassium — 4.3

Nursing Interventions
(use only those that apply; list in priority order)

- Weigh client daily.
- Take vital signs every 4 hours.
- Auscultate heart and lung sounds.
- Check mental status.
- Perform ROM exercises each shift.
- Administer antianxiety/sedatives as ordered.
- Apply antiembolism stockings. Check for calf pain and tenderness.
- Monitor, describe, and record vital signs and hemodynamic status.
- Administer diuretics as ordered.
- Insert Foley catheter.
- Monitor intake and output every hour.
- Administer oxygen as needed.
- Provide bed rest and quiet environment.

NCLEX-PN® Exam Preparation

1 The nurse, caring for a client with fluid collecting in the pericardial space, recognizes that the primary risk to heart function for this client is:

1. Hypovolemia.
2. Inability of the heart to fill and pump effectively.
3. Damage to the pericardium.
4. Arterial-septal damage.

2 Which of the following clients does the nurse consider at greatest risk for heart disease?

1. The client who is paraplegic, smokes, and has elevated lipid levels.
2. The client with hyperlipidemia and hypertension who is employed as a lifeguard.
3. The woman who is under a great deal of stress, takes oral contraceptives, and smokes.
4. The diabetic client who has a family history of early onset heart disease who smokes and has elevated blood pressure.

3 The nurse is caring for a client who is asymptomatic but is suspected of having narrowing of the coronary artery. Which of the following tests would the nurse anticipate to confirm this diagnosis?

1. ECG
2. Echocardiogram
3. Thallium stress test
4. PET scan

4 The nurse admits a client with a diagnosis of angina. When asked about angina pain experience, the client describes pain that comes on with any activity and can even occur at rest. The client says the pain seems to be getting worse and more frequent and nitrates do not always treat it successfully. The nurse recognizes the client is describing what type of angina?

1. Stable
2. Unstable
3. Prinzmetal's
4. Paroxysmal

5 The nurse is assessing the client's heart sounds. To auscultate for the presence of an S_3 sound, the nurse places the client into what position?

1. Fowler's
2. Right side lying
3. Prone
4. Left lateral or supine

6 The nurse is caring for a client diagnosed with congestive heart failure. The client asks, "I know my heart doesn't work effectively, but why do I get so short of breath?" The nurse's best response would be:

1. "It is because of the stress and anxiety you feel about your heart disease, which causes your bronchi to spasm resulting in shortness of breath."
2. "The left ventricle of your heart does not pump blood effectively so it gets backed up in the lungs, allowing fluid to leak into the air sacs and reducing the amount of functioning lung space."
3. "It is because your heart has damaged your kidneys causing increased potassium excretion, which results in reduced muscle function making it harder to breathe."
4. "Reduction in function of the right side of your heart causes blood to back up in the lungs causing shortness of breath."

7 The nurse admits an elderly client who reports having rheumatic fever in his teens. The nurse recognizes this client is at risk for:

1. Valvular disease of the heart.
2. Myocardial infarction.
3. Strep throat.
4. Pericarditis.

8 The nurse, working in a long-term care facility, assesses that the client has an irregularity to the pulse that has not been noted before. The client is asymptomatic at this time. The nurse anticipates which of the following orders?

1. Call 911.
2. Obtain cardiac isoenzymes.
3. Perform an ECG.
4. Prepare for a pericardiocentesis.

9 The nurse admits a client with a medical diagnosis of arteriosclerosis. The client describes cramping and weakness in the calves of the legs while walking that goes away with rest. The nurse recognizes the client is describing:

1. Deep vein thrombosis.
2. Venous insufficiency.
3. Arteriosclerosis obliterans.
4. Intermittent claudication.

10 The nurse administers a calcium channel blocker to a client diagnosed with hypertension and anticipates which of the following therapeutic effects of the medication?

1. Increased urine output
2. Decreased urine output
3. Increased pulse
4. Decreased pulse

Answers and rationales for Review Questions appear in Appendix I.

Chapter 34

Clients with Hematologic and Lymphatic System Disorders

LEARNING Outcomes

After completing this chapter, you will be able to:

1. Identify the structure and function of blood and of lymph.
2. Name common diagnostic tests for hematologic or lymphocytic disorders.
3. List the compatible cross-matches for different types of blood donors and recipients.
4. Name and compare types of anemia, treatment, and nursing care.
5. Identify platelet and coagulation disorders and discuss nursing interventions for them.
6. Discuss white blood cell disorders, including leukemia, and treatment for them.
7. Name and describe four types of lymphatic disorders.
8. Identify nursing considerations for clients with lymphatic disorders.

Clinical Objectives

9. Collect subjective and objective assessment data for clients with disorders related to the hematologic and lymphatic systems.
10. Provide appropriate nursing care for clients undergoing diagnostic tests to evaluate the hematologic and lymphatic systems.
11. Participate in interdisciplinary care of clients with hematologic or lymphatic disorders, including diagnostic tests and commonly prescribed medications.

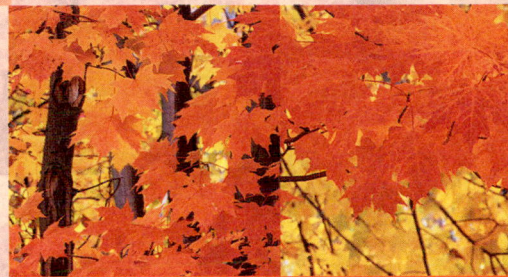

BRIEF Outline

KEY TERMS

Use the audio glossary feature on the MyNursingKit Website to hear the correct pronunciation of the following key terms.

agranulocytosis 894

anemia 889

erythrocytes 886

graft versus host disease 896

hemostasis 892

leukocytes 886

leukopenia 887

lymph 897

lymphadenopathy 897

lymphangitis 897

lymphedema 897

pancytopenia 892

plasma 886

platelets 887

sickle cell anemia 891

sickle cell crisis 891

sickle cell disease 890

sickle cell trait 891

stem cell 886

thrombocytes 886

thrombocytopenia 887

thrombopoietin 887

transfusion reaction 888

The hematologic (also called *hematopoietic*) system and lymphatic system are discussed together in one chapter because of the ways they interact. (Hematopoietic comes from *hematopoiesis*, which means the production and maturation of blood cells.) Therefore, the hematologic system creates new blood cells and alters the composition of blood to support body function and fight off infections. The lymphatic system is a primary means for the body to isolate and clear infectious waste. This chapter will discuss the anatomy and physiology of each system and their common disorders and treatments.

Structure and Function of the Hematologic and Lymphatic Systems

The hematologic system includes components of both the blood formation system and the lymphatic system (Figure 34-1 ■). All systems of the body are dependent on the hematologic system, because this system provides the nutrients that allow the organs of the body to live and function normally. The function of blood is to transport substances throughout the body, and these substances are oxygen, carbon dioxide, food molecules (glucose, lipids, and amino acids), ions, wastes, hormones, and heat. The blood also functions to defend the body against infections and other foreign materials.

Blood is considered a connective tissue because it shares many characteristics with other connective tissue. However, the cells in blood move freely and are not fixed.

The process of blood formation begins in the bone marrow. It produces red blood cells (RBCs), which are also known as **erythrocytes,** white blood cells (WBCs), called **leukocytes,** and platelets, called **thrombocytes.** It is also made up of **plasma,** which is a clear yellow, protein-rich fluid. Many plasma proteins are formed in the liver. Disorders of the hematologic system will be discussed under each type of cell.

All blood cells begin as **stem cells.** These are immature cells that have the ability to change into any of the blood cells depending on what the body needs at the time.

Red blood cells make up most of the cellular portion of the blood. A healthy red blood cell lives for approximately 120 days. The bone marrow is continually producing red blood cells to replace those that are expiring. The growth factor *erythropoietin* is necessary for the production and regulation of red blood cells. It gives the signal to the stem cells to produce red blood cells. Erythropoietin is produced by the liver in the fetus; at birth the kidneys produce erythropoietin.

Erythropoietin is produced by the kidney and stimulates the formation of the red blood cells to replace those red blood cells that are aging and will be destroyed. Low oxygen content in the blood (*hypoxia*) also stimulates red blood cell formation. Because red blood cells transport oxygen, hypoxia sends the signal that more red blood cells are needed to compensate for the lowered oxygen content of the blood. Old red blood cells are trapped by the liver and spleen where they are destroyed, though the iron contained in the destroyed red blood cell is retained and used in the formation of new red blood cells. The iron in the red blood cell is required for the formation of *hemoglobin*, which gives blood its red color. It allows the hemoglobin molecule to transport oxygen. This makes iron critical to the oxygen-transporting function of the red blood cell.

White blood cells or leukocytes are critical in the fight against inflammation and infection. White blood cells are divided into two types:

1. *Granulocytes.* The granulocytes are further differentiated into neutrophils, eosinophils, and basophils. Approximately two-thirds of all white blood cells are *neutrophils*. They have a very short life span (about 10 hours), so the bone marrow is constantly replacing them. The neutrophils increase in number in response to inflammation in the body and defense against bacterial

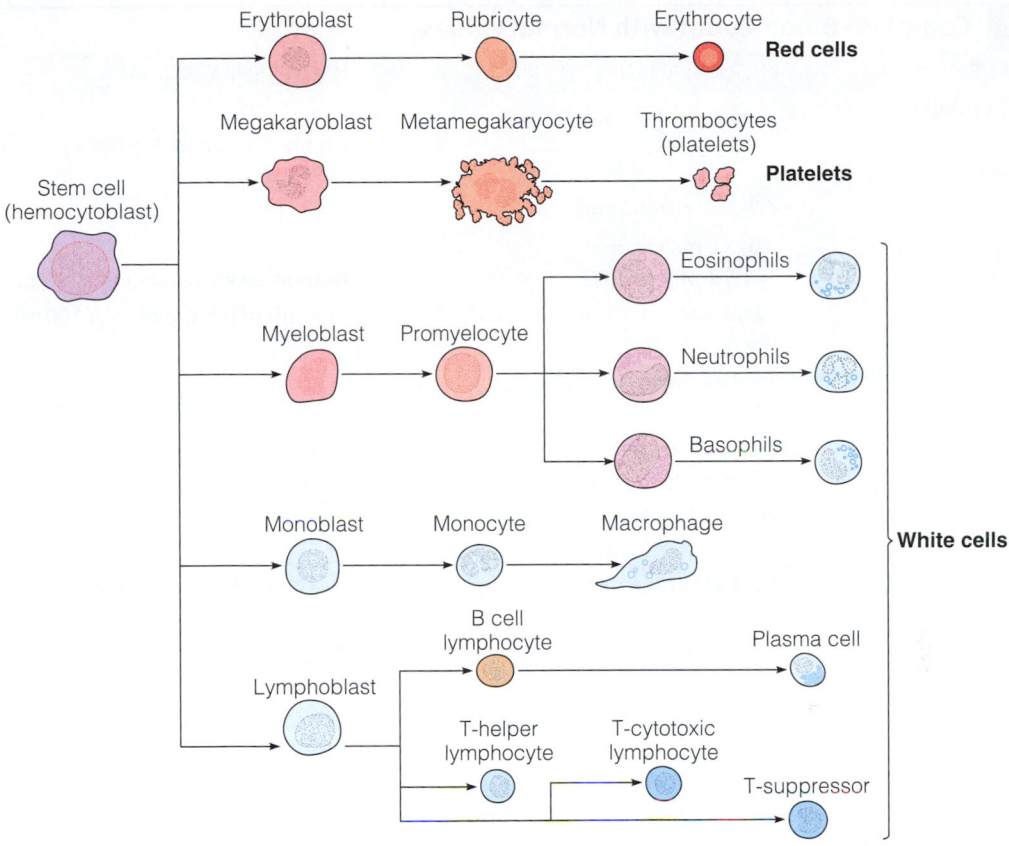

Figure 34-1. ■ The formation of different types of blood cells from the stem cell. The stem cell differentiates into one of five types of blast cells, which then mature into red blood cells (erythrocytes), platelets (thrombocytes), or white blood cells (leukocytes).

infections. The *eosinophils* and *basophils* respond primarily to allergic reactions.

2. *Agranulocytes.* The agranulocytes are divided into monocytes and lymphocytes. The *monocytes* are transformed into macrophages, which kill bacteria and respond to the presence of foreign materials in the body. The *lymphocytes* are formed in lymphatic tissue and are needed for a healthy immune system. They are divided into B lymphocytes, which provide immunity by producing antibodies, and T lymphocytes, which provide cellular immunity.

Platelets are elements in the blood that are necessary for proper blood coagulation. They have a life span of approximately 7.5 days. They are manufactured in the red bone marrow. When an injury is sustained to a blood vessel, platelets move to that site. The production of platelets is controlled by **thrombopoietin** (a protein manufactured by the liver, the kidney, the smooth muscle, and the bone marrow). The release of thrombopoietin is controlled by the number of platelets present in the blood. Table 34-1 ■ provides normal values for a complete blood count.

Laboratory Tests for Hematologic or Lymphatic Disorders

There are many laboratory tests that can indicate disorders of the hematologic and lymphatic systems. All clients will first have a *complete blood count* (CBC). This blood test measures the red cell count, white cell count, platelet count, hemoglobin, and hematocrit, and provides a detailed description of the types of white blood cells in the sample. This simple test can indicate the presence of anemia, **leukopenia** (low number of white blood cells), and **thrombocytopenia** (low levels of platelets in the blood). It will also indicate if the levels of any of the types of white blood cells are abnormal, which may indicate leukemia. An *iron level* (Fe level) and *total iron binding capacity* (TIBC) test may be ordered if iron-deficiency

TABLE 34-1	Complete Blood Count with Normal Values	
LABORATORY TEST	**NORMAL VALUES**	**WHAT TEST MEASURES**
RED BLOOD CELLS (RBCs)		
RBC count		Number of circulating RBCs per cubic millimeter of blood
▪ Men	4.2–5.4 million/mm^3	
▪ Women	3.6–5.0 million/mm^3	
Reticulocyte count	1–1.5% of total RBC	Number of immature RBCs in 1 mm^3 of blood
Hemoglobin (Hgb)	(*Note:* about 1/3 the numeric value of the hematocrit)	Amount of hemoglobin in 100 mL (1 dL) of blood
▪ Men	14–16.5 g/dL	
▪ Women	12–15 g/dL	
Hematocrit (Hct)	(*Note:* about 3 times the numeric value of the hemoglobin)	Packed volume of RBCs in 100 mL of blood; reported as a percentage
▪ Men	40–54%	
▪ Women	37–47%	
Mean corpuscular volume (MCV)	85–100 cubic micrometers (µm^3) per cell	Average volume of individual RBCs
Mean corpuscular hemoglobin (MCH)	31–35 g/dL	Weight of the hemoglobin in an average RBC
Mean corpuscular hemoglobin concentration (MCHC)	33.4–35.5%	Average concentration (percent) of hemoglobin within RBC
WHITE BLOOD CELLS (WBCs) AND PLATELETS		
WBC count	5,000–10,000/mm^3	Number of WBCs per cubic millimeter of blood
Differential WBC count:		Number of neutrophils released by bone marrow
▪ Neutrophils	60–70% or 3,000–7,000/mm^3	Active phagocytes; first to respond to inflammation or infection
▪ Eosinophils	1–3% or 50–400/mm^3	Respond to allergic reaction and parasitic infestations
▪ Basophils	0.3–0.5% or 25–200/mm^3	Respond to allergic and inflammatory reactions
▪ Lymphocytes	20–30% or 1,000–4,000/mm^3	Involved in immune reactions
▪ Monocytes	3–8% or 100–600/mm^3	Active in disposing of foreign and waste material, especially in inflammation

anemia is suspected. A *Schilling test* is conducted to determine if a client has a vitamin B$_{12}$ deficiency. A *sickle cell test* is used to identify whether a client has sickle cell disease. When a client is suspected of having some type of bone marrow disorder, a *bone marrow aspiration* or biopsy is performed.

CROSS-MATCHING FOR BLOOD PRODUCT TRANSFUSIONS

Blood product administration is a treatment frequently used when dealing with clients who have hematologic disorders. The administration of blood products can cause serious complications for clients. Each client has a specific type of blood (A, B, AB, or O), and they are called antigens. These letters indicate what antigen is present on the red cell membrane. An antigen is a protein substance that can cause an incompatibility reaction. The presence or absence of these antigens,

which are inherited, therefore determines a person's blood type. A client with an A antigen has type A blood; a B antigen has type B blood; an AB antigen has type AB blood. Having neither antigen means having type O blood.

The Rh factor or D antigen is important as well and is a specific protein on the red blood cell membrane. If the protein is present, the person is Rh positive. If the protein is absent, the person is Rh negative. When blood is transfused, the donor blood must be type and Rh compatible with the recipient's blood.

Each person does develop antibodies that can react with the AB antigens they are lacking. These antibodies in the person's plasma can react with the antigens on the donor's red cells and cause a transfusion reaction. A **transfusion reaction** occurs when the donor's red cells rupture or hemolyze and release their hemoglobin, with dangerous or even lethal results.

TABLE 34-2	Blood and Rh Types and Compatibilities		
TYPE	**COMPATIBILITY**	**CAN DONATE TO**	**CAN RECEIVE FROM**
BLOOD GROUP			
A	Partial	A, AB	A, O
B	Partial	B, O	B, O
AB	Universal recipient	AB	A, B, AB, O
O	Universal donor	O, A, B, AB	O
Rh ANTIGENS			
Rh positive		Rh positive	Rh positive or Rh negative
Rh negative		Rh positive or negative	Rh negative

It is important that the nurse administer blood that is compatible with the client. Prior to administering a blood product, the client will have a blood typing test performed even if the blood type is already known. This test is used to determine that the client's blood and that of the unit of blood product to be administered will not react with one another. Table 34-2 ■ shows the different types of blood components and compatibilities.

HEMATOLOGIC SYSTEM

Red Blood Cell Disorders

ANEMIA

Anemia is a deficiency of red blood cells or hemoglobin caused by decreased production or increased destruction of red blood cells, or by blood loss. All systems of the body may be affected by anemia, because it is red blood cells that deliver oxygen to the tissues (Figure 34-2 ■). Anemia is the most common nutritional deficiency of children in the United States, caused by insufficient amounts of iron.

Hypovolemic Anemia

When there is a sudden loss of a large amount of blood or a gradual loss from small amounts of blood, a low volume of blood results. There are then fewer blood cells circulating. The body responds by increasing production of red blood cells, but they are smaller and have less hemoglobin.

TREATMENT. Treatment will depend on how severe or mild the hypovolemia is. The cause of the anemia needs to be determined. If severe, the client would require a replacement of blood by a blood transfusion. If chronic, treatment may consist of oral, intramuscular (IM), or intravenous (IV) iron.

Iron-Deficiency Anemia

One of the most common causes of anemia is a lack of sufficient iron in the diet. The body does not manufacture its own iron. It is therefore dependent on ingested iron. Iron-deficiency anemia may occur during pregnancy, because the body requires more iron to support the growing fetus. It may appear in infants and toddlers, so screening procedures should be done between 9 months and 24 months.

It is common in childhood and adolescence, because of irregular eating habits. Iron-deficiency anemia caused by chronic blood loss also occurs in women with heavy menstrual flow and in older adults with chronic gastric bleeding.

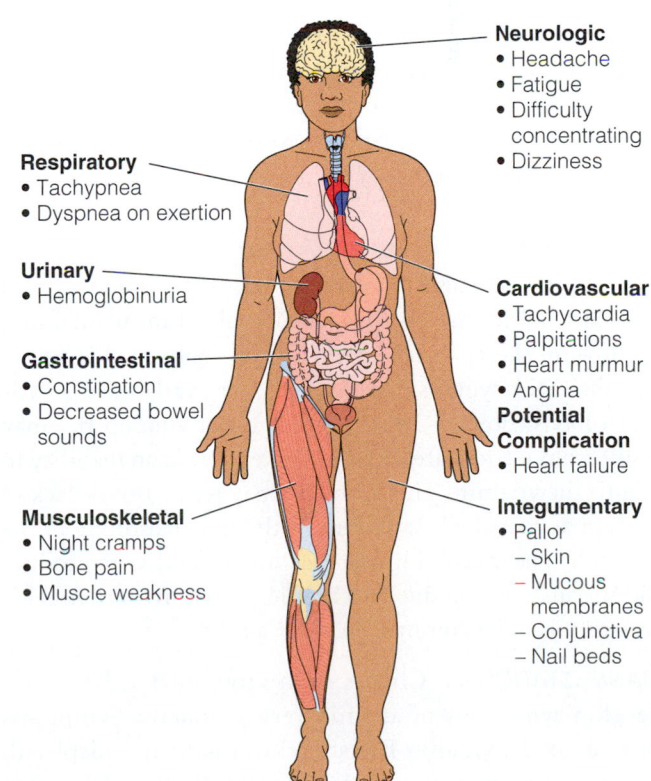

Neurologic
- Headache
- Fatigue
- Difficulty concentrating
- Dizziness

Respiratory
- Tachypnea
- Dyspnea on exertion

Urinary
- Hemoglobinuria

Gastrointestinal
- Constipation
- Decreased bowel sounds

Cardiovascular
- Tachycardia
- Palpitations
- Heart murmur
- Angina

Potential Complication
- Heart failure

Musculoskeletal
- Night cramps
- Bone pain
- Muscle weakness

Integumentary
- Pallor
  - Skin
  - Mucous membranes
  - Conjunctiva
  - Nail beds

Figure 34-2. ■ The multisystem effects of anemia.

BOX 34-1	NUTRITION THERAPY

Common Food Sources of Iron

Liver	Kidney beans	Whole wheat bread
Red meat	Leafy green vegetables	and cereal
Organ meats	Carrots	Raisins
Egg yolks		

BOX 34-2	NUTRITION THERAPY

Common Food Sources of Vitamin B$_{12}$

Liver	Nuts	Green leafy	Citrus fruits
Organ meats	Raisins	vegetables	Brewer's yeast
Dried beans			

TREATMENT. Treatment consists of increasing dietary intake of iron (Box 34-1 ■) or taking oral supplements. Iron may also be administered intramuscularly or intravenously. Parenteral administration may be used to increase creation of red blood cells. Many clients are reluctant to take iron because it may increase problems with constipation. Teach clients who are taking supplemental iron to increase fluid intake and to expect dark, greenish black stools.

clinical ALERT

Client teaching must occur when an infant or child requires iron. Iron, usually ferrous sulfate, is given orally 2 to 3 times a day. It is given between meals with vitamin C and is not given with milk because milk interferes with absorption. Having an iron-fortified formula throughout the first year of life is recommended. Toddlers need solid foods that are rich sources of iron.

If iron is to be administered as an IM injection, it must be given using the Z-track method. The purpose of the Z-track method is to seal medication within the muscle and to prevent staining or irritation to the tissues (see Chapter 27, especially Figure 27-37 ⬤⬤).

Vitamin B$_{12}$ Deficiency Anemia

Vitamin B$_{12}$ is necessary for the utilization of folic acid, and in blood cell formation. It is also involved in maintaining the myelin sheath covering the nerves. Folic acid is necessary for DNA synthesis. Vitamin B$_{12}$ is available in a variety of foods (Box 34-2 ■). A deficiency of vitamin B$_{12}$ may result from inadequate dietary intake or from an inability to absorb the vitamin. This inability may result from a lack of *intrinsic factor*, which is present in the mucosal lining of the stomach. The mucosal lining may lose its ability to produce the intrinsic factor due to chronic gastric irritation. This situation is more common in older adults.

MANIFESTATIONS. Clients with vitamin B$_{12}$ deficiency develop symptoms of anemia very gradually. Symptoms increase as the vitamin B$_{12}$ stored in the body is depleted. Some of the manifestations of vitamin B$_{12}$ deficiency involve the nervous system, because vitamin B$_{12}$ is necessary

for normal nervous system functioning. For example, the client may experience numbness and tingling of the extremities. There may also be complaints of dizziness and problems with balance. The client may be pale, have a very red, swollen tongue, and complain of fatigue.

TREATMENT. When vitamin B$_{12}$ deficiency is due to a lack of intrinsic factor, oral B$_{12}$ replacement will not be effective. Therefore, vitamin B$_{12}$ must be administered parenterally.

Sickle Cell Anemia

Sickle cell disease is an inherited defect in the formation of hemoglobin. Hemoglobin is the oxygen-carrying protein in red blood cells. In sickle cell disease, the cells contain an abnormal form of hemoglobin called hemoglobin S. The membranes of the cells are fragile and can be destroyed, thus reducing their oxygen-carrying ability (Figure 34-3 ■). The shape of the sickled cell makes it difficult to pass through the capillaries. This can cause a clumping up of the cells in small vessels. This clustering may lead to a clot or thrombosis and obstruction of flow of blood.

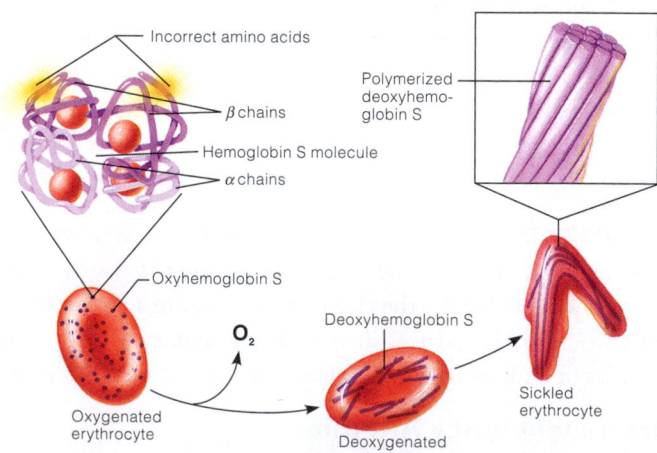

Figure 34-3. ■ Sickle cell anemia is caused by an inherited autosomal recessive defect in hemoglobin (Hgb) synthesis. When sickle cell hemoglobin (HgbS) is oxygenated, it has the same shape as normal hemoglobin. But, when oxygen is released, it crystallizes into rodlike structures (see insert). Clusters of rods form polymers (long chains) that bend the erythrocyte into the characteristic crescent shape of the sickle cell.

There are two types of sickle cell disease: an asymptomatic version called sickle cell trait and a more severe form called sickle cell anemia.

In **sickle cell trait,** the blood of the client contains a mixture of normal hemoglobin (hemoglobin A) and sickle hemoglobin (hemoglobin S). The disease is inherited from only one parent, so the proportion of hemoglobin S is low. Sickle cell trait does not develop into sickle cell disease, but the client is considered a carrier of the trait. Genetic counseling is important when individuals are known carriers. When considering having children, they should be aware of the probability of significant genetic disorders in their children.

In **sickle cell anemia,** both parents must have the sickle cell trait for a child to be born with the disease. It occurs most often among clients of African American descent (Box 34-3 ■) and causes chronic anemia. There is chronic anemia. When the sickled red blood cell becomes lodged in capillaries, occluding blood flow to the affected area, the situation is called a **sickle cell crisis** (Figure 34-4 ■). The client experiences acute pain, infections, and organ damage. The occlusion may lead to death of the involved tissues and may even be fatal.

Because sickle cells can occlude any capillary, damage may occur in any body system. Some of the more common complications are acute chest syndrome (ACS), myocardial infarction, stroke, and splenic sequestration.

Acute chest syndrome refers to a combination of respiratory symptoms. It is caused by inflammation of trapped red blood cells in the lungs. Characteristics of acute chest syndrome are fever, productive cough, chest pain, dyspnea, and hypoxia.

Splenic sequestration happens when sickle cells block the vessels leading out of the spleen. The result is entrapment of large amounts of blood inside the spleen, which causes the spleen to be enlarged and painful. The characteristic symptoms are acute left upper quadrant pain, anemia, and hypotension. Splenic sequestration is serious and potentially life threatening. Circulatory collapse and death can occur within a short time.

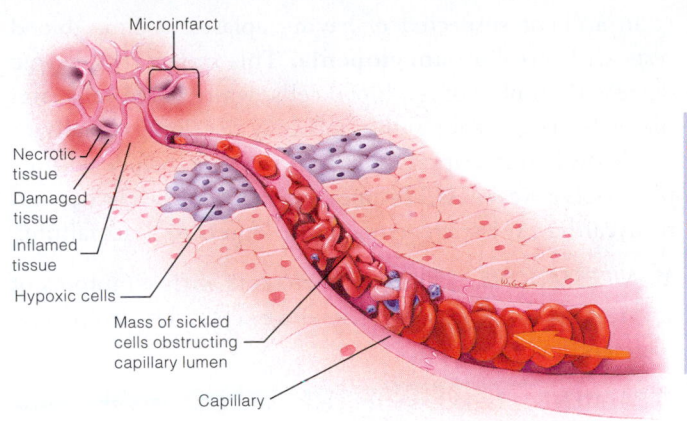

Figure 34-4. ■ Acute painful crises characterize sickle cell disease. Crises are triggered by conditions that demand high tissue oxygen or that affect cellular pH. As the crisis begins, sickled RBCs stick to capillary walls and each other, blocking blood flow and preventing oxygen from reaching tissue cells. Tissue hypoxia and accumulation of acidic metabolic waste products accelerate the process, causing further sickling and cell damage. Sickle cell crises cause microinfarcts in joints and organs that are deprived of oxygen. Repeated crises slowly destroy organs and tissues. The spleen and kidneys are especially prone to sickling damage.

TREATMENT. This disease has no specific treatment. Prevention of infection and dehydration are important goals in the care of a child with sickle cell disease, and the family must learn how to cope with the chronic disease. Encourage older children and adult clients to increase fluid intake to at least 3,000 mL/day and teach that these fluids should have no caffeine or alcohol. Encourage clients to avoid situations that could precipitate a crisis. Teach clients to avoid exposure to individuals with an illness, because any illness may precipitate a crisis in a client with sickle cell disease. Becoming chilled may also precipitate a crisis.

During a crisis, the client receives fluids, oxygen, and pain medication. The nurse supports the client on bed rest during a crisis to reduce oxygen use.

Treatment for acute chest syndrome includes antibiotic therapy, oxygen therapy, and pain medications. Some clients may receive a blood transfusion.

Treatment for sequestration crisis may include the removal of a poorly functioning or nonfunctioning spleen.

Aplastic Anemia

Aplastic anemia occurs when the bone marrow fails to produce stem cells, resulting in a lack of all types of blood cells. The bone marrow is replaced by fatty tissue. In more than 50% of the cases, there is no known cause (idiopathic) for this disorder, but cases have been linked to use of certain medications as well as paint thinner and airplane glue. It also may occur after exposure to radiation or after a severe viral infection.

BOX 34-3   **CULTURAL PULSE POINTS**

Sickle Cell Anemia

Sickle cell trait occurs in about 8 percent of the African American population. The trait occurs when a child inherits the gene from one parent. If both parents are carriers of the trait, the child has a 25% chance of inheriting the gene from both parents and is likely to develop sickle cell anemia. This is a chronic disease that is unpredictable. Genetic testing is particularly important for African American couples prior to deciding to start a family. Hispanics from Central and South America and from the Caribbean may also have the gene related to sickle cell disorder.

In a client suspected of having aplastic anemia, blood tests will reveal a **pancytopenia.** This means they have a decreased number of red blood cells, white blood cells, and platelets. The client's symptoms may develop gradually or suddenly. Manifestations of aplastic anemia include fatigue, progressive weakness, dyspnea on exertion, headache, and tachycardia. Aplastic anemia may progress to heart failure.

MANIFESTATIONS. The client presents with symptoms of severe anemia, possible bleeding episodes from low platelets, and infection.

TREATMENT. Blood, white cells, and platelets are transfused to support the client. The bone marrow may recover on its own, or it may be replaced through bone marrow transplant. Nursing care for aplastic anemia includes protecting the client from infection because of the decreased number of white blood cells. All needle sticks should be avoided because of the decreased platelet count. The nurse encourages the client to conserve energy because of the shortage of red blood cells.

POLYCYTHEMIA

Polycythemia is a disorder in which the number of red blood cells is much greater than normal. This causes the blood to be thicker than normal and it does not flow through the body as it should. When hematocrit is greater than 54%, the blood becomes more sticky. This leads to problems with stasis such as blood clots. The thicker blood is harder to pump, which increases the workload of the heart. The blood vessels dilate in an attempt to handle the thicker blood. Peripheral resistance increases in an attempt to pump the thick blood through the dilated vessels. Individuals who have chronic lung disease or smoke heavily are at risk for developing polycythemia.

Manifestations

The client may experience hypertension and possible chest pain and congestive heart failure. There may also be complaints of intense itching, which is caused by the dilation of blood vessels as well as changes in tissue oxygenation. The client complains of fatigue and may experience weight loss. Often there is enlargement of the spleen and the client is at an increased risk of stroke.

Treatment

There is no therapy that stops the increased red cell production. Treatment is aimed at reducing the number of circulating red blood cells by phlebotomy, which keeps blood volume and viscosity within normal limits. This must be done frequently (as often as five times a week). The nurse encourages clients to increase fluids and administers anticoagulants as prescribed to prevent thrombus formation.

Nursing Considerations

When you care for clients with red blood cell disorders, it is most important to focus on meeting nutritional needs and providing supportive care. Administer iron replacement as ordered for clients with iron-deficiency anemia. Instruct clients to eat foods high in iron such as lean red meats and dark green leafy vegetables. Give Imferon deep IM using Z-track to prevent staining the skin and causing necrosis in the subcutaneous tissue. Give oral liquid iron preparations with a straw to avoid staining the teeth. Also give citrus juices with iron preparations because vitamin C enhances the absorption of iron. Give vitamin B_{12} injections as ordered for clients with pernicious anemia. Clients with low red cell counts are often tired and weak. Assist with ADLs and encourage rest periods during activities. Encourage good nutrition and fluid intake (3,000 mL/24 hours) for clients with sickle cell anemia. Instruct the client to avoid caffeine and alcohol. Provide supportive care during a crisis, focusing on pain management. Administer supplemental oxygen as ordered and maintain bed rest. Clients with polycythemia must be monitored for signs of complications such as stroke, thrombus, and congestive heart failure. Provide support for phlebotomy treatments. Encourage increased fluid intake. Administer anticoagulants as ordered.

Platelet and Coagulation Disorders

HEMOSTASIS

Hemostasis is also known as blood clotting. A platelet has a life span of about 10 days. Platelets are attracted to damage in a blood vessel (Figure 34-5 ■). The platelets rush to the site and release chemicals that cause the damaged blood vessel to constrict, reducing blood flow. The platelets bind with von Willebrand's factor (a coagulation factor produced by the liver) to form a plug at the site of the injury. The plug is stabilized by fibrin. Clients with a decreased number of platelets are at risk of hemorrhaging after a slight injury.

THROMBOCYTOPENIA

Thrombocytopenia is a decrease in the platelet count to lower than 100,000/mL of blood. Thrombocytopenia may result from decreased production or increased destruction of platelets or from storage of platelets in the spleen. It is the most common cause of abnormal bleeding. Primary thrombocytopenia is most often an autoimmune disorder called *idiopathic thrombocytopenia purpura* (ITP). ITP may be either acute or chronic.

Manifestations

Petechiae and purple bruising (*purpura*) develop, especially on the chest, neck, and oral mucous membranes (see Figure 30-6). The client usually experiences bruises on the

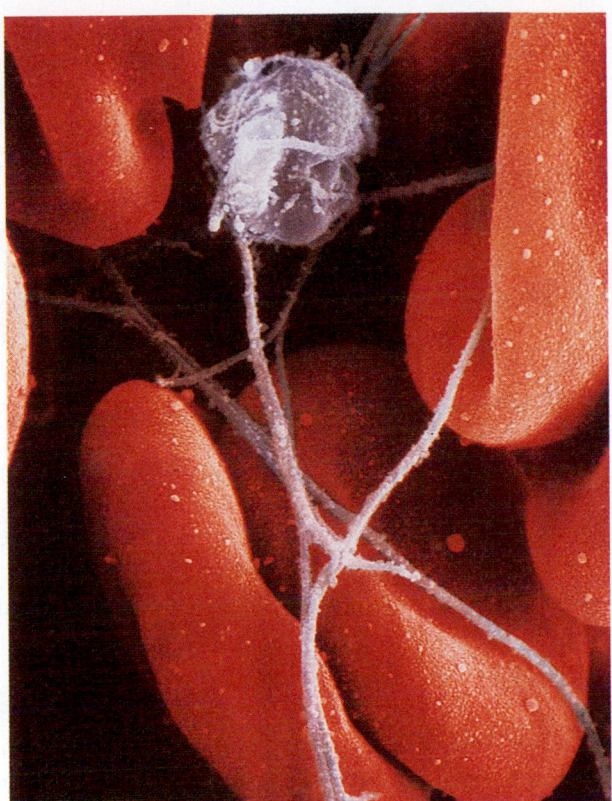

Figure 34-5. ■ Platelets are attracted to damage in a blood vessel. In this scanning electron micrograph, an RBC is trapped in a fibrin mesh. The spherical gray object at the top is a platelet. (*Source:* © Boehringer Ingelheim; photo Lennart Nilsson, Albert Bonniers Förlog AB.)

BOX 34-4	CLIENT TEACHING

Thrombocytopenia

- Client should wear medical identification stating the presence of a low platelet count (important for medical personnel in the case of an accident).
- Only use an electric razor.
- Avoid all skin or body punctures.
- Eat low-roughage foods.
- Avoid the use of all aspirin products.
- Avoid vigorous blowing of the nose.
- Only use a soft toothbrush.

legs and may have nosebleeds. The menstrual periods of women with thrombocytopenia are much heavier and longer than normal.

Treatment

Treatment involves the administration of corticosteroids and platelet transfusions if necessary. The spleen may be surgically removed if it is felt that the spleen is trapping the majority of the platelets. A bone marrow examination may also be ordered.

Secondary thrombocytopenia is caused by conditions such as aplastic anemia, leukemia, or infection. Treatment of the thrombocytopenia is supportive in nature while the primary condition is being treated. The nurse is responsible for helping to educate the client about reducing the risk of bleeding while platelet count is low (Box 34-4 ■).

DISSEMINATED INTRAVASCULAR COAGULATION

Disseminated intravascular coagulation (DIC) is an acute condition that causes widespread disruptions in clotting. It is distinguished by simultaneous bleeding and clotting. It is not considered a disease but a defect in the clotting mechanism.

It is usually precipitated by a severe illness such as sepsis (see Chapter 10 ∞). DIC causes many small clots to form. All of these clots use up all of the clotting factors, which then leads to bleeding at many sites in the body. The bleeding can be minor or excessive.

Manifestations

The clots may result in impaired blood flow to extremities or organs, resulting in tissue necrosis. Box 34-5 ■ lists manifestations of DIC.

Treatment

Treatment is aimed at restoring the clotting capabilities of the body. Platelets, clotting factors, and fresh frozen plasma are administered to the client. IV heparin may be administered if significant clots are impairing circulation. The client with DIC is at high risk for a serious hemorrhage and/or tissue necrosis from abnormal clot formation. Nursing care revolves around constant monitoring for any signs of bleeding and preventing further injury to the client. Frequent assessment of vital signs, level of consciousness, and all distal pulses is necessary. These clients should not receive IM medications or new IV punctures. The nurse encourages the client to rest quietly until clotting returns to normal. The bed should be in a Fowler's to high-Fowler's position to promote maximum chest expansion. It is important to treat

BOX 34-5	MANIFESTATIONS OF DISSEMINATED INTRAVASCULAR COAGULATION

- Cyanosis of extremities
- Dyspnea, tachypnea, bloody sputum
- Hematuria or oliguria, renal failure
- Hemorrhage from incisions
- Increased intracranial pressure
- Mental status changes, anxiety, confusion
- Oozing of blood from IV sites or punctures
- Purpura, petechiae, bruising
- Tachycardia, hypotension

the client's pain adequately, because the client may experience pain due to tissue necrosis. Reassure the client that by performing frequent assessments, further complications can be avoided.

HEMOPHILIA

Hemophilia is a chronic hereditary disease and one of the oldest hereditary diseases known. In hemophilia, the body lacks one or more clotting factors. It is usually diagnosed in childhood (Box 34-6 ■), but the effects of the disease last throughout the client's lifetime. There are four types of hemophilia:

- *Hemophilia A.* Lack of clotting factor VIII. It is the most common type of this disease. It is also known as classic hemophilia. It occurs only in males because it is a genetic defect of the X chromosome. In most cases, bleeding occurs as a result of a minor trauma. Many clients develop deformity in joints because of repeated bleeding episodes. It is treated by giving the client factor VIII replacement or a product called cryoprecipitate. Most clients learn to self-administer the replacement.
- *Hemophilia B.* Lack of clotting factor IX. It is also known as Christmas disease. It is also a defect of the X chromosome and the symptoms are the same as those in classic hemophilia. Treatment is with factor IX replacement.
- *Von Willebrand's disease.* Defective von Willebrand's factor. It occurs in both men and women. The client usually lacks sufficient factor VIII as well. The level of factor VIII can be determined by a blood test called partial thromboplastin time (PTT). Excessive bleeding only occurs after dental procedures or other surgeries. Treatment with platelets, clotting factors, and fresh frozen plasma is used during a bleeding episode.
- *Hemophilia C.* Lack of clotting factor XI. It is most commonly found in people who are Ashkenazi Jews. Bleeding episodes usually follow surgery.

BOX 34-6 PEDIATRIC CONSIDERATIONS

Child with Hemophilia

Hemophilia is usually not apparent in the newborn unless abnormal bleeding occurs at the umbilical cord or after circumcision. Circumcision, heel sticks, and intramuscular injections are delayed to prevent bleeding and tissue injury if the diagnosis is known at birth or there is a family history of hemophilia.

The disease is generally identified early in the child's life. A classic symptom of hemophilia is bleeding into the joints.

Children with hemophilia should have the knees, hips, and elbows of their clothing protected by padding their play outfits. Sport activities should be selected appropriately to avoid potential for injury. If an injury with bleeding occurs, the care includes rest, ice, compression, and elevation.

The child with hemophilia should wear a medic alert bracelet.

It is important to protect the client from injury to prevent bleeding episodes from occurring. This may be frustrating for young people who want to play sports but are prohibited because of the possibility of bleeding. The client's family must also understand the need to let all healthcare professionals know about any clotting factor deficiencies. It is crucial to report any prolonged bleeding episodes prior to dental work or other invasive procedures. All clients with any type of clotting deficiency should be instructed to avoid all aspirin products, because they increase clotting time.

Nursing Considerations

When caring for clients with coagulation disorders, focus your care on prevention of injury and hemorrhage. Assess clients frequently for bleeding from the nose, gums, vagina, and rectum. Report any oozing or active bleeding from these sites to the healthcare provider immediately. Be prepared to administer platelets if ordered. Protect the client from injury by being vigilant during turning and transfers to prevent bumps or scrapes. Do not use or allow the client to use razors other than electric razors. Dental floss may be prohibited to prevent gum bleeding. Use a soft toothbrush. For the client with DIC, protect the client from injury and be prepared to administer heparin, platelets, or both via IV. Do not give IM medications because these can cause additional bleeding.

White Blood Cell Disorders

AGRANULOCYTOSIS

Agranulocytosis is the absence of any white blood cells. It is also referred to as *neutropenia*. It is most commonly seen in conditions such as aplastic anemia or after aggressive chemotherapy. The client is at high risk for infection because there are no white cells to fight infection, especially respiratory infections. The client must be protected from any source of infection. In some cases the client is placed in an environment that is as free of infection as possible. All people who encounter the client with agranulocytosis should wear gloves and masks to protect the client from any outside infectious agents. The client will be treated with colony-stimulating factors that stimulate the production of white blood cells. An example of this is the drug filgrastim (Neupogen).

LEUKEMIA

Leukemia is a malignant disorder in which a type of white cell will begin to overproduce, usually in its immature state. It may be acute or chronic. These abnormal cells leave the bone marrow and infiltrate into other tissues such as the central nervous system, testes, skin, GI tract, lymph nodes, spleen, and liver. Figure 34-6 ■ illustrates the multisystem effects of leukemia.

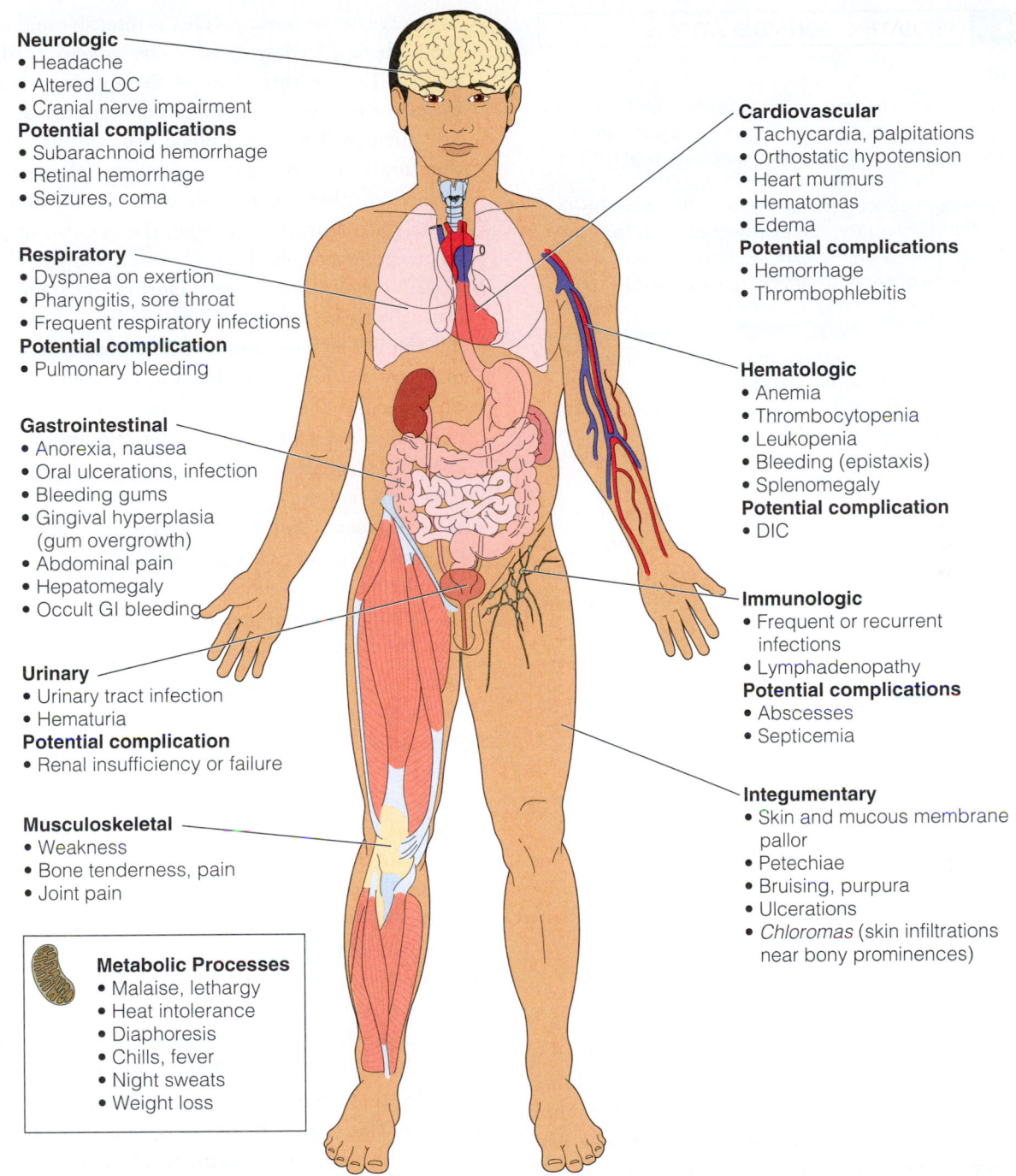

Neurologic
- Headache
- Altered LOC
- Cranial nerve impairment

Potential complications
- Subarachnoid hemorrhage
- Retinal hemorrhage
- Seizures, coma

Respiratory
- Dyspnea on exertion
- Pharyngitis, sore throat
- Frequent respiratory infections

Potential complication
- Pulmonary bleeding

Gastrointestinal
- Anorexia, nausea
- Oral ulcerations, infection
- Bleeding gums
- Gingival hyperplasia
  (gum overgrowth)
- Abdominal pain
- Hepatomegaly
- Occult GI bleeding

Urinary
- Urinary tract infection
- Hematuria

Potential complication
- Renal insufficiency or failure

Musculoskeletal
- Weakness
- Bone tenderness, pain
- Joint pain

Metabolic Processes
- Malaise, lethargy
- Heat intolerance
- Diaphoresis
- Chills, fever
- Night sweats
- Weight loss

Cardiovascular
- Tachycardia, palpitations
- Orthostatic hypotension
- Heart murmurs
- Hematomas
- Edema

Potential complications
- Hemorrhage
- Thrombophlebitis

Hematologic
- Anemia
- Thrombocytopenia
- Leukopenia
- Bleeding (epistaxis)
- Splenomegaly

Potential complication
- DIC

Immunologic
- Frequent or recurrent
  infections
- Lymphadenopathy

Potential complications
- Abscesses
- Septicemia

Integumentary
- Skin and mucous membrane
  pallor
- Petechiae
- Bruising, purpura
- Ulcerations
- *Chloromas* (skin infiltrations
  near bony prominences)

Figure 34-6. ■ Multisystem effects of leukemia.

Leukemia affects more adults than children each year and is more common in adults over age 50. Treatment may include chemotherapy, bone marrow transplant (BMT), stem cell transplant (SCT), or immunotherapy. Research into new drug treatments is opening up options for treatment. There are four different types of leukemia:

- *Acute lymphocytic (or acute lymphoblastic) leukemia (ALL).* This is the most common type of leukemia in children. Treatment is not as successful in adults as it is in children.

- *Acute myelogenous leukemia (AML).* This is the most common type of leukemia in adults. Best treatment is with BMT.

- *Chronic lymphocytic leukemia (CLL).* From 1995 to 2000, the 5-year survival rate was 76.2% (Leukemia-Lymphoma Society, 2008). Most clients live 4 to 10 years.

- *Chronic myelogenous leukemia (CML).* This is the second most common leukemia in adults. New treatments have improved the prognosis of this disease. (See more about care of the client with cancer in Chapter 45 ⬭.)

<table>
<tr><td>

BOX 34-7 PEDIATRIC CONSIDERATIONS

Leukemia

- In children, the most common symptoms of leukemia are low-grade fever, pallor, bruising, leg and joint pain, listlessness, abdominal pain, and enlargement of lymph nodes.
- The treatment of cancer in children is challenging because irradiation, surgery, and chemotherapy often have adverse effects on growth and development.
- The appearance of secondary sex characteristics and menstruation may be delayed in the pubescent client as the result of chemotherapy.
- Chemotherapy can cause bone marrow suppression and families must be taught about infection prevention. Chickenpox can be life threatening to a child who is immunosuppressed.

</td></tr>
</table>

Proliferation of abnormal cells begins in the bone marrow. These abnormal cells then travel to different organs in the body. The excessive white cell production reduces the amount of space available for production of red cells and platelets. The client is anemic and *thrombocytopenic* (lacking normal number of platelets), with excessive numbers of immature white blood cells.

Manifestations

The client generally goes to the physician complaining of fever, fatigue, and bruising. The client often displays petechiae (see Figure 30-6 ∞) on the lower extremities. Pediatric considerations are discussed in Box 34-7 ■.

Diagnosis

Laboratory tests that may be ordered include CBC with WBC differential and platelet count. Leukemia is diagnosed by inspecting the white blood cells for number and maturity. A bone marrow aspiration and biopsy are also performed. In this test the outer aspect of the iliac crest is used. The skin is numbed and a large trocar needle is pushed into the bone. The physician aspirates some bone marrow or actually grabs a piece of bone marrow for examination. At the completion of the test the nurse should hold pressure on the wound for approximately 5 minutes, especially if the client's platelet count is low. This test determines the type of leukemia. The fever is because the immature white blood cells do not adequately protect against infection. The fatigue reflects the anemia, and the bruising and petechiae confirm the thrombocytopenia.

Treatment

All types of leukemia are treated with chemotherapy, though the specific chemotherapeutic drugs are dependent on the type of leukemia being treated. In the acute forms of the disease, treatment is divided into three stages.

- *Stage 1: induction therapy.* This is intensive and aggressive chemotherapy to destroy all of the leukemic cells that are present. During this phase of therapy, it is common for the client to experience severe bone marrow suppression. The client will need red blood cell and platelet transfusions until the bone marrow recovers. Colony-stimulating factors are given to stimulate the production of white blood cells. During this stage, the client is at great risk for infection and bleeding.
- *Stage 2: consolidation therapy.* During this stage, the client is usually treated with the same medications as during induction but at lower dosages. The goal of this stage is to maintain the remission that was attained during induction therapy. The client continues to be at risk for infection and bleeding especially after a round of chemotherapy. This stage may last for 1 to 2 years depending on the treatment regime.
- *Stage 3: maintenance therapy.* This is a milder form of chemotherapy that is used for months to years after the completion of consolidation therapy. The goal is to continue with the remission while weaning the client away from the chemotherapy.

Chemotherapy has many side effects. Most clients develop alopecia (loss of hair), as the chemotherapy attacks all immature cells. Nausea and vomiting are also very common side effects of chemotherapy, though new drugs for nausea have helped to decrease this side effect somewhat. Mouth ulcers and bleeding from the gums, diarrhea, hematuria, and impaired peripheral nerves are not uncommon problems for clients on chemotherapy.

Bone marrow transplant is a very aggressive treatment that replaces the client's diseased bone marrow with the client's own stem cells or with another person's bone marrow. Prior to the transplant, the client is hospitalized and given chemotherapy in an attempt to destroy all of the client's own bone marrow. The client may also receive total body irradiation to remove all malignant cells from the body. The stem cells or transplanted bone marrow is given to the client in the same way as a blood transfusion is given. It will take 2 to 4 weeks for the new bone marrow to engraft into the client's body and begin producing new blood cells. The client is kept in protective isolation until the client can protect himself or herself against infection. A very serious complication of a bone marrow transplant is **graft versus host disease.** In this reaction, the client's own body attacks itself, especially the liver, the skin, and the gastrointestinal tract. Approximately one-quarter to one-half of all BMT clients will develop some symptoms of this disease. To attempt to prevent this complication, the client will take antirejection medications to prevent the body from rejecting the foreign matter. The client will need to take these medications for the rest of his or her life.

If treatment for leukemia is not successful, this disease is fatal. The client usually develops a severe infection or bleeding episode that cannot be reversed.

MULTIPLE MYELOMA

Multiple myeloma is a malignancy of the plasma cells. It is very uncommon in anyone younger than 40 to 50 years of age, and it affects African Americans twice as often as other races. Multiple myeloma is different from leukemia in that, as it develops, the plasma cells multiply uncontrollably and move from the bone marrow into the bone itself, instead of into the circulatory system. As the tumor grows the bone becomes very brittle. The bones may break without any trauma. The disease develops slowly.

Manifestations

The client complains of vague back, pelvis, rib, or bone pain. As the disease progresses, the most common fractures are of the vertebrae, pelvis, and femur.

Diagnosis

On x-ray, the bones look like there are many little punched out holes. A bone marrow biopsy shows too many immature plasma cells. As the disease progresses, the client develops hypercalcemia (see Chapter 25 🔗), because the tumor is pushing the calcium from the bone into the circulatory system. This disease appears to progress slowly, taking many years to run its course. There is no known cure.

Treatment

Treatment consists of medications to boost the body's own immunity combined with chemotherapy to decrease the number of malignant cells. Radiation therapy is often used to treat individual bones. Most clients with multiple myeloma must deal with chronic pain. The nurse must assess the client for any side effects of chemotherapy and also treat the client's pain. It is important for the nurse to work with the client to discover nonpharmacologic means to ease the pain because the client will most likely experience pain during the entire course of the disease. The client is also at increased risk for injury because of brittle bones. The nurse helps the client understand that extra care must be taken to prevent fractures.

Nursing Considerations

When caring for clients with white blood cell disorders, your biggest priorities are to protect them from infection and provide supportive care. Protective precautions may be necessary: Masks and gloves are worn to prevent bringing a potential infection to the client. Clients with leukemia will also have decreased platelets, so precautions for bleeding and infection are used. Take vital signs every 4 hours to detect signs of infection early. Monitor for any open or reddened areas and report them to the healthcare provider immediately to prevent infection. Clients with multiple myeloma not only need protection from infection, but also protection from injury since the bones break very easily. Handle the client with extreme care when turning, and support the client's position with additional pillows. Also, assist with transferring. Provide supportive care for clients with leukemia and multiple myeloma who are undergoing chemotherapy.

LYMPHATIC SYSTEM

Lymphatic System Disorders

The lymphatic system circulates lymph through the body (Figure 34-7 ■). **Lymph** is a fluid that resembles plasma but has less protein. It is the fluid that leaks out of the capillaries into the interstitial tissue but does not return to the venous system. This fluid instead enters the lymphatic system. The lymph nodes, spleen, thymus gland, tonsils, and tissue present in the bone marrow comprise the lymphatic system. Lymph nodes occurring along the lymphatic pathways are used to filter the lymph. Lymph nodes become enlarged (**lymphadenopathy**) due to inflammation, infection, or malignancy. In the case of malignancy, it may indicate a malignancy in the area draining into that lymph node or it may indicate malignancy of the lymph system itself. When assessing the lymph nodes, note the size and density of the node. Also note if there is any tenderness, redness, or warmth to the lymph node.

LYMPHANGITIS

Lymphangitis is an inflammation of a lymphatic vessel. It is usually caused by a bacterial infection. The client will exhibit a red streak along the course of the inflamed lymphatic vessel. The client will complain of pain and chills, and an elevated temperature is possible. The client should rest and elevate the extremity and apply heat. The aim of treatment is to resolve the problem that is causing the lymphangitis. Lymphadenitis is when the lymph nodes become inflamed. The client's complaints are similar to those of lymphangitis.

LYMPHEDEMA

Lymphedema is the inability of the lymph system to remove all the lymph fluid from the interstitial tissues. It may occur because of obstruction, inflammation, or surgical removal of lymph nodes. Lymphedema is usually chronic.

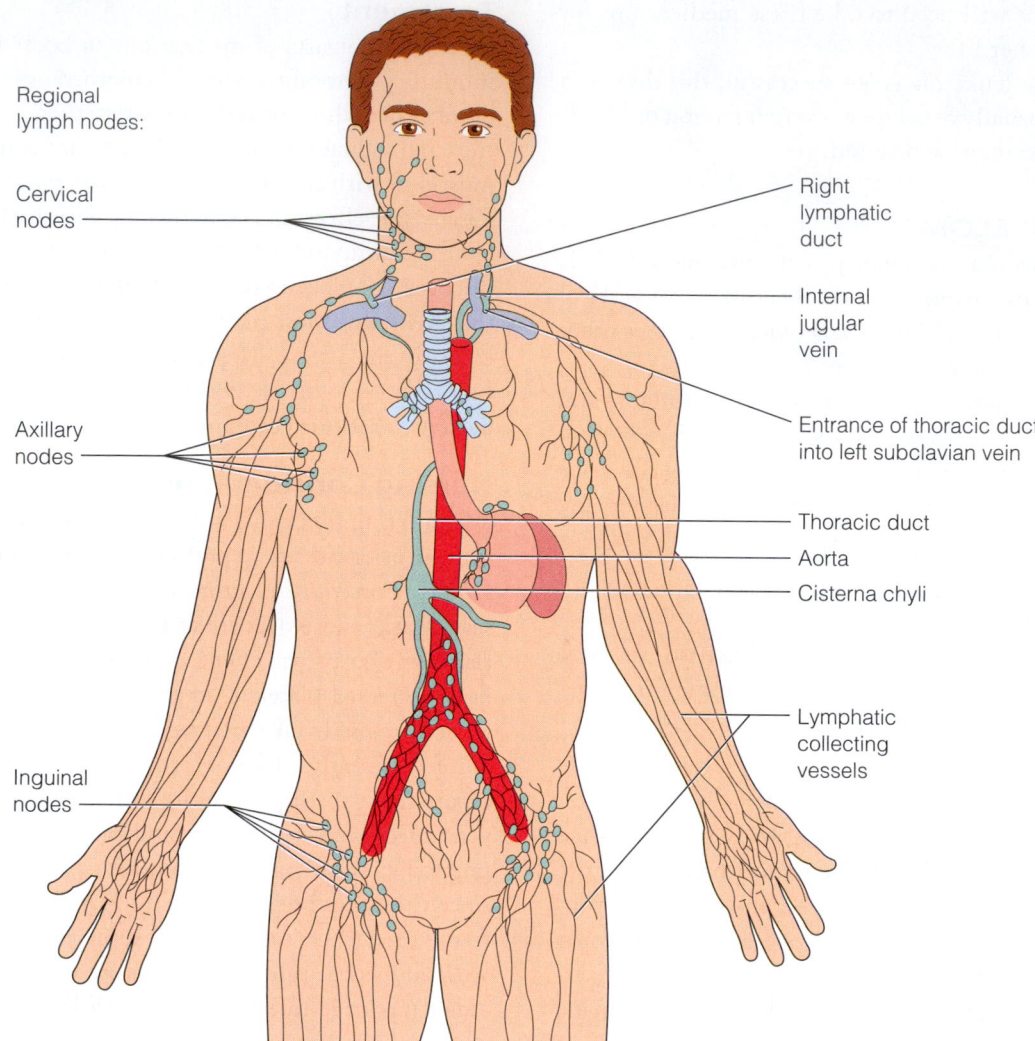

Regional lymph nodes:

Cervical nodes

Axillary nodes

Inguinal nodes

Right lymphatic duct

Internal jugular vein

Entrance of thoracic duct into left subclavian vein

Thoracic duct

Aorta

Cisterna chyli

Lymphatic collecting vessels

Figure 34-7. ■ The lymphatic system.

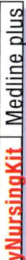

Manifestations

The skin of the edematous tissue changes the longer the edema is present. It becomes hard and tough and the limb resembles a piece of wood (Figure 34-8 ■). The edema in the affected extremity can worsen in warm weather or after standing for long periods of time.

Diagnosis

Lymphedema is diagnosed with ultrasound, CT scans, and MRI. A test using contrast material in the lymphatic system (lymphangiography) may be used to visualize the lymphatic system. This may prove helpful if obstruction of the lymphatic vessel is suspected.

Treatment

Treatment is aimed at resolving the reason for the lymphedema. In many cases, especially those in which a part of the lymph system has been surgically removed, resolving the edema is exceptionally challenging. The client is instructed to keep the limb elevated to allow gravity to assist with

lymphatic drainage. Compression garments are used to force fluid back toward the heart. The client is advised to be very careful with the skin of the affected extremity to prevent injury, and meticulous skin care is essential. It is helpful to apply emollient creams to help soften the skin.

clinical ALERT

It is important to avoid any needle sticks in the affected extremity of someone with lymphedema. This may become a focus for infection. Venipunctures are also avoided because the tourniquet needed to expand the vein may damage the tissue. The nurse should place a sign above the bed of a client with lymphedema to alert other staff to avoid using the affected extremity. Blood pressures should be avoided on an extremity with lymphedema or an at risk extremity, because the squeezing can cause further damage to fragile lymphatics and blood vessels. The lymphedema could worsen with doing this procedure. There is also the possibility of an inaccurate blood pressure reading due to an inappropriate size blood pressure cuff for the size of the extremity.

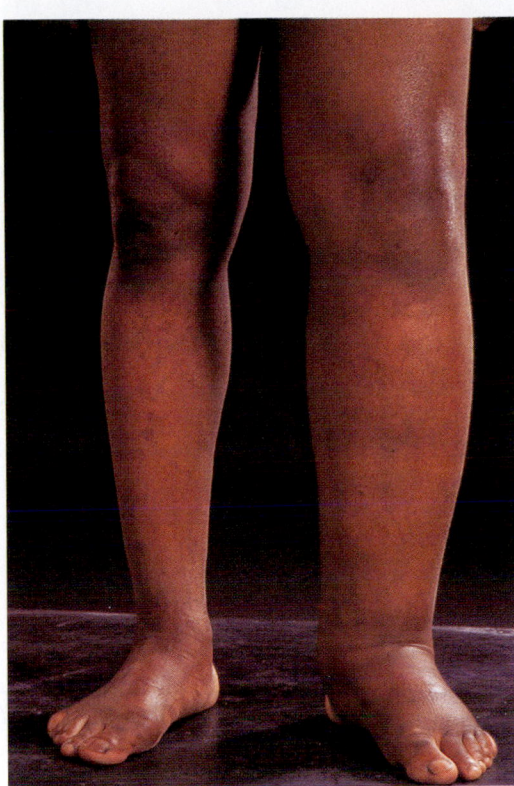

Figure 34-8. ■ Severe lymphedema of the lower extremities.

disease is unknown, but it may be linked to the Epstein-Barr virus. Hodgkin's disease begins in a single lymph node with progressive enlargement and spreads to the entire lymph chain. It may metastasize to the spleen, liver, bone marrow, lungs, or other parts of the body.

MANIFESTATIONS.   The client presents with nontender, enlarged lymph nodes. The nodes are firm but movable. The client may also report fever, fatigue, weight loss, and night sweats.

DIAGNOSIS.   The disease is diagnosed by a biopsy of one of the affected lymph nodes or tissue mass. The diagnosis of Hodgkin's is confirmed if Reed-Sternberg cells are present in the tissue. After Hodgkin's disease has been diagnosed, staging must be determined. The Ann Arbor staging system ascertains the extent of the disease. The classification of staging is from Stage I to IV. The system uses the number and location of involved nodes and client symptoms. The most serious is Stage IV, indicating the disease has metastasized to one or more organs or tissues. The prognosis for Hodgkin's disease depends on the disease's staging at time of diagnosis.

TREATMENT.   Malignant lymphoma is treated with chemotherapy and radiation to the affected nodes.

Non-Hodgkin's Lymphoma

Non-Hodgkin's lymphoma is actually a group of lymphatic malignancies. It is more common than Hodgkin's and does not microscopically look like Hodgkin's disease. It tends to occur in older adults. The prognosis depends on the type of non-Hodgkin's lymphoma that is diagnosed.

MANIFESTATION.   The symptoms are very similar to Hodgkin's disease. There are usually multiple lymph nodes and lymphoid tissue involved.

DIAGNOSIS.   Just as in Hodgkin's disease, non-Hodgkin's is diagnosed with a lymph node biopsy.

TREATMENT.   Treatment with chemotherapy and radiation is similar to that for Hodgkin's. In both types of malignant lymphoma, the physician must first determine the stage of the client's disease. Usually the outcome of non-Hodgkin's lymphoma is not as good as that of Hodgkin's. The extent of treatment is determined by the disease stage.

The client will experience the side effects common to chemotherapy (see Figure 45-8 🔗). The client must also have detailed instructions concerning care of the skin during radiation. The skin in the treated area may be sensitive and must be protected against exposure to sunlight and irritation. The client is instructed not to remove the purple

INFECTIOUS MONONUCLEOSIS

Infectious mononucleosis is a viral infection of the lymph tissue of the nose and throat with the Epstein-Barr virus. The illness is transmitted by droplets in saliva, coughs, sneezes, and direct contact with mucous membranes. The infection is usually benign and self-limiting. The client usually experiences fever, sore throat, cervical lymphadenopathy, and profound fatigue. Enlargement of the liver and spleen may occur. There is no specific treatment for this disease. The symptoms are treated in an effort to make the client more comfortable. The client is encouraged to rest, although the client will most likely feel some degree of fatigue for 1 to 3 months. They should not share eating utensils. If the liver and spleen are enlarged, the client should avoid all vigorous activity until the swelling in the liver and spleen has resolved.

MALIGNANT LYMPHOMA

Malignant lymphoma is a cancerous tumor of lymphoid tissue. There are two types of malignant lymphoma: Hodgkin's disease and non-Hodgkin's lymphoma.

Hodgkin's Disease

Hodgkin's disease occurs most frequently in the late teens and early adulthood and after the age of 50. It is the most curable of all cancers if caught early. The cause of Hodgkin's markings and not to use any creams or ointments on the affected skin unless instructed by the physician. The skin should not be scrubbed during bathing, and no powders should be placed on the affected skin. These measures will prevent further damage to skin affected by radiation treatments. In the client with non-Hodgkin's lymphoma, the disease may become chronic, and the client will need repeated courses of treatment. (See Chapter 45 ⚭ for care of the client with cancer.)

NURSING CONSIDERATIONS. When you care for clients with lymphatic disorders, focus your care on preventing infection and reducing edema. Avoid needle sticks or taking blood pressures in an extremity affected by lymphedema, which is often a complication after surgery to remove lymph nodes. Elevate the affected extremity and apply compression garments as ordered. Provide supportive care for clients with infectious mononucleosis and encourage rest until the liver and spleen have returned to normal size. Assist the client with Hodgkin's or non-Hodgkin's lymphoma through chemotherapy and radiation therapy. Provide nutritional support and skin care. Avoid using creams, lotions, or powders on the skin marked for radiation treatments. Assess the skin frequently for signs of redness or breakdown.

NURSING CARE

PRIORITIZING NURSING CARE

For clients with hematologic or lymphatic disorders, nursing care focuses on protecting the skin and preventing infection. Procedures should be organized together, to allow longer periods of rest. Laboratory tests should be reviewed regularly.

ASSESSING

A thorough assessment of the client with hematologic and lymphatic disorders begins with a detailed history of the client's past medical problems. It is also helpful to determine if any family members have experienced any type of bleeding disorder. The client should be questioned closely concerning prescription and nonprescription medications taken in the past and currently. Question the client about any herbal supplements being used. Bleeding disorders may be aggravated by the use of aspirin and certain herbal supplements. After obtaining a health history, ask the client about the symptoms that brought the client to the physician. Determine when the symptoms began and what appears to make them worse. The nurse should then proceed with a physical assessment. Begin by weighing the client and determining whether there has been any recent weight

loss or gain. Vital signs are an important part of the assessment. Temperature will point to infection and a possible abnormal white blood cell count. The pulse, if elevated, may indicate anemia as the heart beats faster in an attempt to deliver enough oxygenated blood to the body tissues. An elevated respiratory rate and a lowered blood pressure may also indicate anemia as well as infection.

A careful inspection of the skin may reveal pallor, indicating anemia, as well as petechiae and bruising, which indicate thrombocytopenia. The skin should also be inspected for any sign of edema. In lymphatic disorders the skin is tough and rough so it is important also to palpate the skin and see if there is any pitting edema. It is important to palpate for lymph node enlargement, which can occur with infections or malignancies. The abdomen should be inspected for any distention and palpated to detect any increase in size in the liver or spleen.

DIAGNOSING, PLANNING, AND IMPLEMENTING

Some common nursing diagnoses for clients with hematologic or lymphatic disorders are:

- *Risk for Infection*
- *Risk for Injury*
- *Fatigue*

General outcomes for these clients would include:

- Client will maintain adequate immune status.
- Client's coagulation status will be within normal limits.
- Client will experience increased endurance and activity tolerance.

Nursing interventions for clients with hematologic and lymphatic disorders center on the client's fatigue and the need to prevent infection and bleeding. For clients with hematologic or lymphatic disorders, the following interventions apply:

- Organize nursing care to allow the client extended periods of rest. Encourage the client to engage in quiet activities such as reading, watching TV, or listening to music. *This will help the fatigued client.*
- Be meticulous in hand washing. Teach clients and visitors to wash their hands frequently. No one should be in contact with the client who has any signs of infection, and protective equipment should be used (masks, gowns, and gloves) if the client's white blood cell count is extremely low. The client who is at risk for bleeding should be handled very gently during nursing care, especially bathing. *These measures help to prevent infection and bleeding.*
- Check the skin frequently, especially the lower extremities. *The client is also at risk for infections in the tissues. The blood does not adequately deliver nutrients and oxygen to tissue with lymphatic disorders.*

- Turn the client often to keep pressure off the edematous skin. *Clients with lymphatic disorders are at a high risk for impaired skin integrity. Frequent turning will help to prevent skin breakdown.*
- Encourage parents to remain with a child who is receiving a blood transfusion. *The procedure may be frightening for the child, and the presence of a parent will reduce anxiety.*

Assisting Clients Receiving Transfusions

Administration of blood transfusions, like administration of IV medications, requires training and certification that is not part of the core LPN and LVN training in most states. Practical and vocational nurses are expected to obtain such certification early in their careers. Some nursing considerations for blood transfusions are described here.

The unit of blood product is checked to be sure it is the correct one for the specific client. It is the nurse's responsibility to check the unit of blood against the specific client for whom it is ordered. In most institutions, the nurse must check and then verify this information with another professional before administration. A large-gauge IV device is used for blood product administration. The large gauge helps to prevent damage to the blood cells as they travel through the tubing and into the client. Only normal saline solution should be given with blood. The IV site is frequently checked for infiltration. The client is also observed for transfusion reactions, which include itching, chills, rash, fever, and back pain. Circulatory overload is a danger with children. Always use an infusion pump to regulate blood flow.

Once the blood product administration has begun, the nurse must check vital signs frequently to determine if the client is developing a hypersensitivity reaction to the blood product.

clinical ALERT

Hypersensitivity reactions occur when substances in the transfused blood product interact with antibodies in the client's blood. The more blood product transfusions a client has received, the greater the chance of developing a hypersensitivity reaction. The client may complain of itching and hives. If blood is administered that is not the same type as the client's, the client will develop a serious and possibly fatal complication called a *hemolytic reaction*. The client may complain of headache, nausea, flushing, and chest pain. If the client develops any reaction during the transfusion, the transfusion is discontinued immediately and the vein is kept open with normal saline. The nurse then notifies the physician. The blood product unit is returned to the blood bank for testing. The nurse continues to monitor the client's vital signs until they return to normal.

EVALUATING

The nurse collects data for frequent assessment of the client with these disorders to see if treatment is effective. The goal of treatment for clients with hematologic disorders is a return to normal levels of the blood counts. The client's level of energy will return to normal, and the client will be free of infection and bleeding episodes. The client with lymphatic disorders will be free of infection and edema.

NURSING PROCESS CARE PLAN
Client with Iron-Deficiency Anemia

Kay Ford is a 37-year-old woman who has come to the physician because she has no energy. This lack of energy has not begun suddenly but has become worse in the last few weeks. She works as a secretary in a busy law office and lately has had difficulty keeping up with duties she regularly performs. She also reports that she feels "winded" when she walks up the stairs at work. She takes no medications, but does report that she became a vegetarian about 3 months ago. She started a vegetarian diet because she felt it was healthier and she has been anxious to improve her overall health status. That is why she is distressed that her energy level has decreased significantly. She has regular menstrual periods, but she reports that they are consistently heavy and last approximately 7 days.

Assessment

Vital signs: T 98.4, P 112, R 24, BP 98/60. Complete blood count: Hgb 9.1; Hct 30%; WBC 5,900; platelets 400,000; iron level: low; stool is negative for occult blood. The client's skin is pale. Her conjunctiva, mucous membranes, and nail beds are also lacking in color. She states she has a headache and rates her pain as a 3 on a scale of 1 to 10. She denies having any nausea or vomiting. Her only other complaint is that she feels that she has been forgetful lately.

Nursing Diagnosis

The following important nursing diagnoses (among others) are established for this condition:

- *Fatigue* related to anemia
- *Risk for Impaired Gas Exchange* related to low red cell count
- *Risk for Injury* related to weakness

Expected Outcomes

The following expected outcomes are developed for Ms. Ford:

- Will be able to perform usual daily activities with minimal fatigue.
- Memory level will be at level that is normal for the client.
- Will report no pain.

Planning and Implementation

The following nursing interventions are planned and implemented for Ms. Ford:

- Encourage Ms. Ford to rest at regular intervals.
- Instruct Ms. Ford on sources of iron in diet.
- Explain relationship of vegetarian diet to increase in iron deficiency.
- Instruct Ms. Ford to rise from a sitting position carefully to prevent orthostatic hypotension.
- Explain importance of taking medications, especially iron (Fe), as ordered.
- Instruct Ms. Ford that bowel movements will be dark and tarry.
- Encourage Ms. Ford to increase fluid intake.

Evaluation

Ms. Ford begins to take Fe on a daily basis. In approximately 2 weeks the client reports that she is less fatigued and her memory is improving. After nutritional counseling, she has decided to modify her strict vegetarian diet and eat red meat until the anemia is under control. She reports she no longer has a headache.

Critical Thinking in the Nursing Process

1. How could Ms. Ford modify her work environment to allow her to conserve her energy?
2. Develop a diet plan for Ms. Ford to maximize her intake of iron from food sources.
3. What information would you give Ms. Ford to minimize side effects of an iron supplement?

Note: Discussion of Critical Thinking questions appears on the MyNursingKit Website.

Note: The references and resources for all chapters have been compiled at the back of the book.

Chapter Review

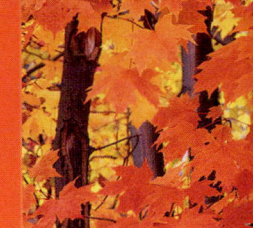

KEY Points

- Anemia may develop over an extended period of time. The client may not be aware of the symptoms until they are significant.
- Clients with white blood cell deficiencies are always at risk for infection. All healthcare personnel should practice meticulous hand washing.
- Clients with clotting disorders must be protected from even the possibility of injury because a minor injury could cause a potentially fatal hemorrhage.
- Most clients with bone marrow and lymphatic system cancers treated with chemotherapy will develop some degree of bone marrow suppression.
- Blood product transfusions require vigilant nursing attention.
- Leukemia is a cancer of the white blood cells and the bone marrow is almost totally filled with leukemic cells. They multiple rapidly but do not function like normal WBCs.
- Multiple myeloma is a malignancy of plasma. The cells replace the bone marrow and infiltrate the bone itself.
- Hodgkin's disease involves one or more lymph nodes. It occurs more often in the younger population. It progresses in an orderly way. Hodgkin's disease will present with systemic symptoms at the time of diagnosis but not at a late stage. Itching or pruritus is often one of the manifestations of Hodgkin's disease and is the result of release of histamines. Some relief can be gained by using cooling baths, mild detergents for bed linens, lightweight cotton blankets and clothing, and systemic and topical medications.

- Non-Hodgkin's involves multiple lymph nodes and lymphoid tissue in other body tissues. It occurs more often in the older population and is more common than Hodgkin's disease. It is less predictable in its course than Hodgkin's disease. It usually will not present with systemic symptoms at time of diagnosis and will likely present at a later stage. If itching results, it is due to abnormalities in the immune system. The treatment for relief of itching is the same as for Hodgkin's disease.

FOR FURTHER Study

Sepsis is discussed in more detail in Chapter 10.

For more information on hypercalcemia, see Chapter 26.

See Chapter 27 for information on Z-track injection.

Petechiae and purple bruising (purpura) are illustrated in Chapter 30.

For additional information about the client with cancer and side effects common to chemotherapy, see Chapter 45.

EXPLORE PEARSON **mynursingkit**™

MyNursingKit is your one stop for online chapter review materials and resources. Prepare for success with additional NCLEX®-style practice questions, interactive assignments and activities, web links, animations and videos, and more!

Register your access code from the front of your book at **www.mynursingkit.com**

Critical Thinking Care Map

Caring for a Client with Thrombocytopenia

NCLEX-PN® Focus Area: Physiologic Integrity

Case Study: Lilly Fantor, age 28, has gone to the physician because of a sudden onset of large bruises. She has multiple areas of purpura as well as petechiae on both legs and torso. The physician suspects idiopathic thrombocytopenic purpura and admits Ms. Fantor to the hospital. She states, "I feel OK, I don't know what all the fuss is about. Am I really that sick?"

Nursing Diagnosis: *Impaired Tissue Integrity*

COLLECT DATA

Subjective	Objective
_____	_____
_____	_____
_____	_____
_____	_____
_____	_____
_____	_____
_____	_____

Would you report this? Yes/No

If yes, report to: _____

What would you report? _____

Nursing Care

_____
_____
_____
_____
_____
_____
_____
_____
_____
_____

How would you document this? _____
_____
_____
_____

Compare your answers and documentation to those provided on the MyNursingKit Website.

Data Collected
(use only those that apply)

- Works as a nanny.
- VS: T 99, P 90, R 16.
- Multiple bruises.
- Hgb 10.3.
- WBC 7,500.
- Platelets 45,000.
- Appears anxious.
- No complaints of pain.
- On high-protein diet.
- Petechiae on legs.
- Has three dogs.
- Works out regularly.

Nursing Interventions
(use only those that apply; list in priority order)

- Use soft toothbrush.
- Give PO meds only.
- No chips or popcorn.
- Use electric razor.
- Wear shoes when walking.
- Apply ice to purpura.
- Avoid IM injections.
- Test stool for blood.
- Bed rest.
- Eat leafy, green veggies.
- Do not drink hot beverages.
- Whisper only.

NCLEX-PN® Exam Preparation

1 When assessing the client's white blood cell count with differential, the nurse anticipates the greatest number of white cells will be:

1. Basophils.
2. Eosinophils.
3. Neutrophils.
4. Monocytes.

2 The nurse is providing dietary teaching for a client diagnosed with anemia requiring increased iron intake. The nurse recognizes the need for further teaching when the client mistakenly identifies which of the following as containing large amounts of iron?

1. Kidneys
2. Shrimp
3. T-bone steak
4. Egg yolks

3 When caring for a 31-year-old client diagnosed with sickle cell anemia, the nurse identifies which of the following as essential client teaching to reduce the risk of sickle cell crisis?

1. Always keep the room temperature below 70 degrees.
2. Eat red meat every day.
3. Never get a flu shot.
4. Drink 3,000 mL of fluid every day.

4 When caring for a client diagnosed with hemophilia A, the nurse instructs the client to avoid which of the following in order to avoid bleeding episodes?

1. Loose cords and wires on the floor
2. Singing in the church choir
3. Getting out of the car without assistance
4. Weeding the garden

5 Which nursing diagnosis would have the highest priority for a client with a WBC of 1,000?

1. *Risk for Injury*
2. *Fatigue*
3. *Risk for Infection*
4. *Risk for Bleeding*

6 The nurse is caring for a client with a hemoglobin of 14.5 g/dL and a hematocrit of 53%. The nurse recognizes these lab results could indicate the client is:

1. Anemic.
2. At risk for infection.
3. Dehydrated.
4. At risk for bleeding.

7 The nurse is caring for a client with type A+ blood. Which of the following blood types would be appropriate to administer to this client in an emergency?

1. AB+
2. B+
3. A−
4. O+

8 The nurse takes precautions to reduce the risk of lymphedema for which of the following clients?

1. A woman who had a modified radical mastectomy for breast cancer
2. A man who had surgery to repair a fractured femur
3. A client diagnosed with diabetes mellitus
4. A client diagnosed with prostate cancer

9 The nurse is caring for a client with a medical diagnosis of Hodgkin's disease who is complaining of pruritus. Which of the following would be appropriate nursing actions? (Select all that apply.)

1. Giving cooling baths
2. Washing clothing and linen in mild detergents
3. Advising the client to buy wool and polyester clothing
4. Avoiding the use of blankets and comforters
5. Giving frequent hot baths

10 Prior to administering a blood product, an essential nursing action is to:

1. Reassure the client that it will only take a few minutes to receive the blood and there is little risk of complications or problems.
2. Start a small-gauge IV (24-gauge) ideally in a hand vein.
3. Verify the client's identification and the number of the unit of blood product with another licensed professional.
4. Maintain the client in high-Fowler's position until the blood infusion is completed and the tubing is flushed with normal saline.

Answers and rationales for Review Questions appear in Appendix I.

Chapter 35

Caring for Clients with Immune System Disorders

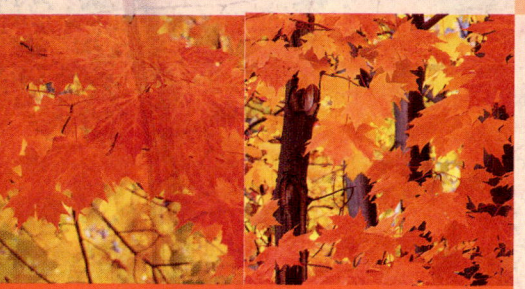

BRIEF Outline

Structure and Function of the Immune System
Major Immune System Disorders
Organ Transplantation
Autoimmune Disorders
Allergies

LEARNING Outcomes

After completing this chapter, you will be able to:

1. Discuss the components of the immune system and their function.
2. Discuss the relationship between antigens and antibodies.
3. Differentiate between active immunity and passive immunity.
4. List factors that affect immunity and tests used to determine the status of the immune system.
5. Identify types of immunizations and nursing considerations when providing them.
6. Describe anaphylaxis, its treatment, and nursing care of a client with anaphylactic shock.
7. Discuss the care of clients with HIV/AIDS.
8. Identify important aspects of care for clients with organ transplantation.
9. Discuss the care of clients with autoimmune disorders.
10. List the manifestations of the four levels of hypersensitivity reaction and discuss treatment and nursing considerations for clients with allergies.

Clinical Objectives

11. Provide care for a client in protective isolation.
12. Provide emergency treatment for a client experiencing a hypersensitivity reaction.
13. Observe a client undergoing allergy testing.
14. Provide teaching for a client with an autoimmune disorder, including the need for rest, self-care, and monitoring signs of a flare-up.

KEY TERMS

Use the audio glossary feature on the MyNursingKit Website to hear the correct pronunciation of the following key terms.

acquired immune deficiency syndrome (AIDS) 915

active immunity 910

allograft 921

anaphylaxis 914

antibodies 909

antigen 907

attenuated 912

autograft 921

autoimmune disease 907

autoimmune disorders 922

autologous 917

calcinosis 926

granulocytes 907

histocompatibility 921

human immunodeficiency virus (HIV) 915

human leukocyte antigens 910

humoral 907

immunotropic 915

indicator diseases 918

isograft 921

leukocytosis 907

leukopenia 907

lymphocytes 907

monocytes 907

neurotropic 915

passive immunity 911

ptosis 924

Raynaud's phenomenon 926

retrovirus 915

rheumatologist 925

sclerodactyly 926

scleroderma 925

seroconversion 915

seropositive 918

telangiectasis 926

thymoma 924

tissue typing 921

toxoid 913

vaccines 912

xenograft 921

The immune system is the body's protective force. Bacteria, viruses, fungi, and parasites are continually attempting to invade the body's structure either through the skin or through mucous membranes. Abnormal cells assault the body and cause illness or tumors.

The immune system prevents most foreign substances from entering the body. If access is gained, the immune system terminates the invaders. In some instances, the body perceives a portion of itself as foreign and responds accordingly. This is called **autoimmune disease**. When *antigens* (foreign substances) invade the body, they produce an immune system reaction.

The immune system is organized in an efficient manner, with protective forces constantly watching over the body. The components of the immune system include cells and organs involved in nonspecific immunity, specific immunity, or a combination of both.

Structure and Function of the Immune System

CELLS OF THE IMMUNE SYSTEM

Leukocytes (white blood cells or WBCs) are the main components of nonspecific and specific immune responses. Leukocytes begin as stem cells from the bone marrow and circulate in the blood throughout the body where they detect and destroy foreign substances (Figure 35-1 ■). (Normal laboratory blood values are provided in Table 34-1 ⊙⊙.) When an infection occurs, increased WBCs are released from the bone marrow to assist in the fight against the infection. **Leukocytosis** is the term for elevated WBCs. **Leukopenia** is the term that describes insufficient WBCs.

The three major groups of WBCs are granulocytes, monocytes, and lymphocytes.

Granulocytes are involved in the inflammatory response. They make up the largest number of normal blood leukocytes. **Monocytes** are also involved in the inflammatory response; they are the largest in size. Monocytes mature into *macrophages*, trapping and consuming foreign substances through the process known as *phagocytosis* (Figure 35-2 ■).

Lymphocytes (Figure 35-3 ■) are found in the blood and lymph and are involved in the immune capability of the body. They are divided into B-cell lymphocytes, T-cell lymphocytes, and natural killer (NK) cells.

B-Cell Lymphocytes

B-cell lymphocytes are responsible for *antibody-mediated immunity* or **humoral** immunity (meaning immunity occurring in the plasma). Figure 35-4 ■ illustrates antibody-mediated immunity. B-cell lymphocytes are involved in antibody production. B cells mature in the bone marrow and recognize the foreign **antigen** (substance that induces sensitivity or immune response). They are stimulated by helper T cells to produce and differentiate. Some B cells produce antibodies against a foreign antigen. Other B cells have memory; they recall an antigen and induce a quick response.

T-Cell Lymphocytes

T-cell lymphocytes involve *cell-mediated immunity* (specific responses). Figure 35-5 ■ illustrates a cell-mediated response. They start their journey as immature cells from the spleen, lymph nodes, and bone marrow. They take a path to the thymus gland, where reaction with the hormone

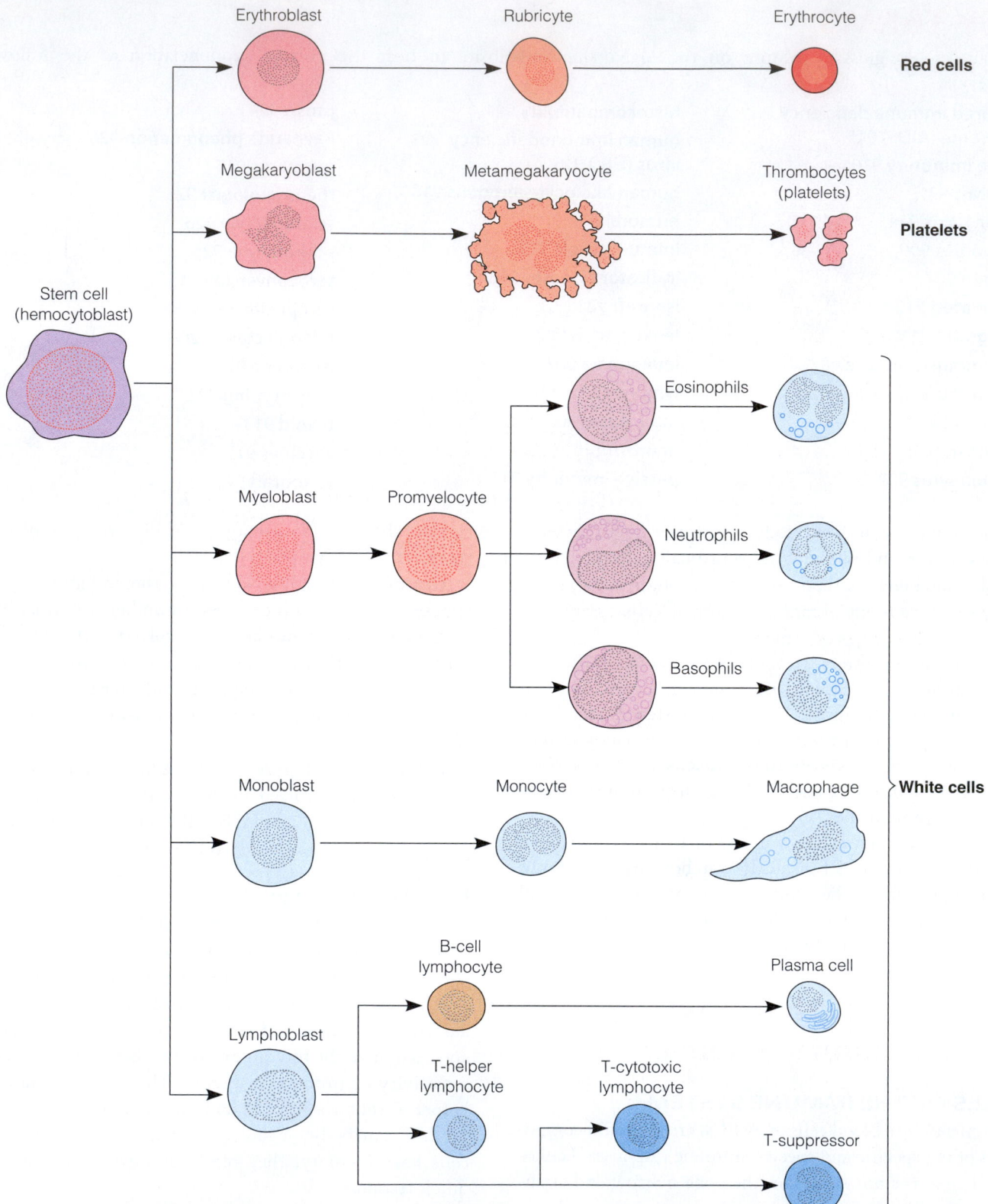

Figure 35-1. ■ Formation of different types of blood cells from the stem cell. The stem cell differentiates into one of five types of blast cells, which then mature into red blood cells (*erythrocytes*), platelets (*thrombocytes*), or white blood cells (*leukocytes*).

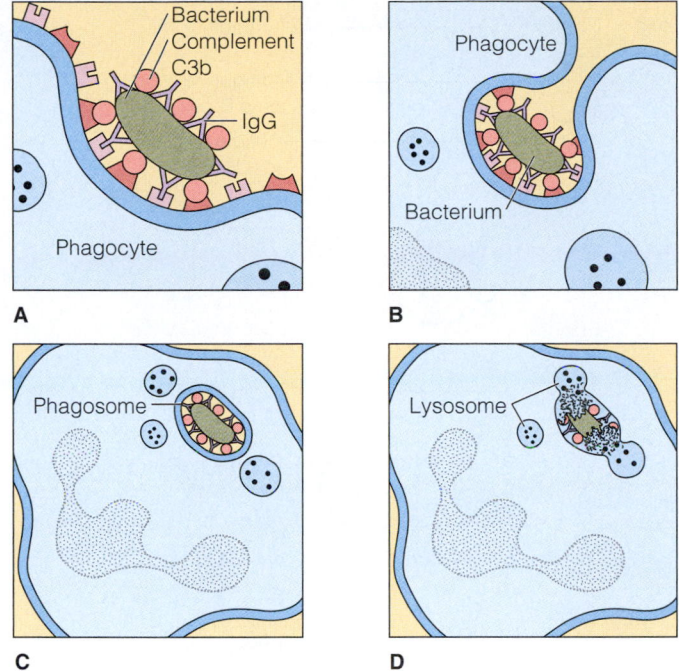

A

B

C

D

Figure 35-2. ■ The process of phagocytosis. **A.** Opsonization coats the surface of the bacterium with IgG (an antibody) and complement. **B.** The bacterium is bound to and engulfed by the phagocyte. **C.** The phagosome is ingested into the cytoplasm of the phagocyte. **D.** The lysosomes fuse with the phagosome, releasing digestive enzymes and destroying the antigen.

thymosin matures the T-cell lymphocytes. T-cell lymphocytes are subdivided into three sets of cells:

- *Helper T cells* (also referred to as *CD4+ cells*) initiate the immune system response, including allergic responses.
- *Suppressor T cells* turn off the immune response. They are important in autoimmune disorders because they prevent the body from self-destruction.
- *Cytotoxic T cells* kill tumor, viral, and foreign cells.

Natural Killer Cells

Natural killer cells are groups of lymphocytes that kill many diverse types of cancer and virus-infected cells. They demonstrate a nonspecific response.

ANTIBODIES

Antibodies, known as immunoglobulins (Ig), are large molecules of proteins produced in reaction to antigens. Each antibody attaches itself specifically to an antigen, labeling it for elimination. B cells have the ability to produce many different antibodies in order to connect to various antigens. The effectiveness of the immune system depends on whether the body is able to distinguish between its own body tissues and foreign tissue. It is thought that the B cells producing antibodies against oneself are usually destroyed in early development, stopping the attack on the body's own cells.

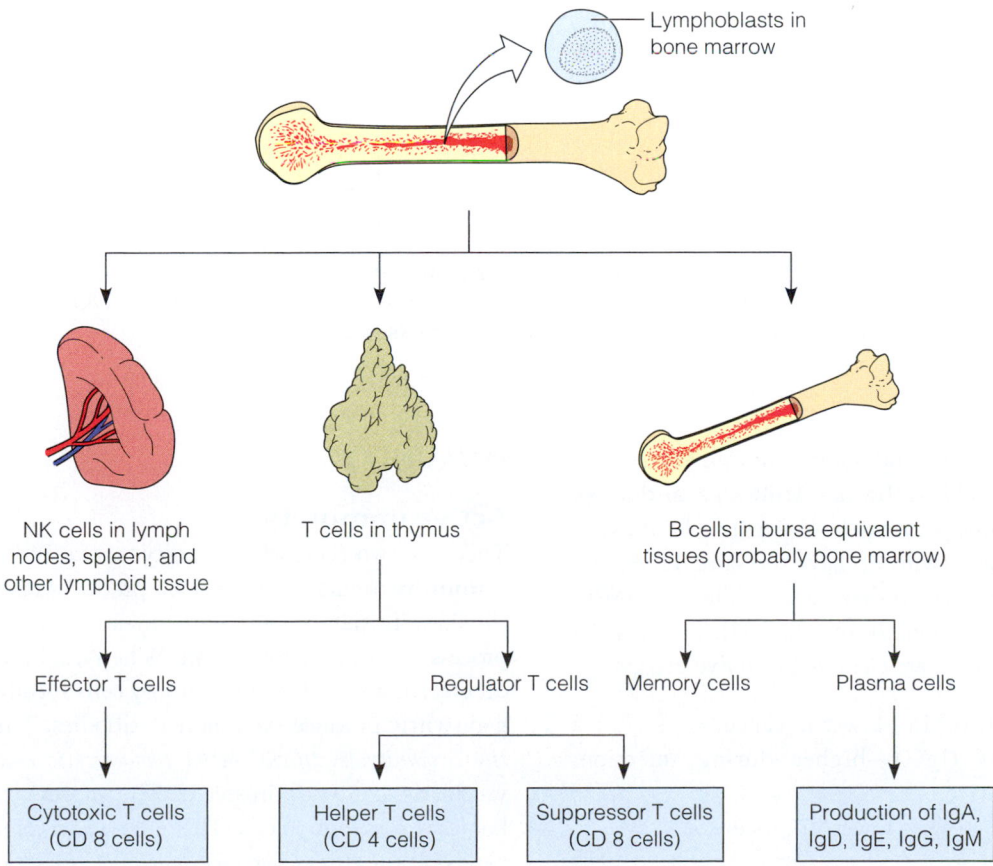

Figure 35-3. ■ The development and differentiation of lymphocytes from the lymphoid stem cell (*lymphoblasts*).

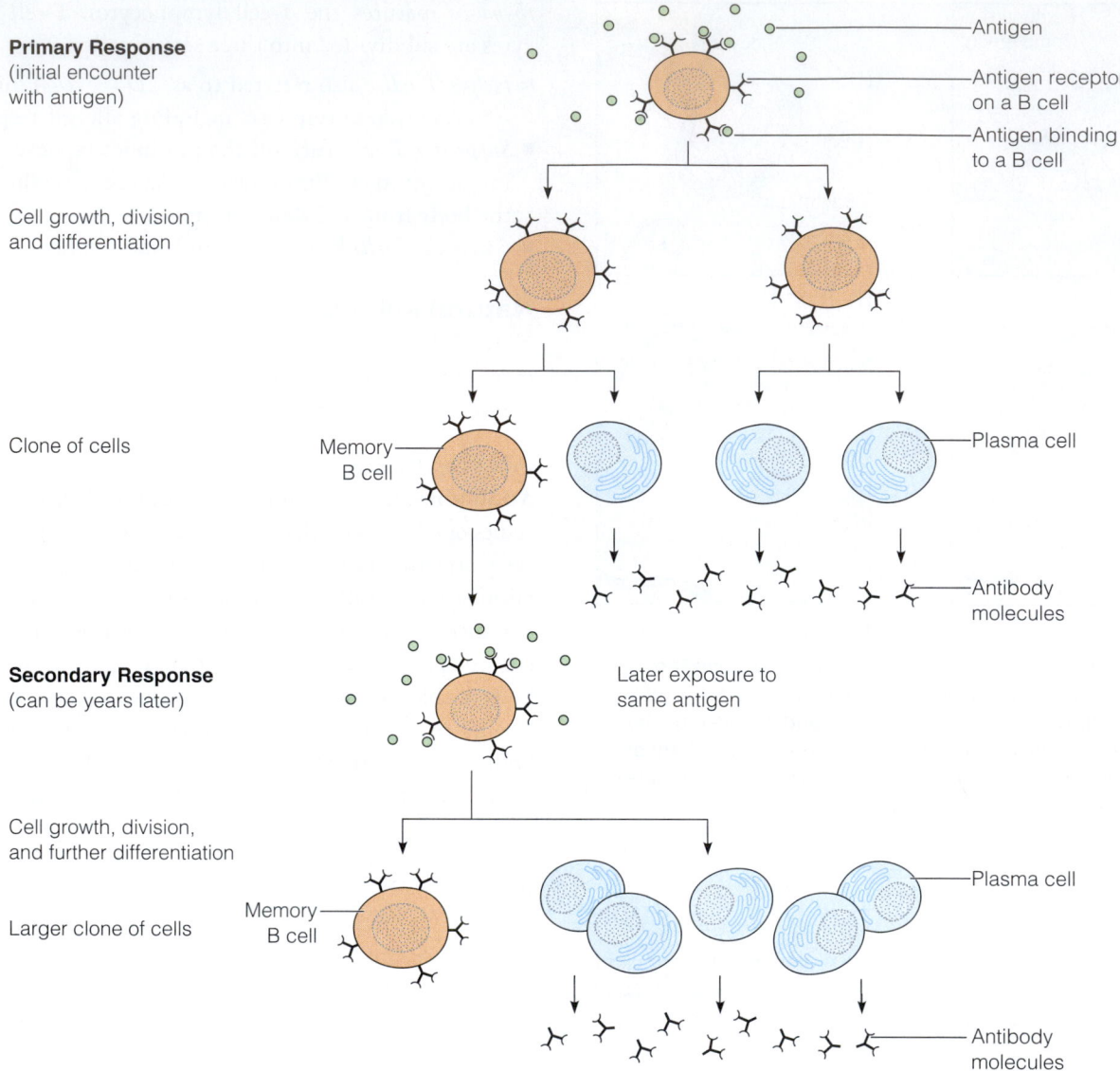

Primary Response
(initial encounter
with antigen)

Antigen

Antigen receptor
on a B cell

Antigen binding
to a B cell

Cell growth, division,
and differentiation

Clone of cells

Memory
B cell

Plasma cell

Antibody
molecules

Secondary Response
(can be years later)

Later exposure to
same antigen

Cell growth, division,
and further differentiation

Larger clone of cells

Memory
B cell

Plasma cell

Antibody
molecules

Figure 35-4. ■ Antibody-mediated (*humoral*) immunity. On initial exposure to the antigen, B cells with appropriate receptor sites are activated to become plasma cells and produce antibodies or memory cells. This is known as the *primary response*. With subsequent exposures, memory cells respond rapidly with antibody production. This is known as the *secondary response*.

Each cell has receptor sites and markers unique to the individual that are known as HLA (**human leukocyte antigens**). It is extremely rare for one person to have the same HLA as another. However, identical twins do have the same HLA, and siblings may have similarly coded genes. When an organ transplant is performed, a closely matched HLA lowers the risk of rejection. Antibodies are classified into five groups:

- Immunoglobulin M (IgM)—lower in cancer
- Immunoglobulin G (IgG)—higher during infection, lower in cancer
- Immunoglobulin A (IgA)—lower in cancer
- Immunoglobulin E (IgE)
- Immunoglobulin D (IgD)

IMMUNITY

Active Immunity

There are two types of immunity: active and passive. **Active immunity** occurs when a person produces his or her own antibodies. Initial contact with an antigen begins the slow process of antibody formation. When a subsequent exposure occurs, the antibodies and memory cells specific for that antigen swiftly produce even more antibodies. This is *natural active immunity*. *Artificial active immunity* is established when vaccinations are administered. The vaccine stimulates antibodies and memory cells. The length of active immunity depends on the disease or vaccination. It may be limited, such as with the flu vaccine, or lifelong, such as with the hepatitis

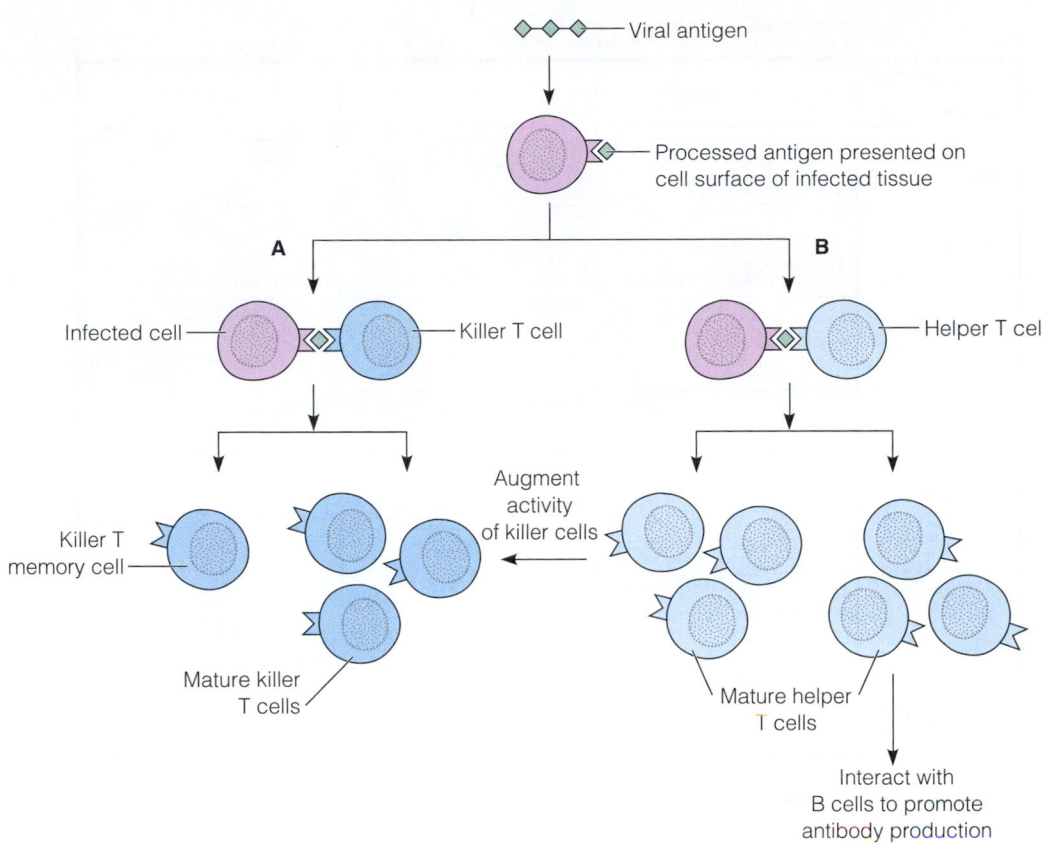

Figure 35-5. ■ Cellular immune response. **A.** An infected cell, a normal cell, or phagocyte presents antigen on its surface that binds with a receptor site on a killer T cell or a helper T cell. The killer T cell is activated to proliferate into memory cells or mature cytotoxic cells. **B.** The helper T cell is activated to augment a cytotoxic response and stimulate the antibody-mediated immune response.

B vaccine. Currently booster shots are being considered to bolster the effect of some vaccinations. Figure 35-6 ■ shows recommendations for adult immunizations and boosters.

Passive Immunity

Passive immunity occurs when a person is given antibodies from another source. Antibodies passed by the mother to the fetus by way of the placenta or to a baby via breast milk are examples of *natural acquired immunity*, one type of passive immunity. *Artificial acquired passive immunity* begins with immunization of preformed antibodies, in an attempt to prevent disease after exposure. An example of this is the immunization for the hepatitis A virus. This immunity is temporary, because these antibodies eventually break down.

Factors that Affect Immunity

There are several factors that influence an individuals' immunity such as age (being very young or very old) and gender (women are more susceptible to autoimmune disorders and men are more susceptible to immunosuppressant disorders). Poor nutrition and nutritional imbalances do not provide adequate support to the bodies' attempts to fight off invaders. Other factors that may impact immunity include

alcohol use or abuse, smoking, and an individuals' level of physical fitness. There is correlation that a healthy diet and active lifestyle helps to maintain a healthy immune system. Those individuals who live in urban environments, experience high stress in their jobs, commute to work, and breathe in air pollution often have higher incidences of immunological disorders. Rural environments may also have stressors, exposure to chemicals and pollutants, as well as limited options for health care.

COLLABORATIVE CARE

Diagnostic Tests

Diagnostic and laboratory tests are commonly performed to determine immune system status. A *complete blood count* (CBC) is usually ordered first. A *sedimentation rate* (sed rate) measures the red blood cell (RBC) descent in the test tube after being in normal saline for 1 hour. If abnormalities are found, further testing is done to identify the disorder. The levels of immunoglobulin (IgA, IgD, IgE, IgG, and IgM) are measured. Higher levels of IgG are found during an infection. Lowered levels of IgG, IgA, and IgM are found in cancer. *Antibody titer testing* identifies whether the client is

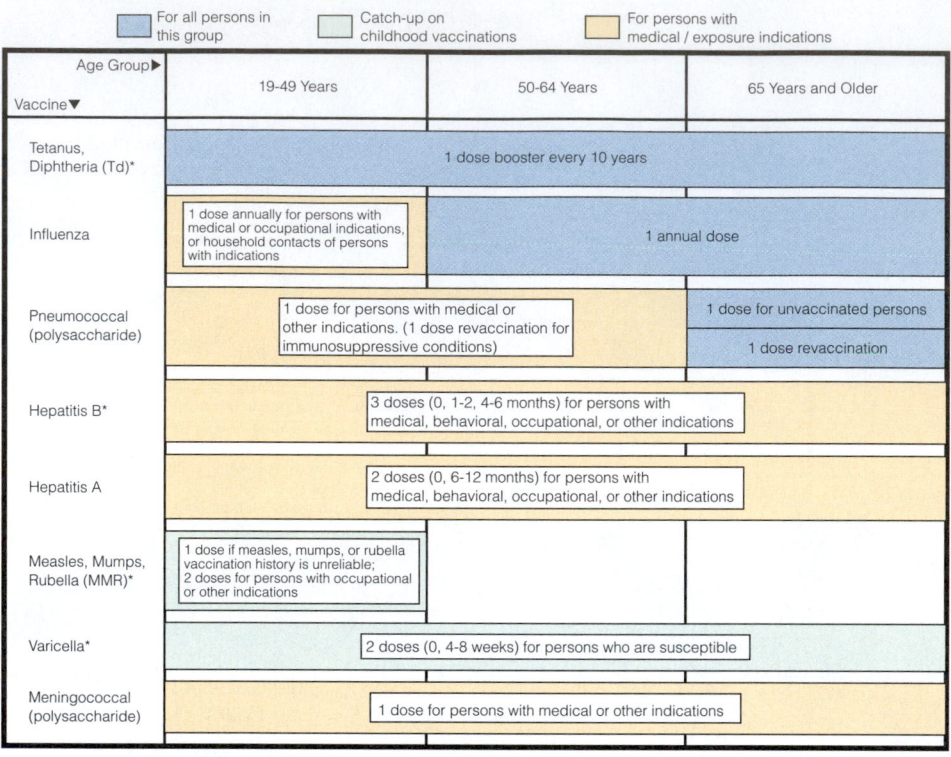

| | For all persons in this group | Catch-up on childhood vaccinations | For persons with medical / exposure indications |

Age Group ▶ Vaccine ▼	19-49 Years	50-64 Years	65 Years and Older
Tetanus, Diphtheria (Td)*	1 dose booster every 10 years		
Influenza	1 dose annually for persons with medical or occupational indications, or household contacts of persons with indications	1 annual dose	
Pneumococcal (polysaccharide)	1 dose for persons with medical or other indications. (1 dose revaccination for immunosuppressive conditions)		1 dose for unvaccinated persons 1 dose revaccination
Hepatitis B*	3 doses (0, 1-2, 4-6 months) for persons with medical, behavioral, occupational, or other indications		
Hepatitis A	2 doses (0, 6-12 months) for persons with medical, behavioral, occupational, or other indications		
Measles, Mumps, Rubella (MMR)*	1 dose if measles, mumps, or rubella vaccination history is unreliable; 2 doses for persons with occupational or other indications		
Varicella*	2 doses (0, 4-8 weeks) for persons who are susceptible		
Meningococcal (polysaccharide)	1 dose for persons with medical or other indications		

*Covered by the Vaccine Injury Compensation Program. For information on how to file a claim call 800-338-2382. Please also visit www.hrsa.gov/osp/vicp To file a claim for vaccine injury write: U.S. Court of Federal Claims, 717 Madison Place, N.W.,Washington D.C. 20005. 202 219-9657.

This schedule indicates the recommended age groups for routine administration of currently licensed vaccines for persons 19 years of age and older. Licensed combination vaccines may be used whenever any components of the combination are indicated and the vaccine's other components are not contraindicated. Providers should consult the manufacturers' package inserts for detailed recommendations.

Report all clinically significant post-vaccination reactions to the Vaccine Adverse Event Reporting System (VAERS). Reporting forms and instructions on filing a VAERS report are available by calling 800-822-7967 or from the VAERS website at www.vaers.org.

For additional information about the vaccines listed above and contraindications for immunization, visit the National Immunization Program Website at www.cdc.gov/nip/ or call the National Immunization Hotline at 800-232-2522 (English) or 800-232-0233 (Spanish).

Approved by the Advisory Committee on Immunization Practices (ACIP), and accepted by the American College of Obstetricians and Gynecologists (ACOG) and the American Academy of Family Physicians (AAFP)

Figure 35-6. ■ Centers for Disease Control and Prevention schedule for recommended adult immunizations by age group.

developing antibodies in response to an antigen, such as an infectious process or vaccination response. An elevated titer indicates antibody production.

Skin testing is another method used to detect impaired cell-mediated immunity. Antigens such as *Candida*, tetanus, or tuberculosis (TB) purified protein derivative (PPD) are injected intradermally. The site is assessed in 48 hours for signs of redness and *induration* (area of hardened raised tissue). If the area is greater than 10 mm in diameter, it is considered positive. A positive reaction indicates depressed cell-mediated immunity, which means that the person has been exposed. It does not mean there is active TB. If the PPD test is positive, the client is referred for a chest x-ray.

Radiographic tests include a routine chest x-ray to determine the lung status and a brief look at the adjacent structures. Magnetic resonance imaging (MRI) or computerized tomography (CT) is also used to assess and identify density

of structures. The size and shape of abnormalities may also be detected. A *biopsy* may be ordered by the physician to aid in the diagnosis of an immune disorder.

Immunizations

Immunizations, or **vaccines,** can cause a person to develop active immunity against a specific organism. Immunizations may be given by injection or as an oral suspension. Some aerosol and powder forms have also been developed that are administered by inhalation. Most immunizations contain a weakened (**attenuated**) or a dead pathogen.

Other types of immunizations contain *inactivated* pathogens. An example would be the influenza (flu) vaccine. The influenza vaccine elicits a weaker immune response and must be repeated yearly. Also, flu strains may differ from year to year, so the vaccine is developed according to the strain that is expected to predominate.

BOX 35-1 NURSING CARE CHECKLIST

Caring for Clients after Immunizations

☑ Remind clients that allergic reactions are most common within the first 24 hours after administration. They should report any signs or symptoms of anaphylaxis such as shortness of breath, swelling of the tongue or airways, or wheezing.

☑ Observe for local reactions such as redness, edema, swelling, and tenderness. Apply warm compresses if these reactions occur to increase blood flow to the area and decrease inflammation.

☑ If the client complains of arm discomfort after immunization in the deltoid, encourage continued movement of the arm to help absorb the vaccine, which will also help decrease the pain.

☑ Clients may complain of fever or malaise after vaccination. This is not unusual, but the client should report any signs or symptoms of anaphylaxis such as shortness of breath, swelling of the tongue or airways, or wheezing.

☑ Reinforce the instruction provided by the public health nurse regarding purpose, timelines of immunizations, and side effects. It is the responsibility of the nurse to assist in preventing the spread of communicable diseases.

☑ Before administering an immunization, check the bottle for the expiration date to ensure that the vaccine is fully potent. Determine the correct site, dosage, and route to ensure proper administration and absorption of the vaccination. Be aware of the client's current health status and avoid administering an immunization when a client has an infectious illness.

Some vaccinations are combined to guard against multiple diseases. Examples of this are MMR (measles, mumps, and rubella) and DTP (diphtheria, tetanus, and pertussis). See Figure 35-6, which shows recommendations for adult immunizations and boosters. (See Table 59-5 ⚭ for recommended immunizations for children.)

Pathogens grown in a laboratory situation are less virulent and are referred to as *live, attenuated vaccines*. A **toxoid** is a toxin that has been treated so that its toxic property is destroyed, but its ability to stimulate production of antibodies remains. Heat and chemicals are used to reduce the potency of the toxin. *Recombinant genetic engineering* is a newer development in vaccine preparation. In this process some vaccines are made from components of the antigen.

Immunizations protect the health of the community. Hepatitis B vaccine is recommended for healthcare workers. People traveling outside U.S. borders are advised to receive immunizations appropriate to the region they are visiting. (A skin test before receiving the immunization may be done at the physician's discretion if a client has allergies.) Many college students are required to receive meningitis vaccination, or to sign a waiver, before they are admitted to a dorm.

Side effects related to immunizations can be mild to anaphylactic. Box 35-1 ■ provides nursing guidelines for clients after immunizations.

HYPERSENSITIVITY AND ANAPHYLACTIC SHOCK

Hypersensitivity is an excessive response of the immune system to a stimulus or antigen. The body responds as it would to a foreign protein or other sensitizing agent. The B lymphocytes produce antigens in response to the allergen; B cells with memory may recall the antigen and quickly respond. The CD4 (helper T cells) begin the immunologic response to the antigen by attaching specifically to that antigen, and working to eliminate the threat. A delayed reaction or cellular reaction, mediated by the cells and T lymphocytes, may occur. A reaction mediated by B lymphocytes causes a humoral reaction, such as anaphylaxis. The more immediate the reaction, the more severe the sensitivity to the allergen.

Upon subsequent exposure to the antigen, an allergic reaction occurs. Mast cells release histamine, which constricts the airways, causing shortness of breath and wheezing. Gastrointestinal symptoms may include cramps, vomiting, and diarrhea, as well as abdominal pain. Urticaria and pruritus may occur.

Hypersensitivity reactions may occur as a result of exposure to pollen, animal dander, chemicals, and certain foods. Box 35-2 ■ provides a list of common foods that trigger reactions. Factors that influence a hypersensitivity reaction are provided in Box 35-3 ■.

Blood vessels dilate and increase the permeability of their cell membranes, allowing intracellular fluid to move into interstitial spaces, decreasing circulating blood volume

---

BOX 35-2 PEDIATRIC CONSIDERATIONS

Foods to Avoid in Children Under 2

Certain foods carry a higher risk of causing allergic reactions. Since the immune system in children younger than 2 years is not fully developed, it is recommended that parents avoid giving the following foods to children under the age of 2:

Nuts (especially peanuts, cashews, and pecans)
Shellfish
Eggs
Chocolate
Strawberries
Cow's milk (if family history of lactose intolerance)

In infants, introduce rice cereal first before wheat or oat because rice has the lowest incidence of allergic reaction.

BOX 35-3	FACTORS THAT INFLUENCE HYPERSENSITIVITY

- Type of allergen
- Entry route of allergen
- Body's response to allergen
- Amount of exposure to the allergen
- Repeated exposure to the allergen

and leading to anaphylactic shock. An adult has approximately 32 L of extracellular fluid and 16 L of intracellular fluid. Six (6) L of blood is within the blood vessels. During a hypersensitivity reaction, one-third of the fluid may leak into the interstitial spaces, causing a drop in blood pressure

and leading to anaphylactic shock. **Anaphylaxis** literally means "a lack of protection," meaning the body cannot compensate for the allergic response (Figure 35-7 ■).

As the intracellular fluid continues to leak into the tissues, the lungs may also become filled with fluid, causing pulmonary edema. The client experiences shortness of breath; a rapid, weak pulse; syncope; confusion; and a sense of impending doom. Other signs and symptoms of anaphylactic shock include nasal congestion, palpitations, erythema, pruritus, a wet-sounding nonproductive cough, and slurred speech.

Immediate medical intervention is necessary. For both hypersensitivity and anaphylaxis, epinephrine in a 1:1000 concentration is used for severe urticaria. Epinephrine is

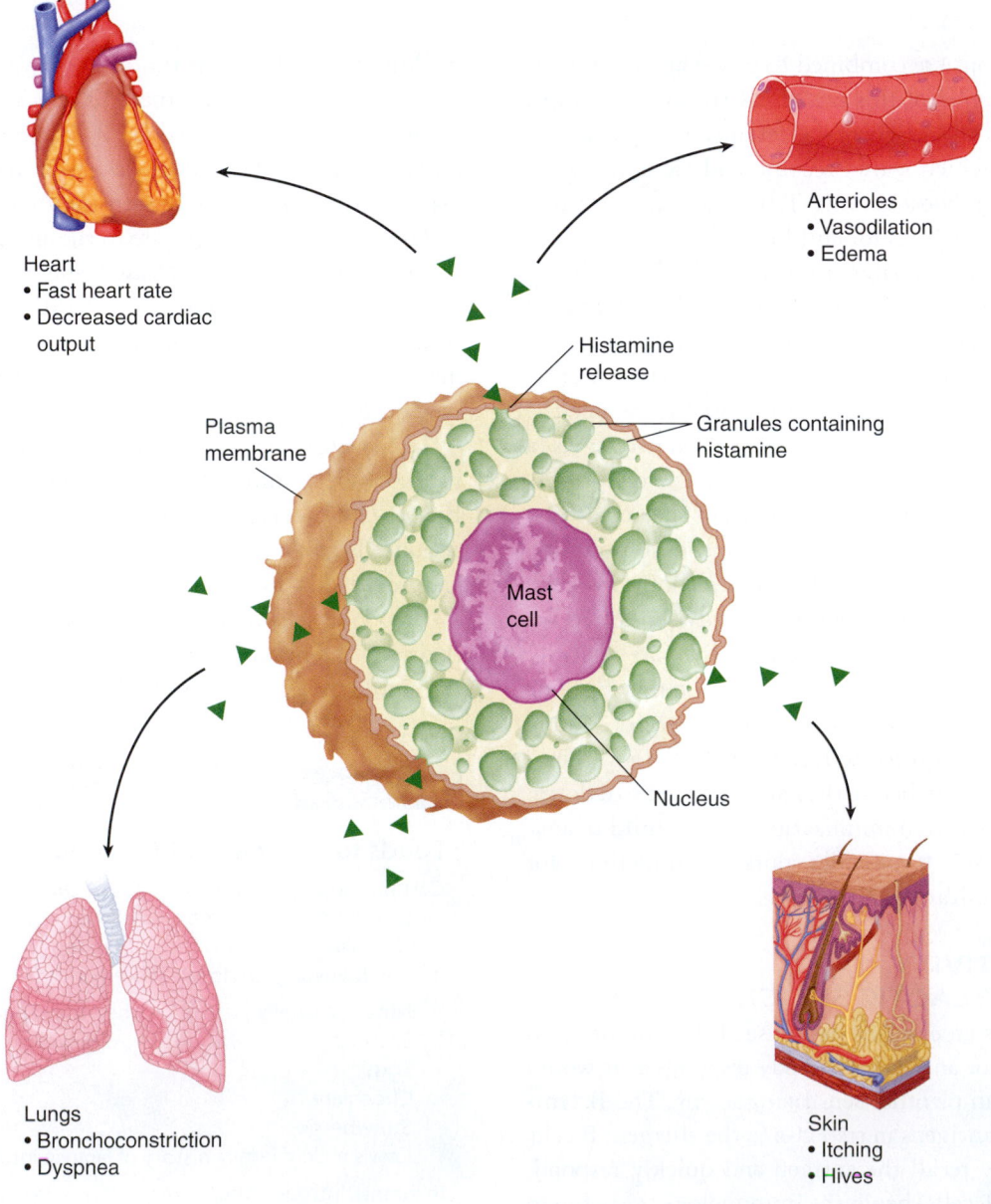

Heart
- Fast heart rate
- Decreased cardiac output

Arterioles
- Vasodilation
- Edema

Plasma membrane

Histamine release

Granules containing histamine

Mast cell

Nucleus

Lungs
- Bronchoconstriction
- Dyspnea

Skin
- Itching
- Hives

Figure 35-7. ■ Anaphylactic shock.

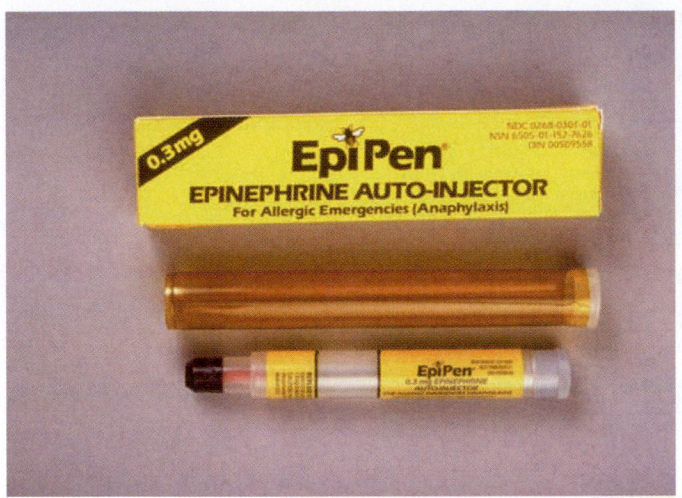

Figure 35-8. ■ EpiPen.

administered subcutaneously in abdominal fat, using a 1/2″ or 5/8″ needle. Subcutaneous injections may also be given in the upper arm. Epinephrine may also be administered IM in the anterolateral portion of the thigh, through clothes if necessary, with an EpiPen (Figure 35-8 ■). Briskly massage the injection site to speed up the drug action. In some cases of anaphylaxis, epinephrine may need to be administered every 10 to 15 minutes until the urticaria has resolved.

clinical ALERT

Use a 1:1000 concentration of epinephrine for hypersensitivity and anaphylactic reactions. NEVER inject 1:100 epinephrine intended for inhalation use; the results can be fatal. Always check with the physician before administration of a pediatric dose of epinephrine as the dose is not the same as for an adult. Pediatric doses of epinephrine are usually administered in the vastus lateralis muscle due to the lower amount of muscle mass in the deltoid.

Nursing Considerations

Elevate the client's feet, and keep the client warm. (Do not position the client in Trendelenburg position; it puts too much pressure on an already compromised circulatory system.) Administer oxygen if needed. Antihistamines, such as diphenhydramine (Benadryl) and corticosteroids (prednisone), may be ordered to boost the effect of epinephrine. The client should be instructed to wear a medical alert bracelet or necklace identifying the allergy, and to carry epinephrine with them (an EpiPen). EpiPens should not be stored in the glove box of a car. Areas of high heat, light, or air can break down the active components of the medication. Additionally, the EpiPen should not be left at home, stored in the refrigerator. Instruct clients to keep the EpiPen with them at all times, and to avoid the allergen if

possible. Anaphylaxis is a medical emergency; dial 9-1-1. With prompt medical treatment, a positive outcome may be achieved; without treatment, death may occur.

Major Immune System Disorders

HUMAN IMMUNODEFICIENCY VIRUS AND ACQUIRED IMMUNE DEFICIENCY SYNDROME

Acquired immune deficiency syndrome (AIDS) was first reported in the United States in 1981. The Centers for Disease Control and Prevention (CDC) reported the presence of a new infection that affected the immune system. Homosexuals were the primary population afflicted. We have since learned that AIDS affects any age, gender, sexual preference, and nationality. It has become a major epidemic, increasing most rapidly among heterosexual women. AIDS is the final stage of disease caused by the **human immunodeficiency virus (HIV),** a virus that damages and destroys cells of the body's immune system. The virus is **immunotropic** (targets the immune system) and **neurotropic** (targets cognitive functioning).

HIV is a **retrovirus,** living and replicating within the host. The genetic material RNA replicates in reverse. It copies RNA into DNA to divide and multiply, instead of the normal cell pattern of copying the DNA into the RNA. The virus endures for extended periods of time, attacking the T cells (CD4 or helper cells). Proteins on the cell surface become a target. HIV infects the CD4 cell most often (Figure 35-9 ■). The virus becomes part of the cell and develops into an HIV factory, replicating the virus. Once a person is exposed to HIV, the replication process begins. Within 6 to 12 weeks of infection there are usually detectable levels of antibodies against the virus in the blood (known as **seroconversion**). It is possible to test positive after 2 weeks, but it can take up to 6 months or longer for the disease to appear on testing. In rare instances, it may take up to 2 years to produce antibodies. During this "window period" a person can test negative even if he or she is infected with HIV. The person can infect others even though a result of the test is negative. When someone has become infected with HIV for an extended time, the number of CD4 cells diminishes. This weakens the immune system. The lower the T-cell or CD4 count is, the more likely the person is to be at risk for opportunistic infections.

Worldwide it is estimated that in 2007, between 33 and 36 million people were living with HIV or AIDS, and in some African nations more than one-fourth are infected (WHO, 2007). Box 35-4 ■ shows data about the incidence of AIDS in the United States at the end of 2006.

MyNursingKit | HIV, AIDS

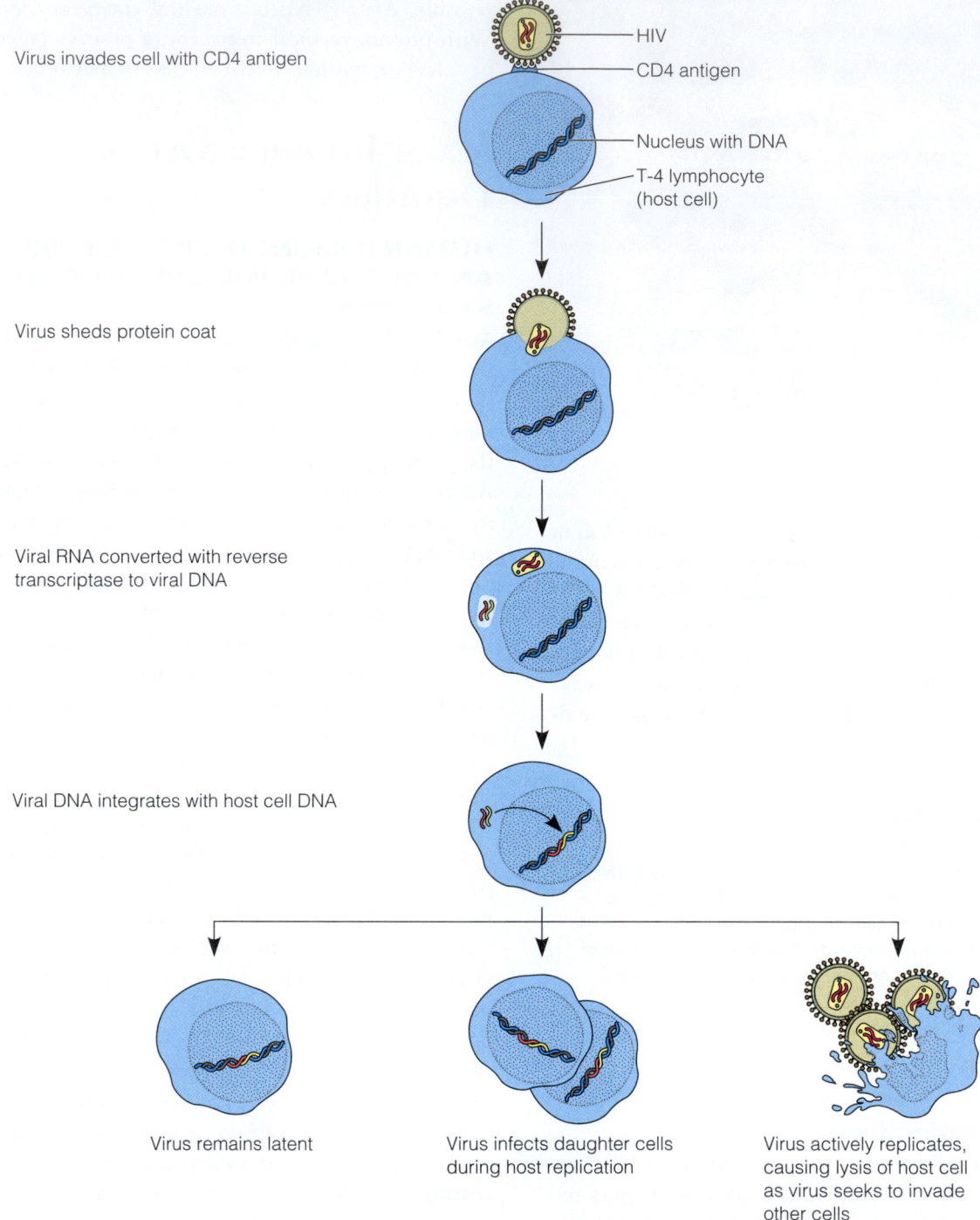

Virus invades cell with CD4 antigen

HIV
CD4 antigen
Nucleus with DNA
T-4 lymphocyte
(host cell)

Virus sheds protein coat

Viral RNA converted with reverse transcriptase to viral DNA

Viral DNA integrates with host cell DNA

Virus remains latent

Virus infects daughter cells during host replication

Virus actively replicates, causing lysis of host cell as virus seeks to invade other cells

Figure 35-9. ■ How HIV affects and destroys CD4 cells.

The main routes of HIV transmission are:

- Sexual contact with an infected person.
- Injection with contaminated blood or blood products.
- Use of contaminated needles.
- Transmission from the mother to her fetus.

HIV is transmitted through blood, semen, vaginal secretions, the placenta, breast milk, and artificial insemination.

Intravenous drug use, prostitution, oral sex, anal sex, and vaginal intercourse increase the risk for passage of the infection through broken skin or mucous membranes. A person who received blood transfusions before effective screening was in place (between 1978 and 1985) is also at risk. People who receive organ transplants or are artificially inseminated can also be at risk.

BOX 35-4   **POPULATION FOCUS**

HIV/AIDS Incidence in the United States

The CDC (2008) reported these estimated figures for the United States and the District of Columbia at the end of 2006:

Newly infected with HIV in 2006	56,300
Cumulative cases of AIDS through 2006	982,498
Adults/adolescents in the United States	973,352
Male cases in the United States	783,786
Female cases in the United States	189,566
Children under age 13 in the United States	9,144

Risk reduction behaviors have been recognized as preventive measures for HIV infection. Sexual abstinence provides 100% protection. Postponing sexual activity or abstaining after one has been sexually active is effective in protecting oneself against infection. A monogamous relationship with an uninfected partner reduces the risk substantially. Note, though, that a large part of our population may not consider abstinence an option. The nurse needs to be nonjudgmental and aware of the needs of all people in the community. It is the nurse's job to give accurate health information when people seek it and to present all options.

Protection from HIV

The CDC reports that latex blocks the passage of viruses. Therefore, safe sex discussions should include information about latex condoms. Although they can provide a 95% to 97% protection against pregnancy, the failure rate with condoms is 12%. This failure rate is usually due to nonuse or incorrect use rather than to condom quality. There is less than a 2% chance of condoms breaking when they are used correctly.

Client teaching is needed to ensure effectiveness of latex condoms. Some people are allergic to latex. If the skin reacts to latex, the client should discontinue use. Oils break down the latex material, so a water-based lubricant should be used if needed, not an oil-based one. Condoms must be stored away from excessive heat or cold (not in a wallet or in the glove compartment of the car). Clients should inspect the expiration date and check packages for damage. Remind the client that, to be effective, condoms must be put on prior to genital contact.

The use of nonoxynol-9, an ingredient found in spermicides, has been shown to kill HIV in laboratory studies. Female condoms have the same effectiveness as male condoms. Dental dams can be used as a latex barrier during oral sex. (See also other contraceptive methods in relation to sexually transmitted infections in Table 40-6 ⚭.)

Alcohol and other drugs impair decision making and judgment. Explain refusal skill techniques. If a client is injecting drugs, teach the importance of not sharing needles, or of cleaning needles if they are being shared. (Needles should be cleaned twice using a bleach solution.) Caution clients to ensure that needles used in tattooing, acupuncture, and body piercing are sterile. Remind the public to use latex gloves when coming in contact with blood. It is also suggested and recommended that clients donate their own blood ahead of time when they are scheduled for elective surgeries (**autologous** blood).

Manifestations

Initial HIV infection can range from no noticeable symptoms to flulike complaints. Fatigue, fever, weight loss, and swollen lymph nodes may be found.

COMMON INDICATOR DISEASES (OPPORTUNISTIC DISEASES). As HIV disrupts clients' immune system, clients become more prone to develop infections that a healthy system would be able to reject. Several such opportunistic diseases are commonly seen in clients with HIV and AIDS.

***Pneumocystis jiroveci* Pneumonia.** *Pneumocystis jiroveci* (formerly called *carinii*) pneumonia (PCP) has been classified as a disease caused by a protozoa (one-celled animal). However, recent evidence suggests that it is a fungus. *Pneumocystis jiroveci (carinii)* is found in the environment and does not affect persons with a normal immune system. People whose immune systems are compromised are unable to fight off the disease. PCP is the most common of the indicator diseases, occurring in 85% of HIV-infected adults. This disease affects the pulmonary alveoli. It results in consolidation of the pulmonary parenchyma (functioning tissue).

Signs and symptoms include a dry hacking cough, fevers, clear breath sounds, shortness of breath, dyspnea, and occasional chest pain. The treatment of choice is the antibacterial Bactrim/Septra. Some AIDS clients have severe adverse reactions to Bactrim including rash, fevers, and leukopenia. Pentamidine, an antiprotozoal drug, is the next option, but it also can have severe side effects. Adverse reactions include impaired glucose metabolism, renal damage, and bone marrow suppression. Another drug used is dapsone (diaminodiphenyl sulphone, DDS), a leprostatic medication (antileprosy drug).

Kaposi's Sarcoma. Kaposi's sarcoma is a cancer that involves the endothelial layer of blood and lymphatic vessels. The symptoms include pinkish-blue macules that develop into reddish purple or dark reddish brown, painful lesions over the body (Figure 35-10 ■). Diagnosis is confirmed by a biopsy. Treatment includes radiation therapy. However, recurrence is quite common. Chemotherapy using drugs such as vinblastine, Adriamycin, bleomycin, or methotrexate is another alternative treatment.

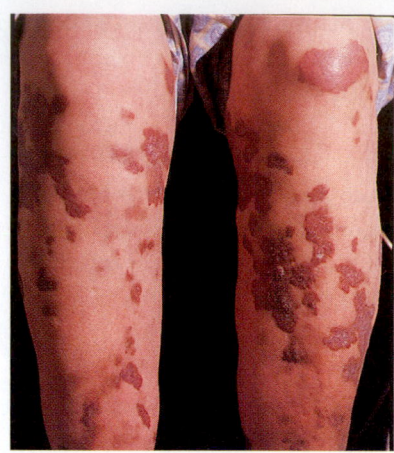

Figure 35-10. ■ Kaposi's sarcoma. (*Source*: Zeva Oelbaum/Peter Arnold, Inc.)

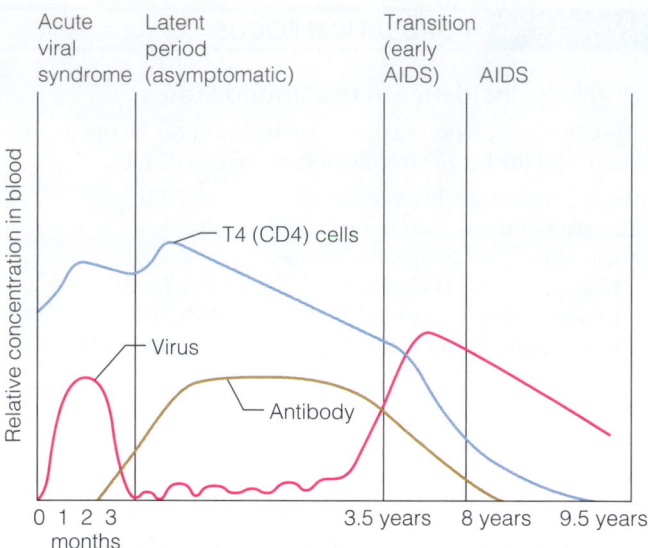

Figure 35-11. ■ The progression of HIV infection in the blood. Acute illness develops shortly after the virus is contracted, corresponding with a rapid rise in viral levels. Antibodies are formed and remain present throughout the course of the infection. Late in the disease, viral activation results in a marked increase in virus, while CD4 (T4) cells diminish as they are destroyed with viral replication. Antibody levels gradually decrease as immune function is impaired.

Cryptosporidium. Cryptosporidium is caused by protozoa and linked to the municipal water supply. When there is an outbreak, water should be boiled or the compromised client should be encouraged to drink filtered water. The symptoms include severe watery diarrhea, nausea, vomiting, abdominal cramping, fever, and weakness. Symptomatic treatment includes antidiarrheal medication and intravenous fluid replacement. There is currently no effective chemoprophylactic agent against cryptosporidium.

Oral candidiasis. Oral candidiasis or "thrush" is another example of an opportunistic infection (see Figure 59-7 ⊙⊙). Candidiasis may cause white patches on the tongue, larynx, or mucous membranes that may bleed when the white patches are removed. Thrush may erupt when the immune system is depressed, the client is recovering from chemotherapy; has diabetes, leukemia, HIV or AIDS, or has taken steroids or antibiotics for a long period of time.

Diagnosis

Diagnostic testing for HIV begins with an *enzyme-linked immunosorbent assay* (ELISA), which usually detects antibodies 6 to 12 weeks after exposure. (As mentioned, some persons do not experience seroconversion or detection for 6 months or longer.) If a person's blood contains antibodies for HIV, it is said to be **seropositive.** The ELISA test can deliver a false positive in a female who has had multiple births. Clients who are high-risk individuals should be reevaluated after several months. Clients who are low risk and test positive should be retested.

If the client is positive, the next test ordered is the *Western blot test*. This test is more specific for HIV and eliminates the false-positive result sometimes found with the ELISA.

The PCR test or the *polymerase chain reaction test*, also called the *viral load test*, measures the HIV RNA, which is increased with an initial HIV infection. The PCR level

decreases after the initial infection due to the body's immune response. (The immune system is somewhat effective but is being worn down.) The majority of the virus is produced during the first few weeks of infection. Figure 35-11 ■ illustrates the progression of HIV virus in the blood.

Diagnosis is based on the client's clinical history, laboratory findings, and the identification of risk factors. The physician performs a physical examination and assesses laboratory evidence of immune function for the presence of HIV antibodies. Other tests that may be ordered include a *CBC, blood chemistries, liver function tests, tests for other sexually transmitted diseases, hepatitis, tuberculosis*, and *toxoplasmosis*. The physician observes for signs and symptoms of opportunistic diseases, also known as **indicator diseases.**

Treatment

Currently, no cure for HIV infection exists. However, highly active antiretroviral therapy (HAART) has been found to prolong life for those afflicted with HIV. It is now possible for a person with HIV infection to live many years without developing AIDS. AIDS is the final stage of the infection. It weakens the immune system and increases the risk of developing cancers, opportunistic disease, and neurologic disorders.

Treatment is usually started if the client is experiencing severe symptoms of HIV infection or has been diagnosed with AIDS. Treatment is initiated if the following two values are found:

- The viral load test (PCR) reaches 55,000 copies/mL or more.
- The CD4 count is 200 to 350 cells/mm^3 or less.

The U.S. Food and Drug Administration (FDA) has approved 20 anti-HIV medications for adults and adolescents. The U.S. Department of Health and Human Services provides HIV treatment and guidelines to physicians and clients. It is recommended that the client take a combination of three or more medications in a regimen (HAART). Taking only one or two drugs is not recommended, because any decrease in the viral load is almost always temporary without three or more drugs. Once treatment has been initiated, clients may need to continue taking anti-HIV medications for the rest of their lives. If the virus is not suppressed completely, drug resistance can develop, limiting future treatment options. (HIV can mutate while a client is taking a drug, decreasing the effectiveness of the medication.) A pregnant woman with HIV would be an exception to the recommendation of three or more medications. She may take Retrovir alone or with other drugs to diminish the risk of passing HIV to the infant.

clinical ALERT

Antiretroviral medications do not cure HIV infection. Individuals taking these medications can still transmit HIV to others.

The FDA has approved four classes of anti-HIV medications:

- *Nucleoside reverse transcriptase inhibitors* (NRTIs) block reproduction of HIV. The most common antiretroviral medications are Retrovir, zidovudine, or azidothymidine (AZT). NRTIs slow virus replication and allow the T cells to recover, multiply, and regain immunologic function. There are side effects, such as bone marrow suppression and hemolytic anemia (see Chapter 34 ⊙⊙).
- *Non-nucleoside reverse transcriptase inhibitors* (NNRTIs) bind to and disable reverse transcriptase, a protein that the HIV needs to make more copies of itself. Delavirdine (DLV) and nevirapine (NVP) are examples.
- *Protease inhibitors* (PIs) disable protease, a protein that HIV needs to replicate itself. Ritonavir (RTV), saquinavir (SQV), and indinavir (IDV) are examples.
- *Fusion inhibitors* prevent HIV entry into cells.

AIDS vaccines are designed to teach the immune system to recognize and defend against disease-causing microorganisms. Currently no HIV/AIDS vaccines are approved for use. However, many are in clinical trial studies. The vaccine is given before exposure to HIV. Its purpose is to help the body rid itself of the virus or to help control HIV enough to prevent disease progression or transmission to others.

The U.S. Department of Health and Human Services lists the following goals for HIV therapy:

- Restore or preserve the immune system.
- Improve the client's quality of life.
- Reduce sickness and death due to HIV.

NURSING CARE

PRIORITIZING NURSING CARE

When caring for clients with HIV and AIDS, focus your care on preventing exposure to pathogens and providing physical and emotional support. Be vigilant about careful hand washing and follow protective measures to prevent bringing pathogens to the client. Remember that when a client's immune system is compromised, microorganisms from a cough or sneeze can cause life-threatening illnesses. Educate friends and family members about protective measures such as wearing a mask if they have a cold and are visiting the client.

Be careful not to make judgments about the client's lifestyle or choices that may have resulted in HIV exposure. The client is a human being with a life-threatening illness. As nurses, we are there to give care and support. Allow clients to talk about their feelings and frustrations. Avoid taking anger or hostility personally, since clients may be working through the grief process. Encourage the client to identify and turn to supportive people. Referral to community support groups may also be helpful.

ASSESSING

Clients with HIV and AIDS should be assessed for signs and symptoms of opportunistic infections. The nurse should do a careful head-to-toe assessment and note any breaks in the skin, since the immune system is compromised. During the assessment, the nurse should also determine the members of the client's support system, so they can be included in planning care. Auscultate lung sounds bilaterally for evidence of pneumonia or decreased breath sounds. Assess height and weight to determine nutritional status and document improvement in nutrition.

DIAGNOSING, PLANNING, AND IMPLEMENTING

Possible nursing diagnoses for clients with HIV and AIDS include:

- *Risk for Infection*
- *Imbalanced Nutrition: Less than Body Requirements*
- *Risk for Impaired Skin Integrity*
- *Impaired Physical Mobility*
- *Impaired Gas Exchange*

- *Acute Confusion*
- *Powerlessness*

Client outcomes for clients with HIV or AIDS include, but are not limited to, the following:

- Client avoids situations that increase the risk for infection.
- Client follows regimen for maintaining nutrition.
- Client maintains intact skin.
- Client expresses feelings about condition and identifies ways of coping.
- Client's support network is included in planning.

Care of clients with HIV or AIDS is supportive. Great care is taken not to expose the client to further infection.

- A primary risk for the client is infection with an opportunistic disease. Follow Standard Precautions and use good handwashing techniques before and after care. *This protects the client from nosocomial infection.*
- Monitor for signs and symptoms of infection (redness, tenderness, chills, sweating, drainage from wounds, and shortness of breath) including WBC levels. *Early detection of signs of infection helps the physician institute treatment as soon as possible.*
- Culture drainage from lesions and monitor lab tests including urinalysis and blood cultures. *Culture will identify causative organisms and resistance to treatment.*
- Administer antiretroviral and anti-infective medications as ordered. *These medications are essential to help the client fight infections.*
- Maintain adequate nutrition, monitor weights, and monitor for fluid and electrolyte imbalances. *Clients with HIV may have difficulty maintaining weight and can suffer muscle wasting (Figure 35-12 ■). Imbalances can result from episodes of diarrhea.*
- Provide small, frequent meals. Offer soft foods. *Small meals may be better tolerated and can help to increase nutritional intake. Soft foods are easier to eat and digest.*

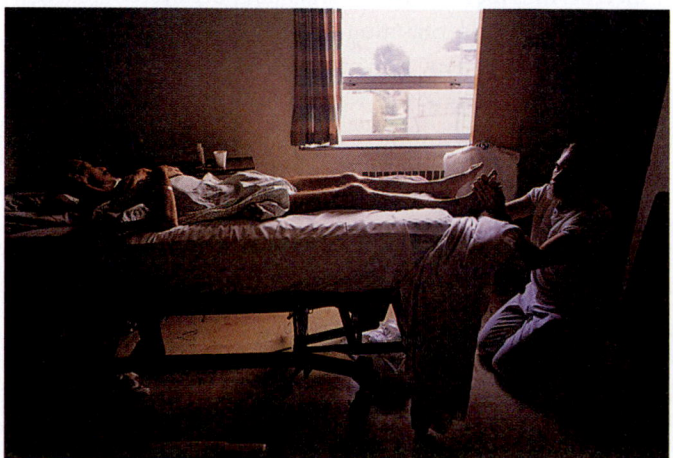

Figure 35-12. ■ Wasting syndrome in a client with AIDS.

- Give good oral hygiene. *Oral hygiene improves the client's comfort and desire to eat.*
- Observe for mouth lesions. Use topical anesthetics such as viscous Xylocaine. *Mouth lesions may be a side effect of medications. Anesthetics can numb the area for a time.*
- If ordered, administer appetite stimulants to enhance dietary intake. Encourage the family and friends to bring in foods that the client enjoys. *Dietary supplements and vitamins can help improve the client's nutritional status. Clients may eat more if provided with their favorite foods.*
- Provide antiemetics and antidiarrheals as ordered by the physician. *These help decrease food and fluid loss.*
- Turn the client frequently and provide devices that decrease pressure to bony prominences. Use mild soap to wash the client and pat skin dry. Keep the perianal area clean, dry, and apply ointment to protect the tissues from skin breakdown due to diarrhea. Treat open blisters/superficial lesions with a transparent film. *These measures decrease the risk for skin breakdown. Friction may cause skin abrasion. Covering lesions protects the area from infection.*
- Encourage ambulation and provide passive and active range-of-motion exercises as appropriate. Encourage the client to avoid fatigue. *Exercise and ambulation increase circulation and muscle tone and strengthen muscles and joints. Rest periods preserve the client's energy.*
- Assess lung sounds for changes. Monitor pulse oximetry and provide supplemental oxygen as ordered *to support respiratory effort.* Encourage the client to turn, cough, and deep breathe *to prevent atelectasis.* Assist the client to a semi-Fowler's position *to allow for lung expansion and abdominal pressure reduction.*
- Medicate with anti-infective medications as per physician order *to decrease incidence and severity of respiratory infections.*
- Use short sentences when giving directions and reorient the client as needed to promote understanding. Limit stimulus in the client's room to avoid confusion and agitation. Encourage the family to visit and socialize to provide familiar contact and orientation. *The neurologic and cognitive functioning of the client may be altered due to the effect of the disease on the brain.*
- Deliver care with a nonjudgmental attitude. Remember that confidentiality is a client's right and must be upheld by the nursing staff. Allow the client to verbalize inner feelings while actively listening. *The client is a human being with an illness. Listening promotes therapeutic communication and trust.*
- Assist the client to understand the regimen and to take medications correctly. *Adherence to the medication regimen maximizes effectiveness of the treatment.*

- Provide the client with information on prevention, and lifestyle and behavior changes. *Client education can help prevent further spread of the disease.*
- Determine the strength of the client's support system. Discuss previous coping measures that have been successful in the past and develop strategies to assist the client and family. *A strong support system and effective coping strategies are essential for effective treatment.*

EVALUATING

The client with HIV or AIDS should be evaluated for improvement in immune system function and positive coping skills. Knowledge about how to contain the disease should be evaluated along with ways to avoid exposure to infection.

Organ Transplantation

Organ transplants were once considered experimental procedures but have become much more commonplace. Acceptability of organ donation or transplantation often depends on a client's culture or religion. Table 44-1 ⬤⬤ provides information about cultural views of organ donation.

Some types of transplants (skin, cornea, bone, and heart valve) are done frequently. Kidney, heart, and liver transplants are seen with regularity in larger hospitals. These procedures are quite expensive, as is the medication required afterward to prevent infection.

Transplants may be performed for clients when organs are failing. In addition, healthy stem cells can be used to stimulate new cells (for example, in the client with leukemia). Skin may be transplanted to cover a large burn area to prevent electrolyte loss and provide a barrier for infection. (Skin grafts for burns are discussed in Chapter 47 ⬤⬤.)

Whenever a transplant is done, it is extremely important for the donor to have closely matched HLA to promote a high success rate. An identical twin is the best matching donor; siblings are the next best match. Organ transplants on average last about 10 years, but the variations can be very individual.

Autograft is the transplant of the client's own tissue and is the most successful type of graft. Skin grafts are the most common type of autograft. *Autologous* (self-donated) blood transfusion or bone marrow transplants are more frequently being done to lower the immune reaction. An **isograft** (identical twin) transplant has a good success rate. An **allograft** is a tissue and organ transplants that are from the same species. Living donors and cadavers are used; whole or partial organs are donated to fill the shortage of donors. A cadaver donation must meet certain criteria developed by the United Network for Organ Donation. A **xenograft** is a transplant from an animal species to a human. *Porcine* (pig) skin is used in a large burn as a temporary covering.

Tissue typing is a process that determines the ability of the cells to be compatible and lessens the risk of rejection. The HLA type is identified along with blood typing of the donor and recipient.

COLLABORATIVE CARE

Diagnostic and laboratory tests are carefully monitored and analyzed to identify a donor and bring about a successful transplant. Routine tests include *CBC with differential, urinalysis, chemistry levels, blood type, Rh factor,* and *coagulation tests. Blood gases* and *electrocardiograms* are ordered to ensure that the donor is in optimum health. A *chest x-ray* assesses the lung status of the donor prior to the surgical procedure. Specific tests related to the transplant recipient include the *blood type* and *Rh factor. Cross-matching* identifies preformed antibodies, *HLA testing* types donors that are closely matched. *MLC (mixed lymphocyte culture) assay* testing determines histocompatibility between the donor and the recipient. (**Histocompatibility** is immunologic similarity that permits successful homograft transplantation.)

Reverse isolation techniques will be in place following the transplant. With reverse isolation, access to the client room is restricted. Every person who enters must wear a gown, gloves, and mask. All equipment must be carefully disinfected before being brought into the client's room.

TRANSPLANT REJECTION

Transplant rejection is a humoral and cell-mediated response. It occurs about 24 hours after the transplant. However, it can arise immediately post-transplant.

Classification and Manifestations

A *hyperactive rejection* usually begins with a healthy organ transplant. Then the organ loses color, softens, and is rejected.

An *acute rejection* starts with an inflammatory response and elevated laboratory values (BUN, creatinine, liver and cardiac enzymes, bilirubin levels) with cardiac collapse.

A *chronic rejection* develops as antibodies and complement are deposited in the walls of the organ blood vessels. The vessel lumen narrows, resulting in diminished blood flow to the transplant. The organ loses functional ability and fails.

Graft versus host disease (GVHD) is a complication associated with bone marrow transplants (see Chapter 34 ⬤⬤). Cells in the grafted tissue begin to attack other tissues in the body (see Figure 35-5). Acute GVHD is typically found 100 days post-transplant. Urticaria develops on the palms of the hands and the soles of the feet. The rash sometimes becomes generalized, causing shedding of the epidermis.

Diagnosis

Signs of rejection are detected by various tests. *Ultrasonography* and *MRI* can identify changes in the size of the organ, perfusion, and function. *Tissue biopsy* is done to confirm rejection.

MyNursingKit | TransWeb

Treatment

Medications used to prevent infection may be ordered prior to and after the transplant. Both antibiotics and antiviral medications may be used. Following the transplant, immunosuppressive drugs are prescribed to prevent rejection. Typical immunosuppressive medications are anti-inflammatories such as corticosteroids (prednisone, Solu-Medrol). These medications have serious side effects, including poor wound healing, increased susceptibility to infection, and fluid retention. Cytotoxic medications such as Imuran or cyclosporine are instrumental in preventing rejection of a transplanted organ or tissue.

NURSING CARE

PRIORITIZING NURSING CARE

When caring for clients with organ transplants, focus your care on preventing infection and early detection of rejection. Use aseptic technique at all times and sterile technique as ordered to help prevent infection. Inform family and visitors of restrictions, such as reverse isolation, if ordered. Monitor the client closely for signs of tissue rejection: elevated lab values (BUN, liver and cardiac enzymes, and bilirubin levels), decreasing blood pressure and increasing heart rate, or loss of function of the transplanted organ. Report significant lab changes immediately. Monitor for skin changes several months after a transplant and report immediately any rashes, hives, or peeling skin.

ASSESSING

The transplant client is assessed for signs and symptoms of potential rejection. Vital signs and laboratory texts are monitored closely, and any changes are reported to the physician. The incisional site is assessed for drainage, redness, edema, and pain.

DIAGNOSING, PLANNING, AND IMPLEMENTING

Possible nursing diagnoses for the client with an organ transplant include:

- *Risk for Fluid Volume Imbalance*
- *Risk for Infection*
- *Impaired Skin Integrity*

Outcomes for clients with organ transplants include the following:

- Client will maintain normal fluid balance.
- Client will be free from infection.
- Client will maintain intact skin.

Clients who have had transplant surgery require careful, attentive nursing care, including the following interventions:

- Document drainage from the incisional site, pain, and signs of inflammation. *Medications such as steroids may mask the signs of inflammation, so the first sign of infection should be reported immediately.*
- Ensure that staff maintains handwashing and aseptic technique during the delivery of client care. *The client has a lowered resistance to disease. Transfer of pathogenic organisms can easily result.*
- Institute reverse isolation if ordered. *Reverse isolation may be considered to safeguard the client's environment.*
- Institute routine postoperative care including turning, deep breathing and coughing, and early ambulation. *These measures help to avoid pulmonary complications.*
- Encourage a nutritious diet with supplements. *The client needs to meet increased energy requirements to heal.*
- Continue to observe for side effects of medications. *Side effects could interfere with healing and the success of the transplant.*

EVALUATING

The client who has undergone a transplant is continuously evaluated for any signs of infection and organ rejection. Observations regarding organ function and laboratory value changes are essential. The client's understanding of his or her medication regime will promote compliance. Knowledge about ways to avoid exposure to infection promotes healing and the transplant's continued function.

Autoimmune Disorders

In **autoimmune disorders** the body is unable to recognize normal cells and perceives them as foreign. It initiates an immune response and targets normal cells to be destroyed. Autoantibodies attack the body, causing inflammation and damage to the cells, tissues, and organs. A systemic autoimmune disorder causes multiple organ involvement.

Autoimmune diseases are more prevalent in females, and prevalence increases with age. In some diseases there is a familial connection, and clients can develop more than one disorder. Some common autoimmune disorders are rheumatoid arthritis (see Chapter 61), systemic lupus erythematosus (SLE), myasthenia gravis (see Chapter 36), and scleroderma, all discussed later in this chapter.

The pathophysiology of autoimmune disorders is unknown. Non-Western clients may have ideas about the cause of their symptoms that challenge Western thinking (Box 35-5 ■).

Manifestations

Symptoms are characteristic of the organ and cells being attacked. Therefore, symptoms can be insidious and vague, often leading to delayed diagnosis or misdiagnosis. Some

Epidemiology or Evil Eye

Western medicine studies the distribution and causes of disease (who gets a disease and what causes it?) and calls this *epidemiology*. We search for the cause of disease (the agent) and try to learn about the relationship among the host, agent, and the environment to understand how disease spreads. We never describe the causative agent as a person.

Some cultures, though, have a traditional view of epidemiology. To them, illness is caused by "soul loss" or "spells." You may encounter clients who cannot accept the idea of a malfunction of the immune system, but who blame their illness on witchcraft, voodoo, or some other form of magic. To people with this worldview, the way to prevent illness is not to provoke the wrath of one's friends, neighbors, and enemies.

The nurse needs to be aware that Western teaching about how a client acquires a disease may fall on deaf ears. For clients with traditional health beliefs, the "evil eye" is a contributing factor that is as real as bacteria and viruses. The healthcare provider must keep an open mind in order to provide useful care to the client who retains traditional beliefs.

common symptoms observed are fever, pain, and fatigue. Acute episodes (*exacerbations*) can then be followed by asymptomatic periods (*remissions*). Lengths of remission time diminish as the disease progresses. There is currently no cure. The goal of care is to control the disease.

Diagnosis

Diagnosis of autoimmune disorders is made based on lab tests such as serum assays to determine the level of antibodies in the body. An *ANA (antinuclear antibody) test* is ordered to screen for SLE. An *LE prep* (lupus erythematosus) is used to detect SLE and to monitor treatment. A positive LE prep may also be seen in rheumatoid arthritis. *RF (rheumatoid factor)* is present in 80% of those afflicted with rheumatoid arthritis.

Treatment

Treatment for autoimmune disorders is based on relieving symptoms and delaying the progression of the disease. A variety of anti-inflammatory medications may be ordered. Aspirin, nonsteroidal anti-inflammatory drugs (NSAIDs), and corticosteroids decrease inflammation. COX-2 inhibitors work to block enzymes released during inflammation. Celecoxib (Celebrex) is used as an anti-inflammatory and is known to relieve pain with one dose for up to 24 hours. Celebrex came under intense scrutiny in 2004 by the FDA because of the COX-2 inhibitor investigations. Another popular medication (rofecoxib or Vioxx) was recently voluntarily withdrawn from the market because of studies showing an increased incidence of heart attack and stroke in clients using the drug. Antirheumatics are used for clients with rheumatoid arthritis and include Plaquenil (hydroxychloroquine)

and gold salts. Cytotoxic medications are used to treat cancers and prevent organ transplantation rejection.

MYASTHENIA GRAVIS

Myasthenia gravis (MG) is a chronic autoimmune neuromuscular disease. The name literally means "grave muscle weakness." MG is characterized by varying degrees of voluntary or striated muscle weakness, which increases during periods of activity and improves with periods of rest. The muscles that control breathing, as well as neck and limb muscles, may be affected. Most people with MG have an average life span. MG occurs in all ethnic groups and both genders. It most commonly affects young women under age 40 and men over age 60. However, it can occur at any age. MG is not directly inherited nor is it contagious. Some clients may have a family history of the disease.

Myasthenia gravis is caused by a defect in nerve impulse transmission to the muscles (see discussion in Chapter 36). Normal communication between the nerve and muscle is interrupted at the *neuromuscular junction*, the place where nerve cells connect with the muscles they control. In MG, antibodies produced by the body's immune system block the acetylcholine receptors at the neuromuscular junction, preventing muscle contraction. One possible explanation for this is that the thymus gland is sending inaccurate messages about the acetylcholine receptor antibodies, so the body mistakenly attacks itself.

Manifestations

Signs and symptoms of MG may occur abruptly and may not be recognized as MG immediately. The first muscles that may be affected control the eyes, eyelid movement, facial expression, and swallowing. Slurred speech may be the first sign of the disorder. The degree of muscle weakness varies greatly, from a localized form that affects the eyes to a generalized form that includes the larger muscles that control breathing. Eye drooping (ptosis), blurred vision, and double vision (diplopia) may be noted (see Figure 36-24). Other symptoms include an unstable gait; weakness in arms, hands, fingers, legs, and neck; changes in facial expression; and shortness of breath. The client experiences periods of remission and exacerbation. Exacerbations may be triggered by emotional upset, trauma, and major health changes (pregnancy, secondary illness, surgery). Drugs (including muscle relaxants, magnesium, and some aminoglycoside antibiotics) can block nerve transmission at the neuromuscular junction.

Major complications occurring with MG include aspiration, respiratory infections, and respiratory failure. *Myasthenic crisis* (see Chapter 36) can result from medication noncompliance or ineffective dosages of prescribed medications (too little or too much). When myasthenic crisis occurs, the client can go into respiratory failure and be unable to speak or swallow. Overmedication can result in cholinergic crisis. Both of these crises are medical emergencies. The symptoms of cholinergic crisis are similar to those for myasthenic crisis.

Diagnosis

MG is difficult to diagnose because weakness is a general symptom of many disorders. The physician assesses any changes in eye movements or muscular weakness. A simple *eye exam* tests the client's ability to look upward for 2 to 3 minutes. If an increase of **ptosis** (drooping of the eyelid) occurs, MG is a probable diagnosis. With rest the client is able to open eyelids normally. An *intravenous injection of Tensilon* (anti-cholinesterase) is administered in one test for MG. If muscle strength improves dramatically, MG is diagnosed. Unfortunately, this improvement is a temporary situation. If the client's symptoms get worse after the injection of Tensilon, a cholinergic crisis can occur. A laboratory *blood test* is performed to check for the presence of acetylcholine receptor antibodies. These antibodies are found in a large percentage of clients with MG, although they may not always be seen in clients suffering from ocular forms of MG.

Electromyography (EMG) is ordered to rule out other disorders. A *nerve conduction test* records weakening muscle responses when the nerves are stimulated repeatedly. A *CT* scan and *MRI* tests are used to identify thymus gland changes or presence of a **thymoma** (a tumor in the thymus gland). *Pulmonary function tests* are used to measure breathing strength and help predict respiratory failure that can lead to myasthenic crisis.

Treatment

Treatment is focused on controlling the disease. Currently there is no cure. Therapies are aimed at reducing and improving muscle weakness. Medications used to treat the disorder are anticholinesterase agents such as neostigmine and pyridostigmine that improve neuromuscular transmission and increase muscle strength. Immunosuppressive drugs include prednisone, cyclosporine, and azathioprine. They are also used to improve muscle strength by suppressing the production of antibodies.

A *thymectomy* is a surgical procedure to remove the thymus gland. A thymectomy improves symptoms approximately 50% of the time. *Plasmapheresis* is a procedure in which antibodies are removed from the blood. This therapy offers relief for a few weeks. A high dose of intravenous immune globulin (IVIG) is given to infuse normal antibodies from donated blood. Most clients with MG who follow treatment regimens can expect to lead normal or nearly normal lives. Some cases go into remission temporarily, and muscle weakness may disappear completely for some time.

Nursing Considerations

When caring for a client with myasthenia gravis, focus your care on preventing complications. Monitor respiratory status closely, reporting signs of infection or aspiration. Monitor pulse oximetry to determine effectiveness of respiratory function. Assess the client carefully for signs of myasthenic crisis, which can be caused by medications. If the client has difficulty breathing, swallowing, or speaking, institute emergency measures immediately.

SYSTEMIC LUPUS ERYTHEMATOSUS

Systemic lupus erythematosus (SLE) gets its name from a facial rash that resembles a wolf bite. (*Lupus* is a Latin word meaning "wolf." The term *erythematosus* means "reddened skin.") The reddened facial rash appears in a butterfly-shaped pattern across the bridge of the nose and cheeks (Figure 35-13 ■). SLE is thought to be an autoimmune disease because autoantibodies are produced. These antibodies and corresponding antigen formation are then released in the connective tissue of the blood vessels, lymphatic system, and other tissues. Any body system or organ can be affected. Early symptoms mimic those of rheumatoid arthritis, with client complaints of joint pain. This disease was at one time called "the great imitator" because many of its symptoms are similar to those of other diseases. For example, clients with the skin disorder *rosacea* also display a rash similar to the characteristic butterfly rash of SLE. The client experiences remissions and exacerbations of the symptoms. Lupus can be drug induced. Symptoms similar to those of SLE typically reverse when the drug is discontinued.

SLE is a chronic inflammatory connective tissue disease. The cause is unknown. However, familial, environmental, and hormonal factors may play a role in disease development. SLE is found more commonly in young women than

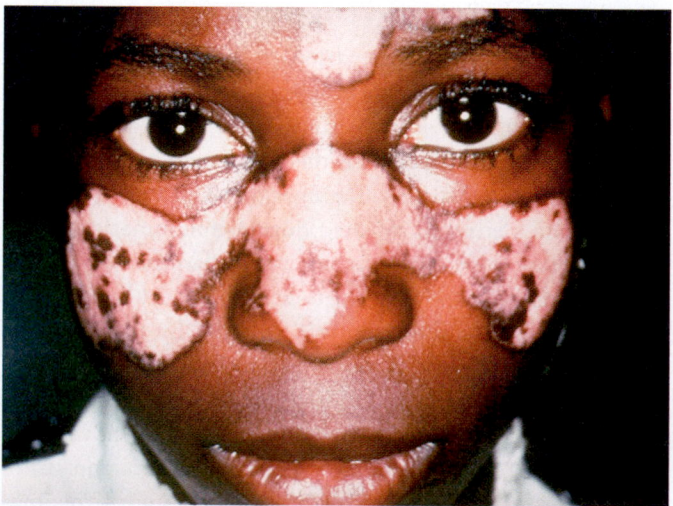

Figure 35-13. ■ The butterfly rash of systemic lupus erythematosus.

in men. It affects those of Hispanic, Asian, and African ethnicity more often. Systemic lupus affects major body organs and systems. It is a progressive disorder and can be life threatening if not treated. *Discoid lupus erythematosus* (DLE) affects only the skin and is not life threatening. The mortality rate for clients with SLE has improved, and life expectancy is normal with treatment.

Manifestations

The symptoms, other than the butterfly mask-like rash and joint pain already mentioned, can range from mild to severe. Fever, anorexia, malaise, weight loss, chest pain, joint stiffness, and inflammation can be found. *Raynaud's phenomenon* can cause the client to have pale or purple fingers or toes due to cold or stress. The clients are photosensitive and develop skin rashes on areas that are exposed to the sun. Exacerbations can be triggered by sun exposure, as well as by physical and emotional stress. Because SLE is systemic, the disease may affect many body systems. The kidneys, lungs, central nervous system, blood vessels, and cardiovascular system can be affected. Approximately 50% of clients with SLE will develop renal problems such as proteinuria or nephrotic syndrome.

Diagnosis

Diagnosis is based on the client's history and symptoms, as well as on diagnostic testing. Diagnosis includes ruling out other possible disorders such as rheumatoid arthritis or rosacea. Typically, an antinuclear antibody (*ANA*) test is done first. Clients with SLE test positive, although many persons who have a positive ANA do not have SLE. An *anti-DNA antibody* test is usually positive and is more specific for SLE. The *erythrocyte sedimentation rate (ESR)* is often increased, indicating inflammation. A *CBC* may show anemia, leukopenia, and low platelets (thrombocytopenia). Other tests may be performed specific to the organ function that is affected. *Biopsy* of skin lesions and kidneys may be done for signs of inflammation.

Treatment

There is no specific treatment for SLE. Most treatments are aimed at reducing the inflammatory effects of the disease and treating symptoms. Treatments for SLE have to be individualized to the client's needs and often change as the disease progresses. A **rheumatologist,** a physician specializing in inflammatory disorders, is often the specialist treating immune system disorders. Other physicians may be consulted as the disease affects the different organs and systems. The goals of treatment are to prevent exacerbations, to treat them as they occur, and to minimize organ damage and complications.

Medications such as NSAIDs have been shown to decrease fever and joint and chest pain. NSAIDs can be used alone or in combination with other medications to control pain and swelling in the joints. Antimalarials are another type of drug used to treat lupus. Hydroxychloroquine (Plaquenil) is the most common drug used to combat joint pain, skin rashes, and inflammation of the lungs. With continuous treatment, Plaquenil has been found to extend periods of remission and limit the length of an outbreak. Corticosteroids (such as prednisone and Medrol) work by rapidly suppressing inflammation and are a commonly prescribed treatment during acute episodes. These drugs are very potent and are used cautiously at a low dose to avoid severe side effects. Immunosuppressives such as azathioprine (Imuran) may be ordered to block the immune system. Methotrexate has an antirheumatic action (it is also an antineoplastic but in this disease its effect is antirheumatic) and may be used to control the condition. Chiropractic and homeopathy are alternative forms of treatment.

Nursing Considerations

When caring for a client with SLE, focus your care on helping the client manage the symptoms. Instruct the client to avoid sun exposure to help prevent the facial rash. Encourage the client to find ways to manage stress and to get plenty of rest to help control symptoms. Monitor the client for changes in vital signs and signs of inflammation such as redness, swelling, and elevated WBC levels. Protect the client with impaired immune function from exposure to pathogens. Help the client identify a treatment plan that keeps joint pain under control. This may include exercise, medication, and hydrotherapy. Assess the client for signs of cardiac or lung involvement, such as pleuritic pain, shortness of breath, or tachycardia. Report any of these findings to the physician.

PROGRESSIVE SYSTEMIC SCLEROSIS (SCLERODERMA)

Progressive systemic sclerosis (PSS) is more often known as scleroderma and is derived from the Greek words *sklerosis,* meaning "hardness," and *derma,* meaning "skin." **Scleroderma** literally means *hard skin.* It involves the abnormal growth of connective tissue that supports the skin and internal organs. It is characterized by hardened, tight, shiny skin. It is likely to be an autoimmune disease, because abnormal antibodies damage healthy tissue. In some clients, only the skin is involved. Other clients have symptoms similar to lupus, because it also affects the blood vessels and internal organs, including the heart, lungs, and kidneys.

PSS is not as common as lupus, but the mortality rate is higher. It affects women four times more often than men and usually is diagnosed between the ages of 30 and 50. Remissions and exacerbations are common. Research suggests that exposure to environmental factors may trigger the disease. Viral infections, adhesive and coating materials, and organic solvents may activate the disease. Silicon was also suspected when it was used for breast implants, but no concrete evidence has surfaced to provide a connection.

Manifestations

The first symptoms that clients with PSS may complain of are arthritis, fatigue, and pitting edema. As the disease progresses, they may have all or some of the symptoms that doctors refer to as CREST (**c**alcinosis, **R**aynaud's, **e**sophageal dysfunction, **s**clerodactyly, **t**elangiectasis):

- **Calcinosis,** the formation of calcium deposits in the connective tissue, is usually found in fingers, hands, face, trunk, and on the skin above the elbows and knees. These calcium deposits break through the skin, causing painful ulcers.
- **Raynaud's phenomenon,** a condition that causes the small blood vessels of the hands and feet to contract in response to cold or anxiety, results in the hands or feet turning white and cold, and then turning blue. (See discussion in Chapter 33 ⬤⬤.) As the blood flow returns, extremities become red, and the fingertips can suffer damage, leading to ulcers, scars, and gangrene.
- **Esophageal dysfunction** occurs when the smooth muscles lose normal peristalsis. If found in the upper esophagus, it can cause swallowing difficulties. When it is in the lower esophagus, it causes heartburn and inflammation.
- **Sclerodactyly** results from deposits of excess collagen with the skin layers. The skin appears thick, tight, shiny, and can be darkly pigmented. The facial skin loses elasticity and is pulled taut, becoming expressionless and masklike. Sclerodactyly causes difficulty bending and straightening the fingers.
- **Telangiectasis** also occurs, which is the development of small, painless, red spider-like spots on the hands and face caused by the swelling of tiny capillaries.

Diagnosis

Diagnosis is largely based on medical history and findings from the physical examination. Two antibodies might be found in the blood of clients with PSS, *anti-Scl-70* and *anticentromere*. However, not all people with the antibodies have scleroderma, and lab test results alone are not conclusive. A *skin biopsy* may be ordered, although the biopsy cannot distinguish between localized and systemic disease.

Treatment

Treatment is focused on delaying the progression of the disease process. Steroids and immunosuppressant drugs are used in large doses when exacerbation is evident. Treatment is symptom driven and is managed as the need arises.

Nursing Considerations

When caring for clients with PSS, focus your care on managing the client's symptoms. Keep skin clean and dry,

applying mild moisturizers. Take special care to prevent skin tears, cuts, or ulcerations. Any open area should be reported immediately and orders obtained for treatment. Encourage clients to avoid exposure to cold to help decrease Raynaud's phenomenon. Offer frequent small meals of bland foods to avoid esophageal irritation.

NURSING CARE

PRIORITIZING NURSING CARE

Monitor and report signs and symptoms, including hypertension, vascular insufficiency, and gastrointestinal distress. Monitor labs, especially renal and respiratory function, as well as antinuclear antibodies (often elevated in PSS). Make sure anti-inflammatory and immunosuppressant medications are administered as ordered. Teach the client to avoid sun exposure. Remind client not to smoke. Avoid prolonged exposure to cool or cold temperatures. Remind client to report numbness, tingling, and pain in the extremities. Stress the importance of physical therapy and moderate activity to maintain function and mobility. Encourage support group participation. Death usually occurs as a result of cardiac, pulmonary, or renal failure.

ASSESSING

Clients with immune disorders are assessed for symptoms of fatigue, muscle pain, and muscle weakness, as well as for specific symptoms of individual diseases. It is also important to assess the client's stress level and coping strategies because autoimmune disorders can be exacerbated by stress. The client's level of pain should be determined, as well as the effectiveness or ineffectiveness of previously used pain relief measures.

DIAGNOSING, PLANNING, AND IMPLEMENTING

Possible nursing diagnoses for clients with autoimmune disorders include:

- *Acute Pain*
- *Impaired Physical Mobility*
- *Risk for Aspiration*
- *Risk for Infection*
- *Risk for Impaired Skin Integrity*
- *Disturbed Body Image*
- *Ineffective Coping*

Examples of desired outcomes for these clients might include:

- Client states pain is controlled with medication.
- Client is able to perform activities of daily living (ADLs) with assistive devices.
- Client is able to maintain patent airway.

For All Clients with Autoimmune Disorders

The LPN/LVN assists the registered nurse in providing support to the client.

- Focus instruction on stress reduction, nutrition, and medication. Encourage the client to include rest periods during the day. *It is important to reduce stress and maintain good nutrition in order to promote stability of the disease. The client will be better able to avoid exacerbations if he or she avoids fatigue.*
- Provide consistent pain management. *Consistent pain management allows the client to continue performing ADLs.*
- Encourage exercises that suit the level and tolerance of the client. *Exercise keeps mobility at an optimal level and promotes self-esteem.*
- Allow the client to verbalize anxiety and discuss past coping strategies that have been successful. *Verbalizing successes of the past will help the client develop new ways of coping.*
- Keep nonverbal communication neutral. *A neutral manner will avoid causing the client to feel self-conscious about appearance.*
- Instruct clients to avoid people with infections. *Infections are a threat to the client's compromised immune system.*
- If possible, refer the client and family to local support groups. *Support groups can provide valuable assistance in coping with the long-term effects of the illness.*
- Teach the client and family about the disease process. *Knowledge empowers them to make informed decisions.*

For Clients with Myasthenia Gravis

- Assess the client for changes in muscle weakness, slurred speech, swallowing difficulties, and vision. Direct care at decreasing or preventing respiratory and swallowing difficulties. *Muscles used in breathing and swallowing are affected by the disease.*
- Encourage the client to reduce stress and fatigue. *This helps avoid exacerbations of MG.*
- Explore coping strategies with the family and client. *Stress can contribute to exacerbations.*
- Encourage family members to learn how to perform CPR and understand the importance of quick intervention. *They may need to provide immediate intervention in the event of respiratory failure or crisis.*
- Instruct the client to adhere strictly to the scheduled medication program. *Following the medication regimen closely will improve disease control.*
- Advise client to wear a medic alert bracelet or necklace. *The bracelet will signal healthcare workers of the special need of the client so that they can provide appropriate care.*

For Clients with SLE

The nurse plans care that is individualized and is dependent on the organ and system that is affected.

- Skin lesions are common symptoms of lupus that can be disfiguring. Encourage the client to avoid the sun and use a sunscreen with a sun protective factor (SPF) of 15 or greater, and to wear long sleeves and hats when outside. *These measures help to minimize sun exposure, which can cause exacerbations of skin lesions and symptomatic symptoms.*
- Discuss the client's fears and anxieties. Actively listen to the client's needs and questions. (Review listening skills in Chapter 11 ⬭ .) *Therapeutic listening decreases anxiety.*
- Instruct the client and family members about increased susceptibility to infections. *This information enables all visitors and staff to institute good handwashing and other policies to prevent spread of infection.*
- Use aseptic technique when performing procedures and wound care. *Aseptic technique decreases the chance of nosocomial infection.*
- Monitor vital signs and signs of inflammation. *Early detection allows for early intervention.*
- Observe for changes in laboratory values such as WBC levels, liver function, kidney function, and cardiac enzymes. *Changes in lab values could indicate worsening of the disease.*
- Institute reverse isolation if it is ordered. *Reverse isolation can protect the client from nosocomial infections.*
- Encourage adequate nutritional intake. *Client has an increased need for nutrition to assist with healing and immune function.*
- Provide oral hygiene. *This may improve the client's appetite and reduce the risk of oral infections.*

For Clients with PSS

- Focus care on maintaining skin integrity. Use mild soaps and moisturizers. Turn the client every 2 hours and use devices to prevent pressure to bony prominences. *These measures maintain integrity of the skin and prevent skin breakdown.*
- Monitor any skin wounds for healing. *This allows you to detect and report complications early.*
- Provide adequate nutrition. Determine the client's preferences, and have the family bring in favorite foods. *Adequate nutrition helps the body meet its energy needs.*
- Provide smaller, more frequent, bland meals. *Bland foods in small amounts will minimize any esophageal problems.*
- Institute effective pain management techniques such as distraction, medication, and imagery. *The client may need to use several techniques to relieve pain from Raynaud's phenomenon and vasculitis.*
- If foot pain is a problem, avoid placing heavy covers on the feet, and use a foot board or bed cradle. (See Figure 33-24 ⬭ .) *These devices help prevent extra pressure on the feet.*

- Keep the client's hands and feet warm with gloves and socks. *Keeping warm will decrease constriction of the blood vessels.*
- Administer medications as ordered to alleviate heartburn and reflux. *This decreases discomfort.*
- Communicate with physical and occupational therapy departments. *The nurse collaborates with these departments to help the client perform ADLs.*

EVALUATING

The client with SLE is evaluated for fatigue, pain, skin integrity impairment, and body image disturbances. The client with MG is evaluated frequently for respiratory distress, swallowing difficulties, medication compliance, and the reduction of fatigue and stress techniques. When evaluating the client with PSS, the nurse observes for CREST syndrome and the client's compliance with medication regime. Pain associated with Raynaud's phenomenon and diet modifications are reviewed for individualized results.

NURSING PROCESS CARE PLAN
Client with Systemic Lupus Erythematosus

Donna M. Harrison is a 24-year-old woman of Mexican descent. She has had complaints of joint pain and stiffness, which are also associated with swelling in the hands. She recently developed a facial rash covering the bridge of her nose and cheeks. Her face is reddened. Her coworkers keep asking if she has been out in the sun. Donna also complains that she is always tired and is concerned she may be anemic. Her primary physician ordered an ANA test and CBC with a sed rate. She was told that her ANA is positive, and she has a low RBC, WBC, and platelet count. The physician told her that she may have lupus and is going to refer her to a rheumatologist.

Assessment
Miss Harrison has exhibited some typical signs of systemic lupus erythematosus. Joint pain, inflammation, and the butterfly rash are consistent with SLE. SLE is commonly diagnosed in young women and commonly affects people of Hispanic, Asian, and African ancestries. Nearly all clients who have SLE are ANA positive. The CBC reflects a lowered RBC, which may provide the cause of Miss Harrison's fatigue and anemia. A rheumatologist specializes in the care of clients with systemic lupus erythematosus.

Diagnosis
The following important nursing diagnoses (among others) are established for this condition:

- *Deficient Knowledge* related to autoimmune disease and SLE
- *Anxiety*
- *Fatigue*

Expected Outcomes
The expected outcomes specify that Miss Harrison will:

- Be able to describe the pathology occurring in autoimmune disease.
- Identify basic signs and symptoms related to SLE.
- Understand the relationship between the sun's exposure and skin manifestations.
- Discuss the multisystem effects of SLE on body organs.
- Be able to describe signs of infection.
- Discuss strategies to avoid fatigue.

Planning and Implementation
The following nursing interventions are planned and implemented:

- Instruct the client regarding autoimmune disease and SLE.
- Provide the client with materials that she can read to supplement instruction.
- Ask the client questions to check for understanding.
- Discuss the photosensitivity effect of SLE and skin manifestations.
- Develop a plan to avoid fatigue and schedule activities when the client has rested beforehand.

Evaluation
A rheumatologist confirmed SLE. At follow-up, client says the written materials helped her understand SLE better. She is aware of the connection between sun exposure and the butterfly rash. She enlisted family to help with some of her errands so she can get more rest. She correctly named warning signs that could indicate infection. Referral to local support group provided.

Critical Thinking in the Nursing Process

1. Why should the client understand the pathophysiology involved in autoimmune disorders and SLE?
2. Why is it necessary for the client to be able to identify the signs and symptoms associated with SLE?
3. Why is the client with SLE protected from the sun?

Note: Discussion of Critical Thinking questions appears on the MyNursingKit Website.

Allergies

Although the immune system normally protects the body against foreign substances, sometimes it fails. Hypersensitivity to an antigen causes a harmful response in the client. Typical hypersensitivity may be mild, such as the runny nose and itchy eyes of hay fever. Extreme hypersensitivity may be severe, such as blood transfusion reactions and organ transplant rejections. There are four classes of hypersensitivity reactions:

- Level I is an *immediate response* related to foods, pollens, and insect bites. The body cells release histamine, which constricts smooth muscle and causes peripheral vasodilatation. This may lead to mild symptoms such as a rash or hives, or to severe symptoms such as anaphylaxis (see Chapter 47 ⬀⬀).
- Level II is *cytotoxic hypersensitivity* due to an incompatible blood transfusion. This triggers autoimmune destruction of the target cells and causes a systemic reaction.
- Level III is an *immune hypersensitivity* to horse antitoxin, bacteria, fungi, and viruses. An inflammatory process begins to form in the blood. Examples include serum sickness, SLE, and rheumatoid arthritis.
- Level IV is a *delayed hypersensitivity* response that is caused by chemicals or plants, fungi, and mycobacteria. The inflammatory response is activated but may be delayed for 24 to 72 hours after exposure. Examples of this include tissue transplant reaction and tuberculin skin test.

LATEX ALLERGY

A unique allergy that has had a profound effect on some healthcare workers as well as the general population is a hypersensitivity to latex. The chemicals used in processing the latex cause the reaction.

Manifestations

The client can have a Level I reaction (resulting in a reaction within minutes) or a Level IV reaction (resulting in delayed hypersensitivity). Symptoms may be mild, such as redness, hives, and itching, or they may be severe, including local symptoms and systemic signs (laryngospasm, wheezing, cardiac arrest, or anaphylaxis).

Diagnosis

To make the diagnosis of allergies, laboratory tests, such as a *radioallergosorbent test (RAST)*, are done to measure IgE levels of specific allergens. *Skin tests* (Figure 35-14 ■) may be used to identify specific allergens that cause hypersensitivity. The physician uses the client's history to determine which allergens to test. The allergen is applied to the skin through various methods, and the skin is then observed for a reaction. For a skin puncture test, a drop of the allergen is placed on the skin and then the skin is punctured or pricked. A positive reaction occurs when redness and wheal formation occur within 15 to 20 minutes. For an intradermal test, an injection of a small amount of solution containing the allergen is administered, usually on the forearm. It is monitored at specific intervals. A positive reaction is similar to the skin puncture reaction. A patch containing the allergen may also be secured to the skin for 48 hours. A positive reaction could range from redness to papules or vesicles.

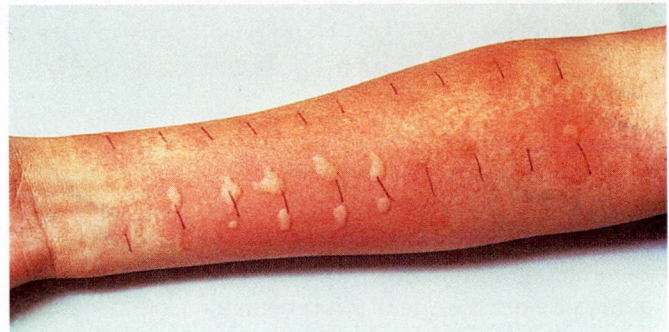

Figure 35-14. ■ Skin testing on the forearm showing induration and erythema typical of a positive response to an antigen. (*Source:* Southern Illinois University/Photo Researchers, Inc.)

Treatment

Once the offending allergens are identified, clients can try to avoid contact with them. Some medications can offer relief. Antihistamines block histamine receptors, alleviating runny nose (rhinitis), itchy eyes, hives, and other symptoms. Decongestants help open air passages. (*Note:* Overuse of decongestant nasal sprays can result in rebound congestion, making the medication ineffective.)

Corticosteroids are used systemically as well as topically for allergic responses (although the anti-inflammatory effect also masks inflammation, so they must be used cautiously). Epinephrine is used in severe reactions.

Allergy injections may be given to decrease sensitization. Small doses of the allergen are given on a routine schedule, allowing the body to develop antibodies to block the allergic response. This can be a lengthy process.

Nursing Considerations

The nurse gathers a detailed allergy history and directs care toward helping the client learn to avoid allergy reactions. The nurse documents the allergy and communicates data to the interdisciplinary healthcare team.

clinical ALERT

When medicating the client who is hypersensitive, the nurse must be attentive because the possibility of allergic response is heightened. Report symptoms of redness, hives, or respiratory distress immediately to the physician.

A second exposure increases the severity of a reaction. Treatment is implemented promptly. An anaphylaxis kit may be prescribed for the client to use when needed. Discharge instruction is reinforced with the client and family. A return demonstration ensures that the client and family member are proficient in proper use of the anaphylaxis kit in the home. Encourage the client to wear a medic alert bracelet or tag.

Note: The references and resources for all chapters have been compiled at the back of the book.

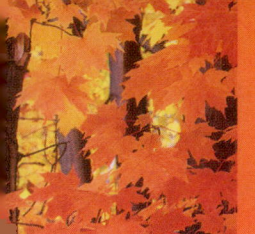

Chapter Review

KEY Points

- The immune system is a network of cells and organs that protects the body against infection and other foreign substances.

- The immune system does not work equally well throughout life. Before the age of 2 it is immature; in older adults, the immune system weakens. Some people have immune systems weakened by disease or stress.

- Autoimmune diseases occur when the body's own cells are not recognized properly and are perceived as foreign. The body then attacks the cells.

- There are two types of immunity: passive and active. Active immunity is acquired by developing the disease or through immunization. Passive immunity occurs when the client is injected with antibodies from animals or humans.

- HIV is caused by a retrovirus, meaning it reproduces in a reverse manner. Diagnosis of HIV infection depends on the client's history, risk factors, physical exam, and laboratory results. Nursing care is based on prevention, health maintenance, education, medication compliance, and support.

- Anaphylaxis is a medical emergency. Call 9-1-1. Keep the client calm and remain with the person until help arrives. If an EpiPen (epinephrine) is available, administer as ordered.

- Nursing care for the client with SLE focuses on maintenance of skin integrity and minimizing disfigurement, protection against infection, and health maintenance.

- Allergic reactions are a result of hypersensitivity to an antigen. Four response levels have been identified: immediate, cytotoxic, immune, or delayed.

∞ FOR FURTHER Study

For a review of listening skills, see Chapter 11.

See Chapter 33 for explanation of Raynaud's phenomenon.

Figure 33-24 shows an example of a bed cradle.

Normal laboratory blood values, bone marrow suppression, and hemolytic anemia are discussed in Chapter 34.

The eye drooping of myasthenia gravis is illustrated in Figure 36-24.

See Table 44-1 for cultural considerations in response to organ donation.

Skin grafts for burns and anaphylaxis are discussed in Chapter 47.

Contraceptive methods and their ability to protect against STIs are listed in Table 40-6.

See Table 59-5 for recommended immunizations for children and Table 59-7 for an example of oral candidiasis.

Rheumatoid arthritis is discussed in Chapter 61.

Caring for the Client with Myasthenia Gravis

NCLEX-PN® Focus Area: Physiologic Adaptation

Case Study: Deborah Joy French is a 25-year-old woman with a recent diagnosis of myasthenia gravis. She has been admitted to the hospital in myasthenic crisis. Miss French has complained of burning on urination for the past 3 days. She has felt hot but did not take her temperature. Today she had an increase in muscle weakness and has fallen down. She is having some trouble breathing and swallowing.

Nursing Diagnosis: *Ineffective Airway Clearance*

COLLECT DATA

Subjective	Objective
_____	_____
_____	_____
_____	_____
_____	_____
_____	_____
_____	_____
_____	_____

Would you report this? Yes/No

If yes, report to: _____

What would you report? _____

Nursing Care

_____
_____
_____
_____
_____
_____
_____
_____
_____
_____

How would you document this? _____
_____
_____
_____

Data Collected
(use only those that apply)

- VS: T 102.8, P 90, R 30, BP 140/88
- Height 5' 50
- Weight 105 lbs
- Skin pale, hot to the touch, cheeks red
- Urinary frequency, burning on urination
- Nasal flaring, dyspnea, use of accessory muscles
- Anxiety is noted
- WBC 15,500
- O_2 saturation at 86%
- Fatigue and weakness

Nursing Interventions
(use only those that apply; list in priority order)

- Place client in high-Fowler's position.
- Administer O_2 as ordered and monitor pulse oximetry.
- Auscultate breath sounds and monitor respiratory rhythm and rate.
- Monitor intake and output, documenting color, odor, and concentration.
- Assess pain levels.
- Turn every 2 hours.
- Use active ROM.
- Assess client for necessary ventilation assistance.
- Monitor VS every 4 hours and prn.
- Administer antipyretic for temperature/comfort.
- Assess the client's swallowing ability.
- Encourage fluids.
- Encourage client to turn, cough, and deep breathe.
- Monitor for restlessness and anxiety.
- Take daily weights.
- Suction as needed and document secretions.
- Provide emotional support.
- Monitor ABGs and WBC labs.
- Encourage ambulation.

Compare your answers and documentation to those provided on the MyNursingKit Website.

NCLEX-PN® Exam Preparation

1 The nurse, while conducting a class for staff nurses, explains that the primary component of the nonspecific and specific immune response begin as:

1. Stem cells from the bone marrow.
2. Leukocytes in the bloodstream.
3. White blood cells from the spleen.
4. Granulocytes from the bone marrow.

2 When a client has a positive reaction to an enzyme-linked immunosorbent assay (ELISA), the nurse anticipates the doctor will order:

1. Medications to treat HIV.
2. A second ELISA test.
3. A Western blot test.
4. Further testing for contagious diseases.

3 The nurse recognizes which of the following diagnoses as an indicator of possible HIV?

1. Kaposi's sarcoma
2. Cryptosporidium
3. Influenza
4. *Pneumocystis jireveci (carinii)* pneumonia

4 The nurse is caring for a client with an infection and anticipates which of the following?

1. Lower IgM
2. Lower IgA
3. Elevated IgG
4. Normal IgG and elevated IgA

5 While caring for a client following a bone marrow transplant, the nurse recognizes which of the following symptoms as a possible indication of graft versus host disease?

1. Urticaria on the palms of the hands and the soles of the feet
2. Nausea and vomiting that do not respond to treatment
3. Acute sporadic pain in the left upper abdominal quadrant
4. Swollen glands in the neck, axillae, and groin areas

6 The client develops influenza. After the client has recovered from the virus, the nurse explains to the client that he or she now has:

1. Natural active immunity.
2. Artificial active immunity.
3. Natural acquired immunity.
4. Artificial acquired passive immunity.

7 The nurse, working in a physician's office, administers an immunization to a child via parenteral injection. The parent is instructed to wait in the office for 20 minutes. Ten minutes after receiving the immunization, the nurse recognizes which of the following symptoms as requiring immediate intervention?

1. Hives over the extremities with complaints of pruritus
2. Numbness and tingling of the lips and tongue
3. Rhinorrhea and watering eyes
4. Complaints of pain at the injection site without edema or erythema

8 Shortly after the nurse begins administering a blood transfusion, the client shows signs and symptoms of a hypersensitivity reaction. The nurse recognizes this reaction as what level of hypersensitivity?

1. Level I
2. Level II
3. Level III
4. Level IV

9 The client complains of arm pain after the nurse administers an immunization intermuscularly in the deltoid muscle. The nurse's priority response would be to:

1. Tell the client the discomfort will go away shortly.
2. Encourage the client to exercise the arm lightly.
3. Put ice packs on the injection site.
4. Advise the client that discomfort indicates the immunization was effective.

10 The nurse is teaching a class on progressive systemic sclerosis and correctly explains that:

1. This disease only affects the skin.
2. Scleroderma is more common than lupus and is underdiagnosed.
3. The mortality rate for scleroderma is higher than that for lupus.
4. Scleroderma does not go into remission once symptoms begin.

Answers and rationales for Review Questions appear in Appendix I.

Chapter 36

Clients with Neurosensory System Disorders

LEARNING Outcomes

After completing this chapter, you will be able to:

1. Describe the structure and function of the central and peripheral nervous systems.
2. Identify common tests and procedures for diagnosis and treatment of clients with neurosensory disorders.
3. Name important considerations in collecting data about neurologic disorders.
4. Identify important considerations in nursing care of clients with neurosensory disorders.
5. Name signs and symptoms of increased intracranial pressure.
6. Describe nursing interventions for clients with increased intracranial pressure.
7. Identify common types of cerebrovascular disorders and nursing care.
8. Name the types of seizures and describe nursing care for a client with seizures.
9. Describe infections of the nervous system and nursing care for them.
10. Identify common injuries to the neurologic system, treatment, and nursing care.
11. Review common tumors and discuss treatment and nursing care.
12. Name four major degenerative neurologic diseases and discuss their nursing care.
13. Identify the manifestations and nursing care for peripheral and cranial nerve disorders.
14. Identify common visual and hearing disorders and their treatments.

Clinical Objectives

15. Implement nursing care for the client having a seizure.
16. Provide care for a client during the acute stage of a CVA.
17. Observe a client following TPA administration.
18. Assist a client with a brain injury to use alternative communication.

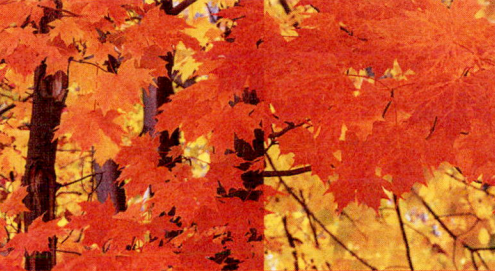

BRIEF Outline

Structure and Function of the Nervous System
Neurologic Testing
Increased Intracranial Pressure
Cerebrovascular Disorders
Seizure Disorders
Infections of the Neurologic System
Neurosensory Trauma and Tumors
Degenerative Neurologic Disorders
Peripheral Nervous System Disorders
Cranial Nerve Disorders
Disorders of Vision and Hearing

Use the audio glossary feature on the MyNursingKit Website to hear the correct pronunciation of the following key terms.

The nervous system is composed of complex structures that transmit electrical and chemical signals between the brain and the body's many organs. It is responsible (1) for the body's ability to interact with the environment and (2) for regulating functions involving internal organs. Although the nervous system functions as a unified whole, it is easier to study by dividing it into structural and functional classifications. Once these groups of structures and functions are understood, it is quite easy to understand (or picture) what the different neurologic disorders are and how they affect the body.

Structure and Function of the Nervous System

Structurally the nervous system is divided into the **central nervous system** (CNS) and the **peripheral nervous system** (PNS). The central nervous system is composed of the brain and the spinal cord, which act as the command and integration centers of the nervous system (Figure 36-1 ■). The CNS is where information or stimuli are analyzed and responses generated. The CNS is also the site of thought, reasoning,

and memory. The information that the CNS receives comes from the PNS. The peripheral nervous system is divided into the cranial nerves and the peripheral, or spinal, nerves (Figure 36-2 ■). The cranial nerves convey impulses to and from the brain. The peripheral nerves convey impulses to and from the spinal cord. Both sets of nerves serve as communication lines linking all parts of the body to the central nervous system. They carry impulses from the sensory receptors to the CNS and from the CNS to the appropriate glands or muscles. The PNS has a vast number of receptors, which are used to gather information about the outside world.

Peripheral nerves are divided into **sensory** (or **afferent**/ascending) pathways that carry impulses toward the CNS and **motor** (or **efferent**/descending) pathways that carry impulses from the CNS to skeletal muscles, glands, and effector organs. *Effector organs* are organs such as the heart or pancreas that are innervated by specific components of the nervous system.

Functionally the peripheral nervous system is divided into the somatic nervous system and the autonomic nervous system. The **somatic nervous system** consists of pathways that regulate *voluntary* control (such as that needed to lift this

(Text continues on p. 937.)

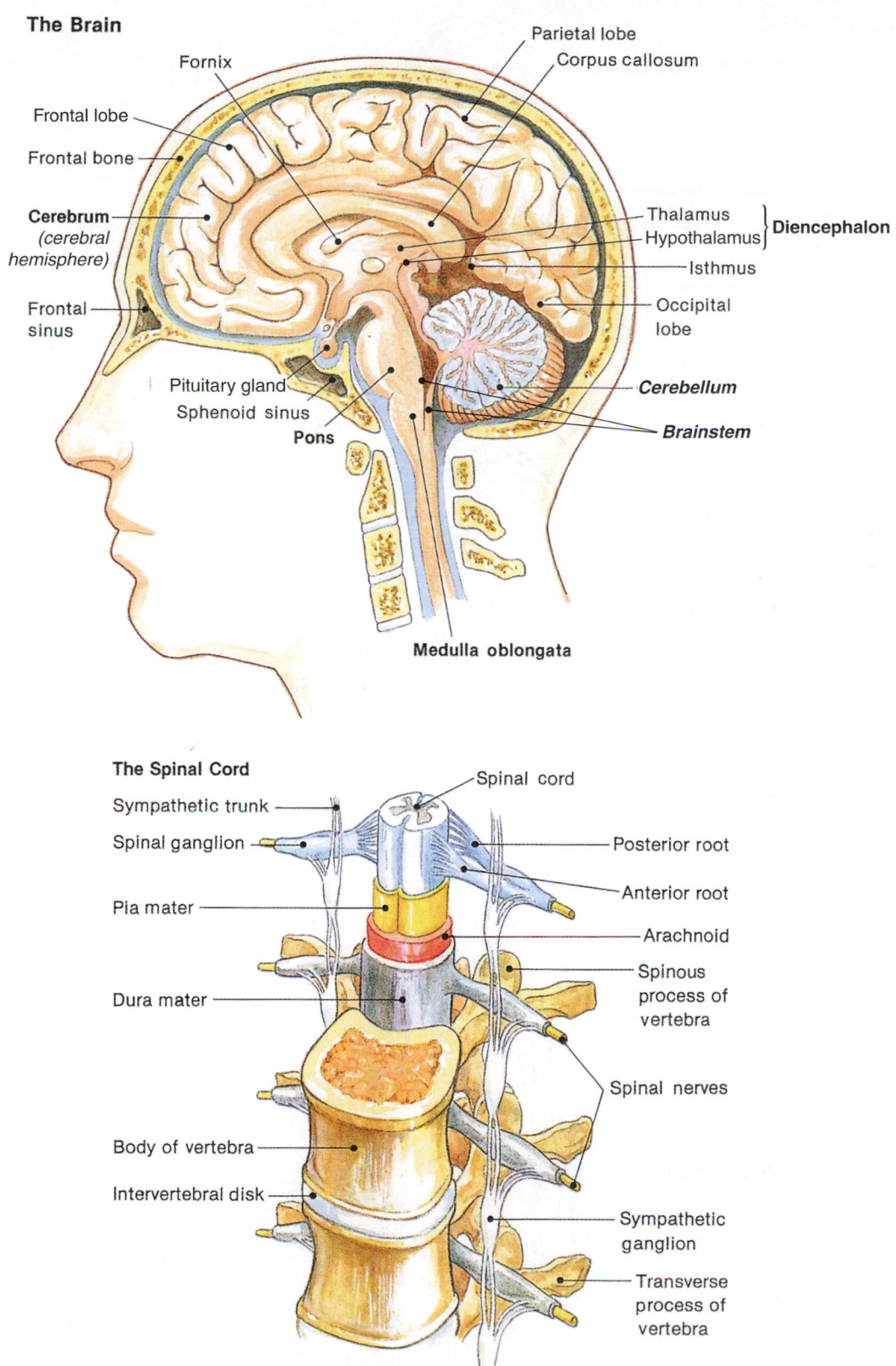

Figure 36-1. ■ The central nervous system is composed of the brain and the spinal cord, which act together to control the nervous system.

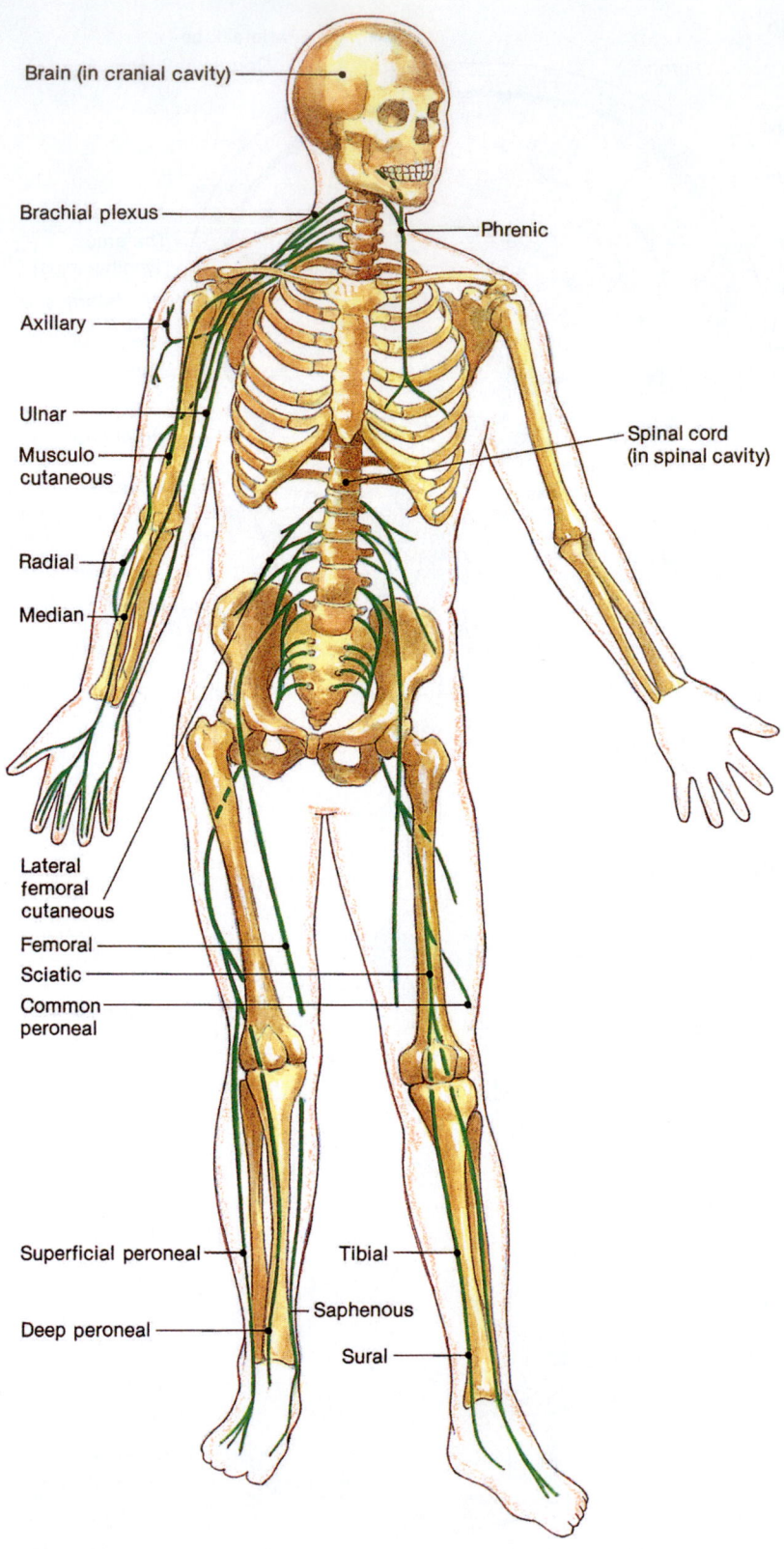

Brain (in cranial cavity)

Brachial plexus

Phrenic

Axillary

Ulnar

Musculo cutaneous

Spinal cord (in spinal cavity)

Radial

Median

Lateral femoral cutaneous

Femoral

Sciatic

Common peroneal

Superficial peroneal

Tibial

Saphenous

Deep peroneal

Sural

Figure 36-2. ■ Nerves of the body. Peripheral nervous system.

book) of skeletal muscles. The **autonomic nervous system** regulates automatic or *involuntary* control of organ systems (such as cardiac muscle and glands). The autonomic nervous system can be further subdivided into the sympathetic and parasympathetic nervous systems (discussed further below).

NERVOUS TISSUE

Two principal types of cells make up nervous tissue: neurons and supporting cells.

Neurons

Nerve cells are called **neurons** and are specialized to transmit nerve impulses (messages) from one part of the body to another. They work alone or in units to detect environmental changes and to initiate body responses to maintain an active, steady state. Neurons differ structurally, yet have common features (Figure 36-3 ■). All neurons consist of:

- A *cell body*, which contains the nucleus that regulates the function of the cell, and one or more processes or fibers extending from the cell body.
- **Dendrites,** neuron processes that conduct electrical currents toward the cell body.
- **Axons,** single fibers that carry nerve impulses away from the cell body.

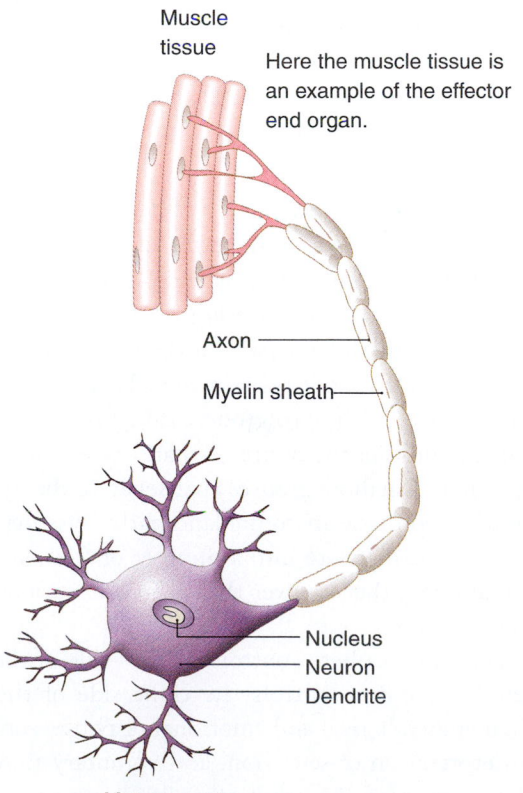

Muscle tissue

Here the muscle tissue is an example of the effector end organ.

Axon

Myelin sheath

Nucleus
Neuron
Dendrite

Motor neuron

Figure 36-3. ■ Structures of the neuron. The *dendrites* bring information to the nucleus. The *axon* carries messages away from the nerve cell.

Neurons have only one axon, but they may have hundreds of branching dendrites, depending on their type. The axons may occasionally give off a collateral branch along their length but all end in multiple branches known as *axonal terminals*. When an impulse reaches the axonal terminals, it stimulates the release of chemicals into the extracellular space (the synapse). These chemicals are called neurotransmitters. They either help an impulse to cross the synapse or stop it from crossing. Neurons are very close together but never actually touch each other. The tiny space that separates them is called the *synaptic cleft*. The **synapse** is the functional junction that "joins" one neuron to another (see discussion of neurotransmitters later). It is usually a chemical type of synapse. However, some neurons are physically joined by gap junctions, where electrical currents are able to flow directly from one neuron to the next.

Supporting Cells

The supporting cells in the central nervous system are **neuroglia.** They generally support, insulate, and protect the neurons. Each type of neuroglia has special functions.

Myelin is the whitish, fatty material that covers most long nerve fibers. It protects and insulates the fibers and increases the transmission rate of nerve impulses. Axons outside of the CNS are myelinated by Schwann cells (forming the myelin sheath). The **neurilemma** is the part of the Schwann cell (cell cytoplasm that ends up beneath the outermost part of the plasma membrane) external to the myelin sheath. The myelin sheath has indentations called nodes of Ranvier, which are formed by the many individual Schwann cells. The neurilemma plays an important role in fiber regeneration if it remains intact when a peripheral nerve fiber is damaged. The velocity of nerve impulses increases where myelin is present. The increased speed occurs because the myelin acts as an insulator that allows ions to flow between segments rather than along the entire length of the membrane. Disorders of the myelin sheath such as multiple sclerosis and Guillain-Barré syndrome, discussed later in the chapter, provide examples of the important role myelin plays in nerve function.

Neuroglia are structurally very similar to neurons. However, they are not able to conduct nerve impulses and they never lose their ability to divide. Because they can divide, most brain tumors are formed by neuroglia and are known as *gliomas*.

The Schwann cells and the satellite cells are the primary supporting cells of the peripheral nervous system. The Schwann cells form the myelin sheaths around nerve fibers found in the PNS, and the satellite cells protect and cushion cells.

Clusters of neuron cell bodies found in the CNS are called *nuclei*. They are well protected within the bony skull or vertebral column. This protection is essential since these neurons do not undergo cell division after birth. The cell body carries out most of the metabolic functions of these neurons. If the cell body is damaged and dies, it is not replaced. **Ganglia** are small collections of cell bodies found outside the CNS in the PNS. (See illustration of ganglia in Figure 36-1.) **Tracts** are bundles of nerve fibers that run through the CNS. These bundles are called nerves in the PNS. **White matter** is composed of dense collections of myelinated tracts. **Gray matter** consists mostly of unmyelinated fibers and cell bodies.

Functionally, neurons are classified according to the direction the nerve impulse is traveling in relation to the CNS. As mentioned earlier, sensory or afferent neurons carry impulses from sensory receptors in the internal organs or the skin to the CNS. The pain receptors are the least specialized. Cutaneous receptors are the most numerous and are actually bare dendrite endings.

Motor or efferent neurons carry impulses from the CNS to the viscera and/or muscles and glands. The motor neuron cell bodies are always located in the CNS. Association neurons or interneurons connect motor and sensory neurons in the neural pathways. Like motor neurons, their cell bodies are always located in the CNS.

Nerve Impulses

Electrical and chemical impulses are generated and conducted by neurons, which selectively change the electrical potential of the plasma membrane and influence other nearby neurons by the release of neurotransmitters (Figure 36-4 ■). A nerve impulse is a self-propagated electrical charge transmitted along the membrane of a nerve fiber. It is much like the electrical impulses that are carried along a telephone wire (Figure 36-5 ■). More than 30 neurotransmitters have been identified. Common selected neurotransmitters are described in Table 36-1 ■.

For electrical impulses to flow through the nervous system, a stimulus must occur. The stimulus raises a potential response (called the **action potential;** see Figure 36-5). If the stimulus is too weak, the membrane remains at rest (unexcited). This is often referred to as the *all-or-none response*—it either is conducted over the entire axon or it does not happen at all. The events that involve nerve impulse are:

- Polarization, which is the normal state of the resting neuron.
- Depolarization and generation of the action potential.
- Repolarization.

These three steps describe the movement of a nerve impulse along unmyelinated fibers. Fibers that have a myelin sheath conduct impulses much faster. The nerve impulse literally leaps from node to node along the length of the fiber.

Reflex Arc

Reflexes are rapid, predictable, and involuntary responses to stimuli. Once initiated, a reflex always goes in the same direction and occurs over neural pathways called *reflex arcs* (Figure 36-6 ■).

Reflexes can be classified as either autonomic or somatic reflexes. *Autonomic reflexes* regulate the activity of smooth muscles, the heart, and glands. Autonomic reflexes regulate body functions such as digestion, elimination, blood pressure, and sweating. The **sympathetic nervous system** responds, that is, activates the "fight-or-flight" response, to get the body moving in emergency or exciting situations. The **parasympathetic nervous system** calms and restores the body. The sympathetic nervous system assists the body in "fight-or-flight" situations. The parasympathetic nervous system returns the body to normal balance. Figure 36-7 ■ illustrates effects on organs of the sympathetic and parasympathetic nervous system. *Somatic reflexes* are the reflexes that stimulate the skeletal muscles.

clinical ALERT

Testing of reflexes is a valuable assessment tool in evaluating the condition of the nervous system. Nervous system disorders are indicated whenever reflexes are exaggerated, distorted, or absent. Often reflex changes occur before the pathologic condition has become obvious in other ways.

BRAIN

Cerebral Hemispheres

The brain can be discussed in terms of its four major regions: cerebral hemispheres, diencephalon (interbrain), brainstem, and cerebellum (see Figure 36-1). The cerebral hemispheres are the largest parts of the brain and cover the diencephalon and part of the brainstem. There is a right and a left hemisphere with deep grooves called *fissures* that separate large regions of the brain. *Gyri* are the elevated ridges and *sulci* are the shallow grooves that separate the gyri. Fissures and gyri provide anatomic landmarks. Fissures divide each cerebral hemisphere into a number of *lobes* named for the cranial bones that lie over them: frontal, parietal, temporal, and occipital.

The right hemisphere controls the left side of the body. The left hemisphere controls the right side of the body. Speech, memory, logical and emotional response, consciousness, interpretation of sensation, and voluntary movement are all functions of the cerebral cortex neurons. The left hemisphere is responsible for speech, problem solving, reasoning, and calculations. The right hemisphere controls the visual or spatial information such as art, music, and the

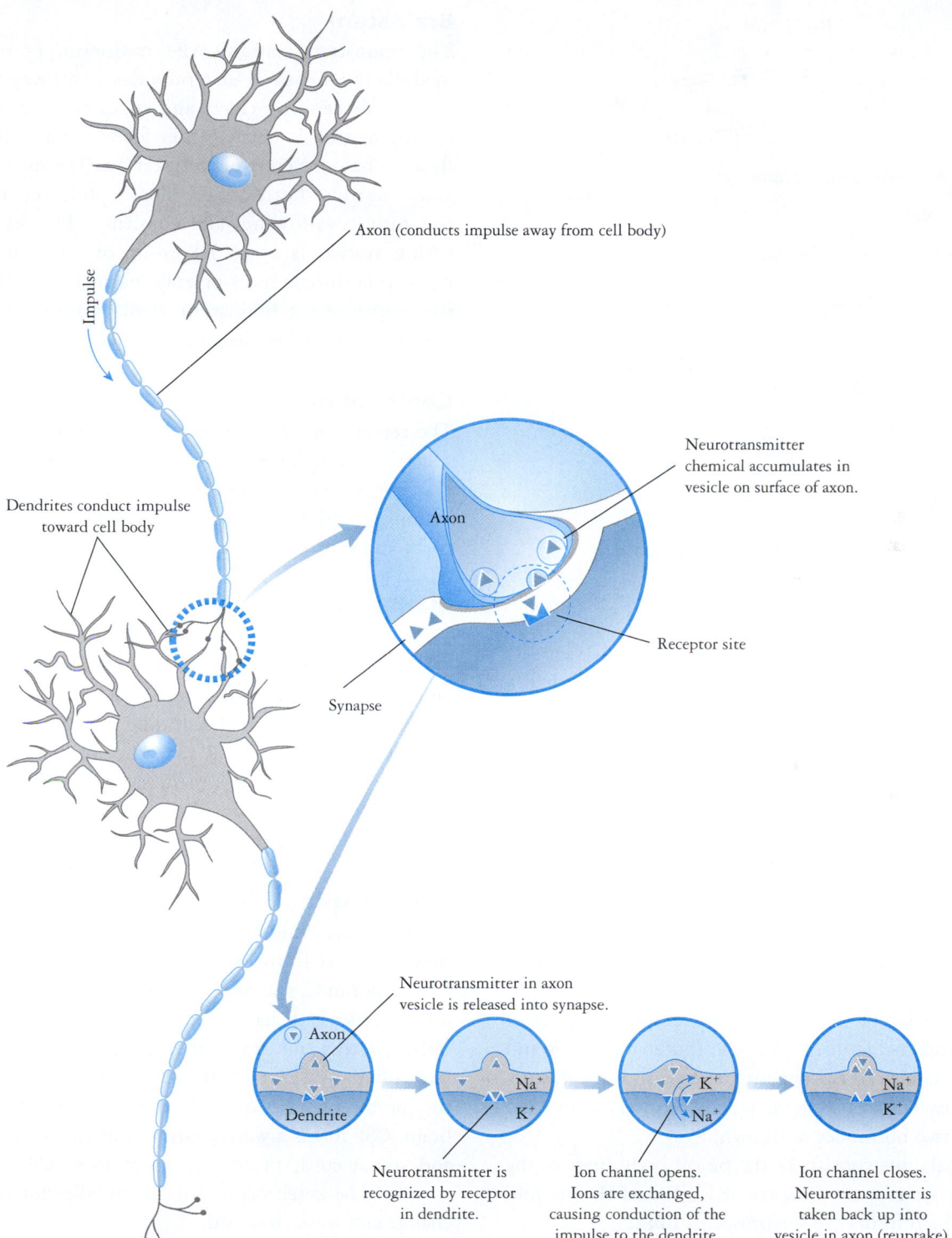

Axon (conducts impulse away from cell body)

Impulse

Dendrites conduct impulse toward cell body

Neurotransmitter chemical accumulates in vesicle on surface of axon.

Axon

Receptor site

Synapse

Neurotransmitter in axon vesicle is released into synapse.

Axon

Dendrite

Na^+

K^+

K^+

Na^+

Na^+

K^+

Neurotransmitter is recognized by receptor in dendrite.

Ion channel opens. Ions are exchanged, causing conduction of the impulse to the dendrite.

Ion channel closes. Neurotransmitter is taken back up into vesicle in axon (reuptake).

Figure 36-4. ■ Neurotransmission. The larger inset shows the synapse. The smaller insets illustrate steps in neurotransmission.

surrounding physical environment. In all individuals one side or the other is dominant.

The functions described above take place in the outermost gray matter of the cerebrum, called the *cerebral cortex*. Small portions of gray matter called *basal nuclei* can also be found buried deep within the white matter. Cerebral white matter is deeper in the hemisphere. It is composed of fiber tracts carrying impulses to or from the cortex. One very large tract, the *corpus callosum*, connects the two hemispheres and enables them to communicate with each other.

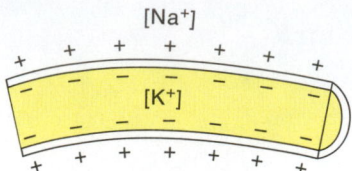

A Resting membrane

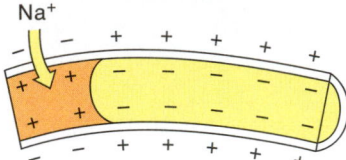

B Depolarization and generation of the action potential

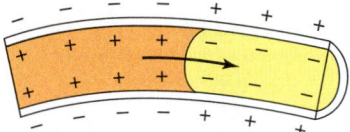

C Propagation of the action potential

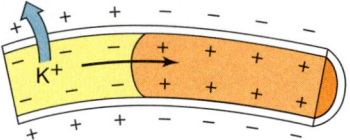

D Repolarization

Figure 36-5. ■ Nerve impulse causing and transmitting an action potential.

Diencephalon

The *diencephalon* or interbrain is located on top of the brainstem and consists of the thalamus, hypothalamus, and the epithalamus:

- The thalamus relays sensory impulses upward to the sensory cortex.
- The hypothalamus regulates body temperature, water balance, and metabolism. It is the center for drives and emotions such as thirst, appetite, sex, pain, and pleasure. The hypothalamus also regulates the pituitary gland and produces two hormones of its own.
- The epithalamus consists of the pineal body (part of the endocrine system; see Chapter 38 ⚭) and the choroid plexus, which forms the cerebrospinal fluid.

Brainstem

The brainstem contains the midbrain, pons, and the medulla oblongata. It also provides a pathway for ascending and descending tracts and contains many small areas of gray matter. It is the center for visual and auditory reflexes. The pons controls respiration. The medulla oblongata controls heart rate, blood pressure, respiration, coughing, swallowing, and vomiting. The reticular activating system is a special group of reticular formation neurons (a diffuse mass of gray matter) extending the entire length of the brainstem. It plays a role in consciousness and the awake–sleep cycles.

Cerebellum

The cerebellum, like the cerebrum, consists of two hemispheres, a convoluted surface, an outer cortex made up of gray matter, and an inner region of white matter. The cerebellum provides the precise timing for skeletal muscle activity and controls balance, posture, and equilibrium.

Meninges

Three protective membranes (the **meninges**) cover the brain and spinal cord (Figure 36-8 ■). The *dura mater* is the outer layer and is double layered where it covers the brain. The *arachnoid mater* is the middle meningeal layer. It has threadlike extensions that span the subarachnoid space to attach it to the innermost membrane, the *pia mater*. The pia mater follows every fold of the brain and the spinal cord, clinging tightly to their surfaces.

Cerebrospinal Fluid

Cerebrospinal fluid (CSF) is similar to the blood plasma from which it forms, except that it contains less protein, more vitamin C, and has a different ion composition. CSF is high in glucose. It has very few white cells and no red blood cells. It forms and drains at a constant rate so that its normal volume is 125 to 150 mL. It is continually formed by the choroid plexuses found in the four ventricles within the brain. CSF forms a watery cushion in and around the brain and spinal cord, protecting them from blows and other trauma. The cerebrospinal fluid provides for nutrient exchange and waste removal.

TABLE 36 -1	Selected Common Neurotransmitters	
TRANSMITTER	**LOCATION**	**ACTION**
Acetylcholine	CNS, autonomic nervous system (ANS), neuromuscular junctions	Excitation—speeds impulse transmission
Serotonin	CNS	Inhibition—controls body heat, hunger, behavior, and sleep
Dopamine	CNS, ANS	Inhibition—controls behavior and fine movement
Norepinephrine	CNS, ANS	Excitation—chief transmitter of sympathetic nervous system

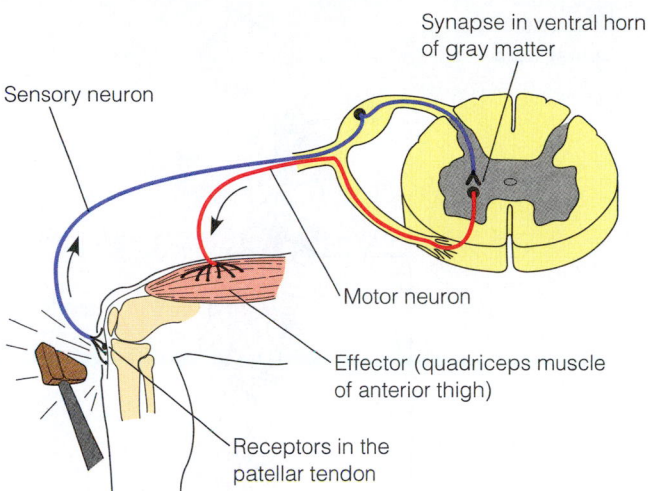

Figure 36-6. ■ A typical reflex arc of a spinal nerve. In the two-neuron reflex arc, the stimulus is transferred from the sensory neuron directly to the motor neuron at the point of synapse in the spinal cord.

Blood–Brain Barrier

The blood–brain barrier is composed of the least permeable capillaries in the whole body. The barrier protects the brain, which does not tolerate changes in its environment. Only water, glucose, and essential amino acids pass through these capillaries easily. Urea, toxins, proteins, and most drugs are prevented from entering the brain tissue.

SPINAL CORD

The spinal cord is a continuation of the brainstem. It extends to the first or second lumbar vertebra and ends in the cauda equina, a collection of spinal nerves. It has 31 pairs of spinal nerves that arise in the cord and exit from the vertebral column to serve the body area close by it (Figure 36-9 ■). The areas of skin innervated by branches of a single spinal nerve are called **dermatomes** (Figure 36-10 ■).

A cross-section of the spinal cord (see Figure 36-1) shows the gray matter in the pattern of an H or butterfly surrounded by white matter. The posterior, or dorsal, horns contain sensory neurons. The anterior, or ventral, horns contain motor neurons. The lateral horn contains sympathetic neurons. The white matter is composed of myelinated fiber tracts (ascending sensory and descending motor pathways carrying messages to and from the brain).

PERIPHERAL NERVOUS SYSTEM

Spinal Nerves

Spinal nerves, cranial nerves, and ganglia make up the peripheral nervous system. They connect the central nervous system with the rest of the body. The 31 pairs of spinal nerves are named according to their location (see Figure 36-9):

Cervical, 8 pairs	Lumbar, 5 pairs
Thoracic, 12 pairs	Sacral, 5 pairs

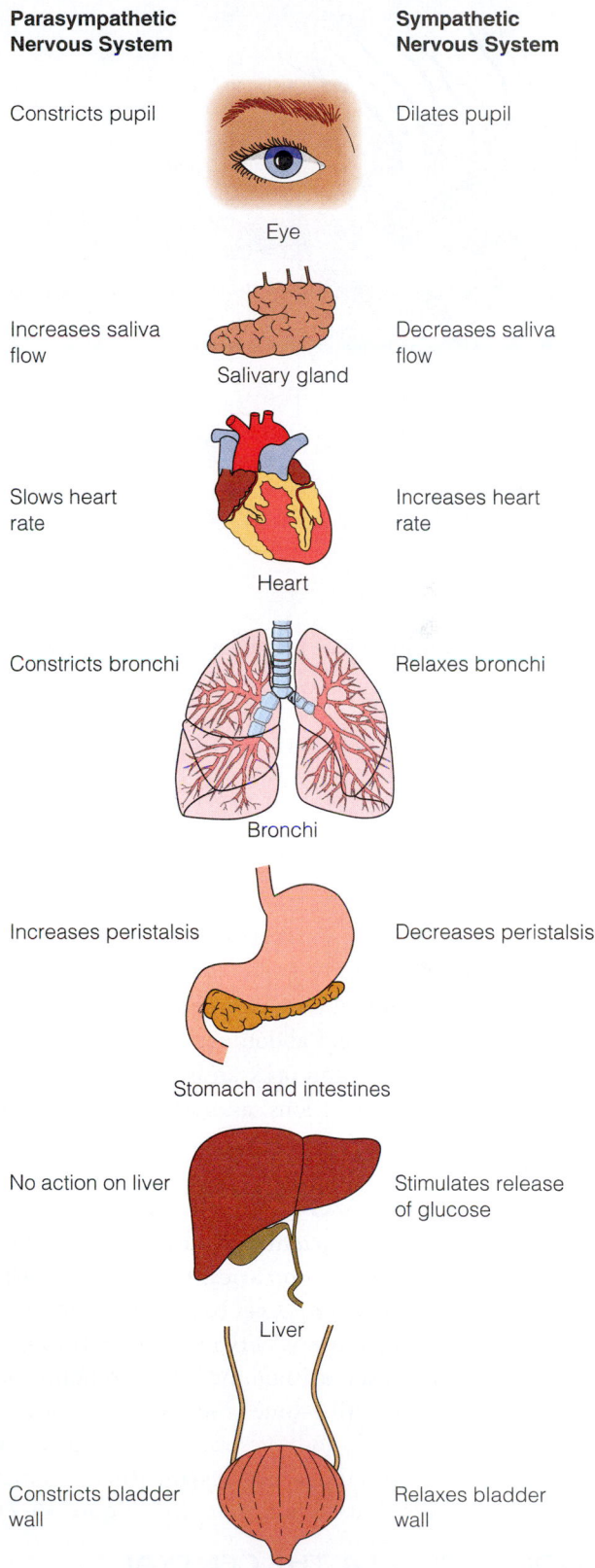

Parasympathetic Nervous System		Sympathetic Nervous System
Constricts pupil	Eye	Dilates pupil
Increases saliva flow	Salivary gland	Decreases saliva flow
Slows heart rate	Heart	Increases heart rate
Constricts bronchi	Bronchi	Relaxes bronchi
Increases peristalsis	Stomach and intestines	Decreases peristalsis
No action on liver	Liver	Stimulates release of glucose
Constricts bladder wall		Relaxes bladder wall

Figure 36-7. ■ Effects on organs of the parasympathetic and sympathetic nervous systems.

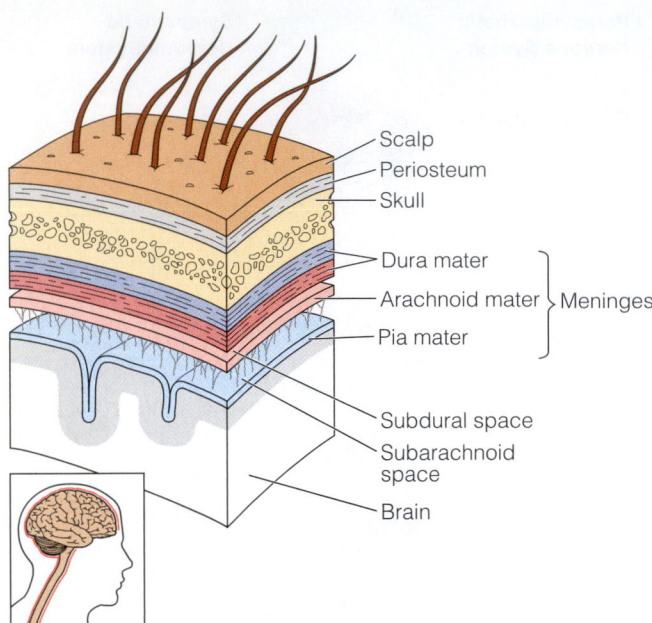

Figure 36-8. ■ Structure of the meninges covering the brain and spinal cord.

Each spinal nerve contains sensory and motor fibers. The sensory fibers are in the dorsal root and the motor fibers are in the ventral root. Both the dorsal and the ventral root of each spinal nerve attach it to the spinal cord.

Cranial Nerves

There are 12 pairs of cranial nerves, which begin in the brain or in the brainstem (Figure 36-11 ■). They are sensory, motor, or both. Except for the vagus nerve, which extends into the thoracic and abdominal areas, they control the function in the head and neck areas. Table 36-2 ■ lists the cranial nerves and functions, assessment tests, and abnormal findings.

AUTONOMIC NERVOUS SYSTEM

The autonomic nervous system is a subpart of the PNS. It controls body activities automatically and is responsible for maintaining the body's internal balance (*homeostasis*). It is also called the involuntary nervous system because it functions without conscious thought. The autonomic nervous system constantly fine-tunes the body's responses to all the input to the CNS to best support the body activities. The sympathetic and the parasympathetic systems were briefly discussed under reflex arc (see Figure 36-7).

BLOOD SUPPLY OF THE CENTRAL NERVOUS SYSTEM

Brain

The brain receives its arterial supply from the internal carotids and the vertebral arteries. The internal carotids supply the greater amount of blood flow. They branch off the common

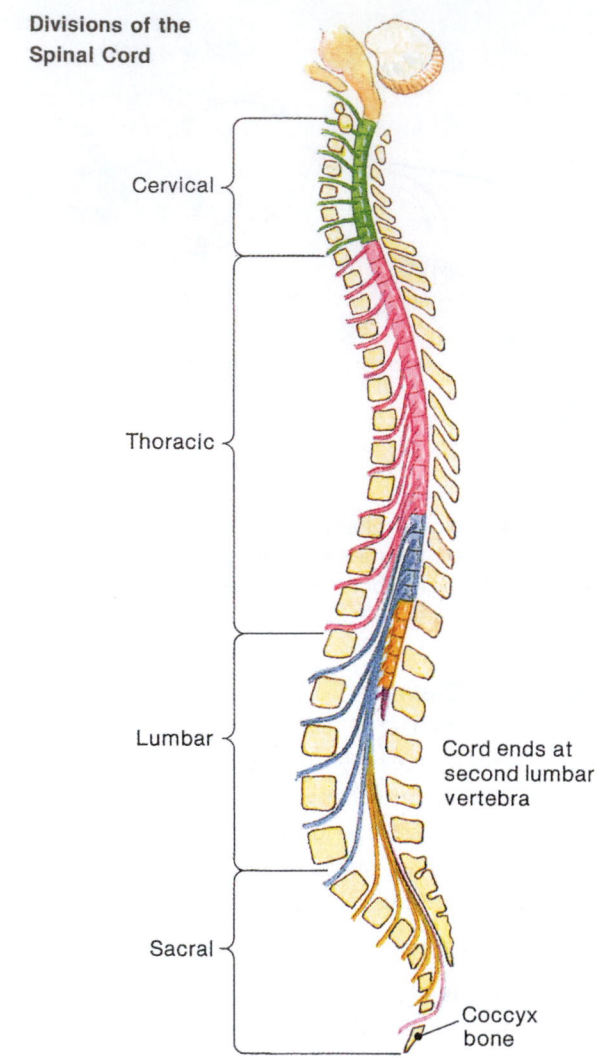

Divisions of the Spinal Cord

Figure 36-9. ■ The 31 pairs of spinal nerves are named according to their location. The four main areas of the spinal cord are cervical, thoracic, lumbar, and sacral.

carotid arteries and enter the cranium through the base of the skull. The vertebral arteries join to form the basilar artery at the base of the pons and medulla. The basilar artery divides to form paired posterior cerebral arteries. The circle of Willis provides an alternate route for blood flow when one of the contributing arteries is obstructed (Figure 36-12 ■).

Spinal Cord

The blood supply for the spinal cord branches off the vertebral arteries and from various regions of the aorta. The anterior spinal arteries and the paired posterior spinal arteries branch off the vertebral artery at the base of the cranium and descend alongside the spinal cord.

Neurologic nursing is concerned with problems of the nervous system that spring from a variety of causes. Manifestations of neurologic disorders may result from damage to a part of the nervous system or from other parts of the system

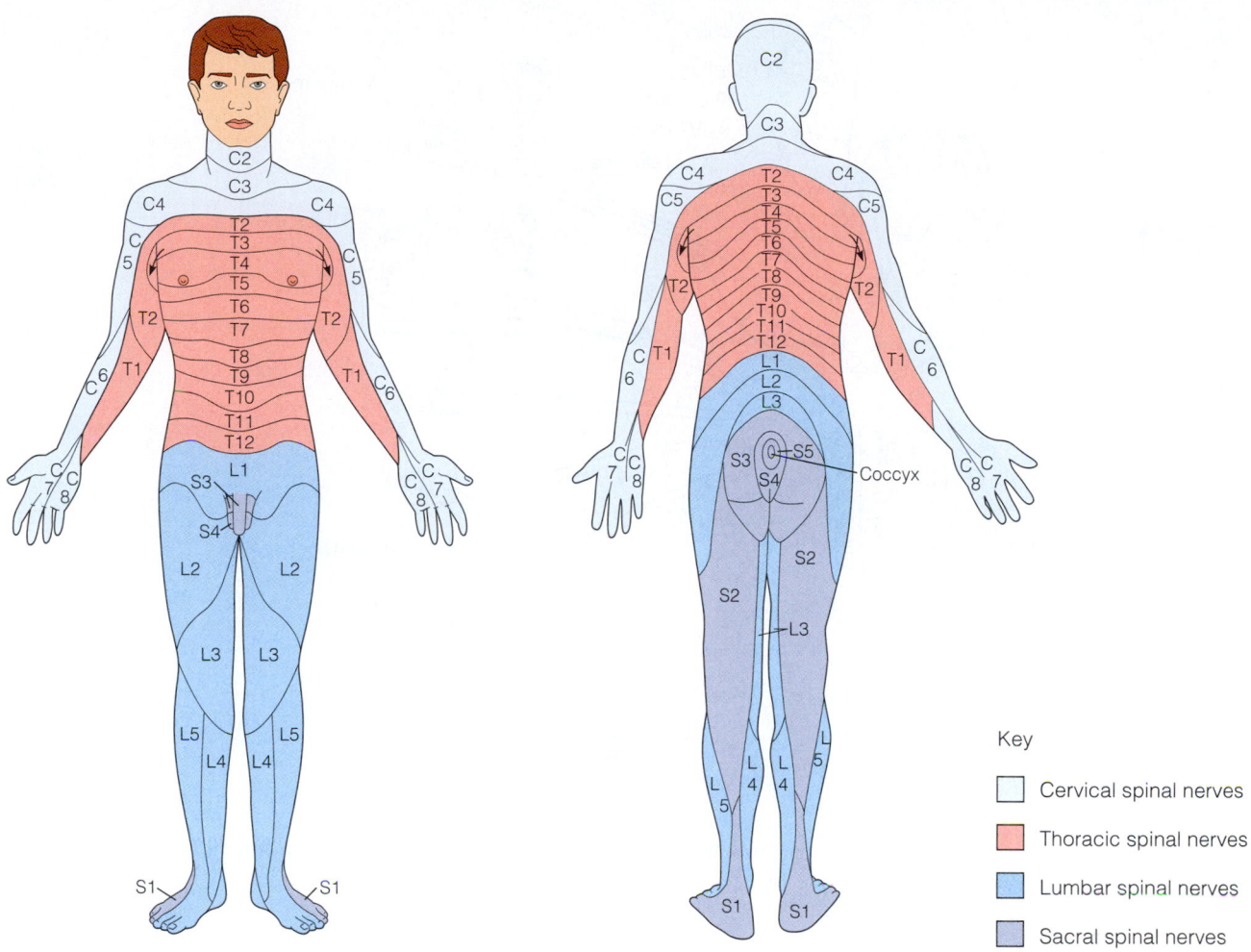

Key
- ☐ Cervical spinal nerves
- ☐ Thoracic spinal nerves
- ☐ Lumbar spinal nerves
- ☐ Sacral spinal nerves

Figure 36-10. ■ Each area of the skin is labeled with the spinal segment that governs skin sensation. Injuries to the spinal cord cause impairment to the region below the affected vertebral segment.

that are affected by the damaged site. It may be difficult to determine the source of the problem. For example, if the cerebellum (which controls coordination) is damaged, a person may lack muscle control and balance. But these symptoms could also occur in a client with damage to the middle ear, or in a person with multiple sclerosis (discussed later in this chapter), which destroys the myelin sheath.

Neurologic Testing

Diagnosis and treatment of neurologic and neurosensory disorders may involve extensive testing. Imaging techniques play a major role in identifying the etiology of a disorder. Laboratory studies are also used. The family of a client who exhibits signs and symptoms of neurologic disorders can play a key role in identifying new symptoms or changes. They can state what is normal for the client, especially in speech and movements, particularly if the client has had a previous traumatic brain injury or neurologic disorder. Informed consent forms must be signed before any type of invasive study.

IMAGING TECHNIQUES

X-Rays of the Head and Vertebral Column

Skull/facial x-rays are performed to determine the configuration, size, and shape of cranial and facial bones; unusual calcifications; evidence of a skull fracture; the integrity of the bony architecture; degenerative changes; the position of the pineal body; or hyperostosis. Some of the pathologic findings may include the presence of fracture or bone erosion suggestive of intracranial or intraosseous lesions. Vertebral column x-rays are ordered for those who have experienced spine injury and those who have back or neck pain. Vertebral fractures, traumatic dislocation, subluxation, a herniated disk (Figure 36-13 ■) or other lesions, and collapsed vertebrae are some of the pathologic findings. Degenerative changes noted might be scoliosis, spondylosis, spondylolisthesis, and foraminal stenosis.

Computed Tomography

A head computed tomography (CT) scan is a scanning of the head in successive layers (or slices, as termed by the imaging technicians) by narrow x-ray beams that pass

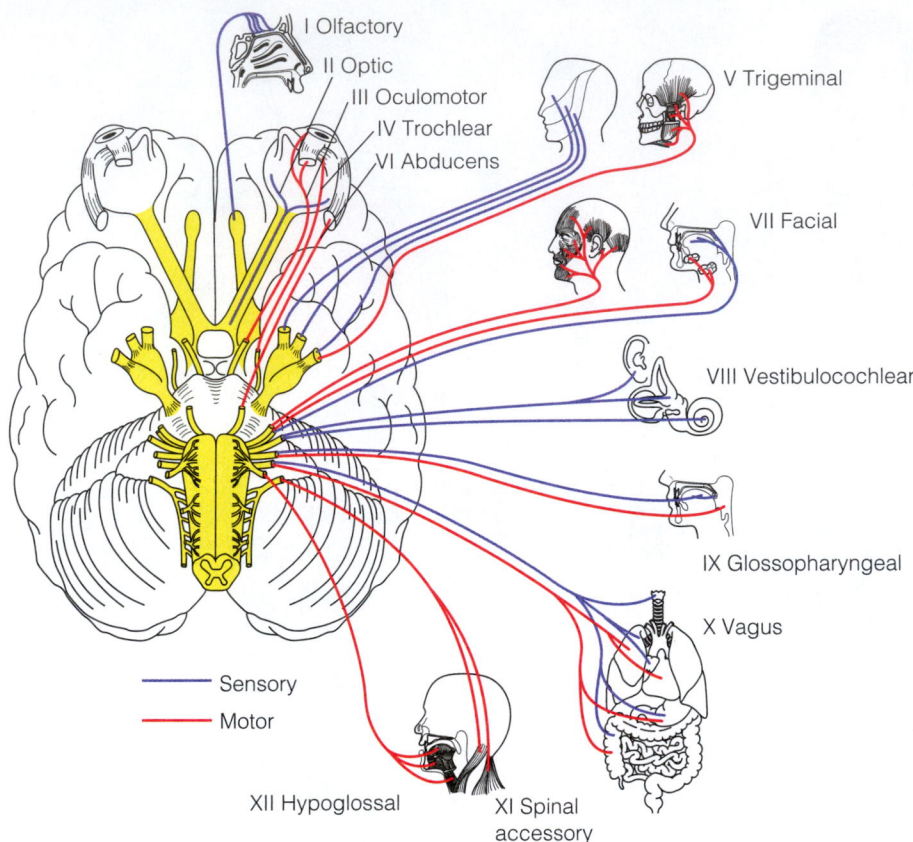

Figure 36-11. ■ There are 12 pairs of cranial nerves, which begin in the brain or in the brainstem. They govern messages to and from the brain.

TABLE 36-2	Assessment of Cranial Nerve Function		
NERVE	**FUNCTION**	**ASSESSMENT**	**ABNORMAL FINDINGS**
I Olfactory	Sensory—smell	Identify odors, e.g., peppermint, cloves; no irritating odors, e.g., ammonia	Anosmia—loss of sense of smell
II Optic	Sensory—vision	Visual acuity; determine visual fields: light flashed in affected eye; light flashed in normal eye; bring hand suddenly toward eye from the side	Loss of both direct and consensual (together) pupillary constriction; direct consensual pupillary constriction; absence of the blink reflex indicates
III Oculomotor	Motor—pupil constriction; elevate upper eyelid; extraocular movement	Eyes tested together for extraocular movements; also pupil reflex for cranial nerve II	Dilated pupil; ptosis. Direct pupil reflex present, consensual reflex absent
IV Trochlear	Motor—downward/inward eye movements	Tested with cranial nerves III and VI	Eye fails to move down and out
V Trigeminal	Motor—jaw movement Sensory—facial sensation of mouth, nose, surface of eye	Motor—bite down or say "cheer" Sensory—light touch, sharp/dull pain	Palpated masseter and temporalis muscle fail to contract Loss of sensation of pain and touch Paresthesia
VI Abducens	Motor—lateral eye movements	Look to the right, look to the left	Affected eye fails to move laterally Diplopia on lateral gaze
VII Facial	Motor—facial muscles; lacrimal and salivary glands	Wrinkle forehead	Paralysis of face muscles—eyelid remains open, angle of mouth droops, forehead fails to wrinkle
			(continued)

TABLE 36-2	Assessment of Cranial Nerve Function (continued)		
NERVE	**FUNCTION**	**ASSESSMENT**	**ABNORMAL FINDINGS**
	Sensory—sense of taste anterior $^2/_3$ of tongue; sensation to external ear	Place sugar on tip of tongue, sour on sides, and salty over most of tongue	Failure to identify tastes
VIII Acoustic (vestibulo-cochlear)	Sensory—hearing (cochlear) Balance—vestibular	Cover one ear and whisper from a few feet away Balance not tested unless problem evident	Sound not heard in affected ear Unable to maintain upright position
IX Glosso-pharyngeal	Sensory—pharynx and larynx, taste posterior $^1/_3$ of tongue, pressure receptors of carotid artery Motor—pharynx	Identification of bitter taste posterior $^1/_3$ of tongue Cotton applicator to soft palate	Loss of taste posterior $^1/_3$ of tongue Loss of sensation affected side of soft palate Gag reflex; uvula movements; hoarseness
X Vagus	Sensory—palate Motor—palate, pharynx and larynx; smooth muscles of abdominal organs: heart, stomach, bronchioles, small and large intestine, arterioles and glands	Usually tested with cranial nerve IX	Sagging of soft palate; deviation of uvula to normal side; hoarseness from paralysis of vocal cord
XI Spinal accessory	Motor—sternocleidomastoid and upper trapezius muscles	Push chin against hand; shrug shoulders; stretch out hands	Palpated sternocleidomastoid fails to contract Upper trapezius fails to contract Affected arm seems longer
XII Hypoglossal	Motor—tongue	Stick tongue out	Tongue protrudes toward affected side Dysarthria (impairment or clumsiness in uttering words)

through the head and are absorbed and/or transmitted, depending on the density of tissue (Figure 36-14 ■). The use of a radiopaque contrast medium (dye) increases the sharpness of the image. The CT scan is used in neurologic clients to obtain noninvasive images of the brain and spinal cord. The CT scan is best for rapid diagnosis of type, location, and extent of injury. A dual diagnosis of head and spinal injury can be determined or ruled out with both a head and neck

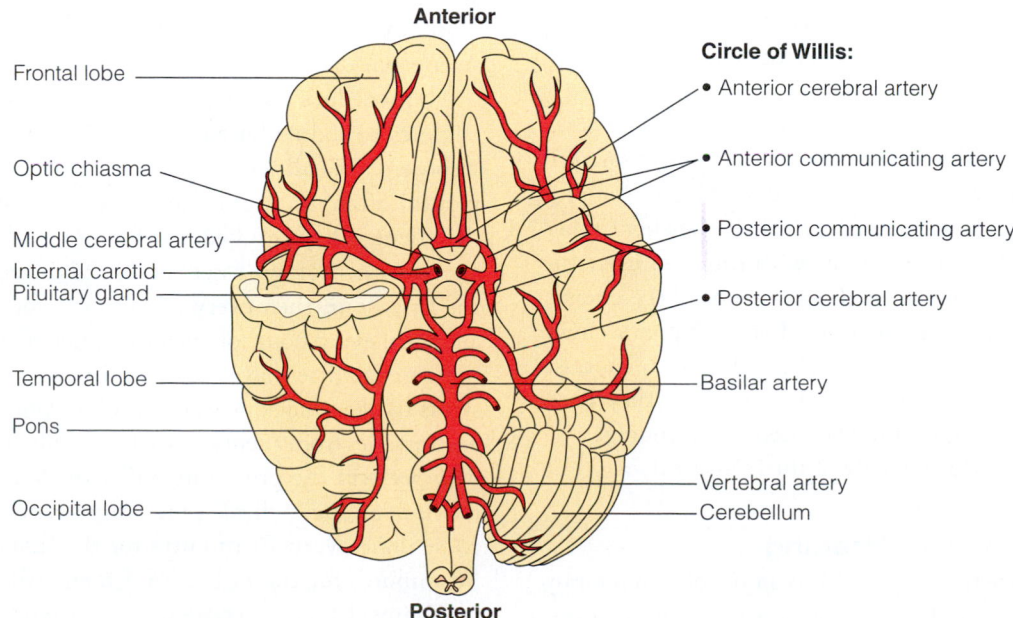

Figure 36-12. ■ Major arteries serving the brain and the circle of Willis.

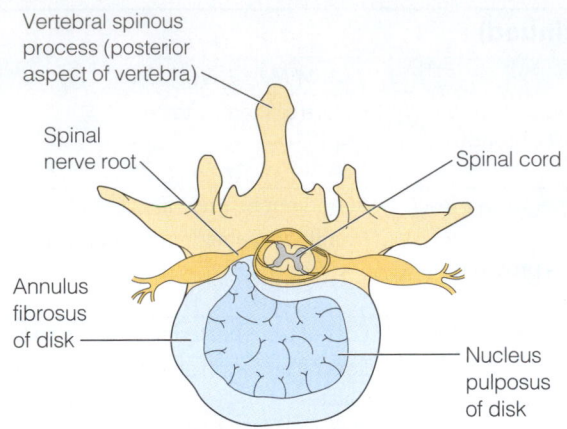

Figure 36-13. ■ A herniated intervertebral disk. The herniated nucleus pulposus is pressing against the nerve root.

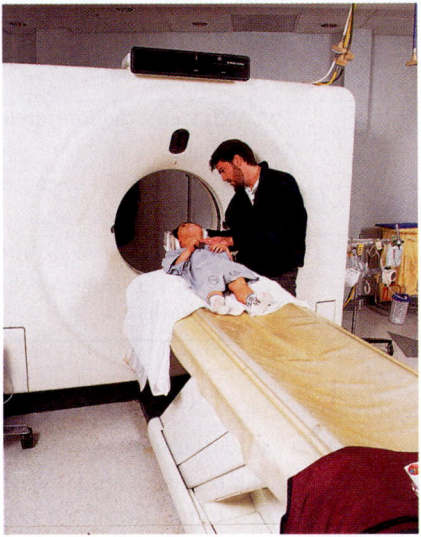

Figure 36-14. ■ A CT scan takes successive layers of x-rays. Such scans are painless but can be frightening for children and adults alike because of the close confinement of the chamber.

CT. Depending on the client's clinical presentation, CT scanning may be repeated every 2 to 3 days. Client teaching prior to the procedure is necessary, because the client must lie completely still on the CT table with the head immobilized during the test. A thorough assessment of the client's allergies is important preprocedure. For example, a client who is allergic to shellfish is probably allergic to contrast materials used in radiographic studies, because they both contain iodine. Postprocedure the client is encouraged to drink fluids to help rid the body of the contrast dye.

Magnetic Resonance Imaging

Magnetic resonance imaging (MRI) is a type of tomography based on the magnetic behavior of protons (hydrogen nuclei) in body tissues. An MRI is better than other types of imaging (e.g., CT or x-ray) at providing better definition of mass lesions, better visualization of the posterior fossa and brainstem, and an increased ability to detect subtle changes in tissue water content. It is superior for supplying detailed cross sections of anatomic structures. MRI takes more time than the CT scan and is not usually performed in acute or unstable clients who are at high risk during scanning. A contrast medium can also be used with an MRI.

Because of the strong magnets used, MRI is contraindicated for clients with pacemakers, implanted insulin pumps, transcutaneous nerve stimulators, spinal cord stimulators, cochlear implants, staples from prior surgeries, and penile prostheses. Clients who have a history of foreign bodies in the eyes, especially from grinding, will be x-rayed prior to the scan to determine the presence of metal embedded in the eyes. If the metal is found, then the MRI scan will not be performed. It is important to review these contraindications with the client, as well as the client's allergies to contrast medium.

Clients may exhibit anxiety during the procedure from fears of the noise or claustrophobic feelings from being enclosed in the "tube." If the option of an open MRI scan is not available, the client may need to be mildly sedated prior to the procedure. Also, if the client is in pain, remember to medicate prior to the scanning.

Cerebral Angiography

Cerebral angiography is the infusion of a radiopaque substance into the cerebral arterial system via the femoral artery. It provides important diagnostic information regarding the patency, size, irregularities, and/or occlusion of the cerebral vessels. It is used to evaluate cerebral aneurysms and arteriovenous malformations and is considered to be the most accurate imaging technique for evaluating carotid artery stenosis.

Preprocedure teaching includes the determination of any allergies to iodine-based dye, and/or a history of bleeding disorders. Usually the client is kept NPO (nothing by mouth) after midnight preceding the test. Postprocedure the client is kept on bed rest for 12 to 24 hours with vital signs and neurologic assessments done every 15 minutes for the first hour, then every 30 minutes for the second hour, and then every hour for the next 4 hours.

Some facilities have the capability to insert carotid artery stints to open blockages or to prevent pressure on the weakened arteries from aneurysms. The neurologists or radiologists who perform the procedure will write specific orders to include neurologic checks, vital signs, and site observations to be done every 15 minutes for the first hour, then every 30 minutes for the next 2 to 4 hours, then hourly, and so on. If any changes are noted, the physician must be notified immediately.

Lumbar Puncture

Lumbar puncture (LP) is the introduction of a hollow needle with a stylet into the lumbar subarachnoid space using strict aseptic technique (Figure 36-15 ■). Lidocaine is used to anesthetize the puncture area to reduce discomfort during the actual spinal needle puncture. The client will feel pressure, but should not feel any discomfort. In the adult, the needle is placed between the L3 and L4 or the L4 and L5 vertebrae. This procedure is done to measure the CSF pressure; to examine the CSF for blood; to collect CSF for laboratory testing (the most common being RBCs, WBCs, protein, glucose, culture and sensitivity {C & S]); to visualize parts of the nervous system by injection of air, oxygen, or radiopaque material; and to evaluate spinal dynamics for signs of blockage or CSF flow.

Preprocedure the client should be well hydrated. The client is placed on the side with both knees and head flexed at an acute angle. This position ensures the most space for insertion of the needle (interspinous space) between the lumbar vertebrae. Occasionally clients may be positioned sitting up and leaning over the bedside table. Postprocedure the client will lie flat for 6 to 12 hours. The nurse monitors neurologic and vital signs, encourages fluids, and administers analgesics for postprocedure headache.

Treatment for postprocedure headache from a slow CSF leak may include increasing oral fluid or IV fluid intake with analgesics and antiemetic medications, as well as bed rest. If medications and rest do not improve the condition, the physician may request a neurologist or anesthesiologist to perform a "blood patch" to seal the CSF leakage.

Myelography/Myelogram

A myelography combines fluoroscopy and radiography to visualize the spinal subarachnoid space, the lumbar, thoracic, or cervical area, or the whole spinal axis. It is used to diagnose a spinal cord tumor, a herniated intervertebral disk, or a ruptured disk. A lumbar puncture must be performed and 10 mL of spinal fluid removed. Then a radiopaque solution is injected and distributed to various tissues and structures to be examined.

The meal prior to the myelogram is omitted. Preprocedure the client should be well hydrated. Force fluids up to 3 liters in the 24 hours following the procedure.

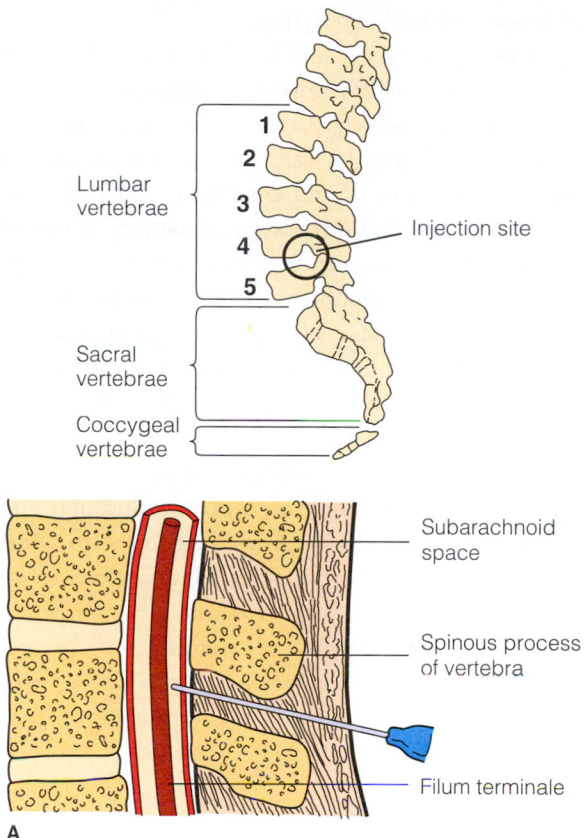
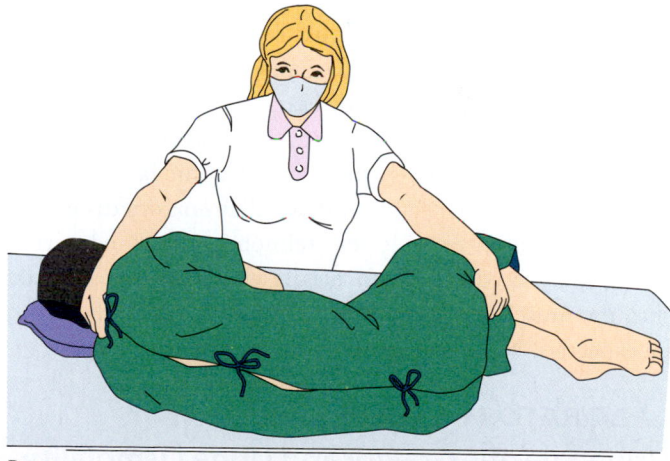
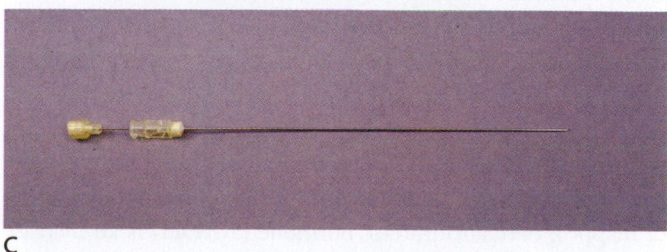

Figure 36-15. ■ **A.** Diagram of the vertebral column, indicating a site of insertion of the lumbar puncture needle into the subarachnoid space of the spinal canal. **B.** Client positioned for lumbar puncture. **C.** A spinal needle with the stylet protruding from the hub.

Electroencephalography

An electroencephalogram (EEG) is a graphic record of brain wave activity. It provides important diagnostic data about abnormal electrical activity in the brain and is used to diagnose epilepsy; to determine cerebral death; to evaluate drug and alcohol intoxication and cerebral blood flow; and to identify trauma and brain irritation secondary to infection.

Preprocedure teaching includes educating the client regarding the procedure. Generally 17 to 21 electrodes are attached with collodion to the client's head at corresponding areas over the prefrontal, frontal, temporal, parietal, and occipital lobes. Withhold stimulants, antidepressants, tranquilizers, and anticonvulsants for 24 to 48 hours prior to the test as prescribed. The recordings may be made while the client is asleep or when sleep deprived. The client must remain quiet during the procedure with his eyes closed without moving unless requested to hyperventilate for a short period of time to accentuate abnormalities. No postprocedure care is required.

Technology is evolving in the neuroscience laboratories. Portable EEG machines are available in some facilities to monitor the client's brain waves on an outpatient basis for 24 hours to several days.

Electromyography

Electromyography (EMG) measures and records the electrical properties of skeletal muscle and nerve conduction. It is performed with the skeletal muscle at rest and with voluntary muscle contraction. It provides important diagnostic data about neuromuscular diseases and other pathologic conditions that affect neuromuscular transmission. For example, EMG is used to evaluate amyotrophic lateral sclerosis, myasthenia gravis, and muscle inflammatory disorders.

Preprocedure, provide or reinforce client education about the procedure. Small needle electrodes are inserted into the muscle to be examined, and some discomfort is to be expected. No special postprocedure care is necessary.

LABORATORY STUDIES

Urine Specific Gravity and Urine Osmolality

Urine specific gravity measures waste and electrolyte concentration in the urine. The range is usually 1.010 to 1.025 but can range from 1.005 to 1.303. A high specific gravity indicates highly concentrated urine and a low specific gravity indicates dilute urine. Radiographic dyes, dextran, sucrose, and diuretics will distort test results. An abnormal finding that indicates dehydration, pituitary tumor, or tumor that causes the syndrome of inappropriate antidiuretic hormone (SIADH) is an increase to a reading over 1.020. Levels greater than 1.030 indicate a decrease in renal blood flow and fever. Decreased levels of less than 1.005 indicate overhydration and diabetes insipidus (DI); and levels of 1.001 to 1.005 indicate renal failures and hypothermia. (See further discussion in Chapters 21 and 39 ⚭.)

A urine osmolality test measures the osmotic pressure of urine and is used to monitor electrolyte and water balance and to evaluate dehydration. It is a more accurate test than specific gravity in determining urine concentration. It is especially useful in the workup of individuals with renal disease, SIADH, or DI. Substances that interfere with this test are diuretics, radiocontrast dye, barbiturates, morphine, and anesthetics. It should always be evaluated in conjunction with plasma osmolality.

Serum Osmolality

Serum osmolality is an indicator of serum concentration and measures the amount of dissolved particles in the serum such as electrolytes, urea, or sugar. A cerebrovascular accident or brain tumor can interfere with accurate test interpretation. Abnormal findings include SIADH and DI.

NURSING CONSIDERATIONS FOR CLIENTS WITH NEUROSENSORY DISORDERS

To work with clients who have neurologic disorders, nurses must understand problems of the nervous system that have a variety of causes. No matter what the source of the disorder is, symptoms occur that are related to both organic and functional causes. Clinical manifestations will appear that are related to the site affected. Other manifestations will appear that result not from the damaged site itself, but from other parts of the nervous system that are affected by the damaged site. An example of this is the lack of control or regulation in Parkinson's disease. The disease occurs in the brain, but it affects balance, coordination, and movement.

The nurse must recognize that clients with neurologic problems may have to make significant changes in lifestyle and adaptation. Neurologic disorders can affect the whole person, the psyche and the body, and often there is no clearcut distinction of symptoms. The individual is an open system with many interacting subsystems.

Although the client may be the focus of the teaching and learning activities about neurologic disorders, it is important to include the client's family members and significant others in a supportive or caregiver role. The same information may need to be shared many times, using various teaching methods, in order for the client to learn self-care skills adequately. (See more about client communication in Chapter 11 and client teaching in Chapter 12 ⚭.)

NURSING CARE

PRIORITIZING NURSING CARE

Clients may present with multiple alterations in their physical and emotional status. The first priority is always the client's ABCs, before any data about neurologic deviations are collected. Neurologic functions are determined to establish a baseline of the client's functions and cognition. Frequent monitoring of the client's neurologic status and vital signs are imperative to detect any significant changes that have occurred or about to occur in the client's physical and neurologic status. Report any deviations to the charge nurse or physician immediately to prevent further disability in the client and/or brain tissue death.

ASSESSING

A complete neurologic assessment is usually performed in phases, depending on the condition of the client and the urgency in collecting the data. (See Procedure 19-1 ⚭, for a focused health assessment.) It is normally performed by the interdisciplinary team (physician, nurse clinician, and LPN or LVN). It includes a history and neurologic examination. A neurologic examination of the conscious adult includes the following:

- *Mental status.* Level of consciousness is the most important assessment. Box 36-1 ▪ describes terms related to level of consciousness (LOC); see also Table 19-2 ⚭, the Glasgow Coma Scale. Also included are orientation, mood and behavior, knowledge, vocabulary, and memory. Any significant deviation from normal should be reported promptly to the charge nurse.
- *Cranial nerve function* (see Table 36-2).
- *Language and speech.* The ability to speak requires interplay between anatomic structures and the cerebrum and brainstem. Dysfunction may be related to a decreased level of consciousness or CNS dysfunction. Specific assessment techniques emphasize the client's ability to understand and use language appropriately. For example, is the

person's speech clear and coherent, or is speech slurred or garbled? Is the person *aphasic* (unable to speak)? Assessment information should include identification by a family member of any changes in the client's speech patterns. Clients with previous speech alterations need to be identified to establish a baseline.

- *Meningeal signs* (see Intracranial Infections later in this chapter).
- *Sensory status.* Touch, pain, temperature, proprioception (awareness of posture, movement, and changes in equilibrium).
- *Motor status.* Gait and stance, muscle strength ("Squeeze my hand," "Push/pull against my hand"), muscle tone, coordination, involuntary movements, and muscle stretch reflexes.
- *Intracranial pressure.* In infants, increased intracranial pressure is visible through bulging fontanels (see Chapter 16, Figure 16-4 ⚭). Once the cranial plates have fused, increased pressure inside the brain can lead to a wide range of symptoms including headache, blurred vision, and even death. Increased intracranial pressure is discussed separately in this chapter.

Certain features of the neurologic examination have been identified as the most important. (For review of a focused assessment, see Part A of Procedure 19-1 ⚭ in the health assessment chapter.) Aspects of a neurologic examination are LOC, pupillary reaction, motor function, cerebellar function, sensory functions, and vital signs. See also Box 31-3 ⚭ for review of a neurovascular assessment.

DIAGNOSING, PLANNING, AND IMPLEMENTING

Many nursing diagnoses apply to clients with neurologic deficits regardless of the underlying cause of the deficit. Some common ones are:

- *Ineffective Airway Clearance* related to decreased LOC and/or cranial nerve deficits
- *Impaired Physical Mobility* related to injury, paralysis, bed rest, or unresponsive state
- *Disturbed Sensory Perception*
- *Risk for Injury*
- *Ineffective Coping*

Examples of client outcomes for clients with neurologic deficits would include the following:

- Client will maintain patent airway.
- Client will maintain mobility on left side.
- Client will express an understanding of the disorder and of the need to use mobility devices to prevent falls.
- Client and significant others will plan assistance for activities of daily living as needed.

BOX 36-1	TERMS DESCRIBING LEVELS OF CONSCIOUSNESS

The following terms describe different levels of consciousness:
- *Alert*—Responds immediately to minimal external stimuli.
- *Confused*—Disoriented to time or place but usually oriented to person, with impaired judgment.
- *Delirious*—Disoriented to time, place, and person with loss of contact with reality; often has auditory or visual hallucinations.
- *Lethargic*—Displays a state of drowsiness or inaction in which an increased stimulus is needed to arouse.
- *Obtunded*—Displays dull indifference to external stimuli, and response is minimally maintained. Questions are answered with a minimal response.
- *Stuporous*—Can be aroused only by vigorous and continuous external stimuli. Motor response is often withdrawal or localizing to stimulus.
- *Comatose*—Vigorous stimulation fails to produce any voluntary neural response.

Nursing interventions for clients with neurologic deficits are supportive:

- Monitor airway status and check for airway patency. Suction excess secretions if swallowing is impaired or client is unable to handle them normally. Monitor oxygen saturation and administer oxygen as ordered. *Clients with altered LOC may be at risk for choking on excess saliva or their own tongues. Proper positioning is crucial to safety.*

- Evaluate orientation and level of consciousness regularly. *The person's orientation to person, place, time, and environment should be checked often. Usually people are described as disoriented or confused if they are not oriented to person (their name), place (where they are), and time (year, month, and/or day). They are said to be oriented times 2 if they get two of the three questions correct (Note: Clients are considered to be oriented times 3 if they answer all three questions correctly each time they are asked.)*

- When possible, encourage client to do as much as possible for self. *Participation in activities of daily living (ADLs) allows the client to achieve maximum rehabilitation and promotes self-esteem.*

- Keep environment clutter free and well lighted. Bed should be in the low position and side rails up as necessary. Items should be placed within reach on client's unaffected side. Avoid use of cooling/heating pads, which can injure sensory-deprived tissues. *All of these measures promote client safety and prevent injury from falls.*

- If client has impaired mobility, position client for proper alignment. Turn client on a regular schedule. Maintain body alignment, keeping the hands and feet in functional positions. *Turning and aligning the client help to prevent contractures and skin breakdown.*

- Provide or reinforce teaching. Include family and support people in learning how to care for the client. *Neurologic deficits often require long-term care and rehabilitation. The change in a person's life because of a neurologic disorder may be profound. It may be hard to absorb new information while learning to cope with the diagnosis. Clients and families may need to hear instructions several times before they feel secure in their understanding.*

EVALUATING

The effectiveness of the nursing care plan needs to be evaluated continuously; each problem and preventive measure should be assessed. The client's cognitive, adaptive, and emotional behaviors must be monitored regularly and compared to previous assessments to determine the improvement or deterioration of the client's condition.

Continuity of Care

The client may need assistance to regain and build or maintain independent ADLs such as speaking, ambulating, eating, drinking, bathing, and performing personal hygiene. It may be difficult to bridge the gap from dependence to independence and rehabilitation. Rehabilitation can be a long, slow process and is probably the most challenging phase for clients and their families. The key nursing goal is to assist both client and family in identifying and utilizing all coping resources. The nurse can help improve the client's self-esteem by assisting with the identification of realistic goals that capitalize on the client's strengths and resources.

Increased Intracranial Pressure

Intracranial pressure is the pressure normally exerted by the cerebrospinal fluid that circulates around the brain and spinal cord and within the cerebral ventricles. Increased intracranial pressure is a finding common to many neurologic disorders and it can be life threatening. Therefore, it is discussed here separately.

Intracranial pressure (ICP) is determined by the ratio of the brain tissue, CSF, and intravascular blood. Compensatory mechanisms maintain intracranial pressure within normal limits—0 to 15 mm Hg—so that an increase in one component causes a decrease in another. The intracranial pressure starts to rise when a state of equilibrium can no longer be maintained by the compensatory mechanisms. This rise in pressure is known as increased intracranial pressure (IICP). **Cerebral edema** is the abnormal accumulation of fluid or water in the intracellular space, extracellular space, or both.

Many neurologic disorders result in IICP. IICP causes decreased cerebral blood flow, leading to ischemia. If ischemia in the brain lasts more than 5 minutes, irreversible brain damage will occur.

Manifestations

Whatever the underlying cause, IICP causes neurologic changes in the level of consciousness, pupil response, speech, motor functions, and vital signs. These changes may develop slowly or rapidly and may be labeled as early or late signs. Box 36-2 ■ lists information to collect about clients with IICP. Table 36-3 ■ contrasts early and late manifestations of IICP.

Diagnosis

The client's vital signs and neurologic assessments are monitored for changes to detect increasing intracranial pressures. The health history and complete physical assessment will direct the healthcare provider in determining which diagnostic study is appropriate for the client. Lab studies will be ordered to establish baselines to compare with future studies to determine electrolyte imbalances, infections, and renal functions. CT/MRI scanning is used to determine the region of the injury or disorder that is the cause of concern or the cause of the IICP.

BOX 36-2   DATA COLLECTION

Increased Intracranial Pressure

Subjective Data

- Determine present health status:
  - When did change in LOC or memory occur first; onset slow or rapid?
  - Presence of headache, nausea, or vomiting
  - Visual changes such as double vision or blurring
  - Ringing in the ears; dizziness, or feeling faint
  - Any numbness or tingling in extremities
- Ask about past medical history:
  - History of trauma, infection, cranial surgery, seizures, or loss of consciousness
  - Medications to include prescriptions, over-the-counter medications (OTC), alcohol, and abused substances

Objective Data

- Check blood pressure, pulse, respirations, temperature.
- Observe for memory lapses or altered thought processes.
- Assess orientation to time, place, and person and LOC. If client is unconscious, use the Glasgow Coma Scale (see Table 19-2 ⚭).
- Check pupil response to light by using a penlight. Normal response should be PERRLA: pupils equal, round, reactive to light, and accommodation.
- Assess strength of hand grip and movement of extremities. Ask client to:
  1. Squeeze your hands.
  2. Push his or her feet against the resistance of your hands.
  3. Raise both legs off the bed.
- Note nausea or vomiting.
- Note color and amount of drainage from ears and nose; presence of "raccoon eyes" or Battle's sign (extravasation of blood into the skin over the mastoid process behind the ear).

Additional Data for Unconscious Clients

- Note any change in breathing pattern.

- Assess for the *Babinski's reflex* (see Chapter 56 ⚭) by stroking the bottom of the foot. An abnormal response in adults is when the big toe flexes upward and the other toes fan out.
- Assess corneal reflex by touching the corneal surface with a wisp of cotton. Normally the client blinks.
- Assess the gag reflex by touching the back of the client's throat gently with a tongue blade. Normally the client will show a gag reflex.
- Assess for abnormal posturing:
  - Decorticate posturing (see Figure 36-16A ▪)
  - Decerebrate posturing (see Figure 36-16B)

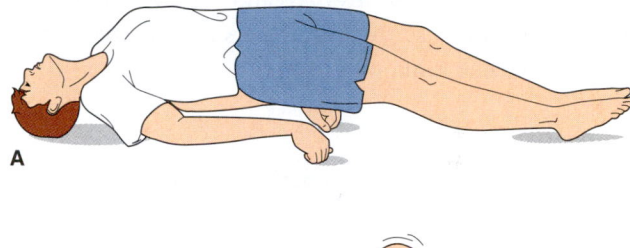

A

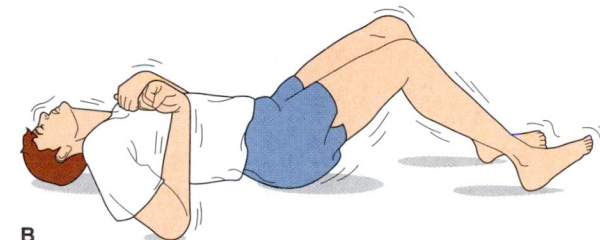

B

Figure 36-16. ▪ Contractions in grand mal seizures. **A.** Tonic phase shows decorticate posturing. **B.** Clonic phase shows decerebrate posturing.

Source: Burke, K., LeMone, P., & Mohn-Brown, E. (2007). *Medical-Surgical Nursing Care* (2nd ed.). Upper Saddle River, NJ: Prentice Hall.

TABLE 36-3   Manifestations of Increased Intracranial Pressure

	EARLY	LATE
Level of consciousness	Irritability; personality changes; restlessness; short-term memory changes; disorientation to time, then to place and person; confusion	Decreasing LOC that progresses to coma; no response to painful stimuli
Pupils	Pupils equal, round, and reactive to light and accommodation	Pupils sluggish in response to light; then fixed pupils First, pupils may be dilated on one side (ipsilateral), then progress to bilateral dilation
Vision	Decreased visual acuity, blurred vision, diplopia	Cannot assess due to decreasing LOC or coma
Motor function	Weakness in one extremity or side; hemiplegia on the opposite side	Decorticate or decerebrate positioning
Speech	Difficulty speaking	Cannot assess due to decreasing LOC or coma
Blood pressure	Elevated blood pressure	*Cushing's triad:* increased systolic blood pressure, widening pulse pressure, bradycardia

(continued)

TABLE 36-3	Manifestations of Increased Intracranial Pressure (continued)	
	EARLY	**LATE**
Pulse	Slightly elevated pulse	
Respiration	Rate may increase	Decreased respiratory rate with altered respiratory patterns (e.g., Cheyne-Stokes)
Temperature	May be increased or decreased	Significantly elevated
Other symptoms	Headache worse on rising in the morning and with position changes	Continual headache; projectile vomiting; loss of pupil, corneal, gag, and swallowing reflexes

Major hospitals can monitor intracranial pressure with a ventriculostomy monitor in the intensive care unit. The monitoring systems are invasive and require strict aseptic management, because the transducers are inserted into the ventricles of the brain.

Treatment

Treatment depends on the underlying cause of IICP, and is aimed at reducing the chance of multiple neurological deficits, coma, or death. Medications such as Mannitol or Decadron might be used to reduce swelling in the brain to decrease the ICP. Other medications might include antiemetics, analgesics, and antibiotics. Surgery may be performed (craniectomy after tumor removal, for example) to relieve excess pressure. If the client is comatose, consider TPN or gastric tube feedings to maintain nutritional status.

Nursing Considerations

The following are suggested nursing interventions for the client with IICP:

■ Monitor VS, neurologic checks, and pain every 15 minutes initially then progress to every 2 hours when stable.
■ Elevate the head of the bed to 30 degrees at all times, unless contraindicated by the healthcare provider's orders.
■ Monitor IV fluids carefully. An overdose of fluids can cause IICP and further injury to the client.
■ Administer anticonvulsants as ordered to prevent seizure activity or to reduce the chances of seizure activity from the injured area in the brain.
■ Keep the room quiet and darkened to reduce stimuli. The increase in stimuli increases the metabolic needs of the brain and may cause further injury if the needs are not met. The increase in stimuli may increase agitation in the client and result in changes in behavioral control and possibility of seizures.
■ Limit visitors to room of client with IICP or brain injuries to reduce the stimuli. Also, limiting the number of visitors in the room will decrease the chances of infections from those with flu symptoms or viral illnesses.

Cerebrovascular Disorders

Cerebrovascular disease is the most frequently occurring neurologic disorder and the third leading cause of death in the United States. A cerebrovascular disease is any abnormality of the brain caused by a pathologic process in the blood vessels. Certain risk factors predispose an individual for a transient ischemic attack (TIA) or cerebrovascular accident (CVA).

TRANSIENT ISCHEMIC ATTACK

A **transient ischemic attack** (TIA) is, as the name implies, a temporary loss of blood supply (oxygen) to an area of the brain. This brief episode of reversible neurologic deficits can present as mildly as a brief loss of vision in one eye to a full stroke syndrome that completely clears in 24 hours with no residual dysfunction. It should be considered as a warning signal for a future brain attack, because an individual who experiences a TIA is 10 times more likely to have a stroke than a person who has not had a TIA. Interventions would include lowering high blood pressure, cholesterol levels, and weight.

CEREBROVASCULAR ACCIDENT

A **cerebrovascular accident** (also called CVA, **stroke,** brain attack) is a sudden, nonconvulsive focal neurologic deficit. It is the common clinical manifestation of cerebrovascular disease. **Brain attack** (the newest term for CVA or stroke) is considered a medical emergency. It is treated with the same urgency as a heart attack. Certain risk factors predispose an individual for a TIA or CVA (Box 36-3 ■).

A cerebrovascular accident occurs when a cerebral blood vessel is occluded by a thrombus or emboli, or when hemorrhage occurs. All three events result in ischemia, because they decrease the oxygen to the area of the brain supplied by the damaged vessel. Table 36-4 ■ provides more details about the different types of CVAs.

Manifestations

When the blood supply to the brain is altered, there is temporary or permanent loss of neurologic function. The warning signals of a stroke are numbness, speech difficulties, blurred vision, headache, dizziness, loss of consciousness,

<table>
<tr><td colspan="2">

BOX 36-3   RISK FACTORS FOR CEREBROVASCULAR ACCIDENT

Modifiable Risk Factors

- Hypertension
- Atherosclerosis
- Cardiac disease
- High cholesterol
- Obesity
- Diabetes mellitus
- Smoking
- Excessive use of alcohol
- Drug use (cocaine)
- Oral contraceptives

Unmodifiable Risk Factors

- Persons over 65 years of age
- African Americans (twice the risk of Caucasians)
- Male gender (slightly higher risk than females)

</td></tr>
</table>

and/or **hemiplegia** (one-sided paralysis). Factors influencing the signs and symptoms are the area of the brain involved, the size of the area, and collateral blood flow.

clinical ALERT

An easy way to determine the possibility of a stroke is to think of the first four letters of the word, and ask the client to:

S – **s**mile.
T – **t**alk clearly. (Ask the client to repeat a simple sentence.)
R – **r**aise both arms.
O – stick **o**ut the tongue. (Deviation to one side may indicate stroke.)

If any of these indicators exist, call 9-1-1.

Diagnosis and Treatment

The diagnosis of CVAs will include a thorough history and physical examination of the client. Additional diagnostic testing will be determined from the finding of the examination, including CBC, metabolic panels, coagulation studies, cerebral arteriography, or CT/MRI scan with and/or without contrast medium. On rare occasions, a lumbar puncture may be performed.

Prompt treatment with thrombolytics (fibrinolytics) is important. If the area experiences a lack of oxygen, that is, *anoxia*, for more than 10 minutes, the brain cells die. The damage to the brain is irreversible. The amount of damage that occurs can be reduced by adequate collateral circulation if there is any. Severe disability or death is the result of a large area of infarction. Usually thrombolytic protocols are established in major facilities, otherwise the attending physician will call a referring agency to arrange for transfer of the client for further treatment.

Nursing Considerations

When caring for clients with TIA or CVA (from hemorrhage or clot), focus your care on early detection of changes in neurologic status. The earlier changes are detected and reported, the better the chance for intervening and preventing more damage. Do neurologic checks every 2 hours on unstable clients. Report immediately any decrease in level of consciousness, changes in pupil size and response, and/or decreases in strength or movement of extremities. For a client with cerebral aneurysm, prepare the client for surgery. Once the client is stable, focus your care on encouraging rehabilitation activities and praising gains, however small.

Supportive care for the client should include turning the client every 2 hours, suctioning the upper airway if needed, inserting a Foley catheter, and encouraging family members to talk with the client. Because of the client's condition, advanced directives should be understood by the family and supported by the healthcare team. Family members will need emotional support from the staff, clergy, or social worker that correct decisions were made. They may feel guilt for not pursuing drastic surgical procedures.

TABLE 36-4	**Types of CVA (Brain Attack or Stroke)**		
TYPE	**CAUSE**	**ONSET**	**PATHOPHYSIOLOGY**
Thrombotic	Atherosclerosis of large cerebral arteries	During or after sleep	Atherosclerosis causes plaque to build up in cerebral arteries. If plaque is not removed or treated, a thrombus or clot develops. This leads to ischemia in the brain tissue supplied by the vessel.
Embolic	Atrial fibrillation, congestive heart failure (CHF), rheumatic heart disease, mitral valve disease, endocarditis	Sudden onset with immediate deficits	Embolus travels to a cerebral artery from a distant site, especially the heart. It usually lodges in a narrow portion of a cerebral artery, causing necrosis.
Hemorrhagic	Hypertension	Occurs suddenly, often during some activity	Hypertension weakens a cerebral blood vessel, causing it to rupture. This leads to bleeding into the brain tissue or subarachnoid space.

CEREBRAL ANEURYSM

A cerebral aneurysm is an abnormal out-pouching or dilatation of a cerebral artery that develops secondary to a weakness in the arterial wall. The weakness is a result of atherosclerosis, hypertension, or a congenital defect. They are usually found in the circle of Willis (see Figure 36-12) and are the most common cause of nontraumatic subarachnoid hemorrhage. There are several types of aneurysms (see Figure 33-22 ⬯). Aneurysms are frequently asymptomatic.

Manifestations

Clinical manifestations may occur if the aneurysm is putting pressure on a cranial nerve. The signs and symptoms vary depending on the size and location of the aneurysm. Unfortunately, the first indication of the presence of an aneurysm is often an acute subarachnoid hemorrhage, intracerebral hemorrhage, or a combination of the two.

Diagnosis and Treatment

Immediate recognition that the client has a cerebral aneurysm is very important. The client's history and physical examination will determine the testing to be completed. The diagnostic testing that can be expected will be the routine CT scan of the brain and possibly a cerebral arteriogram. Baseline laboratory studies will be done as well.

Surgical management is the treatment of choice for an aneurysm. The location and size of the aneurysm and the individual's clinical status determine whether or not surgical intervention is possible. In some cases the client might be a candidate for a surgical procedure to clip or correct the aneurysm. With a large cerebral hemorrhage, supportive care is given by the nursing staff, because surgical procedures may not be possible to correct the defect and the client would not survive the procedure.

HEADACHES

Headaches are an exceptionally common occurrence affecting almost everyone at some time. Headache can be a single primary disorder, or it may be a symptom of an underlying organic problem. The intensity can be just as great in either case. Headaches may be caused by sinus infections or congestion due to allergic reactions. Life-threatening illnesses of which headache may be a sign are brain tumor, cerebral hemorrhage, or meningitis. Most headaches are *benign* (not life threatening).

Determining the type of headache is key to providing appropriate treatment and client education. The International Headache Society has classified migraine, tension-type, and cluster headaches as the three most common primary headaches.

Secondary headaches are headaches associated with other conditions such as head trauma, cerebrovascular disorders, substance use or withdrawal, infection, and disorders of the cranium and neck.

clinical ALERT

A pattern of taking headache medications too often or in excessive amounts can lead to a condition known as **rebound headache.** With rebound headache, the medications stop relieving pain and actually begin to cause headaches. Regular overuse can increase the potential for serious side effects. Treatment for this condition is a tapering of the medication being used or substitution of a different type of treatment or medication.

Migraine Headache

Many people who experience regular headaches are suffering from migraine headaches. Migraines severely affect quality of life although they are not life threatening. Individuals with migraines have nervous systems that are unusually sensitive to environmental and internal factors, including light, odors, sound, hormonal fluctuations, weather changes, irregular sleep, certain foods, and skipped meals.

When the migraine-prone individual reacts to change or stress, there are dips in the brain's neurotransmitter levels (especially serotonin), which may stimulate the "migraine center." The migraine center sends impulses to the trigeminal nerves, resulting in vasodilatation of blood vessels in the scalp and face, inflammation, and pain.

In the United States more than 23 million people suffer from migraine headaches. Migraine is more prevalent in females than in males and in Caucasians more than in African Americans or Asian Americans.

The typical migraine is initially unilateral and localized in the frontotemporal and ocular area (often confusing it with sinus headache). Then over a period of 1 to 2 hours the pain or throbbing progresses posteriorly and becomes diffuse. It lasts from several hours to a whole day. The pain intensity is moderate to severe and intensifies with routine physical activity. About 15% to 20% of sufferers experience a migraine **aura** (a transient neurologic event lasting 5 to 30 minutes and consisting of a visual disturbance, e.g., flashing lights, blind spots) and one-sided numbness or tingling. Associated symptoms include anorexia, nausea, vomiting, blurred vision, skin pallor, **photophobia** (sensitivity to light), **phonophobia** (sensitivity to sound), and light-headedness. The headache subsides gradually within a day and after a period of sleep.

Tension-Type Headache

A tension-type headache is associated with chronic contraction of the muscles of the neck and scalp. It may be brought about by emotional or physical strain. The pain is bilateral, mild to moderate in intensity, and often described as a feeling of tightness, pressure, or constriction or a viselike feeling around the head. It is not accompanied by nausea nor does it intensify with routine physical activity. The duration is from 30 minutes to 7 days with the more chronic form lasting at least 15 days.

Cluster Headache

The cluster headache is seen primarily in men age 20 to 40. The pain is extremely severe, unilateral, recurring, and located behind or around the eye on the affected side. The pain lasts from 15 minutes to 3 hours and comes in clusters of 1 to 8 daily lasting for several weeks or months, and followed by remission of months or years. The headache occurs during the night after 1 to 2 hours of sleep, awakening the person and often accompanied by tearing, nasal congestion, or runny nose. It can be triggered by alcoholic beverages or other vasodilatation agents, such as nitroglycerin.

Diagnosis and Treatment

There is no specific testing done to make a diagnosis for a headache, but the healthcare provider may order diagnostic studies to rule out the possibility of tumors, hemorrhage, or other pathology that may be causing the headache. The client and the family can become very frustrated with the debilitation this disorder can cause.

Once the type of headache is diagnosed or its underlying cause is identified, the appropriate treatment can be given (Table 36-5 ■). The treatment may include client teaching about headaches, control of precipitating factors, stress management, biofeedback and relaxation techniques, and pharmacologic therapies. Pharmacologic therapies are aimed at treating the immediate pain and accompanying symptoms such as nausea and vomiting, as well as preventing the attacks with prophylactic therapies.

The client may be asked to keep a diary of headaches with notes on the weather, possible food triggers, and stressors. This record can help the provider determine a treatment plan, which may include environmental and behavior lifestyle changes.

Nursing Considerations

When caring for clients with headache, the nurse focuses on pain management techniques including distraction, massage, and environmental management. Keep the environment quiet with lights low if the client is photophobic. Encourage the client to identify stressors in life and effective ways to manage stress. Teach relaxation techniques, such as focusing on one muscle group at a time starting at the toes, and have the client contract and relax each muscle group. Assess neurologic status every 2 to 4 hours to ascertain that the headache is not a symptom of a brain disorder. Be careful not to judge the client's pain experience, but rather work toward managing the pain with the client.

HYDROCEPHALUS

Hydrocephalus is excess fluid within the cranial vault, subarachnoid space, or both. It can be congenital (see discussion in Chapter 57 ⬭) or be due to a variety of conditions. It occurs because of interference with CSF flow due to increased fluid production, obstruction within the ventricular system, or defective reabsorption of the fluid. It occurs after a subarachnoid hemorrhage in 19% to 43% of all cases. The most common type of hydrocephalus found in adults is the communicating type. In this type, there is normal communication between the fourth ventricle and subarachnoid space, but absorption is impaired secondary to:

- Adhesions from inflammation such as meningitis, brain abscess, or subarachnoid hemorrhage.
- Compression of the subarachnoid space by a mass.
- Congenital abnormalities of the subarachnoid space.
- High venous pressure with the sagittal sinus.

Manifestations

Manifestations may be noticed by a parent or caregiver. Signs or symptoms may include a change in behavior, complaints of headache, visual disturbances, or bulging fontanels in infants.

Diagnosis and Treatment

Diagnosis of hydrocephalus can be determined by performing CT/MRI scans to show the increased CSF and enlargement of the ventricles. Infants and toddlers will be monitored by frequent measuring of their head circumference.

TABLE 36-5	Headaches		
TYPE	**DESCRIPTION**	**CAUSE**	**TREATMENT**
Migraine	Unilateral, frontotemporal and ocular area; ache progresses to throbbing pain associated with nausea, vomiting, blurred vision, skin pallor, photophobia, phonophobia, and light-headedness; may or may not have aura	Stress; reduction in neurotransmitter levels in brain (serotonin)	Sleep; stress management; simple analgesics, e.g., aspirin, NSAIDs, caffeine; adjuvant compounds: antiemetic; Sumatriptan, narcotics for severe pain
Tension	Bilateral, contracted scalp and neck muscle, viselike constriction around head	Emotional or physical strain	Simple analgesics, e.g., aspirin, ibuprofen, acetaminophen
Cluster	Severe, unilateral, nocturnal, recurring; located behind or around eye	Unknown	Oxygen, Ergotamine, Dihydroergotamine (DHE), Sumatriptan

Treatment is determined by the underlying cause and can include a diuresis regimen (see Chapter 39 ⊛), external ventricular drainage, ventriculoperitoneal shunt, and/or removal of the cause.

Seizure Disorders

A **seizure** is a sudden, explosive, disorderly discharge of cerebral neurons characterized by an abrupt, transient alteration in brain function. Seizures usually involve motor, sensory, autonomic, or psychic clinical manifestations. They also involve a temporarily altered level of arousal. Seizure disorders are not a specific disease entity; they are a symptom or represent a syndrome. Seizure activity can be from one or more focal areas in the brain that become irritated due to congenital factors, trauma, or medication toxicity.

Manifestations

Some seizures are termed *convulsions*, which refers to **tonic-clonic** (jerky, contract–relax) movement (Figure 36-16). **Epilepsy** is a general term for the primary condition that causes seizures. In epilepsy, no underlying correctable cause for the seizures is found, and without treatment, the seizure activity recurs.

There are several ways to classify seizures: clinical manifestations, site of origin, EEG correlates, or response to therapy. Epileptic seizures can be classified as partial, generalized, or unclassified. Table 36-6 ■ provides more information on the types of epileptic seizures and their manifestations.

Partial seizure disorders begin with focal or local discharges in one part of the brain, unilaterally. They usually originate from the cortical brain tissue, thus having a superficial focus. If the individual remains awake, the seizure is considered simple and partial. If impairment or loss of consciousness occurs after a focal seizure, the syndrome is classified as complex and partial. **Generalized seizures** involve neurons bilaterally; they often do not have a focal onset and they usually originate from a subcortical or deeper brain focus. Impaired or loss of consciousness always occurs with a generalized seizure. Box 36-4 ■ provides more important terms and definitions about seizures.

Unclassified seizures are those that cannot be classified as partial or generalized. An example would be neonatal seizures (Box 36-5 ■).

Status epilepticus is prolonged partial or generalized seizures without recovery between attacks, while still in the postictal phase, or a single seizure that lasts more than 30 minutes. The resulting cerebral hypoxia makes this condition a medical emergency. Status epilepticus can be the result of abrupt discontinuation of seizure medications, untreated or inadequately treated seizure disorders, head trauma, or hypoxia.

BOX 36-4	TERMS RELATED TO SEIZURES

Aura—a partial seizure experienced as a peculiar sensation preceding the onset of a generalized seizure—may be *gustatory* (related to taste), visual, or auditory; a feeling of dizziness or numbness; or just "a funny feeling"

Prodroma—early clinical manifestations, such as malaise, headache, or a sense of depression, that occur hours to a few days before seizure

Myoclonic seizure—single jerk of one or more muscle groups; lasts only 1 second

Tonic phase—a state of muscle contraction with excessive muscle tone; stiffening

Clonic phase—a state of alternating contraction and relaxation of muscles; jerking

Tonic-clonic phase—starts with the stiffening or tonic phase followed by the jerking or clonic phase; unconsciousness, tongue biting, bowel and bladder incontinence occur

Atonic seizure—drop attack or abrupt loss of muscle tone

TABLE 36-6	Classification of Epileptic Seizures	
TYPE	**SUBTYPE**	**SYMPTOMS**
Partial—seizures beginning locally, simple	Focal motor; Jacksonian march	Simple without loss of consciousness. With motor signs—movement of eye, head, and body to one side, stopping of movement or speech; special sensory or somatosensory symptoms—tingling, numbness of body part; visual, auditory, olfactory, or taste sensations; autonomic symptoms or signs—pallor, sweating, flushing, piloerection, pupillary dilation; psychic symptoms—overly familiar, dysphagia, dream states, distortion of time sense, fear, illusions, hallucinations.
Partial—complex	Temporal lobe or psychomotor seizures	Impaired consciousness, automatisms, antisocial or aggressive behavior if restrained.
Generalized—bilaterally symmetric and without local onset	Limited grand mal, grand mal, petit mal	Tonic, clonic, or tonic-clonic. Simple—loss of consciousness only; complex—with brief tonic, clonic, or automatic movements.

BOX 36-5 PEDIATRIC CONSIDERATIONS

Febrile Seizures

Children under the age of 3 years are susceptible to febrile seizures and require a septic workup for the etiology of the fever. This workup should include a CBC, blood culture, urinalysis and culture, as well as metabolic panels. The physician may elect to perform a lumbar puncture if the diagnostic tests are inconclusive.

Diagnosis and Treatment

Accurate documentation of the events that are observed by the nurse or healthcare providers include any sounds; length of seizure activity; movements of extremities, mouth, eyes, and head; as well as urine or stool incontinence. An EEG is ordered and is interpreted by the neurologist to locate the focal area of the seizure activity. In the case of a new-onset seizure, CT/MRI scans may be ordered to determine whether the client has a tumor or injury to the brain. The client may experience a period of deep sleep after the seizure activity; this is known as a *postictal state*. The period of deep sleep can last from a few minutes to hours.

Treatment for the client will include monitoring the airway, administering oxygen, and providing safety to prevent injury during seizure activity. Safety procedures can include moving the client to the floor, or if in a bed, laying the client in a supine position or on the side to facilitate drainage of oral secretions during the seizure. Loosen any tight-fitting clothing and allow the client some privacy if the seizure occurs in a public place. During the seizure the healthcare provider may order a benzodiazepine, such as diazepam or lorazepam, to stop the seizure activity. If this medication is administered to the client (by IV or rectally), airway and respirations will need to be monitored carefully, because these medications may cause respiratory depression or apnea.

Anticonvulsant medications will be prescribed to control the seizure activity and will be monitored by periodic serum blood levels to assess the dosage to keep the drug level within the therapeutic ranges.

clinical ALERT

A client should never be physically restrained during seizure activity as joint, skeletal, or muscular injury may occur.

Status Epilepticus

Seizure activity that continues for a longer period of time (greater than 10 minutes) or that occurs in sequential episodes is considered to be status epilepticus. Increased seizure activity raises the risk of aspiration, respiratory difficulty leading to reduced oxygen to the brain, and possible death. Status epilepticus activity requires emergency treatment with medications. Intubation may be necessary because higher doses of medication can result in respiratory depression and the client may require mechanical ventilation.

NURSING CARE

PRIORITIZING NURSING CARE

When caring for clients with seizures, focus your care on preventing complications and protecting the client from injury. Move furniture or other items that the client may hit against away from the immediate area. Time the seizure from the onset to the end. Be prepared to suction the oral cavity afterward to clear the airway. Always reassure the client after a seizure, and reorient the client to time, place, and person. Some clients may be confused and combative after the seizure activity, so safety precautions for the client and the healthcare team are very important. Be alert for another seizure to occur quickly if the client is at risk for status epilepticus or uncontrolled seizure activity.

ASSESSING

The LPN/LVN assists the RN in assessing the client with neurovascular disorders. A thorough history includes information about what was occurring prior to the incident (CVA, TIA, seizure, etc.) and what symptoms the client exhibited. The duration of symptoms, especially seizure activity, is obtained and documented. It is also important to determine which risk factors, if any, are a part of the client's lifestyle, such as substance abuse, or an occupation in a high-risk arena, such as exposure to agricultural sprays and chemicals. Assess the client for level of consciousness (see Box 36-1) for changes in responsiveness. Assess pupil response for equality and reactivity to light. Assess the client's ability to move all extremities and to respond to commands.

DIAGNOSING, PLANNING, AND IMPLEMENTING

Possible nursing diagnoses for the client with neurovascular disorders might include:

- *Acute Confusion*
- *Risk for Disuse Syndrome*
- *Impaired Physical Mobility*
- *Risk for Injury*
- *Risk for Impaired Skin Integrity*
- *Dressing Self-Care Deficit*

Examples of outcomes for these clients would include:

- Client will remain oriented × 3.
- Client will remain free of injury.
- Client will participate in ADLs.

Nursing interventions for clients with neurovascular accidents include:

- Orient clients to person, place, and time as necessary. Explain what has happened and reassure the client that she is in a safe place and is being cared for. *This decreases anxiety and fear.*
- Reevaluate the client's orientation to person, place, and time every shift, noting improvement in the client's confusion. *Expect improvement in orientation to occur as client recovers from CVA.*
- Assist client in active range-of-motion (ROM) exercises at least three times a day. *This helps retain normal range of motion and restores strength to affected extremities.*
- Assist client in learning to perform ADLs with limitations. *Reduces sense of helplessness and gives sense of accomplishment and of independence.*

For Clients with CVA

- Encourage clients to be aware of the affected side after a CVA. As part of this awareness, encourage clients to bathe the affected side and to do passive ROM exercises with the affected limbs. *This helps prevent unilateral neglect.*
- Clients who are unable to turn themselves must be turned every 2 hours while in bed. When clients with paresis or paralysis are sitting up in a chair or wheelchair, assist them to reposition themselves every 2 hours. *This helps to prevent pressure ulcer formation.*
- Evaluate the client's ability to perform ADLs and assist as needed with bathing, grooming, dressing, feeding, and toileting. Teach clients how to overcome limitations due to paresis or paralysis using adaptive equipment for eating and dressing.
- Encourage clients to do as much as possible for themselves and celebrate every positive accomplishment. *Loss of independence is devastating to adults, and regaining independence is the goal of rehabilitation after CVA.*

For Clients with Seizures

- When the seizure occurs, time any seizure activity. Document the types of movements and the length of time the activity lasts. *Documentation will help the physician determine appropriate medications.*
- Protect the client who is having a seizure. Move furniture or other objects out of the way, and pad the side rails with blankets. If the jaw is clenched, do not attempt to place anything in the client's mouth. Loosen any tight clothing

to prevent airway restriction during the seizure. *Taking appropriate measures ensures that the client does not injure himself during tonic-clonic seizure activity.*

- Prepare to suction the throat if needed to clear the airway after a seizure. *After the seizure, check for injuries and turn the client to one side. The tongue and oral cavity may sustain bite injuries during the clonic phase of the seizure. Positioning the client on one side allows drainage of secretions from the mouth.*
- Keep the environment calm and quiet. *This can help to prevent further seizures.*
- Encourage the client to take seizure medications exactly as prescribed. *Medications help keep seizure activity under control.*
- Evaluate the client's memory and experiences prior to the seizure. Ask if an aura was felt, smelled, heard, or seen prior to the seizure. *This information can be helpful in helping the client know when a seizure is about to occur.*
- Offer support and reassurance to the client. *The nurse can prevent fear and embarrassment by providing an accepting, caring attitude.*

EVALUATING

In clients with cerebrovascular disorders, evaluate orientation and LOC frequently to determine client status. Attention to changes and prompt reporting are an important part of the nurse's role. Skin integrity is a major concern. The nurse can gather important information about how the client is coping and about client's ability to perform ADLs. In clients with seizures, safety, skin integrity, and adherence to the medical regimen are important items to evaluate.

NURSING PROCESS CARE PLAN
Client with Cerebrovascular Accident (Stroke)

Martha Wagner, 78 years old, collapsed while fixing her lunch. When discovered several hours later by her daughter, Martha was awake, drooling, and unable to move her extremities on the left side. The paramedics were called and transported her to the local hospital.

Assessment

BP 260/188, P 80, R 24. Her speech is garbled and she continues to drool. She is paralyzed on the left side. Oxygen is administered by face mask. CT scan shows hemorrhagic bleed in the right cerebral hemisphere. An IV with a labetalol drip is started to reduce her BP.

Nursing Diagnosis

The following important nursing diagnoses (among others) are established for this client:

- *Impaired Swallowing* related to neuromuscular impairment
- *Impaired Physical Mobility* related to left-sided paralysis
- *Impaired Verbal Communication*
- *Ineffective Cerebral Tissue Perfusion* related to interruption of blood flow due to hemorrhage

Expected Outcomes

The expected outcomes for the plan of care for Ms. Wagner are:

- Prevent aspiration.
- Maintain/increase strength and function of affected extremities.
- Establish method of communication in which needs can be met.
- Demonstrate stable vital signs.

Planning and Implementation

The following interventions are planned and implemented for Ms. Wagner:

- Perform neurologic assessment and vital signs every 15 minutes for 1 hour then every hour.
- Place client in upright position during and after feeding.
- Promote effective swallowing by adding thickener to all liquids.
- Change position every 2 hours.
- Use arm sling when client is in an upright position.
- Administer O_2.
- Provide alternative methods of communication, e.g., writing or felt board.

Evaluation

One week after admission Ms. Wagner communicates with difficulty. Must be careful with liquids and needs thickener in food. She ambulates in the hall with physical therapy but has not regained her strength in or use of her left arm. Ms. Wagner is stable and continues to improve but will be placed in a long-term care facility for rehabilitation.

Critical Thinking in the Nursing Process

1. Why is Ms. Wagner not considered a candidate for fibrinolytic treatment?
2. Why is it important to control Ms. Wagner's hypertension?
3. How do you answer Ms. Wagner's daughter when she asks if her mother will have to stay in long-term care for the remainder of her life?

Note: Discussion of Critical Thinking questions appears on the MyNursingKit Website.

Infections of the Neurologic System

The bones of the skull and vertebral column, the meninges, and the blood–brain barrier all protect the brain and the spinal cord from infective agents. When infection does occur, it usually presents as an acute clinical situation and most commonly has invaded through the blood. Other routes of invasion include extension along cranial and spinal nerves, cerebrospinal fluid, direct extension from a primary site such as a skull fracture, and the mouth and nasopharynx. The causative agent may be bacterial, viral, or miscellaneous (fungal, protozoal).

clinical ALERT

CNS infections are uncommon, but they are a serious cause of morbidity and mortality. When CNS infection is a possibility, prompt diagnosis and treatment are crucial to survival.

MENINGITIS

Meningitis is an inflammation of the meninges of the brain and spinal cord. The three major organisms causing bacterial meningitis in children and adults are found in the nasopharynx; however, a predisposing factor such as a prior upper respiratory infection must be present before the bacteria become bloodborne. The bacteria are pneumococcal meningitis, *Haemophilus influenzae* meningitis, and meningococcal meningitis.

In *bacterial meningitis*, the pia mater and arachnoid, the subarachnoid space, the ventricular system, and the cerebrospinal fluid are infected. The cerebrospinal fluid is thickened with an exudate caused by neutrophils (blood cells). The exudate may interfere with or obstruct CSF flow. *Viral meningitis* is less severe than bacterial meningitis, because inflammation is limited to the meninges and is non-purulent. Table 36-7 ■ describes common types of intracranial infections.

Manifestations

Although several different organisms can cause meningitis, they cause similar signs and symptoms. The symptoms of meningitis are headache, fever, nuchal rigidity (stiff neck), altered mental status (confusion, irritability, altered LOC), nausea and vomiting, and photophobia. (*Note:* With meningococcal meningitis a skin rash with petechial hemorrhage is evident.)

An early sign of meningeal irritation is a stiff neck. Active or passive flexion of the neck proves difficult and painful. Two additional signs of meningeal irritation are Kernig's and Brudzinski's signs (see Figure 62-5 ⬤⬤). *Kernig's sign* is the inability to extend the leg when the hip

TABLE 36-7	Intracranial Infections	
INFECTION	**CAUSATIVE ORGANISM**	**SUSCEPTIBLE CLIENTS**
Bacterial meningitis		
Pneumococcal	*Streptococcus pneumoniae*	Young adults and those over age 40
Haemophilus influenzae	*Haemophilus influenzae*	Young children: 2 months to 7 years
Meningococcal	*Neisseria meningitides*	Children under 5, adolescents, young adults: 18 to 25 years; higher incidence in males
Viral (aseptic) meningitis	Herpes simplex and zoster; mumps, Epstein-Barr virus; cytomegalovirus	All ages
Encephalitis	St. Louis encephalitis virus, eastern and western equine virus transmitted by ticks and mosquitoes; herpes simplex; rabies; after vaccination with measles, mumps, or rubella	All ages
Brain abscess	Secondary infection from streptococci, staphylococci, pneumococci; complication of AIDS	30 to 40 years old; higher incidence in males

is flexed at a 90-degree angle. In *Brudzinski's sign*, neck flexion also causes the knees and hips to flex.

Diagnosis and Treatment

Diagnosis is based on history, laboratory tests, and physical examination.

Specific treatment for the causative organism must be used. However, antibiotic treatment for infectious meningitis is started immediately in order to save life and reduce complications. Some of the complications include seizures, sepsis, cranial nerve dysfunction, cerebral infarction, coma, and death. Residual effects of meningitis may be visual impairment, hearing loss or deafness, cranial nerve palsies, or paralysis.

clinical ALERT

If bacterial meningitis is suspected, the client will need to be placed in strict isolation until antibiotics have been administered for at least 24 hours. This will prevent spread of the bacteria to the staff caring for the client.

ENCEPHALITIS

Encephalitis is an inflammation of the gray and white matter of the brain and the spinal cord. It ranges from a mild infection to a serious one that can be fatal. It is usually caused by a virus but can also be caused by bacteria, fungi, or parasites. It can also be an aftereffect of systemic viral diseases such as measles, mumps, and influenza. Many of the viruses are endemic to particular geographic areas and certain seasons of the year and can be transmitted by ticks or mosquitoes.

Manifestations

Signs and symptoms vary widely, depending on the neurologic area infected. Common signs and symptoms are fever, headache, seizures, stiff neck, and a change in level of consciousness.

Diagnosis and Treatment

Diagnosis is made on the clinical signs and diagnostic tests, and must be differentiated from meningitis.

There is no specific treatment, except when it is caused by the herpes simplex virus. Then acyclovir seems to be an effective treatment. For other viruses, treatment is supportive care and control of increased intracranial pressure.

clinical ALERT

Older adults, young children, and others with depressed immune responses are at greatest risk of contracting encephalitis.

BRAIN ABSCESS

A **brain abscess** is an infection that has extended into the cerebral tissue or that is caused by organisms carried from other sites in the body. It most commonly occurs secondary to middle ear infections, nasal sinuses, face or skull infections, or from penetrating wounds. It may also be *metastatic* (that is, the infection comes from some other part of the body). Individuals who are immunosuppressed, particularly those with acquired immunodeficiency syndrome (AIDS), are susceptible to brain abscesses.

Manifestations

The initial signs and symptoms of a brain abscess are headache, chills and fever, malaise, irritability, seizures, or paralysis. Later signs and symptoms are a recurrent headache that becomes severe, confusion, drowsiness and stupor, focal or generalized seizures, and increased intracranial pressure. Location of the abscess determines the signs and symptoms.

Diagnosis and Treatment

The healthcare provider will determine the type of abscess that is present through CT/MRI brain scans, lumbar punctures, surgical debriding, and cultures of the operative region.

A complete health history and physical examination are important to determine the entry of the bacteria to form the abscess.

Treatment is based on the underlying infection. Treatments include antibiotics, drainage, and/or surgical removal of encapsulated abscess.

Nursing Considerations

When caring for clients with brain infections or abscesses, focus care on detecting complications quickly. One major complication is an increase in intracranial pressure. Perform neurologic checks every 2 hours and report any changes in level of consciousness, pupil size and reaction, speaking ability, or movement. When edema occurs in the brain, it can increase quickly and cause damage to vital brain centers.

LYME DISEASE

Lyme disease is caused by a spirochete transmitted by the bite of an infected tick found on white-tailed deer and other wild animals.

Manifestations

There are three stages to the progression of Lyme disease. In the first stage there usually is a characteristic rash called *erythema chronicum migrans*. This rash resembles a bull's-eye, with a red ring at the site of the tick bite that expands to leave a clear center. The rash fades in 3 to 4 weeks; during which there may be signs of meningitis, radiculitis, and neuritis without a fever. During the second stage, complications may develop such as atrioventricular block, Bell's palsy, meningitis, encephalitis, polyradiculitis, or inflammation of the eyes. In the third stage, which may occur 4 weeks to years after the bite, arthritic symptoms occur that affect the large joints and cause chronic joint pain.

Diagnosis and Treatment

The healthcare provider will obtain a thorough health assessment to include a history of pets, traveling, camping, hiking, and hunting. Other information gathered will include signs and symptoms of the disease. Diagnosis is made on history of a bite and after 4 weeks an elevated titer to Lyme disease, determined by a serum antibody study.

The best prevention is prompt removal of the ticks from the skin before they become attached or gain access to the bloodstream (generally within 24 hours). Persons who frequent or live in infested areas may want to discuss with their healthcare provider the possibility of receiving a recombinant vaccine, which may help prevent Lyme disease. Treatment consists of various antibiotics during the first two stages. If antibiotics are started as soon as the diagnosis is made, the disease may be cured. The use of antibiotics in the third stage is controversial.

WEST NILE VIRUS

West Nile virus (WNV) is a virus that is transmitted from birds to humans, usually by mosquitoes. It causes viral encephalitis, which can range from mild to fatal. Initial symptoms may be a mild fever, headache, body ache, skin rash, and swollen lymph glands. In more severe infections there is a headache, high fever, neck stiffness, stupor, disorientation, coma, tremors, convulsions, muscle weakness, and paralysis.

Blood tests identify the virus antibodies. Tests are done if indicated when the client has flulike symptoms and lives in an area where the virus exists or the client has been exposed. At present there is no treatment or vaccine for West Nile virus. The Center for Disease Control recommends reporting any dead birds to the local health department, and avoiding handling them. Any client with severe signs and symptoms of the disease needs to seek medical care and possibly hospitalization. The care of the client will be supportive, and treatments will be directed for alleviation of the signs and symptoms, especially confusion and respiratory depression.

The Center for Disease Control recommends the following to prevent spread of West Nile virus:

- Coordinating a nationwide electronic database through which states share information about WNV
- Helping states develop and carry out improved mosquito prevention and control programs
- Developing better, faster tests to detect and diagnose WNV
- Creating new education tools and programs for the media, the public, and health professionals
- Opening new testing laboratories for WNV
- Working with partners on the development of vaccines

NURSING CARE

PRIORITIZING NURSING CARE

When collecting data on clients for Lyme disease or West Nile virus, the main focus should be the health history and possibility of exposure to the viruses. Observation for skin changes, headache, fever, confusion, and joint discomforts will help determine the diagnosis of the disease. Clients in humid and hot regions should be instructed on prevention of the disease through use of proper insect repellents and following the recommended guidelines from the Center for Disease Control.

ASSESSING

Perform the routine neurologic examination of level of consciousness, pupillary evaluation, neuromuscular response, and vital signs frequently to determine further deterioration or the onset of complications.

DIAGNOSING, PLANNING, AND IMPLEMENTING

Possible nursing diagnoses for the client with neurologic infections include:

- *Altered Cerebral Tissue Perfusion* related to increased ICP
- *Ineffective Breathing Pattern* related to depression of the respiratory center
- *Acute Pain* related to irritation of meninges and increased ICP
- *Risk for Injury* related to confusion, seizures, restlessness
- *Fluid Volume Deficit* related to vomiting and fever
- *Risk for Disuse Syndrome* related to bed rest

Outcomes for these clients would include the following:

- Client's breathing will remain within normal limits.
- Client will remain free of injury.

Nurses must be vigilant in caring for clients with infections of the CNS:

- Elevate the head of the bed as ordered. *Helps reduce increased ICP.*
- Instruct client to avoid coughing and to not hold his breath during turning. *These behaviors increase ICP.*
- Monitor the respiratory status and gag and swallowing reflexes. *Ensure patent (open) airway.*
- Assess the location and severity of any discomfort and administer analgesics as ordered. *Reduces and/or alleviates pain increasing client's comfort level.*
- Keep bed in low position, with side rails padded and raised. *Helps protect the client in the event of a seizure.*
- Monitor intake and output. *To determine if client is adequately hydrated.*
- Perform range of motion as tolerated. *Promotes muscle tone and maintains flexibility.*

EVALUATING

In clients with neurologic infections, evaluate orientation and level of consciousness frequently to determine mental status. Clients can deteriorate rapidly, so prompt reporting of changes to the charge nurse is critical. The expected outcomes would be that the ICP would return to normal and that the client would maintain a patent airway, pain and discomfort would decrease as the infection recedes, the client would not harm self during a seizure, fluid volume would be adequate, and neurologic deficits would be minimal to none.

Neurosensory Trauma and Tumors

TRAUMATIC BRAIN INJURY

Traumatic brain injury (TBI) is defined as a traumatic injury to the brain that is capable of producing physical, intellectual, emotional, social, and vocational changes. It is one of the leading causes of disability and death in the United States. Traumatic brain injury occurs three times more often in males than in females. The average client age at injury is between 15 and 30 years. Motor vehicle accidents are the major source of TBIs, followed by falls, sports injuries, and violent assaults. Most instances of TBI occur during evenings, nights, and weekends.

Traumatic brain injuries can be classified as blunt injuries or penetrating injuries. The outcome is affected by the mechanism of injury:

- **Deceleration** *forces*—injuries that occur when the head hits an immovable object
- **Acceleration** *forces*—injuries that occur when a moving object hits the head
- *Acceleration–deceleration forces*—injuries that occur when the head is hit with a moving object and hits an immovable object, moving the brain within the cranium
- *Rotational forces*—movement of the brain in a side-to-side, twisting motion inside the cranium, which often occurs with acceleration–deceleration forces
- *Deformation forces*—injuries that occur due to direct blows to the head that change the shape of the head
- *Penetrating injuries*—caused by nail/air guns, gunshot wounds, stab wounds, and other types of impalement injuries. Gunshot wounds are the most lethal of all injuries to the brain.

A focal cerebral injury directly under the area of impact is called a **coup** injury, and a cerebral injury that occurs opposite the point of impact is called a **contrecoup** injury (see Figure 47-10).

Mild Brain Injury

A mild TBI may result in a concussion. A mild concussion affects attention span and memory without the loss of consciousness. Manifestations may range from temporary confusion and disorientation to more persistent confusion that lasts several minutes. The signs and symptoms of mild brain injury may involve loss of consciousness that usually lasts less than 6 hours. The duration of unconsciousness is an indicator of the severity of the concussion.

The symptoms of postconcussive syndrome are headache, dizziness, irritability, emotional lability, fatigue, poor concentration, decreased attention span, memory difficulties, and intellectual dysfunction. These symptoms may occur from 1 week to 1 year after the initial injury.

Moderate to Severe Brain Injury

Moderate to severe brain injury usually results in a cerebral contusion (bruising of the surface of the brain). The sites of injury are predictable with acceleration–deceleration injuries: They are located where the brain impacts on the bony protuberances of the skull.

Manifestations

Contusions are associated with loss of consciousness, stupor, and confusion. The outcome depends on the area and severity of the injury. If the contusion is located in the deeper structures of the brain, the prognosis is poor due to hemorrhage and destruction of the reticular activating fibers for arousal.

The client with a traumatically injured brain may experience a period of unconsciousness following the trauma that lasts for minutes, days, weeks, or even years. Coma is the deepest form of unconsciousness and is a symptomatic response to an underlying cause. It is a very serious symptom and often has a fatal outcome. In the comatose state the individual lies with eyes closed and does not make an attempt to avoid noxious stimuli. There may be a display of various forms of reflex posturing (see Figure 36-16). A prolonged period of unconsciousness (a **coma**) creates many complications related to the client's inactive and bedridden status.

Diagnosis and Treatment

Diagnosis is based on the findings from the history and physical examination and includes the findings of the CT/MRI scan.

Treatment is based on the client's signs and symptoms. The priority will be the management of the airway, respirations, and nausea/vomiting. Medications may be prescribed for seizure prevention, headache, and increased intracranial pressure. The head of the bed will be maintained at least 30 degrees elevated. The room will be darkened and quiet to reduce stimulation. Occasionally, the client will have behavior problems related to confusion, such as repetitive questioning or forgetfulness. The plan of care will need to be altered to accommodate the changes in client behavior.

HEMATOMA

Epidural, subdural, and intracerebral are the three main types of hematomas that result from trauma. Hematoma is a complication in one-third to one-half of all TBIs. One-fourth of all skull fractures develop a surgically significant hematoma (Figure 36-17 ■). Hematomas are frequently associated with a cerebral contusion.

Epidural Hematoma

Epidural hematomas evolve from bleeding into the epidural space between the skull and the dura mater. A fracture in the temporal bone may cause a tear in the middle meningeal artery, resulting in an epidural hematoma. The middle meningeal artery is located in a groove in the temporal bone, which is the thinnest bone of the skull.

clinical ALERT

An injury indicating an epidural hematoma is a neurologic emergency. The client needs immediate interventions.

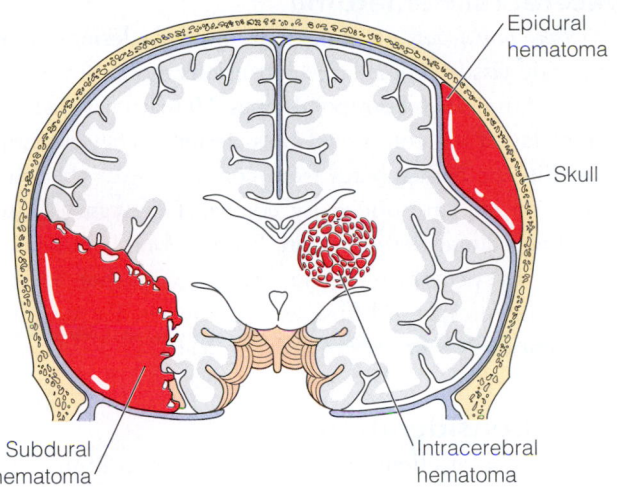

Figure 36-17. ■ Three types of hematomas: epidural, subdural, and intracerebral.

Subdural Hematoma

Subdural hematomas, besides having the highest mortality rate, are also the most common type of hematoma. The bleeding into the subdural space between the dura mater and the arachnoid is usually caused by the rupture of the bridging veins that cross the subdural space.

Subdural hematomas are usually found around the top and sides of the head and are associated with contusions and intracerebral hematomas. There are three types of subdural hematomas:

- *Acute subdural hematoma*—presents within 48 hours postinjury; usually with cortical or brainstem injury and represents a mass lesion. Signs and symptoms mimic rapidly expanding lesion or increased ICP. Significant mortality rates result because brain tissue is damaged and a mass effect is caused by hematoma. Mortality decreases with surgical intervention within 4 hours.

- *Subacute subdural hematoma*—occurs between 24 and 48 hours to 2 weeks postinjury; associated with moderate traumatic brain injury. The individual may show a steady decline in level of alertness. Surgical evacuation of the hematoma may be performed to improve the individual's level of consciousness.

- *Chronic subdural hematoma*—occurs 2 weeks to several months postinjury and is often the result of a low-impact injury such as falling or bumping of the head. Older adults, chronic alcohol abusers, or those on anticoagulant warfarin have higher incidence of this injury. This type of hematoma acts as a space-occupying lesion that progressively enlarges. The damage is often bilateral. Treatment is usually with burr holes for gradual drainage of the hematoma to prevent recurrence or to prevent further brain injury to the individual.

Intracerebral Hematoma

Intracerebral hematomas are single or multiple lesions deep within brain tissue. These large contusions most commonly occur in the frontal and temporal lobes. Hematomas that are 25 mL or larger are considered mass lesions. They develop deep within the hemispheres from contused areas that run together and are surrounded by edema. They can lead to IICP and neurologic deterioration. Intracerebral hematomas are caused by penetrating wounds, e.g., gunshot, deep-depressed fractures, and diffuse axonal injuries. Early surgical intervention is necessary to prevent death.

Nursing Considerations

When you care for clients with traumatic brain injuries or hematomas of the brain, your focus is once again detecting increasing intracranial pressure early so it can be treated before it causes brain damage. Check neurologic signs every 15 minutes to 2 hours depending on the stability of the client. Be very thorough in your assessment and note even small changes. Report any changes promptly so changes in treatment can be initiated as needed. As the client recovers from the condition and becomes more stable, you will focus care on rehabilitation and recovery of cognitive function.

SPINAL CORD INJURY

Spinal cord injuries (SCIs) generally result from vertebral injuries, which usually occur due to acceleration, deceleration, or deformation forces most frequently applied at a distance. Damage occurs to the vertebral or neural tissues by compressing the tissues, pulling or exerting a traction or tension on the tissues, or shearing tissues so that they slide into one another. These forces may be exerted on the vertebral and neural tissues by hyperextension, hyperflexion (Figure 36-18 ■), vertical compression, or rotation of the spine.

Manifestations

Microscopic hemorrhages and edema are the first manifestations, and are greatest at the level of injury, and for two segments above and below it. This localized hemorrhaging and edema are followed by reduced vascular perfusion and development of ischemic areas.

Damage to the cord is described as complete or incomplete. A complete spinal cord injury results in a total loss of motor and sensory functions below the level of injury (see also Box 31-3 ⟳). An incomplete injury results in varying degrees of loss of function below the level of injury. The level of injury determines whether or not the individual develops paraplegia or tetraplegia (formerly referred to as quadriplegia). Figure 36-19 ■ illustrates different types of paralysis.

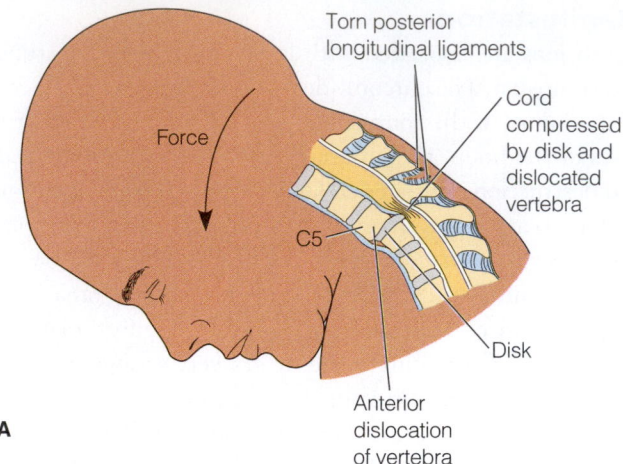

A

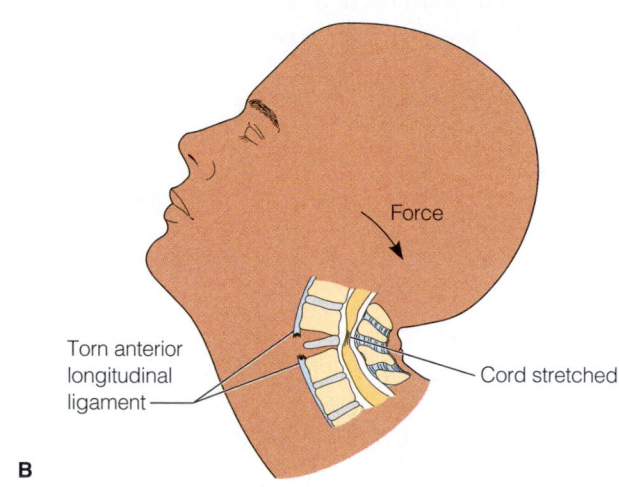

B

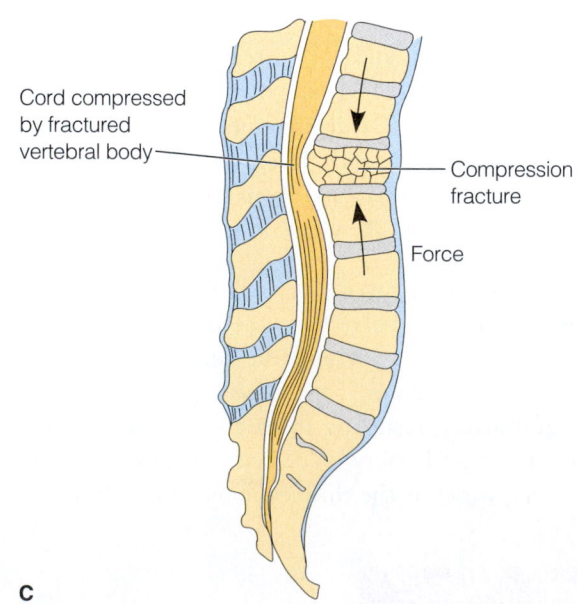

C

Figure 36-18. ■ Spinal cord injury can occur through several mechanisms: **A.** hyperextension. **B.** hyperflexion. **C.** axial loading (compressive force).

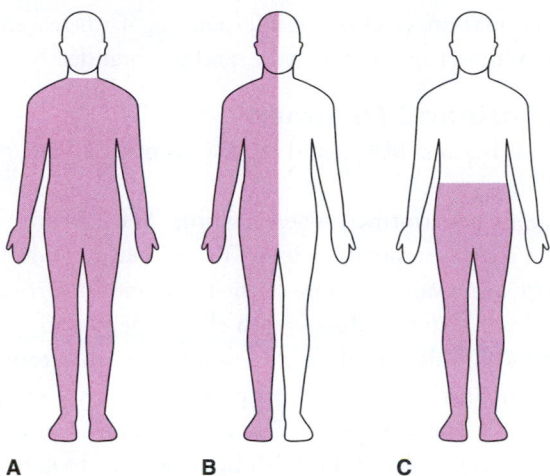

Figure 36-19. ■ Types of paralysis. **A.** Tetraplegia is complete or partial paralysis of the upper extremities and complete paralysis of the lower part of the body. **B.** Hemiplegia is paralysis of one-half of the body when it is divided along the median sagittal plane. **C.** Paraplegia is paralysis of the lower part of the body.

Complications

Paraplegia is paralysis of the lower part of the body as a result of damage done at the thoracic level (see Box 36-1). Tetraplegia is paralysis of the arms, trunk, legs, and pelvic organs due to high cervical injuries. In either case, complications can occur immediately after injury or later.

SPINAL SHOCK. The temporary loss of reflex activity below the level of spinal cord injury is known as **spinal shock.** It usually occurs within 30 to 60 minutes after a complete SCI. In spinal shock there is a loss of motor function, sensation, spinal reflexes, and autonomic function. It can last for 1 to 6 weeks when reflex activity returns.

AUTONOMIC DYSREFLEXIA. An exaggerated sympathetic response in spinal cord injuries at or above the T6 level is known as **autonomic dysreflexia.** It may occur at any time after spinal shock resolves and is a medical emergency that must receive immediate treatment or it may result in seizures, a cerebrovascular accident, or death. It is triggered by a full bladder or fecal impaction resulting in a hypertensive crisis. Systolic pressure goes up to 300 mm Hg and may be accompanied by a severe headache, blurred vision, sweating with flushing of the skin above the level of the lesion and pale, cold, dry skin below it, goose bumps, and bradycardia (heart rate of 30 to 40 bpm).

clinical ALERT

If autonomic dysreflexia occurs, the head of the bed should be elevated 45 degrees to lower the blood pressure, and antihypertensive medications should be administered as ordered. Usually emptying the bladder or bowel relieves the response.

Diagnosis and Treatment

Diagnosis of the spinal cord injury and the level of the injury is made from a complete physical assessment and diagnostic studies, such as CT/MRI scan. The injured area is also investigated with a surgical procedure to either stabilize the fractured vertebrae or remove a foreign body, such as a bullet or knife blade.

Treatment will be supportive and will be determined by the client's symptoms. The priority nursing interventions are focused on the airway and breathing. Secondary priorities are the skin, bowels, and bladder to prevent complications of autonomic dysreflexia. Beware of weakened respiratory and intercostal muscles with injuries in the lower cervical and thoracic spinal regions.

Medical care of the client will initially include a large dose of methylprednisolone to reduce the edema of the injured cord. The healthcare provider will order bowel instructions and a Foley catheter. This will later be reduced to intermittent catheterization for bladder training, and supportive treatments.

The client will have periods of grieving throughout acute stages of care, so the nursing care plans will need to be altered as behaviors change. As the client progresses, the treatment plans developed by a healthcare team will be changed to accommodate the client's progression and goals. The rehabilitation process starts as soon as the client is admitted to the unit of care. (See more on rehabilitation in Chapter 46 ⬀.)

Psychosocial support to the client and the family is crucial. Maintaining a positive attitude will help the client and family as they cope with the possibility of limited functioning in the future. As soon as possible, the goal is for the client to return to society and be functional in ADLs. Rehabilitation and occupational therapy are begun when the client is stable enough to perform physical exercise and to tolerate being in the upright or sitting position for longer periods of time.

Nursing Considerations

When caring for clients with spinal cord injuries, focus your care on preventing further injuries and complications. Because sensation is decreased or absent below the level of the injury, clients may have serious infections or ulcerations and not feel them. Skin integrity is a priority. Clients' position must be shifted every 2 hours while they are in bed; it is also important to ensure position changes when the client is sitting to prevent pressure ulcer formation.

Be vigilant about monitoring bowel activity and keeping the bladder drained to prevent autonomic dysreflexia. Monitor vital signs every shift and more frequently if signs of autonomic dysreflexia appear. If these symptoms occur, take immediate action by elevating the head of the bed to

45 degrees, administering antihypertensive medications, and relieving bowel or bladder blockage. Report symptoms immediately to an RN or physician.

BRAIN TUMORS

Intracranial tumors, or brain tumors, include both benign space-occupying and malignant lesions. Brain tumors can occur in any structural area of the brain and in all age groups with peak incidences in early childhood and in the fifth, sixth, and seventh decades of life. The growth rates vary from the rapid growth of glioblastomas (Figure 36-20 ■) to the almost imperceptible changes of some meningiomas. Brain tumors are named for the tissues in which they arise. Primary brain tumors originate from the cells and structures found within the brain. Metastatic brain tumors originate in structures outside of the brain such as tumors of the lungs, breast, gastrointestinal tract, and genitourinary tract and are classified as secondary tumors. Tumors that are benign but that are surgically inaccessible may offer a worse prognosis than a malignant tumor that is surgically accessible.

Manifestations

Whether benign or malignant, the signs and symptoms of brain tumors reflect neurologic deficits caused by focal disturbances and increased intracranial pressure. The destruction of neural tissue due to increasing compression of brain tissue and the infiltration or direct invasion of brain parenchyma causes focal disturbances. The size and location of a tumor can cause shifts of brain tissue, with associated brain herniation syndromes. Herniation, if untreated, can result in infarction, hemorrhage, and cerebral death.

Diagnosis and Treatment

X-rays, CT scans, MRIs, and PET scans may be used to obtain a diagnosis.

Surgery is performed when possible. Specialized microsurgical techniques may be used. Traditional chemotherapy has little or no value because of the blood–brain barrier, but slow-release wafers suffused with chemotherapeutic agents may be surgically implanted. There has been steady improvement in the strength and precision of laser radiation (such as the gamma knife). The gamma knife can destroy deep or inaccessible lesions with little damage to surrounding tissue.

SPINAL CORD TUMORS

Tumors of the spinal cord are comparatively rare. They are named to reflect their cell type, growth rate, and structure of origin, and are classified as intramedullary and extramedullary tumors. Table 36-8 ■ describes brain and spinal cord tumors. The tumor's rate of growth and degree of compression determine the severity of neurologic symptoms. The spinal cord can accommodate slower growing tumors by compressing into a slender, ribbon-like tissue.

Manifestations

A slow-growing tumor may produce minimum deficits, whereas a fast-growing tumor may produce sudden cord compression, edema, and severe neurologic deficits.

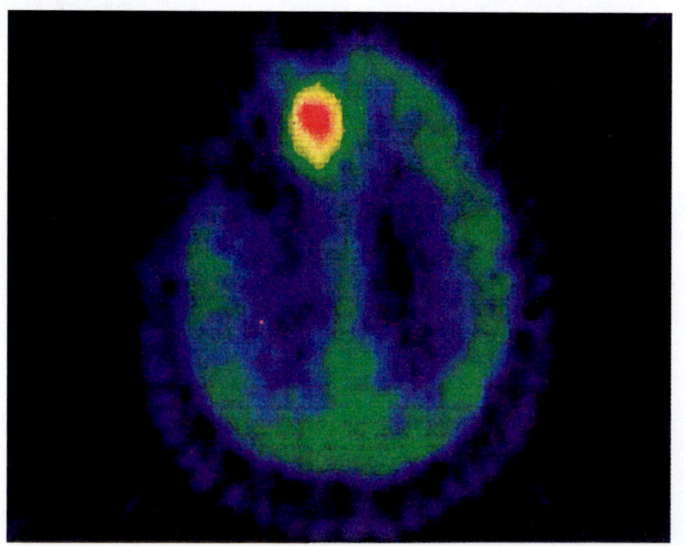

A

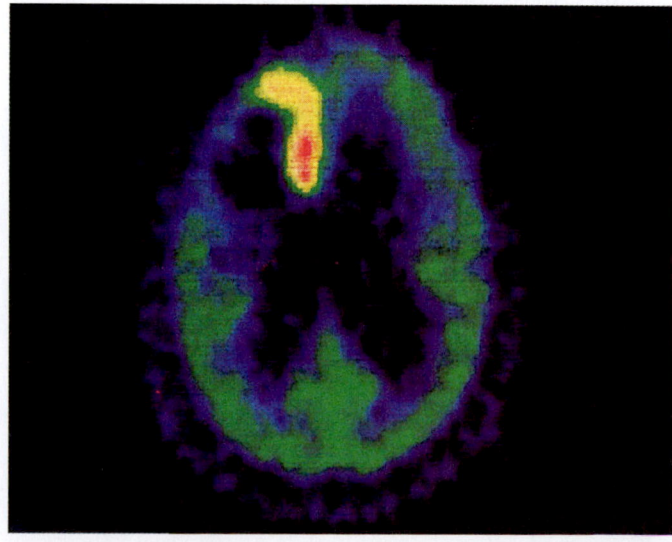

B

Figure 36-20. ■ Glioblastoma multiforme, an actively growing tumor, is shown. **A.** Note the large red area of the tumor. **B.** The same tumor at a different level in the brain. (*Source:* Courtesy of Dr. Giovanni DiChiro and Dr. Ramesh Raman of the Neuroimaging Branch, National Institute of Neurological Disorders and Stroke, National Institutes of Health.)

TABLE 36-8	Common Spinal Tumors
TYPE	**CHARACTERISTICS**
EXTRADURAL TUMORS	
Metastatic tumors: lung, breast, prostate, lymphoma, renal cell, plasmacytoma	Usually invade the bony spine and compress spinal cord or nerve roots. Lymphoma usually is a "dumbbell" mass originating in the paraspinal tissues. Dura acts as a barrier between tumor and spinal cord.
Chordoma	Arises from notochordal remnants and invades bone.
INTRADURAL—EXTRAMEDULLARY TUMORS	
Schwannoma	Benign tumor composed of Schwann cells, arising from the dorsal (sensory) root of spinal or cranial nerves.
Neurofibroma	Benign tumor composed of Schwann cells, fibroblasts, and perineural cells, arising from the dorsal root of spinal or cranial nerves. May be multiple in von Recklinghausen's neurofibromatosis.
Meningioma	Usually benign and arises from the arachnoid villi of the dura.
Ependymoma	Arises from ependymal cells. Fifty percent arise in the intradural portion of the filum terminale.
INTRADURAL—INTRAMEDULLARY TUMORS	
Astrocytoma	Arises from astrocytes.
Hemangioblastoma	Benign tumor composed of a mixture of capillaries and lipid-laden stromal cells. Usually cerebellar.
Metastases: lung, breast, colorectal, melanoma, lymphoma	Presents with pain (radicular or nonradicular), weakness, paresthesias, and sphincter dysfunction.

Diagnosis and Treatment

Unfortunately, a majority of brain tumors are not diagnosed until the client manifests delayed symptoms, including syncope, confusion, loss of vision, ataxia, or headache not relieved with regular medications. The complete health history and a neurologic examination of the client help the neurologist or neurosurgeon to determine the location of the tumor in the brain. After reviewing the CT/MRI scan, the surgeon determines whether the tumor is primary or secondary. Surgical intervention may be necessary to determine the specific tumor as well.

Surgery, radiation, and chemotherapy are all possible interventions depending on the location and extent of the lesion, determined by the results of the CT/MRI scans. Some newer interventions include instillation of radioactive seeds in the brain near or on the lesion to reduce the swelling and potential complications. Anticonvulsants are administered to decrease the incidence of seizure activity from tumor growth or irritation of the brain. Also anticipate the use of glucosteroids to reduce the swelling and pressure from the tumor, especially in the clients that have inoperable tumors.

Nursing Considerations

Priority nursing care for the client with a new diagnosis of a brain tumor will be emotional support. The client and family will be devastated and grieve through the process. The main focus for nursing interventions will be safety, observation of the client for changes in mood and behavior, alterations in level of consciousness, signs or symptoms of IICP; altered vision, and seizure activity. Immediately postoperatively, the client will have vital signs and neurologic checks every 15 minutes, progressing to every 2 hours as the client improves. Any changes indicating deterioration of the client's condition need to be reported to the physician immediately.

As the client deteriorates, the family and client may not feel capable of making a decision. Discussions need to be initiated by the healthcare team to determine the continuation of the treatment plan or any changes in the treatment plan. The advance directives of the client will need to be honored. Hospice services are often beneficial to the client and family when the diagnosis and treatment plans are no longer an option for the client.

NURSING CARE

PRIORITIZING NURSING CARE

Priority nursing interventions for the client with a diagnosis of brain tumor should include airway and breathing, and comfort. If the diagnosis is new for the client, the grieving process of accepting the diagnosis may be the priority for the client and their family. Dangers from self-harm and potential seizure activity increase as the client's health deteriorates. Medications will be administered as ordered by the healthcare provider, and the client's responses to these are monitored. Any deviations from the baseline need to be reported to the RN or physician as soon as possible.

ASSESSING

Level of consciousness is the most important assessment made with traumatic brain injury, and is also a priority with brain tumors. (See Box 36-1 for terms describing levels of consciousness.) After collecting data about level of consciousness, it is important to assess the pupils and determine whether there is lateralized weakness or loss of function of the extremities. The Glasgow Coma Scale (see Table 19-2 ⬤⬤) is used universally to assess level of consciousness.

DIAGNOSING, PLANNING, AND IMPLEMENTING

Many nursing diagnoses may be appropriate for the client with neurosensory trauma or tumors, including:

- *Risk for Decreased Cerebral Tissue Perfusion*
- *Impaired Verbal Communication* related to effects of hematoma (or tumor) on brain tissue
- *Disturbed Sensory Perception* related to impaired conduction of sensory information
- *Impaired Physical Mobility* and *Self-Care Deficits* related to motor disturbances and impaired cognition
- *Ineffective Coping* and *Disabled Family Coping* related to life-threatening trauma/disease, changes in behavior and function

Client goals in the planning stage of the nursing process include:

- Client will adapt to altered thinking; improved mental orientation.
- Client will recognize sensory-perception alterations.
- Client will participate in ADLs and maintain maximum possible mobility.
- Client will maintain skin integrity.
- Client will verbalize steps to begin coping with the event.

To achieve these goals, the nurse provides various interventions. Some of those interventions might include:

- Monitor level of consciousness frequently. *The earliest sign of increasing ICP is a change in the level of consciousness.*
- Monitor for changes in cognitive function. *Expression of thoughts and the ability to concentrate may be hindered and could result in anxiety for the client.*
- Implement safety measures as needed to prevent injury. *Impaired vision or sensation can lead to injury due to reduced awareness of environment.*
- Encourage client to perform ADLs and assist as needed. *Client has a sense of control and independence if doing things for self.*

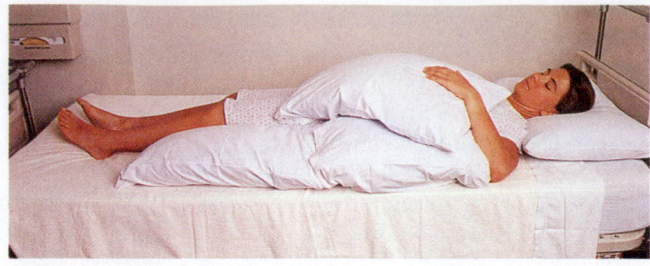

A

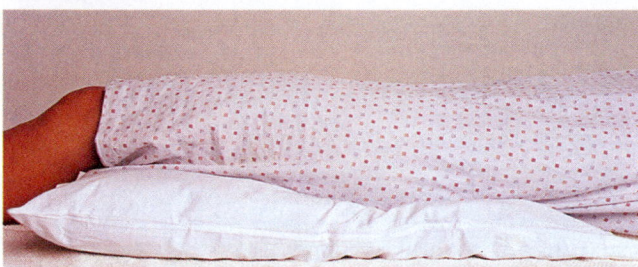

B

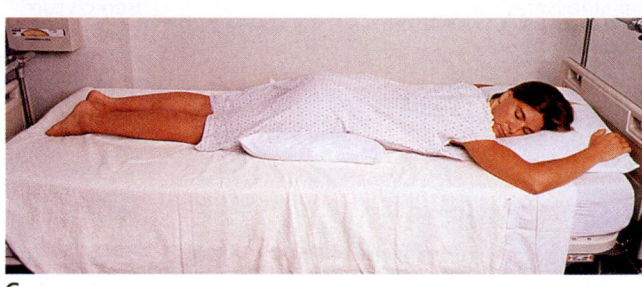

C

Figure 36-21. ■ Positioning the client with hemiplegia is important in preventing deformity of the affected extremities. **A.** With the client in a supine position, place a pillow in the axilla (to prevent adduction) and under the hand and arm, with the hand higher than the elbow (to prevent flexion and edema). **B.** When the client is lying supine, use a pillow from the iliac crest to the middle of the thigh to prevent external rotation of the hip. **C.** When the client is in the prone position, place a pillow under the pelvis to prevent hip hyperextension.

- Position client to maintain skin integrity (Figure 36-21 ■). Turn client often. *Pillows are often needed to support limbs in clients with immobility. Turning client on a regular schedule maintains intact skin.*
- Assist client and family in dealing with a difficult diagnosis. *Neurosensory trauma is life altering and the road to rehabilitation is long.*

EVALUATING

The nurse revises care plan until the expected outcomes are achieved or revised. The expected outcomes for a client with neurosensory trauma include the following:

- Level of consciousness is improved.
- Mental orientation and thinking are improved.

- Client does not experience further injury.
- Client performs ADLs to maximum ability.
- Client and family begin to accept diagnosis and cope effectively.

Degenerative Neurologic Disorders

PARKINSON'S DISEASE

Parkinson's disease is a commonly occurring, slowly progressive, degenerative disorder caused by dopamine deficiency. Dopamine carries messages that tell the body how and when to move. Shortage of dopamine causes movement to become more difficult.

Manifestations

There is a decrease in spontaneous movements, gait difficulty, postural instability, rigidity, and tremors. A "pill-rolling" action of the thumb and forefinger is the most distinctive tremor, though it is the least disabling symptom. Tremors occur at rest and lessen with movement. Tremors commonly occur unilaterally but can spread to involve other body segments. Stress and anxiety increase all tremors.

Rigidity is usually present and is attributed to an increase in muscle tone at rest. The trunk, head, and shoulders are stiff and there is a lack of arm swing when walking. The rigidity (called cogwheel rigidity because of the stiffness and jerky quality of motion) impedes active and passive movement. The first symptoms may be painful muscle cramps in the toes or hands, and then the limb feels stiff, heavy, tired, or aching.

Akinesia/bradykinesia is difficulty in initiating a movement, then moving very slowly. Because they have difficulty rising from a chair, getting in or out of a car, and performing ADLs, individuals with Parkinson's disease sit and lie motionless for long periods. This slowness or lack of movement puts them at risk for pneumonia, deep vein thrombosis, constipation, and pressure ulcers.

Postural abnormalities are caused by the loss of normal postural reflexes. There is an involuntary flexion of the head and neck. The individual is unable to maintain an upright position of the trunk while standing or walking. The small, shuffling steps are an attempt to remain in an upright position while walking. Once movement is initiated, it accelerates and the individual is at risk of falling.

Secondary manifestations are difficulty with fine motor function, monotonic voice, masklike face, general weakness and muscle fatigue, cognitive changes, and depression. There are also many signs and symptoms associated with autonomic dysfunction such as drooling, seborrhea, dysphagia, excessive perspiration, constipation, orthostatic hypotension, and urinary hesitation and frequency.

Diagnosis and Treatment

Parkinson's disease is diagnosed with a complete health assessment, medical history, and complete neurologic examination. The healthcare provider might consider doing diagnostic studies to rule out pathology that can cause changes in the neurologic assessment.

Parkinson's disease cannot be cured or arrested but symptoms can be controlled with drug therapy. Levodopa (a dopaminergic drug) is administered, along with dopamine agonists, anticholinergic drugs, antihistamines, and amantadine. These are used to decrease the akinesia. However, because of side effects and a decreased responsiveness after 5 years, they are not initiated until the symptoms become incapacitating. The signs and symptoms the client displays will be monitored for improvement or deterioration with the use of medication. As the client's condition deteriorates, the medications may be adjusted or altered to seek improvement or stabilization of the symptoms.

Treatment with levodopa does not prevent the progressive changes that are typical of Parkinson's disease. Also, the drug may produce side effects in some people. Some new drugs have been approved, offering a wider choice of medications. Others are under investigation.

MULTIPLE SCLEROSIS

A relatively common disorder that involves the central nervous system myelin is multiple sclerosis (MS). It is a chronic, progressive, degenerative disease that affects the myelin sheath and the conduction pathways of the CNS (the peripheral nervous system is not involved) (Figures 36-22A–C ■). Multiple sclerosis is currently described as being preceded by a viral insult to the nervous system with a subsequent abnormal immune response in the central nervous system. It is also generally accepted that MS occurs in individuals who are genetically susceptible. Women are affected slightly more often than men. The onset of symptoms usually occurs between the ages of 20 and 40 years of age, and the severity, duration, and prognosis vary. However, in the general population, the survival rate of individuals with multiple sclerosis is 85 percent. The clinical course determines the classification of MS:

- *Relapsing/remitting disease*—65% of cases relapse, develop over 1 to 2 weeks, resolve over 4 to 8 weeks, and return to baseline.
- *Relapsing/progressive disease*—15% of cases are similar to the relapsing/remitting form but with less recovery (baseline not returned to), and individual is left with significant residual disability.
- *Chronic progressive disease*—20% of cases are characterized by spinal cord and cerebellar dysfunction; symptoms of the spinal cord and cerebellum are the initial manifestations.
- The term *stable MS* is sometimes used for individuals who have had no active clinical disease or any subjective deterioration in their condition during the last year.

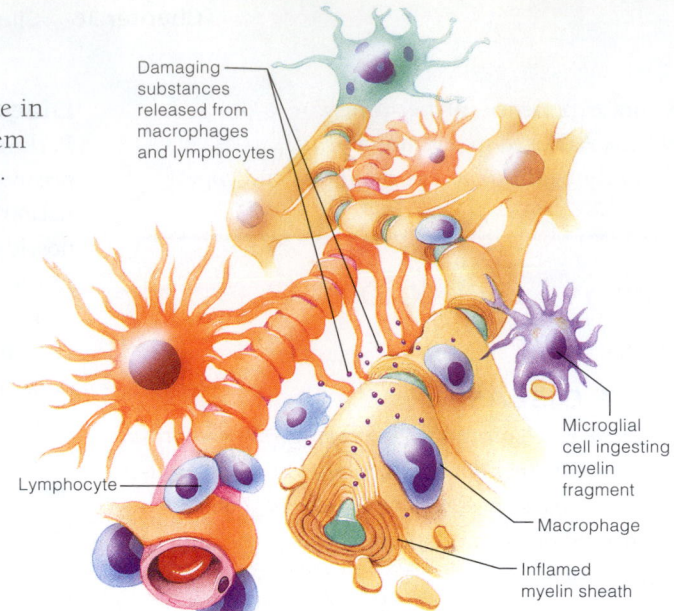

A
Acute Attack

Multiple sclerosis (MS) is a demyelinating disease in which axonal myelin in the central nervous system is eroded, destroyed, and replaced by scar tissue.

An autoimmune process apparently triggered by genetic and environmental factors is believed to cause inflammation of venules in the CNS. This disrupts the blood–brain barrier, allowing lymphocytes to enter CNS tissue. These lymphocytes proliferate and produce IgG, an antibody that attacks and damages myelin and causes the release of inflammatory chemicals and edema. As the inflammation subsides, the myelin regenerates and manifestations of the disease subside.

Damaging substances released from macrophages and lymphocytes

Microglial cell ingesting myelin fragment

Lymphocyte

Macrophage

Inflamed myelin sheath

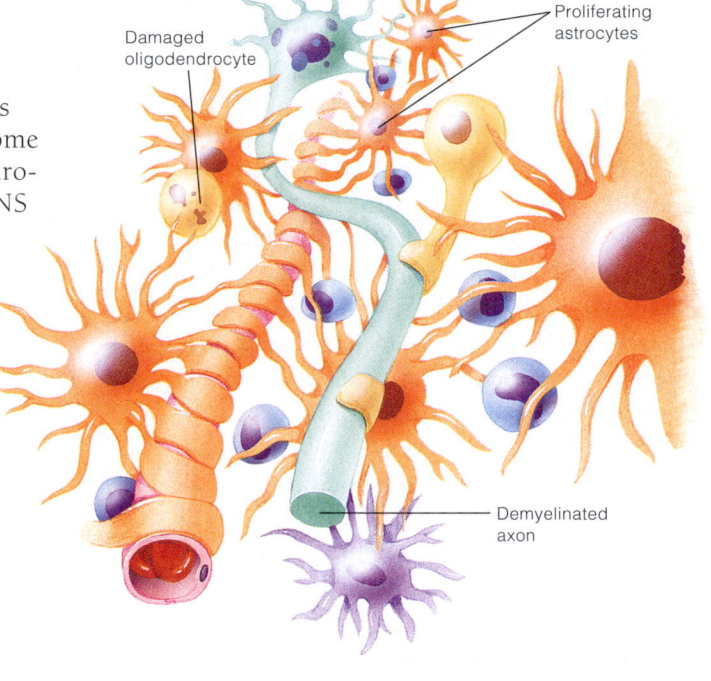

B
Chronic Lesion

After repeated inflammatory attacks, myelin is irreparably damaged. Segments of axons become totally demyelinated and may degenerate. Astrocytes proliferate in damaged regions of the CNS (a process call *gliosis*), forming plaques. The plaques are scattered throughout the CNS, appearing as gray or pinkish lesions. The relapsing-remitting character of MS and the scattered areas of damage within the CNS account for the variable nature of MS manifestations.

Damaged oligodendrocyte

Proliferating astrocytes

Demyelinated axon

C

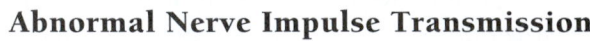

Abnormal Nerve Impulse Transmission

In an undamaged neuron, nerve impulses travel down the axon by "leaping" from one node of Ranvier to the next, thus greatly increasing the speed of impulse transmission. When nerve impulses travel down an axon damaged by MS, they are significantly slowed and weakened as they pass across the surface of demyelin-ated areas. Impulses may be blocked entirely when axons degenerate. The weakening or interruption of the transmission of nerve impulses and plaque formation within the CNS cause the manifestations of MS, including extremity weakness, paresthesias, visual disturbances, bladder dysfunction, and vertigo.

Figure 36-22. ■ Pathophysiology of multiple sclerosis. **A.** Acute attack. **B.** Chronic lesion. **C.** Abnormal nerve impulse transmission.

The conduction of normal nerve impulses is prevented in demyelinated areas since they are scattered throughout the white matter of the brain and spinal cord. The destruction of the myelin sheath leaves patches of sclerotic tissue. The healing of the demyelinated areas with sclerotic tissue results in the remission of symptoms. Ultimately, the nerve fibers may degenerate and the disabilities increase and become permanent.

Manifestations

The signs and symptoms are varied between individuals and may appear singularly or in combination. They fall into four categories: sensory, motor, cerebellar, and miscellaneous. The sensory symptoms include **paresthesia** (numbness, burning, prickling, tingling, pain) and decreased **proprioception** (decreased sense of temperature, depth, and vibration). Motor symptoms include paresis, paralysis, dragging of the foot, spasticity, diplopia, and incontinence or retention of bladder and/or bowel. Cerebellar symptoms include ataxia, loss of balance and coordination, nystagmus, speech disturbances, tremors, and vertigo. Miscellaneous symptoms include fatigue, sexual dysfunction such as impotence or decreased genital sensation, and neurobehavioral disorders such as depression or euphoria.

Diagnosis and Treatment

MS is difficult to diagnose because there is no definitive test; the diagnosis must be made based on clinical history, presentation of symptoms, and the elimination of other neurologic deficits.

Treatment is aimed at treating acute attacks, and decreasing the number of attacks and subsequent neurologic disabilities. Some of the drugs used are corticosteroids, interferon, and Imuran.

Nursing Considerations

When caring for clients with Parkinson's disease and multiple sclerosis, focus care on preventing injuries and complications. Safety is a major concern with these clients. Remove anything in the environment that could lead to falls, such as electrical cords and throw rugs that can slip. Be patient, giving clients ample time to accomplish tasks for themselves if they are able to do so. Assess clients frequently for respiratory complications such as crackles in the lungs. Encourage activity as tolerated to prevent complications of immobility. Encourage clients to do as much as possible for themselves to promote independence.

AMYOTROPHIC LATERAL SCLEROSIS

Amyotrophic lateral sclerosis (ALS) is a degenerative disease of the upper and lower motor neurons that is rapid in its progression. Also known as Lou Gehrig's disease, ALS results in progressive muscle weakness that leads to respiratory failure and death 2 to 5 years after onset of symptoms. Involvement of both the upper and lower motor neurons differentiates ALS from other motor neuron disorders. Also, the degeneration is not accompanied by inflammation. The lower motor neuron component of the syndrome involves progressive muscle wasting (the name *amyotrophic* means "without muscle nutrition"). The term *lateral sclerosis* refers to the scarring that takes place in the lateral column of the spinal cord, which is the upper motor neuron component of the syndrome.

Manifestations

Often muscle weakness and fatigue of a single muscle group are the initial symptoms. Usually muscles of the hand are affected, appearing as clumsiness. Next the shoulder and upper arm muscles are affected. The lower limbs are usually affected last, feeling heavy and subject to fatigue and easy cramping. Other symptoms may include:

- Muscle spasticity and hyperreflexia
- **Fasciculations** (involuntary contraction or twitching of muscle fibers)
- Brainstem signs evidenced by atrophy of the tongue and causing dysarthria
- Dyspnea, if the respiratory muscles are involved
- Fatigue
- Urinary and bowel dysfunctions (usually affected very late in the disease)

Intellectual ability, sensory function, vision, and hearing are not affected.

Diagnosis and Treatment

ALS is diagnosed primarily on the history and a neurologic examination that demonstrates upper and lower motor neuron disease. An electromyelogram will demonstrate fibrillations, which are signs of denervation, muscle wasting, and atrophy. The blood creatine phosphokinase (CPK) may be elevated. Also a myelogram may be done to rule out other diseases. A muscle biopsy confirms the diagnosis but is not usually necessary.

There is no known cure for ALS. However, an antiglutamate—Rilutek (riluzole)—is used to slow the deterioration. Treatment is directed at relieving symptoms, preventing complications, maintaining maximal function, and supporting quality of life. New medications have arisen to help lessen the signs and symptoms of the disease, and may prolong the client's life. As the client weakens, the client may have a tracheostomy tube and be placed on mechanical ventilation. These clients usually succumb to pneumonia, or sepsis from UTIs or skin breakdown.

Nursing Considerations

When caring for clients with ALS, focus care on preventing complications. These clients are at risk for aspiration and pneumonia. If the client is able to eat, feed very carefully to prevent choking. Have suction equipment at the bedside ready for use. If the client is tube fed, check placement of the tube before every feeding and watch closely during the feeding for signs of aspiration. Tube feeding formula may have food coloring added to help determine if it is being aspirated. When this occurs, the formula is then suctioned from the trachea. These clients have difficulty communicating, so keep paper and pencil or a "magic slate" at the bedside. Do not use bedside intercoms for communication if the client is unable to speak. Make notations of this on the intercom system to remind others of the problem.

DEMENTIA

Dementia is the progressive loss of cognitive and intellectual functions without impairment of perception or consciousness. It may be caused by various disorders, usually structural brain disease. Dementia affects brain function, learning capacity, language, and judgment. The ability to calculate is lost in clients with dementia.

Older adults sometimes have a particular type of dementia called sundowning or *sundowner's syndrome*. **Sundowning** is the onset of delirium during the evening or night with disappearance of delirium during the day, most often seen in mid- or later stages of dementia. Clients exhibit acute confusion, agitation, time disorientation, wandering behavior, and sometimes aggression related to the onset of darkness at the end of the day.

ALZHEIMER'S DISEASE

Alzheimer's disease (AD) is a chronic neurologic disorder that involves progressive and selective degeneration of neurons in the cerebral cortex and certain subcortical structures (Figure 36-23 ■). Although Alzheimer's can occur in persons as early as the age of 40, it is most common in those over the age of 65 years. The disease affects both sexes, but is more common in women. Alzheimer's disease is the most common form of severe cognitive dysfunction/dementia in older persons in the United States. The disease is very slow in its onset with a generally progressive deteriorating course.

Manifestations

The initial signs are progressive impairment of short- and long-term memory. At first the individual and the family may easily dismiss the forgetfulness. Eventually the individual is no longer able to compensate for the memory loss with notes and reminders and begins to lose the ability to perform ADLs. Impaired abstract thinking, impaired judgment, and personality change are indications of the individual's loss of global cognitive functions. In the end stages the individual becomes bedridden, emaciated, *aphasic* (unable to communicate) and *apraxic* (unable to make purposeful movement), and loses control of

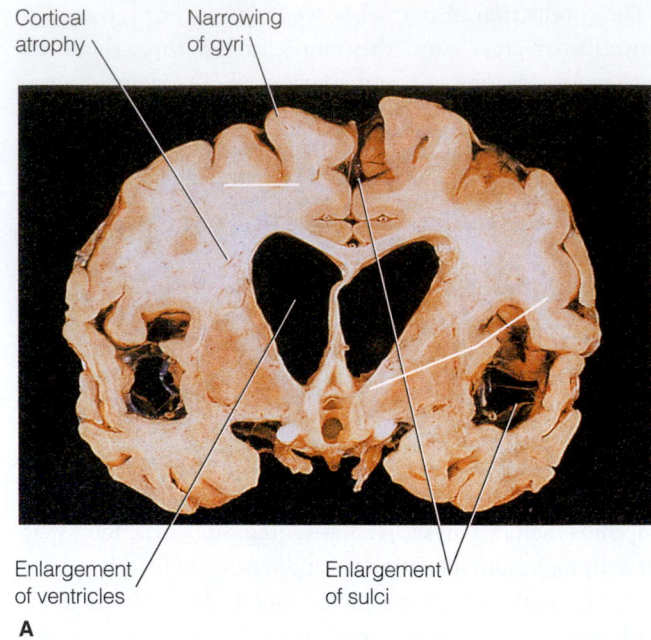

Cortical atrophy — Narrowing of gyri

Enlargement of ventricles — Enlargement of sulci

A

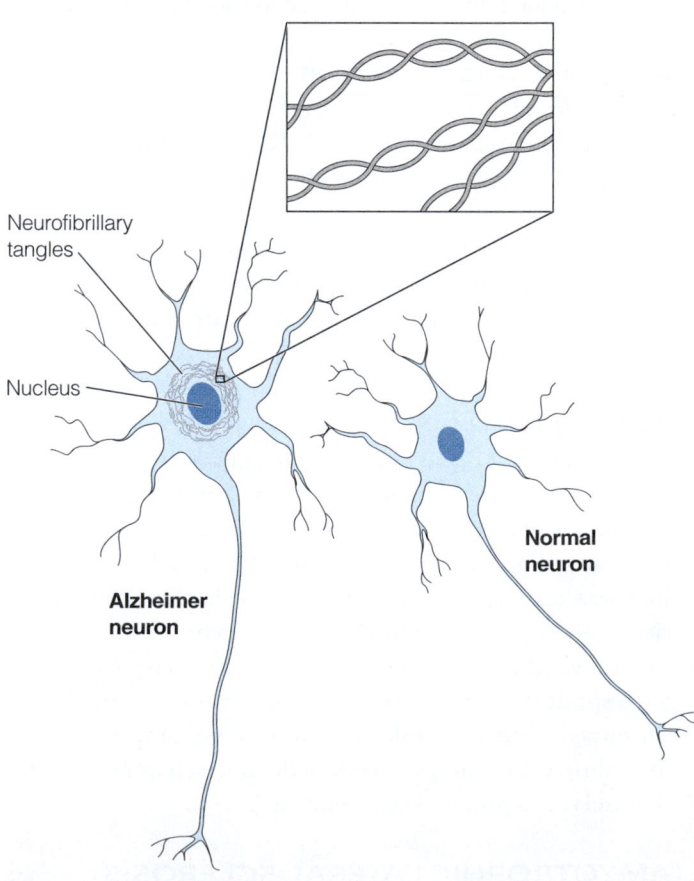

Neurofibrillary tangles

Nucleus

Alzheimer neuron

Normal neuron

B

Figure 36-23. ■ Alzheimer's disease causes changes in neuroanatomy, as shown here. **A.** Note areas of cortical atrophy, narrowing of the gyri, enlargement of sulci, and ventricular dilation. **B.** Note the neurofibrillary tangles in the neuron, found in Alzheimer's disease.

TABLE 36-9	Stages of Alzheimer's	
STAGE	**SIGNS AND SYMPTOMS**	**NURSING INTERVENTIONS**
Stage I (early) Approximately 1 to 3 years duration	Short-term memory loss Forgetful—subtle at first Difficulty learning or processing new information and making decisions Unable to concentrate well Can become angry or depressed or irritable	Remind client frequently of appointments or plans for the day; may use lists and notes. Introduce new information slowly with frequent reminders of changes in medications or treatments. Allow plenty of time for client to make decisions or respond to questions. Limit choices to two or three when asking client to make a decision. Anticipate frustration and reassure client that forgetfulness is expected and accepted.
Stage II (middle) Approximately 2 to 10 years duration	Profound memory loss Significant impairment of other thought processes Severe impairment of judgment Indifference and apathy	Provide missing information, reminders. Do not ask client to perform cognitive skills beyond her ability. Do not expect client to make decisions; provide daily routine. Provide social interactions that are one on one rather than groups.
Stage III (end) Approximately 8 to 12 years duration	Severe impairment of all thought processes Weight loss due to lack of eating Does not recognize family Unsteadiness, repeated falls: limb rigidity, flexion posture; finally loses ability to stand and becomes bedridden Seizures Urinary and fecal incontinence Death usually due to aspiration pneumonia	Supervise in a safe environment; use one-step commands ("bend your knees"). Provide for client's nutritional needs. Provide emotional support to family and refer to support group. Provide supervision to protect from injury. Pad bed rails and have in up position. Establish routine toileting schedule; monitor for constipation.

the body, including sphincters. There is complete loss of cognitive function and emotional responses. The actual cause of death is usually an infection such as aspiration pneumonia.

Diagnosis and Treatment

Because there is no conclusive, identifying diagnostic test for Alzheimer's, the diagnosis is made based on history, physical examination, and laboratory tests. On autopsy, cerebral atrophy (Figure 36-23) and cellular degeneration are the major neuropathologic features noted. There are neurofibrillary tangles and amyloid plaque deposits found primarily in the temporoparietal and anterior frontal regions.

There is no specific treatment for Alzheimer's. Cognex (tacrine hydrochloride) is a drug being used for Alzheimer's clients. It increases brain acetylcholine levels, which is thought to slow mental deterioration. Aricept (donepezil) is a cholinesterase inhibitor. When Aricept is prescribed in the early stages of mild to moderate AD, some clients have shown improvement in memory, language, attention span,

and reasoning skills. Risperdal (risperidone) and Seroquel (quetiapine) are used for the management of psychotic disorders related to AD. Otherwise, treatment is supportive for the client and family. Table 36-9 ■ describes the early, middle, and late stages of Alzheimer's.

NURSING CARE

PRIORITIZING NURSING CARE

Caring for clients with Alzheimer's disease requires a great deal of patience and understanding. Care is focused on safety and quality of life. Because these clients are easily confused, keep the routine as unvaried as possible. Place visual cues in the environment such as large clocks and calendars showing the time and date. Identify the client's room with a unique picture or words if wandering is a problem. If clients become agitated and hostile, try distracting them by helping them do a familiar task, or remove the stimulus causing the agitation.

ASSESSING

The assessment of the client with degenerative neurologic disorders is related to maintaining mobility, preventing injury, and assessing how the disease is affecting the client's ADLs.

DIAGNOSING, PLANNING, AND IMPLEMENTING

Many of the nursing diagnoses that affect other disorders of the neurologic system apply to the degenerative disorders as well. The nursing diagnoses that may be included are as follows:

- *Impaired Physical Mobility*
- *Impaired Verbal Communication*
- *Imbalanced Nutrition: Less than Body Requirements*

Client goals in the planning stage of the nursing process include:

- Client participates in self-care as much as possible.
- Client communicates with others and makes needs known.
- Client maintains stable body weight.

To achieve these goals, the nurse provides various interventions. Some of those interventions might include:

- Encourage client to participate in prescribed exercise program, such as ROM exercises, at least twice a day. *ROM exercises and physical therapy exercises promote joint function, strengthen muscles, and prevent contractures.*
- Encourage client to perform self-care within abilities. *Self-care promotes self-esteem and a sense of independence.*
- Allow time for the client to communicate, and try to anticipate the client's needs. *Clients with degenerative disorders may need more time to verbalize. Rushing them would increase their frustration. Anticipating some needs of the client will assist the communication.*
- Provide a communication board or paper pad and pen. *Facilitating options for communication decreases anxiety, frustration, and isolation.*
- Place client in upright position for all meals and keep suction equipment at the bedside. *This decreases the risk of aspiration.*
- Assist client to eat and/or provide utensils that facilitate self-feeding. *This encourages the client to eat and promotes nutrition.*
- Weigh the client daily. *Weighing the client helps identify fluctuations of weight and adequacy of nutrition.*

EVALUATING

The nurse revises care until the expected outcomes are achieved or revised. The expected outcomes for a client with a degenerative neurologic disorder include:

- Client maintains mobility for as long as possible.

- Client is able to communicate with others effectively by self and/or with assistive devices.
- Client's weight is stable with adequate nutrition.

Peripheral Nervous System Disorders

PERIPHERAL NEUROPATHY

A **neuropathy** is any disease of the nerves, and **peripheral neuropathy** is any syndrome causing muscle weakness, paresthesias, impaired reflexes, and autonomic symptoms in the hands and feet. Peripheral neuropathy occurs as a complication of another disease process, such as diabetes mellitus, renal or hepatic failure, alcoholism, or as a complication of certain drugs, such as phenytoin and isoniazid. It may also be called *polyneuritis* or *polyneuropathy*.

Diabetes mellitus is the most common cause of metabolic neuropathy. Metabolic, or toxic, neuropathies are chronic, progressive diseases. Alcoholism causes the most common nutrition-related neuropathy.

Diagnosis and Treatment

Complete health history, medications, and physical examination will help conclude the diagnosis of neuropathy. The healthcare provider may order an EMG to determine the nerve conduction.

Treatment varies by underlying cause. Most drug-induced neuropathies will reverse when the drug is stopped. The most common causes are diabetes and alcoholism, so treatment is often aimed at these underlying conditions.

MYASTHENIA GRAVIS

Myasthenia gravis (MG) is a chronic autoimmune disease that affects the transmission of nerve impulses to muscles. Normally when impulses travel down the nerve, the nerve endings release the neurotransmitter acetylcholine. In MG, antibodies produced by the body's own immune system block, alter, or destroy the receptors for acetylcholine. MG affects all striated muscles, especially the oculomotor, facial, laryngeal, pharyngeal, and respiratory muscles.

The peak occurrence of MG is age and gender specific. The peak in women is between 20 and 30 years; the peak in males occurs primarily between 60 and 70 years.

Manifestations

Initial signs and symptoms are intermittent double vision (diplopia) and droopy eyelids (ptosis) (Figure 36-24 ■). The ptosis may be unilateral or bilateral and becomes worse when looking upward. Facial weakness with difficulty chewing, swallowing, and speaking also occur. The weakness increases with repeated activity and improves with rest.

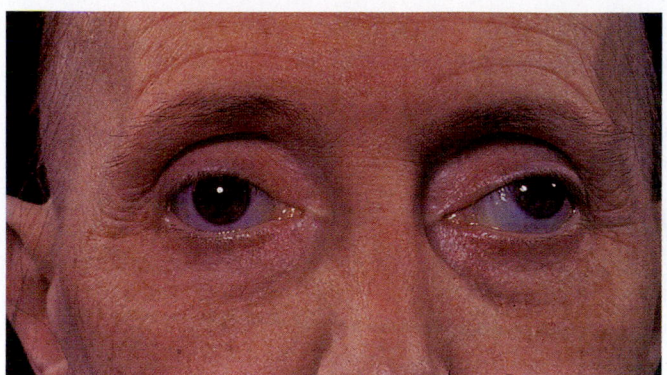

Figure 36-24. ■ In myasthenia gravis, the client experiences unilateral weakness of the facial muscles. Note the drooping of one eyelid. (*Source:* Custom Medical Stock Photo, Inc.)

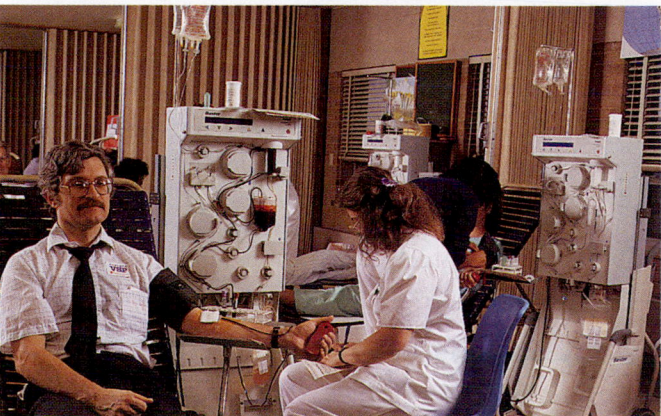

Figure 36-25. ■ Plasmapheresis is a procedure used to separate the blood's cellular components from the plasma. About 50 mL per minute is withdrawn to the centrifuge in the plasmapheresis machine. The plasma is replaced with donor plasma or colloids and returned to the client. (*Source:* Courtesy of Baxter Healthcare Corporation.)

Mobility and expression of the face are altered because the facial muscle is affected. The smile may look more like a snarl. The voice is often nasal and weak, fading with talking. Because swallowing is difficult, saliva may accumulate, causing the individual to drool. Food must be eaten slowly to prevent aspiration. Later, weakness of the neck and limbs frequently develops. If the intercostal muscles or diaphragm are involved, the first sign may be breathlessness, and mechanical ventilation may become necessary. Rapidly progressing weakness leading to respiratory failure is called myasthenia crisis. (See also Chapter 35 ⦿⦿ .)

clinical ALERT

Myasthenia crisis can be life threatening. It may be attributed to worsening of the disease or to overdoses of anticholinesterase medication. Other medications, such as gentamicin, can cause the client to go into myasthenia crisis. It is characterized by severe generalized and rapidly increasing weakness, dysphagia, anxiety, restlessness, and/or respiratory failure. The most important principles in the treatment of crisis are recognizing respiratory failure, maintaining gas exchange, and managing secretions.

There are two types of crisis with MG: myasthenic and cholinergic.

- Myasthenic crisis is caused by an insufficiency of acetylcholine. It can be triggered by a change or withdrawal of medications, emotional or physical stress, infection, or surgery.
- Cholinergic crisis is triggered by an excess of acetylcholine, usually due to drug overdose.

The symptoms of each are very similar: acute weakness of respiratory muscles, generalized muscle weakness, apprehension, and restlessness. Differentiation between the two is done with the Tensilon test. Tensilon (edrophonium chloride) is given intravenously, and the individual is observed for muscle tone

improvement. If improvement occurs, the test is positive and the crisis is myasthenic. If there is no improvement in muscle tone, the test is negative and the crisis is cholinergic.

Diagnosis and Treatment

Myasthenia gravis is diagnosed based on history, physical examination, and laboratory tests. The laboratory tests that confirm MG are cholinesterase inhibitor drug test, repetitive nerve stimulation, antibody titer for anti-acetylcholine receptors (anti-AChRs), and single-fiber electromyography.

No single treatment is best or ideal for all individuals with MG. Therefore, an individualized management plan needs to be developed. The goal is to achieve as much as possible a symptom-free quality of life. Current treatment includes cholinesterase inhibitor drugs, long-term immunosuppression, intravenous immune globulin, and **plasmapheresis** (the complete exchange of plasma; Figure 36-25 ■). The drug protocols are planned to interfere with the autoimmune process that is the basis of MG. Thymectomy (surgical removal of the thymus gland) is helpful in some cases.

Nursing Considerations

When caring for clients with myasthenia gravis, focus on preventing complications and on early detection of myasthenia crisis. Assess respiratory status and vital signs every 4 hours. Monitor for muscle weakness, restlessness, shortness of breath, and increasing anxiety. Report changes immediately. Be prepared to assist with ventilation if required (oropharyngeal airway placement, Ambu bag, and/or intubation).

GUILLAIN-BARRÉ SYNDROME

Guillain-Barré Syndrome (GBS) is an acute inflammatory *polyneuropathy* thought to be an autoimmune response to a viral infection. It is a rapidly progressive disorder that mainly affects the motor component of peripheral nerves, including the cranial nerves. A nonspecific infection such as an upper respiratory infection, viral pneumonia, or gastrointestinal infection usually precedes GBS 10 to 14 days before onset. It affects individuals at any age and occurs in both sexes. The myelin sheath is destroyed accompanied by edema and inflammation of the peripheral nerves. The remyelination process occurs slowly and may take up to 2 years for maximal improvement. Complete functional recovery occurs in 85% of those affected.

Manifestations

The severity of the symptoms may vary. Usually lower extremity weakness progresses in an ascending pattern to the upper extremities and face. Complete **flaccid** (relaxed) paralysis with respiratory failure can occur within 48 hours, but usually occurs symmetrically over 2 to 3 weeks. Sensory loss is less common than motor loss. Sympathetic and parasympathetic nervous system involvement causes autonomic dysfunction. This is manifested by hyper-hypotension, dysrhythmias, and circulatory collapse.

Diagnosis and Treatment

Client with signs and symptoms of GBS are monitored very carefully for worsening of the condition. As weakening of the muscles ascends up the torso, the respiratory rate and breathing will be impaired. Monitoring of the client's respiratory functions with a bedside spirometry may be necessary frequently. The health history from the client or family may indicate the client had a viral illness as much as 2 weeks prior to the development of the symptoms.

Treatment focuses on preventing complications of immobility, infection, and respiratory failure. Mechanical ventilation may become necessary. In some cases when motor strength does not return as anticipated, plasmapheresis may be performed to remove abnormal antibodies affecting the myelin sheath. Emotional support to the client and the family is very important. Maintain a positive attitude that will convey that improvement and complete functional recovery are possible.

Nursing Considerations

Because this disorder is self-limiting, focus care on immediate respiratory needs and on longer term issues such as preventing complications of immobility. Offer emotional support to the client and family during the crisis period of the illness. As the client stabilizes, reassure the family that the client will show improvement, even though it may be slow. Encourage the client and family during the rehabilitation process by celebrating even small gains.

HUNTINGTON'S DISEASE

Huntington's disease (HD) is also known as *Huntington's chorea* because **chorea** (involuntary dancing or writhing of the limbs or facial muscles) is the most common presenting symptom. Dementia and behavioral changes accompany the chorea. Huntington's disease is an inherited, relatively rare, degenerative disorder. The onset of the disease is usually between 30 and 50 years of age, with death usually occurring more than 15 years after diagnosis.

Manifestations

Early symptoms of the disease are mood swings; depression; irritability; or trouble driving, learning new things, remembering facts, or making decisions. The signs and symptoms of HD include abnormal movement and progressive dysfunction of intellectual and thought processes. The *choreiform* (dancing, writhing) movements usually begin in the face and arms, and eventually affect the entire body. Frontal lobe dysfunction is manifested by loss of working memory; reduced capacity to plan, organize, and sequence; slow thinking (*bradyphrenia*); and apathy. Restlessness and irritability are common. *Euphoria* (a heightened state of well-being) or depression may be present.

Diagnosis and Treatment

The diagnosis is based on family history and clinical presentation of the disorder. Genetic testing can isolate the gene for Huntington's disease. Couples wanting to start a family should undergo counseling about the disease. Each child of an HD parent has a 50% chance of inheriting the HD gene. Anyone who inherits the gene will eventually develop the disease.

There is no known treatment to stop or arrest the degeneration process. However, dopamine agonist drugs (i.e., haloperidol or risperidone) can help control the movement disorder. These drugs must be used carefully because of the potential risk of movement-related side effects.

Nursing Considerations

When caring for clients with HD, focus on the emotional support of the client and family. Choreiform movement is exhausting for the client and difficult for the family to watch. The client may be moody, irritable, and depressed, as well as exhausted. The family must deal with possible inheritance of the disorder, as well as caring for the client. Encourage counseling and group support for the client and family.

NEUROFIBROMATOSIS OR VON RECKLINGHAUSEN'S DISEASE

Neurofibromatosis is a group of genetic disorders that affects the cell growth of neural tissues. It is also known as von Recklinghausen's disease. There are basically two types.

Type 1 can vary from a few harmless coffee-colored spots on the skin to numerous nonmalignant or malignant neurofibromas, scoliosis, seizures, gliomas, neuromas, hypertension, and mental retardation. In about 2% to 5% of individuals affected, tumors become malignant. There is no cure for von

Recklinghausen's disease, and treatment varies with the placement of the tumors and their severity. Radiation therapy and surgery can be beneficial. The condition can be mild enough that it is not recognized until the individual's child exhibits a more severe form.

Type 2 causes intracranial and spinal tumors. The eighth cranial nerve is especially susceptible. Treatment is *palliative* (reducing intensity) but does not cure the disease.

NURSING CARE

PRIORITIZING NURSING CARE

Nursing interventions should be related to the comfort of the client. The following are priority:

- Pain
- Safety with visual changes and possibility of seizures
- Skin care
- Urinary/bowel elimination
- Nutrition
- Self-image with the darkened areas on the skin

ASSESSING

Nursing management includes assessment of the client's signs and symptoms to determine the type of care needed.

DIAGNOSING, PLANNING, AND IMPLEMENTING

The nurse is able to identify many nursing diagnoses for the client with degeneration of the nervous system. Some of the nursing diagnoses appropriate for this type of client are:

- *Risk for Powerlessness* related to physiologic changes; psychologic conflicts
- *Impaired Physical Mobility* related to decreased strength/endurance and/or perceptual or cognitive impairment
- *Imbalanced Nutrition: Less than Body Requirements* related to altered ability to ingest nutrients and/or weakness of muscles required for chewing and swallowing
- *Caregiver Role Strain* related to keeping the client confined to a safe environment

Client goals in the planning stage of the nursing process include the following:

- Maintain optimal functioning.
- Assist with/provide for maintenance of ADLs.
- Provide adequate nutrition.
- Obtain respite care for family.

To achieve these goals, the nurse provides various nursing interventions. Nursing interventions for clients with nerve degeneration include client and family teaching, assisting in ADLs, providing a safe environment, and giving emotional support to client and family. The following list of nursing interventions with rationales is appropriate for most clients with degeneration of the nervous system. Other nursing interventions should also be considered in an effort to individualize nursing care.

- Orient the client to person, place, and time frequently; place large, easy-to-read calendars and clocks within client's line of vision. *Orientation promotes reality and reduces confusion.*
- Assess the client's mobility and ability to perform self-care. Provide assistance as needed but encourage client to do as much as possible for self. *This helps client to maintain independence in self-care as long as possible, and aids in maintaining self-esteem.*
- Position client comfortably with head elevated for meals to promote ease of swallowing. *This will aid in preventing aspiration.*
- Encourage family to discuss plans in caring for client. *Aids in realistic planning and gives emotional support.*

EVALUATING

The nurse revises care until expected outcomes are achieved. The expected outcomes for a client with degeneration of the nervous system include:

- Mental confusion will be minimized.
- Client will retain independence for as long as possible.
- Client will not choke while eating.
- Client will maintain weight.
- Family will be able to plan for present and future realistically and obtain help in caring for client.

Cranial Nerve Disorders

BELL'S PALSY

Bell's palsy is acute paralysis of the facial cranial nerve VII (Figure 36-26 ■). Bell's palsy is of unknown origin in about 75% of the cases but is thought to be caused by an inflammatory reaction. It is a common disorder of the facial nerve affecting individuals of all ages and both sexes. It is reported to occur most frequently with young adults, older adults, and individuals with diabetes, hypertension, and lipid abnormalities. It has also been associated with Lyme disease.

Manifestations

Bell's palsy usually occurs suddenly, with unilateral facial paralysis that peaks within 2 to 5 days and resolves gradually over 1 to 2 months. Some individuals report pain behind the ear on the affected side 1 to 2 days prior to the paralysis. The sensory fibers are also involved, impairing taste for up to 2 weeks. Muscles that are connected to the ear are sometimes involved, causing a distortion of sound. The eye does not close and the forehead does not wrinkle;

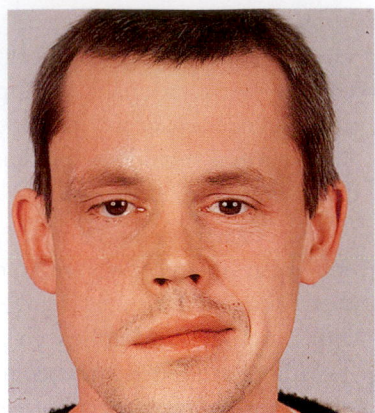

Figure 36-26. ■ Client with Bell's palsy showing typical drooping of one side of the face.

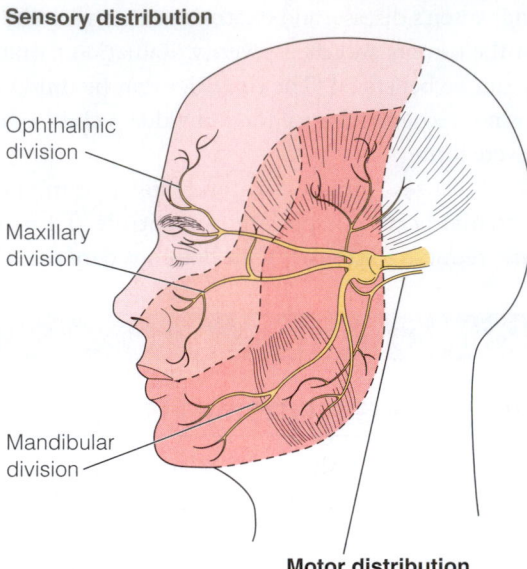

Sensory distribution

Ophthalmic division

Maxillary division

Mandibular division

Motor distribution

Figure 36-27. ■ Sensory and motor branches of the trigeminal nerve. The three sensory branches are ophthalmic, maxillary, and mandibular. Pain of trigeminal neuralgia can be intense.

the individual cannot smile, whistle, or grimace. The paralyzed side of the face is masklike and sags, with constant tearing of the eye, and possible drooling.

Diagnosis and Treatment

The diagnosis is made based on history and a clinical picture of seventh cranial nerve unilateral deficits.

Treatment with prednisone is helpful for the first week after the onset of symptoms. Analgesics are given for pain. Other common methods of treatment are gentle massage, moist heat, and electrical stimulation of the nerve. As muscle tone begins to improve, exercises can be helpful. Grimacing, wrinkling the brow, forcing the eyes closed, whistling, and blowing out air from the cheeks should be practiced for 5 minutes in front of a mirror three or four times a day. Recovery depends on nerve regeneration and is complete in 80% of those affected.

TRIGEMINAL NEURALGIA

The fifth cranial or trigeminal nerve is a mixed nerve of both motor and sensory fibers. Therefore, disorders involving it can present as sensory abnormalities, motor weakness, or both. The most common of these disorders is **trigeminal neuralgia** or **tic douloureux.** The trigeminal nerve has a wide anatomic distribution and for this reason complete disruption of function rarely occurs. However, disorders of isolated parts of the nerve, especially the sensory branch, are common.

Manifestations

Trigeminal neuralgia is characterized by excruciating pain in the area of the maxillary and/or mandibular division of the trigeminal sensory root (Figure 36-27 ■). The pain occurs episodically and is initiated when stimulation occurs somewhere in the distribution of the involved nerve division. The stimuli may be light touch; facial movements, such as chewing, talking, yawning, tooth brushing, shaving, or a light breeze to the face. The face may appear contorted during the painful attack, and remains this way until the pain eases.

The painful episodes are unilateral and generally last less than 2 seconds, but can recur. Frequent recurrences may incapacitate the individual for hours. The anxiety associated with the anticipation of another attack may also compromise the individual's ability to cope with the disorder. The bouts of pain may occur for several weeks or months, followed by a spontaneous remission that may last from days to years. With aging, the length of the remission seems to shorten. Activities of daily living may be affected as the fear of triggering the pain keeps the individual immobilized.

Diagnosis and Treatment

The diagnosis is made based on history, because the neurologic examination is entirely normal.

Initial treatment is drug therapy (Tegretol). Other treatments are tried if the drug therapy is ineffective, starting with the injection of alcohol or phenol into the nerve to block its motor and sensory functions. The final option is surgery, when the nerve is clipped. In this case, the nerve will not be able to send or receive messages from the brain.

GLOSSOPHARYNGEAL NEURALGIA

Glossopharyngeal neuralgia is similar to trigeminal neuralgia but is more rare.

The neuralgias are similar in that they both have attacks of **paroxysmal** (intense, sudden, and repeating) pain, pain triggered by certain activities, no sensory or motor loss of the cranial nerve, and unclear etiology. In glossopharyngeal neuralgia, pain originates in the throat around the tonsil area. The pain may also be localized in the ear or radiate from the throat to the ear. Several nerves may be responsible and since the treatment is the same, it is not necessary to isolate which one is causing the pain.

The diagnosis is based on history. Treatment is drug therapy with phenytoin or carbamazepine or spraying the throat with a topical anesthetic. For long-term relief, an intracranial surgical procedure may be necessary.

ISAAC'S SYNDROME

Isaac's syndrome is also known as *neuromyotonia* and *continuous muscle fiber activity syndrome*. It is a rare neuromuscular disorder caused by continuous signaling of the end regions of peripheral nerve fibers that activate muscle fibers.

The symptoms (which include progressive muscle stiffness, continuous vibrating or twitching of muscles, cramping, increased sweating, and delayed muscle relaxation) can occur even during sleep or when under general anesthesia. Often, clients develop weakened reflexes and muscle pain. In most individuals the stiffness is most prominent in limb and trunk muscles, although symptoms may be limited to the cranial muscles. If the pharyngeal or laryngeal muscles are involved, speech and breathing may be affected. There are hereditary and acquired forms of the disorder. The acquired form may occur in association with peripheral neuropathies or as an autoimmune condition. In the autoimmune-mediated disorder, antibodies are produced that bind to ion channels on the motor nerve fibers. When confusion, hallucinations, and insomnia are associated with this condition, it is known as *Marfan's syndrome*.

MRI scans and EMGs are used to diagnose this disorder. The healthcare provider will need to take an extensive health history, family history, and complete neurologic examination to develop a treatment plan for the client.

The anticonvulsants phenytoin and carbamazepine provide significant relief from the stiffness, muscle spasms, and pain associated with Isaac's syndrome. Plasma exchange may provide short-term relief with some forms of the acquired disorder. There is no cure, and the long-term prognosis is uncertain.

TOURETTE'S SYNDROME

Tourette's syndrome may be chronic or transient. It is considered an inherited disorder. Abnormal metabolism of dopamine and serotonin or other neurotransmitters may be involved. The gene thought to cause Tourette's has not yet been isolated.

Its primary manifestations are repetitive motor and verbal tics (sudden, involuntary movements or vocalizations). Motor tics can include shoulder shrugging, eye blinking, head jerking, hand movements, lip licking, and grimacing. Common vocal tics include sniffing, throat clearing, grunting, making loud sounds, or saying words.

There is no specific test to diagnose this disorder. Monitoring and observing the behaviors of the client with this disorder may become very frustrating for the family members. School performance and social activities need to be included in the health history.

Note: In the past, parental substance use or abuse was thought to be associated with Tourette's, but this is no longer thought to be the case.

Conservative, symptomatic treatment is tried first, because in some cases symptoms resolve without therapy. Non-neuroleptic drugs, such as Catapres and Klonopin, are the first drugs tried. If those are not successful, neuroleptic drugs, such as Haldol, Prolixin, and Risperdal, are prescribed to help control the tics.

MÉNIÈRE'S DISEASE

Ménière's disease is a disorder of the eighth cranial nerve involving both the vestibular and cochlear branches.

Ménière's disease is characterized by recurrent attacks of vertigo accompanied by **tinnitus** (ringing in the ears) and gradual deafness. Hearing is lost until there is complete unilateral deafness. In 10% of the individuals affected there is bilateral deafness. Ménière's disease affects both sexes with equal frequency and most often occurs in the fifth decade of life.

Ménière's is associated with rotational or whirling **vertigo** (acute dizziness and lack of balance). Vertigo may last a few minutes to hours and be so severe that the individual is unable to stand or walk. Nausea, vomiting, a full feeling in the ears, and rotational or horizontal **nystagmus** (involuntary movement of the eyes) with slow movement on the *ipsilateral side* (same side) are accompanying symptoms. The attacks vary in frequency and severity. Remission may occur between a series of bouts. In most individuals the vertigo ceases with complete deafness.

Diagnosis is based on history and clinical findings of fluctuating, progressive hearing loss leading to deafness; episodes of vertigo; and significant tinnitus. Diagnostic testing includes audiometry and caloric testing. Caloric testing involves irrigating the ear canal with warm water for 30 seconds, then irrigating with cold. The normal reaction to the warm water is rotatory nystagmus to the side being irrigated. Cold water produces the opposite reaction. In clients with Ménière's, the reaction is blunted or absent.

The priority treatment for an "attack" is bed rest. The client might try various recumbent positions for comfort and to minimize the vertigo symptoms. Once the nausea and vomiting have subsided a salt-restricted diet may be helpful to reduce the vertigo and ataxia. Medications such as diuretics and vestibular suppressants (e.g., meclizine) are also used in treating the vertigo. Some clients will experience hearing problems during the attacks and hearing will return to baseline once the attack is resolved. After many reoccurring attacks the hearing may worsen and not fully rebound. In severe cases surgical destruction of the labyrinth may be performed.

NURSING CARE

PRIORITIZING NURSING CARE

Interventions that are priority to care for a client with cranial nerve disturbances should include the following: safety measures, encouraging self-care activities, and communication with the client.

ASSESSING

An adequate assessment is a critical element of maintaining and restoring client health. The nurse is responsible for collecting the health history to assist in determining the symptoms related to cranial and peripheral nerve disorders.

DIAGNOSING, PLANNING, AND IMPLEMENTING

The nurse is able to identify many nursing diagnoses appropriate for the client diagnosed with a cranial or peripheral nerve disorder. Some of the nursing diagnoses that are appropriate for this type of client are:

- *Acute Pain* related to disease process
- *Self-care Deficit* related to debilitating pain
- *Fear* related to anticipated painful episodes
- *Deficient Knowledge* related to the disease, prognosis, and treatment

Client goals in the planning stage of the nursing process include:

- Achieve adequate pain relief.
- Accomplish self-care activities.
- Reduce fear.
- Make sure client understands condition and treatment.

To achieve these goals, the nurse provides various nursing interventions. Nursing interventions for clients with cranial or peripheral nerve disorders include the following interventions with rationales. Other nursing interventions should also be considered in an effort to individualize nursing care.

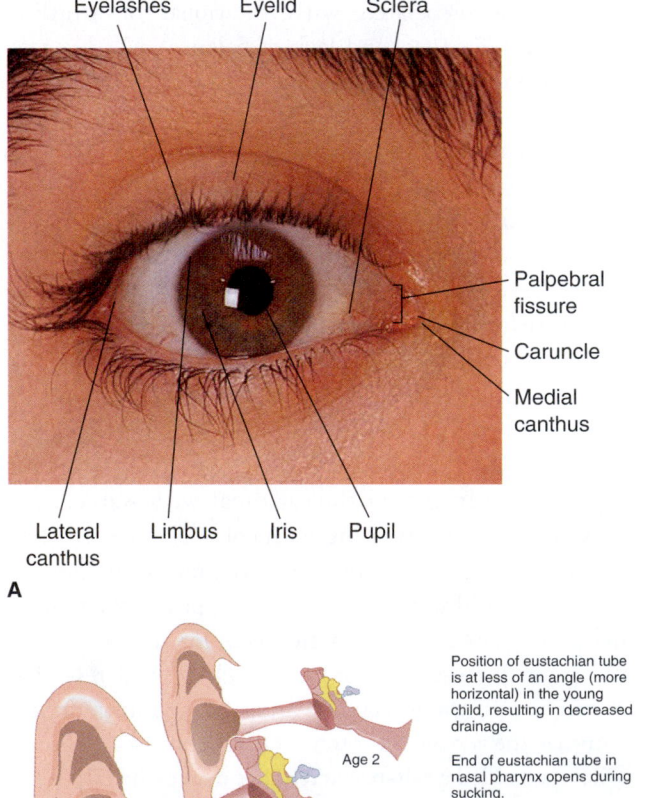

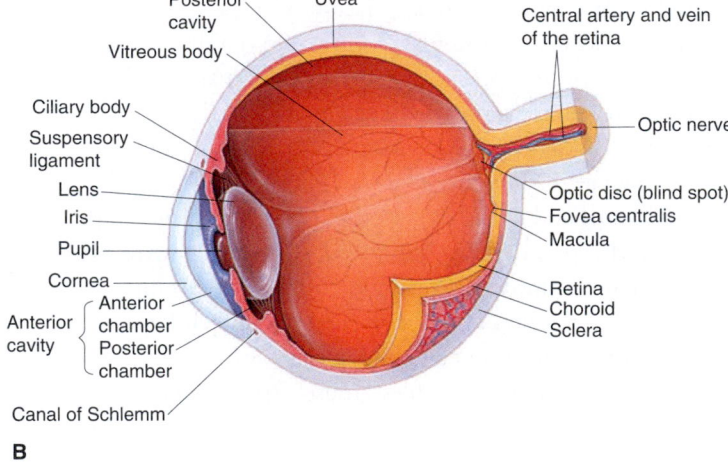

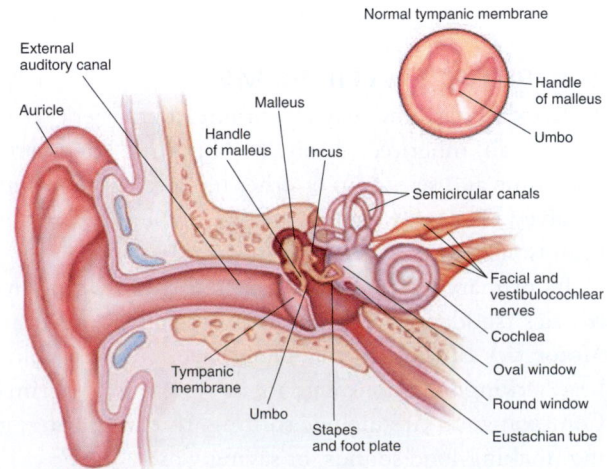

Figure 36-28. ■ **A.** External eye. **B.** Internal structures of the eye. **C.** External ear. **D.** Internal structures of the ear.

- Manage pain by administering analgesics as ordered. *Giving analgesics on a scheduled basis help to minimize the pain.*
- Help the client identify pain triggers. *Avoiding pain triggers minimizes the pain and reduces the amount of analgesic needed.*
- Encourage client to discuss fear. *Assists client in identifying and gaining control of fear.*
- Teach the client guided imagery or realization therapy. *Assists the client in developing alternative strategies for pain relief.*
- Follow up with referrals as needed. *Clients may need to see several specialists in order to identify the cause of the disorder.*

EVALUATING

The nurse revises care until expected outcomes are achieved. The expected outcomes for a client with a cranial or peripheral nerve disorder include:

- Reduced frequency and severity of attacks.
- Self-care activities accomplished.
- Fear is reduced.
- Understanding of condition and treatment is verbalized.

Disorders of Vision and Hearing

Normal anatomy of the eye and ear are shown in Figure 36-28 ■. Vision and hearing are two senses that contribute tremendously to social functioning and quality of life. Therefore, screening for deficits in vision and hearing begins at birth and is repeated periodically through the school years and as needed in adulthood. Vision and hearing screenings are often performed in community

BOX 36-6   CULTURAL PULSE POINTS

Variations in Hearing and Vision

There are ethnic variations with both hearing and vision. Hearing gradually declines after age 40, especially at the higher frequencies. African Americans have better hearing at high and low frequencies and are less susceptible to noise-induced hearing loss.

Visual acuity differs among cultural groups and differences can be clinically significant. African Americans have poorer visual acuity than Hispanic Americans, Caucasians, and Native Americans. Asian Americans (especially Japanese and Chinese) have the poorest corrected visual acuity due to the high incidence of myopia in these populations.

settings (see Chapter 48, Procedures 48-8 and 48-9 ⬭). Vision and hearing disorders are common and are generally diagnosed at an early age. Interestingly, disorders of the eye can vary by racial and ethnic groups, as discussed in Box 36-6 ■.

Vision occurs as the retina, the light-sensitive layer of tissue that lines the inside of the eye, sends messages through the optic nerve to the brain (see Table 36-2). Various disorders of the eye affect the brain's ability to perceive and decode visual messages. Total lack of function of the optic nerve results in blindness. Table 36-10 ■ provides an overview of common visual and hearing disorders, causes, and corrections.

Infections like conjunctivitis (Figure 36-29 ■) are most often seen in children, and are discussed further in Chapter 60 ⬭. Disorders of the eye that generally occur in older adults are discussed in Chapters 42 and 43 ⬭.)

TABLE 36-10	**Visual and Hearing Disorders, Definitions, Causes, and Corrective Actions**		
TYPE OF DISORDER	**DEFINED**	**CAUSE**	**CORRECTIVE ACTION**
VISUAL DISORDERS			
Blindness	Complete lack of function of the optic nerve (cranial nerve II)	Congenital, disease process, or trauma	None unless optic nerve is still functioning after trauma, when corneal transplant can correct the disorder
Amblyopia (lazy eye)	Reduced vision not correctable by glasses or contact lenses	Unknown; the brain, for some reason, does not fully acknowledge the images seen by the amblyopic eye	Glasses, drops, exercises, and/or patching
Myopia (nearsightedness)	Affects the ability of individuals to perceive objects at a distance	Images are focused in front of the retina instead of directly	Glasses, contacts, or surgery
Hyperopia (farsightedness)	Inability to see objects that are near to the individual	Develops due to a defect in the eye in causing images to be focused behind the retina	Glasses, contacts, or surgery
Presbyopia (literally means "old vision")	Distortion of the vision	Disorder of older persons in which the lens hardens	Glasses, contacts, or surgery
Nystagmus	An involuntary movement of the eye because the eye cannot focus properly	May be congenital or can arise as a complication of various neurologic disorders	Treatment of the underlying neurologic causes of the disorder

TABLE 36-10 Visual and Hearing Disorders, Definitions, Causes, and Corrective Actions (continued)

TYPE OF DISORDER	DEFINED	CAUSE	CORRECTIVE ACTION
Astigmatism	Blurring or distorting of visual images	Abnormally shaped cornea or lens of the eye	Glasses, contacts, or surgery
Color blindness	Affecting ability to distinguish colors, occurs mostly in males	Caused by a defect in the retina or in other nerve portions of the eye	No treatment
Computer vision syndrome	Headache, tired and achy eyes; dry, gritty or usually watery eyes; blurred or double vision; difficulty in focusing after working for long on computers	Dry eyes, eye coordination, and focusing issues that are not apparent in other activities become an issue when using the computer; computer typeface may be too small; glare from nearby lights or windows; monitor placed higher than is natural for your eyes	Most of the eye symptoms clear up after a few hours away from the keyboard
Strabismus	A condition in which the eyes deviate when looking at an object	Poor accommodation or eye muscle coordination	Patching, glasses, vision therapy, or surgery
Macular degeneration	Interferes with the individual's central vision; ability to focus the eyes on objects and to see detail is lost; disease is progressive	Gradual disintegration of the macula, part of the retina on which light is focused by the eye; the disorder is usually found in older persons	Incurable; antineoplastic agents injected into eye can sometimes slow or stop degeneration
Cataract	Cloudy or opaque area in ocular lens	Aging, infection, trauma, drugs, diabetes mellitus	Surgical removal of lens (replacement with artificial lens)
Glaucoma: open angle	Loss of peripheral vision with decreased accommodation; increased intraocular pressure greater than 21 mm Hg; difficulty adapting to light changes; painless; leads to blindness	Amount of aqueous humor in the eye increased due to obstruction of the canal of Schlemm; medication induced; congenital; or aging process	Miotics; beta-blockers; ocular steroid; laser trabeculoplasty and cyclocryotherapy when medication therapy is unsuccessful
Glaucoma: angle closure	Medical emergency; rapid onset of elevated intraocular pressure; decreased or blurred vision; severe pain; photophobia; fixed pupil	The angle between the cornea and iris closes completely blocking the drainage of aqueous humor from the eye; medication or herbal use (kawakawa) induced	Miotics; beta-blockers; IV Mannitol, ocular steroids; laser iridotomy
Detached retina	Separation of the retina from the choroid; painless; floaters or flashes of light; diabetic clients at risk	Trauma or a spontaneous occurrence; aging process	Laser therapy or cryotherapy; scleral buckling
Conjunctivitis (see Figure 36-29)	Inflammation of the membrane lining the eye	Infection from germs, allergies, or other sources and is highly contagious	Treated with antibiotics
HEARING DISORDERS			
Deafness	Complete lack of function of the acoustic nerve (cranial nerve VIII)	Congenital or result of meningitis or Ménière's disease	If congenital, surgery may be performed to place a cochlear implant (see Chapter 59); no treatment for loss caused by meningitis or Ménière's
Otitis media	Infection of the middle ear	Infection generally transmitted through the Eustachian tube	Antibiotic therapy
Tinnitus	Ringing in the ears	Age-related, Ménière's disease, sometimes side effect of medications	Depends on cause; if pharmacologic, discontinuation of medication
Otosclerosis	Abnormality in which the stapes become fixed or immobile	Abnormal bone formation in the bony labyrinth with hereditary cause	Hearing aid or surgery

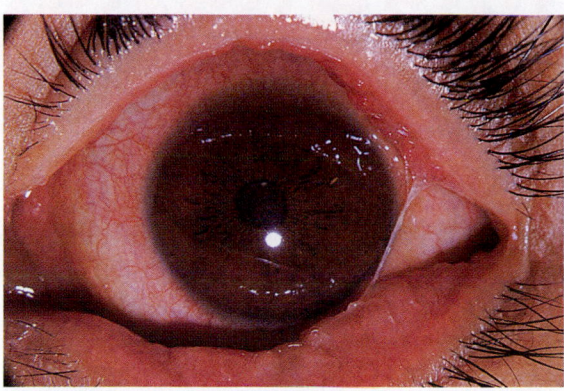

Figure 36-29. ■ Acute conjunctivitis.

Hearing occurs as sound enters the external ear, vibrates the tympanic membrane, passing sounds waves to the malleus, incus, and stapes, and the nerve endings of the cochlea, which transmits impulses to the brain. Review Figures 36-28C and 36-28D for these structures.

In the past, deafness was a permanent condition, and the deaf essentially lived in a culture of their own, using sign (which few others knew) as the mode of communication. Today, however, a child born deaf may have a *cochlear implant* (see Chapter 59 ⬭), a device that, with training, will allow him or her to communicate through speech and hearing.

Some loss of hearing with age is considered normal (see Chapter 42 ⬭), and there is a wide variety of hearing aids now available to augment sound for age-related hearing loss. Unfortunately, hearing loss related to disorders such as meningitis or Ménière's disease is not reversible.

Note: The references and resources for all chapters have been compiled at the back of the book.

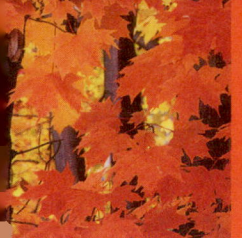

Chapter Review

KEY Points

- Neurologic disorders affect the whole person, as well as his or her support system.

- Deviations from a client's baseline need to be monitored closely and reported to the primary care provider.

- IICP is detected by neurologic changes in the level of consciousness, pupil response, speech, motor functions, and vital signs. IICP treatment is aimed at reducing the chance of multiple neurological deficits, coma, or death, and is dependent on the underlying cause.

- Many of the risk factors for transient ischemic shock (TIA) and cerebrovascular accidents (CVAs) are modifiable. Early detection of these conditions is key.

- Nursing care for seizures is focused on preventing complications and injuries.

- Because the nervous system is well protected, when infections occur, they are acute and have usually invaded through blood. Treatment is immediate and determined by the causative organism.

- Injuries to the neurologic system are usually the result of accidents. Treatment is based on the signs and symptoms.

- Parkinson's, MS, ALS, dementia, and Alzheimer's are degenerative neurologic diseases; nursing care focuses on prevention of injuries, and treatment is most commonly drug therapy.

- For peripheral and cranial nerve disorder, nursing care focuses on preventing complications.

- Many visual and hearing disorders can be detected early by routine screening. Medical advances have greatly improved the outcomes for people who are diagnosed with these disorders.

∞ FOR FURTHER Study

Client communication is discussed in depth in Chapter 11.

Client teaching is the focus of Chapter 12.

Fontanels are illustrated in Chapter 16.

The Glasgow Coma Scale is given in Table 19-2; Part A of Procedure 19-1 in the Health Assessment chapter contains a focused neurologic assessment.

Vital signs are addressed in Chapter 21.

Box 31-3 reviews the neurovascular assessment.

For more information about cerebral aneurysms, see Chapter 33. For an illustration of aneurysms, see Figure 33-22.

For more on myasthenia crisis, see Chapter 35.

For an in-depth discussion of the endocrine system, see Chapter 38.

For discussion of renal failure and diuresis, see Chapter 39.

Normal changes of the eyes and ears in older adults are discussed in Chapter 42.

Disorders of the eye that occur primarily in older adults are discussed in Chapter 43.

See more on rehabilitation in Chapter 46.

For an illustration of coup and contrecoup, see Figure 47-10.

Community Health Nursing is found in Chapter 48.

For discussion on congenital conditions and hydrocephalus, see Chapter 57.

Babinski's reflex in neonates is discussed in Chapter 56.

Cochlear implants are discussed in Chapter 59.

For conjunctivitis, see also Chapter 60.

For more information about Kernig's and Brudzinski's signs, see Figure 62-5.

Critical Thinking Care Map

Caring for a Client with Epilepsy
NCLEX-PN® Focus Area: Physiologic Integrity

Case Study: Lola Brinks is a 34-year-old with a history of epilepsy. She is brought to the emergency department in status epilepticus. History reveals that Lola is usually well controlled on antiepileptic medications. However, due to recent financial difficulties, Lola has reduced her medication and/or skipped taking it. Between seizures Lola appears dazed and says, "Just let me sleep. I'm so tired."

Nursing Diagnosis: *Risk for Trauma/Suffocation*

COLLECT DATA

Subjective	Objective
_____	_____
_____	_____
_____	_____
_____	_____
_____	_____
_____	_____
_____	_____

Would you report this? Yes/No

If yes, report to: _____

What would you report? _____

Nursing Care

_____
_____
_____
_____
_____
_____
_____
_____
_____
_____

How would you document this? _____
_____
_____
_____

Compare your answers and documentation to those provided on the MyNursingKit Website.

Data Collected
(use only those that apply)

- Height: 67"
- Weight: 195 lbs
- States "Just let me sleep. I'm so tired."
- VS: T 98.8° F, P 86, R 16, BP 150/90
- Reports reducing or skipping medication
- Diagnostic data: phenytoin level 2 mg (normal 10–20 mg); CBC, finger-stick blood glucose, urinalysis all negative

Nursing Interventions
(use only those that apply; list in priority order)

- Assess airway, breathing, circulation.
- Maintain strict bed rest.
- Stay with client during/after seizure.
- Perform finger-stick blood glucose test.
- Turn head to side/suction airway as indicated.
- Perform neurologic/vital sign check after seizure, e.g., level of consciousness, orientation, ability to comply with simple commands.
- Administer medications as indicated.
- Administer oxygen and monitor cardiac rhythm, oxygen saturation.
- Establish an IV line with normal saline.
- Insert Foley catheter.

NCLEX-PN® Exam Preparation

TEST-TAKING TIP   Look for the textbook answer to the question, not what you see practiced in the clinical setting.

1 The nurse recognizes the most common source of neurologic tumors is:
1. Microglia.
2. Neuroglia.
3. Ependymal cells.
4. Oligodendrocytes.

2 When performing a complete neurologic assessment, it is best to collect data by:
1. Assessing all neurologic functioning at the same time.
2. Assessing neurologic functioning in phases.
3. Assessing mental status, cranial nerve function, language, and sensory status together.
4. Performing a head-to-toe assessment of all neurologic functioning.

3 A client presents at the emergency department with right-sided hemiplegia and slurred speech lasting for the past 3 days. The family reports they thought it was a TIA, which the client has experienced frequently in the past. After providing family teaching, the family indicates they understand the reality of the situation when they ask:
1. "Will these symptoms go away like the other TIAs he has had?"
2. "If it is a stroke, can he be given TPA to dissolve the clot?"
3. "When does the rehabilitation process begin, and what resources are available to help him?"
4. "Will he have to stay in the hospital overnight?"

4 A client presents with the complaint of weakness in his hands and arms and is being examined for a degenerative neurologic disorder. The nurse interprets these symptoms as compatible with:
1. Multiple sclerosis.
2. Myasthenia gravis.
3. Parkinson's disease.
4. Amyotrophic lateral sclerosis.

5 When teaching the client about strategies to minimize episodes of trigeminal pain, the nurse would correctly instruct the client to:
1. "Wash your face with cotton pads."
2. "Eat food that is neither very warm nor very cold."
3. "Chew your food on the unaffected side."
4. "Rinse your mouth after eating if tooth brushing is too painful."

6 A client is experiencing increased intracranial pressure (IICP). Which of the following procedures does the nurse anticipate will be performed in order to reduce the pressure?
1. Burr holes
2. Craniotomy
3. Craniectomy
4. Stereotaxis

7 In preparing clients for any diagnostic test using contrast medium or dye, such as an angiogram or CT scan with contrast, the nurse's priority action is to determine whether the client:
1. Is claustrophobic.
2. Has a pacemaker.
3. Is allergic to salmon.
4. Is allergic to shellfish.

8 After admitting a client diagnosed with traumatic brain injury, the nurse's priority assessment to determine neurologic status change would be:
1. Vital signs.
2. Pupil reaction.
3. Speech and language.
4. Level of consciousness.

9 The nurse observes a client fall to the floor unconscious. The client stiffens and then begins to contract and relax the muscles. While this is occurring, the client is incontinent of urine. The nurse calls the charge nurse and reports the client had a/an:
1. Atonic seizure.
2. Myoclonic seizure.
3. Grand mal seizure.
4. Partial seizure.

10 The nurse is caring for a client diagnosed with meningitis who is unable to extend the leg when the hip is flexed at a 90-degree angle. The nurse documents a positive:
1. Kernig's sign.
2. Brudzinski's sign.
3. Babinski's reflex.
4. Decorticate posturing.

Answers and rationales for Review Questions appear in Appendix I.

Chapter 37

Clients with Gastrointestinal System Disorders

LEARNING Outcomes

After completing this chapter, you will be able to:

1. Describe the structure and function of the gastrointestinal (GI) system.
2. Identify oral cavity and esophageal disorders and nursing care for them.
3. Discuss common gastric disorders, including prevention, treatment, and nursing care.
4. Describe tests used to diagnose gastrointestinal disorders and the nursing care required before and after those tests.
5. Identify factors that affect defecation and nursing care for common elimination disorders.
6. Identify common infectious or inflammatory disorders and nursing considerations when caring for clients with these disorders.
7. Describe structural disorders of the GI system and their treatment.
8. Explain the nursing interventions that are used to assist clients with colorectal cancer and other disorders of the lower GI tract.
9. Identify common accessory organ disorders, their treatment, and nursing care.
10. Describe important procedures for clients who have undergone surgery for disorders of the gastrointestinal tract.

Clinical Objectives

11. Administer an enema for constipation or diagnostic test preparation.
12. Demonstrate the procedure for changing a colostomy appliance.

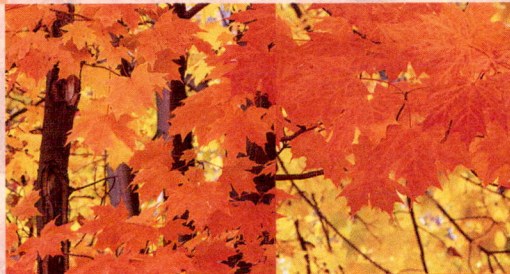

BRIEF Outline

KEY TERMS

Use the audio glossary feature on the MyNursingKit Website to hear the correct pronunciation of the following key terms.

achalasia 994

adhesions 1019

anastomosis 1005

ascites 1031

asterixis 1031

autodigestion 1034

bile 991

borborygmi 1007

caries 992

cathartics 1010

cholecystitis 1027

cholecystokinin 991

cholelithiasis 1027

cirrhosis 1029

colostomy 1021

constipation 1009

decompression 1003

diarrhea 1012

diverticulosis 1018

diverticulum 994

dumping syndrome 1003

dyspepsia 992

dysphagia 992

effluent 1021

emesis 998

enema 1010

enteritis 1013

eructation 992

fecal impaction 1011

fistula 1016

flatulence 992

food poisoning 999

gastric bypass 1006

gastritis 1000

gastroesophageal reflux disease 994

gastroplasty 1006

gavage 1004

gingivitis 993

guaiac test 1014

hematemesis 992

hepatic encephalopathy 1033

hepatitis 1029

hernia 1018

herniorrhaphy 1018

hiatal hernia 995

ileostomy 1021

incontinence 1013

intussusception 1019

lavage 1004

laxative 1010

leukoplakia 993

melena 1000

morbid obesity 1005

Murphy's sign 1027

nausea 996

obesity 1005

ostomy 1021

pancreatitis 1034

paracentesis 1032

peristalsis 989

peritonitis 1015

pilonidal cyst 1024

polyphagia 992

pyloroplasty 1002

pyrosis 992

rebound tenderness 1014

retching 992

Rovsing's sign 1014

rugae 990

sphincters 990

steatorrhea 1003

stomatitis 992

tenesmus 1013

thrush 992

Valsalva maneuver 1009

volvulus 1019

vomiting 992

The human body is a remarkable machine. It requires a continuous source of energy to function properly. This energy comes from the food we eat. Because food cannot enter the bloodstream directly, it needs to be prepared by the digestive system. Food is broken down through mechanical processes (chewing) and chemical processes (enzymes) into a form that can enter the blood. The passage that food goes through is known as the *alimentary canal*, from the Latin word meaning "to nourish" (Figure 37-1 ■). The alimentary canal includes the mouth, pharynx, esophagus, stomach, small intestine, and large intestine. It is approximately 26 to 30 feet long. The teeth, tongue, salivary glands, liver, gallbladder, and pancreas play accessory roles in the process of digestion.

If you were assigned to care for a client with cancer of the pancreas that had spread to the liver and stomach, you would want to better understand the client's problems with digesting and absorbing food. The following review of the anatomy and physiology of the gastrointestinal system will help you see the normal structure and function that are affected when your client has a GI disorder.

Structure and Function of the Gastrointestinal System

The mouth receives food, prepares it for digestion, and aids in the mechanics of speech. The tongue, a thick muscular organ, is anchored to the mouth by the frenulum. It assists in the processes of mastication (chewing), deglutition (swallowing), and speech. The taste buds on the tongue differentiate between bitter, sweet, sour, and salty flavors. Rough projections, called papillae, provide friction to help move the food through the mouth.

The teeth are necessary for mastication. Each tooth rests in a socket in the gums that provides a blood and nerve supply. The front teeth, known as the incisors, are used for cutting food. The more pointed teeth next to the incisors, called canines, are used for tearing food. The molars are and mouth clean. The parotid glands are the largest, located just opposite the upper second molars. The submandibular glands are found on the floor of the mouth. The sublingual glands are the smallest and are located under the tongue. Saliva is the secretion made by the salivary glands. It is 99% water and 1% salts and proteins. Saliva also contains mucus and enzymes. The saliva contains salivary amylase, or ptyalin, which is an enzyme that begins the process of converting starch to sugars, and lysozyme, which destroys bacteria that cause tooth decay and infections.

The pharynx is the cavity located behind the mouth and is a passageway that assists in swallowing. There are three parts: the nasopharynx, which lies behind the nasal cavities; the oropharynx, which is behind the mouth; and the laryngopharynx, which is behind the larynx (voice box) (Figure 37-2 ■). The act of swallowing occurs as the soft palate rises to protect the nasal cavity. The tongue rises to seal the back of the oral cavity and the trachea is guarded by the epiglottis to allow swallowing. The palatine and pharyngeal tonsils are found here. They are made of lymph tissue and help protect the throat from microorganisms that can cause infection.

The esophagus is a muscular tube about 10 inches long that connects the laryngeal pharynx to the stomach. The esophagus lies behind the trachea. No chemical digestion of food occurs in the esophagus. However, glands secrete mucus and **peristalsis** (wavelike progressive movement) facilitates the movement of food. The esophagus passes through an opening in the diaphragm and connects to the stomach just below the diaphragm.

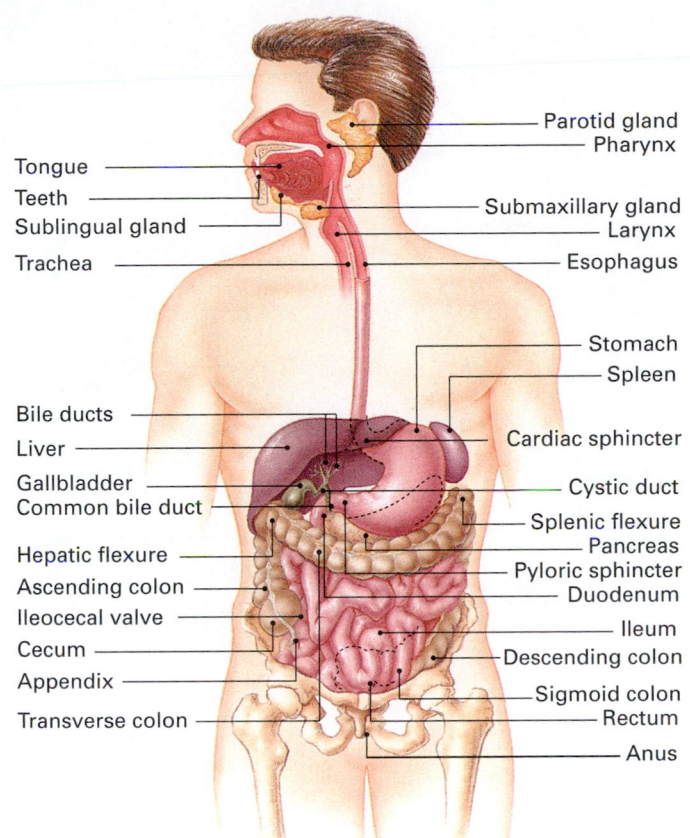

Figure 37-1. ■ Organs of the digestive system.

located along each side to the back of the mouth and grind the food. There are 32 permanent teeth.

Three pairs of salivary glands moisten the food, which facilitates chewing, swallowing, and keeping the teeth

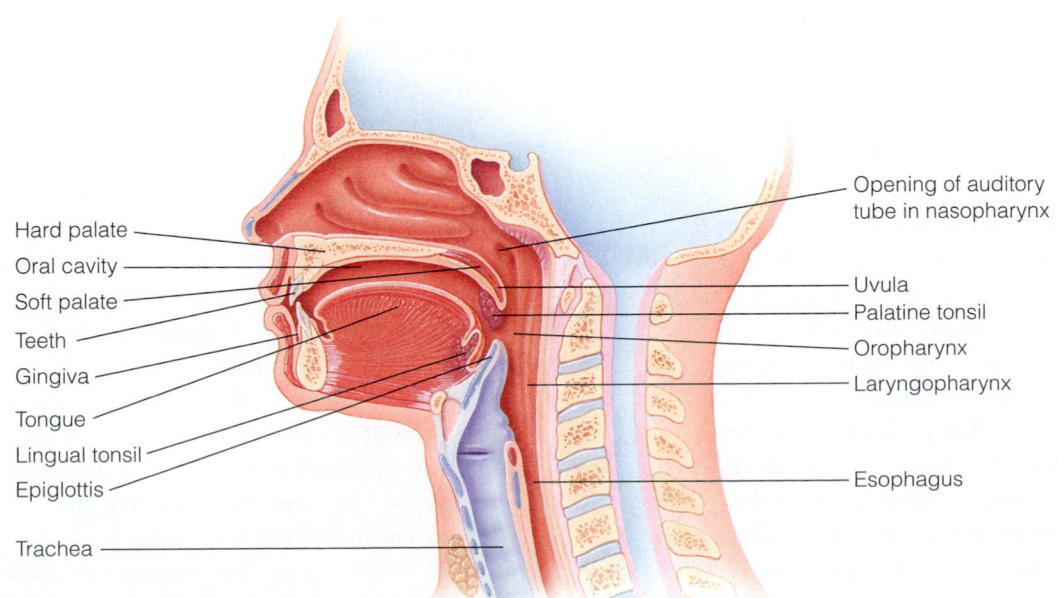

Figure 37-2. ■ Structures of the mouth, the pharynx, and the esophagus.

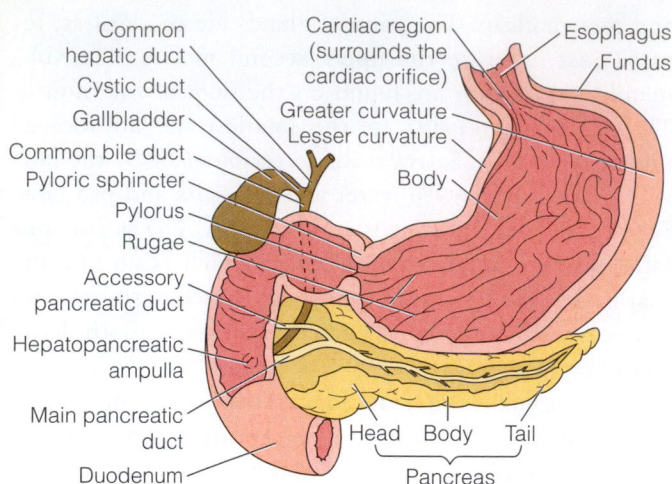

Figure 37-3. ■ The internal anatomic structures of the stomach, including the pancreatic, cystic, and hepatic ducts; the pancreas; and the gallbladder.

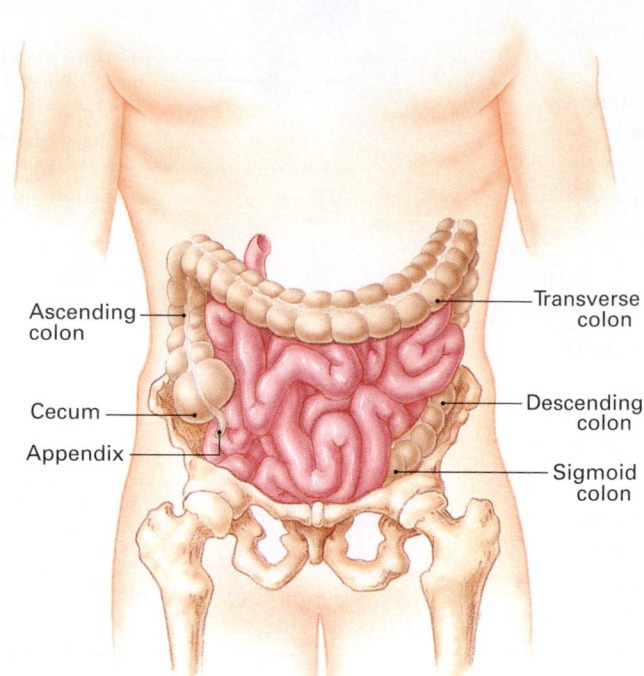

Figure 37-4. ■ The small intestine and large intestine.

The stomach is a J-shaped organ that forms a pouch to hold food for digestion (Figure 37-3 ■). There are two openings:

■ The cardiac (upper) sphincter is located closest to the heart, connecting the esophagus to the stomach.

■ The pyloric (lower) sphincter connects the stomach to the small intestine.

Sphincters are round muscles that allow food and digestive juices to pass through them when they are relaxed. When constricted, they hold food and fluids in the stomach. The folds found in the stomach (**rugae**) allow it to expand when necessary.

Mechanical digestion and chemical digestion take place in the stomach. *Mechanical digestion* occurs when the muscles in the walls of the stomach contract, causing food to mix with digestive juices so chemical digestion can occur. During *chemical digestion*, chemicals break down foods into smaller particles and more digestible forms, such as glucose, amino acids, and fatty acids.

The vagus nerve goes to the stomach, and when the parasympathetic nervous system is stimulated it causes the stomach to secrete gastric juices. The stomach secretes enzymes to break down foods for digestion. Pepsin begins the breakdown of proteins, lipase begins the breakdown of fats, and rennin, found in infants and children, coagulates milk protein, making it more readily acted on by pepsin. The mucous cells of the stomach secrete mucin, which protects the lining of the stomach. The parietal cells secrete hydrochloric acid and the intrinsic factor, which enables the body to absorb vitamin B_{12}. The semiliquid material that moves into the small intestine from the stomach is called *chyme*.

The small intestine extends from the pyloric valve to the ileocecal valve, where it joins the large intestine (Figure 37-4 ■). It is the longest and most coiled part of the intestine averaging 21 feet. The primary functions of the small intestine are digestion and absorption. The small intestine is divided into three areas: the duodenum, jejunum, and ileum.

The duodenum is C shaped; glands secrete mucus to protect it from the acid chyme that is received from the stomach. Enzymes from the pancreas and bile from the gallbladder enter the duodenum where they mix with chyme to further break the food down into absorbable nutrients. Numerous tiny projections, called *villi*, increase nutritive absorption. The pancreas secretes sodium bicarbonate to neutralize stomach acid and stimulate the secretion of bile by the liver.

The jejunum and ileum are the remaining portions of the small intestine. Although no distinct separation of these two sections exists, the diameter is greater, the walls are thicker and more vascular, and the peristaltic activity is greater here than in the duodenum.

The walls of the small intestine absorb nutrients and secrete hormones, mucus, and enzymes. Villi increase the absorptive surface area. The muscles in the walls of the intestines contract to push food through the tube, an action called *peristalsis*. The *peritoneum* is a double-layered serous membrane that separates to cover the organs in the abdomen and to line the abdominal wall, allowing the organs to slide freely against one another. The parietal membrane lines the abdominal cavity. The visceral membrane covers the organs.

The large intestine (*colon*) is about 5 feet long and secretes mucus to protect its lining. The colon's functions are to absorb water, nutrients, and electrolytes; to manufacture certain vitamins; and to store and eliminate feces. The large intestine is divided into five sections. The ileocecal valve connects the small intestine to the large intestine and prevents backflow of intestinal contents. The ileum empties into the *cecum*. The cecum is a pouch; the vermiform appendix attaches to it. The appendix is made of lymphatic tissue, which is believed to help fight intestinal infections. The colon has four parts:

- Ascending colon
- Transverse colon
- Descending colon
- Sigmoid colon

The sigmoid colon is S shaped and bends left. Normally, food takes 3 to 5 days to pass through the colon. The *rectum* is a holding pouch for feces; it contains both an internal and external sphincter made of voluntary muscle (Figure 37-5 ■). The *anus* is the opening at the end of the alimentary canal.

The stool (feces) contains undigested fiber, bile pigments, bacteria, small amounts of salts, and debris from the intestinal epithelium.

PHYSIOLOGY OF DEFECATION

Elimination of the waste products of digestion from the body is essential to health. The excreted waste products are referred to as *feces* or *stool*.

Defecation or bowel movement is the expulsion of feces from the anus and rectum. The frequency of defecation is highly individual, varying from several times per day to two or three times per week. The amount defecated also varies from person to person. When peristalsis moves the feces into the sigmoid colon and the rectum, the sensory nerves in the rectum are stimulated and the individual becomes aware of the need to defecate.

Expulsion of the feces is assisted by contraction of the abdominal muscles and the diaphragm. This maneuver causes an increase in abdominal pressure, which moves the feces through the anal canal. People who ignore the defecation reflex or who consciously inhibit it may eventually lose sensitivity to the defecation response. Constipation can be the end result.

ACCESSORY ORGANS

The liver is a reddish brown organ supplied with blood via the portal vein and hepatic artery (Figure 37-1). One and one-half quarts of blood pass through the liver every minute. The liver is located in the upper right quadrant just below the diaphragm and is comprised of two lobes. The right lobe is larger than the left. The liver has more than 100 functions. Some major functions are:

- Storage of glycogen
- Production of bile to break down fats
- Modification of fats
- Detoxification of alcohol and drugs
- Storage of vitamins
- Synthesis of urea
- Formation of blood protein plasma
- Destruction of old blood cells

The gallbladder, a pear-shaped organ that lies on the inferior surface of the liver, stores and concentrates the bile from the liver. **Bile** is a greenish-brown liquid that consists of water, bile salts, bile pigment, cholesterol, and inorganic salts and is needed to emulsify (break apart) lipids for digestion. The gallbladder is connected to the liver by the hepatic duct and releases bile into the cystic duct. When fats are present, bile flows through the common bile duct into the duodenum. The gallbladder contracts and releases bile as a response to the hormone **cholecystokinin.**

The pancreas secretes digestive fluids containing enzymes to help break down food for absorption. It also makes

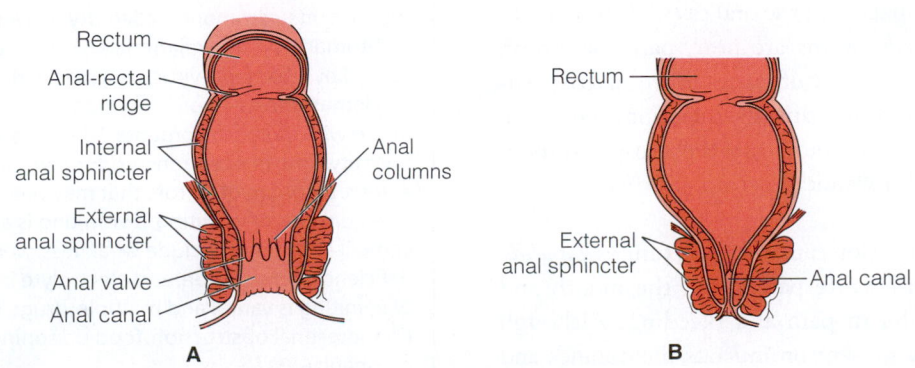

Figure 37-5. ■ The rectum, anal canal, and anal sphincters: **A.** Open. **B.** Closed.

the hormone *insulin*, which circulates through the blood to help the body metabolize glucose. The head of the pancreas lies in the curve of the duodenum; the tail extends to the spleen (see Figure 37-1). The exocrine function of the pancreas is the release of enzymes to the duodenum. The primary enzymes released are:

- *Amylase*, for breaking down carbohydrates to sugar.
- *Lipase*, for breaking down fats.
- *Trypsin*, for breaking down proteins.

Sodium bicarbonate is released to neutralize the acids in the duodenum.

Once the food is broken down into amino acids, fatty acids, and simple sugars, these nutrients enter the villi in the small intestine where they pass into the bloodstream. The mesenteric veins carry the nutrients from the villi to the portal vein, which takes them to the liver. Some nutrients are stored by the liver. The remaining nutrients circulate through the blood to the body cells.

As you care for clients with upper gastrointestinal conditions, you will need to know about the symptoms and treatment of each disorder so you can anticipate the clients' needs and know how to meet them.

UPPER GI DISORDERS

Upper GI conditions are quite common in everyday life. The terminology to describe client complaints is important to know. Box 37-1 ■ lists common digestive disorders and symptoms.

Disorders of the Oral Cavity

DENTAL CONDITIONS

The condition of the client's teeth has a great influence on nutritional status. Teeth that are broken, painful, or missing and ill-fitting dentures can affect the types of foods the client is able to eat. Lesions and inflammation of the oral cavity also affect eating habits.

Dental **caries** (cavities) usually develop in a hard to reach area of the tooth. The cavity begins as a small hole in the tooth and, if left untreated, breaks through the enamel, finally entering the dentin and the pulp. The pulp contains the blood, lymph vessels, and nerves. When the decay has gone this far, the client is suffering pain and may have developed an abscess. The face is swollen and antibiotics may be required to relieve the inflammation. A tooth extraction can be the next step to resolve the problem.

ORAL INFECTIONS

An infection or inflammation in the oral cavity is referred to as *stomatitis*. General symptoms are heat, pain, or mouth soreness. There can be a variety of causes of stomatitis: sensitivity to toothpaste and mouthwash, infection, trauma to the oral cavity, and oral irritants are the most common. Clients with decreased immune function are very susceptible to stomatitis.

Thrush is an oral infection caused by the fungus *Candida albicans*. It causes small white patches on the mouth and tongue. Removal results in pain and bleeding. Although the fungus is normally present on mucous membranes and skin, some clients are susceptible to thrush because their

immune systems are compromised. These include infants and those taking steroids, antibiotics, and chemotherapy.

BOX 37-1	COMMON TERMS FOR DIGESTIVE DISORDERS

Dyspepsia—also known as *indigestion*, is an upper gastrointestinal regurgitation of gastric contents. Clients complain of cramps, burning sensation, fullness, and distention. The pain can be associated with eating, either during or following a meal. Eating spicy and/or fatty foods may contribute to indigestion. Emotional stress may also be associated with this problem.

Pyrosis—also known as *heartburn*, is pain near the heart that results from reverse peristalsis of gastric acids. Antacids are used to neutralize stomach acids.

Dysphagia—difficulty swallowing.

Polyphagia—a voracious appetite.

Eructation—the expelling of gas from the stomach through the mouth, commonly called belching. When the client swallows air while eating, drinking through a straw, or drinking carbonated beverages, it forms gas in the stomach.

Flatulence—expelling of gas from the rectum.

Vomiting—the forceful expulsion of stomach contents through the mouth. Prior to vomiting, the client may experience sweating, a rapid pulse, and pallor.

Retching—the action of vomiting without expelling gastric contents, commonly called dry heaves.

Stomatitis—the inflammation of the oral cavity; may be caused by a bacteria, virus, or systemic disease.

Hematemesis—vomiting blood, which may be clotted and mixed with stomach contents. The nurse should observe the quantity, time of occurrence, odor, color, and frequency of emesis. Be aware of factors that may precipitate and aggravate episodes of vomiting. If vomiting is allowed to continue, complications may include weakness, weight loss, nutritional deficiency, dehydration, and electrolyte imbalance. The cause of vomiting is varied and multiple: drugs, GI or systemic infection, intestinal obstruction, food poisoning, stress, uremia, and pregnancy.

Thrush can be spread easily, so it is very important for nurses and other caregivers to use thorough hand washing. When infants with thrush are breastfed, mothers must wash their breasts and nipples carefully to prevent further infection.

PERIODONTAL DISEASE

Pyorrhea (purulent discharge) is a condition that affects the gums, bone, and supporting structures of the teeth.

Initially, symptoms are few, but later bleeding, gum recession, loosening of the teeth, and infection may develop. Teeth may fall out or need extraction. In **gingivitis** (inflamed gums), the gums are reddened, swollen, and bleed easily, although there is little to no discomfort. Inadequate oral hygiene is the cause of gingivitis, and it can be reversed with treatment and good oral care. However, untreated gingivitis can lead to periodontal disease.

As periodontal disease progresses, the bacteria produce toxins that invade and irritate the gums. The tissues and bone supporting the teeth deteriorate. Pockets of infection form, causing teeth to loosen and fall out. Alcohol and tobacco use contribute to periodontal disease. Other risk factors include diabetes, stress, and hormonal changes of puberty and pregnancy.

Preventive care is essential to detect periodontal disease early. Dentist visits twice a year are recommended. Treatment of periodontal disease may include pocket reduction, soft tissue grafts, regenerative procedures, and dental implants.

LEUKOPLAKIA

Leukoplakia is the name given to smooth irregular white patches found on the tongue, lips, cheeks, or oral mucosa. The patches can be rubbed off with force. They are usually painless, but are considered a precursor to oral cancer. If a leukoplakic patch lasts more than 2 weeks, it is generally recommended that it be biopsied.

ORAL CANCER

Oral cancer occurs in the mouth (Figure 37-6 ■), buccal cavity (cheek pouch), or pharynx. It has a high rate of cure when detected and treated early. It is painless and accounts for 3% of all cancer deaths in the United States, affecting men twice as often as women. A physician should assess any oral lesion that doesn't heal within 2 to 3 weeks. Use of alcohol, heavy smoking, and smokeless tobacco increase the risk for oral cancer.

Manifestations

The client may complain of difficulty chewing, swallowing, and speaking. The client may also have swollen areas in the mouth, numbness in the mouth, or constant pain in the mouth or ear. Swollen cervical lymph nodes may be palpated.

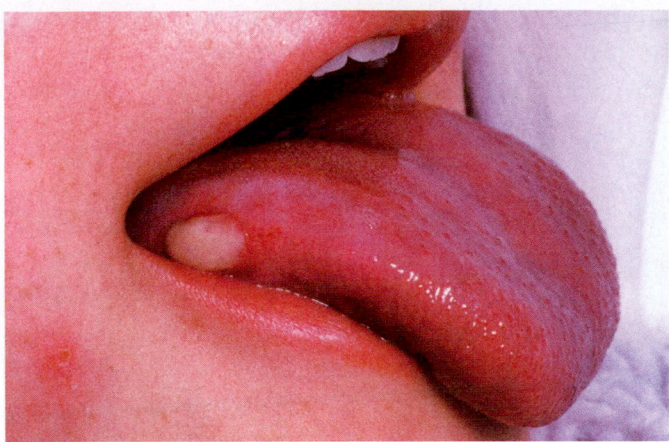

Figure 37-6. ■ Oral cancer.

Diagnosis and Treatment

Diagnosis is confirmed with a biopsy. Oral cancer may be treated with surgery alone, or in conjunction with radiation therapy and chemotherapy (discussed in Chapter 45 ⌾⌾). A modified neck dissection may be required to remove all areas affected by the cancer. Muscles, blood vessels, glands, and possibly a section of the thyroid may be removed in addition to the tumor and surrounding lymph nodes. A tracheostomy may be required and it is important to prepare the client for this. A drain may be placed to remove accumulated serosanguineous fluid. A nasogastric tube may be inserted to prevent gas accumulation and vomiting postoperatively. (Review nasogastric tube insertion in Chapter 25 ⌾⌾ .) It is extremely important for the client to be able to verbalize fears and feelings about changes in appearance and speaking ability.

clinical ALERT

When cancer of the mouth or pharynx exists, maintaining a patent airway is the first priority. Suction and clean the tracheostomy to prevent obstruction. Place the client in a Fowler's position to facilitate breathing, increase drainage, and decrease swelling. Observe for signs of respiratory distress: dyspnea, restlessness, cyanosis, and respiratory rate changes. Keep the client in a room adjacent to the nursing station for quick access. Answer the call light immediately to alleviate the client's fear of being unable to relate his or her needs.

The prognosis for clients with oral cancer is influenced by several factors. The tumor's size and spread (either to lymph nodes or surrounding structures) and the client's immunocompetence and general condition all affect the outcome.

NURSING CONSIDERATIONS FOR ORAL CAVITY DISORDERS

Now that you know the symptoms and treatment for clients with disorders of the oral cavity, you know that you need to focus on maintaining an open airway and promoting food and fluid intake when you care for them. Although each situation may be different, maintaining an open airway will involve positioning the client with the head of the bed elevated, suctioning as needed to clear the airway, and assisting the client to remove secretions or drainage from the throat. The nurse will need to check the client frequently for bleeding or hoarseness that could indicate swelling of the throat. Encourage the client to eat and drink as they are able. Soft foods and nourishing liquids may be better tolerated than regular diets. Give oral care every 2 hours to keep the oral cavity clean. A Water Pik or syringe is used to irrigate the cavity if foam brushes or oral swabs cause pain. Clients with oral cancers may also be dealing with fears about treatment and the diagnosis, as well as with disfigurement of the face after surgery. Providing emotional support by listening and encouraging is a valuable nursing intervention for these clients.

Esophageal Disorders

There are a few conditions of the esophagus that require medical attention. Foreign bodies, such as partial dentures, a large piece of meat, a bone, pins, or coins, can become lodged in the esophagus, causing an obstruction and tissue injury. The foreign bodies are removed with the aid of an esophagoscope. If the foreign body is small and unlikely to puncture the tissue, it may be allowed to pass through the digestive system. If a piece of meat is causing the obstruction, it can be removed or dissolved with proteolytic enzymes (meat tenderizer).

clinical ALERT

Perforation of the esophagus is a rare but serious occurrence. Manifestations include chest pain, elevated temperature, and difficulty breathing. Rupture is associated with a high mortality rate related to respiratory impairment, shock, or sepsis.

ESOPHAGITIS

Esophagitis is an inflammation of the esophagus, and usually occurs as a result of swallowing irritants or reflux of stomach acid into the esophagus. The classic symptom is burning pain in the epigastrium that may progress up the esophagus.

ACHALASIA OF THE ESOPHAGUS

Achalasia occurs when the cardiac sphincter of the stomach does not relax to allow food to pass into the stomach. The lower end of the esophagus then dilates, sometimes enough to hold one or more liters of food. The client complains of feeling full, of food not going down, and eventually experiences regurgitation.

Achalasia of the esophagus is treated several ways. Medications may help relax the sphincter so a balloon can be inserted in the sphincter and slowly inflated. This helps dilate the tightened sphincter and narrowed area around it. Often dilation has to be repeated periodically. Surgical treatment, called *esophagomyotomy*, is a procedure to cut into the muscle layers of the sphincter to allow it to open.

Pyloric stenosis, a thickening of the pyloric sphincter and narrowing of the opening between the stomach and the duodenum, is most commonly seen in 5-week-old boys. This disorder is discussed in Chapter 59 in the Pediatric Unit.

GASTROESOPHAGEAL REFLUX DISEASE

Gastroesophageal reflux disease (GERD) is a fairly common disorder that results when gastric contents splash into the lower end of the esophagus. This *reflux* (backward movement) of gastric contents causes inflammation and scarring in the esophagus. Normally, the lower esophageal sphincter prevents this reflux. When acid from the stomach refluxes into the esophagus (Figure 37-7 ■), GERD results.

Manifestations

Heartburn that is worse after meals and is aggravated by lying down or bending over is a common symptom of GERD. Other symptoms include sore throat, dysphagia, or chest pain.

Treatment

Treatment for GERD includes medications such as Tagamet, Pepcid, and Prilosec to decrease stomach acid production and promote healing of the esophagus. Clients are instructed not to lie down for 3 hours after eating and to raise the head of the bed on blocks or to sleep on a foam wedge to keep the head elevated. Alcohol and tobacco use increase gastric reflux. Other lifestyle changes to improve or eliminate the symptoms of GERD include weight loss if the client is overweight; eating smaller, more frequent meals; and avoiding foods that are high in acid. Other foods that relax the lower esophageal sphincter are those high in fat, peppermint, and chocolate. Clients with GERD should also avoid alcohol, aspirin, and NSAIDs to prevent worsening of symptoms. (See Chapter 59 for more information about GERD.)

ESOPHAGEAL DIVERTICULUM

A **diverticulum** is an outpouching or protrusion of the inner tissue layers (mucosa and submucosa) through a weakness in the muscular wall of the esophagus. The client may complain of regurgitation, especially when lying down. The diverticulum may become distended with foods or fluids

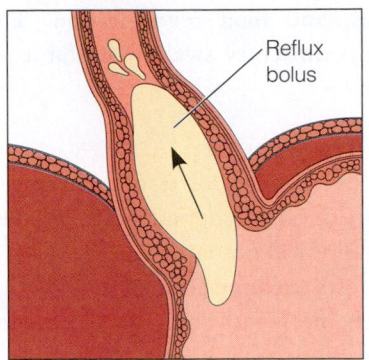
Transient lower esophageal sphincter relaxation

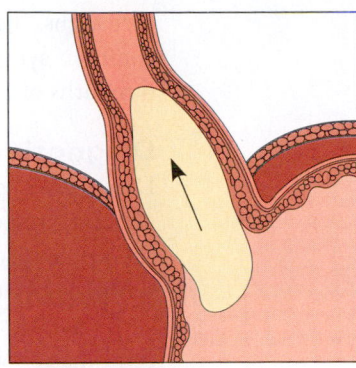
Incompetent lower esophageal sphincter

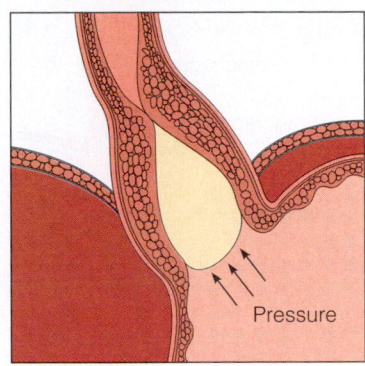
Increased intragastric pressure

Figure 37-7. ■ Mechanisms of gastroesophageal reflux.

and can become inflamed to the point that the esophageal wall can perforate.

Manifestations

The client may complain of regurgitation, especially when lying down. Other manifestations include difficulty swallowing, eructation or regurgitation, halitosis, and a sour taste in the mouth.

Treatment

Treatment for esophageal diverticuli includes intake of soft, easily chewed foods. The head of the client's bed should be in high-Fowler's position, and the client is encouraged to sit upright for 2 hours after eating. If the condition is more severe, a feeding tube may be inserted to allow for healing. If the client does not respond well to this treatment, surgery is done to remove the diverticulum. *Stricture* (narrowing) of the esophagus may occur as a complication of this surgery.

clinical ALERT

Be alert for any difficulty swallowing or vomiting, which might indicate a narrowing of the esophagus.

HIATAL HERNIA

A **hiatal hernia** occurs when part of the stomach moves through an opening in the diaphragm into the chest cavity. The two types are *sliding* and *paraesophageal* (Figure 37-8 ■). Sliding hernia is more common. In this situation, the top portion of the stomach slides through an enlarged opening in the diaphragm through which the esophagus passes. This happens when the client reclines. When the client stands, the stomach slides back into its normal position. With paraesophageal hernia, part of the stomach pushes through a weakness in the diaphragm and lodges beside the diaphragm.

Manifestations

Small hiatal hernias are asymptomatic and often go undetected until the client has an x-ray that reveals the hernia. Larger hernias may cause complaints of *pyrosis* (heartburn) and a feeling of fullness in the lower chest. Regurgitation and reflux occur. Reflux of stomach acids into the esophagus causes irritation and bleeding. The client may hear a

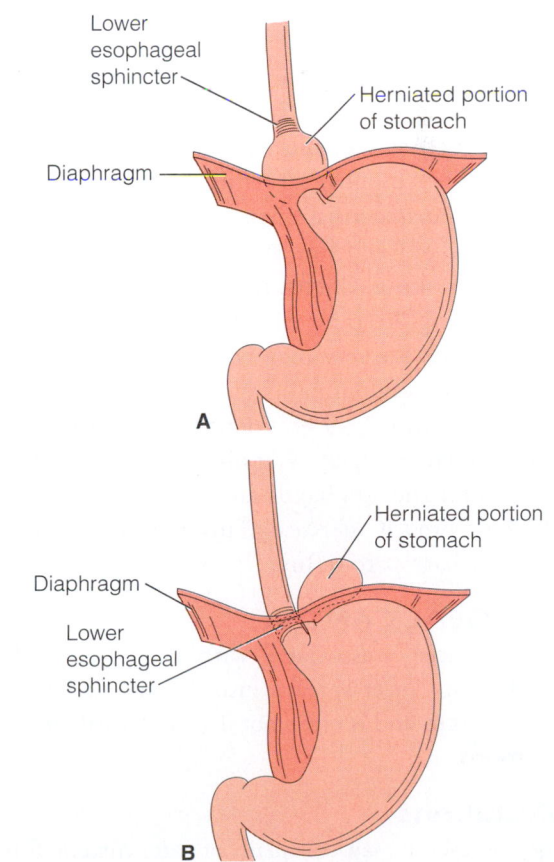

Figure 37-8. ■ Hiatal hernias: **A.** Sliding hiatal hernia. **B.** Paraesophageal hiatal hernia.

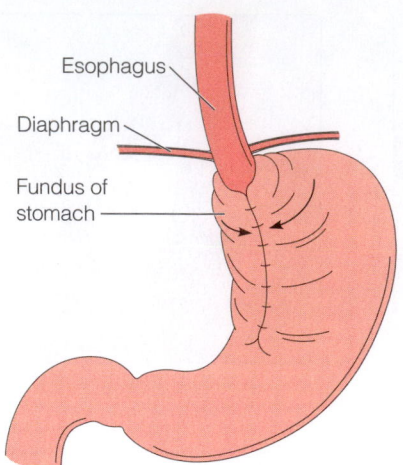

Esophagus

Diaphragm

Fundus of
stomach

Figure 37-9. ■ Nissen fundoplication. The fundus of the stomach is wrapped around the lower esophagus and the edges are sutured together.

splashing sound in the substernal area if the hernia is large. Esophagitis and pain can occur from the sliding of the stomach against the wall of the esophagus.

Treatment

Small asymptomatic hernias are not treated. The head of the bed is elevated or the client is instructed to sit upright for 30 minutes after eating. If the hernia is a sliding type, Fowler's position will help prevent reflux or regurgitation. Antacids are recommended to control gastric irritation. Medications such as Tagamet, Pepcid, Zantac, and Axid are used to control esophageal reflux. Nutritional management includes instructing clients to eat small frequent meals and to avoid bedtime snacks, spicy foods, alcohol, caffeine, and smoking. Clients may also benefit from wearing loose clothing, keeping their weight down, and avoiding heavy lifting. Surgery may be indicated to secure the stomach in the abdominal cavity. In severe cases, a *fundoplication* (Figure 37-9 ■) is done to secure the stomach in the abdominal cavity by wrapping the upper end of the stomach around the esophagus and suturing it onto itself to hold the stomach in place. This restores an effective high-pressure barrier to reflux.

ESOPHAGEAL CANCER

Esophageal cancer is associated with alcohol and tobacco use. Esophageal cancer spreads into the muscle layers and the lymph system and is often not detected until late in the disease process.

Manifestations

Initially, the client may complain of intermittent fullness in the chest area, pain, and difficulty swallowing. The client experiences progressive weight loss, excessive salivation,

hiccoughs, halitosis, and food regurgitation. The most common symptom is difficulty swallowing for a period of 6 months or longer.

Diagnosis and Treatment

Diagnosis is made by a variety of tests including esophagogram, upper GI (UGI), esophagogastroduodenoscopy (EGD), biopsy, and physical presentation. (Table 37-1 ■ describes a variety of tests used for GI disorders.)

Radiation and chemotherapy may be used alone or in combination with surgery (see Chapter 45 ⊙⊙).

To relieve dysphagia, the esophagus may be dilated or stents placed to keep the esophagus open for food to pass through. Esophageal resection with grafting using a section of the colon or a Dacron graft is the surgical procedure used when the cancerous portion of the esophagus is removed.

For coverage of pyloric stenosis and other gastrointestinal disorders primarily affecting the newborn, see Chapter 59 ⊙⊙ .

NURSING CONSIDERATIONS FOR ESOPHAGEAL DISORDERS

By knowing the causes, symptoms, and treatment of esophageal disorders, the nurse can better understand how to care for clients with these disorders. Monitoring the client's ability to swallow and intake nutrition is a priority. Check for problems such as vomiting or regurgitation, hoarseness, and iron-deficiency anemia. Monitor intake and output and daily weights, and assess for signs of dehydration to evaluate the client's nutritional status. In addition, you will want to help alleviate pain, burning, and discomfort in the chest area due to esophageal disorders. Often, medications can relieve these problems. It may be necessary to assist clients in determining which foods and beverages cause them distress. Be aware that clients with esophageal disorders sometimes think that they are having a heart attack because of the location and intensity of the pain. Reassure clients when it is appropriate to do so. Explain why they are experiencing such discomfort and how it relates to the esophagus and stomach; this can relieve the client's mind.

Stomach Disorders

NAUSEA AND VOMITING

Nausea and vomiting (N&V) are common symptoms of gastrointestinal diseases. **Nausea** is the uncomfortable wavelike sensation that may or may not lead to vomiting. Vomiting is the forceful ejection of stomach contents through the mouth. Vomiting occurs by voluntary and involuntary contraction of the diaphragm and abdominal muscles. The cardiac sphincter opens up and the contents of

TABLE 37-1	Diagnostic Tests for Gastrointestinal Disorders		
DIAGNOSTIC TEST	**PURPOSE**	**CLIENT PREPARATION**	**POSTTEST CARE**
Barium swallow/UGI series and small bowel follow-through	To detect hiatal hernia, diverticula, pyloric valve malfunction, and esophageal varices. To diagnose strictures, ulcers, tumors, motility disorders, and the rate at which the stomach empties.	NPO after midnight. No smoking because it stimulates gastric motility. A laxative may be ordered the night before. The morning of the test the client drinks 16 to 20 oz of barium sulfate solution. The barium fills the alimentary canal, making it visible on x-rays. The test can take from 2 to 6 hours to complete.	When the client returns from the test, check with x-ray to determine if the tests are complete. A routine laxative/cathartic is ordered because barium is very constipating. Explain to the client that the stool will be lightly colored for 24 to 48 hours due to elimination of the barium.
Barium enema	To diagnose colorectal cancer, inflammatory bowel disease, diverticulum, polyps, or lesions in the large bowel.	Laxatives and enemas until clear may be ordered. Stool in the colon can obscure the clarity of the x-ray. A low-residue diet may be ordered 1 to 3 days prior to the test and clear liquids the day before the test. The client is NPO after midnight and until the procedure is completed. Barium sulfate is instilled by enema and retained while the x-ray is taken.	Same as UGI, may include a cleansing enema to remove barium.
Gastric analysis	To estimate the amount of gastric activity, determine composition of stomach secretions or retention of gastric secretions, and diagnose possible intestinal obstruction. It is diagnostic for pernicious anemia and cancer.	Client is NPO; smoking is restricted for 8 hours prior to test. A nasogastric tube is inserted and the stomach contents are aspirated by syringe or low suction.	Discontinue nasogastric tube if appropriate.
Gastric acid stimulation test	This test is done in conjunction with a gastric analysis and stimulates gastric acid contents; used to diagnose pernicious anemia, ulcers, gastritis, and gastric cancer.	Histalog or histamine injection is given. The client may feel flushed. The nurse monitors the blood pressure and pulse. Epinephrine and Benadryl are available in case of emergency. Gastric specimens are taken every 15 minutes for 1 hour. Label and time the specimen. Indicate medication used and initial.	None
Esophagogastroduodeno-scopy (EGD)	Procedure to directly visualize the interior of the esophagus, stomach, and duodenum using an endoscope.	Client will be NPO prior to procedure and will undergo conscious sedation during procedure.	Withhold all food and fluids until gag and swallow reflexes have returned; assess for signs of complications such as bleeding, pain in abdomen or back, dyspnea, fever, or dysphagia.
CAT (computerized axial tomography) scan	A narrow x-ray beam is used to detect the density differences from very small cubes of tissue. Sections of the body are shown on the scanner's monitor. This test detects and diagnoses liver, spleen, kidney, pancreatic, and pelvic organ diseases.	Painless and noninvasive. The client may be instructed to hold the breath briefly to avoid movement.	None

(continued)

TABLE 37-1	Diagnostic Tests for Gastrointestinal Disorders (continued)		
DIAGNOSTIC TEST	PURPOSE	CLIENT PREPARATION	POSTTEST CARE
Ultrasound (US)	High-frequency sound waves that pass into the body structures and are then bounced back much like a reflection. This test detects neoplasm, cysts, liver, pancreatic abscesses, liver cancer, and obstructive and nonobstructive jaundice. It is diagnostic for cholelithiasis and cholecystitis.	Noninvasive procedure. A clear, water-based gel is used as a conducting agent over the skin that is to be examined.	None
Magnetic resonance imaging (MRI)	This test is used as a supplement to US and CAT scans. The client lies in a cylindrical machine that produces a static magnetic field. The field interacts with certain nuclei to send a signal that contains information necessary to reconstruct an image. The test can take from 30 to 90 minutes. There is no specific preparation. The client is NPO for 6 hours with an abdomen or pelvic exam. Contraindications are clients with metal plates or pins.	Open MRI machines have served to assist clients who experience claustrophobia. Clients must remain motionless for a quality image. The time may range from 30 to 90 minutes. Contraindications to MRI are pacemakers, metallic clips, and prostheses.	None
Urea breath test	To detect the presence of *H. pylori*.	Tell the client that the test involves drinking a colorless, odorless mixture of water and urea and then exhaling into a machine that detects the enzyme urease. Urease is produced when *H. pylori* is present.	None

the stomach are propelled up and out, causing a reverse peristalsis. Vomiting is a complex reflex coordinated by the vomiting center, the medulla oblongata.

The cause of nausea and vomiting varies. Vomiting can be induced by seeing someone else vomit. Much of the time nausea and vomiting do not require urgent treatment. Excessive vomiting can cause dehydration, however; it is often associated with diarrhea. See the following for possible causes:

- Bacterial or viral infections
- Bulimia
- Cerebral tumors
- Food poisoning
- Food allergies
- Ear infections
- Medications/chemotherapy
- Migraine headaches
- Motion sickness/seasickness
- Morning sickness in pregnancy
- Toxins

Manifestations

Nausea is a subjective symptom and is described by clients as a stomachache or indigestion. Nausea may be accompanied by diaphoresis, pain, and excessive salivation. The client may complain of weakness, being bloated, or having waves of nausea and dizziness. **Emesis** or vomit can consist of undigested food and gastric juices, or it may be green from bile or clear fluid. Bright red emesis indicates fresh bleeding. Dark red vomitus, referred to as *coffee ground emesis*, suggests old blood. Medications can alter the color of the emesis expelled. When excessive amounts of fluids are lost through vomiting, dehydration can occur. Symptoms include dry mouth, decreased urination, poor skin turgor, sunken eyes, and thirst. Loss of electrolytes can result in metabolic alkalosis. If not treated this leads to vascular collapse and death.

BOX 37-2	COMPLEMENTARY THERAPIES

Ginger to Relieve Nausea

Ginger has been used for centuries for stomachaches, nausea, menstrual cramps, and diarrhea. Ginger ale is a common home remedy for an upset stomach. Ginger is often recommended as a safe way for pregnant women to relieve morning sickness. The nausea associated with chemotherapy, or even motion sickness, can also be treated with ginger.

There are some claims that ginger can interfere with blood clotting, so clients with cancer or postsurgical clients should confer with their primary care provider about its use.

Ginger is found in fresh or dried root, tablet, capsule, liquid extract, and tea forms. Dried "candied" ginger is also available. Dosages depend on the form taken.

Treatment

The focus of treatment is to eliminate the cause when possible. Certain techniques can help clients alleviate nausea and vomiting. Eating soda crackers or sucking on a piece of hard candy will sometimes settle the nausea sensation. Soft, bland foods and dry toast may help. Ginger (Box 37-2 ■) is one natural aid for reducing nausea.

Smells often trigger nausea, so avoiding strong fragrances is helpful. Distraction methods for someone with persistent nausea are beneficial. Oral care will freshen the mouth and eliminate the acid taste. The nurse should make sure to recognize clients at risk for aspiration and to turn them to the side to protect the airway.

Vomiting is monitored for amount, frequency, odor, and color. For prolonged vomiting, IV therapy or TPN may be initiated. With excessive vomiting a nasogastric tube attached to suction may be ordered. If the amount of fluid return is increased, the physician will sometimes order that fluid be replaced via IV. The nurse monitors intake and output, vital signs, and weights.

Nausea and vomiting are also treated with a variety of antiemetics. Phenothiazines such as Reglan (metoclopramide) or Compazine (prochlorperazine) are frequently prescribed. Antihistamine and anticholinergic drugs such as Dramamine (dimenhydrinate), Antivert (meclizine), Vistaril (hydroxyzine), and Benadryl (diphenhydramine) are commonly used. A suppository may be used to avoid having the medication be vomited. An example of an antiemetic in suppository form is Tigan (trimethobenzamide).

FOODBORNE ILLNESS

It is estimated that 76 million cases of foodborne illness occur every year in the United States. Most are mild and resolve in a day or two. Others are more serious, sending 325,000 to the hospital and resulting in 5,000 deaths per year.

Consumption of contaminated foods or liquids that cause foodborne illness is commonly called **food poisoning.** There are many types of pathogens, bacteria, viruses, and parasites that contaminate foods, so there are many different types of foodborne infections. Additionally, poisonous chemicals can become harmful when present in food that is eaten.

After eating the pathogen there is an incubation period before symptoms appear. This incubation period can vary from hours to days. The toxins pass through the stomach and into the intestine, multiplying and beginning to enter the bloodstream. Many organisms cause similar symptoms. The most common bacteria found in foodborne infections are *Campylobacter, Salmonella*, and *E coli*. A common virus called Calicivirus, also known as Norwalk, can also be the causative organism.

Manifestations

Typically the symptoms of food poisoning include nausea and vomiting, diarrhea, and painful abdominal cramping. The client may exhibit temperatures higher than 101.5 F orally. There may be blood in the stool or emesis. Signs of dehydration should be monitored closely with continued vomiting and diarrhea. Anal irritation occurs due to persistent diarrhea.

Diagnosis and Treatment

Blood and stool cultures are commonly ordered to determine organisms and verify sensitivities. History and physical symptoms are also taken into consideration when determining a diagnosis. Blood for electrolyte levels will be sent to the lab to determine replacement needs. Some illnesses may go undiagnosed and unreported.

Initially, fluids need to be replaced orally or intravenously. Electrolyte balance is very carefully monitored. Intake and output is accurately measured. Both emesis and diarrhea should be measured and documented. Antidiarrheals and antiemetics may be ordered for symptomatic relief. Antibiotics may be ordered for bacterial infections. Daily weights will also assist in evaluating treatment. Enteric isolation may be indicated.

Prevention

Client education regarding foodborne illness should occur prior to discharge. Reminding the client to cook meat, poultry, and eggs thoroughly can prevent undercooked foods from harboring bacteria. Avoid cross-contaminating foods by washing hands, utensils, and cutting boards after contact with raw meat or poultry and before touching other foods. Refrigerate leftovers promptly; bacteria can grow at a fast rate at room temperature. Clean and wash produce with running water, remove and discard outer leaves. Handwashing prior to food preparation is an essential precaution for everyone.

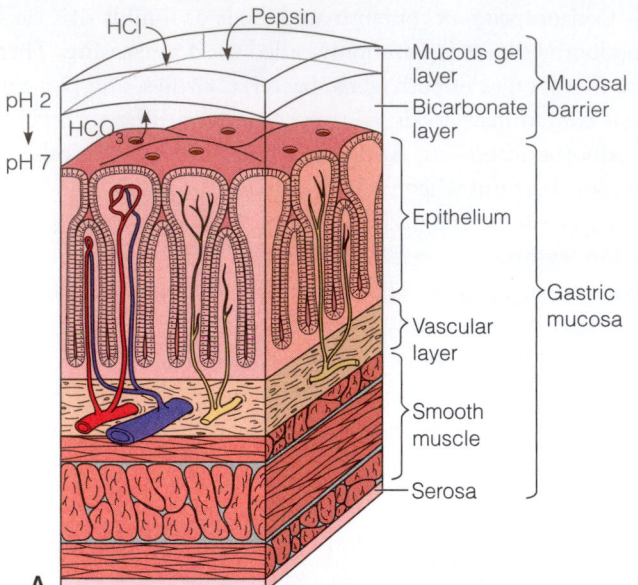

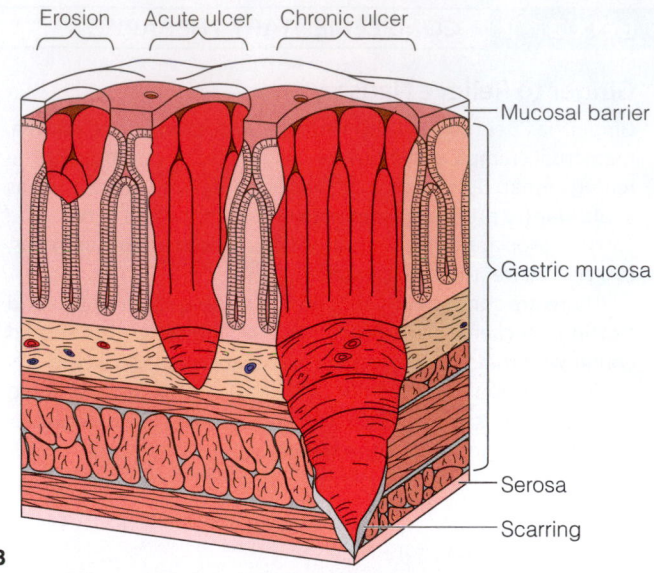

Figure 37-10. ■ **A.** The gastric mucosa and mucosal barrier. The mucous gel and bicarbonate of the mucosal barrier protect the gastric mucosa (the epithelial, vascular, and smooth muscle layers) from damage by the digestive substances such as hydrochloric acid and pepsin. **B.** Erosion and ulcerations of the upper GI tract.

ACUTE GASTRITIS

Acute **gastritis** is an inflammation of the stomach caused by chemotherapy, radiation therapy, food contaminated with toxins, significant alcohol intake, or food allergies. Medications, such as NSAIDs (ibuprofen) and salicylates (aspirin), can also irritate the lining of the stomach (Figure 37-10 ■). Stress-induced gastritis is caused by severe trauma from burns, shock, multisystem trauma, surgery, etc. The inflammation causes scarring and may cause pyloric obstruction. If the inflammation continues, erosion can develop and then perforate the abdominal wall, causing peritonitis.

Manifestations

Pyrosis (heartburn) and indigestion are typical symptoms of gastritis. Abdominal distention, pain, nausea, and vomiting often accompany gastritis. *Hematemesis* (vomited blood) and **melena** (blood in stools) can develop with continued inflammation.

Treatment

Eliminating the cause of irritation usually alleviates the problem. A bland diet of soft foods and liquids is more easily digested. Antacids are given to neutralize gastric acids. The client normally recovers quickly. Stress gastritis is treated with intravenous medication (Tagamet).

CHRONIC GASTRITIS

Chronic gastritis is a progressive disorder, resulting in changes in the mucosal cells of the stomach. One type, known as type A, causes the stomach to be unable to secrete the intrinsic

factor needed to absorb vitamin B_{12} from ingested food. (Lack of intrinsic factor leads to pernicious anemia; see Chapter 34 ●●.)

Manifestations and Treatment

The client may be asymptomatic or complain of weakness, GI upset, vague discomfort following meals, anemia, and fatigue. The client is given B_{12} injections at regular intervals to replace the vitamin since the body no longer absorbs it. Another type of anemia, known as type B, causes pyrosis, *eructation* (belching or burping), poor appetite, nausea, and vomiting. It is due to chronic lower stomach irritation linked to the *Helicobacter pylori (H. pylori)* bacterium and is treated with antibiotics.

PEPTIC ULCER DISEASE

Peptic ulcer disease (PUD) was once thought to be caused by diet, stress, caffeine, tobacco, and alcohol. When Dr. Barry Marshall discovered the *H. pylori* bacterium, he found it could cause ulcers. Research has found that 80% to 90% of ulcers are caused by this bacterium, which may be transmitted by the oral–fecal route. This discovery has altered the treatment and cure of ulcers.

Peptic ulcers are found in the stomach, duodenum, and esophagus. The microorganism causes irritation and erosions in the mucosa that lead to ulceration (Figure 37-11 ■). The crater is further irritated by the gastric acids and enzymes produced in the stomach and duodenum. Some ulcers are related to the acid level in the stomach or a deficiency of buffers in the stomach and duodenum. Some

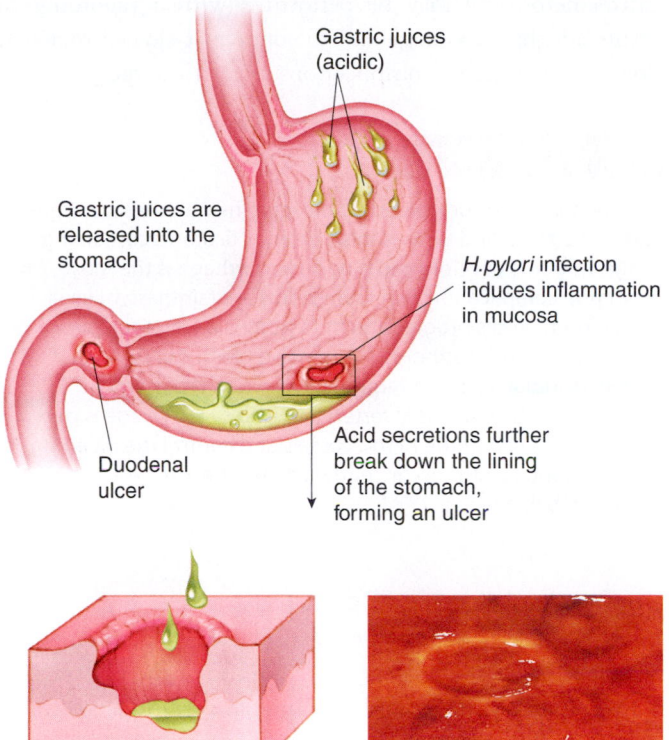

Gastric juices (acidic)

Gastric juices are released into the stomach

H.pylori infection induces inflammation in mucosa

Duodenal ulcer

Acid secretions further break down the lining of the stomach, forming an ulcer

A   B

Figure 37-11. ■ **A.** Mechanics of peptic ulcer formation. **B.** A superficial peptic ulcer. (*Source:* A. Pearson Education/PH College. B. SLP/Photo Researchers, Inc.)

cultural groups are more prone to PUD and other gastric disorders than others (Box 37-3 ■).

Manifestations

Clients with ulcers commonly complain of pain or a burning sensation in the midsternum with radiation to the back or a dull, gnawing pain and a feeling of emptiness. The pain is caused by food and acid contacting the lesion. The acid stimulates smooth muscle contraction. *Dyspepsia* is a term used to describe the combination of nausea, distention, and burping seen with ulcers. Vomiting is another symptom, which is caused by pyloric obstruction due to scarring and swelling. If GI bleeding occurs, the client will vomit blood (hematemesis) and have either occult or frank blood in the stool.

The symptoms differ in timing and location for gastric and duodenal ulcers. The pain of a gastric ulcer often follows meals and may not respond to antacids. Pain is frequently reported to the left of midline in the upper epigastrium. In contrast, the pain of duodenal ulcers is felt when the client has an empty stomach and may awaken the client at night. Pain is localized to the right epigastrium. It is relieved by food or antacids. The LPN/LVN needs to make careful observations about the pain location, where it radiates, timing, relief, and how the client describes the discomfort.

Diagnosis and Treatment

To diagnose peptic ulcer disease, an upper GI series, gastroscopy, gastric analysis, and client symptoms are considered. A urea breath test can be performed to detect the presence of *H. pylori* (see Table 37-1). Blood can be tested for antibodies confirming the bacterium. A biopsy can be taken during an EGD to verify the presence of *H. pylori*.

Medical management includes a 2-week regimen of two antibiotics (tetracycline, metronidazole, amoxicillin) and a proton pump inhibitor (omeprazole and lansoprazole), or a histamine antagonist (ranitidine, cimetidine, famotidine). Pepto-Bismol is used as adjunct therapy.

Additional treatment is aimed at controlling and neutralizing gastric acid. Nutritional considerations include avoiding foods that cause pain, spicy foods, alcohol, fried foods, and caffeine. Use of tobacco or aspirin can increase irritation of the stomach lining. Frequent small meals may be better tolerated than three larger ones. Medications prescribed to treat PUD

BOX 37-4	SELECTED DRUGS USED TO TREAT PEPTIC ULCER DISEASE

- Antacids
  Calcium carbonate (Tums)
  Magnesium hydroxide and aluminum hydroxide (Maalox)
  Magnesium trisilicate and aluminum hydroxide (Gaviscon)
  Sodium bicarbonate (Alka Seltzer)
- Histamine-blocking agents
  Cimetidine (Tagamet)
  Ranitidine (Zantac)
  Famotidine (Pepcid)
- Proton pump inhibitors
  Omeprazole (Prilosec)
  Lansoprazole (Prevacid)
- Rabeprazole sodium (AcipHex)

include antacids, histamine blocking agents, and proton pump inhibitors (Box 37-4 ■), anticholinergics, antispasmodics, sedation, and barrier protectants such as Pepto-Bismol.

Clients with peptic ulcer may be advised to stop smoking and avoid alcohol to prevent further problems with ulcers. In addition, they may be advised to eat six small meals per day rather than three larger ones, to decrease the amount of time the stomach is empty.

Surgical procedures (Table 37-2 ■) may be needed to treat ulcers. A vagotomy may be performed to treat severe, chronic ulcers. A *vagotomy* is the cutting of the vagus nerve. When this nerve is severed, the stomach produces less hydrochloric acid in response to stimulation of the parasympathetic nervous system. In addition, motility is slowed, which can lead to gastric atony. Surgery to enlarge the pylorus (**pyloroplasty**) or

gastroenterostomy may be performed with a vagotomy to ensure adequate drainage and to counteract slowed motility. Box 37-5 ■ describes complications of gastric surgery.

clinical ALERT

The primary signs of a bleeding ulcer are hematemesis, coffee-ground emesis, and tarry stools (melena), or stools containing large amounts of bright red blood. Hemorrhage is the most common complication. Early symptoms are faintness, nausea, and bloody stools progressing to hypotension, thready pulse, palpitations, and diaphoresis. A massive bleed can result in 1,000 mL blood loss and require rapid blood replacement. A nasogastric (NG) tube is inserted and iced saline lavage is performed to constrict the blood vessels and control the bleeding. An intravenous infusion or central line will be inserted to maintain fluid balance.

Perforated Peptic Ulcer

A peptic ulcer can become so deep that it perforates the stomach lining and allows the contents of the GI tract to seep out and cause peritonitis. This can occur unexpectedly.

The client suddenly complains of severe upper abdominal pain that becomes increasingly worse. Referred pain to the right shoulder may occur, because the phrenic nerve in the diaphragm is irritated by the gastric contents when they are released into the abdomen. Other symptoms include fever, diaphoresis, vomiting, rapid shallow breathing, and signs of shock. The abdomen may be rigid or boardlike.

The client is sent to surgery immediately. Peptic ulcers may also cause slower gastric bleeding with scar tissue formation that can lead to obstruction.

TABLE 37-2	Surgical Procedures for Stomach Disorders
PROCEDURE	**PURPOSES AND POSSIBLE COMPLICATIONS**
Vagotomy Severs vagal innervation to the stomach to remove the autonomic stimulus that causes parietal cells to produce hydrochloric acid.	Reduces gastric acid production. May cause delay in gastric emptying; increased risk of diarrhea and gallstone formation.
Pyloroplasty Surgical enlargement of the pylorus or gastric outlet. Done to improve gastric emptying in clients with obstruction or who have had a vagotomy that interferes with emptying.	Relieves obstruction and improves gastric emptying; relatively easy procedure with low surgical risk. May contribute to dumping syndrome; ulcers may recur.
Billroth I (gastroduodenostomy)	Removes damaged mucosa; reduces number of gastrin- and acid-producing cells; reduces ulcer recurrence. Decreases size of the stomach, causing problems with absorption and emptying.
Billroth II (gastrojejunostomy) Removal of the distal portion of the stomach with anastomosis to the proximal jejunum. Vagotomy done at the same time.	Same as Billroth I.

BOX 37-5   COMPLICATIONS OF GASTRIC SURGERY

Hemorrhage postsurgery is uncommon but can occur when a suture slips. Keep diligent watch on vital sign changes and nasogastric tube output to detect bleeding problems. Spontaneous vomiting of bright red blood may be the first sign of hemorrhage. Additional signs are increased pulse, increased respirations, and lowered blood pressure. The client may exhibit restlessness. Notify the RN and physician immediately.

Gastric distention can occur if the nasogastric tube becomes obstructed. Signs and symptoms are increasing abdominal girth, pain, fullness, and hypotension. Vomiting and belching may be seen. Observe for signs of tube patency, do not irrigate or reposition the tube, and notify the RN and physician. The physician will determine the appropriate action.

Steatorrhea means "fatty stools" and occurs when there is inadequate breakdown of fats. The rapid emptying of food prevents pancreatic enzymes and bile from breaking down the fats as in normal digestion. Limiting fat intake can diminish steatorrhea and its odor.

Dumping syndrome occurs when food passes rapidly into the intestines. When the digestive process is altered, such as after gastric surgery, foods high in carbohydrate and electrolytes are diluted by drawing fluids from the intestine. This shift of fluids causes a decrease in the blood volume 5 to 30 minutes after eating. Dizziness, faintness, weakness, and palpitations are a result of the fluid shift. Other signs include abdominal fullness, diaphoresis, cramping pain, and diarrhea. A sudden rise in the blood glucose causes increased insulin production and symptoms of pallor, shakiness, sweating, and palpitations. The client may complain of headache and dizziness.

Eating smaller, more frequent meals that are low in carbohydrates and high in proteins with moderate fat helps alleviate dumping syndrome. Avoid drinking fluids with the meal and 1 to 2 hours before and after the meal. A semirecumbent position is encouraged for 30 minutes after eating to delay gastric emptying. Symptoms diminish with time.

diagnosis. A biopsy may be performed. Pain level, location, and time related to meals are documented.

An NG tube is inserted for **decompression** (the removal of stomach contents and gas from the stomach and intestines). Histamine antagonists are given to inhibit gastric acid secretion, and antacids are given to neutralize and coat the stomach. Surgical intervention may be averted with prompt treatment.

PYLORIC OBSTRUCTION

The valve and opening in the pylorus may become scarred and *stenosed* (narrowed) from edema due to chronic irritation. This leads to obstruction of the pylorus.

Manifestations

Symptoms include nausea and vomiting, constipation, epigastric fullness, loss of appetite, spasm, and weight loss.

Diagnosis and Treatment

History and physical signs and symptoms are noted. A gastric fluid retention test may be administered. The amount and times of emesis and projectile vomiting are documented.

An NG tube may be inserted for gastric decompression (see Procedure 29-5 ⏴⏵). A test may be conducted to determine the amount of fluid that remains in the stomach after 750 mL of fluid has been instilled through the NG tube. If more than 200 mL of stomach contents is obtained after a specified period of time, the finding is suggestive of an obstruction. Intravenous fluids and total parenteral nutrition may be ordered. Pyloroplasty may be performed to provide effective drainage from the stomach to the duodenum (Figure 37-12 ■).

Stress Ulcer

Stress ulcer is a term given to a group of duodenal or gastric ulcers that occur following a traumatic event. Traumas such as burns, shock, severe sepsis, or a multiple organ trauma precipitate the formation of these ulcers. The body compensates by decreasing the blood supply to the stomach and duodenal mucosa and directing the circulation instead to vital organs. Hydrochloric acid increases and compromises the stomach lining.

Erosions can be observed 24 hours after a stressful situation, and they progressively worsen. When acute stress is combined with nervous system trauma, the ulcers are often very deep, and perforation is a major problem.

History and physical manifestations and symptoms are used in conjunction with a UGI series, gastric analysis, endoscopy, or esophagogastroduodenoscopy (EGD) to make a

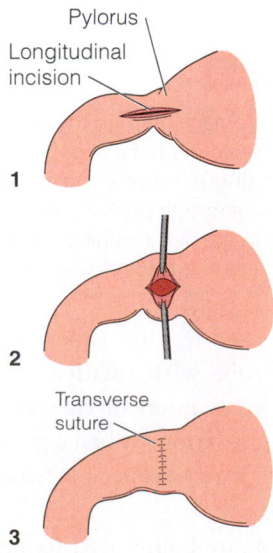

Figure 37-12. ■ Pyloroplasty.

If peristalsis is not working well, the abdomen becomes distended and painful. Vomiting may also occur. The NG tube is inserted through the nose and into the stomach. (Procedure 25-2 ⊙⊙ provides steps for inserting NG tubes.) A nasoenteric tube is inserted through the nose and into the intestines. Nasogastric tubes may also be inserted for **gavage** (feeding through the tube) and **lavage** (washing out the stomach through the tube). To decompress the stomach, an NG tube is inserted and attached to suction (see Procedure 29-5 ⊙⊙). Another type of NG tube, called a Sengstaken-Blakemore tube, is used to apply pressure to bleeding vessels in the esophagus (*esophageal varices*) or at the entrance to the stomach. The tube is inserted like an NG tube, but has a long balloon on the outside of the tube that can be inflated to place direct pressure on oozing blood vessels.

A *single-lumen tube* (one with only one central opening within the tube) is used as a feeding tube or for decompression when attached to intermittent suction. The purpose of using only intermittent suction is to prevent the end of the tube from becoming fixed against the wall of the stomach. A *double-lumen tube* (one with two central openings) is used to decompress the stomach or intestines with continuous suction. It has an air vent (often referred to as a pigtail). The purpose of the pigtail is to prevent high suction (greater than 25 mm) from causing the tube to adhere to the stomach wall. Medications can be administered through NG tubes with a physician's order. It is best to use liquid forms of medications or to crush the medicine thoroughly (if crushing is not contraindicated) and dilute it with water before administering it through the tube. Flush tube with 20 to 30 mL of water after instilling medication. Turn off the suction and clamp the tube for 15 to 30 minutes after administering the medications. Then reconnect to the suction.

clinical ALERT

To prevent reflux of stomach fluids in the air vent, keep the pigtail above the client's midline. If the vent becomes wet, you can dry the tube by inserting 10 mL of air into the pigtail. Some air vents have an attachment that prevents reflux from occurring. Do not make a knot in the pigtail tube or attach a glove to catch the fluid. The vent needs to remain open to the air.

Many manufactured feeding tubes have single lumens. They are a softer tube with smaller lumens. Some tubes require a guide wire to insert or they may be weighted at the tip to facilitate insertion. When a guide wire is used, an x-ray is required to verify proper placement prior to use of the tube.

When NG tubes are being used to gavage, it is the responsibility of the nurse always to check for placement

and residuals. In checking placement the best practice is for the nurse to aspirate gastric secretions and test the acidic level. The pH should be below 6. Although no longer recommended, an alternate method is to insert 10 to 30 mL of air into the tube and to listen with a stethoscope to hear the sound of the air being pushed into the stomach. A chest x-ray is accepted as the best method to determine tube placement.

Determining residuals is necessary before a bolus feeding and also routinely prior to mealtimes or medication administration in a continuous feeding. When the gastric contents are aspirated and the amount is greater than 100 mL, delay feeding and reassess in 2 hours. Document the residual and notify the physician if this pattern continues. If the amount is less than 100 mL, return the aspirate to the client's stomach and resume the feeding. Flush the tube after a bolus feeding or medication administration, and place clients in the semi-Fowler's position. Assess the skin around the insertion site for irritation or breakdown.

A gastrostomy tube is a direct-route tube for administration of a liquid feeding. The tube is inserted into the stomach by an incision made into the stomach. It can also be placed by endoscopy. A percutaneous endoscopic gastrostomy (PEG) is performed in the GI lab.

Common complications from a direct-route feeding include diarrhea and dumping syndrome. *Dumping syndrome* (Box 37-5) is a complex reaction due to a rapid emptying of gastric contents. The signs and symptoms include nausea, weakness, diaphoresis, palpitations, syncope, and diarrhea. Treatment consists of diluting the feeding to a 50% solution and adjusting the rate of the feeding. High-protein, low-carbohydrate, and moderate fat feeding solutions aid in controlling dumping syndrome.

Total parenteral nutrition (TPN), also called hyperalimentation (HAL), is administered intravenously by a central line, often via the subclavian vein. The catheter tip terminates at the superior vena cava within 3 to 4 cm of the vena cava and right atrium junction. This procedure is done when the client's intake of nutrients is less than body requirements. The intravenous solutions are high in sugar content ($D_{50}W$, $D_{25}W$, $D_{10}W$) when the client needs to improve nutritional status, advance weight gain, and develop stronger healing ability. Depending on the sugar content, a standing physician order may include glucose monitoring.

GASTRIC CANCER

Cancerous lesions found in the stomach are the second leading cause of cancer-related deaths in the world (NCI, 2007). Gastric cancer affects people over the age of 40 and is seen more often in men than in women. Risk factors for the development of gastric cancer include heredity, chronic gastritis, *H. pylori* infection, and pernicious anemia. Exposure to substances such as lead, grains, and leaded gasoline add to the risk for developing gastric cancer. A diet high in meat and fish is also a risk factor. Stomach cancer often has already metastasized by the time it is diagnosed. The prognosis for this disease is poor.

Manifestations

The client with gastric cancer complains of weight loss, lack of appetite, and weakness. Lab findings include anemia and blood in the stool. The client may have vomiting with coffee-ground emesis. The vomiting may occur after eating or drinking. As the disease progresses, jaundice may be present because the cancer affects surrounding organs. Due to the client's inability to take in nutrients, emaciation and *cachexia* (general weight loss and wasting) develop.

Diagnosis and Treatment

Gastric cancer is diagnosed through gastric analysis and biopsy via endoscopy.

When this cancer is diagnosed early, immediate surgical intervention is advised. A subtotal gastrectomy involves removal of part of the stomach, usually the antrum and pyloric area. Two subtotal gastrectomy procedures utilized are Billroth I and II (Figure 37-13 ■).

If gastric cancer has metastasized, chemotherapy, radiation therapy, and palliative measures are taken. A gastrostomy or jejunostomy tube, known as a direct feeding tube, may need to be placed to provide nutrition (see Chapter 25 ⬭). In some cases, TPN may be required postoperatively. When the cancer is pervasive, a total gastrectomy (removal of the stomach) and **anastomosis** (alignment and suturing) of the esophagus to the jejunum is performed.

Billroth I, also called a gastroduodenostomy, is a procedure performed to remove the distal portion of the stomach and anastomose the stomach to the duodenum. A

different surgery, called Billroth II, or gastrojejunostomy, is a procedure performed to remove 50% of the stomach and anastomose it to the jejunum, bypassing the duodenum. The duodenum continues to receive pancreatic enzymes and bile necessary for digestion. These surgeries (see Table 37-2) can be used to treat gastric disorders, ulcers, and gastric cancer.

NURSING CONSIDERATIONS FOR GASTRIC DISORDERS

When you care for clients with gastric disorders, you will focus care on the most important client needs. If a client is experiencing gastrointestinal bleeding, one major focus of care is fluid and blood loss with possible resultant shock. Monitor fluid balance closely—assess for dehydration, output of less than 30 mL per hour, and color and clarity of output. Check the function of the NG tube, and test stomach contents for the presence of occult blood. Check vital signs often and note pattern of decreasing blood pressure that could indicate impending shock. Another priority in your care would be the client's anxiety. Always explain what you are doing and why before you begin a procedure. Listen carefully to verbal concerns and watch for nonverbal indications of anxiety. Teach the client about self-care to prepare him or her for discharge.

OBESITY

Obesity is defined as being 20% over normal healthy weight. One-third of adult Americans are obese and 60% are overweight. A person with **morbid obesity** is one who is 100 lb or more over normal weight for age, height, and build. Obesity is caused by consumption of more calories than are burned through daily activities. Sedentary lifestyles and fast foods have contributed to the obesity in America. Emotional pain and self-esteem issues can contribute to overeating of comfort foods. There seems to be a link between stress and rates of overeating, overweight, and obesity. A relatively small percent is caused by malfunctioning thyroid or pituitary glands.

Obesity in children is also a concern. Increased consumption of non-nutritional snacks, lack of exercise, and replacement of outdoor activity with electronic games and entertainment are contributing factors. See Chapter 25 ⬭ for age-specific nutrition and weight concerns. See Chapter 50 ⬭ for the eating disorders anorexia nervosa and bulimia.

Associated Manifestations

People who are severely overweight may experience shortness of breath on exertion, poor exercise tolerance, diaphoresis, cardiac complications, and peripheral vascular disease. Diabetes mellitus (see Chapter 38 ⬭), hypertension, osteoarthritis, cancer, gallbladder disease, sleep apnea, and

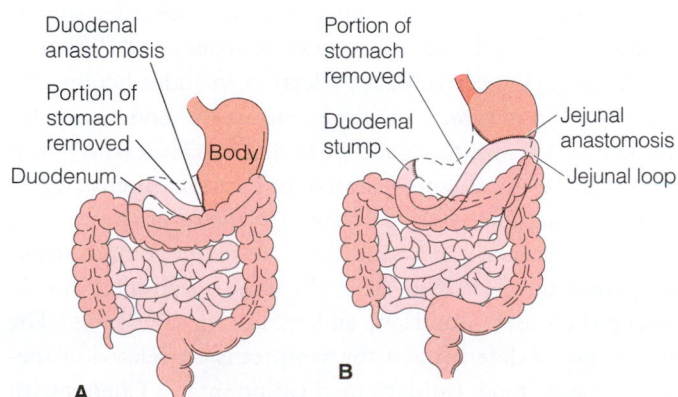

Figure 37-13. ■ A. Billroth I (gastroduodenostomy). B. Billroth II (gastrojejunostomy).

atherosclerosis are commonly associated with obesity. (See discussion of eating disorders in Chapter 50 ⊙⊙.)

Diagnosis and Treatment

Obesity is diagnosed when weight is 20% or more over normal healthy weight and endocrine or other disorders are ruled out.

Clients are given a dietary regimen with a decrease in calories and educated about healthier food choices. Consistent exercise helps burn unnecessary calories, relieves stress, and increases self-esteem. The client's motivation is inherent to success. Psychotherapy and behavioral modification may assist the client to formulate realistic goals. Support groups and centers for weight loss can be found locally. Caution is required with the use of over-the-counter weight loss medication because they can increase blood pressure and heart rate.

Clients who are unresponsive to prescribed treatment may be candidates for surgical intervention. In **gastroplasty**, also known as gastric stapling, the stomach is stapled, creating a small pouch. Restrictive operations lead to weight loss in most clients, although some may regain weight if they fail to make behavioral adjustments. Success depends on making changes and adopting a long-term plan of healthy eating and exercise. A common side effect is vomiting because of the stretching of the stomach by food that hasn't been chewed properly.

ROUX-EN-Y GASTRIC BYPASS. Roux-en-Y **gastric bypass** (RGB) is the most common GI surgery for weight loss (Figure 37-14 ■). A small stomach pouch is created to restrict food intake, then a Y-shaped portion of the small intestine is attached to the pouch. This allows the food to bypass the lower stomach, duodenum, and part of the jejunum, limiting absorption of nutrients and reducing calories. This type of surgery produces more weight loss than restrictive surgeries such as gastroplasty. However, there is greater risk for nutritional and electrolyte imbalances. Anemia and calcium deficiencies in women may occur due to decreased absorption of these nutrients. Dumping syndrome occurs due to the rapid movement of stomach contents. Lifelong supplements, vitamins, medications, and follow-up care are essential. A client considering

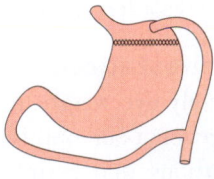

Gastric bypass

Figure 37-14. ■ Surgical procedure to treat obesity.

weight loss surgery should consider both benefits and risks and discuss them with their physician.

Nursing Considerations

When the nurse cares for clients with obesity, the focus is on restoring a healthy weight, lifestyle, and body image. Clients who lose large amounts of weight in a short period of time may need counseling to adjust to their new body image. Although it is a positive change, it is still a change in body image. Clients contemplating weight reduction surgery need support for their decision, either for or against the surgery.

NURSING CARE

PRIORITIZING NURSING CARE

The nurse observes for objective symptoms that the client with an upper GI disorder may exhibit such as nausea, vomiting, dysphagia, and weight loss. Measuring and recording intake and output will determine fluid losses and replacement needs. Monitor electrolyte levels for changes. Assessing dietary intake and daily weights provides information regarding the client's progress. Provide symptomatic relief for pain, nausea, and vomiting by administering prescribed medication and monitoring effect. Additionally, identifying and avoiding triggers that aggravate nausea and vomiting should be implemented. Observation of the client's swallowing ability may indicate the need for a swallowing evaluation to determine further nursing care. If surgical intervention is necessary, the nurse will monitor vital signs and lung sounds. Observation and documentation of wound healing provide information of the client's progress. The nurse will provide ongoing client education regarding disease, treatment, and discharge instruction.

ASSESSING

The client with an upper gastrointestinal disorder should be assessed for subjective data such as nausea and difficulty swallowing. Objective data collection includes height and weight, skin turgor, and inspection of the oral cavity for broken or missing teeth and gum disease. The client's pain must also be thoroughly assessed for location, intensity, and duration. Remember that a change in the severity or nature of epigastric pain can be indicative of major complications of peptic ulcer disease. The client is questioned closely about the onset, duration, and nature of symptoms. The nurse should determine if the symptoms are related to specific types of food, fluid, or medication intake. Clients with upper GI symptoms should always be evaluated for present or recent signs of blood in the stools or emesis.

Assess vital signs for baseline and changes that could indicate infection or blood loss. When checking blood pressure, evaluate sitting and standing BP to detect orthostatic hypotension. Measure and document the color and consistency of any emesis or stools.

Inspect the abdomen. Observe the contour and any scars, masses, and areas of distention. Peristalsis is not normally visible but may be observed in an extremely thin client.

Auscultate the abdomen with a stethoscope, in a systematic clockwise rotation including all four quadrants. Listen for the frequency and character of soft clicks and gurgles produced by air movement, peristalsis, and flatus. Bowel sounds that are absent or infrequent may indicate hypoperistalsis or a paralytic ileus (slow or absent movement of the intestines). If there is an absence of bowel sounds, palpate lightly or have the client eat, drink, or ambulate to stimulate peristalsis. A full bladder can obscure audible bowel sounds. Document the absence of sounds after listening for 5 minutes and report to the charge nurse or physician if this is a new occurrence and not related to the first day or two after surgery. Abnormally loud, intense, frequent bowel sounds usually caused by hunger are called **borborygmi.** Bowel sounds are described as audible, hyperactive, inaudible, or hypoactive. Observe for abdominal distention. Measuring the abdominal girth on admission gives a baseline for comparison of girth measurements.

Percussion is used to identify masses, fluid, and air and is performed by the physician or the nurse clinician. Palpation notes muscular resistance, tenderness, organ enlargement, rigidity, distention, and rebound tenderness.

DIAGNOSING, PLANNING, AND IMPLEMENTING

Nursing diagnoses for clients with upper GI disorders include:

- *Acute Pain*
- *Imbalanced Nutrition: Less than Body Requirements*
- *Ineffective Coping*
- *Deficient Knowledge*
- *Nausea*

Expected outcomes for clients with upper GI disorders include:

- Pain is controlled or relieved.
- Nutritional intake will increase, with corresponding weight gain and improved skin turgor.
- Coping skills will improve with information about condition, modified diet, and decreased pain.
- Client is knowledgeable about disease process, aggravating factors, medication regimen, and signs/symptoms to report immediately.
- Client voices decreased or absent nausea with treatment and medications.

Preoperative Care

Nursing care involves the following:

- Monitor vital signs, pulse oxygenation, and lung sounds. Calculate and record intake and output. *These measures indicate how well body systems are functioning. I&O records help in maintaining fluid balance.*
- Assess the intravenous catheter for patency and the insertion site for redness or swelling. *Regular attention to the IV ensures that the client is receiving necessary fluids and/or nutrition. Redness or swelling at the insertion site could signal infection.*
- When the esophagus is affected, supervise the client during mealtimes. *It is possible for these clients to aspirate their food. Have oral suction available in the event of aspiration.*
- Measure daily weights and involve the dietitian to assess calories. Offer supplemental high-protein drinks between meals for clients who are taking in less than the body requires. *Daily weights provide a good record of weight maintenance or change. Offering supplements between meals helps clients who are undernourished to take in more calories.*
- If an NG tube is in place, observe for patency. Do not reposition or irrigate the NG tube if the client has had surgery. *It is the nurse's responsibility to check that the tube is functioning properly. Pressure to the incisional site can compromise the surgery.*
- Notify the physician of bleeding and abnormal amounts of drainage. Note abdominal distention and girth measurements. *Any of these signs indicate possible complications.*
- Instruct the client who is having a partial or total gastrectomy about dietary requirements and the need for lifelong vitamin B_{12} injections. *A client who has had gastrectomy will also have pernicious anemia. With the removal of part or all of the stomach, the intrinsic factor secretion is diminished or absent. The absorption of vitamin B_{12} depends on the intrinsic factor to protect the vitamin B_{12} molecules from the digestive juices until they reach the intestine.*
- Allow the client to verbalize fears and emotions. Develop a therapeutic relationship of trust using communication skills and techniques. *The client with upper GI cancer is on a roller coaster of emotions. He or she may fear death related to the cancer and be concerned about body image changes with the incision, tubes, drains, and tracheostomy.*

Postoperative Care

Following surgery the nurse observes for airway patency and signs of aspiration in the client with oral or esophageal surgery. Assess vital signs and respiratory rate. Encourage the client to cough, turn, and deep breathe frequently. Encourage the client and family to verbalize feelings and fears.

Postoperatively some clients will be NPO, with an NG tube to suction for decompression while allowing the operative area to heal. Intravenous fluids and antibiotics are ordered. Continued symptoms suggest abscess formation or paralytic ileus. The nurse assesses vital signs frequently and then every 4 hours, monitoring temperature and lab values (such as white blood cell counts and electrolytes). Evaluate signs of bowel activity and wound healing. Auscultate lung sounds every shift or more often as indicated. Early ambulation and diligence in turning, coughing, and deep breathing will prevent respiratory complications.

Assess the client's pain level and medicate as needed. Promote use of spirometer treatments hourly. Observe incision for signs of inflammation, infection, drainage, and bleeding. Document wound healing and dressing changes. Instruct the client in splinting the wound when ambulating or coughing. Give instruction in dressing changes and wound care to client and family. Explain and document follow-up appointments and activity restrictions.

Dietary needs for the postoperative client are important and a focus for client instruction. The client will be NPO for up to 48 hours without an NG tube or with a tube hooked to intermittent suction. Oral care will relieve mouth dryness. IV fluids are administered to prevent dehydration and may include total parenteral nutrition. When bowel sounds are audible, the physician will discontinue the NG tube and order a diet. Initially ice chips are ordered, followed by sips of water and then a clear liquid meal. The LPN/LVN observes for diet tolerance and records intake and output. The diet is advanced slowly, keeping in mind that the stomach intake is limited. The client may complain of lack of appetite, quick satiety, and nausea. Dietary supplements needed after gastric surgeries include vitamin B_{12}, vitamin D, folic acid, and calcium. (See Box 37-5 for a discussion of complications of gastric surgery.)

EVALUATING

Evaluation of the client with upper GI disorders includes observing for improved nutritional status, decreased nausea, and controlled or resolved pain. Clients with these disorders often need nutritional counseling and the services of a dietitian to help identify foods and fluids that cause them problems. The nurse also evaluates the client for complications that can result from ulcers or gastrointestinal surgery.

Continuity of Care

Clients with upper GI disorders should be provided with the following information to help them prevent recurrences or complications:

- Foods and spices to avoid, as well as when to eat and positioning after eating
- Medications, such as ibuprofen and aspirin, that can contribute to ulcer formation and bleeding
- Signs and symptoms to report immediately: increasing or severe epigastric pain, blood in stools or emesis, black and tarry stools, dizziness, fainting

LOWER GI DISORDERS

Elimination Disorders

Elimination disorders are a common problem, and many factors that cause these disorders can be controlled by the client. The nurse plays an important role in helping clients identify causes of elimination problems and changes they can make to correct them. Box 37-6 ■ lists some factors that affect bowel elimination (defecation).

Healthy defecation habits can be supported by (1) privacy, (2) having a regular time for defecation, (3) high-fiber foods in the diet and fluid intake of 2,000 to 3,000 mL a day, (4) regular exercise, (5) correct positioning, and (6) avoidance of over-the-counter medications to treat irregularity.

FLATULENCE

Flatulence is the presence of excessive *flatus* (or gas) in the intestines. It leads to stretching and inflation of the intestines (intestinal *distention*). Large amounts of air and other gases can accumulate in the stomach, resulting in gastric distention. The three primary causes of flatus are action of bacteria on the chyme in the large intestine, swallowed air, and gas that diffuses from the bloodstream into the intestine.

Manifestations

Most gases that are swallowed are expelled through the mouth by *eructation*. Flatulence occurs in the colon, and results from a variety of causes, such as foods (e.g., cabbage, onions), abdominal surgery, or narcotics. If the gas is propelled by increased peristalsis, it may be expelled through the anus.

Diagnosis and Treatment

Clients may present with a complaint of excessive flatulence. They may have used over-the-counter agents (agents that coalesce gas bubbles and facilitate their passage by belching through the mouth or expulsion through the anus). If excessive gas cannot be expelled through the anus, it may be necessary to insert a rectal tube or to provide a return flow enema (also called a Harris flush) to remove it. Procedure 37-2 ■ describes how to insert a rectal tube. Enemas are discussed later in the chapter.

CONSTIPATION

When taking data from clients be aware that they may be reluctant to discuss bowel habits and elimination. Determine the usual pattern of bowel elimination; inquire

BOX 37-6 FACTORS THAT AFFECT DEFECATION

Age and Development

- Defecation material and patterns change dramatically from birth to 2$1/2$ years.
- Bowel patterns are established at an early age and are maintained throughout most of life.

Diet

- Fiber and regular eating patterns stimulate peristalsis and promote regularity.
- Low-residue foods (rice, eggs, and lean meats, cheese and pasta) need to be accompanied by extra fluid to increase their rate of movement.
- Other diet-related factors:
  - Gas-producing foods include cabbage, onions, cauliflower, bananas, and apples.
  - Laxative-producing foods include bran, prunes, figs, chocolate, and alcohol.
  - Constipation-producing foods include cheese, pasta, eggs, and lean meat.

Fluids

- Daily fluid intake should be 2,000 to 3,000 mL.
- When fluid intake is inadequate or output is excessive, the feces become hardened and drier than normal.
- If chyme moves abnormally quickly through the large intestine, there is less time for fluid to be absorbed into the blood, so feces are soft or even watery.

Activity

- Activity stimulates peristalsis, helps move chyme along the colon.

- When abdominal and pelvic muscles are weak from lack of exercise, immobility, or impaired neurologic functioning, it is difficult for the client to defecate or to control defecation.

Psychological Factors

- Anxiety and anger stimulate bowels.
- Depression slows bowel functioning.

Medications

- Constipation-causing medications include tranquilizers, iron tablets, morphine, and codeine.
- Diarrhea-causing medications include antacids, nutritional supplements that contain magnesium, NSAIDs.
- Constipation-treating medications include laxatives, cathartics, stool softeners.
- Diarrhea-treating medications include dicyclomine hydrochloride (Bentyl).
- Some drugs will affect the coloring of or cause bleeding in stools.

Hospitalization

- Clients may be restricted from eating prior to some procedures.
- Cleansing enemas may be given before procedures.
- Anesthetics, spinal cord injuries, head injuries, direct handling of intestines may slow or cease bowel movement.
- Embarrassment, inability to get to the lavatory when needed, and pain may all result in constipation for the client.
- Anal sphincters that are functioning poorly may cause fecal incontinence.

---

regarding frequency, time of day, description, usual stool characteristics, amount, consistency, shape, color, and odor.

Manifestations

Constipation is defined as fewer than three bowel movements per week. Constipation is associated with difficult evacuation of stool and increased effort or straining of the voluntary muscles of defecation, rather than a specific number of bowel movements in a set time. Constipation occurs when the movement of feces through the large intestine is slow, allowing time for additional reabsorption of fluid from the large intestine. Assessment of the person's habits is necessary before a diagnosis of constipation is made. Box 37-7 ■ lists manifestations of constipation.

Diagnosis and Treatment

The client presents with complaints of small, dry, hard stool or passes no stool for a period of time. In addition, other physical complaints include feeling bloated, nausea, vomiting, and general malaise. When expelling constipated stool it may be painful and cause bleeding.

Constipation can be hazardous to some clients. Straining to have a bowel movement accompanied by holding the breath (**Valsalva maneuver**) causes increased intrathoracic and intracranial pressure. To some degree, this pressure can be reduced if the person exhales through the mouth while straining. The Valsalva maneuver can present serious problems to people with heart disease, brain injuries, or respiratory disease. Also, clients who have had eye, ear, nose, or cranial surgery should avoid straining. Avoiding straining is the best precaution for clients with these disorders. Determining laxative use by the client

BOX 37-7 MANIFESTATIONS OF CONSTIPATION

- Decreased frequency of defecation
- Hard, dry, formed stools
- Straining at stool; painful defecation
- Reports of rectal fullness, pressure, or incomplete bowel evacuation
- Abdominal pain, cramps, or distention
- Use of laxatives
- Decreased appetite
- Headache

helps the nurse identify laxative abuse, which can lead to muscle atony and thickening and peristaltic slowing, contributing to further constipation.

Laxative abuse is believed to be a common problem. Older adults in particular often use laxatives improperly. Continual use of laxatives weakens the bowel's natural responses to fecal distention, resulting in chronic constipation. The physician or nurse should examine the client's medication regimen to see whether it could contribute to constipation.

To improve bowel regularity, it is important to establish a bowel elimination routine, increase physical activity, increase fluid intake, and maintain a diet high in fiber. Clients need instruction about which medications cause decreased motility in the bowel. Some medications, such as cathartics and laxatives, help relieve constipation. **Cathartics** are drugs that induce defecation. They can have a strong, purging effect. A **laxative** is milder and produces frequent soft or liquid stools, sometimes accompanied by abdominal cramps. Table 37-3 ■ describes different types of laxatives. Some laxatives, given as suppositories, act by softening the feces, by releasing gases such as carbon dioxide to distend the rectum, or by stimulating the nerve endings in the rectal mucosa.

ENEMAS. An **enema** is a solution introduced into the rectum and large intestine. The purpose of an enema is to distend the intestine and sometimes to irritate the intestinal mucosa in order to increase peristalsis and excretion of feces and flatus.

Enemas are classified into three groups: cleansing, retention, and return-flow.

Cleansing Enemas. *Cleansing enemas* are intended to remove feces. They are given chiefly to:

- Prevent the escape of feces during surgery.
- Prepare the intestine for certain diagnostic tests such as x-ray or visualization tests (e.g., colonoscopy).
- Remove feces when there is constipation or impaction.
- Establish regular bowel function as part of a bowel training program.

See Table 37-4 ■ for commonly used enema solutions.

Cleansing enemas may be high or low:

- A *high enema* is given to cleanse as much of the colon as possible.
- A *low enema* is used to clean the rectum and sigmoid colon only.

TABLE 37-3	Types of Laxatives		
TYPE	**ACTION**	**EXAMPLES**	**PERTINENT TEACHING INFORMATION**
Bulk forming	Increases the fluid, gaseous, or solid bulk in the intestines.	Psyllium hydrophilic mucilloid (Metamucil)	May take 12 or more hours to act. Sufficient fluid must be taken.
Emollient/stool softener	Softens and delays the drying of the feces; permits fat and water to penetrate feces.	Docusate sodium (Colace, Surfak)	Refrigerated oil has less odor. Mixing with fruit juice decreases unpleasant taste.
Wetting agents	Lowers the surface tension of the feces, thus helping water to penetrate the feces.	Docusate sodium (Colace)	Slow acting, may take several days.
Stimulant/irritant	Irritates the intestinal mucosa or stimulates nerve endings in the wall of the intestine, causing rapid propulsion of the contents.	Bisacodyl (Dulcolax)	Acts more quickly than bulk-forming agents. Fluid is passed with the feces. May cause cramps. Prolonged use may cause fluid and electrolyte imbalance.
Lubricant	Lubricates the feces in the colon.	Mineral oil (Haley's M-O)	Prolonged use inhibits the absorption of some fat-soluble vitamins.
Saline/osmotic	Draws water into the intestine by osmosis, distends bowel, and stimulates peristalsis.	Epsom salts, magnesium hydroxide (Milk of Magnesia), magnesium citrate sodium phosphate (Fleet enema)	May be rapid acting. Can cause fluid and electrolyte imbalance, particularly in elderly people and children with cardiac and renal disease. Should not be used by elderly clients. Prolonged use inhibits the absorption of some fat-soluble vitamins.

TABLE 37-4	**Commonly Used Enema Solutions**			
SOLUTION	**CONSTITUENTS**	**ACTION**	**TIME TO TAKE EFFECT**	**POTENTIAL ADVERSE EFFECTS**
Hypertonic	90–120 mL of solution (e.g., sodium phosphate)	Draws water into the colon.	5–10 min	Retention of sodium
Hypotonic	500–1,000 mL of tap water	Distends colon, stimulates peristalsis, and softens feces.	15–20 min	Fluid and electrolyte imbalance; water intoxication
Isotonic	500–1,000 mL of normal saline (9 mL NaCl to 1,000 mL water)	Distends colon, stimulates peristalsis, and softens feces.	15–20 min	Possible sodium retention
Soapsuds	500–1,000 mL (3–5 mL soap to 1,000 mL water)	Irritates mucosa, distends colon.	10–15 min	Irritation of mucosa and possibly damage to mucosa
Oil (mineral, olive, cottonseed)	90–120 mL	Lubricates the feces and the colonic mucosa.	30–60 min	

When administering an enema, it is important to realize that the force of the solution flow is influenced by the height of the solution container, the size of the tubing, the viscosity of the fluid, and the resistance of the rectum. The higher the solution container is held above the rectum, the faster the flow and the greater the force (pressure) in the rectum. During most adult enemas, the solution container should be no higher than 30 cm (12 in.) above the rectum. During a high cleansing enema, the solution container is usually held 30 to 45 cm (12 to 18 in.) above the rectum. This instills the fluid farther to clean the entire bowel.

Retention Enemas. A *retention enema* introduces oil into the rectum and sigmoid colon. The oil is retained for 1 to 3 hours. It softens the feces and lubricates the rectum and anal canal, thus facilitating passage of the feces.

Return-Flow Enema (Harris Flush). A *return-flow enema* (or *Harris flush*) is used occasionally to help the client expel flatus. A flow of 100 to 200 mL of fluid into the rectum and sigmoid colon is alternated with lowering the enema bucket or bag to a point below the rectum, allowing gas to escape and stimulating peristalsis. This process is repeated five or six times until the flatus is expelled and abdominal distention is relieved.

Commercially prepared, low-volume, disposable enema kits are commonly used. The kit includes a flexible bottle of solution with a prelubricated, firm tip. Procedure 37-1 ■ at the end of this chapter describes how to administer a cleansing and retention enema.

FECAL IMPACTION

A **fecal impaction** is a mass or collection of hardened, putty-like feces in the folds of the rectum. It results from prolonged retention and accumulation of fecal material.

Manifestations

Fecal impaction is recognized by liquid fecal seepage and no normal stool. The liquid portion of the feces seeps out around the impacted mass (Figure 37-15 ■). The client may experience a frequent but nonproductive urge to defecate, rectal pain, and a generalized feeling of illness. Eventually, the client becomes anorexic, the abdomen becomes distended, and nausea and vomiting may occur.

Poor defecation habits and constipation are the usual causes of fecal impaction. Certain medications affect elimination and can contribute to impactions.

clinical ALERT

Barium, which is used in radiologic examinations of the upper and lower GI tracts, can cause an impaction because it hardens in the intestines. This is why it is so important to give ordered laxatives after barium studies.

Diagnosis and Treatment

To assess for impaction, the nurse performs a digital examination of the rectum, during which the hardened mass can often be palpated.

Once a fecal impaction occurs, digital removal of impacted feces is sometimes necessary. When fecal impaction is suspected, the client is often given an oil retention enema, a cleansing enema 2 to 4 hours later, and daily additional cleansing enemas, suppositories, or stool softeners. If these measures fail, manual removal is often necessary.

DIGITAL REMOVAL OF A FECAL IMPACTION. To remove an impaction, the nurse breaks up the fecal mass with a gloved finger and removes it from the rectum in portions. This procedure can be painful and should be done very gently

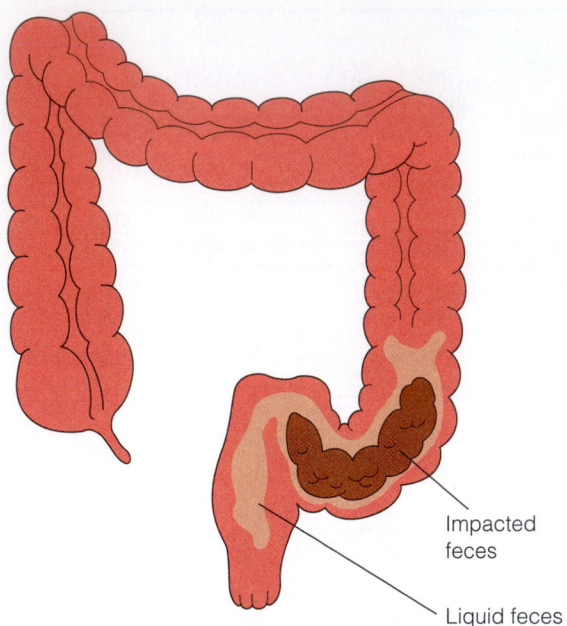

Impacted feces

Liquid feces

Figure 37-15. ■ A fecal impaction with liquid feces passing around the impaction.

and carefully, because stimulating the vagus nerve in the rectal wall can slow the client's heart. Insert your well-lubricated, gloved finger into the anal canal as far as you can reach. Loosen and dislodge stool by gently massaging around it. Break up stool by working the finger into the hardened mass, taking care to avoid injury to the mucosa of the rectum. Carefully work stool downward to the end of the rectum and remove it in small pieces.

DIARRHEA

Diarrhea is the term used for liquid feces and increased frequency of defecation. It is due to rapid passage of chyme through the intestines, reducing reabsorption of water and electrolytes.

Manifestations

The person with diarrhea finds it difficult or impossible to control the urge to defecate and experiences spasmodic cramps. Sometimes the client passes blood and excessive mucus; nausea and vomiting may also occur. With persistent diarrhea, irritation of the anal area, perineum, and buttocks generally results. Fatigue, weakness, and dehydration with possible electrolyte imbalance are the results of prolonged diarrhea. On assessment, bowel sounds are hyperactive.

Acute diarrhea is commonly caused by a bacterial or viral infection. When irritants are present in the intestinal tract, diarrhea is a protective mechanism to remove them from the body. However, it can create serious fluid and electrolyte losses. Table 37-5 ■ lists some of the major causes of diarrhea and the physiologic responses of the body. Acute diarrhea usually resolves within a week.

Diagnosis and Treatment

The client presents with loose watery feces with an increase in frequency and urgency of defecation. The episodes of diarrhea may be uncontrollable. The client may show symptoms of dehydration. The physician may test the stool for culture and sensitivity to determine the organism causing the diarrhea. There may be a temperature and WBC elevation. The anus can become reddened and irritated.

Inflammatory disease such as Crohn's, ulcerative colitis, and irritable bowel syndrome cause chronic diarrhea. Inflammatory diseases affect nutritional absorption, and hyperperistalsis results in liquid stools.

For most clients with diarrhea, treatment is supportive. Therapy focuses on fluid replacement. Box 37-8 ■ provides client teaching information for managing diarrhea.

clinical ALERT

Teach clients that misuse of laxatives prevents absorption of water and nutrients and can produce diarrhea.

TABLE 37-5	**Major Causes of Diarrhea**
CAUSE	**PHYSIOLOGIC EFFECT**
Psychologic stress (e.g., anxiety)	Increased intestinal motility and mucous secretion
Medications	
Antibiotics	Inflammation and infection of mucosa due to overgrowth of pathogenic intestinal microorganisms
Cathartics	Irritation of intestinal mucosa
Allergy to food, fluid, drugs	Incomplete digestion of food or fluid
Intolerance of food or fluid	Increased intestinal motility and mucous secretion
Diseases of the colon (e.g., malabsorption syndrome, Crohn's disease)	Reduced absorption of fluids
	Inflammation of the mucosa often leading to ulcer formation
Surgical operations	Variable

Managing Diarrhea

Drink at least eight glasses of water per day to prevent dehydration.

Avoid alcohol, beverages with caffeine, and excessively cold fluids, which aggravate the problem.

Ingest foods with sodium and potassium. Most foods contain sodium. Potassium is found in dairy products, meats, and many vegetables and fruits.

Limit foods containing insoluble fiber, such as whole-wheat and whole-grain breads or cereals, raw fruits, and raw vegetables.

Eliminate foods that trigger diarrhea.

Increase foods containing soluble fiber, such as oatmeal and skinless fruits and potatoes.

Limit fatty foods (e.g., dairy products and packaged processed meats).

After passing stool, thoroughly clean and dry the perianal area to prevent skin irritation and breakdown. Use soft toilet tissue. Apply a moisture-barrier cream such as zinc oxide or petrolatum as needed.

Discuss medications that cause diarrhea with the primary care provider and ask for an alternative.

When diarrhea has stopped, reestablish normal bowel flora by eating fermented dairy products, such as yogurt or buttermilk.

Once the cause of the diarrhea has been determined, prescription or over-the-counter medication may be administered to address the underlying cause. Antidiarrheal medications are usually reserved for treatment of chronic diarrhea (more than 3 to 4 weeks). They slow the motility of the intestine or absorb excess fluid in the intestine.

BOWEL INCONTINENCE

Bowel incontinence, also called fecal incontinence, is the loss of voluntary bowel control. It may occur at specific times, such as after meals, or it may occur irregularly. Bowel incontinence is generally due to problems with the anal sphincter or its nerve supply. Certain neuromuscular diseases, spinal cord trauma, and tumors of the external anal sphincter muscle may impair the anal sphincter.

Manifestations

Physical symptoms of incontinence are evident with the loss of voluntary control of bowel movements. Episodes may occur after meals or without warning.

Diagnosis and Treatment

The client presents with complaints of involuntary loss of bowel control. Diagnostic tests for detecting tumors or other diseases may be ordered.

Incontinence (loss of ability to control elimination) is an emotionally distressing problem that can lead to embarrassment and social isolation. When a client is incontinent of feces, the acid and digestive enzymes in the fecal material are highly irritating to skin.

The nurse should keep the perineal area clean and dry and apply a moisture barrier ointment, such as zinc oxide, to avoid skin breakdown.

BOWEL TRAINING PROGRAMS. For clients who have chronic constipation, frequent impactions, or fecal incontinence, bowel training programs may be helpful. The program is based on factors within the client's control and is designed to help the client establish normal defecation. Such matters as food and fluid intake, exercise, and defecation habits are all considered. Before beginning such a program, clients must understand it and want to be involved. When a client is on a bowel training program, the nursing staff assists the client to the bathroom or bedside commode at specific intervals or as outlined in the training plan.

NURSING CONSIDERATIONS FOR ELIMINATION DISORDERS

When the nurse provides care for clients with any medical-surgical disorder, it may be necessary to address an elimination disorder as well. Clients who have restricted activity levels or have had abdominal surgery are at risk for constipation. Pain medicines often cause constipation. Other medications, such as antibiotics, may contribute to diarrhea. Postoperative clients often have difficulty with flatus and become very uncomfortable due to it. Focus on client's bowel elimination early, before it becomes a problem. You may be able to prevent constipation, or at least make it less severe, by encouraging the client to drink extra water and fruit juices.

Infectious or Inflammatory Disorders of the Intestines

ENTERITIS

Inflammation of the intestines due to pathogenic organisms is referred to as **enteritis.** Pathogens that cause enteritis generally enter the intestines via food and fluids. Common pathogens causing enteritis include *Salmonella* found in eggs and dairy products, *Clostridia*, secondary infections with a variety of organisms due to antibiotic therapy, and pathogens contaminating mushrooms or fish.

Manifestations

Symptoms of enteritis include vomiting, diarrhea, severe abdominal cramping, and **tenesmus** (painful straining due to the constant urge to defecate). Dehydration and poor nutritional absorption are common complications of enteritis.

BOX 37-9	NURSING CARE CHECKLIST

Obtaining Stool Specimens

When obtaining stool samples:

- ☑ Follow medical aseptic technique.

- ☑ Wear disposable gloves to prevent contamination of the hands or of the outside of the specimen container.

- ☑ Use clean tongue blades to transfer the specimen to the container and then dispose of them in the waste container.

- ☑ Collect the amount of stool required. Usually about 1 in. of formed stool or 15 to 30 mL of liquid stool is adequate. For some timed specimens, the entire stool passed may need to be sent.

- ☑ Include visible pus, mucus, or blood in sample specimens.

- ☑ For a stool culture, dip a sterile swab into the specimen, preferably where purulent fecal matter is present. Using sterile technique, place the swab in a sterile test tube.

- ☑ Send the specimens to the laboratory immediately (fresh specimens provide the most accurate results). In some instances refrigeration is indicated, because bacteriologic changes take place in stool specimens left at room temperature.

BOX 37-10	CLIENT TEACHING

Testing Stool for Occult Blood

- Avoid restricted foods, medications, and vitamin C for the period recommended by the manufacturer and during the test.
- Label the specimens with your name, address, age, and date of specimen. Three specimens are collected from consecutive and different bowel movements to confirm negative results and avoid false-positive results.
- Avoid collecting specimens during your menstrual period and for 3 days afterward, or if you have bleeding hemorrhoids or blood in your urine.
- Avoid contaminating the specimen with urine or toilet tissue. Empty your bladder before the test. To facilitate specimen collection, transfer the stool to a clean, dry container. Wear disposable gloves.
- Use the tongue blade provided to transfer the specimen to the test folder or tape. Only a small amount of stool is required. Take the sample from the center of a formed stool to ensure a uniform sample.
- For a Hemoccult test, a thin layer of feces is smeared over the boxes inside the envelope, and a drop of developing solution is applied on the opposite side of the specimen paper. For the Hematest, a thin layer of feces is smeared onto guaiac filter paper, a tablet is placed in the middle of the specimen, and two or three drops of water are added to the tablet.

Diagnosis and Treatment

The client presents with complaints of vomiting, diarrhea, and painful abdominal cramping. Dehydration may also be evident with poor skin turgor. The physician may order a culture of the feces. See Box 37-9 ■ for instructions on obtaining stool specimens.

Treatment is aimed at preventing dehydration and supporting nutrition.

TESTING FECES FOR OCCULT BLOOD

Stool is tested for occult blood to detect gastrointestinal bleeding that is not visible to the eye. Bleeding can occur as a result of ulcers, inflammatory disease, or tumors. The test for occult blood, often referred to as the **guaiac test** (which uses blood-sensitive guaiac paper), can be readily performed by the nurse in the clinical area or by the client at home. Refer to Box 37-10 ■ for client instructions in testing the stool for occult blood.

Certain foods, medications, and vitamin C can produce inaccurate test results. False-positive results can occur if the client has recently ingested (1) red meat; (2) raw vegetables or fruits, particularly radishes, turnips, horseradish, and melons; or (3) certain medications that irritate the gastric mucosa and cause bleeding, such as aspirin, iron preparations, and anticoagulants.

APPENDICITIS

The vermiform appendix is a finger-like structure attached to the cecum in the right lower quadrant (see Figure 37-1). *Appendicitis* is an inflammation of this structure. It is the most common cause of emergency abdominal surgery in the United States and is especially seen in adolescents and young adults. It is generally more frequent in males than females.

The lumen of the appendix is narrow and can easily fill with feces and become obstructed. The stool irritates the tissue, developing an inflammation, but the sac remains intact. If appendicitis is not diagnosed early, the appendix can become distended and rupture, emptying fecal material into the abdominal cavity. This results in peritonitis (discussed under Peritonitis).

Manifestations

The pain of appendicitis usually starts as a generalized abdominal pain but then localizes to the right lower quadrant at McBurney's point (Figures 37-16A and B ■) and intensifies. Nausea, vomiting, loss of appetite, and a slight temperature may develop. The physician tests for **rebound tenderness** with a deep palpation and quick release to the right side. If the test is positive, the client experiences pain on release. Another test used is **Rovsing's sign,** which is positive if the client extends the right hip and experiences increased pain.

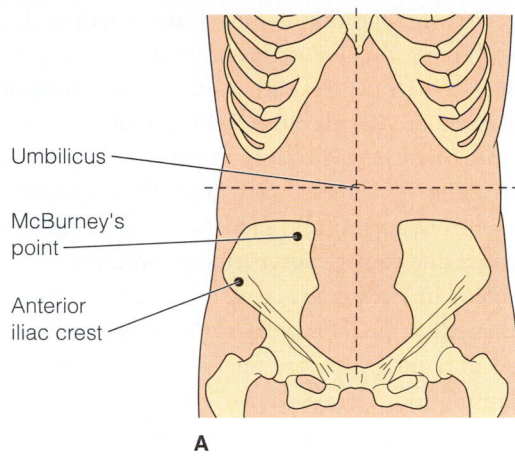

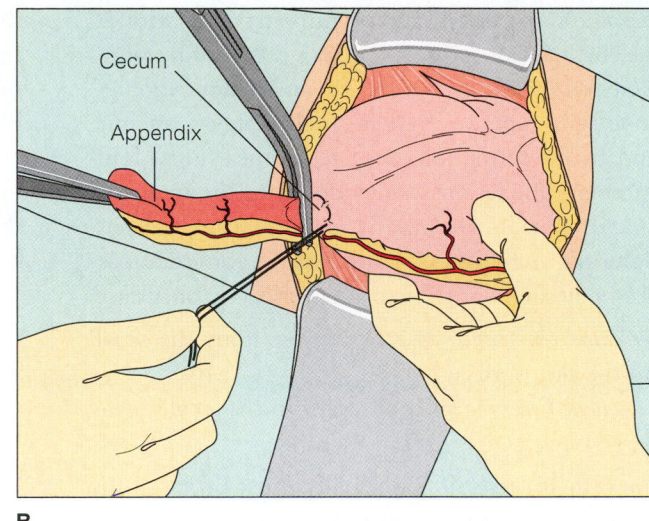

Figure 37-16. ■ **A.** McBurney's point, located midway between the umbilicus and the anterior iliac crest in the right lower quadrant. It is the usual site for localized pain and rebound tenderness due to appendicitis. **B.** Appendectomy. The appendix and cecum are brought through the incision to the surface of the abdomen. The base of the appendix is clamped and ligated; the appendix is then removed.

Diagnosis and Treatment

Diagnosis of appendicitis is based on physical signs and symptoms, as well as results of examination. Diagnostic tests such as an abdominal ultrasound and CAT scan would show an enlarged appendix. The white blood cell (WBC) count and temperature may be slightly elevated.

clinical ALERT

The physician does not order narcotics, laxatives, or enemas for a client with suspected appendicitis. Heating pads should also not be used. Narcotics mask the symptom of pain and rebound tenderness, which could lead to delayed treatment and perforation (rupture) of the appendix. Laxatives and enemas increase the chance of rupture in acute appendicitis, so they are never ordered for this condition. Narcotics are ordered for pain management after a firm diagnosis of appendicitis is made.

When appendicitis is diagnosed, immediate surgery is performed. The client is NPO and intravenous fluids are initiated. If it is suspected that the appendix has ruptured, intravenous antibiotics are ordered. When the client is febrile, the physician may order treatment with Tylenol or aspirin. When an intact appendix is removed, the client will be discharged within a day or two of surgery.

Peritonitis

The most common complication associated with appendicitis is **peritonitis** (infection of the peritoneal cavity), which occurs when the appendix perforates. Signs and symptoms of this condition include a brief reduction in pain, followed by increasing abdominal pain and abdominal rigidity. Bowel sounds are absent. Vital sign changes include increased pulse, fever, rapid, and shallow respirations. The client may become septic and hypotensive.

Treatment for a perforated appendix includes IV antibiotics and fluids. Emergency surgery is performed to clean out the abdominal cavity and repair the perforated area. The client may return from surgery with an NG tube to suction to allow for the bowel to rest.

CROHN'S DISEASE (REGIONAL ENTERITIS)

Crohn's disease is also called *regional enteritis*. It causes patchy lesions that can develop anywhere along the intestine but usually are found in the terminal ileum (last section of small intestine before the cecum). Although the cause is unknown, contributing factors include heredity, autoimmune disease, infection, and environmental exposures. It affects more women than men and is usually diagnosed between the ages of 10 and 30. It is found in higher numbers among the Jewish, Caucasian, and urban populations.

Manifestations

Crohn's disease is characterized by exacerbations and remissions. During exacerbations, the client complains of severe abdominal cramps unrelieved by defecation. The patchy inflammatory lesions cause constant drainage and irritation in the bowel leading to diarrhea, reduced nutritional absorption, and electrolyte imbalance. The number and consistency of stools each day should be evaluated when Crohn's is suspected.

Fatigue, weakness, and dehydration commonly occur with diarrhea. The client avoids eating because of the painful cramps and therefore has significant weight loss and malnutrition.

Objective symptoms to evaluate include fever, anemia, fissures and fistula formation, and steatorrhea (fatty, foul-smelling stools). The lesions can extend into the intestinal wall causing ulceration, fissures, fistula formation, and possible perforation. A **fistula** is defined as an abnormal passage from a body cavity or tube to another cavity or surface.

- An *enterocutaneous fistula* is an opening from the small bowel to the skin surface.
- An *enterocolonic fistula* is an opening from the small bowel to the large bowel.

Fistulas are difficult to heal and usually must be surgically repaired. *Fissures* (cracklike openings) can occur in the anorectal area due to the constant moisture and irritation of diarrhea. Bacteria in the feces can invade the fissure, leading to abscess formation.

Chronic exacerbation of Crohn's may increase the client's risk for intestinal cancer. As the lesions heal, scar tissue forms and the lumen of the bowel narrows, the muscle thickens and the risk for partial or complete obstruction occurs (Figure 37-17 ■).

In addition to fistula and fissure formation, clients with Crohn's may also develop additional complications. Vitamin B_{12} absorption is diminished, which can lead to pernicious anemia. Dehydration and electrolyte imbalance, as well as acid-base imbalance, can occur due to fluid loss.

Diagnosis and Treatment

Barium studies of the upper GI and colon are diagnostic for Crohn's disease, and are usually performed during a remission to avoid exacerbation of symptoms. The studies identify the classic string sign that demonstrates a narrowing of the intestinal lumen. A colonoscopy and sigmoidoscopy may be performed to identify lesions in the lower intestine and biopsy the region. An elevated WBC count and sedimentation rate are consistent with inflammation. Bowel sounds are hyperactive due to increased peristalsis. Stool specimens may show steatorrhea and occult blood. Serum albumin level may be decreased due to poor absorption of protein.

Management is directed at alleviating symptoms. Antidiarrheal medications and sedatives slow peristalsis. Antibiotics and anti-inflammatory agents are used for infection and inflammation. Steroids may be used initially as an anti-inflammatory but are reduced as the inflammation decreases due to the possibility of masking infection and delayed healing. Infliximab (Remicade) infusion may be used in resistant cases.

Clients are advised to reduce stress, rest, and follow a nutritional plan. If lactose intolerance is a problem, clients should avoid dairy products. Foods high in roughage such as broccoli, asparagus, cauliflower, Brussels sprouts, and cabbage should be avoided. Sugarless food, gum, and mints sweetened with sorbitol should also be avoided. The client may have difficulty tolerating highly seasoned or high-fat foods, and beverages that are carbonated, concentrated (such as fruit juices), and those containing alcohol and caffeine. An *elemental diet* may be ordered. The client is given preparations containing foods that have already been broken down to nutritional elements such as amino acids, fatty acids, and glucose. Examples of these preparations include Criticare and Travasorb-HN. Clients with Crohn's disease tolerate these preparations well because they contain little fiber and do not require digestion.

Surgical intervention may be indicated to remove areas of inflammation. A bowel resection and anastomosis is performed. Depending on the extent of the lesions, a colectomy may be performed with a resulting ileostomy (discussed later in the Colorectal Cancer section).

ULCERATIVE COLITIS

Ulcerative colitis affects the mucosal and submucosal layers of the intestine. It usually begins in the rectum and moves upward into the colon. The lining of the colon becomes inflamed and edematous with multiple ulcerations that cause bleeding. Ulcerative colitis is most often diagnosed between the ages of 15 and 40, but it is also seen in older clients. It is most commonly seen in Caucasians. The cause, like Crohn's disease, is unknown, with contributing factors such as heredity, autoimmune disease, infection, and environmental exposures. There is a familial connection. It was once thought to be caused by psychologic issues, but now those anxieties and concerns are described as consequences of the disease. There is an increased risk for colon cancer because of constant irritation to the bowel.

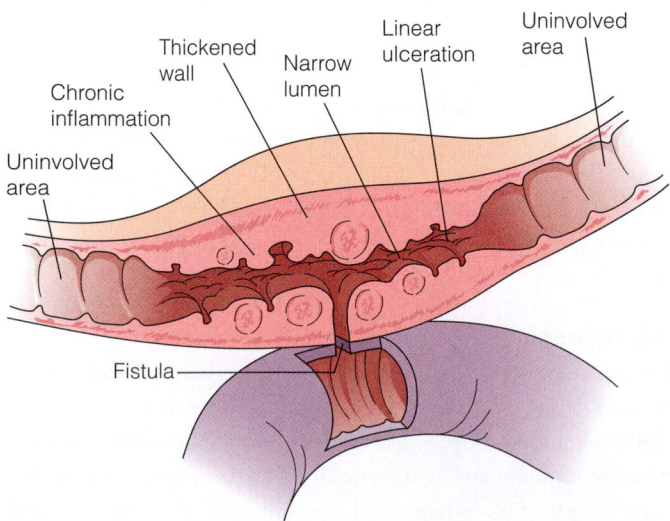

Figure 37-17. ■ An illustration of the major characteristics of Crohn's disease in the small intestine.

Labels: Chronic inflammation, Thickened wall, Narrow lumen, Linear ulceration, Uninvolved area, Uninvolved area, Fistula

Manifestations

Clients with ulcerative colitis typically experience severe changes in bowel habits, weight loss, and symptoms of infection (elevated temperature, elevated WBC count, and increased heart rate). As the intestinal mucosal wall becomes inflamed, it ulcerates, causing bleeding and mucus in watery stools. The intestinal wall heals, scars, and the muscle thickens. Ulcerative colitis can affect the entire colon or just the rectosigmoid area. The most prevalent symptom is painful, severe diarrhea with bleeding and mucus in the stool. The client may have 10 to 20 stools per day, accompanied by straining, cramping, and vomiting. The client loses weight due to diarrhea and malabsorption of nutrients. Fluid and electrolyte imbalance occurs with decreased calcium and albumin levels. Anemia develops due to the blood loss. Scarring of the bowel can occur, which leads to further incontinence. Fatigue and a weakened condition persist. Understandably the client may appear withdrawn, anxious, and depressed with this enormous loss of bowel control. Periods of remission can last from months to years.

The deep ulcerations in the intestine can cause perforation, leading to peritonitis. This is a major cause of death. Hemorrhaging from the lesions can also occur. *Megacolon* (enlarged colon) develops if the bowel is greatly distended. Peristalsis then stops, and shock can occur. Arthritis is commonly associated with both Crohn's and ulcerative colitis.

Diagnosis and Treatment

To diagnose ulcerative colitis, the physician orders a sigmoidoscopy or colonoscopy with biopsy. A CT scan may also be used to identify the extent of the disease. A barium enema may be ordered during a stage of remission. Stool specimens, complete blood count, and electrolyte levels are also ordered. In ulcerative colitis, frank or occult blood is usually seen in the stool. Hemoglobin and hematocrit levels are decreased due to bleeding; the WBC count is elevated due to infection; electrolytes are diminished due to the fluid loss. Dehydration may be evident with poor skin turgor.

Clients should identify and avoid foods that cause diarrhea. A low-residue diet is ordered to decrease peristalsis. Avoiding milk products and highly spiced foods is helpful to some clients. If the client is poorly nourished, foods that are high in protein and calories are recommended. Intravenous fluids and parenteral nutrition may be needed. Vitamin and nutritional supplements are suggested. Stress management and lifestyle changes may be needed because stress increases the symptoms of ulcerative colitis. Medications used are similar to those for Crohn's disease. Surgery is recommended when medical treatment is unable to provide the necessary relief. A colectomy is performed with creation of an ileostomy.

IRRITABLE BOWEL SYNDROME

Irritable bowel syndrome (IBS) is a disorder that inhibits the normal functioning of the large intestine. It affects more women than men and begins around the age of 20. The cause is unknown. The symptoms are uncomfortable and cause distress, yet there is no permanent damage to the colon or bleeding.

Manifestations

Abdominal discomfort is the most prevalent symptom. The symptoms vary with individual clients. Constipation or diarrhea may be the prominent symptom and some clients have alternating constipation and diarrhea. Bloating and abdominal fullness are common complaints. Stools often contain mucus or blood. Spasmodic movement of the bowel promotes the stool to move very quickly through the intestine, or peristalsis temporarily stops, causing an accumulation of gas. Abdominal distention is frequently observed. Bowel sounds are more hyperactive due to spasms of the intestines. Stressful and emotional situations can strongly affect the intestine. Certain foods can also trigger a response. Foods such as wheat, rye, barley, chocolate, milk products, and caffeine may aggravate symptoms. Women suffering from IBS may have more symptoms during their menses, because reproductive hormones may intensify IBS. Fever, weight loss, severe pain, and bleeding are not symptoms of IBS.

Diagnosis and Treatment

Diagnosis of IBS is based on medical history and physical examination. An accurate description of symptoms assists in identification of the disease. Most testing is done to rule out other disorders. Stool and serum examination, x-rays, and sigmoidoscopy or colonoscopy may be completed. The criteria used for diagnosis consists of the client experiencing abdominal pain or discomfort for at least 12 weeks out of the previous 12 months.

Treatment of IBS is focused on controlling symptoms. Medications are prescribed to relieve constipation or diarrhea, as well as antispasmodics and tranquilizers. A diet either high in fiber (for constipation-dominant IBS) or low residue (for diarrhea-dominant IBS) is suggested. Lifestyle changes to reduce stress can diminish the intestine reactions. There is currently no treatment that completely cures IBS. Suggestions that may help decrease symptoms are documenting food intake and bowel activity to determine which foods aggravate the condition. Recognizing triggers for the symptoms, such as foods, beverages, hormones, and stress, can help the client avoid them.

NURSING CONSIDERATIONS FOR INFECTIOUS OR INFLAMMATORY DISORDERS OF THE INTESTINES

When caring for clients with inflammatory and infectious intestinal disorders, your priorities will involve managing pain and diarrhea. Use pain management techniques and administer antispasmodics and analgesics as ordered. Assist the client in identifying foods and fluids that trigger pain, cramps, and diarrhea. Assess pain for location, intensity, character, and duration. Note escalating pain and report it to the physician immediately since it could indicate impending rupture of the appendix or diverticula. Give antidiarrheal medications as ordered. Be diligent in skin care for clients with diarrhea. Cleanse the perineal area often using a gentle cleanser such as perineal cleansing spray. A barrier cream, such as zinc oxide, may be helpful in protecting the skin from frequent diarrhea. Check electrolyte levels frequently to detect a pattern of falling potassium due to fluid loss.

Structural Disorders

ABDOMINAL HERNIAS

A **hernia** is a protuberance of an organ through a defect in the wall of the abdomen. Abdominal hernias usually contain a loop of intestine or omentum in a sac formed by the peritoneum and intestine (Figure 37-18 ■). An *acquired hernia* may be formed due to the pressure from coughing, straining, or strenuous lifting. Pregnancy, ascites, and obesity can cause enough intra-abdominal pressure to create a protrusion.

The types of hernias are related to their location. *Inguinal hernias* are found in the groin. This is the most common type and is also referred to as an *indirect hernia*. A *direct*, or *abdominal*, hernia occurs with a weakness in the abdominal wall. (When it occurs after surgery, it is called an *incisional hernia*.) An *umbilical hernia* occurs when the umbilical orifice does not close completely, allowing intestine to protrude through the opening. It is often seen in small children and obese women.

Manifestations

Hernias are often asymptomatic and only detected during a physical examination. Some clients may complain of pain or pressure in the herniated area. A bulge or swelling is noted when the client strains and disappears when the client is supine. A *reducible hernia* is one that can easily be placed manually positioned back into the abdominal cavity.

An *incarcerated hernia* is one that cannot be positioned back into the abdomen; it has become fixed in place. Fecal material can no longer pass easily through the hernia, leading to a partial or complete bowel obstruction. It becomes a *strangulated hernia* when the blood supply to the area is compromised, and the intestinal contents are trapped in the hernia. Gangrene and/or perforation may follow. The bowel is distended and the client complains of severe colicky pain with nausea and vomiting and requires emergency surgery.

Diagnosis and Treatment

The client will present with a physical bulge that is palpable, with or without symptoms. The physician may order an abdominal x-ray. Elective surgery may be suggested if the client is experiencing symptoms. If the hernia is strangulated, symptoms can include nausea and vomiting. A gangrenous hernia may perforate and then the client presents with a rigid abdomen. A CBC will be ordered and the client may have elevated temperature and WBC. Emergency surgery is ordered.

A **herniorrhaphy** is the repair of a hernia. The surgery involves removal of the hernia sac, replacement of the contents, and closing of the opening. When a hernioplasty is done with a herniorrhaphy, a meshlike material is placed to reinforce the abdominal wall and prevent the hernia from recurring. Simple hernia repairs are commonly performed on an outpatient basis. If the client is unable to undergo surgery, an abdominal binder will exert enough pressure to reduce the hernia. The client can manually reduce the hernia by pushing the bulge back into place. Emergency surgery is required when the hernia is strangulated or perforated.

DIVERTICULOSIS/DIVERTICULITIS

Diverticulosis is defined as an outpouching or pocket herniation of the bowel's mucosa (diverticula). Food and bacteria become trapped in these pockets, causing inflammation and infection (*diverticulitis*) (Figure 37-19 ■). Constipation causes pressure in the bowel, which in turn develops pocket herniations in a weakened area of the bowel. Another possible

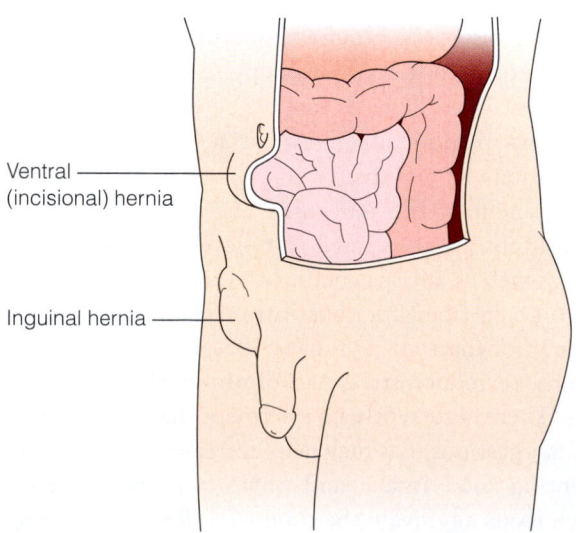

Ventral (incisional) hernia

Inguinal hernia

Figure 37-18. ■ An abdominal wall (ventral or incisional) hernia and an inguinal hernia.

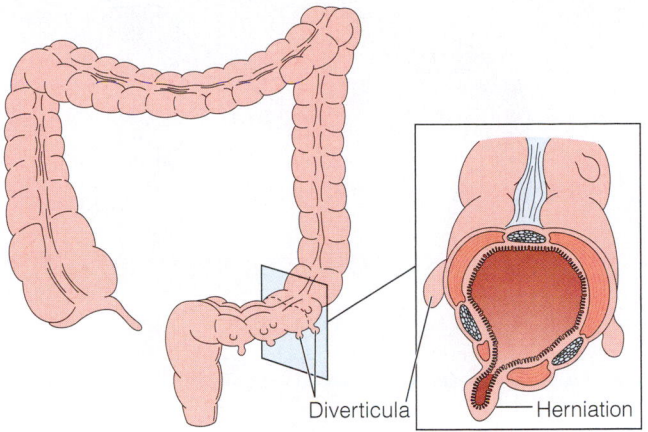

Figure 37-19. ■ Diverticula of the colon.

cause of this disorder may be low fiber intake. Diverticula can occur anywhere along the GI tract. It usually affects men and women over 40 years of age, developing gradually, most commonly in the sigmoid colon.

Manifestations

A client with diverticulosis is asymptomatic and may be un-aware of the disorder. When diverticulitis occurs, the client may experience alternating constipation and diarrhea, with crampy pain in the left lower quadrant. A low-grade fever may accompany the inflammation. As the condition pro-gresses, bleeding, anemia, increased constipation, weakness, and fatigue occur. The client may have narrow stools, be-cause the infection can thicken the walls of the bowel and re-duce the size of the lumen of the colon.

Diagnosis and Treatment

To diagnose diverticulosis and diverticulitis, a barium en-ema may be done first to identify narrowing of the colon, followed by colonoscopy or sigmoidoscopy to confirm the presence of diverticuli. Stool specimens that contain frank or occult blood are another indication of disease.

To manage diverticulosis, the client must avoid consti-pation to prevent the diverticula from becoming impacted with food and bacteria. So, a diet high in fiber is recom-mended. If the client exhibits diarrhea, it is treated sympto-matically with antidiarrheal agents and a low-residue diet. Diverticulitis is treated with antibiotics, antispasmodics, tranquilizers, and sedatives. Pain medication may be indi-cated. Medications that soften the stool (such as Surfak) or provide bulk (such as Metamucil) are given to promote peristalsis. Mineral oil may be used to lubricate the stool. Dulcolax suppositories assist in the evacuation of the stool.

If an acute attack of diverticulitis requires hospitaliza-tion, pain control is initiated and an NG tube for suction is placed to relieve nausea and vomiting. Intravenous fluids

and antibiotics are started to maintain fluid and electrolyte levels and fight infection. If perforation of the diverticula occurs, it results in peritonitis. Surgery is performed imme-diately. A bowel resection of the area and anastomosis are performed. If the client has repeated episodes of diverticuli-tis, the surgeon may suggest a diverticula resection with a temporary colostomy to allow the bowel time to rest and heal. One type of temporary colostomy used in this situa-tion is a *Hartman's pouch procedure*. In this procedure, the proximal end of the colon is brought out through the skin to form a temporary colostomy. The distal portion of the colon is allowed to heal, then reconnected (reanastomosed).

INTESTINAL OBSTRUCTION

A bowel obstruction occurs when the intestinal contents are unable to flow normally along the intestinal tract due to some type of barrier. An obstruction can be partial or com-plete and can be found in any part of the intestine.

A mechanical obstruction blocks intestinal flow. The most common reason for mechanical obstructions is **adhesions** (scar tissue that can cause a kinking of the intestine). Other causes include strangulated hernia, tumors, fecal impaction, foreign bodies, volvulus, and intussusception. An obstruction by a **volvulus** occurs when the bowel twists on itself, occlud-ing the flow. An **intussusception** (see also Chapter 59 🔗) is a telescoping of the bowel into itself, diminishing the lu-men of the bowel. Intussusception occurs most commonly by peristalsis in the ileum of the small bowel.

A *functional*, or nonmechanical, *obstruction* is found when the lumen remains open but peristalsis is absent. It is known as a *paralytic ileus* or *adynamic ileus*. This condition results from trauma or toxins that affect the nerves regulating intestinal movement. Gastrointestinal surgery, peritonitis, and narcotics can cause a functional obstruction.

Manifestations

In small-bowel obstruction, the client complains of wave-like pains and vomiting. The client may pass blood and mucus but no flatus or stool is passed. In a mechanical obstruction the bowel sounds are high pitched proximal to the obstruc-tion and absent below the barrier. In functional obstruction, bowel sounds are absent. As the problem continues, the client's peristaltic waves become extremely vigorous in an attempt to pass the contents. When that fails, the body re-verses the peristalsis, causing fecal emesis. Dehydration and electrolyte imbalance occur as complications.

In large-bowel obstruction, the client complains of cramping abdominal pain. The bowel may empty for a short time to remove fecal contents distal to the obstruction. Fecal vomiting also occurs. Bowel sounds are absent in complete intestinal obstruction. If the condition is untreated, shock and death may result. When a bowel obstruction is complete, the client exhibits vomiting, abdominal pain, a distended abdomen, dehydration, and decreased blood pressure.

ONSET OF MANIFESTATIONS. Onset of a small-bowel obstruction is rapid due to the size of the bowel. The bowel distends with gas and fluid, leading to possible necrosis, perforation, and peritonitis. Unrelieved obstruction can lead to hypovolemic shock and can cause death.

Large-bowel obstruction symptoms develop more slowly. The colon traps gas and fecal material, resulting in abdominal distention. The intestinal loops may even be visible.

Diagnosis and Treatment

X-rays of the abdomen confirm the bowel obstruction, along with physical symptoms. Contrast medium may be used to enhance vision of the area.

Relief of the obstruction is the focus of treatment. The client is NPO and the physician may order a gastrointestinal tube in an attempt to clear the obstruction. It is attached to low suction for gastrointestinal decompression to remove gas and contents. Intravenous fluids and electrolyte replacement are initiated. Surgery is necessary when medical treatment does not resolve the problem and for complications of perforation, necrosis, and peritonitis.

NURSING CONSIDERATIONS FOR STRUCTURAL DISORDERS OF THE INTESTINES

When you care for clients with structural disorders of the intestines, your primary focus will be on promoting bowel function and detecting lack of function. Auscultate the abdomen for bowel sounds every 4 hours or more often if indicated. Be aware of any pattern of decreasing bowel sounds in one or more quadrants or of a change in the hypoactivity of bowel sounds. Be prepared to insert an NG tube (see NG insertion procedures, Chapter 25 ⛓) for gastric decompression and connect it to intermittent suction. Observe the function of the NG tube to be sure decompression is occurring. Stomach contents will be suctioned slowly through the tube and into the suction container. If the client complains of nausea or experiences vomiting with the NG tube in place, decompression is unsuccessful. Irrigating the NG tube with normal saline helps remove mucus or clots that may be blocking the suction. You will also focus on comfort for your client, which may involve pain medications, positioning, distraction, and administration of stool softeners and laxatives once bowel function has been restored.

Colorectal Cancer

Tumors of the small intestine are rare; however, tumors of the colon are fairly common. Colorectal cancer is the second most common cancer in the United States (NCI, 2007)

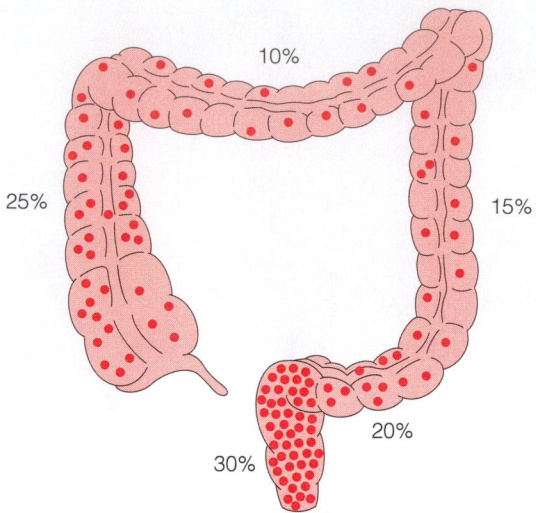

Figure 37-20. ■ The distribution and frequency of cancer of the colon and rectum.

(Figure 37-20 ■). Clients who have a history of inflammatory bowel disease, family/personal background of colon cancer, or a history of rectal polyps are at higher risk for colon cancer. Colorectal cancer risk increases with age. Risk factors for colon cancer include diets high in fat and low in fiber, diets lacking in fruits and vegetables, and cigarette smoking. Lack of folate and calcium in the diet may also increase colon cancer threat.

Manifestations

An early sign of colon cancer is occult blood in the stool. Testing for occult blood helps detect cancer before other symptoms occur. Other symptoms include changes in bowel habits, such as diarrhea or constipation. The shape of the stool may become narrower. The client may complain of gas pains, fullness, distention, and cramps. Weight loss, malaise, nausea, and vomiting may be evident. The client may or may not complain of abdominal and rectal pain. Colon cancer may lead to anemia, bowel obstruction, and perforation.

Diagnosis and Treatment

Screening for colon cancer is advised for men and women age 50 and older. Sigmoidoscopy and colonoscopy are done to identify polyps and tumors. Polyps (Figure 37-21 ■) are removed and the tissue is examined for cancer cells. A digital rectal examination is usually performed with a physical to detect abnormal changes in the rectal area. If cancer is diagnosed, the physician determines the stage or extent of disease. A blood test, known as CEA (carcinoembryonic antigen), is performed to provide information about prognosis in certain types of tumors. A CAT scan can be utilized to determine metastasis.

Chemotherapy, radiation therapy, and surgery have been used separately or in combination to treat colon

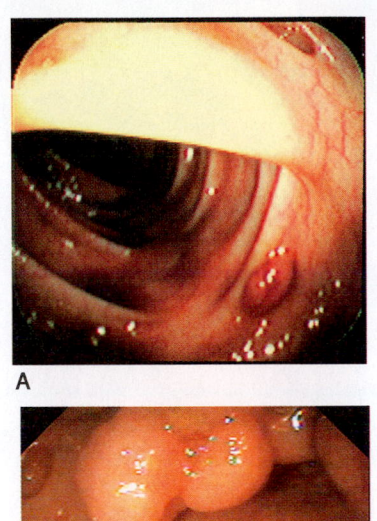

A

B

Figure 37-21. ■ **A.** Single polyp on wall of colon, revealed in colonoscopy. *Source:* Phototake NYC. **B.** Familial *polyposis,* an inherited disorder. Hundreds of polyps on the lining of the colon may cause intestinal bleeding and diarrhea, and almost always turn cancerous later in life. *Source:* Photo Researchers Inc.

cancer. Cancer staging, chemotherapy, and radiation therapy are discussed in Chapter 45 ◗◗ . Surgical tumor removal is the most common treatment for colorectal cancer (Figure 37-22A–D ■). Preparation for this surgery involves cleansing the bowel. The client is on a liquid diet for several days, then takes laxatives and GoLYTELY to empty the bowel. Enemas may be ordered. Antibiotics are given to prevent infection. During this surgery, adjoining bowel and lymph nodes are excised, the tumor is resected, and the remaining bowel is anastomosed when possible. If necessary, a colectomy is performed and an ileostomy is created. Rectal cancers require an *abdominal-perineal resection* resulting in the removal of sigmoid colon, rectum, and anus. A permanent colostomy is formed for fecal elimination. A perineal wound may be packed and have a Penrose drain in place. Ostomy care is discussed later in this chapter.

Complications of colon surgery include urinary retention and paralytic ileus. Urinary retention may result from bladder nerve damage during the surgery. Paralytic ileus is a complication of any abdominal surgery. Should paralytic ileus occur, the nurse would obtain an order and insert an NG tube to suction, maintain NPO status, and increase ambulation to increase peristalsis.

FECAL DIVERSION OSTOMIES. An **ostomy** is an opening in the abdominal wall for the elimination of feces or urine. An **ileostomy** is an opening into the *ileum* (small bowel). A **colostomy** is an opening into the *colon* (large bowel). The purpose of bowel ostomies is to divert and drain fecal material. Bowel diversion ostomies are often classified according to (1) status (permanent or temporary), (2) location (Figure 37-23 ■), and (3) the construction of the stoma.

Ostomy Management. Clients with fecal diversions need considerable psychologic support, instruction, and physical care. Many agencies contract with enterostomal therapy nurses to assist these clients.

Stoma and Skin Care. Fecal material (effluent) from a colostomy or ileostomy is irritating to the skin around the stoma (peristomal skin). Ileal effluent is especially irritating because it contains digestive enzymes. The nurse assesses the peristomal skin for irritation each time the appliance is changed. Box 37-11 ■ describes assessment data for stomas. Any skin irritation or breakdown needs to be treated immediately.

The skin is kept clean by washing off any effluent and drying the skin thoroughly. An *appliance* (pouch or bag) is then fitted securely to the stoma. Drying the skin before attaching the appliance is crucial, because pouches do not adhere to moist skin and effluent will leak out. All appliances have three features in common: a pouch to collect the effluent, an outlet at the bottom for easy emptying, and a faceplate. The faceplate is an adhesive ring placed on the client's skin; the pouch attaches to the faceplate. Procedure 37-3 ■ at the end of this chapter explains how to change a bowel diversion ostomy device. Procedure 37-4 ■ describes the proper method for irrigating a colostomy.

Disposable ostomy appliances can be used for up to 5 to 7 days. They need to be changed whenever the **effluent** (liquid fecal material) leaks onto the peristomal skin or when effluent cannot be rinsed completely away. The bag should be monitored for drainage and emptied when it is one-third full. This prevents the weight of the feces from pulling on the appliance and causing accidental soiling. If the skin is erythematous (red), eroded, denuded, or ulcerated, the appliance should be changed every 24 to 48 hours to allow appropriate treatment of the skin. If the client complains of pain or discomfort, inspect the area carefully.

Odor Control. Odor control is essential to clients' self-esteem. Selecting the appropriate kind of appliance promotes odor control. An intact appliance contains odors. The appliance should be rinsed thoroughly when it is emptied. Deodorizers can be placed in the pouch of the appliance.

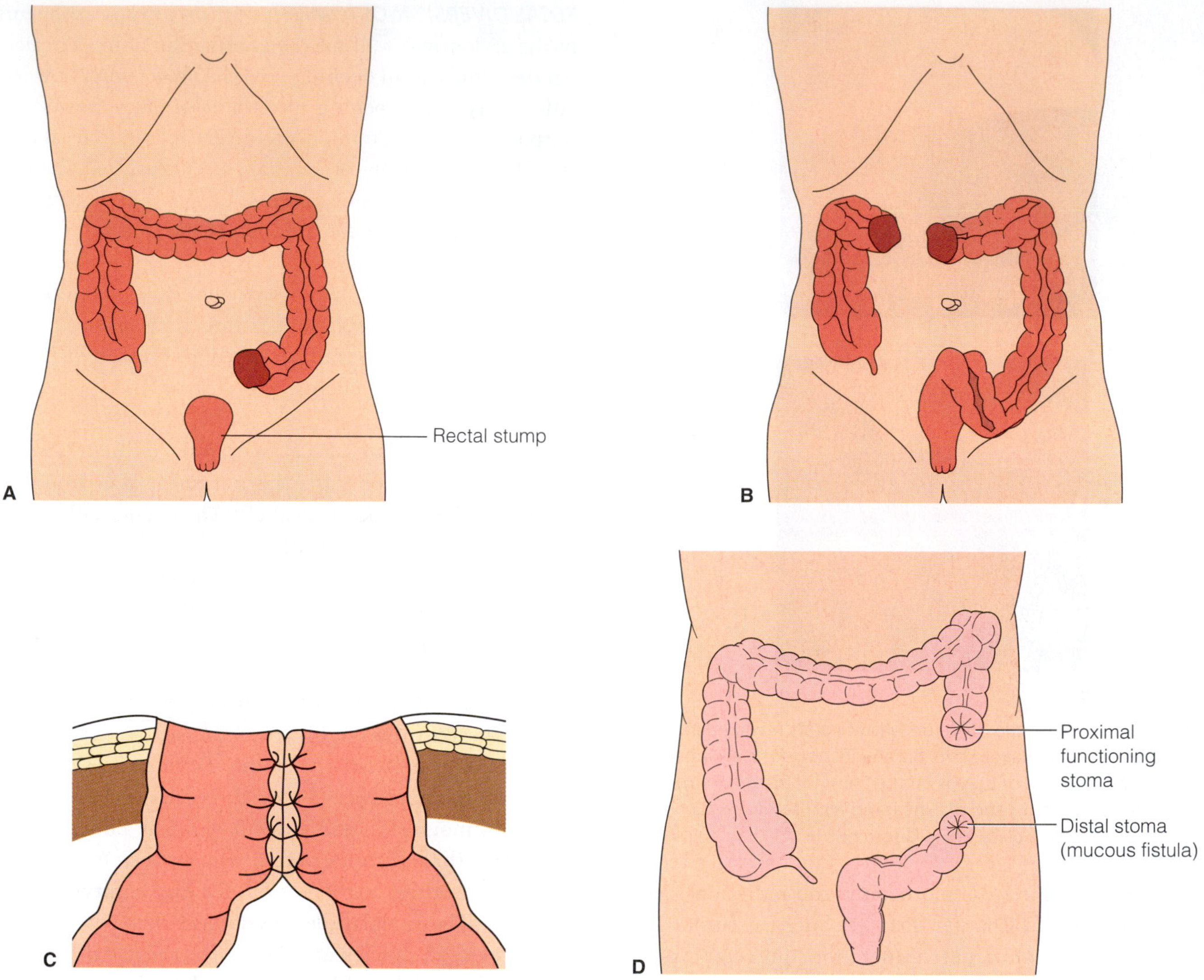

— Rectal stump

A

B

C

— Proximal functioning stoma

— Distal stoma (mucous fistula)

D

Figure 37-22. ■ **A.** End colostomy; the disease portion of bowel is removed and a rectal pouch remains. **B.** Divided colostomy with two separated stomas. **C.** Double-barrel colostomy. **D.** The proximal stoma is the functioning stoma; the distal stoma expels mucus from the distal colon.

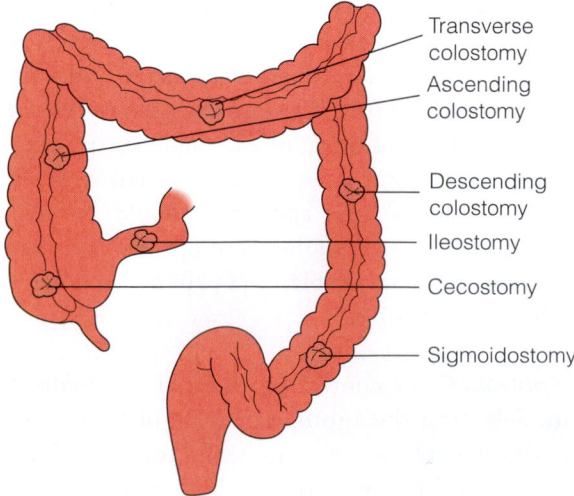

Transverse colostomy
Ascending colostomy
Descending colostomy
Ileostomy
Cecostomy
Sigmoidostomy

Figure 37-23. ■ The locations of bowel diversion ostomies.

Oral intake of bismuth subcarbonate can be prescribed by the physician to help control odor.

NURSING CONSIDERATIONS FOR COLORECTAL CANCER

When you care for clients with cancer of the lower gastrointestinal tract, focus on physical and emotional support for the client during treatment of the disease. Provide foods and fluids the client can tolerate after surgery and during chemotherapy and/or radiation therapy. If a colostomy is performed, focus on helping the client accept this change in body image and manage self-care. The client will need time to accomplish all of this. Observe the stoma for color changes that might indicate impaired circulation and for drainage or odor that could indicate infection. Observe the skin around the stoma for irritation and apply appropriate

BOX 37-11 COLLECTING DATA ABOUT A STOMA

- *Stoma color.* The stoma should appear red, similar in color to the mucosal lining of the inner cheek. Very pale or darker colored stomas with a bluish or purplish hue indicate impaired blood circulation to the area.
- *Stoma size and shape.* Most stomas protrude slightly from the abdomen. New stomas normally appear swollen, but swelling generally decreases over 2 or 3 weeks or as long as 6 weeks. Failure of swelling to recede may indicate a problem, such as blockage.
- *Slight bleeding.* Initially, the stoma bleeds slightly when it is touched, but other bleeding should be reported.
- *Status of peristomal skin.* Any redness and irritation of the peristomal skin—the 5 to 13 cm (2 to 5 in.) of skin surrounding the stoma—should be noted.
- *Amount and type of feces.* For ileal effluent and feces (effluent from a colostomy), assess amount, color, odor, and consistency. Inspect for abnormalities, such as pus or blood.
- *Complaints.* Complaints of a burning sensation under the faceplate may indicate skin breakdown. The presence of abdominal discomfort or distention also needs to be determined.

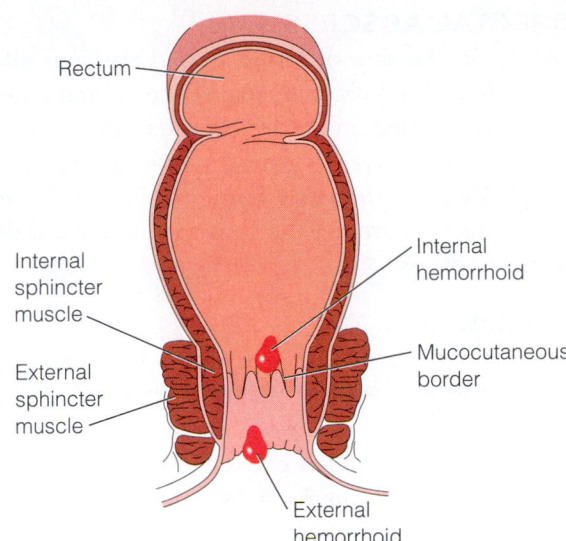

Figure 37-24. ■ The locations of internal and external hemorrhoids.

skin protection as needed. Another focus for these clients involves dealing with the diagnosis of cancer. Listen when clients want to talk and allow them to ventilate fear, anger, and anxiety. Often clients do not feel they can be honest with their friends and family, but they may feel the freedom to be honest with the nurse.

Anorectal Disorders

HEMORRHOIDS

Hemorrhoids are varicose veins that develop in the anal canal (Figure 37-24 ■). They can be located either internally above the sphincter or externally below the sphincter. Constipation, diarrhea, pregnancy, prolonged sitting or standing, and venous congestion due to congestive heart failure or portal hypertension can all cause hemorrhoids.

Manifestations

Anal itching is a common symptom of hemorrhoids, along with bleeding during a bowel movement. Hemorrhoids that are internal are usually painless. If the hemorrhoid prolapses or is *thrombosed* (contains clotted blood), the client usually complains of pain and discomfort. Edema and inflammation of the thrombosed hemorrhoid can result in infection and severe pain. When the hemorrhoid distends and enlarges, it *prolapses* (protrudes through the anus). Hemorrhoids may cause rectal bleeding and constipation, which are also symptoms of rectal cancer. Clients should be evaluated for cancer when these symptoms occur, rather than assuming they are due to hemorrhoids.

Diagnosis and Treatment

Diagnosis is by visual examination of the anorectal area. Examination of the rectal area to treat or assess hemorrhoids can be embarrassing for the client. To minimize embarrassment, be direct and factual while showing concern for the client.

Medications such as stool softeners to prevent constipation and bulk-forming laxatives to reduce straining are prescribed. A *hemorrhoidectomy* is the surgical removal of the hemorrhoid, usually performed on an outpatient basis. *Sclerotherapy* is used to shrink the hemorrhoid by an injection of a sclerosing (hardening) agent. *Cryotherapy* freezes the hemorrhoid tissue. Rubber band ligation involves utilizing rubber bands around the hemorrhoid, which cause necrosis of the tissue by curtailing the circulation to the tissue. A high-fiber diet helps promote peristalsis. Foods high in fiber include whole grains, fresh fruits, and vegetables. Clients with hemorrhoids should be encouraged to drink 10 glasses of water per day to help prevent constipation. Sitz baths relax and increase circulation in the area. Topical medication such as witch hazel and steroids reduce anal irritation.

ANAL FISSURE

An anal fissure is defined as a cracklike ulcer in the anal canal. The ulcer is commonly associated with diarrhea, anal irritation, or constipation. The client may experience bleeding and may delay having a bowel movement to avoid anal pain, which adds to constipation. Treatment is similar to that for hemorrhoids. Surgical excision may be necessary.

ANORECTAL ABSCESS

An opening in the skin or tissue around the anus allows bacteria such as *Escherichia coli*, staphylococci, and streptococci to enter, causing an abscess. Purulent drainage, redness, swelling, and fever are general symptoms found with an abscess. An *anal fistula* may form, causing an abnormal opening in the skin around the anus to develop and drain pus from the abscess.

Manifestations

The client complains of pain that increases with walking and sitting. There is usually inflammation at the site with redness and edema. In an abscess there may be drainage with increasing amounts. The client will exhibit a fever and there will be an increase in the WBC.

Diagnosis and Treatment

A culture is taken of the drainage to identify the organism and antibiotic needed.

An incision and drainage (I&D) may be necessary to surgically open the area. The wound may require packing or a drain. Dressing changes, irrigation, and sitz baths can promote cleanliness and increase circulation and healing. Local anesthetics such as Nupercainal cream or Tucks pads help relieve pain.

PILONIDAL CYST

A **pilonidal cyst** is a sinus tract that is found at the upper end of the intragluteal cleft. It is formed by a congenital defect that allows a fold of skin to turn inward, forming a pouch. A cyst then forms, which may have hair growing in or out of it. It usually affects hirsute males. If the cyst becomes infected, the client complains of pain, tenderness, swelling, and drainage. Inspection reveals a reddened, edematous area draining pus. It is treated with antibiotics for the infection. If the cyst repeatedly becomes infected, it is treated by surgical removal and closure.

NURSING CONSIDERATIONS FOR ANORECTAL DISORDERS

When caring for clients with anorectal disorders, focus on relieving pain and maintaining rectal function. Some clients are fearful that a bowel movement will be painful and delay elimination due to rectal discomfort. This can then lead to constipation and fecal impaction. Encourage clients to drink water and fruit juices and eat high-fiber foods to keep the feces soft as they pass through the rectum and anus. Administer topical analgesics and anesthetics as ordered to relieve localized pain. Because fecal material is in constant contact with the rectum, infection is a constant concern. Observe for drainage, redness, swelling, and tenderness. Look for an increase in temperature and WBC count that would indicate infection is developing.

NURSING CARE

PRIORITIZING NURSING CARE

The main nursing priorities when caring for the client with lower GI disorders include monitoring pain levels and observing for symptoms of nausea, vomiting, and diarrhea or constipation. Rating pain levels assists the nurse to determine changes and allows early intervention. Nausea, vomiting, and diarrhea can lead to a secondary complication such as dehydration. Accurate intake and output monitors fluid losses and replacement needs. Monitor electrolyte levels for abnormalities. Bowel sounds should be auscultated frequently to provide information about hyperperistalsis, hypoperistalsis, or absent bowel sounds. Stools should be observed for abnormalities including blood, steatorrhea, parasites, and changes in shape and color. It is important for the nurse to provide skin care and perianal hygiene for client's with diarrhea. If the client requires surgical intervention, the nurse monitors vital signs and lung sounds. Observation and documentation of the wound site or ostomy care provides information about the healing process.

ASSESSING

The nurse obtains data from the client regarding bowel habits and problems with elimination, including foods or fluids that cause bowel distress. Evaluation of pain includes location, severity, and intensity. The nurse should identify foods or activities that increase or decrease the client's pain. Inspection of the feces for color, consistency, shape, amount, and odor is done.

The nurse performs a physical examination of the abdomen, rectum, and anus. Bowel sounds are auscultated using a stethoscope. It is important to listen for bowel sounds in all four quadrants for several minutes. Absence of bowel sounds in any quadrant or the presence of hypoactive (sluggish) bowel sounds should be noted and reported, because abnormal bowel sounds can indicate bowel obstruction or paralytic ileus. Palpation follows auscultation. The abdomen is evaluated for distention, firmness, tenderness, and masses.

DIAGNOSING, PLANNING, AND IMPLEMENTING

Possible nursing diagnoses for clients with lower gastrointestinal disorders include:

- *Constipation*
- *Diarrhea*
- *Risk for Imbalanced Fluid Volume*

- *Bowel Incontinence*
- *Acute Pain*
- *Anxiety*

Major goals for clients with lower gastrointestinal disorders include:

- Maintain or restore normal bowel elimination pattern.
- Maintain or restore normal stool consistency.
- Prevent risks of fluid and electrolyte imbalance.
- Restore or increase bowel elimination control.
- Client will verbalize pain relief or management.
- Client will be knowledgeable about self-care and prevention of further episodes.

To achieve these goals, the nurse provides various interventions. Some of those interventions might include:

- Monitor pain and pain management by asking clients to rate their pain before and after pain medications and other management tools are used. When pain management is ineffective, report the problem and use other ordered medications and management techniques. *Rating pain gives the nurse a basis for change in condition and determines the effectiveness of pain management.*
- Evaluate the location and severity of the pain as a possible indication of inflammation or infection such as appendicitis or diverticulitis. *Location and severity of pain may require a reevaluation of pain control and may assist in determining the cause of the pain.*
- Keep in mind that stress and anxiety can contribute to lower gastrointestinal disorders. *Unmanaged pain increases stress and anxiety for the client.*
- Assess for bowel sounds and abdominal distention frequently. *Frequent assessment detects changes and promotes early intervention.*
- Monitor stools for frank or occult blood. Observe stools for changes in shape, such as becoming narrowed, because changes can indicate edema of the colon. *Narrowed stool results from intestinal lumen changes.*
- Place the client in semi-Fowler's position to reduce abdominal tension. *A sitting position decreases stress to the abdomen.*
- If the abdomen becomes rigid, it is an indication that perforation of the intestine has occurred. This is a medical emergency and must be reported and treated immediately. A rigid abdomen is different than a distended one. When the abdomen is distended, it is rounded, firm, and hollow sounding. When the abdomen is rigid, it is hard and boardlike. *Abdominal rigidity occurs as a result of abdominal perforation. The intestinal contents entering the peritoneal cavity cause irritation to the peritoneum.*
- If clients are experiencing diarrhea, assess for fluid volume deficit and monitor fluid replacement. *Diarrhea can lead to dehydration and poor skin turgor. Output may exceed intake. Document I&O for early intervention.*

- Encourage rest to decrease hyperperistalsis. *Movement increases peristalsis.*
- Give good skin and perianal hygiene to prevent breakdown and excoriation from the diarrhea. *Constant irritation of liquid stool can lead to skin irritation and ulceration.*
- Clients with lower gastrointestinal disorders generally need to adhere to dietary plans. *Some foods may be tolerated poorly and manifest in diarrhea or constipation.*
- Reinforce the need for a balanced diet with vitamin supplements as ordered. Some clients, such as those with irritable bowel syndrome, may need to avoid certain foods that trigger their symptoms. *Avoiding foods that exacerbate symptoms can diminish the severity of spasms and diarrhea.*
- Provide emotional support for the client. Body image changes can trigger emotional responses such as depression, anxiety, fear, and grief. Sexual function can be affected by the surgery. Encourage the client to express feelings and ask questions. Explore with the client past coping measures and involve family support systems to provide strategies for client. Cancer and ostomy support group referrals provide the client with outside resources and additional support from others living with the same disease. *Support systems reinforce teaching and sharing experiences provides the client with an outlet for feelings and coping strategies. Social services and counseling are other potential sources of assistance. Stress reduction techniques, support, and relaxation training can help clients control the symptoms of some disorders such as irritable bowel syndrome.*
- Reinforce client teaching regarding dressing changes for home care. Ostomy care instruction is initiated during care and continued throughout the hospitalization. Involve the family when teaching care to assist the client at home and provide additional support. Observe the client and family member demonstrating care and provide encouragement and support. Emphasize follow-up care and the importance of scheduled physical examinations. *Knowledge of disease, treatment, and procedures allows the client to make informed decisions and increases compliance with the medical regimen.*

Postoperative Care

- Monitor NG tube patency and output. *NG tube reduces gastric/intestinal pressure. Monitoring output provides a baseline for changes in fluid balance.*
- Frequently assess bowel sounds and vital signs for baseline changes. *Changes in bowel sounds and VS can indicate complications.*
- Observe incisional dressings for increased drainage and provide drain care as needed. Often a Penrose drain will be in place. Assess drainage frequently for amount, color, and odor. *Increased drainage and changes in color, odor are indicative of potential infection.*

- Observe wound for signs of dehiscence or evisceration of the incision site. *Frequent observation of the wound promotes early intervention for complications.*

Patient-controlled analgesia (PCA) may be ordered, allowing the patient to self-administer a regulated amount of pain medication (see Chapter 22 ⦾). Observe for the effectiveness of the administered analgesia; monitor for side effects and document. Coordinate activities with medication administration to gain maximum benefit during ambulation or dressing changes. If pain increases or continues beyond a few days postop, it could indicate that an abscess is forming, which could lead to sepsis. Septicemia is defined as bacteria entering the bloodstream. If allowed to continue, it can result in shock and death. Encourage the client to turn, cough, and deep breathe while splinting the incision to prevent respiratory complications. Early ambulation is essential to the recovery process.

Document daily weights, skin turgor, and intake and output to evaluate for signs of dehydration. Give oral care frequently if the client is NPO. Observe urinary output, because clients may experience urinary retention postoperatively. Administer analgesics as ordered to assist the client in early ambulation. Diet is advanced as tolerated. A mild laxative may be ordered to prevent straining. Discuss proper body mechanics and reinforce lifting restrictions for up to 8 weeks per physician order.

After surgery for an inguinal hernia, the scrotum may become edematous and extremely painful. Elevate the scrotal area with a rolled towel, or a scrotal support may be ordered. Apply ice to the area as ordered to decrease swelling and pain.

After surgery to remove colon cancer, such as an abdominal-perineal resection, monitor the perineal wound for amount, odor, and color of drainage. The wound may require irrigation and dressing changes or packing per physician order.

EVALUATING

The nurse evaluates the client with lower gastrointestinal disorders by determining if pain and dysfunction have been improved or resolved. The client may have an ostomy for cancer or trauma, including diverticulosis. Repair of diverticuli and hernias should resolve those disorders. Clients are also evaluated for management of stress, anxiety, and nutrition, all of which are influential in staying well after lower gastrointestinal disorders.

Continuity of Care

It is important that clients be able to perform self-care or a family member be able to perform care of ostomy appliances. Home health referrals can help clients and families manage at home. Other discharge considerations include:

- Teach clients/families effects and side effects of medications, including when to report side effects to the physician. *Client understanding of medications increases compliance with the medical regimen.*
- Teach clients/families signs and symptoms of serious lower gastrointestinal disorders such as increasing abdominal pain, blood in the stools, high fever, lack of bowel movement over several days, and vomiting. *These signs are indicative of complications requiring early intervention.*
- Teach clients ways to manage stress and anxiety, which contribute to intestinal symptoms. Referral to community mental health agencies for counseling may be appropriate. *Decreasing stress can alleviate anxiety and its accompanying GI symptoms.*
- Teach clients/families appropriate diet to follow and reasons for any dietary restrictions. *Avoid foods that cause intestinal distress.*

NURSING PROCESS CARE PLAN
Client with Constipation

Mrs. Emma Brown is a 78-year-old widow of 9 months. She lives alone in a low-income housing complex for older people. Her two children live with their families in a city 150 miles away. She has always enjoyed cooking. However, now that she is alone, she does not cook for herself. As a result, she has developed irregular eating patterns and tends to prepare soup-and-toast meals. She gets little exercise and has had bouts of insomnia since her husband's death. For the past month, Mrs. Brown has been having a problem with constipation. She states she has a bowel movement about every 3 to 4 days and her stools are hard and painful to excrete.

Assessment
VS: T 98.6° F, radial pulse 78, R 22, BP 130/84. She complains of lack of appetite, and her abdomen is bloated. Bowel sounds are diminished.

Nursing Diagnosis
The following important nursing diagnoses (among others) are established for this condition:

- *Constipation*
- *Risk for Loneliness*
- *Imbalanced Nutrition: Less than Body Requirements*
- *Acute Pain*

Expected Outcomes
The expected outcomes for the plan of care are as follows:

- Establish an elimination pattern suitable to lifestyle.
- Examine possible community resources and seek referrals for coping with loneliness.
- Understand fluid importance in stool consistency.

- Participate in planning a routine diet regimen that includes high-fiber foods to decrease constipation.
- Control pain associated with bowel movements.
- Increase routine physical activity.

Planning and Implementation

The following nursing interventions are planned and implemented for Mrs. Brown:

- Review bowel pattern and lifestyle.
- Provide resources to client for senior interaction and activity.
- Increase fluid intake and exercise.
- Provide information regarding intestinal physiology.
- Offer a variety of easy-to-prepare diet menus high in fiber.
- Discuss aids to soften stool.
- Identify pain level associated with bowel movements.

Evaluating

Mrs. Brown has joined a senior center and signed up for an exercise class. She is drinking more fluids. Her diet has more fiber and bran. Mrs. Brown has established a morning routine that provides a relaxing, unhurried time in the bathroom. She heeds the urge to defecate rather than delaying the process. She is preparing a greater variety of foods at scheduled times.

Critical Thinking in the Nursing Process

1. Describe the process of defecation.
2. Teach Mrs. Brown the measures and rationales that will assist her to prevent constipation.
3. Determine what types of foods will help Mrs. Brown avoid becoming constipated.

Note: Discussion of Critical Thinking questions appears on the MyNursingKit Website.

ACCESSORY ORGAN DISORDERS

Gallbladder Disorders

CHOLECYSTITIS, CHOLELITHIASIS, CHOLEDOCHOLITHIASIS

An inflammation of the gallbladder is called **cholecystitis;** it can be acute or chronic. The cause of cholecystitis is irritation from stones or bile, or an obstruction of the cystic duct or common bile duct. Chronic cholecystitis is caused by repeated episodes of acute cholecystitis. **Cholelithiasis** is the formation of gallstones. *Choledocholithiasis* is the formation of gallstones in the common bile duct.

Calculi (gallstones) are made of cholesterol, bile pigments, calcium salts, and inorganic salts (Figure 37-25 ■). Gallbladder disease occurs more commonly in females and in people who are 40 years or older. The risk increases with age, obesity, family history, a diet high in fat, pregnancy, or chronic indigestion. Excessive cholesterol intake combined with an inactive lifestyle also contributes to gallbladder disease. Medications that lower cholesterol in the blood increase the amount of cholesterol in the bile, adding to the risk of cholesterol calculi.

Manifestations

The primary symptom of gallstones is epigastric pain with sudden nausea and vomiting following a high-fat meal. The pain is located in the right upper quadrant and may radiate to the back and shoulder. Nausea, vomiting, and fever can occur. The client complains of lack of appetite, indigestion, flatulence, and eructation. As the body tries to move the stone, the pain becomes colicky and spasmodic. If a stone is in the common bile duct and blocks the drainage of the bile

(Figure 37-25B and C), it can back up into the liver and jaundice may result (obstructive jaundice). Clay-colored stools may occur due to the absence of bile. Urine may be dark amber, indicating an increase in urobilinogen. Temperature and WBC counts will be elevated.

If cholecystitis and cholelithiasis are untreated, necrosis, gangrene, and perforation of the gallbladder can occur. Peritonitis is a further complication of perforation. Infection, fistula formation, and cancer are less common complications.

Diagnosis and Treatment

Abdominal ultrasound, CAT scan, and oral cholecystogram are common diagnostic tests. **Murphy's sign** (when the client is unable to take a deep breath while the physician applies pressure under the ribs on the right side) is characteristic of gallstones. WBC counts and serum amylase may be elevated with cholecystitis.

Nonsurgical treatment of gallstones includes controlling pain, administering antibiotics, and encouraging compliance with a low-fat diet when tolerated. The client must avoid high-fat foods such as those that are fried, nuts, peanut butter, gravy, pastries, dairy products that are not reduced in fat, and chocolate. Antispasmodic medication may be ordered for the biliary colic pain. For severe pain, the physician may order meperidine (Demerol). Morphine sulfate is contraindicated because it can cause spasms of the sphincter between the common bile duct and the duodenum, leading to more severe pain. Total parenteral nutrition may be instituted when a diet is not tolerated. Actigall and Chenix are oral drugs used in dissolving gallstones, but they can take months

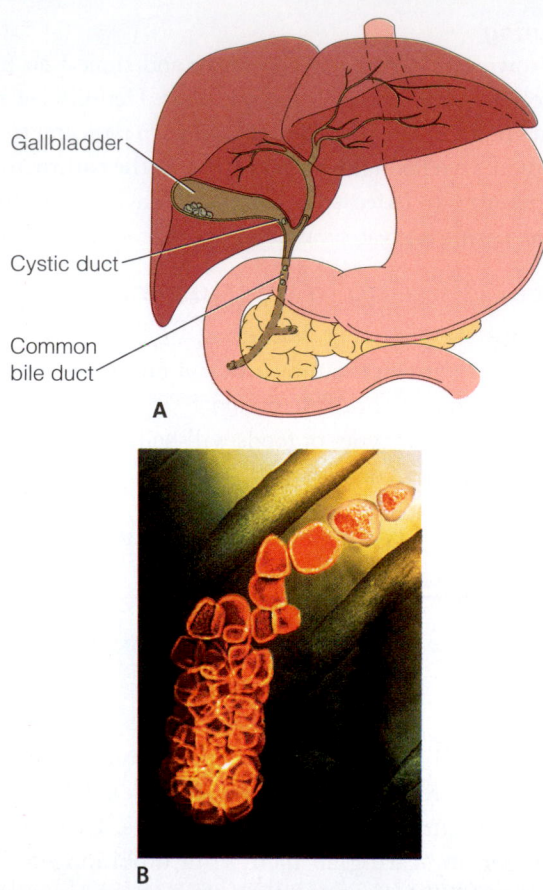

A

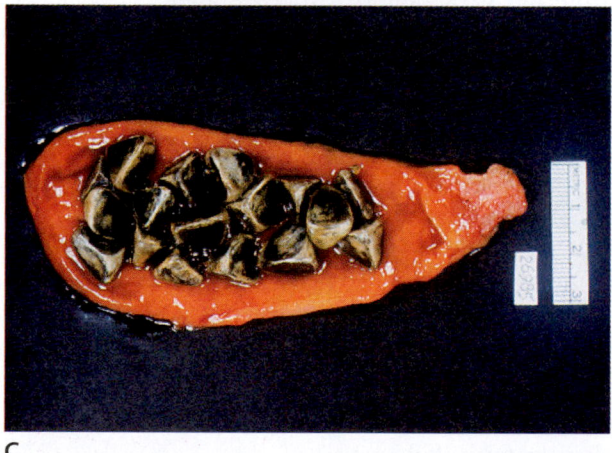

B

C

Figure 37-25. ■ **A.** Common location of gallstones. **B.** X-ray of the gallbladder (*cholecystogram*) showing gallstones. *Source:* Phototake NYC. **C.** Several dark gallstones appear within a dissected gallbladder in cross section. *Source:* Phototake NYC.

to years to be effective. A contact dissolution drug called monoctanoin (Moctanin) can be injected directly into the common bile duct to dissolve stones in 1 to 3 days. The toxicity of this drug must be considered before use. *Extracorporeal shockwave lithotripsy* (ESWL) may be used to break up stones. Biliary *colic* (spasmodic pain) is common following this treatment. *Endoscopic retrograde cholangiopancreatography* (ERCP) is

used to visualize the esophagus, stomach, duodenum, common bile duct, and the pancreatic duct with a scope. Gallstones can be removed with this procedure by basketing the stone and withdrawing it.

Surgery to remove the gallbladder (*cholecystectomy*) is done when the inflammation is persistent or is recurrent. If the inflammation is severe, it is treated with antibiotics to decrease the infectious process and the client returns to have surgery at a later date. A laparoscopic cholecystectomy is performed using endoscopy. Three or four small incisions (sometimes referred to as stab wounds) are made in the abdomen and instruments are passed to visualize the site. The diseased gallbladder is removed using a laser. The client's hospitalization is shorter than if an open surgery is performed. After surgery, the client will be on a clear liquid diet. If that is tolerated well, the diet will be advanced to a low-fat, soft diet.

An open abdominal cholecystectomy involves an incisional opening under the ribs on the right. The abdomen is opened and the gallbladder visualized and removed. A drain may be required, as well as a T-tube. A T-tube is placed in the common bile duct if the duct is edematous to maintain patency and drain bile (Figure 37-26 ■). The T-tube also can be used to inject dye after the surgery (postoperative *cholangiogram*) to be certain all stones have been removed. When a T-tube is placed, it is connected to a drainage bag, which is kept below the level of the incision for gravity drainage. Up to 500 mL may drain the first postoperative day, then the amount decreases until it has nearly stopped. The T-tube is then removed by the physician. As the client starts eating, the T-tube may be ordered to be clamped for 1 to 2 hours before and after meals so bile is available to break down foods. Emergency surgery is done if gangrene, necrosis, perforation, or peritonitis occurs. When the gallbladder

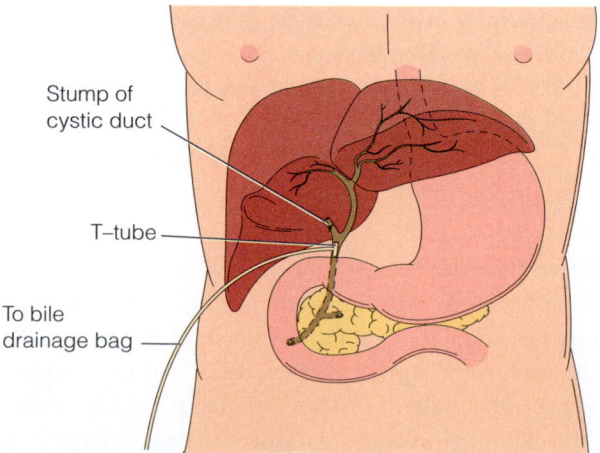

Figure 37-26. ■ T-tube placement in the common bile duct. Bile fluid flows with gravity into a drainage collection device below the level of the common bile duct.

is removed, the bile will drain out of the liver into the common bile duct and may cause diarrhea. The body adjusts to the change and side effects are minimal. Clients must experiment with different foods and fluids to determine which ones cause them nausea or cause intestinal gas. As time passes, the client will be able to tolerate more foods.

Nursing Considerations

Caring for clients with gallbladder disease involves focusing on pain relief, diet modifications, and postoperative care. The pain of an acute gallbladder attack is severe, and because the pain can refer to the back or the chest and be accompanied by nausea and vomiting, clients may believe they are having a heart attack. It is important to help relieve anxiety while taking steps to relieve pain. Administer pain medications as ordered and position the client for comfort. Sometimes clients opt to change their diet and lifestyle rather than have surgery right away if the situation is not an emergency. Encourage clients to avoid high-fat meals and to eat lower fat foods in moderate amounts. Repeated attacks generally require surgical removal of the gallbladder. Care for the client as you would any postoperative client. If a T-tube is present, assess the amount and color of the drainage. Clamp as ordered. Notify the physician if the drainage becomes purulent or the insertion area appears red or swollen.

Liver Disorders

HEPATITIS

Hepatitis is inflammation of the liver, with a multitude of causes. The primary cause is a viral infection. However, other risk factors include bacterial infections, alcohol use, drug use, and autoimmune disorders. Hepatitis generally causes some loss of liver function because the liver cells degenerate and die. The loss of liver cells decreases liver function. Liver cells can regenerate with rest, nutrition, and alcohol abstinence, and when there are no further complications. In viral hepatitis there are six viruses identified. The three most common types are hepatitis A, which is transmitted through the fecal–oral route. It can cause epidemics and often occurs under unsanitary and crowded conditions. Contaminated food, water, or shellfish have been identified as the cause. Hepatitis B is transmitted by blood, needles, sexual contact, and infected mother to fetus. Healthcare workers are at risk for hepatitis B, and they are encouraged to receive the hepatitis B vaccine for protection. In hepatitis C, blood and contaminated needles are the source of transmission. Hepatitis C leads to chronic liver disorder and ultimately a liver transplant. Table 37-6 ■ compares the different types of hepatitis.

Chronic hepatitis is either persistent or active. Chronic persistent hepatitis has mild symptoms associated with fatigue and an enlarged liver. It usually follows an attack of hepatitis B or C. Chronic active hepatitis has a quicker onset, progressing to cirrhosis and liver failure.

Noninfectious hepatitis is either chronic or acute but is caused by alcohol abuse. It can lead to liver cell necrosis, but is most commonly the cause of cirrhosis. A variety of toxins can lead to *toxic hepatitis* with exposure or ingestion of heavy metals such as mercury, arsenic, and copper. Carbon tetrachloride, chloroform, pesticides, and some medications (e.g., Tylenol, oral contraceptives, phenobarbital) also add to the list of toxic materials that are hazardous to the gastrointestinal system.

Manifestations

Symptoms of hepatitis resemble those of influenza. Liver damage, hepatomegaly, liver failure, and cancer can occur as complications of hepatitis. Peritonitis can occur when fluid in the abdomen becomes infected. Esophageal varices can be a complication of portal hypertension caused by hepatitis. Fifty percent of hepatitis C clients develop chronic liver disease.

Those most at risk for contracting hepatitis include people who work in health care, people who use IV drugs and have multiple sex partners because they are at high risk for blood and body fluid contact, and infants of mothers who are positive for hepatitis B. Prevention of hepatitis A includes using good hand washing after oral and fecal contact, using gloves and enteric precautions when caring for clients diagnosed with the illness, and getting vaccinated if appropriate.

Prevention

Prevention of hepatitis B includes use of all blood and body fluid contact precautions. When splashing is anticipated, gown, gloves, mask, and face shield must be worn. The hepatitis B vaccine requires a series of specifically spaced injections. To obtain immunity, all injections must be given at the correct intervals.

Treatment

Some types of hepatitis are reversible if the client is compliant with the prescribed medical regimen. Although there is no specific treatment for viral hepatitis, rest allows the liver to regain function. Clients are observed closely for signs of complications, including liver failure. Vitamin supplements and nutrition are emphasized. A diet low in fat and high in carbohydrates is prescribed. Added vitamins such as B and C are administered IV. If blood clotting is a problem, a supplemental vitamin K injection may be ordered. Fluids are encouraged; abstaining from alcohol is imperative to regaining health, because alcohol is toxic to the liver.

CIRRHOSIS OF THE LIVER

Cirrhosis is a chronic disease that leads to the development of scar tissue (fibrous connective tissue) in the liver. This

TABLE 36-6	Types of Viral Hepatitis					
VIRUS	HEPATITIS A (HAV)	HEPATITIS B (HBV)	HEPATITIS C (HCV)	HEPATITIS D (HDV OR DELTA HEPATITIS)	HEPATITIS E (HEV)	HEPATITIS G (HGV)
Incubation (in weeks)	2–6	8–24	5–12	3–13	3–6	Unknown
Onset	Abrupt	Slow	Slow	Abrupt	Abrupt	Abrupt or slow
Transmission	Fecal–oral	Blood and body fluids; perinatal	Blood and body fluids	Blood and body fluids; possibly perinatal	Fecal–oral	Blood
Communicability	1 wk before onset; minimal after onset of jaundice	1–2 mo. before symptoms; when HBsAg present in blood	When HCV present in blood	When HDVAg present in blood	Rarely spread person to person	Unknown
Carrier state	No	Yes	Yes	Yes	Yes	Probable
Possible complications	Rare	Chronic hepatitis, cirrhosis, liver cancer	Chronic hepatitis, cirrhosis, liver cancer	Chronic hepatitis, cirrhosis, fulminant hepatitis	May be severe in pregnant women	Chronic viremia
Laboratory findings	Anti-HAV antibodies	Positive HBsAg; anti-HBV antibodies	Anti-HCV antibodies	Positive HDVAg early; anti-HDV antibodies later	Anti-HEV antibodies	Anti-HGV antibodies
Prevention	Hepatitis A vaccine (primary dose + booster in 6–12 mo.)	Hepatitis B vaccine (HBV) (primary dose + second 1–2 mo. later + third 2 mo. after second)	None	HBV vaccine	None	None
Prophylaxis	Standard immune globulin before or within 2 wk of exposure	Hepatitis B immune globulin (HBIG) within 1–2 days of exposure; second dose 28–30 days after exposure	None	See hepatitis B prophylaxis	None	None

Source: From Medical-Surgical Nursing Care (2nd ed.). (Table 25-1, p. 477), by K. Burke, P. LeMone, and E. Mohn-Brown, 2007, Upper Saddle River, NJ: Pearson/Prentice Hall.

scarring replaces normal liver cells, blocking the blood that passes through the organ.

Cirrhosis has many causes; alcoholic liver disease and hepatitis C are the most common ones. Primary biliary cirrhosis is caused by destruction of the common bile ducts, and secondary biliary cirrhosis is caused by liver damage due to obstructed bile flow by gallstones or tumors. *Postnecrotic cirrhosis* is caused by exposure to toxins and infections. Cirrhosis due to alcohol consumption (*Laënnec's cirrhosis*) usually develops after years of drinking heavily, which injures the liver by inhibiting the normal metabolism of proteins, fats, and carbohydrates. It is important to note that not all clients who have cirrhosis are alcoholics. For example, the chronic inflammation in hepatitis damages the liver over time. Cirrhosis has a profound negative effect on body systems (Figure 37-27 ■).

Manifestations

When liver function deteriorates, the client experiences fatigue, loss of appetite, nausea, weakness, weight loss, and abdominal pain. *Spider angiomas* (telangiectasis) develop on the skin. The liver normally manufactures clotting factors from vitamin K absorbed from the diet. When the liver is damaged by cirrhosis, it does not absorb and use vitamin K, which causes the client to bleed easily and experience epistaxis, bruising, and petechiae. Vitamin deficiencies, hepatomegaly, and splenomegaly can occur. **Ascites** (fluid accumulations in the abdomen), umbilical hernia, and dyspnea occur due to the pressure from the enlarged abdomen. As the disease progresses, mental dullness and decreased level of consciousness become evident. A unique flapping tremor of the hands with a rapid nonrhythmic extension and flexion in the wrist and fingers develops. It is known as **asterixis.** *Jaundice* occurs most often in relationship to hepatitis. It occurs because the liver is not functioning normally, so large amounts of bilirubin continue to circulate in the blood, causing yellowish pigment in the skin, mucous membranes, and sclera.

The portal vein normally drains blood from the GI tract and brings it to the liver. *Portal hypertension* occurs when the circulation from the liver through the portal vein slows, due to the presence of fibrous connective tissue in the liver. The pressure in the veins increases, causing hypertension, and forces

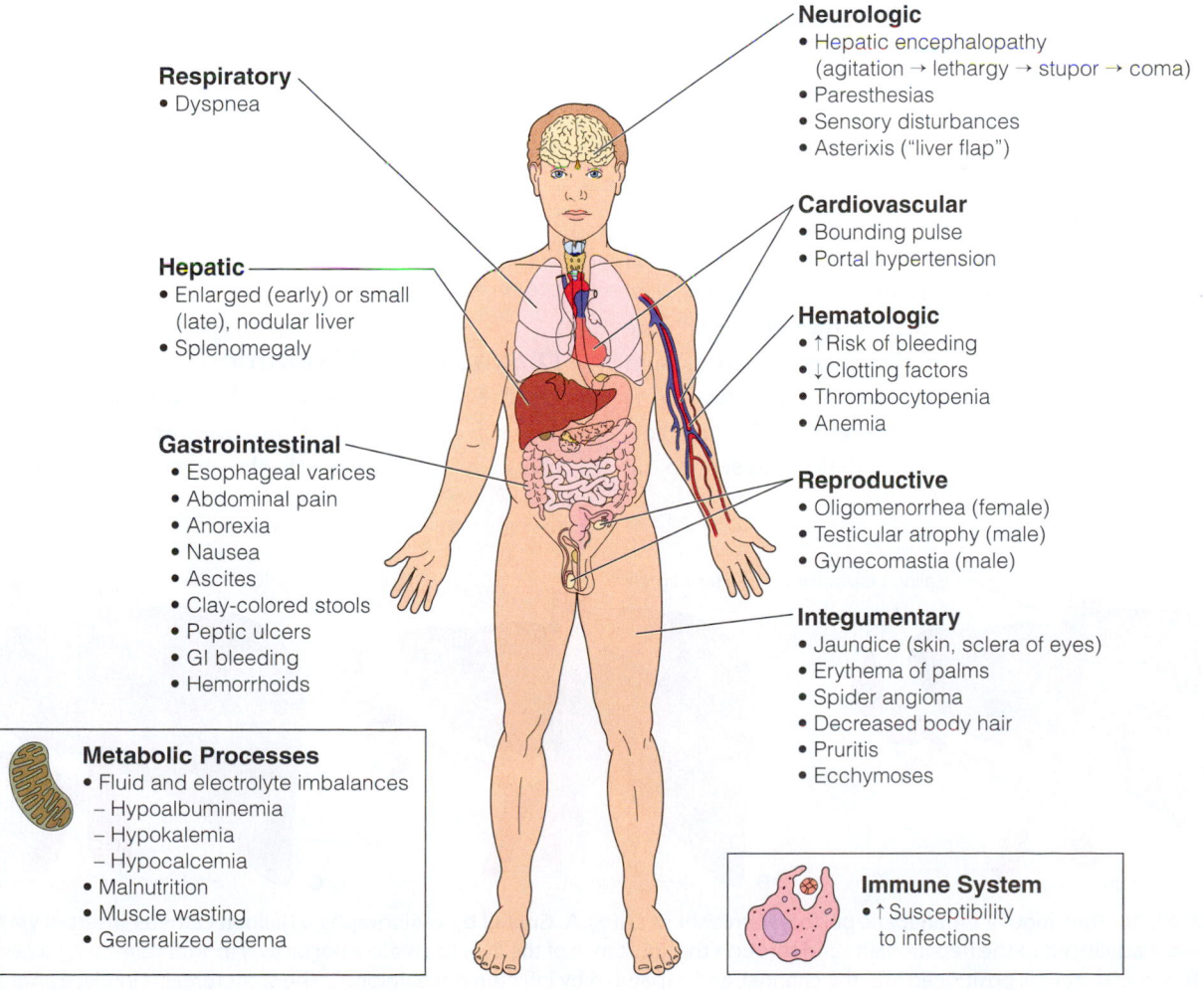

Figure 37-27. ■ The multisystem effects of cirrhosis.

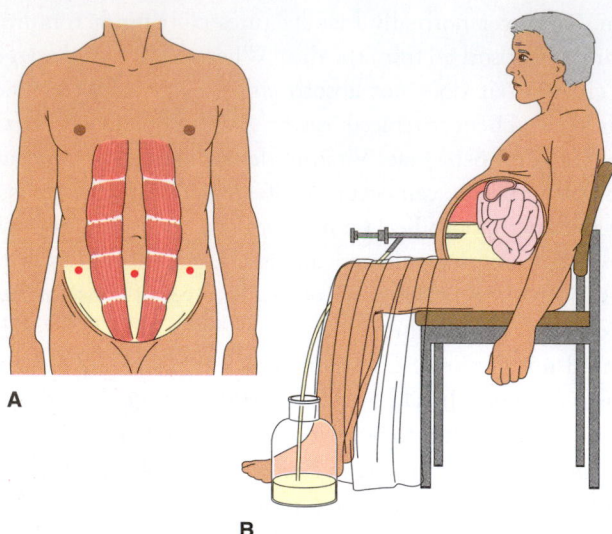

A

B

Figure 37-28. ■ Sites and position for paracentesis. **A.** Potential sites of needle of trocar insertion to avoid abdominal organ damage. **B.** The client sits comfortably; in this position, the intestines float back and away from the insertion site.

fluids out of the vessels and into the abdominal cavity (ascites). The abdomen distends with the accumulation of fluid, and this distention is often seen as a complication of cirrhosis and portal hypertension. Congestion of blood also occurs in blood vessels of the esophagus, abdomen, and rectum.

To alleviate ascites, a **paracentesis** may be performed. This procedure involves the insertion of a needle through the abdominal wall to drain the fluid. The needle is connected to tubing that drains into a collection bottle. This is done in severe cases when respirations are impaired. The client is in sitting position in a chair at the bedside (Figure 37-28 ■). The nurse monitors the client for vital sign changes, particularly the blood pressure. A dressing is placed over the insertion site and observed for drainage following the procedure. Specimens are labeled and sent to the

laboratory. Removing the fluid improves the condition temporarily; the fluid will continue to accumulate.

Esophageal varices are enlarged veins that occur in the esophagus related to the decreasing blood flow through the liver causing *portal hypertension*. The blood from the intestines and spleen starts to back up. Then congestion of the blood vessels in the stomach and esophagus occurs. As the vessels enlarge and the walls become thin, the increasing pressure can cause rupture and bleeding. Upper GI bleeding is a common complication of cirrhosis. Treatment includes portosystemic shunts (Figure 37-29 ■) that reroute the venous circulation to bypass the congested veins and decrease the pressure and risk for rupture and bleeding.

If rupture occurs, large amounts of blood escape into the esophagus and stomach, causing hematemesis and melena. The client is at risk for shock and death due to blood loss. Treatment once the rupture occurs is focused on stopping the hemorrhage and preventing shock. IV vasopressin is administered to constrict blood vessels. A *Sengstaken-Blakemore esophageal tube* (Figure 37-30 ■) can be inserted. (See Procedure 29-5 ⟳ for steps in performing gastric suctioning.) This tube contains a long balloon that can be inflated against the bleeding varices to apply pressure and stop the bleeding. Sclerosing agents may be injected to harden the varices and prevent further bleeding. Iced saline is given by lavage via a nasogastric tube to constrict blood vessels. Blood transfusions and fluid replacement are monitored by the licensed nurse.

Hepatorenal syndrome causes oliguria, sodium retention, and decreasing urine output. It is associated with the final stages of cirrhosis. Though the cause is unknown, the prognosis is poor.

Diagnosis and Treatment

Liver serum enzymes, serum bilirubin, and ammonia levels are increased and clotting times are prolonged when the client has cirrhosis of the liver. Albumin levels are

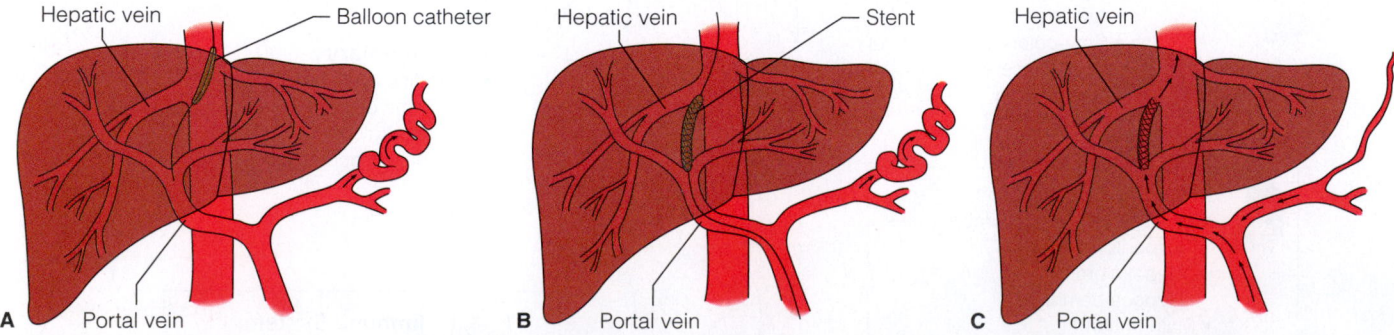

A Portal vein   B Portal vein   C Portal vein

Figure 37-29. ■ Transjugular intrahepatic portosystemic shunt (TIPS). **A.** Guided by angiography, a balloon catheter inserted via the jugular vein is advanced to the hepatic veins and through the substance of the liver to create a portacaval (portal vein-to-vena cava) channel. **B.** A metal stent is positioned into the channel, and expanded by inflating the balloon. **C.** The stent remains in place after the catheter is removed, creating a shunt for blood to flow directly from the portal vein into the hepatic vein.

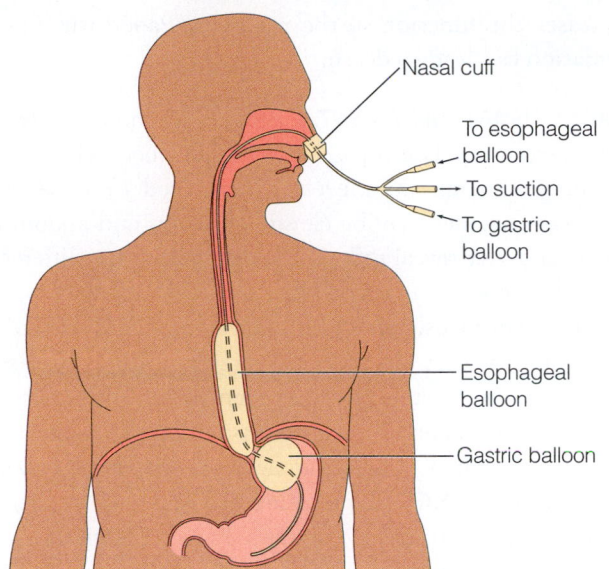

Figure 37-30. ■ Triple-lumen nasogastric tube (Sengstaken-Blakemore) used to control bleeding esophageal varices.

Labels: Nasal cuff; To esophageal balloon; To suction; To gastric balloon; Esophageal balloon; Gastric balloon

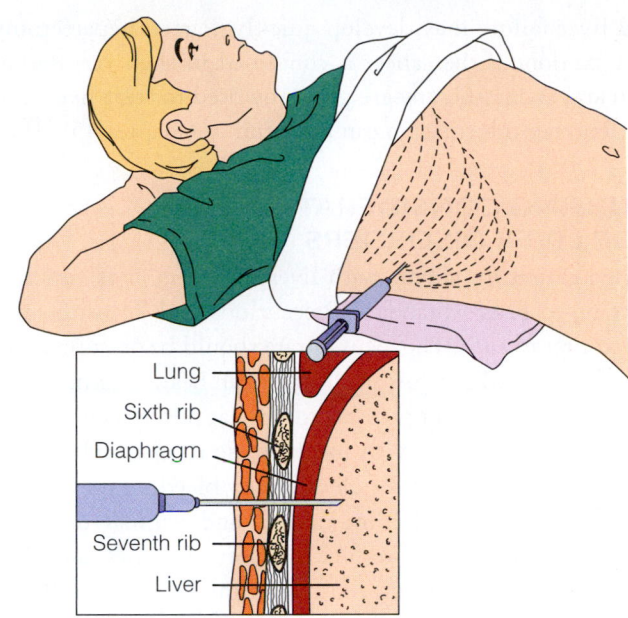

Figure 37-31. ■ A common site for a liver biopsy.

Labels: Lung; Sixth rib; Diaphragm; Seventh rib; Liver

decreased because of altered protein synthesis. Glucose levels may be affected related to glycogen function. An upper GI study visualizes problems occurring in the esophagus and stomach. An EGD (see Table 37-2) may be ordered to detect bleeding.

Liver scans and ultrasound will reveal liver abnormalities. A liver biopsy may be performed to examine tissue and determine extent of liver damage (Figure 37-31 ■).

Treatment for cirrhosis is focused on preventing further liver damage. If alcohol abuse is the cause of cirrhosis, a plan to prevent alcohol dependence is necessary. If hepatitis is the cause of cirrhosis, the treatment is the same as for hepatitis. A healthy diet and bed rest allows the liver to rest and prevents further damage. When all other options are exhausted, liver transplant may be considered.

Complications

HEPATIC COMA OR HEPATIC ENCEPHALOPATHY. As the liver damage progresses and the liver is unable to metabolize and detoxify substances, the toxins build up in the bloodstream. When ammonia and nitrogen levels in the blood affect the central nervous system, the client is diagnosed with *hepatic coma* or **hepatic encephalopathy.** This condition is reversible with prompt treatment.

Manifestations. The symptoms of hepatic coma include confusion, delirium, dementia, mood changes, increased sleepiness, and coma. Asterixis (flapping tremor, especially of the hands) is observed; seizures are rare but may occur. Jaundice is seen with increasing bilirubin levels.

Treatment. Treatment is aimed at preventing further damage and preserving the energy of the client. The client is placed on a high-protein, high-carbohydrate, low-sodium diet if there is no evidence of ascites. Lactulose, a laxative that decreases bowel pH and ammonia levels, is given by mouth or by enema. Antibiotics such as neomycin and kanamycin may be needed. They work locally and reduce microorganisms in the bowel.

If the client complains of lack of appetite, offer small semisolid or liquid meals that are easily digested. Supplemental vitamins are needed; TPN may be necessary, depending on the client's nutritional intake. Dietary needs may change depending on ammonia levels. If ammonia levels increase, proteins are omitted from the diet because proteins produce ammonia during digestion. Restrict fluid to 1,500 mL per day. Take accurate intake and output measurements. Observe stools for color, amount, and consistency. Provide detailed documentation. Assess abdominal girth daily. Residual protein can be removed by laxatives or enemas.

LIVER CANCER

Liver cancer is usually the result of spread from a primary site to the liver. Chronic hepatitis B or C and cirrhosis of the liver are risk factors for liver cancer. Symptoms of liver cancer include a painful mass in the right upper quadrant, weight loss, loss of appetite, and fever. Ascites, jaundice, and liver failure may develop quickly. Partial hepatectomy may be done if the cancer is contained in the liver. Radiation and chemotherapy are generally used to treat liver cancer. Further information can be found in Chapter 45 ⊙.

NURSING CONSIDERATIONS FOR LIVER DISORDERS

When caring for clients with liver disorders, it is very important to follow Standard Precautions and Transmission-based Precautions. The focus of care should be on supportive care for rest and comfort so the liver can heal. Another focus must be observing for possible complications of liver disease. Encourage the client with liver disease to rest and explain the importance of this. Be alert for any bleeding tendencies; report nosebleeds, bleeding gums, and vaginal or rectal bleeding. Monitor lab results for clotting times and electrolytes. The nurse may need to administer AquaMEPHYTON, an injectable form of vitamin K. Measure abdominal girth daily to assess ascites. Clients with ascites are very uncomfortable and have respiratory difficulty. Elevate the head of the bed to help the client breathe more easily. Be prepared to assist with paracentesis to remove ascites if indicated.

Pancreatic Disorders

PANCREATITIS

Pancreatitis is inflammation of the pancreas and can be acute or chronic. *Acute pancreatitis* may occur when the pancreatic duct is blocked by gallstones, after blunt trauma to the area, and in the presence of alcoholism. The pancreatic enzymes accumulate in the pancreas, causing autodigestion in the pancreas. Bile from the liver may back up into the pancreas causing irritation. The onset of acute pancreatitis is rapid.

Acute Pancreatitis

MANIFESTATIONS. The client with acute pancreatitis complains of severe epigastric pain coupled with abdominal pains that radiate to the back. The client may assume a position of comfort by leaning forward to take the weight of the stomach off of the pancreas. The client is nauseated with vomiting. The abdomen is distended with hypoactive bowel sounds. Temperature is mildly elevated. Jaundice may be present in the skin and sclera. The client may have weight loss. Hypotension, tachycardia, and shock may occur.

Internal bleeding may occur. Bruising over the flanks bilaterally (*Turner's sign*) and bruising around the umbilicus (*Cullen's sign*) are noted. Pancreatic pseudocysts develop within the pancreas. They may be surgically drained but if untreated can rupture, causing peritonitis. Scarring

decreases the function of the pancreas. Pancreatic abscess formation can lead to death.

DIAGNOSIS AND TREATMENT. Blood tests show highly elevated serum amylase, lipase, and white blood cells. Serum calcium and magnesium levels are decreased. Glucose levels and liver enzymes may be elevated. X-rays and abdominal ultrasound may reveal inflammation. A CAT scan differentiates between acute and chronic pancreatitis.

Treatment focuses on elimination of the cause and reducing pancreatic secretions to minimize **autodigestion** (self-digestion). Antihistamines are given to inhibit pancreatic enzyme secretion and gastric acid production. Medications are given to control pain and anxiety. The client is NPO and may require an NG tube to allow intermittent suction to decompress the stomach, rest the GI tract, alleviate nausea and vomiting, and prevent stimulation of the pancreas to produce digestive enzymes. Intravenous fluids and total parenteral nutrition may be ordered. TPN allows the pancreas to rest while providing nutrition and hydration. Antibiotics are ordered to either prevent or treat infection. Diet is advanced gradually from clear liquids to a bland, low-fat diet as tolerated. Increased carbohydrates and calories may be needed to promote healing. Clients with pancreatitis should avoid caffeine in foods and fluids to recover completely from the illness because caffeine increases pancreatic secretions and pain.

Chronic Pancreatitis

Chronic pancreatitis may follow acute pancreatitis and continues the process of pancreatic deterioration. The inflammatory process destroys normal pancreatic tissue and replaces it with fibrous tissue. Damage to the pancreas becomes irreversible. The pancreatic ducts become obstructed, dilated, and atrophied. Pancreatic pseudocysts appear, causing further damage and decreasing the function of enzymes.

MANIFESTATIONS. Chronic pancreatitis is characterized by recurrent pancreatic inflammation. Many of the symptoms are the same as acute pancreatitis although less severe. Additional symptoms include flatulence, malabsorption, diarrhea, and steatorrhea. As the disease progresses, the client may develop diabetes mellitus and become insulin dependent. Abscess, fistula, and pseudocyst formation can occur.

DIAGNOSIS AND TREATMENT. Serum amylase and lipase levels decrease due to the poorly functioning pancreas. Abdominal CAT scan and ultrasound are used to identify the changes in the pancreas. *Endoscopic retrograde cholangiopancreatography* (ERCP) is a test that allows visualization of obstructions and evaluation of ductal leakage.

The focus of treatment is pain management, nutrition, and replacement of enzymes and hormones. Pancreatic pseudocysts may be surgically drained. The client is medicated for pain. Histamine blockers are administered to inhibit gastric secretions. Surgery to remove a portion of the pancreas may be necessary.

PANCREATIC CANCER

Cancer of the pancreas is the fourth leading cause of cancer deaths in men and the sixth leading cause of cancer deaths in women. Because it is so difficult to diagnose, it has often progressed greatly by the time it is diagnosed. It may be primary to the pancreas or may have metastasized from nearby structures such as the stomach, lung, or gallbladder.

Those at risk for pancreatic cancer include smokers, diabetics, those who have chronic pancreatitis, and those with a diet high in fat, meat, and coffee.

Manifestations

Symptoms of pancreatic cancer are vague at first and include complaints of loss of appetite, fatigue, flatulence, nausea, and a steady dull pain in the epigastrium that may radiate to the back. Objective symptoms of pancreatic cancer include gradual, progressive weight loss, progressive jaundice, clay-colored stools, and dark urine. A recent onset of diabetes mellitus is significant.

Diagnosis and Treatment

Diagnosis may be by CAT scan, biopsy, or cytologic study of aspirate. Serum levels may assist but are not diagnostic.

Surgery may be performed to remove the head of the pancreas, the duodenum, the distal third of the stomach, a portion of the jejunum, and part of the common bile duct. The common bile duct is then sutured to the end of the jejunum, and the remaining portions of the pancreas and stomach are sutured to the jejunum. This surgery is known as *Whipple's procedure* (Figure 37-32 ■).

Postoperatively, the client must be monitored for fluid and electrolyte imbalance, respiratory function, blood sugar stability, and signs of hemorrhage. In addition, the client must take enzymes to promote digestion of food. Pancreatic cancer is further discussed in Chapter 45 .

NURSING CONSIDERATIONS FOR PANCREATIC DISORDERS

When you care for clients with pancreatic disorders, the focus of care should be on nutritional needs, managing pain, and preventing complications. Monitor finger-stick blood sugars every 4 hours or as ordered, since the pancreas secretes insulin. When the pancreas is compromised, blood sugar is often high. Evaluate the client's ability to eat and keep food down. Carefully monitor TPN if it is in

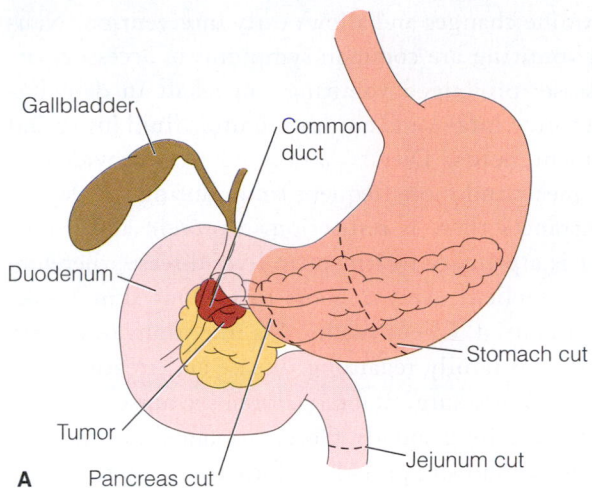

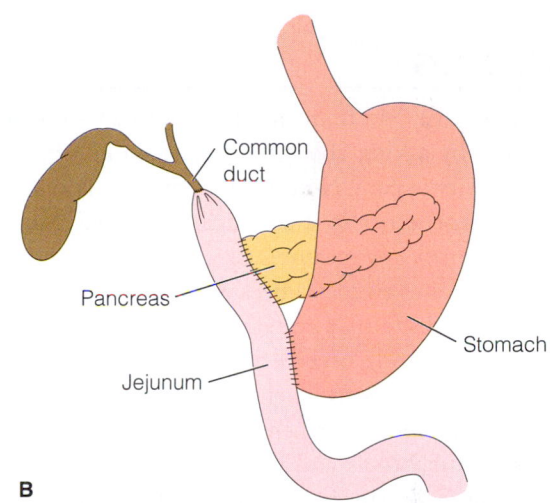

Figure 37-32. ■ Whipple's procedure. **A.** Areas of resection. **B.** Appearance following resection.

use. Be diligent in the use of sterile technique when changing dressings and tubing. Monitor daily weights for evidence that nutrition is adequate. Pain is often severe in pancreatic disorders. Give pain medications and other medications as ordered to prevent severe discomfort. Treat nausea and vomiting with medications or an NG tube as ordered. If an NG tube is in place, monitor for function and irrigate as necessary.

NURSING CARE

PRIORITIZING NURSING CARE

The main nursing priorities when caring for the client with an accessory organ disorder in the GI system include monitoring pain levels and observing for symptoms of nausea and vomiting. Rating pain levels assists the nurse to determine changes and allows early intervention. Nausea and vomiting are common symptoms of accessory organ disease; prolonged vomiting can result in dehydration. Accurate intake and output monitors fluid losses and replacement needs. Dietary intake may be provided in smaller meals and more frequent times during the day. In some instances there is restriction in protein and fluids. Bed rest is a primary treatment in liver disease, therefore turning the client every 2 hours to prevent skin breakdown is essential. Client teaching is important to inform the client and family regarding disease and treatment. If the client requires surgical intervention, the nurse monitors vital signs and lung sounds. Observation and documentation of the wound site provides information regarding the healing process.

ASSESSING

Gather subjective data from the client with an accessory organ disorder by asking about the location, duration, intensity, and severity of pain. Note whether the pain is aggravated by meals and whether it is accompanied by nausea and/or vomiting. Identify any measures the client uses to relieve the pain and their effectiveness. Because loss of appetite, pain, nausea, and vomiting may keep the client from being able to take in food and fluids, observe for signs of malnutrition and fluid volume deficit. Some clients may also complain of flu-like symptoms, especially when hepatitis is a concern.

Assess clients' stools and urine for unusual color: clay-colored stools, or frothy, fatty, stools, and dark urine. When the liver is not functioning effectively, the client's blood will not clot normally. Be alert to any signs of abnormal bleeding from the gums, nose, vagina, or rectum and blood in vomit, urine, or stool.

Observe the skin and sclera for jaundice. Assess the skin for bruising, spider nevi, dryness, and abrasions from scratching.

Assess the abdomen for distention and ascites. When ascites is present, the abdomen is enlarged and fluid filled. The pressure of the fluid compromises the client's respiratory status. Assess for shortness of breath at rest or with minimal exertion, and dilated visible veins in the neck. Measure the client's abdominal girth each shift to assess for an increase in ascites.

Palpate the abdomen for tenderness or masses. When gallbladder disease is a concern, tenderness and guarding may be noted in the right upper quadrant. When cirrhosis is present, the liver may be enlarged and palpable as a firm mass in the right upper quadrant. When pancreatitis is a concern, the abdomen may be tender in the epigastric region with pain radiating to the back.

It is important to assess the mental status and level of consciousness of clients with accessory organ disorders. As the liver fails, toxins remain in the bloodstream, affecting mental function and awareness. Changes in level of consciousness should be reported at once.

DIAGNOSING, PLANNING, AND IMPLEMENTING

Possible nursing diagnoses for clients with accessory organ disorders include:

- *Activity Intolerance*
- *Imbalanced Nutrition: Less than Body Requirements*
- *Acute Pain*
- *Nausea*
- *Excess Fluid Volume*
- *Risk for Injury/Infection*

Major goals for clients with accessory organ disorders include:

- Client will have increased ability to be active without shortness of breath, pain, or discomfort.
- Client will increase nutritional intake of a balanced diet and vitamin supplements as needed.
- Client will state that pain is resolved or managed with medication and management techniques.
- Client will report nausea is resolved and client is able to eat and drink without discomfort.
- Client will have balanced fluid intake and output without edema, ascites, or shortness of breath.
- Client will maintain intact skin and vital signs within normal limits.

Providing nursing care to clients with accessory organ disorders will include the following interventions:

- Monitor pain and pain management by asking clients to rate their pain before and after pain medications and other management tools are used. When pain management is ineffective, report the problem and use other ordered medications and management techniques. Evaluate the location, duration, intensity, and severity of the pain. *The client's report about pain relief or continued pain is the most important factor in assessing pain management. Analgesics are given for pain. However, drugs that have hepatotoxic (liver-damaging) effects should be avoided.*
- Teach clients with liver dysfunction to avoid alcohol and drugs. *Alcohol and drugs are damaging to the liver.*
- Offer small meals several times throughout the day. If clients are nauseated, give antiemetics as ordered. *Clients with accessory organ disorders often have difficulty with digestion and metabolism of certain foods. When the liver is affected, the client may be on a high-protein, high-calorie, high-carbohydrate, low-fat diet, especially after hepatitis. When cirrhosis is a problem, protein, sodium, and fluids are restricted. Many times clients are able to tolerate small meals more frequently rather than three large meals in a day.*

- If the client is on bed rest, be consistent in turning the client every 2 hours and observe skin integrity. Nails should be kept short and clean to prevent secondary infection from scratching. Administer antihistamines for relief of itching. *When clients are jaundiced due to liver dysfunction, skin care is imperative. Jaundice can cause pruritus, and antihistamines may be ordered to ease the itching.*

- Observe changes in vital signs and administer medications such as diuretics as ordered by the physician. Be prepared to assist the physician during a paracentesis (discussed earlier in the Cirrhosis of the Liver section). Maintain fluid restriction as ordered and document accurate intake and output. Monitor daily weights and abdominal girths. Check for peripheral edema. Monitor lab reports daily for electrolyte imbalance. *Clients with cirrhosis often experience ascites and other types of fluid overload. Careful monitoring is necessary. Report significant changes to the team leader.*

- Instruct the client to use electric razors rather than safety razors. Treat any skin tears or skin punctures with a pressure dressing to prevent excessive bleeding or oozing. *Because the liver is unable to manufacture needed clotting factors, the client is at risk for bleeding disorders.*

- If the client has mental changes due to liver dysfunction, it is very important to check the client's level of consciousness frequently and report changes immediately. Keep safety in mind when caring for confused clients. *Changes in cognition can indicate worsening liver failure. Keep bed rails raised to prevent a fall.*

- Help the client find diversional activities that can be done while resting. Encourage rest after activity. Explain that the client's energy level will be decreased for some time. The client should be taught conservation of energy, as well. *When the liver or pancreas is affected, rest is an important part of recovery.*

- Administer pancreatic enzyme supplement as ordered. Perform glucose monitoring and observe for classic symptoms of diabetes (see Chapter 38 ⟳). Instruct the client to avoid alcohol. Teach the client to look for steatorrhea, weight loss, and vitamin deficiencies. Report sudden changes in pain or breathing difficulty. *A sudden change in the intensity of the pain and breathing difficulties may be indicators of pancreatic cysts, abscesses, or fistula formation and should be reported to the physician immediately. When the client is diagnosed with chronic pancreatitis, pancreatic enzyme supplement is ordered, which may affect blood glucose levels. Careful glucose monitoring is done for early detection and interventions for diabetes mellitus.*

Postoperative Care

- Observe the patency of the NG tube and the amount of drainage. *Ensuring the function of the NG tube prevents the client from becoming distended and vomiting. The amount of drainage is collected and documented in order to determine fluid losses and possible replacement needs.*

- Provide frequent oral care. *Oral care will relieve the dryness associated with being NPO.*

- Monitor fluid and electrolyte balance; accurately record intake and output. *This provides a baseline for changes in condition and early appropriate intervention.*

- Sit the client in an upright position for comfort. *This avoids putting undue pressure on the peritoneum or stretching it.*

- Weigh daily, record bowel movements, and describe the color, amount, and frequency of stool. *Weight loss is a common symptom of fluid loss and other diseases. Monitoring weight loss provides a baseline for changes and early intervention. The color, amount, and frequency of stool may indicate the cause.*

- Auscultate bowel sounds for peristaltic movements. *Diseases of the accessory organs can affect bowel sounds, hypoactive, hyperactive, or inactive. Maintaining a baseline will provide the physician with information to provide treatment.*

- Monitor laboratory tests: amylase, lipase, WBC, and glucose levels. *Increasing amylase, lipase, WBC, and glucose levels are indication of organ disease.*

- Observe for changes in the vital signs. Observe the incisions for signs of inflammation. *Changes in vital signs may indicate an infection or inflammation. The temperature can be elevated and the pulse may be rapid. Observations of the incision can indicate changes in the condition and provide for early intervention.*

EVALUATING

Clients with accessory organ disorders should be evaluated for response to pain management and improvement in nutritional/hydrational status. These clients often have chronic problems that must be monitored carefully. Clients with gallbladder disorders usually improve after surgery and are able to resume normal activities and diet in a short time. Clients with hepatic and pancreatic disorders, however, must be continually evaluated for complications.

Continuity of Care

Discharge considerations for clients with hepatic and pancreatic disorders include:

- Instruction regarding the signs and symptoms of a worsening condition that should be reported immediately. This includes abdominal distention, shortness of breath, increasing pain, increasing weight, and edema.

- Provision of follow-up home care where appropriate for clients who have the potential for numerous complications.

- Instruction regarding appropriate diet, vitamin supplements, and the reason for both.

- Instruction for the family regarding precautions needed when a family member has hepatitis.

Note: The references and resources for all chapters have been compiled at the back of the book.

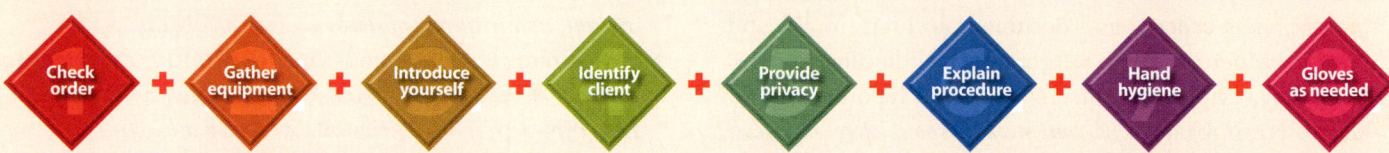

PROCEDURE 37-1 | Administering an Enema

Purposes

- To prepare the bowel for a procedure
- To relieve constipation

Equipment

- Disposable underpad
- Bath blanket
- Bedpan or commode
- Disposable gloves
- Water-soluble lubricant if tubing not prelubricated
- Solution container with tubing of correct size and tubing clamp
- Correct solution, amount, and temperature
- Prepackaged container of enema solution with lubricated tip

Check order ✚ Gather equipment ✚ Introduce yourself ✚ Identify client ✚ Provide privacy ✚ Explain procedure ✚ Hand hygiene ✚ Gloves as needed

MyNursingKit | Enema

Interventions and Rationales

1. Perform preparatory steps (see icon bar above).

2. Prepare the client.
   - Explain the procedure to the client. Indicate that the client may experience a feeling of fullness while the solution is being administered.
   - Assist the adult client to a left lateral position, with the right leg as acutely flexed as possible (Figure 37-33 ■). *This position facilitates the flow of solution by gravity into the sigmoid and descending colon, which are on the left side. Having the right leg acutely flexed provides for adequate exposure of the anus.*
   - Place the underpad under the client's buttocks to protect the bed linen, and drape the client with the bath blanket.

3. Prepare the equipment.
   - Lubricate about 5 cm (2 in.) of the rectal tube (some commercially prepared enema sets already have lubricated nozzles). *Lubrication facilitates insertion through the sphincters and minimizes trauma.*
   - Run some solution through the connecting tubing of a large-volume enema set and the rectal tube to expel any

air in the tubing; then close the clamp. *Air instilled into the rectum, although not harmful, causes unnecessary distention.*

4. Wear gloves, and insert the rectal tube.
   - For clients in the left lateral position, lift the upper buttock to ensure good visualization of the anus.
   - Insert the tube smoothly and slowly into the rectum, directing it toward the umbilicus (Figure 37-34 ■). *The angle follows the normal contour of the rectum. Slow insertion prevents spasm of the sphincter.*
   - Insert the tube 7 to 10 cm (3 to 4 in.) in an adult. *Because the anal canal is about 2.5 to 5 cm (1 to 2 in.) long in the adult, insertion to this point places the tip of the tube beyond the anal sphincter into the rectum.*
   - If resistance is encountered at the internal sphincter, ask the client to take a deep breath, then run a small amount of solution through the tube to relax the internal anal sphincter.
   - Never force tube entry. If resistance persists, withdraw the tube, and report the resistance to the nurse in charge.

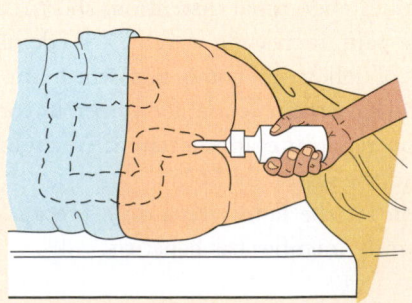

Figure 37-33. ■ Assuming a left lateral position for an enema. Note the commercially prepared enema.

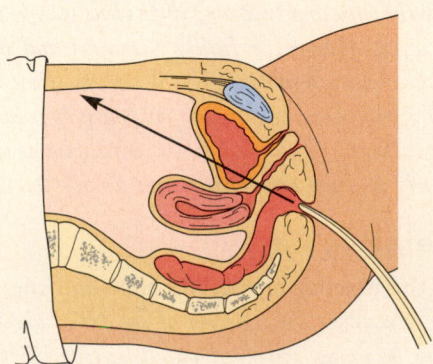

Figure 37-34. ■ Inserting the rectal tube following the direction of the rectum.

5. Slowly administer the enema solution.
   - Raise the solution container, and open the clamp to allow fluid flow.
   OR
   - Compress a pliable container by hand.
   - During most adult low enemas, hold the solution container no higher than 30 cm (12 in.) above the rectum. *The higher the solution container is held above the rectum, the faster the flow and the greater the force (pressure) in the rectum.* During a high enema, hold the solution container a little higher (e.g., 45 cm [18 in.]). *The fluid must be instilled farther to clean the entire bowel.*
   - Administer the fluid slowly. If the client complains of fullness or pain, use the clamp to stop the flow for 30 seconds, and then restart the flow at a slower rate. *Administering the enema slowly and stopping the flow momentarily decrease the likelihood of intestinal spasm and premature ejection of the solution.*
   - If you are using a plastic commercial container, roll it up as the fluid is instilled. *This prevents subsequent suctioning of the solution* (Figure 37-35 ■).
   - After all the solution has been instilled or when the client cannot hold any more and wants to defecate (the urge to defecate usually indicates that sufficient fluid has been administered), close the clamp, and remove the rectal tube from the anus.
   - Place the rectal tube in a disposable towel as you withdraw it.
6. Encourage the client to retain the enema.
   - Ask the client to remain lying down. *It is easier for the client to retain the enema when lying down than when sitting or standing, because gravity promotes drainage and peristalsis.*
   - Ensure that the client retains the solution for the appropriate amount of time, for example, 5 to 10 minutes for a cleansing enema or at least 30 minutes for a retention enema.

7. Assist the client to defecate.
   - Assist the client to a sitting position on the bedpan, commode, or toilet. *A sitting position facilitates the act of defecation.*
   - Ask the client who is using the toilet not to flush it. *The nurse needs to observe the feces.*
   - If a specimen of feces is required, ask the client to use a bedpan or commode.
8. Record and report relevant data.
   - Record administration of the enema; type of solution; length of time solution was retained; the amount, color, and consistency of the returns; and the relief of flatus and abdominal distention.

VARIATION: ADMINISTERING AN ENEMA TO AN INCONTINENT CLIENT

- Occasionally, a nurse needs to administer an enema to a client who is unable to control the external sphincter muscle and thus cannot retain the enema solution for even a few minutes. In that case, the client assumes a supine position with knees flexed on a bedpan. The head of the bed can be elevated slightly, to 30 degrees if necessary for easier breathing, and the client's head and back are supported by pillows. Pressing the buttocks together may help the client to retain the solution. The nurse wears gloves to prevent direct contact with the solution and feces that are expelled over the hand into the bedpan during the administration of the enema.

VARIATION: ADMINISTERING A RETURN-FLOW ENEMA OR HARRIS FLUSH

- For a return-flow enema, the solution (100 to 200 mL for an adult) is instilled into the client's rectum and sigmoid colon. Then the solution container is lowered so that the fluid flows back out through the rectal tube into the container. The inflow–outflow process is repeated five or six times (to stimulate peristalsis and the expulsion of flatus), and the solution is replaced several times during the procedure if it becomes thick with feces.

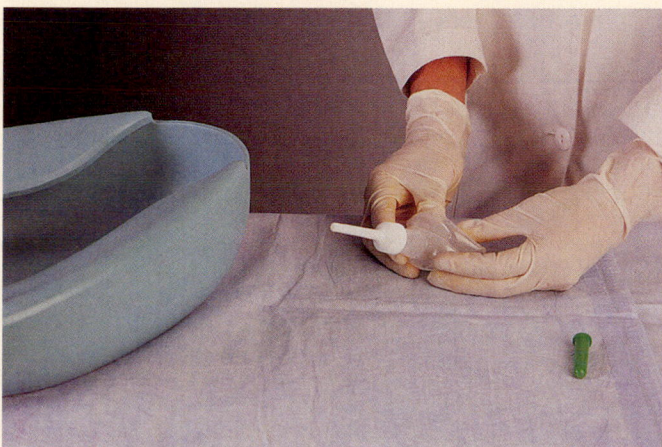

Figure 37-35. ■ Rolling up a commercial enema container. (*Source:* © Elena Dorfman.)

SAMPLE DOCUMENTATION	
[date]	D—No BM × 3 days
[time]	A—Cleansing enema given, client tolerated 750 mL of tap water. R—Returned soft brown stool and water. Client tolerated procedure well. _____
	_____ D. Haus, LVN

PROCEDURE 37-2 ## Inserting a Rectal Tube

Purpose

- To promote removal of flatulence following abdominal surgery or for clients who have swallowed excessive air

Equipment

- Rectal tube, 22–30 Fr. (12–18 Fr. for children)
- Plastic bag or stool specimen container
- Hypoallergenic tape
- Water-soluble lubricant
- Bed protector
- Clean gloves

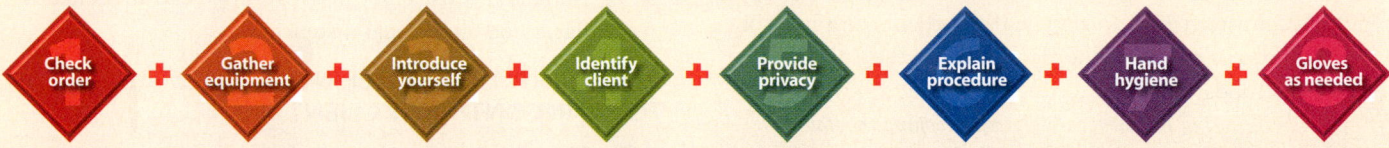

Check order + Gather equipment + Introduce yourself + Identify client + Provide privacy + Explain procedure + Hand hygiene + Gloves as needed

Interventions and Rationales

1. Perform preparatory steps (see icon bar above).

2. Position the client on the left side in a recumbent position and drape. *This position facilitates insertion of the tube following normal curve of rectum and sigmoid colon.*

3. Tape a plastic bag around the distal end of the rectal tube or place it in the specimen container and vent the upper side of plastic bag. *Venting will prevent inflation of the plastic bag.*

4. Lubricate proximal end of rectal tube with water-soluble lubricant. *To ease the insertion of the tube into the rectum.*

5. Gently separate buttocks and ask client to take a deep breath. *Taking a deep breath relaxes the anal sphincter and prevents tissue trauma during tube insertion.*

6. Gently insert tube into client's rectum, past the external and internal sphincters (approximately 5 in.). *To allow tube to reach area where flatus is trapped.*

7. Gently tape tube in place with paper tape. *To maintain proper position of the tube.*

8. Leave tube in place no longer than 20 minutes. *Prolonged stimulation of the anal sphincter may result in loss of*

neuromuscular response. Prolonged presence of the catheter may cause pressure necrosis of mucosa.

9. Remove tube and provide perianal care as needed.

SAMPLE DOCUMENTATION

[date]	D—P 68. Abdomen distended
[time]	and hard. Client states "Unable to pass gas."
	A—30 French rectal tube inserted without difficulty.
1550	R—Tube removed; abdomen soft, nondistended; client admits to feeling more comfortable. P 72. Tolerated procedure well. _____
	_____ C. Lasko, LVN

PROCEDURE 37-3

Changing a One-Piece, Drainable Bowel Diversion Ostomy Appliance

Purposes

- To assess and care for the peristomal skin
- To collect effluent for assessment of the amount and type of output
- To minimize odors for the client's comfort and self-esteem

Equipment

- Disposable gloves
- Electric or safety razor
- Bedpan
- Solvent (presaturated sponges or liquid)
- Moisture-proof bag (for disposable pouches)

- Cleaning materials, including tissues, warm water, mild soap (optional), washcloth or cotton balls, towel
- Tissue or gauze pad
- Skin barrier (paste, powder, water, or liquid skin sealant)
- Stoma measuring guide
- Pen or pencil and scissors
- Clean ostomy appliance, with optional belt
- Tail closure clamp
- Special adhesive, if needed
- Stoma guide strip, if needed
- Deodorant (liquid or tablet) for a non-odor-proof colostomy bag

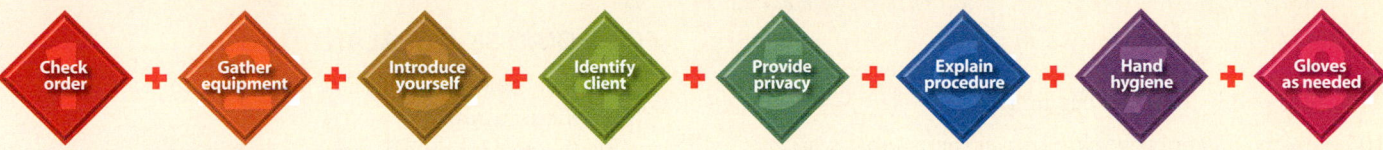

Check order + Gather equipment + Introduce yourself + Identify client + Provide privacy + Explain procedure + Hand hygiene + Gloves as needed

Interventions and Rationales

1. Perform preparatory steps (see icon bar above).

2. Determine the need for an appliance change.
   - Assess the used appliance for leakage of effluent. *Effluent can irritate the peristomal skin.*
   - Ask the client about any discomfort at or around the stoma. *A burning sensation may indicate breakdown beneath the faceplate of the pouch.*
   - Assess the fullness of the pouch. *Pouches need to be emptied when they are one-third to one-half full. The weight of an overly full bag may loosen the faceplate and separate it from the skin, causing the effluent to leak and irritate the peristomal skin.*
   - If there is pouch leakage or discomfort at or around the stoma, change the appliance.

3. Select an appropriate time.
   - Avoid times close to meal or visiting hours. *Ostomy odor and effluent may reduce appetite or embarrass the client.*
   - Avoid times immediately after the administration of any medications that may stimulate bowel evacuation. *It is best to change the pouch when drainage is least likely to occur.*

4. Prepare the client and support people.
   - Explain the procedure to the client and support people. *Changing an ostomy appliance should not cause discomfort, but it may be distasteful to the client. Support persons are often more supportive if properly informed.*
   - Communicate acceptance and support to the client. *It is important to change the appliance competently and quickly.*

- Provide privacy, preferably in the bathroom, where clients can learn to deal with the ostomy as they would at home.
- Assist the client to a comfortable sitting or lying position in bed or (preferably) a sitting or standing position in the bathroom. *Lying or standing positions may facilitate smoother pouch application, that is, avoid wrinkles.*
- Don gloves, and unfasten the belt if the client is wearing one.

5. Shave the peristomal skin of well-established ostomies as needed.
   - Use an electric or safety razor on a regular basis to remove excessive hair. *Hair follicles can become irritated or infected by repeated pulling out of hairs during removal of the appliance and skin barrier.*

6. Empty and remove the ostomy appliance.
   - Empty the contents of the pouch through the bottom opening into a bedpan. *Emptying before removing the pouch prevents spillage of effluent onto the client's skin.*
   - Assess the consistency and the amount of effluent.
   - Peel the bag off slowly while holding the client's skin taut. *Holding the skin taut minimizes client discomfort and prevents abrasion of the skin.*
   - If the appliance is disposable, discard it in a moisture-proof bag.

7. Clean and dry the peristomal skin and stoma.
   - Use toilet tissue to remove excess stool.
   - Use warm water, mild soap (optional), and cotton balls or a washcloth and towel to clean the skin and stoma.

Check agency practice on the use of soap. *Soap is sometimes not advised because it can be irritating to the skin.*

■ Use a special skin cleanser to remove dried, hard stool. *This emulsifies the stool, making removal less damaging to the skin.*

■ Dry the area thoroughly by patting with a towel or cotton balls. *Excess rubbing can abrade the skin.*

8. Assess the stoma and peristomal skin.

■ Inspect the stoma for color, size, shape, and bleeding.

■ Inspect the peristomal skin for any redness, ulceration, or irritation. *Transient redness after the removal of adhesive is normal.*

■ Place a piece of tissue or gauze pad over the stoma, and change it as needed. *This absorbs any seepage from the stoma.*

9. Apply paste-type skin barrier if needed.

■ Fill in abdominal creases or dimples with paste. *This establishes a smooth surface for application of the skin barrier and pouch.*

■ Allow the paste to dry for 1 to 2 minutes or as recommended by the manufacturer.

10. Prepare and apply the skin barrier (peristomal seal).

FOR A SOLID WAFER OR DISK SKIN BARRIER

■ Use the guide (Figure 37-36 ■) to measure the size of the stoma.

■ On the backing of the skin barrier, trace a circle the same size as the stomal opening.

■ Cut out the traced stoma pattern to make an opening in the skin barrier. Make the opening no more than 0.3 to 0.4 cm (1/8 to 1/6 in.) larger than the stoma. *This minimizes the risk of effluent contacting peristomal skin.*

■ Remove the backing to expose the sticky adhesive side.

■ Center the skin barrier over the stoma, and gently press it onto the client's skin, smoothing out any wrinkles or bubbles (Figure 37-37 ■).

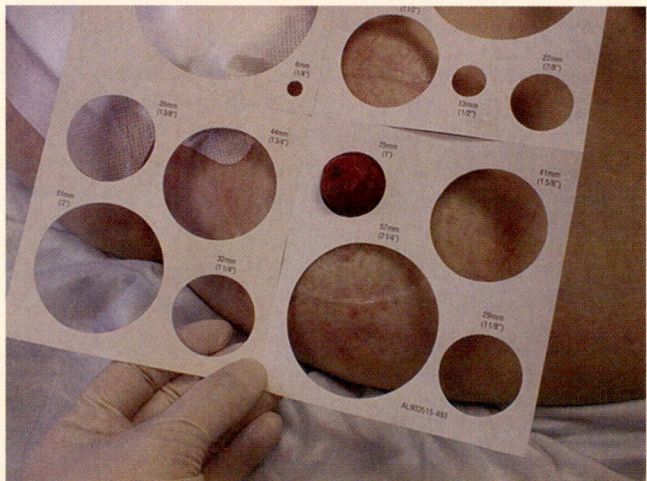

Figure 37-36. ■ A guide for measuring the stoma.

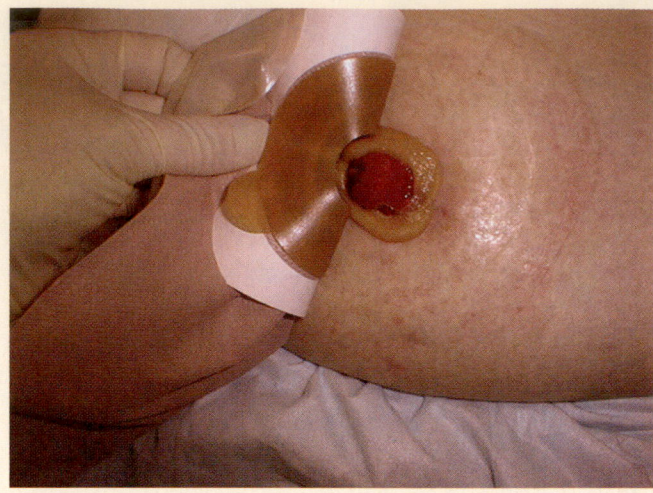

Figure 37-37. ■ Centering the skin barrier over the stoma.

FOR LIQUID SKIN SEALANT

■ Cover the stoma with a gauze pad. This prevents contact with the skin sealant.

■ Either wipe or apply the product evenly around the peristomal skin to form a thin layer of the liquid plastic coating to the same area.

■ Allow the skin barrier to dry until it no longer feels tacky.

11. Fill in any exposed skin around an irregularly shaped stoma.

■ Apply paste to any exposed skin areas. Use a non-alcohol-based product if the skin is excoriated. *Alcohol may cause stinging and burning.*

OR

■ Sprinkle peristomal powder on the skin, wipe off the excess, and dab the powder with a slightly moist gauze or an applicator moistened with a liquid skin barrier. *This creates a barrier or seal.*

12. Prepare and apply the clean appliance.

■ Remove the tissue over the stoma before applying the pouch.

FOR A DISPOSABLE POUCH WITH ADHESIVE SQUARE

■ If the appliance does not have a precut opening, trace a circle 0.3 to 0.4 cm (1/8 to 1/6 in.) larger than the stoma size on the appliance's adhesive square. *The opening is made slightly larger than the stoma to prevent rubbing, cutting, or trauma to the stoma.*

■ Cut out a circle in the adhesive. Take care not to cut any portion of the pouch.

■ Peel off the backing from the adhesive seal.

■ Center the opening of the pouch over the client's stoma, and apply it directly onto the skin barrier (Figure 37-38 ■).

■ Gently press the adhesive backing onto the skin and smooth out any wrinkles, working from the stoma

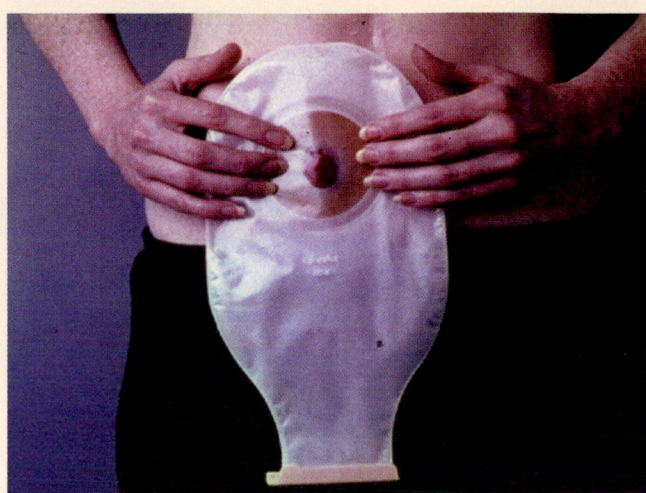

Figure 37-38. ■ Applying the disposable pouch.

outward. *Wrinkles allow seepage of effluent, which can irritate the skin or soil clothing.*

■ Remove the air from the pouch. *Removing the air helps the pouch lie flat against the abdomen.*

■ Place a deodorant in the pouch (optional).

■ Close the pouch by turning up the bottom a few times, fanfolding its end lengthwise, and securing it with a tail closure clamp.

■ Adjust the teaching plan and nursing care plan as needed. Include on the teaching plan the equipment and procedure used. *Client learning is facilitated by consistent nursing interventions.*

VARIATION: APPLYING THE SKIN BARRIER AND APPLIANCE AS ONE UNIT

■ If a disk- or wafer-type skin barrier is used, the skin barrier and appliance can be applied as one unit. *Applying the skin*

barrier and the appliance together not only is quicker but also is thought to reduce the chance of wrinkles. It also is easier for the client to apply without help.

■ Prepare the skin barrier by measuring the size of the stoma, tracing a circle on the backing of the skin barrier, and cutting out the traced stoma pattern to make an opening in the skin barrier.

■ Prepare the appliance by cutting an opening 0.3 to 0.4 cm (1/8 to 1/6 in.) larger than the stoma size (if not already present) and peeling off the backing from the adhesive seal.

■ Center the opening of the pouch over the skin barrier.

■ Remove the skin barrier backing to expose the sticky adhesive side.

■ Center the skin barrier and appliance over the stoma, and press it onto the client's skin.

SAMPLE DOCUMENTATION

[date]
[time]

D—Ostomy is brick red in color, no bleeding noted. Effluent dark brown, watery. Peristomal skin clean and dry.

A—Ostomy measured, appliance applied. Procedure demonstrated for client. Bag secured with ostomy by client.

R—Tolerated procedure well and demonstrated understanding of clamping instructions. _____
_____ D. Haus, LVN

PROCEDURE 37-4   **Irrigating a Colostomy**

Purpose

■ To manage regular bowel elimination

Equipment

■ Solution container
■ 1,000 mL warm water
■ Irrigating tube with cone

■ Irrigating sleeve long enough to reach water level in the toilet
■ Washcloths or gauze sponges to clean skin and stoma
■ IV pole
■ Water-soluble irrigant
■ Plastic bag for disposing used pouch
■ Clean gloves
■ Replacement clean pouch and closure

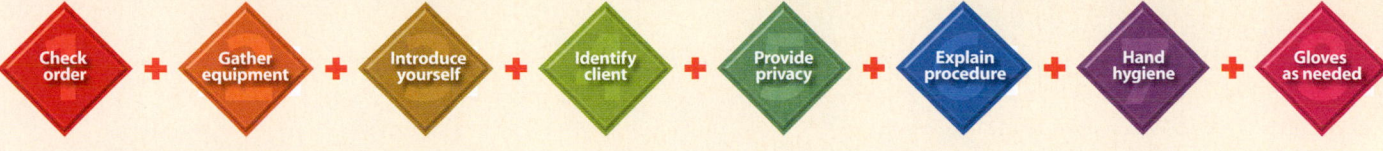

Interventions and Rationales

1. Perform preparatory steps (see icon bar).

2. Remove used pouch and dispose of it in the plastic bag. *Proper disposal of body waste is done for infection control.*

3. Assess pulse and blood pressure. *Assess pulse and BP for client susceptible to vagal response before procedure and monitor closely for early signs of hypotension, bradycardia, or loss of consciousness.*

4. Clean stoma and skin with warm water and soft cloth. *To remove any feces from the area around the stoma.*

5. Assess for signs of irritation or breakdown. *To prevent skin breakdown and to provide timely treatment for skin problems.*

6. Prepare irrigation solution: Fill the container with 750 to 1,000 mL of lukewarm water solution at 105° to 110°F (40.6° to 43.3°C). *Solutions that are too hot or cold can cause cramping.*

7. Hang the container on IV pole next to the toilet or commode. *Solution is positioned 18 in. (45.7 cm) above the insertion site to promote gravity flow.*

8. Allow solution to run through the tubing so that air is removed. Clamp tube. *If air is instilled during procedure, the client may experience discomfort as a result of distention of colon.*

9. Assist client to sit on the toilet/commode or on a chair in front of the toilet.

10. Place sleeve between client's thighs and direct end into toilet. *To prevent soiling the client or the floor.*

11. Lubricate cone tip with water-soluble lubricant. *Danger of perforation of the colon is greater when using a catheter for irrigation. Use of an irrigation cone is safer and results in better water flow.*

12. Position cone in sleeve by placing top through opening. If cone cannot be inserted easily, do not force. Hold cone snugly against the stoma. *This prevents solution backflow.*

13. Remove cone and close off or fold over top of sleeve after solution is instilled.

14. Allow client to remain seated while majority of stool and solution returns, usually 10 to 15 minutes.

15. Clean client's skin and stoma with warm water. Dry thoroughly.

16. Apply skin barriers and clean pouch.

SAMPLE DOCUMENTATION

[date]	750 mL of warm water instilled.
[time]	Large amount of soft brown, semisoft stool returned with solution. Stoma and peristomal skin intact with no signs of bleeding or excoriation. Skin barrier and pouch reapplied. Client assisted back to bed. Tolerated procedure well. P 72, BP 122/70. _____ _____ S. Ceaders, LPN

Chapter Review

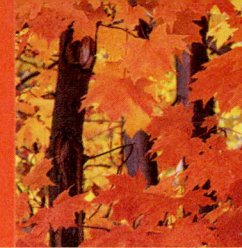

KEY Points

- The function of the gastrointestinal system is to process nutrition and eliminate waste products.
- For clients with disorders of the oral cavity, the nursing focus is on maintaining an open airway and promoting food and fluid intake.
- For esophageal disorders, promote swallowing and monitor all factors that affect nutrition and hydration. Provide pain medications, and reassure clients (if appropriate) that the pain is not from a heart attack.
- If a client is experiencing loss of fluid through vomiting, diarrhea, or gastrointestinal bleeding, fluid and blood loss are a major concern. Dehydration and shock could occur. Decreasing blood pressure could indicate impending shock. Anxiety of the client is an important nursing consideration.
- When you care for clients with obesity, focus on restoring a healthy weight, lifestyle, and body image.
- For clients with structural disorders of the intestines, the primary nursing focus is promoting bowel function and detecting lack of function. Regular auscultation of the abdomen and detection of any pattern of decreasing bowel sounds is important.
- When you care for clients with any medical-surgical disorder, you may need to address an elimination disorder as well.
- When you care for clients with inflammatory and infectious intestinal disorders, your priorities will involve managing pain and diarrhea. Assist the client in identifying foods and fluids that trigger pain, cramps, and diarrhea.
- For clients with cancer of the lower gastrointestinal tract, the nursing focus is on physical and emotional support for the client during treatment. The nurse also helps the client to accept this change in body image and to manage self-care.
- When caring for clients with anorectal disorders, focus on relieving pain and maintaining rectal function.
- Caring for clients with gallbladder disease involves focusing on pain relief, diet modifications, and postoperative care. Clients may need teaching about how to change diet and lifestyle to avoid surgery.

- For liver disorders, follow Standard Precautions and Transmission-based Precautions. Measure abdominal girth daily to assess ascites. For clients with ascites, the head of the bed should be elevated to help them breathe more easily.
- The focus of nursing care for clients with pancreatic disorders should be on nutritional needs, managing pain, and preventing complications. Monitor finger-stick blood sugars as ordered, and monitor TPN if it is in use. Take daily weights. If an NG tube is in place, monitor for function and irrigate as necessary.
- There are a number of radiologic and nuclear studies that can be used to accurately diagnose gastrointestinal disorders.

⬯ FOR FURTHER Study

For more about pain and use of the PCA pump, see Chapter 22.

Steps for inserting and removing a nasogastric tube are provided in Procedure 25-2.

Procedure 29-5 describes gastric suctioning.

See Chapter 34 for information related to lack of intrinsic factor and pernicious anemia.

For a full discussion of diabetes mellitus and other forms of diabetes, see Chapter 38.

See Chapter 45 for cancer staging and care of the client with cancer.

Eating disorders are discussed further in Chapter 50.

Pyloric stenosis, intussusception, and GERD are discussed in Chapter 59.

Critical Thinking Care Map

Caring for a Client with Ulcerative Colitis
NCLEX-PN® Focus Area: Physiologic Adaptation

Case Study: Mrs. Dora Davis is a 60-year-old client being treated for ulcerative colitis. She was hospitalized for a colectomy; she has a permanent ileostomy. Today marks her third postoperative day. She continues to have pain. When you empty her ileostomy bag, she throws the cover over her head. She is due for discharge in 2 days. The enterostomal nurse has visited and initiated teaching care of the ostomy. Mrs. Davis worries that the bag will break when she gets up. She has confided that she is fearful that her husband will find her unattractive.

Nursing Diagnosis: *Deficient Knowledge*

COLLECT DATA

Subjective	Objective
_____	_____
_____	_____
_____	_____
_____	_____
_____	_____
_____	_____
_____	_____

Would you report this? Yes/No

If yes, to: _____

What would you report?_____

Nursing Care

_____
_____
_____
_____
_____
_____
_____
_____
_____
_____

How would you document this? _____
_____
_____
_____

Data Collected
(use only those that apply)

- Ileostomy right abdomen
- Stoma brick red
- Effluent watery, dark brown, flecks of blood
- Refuses to look at the ileostomy
- Pain
- Anxious
- Fearful
- Peristomal area reddened
- Weight 110 lbs
- Hemoglobin 10
- WBC 12,000
- Gait steady
- UA shows 2 + bacteria
- BP 120/86
- 99.4°F
- Skin turgor slow

Nursing Interventions
(use only those that apply; list in priority order)

- Monitor intake and output.
- Take daily weights.
- Increase fluid intake.
- Assess stoma.
- Inspect peristomal skin.
- Monitor lab values.
- Take VS every 4 hours.
- Assess skin turgor.
- Assess coping mechanisms.
- Provide referrals to Ostomy Association.
- Include family in teaching.

Compare your answers and documentation to those provided on the MyNursingKit Website.

NCLEX-PN® Exam Preparation

1 When caring for a client with type A chronic gastritis, the nurse would anticipate which of the following orders?

1. A diet high in iron
2. Vitamin B_{12} injections at regular intervals
3. A test for *H. pylori* bacteria
4. Antibiotics administered IV for 5 days

2 A client diagnosed with peptic ulcer disease begins to have emesis that looks like coffee grounds. The nurse anticipates which of the following changes in vital signs?

1. Hypotension and thready pulse
2. Hypertension and bradycardia
3. Increased respirations and elevated temperature
4. Lowered temperature and tachycardia

3 The nurse assesses the client who had abdominal surgery yesterday and finds bowel sounds are absent. The nurse attributes this to:

1. Constipation.
2. Volvulus.
3. Ulcerative colitis.
4. Paralytic ileus.

4 The nurse is caring for a client with a fecal impaction. The nurse's priority intervention would be to:

1. Insert a rectal tube.
2. Administer a Harris flush.
3. Administer an oil-retention enema.
4. Administer a cathartic.

5 A client with an ileostomy asks why the skin around the stoma turns red and oozes if the effluent from the ostomy comes in contact with the skin. The nurse's best explanation is that the effluent contains:

1. Digestive enzymes that act on the skin.
2. Electrolytes that are toxic to the skin.
3. Bile that attempts to dissolve the skin.
4. Organic salts that irritate the skin.

6 When caring for a client with possible colon cancer, the nurse would anticipate which of the following orders?

1. Stool specimen for culture and sensitivity
2. Guaiac stool specimen for blood
3. Steatorrhea test
4. Test for presence of albumin in stool

7 The nurse is caring for a client diagnosed with AIDS and notes small white spots on the tongue. The nurse suspects the client has:

1. Thrush.
2. Kaposi's sarcoma.
3. *Pneumocystis carinii*.
4. Periodontal disease.

8 The nurse explains the reason for auscultating the abdomen is to listen for bowel sounds caused by peristalsis. The client asks where peristalsis begins. The nurse's best response would be that peristalsis begins in the:

1. Duodenum.
2. Stomach.
3. Esophagus.
4. Ileum.

9 A client with cirrhosis of the liver complains of increasing shortness of breath. The nurse's priority assessment related to the client's complaint would be to:

1. Examine the client for bleeding from mucous membranes and bruising.
2. Determine the client's mental orientation.
3. Observe the hands and wrists of the client for asterixis.
4. Measure the abdominal girth and compare it to previous measurements.

10 The physician suspects the client may have a hiatal hernia. Which of the following tests, ordered by the physician, would the nurse recognize as useful in confirming this diagnosis?

1. Barium swallow
2. Barium enema
3. Gastric analysis
4. Esophagogastroduodenoscopy (EGD)

Answers and rationales for Review Questions appear in Appendix I.

Chapter 38

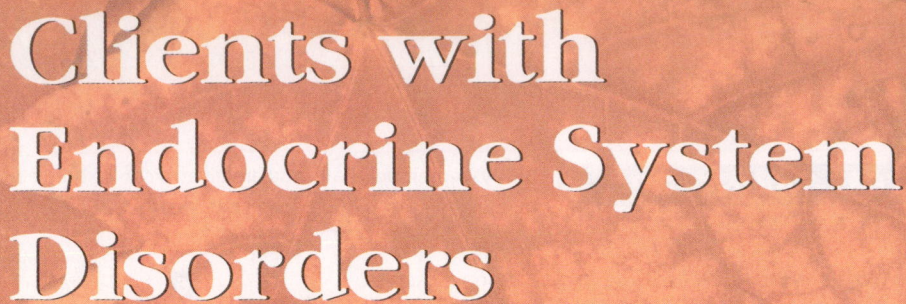

Clients with Endocrine System Disorders

LEARNING Outcomes

After completing this chapter, you will be able to:

1. Define homeostasis and negative feedback mechanisms.
2. Describe the structure and function of the endocrine system.
3. List disorders of the pituitary gland and nursing interventions for clients with pituitary disorders.
4. Explain thyroid and parathyroid disorders.
5. Identify nursing care needed for clients with thyroid and parathyroid disorders.
6. Differentiate between types of diabetes mellitus and treatment for each.
7. Identify topics to include when teaching clients with diabetes mellitus about self-care.
8. Explain complications of diabetes and how to decrease the risk for them.
9. Discuss disorders of the adrenal glands and nursing care needed for these clients.

Clinical Objectives

10. Demonstrate competency in blood glucose monitoring.
11. Demonstrate an understanding of normal lab values when assessing clients with an endocrine disorder.
12. Provide nursing interventions to prevent complications of diabetes mellitus.
13. Develop teaching care plans for clients with endocrine disorders.
14. Demonstrate competence in postoperative care of a thyroidectomy client.
15. Demonstrate competence in the care of a client who has undergone a parathyroidectomy.

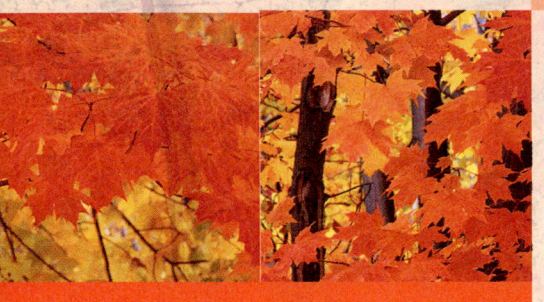

BRIEF Outline

Structure and Function of the Endocrine System
ENDOCRINE DISORDERS
Pituitary Disorders
Thyroid Disorders
Parathyroid Disorders
Diabetes Mellitus
Adrenal Gland Disorders
Gonads

KEY TERMS

Use the audio glossary feature on the MyNursingKit Website to hear the correct pronunciation of the following key terms.

acromegaly 1055
Addisonian crisis 1078
cardiomegaly 1055
Chvostek's sign 1059
cretinism 1060
dawn phenomenon 1073
diabetic ketoacidosis 1074
dwarfism 1056
endocrine glands 1049
exocrine glands 1049
exophthalmos 1058
gigantism 1055
goiter 1060

gonadotropins 1054
hepatomegaly 1055
homeostasis 1049
hormones 1049
hyperglycemia 1064
hyperosmolar hyperglycemic nonketotic coma 1069
hypoglycemic 1055
insulin resistance 1067
ketones 1074
myxedema 1060
myxedema coma 1060
negative feedback 1052

pheochromocytoma 1080
polydipsia 1056
polyphagia 1067
polyuria 1056
somatotropin 1054
Somogyi effect 1073
target cells 1049
tetany 1059
thyroid storm 1058
thyrotoxicosis 1058
tropic hormones 1052
Trousseau's sign 1059

The endocrine glands regulate and integrate all body functions. Disorders result from a hypersecretion or hyposecretion of the hormones released by the glands. Many factors can influence hormonal imbalance such as tumors, infections, surgical removal, and overstimulation or understimulation by an indirect hormone.

Structure and Function of the Endocrine System

The endocrine system is made up of small glands that maintain and achieve **homeostasis** (balance) in the body. From the 4-ounce pancreas to the pea-sized pineal, these glands work with the circulatory and nervous systems to control the body. The endocrine glands include the pituitary, pineal, thyroid, parathyroids, thymus, pancreas, adrenals, ovaries, and testes (Figure 38-1 ■). Table 38-1 ■ lists the endocrine organs and their function. *Note:* The gonads (ovaries and testes) are discussed in depth in separate chapters. Chapter 40 ∞ covers the reproductive system and its disorders.

Glands are categorized into two groups: endocrine and exocrine glands. The ductless **endocrine glands** secrete substances directly into the blood, which circulate to target cells in the body. These substances, called **hormones,** are chemical messengers that function individually, in conjunction with another hormone, or as part of interconnected actions. **Target cells** are cells found in target organs that are influenced either by neurotransmitters or hormones. An example of an endocrine gland is the thyroid gland, which secretes thyroid hormones directly into the bloodstream. The hormones then affect target cells in various tissues throughout the body. **Exocrine glands** secrete substances through ducts that reach the epithelial surface inside the

body or on the skin. An example of an exocrine gland is a sweat gland. It produces fluid that is secreted through ducts to the surface of the skin. Some glands function as both endocrine and exocrine glands. An example of this is the pancreas. The pancreas releases pancreatic enzymes through a

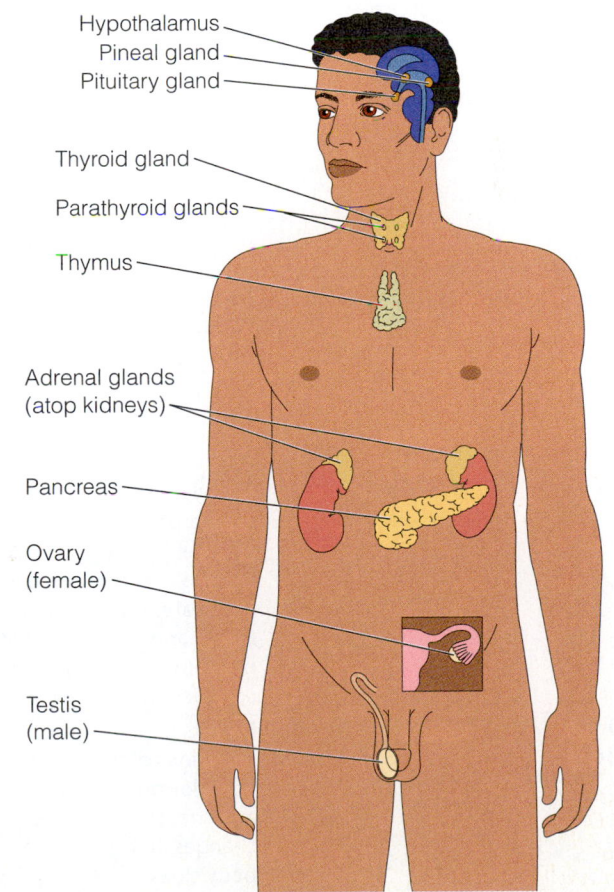

Hypothalamus
Pineal gland
Pituitary gland
Thyroid gland
Parathyroid glands
Thymus
Adrenal glands (atop kidneys)
Pancreas
Ovary (female)
Testis (male)

Figure 38-1. ■ Location of the major endocrine glands.

TABLE 38-1		Endocrine Glands and Functions		
GLAND	**HORMONE**	**FUNCTION**	**HYPERSECRETION**	**HYPOSECRETION**
Pituitary gland	**Anterior pituitary:** *Indirect-acting hormones*			
	Thyroid-stimulating hormone (TSH)	Stimulates the thyroid gland to release T_3, T_4	Hyperthyroidism	Hypothyroidism
	Adrenocorticotropic hormone (ACTH)	Stimulates the adrenal cortex to release cortisol and aldosterone	Cushing's syndrome—muscle weakness and wasting, osteoporosis; thin, easily bruised and infected skin, poor wound healing, ecchymosis, purple striae, hirsutism, emotional lability, psychoses, peptic ulcer, hypertension, renal calculi, polyuria, polydipsia, glycosuria, hypokalemia, hypernatremia, truncal obesity, oligomenorrhea or amenorrhea, impotence, decreased libido	Addison's disease—delayed wound healing, hyperpigmentation, postural hypotension, arrhythmias, tachycardia, lethargy, tremors, emotional lability, confusion, weakness, muscle wasting, joint and muscle pain, anorexia, nausea and vomiting, diarrhea, menstrual changes, hyperkalemia, hyponatremia, hypoglycemia
	Follicle-stimulating hormone (FSH)	Stimulates the ovaries and testes to release hormones		Inhibits sexual development and causes sterility
	Luteinizing hormone (LH)	Stimulates the ovaries and testes to release hormones		Inhibits sexual development and causes sterility
	Direct-acting hormones			
	Growth hormone (GH)	Stimulates body growth, bones, muscles, and tissues	Gigantism, abnormally tall, body is normally proportioned Acromegaly—enlarged extremities, peripheral nerve damage, headaches, hypertension, congestive heart failure, seizures and visual disturbances, impaired glucose tolerance, and diabetes may occur; arthralgia	Growth retardation and short stature
	Prolactin (PRL)	Stimulates breast milk production	Irregular or absent menses, difficulty in becoming pregnant and decreased libido, postpartum female failure to lactate Men—decreased libido, impotent	
	Posterior pituitary:			
	Antidiuretic hormone (ADH)	Stimulates reabsorption of water by the kidneys	SIADH fluid volume excess, hyponatremia, brain cells swell causing headaches, changes in mental status or personality, lethargy, irritability	Diabetes insipidus, fluid volume deficit
	Oxytocin	Stimulates the uterus and prostate contraction	Causes inappropriate ejection of milk in lactating women	May cause prolonged or difficult labor and delivery
Pineal gland	Melatonin	Inhibits the secretions of the gonadotropins and affects changes in the body clock mechanism	Causes winter depression	

TABLE 38-1	Endocrine Glands and Functions (continued)			
GLAND	HORMONE	FUNCTION	HYPERSECRETION	HYPOSECRETION
Thymus gland	Thymin	Blocks the transmission of neuromuscular nerve impulses	Severe muscle weakness	
	Thymosin	Develops the immune system		Depressed immune system
Thyroid gland	Thyroxine (T_4)	Regulates the rate of metabolism	Hyperthyroidism, Graves' disease	Preadult cretinism, (adult) myxedema, goiter
	Triiodothyronine (T_3)	Regulates the rate of metabolism, principal hormone	Goiter; dyspnea, nausea/vomiting, diarrhea, abdominal pain, muscle wasting, fatigue, hand and eye tremors, nervousness, insomnia, emotional lability, hyper-reflexive, blurred vision, photophobia, lacrimation, exophthalmos (Graves' disease), hypertension, tachycardia, palpitations, amenorrhea/decreased fertility (women), decreased libido/impotence (male); fine, thin hair; flushed, moist skin; hyperthermia, diaphoresis, hunger, weight loss, fluid volume deficit	Goiter, pleural effusion, constipation, muscle stiffness, weakness, fatigue, hand and foot paresthesias, lethargy, somnolence, confusion, decrease reflexes, slow speech, memory impairment, periorbital edema, hypotension, bradycardia, dysrhythmia, enlarged heart, anemia, hair loss, brittle nails, coarse dry skin, nonpitting edema, hypothermia, anorexia, weight gain, systemic edema, menorrhagia/infertility (female), decreased libido (male)
	Calcitonin	Decreases calcium in the blood by redirecting it back into the blood	Hypocalcemia	Hypercalcemia
Parathyroid gland	Parathormone (PTH)	Maintains calcium and phosphate balance in the body	Bone pain (back, joints, shins), pathological fractures (women), muscle weakness, muscle atrophy, renal calculi, polyuria, polydipsia, abdominal pain, peptic ulcer, pancreatitis, nausea, constipation, dysrhythmias, hypertension, paresthesias, depression, psychosis, acidosis, weight loss	Muscle spasm, facial grimacing, carpopedal spasms, tetany or convulsions, brittle nails, hair loss, dry, scaly skin, abdominal cramps, malabsorption, dysrhythmias, paresthesias (lips, hands, feet), irritability, depression, anxiety, hyperactive reflexes, psychosis, intracranial pressure
Adrenal gland	**Cortex:**			
	Glucocorticoids (cortisol)	Involved in carbohydrates (CHO), protein, and fat metabolism and the body's reaction to stress	Cushing's syndrome	Addison's disease
	Mineralocorticoids (aldosterone)	Regulates how electrolytes are processed	Increased water retention	Abnormal water loss or dehydration
	Gonadocorticoids	Secretes sex hormones in small amounts		
	Medulla:			
	Epinephrine	Increases body metabolism rate, fight-or-flight reaction	Causes effects of stress	No significant effect

(continued)

TABLE 38-1	Endocrine Glands and Functions (continued)			
GLAND	**HORMONE**	**FUNCTION**	**HYPERSECRETION**	**HYPOSECRETION**
	Norepinephrine	Contracts the blood vessels, increases the blood pressure, slows the GI tract, and dilates the pupils		
Pancreas	Insulin	Moves glucose out of the blood and into the cells	Severe insulin shock hypoglycemia	Diabetes mellitus
	Glucagon	Targets the liver to release glycogen	Uncertain	Uncertain
	Somatostatin	Interferes with the release of GH and glucagon		
Ovaries	Estrogen	See Chapter 40 🔗	Premature sexual development in females and infertility	Lack of sexual development, infertility, and osteoporosis
	Progesterone			Sterility
Testes	Testosterone	See Chapter 40 🔗	Premature male sexual development and muscle hypertrophy	Lack of sexual development in males

duct into the duodenum to break down foods for digestion. It also releases insulin directly into the bloodstream to help the body use glucose.

Tropic hormones (indirect-acting hormones) are secreted by one gland and target another endocrine gland, stimulating growth and secretion. For example, thyroid-stimulating hormone is secreted by the pituitary. It is *thyrotropic* (stimulates the target cells in the thyroid gland to release the thyroid hormones). Direct-acting hormones are ones that have a specific local effect. For example, the pancreas releases insulin specifically to affect the level of glucose in the blood.

HYPOTHALAMUS

Although the pituitary gland has been called the "master gland" of the endocrine system, it is itself controlled by the hypothalamus, located at the base of the brain. The hypothalamus is the command center for the autonomic nervous system, which influences involuntary activities. The hypothalamus is joined to the pituitary by nerve fibers and blood vessels. It also produces the hormones vasopressin and oxytocin and then stores them in the posterior pituitary.

Negative feedback is a method by which hormone production is decreased. Generally endocrine glands have a tendency to oversecrete hormones. Then, when the desired effect has been achieved, information is sent back to the gland that enough hormone has been produced. The gland then slows (*inhibits*) further secretions. For example, when the blood level of a certain hormone is high, the hypothalamus

sends the message to decrease the production of that hormone. The endocrine gland responds to that inhibiting factor, and the correct blood level of the hormone is maintained. If the hormone level is low, the hypothalamus sends a message to release more of the hormone.

PITUITARY GLAND (HYPOPHYSIS)

The pituitary, also referred to as the *hypophysis,* is a small but powerful gland. It is well protected, sitting at the base of the skull behind the base of the nose in the sella turcica (Figure 38-2 ■). The pituitary is connected by a projection to the hypothalamus. It has two parts:

- *Anterior pituitary (adenohypophysis),* consisting of 75% of the gland
- *Posterior pituitary (neurohypophysis)* encompassing the remaining 25%

A strip of tissue between the anterior and posterior pituitary is called the pars intermedia.

Anterior Pituitary (Adenohypophysis)

Four tropic hormones secreted by the anterior pituitary are:

- Thyroid-stimulating hormone (TSH), whose target organ is the thyroid gland.
- Adrenocorticotropic hormone (ACTH), which stimulates the adrenal gland.
- Follicle-stimulating hormone (FSH), which targets the ovaries.
- Luteinizing hormone (LH), which targets the testes.

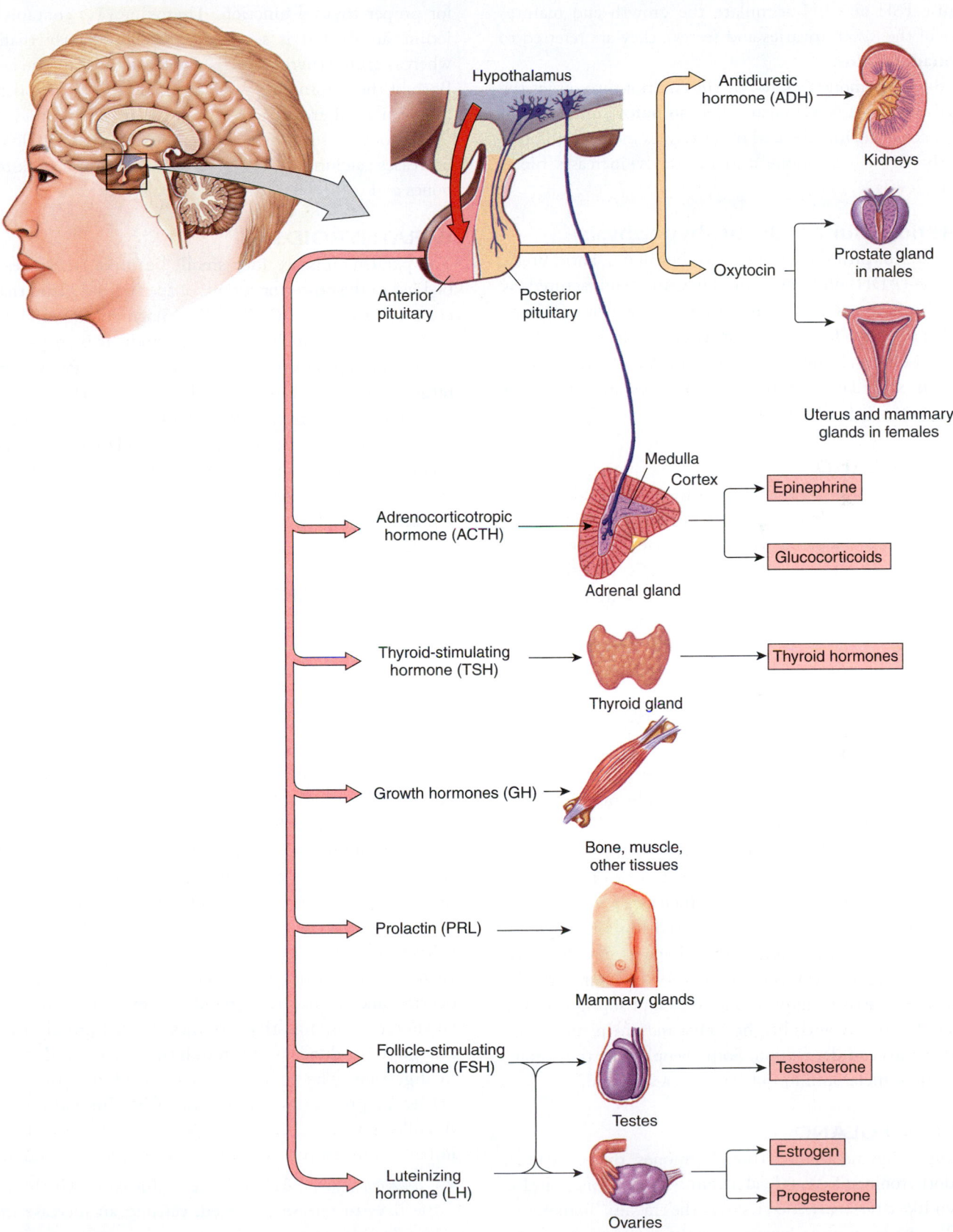

Figure 38-2. ■ Hormones associated with the pituitary gland. (*Source:* Pearson Education/PH College.)

Because FSH and LH stimulate the growth and maintenance of the *gonads* (ovaries and testes), they are referred to as **gonadotropins.**

A direct hormone secreted by the anterior pituitary is the growth hormone (GH) (also called **somatotropin**), which influences bone, muscle, and other tissues included in body growth. Growth hormone also indirectly increases blood glucose levels.

Posterior Pituitary (Neurohypophysis)

The posterior pituitary releases two hormones, antidiuretic hormone (ADH) and oxytocin. They are manufactured by the hypothalamus and stored in the posterior pituitary. ADH is necessary for the reabsorption of water by the distal renal tubules and collecting ducts found in the kidneys. Oxytocin stimulates the prostate in males and the uterus and mammary glands in females.

PINEAL GLAND

The pineal gland is the smallest of the endocrine glands and secretes melatonin. It is a pinecone-shaped gland, approximately the size of a pea. It is thought that the pineal gland affects the thyroid, adrenal cortex, gonads, and the pituitary. Additionally, this tiny gland may secrete as many hormones as the pituitary. However, research continues to determine its exact functions. The pineal gland acts as a matrix for calcium and becomes partially calcified, although this does not affect the hormone secretion.

Hormones secreted by the pineal gland inhibit the secretions of gonadotropins. Hypersecretion of these hormones causes a delay in puberty, whereas hyposecretion results in early puberty. A woman's menstrual cycle may be influenced by pineal gland secretions.

The pineal gland also has an effect on the body clock mechanism, with photoreceptors that react to light filtering through the retina of the eye. Increasing sunlight decreases melatonin production. Decreased sunlight increases melatonin secretion, making the client sleepy. Seasonal affective disorder (SAD) (see Chapter 49 🔗) may be the result of increased melatonin due to lack of sunlight in the winter. Treatment with bright lights may help counteract mood swings and depression. Some people take the dietary supplement melatonin for jet lag or as a sleep aid.

THYROID GLAND

The thyroid gland secretes three hormones: thyroxine (T_4), triiodothyronine (T_3), and calcitonin. The thyroid gland is shaped like a butterfly and sits over the trachea. To make T_3 and T_4, the body must have iodine. In the past, this was a problem for people who lived in areas where the soil was deficient in iodine. However, now iodine is added to table salt. This "iodized salt" supplies the iodine needed by the body

for proper thyroid function. Thyroxine (T_4) contains four iodine atoms and is secreted more abundantly than T_3, whereas triiodothyronine (T_3) contains three iodine atoms. Both of these hormones regulate the rate of metabolism, as well as normal growth and development. The thyroid gland stores hormones and releases them when needed. Calcitonin decreases calcium in the blood by redirecting it back to the bones and is discussed more in the next section.

PARATHYROIDS

The parathyroids are four small, beanlike structures embedded in the posterior surface of the thyroid gland that secrete parathormone (PTH). This hormone maintains calcium and phosphate balance in the body. It is an antagonist to calcitonin produced by the thyroid gland. Parathormone targets the bones, kidneys, and intestinal cells to increase the calcium level in the blood. PTH targets the kidneys to increase phosphate excretion. When PTH levels rise, phosphate is excreted and the blood level of phosphate decreases. Calcium is needed for normal neuromuscular activity, cell permeability, blood clotting, and certain enzyme functions.

THYMUS GLAND

The thymus gland consists of two lobes located in the mediastinum beneath the sternum. This gland is larger and more active in children and then begins to atrophy at puberty. The thymus produces two hormones: thymosin and thymin. *Thymosin* has an essential role in the development of the immune system. Immature T-lymphocytes migrate to the thymus gland from the bone marrow, spleen, and lymph nodes. There, the thymosin causes the T-lymphocytes to mature. The second hormone, *thymin,* blocks the transmission of neuromuscular nerve impulses. Increased levels of thymin produce the severe muscle weakness that is found in myasthenia gravis (discussed in Chapters 35 and 36 🔗).

PANCREAS

As mentioned earlier, the pancreas functions as both an endocrine and an exocrine gland. Its exocrine function involves secreting digestive enzymes and sodium bicarbonate that go to the duodenum through the pancreatic duct to aid in digestion. The endocrine function of the pancreas involves the production and release of insulin and glucagon. A collection of cells, called the islets of Langerhans, is imbedded in the pancreas and secretes three hormones:

- *Glucagon.* The *alpha cells* secrete glucagon, which targets the liver to release glycogen, causing an increase in the blood sugar.
- *Insulin.* The *beta cells* produce insulin, which moves glucose out of the blood and into the cells. Insulin is an antagonist to glucagon.

■ *Somatostatin.* A lesser known hormone is somatostatin, which causes a **hypoglycemic** (lowered blood sugar) effect by interfering with release of the growth hormone and glucagons.

ADRENAL GLANDS

The adrenal glands (also known as the suprarenals) sit on top of the kidneys. The outer portion is the adrenal cortex, and the inner core is the adrenal medulla. Even though they are one gland, the two portions function very differently. The adrenal cortex secretes three groups of hormones, known as the *corticosteroids*.

The glucocorticoids, mainly cortisol (hydrocortisone), are involved in carbohydrate, protein, and fat metabolism and the body's reactions to physical and mental stress. Glucocorticoids also stimulate the liver to release glucose when energy is needed. Glucocorticoids are targeted by ACTH from the anterior pituitary gland. The mineralocorticoids, mainly aldosterone, regulate how electrolytes are processed, and gonadocorticoids (sex hormones), both male and female hormones, are produced in small amounts.

The adrenal medulla secretes *epinephrine* (adrenalin) and *norepinephrine* (noradrenalin). These hormones, also referred to as *catecholamines,* are neurotransmitters. They are released during the "fight-or-flight" reaction when the brain perceives a threat to the body. Approximately 75% of the secretion is epinephrine; the remaining 25% is norepinephrine.

The chief function of epinephrine is to increase body metabolism. It can produce a dramatic jump in the metabolic rate. It causes rapid gluconeogenesis to raise the blood glucose for energy needs. It inhibits gastrointestinal activity, constricts arterioles in the skin causing pallor, but dilates the blood vessels to the muscles, liver, and bronchus. Vasodilatation of the cardiac vessels allows increased activity and cardiac output. People sometimes say, "That got my adrenalin going!" when there is a sudden loud noise or they narrowly avoid an accident. Adrenalin (epinephrine) works very quickly in such situations to allow for "fight or flight."

Norepinephrine causes contraction of blood vessels and an increase in the blood pressure. It also increases heart activity, inhibits gastrointestinal (GI) action, and dilates the pupils for a wider vision range. The effects of norepinephrine last about 10 times longer than epinephrine because it is more slowly removed from the blood. The adrenal glands and their secretions are essential to life.

ENDOCRINE DISORDERS

Endocrine disorders are basically an imbalance of the hormones. These diseases result from a hyposecretion or hypersecretion of hormones from the glands. Factors that can produce imbalance of the hormones include tumors, infections, surgery involving a gland, congenital disease, and increased or decreased stimulation of the target gland by the anterior pituitary.

Pituitary Disorders

ANTERIOR PITUITARY DISORDERS

Hyperpituitarism

When the pituitary secretes too much growth hormone, it results in changes to the skeleton. If this occurs prior to closure of the epiphyses in the bones, the child will have a condition referred to as **gigantism.** Its cause is usually a tumor of the pituitary or malfunction of the hypothalamus.

MANIFESTATIONS. The characteristic symptom of this disorder is that the person reaches a height of 7 feet or taller. Accelerated skeletal growth causes pain, headache, and muscle weakness. The increased amounts of growth hormone also cause **cardiomegaly** (enlarged heart) and **hepatomegaly** (enlarged liver).

If the secretion of too much growth hormone occurs after the client is an adult, the condition is referred to as **acromegaly.** Acromegaly is usually caused by a benign tumor or hypothalamic malfunction. The adult's height does not change because the epiphyses have closed, but the long bones widen and the feet and hands enlarge. The face takes on a coarse appearance with a bulbous nose, thickened lips, and protruding forehead and jaw. Internal organs become enlarged and the client may complain of muscle weakness and arthritis symptoms. The client may have difficulty chewing and swallowing. Visual disturbances and headaches may occur if a tumor is present. Male impotence and female amenorrhea may also occur. Diabetes is a secondary condition that may result because growth hormone increases blood glucose levels.

DIAGNOSIS AND TREATMENT.   These conditions are diagnosed by testing serum levels of growth hormone, and using x-rays and scans to detect a pituitary tumor. If a tumor is found, it may be irradiated to decrease the size. If surgery is required, the tumor is removed through the sphenoid (the procedure is called a *transsphenoidal hypophysectomy*). If the whole pituitary gland must be removed, the client will need lifelong hormone therapy. Surgical removal of the tumor stops soft tissue changes, but the bone changes are permanent. Bromocriptine (Parlodel) may be used to decrease the GH levels but has no effect on the tumor size.

Hypopituitarism

When the pituitary does not secrete enough growth hormone, the resulting condition is **dwarfism.** The child's growth is stunted but the body is proportional. This condition is most often caused by a tumor of the pituitary gland.

MANIFESTATIONS. With hypopituitarism, the child grows to be 3 to 4 feet tall without treatment. Sexual development may be delayed.

DIAGNOSIS AND TREATMENT. To diagnose this condition, serum GH levels are checked and x-rays and scans done to detect the presence of a tumor. A GH stimulation test may be done to observe a response to induced hypoglycemia. Hypopituitarism is treated by replacing growth hormone with a synthetic form. The injections are given until the client reaches a short average stature. Surgery to remove the tumor may be indicated.

Nursing Considerations

When caring for clients with hypo/hyperpituitarism, keep in mind that the conditions are opposites. Assess children for appropriate growth and development whenever health care is given. Report any deviations from normal. Assess adults for symptoms of acromegaly: headache, visual changes, diabetes mellitus, and difficulty chewing and swallowing. Administer injections of growth hormone or pituitary hormone as ordered. Provide emotional support for clients and families because these conditions affect appearance and self-esteem.

POSTERIOR PITUITARY DISORDERS

Syndrome of Inappropriate Antidiuretic Hormone

When the posterior pituitary gland secretes too much antidiuretic hormone (ADH), it causes too much water to be reabsorbed by the kidneys into the bloodstream. This fluid overloads the bloodstream, diluting the blood and decreasing the osmolarity. This condition is known as the syndrome of inappropriate ADH (SIADH). Often, SIADH is caused by a brain tumor that increases ADH secretion. However, certain types of cancers in the lung, duodenum, and pancreas can release an ADH-like substance and cause SIADH. It can also be caused by some medications, such as tricyclic antidepressants. A client who has head trauma or had brain surgery may have a temporary increase in ADH production.

MANIFESTATIONS. Clients with SIADH gain weight without edema. Because the blood is so dilute due to excess fluid, even normal sodium levels look like hyponatremia.

The client may have symptoms associated with hyponatremia, such as increased blood pressure, muscle weakness, nausea, and headache. Urine is concentrated because the kidneys are reabsorbing more fluid than is needed, and urine output is decreased. The urine specific gravity is very high, at 1.030 or above. The excess circulating fluid affects the brain, causing cerebral edema, lethargy, seizures, coma, and even death.

DIAGNOSIS AND TREATMENT. To diagnose SIADH, serum and urine levels of sodium are tested. Osmolarity concentrations are calculated. A "water load test" may be conducted and will show retention of water when SIADH is present. The client is checked for other possible sites of ADH secretion.

The client with SIADH must be on a strict fluid restriction. Hypertonic saline fluids are ordered to counteract hyponatremia. Diuretics, such as Lasix, are ordered and Declomycin may be ordered to block the action of ADH. If a tumor is discovered, it may be removed surgically.

Diabetes Insipidus

When the posterior pituitary does not secrete enough antidiuretic hormone, the condition is known as diabetes insipidus (DI). Without enough ADH, the kidneys do not reabsorb enough water, resulting in large amounts of dilute urine output. Diabetes insipidus may be caused by a tumor in the pituitary gland, intake of glucocorticoid medications, or intake of alcohol. Head trauma can induce diabetes insipidus, but it can be reversed with treatment. When clients with DI are treated with ADH replacement therapy, a side effect can be the symptoms of SIADH.

clinical ALERT

Avoid confusing diabetes insipidus with diabetes mellitus. Although they both contain the word *diabetes* and both have **polyuria** (excessive urination) as a symptom, they are very different disorders. Diabetes insipidus is caused by lack of ADH, produced by the posterior pituitary gland. Diabetes mellitus is caused by a lack of insulin, produced by the pancreas.

MANIFESTATIONS. Clients with DI may urinate from 3 to 15 liters in a 24-hour period. They drink large amounts of fluid (**polydipsia**) and may have an intense desire for ice water. Urine osmolarity is low, while serum osmolarity is high. The urine specific gravity is so dilute it resembles water at 1.000. (See normal characteristics of urine in Table 39-2 .) Signs of dehydration, such as hypotension, weakness, tachycardia, dry skin, dry mucous membranes, and skin turgor tenting, may occur with increased fluid loss. If the client is not treated, hypovolemic shock may ensue and result in death.

DIAGNOSIS AND TREATMENT. Diabetes insipidus is diagnosed based on symptoms exhibited and serum osmolarity levels. Urine specific gravity levels of less than 1.005 are an indication of DI. Scans are done to diagnose a pituitary gland tumor. A "water deprivation test" may be performed. The client takes in no fluids for 8 hours. If DI is diagnosed, the client will continue to lose weight and will have dilute urine even without fluid intake.

Replacement of ADH is the treatment of choice for DI. It is given as aqueous vasopressin (Pitressin), a synthetic form, or desmopressin (DDAVP), a nasal spray. Sodium is restricted. Electrolytes and fluids are replaced by intravenous infusion, using 0.45% sodium chloride. If the pituitary is partially secreting ADH, the medication Diabinese (chlorpropamide) is used to stimulate further ADH production.

OXYTOCIN DISORDERS

Oxytocin initiates contraction of the muscles in the uterus during labor and in the mammary gland in lactation. Hypersecretion is rare; hyposecretion is countered with synthetic Pitocin to induce contraction during labor.

NURSING CARE

PRIORITIZING NURSING CARE

When you care for clients with posterior pituitary disorders, focus your care on maintaining fluid balance. Measure intake and output immediately using a graduated container for accuracy. Assess clients frequently for signs of dehydration (concentrated urine, dry skin, cracked lips) or overload (edema, crackles in the lungs, weight gain). Check the client's level of consciousness every 4 hours and report a decrease in responsiveness immediately.

ASSESSING

On admission, a thorough history will be taken to determine problems with weight gain or loss, fluid intake, amount of output, and signs of pituitary tumor including headaches and visual disturbances. Measure children's height and weight and compare them to growth charts. Ask clients about menstrual irregularities or problems with impotence that may suggest hormonal imbalance. Note the appearance of adults, especially enlargement of the skull, hands, and feet (acromegaly). Collect data on vital signs, noting any abnormal findings.

DIAGNOSING, PLANNING, AND IMPLEMENTING

Nursing diagnoses common to clients with pituitary disorders are:

- *Deficient (or Excess) Fluid Volume*
- *Risk for Disproportionate Growth*
- *Delayed Growth and Development*
- *Impaired Urinary Elimination*
- *Ineffective Coping*

Desired outcomes for clients with pituitary disorders might include:

- Client will maintain fluid volume balance.
- Client will experience appropriate growth and development for age.
- Client's urinary elimination will reach normal levels with medication.
- Client will express an understanding of disorder and medical regimen.

Monitoring of clients with pituitary disorders is an important nursing function. Other interventions for these clients include:

- Measure client's weight gain or loss daily. *Weight gain or loss indicates fluid volume deficit or excess.*
- Monitor intake and output closely and document carefully. *I&O is important data and is also a measurement of the effectiveness of treatment.*
- Implement safety measures for clients with visual disturbances, eating difficulties, and muscle weakness. *The nurse is responsible for client safety.*
- Monitor blood glucose levels and check for changes in neurologic status every 2 to 4 hours. *The client's status may change rapidly.*
- If clients have had surgery to remove a tumor through the sphenoid (transsphenoidal hypophysectomy), assess postoperatively for neurologic changes and monitor the nasal dressing for increased drainage. Teach the client to avoid sneezing, coughing, bending, or straining to have a bowel movement. Provide stool softeners and medication to control coughing as ordered. *These activities could cause increased pressure to the surgical site.*

For Clients with SIADH

- Auscultate lung sounds and measure weight as ordered. *Weight gain and moist lung sounds can alert the nurse to fluid volume excess.*
- Maintain the physician orders for fluid restriction. Monitor serum sodium and urine values, urine specific gravity, and osmolarity. If the client is on fluid restriction, offer frequent oral care, ice chips, and hard candy. *These can alleviate thirst while keeping fluid intake low.*
- If the client requires sodium, offer broth, soft drinks, and tomato juices. *Foods and fluids high in sodium can be used to counteract hyponatremia.*
- Be alert for diminishing level of consciousness (LOC) or seizure activity. Promote safety measures. *Clients with decreasing LOC and seizures can be easily injured.*
- Observe for polyuria and polydipsia. *Symptoms of diabetes insipidus can result when treatment is given to suppress ADH.*

- Determine the client's knowledge level about disease, compliance, and treatment. *Client teaching starts at the client's current level of knowledge. Client understanding about the disease is important to long-term health.*

For Clients with Diabetes Insipidus

- Observe for poor skin turgor and dry skin and mucous membranes. *Dehydration is a frequent problem for clients with DI.*
- Check vital signs frequently for decreasing blood pressure and increasing heart rate. *Hypovolemic shock can result from excess fluid loss.*
- Monitor urine specific gravity, urine and serum osmolarity, and electrolytes, keeping the physician informed of changes. Observe for changes in the level of consciousness. *Such changes indicate a worsening condition.*
- Reinforce the necessity of a low-sodium diet. *Decreasing sodium helps decrease hypernatremia.*
- Determine the client's level of understanding of the DI disease process and treatment. *Client teaching is essential to compliance.*
- Clients with pituitary disorders often have symptoms that are noticeable to everyone. This can result in a lack of coping skills if the clients feel socially isolated. Allow clients to verbalize and discuss feelings. Provide support and comfort measures. Assist the client and family to cope and understand the medication plan, and develop strategies to increase self-esteem and positive body image. Provide the client and family with information regarding support groups. *The nurse may be the person the client and family turn to for emotional support and coping strategies.*

EVALUATING

The nurse reviews the client outcomes to determine which have been met. Close and frequent evaluation is necessary, because client condition can change rapidly. Promptly report changes in LOC or electrolyte balance. Inquire whether client and/or family have been referred to local support groups.

Thyroid Disorders

HYPERTHYROIDISM (GRAVES' DISEASE)

Primary hyperthyroidism is due to oversecretion of T_3 and/or T_4, which in turn increases the client's metabolic rate. Hyperthyroidism can be caused by a tumor, goiter (enlarged thyroid), or autoimmune disorder. Treatment of hypothyroidism with thyroid hormones can cause symptoms of hyperthyroidism if the dose is too high. Untreated, hyperthyroidism can lead to cardiac dysrhythmias or even cardiac arrest.

Manifestations

Hyperthyroidism can have a wide range of signs and symptoms (Figure 38-3 ■). Due to an increased metabolic rate, the client may experience cardiovascular symptoms of tachycardia, palpitations, hypertension, and dysrhythmias. Other symptoms include heat intolerance, nervousness, tremor, and emotional lability. The most visible sign is **exophthalmos** (bulging eyes) resulting from enlarging tissue behind the eyes (Figure 38-4 ■). The client may not be able to close the eyelids over the eyes, leading to possible infection, corneal dryness, or ulceration. Although the appetite increases, the client continues to lose weight. The client may also experience fatigue, weakness, diarrhea, and diaphoresis.

Diagnosis and Treatment

Serum levels of T_3 and T_4 are elevated in hyperthyroidism. TSH is low in primary hyperthyroidism. A *thyroid scan* may be performed to detect a tumor.

To reduce the excessive secretion of thyroid hormones, antithyroid medications (such as Tapazole) are used to inhibit thyroid hormone production. However, Tapazole cannot affect hormones already stored for release. Iodine medications, such as potassium iodide, suppress the release of thyroid hormones and decrease the vascularity of the gland. Potassium iodide is given to ready the gland for surgery. Beta-adrenergic blockers, such as Inderal, are used to relieve thyrotoxicosis (a severe form of hyperthyroidism). Radioactive iodine (RAI or I-131) may be used to irradiate the gland and destroy thyroid cells, thereby decreasing thyroid hormone production. After this type of therapy, the client may become hypothyroid and require lifelong hormone replacement therapy.

If medications are unable to control hyperthyroidism, surgery may be indicated. Table 38-2 ■ lists common thyroid medications. Before surgery, antithyroid medications and iodine are given to suppress the thyroid to normal hormone production. The most common surgical procedure is a subtotal *thyroidectomy*. A subtotal removal allows the gland to continue to produce thyroid hormones. However, a total thyroidectomy may be performed if the tumor is large. When a total thyroidectomy is performed, lifelong hormone replacement is necessary.

Complications of Thyroid Surgery

Thyrotoxicosis (**thyroid storm** or *thyroid crisis*) is a severe form of hyperthyroidism that can occur when clients' hyperthyroidism is left untreated or after thyroid surgery. The manipulation of the thyroid gland during surgery causes it to dump a large amount of thyroid hormone into the bloodstream at one time, causing extreme symptoms (*thyrotoxicosis*). The symptoms of thyrotoxicosis include tachycardia, hypertension, and elevated temperature.

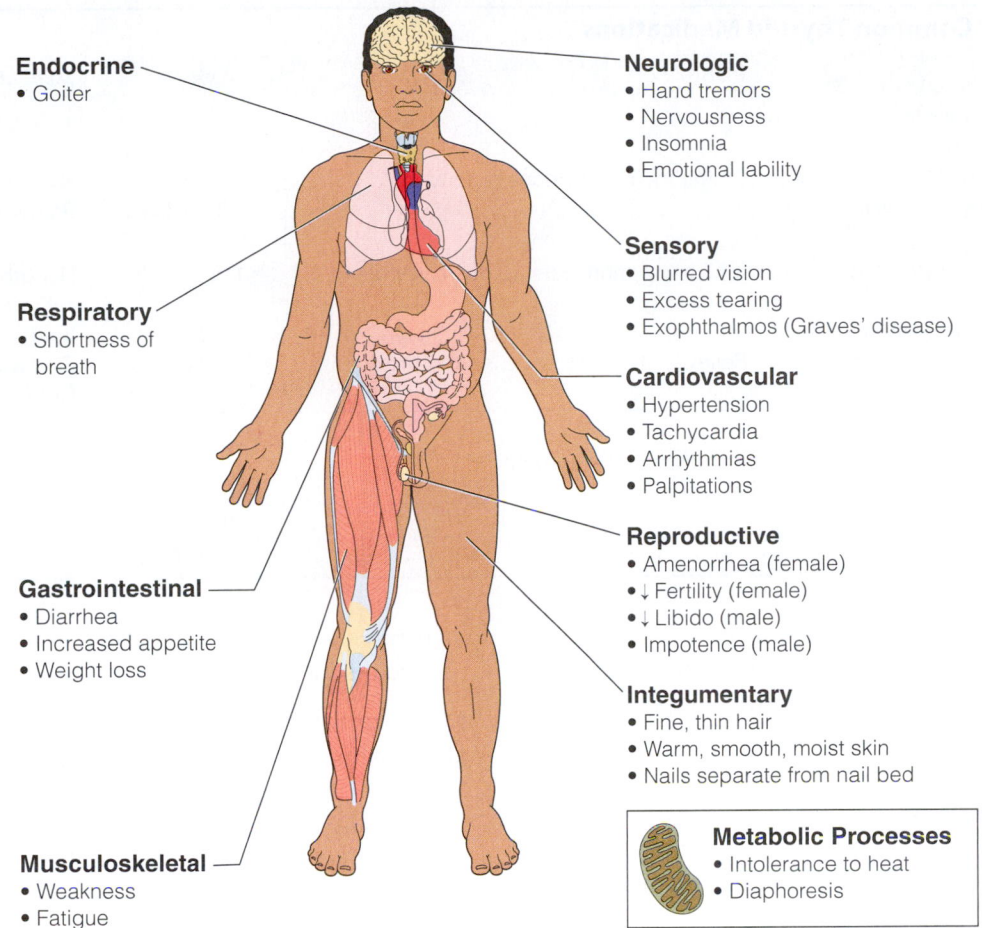

Endocrine
- Goiter

Respiratory
- Shortness of breath

Gastrointestinal
- Diarrhea
- Increased appetite
- Weight loss

Musculoskeletal
- Weakness
- Fatigue

Neurologic
- Hand tremors
- Nervousness
- Insomnia
- Emotional lability

Sensory
- Blurred vision
- Excess tearing
- Exophthalmos (Graves' disease)

Cardiovascular
- Hypertension
- Tachycardia
- Arrhythmias
- Palpitations

Reproductive
- Amenorrhea (female)
- ↓ Fertility (female)
- ↓ Libido (male)
- Impotence (male)

Integumentary
- Fine, thin hair
- Warm, smooth, moist skin
- Nails separate from nail bed

Metabolic Processes
- Intolerance to heat
- Diaphoresis

Figure 38-3. ■ Multisystem effects of hyperthyroidism.

clinical ALERT

Thyrotoxicosis is a life-threatening situation and is treated immediately with antithyroid medications, beta-adrenergic blockers for hypertension, and antipyretic medication for the fever. The client with thyrotoxicosis can progress quickly to seizures and coma.

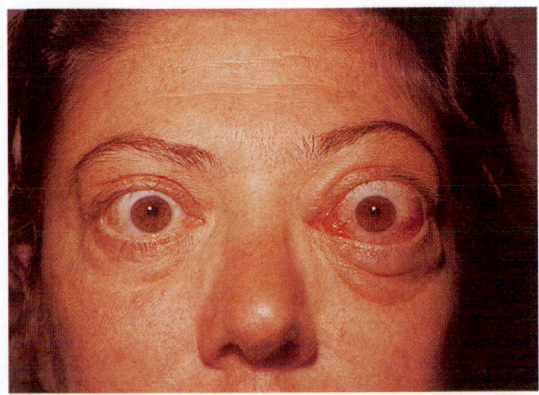

Figure 38-4. ■ Exophthalmos in a client with Graves' disease. The disease causes edema of fat deposits behind the eye and inflammation of the extraocular muscles. The accumulating pressure forces the eyes outward from their orbits. (*Source:* University of Illinois, Custom Medical Stock Photo, Inc.)

Respiratory distress may occur after thyroid surgery due to edema or internal bleeding. The client may have unstable vital signs, with respiratory effort being especially increased. Changes in respiratory rate and depth, along with restlessness, are indications of respiratory distress. It may be necessary for the physician to perform an emergency tracheostomy at the bedside if this occurs.

Clients who hemorrhage after thyroid surgery usually do so within the first 48 hours. Signs of shock and excessive bleeding on the dressing or behind the head may be the first indications of hemorrhage.

Laryngeal nerve damage can occur as a result of the surgery. The client will experience changes in voice quality and hoarseness if laryngeal nerve damage has occurred.

Because the parathyroid glands are very close to the thyroid, one or more may be accidentally removed with thyroid tissue during surgery. Because the parathyroids regulate calcium levels, their removal causes hypocalcemia. **Tetany** (muscle spasms) is the cardinal sign that removal of parathyroid glands has occurred. **Chvostek's sign** (lip and facial spasm occurring when the facial nerve is tapped) and **Trousseau's sign** (carpal spasm occurring

TABLE 38-2	Common Thyroid Medications		
DRUG	**PURPOSE**	**DOSAGE**	**SIDE EFFECT**
Treatment of Hyperthyroidism			
Antithyroid Medications			
Tapazole (methimazole)	Inhibit thyroid hormone production	15–60 mg	Hypothyroidism
Propyl Thyracil (propylthiouracil)		300–900 mg	Bradycardia
Iodine			
SSKI/potassium iodide, saturated solution	Inhibits hormone release, decreases gland vascularity	1–5 gtt	Hypothyroidism Fatigue, weight gain
Lugol's solution/iodine solution		50–250 mg	Bradycardia
Beta-Adrenergic Blockers	Relieves thyroid storm/crisis/thyrotoxicosis	40–240 mg	Bradycardia
Inderal (propranolol)			Fatigue, weakness
Treatment of Hypothyroidism			
Thyroid Drugs	Increase thyroid hormone blood levels		
Synthroid (levothyroxine)		50–125 mcg	Hyperthyroidism
Levothroid		50–60 mcg	Insomnia, palpitations
Cytomel (liothyronine sodium)		25–50 mcg	Nervousness, weight loss

when the blood flow is constricted to the lower arm) are indicators of low calcium levels (Figure 38-5 ■). Intravenous calcium gluconate or calcium chloride is kept available in case of emergency.

HYPOTHYROIDISM

When the thyroid gland does not make enough thyroid hormone, the condition is known as hypothyroidism, or **myxedema.** When this condition occurs in infancy, it is called **cretinism.** Hypothyroidism may be due to a congenital anomaly when it occurs in infants. In adults, it can be the result of an autoimmune disorder (Hashimoto's thyroiditis), iodine deficiency, antithyroid medications, or thyroidectomy. Primary hypothyroidism is most common in women between 30 and 60 years of age. **Goiter** is enlargement

(hyperplasia) of the thyroid gland, which is working overtime to produce thyroid hormones (Figure 38-6 ■).

Manifestations

Hypothyroidism slows the body's metabolism, causing lethargy, personality changes, dull facial expressions, and *periorbital edema* (edema around the eyes). Weight gain, constipation, weakness, hair loss, and nonpitting edema are noted. In fact, the symptoms are the opposite of those of hyperthyroidism. Bradycardia, hypotension, and dysrhythmias occur due to cardiac involvement. The client is intolerant of cold.

MYXEDEMA COMA.   **Myxedema coma,** a severe form of hypothyroidism, occurs more often in winter and affects clients older than 60. It can be life threatening and requires

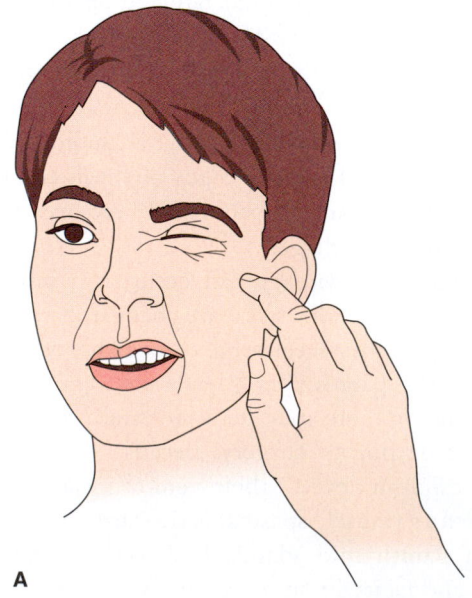

A

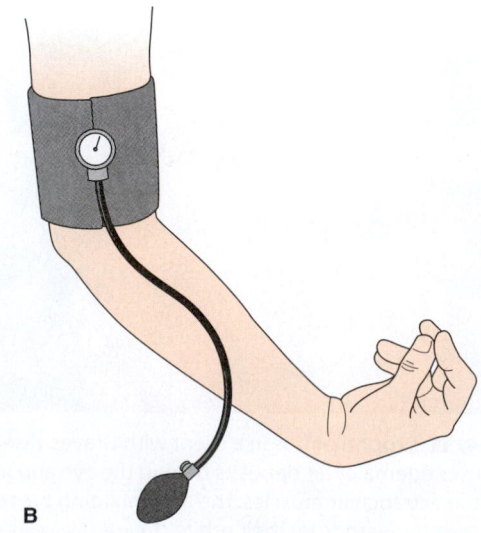

B

Figure 38-5. ■ **A.** Positive Chvostek's sign. **B.** Positive Trousseau's sign. Both of these signs indicate a calcium imbalance.

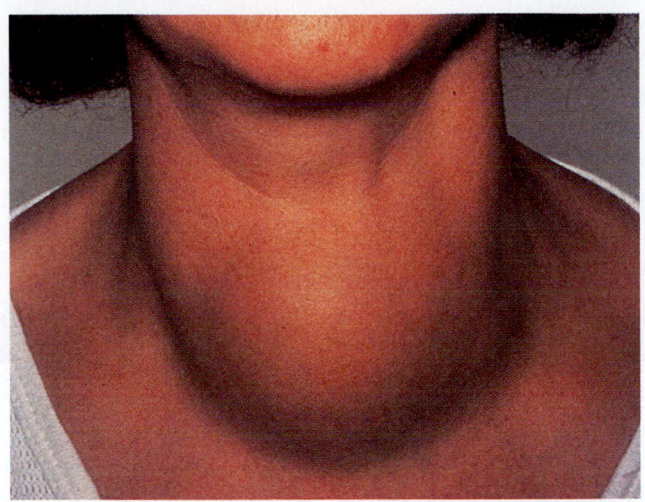

Figure 38-6. ■ Toxic multinodular goiter. The formation and growth of numerous nodules in the thyroid gland cause the characteristic massive enlargement of the neck. (*Source:* Custom Medical Stock Photo, Inc.)

immediate medical intervention. Lethargy progresses to hypothermia and coma. If untreated, the major body systems begin to shut down. Immediate treatment involves establishing a patent airway, providing cardiac support, and administering intravenous hormone replacement.

Diagnosis and Treatment

Diagnosis of myxedema is made by determining serum levels of T_3 and T_4, which are low. TSH is elevated because the pituitary is attempting to stimulate the thyroid to secrete hormones. Cholesterol levels should be monitored for changes. Hypothyroidism is treated with thyroid replacement hormone (levothyroxine). Doses usually start low and progress to a dose that eliminates the symptoms of hypothyroidism.

HASHIMOTO'S THYROIDITIS

Hashimoto's disease is an autoimmune disorder that causes an inflammation of the thyroid gland. The immune system creates antibodies that inappropriately attack the thyroid gland, damaging the cells and causing an imbalance of chemical reactions of the thyroid hormones. Some scientists believe that a virus or bacterium might trigger this response, whereas others think it is a genetic disorder. It is thought that more than one factor may be involved, such as heredity, sex, and age. This disease is common in middle-aged women and tends to be familial. Also known as chronic lymphocytic thyroiditis, it leads to an underactive thyroid gland. Hashimoto's is the most common cause of hypothyroidism in the United States.

Manifestations

Signs and symptoms progress slowly over a number of years and are the same as hypothyroidism. Fatigue and sluggishness are many times attributed to aging but are the initial

symptoms. Forgetfulness, slowed thought processes, and depression may ensue.

Diagnosis and Treatment

Screening and diagnosis involve checking TSH, which is usually elevated, whereas T_3 and T_4 are lowered. A blood antibody test will be performed. Treatment is replacement therapy with the thyroid hormone. Without treatment, the thyroid gland may become hypertrophied, causing goiter (enlargement of the thyroid gland). Other complications include heart disease, mental health changes, and myxedema, a life-threatening condition related to long-term hypothyroidism that can result in a coma. Babies born to women with untreated hypothyroidism have a higher risk of birth defects.

THYROID CANCER

Thyroid cancer is a rare disorder but the risk for it increases with age. It is treated with surgery to remove the gland, and lifelong hormone replacement therapy is necessary. See Chapter 45 ⚭ for information about cancer and its treatment.

NURSING CONSIDERATIONS

When you care for clients with thyroid disorders, focus your care on nutritional needs and comfort. Encourage appropriate food intake: frequent intake of high-calorie, high-protein foods for hyperthyroidism, and high-fiber, low-calorie foods for hypothyroidism. Remember these disorders are exact opposites. Institute comfort measures: a cool, calm environment for hyperthyroidism, and a warmer, more stimulating environment for hypothyroidism. Another major focus of care is detecting symptoms of overtreatment that cause manifestations of the opposite disorder.

Parathyroid Disorders

HYPERPARATHYROIDISM

Overactivity of the parathyroids and increased secretion of PTH results in hyperparathyroidism. Calcium levels are increased and phosphorous levels are decreased in the blood. Calcium moves out of the bones and into the bloodstream. Parathormone promotes the excretion of phosphorus in the urine. The cause of hyperparathyroidism is typically a benign tumor or hyperplasia of the gland. This disease occurs more often in older adults and is more common in women than men.

Manifestations

Clients with hyperparathyroidism complain of low back pain, pathologic fractures, and renal calculi related to the decalcification of the bone and increased blood calcium. High calcium levels cause decreased muscle tone and increased muscle weakness. Polyuria, abdominal pain, nausea, vomiting, and constipation may be reported. Depression, psychosis, and coma can also be present. Arrhythmias and hypertension may be noted and can even progress to cardiac arrest.

Diagnosis and Treatment

The condition is diagnosed when high levels of calcium and PTH along with low levels of phosphorus are found in the blood. X-rays may show bone density changes.

Treatment of hyperparathyroidism involves decreasing calcium levels in the blood. Intravenous and oral fluids are given to dilute the blood, thereby lowering the calcium level. Diuretics such as Lasix may be given to increase excretion of calcium in the urine. Calcitonin may be given to prevent calcium release from the bones into the blood. Mithramycin is also used to lower serum calcium levels; only three doses are given because of the toxicity of this drug. If a tumor is present, surgery may be necessary. If possible, a single parathyroid gland is left to secrete adequate levels of PTH.

HYPOPARATHYROIDISM

In hypoparathyroidism, the production of parathormone by the parathyroid glands is deficient. When PTH is low, the calcium levels in the blood are also low (*hypocalcemia*), but the phosphate level rises (*hyperphosphatemia*). Lowered levels of PTH affect kidney regulation of calcium and phosphates. Absorption of calcium through the intestines is decreased.

The common cause of hypoparathyroidism is the accidental removal of the parathyroids during a thyroidectomy.

Manifestations

Hypocalcemia causes *tetany* (continuous muscle spasms), tremors, tingling, and numbness in the lips, hands, and feet. The client may complain of abdominal cramps, hair loss, dry skin, and depression. Cardiac arrhythmias may be noted. As the disease progresses, muscle spasms can result in bronchospasms, laryngeal spasms, convulsions, and death.

Diagnosis and Treatment

Hypoparathyroidism is diagnosed when serum levels of calcium and PTH are low and phosphate levels are high. The normal calcium range is between 8.5 and 10.0 mg/dL and the phosphorous range is between 3.0 and 4.5 mg/dL of blood. Positive Chvostek's and Trousseau's signs are found.

Hypoparathyroidism is treated with intravenous calcium gluconate, oral calcium, and vitamin D supplements. Thiazide diuretics may also be used to reduce calcium excretion in urine. One temporary way to stabilize the calcium level is to have the client breathe into a paper bag, causing acidosis and increasing serum calcium ionization.

NURSING CONSIDERATIONS

When caring for clients with parathyroid disorders, focus on monitoring vital signs and electrolyte levels, especially calcium. Check vital signs every 4 hours (or more frequently if the client is unstable). Watch for foods high in phosphorus and low in calcium for clients with hyperparathyroidism. Monitor intake for foods high in calcium and low in phosphorus for clients with hypoparathyroidism.

NURSING CARE

PRIORITIZING NURSING CARE

Be ready for emergencies. Have IV calcium and a tracheostomy set at the bedside of every client who has had thyroid surgery. Keep IV calcium at the bedside for clients who have a diagnosis of hypoparathyroidism.

ASSESSING

On admission, a thorough history will be taken to determine problems with sleeplessness, restlessness, heat or cold intolerance, unexplained weight gain or loss, fatigue, back pain, kidney stones, pathologic fractures, muscle weakness, or depression. The nurse takes vital signs to assess for irregular pulse, tachycardia, bradycardia, hypotension, or hypertension. Observe clients for evidence of periorbital edema or exophthalmos. Ask about muscle spasms, numbness, or tingling in the extremities. Check lab work for hypercalcemia or hypocalcemia and hyperphosphatemia or hypophosphatemia, as well as for increased or decreased hormone levels of T_3, T_4, and PTH. If a client has had a subtotal or total thyroidectomy, observe closely for signs of hypoparathyroidism. Assess for positive Chvostek's and Trousseau's signs (see Figure 38-5).

DIAGNOSING, PLANNING, AND IMPLEMENTING

Potential nursing diagnoses for clients with thyroid and parathyroid disorders include:

- *Risk for Decreased Cardiac Tissue Perfusion*
- *Risk for Imbalanced Body Temperature*
- *Imbalanced Nutrition: Less than Body Requirements*
- *Imbalanced Nutrition: More than Body Requirements*
- *Risk for Injury*

Client outcomes for individuals with thyroid and parathyroid disorders might include the following:

- Client will remain free of arrhythmias.
- Client will express that cold intolerance has decreased.
- Client will maintain balanced electrolytes.
- Client will remain free of injury from fractures or falls.

Imbalances of the thyroid and parathyroid glands can have serious consequences. The nurse must remain alert when caring for these clients. Various interventions include the following:

- Monitor vital signs for changes and heart sounds for arrhythmias. *Thyroid and parathyroid imbalances affect vital signs, heart rhythm, and cardiac output.*
- Monitor lab values daily and report abnormal values. *Changes in hormone levels can occur rapidly with hormone replacement therapy or overproduction of hormones.*
- Weigh clients daily. *This helps the healthcare team determine if the client's intake meets or exceeds energy needs.*
- Check environment often to see that the temperature is comfortable for the client. *Heat or cold intolerance is typical of thyroid disorders.*

For Clients with Hyperthyroidism

- Monitor intake and offer frequent high-calorie, high-protein diet and snacks. *This is done to counteract the severe weight loss.*
- Instruct client to avoid high-roughage foods and caffeine. *These foods increase GI motility.*
- Monitor and limit stimulation, and provide rest periods during the day and between activities. *The client needs to conserve energy as much as possible.*
- Offer cool showers and a change of clothing when perspiration is excessive. *Hyperthyroidism often causes heat intolerance.*
- Instruct in relaxation techniques. *This helps the client slow activities and be calm.*
- Determine the extent of visual disturbance and discomfort and report to the physician and RN. *Exophthalmos can cause many visual complications.*
- Reinforce instruction regarding disease, treatment, and medications. *The client will need frequent reminders and explanations regarding her diagnosis and care.*
- Allow the client to verbalize feelings and anxieties. *The nurse is often a major support person during diagnosis and illness.*
- If the client is treated with RAI, increase fluid intake. Limit client contact during this treatment, and explain to the client why this is necessary. *Increased intake helps flush the RAI from the body. It is necessary for nurses to protect themselves from undue exposure to the radiation.*
- Instruct the client to flush the toilet twice after use. Nurses should do the same when emptying bedpans. Plastic utensils and disposable dishes are used. *These precautions help reduce any chance of radiation contamination.*

For Clients with Hypothyroidism

- Offer a high-fiber, low-calorie diet with adequate fluids. *This will combat weight gain and the constipation symptoms of hypothyroidism.*
- Administer stool softeners and laxatives as ordered. *This helps maintain regular GI elimination.*

- Promote activity to the level of the client's ability. Alternate activity and rest periods. *These precautions help avoid cardiac stress.*
- Monitor the client's orientation level, and reorient as needed. *Hypothyroidism can affect mental status.*
- Instruct the client to be alert for signs and symptoms of hyperthyroidism. *These symptoms can occur when the client is taking an increased dose of hormone replacement medication.*
- Reinforce client instruction about lifelong hormone therapy, disease, and treatment. *When the client understands the treatment plan, compliance improves.*

For Clients with Hypoparathyroidism

- Monitor serum calcium and phosphorous levels. *Instability of these levels can indicate worsening of the condition.*
- Observe for signs and symptoms of tetany, and assess for positive Chvostek's and Trousseau's signs. *These tests help detect hypocalcemia early.*
- Provide instruction in a high-calcium diet. Be aware that some foods high in calcium are also high in phosphorus, such as milk and milk products. Foods such as green leafy vegetables, soybeans, and cauliflower are good sources of calcium without raising phosphorous levels. *Clients with hypoparathyroidism need to raise calcium levels without raising phosphorous levels.*
- Listen to respirations for signs of laryngospasm and bronchospasm. *Either of these complications can lead to respiratory arrest.*

clinical ALERT

Ensure that IV calcium and a tracheostomy set are available for use in an emergency situation. *If the client goes into laryngospasm or tetany, immediate treatment is required.*

- Administer oral calcium and vitamin D as ordered. *Calcium cannot be absorbed from the GI tract without the presence of vitamin D.*
- Provide instruction about disease, treatment, and compliance. *When the client understands the treatment plan, compliance improves.*

For Clients with Hyperparathyroidism

- Carefully monitor for safety measures related to muscle weakness and pathologic fractures. *Clients with hyperparathyroidism are at risk for injury.*
- Encourage rest periods. *The client may be weak and will need to rest.*
- Offer frequent oral fluids and record intake and output. *Fluid volume deficit can be a problem.*
- Observe serum calcium and phosphorous levels for changes. *Changes in these lab values can indicate improvement or worsening of the disease.*

- Provide instruction in a diet high in phosphorus and low in calcium. *Clients with hyperparathyroidism need to increase phosphorus without raising calcium levels.*
- Medicate the client for nausea and pain as ordered. *These side effects may interfere with fluid and food intake.*
- Assess the client for changes in mental status. *Changes in LOC can indicate worsening hyperparathyroidism.*

Care after Thyroid Surgery

- Monitor vital signs frequently, paying particular attention to respiratory rate, depth, and effort. Observe for restlessness, which is an early sign of respiratory distress. Provide oxygen therapy and humidification as ordered. *Edema after thyroid surgery can cause respiratory distress and even arrest.*
- Assess the throat dressing for drainage. Check the back of the neck for drainage. *Bleeding from the throat dressing may pool there and go undetected.*
- Instruct the client to move the head with support to prevent hyperextending the neck. *This can cause pressure on the suture line.*
- Monitor serum calcium levels. *Normal values are 8.5 to 10 mg/dL of blood.*
- Monitor closely for tetany, numbness, and tingling of the extremities. *These symptoms could indicate that the parathyroid(s) have been accidentally removed.*

---

clinical ALERT

Have IV calcium at the bedside in case it is needed immediately. *It will be used to reverse tetany.*

- Always have a tracheostomy set at the bedside. *It will be used immediately if laryngeal edema develops that can block the airway.*

EVALUATING

The client with thyroid/parathyroid disorders will have normal levels of thyroid and parathyroid hormones. The client will also verbalize relief of pain, discomfort, and heat or cold intolerance. Weight will be within normal limits, without unexplained gain or loss.

Diabetes Mellitus

As mentioned, the pancreas is both an exocrine and an endocrine gland. It releases pancreatic enzymes through a duct into the duodenum to break down foods for digestion (exocrine function). It also releases insulin directly into the bloodstream to help the body use glucose (endocrine function). Figure 38-7 ■ illustrates how the hormones of the pancreas work to regulate blood glucose.

Diabetes comes from a Greek word meaning "to siphon" and refers to a primary symptom of the disease, polyuria.

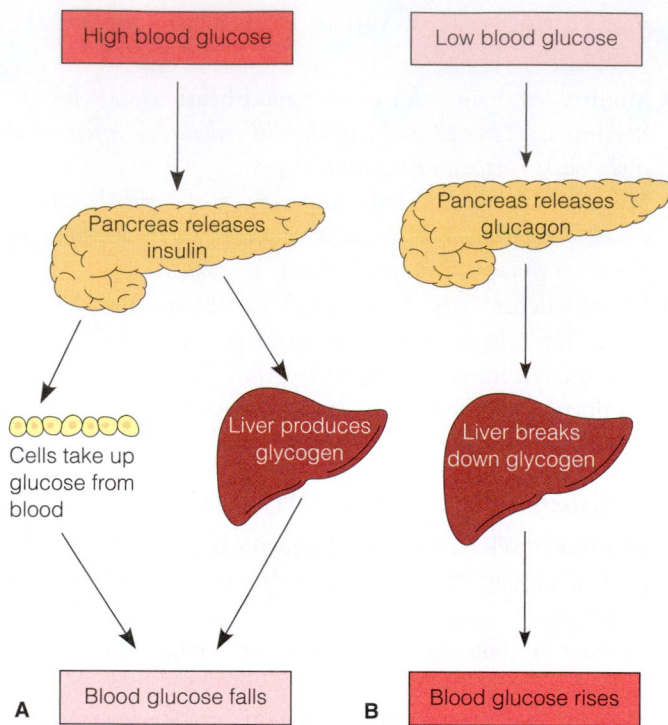

Figure 38-7. ■ Regulation (homeostasis) of blood glucose levels by insulin and glucagons. **A.** High blood glucose is lowered by insulin release. **B.** Low blood glucose is raised by glucagon release.

Mellitus is a Latin word for "sweet" or "honey," referring to sugar in the urine. Diabetes mellitus is described as a group of disorders, with a collection of symptoms that affect multiple body systems (Figure 38-8 ■). The body is unable to metabolize carbohydrates, proteins, fats, and insulin correctly, and this results in glucose intolerance. **Hyperglycemia** (high blood sugar) is caused by lack of an adequate amount of insulin or insufficient insulin action. There is no cure for diabetes, but the ability to control the disease can stop or delay severe complications.

According to the American Diabetes Association, 7% of the population has diabetes mellitus. One-third of these people are undiagnosed. The incidence of diabetes increases with age and is more prevalent in certain groups (Box 38-1 ■). The risk for death in clients with diabetes is twice that of persons without the disease.

OBESITY AND DIABETES

According to the U.S. Department of Health and Human Services, in 1999 13% of children aged 6 to 11 years old and 14% of adolescents from 12 to 19 years of age in the United States were overweight. These figures have doubled in the last 20 years. Type 2 diabetes mellitus was thought to be more of an adult disease; recently there have been dramatic increases in children and adolescents. Obesity and being overweight are closely linked to Type 2 diabetes. Obesity in childhood often precedes insulin resistance syndrome, and

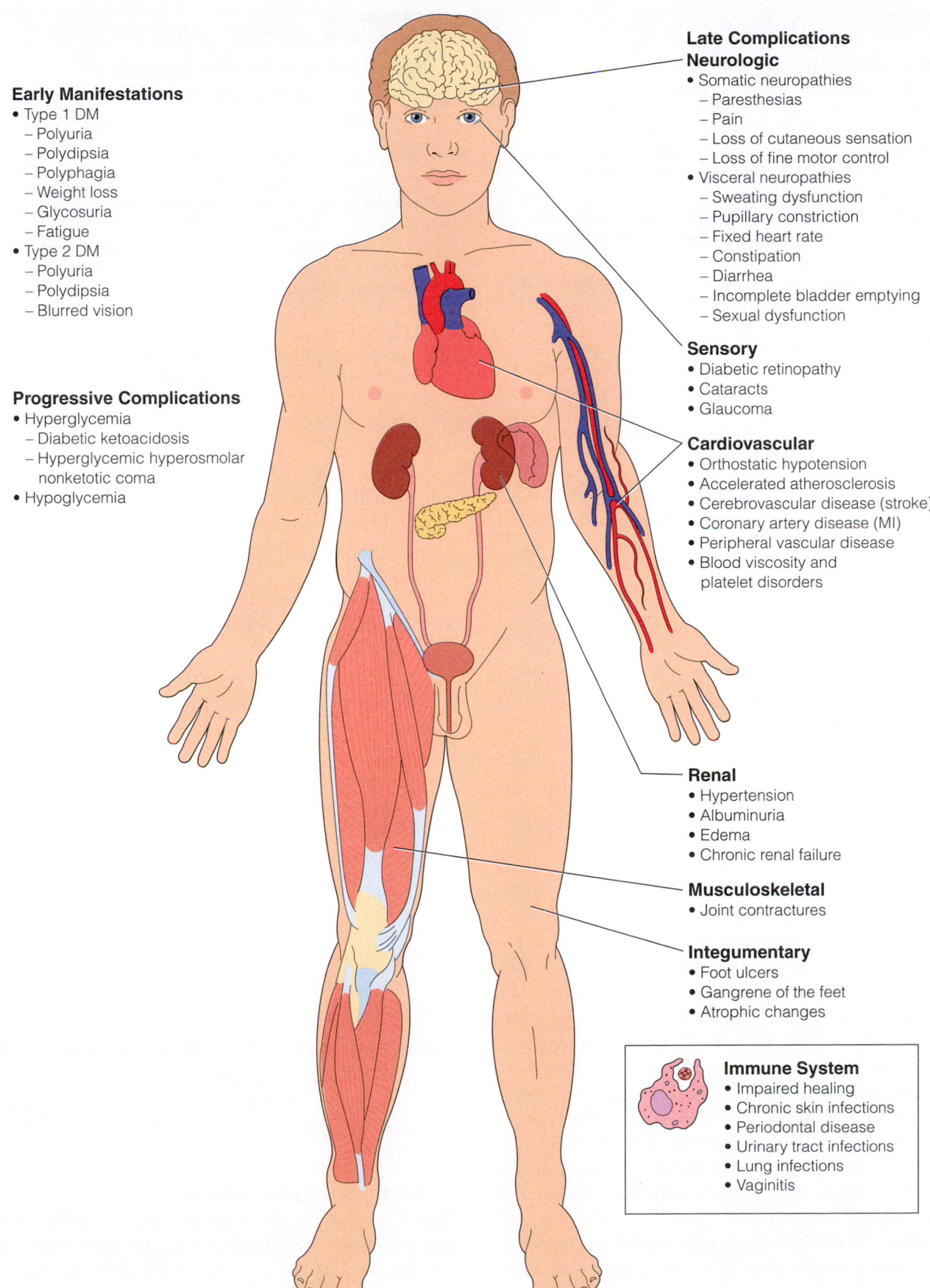

Early Manifestations
- Type 1 DM
  - Polyuria
  - Polydipsia
  - Polyphagia
  - Weight loss
  - Glycosuria
  - Fatigue
- Type 2 DM
  - Polyuria
  - Polydipsia
  - Blurred vision

Progressive Complications
- Hyperglycemia
  - Diabetic ketoacidosis
  - Hyperglycemic hyperosmolar nonketotic coma
- Hypoglycemia

Late Complications
Neurologic
- Somatic neuropathies
  - Paresthesias
  - Pain
  - Loss of cutaneous sensation
  - Loss of fine motor control
- Visceral neuropathies
  - Sweating dysfunction
  - Pupillary constriction
  - Fixed heart rate
  - Constipation
  - Diarrhea
  - Incomplete bladder emptying
  - Sexual dysfunction

Sensory
- Diabetic retinopathy
- Cataracts
- Glaucoma

Cardiovascular
- Orthostatic hypotension
- Accelerated atherosclerosis
- Cerebrovascular disease (stroke)
- Coronary artery disease (MI)
- Peripheral vascular disease
- Blood viscosity and platelet disorders

Renal
- Hypertension
- Albuminuria
- Edema
- Chronic renal failure

Musculoskeletal
- Joint contractures

Integumentary
- Foot ulcers
- Gangrene of the feet
- Atrophic changes

Immune System
- Impaired healing
- Chronic skin infections
- Periodontal disease
- Urinary tract infections
- Lung infections
- Vaginitis

Figure 38-8. ■ Multisystem effects of diabetes mellitus.

BOX 38-1	CULTURAL PULSE POINTS

Deaths from Diabetes Mellitus

Although an estimated 20.8 million people in the United States have diabetes, only 14.6 million people have been diagnosed. Most people affected (20.6 million) are adults over the age of 20. More than half of the people afflicted with diabetes are women. Estimated diabetes costs in the United States in 2002 totaled $132 billion dollars.

Diabetes greatly increases the health risks in people with other disorders. In clients with diabetes, death from heart disease is two to four times higher than in adults without diabetes. Risk of stroke is two to four times higher among people with diabetes than in those without. Diabetes is the leading cause of new cases of blindness among adults 20 to 74 years of age. It is also the leading cause of treated end-stage renal disease with 44% of new cases of ESRD in 2002. Nervous system damage occurs in 60% to 70% of people with diabetes. Sixty percent of nontraumatic lower limb amputations occur among people with diabetes. Diabetes was the sixth leading cause of death on U.S. death certificates in 2002.

Diabetes and deaths related to the disease have some alarmingly high rates in particular cultural groups. Native Americans and Alaskan natives have death rates for diabetes 231% higher than that of the general population. Among Asian/Pacific Islanders, diabetes is the seventh leading cause of death. In African Americans as well as Hispanics, it ranks number 6. Clients from these cultures may look at the disease as an inevitable death sentence. However, with proper care, adherence to diet, and health education, they can live a full life. As with most chronic illnesses, health education is the key.

Source: Data from *National Diabetes Fact Sheet 2005*, American Diabetes Association/CDC.

BOX 38-2	PEDIATRIC CONSIDERATIONS

Healthy Eating to Prevent Diabetes

- Guide family healthy food choices; do not dictate.
- Encourage children to eat when hungry and to eat slowly.
- Eat meals together as a family.
- Decrease fat intake and calories.
- Do not put a child on a restrictive diet.
- Avoid using food as a reward.
- Avoid withholding food as a punishment.
- Encourage the child to drink water and limit beverages with high sugar content.
- Plan for healthy snacks.
- Stock fat-free or low-fat milk, fresh fruit, and vegetables.
- Discourage eating meals or snacks in front of the TV.
- Start the day with a healthy breakfast.

there is an association with hypertension and abnormal lipid levels. Data has shown that weight loss by obese children and adolescents results in a decrease in insulin concentration and improvement in insulin sensitivity.

Overweight adolescents have a 70% risk of becoming overweight or obese adults. That increases to 80% when there is one or more parent that is overweight or obese. This also leads to social discrimination, poor self-esteem, and depression in children and adolescents. The causes of being overweight or obese in the Western world are related to the lack of physical activity, poor eating patterns, or a combination of the two. Genetics and lifestyle are factors that must also be considered. Today's society has become sedentary with television, computers, and video games as the main attractions or distractions for our youth. It is estimated that 43% of adolescents watch 2 hours or more of television per day. Children and especially girls become less active as they progress through adolescence.

The physician will determine whether the child's or adolescent's weight is unhealthy or obese. A tool used is the body mass index (BMI). The BMI is calculated from measurements of height and weight; the physician will also consider age and growth patterns. Testing is recommended for children at significant risk for Type 2 diabetes: children who are overweight, have a family history of diabetes, are predisposed based on race/ethnicity, and display signs of insulin resistance.

It is important to remind parents to tell their children that they are valued and loved whatever their weight is. Children who are overweight need support, encouragement, and acceptance. It is important to focus on the child's positive attributes and health. It is also necessary for the parents to be role models in choosing healthy foods and exercise activities. Box 38-2 ■ lists some guidelines for healthy eating to prevent diabetes in children.

When a child is overweight and still growing, the child doesn't need to lose weight but needs to reduce the rate of weight gain. A diet should be low in calories but not in essential nutrients. Any weight loss program should be gradual and monitored by a physician. It is important to remember that weight lost during a diet is frequently regained unless there are behavior changes, including exercise activities. For many people controlling weight is a lifelong struggle.

CLASSIFICATIONS OF DIABETES MELLITUS

Several types of diabetes mellitus exist. Most common are Type 1 and Type 2 diabetes, but other types include prediabetes, gestational diabetes (see Chapter 52), and secondary diabetes.

Type 1 Diabetes Mellitus

Type 1 is known as *insulin-dependent diabetes mellitus (IDDM)* and was once called *juvenile diabetes*. The term *brittle diabetic* has also been used to describe the client who has wide fluctuations in blood sugars (Figure 39-9 ■). Type 1 affects 5% to 10% of the diabetic population and is usually diagnosed

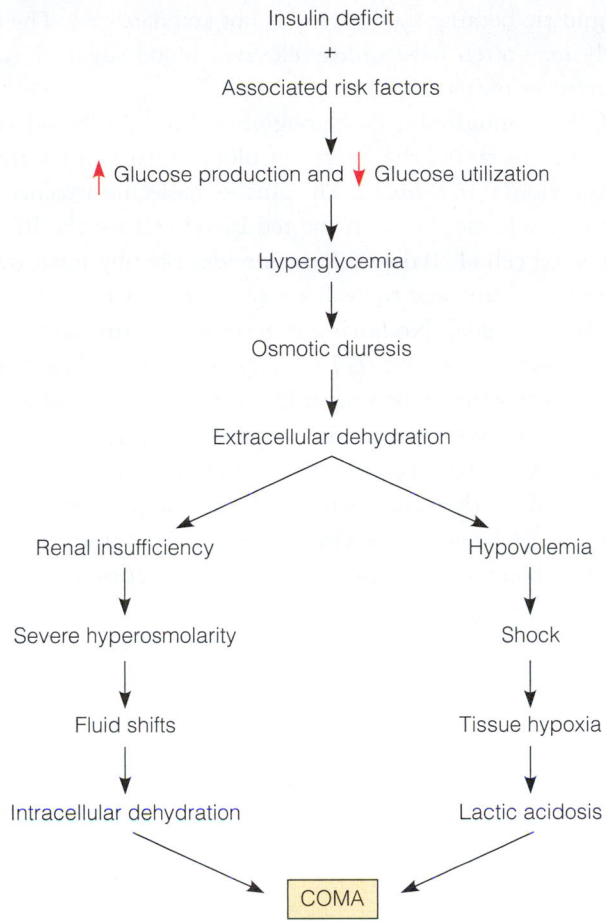

Insulin deficit
+
Associated risk factors

↑ Glucose production and ↓ Glucose utilization

Hyperglycemia

Osmotic diuresis

Extracellular dehydration

Renal insufficiency   Hypovolemia

Severe hyperosmolarity   Shock

Fluid shifts   Tissue hypoxia

Intracellular dehydration   Lactic acidosis

COMA

Figure 38-9. ■ Pathophysiologic results of Type 1 diabetes mellitus.

in clients under age 20, but it can occur at any age. Possible causes of Type 1 diabetes include a virus, an autoimmune reaction, and heredity. The onset is usually abrupt and many times follows a viral infection. These individuals will require lifelong insulin injections.

Type 2 Diabetes Mellitus

Type 2 is known as *non-insulin-dependent diabetes mellitus (NIDDM),* and was once called *mature-onset diabetes.* NIDDM affects 90% of the diabetic population and occurs more frequently in adult females over 40 years of age. However, it can occur at any age, even in children. Heredity and obesity play strong roles in the development of Type 2 diabetes. It develops more slowly than Type 1. The pancreas continues to make insulin but the body's cells are affected by the increased weight and are unable to use the insulin. This is known as **insulin resistance.** Symptoms may go undetected until a routine urinalysis reveals glucose in the urine and further tests are requested. Type 2 diabetes mellitus is usually treated with oral hypoglycemics, although insulin may also be required. Clients with a family history of diabetes are at higher risk for developing diabetes.

PREDIABETES

In the past, the term *borderline diabetic* was used to describe the person with an *impaired glucose tolerance,* now referred to as *prediabetes.* This condition happens when the person's blood sugars are higher than normal but not enough to be diagnosed with Type 2 diabetes; 54 million Americans have prediabetes. Diagnostic findings for this condition include fasting blood sugars that range between 100 and 125 mg/dL on two occasions. The client is most often found to be overweight and have mild hyperglycemia and insulin resistance. This condition is treated by diet modifications that limit carbohydrates and sugars.

GESTATIONAL DIABETES

Gestational diabetes occurs in pregnancy during the final trimester. This may be due to weight gain during pregnancy, resulting in insulin resistance. The disease is usually mild and controlled with diet, however, insulin is occasionally required. Some clients may be asymptomatic and the condition is found in prenatal screening. The incidence of fetal and perinatal complications is increased when the mother has gestational diabetes. Babies may have higher birth weights. Following the pregnancy, the blood sugar returns to normal. The client with gestational diabetes is at increased risk for developing diabetes later in life. Gestational diabetes is discussed further in Chapter 52 ⦿.

SECONDARY DIABETES

Secondary diabetes may result from trauma or disease to the pancreas, such as pancreatitis, pancreatectomy, and cystic fibrosis. Hormonal causes may include acromegaly and Cushing's disease (discussed in this chapter), which affect the blood sugar. Certain drugs such as Dilantin, birth control pills, and steroids may induce diabetes.

Manifestations

Whatever the type of diabetes mellitus, the symptoms and laboratory findings are the same. The most common symptoms are known as the "three Ps":

- *Polyuria* (excessive urination) occurs as the body is trying to eliminate the excess sugar in the blood. Sodium, magnesium, calcium, chloride, potassium, and phosphate are all excreted in the urine in larger amounts than normal.
- *Polydipsia* (excessive thirst) occurs because the body is attempting to counteract the excessive loss of urine. Also, blood viscosity increases as the blood sugar rises, so the body begins to draw fluid from the cells.
- **Polyphagia** (voracious hunger) occurs as the body recognizes the need for energy and demands fuel. The person loses weight because the body is unable to utilize glucose for energy and starts to use the body's fat and protein stores.

Hyperglycemia results from the lack of insulin production. The body feels weak and lacks energy because of the lack of glucose utilization. Blurred vision and headache are other frequent symptoms. Females may experience vulval itching.

The client with Type 2 diabetes may have more symptoms of the complications of diabetes than symptoms of diabetes. For example, it may be complaints of poor vision, leg pain, or impotence that cause the person to seek medical attention. Symptoms such as fatigue, drowsiness after a meal, and irritability develop slowly (Figure 38-10 ■).

Diagnosis and Treatment

Diabetes mellitus is diagnosed with a *fasting blood sugar (FBS)* test done after the client fasts for 8 to 12 hours. The client is instructed not to take medications until after the test is taken. An acceptable FBS level is between 70 and 130 mg. A *postprandial blood sugar* is a measurement taken 2 hours after a regular meal. A range between 140 and 160 mg suggests good blood sugar control. This test is not

diagnostic because food intake is not standardized. The elderly may often have mildly elevated blood sugars 1 to 2 hours after meals.

Glycohemoglobin, or hemoglobin AIc, is a blood test done to determine the degree of blood sugar control from the previous 6 to 8 weeks. The glucose molecule attaches itself to the hemoglobin in the red blood cell for the life of the blood cell (120 days). This provides the physician with a more accurate way to evaluate treatment. A range of 4% to 7% is the goal. No fasting is necessary for this test.

A *glucose tolerance test (GTT)* is an older type of blood test done to determine blood sugar fluctuations. The client eats a high-carbohydrate diet for 3 days prior to the test and limits activity. A fasting blood sugar and urine test is performed for baseline data, then the client drinks a concentrated glucose solution. Blood and urine samples are collected at intervals of one-half hour, at 1, 2, and 3 hours, and sometimes at 4 and 5 hours after ingestion. Medications should not be given during the test. Light activity during this time is recommended.

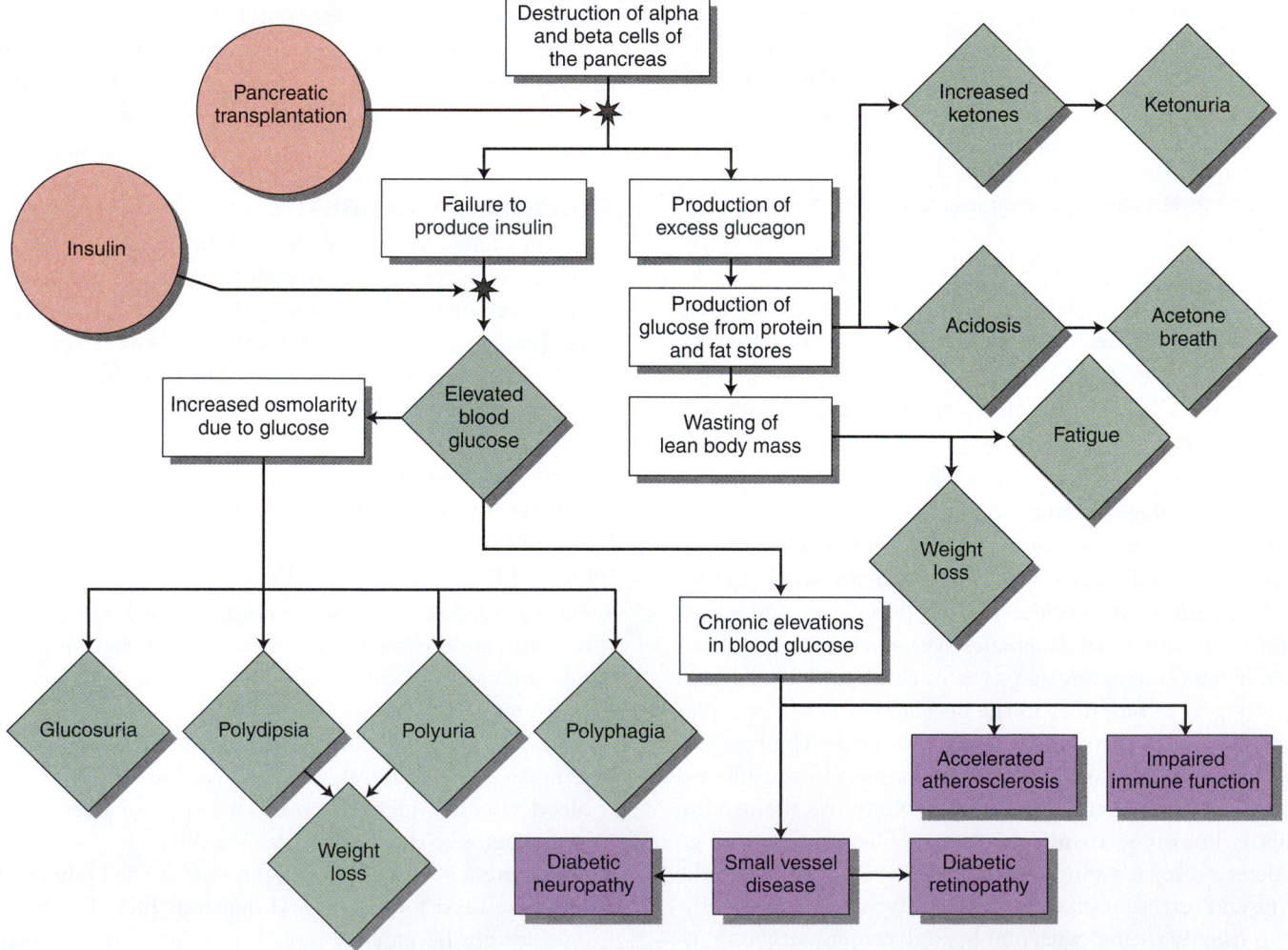

Figure 38-10. ■ Pathophysiology of diabetes mellitus. (*Source:* Adapted from *Medical-Surgical Nursing: Clinical Management for Continuity of Care* [5th ed., p. 1958], by J. M. Black and E. Matassarin-Jacobs, 1997, Philadelphia: Saunders.)

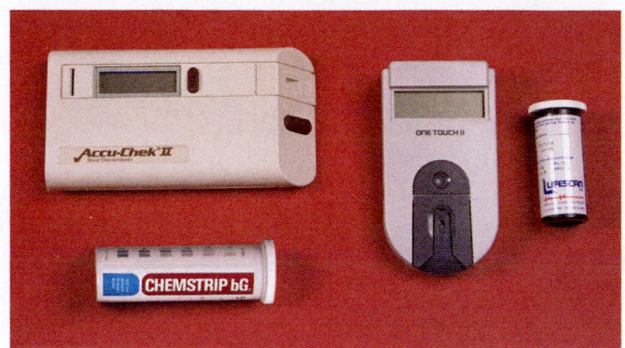

Figure 38-11. ■ Determination of blood glucose levels by visual reading.

A newer and more effective way to determine blood sugar fluctuations is *glucose monitoring,* which is a direct measurement of current glucose control. Procedure 38-1 ■ at the end of this chapter lists the steps in obtaining a blood glucose reading. Physicians are able to adjust the treatment regimen in order to obtain optimal control based on blood sugar readings. The client pricks a finger and obtains a drop of blood, which is placed on a reagent strip and inserted into a glucometer. The blood sugar is displayed in digital readout (Figure 38-11 ■). The newer glucometers are less complex and more operator friendly than those used in the past.

When glucose is found in the urine, it is not a direct measure of the blood sugar. For the glucose to spill into the urine, the blood sugar must be above 180 mg. This is known as the renal threshold. A sugar and acetone (S&A) test may be done on the urine to determine ranges of sugar and identify acetones or fat breakdown. A double-voided urine specimen is used when testing to get the best results. The client is then referred to his or her physician for more specific testing.

The client with Type 2 diabetes is usually overweight, and losing weight becomes part of the treatment plan. Losing weight will lower the blood sugar, blood pressure, and cholesterol. It will also increase the sensitization of the insulin receptor sites, so the client will require less medication. The client with Type 2 diabetes may require insulin in periods of stress, infection, surgery, and illness. **Hyperosmolar hyperglycemic nonketotic coma** (HHNC) occurs when the client with Type 2 diabetes has extreme hyperglycemia.

Diabetes is treated by balancing *food, exercise,* and *medication.* Diet management is a key to diabetic control. The dietitian is a vital member of the interdisciplinary team and works with the physician to determine an individualized diet plan for the client. Diets are based on creating a plan that allows the client to make modifications during times of exercise, illness, pregnancy, and periods of special growth for teens. Type 2 diabetics may need to lose weight and have a calorie restriction. The timing of diet and snacks must coincide with medication action. The client is instructed to avoid skipping or delaying meals and snacks.

A common diet seen in the clinical setting is an 1,800-calorie ADA (American Diabetes Association) diet.

BALANCING FOOD. The exchange system uses the Food Guide Pyramid and includes the six food groups with the needed nutrients to maintain a healthy diet. An exchange is a measured amount of food selected from within one food group. Clients can "exchange" one-half cup of potatoes for one slice of bread. It is important for clients to understand that they can exchange within the food groups but not between the groups. For example, clients cannot exchange one-half cup of potatoes for 3 ounces of meat. All the food groups are needed to provide a healthy nutritious diet. The ADA provides an exchange list of foods to make substitutions and food choices easy.

Foods high in carbohydrates, such as sugars and starches, are broken down by the body to their simplest form, which is glucose. Proteins and fats break down to amino acids and lipids. Dietetic foods, although they are advertised to be low in sugar, may contain more calories than the nondietetic versions. Encourage clients to read nutrition labels on food products and help clients understand what foods increase the blood sugar when metabolized by the body. Nutrition facts found on food products tell the client about the serving size, amount of various nutrients such as total fat, saturated fat, cholesterol, sodium, and fiber per serving. Many noncaloric sweeteners are available that contain very few calories and can be used as desired.

"Free foods" are those that contain 15 to 20 calories per serving. Examples of free foods are dill pickles, sugar-free gelatin, artificially sweetened drinks, and seasonings. "No sugar added" foods may not have sugar added during processing but may still be high in carbohydrates, which ultimately turn into sugar with digestion. Alcohol may cause hypoglycemia because it prevents the body from putting new glucose or sugar into the blood from storage sites in the liver. Clients should not mix alcohol with some oral hypoglycemic medications because it may cause adverse reactions.

Contrary to popular belief, some "fast foods" can be nutritious. Avoid foods high in fat, such as cheeseburgers and French fries. Instead, the client with diabetes can order a salad, diet drink, and a baked potato with light toppings, for example. Many restaurants provide calorie counts for their meals, helping diabetics to make healthy choices. The LPN/LVN reinforces the dietary regimen and focuses education at helping the clients and their families make healthy food choices. Clients need to know that being diabetic does not mean they have to give up all the foods they like, but they must pay attention to the foods they choose to eat.

An alternative diet plan is the glycemic-index (GI) diet. It is a guide in selecting foods, particularly carbohydrates, in meal planning. The glycemic index ranks carbohydrate-containing foods based on the effect on the blood sugar level. Foods with a high glycemic-index value tend to increase the blood sugar more quickly than foods with a lower value. The glycemic-index diet is complicated and there are many factors that affect the value of certain foods, including preparation and what foods are eaten with it. For these reasons the ADA is not recommending this diet at this time.

BALANCING EXERCISE. Exercise is the second important step toward maintaining blood sugar control. For the Type 2 diabetic, exercise coupled with weight loss may be enough to control blood sugar levels. During exercise, body cells become more sensitive to insulin and glucose. The body then burns the sugar for energy and needs less insulin.

Exercise has many benefits, including decreased blood pressure, decreased stress, and lowered heart rate (Box 38-3 ■). Clients with diabetes should discuss their exercise plan with their physician and be consistent in their exercise regimen.

MANAGING DIABETES DURING ILLNESS. There are times when the client with diabetes should avoid exercising and activities. When ill, the person with diabetes will often have increased glucose blood levels, even if not eating. It is important at these times not to omit insulin or oral hypoglycemic medicine. Blood glucose should be monitored every 4 hours, and urine should be tested for ketones if readings are greater than 250 mg/dL. Regular intake of food and fluids is needed: 8 to 10 ounces of fluid each waking hour, and 10 to 15 g of carbohydrate every 1 to 2 hours. If vomiting or diarrhea last more than 6 hours, or the client is unable to eat for more than 24 hours, the client should notify the physician.

BALANCING MEDICATIONS. The third cornerstone to diabetic control is in two medication categories: insulin and oral hypoglycemics. Type 1 diabetics require insulin each

day; Type 2 diabetics may need insulin during times of illness, increased stress, and trauma, but then may return to oral medications alone. The client may be on a combination of different types of insulin. See Table 38-3 ■ for the differences with each type in peak, duration, and use.

In the United States, insulin strength is U 100. This equates to 100 units of insulin in 1 mL. The LPN/LVN must note that there is a specific syringe called an insulin syringe. The U 100 syringe must match the U 100 insulin. Because insulin is inactivated by the digestive juices, it must be injected into the subcutaneous tissue. Directions for administering insulin are provided in Chapter 27. See Procedure 27-2 ⊙⊙ , Preparing Medications, for steps in giving single insulin and mixing two insulins. Injection sites are rotated to prevent induration of the skin (Figure 38-12 ■).

clinical ALERT

Opinions differ about aspirating with insulin. There are blood vessels in the subcutaneous tissue, so the potential for injecting insulin into a blood vessel exists. However rare it might be, such an event would change the effect of the medication. The time it takes to aspirate quickly is worth the precaution. Follow hospital policy when in doubt. When the LPN/LVN is giving insulin, it is a safe practice always to check the dose and amount with another licensed nurse before administering.

The LPN/LVN must know about different insulins and understand the onset, peak, and duration of the insulin that the physician has ordered for the client (Figure 38-13 ■). *Onset* refers to when the insulin begins to take effect. The *peak time* occurs when the medication is most effective and a hypoglycemic reaction is most likely to occur. *Duration* is the length of time that the insulin effect lasts. Rapid-acting insulin, such as lispro insulin or glulisine insulin begin to work about 5 minutes after injection and peaks in one hour, then continues to work for 2 to 4 hours. Regular or short-acting insulin is a clear liquid and may be given subcutaneously or, for faster action, intravenously. This insulin reaches the blood within 30 minutes after injection, peaks anywhere from 2 to 3 hours, and is effective for 3 to 6 hours. Intermediate-acting insulins, such as NPH, have a cloudy appearance and are given subcutaneously. This insulin reaches the bloodstream about 2 to 4 hours after injection, peaks from 4 to 12 hours, and is effective for 12 to 18 hours. Long-acting insulins, such as protamine zinc or ultralente, are not as common as the others. These insulins reach the bloodstream about 6 to 10 hours after injection and are effective 20 to 24 hours. In addition there are combination or premixed insulin: Regular and intermediate-acting insulin are combined in a 70% intermediate-acting and 30% fast-acting ratio. This type of insulin has a quick and

BOX 38-3	BENEFITS OF EXERCISE IN DIABETES

- Reduces blood pressure
- Reduces blood sugar
- Increases circulation
- Increases energy
- Increases lung capacity
- Increases self-esteem
- Lowers the amount of medication needed
- Slows resting heart rate
- Strengthens the heart
- Reduces stress
- Aids in weight loss
- Aids in weight maintenance

TABLE 38-3	Types of Insulin		
INSULIN TYPE	**PEAK**	**ONSET/DURATION**	**USE**
Regular Humanulin R, Novolin R	2–3 hrs	Onset = 0.5–1 hr Duration 5–7 hr	Emergency treatment of diabetic ketoacidosis or coma, used in combination with intermediate-acting or long-acting insulin
Insulin Aspart NovoLog (recombinant analog); faster absorption than regular human insulin	45–90 min	Onset = 15 min Duration 3–5 hrs	Diabetes mellitus
Insulin glargine (Lantus) (recombinant human insulin analog long acting)		Duration 10.4–24 hrs	Bedtime dosing of adults and children with Type 1 or adults with Type 2
Insulin injection concentrated Iletin II Regular	2–3 hrs	Onset = 0.5–1 hr Duration = 5–7 hrs	For occasional client who develops insulin resistance or requires a dose greater than 200u per day
Insulin, Isophane NPH Human N, Novolin N, Novolin 70/30	4–12 hrs	Onset = 1–2 hrs Duration = 18–24 hrs	Control hyperglycemia in diabetic clients
Insulin Lispro Humalog	0.5–1 hr	Onset = <15 min Duration = 3–4 hrs	Treatment of diabetes mellitus—rapid acting
Insulin Protamine Zinc Lenti II	14–24 hrs	Onset = 4–8 hrs Duration = 36 hrs	Diabetes mellitus clients who are not adequately controlled by unmodified insulin
Insulin Zinc Suspension Lente	8–12 hrs	Onset = 1–2 hrs Duration = 1–24 hrs	Hyperglycemia in diabetic clients allergic to other preparations of insulin
Insulin Zinc Suspension extended (Ultralente)	16–18 hrs	Onset 4–8 hrs Duration 36 hrs	DM Type 1
Insulin Zinc Suspension Prompt (Semilente)	4–7 hrs	Onset = 0.5–1 hr Duration 12–16 hrs	Supplement intermediate- and long-acting insulins

longer-term effect for stabilizing blood sugar. Pramlintide is a new synthetic form of the hormone amylin, which is produced along with insulin by the beta cells in the pancreas. Amylin and glucagons work in a related fashion to maintain normal blood glucose levels. Pramlintide injections are taken with meals and have been found to improve amylin insulin cellular (AIC) levels and promote a modest weight loss in clients. Pramlintide must be injected separately and is recommended for Type 1 diabetics who are not achieving their goal AIC levels and for Type 2 insulin-dependent clients who are not achieving glycohemoglobin A1c goals. The first inhalable insulin is coming soon; Exubera has been approved by the FDA. Exubera is a mealtime insulin in powdered form that is taken 10 minutes prior to eating. A capsule is inserted into an inhaler, and the insulin is released from the capsule and inhaled. Exubera takes the place of a rapid-acting insulin only. The client would still need to take longer-acting insulins by injection.

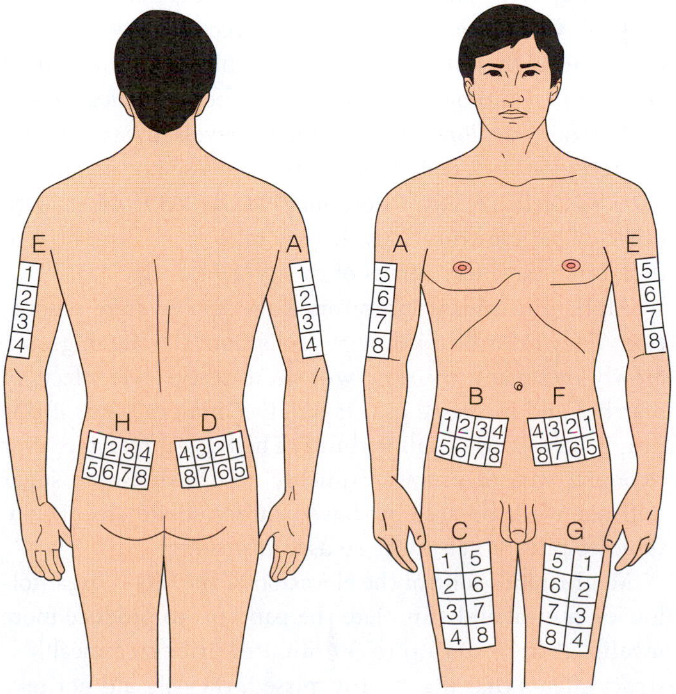

Sliding Scale Insulin. Sliding scale insulin may be ordered in addition to routine morning and evening doses. The insulin given in a sliding scale is always fast-acting (regular) insulin. The nurse checks the blood glucose level with a glucometer and then checks the ordered sliding scale. For example, if a client's blood sugar is 220, and the sliding scale order is for 10 units of regular for a blood sugar between 201 and 250, the nurse would give the client 10 additional units of regular insulin. Glucose monitoring with sliding scale insulin is usually ordered before meals and at bedtime, but it can be used at any time to check the blood sugars. The physician orders the amount of insulin to give depending on the blood sugar level. This is done most often when the client's blood sugar is not well controlled due to illness or stress. An example of a sliding scale is given in Box 38-4 ■.

Figure 38-12. ■ Sites of insulin injection are rotated.

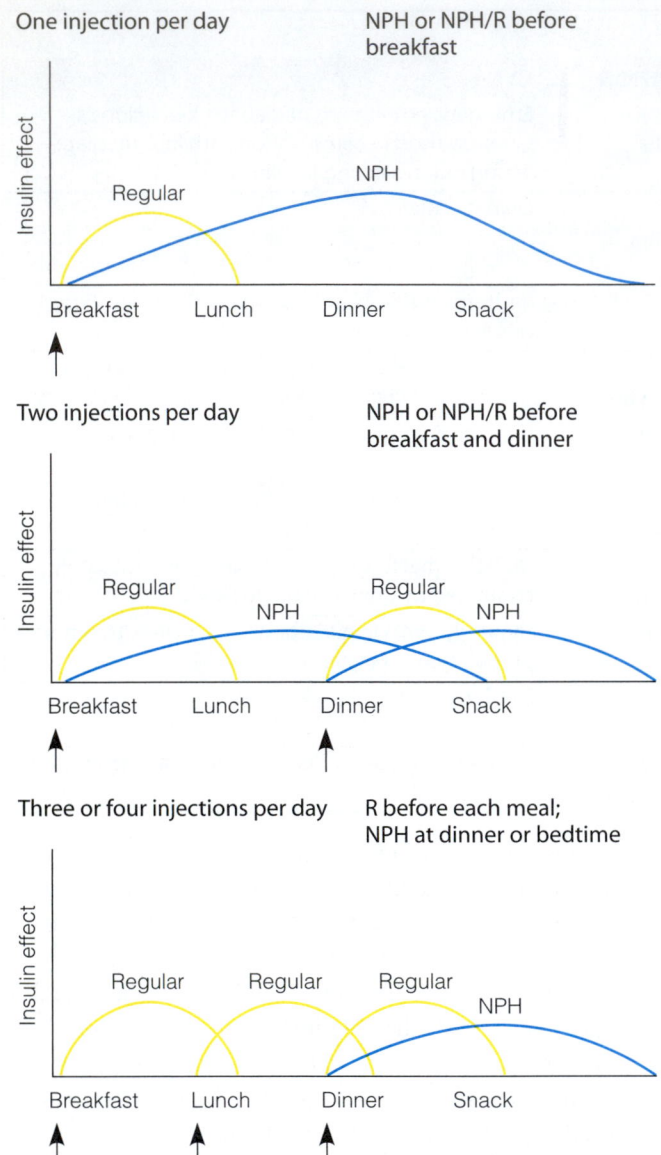

One injection per day   NPH or NPH/R before breakfast

Two injections per day   NPH or NPH/R before breakfast and dinner

Three or four injections per day   R before each meal; NPH at dinner or bedtime

*Insulin types are abbreviated as follows: NPH = intermediate acting, R = regular, rapid acting.

Figure 38-13. ■ Types of insulin regimens. *Top:* NPH (intermediate-acting insulin) *or* NPH with regular insulin are given before breakfast. Afternoon hypoglycemia may result. *Middle:* NPH *or* NPH with regular or premixed insulin is administered before breakfast and before dinner. This regimen, while similar to the body's natural healthy pattern, requires closely regimented eating and exercise. *Bottom:* Regular insulin is administered before each meal. NPH is given at dinner or before bedtime. This regimen allows greater flexibility in exercise and mealtimes, but testing must be done before each mealtime dose.

Insulin Pump. An insulin pump is a portable continuous insulin infusion. It is a battery-operated system the size of a pager and is worn 24 hours a day. A one-day supply of basal insulin is delivered to the body through a butterfly needle inserted under the skin in the subcutaneous tissue. The needle is changed every 1 to 3 days. Additional insulin is given as a bolus at mealtimes. Glucose monitoring is done frequently and the insulin is adjusted to meet the body's

BOX 38-4	SLIDING SCALE EXAMPLE

Accu-Chek AC/HS
0700–1130–1730–2100
Blood glucose under 50 or over 450, call MD
Order Stat Lab B. G.
Sliding Scale Humulin Regular Insulin subQ as follows:
  BG 0–150 mg: no insulin
  BG 151–200 mg: 2 units Humulin R
  BG 201–250 mg: 4 units Humulin R
  BG 251–300 mg: 6 units Humulin R
  BG 301–350 mg: 8 units Humulin R
  BG 351–400 mg: 10 units Humulin R
  BG 401–450 mg: 12 units Humulin R

needs. Studies conclude that diabetics using the insulin pump maintain better blood sugar control.

Clients with Type 2 diabetes are given oral medications if diet and exercise do not control the blood sugar. For these medications to work, the pancreas must produce some insulin.

Oral Medications. Oral medications are not a form of insulin. Rather, they stimulate the pancreas to produce insulin. Oral hypoglycemics also make the cell receptor sites more sensitive to the insulin produced. Sulfonylureas are in the sulfa category and can elicit an allergic reaction. Minor side effects include anorexia, nausea, vomiting, urticaria, and hypoglycemia. If mixed with alcohol Diabinese produces an uncomfortable reaction: face flushing, warm tingling, and burning sensations of the face. Biguanides lower the blood sugar by interfering with the glycogen released by the liver. Glucophage should not be used for a client with poor liver and kidney function. Alcohol should be avoided. Glucophage will lower triglycerides, total cholesterol, and LDL, but increases HDL. This drug can be used alone or in combination with other diabetic medication.

Thiazolidinediones lower glucose levels by sensitizing the receptor sites and allowing the glucose and insulin to enter the cells. A lower dose may be needed if taken with other diabetic medications. It may take up to 3 months to determine the effectiveness of this type of drug.

Alpha-glucosidase inhibitors slow carbohydrate absorption. They must be taken with foods from the starch group. Slowly increasing the dose will decrease the side effects of diarrhea and increased gas. Hypoglycemia can occur if this drug is used with a sulfonylurea. The typical treatment for hypoglycemia of giving a quickly absorbed simple sugar will not work because of slowed carbohydrate absorption. Glucose pills or gels must be used instead.

Meglitinides control the elevation of the blood sugar following a meal and stimulate the pancreas to produce more insulin. Administer up to 30 minutes prior to a meal. Instruct clients that if a meal is missed, they should not take the medication for that meal.

TABLE 38-4	Common Oral Hypoglycemics	
TRADE/GENERIC	DOSAGE (MG)	DURATION (HOUR)
Sulfonylureas		
Diabinese/chlorpropamide	100–250	36+
Tolinase/tolazamide	100–500	12–24
Orinase/tolbutamide	250–500	6–12
Micronase/DiaBeta/ glyburide	1.25–5	24
Glucotrol/glipizide	5–10	40
Biguanides		
Glucophage/metformin	500–1,000	6
Thiazolidinediones		
Avandia/rosiglitazone	2–8	12–24
Actos/pioglitazone	15–45	24
Alpha-Glucosidase Inhibitors		
Precose/acarbose	25–100	2
Meglitinides		
Prandin/repaglinide	0.5–2	1.4

Table 38-4 ■ lists commonly used oral hypoglycemics. Hypoglycemia is a common side effect for many of the drugs discussed (see the later section on Hypoglycemic Reactions).

SHORT-TERM OR ACUTE COMPLICATIONS

Common Blood Sugar Fluctuations

It is difficult to balance the blood glucose and insulin levels. When the client with diabetes is more active than usual, eats less than usual, or eats more than usual, blood sugar control is affected. Likewise, when a client is under extra stress, has surgery, illness, or trauma, blood sugar levels are affected.

Somogyi Effect

The **Somogyi effect** is a normal occurrence. A sudden drop in the blood sugar is followed by a rebound hyperglycemic reaction. The difficulty for the diabetic arises because the treatment for hypoglycemia is sugar that is absorbed quickly. The hyperglycemia is then treated with insulin, causing a yo-yo effect for the client. The treatment is to adjust the insulin amount gradually until the appropriate level is reached.

Dawn Phenomenon

Possibly due to a surge in growth hormone, the blood sugar elevates at approximately 3 A.M. This is referred to as **dawn phenomenon.** The nurse may be ordered to check glucose levels at night, at 3 A.M., and on awakening. The physician makes insulin adjustments and may delay the dinner insulin dosage to an evening dose in an attempt to better control the blood sugar.

Hypoglycemic Reactions

Low blood sugar is also referred to as *hypoglycemia, insulin reaction,* or *insulin shock*. This happens when the blood sugar level drops rapidly or drops to below 60 mg/dL of blood. Hypoglycemia can result from taking too much insulin, not eating enough, or delaying or skipping a meal/snack. Vigorous excessive or unexpected exercise will also lower the blood sugar. A hypoglycemic reaction can occur as a side effect of both insulin and oral hypoglycemics.

MANIFESTATIONS.   The symptoms usually have a rapid onset. The diabetic can experience a few or many of the symptoms. Early signs are cold sweats, clammy skin, shakiness, weakness, and dizziness. The client may be irritable, nervous, and hungry. Numbness and tingling in the tips of the fingers and lips can occur. Headache and blurred or double vision are common.

The brain needs glucose to function effectively. When a hypoglycemic reaction occurs, the client becomes confused, speech is slurred, and personality changes may develop. If untreated, seizures and unconsciousness can occur.

clinical ALERT

The LPN/LVN should report changes signaling a hypoglycemic reaction to the charge nurse and should check the blood sugar immediately. Often diabetics know when they are having a reaction, so be sure to listen to your client.

TREATMENT.   To treat a hypoglycemic reaction, give simple sugars that are absorbed quickly, such as orange, apple, and grape juices. Do not add additional sugar, because it can cause the blood sugar to rise too high too quickly, and then have to be treated with insulin. Regular soda will also elevate the blood sugar. Clients with diabetes should carry a simple sugar to counteract a hypoglycemic reaction. Box 38-5 ■ lists forms of fast sugars. Once the symptoms of hypoglycemia subside, the client should eat a complex carbohydrate such as a sandwich to supply sustained carbohydrates. If the hypoglycemic client is unconscious, do not give oral fluids. The physician may order intravenous dextrose or a glucagon injection. Limit activity to stop energy demands.

BOX 38-5   FORMS OF FAST SUGARS

- Hard candy (Lifesavers, gumdrops, jelly beans)
- Fruit juices (orange, apple, grape)
- Sugar
- Regular soda
- Honey
- Milk
- Cake decorating gel
- Glucose tablets

Diabetic Ketoacidosis

When the blood sugar reaches a very high level, the body begins to form **ketones** as a waste product of breaking down fats for energy. When ketones build up in the blood, the result is **diabetic ketoacidosis** or diabetic coma (see Figure 38-10). This is most commonly seen in Type 1 diabetes. The client experiences nausea and vomiting along with abdominal cramps. Many clients think they have some type of flu. However, as the glucose and ketones in the blood continue to rise, the client develops deep, rapid respirations (Kussmaul respirations) and a fruity smell on the breath due to acetone. If this condition is left untreated, the client can go into a diabetic coma, and death can result.

Hyperosmolar Hyperglycemic Nonketotic Coma

This complication affects Type 2 diabetics between 50 and 70 years of age. Type 2 diabetes is normally mild, but hyperosmolar hyperglycemic nonketotic coma is precipitated by an acute event such as pneumonia, heart attack, and stroke. HHNC can also follow a therapeutic procedure such as dialysis or central line insertion.

MANIFESTATIONS. Hyperosmolar hyperglycemic nonketotic coma causes severe hyperglycemia, altered sensorium, and minimal ketosis. A history of polyuria, inadequate fluid intake, and confusion is noted. If untreated, this condition can lead to coma.

DIAGNOSIS AND TREATMENT. The blood is viscous due to the high level of sugar and ineffective insulin. The hyperglycemia causes osmotic diuresis, resulting in fluid and electrolyte losses and imbalance.

Management involves correcting the fluid volume and electrolyte depletion with intravenous hypotonic saline solution and added electrolytes. Monitor electrocardiograms, telemetry readings, heart rate, and rhythm because these can all be affected by electrolyte imbalances. Insulin is used to control the severe hyperglycemia; the physician may order a sliding scale.

The nurse should observe for signs of hypoglycemia. A client whose blood sugar drops from a high level to a lower level can exhibit signs and symptoms of hypoglycemia even if the blood sugar is not less than 60 to 70 mg/dL.

NURSING CONSIDERATIONS

When you care for clients with diabetes mellitus, make your priorities the monitoring of blood sugar and prevention of complications. Check finger-stick blood sugar (FSBS) before meals and at bedtime or as ordered. Administer sliding scale insulin for elevated FSBS according to orders. Be alert for symptoms of hypo/hyperglycemic reactions. Check finger-stick blood sugar to confirm suspicions

and contact the physician immediately. Keep concentrated sugar on hand to treat hypoglycemia. Be aware of the client's food intake and exercise level when measuring FSBS. Anticipate changes due to imbalances in food, exercise, and medication. Instruct clients with diabetes mellitus about self-care when appropriate.

CHRONIC COMPLICATIONS OF DIABETES MELLITUS

High blood sugar over extended periods of time causes damage to body tissues in the circulatory, renal, and nervous systems, as well as the eyes, teeth, skin, and feet (Figure 38-14 ■). By controlling blood sugar the client can stop, delay, or lessen the severity of chronic complications that accompany diabetes.

Heart and Blood Vessel Complications

Two out of three diabetics die from heart disease and strokes. Heart attacks and decreased circulation to the legs and feet are a primary concern for clients with diabetes. Uncontrolled blood sugar contributes to atherosclerosis at an early age that can progress to circulatory compromise and amputation for lower extremities. Impaired circulation causes paleness of the lower extremities, reduced pedal pulses, and poor capillary refill. There may be loss of hair on the dorsal side of the foot. The toenails are thickened and brown spots are noted on the skin of the legs.

Renal Complications

The kidneys have an extensive vascular system and elevated blood sugar causes extra work for the kidneys, leading to damage and leakage in the glomeruli. Stress and overwork can cause the kidneys to lose their filtering ability. Waste

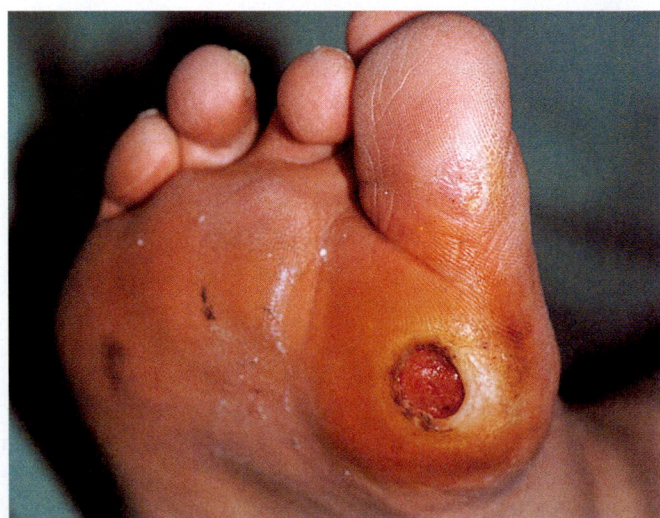

Figure 38-14. ■ Ulceration following trauma in the foot of the person with diabetes. (*Source:* Harry Przekop, Medichrome/The Stock Shop, Inc.)

products can then build up in the blood. If kidney disease is found early, damage can be prevented with treatment. When found in the later stages, treatment may range from dialysis to renal transplant. Forty-three percent of new cases of end-stage renal disease (ESRD) are attributed to diabetes. Studies indicate that effective blood sugar control reduces the risk of renal disease by one-third.

Nervous System Complications

Diabetic neuropathy is a common nervous system complication (see Figure 38-8). *Neuropathy* means nerve damage or disease. Burning, tingling, and numbness in the hands, feet, and legs are symptoms of neuropathy. When the sensory nerve fibers are affected, the client may lose feeling in the extremities and the ability to tell the difference between hot and cold. Dizziness, double vision, ringing, or buzzing in the ears can occur. The male may suffer impotence and the libido may be decreased for both genders. The client may also complain of inability to completely empty the bladder. If the autonomic fibers are damaged, digestion may be affected. A client may complain of pain even though many nerve fibers have been compromised. The reason that high glucose levels cause nerve damage is not fully understood.

Eye Complications

People with diabetes have an increased risk for cataracts and glaucoma with earlier onset of symptoms. When the cataract is mild, the client may be instructed to wear sunglasses more often to protect the eyes. Eventually, most cataracts have to be removed surgically and lens implants done. Forty percent of diabetics will suffer from glaucoma.

Treatment may include eye drops to decrease intraocular pressure, or surgery to relieve this pressure. Diabetic retinopathy occurs when small blood vessels in the retina develop pouches that rupture, causing tissue damage and scarring. Retinopathy is the leading cause of blindness in diabetics. Routine yearly exams are necessary to monitor eye conditions. Early diagnosis and treatment of retinopathy has resulted in more successful treatment and prognosis. Blurred vision occurs when the client suffers from hyperglycemia or hypoglycemia.

Periodontal Complications

Diabetics are at increased risk for periodontal disease, which usually progresses more rapidly and occurs at a younger age in the diabetic. Periodontal disease affects the gums, causing loose teeth, infection, and bone deterioration.

Skin and Foot Complications

Bacteria, yeast, and fungus are organisms normally found on the skin and they thrive in dark moist areas. The groin, vagina, axilla, and under the breast are areas that are susceptible to skin breakdown and invasion by these organisms.

BOX 38-6	NURSING CARE CHECKLIST

Care of the Feet with Diabetes

☑ Teach client to inspect the feet daily. *Clients with neuropathy are unable to feel a painful area.*

☑ Wash the feet using warm water and a mild soap. Remind the client to dry between the toes. Apply lotion to soften the skin. *Careful care of the feet will prevent irritation, cracking, or athlete's foot.*

☑ Toenails should be clipped straight across, and ingrown toenails, corns, and calluses should be treated by a podiatrist. *Any small cut or nick in the toes or around the toenails can lead to infection and gangrene.*

☑ Teach client to wear shoes at all times. Shoes should be fitted correctly and be comfortable. *This will prevent stubbing toes and will protect the feet.*

☑ Instruct the client to wear white cotton socks, and avoid socks or nylons that pinch or roll. *White cotton socks are least irritating to the skin. The rolling or tightness can cause constriction of the circulation to the feet.*

☑ Use foot powder as needed. *Powder will decrease perspiration and dampness in shoes.*

☑ Remind clients to avoid home remedies for foot problems. Encourage them to consult their physician or podiatrist when there is a question. *Clients may cause damage to the skin or nails when treating problems themselves.*

☑ Remind the client to inspect the feet daily. *Clients may not feel a blister developing or a small rock in their shoe that could potentially lead to infection, gangrene, or amputation.*

FOOT CARE.   The client with diabetes must be especially diligent in the care of the feet (Box 38-6 ■). Because many clients have neuropathy, they do not feel injuries to the toes or foot. Because the circulation to the feet is often decreased, it is easy for infection to invade the feet and spread unchecked. A small sore from a rubbing shoe or a stubbed toe in a diabetic client can lead to gangrene and amputation of the leg.

NURSING CARE

PRIORITIZING NURSING CARE

Explain causes of complications such as poor skin care, going barefoot, and noncompliance with diet and medications. Instruct clients to report changes that could indicate complications such as changes in eyesight, sores that do not heal, loss of feeling or numbness in the feet and legs, decreased urine output, and weight gain or loss.

ASSESSING

On admission a thorough history is taken to determine problems with polydipsia, polyphagia, and polyuria. Ask about wounds that do not heal well or become infected easily. Check the blood glucose level using a finger-stick device and glucometer to determine the current level. Evaluate circulation to the feet by palpating pedal pulses and checking for capillary refill and bilateral warmth. Ask about problems with vision, including blurred vision, cataracts, and glaucoma. Evaluate the gums for periodontal disease and the feet for wounds or reddened areas.

DIAGNOSING, PLANNING, AND IMPLEMENTING

Possible nursing diagnoses for clients with diabetes mellitus include:

- *Risk for Infection*
- *Risk for Imbalanced Nutrition: More than Body Requirements*
- *Risk for Impaired Skin Integrity*
- *Delayed Surgical Recovery*
- *Ineffective Peripheral Tissue Perfusion*
- *Impaired Dentition*
- *Ineffective Health Maintenance*

Outcomes and goals include the following:

- The client will be able to recognize the signs and symptoms of infection and seek treatment.
- The client will understand the need to maintain a diet with consistent amounts of CHO, proteins, and fats as prescribed by the physician.
- The client will perform daily inspections of his or her skin for redness or skin breakdown.
- The client will maintain routine oral hygiene and visit a dentist two times a year.
- The client will maintain control of blood sugar levels.

Clients with diabetes mellitus are at risk for a number of complications. Nursing interventions aimed at preventing these complications include the following:

- Monitor closely for signs and symptoms of hypoglycemia, such as pallor, weakness, diaphoresis, trembling, nausea, and headache. Monitor carefully for symptoms of hyperglycemia such as flushed, hot skin, nausea, or vomiting, Kussmaul respirations, acetone breath, and decreasing level of consciousness. Monitor finger-stick blood sugars with sliding scale insulin when ordered before meals and at bedtime. *The blood sugar level can increase or decrease quickly and interventions must be started quickly to prevent shock or coma.*
- Be vigilant about preventing infections and protecting the client from bumps, bruises, and trauma. *Any small skin opening can lead to infection and gangrene.*

- Inspect skin daily. *This helps reveal areas of concern as soon as possible.*
- Monitor the client for symptoms of circulatory compromise and advise the client to avoid sitting with legs hanging down for long periods of time. Instruct the client to avoid crossing legs. *This causes decreased circulation to the legs and feet.*
- Instruct the client in the dangers of smoking. *Nicotine damages the walls of the blood vessels subsequently resulting in narrowed arteries and, hence, reducing the blood flow to the body.*
- Instruct the client to avoid alcohol and tobacco. *Both of these can cause further damage to the nerves.*
- Monitor urinary output for at least 30 mL per hour. *This is the minimum output of kidneys that are working correctly.*
- Monitor vital signs, especially blood pressure. *Elevated blood pressure can lead to further complications for diabetics.*
- Reinforce the need to see the dentist twice a year for dental checkups and cleaning. *Periodontal disease can be treated more effectively if detected early.*
- Protect the client's skin to prevent cuts, cracks, and sores. *These may be a potential port of infection.*
- Inspect the skin during the bath to identify areas that might pose a problem for the client. *Early treatment in collaboration with the health team helps prevent further complications.*
- Assist the client in making appropriate dietary choices and reinforce teaching about food exchanges. *Diabetic diets may be unfamiliar to newly diagnosed clients.*
- Observe the client's tray to be sure that all foods are being eaten. Report any food not eaten, so that calorie adjustments can be made. Serve all snacks to clients with diabetes and report any snacks not eaten. *When food intake is less than normal, insulin or oral hypoglycemic medication dosages may need to be adjusted.*
- Foot care is another major area of concern for the diabetic (see Box 38-6). Refer the client to a diabetic educator and/or diabetic education classes if available. *Group support and scheduled topics ensure that the client receives complete education regarding diabetes.*

Caring for Surgical Clients with Diabetes

There are special considerations when caring for the diabetic client undergoing a surgical procedure. The LPN/LVN in coordination with the RN identifies potential and actual problems that may affect the client preoperatively and postoperatively. Vascular disease will delay healing ability. The client has a decreased resistance to infection. Stress or illness increases the blood sugar, which in turn changes insulin requirements. As the body copes with stress, steroids and epinephrine release increasing glucose levels. Hospital routines affect normal eating habits and the client may be NPO for a period of time.

- Anesthesia increases blood sugar and ketosis. Continue to monitor blood sugar and do routine glucometer checks to assess glucose fluctuation and insulin effectiveness. *The stress of surgery and some medications can increase blood glucose. Hormones are released as a result of stress. The body attempts to cope by increasing glucose to meet energy needs.*
- Preoperative management includes ensuring that the client has as controlled a blood sugar as possible. Report blood sugar readings that are *not* within normal limits. *This helps establish when the client's blood sugar is controlled for surgery.*
- Assess fluid and electrolyte balance and review lab values prior to surgery. Report abnormalities to the physician. *Any imbalance in electrolytes or lab values may need to be treated before surgery is performed.*
- Monitor vital signs preoperatively. *This provides a baseline for changes postoperatively.*
- Monitor glucose before meals and at bedtime. *This also provides a baseline to compare to postoperative readings.*
- Postoperatively, observe the client for signs and symptoms of hypoglycemia. *Clients may not be able to recognize the symptoms or be able to verbally express their needs.*
- Monitor glucose levels and administer sliding scale insulin as ordered. *Blood glucose levels often rise after surgery.*
- Monitor intravenous fluids, especially if a D_5W solution is being administered at a higher rate than "keep vein open." *Moderate amounts of D_5W may increase the blood sugar.* Collaborate with the RN to notify the physician. *The order may be changed to normal saline solution.*
- Observe the incision for healing. Assess for signs and symptoms of infections; monitor WBC and temperature readings. *Clients with diabetes may have delayed healing and their resistance to infection is lowered.*
- Monitor the client for chest pain and level of consciousness. *Potential vascular complications include heart attack and stroke.*

EVALUATING

The client with diabetes mellitus who is in good control will have a stable blood sugar that remains within normal limits for postprandial or fasting situations. The medications, whether oral hypoglycemics or insulin injections, are effective when the blood sugar remains stable. The client will have few, if any, hypoglycemic reactions unless usual routines are not followed.

The client with diabetes must learn a great deal of self-care and when to report a problem before it becomes a major complication. Teaching must be done to help the client learn all the information needed to control diabetes. Client teaching has been successful when the client can demonstrate a skill, such as giving oneself an insulin injection, correctly back to you. The teaching has also been successful when the client can answer your questions about diet, exercise, medications, and complications. (See Chapter 11 and Chapter 12 ⚭ to review client communication and teaching skills, respectively.)

NURSING PROCESS CARE PLAN
Client with Diabetes Mellitus

Della A. Williams, a 45-year-old woman, has been newly diagnosed with diabetes mellitus that is not controlled. She has a family history of diabetes mellitus, is overweight, and has three children. She has complained that she has a blister on her big toe and it seems to be taking a long time to heal. She has stated that she is always tired and finds it difficult to keep up with her children's daily schedule. The nurse notices that when the client is undressing she is wearing knee-highs that are binding around her calves. The client expressed fear of being a burden to her family.

Assessment
VS: T 100, Pulse 84, R 18, B/P 130/90, blood sugar 452, and WBC 11,000. The blister is quarter size, 1×1 inch across with scant serous sanguineous drainage. The client acknowledged that she has felt some numbness in her feet.

Nursing Diagnosis
The following important nursing diagnoses (among others) are established for this client:

- *Impaired Skin Integrity*
- *Risk for Infection* related to blister formation
- *Risk for Peripheral Neurovascular Dysfunction*
- *Ineffective Coping*
- *Deficient Knowledge* related to diabetes mellitus
- *Fatigue*
- *Fear*

Expected Outcomes
The expected outcomes for the plan of care for Ms. Williams are as follows:

- Skin integrity will be effectively managed.
- Blister will be effectively managed without evidence of infection.
- Client will verbalize a basic understanding of diabetes mellitus.
- Client will demonstrate skills needed to check blood sugar levels and continue medication regimen.
- Client will express understanding of diet and exercise management in the care of diabetes mellitus.
- Client will participate in planning care and make decisions regarding care and treatments when possible.

- Family members will be included during diabetic instruction.
- Client will verbalize fears and concerns.
- Client will learn to balance activity and rest periods.

Planning and Implementation

The following interventions are planned and implemented for Ms. Williams:

- Monitor stage II ulceration (blister) with measurements and documentation. *Clients with diabetes may have delayed healing and be at risk for infection. Early intervention can prevent further complications.*
- Maintain glucose levels and medication compliance. *Monitoring glucose levels and medication effectiveness provides a balance for diabetic control.*
- Reinforce the teaching plan developed by the RN. *Reinforcement of the teaching plan assists the client to make informed choices in regard to care.*
- Encourage the client to practice skills needed prior to discharge with supervision. *Practicing skills prior to discharge allows the client to ask questions and be reassured that he/she can manage at home.*
- Observe for signs and symptoms of hypoglycemia. *Hypoglycemia has a quick onset; recognizing signs and symptoms promotes early intervention and treatment.*
- Refer client to continued diabetes education classes. *Ongoing classes reinforce previously learned information and keep the client informed of new treatment options or changes in diabetic research.*
- Encourage increasing activity without the client becoming fatigued. *Exercising moderately maintains health; if the client complains of fatigue; exercise regimen should be evaluated.*
- Reinforce diet instruction per dietitian. *Emphasize compliance with diet regimen that promotes blood sugar control.*

Evaluation

Ms. Williams is discharged home. She is taking an oral hypoglycemic medication b.i.d. Her glucose levels range from 140 to 160 mg. She is feeling less fatigued and is trying to follow a routine of walking around the block with her husband in the evening. She is having difficulty maintaining her diet and changing the way she cooks for her family. She has made contact with the dietitian and was directed to classes on diet management. Her Stage II ulceration is healing slowly and has diminished to the size of a dime without drainage. She is avoiding the use of knee-high stockings and inspecting her feet every evening. Ms. Williams has demonstrated motivation to comply with medication, exercise, and diet regimens. She is making a follow-up appointment with her primary physician for a referral to an endocrinologist for diabetic control.

Critical Thinking in the Nursing Process

1. Develop a teaching plan for a newly diagnosed diabetic.
2. List the signs and symptoms of diabetes and the physical rationale for why they occur.
3. Devise a nursing care plan for a diabetic with a new diagnosis of retinopathy.

Note: Discussion of Critical Thinking questions appears on the MyNursingKit Website.

Adrenal Gland Disorders

Remember that the adrenal glands essentially have two separate endocrine functions. Corticosteroid hormones, such as hydrocortisone, are secreted from the cortex and the medulla secretes adrenaline and norepinephrine.

ADDISON'S DISEASE

When the adrenal glands do not secrete enough corticosteroids, a condition called Addison's disease results. It occurs mostly in women between 30 and 50 years of age. The adrenal cortex becomes atrophied and is unable to produce adequate amounts of the hormones. It is thought that Addison's may be an autoimmune disorder because the adrenal cortex seems to attack itself, causing destruction of the gland. It can also be the result of an adrenalectomy. The onset of Addison's is slow and more than 90% of the gland must be destroyed to develop symptoms of insufficiency.

Manifestations

One of the most notable symptoms is a bronze color of the skin, similar to a deep suntan. It is especially prevalent on the hands, elbows, and knees. Due to decreased aldosterone, the blood pressure falls and tachycardia ensues. Decreased cortisol causes hypoglycemia, weakness, and fatigue, and the body is unable to stimulate liver gluconeogenesis to increase the blood sugar. GI symptoms such as nausea, vomiting, and anorexia result from electrolyte imbalances. Depression and psychosis may be evident.

ADDISONIAN CRISIS. **Addisonian crisis** (adrenal crisis) is a severe form of Addison's disease that causes a life-threatening medical situation. Major stressors can precipitate the crisis in the client with Addison's. This condition can also be induced when a client is abruptly taken off steroid medications rather than being weaned off. Signs and symptoms include hypotension, weakness, rapid weak pulse, fluid volume deficit, and dehydration. Potassium is retained, which can lead to cardiac arrhythmias and arrest. Circulatory collapse and shock can result, requiring immediate treatment. Intravenous fluids, sodium replacement, glucose, and glucocorticoids, mineralocorticoids, and cardiac support are given. The client is kept in a calm quiet environment on bed rest until the crisis is resolved. Once the client has recovered, instruction is given regarding avoiding stressful situations and which symptoms indicate impending crisis and should be reported.

Diagnosis and Treatment

Clients with Addison's disease have lowered blood levels of glucocorticoids and mineralocorticoids and increased levels of ACTH. Elevated potassium levels and lowered glucose and sodium levels are consistent with Addison's. A 24-hour urine test for ketosteroids and 17-hydroxycorticosteroids may be ordered to diagnose the condition. Those findings will be elevated in a 24-hour period. MRI and CT scans are done to identify adrenal gland atrophy.

Addison's is treated with the lifelong replacement of glucocorticoids and mineralocorticoids. Hydrocortisone and fludrocortisone are commonly used. A high-sodium, low-potassium diet may be ordered. During periods of high stress the physician may increase medication doses up to three times the normal dose.

CUSHING'S DISEASE

Cushing's disease is caused by overproduction of the hormone cortisol. Women between 30 and 50 years of age experience it more often than do women of other ages. Cushing's syndrome is the term used to describe the set of symptoms exhibited by the client with this disorder. The causes of Cushing's can be varied. It may be due to a tumor in the adrenal gland that increases secretion of cortisol or to a pituitary tumor that increases ACTH production and thereby increases secretion of cortisol. Chronic steroid therapy can induce symptoms of Cushing's disease. Ectopic release of ACTH from lung and pancreatic tumors can also induce disease. Excess levels of aldosterone and androgens (sex hormones) are also seen.

Manifestations

A common symptom of Cushing's syndrome is weight gain in the truncal area with thin arms and legs. A "buffalo hump" appears as a thickened area below the back of the neck. The face takes on a round "moon face" look because of fatty tissue deposits (Figure 38-15 ■). Increased glucose levels occur as gluconeogenesis in the liver is stimulated. The pancreas may not be able to secrete enough insulin to meet this demand, leading to diabetes mellitus. Muscle wasting, purple striae, easy bruising, and thin skin are noticeable. Lowered calcium absorption leads to osteoporosis, fractures, and back pain. Water and sodium retention from aldosterone increases the blood pressure and produces edema. Potassium is lost in the urine. Cortisol has an anti-inflammatory effect and can mask symptoms of infection. The client may have infection without realizing it until it

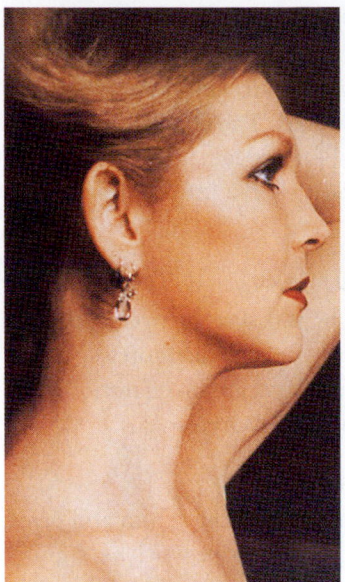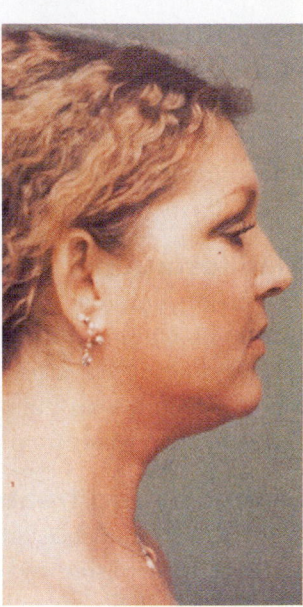

Figure 38-15. ■ A woman before and after developing Cushing's syndrome. In the photo at right, notice the swollen facial features. (*Source*: Courtesy of Dr. Charles Wilson, University of California, San Francisco.)

is overwhelming. Healing is delayed with high cortisol levels. Mental changes occur including irritability and psychosis. The effects of increased sex hormones include acne, hirsutism, and amenorrhea in women.

Diagnosis and Treatment

When a client has Cushing's disease, the serum cortisol, mineralocorticoids, and androgen levels are increased, but ACTH is low. Sodium and glucose levels are elevated, whereas potassium is low. A 24-hour urine test for ketosteroids and 17-hydroxycorticosteroids is positive for high levels of cortisol.

Cushing's disease is treated with medication, radiation therapy, and surgery. The use of medication does not cure it but helps control the disorder. Mitotane or ketoconazole blocks the production of the adrenal steroids. The client is then monitored for signs of decreased adrenal function. If the disease is related to steroid medications, alternative dosing or tapering off of the medication may resolve the symptoms. Abruptly discontinuing steroid medications can result in adrenal crisis. When a tumor is present, radiation therapy can be used to diminish the size of the tumor. However, high doses of radiation may destroy the adrenal cortex, resulting in the need for lifelong cortisol replacement. Surgery is performed to remove a tumor, and an adrenalectomy is performed if necessary. If both glands are involved, bilateral adrenalectomy is necessary, requiring lifelong hormone replacement.

PHEOCHROMOCYTOMA

Pheochromocytoma is a benign tumor located in the adrenal medulla. It causes excessive amounts of epinephrine and norepinephrine to be produced. The effects can be continuous or intermittent and the symptoms may be mild or severe. If not treated, this condition can lead to death.

Manifestations

The major symptom of pheochromocytoma is marked hypertension ranging from 200 to 300 systolic over 150 diastolic. Pounding headache, tachycardia, diaphoresis, flushing, and palpitations can occur. Myocardial infarction (MI) and stroke can result from pheochromocytoma.

Diagnosis and Treatment

When a client has pheochromocytoma, the serum and urine levels of epinephrine and norepinephrine will be significantly elevated. Scans can identify the location and extent of an adrenal tumor.

Adrenalectomy to remove the tumor surgically is the common treatment. Preoperatively the physician will focus on stabilizing the blood pressure to reduce the risk of MI or stroke.

NURSING CARE

PRIORITIZING NURSING CARE

When you care for clients with adrenal disorders, focus your care on monitoring fluid balance, level of consciousness, vital signs, and laboratory tests. Measure intake and output carefully. Use a graduated container to obtain the most accurate measurements of output. Assess the client's level of consciousness and orientation every 2 to 4 hours to determine changes quickly, because such changes can indicate worsening of the condition. Check lab tests for changes in levels of sodium, potassium, glucose, and cortisol. Vital signs are also a major nursing focus since clients with pheochromocytoma can have markedly elevated blood pressure. Clients with Addison's disease develop hypotension and weak pulse when going into an Addisonian crisis.

ASSESSING

On admission of a client with an adrenal disorder, a thorough history will be taken to determine problems with weight gain, weakness, low or high blood sugar, or changes in skin color or facial appearance. Ask about problems with depression or psychosis that may be related to adrenal malfunction. Observe the client for bronzed skin, "moon face" or "dowager hump," bruising, or purple striae that would indicate hypo- or hyperadrenal function. Collect vital sign data for tachycardia, hypertension, or other abnormal

findings. Marked hypertension may indicate pheochromocytoma and should be reported to the physician immediately.

DIAGNOSING, PLANNING, AND IMPLEMENTING

Possible nursing diagnoses for clients with adrenal disorders include:

- *Excess or Deficient Fluid Volume*
- *Imbalanced Nutrition: Less than Body Requirements*
- *Acute Confusion*
- *Risk for Injury*
- *Risk for Infection*
- *Fatigue*
- *Disturbed Body Image*

The goals for this client include the following:

- The client will maintain a balanced intake and output.
- The client will maintain a balanced diet and maintain weight.
- The client will be aware of and recognize changes in thinking and behavior.
- The client will be free of injury.
- The client will recognize signs and symptoms of infection.
- The client will report improved sense of energy.
- The client will verbalize understanding of body image changes.

To achieve these goals, the nurse provides various interventions, including the following:

- Monitor intake and output, and measure weight daily. Record this information accurately. *These measures indicate fluid volume excess or deficit.*
- Evaluate level of consciousness frequently, as well as orientation to time, place, and person. *Adrenal disorders can lead to confusion and disorientation.*
- The client's body image may be altered due to fat redistribution and androgen symptoms, or changes in skin color. Allow the client to vent feelings. *The nurse may be the first support person the client turns to for comfort.*
- Measure vital signs every 4 hours or more frequently if ordered. *Vital sign changes can indicate changes in fluid balance and adrenal status.*

For Clients with Addison's Disease

- Assess for signs and symptoms of dehydration, poor skin turgor, thirst, and dry skin and mucous membranes. *These indicate the need for more hydration.*
- Offer oral fluids frequently. *This helps counteract the client's high urinary output.*
- Monitor vital signs every 4 hours, or more frequently. Check the lab results of sodium, potassium, and glucose

levels and report changes to the physician. *Changes in vital signs and lab values can indicate a rapid change in the client's condition.*

- Provide a diet high in calories and sodium, but low in potassium. Frequent meals may be less tiring than large meals at one time. Reinforce dietary compliance. *This diet is important in helping the client's body meet energy and sodium needs.*

- Assist the client in performing activities of daily living to prevent stress and maintain bed rest. Increase activity slowly until the client's hormonal treatment has reached an adequate level. *Clients with Addison's disease do not have body stores to handle stress and activity until hormone replacement is adequate.*

- Client teaching includes information on disease, treatment, and compliance. The client should carry an identifying bracelet or necklace in case of emergency. *Addison's disease is not easily recognized and Addisonian crises can occur, especially in response to an emergency situation.*

For Clients with Cushing's Disease

- Auscultate lung sounds frequently for crackles. *This indicates the client is retaining fluid and could be a sign of pulmonary edema.*

- Restrict fluids as ordered. *This measure is designed to prevent fluid overload.*

- Safety is a concern for the client with evidence of muscle atrophy, osteoporosis, and fractures. Assist the client in the use of assistive devices, and encourage the client to call for help when needed. *Safety is the nurse's responsibility.*

- Rest periods may be necessary to avoid fatigue. *Clients with Cushing's disease may be short of breath with exertion.*

- Minimize exposure by the use of a private room if possible, and limit visitors. *This client is at risk for infection.*

- Observe wounds frequently for signs and symptoms of infection. Assess skin integrity for potential areas of breakdown, change client's position frequently, and use protective measures when appropriate. *Due to high cortisol levels, signs of infection may be masked until the infection is overwhelming.*

- Monitor lab values such as glucose, sodium, and potassium levels. *Elevated cortisol levels cause elevation in other lab values.*

- Provide instruction about the disease and its treatment and complications. *Clients who understand the treatment plan are more compliant with it.*

For Clients with Pheochromocytoma

- Monitor the blood pressure every hour or more frequently if ordered. Report blood pressure increases immediately. *The markedly elevated blood pressures found with pheochromocytoma can lead to complications of MI and stroke.*

- Administer intravenous antihypertensive medication as ordered and observe closely for hypotension. *Anti-hypertensive medications given IV may cause the blood pressure to drop too low.*

- Give routine postoperative care. *Once the tumor is removed, blood pressure should decrease.*

EVALUATING

Clients with adrenal disorders are evaluated for vital signs within normal limits, balanced fluid volume, stable weight, and rational thought processes. Because these conditions usually involve lifelong medications or surgery, follow-up care is essential to be sure the adrenal hormones stay balanced.

Gonads

The primary sex organs in the male and female are the testes and ovaries, respectively. The testes produce testosterone and are responsible for the growth and development of the male characteristics. They stimulate sperm production and are stimulated by both FSH and LH from the pituitary gland. The ovaries produce estrogens and progesterone. Estrogen promotes the growth and development of the female characteristics. In conjunction with other hormones it is responsible for breast development and the menstrual cycle. Progesterone is chiefly responsible for the secretion of the corpus luteum and maintenance of the lining of the uterus in pregnancy. The ovaries are stimulated by the gonadotropins FSH and LH. The reproductive system is discussed in depth in Chapter 40.

Note: The references and resources for all chapters have been compiled at the back of the book.

PROCEDURE 38-1 Monitoring Blood Glucose

Purposes

- To determine the client's blood glucose level
- To provide data for administering insulin in clients with diabetes mellitus

Equipment

- Chemical strips for reading glucose measurement
- Glucose monitor
- Lancet mechanism for obtaining blood
- Gloves
- Insulin sliding scale

Check order ✛ Gather equipment ✛ Introduce yourself ✛ Identify client ✛ Provide privacy ✛ Explain procedure ✛ Hand hygiene ✛ Gloves as needed

Interventions and Rationales

1. Perform preparatory steps (see icon bar above).

2. Prepare the client. Explain that a drop of blood is needed to determine the client's blood glucose level. *This promotes cooperation.*

3. Confirm the correct chemical strips with the machine code. *Matching the codes prevents an inaccurate reading.*

4. Remove chemical strip from container and place it in the machine.

5. Prepare the lancet for puncture.

6. Don gloves. *This supports infection control.*

7. Hold chosen finger downward and squeeze gently from lower digits to fingertip. *This brings blood to the tip of the finger.*

8. Wipe puncture site (lateral pads of fingers) per hospital protocol. *Using the side of the finger lessens pain to the finger pad. Avoid using the thumbs.*

9. Place lancet firmly against side of finger and release spring or stick finger with darting motion (Figure 38-16).

10. Allow drop of blood to accumulate onto chemical strip.

11. Activate timing device if monitor is not equipped with automatic timing. *Monitors may require a certain amount of time to provide an accurate reading.*

12. Apply pressure to puncture site. *This stops the bleeding at the site.*

13. Allow the appropriate time for a digital readout.

14. Obtain results from the digital reading.

15. Discard soiled materials and gloves in proper containers. *The nurse must always maintain a clean environment to protect against transmission of infection.*

16. Position client for comfort with the call bell within reach. *This reassures client that help will be available if needed.*

17. Document appropriate dose of regular insulin from sliding scale if provided. *Medications will be based on readings. Documentation provides a legal record of care.*

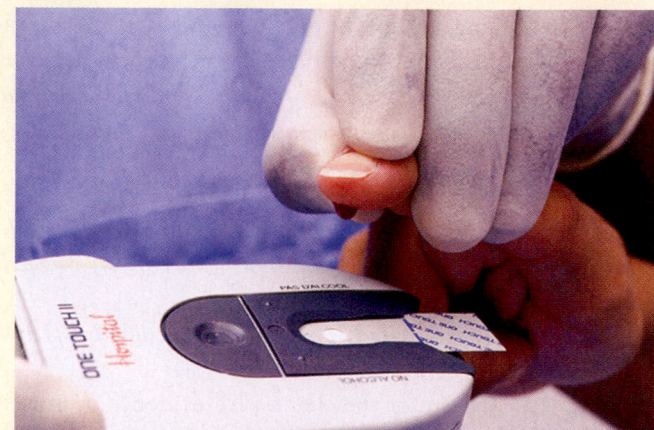

A

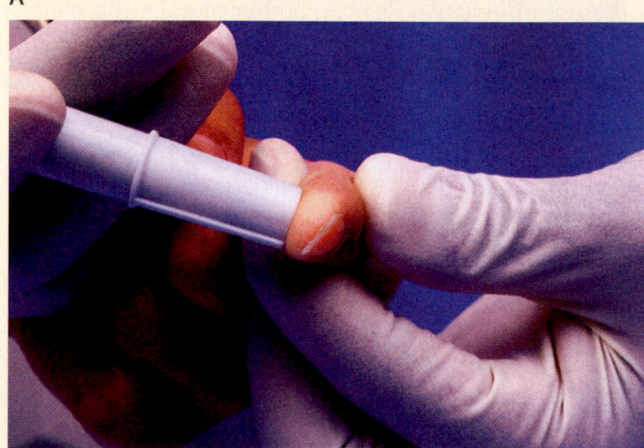

B

Figure 38-16. ■ **A.** Place the injector perpendicular to the site. **B.** Gently squeeze a large drop of blood onto the chemical strip.

SAMPLE DOCUMENTATION

[Date]	BG: 250; 0740 Reg. Insulin
[time]	5 U given SC per sliding scale.
	_____ N. Albamonti, LPN

Chapter Review

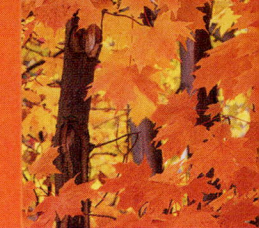

KEY Points

- The endocrine system maintains homeostasis in the body.

- Hormones are chemical messengers that function individually or in conjunction with another hormone to cause a direct action. Endocrine glands secrete hormones directly into the blood.

- One of the factors that produce an imbalance of hormones is increased or decreased stimulation of the target gland by the anterior pituitary.

- Negative feedback is a method by which hormonal production is decreased.

- Thyroid disorders are caused by either oversecretion or undersecretion of the thyroid hormones T_3 and T_4, affecting metabolism rates.

- The causes for hyperthyroidism can be related to tumor or an autoimmune disorder. If left untreated, the client can experience cardiac dysrhythmias or cardiac arrest.

- Hypothyroidism can be the result of a congenital disorder or an autoimmune response. Untreated, the client has bradycardia, hypotension, and dysrhythmias, or cardiac arrest.

- Diabetes mellitus has become one of the most prevalent diseases found today.

- Diabetes increases with age and can strike at any age. The treatment includes diet, medication, and exercise. Nursing measures include maintaining normal blood glucose levels.

- Controlling blood glucose levels can delay or stop diabetic complications. The risk for death in diabetic clients is twice that of persons without the disease.

- When the adrenal gland does not secrete enough corticosteroids, a condition called Addison's results. An overproduction of the hormone cortisol results in Cushing's disease.

FOR FURTHER Study

See Chapter 11 for a discussion about client communication.

Chapter 12 covers client teaching.

Directions for administering insulin are provided in Chapter 27. See Procedure 27-2.

Myasthenia gravis is discussed in Chapters 35 and 36.

The normal characteristics of urine are listed in Table 39-2.

Chapter 40 covers the reproductive system and disorders.

For additional information on cancer, see Chapter 45.

For more on seasonal affective disorder, see Chapter 49.

Gestational diabetes is discussed further in Chapter 52.

PEARSON

EXPLORE **mynursingkit**™

MyNursingKit is your one stop for online chapter review materials and resources. Prepare for success with additional NCLEX®-style practice questions, interactive assignments and activities, web links, animations and videos, and more!

Register your access code from the front of your book at **www.mynursingkit.com**

Critical Thinking Care Map

Caring for a Client with Impaired Physical Mobility

NCLEX-PN® Focus Area: Physiologic Integrity

Case Study: Elsa Gray is a 73-year-old resident of a nursing home who has a stasis ulcer on her left heel. She is refusing to get out of bed to ambulate or sit in her chair, stating her foot hurts worse when it is dependent. Eschar is visible on the ulcer, which has a foul odor.

Nursing Diagnosis: *Impaired Physical Mobility related to pain from stasis ulcer*

COLLECT DATA

Subjective	Objective
_____	_____
_____	_____
_____	_____
_____	_____
_____	_____
_____	_____
_____	_____

Would you report this? Yes/No

If yes, report to: _____

What would you report? _____

Nursing Care

_____
_____
_____
_____
_____
_____
_____
_____
_____
_____

How would you document this? _____
_____
_____
_____

Compare your answers and documentation to those provided on the MyNursingKit Website.

Data Collected
(use only those that apply)

- Complains of burning pain in area of wound
- Eschar visible in wound bed
- Foul odor from wound
- States "It hurts to walk; it even hurts to sit!"
- Foot is cold to touch
- WBC elevated, T 102F
- Edema around wound, feet are swollen (+2 pitting)
- States "It hurts less if I stay in bed."
- Reactive hyperemia visible over coccygeal area
- Type II—NIDDM controlled with diet

Nursing Interventions
(use only those that apply; list in priority order)

- Administer analgesics prior to getting client to ambulate or sit in a chair.
- Report reactive hyperemia and edema.
- Look for hazards in the environment.
- Consult with physical therapist about positioning and ambulation.
- Provide wound care as ordered.
- Provide blanket to keep feet warm.
- Increase turning schedule to once per hour.
- Keep the wound uncovered.
- Apply a boot to keep the heel off the bed.
- Teach client about the importance of ambulating.
- Consult with dietitian regarding diet.
- Keep the leg immobilized.

1 The client asks the nurse why he was instructed to buy salt with iodine. The nurse explains that iodine is needed for production of which of the following hormones?

1. Thymosin and thymin
2. Aldosterone and cortisol
3. Epinephrine and norepinephrine
4. Thyroxine and triiodothyronine

2 The client asks the nurse about the purpose of the hormones produced by the thymus gland. The nurse explains the thymus gland hormones:

1. Play an essential role in the development of the immune system.
2. Regulate water reabsorption by the distal renal tubules.
3. Regulate the rate of metabolism and normal growth and development.
4. Maintain calcium and phosphate balance in the body.

3 The nurse is teaching a class for other nurses on the endocrine system. When the nurse explains that glands stop secreting hormones when they receive information that the desired effect has been achieved, the nurse is describing:

1. Positive feedback.
2. Negative feedback.
3. Hormone secretion.
4. Chvostek's sign.

4 Which of the following would be appropriate for the nurse to teach the client who has had surgery to remove a tumor through the sphenoid (transsphenoidal hypophysectomy)?

1. Cough and deep breathe every 2 hours.
2. Hold the dressing in place when sneezing.
3. Avoid straining to have a bowel movement.
4. Bend slowly from the waist if the client needs to bend.

5 When assigned to care for a client who has just arrived from the recovery room after thyroid surgery, the nurse would consider which of the following essential to keep at the bedside?

1. Nasal oxygen setup
2. Suture removal kit
3. Tracheostomy tray
4. Oropharyngeal airway

6 Which of the following statements made by the nurse would best describe the Somogyi effect seen in clients with diabetes?

1. A sudden drop of blood sugar followed by a rebound hyperglycemic reaction
2. An elevation of blood sugar at approximately three o'clock in the morning

3. An unexplained periodic resistance to insulin requiring larger doses
4. A sudden rise in blood sugar following a period of increased exercise

7 When assessing a client who has diabetes, what symptoms would most cause the nurse to suspect that the client is having a hypoglycemic reaction?

1. Nausea, deep rapid respirations, and a fruity breath
2. Cold sweats, clammy skin, and shakiness
3. Skin hot and dry to the touch and abdominal cramps
4. Slow onset of pallor of the skin and fainting

8 The nurse is caring for a client diagnosed with pheochromocytoma and recognizes which of the following as a major manifestation of the disease?

1. Bronze color of the skin, similar to a deep suntan
2. Hypertension ranging from 200 to 300 systolic over 150 diastolic
3. Elevated red blood cell count
4. Weight gain in the truncal area

9 The nurse, caring for a client with a diagnosis of Addison's disease, recognizes which of the following as a priority goal for this client?

1. Identify potential stressors and ways to deal with them.
2. Demonstrate 100% adherence to the prescribed diet.
3. Verbalize an understanding of the causes of Addison's disease.
4. Exercise for 30 minutes three or more times each week.

10 The nurse is assisting with teaching the client newly diagnosed with Type 2 diabetes mellitus when the client asks, "What can I do to manage my diabetes in a way that will keep me healthy?" The nurse's responses would include which of the following strategies? (Select all that apply.)

1. Diet management is key to diabetic control.
2. Exercise, coupled with maintaining a healthy weight, may help to control blood sugar levels.
3. Monitor blood sugar levels as your doctor recommends.
4. Inject insulin before every meal.
5. Inspect the feet daily.

Answers and rationales for Review Questions appear in Appendix I.

Chapter 39

Clients with Urinary System Disorders

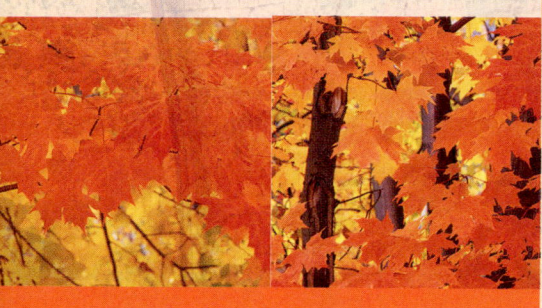

BRIEF Outline

LEARNING Outcomes

After completing this chapter, you will be able to:

1. Review the structure and function of the urinary system and factors that affect urinary function.
2. Describe the characteristics of normal and abnormal urine.
3. Identify factors associated with altered urinary elimination.
4. List and describe tests of renal function and basic nursing skills for urinary care.
5. Describe collection of data related to urinary function.
6. Identify manifestations, diagnosis, treatment, and nursing care for disorders of the kidneys.
7. Explain treatment and nursing care for clients with renal failure and end-stage renal disease.
8. Name common disorders of the ureters, bladder, and urethra, their treatment, and nursing care.

Clinical Objectives

9. Demonstrate care for clients undergoing renal studies.
10. Demonstrate competence in urine collection techniques.
11. Demonstrate male and female urinary catheterization, including selection of proper catheter, and emphasizing strict sterile technique.
12. Demonstrate competence in catheter irrigation.
13. Demonstrate competence in applying a condom catheter.
14. Demonstrate the procedure for documenting intake and output.
15. Care for a client with a renal disorder.
16. Complete health history questions pertaining to renal function.
17. Create a plan of care for a client with end-stage renal disease.

Urinary elimination is essential to health, and voiding can be postponed for only so long before the urge becomes too great to control. Urinary elimination depends on effective functioning of four urinary tract organs: kidneys, ureters, bladder, and urethra. In males, the urethra also plays a central role in reproduction.

The main purpose of the urinary (or *renal*) system is to eliminate waste products and excess water from the body. The organs of this system include the kidneys, ureters, urinary bladder, and the urethra (Figure 39-1 ■). Additionally, the urinary system aids in acid-base balance and electrolyte composition of body fluids. See more about fluid and electrolyte balance in Chapter 26 ⬡.

Structure and Function of the Urinary System

KIDNEYS

The paired kidneys are situated on either side of the spinal column, behind the peritoneal cavity. They are the primary regulators of fluid and acid-base balance in the body. Blood from the abdominal aorta enters the renal artery, which branches extensively within the kidney. The functional units of the kidneys, the **nephrons,** filter the blood and remove metabolic wastes. In the average adult, 1,200 mL of blood pass through the kidneys every minute. Each kidney contains about 1 million nephrons. Each nephron has a *glomerulus* and a tuft of capillaries surrounded by *Bowman's capsule* (Figure 39-2 ■). The glomerular capillaries are porous, allowing fluid and solutes to move across this membrane into the capsule.

From the Bowman's capsule, the filtrate moves into the tubule of the nephron. In the proximal convoluted tubule, most of the water and electrolytes are reabsorbed. Solutes are reabsorbed in the *loop of Henle*, but in the same area

other substances are secreted into the filtrate, concentrating the urine. In the distal convoluted tubule, additional water and sodium are reabsorbed under the control of hormones such as antidiuretic hormone (ADH) and aldosterone. When fluid intake is low or the concentration of solutes in the blood is high, more water is reabsorbed in the distal tubule, and less urine is excreted. The processes of *controlled reabsorption* specifically regulate fluid and electrolyte balance in the body.

URETERS

Once the urine is formed in the kidneys, it moves into the renal pelvis and from there into the ureters (Figure 39-3 ■). The *ureters* are 25 to 30 cm (10 to 12 in.) long and about 1.25 cm (0.5 in.) wide in adults. The ureter is funnel shaped as it enters the kidney. The lower ends of the ureters enter the bladder at the posterior corners of the floor of the bladder (see Figure 39-1B). At the junction between the ureter and the bladder, a valve prevents *reflux* (backflow) of urine up the ureters.

BLADDER

The urinary *bladder* is a hollow, muscular organ that serves as a reservoir for urine and as the organ of excretion. In males the bladder lies in front of the rectum and above the prostate gland. In females it lies in front of the uterus and vagina (Figure 39-4 ■). The base of the bladder is a triangular area marked by the ureter openings at the posterior corners and the opening of the urethra at the anterior inferior corner. Urine exits the bladder through the urethra.

The bladder is able to stretch because of *rugae* (folds) in the mucous membrane lining and because of the elasticity of its walls. When full, the bladder may extend above the symphysis pubis. In extreme situations it may extend as high as the umbilicus.

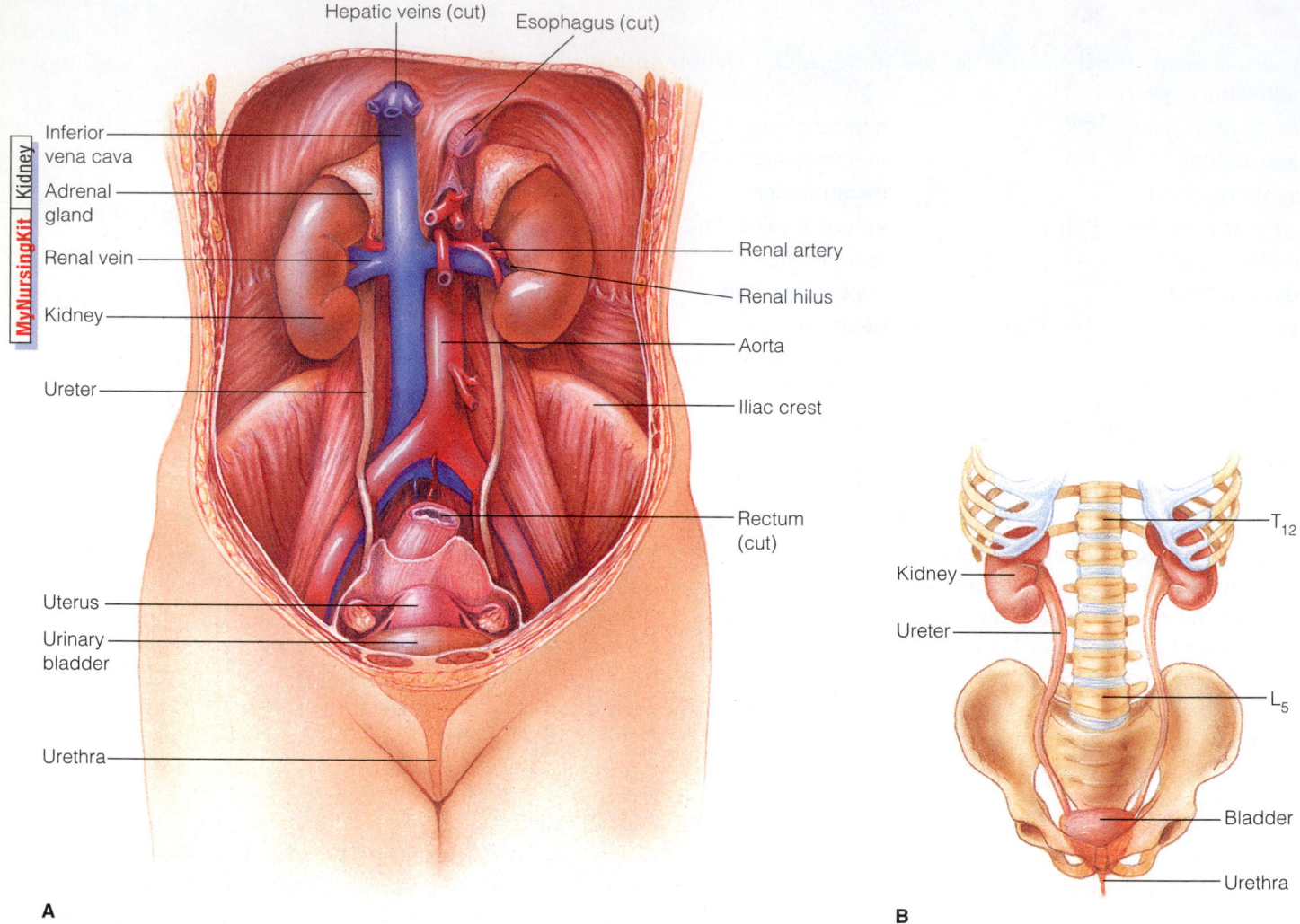

Figure 39-1. ■ Urinary system: **A.** Anterior view of the urinary system in a female. **B.** Kidneys are shown in relation to the vertebrae and ribs.

URETHRA

The *urethra* extends from the bladder to the urinary meatus. The **meatus** is an opening in the external body that serves as a passageway for the elimination of urine. The female's urinary meatus is located between the labia minora, in front of the vagina and below the clitoris. The male urethra is about 10 cm (8 in.) long and serves as a passageway for semen as well as urine (see Figure 39-4A). The male's urinary meatus is located at the distal end of the penis.

The *internal sphincter* muscle situated at the base of the urinary bladder is under involuntary control (Figure 39-5 ■). The *external sphincter* muscle is under voluntary control, allowing the individual to choose when urine is eliminated.

In both males and females, the urethra has a mucous membrane lining that is continuous with the bladder and the ureters. This structure facilitates the spread of an infection of the urethra throughout the urinary tract to the kidneys. Women are particularly prone to urinary tract infections because of their short urethra and the proximity of the urinary meatus to the vagina and anus (see Figure 39-4B).

URINATION

Micturition, *voiding,* and *urination* all refer to the process of emptying the urinary bladder. Urine collects in the bladder until pressure stimulates special sensory nerve endings in the bladder wall called *stretch receptors.* These receptors respond when the adult bladder contains between 250 and 450 mL of urine. They transmit impulses to the spinal cord, causing the internal sphincter to relax and stimulating the urge to void. The conscious portion of the brain relaxes the external urethral sphincter muscle, and urination takes place. If the time and place are inappropriate, voluntary controls allow the micturition reflex to subside until the bladder becomes more filled and the reflex is involuntarily stimulated again.

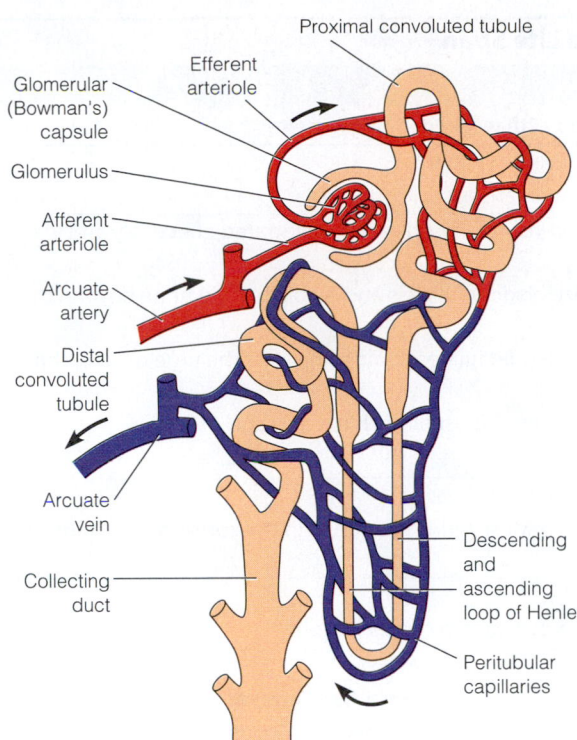

Figure 39-2. ■ The nephrons of the kidney are composed of six parts: the glomerulus, Bowman's capsule, proximal convoluted tubule, loop of Henle, distal convoluted tubule, and collecting duct.

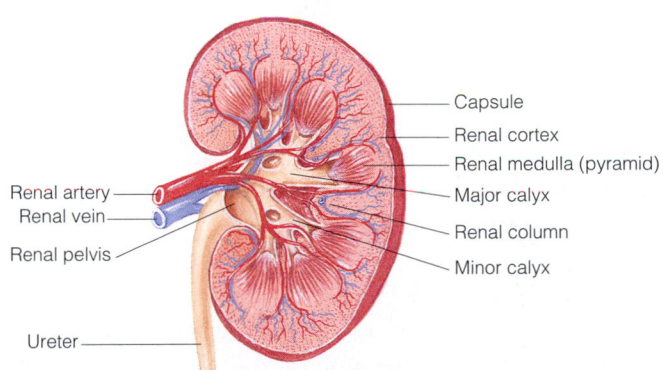

Figure 39-3. ■ Internal anatomy of the kidney.

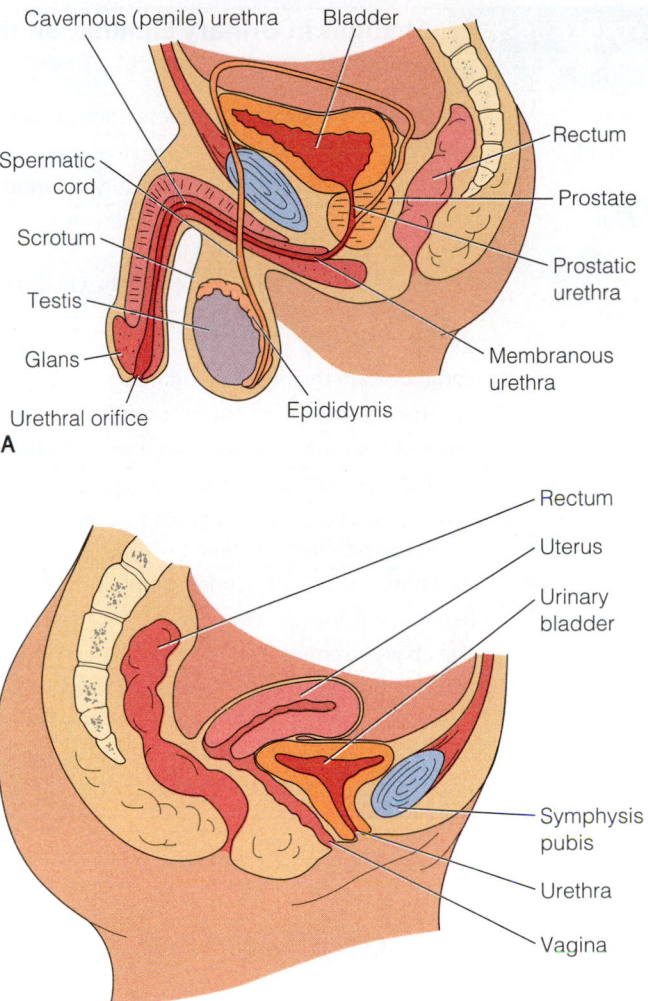

Figure 39-4. ■ **A.** The male urogenital system. **B.** The female urogenital system.

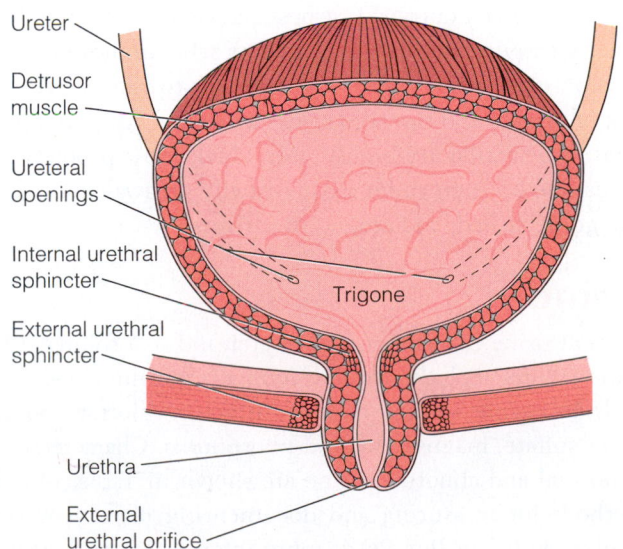

Figure 39-5. ■ Internal view of the urinary bladder and trigone.

Voluntary control of urination is possible only if the nerves supplying the bladder and urethra, the neural tracts of the cord and brain, and the motor area of the cerebrum are intact. An individual must be able to sense that the bladder is full. Injury to any part of the nervous system above the level of the sacral region results in intermittent involuntary emptying of the bladder. Older people whose cognition is impaired may not be aware of the need to urinate or able to respond appropriately to nervous system stimulus.

TABLE 39-1	Changes in Urinary Elimination through the Life Span
STAGE	**VARIATIONS**
Fetus	The fetal kidney begins to excrete urine between the 11th and 12th weeks of development.
Infant	Ability to concentrate urine is minimal; therefore, urine appears light yellow.
	Because of neuromuscular immaturity, voluntary urinary control is absent.
Child	Kidney function reaches maturity between the first and second year of life; urine is concentrated effectively and is a normal amber color.
	Between 18 and 24 months of age, the child starts to recognize bladder fullness and is able to hold urine beyond the urge to void.
	At approximately 2½ to 3 years of age, the child can perceive bladder fullness, hold urine after the urge to void, and communicate the need to urinate.
	Full urinary control usually occurs at age 4 or 5 years; daytime control is usually achieved by age 3 years.
	The kidneys grow in proportion to overall body growth.
Adult	The kidneys reach maximum size between 35 and 40 years of age.
	After 50 years the kidneys begin to diminish in size and function. Most shrinkage occurs in the cortex of the kidney as individual nephrons are lost.
Older adult	An estimated 30% of nephrons are lost by age 80.
	Renal blood flow decreases because of vascular changes and a decrease in cardiac output.
	The ability to concentrate urine declines.
	Bladder muscle tone diminishes, causing increased frequency of urination and nocturia (awakening to urinate at night).
	Diminished bladder muscle tone and contractibility may lead to residual urine in the bladder after voiding, increasing the risk of bacterial growth and infection.
	Urinary incontinence may occur due to mobility problems or neurologic impairments.

Factors Affecting Urinary Function

Numerous factors affect the volume and characteristics of the urine produced and the manner in which it is excreted. These changes include age, activity level, food and fluid intake, medications, muscle tone, and developmental level. See Table 39-1 ■ for a summary of developmental changes affecting urinary output. Psychosocial factors can also affect urinary activity. For example, clients who are hospitalized and confined to bed may find it difficult to void because of lack of privacy and the need to use a bedpan. Although patterns of urination are highly individual, most people void about five to seven times a day: usually on awakening, before going to bed, and around mealtimes.

Urine Characteristics

Normal urine consists of 96% water and 4% solutes. Organic solutes include urea, ammonia, creatinine, and uric acid. Inorganic solutes include sodium, chloride, potassium, sulfate, magnesium, and phosphorus. Characteristics of normal and abnormal urine are shown in Table 39-2 ■. Methods for measuring and documenting urinary output were provided in Box 26-4; more information about fluid balance can be found in Chapter 26 ⚭.

Altered Urinary Elimination

Despite normal urine production, a number of factors or conditions can affect urinary elimination. Selected factors associated with altered patterns of urinary elimination are identified in Table 39-3 ■. Chapter 42 ⚭, Health Promotion for Older Adults, discusses maintenance and restoration of urinary function.

DIAGNOSTIC TESTS

Blood levels of urea and creatinine are routinely used to evaluate renal function because they are eliminated by the kidneys through filtration. One test, blood urea nitrogen (BUN, normal value 8–21 mg/dL), measures the amount of urea in the blood. Creatinine (normal value 0.6–1.2 mg/dL) is produced in relatively constant quantities by the muscles. The *creatinine clearance test* uses 24-hour urine and serum creatinine levels to determine the glomerular filtration rate (GFR), a sensitive indicator of renal function.

Visualization procedures also may be used to evaluate urinary function. An x-ray of the kidneys, ureters, and bladder is referred to as a *KUB. Intravenous pyelography (IVP)* is a radiographic study used to evaluate the urinary tract. For an intravenous pyelogram test, contrast medium is injected through a vein, then x-rays are taken to evaluate urinary tract structures. A *computed tomography (CT) scan* is done to distinguish minor

TABLE 39-2	Characteristics of Normal and Abnormal Urine		
CHARACTERISTIC	NORMAL	ABNORMAL	NURSING CONSIDERATIONS
Amount in 24 hours	1,200–1,500 mL	Less than 1,200 mL More than 1,500 mL	Urinary output normally is approximately equal to fluid intake (adult). Output of less than 30 mL/hr may indicate decreased blood flow to the kidneys and should be reported immediately.
Color, clarity	Straw, amber Transparent	Dark amber Cloudy Dark orange Red or dark brown Mucous plugs, viscid, thick	Concentrated urine is darker in color. Dilute urine may appear almost clear, or very pale yellow. Some foods and drugs may color urine (e.g., beets, carrots, phenazopyridine, phenytoin). Red blood cells in the urine (**hematuria**) may be evident as pink, bright red, or rusty brown urine. Menstrual bleeding can also color urine but should not be confused with hematuria. White blood cells, bacteria, pus, or contaminants such as prostatic fluid, sperm, or vaginal drainage may cause cloudy urine.
Odor	Faint aromatic	Offensive	Some foods (e.g., asparagus) cause a musty odor; infected urine can have a fetid odor; urine high in glucose has a sweet odor.
Sterility	No microorganisms present	Microorganisms present	Urine specimens may be contaminated by bacteria from the perineum during collection.
pH	4.5–8	Less than 4.5 Greater than 8	Freshly voided urine is normally somewhat acidic. Alkaline urine may indicate a state of alkalosis, urinary tract infection, or a diet high in fruits and vegetables. More acidic urine (low pH) is found in acidosis, starvation, diarrhea, or with a diet high in protein foods or cranberries.
Specific gravity	1.010–1.025	Less than 1.010 Greater than 1.025	Concentrated urine has a higher specific gravity; diluted urine has a lower specific gravity.
Glucose	Not present	Present	Glucose in the urine indicates high blood glucose levels (more than 180 mg/dL), and may be indicative of undiagnosed or uncontrolled diabetes mellitus.
Ketone bodies	Not present	Present	Ketones (acetone bodies), the end product of the breakdown of fatty acids, are not normally present in the urine. They may be present in the urine of clients who have uncontrolled diabetes mellitus, are in a state of starvation, or who have ingested excessive amounts of aspirin.
Blood	Not present	Occult (microscopic) Bright red	Blood may be present in the urine of clients who have urinary tract infection, kidney disease, or bleeding from the urinary tract.

differences in the density of tissues. *Renal ultrasonography* is a noninvasive test that uses reflected sound waves to visualize the kidneys. During a *cystoscopy*, the bladder, ureteral orifices, and urethra can be visualized using a cystoscope, a lighted instrument inserted through the urethra.

FLUID INTAKE

Increasing fluid intake increases urine production, which in turn stimulates the micturition reflex. A normal daily intake averaging 1,500 mL of measurable fluids is adequate for most adult clients.

Many clients have increased fluid requirements that require a higher daily fluid intake. For example, clients who are perspiring excessively (have diaphoresis) or who are experiencing abnormal fluid losses through vomiting, gastric suction, diarrhea, or wound drainage require fluid to replace these losses in addition to their normal daily intake requirements.

Clients who are at risk for urinary tract infection or urinary calculi (stones) should consume 2,000 to 3,000 mL of fluid daily. Dilute urine and frequent urination reduce the risk of urinary tract infection as well as stone formation.

Increased fluid intake may be contraindicated for some clients such as people with kidney failure or heart failure. For these clients, a fluid restriction may be necessary to prevent fluid overload and edema.

It is important for overall health to maintain voiding patterns even when ill. Nurses often assist clients who are partially or totally confined to bed. See Chapter 42 ⚭ for nursing guidelines to help clients maintain normal voiding habits.

Clients with *incontinence* (inability to control functions of elimination) also become quite susceptible to skin breakdown. Skin that is continually moist becomes

TABLE 39-3	Selected Factors Associated with Altered Urinary Elimination
PATTERNS	**SELECTED ASSOCIATED FACTORS**
Polyuria (diuresis; eliminating abnormally large amounts of urine)	Ingestion of fluids containing caffeine or alcohol
	Prescribed diuretic
	Presence of thirst, dehydration, and weight loss
	History of diabetes mellitus, diabetes insipidus, or kidney disease
Oliguria, anuria (low amounts of urine or no urine)	Decrease in fluid intake
	Signs of dehydration (see Chapter 26 ⬮⬮)
	Presence of hypotension, shock, or heart failure
	History of kidney disease
	Signs of renal failure such as elevated blood urea nitrogen (BUN) and serum creatinine, edema, hypertension
Frequency (voiding more than usual), **nocturia**—voiding two or more times at night)	Pregnancy
	Increase in fluid intake
	Urinary tract infection
	Any known contributing or initiating causes, such as stress
	Small quantities voided (50–100 mL)
Urgency (feeling that voiding must occur immediately)	Presence of psychologic stress
	Urinary tract infection
Dysuria (painful or difficult urination)	Urinary tract inflammation, infection, or injury
	Presence of other signs that may accompany dysuria, such as hesitancy, hematuria, pyuria (pus in the urine), and frequency
	Burning may accompany or follow voiding
Enuresis (involuntary discharge of urine after voluntary control has normally been reached)	Family history of enuresis
	Difficult access to toilet facilities
	Home stresses
Incontinence (inability to control excretion) (see Chapter 42 ⬮⬮ for coverage of causes and treatment of incontinence)	Bladder inflammation or other disease
	Difficulties in independent toileting (mobility impairment)
	Leakage when coughing, laughing, sneezing
	Cognitive impairment
Retention	Distended bladder on palpation and percussion
	Associated signs, such as pubic discomfort, restlessness, frequency, and small urine volume
	Recent anesthesia
	Recent perineal surgery
	Presence of perineal swelling
	Prescribed medications
	Lack of privacy or other factors inhibiting micturition
Neurogenic bladder (dysfunction of nerves supplying the bladder)	Lesions of the central nervous system or of nerves supplying the bladder

macerated (softened by soaking). Urine that accumulates on the skin converts to ammonia and irritates skin further. So, the incontinent person requires meticulous skin care. Mild soap and water are used; the skin is dried gently but thoroughly; and clean, dry clothing or bed linen is provided. If the skin is irritated, the nurse applies a barrier cream. Bed pads that absorb wetness and leave a dry surface in contact with the skin are utilized. See Chapter 20 ⬮⬮ for perineal care and more information on providing hygiene.

Incontinence is not a normal part of aging. Many times a physical condition can cause urinary incontinence. Bladder training (see Box 42-2 ⬮⬮) can help clients to recover continence once the physical condition is resolved.

Basic Skills for Urinary Care

Some basic skills that nurses perform frequently when caring for clients with urinary disorders include collecting urine specimens, testing urine, measuring residual urine, applying condom catheters, inserting straight and retention catheters, removing retention catheters, and irrigating catheters.

COLLECTING URINE SPECIMENS

The nurse is responsible for collecting urine specimens for a number of tests: clean voided specimens for routine urinalysis; clean-catch or midstream urine specimens for urine culture; and timed urine and indwelling catheter specimens for a variety of tests, depending on the client's specific health problem.

Clean Voided Specimen

Many clients are able to collect a clean voided specimen and provide the specimen independently with minimal instruction. Male clients generally are able to void directly into the specimen container. Female clients usually sit or squat over the toilet, holding the container between their legs during voiding. About 120 mL (4 oz) of urine is generally required for this specimen. Clients who are seriously ill, physically incapacitated, or disoriented may need to use a bedpan or urinal in bed; others may require supervision or assistance in the bathroom. Whatever the situation, explicit directions are required:

- Keep the specimen free of fecal contamination.
- Female clients should discard the toilet tissue in the toilet or in a waste bag rather than in the bedpan.
- Tighten the lid on the container to prevent spillage and contamination of other objects.

Label the specimen container and complete the laboratory requisition correctly, then securely attach it to the specimen.

Clean-Catch or Midstream Specimen

Clean-catch or midstream voided specimens are collected when urine culture is ordered to identify microorganisms causing urinary tract infection (UTI). In these specimens, the client allows some passage of urine to clear the urethra, then collects the specimen in the middle of the urinary flow (hence, the term *midstream*). Care is taken to ensure that the specimen is as free as possible from contamination by microorganisms around the urinary meatus. Clean-catch specimens are collected in a sterile specimen container with a lid. Disposable clean-catch kits are available (Figure 39-6 ■).

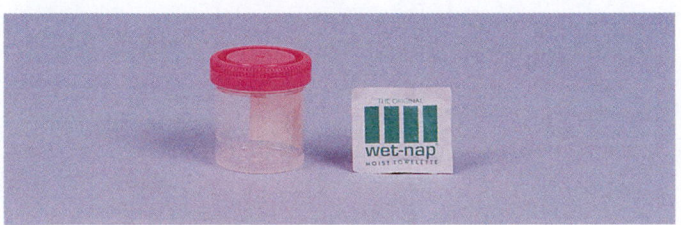

Figure 39-6. ■ Disposable clean-catch specimen equipment. (*Source:* © Jenny Thomas.)

Procedure 39-1 ■ at the end of this chapter explains how to collect a clean-catch urine specimen.

Timed Urine Specimen

Some urine examinations require collection of all urine produced and voided over a specific period of time, ranging from 1 to 2 hours to 24 hours. Timed specimens are generally refrigerated, placed on ice, or contain a preservative to prevent bacterial growth or decomposition of urine components. See Procedure 39-1 for specific steps in collecting a timed specimen.

Indwelling Catheter Specimen

Sterile urine specimens can be obtained from closed drainage systems by inserting a sterile needle attached to a syringe through a drainage port in the tubing. Aspiration of urine from catheters can be done only with self-sealing rubber catheters. When self-sealing rubber catheters are used, the needle is inserted just above the place where the catheter is attached to the drainage tubing.

URINE TESTING

Several basic urine tests are often performed by nurses. These include tests for specific gravity, pH, and the presence of abnormal constituents such as glucose, ketones, protein, and occult blood.

Specific Gravity

The specific gravity of urine is a measure of its concentration, or the amount of solutes present in the urine. The specific gravity of distilled water is 1.000. The specific gravity of urine normally ranges from 1.010 to 1.025. It increases when urine is concentrated (as in dehydration) and decreases when urine is dilute (as in diuresis). A urinometer or hydrometer in a cylinder of urine (Figure 39-7 ■) or a spectrometer or refractometer may be used to measure the specific gravity. Steps to measure specific gravity are outlined in Box 39-1 ■.

Other tests, such as pH and the presence of glucose, ketones, protein, and occult blood, are performed using reagent strips known as *dipsticks*. The strip is dipped into urine in a specimen cup. The nurse waits for a prescribed amount of time, then reads the reagent pad for changes in color to indicate the presence or absence of abnormal constituents or the pH. The reagent pad is compared to a color chart for the most accurate reading.

Urinary pH

Urinary pH is measured to determine the relative acidity or alkalinity of urine and to assess the client's acid-base status. Urine normally is slightly acidic, with an average pH of 6 (7 is neutral, less than 7 is acidic, greater than 7 is alkaline).

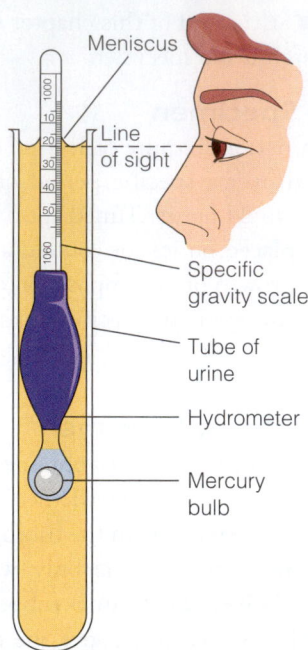

Meniscus

Line of sight

Specific gravity scale

Tube of urine

Hydrometer

Mercury bulb

Figure 39-7. ■ A urinometer measurement of the specific gravity of the urine is taken at the base of the meniscus.

BOX 39-1	**NURSING CARE CHECKLIST**

Measuring Specific Gravity of Urine

To Measure with a Urinometer

☑ Wear gloves and pour at least 20 mL of a fresh urine sample into the glass cylinder, or fill the cylinder three-quarters full.

☑ Place the urinometer into the cylinder and give it a gentle spin to prevent it from adhering to the sides of the cylinder.

☑ Hold the urinometer at eye level and read the measurement at the base of the meniscus at the surface of the urine (see Figure 39-7). The depth to which it sinks indicates the specific gravity.

To Measure with a Spectrometer or Refractometer

☑ Be sure to follow the manufacturer's directions.

☑ Don gloves, and place one or two drops of urine on the slide.

☑ Turn on the instrument light, and look into the instrument. The specific gravity will appear on a scope.

☑ Write down the number, then turn off the instrument.

☑ Remove the urine with a damp towel or gauze.

Following the Test

☑ Discard the urine. Clean the equipment with soap and water. Remove gloves.

☑ Document the results of the test on the client's record.

Glucose

Urine is tested for glucose to screen clients for diabetes mellitus and to assess clients for abnormal glucose tolerance during pregnancy. Normally, the urine does not contain any measurable glucose. The most accurate measurement for blood glucose is done with a glucometer.

Ketones

Ketone bodies, products of the breakdown of fatty acids, normally are not present in the urine but are found in the urine of clients with poorly controlled diabetes, or those who are alcoholic, fasting, starving, or consuming high-protein diets.

Protein

Protein molecules normally are too large to escape from glomerular capillaries into the filtrate. If the glomerular membrane has been damaged, proteins are allowed to escape.

Occult Blood

Normal urine is free from blood. When blood is present, it may be clearly visible or not visible (*occult*).

MEASURING RESIDUAL URINE

Residual urine (urine remaining in the bladder following the voiding) is normally not present or consists of only a few milliliters. If clients are retaining urine, they may void frequently in small amounts (e.g., less than 100 mL in an adult). Residual urine is measured to assess the amount of retained urine after voiding and to determine the need for interventions.

To measure residual urine, the nurse catheterizes the client immediately after voiding. The amount of urine voided and the amount obtained by catheterization are measured and recorded. An indwelling catheter may be ordered if the residual urine exceeds a specified amount.

EXTERNAL URINARY DRAINAGE DEVICES

The application of a condom or external catheter connected to a urinary drainage system is commonly prescribed for incontinent males. Use of a condom appliance is preferable to insertion of a retention catheter because the risk of urinary tract infection from a condom catheter is minimal.

Procedure 39-2 ■ at the end of this chapter describes how to apply and remove a drainage condom.

URINARY CATHETERIZATION

Urinary catheterization is the introduction of a catheter through the urethra into the urinary bladder. It is usually performed only when absolutely necessary because the danger exists of introducing microorganisms into the bladder, ureters, and kidneys. Strict sterile technique is used for catheterization. Box 39-2 ■ provides guidelines to prevent catheter-associated urinary infections.

BOX 39-2 NURSING CARE CHECKLIST

Preventing Catheter-Associated Urinary Infections

☑ Have an established infection control program.

☑ Catheterize clients only when necessary, by using aseptic technique, sterile equipment, and trained personnel.

☑ Maintain a sterile closed-drainage system.

☑ Do not disconnect the catheter and drainage tubing unless absolutely necessary.

☑ Remove the catheter as soon as possible.

☑ Follow and reinforce good handwashing technique.

☑ Provide routine perineal hygiene, including cleansing with soap and water after defecation.

☑ Prevent contamination of the catheter with feces in the incontinent client.

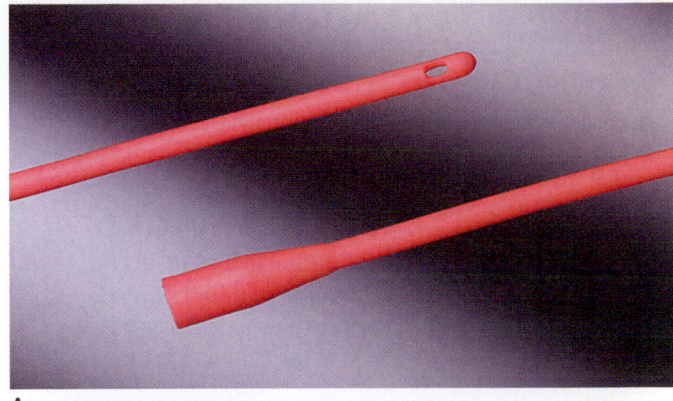

A

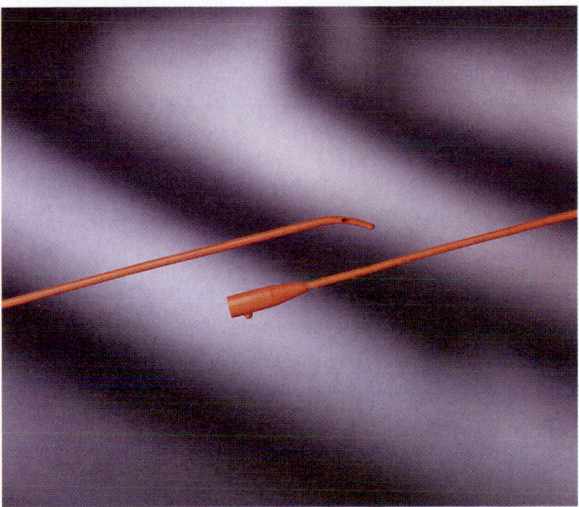

B

Figure 39-8. ■ Two types of straight catheters: **A.** Red-rubber or Robinson catheter. **B.** Coudé catheter. (Courtesy of Bard Medical Division.)

Catheters are commonly made of rubber, plastic, latex, or silicone. They are sized by the diameter of the lumen, using the French (Fr) scale: the larger the number, the larger the lumen.

The straight catheter is a single-lumen tube with a small eye or opening about 1.25 cm (1/2 in.) from the insertion tip (Figure 39-8A ■). It is inserted to drain the bladder, then immediately removed. The coudé catheter, a variation of the straight catheter, is more rigid and has a tapered, curved tip (Figure 39-8B). It is designed for use with men with prostatic hypertrophy because it is more easily controlled and less traumatic on insertion than a straight catheter. Catheterization of females and males using straight catheters is described in Procedures 39-3 and 39-4 ■, respectively, at the end of this chapter.

The retention, or Foley, catheter is a *double-lumen* (double-tube) catheter. The larger lumen drains urine from the bladder. A second, smaller lumen is used to inflate a balloon

near the tip of the catheter to hold the catheter in place within the bladder (Figure 39-9A ■). Clients who require continuous or intermittent bladder irrigation may have a three-way Foley catheter (Figure 39-9B). The three-way

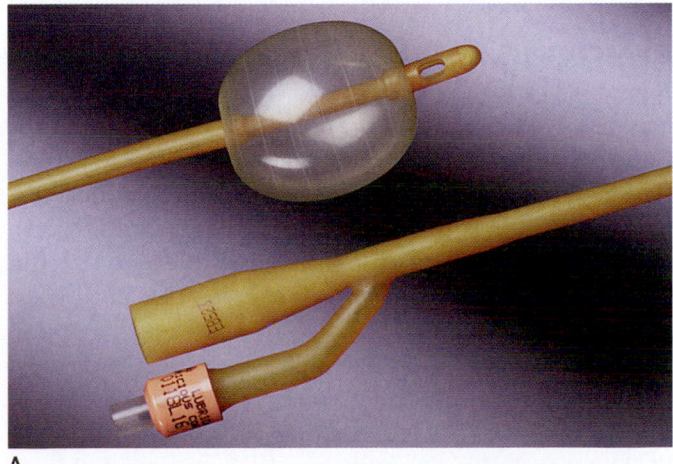

A

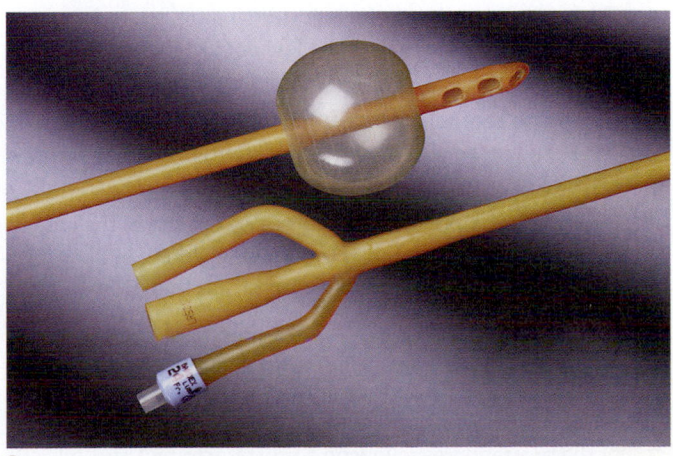

B

Figure 39-9. ■ **A.** Retention (Foley) catheter with the balloon inflated. **B.** Three-way Foley catheter. (Courtesy of Bard Medical Division.)

catheter has a third lumen through which sterile irrigating fluid can flow into the bladder. The fluid then exits the bladder through the drainage lumen, along with the urine. Procedure 39-5 ■ outlines how to insert and remove a retention catheter, and Box 39-3 ■ provides guidelines for assessing clients with retention catheters.

The balloon on a retention catheter is sized by the volume of fluid used to inflate it. The two most common balloon sizes are 5 and 30 mL. The size of the balloon is indicated on the catheter along with the diameter, for example, "#18 Fr—5 mL." Box 39-4 ■ provides guidelines for catheter selection.

Retention catheters usually are connected to a closed gravity drainage system. This system consists of the catheter, drainage tubing, and a collecting bag for the urine. A *closed system* cannot be opened anywhere along the system, from catheter to collecting bag, to reduce the risk of microorganisms entering the urinary tract. Urine drains via gravity from the bladder to the collecting bag.

Encourage the client with a retention catheter to drink up to 3,000 mL per day if permitted. Large amounts of fluid increase urine output, keeping the bladder flushed out and decreasing urinary stasis and subsequent infection and minimizing the risk of sediment or other particles obstructing the drainage tubing. Accurate recording of fluid intake and output is discussed in Chapter 26 🔗.

To acidify the urine of clients with a retention catheter, encourage foods such as eggs, meat and poultry, whole grains, cranberries, plums, and tomatoes. These foods tend to increase the acidity of urine and may reduce the risk of UTI and calculus formation.

Clean the perineal area with soap and water twice daily for the client with a retention catheter to keep the area clean and free from fecal contamination. No special meatal care is recommended. The nurse should check agency practice in this regard.

Routine changing of the catheter and tubing is not recommended. However, they should be changed when sediment collects in the catheter or tubing and impairs urine drainage. When this occurs, a new sterile catheter with a closed drainage system is inserted to prevent obstruction of the catheter and drainage tubing by sediment. Guidelines for assessing clients with retention catheters are given in Box 39-3.

Instruct the client and family to keep the drainage tubing and bag lower than the bladder at all times. This prevents reflux of contaminated urine back into the sterile bladder. Explain how to avoid tension on the catheter tubing, kinks in the drainage tubing, and lying on the tubing to prevent blockage of urine drainage.

REMOVING RETENTION CATHETERS

Retention catheters are removed after their purpose has been achieved, usually on the order of the physician. If the catheter has been in place for a short time (e.g., a few days), the client usually has little difficulty regaining normal urinary elimination patterns. Swelling of the urethra, however, may initially interfere with voiding, so the nurse should regularly assess the client for urinary retention until voiding is reestablished.

Clients who have had a retention catheter for a prolonged period may require bladder retraining to regain bladder muscle tone. With an indwelling catheter in place, the bladder muscle does not stretch and contract regularly as it does when the bladder fills and empties by voiding. A few days prior to removal, the catheter may be clamped for specified periods of time (e.g., 2 to 4 hours), then released to allow the bladder to empty. This allows the bladder to distend and stimulates its musculature. See Procedure 39-5 for steps to remove a retention catheter.

URINARY IRRIGATIONS

An irrigation is a flushing or washing-out with a specified solution. A bladder irrigation is carried out on a physician's order, usually to wash out the bladder and sometimes to apply a medication to the bladder lining. Sometimes this is the RN's responsibility; check facility policy. Catheter irrigations may be performed to maintain or restore the patency of a catheter, for example, to remove blood clots blocking the catheter.

The closed method is the preferred technique for catheter or bladder irrigation because of the lower risk of urinary tract infection (Figure 39-10 ■). Closed catheter

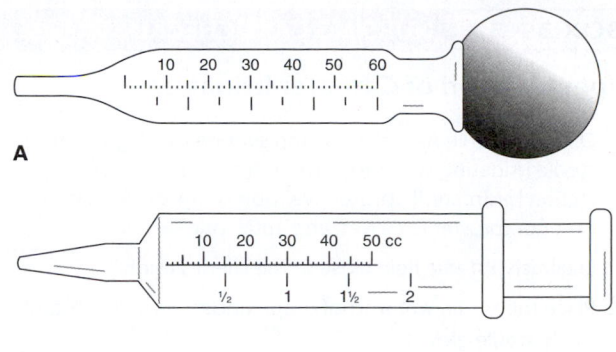

Figure 39-11. ■ Two common irrigation syringes: **A.** Asepto. **B.** Piston syringe.

irrigations may be either continuous or intermittent. A three-way, or triple lumen, catheter generally is used for closed irrigations. Techniques for setting up and maintaining a continuous or intermittent closed catheter irrigation are outlined in Procedure 39-6 ■ at the end of the chapter.

Occasionally, an open irrigation may be necessary to restore catheter patency. The risk of injecting microorganisms into the urinary tract is greater because the connection between the indwelling catheter and the drainage tubing is broken. Strict precautions to maintain the sterility of the drainage tubing connector and interior of the indwelling catheter must be taken to minimize this risk.

A sterile Asepto or piston syringe is used for open irrigation (Figure 39-11 ■) to wash out blood clots and mucous fragments that occlude the catheter, or when it is undesirable to change the catheter. The steps involved in performing an open method of irrigation are shown in Box 39-5 ■.

SUPRAPUBIC CATHETER CARE

A suprapubic catheter is inserted through the abdominal wall above the symphysis pubis into the urinary bladder (Figure 39-12 ■). The physician inserts the catheter using local anesthesia or during bladder or vaginal surgery. The catheter may be secured in place with sutures, with a body seal, or with both sutures and a body seal. The catheter is then attached to a closed drainage system.

Care of clients with a suprapubic catheter includes regular assessments of the client's urine, fluid intake, and comfort; maintenance of a patent drainage system; skin care around the insertion site; periodic clamping of the catheter preparatory to removing it; and measurement of residual urine. Orders generally include leaving the catheter open to drainage for 48 to 72 hours, then clamping the catheter for 3- to 4-hour periods during the day until the client can void satisfactory amounts. Satisfactory

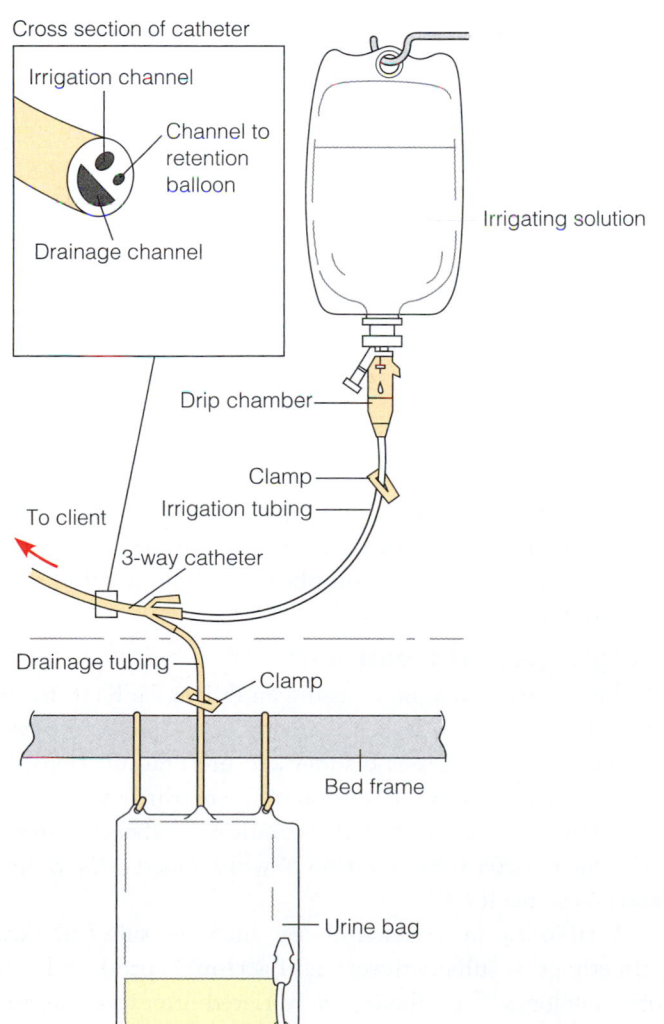

Figure 39-10. ■ A closed catheter or bladder irrigation system.

Open Method of Catheter Irrigation

- ☑ Obtain a sterile Asepto or piston syringe (see Figure 39-11), sterile irrigating solution at room temperature, sterile collection basin, sterile protective tubing cap, sterile waterproof drape, sterile gloves, and antiseptic swabs.
- ☑ Establish a sterile field close to the client's thigh.
- ☑ Place the sterile waterproof drape under the catheter and apply sterile gloves.
- ☑ Clean the junction between the catheter and the drainage tubing with antiseptic swabs.
- ☑ Disconnect the catheter and drainage tubing. Hold the catheter and tubing about 2.5 cm (1 in.) from their ends and place them on a sterile surface to avoid contaminating them. Cover the open end of the drainage tubing with the sterile protective tubing cap.
- ☑ Draw irrigation fluid into the syringe and instill it slowly into the catheter.
- ☑ Remove the syringe and allow the irrigating solution to drain by gravity from the catheter into the collection basin.
- ☑ Repeat irrigations depending on the amount of solution to be instilled or until urine runs freely through the catheter and drainage is clear.
- ☑ Reconnect the catheter and drainage tubing, maintaining the sterility of the ends of the tubing and the inside of the catheter.
- ☑ Remove gloves.
- ☑ Assess and document the irrigation returns.

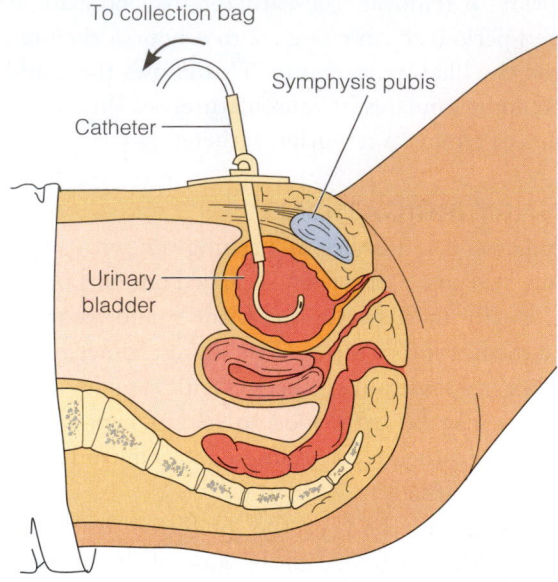

Figure 39-12. ■ Suprapubic catheter in place.

voiding is determined by measuring the client's residual urine after voiding.

Dressings around the suprapubic catheter are changed using sterile technique whenever they are soiled with drainage to prevent bacterial growth and reduce the potential for infection. Procedures for cleaning wounds and changing dressings are discussed in Chapter 24 ∞. Any redness and discharge around the insertion site must be reported.

KIDNEY DISORDERS

Pyelonephritis

Pyelonephritis is an inflammation that affects the kidney pelvis and parenchyma. It can be an acute episode or become a chronic condition. It can present abruptly as with a bacterial infection or be chronic, associated with other disease processes. Factors that cause increased risk are obstruction, pregnancy, and congenital malformations. *Escherichia coli* is commonly the offending organism, spreading the inflammation and affecting the renal pelvis and cortex areas. The kidney becomes edematous with abscesses forming, causing kidney damage.

Manifestations

Signs and symptoms occur quickly with an acute incident manifesting with elevated temperature, chills, malaise, and vomiting. The client may complain of flank pain. Symptoms similar to cystitis may become evident (see the section on Bladder Disorders). Chronic pyelonephritis progresses, with scarring and fibrosis occurring within the renal pelvis and adjoining structures. Complications include chronic renal failure.

Diagnosis and Treatment

Pyelonephritis is diagnosed using an IVP and a KUB to visualize the kidneys, ureters, and bladder. A voiding cystourethrography assesses bladder and urethral functions. A cystoscopy is direct visualization of the urethra and bladder and assists in diagnosis of the condition. Laboratory tests are done to determine elevation of white blood cells, BUN, and creatinine levels.

Antibiotics or antimicrobials such as sulfonamides, trimethoprim-sulfamethoxazole (Bactrim, Septra), and fluoroquinolones (Ciprofloxin) are initiated prior to urine culture results because of their effectiveness in fighting the usual organisms. In acute pyelonephritis, response to the medication is quick. When chronic pyelonephritis is diagnosed, a 21-day antibiotic treatment is necessary. Intravenous doses of antibiotics may be required depending on the extent of infection. Urinary anti-infectives are used for resistant or recurring infections.

Polycystic Kidney Disease

Polycystic kidney disease is a familial disease characterized by an enlarged kidney with multiple fluid-filled cysts (Figure 39-13 ■). It is found in both children and adults of all ages. As the cysts fill and expand, the kidney accommodates the growing cysts by enlarging. The cysts slowly begin to damage the functional units of the kidney. Cysts may also form in other organs, causing further functional deterioration.

Manifestations

Signs and symptoms include kidney pain in the flank area. Hematuria, proteinuria, and polyuria may be observed. Hypertension, urinary tract infection, and stones may occur. The enlarged kidneys are palpable. As the disease progresses, renal failure may result.

Diagnosis and Treatment

A renal ultrasound is used to diagnose the kidney cysts.

Maintaining renal function and preventing further damage are the primary goals of treatment. Increasing fluid intake to 2,500 mL per day helps prevent urinary tract infections and calculus formation. Antihypertensive medications may be ordered for elevated blood pressure readings. As the disease progresses, clients may require hemodialysis and need kidney transplantation. See the Renal Failure section later in this chapter.

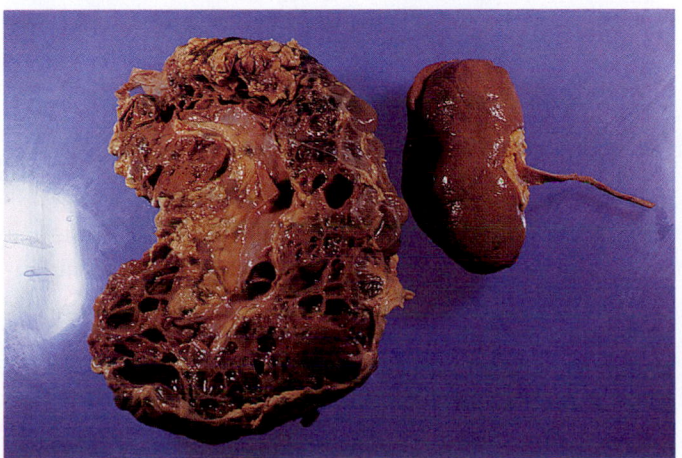

Figure 39-13. ■ A polycystic kidney. The functional tissue of the kidneys is gradually destroyed and replaced with fluid-filled cysts. (*Source:* A. Glauberman/Photo Researchers, Inc.)

Glomerulonephritis

Glomerulonephritis is described as an inflammatory disease of the glomerulus affecting kidney function. It can be acute or chronic. The glomerulus capillaries trap the antigen/antibody (immune response to the infection), causing inflammatory kidney damage. The capillary membrane is compromised, changing the ability to be selectively permeable and allowing RBCs and protein to spill into the urine.

Manifestations of Acute Glomerulonephritis

Acute glomerulonephritis occurs abruptly and sometimes follows an upper respiratory infection (usually one caused by a streptococcal organism). It is most commonly found in young boys 3 to 7 years of age but does affect all ages.

Signs and symptoms include proteinuria, hematuria, azotemia, and oliguria (less than 400 mL of output in 24 hours). Fatigue, headache, hypertension, nausea, and vomiting are common complaints. There is pain over the kidney area as well as generalized edema and facial puffiness, including periorbital edema. Symptoms can subside within 2 weeks, with the client making a full recovery. Others develop chronic glomerulonephritis with recurring renal impairment.

Manifestations of Chronic Glomerulonephritis

Chronic glomerulonephritis is defined as a slow, progressive inflammation resulting in sclerosis, scarring, and damage to the glomeruli with the loss of some nephrons. The kidneys begin to atrophy, becoming granular and losing function. Chronic glomerulonephritis is usually the consequence of systemic disease. In some cases there is no history of previous kidney disease.

Signs and symptoms also develop slowly and are not easily diagnosed until renal failure signs become apparent. Diabetic nephropathy (see Chapter 38 ⌾) occurs in the later stage of the disease; microproteinuria is noted as glomerular filtration is impaired. Clients with systemic lupus erythematosus (see Chapter 35 ⌾) present with nephritis, proteinuria, hematuria, and renal failure.

Diagnosis and Treatment

Laboratory studies assist in the diagnosis and determination of the cause of glomerulonephritis. Studies include BUN, serum creatinine levels, urine creatinine clearance, and electrolytes. Serum albumin and urine protein levels are also monitored. A kidney biopsy may be ordered.

The treatment goal of both acute and chronic glomerulonephritis is to treat the disease process and protect renal function. Medications used include steroids to reduce the inflammation and antibiotics for poststreptococcal infection. Antihypertensives and diuretics may be needed to reduce blood pressure and edema. Daily weights, I&O readings, and a diet low in sodium and protein, with increased carbohydrates and high in iron, will be needed.

Renal Cancer

Tumors can occur anywhere along the urinary tract, although the most common site is the bladder. Risk factors for renal cancer include smoking, obesity, dialysis, and exposure to industrial pollution. The renal system is highly vascular and increases the risk for metastasis. If the tumor is in the kidney, it can become quite large before symptoms are evident. Often, the cancer has metastasized before a diagnosis is made. Wilms' tumor is a highly metastatic tumor of the kidney that may affect children. Box 39-6 ■ provides more information about Wilms' tumor.

See the section on Bladder Disorders for more information about bladder cancer.

Urinary Obstruction

Urinary obstructions can occur anywhere in the urinary tract. Common causes include tumors, stones (renal calculi or nephrolithiasis), cysts, kinked ureter or stenosis, ureter spasms, enlarged prostate, and congenital strictures. Obstructions can occur as a result of surgical intervention or trauma. Complications include **hydronephrosis** (urine backing up into the kidney), which causes kidney distention. Waste products begin to accumulate in the blood, damaging the kidney. When the blockage occurs distal to the kidney, it takes the kidney longer to distend, thus delaying diagnosis. (See the Ureteral Disorders section for information about renal calculi.)

Renal Failure

Renal failure is a condition in which the kidneys are unable to carry out the normal functions necessary to eliminate waste products and maintain fluid and electrolyte balance. Other kidney functions that can be affected include acid-base balance (see Chapter 26 ⬤⬤), red blood cell (RBC) formation (see Chapter 34 ⬤⬤), calcium regulation, and blood pressure regulation (see Chapter 33 ⬤⬤). Renal failure is characterized by:

- **Uremia** (a toxic state marked by an accumulation of urea and other nitrogenous wastes in the blood).
- **Azotemia** (increased nitrogenous wastes in the blood including urea and creatinine).

ACUTE RENAL FAILURE

Acute renal failure (ARF) is described as a sudden decrease in or total lack of kidney function. It can be reversed with prompt treatment. Kidney damage causes toxins to

| BOX 39-6 | PEDIATRIC CONSIDERATIONS |

Wilms' Tumor

Wilms' tumor is one of the most common childhood tumors of the abdomen, and the most common type of kidney tumor. The exact cause of this tumor in most children is unknown. The disease is estimated to occur in about 1 out of 200,000 to 250,000 children. The peak time of occurrence is at 3 years old, and Wilms' tumor is rare after the age of 8 years.

Manifestations

The client may present with abdominal pain, swelling in the abdomen, fever, loss of appetite, nausea and vomiting, or general malaise. There may be blood in the urine (less than $1/4$ of children), or urine may have an abnormal color. Other manifestations are high blood pressure, constipation, or increased growth on one side of the body.

clinical ALERT

The tumor sheds cells easily, leading to tumor metastasis. Avoid palpation of the abdomen, and use care during bathing and handling to avoid injury to the tumor site.

A history and physical examination are done, including questions about a family history of cancer or birth defects in the child. Tests include a CBC (may show anemia), BUN, creatinine, and creatinine clearance (may be decreased). Urinalysis may show blood or protein in the urine. Visualization tests include ultrasound or x-ray; a CT scan of the abdomen, which would show a mass arising from the kidney; a chest x-ray (to look for metastases); and an intravenous pyelogram (to look for kidney distortion). Other tests may be required to determine if the tumor has spread.

When Wilms' tumor is confirmed, surgical exploration and *radical nephrectomy* (removal of the tumor) are scheduled as soon as possible. Radiation therapy and chemotherapy will often be started after surgery, depending on the stage of the tumor.

With treatment, the disease has a high cure rate. Children with a localized tumor have a 90% cure rate when treated with surgery and chemotherapy; or with surgery, radiation, and chemotherapy combined.

Spread of the tumor to the lungs, liver, bone, or brain is the most worrisome complication. High blood pressure and kidney damage may occur as the result of the tumor or its treatment. If Wilms' tumor is present in both kidneys, removal may leave the client with borderline kidney function.

accumulate in the blood. ARF affects 10,000 people per year. Some factors that increase the risk for acute renal failure include renal trauma, surgery, urinary tract obstruction, and infection. Three categories have been identified to describe the causes of acute renal failure:

1. *Prerenal failure* is associated with kidney ischemia that may be precipitated by hypotension related to dehydration or fluid volume deficit. Heart failure and shock can also prompt an episode of acute renal failure. When

the blood supply to the nephrons is inadequate, the ability to produce urine and remove waste products is impaired.

2. *Intrarenal failure* is linked to damaged nephrons and kidney tissue. Common causes include diabetes mellitus, glomerulonephritis, nephrotoxin exposure, and allergic reactions to contrast dyes and medications.

3. *Postrenal failure* is connected to urinary obstruction. The blood supply to the kidneys may be adequate initially but as the urine backs up into the kidney, the nephron function is impaired. Obstructions include renal calculi, tumors, and prostate enlargement.

Manifestations

Characteristic signs include a sudden decrease in urine output to less than 400 mL in 24 hours. Confusion and disorientation occur as azotemia becomes evident. Fluid volume excess is demonstrated with elevated sodium levels, water retention, and edema. Hypertension and heart failure (see Chapter 33) can result. Hyperkalemia is manifested by nausea, vomiting, cardiac dysrhythmias, and muscle weakness. Metabolic acidosis and anemia can occur (see Chapters 26 and 34). Laboratory tests show elevated BUN and creatinine levels.

CHRONIC RENAL FAILURE

Chronic renal failure (CRF) is a slow, progressive deterioration in kidney function. Seventy-five thousand people are affected by CRF in the United States. The functional loss cannot be reversed. Symptoms may go undetected. However, the destruction of the nephrons continues to progress. When the kidneys ultimately lose the ability to excrete waste products and regulate fluid and electrolytes, the client is said to be in **end-stage renal disease** (ESRD). There are many causes of CRF such as polycystic kidney disease, lower urinary tract obstruction that leads to hydronephrosis, glomerulonephritis, chronic pyelonephritis, and renal tumors. Systemic diseases contribute to the development of CRF. Diabetes mellitus leads to nephropathy (see Chapter 38). Autoimmune disease such as systemic lupus erythematous and chronic hypertension result in nephrosclerosis (see Chapter 35).

Manifestations

Symptoms of urinary insufficiency begin to develop when 75% of nephron function is lost. Symptoms in the early stages of CRF include polyuria, lowered specific gravity, and polydipsia. In CRF, the kidneys may be able to maintain some urine output without maintaining urine concentration. As more nephrons become damaged, the remaining nephrons compensate by working harder and, hence, become enlarged.

Anuria, oliguria, weight gain, hypertension, and pulmonary edema can develop. Signs and symptoms of congestive heart failure (CHF), dyspnea, and hypervolemia may be observed. Uremia may be manifested by nausea, fatigue, apathy, and general weakness.

Diagnosis and Treatment

When renal failure is the diagnosis, lab tests indicate highly elevated BUN and serum creatinine levels. A creatinine clearance test is ordered to evaluate the glomerular filtration rate (GFR). Serum electrolytes, complete blood count (CBC), blood gases, and urinalysis, including specific gravity readings, are used to monitor renal function. Subjective data such as confusion and disorientation may indicate uremia and must be documented. In chronic renal failure, a biopsy of the kidney may be done to identify the extent of kidney damage. A fluid restriction will be ordered depending on the amount of kidney function.

Sodium is restricted in the diet to regulate fluid balance. Sodium levels may appear normal due to increased water retention, which dilutes the blood. Increased calorie intake and low protein intake may also be part of the diet. Diuretics are ordered to assist in water excretion. Vitamin supplements and iron may be needed to combat anemia.

DIALYSIS

When medical management of renal failure is insufficient, dialysis may be required. **Dialysis** is a process for eliminating nephrotoxins and retained fluid from the body. It must be done at regular intervals, from daily to three times a week, depending on the buildup of toxins. Because of this schedule, clients on dialysis often feel a lack of control and the inability to perform usual activities. Many times these clients suffer from depression. There are two types of dialysis: hemodialysis and peritoneal dialysis (Figures 39-14A and B ■).

Hemodialysis

Hemodialysis is a process of removing waste products, excess fluids, and electrolytes from the blood. Blood, containing large amounts of nitrogenous waste, passes through a dialysate solution. These highly concentrated waste molecules move to a lowered concentration in the dialysate and are removed from the blood cells. Water and ions can pass through the semipermeable membrane of the hemodialysis machine, but blood cells and proteins are unable to pass through. Hemodialysis is usually performed at an outpatient dialysis center or in the hospital setting. An arteriovenous (AV) fistula is created surgically by joining an artery and a vein, usually in the forearm, with graft tubing. This fistula is used to access the vein and artery to connect the client to

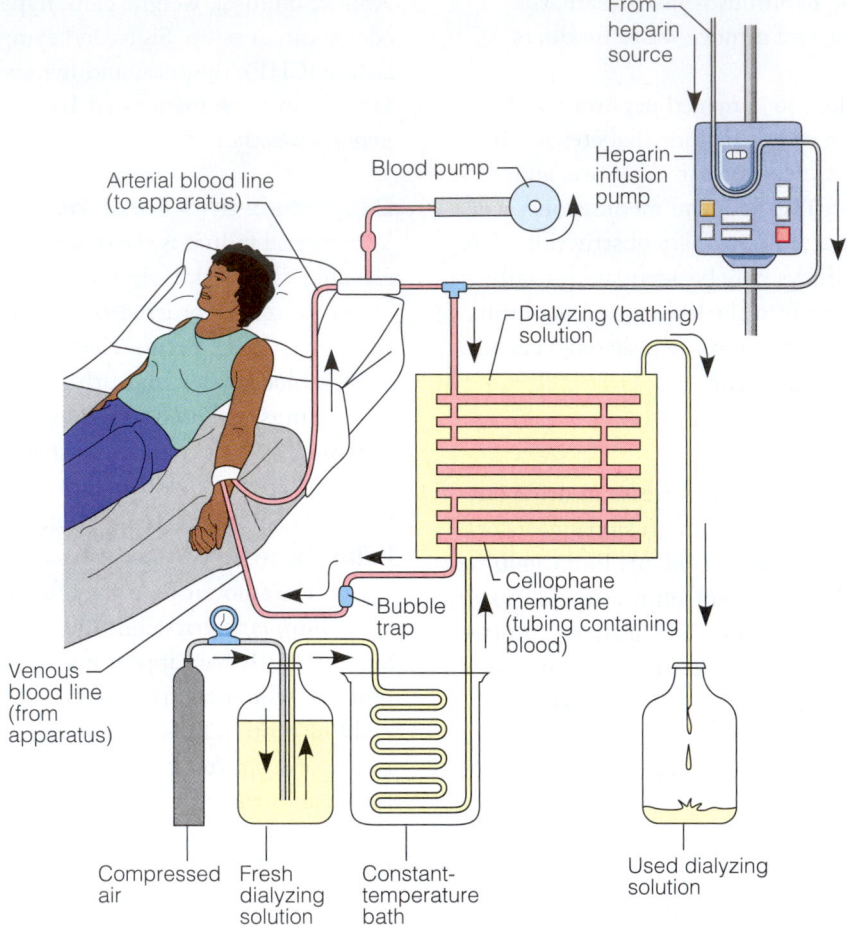

Arterial blood line (to apparatus)

Blood pump

From heparin source

Heparin infusion pump

Dialyzing (bathing) solution

Cellophane membrane (tubing containing blood)

Bubble trap

Venous blood line (from apparatus)

Compressed air

Fresh dialyzing solution

Constant-temperature bath

Used dialyzing solution

A

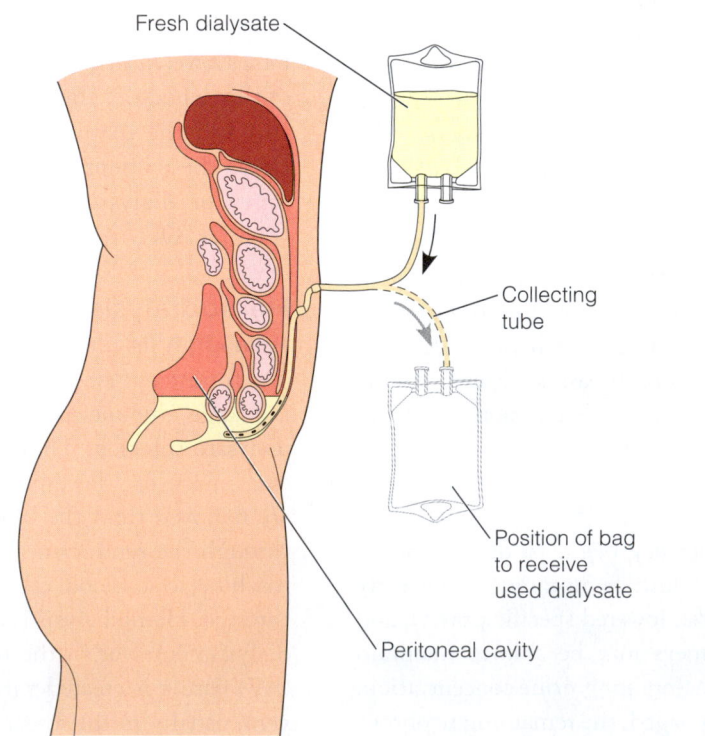

Fresh dialysate

Collecting tube

Position of bag to receive used dialysate

Peritoneal cavity

B

Figure 39-14. ■ **A.** A hemodialysis system. **B.** Peritoneal dialysis.

the hemodialysis machine. Hypotension is a common complication of dialysis, so the nurse often holds blood pressure medications prior to dialysis per the physician's orders.

Peritoneal Dialysis

Peritoneal dialysis is a process to remove extra fluid and waste products, but it differs from hemodialysis because the dialyzing solution is instilled directly into the abdomen (see Figure 39-14B). The peritoneum serves as the semipermeable membrane. Excess concentrations of electrolytes, uremic toxins, and water move across the peritoneal membrane into the dialysate. A peritoneal catheter is inserted into the abdomen and the dialysate is infused through it. Medication may also be added to the dialysate. The fluid remains in the abdomen for an ordered amount of time, usually between 6 and 8 hours (dwell time). The fluid is then drained from the abdomen into a sterile bag. This procedure must be done five to six times per week. Continuous ambulatory peritoneal dialysis (CAPD) is the most common form of peritoneal dialysis. Peritoneal dialysis is less costly and less effective than hemodialysis but can be performed in the home with proper training. However, one serious complication is the risk of peritonitis.

KIDNEY TRANSPLANT

Kidney transplant (Figure 39-15 ■) is the treatment for end-stage renal disease. Some transplants (about 30%) are donated by a living donor. The remaining transplants come from cadavers. The client is placed on a recipient list and counseled regarding the risks and complications of the procedure. The average kidney transplant can last approximately

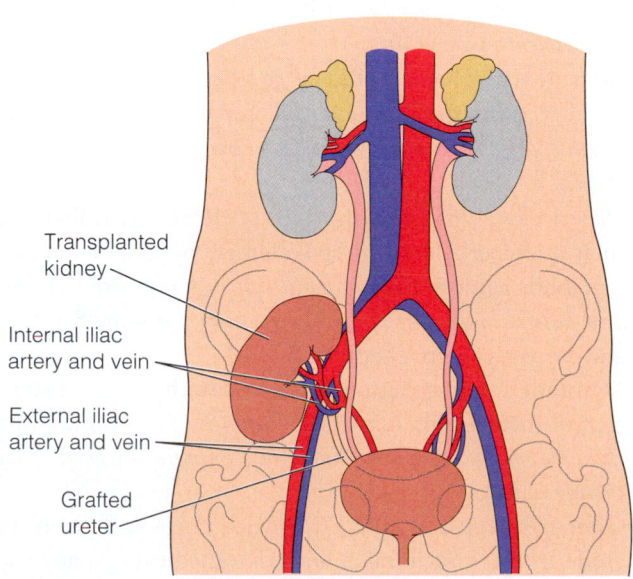

Transplanted kidney

Internal iliac artery and vein

External iliac artery and vein

Grafted ureter

Figure 39-15. ■ Placement of a transplanted kidney in the iliac fossa with anastomosis to the hypogastric artery, iliac vein, and bladder.

10 years, although some last longer. The risk for rejection is the major complication for the transplant client. The body's normal immune system produces an inflammatory response against the transplanted kidney, which it recognizes as foreign tissue. Immunosuppressive drugs and steroids are administered to overcome rejection. However, these medications also increase the client's vulnerability to infections. The WBC count, vital signs, and urinary output are monitored. Signs and symptoms of rejection include fever, swelling, and tenderness over the transplanted kidney site with a decline in urine output and renal function.

NURSING CARE

PRIORITIZING NURSING CARE

When caring for clients with renal disorders who are not in renal failure, your focus of care is preserving renal function and fluid balance. Closely assess clients with kidney infections for signs of worsening infection: elevating temperature, increased WBCs, and decreasing urine output. Monitor for signs of fluid overload, which would indicate lack of kidney function. Signs of fluid overload include less than 30 mL of urine output per hour, crackles in lungs, and edema of feet, hands, and face. Measure intake and output accurately, observing urine for blood, mucus, or cloudiness. Watch IV fluids carefully to be sure that they do not exceed the ordered rate, which could cause the client to go into fluid overload.

When caring for clients who are in acute or chronic renal failure, your focus is to alleviate complications and promote comfort. Be vigilant about dialysis shunts—*do not* take blood pressure or perform venipuncture in the arm where the shunt is located. Measure all intake carefully and record it promptly. When fluid restriction is ordered, follow it exactly for your shift.

ASSESSING

The LPN/LVN is responsible for assessing the client's urinary function by collecting data and collaborating with the RN. The nurse determines the client's normal voiding pattern and frequency, appearance of the urine and any recent changes, any past or current problems with urination, the presence of an ostomy, and factors influencing the elimination pattern. The nurse observes for hematuria and changes in the urine and urinary patterns.

Complete physical assessment of the urinary tract (completed by the RN) usually includes palpation of the kidneys to detect areas of tenderness and palpation of the bladder. The urethral meatus of both male and female clients may be inspected for swelling, discharge, and inflammation. It is important to note a history of recent upper respiratory infection for clients with systemic disease since treatment methods may be influenced by this information.

Because problems with urination can affect the elimination of wastes from the body, it is important that the LPN/LVN observe the skin for color, texture, and tissue turgor as well as for the presence of edema. If incontinence, dribbling, or dysuria are noted in the history, the skin of the perineum should be inspected for irritation, because contact with urine can excoriate the skin.

DIAGNOSING, PLANNING, AND IMPLEMENTING

Possible nursing diagnoses for clients with kidney disorders include:

- *Impaired Urinary Elimination*
- *Excess Fluid Volume*
- *Risk for Infection*
- *Risk for Impaired Skin Integrity*
- *Pain, Acute or Chronic*
- *Anxiety*
- *Readiness for Enhanced Nutrition*
- *Fatigue*
- *Deficient Knowledge* related to medications and treatment

Outcomes for clients with kidney disorders might include the following:

- Client will maintain normal amount and quality of urine output.
- Client will remain free of infection.
- Client will report pain managed with medications.
- Client will be able to describe medication and treatment regimen.

Nursing interventions for clients with kidney disorders include, but are not limited to, the following:

- Assess vital signs, particularly temperature, every 4 hours and palpate the abdomen for areas of tenderness. *These methods can detect signs of infection.*
- Monitor blood pressure every 4 hours for hypertension. *Hypertension can indicate fluid volume excess.*
- Monitor intake and output and observe the color, clarity, character, and odor of the urinary output. *This helps determine kidney function and urine abnormalities.*
- Encourage increased fluid intake *to flush the urinary tract* unless contraindicated.
- Assess the client's access to the bathroom and determine if the client needs a commode, bedpan, or urinal. *This helps prevent falls, especially if the client is experiencing urinary urgency and/or frequency.*

- Monitor laboratory tests for elevated WBCs, *indicating infection,* or elevated BUN and creatinine, *indicating loss of kidney function.*
- Obtain urine specimens for testing as ordered. Test urine samples for pH levels and for the presence of abnormal constituents. *Urine tests help reveal effectiveness of kidney function.*

For Clients with Renal Failure

- Monitor blood pressure and administer antihypertensive medication as ordered. *Renal failure leads to extremely elevated blood pressure.*
- Check ordered medications for nephrotoxicity and ask for alternative medications when possible. *Many medications are eliminated through the kidneys; those that are damaging to kidneys can shut down kidneys that are poorly functioning.*
- Maintain skin integrity and encourage frequent position changes. Inspect for potential areas of skin breakdown. *Clients with renal dysfunction may be on bed rest and therefore be at risk for complications of immobility.*
- Monitor for edema and weight gain. *Edema and weight gain can indicate poor kidney function and fluid volume excess.*
- Monitor intake and output each shift or more often if ordered. *This alerts the nurse to fluid gain and diminishing urine excretion.*
- Auscultate lung and heart sounds every four hours or as ordered and encourage the client to sit in a Fowler's position. *This position increases lung expansion and helps detect early pulmonary and cardiac complications.*
- Encourage client to turn, cough, and perform deep breathing exercises every 2 hours. *Pulmonary complications are frequent causes of death.*
- Administer oxygen as ordered to help relieve fatigue, respiratory difficulty, and anemia. *Supplemental oxygen helps decrease fatigue and helps increase circulating oxygen in the blood.*
- Observe for signs and symptoms of electrolyte imbalances such as hyperkalemia, hypokalemia, hypocalcemia, and metabolic acidosis. *The kidneys' role in fluid, electrolyte, and acid-base balance is compromised in kidney disease.* See fluid and electrolytes in Chapter 26 🔗.
- Maintain fluid restriction as ordered with careful observation of intravenous infusions. *Rapid IV infusions can cause fluid volume excess, which cannot be eliminated by poorly functioning kidneys.*
- Offer frequent oral care. When ice chips are given, include in the total intake, and give medications at mealtimes to use the fluids given with meal to take medications. Accurately measure all intake and output. *This helps keep fluids at a manageable level for clients on dialysis.*

- Cognitive changes may indicate uremia and azotemia. *When waste products are retained in the blood, brain function is affected.*
- Reinforce instruction regarding medication compliance and the importance of completing the antibiotic regimen as ordered when infection is detected. *Clients with acute or chronic kidney disorders need instruction regarding disease, treatment, and compliance.*
- Arrange consultation with a dietitian for diet planning along with low sodium and possible protein restrictions. Reinforce instruction and teaching. *Clients who face a need to change their lifestyles may not be able to absorb all the information at first. Reinforcement and repetition will help them learn what changes they must make and will assist them in coping.*
- Reinforce dietary restrictions. *These help decrease the kidneys' workload.*
- Have the client conserve energy by having rest periods. Observe the client's activity levels. *Clients with renal impairment will tire easily due to waste products in the blood.*
- Offer frequent small meals to clients who are fatigued. *This helps ensure adequate intake and adequate rest.*
- Offer the client the opportunity to ventilate inner feelings and concerns. Encourage the client and family to get involved with a support group. Allow the client to participate in decisions that affect care. *These interventions allow the client some control and provide support for coping with end-stage renal disease.*

For Clients on Dialysis

- Assess the AV fistula site for patency by auscultation of the *bruit* (audible blood flow through the shunt). Palpate the site for a strong pulsation (*thrill*). *Absences of bruit may indicate vessel damage and failure of AV fistula.*
- Notify the physician if there is an absence of the bruit or pulsation. *This indicates a problem with access for dialysis.*
- Monitor the access site for bleeding and infection every shift. *These can indicate complications of dialysis.*
- Arrange for rest periods after dialysis. *The client is often fatigued after the treatment.*

clinical ALERT

Blood pressure readings and venipunctures may not be performed on the same side as a dialysis access device. Always take readings on the opposite extremity.

EVALUATING

Assessing the effect of nursing interventions for the client with kidney disorders includes the accuracy of data collection, goal setting, and nursing care implementation. Fluid volume status, weight gain, blood pressure control, edema, and urine output reflect control of the condition. Evaluate diet, medication, and disease knowledge including compliance. A lowered value of laboratory tests (BUN, creatinine) indicates increasing renal function.

URETERAL, BLADDER, AND URETHRAL DISORDERS

Calculi (Urinary Stones)

Calculi form when salts in the urine precipitate or there is an increased saturation of glomerular filtrate. Urine that is consistently acidic or alkaline increases the risk for stone formation. When a client is immobile, calcium is released from the bone into the blood, adding to the potential for calculi formation. Dehydration, infection, obstruction, and a diet high in purine (uric acid), calcium, or phosphate are factors in calculi formation.

Manifestations

The amount of pain is related to the size of the stone. A small stone may pass without symptoms. A larger stone may occlude the ureter, causing it to spasm. This causes excruciating pain known as *renal colic*. Flank pain may indicate kidney or upper ureter stones. A client may complain of a deep dull aching when stones are in the ureters and spasm does not occur. Nausea and vomiting can accompany

renal colic. Hematuria occurs due to trauma as the stone moves forward and tears the lining of the ureter. The client may experience an elevated temperature, chills, and hypotension. **Pyuria** (pus in the urine) may also be present. Anuria and urine retention can result from calculi causing urinary obstruction. Other urinary changes may include dysuria, hesitancy, frequency, dribbling, nocturia, and decreasing urinary force.

Diagnosis and Treatment

Radiology tests can identify the stone location and approximate size. KUB, IVP, and CT scan may also be used to determine information about the stone(s). A renal ultrasound can be used as an alternate choice to avoid the risk of using contrast medium. Usual laboratory tests include a urinalysis, BUN and creatinine levels, and serum levels of calcium, phosphate, and uric acid.

Medications are ordered for pain, nausea, and vomiting. Ambulation encourages peristalsis and stone movement.

Removal of the stones is also a focus of treatment. Large stones are removed using surgical incisions into the renal pelvis (*pyelolithotomy*), ureter (*ureterolithotomy*), or kidney (*nephrolithotomy*) to remove the stones. A suprapubic incision may be used to remove calculi from the bladder. Transurethral lithotripsy can be performed. A bladder stone can be removed with an instrument known as a *lithotripter* (stone crushing tool). This is less invasive than surgery and is performed transurethrally. Stones in the ureter can be removed using a cystoscope or retroscope. A collapsible basket is used to withdraw the stone. Another way to remove the calculi is to crush them using percutaneous ultrasonic lithotripsy. The probe breaks up the stone by vibration and suctions the fragments from the kidney. Another type of lithotripsy is done using extracorporeal shock wave lithotripsy (Figure 39-16 ■). This machine uses high-energy shock waves from outside of the body to break up the calculi. The small particles that are left are passed through the urethra without difficulty.

A variety of medications may be ordered to prevent further stone formation. Potassium citrate is given to promote urine alkalinity. Allopurinol is prescribed to decrease uric acid. *Cellulose phosphate* blocks calcium absorption. Aluminum hydroxide is used to prevent phosphorous absorption. If the parathyroid hormone is the cause of the stone formation, thiazide diuretics may be ordered. Diet modification may be advised to prevent further calculi formation. Foods that contribute to stone formation may be restricted such as calcium, oxalate, and purines.

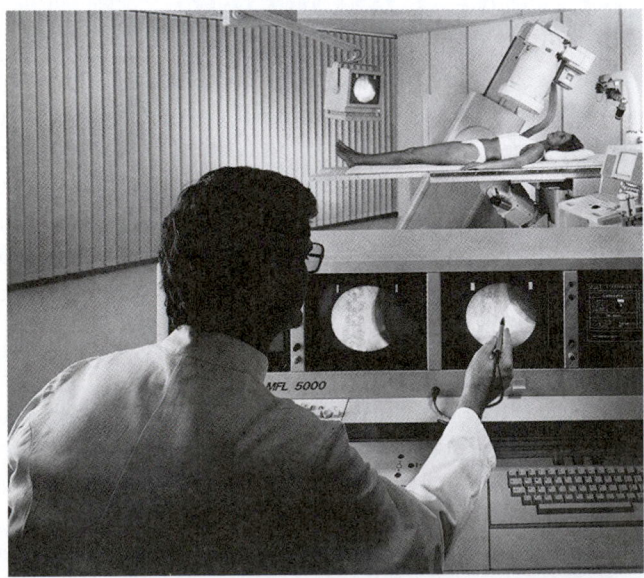

Figure 39-16. ■ Extracorporeal shock wave lithotripsy. Acoustic shock waves generated by the machine travel through soft tissue to shatter the urinary stone into fragments, which are then eliminated in the urine.

Urinary Diversions

A urinary diversion is the surgical rerouting of urine from the kidneys to a site other than the bladder. Urinary diversions are usually created when the bladder must be removed, for example, because of cancer or trauma. The ureters are brought directly to the surface of the skin to form small stomas (cutaneous ureterostomy). The client with cutaneous ureterostomy wears one or two urostomy appliances over the stoma(s).

The most common urinary diversion is the ileal conduit or ileal loop (Figure 39-17 ■). In this procedure, a segment of the ileum is removed and the intestinal ends are reattached. One end of the segment is closed with sutures to create a pouch, or a reservoir for urine. The other end is brought out through the abdominal wall to create a stoma. The ureters are then implanted into the ileal pouch. The mucous membrane lining of the ileum also provides some protection from ascending infection. Urine drains continuously from the ileal pouch. The client with an ileal conduit must wear a urostomy appliance at all times.

Highly motivated clients may be candidates for a continent urinary diversion. The *Kock pouch* (see Figure 39-17B), or continent ileal bladder conduit, also uses a portion of the ileum to form a reservoir for urine. A valve is created to contain the urine inside the reservoir. The client empties the pouch by inserting a clean catheter approximately every 4 hours. A small dressing is worn to protect the stoma and clothing.

> ### clinical ALERT
> In clients with ileal diversions, mucous shreds are commonly seen in the urine and are considered normal.

NURSING CARE

PRIORITIZING NURSING CARE

For all clients with ureteral disorders, monitor closely for signs of urinary tract infection, such as cloudy, foul-smelling urine, hematuria, or pyuria. Report such symptoms to the healthcare provider immediately.

When caring for clients with renal calculi, your focus of care is maintaining adequate urinary output, preventing infection, and managing pain. When a client has kidney stones in the ureters, they are passing from the kidney to the bladder. The ureter is small in diameter and stones cause great pain as they go through. Administer pain medication as ordered, as well as antiemetics. Sometimes clients are more comfortable lying on one side, splinting the ureter. Assist the client to the most comfortable position and assure them that the pain will be managed. Strain all the urine to isolate stones and large sediment. Any stones should be sent

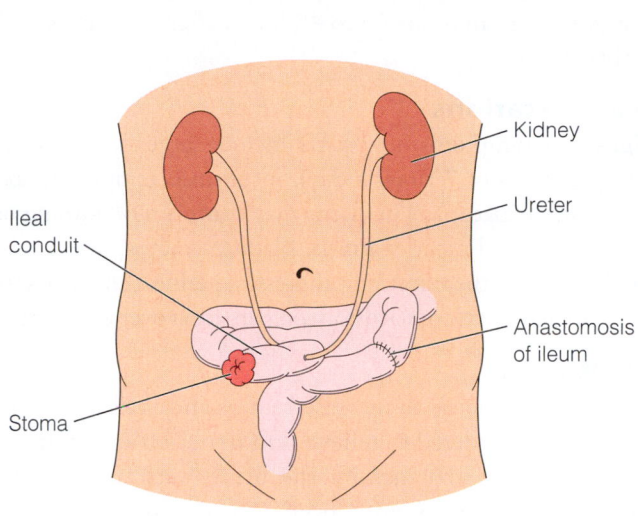

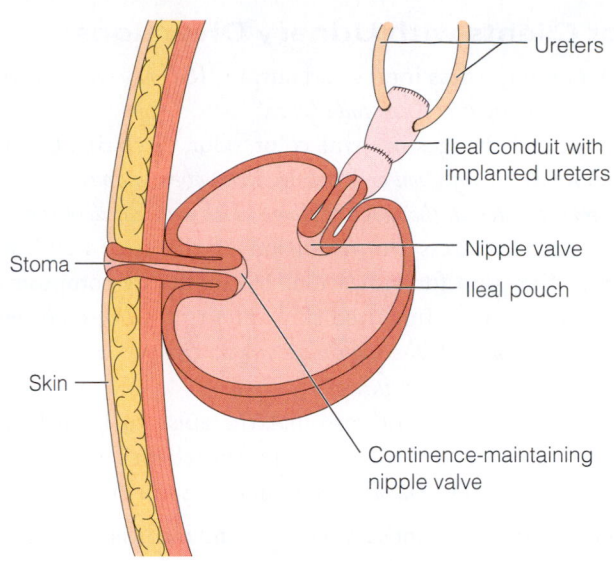

A

B

Figure 39-17. ■ Common urinary diversion procedures: **A.** Ileal conduit. A segment of the ileum is separated from the small intestine and formed into a tubular pouch with the open end brought to the skin surface to form a stoma. Ureters are connected to the pouch. **B.** A continent urinary diversion. A segment of the ileum is separated from the small intestine and formed into a pouch. Nipple valves are formed at each end of the pouch by *intussuscepting* (folding) tissue backward into the reservoir to prevent leakage (Kock pouch).

to the lab for analysis, because the client may be able to alter diet or receive medications to reduce the incidence of calculi.

Clients with ureteral diversions need meticulous skin care to prevent urinary leakage from irritating the skin. Ensure that ureterostomy appliances fit well and do not leak. If the client has a Kock pouch, use aseptic technique to insert the Foley to drain the pouch.

ASSESSING

Nursing assessment is performed in collaboration with the RN and begins with determining the pain level, onset, location, character, and whether the pain radiates. Data are gathered about other symptoms associated with the pain, including nausea and vomiting. Client history and other factors that may be related are documented. Objective and subjective data are gathered.

DIAGNOSING, PLANNING, AND IMPLEMENTING

Possible nursing diagnoses for clients with ureteral disorders include:

- *Acute Pain*
- *Risk for Infection*
- *Risk for Impaired Skin Integrity*
- *Impaired Urinary Elimination*

Expected outcomes for these clients include:

- Client will report pain controlled with medication.
- Client will remain free of infection.
- Client will maintain skin integrity.
- Client will have urinary elimination within normal range.

Nursing interventions for clients with urinary diversions include, but are not limited to, the following:

- Give pain medication as ordered. *Medication decreases the discomfort of renal colic.*
- Fluid intake is increased to 3,000 mL per day unless contraindicated. *Fluids help prevent further stone formation from static urine.*
- Encourage ambulation. *Ambulation increases peristalsis to help move stones through the urinary tract.*
- Monitor intake and output. *I&O measurement helps to ensure adequate fluid balance.*
- Strain all urine for evidence of stones. *Stones that are passed are sent to the lab for analysis. Once the composition of the stones is known, the client can alter the diet to help prevent stone formation.*
- Monitor for hematuria, dysuria, urinary frequency, pyuria, and anuria. *All of these can be complications of urinary stones.*
- Maintain patency of urinary drainage devices. *If a drainage device slows or is blocked, new stones can form. Patency prevents stasis of urine.*
- Reinforce teaching about diet modifications. *When clients understand ways to prevent further stone formation, they are empowered to try to control the condition. Having knowledge about one's health builds self-esteem.*
- Monitor and evaluate pain medication effectiveness. *If the medication is not effective, the physician can make changes in order to keep the client comfortable.*
- Observe for changing urinary output patterns. *Changes might indicate complications.*
- Following a stone removal procedure, monitor for wound healing, vital signs, and urinary drainage. *Monitoring can detect any problems in recovery before complications occur.*

For Clients with Urinary Diversions

- Accurately assess intake and output. *I&O measurements help detect any signs of fluid imbalance.*
- Note any changes in urine color, odor, or clarity. *Changes may indicate infection or bleeding. Remember, mucous shreds are commonly seen in the urine of clients with an ileal diversion.*
- Frequently assess the condition of the stoma and surrounding skin for indications of circulatory compromise to the stoma or impaired skin integrity. *Clients who must wear a urine collection appliance are at risk for impaired skin integrity because of irritation by urine.*
- Consult with an enterostomal therapist to identify the most appropriate appliance for the client's needs. *It is often difficult to contain urine in ostomy appliances.*
- Determine the client's level of pain and medicate as ordered. If surgery is required, implement routine preoperative and postoperative care. If a urinary diversion is performed (see discussion below), assess the stoma for signs of impaired circulation, and monitor the amount and color of urinary output through the stoma. *A stoma that is not pink and moist indicates impaired blood supply to the tissue. Urine may be pink after surgery, but output should be 30 mL per hour or greater.*
- If a retention catheter is in place, give routine catheter care. *This prevents likelihood of infection due to catheter placement.*
- Encourage the client to participate in self-care activities and refer both client and family to local support groups. *These measures provide for improved self-esteem and continuity of care.*
- Reinforce instruction regarding disease, treatment, and compliance. *Clients who understand the disease, its complications, and their treatment regimens are more likely to follow the treatment plan.*

EVALUATING

The nurse reviews desired outcomes to determine whether goals have been met. Effectiveness of pain medication is assessed. The nurse confirms client understanding of the value of increasing liquids and ambulation as a way to prevent kidney stones. Any signs of infection and bleeding are reported.

Cystitis

One of the most common bladder disorders is infection, occurring most frequently in women. The rate of *urinary tract infection (UTI)* in women is about 20% yearly compared with a rate of 0.1% in men. UTI accounts for 40% of all nosocomial infections. Most UTIs are caused by intestinal bacteria, such as *E. coli.* Women are particularly at risk because of the short urethra and its proximity to the anal and vaginal areas. Often, bacteria enter the bladder through the urethra and, if not treated effectively, can spread up the ureters to the kidneys.

Cystitis is infection and inflammation of the bladder. Bacteria reach the bladder by way of infected kidneys, lymph, or more commonly through the urethra. An ascending infection can occur 36 to 48 hours after intercourse or a catheter insertion.

Manifestations

Signs and symptoms of cystitis include urgency, frequency (every 2 hours or 7 times a day), incontinence, dysuria, nocturia, and hematuria. The client may complain of burning on urination, a feeling of warmth, bladder cramps, and a low-grade fever. As the infection progresses, perineal and suprapubic pain may develop, with pain on palpation over the bladder.

Treatment

Cystitis is treated with increased fluids and antibiotics. Sitz baths may be ordered to relieve skin irritation and maintain hygiene. Fluids that acidify the urine, such as cranberry juice, help prevent bacteria from attaching to the lining of the bladder. Urinalysis and urine cultures identify the infecting microorganism and its sensitivity or resistance to antibiotics. Elevated temperature and WBC levels indicate the extent of the infection.

Nursing Considerations

When caring for clients with urinary tract infections, focus your care on managing pain and promoting normal bladder function. Administer pain medications as ordered and report their effectiveness. Note whether the analgesic effects are lasting the prescribed length of time. Encourage clients with UTIs to take steps to prevent recurrences. Encourage the client to drink 8 ounces of fluid every hour or two (unless contraindicated). Find out what fluids the client likes and offer those. Keep in mind that carbonated beverages may be contraindicated in urinary tract infections.

Bladder Cancer

Bladder cancer is the sixth most common type of cancer. It affects people over 50 and occurs more often in men than in women. Risk factors include smoking, obesity, dialysis, and exposure to industrial pollution.

Manifestations

The most frequent symptom of bladder cancer (Figure 39-18 ■) is painless hematuria. Urinary frequency, urgency, and dysuria may also occur. If the cancer is also in the kidney, the classic signs are painless hematuria, dull pain in the flank area, and a mass in the kidney.

Treatment

Treatment for cancer may include chemotherapy, radiation therapy, immunotherapy, and surgery. A *cystectomy* (removal of the bladder) may be required with urinary diversion. See information on urinary diversions in the Ureteral Disorders section of this chapter. (Cancer and its treatment are discussed in depth in Chapter 45 .)

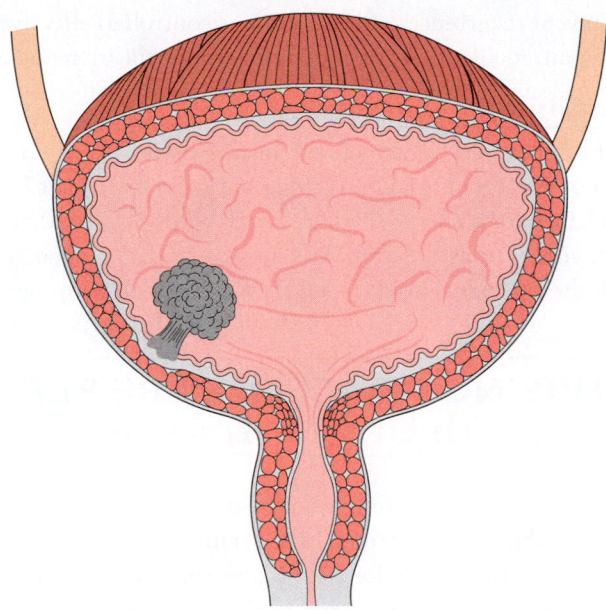

Figure 39-18. ■ A papillary transitional cell carcinoma of the urinary bladder with minimal invasion of the bladder wall.

During cystectomy, adjacent muscles and tissues may be excised. In the male, impotence is a complication of the surgical procedure. The female may also experience sterility.

Urinary Retention

Urinary retention is the inability to empty the bladder completely. Cholinergic drugs such as bethanechol chloride (Urecholine) may be ordered to stimulate bladder contraction and facilitate voiding. When all measures fail to initiate voiding, urinary catheterization may be necessary to empty the bladder completely. An indwelling Foley catheter may be inserted until the underlying cause is treated. Intermittent straight catheterization (every 3 to 4 hours) may be ordered, because it may carry less risk of urinary tract infection than an indwelling catheter.

Another type of catheter that is used with bladder disorders is the suprapubic catheter. It is inserted through a surgical incision made just above the symphysis pubis and is placed through the abdominal wall into the urinary bladder (see Figure 39-12). The physician inserts the catheter using local anesthesia or during bladder or vaginal surgery. This type of catheter keeps the bladder from distending and is especially important when the physician does not want pressure from urine on sutures inside the bladder. The catheter may be secured in place with sutures, with a body seal, or with both sutures and a body seal. The catheter is then attached to a closed drainage system.

NURSING CARE

PRIORITIZING NURSING CARE

When caring for clients with bladder disorders, your care priorities should be regaining normal urinary elimination and managing pain. The client may be unable to empty the bladder at all or unable to empty it completely. Anticipate orders to straight-catheterize the client for residual urine or to empty the bladder. Record and report the amount of residual urine in the bladder. (The physician will use this information to make decisions about the need for an indwelling catheter.) Always use sterile technique when you insert a urinary catheter for any purpose. Be aware, however, that when a client must self-catheterize due to injury or disease process, the client will use clean technique in the home.

ASSESSING

Nursing assessment is performed in collaboration with the RN and begins with determining the symptoms and onset of the illness. Determine the client's history of urinary tract infections; inquire regarding pregnancy possibilities or new sexual relationships. Discuss hygienic practices with the client who has repeated urinary tract infections. Collect data about urinary symptoms, especially hematuria, urinary urgency, frequency, or dysuria. Determine whether retention is a problem by asking about amounts and frequency of voiding. Palpate over the bladder area for distention or tenderness.

DIAGNOSING, PLANNING, AND IMPLEMENTING

Possible nursing diagnoses for clients with bladder disorders include:

- *Urinary Retention*
- *Acute Pain*
- *Impaired Urinary Elimination*
- *Deficient Knowledge* related to prevention of recurring UTIs

Desired or expected outcomes will include:

- Client will achieve bladder emptying every 3 to 4 hours.
- Client will report pain controlled by medication.
- Client will verbalize understanding of causes of recurring UTIs and steps to prevent them.
- Client will demonstrate ability to perform self-catheterization if needed to empty the bladder.

Nursing interventions for clients with bladder disorders include, but are not limited to, the following:

- Monitor clients for frequency of urination and amount of output. *I&O data help determine whether the bladder is emptying completely.*

- Gently palpate over the bladder for a firm rounded mound. *This would indicate bladder distention.*
- Notify physician if a client does not void within an 8-hour period. *Catheterization may be necessary to empty the bladder.*
- Keep accurate records of intake and output. Inspect voided urine for hematuria and test with dipsticks for occult blood as ordered. *Accurate I&O records can detect fluid imbalance early. Hematuria can indicate infection or bladder cancer.*
- Administer pain medications as ordered for clients with bladder cancer. Evaluate the effectiveness of the medication and report any problems to the physician. *Pain medications can be changed to elicit the most effective pain management for the client.*
- Instruct clients on self-catheterization using aseptic technique if necessary to empty the bladder. *Clients with nerve damage may be unable to voluntarily relax the urinary sphincter to empty the bladder.*
- It is important to teach clients how to prevent recurring cystitis. Guidelines for this instruction are listed in Box 39-7 ■. Although these instructions are especially important for women who have already experienced a UTI, they are useful for anyone. Additionally, clients should be instructed regarding hygiene and diet. *Clients can prevent many recurrences of UTI by following these guidelines.*

EVALUATING

The nurse reviews desired outcomes to determine whether goals have been met. Effectiveness of anti-infective therapy is assessed. The nurse confirms client understanding of ways to prevent recurrences of UTIs. Pain is controlled effectively with pain medication. Any signs of hematuria are reported.

Continuity of Care

UTI can be a recurrent problem for many women. The nurse plays an important role in teaching measures to prevent UTI. Guidelines for nurses to share are listed in Box 39-7. Although these instructions are especially important for women who have already experienced a UTI, they are useful for anyone.

NURSING PROCESS CARE PLAN
Client with Urinary Tract Infection

Mrs. Kennedy, 48, is recovering from an automobile accident in which she sustained blunt trauma to her abdomen. She has a mild concussion. An indwelling urinary catheter will be left in place until she is able to communicate her need to urinate. Upon entering Mrs. Kennedy's room to collect a urine specimen ordered for culture and sensitivity, you note that Mrs. Kennedy is restless and moaning. Her abdominal dressing is dry and intact and her urinary bag contains about 200 mL of golden-colored urine. Her abdomen is tender and distended. When questioned, Mrs. Kennedy is able to communicate that she is in pain but is unable to communicate the specifics of her pain.

Assessment

VS: T 99.6°F, radial pulse 86, R 24. BP 130/90. WBC is 15,000. Her catheter is patent and urine is clear, amber colored. IV is infusing with D$_5$W at 75 mL/hr. She has an abdominal incision that is clean and dry, no redness noted.

Nursing Diagnosis

The following important nursing diagnoses (among others) are established for this condition:

- *Acute Pain*
- *Impaired Skin Integrity*
- *Impaired Urinary Elimination*
- *Anxiety*
- *Impaired Verbal Communication*
- *Risk for Infection*

Expected Outcomes

The expected outcomes for Mrs. Kennedy's plan of care are as follows:

- Pain will be controlled.
- Skin integrity will be effectively managed.
- Urinary output will be within normal limits.
- Client will be informed about procedures.
- Body language will be assessed for communication.
- Wound and catheter will be maintained without evidence of infection.

BOX 39-7	**CLIENT TEACHING**

Preventing Urinary Tract Infections in Women

- Drink eight 8-ounce glasses of water per day.
- Practice frequent voiding (every 2 to 4 hours) to flush bacteria out and prevent organisms from ascending into the bladder. Void immediately after intercourse.
- Avoid use of harsh soaps, bubble bath, powder, or sprays in the perineal area.
- Avoid tight-fitting pants or other clothing that creates irritation to the urethra and prevents ventilation of the perineal area.
- Wear cotton rather than nylon underclothes. Accumulation of perineal moisture facilitates bacterial growth, and cotton enhances ventilation of the perineal area.
- Girls and women should always wipe the perineal area from front to back following urination or defecation.
- If recurrent UTIs are a problem, take showers rather than baths.
- Increase the acidity of urine through regular intake of vitamin C and by drinking two to three glasses of cranberry juice daily or taking cranberry tablets.

Planning and Implementation

The following interventions are planned and implemented for Mrs. Kennedy:

- Implement pain control measures.
- Monitor and document wound healing.
- Maintain and measure urinary output.
- Instruct client regarding procedures.
- Observe for body language communication.
- Monitor for signs and symptoms of infection.
- Maintain catheter care.

Evaluating

Mrs. Kennedy will remain in the hospital for a week to determine the status of her concussion and results of tests. Her abdominal incision is approximated and healing without signs of infection. She is able to communicate her level of pain on a pain scale. Urinary output is adequate and is a clear straw color. The urinary C&S was positive for organisms and treated with antibiotics. She is ambulating with assistance.

Critical Thinking in the Nursing Process

1. What precautions should be taken when collecting a urine sample from a person with an indwelling urinary catheter and why?
2. What measures can be taken to prevent Mrs. Kennedy from developing a UTI if one is not already present?
3. Develop a care plan for a client with UTI.

Note: Discussion of Critical Thinking questions appears on the MyNursingKit Website.

Urethral Disorders

URETHRITIS

Urethritis is defined as an inflammation of the urethra and causes redness, irritation, edema of the mucosa, and urethral discharge. In men it usually is caused by an infection from the prostate. In women it is associated with gonorrhea and chemical irritants (bubble baths, feminine hygiene products). The cause is a nonspecific organism other than gonorrhea. In some cases the inflammation is secondary to trichomonal and monilial infections or instrumentation (catheter insertion).

Manifestations

Signs and symptoms include dysuria and urethral discharge. When it is associated with a sexually transmitted disease, the drainage is thick and purulent and appears 2 to 3 days after contact. Pruritus may also be present. See Chapter 41 ⚭ for more information about sexually transmitted infections (STIs).

Treatment

Urethritis is treated with antibiotics, increased fluid intake, analgesics, and sitz baths. The nursing care for clients with urethritis is the same as for those with cystitis.

Urethral obstruction results in bladder distention and diverticula formation. Urine becomes trapped in the diverticula, stagnates, and is a medium for bacterial growth.

Nursing Considerations

When caring for clients with urethral disorders, be vigilant about using sterile technique while inserting catheters. Report urethral redness, swelling, irritation, or discharge. Observe the area for improvement after the client is started on antibiotics. Encourage 8 ounces of fluid intake every 2 hours, unless contraindicated. Evaluate the effectiveness of sitz baths and analgesics in relieving discomfort. When it is painful to urinate, clients sometimes try to delay voiding. This can lead to bladder spasms and incomplete bladder emptying.

Note: The references and resources for all chapters have been compiled at the back of the book.

Collecting a Urine Specimen for Culture and Sensitivity by Clean Catch

Purpose

■ To determine the presence of microorganisms, the type of organism(s), and the antibiotics to which the organisms are sensitive

Equipment

■ Disposable or sterile gloves
■ Antiseptic towelette, such as povidone-iodine
■ Sterile cotton balls or 2 × 2 gauze pads
■ Sterile specimen container
■ Specimen identification label
■ Completed laboratory requisition form
■ Urine receptacle, if the client is not ambulatory
■ Basin of warm water, soap, washcloth, and towel for the nonambulatory client

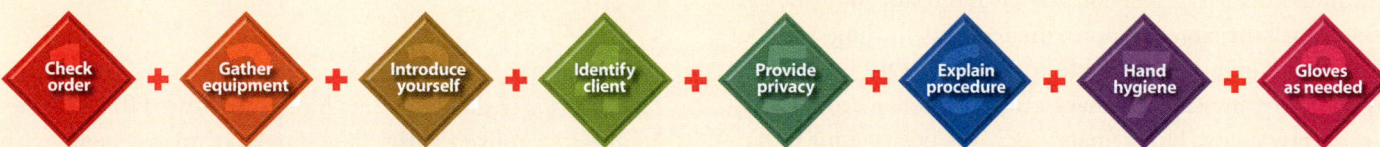

Interventions and Rationales

1. Perform preparatory steps (see icon bar above).

2. Instruct and assist the client appropriately.
   ■ Inform the client that a urine specimen is required; give the reason, and explain the method to be used to collect it.

3. For an ambulatory client who is able to follow directions, instruct the client on how to collect the specimen.
   ■ Direct or assist the client to the bathroom.
   ■ Ask the client to wash and dry the genital and perineal area with soap and water. *This removes microorganisms that could contaminate the specimen.*
   ■ Instruct the client on how to clean the urinary meatus with antiseptic towelettes.

FOR FEMALE CLIENTS

■ Use each towelette only once. Clean the perineal area from front to back, and discard the towelette. Use all towelettes provided (usually two or three). *Cleaning from front to back cleans the area of least contamination to the area of greatest contamination.*

FOR MALE CLIENTS

■ If uncircumcised, retract the foreskin slightly to expose the urinary meatus.
■ Using a circular motion, clean the urinary meatus and the distal portion of the penis. Use each towelette only once, then discard. Clean several inches down the shaft of the penis. *This cleans from the area of least contamination to the area of greatest contamination.*

4. For a client who requires assistance, prepare the client and equipment.
   ■ Wash the perineal area with soap and water; rinse and dry. Assist the client onto a clean commode or bedpan.

If using a bedpan or urinal, position the client as upright as allowed or tolerated.
■ Open the clean-catch kit, taking care not to contaminate the inside of the specimen container or lid.
■ Wear clean gloves.
■ Clean the urinary meatus and perineal area as described in step 3.

5. Collect the specimen from a nonambulatory client or instruct an ambulatory client on how to collect it.
   ■ Instruct the client to start voiding. *Bacteria in the distal urethra and at the urinary meatus are cleared by the first few milliliters of urine expelled.*
   ■ Place the specimen container into the stream of urine and collect the specimen, taking care not to touch the container to the perineum or penis. Avoid contaminating the interior of the specimen container and the specimen itself.
   ■ Collect 30 to 60 mL of urine in the container.
   ■ Cap the container tightly, touching only the outside of the container and the cap (see Figure 39-6).
   ■ If necessary, clean the outside of the specimen container with disinfectant.
   ■ Remove gloves. Wash hands. *This prevents the spread of infection.*

6. Label the specimen and transport it to the laboratory.
   ■ Ensure that the specimen label and the laboratory requisition carry the correct information. Attach them securely to the specimen. *This prevents errors from occurring and ensures good continuity of care.*
   ■ Arrange for the specimen to be sent to the laboratory immediately. *Bacterial cultures must be started immediately, before any contaminating organisms can grow, multiply, and produce false results.*

7. Document pertinent data.
   - Record collection of the specimen, any pertinent observations of the urine in terms of color, odor, or consistency, and any difficulty in voiding that the client experienced.

VARIATION: COLLECTING A TIMED URINE SPECIMEN

1. Obtain a specimen container with preservative (if indicated) from the laboratory. Label the container with identifying information for the client, the test to be performed, time started, and time of completion.

2. Provide a clean receptacle for collecting urine (bedpan, commode, or toilet collection device).

3. Post signs in the client's chart, Kardex, room, and bathroom alerting personnel to save all urine during the specified time.

4. At the start of the collection period, have the client void and discard this urine.

5. Save all urine produced during the timed collection period in the container, refrigerating or placing the container on ice as indicated. Avoid contaminating the urine with toilet paper or feces.

6. At the end of the collection period, instruct the client to empty the bladder completely and save this voiding as part of the specimen. Take the entire amount of urine collected to the laboratory with the completed requisition.

7. Record collection of the specimen, time started and completed, and any pertinent observations of the urine on appropriate records.

VARIATION: COLLECTING A SPECIMEN FROM A FOLEY (RETENTION) CATHETER OR A DRAINAGE TUBE

1. Wash hands.

2. Wear disposable gloves.

3. If there is no urine in the catheter, clamp the drainage tubing for about 30 minutes. This allows fresh urine to collect in the catheter.

4. Wipe the area where the needle will be inserted with a disinfectant swab. The site should be distal to the tube leading to the balloon to avoid puncturing this tube. Disinfecting the needle insertion site removes any microorganisms on the surface of the catheter.

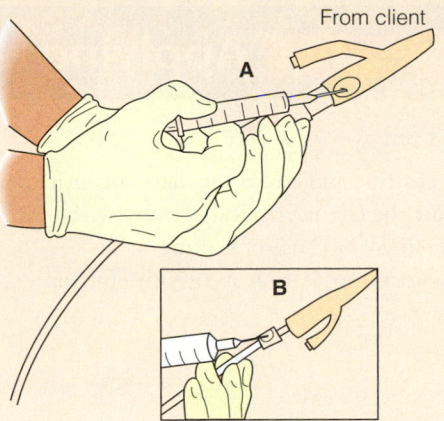

Figure 39-19. ■ Obtaining a urine specimen from a retention catheter: **A.** From a specific area near the end of the catheter. **B.** From an access port in the tubing.

5. Insert the needle at a 30- to 45-degree angle (Figure 39-19 ■). This angle of entrance facilitates self-sealing of the rubber.

6. Unclamp the catheter.

7. Withdraw the required amount of urine, for example, 3 mL for a urine culture or 30 mL for a routine urinalysis.

8. Transfer the urine to the specimen container. Make sure the needle does not touch the outside of the container if a sterile culture tube is used.

9. Without recapping the needle, discard the syringe and needle in an appropriate sharps container.

10. Cap the container.

11. Remove gloves and discard appropriately and wash hands.

12. Label the container, and send the urine to the laboratory immediately for analysis or refrigeration.

13. Record collection of the specimen and any pertinent observations of the urine on the appropriate records.

SAMPLE DOCUMENTATION

[date] [time]	Urine C&S to lab. Urine straw colored, clear and free from odor. No abnormal constituents noted. Client voided freely without complaints of difficulty.
	_____ D. Haus, LVN

PROCEDURE 39-2 Applying a Condom Catheter

Purposes

- To collect urine and control urinary incontinence
- To permit the client physical activity without fear of embarrassment because of leaking urine
- To prevent skin irritation as a result of urinary incontinence

Equipment

- Leg drainage bag with tubing or urinary drainage bag with tubing
- Condom sheath
- Bath blanket
- Disposable gloves
- Basin of warm water and soap
- Washcloth and towel
- Elastic tape or Velcro strap

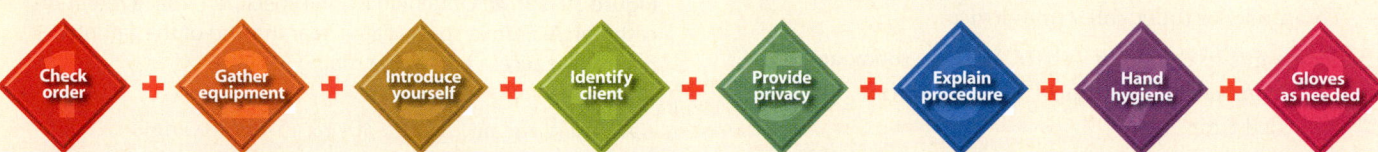

Check order + Gather equipment + Introduce yourself + Identify client + Provide privacy + Explain procedure + Hand hygiene + Gloves as needed

Interventions and Rationales

1. Perform preparatory steps (see icon bar above).
2. Prepare the equipment.
   - Assemble the leg drainage bag or urinary drainage bag for attachment to the condom sheath.
   - Roll the condom outward onto itself to facilitate easier application. *On some models an inner flap will be exposed. This flap is applied around the urinary meatus to prevent the reflux of urine (Figure 39-20 ■).*
3. Position and drape the client.
   - Position the client in either a supine or a bed-sitting position.
   - Drape the client appropriately with the bath blanket, exposing only the penis. *This provides privacy and comfort.*
4. Inspect and clean the penis.
   - Don gloves.
   - Inspect the penis for skin irritation (contact dermatitis), excoriation, swelling, or discoloration. *The nurse needs to obtain baseline data for use later.*

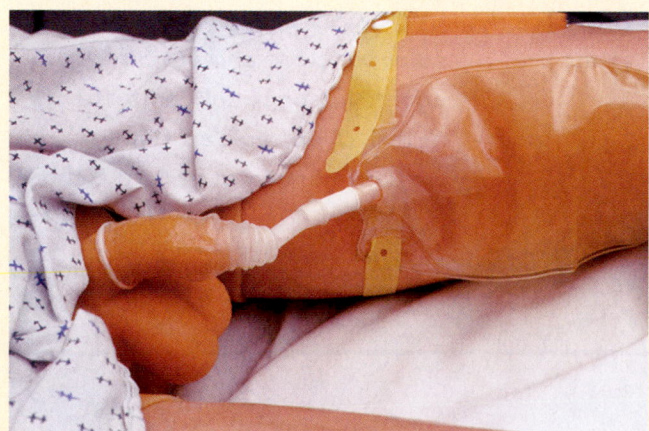

Figure 39-20. ■ Rolling the condom over the penis.

- Clean the genital area, and dry it thoroughly. *This minimizes skin irritation and excoriation after the condom is applied.*

5. Apply and secure the condom.
   - Roll the condom smoothly over the penis, leaving 2.5 cm (1 in.) between the end of the penis and the rubber or plastic connecting tube (see Figure 39-20). *This space prevents irritation of the tip of the penis and provides for full drainage of urine.*
   - Secure the condom firmly, but not too tightly, to the penis by wrapping a strip of elastic tape or Velcro around the base of the penis over the condom. *The elastic or Velcro strip should not come in contact with the skin and should hold the condom in place without impeding blood circulation to the penis.*

6. Securely attach the urinary drainage system.
   - Make sure that the tip of the penis is not touching the condom and that the condom is not twisted. *A twisted condom could obstruct the flow of urine.*
   - Attach the urinary drainage system to the condom.
   - Remove gloves.
   - If the client is to remain in bed, attach the urinary drainage bag to the bed frame.
   - If the client is ambulatory, attach the bag to the client's leg (Figure 39-21 ■). *Attaching the drainage bag to the leg helps control the movement of the tubing and prevents twisting of the thin material of the condom appliance at the tip of the penis.*

7. Teach the client about the drainage system.
   - Instruct the client to keep the drainage bag below the level of the condom and to avoid loops or kinks in the tubing.

8. Document pertinent data.
   - Record the application of the condom, the time, and pertinent observations, such as irritated areas on the penis.

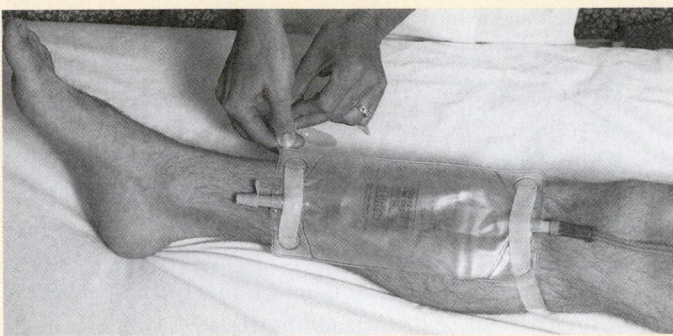

Figure 39-21. ■ Attaching the urinary drainage bag to the leg.

9. Inspect the penis 30 minutes following the condom application, and check urine flow.
   - Assess the penis for swelling and discoloration. *These indicate that the condom is too tight.*

10. Change the condom daily, and provide skin care.
    - Remove the elastic or Velcro strip and roll off the condom.
    - Wash the penis with soapy water, rinse, and dry it thoroughly (see Chapter 20 🔗).
    - Assess the foreskin for signs of irritation, swelling, and discoloration.

SAMPLE DOCUMENTATION

[date]
[time]

Condom catheter applied and attached to gravity drainage. Client tolerated procedure well, no complaints of pain. Urine clear, straw colored. _____
_____ D. Haus, LVN

PROCEDURE 39-3

Female Urinary Catheterization Using a Straight Catheter

Purposes

- To relieve discomfort due to bladder distention or to provide gradual decompression of a distended bladder
- To assess the amount of residual urine if the bladder empties incompletely
- To obtain a urine specimen
- To empty the bladder completely prior to surgery

Equipment

- Flashlight or lamp
- Mask, if required by agency policy
- Bath blanket or drape
- Soap, a basin of warm water, a washcloth, and a towel
- Disposable gloves
- Bladder ultrasound device (optional)

- A sterile catheterization kit containing:
  Water-soluble lubricant
  Sterile gloves
  Sterile drapes, fenestrated drape (optional) to place over the perineum
  Antiseptic solution
  Cotton balls or gauze squares
  Forceps
  Basin for urine (base of kit can be used)
- Sterile catheter of appropriate size (e.g., for an adult, #14 or #16 is often used)
- Specimen container as required
- Bag or receptacle for disposal of the cotton balls

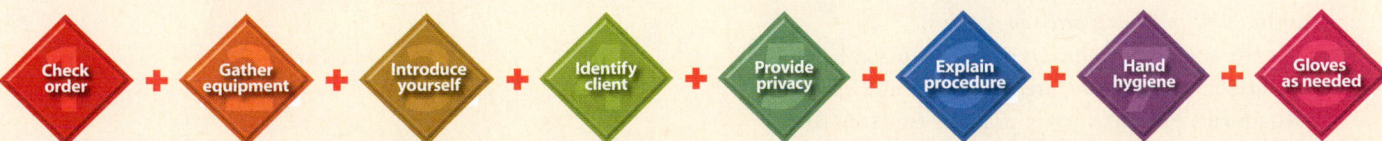

Interventions and Rationales

1. Perform preparatory steps (see icon bar above).
2. Assess for urinary retention.

- To palpate the bladder, indent the skin more than 1.3 cm (0.5 in.) just above the pubic symphysis by pressing the fingers of one hand on the fingers of the other. *This increases the pressure for palpation.*

3. Prepare the client.
   - Explain the catheterization to the client, and provide privacy. *Exposure of the genitals is embarrassing to most clients. Some people fear that the procedure will be painful; explain that normally a catheterization is painless and that there may be a sensation of pressure.*
   - Assist the client to a supine position, with knees flexed and thighs externally rotated. Pillows can be used to support the knees and to elevate the buttocks. *Raising the client's pelvis gives the nurse a better view of the urinary meatus and reduces the risk of contaminating the catheter.*
   - Drape the client. *This maintains comfort and prevents unnecessary exposure.* Cover the client's chest and abdomen with a bath blanket. Pull the client's gown up over her hips. Cover her legs and feet as for perineal care.
   - Wear disposable gloves. *This prevents transmission of microorganisms.*
   - Wash the perineal-genital area with warm water and soap. *Cleaning reduces the number of microorganisms around the urinary meatus and the possibility of introducing microorganisms with the catheter.*
   - Rinse and dry the area well. *Rinsing removes soap that could inhibit the action of the antiseptic if used later.*
   - Remove disposable gloves.
   - Obtain assistance if the client requires help in maintaining the required position. *The client must remain still throughout the procedure to maintain a clear view of the urinary meatus and prevent contamination of the sterile field.*

4. Prepare the equipment.
   - Adjust the light to view the urinary meatus. It may be necessary to use a flashlight or to place a gooseneck lamp at the foot of the bed.
   - Put on a mask, gown, and cap if required by agency policy.

5. Create a sterile field.
   - At the client's bedside, open a sterile kit and the catheter, if it is packaged separately, and put on the sterile gloves.
   - Drape the client with the sterile drape, being careful to protect its sterility and the sterility of your gloves. Place the drape under the buttocks while keeping the edges cuffed over your gloves. *This prevents contamination of the gloves against the client's buttocks.* If a fenestrated drape is provided, place it over the perineal area, exposing only the labia.
   - Place the sterile kit on the drape between the client's thighs. *This facilitates access to supplies.*
   - Pour the antiseptic solution over the cotton balls, if they are not already prepared and if meatal cleansing with an antiseptic is agency practice (see step 6).
   - Lubricate the insertion tip of the catheter liberally, and place it in the sterile container ready for use. *Water-soluble lubricant facilitates insertion of the catheter by reducing friction. Lubrication is done at this point because the nurse will subsequently have only one sterile hand available.*

- Open the urine specimen container, and keep the top sterile. *This prepares the container for specimen collection.*

6. Clean the meatus with antiseptic (if recommended by agency).
   - Check agency protocol about cleaning the meatus. *There is controversy regarding the value of meatal cleaning using antiseptics before catheterization.*
   - Using the nondominant hand, separate the labia minora with your thumb and one finger or another two fingers. Expose the urinary meatus adequately by retracting the tissue of the labia minora in an upward (anterior) direction (Figure 39-22A ■). Clean first from the meatus downward and then on either side, using a

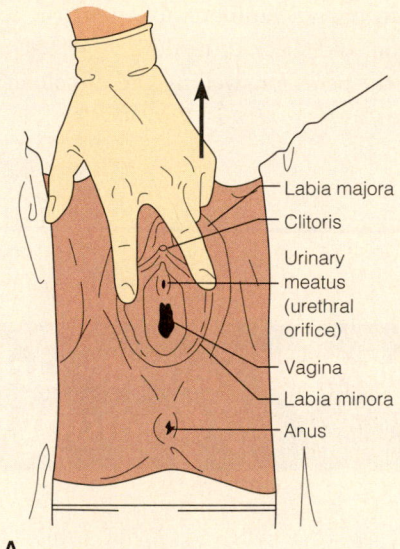

Labia majora
Clitoris
Urinary meatus (urethral orifice)
Vagina
Labia minora
Anus

A

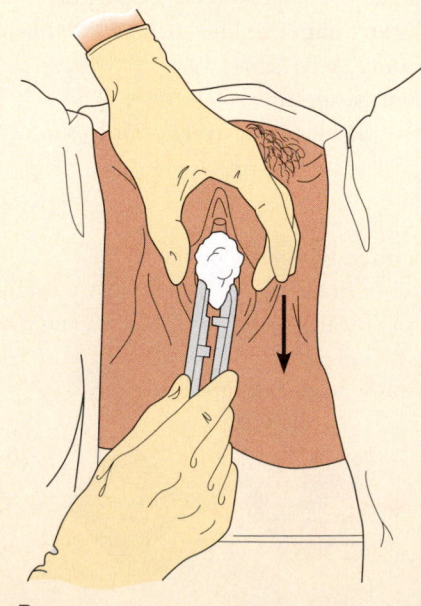

B

Figure 39-22. ■ **A.** To expose the urinary meatus, separate the labia minora and retract the tissue upward. **B.** When cleaning the urinary meatus, move the swab downward.

new swab for each stroke (Figures 39-22B). Once the meatus is cleaned, do not allow the labia to close over it. *Keeping the labia apart prevents the risk of contaminating the urinary meatus. Note: Your hand that touches the client becomes unsterile. It remains in position exposing the urinary meatus, while your other hand remains sterile holding the sterile forceps.*

7. Inspect the meatus.
   - With the urinary meatus exposed (see Figure 39-22A), assess any signs, such as excoriation of the tissues surrounding the urinary meatus, swelling of the urinary meatus, or the presence of discharge around the urinary meatus. *This assessment provides baseline data.* If any discharge is present, obtain a culture swab.

8. Insert the catheter until urine flows.
   - Place the drainage end of the catheter in the urine receptacle. Pick up the insertion end of the catheter with your uncontaminated, sterile, gloved hand, holding it about 5 cm (2 in.) from the insertion tip. *Because the adult female urethra is approximately 1.5 inches long, the catheter is held far enough from the end to allow full insertion into the bladder and to maintain control of the tip of the catheter so it will not accidentally become contaminated.*
   - Gently insert the catheter into the urinary meatus until urine flows. Insert the catheter in the direction of the urethra. If the catheter meets resistance during insertion, do not force it. *Forceful pressure against the urethra can produce trauma.* Ask the client to take deep breaths. *This helps relax the external sphincter.* If this does not relieve the resistance, discontinue the procedure and report the problem to the nurse in charge. Exercise caution to prevent the catheter tip from becoming contaminated. If it becomes contaminated, discard it.
   - When the urine flows, transfer your hand from the labia to the catheter to hold it in place. *This prevents its expulsion by a possible bladder contraction.*

9. Collect a urine specimen.
   - Pinch the catheter, and transfer the drainage end of it into the sterile specimen bottle. Usually, 30 mL of urine is sufficient for a specimen. Securely place the top on the specimen container, and set it aside for labeling later.

10. Empty or partially drain the bladder, and then remove the catheter.
    - For adults experiencing urinary retention, some orders limit the amount of urine drained to 1,000 mL.

Limiting the amount of urine drained has been a controversial issue. Rapid removal of large amounts of urine was once thought to induce engorgement of the pelvic blood vessels and hypovolemic shock. However, retained urine may serve as a reservoir for microorganisms to multiply. Usually agency policy or the physician indicates the amount to be removed and times at which the remaining urine is to be withdrawn. Research findings support the premise that complete drainage of a distended bladder is likely to be more comfortable and certainly seems as safe as threshold clamping.
   - Pinch the catheter. *This prevents leakage of urine.* Remove the catheter slowly.

11. Promote client comfort.
    - Dry the client's perineum with a towel or drape. *Excess lubricant and solution in the area can irritate the skin.*

12. Assess the urine.
    - Inspect the urine for color, clarity, odor, and the presence of any abnormal constituents, such as blood. Measure the amount of urine.

13. Document the catheterization.
    - Include assessments before and after the procedure, type and size of catheter inserted, time, characteristics and amount of urine obtained, whether a specimen was sent to the laboratory, and client response to the procedure.

SAMPLE DOCUMENTATION

[date]
[time]   Client c/o inability to empty bladder fully. Urinary bladder palpable. Urinary straight #14 catheter inserted, urine returned spontaneously 300 mL, clear and straw colored. Urinalysis and C&S to lab. Catheter removed. Client tolerated procedure well.

_____ D. Haus, LVN

Male Urinary Catheterization Using a Straight Catheter

Purposes

- To relieve discomfort due to bladder distention or to provide gradual decompression of a distended bladder
- To assess the amount of residual urine if the bladder empties incompletely
- To obtain a urine specimen
- To empty the bladder completely prior to surgery

Equipment

- See Procedure 39-3. (A #16 or #18 catheter is often used for an adult male).

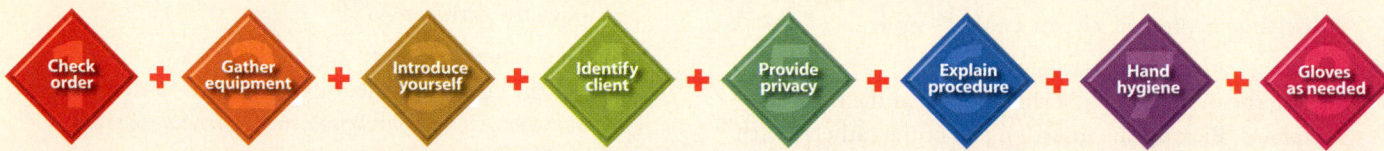

Check order + Gather equipment + Introduce yourself + Identify client + Provide privacy + Explain procedure + Hand hygiene + Gloves as needed

Interventions and Rationales

1. Perform preparatory steps (see icon bar above).
2. Assess for urinary retention.
   - Palpate the bladder.
3. Prepare the client.
   - Explain the catheterization, as in Procedure 39-3. Assist the client to a supine position, with the knees slightly flexed and the thighs slightly apart. *This allows greater relaxation of the abdominal and perineal muscles and permits easier insertion of the catheter.*
   - Drape the client by folding the top bedclothes down so that the penis is exposed and the thighs are covered. Use a bath blanket to cover the client's chest and abdomen.
   - Wear disposable gloves.
   - Wash the penis and dry it well.
   - Remove disposable gloves.
4. Create a sterile field.
   - Open the sterile tray, and apply the sterile gloves.
   - Place a drape under the penis and a second drape above the penis over the pubic area. If a fenestrated drape is available, place it over the penis and pubic area, exposing only the penis.
   - Place the sterile kit on the sterile drape over the client's thighs or next to the thigh.
   - Pour the antiseptic solution over the cotton balls, if they are not already prepared.
   - Lubricate the insertion tip of the catheter liberally for about 5 to 15 cm (2 to 6 in.). Place it in the sterile container ready for insertion. *Water-soluble lubricant facilitates insertion of the catheter by reducing friction. This step is done before cleaning because the nurse will subsequently have only one sterile hand available.*
5. Clean the urinary meatus with antiseptic (if recommended by the agency).
   - Grasp the penis firmly behind the glans with the nondominant hand, and spread the meatus between the thumb and forefinger. Retract the foreskin of an uncircumcised male. The hand holding the penis is now considered contaminated. Grasp the penis firmly to avoid stimulating an erection.
   - With the dominant hand, use sterile forceps to pick up a swab. Clean the meatus first, and then wipe the tissue surrounding the meatus in a circular motion. Discard each swab after only one wipe. *Using forceps maintains the sterility of your gloves.*
6. Insert the catheter.
   - Place the drainage end of the catheter in the urine receptacle. Then pick up the insertion end of the catheter with your uncontaminated, sterile, gloved hand, holding it about 7.5 to 10 cm (3 to 4 in.) from the insertion tip for an adult or about 2.5 cm (1 in.) for a baby or small boy. *In some agencies, the catheter is picked up with forceps.* The male urethra is approximately 20 cm (8 in.) long. Holding the catheter far enough from the end to maintain control of the tip of the catheter avoids accidental contamination.
   - Lift the penis to a position perpendicular to the body (90-degree angle), and exert slight traction (pulling or tension upward). Insert the catheter steadily about 20 cm (8 in.) or until urine begins to flow. *Lifting the penis so that it is perpendicular to the body straightens the downward curvature of the urethra.*
   - To bypass slight resistance at the sphincters, twist the catheter, or wait until the sphincter relaxes. Ask the client to take deep breaths or try to void. If difficult resistance is met, discontinue the procedure and report the problem to the nurse in charge. *Slight resistance is normally encountered at the external and internal urethral sphincters. Deep breathing can help to relax the external sphincter. Forceful pressure exerted against a major resistance can traumatize the urethra.*

- While the urine flows, lower the penis, and transfer your hand to hold the catheter in place at the meatus.

7. Drain the urine from the bladder.
   - Collect a urine specimen (if required) after the urine has flowed for a few seconds. Pinch the catheter, and transfer the drainage end of the catheter into the sterile specimen bottle, taking care not to contaminate the specimen container. Usually, 30 mL of urine is sufficient for a specimen.
   - Empty the bladder, or drain the amount of urine specified in the order. See Procedure 39-3, step 10.

8. Make the client comfortable.
   - Dry the penis with a towel or drape.
   - Replace the foreskin. *This prevents a mechanical phimosis (constriction), which may compromise circulation to the glans.*

9. Assess the client and the urine, as in Procedure 39-3, step 12, and document the procedure and the assessments.

SAMPLE DOCUMENTATION

[date]	Client c/o discomfort
[time]	due to bladder fullness. Client unable to empty bladder completely. Residual urine obtained after client voided per physician order. Straight #16 catheter inserted without difficulty. Urine C&S sent to the lab. Urine cloudy, with occasional mucous threads. Client tolerated procedure well.

_____ D. Haus, LVN

PROCEDURE 39-5

Inserting and Removing a Retention (Indwelling) Catheter

Purposes

- To facilitate accurate measurement of urinary output for critically ill clients whose output needs to be monitored hourly
- To provide for intermittent or continuous bladder drainage and irrigation
- To prevent urine from contacting an incision after perineal surgery
- To manage incontinence when other measures have failed

Equipment

In addition to the equipment used for a straight catheterization, the following equipment is needed:

- Sterile retention catheter kit (Figure 39-23 ■) (#14 or #16 for adults, #8 or #10 for children are often used)
- Prefilled syringe (sterile water is often used)
- Nonallergenic tape or a catheter stabilizing or strapping device (e.g., urologic cath-strap)
- Safety pin or clip
- Urine collection bag and tubing (the tubing may be attached to the retention catheter if a closed drainage system is used)

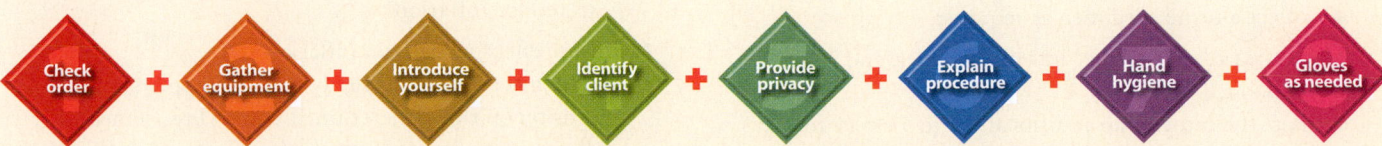

Check order + Gather equipment + Introduce yourself + Identify client + Provide privacy + Explain procedure + Hand hygiene + Gloves as needed

Part A: Inserting a Retention Catheter
Interventions and Rationales

1. Perform preparatory steps (see icon bar above).

2. Prepare the client and the equipment.
   - Explain to the client why the retention catheter is to be inserted, how long it will be in place, and how the urinary drainage equipment needs to be handled to maintain

and facilitate the drainage of urine. Reassure the client that the procedure is painless. *Some clients experience the urge to void during insertion of the catheter and for a short time after the catheter is in place. Reassure these clients that the catheter drains the urine and that the urge to void will disappear.*

   - Follow the procedure for straight catheterization up to and including creating a sterile field.

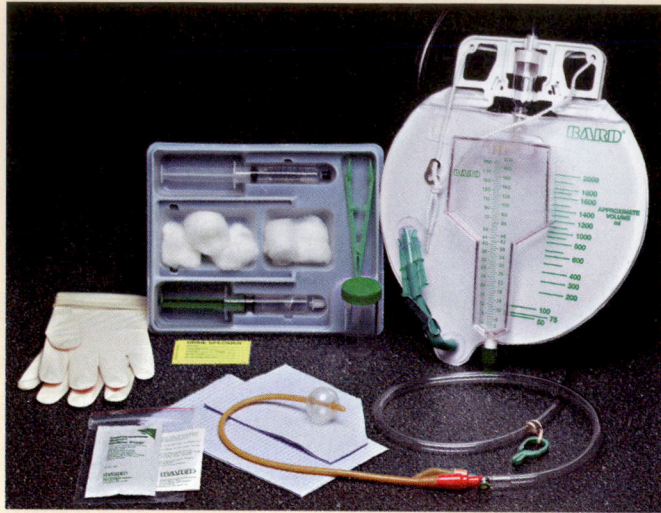

Figure 39-23. ■ Catheter insertion kit.

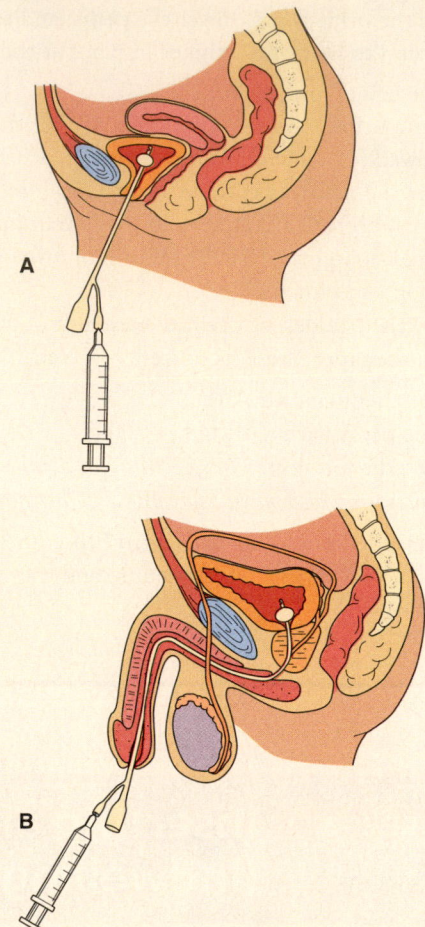

Figure 39-24. ■ Placement of retention catheter and inflated balloon: **A.** Female client. **B.** Male client.

3. Test the catheter balloon.
   - Attach the prefilled syringe to the balloon valve, and inject the fluid. *Sterile water rather than sterile saline should be used because the saline can crystallize and prevent complete deflation of the balloon.* The balloon should inflate appropriately and not leak. Withdraw the fluid, and set aside the catheter with the syringe attached for later use. If the balloon leaks or does not inflate adequately, replace the catheter. In such a case, withdraw the fluid, and detach the syringe for later use. Ask another nurse to obtain a second catheter and open the package for you, then test the new balloon, or remove the equipment and obtain another catheter; then start again with the new sterile equipment. *This prevents contamination of the urethra.*

4. Follow steps as for straight catheterization.
   - Lubricate the insertion tip of the catheter.
   - Remove the sterile cap from the specimen container.
   - Expose and clean the urinary meatus and surrounding tissues with antiseptic if recommended.
   - Insert the catheter and inflate the balloon.
   - Collect a urine specimen as required.

5. Move the catheter farther into the bladder, and inflate the balloon.
   - Insert the catheter an additional 2.5 to 5 cm (1 to 2 in.) beyond the point at which urine began to flow. *The balloon of the catheter is located behind the opening at the insertion tip, and sufficient space must be provided to inflate the balloon. This ensures that the balloon is inflated inside the bladder and not in the urethra, where it could produce trauma.*
   - Inflate the balloon by injecting the contents of the prefilled syringe into the valve of the catheter (Figure 39-24A ■). Placement of the catheter and balloon in a male client is shown in Figure 39-24B. If the client

complains of discomfort or pain during the balloon inflation, withdraw the fluid, insert the catheter a little farther, and inflate the balloon again. Insert no more fluid than the balloon size indicates (e.g., 5 or 30 mL), and remove the syringe. A special valve prevents backflow of the fluid out of the catheter. Follow agency policy when using a 30-mL balloon. Some agency policies state that only 15 mL of fluid is injected for inflation.

6. Ensure effective balloon inflation.
   - When the balloon is safely inflated, apply slight tension on the catheter until you feel resistance. *Resistance indicates that the catheter balloon is inflated appropriately and that the catheter is well anchored in the bladder.*
   - Then move the catheter slightly back into the bladder. *This keeps the balloon from exerting undue pressure on the neck of the bladder.*

7. Anchor the catheter.
   - Tape the catheter with nonallergenic tape to the inside of a female's thigh or to the thigh or abdomen

of a male client (Figures 39-25A and B ■). Some nurses prefer taping the male catheter to the abdomen whenever there is increased risk of excoriation at the penile-scrotal junction. *Taping restricts the movement of the catheter, thus reducing friction and irritation in the urethra when the client moves. It also prevents skin excoriation at the penile-scrotal junction in the male.*

8. Establish effective drainage.
   - Ensure that the emptying base of the drainage bag is closed.
   - Secure the drainage bag to the bed frame, using the hook or strap provided. Suspend the bag off the floor, but keep it below the level of the client's bladder. *Urine flows by gravity from the bladder to the drainage bag. The bag should be off the floor so that the emptying spout does not become grossly contaminated.*
   - Coil the drainage tubing loosely beside the client, so that the remaining tubing runs in a straight line down to the drainage bag. Fasten the vertical tubing to the bedclothes with tape, a tubing clamp, or a safety pin and elastic band. *The drainage tubing should not loop below its entry into the drainage bag, which would impede the flow of urine by gravity.*

9. Document pertinent data.
   - Record the time and date of the catheterization; the type and size of catheter; the reason for catheterization; how much fluid was used to inflate the balloon; assessments before and after the procedure, including amount, color, and clarity of urine obtained; whether a specimen was taken and sent to the laboratory; whether all urine was emptied from the bladder; and the client's response.

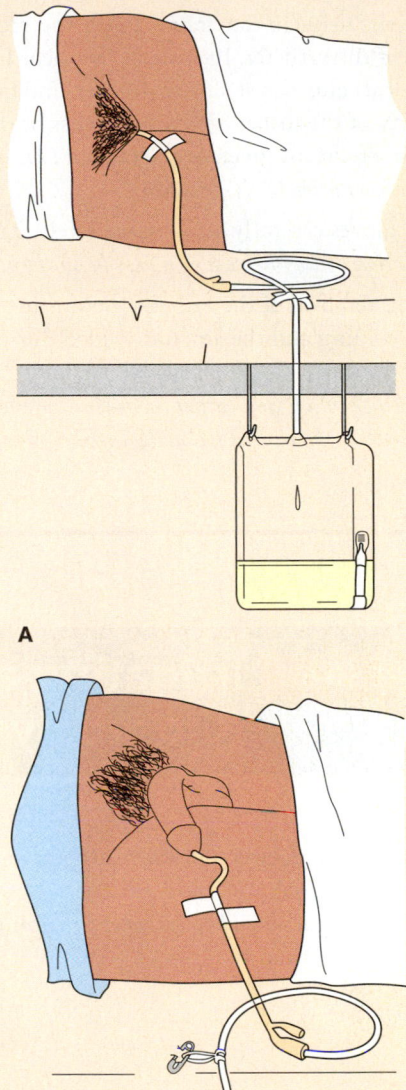

Figure 39-25. ■ **A.** Tape the catheter to the inside of a female's thigh. **B.** Tape the catheter to the thigh or abdomen of a male client.

Part B: Removing a Retention Catheter
Interventions and Rationales

1. Obtain a receptacle for the catheter (e.g., a disposable basin); a clean, disposable towel; disposable gloves; and a sterile syringe to deflate the balloon. The size of the balloon is indicated on the label at the end of the catheter. *This helps to maintain standard precautions and prevent infection.*

2. Ask the client to assume a supine position as for a catheterization. *In this position the catheter can be removed with minimal discomfort for the client.*

3. *Optional:* Obtain a sterile specimen before removing the catheter. Check agency protocol. *Obtain a sterile specimen if needed.*

4. Remove the tape attaching the catheter to the client, apply gloves, and then place the towel between the legs

of the female client or over the thighs of the male. *The towel protects the client and nurse from possible urine leakage.*

5. Insert the syringe into the injection port of the catheter, and withdraw the fluid from the balloon. If not all the fluid can be removed, report this fact to the nurse in charge before proceeding. *Removal of fluid helps prevent discomfort and injury to urethra.*

6. Do not pull the catheter while the balloon is inflated. *Doing so may injure the urethra.*

7. After all the fluid is withdrawn from the balloon, gently withdraw the catheter, and place it in the waste receptacle. *This prevents discomfort to the client and eliminates a potential source of infection.*

8. Dry the perineal area with a towel. *Patting the skin dry helps remove any urine and prevents skin irritation.*

9. Measure the urine in the drainage bag and record the removal of the catheter. Include in the recording (a) the time the catheter was removed; (b) the amount, color, and clarity of the urine; (c) the intactness of the catheter; and (d) instructions given to the client. *This data provides proper documentation of the procedure.*

10. Remove gloves carefully and discard safely. *This prevents contamination by any urine which may be on the gloves.*

11. Following removal of the catheter, determine the time of the first voiding and the amount voided during the first 8 hours. Compare this output to the client's intake. *Comparison of intake and output ascertains the client's ability to void sufficient quantities following catheter removal.*

SAMPLE DOCUMENTATION

[date] Retention catheter #16
[time] inserted per physician order,
        5-mL balloon inflation. Urine
        spontaneously returned with
        300 mL, clear and straw
        colored. Client tolerated
        procedure well. _____
        _____ D. Haus, LVN

PROCEDURE 39-6

Irrigating a Catheter or Bladder (Closed System)

Purposes

- To maintain the patency of a urinary catheter and tubing (continuous irrigation)
- To free a blockage in a urinary catheter or tubing (intermittent irrigation)

Equipment

- Disposable gloves
- Disposable water-resistant sterile towel
- Three-way retention catheter in place
- Sterile drainage tubing and bag (if not in place)
- Sterile antiseptic swabs
- Sterile receptacle
- Sterile irrigating solution warmed or at room temperature
- Infusion tubing
- IV pole

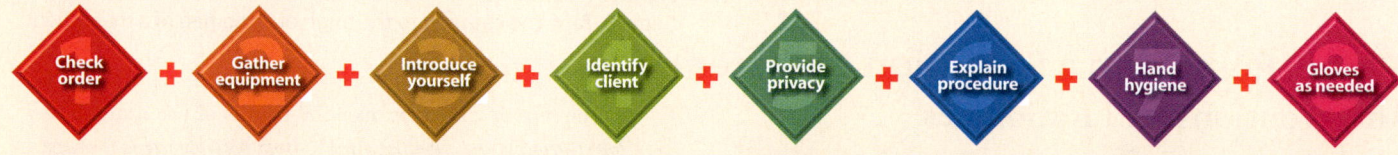

Check order + Gather equipment + Introduce yourself + Identify client + Provide privacy + Explain procedure + Hand hygiene + Gloves as needed

Interventions and Rationales

1. Perform preparatory steps (see icon bar above).

2. Prepare the client.
   - Explain the procedure and its purpose to the client.
   - Provide for privacy and drape the client as needed to allow access to the retention catheter.
   - Wear clean gloves.
   - Empty, measure, and record the amount and appearance of urine present in the drainage bag. Discard urine and gloves. *Emptying the drainage bag allows more accurate measurement of urinary output after the irrigation is in place or completed. Assessing the character of the urine provides baseline data for later comparison.*

3. Prepare the equipment.
   - Wash hands.
   - Connect the irrigation infusion tubing to the irrigating solution and flush the tubing with solution.
   - Connect the irrigation tubing to the input port of the three-way catheter. Connect the drainage bag and tubing to the urinary drainage port if not already in place.

4. Irrigate the bladder.
   a. For continuous irrigation, open the flow clamp on the urinary drainage tubing (if present). *This allows the irrigating solution to flow out of the bladder continuously.*
      - Open the regulating clamp on the irrigating tubing and adjust the flow rate as prescribed by the physician

or to 40 to 60 drops per minute if not specified. Assess the drainage for amount, color, and clarity. The amount of drainage should equal the amount of irrigant entering the bladder plus expected urine output.

b. For intermittent irrigation, determine whether the solution is to remain in the bladder for a specified time.

- If the solution is to remain in the bladder (a bladder irrigation or instillation), close the flow clamp on the urinary drainage tubing. *Closing the flow clamp allows the solution to be retained in the bladder and in contact with bladder walls.*

- If the solution is being instilled to irrigate the catheter, open the flow clamp on the urinary drainage tubing. *This allows irrigating solution to flow through the urinary drainage port and tubing, removing mucous threads or clots.*

- Open the flow clamp on the irrigating tubing, allowing the specified amount of solution to infuse. Clamp the tubing.

- After the specified period the solution is to be retained has passed, open the drainage tubing flow clamp and allow the bladder to empty.

5. Assess the client and the urinary output.
- Assess the client's comfort.
- Assess the amount, color, and clarity of drainage; note any abnormal constituents such as blood clots, pus, or mucous threads.
- To document urine output, empty the drainage bag and measure the contents. Subtract the amount of irrigant instilled from the total volume of drainage to obtain urine output.

6. Document the irrigation.
- Include all assessments obtained before and after performing the irrigation.

VARIATION: CLOSED IRRIGATION USING A TWO-WAY INDWELLING CATHETER

1. Assemble the equipment, including:
- Clean disposable gloves
- Disposable, water-resistant towel
- Sterile irrigating solution
- Sterile basin
- Sterile 30- to 50-mL syringe with an 18- or 19-gauge needle
- Sterile antiseptic swabs

2. Prepare the client (see step 2 of main procedure for catheter irrigation).

3. Prepare the equipment.
- Wash hands and wear gloves.

- Place the disposable, water-resistant towel under the catheter.
- For a bladder irrigation or instillation, clamp the drainage tubing distal to the injection port on the tubing or catheter. *Clamping prevents the urine and solution from draining into the drainage bag.* For a catheter irrigation, leave the tubing unclamped.
- Using aseptic technique, open supplies and pour the irrigating solution into the sterile basin or receptacle. *Aseptic technique is vital to reduce the risk of instilling microorganisms into the urinary tract during the irrigation.*
- Remove the cap from the needle and draw the prescribed amount of irrigating solution into the syringe, maintaining the sterility of the syringe and solution. Using the antiseptic swab, clean the port on the catheter or drainage tubing through which the solution will be instilled.

4. Irrigate the bladder.
- Insert the needle into the port.
- Gently inject the solution into the catheter. In adults, about 30 to 40 mL generally is instilled for catheter irrigations; 100 to 200 mL may be instilled for bladder irrigation or instillation. Smaller amounts are used for children.
- When the total amount to be instilled has been injected (or for catheter irrigation, when urine is flowing freely), remove the needle from the port and discard the syringe and uncapped needle in an appropriate receptacle (sharps container).
- After the prescribed dwelling time for a bladder irrigation, remove the clamp from the drainage tubing and allow the urine and irrigating solution to drain into the drainage bag.
- Assess the drainage for amount, color, and clarity. *The amount of drainage should equal the amount of irrigant entering the bladder plus expected urine output.*

5. Assess the client and the urinary output and document the procedure as previously noted.

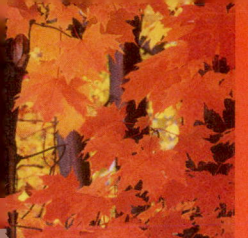

Chapter Review

KEY Points

- Urinary elimination depends on normal functioning of the urinary, cardiovascular, and nervous systems. Alterations in function have physical, social, and emotional effects.

- The normal process of urination is stimulated when sufficient urine collects in the bladder to stimulate stretch receptors.

- Alterations in urine production and elimination include polyuria, oliguria, anuria, frequency, nocturia, urgency, dysuria, enuresis, hematuria, incontinence, and retention.

- Assessment of a client's urinary function includes (1) normal voiding patterns, recent changes, past and current problems with urination, and factors influencing the elimination pattern; (2) a physical assessment of the genitourinary system; (3) inspection of the urine for amount, color, clarity, and odor; and, if indicated, (4) testing of urine for specific gravity, pH, and the presence of glucose, ketone bodies, protein, and occult blood.

- Clients with urinary retention are at risk of urinary tract infection. Urinary catheterization is frequently required for clients with urinary retention.

- The most common cause of urinary tract infection is an invasive procedure such as catheterization or cystoscopic examination. Females in particular are prone to ascending urinary tract infections because of their short urethras.

- Care of clients with indwelling catheters is directed toward preventing infection of the urinary tract and encouraging urinary flow through the drainage system.

- When the urinary bladder must be removed, a urinary diversion is formed to allow urine to be eliminated from the body. The client must wear a urine collection device continually over the stoma.

- When medical management of renal failure is no longer sufficient, the client will be placed on dialysis.

- Glomerulonephritis is an inflammatory disease of the glomerulus and may be either chronic or acute.

- When caring for a client with renal calculi, focus on maintaining adequate urinary output, preventing infection, and managing pain.

FOR FURTHER Study

See Chapter 20 for perineal care and more information on providing hygiene.

For more information about cleaning wounds and changing dressings, see Chapter 24.

See Chapter 26 for a discussion of fluids, electrolytes, and acid-base balance.

Refer to Chapter 33 for more information on hypertension, blood pressure regulation, and heart failure.

See Chapter 34 for information on RBC formation and anemia.

See Chapter 35 for information on systemic lupus erythematosus.

See Chapter 38 for information on nephropathy.

See Chapter 41 for more information about STIs.

Chapter 42 describes ways to help clients maintain normal voiding habits or retrain the bladder.

Discussion of cancer and its treatments is mainly in Chapter 45.

Critical Thinking Care Map

Caring for a Client with Impaired Urinary Elimination
NCLEX-PN® Focus Area: Physiologic Integrity

Case Study: Mr. Lee Jay is a 54-year-old client being treated for Type 1 diabetes that is out of control. He is incontinent of foul-smelling urine. He complains of thirst and frequent urination. He is 6' 3" and weighs 200 lbs. He states, "I try to maintain my diabetic diet but I'm on a fixed income." Mr. Jay is alert and oriented to person, place, and time. He monitors his glucose about once a week and gives himself insulin injections. He has diminished pedal pulses, and his feet are cool to the touch. The physician has ordered lab tests and an indwelling catheter.

Nursing Diagnosis: *Impaired Urinary Elimination*

COLLECT DATA

Subjective

_____
_____
_____
_____
_____
_____

Objective

_____
_____
_____
_____
_____
_____

Would you report this? Yes/No

If yes, report to: _____

What would you report? _____

Nursing Care

_____
_____
_____
_____
_____
_____
_____
_____
_____
_____
_____

How would you document this? _____
_____
_____
_____

Compare your answers and documentation to those provided on the MyNursingKit Website.

Data Collected
(use only those that apply)

- Diabetes out of control
- Incontinent
- Foul-smelling urine
- Cloudy urine
- Mucous threads in urine
- Alert and oriented
- Weakened
- Diminished pedal pulses
- Glucose 440
- T 99°F
- BP 140/80
- Lethargic
- Catheter to gravity drainage
- Thirst
- Diabetic care compliance

Nursing Interventions
(use only those that apply; list in priority order)

- Monitor lab tests.
- Observe urine for output.
- Assess urine for abnormal constituents.
- Assess pedal pulses.
- Maintain catheter asepsis.
- Ambulate client three times a day.
- Monitor vital signs every 4 hours.
- Record daily weights.
- Observe stool.

NCLEX-PN® Exam Preparation

TEST-TAKING TIP   Do not read more into the question than what it asks.

1 The nurse, working in a physician's office, is caring for a woman who has had recurrent urinary tract infections. The client asks why women get more UTIs than men. The nurse explains it is because of the difference in the size of men's versus women's:

1. Ureters.
2. Urethra.
3. Renal pelvis.
4. Glomeruli.

2 The nurse is caring for a client who is producing abnormally large amounts of urine and calls the physician to notify her that the client is demonstrating:

1. Oliguria.
2. Anuria.
3. Polydipsia.
4. Diuresis.

3 The nurse begins the shift at a long-term care facility and enters the room of a client with a retention catheter. The nurse gathers data about which of the following related to the catheter? (Select all that apply.)

1. Color, clarity, and quantity of drainage in the collection bag
2. Tubing is intact without kinks or obstructions
3. Collection bag is hanging at the level of the bladder
4. Connections of tubing are free of leaks
5. Appearance of urinary meatus

4 The nurse enters the client's room to collect a urine culture when the client asks why it is needed. The nurse explains the purpose of a urine culture is to determine:

1. If microorganisms are present in the urine.
2. Urine glucose level.
3. Urine concentration.
4. The presence of occult blood in the urine.

5 The nurse instructs the client on the procedure for collecting a 24-hour urine specimen. When the client demonstrates understanding, the nurse's first action is to:

1. Determine the specific gravity of the first voided specimen.
2. Discard the first void and begin collecting the 24-hour urine specimen.

3. Test the urine for glucose.
4. Instruct the client to begin collecting urine with the first voided urine.

6 The client presents to the physician's office complaining of sudden onset of fever, chills, vomiting, right flank pain, urinary frequency, and dysuria. The nurse suspects a diagnosis of:

1. Pyelonephritis.
2. Polycystic kidney disease.
3. Acute renal failure.
4. Glomerulonephritis.

7 The nurse would assess the client's hydration status if the specific gravity was found to be outside what range?

1. 1.000 to 1.005
2. 1.010 to 1.025
3. 1.025 to 1.030
4. 1.030 to 1.050

8 The nurse anticipates an order for fluid restriction when admitting a client with a medical diagnosis of:

1. Diabetes.
2. Renal calculi.
3. Kidney failure.
4. Urinary tract infection.

9 Which of the following instructions would the nurse give a client to prevent recurrence of a UTI?

1. Limit water intake.
2. Use nylon underclothes.
3. Bathe frequently.
4. Drink cranberry juice and take vitamin C.

10 The client, diagnosed with benign prostatic hypertrophy (BPH), asks the nurse why he has to void so frequently. The nurse explains that the enlarged prostate:

1. Surrounds and applies pressure on the ureter, preventing urine from entering the bladder.
2. Surrounds and applies pressure to the Cowper's glands, preventing urine production.
3. Surrounds and applies pressure to the urethra, preventing complete emptying of the bladder.
4. Invades the epididymis, causing decreased sperm and urine production.

Answers and rationales for Review Questions appear in Appendix I.

Chapter 40

Clients with Reproductive System Disorders

LEARNING Outcomes

After completing this chapter, you will be able to:

1. Review the structure and function of the female and male reproductive systems.
2. Identify points to cover in obtaining a comprehensive sexual history.
3. Describe the normal sexual response cycle and list possible causes of reproductive issues.
4. Discuss common breast disorders, treatment, and nursing interventions.
5. Identify common uterine disorders and changes with menopause, as well as treatment and nursing care for them.
6. Discuss tumors of the female reproductive system, their treatment, and appropriate nursing care.
7. Identify other disorders of the female reproductive system and appropriate nursing care.
8. Describe common disorders of the male reproductive system, treatment, and nursing interventions.
9. Name three infectious disorders that have an impact on family planning issues.
10. Discuss common contraceptive methods and the effectiveness of each.
11. Describe some of the issues involved in infertility and possible methods of treatment.

Clinical Objectives

12. Provide client teaching in basic anatomy and physiology appropriate to self-care needs.
13. Care for a male or female client with a reproductive disorder.
14. Provide psychosocial support for a client with reproductive issues.
15. Demonstrate breast and testicular self-examination to a client.
16. Provide nursing interventions for a client undergoing reproductive system surgery, and create a plan of care.
17. Provide a client with contraception information.

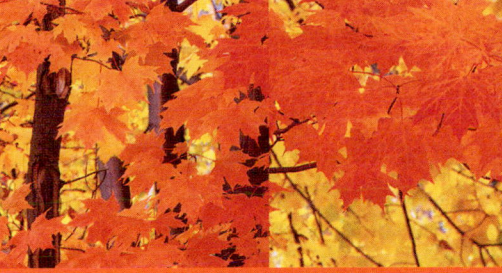

BRIEF Outline

KEY TERMS

Since the mid-1960s, more emphasis and support have been placed on reproductive issues than at any other time in recent history. Many of these issues carry with them emotional, moral, and ethical concerns. This chapter presents common reproductive issues and currently accepted interventions. Disorders of the reproductive tract may affect fertility, childbearing (see Unit IX), sexuality, self-esteem, and general health. To provide effective care, the nurse must have a basic understanding of the anatomy and physiology of the male and female reproductive systems as well as the pathophysiology, etiology, and medical management of reproductive disorders.

Reproductive Structure and Function

FEMALE REPRODUCTIVE SYSTEM

The female reproductive tract consists of the internal and external structures. The external structures (Figure 40-1 ■) include the mons pubis, the labia majora and minora, the

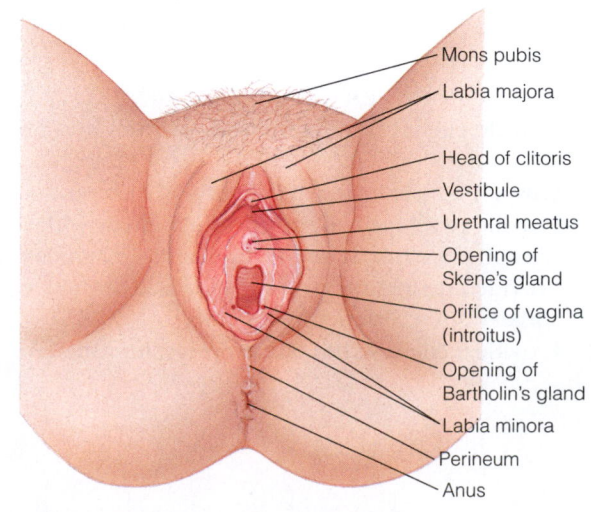

Figure 40-1. ■ External female genitalia structures.

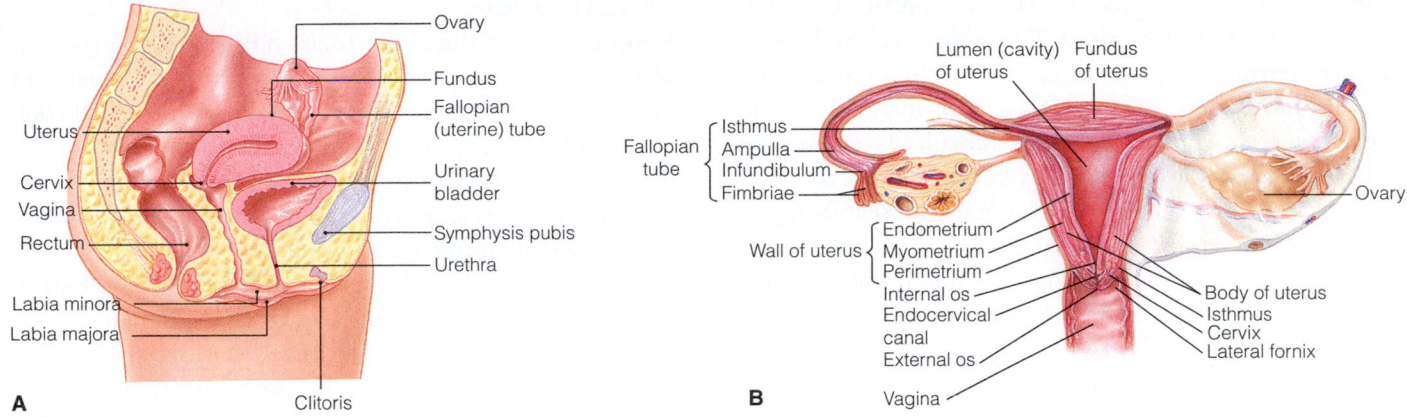

Figure 40-2. ■ Internal female structures: **A.** Cross section of the female reproductive system. **B.** Internal organs of the female reproductive system.

clitoris, the opening of the Skene's and Bartholin's glands, vaginal introitus, perineum, and the breast. The internal structures (Figures 40-2A and B ■) include the uterus, ovaries, and fallopian tubes. The breasts (Figure 40-3 ■) are also considered part of the female reproductive system.

External Structures

Vulva is the collective term used for the external structures of the female reproductive system. The *mons pubis* is a pad of adipose tissue anterior to the symphysis pubis. After puberty, coarse hair, distributed in a triangular pattern, covers this area. The *labia majora* is two folds of skin and adipose tissue, covered with hair, on either side of the vaginal vestibule. The labia majora contains sweat and sebaceous glands. The *labia minora* lies interior to the labia majora. It consists of two thin soft folds of skin and adipose and erectile tissue and covers the vestibule. The *clitoris* is a small erectile

body located in the anterior portion of the labia minora. The clitoris contains highly sensitive tissue and serves a primary role in sexual stimulation for women.

Between the labia majora and labia minora lies the *vestibule*. The vestibule contains the urinary meatus, vaginal introitus, hymen, and the Bartholin's and Skene's glands. The *urinary meatus* is the external orifice of the urethra and is located below the clitoris. The **vaginal introitus** is the external opening of the vaginal canal. It is surrounded by a thin layer of connective tissue called the *hymen*. *Bartholin's* and *Skene's glands* are located on each side of the vestibule. They provide lubrication to the vaginal introitus during sexual activity. Below the vestibule, above the anus, is the **perineum** (area between the thighs extending from the pubis to the coccyx). The muscles, fascia, and ligaments of the pelvis are anchored here. The **true perineum** is the tissue between the vaginal opening and the anus.

Internal Structures

The **vagina** is a tubular structure composed of muscle and membranous tissue connecting the vulva with the uterus. It is approximately 8 to 10 cm (3 to 4 in.) in length. The *rugae* (folds) allow the vagina to stretch for childbirth. The vagina has several purposes including access for intercourse, an outlet for menstrual flow, and as an outlet for birth. In adulthood the vagina has an acidic pH, which serves as protection against infections.

The **uterus** is a hollow organ where the fertilized ovum is implanted and the embryo and fetus develop. It is pear shaped and weighs about 2 ounces (60 grams). It measures 7.5 cm (3 in.) by 5 cm (2 in.) and is 2.5 cm (0.4 to 1 in.) thick. The uterus lies between the rectum and the bladder (see Figure 40-2A). It is supported by the round and broad ligaments. The uterine arteries include the hypogastric or internal iliac and the ovarian arteries, which branch off the descending aorta. The autonomic nervous system innervates the uterus. The uterus is made up of three sections: the

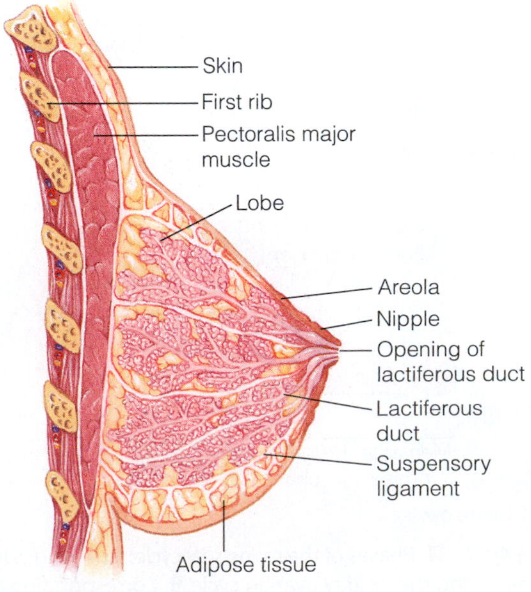

Figure 40-3. ■ Structures of the female breast.

fundus (upper portion), the *corpus* (middle portion or body), and the **cervix** (lower portion). The uterus has three layers: the perimetrium, myometrium, and endometrium. The perimetrium is the serosal layer (layer that lines the outside of the uterus), myometrium is the muscular layer, and the endometrium is the mucosal layer. The cervix connects the vagina and uterus through the lower uterine segment. The opening of the cervix is called the **cervical os.** The cervix serves as a protection against introduction of foreign substances into the uterus and also dilates to allow passage of the fetus during childbirth.

The **fallopian tubes** are the structures that allow passage of the ovum to the uterus. They are connected to the uterus by the ovarian ligament (see Figure 40-2B). The interstitial portion runs into the uterine cavity, the isthmus at the junction between the tubes and the uterus, the *ampulla* (the wider area that is the site for fertilization), and the infundibulum, the funnel-like end of the structure. The end is covered with *fimbriae* (finger-like projections).

The **ovaries** are flat almond-shaped glands located below the ends of the fallopian tubes. The ovaries produce the female hormones estrogen, progesterone, and androgens and store immature ova called *oocytes.* Estrogens are necessary for the development and maintenance of the secondary sex characteristics. They also ready the reproductive tract; maintain skin, bone, and blood vessels; affect serum cholesterol and high-density lipoprotein levels; enhance blood clotting; and alter sodium and water balance. Progesterone primarily affects breast glandular tissue and the endometrium. During pregnancy progesterone releases smooth muscle to decrease uterine contractions and increase body temperature. Androgens are responsible for normal hair growth patterns at puberty and also have a metabolic effect.

During early adolescence (usually 11 to 13 years), primary and secondary sex characteristics develop. Development of the genitals to adult size takes about 5 to 6 years. The hips broaden, the breast tissue develops, pubic hair grows, sebaceous glands become active, and vaginal secretions become "milky" and change from an alkaline to an acid pH.

Breasts

The breasts, though not necessary for reproduction, are considered an important part of the female reproductive system. The breasts contain the **mammary glands,** a network of ducts that carry the milk to the nipple (see Figure 40-3). Each gland has 15 to 20 lobes divided by adipose tissue. The adipose tissue determines the size of the breast but not milk production. **Prolactin,** the hormone produced by the anterior pituitary gland, stimulates milk production. The breast also contains blood vessels and a lymphatic system (axillary and internal mammary lymph nodes) that drain into the breast (see Figure 40-3).

Menstruation

Menarche occurs when menstruation begins during puberty. Menstruation occurs when an **oocyte** (egg cell) is released from the ovary. At puberty the female has approximately 300,000 oocytes. One is released each month following puberty due to the influence of the luteinizing hormone. If the oocyte is not fertilized by the male sperm, the uterine or endometrial lining is shed, defining menstruation (Figure 40-4 ■).

The ovarian cycle has three phases lasting about 28 days. The follicular phase lasts from the 1st through the 10th day. The ovulatory phase lasts from the 11th through 14th day ending with ovulation. The luteal phase lasts from the 14th day through the 28th day. Clients who use the rhythm method of contraception (see discussion later in the chapter) follow the ovarian cycle as a guide.

Each ovary contains follicles. Each follicle contains an immature ovum. Each month several follicles mature and are stimulated by follicle-stimulating hormone (FSH) and luteinizing hormone (LH). The mature follicles (*graafian follicles*) produce estrogen, which stimulates development of endometrium. When the estrogen level is high enough to stimulate the anterior pituitary gland, a surge of LH is produced. LH stimulates the development of the oocyte into a mature ovum and causes the ovarian follicle to rupture, releasing the ovum. This is **ovulation.** The ruptured follicle then becomes a **corpus luteum,** which produces estrogen and progesterone to support the endometrium until conception occurs or the cycle begins again. If pregnancy does not occur, the corpus luteum degenerates and its hormone production ceases. Falling progesterone and estrogen levels allow LH and FSH levels to increase, and a new cycle begins.

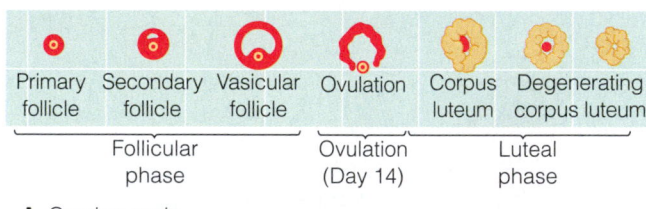

Primary follicle | Secondary follicle | Vasicular follicle | Ovulation | Corpus luteum | Degenerating corpus luteum

Follicular phase | Ovulation (Day 14) | Luteal phase

A Ovarian cycle

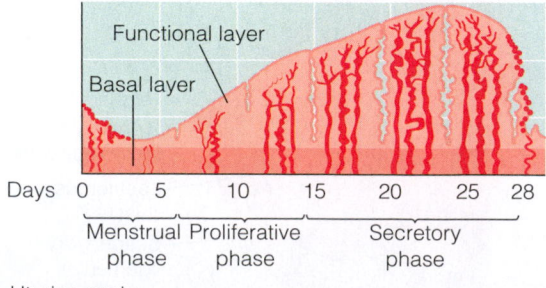

Functional layer

Basal layer

Days 0 5 10 15 20 25 28

Menstrual phase | Proliferative phase | Secretory phase

B Uterine cycle

Figure 40-4. ■ Phases of the menstrual cycle: **A.** Changes in ovarian follicles during the 28-day ovarian cycle. **B.** Corresponding changes in the endometrium during the menstrual cycle.

The menstrual cycle has three phases: the menstrual phase, the proliferative phase, and the secretory phase. During the menstrual phase, the endometrial layer sloughs off and is shed. During the proliferative stage, the endometrial layer thickens and is repaired. Spiral arteries proliferate and tuberal glands form. Cervical mucus is thin and allows the passage of the sperm. During the secretory phase, progesterone increases endometrial vascularity to prepare for the fertilized ovum. Cervical mucus thickens. If fertilization does not occur, hormone levels fall. Spasm of the spiral arteries causes degeneration and sloughing of the endometrial layer.

MALE REPRODUCTIVE SYSTEM

The male reproductive organs can be divided into two groups: primary and accessory organs (Figure 40-5 ■). The *primary reproductive organs* (gonads) are responsible for producing the gametes. The gonads of the male are the **testes.** The *accessory reproductive organs* are those structures that transport, protect, and nourish the gametes after they leave the gonads. In the male, the accessory organs include the epididymis, ductus deferens, seminal vesicles, prostate gland, bulbourethral glands, scrotum, and penis.

The testes are two oval-shaped glands suspended in a pouch known as the *scrotal sac.* The left testis is generally 1 cm lower in the scrotal sac than the right testis. The testes are attached to the perineum by the spermatic cords and scrotal tissue. The vas afferens (blood vessels) reach the testes by passing through the spermatic cord (which encloses the vas deferens, blood vessels, lymphatics, and nerves). The primary functions of the testes are to produce spermatozoa (**sperm**) called male gametes or reproductive cells. The seminiferous tubules produce sperm.

In males, follicle-stimulating hormone (FSH) and interstitial cell-stimulating hormone or luteinizing hormones (ICSH/LH) are the indirect stimulating hormones from the anterior pituitary gland. They stimulate the testes to secrete testosterone (androgen). Testosterone is also responsible for the development of *secondary sex characteristics* (traits associated with gender but not directly necessary for reproduction). These characteristics include a deeper voice, broader shoulders, and more muscle mass.

The **epididymis** is an enclosed single coiled tube that serves as a duct through which the sperm passes from the testis to the outer surface. It also contributes to sperm maturation and secretes seminal fluid. The vas deferens is an extension of the epididymis connecting to the ejaculatory duct. Sperm can remain in the vas deferens for a month without fertility loss. Two short ejaculatory ducts pass through the prostate gland and end in the urethra. The urethra serves the male in two ways: for urine elimination and for the delivery of sperm in the reproductive system.

The **seminal vesicles** are pouches along the lower posterior surface of the bladder. They secrete a viscous alkaline fluid high in sugar content. This provides an energy source for sperm motility after ejaculation. It also contains prostaglandins that influence chemical reactions within the cell. Secretions depend on adequate levels of testosterone production.

The **prostate** gland is found in the male below the bladder and surrounds the urethra. Ducts from the prostate enter the urethra and serve as a pathway for semen on ejaculation. **Semen** is an alkaline fluid that contains sperm. The alkaline secretion neutralizes the acidity of the vaginal tract and enhances the motility of the sperm. Urine is prevented from mixing with semen during ejaculation by the closure of a sphincter at the bladder's opening.

The *bulbourethral glands* (also called *Cowper's glands*) resemble the shape and size of a pea. They are located proximal to the prostate gland and are connected by a duct to the penis and urethra. These glands secrete an alkaline fluid similar to what the prostate and seminal vesicles produce, neutralizing the acid found in the male urethra and female vagina. Mucus is formed and lubricates the urethra.

The **scrotum** is the pouch suspended from the perineal area; it is divided into two sacs. It contains the testes, epididymis, and distal part of the spermatic cord. The contraction of the dartos and cremaster muscle results in the elevation of the testes, which occurs with sexual arousal and cold temperatures. This brings the testes close to the perineal wall, increasing the temperature. For adequate sperm formation the temperature needed is below normal body temperature, rationalizing the normal suspension of the testes outside the body.

The **penis** is the cylindrical external structure that encloses the urethra and contains erectile tissue. The distal end of the penis described as a bulging formation is called the glans penis. A retractable loose skin is known as the *prepuce* or foreskin. The surgical removal of the prepuce is called a *circumcision* and

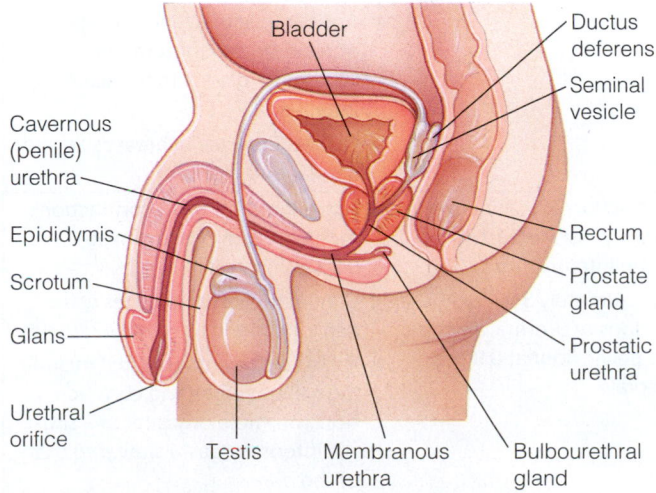

Cavernous (penile) urethra — Bladder — Ductus deferens — Seminal vesicle — Epididymis — Scrotum — Glans — Rectum — Prostate gland — Prostatic urethra — Urethral orifice — Testis — Membranous urethra — Bulbourethral gland

Figure 40-5. ■ Male reproductive system.

is performed based on religious or cultural premises. The opening at the tip of the glans penis is the *urinary meatus*. The functions of the penis are urinary excretion and serving as a reproductive tract. The erectile tissue becomes engorged with blood during sexual arousal. The enlargement and firmness of the penis allows penetration during sexual intercourse.

SEXUAL RESPONSE CYCLE

As anatomic and physiologic maturity occurs, sexual responses become more prevalent and sexual activity may begin. In 1966 Masters and Johnson described the four phases of sexual response: excitement, plateau, orgasm, and

resolution. Table 40-1 ■ summarizes changes in the female and male sexual response cycle.

OBTAINING A COMPREHENSIVE SEXUAL HISTORY

Obtaining a comprehensive sexual history is important in determining reproductive health. The nurse is vital in gathering the data necessary to make a proper assessment. A nonjudgmental, nonthreatening environment is critical to eliciting this data. The client should feel comfortable and privacy should be honored. The nurse should speak in a language that is understandable to the client. Nurses must be

TABLE 40-1	Physiologic Changes Associated with the Sexual Response Cycle		
PHASE OF THE SEXUAL RESPONSE CYCLE	**SIGNS PRESENT IN BOTH SEXES**	**SIGNS PRESENT IN MALES ONLY**	**SIGNS PRESENT IN FEMALES ONLY**
Excitement	■ Increased muscle tension ■ Moderate increase in heart rate, respirations, and blood pressure ■ Sex flush (less prevalent in men than in women; present in 75% of women) ■ Nipple erection (60% of men and most women)	■ Enlargement and erection of penis ■ Scrotum thickens ■ Testicles rise toward the body	■ Enlargement of the clitoris ■ Vaginal lubrication ■ Widening and lengthening of vaginal barrel ■ Separation and flattening of the labia majora ■ Reddening of the labia minora and vaginal wall ■ Breast *tumescence* (enlargement) and enlarged areolae
Plateau	■ Increased voluntary and involuntary myotonia ■ Abdominal, intercostal, anal, and facial muscle contraction ■ Accelerated heart rate and respiratory rate, and increased blood pressure ■ Sex flush (appearance in some men late in the phase; spread over the entire body in women)	■ Ridge of glans becomes more prominent ■ Cowper's glands secrete preejaculatory fluid ■ Testicles remain close to the body	■ Retraction of the clitoris under the hood ■ Appearance of the orgasmic platform (increase in the size of the outer one-third of the vagina and the labia minora) ■ Slight increase in the width and depth of the inner two-thirds of the vagina ■ Further reddening of the labia minora ■ Appearance of a few drops of mucoid secretion from the Bartholin's glands to lubricate inner labia ■ Further increase in breast size and areolar enlargement
Orgasmic	■ Involuntary spasms of muscle groups throughout the body ■ Diminished sensory awareness ■ Involuntary contractions of the anal sphincter ■ Peak heart rate (110–180 bpm), respiratory rate (40/min or greater), and blood pressure (systolic 30–80 mm Hg and diastolic 20–50 mm Hg above normal)	■ Contraction of ejaculatory duct in prostate pushes semen into urethra ■ Approximately 3–6 contractions of urethra, anus, and pelvic floor at 0.8-sec intervals	■ Approximately 5–12 contractions in the orgasmic platform at 0.8-sec intervals ■ Contraction of the muscles of the pelvic floor and the uterine muscles ■ Varied pattern of orgasms, including minor surges and contractions, multiple orgasms, or a simple intense orgasm similar to that of the male

TABLE 40-1	Physiologic Changes Associated with the Sexual Response Cycle (continued)		
PHASE OF THE SEXUAL RESPONSE CYCLE	**SIGNS PRESENT IN BOTH SEXES**	**SIGNS PRESENT IN MALES ONLY**	**SIGNS PRESENT IN FEMALES ONLY**
Resolution	■ Reversal of vasocongestion in 10–30 min; disappearance of all signs of myotonia within 5 min ■ Genitals and breasts return to their preexcitement states ■ Sex flush disappears in reverse order of appearance ■ Heart rate, respiratory rate, and blood pressure return to normal ■ Other reactions include sleepiness, relaxation, and emotional outbursts such as crying or laughing	■ Refractory period from 5 min to 24 hrs in which erection is impossible	■ May move back to plateau stage for multiple orgasms without resolution

aware of and sensitive to the sexual concerns of people from non-Western cultural backgrounds (Box 40-1 ■).

When conducting an interview for sexual information, open-ended questions should be used. This type of question is less threatening to clients. Box 40-2 ■ provides sample questions to use when obtaining a sexual health history.

CAUSES OF REPRODUCTIVE ISSUES

Most reproductive disorders can be categorized as infections, blockage or structural changes, or tumors. Although tumors and some structural changes cannot be prevented, infections and scar tissue formation in reproductive tubules often can be prevented. Nurses can play a significant role in providing teaching to men and women of all ages about issues related to the reproductive system.

BOX 40-1   CULTURAL PULSE POINTS

Issue of Female Circumcision
Mutilation of the female genitalia, sometimes called *infibulation* or female circumcision, is practiced in some African countries, Malaysia, India, Yemen, and Oman. There are several types of female circumcision. Most involve excision of the clitoris, and may include removal of the labia majora and minora, with the excised edges being sewn together. The practice in these cultures is associated with womanhood and sexuality. Complications of this procedure include hemorrhage, infection, dyspareunia, painful childbirth, menstrual difficulties, anxiety, and depression. The nurse must respect the culture, while at the same time creating an open environment where the client feels comfortable discussing her concerns about this condition.

BOX 40-2   DATA COLLECTION

The following questions may be used to elicit information about a client's reproductive and sexual history and activity:
- When did your menstrual period first begin, and when did you have your last menstrual period?
- What is the usual length of your period in days and usual amount of bleeding?
- What are your concerns about the amount or regularity of your menstrual flow?
- If periods are irregular, problematic, or have stopped: Tell me about any evaluations for this change or what you have done to deal with it.
- Are you having any burning with urination, any vaginal itching or discharge, midcycle spotting, pain with intercourse, or any other problems?
- Have you ever been pregnant? (Explore number and outcome of pregnancies, including miscarriages and induced abortions.)
- How often do you do breast self-examination?
- Is there a history of breast or ovarian cancer in your family?
- When did you have your last Pap test and mammogram? What were the results?
- Are you currently sexually active?
- What do you do to protect yourself from infection when you are sexually active?
- Have you ever had a sexually transmitted infection? Which one? Treatment?
- Has any disease, injury, surgery, medication, or other situation affected your sexual health and happiness or your feelings about yourself as a woman or man?
- Do you have any questions about your sexual health or functioning, or is there anything else we have discussed that you would like clarified or explained?

FEMALE REPRODUCTIVE HEALTH ISSUES

Throughout her life, a woman faces many reproductive system issues. Some are minor, easily treatable conditions. Others are major life-threatening disorders. Some disorders affect the woman's ability to conceive, carry a pregnancy to term, or breastfeed the infant. Some disorders may occur early in life but have an impact on the woman's ability to reproduce years later.

Breast Disorders

Breast disorders may be detected by the woman during a monthly breast self-examination (BSE), during a physical examination by the primary care provider, or by **mammography** (diagnostic x-ray of the breast). Because early detection is critical to the treatment of malignancy, women should be taught the BSE technique and encouraged to seek annual physical examination and mammogram. Procedure 40-1 ■ describes steps in performing a BSE. To become familiar with the size and consistency of her breast, a woman should perform BSE beginning in her 20s. Breast cancer is uncommon in young women but the risk increases with age. Therefore, women should have an annual screening mammogram beginning at age 40. If the woman is at an increased risk for breast cancer due to family history or defective genes, she should be encouraged to have screening mammograms at an earlier age.

NONMALIGNANT BREAST DISORDERS

Nonmalignant (benign) disorders of the breast include fibrocystic disease (Figure 40-6 ■), fibroadenoma, and intraductal papillomas.

Fibrosis is the replacement of inflamed or damaged tissue with connective or scar tissue. In the breast, the result is a painless encapsulated tumor or fibroid. Frequently the fibroid degenerates, accumulating fluid in the process. This fluid-filled mass or **fibrocyst** puts pressure on surrounding tissue and becomes painful. Commonly, more than one fibrocyst forms in each breast, resulting in breast irregularities or "lumpiness." Occasionally, the cyst will drain into the nipple.

Fibrocystic breast disease is most common in women between 30 and 50 years of age. Fibrocystic changes in the breast are an excessive response to cyclic hormonal changes. After menopause, these breast changes usually decrease. If cell growth occurs in conjunction with cyst formation, the woman is at a greater risk for breast cancer. Oral intake of caffeine found in coffee, tea, cola, and chocolate may contribute to fibrocystic breast disease. Medical management of fibrocystic breast disease focuses on diagnosis, screening for malignancy, and suppressing estrogen while stimulating progesterone. Aspirated fluid from the cysts is used for diagnosis as well as for relieving pressure and discomfort. There is no evidence that fibrocystic breast disease prevents breastfeeding.

Fibroadenoma is a freely movable, rounded mass with well-defined borders and a solid rubbery texture. These nontender masses are most common in women in their teens and early twenties. Diagnosis is by history and fine-needle biopsy. Excision may be indicated, but caution is exercised to prevent damage to the developing breast structure. Fibroadenomas are not associated with breast cancer.

Intraductal papillomas are tumors growing in a mammary duct. They most commonly occur during menopause. Although they are not malignant, they have the potential of becoming cancerous. These small ball-like tumors are often not palpable but are found on mammography. If they occur near the nipple, a serosanguineous or brownish-green discharge may be present. Because of the risk for malignancy, papillomas are usually removed surgically.

Diagnosis and Treatment

Diagnosis of these conditions is made by examination, mammography, and fine-needle aspiration. Medical management includes aspirin, ibuprofen, vitamin E, dietary changes, danazol, oral contraceptives, and bromocriptine. Women are encouraged to receive regular clinical breast exams, perform monthly BSE, and schedule regular mammograms. Fibroadenomas and intraductal papillomas may be surgically removed. Table 40-2 ■ describes symptoms and treatment of fibrocystic and other breast disorders.

BREAST CANCER

Breast cancer is defined as growth of abnormal or cancerous cells within the breast tissue. One in eight women in the United States develops breast cancer. As a woman ages, her risk for acquiring breast cancer increases. Breast cancer is the second leading cause of cancer-related deaths among women. The most significant risk factor is the woman's age, with most breast cancer occurring after 50. Box 40-3 ■ describes breast cancer risk factors. The 5-year survival rate when breast cancer is detected early is 72% for African American women and 87% for Caucasian women.

Risk Factors

Factors predisposing to breast cancer are being female, older than 50 years, and personal or family history. The defective genes BRCA1 and BRCA2 are associated with an increased incidence of developing breast cancer. Alcohol consumption equal to two drinks per day of any type of alcoholic beverage, early menarche, late menopause, obesity, no children or

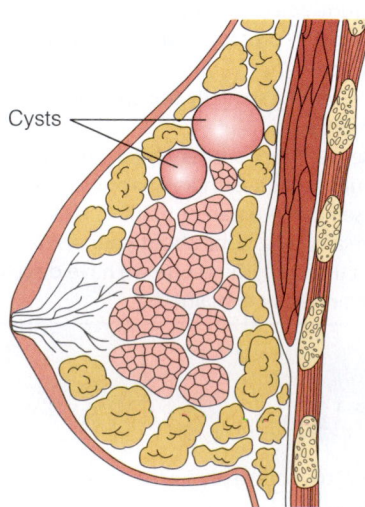

Cysts

Figure 40-6. ■ Fibrocystic breast changes.

TABLE 40-2	Breast Disorders: Manifestations, Treatment, and Nursing Considerations		
DISORDER	**MANIFESTATIONS**	**DIAGNOSIS/TREATMENT**	**NURSING CONSIDERATIONS**
Fibrocystic breast disease	Fluid-filled movable mass Drainage from nipple Localized pain No skin retraction	Diagnosed by history, mammography, aspiration Medication to suppress estrogen and stimulate progesterone Mild analgesic	Teach BSE. Encourage to limit caffeine in diet. Provide emotional support.
Fibroadenoma	Freely movable mass with well-defined edges Rubbery in texture Nontender mass Most common in teens and early twenties	Fine-needle biopsy Excision with caution to prevent structural damage	Teach postoperative wound care. Provide emotional support.
Intraductal papillomas	Small ball-like nonpalpable mass May have nipple drainage of serosanguineous or brownish-green fluid	Found on mammogram Potential for malignancy Surgical removal	Reinforce teaching by healthcare provider. Provide emotional support. Provide referral to support group as appropriate.
Breast cancer	Small, hard painless lump, change in the size or shape of the breast, nipple Discharge, dimpling, pulling, or retraction of the skin of the breast resembling an orange peel	BSE, mammography, biopsy Surgical removal, chemotherapy, radiation Long-term therapy with tamoxifen	Reinforce teaching by healthcare provider. Teach postoperative care. Teach medication use and side effects. Provide emotional support. Provide referral to support group as appropriate.

children after age 30, never breastfeeding, exposure to high dose radiation to the chest, upper socioeconomic status, and use of oral contraceptives or hormone replacement therapy or greater than 5 years are all risk factors. Women who have never had functioning ovaries and who have never had estrogen replacement do not develop breast cancer.

Manifestations

Signs and symptoms of breast cancer include nontender lump in the breast (most often in the upper outer quadrant), bloody discharge from the nipple or a change in its position, dimpling of the skin, retraction of the nipple, and

difference in size of the breasts. Peau d'orange (orange peel) appearance of the skin may be present with inflammatory carcinoma of the breast (Figure 40-7 ■).

clinical ALERT

With inflammatory breast disorder, the skin may appear slightly roughened. The condition may initially be misdiagnosed as an insect or a spider bite. However, if the skin appearance does not resolve quickly, the woman should seek further medical attention. Pain is a late symptom that often prompts the client to seek treatment. If untreated, the cancer will spread to the axillary lymph nodes, and therefore, to other organs such as the lungs, liver, brain, and bone (Figure 40-8 ■).

BOX 40-3	BREAST CANCER RISK FACTORS

- *Personal Data:* Female, over 50
- *Race:* White
- *Family History:* Mother or sister with breast cancer
- *Genetic History:* Defective genes BRCA1 and BRCA2
- *Medical History:* Cancer of breast, endometrial cancer, proliferative fibrocystic breast changes
- *Menstrual/Reproductive History:* Early menarche (before age 12), late menopause (after age 50), first birth after age 30, use of estrogen replacement therapy more than 5 years
- *Radiation Exposure:* Multiple chest x-rays or fluoroscopic exams, particularly before age 30
- *Lifestyle:* More than two alcoholic drinks daily, obesity, smoking, high economic status, breast trauma

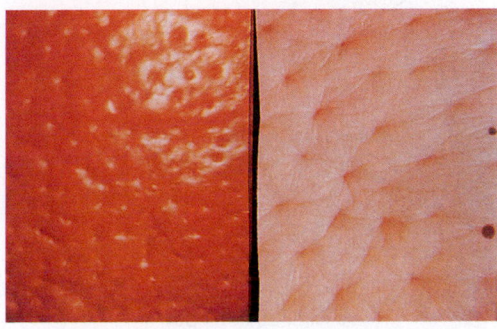

Figure 40-7. ■ *Left:* Orange peel. *Right:* Peau d'orange skin that signals *inflammatory breast disease,* a type of breast cancer.

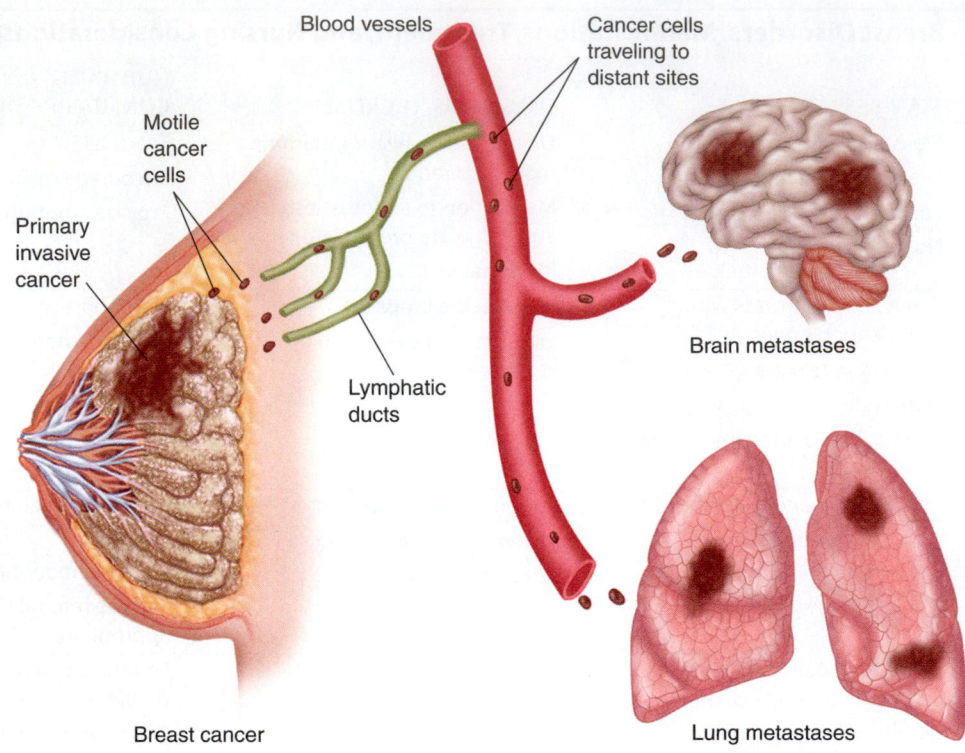

Blood vessels

Cancer cells traveling to distant sites

Motile cancer cells

Primary invasive cancer

Brain metastases

Lymphatic ducts

Breast cancer

Lung metastases

Figure 40-8. ■ Invasion and metastasis by cancer cells. (*Source:* Holland, Adams: Core Concepts in Pharmacology. 2003. Upper Saddle River, NJ: Prentice Hall.)

Diagnosis and Treatment

Mammograms often detect breast lesions at their earliest stage. Biopsy (Figure 40-9 ■) and microscopic exam can confirm the diagnosis. BSE is very important as well and should be performed monthly as discussed earlier in this chapter.

Noninvasive (also called *in situ*) malignancies develop within the ducts or lobes of the breast without invading the surrounding tissue. Diagnosis of these tumors, which often lie under the areola and nipple, is usually made by mammography rather than palpation.

Invasive tumors grow from the intermediate ducts of the breast. Tumors are classified by cell type. However, prognosis and treatment depend on the progression of the disease (stage of development). Breast cancer can metastasize to the ribs, sternum, or lungs. In this case, the woman may also exhibit pain, spontaneous bone fractures, and respiratory symptoms such as labored breathing, cough, and **hemoptysis** (bloody sputum).

Medical management depends on the stage of cancer and a woman's age. Surgery, chemotherapy, hormone therapy,

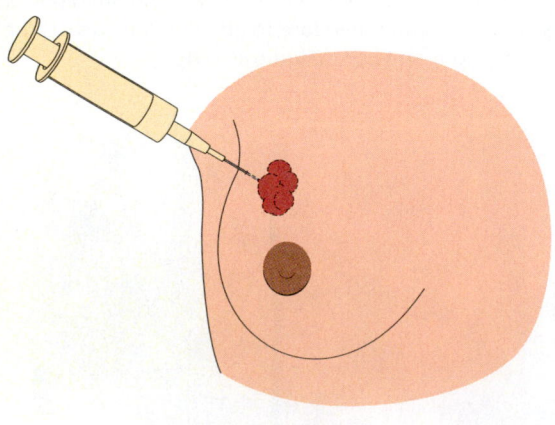

A Aspiration biopsy

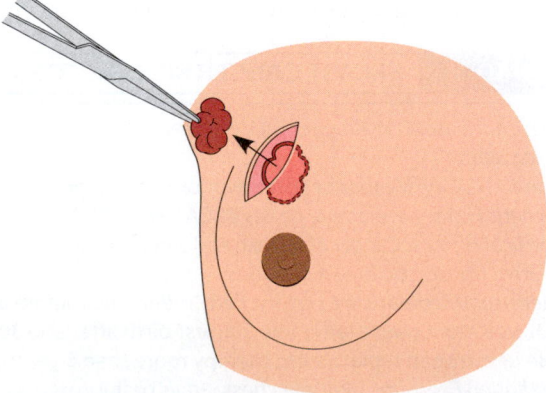

B Excisional biopsy

Figure 40-9. ■ Types of breast biopsies: **A.** In an aspiration biopsy, a needle is used to aspirate tissue or fluid from the breast. **B.** In an excisional biopsy, the breast lesion is removed surgically, and its tissue is examined.

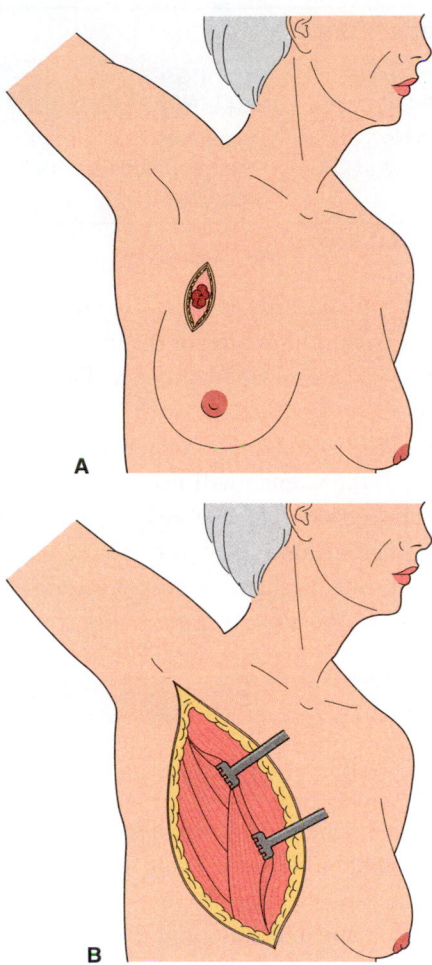

A

B

Figure 40-10. ■ Surgery for breast cancer: **A.** In a lumpectomy, the tumor and a small margin of surrounding tissue are removed. **B.** In a modified radical mastectomy, the entire breast and axillary lymph nodes are removed.

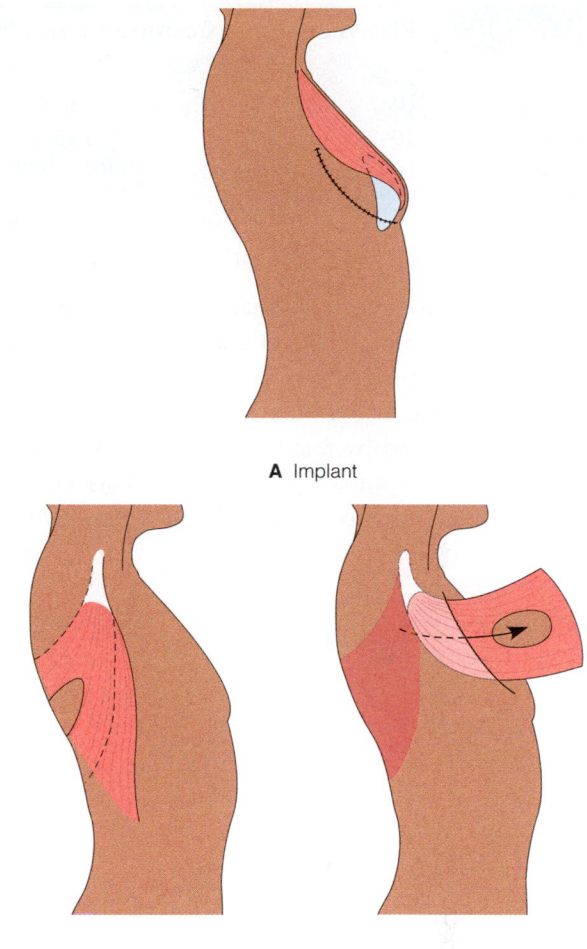

A Implant

B Latissimus dorsi myocutaneous flap

Figure 40-11. ■ Breast reconstruction surgeries: **A.** An implant is inserted under the pectoris muscle. **B.** A latissimus dorsi flap is used to reconstruct the breast.

and radiation are typical regimens. Surgical intervention may include a **lumpectomy** (removal of the lump), breast-conserving surgery (removal of the tumor, a disease-free margin surrounding the tumor, and adjacent lymph nodes), simple **mastectomy** (removal of the breast), or radical mastectomy with removal of the breast, surrounding lymph nodes, and underlying muscle structure. Figure 40-10 ■ illustrates a lumpectomy and a modified radical mastectomy. The client may choose breast reconstruction surgery (Figure 40-11 ■) or a prosthesis. See Chapter 29 ⊂⊃ for care of clients undergoing surgery.

Radiation therapy may be initiated following surgery if the lymph nodes are involved, the chest wall is involved, or the tumor is larger than 5 cm. Palliative radiation may give the client relief from pain and assist in preventing fractures associated with bone metastasis. Adverse effects of radiation include fatigue, skin redness, minor discomfort, or pain.

Chemotherapy may also be used to shrink and destroy the cancer cells. Chemotherapeutic agents most commonly

used to treat breast cancer are mifepristone (RU-486), testolactone (Teslac), cyclophosphamide (Cytoxan), doxorubicin (Adriamycin), 5-fluorouracil (5-FU), methotrexate (Trexall), and prednisone (Deltasone). Usually drugs are given in combination for effectiveness. See more on cancer and its treatment in Chapter 45 ⊂⊃.

Hormone therapy for the treatment of breast cancer is usually recommended (Table 40-3 ■). Tamoxifen (Nolvadex) is an antiestrogen drug that inhibits tumor growth. It may also be used as a preventive measure for high-risk women.

SURGICAL BREAST ALTERATIONS

Surgery on the breast can be done for several reasons. As mentioned, surgery can be performed to remove a tumor or the entire breast and surrounding tissue due to a malignancy. Breast reconstruction (**mammoplasty**) may be performed at the time of the mastectomy or at a later date if extensive therapy is required.

TABLE 40-3	Pharmacology: Common Drug for Clients with Breast Cancer			
DRUG	**USUAL ROUTE/DOSE**	**CLASSIFICATION**	**SELECTED SIDE EFFECTS**	**DON'T GIVE IF (CALL HEALTHCARE PROVIDER IF)**
Tamoxifen (Tamofen, Tamone)	10–20 mg once or twice a day for 5 years	Antiestrogen, antineoplastic	Bone pain, blood clot formation, alteration in CBC, GI upset	Suspected blood clots, signs of thrombophlebitis, or pulmonary embolism

Some women have breasts that are large and heavy, putting strain on the shoulders and upper back. These women sometimes request that a *reduction mammoplasty* be performed. In women of childbearing age, the size of the breast will be reduced by removing fat tissue with an attempt to leave the mammary glands intact. This would allow the woman to breastfeed if she desires. In older women, the breast may be reduced by removing mammary glands and fat tissue.

Some women have smaller breasts. The ability to breastfeed is not related to the size of the breast. However, *breast augmentation* (insertion of implants to create larger breasts) may help these women improve their self-image. Implants contain either saline or silicone. In recent years, there has been controversy over the safety of silicone implants. Continued research should resolve this controversy.

Postoperatively, the woman may have drains leading away from the surgical site. The dressings are usually large and may be cumbersome. It will take 1 week or more for the swelling and bruising to subside. Before discharge, the woman should be taught to care for the incision, apply dressings, and empty the drainage container. During this time, she should be encouraged to look at the breast with a mirror and to begin to adjust to her new image. If a mastectomy has been performed, the woman will need to perform arm exercises on the affected side to facilitate lymphatic drainage and achieve full range of motion (Figure 40-12 ■). Due to the change in body image, she may need additional emotional support and referral to a mastectomy support group.

NURSING CARE

PRIORITIZING NURSING CARE

When caring for clients with breast disorders, focus your care on managing pain and anxiety. Evaluate the effectiveness of pain treatments and notify the physician when the treatments are not adequate. Positioning may help relieve breast

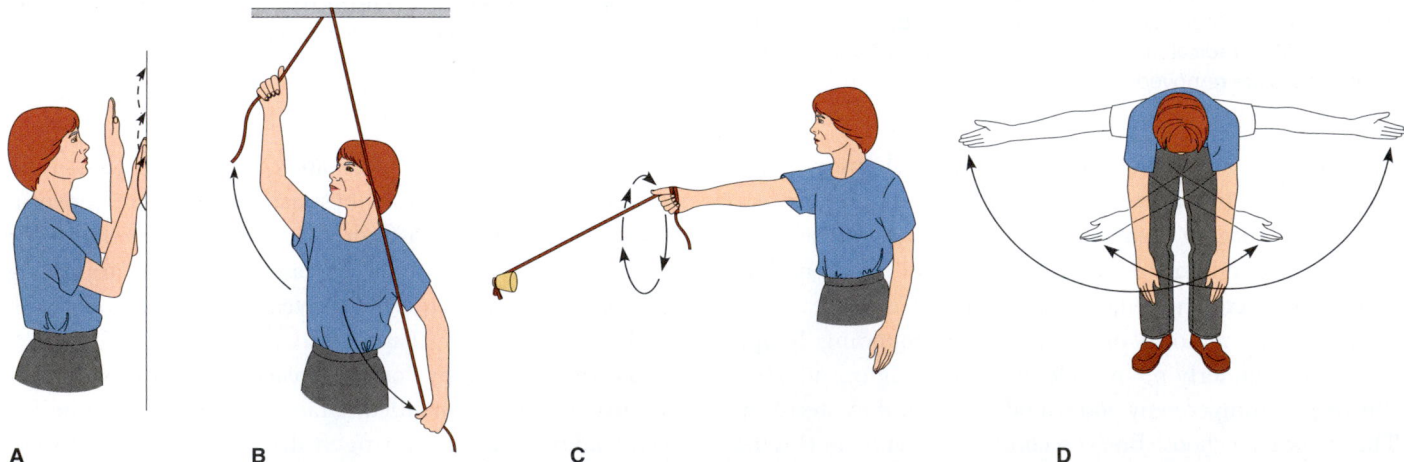

A   B   C   D

Figure 40-12. ■ Postmastectomy exercises: **A.** Wall climbing: Stand facing wall with toes 6 to 12 inches from wall. Bend elbow and place palms against wall at shoulder level. Gradually move both hands up the wall parallel to each other until incisional pulling or pain occurs. (Mark that spot on wall to measure progress.) Work down to shoulder level. Move closer to wall as height of reach improves. **B.** Overhead pulley: Using operated arm, toss 6-foot rope over shower curtain rod (or over top of a door that has a nail in the top to hold the rope in place for exercise). Grasp one end of rope in each hand. Slowly raise operated arm as far as comfortable by pulling down on the rope on opposite side. Keep raised arm close to your head. Reverse to raise unoperated arm by lowering the operated arm. Repeat. **C.** Rope turning: Tie rope to door handle. Hold rope in hand of operated side. Back away from door until arm is extended away from body, parallel to floor. Swing rope in as wide a circle as possible. Increase size of circle as mobility returns. **D.** Arm swings: Stand with feet 8 inches apart. Bend forward from waist, allowing arms to hang toward floor. Swing both arms up to sides to reach shoulder level. Swing back to center, then cross arms at center. Do not bend elbows. If possible, do this and other exercises in front of a mirror to ensure even posture and correct motion.

pain, so assist the client to the most comfortable positions. Encourage clients to talk about their fears and insecurities regarding breast disease. Be supportive and an active listener. Keep in mind that many women strongly connect their sexuality and desirability to the appearance of their breasts. Provide emotional support and encouragement when the client looks at her incision and responds to the feelings it invokes.

ASSESSING

A critical element of maintaining and restoring client health is an adequate assessment. The nurse is responsible for collecting the health history to assist in determining the cause and symptoms related to disorders of the breast. An important question to ask the client is how long the lump has been present. Be sure to assess the client's emotional status and coping skills.

DIAGNOSING, PLANNING, AND IMPLEMENTING

The nurse is able to identify many nursing diagnoses appropriate for the client diagnosed with a breast disorder. Because nursing care is holistic, the nurse must concentrate on physical as well as emotional nursing diagnoses.

Physical nursing diagnoses include Risk for *Acute Pain* related to tumors of the breast. The surgical client may also be at *Risk for Injury*, especially those who have had lymph nodes removed. These clients may experience lymphedema. *Risk for Infection* related to surgical wound is also an appropriate nursing diagnosis.

Emotional nursing diagnoses include *Anxiety* related to possibility of a life-threatening disease. The client may also experience *Disturbed Body Image* related to breast wounds or the removal of one or both breasts. Other emotional nursing diagnoses could include *Grieving, Decisional Conflict*, and *Powerlessness*.

Client goals in the planning stage of the nursing process include:

- Adequate pain relief will be provided.
- Complications of surgery will be avoided.
- Anxiety levels will be reduced.
- Positive body image will be restored.
- Feelings of grief will be expressed and positive measures initiated to deal with the grief.

To achieve these goals, the nurse provides various nursing interventions. Nursing interventions for clients with breast disorders include client teaching, assisting in screening, ensuring proper diagnosis and treatment, and reviewing risks for complications. The following nursing interventions with rationales are appropriate for most clients with breast disorders. Other nursing interventions should also be considered in an effort to individualize nursing care.

- Provide nonpharmacologic and pharmacologic pain relief methods. *Nonpharmacologic pain relief measures often complement or reduce the amount of pharmacologic pain medications.*
- Avoid intravenous infusions and blood pressure monitoring on the surgical side. *Increased pressure on the surgical side may contribute to lymphedema.*
- Without abducting the arm, elevate the arm on the surgical side with hand higher than elbow. *Lymph drainage is encouraged, edema is prevented, and circulation is promoted through the force of gravity.*
- Perform passive range-of-motion exercises and encourage active range-of-motion exercises of the arm on the surgical side. *Promotes collateral drainage.*
- Use therapeutic techniques to encourage the client to express concerns and fears. *Expression of concerns and fears allows the nurse to dispel myths and teach facts regarding the client's condition. Emotional relief is often enhanced through verbal expression of concerns and fears.*
- Encourage the client to view her incision site as quickly as possible and maintain a physical presence when she decides to do so. *The imagined view of the surgical site is often worse than reality.*
- Explain the process of wound healing and the stages the client may experience. *Knowledge that the wound will heal without redness and swelling may hasten acceptance of her physical alteration.*
- Refer the client to a local support group if she desires. *Speaking with other women who have experienced breast cancer can bring about knowledge and acceptance of the disease.*
- Explain the normalcy of depression, anger, denial, and fear following a diagnosis of breast cancer and the resulting surgery. *Giving permission to the client to express expressions of grief in an appropriate manner can facilitate recovery.*
- Include the client and her support system, if appropriate, in decisions relating to her care. *Giving the client an opportunity to be involved in decision making returns control and power to her.*

EVALUATING

The nurse revises care until expected outcomes are achieved. The expected outcomes for a client with breast cancer include:

- Pain is avoided and adequate pain relief is maintained.
- No complications of surgery noted.
- Anxiety levels are reduced.
- Positive body image is restored.
- Expresses feelings of grief and initiates positive measures to deal with the grief.

Ovarian Disorders

Cysts (fluid-filled sacs) commonly form in the ovary, whether from the graafian follicle or from the corpus luteum. Most cysts regress spontaneously in two to three menstrual cycles. Some cysts become so large that they rupture and drain into the pelvis. Bleeding and a surgical emergency could occur.

Polycystic ovary syndrome (PCOS) results from numerous follicular cysts. This endocrine disorder is characterized by higher than normal LH, estrogen, and androgen levels, and low FSH levels. This hormone imbalance results in irregular menstrual cycles, **hirsutism** (excessive hair growth), acne, obesity, and infertility. The woman may develop Type 2 diabetes mellitus and has an increased risk for endometrial cancer, hypertension, and high cholesterol.

Diagnosis of ovarian cysts is made by pelvic ultrasound. Hormone levels are evaluated to diagnose PCOS. Laparoscopic surgery may be necessary to drain large cysts or control bleeding. Hormone therapy may be useful to prevent cyst formation.

Ovarian cancer is discussed under Tumors and Ectopic Disorders later in the chapter.

Uterine Disorders

The average woman who has a regular menstrual cycle will have approximately 450 periods in her lifetime. Occasionally, women may experience altered courses of their menstrual cycles. These alterations include premenstrual syndrome, dysmenorrhea, amenorrhea, menorrhagia, metrorrhagia, and menopause.

Most women experience minor discomforts just prior to and during menstruation. These include bloating, breast tenderness, cramping, and backache. Other effects can be symptoms of more serious disorders.

PREMENSTRUAL SYNDROME

Premenstrual syndrome (PMS) is a group of symptoms occurring 3 to 14 days prior to menstruation and is relieved by the onset of menses. PMS is linked to an imbalance of estrogen and progesterone, as well as increased prolactin and aldosterone levels. Rising aldosterone causes sodium and water retention. The neurotransmitters monoamine oxidase (MAO) and serotonin may also play a role in PMS. It is most common in women ages 30 to 40 and about 25% to 30% of menstruating women report symptoms.

Manifestations

Symptoms include headache, irritability, depression, edema of extremities, abdominal fullness, and breast swelling and tenderness. Fatigue, lethargy, anxiety, and crying may also occur. The manifestations of multisystem effects of PMS vary for each client and each month. They are described in Box 40-4 ■.

Diagnosis and Treatment

There is no specific diagnostic test for identifying this syndrome. Diagnosis is based on the presence of symptoms for at least 3 months.

BOX 40-4	EFFECTS OF PREMENSTRUAL SYNDROME

Premenstrual syndrome (PMS) can have a wide range of manifestations that vary by person. It can affect many systems.

- *Neurologic:* syncope, dizziness, paresthesias, headache, inability to concentrate, depression, irritability, anxiety, mood swings, anger, aggressive behavior
- *Sensory:* conjunctivitis, visual disturbances
- *Cardiovascular:* bruising, palpitations
- *Integumentary:* acne, herpes recurrence, urticaria
- *Urinary:* cystitis, oliguria
- *Gastrointestinal:* constipation, nausea, vomiting
- *Musculoskeletal:* backache, pelvic stiffness
- *Immune:* increased susceptibility to infection, asthma, increased allergic reactions
- *Metabolic processes:* breast tenderness, edema, transient weight gain, food cravings

---

Medical management of PMS focuses on diet, exercise, and relaxation techniques to reduce stress. A diet high in complex carbohydrates with limited simple sugars, sodium, caffeine, and alcohol is recommended. Restriction of tobacco is also recommended. An increased intake of calcium, magnesium, and vitamin B_6 may be helpful. A balance between exercise and rest can also help reduce irritability. Relaxation techniques and stress management include muscle relaxation, deep abdominal breathing, guided imagery, and meditation. Ibuprofen, diuretics, and antidepressants may be helpful. If symptoms interfere with activities of daily living, low-dose birth control pills may be helpful.

DYSFUNCTIONAL UTERINE BLEEDING

There are several disorders related to menstruation. They may be associated with excessive discomfort or classified as *dysfunctional uterine bleeding* (DUB). **Dysmenorrhea** (painful menses) may be primary (occurring without pelvic pathology) or secondary (with pelvic pathology). Primary dysmenorrhea is due to an excessive production of prostaglandins, causing uterine muscle contractions during ovulatory cycles. These contractions cut off oxygen to uterine tissue (ischemia). They result in pain varying from mild cramping to severe uterine pain. Secondary dysmenorrhea may be related to endometriosis, fibroid uterine tumors, pelvic inflammatory disease, ovarian cancer, or the use of an IUD.

DUB is characterized by *anovulatory* cycles in which the uterine blood flow occurs in abnormal amounts, for varying lengths of time, and without regard to the typical time of occurrence. Types of DUB include menorrhagia, metrorrhagia, and amenorrhea.

Menorrhagia is defined as repetitive, excessive, or prolonged menstruation flow. It may be related to thyroid disorders, endometriosis, uterine fibroids, clotting disorders, or anticoagulant use. Menorrhagia can lead to excessive blood loss, fatigue, anemia, hemorrhage, and sexual dysfunction.

Metrorrhagia is bleeding between periods. Causes of metrorrhagia include hormonal imbalances, oral contraceptive use, subdermal implant use, pregnancy, ectopic pregnancy, endometriosis, sexually transmitted infections, cervical or uterine polyps, fibroids, or cancer.

Amenorrhea is defined as absence of menstruation. Primary amenorrhea exists when the client has not had menstruation by age 16 or age 14 if secondary sex characteristics have not appeared. This may be related to hormonal imbalances, structural abnormalities, polycystic ovarian disease, imperforate hymen, anorexia nervosa, bulimia nervosa, or excessive athletic training. Secondary amenorrhea is the absence of menses for at least 6 months in women who have previously had a regular menstrual cycle. It is caused most often by pregnancy, or by breastfeeding, weight loss, hormonal imbalances, anorexia nervosa, excessive athletic training, ovarian tumors, menopause, or premature ovarian failure.

Diagnosis and Treatment

Disorders of DUB require diagnostic testing including thyroid function studies, endocrine studies, and progesterone levels. A CBC is drawn to determine systemic disease, and a pelvic ultrasound may be used to identify structure abnormalities. An endometrial biopsy may be necessary to examine the uterine cellular structure.

Medical management is determined by the cause. Often these disorders require hormone therapy such as oral contraceptives. Iron supplements and possibly blood transfusions may be needed if the hemoglobin and hematocrit are low from blood loss. Therapy might involve **dilatation and curettage** (D & C) (opening of the cervix and scraping of the lining of the uterine walls). Endometrial ablation and hysterectomy may be necessary if continued anemia and blood loss occur.

Menopause

Menopause (climacteric), the permanent cessation of menstruation, occurs between 35 and 58 years of age. Menses may stop suddenly, may decrease in volume until cessation occurs, or may occur at longer and longer intervals until they stop. Women who have short menstrual cycles or who smoke usually experience menopause 1 to 2 years sooner than women with longer menstrual cycles or women who do not smoke.

Manifestations

Symptoms of menopause begin shortly after the ovaries stop functioning whether menopause occurs naturally or due to surgical removal of the ovaries (**oophorectomy**). Symptoms include hot flashes, irritability, fatigue, apathy, depression, crying episodes, palpitations, vertigo, and vaginal dryness.

Long-term physical changes associated with menopause include *osteoporosis* (decalcification of bones), coronary artery disease, and tendency toward increased weight.

Diagnosis and Treatment

Diagnosis is generally made by a review of symptoms. If diagnosis is questionable, a test to help diagnose menopause is a FSH level greater than 40 to 170 mU/mL.

Hormone replacement therapy (HRT) may be recommended for many women to ease the menopausal symptoms and promote bone health. In recent years, much study has been conducted on the long-term effects of HRT on a woman's health. There is some indication that the risk associated with HRT may outweigh the benefits (Writing Group for the Women's Health Initiative Investigators, 2002). Other studies (Stefanick et al., 2006; Manson et al., 2007) indicate a decreased risk of breast cancer and coronary artery calcification in posthysterectomy women taking HRT. It is essential that each woman's history be reviewed and individual risk be identified prior to initiating HRT. Some women choose complementary herbal or food-based supplements instead of HRT (Box 40-5 ■).

NURSING CARE

PRIORITIZING NURSING CARE

When caring for clients with menstrual disorders, focus your care on managing symptoms and reassuring clients. Evaluate pain and discomfort using a scale, and evaluate the effectiveness of pain management. Ensure that the client truly understands the causes and treatment of the disorder and what effect, if any, it could have on fertility. Explain the interactions of hormones and emotions to help reassure clients about possible causes of mood changes.

BOX 40-5   COMPLEMENTARY THERAPIES

Alternative Therapy for Menopausal or Menstrual Symptoms

Some women prefer to use natural substances to assist with symptoms of menopause. Complementary therapies include creating a cool environment, reducing caffeine and alcohol, practicing stress management, taking a daily supplement of vitamin E, Kegel exercises, use of a water-soluble lubricant for intercourse, a balanced diet, and regular exercise.

Phytoestrogens are plant substances that have an effect like estrogen. Phytoestrogens are found in agnus castus, dong quai, licorice, red sage, soy, tofu, Mexican yam, flax seed, and other plants. However, research (Krebs, Ensrud, MacDonald, & Wilt, 2004) indicates phytoestrogens do not improve hot flashes or other menstrual symptoms.

When caring for clients in perimenopause, focus your care on client teaching and managing the effects of the condition. Encourage clients to take responsibility for managing symptoms of menopause and determining what works and does not work for them. Encourage clients to see this phase of life as normal, natural, and manageable. Be alert for indications of emotional distress and refer clients to mental health professionals as appropriate.

ASSESSING

A critical element of maintaining and restoring client health is an adequate assessment. The nurse is responsible for collecting the health history to assist in determining the cause and symptoms related to disorders of menstruation. Review Box 40-2 for questions to ask to determine the client's reproductive and sexual history.

DIAGNOSING, PLANNING, AND IMPLEMENTING

The nurse is able to identify many nursing diagnoses appropriate for the client diagnosed with a menstrual disorder. Because nursing care is holistic, the nurse must concentrate on physical as well as emotional nursing diagnoses.

Physical nursing diagnoses include *Risk for Pain* related to declining ovarian function. The client is also at *Risk for Injury* related to the many complications of menstrual disorders such as osteoporosis or coronary heart disease. *Impaired Urinary Elimination* related to incontinence may also be diagnosed for the client with a menstrual disorder.

Emotional nursing diagnoses include *Anxiety* related to undiagnosed menstrual disorder. A client with a menstrual disorder may also have *Deficient Knowledge* related to management of perimenopause. Other emotional nursing diagnoses that may result are *Sexual Dysfunction, Fear,* and *Ineffective Coping.*

Client goals in the planning stage of the nursing process include:

- Adequate pain relief will be achieved.
- Measures will be implemented to prevent complications.
- A decrease in anxiety will be reported.

To achieve these goals, the nurse provides various nursing interventions. Nursing interventions for clients with menstrual disorders include client teaching, assisting in screening, ensuring proper diagnosis and treatment, and reviewing risks for complications. The following nursing interventions with rationales are appropriate for most clients with menstrual disorders. Other nursing interventions should also be considered in an effort to individualize nursing care.

- Teach nonpharmacologic and pharmacologic pain relief measures. *Nonpharmacologic pain relief measures often complement or reduce the amount of pharmacologic pain medications.*

- Assess ADLs with client to evaluate the need for activity versus rest. *Rest increases energy and decreases oxygen requirements. This may in turn lower the client's pain level.*
- Teach the client to implement measures for preventing complications of menstrual disorders such as calcium and vitamin E supplementation, a diet low in fat and high in fiber, and a regular cardiovascular, weight-bearing exercise program. *These prevention methods may be effective in helping the client to avoid osteoporosis and coronary heart disease.*
- Instruct the client about the causes, treatments, risks, and prognosis of the diagnosed menstrual disorder. *Allows for effective communication about the client's state of health and encourages the client to assume responsibility for her health care.*
- Discuss stress management techniques. Provide teaching as necessary. *Stress management techniques can assist the client in reducing and preventing anxiety.*

EVALUATING

The nurse revises care until expected outcomes are achieved. The expected outcomes for a client with a menstrual disorder include:

- Client reports that pain level is decreasing.
- Complications are avoided.
- Client reports anxiety decreased due to stress management techniques.

NURSING PROCESS CARE PLAN
Client with Amenorrhea

Kallie, 13 years old, is training as a gymnast with the hope of becoming an Olympic athlete. Her exercise and training regime includes running 5 miles, 100 sit-ups, and 30 minutes of weight training in the morning. She eats a light breakfast and trains in the gym until supper. After a vegetarian meal she returns to the gym for dance and rhythm class. Kallie's menarche was at age 11, with periods every 32 days, lasting 5 days. She had difficulty with dysmenorrhea that was managed by over-the-counter analgesics. During a pre-event physical she reports to the nurse practitioner that she has not had a period in 7 months. This truly concerns her because her mother died of ovarian cancer shortly after Kallie's eighth birthday. She reports that she is not sexually active.

Assessment
Initial vital signs: BP 106/72, P 60, R 18 and even. After discussing her condition, Kallie began to breathe rapidly and deeply. She reported tingling of her lips and fingers. Her pulse increased to 90 bpm. Height: 4 feet, 10 inches. Weight: 98 pounds. Small frame. Pregnancy test negative. CBC and thyroid function studies were within normal

limits (WNL). Vaginal ultrasound was performed without significant findings.

Nursing Diagnosis

The following important nursing diagnoses (among others) are established for this condition:

- *Deficient Knowledge* related to causes and complications of amenorrhea
- *Anxiety* related to lack of menstrual activity
- *Imbalanced Nutrition: Less than Body Requirements* related to deficient protein intake

Expected Outcomes

The expected outcomes for the plan of care are that Kallie will:

- Relate aggressive athletic training and poor nutrition to her amenorrhea. Kallie should acknowledge that ovarian cancer is not related to amenorrhea, but she should relate that osteoporosis, infertility, increased risk of injury, cardiovascular disease, and endometrial cancer are associated with amenorrhea.
- Report reduced anxiety as evidenced by implementation of stress-reducing activities and reduced episodes of hyperventilation.
- Plan a diet that will include more calories and increased protein.

Planning and Implementation

The following nursing interventions are implemented for Kallie:

- Teach Kallie that the cause of her amenorrhea is excessive exercise combined with a diet low in calories and protein.
- Teach Kallie the complications associated with amenorrhea.
- Provide Kallie with anxiety-reducing techniques such as abdominal breathing and guided imagery.
- Assess members of Kallie's support system and discuss with them the need to assist Kallie in reducing her anxiety.
- Encourage Kallie to eat a diet with at least 2,500 calories per day.
- Teach Kallie about the importance of adequate calcium and protein and the food sources containing these nutrients.

Evaluation

At the 3-month follow-up clinic visit, Kallie's vital signs are BP 110/78, P 64, R 18, T 98.6° F. Wt 103 pounds. Kallie stated that she had a better understanding about the reason she experienced amenorrhea. She had altered her training schedule and increased her daily calories and protein intake slightly. She had not had a menstrual cycle yet but reported slight abdominal bloating, breast tenderness, and irritability which occurred for the first time 2 days ago.

Critical Thinking in the Nursing Process

1. How would you avoid discouraging Kallie with regard to achieving her Olympic dream while at the same time presenting to her the importance of a balanced nutrition and exercise regime?
2. Plan a relaxation technique to assist in the reduction of Kallie's anxiety.
3. Design a meal plan that would be appropriate for Kallie.

Note: Discussion of Critical Thinking questions appears on the MyNursingKit Website.

Female Structural Abnormalities

UTERINE DISPLACEMENT AND UTERINE POSITIONS

Uterine displacement is a change of placement of the uterus within the pelvic cavity or descension of the uterus in the vaginal canal. Uterine positions include anteversion, retroversion, anteflexion, and retroflexion (Figure 40-13A–D ■). These conditions can be congenital or acquired.

When the uterus descends into or out of the vaginal canal, the condition is called **uterine prolapse** (Figure 40-13E). Childbirth usually is the cause of prolapse, but obesity or tumors can also cause it. Uterine prolapse occurs because of stretching of the uterine ligaments or increased intra-abdominal pressure.

Manifestations

Signs and symptoms of positioning conditions include dysmenorrhea, dyspareunia, and backache. Manifestations of uterine prolapse include a heavy or dragging feeling in the groin or lower back that may be relieved by lying flat. The woman may feel a mass protruding from the vagina when bearing down or with heavy lifting. Constipation, urinary incontinence, hemorrhoids, and dyspareunia are common.

Treatment

Most uterine positions do not need medical management. Medical management of uterine prolapse may include Kegel exercises (see Chapter 54 🔗), use of a **pessary** (a plastic device shaped like a ring, arch, or ball that is placed in the vagina to support the uterus), and physical therapy. Surgery may be done to shorten and suspend uterine ligaments. If the client is postmenopausal or does not want children, a hysterectomy may be recommended.

Tumors and Ectopic Disorders

UTERINE TUMORS

Common uterine tumors include nonmalignant fibroids, endometrial cancer, and cervical cancer. Fibroid tumors of the uterus, common among women of all ages, are classified by their location within the uterus (Figure 40-14 ■). Although the exact cause of fibroid uterine tumors is

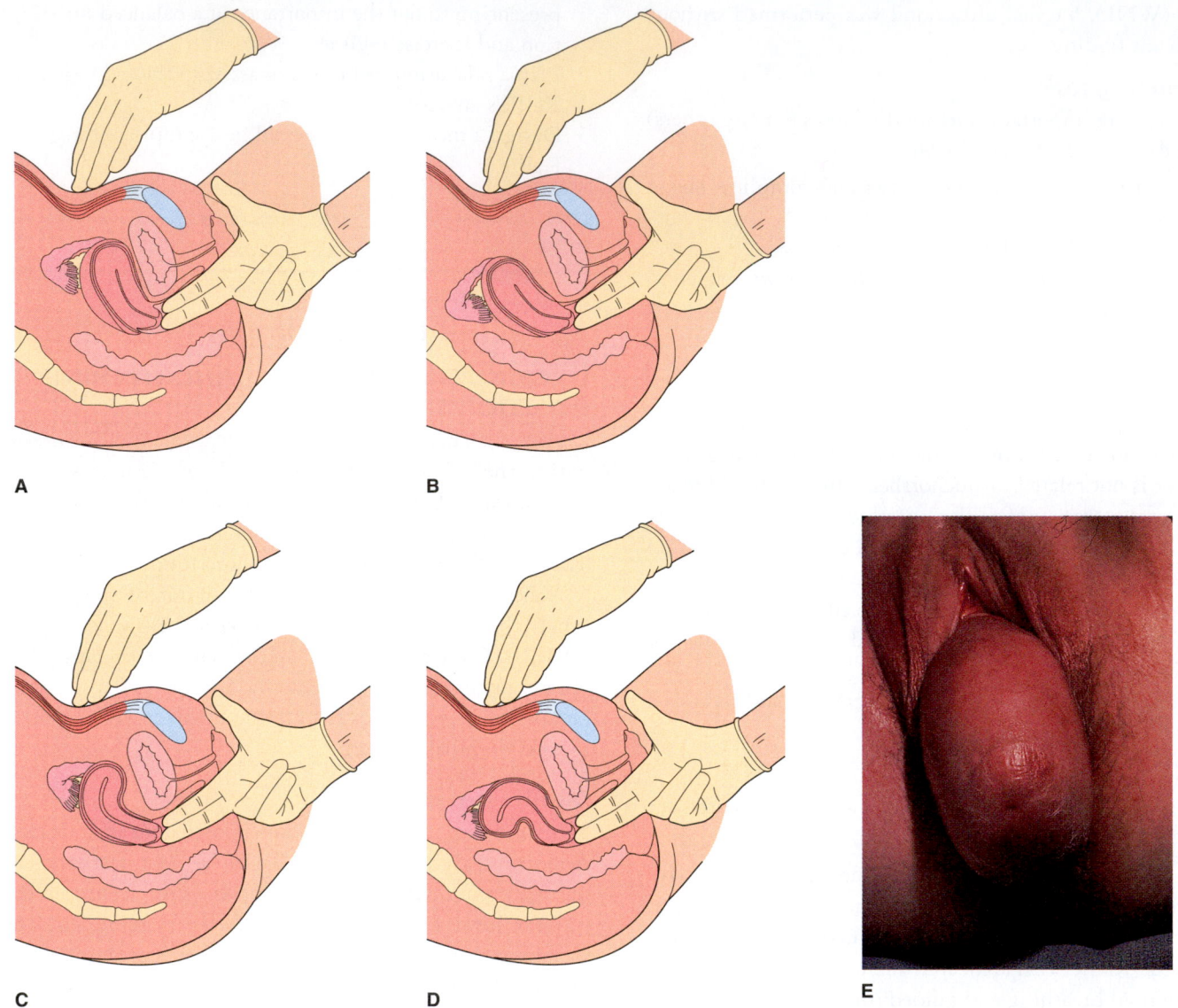

Figure 40-13. ■ Common uterine positions: **A.** Anteversion. **B.** Retroversion. **C.** Anteflexion. **D.** Retroflexion. **E.** A fully prolapsed uterus.

unclear, they are probably related to estrogen secretion. Small tumors may go unnoticed for some time. Large tumors can enlarge the uterus, cause menorrhagia, put pressure on surrounding tissues, and cause lower abdominal and pelvic pain. In asymptomatic women who want to bear children, the fibroid tumors are monitored. In some cases, a laparoscopic **myomectomy** (removal of tumor and surrounding myometrium) may be performed. If tumors are large, a **hysterectomy** (surgical removal of the uterus) may be necessary.

Hysterectomy

Hysterectomy may be necessary due to uterine tumors, severe endometritis, uterine hemorrhage, or uterine prolapse. Often removal of the fallopian tubes (**salpingectomy**) and ovaries (*oophorectomy*) are done at the same time. Hysterectomy can be

accomplished through a lower abdominal incision (open hysterectomy), or a vaginal incision. Often a vaginal incision is used with the assistance of a laparoscope to secure intra-abdominal structures.

A new technique using a *da Vinci robot* is being done in many areas of the country. Through use of a tiny camera and robotic arms with surgical tools, the da Vinci robot allows surgery with smaller incisions, leading to reduced client pain and faster recuperation time.

In all instances the postoperative care is similar. See Chapter 29 ⬭ for routine postoperative care. The client will have IV fluids, a Foley catheter, and surgical dressing. The surgeon will pack the vagina to control bleeding. Pain medication will be administered as needed. Vaginal packing and Foley catheter are usually removed in 12 to 25 hours. It is important to observe for excessive vaginal

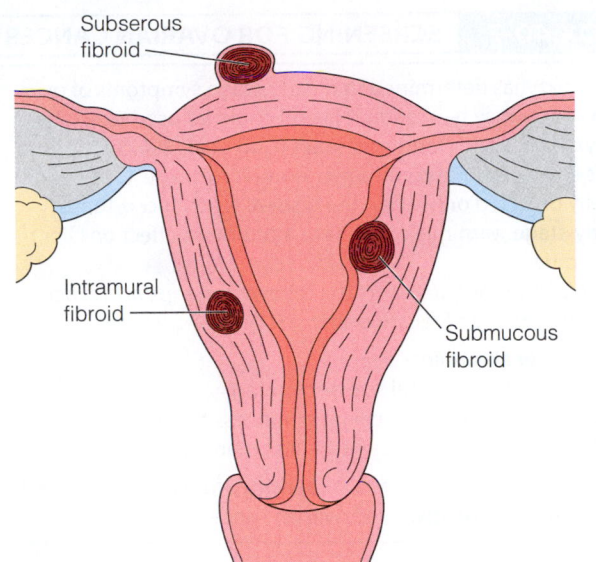

Subserous fibroid

Intramural fibroid

Submucous fibroid

Figure 40-14. ■ Sites of uterine fibroid tumors.

drainage. Some women have difficulty voiding after the catheter is removed so urinary output must be measured and recorded. At times the woman is discharged with a Foley catheter in place. Discharge teaching should include perineal care with each voiding and stool to prevent infection, care of the Foley catheter if necessary, taking pain medication as ordered, and limiting activity including avoiding sexual intercourse until approved by the surgeon.

ENDOMETRIAL CANCER

The most common malignant disorder of the pelvis is cancer of the endometrium, affecting women between 50 and 70 years of age. These slow-growing tumors begin with endometrial **hyperplasia** (excessive proliferation of normal cells). The tumor usually begins in the fundus, spreads to the myometrium, and invades the entire female reproductive system. Metastasis occurs through the lymphatic system, with common sites being lungs, liver, and bone.

Manifestations

Bleeding in the postmenopausal woman is the most common symptom. Abdominal pain and pressure are late symptoms. Risk factors include an early menarche, late menopause, use of estrogen preparations without progestin for prolonged periods, obesity, and diabetes.

Diagnosis and Treatment

Diagnosis is usually made by a Pap smear or endometrial biopsy or D & C. Treatment of choice for endometrial cancer is a TAH with bilateral salpingo-oophorectomy (BSO). This stands for *total abdominal hysterectomy* (surgical removal of the uterus) with *bilateral salpingectomy* (surgical removal of the fallopian tubes) and *oophorectomy* (surgical removal of

the ovaries). Chemotherapy or radiation may be recommended if cancer has spread beyond the uterus. See more about cancer and its treatment in Chapter 45 .

CERVICAL CANCER

Cervical cancer is, in most cases, a slow-growing squamous cell carcinoma of the cervical epithelium. Cancer of the cervix generally occurs in women ages 35 to 50. Some of the risk factors of cervical cancer are listed in Box 40-6 ■.

Most cervical cancers result from an infection by the human papillomavirus (HPV). Other risk factors also include early sexual intercourse, unprotected sex, multiple sex partners, HIV infection, smoking, and poor diet. Early detection and intervention have reduced the incidence of invasive cervical carcinoma. See discussion of sexually transmitted infections later in this chapter. Immunization with Gardasil® can prevent HPV infection.

Manifestations

Most cervical cancers begin as **cervical dysplasia** (abnormal changes in the tissue of the cervix) or cervical intraepithelial neoplasia (CIN), including changes in the squamous cells of the cervix. Over time these cellular changes develop into carcinoma *in situ*, a localized cancer that becomes invasive if not treated. Prior to invasion of the vaginal wall, pelvic wall, bladder, and rectum, cervical cancer is asymptomatic.

Cervical cancer invades the surrounding tissue, including the vagina, urethra, bladder, and rectum. Invasive cervical cancer may be characterized by back or thigh pain, hematuria, occult blood in the stool, anemia, and weight loss.

Diagnosis and Treatment

Diagnosis is made by a "thin prep" or a Papanicolaou (Pap) smear. In these tests, cells and secretions from the cervix are collected and sent to the laboratory for examination. If cancerous cells are identified, magnetic resonance imaging (MRI) or a computed tomography (CT) scan of the pelvis, abdomen, and bones may be ordered to determine the extent of invasion.

BOX 40-6	RISK FACTORS FOR CERVICAL CANCER

- Human papilloma virus (HPV)
- Multiple sexual partners and sex partners with multiple partners, early intercourse, especially when younger than 16 years
- Use of oral contraceptive for longer than 5 years
- Smoking
- Poor nutritional status
- History of HPV infection
- History of chemotherapy
- History of HIV
- History of dysplasia

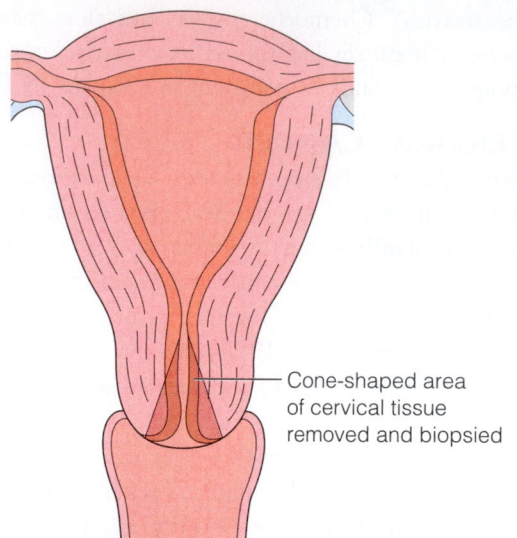

Cone-shaped area
of cervical tissue
removed and biopsied

Figure 40-15. ■ Conization of the cervix.

When the tumor is localized within the cervix, it may be removed by laser, heated or cooled probes, or cauterization. A **conization** (removal of a cone-shaped wedge of cervical tissue) may be done if lesions extend into the endocervical canal (Figure 40-15 ■). If the client becomes pregnant, it is important for her to discuss the cervical conization with her healthcare provider. As the pregnancy progresses, the cervix may dilate under pressure, and premature delivery may result. If the cancer has spread to surrounding organs, **pelvic exenteration** (surgical removal of the bowel, uterus, ovaries, fallopian tubes, vagina, and bladder) or hysterectomy may be needed. Depending on lymph node involvement, radiation therapy (including radium implants) or chemotherapy may be done. See more about cancer and its treatment in Chapter 45 ⚭ .

OVARIAN CANCER

Approximately 70% to 80% of ovarian tumors are benign. However, ovarian cancer is the second most common gynecologic cancer in women over 40 and is the most lethal of all female reproductive cancers. It may appear as epithelial tumors, germ cell tumors, or gonadal tumors. These tumors shed cells that spread the cancer to organs of the peritoneal cavity.

Manifestations

Ovarian cancer is difficult to diagnose because the client either is asymptomatic or experiences vague symptoms. These might include abdominal bloating, pelvic pressure, slight constipation, and increasing abdominal girth. Abnormal vaginal bleeding and dyspareunia may also develop. Some progress is being made in early detection. Box 40-7 ■ provides a list of early warning signs that may signal ovarian cancer.

BOX 40-7	SCREENING FOR OVARIAN CANCER

Research has determined that early-stage symptoms of ovarian cancer may be identifiable and could be used to establish a symptom index for that disease (Goff et al., 2007). Because this cancer is quite common in women over age 40 and is normally detected only when the disease is advanced, these early-stage warnings could have a profound effect on client outcome.

Teach women to report the following symptoms, especially if recurrent and of recent onset:

- Pelvic or abdominal pain
- Increased abdominal size or bloating
- Difficulty eating, or a feeling of fullness that is present more than 12 days a month and for less than a year

This set of symptoms was 57% sensitive for early disease and 80% sensitive for advanced ovarian cancer.

Risk factors for ovarian cancer include older age, early menarche, late menopause, history of infertility, treatment of infertility with Clomid (clomiphene), and a history of breast or ovarian cancer.

Once identified, the tumor may be palpable to the examiner and may be tender or nontender.

Diagnosis and Treatment

Diagnosis is made by transvaginal or abdominal ultrasound, or by CT scan. Laparoscopy (Figure 40-16 ■) may be used to reach a diagnosis. Tumor marker antigens, CA125, alpha-fetoprotein, and carcinoembryonic antigen may be tested.

Medical management includes unilateral oophorectomy or TAH with BSO. Chemotherapy or radiation may be used as palliative measures; at or after Stage 2 they are not curative. See more about cancer staging and treatment in Chapter 45 ⚭ .

ENDOMETRIOSIS

Endometriosis occurs when endometrial tissue grows outside the uterine cavity (Figure 40-17 ■). Although the exact cause is unknown, it is theorized that endometrial cells migrate to deeper uterine tissue (myometrium) during fetal development or are washed through the fallopian tubes during menstruation. Endometrial cells can also be picked up in the lymph vessels and transported throughout the body. Endometrial cells that are **ectopic** (outside) the uterus respond to cyclic hormone influence just as uterine endometrium does. The cyclic bleeding results in inflammation, scar tissue formation, adhesions, and occlusions. Endometriosis may lead to infertility.

No single symptom is diagnostic of endometriosis. Often the client will complain of dysmenorrhea with pelvic pain or premenstrual **dyspareunia** (painful intercourse).

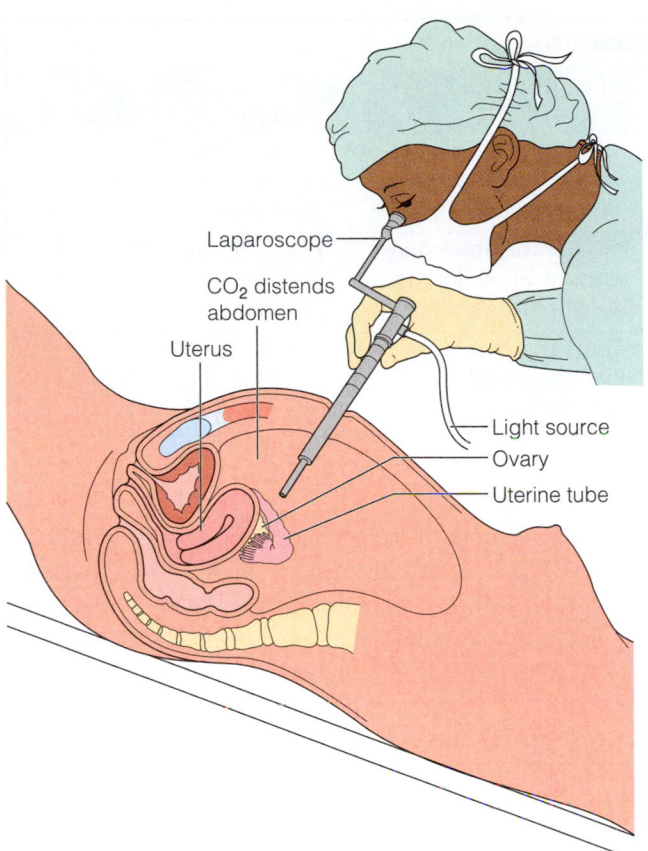

Figure 40-16. ■ Laparoscopy. A flexible, lighted instrument (laparoscope) is inserted through a small incision to visualize the abdominal and pelvic cavities.

Dysuria may indicate involvement of the urinary bladder. Premenstrual **tenesmus** (painful straining to defecate) and diarrhea may indicate colon involvement. Diagnosis is made by laparoscopic examination and biopsy of suspected tissue.

The goal of treatment is to preserve fertility for as long as possible. The woman who wants to have children is encouraged to become pregnant as soon as she can. Hormones may be prescribed to cause endometrial atrophy. Table 40-4 ■ identifies common medications used to treat endometriosis.

Surgical treatment may include endometrial obliteration with a laser or electrocautery via a laparoscope. If adequate symptom relief is not achieved, a hysterectomy with bilateral salpingo-oophorectomy may be required.

CANCER OF THE VULVA

Cancer of the vulva usually occurs after age 60. Vulvar cancers are epidermoid or squamous cell carcinomas found on the labia majora or minora or clitoris. Metastasis occurs by direct invasion or through the lymphatic system. Its incidence is associated with human papillomavirus (HPV), melanoma, and Paget's disease.

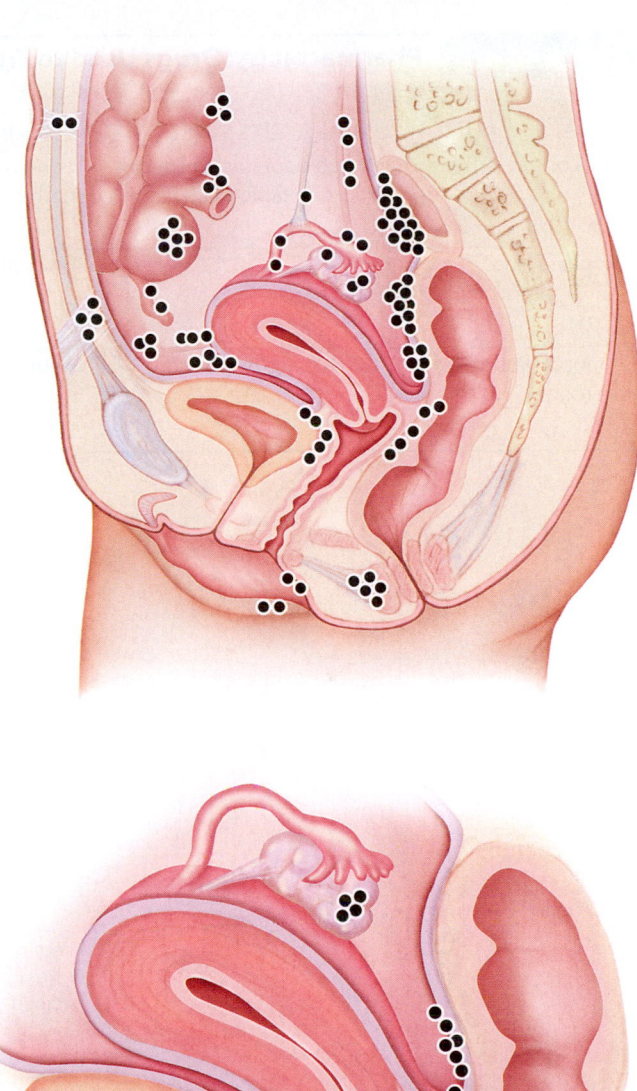

Figure 40-17. ■ Common sites of endometriosis.

Manifestations

Symptoms may not be present, or the client may report pruritus or the presence of a flat red or white lesion. These lesions are typically painless.

Diagnosis and Treatment

Diagnosis of vulvar cancer is based on the physical examination, a biopsy of the lesion, and various methods to determine metastasis. Laser surgery, cryosurgery, electrocautery, or a **vulvectomy** (surgical removal of the vulva, labia majora

TABLE 40-4	Pharmacology: Drugs Used to Treat Endometriosis			
DRUG	USUAL ROUTE/DOSE	CLASSIFICATION	SELECTED SIDE EFFECTS	DON'T GIVE IF (CALL HEALTHCARE PROVIDER IF)
Oral contraceptives	mg/tab depends on specific drug, one tablet daily	Contraceptive hormone	GI upset, depression, increased blood clotting, weight change	History of blood clotting disorders Pregnancy
Progesterone	Individual	Hormone	GI upset, depression, increased blood clotting, weight change	History of blood clotting disorders Pregnancy
Danozol (androgen hormone)	100–400 mg twice daily	Androgen hormone	Decreased breast size, decreased libido, emotional lability	Pregnancy

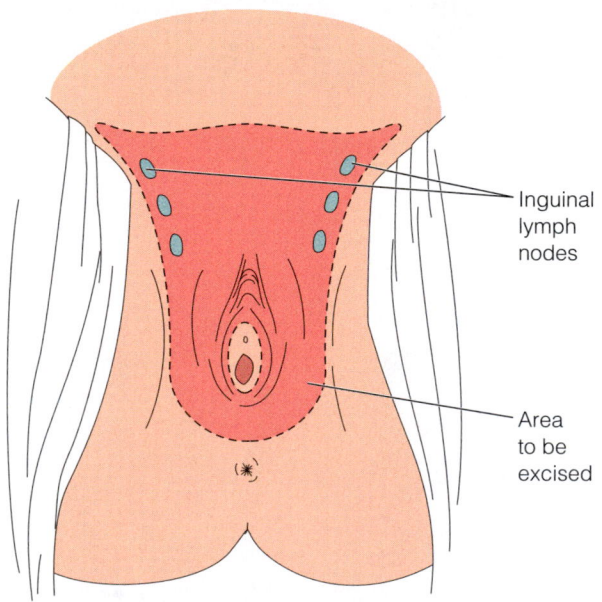

Inguinal lymph nodes

Area to be excised

Figure 40-18. ■ Vulvectomy for cancer of the vulva.

and minora, clitoris, and prepuce) may be indicated (Figure 40-18 ■). Chemotherapy and radiation may be used if metastasis has occurred. See more about cancer and its treatment in Chapter 45 ⬭.

Nursing Considerations

Provide nursing care as for clients with other reproductive cancers. Emotional support is an important aspect of nursing care, since body image may be profoundly affected.

NURSING CARE

PRIORITIZING NURSING CARE

When caring for clients with cancer of the female reproductive organs, focus your care on emotional support and management of symptoms. Be attentive to clients' complaints of pain, pressure, and menstrual irregularities. Emotional

needs of women with reproductive cancer are great. Be supportive and a willing listener to clients who are sorting through their feelings about surgical removal of female organs, end of reproductive function, as well as a diagnosis of cancer and the possibility of dying.

ASSESSING

Nursing management includes assessment of the client's past and present history, risk factors, and signs and symptoms. The client's understanding of her condition is critical and the nurse should assess the client's knowledge level.

DIAGNOSING, PLANNING, AND IMPLEMENTING

The nurse is able to identify many nursing diagnoses appropriate for the client diagnosed with a structural abnormality of the uterus or abnormal growths within the female reproductive system. Because nursing care is holistic, the nurse must concentrate on physical as well as emotional nursing diagnoses.

Physical nursing diagnoses include *Acute Pain* related to pressure secondary to tumors, uterine displacement, or growth of endometrial tissue outside of the uterus. The client may also experience *Urge Urinary Incontinence* related to uterine displacement. *Impaired Tissue Integrity* related to vulvar lesions or surgical wounds is appropriate for these disorders.

Emotional nursing diagnoses include *Powerlessness* related to client's inability to control her current health status. A client with these disorders may also have *Grieving* related to a medical diagnosis of cancer. Other emotional nursing diagnoses that may result are *Disturbed Body Image, Fear,* and *Ineffective Coping.*

Client goals in the planning stage of the nursing process include:

■ Achieve adequate pain relief.
■ Demonstrate a regular pattern of urinary elimination.

- Wounds and lesions will have evidence of healing.
- Demonstrate control over various aspects of healthcare regime.
- Express resolution of the grieving process.

To achieve these goals, the nurse provides various nursing interventions. Nursing interventions for clients with structural disorders and abnormal growths of the female reproductive system include patient teaching, assisting in screening, ensuring proper diagnosis and treatment, and reviewing risks for complications. The following nursing interventions with rationales are appropriate for most clients with these disorders. Other nursing interventions should also be considered in an effort to individualize nursing care.

- Encourage regular ambulation. *Ambulation facilitates expulsion of flatus.*
- Apply heat to abdomen or back. *Through dilation of the blood vessels, blood supply, and therefore, oxygen to the tissues is improved.*
- Encourage the use of Kegel exercises (see Chapter 54 🔗). *Kegel exercises improve the perineal musculature and assist the client in improving urinary continence.*
- Encourage increased hygiene. *Frequent cleansing and changing of perineal pads can assist the client in avoiding urinary tract infections.*
- Encourage a diet high in protein and vitamin C. *These nutrients encourage wound healing.*
- Teach the client to assess for improved wound healing. *Clients who learn what a healing wound looks like will be able to report difficulties and receive proper treatment.*
- Allow the client to participate in healthcare choices. *Giving women a choice in their healthcare will increase their perceived control over the situation.*
- Provide the client with an opportunity to express her grief in an unhurried situation. *Clients dealing with potential end-of-life issues need a safe environment in which to express their thoughts, fears, and concerns.*
- Refer client to a support group. *Established support groups provide clients companionship with individuals who have had similar experiences.*

EVALUATING

The nurse revises care until expected outcomes are achieved. The expected outcomes for a client with a menstrual disorder include:

- Pain levels diminish progressively.
- Episodes of urinary incontinence decrease.
- Wounds or lesions are intact, without purulent drainage, and dry.

- Client actively participates in healthcare decisions.
- Client shows adequate progression through the stages of grief.

Pelvic Floor Disorders

Relaxation or damage of the pelvic muscles may result in prolapse or displacement of pelvic organs, including the urinary bladder, uterus, and rectum. A **cystocele** develops when the ligaments supporting the urinary bladder are damaged allowing the bladder to prolapse into the vagina. A **rectocele** develops when the anterior rectal wall protrudes into the vagina. Uterine prolapse (see Figure 40-13E) develops when the ligaments supporting the uterus in the pelvic cavity are stretched or damaged, allowing the uterus to slip into the vagina. All three conditions are caused by stretching supporting ligaments, thinning of tissue with aging, and damage during vaginal birth.

Manifestations

Manifestations of prolapse of pelvic organs include stress incontinence, urgency, difficulty emptying the bladder, a heavy or dragging sensation in the pelvis, constipation, and dyspareunia. A woman may be able to feel or see the cervix or entire uterus protrude from the vagina, especially after bearing down or heavy lifting. Frequent bladder infections may develop. The woman may need to push up on the perineum or press against the back wall of the vagina to assist proper bowel alignment for defecation.

Treatment

Kegel exercises may be ordered to strengthen the pelvic muscles (see Chapter 54 🔗). Pelvic organ prolapse is often treated with surgery to shorten the muscle and supportive ligaments, and resuspend the pelvic organs in their natural position. In postmenopausal women, a hysterectomy is the preferred treatment for significant uterine prolapse. When surgery is contraindicated, the uterus and bladder may be supported with a vaginal pessary (device for holding the uterus in place). The pessary must be removed, cleaned, and reinserted at regular intervals.

Rape Trauma Syndrome

Rape is forced sexual intercourse that involves vaginal, anal, or oral penetration. The rape can be forced by physical or psychological coercion, and drug or alcohol ingestion may be used to decrease the woman's awareness of the situation.

The rapist can be a stranger, friend, or relative. **Incest** is sexual intercourse between close blood relatives and may or may not be consensual.

Sexual abuse affects the woman physically and mentally. Rape can cause trauma to the reproductive organs and lead to infection and scarring. Scarring may result in painful intercourse and may prevent future pregnancy. Following a rape, many women have a strong urge to shower and "wash away" all traces of the experience. Showering can actually destroy vital evidence the police will need to apprehend and prosecute the offender. It is, therefore, important for the woman to seek help from police and medical personnel prior to cleaning herself.

The psychological trauma is as great as or greater than the physical trauma. (See also Chapter 17 ⊂⊃ .) The woman may feel guilty that she allowed the sexual abuse to occur, that she might have done something to encourage the assailant, or that she could not defend herself. She may be afraid that sexual abuse will recur with the same person or another person. The woman may be asked to testify in court regarding the sexual abuse, which could open her past sexual relationships to public scrutiny. Following this emotional trauma, it may be difficult for her to develop trusting relationships and enjoy future sexual encounters.

A woman might present in the emergency department or clinic stating that she has been raped, or she might present with physical trauma suspicious of a violent sexual encounter. The nurse's responsibilities are to provide emotional support and assist in data collection. Most facilities have a "rape kit" containing specimen containers, comb, slides, and other supplies necessary to collect evidence. It is important that all evidence be collected and secured according to legal standards. Guidelines and procedures for collecting this evidence should be outlined in a facility's policy and procedure manual.

Before collecting data, the woman needs to sign an informed consent form (see Chapter 4 ⊂⊃ for legal responsibilities of the nurse). A detailed history is obtained using the woman's own words to describe the events. The caregiver should use a nonjudgmental approach and must avoid coaching or leading the woman. The collecting of physical evidence serves the purpose of:

- Confirming recent sexual contact.
- Showing that force or coercion was used.
- Identifying the assailant.
- Collaborating the woman's story.

The woman will be asked to remove all her clothing, and each item will be placed in a separate paper bag and labeled. Samples of stains and body fluids will be obtained for sperm analysis. The absence of sperm does not mean that a rape did not occur; the assailant could have used a condom or might not have ejaculated. Hair samples will be pulled from the woman's head and pubic area to compare with other hair found on her body. The pubic hair will be combed to check for loose hairs that may have been transferred from the assailant. Debris will be collected from under her fingernails to check for blood or tissue from the assailant. Photographs should be taken of any injuries. A colposcope with photographic capability can be used to photograph intravaginal injury. All evidence must be labeled, placed in a paper bag, and remain in the possession of a professional until it is turned over to the police.

Because the psychological trauma during a rape is so great, the woman should receive counseling immediately. Many areas have rape crisis centers and personnel trained to provide the psychological support and counseling required in this situation. The psychological response to rape can be described in a series of overlapping phases. The acute phase begins during the rape and can last for a few days or longer. The woman feels fear, shock, disbelief, powerlessness, or helplessness. She may feel angry, humiliated, and unclean. She may suppress her feelings or exhibit an outward response in the form of crying or being tense and restless. She may experience alterations in sleep patterns such as insomnia or nightmares.

Within a few weeks, the woman may appear calm and composed as though she has adjusted to the situation. Frequently, however, these are outward signs of denial. She may go about her daily activities and return to work or school. This resumption of routine is important for her to regain a sense of control over her life. She may seek some forms of self-protection such as installing extra locks on her doors, taking a self-defense course, or buying a weapon. These activities do not resolve the emotional trauma. Instead, they give the impression to her support system that she is "over it." The support system may then withdraw.

However, denial does not last long. She may become depressed and anxious. She may want to talk about the rape. She may develop phobias, especially to situations similar to those in which the rape occurred. For example, if she was attacked at night, she may fear leaving her home after dark. If the rape occurred in her home, she may fear returning to an empty house. If her attacker was a stranger, she may fear crowds. She may continue to have nightmares in which she relives the rape. She may replay the incident repeatedly until she finally resolves that the attack was out of her control. It is important for the nurse to be a good, nonjudgmental listener and to make appropriate referrals to the registered nurse, physician, or counselor.

MALE REPRODUCTIVE HEALTH ISSUES

Disorders of the Testes, Scrotum, and Penis

Two fairly common disorders of the testes, present at birth, are cryptorchidism and hydrocele. *Cryptorchidism* occurs when one or both of the testes do not descend into the scrotum prior to birth. This condition can be corrected surgically if the testes do not descend spontaneously after 1 year. The surgery is done prior to the age of 3 to preserve fertility. See Chapter 59 for further discussion of this childhood disorder.

Hydrocele (Figure 40-19 ■) occurs when fluid enters the scrotum. The fluid in the scrotum is a round, nontender mass. This condition may resolve spontaneously or surgical removal of fluid may be required.

Two disorders of the penis and urethra, also present at birth, are known as hypospadias and epispadias and are discussed in Chapter 59 .

TESTICULAR CANCER

Testicular cancer is the most common cancer in younger men, ages 15 to 35. It is seen most often in men with cryptorchidism. There is also a link between testicular cancer and men whose mothers took hormones during pregnancy.

Manifestations

Testicular cancer can be detected through self-exam (Box 40-8 ■ with Figure 40-20 ■), when thickened tissue or a lump is felt. It is very important that men in this age group be taught to perform self-exam because the earlier the diagnosis is made, the more positive the outcome.

Diagnosis and Treatment

This type of cancer is diagnosed using ultrasound after a lump or thickening is found. Elevated serum acid or alkaline phosphatase is found with testicular cancer. Biopsy is not done because it increases the chance for the cancer to spread.

Testicular cancer is treated surgically, with the removal of the testis, epididymis, and spermatic cord. Nearby lymph

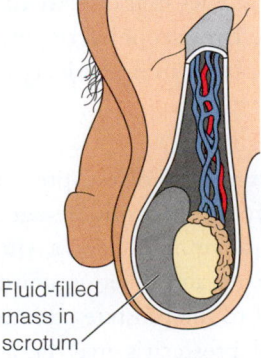

Figure 40-19. ■ Hydrocele.

Fluid-filled mass in scrotum

BOX 40-8	CLIENT TEACHING

Testicular Self-Examination

- Examine your testicles during or just after a warm shower or bath. Soap on your hands and scrotum allows easy manipulation of tissue.
- Gently roll each testicle between your thumb and fingers. The testicles normally feel smooth, rounded, walnut sized, and freely movable.

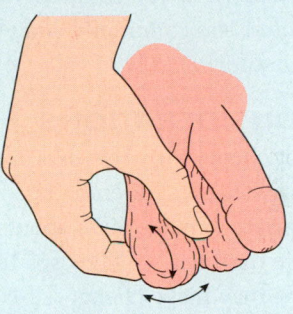

Figure 40-20. ■

- If one testicle is significantly larger than the other, or if you feel any hard lumps, contact your healthcare provider immediately.
- Examine your testicles on the same day of each month (e.g., the first day of the month) to help you remember.

Source: Burke, K. M., LeMone, P., Mohn-Brown, E. L. *Medical surgical nursing care* (2nd ed.). (2007). Upper Saddle River, NJ: Prentice Hall. P. 828, Box 34-8.

---

nodes are tested for cancer and removed if indicated. Chemotherapy may be prescribed after surgical treatment. (See Chapter 45 for more information about caring for clients with cancer.)

ERECTILE DYSFUNCTION

Erectile dysfunction, or impotence, can have several causes. The cause is determined before treatment is prescribed. Some antihypertensive, antidepressant, and cardiac medications may have side effects of erectile dysfunction. Chronic diseases such as diabetes mellitus, chronic obstructive pulmonary disease, and cardiac disease can affect erectile function.

Treatment

Two newer oral medications are available to treat erectile dysfunction. They work by allowing the smooth muscle in the penis to relax, increasing blood flow into the erectile tissue during sexual stimulation. Sildenafil citrate (Viagra) was the first of the medications on the market. It is prescribed in 50-mg doses (25 mg for older men), to be taken approximately 1 hour before engaging in sexual activity. An even newer oral medication is vardenafil hydrochloride (Levitra), which is prescribed in 2.5-, 5-, 10-, and 20-mg dosages. It can be taken several hours before engaging in sexual activity, but should be taken no more than one time per day. Contraindications for both of these oral medications include mixing them with nitrates or alpha-blockers (certain types of antihypertensives). Both can cause severe hypotension as a side effect.

Alprostadil is an injectable medication used for erectile dysfunction. It is injected at the base of the penis or inserted into the penis as pellets. Because this medication acts locally, it does not absorb into the bloodstream as much as oral medications and so has fewer side effects.

Penile implants can also be used to treat erectile dysfunction. These are usually in the form of vacuum devices or pumps, but are used less commonly since oral medications have become available.

NURSING CONSIDERATIONS

When you care for clients with disorders of the penis or testicles, be very sensitive to possible embarrassment to the client. It is never appropriate to make jokes about medications prescribed for erectile dysfunction. Hypospadias and epispadias are anomalies that may make clients self-conscious. Be very professional when dealing with these clients and avoid making comments that could embarrass them.

Prostate Disorders

BENIGN PROSTATIC HYPERTROPHY

The prostate gland may enlarge beginning around age 50. The enlargement is benign (noncancerous) and gradually causes obstruction of urine flow. The urethra is narrowed, causing urinary retention (Figure 40-21 ■). Because the bladder does not empty completely, urine can back up into the kidney, causing hydronephrosis.

Manifestations

Signs and symptoms of benign prostatic hypertrophy (BPH) include urinary pattern changes, difficulty in starting urinary stream, and decreasing urine force. The client

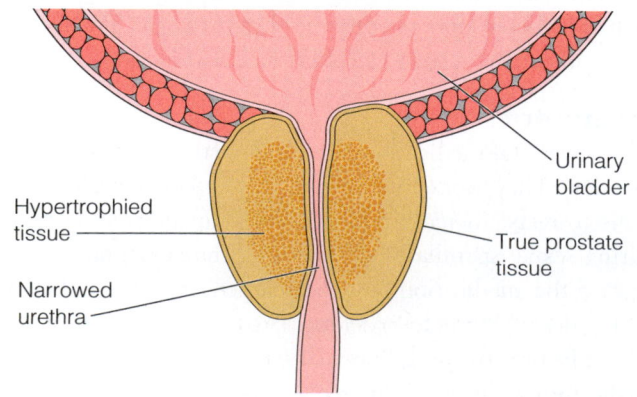

Hypertrophied tissue

Narrowed urethra

Urinary bladder

True prostate tissue

Figure 40-21. ■ Benign prostatic hyperplasia.

may feel that the bladder does not empty fully. Leaking, dribbling, and incontinence of urine may become a problem as the disease progresses. Other possible symptoms include urgency, **dysuria** (pain on urination), **hematuria** (blood in the urine), and **nocturia** (excessive nighttime urination).

Diagnosis and Treatment

A laboratory test for prostate-specific antigen (PSA) is done. An elevated PSA is considered indicative of prostate cancer. Other blood work such as BUN and serum creatinine may be ordered. The physician assesses the prostate gland for enlargement by performing a digital rectal examination (DRE). Other diagnostic tests include a urodynamic flow study to determine bladder function, ultrasound, biopsy, and cystoscopy.

Medical treatment is initiated when the symptoms cause discomfort. Medications are ordered to relax the smooth muscles of the prostate and bladder sphincter to increase urine flow. Finasteride (Proscar) blocks the secretion of testosterone, which is believed to increase hypertrophy. An herbal therapy is thought to have a similar action as Proscar.

Surgical treatment for BPH is the removal of the prostate tissue that is compressing the urethra. The most common procedure is transurethral resection of the prostate (TURP) (Figure 40-22 ■). In this procedure, a resectoscope inserted into the urethra removes sections of the prostate. The client returns from the recovery room with an indwelling three-way catheter that has a port for urinary drainage, an irrigating port (to flush the surgical site), and the balloon port. Transurethral incision of the prostate (TUIP) is a procedure in which incisions are made into the gland to relieve the obstruction.

Transurethral ultrasound guided laser-induced prostatectomy is an alternate procedure that may be used. In this procedure, laser incisions are made into the prostate gland. A suprapubic, retropubic, or perineal resection can also be done to access the prostate gland and remove the obstruction. These procedures involve abdominal incisions or incisions into the perineal area for gland removal.

A nonsurgical treatment, called transurethral microwave antenna (TUMA), applies heat directly to the prostate gland to help destroy the hypertrophied tissue. Prostatic balloons and stents may be placed to ease urinary obstruction.

PROSTATITIS

Prostatitis is inflammation of the prostate gland. It commonly occurs in young and middle-aged men. Prostatitis can be an acute inflammation or a chronic nonbacterial disease. *Escherichia coli* and other organisms that ascend the urethra and spread to the prostate often cause acute prostatitis. Nonbacterial prostatitis may be a result of viruses, chlamydiae, mycoplasmas, or an unknown cause. It may

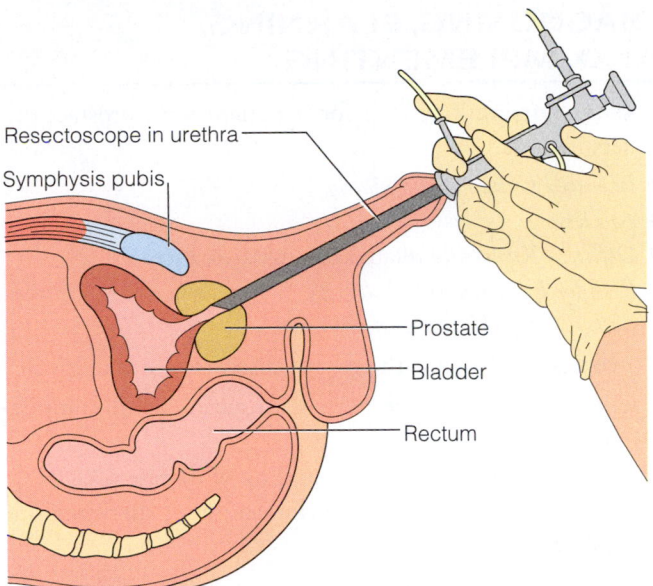

A Transurethral resection of the prostate

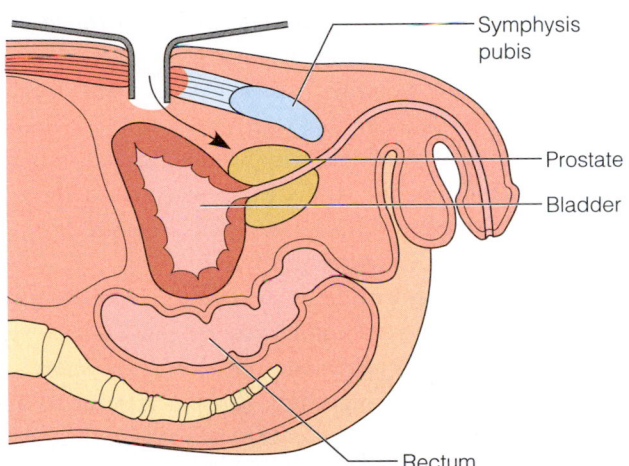

B Retropubic prostatectomy

Figure 40-22. ■ **A.** In a transurethral resection of the prostate (TURP), a resectoscope is inserted through the urethra to remove excess prostate tissue. **B.** In a retropubic prostatectomy, prostate tissue is removed through an abdominal incision.

also be caused by an autoimmune disease or a sexually transmitted infection.

Manifestations

Signs and symptoms of prostatitis include fever, chills, frequency, and nocturia. The client complains of back pain, dysuria, urgency, and obstruction. Pain after ejaculation may also occur.

Diagnosis and Treatment

Diagnostic tests for prostatitis include CBC and urinalysis. Urine cultures are done to determine the causative organism. Prostatic secretions are also tested. DRE is performed.

Prostatitis caused by bacteria is treated with antibiotics. For severe infections, the treatment can last from weeks to months. Nonbacterial prostatitis is treated symptomatically. To eliminate prostate gland congestion, frequent ejaculation is suggested. Anti-inflammatory medications are ordered for pain. Anticholinergic medications may be given to reduce voiding difficulties. Stool softeners and sitz baths may be ordered to decrease pain and irritation caused by urination and defecation.

PROSTATE CANCER

Prostate cancer is the second leading cause of death after lung cancer. Factors that contribute to the development of prostate cancer are age, family history, high-fat diet, occupational chemical exposure, and increased testosterone levels. There is a high incidence of prostate cancer among African American men (Box 40-9 ■). Early diagnosis and intervention increase survival rates. Prostate tumors are typically adenocarcinomas that enlarge and then compress the urethra, causing voiding difficulties. Prostate cancer may spread to the seminal vesicles, bladder, pelvic lymph nodes, pelvic bones, spinal column, liver, and lungs. Cancer and its treatment are discussed in Chapter 45 ⬭ .

Manifestations

Initially the client may be asymptomatic or have vague symptoms. As the disease progresses, signs of urinary obstruction such as dysuria, hesitancy, frequency, and nocturia develop. During DRE, the physician finds a hardened prostate gland. The client may complain of bone pain, backaches, or bowel and bladder problems.

Diagnosis and Treatment

Men aged 50 and older should have annual physical exams to help detect and diagnose prostate cancer. DRE and PSA are used as screening tools. Ultrasound, needle biopsy, bone scan, CT scan, and MRI are performed to diagnose and identify metastasis.

BOX 40-9	CULTURAL PULSE POINTS

Urinary or Male Reproductive System Disorders
African American males have a higher incidence of prostate cancer than any other race. They are also more likely to die from prostate cancer. Their mortality rate is more than double that of any other racial or ethnic group. Education about prevention and screening procedures is particularly important in the African American community, especially with young adult males. This age group does not routinely see a healthcare provider unless ill or injured.

Because of the high incidence of prostate cancer, it is recommended that all African American males have a yearly digital rectal examination and a prostate-specific antigen screening after the age of 40.

Treatment for prostate cancer is determined by biopsy and cytology. Hormone therapy is prescribed to inhibit cancer growth. To reduce testosterone levels, which promote prostate cancer growth, a bilateral orchiectomy (removal of the testes) may be performed. Prostatectomy is the surgical removal of the prostate gland (simple prostatectomy). A radical prostatectomy removes the prostate, seminal vesicles, and a section of the bladder neck. Side effects of the surgery include urinary incontinence and impotence. Radiation or radioactive seed implantation may be used. Cryosurgery, an alternative treatment, destroys the prostate by freezing and thawing tissue. Complications of cryosurgery may include bladder outlet injury, incontinence, impotence, and rectal impairment.

NURSING CARE

PRIORITIZING NURSING CARE

When caring for clients with prostate disorders, focus your interventions on maintaining urine output, preventing skin breakdown, managing pain, and preserving the client's dignity. For clients who have had prostate surgery (TURP), frequently assess the color and clarity of the output from the three-way catheter. Flush the tubing with increased irrigation fluid whenever the urine looks bloody or clots are present. Pink-colored urine is normal for the first 24 to 48 hours after surgery. Use aseptic technique when changing irrigation bags. Empty the urinary drainage bag frequently; it fills quickly with irrigation fluid. Record all output on the I&O sheet. Record the amount of irrigation fluid used each shift so that it can be subtracted from the output.

Give medication to manage pain from surgery or prostatitis, and evaluate its effectiveness. Urinary incontinence or dribbling may be a problem after prostate surgery. Be matter of fact when assisting clients who have had accidents. Be kind and supportive, so the client does not feel embarrassed or ashamed. Assess skin frequently for reddened or open areas. Wash the area thoroughly with gentle soap or periwash and water to prevent skin breakdown due to urine contact.

ASSESSING

The LPN/LVN in collaboration with the RN records and documents the client's signs and symptoms, which can include dysuria, urinary force, starting urine stream, and frequency. It is essential to monitor urine output, color, character, and amount. Determine the severity of incontinence, if present, and the effect on the client's lifestyle.

DIAGNOSING, PLANNING, AND IMPLEMENTING

Possible nursing diagnoses for the client with prostate disorders include:

- *Impaired Urinary Elimination*
- *Anxiety*
- *Deficient Knowledge* related to prostate cancer
- *Risk for Impaired Skin Integrity*
- *Risk for Urge Urinary Incontinence*

Outcomes for clients with prostate disorders are as follows:

- Client will experience normal urination with complete emptying of the bladder.
- Client will verbalize understanding of disease process.
- Client will be continent of urine and not experience skin breakdown.

The following interventions apply to care of clients with prostate disorders:

- Encourage fluid intake up to 2 to 3 liters per day if not contraindicated for the client. *This amount of liquid helps flush out the genitourinary system.*
- Assess for fluid volume excess. *Excess could indicate hyponatremia.*
- Observe for fluid retention, weight gain, intake and output; restrict fluids and assess pulmonary status. *Clients with prostate problems could go into fluid volume excess with cardiac and respiratory compromise.*
- Assess pain level and medicate as ordered. Nonpharmacologic measures to increase comfort are taught. *The client must have pain controlled to be able to understand and process instruction.*
- Reinforce instruction regarding disease, treatment, and follow-up care. *Clients who understand instructions and the reasons for them are more likely to comply with them.*
- Be sensitive to sexual concerns of the client and provide referrals as needed. *Clients may be embarrassed to talk about these concerns.*
- Encourage the client to verbalize feelings and promote discussion with spouse and physician. *Communication regarding sexual or urinary problems helps all those involved be aware of the issues and take steps to solve them.*

For Clients with BPH

- Administer routine postoperative care. Monitor the three-way catheter irrigating solution. *This will ensure appropriate use and function.*
- Subtract the inflow from the client's urinary output. *Irrigation fluid cannot be counted as urine output, but is contained in the catheter drainage bag.*
- Observe for blood clots, frank bleeding, and diminishing urine output postoperatively. *These can indicate blockage or potential blockage of the three-way catheter. Frank bleeding may indicate lack of clotting at the surgical site.*

- Medicate as ordered if the client complains of bladder spasms. *Medications relieve discomfort and allow adequate irrigation.*
- Maintain the patency of the catheter and tubing. *This allows for adequate irrigation.*
- Monitor for transurethral syndrome or fluid volume excess. *The large amount of irrigating fluid being used could lead to electrolyte imbalance.*
- Increase fluid intake unless contraindicated. *Increased fluids help flush the wound site.*

For Clients with Urinary Incontinence

- Instruct in the use of Kegel exercises. *Strengthening the tone of muscles of the pelvic floor can increase urine retention.*

- Increase fluid intake during the daytime hours and restrict it at night. *This helps prevent incontinence while sleeping.*
- Suggest the use of absorbent pads to control wetness. *This measure aids self-esteem.*

EVALUATING

Assessing the effect of nursing interventions for the client with prostate disorders includes the accuracy of data collection, goal setting, and nursing care implementation. Data assessed include urine output, urine character, urgency, and frequency. Evaluate the client's knowledge of disease, treatment, and surgical interventions.

FAMILY PLANNING ISSUES

Infections

Infections of the reproductive system can impair a person's ability to conceive. Most reproductive infections are sexually transmitted, and are discussed in Chapter 41 ⊙⊙.

CANDIDIASIS

Candidiasis (monilia or yeast infection) is a common organism that causes vaginitis. Characteristics of a yeast infection are thick white patches resembling cottage cheese adhering to the cervix, vaginal wall, and labia. There is intense itching of the vulva and vagina. The mucous membrane is red and inflamed. When a specimen is viewed under the microscope, *hyphae* (threadlike filaments) and spores may be seen. *Candida* can also grow on the foreskin, glans, and outer skin of the penis.

Treatment includes medicated creams, vaginal tablets, or suppositories. The sexual partner should be treated. The client should be taught to wear cotton, not synthetic underpants, because synthetic underclothes do not "breathe" and so create an environment where microorganisms can multiply rapidly.

TOXIC SHOCK SYNDROME

Toxic shock syndrome (TSS) is a condition in women caused by a bacterial toxin (usually *Staphylococcus aureus*) entering the bloodstream. The cause is unknown. However, about 70% of cases are associated with menstruation and infrequent change of tampons. Conditions other than tampon use related to TSS include infected surgical wounds, subcutaneous abscesses, and improper use of a diaphragm. TSS has a high mortality rate.

Manifestations

Signs and symptoms include sudden fever of greater than 102°F (38.8°C), vomiting, and diarrhea leading to hypotension and shock within 72 hours of onset. A rash of the trunk may develop 1 to 2 weeks after onset, with desquamation (sloughing) of the palms and soles. There may be sore throat, headache, or myalgia.

Diagnosis and Treatment

Diagnostic testing includes blood, urine, throat, vaginal, cervical, and cerebrospinal fluid cultures. Testing is done to rule out tick-borne diseases, meningitis, Epstein-Barr, or coxsackievirus. Routine lab work is also done, including the CBC, electrolytes, BUN, and creatinine.

Medical management includes IV therapy with fluid replacement. Dopamine may be used to maintain blood pressures. Antibiotics, usually the cephalosporins, are administered. Antipyretics may be ordered for fever.

PELVIC INFLAMMATORY DISEASE

Pelvic inflammatory disease (PID) is an infection usually involving the fallopian tubes, ovaries, cervix, uterus, and peritoneum. A few of the causative agents are *Neisseria gonorrhoeae, Chlamydia trachomatis*, or streptococci. PID often begins as a cervical infection that spreads to the endometrium, fallopian tubes, and peritoneal cavity. Risk factors include multiple sex partners and early sexual activity, or rarely IUD, therapeutic abortions, cesarean sections, and hysterosalpingograms.

Manifestations

PID is characterized by pain in the pelvic area, fever, purulent cervical discharge, vaginal bleeding or spotting, nausea, vomiting, dysuria, and urinary frequency.

Diagnosis and Treatment

Diagnosis is made by clinical exam, endocervical or cervical culture, or laparoscopy. WBCs will be elevated and sedimentation rate will be elevated.

Medical management includes a combination of antibiotics (tetracycline, penicillin, quinolones, or cephalosporins) usually IV for 24 hours then orally. The client may be on bed rest for 1 to 3 days. Surgical management may be needed if the client has an abscess, adhesions, or damage to the fallopian tubes. PID greatly increases the client's risk of ectopic pregnancy (due to scarring of the fallopian tubes) or infertility in the future.

NURSING CARE

PRIORITIZING NURSING CARE

When caring for clients with infections of the reproductive tract, focus your care on managing symptoms and client teaching. Ensure that pain management is a priority, especially for clients with PID. Clients with toxic shock syndrome have a life-threatening condition and all nursing care is focused on reversing shock and stabilizing the client. Instruct clients about potential causes of reproductive infections and how to minimize their own risk. Teach clients to avoid sexual activities that put them at risk for PID. Teach clients about predisposing factors for the development of TSS and how to avoid them. Encourage clients to seek medical attention when pelvic pain, vaginal discharge, and fever are present.

ASSESSING

A critical element of maintaining and restoring client health is an adequate assessment. The nurse is responsible for collecting the health history to assist in determining the cause and symptoms related to infections of the female reproductive system.

DIAGNOSING, PLANNING, AND IMPLEMENTING

The nurse is able to identify many nursing diagnoses appropriate for the client diagnosed with an infection of the reproductive system. Because nursing care is holistic, the nurse must concentrate on physical as well as emotional nursing diagnoses.

Physical nursing diagnoses include *Risk for Injury* related to complications associated with PID or TSS, *Deficient Knowledge* related to understanding or management of the infection, *Impaired Tissue Integrity* related to vaginal discharge, and *Ineffective Sexuality Patterns* related to effects of the infection and the required treatment.

Emotional nursing diagnoses include *Anxiety* related to long-term effects of the infection, *Disturbed Body Image* related to vaginal discharge, and *Impaired Social Interaction* related to required periods of abstinence during treatment.

Client goals in the planning stage of the nursing process include:

- Life-threatening complications will be avoided.
- Knowledge of treatment and infectious process will be communicated properly.
- Tissue integrity will be restored.

- Healthy sexual patterns will be verbalized.
- Anxiety levels will be reduced.
- Positive body image will be restored.
- Increased incidences of social interactions will be reported.

To achieve these goals, the nurse provides various nursing interventions. Nursing interventions for clients with an infection of the reproductive system include client teaching, assisting in screening, ensuring proper diagnosis and treatment, and reviewing risks for complications. The following nursing interventions with rationales are appropriate for most clients with an infection of the reproductive system. Other nursing interventions should also be considered in an effort to individualize nursing care.

- Administer antibiotic therapy as ordered. *For proper treatment and cure of the infection, antibiotics need to be administered precisely.*
- Explain transmission methods of the infection, prevention methods, and the treatment regime. *Understanding these can improve treatment compliance and prevent further infections.*
- Teach the client characteristics of a healing wound, including color, drainage, and edema. *Encouraging self-assessment of the wound will enhance compliance.*
- Discuss safe sexual practice. *Serves to assist the client in avoiding future infections.*
- Ensure that the client understands that these infections of the reproductive system can be treated effectively. *Knowledge of effective treatment can decrease a client's worry and fears.*
- Communicate with the client in a nonjudgmental manner, respecting privacy and confidentiality. *Therapeutic communication allows the client to trust the nurse and discuss issues that may be of concern.*

EVALUATING

The nurse revises care until expected outcomes are achieved. The expected outcomes for a client with an infection of the reproductive system include:

- Life-threatening complications are avoided.
- Knowledge of treatment and infectious process is communicated effectively.
- Tissue integrity is restored.
- Healthy sexual patterns are verbalized.
- Anxiety levels are reduced.
- Positive body image is restored.
- Increased incidences of social interactions are reported.

Contraception

Contraception is the prevention of pregnancy. Although several methods are addressed here, it is important to encourage teens and others to discuss methods of contraception with their healthcare provider (Figure 40-23 ■). Some methods

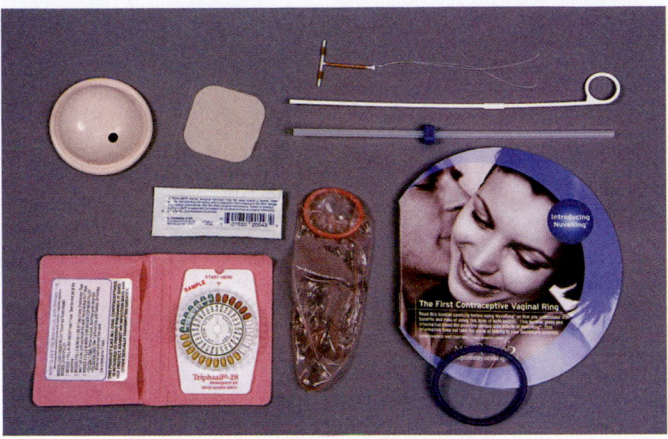

Figure 40-23. ■ Methods of contraception.

may not be recommended with certain physical disorders. Table 40-5 ■ lists facts about conception and contraception.

Male clients have limited choices when it comes to contraception. Condoms are used to help prevent the transmission of sexually transmitted infections. They can be effective for contraceptive purposes if maintained (not exposed to high heat or to light; not used if old or cracked) and if applied according to proper guidelines. Condoms must be used carefully and appropriately to provide protection against STIs. Research is ongoing for more temporary contraceptive choices for men.

FERTILITY AWARENESS

Fertility awareness is contraception planning based on the assumption that ovulation occurs at the same time each month. By collecting data regarding physical changes that take place throughout the menstrual cycle, the time of ovulation can be identified. The couple then abstains from intercourse or uses other methods of contraception during ovulation. Objective data to identify ovulation include a **basal body temperature** taken every morning before activity and assessment of cervical mucus (*spinnbarkeit*) (Figure 40-24 ■). Subjective data include increased libido, bloating, and breast changes. Some women may also experience *mittelschmerz* (abdominal pain with ovulation). Once the data are collected for several months, patterns can be identified. Abstinence is generally recommended for several days prior to ovulation and until 3 days after ovulation. The calendar method is the least effective method of contraception.

SPERMICIDES

Spermicides are chemicals in the form of creams, foams, jellies, or suppositories that are inserted into the vagina prior to sexual intercourse. They destroy the sperm or prevent sperm mobility. The chemical must be inserted deep in the vagina and come in contact with the cervix. Suppositories may take up to 30 minutes to dissolve, and they will not offer protection until then. The spermicide must be inserted before each ejaculation.

TABLE 40-5	Facts about Conception and Contraception	
DATE	**EVENT**	**DESCRIPTION**
1500 BC	First record of vaginal contraception	One of the earliest mentions of contraceptive vaginal suppositories appears in the Ebers Medical Papyrus. The guide suggests that a fiber tampon moistened with an herbal mixture of acacia, dates, colocynth, and honey would prevent pregnancy. The fermentation of this mixture can result in the production of lactic acid, which today is recognized as a spermicide.
16th century	Male condom	The condom was first created out of sheep intestines by a physician in the court of King Charles II of England. The condom became widely used as a birth control device after the vulcanization of rubber in 1844.
1838	Barrier methods of contraception—female; diaphragm and cervical cap	The modern diaphragm was invented by a German physician. The cervical cap was invented in 1860, but it did not receive the approval of the U.S. Food and Drug Administration for use in the United States until the late 1980s, despite its widespread use in Europe.
1921	Margaret Sanger	An advocate for birth control in the United States, she founded the American Birth Control League, which became the Planned Parenthood Federation of America in 1942.
1960	Gregory Pincus	Developed an oral contraceptive.
1965	Birth control pills or oral contraceptives	First approved for use in the United States. These early pills, known as combination pills, contained both estrogen and progestin (a synthetic form of progesterone). In 1973, progestin-only pills also became available.
1980s	Artificial insemination	Initiated as a means of fertilization. Many couples now resort to various methods of *in vitro* fertilization ("test tube" babies) or transplantation of fertilized ova from one womb to another.

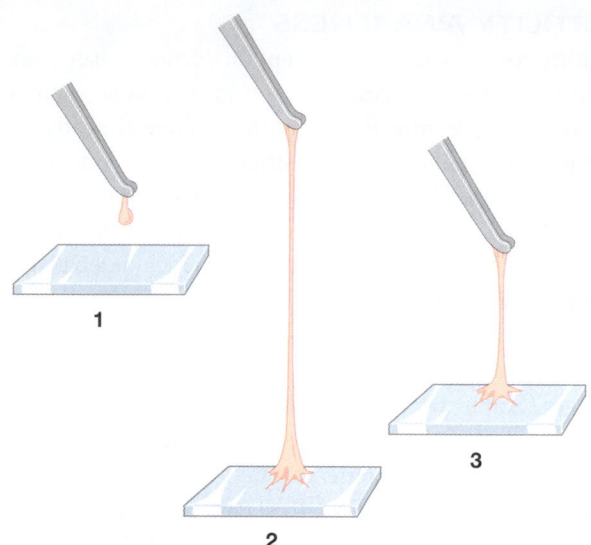

Figure 40-24. ■ *Spinnbarkeit,* a density and elasticity of vaginal secretions that correlates with ovulation. **1.** Three days before ovulation. **2.** Day of ovulation. **3.** Day after ovulation.

clinical ALERT

It is important to teach clients that spermicides do not prevent STIs.

BARRIERS

Barriers, including male and female condoms, vaginal diaphragms, and cervical caps, are devices placed in the vagina or over the penis to prevent sperm from entering the cervix. To be effective, these devices must be correctly applied. The use of spermicide increases their effectiveness.

The male condom is applied to the erect penis before contact with the vulva or vagina. A small space must be available at the end of the condom to contain the ejaculate. After ejaculation, the man should withdraw the penis from the vagina while it is still erect and hold the rim of the condom to prevent spillage. Figure 40-25 ■ illustrates correct male condom use.

The female condom contains a ring at the closed end. It is inserted into the vagina so the ring rests around the cervix. The open end extends from the vagina and partially covers the vulva. The female condom can be inserted up to 8 hours prior to intercourse. A fresh condom must be used with each sexual episode. Figure 40-26 ■ illustrates application of a female condom.

The vaginal diaphragm consists of a metal ring covered with rubber. When inserted high in the vagina, the rubber covers the cervix (see Figure 40-23). The cervical cap is a similar device: a small ring covered with rubber that fits over the cervix. Both the vaginal diaphragm and cervical cap are most effective when spermicide is applied to the inner surface and rim before being placed next to

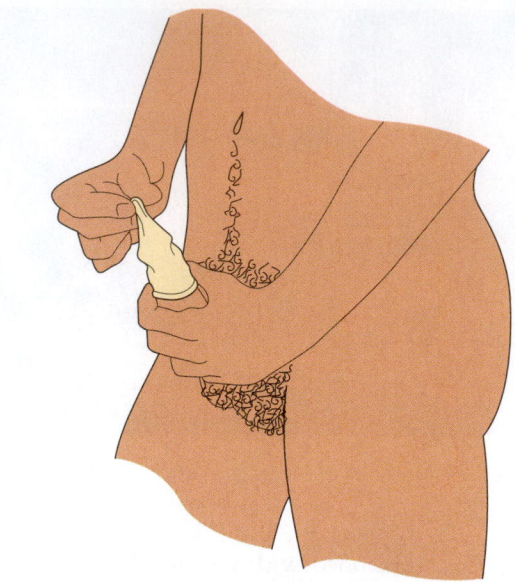

Figure 40-25. ■ Method for applying a male condom.

the cervix. The devices should be left in place for 6 hours after intercourse in order to ensure that sperm do not enter the cervix. If intercourse is desired again within 6 hours, the diaphragm or cervical cap should remain in place and another method of contraception should also be used.

INTRAUTERINE DEVICE

The **intrauterine device (IUD)** is a small T-shaped piece of metal covered with copper or levonorgestrel (see Figure 40-23). The exact mechanism of action of an IUD is unclear. It is believed that the copper or levonorgestrel either kills the sperm or alters its motility to prevent conception. The IUD also disrupts the normal turbulence inside the uterus and may prevent implantation of the fertilized egg. The IUD is inserted into the uterus by a qualified health professional so that a string attached to the lower end of the "T" protrudes from the cervix. The woman is instructed to feel the string once a week for the first month and then after each menses to be sure it is in the proper position. If she develops signs of infection or pregnancy, she should consult her healthcare provider immediately. In case of pregnancy, the IUD is generally removed, but its removal could cause a spontaneous abortion.

HORMONAL CONTRACEPTIVES

Hormonal contraceptives are usually a combination of estrogen and progestin. They may be supplied in oral pill form taken once a day for 21 days (followed by 7 days "off"), a dermal patch applied weekly (see Figure 40-23), or an intramuscular injection given every 3 months. Women who smoke or who have a history of clotting disorders, liver disease, hyperlipidemia, hypertension, or diabetes should not

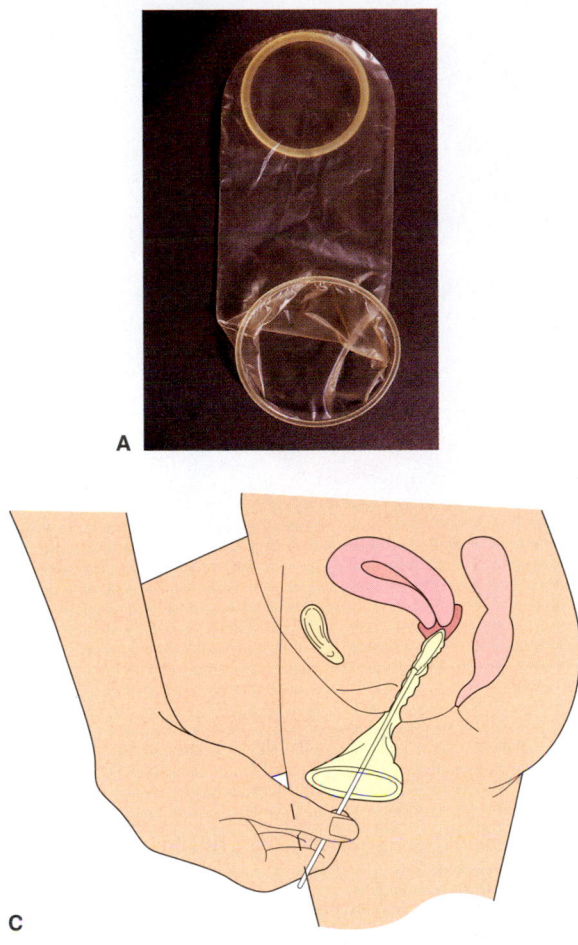

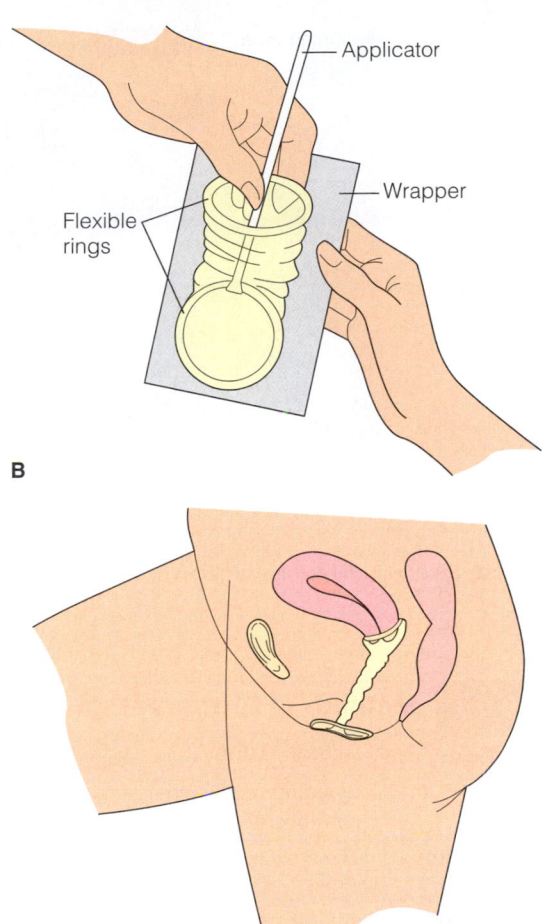

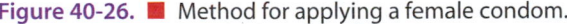

Figure 40-26. ■ Method for applying a female condom.

take oral contraceptives. For further information, please refer to a pharmacology text.

In August 2006, the Food and Drug Administration approved Plan B, an *emergency contraceptive* formulation of progestin (levonorgestrel). Available over the counter to 18-year-olds and by prescription to girls 17 and younger, the drug acts by delaying ovulation and perhaps preventing fertilization and implantation. (It is not effective if an embryo is already implanted; the pregnancy would continue.) One dose of 0.75 mg is taken as soon as possible after unprotected vaginal intercourse, with a second dose of 0.75 mg taken 12 hours later (FDA, 2006). Although it was dubbed the "morning-after" pill, it is effective up to 72 hours after intercourse. As with all hormonal contraceptives, Plan B does not provide protection against STIs.

SURGICAL STERILIZATION

Surgical sterilization—**tubal ligation** or **vasectomy**—is the tying and cutting of the fallopian tubes or vas deferens (Figure 40-27 ■). In rare instances, the procedure can be reversed. However, the couple should understand that the procedure is usually permanent. Following a vasectomy, it

might take six or more ejaculations to clear the vas deferens of sperm. The couple must use other methods of birth control until negative sperm counts are obtained.

A tubal ligation might be performed at the time of a cesarean section delivery, through a laparoscopy following delivery or at another time. The woman is encouraged to abstain from sexual intercourse until her healing is complete. She can then engage in unprotected intercourse.

A vasectomy may be performed to prevent conception. Although the procedure can sometimes be surgically reversed, it is considered permanent and should be undertaken with that understanding. After vasectomy, follow-up sperm counts are extremely important to ensure that sterility has occurred. Another method of contraception should be used until sterilization is confirmed. Table 40-6 ■ provides a review of contraceptive methods, with effectiveness ratings from the Food and Drug Administration.

Infertility Issues

Infertility is the inability to achieve pregnancy after 1 year or more of unprotected intercourse. There are several causes of infertility. The simplest and least invasive diagnostic

(*Text continues on p.1163.*)

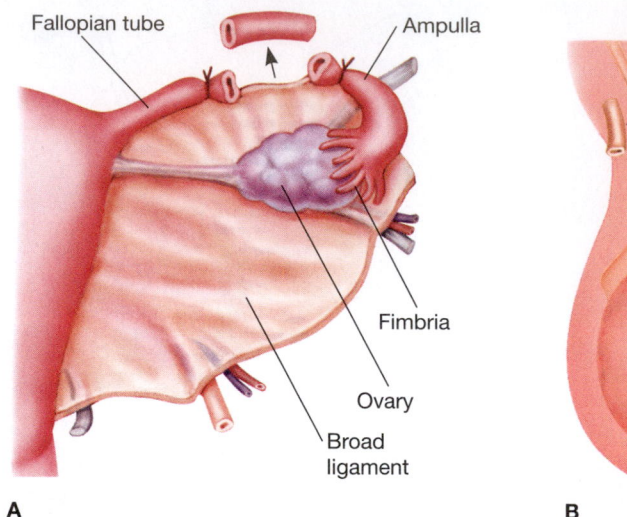
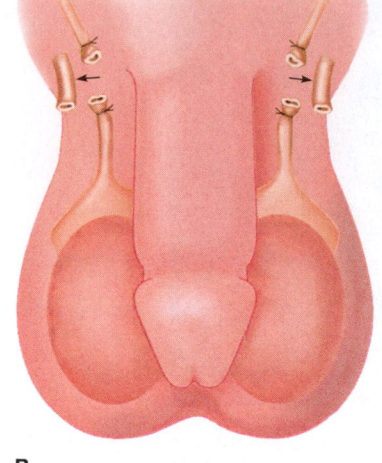

Figure 40-27. ■ Sterilization by tubal ligation or vasectomy.

TABLE 40-6	Methods of Contraception	
METHOD	**DESCRIPTION**	**NURSING MEASURES**
Abstinence	Avoiding sexual intercourse. Abstinence is the only contraceptive method that is 100% effective.	■ Provide support.
Withdrawal or coitus interruptus	The male must withdraw the penis from the vagina prior to ejaculation. Effectiveness is variable and unreliable.	■ Teach client that preejaculatory fluid may contain sperm. ■ Teach client that this method does not provide protection from sexually transmitted infections (STIs).
Natural family planning or fertility awareness, calendar method, or rhythm method	Based on the assumption that fertility rates are higher during ovulation, which occurs 14 days ±2 days before start of the last menstrual period. Abstinence during the fertile period of a woman's menstrual cycle. Effectiveness is variable with 25% pregnancy rate.	■ Teach the client proper recording methods of the menstrual cycle. ■ Teach the client to recognize fertile periods. ■ Teach the importance of abstinence during this time frame.
Ovulation detection methods including basal body temperature (BBT), cervical mucus method (Billings' method), symptothermal method, and predictor tests for ovulation	Women take their temperature every morning for 3–4 months with a basal body thermometer and plot temperatures on a graph. Temperature drops slightly before and rises after ovulation. The cervical mucus method involves assessing for a characteristic change from thin and scanty prior to ovulation to clear and stretchy during ovulation. The symptothermal method combines BBT, the cervical mucus method, and premenstrual symptoms to chart the fertile period. The predictor tests for ovulation detect an LH surge, which occurs 12–24 hours prior to ovulation. These tests are available for home use. Effectiveness is variable with a 25% pregnancy rate.	■ Teach proper use of the basal body thermometer to include charting methods. ■ Teach cervical mucous characteristics. ■ Teach proper use of ovulation predictor kits. ■ Teach the importance of abstinence when ovulation is suspected.
Spermicides (creams, jellies, foams, vaginal films or suppositories)	Substances inserted into the vaginal canal prior to sexual intercourse that destroy sperm or neutralize vaginal secretions. Predicted effectiveness is 94%, but effectiveness with typical use was 74%.	■ Suppositories may take 30 minutes to dissolve and therefore should be inserted prior to sexual activity. ■ Teach client that this method does not provide protection from STIs. ■ Teach client to avoid douching for 6 hours following intercourse.

TABLE 40-6	Methods of Contraception (continued)	
METHOD	**DESCRIPTION**	**NURSING MEASURES**
Male condom	A latex or natural fiber sheath that fits over the erect penis to provide a mechanical barrier to prevent sperm from coming into contact with the ovum. The latex male condom protects against STIs. Effectiveness is 97% when used as directed.	■ Assess for latex allergies. ■ Teach client to check expiration dates and inspect condom for damage. ■ Use in conjunction with water-based lubricant. ■ Apply condom prior to genital contact. ■ Withdraw the penis from the vagina while still erect, holding firmly during withdrawal.
Female condom	Thin polyurethane sheath with flexible rings applied in the vaginal canal. The closed end fits over the cervix and the open end covers a portion of the perineum. It provides a mechanical barrier to prevent sperm from coming into contact with the ovum. The female condom protects against some STIs. Effectiveness is 95% when used as directed.	■ Teach client that condom may be inserted up to 8 hours prior to intercourse. ■ Teach client that condom can only be used once.
Diaphragm	Used in conjunction with spermicide, the diaphragm is a rubber dome with a flexible ring that is placed high in the vagina to cover the cervix. It provides a mechanical barrier to prevent sperm from coming into contact with the ovum. Effectiveness is 94% when used as directed with spermicide.	■ Client must have an initial and annual gynecologic examination to ensure proper fit and insertion method. ■ Diaphragms should be refitted following weight loss or gain, childbirth, or second-trimester abortion. ■ Client may insert up to 6 hours prior to intercourse and leave in place 6 hours following intercourse. ■ Encourage clients to clean diaphragm with mild soap and water, dry thoroughly, and dust with cornstarch.
Cervical cap	A cervical cap is a soft rubber dome that fits over the base of the cervix. It provides a mechanical barrier to prevent sperm from coming into contact with the ovum. Effectiveness is 91% with no previous pregnancies and spermicide. Effectiveness is 74% with prior pregnancies and spermicide.	■ Client must have an initial and annual gynecologic examination to ensure proper fit and insertion method. ■ Instruct client that cap should be left in place at least 8 hours and up to 48 hours following intercourse.
Vaginal sponge	A small, round, one-time-use sponge made of synthetic fibers and containing spermicide placed against the cervix. The vaginal sponge has a loop to assist removal. Effectiveness is 91% when used as directed.	■ Ensure proper application method and use, including moistening prior to use to activate the spermicide; leave in place at least 6 hours and up to 24 hours following intercourse.
Intrauterine device (IUD)	A small device coated with copper or progesterone inserted by a healthcare provider into the uterus and left in place for an extended period. A spermicidal reaction prevents fertilization. There is also a local inflammatory reaction. IUDs can be used in nulliparous as well as parous women. Mirena and ParaGard IUDs may be more effective than tubal ligation. Effectiveness is 98.5% to 99.4% depending on IUD.	■ Assess for history of pelvic inflammatory disease, pregnancy, undiagnosed genital bleeding, genital malignancy, misshapen uterine cavity. ■ Teach client to check for string following menstruation, at ovulation, and prior to each intercourse. ■ Review symptoms of complications: irregular vaginal bleeding or the absence of a period, abdominal pain, dyspareunia, abnormal vaginal discharge, fever, chills, absence or change in string length.
Oral contraception ("the pill")	Oral medication containing synthetic estrogen and progestin that causes suppression of the hypothalamus and anterior pituitary. LH and FSH are inhibited so that follicles do not mature and ovulation does not occur. Other effects include endometrial atrophy and increased viscosity of the cervical mucus. Effectiveness is 99.5%–99.9% depending on specific medication when used as directed.	■ Assess for pregnancy, history of thrombophlebitis or thromboembolic disease, acute or chronic liver disease, estrogen-dependent cancers, uterine bleeding, heavy smoking, gallbladder disease, hypertension, diabetes, and hyperlipidemia. ■ Review dosing regime and procedure for missed dosages. ■ Discuss complications: depression, breast lumps, jaundice, abdominal pain, chest pain, shortness of breath, headaches, vision loss or blurring, and severe leg pain. ■ Assist client in choosing a backup method of contraception. ■ Advise client to use a barrier method to protect against STIs.

(continued)

TABLE 40-6	Methods of Contraception (continued)	
METHOD	**DESCRIPTION**	**NURSING MEASURES**
Transdermal patch	A small transdermal patch that is applied to a client's abdomen, buttocks, upper arm, or trunk for 3 consecutive weeks. During the fourth week the client does not apply a patch and typically experiences menses. See physiologic action of oral contraception. Effectiveness is similar to oral contraception.	■ Assess client weight (contraindicated for weights greater than 198) and for skin disorders. ■ See "Oral contraception."
Vaginal contraceptive ring	A flexible vaginal ring that contains sustained-release combination hormonal contraceptives. The one-time-use ring is inserted by the client, worn for 3 weeks and removed. A new ring is inserted by the client following menses. See physiologic action of oral contraception. Effectiveness is similar to oral contraception.	■ Assess for vaginal prolapse. ■ See "Oral contraception."
Combination injectable contraceptive	A monthly intramuscular injection of combined estrogen and progestin. See physiologic action of oral contraception. Effectiveness is similar to oral contraception.	■ See "Oral contraception."
Depo-Provera (DMPA)	Intramuscular injection of long-acting progestin, administered every 3 months. See physiologic action of subdermal implants. Effectiveness is 97.7% when administered on schedule.	■ Avoid massaging injection site because this could increase absorption and decrease effectiveness. ■ Explain side effects: amenorrhea, irregular bleeding, risk of thrombosis, headache, breast tenderness, weight gain, and depression.
Emergency postcoital contraception	A therapeutic regimen designed to prevent pregnancy following unprotected intercourse, rape, or contraception failure. Taken within 72 hours of unprotected intercourse, emergency contraception may prevent pregnancy in 75%–89% of cases. Methods include high-dose combined oral contraceptives, progestin, or insertion of an IUD.	■ Assess for current pregnancy. ■ Offer antiemetics to minimize nausea. ■ Schedule follow-up visit within 21 days of initiating regime. ■ Provide contraception counseling and risky sexual behavior modification suggestions.
Tubal ligation	A surgical procedure to interrupt patency of the fallopian tube, thereby preventing fertilization. It may be achieved by electrocoagulation, ligation, or banding of the fallopian tubes. Effectiveness is 99.5%.	■ Assess for pregnancy. ■ Ensure client understands the permanency of the procedure. ■ Provide nonpharmacologic and pharmacologic pain management. ■ Assess for and explain complications: internal burns from electrocoagulation, bowel perforation, pain, infection, hemorrhage, adverse effects of anesthesia.
Vasectomy	A surgical procedure to sever the male vas deferens bilaterally, hindering transfer of sperm during ejaculation. Effectiveness is 99.9%.	■ Ensure client understands the permanency of the procedure. ■ Assess for and explain side effects: pain, infection, hemorrhage, anesthetic agent reaction, hematoma, sperm granulomas, spontaneous reanastomosis. ■ Provide nonpharmacologic (ice packs and scrotal support) and pharmacologic pain management. ■ Explain that sterility is not fully achieved until remaining sperm are cleared from the vas deferens (usually 20 ejaculations). Advise client to use contraception during this period. ■ Schedule follow-up appointment for 6–12 months postprocedure.

exam is to obtain a semen sample and analyze the number and quality of sperm. If the sperm count is low, the testes may not be producing enough sperm, or occlusion of the seminiferous tubules or vas deferens may be preventing transport of sperm. Some occlusions of the vas deferens may be correctable with surgery. Spermatogenesis may be stimulated by hormone therapy with varying degrees of success. If the quality of sperm is poor, little can be done to correct the problem.

The male is the infertile partner in about 40% of the cases of infertility, and about 20% of the cases are shared problems with the male and female. Diagnostic tests for the male include semen analysis and hormone levels. A semen analysis tests the quantity and quality of the semen and the sperm cells, as well as the motility and density of the sperm. The scrotum and testes are examined. Sometimes a **varicocele,** or dilated blood vessel in the testis, can increase the temperature of the testes enough to cause sperm death.

Infertility in women is generally easier to treat than infertility in men. Diagnostic tests, including hormone levels and ultrasound of the reproductive organs, are used to determine the exact cause. Hormone therapy may be used to stimulate ovulation. Narrow fallopian tubes can sometimes be enlarged, and pregnancy may then be obtained by natural means.

If the couple remains infertile, other methods may be used to become pregnant. The man's sperm can be obtained, stored, and concentrated to obtain a high sperm count. The semen can then be instilled by artificial insemination. The eggs can be obtained through a laparoscopic procedure, fertilized in the laboratory, and then implanted into the uterus. This process is known as *in vitro* **fertilization.** When pregnancy takes place by *in vitro* fertilization, several fertilized eggs are instilled in an attempt to have at least one embryo implant in the uterus. Hormone therapy, used to stimulate ovulation, frequently results in more than one egg being released from the ovary. Therefore, there is an increased risk of a multifetal pregnancy.

Many treatment options are now available to unite the sperm and egg outside the body and then implant the embryo into the uterus. Donor eggs or donor sperm may also be used.

NURSING CONSIDERATIONS

The nursing responsibilities include emotional support and teaching. When the couple desiring a child learns that one partner is infertile, feelings of sadness, guilt, and blame put strain on the relationship. Counseling may be needed to help the couple explore these feelings and keep lines of communication open. The nurse, working with the obstetrician, can be helpful in clarifying medical and surgical options. The treatment of infertility can be quite costly, and the couple may need assistance in exploring financial resources.

Note: The references and resources for all chapters have been compiled at the back of the book.

PROCEDURE 40-1   **Breast Self-Examination**

Purposes

- To provide instruction in monthly self-examination of the breasts
- To identify abnormalities in the breast tissue

Equipment

- Mirror
- Small pillow or folded towel

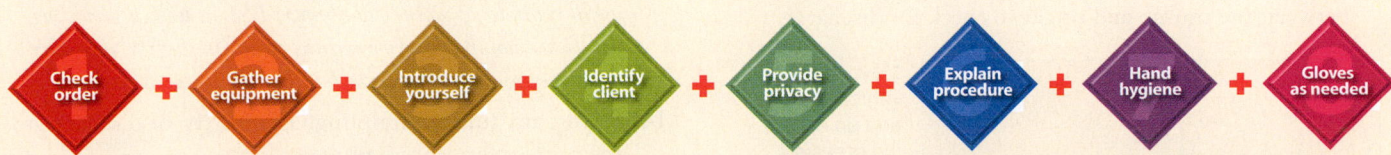

Check order + Gather equipment + Introduce yourself + Identify client + Provide privacy + Explain procedure + Hand hygiene + Gloves as needed

Interventions and Rationales

1. Perform preparatory steps (see icon bar above).

2. Instruction is provided by demonstration, return demonstration, and written material. *Showing the client what to do and then watching her return the demonstration ensures proper technique. Written material is a useful reference when at home.*

3. Stand in front of a mirror in good light with both breasts exposed. *Standing in front of a mirror with good light provides the opportunity to visually inspect all areas of the breast.*

4. Observe the breasts individually for lumps, dimpling, deviation, recent nipple retraction, irregular shape, edema, or discharge. Compare the right and left breast for symmetry. *Tissue should be consistent throughout the breast. Inconsistent tissue could indicate abnormalities.*

5. Observe the breasts in these positions (Figure 40-28 ■). *Changing position allows for adequate inspection.*
   - With her arms relaxed at her sides
   - With her arms lifted over her head
   - With her hands pressed against her hips and leaning forward

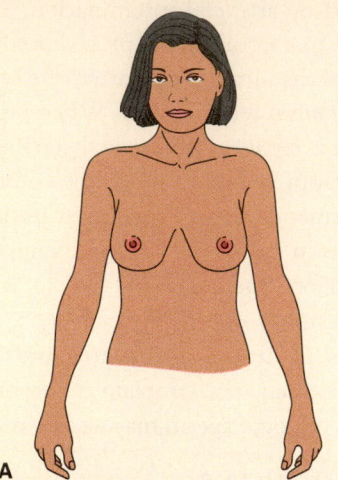 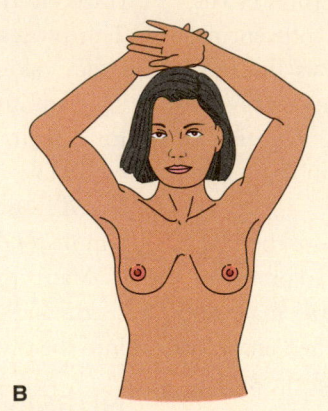 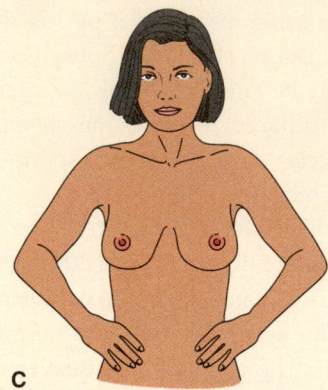

Figure 40-28. ■ Positions for inspection of the breast: **A.** Both arms relaxed at sides. **B.** Both arms above the head. **C.** Both arms on hips while leaning forward.

6. While sitting or standing in the shower, place one hand behind the head. Use the finger pads of the other hand to palpate the breast, moving in small, dime-sized circles. *Soap and water make the skin slick and decrease discomfort.*

7. Palpate the area from the collarbone to below the breasts, and from the middle of the armpit to the breastbone. Gently press the breast tissue against the chest wall, feeling for lumps or thickening of the tissue. *This pattern ensures all areas of the breast are examined.*

8. Repeat on the other side.

9. Position supine with a small pillow or folded towel under one shoulder. Place the arm on that side under the head. *In this position, gravity pulls the breast into a different position, allowing for more complete examination.*

10. Using the pads of the fingers, palpate the breast again as in step 6. Move down and up across the breast, starting at the axilla (Figure 40-29 ■).

11. Repeat on the other side.

12. Palpate the areola and the nipple. Compress the nipple between the thumb and finger to check for discharge

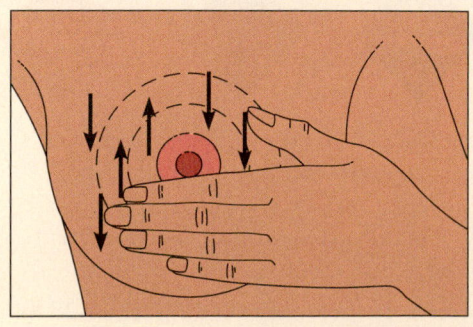

Move the hand vertically down and up across the breasts, starting at the axilla and working toward the center of the body. Press with the finger-pads in small, dime-sized circles to feel the chest wall.

Figure 40-29. ■ Check each breast, moving across the breast in the pattern indicated previously, feeling all parts of the breast. While holding one hand behind your head, palpate your breast.

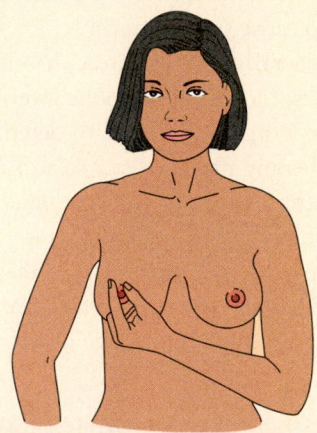

Squeeze your nipple between your thumb and forefinger; look for any clear or bloody discharge.

Figure 40-30. ■ Squeeze the nipple and look for any drainage.

(Figure 40-30 ■). *Gently compressing the nipple forces any drainage from the lactiferous duct.*

13. Use a calendar to record when BSE was performed. BSE should be performed once a month, usually on the fifth day after onset of menses. *Recording when BSE was performed is a useful reminder of when to do the next BSE as well as providing documentation should abnormalities occur. On the fifth day after menses begins, the breast tissue has the least hormonal influence.*

14. Report any lumps, dimpling, asymmetry, or discharge to the primary healthcare provider.

SAMPLE DOCUMENTATION

[date]	Instruction in BSE provided.
[time]	Return demonstration indicates
	appropriate technique. Written
	material provided. _____
	_____ C. Downey, LPN

Chapter Review

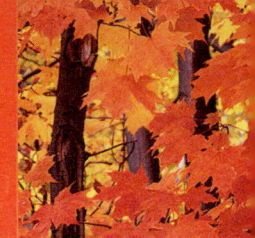

KEY Points

- It is extremely important for the nurse to consider the anatomy and physiology of the female and male reproductive systems each time a history or physical is performed.

- Common disorders of the female reproductive system may be related to the menstrual cycle, structural abnormalities, abnormal growths (including tumors and cysts), infections, and disorders of the breast.

- A common disorder of the male reproductive system is prostate enlargement, which causes a gradual obstruction of urine flow and urinary retention. The treatment can include medications and, ultimately, surgical intervention.

- Members of the healthcare team must work collaboratively to address the many issues related to disorders of the reproductive system.

- Clients diagnosed with a disorder of the reproductive system benefit greatly from teaching about causes of the disorder, treatment regimens, self-care interventions, and follow-up care.

- Many complications related to disorders of the reproductive system may be avoided when the nurse provides adequate teaching about prevention methods such as breast or testicular self-exam, early reporting of symptoms, diet changes, hygiene, and safe sexual practices.

- The nurse caring for clients diagnosed with disorders of the reproductive system uses the nursing process to provide adequate care.

- When caring for clients with reproductive system disorders, it is important to use a straightforward, professional demeanor. This will help to reduce any embarrassment that the client may feel because of the personal nature of the situation.

- The effectiveness of contraceptive methods varies depending on the individual, the specific method, and diligence of following directions for use.

- The nurse should provide verbal and written instruction in the use of contraceptive methods.

- Infertility can cause stress on a couple's relationship. The nurse must provide empathetic, nonjudgmental care for both individuals.

FOR FURTHER Study

For an informed consent form, see Chapter 4.

See Chapter 17 for more on the psychosocial aspects of physical illness.

See Chapter 29 for care of clients undergoing surgery.

For more information on sexually transmitted infections, see Chapter 41.

For more information about caring for clients with cancer, see Chapter 45.

Kegel exercises are described in Chapter 54.

See Chapter 59 for cryptorchidism, hypospadias, and epispadias.

EXPLORE PEARSON **mynursingkit™**

MyNursingKit is your one stop for online chapter review materials and resources. Prepare for success with additional NCLEX®-style practice questions, interactive assignments and activities, web links, animations and videos, and more!

Register your access code from the front of your book at **www.mynursingkit.com**

Critical Thinking Care Map

Caring for a Client after Hysterectomy

NCLEX-PN® Focus Area: Psychosocial Integrity

Case Study: Lisa Greene is a 46-year-old female with endometrial cancer who had a hysterectomy 2 days ago. She is tearful and states to the nurse, "I will never be able to please my husband again." She states, "I know if I have to have chemo I will lose my hair and he will just have to find someone else."

Nursing Diagnosis: *Risk for Impaired Social Interaction*

COLLECT DATA

Subjective	Objective
_____	_____
_____	_____
_____	_____
_____	_____
_____	_____
_____	_____
_____	_____

Would you report this? Yes/No

If yes, report to: _____

What would you report? _____

Nursing Care

_____
_____
_____
_____
_____
_____
_____
_____
_____
_____
_____

How would you document this? _____
_____
_____
_____

Compare your answers and documentation to those provided on the MyNursingKit Website.

Data Collected
(use only those that apply)

- The client works in the insurance department of a large clinic
- States she will never be able to please her husband again
- Is tearful and does not make eye contact
- States she is worried about chemotherapy and alopecia
- States her husband will just have to find someone else
- Has three children in college: ages 19, 20, and 21
- Incision to midline abdomen: clean, dry, intact
- IV of normal saline infusing 100 mL per hour per pump
- Ate 20% of breakfast (regular diet)
- Husband at bedside; stayed both nights and is very attentive
- None of the children have been to visit because they are at college in classes
- All lymph nodes were negative
- Refused to take morphine sulfate 10 mg IVP every 3 to 4 hours that was ordered for pain
- States pain is 8 on scale of 1 to 10

Nursing Interventions
(use only those that apply; list in priority order)

- Encourage the client to express her feelings about the loss of her uterus.
- Discuss the usual feelings of clients who have had a hysterectomy with cancer diagnosis.
- Change client's diet to increase appetite.
- Instruct client in importance of communication with husband to work through feelings of acceptance.
- Discuss available support groups in the community for follow-up (i.e., American Cancer Society).
- Encourage client to discuss sexuality with healthcare provider and support groups.
- Encourage client to take pain medication to decrease pain.

NCLEX-PN® Exam Preparation

1. The client, diagnosed with benign prostatic hypertrophy (BPH), complains of feeling as though he is not adequately emptying his bladder. The nurse recognizes this places the client at risk for:
   1. Bladder hypertrophy.
   2. Urinary tract infection.
   3. Renal calculi.
   4. Bladder pain.

2. When the nurse is collecting data related to a sexual history, which of the following strategies would improve the client's comfort in discussing this topic?
   1. Avoid looking at the client.
   2. Use euphemisms when referring to genitalia.
   3. Write the questions down on paper instead of vocalizing them.
   4. Maintain professionalism and treat the subject in a businesslike manner.

3. The nurse is teaching a community education course on menopause. A student asks the nurse, "Is there any way to avoid hot flashes?" The nurse's best response is:
   1. "Taking hormone replacement therapy is the only way to avoid hot flashes."
   2. "While there is no treatment, they don't last long."
   3. "Turn the thermostat down and avoid caffeine."
   4. "Have one glass of wine and exercise every day."

4. The nurse explains proper technique for a breast self-exam to a client. The nurse evaluates that teaching was effective when the client states:
   1. "I should check my breasts monthly on the day my period starts."
   2. "I should check my breasts monthly 5 days after my period starts."
   3. "I need to check my breasts monthly just before my period starts."
   4. "I need to begin checking my breasts at the same time I need to begin yearly mammograms."

5. A female client, newly diagnosed with endometriosis, asks the nurse what that means. The nurse's priority teaching strategy would be to:
   1. Call the physician and ask her to provide more information to the client.
   2. Ask the client if she was paying attention when the physician explained it.
   3. Use drawings of the female reproductive system to explain the disorder.
   4. Describe the various complications that can occur from the disease.

6. A client who is 16 years old is diagnosed with toxic shock syndrome. What should be included in the nursing teaching plan?
   1. Suggest the use of a diaphragm for birth control.
   2. Proper use of tampons.
   3. Antibiotics can be discontinued after symptoms resolve.
   4. TSS is caused by the bacteria *Chlamydia trachomatis*.

7. The nurse, assigned a client prescribed tamoxifen (Nolvadex), understands that the primary action of the drug is to:
   1. Increase the WBC count.
   2. Accelerate estrogen production.
   3. Destroy bacteria by interfering with cell wall synthesis.
   4. Inhibit growth of cancerous tissue.

8. The nurse is providing information to a client who has a newly implanted IUD. Which of the following is NOT a valid teaching point?
   1. You may go several months without a period.
   2. Check the string frequently for change in length.
   3. Abdominal pain may occur.
   4. Report fever and chills immediately.

9. The nurse, working in a Planned Parenthood clinic, is teaching a class on the sexual response cycle and explains that the clitoris retracts under the hood, the outer one-third of the vagina and labia minora become larger, and there is a slight increase in the width and depth of the inner two-thirds of the vagina during what phase?
   1. Excitement.
   2. Plateau.
   3. Orgasmic.
   4. Resolution.

10. The couple, undergoing fertility testing, has just been told that a varicocele may be at the root of their problems. The clients ask the nurse how a varicocele can impact fertility. The nurse's best response would include what information?
    1. Varicoceles increase the temperature of the testes causing sperm death.
    2. Varicoceles cause a blockage that does not permit entrance of sperm into the ejaculate.
    3. Varicoceles cause a blockage in the fallopian tube preventing fertilization of the ova.
    4. Varicoceles reduce the likelihood of ovulation.

Answers and rationales for Review Questions appear in Appendix I.

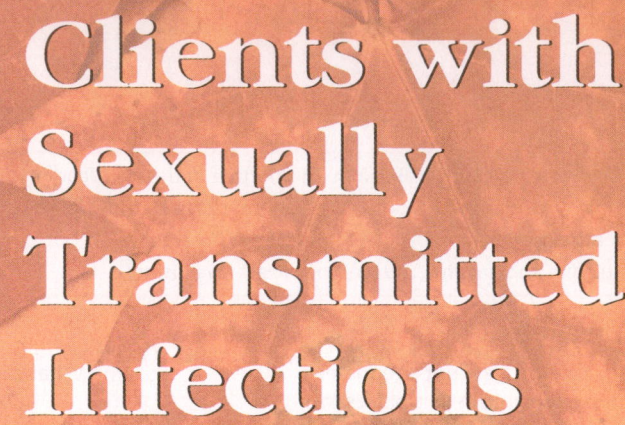

Chapter 41

Clients with Sexually Transmitted Infections

LEARNING Outcomes

After completing the chapter, you will be able to:

1. Describe the prevalence of and risks for STIs.
2. Identify methods of transmission and prevention of STIs.
3. Name diagnostic tests for STIs.
4. Identify common STIs, including their clinical manifestations, potential complications, diagnosis, and treatment.
5. Discuss the nursing care appropriate for clients with STIs using the nursing process.
6. Identify key concepts in client teaching for STIs.

Clinical Objectives

7. Provide appropriate nursing care for clients with STIs.
8. Develop a teaching plan for a client with an STI, including preventing the spread of infection.
9. Assist the client to deal with psychosocial issues related to STIs.

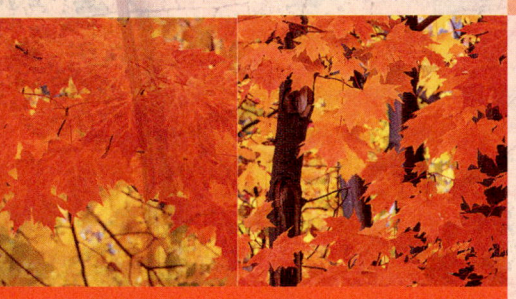

BRIEF Outline

More than 25 diseases have been found to be transmitted through sexual contact. These diseases are most commonly either bacterial or viral. They can also result from a protozoan or parasitic infestation. Nurses play an important role in identifying these diseases, ensuring proper treatment, and providing client education to prevent further transfer of infection.

Incidence

It is estimated that one in four Americans is infected with a sexually transmitted infection (STI). One-fourth of the U.S. population (65 million individuals) lives with the permanent effects of these diseases. The most commonly reported STI is *Chlamydia trachomatis*. Public education and treatment modalities have assisted in the decline of gonorrhea rates in the United States during the 1970s, 1980s, and early 1990s. However, since 1998 these rates have not changed significantly. More than 45 million Americans deal with the lifelong effects of herpes simplex virus type 2. Of men and women in the reproductive stage of life, 75% are estimated to be infected with human papillomavirus (HPV). Of the 40,000 new cases of human immunodeficiency virus (HIV) each year in the United States, half of those infected are younger than 25 years of age. Men are affected with HIV more often than women. However, in some ethnic groups, male gender roles increase the risk of HIV greatly (Box 41-1 ■). These numbers are staggering. It is clear that prevention of STIs should rank high as a nursing priority.

Prevention

RISK FACTORS

STIs are more prevalent among the following groups:

- Individuals with a personal history of STIs or in sexual contact with a partner who has a history of STIs
- People who use oral contraceptives
- Individuals who have unprotected sexual contact
- People with multiple sexual partners
- People with a history of intravenous drug abuse and other substance abuse
- Pregnant women
- Teens and young adults, particularly those with multiple sex partners and those who practice unprotected sexual contact (Box 41-2 ■).

| BOX 41-1 | CULTURAL PULSE POINTS |

Factors that Increase Risk of HIV

Puerto Rico has the highest number of HIV infections of any state or territory. In the United States, Puerto Ricans have the highest incidence of HIV when compared to other ethnic groups. In some states, AIDS is the leading cause of death for Puerto Rican women ages 25 to 44 (Centers for Disease Control and Prevention, 2003). These women become HIV positive mostly through heterosexual contact and/or intravenous drug use (Centers for Disease Control and Prevention, 2001).

Puerto Ricans abide by many socioeconomic and culturally supported gender roles, such as *machismo* and submissive women's roles. These roles foster high-risk behaviors that impede the prevention and increase the transmission of HIV. In traditional Puerto Rican culture, most men are given free will over sexual practices, including the approval and initiation of sex before marriage and extramarital affairs with other women. Some men may perceive that sexual intercourse with males is a sign of virility and sexual power rather than a homosexual behavior. This practice is not viewed positively by Puerto Rican women. Knowledge about HIV, beliefs about health and illness, and beliefs and practices related to condom use are common difficulties encountered by healthcare providers in the prevention and transmission of HIV.

Lack of condom use is perhaps one of the most significant risk behaviors that needs immediate attention and intervention from healthcare providers. Issues such as embarrassment, cost, gender/power struggles, and abuse are among some of the barriers encountered by Puerto Rican women. Some men fear that if they use condoms they will portray a less *macho* image, have decreased sexual satisfaction, or imply that they have a sexually transmitted infection or HIV. Additionally, Catholicism, lower educational levels, lower socioeconomic status, and acculturation are significant variables related to the high rates of AIDS and HIV among Puerto Ricans and other Hispanics. Healthcare providers must be aware of these barriers, assess individual perceptions of high-risk behaviors, and intervene with programs designed to meet the particular needs of clients who are at high risk for HIV infection or other sexually transmitted infections.

TRANSMISSION

Transmission of STIs occurs when clients come in contact with infected body fluids or lesions. This transmission is likely to occur during unprotected oral, genital, or anal sexual contact. Heterosexual and homosexual partners are both at risk of transmitting these infections. Many STIs

---

BOX 41-2 PEDIATRIC CONSIDERATIONS

Prevalence of STIs among Teens

A 2008 CDC study estimates that about 3.2 million adolescent females in the United States are infected with one of the following STIs: human papillomavirus (HPV) infection, chlamydia, herpes simplex virus Type II (HSV-II) infection, or trichomoniasis. The most common STI is HPV (related to cancer and genital warts), followed by chlamydia, trichomoniasis, and HSV-II. Fifteen percent of teens who had an STI had more than one.

The long-term risks of undiagnosed STIs include infertility, cervical cancer, and pelvic inflammatory disease (PID). These statistics reinforce the importance of educational programs for teens. Topics to be discussed in these programs include abstinence, mutual monogamy, and the correct and consistent use of condoms.

In addition, preventive counseling needs to include client-centered discussion of effective risk reduction tailored to the client's needs. Prevention counseling needs to include a thorough sexual history, including partner information (male, female, both, how many); pregnancy prevention (Are you trying to get pregnant? If not, how?); protection from STIs (What are you doing to protect yourself from STIs?); types of sexual practice (vaginal sex [penis in vagina], anal sex [penis in rectum]) and prevention (Do you use a condom? Are you always able to use condoms?); and past history of STIs (client and partner). Abstinence is the only completely sure way to avoid contracting or transmitting an STI. To be effective long term, care must be provided in a matter-of-fact, nonjudgmental manner that allows the teen or teens to express their needs and concerns openly.

Source: Prevalence of Sexually Transmitted Infections and Bacterial Vaginosis among Female Adolescents in the United States: Data from the National Health and Nutritional Examination Survey (NHANES) 2003–2004; National STD Prevention Conference, Chicago, March 10–13, 2008).

(such as herpes and HIV) can be transmitted to the fetus via the placenta during pregnancy or by direct contact with infected body fluids during the birth process or breastfeeding.

METHODS OF PREVENTION

Nurses must be involved in assisting clients to avoid STIs through abstinence (the only 100% effective means) or through careful prevention. Clients should be taught which contraceptives provide some protection against STIs and which do not. Client education and thorough assessment can aid prompt identification and effective treatment of any client exposed to these diseases. Risk factors and transmission methods should be explained to clients. The nurse can assist clients to lower their risk by proper use of barrier contraceptive methods. See the Nursing Care section for more information.

Routine STI screening assists in establishing early treatment. Screening can take place on a regular basis for high-risk clients. Annual male physical examinations and gynecologic examinations are appropriate times for STI screening. The Centers for Disease Control and Prevention (CDC) maintains a national database of STIs and requires healthcare personnel to report identified cases of gonorrhea, syphilis, acquired immune deficiency syndrome (AIDS), and, in some states, chlamydia. Reporting and gathering statistical data adds to the body of knowledge related to STIs. This information will benefit diagnostic, treatment, and prevention methods.

Vaccines for Prevention of STIs

Pre-exposure vaccination is very effective in preventing some STIs. Hepatitis B virus is frequently sexually transmitted. Hepatitis B vaccination has been available for many years. In addition, the hepatitis A vaccine is suggested for uninfected men who have sex with men, as well as for those who use illegal drugs. The HPV vaccine is now available and is licensed for females ages 9 through 26 (Centers for Disease Control and Prevention, 2006).

Diagnostic Tests for STIs

Diagnostic testing for STIs is based on presenting symptoms. Cultures of cervical, urethral, anal, or oropharyngeal tissue may be performed. DNA amplification of urethral or vaginal secretions or of urine may be done. Direct fluorescent antibody testing or enzyme immunoassay may be ordered, or there may be a Gram stain to identify the organism. **Chancre** (hard ulcer) specimens may be examined microscopically with immunofluorescent staining or darkfield microscopy.

Blood tests may include venereal disease research laboratory (VDRL), rapid plasma regain (RPR), or fluorescent treponemal antibody absorption (FTA-ABS) to detect antibodies. The enzyme-linked immunosorbent assay (ELISA) or Western blot is done to test for HIV. Saline wet preparation is used if a protozoal infection (*Trichomona*) is suspected. Discharge is examined for hyphae to rule out *Candida*. Specific testing for individual STIs is provided in Table 41-1 ■.

Chlamydia

In the United States, 1 in 25 men and women is infected with chlamydia. African American women have the highest rate (14%), and African American men have a rate of 11%. Chlamydia is caused by the bacteria *Chlamydia trachomatis*. The incubation period for this disease is 1 to 3 weeks following exposure.

(Text continues on p.1174.)

TABLE 41-1	Manifestations and Potential Complications, Diagnosis, and Treatment of STIs		
DISEASE	**MANIFESTATIONS AND POTENTIAL COMPLICATIONS**	**DIAGNOSTIC TESTS**	**TREATMENTS**
Chlamydia	-Female—may be asymptomatic; vaginal discharge; dysuria; urinary frequency; pelvic pain; possible mild pharyngitis -Complications female: pelvic inflammatory disease (PID), which can lead to chronic pelvic pain, scarring of fallopian tubes, ectopic pregnancy, preterm labor (PTL), infertility -Male—often asymptomatic; urethritis or penile discharge; dysuria; epididymitis; possible mild pharyngitis -Complications male: nongonococcal urethritis, possible scarring of urethral mucosa, prostatitis -Complications fetus/newborn: conjunctivitis, pneumonia, *ophthalmia neonatorum* (eye infection that can result in blindness; see Chapter 56 ⚭)	-Cervical or urethral tissue cultures -Urine samples to detect antibodies using direct fluorescent antibody (DFA), enzyme immunoassay (EIA), or DNA amplification -Often found with gonorrhea	**-Azithromycin** 1 g PO, single dose **-Doxycycline** 100 mg PO, b.i.d. **-Erythromycin base** 500 mg PO q.i.d. **-Erythromycin ethylsuccinate** 800 mg PO, q.i.d. **-Ofloxacin** 300 mg PO, b.i.d. **-Levofloxacin** 500 mg PO for 7 days Both partners must be treated to ensure cure of infection. Reinfection is likely unless clients abstain from sex or use condoms until cure. A second culture will be taken to ensure infection has cleared.
Gonorrhea	-Female—usually asymptomatic; may have vaginal discharge, interruption of menstrual cycle, urinary frequency -Complications female: PID; ectopic pregnancy; infertility; intra-abdominal adhesions resulting in chronic pelvic, abdominal, or menstrual pain -Male—dysuria; urethritis with watery white purulent penile discharge -Complications male: prostatitis, sterility associated with scarring of the seminiferous tubules -Complications fetus/newborn: *ophthalmia neonatorum* (see also Chapter 56 ⚭); pneumonia	-Gram stain smear of exudates to identify organism -Cervical, urethral, anal, or oropharyngeal culture -Urine, vaginal discharge, or urethral secretions using DNA amplification -Often found with chlamydia	**-Cefixime, ofloxacin, gatifloxacin,** or **lomefloxacin** 400 mg PO **-Ciprofloxacin** 500 mg PO **-Norfloxacin** 800 mg PO **-Levofloxacin** 250 mg PO **-Ceftriaxone** 125 mg IM, single dose **-Spectinomycin** 2 g in a single, IM dose Adequate treatment of both partners is essential to cure the infections. Abstinence or condom use is needed to prevent reinfection until cure is achieved. Further cultures must be taken to verify that treatment was successful.
Syphilis	-Female and male— -*Primary syphilis*: single or multiple, painless chancre at site of exposure; may be associated with inguinal **adenopathy** (generalized lymph node swelling) -Complications female and male: if untreated, syphilis progresses through stages resulting in heart failure, blindness, mental illness, and death -*Secondary syphilis*: low-grade fever, malaise, sore throat, headache, anorexia, generalized adenopathy, skin lesions or fine red rash, mucous membrane lesions, **condylomata lata** (flat papules in the anal area and/or skin folds), alopecia -*Tertiary syphilis*: **Gumma** (infectious granuloma) or cutaneous bone lesions; meningitis; dementia; generalized paresis; optic atrophy; aortic aneurysm, coronary artery disease -Complications fetus/newborn: congenital syphilis characterized by muscle wasting, notches of incisor teeth, bowing of tibia; if untreated, deafness, blindness, crippling, or death may result	-Blood tests called venereal disease research laboratory (VDRL), rapid plasma regain (RPR), or fluorescent treponemal antibody absorption (FTA-ABS) to detect antibodies -Chancre specimens to examine microscopically with immunofluorescent staining or dark-field microscopy	**Benzathine penicillin G** 2.4 million units IM in a single dose *Late latent syphilis* or *Latent syphilis of unknown duration* requires **benzathine penicillin G** 7.2 million units, IM, in three doses weekly for 3 weeks

(continued)

TABLE 41-1	Manifestations and Potential Complications, Diagnosis, and Treatment of STIs (continued)		
DISEASE	**MANIFESTATIONS AND POTENTIAL COMPLICATIONS**	**DIAGNOSTIC TESTS**	**TREATMENTS**
Herpes	-Female and male— -Primary episode: fever, headache, malaise, myalgias, dysuria, vaginal or urethral discharge, inguinal lymphadenopathy, painful genital **vesicles** (blisters) that may develop ulcerations -Recurrent episodes: genital vesicles that may be associated with pain and itching. A burning, itching sensation precedes blister formation. When blisters break, they result in painful open lesions that shed the virus and are highly contagious. Lesions heal spontaneously in several weeks. -Complications female: meningitis, encephalitis, cervical cancer; operative (cesarean) birth -Complications male: meningitis, encephalitis, erectile dysfunction, proctitis (inflammation of the rectum) -Complications fetus/newborn: neonatal herpes, which can cause disabilities or be fatal	-Tissue culture of lesion to isolate the virus -Serology to detect antibodies using DFA, EIA, or DNA amplification	-The following inhibit viral replication: **Acyclovir** 400 mg PO, t.i.d. -**Acyclovir** 200 mg PO five times a day -**Famciclovir** 250 mg PO, t.i.d. -**Valacyclovir** 1 g PO, b.i.d. for 7–10 days
Human papillomavirus	Female and male—single or multiple condylomata appearing on genitals or perianal area; may cause discharge, pruritus, or bleeding -Complications female: cervical cancer; operative birth; infection; urinary obstruction; bleeding -Complications male: urinary obstruction; bleeding -Complications fetus/newborn: laryngeal **papillomata** (warts); if large enough these may cause airway obstruction	Cervical specimen to determine dysplasia Serology and cytology to differentiate from other STIs	-**Podofilox 0.5% solution or gel** b.i.d. × 3 days, may be repeated up to 4 cycles -**Imiquimod 5% cream** h.s., three times a week for up to 16 weeks -**Cryotherapy** with liquid nitrogen or cryoprobe; repeat applications every 1–2 weeks -**Podophyllin resin 10–25%**, may be repeated weekly -**Trichloroacetic acid (TCA) or bichloracetic acid (BCA)** 80–90%, may be repeated weekly -**Surgical removal** by scissor excision, shave excision, curettage, or electrosurgery -**Intralesional interferon**
Human immunodeficiency virus (HIV) or acquired immune deficiency syndrome (AIDS)	-Female and male—night sweats, low-grade fever, anorexia, unexplained weight loss, fatigue, enlarged lymph nodes, cough, shortness of breath, persistent colds and infections, diarrhea -Complications female and male: chronic immunosuppression; meningitis; progressive dementia; Kaposi's sarcoma; non-Hodgkin's lymphoma; death (see also Chapter 35 ⌘) -Complications fetus/newborn: transmission of disease may occur *in utero*, during birth, or through breastfeeding	Blood tests to detect antibody development using enzyme-linked immunosorbent assay (ELISA) or Western blot Blood tests to detect antigen development and blood cultures	**Zidovudine** 500–600 mg/day PO, usually for life

TABLE 41-1	Manifestations and Potential Complications, Diagnosis, and Treatment of STIs (continued)		
DISEASE	MANIFESTATIONS AND POTENTIAL COMPLICATIONS	DIAGNOSTIC TESTS	TREATMENTS
Trichomoniasis	-Female—frothy vaginal discharge producing a foul odor; pruritus; lower abdominal pain -Complications female: **salpingitis** (inflammation of the uterine tube) -Male—may be asymptomatic; pruritus; penile discharge; burning on urination -Complications male: urethritis -Complications fetus/newborn: lower birth weights; prematurity	Discharge is examined for protozoa using saline wet preparation	-**Metronidazole** 2 g PO, single dose -**Metronidazole** 500 mg PO, b.i.d. for 7 days *Note:* Flagyl is ***contraindicated*** in the first trimester of pregnancy because it can cause abnormal fetal development. Clotrimazole vaginal suppositories are used during the first 12 weeks of pregnancy for symptom relief, and then Flagyl can be given.
Candidiasis	-Female—thick, curdlike, odorless vaginal discharge; intense pruritus -Complications female: cervical bleeding -Male—thick, curdlike penile discharge; plaque found under the foreskin; pruritus -Complications fetus/newborn: oral thrush; diaper dermatitis	Discharge is examined microscopically for hypha	-**Butoconazole** 2% cream 5 g intravaginally for 3 days **Clotrimazole** 1% cream 5 g intravaginally for 7–14 days -**Miconazole** 2% cream 5 g intravaginally for 7 days -**Nystatin** 100,000-unit vaginal tablet for 14 days -**Tioconazole** 6.5% ointment 5 g intravaginally, single application -**Terconazole** 0.4% cream 5 g intravaginally for 7 days -**Fluconazole** 150 mg PO, single dose

Manifestations

Unfortunately, clinical manifestations are often not apparent, particularly in women. The condition goes undiagnosed until complications occur. Table 41-1 lists manifestations, diagnosis, treatment, and complications of STIs. Clients with chlamydia infection often have gonorrhea also. Therefore, the two diseases may be treated concurrently.

Diagnosis and Treatment

Table 41-1 lists the tests used to diagnosis chlamydia and other STIs. It shows drugs used to treat these infections. Antibiotics are used to treat chlamydia.

Gonorrhea

Gonorrhea, first identified in 1879, was the first STI to be documented. It is caused by a bacteria known as *Neisseria gonorrhoeae*. The incubation period is between 1 and 14 days, with symptoms usually occurring within 10 days. This time frame varies for men and women.

Manifestations

Clinical manifestations are usually gynecologic or urologic but may include pharyngeal symptoms if oral–genital contact occurred. Females may be asymptomatic, or the disease may be exhibited as vaginal discharge, urinary frequency, or interruption of the menstrual cycle. Males are more likely to experience dysuria. There may be watery white penile discharge. See Table 41-1 for possible complications of gonorrhea.

Diagnosis and Treatment

Oral or intramuscular antibiotics are the usual treatment for gonorrhea. Common drugs used in treating gonorrhea are listed with dosage in Table 41-1.

Syphilis

The spirochete *Treponema pallidum* is the cause of syphilis. This type of bacteria is very mobile and spiral shaped; it enters the subcutaneous tissue through fine abrasions that occur during sexual contact. The incubation period ranges from 5 to 90 days.

Classifications and Manifestations

Clinical manifestations generally occur within 3 weeks and are characterized by three stages. *Primary syphilis* occurs as a single, painless lesion (Figure 41-1 ■) or *chancre* (see Chapter 30 ⊙⊙), which heals without treatment in 2 to 8 weeks. *Secondary syphilis* typically presents with flulike symptoms 6 weeks after the initial chancre. Surprisingly, this stage may also heal without treatment in 2 to 10 weeks. *Tertiary syphilis*, also known as **neurosyphilis,** can appear from 1 to 40 years following the onset of the

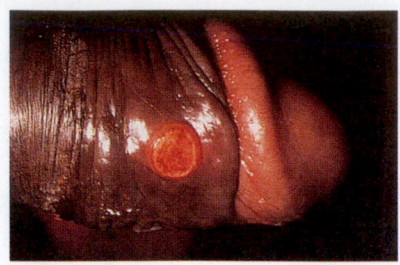

Figure 41-1. ■ *Primary syphilis* chancre on the penile shaft.

infection. There is a high morbidity and mortality rate for clients with tertiary syphilis.

Diagnosis and Treatment

Penicillin is the treatment of choice for syphilis (see Table 41-1). However, many clients are allergic to penicillin and may require desensitization prior to treatment. Due to the rapid destruction of spirochetes during treatment, clients may develop a **Jarisch-Herxheimer reaction.** This reaction, lasting several hours, is characterized by fever, headache, myalgia, and significant chancre changes. Chancres become edematous and brightly colored.

Herpes

Infection with genital herpes (Figure 41-2 ■) has reached epidemic proportions, although herpes is not currently a reportable disease according to the CDC. It is caused by two viral strains of herpes virus (see also Chapter 30 ⊙⊙). Herpes simplex virus type I (HSV-I) causes cold sores and typically occurs above the waist. It is not sexually transmitted. Herpes simplex virus Type II (HSV-II) causes the vast majority of STIs. This disease cannot be cured, and

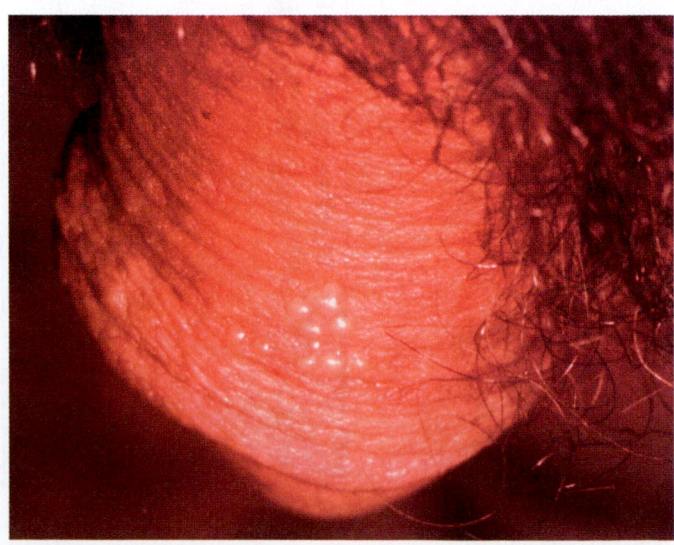

Figure 41-2. ■ Genital herpes blisters.

many clients experience recurrences for the remainder of their lives. The incubation period for this virus varies from 1 to 26 days, but typically symptoms appear in 6 to 8 days.

Manifestations

Primary episodes result in both local and systemic symptoms and last up to 3 weeks. Manifestations include fever, headache, malaise, myalgias, dysuria, vaginal or urethral discharge, inguinal lymphadenopathy, and painful genital vesicles that may develop ulcerations. After the primary episode, recurrent episodes produce only local soreness and sores. Table 41-1 lists possible complications of herpes, the most serious of which is neonatal death.

Diagnosis and Treatment

The goals for treatment of herpes genitalis are to shorten the duration of outbreaks and to reduce viral shedding (see Table 41-1 for drugs that are available). If a woman is pregnant, a further goal is protection of the fetus from exposure; birth in an infected woman is done by cesarean section.

Some newer agents are being developed to prevent the spread of herpes to sexual partners.

CYTOMEGALOVIRUS

Cytomegalovirus (CMV) is a member of the herpes virus family. It is spread through close contact with body fluids, such as urine, saliva, breast milk, blood, tears, semen, and vaginal fluids. A pregnant woman can pass this to her unborn baby. Most infections with CMV are silent, meaning there are no obvious signs or symptoms. Development of a mild illness may mimic many other illnesses, with mild fever, body aches, swollen glands, and sore throat. Blood testing for CMV IgG antibodies can be done but is not 100% reliable. There is no treatment for CMV at this time, although research into the effectiveness of antiviral medications and vaccinations is ongoing.

CMV is the most common virus transmitted to the unborn fetus. Congenital CMV can cause permanent neurologic disabilities, most commonly visual and auditory deficits. Nurses need to teach pregnant women about the need to practice careful hand washing and good hygiene. Minimizing exposure to urine and saliva will decrease the woman's risk of infection while pregnant (New York State Department of Health, 2008).

Human Papillomavirus

HPV is also known as *genital warts*, *venereal warts*, or *condylomata acuminata* (Figure 41-3 ■). The infecting agent is called human papillomavirus. There are more than 40 varieties of these viruses. However, five varieties are thought

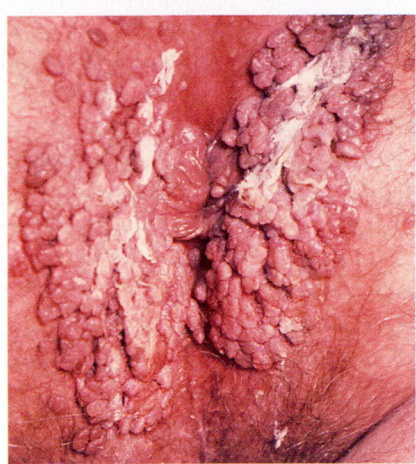

Figure 41-3. ■ *Condylomata acuminata* (genital warts) on the labia.

to be sexually transmitted. The virus has an incubation period of 3 weeks to 9 months. Several types of warts may appear at the point of contact (see Table 41-1).

HPV is associated with an increased risk of cervical cancer, so lesions should be biopsied and treated. A vaccine against several types of HPV is currently being recommended for use in prepubescent and teenage girls (Box 41-3 ■). Treatment for HPV includes applications of chemical compounds and various surgical procedures (see Table 41-1).

Human Immunodeficiency Virus and Acquired Immune Deficiency Syndrome

Compared to the other STIs, HIV and AIDS are relatively new. AIDS was not identified as a separate disorder until 1981. A short 2 years later the retrovirus, HIV, was identified

BOX 41-3	CULTURAL PULSE POINTS

HPV Vaccine for Girls

Currently, the HPV vaccine is licensed to be given to prepubescent and teenage girls, because statistics show that many females are exposed to or infected with a strain of HPV in adolescence. This has led to much debate about mandatory vaccination of young girls before they become sexually active.

Many cultural and religious groups have raised concerns about this vaccine. They object to the assumption that girls will become sexually active in the teen years. They are concerned that the long-term effects of the vaccine are not yet known.

Nurses need to provide careful, factual, nonjudgmental counseling to the clients and families about the vaccine. Follow-up phone contact may be indicated to assess the need for further counseling or information.

as the causative agent. This virus, which destroys the body's immune system, originated in primates in central Africa.

Transmission of the virus can occur through sexual contact, both homosexual and heterosexual. Exposure to infected body fluids may also occur through sharing of needles and syringes and through the maternal placenta to a fetus during birth or through breast milk.

Manifestations

Following exposure to the virus, the antibody response occurs within 6 weeks to 6 months. During this period the client is typically asymptomatic. Development of the disease, AIDS, may not occur for up to 10 years. Clinical manifestations vary but are typically neurologic or related to immunodepression (see Table 41-1).

Diagnosis and Treatment

There is still no cure for AIDS. Current treatment focuses on suppression of the virus and correction of the various diseases afflicting the client (see Table 41-1), and on preventing its spread. *Note:* The main discussion about HIV/AIDS appears in the Immune Disorders chapter (see Chapter 35).

Trichomoniasis

Among young sexually active women, trichomoniasis is the most common, curable STI. *Trichomonas vaginalis* is the protozoan that causes trichomoniasis. The protozoan thrives in warm, moist environments. It has been found alive in warm, moist environments outside of body cavities. It can be transmitted through shared bath facilities, wet towels, and wet swimwear. The incubation period is from 4 to 28 days.

Manifestations

Males and females infected with *T. vaginalis* may be asymptomatic. Symptoms in males are typically urologic. In females, the symptoms are usually gynecologic. Note also that the inflammation caused by trichomoniasis may increase a woman's risk of acquiring or transmitting HIV infection (see Table 41-1).

Diagnosis and Treatment

Pharmacologic treatment with metronidazole is effective against trichomoniasis. To prevent reinfection, both sexual partners must be treated (see Table 41-1).

Candidiasis

Candidiasis (also called monilial vulvovaginitis or candidal vaginitis in women) is a fungal or yeast infection caused by *Candida albicans* (Figure 41-4 ■), a fungus. Candidiasis

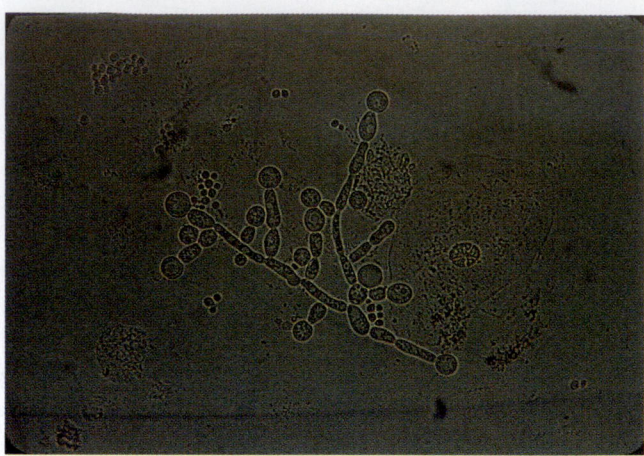

Figure 41-4. ■ *Candida albicans.*

may be found in combination with other STIs. However, transmission of this organism occurs by nonsexual contact as well.

Manifestations

Clinical manifestations of candidiasis are given in Table 41-1.

Diagnosis and Treatment

Creams, ointments, or tablets are instilled vaginally to treat this infection. Length of therapy depends on the level of infection (see Table 41-1).

NURSING CARE

PRIORITIZING NURSING CARE

When caring for clients with STIs, make it a high priority to have nonjudgmental, supportive interactions. Some clients may feel embarrassed or "dirty" when diagnosed with STIs. Others may have frequent infections due to lifestyle choices. In all situations, focus your care on the clients and their health needs. Some clients may be reluctant to share names of all sexual partners so that they can be treated. Sometimes clients do not follow through with treatment plans if they feel they are not treated with respect by the healthcare staff. Your caring attitude will help them overcome fears and objections about divulging information and seeking treatment.

ASSESSING

A critical element of maintaining and restoring client health is an adequate assessment. Identification of clients infected with STIs is an important way to prevent the spread of STIs to uninfected individuals, and to provide

BOX 41-4 DATA COLLECTION

Sample Questions on Sexual Activity

- "This information will remain confidential and may be uncomfortable to discuss but it is important in order to best care for your health. Tell me about how often you engage in sexual activity."
- "Tell me about your sexual partner or partners." (This avoids the bias of homosexuality or heterosexuality. It also allows clients to express issues related to their sexual partners that are important to them.)
- "Many people are concerned about birth control, sexually transmitted infections, or types of sexual practices. Are you concerned about any of these issues?"
- "What other concerns do you have?"

proper treatment for those currently infected. Because STIs may be asymptomatic, the nurse must elicit data beyond clinical manifestations, such as sexual practices that may put the client at risk for STIs.

When taking a sexual history, the nurse must be comfortable with the questions and terms to be used. Developing a trusting relationship with the client, providing privacy, ensuring confidentiality, and using easy-to-understand language will help the client feel more comfortable discussing intimate issues. The nurse should use open-ended questions and a nonjudgmental attitude to encourage discussion. Examples of assessment questions are provided in Box 41-4 ■.

Collecting the necessary information requires the nurse to obtain both subjective and objective data. This can be obtained through client interviews, interviews with sexual partners, and chart review (Chapter 11 ⬭).

Subjective Data

During the nursing history the client should be asked about his or her sexual practices, including knowledge of partners' exposure to STIs and the number of sexual partners. Use and type of contraception should be identified, as well as other medications taken on a regular basis. For female clients, menstrual history and obstetrical history are important. The nurse should inquire about symptoms associated with STIs. This list would include, but not be limited to, vaginal or penile discharge, presence of lesions in the genital or perianal region, flulike symptoms, and *dysuria* (pain on urination).

Objective Data

During the physical examination the nurse gathers much important objective data. Vital signs, particularly temperature, should be measured and recorded. The nurse

should observe for lymphadenopathy, lesions, and vaginal or penile discharge. It is important for the nurse to describe the characteristics of these findings fully. The specific site, size, and presence of tenderness and erythema should be recorded about *lymphadenopathy* (swollen lymph nodes). Lesions should be described according to their type and size. The presence and characteristics of drainage should be noted. The skin surrounding these lesions should also be described. Discharge should be described according to color, viscosity, and odor.

The nurse is responsible for obtaining specimens for laboratory tests used to determine the presence of STIs. It is also important that the nurse review these results and report them to the clinician responsible for making the medical diagnosis. (See Chapters 19 and 39 ⬭ for methods of obtaining specimens.)

DIAGNOSING, PLANNING, AND IMPLEMENTING

The nurse is able to identify many nursing diagnoses appropriate for the client diagnosed with a STI. Because nursing care is holistic, the nurse must concentrate on both physical and psychosocial nursing diagnoses.

Physical nursing diagnoses include *Acute Pain* and *Impaired Tissue Integrity* related to lesions, dysuria, inflammation, or *dyspareunia* (pain associated with sexual intercourse). The client is also at *Risk for Injury* related to the many complications of STIs, especially when they are not treated promptly. *Impaired Urinary Elimination* related to dysuria and urinary frequency may also be diagnosed for the client with a STI.

Emotional nursing diagnoses include *Ineffective Health Maintenance* related to inappropriate sexual practices that led to STIs. A client with a STI may also have *Deficient Knowledge* related to the transmission, treatment, and effects of STIs. Other emotional nursing diagnoses that may result are *Sexual Dysfunction, Anxiety, Fear, Situational Low Self-Esteem*, and *Impaired Social Interaction*.

When planning appropriate nursing care, the nurse should consider the following goals:

- Pain will decrease and comfort will improve.
- Injury from complications will be avoided.
- A normal pattern of urinary elimination will be restored.
- Client will obtain an adequate knowledge base.
- Client will complete treatment and initiate safer sexual practices.
- Client will express restored emotional and psychosocial well-being.

Nursing interventions for clients with STIs include client teaching, assisting in screening, ensuring proper diagnosis and treatment of infections, and identifying sexual partners exposed to STIs. The following nursing interventions with rationales are appropriate for most clients with STIs. Other nursing interventions should also be considered in an effort to individualize nursing care. See also the Continuity of Care section that follows.

- Have the client apply cool compresses to genital lesions. *This is an effective nonpharmacologic pain relief measure that may augment the use of analgesics.*
- Encourage client to choose positions that avoid direct pressure on genital lesions. *Avoiding prolonged pressure promotes circulation and improves healing.*
- Monitor for signs and symptoms of complications related to STIs. *Complications may occur with ineffective treatment. Early identification promotes effective treatment.*
- Encourage fluid intake of at least 2 L/day unless otherwise contraindicated. *Adequate fluid intake assists in restoring normal patterns of urinary elimination.*
- Practice proper hand washing and use universal precautions. *Avoiding contact with infected body fluids will decrease the risk of spreading infection.* For more detailed information on preventing the spread of infection, see Chapter 10 ⚭.
- Develop a nurse–client relationship based on respect of privacy, compassion, and a nonjudgmental attitude. *These characteristics allow trust to develop between nurse and client. As trust develops, the nurse is able to elicit more complete data from the client.*
- Refer clients to appropriate community agencies. *Community agencies and support groups offer clients the opportunity to develop supportive relationships with individuals who may be experiencing similar situations.*

EVALUATING

The care plan is revised until expected outcomes are achieved. To evaluate the effectiveness of interventions, the nurse would gather data concerning:

- Resolution of pain and discomfort.
- Avoidance of complications through proper, prompt treatment of STIs.
- The client's understanding about transmission, treatment, and prevention methods for STIs.
- The client levels of anxiety and fear, self-esteem, and resolution of sexual dysfunction.

Continuity of Care

Discharge teaching is a priority nursing intervention when assisting clients with STIs. Box 41-5 ▪ provides crucial teaching points for the nurse to consider.

BOX 41-5 CLIENT TEACHING

Ongoing Care for Client with STI

- Discuss the presenting symptoms and complications for males and females of all STIs. Also include the importance of prompt reporting of these symptoms.
- Discuss transmission methods of STIs. Be sure to include transmission to fetus/newborn during pregnancy.
- Ensure that the client understands the need to inform all sexual partners to prevent future transmission and avoid complications.
- Explain that the entire course of treatment prescribed must be completed in order to prevent transmission.
- Teach the client the importance of refraining from sexual contact until treatment is completed.
- Be sure that the client understands the need to use latex condoms for sexual activity when treatment is completed. Educate the client on proper use. (Proper use includes choosing a condom that is not old [check expiration date], placing a small amount of spermicide on the inside tip of the condom, and rolling the condom down the penis leaving space at the tip.) Also provide information about proper disposal. (After ejaculation remove the penis while it is still erect, and hold the condom firmly against the base of the penis during removal.) Include teaching about hand washing, to avoid transmission of STIs.
- Discuss with the client the importance of follow-up examinations to determine cure and prevent transmission of the infection.
- Explain to the client the importance of healthcare behaviors that can reduce the risk of transmission of STIs: condom use, hand washing, urinating and bathing following intercourse, abstinence or monogamy, avoiding the abuse of intravenous drugs, and avoiding sexual relations with those who engage in drug use.
- Encourage regular screening for STIs.
- Encourage the client to contact the healthcare clinic for emotional needs as well as physical needs following discharge.

NURSING PROCESS CARE PLAN
Client with Gonorrhea

Mr. West is a 20-year-old college student living in an apartment with two roommates. He is an honor student and treasurer of his fraternity, and he volunteers his time at the campus tutoring center. He reports a monogamous sexual relationship with Ms. Pace whom he has been seeing for 4 months. This morning he makes an appointment at the student health center. For the past 2 days he has been experiencing pain during urination and has noticed a white penile discharge. He reports that his testicles feel swollen and painful.

Assessment

Vital signs: BP 122/78, P 99, R 21 and labored, T 99.3°F. Mr. West rates the testicle pain as 6 out of 10. Weight 178 pounds. Height 6'0". Skin is moist and pink without notable lesions. He is alert, responding appropriately, and states that he is anxious to discover the reason for his symptoms and return to his class schedule. He also asks if this appointment will be kept confidential because he does not want his girlfriend, Ms. Pace, to know he is here. A specimen of the penile discharge is obtained for Gram staining. A blood sample is obtained for screening of other STIs including HIV. The Gram stain is positive for gonorrhea. All other tests are negative.

Nursing Diagnosis

The following important nursing diagnoses (among others) are established for this condition:

- *Deficient Knowledge* related to treatment modalities and the need to contact all sexual partners
- *Acute Pain* related to inflammation of testicles
- *Anxiety* related to status of physical health and threat of social isolation
- *Impaired Urinary Elimination* related to infectious process and dysuria

Expected Outcomes

The expected outcomes for the plan of care are that Mr. West will:

- State correct information regarding treatment modalities including transmission methods and the need to contact all sexual partners before discharge from initial clinic visit.
- Demonstrate a decrease in testicular pain within 48 hours of initiating treatment as evidenced by lower rating on pain scale, no facial grimacing.
- Demonstrate decreased symptoms of anxiety at follow-up clinic visit as evidenced by pulse and respirations within normal limits (WNL) and statement of positive social interactions with sexual partners.
- State return to typical pattern of urinary elimination within 48 hours of initiating treatment as evidenced by urinary output WNL and statement of lack of dysuria.

Planning and Implementation

The following nursing interventions are implemented for Mr. West:

- Discuss transmission of gonorrhea to include risk factors that increase the chance of infection, such as multiple sex partners and unprotected sexual contact. *Client education is*

the first step in prevention of STI. Reinfection with gonorrhea, usually from a person who is asymptomatic, is common. Client education decreases the chance of reinfection and spread of infection.

- Discuss treatment modalities to include medication action, side effects, and the need for follow-up clinic visit. Reinforce the need to finish all prescribed medication for complete treatment. *Client education may decrease anxiety and fear. It increases the likelihood of follow-through with the treatment plan.*
- Inform the client of the importance of communicating the diagnosis of gonorrhea to all recent sexual partners. Provide an opportunity to role play. *All the client's sexual partners are at risk for contracting the infection. The client is at risk for reinfection if infected partners are not treated. Role playing will give the client an opportunity to rehearse what may be difficult conversations.*
- Reassess testicular pain by telephone follow-up call within 48 hours of initiating treatment. *Epididymitis with potential for sterility may occur. If there is no improvement in testicular pain, further assessment or treatment may be needed.*
- Have the client apply moist heat to the groin. *Heat may decrease discomfort from swelling and inflammation; it increases blood flow to the affected area, which will also decrease swelling and inflammation. Use of nonpharmacologic pain control measures reduces the need for medication.*
- Encourage the client to self-administer analgesics prior to pain levels of 5 or above. *Administering pain medication before severe pain occurs will decrease the amount needed for pain control. Controlling pain is one way to help control anxiety, since pain causes anxiety in many clients.*
- Encourage the client to express his feelings and fears related to his diagnosis. Reassess anxiety levels at the follow-up clinic visit. *The client may be anxious about communicating the diagnosis and about potential complications to himself and partners.*
- Encourage and support effective coping behaviors. *Verbalization of anger or anxiety about the diagnosis, the method of contracting the disease, and potential complications of infection may decrease the occurrence of inappropriate behavior.*
- Teach the client to monitor intake and output during treatment. *Urethral swelling and purulent material may impede the flow of urine. Timely reporting of this symptom decreases the chance of further injury.*
- Encourage the use of a discomfort log to record levels of dysuria. *Improvement of pain symptoms suggest treatment is effective. Resistant strains do exist.*
- Encourage increased fluid intake, especially the intake of eight to ten 8-ounce glasses of water per day. *Adequate fluid intake will help to decrease pain on urination and restore normal urinary elimination.*

Evaluation

At the follow-up clinic visit, Mr. West's vital signs are BP 120/80, P 66, R 16, T 98.6°F. He had contacted two sexual partners and given them both contact information where they could receive treatment. He reports that his penile discharge, testicular pain, and dysuria have subsided.

Critical Thinking in the Nursing Process

1. List appropriate questions for collecting data regarding Mr. West's sexual history.

2. What types of personal protection should be recommended to Mr. West and why?

3. Describe the psychologic support necessary for Mr. West.

Note: Discussion of Critical Thinking questions appears on the MyNursingKit Website.

Note: The references and resources for all chapters have been compiled at the back of the book.

Chapter Review

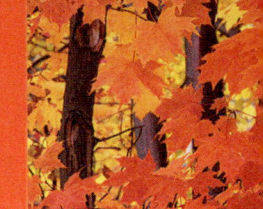

KEY Points

- STIs may be caused by bacteria, viruses, protozoans, or parasites. Bacteria, protozoans, and parasites may be cured with effective treatment, but viruses produce some long-lasting effects on clients.
- Clinical manifestations of STIs may be local (dermatologic changes) or systemic (urinary or gynecologic changes).
- Many women learn of positive HIV status during routine prenatal care. The nurse will need to assist the client during this period, utilizing communication skills, as well as teaching and referring to appropriate resources.
- STIs are preventable diseases. The nurse is responsible for providing teaching to the client to assist in preventing these diseases. Abstinence, safer sexual practices, prompt identification, seeking health care following symptom recognition, and adequate treatment of all infected partners are important client teaching points.
- STIs may cause complications to women, men, unborn fetuses, or newborns. These complications range from local effects to life-altering disabilities and life-threatening systemic diseases.
- Screening, diagnosis, and treatment of STIs can be effective in identifying clients at risk and in preventing the transmission of sexually transmitted diseases.
- Nursing care is vital to the proper identification, prevention, and treatment of STIs.

FOR FURTHER Study

For more detailed information on preventing the spread of infection, see Chapter 10.

Suggestions for conducting a client interview are in Chapter 11.

For more detailed information on health assessment, see Chapter 19.

See Chapter 19 for methods of obtaining specimens.

The main discussion of skin lesions is in Chapter 30.

For discussion of immune disorders and Kaposi's sarcoma, see Chapter 35.

Chapter 39 provides information on collecting urinary specimens.

See discussion of *ophthalmia neonatorum* in Chapter 56.

Critical Thinking Care Map

Caring for a Client with Genital Herpes

NCLEX-PN® Focus Area: Physiologic Integrity

Case Study: Jeanne Coy presents to the family planning clinic with complaints of genital pain, a slight headache, dysuria, and muscle aches. Upon examination, multiple perineal vesicles are identified. Ms. Coy has a temperature of 100.9°F. The tissue culture of the lesion reveals the herpes virus.

Nursing Diagnosis: *Impaired Tissue Integrity*

COLLECT DATA

Subjective	Objective
_____	_____
_____	_____
_____	_____
_____	_____
_____	_____
_____	_____
_____	_____

Would you report this? Yes/No

If yes, report to: _____

What would you report? _____

Nursing Care

_____
_____
_____
_____
_____
_____
_____
_____
_____
_____
_____

How would you document this? _____
_____
_____
_____

Compare your answers and documentation to those provided on the MyNursingKit Website.

Data Collected
(use only those that apply)

- Headache pain level 4
- Genital pain level 7
- States thighs and lower abdomen ache
- Urinary output 100 mL
- Urine characteristics: dark amber with sediments
- Multiple perineal vesicles measuring $\frac{1}{4}$ to $\frac{1}{3}$ inch in diameter
- Labia with diffuse redness

Nursing Interventions
(use only those that apply; list in priority order)

- Assess characteristics of the vesicle.
- Teach the importance of informing all sexual partners.
- Offer foam "doughnut"-type pillow for seating.
- Use mild, hypoallergenic soaps.
- Encourage client to join a herpes support group.
- Encourage diet high in protein and carbohydrates and containing RDA of vitamins and minerals.
- Encourage adequate mobility.
- Avoid restrictive clothing.
- Monitor electrolyte levels.

NCLEX-PN® Exam Preparation

TEST-TAKING TIP Nervous energy and auditory distractions can often interfere with clear thinking while taking a test. Bring a rubber stress ball, modeling clay, or Silly Putty into the test with you. Release nervous energy by squeezing these objects. Use foam ear plugs to block distracting noises. These steps will increase your level of concentration.

1 While teaching the client newly diagnosed with genital herpes the client states, "I'll be glad when this disease is cured." What is the best nursing response?

1. "Genital herpes is a virus that may become dormant but will not be cured."
2. "Genital herpes is a horrible disease that will stay with you for the rest of your life."
3. "Genital herpes is cured by acyclovir only when it is taken properly so be sure to complete all of your prescription."
4. "Once genital herpes is cured, the goal will be not to contract it again."

2 A male client presents to the healthcare clinic concerned about possibly contracting genital herpes because his partner reports being diagnosed with the disease. The nurse assesses for the presence of which of the following symptoms?

1. Thick, curdlike penile discharge; plaque found under the foreskin; pruritus.
2. Multiple genital vesicles, fever, muscle aches.
3. Painless chancre, swelling in the groin.
4. Unilateral scrotal pain, dysuria, and penile discharge.

3 The nurse is teaching a sex education course to a class of 10th-grade females. A student asks the nurse, "Is there any way to completely avoid ever becoming infected with an STI?" The nurse's best response is:

1. "You should have regular screenings for STIs."
2. "Research shows that female condoms are as effective as male condoms."
3. "Abstinence is the only sure way to avoid an STI."
4. "Make sure your partner wears a latex condom."

4 The nurse, working in a gynecology clinic, admits a female client reporting a yellow vaginal discharge. The nurse anticipates which of the following diagnostic tests will be performed?

1. Vaginal culture
2. ELISA
3. VDRL
4. Microscopic exam of discharge

5 A female client, in a monogamous relationship, is diagnosed with a sexually transmitted type of HPV. The client asks, "How could I have contracted this?" The nurse's best response will include which of the following?

1. Inform about the increased risk of cervical cancer.
2. Explain the treatment options for HPV.
3. Inform her of methods of transmission for HPV.
4. Encourage her to speak to her sexual partner about the diagnosis.

6 A client who is 3 weeks postpartum is diagnosed with candidiasis. What complications should be included in the nursing teaching plan?

1. Pelvic inflammatory disease
2. Diaper dermatitis of the newborn
3. Cervical cancer
4. Infertility

7 The nurse is caring for a client diagnosed with gonorrhea. An important factor to include in the client teaching plan is:

1. Use of barrier techniques to prevent another sexually transmitted disease.
2. Avoiding sexual activity for 24 hours.
3. Methods of preventing pregnancy.
4. Need for retesting in 1 week.

8 The nurse has provided hygiene information to a client at risk for contracting an STI. The nurse evaluates further teaching is needed when the client says:

1. "It is important to douche following intercourse."
2. "Hand washing prior to and following intercourse is recommended to reduce my risk of STIs."
3. "Underclothes made of cotton are preferred over synthetic materials."
4. "Voiding is important immediately following sexual intercourse."

9 A male client received an injection of ceftriaxone today for the treatment of gonorrhea. He asks about resuming sexual activity. The most appropriate nursing response is that the client may resume sexual activity:

1. In 7 days.
2. Today.
3. In 24 hours.
4. In 6 weeks.

10 The nurse is caring for a client with an STI. The client expresses embarrassment about the diagnosis. Which of the following would be important strategies for the nurse to employ? (Select all that apply.)

1. A nonjudgmental attitude
2. Care focused on the client's need
3. An expectation that the client must follow the nurse's recommendations
4. Strict confidentiality following HIPAA guidelines
5. A supportive approach to the client's needs

Answers and rationales for Review Questions appear in Appendix I.

Thinking Strategically About...

You are a new grad recently hired on a medical-surgical unit in a hospital where you did much of the clinical during your LPN/LVN program. Today you are assigned three clients. You will be expected to provide them with their medication and treatments and to oversee all of their care. The RN team leader will give any IV medications, although you can hang fluids and monitor the IVs.

Client 1—Jake Reinhardt, a 54-year-old male, was admitted with a diagnosis of Type 2 diabetes mellitus, end-stage renal disease, and gangrenous infection of the left foot. Client is receiving hemodialysis three times per week. Physician's orders on admission are as follows:

- Bed rest
- Lab in A.M.
  - Chemistry panel (chem. 16)
  - Glycohemoglobin level
  - CBC
- Diet: 1,500-calorie carbohydrate-consistent
- Fluid restriction: 1,200 mL per 24 hours
- Glucoscan a.c. and h.s.
- Sliding scale insulin coverage

A.M. Lab Results

	NORMAL VALUES	CLIENT VALUES
Potassium	(3.6–5.0)	5.6
Chloride	(98–107)	94
Creatinine	(0.7–1.5)	10
Blood urea nitrogen	(7–20)	50
Glucose	(70–110)	328

Client 2—Genevieve Morrison, age 60, 1 day post-op after a total hysterectomy. She has an IV of 5% glucose in H_2O. She has a PCA device of morphine sulfate 2mg/hr maximum. Her dressing has a moderate amount of bright drainage. She has not been out of bed since surgery. She is NPO. She may progress to clear liquids once bowel sounds are present and as tolerated. She is wearing thigh-high TED hose. Her hemoglobin and hematocrit (H&H) this A.M. was 10.2 and 34. She has an order for a unit of blood.

Client 3—Mules Brenerman, age 25, is scheduled for an open reduction with application of an external fixator of his right thigh this afternoon. He has been in Buck's traction since he was admitted following a motor vehicle crash 2 days ago.

CRITICAL THINKING

- Why was Mr. Brenerman placed in traction prior to his surgery?
- Before sending Mr. Brenerman to surgery, what procedures should be completed and why?

PRIORITIZING NURSING CARE

You need to prioritize your client's care. Outline your plan of care for each and provide rationales.

MANAGEMENT OF CARE

What procedures and safeguards are necessary when a client is to receive a blood transfusion? What care should be given prior to the transfusion?

COLLABORATIVE CARE

The lab calls the results to the nursing unit for Jake. What should you do about the lab report?

COMMUNICATION

Jake expresses concerns about his self-care when he is discharged. Outline important client teaching points that must be addressed and how you would evaluate Jake's learning and his ability to carry out his self-care.

DELEGATING

What tasks can be delegated to a nursing assistant? What follow-up is necessary?

CLIENT TEACHING

Mr. Brenerman will be discharged in a day or so. Provide him with necessary instructions for pin care once he is discharged. Describe what information he will need to know and what techniques you will use to be certain he understands the instructions.

DOCUMENTING AND REPORTING

What documentation needs to be completed for each of your clients? Write a nurse's note on each client using the Focus charting method.

Gerontology

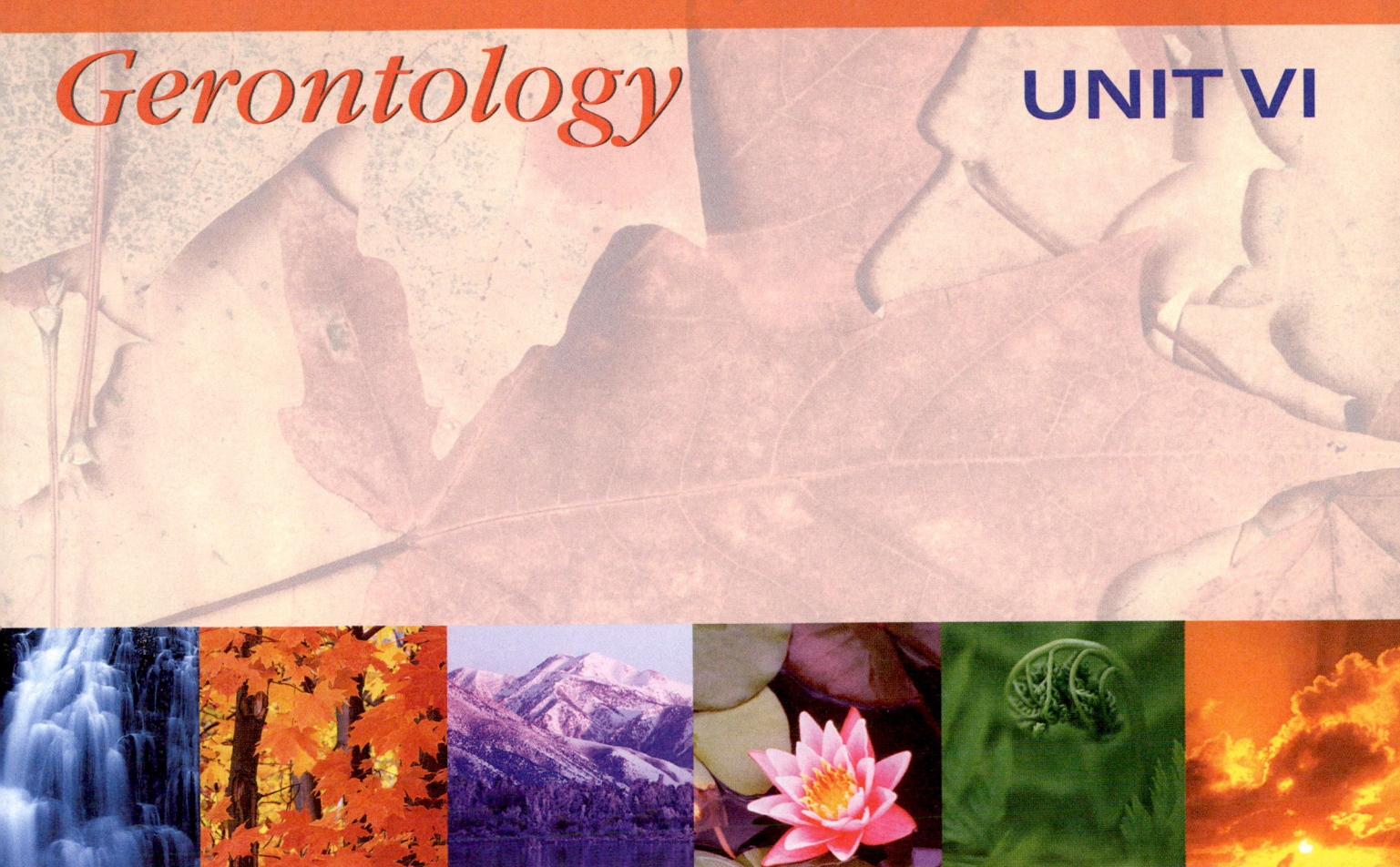

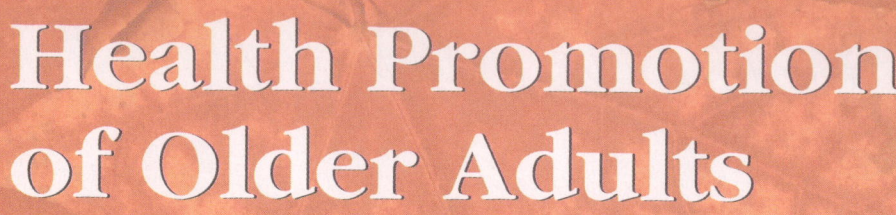

Chapter 42

Health Promotion of Older Adults

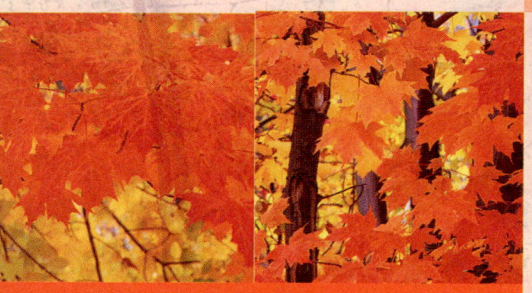

BRIEF Outline

LEARNING Outcomes

After completing this chapter, you will be able to:

1. Define the term *gerontology* and discuss its importance as a specialty.
2. Identify factors that affect the aging process.
3. Discuss normal physiologic changes of older adults by body system, including sensory changes and adaptations.
4. Identify ways of maintaining or restoring urinary continence.
5. Describe psychosocial challenges confronting older adults.
6. Identify special health concerns of older adults.
7. Identify important safety issues of older clients.
8. Discuss caregiver stress, factors that contribute to elder abuse, and client teaching to prevent elder abuse.

Clinical Objectives

9. Facilitate client and family discussion of home safety needs.
10. Provide client/family teaching on special nutritional needs of the older client.
11. Observe an LPN/LVN working in a senior center or adult day care.
12. Interview a well elder and perform a well-elder assessment.

KEY TERMS

Use the audio glossary feature on the MyNursingKit Website to hear the correct pronunciation of the following key terms.

arcus senilis 1190

assisted living facilities 1194

benign prostatic hyperplasia 1192

cataracts 1196

elder abuse 1198

geriatrics 1187

gerontology 1187

health conditions 1187

macular degeneration 1196

nocturnal myoclonus 1190

osteopenia 1196

osteotomy 1195

presbycusis 1191

presbyopia 1190

probiotics 1191

restless leg syndrome 1190

urinary incontinence 1191

Every day, thousands of the 75 million American baby boomers born between 1946 and 1964 turn 50 years old. The growing number of older adults has important implications for nurses. These clients are, and will be, seeking health care in increasing numbers.

Gerontology

The age of the older adult is usually defined as 65 years old and older. **Gerontology** or **geriatrics** is a health specialty that focuses on care of the older adult. It includes many methodologies of care, because older adults may have a wide range of health issues related to lifestyle and aging.

The effects of aging are cumulative. In youth and middle age, it may have been possible to ignore body needs and the importance of balancing work and personal/emotional/spiritual concerns. However, many people who reach older adulthood find that they have paid a price for ignoring those concerns. If they have not exercised and have led a very sedentary life, they are likely to begin to have serious health issues in older adulthood. If they have neglected their personal life in favor of work achievements, they may begin to feel anxiety or bitterness about unfulfilled aspects of life.

Fortunately, it is still possible for most to achieve a healthful lifestyle in older adulthood. Moderate changes that include more healthful foods in the diet, regular amount of enjoyable exercise, and involvement in areas of life that foster creativity can set a person on a path toward better health, no matter when the person begins.

As an individual ages, some slowing of body functioning and processes occurs. It becomes important to listen to and take cues from one's body. On some days a person may feel like 40 again and feel able to keep up with all the grandchildren. On other days, relaxing with a good book may be the right thing to do. Being aware of these different feelings may prevent illness and injury.

Older people require more time to recover from illness, injury, or surgery than they did when they were younger. Nurses should include information on recovery in client teaching, in order to be sure that clients understand this is normal. Also, people need to take extra care as they get older to avoid exposure to infectious or communicable diseases. Flu shots and pneumonia vaccines should be given to all clients 60 years of age and older, unless contraindicated by other health problems.

Factors that Affect the Aging Process

Different factors come into play when discussing the bodily changes that occur. These factors are health conditions, heredity or genetics, and the environment in which the person is living.

The term **health conditions** refers to the way a person has taken care of his or her body. The health conditions of an obese, sedentary smoker and of a lean, active nonsmoker are vastly different from each other. Both activity level and smoking habits have profound effects on the aging process. Inactivity and smoking lead to overweight, poor oxygenation of tissue, poor circulation, inefficient elimination (constipation), and heart problems. A healthy diet and regular exercise lead to a strong heart and lungs, healthy circulation, more efficient metabolism and elimination, and a greater sense of well-being from endorphins released during exercise.

Heredity and genetics play a large role in longevity and in the types of health concerns a person might face. Many health disorders seem to have a genetic link, such as heart disease and diabetes, two of the most prevalent causes of death in the United States. Being aware of the client's family health history can help the nurse to affect lifestyle changes that may lead to positive outcomes.

Environment will also be a factor in a person's aging process. Environment can be defined in many ways: from the physical home to the climate of the community or even to the emotional tone in which the individual lives. The fewer physical and psychological stressors a person encounters, the less likely the environment will adversely affect his or her health. A nurse may be aware of aspects of an aging person's environment that could be changed to increase well-being.

Innovative strides in health care continue to contribute to longevity and activity in the older adult. It is estimated

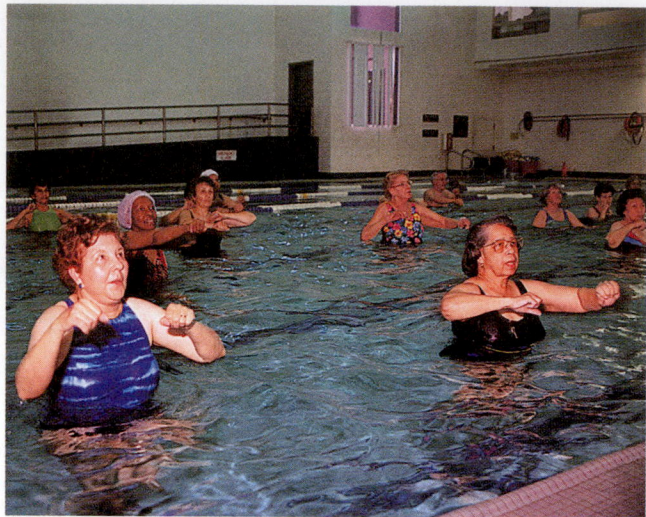

Figure 42-1. ■ Making adaptations in exercise in order to maintain regular physical activity is one way to slow the aging process.

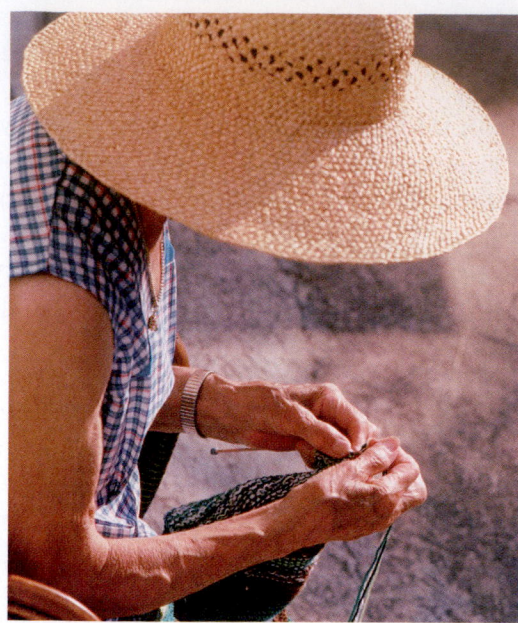

Figure 42-2. ■ Skin changes in the elderly are caused by loss of subcutaneous tissue and loss of elasticity. *Source:* Photo Researchers Inc.

that from 2010 to 2030, the number of adults age 65 and over will rise by 75%, to more than 69 million people. From 2030 to 2050, the number of adults in the over-65 age group will rise to approximately 79 million. Older adults are living longer (Figure 42-1 ■) and healthier existences due to knowledge about healthy lifestyles, exercise, and diet, as well as medical breakthroughs.

Physiologic Changes of Older Adults

The human body begins to change at birth. The older adult has experienced many changes throughout life, and the changes continue with aging. Predicting the time of these *physiologic* (bodily) changes is impossible. Even identical twins can age and experience bodily changes at different rates.

Many predictable changes can be observed in the older adult's physiology and structure. These changes are somewhat dependent on the factors listed above, and nurses can play an active role in promoting physical health among older adults.

Learning about physical changes that occur in the older adult helps the nurse know how to customize client care. The following text provides a system-by-system review of some of the more predictable changes that take place in the older adult.

INTEGUMENTARY SYSTEM

The older adult experiences *drier skin* due to a decrease in both tissue fluid composition and sebaceous gland activity. Older adults sweat less because they have fewer and less active sweat glands. This change in the sweat glands puts older people at risk for heat stroke or heat exhaustion.

The skin of older, light-skinned adults is a paler hue than that of their juniors. The skin becomes more fragile due to the loss of subcutaneous fat and reduced thickness and vascularity of the dermis (Figure 42-2 ■). Many older people feel the cold more readily than their juniors, and they are more susceptible to *hypothermia*.

Reductions in skin elasticity, fluid content, and subcutaneous fat lead to sagging, wrinkled skin. Assessing the older adult for dehydration can often be challenging for the nurse. When checking for skin turgor or "tenting," the nurse has to be innovative and assess areas that are not affected by wrinkling.

"Age spots" (*lentigo senilis*) are areas of brown pigmentation that appear on exposed body parts such as the hands, face, and arms. Skin care companies have a faithful following in the older population who buy products to minimize these skin conditions.

Hair changes as pigment cells are lost from hair bulbs. Hair turns gray or white and becomes thinner. Nails show aging by slower growth and increased thickening. Ridges along the nails are caused by an increase in calcium deposits.

MUSCULOSKELETAL SYSTEM

A gradual loss of calcium in the bone starts in the third to fourth decade of life. (See discussion of the musculoskeletal system and its disorders in Chapter 31 ⊚⊚.) The skeletal bones become thinner and weaker with each decade. Females lose approximately 8% of their skeletal mass with each passing decade. Males lose approximately 3% per decade.

Intervertebral disks shrink as the disks lose some of their fluid or cushioning. Disk shrinkage in the thoracic disks can give the older adult a stooped over appearance. This condition is called *kyphosis* (see Figure 31-13B ⬯). The combination of disk shrinkage and stooped posture results in an overall loss of height.

Reduced elasticity in the connective tissues leads to discomfort and *decreased mobility and flexibility*. Decreased muscle tone leads to a more flaccid appearance, and clothing may not fit as it once did. *Glycogen* (the fuel for muscles) is in reduced supply, so less fuel is available for muscle contraction. Anemia and respiratory problems can restrict available oxygen and lead to a buildup of cellular waste products such as lactic acid and carbon dioxide. These buildups can increase painful *muscle spasms* and *muscle fatigue*, even with minimal exertion. Decreased muscle tone and control can give the older adult the appearance of having a staggering or *unsteady gait*. Maintaining the client's safety is an important nursing intervention because falls contribute to fractures in this age group. Instruct the client and family in simple safety measures. For example, they can remove throw rugs and other objects that may cause the client to trip or fall.

RESPIRATORY SYSTEM

The marked decrease in body fluids in the older adult reduces their *ability to humidify air*. Mucous membranes in the nose are drier. Also, because the number of cilia in the nose is decreased, the body is less able to trap and get rid of debris in the nasal pharynx.

As vocal cords lose their elasticity, *changes in vocal pitch and quality occur*. The voice can develop a characteristic weak or tremulous sound.

The shape and size of the chest cavity is diminished due to musculoskeletal system changes. Cartilage located at the tips of the ribs calcifies, reducing the mobility of the rib cage. The intercostal muscles and diaphragm lose their elasticity, contributing to *decreased lung capacity* and *increased respiratory effort*.

Changes in structure affect overall functioning. Decreased ciliary movement, reduced tissue elasticity in the airway and alveoli, and reduction in the number of capillaries surrounding the alveoli can lead to *impaired gas exchange*. The combination of less elastic lung tissue and reduced physical exercise can cause an increased pooling of secretions in the lungs. This increases the older adult's risk of *respiratory tract infections*. The nurse can play an important role in educating clients to keep physically active. Older adults who remain active can minimize these potentially life-threatening conditions.

CARDIOVASCULAR SYSTEM

Unlike other muscles in the body, the heart does not get smaller or atrophy with aging. Instead, it increases slightly with age, and the left ventricular chamber wall gets thicker. There is reduced cardiac output and stroke volume, especially during unusual demands on the heart (e.g., exercise, excitability). The person may experience shortness of breath with activity, and pooling of the blood in the extremities. The arteries are less elastic (more rigid). *Baroreceptors* (special receptors in the heart) become less sensitive. (See Chapter 33 ⬯ for discussion of cardiovascular disorders.) As a result, diastolic and systolic blood pressures tend to increase. Orthostatic hypotension can occur because the body's circulation is slower and does not respond as quickly to postural or positional changes. (See blood pressure readings in Chapter 21 ⬯ .)

HEMATOLOGIC AND LYMPHATIC SYSTEMS

A decrease in body fluids in older adults causes slight thickening of the *plasma*, which as you remember is the fluid portion of blood and lymph. Bone marrow red and white blood cell production decreases slightly as well.

There are more immature T cells in older adults; this leads to a slower immune response. It also increases the person's risk for acquiring infections, especially urinary and respiratory tract infections. The nurse has many opportunities for teaching the older adult how to avoid these infections, which can lead to severe systemic problems. (Hematologic and lymph disorders are discussed in depth in Chapter 34 ⬯ .)

The changes in the immune response can mask signs and symptoms of infection. Body temperature changes (e.g., fever) may not appear until an infection is in the advanced stages. Furthermore, the older adult may not sense pain as quickly as a younger person because of overall physiologic changes.

IMMUNE SYSTEM

As people age, the immune system becomes less effective. It becomes less able to distinguish self from nonself. As a result, autoimmune disorders become more common. Macrophages destroy bacteria, cancer cells, and other antigens more slowly. This slowdown may be one reason that cancer is more common among older people. T lymphocytes respond less quickly to antigens, and there are fewer lymphocytes capable of responding to new antigens. Thus, when older people encounter a new antigen, the body is less able to recognize and defend against it.

Older people have smaller amounts of complement proteins than younger people, especially during bacterial infections. The amount of antibody produced in response to an antigen and the antibody's ability to attach to the antigen are reduced. These changes may partly explain why pneumonia, influenza, infectious endocarditis, and tetanus are more common among older people and result in death more often. Also, vaccines are less likely to produce immunity in older people. These changes in immune function may contribute to the greater susceptibility of older people to some infections and cancers (Merck Manual, 2003).

NEUROSENSORY SYSTEM

In older adults there is a gradual decrease in the efficiency of the body's temperature-regulating mechanism. This results in a decrease in body temperature and impairment of the body's ability to adapt to environmental temperature. Because of this physiologic change, the elderly are more susceptible to both hypothermia and hyperthermia.

Cellular changes take place in the brain, as in other parts of the body. The size and weight of the brain decrease. Shrinkage of brain tissue is linked to a decrease in circulating functional cortical neurons. There is a *change in mental acuity* as some of these cortical neuron cells are lost or change in function. Fatty deposits in the brain cause a decrease in cerebral metabolism. Elders may report that they "can still think, but it takes more time." (See more about the neurologic system in Chapter 36 ⊂⊃.)

Physiologic changes cause a *decrease in motor responses*. Reflexes become sluggish and slow. Loss of coordination is common. Tasks that require quick responses are harder for the older adult to do safely. Many older adults adapt their activities and lifestyles to avoid situations that could put themselves and others at risk (such as driving a car). As balance and coordination diminish, older adults should avoid climbing ladders or standing on chairs. They may begin using a cane or a walker for stability (see Figure 23-6 ⊂⊃).

Sleep efficiency diminishes with aging and is a common complaint of the older adult. Many clients in this age group complain of feeling tired during the day and are frustrated when they have to take frequent naps. Changes in sleep patterns result in less deep and refreshing sleep. Circadian rhythms also may change with aging, resulting in earlier bedtime and earlier rising. Additionally, the older adult may be awakened by the need to urinate, disturbing sleep even further. Nursing interventions include teaching relaxation techniques and teaching the client about decreasing stimulants (e.g., caffeine) before bedtime.

Insomnia can also be caused by medical conditions, medications, or psychological, environmental, or behavioral factors. Common medical conditions in the older adult that may lead to insomnia are arthritis, bursitis, GI disturbances, chronic obstructive pulmonary disease, congestive heart failure, and sleep apnea, to name a few. Night movement disorders, including **restless leg syndrome** (an uncontrollable movement of the lower extremities) or **nocturnal myoclonus** (sudden, repetitive kicking or jerking movements of the lower extremities), can add to insomnia in older adults.

Vision

The eyes incur many functional and structural changes with aging. The eyelids sag as they lose elasticity and thickness. Eyelashes may thin, become shorter, or even disappear. **Arcus senilis** (a benign grayish haze of the outermost part of the cornea) can sometimes be seen on visual inspection. It is more noticeable in persons with darker corneas.

Older persons often complain of dry, itchy, or burning eyes due to the *decreased tear production*. Without the mechanical and antibacterial protection of tears, debris and even the eyelid can irritate the eyes, and bacterial eye infections can occur more often.

The over-50 population commonly experiences **presbyopia** (difficulty focusing on close objects). Members of this age group often hold reading materials at arm's length. Presbyopia occurs because of decreased elasticity of the muscles of the eye and slower accommodation. Contact lenses, laser surgery, and prescriptive lenses are ways of correcting near- and far-sightedness. Laser surgery does not, however, correct presbyopia. (See more about accommodation in Chapter 19 ⊂⊃ and care of lenses in Chapter 20 ⊂⊃ .)

Astigmatism (blurring of objects seen at any distance) is caused by a malformation of the cornea. Younger persons can usually compensate by refocusing on the object. Older adults cannot compensate as well. This can be the cause of much frustration in the older person, but the condition can be managed with corrective lenses.

Night blindness (inability to see well at night or in diminished lighting, especially when driving) is a common occurrence with aging. Also, peripheral vision and depth perception often decrease with age. The older adult needs to be reassured that these conditions are normal. Clients with night blindness should be encouraged to avoid driving in the dark or in poor light. The condition creates a safety risk to the older person and others.

Clouding of the lens occurs with age, possibly causing a misperception of colors. Darker colors may be mistaken for black and even lighter colors may be misinterpreted.

Older persons often complain of flecks, spots, or crystals in their vision, commonly referred to as *floaters*. These are frustrating but harmless, although they can interfere with common activities such as reading, watching television, or doing hobbies.

It is important to note that a sudden occurrence of eye "floaters," or floaters accompanied by flashes of light or peripheral vision loss, could indicate a serious condition such as diabetic retinopathy, vascular abnormalities, or the beginning of a retinal detachment.

Hearing

The tympanic membranes in the ear become thinner as do other body tissues. The muscles that support the tympanic membrane show atrophic changes related to the aging process.

The older adult's hearing becomes altered. This condition is called **presbycusis.** It affects an estimated 13% of persons over the age of 65, with men affected more than women.

Smell and Taste

A decrease in the number of functional receptors in the nasal cavities and papillae on the tongue occurs with aging. This decrease may result in *altered smell or taste*.

Degeneration and loss of fibers in the olfactory bulb result in diminished sense of smell, which also affects taste. Older adults commonly report that they do not smell as well as before. They may say foods are not salty enough and may add more salt than is healthy to their food. They also may complain about food not having enough flavor or not being sweet enough. Atrophy of taste buds may lead to malnutrition and weight loss due to loss of taste.

Medications can also cause the person to have an altered taste for foods. In these situations, the nurse can reinforce teaching about healthful eating and reassure clients that the changes they are experiencing are normal and what to look for when taking certain medications.

Touch

A decrease in sensory receptors results in a diminished sense of touch; an inability to localize stimuli; and a decrease in appreciation of touch, temperature, and peripheral vibrations. Pain and touch sensations may also be reduced with age. The older adult may not notice a scratch, insect bite, or bump that later becomes a problem.

GASTROINTESTINAL SYSTEM

The bodies of older adults experience a decrease in digestive enzymes, a slower absorption rate, and a reduction in gastric pH. All of these together may contribute to indigestion or flatulence. There is also a tendency for decreased peristalsis and muscle tone of the intestines, causing constipation. (Modifications in the diet, such as relatively more protein and less carbohydrate, reduction in fatty foods, and an increase in fiber, can reduce some of these symptoms. **Probiotics**—foods or supplements containing live beneficial organisms—can help to restore or support healthy digestion.

With aging, there is an alteration in the mechanism that permits the swallowing reflex, causing delayed swallowing time. This can sometimes cause the older adult to experience a feeling like they are choking on their saliva.

Teeth may loosen and food may be harder to bite and chew. Good oral hygiene can slow some of the dental problems that indirectly affect the digestion (such as poorly chewed food).

ENDOCRINE SYSTEM

A normal age-related change in endocrine function occurs when the pituitary gland produces less growth hormone, resulting in decreased muscle mass. Some older adults experience a decrease in the production of thyroid-stimulating hormones manifested by a decreased basal metabolic rate and sensitivity to colder temperatures. The pancreas's function decreases with age but can meet normal body functions in the older adult. Endocrine system disorders (diabetes, hypothyroidism, etc.) are discussed in detail in Chapter 38 🔗.

URINARY SYSTEM

The number of working nephrons decreases in the older adult's renal system. Arteriosclerotic changes in blood flow show up as a reduced filtering ability of the kidneys and *impaired renal function*. (See full discussion of the renal system in Chapter 39 🔗.) The decreased tubular functioning of the kidneys can lead to a less effective concentration of urine. The aging bladder has less capacity and tone, causing *ineffective bladder emptying* and a tendency toward urinary frequency at night (*nocturnal frequency*). Older clients may be taught to stay away from caffeinated drinks and to reduce fluid intake in the evening hours.

Medical therapies often interfere with a client's normal voiding habits. When a client's urinary elimination pattern is adequate, the nurse helps the client adhere to normal voiding habits as much as possible. Guidelines to help the nurse assist clients to maintain normal voiding habits are listed in Box 42-1 ■.

Clients who are weakened by a disease process or are physically impaired require assistance to use the toilet. The nurse should assist these clients to the bathroom and remain with them if the client is at risk for falling. The bathroom should contain an easily accessible call signal to summon help if needed. Clients also need to be encouraged to use handrails placed near the toilet to assist them in standing or keeping their balance.

For clients unable to use bathroom facilities, the nurse positions toileting equipment close to the bedside (e.g., urinal, bedpan, commode) and provides necessary assistance to the client (see Chapter 20 🔗).

Continence Training

It is important to remember that **urinary incontinence** (inability to control urine excretion) is not a normal part of aging and often is treatable. Independent nursing interventions for clients with urinary incontinence (UI) include a behavior-oriented continence training program, prompted voiding, pelvic muscle exercises, positive reinforcement, meticulous skin care, and, for males, application of an external drainage device (condom catheter).

A continence training program requires the involvement of the nurse, the client, and support people. Clients must be alert and physically able to follow the directions in the program. The goal of continence training is to decrease the

---

BOX 42-1	**NURSING CARE CHECKLIST**

Maintaining Normal Voiding Habits

Positioning

☑ Assist the client to a normal position for voiding: standing for males; for females, squatting or leaning slightly forward when sitting. These positions enhance movement of urine through the tract by gravity.

☑ If the client is unable to ambulate to the lavatory, use a bedside commode for females and a urinal for males standing at the bedside.

☑ If necessary, encourage the client to press over the pubic area with the hands or to lean forward to increase intra-abdominal pressure and external pressure on the bladder.

Relaxation

☑ Provide privacy for the client. Many people cannot void in the presence of another person.

☑ Allow the client sufficient time to void.

☑ Suggest the client read or listen to music.

☑ Provide sensory stimuli that may help the client relax. Pour warm water over the perineum of a female or have the client sit in a warm bath to promote muscle relaxation. Applying a hot water bottle to the lower abdomen of both men and women may also foster muscle relaxation.

☑ Turn on running water within hearing distance of the client to stimulate the voiding reflex and to mask the sound of voiding for people who find this embarrassing.

☑ Provide ordered analgesics and emotional support to relieve physical and emotional discomfort to decrease muscle tension.

Timing

☑ Assist clients who have the urge to void immediately. Delays only increase the difficulty in starting to void, and the desire to void may pass.

☑ Offer toileting assistance to the client at usual times of voiding, for example, on awakening, before or after meals, and at bedtime.

For Bed-Confined Clients

☑ Warm the bedpan. A cold bedpan may prompt contraction of the perineal muscles and inhibit voiding.

☑ Elevate the head of the client's bed to Fowler's position, place a small pillow or rolled towel at the small of the back to increase physical support and comfort, and have the client flex the hips and knees. This position simulates the normal voiding position as closely as possible.

---

frequency of UI. A bladder training program may include the following:

- Education of the client and support staff
- Bladder training (Box 42-2 ■), which requires that the client postpone voiding, resist or inhibit the sensation of urgency, and void according to a timetable rather than according to the urge to void
- Delayed voiding, which provides larger voided volumes and longer intervals between voiding
- Pelvic muscle exercises, referred to as Kegel exercises, strengthen pelvic floor muscles and can reduce episodes of incontinence. The client can identify perineal muscles by stopping urination midstream or by tightening the anal sphincter as if attempting to hold a bowel movement. Then the client practices contracting and holding these muscles. Kegel exercises can be performed anytime, anywhere, sitting or standing—even when voiding.

REPRODUCTIVE SYSTEM

Female Reproductive Changes

In the female, significant changes have occurred as part of the aging process. The onset of *menopause* generally has occurred by age 50 as production of estrogen and progesterone decreases (see discussion in Chapter 40 🔗). During menopause the female may experience periods of flushing (*hot flashes*), which can cause her to be irritable, uncomfortable, or embarrassed. The female body stops producing eggs for fertilization, and the drive for procreation ends. External reproductive organs become less elastic, and subcutaneous tissue decreases. The external genitalia (labia) shrink and the amount of pubic hair decreases.

In postmenopausal women, there is less vaginal vascularity. The tissue is drier and more alkaline (instead of acidic as in the younger female). Vaginal secretions decrease and the resultant dryness may cause vulvar soreness and painful intercourse. Hormonal tablets or creams may be used to prevent dryness. Atrophy of the cervix, uterus, ovaries, and fallopian tubes makes them difficult to palpate during a manual examination. Because of the decreased hormone levels, breasts atrophy and sag.

Male Reproductive Changes

The older male adult continues to produce testosterone and sperm, although there is a decrease in the amount that is produced. Men well into their 80s can father children. The penis can still maintain an erection but may take longer to become erect.

The prostate gland enlarges in the older male (**benign prostatic hyperplasia** or BPH). BPH may cause frequent day and night urination, hesitancy, decreased force when urinating, loss of urinary control, increased urinary tract infections (see Chapter 40 🔗), and decreased ejaculatory force.

| BOX 42-2 | NURSING CARE CHECKLIST |

Bladder Training

☑ Determine the client's voiding pattern and encourage voiding at those times, or establish a regular voiding schedule and help the client to maintain it, whether the client feels the urge or not. The stretching–relaxing sequence of such a schedule tends to increase bladder muscle tone and promote more voluntary control.

☑ Encourage the client to inhibit the urge-to-void sensation when a premature urge to void is experienced.

☑ Instruct the client to practice slow, deep breathing until the urge diminishes or disappears. When the client finds that voiding can be controlled, the intervals between voiding can be lengthened slightly without loss of continence.

☑ Regulate fluid intake, particularly during evening hours, to help reduce the need to void during the night.

☑ Encourage fluids about half an hour before the voiding time between the hours of 0600 and 1800.

☑ Avoid excessive consumption of citrus juices, carbonated beverages (especially those containing artificial sweeteners), alcohol, and drinks containing caffeine because these irritate the bladder, increasing the risk of incontinence.

☑ Schedule diuretics early in the morning.

☑ Explain to clients that adequate fluid intake is required to ensure adequate urine production to stimulate the micturition reflex.

☑ Apply protector pads to keep the bed linen dry, and provide specially made waterproof underwear to contain the urine and decrease the client's embarrassment.

☑ Assist the client with an exercise program to increase the tone of abdominal and pelvic muscles.

☑ Provide positive reinforcements to encourage continence.

Psychosocial Changes and Adaptations

According to the philosophy of Erikson, the developmental task for this phase of life is *integrity versus despair*. Clients who are able to complete this task will view life and accomplishments with a healthy attitude and sense of wholeness as they look back on their lives (Figure 42-3 ■). Those who despair look at the past and wish they could change or relive their lives. You, as the nurse, may sense whether clients are dealing with this phase with integrity or despair (depression). (Depression in the older adult is discussed more in Chapter 43 ⬭.)

Older adults face many changes in this phase of their lives. Besides the physical changes, they face major changes economically and socially. Loss of spouse and friends can be a cause for depression, as can feelings of unfulfillment in their lives. Chapters 16 and 17 ⬭ discuss growth and development and psychosocial issues. Chapter 44 ⬭ provides a focused discussion of the care of chronically or terminally ill clients.

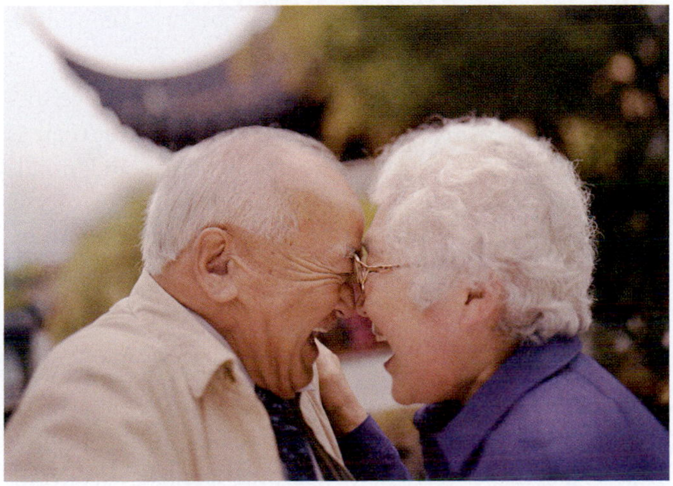

FINANCIAL CHANGES

The majority of older adults over the age of 65 are not employed. But, unlike in the past when people over 65 retired, a considerable number of older adults continue to work on a full- or part-time basis. Work offers an income, sense of fulfillment, socialization, and a dependable routine.

For some, retirement is used as a time to relax, visit family and friends, travel to destinations only dreamed about during their lifetime, and pursue interests they were too busy to pursue while they were raising families and working. This period of their lives can be very fulfilling.

However, the financial situations of older adults can vary greatly. Low retirement benefits or inadequate or nonexistent pensions often put a strain on what were supposed to be the "golden years." Housing, food, and medical costs can produce a huge financial burden. People with fewer financial resources face hardship and may lose independence.

As nurses, we should be familiar with the rising costs of health care and what is available to older adults to help reduce their financial burdens.

INDEPENDENCE AND FAMILY ISSUES

It is very important for older adults to participate in making decisions about their own lives. Their wishes should be respected as much as possible. They should not be ordered around or talked down to as if they were children. As

Figure 42-3. ■ Older adults who are satisfied with the lives they have lived are more likely to enjoy their later years. *Source:* CORBIS-NY.

nurses, we have to acknowledge the older adult's ability to think and to make decisions. Find out the wishes of the client and support that decision whenever possible in order to support the client's well-being.

In their later years, older adults often relocate from their homes. The family home may suddenly be too big for one or two persons. Home maintenance may be burdensome or impossible, and weather extremes may make older people virtual shut-ins.

Leaving familiar neighbors and surroundings can be very traumatic for the older adult. However, it is less traumatic if the older adult makes the decision voluntarily instead of being forced into a move. Loss of independence and related family issues need to be addressed long before changes in residence or level of care is needed.

One related issue in planning for older age is how families participate in care. The 40-to-50 age group has become what is known as the *sandwich generation*. Because of social changes over the past few decades, many adults in their 40s and 50s are "sandwiched" between older parents and offspring, providing care to both. Families have children in the home or are still providing financial and emotional support for offspring in college or graduate school. At the same time, their parents are aging and need or anticipate additional care and support.

Another issue affecting adults as they plan for older age is the care they may be providing to other members of the family. The number of younger grandparents who provide day care or even total parenting for their children's children is on the rise. In some cases, adults in late middle age essentially carry responsibility for four generations (their parents, themselves, their children, and their grandchildren). They also may have full-time employment outside the home. If their parents suddenly are unable to live independently, the family stress can seem insurmountable. Transitions can be smoother if the family has a plan for the future and discusses it with all generations before a crisis strikes.

Issues of this type will only multiply as life expectancy increases and the costs of health care rise for all generations of the family. Long-term care insurance can provide inpatient as well as in-home care for older family members, thus assisting with some day-to-day care and part of the financial burden. Many employers are offering this insurance as a benefit. It is best to begin long-term care insurance during middle age, because rates increase tremendously as retirement age approaches.

ASSISTED LIVING FACILITIES

Many older adults move to assisted living or long-term care facilities. The decision to make such a move usually occurs when older adults can no longer care entirely for themselves.

Assisted living facilities give residents the independence to be in their own apartments or condominiums, but offer nursing or medical care on the grounds. Often, help is offered with housework and other amenities. In these facilities, the older adult has many activities to choose from to maintain their social contacts. Such environments allow older adults to maintain their sense of dignity and self-respect. The nurse and family should encourage them to do as much as possible for themselves. It is important to emphasize safety in their environment (see also Chapter 9 ⊙). Items such as throw rugs and clutter should be removed for their safety.

Assisted living facilities are usually costly and can rapidly drain retirement funds. Some older adults instead move to one of their children's homes until the children are unable to meet their needs for care. Then the decision is usually made to move the parent to a long-term care facility. Nurses often play a role in listening to the concerns of clients and family as they make decisions about assisted living and long-term care (see Chapter 46 ⊙). Review therapeutic communication techniques in Chapter 11 ⊙ for ways to assist clients and families.

FACING DEATH

Many couples experience loss of a lifelong mate in this phase of life. It can be a time of loss, loneliness, and emptiness for the survivor. Grief for their mate can combine with thoughts of their own mortality, a normal feeling in reaction to loss. Many older adults are able to emerge from the grieving process and carry on with life. Others are not. Nurses must watch for signs of extended grieving and depression. Such patterns of behavior are unhealthy for the client. Those who have family and friends, are independent, have outside interests in community happenings and hobbies, and are financially secure have an easier time of adjusting to loss of a loved one. Older adults with strained financial resources and limited social support are most at risk. Nurses can encourage these clients to nurture relationships with children, grandchildren, and others.

Special Health Concerns of Older Adults

People in the United States are living longer than ever before. Many seniors live active and healthy lives. But there is no avoiding this fact: as we age, our bodies and minds change. However, there are things that can be done to stay healthy while aging. Eating a balanced diet, keeping mind and body active, not smoking, getting regular checkups, and practicing safety habits at home and in the car are all actions that help people make the most of life.

Much of the illness, disability, and death associated with chronic disease is avoidable through known prevention measures. Key measures include practicing a healthy lifestyle and use of early detection practices (e.g., screening for breast, cervical, and colorectal cancers, diabetes and its complications, and depression).

Critical knowledge gaps exist in responding to the health needs of older adults. Chronic diseases and conditions such as Alzheimer's disease, arthritis, depression, psychiatric disorders, osteoporosis, Parkinson's disease, and urinary incontinence reach all segments of the older adult population. However, much remains to be learned about their distribution in the population, associated risk factors, and effective measures to prevent or delay their onset.

A person who has been free of chronic or acute health problems until older adulthood may begin to feel that the body's "warranty" has expired. Problems begin to appear, and they need to see their healthcare provider on a more regular basis. Some of the most common health concerns are hypertension, arthritis (or degenerative joint disease), visual and hearing deficits, and osteoporosis. Some of the effects of these conditions can be prevented, and improved treatment can allow the individual to remain active.

HYPERTENSION

Many individuals, especially females who have always had normal or even low blood pressure, begin to experience an elevation in blood pressure. This is due in part to loss of elasticity of the vessels, and in part to the presence of plaque, which requires increased pressure to pump the blood. Adjustments have also been made in the recommended blood pressure levels, so more people are being diagnosed with hypertension. Box 42-3 ■ provides current recommended blood pressure readings.

OSTEOARTHRITIS/DEGENERATIVE JOINT DISEASE

Most of the time, the cause of osteoarthritis (OA) is unknown. It is mainly related to aging, but metabolic, genetic, chemical, and mechanical factors can also lead to OA. The symptoms of OA usually appear in middle age, and almost everyone has some level of OA by age 70. Before age 55, the condition occurs equally in both sexes. However, after age 55 it is more common in women. Very few older adults are able to escape OA completely.

Osteoarthritis can be primary or secondary. Primary OA occurs without any type of injury or obvious cause. Secondary OA is osteoarthritis due to another disease or condition. The most common causes of secondary OA are metabolic conditions, such as *acromegaly* (progressive enlargement of the head, face, hands, and feet caused by excessive secretion of a pituitary hormone), problems with anatomy (for example, being bow-legged), injury, or inflammatory disorders such as septic arthritis.

Manifestations

The symptoms of osteoarthritis include deep aching joint pain that gets worse after exercise or putting weight on it and is relieved by rest, joint swelling, morning stiffness, and limited movement. Clients may have grating of the joint with motion. Many state that joint pain is increased in rainy weather.

Diagnosis and Treatment

Diagnosis of osteoarthritis is by x-ray and clinical symptoms.

The goals of treatment are to relieve pain, maintain or improve joint movement, increase the strength of the joints, and reduce the disabling affects of the disease. The treatment depends on which joints are involved. The most common medications used to treat osteoarthritis are nonsteroidal anti-inflammatory drugs (NSAIDs). They are pain relievers that reduce pain and swelling. Types include aspirin, ibuprofen, and naproxen. Although NSAIDs work well, long-term use of these drugs can cause stomach problems, such as ulcers and bleeding.

Exercise helps maintain joint and overall movement. Water exercises, such as swimming, are especially helpful. Applying heat and cold, protecting the joints, using self-help devices, and resting are all recommended.

Good nutrition and careful weight control are also important. Losing weight reduces the strain on the knee and ankle joints.

Physical therapy can help improve muscle strength and the motion at stiff joints. Therapists have many techniques for treating osteoarthritis. Splints and braces can sometimes support weakened joints. Some prevent the joint from moving; others allow some movement.

Severe cases of osteoarthritis might need surgery to replace or repair damaged joints. Surgical options include:

- Total or partial replacement of the damaged joint with an artificial joint
- Arthroscopic surgery to trim torn and damaged cartilage and wash out the joint
- Cartilage restoration to replace the damaged or missing cartilage in some younger clients with arthritis
- Change in the alignment of a bone to relieve stress on the bone or joint (**osteotomy**)
- Surgical fusion of bones, usually in the spine

Possible Complications

- Decreased ability to walk
- Decreased ability to perform everyday activities, such as personal hygiene, household chores, or cooking

---

BOX 42-3	BLOOD PRESSURE VALUES

Blood pressure can change from minute to minute, with changes in posture, exercise, or wakefulness/sleep. However, blood pressure should normally be less than 120/80 mm Hg (millimeters of mercury) for an adult. Blood pressure that stays between 120–139/80–89 is considered prehypertension. Readings above this level (140/90 mm Hg or higher) are considered high (hypertension).

- Adverse reactions to drugs used for treatment
- Surgical complications

OSTEOPOROSIS

Osteoporosis weakens bones and makes them more likely to break. Anyone can develop osteoporosis, but it is common in older women. As many as half of all women and a quarter of men older than 50 will break a bone due to osteoporosis. (See Chapter 31 ⚭ for main discussion. Effects on older adults are shown also in Chapter 43.)

Risk factors for osteoporosis include getting older, being small and thin, having a family history of osteoporosis, taking certain medications, being a white or Asian woman, or having **osteopenia** (low bone mass).

Osteoporosis is a silent disease. Until a fracture occurs, the client is not likely to be diagnosed with osteoporosis. A *bone mineral density test* is the best way to check for bone health, and screening tests are recommended, especially for women with the risk factors described above.

To keep bones strong, the diet should be kept rich in calcium and vitamin D. Weightbearing exercise is recommended, and clients should be cautioned not to smoke. If needed, weekly or monthly medications to restore bone health are available.

Sensory Changes in Older Adults

VISUAL DEFICITS

Two of the most common visual problems affecting the elderly are cataracts and macular degeneration.

Cataract

A **cataract** is a clouding of the lens in the eye that affects vision. Cataracts are very common in older people. By age 80, more than half of all people in the United States either have a cataract or have had cataract surgery.

A person with cataracts commonly complains of blurry vision, colors that seem faded, and glare. They frequently cannot see well at night. They may have double vision or require frequent prescription changes in eyewear. Diagnosis of cataracts is made by the ophthalmologist or optometrist.

Wearing sunglasses and a hat with a brim to block ultraviolet sunlight may help to delay cataracts. Cataracts usually develop slowly. New glasses, brighter lighting, antiglare sunglasses, or magnifying lenses can help at first. Surgery is also an option. The cloudy lens is removed and replaced with an artificial lens (Figure 42-4 ■).

Age-Related Macular Degeneration

Macular degeneration, or age-related macular degeneration (AMD), is a leading cause of vision loss in Americans 60 years and older. It is a disease that destroys sharp, central vision. Central vision is needed to see objects clearly and to do tasks such as reading and driving.

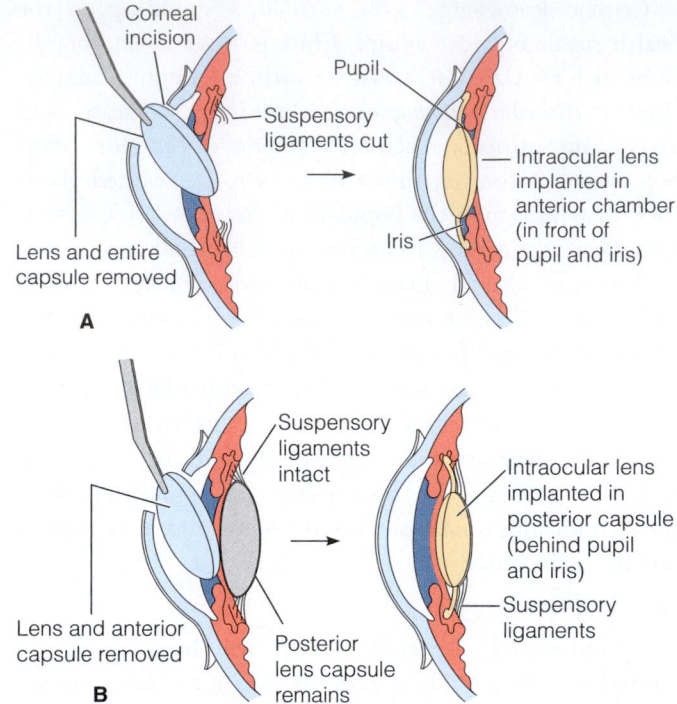

Figure 42-4. ■ Cataract removal with intraocular lens implant. **A.** Intracapsular cataract extraction with removal of the entire lens and capsule. The intraocular lens is implanted in the eye's anterior chamber. **B.** Extracapsular cataract extraction with removal of the lens and anterior capsule. Cataract surgery generally improves vision greatly.

Two types of macular degeneration have been identified, atrophic (dry) and neovascular (wet). The *atrophic form* results from an inadequate nutrient supply to the eye or inadequate waste removal as a result of vascular changes. With this type of macular degeneration, the central visual field is significantly diminished (Figure 42-5 ■). Vision is restricted but not entirely lost. The *neovascular form* of macular degeneration results from abnormal growth of very small blood vessels under the retina. These blood vessels cause leaking of fluid and blood and distortion of the retina from the swelling. This form of macular degeneration can cause severe vision loss. Laser or microsurgery to seal the

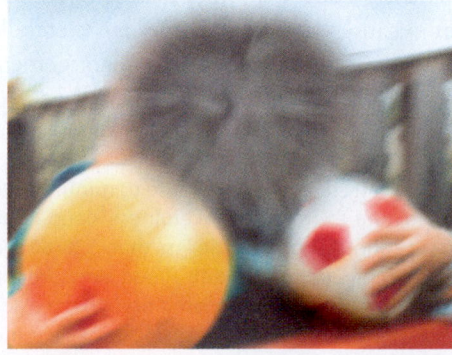

Figure 42-5. ■ Macular degeneration can cause loss of central vision.

leaking vessels is sometimes performed to prevent further loss of vision. Injection of an agent to slow neovascular formation is another commonly used treatment.

Although AMD affects the part of the eye that allows a person to see fine detail (the macula), it does not hurt. In some cases, AMD advances so slowly that people notice very little change in their vision. In others, the disease progresses faster and may lead to loss of vision in both eyes.

Regular comprehensive eye exams can detect macular degeneration before the disease causes vision loss. Treatment can slow vision loss. However, for most people treatment does not restore vision.

HEARING DEFICITS

The popular notion that older people are "hard of hearing" is often true. We are born with a set of sensory cells, and at about age 18 we slowly start to lose them. Because age-related hearing loss (presbycusis) progresses so slowly, most people do not notice any changes until well after age 50. According to the National Institute on Deafness and Other Communication Disorders (NIDCD), part of the National Institutes of Health, about 1 in 3 U.S. adults between the ages of 65 and 75 has a hearing loss. The NIDCD further estimates that about half of people 75 and older have some degree of hearing loss.

Presbycusis, which the NIDCD says usually affects both ears equally, is most commonly caused by gradual changes in the inner ear. As people age, structures of the ear can become less responsive to sound waves.

Hearing problems can make it difficult for older people to hear doorbells, car horns, and alarms. Hearing loss also can make it hard to understand and therefore to follow a doctor's advice or to respond to warnings. Its effect on speech communication can reduce a person's physical, functional, emotional, and social well-being. Isolation and depression often accompany hearing loss. All of this can be frustrating, embarrassing, and even dangerous. Box 42-4 ■ describes causes and manifestations of presbycusis.

Without being aware of it, people with presbycusis may make small adjustments over time. For example, they may stand closer to someone who is speaking, or turn up the TV volume to perceive the sounds and cues they otherwise would miss. At some point, though, the loss may become so severe that these adjustments become ineffective. Because the symptoms of presbycusis may resemble other more serious conditions or medical problems, it is important to consult a physician for a diagnosis.

Many times clients will complain of hearing loss (or hearing loss in a spouse) at a routine office visit. Hearing may be tested at the primary care physician's office with the same audiometer used for hearing screenings. The client may be referred to a specialist where more extensive tests are performed.

> ### BOX 42-4 CAUSES AND MANIFESTATIONS OF PRESBYCUSIS
>
> Presbycusis can be categorized by two types of causes, sensorineural and conductive.
>
> #### Causes of Sensorineural Hearing Loss
>
> The causes of sensorineural hearing loss include:
> - Disorders of the inner ear or auditory nerve
> - Hereditary factors
> - Various health conditions
> - Side effects of some medicines, such as aspirin and certain antibiotics
> - Repeated exposure to noise and loud music
> - Complex changes along the nerve pathways to the brain
> - Changes in the blood supply to the ear because of heart disease, high blood pressure, blood vessel conditions caused by diabetes, or other circulatory problems
>
> #### Causes of Conductive Hearing Loss
>
> Sometimes hearing loss is a conductive hearing disorder, meaning the loss of sound sensitivity is caused by abnormalities of the outer ear, middle ear, or both. Such abnormalities may include reduced function of either the eardrum or the three tiny bones that carry sound waves from the eardrum to the inner ear.
>
> #### Manifestations of Presbycusis
>
> Sounds often seem less clear and lower in volume with presbycusis. Most commonly clients report:
> - Sounds of mumbled or slurred speech by others.
> - Difficulty in distinguishing high-pitched sounds. (The progression of the loss begins with the highest pitches. Loss of the ability to hear high-pitched sounds such as "s" and "th" often makes it more difficult to tell them apart. Later, the ability to hear the lower pitches will be affected.)
> - Difficulty in understanding conversations, particularly when there is background noise.
> - Hearing men's voices more easily than women's.
> - Increased sensitivity to loud noises.
> - **Tinnitus**, a ringing, roaring, hissing, or other sound in one or both ears.

There is no way to reverse age-related hearing loss. Treatment is focused on functional improvement—compensating for the loss as much as possible. Hearing aids are the mainstay of treatment. These devices do not restore hearing to normal, but they do improve people's hearing ability and with it their ability to communicate. Box 42-5 ■ describes common types of hearing aids and the advantages and disadvantages of each.

Hearing aids, telephone amplifiers, and medical evaluations can help individuals with hearing impairment avoid social isolation and other problems associated with hearing difficulties. However, these options are not used by the majority of older people who could potentially benefit—perhaps because of embarrassment, because the hearing loss is underdiagnosed, or because hearing loss is undertreated.

BOX 42-5 | TYPES OF HEARING AIDS

- **Behind-the-ear:** This hearing aid carries sound to the ear through a custom ear mold. Behind-the-ear devices are useful for mild to severe hearing loss. Hearing aids attached to eyeglasses are a type of behind-the-ear hearing aid.
- **In-the-ear:** This hearing aid is custom made to fit in the outer ear. In-the-ear devices are useful for mild to severe hearing loss. No outside wires are visible because they are inside the device.
- **In-the-ear-canal:** This type of hearing aid is custom made to fit in the ear canal. In-the-ear-canal hearing aids help people with all but the worst hearing loss. There are no outside wires or tubes, and the devices are relatively inconspicuous. However, they are difficult to use with telephones.
- **On-the-body:** This hearing aid includes a case with a larger microphone, amplifier, and battery. On-the-body devices are for people with significant hearing loss. The case can be carried in pockets or attached to clothing. The on-the-body device is connected by a wire to an ear receiver attached to an ear mold. (Review illustrations of hearing aids in Figure 20-9 ⚭.)

Safety Issues for Older Adults

PERSONAL SAFETY

The elderly are more vulnerable to personal attacks, both because of their slower movements and reactions, and because of diminished strength and balance. Older persons should not travel alone in unsafe areas, especially at night. Cell phones can be used not only for convenience, but also for safety. The phone can be programmed for one-button access to summon assistance in an emergency. The cell phone's directory contains a number designated "ICE" (**i**n **c**ase of **e**mergency). Police, fire, and first responder personnel have been trained to look for "ICE" to reach the appropriate contact more quickly and efficiently.

Seniors who live alone may want to consider a "life alert" system. With these systems, a person can call for help by activating a button worn around the neck. The services can be customized for each senior's needs. Alert systems can provide seniors living alone with some added independence and give family members peace of mind.

FINANCIAL SAFETY

Some of the most troubling safety issues now facing the older members of our population are fraud, identity theft, and extortion. Elders who live alone are particularly vulnerable because the perpetrator is usually very friendly and provides contact for the individual who may be lonely. Senior citizens' groups and support services do their best to keep their members informed of current schemes aimed at defrauding seniors.

Seniors, like everyone, should guard their personal information. They should be reminded never to give bank account or credit card information to solicitors. If they are interested in a product, it is best to get a number and call back at a later date and time. Many attempts at fraud can be prevented in this manner. Anytime citizens feel threatened or fear that they may have been a victim of fraud, they should report the situation to local law enforcement personnel.

Older people who require hired caregivers in order to stay in their own homes should keep bank books, credit cards, and other financial information in a secure place. It is advisable for a family member, or the bank or other financial institution, to pay bills and manage accounts, rather than giving that responsibility to the caregiver.

As people continue to live independently into their 80s and 90s, there is a greater availability of services to support their independence. Shopping for groceries, prescriptions, and other items can be done by computer, phone, or mail and delivered. Personal services such as hair dressing, massages, cleaning, and alterations can be provided in the home.

ELDER ABUSE

Elder abuse is an action or inaction that results in harm to an elderly person or puts a helpless older person at risk of harm. This includes:

- Physical, sexual, and emotional abuse
- Neglecting or deserting an older person for whom one has responsibility
- Taking or misusing an elderly person's money or property

Elder abuse can happen within a family. It can also happen in settings such as hospitals or nursing homes or in the community. Elder abuse is a serious problem in this country. All 50 states have laws against elder abuse. The laws differ, but all states have systems for reporting suspected abuse.

There are many resources available to professionals and family members related to the prevention of mistreatment of the elderly. The National Center on Elder Abuse (NCEA) serves as a national resource center dedicated to the prevention of elder mistreatment. First established by the U.S. Administration on Aging (AoA) in 1988 as a national elder abuse resource center, the NCEA was granted a permanent home at AoA in the 1992 amendments made to Title II of the Older Americans Act. Since its inception, the NCEA has proved a valuable resource to adult protective services; national, state, and local aging networks; law enforcement; healthcare professionals; domestic violence networks; and others. The NCEA serves as a national clearinghouse of information for elder rights advocates, law enforcement, legal professionals, public policy leaders, researchers, and others working to ensure quality care for older adults.

Manifestations

Manifestations of elder abuse can be nonspecific. They include lack of cleanliness, unexplained weight loss, unexplained injuries or bruising, and/or indications that the client is fearful of his or her caregivers (Box 42-6 ■). The nurse should observe elderly clients closely for any such signs and report them to the supervisor immediately.

BOX 42-6   INDICATORS OF ELDER ABUSE

Physical Abuse Indicators

- Bruises and discoloration on inner arm/thigh, thumb/finger prints, choke marks, presence of old and new bruises in the same place, different colored bruises, and suspicious shapes caused by coins, cords, or belts used as restraints
- Scratches, cuts, pinch marks, cigarette burns, rope burns, and fractures
- Physical injury on head, scalp, or face (e.g, black eye)
- Bruises around breast or genital areas, unexplained vaginal or anal bleeding, or torn, stained, and bloody underclothing
- Physical restraint use not ordered by a doctor and used for the convenience of care provider (e.g., persons tied in bed, strapped into wheelchairs while slumping over, or sitting out of alignment)
- Drowsiness, dry and cracked lips, drooling, vacant stare from overmedication

Neglect Indicators

- Poor hygiene (e.g., unkempt appearance, stained or torn clothes)
- Dirty or uncut finger or toe nails
- Inadequate dental hygiene
- Signs of feces on resident or in bathroom and smell of urine
- Person lying in urine or feces
- Unexplained weight loss, malnutrition, and dehydration

- Person left unattended on the toilet
- Bruising or fractures from rough handling or frequent falls due to lack of attention
- Bedsores on buttocks, heels, elbows, shoulder blades, etc.
- Staffing problems in care facilities lead to neglect (e.g., limited number of staff on nights and weekends, staff inadequately trained or experienced for assignment, and high staff turnover)

Behavioral Abuse Indicators

- Fear, helplessness, resignation
- Implausible stories
- Anger, denial
- Withdrawal, hesitation to talk openly, nonresponsiveness
- Confusion or disorientation
- Depression, anxiety, agitation

Relational Abuse Indicators

- The elder is not given the opportunity to speak for himself or herself.
- Family or care providers restrict activity and outside contacts.
- Family or care providers do not allow the elder to be alone with anyone.
- Family or care providers provide conflicting reports on the condition of the elder.
- Suspicions of substance abuse by the caregiver.

CAREGIVER STRESS

An issue closely related to elder abuse is caregiver stress. Healthcare professionals, especially nurses who have the opportunity to observe interactions between a caregiver and care receiver, need to be aware of signs of caregiver stress. Although it is known that in 90% of all reported elder abuse cases, the abuser is a family member, it is not known how many of these abusive family members are in the caregiver role. Researchers have estimated that anywhere from 5% to 23% of all caregivers are physically abusive. Most agree that abuse is related to the stress associated with providing care.

Characteristics of the care receiver, or the relationship between the caregiver and receiver, can also be the cause of abuse. For example, when the relationship between the caregiver and the care receiver was poor to begin with, the caregiver is more likely to feel stress and to become abusive. Aggression by the care receiver also raises the risk of abuse.

The following should raise the concern of a professional in relation to elder abuse. The caregiver:

- Fears that he or she will become violent.
- Suffers from low self-esteem.
- Perceives that he or she is not receiving adequate help or support from others and views caregiving as a burden.
- Experiences emotional and mental "burnout," anxiety, or severe depression.
- Feels "caught in the middle" by providing care to children and elderly family members at the same time.

- Has "old anger" toward the care receiver that can be traced back to the past relationship.

The nurse would also be concerned if the following traits were seen in the care receiver. There is increased risk of abuse if the care receiver:

- Is aggressive or combative.
- Is verbally abusive.
- Exhibits disturbing behavior such as sexual "acting out" or embarrassing public displays.

Concern about abuse would be heightened if the caregiver and receiver live together, and if they had a poor relationship prior to the onset of the illness or disabling condition. It would also be a concern if the caregiver and receiver are married and have a relationship characterized by conflict. Box 42-7 ■ provides suggestions for reducing the risk of elder abuse.

NURSING CARE

PRIORITIZING NURSING CARE

When caring for elderly clients, focus your care on meeting physical and psychosocial needs. Observe normal and abnormal changes of body systems and report significant departures from the client's normal status. Assist clients as needed with physical care. Create a safe environment for clients who may have difficulty seeing or hearing potential dangers. Make adaptations in personal care to meet the unique needs of the

BOX 42-7   **CLIENT TEACHING**

Reducing the Risk of Elder Abuse

Reducing the risk of elder abuse by caregivers requires effort by the caregivers, professionals and agencies, and the community. Teach caregivers to do the following:

- Get help. *Making use of social and support services, including support groups, respite care, home delivered meals, adult day care, and assessment services, can reduce the stress associated with abuse.*
- Learn to recognize triggers. *Identifying stressors can help the caregiver to avoid, prevent, or seek respite from them.*
- Learn to recognize and understand the causes of difficult behavior. *The caregiver can then learn techniques to deal with these more effectively to lessen stress.*
- Develop relationships with other caregivers. *Caregivers with strong emotional support from other caregivers are less likely to report stress or to fear that they will become abusive.*
- Get healthy. *Exercise, relaxation, good nutrition, and adequate rest have been shown to reduce stress and help caregivers cope.*
- Hire helpers. *Attendants, chore workers, homemakers, or personal care attendants can provide assistance with most daily activities. Caregivers who cannot afford to hire helpers may qualify for public assistance.*
- Plan for the future. *Careful planning can relieve stress by reducing uncertainty, preserving resources, and preventing crises. A variety of instruments exist to help plan for the future, including power of attorney, advanced directives for health care, trusts, and wills.*

Professionals and agencies can:

- Screen caregivers and clients carefully for the risk factors associated with abuse.
- Provide caregivers with information and support to lower their risk.
- Provide instruction to caregivers (through materials, classes, websites, or support groups in conflict resolution and how to deal with difficult behaviors such as violence, combativeness, and verbal abuse).
- Promote better coordination between agencies that offer services for caregivers and those that offer protection of victims.

Individuals can help reduce the risk of elder abuse in the community. Concerned citizens can:

- Lend a hand to a caregiver who needs help.
- Report abuse. *In most communities, Adult Protective Services is the agency that accepts and investigates reports.*
- Advocate for public policies to increase the supply and scope of services available to caregivers.
- Volunteer. *Volunteers can make friendly visits, serve as guardians or bill payers, or provide respite care.*
- Arrange to have speakers make presentations on caregiving at churches, clubs, or civic organizations.

---

elderly client. For example, give routine baths three times a week unless otherwise ordered. The skin of the elderly client is dry, and sweat and oil glands produce fewer secretions than in younger people, so routine bathing is not needed as frequently. Give perineal care frequently for the incontinent client. It should be done each time an incontinence device is changed. Be sure to preserve the client's dignity and self-esteem. Address the client respectfully, and avoid using pet names such as "Gramps," "Grandma," or "Sweetie." Encourage clients to interact with one another to meet social needs. Make it a point to assist clients to activities within the care facility.

ASSESSING

When helping to collect data for assessment of older adults, it is important to keep in mind the physical changes that may affect the situation and the data collected. Ask about vision and hearing deficits early in the interview. A client who has a hearing impairment may need special interventions from the nurse (facing the client directly, modifying voice tone, writing questions on a note pad, etc.).

A number of concerns should be addressed, especially cognition, nutrition, sleep, and safety. If mental changes have occurred (loss of memory, depressed mood), physical causes for these changes should be explored. Weight loss or weight gain should be recorded and reasons for the change should be sought. Many older people have profound changes in sleep patterns. Lack of sleep and daytime drowsiness can lead to falls. Safety in the environment should also be assessed.

DIAGNOSING, PLANNING, AND IMPLEMENTING

- Adapt interventions as needed if the client has sensory deficit or mental acuity changes. *Older adults are more likely to have difficulty hearing, reading small print, and processing new information rapidly. Speaking slowly, using understandable terms, and providing written materials to read later are all good nursing interventions.*
- Inquire directly about physical changes that might be expected for the client's age. *Clients may feel embarrassed or ashamed and may not raise concerns unless asked. Using open communication methods is often effective with the older adult. Allow them time to think about their answers without pressuring them.*
- Allow time for clients to think and respond. *Older adults have reduced reaction time. Even when they are mentally sharp, they may need a little extra time to ask or answer questions.*
- Show respect for the cultural or religious views that older adults hold (Box 42-8 ■). *A person's cultural and spiritual affiliations can be a great source of strength for older adults. They can be a way of maintaining hope and meaning despite physical setbacks.*
- Check skin tenting for older adults on the upper chest. *The chest will provide a more accurate check on dehydration than the arm. Tenting on the arm may be exaggerated by muscle atrophy and wrinkling.*
- Have clients change positions slowly from lying to sitting or sitting to standing. Observe older clients as they come to a standing position. Compare blood pressure readings to the client's baseline. *Older adults are more prone to postural (orthostatic) hypotension and there is a risk for falls with*

BOX 42-8   CULTURAL PULSE POINTS

Cultural Views of Wellness and Illness

Culture influences the way we view aging as well as our views about wellness and illness. Older adults may continue to follow their cultural health practices as a means of preventing illness. They may use prayer, light candles, or wear an amulet. The nurse should find ways to reinforce client's views as they teach and promote other methods of health maintenance and health promotion. It is important for the nurse to address these issues in a nonjudgmental manner and to recognize that many cultural and religious practices and folk remedies actually work.

sudden changes. Blood pressure readings often are higher in older adults (see Table 21-1 ∞). The client's baseline blood pressure should be the reference point.

EVALUATING

Older adults may benefit from follow-up. Written materials or tapes that can provide or review information are very useful. The nurse can provide a great service to older adults who have few resources by informing them of services that are available for free or at little cost.

NURSING PROCESS CARE PLAN
Client with Independence Issues

Elvira Clemens is a 79-year-old widow who has recently moved to an active senior community. The community is about 400 miles away from the home where she raised her children and lived all her married life. Since her husband died 2 years ago, the children have been encouraging her to move closer to them. She has agreed to make the move but decided against living with any of the children. She has delayed selling her home until "I see if I like this place." Renee, Mrs. Clemens' granddaughter, has come today to help her get settled in her new apartment. The granddaughter suggests that they take a walk around the community to see what services and activities are available. Mrs. Clemens reluctantly agreed stating, "I really miss my friends and home. I'm sure there isn't anything going on that would interest me."

Assessment

Client is a 79-year-old female with mild osteoarthritis and mild hearing deficit in the right ear. She wears an in-ear hearing aid. Vision is well corrected with variable lenses. She has no serious health problems, is very alert, and her memory is intact.

Nursing Diagnosis

The following important nursing diagnoses (among others) are established for this client:

- *Risk for Loneliness*
- *Readiness for Enhanced Decision Making*
- *Readiness for Enhanced Spiritual Well-Being*

Expected Outcomes

The expected outcomes for the plan of care include the following:

- Participate in community activities on a weekly basis.
- Participate in a neighborhood get-acquainted tea.
- Meet with financial planner to discuss benefits and disadvantages of home sale.
- Participate in religious activities of her faith.

Planning and Implementation

- Discuss interests, hobbies, and activities that client previously enjoyed. *Thinking of enjoyable activities of the past may encourage the client to renew a past interest.*
- Encourage participation in one or more activities or groups. *Involvement with others will lessen loneliness and begin to build a feeling of community.*
- Verbalize the need to make long-term financial decisions. *Naming a task that needs doing is one way of bringing it into a person's awareness. This allows the person to reflect on what will need to be done.*
- Inquire about available services and activities at community churches. *Churches can be a good source of support.*

Evaluation

Mrs. Clemens attended a Get-Acquainted Tea with new and old residents in her neighborhood. She learned that several of the ladies played bridge, and she was invited to join the group since one of the players was moving away. She found that her next-door neighbor grew up in her hometown, so they planned to get together and reminisce. After a meeting with her financial planner, she decided to rent her home until the real estate market improves. The rent will increase her retirement income and the house will not be vacant, which was a concern for her. Another neighbor invited her to attend church services with her, and later she said, "The little church up the street is so nice. I felt right at home. The service is just like the one at First Church in Glenwood."

Critical Thinking in the Nursing Process

1. Why is it difficult for an elderly widow to leave the family home and familiar surroundings, even if it is to move closer to family members?
2. Why is it important to learn about interests a client has had in the past before suggesting involvement in new activities?
3. How can spiritual distress affect an individual's physical and emotional well-being?

Note: Discussion of Critical Thinking questions appears on the MyNursingKit Website.

Note: The references and resources for all chapters have been compiled at the back of the book.

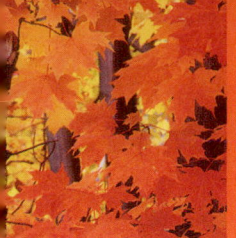

Chapter Review

KEY Points

- Gerontology is a growing healthcare specialty and one that encompasses a variety of methodologies of care, because the older adult may have many health issues due to the effects of lifestyle and aging.
- "Older adult" is usually defined as 65 years or older.
- Health conditions refer to the way a person has taken care of his or her body. Although changes of aging are normal, diet and exercise can retard the inevitable changes.
- Factors that influence body changes are heredity, genetics, and environment.
- Certain predictable changes occur as the human body ages.
- Changes in the immune response can mask signs and symptoms of infection.
- Body temperature changes may not be evident in the older adult until an infection is in the advanced stage.
- The heart does not atrophy with aging as do other muscles in the body; instead, it enlarges.
- Cardiovascular disease is the leading cause of death in the United States and accounts for more than 75% of the deaths in persons over the age of 65.
- Most body systems are less efficient in the older adult.
- Decrease in subcutaneous fat and slowing of circulating blood volume lead to circulatory problems and cold extremities.

∞ FOR FURTHER Study

Safety in the environment is discussed in Chapter 9.

For a discussion of therapeutic communication techniques, see Chapter 11.

Chapters 16 and 17 discuss growth and development and psychosocial issues, respectively.

See more about visual accommodation in Chapter 19.

Review Chapter 20 for care of contact lenses and hearing aids (Figure 20-9), and for providing assistance to clients needing a urinal, bedpan, or commode.

Procedures for taking blood pressure readings and adaptations for orthostatic hypotension appear in Chapter 21. Normal vital signs by age are found in Table 21-1.

Assistive devices such as canes and walkers are shown in Figure 23-6.

Care of clients with musculoskeletal disorders, such as kyphosis (Figure 31-13B), is discussed in Chapter 31.

See Chapter 33 for discussion of cardiovascular and peripheral vascular disorders.

Disorders of blood and lymphatic disorders are discussed in depth in Chapter 34.

See Chapter 36 for disorders of the nervous system.

Endocrine system functions and disorders (diabetes, hypothyroidism, etc.) are discussed in detail in Chapter 38.

Care of clients with renal system disorders is discussed in Chapter 39.

See Chapter 40 for discussion of reproductive disorders.

Depression in the older adult is discussed more in Chapter 43.

Chapter 44 discusses care of the chronically or terminally ill person.

For a description of long-term care, see Chapter 46.

Caring for a Client with Macular Degeneration

NCLEX-PN® Focus Area: Safety

Case Study: Raymond Page is a 93-year-old male retired college professor who until recently continued to guest lecture. He lives in his own home with his wife of 66 years. She is recovering from a stroke and has a daily caregiver who assists with personal care, meals, and housekeeping. Dr. Page was diagnosed with macular degeneration approximately 18 months ago. He is seen by an eye specialist who is treating the macular degeneration with monthly injections. His vision deficit had progressed to the point that he is unable to read even jumbo print text. Several months ago he was seen by a low vision specialist, who prescribed eyeglasses to assist with reading. The treatment has not been completely satisfactory. He has also attempted to use a reader, but finds it difficult to manage. He continues to be quite active and independent. He regularly attends church services and weekly service club meetings. He is able to do all personal care. Handling his medications seems to be the most pressing problem at this time. Because he cannot see, they must be put out for him both morning and night. Though his daughter puts them out for him, he frequently misses doses. This is worse when she is out of town and he gets very confused, missing doses, and ending up in the emergency room with effects of hypertension.

Nursing Diagnosis: *Ineffective Therapeutic Regimen Management*

COLLECT DATA

Subjective	Objective
_____	_____
_____	_____
_____	_____
_____	_____
_____	_____

Would you report this? Yes/No

If yes, report to: _____

What would you report? _____

Nursing Care

_____
_____
_____
_____
_____
_____
_____
_____

How would you document this? _____
_____
_____

Compare your answers and documentation to those provided on the MyNursingKit Website.

Data Collected
(use only those that apply)

- Height 5′11″
- Weight 128 lbs; 5-lb weight loss
- Has a good appetite, eats three full meals daily with one or more snacks
- VS: T 97.8 P 76 R 20 BP 188/90
- Daily medications: Flomax 0.4 mg H.S.; Plavix 75 mg q.d.; Lipitor 20 mg q.d.; Nitro spray 1 X 3 PRN; Restoril 15 mg H.S.; Isordil 40 mg ER; Calan SR 120 mg
- Calcium 1200 mg; multivitamin; vitamin E 400 IU; Occuvite 1 daily
- History of TIA—"I do not remember if I took my medication this morning." "I feel like I am having a stroke."
- Uses walker when going outside; has Life-Alert alarm for safety
- "I just can't see anymore, and I am so forgetful. I just can't seem to get the words out."

Nursing Interventions
(use only those that apply; list in priority order)

- Discuss medication routine with client, family members, and caregiver.
- Explain to caregiver the importance of placing medication and other needed items in the same place so he can easily find them.
- Arrange for home safety assessment.
- Monitor blood pressure weekly.
- Assess client's feelings, values, and reasons for not following plan of care.
- Identify support groups related to the disease process.
- Monitor weight and dietary intake.
- Encourage client to take extra time when expressing thoughts.
- Arrange for home health nurse visit.

NCLEX-PN® Exam Preparation

TEST-TAKING TIP Read each question thoroughly. As you are reading, formulate in your mind the intent of the question, then read all of the answers. Go with the most correct answer and avoid assigning hidden meanings to the questions and answers.

1 The nurse, working on a geriatric unit, anticipates that all of the clients will be over the age of:
1. 60.
2. 65.
3. 70.
4. 72.

2 The nurse recognizes all of the following factors will impact body changes in geriatric clients except:
1. Life choices.
2. Heredity.
3. Genetics.
4. Marital status.

3 The nurse is caring for a geriatric client with new onset of incontinence. Which of the following would the nurse view as potentially contributing to the client's inability to remain continent?
1. Assisting the client to a normal position for voiding.
2. Providing privacy for the client to void.
3. Offering toileting assistance to the client at usual times of voiding.
4. Encouraging the client to delay voiding to build bladder capacity.

4 The nurse is caring for a client who voices sadness at the choices made throughout life and tells the nurse, "I wish I could go back and do things differently." The nurse recognizes that this client is experiencing what Erikson described as:
1. Integrity.
2. Despair.
3. Suicidal ideation.
4. Normal reflective behavior.

5 The client says, "My blood pressure has always been on the low side. Why is it suddenly getting higher and higher as I get older?" The nurse's best response would be:
1. "Perhaps you should drink less fluid."
2. "You are probably eating too much sodium."
3. "As you age your heart doesn't work as effectively so this causes your blood pressure to elevate."
4. "As you age the blood vessels lose elasticity and develop plaque, which increases the pressure required to pump blood."

6 The nurse makes a home visit for a geriatric client at risk for falls and recommends doing which of the following to reduce the client's level of risk?
1. Obtain a life alert system.
2. Keep a cell phone nearby at all times.
3. Remove throw rugs.
4. Never give out bank account or credit card information.

7 The nurse is caring for an elderly client admitted to the facility today. When the admission assessment is performed, the nurse notes which of the following as an indication of possible abuse? (Select all that apply.)
1. Unexplained bruising
2. Unexplained weight loss
3. Fearful attitude toward caretaker
4. Moments of sudden tearfulness
5. Inability to afford their prescription medications.

8 The nurse, working in a physician's office, admits a client diagnosed with Alzheimer's disease accompanied by his daughter. The daughter says, "I am so tired. He doesn't sleep at night and I have to watch him night and day." The nurse recognizes the daughter is experiencing:
1. Sleep deprivation.
2. Caregiver role strain.
3. A dilemma about putting her father in a nursing home.
4. A bad day that will improve with a good night's sleep.

9 Which of the following would be of more concern to geriatric clients than to younger clients?
1. Osteoarthritis
2. Cancer
3. Heart disease
4. Phlebitis

10 Mrs. A asks you the medical name for the brown spots on her hands and arms. You tell her the name of this condition is:
1. Arcus senilis.
2. Lentigo senilis.
3. Osteo senilis.
4. Rosacea.

Answers and rationales for Review Questions appear in Appendix I.

Chapter 43

Nursing Care of Ill Older Adults

LEARNING Outcomes

After completing this chapter, you will be able to:

1. Discuss the role of the LPN/LVN in providing nursing care for ill older adults.
2. Describe common disorders of older adults by body system.
3. Identify specific needs and appropriate nursing interventions for the ill older client with an acute illness.
4. Discuss specific issues related to medication administration for older clients.

Clinical Objectives

5. Carry out the admission procedure for an older client in the hospital.
6. Provide special skin care for an older client.
7. Provide client teaching about multiple medications.
8. Interact with the older client and family members in ways that respect the client's dignity.

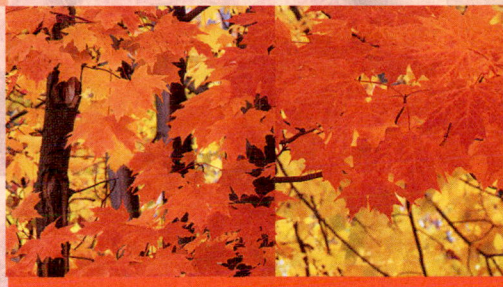

BRIEF Outline

Role of LPNs/LVNs
Abnormal Changes in Older Adults
Special Concerns of the Hospitalized Older Adult

Use the audio glossary feature on the MyNursingKit Website to hear the correct pronunciation of the following key terms.

bunions 1207	**gout** 1207	**polypharmacy** 1214
bursitis 1207	**hammertoe** 1207	**priapism** 1213
cardiomegaly 1208	**hypoglycemia** 1212	**reflux** 1212
congestive heart failure 1208	**malaise** 1214	**retinal detachment** 1211
diabetic retinopathy 1211	**mitral regurgitation** 1208	**rosacea** 1206
diplopia 1210	**mitral valve prolapse** 1208	**sundowning** 1210
glaucoma 1210	**otosclerosis** 1211	

In the United States, more adults are living into old age than ever before, and many have long, healthy lives. However, when illness occurs, a person's age may be a factor both in the speed of recovery and in the care required to reach recovery. This chapter focuses on caring for older adults who experience acute illness. (Chapter 42 ⚭ described health promotion in older adults. Chapter 44 ⚭ will describe care of chronically or terminally ill clients of all ages. Chapter 46 ⚭ will discuss specifics of long-term and rehabilitation care.)

Role of LPNs/LVNs

An LPN/LVN may be assigned to nursing care for older adult clients admitted to the hospital with an acute illness. Basic nursing care duties will not change based on age. (A complete history and physical assessment will be obtained. Medications will need to be administered on schedule, and procedures will be performed according to the established plan of care.) However, the ill older adult may have age-related changes or chronic conditions underlying the acute illness. These conditions make caregiving more complex and require special attention.

The LPN/LVN will often be required to adapt interventions for ill older adults. For example, an older adult with osteoarthritis may require additional time for ADLs, treatments, and procedures. Since loss of independence is an issue for older adults, the nurse will need to balance the need to complete tasks quickly with the client's need to feel a measure of control over his or her life. Also, older adults with cognitive deficits may need extra time and patience when the nurse is providing client teaching.

Abnormal Changes in Older Adults

In addition to the factors mentioned above, some abnormal changes may occur in older adults, and the LPN/LVN must be aware of them. These conditions are reviewed by body system in the following pages.

INTEGUMENTARY SYSTEM

As with other body systems, environmental and genetic factors play a role in skin disorders. *Basal cell carcinoma* (see Figure 30-12A ⚭) is commonly seen in older adults who have spent significant amounts of time outdoors in the sun. Older adults should be taught to examine their skin for suspicious pigmented areas that change in shape or color or that bleed when touched.

Skin infections and inflammation are common in the older adult and mostly occur on exposed skin surfaces such as the face, scalp, hands, arms, and legs. (See Chapter 30 ⚭ for integumentary skin disorders.) Different forms of *dermatitis* are common. Dermatitis can be frustrating to the older adult because it is sometimes difficult to cure. Allergic and contact dermatitis appear as rashes or inflamed areas on the skin. The reaction may be localized or generalized. The offending substance may be difficult to identify, but isolating the cause of the irritation is the only solution to a cure.

Rosacea is an inflammation that appears as reddened dilated blood vessels and small eruptions or pimples on the nose and center of the face. The affected area may spread to cover the chin and cheeks. If this condition is left untreated, it can progress to swelling and enlargement of the nose and may also cause conjunctivitis.

Bruising and skin tears can occur easily in the older adult. If not treated, they can develop into hematomas or infections. Nosocomial infections such as staph or MRSA are a constant concern among ill older adults with decreased immunity. (MRSA and nosocomial infections are discussed in depth in Chapter 10 ⚭. A chart of communicable diseases is provided in Chapter 60 ⚭.)

Pressure ulcers are seen more commonly in the older adult due to the loss of the protective cushioning and decreased circulation. Also, poor nutritional status (especially poor protein intake) can contribute to pressure ulcers. Older persons who are immobile, bedridden, or inactive are prone to pressure ulcers (see full discussion with wound care in Chapter 24 ⚭). Regular attention to the skin of these clients, judicious skin care, and frequent turning reflect good nursing care and can ward off future complications.

Herpes zoster, also known as *shingles*, is a common infection of the nerves that supply certain areas of the skin. (Herpes zoster was discussed with integumentary disorders in Chapter 30 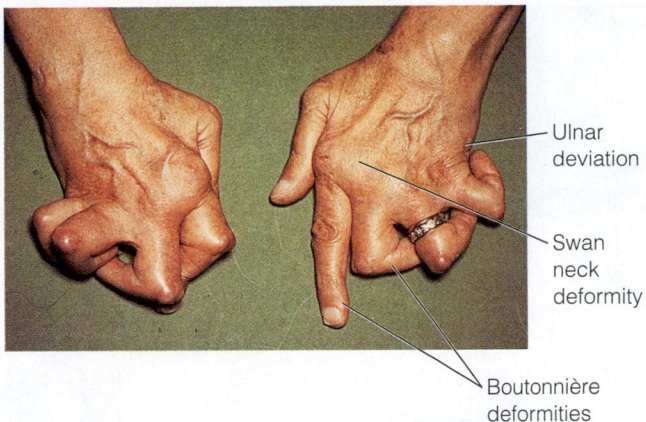.) It causes a painful rash of small, crusting blisters that may persist for months. In fact, the older the client and the more pronounced the rash, the more likely the pain will be severe and persistent. Palliative measures and pain management are the biggest nursing interventions for these clients.

Figure 43-2. ■ Typical hand deformities of late rheumatoid arthritis.

clinical ALERT

The Advisory Committee on Immunization Practices of the Centers for Disease Control and Prevention has recommended that everyone age 60 and older receive the Zostavax vaccine to prevent herpes zoster. This recommendation includes those who have already had shingles.

MUSCULOSKELETAL SYSTEM

Osteoporosis is an excessive loss of calcium from the bone so that the supply of calcium is not enough for the body's demand (Figure 43-1 ■). Postmenopausal women and inactive or immobilized persons are most at risk for osteoporosis. Spontaneous fractures occur because the bones are brittle, fragile, and porous. Common fracture sites are the hip, ribs, arm, and clavicle. Fractured hips and compression fracture of the spine are the two most common types of fracture seen in the older adult. Hip fractures often lead to other complications and even death.

Degenerative joint disease or *osteoarthritis* is a painful condition caused by wear and tear on the joints. This is the most common form of arthritis and is common in the older adult population. The exact cause is unknown but researchers know that genetic, chemical, hormonal, and mechanical factors are involved in this disease process.

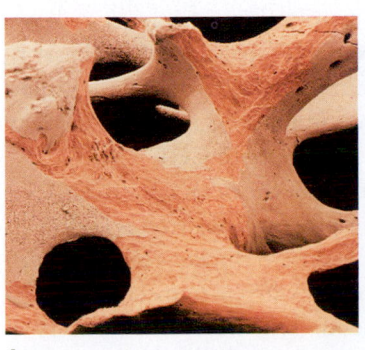 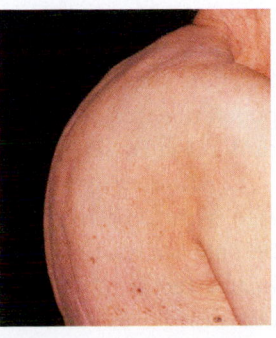

A   B

Figure 43-1. ■ ■ A. Osteoporosis in a hipbone. Note the areas that appear spongy. *Source:* Photo Researchers, Inc. **B.** Excessively curved spine, or kyphosis, seen in an 87-year-old woman suffering from crush fractures caused by osteoporosis. *Source:* Photo Researchers, Inc.

Osteoarthritis is treated with nonsteroidal anti-inflammatory drugs (NSAIDs), corticosteroid injections, heat therapy, and rest. For extreme cases, total joint replacement surgery may be necessary to relieve the pain and improve the quality of the person's life.

Rheumatoid arthritis is an autoimmune disease that strikes mostly women. It is characterized by inflammation of the lining of the joints and/or other internal organs (Figure 43-2 ■). The inflammatory cells release enzymes that digest bone and cartilage, causing pain, heat sensations, redness, swelling, and stiffness. The treatment is the same as osteoarthritis: NSAIDs, corticosteroids, disease modifying antirheumatic medications, and surgery to replace the painful deformed joints.

Bursitis (inflammation of the bursa and the adjoining fibrous tissue) can result from infection or excessive stress and strain on a joint. Common areas where bursitis occurs are the elbow, shoulder, and knee. Bursitis can be very painful and can cause the person to guard the area, leading to restricted movement. It is often treated with NSAIDs. If persistent, corticosteroid injections may be used.

Gout, or gouty arthritis, is caused by an elevation in uric acid levels in the body (see also Chapter 31). Uric acid crystals are deposited in joints and tissues, causing severe joint swelling and pain. The joint most commonly affected is the great toe, making it painful for the person to walk. Fever and chills may also be present. If ignored, gout can result in joint destruction.

Bunions (a firm, fluid-filled pad or bursa), found overlying the inside of the joint at the base of the big toe, and **hammertoe** (a deformity of the toe, usually the second toe, that causes the main toe joint to bend upward like a claw) are both serious problems for the older adult (Figure 43-3 ■). Both can be painful and can contribute to reduced mobility. Corrective shoes and occasionally surgical correction are needed.

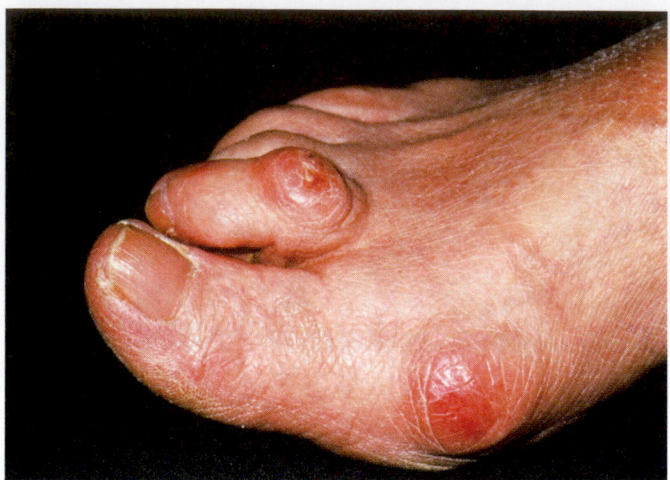

Figure 43-3. ■ Close-up of a 75-year-old woman's foot deformed by a hammertoe and bunions. Hammertoe is usually, as in this case, seen in the second toe where the main toe joint stays bent. A painful corn (of hard, horny skin) has developed on the joint which tends to rub against footwear. A bunion is seen as a deformity (an inflamed joint) at the base of the big toe. A fluid-filled pad has developed (known as a bursa) on this joint, also due to friction. The underlying cause of bunions is hallux valgus, where the joint at the base of the big toe points outward. *Source:* Photo Researchers, Inc.

RESPIRATORY SYSTEM

With all of the changes in the older adult's respiratory system, it is common to see several respiratory disorders. (Respiratory disorders are discussed in depth in Chapter 32 ⦾ .)

A common respiratory disorder in the older adult is *chronic obstructive pulmonary disease* (COPD). COPD is not a single disorder but a set of disorders that include chronic bronchitis, asthma, and emphysema. It is common in persons with a history of smoking or exposure to a high level of pollutants in the environment. The person with COPD has a productive cough, cyanosis because of insufficient air exchange, wheezing, and dyspnea on exertion. Because these persons are at a higher risk of developing respiratory tract infections due to the decreased gas exchange and decreased cilia, their symptoms can easily develop into respiratory failure.

Respiratory tract infections (both upper and lower) can cause serious problems for the older adult. Both the common cold and pneumonia can be deadly to an older adult whose body is already immunocompromised due to the normal aging process or present disease.

Tuberculosis, commonly called TB, was once a major killer. TB is an infectious disease passed from person to person in airborne droplets (produced by coughing and sneezing). It is then breathed into the lungs and causes an inflammatory response, leaving behind a scar. Although today's drugs are very effective in management and prevention of future episodes, drug-resistant strains have developed. The treatment of TB is long and requires careful follow-up to ensure a cure and to prevent increased resistance from developing.

CARDIOVASCULAR SYSTEM

Cardiovascular disease accounts for more than 75% of the deaths in persons over the age of 65. By the seventh decade of life, the older adult has some degree of coronary disease. Coronary arteries carry the blood supply to the heart. If these arteries narrow or become obstructed, the heart may not receive the nutrients and oxygen it needs for adequate functioning. When this happens, the area of the heart affected becomes damaged (*ischemic*). Pain from ischemia (called *angina pectoris*) manifests itself in many different ways. Some clients feel mild to severe pain in the chest, pain down the left or right arm, GI distress, or shortness of breath. Others have no symptoms at all. When one or more coronary arteries are completely blocked, the person has a heart attack or *myocardial infarction* (MI). Symptoms of an MI include chest pain or discomfort, confusion, syncope (fainting), diaphoresis, and jaw or arm/shoulder pain. (See the main discussion of cardiovascular disorders in Chapter 33 ⦾ .)

Coronary artery bypass surgery, stent placement, angioplasty, and laser angioplasty are quite common procedures in older adults. They can be performed if severe atherosclerotic occlusion of the coronary arteries is detected before a total occlusion happens. If the client has an MI caused by an embolus that is rapidly detected, the embolus can be treated using fibrinolytic agents (e.g., streptokinase). These agents can prevent permanent damage to heart muscle but also carry precautions and cannot be used in all clients.

Coronary valve disease is another disorder that may arise in older adults. In coronary valve disease, calcium deposits on the valves prevent them from closing correctly. Coronary valve disease can result in **mitral regurgitation** (backflow of blood from the left ventricle into the left atrium; Figure 43-4 ■), **mitral valve prolapse** (displacement of the mitral valve usually due to benign proliferative changes of the valve leaflets), and congestive heart failure. The client with mitral valve prolapse experiences chest pain, fatigue, dyspnea, and palpitations.

Congestive heart failure (CHF; inability of the heart to function effectively as a pump) mostly affects the aging population (see manifestations in Figure 33-17 ⦾ .) Many cardiovascular diseases can contribute to CHF.

Cardiomegaly (enlargement of the heart) is often associated with CHF. In the aging process, the arteries and veins become less elastic. The left ventricle thickens (*hypertrophies*) in an attempt to improve cardiac output to meet the body's demands for oxygenated blood. The decreased elasticity of arteries and veins causes the heart to work harder. Increased resistance in the pulmonary circulation causes the right side of the heart to enlarge. If one side of the heart weakens, it is inevitable that the other side will weaken due to the added stress placed on it.

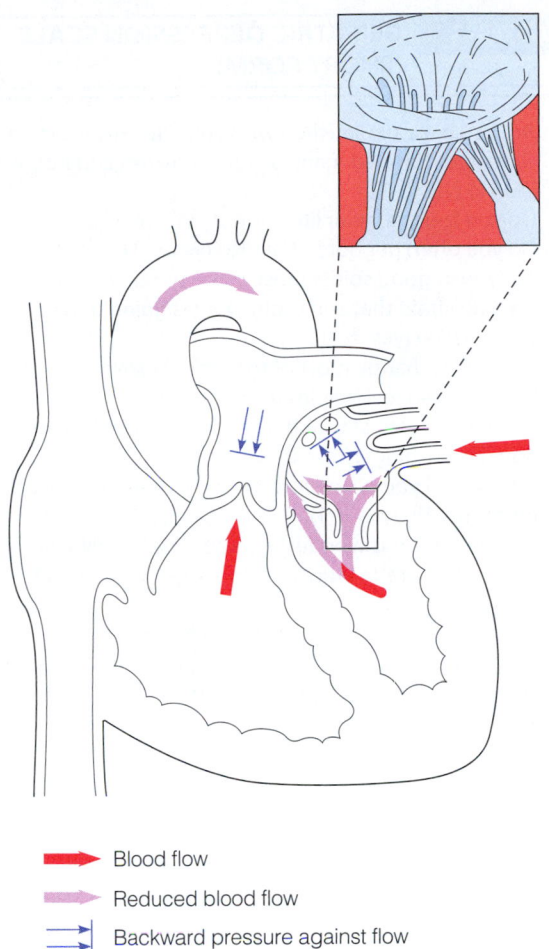

➡️ Blood flow

➡️ Reduced blood flow

⇥ Backward pressure against flow

Figure 43-4. ■ Mitral regurgitation. The mitral valve does not close completely, and blood backs up through the valve into the atrium.

Clotting (*thrombus formation*) in the lumen of a vein is a common problem in older adults who are sedentary or immobile. Thrombi can form quickly because of sluggish blood flow in the blood vessels. Thrombi commonly form in lower extremity veins where they can irritate and inflame the vessel, causing *thrombophlebitis*. (See Chapters 33 and 34 🔗 for discussions on peripheral vascular and blood disorders.) Anticoagulants may be ordered to dissolve the clot(s) and prevent them from traveling to other parts of the body, which could be life threatening.

Peripheral vascular disease is often associated with aging. Weak elasticity and plaque formations in the walls of the arteries hamper the blood flow. If the lumen or diameter of the blood vessel becomes too narrow, blood flow is restricted, especially to the lower extremities. *Arterial occlusive disease* causes diminished circulation and pain. It manifests as cramping in the legs during or after walking (called *intermittent claudication*). If the impairment is severe, causing tissue necrosis, amputation becomes necessary. Venous stasis can occur from immobility or from clients sitting for long periods of time with their legs in a dependent position. Clients

who ride for long periods of time should be taught how to exercise their calves to prevent venous stasis from occurring.

Varicose veins (see Chapter 33 🔗) are seen in clients as a result of blood pooling in the veins. This pooling stretches or dilates the veins. Varicose veins are twisting, often painful superficial veins of the lower extremities. Obese, inactive older adults, as well as older adults who spend a lot of time on their feet, are prone to varicose veins.

Aneurysms are a ballooning out and thinning of any arterial wall (described in Chapter 33 🔗). Aneurysms are more commonly seen in older adults with arteriosclerotic vessel disease than in other groups. Abdominal aortic aneurysms can occur at any age, but are more common in older adults.

Hypertensive disease is common in more than 50% of persons over the age of 65. Stress, obesity, increased cholesterol levels, smoking, and impaired renal, cardiovascular, and endocrine function all contribute to hypertension.

BLOOD AND LYMPHATIC SYSTEMS

Anemia, an inadequate level of red blood cells (RBCs) or hemoglobin, is common in older adults. Older adults are prone to anemic conditions such as:

- Iron-deficiency anemia, which results from an inadequate nutritional intake, malabsorption, blood loss, or increased physiologic demand.
- Pernicious anemia, which is due to a decreased intake or absorption of vitamin B_{12}.
- Folic acid-deficiency anemia, which is commonly caused by poor nutrition, malabsorption syndrome, or chronic alcohol abuse.

Leukemia is another blood condition that is due to an excess production of immature white blood cells (WBCs) (see Chapter 34 🔗). It often accompanies anemia and hemorrhagic conditions. Leukemia may be acute or chronic. Chronic lymphocytic leukemia is the type of leukemia commonly seen in older adults. Approximately 75% of persons diagnosed with this type of leukemia are over age 60.

Bleeding disorders result from a defect in the normal processes that stop bleeding. Imbalances can occur in either clotting or anticlotting blood mechanisms. Medications often affect this balance, so they must be monitored by laboratory results of PTT (partial thromboplastin time), PT (prothrombin time), and INR (international normalized ratio [of PTT to PT]).

NERVOUS SYSTEM

Parkinson's disease is a gradual-onset, degenerative disorder of the central nervous system. (See Chapter 36 🔗 for the main discussion of this and other disorders of the nervous system.) Symptoms include tremors; weakness; a flat, mask-like facial expression; slowed speech; difficulty swallowing;

shuffled, forward leaning gait; and rigidity. Mental as well as physical changes may occur, but the two do not necessarily happen at the same time. About 50% of people with Parkinson's disease suffer from a form of dementia late in the disease process. Medications are available to decrease the symptoms of Parkinson's disease, but the effects of these medications lessen as the disease progresses.

Dementia is a permanent or progressive organic mental disorder characterized by changes in personality; disorientation; diminished mental functioning; and impaired judgment, memory, and impulses. It may be caused by various disorders, usually structural brain disease. This condition can affect younger persons as well as older adults. It can be caused not only by organic means but also by drug overdoses, trauma, or other disease processes.

Ill older adults sometimes have a particular type of dementia called sundowning or *sundowner's syndrome*. **Sundowning** is the onset of delirium during the evening or night with impairment or disappearance during the day, most often seen in mid- or later stages of dementia. Clients exhibit acute confusion, agitation, time disorientation, wandering behavior, and sometimes aggression related to the onset of darkness at the end of the day. (See Chapter 36 ⚭ for this and all neurologic disorders.)

Alzheimer's disease is the most common form of dementia today and is typically seen in older adults. It is a progressive, chronic disease in which brain cells and tissues are affected by atrophy, plaque, and neurofibrillary tangles, and there is a decrease in the neurotransmitter acetylcholine. This decrease in acetylcholine leads to a decreased ability to reason and to retain information. Norepinephrine and dopamine levels are diminished in persons with Alzheimer's disease. The buildup of plaque and neurofibrillary tangles interferes with everyday thought processes. Starting with short-term memory, cognition is gradually reduced. Those affected eventually do not remember their spouses or children. Nursing support for whole families of Alzheimer's clients is necessary because of the client's severely altered abilities and personality.

Transient ischemic attacks (TIAs, or "mini-strokes") are temporary interruptions in the brain's blood supply caused by a piece of atherosclerotic plaque or an embolus. They can occur without warning and can last from minutes to 24 hours. TIAs are often a warning of a future stroke but can recur without a person ever having a stroke.

Strokes, commonly referred to as "brain attacks" or *cerebrovascular accidents* (CVAs), are a disturbance in the brain's blood supply. They may cause temporary or permanent impairment or paralysis. Most strokes are related to one or a combination of atherosclerosis, high blood pressure, or diabetes. Strokes may occur at any age but usually affect persons over the age of 65.

BOX 43-1	GERIATRIC DEPRESSION SCALE (SHORT FORM)

1. Are you basically satisfied with your life? Yes/No (no = 1)
2. Have you dropped many of your activities and interests? Yes/No (yes = 1)
3. Do you feel that your life is empty? Yes/No (yes = 1)
4. Do you often get bored? Yes/No (yes = 1)
5. Are you in good spirits most of the time? Yes/No (no = 1)
6. Are you afraid that something bad is going to happen to you? Yes/No (yes = 1)
7. Do you feel happy most of the time? Yes/No (no = 1)
8. Do you often feel helpless? Yes/No (yes = 1)
9. Do you prefer to stay at home, rather than going out and doing new things? Yes/No (yes = 1)
10. Do you feel you have more problems with memory than most? Yes/No (yes = 1)
11. Do you think it is wonderful to be alive? Yes/No (no = 1)
12. Do you feel pretty worthless the way you are now? Yes/No (yes = 1)
13. Do you feel full of energy? Yes/No (no = 1)
14. Do you feel that your situation is hopeless? Yes/No (yes = 1)
15. Do you feel that most people are better off than you are? Yes/No (yes = 1)

Score_____

Scoring: A score of 5 or more indicates depression.

Depression is a frequent condition of older adults with chronic diseases or impairments. Depression was often overlooked among older adults or considered to be a condition of old age. This is no longer the case. Depression is now commonly treated. The nurse can use tools to determine whether a client has indicators of depression. The geriatric depression scale is one such tool (Box 43-1 ■).

Altered sleep patterns occur in most older adults. Sleep is a fundamental human need, and sleep deprivation is both mentally and physically draining. The older adult gets less sleep at night. Many compensate by having naps during the day.

SENSORY CHANGES

Eyes

The following diseases of the eye (Figure 43-5 ■) are most common in the older adult. However, they may be seen in any age group.

Double vision (**diplopia**) is a condition that may affect older adults for various reasons. It should always be reported to the person's physician to rule out any neurologic disorders.

Glaucoma (see Figures 43-5A and B) is a disease progression in the eye characterized by increased intraocular pressure. The person with glaucoma usually does not experience symptoms, and the disease usually causes damage before it is detected. If left untreated, blindness can occur. Older adults should be encouraged to obtain regular eye examinations, because this and other eye conditions can be

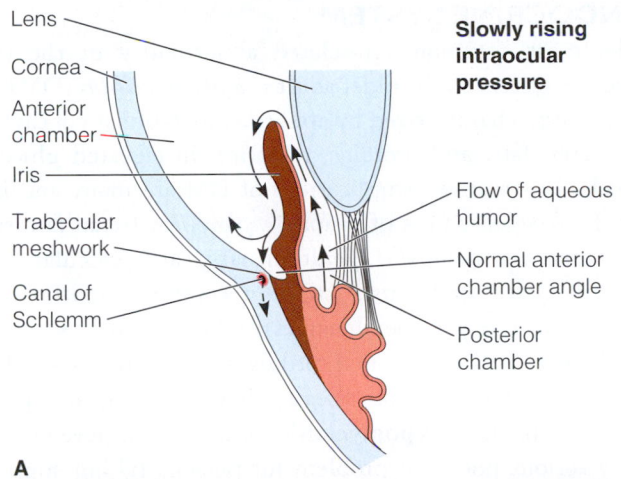

A

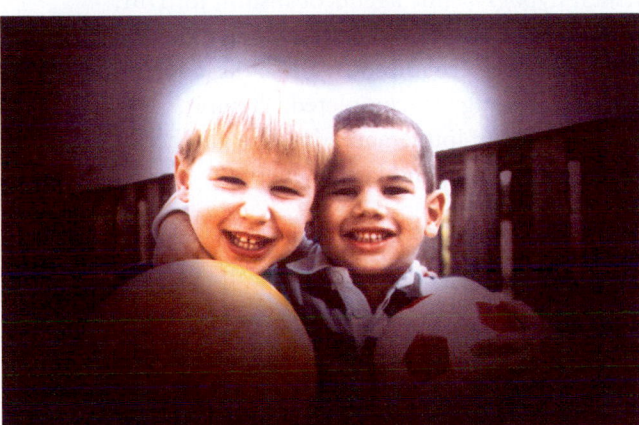

B

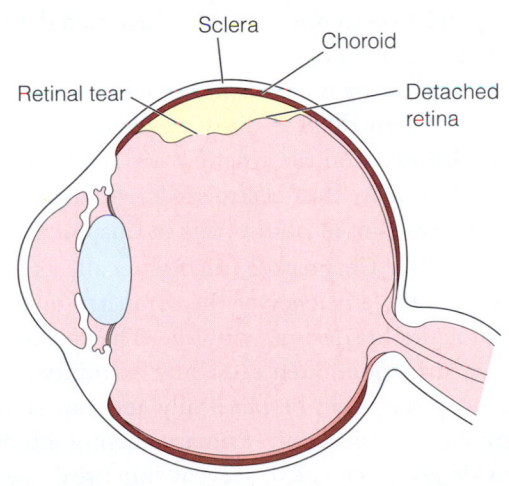

C

Figure 43-5. ■ A. Chronic open-angle glaucoma. B. Untreated glaucoma narrows the visual field. C. Retinal tear and retinal detachment.

detected during a routine exam. Glaucoma can also occur suddenly (called *angle-closure glaucoma*) but *chronic open-angle glaucoma* (Figures 43-5A and B above) is more common.

Diabetic clients are prone to a condition called **diabetic retinopathy.** In diabetic retinopathy circulatory changes occur in the blood vessels of the eye. The small blood vessels

hemorrhage into the vitreous humor of the eye. Like neovascular macular degeneration, this condition may cause blindness. Laser treatment can slow the progression of this disease but does not cure it. Yearly eye examinations are recommended for all adults with diabetes.

Retinal detachment is a separation of the retina from the choroid (see Figure 43-5C). It can be caused by normal shrinkage of the eye in the older adult and changes in the consistency of the vitreous humor in the eye. Retinal detachment can cause loss of peripheral or central vision.

Ears

Hardening of the stapes to the oval window in the ear is a condition referred to as **otosclerosis.** This condition causes an interference with sound wave transmission into the inner ear and can be surgically corrected.

Ringing in the ears (*tinnitus*) is a common complaint of the older adult. It can occur from ear trauma, certain medications, pressure from accumulated earwax (cerumen) against the eardrum, otosclerosis, presbycusis, or Ménière's disease (discussed in the next subsection and in Chapter 36 ∞).

Deafness is another condition seen primarily in the older adult and can be detected in one or both ears. Deafness can be permanent or temporary, depending on the cause. If hearing loss is only partial, hearing aids can help keep the person from becoming socially isolated. (See care of hearing aids in Chapter 20 ∞ ; types of hearing aids were described in Chapter 42 ∞ .)

Ménière's disease is a chronic disorder of the inner ear, more commonly found in persons over age 40. In Ménière's disease there is a progressive distention of the endolymphatic space of the inner ear. Fluid buildup in the inner ear, caused either by overproduction or reduced absorption of the fluid, progressively damages or paralyzes hair cells that are responsible for sensing movement and balance. Clients describe a feeling of fullness in the ear. The person with this condition has frequent dizziness, often with nausea and vomiting. Loss of balance may also occur.

Some antibiotics and viral infections can cause nerve deafness, which occurs when the receptors in the cranial nerves or inner ear are damaged or destroyed. Exposure to loud noises speeds up this process. Many older men who have worked in factories or other high-noise places may have employment-related hearing loss. Employees in these situations today are protected from excessive exposure to loud noises in the workplace by regulations of the Occupational Safety and Health Administration (OSHA).

GASTROINTESTINAL SYSTEM

Gastroesophageal reflux disease (GERD) is a problem that can occur with a condition called hiatal hernia. (See Chapter 37 ∞ for the main discussion of disorders of the GI system.) Hiatal hernias and GERD may result in gastric and duodenal ulcers in older adults. Ulcers can also be caused by stress, trauma, smoking, alcohol, regular ingestion of aspirin or nonsteroidal anti-inflammatory drugs (NSAIDs), or illness.

Diverticula (small pouches that develop from weakness in the intestinal wall) occur in 30% to 40% of persons over age 50. Diverticulitis occurs from inflammation of one or more of the diverticula.

Cancer of the colon increases at age 40 and peaks in older adults between the ages of 60 and 75. Clients over age 40 should be encouraged to have routine screenings for rectal cancer.

Over- and undernutrition are common among older adults. Many older adults experience a decrease in appetite or an increased desire for sweets. Common causes include decreased functioning of taste buds, medications that alter taste, disease processes, swallowing difficulties resulting in choking, or various conditions of the mouth. This last set includes ill-fitting dentures, dental disorders such as cavities, chipped or missing teeth, fillings or crowns with jagged edges that dig into the mouth or gums, or bleeding gums.

Dehydration can happen quickly in the older adult. Various causes such as vomiting, diarrhea, or infections can delete the body not only of essential fluids but also of important minerals such as salt. If the dehydration is severe enough, the client may need intravenous fluids to restore balance and prevent further system involvement.

Inadequate intake of fluids coupled with inactivity can lead to *chronic constipation* in older adults. Medications also can alter digestion and increase constipation. A diet with plenty of fiber may be recommended, and stool softeners may also be prescribed.

Older adults often experience problems with *hemorrhoids* (small internal or external herniations in the rectal area; see Figure 37-24 ∞). Clients who have existing problems with constipation and persons who are overweight commonly have problems with hemorrhoids. Teaching the client about the importance of fiber in the diet can often help alleviate or lessen symptoms of constipation.

Rectal prolapse is a condition in which the rectum bulges through the anus. It occurs most commonly in women over 60 years of age. If this condition causes great distress or discomfort, medical or surgical intervention may be necessary.

Older adults often eat the same foods they did when they were younger, but they cannot properly digest certain foods (such as fatty foods). Complaints of gas, indigestion, and flatulence abound. They are frustrating for the client and often result in anorexia and malnutrition. Nurses have a great opportunity to teach the older adult about proper nutrition and avoidance of irritating foods and drinks. A change in nutritional practices may be all it takes for the older adult to regulate bowel function and experience less GI distress.

ENDOCRINE SYSTEM

The most common age-related abnormality of the endocrine system in the older adult is *diabetes mellitus* (DM). It is a disease characterized by abnormal metabolism of carbohydrates, fats, and proteins, resulting in elevated glucose levels. Progressive complications of DM are many and include *retinopathy* (loss of vision), *nephropathy* (renal failure), *autonomic neuropathy* (GI, genitourinary, cardiovascular, and sexual-related problems), *peripheral neuropathy* (pathologic change in the peripheral nerves), atherosclerotic vascular problems (such as increased cardiovascular, cerebrovascular, and peripheral vascular disease), hypertension, and periodontal disease. **Hypoglycemia** (low glucose levels) is a very serious potential problem for persons taking supplemental hypoglycemic agents or insulin for DM.

Hypothyroidism is a reduced function of the thyroid gland. It may not be recognized in the older adult until thyroid function testing is completed. Symptoms of hypothyroidism are cold intolerance, dry skin and body hair, constipation, depression, and lack of energy.

URINARY SYSTEM

Urinary tract infections (UTIs) occur in approximately 15% of women over the age of 60 and are more prevalent in women than in men. However, if UTIs do occur in men, they generally occur in men who are older. Normal physiologic changes and health problems contribute to the increase in UTIs. Diseases such as diabetes mellitus, stroke, dementia, and hypertension are often associated with persons with frequent UTIs.

Chronic renal failure is increasingly seen in adults over age 70. Different methods of dialysis are available to persons with this disease. Contributing factors are hypertension, chronic UTIs, urinary tract obstructions, and diabetes mellitus. (See discussion of renal disorders in Chapter 39 ∞.)

Incontinence (see Chapter 42 ∞) often affects the older adult, because the efficiency of the sphincter muscles surrounding the urethra declines with age. The uncontrollable, involuntary urination, often caused by an injury or disease of the urinary tract, can be physically and psychologically detrimental to an older adult. Primary nursing intervention is to provide good hygiene to prevent skin breakdown from the ammonia in the urine.

Benign prostatic hyperplasia is a common nonmalignant condition. Potential complications of prostatic enlargement include impeded urinary outflow and urinary **reflux** (backward flow). Symptoms range from blood in urine to complete urinary obstruction and retention.

Prostate cancer is quite common among older adult men. At this stage of life, the cancer generally advances very slowly and usually is treatable if discovered early. (See Chapter 45 ∞ for the methods of treating cancer.)

REPRODUCTIVE SYSTEM

Uterine prolapse (a falling of the uterus from its normal position) into the vagina is a condition sometimes found in older women (see Figure 40-13E 🔗). It is seen more commonly in women who have had many pregnancies or delivered children with minimal medical assistance requiring much straining. Surgical correction may be warranted, especially if the woman is experiencing other annoying signs and symptoms such as urinary frequency and retention, back pain, and constipation. (This and other disorders of the reproductive system were discussed in Chapter 40 🔗.)

A change in vaginal pH in the older woman can lead to increased vaginal infections, specifically *yeast infections.*

The risk of *breast cancer* increases with age. Although men can be victims of breast cancer also, it continues to be a major cause of cancer deaths in women. Aging women should be taught to be aware of any changes in their breasts and to have routine medical examinations. (See Chapter 40 🔗 for a discussion of breast cancer.)

The major form of cancer in men is *prostate cancer*. This cancer does not create noticeable changes in function. Therefore, it is very important for men to have regular examinations for prostate changes (see Chapter 40 🔗 for discussion).

Erectile dysfunction is a fairly common condition among older men. Conditions can range from total or partial failure to attain or maintain an erection (*impotence*) to persistent erection without any sexual desire (**priapism**). Advances in pharmacology treatments have made these treatable conditions for many.

Special Concerns of the Hospitalized Older Adult

LPNs/LVNs will need to collect data carefully from the older adult who is admitted to the hospital, because the assessment provides the basis for nursing interventions. Older adults may be "set in their ways" of how things should be done. They may require time before responding to questions, and they may be slow in performing steps in a process. It will be your job as a nurse to work *with* the client rather than *on* the client in a partnership that encourages and supports the client's individuality and sense of control.

Based on the particular reason for the hospitalization, the older adult's needs will vary greatly. If admission is due to worsening of a chronic condition, pain, anxiety, stress, fear, and depression may require interventions. However, if an independent, healthy older adult falls and is admitted because of a fractured hip, then loss of independence, maybe financial worries, care of spouse still in the home, and placement in rehab may be this client's immediate concerns.

Whatever the reason for hospitalization, older adults have some specific needs:

- Because their immune system is somewhat weakened, older adults are susceptible to nosocomial infections. They need protection from hospital-acquired infections. It will be the nurse's job to make sure that people coming in contact with the client wash their hands first and do not expose them to infectious diseases.
- Because of the thinning of skin and underlying tissue, older adults need careful skin care and frequent position changes. Pressure ulcers (Figure 43-6 ■) are a constant danger for immobilized older adults, especially those whose level of consciousness and/or mobility are impaired by illness.
- They will need reassurance about what is happening. A priority when dealing with older adults is to decrease their level of anxiety by explaining treatments, several times if necessary, so they can understand. Trying to maintain a part of their routine prior to hospitalization will also alleviate stress and anxiety.
- They must have a safe environment and appropriate assistive devices. For example, it takes a certain amount of coordination to be able to walk and push an IV pole without tripping over its legs or wheels. If a client cannot physically manage this, alternatives must be found.
- Older adults need relief of pain *and* protection against overmedication. Good pain management for older adults promotes both physical and psychological healing. When administering pain medications to older adults, remember that their metabolism is slower and their bodies will be slower to clear drugs than a younger person's is. This makes drug toxicity more of a danger.

SEDATION

Occasionally, the LPN/LVN will need to provide an older adult with sedation for various reasons and at various times of the day. Certain sedatives are used in relieving pain.

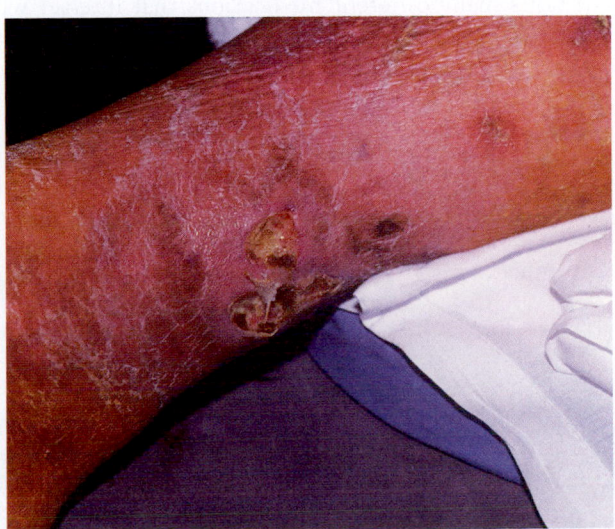

Figure 43-6. ■ Older adults, especially those who are immobile, are in danger of developing pressure ulcers.

Sedation may also be necessary to provide a calming effect in an individual who is exhibiting an acute anxiety or panic attack. Depending on the sedation it could have a twofold outcome, a calming effect and a drowsy state. Research proves that rest and relaxation promotes a faster healing and recovery rate.

clinical ALERT

Some medications cause mental confusion; when these are administered, side rails or restraints may be necessary to prevent injury.

The LPN/LVN needs to remember that the older adult is not accustomed to sleeping in hospital beds or hearing all the noises that go along with being hospitalized (Figure 43-7 ■). The beds for the most part are uncomfortable and generally feel cold and sterile. Common hospital noises include hospital personnel walking and talking, ringing phones, medical monitors beeping, doors opening and closing, and other clients on the unit. These are not conducive to rest, relaxation, or sleep.

DANGERS OF POLYPHARMACY

Pharmacologic remedies are offered for nearly every physical complaint. The trend today is to "take something" for these maladies in order to alleviate pain and increase quality of life. The older adult often takes prescription medications for different disease processes and/or chronic or acute conditions. Many times these prescriptions are from different providers. (The client may see a GI specialist for diverticulitis, a lung specialist for COPD, and so on, and each may prescribe medications.) Many drugs are metabolized in the liver, but like other body organs, liver function declines with age. A condition called **polypharmacy** occurs when a client takes many different medications that interact with

each other and create side effects. Because of decreased body system functioning, the elderly are most susceptible to polypharmacy. This often occurs in the elderly when medications remain in the body longer than intended, interact with each other, and cause a toxic effect. It is estimated that 3% to 16% of hospitalizations occur from polypharmacy in the older adult.

Also, older adults may self-medicate with herbal and vitamin supplements. Older adults especially should be warned of potential side effects of these supplements, especially when taken with prescription medications. For example, the herb ginkgo biloba can interact with prescription medication, causing an increased potential for hemorrhage, seizures, stroke, or even death in sensitive individuals. As nurses, we must encourage our clients to identify all of the medications they are taking *including* supplements and herbal remedies.

clinical ALERT

Many older people think of acetaminophen (Tylenol) as the "safe alternative" to salicylic acid (aspirin). They may not be aware of the dangers of exceeding recommended doses of acetaminophen. In fact, there is a narrow range between therapeutic and toxic dosages of this drug. Overuse of acetaminophen can lead to liver toxicity and death. Yellowing of the skin (*jaundice*) may be an early sign of toxicity.

Indications of adverse effects of polypharmacy include, but are not limited to, the following:

- Nausea or **malaise** (a generalized feeling of being unwell)
- Confusion or irritability
- Fainting
- Jaundice
- Sluggishness
- Changes in elimination

When these signs are noted, the LPN/LVN reports them to the charge nurse or primary care provider.

NURSING CARE

PRIORITIZING NURSING CARE

The unique focus of nursing interventions for the older adult emerges from a care domain rather than a cure domain. Nurses will assist the client to resolve the acute illness or event while providing holistic care for age-related or chronic conditions that cannot be cured.

ASSESSING

Collect data for a head-to-toe assessment, focusing on the area addressed by the presenting problem (e.g., neurological

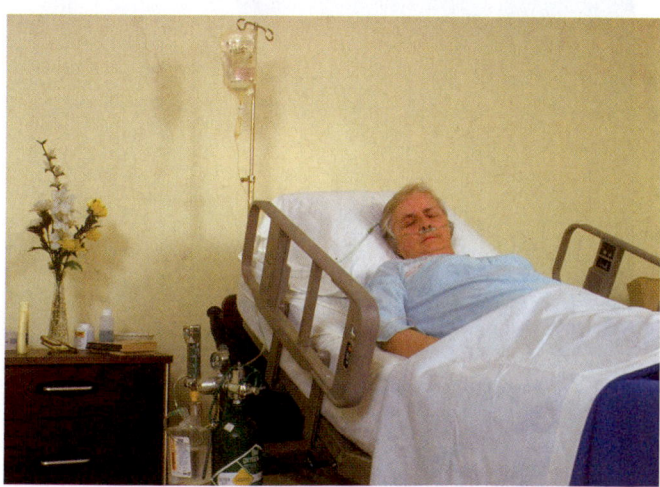

Figure 43-7. ■ Sleep disturbances in institutional settings are common.

if the client is complaining of unilateral weakness, in order to rule-out or confirm a CVA). Compare any abnormal finding to baseline information if available. The ill older adult client may not be the best source of information. Make a note if a family member or caregiver is supplying the information. Accurately determine when the symptoms began, because this may be crucial information in determining the client's eligibility for emergency treatment of CVA or MI.

DIAGNOSING, PLANNING, AND IMPLEMENTING

Possible nursing diagnoses for a client with left-sided weakness, slurred speech, and inability to smile when directed, include:

- *Impaired Verbal Communication*
- *Risk for Injury* (falls)
- *Impaired Swallowing*
- *Functional Urinary Incontinence*, related to inability to transfer to toilet or commode independently
- *Caregiver Role Strain*

Outcomes for these clients would include the following:

- Client will communicate expressively in writing, with head nods, or pointing to express needs and wishes.
- Client will ask for assistance when attempting to get out of bed.
- Client will consume food or fluids safely without aspiration.
- Client will request assistance to commode when experiencing the urge to void.
- Caregiver will maintain personal, physical, and emotional health while caring for the client.

Nursing interventions may include the following:

- Attend closely to and attach significance to client's verbal and nonverbal messages. *The client may not be able to communicate in the normal way.*
- Monitor and manipulate the physical environment to promote safety. *This will prevent falls and injury to client.*
- Use side rails and have call light in reach at all times. *This will help to prevent falls.*
- Answer the call light in a timely manner. *Delay in attention may encourage the client to try to get out of bed independently.*
- Observe the client's ability to swallow. Provide chopped food and thickened liquids as ordered. *This promotes swallowing without choking or aspiration.*
- Feed the client if necessary. *It is important to maintain nutritional status and prevent aspiration.*
- Schedule regular times for commode use. *A regular schedule will help the client maintain continence.*
- Provide incontinent briefs to keep the client and bed dry. *Briefs will prevent skin irritation and odor.*

- Change and clean frequently if necessary. *This will prevent skin breakdown and maintain client dignity.*
- Provide necessary information, advocacy, and support to help the primary caregiver obtain help from someone other than a healthcare professional. *This provides needed support so the caregiver is able to maintain his or her own health.*

EVALUATING

Evaluate client's safety and ability to perform ADLs as well as the caregivers' ability to provide home care.

NURSING PROCESS CARE PLAN
Client with Chronic Obstructive Pulmonary Disease

Mr. H is a 78-year-old man with a 30-year history of smoking approximately one pack of cigarettes a day. He quit smoking 7 years ago but not before his lungs were permanently damaged by the history of smoking. Mr. H, due to emphysema and chronic lung infections, has been taking steroids for the past 5 years and has had several hospitalizations for pneumonia. Due to the long-term steroid use, Mr. H has developed osteoporosis, his skin is extremely fragile, and his lung condition has progressively worsened. He has oxygen delivered to his house because he is on continuous 4 liters of oxygen and wears an oxygen delivery mask (CPAP) during the night. The oxygen is delivered via long oxygen tubing that allows him to move freely about the house and outside. His oxygen saturation is at 92% while on the delivery system. He rapidly *desaturates* (loses blood level oxygen) if he is without his oxygen for short periods.

Mr. H got up from a sitting position and tripped over his oxygen tubing, landing on his right hip. He cried out in pain and the paramedics were called after he was not able to move from the fall. He was transported to the hospital and radiologic studies revealed a fractured right hip. He was deemed a poor surgical candidate because of his COPD and was given pain medication to alleviate his pain. The pain became progressively worse due to the spasms of the large muscles surrounding the hip. Medication could not alleviate his pain and precautions with the medication dosages and interactions with other medications he was taking had to be considered due to his pulmonary status. The decision was made to take Mr. H to surgery but the anesthesiologist cautioned the family about the risks anesthesia and surgery could have on Mr. H. The anesthesiologist also told the family that due to Mr. H's lung condition, Mr. H may not survive the surgery. Mr. H and his family discussed the risks and Mr. H made the decision to have surgery.

Assessment

Vital signs: BP 136/76, P 86, R 24 and shallow, T 99.0, pain assessment is 8/10, weight 119, height 75 inches. Oxygen is being delivered at 6 liters and rales are heard in the bilateral lobes. Nail beds are pale with poor capillary refill. Mr. H has a wet, productive cough. Sputum samples have been collected and sent to the lab for evaluation. His WBC count is elevated. Chest x-ray shows bilateral infiltrates in the lower lobes and diffuse scarring throughout all lung fields. Skin assessment: pale, warm, moist, poor fragile turgor, intact except for area on right arm that tore open when he fell. This area has been dressed with transparent dressing. There is a large ecchymotic area over the right hip and thigh that extends down to the right knee. He is in 5-pound Buck's traction.

Nursing Diagnosis

The following important nursing diagnoses (among others) are established for this condition:

- *Risk for Infection* due to decreased lung capacity, history of pneumonia, and immobility
- *Excess Fluid Volume* (Fluids will have to be monitored due to his COPD.)
- *Impaired Gas Exchange* due to rapid respiratory rate and pulmonary infiltrate
- *Ineffective Airway Clearance* related to pulmonary infiltrate, secretions, and guarded position due to his hip pain
- *Acute Pain* related to fractured hip
- *Risk for Impaired Skin Integrity* due to immobility

Expected Outcomes

The following are the expected outcomes for the plan of care for Mr. H. It is expected that Mr. H will:

- Maintain adequate oxygenation and patent airway.
- Survive the surgical procedure and anesthesia.
- Avoid infection of pulmonary fields and skin.
- Understand and be able to verbalize understanding of the surgical procedure, healing process, and postoperative rehabilitative process.

Planning and Implementation

The following nursing interventions are implemented for Mr. H. Ongoing assessments are performed to monitor his condition preoperatively and postoperatively.

- Monitor respirations and maintain oxygen delivery. Monitor client's oxygen saturation with pulse oximeter.
- Maintain a patent airway.
- Auscultate breath sounds. Encourage deep breathing with incentive spirometer.
- Encourage coughing and expectorating of secretions.
- Document volume, color, and consistency of secretions.
- Prepare for antibiotic administration due to infection.
- Continue steroid therapy.
- Maintain NPO status before and after surgery. Hydration will be continued per IV fluids.
- Position Mr. H in semi-Fowler's position to facilitate breathing and decrease pain in hip.
- Ensure aseptic technique is carried out when caring for Mr. H's surgical site.
- Prepare client for surgery and anticipate possible admission to the intensive care unit (ICU) postoperatively.

Evaluation

Mr. H went to surgery for a right hip pinning and was admitted to the ICU postoperatively on the ventilator. His immobility in the first three postoperative days led to an increase in temperature and diagnosis of pneumonia. Antibiotics were administered and strict pulmonary care was given while he was on the ventilator. He was extubated 2 days after surgery and returned to the nasal cannula for oxygen delivery. His steroids and pain medication were continued along with blood thinning medication, which was started due to the bone fracture and his immobility. Mr. H showed signs of recovery from the pneumonia 1 week after onset but antibiotics were continued prophylactically. He was moved to the medical-surgical floor where he remained for another 5 days. He was able to verbalize relief from the pain and was started on rehabilitation. He was moved to a rehabilitation facility for long-term rehabilitation.

Critical Thinking in the Nursing Process

1. What were some of the challenges encountered in caring for Mr. H?
2. How many body systems were involved in his care?
3. Which of the assessment findings for Mr. H are consistent with signs and symptoms of pneumonia?

Note: Discussion of Critical Thinking questions appears on the MyNursingKit Website.

Chapter Review

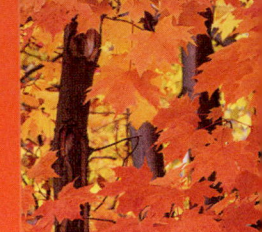

KEY Points

- Basic nursing care duties do not change based on age.
- The ill older adult may have chronic conditions related to age that make caregiving more complex and that require special attention.
- As the client ages all body systems may be affected by the aging process.
- Musculoskeletal problems such as fractures and degenerative joint disease are common among elderly clients and may require a long recovery process.
- CVA may cause major disabilities for older clients and may require long-term care in a facility or a full-time caregiver at home.
- Sundowning is the onset of delirium during the evening or night with impairment or disappearance during the day, most often seen in mid- or later stages of dementia.
- Depression was often overlooked among older adults or considered to be a condition of old age. This is no longer the case. Depression is now commonly treated.
- Over- and undernutrition are common among older adults. Many older adults experience a decrease in appetite or an increased desire for sweets.
- Because the older client's immune system is somewhat weakened, older adults are very susceptible to nosocomial infections. They need protection from hospital-acquired infections.
- Some medications cause mental confusion; when these are administered, side rails or restraints may be necessary to prevent injury.
- Polypharmacy is a major concern for older adults who have a variety of prescriptions. Because the older adult's body is slower to metabolize and excrete medications, drug interactions and drug toxicity can occur.

FOR FURTHER Study

MRSA and nosocomial infections are discussed in depth in Chapter 10.

Care of hearing aids is described in Chapter 20.

The full discussion of wound care is in Chapter 24.

Chapter 30 describes integumentary disorders.

Discussion of gout, or gouty arthritis, is in Chapter 31.

Respiratory disorders are discussed in depth in Chapter 32.

See the main discussion of cardiovascular disorders in Chapter 33.

Chapter 34 discusses peripheral vascular and other blood disorders.

Chapter 36 has the main discussion of disorders of the nervous system.

See Chapter 37 for the main discussion of disorders of the GI system.

See discussion of renal disorders in Chapter 39.

Disorders of the reproductive system are discussed in Chapter 40.

Chapter 42 describes health promotion in older adults, including bladder retraining for incontinence and use of hearing aids.

Chapter 44 describes care of chronically or terminally ill clients of all ages.

Chapter 45 is the main discussion about cancer.

Chapter 46 discusses specifics of long-term and rehabilitation care.

A chart of communicable diseases is provided in Chapter 60.

EXPLORE PEARSON **mynursingkit**™

MyNursingKit is your one stop for online chapter review materials and resources. Prepare for success with additional NCLEX®-style practice questions, interactive assignments and activities, web links, animations and videos, and more!

Register your access code from the front of your book at **www.mynursingkit.com**

Critical Thinking Care Map

Caring for a Client after Coronary Artery Stent Placement

NCLEX-PN® Focus Area: Physiologic Integrity

Case Study: Mr. B, age 59, states that he is worried about his heart since he had stents placed in three of his coronary arteries 3 weeks ago. The three arteries were 90% blocked due to atherosclerotic heart disease. He has come into the clinic for his postprocedure checkup. Mr. B had an uneventful postprocedure period but tells you he is worried about the stents "not working." He has been on various medications since his stent placements and has been instructed to walk as a form of exercise and to quit smoking. He had led a sedentary lifestyle before his stent placements and had smoked one pack of cigarettes a day for more than 25 years.

Nursing Diagnosis: *Anxiety*

COLLECT DATA

Subjective	Objective
_____	_____
_____	_____
_____	_____
_____	_____
_____	_____
_____	_____
_____	_____

Would you report this? Yes/No

If yes, report to: _____

What would you report? _____

Nursing Care

_____
_____
_____
_____
_____
_____
_____
_____
_____
_____
_____

How would you document this? _____
_____
_____
_____

Compare your answers and documentation to those provided on the MyNursingKit Website.

Data Collected
(use only those that apply)

- 59 y/o white male
- Lives with second wife; no children
- Weight 185 lbs, 5-lb weight loss since surgery, height 6 ft
- BP 124/80. (He is taking medication for hypertension.)
- Heart rate 60 and regular
- Pack of cigarettes in shirt pocket
- Respiratory rate 12
- Skin pink, warm, and dry; good capillary refill
- No signs of infection at surgical site
- He tells you he has been walking twice a day and increasing the length of his walk every 2 days. His wife accompanies him on these walks.
- Points to his chest saying, "It just feels different in here." You notice he repeatedly puts his hand on the left side of his chest.
- Both parents died in their early 60s of "heart conditions." Mr. B can't remember specifics.
- Tells you he is wondering if he will die in his early 60s because that is when his parents died.
- Runs own business as a financial advisor

Nursing Interventions
(use only those that apply; list in priority order)

- Assess medications Mr. B is taking and make sure he is taking correct dosages.
- Point out to Mr. B that his vital signs were all within the normal range.
- Encourage Mr. B to ask his physician questions/concerns he may have about the stents.
- Monitor client for signs of anxiety and other defense mechanisms.
- Obtain additional client information about stents to give to him.
- Advise client to follow instructions for medication, diet, and exercise as prescribed.
- Assist client in verbalizing any other concerns about his health and determine if there are other reasons for his concern or if it is a normal response.
- Teach client and his wife about good dietary habits and the value of quitting smoking.
- Identify support groups for people with CV disease and/or stent placements.

NCLEX-PN® Exam Preparation

TEST-TAKING TIP When answering a question, look for words that relate to elements of the Test Plan (e.g., that are asking about the Physiologic Integrity or Safe, Effective Care Environment). These will help you identify the correct answer.

1 The LPN is assigned an elderly client and a young adult. The nurse recognizes that the primary difference in providing care to these two clients is that the elderly client:

1. Requires different basic nursing care duties to be performed.
2. May have more complex caregiving needs as a result of chronic conditions and age-related changes.
3. Is less likely to recover from illness.
4. Is less likely to be able to understand client teaching.

2 The nurse is caring for a client admitted to the acute care facility with a fractured hip. The client reports a history of a fractured ulna after slipping on the ice outside her home and a fractured patella after falling on her cement patio. The nurse recognizes these fractures are likely the result of:

1. Degenerative joint disease.
2. Osteoarthritis.
3. Osteoporosis.
4. Inadequate caloric intake.

3 The client asks the nurse, "What did the doctor mean when he said I had COPD?" Which of the following responses would be incorrect?

1. "COPD is a single disorder that is the result of lung damage."
2. "COPD is a common disorder in persons with a history of smoking."
3. "The person with COPD often displays signs and symptoms such as productive cough, wheezing, and difficulty breathing on exertion."
4. "COPD stands for chronic obstructive pulmonary disease."

4 The nurse is assisting with an in-service for other nurses. The nurse is asked what causes the most deaths in people over the age of 65. The nurse's best correct answer is:

1. Respiratory disorders.
2. Integumentary disorders.
3. Neurological disorders.
4. Cardiovascular disorders.

5 When amending care specific to the needs of an elderly client, the nurse would do which of the following?

1. Administer medications in a timely manner.
2. Provide for daily hygiene needs.
3. Provide careful skin care with frequent position changes.
4. Speak in a loud voice.

6 The nurse is caring for an elderly client requiring narcotic analgesics to control pain. The nurse recognizes that the elderly client is at greater risk for:

1. Inadequate pain relief.
2. Inaccurate reporting of pain level.
3. Drug toxicity.
4. Inadequate healing.

7 The nurse is caring for an elderly client who was alert and oriented on admission but is now demonstrating mental confusion. The nurse suspects this confusion could be the result of which of the following? (Select all that apply.)

1. Medications
2. Unfamiliar environment
3. Alteration in routine
4. Lack of sleep
5. Lack of family involvement

8 The nurse is caring for a client with several chronic diseases. The client reports concerns that the nurse believes may be due to medication interactions, known as:

1. Side effects.
2. Contraindications.
3. Allergies.
4. Polypharmacy.

9 While obtaining a nursing history, the client discloses that she takes acetaminophen (Tylenol) frequently throughout the day to control pain caused by osteoarthritis. Which of the following symptoms would the nurse interpret as possibly related to toxic effects of this medication?

1. Rebound pain
2. Headaches and nausea
3. Jaundice
4. Kidney failure

10 The nurse is providing discharge teaching for a client taking numerous medications. An important teaching point for this client would be to:

1. Talk with the physician about reducing the number of medications prescribed.
2. Remember the names and dosages of all medications.
3. Take as many medications at the same time as possible.
4. Keep an accurate and updated list of medications in their wallet at all times.

Answers and rationales for Review Questions appear in Appendix I.

Thinking Strategically About...

You have been working in a skilled nursing facility since you completed your LPN/LVN program and received your license. The facility is opening an adult day care facility in a nearby community center. You have been asked to be one of the LPNs/LVNs on staff. In addition to you, there will be two nursing assistants, a PT assistant, and a recreational therapist. There will be an activities department with a director and three assistants, as well as two food service workers who will deliver lunch and snacks from the facility's dietary department. You will work two 10-hour days, and one day will be split with the other LPN/LVN for a total of 25 hours per week. The LPNs/LVNs will be expected to cover each other for days off or illness. The center will be closed on weekends and holidays. You have talked it over with your family and feel that having better hours, no weekends, and holidays off would be nice since your children are at the age when they are involved in a lot of activities. The change in hours will not affect your benefit package.

You decided to take the position and today is your first day with clients.

You have six clients:

- Mr. John Gale, 88 years old, has a diagnosis of early stage Alzheimer's and a history of wandering. He takes Aricept 10 mg H.S. He appears to be very tired and needs help with meals.

- Mrs. Lolly Johansen is age 93. She is very independent, and she does not feel she needs a "babysitter." She lives with her daughter and three grandchildren, but is becoming forgetful and has been leaving the stove on when she cooks.

- Mr. Gregory Davis is age 86. His wife died 3 months ago and he has been very depressed. He has lost interest in all of his outside activities; his son travels a lot for work and thought he should get out during the day. Mr. Davis could not go to the community center because he is diabetic and needs blood sugar monitoring prior to lunch. His wife used to help him with his glucose check and insulin.

- Mr. Lamar Wallace, age 80, had a right-side CVA last year. He walks with a walker and feeds himself with his left hand. He needs help cutting food and has limited vision. You will be giving him his medication after he arrives at the center each morning.

- Mrs. Misohi Shu is a 79-year-old female who has recently come from Southeast Asia to live with her daughter and her American husband. Mrs. Shu has limited English. Her family feels that the day care center would be better for her since it is smaller and there are fewer people than at the community center.

- Mrs. Lois Suki is a 75-year-old woman who had an above-the-knee amputation 9 months ago. She lives with her niece and her husband in a two-story house. Mrs. Suki insists on doing chores around the house when the rest of the family is at work. She fell on the stairs while trying to vacuum last week. Her family feels she will be safer at the senior day care center. Mrs. Suki insists that she does not need to be there and will be bored with no work to do all day. Mrs. Suki met her late husband while teaching English in Laos prior to the Vietnam War. She is fluent in French and several Asian dialects.

CRITICAL THINKING

- What other information would be helpful to have before making the decision to accept the position?

PRIORITIZING NURSING CARE

Prioritize your day and the care for each of the six clients.

MANAGEMENT OF CARE

What is the best way to organize your day and communicate the clients' needs on your half day when the other LPN/LVN comes to relieve you?

DELEGATING

What assignments will you give to the two nursing assistants? What kind of follow-up will be needed?

CLIENT TEACHING

The day care center is a perfect place to offer health teaching on various topics. List some appropriate topics and identify the ones you are equipped to teach. Identify other staff members or outside people who might provide client teaching.

CULTURAL CARE STRATEGIES

- What can you do to help Mrs. Shu improve her communication skills, and thus become more socially involved with the other clients?

- Are there other clients who have skills that may help Mrs. Shu become more comfortable with her new surroundings?

DOCUMENTING AND REPORTING

- What activities will require daily documentation?

- What occurrences will need to be reported to the facility administrator?

- What information should be reported to the families or the client's primary physician?

Specialized Nursing Care

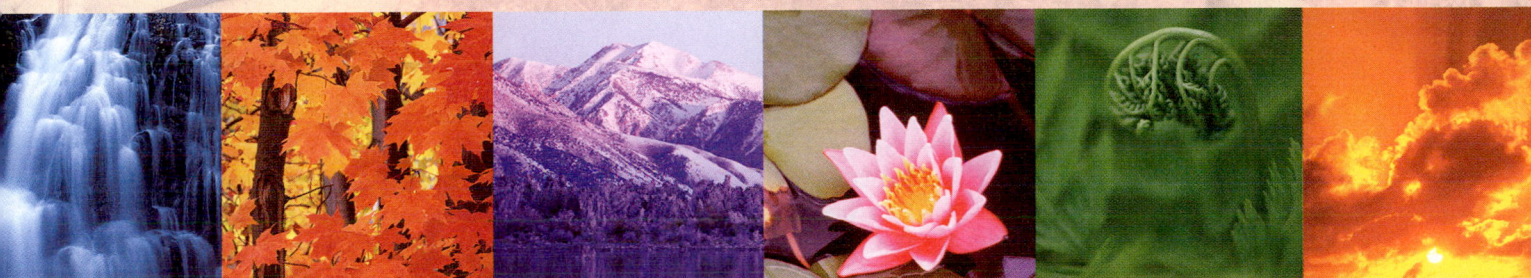

Chapter 44

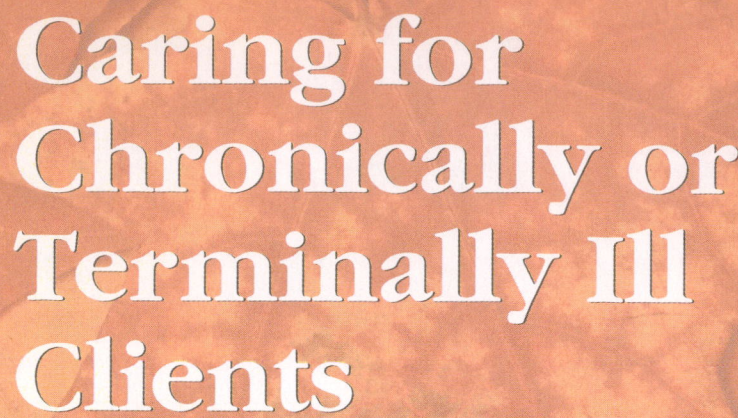

Caring for Chronically or Terminally Ill Clients

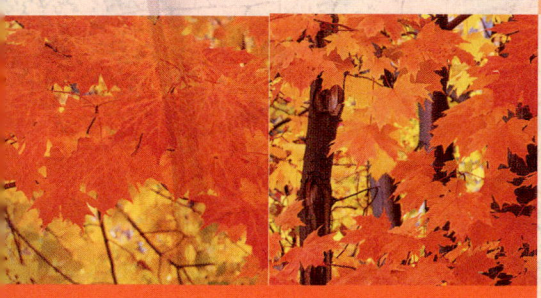

LEARNING Outcomes

After completing this chapter, you will be able to:

1. Name characteristics of chronic illness.
2. Explain factors associated with chronic illness and preventive measures.
3. Describe the role of the LPN/LVN in caring for chronically ill clients.
4. Define terminal illness, palliative care, and hospice.
5. Discuss aspects of the LPN/LVN role in caring for dying clients and their families.
6. List common nursing diagnoses used in end-of-life care.
7. Identify interventions the LPN/LVN can perform in caring for the dying person and the family.
8. List clinical signs of impending death.
9. Identify legal issues in terminal illness, including essential aspects of the Patient Self-Determination Act.
10. List definitions and clinical indications of death.
11. Discuss special pediatric and cultural concerns related to dying.
12. Describe nursing measures for the care of the body after death.

Clinical Objectives

13. Provide client/family teaching on chronic illness remissions.
14. Provide nonpharmacologic comfort measures for a terminally ill client.
15. Assist family members and the client to achieve closure at the time of death.

In the last several decades, life expectancy in the United States has improved dramatically due to medical advances. The "morbidity," incidence or prevalence, of many diseases, such as cancer, heart disease, and chronic respiratory disease, has changed markedly over the years as long-term treatment options have become more available and effective. Along with these changes, the "mortality" or death rates of these same diseases has also changed. This means both that healthy people and the chronically and terminally ill are living longer. LPNs and LVNs play an active role in the long-term care of these groups of people.

CHRONIC ILLNESS

A **chronic illness** has certain characteristics:

1. It is caused by disease that produces symptoms and signs within a variable time.
2. Symptoms persist over a long and variable time.
3. It allows only partial recovery due to the eventual presence of irreversible pathological changes.

Some examples of chronic diseases are chronic obstructive pulmonary disease (COPD), muscular dystrophy, diabetes mellitus, and lupus erythematosus. (These diseases are discussed in depth in Chapters 32, 31, 38, and 35 ⚭, respectively.)

Although the symptoms and general reactions caused by chronic disease may subside with proper treatment and care, the underlying pathology remains. The period during which the disease is controlled and symptoms are not obvious is known as **remission.** Reactivation of the disease and recurrence of symptoms is known as an **exacerbation.** Exacerbations of chronic disease often cause the client to seek medical attention and may lead to hospitalization. Following an acute exacerbation, recovery is often not to pre-exacerbation levels. Rather, the client's overall condition slowly but gradually deteriorates.

Factors Associated with Chronic Illness

There are several factors associated with chronic illness. The first factor is age. Chronic illness can occur at any age, but the elderly are more likely to have long, drawn-out chronic diseases.

The second factor is cultural values. Western culture tends to be cure oriented. Therefore, health care for acute conditions is often more valued than health care for the chronically ill.

Genetic predisposition and environment or lifestyle are the third and fourth factors that influence chronic illnesses. Genetic factors have been implicated in the high cholesterol levels associated with heart disease and hypertension. Lifestyle factors, such as diet and exercise, are also extremely important in both the etiology and treatment of chronic conditions. Chronic diseases tend to be very complex. Factors such as lifestyle and genetics contribute to the predisposition, development, and course of chronic illnesses. Change in just one element does not eradicate or cure the entire disease complex.

A fifth factor is race and ethnicity. There is an association between disease occurrence and race (called *race-specific rates*). Not only are some problems more common among nonwhites, but research also indicates that many nonwhites fail to receive necessary care.

A final factor, the cost of disability, has a great effect on chronic illnesses and the people who have them (Figure 44-1 ■). Chronically ill people and their families are subject to great personal and emotional losses. Some of these are loss of self-esteem, loss of independence, feelings of rejection, feelings of helplessness, and economic deprivation due to the high cost of medical care. Families with a chronically ill child face a lifetime of expenses related to the disease. Box 44-1 ■ discusses particular concerns related to children with chronic illnesses.

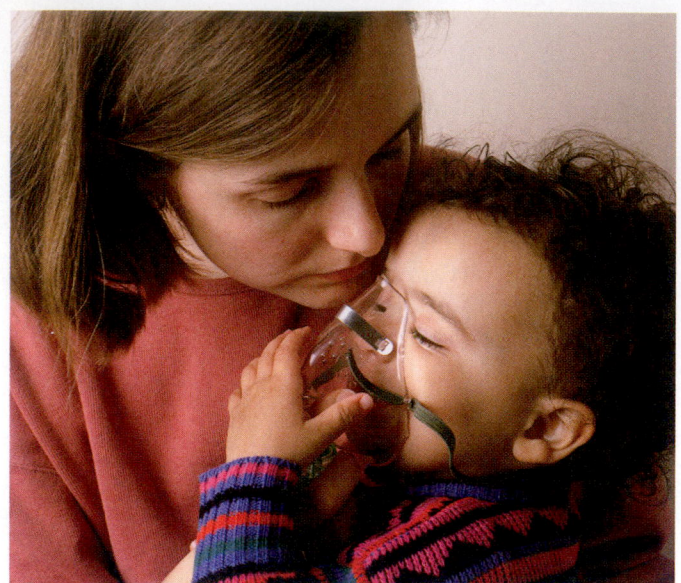

Figure 44-1. ■ The family with a chronically ill child has to structure a life around that child's needs and medical expenses. *Source:* Dorling Kindersley.

BOX 44-1	PEDIATRIC CONSIDERATIONS

Care of the Child with a Chronic Illness

When caring for children with chronic illnesses, the nurse must be alert to developmental stages (see Erikson's developmental stages in Chapter 16 ⚭) and how a child's developmental stage may impact the plan of care. Children born with such chronic conditions as muscular dystrophy and cerebral palsy may never have known any other life. Still, they are often very aware of how they are different from their peers. Programs that focus on allowing "kids to be kids" within the level of their disability can be valuable in providing some degree of normalcy.

Chronically ill children pose many challenges to families. The challenges, both physically and financially, can be overwhelming, placing stress on relationships among family members. Knowledge of the support available through community services is essential. Appropriate referrals are needed so that families can manage care of their children and receive support when they are feeling overburdened.

Prevention of Chronic Illness

Because chronic disease evolves over time and pathologic changes eventually become irreversible, the goal is to detect risk factors as early as possible. Generally, *prevention* means interrupting or stopping the development of a disease before it occurs. **Primary prevention** refers to health promotion and specific protection against diseases. An example of a primary prevention activity would be giving a talk on how to prevent colon cancer. **Secondary prevention** refers to early detection of disease and prompt intervention to halt disease progression. An example of secondary prevention is doing fecal occult blood tests and screening colonoscopies to screen for colon cancers. **Tertiary prevention** refers to rehabilitation (appropriate to the stage of disability), preventing further complications, and restoring functioning to the highest possible level. An example of tertiary prevention would be dietary and lifestyle changes to prevent further cancers from developing.

LPN/LVN Role in Care of Clients with Chronic Illness

Clients with chronic illness are seen in both acute care and long-term care environments. The LPN's/LVN's principal role in either setting is the delivery of excellent basic physical care and emotional support. The nurse focuses on preventing complications (bedsores, contractures, etc.) and encouraging independence so that clients are good candidates for future rehabilitation. There is no substitute for meticulous physical hygiene, repositioning clients at least every 2 hours, and the prevention, reporting, and early treatment of decubiti before they become debilitating.

REHABILITATION

Rehabilitation is the process of assisting individuals with handicaps to realize their particular physical, mental, social, and economic goals. Rehabilitation is an active process and is very different from "maintenance" care. A rehabilitation plan is made after a thorough assessment of a client's disabilities and capabilities. It is based on the potential for improving the client's condition. If improvement cannot be made, then care is directed toward maintaining the client in the current condition and preventing further disability. With each client, rehabilitation reaches a point at which no further progress is possible. Then the focus of care changes to maintaining that optimal level. The purpose or extent of rehabilitation ranges from employment or reemployment for someone with a handicap to the more limited achievement of providing one's own daily self-care. Rehabilitation involves a multidisciplinary approach. Members of the healthcare team use different areas of knowledge and skill to contribute to the client's care (Figure 44-2 ■). (This topic is discussed at greater length in Chapter 46 ⚭.)

Client and family teaching regarding chronic illness should include information about disease remission. Both need to understand that symptoms lessen or may disappear totally because of the prescribed treatments. A remission does not signal the need or opportunity to discontinue medication or other prescribed treatments. The diabetic, for example, who is well-controlled on his or her insulin must not take this as a sign of "cure." Chronic illness is "managed" or controlled through client/family education and involvement; it is not cured.

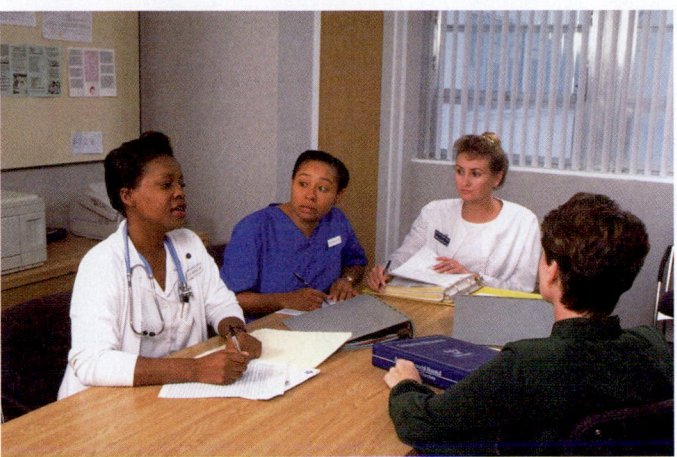

Figure 44-2. ■ The healthcare team works together to restore the client's optimal function.

FACILITIES FOR CONTINUING CARE

As described in Chapter 7 ◑, different types of healthcare institutions include long-term care facilities and home care. With hospital stays being shorter than in the past, a great deal of care for the chronically ill takes place in long-term care facilities (see Chapter 46 ◑), outpatient facilities, and the home.

NURSING CARE

PRIORITIZING NURSING CARE

When caring for clients who are chronically ill, focus your care on a thorough assessment of the client's functional abilities and potential for independence. Clients with chronic conditions often develop creative ways of coping with their unique situations. In addition to allowing them more time to complete tasks, ask clients how they like things done, giving them as much control over their care as possible. Clients who have coped with a disease over time have usually developed ways of managing and coping that fit their disability and lifestyle. Focus on the client's ability to manage the chronic illness; this supports client dignity and control.

Maintain a positive, hopeful attitude about chronically ill clients; this will help them focus on and invest in the often slow process of rehabilitation. The nurse who can point out small but significant gains will do much to motivate clients to keep on trying to achieve their goals.

Pain, "the fifth vital sign" and a factor in many chronic conditions, will interfere with a client's participation in exercise and other rehabilitation activities. Ask about pain and ensure that the client is properly medicated 30 to 60 minutes prior to exercise or activities that require their full attention and stamina. Observe clients who are unable to rate their pain for other signs, such as grimacing and irritability, that may indicate the need for pain relief.

(*Note:* The major discussion of pain, including adult and child pain scales, is in Chapter 22 ◑.)

ASSESSING

Before a plan of care can be devised for the chronically ill person, a thorough assessment of needs and capabilities is carried out. The assessment includes the individual's physical, psychological, social, and financial status.

DIAGNOSING, PLANNING, AND IMPLEMENTING

Nursing diagnoses are determined from all the data gathered about the client. Clients with chronic illness may have a long list of nursing diagnoses related to their disorders (Box 44-2 ■).

Some of the most common nursing diagnoses for the person with a chronic illness are:

- *Activity Intolerance*
- *Impaired Individual Resilience*
- *Ineffective Health Maintenance*
- *Risk for Injury*
- *Deficient Knowledge*
- *Disturbed Body Image*
- *Ineffective Coping*

In caring for the chronically ill person, the nurse has two important goals:

- To prevent and/or reduce disability
- To enable the client to remain a functioning individual across all domains (physical, social, intellectual, and spiritual)

BOX 44-2	NURSING DIAGNOSES RELATED TO CHRONIC DISORDERS

- *Anxiety*
- *Constipation*
- *Ineffective Breathing Pattern*
- *Impaired Verbal Communication*
- *Ineffective Coping*
- *Impaired Home Maintenance*
- *Hopelessness*
- *Impaired Urinary Elimination*
- *Dysfunctional Gastrointestinal Motility*
- *Impaired Physical Mobility*
- *Imbalanced Nutrition*
- *Chronic Pain*
- *Powerlessness*
- *Self-Care Deficit*
- *Disturbed Personal Identity*
- *Ineffective Role Performance*
- *Sexual Dysfunction*
- *Impaired Skin Integrity*
- *Impaired Social Interaction*

Interventions that the nurse can use with clients who are chronically ill include, but are not limited to, the following:

- Keep the person's body in good alignment; maintaining joint range and strength and preventing decubitus ulcers are physical measures that must be done every 2 hours. *Many of the difficulties that limit the chronically ill may not have been caused by the disease itself. Instead, they may have developed because of immobility, and its many complications, during the acute phase of illness.*

- Plan carefully for periods of rest between necessary activities. *Periods of rest will help preserve the client's physical resources.*

- Recognize that what is meaningful to the individual is a primary step toward developing self-care. Physical needs become paramount to chronically ill clients (see Maslow's hierarchy of needs, Figure 6-4 ⚭). *By meeting clients' physical needs, nurses can convey an interest in their progress and welfare, setting the stage for attention to higher level needs.*

- Encourage clients to perform as much of their own care as possible. Clients who have been independent in self-care before hospitalization should not be allowed to regress in their abilities, if at all possible. *Self-care maintains abilities and improves self-esteem.*

- Express warmth and interest in the client. Care of the chronically ill client requires that the nurse utilize all her senses to continually assess the client and his or her progress. Continued warmth and interest are necessary to the well-being of any chronically ill person. Very often a caring and concerned nurse can help a client become motivated and stay motivated. *Nurse–client relationships with the chronically ill develop and continue over a long expanse of time. It is essential that the nurse remain professional in that relationship and resist the temptation to become "friends" with the client.*

- Be prepared to review ideas with the client and to hear stories or concerns more than once. *It may be time-consuming to listen to the same questions and to say the same things over and over, but the nature of chronic illness may require this attention. Responding with warmth and interest is an important nursing intervention. Part of the adjustment to chronic illness is coming to terms with the many and progressive losses that occur as the disease process advances. "Telling the story" of these losses and their impact on the client's life is an essential part of coming to terms with, and making the life adjustments demanded by, chronic illness.*

- Encourage clients to identify coping methods and explore alternative approaches if necessary. *Chronic pain, ongoing medical costs, and difficulty carrying out ADLs all challenge the coping skills of chronically ill clients. Success in learning to adjust to a disability depends on what the person's personality, total life experience, and family relationships were before the illness. It also depends on the client's current behavior and motivation. The nurse can assist greatly by helping clients to recognize their past strengths and to focus on the choices they still can make in their lives.*

EVALUATING

Outcomes for specific chronic diseases are reviewed and adjusted as necessary. The nurse asks the client which interventions have been helpful. The nurse also asks about ongoing support for rehabilitation or maintenance therapy. It is especially important to note what motivates the client or gives the client hope.

Continuity of Care

Clients with chronic conditions require extra support and must plan for the long term. Generally, before discharge from the hospital, clients with chronic disease or their family members should be able to do the following:

- Demonstrate or explain measures that must be taken to avoid further preventable disability.
- Demonstrate or explain self-care activities they will perform.
- Identify activities for which they need help.
- Explain who will be available to help them with those activities and on what basis that help will be available.
- Explain what community resources are available and how to obtain help from them.
- Discuss in reasonable detail their plans for follow-up care and reevaluation.

TERMINAL ILLNESS

Despite amazing advances in science, nursing, and medical knowledge, dying will always be a part of life. **Terminal illness** is defined as an illness from which there is no reasonable expectation of survival (Figure 44-3 ■). When we interact with persons who are known to have a life-threatening disease, we are directly confronted with their dying and with our own mortality. This confrontation can evoke anxiety and cause the nurse to focus on his or her own death. The nurse must guard against **distancing** (eliminating any emotional connection to a client for fear of feeling grief when the person dies). The purpose of this section is to offer general guidelines for providing physical care and comfort to the dying client and family members who are caring for their loved one.

Palliative Care

The term **palliative care** or *palliative management* describes a shift in treatment goals from curing a disease to providing relief from suffering. Palliative care may be provided for

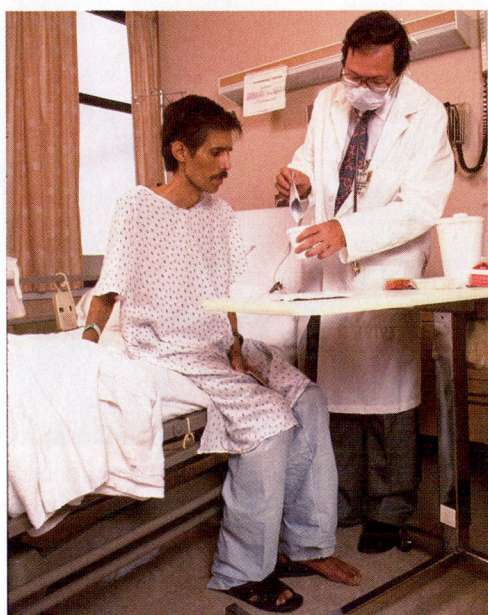

Figure 44-3. ■ A physician prepares treatment for this client in the terminal stages of AIDS. Comfort and emotional support are key nursing measures for terminally ill clients and their families. *Source:* Phototake NYC.

people whether or not they have been classified as "terminally ill." It can occur even in a hospital setting. Palliative care includes the following principles:

■ The overall goal of treatment is to optimize quality of life. Pain and other distressing symptoms are controlled, and the hopes and desires of the client are fulfilled as much as possible.

■ Death is regarded as a natural process, to be neither hastened nor prolonged.

■ Diagnostic tests and other invasive procedures are minimized, unless they are likely to alleviate symptoms or provide information that will facilitate symptom management.

■ Use of "heroic" treatment measures is discouraged.

■ When using analgesics, the right dose is the dose that provides pain relief without unacceptable side effects or toxicity.

■ The client is the "expert" on whether pain and symptoms are adequately relieved.

■ Clients eat if they are hungry and drink if they are thirsty. Feeding and fluids are not forced.

■ Care is individualized and is based on the goals of the client and family.

Relief of suffering in dying clients goes beyond identifying and treating physical symptoms. The emotional, social, spiritual, and existential components of suffering and pain must also be addressed.

Hospice

Hospice is care that incorporates the holistic concepts of palliative care and is provided for terminally ill clients with a prognosis of 6 months or less survival time. All hospice care is palliative in nature, but not all palliative care is hospice. The focus of hospice care is to improve the quality of life rather than to prolong it, although the outcome of improved quality, may indeed result in additional survival time.

The hospice movement was founded by Cecily Saunders, physician, nurse, and social worker, in London in 1967. The modern-day hospice movement came to the United States in 1974 with the opening of a hospice unit at Yale-New Haven Hospital in Connecticut. It grew rapidly after the enactment of the Medicare Hospice benefit in 1983. There are now more than 3,000 hospice programs serving all 50 states in the United States. Hospice care in the United States is significantly impacted by the Medicare system. Medicare pays an all-inclusive "per diem" benefit that provides the client with durable medical equipment (oxygen, hospital bed, etc.) and all medication and treatment related to the terminal illness or symptom management.

In contrast, the Canadian hospice program receives limited funding from Canada's National Health Services, and most of the cost of in-home hospice care is still carried by the dying person's family. The Canadian Palliative Care Association has worked since its founding in 1991 to promote the hospice care movement.

Hospice care can be carried out in a variety of settings. The most common settings are now in the client's home or extended-care facilities. Independent hospice and hospital-based palliative care units are also becoming more available as chronically ill clients are living longer and the demand for services increases.

Hospice programs cover a wide range of services. They are usually comprehensive, addressing the client holistically. Regardless of setting, hospice care is always delivered by an interdisciplinary team of healthcare professionals. The team members generally consist of the dying person, family and caregivers, physicians (including the client's primary care practitioner and the hospice doctor), nurses, aides, chaplains, social workers, bereavement specialists, and volunteers. Spiritual evaluation and support are a mandated part of every hospice program.

Entrance or admission into a hospice program requires a physician's "certification of terminal illness." Typically, the referring physician will discuss the referral with the client and family first and then initiate a hospice referral. If the client is a hospital inpatient, the hospice referral may be made with the assistance of the social worker or discharge planning coordinator. Referral of outpatients may be facilitated by home care agencies or other healthcare personnel, or they may come directly from the client/family. Most hospices try to respond to referrals within 24 hours of their receipt.

The Medicare guideline for admission is a life expectancy of 6 months or less, if the disease takes its natural course. Rather than being put into the uncomfortable position of trying to "predict" death, physicians may be more comfortable with answering the question, "Would you be surprised if the client dies within 6 months?" In many situations, a prognosis is nothing more than a medically educated guess.

Clients may seem terminal because of pain and other distressing symptoms that are not adequately controlled. Once these symptoms have been addressed, clients might enjoy an improved quality of life and live longer than their admitting prognosis. Clients are not denied claims if they live longer than 6 months, as long as they continue to meet the Medicare "conditions of participation" in a hospice. Clients admitted to hospice are evaluated periodically to ensure that they meet the hospice criteria for recertification (two initial 90-day periods followed by unlimited 60-day periods).

LPN/LVN Role in Care of Clients with Terminal Illness

When medical treatments are no longer an option, nurses can care for the family by providing comfort assistance to the client and by maintaining a caring, calm, and patient presence. They can use therapeutic communication to allow the client and family to express their fears, concerns, and anticipatory grief. (See Chapter 11 🔗.) Listening and paying attention to their responses are also important roles. Do not be quick to judge clients who turn to isolation for self-protection. What looks like emotional distance may be a defense against potentially overwhelming feelings.

Every human being has anchors in life that keep them grounded, especially during difficult times. These anchors are uniquely personal and should never be dismissed. Nor should another's faith be dismissed (Figure 44-4 ■). Personal beliefs and values can be a great source of strength.

Nurses keep the family informed about the client's status and let them know what changes (such as mottling of extremities and changes in respirations) indicate impending death. They may need to reinforce information that grieving family members may not have been able to absorb. (The moderate to severe anxiety that may be part of confronting death interferes with comprehension, learning, and memory.) Some clients may require a higher level of patience, which is usually in short supply due to the nurse's own busy life. It is important to remember that we all have hidden frailties and weaknesses. Terminal illness never resolves itself and is constantly attacking the body and spirit. Clients may need to draw from the courage within themselves to deal with their affliction.

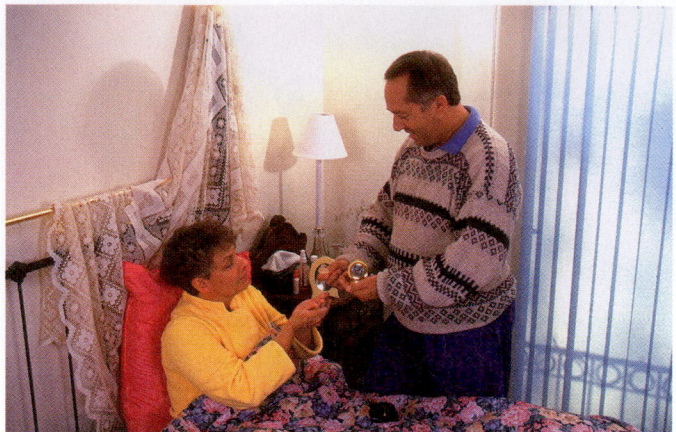

Figure 44-4. ■ Spiritual support in a time of illness can draw on a client's deepest strength. The nurse assists the client to contact those who can be of help. *Source:* PhotoEdit Inc.

Nurses should be aware that families handle approaching death in a variety of ways. Some families may be very open about the fact that the person is dying. Others may deny it and act as though the dying person will recover. Denial can be liberating because it throws off despair and allows the person to focus on what is possible in the time the person has left. Chapter 18 🔗 describes these different types of awareness.

Major goals of care for dying clients are to maintain comfort and dignity (see the Dying Person's Bill of Rights, Figure 18-4 🔗). Dying clients may appear alert, agitated, drowsy, or comatose. Keeping an open mind rather than a closed mind when dealing with these clients and "meeting them wherever they are" is essential to compassionate care of the dying. Dying clients may "see" a person or image that others cannot, and this experience should be treated with respect.

It is important to show kindness and empathy, even if the family seems angry or hostile. They may be angry because their loved one is leaving them or angry with the staff for being unable to save the client. This type of anger is not intentionally directed at nursing or medical staff, and should not be taken personally. Offer tissues, coffee, and a private area where they may grieve. Families should not be limited to regular visiting hours. They should be allowed to be with their dying loved ones as often and as long as they wish to be.

When family members choose to care for a loved one at home, nurses can encourage them to keep a "care journal," documenting the client's condition, medications, new symptoms, and response to various interventions. The journal can be a help to caregivers whose daily routines and sleep patterns are disrupted by the client's illness, and it may be a valuable memento after the person has died.

Care of a dying family member is a stressful event even if the person has lived a long and full life. When the dying

BOX 44-3   PEDIATRIC CONSIDERATIONS

Care of the Terminally Ill Child

The death of a child, whatever the cause, violates the normal order of things and is one of the most stressful events a family can endure. Terminally ill children are usually aggressively treated until shortly before death. Parents, understandably, don't want to abandon curative approaches, always holding out hope for a "miracle" or some new research that will save their child's life. Referrals to hospice, therefore, come even later in the disease process than for adults. Whenever possible, the child should be cared for at home, if parents and the home situation can accommodate this. Hospice's interdisciplinary team can be an invaluable resource before, during, and after the death. Other children in the home can be helped to understand and deal with their grief within their developmental level. While discussing death and assisting children to confront it is never easy, an honest approach, using terms the child can relate to and understand, is essential to facilitating healthy mourning and adjustment. There are many books available to present death in terms a child can understand and to assist adults in supporting grieving children.

person is a child, death is especially challenging. Life takes on a whole new meaning. The nurse can support the family to focus on the road ahead and all it holds rather than on its length. Box 44-3 ■ details some special considerations related to care of a terminally ill child.

The LPN/LVN can provide many helpful interventions for the dying person. Specific details are provided in the following section.

NURSING CARE

PRIORITIZING NURSING CARE

When caring for clients who are terminally ill, focus your care on meeting physiological needs, managing pain, and providing emotional support. Keep the client's skin clean, warm, and dry. Assist to positions of comfort. Offer food and fluids, but be aware that the terminally ill client may refuse them. Take every measure available to manage pain. If a patient-controlled analgesia (PCA) pump is in use, remind the client to push the button, if necessary. Administer ordered pain medications promptly and report breakthrough pain not managed by analgesics.

Dying, although it is a universal experience, is also highly individual in the way that clients and families react to anticipated loss. It is essential for the nurse to be sensitive to each client's need to discuss fears and concerns associated with the end of life. Clients and families will vary in their need to confront the diverse and strong feelings that are a part of coping with death. The nurse must remain supportive, even in the face of strong emotions such as anger and hostility

directed at them. More often than not, these emotions indicate feelings of hopelessness and helplessness that clients and families feel as they confront the realities of death and grief. (See Chapter 18 ⚭ for a full discussion of issues related to grief and loss.) The nurse learns to "reframe" anger by considering what other emotion(s) could be triggering the angry response. Usually negative responses are triggered by emotions that make the client feel vulnerable. Fear is often expressed outwardly as anger. The nurse who is able to recognize and reframe this can be supportive and positive, allowing expression of the underlying concerns and avoiding a response of anger and defensiveness.

ASSESSING

During the routine health care of a client, the nurse poses questions about previous losses and coping techniques. If there are concurrent or recent losses that put the client/family at risk for bereavement overload, more in-depth assessment is needed. (See Chapter 18 ⚭, Loss, Grief, and Death for questions to ask in an interview.)

Body processes slow as a person approaches death, and system imbalances occur that affect comfort and well-being. Some of the common signs and symptoms the dying client can have are:

- Nausea and vomiting due to slowing of GI tract processes and/or advancing disease process
- Pain due to the disease process, skin breakdown, or emotional and spiritual factors
- Decreased appetite and thirst due to the slowing of GI tract processes
- Agitation, confusion, and restlessness due to the disease process or medications
- Hypothermia or hyperthermia due to the brain's inability to regulate temperature
- External hemorrhaging due to certain disease processes
- Skin wounds due to immobility and loss of body tissue
- Dyspnea (shortness of breath) due to the disease process, fluid buildup, anemia, or weakness and inability to cough
- Incontinence of bowel and bladder due to weakness of muscles and declining cognitive processes

DIAGNOSING, PLANNING, AND IMPLEMENTING

Common nursing diagnoses for clients with a terminal illness include:

- *Activity Intolerance*
- *Acute Pain*
- *Ineffective Airway Clearance*
- *Anxiety*
- *Bowel/Bladder Incontinence*
- *Caregiver Role Strain*

- *Impaired Verbal Communication*
- *Ineffective Coping*
- *Fatigue*
- *Interrupted Family Processes*
- *Fear*
- *Grieving*
- *Hopelessness*
- *Imbalanced Nutrition: Less Than Body Requirements*
- *Impaired Oral Mucous Membrane*
- *Powerlessness*
- *Feeding Self-Care Deficit*
- *Impaired Skin Integrity*
- *Disturbed Sleep Pattern*
- *Social Isolation*
- *Risk for Spiritual Distress*

When clients receive a diagnosis of terminal illness, client goals are:

- To be comfortable
- To use positive coping in confronting the death

For the family and loved ones of the dying client, priority outcomes are:

- To maintain a relationship with the dying person
- To support the dying person through the process
- To adjust to the actual or impending loss

(See information about the processes of grief and mourning in Chapter 18 ⊖.)

Nursing interventions for dying clients and their families fall into several categories.

Supporting the Client and Family

- Offer attentive, active listening and presence. *For these clients, your greatest gift is your presence and your caring.*
- Monitor for sensory deficit or overload by adjusting television or radio volume and lights. *This supports a more comfortable environment and shows respect for client preferences.*
- Support clients spiritually if they speak of seeing someone who has passed and/or are speaking with someone who is not visible to others. *This will provide emotional comfort and show respect for the client.*
- Prepare the family of the dying person for impending death. (Box 44-4 ▪ lists signs of impending death.) *Nurses can inform the family and friends of the dying client when signs of approaching death occur. Most hospice programs have educational materials that inform caregivers of these signs.*
- Teach the client and family about the grieving process. *Grief goes hand in hand with dying. It is helpful for the family to learn what to expect in the grieving process. (Review the major discussion of loss, grief, and death in Chapter 18 ⊖.)*
- Encourage family and friends to speak with the dying client. *Hearing is the last of the senses to be lost; this can be a time for loved ones to share their thoughts and feelings.*

BOX 44-4 SIGNS OF APPROACHING DEATH

- Changes in level of consciousness
- Coolness, mottling, and cyanosis of the extremities
- Decreased sensation, taste, and smell
- Decreased, irregular, "noisy" or *Cheyne-Stokes respirations* (deep to shallow breathing pattern, with periods of apnea)
- Decreasing blood pressure
- Decreasing urinary output
- Difficulty talking or swallowing
- Nausea, flatus, abdominal distention
- Restlessness, agitation
- Urinary and/or bowel incontinence, constipation
- Weak, slow, "thready," and/or irregular pulse

- Give nonjudgmental assistance to the family. If family members would like to assist in care, provide teaching. If they need space away from the dying client, provide a private area. *Providing care may give comfort to some family or friends. Others may need a place where they can be, outside of the presence of the dying client.*
- Whenever possible, provide clients with resources to use in the future. The nurse can prepare the family for times of grief by providing information about support groups and counseling. *Bereavement support services are a mandated part of hospice services for 13 months following the client's death. These programs often provide services to both hospice bereaved and others from the community whose loved ones may not have been served by hospice.*

Maintaining Physical Comfort

The nurse can help the dying client maintain a level of comfort.

- Assist client to breathe by positioning client in Fowler's position and encouraging the client to cough if able, and as needed. *This helps mobilize secretions and terminal congestion (death rattle). Suctioning is only used if the client is unable to clear secretions and cholinergic blocking agents (Atropine, scopolamine) have not been successful in lessening secretions. Frequent suctioning can act as a stimulus for further secretion formation. It should, therefore, be used sparingly or not at all, and only if less invasive methods fail.*
- Help control pain by administering medications on time or as needed (for breakthrough pain not managed with scheduled dose).
- Keep the side rails up for safety and also use nonpharmacological techniques that are effective for the client, such as soft music and lighting, guided imagery, and massage. *These will help the client relax and decrease anxiety.*
- Assist with ADLs such as bathing and dressing. *This will help the client feel better physically and will comfort both client and family.*
- Provide frequent turning and repositioning to prevent skin breakdown and pain. If skin breakdown already

exists, provide dressing changes and good skin care along with pain medication. *Skin breakdown can cause infections as well as increase pain. The best intervention is to prevent skin breakdown. However, as a client enters into the active phase of dying, complete body care may become too uncomfortable. If the client is unable to speak, observe nonverbal communication such as facial expressions for grimacing, moaning, and even breathing pattern changes to assess objective cues to client discomfort.*

- Support the client's nutritional needs. Prevent constipation by administering prescribed laxatives or stool softeners and oral fluids as requested. *This will decrease skin breakdown and prevent constipation.*

clinical ALERT

All clients on narcotics for pain relief should be placed on a bowel regimen (stool softener, suppositories, etc.) to prevent constipation.

- Explain to the family that decreased circulation of body fluids can cause bloating and swelling. Tell them that fluids and food will be offered but never forced. *Decreased fluid and dietary intake can be distressing to the family (who may say the facility is "starving the client"). However, forcing food or fluids by feeding tubes and IVs can make the client more uncomfortable. Declining kidney function may not allow excess fluid to be excreted. At some point in the terminal phase of most diseases, nutrients are no longer absorbed and, hence, of no benefit to the client even when put directly into the GI tract with tube feedings.*
- Support urinary elimination by supplying easy access to water and juices as appropriate to client. *This will support intake as desired by client.*
- If the client becomes incontinent of bowel and bladder, place a Foley catheter per standing or physician's order and provide frequent linen changes with extra padding added to the linen. *Incontinence can be distressing and can contribute to skin breakdown. Extra padding can make linen changes easier.*
- For nausea, administer antiemetics such as Compazine, Ativan, or Reglan, on schedule as prescribed. *Antiemetics help promote comfort. Many hospices have access to compounding pharmacists who prepare topical medications in the form of PLO gels. The most notable of these is ABHR gel, an individualized combination of Ativan, Benadryl, Haldol, and Reglan, applied topically to a nonhairy area every 4 to 6 hours for the control of nausea, vomiting, anxiety, and restlessness.*
- Provide natural pain relief measures such as distraction, music, and imagery. Administer prescription medications such as morphine, oxycodone, methadone, Dilaudid, and Duragesic patches around the clock as well as shorter acting medications, when needed, for breakthrough pain. If the client has a PCA pump (see Figure 45-5), ensure that it is working and that the client and family understand its use. See also Chapter 45 . *Cold compresses can help to lessen localized pain. Pain medications are most effective when they are administered regularly to maintain a therapeutic level. Having a PCA device gives the client some control over the pain and so reduces anxiety.*

- If a client is agitated, wrap a warm, moist sheet around the client for short periods of time. Medications such as Ativan, Xanax, Haldol, and Valium (if ordered) also help lessen agitation.
- Provide frequent tepid sponge baths and frequent linen changes for clients with fever. Dress client in light, cotton clothing. Sometimes the fevers will respond to acetaminophen or aspirin as well. *High fevers can be very uncomfortable as the client perspires. Tepid baths and frequent changes of linens and light clothing can promote comfort.*
- If there is external hemorrhaging, put direct pressure and application of ice packs over the bleeding areas. Remain calm. Provide comfort and reassurance. *External hemorrhaging can be very frightening to all present. The use of red towels to absorb blood and control hemorrhage can help to lessen the fears associated with the sight of blood.*
- Administer medications such as morphine and Ativan, if ordered, to control pain, decrease anxiety and intervene in the "anxiety-dyspnea" cycle. Nurses who have been trained can perform chest compressions to help break up fluid collection in the lungs. *Both of these interventions help to ease dyspnea and help the client relax.*
- Atropine drops and scopolamine patches may decrease fluid secretions that contribute to noisy respirations, often referred to as the "death rattle" by laypersons. *These are most frequently treated to ease family concerns. The client is usually semiconscious to comatose at this point, unaware and unbothered by the symptom.*
- Reinforce teaching to family members when the dying person is being cared for in the home. *Hospices usually have standing orders, signed by the primary care physician on admission, for many of the interventions described above. They facilitate prompt attention to distressing symptoms as they arise. When hospice care is in the client's home, a "comfort care pack" is delivered with orders for medications to control fever, restlessness, nausea and vomiting, constipation, incontinence, and increased secretions as they arise. In some states, narcotic pain medication is also allowed in these packets.*

Promoting Positive Coping

The nurse can foster positive coping through the following interventions:

- Provide factual information about diagnosis, treatment, and prognosis. *This reduces fear of the unknown and facilitates realistic end-of-life planning.*

- Instruct the client and caregivers in the use of relaxation techniques. Relaxation techniques assist *with the management of pain and stress.*
- Involve client and family in all decisions about care. *This helps the client and family feel some sense of control over their situation.*
- Provide an atmosphere of caring and acceptance. *This facilitates the expression of feelings.*
- Discourage decision making when the client is under severe stress. *Moderate to severe anxiety interferes with concentration, problem solving, and healthy choices.*
- Assist the client and family to identify a support system. *Keeping caregivers healthy and giving them "time off" is essential to being able to persevere in a caregiving situation that may go on much longer than expected.*
- Foster healthy outlets for anger and hostility. *Healthy outlets for strong emotions help to minimize or manage internal stress and anxiety, leaving energy for more positive coping.*
- Provide a caring atmosphere that encourages and maintains realistic hope. Box 44-5 ■ describes a way to maintain hope in the dying process. *Although hope for a cure of the client's disease may need to be abandoned, the possibility of "healing" (a far more holistic process) continues to exist throughout the dying process and beyond.*

EVALUATING

Evaluating the effectiveness of nursing care for the terminally ill client is difficult because of the many dimensions of end-of-life care. The nurse must evaluate outcomes in the physical, psychosocial, and spiritual dimensions. The holistic nature of end-of-life care challenges the nurse to be proficient in collecting data across all of these domains. Goals are always set by the interdisciplinary team in consultation with the client and family. These are jointly reevaluated and the plan of care adjusted accordingly every 14 days, or more frequently, as changes in the client's condition dictate. This interdisciplinary team approach is the hallmark of palliative and hospice care. With the client and family at the center of care, the team (physician, nurse, social worker, and spiritual care advocate) meets together face-to-face to assess the impact of the plan of care on the client and to adjust goals and interventions as needed.

With the long-term goal of a peaceful death, free from distressing symptoms, in an environment of the client and family's choosing, the team continually evaluates the relevance of short-term goals and interventions in relation to the client's current circumstances.

Pain, for example, is evaluated and assessed on a 10-point scale, with 0 representing no pain and 10, the worst possible pain from the client's perspective. Medication and other pain-relieving measures are ordered based on the degree of comfort desired and the client's desire to remain alert. Some clients request that their pain be kept at 0 and are willing to be sedated to achieve that goal. Others may be willing to tolerate pain of 4 to 5 so they can remain alert and be able to interact with others.

The nurse continually uses active listening and observation to evaluate the client's responses, remaining alert to both verbal and nonverbal cues. Client goals and outcomes vary with the individual and the issues to be confronted.

| BOX 44-5 | HEALING STEPS FOR THE TERMINALLY ILL CLIENT |

Maintaining hope in the face of inevitable death may seem futile or impossible to some. Many, even in the healthcare professions, believe that we give up all hope when someone is dying. Indeed, those who opt for hospice services late in their disease process often say that they didn't call sooner because they "had not given up hope."

An alternate view regarding hope is that we never truly "give up" hope, but that the focus of our hope changes with age, circumstances, and state of health. The client who is healthy hopes to remain so and hopes for a cure when diagnosed with an illness. When the condition, illness, or disease cannot be cured, the shift is to the hope that it can be managed or controlled for as long as possible. As disease progresses to a "terminal" stage, the focus of hope might shift to comfort, a peaceful death, and support for grieving loved ones.

The nurse can facilitate realistic hope for clients and families, regardless of the focus of their hope. The nurse can reassure both client and family that everything possible will be done to control pain and other distressing symptoms. A hospice referral can provide clients and caregivers with much needed support before, during, and after the death.

One of the universal emotional needs of dying clients seems to be the sense that their lives have had meaning; that they "mattered" in some way to at least one other human being. In addition to encouraging families and friends to share this with their loved one, the nurse can provide the "gift" of how a particular client has enriched the nurse's life as he or she was privileged to participate in their care.

The healing of relationships, some of which may have been fractured for years, can add to a more peaceful death and less complicated bereavement period. Dr. Ira Byock (2004), in his book *The Four Things That Matter Most*, addresses themes he has noted while caring for terminally ill clients. The taking care of "unfinished business" contributes to a peaceful death. Unfinished business includes anything that might be left incomplete and unattended to by the client and family.

According to Byock, there are four things that dying clients and families need to hear and/or say: "Please forgive me," "I forgive you," "Thank you," and "I love you." Each statement can be a tool for conveying "forgiveness, gratitude, and love" (Byock, 2004, p. 216).

Criteria for evaluation must be based on goals set by the client and family in consultation with the healthcare team.

To measure the bereaved's accommodation to loss (actual or anticipated), the nurse might ask about his/her participation in therapy sessions, or about whether he/she is now sleeping through the night. If outcomes are not achieved, the nurse needs to help the team explore why the plan was unsuccessful and adjust or renew the plan as appropriate.

NURSING PROCESS CARE PLAN
Client with Metastatic Carcinoma of the Bowel

John Yee, age 63, was diagnosed with metastatic carcinoma of the bowel 4½ months ago. A colostomy was done at that time to relieve a bowel obstruction. No further treatment was available and Mr. Yee was discharged home on hospice.

Assessment
Roger Hadrick, Mr. Yee's hospice nurse, has noted that Mr. Yee has become profoundly weaker over the past week and is no longer able to walk to the bathroom. His abdomen is greatly distended, firm, and tender, and he complains of feeling bloated and nauseated. Bowel sounds are sluggish. Although he complains of having no appetite, his wife has been encouraging him to eat several times a day. Over the past 2 months he has become increasingly jaundiced. Mr. Yee describes his pain as 8 out of 10 even though he is taking a long-acting morphine preparation twice a day. On this visit he tells his nurse, "I know I don't have long to live. Why can't they just give me a big dose of morphine and get it over with?"

Nursing Diagnosis
The following priority nursing diagnoses (among others) are established for this client:

- *Hopelessness* related to deteriorating physiologic condition and uncontrolled distressing symptoms
- *Powerlessness* related to terminal illness
- *Acute Pain* related to increased tumor growth

Expected Outcomes
The expected outcomes specify that Mr. Yee will:

- Participate in self-care activities in accordance with health status.
- Make choices related to care and treatment.
- Maintain physiologic comfort; pain less than 4 out of 10 within 30 to 60 minutes after being medicated, and maintained with a combination of long-acting and breakthrough medications.
- Share values and personal meaning of life.

Planning and Implementation
The following nursing interventions are planned and implemented:

- Encourage client and family to maintain pain diary. *The diary assists the hospice nurse in evaluating the pain medication regimen.*
- Monitor use of breakthrough pain medication. *This allows the supervising nurse to evaluate the need for a possible increase in long-acting pain medication.*
- Evaluate efficacy of pain regimen. *The goal is to maintain constant pain control and prevent exacerbation of pain.*
- Administer antiemetics and antianxiety medications as ordered. *These medications promote comfort and facilitate the client being able to remain active socially, and to participate in care.*
- Teach the client and family about the dying process. *Information lessens anxiety about the unknown and prepares them for the client's eventual death.*
- Instruct the family about the decreased nutritional needs of a dying person. *This helps maintain the client's dignity, comfort, and right to choose or refuse food.*
- Allow the client to verbalize feelings. *Listening provides an emotional outlet for the client and contributes to a more peaceful death.*
- Identify support systems available to client and family. *Support systems lessen the burden on the client and caregivers.*

Evaluation
After 3 days of monitoring and adjusting Mr. Yee's medications, his symptoms are under control. His long-acting morphine has been increased and his wife administers the short-acting morphine at the onset of breakthrough pain, when Mr. Yee requests. Also, his wife has told him to ask for food if he is hungry, rather than offering food and encouraging him to eat. Although he is spending more time sleeping, his waking moments often include short conversations with his wife and children. He no longer expresses a desire to hasten his death.

Critical Thinking in the Nursing Process

1. Why is Mr. Yee's appetite decreased?
2. What is the rationale for giving both long-acting and short-acting preparations of morphine?
3. Why is Mr. Yee's abdomen distended, firm, and tender?

Note: Discussion of Critical Thinking questions appears on the MyNursingKit Website.

Legal Issues in Terminal Illness

The nurse must be familiar with and follow state laws and facility policies about legal issues related to death. Conditions of terminal illness may sometimes raise serious ethical considerations. Nurses should try to prepare themselves for difficult situations by learning about them and by discussing them with other health team members.

DIRECTIVES AND MEDICAL ORDERS

As described in Chapter 18 ⊂⊃, the Patient Self-Determination Act of 1991 requires all healthcare facilities receiving Medicare and Medicaid reimbursement to do the following:

- Check the client's chart and/or ask clients whether they have advance directives.
- Recognize and abide by advance directives.
- Provide written information to clients about their right to declare their personal wishes about treatment decisions, including the right to refuse medical treatment.

Two types of advance medical directives may be implemented as death approaches. The first is the **living will** (a document that provides specific instructions about what medical treatment the client chooses to omit or refuse in the event that he or she is unable to make those decisions); it would be referenced prior to cardiopulmonary resuscitation (CPR), intubation, or ventilatory (breathing) support. Living wills may be ignored if there is no durable power of attorney for health care. The second advance directive that comes into play, the **durable power of attorney for health care** (also called a *healthcare proxy*), provides for a designated person or persons to see that the client's wishes are honored when the client can no longer speak for himself or herself (power of attorney with organ donation form was shown in Figure 4-2 ⊂⊃). Living wills are usually drawn up with the services of an attorney. Durable power of attorney for healthcare decisions may be done without a lawyer, as long as the document is properly witnessed.

As clients reach a stage of terminal illness or expected death, the physician may order "no code," **Do Not Resuscitate** (DNR) orders, or similar orders in their chart. These orders prevent interventions the client does not wish to have performed when death approaches. Usually this is done when the client or surrogate has stated that no resuscitation is to take place in the event of respiratory or cardiac arrest. If this order is not in place, the nurse is required to call a resuscitation team when a client stops breathing.

A *comfort measures only* order would be written to indicate that the goal of treatment is a dignified and comfortable death. No life-sustaining measures would be undertaken when this order was in place.

"Comfort care" for both the client and the family includes the reassuring presence of the nurse or nurse-substitute as death becomes imminent (Figure 44-5 ■).

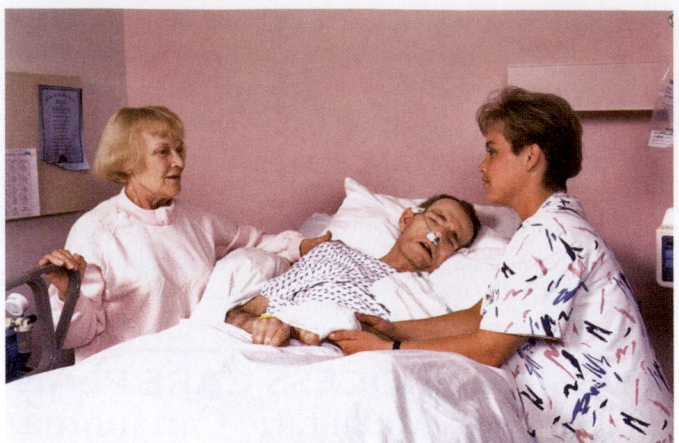

Figure 44-5. ■ The nurse's presence and concern are valuable offerings to the terminally ill client. *Source:* Pearson Education/ PH College

A value inherent in the hospice philosophy is that, if possible, no one should die alone. When family members are not able to be present at the time of death, they derive immeasurable comfort from the knowledge that their loved one's nurse cared enough and took the time to hold their hand and stay with them as they died.

LABELING OF THE DECEASED

Nurses have a duty to handle the deceased's body with dignity and respect and to label the body appropriately. Mishandling can cause tremendous emotional distress to survivors. It can also create legal problems if the body is inappropriately identified and prepared incorrectly for funeral services. In the hospital, the deceased's wrist identification tag is left on, and another tag is tied to the client's ankle or toe, in case one of the tags becomes detached. A third tag is attached to the **shroud** (a large piece of plastic or cotton material used to enclose a body after death). All identification tags should include the client's name, hospital number, and physician's name. In most hospitals this is provided on the Addressograph plate or hospital card, which has the appropriate information already on it. The nurse's last written note in the client's chart must document the disposition of the body, where it was transported (morgue, funeral home), and by whom.

AUTOPSY

An **autopsy,** or postmortem examination, is an examination of the body after death. It is performed to learn more about the cause of death, to learn more about a disease, or to assist in gathering statistical data. Except in cases where criminal activity may be suspected, family/surrogates must give their written permission and pay for an autopsy to be performed.

ORGAN DONATION

Organ donation (discussed in Chapter 18 **⊂⊃**) requires a written statement of the decision to make a gift of all or part of one's own body for medical or dental education, research, advancement of science, therapy, or transplantation.

Nurses may serve as witnesses for people who consent to donate organs or who revoke the organ donor designation. No matter what the decision, organ donation is an emotional issue because it hinges on the death of a loved one. Some families may find it extremely distressing even to be asked about organ donation. Other families may derive peace and satisfaction from the thought that someone else's life has been saved by the donation of their loved one's organ(s). In a sense, their loved one's death "was not in vain." This knowledge can also assist with emotional closure and healthy accommodation to the loss. Specific guidelines are observed to determine that a person has died before organ donation can begin.

Definitions and Signs of Death

Traditionally, clinical signs of death were cessation of the apical pulse, respirations, and blood pressure, also referred to as *heart-lung death*. However, since artificial means were developed to maintain respirations and blood circulation, it has become more difficult to identify death. Box 44-6 ■ lists clinical indications of death.

If a person is connected to life support equipment, death is determined by an absence of brain wave activity (a flat electroencephalogram) for at least 24 hours. Some would also include **cerebral death** (irreversible damage to the cerebral cortex) within the definition of death, even though a person might still be able to breathe. An irreversible state of unconsciousness (**vegetative state** or **coma**) is never used as a defining factor for the determination of brain death. *The one legal standard is the lack of EEG activity tested twice in a 24-hour period*, analyzed and verified by two separate physicians qualified to do so.

Care after Death

After death, the nurse may need to provide postmortem care for the client. Steps for performing this care are given in Procedure 44-1 ■ on page 1237.

The nurse should expect some characteristic physical changes to occur. **Rigor mortis** is the stiffening of the body that begins about 2 to 4 hours after death. It results from a lack of adenosine triphosphate (ATP), which is necessary for muscle fiber relaxation. Without ATP the muscles contract, making the joints rigid. Rigor mortis starts in the involuntary muscles (heart, bladder, etc.), then progresses to the head, neck, and trunk, and finally reaches the extremities. Rigor mortis usually leaves the body about 96 hours after death.

Algor mortis is the gradual decrease of the body's temperature after death. When blood circulation stops and the hypothalamus ceases to function, body temperature falls about 1°C (1.8°F) per hour until it reaches room temperature. Simultaneously, the skin loses its elasticity and can easily be broken when dressings and adhesive tape are removed.

After blood circulation has ceased, the red blood cells break down, releasing hemoglobin, which discolors the surrounding tissues. This discoloration, referred to as **livor mortis,** appears in the lower (most *dependent*) areas of the body.

Tissues after death become soft, and bacterial fermentation eventually liquefies them. The warmer the temperature, the more rapid the change. Bodies are often stored in cool places to delay this process. Embalming delays the process, through injection of chemicals into the body to destroy the bacteria and retard the fermentation process to allow for funeral rituals and viewing the body as desired.

The nurse must be familiar with institutional policies and procedures about care of a body after death. Postmortem care should be carried out according to the policy of the institution. Because care of the body may be influenced by religious law, the nurse should check the client's religion and make every attempt to comply. Table 44-1 ■ describes some cultural traditions related to death and death rituals.

If the deceased's family or friends wish to view the body, it is important to make the environment as clean and pleasant as possible and to make the body appear natural and comfortable. All equipment, soiled linen, and supplies should be removed from the bedside. Some institutions require that all tubes in the body remain in place. In other institutions, tubes may be cut to within 2.5 cm (1 in.) of the skin and taped in place. In still others, all tubes may be removed.

BOX 44-6	**CLINICAL INDICATIONS OF DEATH**

- Total lack of response to external stimuli
- No voluntary muscular movement, especially breathing
- Absent reflexes
- Flat encephalogram

For people on artificial support:

- Absence of electric currents from the brain (measured by an electroencephalogram) for at least 24 hours
- Irreversible destruction of the cerebral cortex (cerebral death or higher brain death); the client may still be able to breathe but is irreversibly unconscious

TABLE 44-1	**Cultural Traditions in Mourning and After-Death Rites**	
RELIGIOUS GROUP	**POSSIBLE RITUALS**	**ORGAN DONATION OR AUTOPSY BELIEFS**
American Indians	Beliefs and practices vary widely. Navajo do not touch the deceased or their belongings. Mourning is done in private.	Varies among tribes.
Baha'i	No embalming or cremation; must be buried within an hour's travel distance of place of death. Body washed and wrapped in shroud. Prayer for the Dead recited.	Decision left to individual.
Buddhism	Last-rite chanting at bedside. Cremation common. Prayers weekly for 49 days to help soul in its transformation and possible rebirth.	Organ donation considered act of mercy, autopsy individual choice.
Catholicism	Sacrament of the sick. Obligated to take ordinary but not extraordinary means to prolong life. Burial preferred in Catholic cemeteries. Cremation allowed, but remains must be interred, not scattered.	Autopsy, organ donation acceptable.
Christian Science	Unlikely to seek medical help to prolong life. Disposal of body and parts decided by family.	Individual decides about organ donation.
Hinduism	No restrictions to right-to-die issue. Religious prayers chanted before and after death. Body washed, wrapped in white cloth, laid in coffin. Cremation common. Men and women display outward grief, do not take part in any rituals for length of mourning period. Thread tied around wrist signifies a blessing, do not remove. No embalming.	Autopsy, organ donation acceptable.
Islam	Attempts to shorten life prohibited. Body is washed only by Muslims of same gender and wrapped in a plain cloth (*kafan*). Only burial is permitted by Islamic law (*Shari'ah*). Prayer for forgiveness recited.	Organ donation acceptable. Autopsy only for medical or legal reasons.
Jehovah's Witness	Use of extraordinary means to prolong life is individual choice. Burial determined by family preference.	Autopsy if required by law. Organ donation forbidden.
Judaism	If death is inevitable, no new procedure needed, but must continue those ongoing. Body ritually washed. Burial as soon as possible, all body parts must be buried together. Seven-day mourning period.	Autopsy permitted in certain circumstances; organ donation is a complex issue.
Mennonite	Do not believe life must be continued at all cost.	Autopsy, organ donation acceptable.
Mormonism	If death inevitable, promote a peaceful and dignified death. Burial in temple clothes. Burial preferred to cremation ("dust to dust").	Autopsy permitted with permission of next of kin. Organ donation is permitted.
Protestantism	Burial or cremation is individual decision.	Autopsy, organ donation are individual decisions.
Seventh-Day Adventist	Follow ethic of prolonging life. Disposal of body and burial are individual decisions.	Autopsy, organ donation acceptable.

Source: Adams, E. D., Towle, M. A. (2008). *Pediatric nursing care.* Upper Saddle River, NJ: Prentice Hall. Table 9-3.

Normally the body is placed in a supine position with the arms either at the sides, palms down, or across the abdomen. One or two pillows are placed under the head and shoulders, or the head of the bed is elevated 30 degrees, to prevent blood from discoloring the face by settling in it. The eyelids are closed and held in place for a few seconds. Often, the eyes and mouth do not remain closed and require the intervention of a *mortician* (an undertaker or funeral director; a person trained in care of the dead).

Soiled areas of the body are washed. However, a complete bath is not necessary, because the mortician will wash the body. Absorbent pads are placed under the buttocks to capture any feces and urine released because of relaxation of the sphincter muscles. A clean gown is placed on the client, and the hair is brushed and combed. All jewelry is removed, except a wedding band in some instances, which is taped to the finger. The top bed linens are adjusted neatly to cover the client to the shoulders. Soft lighting and chairs should be provided for the family to make the surroundings as peaceful as possible.

Viewing the body before it is taken to the morgue or funeral home may be the first opportunity for "closure" to the death event. Some families, due to financial limitations, choose to forgo the formal funeral and calling hours. For them, viewing of the body immediately after death may be the only opportunity to realize that death has actually occurred. This can be an important part of the grieving process and the nurse should be sensitive to this. The body should be prepared with care and made to look as natural as possible. Within reason, family should be allowed as much time as they need to be with the body, with the realization that this may be the last time they will actually see the deceased.

In the hospital, after the body has been viewed by the family, additional identification tags are applied, as discussed earlier. The body is wrapped in a shroud, and identification is placed on the outside. The body is then taken to the morgue if arrangements have not been made to have a mortician pick it up from the client's room. The nurse needs to be familiar with the institutional polices and procedures in order to make these events go as smoothly as possible for the family.

As discussed in Chapter 18 ⚭, cultural groups may wish to retain their native customs in preparing the body for burial or cremation (see Table 44-1).

> **Note:** The references and resources for all chapters have been compiled at the back of the book.

PROCEDURE 44-1 Performing Postmortem Care

Purpose

- To clear and prepare the body of a deceased client for family visitation and for transport to mortuary

Equipment

- Bathing supplies
- Morgue packet
- Identification tags
- Rolled gauze and abdominal pads
- Plastic bag for client's personal belongings
- Gurney or morgue cart
- Clean gloves

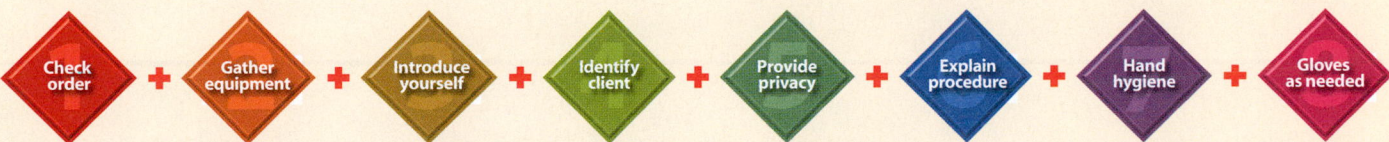

Check order ✚ Gather equipment ✚ Introduce yourself ✚ Identify client ✚ Provide privacy ✚ Explain procedure ✚ Hand hygiene ✚ Gloves as needed

Interventions and Rationales

1. Perform preparatory steps (see icon bar above).
2. If there are other clients or visitors in the room, temporarily ask them to leave if possible, to provide privacy.
3. Follow facility procedures for notification of personnel and other departments:
   a. Follow the client's advance directives on file at the hospital for donor instructions.
   b. Determine if the client has a donor card and/or has made a decision to donate any organs.
   c. Notify appropriate hospital personnel or local procurement organization for assistance with organ donation.
   d. Follow specific procedures for organ transplants according to hospital policy.
4. Don gloves.
5. Maintain proper alignment of the body. When rigor mortis sets in with the body in poor or contracted

alignment, it makes it difficult for the funeral director to dress and prepare the body for possible viewing.

6. Do not replace dentures if they fall out. *As facial muscles relax, dentures can fall out and be lost. Leave dentures in denture cup and send with client to the morgue.*

7. Remove any external objects causing pressure or injury to the skin (e.g., oxygen mask).

8. Convert all IV lines to intermittent infusion devices. *Removing catheter and IV lines can cause fluid to leak into tissues and cause edema and discoloration. Hospital policy may supersede this action; if so, follow hospital policy.*

9. Cleanse the body as needed. *Partial bath may be required to remove secretions, wound drainage, stains.*

10. Close the eyes, if necessary, using paper tape or gauze pads. *You may do this after the family has visited the deceased.*

11. Place protective incontinent pad under the buttocks and between the legs diaper fashion. *Bowel and bladder may continue to release waste.*

12. If the family is to visit the deceased, provide clean linen and gown for client. *This shows respect for the deceased and is a comfort to the family.*

13. Remove equipment used for cleaning the client. *This provides a more pleasing environment.*

14. If previously determined or requested by client or family, notify the appropriate clergy or religious support person. *This will provide spiritual support for the family of the deceased.*

15. After the family and clergy have visited, label the body, attaching ID tags to the great toe, wrist, and shroud or morgue bag, or as determined by standard procedure. *It is important to follow policy carefully to prevent misidentification of the body.*

16. Place arms and hands loosely at side or on abdomen. *This prevents discoloration of the hands.*

17. Place the body in the shroud or morgue bag.

18. Label all personal belongings and place them in a bag. *Belongings will be returned to the family.*

19. Remove gloves and wash hands. *This prevents transmission of microorganisms.*

20. Close the doors to the client's room and clear hallways in preparation for transfer of the body to the morgue. *It is upsetting for other clients and families to see a body being removed.*

21. Transfer the body to the morgue on a gurney or morgue cart. Keep the client's head elevated.

22. Place the client's personal belongings in the appropriate place determined by the facility. *This ensures safe transferal of belongings.*

23. Support family members as needed. *Providing support is an important nursing action at this time.*

clinical ALERT

Inform the funeral home if the client has any infectious disease so that appropriate care can be taken to prevent contamination of personnel or the environment.

SAMPLE DOCUMENTATION

[date]
[time] Without pulse or spontaneous respirations at 0600 assessment. Dr. Smitts notified at 0610. Pronounced by Dr. Owens at 0620. Family notified at 0630. Postmortem care provided. Family and clergy visited. Personal belongings signed for and taken by John Marsh (son). Peace Brothers Mortuary notified. Body transported to the morgue. _____

_____ L. Anderson, LPN

Chapter Review

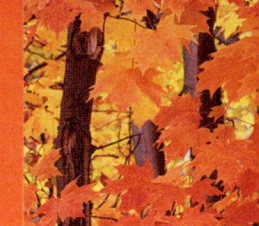

KEY Points

- Nurses help clients deal with all types of chronic illnesses. They help prevent chronic illnesses, and they also help clients live with their chronic illnesses.

- Nurses have two major roles in helping clients with chronic disease processes in rehabilitation. The first is to see that disability is limited as much as possible through the prevention of complications. The second is to plan and implement a rehabilitation program as appropriate for the client.

- The most important contribution to a client's rehabilitation is made by clients themselves.

- Nurses help clients deal with all kind of losses, such as loss of body image, loss of limbs, loss of function, and death.

- Palliative care or palliative management shifts treatment goals from curative to comfort.

- Hospice care is based on the holistic concepts of palliative care and emphasizes quality of life.

- Caring for the dying and bereaved is one of the nurse's most challenging responsibilities. It can also be one of the most rewarding aspects of nursing care.

- Goals of care for terminally ill clients include maintaining comfort and dignity until the person dies.

- Nurses must know their responsibilities in regard to legal and policy issues surrounding death.

- It is important to identify signs of impending death for family members and to explain what these signs mean.

- Anger that is misdirected at nurses or caregivers must be "reframed" with an understanding that the person or persons are upset about the client's death and may be substituting anger for other feelings such as fear and helplessness. The nurse should continue to convey kindness and empathy.

- Dying clients and their families require open communication, physical help, and emotional and spiritual support to achieve a peaceful and dignified death.

FOR FURTHER Study

Chapter 4 has discussion of advance directives.

See Figure 6-4 for Maslow's hierarchy of needs.

Different types of healthcare facilities are described in Chapter 7.

Refer to Chapter 11 for a full discussion on therapeutic communication.

Erikson's developmental stages are discussed in Chapter 16.

See Chapter 18 for a full discussion of loss, grief, and death.

The pain scales are provided in Chapter 22.

Chapter 31 covers muscular dystrophy.

See Chapter 32 for information on COPD.

Chapter 35 provides information on erythematosus.

See Chapter 38 for more on diabetes mellitus.

PCA pumps are illustrated in Chapter 45.

For more information about the multidisciplinary approach, see Chapter 46.

Critical Thinking Care Map

Caring for the Client with End-Stage COPD

NCLEX-PN® Focus Area: Physiological Integrity: Basic Care and Comfort; Pharmacological Therapies

Case Study: Mr. Wilkins, a 75-year-old Caucasian male, with a 25-year history of COPD, discharged on December 18 to home hospice care with wife after a 10-day hospital stay for pneumonia. He wants to be home and "hopes that he lives to see one more Christmas." Physician states a prognosis of 1 to 3 weeks.

Nursing Diagnosis: *Chronic Fatigue* related to inadequate oxygenation secondary to COPD and "cor pulmonale"

COLLECT DATA

Subjective	Objective
_____	_____
_____	_____
_____	_____
_____	_____
_____	_____
_____	_____
_____	_____

Would you report this? Yes/No

If yes, report to: _____

What would you report? _____

Nursing Care

_____
_____
_____
_____
_____
_____
_____
_____
_____
_____
_____
_____

How would you document this? _____
_____
_____
_____

Compare your answers and documentation to those provided on the MyNursingKit Website.

Data Collected
(use only those that apply)

- S.O.B. at rest
- Increased S.O.B. with exertion
- Consumes less than 30% of meals
- Weighs 170 lbs
- AP=120 at rest
- R=40, rapid, labored
- Lethargic
- "Tired all the time"
- "Can't catch my breath"
- Nail beds cyanotic
- Orthopnea
- Self-care deficit: all ADLs
- Wife is the sole caregiver and in "good health"
- PO2 = 80% on room air
- BP = 160/90
- Temp 97.6 orally
- Discharged to home via ambulance
- Looks older than stated age

Nursing Interventions
(use only those that apply; list in priority order)

- Administer oxygen at 3 L/min per physician's order.
- Position for comfort: Fowler's or orthopneic position.
- Encourage ambulation 4x/day with minimal assist.
- Humidifier prn.
- Complete bed bath.
- Monitor cardiorespiratory status/response to exertion.
- Monitor sleep patterns.
- Monitor nutritional intake.
- Fan in room.
- Vital signs every 8 hours and prn, changes in status.
- Encourage self-care.

NCLEX-PN® Exam Preparation

1 The nurse recognizes which of the following as an important component of a chronic disease?

1. The disease condition produces signs and symptoms suddenly.
2. The disease condition produces signs and symptoms gradually.
3. Only partial recovery occurs due to the eventual presence of irreversible pathological changes.
4. The signs and symptoms never go away.

2 The role of the LPN/LVN in caring for the chronically ill client includes which of the following? (Select all that apply.)

1. Preventing complications
2. Providing basic physical care
3. Creating a rehabilitation plan
4. Encouraging client independence
5. Providing emotional support

3 The LPN/LVN is caring for a terminally ill child whose parents asked the nurse how God could let a child suffer like this. When the nurse is asked to assist the RN with creating a plan of care for this client, the nurse would consider which nursing diagnosis appropriate as a result of this conversation with the parents?

1. *Anticipatory Grieving*
2. *Spiritual Distress*
3. *Powerlessness*
4. *Hopelessness*

4 The nurse, caring for a client with a terminal illness, would interpret which of the following as a sign of impending death? (Select all that apply.)

1. Client is alert, oriented, and asking when family will arrive.
2. Extremities are cool, mottled, and cyanotic.
3. Glasgow coma scale increases from 6 to 10.
4. Pulse becomes weak and thready.
5. Respirations are irregular.

5 A terminally ill client is aware of his surroundings but death seems imminent. He does not want any measures to prolong his life. What is the nurse's priority action at this time?

1. Sit quietly and hold the dying client's hand.
2. Move the client to the hall so he can be observed.
3. Place him in a single room near the nursing station.
4. Tell him to put on his call light if he needs anything.

6 During morning care, the client tells the nurse that he knows that he is dying and does not want anything done to prolong his life. The nurse advises the client to discuss his wishes with the physician who can write an order to that effect. The nurse calls the physician, who says she will discuss the DNR order with the client at rounds the next morning. Later in the day the nurse finds the client pulseless and not breathing. The nurse will:

1. Respect the client's wishes.
2. Call the family and ask them what they would like done.
3. Call the physician and ask for orders.
4. Call the resuscitation team and inform the lead physician of the client's wishes.

7 A client has terminal cancer and the physician has recommended hospice care to the family. The most appropriate explanation of hospice is:

1. "Hospice nurses give better care than the hospital nurses."
2. "Hospice care is cheaper than hospital care."
3. "Hospice allows terminal clients to be cared for in an environment of their own choosing."
4. "Hospice uses specialized equipment not available in the hospital."

8 The nurse recognizes which of the following criteria as essential in order for the physician to pronounce the client dead who is on life support?

1. The family must agree to discontinuance of life support.
2. Brain activity must be absent for at least 24 hours.
3. The client may still be able to breathe but is irreversibly unconscious.
4. A court order was provided to discontinue life support.

9 The nurse is caring for a Muslim client after death. Understanding the client's cultural needs, the nurse instructs the unlicensed assistive personnel to:

1. Bathe the client but do not wrap the body in a shroud until the family arrives.
2. Cover the client's face with a white sheet until the family arrives.
3. Wait for the family to arrive to bathe the body.
4. Take the client to the morgue without bathing the body.

10 After the client dies, the nurse places the body in which of the following positions?

1. Supine with the arms crossed across the chest
2. With head elevated 30 degrees with a coin on each eye to maintain closure
3. Supine with head and shoulders placed on two pillows (at a 30-degree angle), with arms straight at the side
4. Side lying with arms folded over abdomen and mouth closed using a string around the head and chin

Answers and rationales for Review Questions appear in Appendix I.

Chapter 45

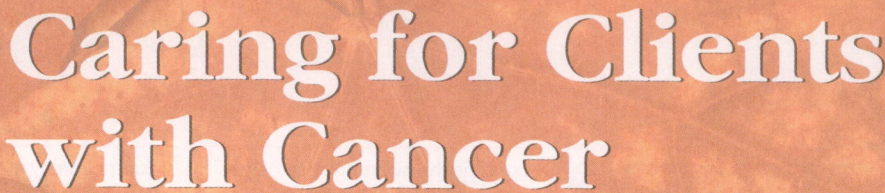

Caring for Clients with Cancer

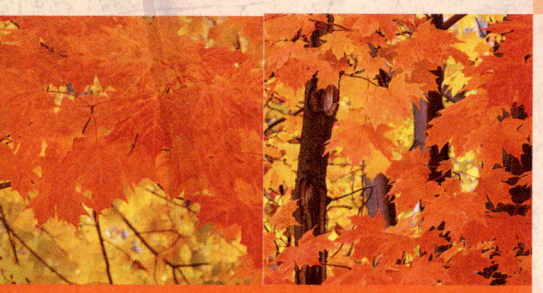

LEARNING Outcomes

After completing this chapter, you will be able to:

1. Define basic terms for what cancer is and does.
2. Differentiate between normal and malignant cells.
3. List important concepts in cancer prevention.
4. Identify factors that affect a client's choice of evaluation for cancer.
5. Describe nursing concerns when caring for clients receiving a cancer diagnosis.
6. Identify ways of classifying and staging cancer and tests used to determine whether a client has cancer.
7. Discuss the treatments for cancer and their common effects on the client.
8. Describe nursing interventions for clients receiving cancer treatment.
9. Name important considerations when caring for very young or very old clients with cancer.

Clinical Objectives

10. Provide care for clients who have been treated for cancer by surgery, radiation, or chemotherapy.
11. Provide client and family teaching with a cancer diagnosis.
12. Identify common nursing interventions for clients receiving cancer treatment.

KEY TERMS

Use the audio glossary feature on the MyNursingKit Website to hear the correct pronunciation of the following key terms.

adjuvant chemotherapy 1243

adjuvant therapy 1243

anaplastic 1243

anemia 1243

apheresis 1258

biological response modifiers 1258

biopsy 1249

biotherapy 1249

cachexia 1244

cancer 1243

cancer suppressor genes 1243

carcinogenesis 1243

differentiation 1245

leukopenia 1243

limb salvage 1250

metastasis 1243

nadir 1243

neoplasm 1243

neutropenia 1243

oncogenes 1243

oncology 1243

primary tumor 1243

second primary tumor 1243

simulation 1253

tumor 1243

unknown primary tumor 1243

Cancer is a complex disease process that may affect any body organ or system. **Oncology** (the study of cancer) has a language of its own. Important terms related to cancer are defined in Box 45-1 ■.

BOX 45-1 | **IMPORTANT TERMS IN STUDYING CANCER**

Adjuvant chemotherapy—Chemotherapy used to enhance the result of another therapy; for example, chemotherapy following surgery

Adjuvant therapy—A treatment used to enhance the result of another therapy; for example, radiation therapy following surgery

Anaplastic—Lacking structural differentiation

Anemia—A decrease in the number of red blood cells with a resultant decrease in the hemoglobin and hematocrit

Cancer—Malignant tumor capable of metastasis and invasion, characterized by uncontrolled growth

Cancer suppressor genes—Genes with the opposite function of oncogenes; they "turn off" cell division and inhibit malignant growth

Carcinogenesis—The production of cancer; carcinogenic substances increase the likelihood of developing cancer

Leukopenia—A decrease in the number of white blood cells

Metastasis—Cancerous cells that have traveled from the primary site to a distant site

Nadir—The lowest point that the blood cell counts reach before they begin to rebound following chemotherapy

Neutropenia—A decrease in the number of a specific type of white blood cells, called neutrophils

Neoplasm—Any abnormal growth of new tissue that may be harmless (benign) or cancerous (malignant)

Oncogenes—Genes found in the chromosomes of tumor cells

Primary tumor—Original histologic site of tumor; tissue where tumor originated

Second primary tumor—New, histologically separate malignant neoplasm in a person with a primary tumor

Tumor—Mass of tissue that may be benign or malignant

Unknown primary tumor—Cells that are markedly anaplastic, making it impossible to determine tissue of origin

---

A *neoplasm* is any abnormal growth of new tissue that may be harmless (benign) or cancerous (malignant). *Cancer* is a general term for a malignant tumor or forms of new malignant cells that lack a controlled growth pattern. *Cancer epidemiology* is the study of the frequency of cancer in populations, its risk factors, and the interrelationships between host and environment. Box 45-2 ■ describes some of the factors that have been linked to increased likelihood of getting some types of cancer. Figure 45-1 ■ shows how these factors can link together to increase the likelihood of developing cancer.

In carcinogenesis (see Box 45-1), oncogenes are activated. Oncogenes hold the code for cellular growth. Alterations by carcinogens (such as viruses, chemicals, and radiation) "turn on" cell division, leading to neoplastic growth. Normal cells are converted into cancer cells. Anti-oncogenes (*cancer suppressor genes*) "turn off" cell division and inhibit malignant growth. Cancers occur when these factors exist:

1. Cancer suppressor genes are absent.
2. Abnormal products of oncogenes are present.

Normal Cells versus Cancer Cells

DIFFERENCES IN GROWTH

Normal cells are carefully regulated and kept under control, meaning that the number of new cells formed in tissues equals the number lost by cell death or injury. The primary feature of cancer cells, however, is uncontrolled growth. In cancer, cells continue to divide without regard to the needs of the host. The number of new cells is greater than the number of cells lost, resulting in tumor mass. Uncontrolled growth of tumors occurs because of:

- *Cancer cell immortality.* Most normal cells divide only 50 to 60 times before they die, but cancer cells are not limited in the number of times they divide.
- *Loss of contact inhibition.* When grown in a petri dish, normal cells divide until they form a single layer on the bottom. Cancer cells do not stop dividing; they grow out

BOX 45-2 RISK FACTORS FOR CANCER

Tobacco	Cigarette smoking causes 90% of lung cancers
Diet	Contributing factor in 20% to 70% of cancer deaths
Alcohol	Associated with cancers of the oral cavity, pharynx, larynx, esophagus, and liver
Occupational exposure to carcinogens such as asbestos or oil refinery chemicals	Related primarily to lung cancers
Pollution	Related primarily to lung and skin cancers
Reproductive factors and sexual behavior	Cervical cancer can be related to number of sexual partners
Viruses	Hepatitis B, Epstein-Barr, human papillomavirus
Radiation	Responsible for 3% of cancer deaths
Antineoplastic drugs (anticancer drugs)	Second malignancy is late effect of resulting cell damage
Aging	Individuals over age 65 are 10 times more likely to develop cancer due to lifetime exposure to cancer-inducing agents
Genetic predisposition	Familial polyposis, BRCA1, BRCA2
Ethnicity and race	Biological and cultural factors cause differences in incidence and mortality
Socioeconomic status	Strongly associated with lifestyle

and up. They can also invade neighboring cells and travel to new sites (Figure 45-2 ■; see Figure 40-8 for an illustration of metastasis from breast cancer to brain and lung).

■ *Diminished growth factor requirements.* Cancer cells have the ability to rob the body of nutrients to support their growth, which can lead to **cachexia** (physical wasting and weight loss). However, cancer cells appear to divide without serum growth factors (or they may make their own growth factors, which is why someone who is

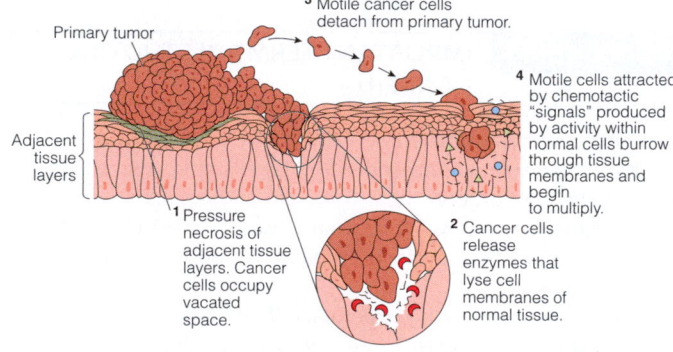

A

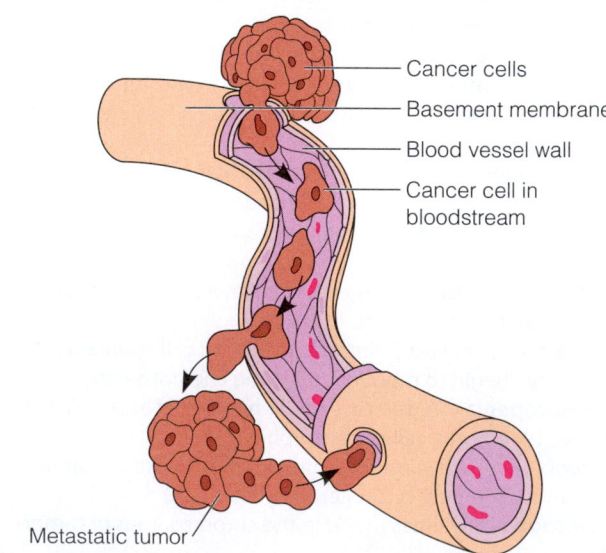

B

Figure 45-2. ■ **A.** Cancer cells can invade neighboring cells. **B.** Metastasis occurs when cancer cells break off and travel through lymph or blood to new sites. In the blood, only about 1 cell in 1,000 escapes immune detection, but that can be enough. The tumor cells may move "downstream" from the original tumor, or a chemical attraction may cause them to target a specific site. In the new site, malignant cells multiply and establish a metastatic tumor.

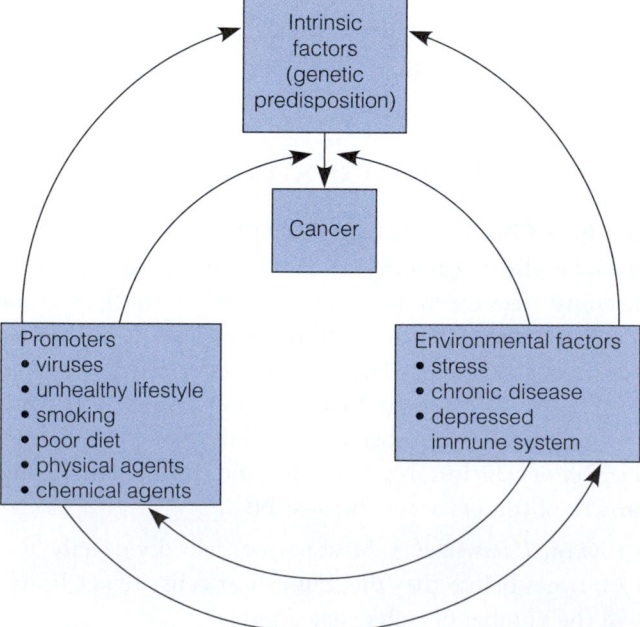

Figure 45-1. ■ Preventable and unpreventable factors can link together to increase the likelihood of developing cancer. Any combination of these factors may exist.

severely malnourished can continue to have cancer cell growth).

- *Ability to divide without anchoring to a surface.* Most normal cells will not divide in liquid medium; they require anchorage. In contrast, cancer cells can grow in suspension or in gel.
- *Lack of resting phase in cell cycle.* Cancer cells never enter the resting phase.

DIFFERENCES IN APPEARANCE

Normal cells have a well-organized and extensive cytoskeleton that provides structure and shape. Transformed cells have variable sizes and shapes, darker staining and larger nuclei, and a variety of other abnormal features.

DIFFERENCES IN DIFFERENTIATION

Differentiation is the process by which cells become adapted for specific functions. This occurs by turning certain genes "on and off." The more differentiated a cell, the more its potential is restricted. Fully differentiated cells are often incapable of replicating (reproducing). Because of differentiation, it is possible to distinguish a skin cell from a brain cell through *histologic examination* (examination of cells under a microscope to determine their exact anatomic location or source).

Cancer cells can arise at any stage in differentiation. They tend to be less differentiated than cells from normal tissue. *Anaplasia* occurs when cancer cells are so undifferentiated that the tissue of origin cannot be identified.

Cancer Prevention and Cancer Screening

Although some risk factors cannot be prevented (such as hereditary risk), there are some things we can all do to reduce the risk of certain cancers. According to the 2004 Harvard Center for Cancer Prevention at the Harvard School of Public Health website, up to 50% of cancers can be prevented by things over which we have control. Table 45-1 ■ provides tips for preventing cancer.

TABLE 45-1	Cancer Prevention Tips for Adults and Children	
WAY TO PREVENT CANCER	**FOR CLIENTS**	**FOR CHILDREN**
Reach and maintain a healthy weight.	Teach the importance of being physically active. Balance the amount of food eaten with the amount of energy used in a day.	Limit the amount of time children sit around the house. Encourage healthy snacking on fruits and vegetables.
Get at least 30 minutes of physical activity every day. Being physically active lowers the risk of colon cancer and may lower the risk of breast cancer.	Encourage physical activity, at home and at work. Try walking, jogging, or dancing—whatever activity is enjoyable. Teach that any amount of physical activity is better than none. In general, the more a person does, the better.	Do physically active things with children on a regular basis, beginning when they are very young. Encourage children to play outside (when safe) and participate in organized sports or other physical activities such as dancing or aerobics.
Do not smoke. If you already smoke, quit for good as soon as you can. Tobacco use (including cigarettes, pipes, cigars, and chewing tobacco) is linked to cancers of the lung, throat, pancreas, kidney, bladder, cervix, prostate, colon, and rectum.	Be positive about client's ability to quit. Quitting is tough but not impossible. More than 1,000 Americans stop for good every day. Recommend the client talk to a healthcare provider for help or join a quit-smoking program. The person's employer may offer quit-smoking programs for employees.	Teach parents that if they smoke, their children will also be more likely to smoke. Tell them not to smoke in the house or car. Children who breathe in smoke have a higher risk of breathing problems and lung cancer. Encourage conversations about the dangers of smoking and chewing tobacco. A healthcare professional or school counselor can help.
Eat a healthy diet. A healthy diet lowers the risk of cancers of the prostate, breast, lung, colon, rectum, stomach, and pancreas.	Recommend client make fruits and vegetables a part of every meal. Adding fruit to cereal or vegetables to a snack are easy ways to increase intake. Teach clients to choose chicken, fish, or beans, instead of red meat and to include more whole grains, fiber, and whole wheat bread in their diets.	Encourage parents to have a bowl of fruit out all the time for children to eat as snacks. At fast-food restaurants, offer broiled chicken sandwiches rather than burgers. Make sandwiches using whole wheat bread.

(continued)

TABLE 45-1	Cancer Prevention Tips for Adults and Children (continued)	
WAY TO PREVENT CANCER	**FOR CLIENTS**	**FOR CHILDREN**
Drink less than one alcoholic drink a day. One drink is a glass of wine, a bottle of beer, or a shot of hard liquor. Limiting alcohol lowers the risk of cancers of the breast, colon, rectum, mouth, throat, and esophagus.	Encourage nonalcoholic beverages at meals and parties. Avoid occasions centered on alcohol. Teach clients to talk to a healthcare professional if they feel they have trouble limiting alcohol. Avoid making alcohol an essential part of family gatherings.	Discuss the dangers of drug and alcohol abuse with children. Obtain help from a healthcare professional or school counselor.
Protect yourself from the sun. Sunlight is linked to skin cancer.	Teach clients to stay out of direct sunlight between 10:00 A.M. and 4:00 P.M. (peak burning hours). Teach them to avoid getting sunburned and not to use sun lamps or tanning booths. Encourage use of hats, shirts, and sunscreens with SPF 15 or higher.	Make sure children are properly protected from the sun with hats, long-sleeved shirts, and SPF 15 sunscreens or higher. Serious skin cancer is caused by sunburns in childhood.
Protect yourself and your partner(s) from sexually transmitted infections. Sexually transmitted infections are linked to cancers of the cervix, vagina, anus, and liver.	Teach client not to have casual unprotected sex. Abstinence is the safest protection. Teach clients always to use a condom and follow other safe sex practices when sexually active. Teach clients not to rely on a partner for protection but to be in charge and be prepared. Inform young women about the HPV vaccine for preventing certain types of cervical cancer.	When appropriate, discuss with children why abstinence or practicing safe sex is important. A healthcare professional or school counselor can help.

BOX 45-3	CLIENT TEACHING

Early Warning Signs of Cancer

The acronym CAUTION can be used to help clients remember cancer's early warning signs:
- Change in bowel or bladder habits
- Any sore that does not heal
- Unusual bleeding or discharge
- Thickening or lump in breast or elsewhere
- Indigestion or difficulty in swallowing
- Obvious change in wart or mole
- Nagging cough or hoarseness

Manifestations

With cancer, early detection and treatment are keys to survival. It is crucial to try to treat cancer before it has completely overwhelmed the body's immune system and spread from its site of origin. Nurses play an important role in teaching about cancer prevention and early detection. The seven warning signals of cancer are listed in Box 45-3 ■. A good way to remember the warning signs of cancer is the acronym, CAUTION.

The major goals of diagnostic evaluation are to determine:

- Tissue type (skin, bone, etc.).
- Primary site (breast, pancreas, etc.).

- Extent of disease (in primary site only [*in situ*] or extended).
- Potential for recurrence.

Factors Affecting Choice of Diagnostic Evaluation

There are many choices of diagnostic evaluation for a cancer client. Various laboratory and radiologic testing methods are available, and the approach to diagnostic evaluation depends on many factors. The first is the client's presenting symptoms. Frequently, these symptoms include complaints of weight loss, persistent pain, unexplained fever, fatigue, or one of the seven warning signs (see Box 45-3). Unfortunately, many clients who are at greatest risk for developing cancer do not understand the importance of early detection of symptoms. As a result, they are diagnosed in a late stage of disease.

The second factor is the client's clinical status. The client's history of coexisting (*comorbid*) conditions, such as heart disease, lupus, or renal failure, has a profound effect on the ability to tolerate cancer treatment. It can be a deciding factor in determining the extent of diagnostic testing to be done.

The third factor in diagnostic evaluation is the client's tolerance of invasive tests. For example, a client may not be able to tolerate an invasive test such as a spinal tap or anesthesia for a biopsy. This factor would limit diagnostic testing and reduce the likelihood of a favorable outcome from treatment.

The fourth factor is the anticipated goal of treatment. The diagnostic testing done for an anticipated curative goal is much more aggressive than that done for a goal of palliative treatment.

The fifth factor for diagnostic evaluation is the biological characteristics of the tumor. For example, if the cancer is a microscopic metastasis, it will not be detected using a computerized tomography (CT) scan. The only diagnostic method available for this situation would be a surgical biopsy and microscopic examination.

The availability of diagnostic equipment also plays a role in the physician's diagnostic evaluation of disease. For example, positron-emission tomography (PET) (see the Diagnostic Tests section later in this chapter) is an advanced diagnostic method that is available only in certain locations. A rural physician who has diagnosed cancer in a client is unlikely to send the client elsewhere for the technology. Most likely the physician will get by with technology that is readily available.

Last, it is apparent that third-party payers, prospective payment systems, and managed care networks play an important role as gatekeepers in the diagnostic evaluation process. Newer diagnostic technology is usually much more expensive than traditional technology and has not been proven to be better. Therefore, it is often not paid for by insurance. This is the case with PET scans. Once the technology is more widely used and can be proven to be an invaluable diagnostic tool, then insurance companies will consider reimbursement.

Nursing Implications in Diagnostic Evaluation

ROLE OF THE NURSE

The nurse performs several functions in helping the client who is newly diagnosed with cancer. When a cancer diagnosis is suspected, the nurse can help set up an appointment at a diagnostic center. At times, the nurse can alert other caregivers to concerns the family has about hearing the diagnosis; these concerns can vary with culture and lifestyle (Box 45-4 ■). The nurse can also help the client obtain a referral to an oncologist or cancer treatment center with the client's insurance. The nurse can be a source of comfort to the client with newly suspected or confirmed cancer. The client may feel more comfortable showing emotions or discussing fears with the nurse than with the family or the physician. This

---

BOX 45-4	CULTURAL PULSE POINTS

Discussing a Diagnosis of Cancer

The Western medical community increasingly emphasizes two things as a necessary part of ethical practice:

- Full truthful disclosure of cancer diagnosis or prognosis
- Respect for autonomy

However, Japanese, Native American, Korean, Chinese, Mexican, Hispanic, African, and European American cancer clients may consider complete and accurate disclosure of cancer undesirable. In such cases, the physician may use euphemisms to give a true or false diagnosis. All healthcare professionals should be informed about whether the client would like to be informed of a diagnosis and how involved he or she would like family members to be. In addition, an awareness of the psychosocial impact of certain terms, such as *cancer*, is essential. Often, phrases such as *malignant tumor* or *growth* are less inflammatory and are more readily accepted.

---

may be because the nurse is supposed to be easy to speak to and a "source of comfort." The client may not want to burden a family member further, and he or she may feel that the physician is more distant or stoic. The nurse, on the other hand, can be a shoulder to cry on or someone who listens. In addition, the nurse can ease complications of the referral by assisting with the client's appointment and making sure pertinent records get to the referral physician.

PSYCHOSOCIAL ASPECTS OF CANCER

The psychosocial responses to the cancer experience are determined by the:

- Characteristics of cancer.
- Person with, or at risk for, cancer.
- Social system and environment of significance to individual.

Because cancer poses a universal threat and because the disease and treatment are marked with uncertainty, it is among the most feared of all diseases. Stress, anxiety, depression, and hopelessness run high among cancer clients. Nurses can help clients realize the various manifestations of stress and anxiety and help them activate coping strategies to control anxiety levels. Nurses can assist with referrals as appropriate. Nurses can reinforce personal power and ability by including the client in planning care, goals, and schedule. Nurses can also encourage supportive relationships with friends, family, and groups.

The needs of the family going through a cancer experience are:

- *Information*. Nowadays, families have to assume more responsibility than in the past in the care of clients. Therefore, families need to be taught many things such as dressing changes.
- *Communication*. Communication becomes a primary issue among family members as caregiving demands increase.

- *Coping skills.* Roles and relationship rules within the family may need to be modified to meet demands imposed by illness.
- *Support services.* The type and amount of support systems and services needed differ by caregivers of differing age, sex, and socioeconomic status.

RESPONSES OF NURSES TO CLIENTS WITH CANCER

Distancing is an unconscious response of professionals, especially to dying clients. Distancing is especially prevalent when the client is not aware of the truth. This behavior can enhance loneliness and fear in the client.

Getting too close to clients can also pose a problem. Because cancer is a chronic—and often terminal—disease and the treatment of cancer is prolonged, it is very easy for nurses to become attached to and familiar with long-term clients and their families. Familiarity can improve continuity of client care and can be comforting to the client. However, nurses have to be careful not to be too upset by the emotions of those clients who are faring poorly. Although it is difficult, the professional nurse should maintain a caring, action-oriented, positive environment without getting too personally attached to the client. This allows the nurse to maintain his or her own mental health and yet provide a healthy surrounding for the client.

Diagnostic Tests

CLASSIFICATION AND STAGING

It is important to be familiar with the basic terms that are used in discussing cancer (see Box 45-1). *Staging* is a method of classifying a malignancy by the extent of its spread. The objectives of staging tumors are to aid in treatment planning, determine a prognosis, and assist in evaluation of treatment. Staging also helps treatment centers exchange information and compare statistics. In this way, centers can learn which treatments are most successful.

Several staging systems are used:

1. *Tumor-node-metastasis (TNM) staging.* The TNM staging system is an internationally accepted method of staging solid tumors. The $\underline{T}$ refers to the depth of invasion, the surface spread, and the size of the primary tumor. The $\underline{N}$ refers to the absence or presence and extent of regional lymph node metastasis. The $\underline{M}$ refers to the absence or presence of distant metastasis. Numbers appear after the letters in a range from 0 (no cancer cells) to 4 (very large or widespread). For example, a breast tumor that has metastasized to the brain would be designated a Stage IV, T4, N3, M1.

2. *Clark level.* In this staging system, melanomas are staged *histologically* by level of invasion by the primary tumor.
3. *Duke's staging system.* Colorectal cancer is classified by depth of invasion and by the presence of nodal metastasis.

LABORATORY STUDIES

Biochemical analysis of blood and urine may be performed to rule out or diagnose cancer. Analysis can identify *tumor markers* (chemicals produced by the tumor or by other cells in response to tumor), which can be used to detect cancer or monitor response to therapy. An example of a tumor marker is carcinoembryonic antigen (CEA). Its presence can help detect cancers of the colon-rectum, stomach, pancreas, prostate, lungs, and breast. Another common tumor marker is prostate-specific antigen (PSA), which helps detect prostate cancer.

Alpha-fetoprotein (AFP) may be found in higher levels in the presence of liver, testicular, or breast cancer. CA 125 may be found in higher levels in the presence of ovarian cancer. Lastly, the tumor markers CA 15-3 and CA 27-29 may be used to monitor for recurrence or in the presence of advanced breast cancer.

TUMOR IMAGING

Nuclear medicine techniques involve the intravenous injection or ingestion of radioisotope compounds, followed by camera imaging of those organs or tissues that have concentrated the radioisotopes. Nuclear medicine studies are very sensitive and often can detect sites of abnormal metabolism or early malignancy several months before changes are seen on a radiograph. Gallium scans, for example, are particularly sensitive in detecting bronchogenic carcinomas (cancers of the bronchus or lungs) and lymphomas.

Positron-emission tomography combines properties of conventional nuclear scanning and scanning for radioactive material (radionuclides). PET scans can provide more detailed information about certain tumors' metabolism, blood flow, oxygen, and glucose use. However, because of its expense, it is not widely available.

Ultrasonography is the use of high-frequency sound to make a picture of structures inside the body such as a tumor.

Magnetic resonance imaging (MRI) provides physiologic information and detailed anatomic views of tissues using a superconducting magnet and radio-frequency signals. Computers use the signals to construct detailed sectional images of the body. IV contrast agents are commonly used to allow for basic contrast and tissue signals.

INVASIVE TECHNIQUES

Endoscopy is an invasive technique that makes use of an endoscope. An *endoscope* is a fiber-optic instrument with a lighted lens system that is used for direct visual examination of body organs or cavities (see Chapter 37 ⬮⬮).

A **biopsy** is the surgical removal of living tissue from an organ or other part of the body for microscopic examination in order to establish a diagnosis or follow the course of a disease. There are different types of biopsies:

- An *aspiration biopsy* is made with a fine needle attached to a syringe (see Figure 40-9 ⚭ for breast biopsy).
- A *cone biopsy* is accomplished by surgically removing a cone-shaped piece from the cervix to help make a diagnosis.
- A *needle biopsy* is made by putting a hollow needle through the skin on the surface of an organ or tumor and turning it within the cell layers (Figure 45-3 ▪).

clinical ALERT

When needle biopsy of the liver is performed, the nurse must monitor the client carefully. Bleeding in liver tissue can be profuse and difficult to contain. The nurse maintains pressure on the biopsy site for 5 minutes, and monitors the client for manifestations of hemorrhage (see Chapter 37 ⚭).

- A *punch biopsy* refers to the removal of a sample of tissue (usually skin) by means of an instrument with punch action.
- Finally, tissue removed by scraping the surface of a sore or tumor is called a *surface biopsy* such as the method used, a Pap test, to detect cancer of the cervix. (See a discussion of the Pap test in Chapter 40 ⚭ .)

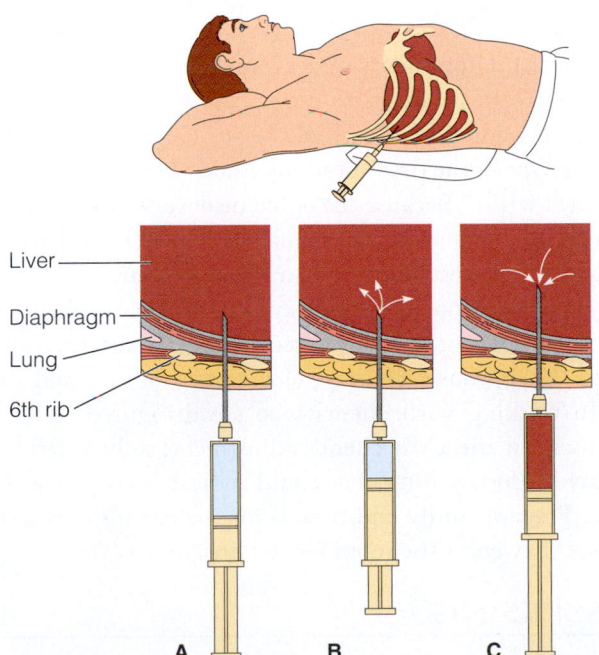

Liver
Diaphragm
Lung
6th rib

A   B   C

Figure 45-3. ▪ Needle biopsy of liver. **A.** The client exhales completely and holds breath, bringing the liver and diaphragm to their highest position. The needle is inserted between the sixth and seventh ribs. **B.** A small amount of saline is injected to clear the needle of blood and tissue. **C.** A tissue sample is aspirated into the needle. The needle is then withdrawn. Pressure is applied to the site.

Treatment Planning

A client's treatment plan involves interdisciplinary decision making based on several factors. The first factor is the aggressiveness of the tumor. If a client has overwhelming comorbid conditions and is older and has a very aggressive tumor, the treatment plan is likely to be much less involved than it would be for a young, healthy client.

The second treatment plan factor has to do with the predictability of the disease's spread. If the biological features of the tumor are proven to cause metastatic spread to certain areas, then usually the treatment plan consists of some type of prophylactic treatment to those areas. For example, a breast cancer with likely microscopic spread to lymph nodes is usually treated with radiation to the lymph nodes in an attempt to prevent spread of the disease.

Also the morbidity and mortality that can be expected from the treatment influence the treatment plan. Again, comorbid conditions can greatly influence the morbidity and mortality of the disease and its treatment. Also, with cancer treatment, the treatment can cause a great number of serious side effects, such as increased susceptibility of infections that can be overwhelming to the client's body.

Another deciding factor is the successful cure rate of the disease. Sometimes, physicians are hesitant to put the client through rigorous treatments if the odds of curing the disease are overwhelmingly not in the client's favor.

Finally, but probably most importantly, the client's wishes must be taken into consideration. Once all the information about the disease, treatment options, side effects, and the consequences of treatment versus no treatment are presented to the client in a manner in which he or she understands, the client needs to make some serious decisions about what is right for him or her.

Major Medical Treatments

There are three major treatments for cancer: surgery, radiation, and chemotherapy. Biotherapy and bone marrow transplantation (discussed later in the chapter) are also treatment modalities but are not used as often. **Biotherapy** refers to the manipulation of the immune system to restore, augment, or modulate its function. Bone marrow transplantation is the replacement of diseased marrow with healthy donor marrow. It is a very high-risk procedure that has limited effectiveness with solid tumors. It is mostly used with hematologic cancers such as *multiple myeloma* (a bone marrow–destroying cancer) and *leukemias* (cancers of blood-forming tissues). The treatment design may include any or all of these types of therapy. Most cancers are treated using multiple treatment modalities.

The goal of therapy needs to be established as:

- *Curative* (complete elimination of cancer).
- *Controlling* (slowing the progression of the disease).
- *Palliative* (providing comfort only).

Combination therapy and more aggressive therapies are appropriate if a cure is possible. If a cure is not possible, the therapy should not create more hardship.

Response to treatment should be evaluated using objective criteria. *Complete response* (CR) shows a complete disappearance of signs and symptoms of disease for at least a 1-month period. A *partial response* (PR) means a 50% or more reduction in all measured lesions for at least a month, with no new lesions appearing. A *minimal response* (MR) is the same as PR but with less than a 50% reduction. A *progression in disease* refers to a 25% or more increase in the total of all measured lesions or new lesions. *Stable disease* refers to a measurable tumor that does not meet criteria for CR, PR, MR, or progression.

SURGICAL THERAPY

Approximately 55% of all individuals with cancer are treated with a surgical intervention. Surgery can be used alone or in combination with other therapeutic modalities. Surgery can be used for:

- *Cancer prevention*. An example would be a *bilateral prophylactic mastectomy* (removal of both breasts to prevent possibility of breast cancer in individuals who have extremely high risk factors).
- *Diagnosis*. An example would be a colonoscopy with biopsies.
- *Definitive treatment*. An example would be a *colectomy* (removal of the colon).
- *Rehabilitation*. An example would be **limb salvage** for sarcoma. In limb salvage, the surgeon is able to save part of the limb, but a significant portion of the limb is removed or some functionality is lost. Physical rehabilitation is needed to restore function to the greatest potential.
- *Palliation*. An example would be removal of a huge mass to improve breathing and mobility in a person with advanced lung cancer.

Many factors influence the decision to take a surgical approach. The benefits of surgery should outweigh the risks. Some of the factors influencing the decision are:

- *Tumor cell kinetics*. The knowledge of tumor cell *kinetics* (movement patterns) has helped to identify tumors best treated with surgery.
- *Growth rate*. Slow-growing tumors with prolonged cell cycles are best for surgical treatment because they tend to be more localized.
- *Invasiveness*. A surgical procedure that is intended to be curative must resect more than the entire tumor mass. It must also remove normal surrounding tissue in order to ensure removal of all the cancer cells.

- *Metastatic potential*. For tumors known to metastasize early, surgery may not be appropriate. However, it may be used to remove all visible tumor in preparation for *adjuvant* (auxiliary) chemotherapy or radiation treatment.
- *Tumor location*. The location and extent of the tumor determine the structural and functional changes after surgery. For example, a limb sarcoma (a tumor arising from soft tissue) can physically change both function and structure if a large amount of the muscle or even the entire limb has to be removed in surgery. In contrast, a small colon tumor may be effectively removed with surgery alone without the need for surgery to divert the colon structurally.
- *Physical status*. Factors identified in the preoperative assessment may increase the risk of surgical morbidity and mortality. For example, coexisting lung disease may alter the client's ability to recover from anesthesia.
- *Quality of life*. The goal of surgical therapy varies with the stage of disease. The quality of the client's life after the surgery should always be considered.

NURSING CARE

The nursing care associated with cancer surgeries depends on the location of the surgical site. The same type of nursing interventions would apply as for any other surgical client. (See Chapter 29 ⚭ for perioperative nursing care.)

PRIORITIZING NURSING CARE

When caring for clients undergoing surgery for cancer, focus your care on meeting immediate postoperative needs and on the emotional needs of the postoperative client with cancer. One of the first questions asked after surgery is "Did they get it all?" Because the outcome of surgery often determines the remaining treatment, the client is understandably anxious. Reassure the client as appropriate. Also, many surgeries to remove cancer may leave clients disfigured—either permanently or until reconstructive surgery can be done. Keep your face and voice matter of fact and calm when working with clients who are disfigured. Your responses can affect the client's adjustment, so be careful not to say or do anything that could indicate a negative reaction. Prepare family and friends for the client's appearance before they enter the room for the first time.

ASSESSING

It is important to obtain information about the client's past history with anesthetics and any problems or complications with any previous surgery. This knowledge can prevent complications. Also, thorough data must be collected about drug allergies and any coexisting conditions that could affect the outcome of surgery.

DIAGNOSING, PLANNING, AND IMPLEMENTING

Some common nursing diagnoses for clients who have or are about to have surgery for cancer are:

- *Acute Pain*
- *Risk for Infection*
- *Risk for Imbalanced Nutrition*
- *Anxiety*
- *Powerlessness*
- *Disturbed Body Image*

Client goals or outcomes would include:

- Will report pain within reasonable limits by second day postoperative.
- Will remain free of infection.
- Will maintain weight in normal range.
- Will demonstrate effective and healthy coping mechanisms.
- Will retain the ability to make decisions about treatment options.
- Will be able to find positive ways to cope with body image issues.

Care of the client after surgery is discussed in depth in Chapter 29 . The following interventions are important for clients with cancer:

- The nurse will ask clients about their pain level at least every 4 hours postsurgery. (See discussion of pain in Chapter 22. See nursing care of clients with chronic or terminal illness in Chapter 44.) *This will help determine effectiveness of pain therapies.*
- The nurse will take the client's vital signs at least every 4 hours postsurgery. *Temperature spikes can indicate an infection.*
- The nurse will keep wounds and dressings clean (see Chapter 24). Surgical drains are common after cancer surgery, so the client or family member will need instructions on how to keep the drain and the skin around the drain clean. The client and family also need instructions on emptying the drain and measuring the fluid from the drain. It is important for the client to understand that he or she should call the physician if the amount of drainage does not taper off or if there are signs of infection. *Proper care of wounds, dressings, and drains can prevent infections postsurgery.*
- The nurse will measure the client's weight daily. *This ensures adequate weight maintenance.*
- The nurse will monitor intake and output (I&O) (see also Chapter 26). *This ensures that adequate nutrition is provided postoperatively.*
- The nurse will measure calorie counts as ordered to ensure adequate caloric intake postsurgery. *Rapidly dividing cancer cells steal nutrients from other body areas and can lead to*

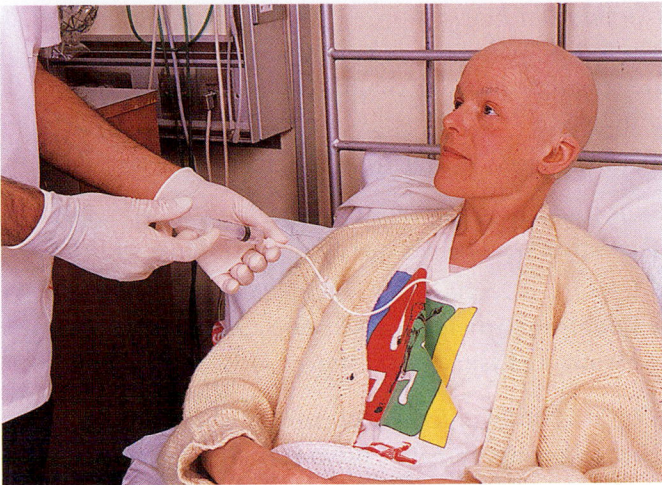

Figure 45-4. ■ The demands of relentlessly growing cancer cells can deprive the body of nutrition. Cancer robs its host of nutrients and increases body catabolism of fat and muscle to meet its metabolic needs. (*Source:* Simon Fraser/SPL/Photo Researchers, Inc.)

malnutrition (Figure 45-4 ■) and an emaciated appearance (called cachexia).

- The nurse will listen to the client and provide emotional support. (Refer to Chapter 17 for a discussion of the psychosocial aspects of physical illness.) *This will assist the client through the grieving process and help the client work through body image disturbances in order to have a healthy coping strategy.*

EVALUATING

Evaluation is based on the individual outcomes identified for each client. Documentation of findings such as the persistence of pain or increase in pain, signs and symptoms of infection, significant changes in weight, and severe inability to cope with body image changes should be reported to the team leader or physician.

NURSING PROCESS CARE PLAN
Client with Pain After Colectomy

Mr. Jones is a 56-year-old male who has just had a large malignant mass removed from his colon. He is complaining of pain at the surgical site. He has just come out of the recovery room to the medical-surgical unit where he did not receive any medication for pain.

Assessment

Mr. Jones rates his pain at 8 out of 10 on the pain scale. He is also guarding his abdomen and grimacing. Once you get him settled in bed you check his orders.

Nursing Diagnosis

The following important nursing diagnoses (among others) are established for this condition:

- *Acute Pain* related to surgical procedure
- *Activity Intolerance* related to discomfort

Expected Outcomes

The expected outcomes specify that Mr. Jones will:

- Report a decrease in pain that is tolerable.
- Be able to participate in self-care activities.
- Maintain physiologic comfort.

Planning and Implementation

The following nursing interventions are planned and implemented:

- Set up a patient-controlled analgesia (PCA) pump (Figure 45-5 ■) for client as ordered.
- Teach the client how the PCA pump works. Older children with cancer can be taught to use the PCA pump (see Figure 45-5B).
- Monitor pain scale consistently.
- Report and record pain that does not improve.
- Use additional methods of pain control such as distraction and guided imagery.
- Encourage the client to participate in self-care activities.

Evaluation

Through the evening, Mr. Jones's pain continues to lessen, and he reports a score of 3 out of 10 on the pain scale. By the next morning, Mr. Jones has rested well and he wants to try to get up to wash his face.

Critical Thinking in the Nursing Process

1. Why is pain control so important?
2. Besides pain control, what is another benefit of using a PCA pump?
3. Why are alternative methods of pain control such as guided imagery and distraction important?

Note: Discussion of Critical Thinking questions appears on the MyNursingKit Website.

RADIATION THERAPY

Radiotherapy may be used alone or in combination with other treatment modalities. Sometimes it is used first. For example, some breast tumors can be shrunk by radiation first in order to make them easier to remove surgically. Other times, the tumor can be surgically removed, and radiation follows to help eradicate microscopic metastatic cells. Some of the cancers that benefit from radiation treatment are breast, lung, and brain cancers. The goal of radiation therapy may be:

- *Cure*, such as when used to treat cancer of the cervix.
- *Control*, such as when used to treat breast cancer.

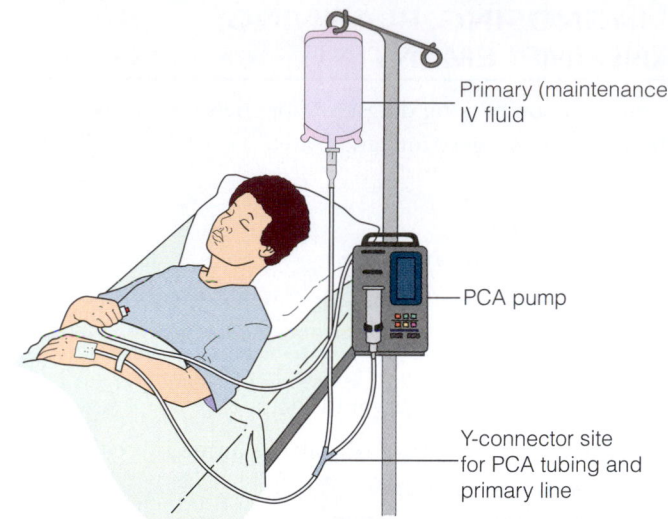

Primary (maintenance) IV fluid

PCA pump

Y-connector site for PCA tubing and primary line

A

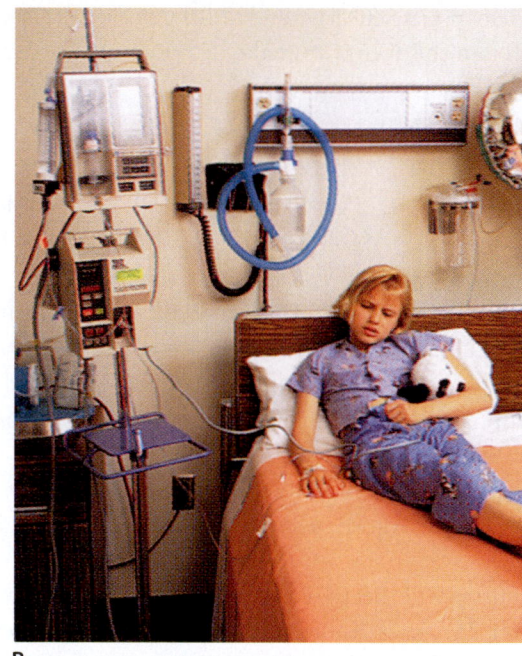

B

Figure 45-5. ■ **A.** PCA pump for postoperative client. The PCA line is introduced into the injection port of a primary line. **B.** An older child is able to regulate a PCA pump for pain control.

- *Palliation*, such as when used to relieve symptoms resulting from spinal cord compression due to metastasis of disease.

Radiation therapy can be delivered two ways:

- External radiation (*teletherapy*), which produces x-rays of varying energies.
- Internal radiation (*brachytherapy*), which uses sealed sources of radioactive material placed within or near the tumor. Brachytherapy is used frequently to treat head and neck tumors, gynecologic tumors, and prostate tumors. (See also Chapter 40 ⬤⬤.)

Safety with Radiation Administration

Three major safety factors should be considered when caring for radiation therapy clients:

1. *Time.* Exposure to radiation is directly proportional to time spent within a specific distance of the source.
2. *Distance.* The amount of radiation reaching a given area decreases as distance increases.
3. *Shield.* A sheet of absorbing material placed between the radiation source and detector decreases the amount of radiation.

Client education should include time, distance, and shielding in order to protect visitors. Also, client education will help clients understand that staff also must limit the time they spend in the client's room.

Simulation

Simulation is a run-through of the radiation procedure. It occurs during the client's first visit to the radiation oncologist. In simulation, the tumor bed is localized, the volume to be treated is defined, and the field of treatment is determined. The radiation therapist will mark the client's skin by tattooing it with India ink to ensure that the radiation is delivered to the exact spot needed. Sometimes the client requires an immobilization device to ensure precise delivery of the radiation to an extremity or to the head and neck. Lead blocks may also be used to protect vital organs and

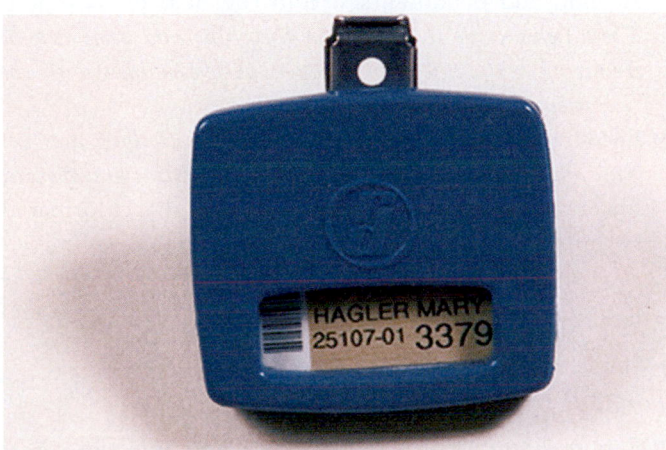

Figure 45-6. ■ Radiation badge alerts the nurse to dangerous levels of exposure.

tissues from damage. These are placed between the radiation beam and the client.

NURSING CARE

PRIORITIZING NURSING CARE

When caring for clients undergoing radiation therapy, focus your care on maintaining nutrition, hydration, energy, and skin integrity. Encourage clients to adapt food and fluid intake as necessary to obtain needed nutrients. Provide liquid meals if solids are not tolerated well, especially for clients who are undergoing radiation to the mouth, esophagus, or stomach. Encourage realistic expectations about rest, conservation of energy, and activity during radiation treatment. Observe skin closely for signs of burns or breakdown in the area of treatment. Report any loss of skin integrity immediately.

ASSESSING

The pretreatment evaluation phase is an information-gathering time. It is important to gather information about the presence of any metal objects in the client's body in order to avoid irradiating them. Irradiation of metal can damage the object, melt the object, or cause a severe burn to the client. A clinical history, and especially information about comorbid conditions, can greatly influence successful treatment outcomes.

Conditions such as cardiac and neurologic status are especially important if the head or heart is in the radiation field of treatment. For example, if the heart is in the radiation field (as with lung or breast cancer), some radiation damage can be caused to the heart. So, it is important to know of any heart disease or condition existing prior to treatment. Neurologic status is important if the spine or the brain is within the radiation field. Most commonly, the brain and spinal cord get radiated in an effort to eliminate or alleviate metastasis to those sites. For the client with cancer, neurologic damage in the form of paralysis or some other loss of function secondary to radiation would be devastating.

DIAGNOSING, PLANNING, AND IMPLEMENTING

Some common nursing diagnoses for clients undergoing radiation treatment are:

- *Acute Pain*
- *Risk of Infection*
- *Risk for Impaired Skin Integrity*
- *Anxiety*
- *Deficient Knowledge* related to treatment

MyNursingKit | Cancer care

Client goals or outcomes would include:

- Will report pain within reasonable limits.
- Will remain free of signs and symptoms of infection.
- Will remain free of skin breakdown surrounding the radiation sites.
- Will exhibit positive coping mechanisms to ease anxiety.
- Will be able to verbalize the steps involved in treatment.

Interventions for clients undergoing radiation for cancer follow:

- In caring for the client undergoing radiation therapy, the nurse reinforces education about exactly what will occur step by step during the radiation treatment. *Being left alone in a room with a big machine and being unable to move can be very frightening to some clients.*
- Ask the client about pain levels at each visit. *This will ensure that the client's comfort is being maintained.*
- Monitor vital signs at each visit. *Changes in vital signs, especially temperature spikes, can indicate the presence of infection.*
- Observe the skin at and around the radiation site to monitor for changes. *Early awareness of changes can help prevent skin breakdown.*
- Explain what the client can expect to experience during a procedure. *Providing information about what the client will experience helps to ease the client's anxiety level.*
- Listen to the client's concerns and fears. *Therapeutic listening (see Chapter 11 ⦾) helps the client maintain a sense of control and reduces anxiety levels.*
- Ask the client questions about the treatment procedure. *In this way, the nurse can determine whether the client has an appropriate level of understanding of the treatment.*

Helping Clients to Overcome Side Effects

The side effects of radiation depend on the site being treated. Side effects can occur in many different body systems, as listed in Table 45-2 ■.

- Encourage clients to get extra rest and to reduce their normal activity levels. Clients can also benefit from delegating tasks to family members and friends. *Clients who experience mild to profound fatigue with treatment may need to be reminded of the importance of rest in the healing process.*
- For esophagitis and dysphagia, instruct clients to replace regular meals with high-calorie, high-protein, high-carbohydrate liquids or soft, bland foods. Dietitians who work specifically with cancer clients can help clients with foods to eat when it is difficult for them to swallow or what foods to eat when they just do not feel like eating. *These meals will provide them with the most nutrition. Bland foods are easiest to tolerate. Cool foods such as sandwiches or applesauce may have less odor and therefore may be more palatable.*

- Encourage clients with nausea and vomiting to delay intake of a full meal until 3 or 4 hours after treatment. Also, taking the tray toppers off of food trays to let the food smells escape and cool off helps minimize nausea and vomiting. *Delaying food ingestion can reduce the incidence of nausea or vomiting.*
- Encourage clients with diarrhea to eat a low-residue diet and to use loperamide hydrochloride as instructed. *Nutritionally, a low-residue diet is best for clients with diarrhea related to radiation treatment. Medication can help to eliminate symptoms.*
- Encourage clients with cystitis or urethritis to have a high fluid intake, especially water. *Liquids can reduce the concentration of urine and decrease irritation of the bladder and urethra.*

For Mucositis

- Instruct clients to avoid irritants such as alcohol, tobacco, spicy or acidic foods, and very cold or hot foods and drinks. *Alcohol and tobacco are irritants. Milder seasonings and moderate temperatures are easiest on mucous membranes.*
- Instruct client to gargle frequently with recommended solution. *Usually clients are instructed not to use commercial mouthwash because it contains alcohol and will worsen irritation in the mouth. Using a half-strength H_2O_2 and H_2O solution is one alternative. Mouthwashes without alcohol are also available commercially.*
- Instruct client to brush teeth with soft-bristled brush several times a day. *Keeping the mouth fresh and free of bacteria improves oral health as well as self-esteem.*

For Skin

- Encourage client to keep skin free from moisture such as sweat. *Skin that is free from moisture such as sweat is least susceptible to breakdown and growth of organisms.*
- Discourage client from using powders, lotions, creams, alcohol, and deodorants within the field of radiation. *These items leave a residue on the skin, and some can be irritating and cause skin damage when combined with the radiation.*
- Encourage loose-fitting garments. *Loose clothing does not chafe and keeps skin drier by allowing perspiration to evaporate.*
- Encourage protection of skin from sunlight, chlorinated swimming pools, and temperature extremes. *Skin must be protected during this period, because it is already being stressed. Sun damage and chemicals such as chlorine can further damage skin.*

For Bone Marrow Suppression

- Report signs of bleeding, anemia, and infection. *Bone marrow suppression can be life threatening and requires prompt follow-up and treatment.*

TABLE 45-2	Side Effects of Radiation on Body Systems
BODY SYSTEMS	**SIDE EFFECTS**
Integumentary system	■ Skin reactions may range from erythema to dryness and then moist *desquamation* (sloughing of the top layer of skin). ■ Healing may be slow in the field of radiation. ■ Radiation of hair follicles, sweat, and sebaceous glands results in temporary loss of hair and decreased gland activity.
Hematopoietic system	■ If large areas of red bone marrow are irradiated (vertebrae, ribs, long bones, skull, sternum), the number of circulating mature blood cells is suppressed. ■ Red blood cells are damaged, causing anemia. ■ White blood cells are damaged, leaving the client more susceptible to infection. ■ Platelets are also damaged, leaving the client's blood less able to clot.
Gastrointestinal system	■ Oral cavity may develop mucositis. ■ Temporary or permanent alterations in taste. ■ Gastritis and esophagitis. ■ Anorexia, diarrhea, and cramping.
Respiratory system	■ Hoarseness. ■ Radiation pneumonitis. ■ Fibrosis in lung tissue.
Reproductive system	■ Temporary or permanent sterility. ■ Early menopause. ■ Genetic damage.
Urinary system	■ Radiation-induced cystitis and urethritis. ■ Nephritis.
Cardiovascular system	■ Thrombosis. ■ Sclerosis.
Nervous system	■ Myelopathy.
Skeletal system	■ Severe effect on growing bones and cartilage, causing deformities and stunting growth.

■ Teach clients to avoid crowded places, anyone who is sick, and children (who often carry viruses). Also teach them to be extra careful to avoid cutting themselves, and to wear gloves if they garden. *Protecting immunosuppressed clients from infections and other diseases is a challenge. Clients are very susceptible to colds, flu, and other viral infections.*

■ If certified, assist with transfusion of blood products as ordered. *LPNs and LVNs must receive training and certification in order to administer blood products (see also Chapter 34* 🔗 *). Follow state nurse practice acts and agency policy. Clients receiving blood must be closely monitored.*

EVALUATING

Evaluation, again, depends on the individualized outcomes identified for the client. However, it is important to document and report the following findings to the team leader or physician:

■ Persistence of or increase in pain
■ Presence of signs and symptoms of infection
■ Signs of skin breakdown
■ Uncontrolled anxiety levels
■ Signs of anemia

Continuity of Care

Teach the client undergoing radiation treatment to report signs of infection (see Chapter 10 🔗) or anemia (see Chapter 34 🔗). Encourage the client to keep follow-up appointments in order to monitor treatment success and side effects of treatment.

CHEMOTHERAPY

Several factors influence chemotherapy's effectiveness against cancer cells. The biological characteristics of tumors have an effect. The more actively dividing cells are most sensitive to chemotherapy. Host (client) characteristics, such as nutritional status and immune system play a role in the effectiveness of chemotherapy. The drug regimen, dose, scheduling, toxicity, route, and drug resistance also affect response to the chemotherapy.

The use of multiple drug agents (or *combination chemotherapy*) with different actions can provide maximum cell kill for resistant cells, minimize the development of resistant cells, and provide maximum cell kill with tolerable toxicity. Measures used to prevent acquired drug resistance include administering intermittent high doses of drugs, alternating

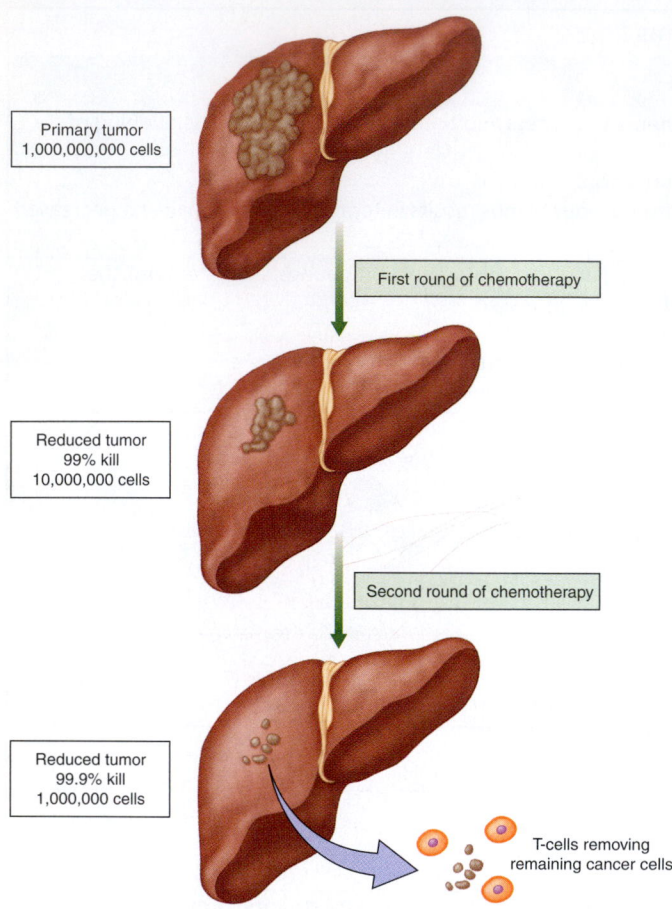

Primary tumor
1,000,000,000 cells

First round of chemotherapy

Reduced tumor
99% kill
10,000,000 cells

Second round of chemotherapy

Reduced tumor
99.9% kill
1,000,000 cells

T-cells removing
remaining cancer cells

Figure 45-7. ■ Cell kill in chemotherapy for liver cancer. (*Source:* Holland, N. and M. P. Adams. *Core Concepts in Pharmacology.* (2003). Upper Saddle River, NJ: Prentice Hall.)

non-cross-resistant chemotherapy regimens, timing the interval between treatments to coincide with normal cell recovery, and maintaining optimum duration of therapy without having to reduce the dosage or delay treatment. Figure 45-7 ■ illustrates cell kill in the liver with chemotherapy.

A *clinical trial* is a scientific study designed to answer clinical and biological questions. It is conducted according to a written guideline or protocol for the study. The trial provides a mechanism to test effectiveness of new therapies. There are four phases of studies. The length of each trial varies depending on the study itself and the drug.

Phase I. Testing is done in clients who may benefit from the drugs and for whom there is no treatment known to be superior. The goals are to evaluate acute toxicities, establish a maximum tolerated dose, and analyze pharmacologic data.

Phase II. The goals of phase II studies are to determine tumor activity, design administration techniques, identify precautions and toxicity, determine dose modifications, and identify the need for supportive care.

Phase III. The goals of phase III studies are to compare drug(s) to standard therapy, evaluate response and duration of response, and evaluate toxicity and quality-of-life issues. *Phase IV.* The goals of phase IV studies are to determine new ways to use the drug(s), and determine the effect of the drug in adjuvant therapy.

Management of Chemotherapy Toxicities

Both acute and long-term toxicities are associated with chemotherapy. They are often the function of the effect the drug or drugs have on rapidly dividing cells. The incidence and severity of toxicities are related to drug dosage, administration schedule, specific mechanism of action, concomitant illness, and measures employed to prevent or minimize toxicities. Figure 45-8 ■ illustrates the multiple effects of chemotherapy on body systems. Clients undergoing chemotherapy may need a great deal of emotional support to maintain hope during this period.

NURSING CARE

PRIORITIZING NURSING CARE

When caring for clients undergoing chemotherapy, focus your care on managing side effects and providing emotional support. Frequently evaluate the effectiveness of treatment for nausea and vomiting. Contact the physician if the treatment is not controlling these side effects. Monitor blood work closely for signs of decreasing red and white blood cells and platelet levels. Report decreases immediately. Instruct the client on protective actions to take to prevent additional problems due to decreasing cell counts. For example, if white blood cells are low, the client should avoid any exposure to viral or bacterial infections. If platelets are low, the client should avoid shaving with a blade, and immediately report bleeding from gums, nose, rectum, or vagina. If red cells are low, the client should rest frequently, taper activities to tolerable levels, and immediately report increasing shortness of breath. Be available for clients to verbalize feelings of discouragement or anguish. The results of the effectiveness of the chemotherapy may not be known for several months, and clients may begin to doubt whether the treatment is worth the discomfort it causes. Allow clients to vent their feelings. Avoid imagining what you would do in the situation. Provide emotional support to clients even if they decide against further chemotherapy. Always preserve the client's hope.

ASSESSING

The nurse will assist in gathering information about the client's past medical history such as known allergies and medications that might interfere or interact with chemotherapy drugs.

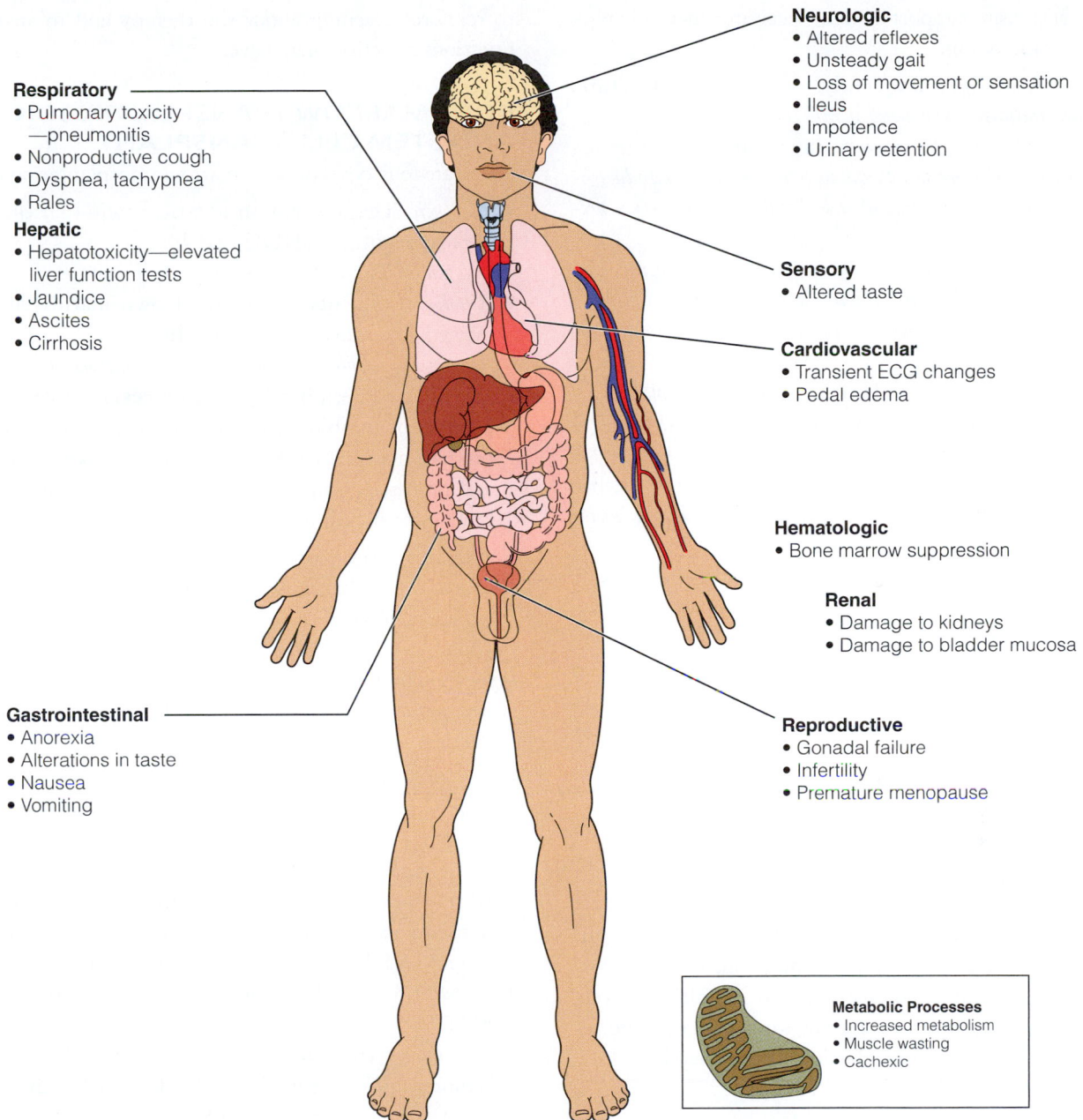

Neurologic
- Altered reflexes
- Unsteady gait
- Loss of movement or sensation
- Ileus
- Impotence
- Urinary retention

Respiratory
- Pulmonary toxicity —pneumonitis
- Nonproductive cough
- Dyspnea, tachypnea
- Rales

Hepatic
- Hepatotoxicity—elevated liver function tests
- Jaundice
- Ascites
- Cirrhosis

Sensory
- Altered taste

Cardiovascular
- Transient ECG changes
- Pedal edema

Hematologic
- Bone marrow suppression

Renal
- Damage to kidneys
- Damage to bladder mucosa

Gastrointestinal
- Anorexia
- Alterations in taste
- Nausea
- Vomiting

Reproductive
- Gonadal failure
- Infertility
- Premature menopause

Metabolic Processes
- Increased metabolism
- Muscle wasting
- Cachexic

Figure 45-8. ■ Multisystem effects of chemotherapy.

DIAGNOSING, PLANNING, AND IMPLEMENTING

The nursing diagnoses for clients undergoing chemotherapy treatment vary with the drugs being administered. Some of the common nursing diagnoses for clients undergoing chemotherapy are:

- *Risk of Infection*
- *Nausea*
- *Anxiety*
- *Fatigue*
- *Disturbed Body Image*

Client goals and outcomes would include:

- The client will not exhibit the signs and symptoms of infection.
- The client will not have a significant drop in lab values.
- The client will not report any nausea or have any vomiting.
- The client will demonstrate healthy, effective coping mechanisms to relieve anxiety.
- The client will be able to maintain energy levels.
- The client will not exhibit signs of drug toxicities.

Nursing actions to support a client receiving chemotherapy include the following:

- Monitor vital signs frequently, especially temperature. *Fever can indicate the presence of infection.*
- Reinforce teaching to prevent infection. *Clients receiving chemotherapy are more susceptible to infection. Good handwashing technique and avoidance of sick children are important prevention strategies.*
- Monitor results of blood work and report any significant drops. *Decreased blood cell counts such as red blood cells and white blood cells (neutrophils in particular) may indicate suppression of bone marrow.*
- Routinely ask the client about nausea. *If the client is nauseous, the nurse will ask the physician for an antiemetic order to help ease nausea and promote client comfort.*
- Ask clients about their anxiety levels and coping mechanisms. *This opens the door for communication and helps identify healthy, effective coping mechanisms.*
- Provide openings for the client to discuss feelings about changes in body image. *Clients adapt better if they can think of body changes as part of the healing process.*
- Ask clients about energy level and offer suggestions to help maintain energy. *Clients can prioritize activities, take naps, and delegate tasks to family members as ways of saving energy they need for healing.*
- Observe for signs of drug toxicity (Box 45-5 ■). *Clients may need help recognizing the signs and symptoms of toxicity.*

EVALUATING

Evaluation always depends on the individual goals set for the client. However, any signs of infection, bone marrow suppression, uncontrolled nausea and vomiting, overwhelming fatigue, or signs of drug toxicity should be reported to the team leader or physician immediately.

BIOTHERAPY

Biotherapy is based on the hypothesis that the immune system can be manipulated to restore, augment, or modulate its function. **Biological response modifiers** (BRMs) are soluble substances capable of stimulating or suppressing the immune system. There are three major categories of BRMs:

- Agents that restore, augment, or modulate a host's immunologic mechanisms
- Agents that have direct antitumor activity
- Agents that have other biological effects (agents interfering with a tumor cell's ability to survive or metastasize; differentiating agents or agents affecting cell transformation)

Nurses obtain client vital signs frequently and provide emotional support during treatment. It may also be necessary to reinforce teaching about the therapy and to answer any questions the client may have.

BONE MARROW TRANSPLANTATION AND STEM CELL TRANSPLANT

There are four types of bone marrow transplantation (BMT):

- *Syngeneic.* The donor is an identical twin (perfect human leukocyte antigen [HLA] match).
- *Allogeneic.* The donor is not a perfect match.
- *Autologous.* Clients receive their own marrow after it is purged to remove malignant cells.
- *Autologous peripheral stem cell transplantation (PSCT).* Cells are collected peripherally by **apheresis** (removal of components of the blood, in this case the stem cells, which produce mature blood cells). Blood is drawn from the arm and processed. Only stem cells are then returned to the body in transfusion.

Candidates and donors require comprehensive clinical and psychologic evaluations. The pretransplant conditioning regimens involve high-dose chemotherapy alone or with total body irradiation. Toxicities and complications are most severe until the marrow graft becomes functional and restores hematocrit and hemoglobin levels.

Some of the acute complications of BMT are:

- *Gastrointestinal toxicity.* Occurs up to 28 days after BMT and manifests as mucositis, nausea and vomiting, or diarrhea. (See GI disorders in Chapter 37 ⬤.)
- *Acute graft versus host disease (GVHD) reaction.* Can occur 10 to 70 days after allogeneic BMT. Clinical manifestations are rash, elevated liver enzymes, diarrhea, and vomiting. (GVHD is discussed in depth in Chapter 35 ⬤.)
- *Chronic GVHD.* Major cause of morbidity after allogeneic BMT.
- *Hematologic complications.* Bleeding from body orifices, hemorrhagic cystitis. (See blood disorders in Chapter 34 ⬤.)
- *Renal insufficiency.* Occurs 1 to 50 days after BMT. Early manifestations include anuria, acid-base imbalances, and doubling of baseline creatinine. (See acid-base imbalance in Chapter 26 ⬤; see renal disorders in Chapter 39 ⬤.)
- *Veno-occlusive disease of liver.* Almost exclusive to BMT. It occurs 6 to 15 days after BMT. The clinical manifestations are fluid retention, sudden weight gain, abdominal distention, hepatomegaly, and encephalopathy.
- *Infection.* The most common sites are the GI tract, oropharynx, lung, skin, and indwelling catheter sites. (See Chapter 10 ⬤ for more on infections.)

An important nursing role is to be aware of the complications associated with BMT and to reinforce teaching in order to prevent them. (See also care of clients with immune disorders, Chapter 35 ⬤.)

| **BOX 45-5** | **COMMON SYSTEMIC TOXICITIES FROM CHEMOTHERAPY** |

Some of the more common systemic toxicities from chemotherapy (see Figure 45-8) are:

- *Bone marrow suppression*—The most common dose-limiting side effect; thrombocytopenia, anemia, and neutropenia are common. A great deal of time should be spent on teaching clients infection prevention measures such as the importance of hand washing and avoiding sick people. Medications such as Neulasta or Neupogen may be considered to stimulate production of white blood cells.

- *Fatigue*—Common and distressing side effect. Interventions to overcome fatigue are energy conservation, rest, setting priorities for activities, and delegating tasks. Fatigue should be discussed with the physicians because medications may be available to treat the underlying cause of fatigue. Procrit and Epogen are examples of medications used to treat the anemia that is usually responsible for fatigue. Insomnia from stress or medications like steroids should also be addressed.

- *Gastrointestinal*—Anorexia can be caused by alterations in food perception, taste, and smell, and can lead to weight loss and a compromised immune status. Consultation with a dietitian is often necessary. Nausea and vomiting occur because the vomiting center in the brain contains neurotransmitter receptors that are sensitive to the chemical toxins of chemotherapy that circulate in blood and cerebrospinal fluid. Acute nausea and vomiting occur 1 to 2 hours after treatment. Delayed nausea and vomiting develop 24 hours after chemotherapy. Anticipatory nausea and vomiting occur as a result of classic operant conditioning from stimuli associated with chemotherapy. The identification of risk factors is an important strategy in keeping the client comfortable. The risk factors include emetic potential of the drug(s), onset and duration of emetic response, dose of drug(s), schedule of drug(s), and anxiety level of the client, which can worsen nausea. Clients should be encouraged to increase their nutritional and caloric intake prior to chemotherapy. After chemotherapy, cool or room temperature foods such as sandwiches or canned fruit often have fewer odors and are therefore more palatable.

Organ Toxicities

- *Cardiotoxicity*—Acute toxicity is characterized by transient electrocardiogram (ECG) changes. Chronic toxicity is characterized by onset of symptoms occurring weeks or months after therapy. The signs and symptoms are a nonproductive cough, dyspnea, and pedal edema. The nursing management is to:
  - Monitor ECGs.
  - Instruct client to conserve energy.
  - Stress minimization of client sodium intake.
  - Administer oxygen as ordered.

- *Neurotoxicity*—May result in direct or indirect damage to CNS, which can produce altered reflexes or unsteady gait. Damage may also occur to the peripheral nervous system, which may cause loss of movement and sensation. Damage can also occur to the autonomic nervous system, which can cause an ileus, impotence, or urinary retention.

- *Pulmonary toxicity*—Chemotherapy can damage endothelial cells, resulting in pneumonitis. The presenting symptoms are dyspnea, unproductive cough, rales, and tachypnea. The nursing management is supporting the client's efforts at conservation of energy.

- *Hepatotoxicity*—Chemotherapy can cause damage to parenchymal cells. Symptoms of hepatotoxicity are elevated liver function tests, jaundice, ascites, and cirrhosis. Obstruction to hepatic blood flow can result in hepatocellular necrosis and veno-occlusive disease. The signs of veno-occlusive disease are weight gain, jaundice, abdominal pain, and hepatomegaly.

- *Hemorrhagic cystitis*—Results from damage to bladder mucosa caused by certain chemotherapeutic drugs such as cyclophosphamide and iphosphamide. Symptoms are hematuria, dysuria, and pubic pain. Nursing management includes hydration, encouraging frequent bladder emptying, and testing urine for occult blood.

- *Nephrotoxicity*—Damage to kidneys is caused either by direct renal cell damage or obstructive nephropathy. The symptoms are increased blood urea nitrogen and creatinine, oliguria, proteinuria, and hyperuricemia. Prevention of nephrotoxicity includes encouraging hydration.

- *Gonadal toxicity*—Chemotherapy can cause gonadal failure, infertility, and premature menopause.

Cancer Care for Special Populations

CHILDREN WITH CANCER

About 9,000 children under the age of 15 in the United States were diagnosed with cancer in 2004 (see Chapter 60 ⟳). The good news is that because of significant advances in therapy, 78% of these children will survive 5 years or more. This is an increase of almost 46% since the early 1960s.

The most common types of cancers that occur in children vary greatly from those seen in adults. Leukemias, brain, and other nervous system tumors, lymphomas, bone cancers, soft tissue sarcomas, kidney cancers, eye cancers, and adrenal gland cancers are the most common in children. Breast, prostate, lung, skin, and colorectal are the most common cancers in adults. Some pediatric cancers are the result of a familial disposition (that is, cancer runs in the family). However, the cause of most childhood cancers is unknown because they cannot be related to lifestyle risk factors such as smoking.

Childhood cancers can be treated with surgery, chemotherapy, radiation therapy, or a combination of two or more of these therapies. Childhood cancers tend to respond well to chemotherapy because they are cancers that grow fast.

Children with cancer and their families have special needs, especially for psychologic coping. These can best be met at children's cancer centers where a team of specialists focuses on the unique needs of children and their families. Besides the traditional medical team, psychologists, social workers, child life specialists, nutritionists, rehabilitation and physical therapists, and educators should be involved in the treatment of a child with cancer. The team provides support to both the child and the entire family. Adaptations are geared toward the developmental level of the child, and facilities are oriented around every child's need to play.

Information regarding chemotherapy or radiation treatment should be geared to the age and development of the child. Children may experience the same side effects of chemotherapy or radiation as adults but may not be able to explain what they feel. Young children can understand that they may feel tired and their hair may thin or fall out. Older children can understand and often want more information. Any teaching about treatment and possible side effects should be given prior to the start of treatment to reduce fear and anxiety later. Children should be encouraged to report symptoms such as nausea, vomiting, pain, or diarrhea so that interventions can be initiated quickly. Parents should be taught about signs or symptoms to report for younger children.

Adequate nutrition is especially important for children undergoing treatment to support growth and development. Frequent small meals may be easier to tolerate. Cold foods may be more palatable than hot foods. Popsicles or slushies may provide liquid to help prevent dehydration. Nutritional supplements in child-friendly flavors may also be used. Changes in nutrition and chemotherapy may cause delays in cognitive and physical development that will resolve following completion of treatment.

Children receiving treatment for cancer may require increased attention and comforting. Parents and family members should be encouraged to participate in the child's care. Siblings or friends should be encouraged to visit as long as it is not medically contraindicated. Comforting objects such as stuffed toys or soft blankets may help some children cope with medical treatments. Play activities may need to be adapted due to the child's illness. School-aged children may want to communicate with classmates and be included in activities to make the transition back into school easier after treatment. School districts may provide tutors to children missing class due to treatment or to children too ill to attend regular classes.

OLDER ADULTS WITH CANCER

The risk of cancer increases with age making it more likely to have cancer in later years. Older adults may have the same side effects from chemotherapy or radiation as younger adults but are more likely to have them. Older adults may have several chronic diseases and take several medications already that may complicate treatment. The overall health status of the client rather than chronologic age is most important in selecting treatment options. Older adults are more likely to be undertreated than younger adults due to age.

Physiological changes occur with aging that may complicate cancer treatment. Decreased hepatic or renal function may cause a decrease in the metabolism or excretion of chemotherapeutic agents. A decrease in lean muscle mass may necessitate a reduction in the dosage of some agents. Drug interactions may occur between medication used to treat cancer and those used for other diseases. Clients with cardiac disease may be excluded from taking chemotherapy that is cardiotoxic. Pain medication may be metabolized differently in older adults causing oversedation or undertreatment. Pain medication may increase the risk of falls in this age group.

Nutrition may be a problem in older adults due to poor dentition, medication side effects, fatigue, or loss of appetite due to chronic disease. Chemotherapy or radiation may further complicate this problem. Monitoring the client's weight on a frequent basis and tracking caloric intake during a calorie count should give information about the nutritional status of the client. Small frequent meals, cool foods, or liquid nutritional supplements may enhance the client's intake. Families should be encouraged to prepare meals that include the client's favorite foods. Meals on Wheels or senior meal programs may also be an option to obtain prepared meals.

Psychosocial concerns facing older adults can have an adverse impact on cancer treatment. Clients living on a fixed income may be overwhelmed with expenses from co-payments, increased medication costs, and hospital bills. Financial concerns may be cited as a reason to decline treatment or fill prescriptions. Older adults may also encounter transportation issues or be dependent on others to provide transportation. A lack of transportation may make it difficult to coordinate appointments and treatments. Public transportation may be an option.

An older client with cancer may also be a caregiver for a spouse or family member. Alternative care providers or respite care can be arranged to allow the client to receive treatment or visit physicians without worry. Previously independent older adults may find it difficult to perform ADLs or maintain their home during illness. In-home assistance with physical care, housekeeping, or other chores may be arranged to help the older adult maintain their independence.

Older adults may experience depression or anxiety following a cancer diagnosis. A change in hygiene, appetite, or sleeping pattern may indicate coping difficulties. Older adults may be hesitant to verbalize these changes to medical practitioners. Family members should be encouraged to report any changes in behavior. Older adults who have lost a spouse or are otherwise alone may feel very isolated following a cancer diagnosis. Older adults are more likely to view a cancer diagnosis as terminal. Medications to treat depression, anxiety, or insomnia may improve the quality of life for clients in this age group.

Note: The references and resources for all chapters have been compiled at the back of the book.

Chapter Review

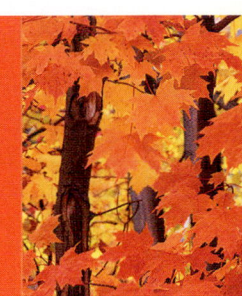

KEY Points

- Cancer is a complex disease process of uncontrolled cell growth. It can affect every body system.
- Cancer treatment consists of multiple treatment modalities, usually used in combination.
- The client can influence some risk factors for cancer such as smoking and diet.
- Care of the client with cancer has a large psychosocial component.
- The treatment plan for the client with cancer involves interdisciplinary decision making that is dependent on several factors such as tumor aggressiveness, morbidity and mortality, and client wishes.
- Cancer treatment modalities carry some severe side effects and toxicities.

⟳ FOR FURTHER Study

For in-depth discussion of infection, see Chapter 10.

See Chapter 11 for additional information on therapeutic listening.

Refer to Chapter 17 for a discussion of the psychosocial aspects of physical illness.

Pain is discussed in full in Chapter 22.

Cleaning of wounds is covered in Chapter 24.

For further information on I&O and acid-base and fluid balance, see Chapter 26.

See Chapter 29 for perioperative nursing care.

Chapter 34 discusses disorders of blood and lymph.

See discussion of the immune system and acute graft-versus-host-disease (GVHD) in Chapter 35.

See Chapter 37 for more information on GI disorders.

Renal disorders are discussed in Chapter 39.

Gynecologic tumors, male reproductive disorders, and other reproductive disorders, including prostate cancer, are discussed in Chapter 40; metastasis of breast cancer cells to brain and lung is shown in Figure 40-8; an aspiration biopsy is shown in Figure 40-9.

Nursing care of clients with chronic or terminal illness is discussed in Chapter 44.

Cancer in young children is discussed in Chapter 60.

Critical Thinking Care Map

Caring for Client with Fatigue

NCLEX-PN® Focus Area: Comfort

Case Study: A 44-year-old female is undergoing radiation and chemotherapy for advanced breast cancer. She has been admitted to the hospital for anemia, extreme fatigue, and weakness.

Nursing Diagnosis: *Fatigue* related to cancer therapy

COLLECT DATA

Subjective	Objective
_____	_____
_____	_____
_____	_____
_____	_____
_____	_____
_____	_____
_____	_____

Would you report this? Yes/No

If yes, report to: _____

What would you report? _____

Nursing Care

_____
_____
_____
_____
_____
_____
_____
_____
_____
_____
_____

How would you document this?_____
_____
_____
_____

Compare your answers and documentation to those provided on the MyNursingKit Website.

Data Collected
(use only those that apply)

- Inability to stay awake and alert
- Inability to concentrate
- General appearance is weak and fatigued
- Decreased red blood cells, hemoglobin, and hematocrit levels
- Increased appetite
- BP 140/90

Nursing Interventions
(use only those that apply; list in priority order)

- Administer blood products as ordered.
- Teach client interventions that assist in management of fatigue such as energy conservation, nutrition, exercise, sleep, and rest.
- Monitor vital signs during blood administration.
- Administer oxygen as ordered.
- Delegate the client's duties to the family members for the client.
- Teach importance of eating three big meals a day.

NCLEX-PN® Exam Preparation

1 You are caring for a client receiving radiation to red bone marrow. The nurse anticipates which of the following as a side effect of this treatment?

1. Reduction in white blood cells, proliferation of red blood cells
2. Anemia and resulting fatigue
3. Risk for thrombosis
4. Increased sebaceous gland production

2 The nurse knows that which of the following should not be a primary reason for choosing a cancer treatment plan?

1. Cost of treatment
2. Aggressiveness of treatment
3. Morbidity
4. Client wishes

3 Which of the following is not a nursing intervention for the treatment of clients with cancer?

1. Preventing infections by using good handwashing technique
2. Monitoring I&O for vomiting, adequate hydration, and adequate kidney function
3. Determining the tissue type of the cancer
4. Listening to a client's fears and being supportive

4 Which of the following clients would the nurse consider at greatest risk for cancer?

1. The female client with a history of breast cancer in her family.
2. The client who smokes, drinks alcohol, and is over the age of 65.
3. The client with a high number of sexual partners.
4. The client who lives in a large city known to have a great deal of air pollution.

5 The client, newly diagnosed with cancer, asks the nurse what the difference is between a regular cell and a cancer cell. The nurse's best response would be:

1. "Cancer cells die fairly quickly compared to normal cells."
2. "Cancer cells divide abnormally and change their appearance."

3. "Cancer cells require something to anchor to in order to grow."
4. "Cancer cells grow quickly in an uncontrolled manner."

6 An individual who recently had an ultrasound-guided percutaneous needle biopsy of the liver must be closely monitored by the nurse for symptoms of:

1. Spinal cord compression.
2. Hematemesis.
3. Headache.
4. Hemorrhage.

7 When caring for a client with distant metastases, the nurse anticipates the focus of treatment will be:

1. Radical surgery.
2. Local control.
3. Combined modality treatment.
4. Palliation only.

8 The nurse is caring for a client diagnosed with colorectal cancer and anticipates what form of staging will be used?

1. Tumor-node-metastasis staging
2. Clark level staging
3. Duke's staging system
4. Surgical staging

9 The nurse is caring for a client receiving chemotherapy who complains of nausea and vomiting following treatments. The nurse would advise the client to:

1. Get extra rest and reduce normal activity levels.
2. Delay intake of meals for 3 to 4 hours after treatments.
3. Increase fluid intake.
4. Eat bland, soft foods.

10 The nurse is working on a pediatric oncology unit and recognizes that, unlike with adults, the healthcare team must also include a/an:

1. Oncologist.
2. Social worker.
3. Psychologist.
4. Educator.

Answers and rationales for Review Questions appear in Appendix I.

Chapter 46

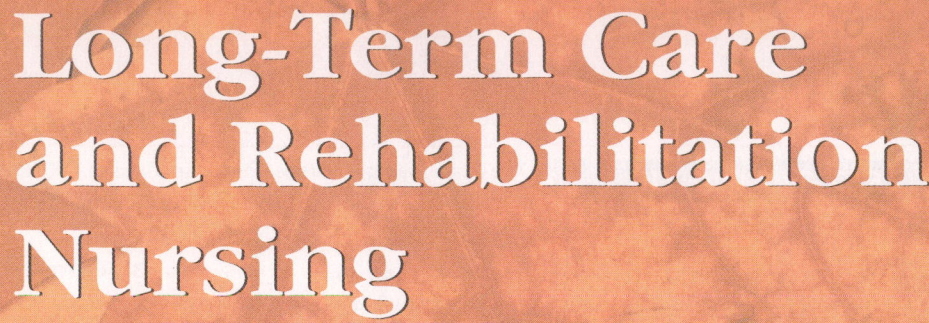

Long-Term Care and Rehabilitation Nursing

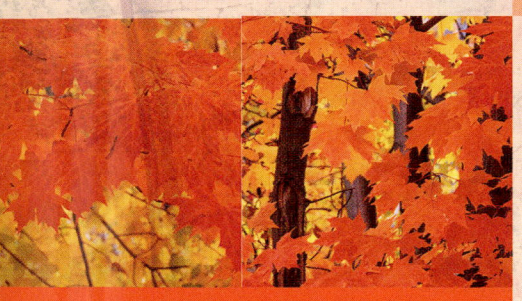

BRIEF Outline

LEARNING Outcomes

After completing this chapter, you will be able to:

1. Differentiate between skilled and custodial care in a long-term care facility and state why these facilities are important.
2. Discuss the roles and responsibilities of the LPN/LVN in long-term care.
3. Identify the LPN/LVN role in supervising and delegating to nursing assistants and aides.
4. Describe the multidisciplinary approach to long-term client care, including the importance of family.
5. Discuss the specialized needs of young adult clients receiving care in a skilled nursing or rehabilitation facility.
6. Discuss the roles of the LPN/LVN in rehabilitation.
7. Identify legal and ethical concerns for long-term care and rehabilitation.
8. Discuss Medicare, Medicaid, and insurance reimbursement for long-term care and rehabilitation.

Clinical Objectives

9. Identify the responsibilities of a charge nurse in a long-term care setting.
10. Function as a medication or treatment nurse in long-term care.
11. Participate in a client care conference.
12. Delegate appropriately to unlicensed personnel.

Because long-term illness occurs most often in the elderly, long-term care facilities have programs that are oriented to the needs of this age group. These facilities can, in effect, become the client's home, and consequently the people who live there are frequently referred to as *residents* rather than patients or clients.

In 1987, **Omnibus Budget Reconciliation Act** (OBRA) was passed to improve nursing homes and extended-care facilities. OBRA requirements for nurse's aide training include a certification program for nurse's aides and competence evaluations of aides.

Specific guidelines govern the admission procedures for clients admitted to an extended-care facility. Insurance criteria, treatment needs, and nursing care requirements must all be assessed beforehand. Many skilled nursing facilities exist as units within a hospital but are regulated by federal, state, and local governmental bodies to make sure they are meeting the requirements for a long-term care facility. If a client in a hospital needs to be transferred to such a unit, the client is discharged from the hospital and then admitted to the long-term care unit. Types of healthcare facilities are discussed in Chapter 7 🔗.

Extended-care and skilled nursing facilities are becoming increasingly popular means for managing the healthcare needs of clients who require additional care but who do not meet the criteria for remaining in the hospital (Figure 46-1 ■). Often, these extended-care facilities have waiting lists for admission. Nurses in extended-care facilities assist clients with their daily activities, provide care when necessary, and coordinate rehabilitation activities.

This chapter focuses on the particulars of long-term care and rehabilitation. Several chapters in this book discuss related topics. Psychosocial issues related to grief, loss, and death are discussed in depth in Chapter 18 🔗. Health promotion of older adults is in Chapter 42 🔗. Nursing care of ill older adults is in Chapter 43 🔗. In-depth discussion about nursing care of chronically and terminally ill clients is in Chapter 44 🔗.

Levels of Care

SKILLED CARE

Skilled-care facilities (also called acute care) are those in which clients require specialized care. This may include tube feedings, IV therapy, frequent dressing changes, at

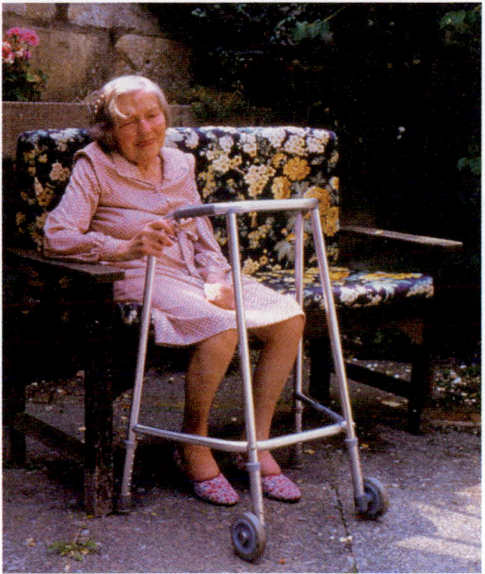

Figure 46-1. ■ As the older adult population increases, many older people will call long-term care facilities home. *Source:* Photo Researchers, Inc.

least one daily nursing assessment, physical therapy, or occupational therapy at least 5 days a week. Skilled care is meant to cure disease, restore prior functioning, or prevent further problems. For example, a fairly independent, elderly client may be in skilled care for IV antibiotic therapy for pneumonia.

CUSTODIAL CARE

Custodial care is ongoing, maintenance care. A client receiving custodial care may require 24-hour nursing care, but is not receiving skilled nursing services. Further progress of the client is not expected, and acute medical treatment is not provided. Clients may be bedridden, have dementia, or have some other physical or mental condition that demands nursing care. They do not have the ability to live independently.

The actual amount of care needed varies among clients. Some clients in custodial care can perform most ADLs independently, but they may have some physical or cognitive deficit that makes it unsafe for them to live alone. (For example, they may be unsteady on their feet, or they might leave the stove on or the front door open.) These clients can usually wash their face and hands when handed a washcloth, feed themselves, dress themselves, or participate in dressing.

Other clients may be unable to perform simple tasks. Many clients need to be bathed, fed, dressed, and undressed. They need to be repositioned every 2 hours in the night and moved into chairs in the day. They may have lost a sense of when they need to urinate or defecate, or they may no longer have the ability to wait until they reach the bathroom, so many are incontinent.

Custodial care involves providing care for those who are dependent and checking that the more independent clients have taken their meds, bathed, put in their teeth or hearing aid, been to the toilet, and washed their hands. Some clients may need light guidance or assistance. For example, if a client has had a stroke, he or she may need clothes buttoned or shoelaces tied.

Roles of the LPN/LVN in Long-Term Care Nursing

Of all the possible work settings, long-term care settings offer LPNs/LVNs the largest role in terms of independence and responsibility. In many such facilities, an LPN/LVN is the charge nurse, coordinating client care, working with physicians, supervising a shift of unlicensed assistive personnel, and holding final responsibility for care of residents. Roles that LPNs/LVNs play in long-term nursing are listed in Box 46-1 ■.

HEAD-TO-TOE DATA COLLECTION

Once per day, the LPN/LVN is responsible for compiling head-to-toe assessment data for each assigned client. However, this does not mean that LPNs/LVNs themselves collect all the data for this assessment. They often rely on assistive personnel for vital signs, skin condition, cognitive changes, and information about intake and output.

SHIFT-CHANGE REPORTS

On entering work, the LPN/LVN would first get change-of-shift report for every client on the unit (or every client who is assigned to care). Report would indicate any changes in client condition. Changes in aide assignments would be done at this time if necessary.

At the start of day shift, any event that might require a call to the primary care or other provider would be listed. For example, if a client had broken his or her glasses, the nurse would make a call to begin the process of repairing or replacing them. There might be a note that the family was planning to pick up the client for an outing at a certain time, so a client would need to be dressed and ready.

DOCUMENTATION

Documentation of any abnormal findings or significant changes is a major role of the LPN/LVN (see documentation discussion in Chapter 13 ⚭). The nurse must judge when to report changes to the primary care provider in order to

---

BOX 46-1	LPN/LVN ROLES IN LONG-TERM CARE

The following are important roles that an LPN/LVN can have in a long-term care facility:

- Head-to-toe assessments of clients
- Documentation of client status and any changes (e.g., a talkative, mobile client now in bed all day; a client suddenly knocking things over or not responding to sound; client seeming confused who is normally lucid)
- Notifying the primary care provider of changes in the client's status or of lack of expected change (e.g., no response to a medication)
- Administering medications (all medications except IV push)
- Providing treatments and doing procedures
- Coordinating and communicating with other healthcare staff through staff meetings and change-of-shift reports
- Maintaining care plans for all residents
- Advocating for the client
- Acting as liaison with the client and family
- Doing rounds with the primary care provider; noting verbal orders and information to share with staff (e.g., client off bed rest, ambulation three times a day, etc.)
- Communicating information from physician's rounds to family and staff
- Taking phone orders
- Faxing new prescriptions to the pharmacy
- Setting up appointments for clients and arranging for transportation as needed
- Delegating tasks to and supervising aides

---

update or alter the plan of care. A client fall always requires reporting. A superficial skin tear would not be reported, but signs of infection in a skin tear warrant a phone call.

The LPN/LVN charts medications and treatments (Figure 46-2 ■). Other data that may be charted (depending on the client) include pain levels, intake and output, scale for food (e.g., 75% of lunch eaten), level of consciousness,

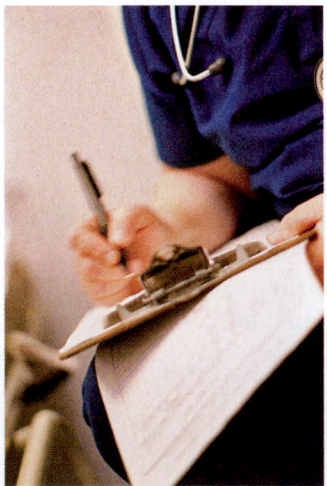

Figure 46-2. ■ Charting medications and treatments is one of many roles of the LPN/LVN in long-term and rehabilitation care. *Source: Getty Images Inc.—Image Bank.*

and general appearance. If a client entered the facility after a surgery, the nurse might record information about a Foley catheter or drainage. (Most facilities with acute surgical clients would be likely to have an RN on each shift.)

MEDICATIONS AND PROCEDURES

Administering Medications

Another major role of the LPN/LVN in long-term care is administration of medications for disease processes as well as for procedures. Some medications require prior collection of data (e.g., blood pressure, pulse, temperature) before the drug is administered. The aides would begin a morning shift by taking readings and providing data to the LPN/LVN as they are collected.

When LPNs/LVNs administer medications, they first observe the client's overall condition for side effects or any manifestations that might contraindicate administration of the drug. Oral medications are generally provided early in the day to be taken with food. Insulin administration is determined by the individual needs of the client.

Medications used in procedures are applied with AM and PM care or as baths are being given. This would include mouthwash for candidiasis, creams to skin tears or decubiti, Fleet's enema, treatment for lice infestation (*pediculosis*), and so on.

LPNs/LVNs may hang IV solutions but do not administer IV push medications. Some larger facilities have a special floor or wing dedicated to clients who are on IV therapy and/or mechanical ventilators. RNs may perform these interventions, or (in some states) LPNs/LVNs may receive special training to work with these clients.

Performing Procedures

LPNs/LVNs perform many procedures in the long-term care setting. (Note: Procedures are described in Units IV and V of this book.) Nursing procedures performed by the LPN/LVN may include, but are not limited to, the following:

- Treatments for bedsores (see Chapter 24 ⚭)
- Enemas or digital fecal disimpaction (see Chapter 37 ⚭)
- Drawing blood for Coumadin (warfarin) levels to be checked (see Chapter 28 ⚭)
- Glucose testing (see Chapter 38 ⚭)
- Checking pacemakers over the phone. (This can often be done by using a cell phone at the client's bedside.) Batteries and pacemakers are checked on a regular schedule.

MAINTAINING CLIENT RECORDS

Besides the change-of-shift reports mentioned above, the LPN/LVN communicates with the full healthcare staff at regularly scheduled staff meetings. At these meetings, the plan of care for each resident is reviewed and updated as needed by the healthcare team. (Note, however, that changes from physician's orders are implemented as they are received.)

In many long-term care facilities, planning meetings are held on a weekly or biweekly basis, and a set of resident care plans is reviewed at each meeting. The care plans for all residents are reviewed each month. All staff except physicians attend these meetings. Physicians sign the reports of these planning sessions when they do rounds.

CLIENT ADVOCACY

Client advocacy is a must for LPNs/LVNs in long-term care. This means taking into account each person's background, culture, end-of-life wishes, and so on. If a resident says he does not want to see a family member who only comes to visit once a month, the nurse would approach the person at the entrance and state the resident's wishes. If the family member insisted, the nurse would have the visitor wait until he or she had informed the resident that the family member insisted on visiting.

The LPN/LVN can advocate for clients in a multitude of big or small ways. For example, it can make a huge difference to a resident if the nurse remembers to request a favorite type of cookie for him or her, or if the nurse reminds the resident about an upcoming visit. Small things done out of caring and respect show that the nurse values the residents' choices. These actions support clients' dignity.

PHYSICIAN'S ROUNDS

Most long-term care facilities do not have a physician in attendance. Instead, in accordance with Medicare and Medicaid guidelines, a physician generally does rounds of residents every 30 days.

The LPN/LVN supervisor attends rounds when the physician makes monthly visits to the long-term care facility. The LPN/LVN listens and may take notes on what the doctor tells clients. This has two purposes. First, clients often need repetition, reinforcement, or clarification about what they hear the physician say. Also, the LPN/LVN makes notes for follow-up. For example, if the physician tells a client, "We'll get you some Cepacol lozenges," but then does not write the order for lozenges before leaving the facility, the nurse can follow up that a verbal order was received.

During physician rounds, the LPN/LVN advocates for the client. For example, if a client refuses a particular medication the physician had prescribed, the nurse would ask the reasons why he or she refused it, and then might ask the physician whether an alternative could be provided.

After the physician's rounds, LPN/LVN supervisors share changes in a client's plan of care with the unlicensed staff. It is the LPN/LVN supervisor's responsibility to do this. Communication may need to be immediate (depending on client's condition), or it can be done at change of shift. Medication changes would be reported to the oncoming LPN/LVN.

Between rounds, the LPN/LVN reports changes in client condition and abnormal vital signs or lab values by phone to the primary care provider. Anything that might require a change in medication or plan of care for the client is reported.

FAMILY LIAISON

The LPN/LVN is the primary communicator with the immediate family. The nurse would convey any pertinent information from the physician's rounds. The nurse might also have to call the designated family member to provide transportation to doctor visits or other events, or to update status. Family would also be called when holidays are approaching to determine whether the client would be leaving the facility for the day.

NOTIFICATION OF DEATH

In the event of a death, there is a checklist of people to notify. The nurse calls the funeral home (the information will be on the client's chart). The LPN/LVN would also notify an aide to do postmortem care, wrap the client, provide a toe tag, and gather the client's belongings. If family is present, the nurse waits for the family to say its goodbyes. The body is then taken to the morgue (or a designated room) until the body is picked up. If there was a DNR order, the nurse does not have to call the coroner. However, if foul play is suspected in a death, or if the family or family physician requests a coroner, the nurse would call the coroner.

OFFICE TASKS

Office tasks such as making phone calls for appointments or referrals or faxing new med orders to pharmacies are tasks the LPN/LVN would perform. LPNs/LVNs in long-term care are allowed to take phone orders from the primary care provider, following state practice acts and facility policy.

DELEGATION TO UNLICENSED ASSISTIVE PERSONNEL

The LPN/LVN in long-term care supervises certified nursing assistants (CNAs) and other unlicensed assistive personnel and so is responsible for the quality of work they perform. It will be the LPN's/LVN's job to give both positive and negative feedback on care that CNAs provide. Some aides will need more guidance than others, and LPNs/LVNs must keep in mind the five rules of delegating when assigning work (Box 46-2 ■). The flow sheet in Figure 63-1 ⊕ illustrates the path to proper delegation.

As an LPN/LVN, you should strive to maintain an open line of communication between yourself and the aides who work with you. They are your eyes and ears when you are not with the clients, and they have major responsibility for clients' personal care. Establishing a mutually supportive relationship is a key aspect of team building.

BOX 46-2	**FIVE RULES OF DELEGATION**

RIGHT TASK: One that is delegated for a specific client.
RIGHT CIRCUMSTANCES: Appropriate client setting, available resources, and other relevant factors considered.
RIGHT PERSON: The *right person* performs the task on the *right person*.
RIGHT DIRECTION/COMMUNICATION: Clear, concise description of the task, including its objective, limits, and expectations.
RIGHT SUPERVISION: Appropriate monitoring, evaluation, intervention as needed, and feedback.

Source: Adapted from Adams, E. D., and Towle, M. A. (2009). *Pediatric nursing care.* Upper Saddle River, NJ: Prentice Hall.

The LPN/LVN supervisor assigns residents to the aides and assistive personnel, balancing workload. Male assistive personnel are generally assigned to male residents. The LPN/LVN supervises the following routine tasks that unlicensed personnel perform for residents in long-term care:

- Vital signs
- Bathing
- Dressing
- Feeding or feeding assistance (opening containers, etc.)
- Range of motion (ROM), usually done when bathing or dressing
- Bed making
- Transferring residents (all levels)
- Changes of position
- Filling water pitchers
- (In some states) glucose readings; follow state practice acts and facility guidelines
- Postmortem care: washing, tagging, and gathering belongings

Nurse's aides do skin checks when they give baths or are dressing or undressing residents. They watch for bruising, skin tears, or any evidence of bedsores and report these to the LPN/LVN. They help the nurse maintain adequate documentation by reporting abnormal vital signs or other significant changes.

At times, evaluation of performance may reveal concerns that are beyond the scope of the role of the LPN/LVN. The LPN/LVN would consult with the supervising RN. Major performance problems (such as suspicion of substance abuse) must be referred to the RN supervisor.

Onsite Healthcare Team

RN

The LPN/LVN in long-term care always has reference to a Registered Nurse supervisor. If anything is outside the scope of the LPN/LVN nurse practice act, the nurse calls the RN.

The LPN/LVN might also get a second opinion from an RN. An example might be if an order is received for a medication and the LPN/LVN thinks that it might be contraindicated for the client. The LPN/LVN could contact the RN for a second opinion before calling the primary care provider.

AIDES/UNLICENSED ASSISTIVE PERSONNEL

Much of the hands-on client care in long-term care facilities is provided by unlicensed staff. Certified nursing assistants (CNAs) and trained aides do everything from taking vital signs to helping residents with ADLs. The role of unlicensed assistive personnel was discussed under Delegation to Unlicensed Assistive Personnel.

FAMILY

The family is an important part of the rehabilitation team. Family members can provide insight and information about the client, especially if the client has some measure of impairment when entering the facility. It is helpful to learn the level of interaction that can be expected by the family. For example, the nurse would ask if family members plan to transport clients to doctor or dentist appointments or whether the client will need another form of transportation.

The nurse gets information from and gives information to the family. If a client cannot speak, for example, the nurse or aids would inform them of recent events (parties, visits, etc.). The nurse would describe any updates in treatment or client condition from the doctor's rounds. The nurse would explain changes in the care plan for the client as well as any pertinent facility policies that might affect the client.

Keep the family informed of changes in the client or in the plan of care. Encourage family members to be as involved as they wish to be in the client's ongoing daily life. Become informed about what roles they will fill (bringing clients to the dentist, visiting or attending a holiday meal, providing new clothing when needed, etc.). Be nonjudgmental and professional in manner in all interactions.

The level of involvement of family in the life of residents may vary widely. Some may stop in every day after work to visit. Others may drop in once a month for 10 minutes. The level of family involvement should not affect the quality of care delivered to the client.

PHYSICAL THERAPIST

The physical therapist is responsible for the progression of exercises in rehabilitative care (Figure 46-3 ■). For example, for a client with left-sided hemiplegia following a stroke, the therapist would initiate passive exercises to prevent muscle contracture. Then, active exercises would be introduced as the client's condition improved. Perhaps initially the client would be asked to move the fingers and would progress to squeezing a tennis ball with the hand. Physical therapy for residents

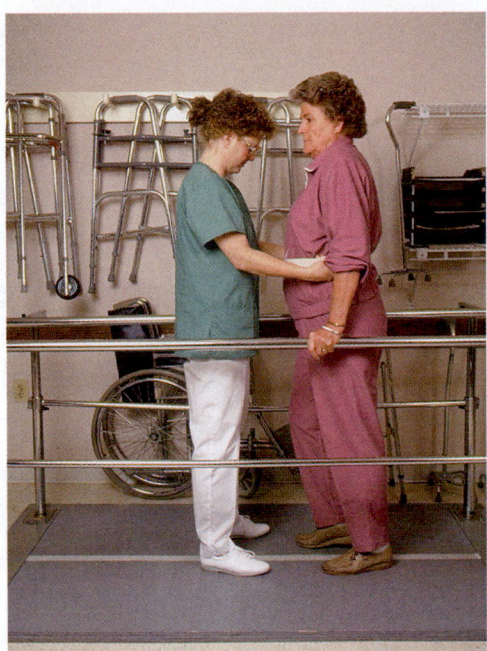

Figure 46-3. ■ The physical therapist is responsible for the progression of exercises in rehabilitative care. *Source:* Pearson Education/PH College.

might only occur twice a week. In staff meetings to review the plan of care, the physical therapist would share what the client should be encouraged to do throughout the day. Then the LPN/LVN or aides could give daily reminders (e.g., hand the client a tennis ball to squeeze 10 times, or encourage the client to try to button his or her shirt in the morning).

The LPN/LVN works with the physical therapist to promote the rehabilitation of the client. An important intervention is to coordinate the pain relief medication schedule so that medication will be effective while the client is engaged in physical therapy.

RESPIRATORY THERAPIST

Some facilities have respiratory therapists on staff to assist clients on ventilators. They may provide respiratory treatments. They might give or oversee oxygen therapy and adjust the concentration level to be given. They would participate in codes. If a client who has a resuscitation order stops breathing, the RT would be available to assist with manual ventilation until mechanical ventilation could be started, and would help with intubation.

OCCUPATIONAL THERAPIST

Occupational therapists provide daily activities to stimulate the mind and to encourage or maintain ADL skills. They assess ADL levels and order adaptive devices (Figure 46-4 ■). They or an activities director would lead games, lay out puzzles, and organize crafts. In staff meetings, the occupational therapist tells aides what ADLs clients should do for themselves, and what actions to encourage.

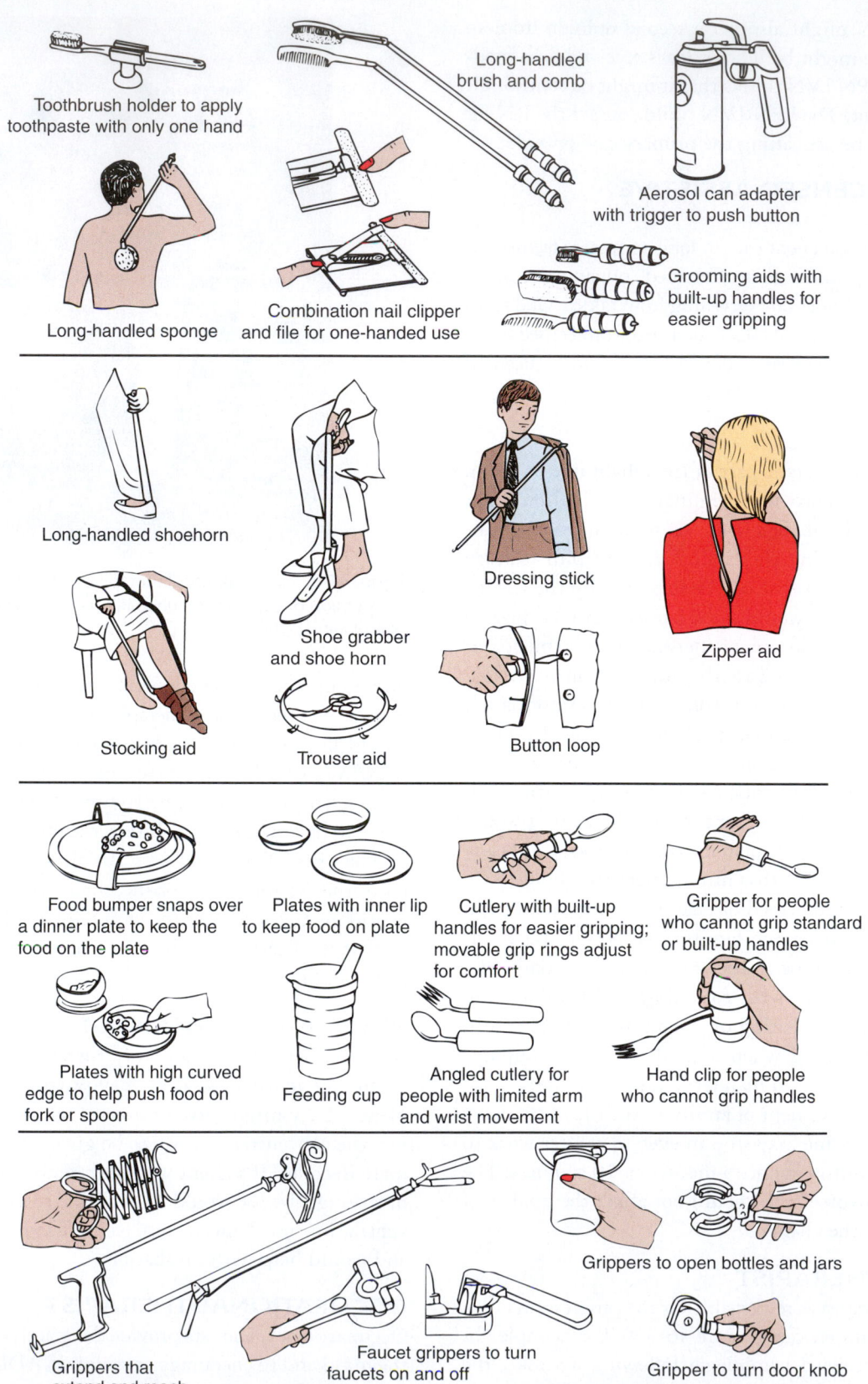

Figure 46-4. ■ Adaptive devices.

The occupational therapist (OT) might attend mealtime to observe a person who has experienced a cerebrovascular accident (CVA or stroke) to determine whether the person requires special assistive devices in order to eat. The OT would inform the charge nurse of the need for special equipment; the LPN/LVN would obtain a physician's order (needed for Medicaid reimbursement for the equipment) and order the equipment from the kitchen.

The OT instructs the resident on how to hold and use the equipment. Then, the aide reinforces teaching and makes sure the stroke bowl and spoon are provided with meals.

SOCIAL SERVICES

Every long-term facility has a social services staff member. It is the responsibility of social services to speak for the client and to advocate when family is not available or when the client lacks funds. For example, social workers might order new eyeglasses or clothing for a client who has no relatives, and would obtain reimbursement. They would help a resident who has been in a private pay facility to find a government-funded facility if the person's funds had run out. Social workers also make funeral arrangements for clients who have died and have no family.

SPEECH THERAPIST

A common outcome of CVA is reduced ability or inability to speak (**aphasia**). Speech therapists work with clients to regain that ability. At staff meetings, the speech therapist shares information about clients and tells staff what the client should be expected or encouraged to say. For example, the speech therapist might tell the aides and the LPN/LVN to ask a client to state what his or her pain level is, not just to grimace. The therapist may say that the client should ask for items, not just point.

Speech therapists also deal with swallowing issues. They test a client's gag reflex and ability to swallow. That leads to the type of food ordered. For example, they would notify the dietitian if a resident cannot chew properly and needs a change to a soft or pureed diet.

PHARMACIST

Many long-term care facilities have a pharmacy that is staffed during the day. The LPN/LVN is responsible for administering all medications. The supervising RN may have access to the pharmacy to get items during the hours the pharmacy is closed. Most orders will be provided by the physician after rounds or by phone. The LPN/LVN faxes these to the pharmacy.

DIETITIAN

Dietitians are an important part of the rehabilitative and long-term care team. Proper nutrition enhances healing and provides a balance of nutrients to support health.

Information about client preferences is obtained from the client or the client's family on admission. Documentation is kept of clients' daily food intake. If aides report that a client who normally eats full meals has eaten only 25% of meals since yesterday, the nurse or dietitian would talk with the client about why he or she is not eating and would make adjustments as needed.

The nurse may initiate a change in diet. For example, if a client's diabetes is not being controlled well, the LPN/LVN would report this to the primary care provider and may obtain an order for a lower-calorie diet.

CLERGY/SUPPORT STAFF

A client's emotional and spiritual health can support physical gains. In contrast, feelings of depression and sadness can slow a person's return to physical health and well-being.

Specialized Needs of Younger Clients in Long-Term Care

For many years, long-term care facilities were referred to as "old people's homes." Rehab and long-term care facilities mostly do support that population. However, at times a child or young adult becomes a resident in long-term care.

When possible, long-term care is provided among peers (e.g., a "home" that specializes in care for children with severe forms of cerebral palsy). Care among peers is helpful for youth, even though it may mean being at some distance from birth family. Schooling can be incorporated into the long-term care environment. Activities and entertainment can be aimed at the appropriate developmental levels (Figure 46-5 ■).

However, when no specialized facility is available, the staff in a long-term care facility must address developmental issues as well as possible. Tutors may be sought to assist the child in continuing schoolwork.

Psychological issues must also be addressed. When most residents are considerably older and in poor health, a child or young adult may find the environment very upsetting. The healthcare team will need to work with the family to provide a caring, positive environment.

Rehabilitation Nursing

Rehabilitation is the set of skills and activities applied to client care to assist the individual to return to his or her maximum level of functioning. The maximal potential may involve chronic impairment and resulting functional disability. The philosophy behind rehabilitation nursing is that each client has unique strengths and abilities that enable that person to live with dignity, self-worth, and independence.

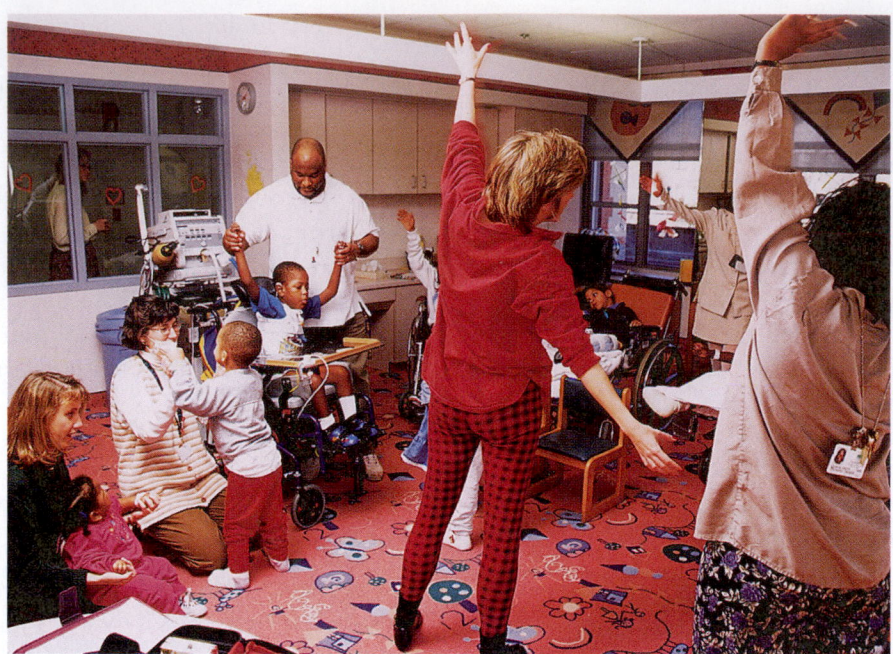

Figure 46-5. ■ Young people require special interventions when they are in long-term care. Ideally, children who require long-term care will be placed in a pediatric long-term care facility.

The terms *handicap, disability*, and *impairment* are often used interchangeably, but they have distinct meanings. **Handicap** is the total adjustment to a disability that limits functioning at a normal level. A **disability** is the degree of observable and measurable impairment. An **impairment** is a disturbance in structure or function resulting from physiologic or psychological abnormalities.

Rehabilitation takes place in a number of settings. It may begin in the acute hospital as soon as the client is stabilized. It may occur in special rehabilitation facilities. It may also occur in long-term care.

Rehabilitation facilities consist of clients, families, primary care providers, physical therapists, occupational and/or speech therapists, unlicensed assistive personnel, dietitians, clergy, and other caregivers. In long-term care, the supervising nurse (LPN/LVN or RN) schedules regular staff meetings to discuss the plan of care for a set of residents. Usually, a subset of residents is discussed at each weekly meeting, and all resident care plans are updated each month. In addition, changes in client condition are discussed as they occur.

ROLE OF THE NURSE IN REHABILITATION

Nurses have two major responsibilities when working with clients who have disabilities. Their first responsibility is to see that disability from disease is limited as much as possible. This is done by:

- Preventing complications through early recognition of symptoms.
- Reviewing the signs and symptoms with the client/family members frequently.

- Preventing deformities by maintaining client's proper body alignment, positioning limbs to prevent contractures, turning the client frequently to prevent skin breakdown (see Chapters 23 and 30 ⚭), and providing adequate nutrition and fluid intake (see Chapter 25 ⚭).

Their second responsibility is to support the nursing plan and to implement an appropriate rehabilitation program. This is accomplished by determining the client's own goals for rehabilitation and by using appropriate nursing interventions based on mutually agreed-on goals. Nursing interventions should encourage the client to assume responsibility for his or her own activities of daily living (ADLs) as soon as possible. Short-term, realistic, attainable goals give the client the most opportunity for success. Assistive devices (see Figure 46-4) can enable a client to bathe or dress even when range of motion and muscle strength are compromised. Positive feedback from the nurse reinforces client progress. The nurse works with other team members to provide a consistent, coordinated plan.

ROLE OF THE CLIENT IN REHABILITATION

Clients themselves make the most important contributions to their rehabilitation. The client, physician, nurse, social worker, occupational therapist, and others can arrive at an ideal plan. However, only the client's attitude, acceptance, and motivation will make that ideal plan work. If the client cannot adjust to the disability, attempts at rehabilitation usually are hindered. Clients make decisions at their own pace. The client's day-to-day behavior is the first indication of positive motivation, so self-care is always encouraged.

When working with chronically ill clients, it becomes evident that life has meaning for the affected individual, even though it may not be readily apparent to others. Nurses look for what motivates each client. For example, a woman who was a classical pianist developed severe arthritis in her hands. She needed to exercise those joints even though it was extremely painful. She decided that every day she would practice Mozart. Because she loved the music so much, she was able to focus on the music, not the pain, until her joints loosened up. When looking for ways to help clients with chronic illnesses, nurses can be sensitive to what clients love to do. This knowledge can help them to support the client in meeting goals.

The mental status of the client has a great impact on success. If the client has given up or is too confused to understand the long-term process or effects, the nurse may find it difficult to gain compliance with the exercise regimen.

Legal and Ethical Concerns in Long-Term Care

In general, legal and ethical concerns are the same as those for any client (see Chapter 4 ⚭). However, in long-term care, some legal and ethical issues are more common.

ADVANCE DIRECTIVES

The facility must maintain a record of advance directives of residents or clients. These records would include living wills, powers of attorney for health care, organ donation records, and so on. Any specific orders about intubation, CPR, or fluids would be part of the resident's file.

CLIENT'S RIGHTS

The client's rights must be respected in long-term care as in other healthcare situations. Clients have the right to refuse medications. Forcing a client to take a medication can result in a charge of battery.

Restraints may need to be used for safety if a resident would fall from a wheelchair. However, the rule of the least restrictive restraint for the least amount of time possible should be maintained.

Informed consent is obtained for procedures. Confidentiality of client information must, of course, be respected.

NEGLIGENCE

The LPN/LVN must be vigilant in supervising and following up on delegated tasks. If unlicensed personnel neglect a client, the person responsible is the LPN/LVN. As mentioned previously, aides and CNAs are responsible for a great deal of the hands-on care of residents and clients. Adequate supervision and open lines of communication play a crucial part in developing a strong, quality healthcare team. Listen to the staff to whom you have delegated client care; they are your eyes and ears.

Medication errors can be especially serious among people in long-term care who already have one or several health deficits. Falls can easily result in fractures in this population.

RESIDENT SEXUALITY

In long-term care facilities, sexual relations among residents may occur. This is a challenging situation because it involves both the privacy and the safety of clients. These situations should be handled with concern and respect. The LPN/LVN would inform the RN supervisor.

ABUSE OR POTENTIAL FOR ABUSE

Abuse can take many forms in institutions and long-term care facilities. It is crucial for administrators to set an expectation that residents will be cared for and kept safe, and that their well-being is the mission of all who work there. LPNs/LVNs who supervise long-term care must promote client health and well-being while being watchful for signs of inadequate care or outright abuse. Box 46-3 ■ provides some guidelines in identifying abuse potential.

BOX 46-3   RECOGNIZING ELDER ABUSE POTENTIAL IN THE WORKPLACE

The LPN/LVN in charge of a long-term care facility carries responsibility for the quality of care given by the staff under his or her supervision. This includes not only the technical quality of getting tasks done on time and accurately, but also the emotional quality of supporting and nurturing individual clients. Unfortunately, some staff may use their work relationships to vent frustration or stress, creating a potentially abusive situation for clients. The nurse in charge must monitor against all forms of staff-to-client abuse. Aspects of employee manner to review when assessing for abuse potential follow. In all instances, suspicion of abuse must be reported.

Physical Abuse

Does the worker use gentle motion and touch in relation to clients? Or, is there unnecessary abruptness or roughness in the worker's manner?

Eye Contact

Does the worker make friendly eye contact with clients? Or, do glances appear angry and indirect? (Note: The level of eye contact may vary, depending on a person's culture and personality. The quality or "message" of eye contact is key.)

Verbal Abuse

Does the worker use language and tone that convey respect and caring? Or, is there minimal or antagonistic verbal interaction? (Note: Is there name calling, either directly or when talking with other workers about a client? Do workers make remarks under their breath as they leave a room?)

Sexual Abuse

Does a client appear excessively anxious in the presence of a particular worker? Does a worker make opportunities to be alone with a client, especially a mentally incompetent client?

Reimbursement for Long-Term Care and Rehabilitation

Sources for funding for long-term care in the United States include Medicare, Medicaid, and private insurance. The sources of funding are shown in Figure 46-6 ■.

The LPN/LVN needs to be aware that documentation is crucial to justifying reimbursement for care. For example, if a client falls often, the LPN/LVN needs to provide documentation so that the restraints to prevent the client from falling out of a wheelchair can be reimbursed. If a client exhibits changes in level of consciousness, those changes must be documented in order to obtain orders to move the client to a more skilled facility.

MEDICARE

Medicare pays for health care for people 65 and over and for those who are disabled. Medicare does not pay for long-term medical service such as assisted living or adult day care. Medicare coverage pays only the first 100 days of skilled care, such as physical therapy or nursing. This accounts for only 5% of all long-term care costs.

To be eligible for Medicare, clients must have been in the hospital for at least 3 days. The personal care provided to these clients must relate to the treatment of an illness or injury. Medicare pays 100% for the first 20 days and all but the first $95 per day for the next 80 days.

Many individuals who are covered by Medicare have assigned their benefits to one of the approved health maintenance organizations or HMOs (see types of plans in Chapter 7 ⭕). HMOs are governed by Medicare laws and regulations, and they have their own provisions as well.

It is important for the covered individual to be aware of what the plan pays. Many clients do not understand their coverage. As a result, they become very frustrated with the facility, feeling they are being denied services that are rightly theirs. The LPN/LVN does not engage in debate about what is covered and what is not. The appropriate response is to refer questions about coverage to the insurance or business office. Staff there can meet with the client or family to provide explanations of coverage.

MEDICAID

Medicaid (known as Medi-Cal in the state of California) pays for health services for the very poor of any age. Qualifications for Medicaid vary by state, but generally the law says that clients must first spend down to the poverty level, using up all but about $2,000 of their assets.

Being eligible for Medicaid does not guarantee placement in a nursing home. There may be long waiting lists for facility care. Unfortunately, depending on the state and facility, Medicaid clients often receive lesser-quality care than clients who are paying on their own. Under Medicaid, nursing home care is essentially the only option. Home care, assisted living facility care, adult day care, outpatient services, and alternate caregiver services are not usually reimbursed under Medicaid.

PRIVATE INSURANCE

The particulars about private insurance are too many to cover in this text. Generally, clients who can afford more coverage have a greater range of options when they require long-term care.

Many people obtain Medicare supplement insurance if their finances allow. Medicare supplement insurance is a private insurance that helps pay for some gaps in Medicare coverage. Plans D, G, I, and J do pay up to $1,600 per year for services to people recovering at home from an illness, injury, or surgery.

Exceptions, Limitations, and Exclusions

Most long-term care insurance policies have limits on when and for how long they will pay benefits. In addition, there are certain conditions under which companies will not pay benefits for any confinement, care, treatment, or service(s). Box 46-4 ■ shows typical exclusions or exceptions for which private insurance would not pay.

NURSING CARE

PRIORITIZING NURSING CARE

When you are caring for clients in long-term care, focus care on their quality of life. Assist them in meeting any psychosocial needs. Allow them to take part as much as possible in ADLs, helping them only when needed. Provide support and encouragement to participate in decisions about their course of treatment.

ASSESSING

On admission, a thorough assessment will be done by the RN or LPN/LVN, depending on state and facility policies.

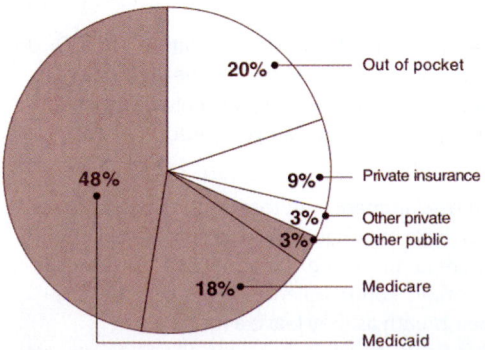

20% — Out of pocket
9% — Private insurance
3% — Other private
3% — Other public
48%
18% — Medicare
— Medicaid

▨ Public payers

Source: GAO analysis of 2003 data from the Centers for Medicare & Medicaid Services and The MEDSTAT Group.

Notes: Amounts do not include unpaid care provided by family members or other informal caregivers. Percentages do not add to 100 percent due to rounding.

Figure 46-6. ■ Sources of reimbursement for long-term care.

BOX 46-4	COMMON EXCEPTIONS, LIMITATIONS, AND EXCLUSIONS OF PRIVATE INSURANCE FOR LONG-TERM CARE

The following exceptions, limitations, or exclusions are generally not covered by private insurance companies:

- Condition that results from attempted suicide or intentionally self-inflicted injury
- Condition that results from voluntary participation in a felony, attempted felony, or illegal occupation
- Condition that results from a sickness or injury for which benefits are provided under any state or federal workers' compensation law
- Treatment provided outside the United States or Canada
- Treatment provided in a government facility (unless otherwise required by law)
- Treatment provided because of alcoholism or drug addiction, or in facilities operated primarily for such treatment
- Treatment provided in facilities operated primarily for the treatment of mental or nervous disorders or disease, other than Alzheimer's disease or dementia

Preexisting Conditions

In addition to the list above, insurance companies might decline to provide insurance if the client already has any of the following condition(s):

- Alzheimer's disease
- Severe arthritis with functional limitations
- Diabetes that is not under control
- Cancer within the past 6 months
- Parkinson's disease
- Stroke within the past 6 months *or* a stroke at any time that has caused functional limitations
- Congestive heart failure within the past 6 months
- Emphysema, if severe or still smoking
- Chronic obstructive pulmonary disease (COPD), if severe or still smoking
- Any conditions that require the assistance of another human being for the basic activities of daily living: bathing, eating, toileting, or transferring in and out of a bed or chair

This will include a detailed history of past medical problems. Family involvement and contacts will be determined. The client's end-of-life wishes are recorded and kept in the front of the client's file. All medications and supplements (prescription, nonprescription, herbal) need to be recorded. A complete physical examination is important for baseline information. Any special needs (such as hearing or vision loss, history of stroke requiring special tools for eating, etc.) are noted at this time.

For daily assessment, data are compiled from information collected by team members. This would include information from CNAs and other personnel who assist with ADLs, as well as data the LPN/LVN collects in person.

DIAGNOSING, PLANNING, AND IMPLEMENTING

Some common nursing diagnoses for clients in long-term care and rehabilitation are:

- *Activity Intolerance*
- *Ineffective Coping*
- *Acute Pain*
- *Risk for Injury*

For this client population, there may be numerous individual nursing diagnoses.

Outcomes that may be identified for the NANDA listings above include, but are not limited to, that the client will:

- Take part in physical care to the extent possible.
- Participate in decision making about care.
- State pain is relieved or within manageable levels.
- Be free from falls and injury.

Common nursing interventions for clients in long-term and rehabilitation care may include the following:

- Review all data provided by assistive personnel and complete your daily head-to-toe assessment of your clients. *Every client requires a complete check each day.*
- Adjust assignments of assistive personnel as necessary. *It is important to divide care among the staff so all clients get the care they need throughout the day.*
- When providing care, allow clients time to think and respond to questions. They may also need time to frame questions they have for you. *Clients in long-term care or rehab may have cognitive deficits or speech delay related to medical condition, medications, or the aging process.*
- Avoid taking over for clients who can provide their own care. *It may be tempting to perform ADLs for clients because you can do them faster. However, this could have adverse effects physically and mentally. Doing tasks the client is capable of doing will ultimately lead to having more full-care clients. A spiral can occur when the nurse "does for" the client of the client doing less, feeling less capable, becoming slower, and needing more done.*
- Show respect for the views of the client. Ask about personal preferences whenever possible. *This action supports self-esteem in the client. You may be one of the few people who speak to the client in the day. Your words and manner will have an impact. Religious and cultural views are an important part of a person's identity and should be valued. Nurses provide a great service to clients in long-term care by helping them keep their dignity intact.*
- Report any significant changes to the appropriate care provider. *This will allow the plan of care to be adjusted as necessary.*
- Document all pertinent data and procedures in the chart. *Maintaining good client records is a key component of quality nursing care.*

EVALUATING

The nurse will evaluate the plan of care daily to see if current treatments are effective. The nurse will also evaluate the safety of the environment and the knowledge and skills of team individuals to ensure quality of care.

NURSING PROCESS CARE PLAN
Client Experiencing Sundowner's Syndrome

Mrs. Mary Rodgers is an 89-year-old female who recently was moved from her home of 37 years to a retirement home. Her husband, John, died about 6 months ago. Her daughter's husband was transferred out of the area, and the family will be moving about 2 hours away at the end of the school year. Mrs. Rodgers did not want to move with them because of friends and connections in her hometown. She agreed to try the retirement home after her children said they felt she should not be living alone with no family member close.

On the third night at Oakdale, Mrs. Rodgers began to exhibit rapid mood changes. Normally she was very pleasant but she lashed out at a favorite grandson when he came to visit. When the LVN came to give Mrs. Rodgers her medication, she was crying. She also has been agitated and pacing in her room. She refused to go to the dining room for dinner because, "If I leave my room someone will steal my belongings." The staff is concerned because of her paranoia. She wandered out of the building, saying she was looking for her car so she could go home. When her daughter came the following morning, she was "her old self" again and did not seem to remember what had happened the evening before.

Assessment
Vital signs: BP 128/76, T 98.2, P – 68 R – 20 and regular. Weight 108 lbs stable at that weight for 6 months. Alert and oriented × 3 at 6 A.M. and 12 noon, confused and combative at 6 P.M. Refused to have vital signs taken at 6 P.M.

Medicated for hypertension Cozaar 100 mg daily; Lasix 20 mg every other day; K-Dur 10 mEq every other day. ASA 81 mg daily and naproxen 200 mg every 12 hours for arthritis pain. Sleeping during day; awake and crying most of night. "I want to go home, John is going to be worried, I never stay out this late."

Nursing Diagnosis
The following important nursing diagnosis (among others) is established for this client:

■ *Disturbed Sleep Pattern*

Expected Outcomes
The expected outcomes specify that Mrs. Rodgers will:

■ Sleep from 11 P.M. until 6 A.M. nightly.

Planning and Implementation
The following nursing interventions are implemented for Mrs. Rodgers:

■ Assess sleep patterns and changes, naps and frequency, amount of activity, sedentary status, number of times of awakenings during night and client complaints of fatigue, and lethargy. *This allows information to structure activities that will encourage activities during the day and sleep at night.*
■ Assess client's complaints of pain or signs of pain, dyspnea, nocturia, or leg cramps. *Pain can affect ADLs, sleep, and mental status.*
■ Monitor client's medication and caffeine ingestion. *Side effects can cause additional problems in sleep patterns.*
■ Ensure a quiet environment that is well ventilated and at a comfortable temperature. *This environment will support nighttime sleep.*
■ Provide ritualistic procedures of warm drink, extra covers, clean linens, and a warm bath at bedtime. *A presleep ritual will support a normal sleep pattern.*
■ Maintain consistent schedule and surroundings. *Routine helps with orientation.*
■ Provide reorientation as appropriate. *This decreases confusion.*

Evaluation
Mrs. Rodgers is sleeping from 12 midnight until 6 A.M. but continues to be confused if awakened during night. More active during day hours; not sleeping but does have a rest period before dinner while listening to music. Willingly went to dining room 4 out of 5 days.

Critical Thinking in the Nursing Process

1. Discuss nursing interventions that may be done to prevent sundowner's syndrome.
2. Recently some facilities have begun to use bright light treatment to decrease the signs and symptoms of sundowner's. What is the rationale behind this treatment?
3. Clients with sundowner's syndrome frequently become wanderers. This can present a real safety problem for the client. What interventions can be used to keep the client safe without the use of chemical or physical restraints?

Note: Discussion of Critical Thinking questions appears on the MyNursingKit Website.

Note: The references and resources for all chapters have been compiled at the back of the book.

Chapter Review

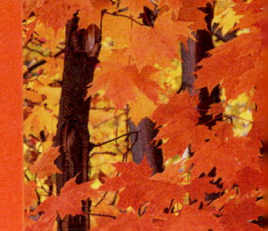

KEY Points

- Nursing in long-term care facilities is either skilled (requiring total care of the client) or custodial care (requiring supportive nursing measures).

- The LPN/LVN in long-term care may have more extensive roles and responsibilities than in other settings, including charge nurse.

- In long-term and rehabilitation settings, the LPN/LVN uses data collected by nursing assistants and aides as part of a full head-to-toe daily assessment of each assigned client.

- In long-term client care, a multidisciplinary approach that involves the entire healthcare team and the family is most effective.

- When a child or young adult enters a skilled nursing or rehabilitation facility, the healthcare team works with the family to provide a caring, positive environment that addresses developmental as well as physical needs.

- In rehabilitation, the LPN/LVN provides assistive devices, gives pain medication prior to therapy sessions, and organizes interventions to allow for periods of activity and rest.

- Legal and ethical concerns for long-term care or rehab include advance directives, client's rights, guarding against negligence, and avoiding potential for abuse.

- Medicare, Medicaid, or private insurance reimbursement for long-term care and rehabilitation may affect the level of care clients receive.

⌘ FOR FURTHER Study

For legal and ethical concerns, see Chapter 4.

Healthcare facilities and HMOs are discussed in Chapter 7.

Documentation is discussed in Chapter 13.

Psychosocial issues related to grief, loss, and death are discussed in depth in Chapter 18.

Treatments for bedsores are discussed in Chapter 24.

Information on drawing blood can be found in Chapter 28.

For more information on enemas or digital fecal disimpaction, see Chapter 37.

For more information on glucose testing, see Chapter 38.

For health promotion of older adults, see Chapter 42.

For care of ill older adults, see Chapter 43.

The main discussion about nursing care of chronically and terminally ill clients is in Chapter 44.

Figure 63-1 illustrates the path to proper delegation.

EXPLORE PEARSON **mynursingkit**™

MyNursingKit is your one stop for online chapter review materials and resources. Prepare for success with additional NCLEX®-style practice questions, interactive assignments and activities, web links, animations and videos, and more!

Register your access code from the front of your book at
www.mynursingkit.com

Critical Thinking Care Map

Client Needing Rehabilitation following Total Hip Replacement

NCLEX-PN® Focus Area: Physiologic Integrity

Case Study: John Simon was admitted to the rehabilitation unit to continue his recovery following total hip replacement surgery on his left hip. He was in the acute hospital for 4 days and is scheduled for 3 weeks of rehabilitation. John is 78 years old. He was very active in his younger days. He was a building inspector for the city and played on the city softball team until he retired 10 years ago. He has a history of several injuries over the years and has been diagnosed with degenerative joint disease. He lives with his wife, who is recovering from a broken wrist 3 weeks ago. They live in a two-story house, so he needs to get to the point where he can independently get around the house. At this point it would be difficult for his wife to assist him. His surgical staples were removed this morning and physical therapy begun.

Nursing Diagnosis: *Impaired Physical Mobility*

COLLECT DATA

Subjective	Objective
_____	_____
_____	_____
_____	_____
_____	_____
_____	_____
_____	_____
_____	_____

Would you report this? Yes/No

If yes, report to: _____

What would you report? _____

Nursing Care

_____
_____
_____
_____
_____
_____
_____
_____
_____

How would you document this? _____
_____
_____
_____

Compare your answers and documentation to those provided on the MyNursingKit Website.

Data Collected
(use only those that apply)

- "I need to get back on my feet so I can take care of my wife."
- Pain 5/10 relieved with Tylenol #4 every 4 hours PRN and 30 minutes prior to therapy
- Surgical incision clean and dry, well approximated healing, Steri-Strips in place
- Weight 169 lb; height 73"
- VS: BP 138/86, T 99.4, P 78, R 24
- Refused pain medication prior to PT: "I don't want to take the pain pill, I think I will get better quicker without them."
- Able to ambulate from bed to bathroom with use of a walker
- Walked 10 feet on parallel bars
- Appears to be in pain, facial grimace
- Difficulty sleeping
- Restoril 15 mg 1 h.s.
- DSS 1 every morning
- H & H INR every 3 days 13.9 / 42 INR 15 SEC
- Lovenox 100 mg daily
- Multi-vitamin with iron, 1 daily

Nursing Interventions
(use only those that apply; list in priority order)

- Client teaching related to need for pain medication prior to therapy.
- Encourage client to follow exercise plan between therapy sessions.
- Assess for signs of depression or mood change.
- Expect client to meet responsibilities; give positive reinforcement.
- Observe client's medication, diet, and caffeine intake. Look for hidden sources of caffeine.
- Identify causes for and observe client's expression of sorrow.
- Advise client to avoid use of alcohol or hypnotics to induce sleep.
- Assist to resolve ambivalent feelings about illness and management of therapeutic regimen.

NCLEX-PN® Exam Preparation

TEST-TAKING TIP Be sure to consider the client's level of care when the question asks the nurse to prioritize interventions.

1 The nurse, working in an acute care facility, is taking care of a client who requires tube feedings and frequent dressing changes along with rehabilitative care. In arranging for the client's discharge, the nurse would arrange for what specific type of facility?

1. Custodial care
2. Skilled care
3. Long-term care
4. Assisted living

2 The LPN/LVN, working in a long-term care facility, finds the role of the nurse is:

1. Expanded in long-term care as opposed to acute care.
2. Less in long-term care than it would be in an acute care facility.
3. About the same in both long-term care and acute care.
4. Different depending on what shift the nurse is working.

3 When delegating a task to unlicensed assistive personnel, the nurse ensures that all of the five rules of delegation are covered, including which of the following? (Select all that apply.)

1. The task delegated is an appropriate task for the UAP to perform.
2. Adequate directions are given for performance of the task.
3. The task is delegated to the right person to perform the task.
4. Responsibility for the task is adequately explained.
5. The nurse provides adequate supervision of the performance of the task.

4 The nurse, working in long-term care as a member of the multidisciplinary team, includes the family as a member of the team because the family:

1. Needs to determine the physical needs of the client.
2. Can provide insight and information about the client.
3. Always speaks for the client.
4. Provides updates in treatment and client condition.

5 When the nurse is helping to determine what long-term care facility is best for the younger client requiring care, the general rule is to:

1. Provide long-term care among peers.
2. Place younger adults with older adults and place pediatric clients in a separate facility.
3. Mix people of different ages in the same facility to simulate real-world conditions.
4. Ask clients what they would prefer.

6 The nurse, working in a rehabilitation facility, is caring for a newly admitted client who fractured his cervical vertebrae and is quadriplegic. What are the nurse's major responsibilities when working with this client? (Select all that apply.)

1. See that disability from the disease is limited as much as possible.
2. Assume responsibility for activities of daily living.
3. Return the client to his prior level of functioning.
4. Support the nursing plan of care.
5. Implement an appropriate rehabilitation program.

7 The nurse makes it a practice to delegate the task of providing hygiene care for a client to an unlicensed assistive personnel (UAP) for several days in a row. The nurse discovers the client was not bathed by the UAP when the family member visits and complains to the nurse. Who is responsible and what are they responsible for?

1. The UAP is responsible for providing poor client care.
2. The nurse is responsible for slander.
3. The nurse is responsible for libel.
4. The nurse is responsible for neglect.

8 The appropriate time for justifying insurance reimbursement for the client is when the nurse:

1. Delivers the care.
2. Tells the family what care was delivered.
3. Charges the client for the required care items.
4. Documents the provision of care.

9 Which of the following clients would the nurse expect to be covered by Medicare?

1. The 32-year-old client who broke her leg and requires rehabilitation to regain her previous level of functioning
2. The 48-year-old client who is quadriplegic as a result of a diving accident
3. The 64-year-old client who required a total knee replacement
4. The 56-year-old client who required an amputation of the distal right foot

10 The LPN/LVN, working in a long-term care facility, is acting as the charge nurse. While operating within this role, additional responsibilities of the position include:

1. Providing client care.
2. Delegating care to unlicensed assistive personnel.
3. Coordinating the smooth functioning of the unit on a given shift.
4. Working with physicians.

Answers and rationales for Review Questions appear in Appendix I.

Emergency Room and Urgent Care Nursing

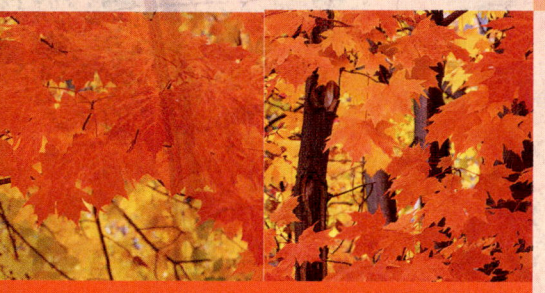

LEARNING Outcomes

After completing this chapter, you will be able to:

1. Identify roles and safety issues for the LPN/LVN in emergency care/urgent care (EC/UC) nursing.
2. Describe the use of triage in the EC/UC setting.
3. List important components involved in initial contact with clients and admission to the EC or UC setting.
4. Describe airway management and CPR in emergency nursing care.
5. List and describe different types of shock and their management.
6. Identify important factors in care of clients with trauma.
7. Name other conditions that would require urgent or emergent care and nursing considerations for each.
8. List important concepts to remember when dealing with the effects of bioterrorist or terrorist attacks in the EC setting.
9. Discuss nursing care for different types of burns in the EC/UC setting.
10. Describe appropriate nursing actions after the death of a client in the EC/UC setting.
11. Explain steps in nursing procedures that might be performed in an EC/UC setting for clients with a sprain or fracture.

Clinical Objectives

12. Carry out the admission procedure for a client in an ER or UC facility.
13. Perform airway management or CPR, including the use of AED in an emergency.
14. Assist the primary care provider in emergency burn treatment and dressing.
15. Provide discharge instructions for a client in an ER or UC facility.
16. Apply a splint.
17. Prepare for and assist in the application of a cast.
18. Measure a client for crutches, cane, or walker.

Use the audio glossary feature on the MyNursingKit Website to hear the correct pronunciation of the following key terms.

ACLS 1289	**eupneic** 1298	**shock** 1289
BLS 1289	**full-thickness burns** 1297	**stat** 1285
cannulation 1282	**hazmat** 1282	**superficial burns** 1296
cardiopulmonary resuscitation 1286	**high acuity** 1281	**third spacing** 1291
cervical spine alignment 1286	**PALS** 1289	**titration** 1285
defibrillator 1288	**partial-thickness burns** 1296	**triage** 1282
DuoNeb 1286	**peak flow test** 1285	**urgent care** 1281
emergency care 1281	**phlebotomy** 1282	

In today's rapidly changing healthcare system, emergent care and urgent care environments are placing increasing demands on nurses and staff. "Emergency rooms across the US are in a state of crisis today" (Institute of Medicine, 2006). This crisis is largely related to increased volume of clients being treated, and the inability of ECs in the United States to afford the newest technology because of costs involved.

Rapid assessment skills, the ability to prioritize demands, and strong interpersonal communication skills (see Chapter 11 ⚭) are essential for ensuring the best client outcomes. This chapter discusses various areas of emergency and urgent care and the role of the LPN or LVN in them.

Emergency Care and Urgent Care

Centers for emergency care (EC) and urgent care (UC) are a vital part of our healthcare system. **Emergency care** (also called ER for emergency room, or ED for emergency department) is a center where staffing is maintained around the clock to provide care for **high acuity** (very urgent and possibly life-threatening) cases, such as trauma. It is also a place where a variety of clients receive primary care through a milieu of primary care providers (PCP). The primary care provider within the EC and UC settings can be a physician, primary care provider assistant, advanced practice RN, a nurse practitioner, and more. The affordability and insurance of the client can affect the outcome for the client in today's cost-saving healthcare environment. This includes clients who have insurance for Preferred Provider Organizations (see Chapter 7 ⚭), those receiving medical assistance, and those who are uninsured or underinsured (Box 47-1 ■).

The **urgent care** center offers care for minor injuries and acute illnesses (e.g., strep throat) when clients cannot see their primary care provider (PCP), or if they do not have a designated healthcare provider. Today, there are more UC centers throughout the United States that are not attached directly to an EC facility than in the past. The EC need to "triage" client care created a demand for UC settings that could operate independently, improve client waiting time,

and allow for cost savings to insurance companies and clients. The UC environment has services similar to the EC setting. Major medical events and emergencies are still transferred from the UC facility to the EC.

This chapter focuses primarily on the emergency care environment. Important differences in UC settings will be noted.

ROLE OF THE LPN/LVN

LPNs/LVNs are a valuable part of the healthcare team in the emergent or urgent care setting (see Chapter 7 ⚭). They are primarily responsible for data collection, administering nursing interventions, and assisting the RN in discharge planning (if applicable). Several states use certified LPNs/LVNs in more advanced roles. As the need for advanced practice protocols and sophisticated technology within the EC and UC settings has emerged, facilities have developed effective preimplementation training and structured processes for bringing new equipment online.

BOX 47-1	CULTURAL PULSE POINTS

Underserved Populations in the Emergency Care or Urgent Care Setting

Much of the health care for minority populations is delivered in emergency care or urgent care centers, especially in large urban areas. This perhaps is partially due to an increasing number of uninsured and underinsured clients. Lack of access to care is one reason for the increased use of the EC.

Not having a regular healthcare provider makes follow-up and preventive health care almost impossible. Uninsured or underinsured clients in the EC or UC must receive clear discharge instructions, including the need for follow-up. The EC or UC nurse can be a source of referrals for future care. Referral information can be included in the teaching carried out at the end of the visit.

It is important for the nurse who is working in either of these areas to consider the cultural needs of clients and their families. The triage nurse in the EC unit must be able to explain why clients with nonurgent problems must wait, without making them feel that they do not deserve health care. The need for improved ability to "triage" clients has intensified with increases in EC visits, and many EC rooms nationally have closed. Community clinics may be a real alternative for people without a primary healthcare provider.

The need for the LPN/LVN to achieve training and competency in the areas of technology and documentation is critical. Today's LPN/LVN who is administering care within the EC and UC settings must learn to use *computerized physician order entry* (CPOE), electronic documentation, and *emergency data information systems* (EDIS) for laboratory and radiology. EDIS reduces potential errors of transcription and misinterpretation among the RN and LPN/LVN staff within the EC and UC environments.

The complexity of the client population, coupled with the need for advanced technology and standards of practice, makes caring for the client in the EC or UC a challenge for the nurse.

LPNs/LVNs in the EC/UC must recognize the fast pace and acuity of clients for whom they provide care. An LPN/LVN may be called on to check client's vital signs, administer medications as ordered, and reinforce teaching. The EC environment invites continuous assessment and data collection by the nurses. A high level of expertise in all disciplines is necessary in order to meet the demands of this much-accelerated healthcare environment.

Nurses can acquire specialized training in many areas to improve their practice of nursing within the EC and UC environments. Once nurses have received special certification, they can perform such tasks as intravenous (IV) **cannulation** (the insertion of an IV needle into the body), **phlebotomy** (drawing and dispensing blood), IV piggyback medication administration (see Chapter 28 ⚭), and application of dressings. The LPN/LVN *always* works under the supervision of the primary care provider in the EC and UC settings.

clinical ALERT

The LPN or LVN may not be able to accept *verbal orders* in the EC setting. This is determined by the state's nurse practice act, the state board of nursing where the nurse is licensed, and facility policy. For their own and their clients' safety, nurses must identify and follow facility procedures and the guidelines of their state's nurse practice act. Today's practicing LPN/LVN will be directly involved in meeting plan-of-care outcomes in both the UC and EC setting with the use of CPOE and EDIS technology. Standard nursing clinical pathways are often used, helping the nurse to meet accepted healthcare guidelines and clinical practices for clients seeking medical care.

SAFETY ISSUES

The EC and UC settings create safety concerns for clients and staff. Clients may present with life-threatening conditions or highly contagious diseases. Client risk for infection may be heightened by diseases or open wounds. Risk for falls is increased with fainting, loss of blood, or fractures.

First and foremost, nurses must use Standard Precautions at all times in the EC and UC settings (see Figure 10-4 ⚭). Standard Precautions include gloves, gown, masks, protective eyewear, face shields, and, of course, meticulous hand hygiene. The Centers for Disease Control and Prevention mandate clinical guidelines for safe practice.

The careful and sensible use of Standard Precautions is especially important in the care of combative and confused clients. Such clients may be unable to identify areas of the body or body fluids that could transmit disease or pathogens with initial contact. Without Standard Precautions, nurses or other staff could become infected and perhaps cause infection to others via a nosocomial infection.

OTHER RISKS IN THE EC AND UC SETTING

Healthcare professionals are at high risk for back injuries due to lifting or handling clients in an emergency situation. They must adhere to good body mechanics (see Chapter 9 ⚭) in order to prevent harm to themselves.

Healthcare professionals are also the "front line" in providing care in bioterrorism, weather emergencies, and hazardous material (**hazmat**) situations. They must be familiar with the use of protective equipment. Safety and readiness for unexpected situations must be primary concerns for the healthcare professional at all times.

Initial Contact

TRIAGE AND DISASTER PLANNING

The EC setting can become overwhelmed with clients at a moment's notice. Today's ECs and UCs have longer wait times for clients because of increased client need. An efficient response to increased client numbers and high-acuity levels requires triage. **Triage** is the process used by healthcare providers to determine which person has the most *emergent* (pressing) problem. Triage is used routinely in the EC and UC settings. Usually, clients are prioritized by ABCD:

Airway
Breathing
Circulation
Deformity

With triage, clients' conditions are prioritized in a range from critical to stable.

Note: In the event of a disaster internal or external to the EC (Figure 47-1 ■), the nurse would require additional assistance to manage the number of clients created by the situation. (Part of staff training as an employee in this setting would be to know how to react in case of a major event.) The EC department would initiate a disaster plan or critical incident plan. This allows each individual within the EC and ancillary departments to prepare and assist a larger number of clients. It also allows various personnel from within and outside the facility (emergency medical staff, community law enforcement officials, etc.) to respond so that safe, effective care can be given to a large number of

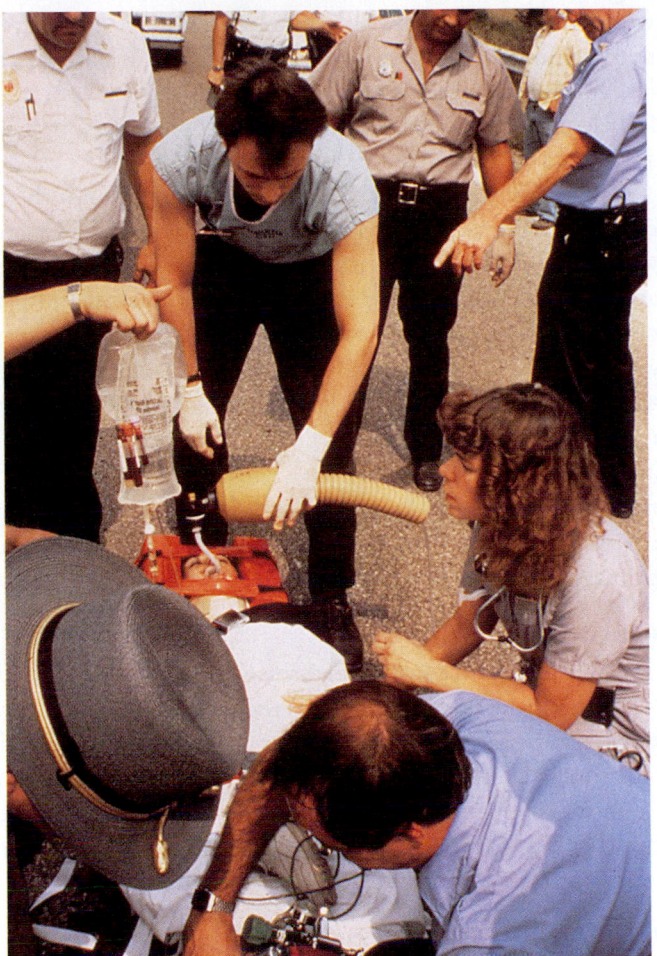

Figure 47-1. ■ Emergency medical technicians often provide the first treatment to victims outside the healthcare environment. (Courtesy of University Air Core/University of Cincinnati Hospital.)

clients. Training and practice for disaster situations and knowing how to work with an incident command system are essential to handling a disaster effectively. It is also essential to understand facility policy and emergency codes for such an event.

PRIORITIZING URGENT CARE

Urgent care requires continuous monitoring of clients for acute changes. However, urgent care clients are generally treated on a first-come, first-served basis. Today there are increased numbers of UC centers, either attached to the EC setting or operating independently of the acute care facility. Clients are triaged for severity of illness in the UC setting. However, the first-come, first-served rule is usually carried out for medical treatment.

LEGAL ISSUES IN EC AND UC

Confidentiality

Prior to receiving treatment in the EC or UC setting, the client must sign consent for treatment and confidentiality forms. If the client is unable to sign, a legal responsible

party or power of attorney may sign consent forms for the client. Consent for treatment includes forms for valuables, procedures, and the Health Insurance Portability and Accountability Act (HIPAA) (described in detail in Chapter 14 ⚭). All forms must be signed and documented in the client's chart. The staff is responsible for following protocols for standards of privacy and consent for treatment. The nurse must be mindful of who has a legal right to information obtained in the EC and UC setting.

clinical ALERT

Privacy for EC and UC clients remains a special challenge for the healthcare staff. The healthcare professional must not forget that the EC and UC client has rights to privacy. All members of the healthcare team must follow HIPAA regulations. Questions should be asked in a private area, away from others at all times, so HIPAA may not be violated, and confidentiality may be assured for the client.

Consent for Minors

In most cases, the nurse obtains the consent for minors from a parent or guardian. Exceptions to this rule are the following: a life-threatening situation, sexually transmitted infections, drug or alcohol abuse, or pregnancy. If no parent or guardian is present, then the decision to treat is really up to the primary care provider. Follow your facility's policy for treating minors without a consenting adult present. Many times, if an adult's consent is needed but the adult can only be reached by phone, two nurses will listen to the adult give consent. Documentation on the client's chart must reflect the decision process and methodology for obtaining verbal consent that the nurse used.

clinical ALERT

When verbal telephone consent is obtained, BOTH registered nurses must document it in the chart. Depending on the state's nurse practice act, the LPN/LVN may not be allowed to accept telephone or verbal orders in the EC or UC settings.

Admission to EC or UC

BASIC DATA COLLECTION

On entering the EC, the client's basic data information will be obtained. Height and weight, vital signs, and, of course, the level of pain as the fifth vital sign must be obtained. (*Note:* Height is important because peak flow meter ranges are based on age and height. It is also helpful in determining growth and development norms.) Accuracy of data in an emergency situation is especially important. (See Figure 14-1 ⚭ for an adult admission assessment form.) Data collection is a systematic gathering of information about the client. The client is the primary source of information. Secondary sources of information include the client chart, family, and health team members. The nurse gathers subjective and objective data. *Subjective data* is the information the client or the caretaker tells the nurse during the nursing assessment. Subjective data can be called *symptoms*. *Objective data* is information collected by using the senses. Objective data may be obtained through the following methods: inspection, auscultation, percussion, and palpation. Objective data can be called *signs*. So subjective (S) data is what the client says (S), and objective data (O) is what the nurse observes (O).

Data collection includes taking a health history by obtaining biographical data, the chief complaint, present illness, past history, current health information, and family history. Depending on the acuity of the client's condition, a more focused collection of data may occur.

History

Medication history, allergies, over-the-counter (OTC) medications, vitamins, cultural treatments, and complementary medicines are vitally important information (see Chapter 8 ⊕). Sometimes an OTC or herbal treatment can be the cause of the client's problem. However, clients often do not mention these products without prompting, because they do not think of them as medicine. Women using birth control may forget to mention that they are taking pills or injections. This information can be very important when reviewing test results or initiating a treatment. Most forms for emergency departments and urgent care centers have fill-in spaces for last menstrual period, medications, and contraceptives. Proper documentation of the client's medications is extremely important for the nurse to do, because outcomes and treatments by the primary care provider are based on the history of problems and illness.

Obtaining medication information during the data collection process is critical. This includes all medications routinely and occasionally taken by the person. Cardiac medications such as calcium channel blockers, digoxin, and diuretics are often heavily documented in cases of cardiac clients. Antibiotic use and pain medicines are also important to note, so that a complete evaluation by the primary care provider can be performed.

A brief history of events, including the reason for admission, or chief complaint (C), is obtained and documented. Information should be obtained from the client, but may be obtained from family or friends if the client is unable to respond. Remember, the provider will treat the client according to the information obtained by the nurse. Information must be accurate and nonjudgmental.

At this time a complete review of systems should be performed, with the client answering questions about each system. This information is used to determine what to include in the head-to-toe physical exam. The healthcare provider

will complete the physical assessment. The review of systems includes head and neck, respiratory, cardiovascular, integumentary, gastrointestinal, genitourinary, musculoskeletal, neurologic, reproductive, psychological, spiritual, social, and developmental information.

The charge nurse will triage the clients and inform them of the EC procedures and protocols. Oftentimes ECs are overloaded with clients with various needs. Waiting times are often long due to the high volume of clients, limited client care areas, limited number of staff, and the *urgency* (acuity level) of client needs. The nurse should explain to the client that the waiting time to be seen may be from minutes to hours. The nurse must ask for patience and reassure clients that they will be seen. The nurse must also monitor previously admitted clients for acute changes and determine whether they need to be evaluated sooner by the primary care provider.

Physical Examination

The physical examination and assessment will be performed by the healthcare provider, such as the primary care provider, nurse practitioner, or primary care provider's assistant. At this time a complete head-to-toe examination or a focused exam may be performed. The information obtained in the health history, including the review of systems, aids the healthcare provider in the head-to-toe examination.

INITIAL PROTOCOLS

Depending on the nature of the problem causing admission to the EC, the nurse may initiate treatment while the client is in the waiting room, before evaluation by the primary care provider. Examples include hot/cold packs to an injured area or bandages applied to minimal wounds (see Chapter 24 ⊕). The nurse utilizes the various treatment protocols and standing orders and clinical pathways (if in place) to initiate nursing care, and also communicates with the attending PCP.

clinical ALERT

Personnel should *always* follow Standard Precautions. Many times healthcare providers use poor judgment and do not protect themselves from body fluids from clients. There is no need to be heroic or a martyr. Use the necessary precautions and do not worry about what other professionals are doing. Remember, by following Standard Precautions you are protecting both yourself and your loved ones. Failure to adhere to suggested protocols for safety may place the nurse and EC or UC at risk for a violation and fine against the hospital, based on the Centers for Disease Control (CDC) guidelines.

Depending on facility policy, the nurse may administer certain medications to clients (usually to reduce fever) before the provider examines them. Fever is a sign of infection, and it is not necessary for clients to prove that they have a fever.

(This depends on standing or routine orders and the agency protocols.) Of course, it is important to find out what medicine and what dose was used and when, before administering medication. Medications for fever are usually administered according to weight and age in children (see Chapter 27 ⊚⊙).

Note: In case of trauma, the nurse does not routinely administer pain medication prior to examination by the primary care provider.

COLLABORATIVE CARE

Continuous communication and updating of client services and information are necessary to ensure quality of care for the EC client. The management of the client in the EC setting often requires communication with ancillary department staff. The use of radiography, laboratory, and pharmacy consultation of healthcare professional/specialists results in a valuable network of services that assists in the care of the EC client.

Electronic documentation may require follow-up with other departments, because computers may be "down" and electronic communication may be impaired at times. Continuous awareness of the "plan of care" for each client is still the responsibility of the nurse in each of the settings.

Laboratory and Diagnostic Tests

Depending on the medical diagnosis of a client, laboratory tests may be ordered. For example, if a person presents with airway difficulty, a peak flow test may be ordered. A **peak flow test** evaluates maximum airflow during forced expiration and monitors bronchospasm in asthmatic clients. A nebulizer or metered-dose inhaler allows medication to be given via aerosol and inhaled for rapid treatment of airway difficulties. Peak flow measurements would be taken before and after use of the handheld nebulizer (Figure 47-2 ■). (See more about care of respiratory disorders in Chapter 32 ⊚⊙.)

If chest pain is present, an electrocardiography (ECG) monitor would be attached. **Stat** (immediate) labs for chest pain would include cardiac labs such as troponin levels, CPKs, LDH, and electrolytes.

Tests for trauma would include imaging techniques such as x-rays, positron-emission tomography (PET) scans, computerized tomography (CT) scans, and magnetic resonance imaging (MRI) if available in the EC. With today's technology, it is possible to transmit electronic 12-lead ECGs from emergency medical staff (EMS) directly to the EC setting. Electronic transmissions allow immediate treatment for heart attacks or brain attacks to be implemented even before the client arrives at the EC.

Tests for infectious diseases would include a complete blood count with a differential count. Sedimentation rates are often helpful in pinpointing inflammation and infectious disease parameters.

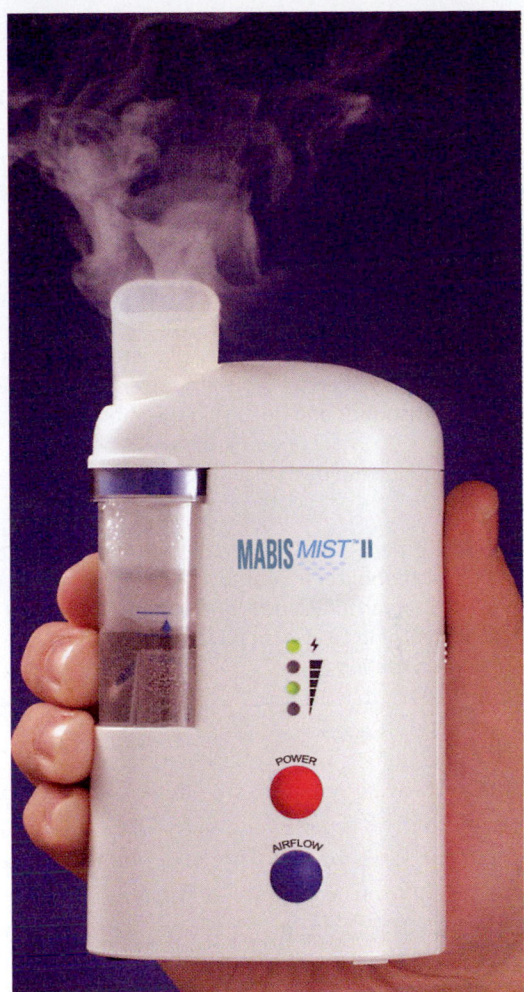

Figure 47-2. ■ A handheld nebulizer is used to assist the client. (Courtesy of Mabis.)

Other tests would be ordered according to client symptoms. Box 47-2 ■ lists tests and treatments commonly performed in the EC setting.

Airway Management and CPR

The primary concern for any client in the EC setting is airway management. The nurse is responsible for assessing changes in the client's respiratory or breathing pattern at all times. Oxygen therapy and adjuncts are frequently utilized in maintaining airways. Apparatuses from oral and nasal airways, low-flow devices (nasal cannulas, Venturi masks, and simple face masks), and high-flow devices (non-rebreather, bag-valve-mask units, endotracheal tubes) are most often used. (See respiratory disorders and procedures for administering oxygen in Chapter 32 ⊚⊙.) Saturation readings for O_2 are done frequently with clients requiring O_2, to monitor changes and to assess oxygen **titration** (determination of the correct volume for administration). Oxygen therapy is not routinely given in the UC setting. However, should a client need a breathing

---

BOX 47-2   COMMON EC TESTS AND TREATMENTS

Lab Tests

CBC, chemistry, cardiac enzymes, troponin levels, BMPs, PT, PTT, liver enzymes, ALT, ASTs for GI, BMPs, ABGs, Chlamydia, STI profiles

Diagnostics

ECGs

    Coaxial radiology (CXR), CT scans, MRI if CT scans are not revealing

    Abdominal flat plate, and bone-specific x-rays related to mechanism of injury or area of concern

    Doppler ultrasounds and deep vein thrombosis (DVT) Dopplers

    Urine pregnancy, rapid strep cultures, etc.

Treatments

Respiratory treatments, **DuoNeb** (two-medication broncho-dilator given via nebulizer for improved gas exchange in cases of respiratory insufficiency), or albuterol treatments (respiratory breathing treatments), O₂ therapy

    Suturing and casting

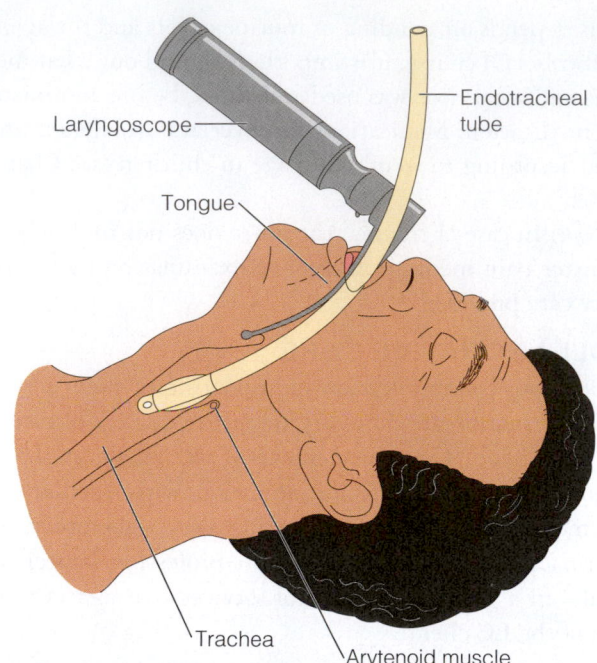

Figure 47-3. ■ Endotracheal intubation maintains a patent airway for oxygen administration.

treatment for wheezing, and the client is stable, oxygen may be given by the nurse.

As mentioned, an initial survey of the ABCs (airway, breathing, circulation) is always conducted on a client who presents in the EC. The airway must be maintained for *patency* (openness), airflow, and adequate ventilation.

In cases of trauma, a client must have **cervical spine alignment** (*C spine*) performed. A C spine is a manual maneuver performed by an individual to maintain the client in proper spinal alignment. At times, this may include application of a cervical stabilizing collar device. (A soft collar is not recommended because it is not effective in stabilizing a C spine.) Once any stabilizing device is in place, an x-ray should be taken to "clear" the client before immobilization devices can be safely removed. (Care of the client with spinal trauma is discussed in detail in Chapter 36 🔗.)

A chin-lift or modified jaw-thrust maneuver (discussed later in the CPR section) must be performed with clients who have experienced trauma. The mouth is inspected for bleeding, loose teeth, dentures, foreign objects, and emesis.

The nurse needs to observe for signs and symptoms of respiratory distress, as evidenced by decreased O₂ saturation, dyspnea, increased respirations (tachypnea), and cyanosis. If the nurse witnesses distress behaviors, the nurse should report to the primary care provider so that airway management may be performed.

To keep the airway open, an apparatus may be placed into the nasopharyngeal or oral cavity. Endotracheal intubations (Figure 47-3 ■) may also be done. In severe cases a *cricothyroidectomy* (an incision into the trachea) may be

performed by a primary care provider or licensed professional in emergency care to make a direct opening into the trachea.

Breathing must be evaluated for rate, rhythm, and quality. Oxygen adjunct devices that deliver high-flow O₂ (nonrebreather, bag-valve-mask unit, endotracheal tube via intubation) may be used. Low-flow devices such as nasal cannulas, Venturi masks, and face masks can also support ventilation in minor cases of compromise.

CARDIOPULMONARY RESUSCITATION

In clients with trauma and altered levels of consciousness (LOC), the carotid pulse is evaluated for presence, rate, and quality. **Cardiopulmonary resuscitation** (CPR, a combination of oral resuscitation and external cardiac massage) is always performed on clients in the EC who have an absent pulse. During times of inadequate tissue perfusion during cardiac arrest, CPR offers a small percentage of core circulation to the vital organs in order to sustain life during times of pulselessness.

CPR can be administered to people of any age from newborn to geriatric (Figure 47-4 ■). However, CPR technique varies in compressions, depth, and ratio in the adult, child, and infant. See general guidelines for adults in Box 47-3 ■.

Specific training is provided by the American Heart Association (AHA) and the Red Cross for certification in CPR. Nurses must obtain continued education and training updates as an important part of providing quality, professional care.

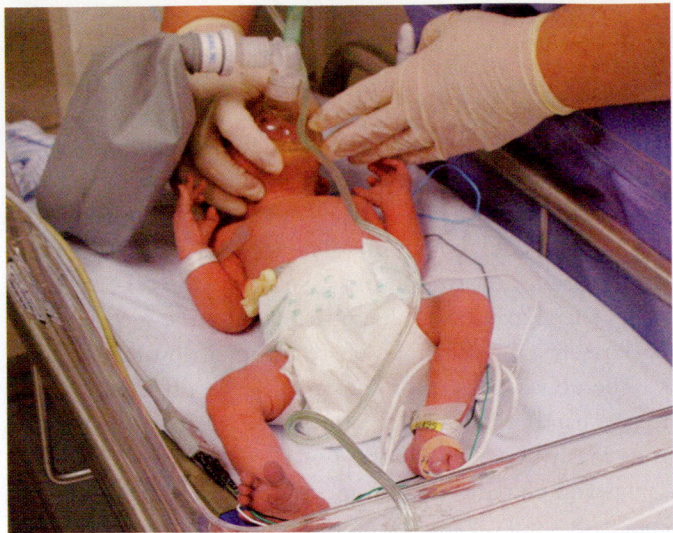
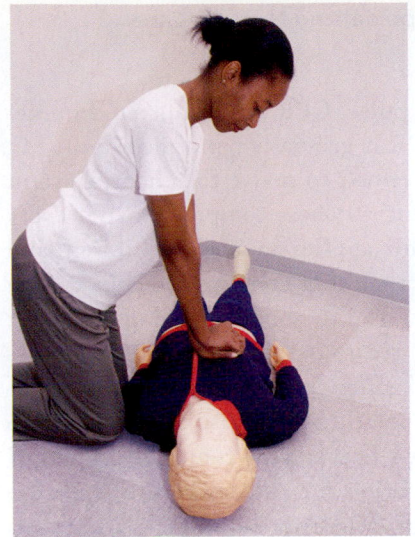

A   B

Figure 47-4. ■ **A.** Specialized training is required to perform CPR on a neonate. **B.** Locate the compression site by following the edge of the rib cage to the notch where the ribs join the sternum. Apply chest compressions with your arms vertical over the victim.

BOX 47-3   FIRST STEPS TO PREPARE FOR ADULT CPR

The following steps are based on instructions from the American Heart Association. The AHA updates its procedures on an ongoing basis, and the nurse MUST maintain up-to-date training and accreditation according to agency and institutional guidelines.

1. **Check for responsiveness.** Shake or tap the person gently. See if the person moves or makes a noise. Shout, "Are you OK?"
2. **Call 911 if there is no response.** Shout for help and send someone to call 911. If you are alone, call 911 even if you have to leave the person. Retrieve the automated external defibrillator (AED) and emergency equipment, if available. AED equipment may be utilized and brought to the EC and changed to a defibrillator. CPR steps would continue according to the PCP's instructions and client condition.
3. **Carefully place the person on his or her back.** If there is a chance the person has a spinal injury, two people are needed to move the person without twisting the head and neck.
4. **Open the airway.** Lift up the chin with two fingers. At the same time, push down on the forehead with the other hand.
5. **Look, listen, and feel for breathing.** Place your ear close to the person's mouth and nose. Watch for chest rise and fall. Feel for breath on your cheek.
6. **If the person is not breathing:**
   - Cover the person's mouth tightly with your mouth.
   - Pinch the nose closed.
   - Keep the chin lifted and head tilted.
   - Give two slow, full breaths.
   - Use bag-mask unit with oxygen or barrier device whenever possible.
7. **If the chest does NOT rise, try the head-tilt/chin-lift maneuver again, and give two more breaths.** If the chest still doesn't rise, check to see if something is blocking the airway and try to remove it.

8. **Look for signs of circulation.** These signs include normal breathing, coughing, or movement. If these signs are absent, begin chest compressions.
   If there is circulation but no breathing:
   Provide rescue breathing (one breath every 4 to 5 seconds).
   If no pulse or signs of circulation are present:
   If AED is available: power on, attach electrodes, and follow prompts.
   IF no AED, perform chest compressions.
9. **Perform chest compressions:**
   - Place the heel of one hand on the breastbone, right between the nipples.
   - Place the heel of your other hand on top of the first hand.
   - Position your body directly over your hands. Your shoulders should be in line with your hands. DO NOT lean back or forward. As you gaze down, you should be looking directly down on your hands.
   - Give 30 chest compressions. Each time, press down about 2 inches into the chest. These compressions should be FAST with no pausing. Count the 30 compressions quickly: "a, b, c, d, e, f, g, h, i, j, k, l, m, n, off."
10. **Give the person two slow, full breaths.** The chest should rise.
11. Continue cycles of 30 chest compressions followed by two slow, full breaths.
12. After about 2 minutes (five cycles of 30 compressions and two breaths), recheck for signs of circulation.
13. Repeat steps 11 and 12 until the person recovers or help arrives.

If the person starts breathing again, place him or her in the recovery position. Periodically recheck for breathing and signs of circulation until help arrives. **Remember, it is the nurse's responsibility to become certified and to maintain updated training in CPR.**

Source: Adapted from the *2005 American Heart Association Guidelines for Cardiopulmonary Resuscitation and Emergency Cardiovascular Care.*

If the client has no pulse, CPR is administered immediately. Two-person CPR is generally performed in the EC, as staff participates in efforts to revive the client. Current AHA guidelines call for 30 chest compressions for every two rescue breaths. This applies to adults, children, and infants. Studies show that this creates more blood flow from the heart to the rest of the body until a defibrillator is available (American Heart Association, 2005). The revised guidelines also recommend that emergency personnel cool the body temperature of cardiac arrest clients to 90 degrees for 12 to 24 hours. This results in improved survival and brain function for those who are comatose after initial resuscitation. Also, high-flow O_2 is always administered with a bag-valve-mask unit while compressions are performed.

Intravenous cannulation with a large-bore IV is initiated by a member certified with the EC to perform the function. IV lifelines provide access for medications to be administered hemodynamically, to improve the client's chances of survival. Should life-threatening dysrhythmia occur in cardiac arrest, a defibrillator may be used. A **defibrillator** is an instrument that provides various voltages of electricity (measured in joules) to trigger the electrical impulses of the heart (Figure 47-5 ■). If the client has a pulse initially, circulation is carefully monitored with frequent vital signs so that changes may be reported to the primary care provider.

HEIMLICH MANEUVER

The Heimlich maneuver (see also Chapter 9 ⬤) is necessary for clients who have an airway obstruction due to ingestion of a foreign object. Food (such as a bolus of meat) is a common cause of choking. The tongue is the most common cause for obstruction in the unconscious client. Many times the relaxation of the muscle allows the tongue to fall back in the client's throat, obstructing airflow.

The universal sign for choking is typically demonstrated by the hand or hands at the throat, for an individual who is consciously choking (Figure 47-6 ■). Victims who are conscious and choking should not be touched if they can talk, cough, or speak in a high-pitched tone. If a client asks for assistance or becomes unconscious, abdominal thrusts are administered. Abdominal thrusts are given at the level of the midepigastric region, and below the xiphoid process (see Figure 47-6). If the client does not expel the object and becomes unresponsive, he or she should be assisted to the ground carefully. Examination of the mouth is done to see whether the airway has become patent from the position change. This examination is done again after a sequence of abdominal thrusts to determine whether the object has moved or the airway has become patent. Abdominal thrusts serve the purpose of an artificial cough. They produce force within the trachea to expel the object that is blocking the airway.

Within the EC setting, medical instruments such as Magill forceps may be used by the primary care provider to remove objects in the airway if necessary. Suction should be readily available. The nurse should be prepared to assist with suctioning

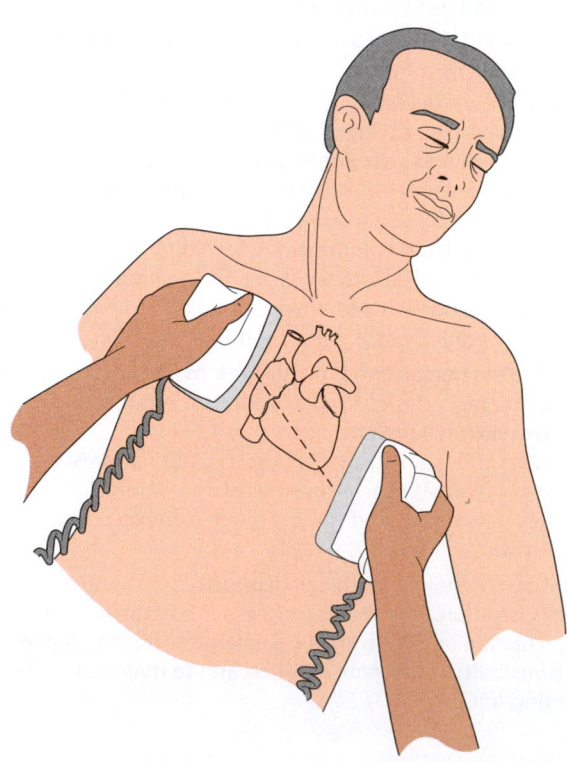

Figure 47-5. ■ Defibrillation.

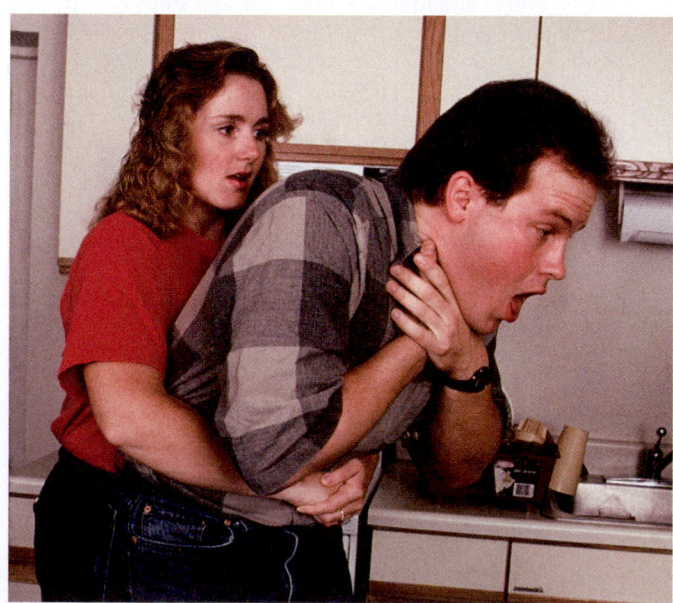

Figure 47-6. ■ This person is using the universal sign of choking. Hands are positioned below the xiphoid process and above the umbilicus before applying the thrust. *Source:* Photo Researchers, Inc.

during the procedure. On successful removal of the object, oxygen therapy and airway management are always performed by the healthcare team until the client becomes stable.

Primary nursing diagnoses for these clients include *Ineffective Airway Clearance, Risk for Aspiration, Acute Confusion, Impaired Gas Exchange*, and *Ineffective Tissue Perfusion*. LPNs/LVNs monitor airway, breathing, and circulation, and assist as noted earlier.

SKILL CERTIFICATIONS AND STAT TESTS

Because of the severity and acuteness of client conditions in the EC setting, the nurse and other healthcare professionals are required by institutions to maintain standards of practice and certification in skill and competence. Certification is standardized by the American Heart Association and must be maintained in:

- **ACLS** (advanced cardiac life support), which is a specialized training course that prepares the healthcare professional to perform advanced lifesaving skills or techniques on the client. This is standardized by the American Heart Association.

- **BLS** (basic life support), which is a specialized training course that prepares the healthcare professional to perform basic lifesaving skills or techniques (CPR, Heimlich maneuver, defibrillation, etc.).

- **PALS** (pediatric advanced life support), which is a specialized training course that prepares the healthcare professional to perform advanced lifesaving skills or techniques on the pediatric client.

All licensed professional healthcare providers are required to maintain proficiency in these areas while employed in the EC and sometimes the UC setting.

During a critical situation such as trauma or myocardial infarction, the ACLS, PALS, or BLS protocols are utilized. Twelve-lead ECGs are performed on clients to diagnose cardiac status and dysrhythmia so that appropriate treatments can be administered.

In cases of myocardial infarction (MI), cardiac labs (mentioned earlier under Collaborative Care) are often ordered in conjunction with diagnostics to verify a medical diagnosis. Most often labs are ordered *stat* (immediately) in the EC so that treatments can be given in a rapid sequence.

Shock

In the EC setting clients can have an array of wounds or injuries. One of the most urgent concerns is **shock** (life-threatening condition of inadequate tissue perfusion). Depending on the nature of the wound and the amount of blood or fluid volume loss, the nurse must identify changes in vital signs that indicate suspicion of shock. Vital signs include

tachycardia, tachypnea, and hypotension. Figure 47-7 ■ shows the numerous effects of shock on body systems. The nurse must also monitor the possible effects of shock on the endocrine system, including decreased insulin production, increased blood sugar, and polyuria.

HYPOVOLEMIC SHOCK

Different types of shock can occur as a complication of trauma. Hypovolemic shock occurs when the body has sustained a severe amount of fluid deficit or loss. Reasons may include bleeding, burns, fluid and electrolyte imbalances related to excessive diarrhea or vomiting, or sepsis from trauma or injury. Signs and symptoms generally reveal pallor, *diaphoresis* (sweating), hypotension, tachycardia, tachypnea, and decreased urine output (*oliguria*). There may also be changes in LOC. The symptoms may gradually become worse as fluid loss becomes greater, therefore creating obvious clinical manifestations. A pneumatic antishock garment (Figure 47-8 ■) or military antishock trousers (MAST) might be used to help maintain blood pressure. Hemorrhagic shock is a type of hypovolemic shock in which the client has lost a significant amount of blood.

MAST (military antishock trouser) or PASG (pneumonic antishock garment) may also be used with hypovolemic shock, trauma, and other types of prehospital emergencies for improving perfusion to the client's core circulation. During times of severe bleeding/hemorrhage, MAST increases the venous return to the heart by constriction. The device is used to facilitate blood flow from the lower extremities to the core circulation, including the heart, brain, and lungs.

The nurse must understand the protocol for MAST/PASG so that the garment is not deflated without a primary care provider order or the agency's or institution's guidelines. Removal of the MAST is done under protocol and PCP order.

CARDIOGENIC SHOCK

Cardiogenic shock occurs when the heart sustains an injury or trauma resulting in pump failure. Acute MI, CHF, dysrhythmia, and blunt and penetrating chest trauma are known causes of cardiogenic shock. Signs and symptoms are similar to those for hypovolemic shock. In addition, clients may have pulmonary edema and distended (swollen) neck veins.

ANAPHYLACTIC SHOCK

Anaphylactic shock occurs in clients who experience hypersensitivity reactions to various antigens. It is a severe allergic reaction that can involve the entire body (American Academy of Allergy, 2007). Exposure to a substance

MyNursingKit | Shock

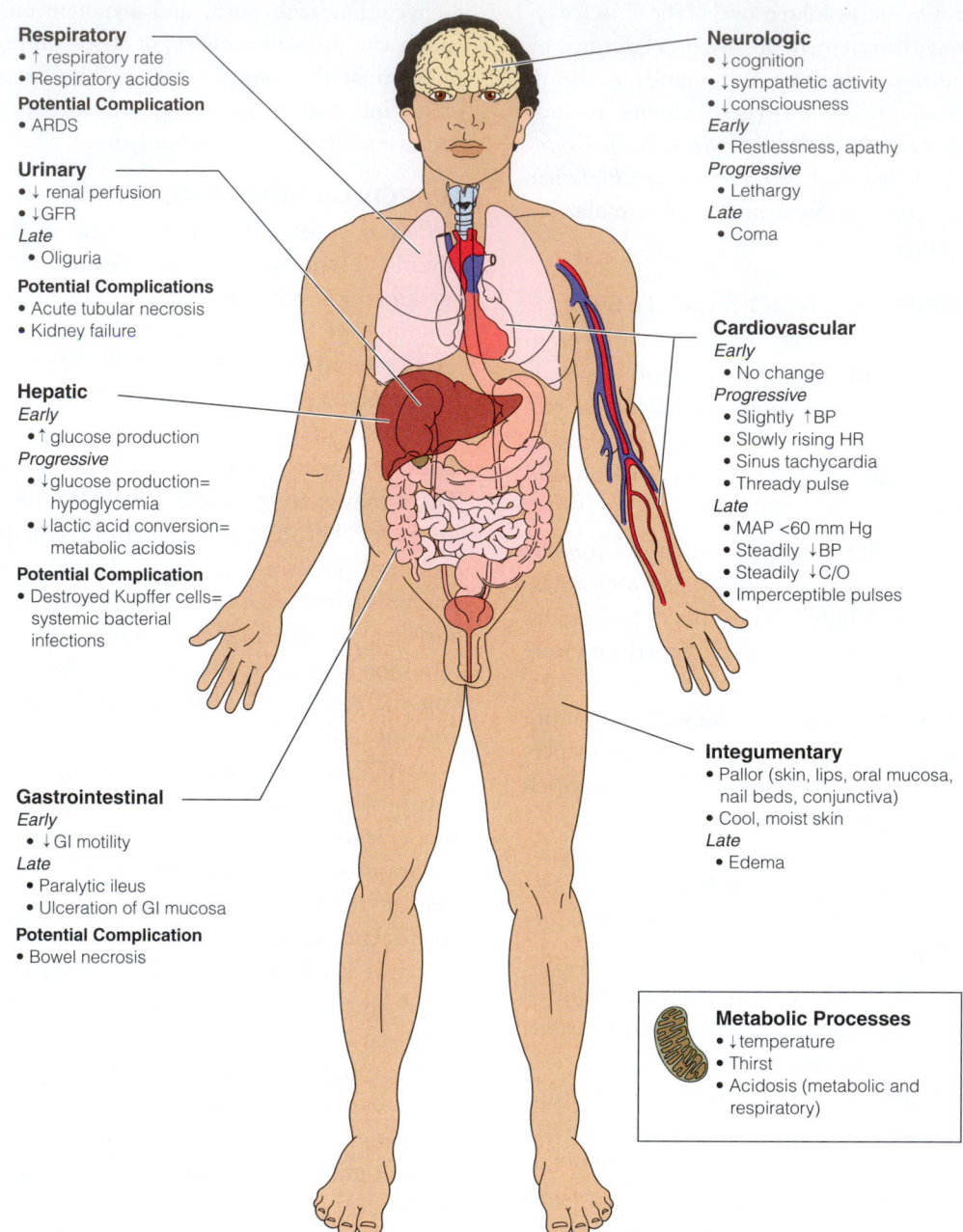

Respiratory
- ↑ respiratory rate
- Respiratory acidosis

Potential Complication
- ARDS

Urinary
- ↓ renal perfusion
- ↓GFR

Late
- Oliguria

Potential Complications
- Acute tubular necrosis
- Kidney failure

Hepatic
Early
- ↑ glucose production

Progressive
- ↓glucose production= hypoglycemia
- ↓lactic acid conversion= metabolic acidosis

Potential Complication
- Destroyed Kupffer cells= systemic bacterial infections

Gastrointestinal
Early
- ↓GI motility

Late
- Paralytic ileus
- Ulceration of GI mucosa

Potential Complication
- Bowel necrosis

Neurologic
- ↓cognition
- ↓sympathetic activity
- ↓consciousness

Early
- Restlessness, apathy

Progressive
- Lethargy

Late
- Coma

Cardiovascular
Early
- No change

Progressive
- Slightly ↑BP
- Slowly rising HR
- Sinus tachycardia
- Thready pulse

Late
- MAP <60 mm Hg
- Steadily ↓BP
- Steadily ↓C/O
- Imperceptible pulses

Integumentary
- Pallor (skin, lips, oral mucosa, nail beds, conjunctiva)
- Cool, moist skin

Late
- Edema

Metabolic Processes
- ↓temperature
- Thirst
- Acidosis (metabolic and respiratory)

Figure 47-7. ■ Multisystem effects of shock.

or foreign body can trigger anaphylaxis. Examples of triggers include medications, blood products, natural rubber latex, foods, and bee stings (discussed later in this chapter). The anaphylactic reaction involves compromise of the respiratory and immune systems. Dyspnea, laryngeal spasm and edema, and bronchospasm are often witnessed within minutes of onset. Clients will become extremely anxious and require immediate airway management to ensure safety. (Anaphylaxis is discussed further in Chapter 35 ⬭.)

clinical ALERT

To prevent loss of life, the nurse must ensure that any client receiving an injection remain at the facility for 20 to 30 minutes, to observe for signs and symptoms of anaphylactic shock. Note that a localized reaction at the site on injection could lead to a systemic reaction and overall anaphylaxis. The client can wait in the waiting room if appropriate and report back to the nurse after the waiting period. Documentation of the person's condition at discharge and the time of discharge is crucial.

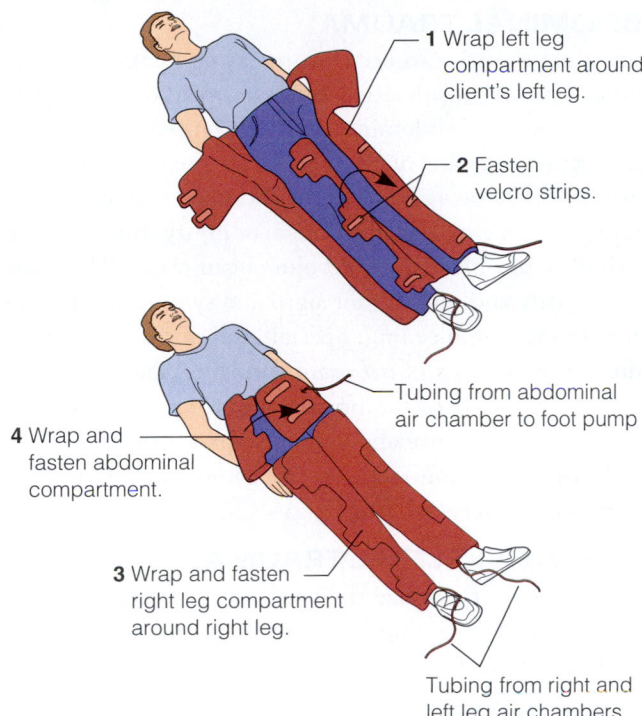

1 Wrap left leg compartment around client's left leg.

2 Fasten velcro strips.

Tubing from abdominal air chamber to foot pump

4 Wrap and fasten abdominal compartment.

3 Wrap and fasten right leg compartment around right leg.

Tubing from right and left leg air chambers

Figure 47-8. ■ Pneumatic antishock garment provides rapid, emergency treatment of shock.

SEPTIC SHOCK

Septic shock is a condition that occurs from a systemic reaction and infection in the body. The body becomes overwhelmed with poisons (*endotoxins*) that cause the blood vessels to dilate. The body attempts to compensate for the fluid loss and *interstitial spacing* or **third spacing** (shunting of fluids into the extracellular space). Most often the causes are pathogens, such as gram-negative bacteria or viruses.

Septic shock is known for two phases of signs and symptoms. The first phase has normal BP, pulse, and urine output. Oftentimes the client becomes febrile with flushed skin tones and diaphoresis. The second phase reveals more obvious latent signs of shock: hypotension, bradycardia, oliguria, cold, clammy extremities, and a normal temperature (*afebrile*).

NEUROGENIC SHOCK

Neurogenic shock occurs when there is trauma or malfunction to the nervous system. Most frequently known as *spinal shock*, neurogenic shock is related to gross injury to the spinal column. Motor vehicle crashes, household injuries, and falls are primary reasons for neurogenic shock. Changes in level of consciousness are observed.

Some signs and symptoms of neurogenic shock are similar to those of hypovolemic shock. However, in neurogenic shock, the skin is warm and dry and the heart rate falls

(bradycardia). In addition, paralysis or limited extremity movement below the area of injury is seen.

NURSING CONSIDERATIONS

When caring for clients in shock, you must focus on recognizing the signs rapidly and implementing emergency measures quickly. Monitor vital signs in clients with suspected shock every 15 minutes or more often if the condition is changing rapidly. Position the client with shock in modified Trendelenburg position unless the client is in cardiogenic shock. This helps return blood to the heart. Be prepared to assist with immediate administration of IV fluids to increase blood volume and blood pressure. Be ready to obtain plasma expanders as ordered to keep blood volume increased. Administer oxygen as ordered to increase oxygen delivery to the brain, heart, and other vital organs. Maintain an open airway, especially if the client loses consciousness.

Trauma in the Emergency Center

Trauma is one of the most common reasons for visits to the EC setting. Two types of mechanisms of injury can be linked to life-threatening conditions and death if not treated promptly: penetrating trauma and blunt trauma. Penetrating trauma (Figure 47-9 ■) can be from a sharp object that enters the body rapidly. It can range from minor (stepping on a nail) to life threatening (being stabbed with a knife).

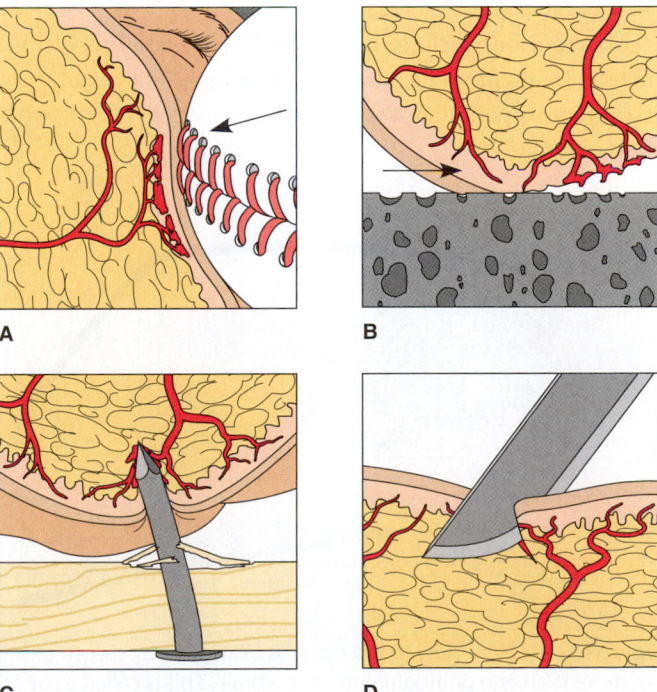

A

B

C

D

Figure 47-9. ■ Traumatic injuries to the skin: **A.** contusion; **B.** abrasion; **C.** puncture wound; **D.** laceration.

Blunt trauma (also called *closed injury*) is an injury that causes impact to an area (bone, tissue, organ), leading to internal bleeding or gross trauma at the point of origin. A blow from a baseball (see Figure 47-9A) or impact with a steering wheel in an automobile collision are two examples of blunt trauma.

HEAD TRAUMA

Trauma to the head can result in intracranial bleeding, intracranial pressure, and edema. Death may result if the client is not treated immediately. Assessment of the mechanism of injury is of utmost importance in determining how severe the injury is. Figure 47-10 ■ illustrates the double head injury that can occur in a car crash. Chapter 36 ⊘ discusses hematomas and concussions.

With head trauma, careful continuous monitoring of LOC is essential. The EC uses the Glasgow Coma Scale to evaluate level of consciousness (see Table 19-2 ⊘). The test scores range from 15 (alert and oriented) to 0. A score of less than 13 with head trauma is cause for concern and intervention. Lower scores may indicate increased intracranial pressure (IICP) and a potentially life-threatening situation for the client.

CHEST TRAUMA

Chest trauma occurs from injury to the thorax and mediastinal areas. Motor vehicle crashes, stab wounds, gunshot wounds, and sport injuries, for example, can cause chest trauma. Any type of injury to the chest area can result in a life-threatening situation. Complications of injuries to the chest area can include pneumothorax, hemothorax, and flail chest (see Chapter 32 ⊘).

Interventions include high-flow O_2, IV administration/lifeline, frequent vitals, and O_2 saturations. The respiratory assessment is paramount in ensuring success in clients with chest trauma.

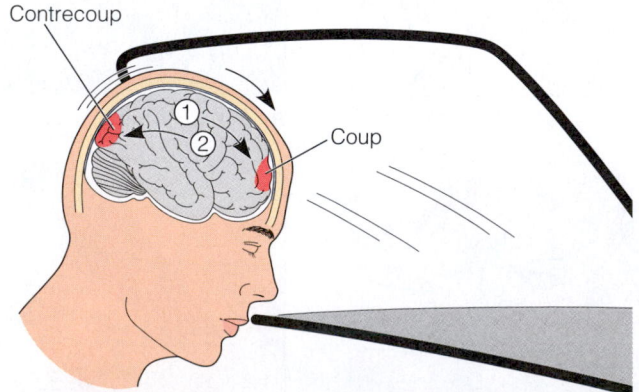

Figure 47-10. ■ A blow to the head, as from a car crash, can create more than one point of injury in the brain. This is called a *coup-contrecoup injury.* Following the initial injury (the coup), the brain rebounds within the skull and receives a second injury (contrecoup) in the opposite part of the brain.

ABDOMINAL TRAUMA

Abdominal trauma can occur in the same manner as chest trauma. Careful consideration and assessment of vital organs must be done. The abdominal cavity encompasses many vascular organs that are not protected by bone structure, so injury can more easily occur in the abdomen than chest. Depending on the type and mechanism of injury (blunt or penetrating), rapid blood loss or volume can occur. The nurse must identify and monitor for signs and symptoms of shock that may indicate bleeding. Special attention is paid to the abdomen. Any signs of *ecchymosis* (bruising) and distention should be reported to the primary care provider. Pregnant women who experience abdominal trauma may develop internal bleeding or contractions strong enough to result in a precipitous delivery (see Chapter 53 ⊘).

MUSCULOSKELETAL TRAUMA

The nurse must recognize the need for immediate first aid and collaborate in giving care to the client for the area of sustained injury.

SPINAL INJURY

Spinal cord injuries are discussed in detail in Chapter 36 ⊘ . Stabilization and immediate treatment are crucial to client outcomes.

Fractures

Other procedures that the LPN/LVN may be required to know include caring for fractures, assisting with lacerations and stitching, splinting (Procedure 47-1 ■, page 1300), and casting (Procedure 47-2 ■). Procedure 47-3 ■ provides steps for measuring crutches, canes, and walkers. Because a large number of x-rays are taken in the emergency setting, x-ray knowledge and safety are important.

First Aid

First aid procedures are still heavily used within the EC and home care settings on a daily basis. First aid consciousness in the client care environment is a critical entity for the healthcare professional. The following acronym is a reminder of basic first aid nursing interventions in the EC, UC, and home care environments. Box 47-4 ■ provides a mnemonic for first aid for the nurse.

SOFT-TISSUE INJURY

The care and management of soft-tissue injuries in the EC or UC are common. The injuries are designed by classification from mild or moderate to severe (Class I, II, III).

Common areas for soft-tissue injuries are the extremities, specifically the rotator cuff, knees, ankles, feet, and hands. The signs and symptoms are pain, edema, tenderness, ecchymosis, and at times (depending on the severity) hematoma. The acronym RICE is used for treating soft-tissue injuries:

  R—Rest the injured area
  I—Ice for 48 to 72 hours

BOX 47-4	FIRST AID REMINDERS FOR THE NURSE

F- Fever that is prolonged needs to be reported to the primary care provider.

I- Ice should be used for injuries, bruises, falls, soft tissue.

R- Recognize ABCs and start CPR in an emergency.

S- Standard precautions are to be used during exposure to body fluid, etc.

T- Triage clients with medical emergencies from severe to nonthreatening.

A- Activate EMS/911 in times of emergency outside the EC or UC setting.

I- Initiate care promptly and report changes to the primary care provider.

D- Document all interventions on client care after initiating them.

C—Compression via splint, bandage, cast

E—Elevate the extremity above heart

The ability to obtain data information through a complete history and mechanism of injury for the client will assist in the PCP ruling out a differential diagnosis. Radiography and arthroscopy may be ordered to assist in creating a definitive diagnosis.

TRAUMA TO EYES, EARS, OR NOSE

Any eye problem requires a visual acuity exam on a Snellen or other type of eye chart. Most providers want documentation of the best corrected vision. If the client has contact lenses (and if the contacts are not part of the urgent problem), test the eyes before having the client remove them. Clients who wear glasses for distance vision (myopia) would wear them for the exam.

The top number to the left of the line of letters on an eye chart is the number of feet the client should stand from it. Most eye charts are 20-foot charts. The bottom number indicates how far (in feet) a person with normal vision could be from the chart and still read the line. There is usually a line or some other type of indication on the wall or floor near the eye chart that indicates distance. Check for this line so that you can avoid guessing at the distance. The client stands at the proper distance, covers the eye with an eye occluder or a solid object such as a piece of clean paper, and reads each line starting at the top. See Procedure 48-8 🔗 in the next chapter for steps in performing an eye examination.

clinical ALERT

Never have a client use the hand or fingers as an occluder. If an eye occluder is available, remember to clean it between uses to prevent transfer of eye infections or even foreign material from one client to another.

Check the right eye first, then the left eye, and finally both eyes. Stay with the same routine. *Note:* The Joint Commission that grants accreditation to healthcare organizations (formerly JCAHO) states that documentation for eye tests must spell out "left eye, right eye, and both eyes." The abbreviations for eyes (OS, OD, and OU) are not to be used in charting in accredited institutions.

If a client presents with a chemical or foreign substance in the eye, an eye kit will need to be obtained. The eye kit includes a topical eye anesthetic (located in the refrigerator most often), a Wood's black light, fluorescing drops or strips, sterile needles, sterile applicators, a solution for flushing the eye such as Dacriose, a device to do a continuous irrigation when hooked to an IV line, ointments and drops, and eye patches.

Ear Lavage

Clients may present with otitis media, impacted cerumen, foreign body in the ear, or trauma. The client may need an ear lavage after the provider examines the client. Ear lavage is also a common procedure in young children. It is described in Chapter 60, Procedure 60-1 🔗.

Foreign Object in the Nose

Children especially can put items in places where they will become trapped. If a child has a foreign body caught in the nose, the provider will need equipment necessary for viewing the site of the foreign object. Tweezers or small forceps may also be required for extraction of the object.

Epistaxis

Nosebleeds can occur spontaneously without cause or because of blunt trauma to the face. *Epistaxis* (nosebleed) is common in all ages. Symptoms to report include how long the bleeding lasted after initial treatment was ordered. Epistaxis is generally treated with cold packs to the nose and cheek areas for 10 to 20 minutes. The cold will constrict the blood vessels in the immediate region and reduce blood flow to the area. Pinching the nostrils and blowing any clots are also advised. Standard precautions are to be taken by the nurse while treatment is involved. The LPN/LVN should monitor and report changes in the condition of epistaxis in the UC environment.

Near-Drowning

Near-drowning injuries are another type of emergency that can be life threatening. Different electrolyte imbalances may occur, depending on whether the event occurred in fresh or in salt water. Submersion in water or fluid impairs the ability of the individual to breathe. Wet drowning (known as *aspiration*) can happen when fluid enters the lungs.

"Dry drowning" is laryngeal spasm without aspiration of fluid. Asphyxiation causes hypoxemia for the client, requiring a rapid response for airway management. Oxygen therapy with high-flow O_2 and ventilatory support is needed. Should oxygen demands be unmet, the client can suffer central nervous system damage. Multisystem failure and death can also accompany drowning of any type (Verve, 2007).

The treatment includes prehospital care (if applicable), ABCs, and oxygen therapy to correct the potential acidosis. Careful management of cardiac dysrhythmias, electrolytes, IV lifeline, and blood pressure for shock are also aspects of care by the healthcare team.

Poisoning and Bites

INGESTED OR INHALED POISONS

Poisonings require rapid assessment and medical intervention within minutes. Poisoning can occur at any age. Poisons can be introduced into the body by inhalation, ingestion, and absorption and by venomous bites.

One of the primary concerns of assessment is to identify and report the method of exposure. A history of events must be taken and vital signs recorded.

Ingested poisons require rapid removal of the poison by two medications. Syrup of ipecac (for ingested poisons that will not erode the GI tract and that are not petroleum based) is administered by mouth. The standard recommended dose is 15 mL for children ages 1 to 5 and 30 mL for clients older than 6 years of age. Syrup of ipecac induces vomiting, and its administration is followed with large amounts of water.

Another modality used today is activated charcoal. Activated charcoal is administered for medication overdoses and poisons that can cause esophageal damage if regurgitated. The dosage is normally 50 g by mouth or by nasogastric tube (if needed).

A secondary method for treatment of ingested poisons is gastric lavage. Lavage flushes the GI tract and may evacuate any remaining ingested poison.

Inhaled poisons require treatment with oxygen therapy and airway management.

A mnemonic for the care of poisoning injuries is SIRES:

S-Stabilize the client.   **E**-Eliminate the poison.
I-Identify the poison.   **S**-Support vital functions.
R-Reverse the effects.

INJECTED POISONS AND SNAKEBITES

Injected poisons or snakebites are serious situations that require rapid intervention. The source of the bite must be identified immediately if possible. These injuries can cause anaphylactic and respiratory impairment, as well as localized reaction in the immediate area, which can impair circulation to the extremity or area involved. If snakebites are poisonous, treatment must focus on airway management and circulatory stabilization of the area of the body. Tourniquets are used to reduce blood flow or circulation to the involved area. However, tourniquets must not cut off circulation to a body part. The nurse should anticipate the need for antivenom and have it ready for use after initial airway stabilization and IV lifeline insertion by the healthcare team. Antivenom can be very costly for clients. Clients may experience serum sickness from antivenom. If the immune system rejects the antivenom, treatment and follow-up in the critical care unit may be required. Careful monitoring by the nurse and healthcare team is crucial for successful client outcomes.

BITES OF ANIMALS OR INSECTS

Animal and insect bites are another urgent situation, depending on the amount, location, and animal or insect involved. The nurse needs to control any bleeding, minimize the risk for infection or anaphylaxis, and provide pain management as focal points for management. The initial treatment and care of the client are similar in nature for a variety of bites. However, the severity and the mechanism of injury determine placement of the client in the EC or UC setting. If an animal is potentially infected with rabies, rabies treatment is initiated until it is determined whether or not the animal has the disease.

Psychiatric Emergencies

The nurse must be prepared for psychiatric emergencies, which have increased in number within the EC today. Conditions such as suicide, substance abuse or overdose, depression, violence, and rape are often seen in the EC setting. Initial care of the client requires emergency crisis intervention and stabilization of the client to prevent harm. Treatment for these emergencies will vary according to the presenting signs and symptoms. However, the primary care provider's ability to intervene and begin a rapid treatment sequence is critical for success. The outcome for psychiatric emergencies is to stabilize any life-threatening condition and to refer the client to a psychiatric facility or provider so that best practices can be achieved. Brief psychotherapy may occur acutely in the EC setting, as well as physical treatment of any presenting symptoms that require immediate attention by the healthcare team. The goal of the team is to recognize the problem, gather pertinent data, and formulate goals for a specific outcome. If medication or substance overdose is involved, the priority is to identify the drug so that appropriate medical intervention can occur.

Rape

Rape is both a physical and a psychological assault on another person. It is also a crime. When caring for a person who has been raped, evidence of the crime must be obtained at the same time as physical and emotional care are provided. For this reason, many EC centers now have special personnel called Sexual Assault Nurse Examiners (SANE). The SANE nurse is a specially certified RN who assists the PCP in collecting high-quality forensic evidence from rape victims (see Chapter 40 ⚭). SANE nurses are also trained and educated to treat rape victims and to obtain physical and emotional evidence from them during the rape examination. The healthcare team works collaboratively with SANE nurses in the EC to achieve positive client outcomes after cases of rape, whatever the victim's age or gender (Cole, 2007).

Bioterrorism and Terrorist Attacks

The need for careful planning and preparedness in the EC has escalated since the 9/11 attacks. Biological and chemical weapons can create a mass disaster among a population and impact the EC setting at any moment. Various agents can be used during a bioterrorism attack. Common bacteria include the following:

- *Bacillus anthracis* (anthrax)
- *Brucella* organism (brucellosis)
- *Yersinia pestis* (plague)
- *Francisella tularensis* (tularemia)

Common viruses that have been named as potential bioterrorist agents are smallpox, Ebola, and Lassa fever.

Nursing diagnoses for bioterrorism include *Risk for Trauma, Powerlessness, Ineffective Coping: Community, Anxiety* (mild, moderate, severe, panic), *Fear, Post Trauma Syndrome, Hopelessness*, and *Environmental Interpretation Syndrome*.

In a bioterrorist attack, the guidelines for nursing responsibilities would be the same as with other large-scale disasters. It is important to know the facility policy and protocols and to follow them in the event of an attack or emergency.

RADIATION AGENTS

Radiation injury is a potential hazard. Radioactive agents can affect clients in the EC through inhalation, gastrointestinal absorption, or skin exposure. First responders must

be prepared to use first aid and adhere to Standard Precautions when following the disaster plan within the EC.

The nurse must treat victims with life-threatening injuries first, triage others using the disaster plan, and follow the facility's Emergency Operations Plan (EOP). The LPN/LVN must communicate with the healthcare team and RN charge nurse for specific interventions and protocols to be utilized in the event of a disaster. Understanding and preparation are initial actions for the nurse during natural disasters or chemical, radiological, or bioterrorist attacks.

NURSING CARE

PRIORITIZING NURSING CARE

When caring for clients in the EC, maintain the order established by triage. Recall that the priority is to establish an airway and monitor breathing and circulation. Focus your care on controlling external bleeding and monitoring for internal bleeding. Check vital signs every 15 to 30 minutes. Monitor for signs of shock and changes in LOC. Give emotional support to the client and family, because traumatic injuries are generally grave in nature and extremely upsetting to those who witness them. Give family members a private place to meet and support one another. Be aware of the importance of the family. The primary care provider will update the family with the condition of the client as changes occur.

ASSESSING

The treatment and management of emergent clients in the EC include rapid assessment and interventions for life-threatening situations. The LPN/LVN should be able to assist the EC healthcare team in the initial stages until the client's condition has stabilized. Airway management, breathing, and circulation control ("the ABCs") are essential initial treatment. It is crucial to be ready to assist the RN in prioritizing and triaging the situation. The ability to obtain vital signs in a life-threatening situation is also a requirement for the LPN/LVN in the EC setting. Monitoring treatments for responses and assisting the healthcare team in the immediate recovery are paramount in the role of LPN/LVN within the EC.

> **clinical ALERT**
>
> Clients in nursing units may go into shock. In fact, the LPN/LVN is often one of the first to recognize signs of shock, take immediate action to support the client's circulatory status, and call for help. Recognition of the signs and symptoms of shock are of utmost importance in the immediate treatment and management of the client.

DIAGNOSING, PLANNING, AND IMPLEMENTING

Some common nursing diagnoses for clients with shock include the following:

- *Ineffective Airway Clearance*
- *Decreased Cardiac Output*
- *Impaired Gas Exchange*
- *Deficient Fluid Volume*
- *Ineffective Peripheral Tissue Perfusion*

Outcomes for clients in the EC include, but are not limited to, the following:

- The client will remain free from signs and symptoms of further hypoxia or respiratory distress.
- The client will remain free from aspiration.
- The client will maintain vitals within normal limits.
- The client will remain at 95% O_2 saturation level at all times.
- The client will maintain eupneic respirations at 95% O_2 saturation or greater.
- The client will maintain fluid and electrolyte balance.
- The client will maintain adequate circulation at all times as evidenced by blood pressure within normal limits (WNL).
- The client will remain free from signs and symptoms of inadequate circulation.

The nurse must give close attention to clients. Shock is one of the most dangerous complications. Common interventions for all types of shock follow:

- Except for cardiogenic shock, place client in modified Trendelenburg position (supine with head of bed elevated 10 degrees and foot raised 20 degrees) (Figure 47-11 ■). *This position maintains blood flow to vital organs.*
- Monitor changes in level of consciousness. *These changes can signal further underlying changes that require medical attention. Report changes in LOC to the team leader or charge nurse.*
- Administer oxygen and monitor breathing. Monitor cardiac circulatory status. *The ABCs are of primary importance in a client with shock.*

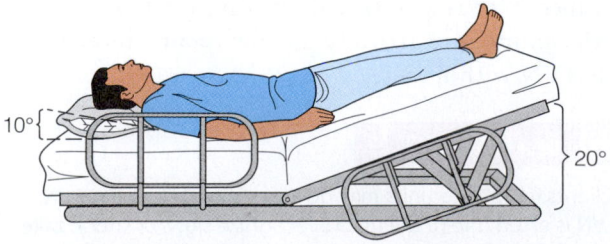

Figure 47-11. ■ Positioning of client for hypovolemic shock. The client in shock should be positioned with the lower extremities elevated about 20 degrees (knees straight), trunk horizontal, and the head elevated about 10 degrees.

- Monitor IV fluids. *Increasing fluids helps replace blood volume and raise blood pressure. Clients with cardiac compromise may not be able to tolerate rapid fluid administration, so the nurse must monitor for signs of respiratory congestion. Vocational and practical nurses working in this environment can obtain a certification that qualifies them to administer IV fluids.*
- Report changes in vital signs stat! *In the severely compromised client, changes can occur rapidly. Prompt reporting can save a life.*
- Monitor I&O for deficits, especially urine decrease. *Reduction in the amount of urine may signal third spacing.*
- Treat symptoms appropriately and in a timely way as ordered by primary care provider. Report all findings to the primary care provider stat. *Communication among the emergency or urgent care staff is crucial to ensuring the best client outcomes.*

EVALUATING

The nurse checks vital signs, I&O, and LOC to determine whether the client's condition has become or remains stable. All changes must be reported promptly to the primary care provider.

Burns

Burns are a type of injury that is frequently seen in the EC setting. The three types of burns that can inflict injury are thermal, chemical, and electrical. Thermal burns are most common. They occur from everyday events, household scalds, fire, hot temperature contact with a substance or object, and even sun exposure. Chemical burns can occur within the household or outside environment. Chemical burns are either alkaline or acidic in pH, burning the mucous membranes on contact or exposure. Electrical burns can be caused by exposure to either high or low voltage or to a lightning strike while outdoors.

CLASSIFICATION OF BURNS

Burns are classified according to their thickness (Figure 47-12 ■). **Superficial burns** (also called first-degree burns) injure only the epidermis and may be caused by everyday events such as touching a hot element on the stove. Superficial burns may be pink and painful, but they generally heal within 3 to 6 days. **Partial-thickness burns** (also called second-degree burns) may be superficial or deep. If they are *superficial partial-thickness burns*, they involve the epidermal layer. They are generally painful to touch and are red in appearance.

Deep partial-thickness burns involve more injury to the skin. The areas involved include both the epidermis and dermis. The burn remains red in appearance. Blistered areas may lack some sensation but have a painful area of injury surrounding them.

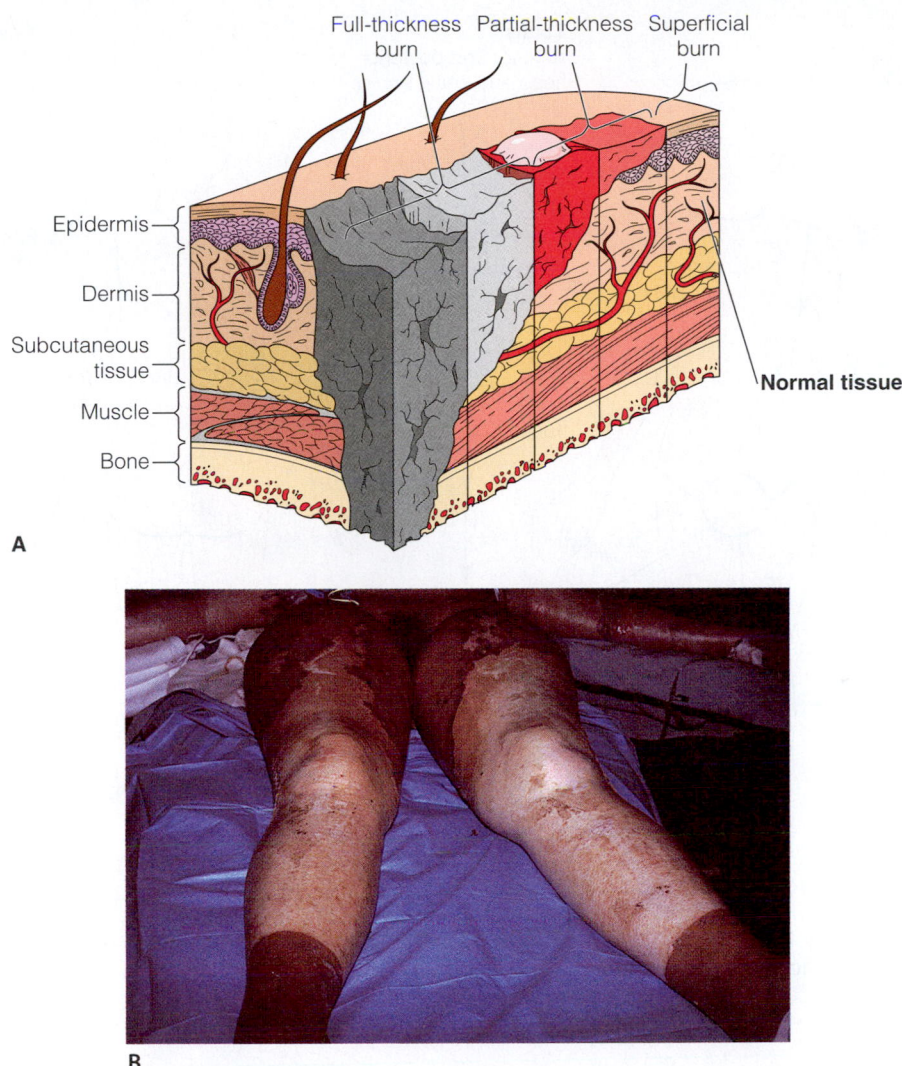

Figure 47-12. ■ **A.** Burn levels from superficial to full thickness. **B.** Client with a partial-thickness burn.

Full-thickness burns (also called third-degree burns) are the most severe. The layers of the skin (dermis, epidermis, subcutaneous) are totally involved. The appearance is blackened, charred, and white to leathery. Full-thickness burns are painless, because the nerve endings have been destroyed. The surrounding tissues that may be partially burned may have some nerve sensation causing pain. However, the full-thickness burns do not generate discomfort. Skin affected by full-thickness burns may not recover from damage. Extensive skin grafting may be required.

The "rule of nines" is a measure of the total body surface area (TBSA) and is used to calculate an approximate percentage amount of burned area. The areas are divided into or are multiples of 9% (Figure 47-13 ■). Full-thickness burns and some partial-thickness burns are assessed and calculated to determine the TBSA involved.

Clients sustaining burns may be transported to a burn unit if the EC staff determines such a move would be beneficial for them. Burn centers specialize in the recovery and rehabilitation of severe burns. Treatment for clients with major burns includes aseptic technique for wound care and protective isolation. Burn centers provide the very specialized care needed to support wound healing, such as removing necrotic tissue (*debridement*; see also Chapter 23 ⊗) and skin grafting.

NURSING CARE

PRIORITIZING NURSING CARE

When caring for clients with burns, use meticulous aseptic technique to prevent infection. Monitor respiratory status and circulatory status closely, especially if the head and neck are burned. Take vital signs every 15 to 30 minutes and watch for signs of shock. Administer pain medications as ordered and evaluate their effectiveness. The client with burns is generally in a great deal of pain and does not lose consciousness.

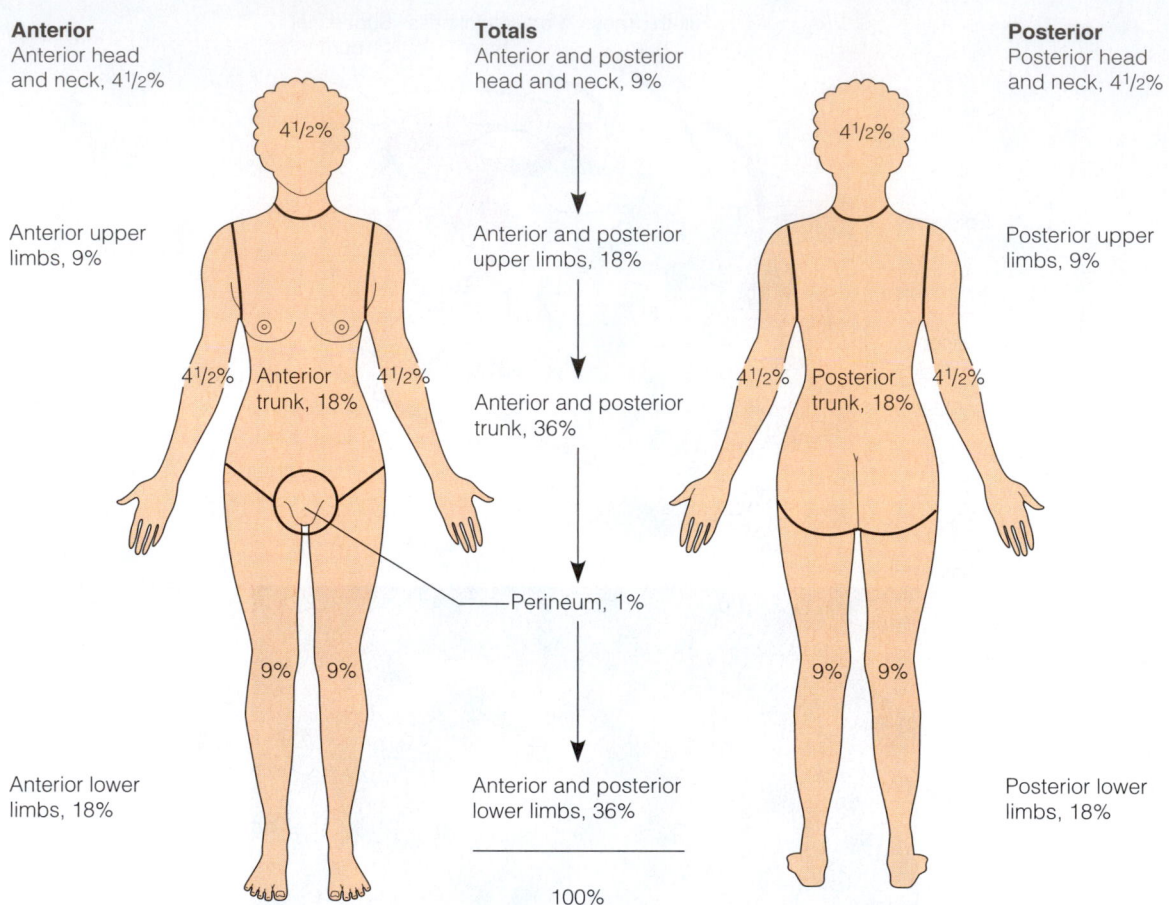

Anterior
Anterior head and neck, 4½%

4½%

Anterior upper limbs, 9%

4½% | Anterior trunk, 18% | 4½%

Perineum, 1%

9% | 9%

Anterior lower limbs, 18%

Totals
Anterior and posterior head and neck, 9%

Anterior and posterior upper limbs, 18%

Anterior and posterior trunk, 36%

Anterior and posterior lower limbs, 36%

100%

Posterior
Posterior head and neck, 4½%

4½%

Posterior upper limbs, 9%

4½% | Posterior trunk, 18% | 4½%

9% | 9%

Posterior lower limbs, 18%

Figure 47-13. ■ The "rule of nines" for estimating the percentage of TBSA affected by a burn injury. This method is quick and useful in emergency situations, but it is not accurate for short, obese, or very thin adults.

ASSESSING

In clients with burns, especially burns to the face and neck, it is crucial to focus on airway, breathing, and circulation. Increased edema and burns to the airway may be invisible, but they can be life threatening and critical to determine.

DIAGNOSING, PLANNING, AND IMPLEMENTING

Depending on the extent and location of the burn, the following nursing diagnoses might apply to a client with burns:

- *Impaired Skin Integrity*
- *Risk for Infection*
- *Ineffective Airway Clearance*
- *Ineffective Peripheral Tissue Perfusion*
- *Acute Pain*
- *Deficient Fluid Volume*
- *Imbalanced Nutrition: Less than Body Requirements*
- *Disturbed Body Image*
- *Ineffective Coping*

Outcomes for clients with burns include, but are not limited to, the following:

- Respirations will remain within normal range and clear (**eupneic**).
- O_2 saturation will remain above 95%.
- Pain will be controlled by regularly administered medication.
- Client will maintain weight.
- Client will verbalize feelings about the injury and identify sources of support.

A client with a burn has lost the first line of defense against infection. Depending on the extent of the burn injury, a topical antimicrobial agent (silver nitrate, silver sulfadiazine, or mafenide acetate) and closed dressing may be applied (Figure 47-14 ■).

If the wound area is large, the client is also at risk for loss of fluid and loss of body heat (*Ineffective Thermoregulation*). Damage to tissues may interfere with circulation, leading to loss of fluid and decreased tissue perfusion. Increased demands for nourishment may cause imbalanced

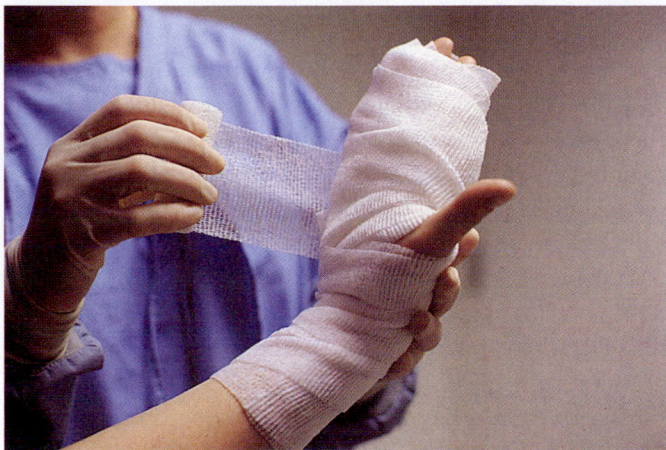

Figure 47-14. ■ Closed method of dressing a burn.

nutrition. In addition, the pain, trauma, and visible damage done to the body result in increased stress and psychosocial strain for the client. In the EC or UC setting, the primary concerns are airway, breathing, and circulation.

- In the EC or UC, the nurse's most important interventions support the client's ABCs. *Airway management and securing the airway when burns to the face and neck areas have been sustained are critical.*
- The nurse monitors O_2 administration and saturation whenever there are burns to the face and neck. *Edema and damage to the airway can be life threatening.*
- Monitor IV therapy/lifeline. *A 16- to 18-gauge IV is routinely established in case of third spacing and shock.*
- Take vital signs frequently and monitor LOC for changes. These can be subtle. *The first sign is often missed. Changes may indicate impending shock.*
- Provide clients with sterile blankets or gowns if the percentage of estimated burns is severe and if heat loss occurs. *Full-thickness burn areas have lost the ability to retain or create heat related to the loss of skin; therefore, the nurse must keep the client's body temperature warm.*
- Maintain infection precautions. *The client's first line of defense has been injured or destroyed. Clients with burns are at risk for sepsis, infection, and death.*
- Provide or assist in treatment for minor burns including pain management, anti-infective medications (Silvadene, Flamazine), and wound care for the client (see Figure 47-14). Teaching is an important function in these cases. *The client, parent, or family member must continue treatment until the wound is healed. The nurse plays an important role in teaching the client what normal healing and trouble signs look like. The nurse also provides client education about ways to prevent future injuries.*

EVALUATING

The nurse evaluates the client's status frequently to be sure ABCs are stable. Changes in client condition are always reported stat to the primary care provider.

NURSING PROCESS CARE PLAN
Client with Burns

You are the practical nurse planning in the care of a 51-year-old client admitted to the EC with burns to the face and neck. The nares (nostrils) are also singed. On review, the client complains of difficulty breathing and severe discomfort to the affected areas.

Assessment

VS: T 98.7, P 100, R 26, BP 110/60. The client is oriented to person, place, and time. Pain is rated an 8 on a scale of 0 to 10.

Nursing Diagnosis

The following important nursing diagnosis (among others) is established for this client:

- *Ineffective Airway Clearance* related to burns to the face, neck, and nares

Expected Outcomes

The outcomes for this client will include the following:

- Respirations will remain within normal range.
- O_2 saturation will remain above 95%.
- Breath sounds will be clear and equal to auscultation.
- Pain will be managed at a mild level (i.e., less than a rating of 3).

Planning and Implementation

The following interventions are planned and implemented for the client:

- Administer O_2 as ordered; titrate as necessary via nonrebreather mask. *O_2 high flow improves oxygen saturation levels for ABC and sustaining life.*
- Monitor respirations every 5 to 10 minutes for acute changes and report. *The nurse must watch for changes in LOC and O_2 as a sign or symptom of shock and client decompensation.*
- Monitor O_2 saturations for changes in conjunction with respiratory rate, and report stat to primary care provider. *Communication of changes in the client's condition to the primary care provider are important so that orders for improved outcomes can be achieved in a timely manner.*
- Administer analgesia for pain as ordered. *Client's pain must be relieved so that increased O_2 consumption will be reduced, and pain will be alleviated.*

- Evaluate lung sounds every hour and prn for changes and report. *Reporting changes in lung sounds to the primary care provider allows for improved outcomes for the client who is in respiratory compromise.*
- Assist ventilation via bag-valve-mask (BVM) unit if *bradypnea* (low respiration rate) occurs. Notify primary care provider stat. *Maintaining adequate ventilation is necessary when the clients are bradypneic and hypoxic. The BVM is a device that fosters high-flow O_2 and improved oxygen levels when used on clients with hypoxia.*

Evaluation

Client demonstrates ability to maintain safe effective respirations and rate. O_2 saturation level remains greater than 95%. Breath sounds are clear bilaterally. Pain management interventions effective; pain is controlled and reduced to a 2 at this time.

Critical Thinking in the Nursing Process

1. Identify factors that place client at risk for airway ineffectiveness.
2. Discuss why pain management may be indicated with burns to the face and neck. Identify possible medications that may be administered for the client.
3. What are the potential risks the client may face during the rehabilitation process with burns to the upper torso? List three nursing diagnoses that may be applicable.

Note: Discussion of Critical Thinking questions appears on the MyNursingKit Website.

Death in the EC

The role of the nurse when dealing with death in the EC is difficult. Death is often sudden and unexpected in the EC, as client problems overwhelm attempts at treatment. The nurse must be prepared to deal with death of clients of any age from very young to very old. Emotional, physical, cultural, and legal issues are involved when a death occurs in the EC setting.

If a client has died and you must notify a family member by phone, it is best to say, "There has been an accident." Ask the person to come to the EC, and do not tell them of the death over the telephone.

Assisting the grieving family is a responsibility of the healthcare team in the EC environment. The nurse must recognize and implement involvement of the interdisciplinary team (social service, chaplains, and case management).

Depending on the reason for death, certain policies and procedures must be carried out by the team. These can include preparing for donation of life organs and postmortem care for the client.

Sensitivity and awareness by the nurse are expected during times of death. Counseling and assisting the family are of the utmost importance during a crisis or after the death of a loved one. The nurse and healthcare team must document interventions and outcomes.

> **Note:** The references and resources for all chapters have been compiled at the back of the book.

PROCEDURE 47-1 Applying a Splint

Purpose

- To immobilize an injured extremity to prevent further injury until swelling decreases and a cast can be applied

Equipment

- Ready-made or customized splint appropriate for the area of injury
- Velcro® straps or elastic bandage
- Clips or tape

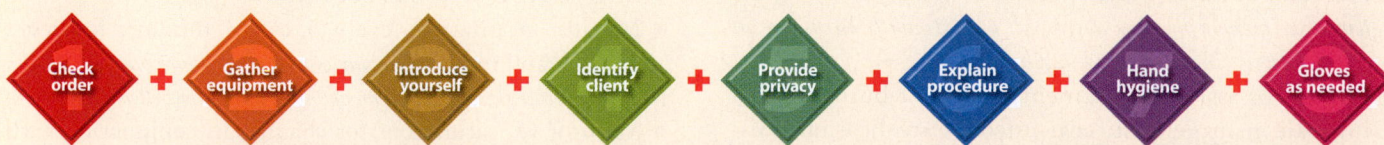

Check order + Gather equipment + Introduce yourself + Identify client + Provide privacy + Explain procedure + Hand hygiene + Gloves as needed

Interventions and Rationales

1. Perform preparatory steps (see icon bar above).
2. Assist the client to the examination table. Place in a comfortable position supporting injured extremity. *In order for the splint to be applied properly, the client must be seated or lying down. Supporting the extremity can lessen the pain.*
3. Pad the inside of the splint (if necessary) and check for proper fit on the extremity. Ready-made splints (Figure 47-15 ■) are already padded. *On a custom splint the padding will need to be added to support the extremity properly.*
4. Fasten the Velcro straps, or wrap splint and extremity evenly and snug enough to provide support but not

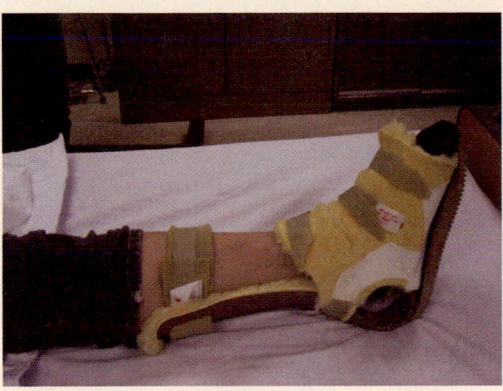 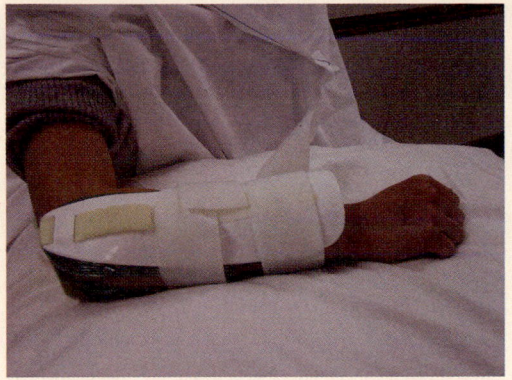

Figure 47-15. ■ Ready-made leg and arm splints.

enough to impede circulation of the limb, with an elastic bandage and fasten with clips or tape. *The splint and straps or wrapping should be only tight enough to immobilize the injured extremity. Wrapping that is too tight can impede circulation and increase swelling.*

5. Instruct the client to keep the extremity elevated and apply ice. *Elevating the extremity above the level of the heart and applying ice aid in decreasing swelling.*

6. Apply a sling for an arm splint (Figure 47-16 ■). *The sling will help the client support the injured arm and keep it elevated.*

7. If a leg splint has been applied, provide client with crutches and instructions for use. An elderly client may need a wheelchair rather than crutches. *The client should not bear weight on the splinted leg. Crutches can be used if the client is agile enough to use them to keep weight off the injured extremity. Otherwise the client should use a wheelchair until the limb is casted and weight bearing is allowed.*

8. Provide verbal and written instructions for follow-up care. *Instructions need to be given that include when the follow-up visit for casting is scheduled and how to care for injury until that time. Written instructions serve as a reminder when the client is at home.*

9. Document procedure.

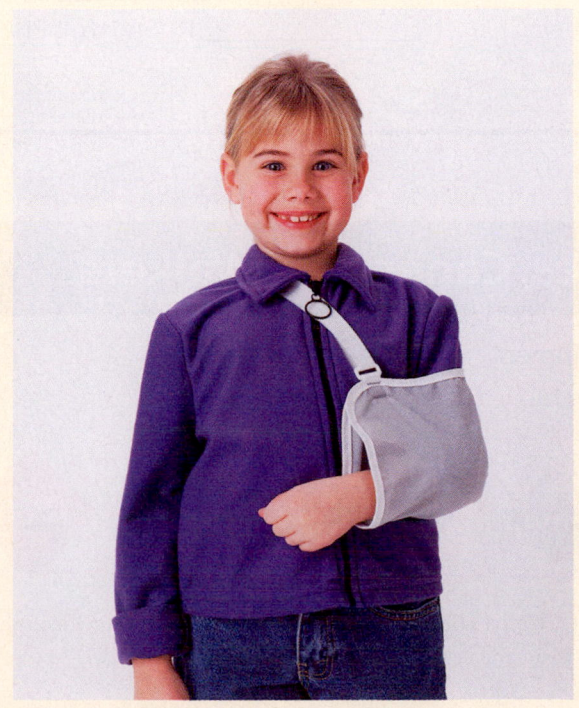

Figure 47-16. ■ Arm sling.

SAMPLE DOCUMENTATION

| [date] [time] | Splint applied to right lower leg and wrapped with elastic bandage, per Dr. Morrison, following x-ray that revealed tibia/fibula fracture. To return to orthopedic clinic on [date] for application of a cast. Verbal and written instructions given and client verbalized understanding. Crutches measured and fitted by PT and instructions for use given. Rx for Motrin 600 mg every 4 h prn pain. _____ _____ B. Rodgers, LVN |

PROCEDURE 47-2 Applying a Cast

Note: Cast application will be done by the healthcare provider unless you are specially trained to assist.

Purpose

- To prepare the materials for casting and application

Equipment

- Casting material, stockinette, padding, water, protective coverings (if needed)

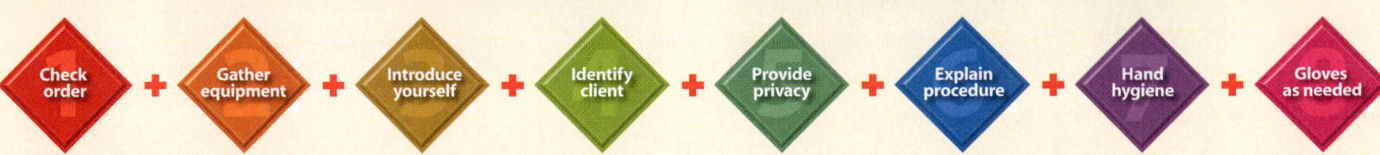

Interventions and Rationales

1. Perform preparatory steps (see icon bar above).

2. Determine the type of material the primary care provider or technician will be using.

3. Gather supplies and cover area with protective covering if needed.

4. Position client supporting the extremity to be cast. *Position will be determined by type of cast and area.*

5. Explain the procedure and tell the client that the cast may feel warm after application. Explain that no pressure should be put on the cast until it is dry. *Explanations will help the client understand what to expect and encourage cooperation. The cast is elevated on pillows until dry. Putting pressure (fingertips, edge of table) against the cast can cause an area of impaired circulation.*

6. Assist the primary care provider or technician during application by handing materials and holding the extremity.

7. When completed provide client and family with home care instructions. *To ensure compliance with treatment plan.*

SAMPLE DOCUMENTATION

[date] [time]	Short arm fiberglass cast applied to left arm, to treat Colles fracture. Home care instruction given. Client to report increased pain, swelling, or lack of circulation to primary care provider. _____ _____ R. Smith, LPN

PROCEDURE 47-3 Measuring for Crutches, Canes, and Walkers

Purpose

- To ensure proper fit for ambulation assistive devices

Equipment

- Measuring tape; hard sole street shoes

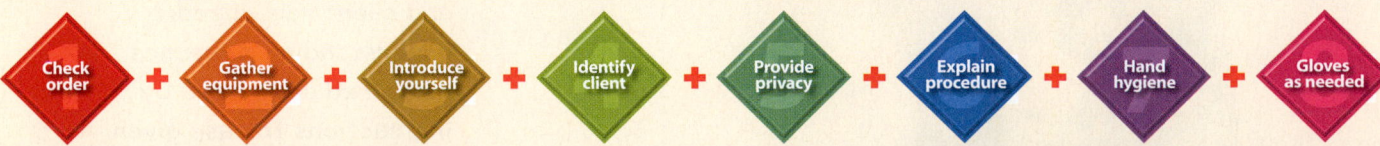

Interventions and Rationales

Crutches

1. Perform preparatory steps (see icon bar above).

2. Explain the procedure to the client. *Explanation will help gain cooperation from the client.*

3. Have the client put on the shoes that will be worn when using the crutches. *This ensures that crutches will be the proper length.*

4. Ask client to lay flat in bed with hands at side. *This permits measuring without requiring the client to bear weight.*

5. Measure the distance from the client's axilla to a point 15 to 20 cm (6 to 8 in.) out from the heel. *This will determine the length of the crutch.*

6. Adjust the hand bar on the crutches so that the client's elbows are always slightly bent. *This is proper position for the elbows when crutch walking.*

7. Have client stand with crutches under the arm. *This allows the nurse to check length.*

8. Measure the distance between the client's axilla and the crutch bar. *Crutches that do not fit the client correctly or crutches that are used incorrectly can damage the brachial plexus and cause paralysis of the arms.*

Variation for Canes

1. One cane. *A single cane is indicated for mild balance problems, fatigue with walking long distances, or increased weakness in one leg.*

2. Two canes. *Two canes are beneficial for further balance problems or increased weakness in both legs.*

3. Place the device 15.2 cm (6 in.) away from the side of foot and with arm relaxed, adjust the device so it is even with the crease on the inside of the wrist, with a 25° elbow flexion. *This is done to make sure the cane fits correctly.*

Variation for Walkers

Walkers help with more severe balance problems, progressive leg weakness in one or both legs, or fatigue.

1. Measure a walker in the same manner as a cane. *This will provide correct size.*

2. Confer with client and therapist on the appropriate type of walker. *Different types of walkers are prescribed depending on the client's physical needs and environment.*

SAMPLE DOCUMENTATION

[date]	Crutches measured according to
[time]	procedure; with client supine
	and standing. Hand bar adjusted.
	Crutch bar two finger widths
	from axilla. _____
	_____ S. Powell, LVN

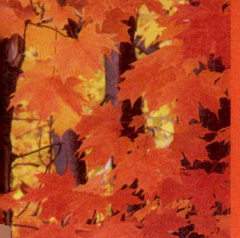

Chapter Review

KEY Points

- Triage is always performed in the EC setting. Triage is used to identify clients who should be treated as a priority. The UC setting generally treats clients on a first-come, first-served basis. The acuity of clients in the UC is less severe; clients who need emergency care are transferred to the EC.

- The LPN/LVN assists the RN in the treatment and care of clients in the EC setting. The ability of the LPN to collect data and perform assigned interventions is of critical importance. LPNs/LVNs are a valuable part of the healthcare team within the EC setting.

- Inadequate tissue perfusion can be an outcome of all types of shock. Changes in level of consciousness are generally the first sign of impending shock.

- The rule of nines is used in the EC setting to calculate percentage of burns and estimate outcomes.

- The identification of the substance responsible for a poisoning is the primary concern in determining positive treatment and outcomes for clients.

- If rabies is suspected in an animal bite, treatment is started and continued until rabies is ruled out.

- In cases of emergency, natural disaster, or acts of terrorism, the nurse follows established protocol to help support safety in the environment.

FOR FURTHER Study

Chapter 7 discusses the various types of healthcare systems.

Complementary medicines are discussed in Chapter 8.

For body mechanics, choking, and Heimlich maneuver information, see Chapter 9.

For Standard Precautions, see Figure 10-4.

See Chapter 11 for a discussion of interpersonal communication skills that can ensure the best client outcomes.

An adult admission form, a consent form for valuables, and details about HIPAA are shown in Chapter 14.

The Glasgow Coma Scale is shown in Table 19-2.

For more on wound care, see Chapter 23.

For more on hot/cold packs to an injured area, see Chapter 24.

Medication administration is discussed in Chapter 27.

IV piggyback medication administration and other IV procedures are discussed in Chapter 28.

The main discussion of respiratory disorders and their care is in Chapter 32.

Anaphylaxis is discussed further in Chapter 35.

Spinal cord injury, hematomas, and concussions are in Chapter 36.

For more information on rape, see Chapter 40.

Procedure 48-8 gives steps for performing an eye examination.

Guidelines for assisting pregnant women who have precipitous delivery are provided in Chapter 53.

The ear lavage procedure is common in young children and is described in Chapter 60.

Critical Thinking Care Map

Caring for a Client with Hypovolemia
NCLEX-PN® Focus Area: Physiological Integrity

Case Study: Max Bayer is a 64-year-old male admitted to the EC with excessive nausea, vomiting, and diarrhea for 3 days. He is unable to tolerate PO fluids and is extremely weak with malaise. An IV of 1,000 mL of 0.9 normal saline is infusing via a 16-gauge catheter at 100 mL/h in his left arm.

Nursing Diagnosis: *Deficient Fluid Volume*

COLLECT DATA

Subjective	Objective
_____	_____
_____	_____
_____	_____
_____	_____
_____	_____
_____	_____
_____	_____

Would you report this? Yes/No

If yes, report to: _____

What would you report? _____

Nursing Care

_____
_____
_____
_____
_____
_____
_____
_____
_____

How would you document this? _____
_____
_____
_____

Compare your answers and documentation to those provided on the MyNursingKit Website.

Data Collected
(use only those that apply)

- VS: T 99.2, P 92, R 22, BP 90/58
- "I feel so weak, yet I'm hungry."
- "I'm so worried, my daughter hasn't called all day."
- Skin turgor greater than 3 seconds
- Complains of nausea
- Mucous membranes dry and cracked
- Increased thirst
- K^+ 3.5 mEq/L
- Complains pain at 8 (on a scale of 0 to 10) one-half hour before medication scheduled
- Decreased appetite

Nursing Interventions
(use only those that apply; list in priority order)

- Monitor vital signs every 15 min.
- Encourage PO fluids.
- Instruct client on signs/symptoms of dehydration.
- Monitor IV site for infiltration.
- Notify primary care provider regarding K^+ level.
- Administer antiemetics as ordered.
- Notify clergy.
- Assist PT with ambulation.
- Administer high-flow O_2.
- Order chest x-ray stat.
- Record I&O every shift.

NCLEX-PN® Exam Preparation

1 A nurse, working in the emergency department, is caring for a client after defibrillation from cardiac dysrhythmia. Which of the following observations is the highest priority for the nurse?

1. O_2 flow rate
2. Airway management
3. Changes in cardiac rhythm
4. Level of consciousness

2 A nurse, working in the emergency department, is preparing a client for discharge. When teaching the client about a new prescription for daily digoxin (Lanoxin), the nurse evaluates a need for further teaching when the client says:

1. "I should call my doctor if my pulse goes outside the range you gave me."
2. "I should be careful not to mix these up with my other medications."
3. "If I forget to take my pill, I'll just take two the next day."
4. "I know to call the doctor if I have any questions."

3 The nurse, working in the emergency department, is caring for a client with a partial-thickness burn to the face and neck areas. The priority nursing concern would be:

1. Airway management.
2. IV lifeline placement.
3. Sterile dressing application.
4. Maintenance of protective isolation.

4 A 42-year-old female is admitted to the emergency department with a medication overdose. Vital signs are BP 118/70, P 84, R 20. Which of the following nursing interventions is of highest priority for this client?

1. Insertion of a gastric lavage tube.
2. Identification of the medication taken and reporting it to the physician.
3. Administering syrup of ipecac as ordered.
4. Monitoring vital signs.

5 The nurse is gathering data for the triage nurse and admits a combative, confused client in the emergency department. The client states he has been consuming alcohol and has a severe headache. He has an abrasion over the left temple. The client is demanding pain medication for the headache. The nurse's best response is:

1. "You are fourth on the triage list; it'll only be forty-five minutes longer."
2. "I will need to take your vital signs and report to the doctor first."
3. "What type of pain medicine do you normally take?"
4. "I know your headache is causing you discomfort. I will give you your pain medicine as soon as I talk to the doctor."

6 The nurse is working in the emergency department when the department receives notification of a mass casualty event caused by an unknown biological agent. The nurse would respond to this event by:

1. Following the facility's Emergency Operations Plan.
2. Following routine policies for care of clients within the department.

3. Discharging all clients currently in the department to make room for the mass casualty clients.
4. Obtaining additional assistance from other departments.

7 The nurse admits a client to the emergency department who is diagnosed with a simple closed fracture of the left ulna. When providing discharge teaching for the newly casted client, the nurse would instruct the client to: (Select all that apply.)

1. Apply ice to the arm for 24 to 48 hours.
2. Notify the family physician if the client notes any loss of sensation or tingling in the fingers.
3. Elevate the arm above the level of the heart by propping it on a table next to the client's bed.
4. Avoid getting the plaster cast wet by placing a plastic bag around the cast when bathing.
5. Do not insert anything sharp into the cast if the client experiences itching, but use ice or a hair dryer set to cool.

8 After the death of a client brought to the emergency department following trauma, the nurse is asked to notify the parents and ask them to come to the hospital. The nurse would notify the parents by saying:

1. "I'm sorry to tell you your son was involved in a motor vehicle crash and passed away. Can you come to the emergency department immediately to identify the body?"
2. "Is there anyone at home with you? I'm afraid your son died in a motor vehicle crash. Please have someone drive you to the hospital emergency department immediately."
3. "Your son was involved in a motor vehicle crash and we need you to get to the hospital as soon as possible."
4. "Your son was involved in a motor vehicle crash. Is there someone who could bring you to the hospital? Please, drive safely and do not exceed the speed limits but come to the hospital as soon as you can."

9 The nurse admits a 24-month-old child with a diagnosis of insulin dependent diabetes mellitus who was found to be unresponsive after his nap. The child's vital signs are T 97.2 axillary, R 130, P 60, BP 70/38 with an oxygen saturation of 67%. The mother reports the child's blood sugar was 396 and this is confirmed by the nurse after performing a fingerstick blood glucose. The nurse's priority action is to:

1. Administer O_2.
2. Initiate an IV line.
3. Begin cardiopulmonary resuscitation.
4. Insert a Foley catheter for urine sample.

10 The nurse, working in the emergency department, admits an unresponsive client from a long-term facility in shock. The client has had a Foley catheter and is currently taking antibiotics for a urinary tract infection. She has not been feeling well for 5 days. The nurse anticipates the client is demonstrating what type of shock?

1. Hypovolemic
2. Cardiogenic
3. Septic
4. Neurogenic

Answers and rationales for Review Questions appear in Appendix I.

Chapter 48

Community Nursing

LEARNING Outcomes

After completing this chapter, you will be able to:

1. Identify common community nursing care settings.
2. Describe the LPN/LVN scope of practice in a physician's office or outpatient surgery center.
3. List important aspects of nursing care in a school health office or clinic.
4. Identify nursing responsibilities in home care and hospice.
5. Describe the client admission process and preparation of a client for examination in a physician's office or clinic.
6. List ways the LPN/LVN can assist with office surgical procedures.
7. Explain how to perform or assist with office screening and testing procedures.

Clinical Objectives

8. Admit a new client in a physician's office.
9. Prepare a client for a physical examination.
10. Assist a physician with an office surgical procedure.
11. Perform a 12-lead ECG.
12. Perform a venipuncture.
13. Obtain a capillary blood sample.
14. Assist a physician with a sigmoidoscopy.
15. Measure visual acuity and test for color blindness.
16. Conduct audiometric testing.
17. Perform a test for scoliosis screening.

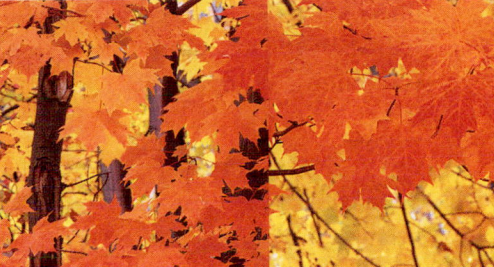

BRIEF Outline

Community Care Settings
Other Practice Areas

KEY TERMS

Use the audio glossary feature on the MyNursingKit Website to hear the correct pronunciation of the following key terms.

adult day care facility 1310

ambulatory care nursing 1310

assisted living facility 1310

clinics 1310

correctional nurse 1310

mental health clinic 1310

same-day surgery clinic 1310

school-based health clinic 1310

school health office 1310

scoliometer 1312

summer day camp 1310

traveling nurse 1310

urgent care office 1310

The opportunities for the LPN/LVN to deliver nursing care in the community have increased during the past few years. In the not so distant past, LPN/LVN students could only look forward to jobs in skilled nursing facilities or in medical-surgical units of acute hospitals. Today, with the nursing shortage and higher client acuity, many other opportunities have become available. These practice settings require the ability to think critically and to function at times without direct supervision of a registered nurse. In this chapter you will learn about opportunities to use your nursing skills in community settings.

Community Care Settings

When ambulatory care nursing is considered, the primary location that comes to mind is the physician's office. In addition, you may wish to consider clinics, urgent care offices (see Chapter 47 ⬭⬭ for full coverage of urgent care nursing), school health offices, child and adult day care, medical research offices, outpatient or same-day surgery clinics, cardiac rehab centers, physical and occupational therapy centers, dialysis centers, home care, and traveling and/or companion nursing (Figure 48-1 ■). A description of selected ambulatory settings is provided in Box 48-1 ■.

The scope of practice of LPNs and LVNs in these settings is delineated by the state board of nursing in the state where you are delivering care. It is described in the state's nurse practice act.

PHYSICIAN'S OFFICE

When the LPN/LVN is employed in a physician's office, he or she will be supervised by the physician or by a registered nurse. In smaller offices, there may not be a registered nurse. A medical assistant should not be given the authority to supervise the licensed nurse. Although the medical assistant may be designated as an office manager, in matters related to client care the LPN/LVN is responsible to the RN or directly to the physician. It is very important that the LPN/LVN understand the scope of practice and adhere to it at all times.

Some of the duties that the LPN/LVN may be called on to perform in the office are:

- Admitting new clients (Figure 48-2 ■; see the admitting steps in Procedure 48-1 ■ later in this chapter)

- Preparing clients for examination by the physician or nurse practitioner (Procedure 48-2 ■)
- Assisting with diagnostic and surgical office procedures (Procedures 48-3 ■ and 48-6 ■)
- Conducting electrocardiograms (Procedure 48-4 ■)
- Performing lab tests (Procedure 48-5 ■)

(Step-by-step procedures appear at the end of this chapter.)

With the exception of the receptionist, the person who escorts the client from the waiting room to the exam room is responsible for the impression the entire experience has on the new client. As a nurse, you are responsible for maintaining not only your reputation, but also the reputation of the physician for whom you are working. New clients should always be greeted warmly, using their title and last name. During the admission period you may ask how the client wishes to be addressed. If the client prefers to be addressed less formally, she or he will let you know at that time.

It is common procedure to weigh clients prior to seating them in the exam room. Many clients are self-conscious about their weight. If the scale is in the hallway, be discrete if other staff or clients are in the area.

Although the physician's office may be very busy, when possible take a few minutes to introduce yourself, describe the office, and get to know the new client prior to beginning your assessment. Make the client comfortable and perform as much of the assessment as possible prior to having the client disrobe. This is an important consideration if there may be a delay before the physician sees the client.

Once the client has disrobed, be sure to inquire if he or she is warm enough. If the client is cool, provide a blanket.

After the physician has completed the consultation and examination, assist the client to dress if necessary. Be sure that the client has all prescriptions, referrals, and instructions prior to leaving the office.

Follow-Up

It is important that the client be notified of the results of any tests or lab work conducted during the visit. Inform the physician when results have been received. The physician decides who will contact the client with results. If office protocol demands it, the client will be contacted and instructed to make an appointment.

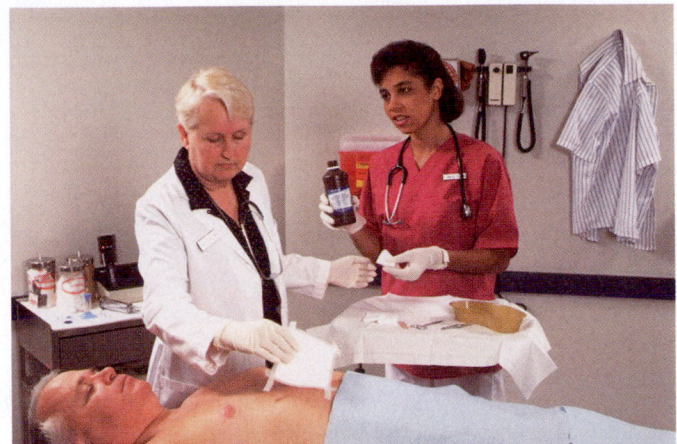
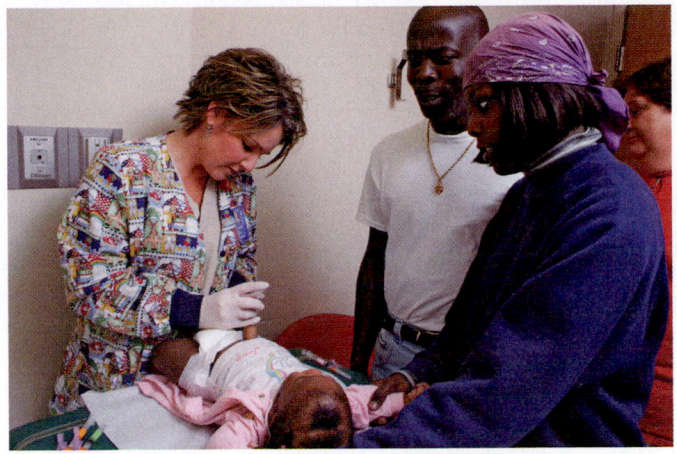
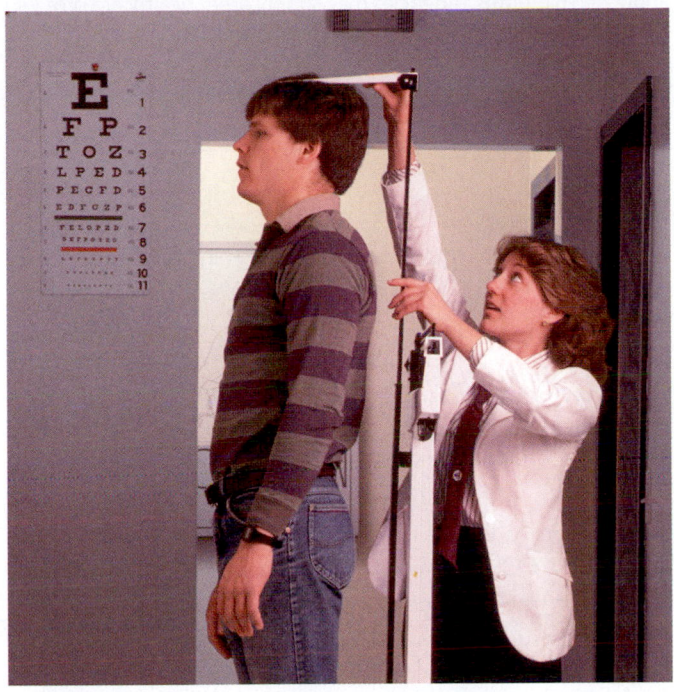
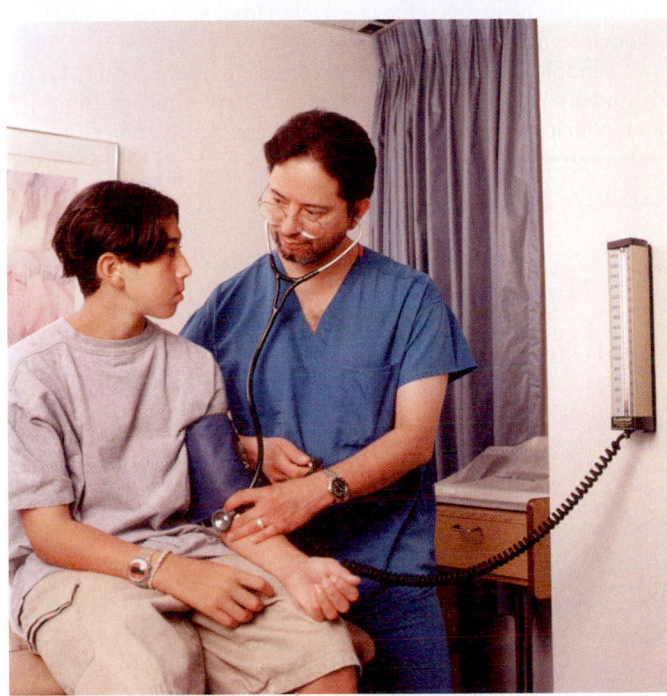

Figure 48-1. ■ Examples of alternate care settings in which LPNs/LVNs can practice.

Confidentiality

The LPN/LVN employed in the physician's office must protect the client's privacy. This may be more difficult to ensure than in the hospital setting. Because the waiting room may be small and crowded, it is inappropriate to ask a client questions while standing at the reception window. If the receptionist or billing clerk is overheard discussing treatment or insurance issues where others can overhear the conversation, mention this to the office manager or physician.

HIPAA requirements apply to physicians' offices, just as they do to in-client settings. If you are responsible for calling test results to the client, take care not to leave private information on a home answering machine, on office voice mail, or with another person, not even a family member. If a message must be left, you could say something similar to

this: "Mrs. Alvarez, this is Marie. Would you please call me at 555-1345 between 9 A.M. and 5 P.M. concerning your appointment." Be sure to inform the client during the office visit that you will be calling him or her with the results and how you will be leaving the message, so that your call is not confused with a telemarketing call. To adhere to HIPAA regulations, the office will provide information to new clients that outlines rules governing release of information. For additional information concerning HIPAA, see Table 14-1 ⚭ .

OUTPATIENT SURGERY CENTERS

Outpatient or same-day surgery centers have become very popular in many areas of the country. The client arrives early in the morning and returns home after he or she is fully recovered from the anesthesia. Although registered

BOX 48-1   SELECTED AMBULATORY CARE SETTINGS

Ambulatory care nursing: Care provided to clients in a physician's office or clinic, in which the client obtains some medical service before returning home the same day

Clinics: Walk-in medical facilities where clients can obtain diagnostic testing or treatment before returning home the same day; also known as ambulatory care centers

Urgent care office: Walk-in medical facility where clients can obtain treatment for minor injuries and acute illnesses; may be connected to or affiliated with a hospital

School health office: Room or area within a school where medications and first aid supplies are kept and distributed by qualified personnel

Same-day surgery clinic: Health facility in which the client arrives early in the day, has a surgical procedure, and returns home after he or she is fully recovered from anesthesia; also known as an outpatient surgical center

School-based health clinics: Ambulatory care centers, located in a number of intercity school districts, which perform a higher level of care than the typical school nurse office

Summer day camp: A daytime program for children where LPNs/LVNs may obtain work; staff must be trained in first aid and CPR

Mental health clinic: Medical facilities whose focus is on psychosocial issues and mental health status of its clients

Adult day care facility: Center that provides health and social services to the older adult who is still living at home

Assisted living facility: Facility that meets the needs of the ambulatory older adult; various degrees of personal care assistance may be provided

Traveling nurse: Companion nurse; a licensed nurse who works for a company that contracts with healthcare agencies to provide them with staff. The "traveler" may be provided with housing and traveling expenses. The assignments vary in length, usually about 4 to 6 months. (Agencies may supply other healthcare professionals also, such as physical and occupational therapists.)

Correctional nurse: Nurse who provides for the health care of inmates in correctional facilities such as juvenile offender homes, jails, prisons, and penitentiaries

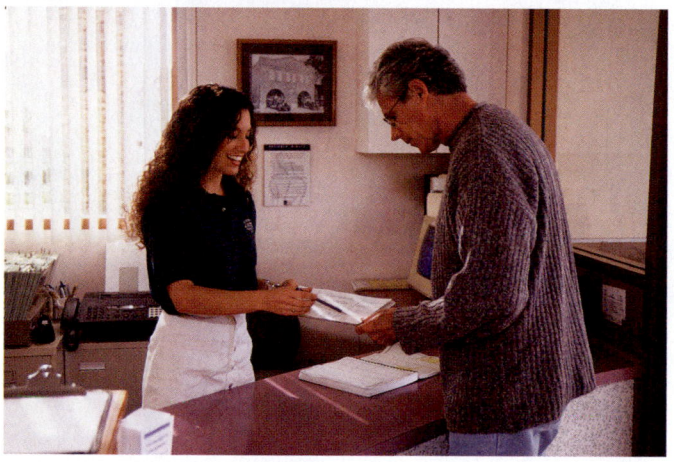

Figure 48-2. ■ The nurse in the physician's office greets the client and sets a positive tone for the visit. *Source:* PhotoEdit Inc.

nurses serve as the circulating nurse during surgery and in the postop recovery area, LPNs/LVNs are in demand for the admission area. In some states LPNs/LVNs are also trained to assist in surgery as scrub techs.

In the admission area, the LPN/LVN would be responsible for completing the admission paperwork with the surgical client. (See the perioperative chapter, Chapter 29 ⊙⊙, for an example of a preop checklist.) After the client is undressed and wearing the hospital gown, ask the client if he or she needs to use the restroom. The client will then be assisted onto the gurney or a lounge chair so that the nurse can obtain vital signs and any other required assessment. Any collected data that is outside the normal parameters should be reported to the charge nurse, anesthesiologist, or

surgeon immediately, because surgery may need to be postponed. (Procedures for collecting vital sign measurements are found in Chapter 21 ⊙⊙.)

The LPN/LVN will also inquire about the last time clients ate or drank and if they have taken any medications this morning. Although the admission area can be fast paced due to the large number of early admissions, it is important that you take time to answer all the client's or family members' questions and inform them of all department procedures. Once the client is ready for surgery, document all of your findings and inform the clerk of transportation that the client is ready.

An LPN/LVN who is hired to work in the surgery suite or recovery area will be given additional training. Check with your state board of nursing to determine if the duties you will be performing are within your scope of practice.

SCHOOL HEALTH OFFICE OR CLINIC

In addition to physician's offices and surgery centers, LPNs/LVNs have been employed as health aides in school health offices or clinics. Many school districts are unable or unwilling to staff the health office at each school with a registered nurse. The district school nurse would serve as the supervisor for the LPN/LVN health aide. (The title of health technician or health clerk is also frequently used.) The school district will also retain a physician, who will serve as the medical director and will sign protocols for the school health office.

In this capacity the LPN/LVN administers basic first aid and conducts health screenings (discussed later in the chapter). He or she would also monitor health records such as immunizations. Having a licensed nurse on campus can offer the opportunity for health teaching for students as well as staff.

Working with minors in a school situation requires extra care in record keeping. A licensed nurse, no matter what the level of education, may not provide even over-the-counter medication to students without parental permission and physician's instructions. The LPN/LVN must follow office protocols that have been set up by the credentialed school nurse. This nurse will supervise the LPN/LVN who is employed as a health clerk or aide. The health aide should always contact the supervising nurse when an issue outside protocol presents itself.

A number of intercity school districts have school-based health clinics that perform a higher level of care. In many of these clinics a pediatric nurse practitioner is in charge of the clinic, and he or she follows the standards and protocols set forth by the medical director. When a high school has a health clinic, potential legal and ethical issues can arise. Students relate many of these issues to their involvement in sexual activity. The nurse must be aware of state laws and school district policies for providing information or treatment for sexually transmitted infections and referrals for pregnancy. The adolescent client may confide in the health clinic nurse. This presents ethical issues involving privacy and confidentiality, as well as the need for parent involvement in health issues of a minor.

School health clinic and health office staffs encounter many opportunities for preventive health education for both students and families. Involvement of the family in health education programs can provide a forum for students to communicate with parents on personal health issues they have previously been reluctant to discuss. Many parents do not know how to approach their teen about sexual activity and drug, alcohol, and tobacco use. The school nurse can provide training in this area for parents. The school health staff can be proactive in establishing communication about good health habits in the students and their families.

Nurses in a school setting often must provide initial care for injuries sustained on the playground. This might involve ice for a strain or sprain (see Heat and Cold Applications in Chapter 24). It might also include first aid for an abrasion or splinting to immobilize a limb (see Chapter 47 for emergency and urgent care).

Administering Medication in School Settings

Health issues in the schools are becoming more complex. There has been an increase in the number of students of all ages who require blood glucose monitoring, carbohydrate counting, and insulin administration. Students as young as 9 years old are managing their own care with supervision of

the school nurse, while most high school students are completely independent. Many school districts are pushing for unlicensed staff to supervise students' diabetic care. The School Nurse Association as well as the ANA have policies against such practices and have filed a suit against the Superintendent of Public Instruction to prevent this dangerous practice in California. In addition to diabetic care, asthma has become another serious health care concern in the schools. Students with a diagnosis of asthma should have medication via inhaler available at school. Depending on the school district or state policy, the inhaler will be carried by the student or kept in the school health office. No matter where the medication is kept, the school must have a parental release and a physician's prescription on file.

On occasion, medication may not be available or may not be effective. In that case the school nurse, licensed health technician, and unlicensed staff must know the procedures to be followed. Box 48-2 ■ provides emergency procedures for an asthma episode.

clinical ALERT

When medication is not available, *mild* symptoms may be alleviated by having the student drink a room-temperature cola drink.

The nurse must be alert to the danger of *nonwheezing asthma*. Deaths have been associated with this condition, when nurses failed to provide inhalers because students were not wheezing.

Preventing Spread of Infection

Infections in the school are also an increased concern. In the fall of 2007 media attention about CAMRSA (community acquired methicillin-resistant *Staphylococcus aureus*) caused panic in many school districts. Chapter 10 provides complete information on CAMRSA in schools.

Meningitis is a grave concern when it appears in the community, especially in schools. Colleges now require

---

BOX 48-2	EMERGENCY PROCEDURES FOR ASTHMA CARE

- Do not leave the student alone.
- Keep the student in a sitting position.
- Administer fast-acting inhaler (if available).
- Give the student room-temperature water to drink.
- Call 911 or take the student to the nearest emergency facility if the student has
  - An uncontrollable cough.
  - Difficulty speaking.
  - Cyanosis.
- Be sure a parent or emergency contact is notified.

incoming students living in dorms to be vaccinated against meningitis.

More common infections such as chickenpox or conjunctivitis are highly contagious. Students with evidence of these diseases are excluded from school until they have been cleared by the doctor or are symptom free.

Providing Screenings

SCOLIOSIS SCREENING. Scoliosis, a lateral curvature of the spine (Figure 48-3 ■), can be detected in children during the growth spurt period between the ages of 10 and 15 years. Girls are affected more often than boys. About 2 in 100 people have a mild form of scoliosis. Scoliosis can be relatively easily detected by performing a 30-second scoliosis screen. If scoliosis is detected early, then treatment can be started before it becomes a physical or emotional disability. State requirements provide a method to ensure that all school-age children are screened for scoliosis, and to ensure that all children who fail the screening are referred for appropriate medical follow-up. The steps for scoliosis screening are provided in Procedure 48-7 ■ on page 1328).

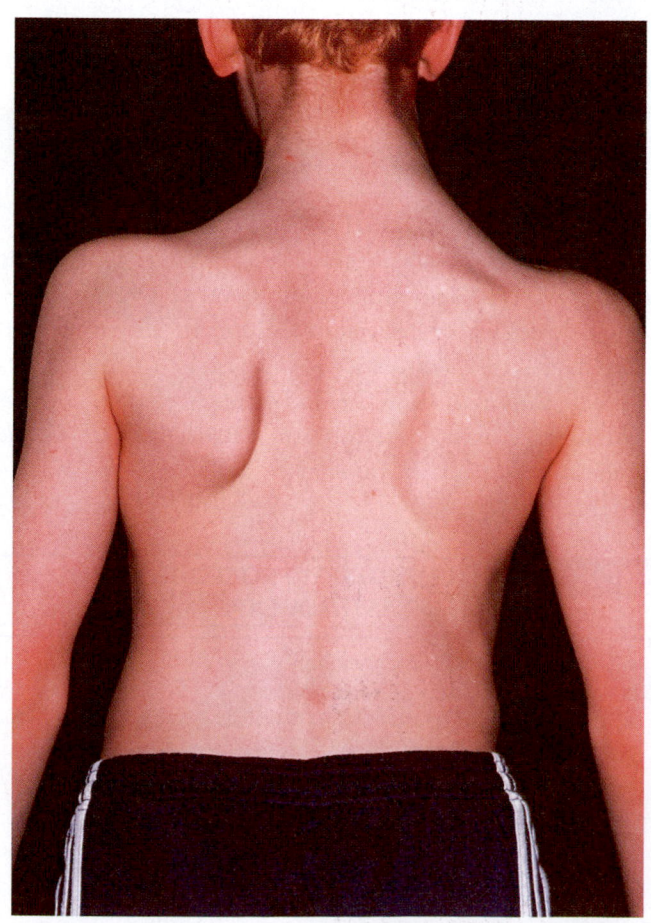

Figure 48-3. ■ Scoliosis.

Guidelines of Scoliosis Screening Program

- *Qualifications of screeners:* Screeners shall be licensed physicians, individuals trained by a certified scoliosis screening instructor. School health personnel, volunteers, and other school employees will not perform scoliosis screening.
- *Guidelines for screening:* Girls in the 5th grade through the 10th grade should receive a scoliosis screening every year. Boys receive a scoliosis screening every other year from the 6th grade through the 10th grade.
- *Screening procedure:* The scoliosis screening procedure is used as the first stage of screening. If the scoliosis screening procedure indicates positive findings for possible scoliosis, the **scoliometer** (a device for measuring the amount of abnormal spinal curvature) will be used as the second stage of screening.
- *Recommendation for referral:* Refer a child with an abnormal screening and/or scoliometer reading of 7 degrees or more to a licensed physician. It is highly recommended that a child with a scoliometer reading of more than 8 degrees be referred to an orthopedist.
- *Referral system:* A certified scoliosis screening instructor or school health nurse shall contact the parents of a child who fails the screening by letter, telephone call, or in person to:
  1. Explain the findings.
  2. Define and discuss scoliosis.
  3. Discuss the need for referral to a licensed physician.
- The school provides a scoliosis screening report to the parent to take to the licensed physician. (Regulations of the Commissioner of Education Section 136.1–3 March 2006.)

Directions for Use of a Scoliometer. An *inclinometer* (scoliometer) measures distortions of the torso. The client is asked to bend over, with arms dangling and palms pressed together, until a curve can be observed in the thoracic area (the upper back). The scoliometer is placed on the back and used to measure the *apex* (the highest point) of the curve. The client is then asked to continue bending until the curve in the lower back can be seen; the apex of this curve is then measured.

The measurements are repeated twice, with the client returning to a standing position between repetitions. The results of the scoliometer can indicate problems, and some experts believe it is a useful device for widespread screening. Scoliometers, however, measure rib cage distortions in more than half of children who turn out to have very minor or no sideways curves. Scoliometers are not accurate enough to guide treatment. If results show a deformity, x-rays need to be performed.

Follow-Up. Students who were not screened because of absence should be scheduled within 90 days after the missed screening. Any reason for exclusion from the screening is documented.

The school shall recontact the parents of students who failed the screening and were referred, but then missed that appointment. This contact is made by letter, telephone call, or in person at least one additional time to discuss the importance of follow-up. Refer to Procedure 48-7 for the scoliosis screening procedure.

VISUAL AND HEARING ACUITY SCREENINGS. The LPN/LVN in the school setting is also asked to perform visual and hearing tests on school children according to established state and school policies. Visual acuity tests for school children are described in Procedure 48-8 ■ on page 1329. Screening tests for hearing are described in Procedure 48-9 ■.

Immunizations

The school nurse or health clerk is also responsible for keeping records of students' immunizations. An immunization record should be on file for each student in the school (Figure 48-4 ■). Students who do not have up-to-date immunizations may be excluded from school. Some students cannot be immunized because of a compromised immune system (e.g., a child receiving chemotherapy). In the event of an identified case of measles, mumps, rubella, or chickenpox, these children would be excluded from school to protect them from exposure and possible health complications.

Parents may sign a waiver for their child because of religious reasons or personal objection to immunizations. The school will honor the waiver, but the parents are informed in writing that their child may be excluded from school in the event that their lack of immunizations presents a health risk to students or staff. The American Academy of Pediatrics frequently reviews and updates the immunization schedules. Table 48-1 ■ illustrates such an immunization schedule.

Immunizing School-Aged Children for Influenza. In recent years there was some thought that it might not be necessary to immunize children over the age of 2 against influenza unless they suffered from a chronic illness. Although influenza may not be serious for healthy children in the elementary school-age group, infected children are a risk to others. Elementary school children are notorious "spreaders and shedders" of infection. Their lack of good hand hygiene and poor control of sneezing and nasal discharge, as well as the fact that they are contagious for up to 4 days before and 14 to 20 days after signs and symptoms appear, have increased the need for them to be immunized.

It is also recommended that, in the first year a child is immunized, the child should receive an additional dose of the vaccine 4 to 6 weeks after the first dose.

HOME CARE AND HOSPICE

Until a few years ago, home care and hospice agencies would not employee LPNs/LVNs until they had completed 2 or more years of acute hospital experience. The nursing shortage has resulted in some allowances being made in this area. A new graduate may be hired and be given on-the-job training under the direction of a case manager RN. An LPN/LVN with previous experience as a home health aide or a hospice caregiver may have more opportunities to be hired once licensed. Working in home care or home-based hospice care requires the nurse to have well-developed observational and critical thinking skills. Although the case manager is available by phone, home care requires the nurse to assess the client and the situation independently. When a client is admitted to home care or hospice, a registered nurse makes an initial visit to do the admission. An RN case manager will make occasional visits, but regular visits may be assigned to an LPN/LVN or an aide to carry out. The decision to assign a licensed nurse rather than a home health aide will depend on the level of care required.

The decision to work in hospice is one that needs to be considered carefully. The LPN/LVN working in this area must have well-developed communication skills and the ability to provide empathic care in crisis situations. Hospice agencies provide ongoing training and support for staff, to assist them in providing quality care to clients who may not have long to live. Hospice care can be given in the client's home, but it can also continue if the client needs to be admitted into a skilled nursing facility. A nurse may see clients in both settings. The client's physician will certify the diagnosis and refer the client for admission. For additional information about hospice and end-of-life care, see Chapter 44 ∞.

Other Practice Areas

Opportunities for LPNs/LVNs to use their skills are varied and interesting. With research and investigation, nurses can find a career opportunity that will interest and excite them. A few of these opportunities are described here.

The correctional nurse provides for the health care of inmates in correctional facilities such as juvenile offender homes, jails, prisons, and penitentiaries. An LPN/LVN would work under the supervising correctional nurse who is an RN.

Some of the health problems that will be addressed are trauma, influenza, and chronic health problems, including AIDS, substance abuse, mental illness, renal failure/dialysis, respiratory diseases, and terminal cancer. An LPN/LVN who has been trained to draw blood may be employed in an intake center. A nurse who has a desire to make a difference and establish long-term relationships can be rewarded with

(Text continues on p.1316.)

Vaccine Administration Record for Children and Teens

Client name: _____

Birthdate: _____

Chart number: _____

Vaccine	Type of Vaccine[1] (generic abbreviation)	Date given (mo/day/yr)	Source (F,S,P) [2]	Site[3]	Vaccine		Vaccine Information Statement		Signature/ initials of vaccinator
					Lot #	Mfr.	Date on VIS [4]	Date given [4]	
Hepatitis B[5] (e.g., HepB, Hib-HepB, DTaP-HepB-IPV) Give IM.									
Diphtheria, Tetanus, Pertussis[5] (e.g., DTaP, DTaP-Hib, DTaP-HepB-IPV, DT, Tdap, Td) Give IM.									
Haemophilus influenzae **type b**[5] (e.g., Hib, Hib-HepB, DTaP-Hib) Give IM.									
Polio[5] (e.g., IPV, DTaP-HepB-IPV) Give IPV SC or IM. Give DTaP-HepB-IPV IM.									
Pneumococcal (e.g., PCV, conjugate; PPV, polysaccharide) Give PCV IM. Give PPV SC or IM.									
Rotavirus (Rv) Give oral (po).									
Measles, Mumps, Rubella[5] (e.g., MMR, MMRV) Give SC.									
Varicella[5] (e.g., Var, MMRV) Give SC.									
Hepatitis A (HepA) Give IM.									
Meningococcal (e.g., MCV4; MPSV4) Give MCV4 IM and MPSV4 SC.									
Human papillomavirus (e.g., HPV) Give IM.									
Influenza[5] (e.g., TIV, inactivated; LAIV, live attenuated) Give TIV IM. Give LAIV IN.									
Other									

1. Record the generic abbreviation for the type of vaccine given (e.g., DTaP-Hib, PCV), **not** the trade name.
2. Record the source of the vaccine given as either F (Federally-supported), S (State-supported), or P (supported by Private insurance or other Private funds).
3. Record the site where vaccine was administered as either RA (Right Arm), LA (Left Arm), RT (Right Thigh), LT (Left Thigh), IN (Intranasal), or O (Oral).
4. Record the publication date of each VIS as well as the date it is given to the patient.
5. For combination vaccines, fill in a row for each separate antigen in the combination.

Technical content reviewed by the Centers for Disease Control and Prevention, Nov. 2006.

www.immunize.org/catg.d/p2022b.pdf • Item #P2022 (11/06)

Immunization Action Coalition • 1573 Selby Ave. • St. Paul, MN 55104 • (651) 647-9009 • www.immunize.org • www.vaccineinformation.org

Figure 48-4. ■ Sample immunization record for children and teens. (Courtesy of Immunization Action Coalition, St. Paul, MN.)

TABLE 48-1	Childhood Immunization Schedule	
CHILD'S AGE	**VACCINE AND DOSE**	**PROTECTS AGAINST**
Birth to 2 months	Hepatitis B Dose 1 of 3	Hepatitis B virus (chronic inflammation of the liver, lifelong complications)
1 to 4 months	Hepatitis B Dose 2 of 3	Hepatitis B virus (chronic inflammation of the liver, lifelong complications)
2 months (part of well-baby visit)	DTaP Dose 1 of 5 Hib Dose 1 of 4 Polio (IPV) Dose 1 of 4 Pneumococcal conjugate (PCV7) Dose 1 of 4	Diphtheria, tetanus, whooping cough (pertussis) Infections of the blood, brain, joints, or lungs (pneumonia) Polio Infections of the blood, brain, joints, and inner ear
4 months (part of well-baby visit)	DTaP Dose 2 of 5 Hib Dose 2 of 4 Polio (IPV) Dose 2 of 4 Pneumococcal conjugate (PCV7) Dose 2 of 4	Diphtheria, tetanus, whooping cough (pertussis) Infections of the blood, brain, joints, or lungs (pneumonia) Polio Infections of the blood, brain, joints, and inner ear
6 months (part of well-baby visit)	DTaP Dose 3 of 5 Hib Dose 3 of 4 Pneumococcal conjugate (PCV7) Dose 3 of 4	Diphtheria, tetanus, whooping cough (pertussis) Infections of the blood, brain, joints, or lungs (pneumonia) Infections of the blood, brain, joints, and inner ear
6 to 18 months	Hepatitis B Dose 3 of 3 Polio (IPV) Dose 3 of 4	Hepatitis B virus (chronic inflammation of the liver, lifelong complications) Polio
6 to 23 months	Influenza 1 dose every year	Flu and complications
12 to 15 months	Hib Dose 4 of 4 Pneumococcal conjugate (PCV7) Dose 4 of 4 MMR Dose 1 of 2	Infections of the blood, brain, joints, or lungs (pneumonia) Infections of the blood, brain, joints, and inner ear Measles, mumps, and rubella (German measles)
12 to 18 months	Varicella Dose 1 of 1	Chickenpox
15 to 18 months	DTaP Dose 4 of 5	Diphtheria, tetanus, whooping cough (pertussis)
2 to 5 years	Pneumococcal polysaccharide (PPV23) Dose 1 of 2 (*high risk only*)	Infections of the blood, brain, joints, and inner ear
5 years through 18 years	Pneumococcal polysaccharide (PPV23) Dose 2 of 2 (follows 3–5 years after dose 1 if needed)	Infections of the blood, brain, joints, and inner ear

TABLE 48-1	Childhood Immunization Schedule (continued)	
CHILD'S AGE	**VACCINE AND DOSE**	**PROTECTS AGAINST**
2 to 18 years	Hepatitis A Dose 1 of 2	Hepatitis A (inflammation of the liver)
2 ½ years or older	Hepatitis A Dose 2 of 2 (follows 6 months after dose 1)	Hepatitis A (inflammation of the liver)
4 to 6 years	DTaP Dose 5 of 5	Diphtheria, tetanus, whooping cough (pertussis)
	Polio (IPV) Dose 4 of 4	Polio
	MMR Dose 2 of 2	Measles, mumps, and rubella (German measles)
11 to 12 years	Td booster 1 dose every 10 years	Tetanus and diphtheria

client gratitude. The age of the clients can range from young children to older adults.

The presence of guards, difficulty in establishing trust and confidential relationships, and bureaucratic red tape can be frustrating and would be considered the drawbacks of this type of job. An LPN/LVN who has medical-surgical, emergency, and trauma skills and who can function without direct supervision would be a good candidate for this job. Positions as correctional nurses are often appealing to male nurses.

Traveling nurse positions have become available to the LPN/LVN in recent years. Assignments vary in length; the normal assignment is 13 weeks. Traveler assignments can provide the nurse with an opportunity to assess a new location prior to making a commitment for a permanent move. Most traveler nurses do not have family ties or responsibilities, although it could provide an opportunity to be assigned to a location near a family member who is in the military or college. Traveler positions are obtained through employing agencies that provide benefits, relocation expense reimbursement, and a housing allowance. Travel assignments may sound really exciting, but the prospective traveler needs to consider whether living and working in an unfamiliar area away from family and friends is desirable.

Adult day care or assisted living facilities may not be required by law to have a licensed nurse on duty, but many employ LPNs/LVNs to have a qualified person to oversee the health and safety of their clients. A nurse who enjoys interacting with elders would be well suited to such a position.

Summer day camps can be a summer job opportunity for an LPN/LVN who works during the year in a school health office or clinic. Good first aid and CPR skills are a must. Many camps will allow a staff member's children to attend at a reduced rate, so this job could provide a summer income as well as summer activities for the nurse's children.

Some states have licensed psychiatric technicians who are employed in mental health facilities and clinics. In other locations, other jobs in these facilities are open to LPNs/LVNs. Nurses with an interest in psychosocial health care could find working with these clients very rewarding. Mental health nursing courses in LPN/LVN programs are usually not comprehensive enough to prepare the LPN/LVN to work in a psychiatric facility without additional training, although many facilities provide the necessary training. Geropsych units (an inpatient specialized unit, normally in a skilled nursing facility, that deals with the multiple aspects of normal and abnormal changes in cognition, personality, well-being, and mental health that occur with aging in the later years of life) and facilities that care for children with developmental disabilities do have positions for the LPN/LVN. These are attractive positions, especially if they are state-supported institutions, because compensation and medical and retirement benefits are usually excellent.

The LPN/LVN who is considering advancing on the career ladder in the future may feel that acute hospital experience is essential. Opportunities are available although many hospitals are leaning toward all-RN staffs to meet state-imposed nursing ratios. Good experience can be obtained in sub-acute units and skilled nursing facilities that take Medicare clients. Hospital staff mixes change frequently due to supply and demand, so do not become discouraged if that "perfect" job seems to be eluding you as a new graduate. The LPN/LVN has a contribution to make to health care, and there are many opportunities available for the nurse who "looks outside the box" and is willing to stretch a bit and try something new.

NURSING PROCESS CARE PLAN
Same-Day Surgery Client

Dory Page is an 89-year-old female who lives with her husband in a retirement community. They have a homemaker aide four mornings per week to assist with showering, laundry, and light housekeeping. During the week they have senior meals delivered for lunch and dinner. One daughter lives locally, and she assists with shopping on weekends and takes them out for meals when they are up to it.

Mrs. Page also has a cataract on her left eye that will be removed surgically at a later date. Her daughter is present for discharge instructions and will provide transportation home.

Assessment
VS: T 97.8, P 84, R 28, BP 132/88. She is awake and stable. An eye patch/shield is in place over right eye. She has been up to the bathroom and has eaten half a sandwich and a cup of tea. Client has no c/o of pain. She is now ready for her instructions and discharge.

Nursing Diagnosis
The following important nursing diagnoses (among others) are established for this client:

- *Ineffective Coping* related to surgical experience
- *Risk for Injury* related to visual impairment
- *Deficient Knowledge* regarding home care related to unfamiliarity with information

Expected Outcomes
The expected outcomes for the plan of care are as follows:

- Demonstrates knowledge of psychological responses to surgical procedures.
- Free from signs and symptoms of physical injury.
- Communicates purpose, dosage, route, and possible side effects of medication; provides return demonstration on proper medication administration; communicates proper storage of medication.
- Communicates concerns related to surgical procedure, next planned visit to healthcare provider, goals in realistic terms, sequence of postoperative events, and activities related to her care.

- Communicates sequences of wound healing related to surgical procedure; concerns about healing, dressing care, and wound management techniques; and goals of wound healing.

Planning and Implementation
The following nursing interventions are planned and implemented for Mrs. Page:

- Assess coping mechanisms based on psychological status.
- Identify individual's values and wishes concerning care.
- Note the following sensory impairments: Ask what the client can see with each eye. Implement protective measures to prevent injury. Orient the client to the environment and remove potential hazards.
- Evaluate environment for home care.
- Identify potential hazards such as throw rugs or extension cords and instruct family member to remove them.
- Provide instructions about prescribed medications.
- Identify expectations for home care; leave eye shield in place for 12 to 18 hours; put nothing into the eye unless instructed by surgeon; have companion stay with client; and contact physician if vision, pain, or nausea worsens or if vomiting occurs.
- Evaluate response to instructions.

Evaluation
Mrs. Page returns to the surgeon's office on the morning following surgery. She is free of any signs and symptoms of physical injury. She demonstrates proper procedures for instilling medication into eye and doing the dressing change. She demonstrates no psychological reaction to surgical procedure and is looking forward to having the other cataract removed, since her vision in her right eye has been poor since she was a child.

Critical Thinking in the Nursing Process

1. Discuss reasons for avoiding general anesthesia in a client of Mrs. Page's age.
2. Provide Mrs. Page and her daughter with discharge instructions for cataract removal.
3. Why was it recommended to first remove the cataract in the eye with the poorest vision?

Note: Discussion of Critical Thinking questions appears on the MyNursingKit Website.

Note: The references and resources for all chapters have been compiled at the back of the book.

PROCEDURE 48-1 — Admitting a New Client in the Physician's Office

Purpose

- To complete a medical history form and gather necessary information for the physician

Equipment

- Medical history form
- Black and red pens
- Vital sign equipment

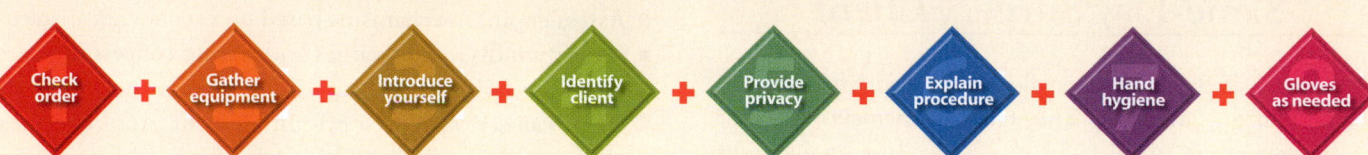

Check order + Gather equipment + Introduce yourself + Identify client + Provide privacy + Explain procedure + Hand hygiene + Gloves as needed

Interventions and Rationales

1. Perform preparatory steps (see icon bar above).

2. Review the medical history form and client's chart. *Be familiar with the order of the questions and the type of information required and the information already given by the client, in order to facilitate communication.*

3. Sit across from the client at eye level and make frequent eye contact. *Standing above the client may be perceived as threatening and hinder communication.*

4. Introduce yourself and explain the purpose of the interview. *This will establish professional rapport with the client.*

5. Using language that the client can understand, ask appropriate questions and document the responses. *To obtain complete information for physician.*

6. Listen actively and look at the client when he or she is speaking. *Client can sense when the nurse is not listening, so be sure to show interest in what the client is saying.*

7. Regardless of the confidence the client shares, avoid displaying a judgmental attitude with words or actions. *Maintains professionalism and ensures the client's trust.*

8. Using open-ended questions, determine why the client is seeking medical care. *This will allow the client to explain his or her chief complaint (CC) in his or her own words.*

9. Determine the present illness (PI) using open-ended and closed-ended questions. *Use closed-ended questions to obtain specific data only after the client has responded to open-ended questions.*

10. Obtain client's vital signs (see Procedures 21-1 through 21-4 ⬤⬤ for complete steps).

11. Document the CC, PI, and complete vital signs on the progress sheet in the client's chart. *Documentation should include date, time, CC, PI, TPR, BP, weight, and any other information obtained from the client and your signature and title. Use correct medical terminology and approved abbreviations.*

12. Thank the client for cooperating and explain that the physician will be in shortly to examine the client. *Courtesy encourages a positive attitude about the office. If you indicate a time frame in reference to the physician coming into the examination room, be honest.*

SAMPLE DOCUMENTATION

[date] [time]	CC: C/o headache and nausea ×3 days. Has taken 6 200-mg tablets per day of OTC ibuprofen for the pain with minimal relief. The pain is a "dull ache" in the frontal area of the head and face. No emesis. Face flushed, skin warm and dry. T 99.4, P 88, R 16, BP 186/100 [L] sitting. Weight 186. _____ _____ R. Smith, LPN

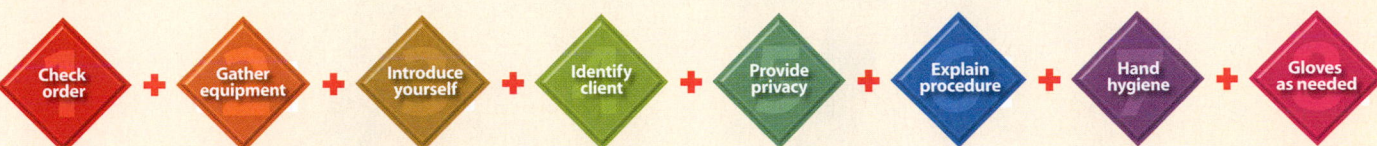

| PROCEDURE 48-2 | **Preparing a Client for Examination by the Physician or Nurse Practitioner** |

Purpose

■ To prepare the client for examination

Equipment

■ Stethoscope
■ Ophthalmoscope
■ Otoscope
■ Penlight
■ Tuning fork
■ Nasal speculum
■ Tongue blade
■ Percussion hammer
■ Gloves
■ Client gown and draping

Check order + Gather equipment + Introduce yourself + Identify client + Provide privacy + Explain procedure + Hand hygiene + Gloves as needed

Interventions and Rationales

1. Perform preparatory steps (see icon bar above).

2. Prepare the examination room and assemble the equipment (Figure 48-5 ■). *A clean room free of contamination prevents transfer of microorganisms.*

3. Greet the client by name and escort him or her to the examination room. *Identifying the client by name prevents errors.*

4. Explain the procedure. *This reduces anxiety and helps ensure compliance.*

5. Obtain and record the medical history and chief complaint. *This provides information for the examiner.*

6. Take and record vital signs, height, weight, visual acuity, and an audiogram if ordered. *The vital signs and other measurements give the examiner an overall picture of the client's health.*

7. If the physician requires it, instruct the client in the correct method of obtaining a urine specimen, then escort the client to the bathroom. *Even if the urine specimen is not a part of the physical examination, an empty bladder makes the abdominal examination more comfortable.*

8. Once the client has returned from the bathroom, instruct him or her in disrobing and how to put on the gown (open in the front or back). Leave the room while the client disrobes unless he or she needs assistance. *The gown must be open in the direction that provides accessibility for the examination. Older people and people with disabilities may need help disrobing and putting on the gown.*

9. Help the client sit on the end of the exam table and cover lap and legs with the drape. *The sitting position is often the first position used by the examiner.*

10. Place the medical record outside the examination room and notify the physician or RN practitioner that the client is ready. *Alerting the examiner helps prevent delays.*

11. Assist the examiner by handing him or her the instruments as needed and positioning the client appropriately. *Anticipating the examiner's needs promotes efficiency and saves time.*

   ■ Begin by handing the physician the instruments necessary for examining the following:
   a. Head and neck—stethoscope
   b. Eyes—ophthalmoscope (Figure 48-6A ■), penlight
   c. Ears—otoscope (see Figure 48-6B), tuning fork, audioscope
   d. Nose—penlight, nasal speculum
   e. Sinuses—penlight
   f. Mouth—tongue blade, penlight
   Hold the tongue blade in the middle when giving it to and receiving it from the primary care provider. This prevents transmission of microorganisms between your hand and the client's mouth.
   g. Throat—gloves, tongue blade, laryngeal mirror, penlight
   Only the part of the body being examined should be exposed. Always preserve the client's privacy and keep the client covered as much as possible.

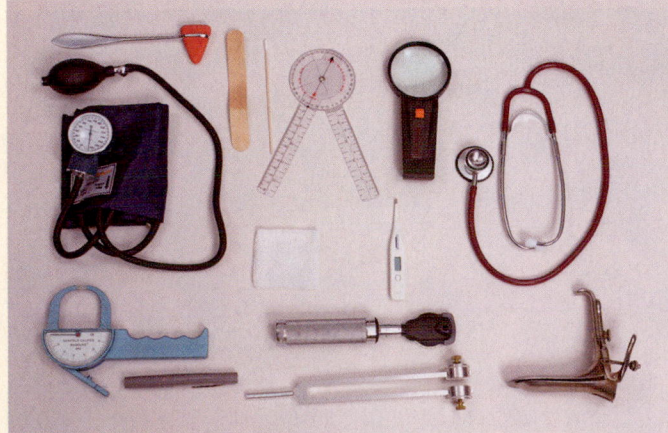

Figure 48-5. ■ Common equipment used in an adult physical examination.

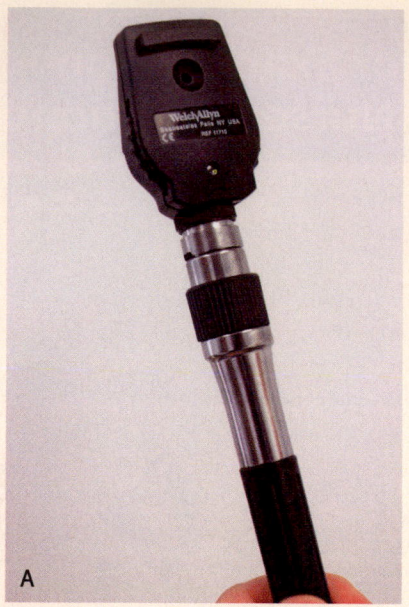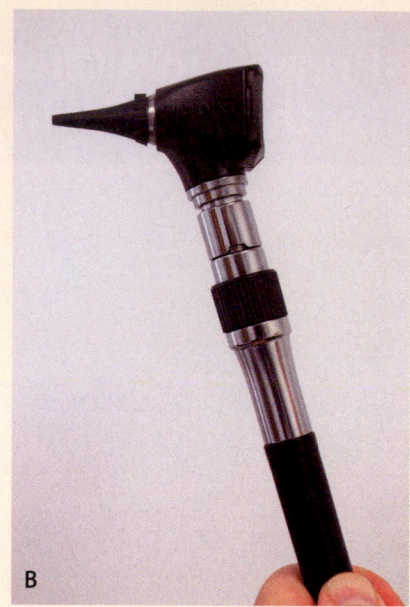

Figure 48-6. ■ **A.** Ophthalmoscope. **B.** Otoscope.

- Help the client drop the gown to the waist for examination of the chest and upper back. Hand the examiner the stethoscope.
- Help the client to pull up the gown and remove the drape from the legs so the examiner can test reflexes. Hand the examiner the reflex hammer.
- Help the client to lie supine, opening the gown at the top to expose the chest again. Place the drape to cover the waist, abdomen, and legs. Hand the physician the stethoscope.
- Cover the client's chest and lower the drape to expose the abdomen. Hand the physician the stethoscope.
- Assist with the genital and rectal examinations. Hand the client a tissue following the examinations. *Tissue may be used to wipe off excessive lubricant.*

FOR FEMALES

a. Assist the client to the lithotomy position and drape appropriately.

b. For examination of the genitalia and internal reproductive organs, provide a glove, lubricant, speculum (Figure 48-7 ■), microscope, slide or prep solution, and spatula or brush.

c. For the rectal exam, provide a glove, lubricant, and fecal occult blood test slide.

FOR MALES

a. Help the client to stand and have him bend over the examination table for a rectal and prostate examination.

b. For a hernia examination, provide a glove.

c. For a rectal examination, provide a glove, lubricant, and fecal occult blood test slide.

d. For a prostate examination, provide a glove and lubricant.

- With the client standing, the examiner can assess legs, gait, coordination, and balance.

12. Help the client sit on the edge of the exam table. *The physician often discusses findings with the client at this time and may provide instructions.*

13. Perform any follow-up procedures and treatments.

14. Leave the room while the client dresses unless the client needs assistance. *Leaving the room provides privacy for the client.*

15. Return to the examination room when the client has dressed to answer any questions, reinforce instructions, and provide client education. *Compliance depends on full understanding of the treatment plan. Client education is the responsibility of all healthcare workers.*

16. Escort the client to the front desk. *You can clarify the appointment scheduling or billing issues.*

17. Properly clean or dispose of the equipment and supplies. Clean the room with a disinfectant and prepare for the

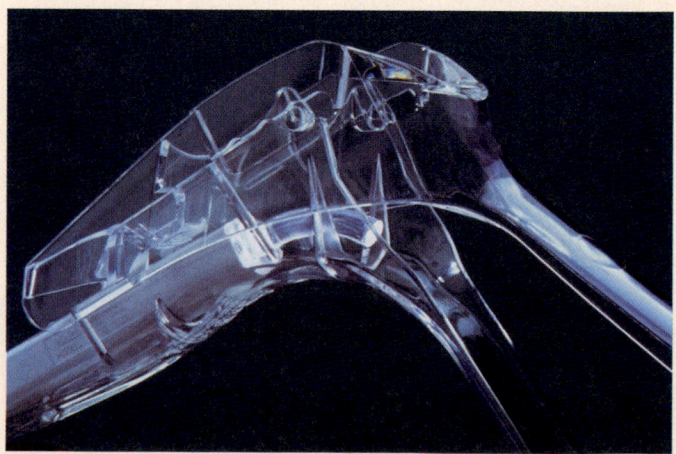

Figure 48-7. ■ Vaginal speculum.

next client. *All instruments, supplies, and equipment that came into direct contact with the client must be appropriately decontaminated or disposed.*

18. Perform hand hygiene and record any instructions from the physician. Also note any specimens and indicate the results of the tests or the laboratory where the specimens are being sent for testing. *Procedures and instructions are considered not to have been done if they are not recorded.*

PROCEDURE 48-3   Assisting with Office Surgical Procedures

Purpose

- To prepare for and assist with procedure while maintaining sterile technique

Equipment

At-the-side equipment:

- Sterile gloves
- Local anesthetic
- Antiseptic wipes
- Adhesive tape
- Specimen container
- Completed laboratory request

Sterile field containing:

- Basin for solutions
- Gauze sponges and cotton
- Antiseptic solution
- Sterile drape
- Dissecting scissors
- Disposable scalpel
- Blade of physician's choice
- Mosquito forceps
- Tissue forceps
- Needle holder
- Suture and needle of physician's choice

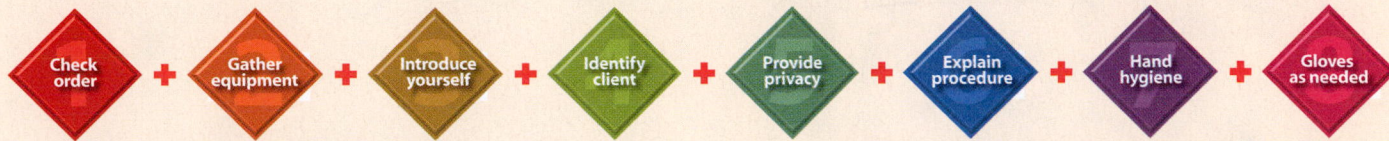

Check order + Gather equipment + Introduce yourself + Identify client + Provide privacy + Explain procedure + Hand hygiene + Gloves as needed

Part A: Excisional Surgery
Interventions and Rationales

1. Perform preparatory steps (see icon bar above).

2. Greet and identify client, explain procedure, and answer any questions. *This prevents errors in treatment, helps gain compliance, and eases anxiety.*

3. Set up a sterile field on a surgical stand with the at-the-side equipment close at hand. *Keeps sterile items separate and all items within easy reach.*

4. Position the client appropriately. *The required position depends on the location of the lesion.*

5. Put on sterile gloves or use sterile transfer forceps and cleanse the client's skin. *The antiseptic discourages the entrance of microorganisms into the wound. After cleansing skin, remove the gloves if used and perform hand hygiene.*

6. As the physician performs the procedure, you may be asked to assist by adding supplies as needed. Watch closely for opportunities to assist the physician and comfort the client. *It is not necessary for you to wear sterile gloves during the procedure unless the physician requires you to handle sterile instruments or supplies.*

7. For lesions being referred to pathology for analysis, assist with collecting the specimen in the appropriate container. *Always follow Standard Precautions, wearing examination gloves when handling specimens. Have the container ready to receive the specimen.*

8. At the end of the procedure, perform hand hygiene and dress the wound using sterile technique (according to Procedure 24-1 ⚭). *The wound must be covered to protect the incision from contamination.*

9. Thank the client and give appropriate instructions for care of the operative site, changing the dressing, postoperative medications, and follow-up visits as ordered by the physician. *Courtesy encourages the client to have a positive attitude about the physician's office, and giving necessary instruction will ensure compliance from the client.*

10. Don gloves. Clean the examination room in preparation for the next client. Discard all used disposable items in appropriate biohazard containers. Return unused items to their proper place. Remove gloves and perform hand hygiene. *Standard Precautions must be followed.*

11. Record the procedure. *Procedures must be documented to be considered done. Documentation of the procedure requires postoperative vital signs, care of the wound, instructions on postoperative care, and processing of any specimens.*

Part B: Incision and Drainage (I&D)

Additional Equipment

- Packing gauze (Figure 48-8 ■)
- Culture tube
- Probe

Interventions and Rationales

Follow the steps for excisional surgery. After the procedure, the wound must be covered to avoid further contamination and to absorb drainage. *The exudate is a hazardous body fluid requiring Standard Precautions.*

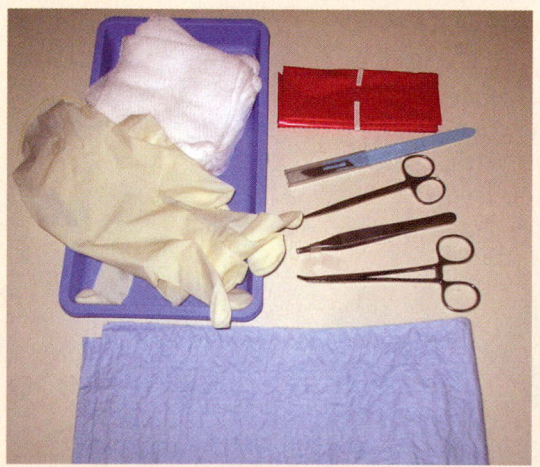

Figure 48-8. ■ Inicision and drainage (I&D) surgical tray set up.

PROCEDURE 48-4   # Performing a 12-Lead Electrocardiogram

Purpose

■ To prepare client for and obtain a 12-lead ECG that is free of artifacts

Equipment

■ ECG machine with cable and lead wires
■ ECG paper
■ Disposable electrodes that contain coupling gel
■ Gown and drape
■ Skin preparation materials including razor and antiseptic wipes

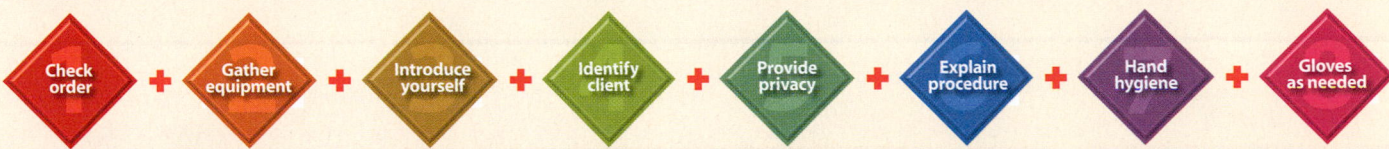

Check order + Gather equipment + Introduce yourself + Identify client + Provide privacy + Explain procedure + Hand hygiene + Gloves as needed

Interventions and Rationales

1. Perform preparatory steps (see icon bar above).

2. Turn the machine on and enter appropriate data, including the client's name and/or identification number, age, sex, height, weight, blood pressure, and medications. *Information will assist the physician in determining a proper diagnosis.*

3. Instruct the client to disrobe above the waist and provide a gown for privacy. Female client should also be instructed to remove any nylons or tights. *Clothing may interfere with proper placement of the leads. Clients wearing pants do not have to remove them if they can be pulled up to expose the lower legs.*

4. Position the client comfortably supine with pillows as needed for comfort. Drape the client for warmth and privacy. *If the client is uncomfortable, too cool, or improperly draped, movement is likely, which will result in artifacts on the ECG tracing.*

5. Prepare the skin as needed by wiping away skin oils or lotions with antiseptic wipes or shaving any hair that will interfere with good contact between the skin and the electrodes. *Skin preparation ensures properly attached leads and helps avoid improper readings and lost time repeating the test.*

6. Apply electrodes snugly against the fleshy, muscular part of the upper arms and lower legs according to the manufacturer's directions. Apply the chest electrodes, V_1 through V_6. In case of an amputation or otherwise inaccessible limb, place the electrode on the uppermost part of the existing extremity or on the anterior shoulder (upper extremity) and groin (lower extremity). *Electrodes that are not snug against the skin or are on bony prominences may cause improper reading and artifacts.*

7. Connect the lead wires securely according to the color-coded notations on the connectors (RA, LA, RL, LL, V_1–V_6). Untangle the wires before applying them to prevent electrical artifacts. Each lead must lie unencumbered along the contours of the client's body to decrease the likelihood of artifacts. Double check placement. *Improperly placed leads will result in time lost to an inaccurate reading and retesting.*

8. Determine the sensitivity, or gain, and the paper speed settings on the ECG machine before running the test. Set sensitivity or gain on 1 and paper speed on 25 mm/second. *A sensitivity setting of 1 and a paper speed of 25 mm/second are necessary to obtain an accurate ECG. These settings should not be changed without a direct order from the primary care provider; the changes would be noted on the ECG tracing.*

9. Depress the automatic button on the machine to obtain the 12-lead tracing. The machine will automatically move from one lead to the next without your intervention. *If the primary care provider wants only a rhythm strip tracing, use the manual mode of operation and select the lead manually.*

10. When the tracing is complete and printed, check the ECG for artifacts and the standardization. *With sensitivity set on 1, the standardization mark should be 2 small squares wide and 10 small squares high. The standardization mark documents accuracy of operation and provides reference points.*

11. If the tracing is adequate, turn off the machine and remove and discard the electrodes. Assist the client to a sitting position and help with dressing if needed. *Some clients become dizzy while lying supine.*

12. If a single-channel machine was used (each lead produced on a roll of paper, one lead at a time), carefully roll the ECG strips without using clips to secure the roll. The ECG must be mounted on 8½ × 11-inch paper or a form before going into the medical record according to the office policy and procedure. *Folding the ECG tracing or applying clips may make marks on the surface, obscuring the reading. Special forms may be purchased specifically for*

mounting a single-channel ECG strip and placing it in the medical record.

13. Record the procedure in the client's medical record. *Procedures need to be documented in order to be considered done.*

14. Place the ECG tracing and the client's medical record on the primary care provider's desk or give it directly, as instructed.

SAMPLE DOCUMENTATION

[date]	Preop 12-lead ECG obtained and
[time]	placed in chart. Given to
	Dr. Crane for evaluation.
	Discharged, no follow-up
	required at this time.
	_____ S. Tensor, LPN

PROCEDURE 48-5 — Obtaining a Capillary Blood Sample by Skin Puncture

Purpose

- To obtain blood for diagnostic purposes and/or monitoring of prescribed treatment

Equipment

- Sterile disposable lancet or automated skin puncture device
- 70% alcohol or other antiseptic
- Sterile gauze pad
- Micro-collection tubes or containers
- Heel-warming device (when obtaining sample from the heel of an infant)
- Appropriate biohazard barriers (gloves, gown, face shield, sharps container)

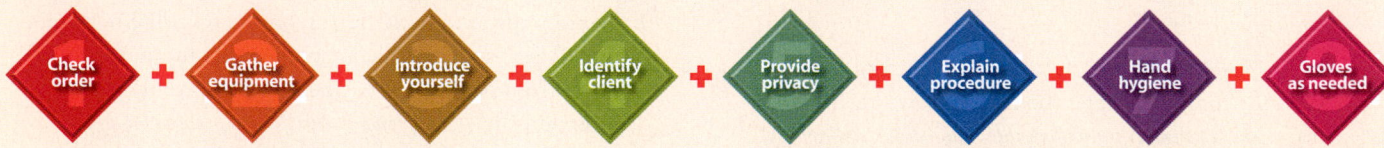

Check order + Gather equipment + Introduce yourself + Identify client + Provide privacy + Explain procedure + Hand hygiene + Gloves as needed

Interventions and Rationales

1. Perform preparatory steps (see icon bar above).

2. Select the puncture site (the lateral portion of the tip of the middle or ring finger of the nondominant hand; lateral curved surface of the heel or the great toe of an infant). The puncture should be made in the fleshy central portion of the second or third finger, slightly to the side of center, and perpendicular to the whorls of the fingerprint (Figure 48-9 ■). Perform heel puncture only on the plantar surface of the heel, medial to an imaginary line extending from the middle of the great toe to the heel, and lateral to an imaginary line drawn from between the fourth and fifth toes to the heel (Figure 48-10 ■). *Note:* When using the heel of an infant, apply a warm washcloth or heel warmer to the heel 10 to 15 minutes prior to procedure to stimulate blood flow. Use the appropriate puncture device for the site selected (Figure 48-11 ■). *The ring and middle finger are less calloused than the forefinger. The lateral tip is the least sensitive part of the finger. A puncture made across the fingerprints will produce a round, large drop of blood. In an infant skin puncture, the area and the depth designed reduce the risk of puncturing the bone.*

3. Make sure the site selected is warm and not cyanotic or edematous. Gently massage the finger from the base to the

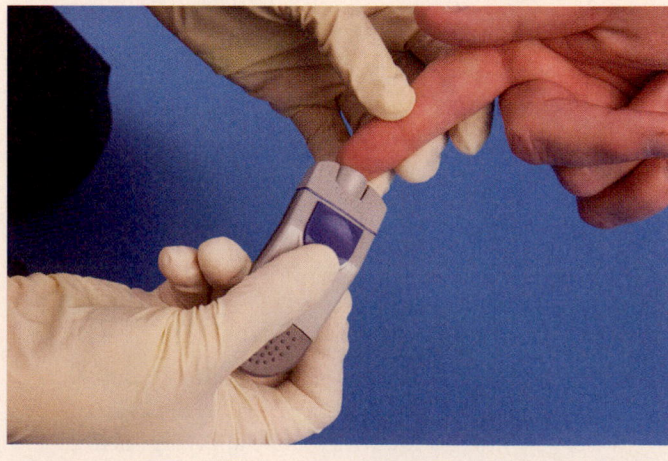

Figure 48-9. ■ Recommended site and direction of finger puncture.

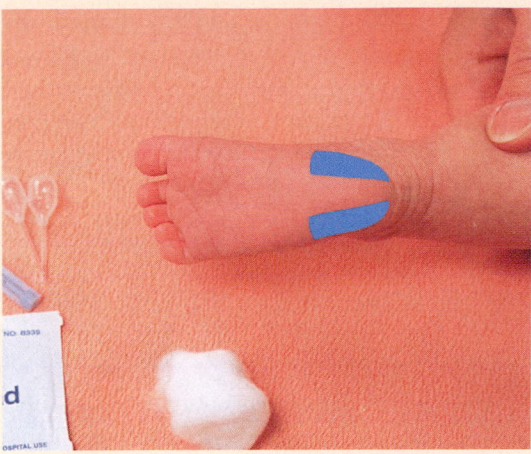

Figure 48-10. ■ Acceptable areas for heel puncture on newborns.

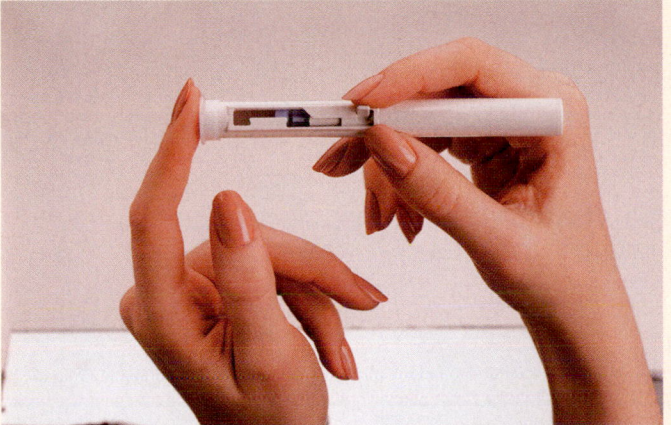

Figure 48-11. ■ Finger puncture lancets. Client obtained self sample.

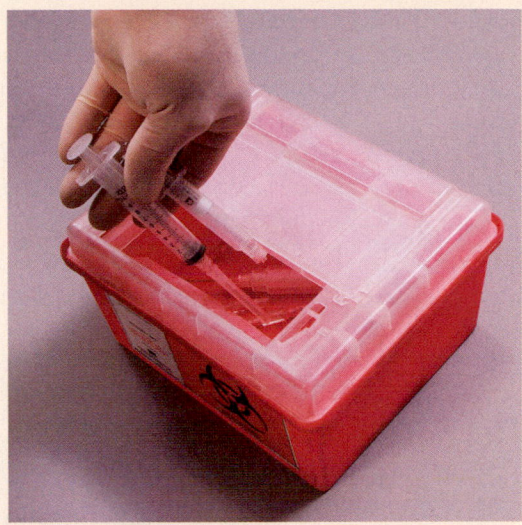

Figure 48-12. ■ Proper disposal of used venipuncture supplies.

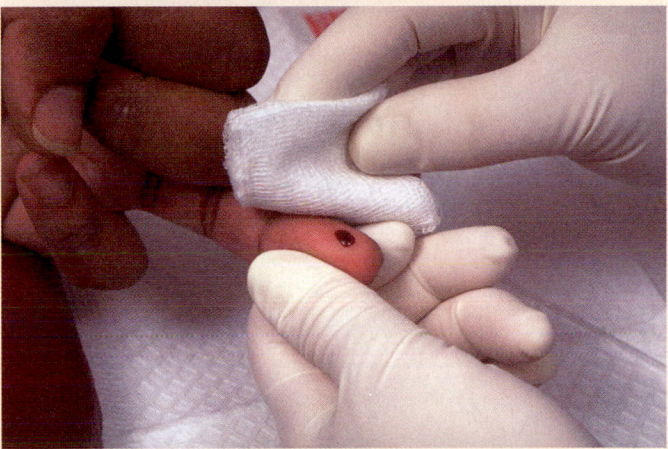

Figure 48-13. ■ Wipe away first drop of blood.

tip. *Massaging the area increases the blood flow. Good circulation at the chosen site yields a better blood sample for analysis.*

4. Grasp the finger firmly between your nondominant index finger and thumb, or grasp the infant's heel firmly with your index finger wrapped around the foot and your thumb wrapped around the ankle. Cleanse the selected area with 70% isopropyl alcohol and wipe dry with a sterile gauze pad or allow to air dry. *Maintaining your hold at the site prevents the client from contaminating the cleansed puncture area and allows you to have control of the puncture site. The area must be dry to eliminate alcohol residue, which can cause the client discomfort and interfere with test results.*

5. Hold the client's finger or heel firmly and make a swift, firm puncture. Perform the puncture perpendicular to the whorls of the fingerprint or footprint. Dispose of the used puncture device in a sharps container (Figure 48-12 ■).
   ■ Wipe away the first drop of blood with sterile dry gauze (Figure 48-13 ■). *The first discarded drop may be contaminated with tissue fluid or alcohol residue.*
   ■ Apply pressure toward the site but do not milk the site. *Milking the site will dilute the specimen with tissue fluid.*

6. Collect the specimen in the chosen container or slide. Touch only the tip of the collection device to the drop of blood (Figure 48-14 ■). Blood flow is encouraged if the

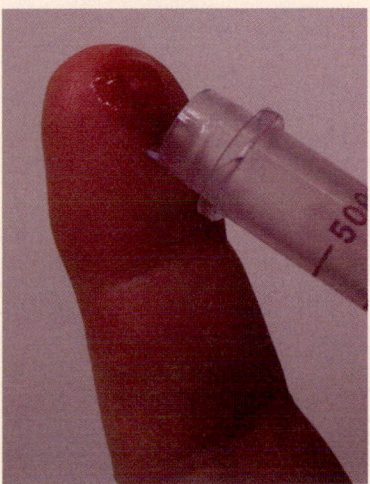

Figure 48-14. ■ Touch only the tip of the collection tube to the drop of blood.

puncture site is held downward and gentle pressure is applied near the site. Cap micro-collection tubes with the cap provided and mix additives by gently tilting or inverting the tube 8 to 10 times. *Scraping the collection device on the skin activates platelets and may cause hemolysis. Touching the tube to the site may cause contamination. Mixing the specimens prevents clotting.*

7. When collection is complete, apply clean gauze to the site with pressure (Figure 48-15 ■). Hold pressure or

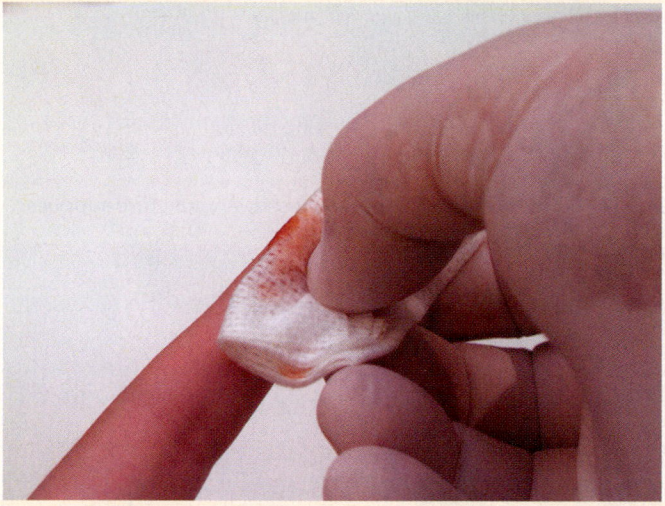

Figure 48-15. ■ Apply pressure with clean gauze.

have the client hold pressure until bleeding stops. Label the containers with the proper information. Do not apply a dressing to a skin puncture of an infant under 2 years of age. Never release a client until the bleeding has stopped. *Proper labeling prevents mixing up specimens. Younger children may develop skin irritation from the adhesive bandage. Also young children may put the bandage in their mouths and choke.*

8. Thank the client. Instruct the client to leave the bandage in place for at least 15 minutes. *Courtesy helps the client have a positive attitude about the procedure and the facility.*

9. Properly care for or dispose of equipment and supplies. Clean work area. Remove gloves and perform hand hygiene. *Standard Precautions must be followed throughout the procedure.*

10. Test, transfer, or store specimen according to the facility policy.

11. Document the procedure.

SAMPLE DOCUMENTATION

[date]	OP fingerstick for prothrombin
[time]	time per Dr. Rubin. _____
	_____ C. Wasson, LPN

PROCEDURE 48-6 **Assisting with a Sigmoidoscopy**

Purpose

■ To prepare the client and assist with an endoscopic colon procedure

Equipment

■ Flexible or rigid sigmoidoscope
■ Water-soluble lubricant
■ Gown and drape
■ Cotton swabs
■ Suction if not part of the scope
■ Biopsy forceps
■ Specimen container and preservative
■ Completed lab requisition form
■ Personal wipes or tissue
■ Equipment for assessing vital signs
■ Examination gloves

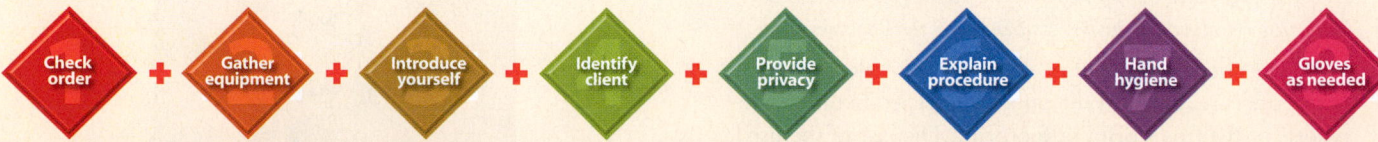

Check order + Gather equipment + Introduce yourself + Identify client + Provide privacy + Explain procedure + Hand hygiene + Gloves as needed

Interventions and Rationales

1. Perform preparatory steps (see icon bar above).

2. Check the light source if a flexible sigmoidoscope (Figure 48-16 ■) is being used. Turn off the power after checking for working order to avoid a buildup of heat in

the instrument. *If heat is permitted to build up in the scope, the client may be burned.*

3. Greet and identify the client and explain the procedure. Inform the client that a sensation of pressure or need to defecate may be felt during the procedure and that

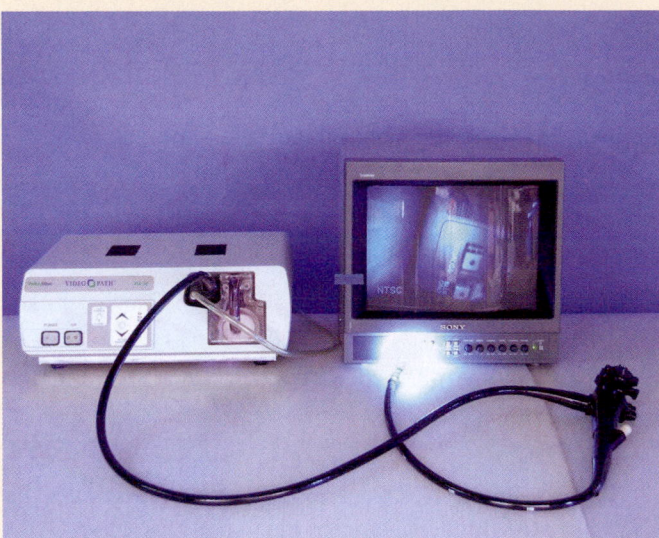

Figure 48-16. ■ A flexible sigmoidoscope.

pressure is from the instrument and will ease. The client may also feel gas pressure when air is insufflated during the sigmoidoscopy. *Note:* The client may have been ordered to take a mild sedative before the procedure. *Identifying the client prevents errors in treatment. Explaining the procedure helps to ease anxiety and ensure compliance.*

4. Instruct the client to empty the urinary bladder. *Pressure from the instrument may injure a full bladder. Urine in the bladder increases discomfort.*

5. Assess the vital signs and record in the medical record. *Colon examination procedures may cause cardiac arrhythmias and change in blood pressure in some clients. Baseline vital signs will allow you to detect variations from the client's normal vital signs.*

6. Have the client undress completely from the waist down and put on a gown. Drape appropriately.

7. Assist the client on to the examination table. If a fiber-optic device is being used, Sims' position is the most comfortable for the client (Figure 48-17 ■). If a rigid instrument is used, the client will be placed in the

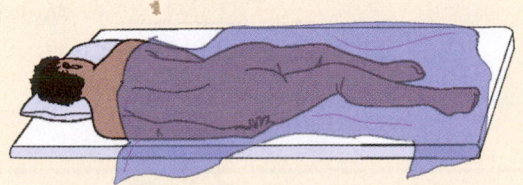

Figure 48-17. ■ Sims' position.

knee–chest position when the physician is ready to begin. *These positions facilitate the procedure by moving the abdominal organs up into the abdominal cavity rather than the pelvis.*

8. Assist the physician as needed with lubricant, instruments, power, swabs, and specimen container.

9. During the procedure, monitor the client's response and offer reassurance. Instruct the client to breathe slowly through pursed lips to aid in relaxation if necessary.

10. When the physician is finished, assist the client to a comfortable position and allow a rest period. Offer personal cleaning wipes or tissues. Take the vital signs before allowing the client to stand and assist the client from the table and with dressing as needed. Give the client any instructions regarding care after the procedure and follow-up as ordered by the physician. *A drop in blood pressure on standing is common after lying in any of these positions for an extended period. If clients complain of dizziness or light-headedness after sitting up, have them lie down again. If any biopsy samples were taken, the client may have slight rectal bleeding.*

11. Clean the room and route the specimen to the laboratory with the requisition. Disinfect or dispose of the supplies and equipment as appropriate and wash your hands. *Follow Standard Precautions throughout the procedure.*

12. Document the procedure.

SAMPLE DOCUMENTATION

[date] [time]	VS: T 98.4, P 100, R 22, BP 144/84. Sigmoidoscopy performed by Dr. Narang and specimen obtained. Procedure tolerated well. Specimen to Quest Laboratories, VS after procedure: P 112, R 24, BP 146/86. Denies dizziness after procedure. Discharged per Dr. Narang with verbal and written instructions on procedural care. Client verbalizes understanding. _____ _____ S. Lewan, LPN

PROCEDURE 48-7 Screening for Scoliosis

Purpose

- To meet school health guidelines for scoliosis screening and identify students who need medical evaluation for spinal curvature

Equipment

- Scoliometer

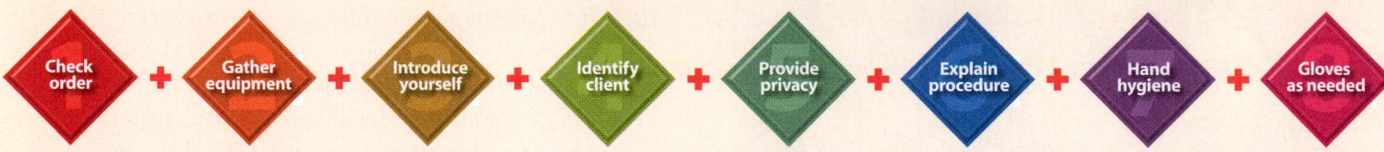

Interventions and Rationales

1. Perform preparatory steps (see icon bar above).

2. Explain the procedure to the group or each student individually. *A general explanation can be given class by class as long as the student is given the opportunity to ask questions privately.*

3. Have child remove outer garments. *Deformity, if any, will be easier to identify through a t-shirt.*

4. Instruct student to bend over with arms dangling while standing with feet together and knees straight. *The curve of structural scoliosis is more apparent when bending over.*

5. Observe an imbalanced rib cage, with one side being higher than the other. *The lateral curve of scoliosis will cause ribs to be asymmetrical.*

6. Observe for other deformities if present. *The hip opposite the deviation will be higher with scoliosis, resulting in what appears to be unequal leg lengths.*

7. Confirm diagnosis using additional physical test. The student is requested to walk on the toes, then the heels, and then is asked to jump up and down on one foot. *Such activities indicate leg strength and balance.*

8. Additional screening can be performed with the inclinometer (scoliometer). An inclinometer, also known as a scoliometer, measures distortions of the torso. The procedure is as follows:
   - The student bends over, arms dangling and palms pressed together, until a curve can be observed in the *upper* back (thoracic area).
   - The scoliometer is placed on the back and measures the apex (the highest point) of the upper back curve.
   - The student continues bending until the curve can be seen in the *lower* back (lumbar area). The apex of this curve is also measured.

   Some experts believe the scoliometer would make a useful device for widespread screening. Scoliometers, however, indicate rib cage distortions in more than half of children who turn out to have very minor or no sideways curves. They are therefore not accurate enough to guide treatment.

9. Document findings and notify parent if medical follow-up is needed. *Provide parents with result of screening to take to family physician.*

SAMPLE DOCUMENTATION

[date] [time]	Fifth-grade female examined using the Adams forward bend test. Exam revealed a right deviating lateral curve of approximately 30°, confirmed with scoliometer. Parent contacted and instructed to follow up with private physician. _____ G. Miller, LPN—School Health Clerk

Measuring Visual Acuity (Distance, Near, and Color)

Purpose

- To assess and document the distance visual acuity of a student in both eyes, with or without corrective lenses, according to required health assessment timelines

Equipment

- Snellen eye chart
- Paper cup or eye paddle
- Titus machine or handheld charts (for near vision testing)
- Plus lens glasses (for near vision testing)
- Ishihara Color Test Plates *or* the Hardy-Rand Rittler Pseudoisochromatic Plates (for color vision testing)

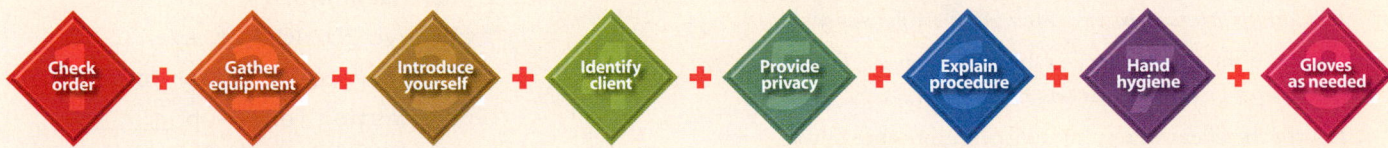

Check order + Gather equipment + Introduce yourself + Identify client + Provide privacy + Explain procedure + Hand hygiene + Gloves as needed

Part A: Testing Distance Vision

Interventions and Rationales

1. Perform preparatory steps (see icon bar above).

2. Prepare the examination area. Make sure the area is well lighted, a distance marker is placed exactly 20 feet from the Snellen chart (Figure 48-18 ■), and the chart is at eye level. *All distance visual testing is done at 20 feet for consistency of results.*

3. Greet and identify the student and explain the procedure. *A student who understands the procedure is likely to be compliant and produce accurate results.*

4. Position the student at the 20-foot mark. *The student may stand or sit as long as the chart is at eye level and 20 feet away.*

5. Observe whether the student is wearing glasses. If not, ask if he or she is wearing contact lenses and mark the results of the test accordingly. *The visual acuity examination is usually performed with students who need corrective lenses wearing them. If that is the case, the record must indicate that the lenses were worn for the test.*

6. Have the student cover the left eye with the paper cup or eye paddle. Instruct the student to keep both eyes open during the test. *The test starts with the left eye covered for consistency. The hand should not be used to cover the eye, because pressure against the eye or peeking through the fingers affects the results. Closing one eye will cause squinting of the other, which changes the vision and skews the findings.*

7. Stand beside the chart and point to each row as the client reads aloud the indicated lines, starting with the 20/200 line. The line numbers are shown on the right side of the chart next to each line. *It is generally best to start about the second or third row to judge the student's response. If these lines are read easily, move down to smaller figures. If the student has difficulty reading the larger lines, inform the parents so student can be taken for follow-up exam.*

8. Record the smallest line that the student can read with either 1 or no errors, according to policy. If line 5 is read with one error with the right eye, it will be recorded as Rt. eye 20/40-1. If no errors are read at 20/40 line, it is recorded as Rt. eye 20/40.

9. Repeat the procedure with the right eye covered and record as in step 8 using left eye.

10. If the student squints or leans forward while testing either eye, record this observation on the health record. *As the health clerk it is important that testing be documented, including the notification to the parent, in order to comply with student health screening requirements.*

11. Perform hand hygiene and document results.

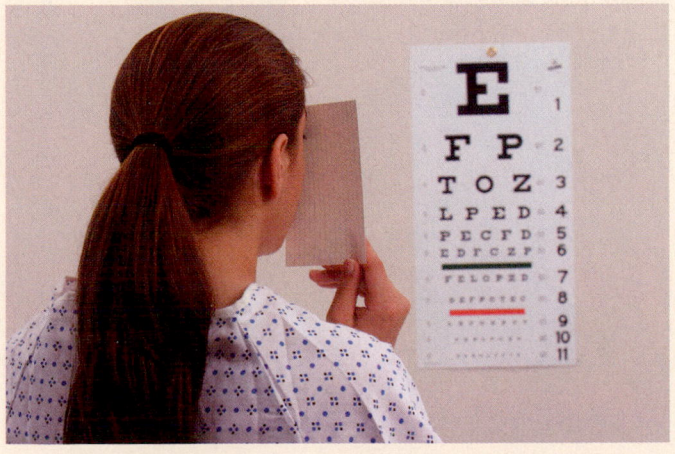

Figure 48-18. ■ Snellen charts used to assess distance vision.

If student is not yet reading or is unable to identify letters, an E chart or picture chart should be used. In step 7 ask the student to use his or her hand to indicate in which directions the legs of the E are pointing on the indicated line or to name the pictures on the indicated line.

Part B: Testing Near Vision

Follow the procedure as for distance vision.

Part C: Testing Color Vision

Interventions and Rationales

1. Hold the plates at approximately 30 inches and at right angles to the client's line of vision. They should be illuminated with cool white fluorescent light. *Use of daylight will cause more individuals to fail the test.*

2. Ask the client to read the numbers or trace the shapes. *This will identify whether the client can identify the number or shape.*

3. Compare the results to the table of responses. *This will identify red-green blindness and red-green weakness.*

4. Inform the client of results and the significance of the results. *There is no cure or treatment for color deficiency. Intervention may include teaching young students to read colors on crayons. Vocational counseling suggesting avoidance of professions requiring color acuity may be appropriate for older students.*

PROCEDURE 48-9 # Conducting Audiometric Testing

Purpose

- To accurately assess and document a hearing test using audiometry and comply with mandated health screening

Equipment

- Audiometer
- Otoscope or audioscope

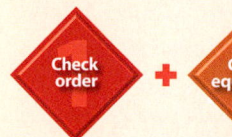 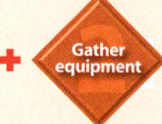 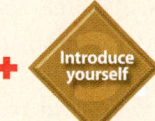     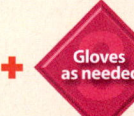

Check order + Gather equipment + Introduce yourself + Identify client + Provide privacy + Explain procedure + Hand hygiene + Gloves as needed

Interventions and Rationales

1. Perform preparatory steps (see icon bar above).

2. Take the student to a quiet room for testing. *A quiet room allows for accurate results without distraction. Determine the signal (raising the hand or saying yes) to indicate that the tones are heard.*

3. Using an otoscope or audioscope with a light source, visually inspect the ear canal and tympanic membrane before testing. *Looking in the ear canal verifies that there are no obstructions, such as cerumen, to interfere with the test. If you see an obstruction, refer the student to have the ear irrigated.*

4. Choose the correct size tip for the end of the audiometer (Figure 48-19 ■). Attach a speculum to fit the student's external auditory meatus, making sure the ear canal is occluded with the speculum in place. *The design of the tip*

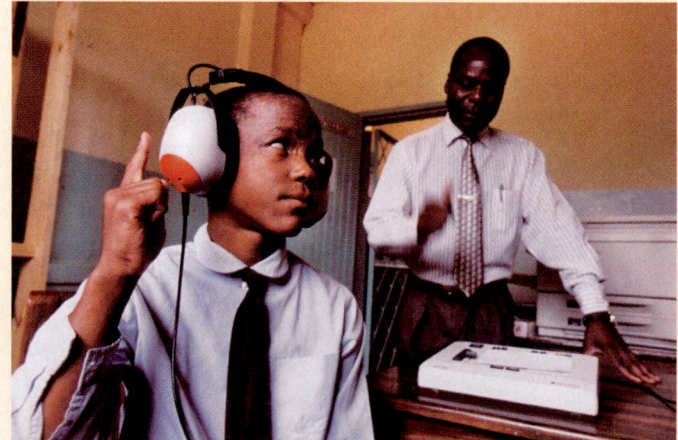

Figure 48-19. ■ Audiometer.

5. With the speculum in the ear canal, retract the pinna, down and back for a child. (For older students, pull pinna up and back.) *Pulling the pinna down and back for a child straightens the ear canal.*

6. Turn the instrument on and select the screening level. There is a pretest tone for practice if necessary. Press the start button and observe the tone indicators and the client's response. *The signal (raising the hand, saying yes) was determined before starting to test. The audiometer will proceed down each tone with a light indicator.*

7. Screen the other ear.

8. If the student fails to respond at any frequency, rescreening is required. If a particular tone does not elicit a response, a second opportunity should be given.

9. If the student fails rescreening, notify the parents so they can take the child to their family physician. *A student who fails to hear one or more tones may need to be referred to an audiologist.*

or speculum obviates bulky earphones; the tip should block any environmental noise during the test.

10. Record the results in the student health record. *Hearing tests are mandated by state law at various grade levels; these need to be recorded in the student's health record.*

SAMPLE DOCUMENTATION

[date]
[time]
Audiometric testing completed as part of 2nd-grade health screening. Rt. ear canal impacted cerumen. Referred to family healthcare provider and scheduled for repeat screening.
_____ L. Sims, LVN— Certified Audiometric Examiner

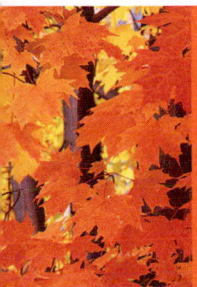

Chapter Review

KEY Points

- A variety of opportunities are available for LPNs/LVNs to use their skills.

- Although a medical assistant may be designated as the office manager in a physician's office, the LPN/LVN never defers to an unlicensed person for treatment questions.

- Privacy and confidentiality are more difficult to ensure in a medical office, but nevertheless all HIPAA regulations must be followed closely.

- School health offices and school-based clinics are providing care for minors, so laws and district policies must be followed.

- School health personnel are a great source of health education for students and families.

- Home care and hospice opportunities are opening up for the LPN/LVN.

- Same-day surgery clinics employ the LPN/LVN to admit clients and prepare them for surgery.

- LPNs/LVNs assist the physician or the nurse practitioner with many procedures in the physician's office.

⊕ FOR FURTHER Study

Chapter 10 provides complete information on CAMRSA in schools.

For additional information concerning HIPAA, see Table 14-1.

Procedures for collecting vital sign measurements are found in Chapter 21.

Heat and Cold Applications are discussed in depth in Chapter 24.

See Chapter 29 for an example of a preop checklist.

See Chapter 44 for information about hospice and end-of-life care.

See Chapter 47 for information about emergency and urgent care nursing, including first aid and splinting a limb.

Critical Thinking Care Map

Caring for a Client with Scoliosis Who Attends School with a Milwaukee Brace

NCLEX-PN® Focus Area: Psychological Integrity

Case Study: J. J. Smith is a 16-year-old male who will be returning to his junior year in high school with a Milwaukee brace for treatment of scoliosis. "JJ" is to wear the brace 23 of 24 hours per day. Last year he was the forward on the water polo team and a competitive swimmer. JJ is reluctant to return to school because the "brace is very visible and I know the guys will make fun of me." He also states that he is "bummed that he won't be on the water polo team, and I am not sure I will be ready to compete for the swim team in the spring." After conferring with his parents, physician, and coach, they are contemplating allowing him to practice with the team as long as he wears the brace the remainder of each day.

Nursing Diagnosis: *Disturbed Body Image* related to Milwaukee Brace

COLLECT DATA

Subjective	Objective
_____	_____
_____	_____
_____	_____
_____	_____
_____	_____
_____	_____
_____	_____

Would you report this? Yes/No

If yes, report to: _____

What would you report? _____

Nursing Care

_____
_____
_____
_____
_____
_____
_____
_____

How would you document this? _____
_____
_____
_____

Compare your answers and documentation to those provided on the MyNursingKit Website.

Data Collected
(use only those that apply)

- Weight: 178 lbs
- Height: 5′ 11″
- 35° lateral spinal curve
- Will not make eye contact
- Wearing Milwaukee brace over t-shirt; reluctant to remove jacket
- C/o pain and requesting to call mother and go home
- VS: T 98.4, P 72, R 24, BP 110/74
- Did not eat lunch, complains that brace is putting pressure on abdomen so he cannot eat

Nursing Interventions
(use only those that apply; list in priority order)

- Assist JJ to develop new interests that he can be involved in while still in a brace.
- Establish a contract with JJ that he will wear brace at all times except during practice and workout in the pool and shower time.
- Regularly monitor height and weight.
- Evaluate brace for pressure areas.
- Consider JJ's developmental level and how wearing the brace at school can affect it.
- Arrange meeting with counselor, coach, parents, and physician to discuss available options.
- Obtain order for pain medication during school as needed.
- Allow JJ to come to health office or see the counselor if he has the need to talk.

NCLEX-PN® Exam Preparation

1 The nurse, working in a physician's office, is asked to perform a specific task. The nurse doesn't know if this task falls within the nurse's scope of practice. The nurse would determine whether it is acceptable to perform this task by consulting:

1. The physician.
2. The office manager.
3. The nurse practice act for the state.
4. The nurse manager of the practice.

2 The LPN/LVN, working in a physician's office, considers which of the following to be the supervisor related to client care issues?

1. The office manager
2. The receptionist
3. The medical assistant with the most seniority
4. The RN

3 At what grade would the school nurse begin screening the male student for scoliosis?

1. 5th
2. 6th
3. 10th
4. 11th

4 The nurse, working for a home health agency that offers hospice services, is asked to explain the requirements for admission to a client considering the service. After explaining the criteria for admission, which of the following statements made by the family would indicate that the nurse needs to provide further clarification?

1. "Our physician is not supporting our decision to seek hospice care, but we want to sign up anyway."
2. "Hospice can provide care to improve the quality of Dad's life for the time he has left."
3. "I know that Dad may have less than 6 months to live, but I want him to be as comfortable as possible."
4. "I am so glad that hospice care can be given in our home or in the nursing home if there comes a time that Dad needs more care than I can give him."

5 The LPN/LVN can perform all of the following duties in a same-day surgery center except:

1. Admission nurse.
2. Scrub tech.
3. Circulating nurse.
4. Recovery room nurse.

6 The nurse, employed at a physician's office, can assume all of the following responsibilities during the office surgical procedure except:

1. Setting up the sterile field and instruments.
2. Positioning the client.
3. Administering the local anesthetic.
4. Completing laboratory requisitions.

7 The nurse is preparing to perform a vision screening test on a 4-year-old child presenting to the pediatrician's office. Because the child does not yet know the alphabet, the nurse would:

1. State on the physical form that visual acuity could not be tested.
2. Assess the child to see what letters she knows and use a line that contains only those letters.
3. Teach the child a few letters required to read the eye chart.
4. Use the Snellen E chart.

8 The nurse is admitting a new client to the physician's office. When gathering information for the medical history form, the nurse would improve the quality of the data gathered and make the client less anxious by doing which of the following? (Select all that apply.)

1. Sitting across from the client at eye level.
2. Making frequent eye contact.
3. Explaining the purpose of the interview.
4. Writing down what the client is saying, as they say it, for accuracy.
5. Reviewing the client's medical history and medical record while sitting with the client.

9 The nurse has decided to work in a community setting and considers all of the following as potential employers except:

1. Prisons.
2. Hospice centers.
3. Physician's office.
4. Long-term care facility.

10 The nurse is working in a school health office checking immunization records for incoming kindergarten students and screening for students who do not have the recommended immunizations. For students to meet the recommended immunization requirements, they should have had how many doses of DTaP, polio, and MMR?

1. DTaP, 5; polio, 3; MMR, 2
2. DTaP, 4; polio, 4; MMR, 2
3. DTaP, 5; polio, 4; MMR, 2
4. DTaP, 5; polio, 4; MMR, 1

Answers and rationales for Review Questions appear in Appendix I.

Thinking Strategically About...

David Screaming Eagle, a 68-year-old Native American, presented in the emergency room with a temperature of 101.4°F and complaints of severe abdominal pain (10 on a scale of 0 to 10). Mr. Screaming Eagle was admitted for a urinary tract infection and urosepsis. Past medical history includes prostate cancer. Client reports incontinence related to long-term indwelling catheter that was removed 1 week ago. The last episode of chemotherapy treatment was completed 2 months ago. A 16-gauge Foley catheter was inserted in the emergency center and produced 30 mL of dark brown urine with no visible blood. A catheter was attached to the collection bag following insertion.

The client's son reports that his father has been refusing to drink liquids, due to discomfort associated with urination. The client has been receiving antibiotic therapy via a saline lock placed in the right forearm. The lock is patent and free of signs of infection. His daughter-in-law is being trained by the home health nurse to administer medications, but she is reluctant to continue since the client seems to be "getting worse." The son reports the client has lost an additional 10 pounds since chemotherapy was completed.

While reviewing the chart to gather data, you notice that the client was given 500 mg of amoxicillin, and the physician's order sheet was for 250 mg of amoxicillin 3 times per day.

CRITICAL THINKING

- Use your critical thinking skills to analyze your finding about the medication.
- Use interpretation to describe what this means.
- Identify what questions need to be answered regarding this situation.
- What conclusions can be drawn from the situation that will affect your decision?

- Describe what to do and why.
- What should a nurse do differently to improve the delivery of care?

PRIORITIZING NURSING CARE

What is the first thing that needs to be done for Mr. Screaming Eagle? Give the rationale for your decision.

MANAGEMENT OF CARE

How often should the client be monitored and what information should you collect when monitoring him?

DELEGATING

What aspects of Mr. Screaming Eagle's care can be delegated to an UAP? What follow-up will be necessary on your part?

CLIENT TEACHING

Devise a teaching plan related to fluid intake and urinary output. Who should be included in the teaching?

CULTURAL CARE STRATEGIES

Mr. Screaming Eagle asks to be discharged from the hospital. He is talking about a trip that he must take to be with the great white chief. When you tell him the physician wants him to stay a few days for observation, he becomes angry and agitated and says the great chief will send the warriors to get him if he does not go. What message do you think he is trying to convey to you and his family? Consider his Native American culture when you answer this question.

DOCUMENTING AND REPORTING

Document Mr. Screaming Eagle's care and treatment while in the emergency room. What findings need to be reported and to whom?

Mental Health Nursing Care

UNIT VIII

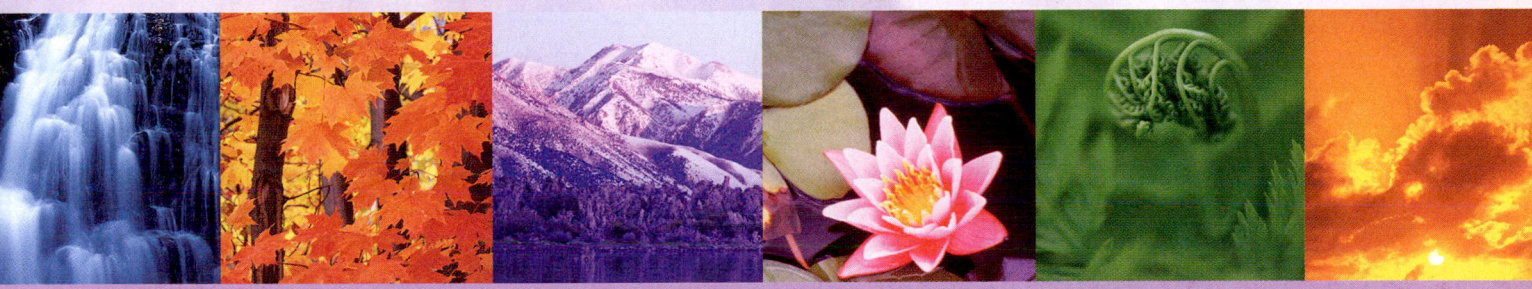

Chapter 49

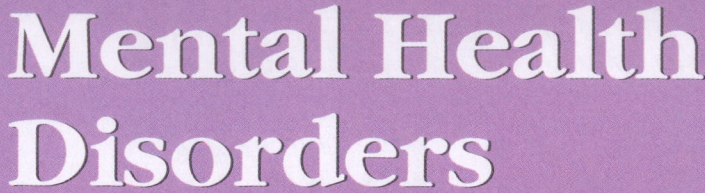

Mental Health Disorders

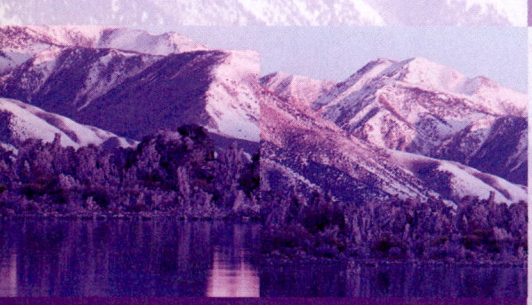

LEARNING Outcomes

After reading this chapter, you will be able to:

1. Identify characteristics of a mentally healthy person.
2. Explain key concepts about mental disorders, including why they are difficult to diagnose and treat.
3. Discuss mental health and mental health disorders in children.
4. List three major types of treatment used for clients with major mental health disorders.
5. Describe the nurse's role in promoting mental health.
6. Identify diagnostic criteria, treatment, and nursing care for clients with schizophrenia.
7. Name several types of mood disorders and describe treatments and nursing care for them.
8. Identify key aspects of personality disorders and describe nursing care for clients with this disorder.

Clinical Objectives

9. Monitor the mental status of clients.
10. Apply the nursing process to the care of clients with schizophrenia.
11. Apply the nursing process to the care of clients with major mood disorders and personality disorders.
12. Safely and effectively care for clients receiving psychotropic medications.

KEY TERMS

Use the audio glossary feature on the MyNursingKit Website to hear the correct pronunciation of the following key terms.

alogia 1346

anhedonia 1346

avolition 1346

catatonic behavior 1346

delusions 1345

depot injection 1351

disorganized behavior 1346

disorganized thinking 1346

executive function 1344

flat affect 1346

hallucinations 1345

insight 1337

kindling 1368

personality 1373

personality disorder 1373

pressured speech 1365

prodromal phase 1347

psychomotor retardation 1355

psychosis 1344

stigma 1339

Wherever you work as a nurse you will encounter clients with psychosocial needs. These needs can fall into several different categories: clients' inability to cope with changes in health status, family problems, anticipatory loss of functioning and ability to support self or family, or spiritual distress. People who are physically ill have anxiety, fear, grief, and learning needs. Likewise, people with mental health disorders become ill and need treatment, have babies in obstetrics units, and bring in their children for pediatric care. Mental disorders are more common than most people realize. In this chapter we will cover the major mental disorders, nursing interventions to help the people who have them, and the nurse's role in promoting mental health.

Mental Health

For many reasons, mental health and mental illness are difficult to define. People are unique and unpredictable. People have different life experiences. Acceptable behavior is not universal. The definition can change as culture and society change their attitudes and expectations (Box 49-1 ■).

There is some agreement, however, about what aspects of thinking, feeling, and acting are considered healthy or unhealthy. Box 49-2 ■ lists seven aspects of a mentally healthy person. All seven are discussed in more detail in the following paragraphs.

BOX 49-1   **CULTURAL PULSE POINTS**

Mental Illness Versus Culturally Supported Behavior

Mental illness is defined as a deviation from normal behavior. Because behaviors are defined differently by different cultures, what one culture views as abnormal may be perfectly acceptable by another. In a culture where independence is valued, any young adult who continues to live in the family home and defers to parents for approval may be seen by some as having issues that need to be worked through in therapy. In cultures that value emotional control, expressiveness may be viewed as a sign of instability. It is very important for healthcare professionals to be able to distinguish between mental illness and culturally supported behavior or personality traits.

BOX 49-2   **CHARACTERISTICS OF MENTALLY HEALTHY PEOPLE**

In general, mentally healthy people share these aspects:
- Accurate evaluation of reality
- Healthy self-concept
- Ability to relate to others
- A sense of meaning in life
- Creativity/productivity
- Control over one's own behavior
- Adaptability to change and conflict

The ability to determine *reality* accurately is a critical part of mental health. It includes being able to tell the difference between what really is and what might be, and being reasonably able to predict the consequences of one's behavior ("If I touch the stove, it will be hot").

A *healthy self-concept* includes a realistic opinion of the self (abilities, function, and appearance) and a positive acceptance of the self as it is. **Insight,** or self-understanding, is important; it allows people to understand why they feel and act the way they do. A person who lacks insight might refuse to take a medication because his or her symptoms are under control and so it is easy to feel there is no longer a need for the medication. This frequently happens with clients on antipsychotics. With insight, a person could decide that he does not like to take the medication, but he will because it helps his mental illness. Insight is critical for problem solving. Without it people often do not realize that they have a mental illness.

Human beings thrive best when they are with others. Love is the most important human emotion. Normal human development is not possible in isolation. People must be able to interact with and *relate to others* in order to flourish. Without the ability to relate to others in a satisfying way, a person cannot be healthy.

Humans seek reasons and *meaning in life*. Many people find a sense of meaning in the world through religion. Others find meaning in nature, philosophy, ethics, or service. This uniquely human spirituality is an important part of what it means to be a person. A fully mentally healthy person will have a sense of what is important in life and what gives life meaning.

A person does not have to be an artist to be *creative*. Healthy people can solve problems creatively. They can interpret experiences abstractly. Some people think *concretely*, meaning literally or without creativity. For example, a concrete thinker may say that the proverb "A stitch in time saves nine" means that if you sew something up in time, you will save nine stitches. A more abstract thinker might say it means that if you put a little bit of work into solving a problem early, you will save a lot of trouble in the long term. Another aspect of healthy creativity is a sense of productivity or contribution. Healthy people want to feel as though they make a difference to others or to the world.

Control of behavior means that mentally healthy people can balance conflicts with their instincts, conscience, and reality before they act. Healthy people do not act out violently just because they are frustrated in the moment. They do not steal something just because they want it. Mentally healthy people can delay gratification. They can act in a way that helps someone else, even if it is difficult for them. The healthiest people have the integrity to act on their values.

Adaptability is critical to success as a person. The one consistent thing around us is change. Healthy people can compromise, plan, and be flexible. They can manage conflict successfully. Learning to change is not easy, but if people are healthy they will manage it. Mental health is really a range of behavior, a relative state instead of an absolute thing. Nobody is at the ultimate level of health in each of the above areas all the time. Whether people have mental disorders or not, they can have anywhere from minimal to maximal mentally healthy behavior. Just as all people are developing throughout their lives, *all people have the potential for growth toward greater mental health*. Because nurses treat clients holistically, an important aspect of nursing is to promote the mental health of clients.

People with chronic physical illnesses such as diabetes or heart disease can still be healthy (within the limits of their abilities) if they take their medications and choose healthy behaviors. Similarly, people with mental illnesses who take their medications and choose healthy behaviors can be relatively healthy also.

Mental Disorders

Mental disorders are chronic illnesses with symptoms related to thinking, feeling, or behavior. They are due to genetic, biological, social, chemical, or psychologic influences. These illnesses result in impairment of functioning and other symptoms.

Much research has been done on mental disorders. The definitive source for psychiatrists and other physicians to use for the diagnostic criteria for mental disorders is the *Diagnostic and Statistical Manual of Mental Disorders*, fourth edition, text revision (*DSM-IV-TR*, American Psychiatric Association [APA],

2000). This book was written by a team of experts from all over the world who created a standard terminology for mental disorders and a set of criteria for diagnosing them. Now a physician in Canada and another in Florida will use the same list of criteria to diagnose their clients, and they will call the disorders by the same names. This standardization is critical as a foundation for research and treatment of mental disorders. Some of the *DSM-IV-TR* diagnostic criteria are included in this chapter. (See further discussion in Chapter 17 🔗.)

The authors of the *DSM-IV-TR* have made a point to say that they are attempting to *classify disorders, not people* (APA, 2000). People are not defined by their illnesses. A person with a disease is just that—a person first, not a diabetic or a schizophrenic, or "the appendectomy in room 222."

Mental disorders are a major problem for people all over the world. The incidence of mental disorders is often underestimated. One reason for this is probably that mental disorders are not recognized for the severe impact they have. In 1996, the Global Burden of Disease Study was done (Murray & Lopez, 1996). The study showed that mental illnesses make up 5 of the 15 leading causes of disability in developed countries. The five most common mental illnesses are:

- Major depressive disorder
- Alcohol abuse
- Schizophrenia
- Self-inflicted injuries
- Bipolar disorder

In the United States, almost half of all people will have a psychiatric or substance abuse disorder at some time in their lives. Box 49-3 ■ provides details about the incidence of mental illness in the United States.

BOX 49-3	FACTS ABOUT MENTAL ILLNESS IN THE UNITED STATES

- In any given year, approximately 1 out of every 4 adults will have a mental disorder.
- About 20% of children under age 18 have a mental illness that causes some functional impairment.
- Six percent of Americans have a substance abuse disorder.
- One-third of the nation's 600,000 homeless people have severe mental illnesses.
- More than 25% of jail inmates have a mental disorder.
- Major depression is the leading cause of disability (measured by the number of years lived with a disabling condition) worldwide among persons age 5 and over.
- Alcohol or mental illness is involved in 94% of all suicides. Suicide is the second leading cause of death in people ages 15 to 24.
- Most medical insurance either does not cover mental illness treatment or covers it at a lower level than general medical illness.

Source: National Institute of Mental Health.

Stigma of Mental Illness

Common terms referring to people with mental illness—*crazy, nuts, bonkers, one-brick-short-of-a-full-load, wacko, goofy,* and *mental*—all have one thing in common. They are all negative, insulting, and demeaning. When we talk about physical illnesses, we do not use such insulting terms. We would never call a person with diabetes an "insulin junkie" or a "sugar fool." These labels are inaccurate and inappropriate.

Simply talking about mental illness often causes people to laugh nervously, because mental illness has a **stigma** (negative cultural attitude that marks people with disgrace). Having a mental illness can make a person feel "labeled" or "marked" for ridicule and judgment. (If a friend asked you "Do you have asthma?" or "Are you mentally ill?" would you feel differently about the two questions?) It can feel so shameful to have a mental illness that people often refuse to seek treatment. People running for political office have dropped out of politics when it became known that they had been treated for mental illness. Even physicians sometimes hesitate to give their clients the diagnosis of a mental disorder for fear that the clients will be "labeled" and treated badly as a result.

Evidence of the stigma against people with mental illness includes the following (Depression Guideline Panel, 1993):

- People are often required to report their mental illnesses when they apply for driver's licenses, jobs, security clearances, and other routine purposes, whereas those with other medical diseases are not (some of this has decreased since passage of the Americans with Disabilities Act).
- Insurance companies reimburse for mental illness treatment at a reduced rate compared with general medical illnesses. There is often a limit on the amount of coverage for mental illness treatment that does not apply to general medical conditions.
- Physicians might not enter the diagnosis of depression into medical records because they want to protect their clients from the stigma.

clinical ALERT

The nurse practice act in many states includes a section on the nurse's competency to practice. Mental health issues as well as substance abuse issues may be addressed.

It is true that people with mental disorders have symptoms and impairment in their functioning (the specifics depend on which disorder they have). However, these disorders are treatable. Affected people can be and often are successful at being politicians (including heads of state), artists, teachers (maybe your teacher), physicians, clergy, bus drivers, nurses, and nursing students. Congress has passed a bill of rights for people with mental health disorders to ensure proper treatment of those affected (Box 49-4 ■).

BOX 49-4   MENTAL HEALTH BILL OF RIGHTS

Congress passed a Mental Health Bill of Rights that requires states to ensure mental health protection and services to people with mental disorders. The following is a summary of its provisions. It states that people with mental health disorders have these rights:

- The right to appropriate treatment and related services in a supportive setting that is not restrictive of liberty beyond what is necessary for the disorder
- The right to an individualized, written, treatment or service plan, with review and revision of the plan as needed
- The right to ongoing participation in one's own plan of care to the extent possible
- The right not to receive a mode or course of treatment without consent unless the matter is an emergency or approved by a court
- The right not to participate in experimentation
- The right to freedom from restraint or seclusion
- The right to a humane treatment environment that affords reasonable protection from harm and appropriate privacy
- The right to confidentiality of such person's records
- The right to access, upon request, to such person's mental health care records (with limited exceptions)
- The right, in the case of a person admitted on a residential or inpatient care basis, to converse with others privately, to have convenient and reasonable access to the telephone and mail, and to see visitors during regularly scheduled hours, unless medically contraindicated
- The right to be informed promptly at the time of admission, and periodically thereafter, of one's rights
- The right to assert grievances with respect to infringement of one's rights
- The right to referral as appropriate to other providers of mental health services upon discharge

---

The stigma against people with mental illnesses is not warranted. As client advocates, nurses should educate the public that mental illnesses should be treated in the same way as physical illnesses. Nurses must base their practice on evidence, not guesses or stereotypes.

Child and Adolescent Mental Health

The future of our country depends on the mental health and strength of our young people. However, many children have mental health problems that interfere with normal development and functioning. In the United States today, one in ten children suffers from a mental disorder severe enough to cause some level of impairment.

The mental disorders affecting children and adolescents include the following:

- Attention Deficit Hyperactivity Disorder (ADHD)
- Autism Spectrum Disorders (Pervasive Developmental Disorders)

- Bipolar Disorder
- Borderline Personality Disorder
- Depression
- Eating Disorders

Children are in a state of rapid change and growth during their developmental years. Diagnosis and treatment of mental disorders must be viewed with these changes in mind. Although some problems are short-lived and do not need treatment, others are persistent and very serious, requiring that parents seek professional help for their children.

Not long ago, it was thought that many brain disorders such as anxiety disorders, depression, and bipolar disorder began only after childhood. We now know they can begin in early childhood. Fewer than one in five of these ill children receives treatment. Perhaps the most studied, diagnosed, and treated childhood-onset mental disorder is attention deficit hyperactivity disorder (ADHD), but even with this disorder there is a need for further research in very young children.

Researchers supported by the National Institute of Mental Health (NIMH) have found that half of all lifetime cases of mental illness begin by age 14, and that despite effective treatments, there are long delays—sometimes decades—between first onset of symptoms and when people seek and receive treatment. The study also reveals that an untreated mental disorder can lead to a more severe, more difficult-to-treat illness, and to the development of concurrent mental illnesses (NIMH, 2005).

PREVALENCE AND AGE OF ONSET OF MENTAL DISORDERS

As mentioned, mental illness begins very early in life (50% of cases begin by age 14; 75%, by age 24). Thus, mental disorders are really the chronic diseases of the young. For example, anxiety disorders often begin in late childhood, mood disorders in late adolescence, and substance abuse in the early twenties. Unlike older people with heart disease or most cancers, young people with mental disorders suffer disability when they are in the prime of life, when they would normally be the most productive.

Although approximately 80% of all people in the United States with a mental disorder eventually seek treatment, untreated psychiatric disorders can lead to more frequent and more severe episodes, and they are more likely to become resistant to treatment. In addition, early-onset mental disorders that are left untreated are associated with school failure, teenage childbearing, unstable employment, early marriage, marital instability, and violence. Treating cases early could prevent enormous disability, before the illness becomes more severe. A disorder is categorized as "serious" if it involves a substantial limitation in daily activities or work disability, a suicide attempt with serious lethal intent, or psychosis. The condition is defined as serious if, for

3 months of the year, the person was unable to carry out normal daily activities.

People with mental or substance abuse disorders are more likely to get treatment from a primary care physician, nurse, or other general medical doctor than from a psychologist or psychiatrist. Because of this, the LPN/LVN needs to be aware of signs and behaviors that may be related to a mental health disorder in a child or adolescent.

Treatment for Mental Health Disorders

Because they are disorders that affect every aspect of clients' lives, mental health disorders require a multifaceted approach to treatment. To be effective, treatment must help the client understand and accept the facts about the disorder, help the client make life changes that will improve overall health and well-being and support the treatment regimen, and treat the underlying chemical condition. Treatment modalities described in Chapter 17 ⚭ (group or individual therapy, behavioral therapy, etc.) may be employed. Therapies discussed here relate to inpatient care for the mental health disorders that are the focus of this chapter.

MILIEU THERAPY

For psychiatric inpatients, the surrounding environment or *milieu* can be used as part of therapy. In mental health settings, an attempt is made to create a safe, structured environment in which to do mental health work. This means a quiet, pleasant environment with no distractions. It is helpful to have consistent nursing staff to promote trust.

Clients have the chance to practice and receive feedback on their behavior in the milieu. Structure offers a predictable environment that reduces stress for clients.

PSYCHOSOCIAL REHABILITATION

The goal of psychosocial rehabilitation is for individuals with mental illness to adjust or readjust to living in the community. Psychosocial rehabilitation begins while a person is still hospitalized and continues in a community mental health program or with ongoing counseling. People with mental illnesses may learn social skills, including ways to deal with other people in a variety of settings. They may learn how to cope with their mental health issues in a day-to-day environment.

Psychosocial rehabilitation also includes learning strategies for preventing relapse of mental illness. Box 49-5 ■ provides some strategies for preventing relapse that nurses can teach to clients. Behavioral techniques are often used. The goal is to improve interpersonal and occupational functioning so people with severe mental illnesses can be successful members of their communities.

BOX 49-5   STRATEGIES FOR PREVENTING RELAPSE OF MENTAL ILLNESS

Discuss the following suggestions with the client for how she or he can reduce the chance of relapse of mental illness:

- Learn from your experience. In the past how did you feel in the weeks before you needed to be hospitalized? What feelings or symptoms did you experience? These are the predictors of relapse for you. Tell your family about them, and watch for these symptoms. When they happen, get help from your psychiatrist who can change your treatment to help prevent or reduce the severity of the relapse.
- How do you feel about your medication? (Look for some positive aspect of client's attitude and repeat it.) What are your goals for the long term? Whatever you want to accomplish (becoming the president, going to Disneyland) will not happen if you do not take your medication. If medication is part of your treatment, take it. It is what keeps you out of the hospital. Tell your prescriber about side effects, most can be treated.
- Do what you can to decrease the stress in your life. Keep it quiet around yourself. Go to a room alone or with one person if you want to. When someone argues with you, go to a quiet place. Know what is most stressful for you. If you know something is really stressful for you, avoid it.

- Know your resources and have a plan. Make a list of people who can give help when you need it. For example: Adam can take me to the pharmacy to refill my prescription. Betty can talk when I am lonely or scared. Carlos can take care of my fish if I am too tired. Dad can call the doctor or the hospital if I need to go, etc. Write down all their phone numbers.
- Think of some things that make you feel better. Write them on a list. Take it out and do them when you start to feel bad. Maybe you feel better when you take a walk, do relaxation techniques, have a snack, paint, draw, take a nap, look at pictures, listen to music, talk to a trusted person, or pet a dog. The list has to be things you would really do.
- Avoid risky situations. Stay away from people who want you to use drugs or alcohol with them. It is too hard to say no. Stay away from negative people who criticize you or make you feel bad about yourself. Avoid situations that increase the voices or your stress.
- Keep healthy. Eat right. Sleep regularly. Stay active with hobbies, work, and exercise.
- Keep hope alive. Remember how life is always changing. Do you agree that some days you feel bad and some days you feel better? Even when you feel your worst, know that this is only temporary. You will feel better again in time.

PSYCHOPHARMACOLOGY

Because mental health disorders are a result of chemical imbalances in the brain, a major modality for their treatment is pharmacology. Specific agents in use will be discussed under particular disorders.

Nurses' Role in Mental Health Promotion

The evidence is clear: Mental illness is a big problem. Many people are affected, and the quality and length of their lives are diminished. What can nurses do? Nurses can make a difference in three areas:

- *Prevention.* Nurses can help prevent healthy people from becoming affected by mental disorders. An example is drug abuse education with children. With *primary prevention*, children avoid drug use and never develop a problem.
- *Treatment in the acute phase of illness. Secondary prevention* involves early diagnosis and treatment for people who have a disorder, to prevent the negative outcomes. An example is depression screening, which identifies depression early before it leads to loss of jobs, despair, or even suicide.
- *Rehabilitation. Tertiary prevention* aims to prevent further disability for people who have mental disorders. An example of tertiary prevention is a community walk-in clinic where people with schizophrenia can come to learn socialization, independent living, and medication management skills. This helps them stay out of institutions and in their homes.

Nurses have an important role in supporting therapy for clients with mental health issues. They establish a positive environment. They can be valuable role models of normal behavior for clients. They demonstrate how to interact with other people, how to dress, how to ask someone to change behavior, and how to participate in group activities.

Nurses can also be aware of risk factors for mental health disorders. The first steps in prevention are to recognize the risk factors and work to minimize them. Some factors, such as biological predisposition, are not modifiable. Others, such as inadequate resources, are modifiable risks. Figure 49-1 ■ depicts the factors that promote mental health or put people at risk for mental illness. Nurses can promote clients' mental health by helping them strengthen the health-promoting factors.

ADVOCACY

People with mental illnesses are among the most vulnerable in our society. They are often too severely affected by their disease processes to be able to speak for themselves effectively. The disheveled mentally ill homeless person stirs less sympathy from charitable contributors than even homeless animals.

The National Alliance for the Mentally Ill (NAMI) is an organization that acts as an advocate for people with mental illnesses and their families. State affiliates of NAMI help families cope with mental illnesses on a local level. They provide support, education, and advocacy.

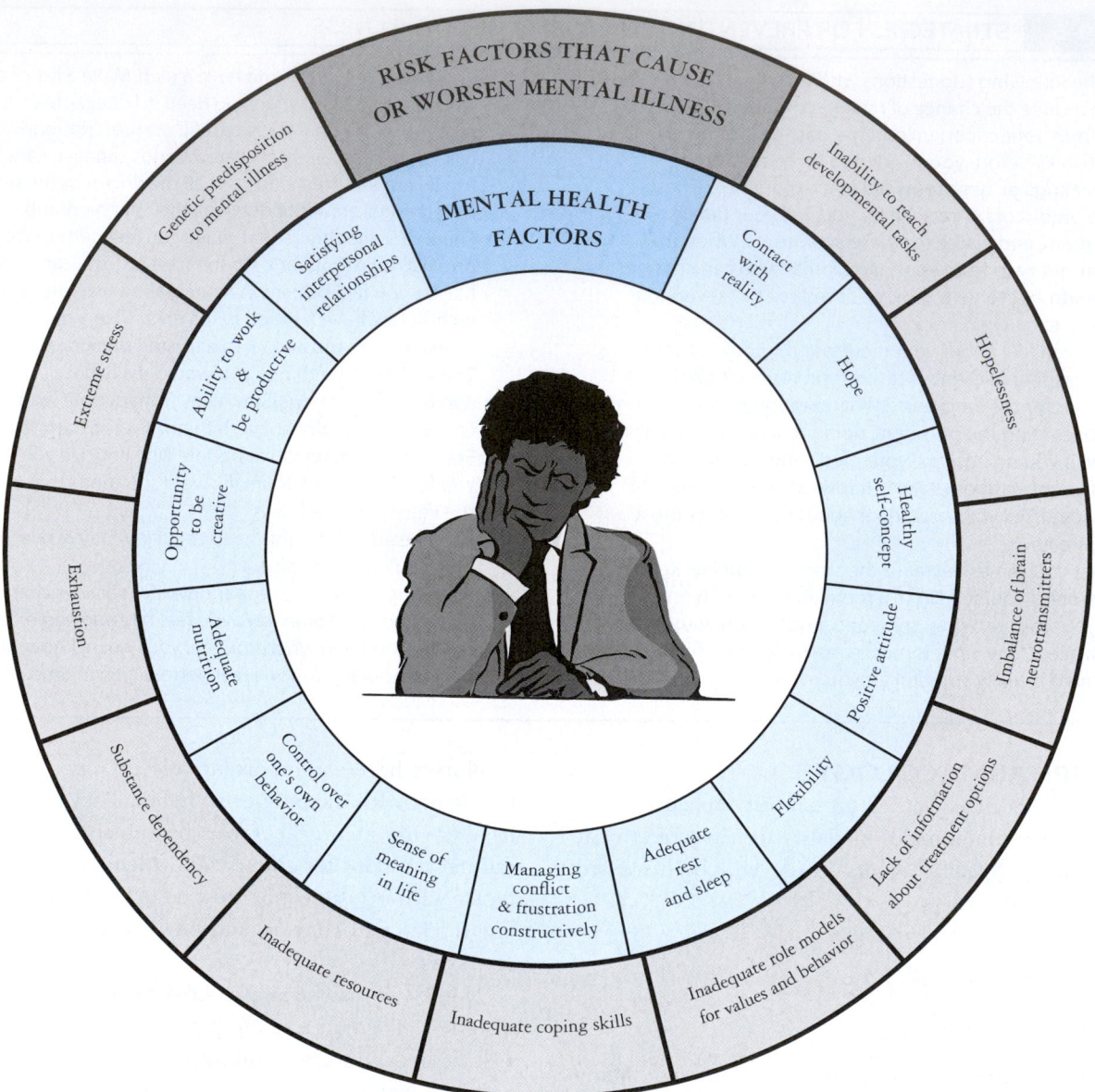

Figure 49-1. ■ Factors that promote mental health or put people at risk for mental illness.

Nurses are client advocates. People with mental illnesses are especially in need of advocacy for access to services, funding for services, and research into new treatment modalities. Nurses can be advocates for these clients by:

- Refusing to participate in stigmatizing people with mental illnesses.
- Providing excellent nursing care for clients with mental illnesses.
- Telling our legislators to change laws and health policies to make mental health services available.
- Contributing to NAMI or to research on treatments for mental disorders.
- Speaking out for people with mental disorders who often need an advocate to receive the simplest of human rights.

This chapter covers three major mental disorders that affect millions of people worldwide: schizophrenia, major depressive disorder, and bipolar disorder. These disorders all affect the thinking, emotions, and behavior of people who have them. They affect people's ability to function and the quality of their daily lives. All are caused by a complicated combination of *nature and nurture*. They all have abnormalities of genetics, brain structure, and neurotransmitter function (the nature part). People with all three disorders are also affected by stress and life experiences (the nurture part). Table 49-1 ■ lists the brain neurotransmitters involved in mental illness and their effects. Psychotropic medications (those that affect the mind) act by affecting these neurotransmitters. Figure 49-2 ■ illustrates categories of psychotropic medications and the symptoms they target.

TABLE 49-1		Neurotransmitters	
NEUROTRANSMITTER	TYPE	PHYSIOLOGIC EFFECTS	RELATIONSHIP TO MENTAL DISORDERS
Acetylcholine (ACh)	Monoamine	Sleep–wake cycle. Signals muscles to become active.	Decreased in Alzheimer's and Parkinson's diseases.
Dopamine (DA)	Monoamine	Controls complex movements, cognition, motivation, and pleasure and regulates emotional responses.	Increased in schizophrenia and mania. Decreased in depression and Parkinson's disease. Some drugs of abuse stimulate dopamine release (cocaine and amphetamines).
Norepinephrine (NE)	Monoamine	Affects attention, learning, memory, and regulation of mood, sleep, and wakefulness.	Reduced activity in depression. Increased in schizophrenia, mania, and anxiety.
Serotonin (5-HT)	Monoamine	Affects sleep and wakefulness, especially falling asleep. Affects mood and thought processes.	Probably plays a role in the thought disorders of schizophrenia (hallucinations, delusions, and social withdrawal). Decreased in depression. Possibly decreased in anxiety and obsessive compulsive disorders.
Gamma-aminobutyric acid (GABA)	Amino acid	Modulates other neurotransmitters.	Decreased in anxiety and in schizophrenia.
Glutamate	Amino acid	Controls opening of ion channels for calcium, affecting neurotransmission.	Implicated in schizophrenia. Neurotoxicity results from overexposure to glutamate (as in Huntington's disease).

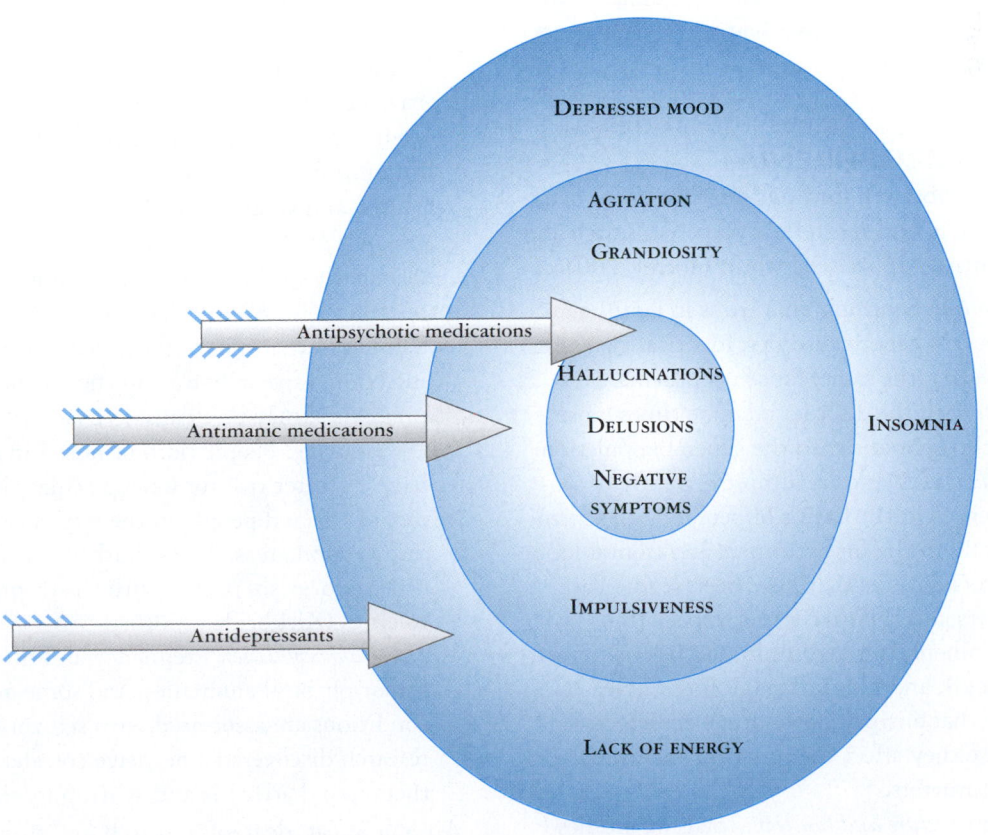

Figure 49-2. ■ Target symptoms of psychotropic medication.

Schizophrenia

Schizophrenia is a complex disorder of the brain. In general, schizophrenia affects a person's thinking, mood, and behavior. **Psychosis** is a major feature of schizophrenia. The major characteristics of psychosis are:

- Abnormal interpretation of reality.
- Decreased ability to relate to self and others.
- Decreased ability to function.
- Disorganized thoughts and behavior.

Other disorders also cause psychosis. *Schizoaffective disorder* (a combination of schizophrenia and a mood disorder), bipolar mania, and depression with psychotic features are three. However, in this chapter schizophrenia serves as a *prototype* (model) for the nursing approach to care of people with thought disorders.

About 2.2 million people in the United States (1% of adults) have schizophrenia (Torrey, 2001). Although it affects women, men, all races, and all socioeconomic classes, it is underrepresented in research funding and in services. Approximately 40% of people with schizophrenia are not receiving treatment at any given time. Worse yet, there are more people with schizophrenia in jail than in the hospital. People with schizophrenia are often homeless. They often are victims of crime. If untreated, they are more likely to be violent. This is the biggest cause of the stigma against the entire group of people. Even though schizophrenia is a major public health issue, public psychiatric treatment services, housing, and rehabilitation services are grossly inadequate (Torrey, 2001).

CAUSES OF SCHIZOPHRENIA

E. Fuller Torrey describes ten findings relating to the cause of schizophrenia. These findings reflect years of research and experience by scientists all over the world (Torrey, 2001):

1. *The disease is familial.* Schizophrenia "runs in families," but it is not a purely genetic disorder. Identical twins are not always *concordant* (the same) for schizophrenia. Siblings of a person with the disorder are nine times more likely to have schizophrenia than the general population.

2. *Neurochemical changes.* There are almost certainly neurochemical differences in the brains of people with schizophrenia, especially in the hippocampus and frontal lobe. The major neurochemicals that have been studied are neurotransmitters and their receptors, especially dopamine, norepinephrine, serotonin, GABA (gamma-aminobutyric acid), and glutamate (Goff & Coyle, 2001). The fact that antipsychotic drugs are effective is probably because they affect the function and availability of neurotransmitters.

3. *Changes in brain structure and function.* Imaging studies have repeatedly shown structural changes in the brains

of people with schizophrenia. These include enlargement of the brain ventricles, decrease in the size of the limbic system, and changes in the cell structure in the hippocampus, amygdala, parahippocampal gyrus, entorhinal cortex, and cingulate.

4. *Cognitive impairments.* Four types of cognitive function are affected by schizophrenia: (1) attention, (2) **executive function** (abstract thinking and problem solving), (3) awareness of the illness (*insight*), and (4) short-term memory. The disease affects some aspects of thinking; others are intact, such as language skills, knowledge of information, judgment, and visual spatial abilities.

5. *Neurologic abnormalities.* The disease can cause abnormal reflexes (such as the grasp reflex found normally only in infants). It can cause confusion between right and left sides of the body, causing an inability to perceive two simultaneous touches on the body (e.g., the examiner touches the palms of each hand simultaneously, but the client is only able to perceive one palm being touched. Abnormal eye movements (rapid eye movement and blinking too frequently or not often enough) have been associated with the disease. Abnormal body movements can be caused by the disease, but also by medications used to treat it.

6. *Brain electrical abnormalities.* People with schizophrenia are more likely to have abnormal electrical activity in the brain (Figure 49-3 ■).

7. *Immunologic and inflammatory abnormalities.* Reduced immune function and an increase in cytokines (interleukin-6), and abnormalities in leukocytes and immunoglobulins have been reported in people with schizophrenia. However, because antipsychotic medications can also affect immune function, it is hard to know what the disease causes, and what the medication causes.

8. *Season of birth.* People with schizophrenia are born more frequently in the winter and spring than in the summer or fall (5% to 8% increase in December through April). Some researchers have theorized that a maternal virus infection, especially during the second trimester of pregnancy, may be a causative factor.

9. *Urban living.* People born or raised in an urban area have a greater risk for having schizophrenia. The birth rate of affected people in the city is twice that of the rate in rural areas. The suburbs have a rate between the other two. Also, people with the disorder tend to move to cities (Kirkbride, 2006).

10. *Other abnormalities.* Pregnancy and birth complications, minor physical anomalies, and some autoimmune conditions are associated with schizophrenia, although research discovered a negative correlation between rheumatoid arthritis and schizophrenia.

After a great deal of research on this debilitating disorder, the current answer is that schizophrenia is caused by

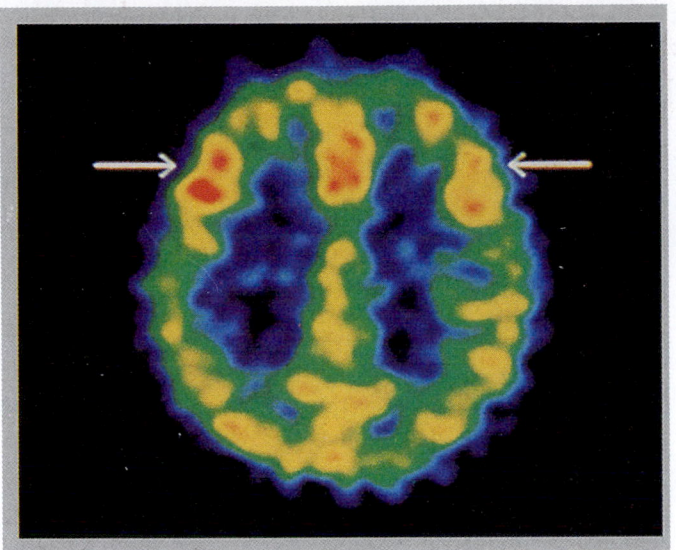
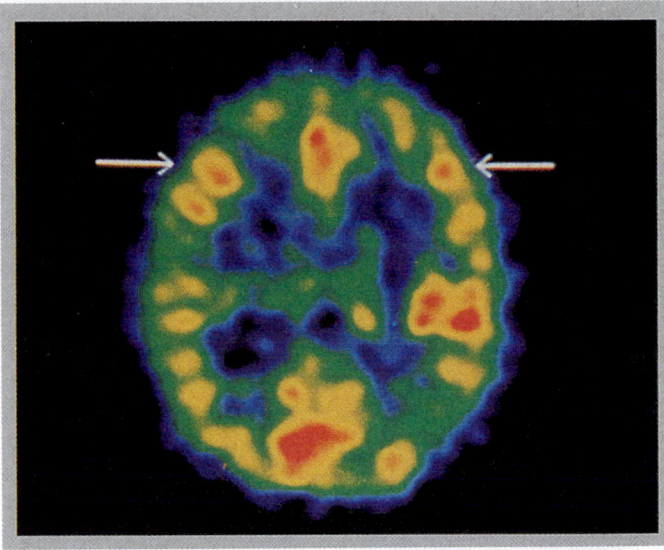

A

B

Figure 49-3. ■ Schizophrenia scans. PET scans of discordant monozygotic twins during a test to provoke activity and measure regions of cerebral blood flow. **A.** Arrows indicate areas of normal blood flow and brain activity in an unaffected twin. **B.** Arrows indicate areas of lower blood flow and brain activity in the twin with schizophrenia. (Courtesy of Dr. Karen F. Berman, Clinical Brain Disorders Branch, National Institute of Mental Health.)

abnormalities in brain structure and function. Schizophrenia is probably more than one distinct disorder, in which similar symptoms arise from different causes.

Manifestations

The symptoms associated with schizophrenia may be placed into three major categories: positive, disorganized, and negative symptoms.

POSITIVE SYMPTOMS. The *positive symptoms* of schizophrenia seem to be an excess or distortion of normal functions (APA, 2000). Positive (also called *psychotic*) symptoms include hallucinations and delusions:

- **Hallucinations** are sensory perceptions that seem very real but occur without external stimulus. The client may or may not realize that they are not real. *Auditory* hallucinations are the most common (clients hearing voices that nobody else hears). About 75% of people with schizophrenia hear voices at some time (Torrey, 2001). *Visual* hallucinations are the next most common. Others are *tactile* (touch), *gustatory* (taste), *olfactory* (smell), or *somatic* (involving body sensations, such as electricity).

- **Delusions** are fixed false beliefs, such as believing you are the king of England. These beliefs persist despite evidence that they are not true. Table 49-2 ■ lists types of delusions.

TABLE 49-2	**Types of Delusions**	
TYPE OF DELUSION	**CONTENT**	**EXAMPLES**
Grandiose	The affected person has beliefs of inflated powers, knowledge, identity, or relationship to a deity or famous person.	"I am Spiderman."
Delusion of reference	Events, objects, or other people in the immediate environment have a particular and unusual significance.	"The TV newsman is talking to me."
Persecutory	The central belief is that the affected person is being conspired against, harassed, cheated, or persecuted.	"The food here is poisoned."
Somatic	The content of the delusion relates to the structure or function of the client's body.	"There is a machine inside my body."
Bizarre	Ideas are clearly improbable and not derived from real-life experiences.	"My neighbor planted a fish inside my brain that tells me when to drink water."
Thought broadcasting	One's thoughts are being transmitted out loud so other people can hear them.	"I don't want to go to the store. Maybe I'll hurt somebody's feelings if I think they are fat or something."
Thought insertion	One's thoughts are not one's own, but are inserted into one's mind.	"You think I'm bad, but it's not me. The devil puts those ideas there."

DISORGANIZED SYMPTOMS. The *disorganized symptoms* of schizophrenia include disorganized thinking and disorganized behavior:

- **Disorganized thinking** is a major feature of schizophrenia. A client's thinking is assessed by observing what the client says. Clients with schizophrenia cannot sort and interpret incoming sensory information, or respond appropriately. Clients may change topics every few words (*incoherent speech*). At its worst, they may throw words together in a "word salad" where words have no relationship to each other ("Dogs, hat, fight, door, happening, machine, quickly"). Loose associations (called *derailment*) can occur, with a person's ideas moving from one track to another frequently (APA, 2000). An example of loose associations is "You know I live in the zoo, I like animals, I plan to wear my new shoes when I go on the walk, are you coming?"

- **Disorganized behavior** lacks goal orientation. Without goals, even activities of daily living (ADLs—personal hygiene or preparing meals) are difficult. Clients may have unusual or purposeless behavior (walk in circles, pace). They may dress oddly (wearing several coats and hats on a hot day). They may have bouts of unpredictable agitation (pacing, shouting, profanity) or display inappropriate personal behavior, such as public masturbation (APA, 2000). They may also have *catatonic behavior* (inability to move or talk).

NEGATIVE SYMPTOMS. The negative symptoms of schizophrenia represent another major source of disability for clients. In contrast to the positive symptoms, the negative symptoms involve a deficit or decrease of normal functions. Negative symptoms include:

- **Flat affect.** *Affect* is the nonverbal expression of emotion. The person experiencing schizophrenia may have decreased (*blunt*) or absent (*flat*) affect. With flat affect, the person does not show any facial expressions or other body language indicating feelings.

- **Alogia.** *Alogia* is decreased amount and richness of speech (poverty of speech). It is thought that reduced speech reflects reduced thinking. A person with alogia has brief verbal responses, with little emotional expression and no abstract ideas (*DSM, IV*, 2000).

- **Avolition.** *Avolition* is a lack of motivation. These clients have difficulty with any goal-directed activities. This symptom can make it difficult for affected people to hold jobs or care for themselves.

- **Anhedonia.** *Anhedonia* means lack of ability to feel pleasure.

DIAGNOSTIC CRITERIA

The diagnostic criteria for schizophrenia are that the client must have (APA, 2000):

1. Two or more of the following symptoms:
   - Delusions
   - Hallucinations
   - Disorganized speech
   - Grossly disorganized or **catatonic behavior** (a marked decrease in response to the environment)
   - Negative symptoms (see text for description)

2. *Social/occupational dysfunction:* The disorder must markedly decrease the person's ability to function at work or school, in interpersonal relations, or in self-care.

3. *Duration:* Continuous signs of the disturbance persist for at least 6 months. Nursing practice is concerned with the client's response to illness, so the client's symptoms are important to nurses. Box 49-6 ■ describes the experience of schizophrenia by the real experts—people who have it and their families.

BOX 49-6	REALITY CHECK ON SCHIZOPHRENIA

- "At first it just sounds like wind in the leaves, rustling and soft. Then it becomes voices, whispering then talking louder. If I concentrate I can hear them more clearly."
- "I am just here [psychiatric hospital] because I had a fight with my brother. There is nothing wrong with me. You are the one who is crazy!"
- "The witches are in my head and after me all the time. I'm never safe. It's OK, they won't get you."
- "An android named Les told me that if I jumped off the bridge I could fly."
- "I am just afraid. I'm always afraid."
- "I talk to the animals, you know, through their bellies. I am a vegetarian. I could never hurt them. I know what it is like to be eaten alive."
- "I must work day and night to keep these demons at bay! It is exhausting."
- "If I listen to heavy metal [music] really loud through the headphones, it drowns out the voices sometimes."
- "The voices are talking to me all the time. They comment on everything, like 'You want that but it's too good for you,' or 'You are so bad,' or 'That man is going to kill you.'"
- "Sometimes I wonder: Is that a real memory, or not? Is that person trying to kill me? Will my thoughts hurt someone? My mother killed herself. I know why."
- "Please. Please, can you or one of your kind tell me what happened to me? Why are my thoughts like this? The last time I saw you, you were blue. Now you're red. I know you're an alien. Please tell me what is wrong with me!"
- "Before the new medication, I spent all of my adult life in the hospital. Now that I'm being discharged I have some new problems I had never considered before, like 'How do I have fun?' and 'How do I prepare food?' These are not such bad problems to have."

COURSE OF THE DISEASE

The onset of schizophrenia is usually between the ages of 16 and 30, although it can affect people of any age (Torrey, 2001). In addition to the thought and neurologic symptoms, schizophrenia affects the person's abilities to relate to self and others, and to function in society. Most people with schizophrenia do not marry, and they are more likely than their parents to be unemployed (APA, 2000).

Like many chronic illnesses, schizophrenia is characterized by *exacerbations* and *remissions* (periods when the client has psychotic and other symptoms, and periods when the symptoms subside, respectively). Many clients experience a **prodromal phase** (warning phase) in which early symptoms occur, before they have a full psychotic episode. If individuals recognize the warning symptoms, it may be possible for treatment with medication to prevent or lessen the psychotic episode that follows. The prodromal phase often starts with negative symptoms. Family members can look back and remember that the client spent a lot of time in bed, or became more distant or isolated before a psychotic episode (APA, 2000).

In the acute phase of the disorder, the affected person may experience the positive symptoms and negative symptoms described earlier. The person is usually not able to pursue normal tasks or even do ADLs while in an acute episode.

Medication appears to improve the long-term prognosis for people with schizophrenia. After 10 years of treatment, 25% of those with schizophrenia have recovered completely, 25% have improved considerably, and 25% have improved moderately. Fifteen percent do not improve, and 10% are dead despite treatment (Torrey, 2001).

People with schizophrenia have a shorter life expectancy than other people do. Females have a 5.6 times greater risk of early death than the general population. Males have a 5.1 times greater risk of early death. Suicide contributes to most excess mortality. People with untreated schizophrenia who are experiencing depression and psychosis are the ones most likely to kill themselves. Other increased risks associated with schizophrenia are accidents, diseases (heart disease, infections, and breast cancer), and homelessness (Torrey, 2001).

The brain disorder in schizophrenia leaves many people unable to understand that they are mentally ill. This is a cruel irony: that people with schizophrenia avoid effective treatments because they lack the insight to use them. Denial is not the problem when people with schizophrenia do not seem to take their disease seriously. In fact, lack of insight is part of the disorder (Amador, 2001).

Early diagnosis and treatment of schizophrenia is important to prevent frequent relapses and rehospitalizations. It may also prevent the worst long-term outcomes of this devastating disorder: homelessness and death (Torrey, 2001).

Dual diagnosis means that the problems of mental illness and substance abuse occur together. (See also Chapter 17 ⚭ .) Substance abuse is particularly common among people with schizophrenia. In combination, the problems of dual diagnosis lead to even more homelessness, disease, violence, incarceration, and death.

Treatment

During acute episodes of schizophrenia, many people require hospitalization.

Milieu therapy is useful and helps to model a healthy environment. For people with psychosis, poor judgment about their own safety, difficulty relating to others, and delusional thinking, the environment should be pleasant, simple, and safe. There should be no background music, loud television, loud talking, or flashing lights. It is helpful to have consistent nursing staff to promote trust. Nurses also can model normal behavior. Nurses demonstrate how to interact with other people, how to dress, how to ask someone to change their behavior, and how to participate in group activities. Clients have the chance to practice and receive feedback on their behavior in the milieu.

To encourage independence, the nurse may give the client a chance to do activities independently first (for example, to comb hair before breakfast). If the client does not comb his or her hair, the nurse will *prompt* (remind) the client to do so. Milieu therapy provides structure for clients' daily living. Meals are served on schedule. There is a schedule of group activities. Unit policies are followed consistently.

Psychosocial Rehabilitation

For clients with schizophrenia, the goal is to adjust to living in the community. Psychosocial rehabilitation begins while a person is still hospitalized, and continues in a community mental health program. People with mental illnesses learn social skills, including ways to deal with other people in a variety of settings. They learn practical skills for living in the community. Skills training may include money management, how to use public transportation, recreation skills, personal hygiene, food preparation, and job skills.

Psychopharmacology

Medication is not the only treatment, but it is a cornerstone in the treatment of schizophrenia. Antipsychotic medications help relieve the hallucinations, delusions, and disordered thinking associated with the disorder.

Antipsychotic medications (also called *neuroleptics*) are used to treat disorders like schizophrenia. They are also used to treat thought disorders sometimes associated with dementia, mania, or major depression with psychotic features (see Figure 49-2). The antipsychotics are grouped as typical (first-generation), atypical (second-generation), or new-generation antipsychotic drugs. Box 49-7 ■ provides a list of antipsychotic medications.

BOX 49-7 ANTIPSYCHOTIC MEDICATIONS

Traditional or Typical Antipsychotics

Chlorpromazine (Thorazine)
Fluphenazine (Prolixin)
Haloperidol (Haldol)
Loxapine (Loxitane)
Mesoridazine (Serentil)
Molindone (Moban)
Perphenazine (Trilafon)
Thioridazine (Mellaril)
Thiothixene (Navane)
Trifluoperazine (Stelazine)

Atypical Antipsychotics

Clozapine (Clozaril)
Olanzapine (Zyprexa)
Quetiapine (Seroquel)
Risperidone (Risperdal)
Ziprasidone (Geodon)

New-Generation Antipsychotics

Aripiprazole (Abilify, Abilitat)

Because schizophrenia affects people differently, individual clients may need to try several different antipsychotics before finding the one that works well. This trial process can be demoralizing.

clinical ALERT

The nurse should explain to clients that each antipsychotic medication may take 3 to 6 weeks to have the desired effect. Tell them that the healthcare team will work with them until the right one is found. Without this knowledge, they might give up hope, and stop taking the medication too soon (Stuart & Laraia, 2001).

The goals of treatment with antipsychotic agents are to:

- Relieve symptoms of psychosis.
- Provide for safety.
- Improve clients' function and quality of life.

Medication compliance is a major problem for clients with schizophrenia. Approximately 80% of those who stop taking their medication after an acute episode have a relapse of psychosis within a year. Even people who continue to take their medications experience relapse at the rate of approximately 30% in a year (Torrey, 2001). Medication clearly improves the quality and quantity of life for people with severe mental illnesses like schizophrenia. Unfortunately, the people who need medications most often do not realize this. Also, certain medications cause side effects that combine with lack of insight to decrease client compliance even further.

TYPICAL (FIRST-GENERATION) ANTIPSYCHOTICS. The typical antipsychotics tend to be effective in treating psychosis or the "positive" symptoms of schizophrenia. They are especially effective in treatment of acute psychosis with agitation.

The "negative" symptoms of schizophrenia (decreased and slowed movement, decreased thought and speech, flattened affect, and avolition) are not very responsive to typical antipsychotic medications.

It may take 2 days to 2 weeks for clients to experience the sedating effects of the typical antipsychotic drugs. Full effect may take 4 weeks or longer.

After approximately 12 to 24 months of stable maintenance on antipsychotic medication, the client can be slowly tapered from the drug to assess whether he or she continues to need this treatment. Some people with schizophrenia who have had more than three episodes in a 5-year period, or those who have chronic symptoms, may require lifetime medication therapy (Stuart & Laraia, 2001).

Psychotic symptoms are thought to be related in part to excess dopamine activity. Typical antipsychotic medications target the dopamine-2 (D_2) receptors in an area of the brain. They act as *antagonists* of the D_2 receptors, meaning they reduce dopamine activity in the brain.

Side effects are common with antipsychotic agents. They are often the reason clients stop taking their medications when they are at home. *Management of side effects is a critical part of the care of clients taking antipsychotic medications.*

Extrapyramidal Side Effects. While antagonism of D_2 receptors causes a reduction in psychosis, it also causes extrapyramidal side effects (also called EPSE or EPS for extrapyramidal symptoms). Box 49-8 ■ lists the extrapyramidal side effects. EPS result from the effects of antipsychotic drugs on the part of the central nervous system (CNS) that controls involuntary movement (*extrapyramidal tracts*). Dopamine and acetylcholine (another neurotransmitter) must be in balance for the client to have normal muscle movement. When the antipsychotic medication first reduces dopamine, it causes an imbalance between acetylcholine and dopamine. Treatment is an anticholinergic drug, which will bring down cholinergic activity, and put dopamine and acetylcholine back in balance.

EPS are very uncomfortable for clients. When a client experiences EPS, the provider may reduce the dose of the antipsychotic medication, prescribe a different antipsychotic, or try an anticholinergic (a medication that blocks the passage of impulses through the parasympathetic nerves) or other medication to treat the symptoms. Anticholinergic medications are usually given orally, but some may be given parenterally in emergent situations. It is the responsibility of the nurse to ask whether the client is uncomfortable and to advocate for the client to obtain relief. Table 49-3 ■ lists drugs used to treat EPS. These medications may be ordered regularly when a client is starting antipsychotic therapy, or on a prn basis to treat EPS as they occur.

BOX 49-8   MANIFESTATIONS OF EXTRAPYRAMIDAL SIDE EFFECTS

- **Dystonia:** Muscular rigidity, abnormal muscle contraction. If tongue or larynx is involved, choking can result. Acute dystonia can be painful and terrifying. It can be mild, such as jaw muscle tightening, or so severe that the client has generalized muscle tightening that results in arching of the entire body. Dystonia occurs in approximately 20% of clients taking typical antipsychotics.
- **Pseudoparkinsonism** or **dyskinesia** (abnormal movement): Stiff, stooped posture; shuffling gait; tremor; slow movements; cogwheel rigidity (jerky, ratchet-like movements of the joints); masklike faces (loss of facial expression). These movement symptoms are caused by the imbalance between dopamine and acetylcholine, not by real Parkinson's disease. Twenty percent of clients taking typical antipsychotics experience either pseudoparkinsonism or dystonia.
- **Akathisia:** Restlessness, intense need to move. The client may report a sense of "jumping out of my skin" or an inability to sit still. Akathisia may cause clients to pace the floor (walk back and forth continuously), to fidget with fingers, or to move arms and legs while sitting. Akathisia can make it

impossible for a client to rest or sleep for days. It is the most common of the extrapyramidal side effects, affecting 25% of clients, and it responds poorly to treatment (Keltner et al., 2003). Akathisia may be so intolerable for clients that they consider suicide.
- **Tardive dyskinesia** (late onset of abnormal movement): Tardive dyskinesia is an extrapyramidal side effect that develops after extended antipsychotic drug therapy (also see Chapter 36 ⊙⊙). The symptoms of tardive dyskinesia (TD) include involuntary movements such as lip smacking, facial grimacing, tongue protrusion, tongue writhing, blinking, or other involuntary movements of the limbs and trunk. The most common TD symptoms involve abnormal involuntary movements of the face and tongue. The symptoms disappear during sleep. Sometimes clients can voluntarily suppress the abnormal movements briefly, but they recur when the client concentrates on something else. TD may be due to development of hypersensitivity to dopamine. It is not caused by the same dopamine-acetylcholine imbalance as the other EPS. It does not respond to anticholinergic medications (Keltner et al., 2003).

clinical ALERT

Tardive dyskinesia can be irreversible. It is important for clients on antipsychotic therapy to be monitored for abnormal involuntary movements. If EPS are identified early, the physician can change the treatment plan to prevent tardive dyskinesia.

Neuroleptic Malignant Syndrome. Neuroleptic malignant syndrome (NMS) is a potentially fatal side effect of antipsychotic drugs. It is an idiosyncratic reaction to antipsychotic drugs. It is not a toxic or allergic effect. High-potency typical antipsychotics are most frequently involved. The major symptoms are high fever, muscle pain and rigidity, autonomic instability (unstable blood pressure, diaphoresis, pale skin), delirium, inability to speak, tremors, and elevated levels of enzymes that indicate muscle damage (CPK). Temperatures may rise as high as 108°F (42.2°C). Less than 1% of people who take antipsychotic drugs develop NMS, but for these it can be fatal. Early diagnosis and treatment are the keys to client survival. Clients are at higher risk for developing NMS if they have dehydration, poor nutrition, or

concurrent medical illness. Treatment involves discontinuing antipsychotic drugs and providing supportive treatment for dehydration and other symptoms.

clinical ALERT

Neuroleptic malignant syndrome can be fatal to clients taking antipsychotic drugs. It usually (but not always) occurs early in therapy. Nurses should monitor for high fever, muscle pain, and unstable vital signs. Report these to the physician immediately!

Endocrine Side Effects. Dopamine inhibits the hormone prolactin, which promotes breast enlargement and milk production. Typical antipsychotics elevate levels of prolactin because they inhibit dopamine. Chronic prolactin elevation can cause decreased libido (sexual drive), breast enlargement (*gynecomastia*), and *galactorrhea* (leakage of milk) in women or men. It can also cause menstrual dysfunction in women.

The incidence of Type 2 diabetes is increased in people who have schizophrenia, even in those who are not obese. Nurses should be alert for signs and symptoms of hyperglycemia in clients taking antipsychotics.

TABLE 49-3	Anticholinergic Drugs Used to Treat Extrapyramidal Symptoms	
GENERIC (TRADE) NAME	**DRUG CLASSIFICATION**	**AVAILABLE IN INJECTABLE FORM?**
Benztropine (Cogentin)	Anticholinergic	Yes
Biperiden (Akineton)	Anticholinergic	Yes
Diphenhydramine (Benadryl)	Antihistamine (has strong anticholinergic side effects)	Yes
Procyclidine (Kemadrin)	Anticholinergic	No
Trihexyphenidyl (Artane)	Anticholinergic	No

BOX 49-9 MANIFESTATIONS OF ANTICHOLIN-
ERGIC SIDE EFFECTS

Dry mouth
Orthostatic hypotension
Constipation
Urinary hesitancy or retention
Pupil dilation (*mydriasis*)
Blurred near vision
Dry eyes
Photophobia (sensitivity to light)
Increased heart rate

Anticholinergic Side Effects. Anticholinergic side effects often result from the use of antipsychotics. Box 49-9 ■ lists anticholinergic symptoms. Clients taking anticholinergic medications for EPS have an increased risk for these side effects.

Weight Gain. Any of the antipsychotics can cause weight gain. Weight gain with antipsychotics is associated with increased appetite, binge eating, carbohydrate craving, decreased satiety, and change in food preferences.

Obesity is common in people with schizophrenia in general. People with schizophrenia are less likely to exercise or eat a healthy low-fat diet. The appetite changes, sedentary lifestyle, and unhealthy food choices all add up to an increased risk for obesity, Type 2 diabetes, and cardiovascular diseases.

Medical opinion is that the therapeutic effects of medication outweigh the importance of weight gain. However, weight gain can be a body image and self-esteem issue for clients. Clients benefit from discussing their concerns with nurses.

The best approach to the risk of weight gain is prevention. Nurses can teach clients and their families about this risk, and about how to reduce the likelihood of obesity with healthy nutrition and exercise.

Orthostatic Hypotension. The hypotension caused by antipsychotics is due to an antiadrenergic effect. In other words, normally the blood vessels can respond to changes in body position by constricting, ensuring adequate blood flow to the brain. With antipsychotics, sympathetic alpha-1 receptors are blocked, and the vessels are prevented from responding automatically to body position changes.

This *orthostatic* (position-related, postural) hypotension happens when the individual stands up or changes position quickly. It can create a safety hazard for the client who becomes dizzy or falls when the blood pressure drops. (See Box 21-10 for a reminder on how to measure for orthostatic hypotension.)

Cardiac Side Effects. Antipsychotics may cause increased heart rate as an anticholinergic side effect. They may also cause prolonged conduction time through the heart's electrical system. On ECG this would be a prolonged QT interval.

Seizures. The antipsychotics tend to decrease the seizure threshold. This means that it would take a smaller stimulus to cause a seizure in a client taking these medications. Epilepsy or a history of seizures is not a contraindication for the use of antipsychotic drugs, but the physician should be notified of any such history. (See further discussion of seizures in Chapter 36 .)

Photosensitivity. Some clients taking antipsychotics experience an increased sensitivity to the effects of the sun (photosensitivity). They may get severe sunburn with minimal sun exposure, whether they are dark skinned or light skinned. Clients should be counseled to avoid prolonged exposure to sunlight and to wear sunscreen whenever they are outdoors.

ATYPICAL ANTIPSYCHOTICS. The atypical antipsychotics have been used since the 1990s to treat schizophrenia and other psychotic disorders. Their mechanism of action differs from that of the typical agents. Where typical agents act largely on one specific type of receptor site (D_2 receptors), the atypical agents influence a variety of dopamine receptor sites, serotonin receptors, muscarinic receptors, alpha-receptors, and histamine receptors. Atypical agents have several important features. The atypical agents (Rankin, 2000):

1. Are effective in treating the negative symptoms of schizophrenia.
2. Cause fewer extrapyramidal side effects.
3. Are effective against the symptoms of schizophrenia for some people who do not respond to typical agents.

Side Effects. EPS are the side effects most commonly cited by clients as their reason for noncompliance with antipsychotic medications at home. As a group, the atypical agents cause less EPS, less prolactin increase, and less tardive dyskinesia. They treat psychosis effectively in some people who are resistant to the typical antipsychotics. Because of their efficacy and more favorable side effect profile, the atypical antipsychotics are currently prescribed more frequently for clients with psychosis. See Box 49-7 for a list of atypical antipsychotic agents.

Individual atypical antipsychotics have some of the same side effects as the typical agents. Examples are the increased risk of weight gain with olanzapine, increased prolactin with risperidone, and the risk of increased heart conduction time with ziprasidone.

Agranulocytosis Even though their side effect profile is favorable, the atypical agents still have side effects. The most notable is that clozapine can cause agranulocytosis, a life-threatening decrease in white blood cell (WBC) production (see Chapter 34). This effect happens to 1% of clients who take clozapine. Because of this serious possibility, clozapine is only used for clients who are resistant to treatment with other antipsychotics. Treatment resistance is established by failure to respond to at least two different antipsychotic agents. Clozapine is effective in treating 25% to 50% of clients whose symptoms do not respond to typical agents (Brown et al., 2002).

clinical ALERT

All clients receiving clozapine should have a WBC count measured once per week during the first 6 months of therapy, and every other week after that, to assess whether their WBC count is stable. If a client's WBC count drops (indicating bone marrow suppression), clozapine should be permanently discontinued.

Diabetes Clients receiving atypical antipsychotics are 9% more likely to have diabetes than people taking typical agents. In one study, the likelihood was significantly increased for clients taking clozapine, olanzapine, or quetiapine. The mechanism may be an increase in insulin resistance in body cells. Clients taking these drugs should be monitored regularly for development of diabetes. Other risk factors, such as African American or Latino ethnicity, obesity, female gender, and family history of Type 2 diabetes increase the client's risk (Brown et al., 2002). (Diabetes is discussed in detail in Chapter 38 ∞.)

NEW-GENERATION ANTIPSYCHOTICS. A new type of atypical antipsychotic is now available. This dopamine system stabilizer is aripiprazole (Abilify, Abilitat). Unlike the other antipsychotic agents, aripiprazole has a stabilizing and modulating effect on brain dopamine. This drug is intended to reduce dopamine transmission when it is too high and to preserve it when it is too low, thus maintaining the dopaminergic-cholinergic balance. The drug is not expected to cause abnormal involuntary movements (EPS).

DEPOT INJECTION AND OTHER DRUG FORMS. Several antipsychotic agents are currently available in long-acting decanoate (depot injection) form. The **depot injection** is an oil-based medication form of the drug injected intramuscularly for the purpose of slow release of the drug over several weeks. Haloperidol (Haldol) and fluphenazine (Prolixin) are the typical agents available in depot form. They are supplied in a sesame oil solution. Haloperidol is repeated every 4 weeks, and fluphenazine every 1 to 4 weeks. Risperidone is the only atypical antipsychotic agent currently in injectable form. It is given intramuscularly in a saline solution every 2 weeks.

The advantages of the long-acting form of antipsychotic drugs relate to compliance with drug therapy. A client may be able to comply with a clinic visit once every few weeks more easily and consistently than he or she can take oral medications daily. Several antipsychotic agents are available in liquid oral concentrate forms. The liquid form can be used to prevent situations in which clients move pills to their cheeks instead of swallowing them and spit them out later. It is also helpful when the client has difficulty swallowing, or prefers liquid to the pill form. The liquid concentrates must be mixed with a small amount of juice or other liquid to improve the taste.

DRUG INTERACTIONS. All antipsychotic agents potentially interact with other CNS agents. There is an additive CNS depressant effect when they are combined with sedatives, narcotics, or alcohol. Antacids can decrease gastrointestinal absorption of the antipsychotics, reducing their effectiveness. Anticholinergic drugs can add to the anticholinergic side effects and decrease the effectiveness of the antipsychotic (Rankin, 2000).

ABUSE POTENTIAL. The antipsychotic medications do not cause euphoria, so there is virtually no abuse potential from these drugs. They also do not cause addiction or dependency. This lack of abuse potential is an important teaching point, because many consumers believe that any drug that affects the mind is addictive.

clinical ALERT

Students as well as nurses often hesitate to give prn medications, perhaps from fear of responsibility for making the decision to give them. If your client has EPS, do not hesitate to give these anticholinergics when they are ordered prn. EPS are very uncomfortable for clients, and are a major reason for noncompliance with antipsychotic medications.

NURSING CARE

PRIORITIZING NURSING CARE

When caring for clients with schizophrenia, focus your interventions on promoting self-care and effective coping skills, as well as safety. Encourage clients to perform ADLs such as personal hygiene, making their beds, doing their laundry, keeping appointments for individual and group therapy, and participating in leisure activities. Give positive reinforcement for appropriate behaviors and interactions, as well as for insight. Be aware of escalating behavior and intervene as appropriate to prevent unsafe situations for client and staff. Provide a quiet environment, the opportunity to talk, medications, and the least restrictive environment possible when behavior begins to escalate.

ASSESSING

In psychiatric nursing the client's potential for violence is assessed first because it is a safety issue. In general, people with mental illnesses are no more violent than the general public, but there are groups of mentally ill people with increased risk for violence toward others (Torrey, 2001). These risk factors for violence are:

- Previous violent acts at home or in treatment.
- History of substance abuse, especially if currently under the influence of substances.
- Paranoid delusions.
- Command hallucinations (commanding the client to hurt someone).
- History of being a victim of violence (violence is a learned behavior).

Certain behaviors suggest that a client is becoming increasingly agitated and more likely to act out violently. These behaviors are clenching fists, talking loud or yelling, threatening, increasing motor activity (was sitting, then walking, then pacing back and forth quickly), hitting walls or furniture, wincing, or looking afraid.

Mental Status Assessment

When asked, "What is the client's mental status?" the nurse will often reply: "Alert and oriented" or "Oriented times 3." The major clinical findings in schizophrenia are not addressed by the "alert and oriented" assessment. A client could say, "I am Linda Eby. I am in the hospital. It is Tuesday at 8:00 P.M." This sounds pretty good, but does it show whether the client is experiencing hallucinations or delusions, or if her thinking is disorganized? When the assessment is charted, does the reader know if the client had flat affect or avolition?

Because most nurses do not read minds, systematic observation of the client's speech and behavior works best for assessing mental status. A complete mental status assessment includes:

- Appearance (dress, grooming, posture, activity)
- Orientation (to person, place, time, situation)
- Mood and affect (depressed, elated, flat, anxious, changeable, angry)
- Speech characteristics (rate, content logical, pressured, loose associations)
- Thought disorder (delusions, obsessions, phobias)
- Hallucinations (auditory, visual, kinesthetic, olfactory)
- Behavior (aggressive, withdrawn, suicidal, homicidal, manipulative, intimidating, confused, intrusive, impulsive)
- Memory (short term and long term)
- Judgment/insight (understands illness, understands need for treatment, able to maintain own safety, able to maintain safety of others)

Cultural Issues

Interpreting the meaning of client behaviors can be difficult if the client is from a different culture from the nurse. Sometimes a client's behavior is accepted in his or her own culture, but may seem abnormal based on the nurse's

experience. An example could be a client from Cuba who talks with her father (who is dead) about how she should solve various problems. In her culture thinking about (and talking to) the spirit of a dead relative is commonly done. In the North American nurse's culture, talking with people who are not present might be interpreted as hallucinating. Nurses must learn to be sensitive to the cultural meanings of clients' behaviors. An interpreter who is from the client's culture and who understands the cultural meaning of the client's behavior is an ideal member of a treatment team.

Physical Assessment in the Psychiatric Setting

A physician or nurse practitioner performs an initial physical assessment as part of the psychiatric client's admission process. Nurses confine the physical data they collect to pertinent illnesses or drug responses by clients. They do not routinely take all readings, such as listening to every client's lungs every shift.

clinical ALERT

The touching involved in physical assessment may have a different meaning for clients in the psychiatric setting. When clients are hallucinating, they may not be sure about what is real and what is not. Physical touching may be perceived as part of a threatening hallucination. Delusional thinking may make even the well-intentioned nurse seem dangerous. Some clients mistake physical touch for sexual advances. Physical assessment may be very stressful for the client. Therefore, only priority physical assessments should be done in the acute psychiatric situation.

Nurses must understand and monitor the desired effects and potential side effects of all medications and treatments received by their clients. Psychiatric clients may not be able to describe clearly what is wrong with them, so careful listening is another important nursing skill. When a client with psychosis says, "The snake is squeezing my chest!" it is possible that this client is experiencing a heart attack.

Obtaining Additional Input from the Family

The client's family is a critical part of psychiatric care. It is important to obtain written permission from clients to communicate with anyone about them, including their family members (see discussion of the Health Insurance Portability and Accountability Act [HIPAA] in Chapter 14 🔗). The client's family is interviewed in terms of who they are, how involved they are in the client's life, what their learning needs are, and what their questions and concerns about the client are. Families can make a big difference as allies in treatment for psychiatric clients. However, healthcare providers often overlook them, out of a mistaken sense of protecting the client's confidentiality. When mental disorders exist, they are important members of the treatment team. (See the discussion of family systems in Chapter 16 ⬮.)

DIAGNOSING, PLANNING, AND IMPLEMENTING

Data about the client's mental status, observation of the client's behavior and interactions with others, physical assessment findings, and information from family all contribute data for establishing nursing diagnoses. In the acute phase of psychosis, treatment should focus on the client's basic needs. Safety, nutrition, and rest are the priorities. Acute symptom management is also important.

Priority nursing diagnoses that often apply to clients with schizophrenia include the following:

- *Risk for Violence*, self-directed or directed at others
- *Impaired Environmental Interpretation Syndrome*
- *Disturbed Sensory Perception* (specify auditory or visual)
- *Ineffective Coping*
- *Impaired Social Interaction*

Desired outcomes for a client with schizophrenia include the following:

- Client will cause no harm to self or others.
- Client will have reality-based thinking.
- Client will use healthy, adaptive coping skills.
- Client will take medications regularly.
- Client will continue to be active (employment, hobbies, exercise).
- Client will have a routine daily and weekly schedule.
- Client will include enjoyable activities in the schedule.
- Client will perform ADLs independently.
- Client will keep in touch with family and important friends.

Risk for Violence (Directed at Self or Others)

- Avoid touching an actively hallucinating client. *Touch may be perceived as part of a threatening hallucination. Client may hit in self-defense.*
- Intervene early as soon as you have identified increased agitation. Reassure clients that they are safe in the hospital. *Agitation can escalate quickly. Early intervention can prevent the situation from getting worse. Fear may motivate agitation. Clients often benefit from reassurance that they are safe.*
- Avoid confronting clients aggressively about their behavior. When inappropriate behavior arises, tell the client simply and calmly that the behavior is not acceptable and redirect the client to another activity. *Clients may not realize that their behavior is inappropriate. Aggressive behavior by the nurse may make them feel defensive.*

- Start with less restrictive interventions for inappropriate behavior: Try to talk first, then redirect, offer meds, isolate or medicate, and restrain only as a last resort. *Clients have an ethical and legal right to the least restrictive treatment that is effective.*
- Maintain a low-stimulation environment. *Clients with psychosis may have difficulty processing multiple stimuli, and extra stimuli may lead to agitation.*
- In advance, talk with clients about signs and symptoms of anxiety and agitation, and the triggers that start these feelings. Discuss options for appropriate behavior and anxiety management techniques. *If clients can recognize anxiety and agitation early, they can notify staff, who can help identify coping mechanisms to prevent violent acting-out. Clients with schizophrenia often have short attention spans and inadequate coping skills and may have impulsive behavior. Cognitive approaches to planning for future episodes are an effective way to help them learn new behavior.*
- When you are talking with an agitated client, turn your body slightly to the side, instead of facing the client directly face to face. *Direct face-to-face interaction can feel like a confrontation to the client. Also, if the client tries to hit the nurse, a blow to the side is much less dangerous than one to the front of the nurse's body.*
- Be aware of your body language. Communicate calmness and confidence. *Your attitude can be contagious. If you act anxious, the client may feel more anxious. Speak softly. Avoid loud, angry talking. Keep your hands in sight, open, and low to communicate that you are not threatening. Show that you are in control of your own behavior, and that you expect the same from the client.*
- Observe people experiencing paranoia or hallucinations closely. *A person who has a nonviolent personality may act out violently when confronted with an apparently life-threatening hallucination, or when terrorized by a paranoid delusion that threatens the person's life. Many people will never be violent unless they are in a life-threatening situation. Imagine how hard it is for a person to live with the constant threat of harm. When people with schizophrenia are violent, usually the violent act is a matter of self-defense from their point of view.*

Box 49-10 ◾ suggests guidelines for interacting with clients who are actively hallucinating.

Disturbed Thought Processes

- Provide antipsychotic medications as ordered and monitor effects. *It is the responsibility of nurses to monitor the client's response to medications for the purpose of evaluating their effectiveness.*
- Look for the client's strengths and abilities when providing nursing care. *When a person has a severe mental illness such as schizophrenia, it is easy to see the pathology. It is important to look for the person's strengths and to acknowledge the*

BOX 49-10 NURSING CARE CHECKLIST

Interacting with a Person Who Is Hallucinating

☑ Only one person should interact with the client at a time. *The client is having difficulty interpreting stimuli, so it will be easier for the client to respond to one person.*

☑ Keep environmental noise to a minimum. Do not speak loudly. *The client is having difficulty filtering sensory stimuli. A low-stimulation environment will make it easier for the client to differentiate real stimuli from the voices.*

☑ Initially, specifically ask the client about the hallucinations (usually voices) and what they are saying or telling the client to do. *It is helpful to know if clients are experiencing voices commanding them to hurt themselves or others.*

☑ Focus on reality. Do not continually ask clients to describe the hallucinations. Do not react to clients' report of hallucinations as if they are real. *Often hallucinations are transitory experiences for clients. Describing the hallucination can form it more clearly in the client's mind and reinforce it. The nurse's role is to help clients recognize reality, not to further confuse them about their hallucinations or delusions. When the nurse keeps the conversation in reality, reality is reinforced and the hallucinations may be minimized.*

☑ Do not argue with the client's experience. Share your own perceptions. Reassure the client that she or he is safe. *The client is truly hearing the voices. The goal is to present reality, not to convince the client that she or he is wrong. Respectful disagreement can help the client understand what is real, such as "I know you hear voices, but I don't hear them." Reassurance may help the client see that she or he is not in danger and does not need to defend herself or himself.*

☑ Avoid touching a person who is actively hallucinating. *During a hallucination, any touch may be perceived by the client as part of the hallucination. If the hallucination is threatening, the client may strike out in self-defense.*

normal parts of the person. *Even psychotic clients have coping skills that the nurse can draw on for the client's benefit.*

- Reinforce reality. Talk about what is really happening. *Conversations about the simple realities of daily life (the weather, doing laundry, meals, etc.) bring the client's attention away from disordered thoughts and into the here and now. The nurse's role is to help clients recognize what is real.*

- Encourage or assist clients to express feelings of fear or anxiety. Validate their feelings. *The sense of losing contact with reality can be frightening. It can be affirming and helpful to express feelings and have the nurse listen to them, accept them without judgment, and validate how difficult the situation must be.*

Ineffective Coping

- Establish a trusting relationship in which clients are safe to express true feelings, especially negative ones. Do not react to client's negative feelings. *Client may feel that only*

positive feelings are appropriate and not know an appropriate way to express negative feelings. A nonthreatening relationship may provide the client with the chance to express unresolved feelings. Reacting strongly to their feelings may suggest rejection.

- Offer medications in a confident way, expecting clients to take them. Clients should be assigned the same nurse each day if possible. *Consistency of staff and a confident approach promote trust and compliance.*

- Model how to interact and disagree with others. Teach clients stress management techniques such as going to their room and doing relaxation exercises. *Role modeling and behavioral approaches are effective ways to teach new coping skills.*

Impaired Social Interaction

- Approach clients with an accepting attitude. Be honest and sincere. *Acceptance, honesty, and sincerity promote trust.*

- Interact with the client individually and model appropriate social behavior (body language, topics). *People with schizophrenia often lack social skills and benefit from role modeling as a way to learn them.*

- Give positive reinforcement for client's voluntary interactions with others. *Positive reinforcement is an effective behavioral approach to behavior change.*

- Encourage clients to attend group activities in the hospital. Accompany them at first if necessary. *Clients may respond positively to encouragement from a trusted nurse. Trust is an important issue for clients with schizophrenia.*

EVALUATING

When evaluating the effectiveness of nursing care for clients with schizophrenia, the nurse looks to the desired outcomes. The nurse will determine whether the client:

- Demonstrates reality-based thinking.
- Demonstrates an understanding of medication management.
- Interacts effectively with others.

Continuity of Care

As the client recovers from psychosis and moves into the rehabilitation phase, the focus changes to teaching and psychosocial rehabilitation issues. Medication teaching, group therapies, self-care skills, and social skills become more important. Clients can learn strategies to decrease the likelihood of relapse of schizophrenia. See Box 49-5 for these strategies. Learning these strategies can give clients more control over their lives and disease processes.

Some people with schizophrenia will still have psychotic (delusional or hallucinatory) thinking when they are discharged. Research has been done in the area of helping people deal with strange thoughts. Strategies include *distraction* (such as listening to music, reading aloud, counting backward from 100, watching television, or describing an object in detail). *Interacting* is another strategy. Clients can tell the voices to stop, talking to the voices while pretending to use a cellular phone, and agree to listen to the voices at certain times. The *activity* strategy for clients includes walking, doing housework, taking a relaxing bath, playing a musical instrument, singing, and exercising. The *social* strategy involves talking to a trusted person, phoning a help line, avoiding people, going to a drop-in center, or going to a favorite place (Mills, 2000).

Clients with schizophrenia tend to have poor social skills. Relating to others is difficult for them. People with schizophrenia often need a network of social contacts when they are living in the community. The hospital nurse can help by assisting the client to write a list of people who could help in a variety of situations. The client's father may give her a ride to clinic appointments. Her neighbor may be able to take care of her cat if she has to stay in the hospital. The pharmacist in the local grocery store may be able to fill prescriptions when they run out. Her sister might be the best person to call if she wants to talk. Preparing a list like this will help clients to think about problem-solving resources they have when they are at home. If the phone numbers are included, they will go home with a practical list of resources to use when a problem arises.

Mood Disorders

MAJOR DEPRESSIVE DISORDER
Because everyone has experienced sadness and a low mood at some time, it seems that it would be easy for people to relate to how it feels to be depressed. The difficulty is that depression takes sadness and lack of energy to a level that is not in the usual experience of unaffected people. A person with depression cannot "cheer up." Low mood is a part of the disease.

Consider the case of Pearl, a 70-year-old woman who lives in a long-term care facility. Pearl had a stroke a year ago and has hemiplegia on her right side. She does not feed herself and has little appetite. She cooperates with having her activities of daily living done for her, but she does not try to help. When she talks, it is only one or two words at a time. Her face always seems to look sad. The nurse thinks Pearl is depressed. In this chapter we hope to prepare nurses to help people like Pearl live with this debilitating brain disorder.

Diagnostic Criteria and Manifestations
According to the APA (2000), an episode of major depressive disorder is diagnosed when a person has five or more of the following symptoms (one of them must be #1 or #2):

1. *Depressed mood* most of the day, nearly every day, as indicated by either subjective report ("I feel sad, or empty") or observation made by others (appears tearful). In children or adolescents, mood can be *irritable*.
2. *Very diminished interest or pleasure* in all, or almost all, activities most of the day nearly every day (*anhedonia*).
3. *Significant weight loss* while not dieting or *weight gain* (change of more than 5% of body weight in a month). Children may fail to make expected weight gains.
4. *Insomnia* or *hypersomnia* (sleeping too much) nearly every day.
5. *Psychomotor agitation* or **psychomotor retardation** (lack of activity) nearly every day (observed by others, not just feeling restless or slow).
6. *Fatigue* or *loss of energy* nearly every day.
7. Feelings of *worthlessness* or *inappropriate or excessive guilt* nearly every day.
8. *Diminished ability to think or concentrate,* or indecisiveness, nearly every day.
9. *Recurrent thoughts of death* (not just fear of dying), recurrent thoughts of suicide, a plan for committing suicide, or a suicide attempt.

The symptoms must cause significant distress or impairment in social, occupational, school, or other important areas of functioning.

Causes and Incidence
Major depressive disorder has a genetic component, a brain physiology component, and a psychosocial component. Each contributes, but none explains the disorder alone. Because multiple factors cause and also affect the disorder, effective treatments must include psychosocial (teaching and counseling) and physiologic (medication) approaches. (See also Chapter 17 .)

Major depressive disorder is 1.5 to 3 times more common among first-degree biological relatives of affected people than among the general population (APA, 2000). A single gene is not implicated in the inheritance of depression. A genetic predisposition may interact with environmental factors to create the disorder. People may inherit the tendency to respond to life stressors with the development of depression.

Recent advances in brain imaging have been used to assess brain function of people with depression. Positron-emission tomography (PET) scans show abnormal function in the prefrontal cortex of the cerebrum and in the limbic system during depressive episodes. There is also evidence that an abnormality in brain neurotransmitter physiology causes depression. Brain neurotransmitters such as serotonin, norepinephrine, dopamine, acetylcholine, and GABA are likely involved. We learned that in schizophrenia, brain neurotransmitters are overactive. In depression, the opposite is true: The neurotransmitters have reduced function. The fact that antidepressant medications are so effective is proof that neurotransmitter function affects mood.

The endocrine system is also involved. The hypothalamus, pituitary, and adrenal glands (together called the *HPA axis*) control the physiologic responses to stress. These glands may be hyperactive in people with depression. The HPA axis also affects the 24-hour day–night cycle of body rhythms (*circadian rhythms*). In both depression and mania, the normal circadian rhythms are disrupted. Circadian rhythms affect many physiologic functions, including sleep and wakefulness, hormone secretion, mental alertness, and body temperature.

Women are twice as likely as men to develop depression. Children show no gender difference in risk, but at puberty women become more likely to be affected. A significant proportion of affected women report a worsening of depressive symptoms in the few days before menstruation. The lifetime risk of having a major depressive episode is 10% to 25% for women and 5% to 12% for men. At any given time, 3% to 5% of people in the United States are experiencing a major depressive episode. Most of these are not diagnosed or treated. The disorder affects people of all ethnicities and socioeconomic groups equally (APA, 2000).

It is common for people with depression to have other disorders at the same time. The disorders that frequently occur with depression include schizophrenia, substance abuse, eating disorders, anxiety disorders, general medical conditions such as diabetes, cerebrovascular accident (CVA or stroke), and other chronic conditions. Depression may be caused by certain medications. Some antibiotics, antifungal, anti-inflammatory, antineoplastic, cardiovascular, and gastrointestinal drugs have been shown to cause depression in some people.

Course of the Disease

The disorder may begin at any age. The average age of onset is in the mid-20s. A major life stressor precedes the first major depressive episode for many people (APA, 2000). However, it is not the stressor itself that causes depression. The person who becomes depressed is probably susceptible to depression after a stressful event.

Some people experience only a single episode of depression. Most people who have one episode of depression continue to have episodes throughout their lives. Yet others experience almost a steady state of depressed mood. An untreated episode of depression can last for years.

Some clients experience psychotic symptoms associated with severe depression, such as hallucinations or delusional thinking. This *psychotic depression* is more disabling and often requires more intensive treatment than a depressive episode without psychotic features.

POSTPARTUM DEPRESSION. Depression after childbirth can range from the "postpartum blues" to psychotic depression. It is very common for women to experience tearfulness, anxiety, impaired concentration, and lack of energy immediately after delivery. This normal case of "the blues" usually starts within 3 to 4 days after delivery and lasts no longer than 2 weeks. It usually resolves without medical treatment. The client may benefit from reassurance by the nurse that the condition is common and will resolve with time, rest, and family support. The client and her family should be encouraged to notify the care provider if the depressive symptoms do not resolve after 2 weeks.

Postpartum psychosis usually develops within 3 weeks of delivery. It is characterized by depressed mood, lack of concentration, guilt, lack of interest in the baby, rejection of the baby, or unreasonable fear that something bad will happen to the baby. Treatment depends on the individual client's symptoms. Women with a history of psychiatric disorders are more likely to develop postpartum psychosis. (See also Chapter 55 ⚭.)

SEASONAL AFFECTIVE DISORDER. Seasonal affective disorder (SAD) is depression that is associated with shortened exposure to daylight. It happens in the fall and winter when the days become shorter. The symptoms are sleepiness, fatigue, lethargy, irritability, and increased appetite. It is thought to be a result of abnormal melatonin metabolism. The treatment is light therapy (*phototherapy*). The client is exposed to bright light each morning and for a prescribed number of hours each day. Light therapy has been effective for clients with mild to moderate seasonal depression (Depression Guideline Panel, 1993).

Clinical Features

Major depressive disorder is a disabling disease that affects occupational and personal functioning. An affected person will have a depressed or low mood every day. A list of symptoms can never fully describe the human consequences of a disease. Box 49-11 ■ gives examples of how people with depression describe their feelings. Figure 49-4 ■ shows the symptoms of a major depressive episode.

Depression causes misery and disability (loss of function) for the people who have the disorder. It also causes difficulty in their relationships with other people. Depression causes people to lose the ability to enjoy the things that used to make them happy. Depressed people miss work, lose their jobs, or have reduced effectiveness and productivity at work. Affected people often cannot continue their family and work responsibilities. They may not be able to do their activities of daily living. Most of the people who commit suicide are depressed at the time.

Depression has a high cost in human suffering as well as a financial cost to businesses that lose productivity. When a person has depression along with a general medical condition (such as diabetes or a stroke), the medical condition is

BOX 49-11   REALITY CHECK ON DEPRESSION

What people with depression have to say:

- "When I am depressed I really don't think very much. I feel sad and lonely and detached."
- "The color, flavor, and spark of life are extinguished."
- "Everywhere is another reason for me to feel sadness and regret. I am so sensitive. Every little thing makes me feel sad. I dwell on feeling bad and what I should have done."
- "I feel like I'm in a deep dark hole and can't even try to get out."
- "Everything worth living for goes out of focus."
- "I've been too tired to chew."
- "People can be overstimulating, especially when they are cheerful."
- "People want me to do things that I should really want to do. I just can't get the motivation for it, and it makes me feel guilty."
- "My arms and legs might as well be trees, they are so heavy."
- "My soul left and was replaced with lead."
- "My kids want me to get up and play. It's not that I don't want to. I wish I could! I can't move. They must hate me."
- "I am a failure in every sense of the word."
- "My job was so important to me, so important, but I got to the point where I couldn't concentrate at work, then I was unable to go to work at all."
- "When I didn't answer your questions, it was because I didn't have the energy to talk."
- "If I don't feel like living, why would anyone else want me to?"

likely to be worse than it would be if the depression were not present (Depression Guideline Panel, 1993). Depression is associated with increased disability and even reduced life expectancy in hospitalized clients with serious medical conditions (Roach et al., 1998). Because of the stigma associated with mental illness (discussed earlier), people are reluctant to seek help when they have the symptoms of depression.

- People with depression are less likely to accept treatment, to comply with treatment recommendations, and to continue treatment than are people with general medical conditions without depression.
- At least 80% of all depression treatment takes place outside the mental health setting.
- Only 12% of people are willing to take medication for depression, whereas 70% would take medication for a headache.

People with depression may fear being stigmatized or discriminated against in hiring, promotion, and other opportunities. Until mental illness is seen on an equal plane with general medical disorders attitudinally, economically, socially, and politically, it will be underreported, underdiagnosed, and undertreated (Depression Guideline Panel, 1993).

SUICIDE

In 1996 the World Health Organization (WHO) urged member nations to create suicide prevention strategies. The U.S. Surgeon General published a call to action in 1999, which included the risks and protective factors for suicide (Box 49-12 ■) and the following statistics.

An average of 85 Americans die from suicide each day. The suicide rate in the United States has remained relatively stable during the last three decades. However, the rates for certain groups have increased significantly. The suicide rate among adolescents and young adults has nearly tripled. (Chapter 62 ⚭ discusses suicide in adolescents in more detail.) Among all persons ages 15 to 19, suicides increased 14% from 1980 to 1996. Among African American males in the same age group, the rate increased 105%. Firearms-related suicides account for almost 100% of this increase in adolescent suicide. In the general population, firearms constitute the most common means of suicide in the United States (59%). More Americans die each year from suicide than from homicide.

Suicide rates are highest among older adults. There is no recent change in the rates for this population. Most elderly

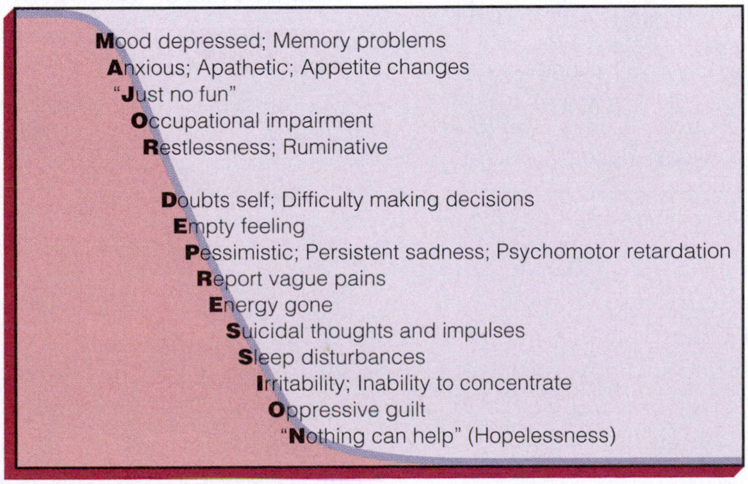

Mood depressed; Memory problems
Anxious; Apathetic; Appetite changes
"**J**ust no fun"
Occupational impairment
Restlessness; Ruminative

Doubts self; Difficulty making decisions
Empty feeling
Pessimistic; Persistent sadness; Psychomotor retardation
Report vague pains
Energy gone
Suicidal thoughts and impulses
Sleep disturbances
Irritability; Inability to concentrate
Oppressive guilt
"**N**othing can help" (Hopelessness)

Figure 49-4. ■ Symptoms of a major depressive episode. (*Source:* From *Contemporary Psychiatric-Mental Health Nursing,* by C. R. Kneisl, H. W. Wilson, and E. Trigoboff, 2004, Upper Saddle River, NJ: Pearson Education. Reprinted with permission.)

BOX 49-12   SUICIDE: RISK FACTORS AND PROTECTIVE FACTORS

Risk Factors

- Previous suicide attempt
- Mental disorders, especially mood disorders such as depression and bipolar disorder
- Co-occurring mental and alcohol or substance abuse disorders
- Family history of suicide
- Hopelessness
- Impulsive and/or aggressive tendencies
- Barriers to accessing mental health treatment
- Relationship, social, work, or financial losses
- General medical illness
- Easy access to lethal suicide methods, especially guns
- Unwillingness to seek help because of the stigma attached to mental and substance abuse disorders, and/or suicidal thoughts
- Influence of significant people—family members, celebrities, peers who have died by suicide—both through direct personal contact or inappropriate media representations

- Cultural or religious beliefs—for example, the belief that suicide is a noble resolution of a personal dilemma
- Local epidemics of suicide that have a contagious influence
- Isolation, a feeling of being cut off from other people

Protective Factors

- Effective and appropriate clinical care for mental, physical, and substance abuse disorders
- Easy access to a variety of clinical interventions and support
- Restricted access to highly lethal methods of suicide
- Family and community support
- Support from ongoing medical and mental health care relationships
- Learned skills in problem solving, conflict resolution, and nonviolent handling of disputes
- Cultural and religious beliefs that discourage suicide and support self-preservation instincts

Source: U.S. Public Health Service. (1999). *The Surgeon General's Call to Action to Prevent Suicide.* Washington, DC: Author.

suicide victims are seen by their primary care provider within a few weeks of their suicide and are experiencing a first episode of mild to moderate depression. This demonstrates a lost opportunity for identifying suicide risk and preventing suicide (U.S. Public Health Service, 1999). Physicians and nurses must assess the elderly for depression and suicide risk. Chapter 43 ⚭ provides the Geriatric Depression Scale, a screening tool for depression. The nurse should report clients who score as depressed on the Geriatric Depression Scale. They should be referred for further assessment.

clinical ALERT

It is a dangerous myth that discussing suicide with someone who is not considering it may suggest the idea. Most people with depression, whether they are contemplating suicide or not, benefit from talking about their feelings. For people who are contemplating suicide, discussion of their feelings may be the only opportunity for prevention. Depression makes it hard for people to identify and explain their own feelings. Talking about and clarifying these feelings can help a depressed person gain perspective, interrupt negative thinking, or work on problem solving. Active listening is a powerful tool for nurses to use. Clients often express gratitude for the opportunity to express their thoughts about suicide (Rives, 1999).

Only when the nurse is aware of a client's suicidal thinking (*suicidal ideation*) can the nurse intervene to help the client. Questions can clarify the dangerousness of the client's suicidal thoughts. Fleeting thoughts such as "I feel so bad, I wish I were dead" are not as dangerous as "I have a gun at home, and as soon as I am discharged I plan to shoot myself."

Imagine yourself asking a client: "Do you ever think about hurting yourself or other people?" This is a hard

question. It is socially inappropriate. It is just not polite to talk about suicide, or to suggest that a person may be thinking about it. So, what should a nurse do?

Remember why you are here. This is not a social relationship. It is a professional one. The nurse is the professional. The nurse's goal is to ensure the client's safety, and to protect the client or others as necessary. It is difficult to ask people if they feel like hurting themselves or others, but if nurses do not ask, they cannot provide appropriate care for the client.

Every client in the psychiatric setting should be asked specifically about suicidal and homicidal ideation as part of a mental status assessment. In the general medical setting every elderly client with a chronic illness, and every client who has the risk factors for suicide listed in Box 49-12 should be asked: "Do you feel like hurting yourself?"

clinical ALERT

The nurse may learn that a client is feeling hopeless. Hope that depression will improve is what keeps many people from self-harm. It is important for the nurse to keep hope alive. The nurse should communicate to the client that depression is very treatable. The treatment team will not give up trying until the client feels better. Suicidal thinking should always be reported to the physician.

COLLABORATIVE CARE

A good reason for hope is that effective treatment for depression is available. Once it is accurately identified, depression can almost always be treated successfully with medications, psychotherapy, or a combination of the two (Depression Guideline Panel, 1993). Clients are individuals and respond to treatment differently. However, when a client does not respond to one therapy, there are others to try. The goals of medical treatment for depression are:

- To decrease the depressive symptoms (depressed mood, decreased interest in daily activities, inability to experience pleasure, worthlessness, sleep disturbances, lack of motivation, inability to concentrate).
- To improve client's functional level.
- To prevent recurrence.

There are five medical treatments for depression:

1. Medication
2. Psychotherapy
3. Combination of medication and psychotherapy
4. Electroconvulsive therapy (ECT)
5. Light therapy (discussed earlier in the Seasonal Affective Disorder section)

Clients experience the best treatment outcomes when their depression is treated with a combination of medications, psychosocial therapy, client and family education, and a treatment plan that includes significant others in the client's life. ECT can also be an effective treatment for depression.

Psychotropic Agents

Medications have been shown to be effective for all types of depression. However, no single medication works for everyone, and no single medication is better or more effective than the others.

Antidepressant medications have limitations. People with depressive symptoms often wait until their symptoms are almost unbearable before they seek help. Then the antidepressants can take 2 to 6 weeks to reach full effect. If the first medication is not effective, the wait for effectiveness of a second or even third drug can seem endless. Some clients experience side effects that they are not willing to tolerate. Some people experience no improvement with antidepressant medications.

The provider often chooses which antidepressant medication to prescribe based on the side effect profile or on which drug has been used effectively by a family member or the client in the past. In some situations, a drug may be chosen because its particular side effects might be useful. For example, the choice of an antidepressant with sedating effects can benefit a client who has trouble sleeping.

As mentioned earlier, depression appears to involve reduced neurotransmitter function in brain synapses and changes in receptors on brain neurons. Figure 49-5 ■ illustrates neurotransmitters in depression and the action of antidepressant drugs. Antidepressants are only given orally. For the most part they act on two major brain neurotransmitters (serotonin [5-HT] and norepinephrine [NE]), which regulate mood. New antidepressants have been developed to act on dopamine also. (*Note:* Although antidepressants are used

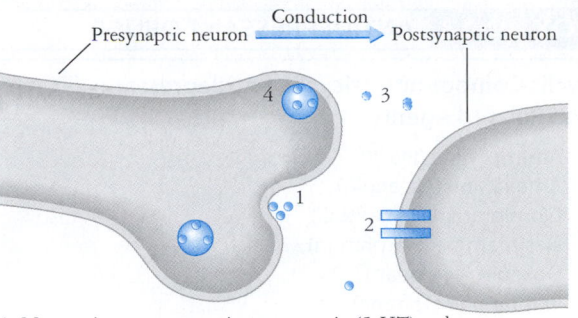

1. Monoamine neurotransmitters serotonin (5-HT) and norepinephrine (NE) are released into synapse.
2. Depression is caused by too little neurotransmitter in synapse to stimulate postsynaptic receptor.
3. Neurotransmitters are broken down by monoamine oxidase.
4. Reuptake of neurotransmitter into vesicle in presynaptic neuron.

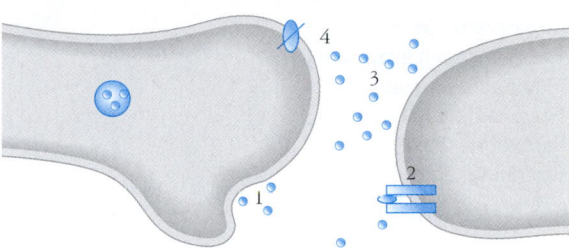

1. Monoamine neurotransmitters (5-HT and NE) are released into synapse.
2. Cyclic antidepressants and MAOIs make receptors more sensitive to 5-HT and NE.
3. MAOIs block breakdown of 5-HT and NE (more neurotransmitters in synapse).
4. SSRIs block reuptake of serotonin, cyclics block reuptake of 5-HT and NE (less goes back into presynaptic cell, leaving more in synapse).

Figure 49-5. ■ Neurotransmitters in depression and the action of antidepressant drugs.

mostly to treat depression, they have other uses as well. They are used to treat obsessive-compulsive disorder, panic disorder, eating disorders, and anxiety disorders. The tricyclic amitriptyline is also used as an adjunctive treatment for chronic pain.)

The antidepressants may be organized into four groups, listed in Box 49-13 ■:

1. Tricyclic antidepressants (TCAs) and related cyclic agents
2. Selective serotonin reuptake inhibitors (SSRIs)
3. Novel antidepressants
4. Monoamine oxidase inhibitors (MAOIs)

Tricyclic and Related Agents

The tricyclic antidepressants (TCAs) were the first-choice treatment for depression from the 1950s until the 1990s, when newer drugs with similar efficacy but fewer side effects were introduced. TCAs block the reuptake of serotonin and norepinephrine, increasing the amount of these monoamine neurotransmitters in brain synapses. See Figure 49-5 for a diagram of antidepressant action.

BOX 49-13   ANTIDEPRESSANT DRUGS

Cyclic Compounds: Tricyclic Antidepressants (TCAs) and Related Agents

Amitriptyline (Elavil)
Amoxapine (Ascendin)
Clomipramine (Anafranil)
Desipramine (Norpramin)
Doxepin (Sinequan)
Imipramine (Tofranil)
Maprotiline (Ludiomil)
Nortriptyline (Pamelor)
Protriptyline (Vivactil)
Trimipramine (Surmontil)

Selective Serotonin Reuptake Inhibitors (SSRIs)

Citalopram (Celexa)
Escitalopram (Lexapro)
Fluoxetine (Prozac)
Fluvoxamine (Luvox)
Paroxetine (Paxil)
Sertraline (Zoloft)

Other, Novel Antidepressants

Bupropion (Wellbutrin, Zyban)—norepinephrine and dopamine reuptake inhibitor (NDRI)
Mirtazapine (Remeron)—nonadrenergic-specific serotonergic antidepressants (NaSSA)
Nefazodone (Serzone) and trazodone (Desyrel)—serotonin antagonists and reuptake inhibitors (SARI)
Reboxetine (Edronax, Vestra)—selective norepinephrine reuptake inhibitor (NRI)
Venlafaxine (Effexor)—serotonin and norepinephrine reuptake inhibitor (SNRI)

Monoamine Oxidase Inhibitors (MAOIs)

Isocarboxazid (Marplan)
Phenelzine (Nardil)
Tranylcypromine (Parnate)

TCAs take 2 to 4 weeks to relieve depression symptoms significantly. This long delay before the drug is effective is explained by the time required to cause a change in the receptors on postsynaptic neurons (Keltner et al., 2003). The four major types of antidepressants act by increasing the availability or activity of monoamine neurotransmitters (serotonin, norepinephrine, or both) in brain synapses.

SIDE EFFECTS.   The cyclic compounds have more side effects than the SSRI antidepressants. As a group the tricyclics tend to cause sedation, orthostatic hypotension, weight gain, and anticholinergic side effects.

ANTICHOLINERGIC EFFECTS.   The tricyclics all carry increased risk for anticholinergic effects. (Review Box 49-9 for a list of these effects.) One of the anticholinergic side effects is *mydriasis* (abnormal or excessive dilation of the pupils).

clinical ALERT

It is important for nurses to know that clients with narrow-angle glaucoma may experience increased eye pressure due to the anticholinergic effects of psychiatric drugs. The nurse should notify the physician of any psychiatric client's history of glaucoma.

More severe anticholinergic effects (agitation, mental confusion, and paralytic ileus) may occur in older adults. Box 49-14 ■ lists considerations for older adults taking antidepressants.

The anticholinergic side effects are the ones most often cited by consumers (clients) as the reason they quit taking TCA medications. Weight gain and sexual dysfunction are also reasons cited for noncompliance.

OVERDOSE AND TOXIC EFFECTS.   Acutely suicidal clients should be hospitalized, and precautions should be taken for clients who are at risk. If a client has significant suicidal thinking, a history of suicide attempts, or impulse control problems, another class of antidepressant is usually prescribed.

The TCAs cause cardiac side effects even in therapeutic doses. Increased heart rate is common. In toxic doses dysrhythmias can cause death.

clinical ALERT

The tricyclic antidepressants can be fatal in overdose. Because suicide is a risk of depression, the healthcare team must consider the possibility of use of antidepressants as a method of suicide.

Amitriptyline is considered the most cardiotoxic antidepressant. Because of this and its increased risk for sedation, orthostatic hypotension, and anticholinergic activity, it should be used with caution in the elderly (Keltner et al., 2003).

BOX 49-14   POPULATION FOCUS

Antidepressants and the Older Adult

Older adults with depression tend to respond well to antidepressant drugs. However, there are some special considerations for this group:

■ Due to slower and less efficient metabolism, the elderly do not clear medications as rapidly as younger people. Therefore, they usually require lower doses of medications.

■ Elders are at increased risk for orthostatic hypotension, which increases their risk for falls and injury.

■ If older adults are dehydrated, they are at increased risk for medication side effects.

Selective Serotonin Reuptake Inhibitors (SSRIs)

The SSRIs are usually the first-choice drugs for the treatment of depression. They have fewer side effects than the earlier antidepressants, and they are just as effective. The SSRIs inhibit the reuptake of serotonin into the presynaptic neuron, increasing the amount of serotonin in brain synapses. See Figure 49-5 for a diagram of antidepressant drug action. The SSRIs are also used to treat obsessive-compulsive disorder (fluvoxamine, fluoxetine), premenstrual dysphoric disorder (fluoxetine), panic disorder (paroxetine), anxiety disorder (paroxetine), posttraumatic stress disorder (sertraline), and bulimia nervosa (fluoxetine).

SSRIs take about 2 to 3 weeks to reduce depression symptoms effectively, and up to 5 weeks to reach peak effect. Like TCAs, these drugs increase serotonin in brain synapses relatively quickly, but the therapeutic effect probably requires receptor changes that take several weeks.

SIDE EFFECTS. Side effects of the SSRIs are less severe than for TCAs or MAOIs. However, they still do cause anticholinergic, cardiovascular, and sedating side effects for some clients. They have a higher incidence of sexual side effects (decreased libido, ejaculatory and orgasmic dysfunction) than the TCAs. They also have more GI effects, such as nausea, loose stools, and weight loss. As with other medications, the dosage of SSRIs should be decreased in the elderly.

The most common side effects of SSRIs are headache, anxiety, nausea, diarrhea, and insomnia. Some SSRIs (such as fluoxetine) tend to be "activating" and have more side effects related to anxiety and insomnia. They may cause weight loss. Others (such as paroxetine) tend to be sedating. These side effects can be considered when the prescriber chooses which SSRI to use for an individual client. SSRIs can cause mild EPS.

The SSRIs have a low potential for harm with overdose. They also have low potential for abuse, because like all antidepressants they do not cause euphoria or physical dependency.

DRUG INTERACTIONS. The SSRIs are highly protein bound. They can increase the circulating levels of other protein-bound drugs that must compete for binding sites. TCA toxicity can result when SSRIs are given in combination with TCAs. When SSRIs are given with lithium, lithium levels increase (causing potential lithium toxicity). When SSRIs are combined with antipsychotics, EPS are increased. The SSRIs interact dangerously with MAOIs. The combination can cause serotonin syndrome.

SEROTONIN SYNDROME. Serotonin syndrome is a serious drug side effect caused by too much serotonin activity. It can result from combining SSRIs with MAOIs, St. John's wort (herbal antidepressant), or tryptophan (an amino acid that is a serotonin precursor). The signs and symptoms of serotonin syndrome include changes in mental status, agitation or restlessness, muscle spasms, hyperreflexia, diaphoresis, shivering, tremor, diarrhea, abdominal cramps, nausea, lack of coordination, and headache (Keltner et al., 2003).

clinical ALERT

Potentially fatal serotonin syndrome can result from combining SSRIs or TCAs with MAOI antidepressants. One drug must be cleared from the body before starting the other. A 2-week "washout" period should occur between the use of these two groups of drugs. If the nurse suspects serotonin syndrome, the SSRI should be held, and the physician notified immediately.

Novel Antidepressants

As their name implies, this group of antidepressants is composed of several unique individual drugs. Bupropion (Wellbutrin, Zyban) is a *norepinephrine and dopamine reuptake inhibitor* (NDRI). It does not act on serotonin, but inhibits dopamine and norepinephrine reuptake. As an activating antidepressant, it is more likely than other antidepressants to cause anxiety, agitation, insomnia, nausea, and weight loss. It also increases the risk of seizures, especially at high doses. This drug is primarily used to help clients stop smoking. Venlafaxine (Effexor) is a *serotonin and norepinephrine reuptake inhibitor* (SNRI), increasing the availability of both major monoamine neurotransmitters. It causes few severe side effects, but can cause nausea, decreased appetite, and insomnia. It may cause elevated blood pressure, especially at high doses. Venlafaxine is also used in panic disorder and obsessive-compulsive disorder.

Mirtazapine (Remeron) is an alpha-2 antagonist with serotonin-2 and serotonin-3 antagonism. Its group is called *nonadrenergic-specific serotonergic antidepressants* (NaSSAs). It increases norepinephrine and serotonin by affecting the presynaptic feedback system. It causes sedation in approximately 20% of clients. Mirtazapine is available in a form called Remeron SolTab, which dissolves on the tongue (Keltner et al., 2003).

Trazodone (Desyrel) and nefazodone (Serzone) make up the class of *serotonin antagonists and reuptake inhibitors* (SARIs). They block a subtype of serotonin-2 on the postsynaptic receptor, and block serotonin reuptake. Trazodone is seldom used as an antidepressant because more effective drugs are available. It is more often used for its sedating effect as a treatment for insomnia. Trazodone does have the potentially serious side effect of *priapism* (prolonged painful penile erection). Nefazodone inhibits serotonin, but it also inhibits serotonin-2. This decreases the likelihood of clients taking nefazodone to have anxiety, sexual dysfunction, and insomnia. The blocking of serotonin-2 probably also inhibits migraine headaches. Rarely, nefazodone has been known to cause life-threatening liver failure (Keltner et al., 2003).

Reboxetine (Vestra) is a selective *norepinephrine reuptake inhibitor* (NRI), which focuses on increasing norepinephrine availability. It is thought that people with severe depression can benefit from agents that promote norepinephrine. It is also expected to be effective against anxiety disorders. Its most common side effects are the anticholinergic effects (Keltner et al., 2003).

Monoamine Oxidase Inhibitors (MAOIs)

The MAOIs are effective antidepressant agents, but they are seldom prescribed because of their serious adverse effects. The MAOIs can cause potentially fatal drug interactions and hypertensive crisis. The MAOIs are usually prescribed for people who have not responded to other antidepressants and who can carefully comply with diet and drug restrictions.

The MAOIs act by inhibiting the breakdown of the monoamine neurotransmitters. They block the enzyme (monoamine oxidase) that breaks down neurotransmitters in brain synapses, causing increases in available serotonin and norepinephrine. The MAOIs take approximately 2 to 4 weeks to have an antidepressant effect.

The MAOIs must be used with extreme caution because they can cause:

■ Hypertensive crisis when combined with foods containing the amino acid tyramine.
■ Potentially fatal drug interactions with SSRIs, other MAOIs, TCAs, meperidine (Demerol), CNS depressants including general anesthetic agents, sympathomimetics (stimulants or anticongestants such as over-the-counter cold, allergy, and weight loss remedies), methylphenidate (Ritalin), bronchodilators, and some antihypertensives.
■ Death in overdose.

clinical ALERT

Symptoms of hypertensive crisis are a throbbing headache, sense of speeding or pounding heart, and stiff neck. If you suspect hypertensive crisis, hold the MAOI drug, take vital signs, and notify the physician.

Clients taking MAOIs must avoid foods high in tyramine. A list of high-tyramine foods is provided in Box 49-15 ■. Keep in mind that not all antidepressants cause these food and drug interactions. The nurse must recognize which type of antidepressant the client is taking. Client education is critical for people taking MAOI drugs.

One of the newer MAOIs, moclobemide (Manerix), is a reversible selective inhibitor of MAO-A. It is shorter acting and lacks the serious hypertensive side effects of the older, irreversible, nonselective MAOIs. It does not require a low tyramine diet. It should not be given with the older MAOIs or with narcotics (Keltner et al., 2003).

BOX 49-15 FOODS TO AVOID WHEN TAKING MAOIs

The following foods are high in tyramine and should be avoided by people taking monoamine oxidase inhibitors:

■ Aged cheeses (all cheese is considered aged except cottage, cream, ricotta, and processed cheese slices)
■ Foods containing aged cheeses, such as pizza and blue cheese dressing
■ Preserved meats, such as pepperoni, sausage, salami, lunchmeats, canned ham, pickled herring, dried fish
■ Liver, other organ meats
■ Broad fava beans, sauerkraut, and banana peel
■ Draft beer (even alcohol-free), red wine
■ Soy sauce, yeast or protein extract (concentrated) products
■ While caffeine does not contain tyramine, large amounts of caffeine can cause a sympathomimetic effect. Coffee, cola, and tea should be used in moderation.

Psychotherapy

Some of the psychosocial problems associated with depression (difficulty relating to others, low motivation, impaired mental concentration) can be resolved by medications. Psychotherapy, however, is usually used in addition to medication therapy for major depression. Psychotherapy may be used to help the client learn to live with a chronic depressive disorder, to manage the specific symptoms that plague the specific client, to promote effective coping skills, or for psychosocial rehabilitation. Clients experiencing a mild to moderate depressive episode without psychotic symptoms may benefit from psychotherapy alone. Figure 49-6 ■ illustrates approaches to psychotherapy based on different theories of personality development.

COGNITIVE THERAPY. Cognitive therapy is the most effective psychotherapeutic approach for depression (Depression Guideline Panel, 1993). For depression, the objective of cognitive therapy is to reduce symptoms by identifying and correcting the client's distorted, negatively biased thinking (Beck & Rush, 1995). According to cognitive theory, depressed people have automatic negative thoughts even in the midst of positive life events. They have negative expectations of their environment, negative perceptions and expectations of self, and negative expectations for the future. Cognitive therapy approaches include identifying the client's negative thinking errors, developing new thinking patterns, and trying new behavior.

BEHAVIORAL THERAPY. Behavioral therapy is often used along with cognitive therapy. The behavioral approach to therapy is based on learning theory. The therapist and client work together to determine what behaviors to change. The client practices new ways to behave that are positive, replacing the old dysfunctional behavior. The principle in behavioral therapy is that clients' thinking and feelings will

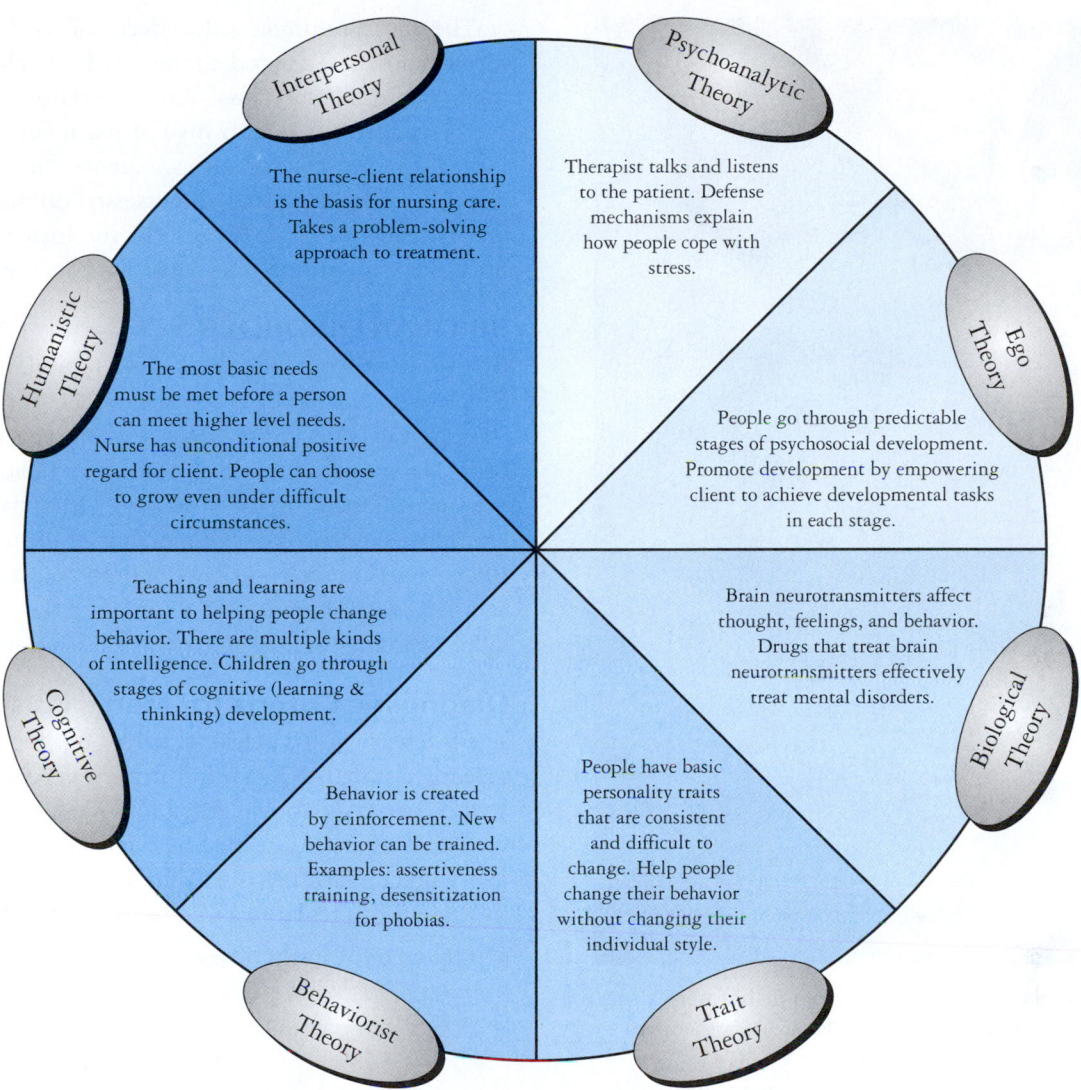

Figure 49-6. ■ Current psychotherapy is based on several theories of personality development.

follow their behavior. When people learn to act in a positive, self-confident way, they will feel positive and self-confident. Reinforcement of the client's successes will promote the persistence of positive effective behavior for coping.

Exercise

Moderate physical exercise has been shown to relieve mild to moderate depressive symptoms. The effects of exercise on depression may be due to the release of endorphins. The difficulty with exercise as a treatment for depression is that depressed people do not feel like exercising. Lack of energy and motivation are part of the disease. Exercise is best used as a preventive strategy. However, it is appropriate to teach clients that it is better to start exercising before they feel like it, rather than waiting until they feel like exercising.

Electroconvulsive Therapy

Electroconvulsive therapy (ECT) is the application of electrical current to the brain, which induces a generalized seizure (Figure 49-7 ■). The procedure is done while the client is under general anesthesia with muscle relaxation. The exact mechanism of action is not known, but ECT does increase circulating levels of brain neurotransmitters, which may be the way it relieves depression.

ECT is not recommended for use as a first treatment for uncomplicated nonpsychotic major depression, because less invasive treatments are available. It is used for clients who have intense, prolonged symptoms with marked disability, especially if the client has not responded to adequate trials with medications, or if psychotic features are present. ECT has been successful in inducing remission in people with severe psychomotor retardation. It may also be used for clients who cannot take medications, or those at imminent risk of suicide or having dangerous delusions. Clients tend to respond more quickly to ECT than they do to medication therapy (Depression Guideline Panel, 1993; Mendelowitz et al., 2003).

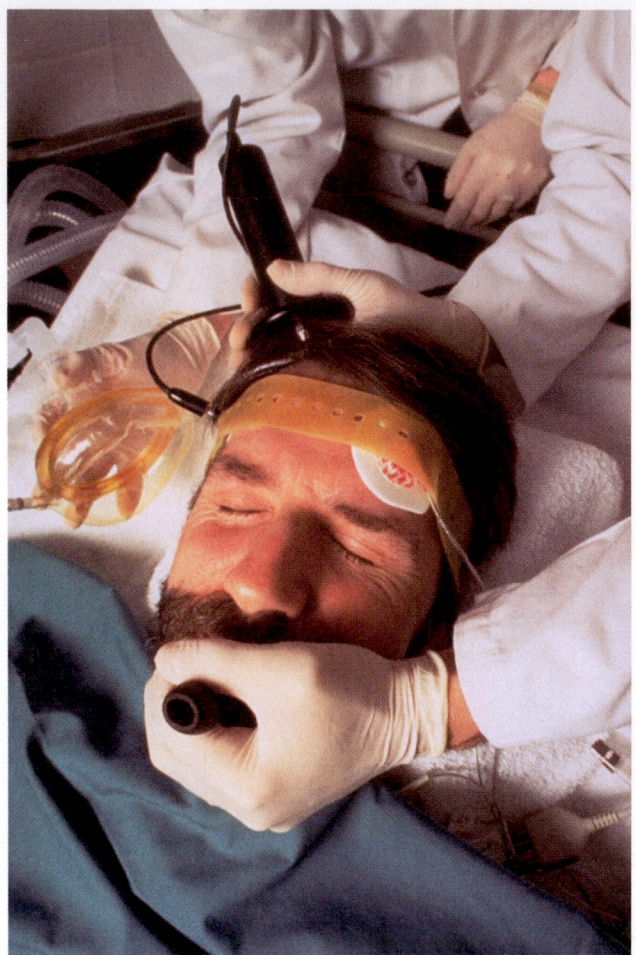

Figure 49-7. ■ A physician prepares a client for unilateral electro-convulsive therapy. (*Source:* W&D McIntyre/Photo Researchers, Inc.)

The most common side effects of ECT are transient memory loss and mental confusion. Some clients have had more severe memory loss. Rare mortality associated with the procedure was due to myocardial infarction, stroke, or cardiac rhythm abnormalities. Clients with cardiovascular disease should be treated and assessed carefully for the appropriateness of ECT. Because of the history of misuse of ECT, there is a stigma associated with its use.

BIPOLAR DISORDER

Bipolar disorder is our other prototypical mood disorder. People with bipolar disorder, also called *manic-depressive disorder*, have experienced at least one manic episode (see criteria below) or one mixed mood episode (with rapid cycling of depression and mania in the same day). Often these individuals have also experienced one or more major depressive episodes. *Bipolar* refers to the experience of both poles of mood: mania and depression. Figure 49-8 ■ compares the client's mood in bipolar disorder to that in major depressive disorder.

Diagnostic Criteria for Manic Episode

The manic client has a distinct period of abnormally and persistently elevated, expansive, or irritable mood, lasting at least 1 week (or any duration if hospitalization is necessary). During the period of mood disturbance, three (or more) of the following symptoms have persisted (four if the mood is only irritable) and have been present to a significant degree (APA, 2000):

- Inflated self-esteem or *grandiosity*
- *Decreased need for sleep* (e.g., rested after only 3 hours of sleep)
- More *talkative* than usual or pressure to keep talking

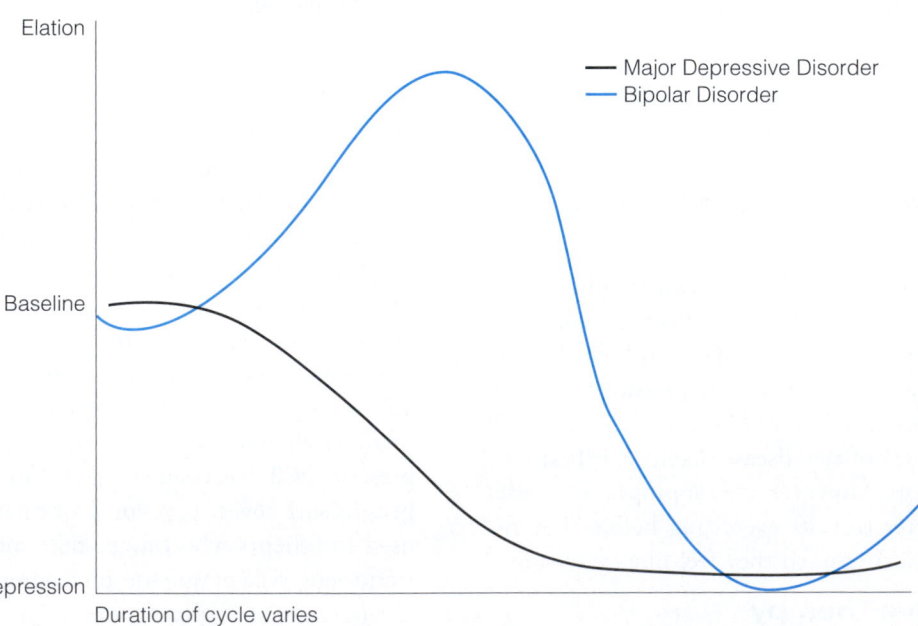

Figure 49-8. ■ Compares the client's mood in bipolar disorder to that in major depressive disorder. (*Source:* From *Contemporary Psychiatric-Mental Health Nursing*, by C. R. Kneisl, H. W. Wilson, and E. Trigoboff, 2004, Upper Saddle River, NJ: Pearson Education. Reprinted with permission.)

- *Flight of ideas* or subjective experience that thoughts are racing
- *Distractibility* (i.e., attention too easily drawn to unimportant or irrelevant external stimuli)
- Increase in *goal-directed activity* (either socially, at work or school, or sexually) or psychomotor agitation
- *Excessive involvement in pleasurable activities* that have a *high potential for painful consequences* (e.g., engaging in unrestrained buying sprees, sexual indiscretions, or foolish business investments)

The mood disturbance in mania causes marked impairment in the individual's occupational or social functioning. It may require hospitalization to prevent harm to self or others. The client may experience psychosis. Mania will not be diagnosed if the client is experiencing similar symptoms due to a reaction to drug use or another illness.

Manifestations

The mood a client feels while in a manic episode may be described as elated, euphoric, high, or unusually good. The mood is characterized by constant enthusiasm. Frequently the person alternates between elation and irritability. An affected person may play basketball enthusiastically for 24 hours, becoming angry when someone tries to take the ball. He or she may go on an extended shopping spree, buying gifts for everyone on credit, or gamble away an entire paycheck without thinking about the consequences. The flurry of activity seems productive to the client, but can be really disorganized and unproductive.

Grandiose delusions are common. The client may believe that he is a famous musician or a successful novelist, without having any skill at music or writing. The client may feel qualified to give advice on any subject, such as how to conduct brain surgery or send a rocket to Mars. The client may believe that she is a superhero. People in mania almost always have a decreased need for sleep. They may awaken several hours earlier than usual, feeling alert and energetic. When mania is severe, the affected person may go for days with no sleep and not feel tired (APA, 2000).

Manic speech is rapid and **pressured speech,** which means that it is so fast and determined that it is hard to interrupt. The person's expressions may be dramatic, or may be related to sounds more than words, such as in rhyming speech. The following is an example: "I went to the store, tell me more, open the door, I like cake, may I have a rake?" If irritability is present, the person may make long speeches about angry subjects, such as why anyone would ever want to do nursing care plans. Rapid speech reflects rapid thinking. The person's thinking may be going so fast that the thoughts are disorganized and incoherent. Box 49-16 ■ describes bipolar disorder in the words of people who experience it.

The affected person is likely to be easily *distractible*. Distractibility is evidenced by an inability to screen out excess

---

BOX 49-16   REALITY CHECK ON BIPOLAR DISORDER

- "Yes, I am feeling better. I am the CEO of Nordstrom. Did you know that I put grocery departments in Nordstrom? You and your family can join all the clients here for free groceries. I will also have free medications for everybody who needs them. Just go to any Nordstrom and mention my name. They'll give you some new clothes for work."
- "I think faster and faster. Sometimes the thoughts fly so fast I can't keep up with them and I am lost in the confusion."
- "Believe me, I have tried every drug I can find. Nothing feels so good as the natural high I get. I am smarter, stronger, quicker, happier, more alive, everything. When I get depressed, I think nothing can feel as bad as that. It is not like being alive. My life is a roller coaster, only more so."

---

sensory stimuli. The person may not be able to distinguish which thoughts are relevant to the situation and which are not. Manic clients may be distracted from a conversation by someone's clothing, colors, sounds, or even furnishings in the room (APA, 2000).

Excess goal-directed activity may involve planning and doing multiple activities, such as having sexual encounters with multiple partners, producing great volumes of work that later turn out to be confusing, or getting involved in multiple financial dealings. Affected people may hold several conversations at the same time, in person and on the phone. They may start many different projects without being able to finish them (APA, 2000).

Unwarranted optimism, grandiosity, and poor judgment characterize their behaviors. Clients may spend an entire paycheck on lottery tickets, gamble, drive recklessly, and engage in unsafe sexual behavior ignoring possible painful consequences. Affected people may spend money they do not have, do illegal things that have serious penalties, or hurt themselves or others in the moment without foreseeing future consequences (APA, 2000).

What may look like an exciting experience at the beginning can be devastating to affected people and their families. Manic episodes impair affected individuals' judgment and ability to function, and may threaten their lives. Excess energy expenditure without adequate rest can lead to exhaustion. Often during a manic episode, people will be too busy to eat, thus decreasing their energy supply even more. Figure 49-9 ■ shows the characteristics of a manic episode.

People in a manic episode frequently lack insight about their illness and its effects on themselves and others. They often resist treatment. Sometimes involuntary hospitalization is necessary to protect clients from their own behavior. Involuntary hospitalization is indicated when a person is dangerous to self or others.

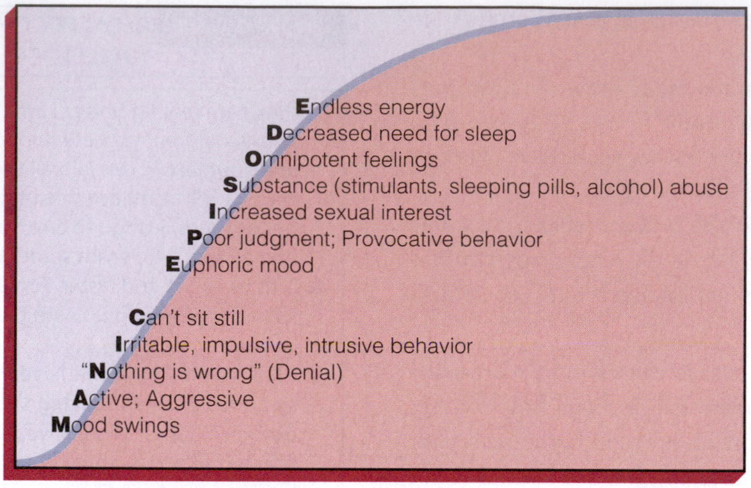

Endless energy
Decreased need for sleep
Omnipotent feelings
Substance (stimulants, sleeping pills, alcohol) abuse
Increased sexual interest
Poor judgment; Provocative behavior
Euphoric mood

Can't sit still
Irritable, impulsive, intrusive behavior
"**N**othing is wrong" (Denial)
Active; Aggressive
Mood swings

Figure 49-9. ■ Characteristics of a manic episode. (*Source:* From *Contemporary Psychiatric-Mental Health Nursing,* by C. R. Kneisl, H. W. Wilson, and E. Trigoboff, 2004, Upper Saddle River, NJ: Pearson Education. Reprinted with permission.)

Cause of Bipolar Disorder

Like major depressive disorder, bipolar disorder has a tendency to recur in families. There is evidence of a genetic etiology, but not of a single gene inheritance. First-degree biological relatives of a person with bipolar disorder have a 4% to 24% chance of having the disease, the same recurrence rate as depression. Any given manic episode is likely to follow a stressor. Disordered sleep (such as that experienced when traveling across time zones or working the night shift) may be a trigger (APA, 2000). The brain neurotransmitters norepinephrine and dopamine are implicated in the cause of manic episodes. The same neurotransmitters that are decreased in depression are increased in mania. Hormones also interact with neurotransmitters in mood disorders. Hypothyroidism is correlated with depression and with rapid cycling of mood between depression and mania.

Mania is considered to be a biological condition. Psychosocial factors are more important in the timing of manic episodes than in their cause. Stressful events may precede manic episodes.

The person with bipolar disorder will probably be taking a mood-stabilizing drug, which prevents and treats the manic aspect of the disorder. In addition to the mood stabilizer, an antidepressant is often prescribed, often in lower doses than for people who have depression alone. The dose is kept low because antidepressant medications can trigger a manic episode in a person with bipolar disorder.

Course of Bipolar Disorder

The average age of onset of a first manic episode is in the early 20s. It affects women and men equally. More than 90% of all individuals who have one manic episode will go on to have more. The exact pattern of recurrence is individual, but without treatment the average rate of manic episodes is four in 10 years. A few individuals have more rapid cycling (four or more episodes per year).

Some children show a history of behavior problems before their first actual manic episode. Like depressive episodes, manic episodes tend to occur following psychosocial stressors. The episodes usually begin suddenly and last from a few weeks to several months. Manic episodes are briefer and end more abruptly than depressive episodes. Fifty to 70% of the time, a major depressive episode will come immediately before or after a manic episode. When a manic episode is accompanied by psychosis (hallucinations and delusions), it is more serious and more likely to lead to aggression or suicide (APA, 2000).

Concurrent Disorders

Disorders of substance abuse occur commonly with bipolar disorder. People with substance abuse disorders who have bipolar disorder tend to experience more rapid cycling between mania and depression and have more *dysphoric* (unpleasant, unhappy) feelings in the manic phase (Sonne & Brady, 1999).

Collaborative Care

In the acute phase of a manic episode, the treatment priorities are ensuring client safety and treating the mood disorder. Medication is the mainstay of treatment for bipolar disorder. Counseling is valuable for helping the client learn to manage the disorder.

PSYCHOTROPIC AGENTS. The desired treatment outcomes for clients with bipolar disorder are to:

- Eliminate the symptoms of the mood episode (either depression or mania).
- Stabilize the mood to prevent cycling between depression and mania.
- Improve the client's self-care ability, function, and quality of life.

The classes of drugs used to treat manic episodes are mood stabilizers (antimanic agents), anticonvulsants (that act as mood stabilizers), benzodiazepines (to decrease anxiety and agitation while the other drugs are starting to work), and antipsychotics (if the client has psychotic symptoms). This chapter focuses on the mood stabilizing, or antimanic, agents.

LITHIUM.   Lithium, a naturally occurring element, is the classic mood-stabilizing drug. It is a first-line treatment for acute mania due to bipolar disorder and for long-term prevention of recurrent episodes. Target symptoms of mania include irritability, euphoria, pressured speech, flight of ideas, motor hyperactivity, aggressive behavior, grandiosity, delusions, impulsiveness, and hallucinations. The symptoms of depression include sadness, anhedonia, guilt, worthlessness, slowed thinking and movement, helplessness, hopelessness, suicidal thinking, and sleep disturbances.

The symptoms of bipolar depression are the same as those in clients who have depression alone (unipolar depression). See Figure 49-4 for symptoms of depression. The depression associated with bipolar disorder does not respond well to antidepressant medications alone. Antidepressants given with a mood stabilizer have been found to be effective in stabilizing mood (Bowden, 2003).

Lithium's mechanism of action is not fully understood. It is thought to affect many neurotransmitter functions. It probably corrects an ion exchange abnormality in the neuron and normalizes neurotransmitter functions.

Before a client starts on lithium therapy, a full history and physical exam should be done. Lithium is excreted by the kidneys and can have toxic effects on renal function. It inhibits several steps in thyroid hormone synthesis and metabolism, so thyroid function should be assessed. Lithium has a narrow therapeutic index, and toxicity is close to therapeutic blood levels.

In acute mania, lithium is effective in 1 to 2 weeks. It may take up to 4 weeks or longer for the symptoms to be fully relieved. A benzodiazepine or other agent may be needed to help the client during acute mania before the lithium becomes fully effective. When the client is on a maintenance dose of lithium, the frequency and severity of both manic and depressive episodes are decreased. For some people lithium offers full symptom relief. For many it is only partially effective. The combination of lithium and one of the anticonvulsants may improve mood stability. Some people are not able to tolerate the side effects of lithium, which can be significant. Box 49-17 ■ lists lithium side effects and toxic effects.

Lithium is a salt. Because of this, the sodium and fluid balance of the body affects lithium levels. The relationship between sodium and lithium is *inverse*. As the client's serum sodium decreases, the lithium level increases because the

---

BOX 49-17	**LITHIUM SIDE EFFECTS AND TOXICITY**

Common Side Effects
   Fine hand tremors
   Polyuria
   Weight gain
   GI discomfort, mild nausea
   Subjective feeling of mental dullness
   Thyroid dysfunction

Early Toxicity (Lithium level is greater than 2.0 mEq/L)
   Nausea/vomiting
   Diarrhea
   Coarse hand tremor
   Slurred speech
   Muscle weakness

Severe Toxicity (Lithium level is greater than 2.5 mEq/L)
   Mental confusion
   Muscle irritability and decreased coordination
   Fever
   Seizures
   Decreased urine output
   Cardiac dysrhythmias (irregular pulse)
   Severe hypotension
   Coma
   Death

---

kidneys conserve lithium as though it is salt. When the sodium increases, lithium levels decrease. Regular serum lithium levels are required to monitor each individual's status.

Treatment Compliance.   Compliance with lithium therapy is an important issue. Clients sometimes find the side effects of the drug to be intolerable. There is a relatively high dropout rate for people on lithium therapy. Tolerability of treatment is especially important in bipolar disorder for two reasons:

■ People with bipolar disorder expect to live full occupational and social lives.
■ Other effective treatments can be used.

Trials of several drug combinations may be required before the most effective and agreeable treatment plan for an individual is found. It is no longer necessary for the treatment team to encourage a client to endure intolerable discomfort in exchange for prevention of mania (Bowden, 2003).

Client Teaching.   Part of client education about lithium therapy is how to maintain consistent lithium and sodium levels. For example, if a person taking lithium played basketball for hours, losing sodium through perspiration, he would be at risk for lithium toxicity unless he replaced the lost sodium, maybe with a sports drink or a salty snack. He would also need to replace the water lost during exercise by drinking at intervals during the basketball game. The

management of lithium therapy is difficult and can be a challenge for clients.

For the client to have the best possible outcomes, the nurse must ensure that the client understands and participates in the treatment plan. Lifestyle changes are necessary to maintain lithium/fluid and electrolyte balance and to prevent toxicity. People taking lithium require ongoing support.

ANTICONVULSANT MOOD STABILIZERS. Because bipolar disorder is so disabling, and lithium has so many side effects, researchers have continued to search for effective therapies with fewer side effects. Some anticonvulsants have proven to be clinically effective both in treating the symptoms of mania and in preventing recurrence of episodes. The anticonvulsant valproate is endorsed as a first-line drug for mood stabilizing in bipolar disorder.

As with lithium, the exact reason the anticonvulsants stabilize mood is not known. The antimanic effect of valproate is probably due to the following actions: decreased nerve cell irritability (less likely to conduct impulses), increase in GABA, increase in postsynaptic membrane response to GABA, and reduced calcium influx into nerve cells (Keltner et al., 2003).

The valproate agents valproic acid (Depakene), sodium valproate (Depacon), and divalproex sodium (Depakote) are especially effective for clients with rapidly cycling bipolar disorder, and for mania caused by a general medical condition. They act quickly and tend to be well tolerated without effects on cognition. With high doses, their side effects include transient hair loss, weight gain, tremors, GI upset, and thrombocytopenia (loss of blood clotting cells) (Keltner et al., 2003).

The anticonvulsant drugs are CNS depressants and should not be combined with other CNS depressants or alcohol. In its liquid form, valproate can be irritating to the mouth, so it should be mixed with juice. It should not be mixed with carbonated beverages because this can make the drug more irritating.

clinical ALERT

Valproate has been known to cause fetal anomalies, and should not be taken by clients during pregnancy or by those who are planning to become pregnant.

Carbamazepine (Tegretol) is another anticonvulsant proven effective for the treatment of bipolar disorder. Carbamazepine is used for clients who do not respond to lithium or valproate. It is thought to stabilize mood by inhibiting the *kindling* process. (**Kindling** is the process of small seizure activity that builds up into a major seizure or manic episode, like small pieces of wood kindle a larger fire.) Like the valproates, carbamazepine increases the amount of stimulus needed to cause seizures or mania.

Carbamazepine can cause bone marrow suppression with decrease in red and white blood cell formation. Clients need to have regular blood cell counts taken while on this drug.

Lamotrigine (Lamictal) is also used as a mood stabilizer. It acts by stabilizing nerve cell membranes, and inhibiting neurotransmitter release. Lamotrigine can cause serious skin reactions, especially in children less than 16 years of age.

PSYCHOTHERAPY. Although bipolar disorder has a largely physiologic cause, psychosocial therapy is still valuable. Living with bipolar disorder is challenging. At some point in a manic episode, the client may feel so wonderful that taking medications to stop this feeling seems absurd. He or she may lack the insight to connect untreated mania with its many negative outcomes. Compliance with medication therapy is challenging, and often a problem for these clients. Psychotherapy, in any of the same styles described under depression, can be a valuable tool to help clients with bipolar disorder. It can assist clients to learn about their disorder, learn to manage and live with it, discuss and organize their feelings about having a chronic mental illness, discuss the dilemma of treatment, and work on development of insight into the real consequences of untreated bipolar disorder.

GROUP THERAPY. When the acute phase of mania or depression has passed, client outcomes shift to coping with the disorder over the long term. Group therapy can be very valuable toward the goal of living with a chronic mental illness (or any chronic illness). The therapy or support group is composed of people who all experience the same chronic mental illness. There may or may not be a mental health professional group facilitator.

The group discusses topics relevant to managing and coping with the disorder. For example, one session may be about dealing with medication side effects. Another may be on what to do if a client is unable to work. A third may cover how to respond to family members. People who have actually experienced these challenges may share with the group what they have learned from their experiences. The newly diagnosed member receives valuable advice from real experts on how to cope. The more experienced members receive the benefit of being able to help others and the validation that comes from being knowledgeable. Local affiliates of the National Alliance for the Mentally Ill have support groups for clients and their families.

NURSING CARE

PRIORITIZING NURSING CARE

When caring for clients with depression, focus your interventions on client safety and promoting social interactions. Intervene if the client reports suicidal thoughts. Never promise a client to keep suicidal ideas confidential—always share such information with the treatment team. Follow orders of one-to-one staffing for clients who are suicidal risks. Work to build rapport and trust with clients by allowing them to discuss suicidal feelings openly. Encourage clients with depression to participate in brief, structured group activities such as listening to music with others. Encourage hope in depressed clients by teaching them about their disorder and treatment plan.

When caring for clients with bipolar disorder, particularly in the manic phase, focus your interventions on encouraging appropriate behavior and on medication compliance. Establish acceptable guidelines for client behavior and inform client of these guidelines. All staff should enforce the same behavioral guidelines. If the client becomes agitated, intervene quickly, using the least restrictive environment, to help the client regain control. These clients may need to be physically active due to their energy levels. Encourage clients to use their energy in a positive way such as exercising or walking. Group activities are not appropriate when the client is in the manic phase. Encourage clients to follow treatment plans, especially compliance with medication schedules. Teach clients that when they feel better, it means the medication is working, so they should continue to take it, rather than to feel they no longer need it.

ASSESSING

Mood is reflected in the client's behavior and speech. When a client has a mood disorder, a mental status assessment is conducted on admission to provide baseline information. Briefer checks can be made on an ongoing basis related to pertinent parts of mental status. They should be compared to the original assessment in the client's chart.

Most cases of depression are not diagnosed or treated. Nurses in every area of specialty work with depressed people. It makes sense for nurses to routinely do screening assessments for depression.

In a depressed client, suicidal thinking must be assessed. The nurse can assess suicidal ideation as follows:

1. Start with an assessment of whether the person has suicidal ideation (thinking): "Are you thinking about hurting yourself?" or "Do you think about killing yourself?"
2. If clients have suicidal ideation, determine whether they have organized their thoughts about it enough to have a plan: "Do you have a plan?"
3. Assess lethality of the plan: "What is your plan?" or "How would you do it?" (more serious if planned means is firearm or hanging).
4. Assess whether the client has access to the planned means of suicide: "Do you have access to a gun? Drugs?" (the means in the client's plan).

5. Inform the treatment team. Failure to report suicidal ideation constitutes breach of the nurse's legal duty to protect the client.

It is the responsibility of the nurse to monitor the client's response to drug therapy for any mood disorder.

Mental Status

Client Self-Assessment

One way to monitor a client's mood over time is to use a mood scale. Ask the client, "Please rate your mood on a scale of one to ten, where one is the lowest and ten is the best possible mood." Although the numbers themselves do not have real measurement value, the client's perception of how she feels may be quantified in this way. The nurse can compare the numbers to see if the client is feeling better or worse. The mood assessment is done at least once per shift and documented in the nurses' notes.

Other aspects of mental status that are pertinent to a person with a mood disorder are appearance, *affect* (nonverbal expression of mood), behavior, motor activity, and thought processes. The appearance of a person with depression may be disheveled, if she does not have the energy to bathe and change clothes. Mania may be expressed with flashy, bright clothing and outrageous makeup and jewelry.

Normal affect is called "broad," meaning that the client can express a broad range of emotions from happiness to sadness. A person with depression cannot usually express the full range of emotions. Depression limits emotions (affect) to sadness. This finding is expressed as "blunted or restricted affect" (blunted affect is more limited than restricted affect). Emotions in mania may be restricted to excitement, elation, rage, or irritability.

Psychomotor Activity

Psychomotor activity would be slow in depression and agitated in mania. The depressed client may have psychomotor retardation, and may lie in bed all day, or sit moving very little. The manic person may be so active that she is in danger of exhaustion.

Documenting Findings

The nurse's assessment should be documented as specifically as possible. It is clearer when the nurse documents the findings that led to a conclusion, rather than the conclusion only. Charting "agitated" is not as clear as "Client has been pacing up and down the halls all night, except when he washed the windows and floors in the lounge with a paper towel, and ran in place near the nurses' station for 30 minutes. He has blisters on the soles of his feet and states that he is fine, not tired, and is ready to run a marathon."

Thought Processes

Clients' thought processes also demonstrate how they are affected by mood disorders, and how they are responding to treatment. Everyone has occasional thought blocking, in which it is difficult to think of a word that you intended to say. However, thought blocking is very common and more severe in . . . uh . . . wait a minute . . . uh . . . umm . . . depression.

Flight of ideas, in which thoughts are moving so fast that the client's speech jumps from one subject to another frequently, is common in mania. Grandiosity is also common in mania. "I am the world's most famous author, and I will be glad to write my next book about you, if you will give me a candy bar" is a grandiose statement that would more likely be used by a person in mania than one in depression.

Thought processes might include psychotic features in either severe depression or severe mania. The content in depressive delusions or hallucinations would likely be frightening, persecutory, or very negative ("My boss hates me and wants to kill me"). In mania, delusions or hallucinations would be expansive and fantastic, such as "I will fly on over to my department store to pick up a new TV. No need for a plane."

The nurse also monitors and documents any side effects from psychotropic medications. Review the section on Psychotropic Agents for side effects of drugs used for mood disorders.

DIAGNOSING, PLANNING, AND IMPLEMENTING

Common nursing diagnoses for clients with either depressive disorder or bipolar disorder include:

- *Risk for Violence* (to self with major depressive disorder, to self or others with bipolar disorder)
- *Impaired Social Interaction*
- *Risk for Imbalanced Nutrition*
- *Hopelessness*

Powerlessness, Chronic Low Self-Esteem, and *Self-Care Deficit* are common among people with depression. *Disturbed Thought Processes* and *Risk for Injury* are common nursing diagnoses for clients with bipolar disorder. Desired outcomes for clients with mood disorders are shown in Figure 49-10 ■. The same interventions listed under schizophrenia for the client experiencing disturbed thought processes related to psychosis would apply.

Nursing care must be personalized for each individual client. The suggested interventions in this chapter are based on common concerns for clients with mood disorders. If a client has different concerns, creativity will be needed. Creativity is one of the cornerstones of nursing.

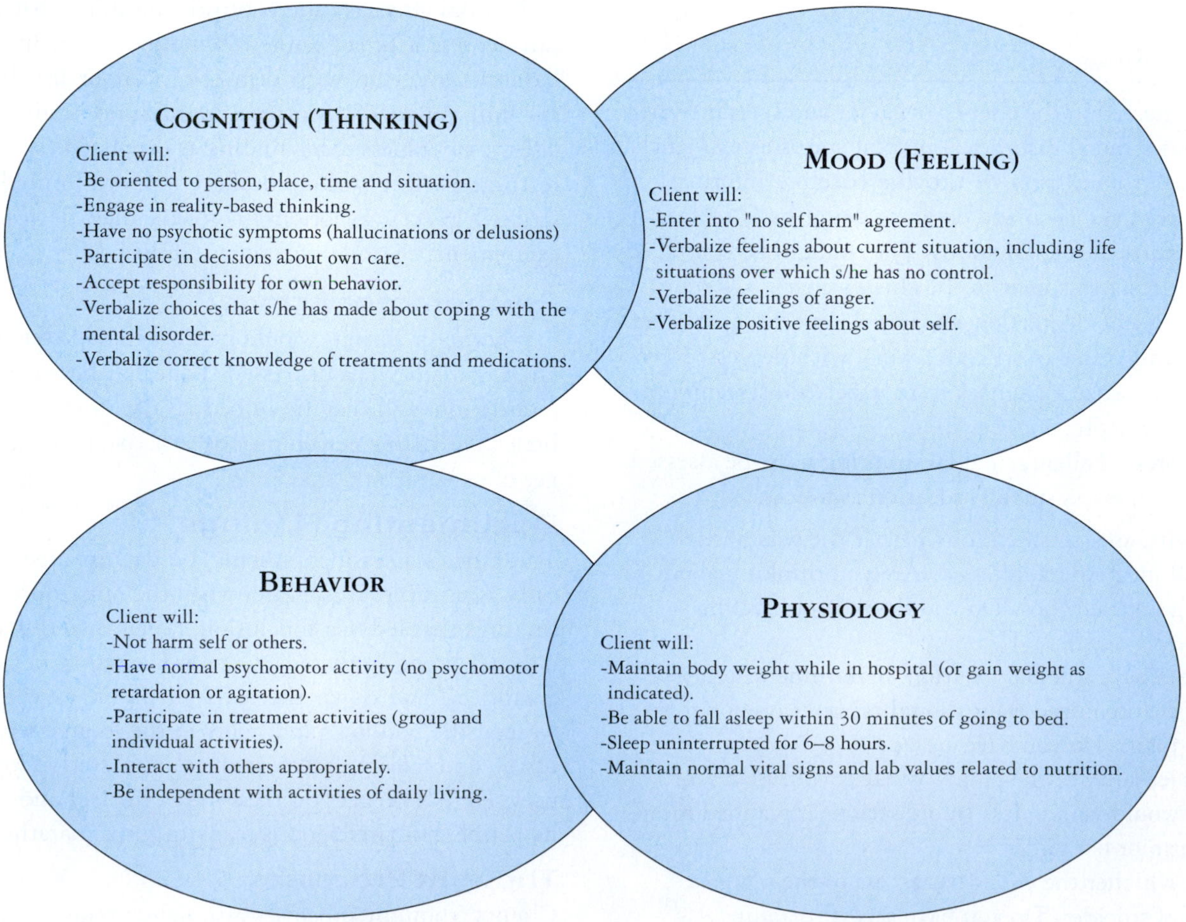

COGNITION (THINKING)
Client will:
-Be oriented to person, place, time and situation.
-Engage in reality-based thinking.
-Have no psychotic symptoms (hallucinations or delusions)
-Participate in decisions about own care.
-Accept responsibility for own behavior.
-Verbalize choices that s/he has made about coping with the mental disorder.
-Verbalize correct knowledge of treatments and medications.

MOOD (FEELING)
Client will:
-Enter into "no self harm" agreement.
-Verbalize feelings about current situation, including life situations over which s/he has no control.
-Verbalize feelings of anger.
-Verbalize positive feelings about self.

BEHAVIOR
Client will:
-Not harm self or others.
-Have normal psychomotor activity (no psychomotor retardation or agitation).
-Participate in treatment activities (group and individual activities).
-Interact with others appropriately.
-Be independent with activities of daily living.

PHYSIOLOGY
Client will:
-Maintain body weight while in hospital (or gain weight as indicated).
-Be able to fall asleep within 30 minutes of going to bed.
-Sleep uninterrupted for 6–8 hours.
-Maintain normal vital signs and lab values related to nutrition.

Figure 49-10. ■ Desired outcomes for clients with mood disorders.

Risk for Violence (Self-Directed)

- Assess mental status, including suicidal ideation. *Mental status assessment includes information about client's mood and whether client has psychosis (increased suicide risk due to abnormal reality testing).*
- If client does have suicidal ideation, ask about the plan, and whether client has the means to complete it. *The client's suicidal plan is more dangerous if the client has a specific lethal plan and the means to complete it.*
- Share information about suicidal thinking with the treatment team. *Team must be involved to ensure client safety.*
- Remove potentially dangerous items from client's area (knives, lighters, razors, belts, shoe laces, glass, etc.). *Removing dangerous items decreases client's opportunity for impulsive self-harm. People experiencing mania have impaired judgment, so the nurse must anticipate the risks and control the environment to promote safety.*
- Assess client safety frequently during the night. *Client may feel unsupervised at night.*
- Remain with a client who is having feelings about harming self. *The nurse's presence shows regard for the client's safety and worth. The nurse can prevent harmful behavior. A client at high risk for suicidal behavior requires close observation.*
- Create a "no self-harm" contract with the client. *Although an agreement by the client not to harm self is not really binding, it suggests that the client is in control and responsible for his behavior. The contract emphasizes the worth of the client and the concern by the staff for his safety.*

Risk for Violence (Directed at Others)

- Provide a low-stimulation environment for a manic client. *People experiencing mania have a reduced ability to filter and process stimuli. The more sensory stimuli, the more difficult it is for the client to determine what is real and to maintain control over behavior.*
- Make expectations for client behavior clear to client as soon as possible. Staff must be consistent in expectations of client. *Having clear, structured expectations can make it easier for client to comply with behavior expectations. Consistency among staff is important to avoid confusion and client manipulation of staff to change expectations.*
- Observe client closely and respond quickly to increasing agitation. Start with least restrictive approach: redirection, prn medication, isolation, finally restraint. *Early intervention may prevent violent behavior and injury to client and others.*
- Minimize group activities for client in mania. *Client in mania becomes easily overstimulated. May have difficulty responding appropriately with multiple people. One-to-one interactions are less stimulating and easier for client to manage.*
- Provide appropriate opportunities for physical activity. Walking is the ideal activity. Client may prefer another activity, such as ping-pong or basketball. *Client may feel compelled to be physically active and would thus find confinement very stressful. Walking is active without being exhausting.*

Impaired Social Interaction

- Establish a trusting relationship with the client. *The nurse–client relationship is the foundation for nursing care and for understanding the client's needs. When the client trusts the nurse he has an opportunity to have a sense of emotional security. A client who feels secure will be more likely to interact positively with others. The nurse provides a role model for how to communicate and behave in an individual relationship.*
- Provide structured activities to allow the client with depression to interact with others. Encourage client to participate (arts and crafts groups, listening to music in a group, walking or exercising in a group, discussing medications, reminiscing, etc.). *The depressed client is more likely to be able to interact with others if the situation is structured, because the demands on the individual are less. Positive interactions with others reinforce socializing.*

Imbalanced Nutrition

- If client is lethargic and overweight, offer lighter foods, snacks, and liquids. Discuss the value of regular exercise in improving one's spirits. Encourage the client to set a plan of regular, light exercise. *The client may be unable to focus on weight loss until depression is resolved, and may be too depressed to think of exercising. It is better to have a regular time for exercise than to try to get up and exercise when the depression is at its worst. Light, brief efforts are more possible to achieve and thus can improve self-esteem.*
- The client may feel too depressed to eat. *Offer fluids frequently, and small amounts of nutritious foods as the client tolerates.*
- If a client is highly active, pacing, or too busy to eat, provide nutritious "finger foods" (sandwiches, fruit, etc.) that the client can eat while walking. Offer food and fluids frequently. *Client has high-energy needs while in a manic phase, and may not be able to meet nutritional needs. Client may be able to eat foods that can be held in his hands when he is unable to sit down for a meal. Client is also at risk for dehydration from excessive activity, especially in hot weather.*

Hopelessness

- Allow client to talk about feelings and life events. Use therapeutic communication techniques to help client see that he has survived difficulties in the past and that he has strengths. *The knowledge that one has overcome obstacles before suggests that it is possible to do so again. When clients recognize their own strengths, it provides a foundation for hope that the current trouble can be overcome.*

- Teach client about the disorder and medications and that the treatment team will not give up hope until the client feels better. Keep hope alive! *Knowledge that the client is likely to have a positive response to treatment is hopeful. It may be beneficial to point out that depression has episodes and that this one will eventually resolve. Many clients worry that the staff will abandon them if they do not respond to treatment.*

EVALUATING

In the evaluation phase, the nurse looks back at the desired outcomes and asks, "Were the outcomes met?" Desired outcomes for clients with mood disorders include that the client will:

- Cause no harm to self or others.
- Perform ADLs and occupational responsibilities independently.
- Eat a balanced diet.
- Participate in appropriate regular exercise.
- Have a realistic sense of hope for the future and a sense of personal efficacy.

Continuity of Care

Clients with mood disorders face many challenges related to their disorder and its treatment. The nurse should reinforce client teaching about medications, side effects, and the interaction between medication and diet or activities. Most clients will need ongoing psychotherapeutic support. Information about support groups, as well as emergency numbers, should be provided. The National Alliance for the Mentally Ill has support groups in many locations.

NURSING PROCESS CARE PLAN
Client with Depression

Remember Pearl from the beginning of this chapter? Pearl G. is a 70-year-old African American widowed woman who is a resident in a long-term care facility. She had a stroke a year ago and has hemiplegia on her right side. She is right handed. She does not feed herself and has little appetite. Ms. G. is alert and oriented to person and place. She cooperates with having her activities of daily living done for her, but she does not try to help. When she talks, it is only one or two words at a time. Her face always seems to look sad. The nurse has worked with Ms. G. for the 11 months since she has been in this facility. The nurse thinks Ms. G. is depressed. The nurse assessed her with the Geriatric Depression Scale. Ms. G. scored 12. In the conversation they had about the depression scale, Ms. G. said that she missed her family.

Assessment

The nurse collected all the assessment findings in the case study above. In addition, the chart stated that Ms. G. had an adult daughter and a married son with one teenage granddaughter living nearby.

Nursing Diagnosis

The following important nursing diagnoses (among others) are established for this condition:

- *Powerlessness* related to disability and impaired communication
- *Self-Care Deficit*, bathing/hygiene, dressing/grooming, feeding, and toileting related to hemiplegia and lack of motivation
- *Impaired Social Interaction* related to lack of motivation and lack of opportunity to socialize with family and peers

Expected Outcomes

The expected outcomes for the plan of care for Ms. G. are as follows:

- Client will identify two areas in which she feels some control.
- Client will assist with all her ADLs, feeding herself independently within 2 weeks.
- Client will interact with the staff, her peers, and her family.

Planning and Implementation

Before beginning to work on independent nursing actions, the charge nurse consulted with Ms. G.'s physician about the possibility of treating her depression. The physician agreed that Ms. G. is depressed. She prescribed fluoxetine 20 mg to be given to Ms. G. PO each morning. The LPN (Kevin) looked up fluoxetine, and found it to be a selective serotonin reuptake inhibitor type of antidepressant drug. The following interventions were planned and implemented:

- Offer simple choices first. *Ms. G. is given a choice of clothes to wear each day. She is asked if she wants to take her shower before or after breakfast, and where she wants to eat lunch (there are three dining rooms in this facility). Ms. G. has some cognitive deficit after the stroke. She is asked which radio station she wants to listen to.*
- Encourage self-care. *The aides who supervised meals were asked to help her use her left hand to feed herself. Self-feeding was tried months before, and it worked until Ms. G. became unwilling to do it.*
- Encourage social contact. *Kevin, the nurse, called each of Ms. G.'s children and encouraged them to visit. He also arranged to visit with Ms. G. for a few minutes each day that he worked. (We know that Kevin would have liked to have had time to talk longer with her, but this a real story.) He had Ms. G. put on the list of residents who attend the news group (where the activity aide reads parts of the newspaper each morning).*

Evaluation

Two weeks after the plan was started, Kevin evaluated its effectiveness. With encouragement, Ms. G. had started to make choices about her clothes, radio stations, social activities, and visitors. Ms. G. assisted in washing herself during her shower. She tried feebly, but was not much help with dressing. She was able to feed herself about 50% of her meals, and was able to call for help to get to the bathroom about 75% of the time.

Within 10 days after starting her new medication, she was smiling, more interested in her surroundings, had more appetite, and was more active. She is more talkative and enjoys visits from her family.

Critical Thinking in the Nursing Process

1. Was outcome 1 (self-efficacy) met, and why was it important for Ms. G.?
2. How successful was outcome 2 (independence with ADLs) of Ms. G.'s plan? How might it be adapted after evaluation?
3. Discuss how the range of social interactions that were set up for Ms. G. increased the likelihood that outcome 3 (social interaction) would be met.

Note: Discussion of Critical Thinking questions appears on the MyNursingKit Website.

Personality Disorders

Personality is the relatively stable way that a person thinks, feels, and behaves. Personality includes the psychosocial (not physical) traits and characteristics that make a person an individual. Personality is affected by genetic predispositions and by life experiences. Culture affects the client's behavior and personality. Naturally, people have a variety of different personality traits.

MANIFESTATIONS

Impaired self-identity is a central problem in disorders of personality. Self-identity includes a combination of social and occupational roles, chosen values and behaviors, beliefs about sexuality and intimacy, gender roles, and life goals. An adequately formed identity is necessary for goal-directed behavior and for satisfying interpersonal relationships. Self-identity is often minimal or absent in personality disorders (Limandri & Boyd, 2002).

Thinking patterns are distorted in personality disorders. The individual's ability to interpret environmental events is impaired. Maladaptive thinking patterns cause individuals to misinterpret the actions of others. The misinterpretations result in maladaptive responses by the affected person.

Emotions, in their intensity and quality, appear to be affected by disorders of personality. The emotional experiences of affected people may be blunted or distorted. They tend to have more negative emotional experiences. Their ability to function in daily life is affected.

Behavior is affected by personality disorders. Personality disorders cause impulsive and inflexible behavior. These disorders appear to make it more difficult for people to predict the consequences of their actions, or to control their impulses despite probable negative consequences. Affected people also tend to be rigid. They are unable to change their usual behavior when circumstances suggest that a change is indicated.

This inflexibility traps the client in *vicious cycles of behavior* that are self-defeating. Inflexibility in personality disorders makes it difficult for people to learn new ways to behave or cope. The inflexibility provokes problems. The clients continue to be inflexible, which creates more problems. The more inflexible they are, the more problems they have. The more problems they have, the more inflexible they are. This vicious circle reduces learning opportunities and alienates other people (Millon & Davis, 1999). See Figure 49-11 ■ for a diagram of this vicious cycle.

DIAGNOSTIC CRITERIA

Although the normal range of human behavior, feelings, and thought is broad, it is possible for personality to be outside the normal range. A **personality disorder** is an enduring pattern of inner experience and behavior that has the following characteristics (APA, 2000):

- It deviates markedly from the expectations of the individual's culture.
- It is pervasive and inflexible.

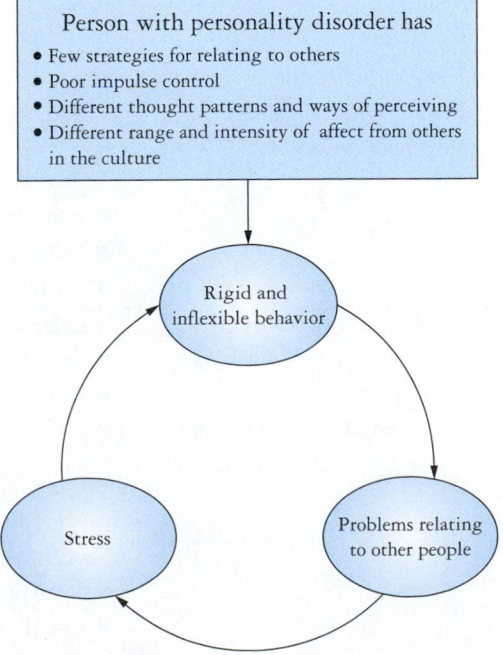

Figure 49-11. ■ Vicious cycle of personality disorders.

- It begins in adolescence or young adulthood.
- It is stable over time.
- It leads to distress for the individual or impairment of functioning.

A person's personality significantly affects how the person responds to life events, including illness. The response a client has to a mental disorder will be affected by that client's personality as well.

Personality disorders are not considered to be the same as mental disorders or diseases. Diagnosing personality disorders requires an evaluation of the person's long-term patterns of functioning. Personality patterns must be persistent to be significant. For a personality disorder to be present, the individual's symptoms cannot be caused by a general medical disorder or by substance abuse. The personality characteristics used for diagnosis must have persisted since the individual was an adolescent or young adult (APA, 2000). The APA describes 10 types of personality disorders. These disorders are grouped into three clusters by their similarities. Table 49-4 ■ provides an outline of the disorders and their features. Therapy is long-term and changes occur slowly.

CHALLENGES FOR NURSES

Nurses often find it frustrating to work with clients who have disorders of personality. These clients can be manipulative, socially inappropriate, and difficult. When nurses see the rigid, inflexible behavior patterns, they often believe that these clients could change if they tried. However, personality represents a *persistent* pattern of thought, emotion, and behavior. Although these clients are responsible for their own behavior, they cannot change their personalities completely. These clients need all the patience and skill nurses have to offer. Remember that the goal of the nurse is to provide professional care, not to be the friend of the client.

NURSING CARE

PRIORITIZING NURSING CARE

When caring for clients with personality disorders, be aware of your own responses. Clients with these disorders are very good at "pushing people's buttons," including those of staff. Be careful to react to the client as a person

TABLE 49-4 Features of Personality Disorders		
CLUSTER A: **ODD-ECCENTRIC DISORDER**	**CLUSTER B:** **DRAMATIC-EMOTIONAL DISORDERS**	**CLUSTER C:** **ANXIOUS-FEARFUL DISORDERS**
Paranoid Personality Disorder ■ Pattern of distrust and suspiciousness ■ Difficulty with relationships ■ Hostility and defensiveness	*Antisocial Personality Disorder* ■ Pattern of disregarding and violating the rights of others ■ Manipulate others for personal gain or pleasure ■ Impulsive, irresponsible behavior ■ No remorse for harming others	*Avoidant Personality Disorder* ■ Pattern of social shyness and feelings of inadequacy ■ Fearful and tense ■ Low self-esteem ■ Preoccupied with thoughts of rejection
Schizoid Personality Disorder ■ Detachment from social relationships ■ Restricted range of emotional expression	*Borderline Personality Disorder* ■ Pattern of intense and unstable relationships ■ Fear of abandonment ■ Impulsive behavior ■ Self-harm ■ Unstable self-image	*Dependent Personality Disorder* ■ Need to be taken care of ■ Difficulty making decisions ■ Take no initiative ■ Powerlessness
Schizotypal Personality Disorder ■ Reduced capacity for relationships ■ Eccentric behavior ■ Inappropriate emotional expression	*Histrionic Personality Disorder* ■ Excessive emotionality ■ Attention-seeking behavior ■ Difficulty forming satisfying relationships	*Obsessive-Compulsive Personality Disorder* ■ Preoccupation with orderliness and control ■ Perfectionism ■ Inflexibility ■ Overly conscientious
	Narcissistic Personality Disorder ■ Need of admiration from others ■ Grandiosity ■ Lack of empathy for others	

with a mental illness, rather than as a person who is baiting you. This can be very difficult. Be professional at all times. If need be, ventilate to other staff if you become irritated with the client's behavior. Encourage and support all positive steps the client makes in using positive behaviors rather than negative ones.

ASSESSING

After the physician or psychiatrist makes the diagnosis of personality disorder, the nurse will help the client deal with the effects of the disorder. Information will be collected about the client's functional ability, mental status, and interpersonal relationships. Because personality is so integral to self-identity, people usually cannot see their own abnormalities. Significant others are a valuable source of information about the client. They can identify how a client behaves or copes with problems at home.

DIAGNOSING, PLANNING, AND IMPLEMENTING

Nursing diagnoses for clients with personality disorders are tailored to the particular type of disorder. Some nursing diagnoses that apply to many different types of personality disorders are:

- *Impaired Social Interaction*
- *Chronic Low Self-Esteem*
- *Ineffective Coping*
- Antisocial and borderline personality disorders also carry *Risk for Violence* to self or others as a nursing diagnosis

Client outcomes for people with personality disorders would include:

- Client will participate appropriately in social activities.
- Client will express awareness that feelings of low self-esteem are part of disorder.
- Client will not cause physical harm to self or others.

Nursing interventions for clients with personality disorders must be individualized to the person and to the disorder. However, certain guidelines generally apply:

- If possible, enlist the family in helping to understand the client. *Personalities develop over years. The client cannot be objective, but the family will have years of experience and insight to help identify coping behaviors, triggers of difficult behavior, and areas of concern.*
- Be matter of fact and professional. Do not ignore a client's suspicions, but do not support irrational fears. *If client has paranoia, a brief, respectful reassurance will probably be more effective than elaborate "proofs." If client is being insulting or manipulative, do not try to be friendly or personal; be confident, and provide professional care.*

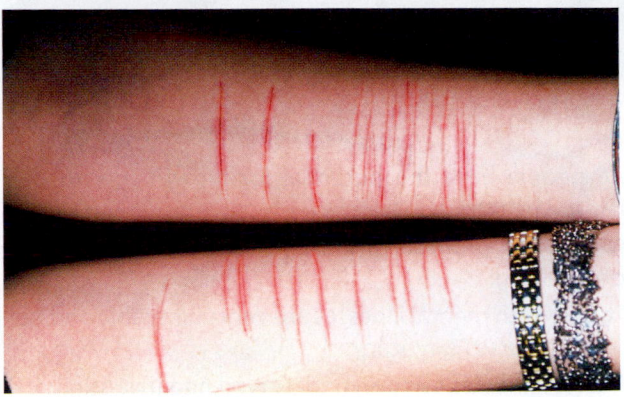

Figure 49-12. ■ Some people with borderline personality disorders engage in recurrent suicidal gestures or self-mutilating behaviors. (*Source: Dr. P. Marozzi/Science Photo Library; Photo Researchers, Inc.*)

- Understand your own reactions to the client with a personality disorder, and behave professionally. *It can be frustrating to work with people with personality disorders. Remember that the behavior is related to a disorder and is not intended to aggravate you or the staff.*
- If there are signs of self-harm, ask about them (Figure 49-12 ■). Help the client identify factors that might have initiated the need to cause self-harm. Teach coping skills for reducing stress. *To treat the disorder, it is necessary to acknowledge it and to identify factors that triggered the episode. Once clients know what began the episode, they can avoid those situations. Skills can be written on a card for the client to carry.*
- Tell clients with a *Risk for Violence* diagnosis to tell the staff if they feel like hurting themselves. *The client who agrees to report feelings of self-harm or harm to others is participating actively in treatment. The nurse encourages the client to examine those feelings and to look at alternatives to violence. The nurse reports client's feelings about injuring self to the treatment team.*
- Help clients to make positive steps with their disorders. *Personalities take years to develop. They cannot be changed in a day or a week. Encourage client attempts to cope with their disorders. Praise positive changes (however small) in the client's way of interacting and coping.*

EVALUATING

Review the desired outcomes for the client. Document client responses to nursing interventions. Report any significant changes, especially those that could indicate ideas of harm to others or self-harm.

Note: The references and resources for all chapters have been compiled at the back of the book.

Chapter Review

KEY Points

- All people have the potential for growth toward better mental health.
- Nurses can promote the mental health of clients in any care setting.
- People with mental illnesses are very vulnerable and benefit from nurses' advocacy.
- Mental illnesses carry an undeserved negative stigma.
- Major mental illnesses are complex disorders caused by functional and structural abnormalities of the brain. Both internal (biological) and external (environmental stress) factors are involved.
- Schizophrenia is among the most devastating of all illnesses to the quality and length of the lives of affected people, yet it is underrepresented in funding for research and client services.
- People with schizophrenia have disordered thinking, decreased motivation, difficulty relating to other people and to themselves, and an increased risk of suicide.
- Families are important members of the treatment team.
- Antipsychotic medications have side effects. Some (NMS and TD) are life threatening or long lasting; others (EPS) cause discomfort and may encourage noncompliance with medication therapy.
- Depression is the most common mental disorder in the world.
- Nurses in every specialty area work with people who have mental disorders, especially depression.
- Most people who commit suicide were depressed.
- People with depression may experience anhedonia, lack of energy, lack of motivation, difficulty relating to other people, and psychomotor retardation, as well as sadness.
- Serious possible side effects are associated with the MAOI antidepressants, including hypertensive crisis when clients combine foods containing tyramine with taking these drugs.

- People with bipolar disorder in the manic phase have several challenges including lack of insight, poor judgment, and impulsive behavior.
- There is hope for people with mental disorders. Most people respond well to treatment.

☯ FOR FURTHER Study

For information about HIPAA, see Chapter 14.

A discussion on family systems is found in Chapter 16.

See Chapter 17 for more information about the *DSM* and psychosocial nursing skills.

See Box 21-10 for a reminder on how to measure for orthostatic hypotension.

See Chapter 34 for more information on hematopoietic and lymphatic system disorders.

See Chapter 36 for further discussion of seizures, tardive dyskinesia, and other neurologic disorders.

Diabetes is discussed in detail in Chapter 38.

See Chapter 43 for the Geriatic Depression Scale.

Postpartum psychosis is discussed further in Chapter 55.

See Chapter 62 for more discussion about suicide in adolescents.

Critical Thinking Care Map

Caring for a Client Experiencing Psychosis
NCLEX-PN® Focus Area: Psychosocial Integrity

Case Study: Bob Goldman is a 40-year-old European American Jewish man who is diagnosed with schizophrenia. He has not been taking his ordered antipsychotic medication at home. He was admitted to the psychiatric unit today with the diagnosis of psychosis due to acute exacerbation of schizophrenia. It is time to give him his oral antipsychotic medication.

Nursing Diagnosis: *Disturbed Thought Processes*

COLLECT DATA

Subjective	Objective
_____	_____
_____	_____
_____	_____
_____	_____
_____	_____
_____	_____
_____	_____

Would you report this? Yes/No

If yes, report to: _____

What would you report?_____

Nursing Care

_____
_____
_____
_____
_____
_____
_____
_____
_____
_____

How would you document this? _____
_____
_____
_____

Compare your answers and documentation to those provided on the MyNursingKit Website.

Data Collected
(use only those that apply)

- History of benign prostatic hypertrophy
- History of suicide attempt at age 18
- BP 130/82
- Client states, "I don't need the medication. I am fine. The doctor is the one who is crazy."
- Weight loss of 15 pounds since last hospitalization 9 months ago
- Client states, "I like cereal for breakfast"
- Client is dirty and has strong body odor
- Client takes the blanket off his bed, rolls it into a log shape, and swings it around
- Client states, "I'll use this log to fight off the attackers!"

Nursing Interventions
(use only those that apply; list in priority order)

- Tell the client, "You are safe here in the hospital."
- Take VS every 2 hours.
- Maintain a low-stimulation environment.
- Tell the client, "Yes you do need the medication, and if you don't take it willingly, we can force you to take it."
- Teach the client about the chemical structure of his medication.
- Tell the client, "This medication will help to straighten out your thoughts. I think you should take it."
- Remove all bed linens from the client's room for the duration of his hospitalization.
- Communicate simply and calmly with the client.
- Say, "I will save you from the attackers."
- Say, "There are no attackers here."
- Ask, "Why don't you bathe?"
- Encourage the client to take a shower.
- Give the client a big hug to reassure him.

NCLEX-PN® Exam Preparation

TEST-TAKING TIP   Some questions will ask about the correct thing for a nurse to say in a given situation. It may seem that you would never really say any of these things. Remember that these are questions illustrating principles of nursing care, not necessarily the exact words you would say. Choose the answer that illustrates caring, respecting the client's right to make his or her own decisions, helping the client express feelings, or validating the client's feelings.

1 The nurse recognizes all of the following as characteristics of a mentally healthy person except for:
1. Accurate evaluation of reality.
2. Healthy self-concept.
3. Control over other's behavior.
4. Creativity and productivity.

2 The nurse expects to find which of the following if the client is experiencing negative symptoms of schizophrenia?
1. Flat affect and little speech.
2. Rigid posture.
3. Excessive purposeless movements.
4. Inappropriate laughter.

3 The nurse has noticed that physicians are reluctant to diagnose clients with a mental illness and the nurse expects this may be due to the:
1. Stigma related to mental illness.
2. The extra paperwork associated with a mental illness diagnosis.
3. The physician's lack of understanding of mental health disorders.
4. The client's preference to diagnose the disorder as a physical disease.

4 The nurse would consider which of the following mental health disorders as rarely occurring in children?
1. Depression
2. Bipolar disorder
3. Borderline personality disorder
4. Schizophrenia

5 The nurse's role in promoting mental health includes all of the following except:
1. Helping prevent healthy people from becoming affected by mental disorders.
2. Assisting with early diagnosis and treatment for people with mental health disorders.
3. Preventing further disability for people who have mental disorders.
4. Reducing the risk of those with genetic and biological predispositions for mental health disorders.

6 The nurse has been studying personality disorders and recognizes that which of the following is not a specific cluster type?
1. Eccentric disorders.
2. Emotional disorders.
3. Fearful disorders.
4. Sociopathic disorders.

7 When assisting the client who is taking an antipsychotic medication, a priority nursing intervention is to:
1. Encourage a high-fat diet.
2. Encourage daily time in the sun.
3. Remind the client to change positions slowly.
4. Remind the client to take the medication with an antacid.

8 The unlicensed assistive personnel asks the nurse why so many people with mental disorders aren't diagnosed as mentally ill. The nurse explains that mental disorders are often underdiagnosed because:
1. Physicians do not recognize the condition.
2. General practitioners feel underqualified to treat a mental disorder.
3. Clients underreport their feelings, for fear of the stigma of being labeled "mentally ill."
4. Physicians do not value the depth of the psychologic feelings a client reports.

9 The nurse administers traditional, or typical, antipsychotic medications to relieve which of the following symptoms of schizophrenia?
1. Anhedonia
2. Flat affect and alogia
3. Hallucinations, delusions, and disordered thoughts
4. Avolition

10 The nurse, working on an inpatient psychiatric unit, would monitor which of the following clients most closely for potentially violent behavior?
1. A client experiencing catatonic symptoms.
2. A client who has been pacing all day and talking loudly to an unseen voice.
3. A client who refuses to participate in the morning arts and crafts activity.
4. A client who has been following you around all day.

Answers and rationales for Review Questions appear in Appendix I.

Chapter 50

Substance Abuse and Eating Disorders

LEARNING Outcomes

After completing this chapter, you will be able to:

1. Discuss issues and terms related to substance abuse and dependency.
2. Identify effects of alcohol and other CNS depressants.
3. Describe effects of commonly abused substances.
4. Identify treatments and nursing interventions for clients with problems related to substance abuse and dependency.
5. Discuss the philosophy of the 12-step programs for treatment of substance abuse.
6. Describe the appropriate response when substance abuse issues impair a colleague at work.
7. Identify three major types of eating disorders.
8. Discuss treatment and nursing care for clients with eating disorders.

Clinical Objectives

9. Collect data for assessment of clients with substance abuse symptoms.
10. Apply the nursing process to clients with problems related to substance abuse.
11. Help families plan strategies for preventing eating disorders in their children.
12. Apply the nursing process to the care of clients with eating disorders.

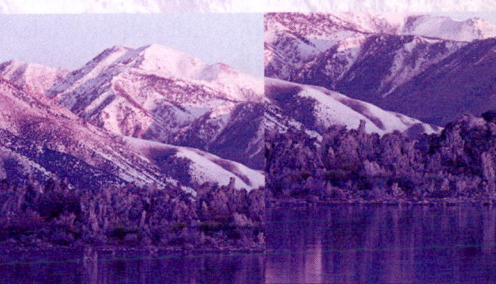

BRIEF Outline

SUBSTANCE ABUSE
Delayed Diagnosis
Substance Abuse and Dependency
Alcohol
Other CNS Depressants
CNS Stimulants
Hallucinogens
Inhalants
Caffeine and Nicotine
Prescription Medication Abuse
Collaborative Care
Substance Dependency among Nurses
EATING DISORDERS
Anorexia Nervosa
Bulimia Nervosa
Binge Eating Disorder
Causes of Eating Disorders
Collaborative Care
Diabulimia
Obesity

abstinence 1386	**dichotomous thinking** 1399	**substance abuse** 1382
binge 1398	**intoxication** 1381	**substance dependency** 1382
body mass index 1400	**Korsakoff's syndrome** 1385	**tolerance** 1382
confabulation 1385	**metabolic syndrome** 1401	**Wernicke's syndrome** 1385
cross-tolerance 1389	**myopathy** 1385	**withdrawal** 1382
denial 1380	**purging** 1397	
diabulimia 1400	**relapse** 1386	

This chapter provides an overview of two serious health problems: substance abuse and eating disorders. As many as 20% of adults in the United States meet the diagnostic criteria for an alcohol- or substance-related disorder (American Psychiatric Association [APA], 2000). Along with alcohol and substance-related disorders, there is also an increase of domestic violence, elder abuse, violent crimes, and traffic fatalities, especially in under-age drinking. Alcohol and substance use is an individual, family, and societal problem that puts a drain on government and healthcare resources. The incidence of eating disorders is increasing in North America and all over the world. The care of clients with both substance abuse disorders and eating disorders is complicated. People with these disorders have both physiologic and psychosocial needs. Nursing care for these clients must be holistic, including the whole person (mind, body, and spirit).

There are some commonalities between substance dependency and eating disorders. In both types of disorders people use behavior that is harmful to their health as a coping mechanism to manage their anxiety. Society often has negative attitudes toward people who have substance abuse and eating disorders. Affected people often hesitate to seek treatment. Nurses can be helpful to people with both types of disorders and their families.

SUBSTANCE ABUSE

People use substances for a variety of reasons: to alter their perceptions; to elevate mood; to relieve pain, fear, anxiety, or boredom; or to aid in religious ceremonies. Although all substance use is not problematic, the abuse of substances can destroy people's lives. Substance use becomes a problem when:

- It interferes with the ability to function at work or at home.
- It puts anyone in danger.
- It continues despite negative consequences.

Alcohol is a factor in many fatal events. Figure 50-1 ■ shows how often alcohol contributes to fatalities in the United States.

Delayed Diagnosis

The reason why the exact number of people with substance abuse and dependency is not known is **denial** (see also Chapter 17). Denial is a common coping mechanism for people with these disorders. Ironically, denial is also common in health professionals who work with these clients. Think about it: 20% of American adults have diagnosable problems with substance abuse. Are 2 out of every 10 clients in the facilities where you work or have clinical courses diagnosed with substance abuse or dependency? Healthcare providers do not assess for it or diagnose it, even though substance abuse and dependency cause significant health effects. Another factor in the many missed cases is that people with substance-related disorders do not tend to seek treatment for these disorders.

Current research suggests that alcohol problems often follow a predictable course. Chronic excessive drinking happens first. Legal, social (relationship), and job problems come later, followed by tolerance, withdrawal symptoms, neurologic problems, and emotional problems. General health problems come last (see, for example, liver cirrhosis in Chapter 37), but most people wait until their health deteriorates before seeking help—years after the alcohol dependency began (Simpson & Tucker, 2002).

The attitudes of health professionals contribute to the tendency of people to be diagnosed late. The *stigma* (negative label) against substance abuse is very strong (see also Chapter 17). Health professionals often hesitate to ask the questions that could determine who is affected by substance use. Sometimes health professionals are not aware of how they can help. This chapter helps nurses identify clients with substance-related disorders and suggests interventions to help them.

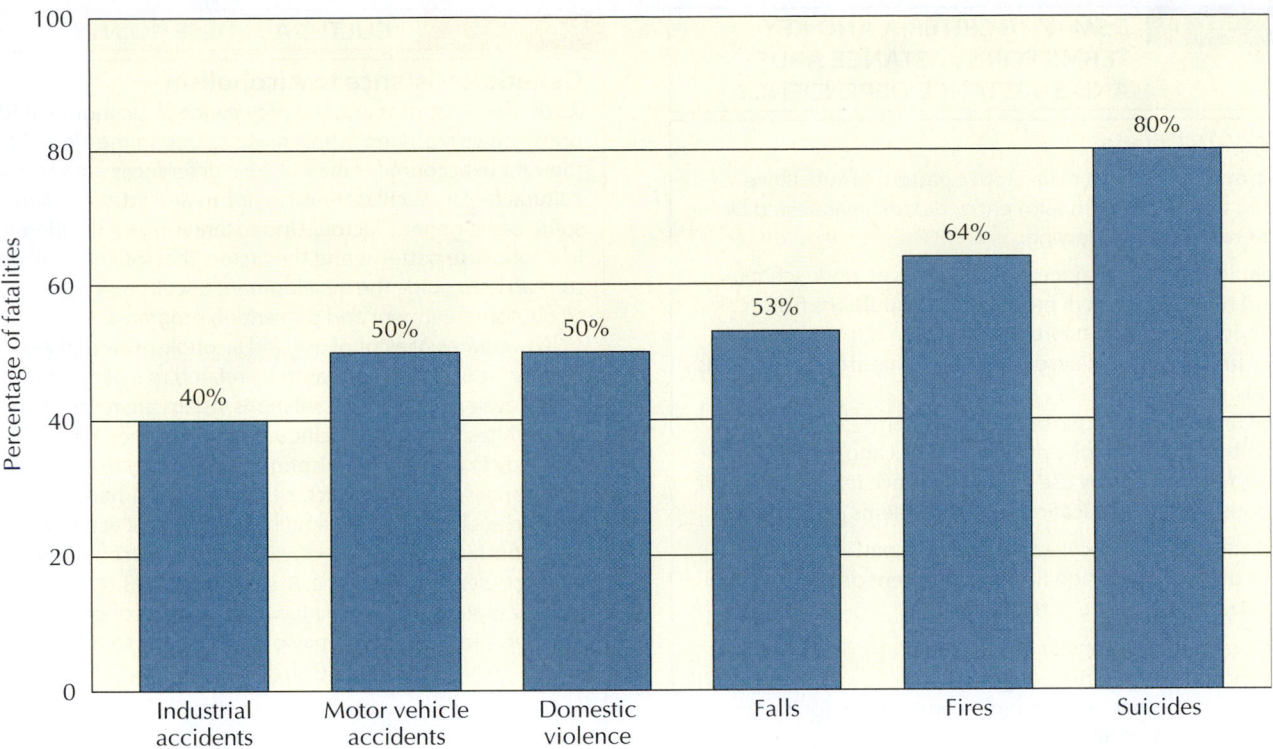

Figure 50-1. ■ Fatal events in which alcohol is a factor. (*Source:* From *Mental Health Nursing*, 5th ed., by K. L. Fontaine, 2003. Upper Saddle River, NJ: Prentice Hall. Reprinted with permission.)

Substance Abuse and Dependency

Initial treatment will depend on the client's level of substance use. *Substance abuse* is a maladaptive pattern of substance use despite adverse outcomes (APA, 2000). Box 50-1 ■ lists key terms related to substance abuse and for the diagnostic criteria according to the *Diagnostic and Statistical Manual for Mental Disorders*, fourth edition, text revision (*DSM-IV-TR*; APA, 2000). People who abuse substances suffer the harmful consequences of repeated use. *Substance dependency* is more severe. It involves *tolerance, withdrawal*, and *compulsive use* (see Box 50-1). *Addiction* refers to psychologic and physiologic dependence and drug-seeking behavior. These definitions apply to all substances of abuse and dependence.

The most commonly abused substances are those that rapidly change a person's mental state, either by stimulating or by depressing the central nervous system (CNS). The *DSM-IV-TR* (APA, 2000) lists 11 substances of abuse:

- Alcohol
- Opioids
- Sedatives, hypnotics, and anxiolytics (antianxiety drugs)
- Cocaine
- Amphetamines and similar drugs
- Hallucinogens
- Phencyclidine (PCP) and similar drugs
- Inhalants
- Cannabis (marijuana)
- Caffeine
- Nicotine

Alcohol

The most commonly abused substance in the world is *beverage alcohol* (ethanol or ethyl alcohol). Alcohol is quickly absorbed into the blood and acts as a central nervous system depressant. Initial symptoms of alcohol **intoxication** (a reversible set of physical, psychologic, and behavioral symptoms caused by use of a substance) are relaxation, loss of inhibition, *euphoria* (an exaggerated feeling of well-being), and decreased mental concentration. With higher doses, symptoms progress to slurred speech, *ataxia* (staggering gait), *labile* (changeable) mood, aggressive behavior, incoherent speech, vomiting, coma, respiratory depression, and death. Physiologic reactions to alcohol are influenced by the individual's genetic makeup (Box 50-2 ■). Blood alcohol concentrations and the symptoms they produce are provided in Table 50-1 ■.

TOLERANCE AND WITHDRAWAL

With continued use, the user develops *tolerance* (see Box 50-1). When an individual regularly drinks large amounts of alcohol, the CNS is repeatedly depressed. To maintain balance (homeostasis) for survival, the CNS increases its own stimulation to keep the person conscious and functioning. As

BOX 50-1 *DSM-IV-TR* CRITERIA AND KEY TERMS FOR SUBSTANCE ABUSE AND SUBSTANCE DEPENDENCY

DSM-IV-TR Criteria

Substance abuse—a maladaptive pattern of substance use leading to significant impairment or distress manifested by one or more of the following:

1. Inability to fulfill major role obligations at work, school, and home (poor work performance, expulsions from school, neglect of children)
2. Recurrent substance use in physically hazardous situations (driving a car, operating a machine)
3. Recurrent legal or interpersonal problems
4. Continued use despite persistent social and interpersonal problems caused by use of the substance (arguments with spouse about intoxication, fights, problems at work)

Substance dependency—a maladaptive pattern of substance use leading to significant impairment or distress, manifested by three or more of the following:

1. Tolerance to the substance
2. Withdrawal syndrome
3. Substance either taken in higher amounts or for longer periods than intended
4. Unsuccessful or persistent desire to cut down or control use
5. A great deal of time spent in obtaining, using, and recovering from effects of the substance
6. Reduction of important social, occupational, or recreational activities due to substance use
7. Continued substance use despite knowledge of a persistent physical or psychologic problem that is likely caused by the substance

Key Terms in Substance Dependency

Tolerance
Defined by either of the following:

a. A need for increased amounts of the substance to achieve the same effect, or
b. Diminished effect with continued use of the same amount of the substance.

Withdrawal
Due to discontinuing or reducing use of a substance that has been heavy and prolonged:

a. A substance-specific withdrawal syndrome develops.
b. The same or related substance is taken to relieve or avoid withdrawal symptoms.
c. Significant distress or impairment in social or occupational functioning occurs.

Compulsive Substance Use

Repetitive substance use behavior for the purpose of reducing distress. Compulsive use is often unwanted and time-consuming.

Source: Adapted from *Diagnostic and Statistical Manual of Mental Disorders*, 4th ed., text revision, 2000 Washington, DC: American Psychiatric Association.

BOX 50-2 CULTURAL PULSE POINTS

Genetic Resistance to Alcoholism

Alcohol use patterns and the prevalence of alcohol-related problems vary among ethnic groups. Among the elements thought to account for these ethnic differences are social or cultural factors such as drinking norms and attitudes and, in some cases, genetic factors. Understanding ethnic differences in alcohol use patterns and the factors that influence alcohol use can help guide the development of culturally appropriate alcoholism treatment and prevention programs.

Lower rates of alcohol use and alcoholism among Asians and Pacific Islanders appear to be related to a genetic variation prevalent in these populations. Asians are more likely than whites to have a specific variant of a gene that causes the body to break down alcohol in such a way that the person experiences symptoms such as facial flushing, nausea, headache, dizziness, and rapid heartbeat—collectively known as the flushing response—after consuming alcohol. Because of the presence of the gene, Asian populations tend to consume less alcohol and have lower levels of alcoholism than other ethnic groups. This may provide Asians some protection against heavy drinking and alcoholism.

Source: From "Drinking patterns and drinking problems among Asian Americans and Pacific Islanders," by K. Makimoto, *Alcohol Health & Research World*, 22, 270–275.

this person's CNS is continually forced to produce excess neurochemical stimulation, the individual will require more alcohol to achieve intoxication.

When the alcohol-dependent individual (*alcoholic*) stops drinking, the homeostatic mechanism that balanced the depressant effects of the alcohol takes time to return to normal. The CNS is still stimulated, and the individual suffers *withdrawal* symptoms.

Manifestations

Alcohol withdrawal syndrome includes elevated vital signs, anxiety, tremors, diaphoresis, slurred speech, GI disturbances (vomiting, cramping, diarrhea), ataxia, nystagmus, disorientation, and, at its most severe, hallucinations, seizures, and death. (See discussion of neurologic disorders in Chapter 36 ⛓ and discussion of GI disorders in Chapter 37 ⛓.) Eventually, after years of alcohol dependency, the individual must drink almost constantly to avoid the distressing symptoms of CNS stimulation that constitute alcohol withdrawal. Figure 50-2 ■ shows a diagram of how the CNS responds to chronic alcohol use with tolerance and withdrawal.

Diagnosis and Treatment

Alcohol withdrawal delirium (*delirium tremens* or DTs) is diagnosed when withdrawal causes severe cognitive symptoms such as confusion, delusions, and terrifying hallucinations. This delirium happens to people with a long (5- to 15-year) history of alcoholism.

TABLE 50-1	Symptoms of Alcohol Intoxication by Blood Alcohol Concentration
BLOOD ALCOHOL CONCENTRATION	**SYMPTOMS**
0.05–0.15 g/dL (0.08–0.10 is legal level of intoxication in most states)	Relaxation, euphoria, decreased inhibitions, impaired judgment, changeable mood, decreased mental concentration, decreased fine motor coordination
0.15–0.3 g/dL	Slurred speech, decreased motor function, ataxia, mood outbursts, aggressive behavior
0.3–0.4 g/dL	Incoherent speech, mental confusion, stupor, vomiting, labored breathing; blood alcohol concentrations above this level are life threatening
0.4–0.5 g/dL	Unconsciousness, coma, death
Greater than 0.5 g/dL	Respiratory depression, death

clinical ALERT

Alcohol withdrawal delirium is a medical emergency. When it is accompanied by seizures, alcohol withdrawal can be fatal.

The symptoms of alcohol withdrawal are generally the opposite of those of alcohol intoxication. The individual repeatedly takes the CNS depressant substance; the CNS stimulates itself to maintain homeostasis and keep the person awake and functioning. When the substance is withdrawn, the CNS is still stimulated. The individual has CNS stimulation symptoms until the CNS eventually regains balance without alcohol, and the symptoms subside. Alcohol withdrawal syndrome usually lasts about 4 days. (Table 50-2 ■ describes the effects, overdose symptoms, and withdrawal symptoms of alcohol and other CNS depressants.) During this time, the client will benefit from a low-stimulation environment.

The alcohol-dependent individual may experience many episodes of withdrawal symptoms that he or she treats with alcohol. The statement "I feel bad (nervous, tired, angry, lonely, etc.); I need a drink," may be evidence that the client is having withdrawal symptoms. Substance withdrawal symptoms are often behind a client's desire to leave the

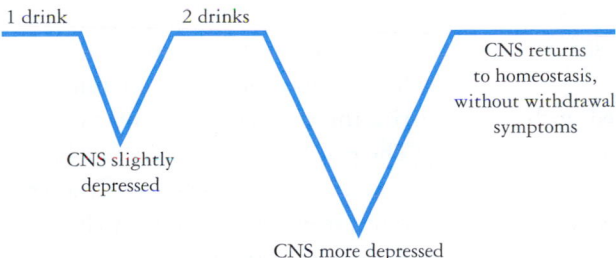

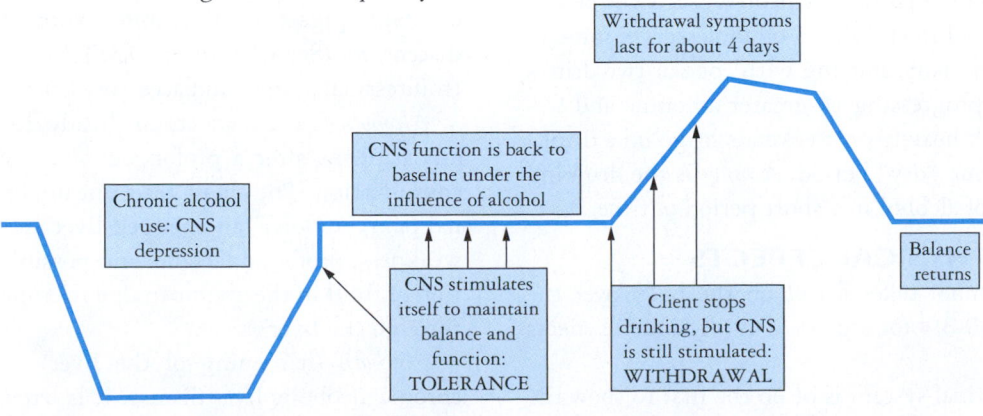

Figure 50-2. ■ CNS response to long-term alcohol use. (*Source:* From *Mental Health Nursing Care* [p. 224], by L. Eby and N. J. Brown, 2005, Upper Saddle River, NJ: Prentice Hall. Reprinted by permission.)

TABLE 50-2	Comparison of Commonly Abused CNS Depressants and Stimulants		
DRUG	EFFECTS OF USE	OVERDOSE SYMPTOMS	WITHDRAWAL SYMPTOMS AND THEIR ONSET (AFTER LAST DOSE)
CNS DEPRESSANTS			
Alcohol, beer, wine, liquor	Euphoria, loss of inhibition, ataxia, lack of coordination, reduced cognition, impaired judgment, nausea	Respiratory depression, mental confusion, unconsciousness, death	6–8 hours; CNS irritability, anxiety, increased vital signs (T, P, R, BP), tremors, ataxia, diaphoresis, slurred speech, GI disturbance, disorientation, hallucinations, seizures, death
Opioids (narcotics) morphine, methadone, hydromorphone, heroin	Analgesia, cough suppression, constipation, constricted pupils, same as alcohol	Same as alcohol	12–72 hours; watering eyes; same as alcohol, less likely to cause death
Sedatives, hypnotics, anxiolytics, barbiturates, benzodiazepines	Sedation; same as alcohol; anxiolytics cause less sedation in low doses	Same as alcohol	Onset depends on type of sedative (short- or long-acting); same as alcohol
CNS STIMULANTS			
Cocaine	Sudden rush of euphoria, elation, energy, talkativeness, anorexia, weight loss, elevated VS, grandiosity	Chest pain, slurred speech, mental confusion, vomiting, hallucinations, myocardial infarction, severe elevation of BP and P, shock, death	Acute depression, craving drug, fatigue, irritability, suicidal thoughts, loss of pleasure (anhedonia), not life threatening
Amphetamines	Same as cocaine	Same as cocaine	As with cocaine, withdrawal severity depends on amount of drug use

hospital against medical advice. Clients who state the desire to leave the hospital against advice should be assessed for withdrawal symptoms.

Alcohol withdrawal symptoms are usually treated with benzodiazepine antianxiety drugs. These medications cause CNS depression. They are used to counteract the CNS stimulation of the withdrawal syndrome, and are only necessary for the approximately 4 days of symptoms.

PATTERN OF USE

Individuals vary in their pattern of alcohol use. Some people start drinking alcohol in childhood or adolescence, some in old age. Some drink daily, starting with "one or two drinks with dinner" and progressing to greater amounts and frequency. Some drink heavily on weekends or go on a drinking binge after a long "dry" period. A *binge* is the drinking of a large amount of alcohol in a short period of time.

LONG-TERM PHYSICAL EFFECTS

Chronic use of alcohol takes a toll on the body over the years. See Figure 50-3 ■ for a picture of physiologic effects of alcoholism.

The gastrointestinal system is often the first to show the effects of chronic alcoholism. Alcohol causes *gastritis* by inflaming the stomach lining. The protective mucous lining of the stomach is damaged, allowing hydrochloric acid to erode the stomach wall. Bleeding can occur. Ulcers may

form in the stomach. Symptoms include gastric distress, nausea, vomiting, black stools, and abdominal distention. Alcohol causes *esophagitis* (inflammation of the esophagus) by irritating the esophagus and by causing frequent vomiting. The primary symptom is esophageal pain.

Pancreatitis (inflammation of the pancreas), either acute or chronic, may also be caused by chronic alcohol use. Chronic pancreatitis leads to malnutrition, weight loss, and diabetes mellitus. Acute pancreatitis happens 1 or 2 days after a binge of drinking alcohol. The symptoms include severe, constant epigastric pain, nausea, vomiting, and abdominal distention. (See Chapter 37 ◯◯ for disorders of the gastrointestinal system and accessory organs.)

Alcoholic hepatitis affects an already damaged liver. It usually happens after a prolonged binge of excessive alcohol consumption. The client has right upper quadrant abdominal pain, jaundice, an enlarged liver and spleen, vomiting, weakness, profound fatigue, and possibly *ascites* (accumulation of fluid in the abdomen due to impaired venous return through the liver).

Cirrhosis (hardening of the liver) is the end stage of chronic alcoholic liver disease. It is irreversible because destroyed liver cells are replaced by scar tissue. Cirrhosis causes portal hypertension, ascites, *esophageal varices* (varicose veins in the esophagus that can rupture and hemorrhage), and hepatic encephalopathy.

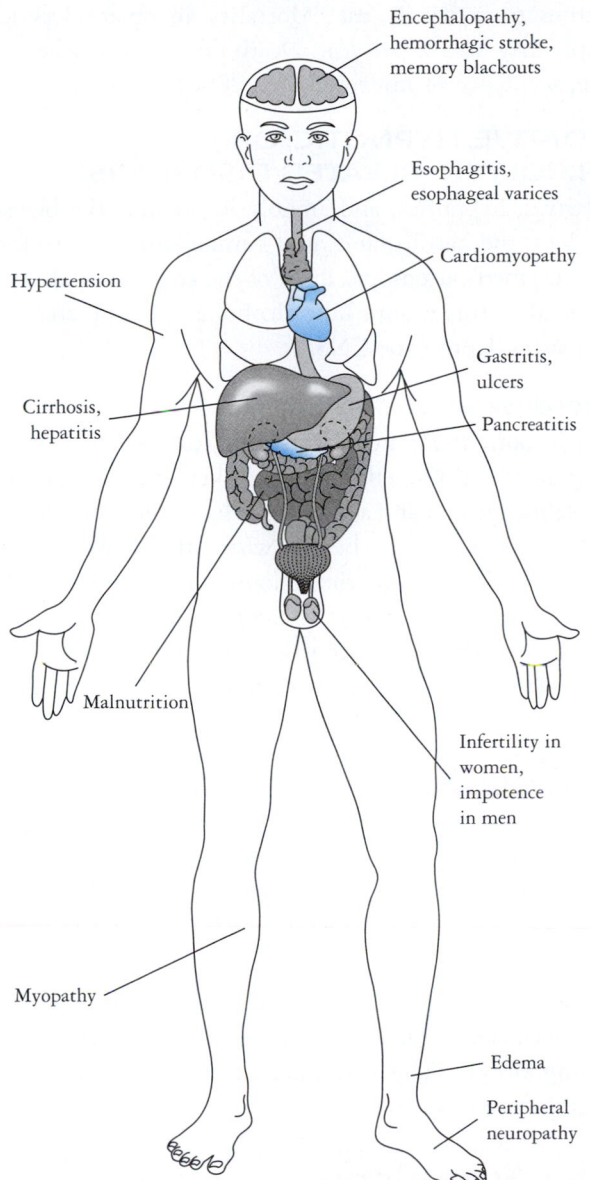

Encephalopathy, hemorrhagic stroke, memory blackouts

Esophagitis, esophageal varices

Cardiomyopathy

Hypertension

Gastritis, ulcers

Cirrhosis, hepatitis

Pancreatitis

Malnutrition

Infertility in women, impotence in men

Myopathy

Edema

Peripheral neuropathy

Figure 50-3. ■ Physiologic effects of alcoholism. (*Source*: From *Mental Health Nursing Care* [p. 226], by L. Eby and N. J. Brown, 2005, Upper Saddle River, NJ: Prentice Hall. Reprinted by permission.)

Hepatic encephalopathy (see Chapter 37 ⬭) is caused by accumulation of ammonia (due to the damaged liver's inability to metabolize protein). It results in impaired mental function and progresses to death.

The cardiovascular system is also affected by chronic alcohol use. *Cardiomyopathy* (weakening and enlargement of the heart), heart failure, and cardiac dysrhythmias may occur (see Chapter 33 ⬭). The risk of *hemorrhagic stroke* is increased. *Hypertension* (especially diastolic elevation), tachycardia, and edema can also occur.

Neurologic changes include *blackouts*, which are an early sign of alcoholism. The affected individual remains conscious and appears to be functioning normally, but is completely unable to remember anything that occurred while intoxicated.

After many years of alcohol abuse, a person may develop Wernicke's syndrome and Korsakoff's syndrome, which affect the entire neurologic system. These syndromes usually occur together, and are often called Wernicke-Korsakoff's syndrome.

Wernicke's syndrome (alcoholic encephalopathy) is the result of severe vitamin B_1 deficiency caused by poor nutrition. It is characterized by ataxia, paralysis of eye muscles, nystagmus (rapid involuntary movement of the eyeballs), and mental confusion. If it is treated early, this brain dysfunction may respond well to large doses of parenteral thiamine. If not treated, Wernicke's syndrome becomes irreversible and fatal.

clinical ALERT

Early treatment of vitamin B_1 deficiency can prevent alcoholic encephalopathy (Wernicke's syndrome) or stop its progression. The nurse should expect to give vitamin B_1 (thiamine) to all clients with alcohol dependency.

Korsakoff's syndrome is a group of symptoms caused by a deficiency in the B vitamins, including thiamine, riboflavin, and folic acid. Clients have amnesia, disorientation to time and place, **confabulation** (filling in gaps in memory with imagined or made-up events), and severe peripheral neuropathy. Symptoms of the neuropathy include tingling; muscle weakness; sore, burning muscles; abnormal sensation; and pain with movement. The extremities are affected, especially the legs. Because of their extreme pain, care must be taken when moving these clients.

The reproductive system is also affected by chronic alcohol use. Men may become impotent. Women may stop menstruating and become infertile. Further, the unborn child of a pregnant woman who abuses alcohol may be seriously affected. Fetal alcohol syndrome gives rise to low birth weight, *microcephaly* (small brain and small head circumference), facial abnormalities, and developmental disorders (learning disabilities, distractibility, poor coordination).

When the musculoskeletal system is affected, osteoporosis can develop. Also, acute or chronic **myopathy** may occur, characterized by muscle cramps of sudden onset and later development of pain, tenderness, and edema of the skeletal muscles, especially of the legs. In chronic myopathy there is wasting and weakness of the skeletal muscles.

Other CNS Depressants

Other CNS depressants are similar to alcohol in their effects on the CNS: intoxication symptoms, tolerance effects, and withdrawal symptoms (see Table 50-2).

OPIATES

Opiates are naturally occurring substances derived from opium (such as morphine), semisynthetics (such as heroin), and drugs that resemble them (such as methadone, meperidine, oxycodone, or codeine). These drugs have alleviated immeasurable human pain, but when abused they have caused immense suffering as well.

Effects of Opiates

Opiate (narcotic) drugs are prescribed to relieve pain or diarrhea, or to reduce cough. Opiates can cause physical dependence (tolerance and withdrawal). Intoxication symptoms are similar to those of alcohol. Common effects include drowsiness, analgesia, euphoria, mood changes, nausea, constipation, and constriction of the pupils. In high doses, opiates cause hypotension by reducing vascular resistance.

Clients who take opiates for severe persistent pain, such as cancer pain, may become tolerant to usual therapeutic doses of narcotics. They will require increasing doses to achieve pain relief. This tolerance is expected, and the increasing dose appropriate. These clients are at less risk for respiratory depression than the "narcotic naive" client, who is new to taking narcotic medications.

Manifestations

Opioids also affect sexual functioning. People who use opioids regularly in high doses have decreased libido (sexual drive) and may have lack of orgasm. Men can have ejaculation abnormalities and impotence. Women often have menstrual irregularities and infertility. *Opiate overdose* is a medical emergency. The client may have pinpoint pupils, depressed (slow, shallow) respiration, seizures, and coma. Death can result from respiratory arrest.

Treatment

The treatment for opiate overdose is a narcotic antagonist drug, such as naloxone hydrochloride (Narcan). This drug competes for opiate receptors and blocks the action of narcotics.

Patterns of Substance Use

Unlike alcohol, opiates are either available only by prescription or are illegal under all circumstances (e.g., heroin). Opiate dependence is often associated with a history of crimes committed to obtain drugs or money to buy them. Healthcare professionals with opiate dependency may steal medications from clients or their employers, write prescriptions for themselves, or manipulate physicians to write prescriptions for them.

Although opioid dependence may begin at any age, problems are most commonly observed in the late teens or early 20s (APA, 2000). Dependence develops over a period of years, with periods of **abstinence** (complete lack of drug use). **Relapse** (return to drug use after abstinence) is very common. Men are more commonly affected than women. People with opiate dependency have increased risk of developing hepatitis B or C, HIV infection, or other bloodborne diseases from needle use. Mortality in opiate-dependent people may be 2% per year. Death often results from overdose, accidents, or injuries (APA, 2000).

SEDATIVE, HYPNOTIC, OR ANXIOLYTIC-RELATED DISORDERS

Sedatives, hypnotics, and anxiolytics include the benzodiazepines, the barbiturates, and similar drugs. Prescription sleeping medications and most of the antianxiety drugs are included in this group. Like alcohol and the opiates, these substances depress the CNS.

Overdose

It is important for nurses to know that CNS depressant drugs have additive effects when taken together. So, when people use alcohol and a sedative drug at the same time, the CNS depressant effect is beyond what either substance would cause alone. Although the amount of sedative may be a usual dose and the amount of alcohol may be what the person usually drinks, the two together could cause fatal respiratory depression. It is not uncommon for people to die as a result of this additive effect.

> ### clinical ALERT
>
> Medications prescribed for pain, sleep, and anxiety often cause CNS depression and are dangerous when taken with alcohol due to additive depression of the CNS. Nurses should teach clients with prescriptions for psychotropic drugs to avoid alcohol completely.

The substance-dependent individual commonly has a drug of choice, but may use a variety of other substances, including alcohol. This combination of abused substances is called *polysubstance abuse*.

CNS Stimulants

AMPHETAMINES AND COCAINE

The clinical usefulness of the amphetamines is limited. They are used for treatment of attention deficit hyperactivity disorder, and occasionally for daytime sleepiness caused by other medications and disorders. Cocaine can be used as a potent topical vasoconstrictor for surgery involving the mucous membranes of the nasopharynx. Cocaine is a popular drug of abuse because it causes immediate euphoria.

Manifestations

Symptoms of intoxication include hyperactivity, talkativeness, grandiosity, anger, aggression, impaired judgment, and possibly hallucinations. Physical effects (see Table 50-2) include elevated blood pressure, nausea, chest pain, dilated pupils, confusion, and cardiac dysrhythmias (see also Chapter 33). Figure 50-4 ■ shows the cycle of cocaine use, which also applies to the other stimulant drugs.

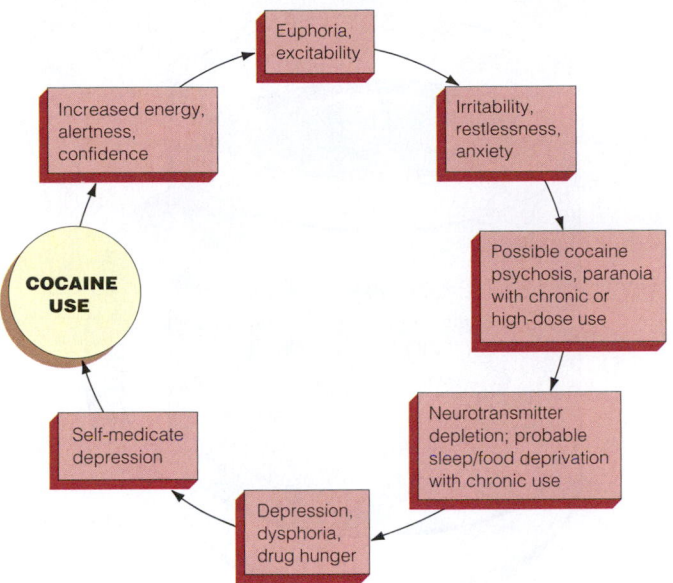

Figure 50-4. ■ Cycle of cocaine use. (*Source:* Reprinted with permission from Mim Landry, Danya International, Silver Spring, MD.)

WITHDRAWAL. Just as the brain elevates its stimulation to balance regular use of depressants, it also depresses its function to balance regular use of a stimulant. When the stimulant-dependent individual abstains from stimulant drugs, the withdrawal syndrome includes CNS depression. The individual feels lethargic and depressed. Withdrawal from stimulants is uncomfortable but not life threatening and may last several days.

Hallucinogens

Hallucinogens distort the user's perception of reality. The most commonly used hallucinogens are LSD, mescaline, and PCP (phencyclidine). The CNS effects are unpredictable and may be influenced by the expectations of the user.

Manifestations

Hallucinations can lead to violent behavior. Some individuals have frightening psychotic experiences. When people with mental illnesses take hallucinogens, the outcome is less predictable. The combination of schizophrenia and hallucinogenic drugs can cause hallucinations that are prolonged and frightening.

There is no withdrawal syndrome associated with hallucinogens. However, flashbacks can occur for months after the last dose is used. During flashbacks, the individual has similar symptoms to those associated with use of the drug. Table 50-3 ■ describes effects of use, overdose symptoms,

TABLE 50-3	Hallucinogens, Inhalants, Cannabis, Caffeine, and Nicotine		
SUBSTANCE	**EFFECTS OF USE**	**OVERDOSE SYMPTOMS**	**WITHDRAWAL SYMPTOMS**
HALLUCINOGENS			
LSD, DMT, mescaline, MDMA (Ecstasy)	Hallucinations and distorted perceptions, distortions of time and space, illusions, emotional instability, tremor, nausea and vomiting	Panic (may be drug reaction, not OD), seizures (rare)	No withdrawal, may experience flashbacks for several months after last dose
Phencyclidine (PCP)	Bizarre perceptions, disorientation, hallucinations, agitation, grandiosity, withdrawn or agitated or both, paranoid, dilated pupils, dry red skin	Seizures, coma, death	No withdrawal
INHALANTS AND CANNABIS			
Inhalants Hydrocarbons: glue, gasoline, aerosol spray, solvents Nitrites: amyl nitrite, nitrous oxide	Hydrocarbons: euphoria, impaired judgment, nystagmus, ataxia, slurred speech, perceptual changes, sense of invulnerability Nitrites: prolong erection or enhance intercourse	Hydrocarbons: stupor, coma, cardiac depression and dysrhythmias, respiratory arrest, renal complications Nitrites: panic, hypotension Both: brain damage	Similar to alcohol
Cannabis, marijuana, hashish	Mild euphoria, pleasure, confidence, grandiosity, relaxation, red eyes, dry mouth, increased appetite	None	No physical withdrawal; may have craving
CAFFEINE AND NICOTINE			
Caffeine	Increased alertness, increased pulse, anxiety, jitters (tremors)	None	Headache, fatigue
Nicotine	Pleasure, alertness, increased BP, P, decreased blood flow to heart muscle	None	Anxiety, depressed mood, anger, craving, increased appetite

and withdrawal symptoms (if any) of hallucinogens and other categories of frequently abused substances.

Synthetic or "designer" drugs have become increasingly popular. MDMA or Ecstasy, for example, is derived from amphetamine and methamphetamine. So, it acts as both a stimulant and a hallucinogen.

Inhalants

Two kinds of inhalants are commonly abused. The hydrocarbons (solvents, glue, and aerosols) produce euphoria, loss of inhibitions, altered sensations, and hallucinations. The hydrocarbons can cause cardiac depression, renal injury, respiratory depression, and death from cardiac dysrhythmias or accidents while intoxicated. Because these inhalants are readily available in stores (in the form of spray paint, certain glues, and even gasoline) they are the drug of choice for many young people who have difficulty buying alcohol (see Table 50-3) (Sullivan, 1995).

The second source of inhalant abuse is the nitrites group. Amyl nitrite, butyl nitrite, and nitrous oxide are included. The nitrites are used to prolong penile erection and to enhance intercourse. They may cause euphoria and perceptual alterations. Some individuals experience panic, nausea, confusion, headache, and hypotension from their use (Sullivan, 1995).

CANNABIS (MARIJUANA)

Delta-9-tetrahydrocannabinol (THC) is thought to be the chemical responsible for the psychoactive effects of marijuana and hashish. Cannabis effects include euphoria, a sense of serenity, and perceptual changes in vision, hearing, taste, touch, or smell (see Table 50-3).

Cannabis is the most widely used illegal substance in the United States. It has been therapeutically used to treat anorexia, nausea, and vomiting associated with AIDS and cancer.

Caffeine and Nicotine

It may be surprising to find caffeine and nicotine listed as substances of abuse. Still, these substances fit the model of substance dependence. Both substances cause tolerance and withdrawal.

Caffeine, the most commonly used stimulant drug, is primarily a performance enhancer. It prolongs the time the user can continue to work (which makes it popular among nurses), improves mental alertness, and elevates mood. However, it also increases anxiety and can cause insomnia, irritability, diuresis, tremors, and tachycardia (see Table 50-3).

The amount and frequency of caffeine use determine its effects and whether tolerance and withdrawal develop. Withdrawal symptoms include headache, fatigue, irritability, and nervousness. Figure 50-5 ■ shows common sources

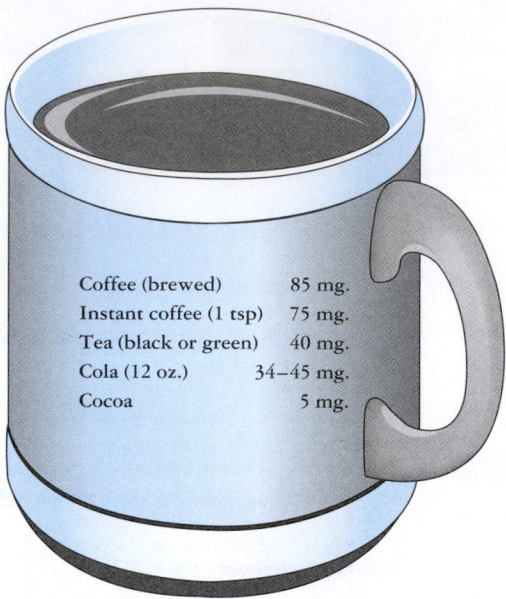

Coffee (brewed)	85 mg.
Instant coffee (1 tsp)	75 mg.
Tea (black or green)	40 mg.
Cola (12 oz.)	34–45 mg.
Cocoa	5 mg.

Figure 50-5. ■ Common sources of caffeine, with doses. (*Source: From* Mental Health Nursing Care *[p. 224], by L. Eby and N. J. Brown, 2005, Upper Saddle River, NJ: Prentice Hall. Reprinted by permission.*)

of caffeine and their doses. The average adult coffee-drinker consumes 360 to 450 mg of caffeine per day. Intake of more than 600 mg of caffeine per day is considered excessive (Kneisl et al., 2004).

Nicotine dependence is the most common substance dependence in the United States (Rosencrans and Karin, 1997). Effects of use include increased performance, decreased appetite, reduced anxiety, and increased alertness initially, followed by relaxation. Smoking is especially common among people who use alcohol and other substances. It is often associated with social acceptance and peer group behavior (Figure 50-6 ■).

The consequences of smoking are due to nicotine and other substances present in tobacco. Cancer of the lungs, oral

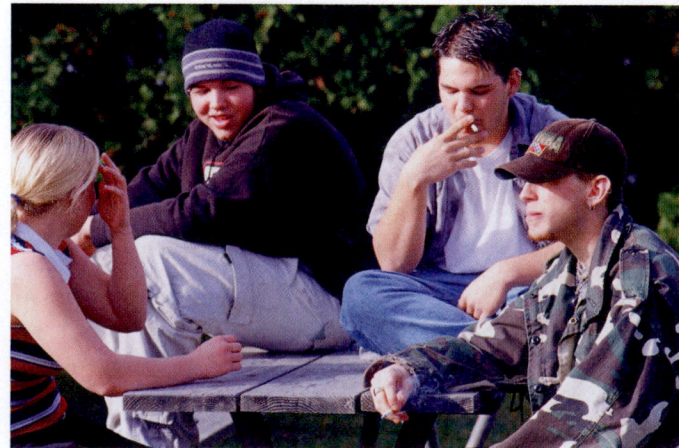

Figure 50-6. ■ About 70% of children have tried smoking by their high school years. Early intervention can begin with discussions about smoking starting at 9 to 10 years of age.

cavity, esophagus, pancreas, and prostate is increased significantly among tobacco users. Chronic obstructive pulmonary disease (COPD and emphysema) is more likely to occur or to be worsened in people who smoke. The risk of cardiovascular disease (stroke, myocardial infarction, and peripheral arterial disease) is increased by tobacco use as well. Accidents related to fire are also a concern (smoking in bed while drinking alcohol can be deadly). Respiratory diseases including cancer, asthma, and COPD are increased in people who do not smoke but live with people who smoke. The exposure to second-hand smoke is dangerous. Nicotine withdrawal symptoms include irritability, restlessness, drowsiness, anxiety, craving, and a transient increase in appetite. Nicotine patches or nicotine gum can help to relieve symptoms.

Hospitalized clients often experience caffeine or nicotine withdrawal. Nurses may find that the headache clients have after surgery is better treated with a cup of coffee than with medication. Some clients may consider checking themselves out of the hospital against medical advice so they can smoke cigarettes. These situations require the nurse's problem-solving skills.

Prescription Medication Abuse

Misuse and abuse of prescription medication is on the rise. Adolescents and young adults have a ready supply in the home medicine cabinet. A dangerous practice is being followed, where young people take medication from a parent's medicine cabinet and dump it into a bowl at a party. Partygoers take pills from the bowl. If a drug interaction or overdose occurs, there is no way to identify what has been ingested or the amount. A person grabbing a handful of unidentified pills and swallowing them may ingest an antidepressant, an antihypertensive, analgesics, or many other lethal combinations. The combined drug actions could result in cardiac or respiratory arrest or coma. By the time the individual is transported to the emergency room, there may not be enough time to identify the substances in order to reverse their effects, and death may result.

In addition to abuse of prescription drugs as a party game, there is also a rise of abuse and overuse of certain prescription drugs. See Table 50-4 ■ for selected prescription drugs with potential for abuse.

Collaborative Care

In the acute phase of withdrawal from alcohol or other drugs, medical treatment focuses on physiologic safety. Priorities are managing symptoms, preventing seizures, stabilizing vital signs, and minimizing the effects of CNS stimulation. In the rehabilitation phase, management is supportive. Nurses, physicians, therapists, social workers, and others cooperate on the healthcare team.

Medical management includes prescription of medications, so drug interactions and cross-tolerance must be considered.

clinical ALERT

Clients who use drugs or alcohol *regularly* are at risk for *withdrawal*. Those who have used drugs or alcohol *recently* are at risk for *additive effects* with prescribed drugs.

A person who is dependent on heroin or alcohol will be tolerant to other CNS depressants as well. This phenomenon of tolerance to several drugs in the same classification is called **cross-tolerance.** The anesthesiologist may find that the tolerant client needs more anesthetic than the nontolerant clients. Physicians and nurses may discover that the client needs a higher than usual analgesic dose to relieve pain.

There are several theories about the causes and best treatment for chemical dependency. Basically, substance dependency is viewed as a chronic, progressive medical illness that (1) is characterized by remissions and relapses and (2) is eventually fatal if untreated. Its etiology is a combination of genetic and cultural influences (nature and nurture).

People with substance dependency have learned to use substances to cope with their problems. They must have new skills to replace the role substances play in their lives. *A promise of abstinence alone is not a long-term solution*. The ultimate goals of substance dependency treatment are:

1. To abstain from substance use.
2. To develop effective coping mechanisms to replace substances as a way to solve problems.

ACUTE PHASE OF TREATMENT

Substance dependency treatment has two major phases: acute and rehabilitation. In the *acute phase*, the person may be in a hospital, a detoxification center, a drug treatment facility, or another inpatient or outpatient setting. The client often enters treatment while intoxicated. *Detoxification*, or removal of the substance from the body, begins the acute phase. The withdrawal syndrome also occurs acutely. Medical and nursing supports are often needed during withdrawal.

Medications are used in the acute phase of treatment to provide safe withdrawal from CNS-depressant drugs and alcohol. Alcohol withdrawal is usually managed with a benzodiazepine antianxiety agent. This agent is given in a decreasing dose over several days to treat the CNS withdrawal symptoms. Clients who abuse alcohol are given vitamin B_1 (thiamine) to prevent alcoholic encephalopathy (Wernicke-Korsakoff's syndrome).

TABLE 50-4	Prescription Drugs with Potential for Abuse		
SUBSTANCES: CATEGORY AND NAME	**EXAMPLES OF COMMERCIAL AND STREET NAMES**	**DEA SCHEDULE/ ROUTE**	**INTOXICATION EFFECTS/POTENTIAL HEALTH CONSEQUENCES**
DEPRESSANTS			
Barbiturates	Amytal, Nembutal, Phenobarbital; barbs, reds, red birds, phennies, tooies, yellows, yellow jackets	II, III, V Oral/injection	Reduces pain and anxiety, feeling of well-being, lowers inhibitions; slows pulse and breathing, lowers BP, poor concentration/confusion, fatigue; impaired coordination, memory, judgment, respiratory depression and arrest, addiction
Benzodiazepines (other than flunitrazepam)	Ativan, Halcion, Librium, Valium, Xanax, candy, downers, sleeping pills, tranks	IV/swallowed	Also, for barbiturates—sedation, drowsiness/depression, unusual excitement, fever, irritability, poor judgment, slurred speech, dizziness
Flunitrazepam	Rohypnol, forgot-me pill, Mexican Valium, R2, Roche, roofies, roofinol, rope, rophies [associated with sexual abuse]	IV/swallowed, snorted	For flunitrazepam—visual and gastrointestinal disturbance, urinary retention, memory loss for the time under the drug's effects
DISSOCIATIVE ANESTHETICS			
Ketamine	Ketalar SV; cat Valium, K Special K, vitamin K	III/injected, snorted, smoked	Increased heart rate and BP; impaired motor function/memory loss; numbness; nausea/vomiting At high doses, delirium, depression, respiratory depression and arrest
OPIOIDS & MORPHINE DERIVATIVES			
Codeine	Empirin with codeine, Fiorinal with codeine, Robitussin A-C, Tylenol with Codeine, Captain Cody, Cody, Schoolboy (with glutethimide), doors & fours, loads, pancakes and syrup	II, III, IV/oral injection	Pain relief, euphoria, drowsiness/respiratory depression and arrest, nausea, confusion, constipation, sedation, unconsciousness, coma, tolerance, addiction Also for codeine—less analgesia, sedation, and respiratory depression than morphine
Fentanyl	Actiq, Duragesic, Sublimaze, Apache, China girl, China White, dance fever, friends, goodfella, jackpot, morder 8, TNT, Tango and Cash	II/injection, smoke, snorted	Same as codeine
Morphine	Roxanol, Duramorph; M, Miss Emma, monkey, white stuff	II, III/injected, swallowed, smoked	Same as codeine
Opium	Laudanum, paregoric; big o, black stuff, block, gum, hop	II, III/injected, swallowed, smoked	Same as codeine
Other opioid pain relievers (oxycodone, meperidine, hydromorphone, hydrocodone, propoxyphene)	Tylox, OxyContin, Percodan, Percocet, oxy 80s, ocycotton, oxycet, hillbilly heroin, percs, Demerol, meperidine hydrochloride; demmies, pain killer Dilaudid; juice, dillies Vicodin, Lortab, Lorcet, Darvon, Darvocet	II, III, V/injected, swallowed, smoked, suppositories, chewed, crushed, snorted	Same as codeine
STIMULANTS			
Amphetamines	Biphetamine, Dexedrine, bennies, black beauties, crosses, heart, LA turn-arounds, speed, truck drivers, uppers	II/injected, swallowed, smoked, snorted	Increased heart rate, BP, metabolism; feelings of exhilaration, energy, increased mental alertness/rapid or irregular heart beat; reduced appetite, weight loss, heart failure

TABLE 50-4	Prescription Drugs with Potential for Abuse (continued)		
SUBSTANCES: CATEGORY AND NAME	**EXAMPLES OF COMMERCIAL AND STREET NAMES**	**DEA SCHEDULE/ ROUTE**	**INTOXICATION EFFECTS/POTENTIAL HEALTH CONSEQUENCES**
			Also for amphetamines—rapid breathing, hallucinations/tremors, loss of coordination; irritability, anxiousness, restlessness, delirium, panic, paranoia, impulsive behavior, aggressiveness, tolerance, addiction
Cocaine	Cocaine hydrochloride, blow, bump, C, candy, Charlie, coke, crack, flake, rock, snow, toot	II/injected, smoked, snorted	For cocaine—increased temperature/ chest pain, respiratory failure, nausea, abdominal pain, strokes, seizures, headaches, malnutrition
Methamphetamine	Desoxyn; chalk, crank, crystal, fire, glass, go fast, ice, meth, speed	II/injected swallowed, smoked, snorted	For methamphetamine—aggression, violence, psychotic behavior/memory loss, cardiac and neurologic damage; impaired memory and learning, tolerance, addiction
Methylphenidate	Ritalin, JIF, MPH, R-ball, Skippy, the smart drug, Vitamin R	II/injected, swallowed, snorted	For methylphenidate—increase or decrease in blood pressure, psychotic episodes/digestive problems, loss of appetite, weight loss
OTHER COMPOUNDS			
Anabolic steroids	Anadrol, Oxandrin, Durabolin, Dep-Testosterone, Equipoise; roids, juice	III/injected, swallowed, applied to skin	No intoxication effects/hypertension, blood clotting and cholesterol changes, liver cysts and cancer, kidney cancer, hostility and aggression, acne, premature stoppage of growth in adolescents
			In males: prostate cancer, reduced sperm production, shrunken testicles, breast enlargement
			In females: menstrual irregularities, development of beard and other masculine characteristics

There is a dangerous assumption that allowing clients to suffer agonizing withdrawal will "teach them a lesson" about why they should stop drinking alcohol or using drugs. In fact, withdrawal causes a person to crave and be preoccupied with the substance. There is no ethical justification for allowing clients to suffer needlessly. Alcohol and barbiturate withdrawals can be life threatening.

REHABILITATION PHASE

Rehabilitation is the second phase of substance dependency treatment. It begins when clients have detoxified and are abstaining from substance use. Rehabilitation continues indefinitely.

Medications

Medications used in the rehabilitation phase are to prevent relapse. Disulfiram (Antabuse) may be prescribed to deter clients from drinking alcohol. It causes a severe, uncomfortable reaction when the client drinks alcohol (flushing, throbbing headache, nausea, and vomiting).

Methadone, a synthetic opiate, is used as a replacement for heroin. A regular oral dose is prescribed, and the client basically trades one dependency for another. The goal is to prevent the physical and psychosocial risks of intravenous drug use and the dangerous behaviors associated with obtaining heroin (prostitution, burglary, robbery, etc.). Many clients on methadone lead productive lives. Methadone can also be used to manage severe chronic pain.

Naltrexone (ReVia) is an opioid antagonist used to treat opiate overdose. It blocks the effects of any opioids used by the client. It has been found to reduce the cravings for alcohol in abstinent clients (Freed & York, 1997).

Clonidine (Catapres) is an antihypertensive drug. It is sometimes given to clients with opiate dependence to prevent some of the symptoms of withdrawal. Nurses should take the client's blood pressure before each dose, and hold the drug (and notify the physician) if the person is hypotensive.

Cognitive Behavioral Therapy

Other approaches to treatment include cognitive behavioral therapy (CBT; see also Chapter 17 ⬭). In CBT, the client is helped to alter the thinking and behaviors associated with addiction. Family therapy is also used, in which the entire family is counseled to see the combination of unhealthy family behaviors that contribute to the identified client's addiction.

The tasks of rehabilitation are:

- To maintain sobriety (abstinence).
- To develop new coping skills.
- To make a plan for relapse prevention.
- To live life with all its responsibilities, joys, and frustrations.

Relapse is common. The best response to relapse is for the person to learn from the experience and to begin rehabilitation again.

Support Groups

Many people with substance abuse and dependency problems respond well to treatment. Alcoholics Anonymous, a fellowship of men and women who share their experience, strength, and hope with each other to help themselves and others to recover from alcoholism, is based on 12 steps. Box 50-3 ■ lists the 12 steps. AA itself is for alcoholics only. Other 12-step programs are based on their principles. In all these anonymous groups, people with similar problems share experiences, strength, and hope. The groups offer a sense of community and unconditional support.

There are thousands of AA groups. Refer clients to their local telephone book or directory assistance to find Alcoholics Anonymous. There are AA meetings for special interest groups, such as people with dual diagnosis, nonsmokers, women, lesbians, and people who want to focus on religious aspects of recovery. Other 12-step programs include Overeaters Anonymous, Narcotics Anonymous, and Cocaine Anonymous.

Al-Anon is a group for family members, especially spouses, of alcoholics. Ala-Teen is a similar group for teenage children of alcoholics (Box 50-4 ■). Substance dependency is certainly a family illness; these groups have helped many family members.

CHILDREN IN FAMILIES AFFECTED BY ALCOHOL

Approximately one in four children in the United States is exposed to family alcohol abuse or alcohol dependence. Alcohol and drug exposure create biological, psychological, behavioral, and social consequences. Children exposed to them are at risk of adverse developmental, social, and health outcomes. The large number of children affected defines one of today's major health problems.

Healthcare practitioners have an important opportunity to help children and adolescents. Box 50-4 provides guidelines for helping children of alcoholics.

BOX 50-3	TWELVE STEPS OF ALCOHOLICS ANONYMOUS

Twelve Steps of Alcoholics Anonymous

We

1. Admitted that we were powerless over alcohol, that our lives had become unmanageable.
2. Came to believe that a Power greater than ourselves could restore us to sanity.
3. Made a decision to turn our wills and lives over to the care of God as we understood Him.
4. Made a searching and fearless moral inventory of ourselves.
5. Admitted to God, to ourselves, and to another human being the exact nature of our wrongs.
6. Were entirely ready to have God remove all these defects of character.
7. Humbly asked Him to remove our shortcomings.
8. Made a list of all persons we had harmed, and became willing to make amends to them all.
9. Made direct amends to such people whenever possible, except when to do so would injure them or others.
10. Continued to take personal inventory and when we were wrong promptly admitted it.
11. Sought through prayer and meditation to improve our conscious contact with God as we understood Him, praying only for knowledge of His will for us and the power to carry that out.
12. Having had a spiritual awakening as a result of these steps, we tried to carry this message to alcoholics and to practice these principles in all our affairs.

Source: Alcoholics Anonymous World Services, 1952. The Twelve Steps are reprinted with permission of Alcoholics Anonymous World Services, Inc. (A.A.W.S.). Permission to reprint the Twelve Steps does not mean the A.A.W.S. has reviewed or approved the contents of this publication, or that A.A.W.S. necessarily agrees with the views expressed herein. A.A. is a program of recovery from alcoholism *only*—use of the Twelve Steps in connection with programs and activities which are patterned after A.A., but which address other problems, or in any other non-A.A. context, does not imply otherwise.

DUAL DIAGNOSIS

The term *dual diagnosis* (see also Chapter 49 ⬭) refers to clients who have both a substance abuse disorder and a serious mental illness. Up to 51% of people with severe mental illnesses also have substance abuse disorders (El-Mallakh, 1998). These individuals have two separate chronic illnesses, and they have greater functional impairment than the general population of people with substance dependency. Both the mental disorder and the substance abuse disorder must be treated together.

People with psychiatric symptoms may self-medicate with alcohol or drugs. Many mentally ill people experience impulsiveness, poor judgment, and difficulty anticipating the consequences of their behavior. Think about the substances of abuse. In the short term they help people forget their problems and make them feel better. Only later will the full consequences of loss of job, family, friends, health, and even life become real.

For a person who is living in the moment, substance abuse may seem to make sense. It may seem to be an effective way to solve problems. For people who are unable to plan beyond the current day, problem solving has a different meaning.

Substance Dependency among Nurses

It may seem unlikely for nurses to have problems with substance use, because they should know better. In fact, many nurses do abuse substances. Some reasons our profession is at especially high risk for substance abuse disorders are as follows:

- Nurses see medications as a solution to problems.
- Nurses have access to drugs at work and to the physicians who prescribe them.
- Nurses often believe that they should work even when they are tired or sick, so they may use drugs to increase their ability to continue working.
- Nurses experience pressure, emotional pain, anger, and frustration, which are symptoms that respond to drugs in the short term.
- Nurses think that if they know about drugs and drug abuse, addiction will not happen to them.

Manifestations

When nurses understand substance dependency, we are able to recognize it earlier in our coworkers and ourselves. Signs of *impaired nursing* (practicing nursing under the influence of intoxicants) include changes in the nurse's behavior such as mood changes, irritability, forgetfulness, isolation from coworkers, and inappropriate behavior (see also Chapter 4 🔗). Work performance may be affected (multiple medication errors, missed deadlines, sloppy charting, inattention to detail, absenteeism, poor judgment, volunteering to give narcotics to other nurses' clients, excessive wasting of narcotics, client complaints that pain medications are not effective, tampering with drug packaging, going to the bathroom after administering narcotics). The nurse may also have signs of drug use or withdrawal (alcohol on breath, heavy use of breath mints and perfume, red eyes, ataxia, restlessness, anxiety, slurred speech, hyperactivity, tremors, runny nose, family problems that interfere with work).

Treatment

Substance dependency is a chronic physiologic and psychosocial illness that requires treatment. Affected nurses deserve to be diagnosed and treated before they hurt their clients or themselves. If you suspect that a peer is impaired, notify a manager or hospital supervisor. The nurse is unlikely to be able to manage the problem alone. Your state board of nursing may have a nurse-monitoring or treatment program that can help affected nurses recover and return to the profession. The manager will notify the state board of nursing, which will refer the impaired nurse to the recovery program.

CLIENT SAFETY

In the acute situation, the nurse's primary responsibility is client safety, including protection from an impaired nurse. In the big picture of mutual respect and caring for colleagues in the profession, your duty is to help your peers get treatment. The intervention to reach each of these outcomes is the same: Tell a supervisor (not just the unit charge nurse for the day), so clients will be safe and the nurse will be treated. A nurse who is so far advanced in substance dependency that she or he is under the influence of substances at work will not be able to stop using just because you say she or he should. The nurse needs treatment. This is no time to engage in denial.

NURSING CARE

PRIORITIZING NURSING CARE

When caring for clients dealing with substance abuse, encourage the use of positive coping mechanisms. Help clients identify ways to relate to others without using substances to feel at ease. Help clients identify triggers for substance use and strategies for avoiding or managing those triggers. Be honest with clients about observations regarding their progress. Establish an atmosphere of trust so clients can be honest with you about their feelings. Give positive reinforcement for any insights into behavior. Encourage clients to take responsibility for their own choices and avoid blaming others.

ASSESSING

Some recent research looked at denial in alcohol-dependent clients. These clients denied to themselves that they had trouble with alcohol for years after problems developed. Then, for years after they recognized the problem, they continued to deny to others that it existed. They tended to postpone seeking treatment until they had severe chronic health problems (Simpson & Tucker, 2002). This research has implications for nurses. If nurses assess all clients for substance abuse problems, these clients can be identified before they are likely to seek help for themselves. Some of these clients may respond positively to the nurse's advice to seek treatment for substance dependency. Confirmation of substance abuse by health professionals can be a powerful tool in the battle against denial.

It is important to assess the substance use history of every client. The nurse can notify the physician of recent use or regular use so appropriate measures can be taken to adjust doses of medications that affect the CNS. Nursing assessment questions are listed in Box 50-5 ■. Note that the substance use assessment does not ask, "Do you drink?" Because alcohol and drug use is associated with strong negative attitudes by society and with guilt by users, the client is most likely to believe that the right answer is "No." People use denial to cope with their substance abuse problems, and they often lie about or underestimate their use. The nurse must present a nonjudgmental attitude

BOX 50-5	DATA COLLECTION

Substance Abuse

This is a screening assessment. A more thorough assessment would be indicated in a substance abuse treatment setting.

- How many cigarettes a day do you smoke?
- How often do you drink alcohol?
- About how much do you drink?
- What kind of drugs do you use that are not prescribed?
- What is your method of use (oral, smoking, inhaling, injecting)?
- Under what circumstances do you drink or use substances? OR What leads to your drinking or drug use? (Do you drink for relaxation, fun, something to do with your friends; to help you get through the day, when you are sad, lonely, frustrated, or angry)?
- Have you had any problems because of drinking or drug use (social, job, or legal)?
- When was the last time you used alcohol or any drug, what was it, and how much?

BOX 50-6	THE "FIVE As" FOR ASSESSMENT AND INTERVENTION WITH CLIENTS WHO SMOKE

These should be used at each clinic or hospital visit (Gordon et al., 2001):

- **Ask** the client about tobacco use.
- **Advise** the client to quit.
- **Assess** the client's willingness to make a quit attempt.
- **Assist** the client to make a quit attempt.
- **Arrange** for follow-up contacts to prevent relapse.

and be accepting of clients as people, whether they use drugs or not.

Notice the assessment question that asks under what circumstances the client drinks alcohol or uses drugs. This question is aimed at determining the purpose the substance serves for this person. People use substances for a variety of reasons. Knowing the reasons increases the nurse's ability to help the client find other choices for coping or entertainment.

Similarly, the nurse can ask direct questions about tobacco use. Box 50-6 ■ contains the "Five As" of assessment and intervention with clients who smoke. Simply having a conversation with the physician or nurse about quitting smoking or other substance use helps many people to begin the process of quitting. Nurses can be a powerful force for healthy behavior change. Use your power!

DIAGNOSING, PLANNING, AND IMPLEMENTING

Nursing interventions for clients with substance abuse disorders often relate to three nursing diagnoses: *Ineffective Protection*, *Deficient Knowledge*, and *Ineffective Coping*. Other nursing diagnoses that commonly apply to people with substance abuse disorders are:

- *Interrupted Family Processes*
- *Chronic Low Self-Esteem*
- *Powerlessness*
- *Fear*
- *Ineffective Denial*
- *Imbalanced Nutrition: Less than Body Requirements*
- *Risk for Injury*
- *Disturbed Sleep Pattern*
- *Social Isolation*
- *Spiritual Distress*
- *Disturbed Sensory Perception*
- *Risk for Violence*

Ineffective Protection

The nursing diagnosis of *Ineffective Protection* is used when a client is experiencing drug or alcohol withdrawal.

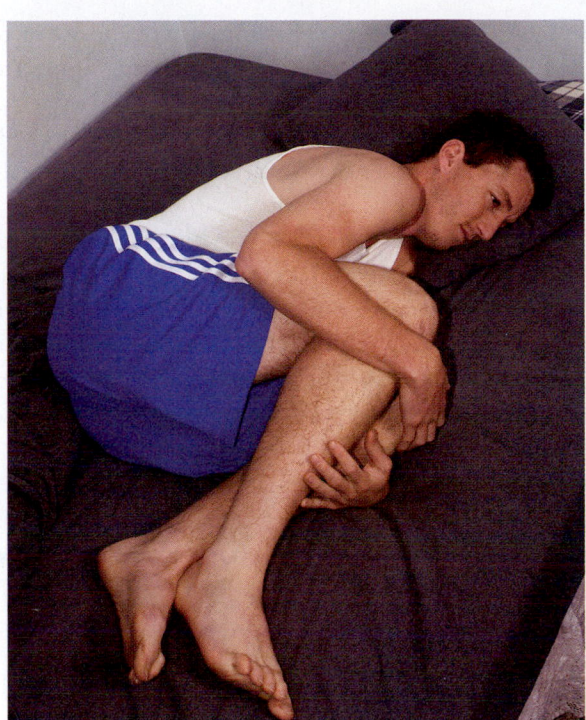

Figure 50-7. ■ A person in withdrawal is in extreme physical and mental distress. *Source:* PhotoEdit Inc.

- Take vital signs frequently. If they are elevated (T, P, R, and BP may be involved), medicate with ordered benzodiazepines according to physician's orders. *Benzodiazepines either treat or prevent symptoms of alcohol withdrawal by balancing the CNS stimulation with a depressant effect until the client's CNS can return to homeostasis without alcohol.*

- Assess for other withdrawal symptoms: anxiety, agitation, sweating, nausea, vomiting, tremors, and ataxia (Figure 50-7 ■). *Treat with prn benzodiazepines as above. If withdrawal is so severe that the client has hallucinations or seizures, call the physician immediately. These are symptoms of life-threatening withdrawal.*

- If the client is nauseated, do not push fluids. Offer small amounts of fluids frequently. Offer high-calorie feedings. *Assess for dehydration. Clients in withdrawal are at risk for fluid and electrolyte disturbances. They are also at risk for inadequate nutrition. It is easier for the nauseated client to take foods and fluids in small amounts than in big meals.*

- Maintain a low-stimulation environment for the client. *Clients in withdrawal are experiencing CNS stimulation. They will be more comfortable and less likely to have a seizure if they are in a quiet room with dim lights.*

- Encourage clients to express their feelings. *People with alcohol dependency often have difficulty understanding their own feelings. Expressing them can begin the process of behavior change.*

Deficient Knowledge

- Assess what clients know and what they need to learn. Teach them about the process of drug abuse and dependency, and how people use drugs for coping, recreation, and company. Reinforce teaching that was done previously. *When people know what the problem is physiologically and realistically, they can begin to do something about it. Reinforcement is helpful because people often forget what they learned under pressure. Maybe the client is ready to learn now.*

- Discuss the consequences to the client of substance abuse. *Because so many people deny the severity of the problem, nurses must be honest about what the consequences are (job loss, divorce, family problems, disease of every body system, etc.). People are more likely to be able to change behavior when they understand the consequences and make the choice to change.*

Ineffective Coping

- Help plan for new healthy coping strategies to replace substance use. *The client may need to meet new people to make new friends if all his or her old friends only get together to drink or use drugs. People need alternatives to substance use when they become too **H**ungry, **A**ngry, **L**onely, or **T**ired. (HALT is an acronym for feelings that lead to relapse into drug use.)*

- Help make a list of fun, recreational activities. *Clients may not even know what to do for fun. Be sure the list is realistic and includes the client's preferences. (Taking a walk, calling a friend on the phone, listening to music, watching or playing sports, hiking, bike riding, outdoor work, reading, community service, pets, spiritual activities, dancing, carpentry, arts and crafts, and appreciating nature are a few ideas.)*

- Help clients identify their resources for various needs and stressful situations (e.g., who could help with a ride to the grocery store or the doctor's office, help care for the dog if the client is in the hospital, or help to refill a medication prescription). His or her sponsor from Alcoholics Anonymous may be the one to call if he or she feels like drinking again, or if he or she wants to talk about how hard life is. *A practical list like this may be the thing the client turns to instead of drinking when he or she has a problem and cannot think of what to do.*

The following strategies for helping people quit smoking may be useful for people who are using other substances as well. The "Five Rs" for smokers who are currently unwilling to quit:

- Provide motivational information that is personally *relevant* to the client.

- Discuss the *risks* associated with smoking and the *rewards* of quitting, such as improvements in functioning and self-efficacy.

- Ask the client about *roadblocks* or barriers to quitting.

- *Repeat* motivational strategies at every clinic visit because most smokers need to make repeated quit attempts to be successful (Gordon et al., 2001).

EVALUATING

To evaluate whether nursing interventions for clients with substance abuse disorders are effective, look at the outcomes. Desired outcomes include:

- Client will have a plan for healthy alternatives to substance abuse for coping.
- Client will identify resources for obtaining help when needed (family, friends, Alcoholics Anonymous, social service agencies).
- Client will identify risk factors for relapse and plan for relapse prevention.
- Client will identify and verbalize feelings.
- Client will assume responsibility for own behavior.
- Client will use peer support to maintain sobriety.

Continuity of Care

When people with substance abuse disorders are discharged from the hospital, there must be follow-up of their substance abuse issues. They may benefit from a written list of telephone numbers for counseling resources, drug abuse treatment, or Alcoholics Anonymous. They may need a referral to the social services department for help with discharge planning. The social worker may be able to obtain a referral for treatment on an outpatient basis.

If a client with a substance abuse history is going to be discharged with sedatives, narcotics, or other medications that could interact with drugs of abuse, the potential risks should be discussed with the physician. When a person is not expected to abstain from substance use, the physician must consider this when prescribing medications for use at home.

Remind clients that they are in control of their own behavior. Give clients resources for outpatient support. A promise "never to use again" will not make the person successful. Provide a list of resources for families as well. See the MyNursingKit Website (www.prenhall.com/ramont) for a list of resources for clients and families.

EATING DISORDERS

Before you begin to care for clients diagnosed with eating disorders, take a look at your own attitudes about eating and body weight. Food and eating have meanings far beyond nutrition. Contemplate the following questions: How do you feel when you see an extremely thin person? What are your feelings about severely obese people? How does your body compare to the people you see in advertising and entertainment? How do you feel about your own body? How do you feel when you have a big holiday meal with your family? What do you eat when you are under stress? Do you ever have problems that chocolate or ice cream can solve?

The above questions relate to personal attitudes about eating and body weight. Beliefs about the meaning and importance of issues like these are learned through our culture. We learn our standards for beauty and our attitudes about food as we learn the values and behaviors of our culture.

When nurses bring their personal opinions and feelings with them to work, these feelings can affect client care behavior. Maybe you feel that thin people are weak physically and should be protected from demands placed on them. Maybe you feel that obese people are weak emotionally and should be challenged to strengthen their personality.

People who have eating disorders suffer deeply both emotionally and physically. These disorders cause low self-esteem, self-hatred, fear, hopelessness, and risks for a variety of physiologic problems (Figure 50-8 ■). Eating disorders can be fatal. Nurses should not underestimate the significance of these disorders.

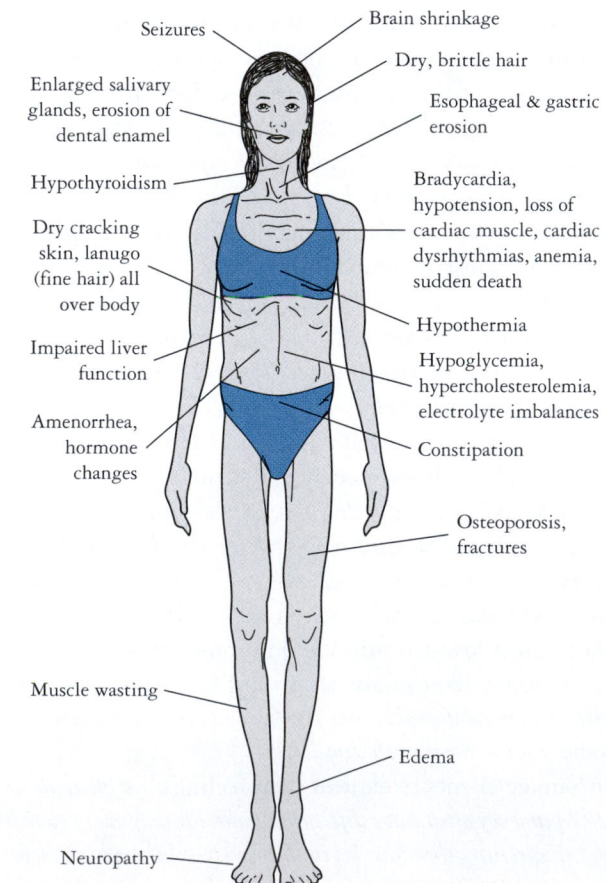

Figure 50-8. ■ Medical complications of anorexia nervosa.
(*Source:* From *Mental Health Nursing Care* [p. 271], by L. Eby and N. J. Brown, 2005, Upper Saddle River, NJ: Prentice Hall. Reprinted by permission.)

Anorexia Nervosa

Diagnostic Criteria and Manifestations

The diagnostic criteria for anorexia nervosa include (APA, 2000):

- Refusal to maintain body weight of at least 85% of minimally normal weight for age and height
- Intense fear of gaining weight or becoming fat, even though underweight
- Disturbance in the way one's body weight or shape is perceived, undue influence of body weight or shape on self-evaluation, or denial of the seriousness of the current low body weight
- Amenorrhea (absence of at least three menstrual periods in a woman after puberty)

The APA (2000) describes two subtypes of anorexia nervosa:

1. *Restricting type* with weight loss through dieting, fasting, or excessive exercise
2. *Binge-eating purging type* in which the individual has regularly engaged in binge eating and purging (or both) during the current episode. Purging involves self-induced vomiting, or abuse of laxatives, diuretics, or enemas. Some people with anorexia nervosa binge and purge and others purge after eating small amounts.

People with anorexia nervosa usually accomplish the weight loss by severely restricting their food intake. They often begin by excluding what they think are high-calorie foods, and progress to a very limited diet. Other methods of weight loss include **purging** (self-induced vomiting or abuse of laxatives or diuretics). People with anorexia nervosa have an intense fear of gaining weight, even when they are *emaciated* (excessively thin, wasted).

Distortion of how they perceive their body size and shape is another characteristic of people with anorexia nervosa (Figure 50-9 ■). Some people feel overweight, even though they are thin. Others know they are thin, but are concerned that parts of their bodies, especially the abdomen, thighs, and buttocks, are too fat. The self-esteem of people with anorexia nervosa is closely tied to body shape and weight. Weight loss is seen as an improvement and a sign of extraordinary self-control. Weight gain becomes an unacceptable failure of self-control. Some people with the disorder admit that they are thin, but they typically deny the serious medical implications of their condition (APA, 2000). The mortality rate of anorexia nervosa is 5% to 10%.

The term *anorexia* is an inaccurate name for this condition. It means "loss of appetite." In fact, people with anorexia nervosa continue to have a normal sense of hunger and appetite.

Usually the affected person is brought to the attention of healthcare providers by parents. Because of clients' denial or lack of insight, the parents may be better sources of

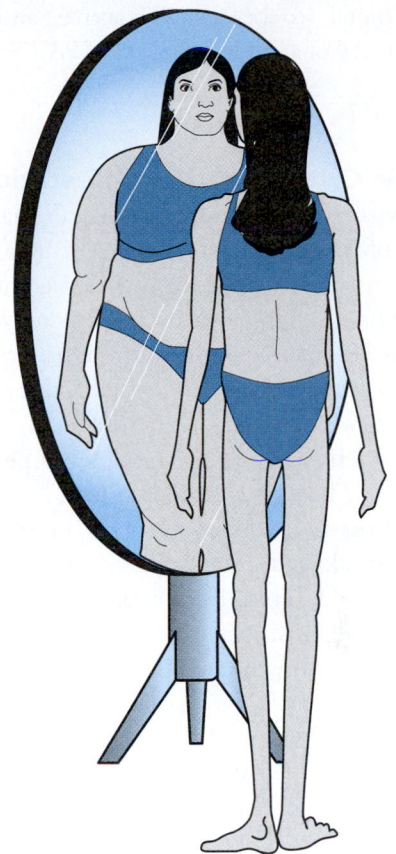

Figure 50-9. ■ Disturbance in body perception.

information about the client's symptom history. Be sure to follow your institution's policy about confidentiality and disclosure of client information before discussing the client's condition with her parents. The parents may provide information to the nurse, but the nurse must be careful about what information is given to the parents without the client's consent.

Ninety percent of individuals who have anorexia nervosa are female. Onset before puberty is rare. It typically begins in mid to late adolescence (14 to 18 years of age), and rarely starts after age 40. Some people recover completely after a single episode. Others have a fluctuating pattern including weight gain followed by relapse. Still others have a chronically deteriorating course over many years (APA, 2000).

Most affected people are preoccupied with thoughts of food. They may collect recipes or hoard food. These symptoms, as well as depression, may be due to the physiologic effects of undernutrition. People with anorexia nervosa may have concerns about eating in public, a strong need to be in control of their environment, inflexible thinking, perfectionism, limited social spontaneity, feelings of ineffectiveness, lack of initiative, and strained emotional expression. Many have a personality disorder as well. Those with the binge eating/purging type are more likely to have other impulse control problems, to abuse alcohol or drugs, to have changeable mood, to be sexually active, and to have a greater frequency of suicide attempts (APA, 2000).

Bulimia Nervosa

Diagnostic Criteria and Manifestations

Bulimia nervosa is more common than anorexia. The essential features of this disorder are binge eating and inappropriate compensatory methods to avoid weight gain. The self-evaluation of individuals with bulimia nervosa is excessively influenced by body shape and weight. The binge eating, which is usually followed by self-induced vomiting, occurs at least twice a week (APA, 2000).

A **binge** is defined as eating in a limited period of time (usually within 2 hours) an amount of food that is definitely larger than most individuals would eat under similar circumstances. Snacking through the day does not constitute a binge. The food typically includes high-calorie, high-carbohydrate foods such as cakes and ice cream. Binge eating is characterized more by the amount of food eaten than by the specific type of food. A binge may or may not be planned in advance, and the food is usually eaten rapidly (APA, 2000).

An episode of binge eating is characterized by a feeling of loss of control. People are often ashamed of their eating behavior, and usually binge secretly. A binge may be triggered by a sad mood, a stressful event, hunger from dieting, or feelings about body image, appearance, or weight. The binge may temporarily relieve the stress or low mood, but shame and self-criticism recur.

The most common method of compensating for binge eating is purging by self-induced vomiting, usually by stimulating the gag reflex. Clients report that the vomiting relieves the sense of physical discomfort and decreases the fear of gaining weight. Some people with bulimia nervosa abuse laxatives and diuretics after binge eating. A few misuse enemas after bingeing.

People with bulimia nervosa may exercise excessively in an effort to lose weight. Exercise becomes excessive when it significantly interferes with other important activities, when it occurs at inappropriate times or in inappropriate settings, or when the individual continues to exercise despite injury.

The binge eating and inappropriate compensatory behaviors occur, on average, at least twice a week for at least 3 months. For people with bulimia nervosa, body shape and weight are the most important factors in determining their self-esteem. People with bulimia are usually within the normal weight range, although they may be slightly above or below it.

The APA (2000) recognizes two subtypes of bulimia nervosa:

- *Purging type*. During the episode of bulimia nervosa, the person has regularly engaged in self-induced vomiting or the misuse of laxatives, diuretics, or enemas.

- *Nonpurging type*. During the episode of bulimia nervosa, the person has used other inappropriate behaviors to compensate for the binge eating, such as fasting or excessive exercise, but has not regularly engaged in self-induced vomiting or the misuse of laxatives, diuretics, or enemas.

There is an increase in the incidence of depression and anxiety in people who have bulimia nervosa. Substance abuse, especially of alcohol or stimulants, is also increased in this group. So is the incidence of *borderline personality disorder* (a disorder that includes a pattern of impulsiveness and instability in interpersonal relationships, self-image, and emotions). Ninety percent of individuals with bulimia nervosa are female. Bulimia nervosa usually begins in late adolescence or early adult life. The course may be chronic or intermittent, and the symptoms of many individuals decrease over time. See Figure 50-8 for a drawing of the medical problems associated with the eating disorders.

Binge Eating Disorder

Diagnostic Criteria and Manifestations

The diagnosis of binge eating disorder is currently under study. It is characterized by episodes of binge eating without the compensatory behaviors used in bulimia (vomiting, laxatives, enemas, excessive exercise).

As in bulimia nervosa, people with binge eating disorder experience marked distress during and after the binge eating episodes. They have feelings of loss of control over the binge eating. They are also concerned with the possible effects of the bingeing. As in bulimia, large amounts of food are consumed quickly, when the individual is not hungry. The individual eats until uncomfortably full, eating alone due to shame, disgust, and guilt about overeating. Unlike people with bulimia, people with binge eating disorder do not regularly purge or abuse laxatives, diuretics, or enemas. To have this diagnosis, the individual must binge at least twice a week for 6 months (APA, 2000).

People with binge eating disorder tend to be overweight, whereas people with bulimia are often normal weight or slightly overweight. People with binge eating disorder often report that their eating or weight interferes with their relationships with other people, their work, and their ability to feel good about themselves. They tend to have more self-loathing, disgust about body size, depression, anxiety, and physical complaints than people of the same weight who do not have the disorder. Females are approximately 1.5 times more likely to have this disorder than males. It typically starts in late adolescence or the early 20s. The first episode may occur after a stressful event (APA, 2000).

MALES WITH EATING DISORDERS

Ten percent of the people with eating disorders are male. The diagnostic criteria for the disorders and the treatment for them are the same as for women. One difference is that males with eating disorders are more likely to be involved in athletics. Males sometimes begin an eating disorder through an effort to "make the weight" for a sport such as wrestling. Males are more likely than females with eating disorders to be obese before the eating disorder begins, and they are less likely to have guilt feelings about episodes of binge eating and purging (Ricciardelli et al., 2001).

People with eating disorders often have difficulty trusting others, whether they are male or female. It can be difficult for adolescent males to express their feelings about eating-related problems. Because of this, it is especially important for the nurse to establish a trusting nurse–client relationship.

Pressure is increasing on adolescent males to measure up to an ideal male physique as depicted in advertising, in the movies, and by professional athletes (many of whom are pressured to use anabolic steroids). If this process continues, the incidence of eating disorders in males may also rise.

Causes of Eating Disorders

What causes eating disorders? This is a good question. An increased incidence among family members suggests a genetic influence. A biological influence is suggested by the fact that reduced serotonin decreases the sense of satiety (fullness) and increases food intake. Depressive symptoms are common in people with eating disorders.

Psychologic theorists suggest that early separation conflicts, a sense of helplessness, difficulty interpreting feelings, intolerance of high emotion, and fear of maturity may predispose a person to an eating disorder. Women who binge report low mood, shame, guilt, and great fluctuations in self-esteem (Greeno et al., 2000).

Environmental factors and experiences may predispose a person to having an eating disorder. Sexual abuse is reported in 20% to 50% of clients with anorexia and bulimia. People with bulimia report more behavior problems and a higher incidence of substance abuse than the general population (Wonderlich et al., 1997).

Control issues have been proposed as a possible cause of anorexia nervosa. The idea is that the person feels a loss of control over the life environment (perhaps from a perfectionist family with unreachable expectations). The person seeks control and satisfaction where she or he can find it, in refusing food. Control of their environment is important to nurses also. Box 50-7 ■ describes some ways that control issues can affect nursing care.

BOX 50-7   CONTROL ISSUES

The nurse's responses to clients with eating disorders can interfere with client care when:

- Feeling overwhelmed by the client's problems, the nurse sets overly rigid rules for the client in order to have some control.
- The nurse, feeling powerless to help the client, becomes resentful and angry with the client.
- The nurse sees other staff feeling frustrated with the client, and creates a hidden alliance with the client instead of working with the staff to improve client care.

The behavior theorists believe that children learn how to relate to food early in life. They may learn that food can provide a certain satisfaction and sense of calm and composure. Learning to use food as a coping mechanism or substitute for affection can lead to obesity. A behavioral approach to anorexia suggests that avoidance of eating relieves anxiety. Behavioral treatment would include practicing and learning new ways to manage anxiety.

Parents who overemphasize athletic performance, reward slimness, or express disapproval of overweight people are placing their children at risk (Chally, 1998). Parents who model unhealthy eating behaviors also put their children at risk, because children learn the behavior that they see. Some examples of unhealthy eating behaviors are overeating under stress, not eating when under stress, and using food as rewards.

The expectations of perfection and maintenance of a slender body shape increase the incidence of eating disorders in certain groups. This pressure, and the competition with others to be the most perfect or thinnest, may be the force behind the increased incidence of eating disorders in people who participate in gymnastics and dance (especially ballet).

Cognitive theorists propose that eating disorders are due to cognitive distortions (distorted thinking). People with anorexia nervosa tend to *catastrophize*, meaning they consider a small event to be a big catastrophe. For example, "If I gain a pound, my clothes won't fit." They also tend to use **dichotomous thinking,** which is similar to black-and-white thinking. For someone with dichotomous thinking, something is either all one way or all its opposite. Examples are "If I am not thin I will be hugely fat" and "If I eat anything I will lose control and gain a hundred pounds." Cognitive therapy focuses on changing the distorted thinking.

People learn their feelings about food and eating as they learn about their culture. Eating can symbolize parental nurturing. It symbolizes celebration and holidays. It can also symbolize loss of control.

Eating disorders involve attitudes and coping mechanisms that are perceived by clients as important parts of

MyNursingKit | Eating disorders

themselves. Therefore, maladaptive eating patterns are very difficult to change. Many people with eating disorders feel threatened by the idea of therapy. They are unable to see alternatives to their behavior that will allow them to cope with their stressors. For these reasons, eating disorder treatment is challenging. It requires long-term effort by clients, their families, and the healthcare team. A combination of strategies should be used to treat eating disorders.

Collaborative Care

MEDICATIONS

Medications have not been found effective for the general treatment of eating disorders. Some clients respond to antidepressant medications. These drugs have been used successfully to decrease the mood and obsessive-compulsive symptoms and to prevent relapse in some people with eating disorders. However, the effects appear to be short term (Zhu & Walsh, 2002). Olanzapine (Zyprexa), an antipsychotic medication, has been used to treat the bizarre body image distortion in anorexia nervosa and because it has a side effect of weight gain.

COGNITIVE BEHAVIORAL THERAPY

A variety of therapeutic approaches to eating disorders are used. Cognitive behavioral therapy, in which clients change their distorted thinking and practice healthy coping mechanisms, has been used successfully with clients who have bulimia nervosa. It has been shown to reduce binge eating and purging (Walsh, 1997). Due to frequent extensive family involvement, family therapy is a popular technique for treatment of anorexia nervosa. A major obstacle to treatment is that insurance companies frequently either do not cover or underfund eating disorder treatment.

Ideally, eating disorders are treated on an outpatient basis, because when lifestyle changes are needed, clients are more successful when they can practice their new behaviors at home. Outpatients have more autonomy, which is important in these disorders. However, there are times when hospitalization is required. Clients who have life-threatening fluid and electrolyte imbalances, organ failure, or complete inability to eat must be hospitalized. Tube feeding and total parenteral nutrition have been used in the short term to treat acute malnutrition.

Diabulimia

A new concern for healthcare professionals treating Type I diabetes, especially in female adolescents, is diabulimia. Box 50-8 ■ describes short-, medium- and long-term symptoms of diabulimia.

Diabulimia refers to an eating disorder in which clients with Type I diabetes deliberately give themselves less insulin for the purpose of weight loss. A person with diabulimia,

---

BOX 50-8	MANIFESTATIONS OF DIABULIMIA

Short-Term Signs and Symptoms
- Constant urination
- Constant thirst
- Excessive appetite
- High blood glucose levels (often over 600)
- Large amount of glucose in urine
- Weakness
- Fatigue
- Inability to concentrate
- Elevated electrolytes
- Severe ketonuria and ketonemia
- Low sodium levels

Medium-Term Signs and Symptoms
- Muscle atrophy
- GERD
- Indigestion
- Severe weight loss
- Proteinuria
- Moderate to severe dehydration
- Edema with fluid replacement
- High cholesterol

Long-Term Signs and Symptoms
- Severe kidney damage
- Blindness
- Severe neuropathy (nerve damage to hands and feet)
- Extreme fatigue
- Edema (during blood sugar controlled phases)
- Hearing problems
- High cholesterol
- Osteoporosis

---

especially if not caught and treated early, is likely to suffer the negative effects on the body of diabetes earlier than a person who manages his or her diabetes in a faithful manner. LPNs/LVNs working in ambulatory settings such as physician's offices, school health clinics, or urgent care need to be alert to the signs and symptoms of this disorder. Type I diabetics in their teen years should be evaluated for psychosocial issues along with the consistent monitoring of their diabetes.

Obesity

Obesity is not considered a mental disorder or eating disorder. Many people with obesity are mentally healthy. However, obesity is covered here because it causes a great deal of physical and emotional suffering, and many of the people it affects are nurses.

The Office of the U.S. Surgeon General reports that the risks of overweight or obesity may soon cause as much disease and death as cigarette smoking. Overweight in an adult is determined by **body mass index** (BMI). BMI is defined as weight in kilograms divided by the square of

BOX 50-9	WEIGHT CATEGORIES BY BMI FOR AGE
Overweight	Greater than 95th percentile
At risk for overweight	85th–94th percentile
Normal range	5th–84th percentile
Underweight	Less than 5th percentile

Example:
A 12-year-old female with a weight of 120 pounds and a height of 58.5 inches is above the 90th percentile for weight and the 25th percentile for stature. To calculate the BMI, the weight is multiplied by 703 and divided by the height twice:

$$120 \times 703 = 84,360 \div 58.5 = 1442.05 \div 58.5 = 24.65 \text{ BMI}$$

height in meters (see Chapter 25). Another way to calculate it is as follows: weight in pounds multiplied by 703 and then divided twice by height in inches (this is easier with a calculator). Overweight is diagnosed when BMI is between 25 and 29.9, and a BMI of 30 or greater indicates obesity. The risk of early death increases as the BMI goes above 30. Twenty-five percent of American adults are obese (Blackburn & Bevis, 2003). BMI is also a useful measurement for identifying weight problems in children and adolescents. The revised CDC growth charts now include calculations and grafting for body mass index. Box 50-9 ■ provides weight categories by BMI.

This is at the 94th percentile, placing the student in the "At risk for being overweight" category. Childhood obesity is fast approaching a major healthcare problem, so it is important to screen at every opportunity. Whenever a child or adolescent comes in contact with a healthcare professional, he or she should be evaluated for possible weight and nutritional issues. This can be done quickly and easily. When issues arise, counseling should be provided to the client as well as adult family members.

Many overweight people have a group of major risk factors that constitute a condition called **metabolic syndrome.** The metabolic syndrome includes:

- Abdominal obesity
- Abnormal serum lipids (increased triglycerides and decreased high-density lipoprotein)
- Elevated blood pressure
- Insulin resistance
- Increased clotting of the blood

This syndrome is caused by improper nutrition and inadequate exercise. The syndrome significantly increases cardiovascular risks, such as heart disease and stroke. Weight loss is the key therapeutic objective. Even modest weight reductions (5% to 10% of initial body weight) cause significant clinical improvements (Blackburn & Bevis, 2003).

Obesity has adverse effects on physical as well as mental health (see also Chapters 37 and 49). Some people with obesity experience low self-esteem, poor body image, depression, and anxiety. Some feel guilt and self-disgust. People with compulsive eating behavior overeat for emotional rather than physical reasons. Food may offer the same relief from anxiety or stress that companionship and nurturing from others might provide. Food becomes a mechanism for coping with stress.

Causes

Obesity has a similar profile to the eating disorders. It runs in families. This is probably due to a combination of predisposing factors and learned behavior. It has behavioral aspects (people learn to overeat because they receive some reinforcement from food) and cognitive components (distorted thinking). Cultural and social factors also lead to obesity. People are increasingly turning to sedentary recreational activities (electronic entertainment). Fast food is readily available and yes, thanks, I will have fries with that.

Treatment

To lose weight, more energy must be spent than is consumed on a daily basis. The chance of success in long-term maintenance of weight loss is improved with the following (Blackburn & Bevis, 2003):

- Realistic weight loss goals (5% to 10% of initial body weight)
- Change in eating patterns to include less high-calorie, low-nutrition foods, and more nutrient-dense, low-energy foods, such as fruits and vegetables
- Social support
- Structured meal plans, to avoid misunderstanding and measurement errors in food amounts
- Record of eating, to keep it conscious
- Moderate physical activity on most, if not all, days

NURSING CARE

PRIORITIZING NURSING CARE

When caring for clients with eating disorders, help them focus on developing healthy lifestyle choices. Encourage openness and discourage secretive behavior. Encourage clients to seek insight into their eating behavior: Does it help them feel some type of control, or is it a way to avoid overwhelming emotions? Support clients as they seek positive ways to cope with emotions other than using or denying food.

Healthier lifestyle changes make a lot of sense, but they are notoriously difficult. Nurses can help by being role models of healthy behavior and by acknowledging the difficulty of the challenge. There is hope. Change is possible, but recognize the challenge, and give the client a lot of support. Once a client begins a regular exercise program, the increased sense of well-being will be very rewarding.

ASSESSING

The assessment of a client with weight loss or gain should begin with subjective information about the client's experience. Imagine that we have two very thin adolescents in the clinic. One states that she is just fine, and could only be improved by a little more weight loss. The second client might say, "I've been so hungry, and I've been eating and drinking everything in sight, but I'm still losing weight." The first client may have anorexia nervosa, and the second may have untreated Type 1 diabetes. Let's not forget that there are general medical conditions that cause weight gain and loss.

Other subjective information to collect includes information about the client's body image. A picture like the one shown in Figure 50-10 ■ is useful for assessing whether a client has a realistic body image. A distorted image of the thin self as obese is very common in anorexia nervosa, but not in bulimia or binge eating disorder. The client's perception of her or his body and attitudes about eating will also demonstrate whether the client has distorted thinking related to body shape and weight.

Another important subjective assessment is about how the eating disorder serves the client. Does it take the focus off unhealthy family dynamics? Does it give the client control in a chaotic situation? Does purging relieve anxiety? Does binge eating give the client some momentary comfort (before the shame and embarrassment)?

Objective findings include the ever-popular vital signs and weight. Expect the provider to order lab values that indicate the client's nutritional status, and whether an eating disorder has affected organ function. A well-documented baseline assessment is important because it provides a point of comparison for evaluating the client's progress in treatment.

Weighing clients with eating disorders can be problematic. Clients with anorexia nervosa may go to great lengths to make it appear that they have gained or maintained weight. Clients have awakened during the night to drink large volumes of water, stuffed their socks with coins, put on extra clothing, and concealed heavy items in their clothing. The nurse's problem-solving skills will be helpful here.

DIAGNOSING, PLANNING, AND IMPLEMENTING

Some common nursing diagnoses for clients with eating disorders include:

- *Imbalanced Nutrition: Less than Body Requirements*
- *Imbalanced Nutrition: More than Body Requirements*

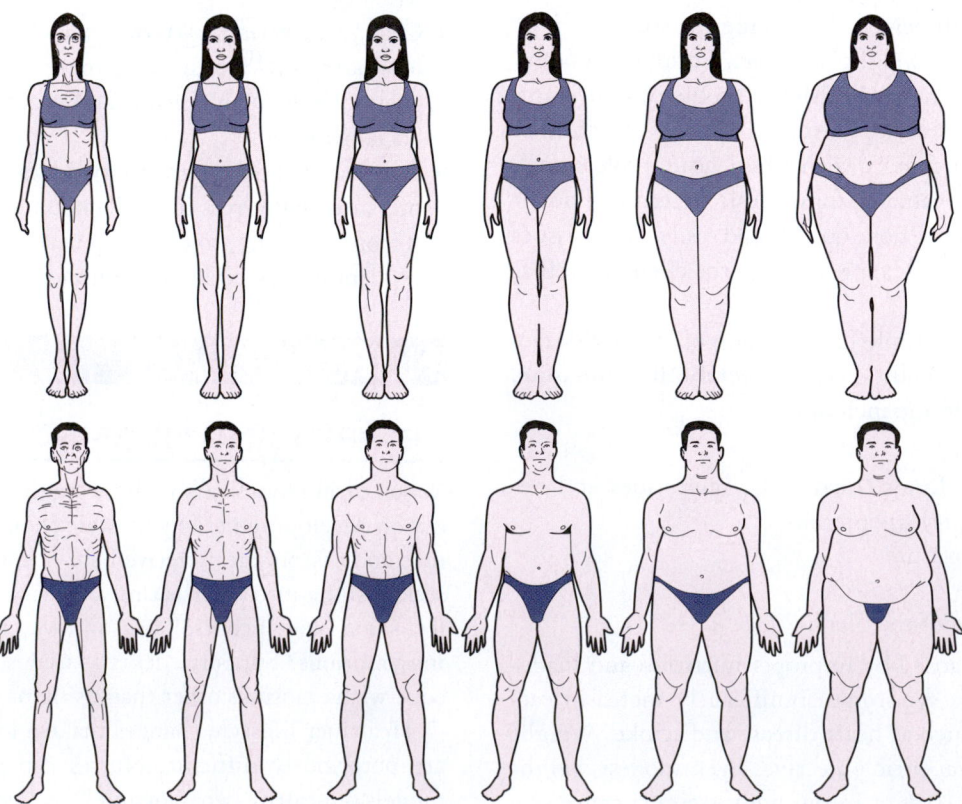

Figure 50-10. ■ Assessment of body image.

- *Ineffective Coping*
- *Chronic Low Self-Esteem*
- *Powerlessness*
- *Disturbed Body Image* (distortion of the mental picture of one's physical self).

Desired outcomes for clients with eating disorders are that the client will:

- Have healthy eating patterns (without binge eating or purging).
- Maintain body weight at least 85% of desired weight for age and height.
- Maintain a body mass index of less than 25.
- Have positive self-esteem separate from physical appearance.
- Make positive statements about self.
- Have a realistic image of own body.
- Have a sense of self-efficacy (power over one's own outcomes).

Ineffective Individual Coping

Clients with eating disorders have ineffective coping skills. They may demonstrate self-destructive behaviors (starving, purging, bingeing, or other self-harm), inability to ask for help, poor impulse control, inability to meet their basic nutritional needs, inability to change their behaviors, denial of illness, or insufficient problem-solving skills. The nurse chooses appropriate interventions for individual clients.

- Encourage the client to express feelings. *Clients with eating disorders often have difficulty expressing their feelings. Verbal expression of feelings can reduce anxiety and decrease the need for purging behavior. Practice with expressing feelings helps the client learn to recognize own feelings.*
- Help the client explore alternate ways of responding to feelings of frustration, anger, or anxiety that do not involve food. *If the client can identify and plan to use behaviors to relieve anxiety that do not involve food or purging (such as talking with a friend), she or he will have a healthy alternative when the trigger feelings arise. It is important to separate feelings from food.*
- Encourage the client to eat with others. *Eating with other people will take the secrecy out of eating and provide role models for normal behavior. This is especially stressful for clients with anorexia nervosa.*
- Help the client explore personal strengths that are not related to eating or appearance. *The client's self-concept can be improved by discovering personal strengths. It is important for the client with an eating disorder to recognize that appearance does not define the character of a person.*
- Help the client identify situations and feelings that trigger binge eating or purging. Encourage the client to notify the nurse when these feelings arise, then discuss problem

solving with the client. *The goal is for the client to understand her or his feelings and to stop the urge to engage in unhealthy behavior, ultimately replacing it with healthy alternatives. The nurse can support the client as she or he works through this process.*

- Be nonjudgmental in your interactions with clients, even when their behavior is inappropriate. *Clients with eating disorders already have feelings of low self-esteem, guilt, and shame. The role of the nurse is to help the client develop healthy behavior, not to punish the client for poor judgment.*

EVALUATING

Evaluation of the effectiveness of the nursing interventions is an ongoing part of the nursing process. The client's body weight goals will be to maintain body weight at least 85% of typical weight for age, with a BMI of less than 25. The behavioral goal is healthy eating patterns, including balanced nutrition without binge eating or purging. The cognitive goals are that clients will have a realistic self-perception, and a positive self-esteem separate from their physical appearance.

Continuity of Care

Nurses can play a leading role in teaching about healthy eating behaviors. The best approach to eating disorders is prevention. Some points the nurse may use for client teaching are provided in Box 50-10 ■. Teaching about healthy eating can be done with clients of any age, or with parents with the goal of preventing eating disorders in their children.

BOX 50-10	CLIENT TEACHING

Strategies for Preventing Eating Disorders

1. Address our cultural obsession with slenderness as a physical, psychological, and moral issue.
2. Help children develop self-esteem in a variety of areas that transcend physical appearance.
3. Discuss the roles of women and men in our society beyond their appearance.
4. Encourage parents to examine their own attitudes about food and think about how these attitudes affect the way they handle food with their children.
5. Teach parents ways to identify their child's hunger behavior, loneliness behavior, and need for nurturance. Discuss the need to respond accordingly with food, companionship, or nurturing (not with food for all needs). Help them to think about the difference between hunger for food and hunger for affection.
6. Advise parents to allow their children to determine their feeding needs and to let go of the need to "clean the plate."
7. Do not make insulting remarks about overweight people.
8. Do not overemphasize success (expecting perfection) in athletics.
9. Be a good role model for healthy eating. Eat a variety of nutritious foods. Avoid overeating or undereating under stress.
10. Emphasize that thinness is not the same as happiness.

NURSING PROCESS CARE PLAN
Client with Obesity

Ruby Red is a 50-year-old European American woman admitted to the general hospital for a total knee arthroplasty (replacement) 2 days ago. She is also obese. She has 2 children and 2 dogs. Ms. Red is concerned about her health, self-image, and recovery from surgery. She would like help to lose weight. She has tried weight-loss diets in the past with no long-term success.

Assessment

Client is 5' 5" tall, 190 lbs. Client states that she eats when she feels nervous; she states that she frequently overeats in the evenings; BP 148/94. Friends bring candy to hospital for client. It is very painful for client to ambulate. Client asks, "Is there a pill that will make me lose weight?" Client states that her physician has never talked with her about losing weight.

Nursing Diagnoses

The following important nursing diagnoses (among others) are established for this condition:

- *Ineffective Coping*
- *Imbalanced Nutrition: More than Body Requirements*
- *Deficient Knowledge* related to weight management

Planning and Implementation

The following nursing implementations are planned and implemented for Ms. Red:

- Discuss with the client her reasons for wanting to lose weight.

- Teach the client about the relationship between dietary intake, calorie burning by exercise and metabolism, and weight.
- Encourage client to accept herself as a person, just as she is, and to lose weight for her health and well-being.
- Discuss strategies for dealing with feelings in ways other than eating.
- Discuss cues for eating that are not related to hunger.
- Encourage increasing physical activity at the client's ability level, keeping goals realistic and surgical pain under control.
- Refer client to the dietitian to determine realistic goals, and to plan a weight loss program.

Evaluation

Ms. Red maintained her admission weight while she was in the hospital. She was very willing to discuss nutrition and exercise plans for when she is at home. She recognizes that she uses food as a way to cope with stress, frustration, and anxiety. She asked her friends who brought candy to give it to the nurses.

Critical Thinking in the Nursing Process

1. What will put Ms. Red at risk for overeating when she is at home?
2. Will the nurse teach this client to exercise strenuously nearly every day when she is discharged?
3. What strategies might the nurse suggest to this client to replace eating when she is under stress?

Note: Discussion of Critical Thinking questions appears on the MyNursingKit Website.

Note: The references and resources for all chapters have been compiled at the back of the book.

Chapter Review

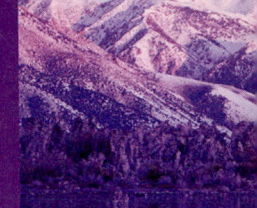

KEY Points

- Substance abuse is a maladaptive pattern of substance use despite adverse outcomes. Substance dependency involves continuing to use the substance despite significant substance-related problems, including tolerance, withdrawal, and compulsive use.

- Substance abuse disorders affect 20% of adults in the United States, but most of these people go undiagnosed.

- Clients use denial about substance use, and so do health professionals.

- There are 11 substances of abuse: alcohol; opioids; sedatives, hypnotics, and anxiolytics; cocaine; amphetamines and similar drugs; hallucinogens; phencyclidine (PCP) and similar drugs; inhalants; cannabis; caffeine; and nicotine.

- The combination of alcohol with other CNS depressants can be fatal due to additive CNS depression.

- Nurses should assess the substance use history of each client on admission.

- When substance abuse and dependency occur among other nurses and healthcare professionals, the first responsibility of the nurse is client safety and the second is to seek help for your colleague. Both are achieved by reporting the situation to the nurse manager.

- The goal of substance abuse treatment is abstinence from substance use and development of skills to replace drug use for coping, enjoyment, or companionship.

- Clients with substance dependency need referral to social services for assistance and follow-up after discharge.

- Eating disorders are serious and can be fatal.

- Eating disorders affect physiologic as well as psychologic function.

- People with eating disorders have ineffective coping skills.

- The cultural attitude that extreme thinness defines beauty and symbolizes success and self-control contributes to the occurrence of eating disorders.

- Obesity is becoming more common, and causes increased cardiovascular risks, arthritis, poor self-esteem, and mortality rates.

- Strategies are available for preventing eating disorders.

- Many people respond well to treatment for substance-related and eating disorders: Keep hope alive.

⚭ FOR FURTHER Study

Refer to Chapter 4 for a discussion of impaired nursing.

For more information on psychosocial nursing, including denial and cognitive behavioral therapy, see Chapter 17.

Body mass index is discussed further in Chapter 25.

See Chapter 33 for a discussion of cardiac dysrhythmias.

Discussion of neurologic disorders appears in Chapter 36.

Read more about GI disorders, including liver cirrhosis, in Chapter 37.

See Chapter 49 for further discussion of dual diagnosis and of stigma related to mental disorders.

Critical Thinking Care Map

Caring for a Client with Substance Dependency
NCLEX-PN® Focus Area: Psychosocial Integrity

Case Study: The client is a hospitalized 43-year-old European American male with hyperglycemia due to Type 2 diabetes and alcoholism. He was admitted 4 days ago after his daughter visited him in his apartment and found him lying on his bed semiconscious. On admission, his blood glucose was 502, he was severely dehydrated, and he had alcohol on his breath. He said: "I need my wine to keep me company." He is thin and underweight for his height. He is taking his oral antidiabetes medication inconsistently. He had alcohol withdrawal symptoms for the first 4 days of his hospitalization. Now he is feeling better, his corticosteroid-binding globulin (CBG) is normal, and his vital signs are stable.

Nursing Diagnosis: *Ineffective Coping*

COLLECT DATA

Subjective	Objective
_____	_____
_____	_____
_____	_____
_____	_____
_____	_____
_____	_____

Would you report this? Yes/No

If yes, report to: _____

What would you report? _____

Nursing Care

_____
_____
_____
_____
_____
_____
_____
_____

How would you document this? _____
_____
_____
_____

Compare your answers and documentation to those provided on the MyNursingKit Website.

Data Collected
(use only those that apply)

- Client states, "Drinking helps me forget my problems."
- Will get up to do ADLs with encouragement
- Eats 90% to 100% of the food on his meal trays
- Has gained 4 pounds since admission
- Takes all meds given to him in the hospital
- Daughter visits client in the hospital
- States, "What else can I do besides drink? It is all I know anymore."
- States, "I can quit when I want. I just don't want to quit."
- He is oriented to person and place. Knows the year and month, not the date
- States, "Let me go home. I can take care of myself."

Nursing Interventions
(use only those that apply; list in priority order)

- Discuss the consequences of the client's drinking when he is able.
- Spend at least 3 hours each day explaining all the details of alcoholism, the theories of the disease, and potential treatments.
- Help him develop a list of his resources for help.
- Help him develop a list of healthier things he could do when he feels like drinking, to prevent relapse.
- Allow the client to spend the majority of his time in his bed.
- Ask why he wants to go home.
- Reinforce teaching about his disorders and meds at his level.
- Spend time with the client each shift. Talk with him or sit beside him.
- Push the client to talk at length about his problems with drinking and diabetes.
- Tell the physician to write an order for the client to go to AA when he is discharged.
- Encourage the client to take his antidiabetes medication.
- Tell the client that he cannot go home until he promises to quit drinking.

NCLEX-PN® Exam Preparation

1 The nurse, after admitting a client with a history of alcohol dependence, anticipates which of the following when planning pain management for this client? This client will:

  1. Need more narcotics because he is tolerant to CNS depressants.
  2. Try to manipulate the staff to obtain drugs.
  3. Be uncooperative with nursing care.
  4. Benefit from the fewest and lowest possible doses of narcotics.

2 The nurse admits a new client to the unit and notes blood pressure, pulse, and respirations are elevated. The client displays tremors and tells the nurse he would really like a beer right now. The nurse suspects this client's symptoms are a result of:

  1. Anxiety secondary to hospital admission.
  2. Lack of compliance with prescribed medication regimen.
  3. Alcohol intoxication.
  4. Alcohol withdrawal.

3 A client is admitted with a history of alcohol abuse for an acute medical problem. The nurse anticipates administering which of the following medications to prevent alcoholic encephalopathy?

  1. Demerol (meperidine).
  2. Valium (diazepam).
  3. Thiamine (vitamin B_1).
  4. Dilantin (phenytoin).

4 When assessing a client for potential substance abuse, the nurse would recognize that which of the following would indicate the client's use of the substance has become a problem? (Select all that apply.)

  1. The client has been convicted of driving under the influence twice.
  2. The client lost her job because she reported to work under the influence.
  3. She drinks one glass of wine almost every evening.
  4. Her ex-husband says he had to divorce her and take the children because her substance use was negatively impacting the children.
  5. The client reports the amount of substance she uses has increased over the last few months.

5 While working on a surgical unit the nurse notices one of the other staff nurses frequently volunteering to administer medications for other nurse's clients and notices slurred speech when this nurse comes back from break. Later that night, when the narcotic count is wrong, the nurse's best action is to:

  1. Confront the nurse with your suspicion of narcotic use.
  2. Assess the nurse for signs, to confirm narcotics use.
  3. Notify the charge nurse that the nurse is impaired.
  4. Notify the nursing supervisor of your observations.

6 The nurse admits a client to the emergency department who admits to drinking alcohol. The client has incoherent speech, has mental confusion, is vomiting, and has labored breathing. Based on these symptoms the nurse anticipates a blood alcohol level of:

  1. 0.05–0.15 g/dL.
  2. 0.15 – 0.3 g/dL.
  3. 0.3–0.4 g/dL.
  4. 0.4–0.5 g/dL.

7 The nurse, conducting a class on alcohol use for college students, is asked by one of the participants, "Why does it seem like it takes more and more beers to get the same effect?" The nurse would answer this question by explaining the principle of:

  1. Abuse.
  2. Dependence.
  3. Addiction.
  4. Tolerance.

8 While caring for an adolescent, the mother of the client approaches the nurse to report concerns about her daughter's recent fasting, exercising excessively to the point of skipping school to work out, obsession with body image, and loss of weight. The mother says the teen frequently claims that she is fat, despite having a measurement of less than average body mass. The nurse's best response would be:

  1. "It is normal for teens to become obsessed with their body image. She'll get over it with maturity."
  2. "It's not serious unless you see that she is also abusing laxatives and vomiting after meals."
  3. "Your daughter may have an eating disorder, and she needs an immediate assessment before she endangers her overall health."
  4. "Your daughter may have an eating disorder, but her weight is not in the dangerous level. Monitor her condition and call your doctor if it gets worse."

9 The nurse admits a client with a medical diagnosis of anorexia nervosa. Which of the following behaviors, if noted, would increase the nurse's level of concern?

  1. Sexually provocative behavior
  2. Suicidal ideation
  3. Staff manipulation
  4. Alcohol and drug use

10 The nurse, working in a substance abuse treatment facility, explains the value of attending support groups such as Alcoholics Anonymous or Narcotics Anonymous as including which of the following? (Select all that apply.)

  1. Sharing problems with others with similar experiences.
  2. A sense of community and unconditional support.
  3. Assisting the substance abuser to gain insight into his or her behavior.
  4. Improve their faith and belief in God.
  5. Cure their substance abuse problem.

Answers and rationales for Review Questions appear in Appendix I.

Thinking Strategically About...

You are a recently licensed LPN/LVN working in a geriatric psychiatry (geropsych) unit in a skilled nursing facility. Today is your first day as charge nurse. Besides you, there is an LPN/LVN treatment nurse and an RN supervisor for the facility. There are four nursing assistants assigned to the 16 clients.

This is the status of the clients: Ten of the clients are in the dining hall awaiting breakfast. Three need to be fed in their rooms. One client, Agnes Reiker, is not feeling well, has a fever of 102, is not taking fluids, and is very congested. You are waiting for a call back from the physician to transfer the client to the hospital to rule out pneumonia. Regina Charles is crying that her mother left her last night and did not return. She is wandering in and out of rooms, calling for her mother. Terry Smyth is dressed and says he is going home. One of the CNAs is arguing with him, telling him that this is home and he is not going anywhere. (Actually, he is scheduled to leave on a day pass to attend his granddaughter's graduation.)

There are two empty beds on the unit, and the admission coordinator tells you that you will be getting two new admissions today: Joanna Wiley, age 70, who was diagnosed with bipolar depression 25 years ago and can no longer take care of herself; and Robert Sinclair, a retired 3-star general of the U.S. Army, who is 90 years old and thinks he has been assigned a new command. The admissions coordinator has warned you that the previous facility said he marched around giving everyone orders. They did not have the facilities to manage a geropsych client, so he is being transferred.

CRITICAL THINKING

- What information will you need to have before making assignments for the nursing assistants?
- If you use criteria other than just number of clients, how will you rationalize this to the nursing assistant who complains that he or she has more work than other CNAs?

PRIORITIZING NURSING CARE

In addition to charge nurse responsibilities, you will also be responsible for passing medications. How will you prioritize your responsibilities?

MANAGEMENT OF CARE

Which clients will you need to monitor closely? How often should you be monitoring the client with possible pneumonia?

DELEGATING

What tasks can be delegated to the nursing assistants? What follow-up will be necessary?

CLIENT TEACHING

Will any of the clients benefit by reality orientation? If so, how should this be accomplished?

CULTURAL CARE STRATEGIES

Three of the four regular CNAs are Filipino and speak to one another in Tagalog while feeding the clients in the dining hall. Is there a problem with this practice? If so, what is the best way to address it with them?

DOCUMENTING AND REPORTING

How does documentation and reporting differ in long-term care versus the acute care setting?

Given no other information about the clients, which ones would you think would require documentation from you today? Write a nurse's note on one or more of the clients who would require documentation today.

NURSING ASSESSMENT

Following the admission assessment of General Sinclair, what should the nurse do to collect further data about the client's mental status?

COMMUNICATION

Mrs. Santos is of Hispanic origin. She is one of the clients who is stable and is able to do her own care with assistance. She is eating in the dining room. Culturally Hispanics have a strong family connection. She wants to go home with them and feels she is able to baby-sit the grandchildren. Her family is very concerned for her welfare as well as the children's safety. They express their fears about taking her home. How could you, as the nurse, facilitate communication in order to relieve the family stress?

COLLABORATIVE CARE

The family feels strongly that they want to care for Mrs. Santos at home. A discharge planning conference is being convened. Your RN team leader has asked you to attend because you have a good relationship with the family and client. Also participating will be the RN, the diabetic educator, the psychiatric social worker, the home care nurse, and the physician. The son and daughter-in-law will also attend. As the LPN/LVN, what input could you give that would help with the transition from hospital to home?

Maternal-Newborn Nursing Care

UNIT IX

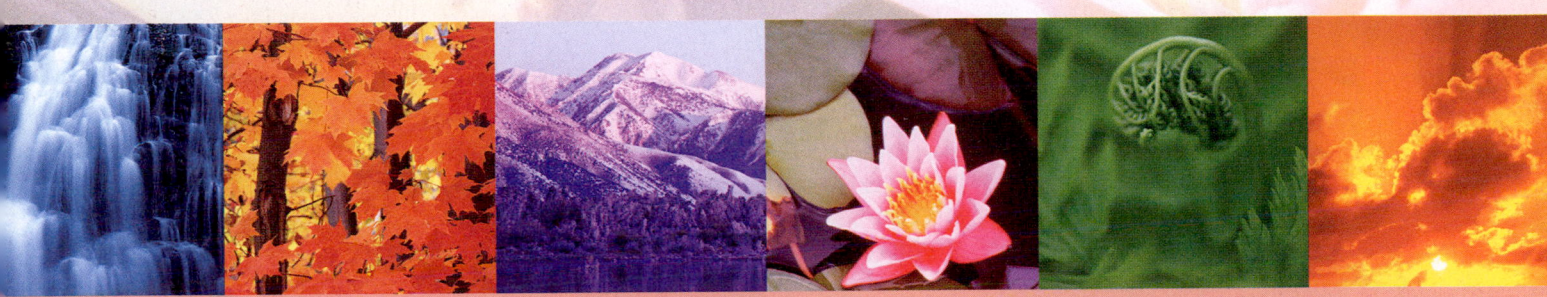

Care of Women during Normal Pregnancy

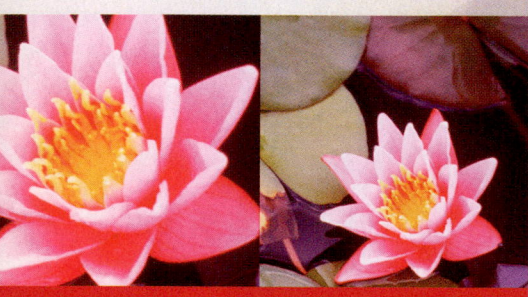

LEARNING Outcomes

After completing this chapter, you will be able to:

1. Identify concerns related to preconception care.
2. Describe fertilization and fetal development.
3. List signs of pregnancy and tests used to determine pregnancy.
4. Identify maternal changes throughout pregnancy.
5. Describe nursing care of a pregnant woman.
6. Discuss common maternal discomforts during pregnancy and their treatment.
7. Discuss client teaching related to prenatal care.
8. Contrast normal with warning signs found during pregnancy.
9. List steps in obtaining a fetal heart rate with Doppler ultrasound.
10. Identify ways to assist with fetal testing procedures.

Clinical Objectives

11. Teach the client how to alleviate the common discomforts of pregnancy.
12. Provide client teaching about the basic concepts of conception when appropriate.

KEY TERMS

Use the audio glossary feature on the MyNursingKit Website to hear the correct pronunciation of the following key terms.

Pregnancy is a powerful and complex time in a woman's life. The woman may be happily looking forward to the birth of a long-awaited first child. She may be wondering how to make adjustments for another of many children. She may be waiting fearfully through the period of pregnancy to give the baby up for adoption. In any case, she will face physical changes and processes that are unique and life altering.

The role of the nurse in caring for pregnant women involves a great deal of emotional support and client education. The nurse can have a powerful impact on the clients' experience, so that women leave the unit with increased self-esteem and stronger self-image.

Preconception

For many years, health professionals have recognized that a healthy pregnancy begins before conception with good health habits. The focus of preconception care is to help the couple identify their pregnancy risk and prepare for conception. Unhealthy lifestyle habits can affect the fetus before the mother even knows she is pregnant. Likewise, good eating patterns and regular exercise can promote early fetal health. Box 51-1 ■ provides a list of foods that are high in nutrients required by pregnant women.

To better understand pregnancy, it is important for the student to review male and female reproductive anatomy and physiology.

MALE CONTRIBUTION

The health of the fetus is not just related to the mother. For example, smoking decreases sperm production and motility. Men who have been exposed to industrial chemicals father more stillborn infants and infants who are small for gestational age. They are involved in more pregnancies that

---

BOX 51-1 | **NUTRITION THERAPY**

Food Sources of Iron, Folic Acid, and Vitamin B_{12}

Iron-Rich Foods
- Beef, chicken, pork loin, turkey, veal, egg yolk
- Bran flakes, oatmeal, brown rice, whole-grain breads
- Clams, oysters
- Dried beans
- Dried fruits
- Greens

Folic Acid Food Sources
- Asparagus, broccoli, green leafy vegetables
- Eggs, liver, milk, organ meats
- Kidney beans
- Wheat germ
- Yeast

Vitamin B_{12} Food Sources
- Eggs, cheese, milk
- Fresh shrimp and oysters
- Meats, organ meats (liver, kidney)

---

end in preterm labor or spontaneously abort. Because production of sperm (*spermatogenesis*) is a continuous process, men can decrease these risks by avoiding smoking and industrial chemicals for 3 to 4 months before conception. Scar tissue inside the vas deferens can block the transport of sperm to the outside. Formation of scar tissue often results from infection by chlamydia, gonorrhea, and other sexually transmitted infections. It is important for men to maintain a healthy lifestyle in order to father healthy children.

FEMALE CONTRIBUTION

To carry a pregnancy with minimal risk, the mother should develop a healthy lifestyle well before conception. A healthy lifestyle begins by eating a well-balanced diet that is low in fat and high in fiber. Because young women are often low in folic acid, a daily multiple vitamin supplement is recommended. Exercising at least three times per week strengthens the heart, helps control cholesterol levels, and is necessary for weight control. The healthy woman begins pregnancy within 15 pounds of her ideal weight. Because pregnancies are not always planned, avoiding unhealthy or risk-taking behavior will help to ensure a healthy infant.

NUTRITIONAL DEFICITS AND HARMFUL CHEMICALS

Smoking, alcohol consumption, and illicit drug use can have a negative effect on a pregnancy. Smoking during pregnancy can cause low birth weight and spontaneous abortion (discussed later). Alcohol, even in moderate amounts, may cause fetal alcohol syndrome, including craniofacial malformation and central nervous system dysfunction. Illicit drugs can cause a variety of anomalies. Infants born to drug-addicted mothers face a life of mental and emotional problems. Clients should be encouraged to stop using these substances prior to and during pregnancy. Some medications, including prescription, over-the-counter, and herbs may interfere with normal pregnancy and should be discussed with the healthcare provider.

A *teratogen* is any chemical that can cause abnormal development to the fetus. Drugs are one from of teratogen. To prevent teratogenic effects, the U.S. Food and Drug Administration (FDA) has established five categories of potential risk for the development of birth defects. Box 51-2 ■ identifies these categories. It is important to recall that herbal medicines are categorized as dietary supplements rather than drugs and therefore the testing, regulation, and standardization of herbs may not be as strict.

Infectious diseases and other disorders can have a negative impact on pregnancy. Routine testing should be done for infections like syphilis, gonorrhea, HIV, chlamydia, human papillomavirus, herpes simplex, and group B *Streptococcus*. See Chapter 41 ⚭ for a discussion of sexually transmitted infections. If

---

| BOX 51-2 | PREGNANCY CATEGORIES FOR MEDICATIONS |

Category A
- Studies do not show a risk to the fetus in the first trimester of pregnancy.
- There is no evidence of risk in the second and third trimesters.
- The possibility of fetal harm appears remote.

Category B
- Animal studies have not proved a risk to the fetus but there are no controlled studies in pregnant woman.
- Animal studies show adverse effects but controlled studies in pregnant woman have not shown risk to the human fetus.

Category C
- Animal studies show an adverse effect on the fetus but there are no controlled studies in humans.
- There are no studies in women or animals available.
- The drug may be used during pregnancy if the benefits of the drug outweigh its possible risks.

Category D
- Evidence shows a risk to the human fetus.
- The potential benefit from the use of the drug may outweigh the risk to the fetus.

Category X
- Studies in animals and humans prove fetal abnormalities, or reports indicate evidence of fetal risk.
- The risks of using these drugs clearly outweigh any possible benefits.

---

the client tests positive, treatment should begin as soon as possible. Infection of the fallopian tubes (**salpingitis**) can cause scarring and narrowing of the lumen. A narrow fallopian tube can lead to infertility or tubal pregnancy. See Chapter 40 ⚭ for disorders of the female reproductive system.

Fertilization and Fetal Development

Fertilization is the process of uniting a sperm and an ovum (egg), each containing 23 chromosomes to form one cell containing 46 chromosomes. **Pregnancy,** *prenatal period*, and *antepartum* are terms for carrying the resulting offspring in the uterus. Pregnancy can be described by a series of events that take place throughout the 40 weeks of intrauterine development.

FERTILIZATION

For pregnancy to occur, sperm from the male must be deposited near the cervix of the female. Although this most commonly occurs with coitus or copulation, sperm can also be deposited by artificial means. Once deposited, the *flagellation* (whip-like motion of the tail) propels the sperm through the mucus inside the cervix, through the uterus,

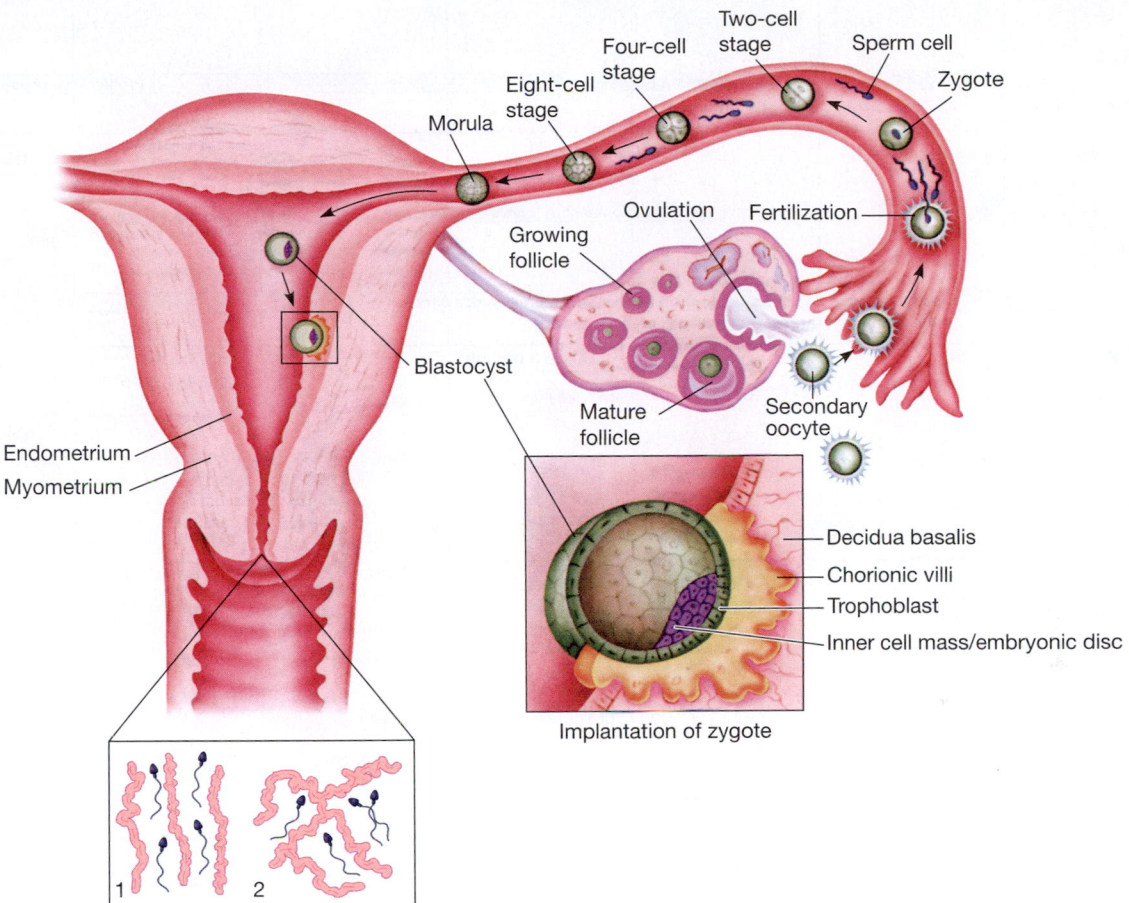

Figure 51-1. ■ Fertilization. During ovulation, the ovum leaves the ovary and enters the fallopian tube. Sperm pass more easily through cervical mucus during ovulation (see *inset 1*) than during the rest of the menstrual cycle (*inset 2*). Fertilization generally occurs in the outer third of the fallopian tube. Subsequent changes in the fertilized ovum from conception to implantation are depicted.

and down the fallopian tube. At the same time, the egg (ovum) must leave the ovary (ovulation) and travel through the fallopian tube (Figure 51-1 ■). The ovum and sperm usually unite in the outer one-third of the fallopian tube. Because sperm and ovum only remain viable for 24 to 36 hours, fertilization or **conception** (the uniting of ovum and sperm) is only possible for a short time.

The fertilized egg is called a **zygote.** The inner layer of the fallopian tube contains thousands of small cilia. The rhythmic movement of the cilia propels the zygote through the fallopian tube. Traveling through the fallopian tube, the zygote divides rapidly to form a many-celled, mulberry-shaped mass called a **morula.** By the time the morula reaches the uterus (4 to 5 days), the cells have formed a two-layer ball called a *blastocyst.* The outer layer (*trophoblast*) will become the placenta and fetal membranes. The inner layer of the blastocyst (*embryonic disk*) will become the **embryo.** By day 9 the blastocyst forms a yolk sac where primitive red blood cells are made until the liver is able to assume this function in week 6. Figure 51-2 ■ illustrates the weeks of embryonic development.

Implantation is the embedding of the blastocyst into the endometrium, or decidua. One area of the trophoblast

develops finger-like projections called *villi* (singular, *villus*) that secure the blastocyst to the uterus.

The villi begin producing the chemical **human chorionic gonadotropin** (hCG) 8 to 10 days after fertilization. The hormone hCG is very important to the success of the pregnancy because it maintains and stimulates the corpus luteum to continue producing estrogen and progesterone for another 11 to 12 weeks. If the corpus luteum stops functioning before the 11th week of pregnancy, spontaneous abortion occurs. By that time, the placenta is developed enough to produce estrogen and progesterone to maintain the pregnancy. In the male embryo, hCG stimulates the interstitial cells in the testes to produce testosterone. A small amount of testosterone causes the formation of male sex organs.

DEVELOPMENT OF SUPPORT STRUCTURES

Fetal Membranes

The chorionic villi develop into the placenta. The remainder of the trophoblast becomes the outer layer of the membranes called the **chorion.** The inner layer of the placenta,

MyNursingKit | Conception

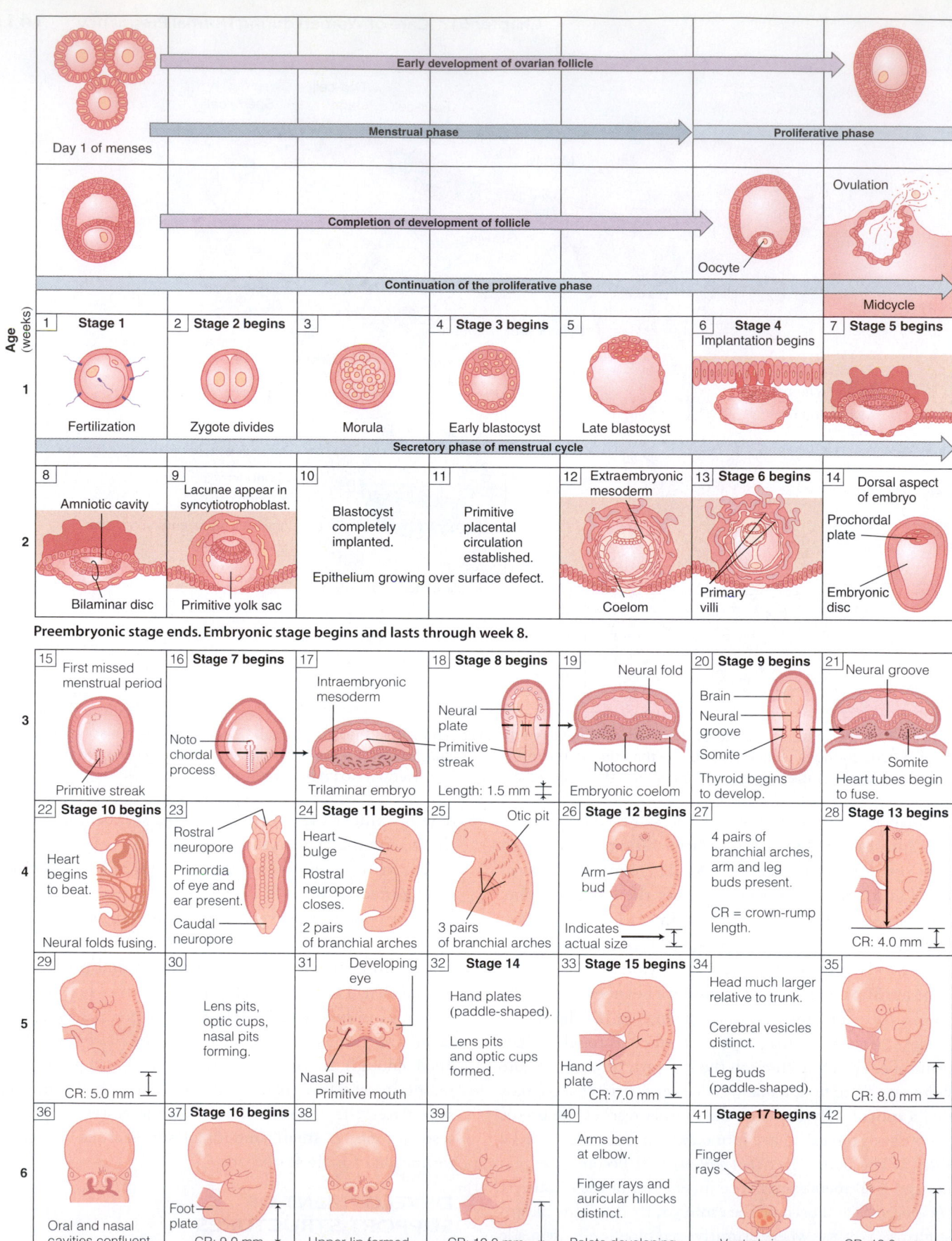

Figure 51-2. ■ **A.** Human prenatal development from conception through 10 weeks. **B.** Human fetal development: 12, 20, 24, and 30 weeks. (*Source*: A: Reprinted from Moore, K.L. [1989]. *The developing human: Clinically oriented embryology* [3rd ed.]. Philadelphia: W. B. Saunders, pp. 2–4, with permission from Elsevier, Inc.)

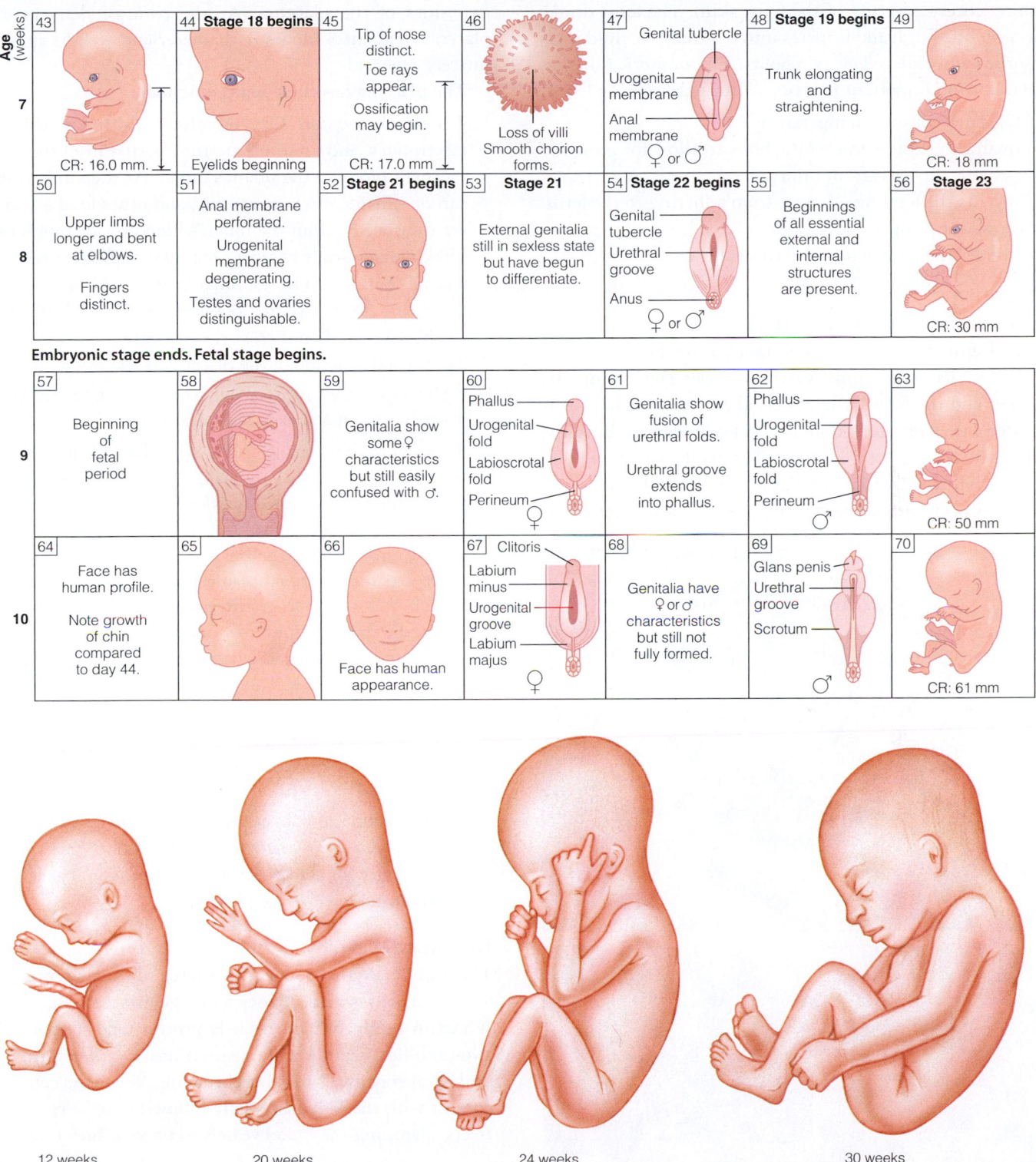

B   12 weeks   20 weeks   24 weeks   30 weeks

Figure 51-2. ■ *Continued.*

the **amnion,** originates from inside the blastocyst. The amnion grows as the fetus grows until it comes in contact with the chorion. Together the two layers form the fetal membranes, also called the *bag of waters.*

Amniotic Fluid

The amniotic fluid is formed by the amnion. About 98% of the amniotic fluid is water, but it also contains glucose, proteins, urea, **lanugo** (fine fetal hair), and **vernix caseosa** (white, cheesy covering of the fetus skin). The fetus drinks the amniotic fluid, and urinates into it. Amniotic fluid is re-absorbed and replaced every 3 hours. The amniotic fluid has the following important functions for the developing fetus:

- Maintains constant temperature.
- Equalizes pressure around the fetus to allow for growth.
- Cushions the fetus from injury.
- Prevents the fetal membranes from adhering to the fetus.
- Allows the fetus to move freely.
- Provides the fetus with fluid to swallow.

Placenta

By the third week after fertilization, the placenta has formed, but it is not fully functional until the 12th week. The placenta is a highly vascular organ connecting the mother and the fetus. The maternal side of the placenta is divided into irregular sections called **cotyledons.** Both the color and texture are like liver. The fetal side of the placenta is white and shiny; the large blood vessels leading to the umbilical cord are visible. Figure 51-3 ■ illustrates the

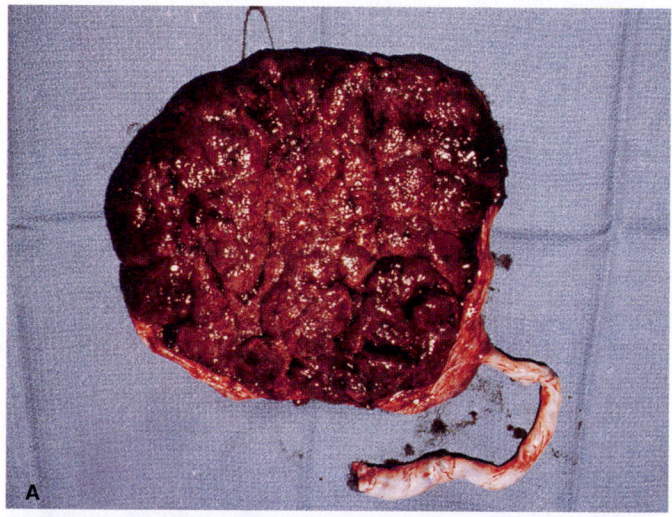

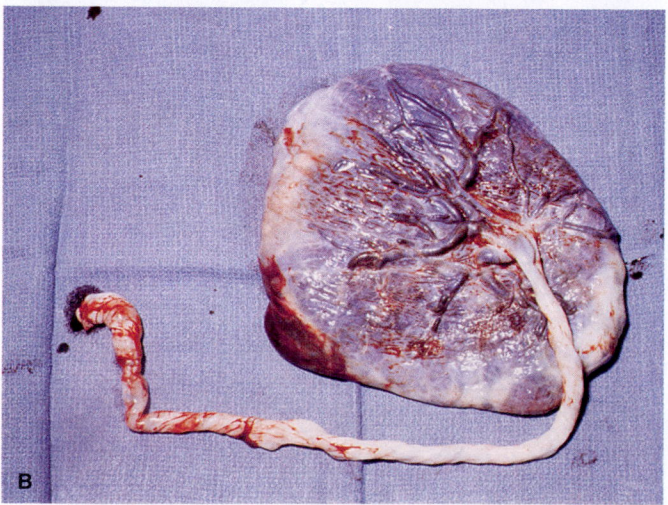

Figure 51-3. ■ Placenta. A. Maternal side. B. Fetal side. (*Source: Courtesy of Marcia London, RNC, MSN, NNP.*)

two sides of the placenta. At the time of delivery, the placenta is about 8 inches in diameter and weighs approximately 1 pound.

The placenta has three main functions:

1. The first is *transport*. Oxygen, glucose, amino acids, electrolytes, and vitamins are transported from the mother's blood to the infant's blood. At the same time, carbon dioxide, urea, creatinine, and other fetal waste are transported from the infant's blood to the mother's blood. Many drugs entering the maternal blood will also be transported to the infant's blood. Although chemicals are transported between mother and infant, the blood cells do not cross the placenta.

2. The second function of the placenta is *hormone production*.

   - *Human chorionic gonadotropin (hCG)*, the basis for pregnancy tests, has already been discussed.

   - *Human placental lactogen (hPL)* stimulates changes in maternal metabolism. This change makes protein, glucose, and minerals more readily available to the fetus. Human placental lactogen is an insulin antagonist; thus, it decreases maternal metabolism of glucose. The mother's body prepares for lactation because of an increase in hPL. The placenta also produces estrogen and progesterone to maintain the endometrium, to stimulate breast development, and to prevent uterine contractions.

   - **Relaxin** is a hormone produced by the placenta that causes softening in the collagen connective tissue of the symphysis pubis and sacroiliac joints. In late pregnancy, these joints become movable, making a larger passageway for the delivery.

3. The third function of the placenta is *production of fatty acids, glycogen, and cholesterol for fetal use*. Enzymes that are necessary for the transport of nutrients to the fetus are also produced by the placenta.

Umbilical Cord

The **umbilical cord** connects the fetus to the placenta. The umbilical cord is made up of a white gelatinous tissue called **Wharton's jelly.** Wharton's jelly protects and supports the two umbilical arteries and one umbilical vein. At term, the umbilical cord is 22 to 24 inches long. When air comes in contact with the Wharton's jelly following delivery, it contracts, clamping the blood vessels to prevent bleeding.

FETAL DEVELOPMENT

Fetal development or gestation is marked in the weeks following conception. Fetal development takes place in three stages:

- Stage I, called the *preembryonic stage*, is from fertilization through 14 days. This is the time when the fertilized ovum travels through the fallopian tube, differentiates into trophoblast and embryonic disk, and attaches to the endometrium.

- Stage II, the *embryonic stage*, is from weeks 3 through 8 (see Figure 51-2). During this stage, all body systems are formed. If the mother consumes any teratogenic chemical during this time, there is great risk of fetal anomalies or malformation.
- Stage III, the *fetal stage*, is from weeks 9 through weeks 38 to 40. During this stage, all body systems are refined and begin to function. Some body systems will take several years to reach their maximum functioning. Consumption of harmful chemicals at this time could result in delayed or abnormal functioning of body systems.

The embryonic disk (Stage I) forms three germ layers from which all body systems develop. Table 51-1 ■ identifies the three germ layers and the body systems derived from each. Development is very systematic, occurring from head to toe (*cephalocaudal*), from proximal to distal, and from general to specific.

Cardiovascular System

The cardiovascular system begins by the development of a series of a tubes, carrying a primitive blood. On day 21, one area of a vessel begins to beat. This area will develop into the heart through a series of foldings, openings, and closings. Most heart anomalies occur during weeks 6 to 8. (See discussion of congenital heart defects in Chapter 57 ⭗ .)

Because circulation in the fetus must carry blood to and from the placenta, and because the fetal respiratory system does not oxygenate blood, several structures are different in the fetus than in the adult. Blood flows from the internal iliac arteries in the fetus to the placenta through two *umbilical arteries*. In the placenta, blood gases are exchanged, waste is removed, and nutrients are received. The fetal blood then flows back to the fetus through one *umbilical vein*. After

TABLE 51-1	Germ Layers
EMBRYONIC (GERM) LAYER	**BODY SYSTEMS**
Endoderm (inner layer)	Respiratory system
	Gastrointestinal system, liver, pancreas
	Bladder and urethra
Mesoderm (middle layer)	Muscular system
	Skeletal system
	Heart, blood, and blood vessels
	Spleen
	Urinary
	Reproductive
Ectoderm (outer layer)	Skin
	Nervous system
	Sense organs
	Mouth and anus

entering the fetal abdomen, the umbilical vein divides into two branches. The umbilical vein carries blood to the fetal liver. The other branch, the **ductus venosus,** carries blood to the inferior vena cava.

Two structures limit the amount of blood going to the fetal lungs. Inside the fetal heart, the **foramen ovale** is an opening in the septum between the right atrium and left atrium. The higher pressure in the right atrium pushes some blood through the foramen ovale into the left atrium. Outside the fetal heart, the **ductus arteriosus** connects the main pulmonary artery to the aorta. Some blood flows from the pulmonary artery to the aorta, thus bypassing the lungs. The small amount of blood actually reaching the lungs is necessary for the development of the respiratory system. Figure 51-4 ■ illustrates fetal circulation. Usually, shortly after birth, these fetal structures close, and the cardiovascular system adjusts to normal functioning.

Fetal blood is initially formed on day 14 in the yolk sac. The liver will not be able to make blood cells until the 6th week, and the bone marrow will not function until the 10th week. Fetal hemoglobin (HgbF) has a greater attraction for oxygen, ensuring that the fetus receives adequate oxygenation. The blood type is determined at the time of conception.

Respiratory System

The respiratory system begins as lung buds during the 6th week of development, and is formed by the 23rd week, but there are not enough alveoli to maintain gas exchange outside the uterus. By weeks 20 to 23 the primitive lungs begin to produce surfactant. *Surfactant* decreases the surface tension of fluid inside the alveoli. By the 24th week, the lungs are capable of borderline support outside the uterus. Therefore, the age of **viability,** or the ability to live outside the uterus, is 24 weeks. An infant born at this time would require intensive nursing care, including ventilation support. Surfactant production matures by the 35th week and the prognosis is more favorable for a baby born after this time. The lungs will continue to add alveoli until adulthood.

Nervous System

The head and brain develop rapidly in the fetus. The brain and spinal column form in the first 25 days after conception. For proper brain formation and spinal column closure, the mother must consume an adequate amount of folic acid. By the 4th week the brain has differentiated into lobes. A week later the cranial nerves are present and function. By the 6th week, the entire central nervous system is present. The peripheral nervous system, however, will not function completely for another 7 to 10 years.

Special Senses

The ears begin to form in the 3rd week, low on the head in the region of the lower jaw. They gradually move upward to

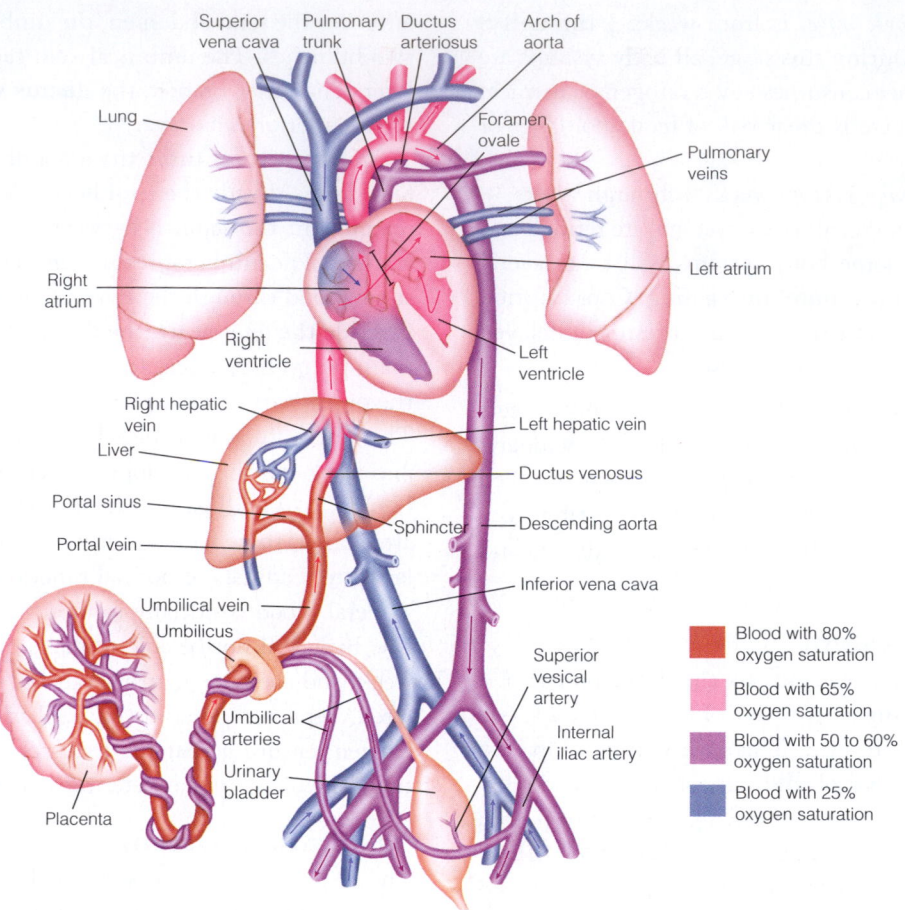

Figure 51-4. ■ Fetal circulation. Blood leaves the placenta and enters the fetus through the umbilical vein. After circulating through the fetus, the blood returns to the placenta through the umbilical arteries. The ductus venosus, the foramen ovale, and the ductus arteriosus allow the blood to bypass the fetal liver and lungs.

their designated place on the head by the 8th week. The fetus can hear and respond to sound by the 12th week.

In the 3rd week the eyes can be seen as large dark disks on the side of the developing head. By the 7th week, eyelids form and seal to protect the developing retina (Figure 51-5 ■). A week later the eyes have moved to the front of the face. The eyelids remain closed until the 28th week of development.

Gastrointestinal System

The gastrointestinal system begins formation in the 4th week. The esophagus, stomach, small intestines, liver, pancreas, and most of the colon are developed from the same germ layer, the endoderm (see Table 51-1). The oral cavity, pharynx, and anus are formed from the ectoderm. Occasionally there is incomplete development in the area where the germ layers meet, resulting in congenital anomalies.

By the 12th week, the fetus swallows amniotic fluid, and the liver makes bile. In the 16th week, **meconium** (the first fetal stool) is made from amniotic fluid, bile, and epithelial cells. Meconium should remain in the colon until after delivery. The passage of meconium prior to delivery signals there has been some type of fetal distress that can cause respiratory problems for the newborn.

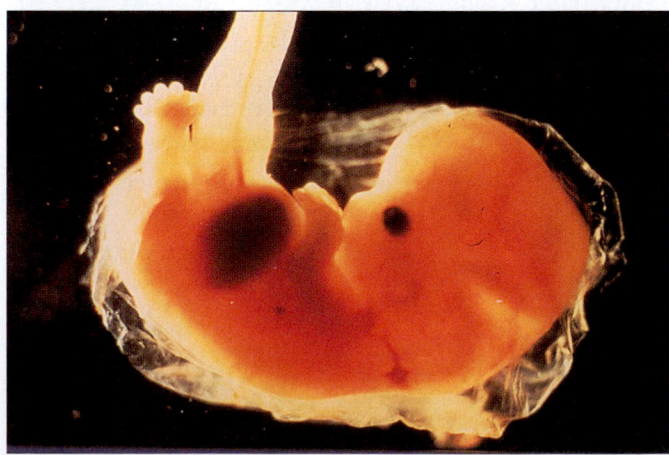

Figure 51-5. ■ The embryo at 7 weeks. The head is round and nearly erect. The eyes have shifted forward and are closer together. The eyelids begin to form.

Urinary System

The urinary system is another system that develops from more than one germ layer (refer to Table 51-1). The kidneys, ureters, and the *trigone*, or lower section of the bladder, develop from the mesoderm. The remainder of the bladder, female urethra, and proximal male urethra develop from the endoderm. The distal male urethra develops from the ectoderm. Any disruption in the development can result in complex anomalies. (See urinary system disorders in Chapter 39 ⌘.)

The kidneys are developed in several stages in the pelvis and ascend to their normal location. The kidneys begin producing urine in the 10th week, and the fetus urinates in the amniotic fluid by the 11th week of development.

Reproductive System

The sex of the fetus is determined at conception. The fetus develops undifferentiated gonads until the 7th week. In the presence of the Y chromosome, testosterone stimulates the gonads to differentiate into testes. Sperm will not be produced until puberty. Testosterone will also stimulate the development of male genitalia. Without testosterone, the gonads develop into ovaries and female genitalia will be formed. Ova will be produced and will remain in the ovaries until puberty. External male and female genitalia can be identified in the 12th week of development.

Musculoskeletal System

Limb buds appear in the 4th week. Cartilage forms a primitive skeleton covered by muscles by the 6th week. A week later fetal movement can be seen on ultrasound, but **quickening,** or the first fetal movements felt by the mother, will not occur until the 16th to 20th week. By the end of the 8th week, ossification in the bones begins, marking the transition from embryo to fetus.

Integumentary System

The skin of the fetus is thin and pink. Lacking fat until the last 4 to 6 weeks, the blood vessels can readily be seen. Fingernails and toenails reach the end of the digit by the 36th week. Lanugo begins to disappear in the 28th week, leaving only hair on the scalp and at times the shoulders and upper back at birth. *Vernix caseosa* covers the skin and protects it from the amniotic fluid. This white cheesy substance is gradually absorbed by the skin, leaving a small amount in the body folds and the lower back. Skin color is determined at conception.

Signs of Pregnancy

During pregnancy, many physiologic changes will be reported by the mother or observed by the healthcare provider. These changes can be categorized by presumptive, probable, and positive signs of pregnancy.

PRESUMPTIVE SIGNS

The subjective signs the mother experiences during pregnancy are **presumptive signs.** They may be indicators of other conditions besides pregnancy, so they are not diagnostic in nature. Presumptive signs include:

- *Amenorrhea:* Absence of menses, or amenorrhea, is usually the first sign a woman notices that may cause her to think she is pregnant. Although pregnancy is the most common cause of amenorrhea, other causes could be hormone imbalance, stress, menopause, or tumors.
- *Nausea and vomiting:* Usually occurring in the morning, but could occur any time, nausea and vomiting are commonly experienced during early pregnancy. Nausea and vomiting are associated with many other conditions as well.
- *Breast changes:* Tenderness, tingling, and enlargement of the breast occurs in early pregnancy. Many women also experience these changes with the monthly period.
- *Urinary frequency:* The enlarging uterus pressing on the bladder gives the woman the feeling of needing to urinate often. Other disorders including urinary infection and abdominal tumor could also elicit this sensation.
- *Fatigue:* Fatigue is most often noted in the first few months of pregnancy, but it could occur for many reasons.
- *Abdominal enlargement:* Abdominal enlargement is noted by the 12th week, but may be earlier in the very thin woman or later in the large woman. Abdominal enlargement may also be noted when tumors are present.
- *Quickening:* Quickening is a fluttering sensation felt as the fetus moves. The sensation begins between 16 and 20 weeks and gradually becomes stronger and more frequent. Other things, such as muscle twitch or intestinal gas can mimic this sensation. Because the mother is experiencing this subjective sensation, quickening is a presumptive sign.

Pregnancy is usually diagnosed before the woman experiences all of the presumptive signs. Denial of pregnancy could keep the woman from noticing the presumptive signs. False pregnancy, also known as **pseudopregnancy,** occurs when the nonpregnant woman so strongly wants to be pregnant that she experiences the presumptive signs. Treatment of pseudopregnancy is by psychiatric means.

PROBABLE SIGNS

The healthcare provider can identify objective signs that could indicate pregnancy. Because these signs could also indicate other conditions, they are not diagnostic. Probable signs include:

- *Positive pregnancy test:* Pregnancy tests screen for the presence of hCG in the urine or blood. Most home tests are based on the amount of hCG in the urine. A test may be positive 8 to 14 days after conception. Some medication, the timing and accuracy of specimen collection, and the presence of hormone-producing tumors can affect the accuracy of the test.

- *Ballottement:* If the examiner puts two fingers into the vagina and pushes upward on the uterus, the fetus will rebound against the fingers. This rebounding is known as **ballottement.** A tumor floating in the uterus could elicit the same response.
- *Uterine changes:* Hegar's sign, Goodell's sign, and Chadwick's sign (discussed below under Maternal Changes) can be observed in the first few weeks of pregnancy. The fundus of the uterus can be palpated just above the pubis at 12 weeks. Tumors can also cause uterine enlargement.

When probable signs are combined with presumptive signs, there is a strong indication of pregnancy.

POSITIVE SIGNS

Positive signs are diagnostic of pregnancy. No other condition can cause these signs. Positive signs of pregnancy include:

- *Hearing fetal heart tones: Fetal heart tones* (FHT), or the fetal heartbeat, can be heard with a Doppler by 10 to 12 weeks of conception (Figure 51-6 ■). Doppler is discussed in Procedure 51-1 ■ later in this chapter. The normal fetal heart rate is 120 to 150 beats per minute (bpm). It is important to distinguish the fetal heart rate from the maternal heart rate. When auscultating the abdomen, a soft blowing sound can be heard. The sound occurring at the same rate as the maternal pulse is called **uterine soufflé** and is caused by increased maternal blood flow to the uterus. The sound occurring at the fetal heart rate is called **funic soufflé** and is caused by fetal blood flowing through the umbilical cord.
- *Visualization of the fetus:* An abdominal ultrasound can detect a pregnancy by the 6th week. An endovaginal ultrasound can detect a trophoblast by the 10th day after

conception. X-ray examination of the pelvis is rarely done due to the risk of radiation exposure to the fetus and maternal reproductive organs.

- *Fetal movement felt by examiner:* The fetus usually does not kick strongly enough for the examiner to feel the movement until the 15th to 16th week.

DIAGNOSTIC TESTS

A variety of tests can be used to assess fetal well-being. *Ultrasound* is used to outline the shape of various organs. Not only is ultrasound used to diagnose pregnancy, but it can also be used to identify some developmental anomalies. *Note:* Some women choose not to have prenatal testing for religious or ethical reasons. For example, a woman may refuse testing on the grounds that a positive result could indicate an abnormality in the fetus and possibly cause the healthcare provider to recommend abortion. The nurse plays an important role as client advocate. In some cases this means supporting the woman's right to refuse testing.

Amniocentesis, the withdrawal of amniotic fluid through a needle inserted into the abdomen and the uterus, is a means of gathering data about the developing fetus. The amniotic fluid and fetal cells contained in the fluid are studied to determine genetic abnormalities, maternal–fetal blood incompatibilities, and the maturity of the fetal lungs. Procedure 51-2 ■ later in this chapter describes the nurse's role in assisting with an amniocentesis and similar tests.

A **nonstress test** (NST) is used to assess fetal movement and fetal heart rate. External fetal monitoring equipment is attached to the client's abdomen and the fetal heart rate is recorded. The client identifies fetal movement. Fetal movement can be stimulated with a low-frequency vibrator. The test is reactive or normal if two episodes of the fetal heart rate increasing by 15 bpm and lasting 15 seconds occur in a 20-minute period.

Biophysical profile is used to assess five variables: fetal breathing, fetal movement, fetal tone, fluid volume, and fetal reaction. To complete a biophysical profile, a combination of ultrasound and NST is used. While an LPN/LVN can be taught to collect the data, a trained registered nurse or physician will interpret the data. A score of 8 or more indicates positive fetal well-being.

Maternal Changes during Pregnancy

Typically, the progression of the pregnancy is described in 3-month blocks of time called **trimesters.** This might seem confusing when fetal development is described by weeks. A normal pregnancy is divided into three trimesters equaling 9 calendar months, or 40 weeks equaling 10 lunar months.

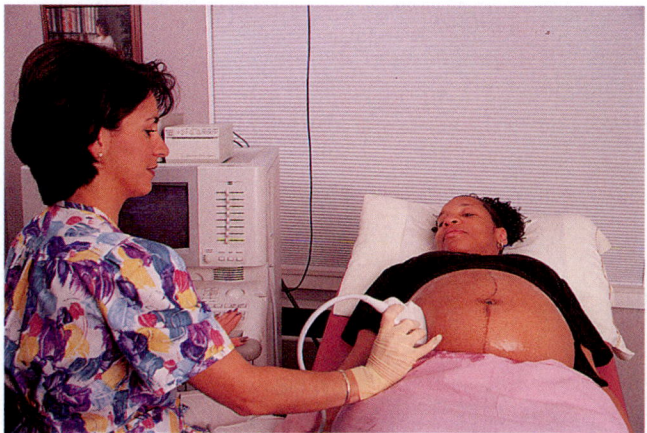

Figure 51-6. ■ Ultrasound scanning permits visualization of the fetus *in utero.* The woman may experience some discomfort as the probe moves over a full bladder.

Pregnancy causes many changes and additional work in each body system. A healthy woman's body can tolerate the additional work, but if disease is present, the additional stress may be harmful or life threatening to the mother.

REPRODUCTIVE SYSTEM

The most obvious changes occur in the reproductive system. Prior to pregnancy, the uterus is a small, pear-shaped, thick-walled organ weighing 60 g (2 oz) with a capacity of 10 mL. By the end of pregnancy, the uterus is a large, thin-walled organ weighing 2 pounds with a capacity of 5 L. The structure of the three muscle layers of the uterus allows the uterus to expand evenly in all directions. Painless contractions called **Braxton-Hicks contractions** occur throughout the pregnancy, but become more noticeable after the 20th week and during periods of rapid fetal growth.

The cervix secretes thick, sticky mucus that plugs the os to prevent microorganisms from entering the uterus. When the cervix dilates prior to delivery, the mucous plug is expelled. Certain signs develop in the presence of estrogen and are present by the 8th week (Figure 51-7 ■):

- **Hegar's sign,** softening of the lower uterine segment
- **Goodell's sign,** a softening of the cervix
- **Chadwick's sign,** a bluish-purple discoloration of the cervix and vagina

The ovaries do not release ova during pregnancy. The corpus luteum produces estrogen and progesterone for approximately 12 weeks until the placenta takes over this function. Ovulation usually returns within 3 months following delivery.

The breasts enlarge due to hormonal influence. The areolae darken, and the nipple becomes more erect. **Colostrum,** a yellowish fluid rich in antibodies, is secreted in the last trimester and the first few days following delivery. The colostrum will be replaced with milk.

CARDIOVASCULAR SYSTEM

The mother's pulse rate increases by 10 to 15 beats per minute by the end of pregnancy. Cardiac output also increases, and there is an increased blood flow to the uterus and kidneys. The blood pressure decreases slightly in the second trimester due to the influence of progesterone on the smooth muscles of blood vessels, but returns to normal during the third trimester.

clinical ALERT

Any increase in blood pressure above the normal range should be monitored and reported to the healthcare provider.

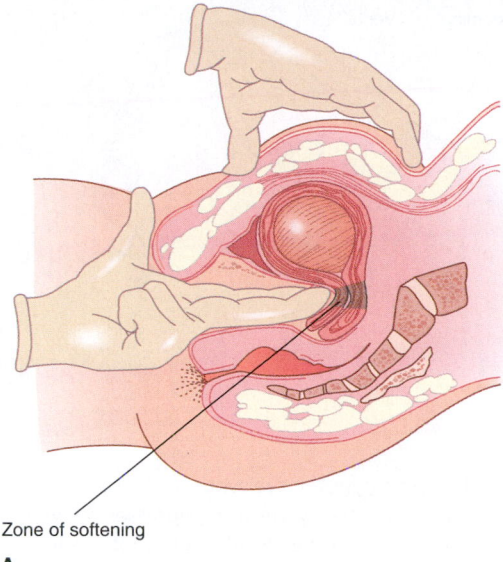

Zone of softening

A

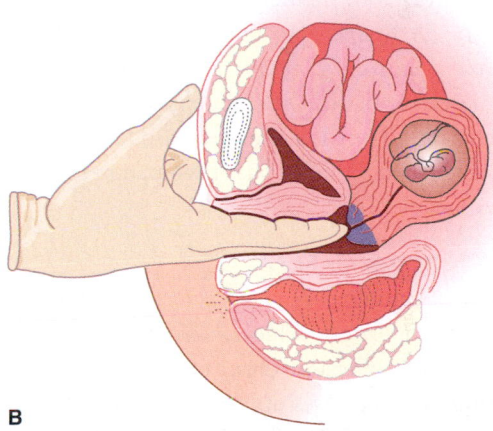

B

Figure 51-7. ■ A. Hegar's sign. **B.** Goodell's sign and Chadwick's sign. (*Source:* Reproduced, with permission, from McGraw Hill Companies, Inc. DeCherney, A. H., & Pernoll. M. L. [1994]. *Current obstetric and gynecologic diagnosis and treatment* [8th ed.]. Norwalk, CT: Appleton & Lange, p. 187.)

Supine Hypotensive Syndrome

The enlarging uterus puts pressure on the deep veins of the pelvis, resulting in venous stasis in the lower extremities. Venous stasis often leads to dependent edema and varicose veins of the legs, vulva, and rectum. *Supine hypotensive syndrome* occurs when the mother lies supine. The heavy uterus presses on the inferior vena cava (Figure 51-8 ■), resulting in reduced blood flow back to the right atrium. The mother will experience low blood pressure, dizziness, and pale skin. The mother should be encouraged to sleep on her side to prevent hypotension.

Physiologic Anemia of Pregnancy

There is an increase in blood volume during pregnancy. The red blood cell count is only slightly elevated, but there is an increase in plasma volume. *Physiologic anemia of*

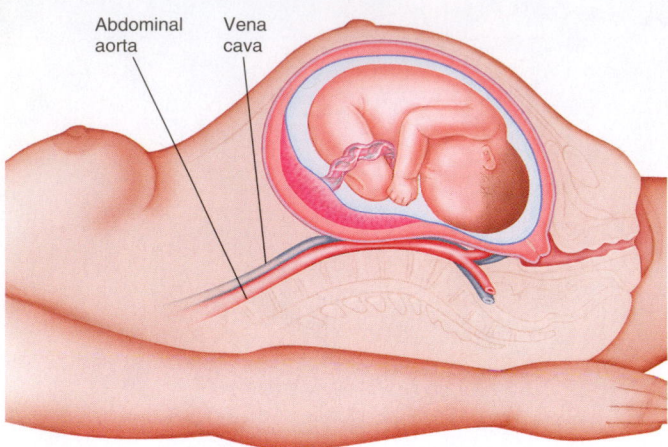

Figure 51-8. ■ Supine hypotensive syndrome. When the woman lies on her back, the large, heavy uterus compresses the vena cava and abdominal aorta against the spinal column, interfering with circulation.

pregnancy results from hemodilution as evidenced by a hematocrit of 34% to 40%. The number of white blood cells increases beginning in the second trimester. An increase in platelets, fibrin, fibrinogen, and other coagulation factors coupled with venous stasis increases the risk of thrombus formation. The pregnant woman needs increased iron to prevent anemia.

RESPIRATORY SYSTEM

Pregnancy causes an increase in oxygen consumption and demand in the heart, lungs, kidneys, uterus, and other organs. It also causes some physical changes that affect breathing. The enlarging uterus presses upward on the diaphragm. The ribs move outward and the diameter of the chest increases. Progesterone relaxes smooth muscles, decreases airway resistance and, hence, allows more oxygen into the lungs. Estrogen may cause swelling of the nasal mucosa. Some women experience epistaxis (see also Chapter 32 ⦾).

URINARY SYSTEM

In the first trimester, urinary frequency is caused by the enlarging uterus pressing on the bladder. During the second trimester, the uterus has elevated out of the pelvis and the pressure on the bladder is relieved. In the third trimester, the infant descends into the pelvis, again pressing on the bladder.

Glomerular infiltration and tubular reabsorption increase to remove the added waste products from the fetus. If the kidneys are unable to reabsorb all of the glucose, glycosuria will result.

clinical ALERT

Any amount of glucose over a trace amount should be reported to the healthcare provider.

GASTROINTESTINAL SYSTEM

"Morning sickness," usually beginning in the 6th week and ending in the 12th week, results from an increase in progesterone. Nausea and vomiting can range from mild to severe and can occur at any time of the day. Prolonged, excessive vomiting, or **hyperemesis gravidarum,** leads to dehydration and electrolyte imbalance. It should be reported to the healthcare provider. (See Chapter 52 ⦾ for a discussion on hyperemesis gravidarum.) Relaxation of the cardiac sphincter can cause gastric reflux. Medication may be prescribed for these discomforts.

The enlarging uterus puts pressure on the stomach and intestines. Progesterone relaxes the smooth muscle of the intestine, resulting in a decrease in peristalsis. Together these two factors result in constipation. Pregnant women should be taught to eat a diet high in fiber (fresh fruits and vegetables).

MUSCULOSKELETAL SYSTEM

The increased size and weight of the uterus cause an alteration in the mother's center of gravity. To compensate, the mother increases the lumbar curve (*lordosis*) and widens her stance. The pelvic joints become more relaxed in preparation for childbirth. These factors result in low backache and waddling gait.

Muscle cramps, especially in the lower legs, result from venous stasis and possible electrolyte imbalance. Low calcium and phosphorous levels are the most common cause. The mother should be encouraged to consume adequate amounts of milk or other calcium-rich products.

INTEGUMENTARY SYSTEM

Changes in skin color result from an increase in maternal hormones. The areolae, nipples, and vulva darken. **Linea nigra** is a dark line on the abdomen from the umbilicus to the pubis. **Chloasma,** or "mask of pregnancy," is a darkening of the forehead, cheeks, and around the eyes. Both are more obvious in later pregnancy.

Striae gravidarum, or "stretch marks," occur when the underlying connective tissue separates during periods of rapid growth. Following pregnancy, these dark red streaks gradually lighten and become white, but they will never disappear.

ENDOCRINE SYSTEM

Prolactin, from the anterior pituitary gland, stimulates the production of milk by the mammary glands. Oxytocin, from the posterior pituitary gland, stimulates uterine contractions, and the **let-down reflex,** or release of milk after delivery.

The placenta hormones are insulin antagonists, which means they counteract insulin. This results in the islets of Langerhans needing to produce more insulin to meet the mother's requirements. If the mother is marginal in meeting the need for more insulin, gestational diabetes results.

NURSING CARE

PRIORITIZING NURSING CARE

Research has shown that prenatal care, beginning as soon as possible, has a dramatic effect on the outcome of the pregnancy (Box 51-3 ■). The goals of prenatal care include:

- A healthy, prepared mother who has minimal discomforts during the pregnancy
- The safe delivery of a healthy fetus
- A prepared family, including father or partner, siblings, grandparents, and any significant others

When caring for clients who are pregnant, focus on early detection of complications and client teaching. Every pregnancy is different, so even multiparas may need instruction and guidance. Instruct clients about signs and symptoms to report immediately such as bleeding, significant cramping, pain, and lack of fetal movement. Instruct clients to observe and report signs and symptoms of preeclampsia such as swelling in the ankles, hands, and face, blurred vision or double vision, and fainting. Encourage clients to make healthy choices for themselves and their babies. Keep in mind that many times women get misinformation from friends and relatives during their pregnancy. Answer questions kindly and listen to fears and concerns patiently. Reassure clients regarding usual feelings and discomforts during pregnancy.

BOX 51-3	CULTURAL PULSE POINTS

Views on Prenatal Care

Western medicine places high value on prenatal care. A frequent complaint of labor and delivery nurses is the lack of prenatal care by many mothers-to-be from other cultures. Many Americans view pregnancy and childbirth as a medical condition and begin to be followed by a physician almost from the day they discover they are pregnant. Women from other cultures, Hispanic as an example, view pregnancy as a normal condition; they do not feel that consultation with a physician is necessary. They depend on older women to supply them with the information and support they need. If the woman does seek prenatal care, it is important to stress the need to continue to see the physician especially if the mother is considered to be a high-risk client.

ASSESSING

The assessment of the pregnant family includes collecting physical data, determining the psychologic response to pregnancy, and evaluating family functioning.

Initial Visit

The initial visit to a healthcare provider can be happy or sad depending on the woman's feelings about being pregnant. A comfortable environment, open communication, and the nurse's attitude are important in putting the woman at ease. At times the father or partner attends the initial visit, and the degree of support from this person should be assessed.

The initial visit is generally longer than subsequent visits. Unless a health history has been obtained prior to pregnancy, it must be done at this time. The health history includes identifying all past medical and health issues that could have an impact on the pregnancy. This includes smoking, use of alcohol or other substances, history of infection (especially sexually transmitted infections), and other factors.

A menstrual history will be obtained including any past pregnancies. (Table 51-2 ■ identifies descriptive terms used to refer to pregnancy.) The woman's gravida, para, the number of deliveries after 24 weeks gestation, and the outcome of past pregnancies will be recorded. Possible outcomes include abortion, preterm, term, postterm, and whether the infant lived. It is important to remember that the word *abortion* is used medically to describe the loss of a pregnancy, whether that is a planned event or a spontaneous occurrence (miscarriage).

A physical assessment, done by the healthcare provider, will include a detailed assessment of the reproductive organs. In most cases, the nurse is present during the physical assessment. This is especially true when the healthcare provider is male. The role of the nurse in this situation is to provide reassurance to the client and to act as a witness of events occurring during the exam. (The nurse's presence also decreases the possibility of accusations of sexual misconduct.)

An ultrasound may be performed to diagnose pregnancy. Blood may be drawn to determine a baseline for future reference.

If pregnancy is diagnosed, the duration of pregnancy will be determined. The *estimated date of delivery* (EDD), the *estimated date of birth* (EDB), or the *estimated date of confinement* (EDC) are terms used to refer to the expected delivery date. The EDD can be determined by several methods. Naegele's rule is the most common. To apply the rule, take the first day of the last menstrual period (LMP), subtract 3 months, and add 7 days. If the LMP were on January 18, the EDD would be October 25. Adjustments to the rule would have to be made if the LMP were July 29. Subtracting 3 months would

TABLE 51-2	Common Terms in Pregnancy
TERM	**DEFINITION**
Abortion	Expulsion from the uterus of an embryo or fetus prior to the stage of viability at about 20 weeks of gestation. May be either spontaneous (occurring from natural causes, commonly called a *miscarriage*) or induced (artificial or therapeutic)
Gravida	A pregnant woman
Multigravida	A woman who has been pregnant several times
Multipara	A woman who has had two or more pregnancies that resulted in viable fetuses, whether or not the offspring were alive at birth
Nulligravida	A woman who has never conceived
Nullipara	A woman who has never borne a viable child
Para	A woman who has produced viable young whether the child was living at birth
Postterm	Delivery after 42 weeks of pregnancy
Preterm	Delivery after 24 weeks and before 38 weeks of pregnancy
Primigravida	A woman pregnant for the first time
Primipara	A woman who has had one pregnancy that resulted in a viable child, regardless of whether the child was living at birth, and regardless of whether it was a single or multiple birth
Term	The period of pregnancy between 38 and 42 weeks gestation

be April, and adding 7 days would be the 36th. April has only 30 days so the EDD would be advanced to May 6. A gestational wheel or chart can be used for quick reference. Figure 51-9 ■ illustrates a gestational wheel that provides expected dates for other pregnancy landmarks as well as the EDD.

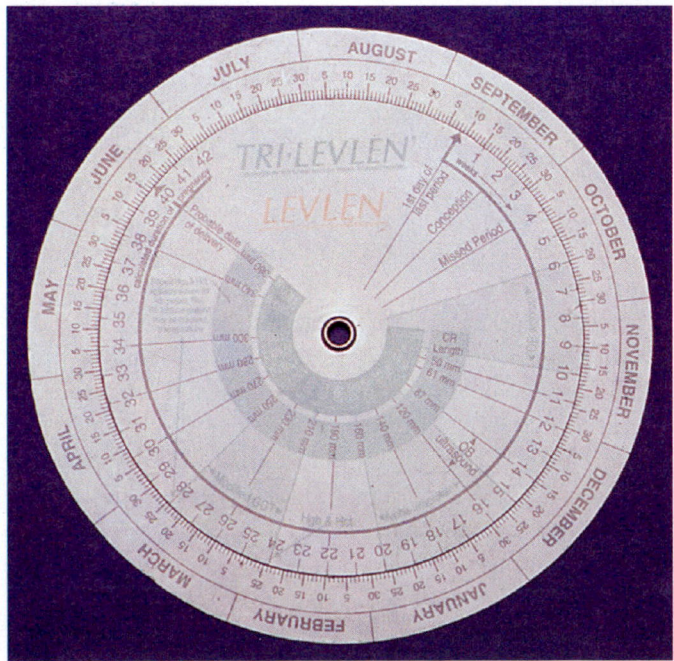

Figure 51-9. ■ EDB (estimated date of birth) wheel can be used to calculate the due date. To use it, place the "last menses began" arrow on the date of the woman's last menstrual period (LMP). Then read the "EDB date" at the arrow labeled 40. In this case, the LMP is September 8 and the EDB is June 17. (*Source:* © Elena Dorfman.)

Follow-Up Visits

The pregnant woman should return to the clinic for follow-up care on a routine basis. The following schedule is a common one:

- Every 4 weeks for the first 28 weeks
- Every 2 weeks during weeks 29 to 36
- Every week after 36 weeks until delivery

If complications develop, more frequent visits will be needed.

During the follow-up visits, the following subjective data should be collected:

- How the client is feeling
- Any discomforts, concerns, questions the client may have
- How the client and family members are coping with the pregnancy (*Note:* Incidents of domestic abuse occur more commonly among pregnant women than otherwise. It is important to be vigilant to possible signs of domestic abuse and to report them immediately to the supervising RN.)

Objective data should be collected and compared with previous data. Objective data include:

- *Blood pressure:* A blood pressure increase of 30 mm Hg systolic and 20 mm Hg diastolic over previous measurement should be reported to the healthcare provider. If a previous blood pressure measurement is not available, a recording of 140/90 or higher should be reported.
- *Weight:* Total weight gain during pregnancy should be 25 to 35 pounds, with the most rapid weight gain being the last half of the pregnancy. From weeks 1 to 12, the client

should gain 3 to 4 pounds. From weeks 13 to 40, she should gain 1 pound per week. Weight gain less than this could indicate poor nutrition and low fetal growth. A weight gain of more than this could indicate improper nutrition or fluid retention.

- *Fundal measurement:* The height of the fundus above the pubis is measured in centimeters. This measurement is compared to previous measurements and the weeks of gestation. The fundus should enlarge 1 cm per week. The fundus not enlarging at this rate would indicate the fetus is not growing at a normal rate. The fundus enlarging more than this rate would indicate the fetus is growing too rapidly or a multiple pregnancy is suspected.

- *Edema:* A small amount of dependent edema is often present in the last few weeks of pregnancy. A large amount of edema in the feet or edema of the calves, thighs, hands, and face should be reported to the healthcare provider.

- *Laboratory tests:* A urine sample is collected at each visit and dipstick tested for glucose, protein, and ketone bodies. A glucose tolerance test might be ordered in the 20th week to determine the presence of gestational diabetes. Gestational diabetes is discussed in Chapter 52 ⚭. Specific blood tests such as complete blood count, hematocrit and hemoglobin, and alpha-fetoprotein (AFP) may be ordered in the 16th week and as indicated by client symptoms. Table 51-3 ■ identifies pregnant and nonpregnant laboratory values.

DIAGNOSING, PLANNING, AND IMPLEMENTING

In planning nursing interventions for the prenatal client, the nurse should consider the woman's knowledge, past experiences, behaviors that increase risk, family support system, and socioeconomic status. Most nursing interventions involve teaching or anticipatory guidance. Specific topics and time frame depend on when prenatal care is begun and complications. Nursing diagnoses might include:

- *Anxiety*
- *Constipation*
- *Readiness for Enhanced Family Coping*
- *Deficient Fluid Volume*
- *Deficient Knowledge* (specify)
- *Disturbed Body Image*
- *Disturbed Sleep Pattern*
- *Excess Fluid Volume*
- *Fatigue*
- *Fear*
- *Imbalanced Nutrition: Less than Body Requirements*
- *Impaired Physical Mobility*
- *Risk for Injury*
- *Sexual Dysfunction*

Much of nursing care for pregnant clients involves client and family teaching.

Environmental Hazards

- Teach the importance of a safe home and work environment for the pregnant client. The home should be inspected for hazards, and corrections made. *In late pregnancy, the woman is at risk for falls. Chemicals, including cleaning supplies, insecticides, and weed control agents, can harm the fetus. These chemicals should be avoided if possible. If the woman must use these chemicals, she should avoid skin contact and inhaling fumes.*

- Teach the client to avoid excessive heat from hot tubs, saunas, or hot humid weather. *It is important to prevent maternal hyperthermia. Even 10 minutes in a tub of water 106°F can cause maternal hyperthermia* (Rogers & Davis, 1995).

Discomforts of Pregnancy

Pregnancy often causes discomforts for many women. Table 51-4 ■ identifies the common discomforts and possible interventions to alleviate or decrease the discomfort.

TABLE 51-3	Pregnant and Nonpregnant Laboratory Values	
TEST	**PREGNANT VALUES**	**NONPREGNANT VALUES**
Hematocrit (%)	32–42	37–47
Hemoglobin (g/dL)	10–14	12–16
Platelets (mm3)	Significant increase 3–5 days after birth	150,000–350,000
White blood cells (mm3)	5,000–15,000	4,500–10,000
Fibrinogen (mg/dL)	Up to 600	175–400
Serum glucose (mg/dL)	65 (fasting) less than 140 (2hr PP)	70–80
Sodium (mEq/L)	135–145	135–145
Potassium (mEq/L)	3.5–5.1	3.5–5.1
Chloride (mEq/L)	100–108	100–108
Bicarbonate (mEq/L)	22–26	22–26
Calcium (mg/dL)	Falls 10% by term	8.5–10.5

TABLE 51-4	Client Teaching for Common Discomforts of Pregnancy
COMMON DISCOMFORT	**CLIENT TEACHING**
Backache related to softening of cartilage in body joints (from ↑ hormones), poor body mechanics, fatigue, increased lumbosacral curve	Rest lying on side Wear low-heeled shoes Use proper body mechanics
Constipation resulting from slowing of bowel as a result of ↑ progesterone, pressure of enlarged uterus, diet, or reduced activity	Increase fiber from fruits and vegetables (raisins, prunes, apples) Daily activity (walking) Increase fluids
Dyspnea related to pressure of the uterus on the diaphragm; faintness	Lie on side or semi-Fowler's position; in third trimester, lie on left side more often than right; change positions slowly
Edema caused by hormonal changes (↑ sodium and water retention), reduced activity level, congestion of lower extremities (see also varicose veins entry); ankle edema, carpal tunnel	Walk several times during the day Rest with feet elevated; reduce repetitive hand motions that aggravate carpal tunnel, or use splints to support wrist Avoid salty foods If edema increases or is routinely present on arising, contact healthcare provider
Flatulence due to hormonal changes (progesterone) and pressure of uterus on abdominal organs	Omit gas-forming foods Increase bulk in diet Have regular bowel movement
Heartburn from pressure of enlarged uterus or relaxing effect of progesterone on the cardiac sphincter	Avoid fried or spicy foods Eat small amounts; avoid overeating Sit up for 30 minutes after eating Take antacids ONLY with healthcare provider's approval
Hemorrhoids caused by pressure of gravid uterus on rectal veins or straining (see also constipation entry)	Prevent constipation Cool compresses Warm sitz bath Topical analgesic ointment
Leg cramps due to imbalance of calcium/phosphorous ratio, poor circulation, pressure of uterus on nerves, fatigue	Increase calcium in diet Frequent rest periods with legs elevated
Mood swings related to hormonal changes, fatigue, psychosocial factors, diet	Express fears, concerns Adequate diet and fluids Adequate rest periods
Nausea and/or vomiting from changes in hormonal level or pressure of the uterus on the stomach	Limit fluids on waking Eat dry toast or crackers Eat small amounts frequently Avoid fried or spicy foods
Urinary frequency from pressure of uterus on bladder in first and third trimesters	Empty bladder frequently Do NOT limit fluids Contact healthcare provider if other signs of urinary infection are present
Vaginal discharge related to ↑ estrogen; may be indicative of infection	Good hygiene If other signs of vaginal infection are present, contact healthcare provider
Varicose veins resulting from congestion in lower veins, hereditary weakness or faulty valves in veins, weight gain, effect of progesterone (relaxation of vessel walls)	Rest with feet elevated Avoid restrictive clothing, crossing legs Wear support hose Walk

<table>
<tr><td>**BOX 51-4**</td><td>**CLIENT TEACHING**</td></tr>
</table>

Health Promotion Topics during Pregnancy

Nutrition, Diet, and Exercise (affecting both mother and fetus)

- Prenatal vitamins and/or foods to supply pregnancy needs
- Importance of fluids
- Hygiene, clothing adaptations, dental care
- Pattern of weight gain, desired weight gain (individualized teaching)
- Referral, if needed, to WIC program or other community assistance
- Alcohol's effects on the fetus
- Limiting or eliminating caffeine

Safety

- Adapting to body changes and changes in balance
- Techniques for relieving physical stresses of pregnancy
- Checking all medications (even OTC) with physician before use
- Smoking cessation
- Pets (especially cats because of the potential for being infected with toxoplasmosis when handling cat feces)
- Toxins and exposure to dangerous chemicals in the home and environment (wearing gloves when gardening)

Work

- Learning to balance work and rest
- Adaptations to jobs requiring long periods of standing

Travel Considerations

- Car travel—seatbelt adjustment
- Air travel—restrictions

Prenatal Classes

- Physical and mental preparation for childbirth and parenting
- Effects of pregnancy on sexuality
- Awareness of possible complications requiring medical aid
- Value of prenatal healthcare visits
- Planning for effects of pregnancy on home life

Nutrition

If the woman is already eating a well-balanced diet, very little change needs to be made during pregnancy. (See Chapter 25 ∞ to review basic nutrition.) However, most women benefit from nutritional teaching. Box 51-4 ∎ lists important teaching topics for pregnant women.

- During pregnancy the woman should add 300 kilocalories (kcal) a day. She should add 500 kcal when breastfeeding. The addition of two milk servings and one meat serving will meet the need for increased calories as well as calcium and protein. Table 51-5 ∎ identifies a food guide to meet the nutritional needs of the woman and developing fetus. *Many women, however, do not eat a well-balanced diet prior to pregnancy, so the nurse must provide them with more*

in-depth information or refer them to a dietitian. Many health-care providers have their clients take a multiple vitamin with calcium and iron.

clinical ALERT

Deficiency in folic acid during pregnancy can result in neural tube defects including **anencephaly** (absence of neural tissue in the cranium) and **spina bifida** (defect with incomplete closure of the vertebra and neural tube). Folic acid supplements taken 1 month before conception and throughout the first trimester of pregnancy can help prevent neural tube defects.

- Teach the importance of adequate fluid intake for pregnant women. *Drinking 1,500 to 2,000 mL of water, milk, or juice every 24 hours is recommended. It is best to limit caffeine-containing beverages.*
- Provide referral to assistance programs like Woman, Infant, and Child (WIC) programs as appropriate. *Women at a low socioeconomic level may not have the financial resources to purchase adequate amounts of milk and high-protein foods. Resources are available.*

Warning Signs of Complications

Teach the client warning signs of possible complications (Table 51-6 ∎). Signs of impending labor should be discussed with the client in the third trimester of pregnancy. *Usually, the sooner interventions are begun, the better the outcome.*

Fetal heart rate is discussed in more detail in Chapter 52 ∞.

Self-Care

Self-care generally involves a minimal adjustment of normal habits.

- Encourage the client to bathe daily. In late pregnancy, the woman may have difficulty rising from a sitting position in the bathtub. Care should be taken to prevent falls in the tub or shower. *Daily bathing is important due to an increase in perspiration and vaginal secretions. Either a tub bath or shower may be used. Douching should be avoided because of the possibility of introducing pathogens.*
- Breast care involves cleaning with water, rubbing the nipple with a washcloth to toughen the tissue prior to breastfeeding, and air-drying the breast. *A properly fitting maternity bra promotes comfort, supports the enlarged heavy breast, and prevents back strain. Leakage of fluid from the nipple is common. This fluid should be rubbed into the nipple to lubricate the skin and promote breast health.*
- The pregnant woman should have regular activity. Fatigue should be avoided. Periods of rest, with the legs elevated, should be scheduled throughout the day. *Walking and swimming are best, and very strenuous activity should be avoided. Activities routinely practiced before pregnancy can*

TABLE 51-5	Food Guide during Pregnancy and Lactation		
		SUGGESTED SERVINGS PER DAY	
FOOD GROUP	**SERVING SIZE**	**DURING PREGNANCY**	**DURING LACTATION**
Grain products (whole-grain breads, cereals, pasta, rice)	1 slice bread ½ bun, bagel ½ cup cereal	6–11	6–11
Vegetables (dark green leafy, deep yellow, dry beans/peas)	1 cup leafy greens ½ cup all others	3–5 (eat dry beans and peas often)	3–5
Fruits (citrus fruits and others)	1 medium apple, banana, orange, etc. ½ cup canned ¾ cup juice	2–4	2–4
Meat/poultry/fish, beans/nuts/eggs (limit peanut butter and nuts due to fat content) Trim fat, remove skin from poultry	½ cup cooked dry beans 1 egg, 1½ tbsp peanut butter = 1 oz meat	Up to 6 oz total	Up to 6 oz total
Milk and milk products	1 cup milk or yogurt 1½ oz cheese	3 or more	4 or more

generally be continued as long as there are no complications and the woman can safely participate.

- Clothing is important for the self-image during pregnancy. Clothing that is attractive, loose fitting, and easy to care for should be selected. Because maternity clothing is only worn for a short time, encourage sharing of clothing among friends or suggest purchasing second-hand clothing, which is more reasonably priced. *Knee-high or thigh-high stockings can interfere with circulation. Low-heeled shoes are generally recommended due to the difficulty of maintaining balance in high-heeled shoes.*

- Encourage dental care throughout pregnancy. The woman should inform her dentist that she is pregnant. X-ray examination should be postponed until after the pregnancy. Bleeding of gums is a common finding and will resolve when pregnancy ends. *Dental hygiene promotes oral health and self-esteem and prevents such problems as gingivitis.*

- Sexual activities may continue throughout the pregnancy unless there are complications. After the fourth month, the woman should not lie flat on her back due to hypotensive syndrome. A pillow can be placed under her right hip or an alternative position can be used. *There may be a*

TABLE 51-6	Warning Signs during Pregnancy
WARNING SIGN	**POTENTIAL RISK OR COMPLICATION**
Abdominal pain, cramping	Ectopic pregnancy, spontaneous abortion, abruptio placenta, labor
Bleeding (any) from vagina	Spontaneous abortion, placenta previa, abruptio placenta
Blurred vision, double vision, seeing spots or flashes of light	Pregnancy-induced hypertension (PIH) also called gestational onset hypertension preeclampsia
Dizziness, fainting, persistent headache	PIH, preeclampsia
Dysuria	Urinary infection
Fetal movement decreased or absent	Fetal distress, fetal death
Fever over 100°F (37.8°C) and chills	Infection
Fluid gushing or leaking from vagina ("water breaks")	Rupture of membranes (leaking urine may appear similar)
Oliguria	Dehydration, PIH
Persistent vomiting	Hyperemesis gravidarum
Swelling of hands, face, legs, feet	PIH, preeclampsia
Vaginal discharge that is thick, white/yellow, irritating	Vaginal infection

decreased desire for sexual activity during pregnancy. The woman should be supported to participate to the level of comfort.

- Provide support for the woman to discuss issues surrounding employment. *The decision to continue employment should be based on several factors. Are there hazards in the workplace that would place additional risk on the pregnancy? Would the woman be under undue physical strain? Would periods of rest be available? Any areas of concern should be discussed with the healthcare provider.*

- Discuss adaptations for travel. *When traveling, the woman should walk for about 10 minutes every 2 hours to prevent venous stasis. The seat belt should be worn snugly, below the abdomen. Travel need not be restricted unless complications develop. Generally the best time to travel is in the second trimester, when there are fewer risks of complications. The woman should be aware that some airlines may not accept passengers past a certain week of pregnancy.*

- Encourage enrollment in a childbirth education class. *Preparation for childbirth usually begins in the third trimester. Many hospitals and birthing centers present childbirth classes. Printed resources are also available to assist in childbirth preparation.*

EVALUATING

Clients should be able to verbalize an understanding of the instructions. A change, or a lack of change, in a client's behavior is also used to evaluate the instruction provided.

NURSING PROCESS CARE PLAN
Client with Hypertension

Mrs. Ross is expecting her first baby in 5 weeks. She comes to the clinic for a routine visit.

Assessment
BP 135/85 (prenatal 125/70). 1+ protein in urine. 2+ pitting edema in ankles. States she has had a headache every day for the past 3 days that is relieved by Tylenol. Denies blurred vision. Reflexes are within normal limits. Wt increased by 3 pounds in last 2 weeks.

Nursing Diagnosis
The following important nursing diagnosis (among others) is established for this client:

- *Ineffective Peripheral Tissue Perfusion* related to hypertension

Expected Outcomes
The expected outcome for Mrs. Ross is:

- Client will experience no adverse reaction to hypertension and will have birth under optimal conditions.

Planning and Implementation
The following nursing interventions are planned and implemented for Mrs. Ross:

- Teach Mrs. Ross to take frequent rest periods lying on side. *Because hypertension and edema increase the workload on the heart and decrease tissue perfusion, adequate rest is needed. The side-lying position prevents pressure on the uterine artery.*

- Encourage her to increase fluid to 8 glasses/day and increase roughage in diet. *Fluid and roughage are needed to prevent constipation.*

- Teach client to avoid salty foods. *Salt can cause fluid retention, making hypertension and edema worse.*

- Teach client to do nonstressful exercise such as walking around the house and to avoid exercise that increases heart rate. *Exercise is important to maintain muscle strength, but additional stress on the heart should be avoided.*

- Encourage diversional activities such as crafts, reading, and puzzles. *These activities can reduce boredom and decrease stress.*

- Encourage family participation in care and household chores. *The household chores need to be completed to prevent additional stress, but the patient with PIH may not be able to tolerate additional activity.*

- Teach symptoms of worsening PIH, including blurred vision, increased edema, and worsening headache. Notify healthcare provider of worsening symptoms. *If treatment is not effective, PIH can increase rapidly and threaten the life of mother and child.*

- Set up a return visit to clinic in 1 week. *Follow-up monitoring is important to ensure the safety of mother and child.*

Evaluation
Blood pressure, weight, edema, proteinuria, and reflexes must be evaluated. Any notable increase in these values must be reported to the physician immediately.

Critical Thinking in the Nursing Process

1. What complications to the fetus might occur if Mrs. Ross does not reduce her hypertension?
2. How frequently should follow-up visits occur between now and delivery?
3. Should Mrs. Ross be warned that she will need to take medication for hypertension for the rest of her life? Why or why not?

Note: Discussion of Critical Thinking questions appears in on the MyNursingKit Website.

Note: The references and resources for all chapters have been compiled at the back of the book.

Assessing the Fetal Heart Rate with Doppler

Purposes

■ To provide information about the status of the fetus
■ To monitor the status of the fetus

Equipment

■ Doppler device
■ Ultrasonic gel

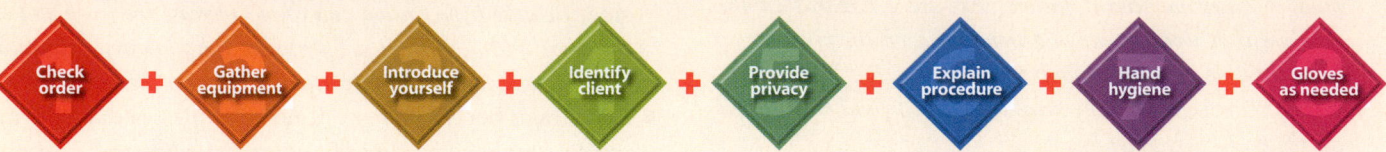

Check order + Gather equipment + Introduce yourself + Identify client + Provide privacy + Explain procedure + Hand hygiene + Gloves as needed

Interventions and Rationales

1. Perform preparatory steps (see icon bar above).
2. Apply gel to the diaphragm of the Doppler. *Gel aids sound transmission and helps maintain contact between the Doppler diaphragm and the abdomen.*
3. Uncover the woman's abdomen. Position the diaphragm in the midline of the woman's abdomen halfway between the umbilicus and symphysis pubis (see Figure 51-6). *This is the most likely position in which to hear the fetal heartbeat.*
4. When pulse is heard, check it against the woman's pulse. If they are the same, reposition the Doppler diaphragm. If the pulse is not heard, move the diaphragm laterally. *If the rates are the same they are probably both the mother's pulse.*
5. If the rates are not the same, count the beats for 1 minute. Count each double rhythm as one beat. *The fetal heart sound has a double rhythm. The beats per minute are the fetal heart rate (FHR).*
6. Auscultate the FHR at each office visit during pregnancy. FHR is also assessed before, during, and for 30 seconds after a uterine contraction during labor. *This can provide information about fetal health or distress.*

7. Follow recommendations for frequency of auscultation and documentation. *The health and risk status of the woman will determine the usual frequency of auscultation.*
   a. FHR should be assessed at each office visit.
   b. FHR should be assessed anytime the mother accesses health care for any reason during the pregnancy.
   c. FHR should be assessed if the woman believes she is in labor. Fetal assessment during labor is discussed in Chapter 53 ∞.

SAMPLE DOCUMENTATION

[date]	FHR 144. Mother reports
[time]	increase in fetal activity the
	past 2 weeks, especially after
	periods of maternal activity.
	Reassured that this is usual
	during the 6th month of
	pregnancy. _____
	_____ K. Doss, LPN

Assisting with Amniocentesis, Umbilical Cord Sampling, or Chorionic Villus Sampling

Purposes

■ To provide information about the genetic makeup of the fetus
■ To provide information about the status of the fetus

Equipment

■ Ultrasound equipment
■ Ultrasonic gel

■ Amniocentesis kit containing skin prep (Betadine), sterile drapes, 22-gauge spinal needle with stylet, and amber colored test tubes. If a kit is not available, the nurse must assemble the supplies from stock. *Amniotic fluid must be protected from light. If amber-colored test tubes are not available, place tape over test tube to protect the specimen.*
■ Sterile gloves
■ Local anesthetic (1% Lidocaine)

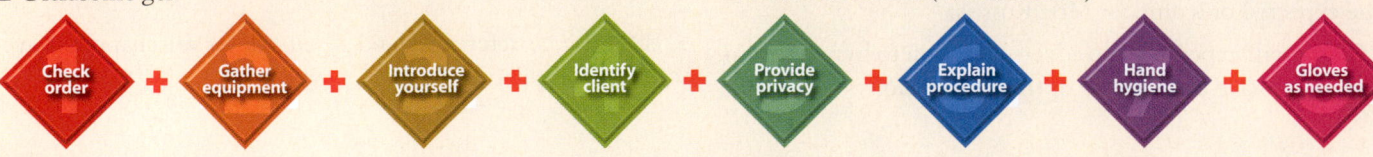

Check order + Gather equipment + Introduce yourself + Identify client + Provide privacy + Explain procedure + Hand hygiene + Gloves as needed

Interventions and Rationales

1. Perform preparatory steps (see icon bar above).

2. Ensure that a signed Informed Consent form is in the chart. If not, inform the care provider. *This procedure requires an informed consent signature.*

3. Obtain the mother's vital signs and the fetal heart rate. Monitor maternal vital signs and FHR every 15 minutes during the procedure and for a minimum of 30 minutes after the procedure. *The first VS and FHR readings provide a baseline. Later readings give information about the status of the mother and the fetus. Changes can signal complications.*

4. Position the woman on her back, with a wedge placed under her right hip to displace the weight to the left side. External fetal monitor may be used during the exam to monitor the fetus. *This position will promote better blood flow and prevent supine hypotension.*

5. The physician uses ultrasound to locate the placenta and fetus. Provide ultrasound gel and assist as needed. *Gel creates a seal between the monitor and the woman's skin and improves the quality of the ultrasound reading.*

6. The physician dons sterile gloves and cleanses the woman's abdomen. *Cleansing the abdomen prior to needle insertion helps prevent infection.*

7. The physician applies sterile drapes, then inserts the needle into the uterus and withdraws a sample of amniotic fluid, umbilical cord blood, or chorionic villi (see Figure 51-10A ■, B, or C, respectively). *Note:* If a sample of the placenta is obtained for chorionic villus sampling or blood is obtained from an umbilical vessel, other specimen containers may be needed. The nurse may be required to assist with continuous ultrasound monitoring. *Sterile technique is essential to prevent infection of the mother and fetus.*

8. Obtain specimen containers from physician, attach proper labels, and send to lab with appropriate lab slips. *It is the nurse's responsibility to be sure materials are labeled properly. Prompt delivery to the lab helps ensure accurate results.*

9. Assist physician to apply a small dressing over puncture site.

10. Monitor the woman and fetus for 30 minutes, paying close attention to the mother's vital signs, FHR, and any contractions she may be having. *Changes from normal may indicate complications that would need to be reported.*

11. Assess the woman's blood type and determine if Rh immune globulin (RhoGam) is needed and administer if necessary (see Chapter 52 ⚭). *To prevent Rh sensitization of an Rh-negative woman during the procedure, Rh immune globulin is administered.*

12. Instruct the woman to report any of the following changes immediately to her primary care provider:
    a. Unusual increase in fetal activity or lack of fetal movement
    b. Vaginal discharge, either clear fluid or bloody drainage
    c. Uterine contractions or abdominal cramping
    d. Fever or chills

    These are signs of complications that will require further medical investigation and treatment.

13. Encourage the woman to engage in only light activity for 24 hours and to increase her fluid intake. *Light activity will decrease uterine irritability. Fluid is needed to replace the amniotic fluid.*

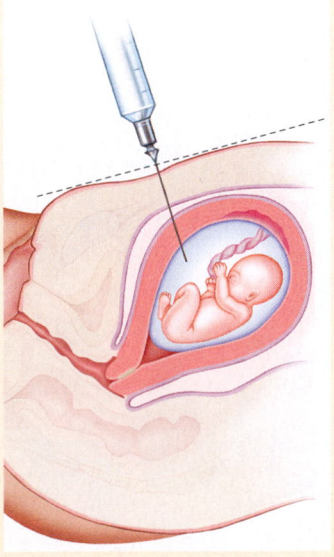
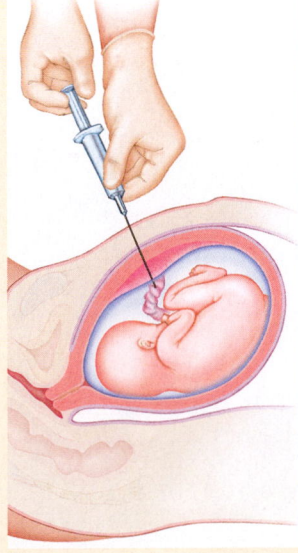
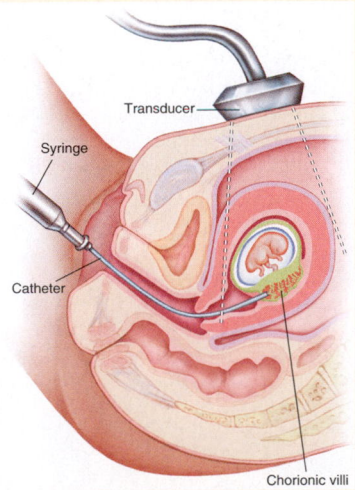

Figure 51-10. ■ **A.** Amniocentesis. **B.** Umbilical cord blood sampling. **C.** Chorionic villus sampling using transcervical approach.

14. **Complete the client record.** *Full documentation includes date and time, vital signs, type of procedure, name of provider who performed the procedure, number of specimens obtained and disposition of specimens, repeat VS and client status, record of discharge teaching and follow-up care.*

SAMPLE DOCUMENTATION

[date] [time]	T 98.2, P 82, R 24, BP 136/72, FHR 150. No uterine contractions noted at this time. Dr. Lopez here. Amniocentesis completed without incident. 3 specimens sent to lab.
[time]	Vital signs have remained stable since amniocentesis. BP 130/70, P 78, R 22, FHR 144–150. No contractions noted on monitor. Written instructions provided and reviewed regarding home care, activity, and warning signs to report to the physician. Instructed to return to clinic in 1 week for follow-up. _____ _____ J. Sole, LPN

Chapter Review

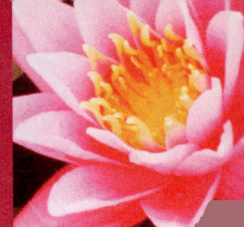

KEY Points

- During fetal development, all body systems are formed in the first 8 weeks.

- Most pregnancies progress as planned. The LPN/LVN is responsible for collecting data and reporting symptoms of complications.

- The key to a healthy pregnancy is prenatal care, including patient teaching and early detection of complications.

- Nurses have a responsibility to teaching good health practices including nutrition, exercise, and eliminating risky behaviors.

- The nurse must know the signs of pregnancy to anticipate data needing to be collected, client teaching needs, and what equipment the primary care provider will need for diagnostic exams.

- The nurse must teach the client about physical and psychological changes that occur during pregnancy.

- The nurse must teach the client common discomforts of pregnancy and methods of lessening them.

- The nurse must provide client instructions in verbal and written format to ensure client understanding.

⬤ FOR FURTHER Study

See Chapter 25 to review basic nutrition.

See Chapter 32 for more about epistaxis.

Urinary system disorders are discussed Chapter 39.

See Chapter 40 for information on treatments such as D&C and for disorders of the female reproductive system.

See in-depth discussion of sexually transmitted infections in Chapter 41.

Hyperemesis gravidarum, Rh factor, and other high-risk issues are discussed in Chapter 52.

FHR during labor is discussed in Chapter 53.

Congenital heart defects are discussed in Chapter 57.

EXPLORE **PEARSON**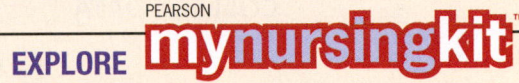

MyNursingKit is your one stop for online chapter review materials and resources. Prepare for success with additional NCLEX®-style practice questions, interactive assignments and activities, web links, animations and videos, and more!

Register your access code from the front of your book at
www.mynursingkit.com

Critical Thinking Care Map

Caring for an Undernourished Pregnant Woman
NCLEX-PN® Focus Area: Physiologic Adaptation

Case Study: Jean, a 17-year-old, comes to the clinic for her first visit. She appears pale and thin. She is 5'10". Her weight is 130 lbs. Her vital signs are within normal limits. Her urine is negative for protein. It is determined she is 10 weeks pregnant. She states she is living with her boyfriend in a one-bedroom basement apartment. Both Jean and her boyfriend have had to drop out of high school to get jobs. They are barely able to pay the rent and buy food. Jean begins to cry, stating she does not know what to do.

Nursing Diagnosis: *Imbalanced Nutrition: Less than Body Requirements*

COLLECT DATA

Subjective	Objective
_____	_____
_____	_____
_____	_____
_____	_____
_____	_____
_____	_____
_____	_____

Would you report this? Yes/No

If yes, report to: _____

What would you report?_____

Nursing Care

_____
_____
_____
_____
_____
_____
_____
_____
_____

How would you document this? _____
_____
_____
_____

Compare your answers and documentation to those provided on the MyNursingKit Website.

Data Collected
(use only those that apply)

- Crying
- States she does not know what to do
- Ht. 5'10"; wt. 130 lbs.
- Vital signs WNL
- Urine negative for protein
- Pale
- Thin
- Money only for rent and food

Nursing Interventions
(use only those that apply; list in priority order)

- Refer to WIC program.
- Teach need for increased protein, lower carbohydrates in diet.
- Refer to therapist for depression.
- Teach need for prenatal vitamins.
- Teach need for milk products.

NCLEX-PN® Exam Preparation

TEST-TAKING TIP Words such as *prepare* or *anticipate* in a question refer to the planning phase of the nursing process. The answer should be consistent.

1. While having blood drawn to test for pregnancy, the client asks the nurse when the chemical they test (hCG) begins to be produced. The most accurate response of the nurse would be:
   1. 8 to 12 hours.
   2. 18 to 36 hours.
   3. 4 to 6 days.
   4. 8 to 10 days.

2. The nurse, working in a gynecologist's office, learns that the client hopes to become pregnant within the next year. The nurse would advise the client to do all of the following except:
   1. Maintain adequate intake of calcium.
   2. Increase intake of folic acid.
   3. Maintain adequate intake of iron to prevent anemia.
   4. Increase intake of vitamin C.

3. While caring for a woman who is 16 weeks pregnant, the nurse notes which of the following as being an abnormal change?
   1. Breast enlargement
   2. Pulse rate increase by 10 to 15 beats per minute
   3. Slight decrease in blood pressure
   4. Increased peristalsis

4. The nurse is providing client teaching to the woman who is 38 weeks pregnant. Which of the following would be a key point for the nurse to discuss at this time?
   1. The importance of taking prenatal vitamins and avoiding alcohol and caffeine
   2. Checking with the physician before taking any medications
   3. Avoiding cat litter box care to reduce the risk of toxoplasmosis infection
   4. Preparing physically and mentally for childbirth

5. The nurse, caring for a newly pregnant woman who is already eating a well-balanced diet, will advise the client to:
   1. Make no changes in her diet.
   2. Add one protein and two milk servings.
   3. Add one fruit and two vegetable servings.
   4. Decrease the amount of carbohydrates.

6. The nurse, caring for a pregnant woman in the last trimester, will advise the client to sleep on her side primarily for the purpose of:
   1. Relieving pressure on the bladder.
   2. Relieving pressure on the fetus.
   3. Facilitating sleep.
   4. Preventing hypotension.

7. The earliest the nurse will be able to hear the fetal heart tones using a Doppler is week:
   1. 2.
   2. 6.
   3. 10.
   4. 20.

8. The client's last menstrual period began on May 6 and ended on May 11. The nurse calculates the client's estimated date of delivery using Naegele's rule as February:
   1. 6.
   2. 11.
   3. 13.
   4. 18.

9. The nurse, working in an obstetrician's office, receives a call from a woman who is 36 weeks pregnant saying she is experiencing headache, blurred vision, and a lot of swelling. The nurse would advise the client to:
   1. Rest and call back if the symptoms do not stop within 24 hours.
   2. Go to the emergency room immediately.
   3. Lie down, put her feet up, and call back if the headache continues for 4 hours.
   4. Come to the office to be seen this morning.

10. The nurse is assisting with the performance of an amniocentesis. Prior to beginning the procedure the nurse's first priority action is to:
    1. Prepare the skin site according to agency policy.
    2. Position the woman on her back with a wedge under the right hip.
    3. Ensure that an Informed Consent is signed and in the chart.
    4. Perform hand hygiene.

Answers and rationales for Review Questions appear in Appendix I.

Chapter 52

Care of Women during High-Risk Pregnancy

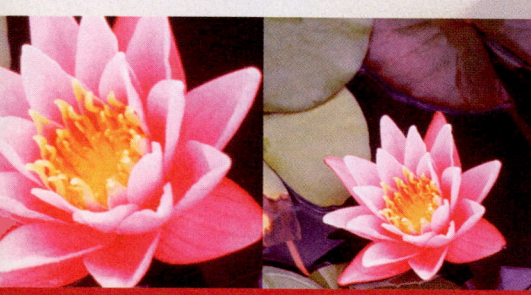

BRIEF Outline

LEARNING Outcomes

After completing this chapter, you will be able to:

1. List risk factors that create a high-risk pregnancy.
2. Identify the physical, psychological, and sociologic risks faced by the adolescent who is pregnant.
3. Describe tests used to assess maternal and fetal well-being.
4. Discuss complications of pregnancy, their treatment, and nursing care.
5. Identify medical conditions that are complicated by pregnancy and appropriate measures to support the pregnant woman.
6. Describe nursing care for the woman with a high-risk pregnancy.

Clinical Objectives*

7. Observe and assist with the care of a client experiencing a high-risk pregnancy.
8. Collect data and report variations on vital signs or status to the RN.
9. Assess deep tendon reflexes and clonus.

*The care of high-risk clients does not usually fall within the scope of the LPN/LVN, although it is important to recognize risks as they occur.

KEY TERMS

Use the audio glossary feature on the MyNursingKit Website to hear the correct pronunciation of the following key terms.

abruptio placentae 1444

cerclage 1442

eclampsia 1446

ectopic pregnancy 1442

gestational diabetes mellitus 1448

gestational hypertension 1446

hydramnios 1448

hydatidiform mole 1444

HELLP syndrome 1446

incompetent cervix 1442

placenta previa 1443

preeclampsia 1445

sequelae 1439

TORCH group 1449

The role of the LPN/LVN is generally one of caring for stable clients, including identifying and reporting signs of complications and teaching clients to prevent them. At times, the RN needs assistance in providing care to clients who are seriously ill. In these cases, the LPN/LVN needs to have a deeper understanding of the pathophysiology and treatment. This chapter contains information about care of the woman at risk for life-threatening complications during pregnancy. Even with the best of prenatal care, complications can happen. With frequent monitoring and evaluation, the severity of complications may be kept to a minimum. If signs of complications are detected, further testing is warranted to evaluate fetal well-being.

Risk Factors in Pregnancy

Factors associated with high-risk childbearing are grouped according to the threat to health and the outcome of the pregnancy. Box 52-1 ■ identifies these risk factors. Figure 52-1 ■ shows likely referrals for various high-risk issues. Risk factors are interrelated and cumulative. Therefore, a pregnant woman who has multiple risk factors is considered to have a high-risk pregnancy even if each risk factor is not major by itself. Risk factors are identified by verbal interview or written survey. The LPN/LVN may help collect data about risk factors.

Ideally, women prepare for pregnancy by maintaining healthy behaviors, including proper nutrition and the avoidance of risky behavior prior to conception. As stated in Chapter 51 ⚭, the woman should obtain prenatal care as soon as she suspects she is pregnant, or within the first 6 to 8 weeks. However, many women do not plan for pregnancy. Some engage in a variety of risk-taking behaviors (large intake of alcohol or other substances, unguarded sexual intercourse with multiple partners, smoking, poor nutritional habits, or fad diets). These behaviors may be part of a woman's lifestyle, and they increase the woman's risk of complications. Figure 52-2 ■ shows teratogenic effects on the fetus at different stages of development.

BOX 52-1   RISK FACTORS FOR HIGH-RISK PREGNANCY

Biophysical Factors

Genetic make-up: Abnormalities may interfere with normal fetal development.

Nutritional status: Normal fetal growth and development cannot progress without adequate nutrients.

Medical and/or obstetric history: Mother's health can lead to complications; examples include history of preterm labor, diabetes, or kidney disease.

Psychosocial Factors

Smoking: Maternal smoking leads to low-birth-weight infants.

Caffeine: Heavy consumption may lead to slight decrease in birth weight.

Alcohol: Consumption of alcohol can lead to fetal disabilities including fetal alcohol syndrome, learning disabilities, and hyperactivity.

Drugs: Many drugs can affect the fetus, including prescription, over-the-counter, and illicit drugs.

Psychologic status: Pregnancy triggers complex psychological responses that affect maternal well-being.

Sociodemographic Factors

Low income: Inadequate financial resources lead to no prenatal care, poor diet, and poor general health.

Lack of prenatal care: Early diagnosis and treatment of complications affect the outcome of the pregnancy.

Age: Adolescents have a higher incidence of complications including anemia, PIH, and difficult labor. The mature woman is at higher risk for low birth weight, macrosomia, chromosomal abnormalities, congenital malformation, and neonatal mortality.

Parity: First pregnancies and multigravida (especially when pregnancies are close together) carry higher risk.

Marital status: Mortality and morbidity rates are higher for the fetus of nonmarried women.

Residence: Residence alone is not a risk factor, but health care in some areas is not available or of poor quality.

Ethnicity: Ethnicity alone is not a risk factor, but it may be impacted by other sociodemographic factors.

Environmental Factors

Many environmental substances can impact the pregnancy including air quality, chemicals such as pesticides, radiation, and stress. These are found in the workplace, the home, and the community.

Early pregnancy risk identification

Medical history/conditions   **Recommended consultation ***

Condition	Consultation
Asthma	
Symptomatic on medication	■
Severe (multiple hospitalizations)	△
Cardiac disease	
Cyanotic, prior MI, prosthetic valve, AHA Class ≥ II	△
Other	■
Diabetes mellitus	
Class A–C	■
Class ≥ D	△
Drug/alcohol use	■
Epilepsy (on medication)	■
Family history of genetic problems (Down Syndrome, Tay Sachs)	△
Hemoglobinopathy (SS, SC, S-thal)	△
Hypertension	
Chronic, with renal or heart disease	△
Chronic, on medication or diastolic ≥ 90	■
Prior pulmonary embolus/deep vein thrombosis	■
Psychiatric disease	■
Pulmonary disease	
Severe obstructive or restrictive	△
Moderate	■
Renal disease	
Chronic, creatinine 3 or above with/without hypertension	△
Chronic, other	■
Requirement for prolonged anticoagulation	△
Severe systemic disease (examples: SLE, hyperthyroidism)	△

Obstetric history/conditions

Condition	Consultation
Age over 35 at delivery	■
Cesarean delivery, prior classical or vertical	■
Incompetent cervix	■
Prior fetal structural or chromosomal abnormality	△
Prior neonatal death	■
Prior stillbirth	■
Prior preterm delivery or preterm PROM	■
Prior low birthweight (less than 2500 g)	■
Second trimester pregnancy loss	■
Uterine leiomyomata or malformation	■

*At the time of consultation, continued patient care should be determined to be by collaboration with the referring care provider or by transfer of care

Initial laboratory

Condition	Consultation
HIV	
Symptomatic or low CD4 count	△
Other	■
Rh/other blood group isoimmunizations (excl. ABO, Lewis)	△

Initial examination

Condition	Consultation
Condylomata (extensive, covering vulva/vaginal opening)	■

Key
- ■ Specialty
- △ Subspecialty

Figure 52-1. ■ Early pregnancy risk identification, showing the likely referral for each condition. Depending on the condition, the client may stay with the original healthcare provider, who would collaborate with the specialist, or the client might be transferred to the specialist for the duration of the pregnancy. (*Source*: Data from Committee on Perinatal Health, 1995.)

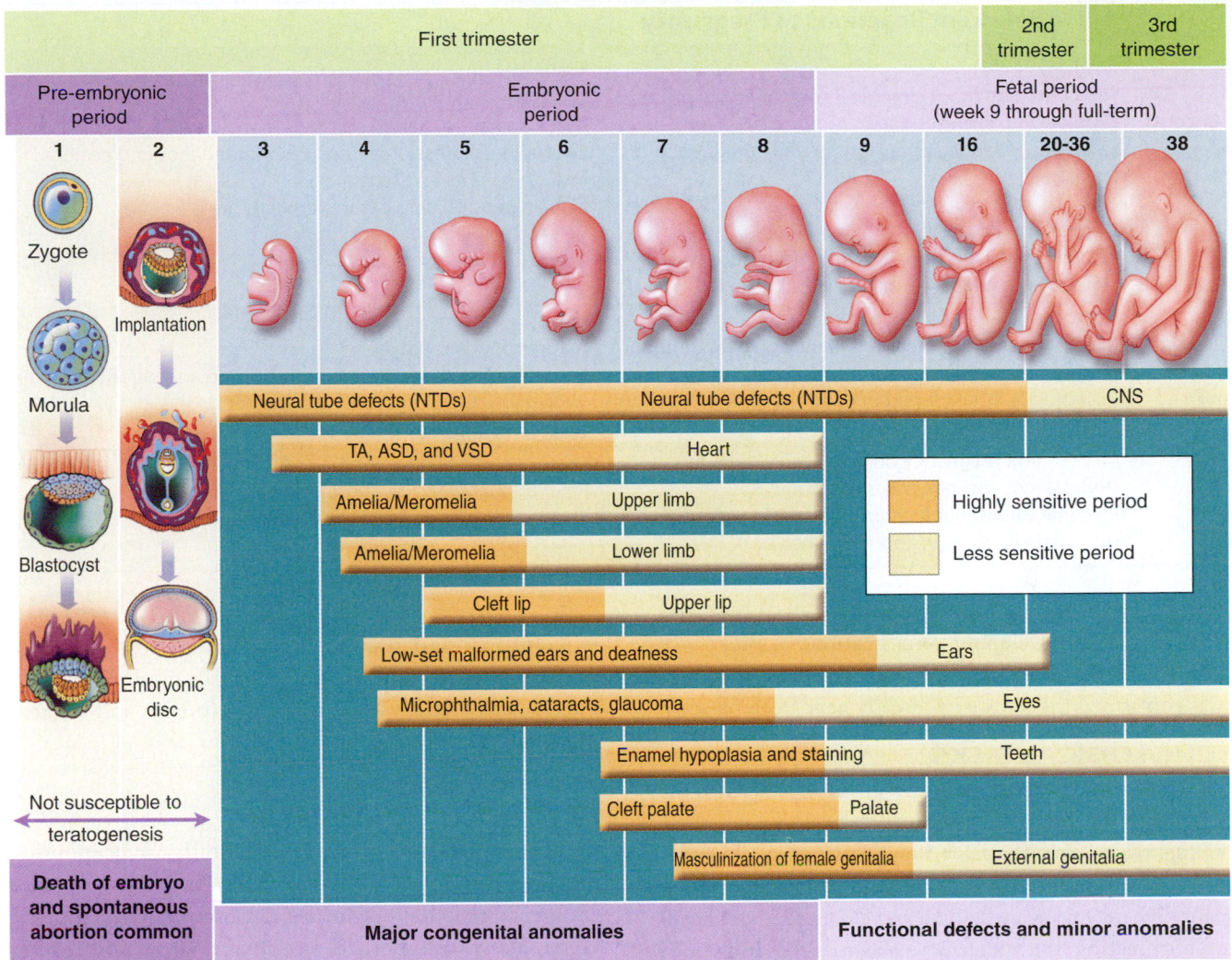

Figure 52-2. ■ There are highly sensitive periods during the embryonic state. For the first 2 weeks after conception, exposure to a teratogen has an all-or-nothing effect. It either disrupts implantation and causes spontaneous abortion or leaves the embryo unharmed. From about the 3rd through the 8th week of pregnancy (when organs form), exposure to a hazardous agent may cause serious anomalies. After organ formation and for the remainder of the pregnancy, exposure to fetal toxins will not cause malformation. However, it can interfere with maturation of the central nervous system and retard intrauterine growth. It may also cause cognitive or behavioral abnormalities.

Increased risk is not limited to behavior. The age of the mother can add risk to the pregnancy. When the adolescent becomes pregnant, she places her own health and the health of the fetus at risk for complications. The woman who becomes pregnant after 35 also places her health and the health of her baby in jeopardy.

Risks of Pregnancy to the Adolescent Mother

PHYSICAL RISKS

The adolescent over age 15 who receives early prenatal care is at no greater risk than the 20 year old. The adolescent under age 15 is at greatest risk during pregnancy. The early adolescent is still growing and physically developing. Because of irregular menstrual periods, the early adolescent may not be aware of the pregnancy for some time. The pregnant adolescent has an increased need for adequate nutrients to maintain their own growth, coupled with the needs of the fetus. Because their bone structure is still developing, the dimensions of pelvis may not be adequate to deliver a baby at term.

Adolescents typically do not seek prenatal care until later in the pregnancy. The risks for the pregnant adolescent are preterm birth, iron deficiency anemia, pregnancy-induced hypertension and the accompanying **sequelae** (a condition occurring because of another condition). Adolescents have a high incidence of sexually transmitted infections. Some vaginal infections are curable with antibiotics; others are not. Vaginal infections during pregnancy greatly increase the risk to the fetus.

Substance abuse is high in many adolescents. Adolescents who smoke cigarettes and use drugs, including alcohol, are

TABLE 52-1	Adolescent Reactions to Pregnancy	
AGE	**REACTION**	**NURSING IMPLICATIONS**
Early adolescent (Under 15)	Self-conscious about changing body of adolescence coupled with changes due to pregnancy Lack of knowledge about signs of early pregnancy Denial Fear of confiding in anyone Dependent on parents Fear of pregnancy, labor, delivery, motherhood Unable to develop maternal role at this time	Use a nonjudgmental approach Focus on needs of adolescent Encourage expression of feelings of pregnancy and options Include parents in discussion Explain physical changes in simple terms Refer to counseling as appropriate
Middle adolescent (15–17 years)	Fear of rejection by peers, parents May seek confirmation of pregnancy on own through pregnancy kits, Planned Parenthood, etc. Possible conflict with parent's and personal values	Use a nonjudgmental approach Assure confidentiality Be aware of state laws regarding abortion and parental consent Encourage communication with parents Refer to counseling as appropriate
Late adolescent (18–19 years)	May confirm pregnancy on own Understands consequences of actions Personal values, relationship with father, and future plans help in decision about pregnancy	Use a nonjudgmental approach Refer to counseling as appropriate Encourage to be realistic about pregnancy

at increased risk of developing complications of pregnancy including abnormalities in the fetus. By the time the pregnancy is confirmed the fetus may already have been harmed.

PSYCHOLOGICAL RISKS

The major psychological risk to the pregnant adolescent is the added pressure on her developmental tasks. Delaying these developmental tasks may have life-long implications. The adolescent may be fearful of telling peers and parents that she is pregnant. She may be overwhelmed and confused about keeping or terminating the pregnancy. She may be frightened about the delivery process. Table 52-1 ■ identifies some initial reactions when pregnancy begins in early, middle, and late adolescence. The nurse should realize that other factors might affect the psychological response of the adolescent. The nurse's role is to be supportive and nonjudgmental. The nurse may need to assist in informing parents of the pregnancy. The nurse may become a mediator should conflict arise.

If the pregnancy has resulted from abuse, the nurse has a responsibility to inform the authorities. If the abuse occurred in the home, the adolescent may be placed in foster care or a home for pregnant adolescents. The adolescent will need support from the nurse to deal with the abuse, the pregnancy, and pending legal actions.

Risks to the Child of an Adolescent Mother

PHYSICAL RISKS

The adolescent mother requires additional nutrition to support her growth as well as the growth of the fetus. The adolescent may have a lack of knowledge of nutritional

requirements and limited financial resources to purchase nutritious foods. Limited nutrition can result in intrauterine growth restriction, premature birth, and increased death rate in the fetus.

PSYCHOLOGICAL RISKS

Because teens are not developmentally or economically prepared to be parents, the children of adolescent mothers are at risk for becoming developmentally disadvantaged. Many teen mothers face adverse social and economic conditions. Children of adolescent mothers have a high rate of abuse and neglect (Koniak-Griffin, Anderson, Verzemnieks, & Brecht, 2000). These children do not do well in school and are less likely to complete high school.

Risks to the Older Mother and Child

The older mother may have more health issues such as hypertension, vascular changes, and obesity. If she has had other pregnancies, her body may not have had time to recover fully before she became pregnant again. This puts additional stress on her reserves. The older mother has an increased risk for preeclampsia and for cesarean birth. The infant of the older mother has an increased risk of congenital anomalies and chromosomal irregularities.

Once the pregnant woman obtains health care and risk factors are identified, teaching can begin and a plan of care can be implemented to decrease the number and severity of complications.

Tests Used to Assess Maternal Well-Being

Besides evaluating fetal well-being, prenatal care must include an assessment of maternal well-being. Recall that routine prenatal maternal assessment includes vital signs, weight, and urine analysis for glucose and protein. Baseline blood tests are usually done during the initial prenatal visit and then repeated as indicated. Refer to Table 51-3 🔗 for normal values during pregnancy.

MATERNAL HEMOGLOBIN

A maternal hemoglobin test is repeated at 7 months to assess for anemia. Recall that hemoglobin, found inside the red blood cell, is the chemical made from iron, which carries oxygen. If the hemoglobin level is low, an increased intake of iron or iron supplements may be necessary. There is a tendency for anemia to occur in certain cultural groups. Box 52-2 ■ describes this tendency further.

INDIRECT COOMBS' TEST

An indirect Coombs' test is done at 28 weeks on an Rh-negative woman. If the indirect Coombs' changes from a normal value of negative to a positive value, it indicates that the woman's blood has been sensitized by fetal Rh-positive blood. RhIgG prophylaxis must be given. More information on this condition is provided later in this chapter.

MULTIPLE MARKER SCREEN

A multiple marker screen (also called triple screen) test, done at 16 weeks, evaluates maternal serum alpha-fetoprotein (MSAFP), unconjugated estriol (UE), human chorionic gonadotropin (hCG), and inhibin-A levels. MSAFP is elevated when the fetus has an open neural tube defect, anencephaly, omphalocele, or gastroschisis, and when there are multiple gestations. Low MSAFP is associated with Down syndrome (Jenkins & Wapner, 2004). High hCG and inhibin-A and a low UE are also seen with Down syndrome. Because inaccurate data is the most common cause of abnormal results, it is important that further testing of amniotic fluid be done. The mother will need encouragement and emotional support.

BOX 52-2	CULTURAL PULSE POINTS

Erythroblastic Anemia

Women of Mediterranean descent are prone to developing thalassemia, a type of erythroblastic anemia. These women may have a chromosomal defect that results in fragile red blood cells. The stress of pregnancy could cause these fragile cells to be destroyed, resulting in anemia.

1-HOUR GLUCOSE SCREEN

A 1-hour glucose screen is a test done at 24 to 28 weeks' gestation. Values above 140 mg/dL indicate gestational diabetes. Values between 110 and 140 mg/dL may indicate further testing, such as a 100-gram oral glucose tolerance test. More information on this condition is provided under Gestational Diabetes Mellitus in this chapter.

VAGINAL CULTURE

Vaginal culture for group B streptococcal infection is a test obtained at 35 to 37 weeks. Beta streptococcus, commonly found in the vagina, is easily treated with antibiotics. If the infection is not diagnosed and treated, it is possible for the fetus to become exposed during vaginal delivery. Sexually transmitted infections can also be identified by vaginal culture.

Assessing Fetal Well-Being

Fetal assessment begins by questioning the mother about her health. If the mother is feeling well, there is a greater possibility the fetus is well. On the other hand, if the mother experiences vomiting and becomes dehydrated, the fetus may become dehydrated, too.

FETAL MOVEMENT

The mother should be able to feel fetal movements (quickening) at 18 to 20 weeks gestation. After that point, the mother should be questioned about fetal activity. A healthy fetus may sleep for 20 to 30 minutes and then become active for some time. As the fetus grows, muscle strength increases and fetal movements become stronger.

Several methods of keeping track of fetal movement have been developed. They all focus on having the mother count the number of fetal movements over a short time period and recording the data. The woman should count for 20 to 30 minutes, at the same time every day, usually 1 hour after a meal. Lying on her side, she should record every fetal movement during the desired time period. If there are fewer than 3 movements in 30 minutes, she should continue to count for 1 hour or more until 10 fetal movements are recorded. She should contact the primary care provider if:

■ There are fewer than 10 movements in 3 hours.
■ It takes longer each day to record 10 movements.
■ Fetal movements are absent.

She should bring the fetal movement record with her to each clinic visit so the primary care provider can review the data.

FETAL HEART RATE

The fetal heart rate (FHR) can be heard by a Doppler (an instrument that uses ultrasound to magnify sound) at 10 to 12 weeks' gestation. A *fetoscope* (an older assessment tool similar to a stethoscope) can be used to obtain the FHR by 14 to 16 weeks. The nurse may perform manual FHR monitoring at most prenatal visits. The normal fetal heart rate is 120 to 150 beats per minute. If complications develop, continuous electronic monitoring of the FHR may be required.

clinical ALERT

If the FHR is less than 100 or greater than 160, the charge nurse and primary care provider should be notified immediately.

Complications of Pregnancy

Complications are grouped here by those that only occur during a pregnancy, and those that are associated with other medical conditions. At times, the pregnant woman may develop more than one complication, placing her health and that of the fetus at greater risk.

HYPEREMESIS GRAVIDARUM

Although "morning sickness" is common in the first 12 weeks of pregnancy, excessive vomiting, or hyperemesis gravidarum, leads to dehydration and electrolyte imbalance. The client vomits everything she tries to eat. She may develop tachycardia, hypovolemia, hypotension, a decrease in urinary output, and an increase in blood urea nitrogen. Lack of nutrition leads to protein and vitamin deficiencies. The embryo or fetus can suffer from lack of nutrients as well.

Treatment

The goal of treatment is to regain fluid and electrolyte balance and maintain adequate nutrition. Hospitalization may be required to administer intravenous fluids and antiemetic medication.

COMPLICATIONS WITH BLEEDING

Bleeding during pregnancy is always a potential life-threatening condition for both the mother and the fetus. It should be evaluated by the healthcare provider. Although bleeding could happen at any time, it more commonly occurs in the first and third trimesters.

Menstruation

Menstruation could occur after conception. If the blastocyst implants a few days late, there may not be enough hCG produced to prevent the breakdown of the corpus luteum. A decrease in progesterone would lead to menstrual bleeding. If this occurs, the blastocyst may become detached and the pregnancy ends before the client knows she is pregnant. However, the blastocyst may remain attached to the endometrium and the pregnancy could continue.

Spontaneous Abortion

Spontaneous abortions, occurring most commonly in the first trimester, can be classified as follows:

- *Threatened:* Bleeding and cramping occur with the cervix closed and membranes intact.
- *Inevitable:* Bleeding and cramping occur with the cervix beginning to dilate. The membranes may or may not rupture.
- *Complete:* All of the products of conception are expelled.
- *Incomplete:* Some of the products of conception are expelled, but the placenta remains attached. Heavy bleeding and severe cramping continue until the placenta is removed.
- *Missed:* The embryo or fetus dies but is not expelled. This situation is often discovered by the physician when no fetal heart tones are present. If the fetus is not expelled within 6 weeks, other complications, including infection and disseminated intravascular coagulation (DIC), can occur.
- *Habitual:* Any of the above occurring in three consecutive pregnancies. In some circumstances, the cervix is weak, dilates in the second trimester, and expels the fetus. This condition is called **incompetent cervix.**

TREATMENT. The treatment of abortion depends on the cause. For a threatened abortion, the client would be placed on bed rest for several days. If the bleeding stops, she should be advised to avoid strenuous activity, fatigue, and sexual intercourse until the pregnancy seems to be progressing normally.

Dilatation and Curettage. If the bleeding does not stop, the fetus may be lost and surgical intervention may be necessary. For an inevitable, incomplete abortion, a scraping of the lining of the uterus called a D & C (for dilatation and curettage) is usually performed under anesthesia. (See discussion of D & C in Chapter 40 ⊙⊙.) The cervix is dilated, a curette is inserted into the uterus, and the endometrium is scraped, removing all products of conception. For a missed abortion, a D & C may be performed or labor may be induced depending on the gestational age of the fetus.

Cerclage. For habitual abortion caused by an incompetent cervix, a **cerclage** (Shirodkar procedure) is used. This procedure, done at 16 weeks of gestation, involves surgically placing a suture in the cervix in a purse-string design to hold the cervix closed (Figure 52-3 ■). The suture can be removed at term and the fetus is delivered vaginally. The suture can remain in place for future pregnancies and the fetus is delivered by cesarean section.

Ectopic Pregnancy

Ectopic pregnancy occurs when the blastocyst implants outside the uterine cavity (Figure 52-4 ■). The most common site for an ectopic pregnancy is the fallopian tube (*tubal pregnancy*). Because the fallopian tubes are not attached to

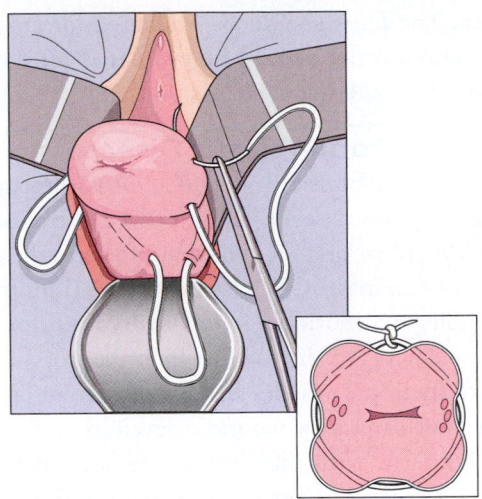

Figure 52-3. ■ A cerclage or purse-string suture is inserted into the cervix to prevent cervical dilation and pregnancy loss. After placement, the string is tightened and secured anteriorly.

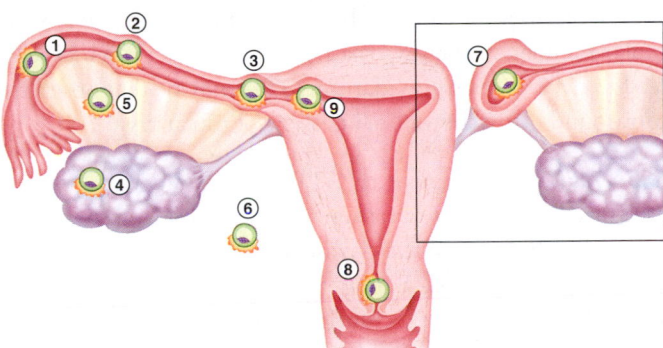

Figure 52-4. ■ Implantation sites of ectopic pregnancy in order of frequency: 1. Ampulla of fallopian tube. 2. Remainder of tube. 3. Interstitial portion of tube. 4. Ovary. 5. Broad ligament. 6. Surface of peritoneum (abdominal). 7. Rudimentary horn. 8. Cervix. 9. Tubouterine junction (angular).

the ovaries, the blastocyst could attach to the ovary or any intra-abdominal structure. The blastocyst could also travel through the uterus and implant in the cervix. As the embryo grows, it damages the organ. In the event of tubal pregnancy, the fallopian tube will rupture, causing bleeding into the abdominal cavity, some vaginal bleeding, and shock. Surgery must be performed immediately to stop the bleeding and save the client's life. In most cases the embryo will not survive an ectopic pregnancy.

Placenta Previa

Placenta previa results from the blastocyst implanting low in the uterus, allowing the placenta to partially or totally grow across the cervical opening. (Placenta previa comes from the Latin for "leading the way." It is called this because the placenta is in front or in the way of the baby as it moves toward the cervical os.) There are three classifications of placenta previa:

- *Marginal or low-lying:* The placenta is near the internal cervical opening, but does not cover it.
- *Partial:* The placenta covers part of the cervical opening.
- *Total or complete:* The placenta totally covers the cervical opening.

Figure 52-5 ■ illustrates placenta previa.

MANIFESTATIONS. During the latter part of pregnancy, the cervix begins to efface and dilate, resulting in the placenta being torn away from the endometrium. This causes the classic symptoms of painless bleeding in the third trimester. The uterus will be relaxed and nontender. Bleeding could be spotting or more profuse, but usually is intermittent. Vaginal exams are contraindicated until diagnosis can be made by ultrasound. If ultrasound is unavailable, the healthcare provider makes preparations for an emergency cesarean section delivery of the fetus. The mother cannot deliver vaginally.

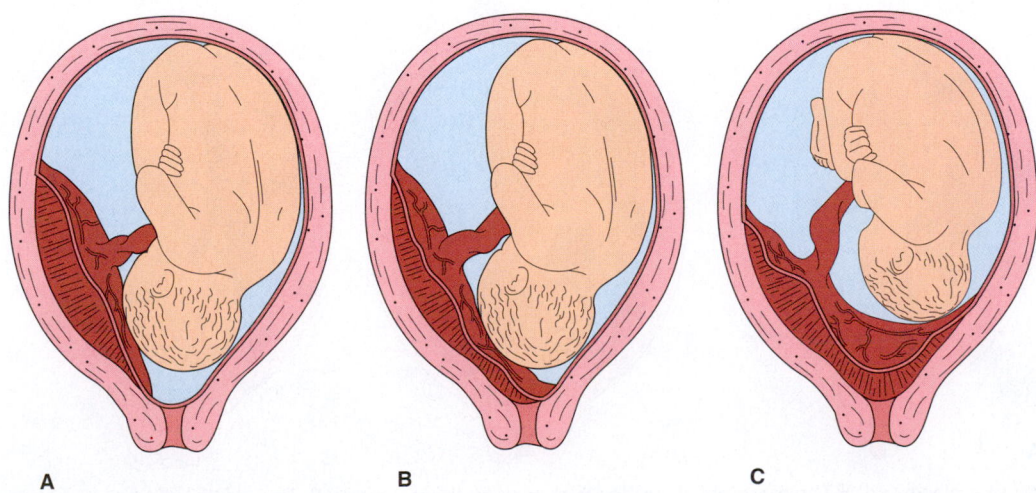

Figure 52-5. ■ Placenta previa. **A.** Lower placental implantation. **B.** Partial placenta previa. **C.** Total placenta previa.

TREATMENT. The goal of treatment for placenta previa is to stop the bleeding, allowing the fetus time to mature. This may be accomplished by placing the client on bed rest. At times, drugs like betamethasone (Celestone) may be given to accelerate fetal lung maturity. If bleeding continues, delivery by cesarean section is begun immediately. The infant and mother should be assessed for anemia.

Abruptio Placentae

Abruptio placentae (premature separation of the placenta) may occur in late pregnancy or during labor. The cause is unknown, but contributing factors include maternal hypertension, multiple pregnancy, smoking, use of alcohol and other illicit drugs, uterine trauma, and pregnancy continuing past the due date. There are three classifications of abruptio placentae:

- *Marginal:* Edge of the placenta separates and bright red vaginal bleeding occurs.
- *Central:* The center of the placenta separates, trapping blood between the placenta and the uterus. There is no vaginal bleeding, but the uterus becomes painful.
- *Complete:* The entire placenta separates, resulting in profuse bleeding. This is a medical emergency that may cause the death of the fetus.

MANIFESTATIONS. If the fetal head is tight against the cervix and maternal pelvis, some blood can be trapped inside the uterus. Bleeding into the myometrium causes a rigid, painful abdomen. After delivery the uterus may contract poorly, resulting in postdelivery bleeding. Figure 52-6 ■ illustrates abruptio placentae.

TREATMENT. The goal of treatment for abruptio placentae is delivery as soon as possible. If the separation is small and there are no signs of fetal distress, labor may be induced and allowed to progress. If the separation is moderate or severe, or if the fetus is in distress, an immediate cesarean section is performed. The fetus should be evaluated for anemia and hypoxia. The mother should be evaluated for continued vaginal bleeding and hypovolemia.

Gestational Trophoblastic Disease

Gestational trophoblastic disease (GTD) is the pathologic increase in trophoblast cells. (Recall that the trophoblast is the outer layer of embryonic cells that produces the placenta and fetal membranes.) GTD includes hydatidiform mole, invasive mole, and choriocarcinoma. A **hydatidiform mole** (molar pregnancy) is a disease in which the trophoblast develops into hydropic vesicles instead of normal embryonic tissue. In some cases a partial mole develops, and a fetal sac (including a fetus with multiple anomalies) may develop. The molar tissue may invade the myometrium (*invasive mole*) or develop into a form of cancer (*choriocarcinoma*).

MANIFESTATIONS. Clinical manifestations of GTD include vaginal bleeding, either a brownish fluid resembling prune juice or bright red bleeding (Figure 52-7 ■). If bleeding is excessive, anemia can result. Serum hCG is higher with molar pregnancy than with a normal pregnancy, which can lead to hyperemesis gravidarum. GTD may be diagnosed by ultrasound or by the vaginal passage of molar tissue.

TREATMENT. Treatment of GTD includes suction evacuation of the mole and curettage of the uterus to remove all fragments. Because of the risk of choriocarcinoma, extensive follow-up is required. Follow-up care includes monitoring serum hCG levels weekly until the woman has normal values for 3 consecutive weeks. Values are then monitored monthly for 6 months, and then every 2 months for another 6 months (Copeland & Landon, 2007).

Malignant GTD develops following molar evacuation in 20% of cases, with secretion of hCG by metastatic cells being a primary indication. If elevated hCG or metastases are

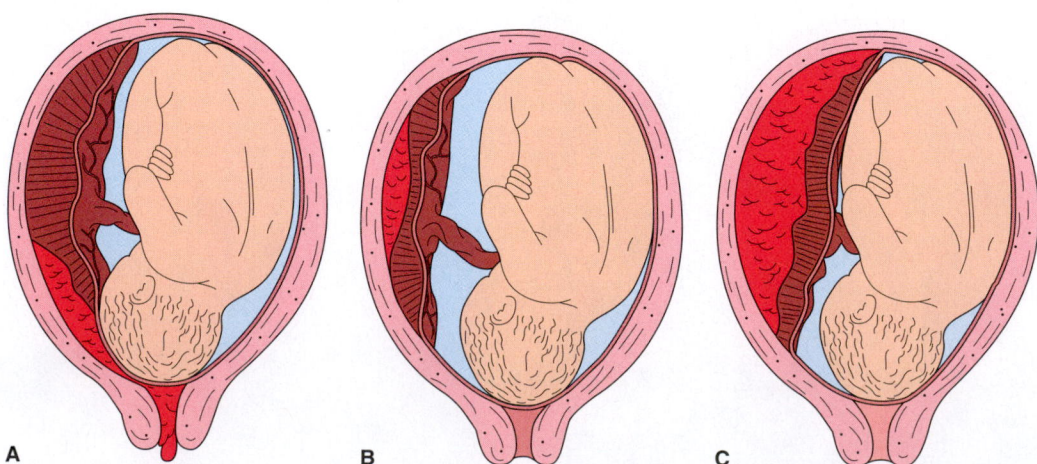

Figure 52-6. ■ Abruptio placentae. **A.** The marginal abruption with external hemorrhage. **B.** The central abruption with concealed hemorrhage. **C.** Complete separation.

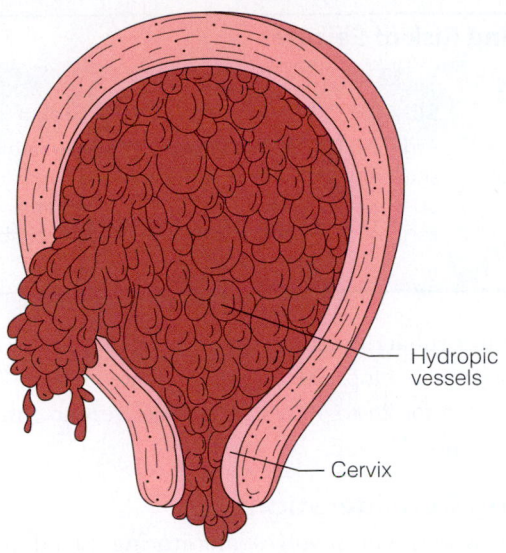

Figure 52-7. ■ Hydatidiform mole. A common sign is vaginal bleeding, often brownish (the characteristic "prune juice" appearance) but sometimes bright red. In this figure, some of the hydropic vesicles are being passed. This confirms the diagnosis of hydatidiform mole.

detected, chemotherapy is begun at once. Therefore, women with GTD are advised to avoid pregnancy for a year after the evacuation of a mole. If the woman has completed her childbearing or if excessive bleeding occurs, a hysterectomy may be recommended.

HYPERTENSIVE DISORDERS

Several hypertensive disorders can occur throughout pregnancy. The National Heart, Lung, and Blood Institute recommends the following classification of hypertensive disorders (Roberts, Pearson, Cutler, & Lindheimer, 2003):

- Preeclampsia/eclampsia
- Gestational hypertension
- Chronic hypertension
- Superimposed preeclampsia on chronic hypertension

Preeclampsia is the most common complication of pregnancy. Although the cause of preeclampsia is unknown, it is most often seen in primigravidas under 20 or over 35 years of age who have a poor nutritional status. Diabetes and multiple pregnancy increase the risk of preeclampsia. The only cure is delivery of the baby.

Manifestations

Preeclampsia is a complex condition that develops after 20 weeks of gestation, during labor, or in the first 48 hours after birth. The classic symptoms include progressive hypertension and proteinuria. Vasoconstriction decreases circulation to the uterus and placenta (Figure 52-8 ■). Blood flow to the kidneys slows, which decreases filtration through the glomerulus, resulting in protein in the urine and altered BUN, creatinine, and uric acid levels. A decreased urinary output leads to fluid overload, cerebral edema, headache, visual disturbances, and hyperactive deep-tendon reflexes. The liver enlarges, resulting in epigastric pain and liver damage.

The disorder ranges from mild preeclampsia to eclampsia and HELLP syndrome (see next paragraph). The blood pressure elevation is obtained on two occasions 6 hours apart. Mild preeclampsia is exhibited by a blood pressure of 30 mm Hg systolic *OR* 15 mm Hg diastolic above the client's normal blood pressure reading *OR* a blood pressure reading of 140/90 or higher. Edema may be seen in the hands and face, but edema alone is not diagnostic as other disorders can also cause edema. The client often has a weight gain of more than 1 pound per week. The urine may show 1+ or 2+ protein on a dipstick. In severe preeclampsia the blood pressure increases to 160/110 or higher. Generalized edema is noted in the hands, face, sacrum, lower extremities,

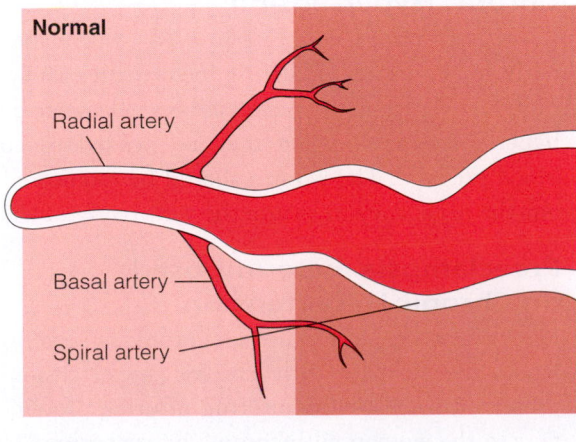

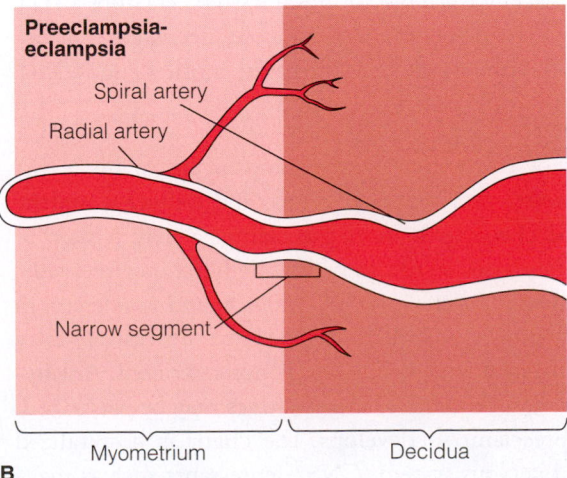

Figure 52-8. ■ **A.** In normal pregnancy, the spiral arteries permit increased blood flow to the placenta. **B.** In preeclampsia, vasoconstriction occurs. This restricts blood flow to the placenta.

TABLE 52-2 **Pharmacology: Drug to Reduce CNS Activity and Risk of Seizures**

DRUG NAME (GENERIC NAME AND CLASS)	USUAL ROUTE/DOSE	CLASSIFICATION AND PURPOSE	SELECTED SIDE EFFECTS	DON'T GIVE IF
Magnesium sulfate (MgSO$_4$)	Loading dose: 6g in 100 mL IV solution over 20 minutes. Maintenance dose 2g/hr via infusion pump.	Mineral/electrolyte used as anticonvulsant and smooth muscle relaxant	Arrhythmias, headache, slurred speech, flushing, absent reflexes, circulatory collapse	Respiratory rate is less than 12, urinary output less than 30 mL/hr, diminished or absent reflexes

and abdomen. Weight gain may be 2 or more pounds in a few days to a week. Protein will be 3+ to 4+ on a dipstick. Urine output may drop to less than 500 mL in 24 hours. The client may exhibit other symptoms including headache, blurred vision, scotoma (spots before the eyes), irritability, hyperreflexes, and epigastric pain. If left untreated, the disorder may progress to **eclampsia** as evidenced by grand mal seizures. The client may slip into a coma. The seizures may reoccur and the client may die. The seizure activity may induce uterine contractions, but the comatose client may be unable to let anyone know about them. Severe preeclampsia with liver damage is characterized by Hemolysis, Elevated Liver enzymes, and Low Platelet count or **HELLP syndrome.** Hemolysis, broken red blood cells (RBCs), occurs when vasospasms cause platelets to aggregate and a fibrin network to form. As RBCs are forced through the fibrin network, they break, resulting in a large decrease in hematocrit. It is thought that elevated liver enzymes (AST and ALT) are due to microemboli in vessels in the liver causing ischemia. A low platelet count of less than 100,000/mm^3 occurs when platelets aggregate in the arteries. HELLP syndrome results in ischemia and tissue damage. The low platelet count may potentiate postdelivery bleeding.

Preeclampsia may cause placental infarction, which in turn may cause intrauterine growth restriction (IUGR) and acute hypoxia in the fetus, leading to intrauterine death. Abruptio placentae is more common with preeclampsia. The fetus may be born preterm due to spontaneous labor or obstetrical induction to save the life of the mother and infant.

Treatment

The goals of treatment of preeclampsia are to lower the blood pressure, prevent convulsions, and deliver a healthy infant. The client with mild preeclampsia may remain at home but is advised to rest in bed while lying on either side. A well-balanced diet, high in protein and moderate in sodium, should be provided for the client. Excessively salty foods should be avoided, but salt is not restricted. Antihypertensive drugs, diuretics, and sedatives may be prescribed. If severe preeclampsia develops, the client is hospitalized and central nervous system (CNS) depressants such as magnesium sulfate (MgSO$_4$) are given by intravenous infusion. A syringe containing calcium carbonate, the antidote for

magnesium sulfate, must be at the bedside in case magnesium toxicity develops. Magnesium sulfate (Table 52-2 ■) is usually given for 24 to 48 hours after delivery to ensure that seizures do not develop.

Nursing Considerations

Nursing assessment involves monitoring blood pressure, urine output, proteinuria, and deep-tendon reflexes. In mild preeclampsia, the client feels healthy and must be encouraged to follow the plan of care. Teaching regarding diet, activity, and medication must be provided. In severe preeclampsia, the client is hospitalized, and fetal and maternal monitoring is more frequent. The nurse should be prepared to assist with induction of labor or cesarean section delivery if the client does not improve. Preeclampsia slowly decreases following delivery, but the client remains at risk for seizure for several days. For this reason, clients usually remain hospitalized and blood pressure, urine protein, and deep-tendon reflexes are frequently monitored.

Gestational Hypertension

Gestational hypertension (GH), formerly called pregnancy-induced hypertension (PIH), is hypertension occurring for the first time in midpregnancy and returning to normal levels by the 12th week after birth. The client does not develop proteinuria.

Chronic Hypertension

Chronic hypertension is the term used to describe the client with hypertension occurring before pregnancy or when high blood pressure persists past 6 weeks after birth. Antihypertensive medication may be needed to control the blood pressure. The woman should be monitored throughout the pregnancy to ensure the well-being of the fetus.

Preeclampsia Superimposed on Chronic Hypertension

Preeclampsia superimposed on chronic hypertension occurs when the woman with chronic hypertension develops preeclampsia. Close monitoring of urine protein is important in the woman with chronic hypertension. The woman with chronic hypertension who develops preeclampsia can rapidly progress to eclampsia. Box 52-3 ■ lists manifestations of preeclampsia and eclampsia.

BOX 52-3 | DATA COLLECTION

Preeclampsia and Eclampsia

Mild Preeclampsia

- Blood pressure of 30 mmHg systolic or 15 mmHg diastolic above the client's normal blood pressure reading *or* BP reading of 140/90
- Possible edema in hands and face
- Weight gain of more than 1 pound per week
- Possible urine output reduction
- Urine may show 1+ protein on a dipstick
- Hyperreflexes
- Complaints of headache, blurred vision, scotoma (spots before eyes), irritability, epigastric pain

Severe Preeclampsia

- Blood pressure increases to 160/110 or higher
- Generalized edema in hands, face, sacrum, lower extremities, and abdomen
- Possible weight gain of 2 or more pounds in a few days to a week
- Urine protein 2+ or more on a dipstick
- Urine output reduced, possibly less than 500 mL in 24 hours

Eclampsia

- Grand mal seizures
- Possible coma
- Initiation of contractions (The seizure activity may induce uterine contractions, but the comatose client may be unable to let anyone know.)
- Death

HEMOLYTIC DISORDERS

Hemolytic disorders are those conditions that cause a breaking of fetal RBCs either during or immediately following delivery. There are two types of hemolytic disorders.

Rh Incompatibility

Rh incompatibility can only happen when the mother is Rh negative and the fetus is Rh positive. The placenta normally keeps the maternal and fetal blood from mixing. However, there could be times when tears occur in the placenta. Examples include abruptio placentae, placental infection, abortion, and birth. At that time fetal blood can enter the maternal circulation. Sometimes a miscarriage occurs without the mother's knowledge, causing her to develop sensitivity to the Rh factor.

The maternal Rh-negative blood produces antibodies against the Rh-positive fetal blood. Because this mixing of blood usually occurs at the time of delivery, this fetus is not harmed. However, the mother has been sensitized to the Rh factor. If the next pregnancy is an Rh-positive fetus, the maternal antibodies will attack the fetus, resulting in hemolysis (Figure 52-9 ■). The infant will develop severe anemia, congestive heart failure, and jaundice. The fetus may need blood transfusion on delivery; in some cases, an intrauterine blood transfusion may be indicated.

DIAGNOSIS. Blood-screening tests done at the first prenatal visit determine the mother's Rh factor and an indirect Coombs' test detects Rh antibodies. The indirect Coombs' test may be repeated throughout the pregnancy as necessary.

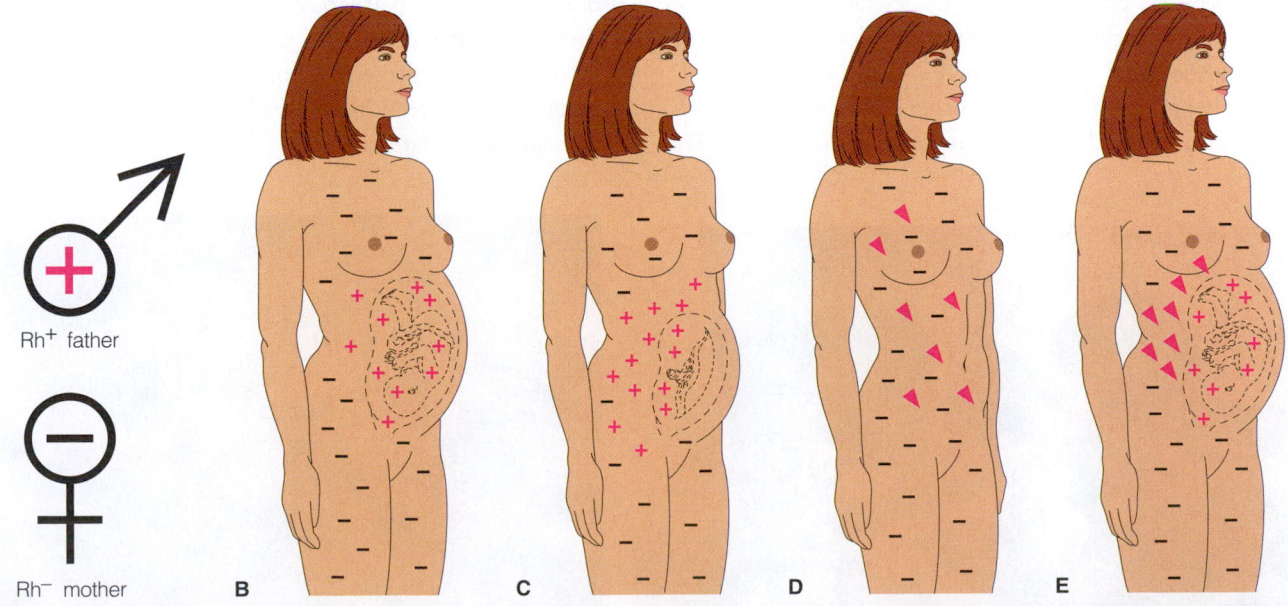

Rh+ father

Rh− mother

A   B   C   D   E

Figure 52-9. ■ Rh isoimmunization sequence. **A.** Rh-positive father and Rh-negative mother. **B.** Pregnancy with Rh-positive fetus. Some Rh-positive blood enters the mother's bloodstream. **C.** As the placenta separates, the mother is further exposed to the Rh-positive blood. **D.** The mother is sensitized to the Rh-positive blood; anti-Rh-positive antibodies (see *triangles*) are formed. **E.** In subsequent pregnancies with an Rh-positive fetus, Rh-positive red blood cells are attacked by the anti-Rh-positive maternal antibodies, causing hemolysis of red blood cells in the fetus.

TABLE 52-3	Pharmacology: Drug for Prevention of Hemolysis				
DRUG NAME (GENERIC NAME AND CLASS)	USUAL ROUTE/DOSE	CLASSIFICATION AND PURPOSE	SELECTED SIDE EFFECTS	DON'T GIVE IF
Rh immune globulin (RhoGAM)	300 mcg at 28 weeks' gestation 300 mcg within 72 hours of delivery	Immune globulin	Injection site irritation, fever myalgia	Mother is Rh positive; infant must be Rh positive if post-partum dose is given

TREATMENT. Every Rh-negative mother following delivery of every Rh-positive fetus should receive Rh immune globulin (RhoGAM) within 72 hours of delivery. It is also recommended that RhoGAM (Table 52-3 ■) be given at 28 weeks' gestation to protect the fetus from hemolysis.

ABO Incompatibility

The second hemolytic disorder affecting the fetus is ABO incompatibility. The most common type of ABO incompatibility occurs when the mother is type O and the fetus is A, B, or AB. The mother's blood contains anti-A and anti-B antibodies. If the mother's blood enters the fetal circulation, these antibodies attack the fetal blood. Because only a small amount of maternal blood enters the fetus, the amount of antibodies is limited. The impact on the fetus is not as severe as Rh incompatibility.

GESTATIONAL DIABETES MELLITUS

Appearing only during pregnancy, **gestational diabetes mellitus** (GDM) is an abnormal glucose metabolism caused by the additional requirement for insulin. Many women who develop GDM will develop diabetes mellitus later in life. The client who develops diabetes prior to pregnancy faces the same risks to the pregnancy as does the client who develops gestational diabetes, but the blood glucose is more difficult to control.

In early pregnancy, the mother's pancreas increases insulin production due to an increase in hormones. The tissue's response to the high insulin level is increased as well. After the 20th week of pregnancy, an increased resistance to insulin develops as a result of increased placental hormones. Fat is more readily metabolized, resulting in ketonuria. Because the maternal glucose provides energy for the developing fetus, balancing blood glucose levels is more difficult. After delivery of the placenta, there is a rapid decrease in the amount of insulin required. The diabetic client is at greater risk for preeclampsia and ketoacidosis than the nondiabetic client (Figure 52-10 ■).

Maternal hyperglycemia can result in *macrosomia* (excessive growth) in the fetus (see Figure 52-10B). Hyperglycemia stimulates fetal insulin production. After birth, the source of glucose is removed, and the infant can develop hypoglycemia within 2 to 4 hours. Gradually the fetus will produce only the amount of insulin needed.

HYDRAMNIOS

Hydramnios (also called *polyhydramnios*) is excessive amniotic fluid. The exact cause is unknown, but it occurs more frequently when the fetus has congenital anomalies (Laughlin & Knuppel, 2003) or in pregnant women with diabetes (Dashe, Nathan, McIntire, & Leveno, 2000). Hydramnios can increase the chance of premature rupture of membranes and preterm labor. Other complications include uterine dysfunction from overdistention, postpartum hemorrhage, and cesarean birth.

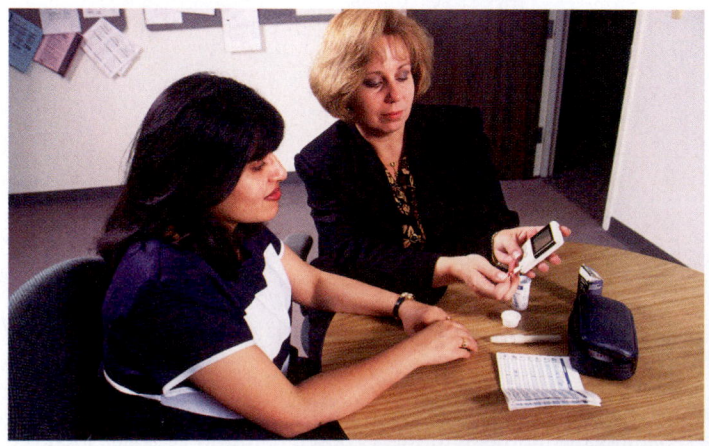

A

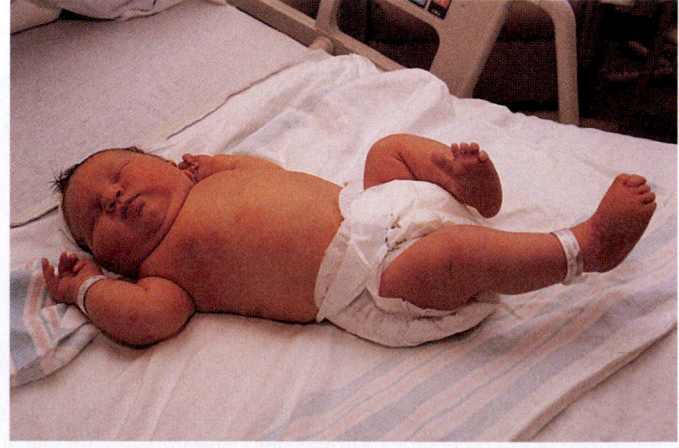

B

Figure 52-10. ■ **A.** Pregnant woman learning to do serum glucose monitoring. **B.** Macrosomia. This infant's mother had diabetes during the pregnancy.

MULTIPLE PREGNANCY

Multiple pregnancy is the carrying of more than one fetus. The most common multiple pregnancy is twin pregnancy. Other multiple pregnancies could occur naturally, but they usually are a result of infertility treatment. *Fraternal twins* result from two ova being fertilized by two sperm. Fraternal twins could be two boys, two girls, or one boy and one girl.

Identical twins result from one ova fertilized by one sperm, dividing into two blastocysts. Because identical twins come from the same fertilized ovum, they must be the same sex.

Conjoined twins result from incomplete separation of the blastocyst.

Multiple pregnancy is suspected when the fundal height is greater than expected in the first few weeks of pregnancy. Diagnosis may be confirmed with an ultrasound. As the uterus enlarges, the discomforts of pregnancy are enhanced.

Preeclampsia, gestational diabetes, and preterm labor are more common with multiple pregnancy. More frequent prenatal monitoring is indicated.

Medical Conditions Complicated by Pregnancy

CARDIAC DISORDERS

Pregnancy puts additional work on the woman's heart. Although the cardiovascular system must be routinely assessed, most young women compensate without undue risk. However, not every young woman has a healthy heart prior to pregnancy. She may have a heart defect or have sustained cardiac damage from a childhood infection, chronic illness, or drug abuse. The added workload on the damaged heart may result in congestive heart failure. The following symptoms are indicative of congestive heart failure and must be reported to the primary care provider:

- Frequent cough with or without hemoptysis (bloody sputum)
- Progressive dyspnea with exertion
- Rales in lung bases
- Progressive generalized edema
- Heart murmur
- Fatigue

The client with cardiac disorders may require constant heart monitoring during labor. Signs of worsening heart failure may necessitate a cesarean section delivery.

URINARY DISORDERS

Pregnancy puts additional work on the urinary system. If the pregnant woman has preexisting renal disorders, such as glomerulonephritis, the additional work on the kidneys may result in further renal damage or renal failure. Signs of worsening renal damage include edema, hypertension, decreased urine output, and increase in serum creatinine and blood urea nitrogen (BUN). The urologist may need to be consulted in the medical management of the pregnant woman with renal complications.

The enlarging uterus can put pressure on the urethra, bladder, and ureters, slowing the flow of urine and increasing the possibility of urinary infection. Signs of urinary infection include burning on urination, cloudy, foul smelling urine, and blood in the urine. If the infection progresses into the ureters and kidneys, flank pain and fever are also common symptoms. Urinary infection in the pregnant woman can stimulate uterine contractions and should be treated with antibiotics.

INFECTIONS

Any infection during pregnancy should be diagnosed and treated. Although many infections are not harmful to the fetus, some can cause preterm labor, fetal infections, congenital anomalies, and death. One group of infections is particularly dangerous during pregnancy and will be discussed here.

Toxoplasmosis

The **TORCH group** of infections includes **to**xoplasmosis, **r**ubella, **c**ytomegalovirus, and **h**erpesvirus type 2.

Toxoplasmosis is caused by a protozoan picked up by eating raw or partially cooked meat and from cat feces. If the mother contracts toxoplasmosis during pregnancy, there is an increased incidence of stillbirth, preterm labor, and neonatal death. If contracted before the 20th week of pregnancy, fetal anomalies involving the CNS may occur. The best treatment is preventing the infection by eating fully cooked meat and avoiding contact with a cat litter box. Infected women may be treated with sulfadiazine (Microsulfon) or pyrimethamine (Daraprim).

Rubella

Rubella, also known as German or 3-day measles, is a highly contagious virus that is transmitted by the airborne route. The earlier in the pregnancy the mother is infected, the more serious the effects are on the fetus. Congenital rubella syndrome in the fetus is characterized by cataracts, deafness, and heart defects. Prevention is the best cure. Rubella immunization prior to pregnancy will allow the client to develop active immunity. Prenatal blood testing for hemagglutination inhibition (HAI) will indicate maternal immunity. A susceptible client should avoid exposure to rubella during pregnancy. The client who becomes pregnant may be counseled regarding a therapeutic abortion.

Cytomegalovirus

Cytomegalovirus (CMV), a member of the herpesvirus group, is found in the saliva, breast milk, urine, cervical mucus, and semen of infected individuals. Antibodies for CMV are found in half of all adults. The fetus may have no noticeable defects or a variety of CNS anomalies. There is no treatment for mother or fetus.

Herpes Genitalis

Herpes genitalis (herpes simplex virus Type II or HSV-II) is exhibited by painful vesicles on the genitals. The lesions appear several hours to 20 days after exposure. The first episode is usually the most severe. While recurrence can happen at any time, stress associated with pregnancy can stimulate a new outbreak. There is no cure, but medications such as acyclovir (Zovirax) can reduce the time the lesions contain live virus and shorten healing time. If an acute outbreak occurs during the first trimester, there is a 50% chance the pregnancy will end in spontaneous abortion or stillbirth. If no lesions are noted at the beginning of labor, a vaginal delivery may be performed. If active lesions are present at the beginning of labor, there is a risk the fetus will be exposed during a vaginal delivery. Therefore, a cesarean section delivery is planned. (See in-depth discussion of sexually transmitted infections in Chapter 41 ⚭.)

AIDS

Acquired immune deficiency syndrome (AIDS), caused by the human immunodeficiency virus (HIV), is discussed here as it relates to the mother and fetus. Further discussion appears in Chapter 35 ⚭. To understand the transmission, pathophysiology, and treatment of HIV/AIDS, refer to a general medical-surgical textbook.

Although AIDS in the United States remains more prevalent in homosexual and bisexual males, the incidence in women is increasing, and rates among some racial and ethnic groups are significantly higher than others (Box 52-4 ■). The number of pediatric cases is declining, with the majority of reported cases being infants born to HIV-positive mothers. The decline is associated with implementing

---

BOX 52-4 | **CULTURAL PULSE POINTS**

Incidence of HIV and AIDS by Ethnic Group

There continues to be an increase in reported cases of HIV/AIDS among heterosexual women in the United States, especially in the regions of the Northeast and the South. A CDC report on AIDS cases in 2003 for females age 13 and older also showed that there were strong racial and ethnic correlations among groups. This study, which encompassed the 50 states and Washington, D.C., documented the actual number of reported cases of AIDS, the percentage of the total number of cases, and the rate per 100,000 population for five groups of women over age 13: White women, Hispanic women, Black women, Asian/Pacific Islanders, and American Indian/Alaska Natives.

The study showed White women as having 1,725 cases of AIDS. This is 15% of all reported cases, and a rate of 2 infected women per 100,000 population.

Hispanic women had almost an equal number of cases of AIDS (1,744), and a similar percentage (16%) of total cases. However, this number indicated a rate six times greater than that in White women: 12.4 per 100,000 population.

Black women had the highest number of AIDS cases (7,551) and the highest percentage (68%). These figures translate to a rate of just over 50 infected women per 100,000 population.

Among Asian/Pacific Islanders, the number of cases of AIDS was 86, representing less than 1% of all cases and the lowest rate (1.6 per 100,000 population).

American Indians/Alaska Natives had the smallest number of reported cases (46) and also less than 1% of all cases of AIDS. However, this number represents a rate three times greater than that of Asian/Pacific Islanders (4.8 per 100,000).

(Source: CDC: National Center for HIV, STD and TB Prevention. AIDS Cases and Rates for Female Adults and Adolescents, by Race/Ethnicity 2003—50 States and D.C.)

---

universal counseling about the risk of transmission from mother to fetus, voluntary testing of pregnant women, birth by cesarean section, and the use of zidovudine (ZDV) therapy for infected women and their infants (Table 52-4 ■).

TABLE 52-4	**Pharmacology: Drugs Used to Treat Infections**			
DRUG NAME (GENERIC NAME AND CLASS)	**USUAL ROUTE/DOSE**	**CLASSIFICATION AND PURPOSE**	**SELECTED SIDE EFFECTS**	**DON'T GIVE IF**
Sulfadiazine (Microsulfon)	PO 2–8 g/d divided dose every 6 hours	Anti-infective	Drug allergy, headache, malaise, anemia	Allergic to sulfa Pregnant Category C drug; use drug with caution Breastfeeding
Pyrimethamine (Daraprim)	PO 50–75 mg/d with sulfadiazine	Anti-infective	Folic acid deficiency GI upset, anemia, skin rash, CNS stimulation including seizure	Dose needed to treat toxoplasmosis near toxic level Administration of folic acid decreases effectiveness Breastfeeding
Acyclovir (Zovirax)	PO 400 mg tid × 7–10 days	Antiviral, anti-infective	Minimal	Breastfeeding
Azidothymidine (AZT) Zidovudine (ZDV)	PO 200 mg every 4 hours	Antiviral, anti-infective	Headache, dizziness, malaise, bone marrow depression	Hematology indicative of toxicity Breastfeeding

Many women who are HIV positive actively avoid pregnancy because of the risk to the infant and the probability of their death before the child can be raised. Some women are asymptomatic and may be unaware of HIV exposure until after they become pregnant.

Pregnancy is not believed to accelerate the progression of AIDS in the woman who is asymptomatic. However, women with low CD4 counts who are symptomatic have been known to have accelerated progression of AIDS. The administration of ZDV (azidothymidine, AZT) greatly reduces the risk of transmission to the fetus. Most medication used to treat AIDS is safe to administer during pregnancy.

HIV transmission can occur during pregnancy and through breast milk, but most transmission occurs during the birth process. The rate of transmission to the infant is less than 2% in women who have been treated with ZDV, who delivered by cesarean section at 38 weeks and prior to rupture of membranes, and who did not breast feed. Following delivery, infants are usually asymptomatic. They may have a positive antibody titer, which indicates passive immunity from the mother. Many of these infants are small for gestational age and are likely to be premature. However, this could be due to socioeconomic conditions and not necessarily HIV. The signs of HIV in infants include failure to thrive, hepatosplenomegaly, and recurrent infections, including Epstein-Barr virus and bacterial infections. Delayed development milestones and loss of acquired skills are common. The prognosis for the infected child is poor.

NURSING CARE

PRIORITIZING NURSING CARE

Priorities of care for the at-risk pregnancy focus on the following:

- Detecting complications at an early stage
- Assisting with implementation of medical treatment
- Evaluating the response to treatment as evidenced by stability of the specific condition

ASSESSING

The assessment of the high-risk mother and fetus consists of frequent monitoring. The time intervals between data collecting vary, depending on the severity of the symptoms and the stability of the client. The data that can be collected without a physician order include:

- Vital signs: mother's temperature, pulse, respiration and blood pressure, and FHR
- Mother's reflexes and clonus
- Amount of protein in mother's urine
- Uterine contractions
- Uterine bleeding

- Cervical changes unless contraindicated by uterine bleeding of unknown cause

Data that may be collected with a physician order include:

- Biophysical profile
- Fetal ultrasound

DIAGNOSIS, PLANNING, AND IMPLEMENTING

The plan of care is based on two goals. The first goal is to maintain the pregnancy for as long as possible to allow the fetus time to grow and mature. The second goal is to deliver in the best circumstances for both the mother and the fetus. The nursing diagnosis would be determined by the specific complication the woman is experiencing. For example, if uterine bleeding is present, the nursing diagnoses might include:

- *Deficient Fluid Volume*
- *Ineffective Peripheral Tissue Perfusion*
- *Deficient Knowledge* related to high-risk pregnancy

Expected outcomes might include:

- The urine output will be at least 50 mL/hr.
- The FHR will remain within normal limits.
- Client will verbalize an understanding of the high-risk disorder.

Medical and nursing interventions might include:

- Administer intravenous fluids including blood transfusion as ordered. *To maintain fluid volume, IV fluids must be administered. The client should be kept NPO in case surgery is needed. If blood loss is excessive, blood replacement will be needed to maintain tissue perfusion to the placenta.*
- Maintain bed rest with bathroom privileges. *Ambulation could cause increase in uterine bleeding. Activity increases the workload on the cardiovascular systems, which puts additional stress on the maternal heart, decreasing tissue perfusion to the placenta.*
- Administer tocolytic medications (drugs used to inhibit contractions). See Chapter 53 ⚭ for discussion of these medications.
- Administer medication to control blood pressure as ordered. *Fluid loss can lead to hypotension. Medication may be needed to maintain blood pressure. When GH is a complication of pregnancy, medication may need to be administered to lower the blood pressure.*
- Provide emotional support. *The mother, her partner, and family members are concerned for the well-being of both the mother and baby. Hemorrhage or hypertension puts both lives at risk. Being professional, remaining at the bedside, and keeping everyone informed of changes provides reassurance.*
- Provide instruction about diagnostic exams, medications, activity, and prognosis. *Providing information about the situation allows the client and family to make informed decisions and reduces anxiety.*

EVALUATING

Evaluating the effectiveness of the treatment for prenatal complications is essential to determine the well-being of both the mother and the fetus. Evaluation consists of a continual process of collecting data and comparing it to older data to determine if the mother and fetus remain stable. If the complication is controlled with treatment, the pregnancy can usually progress to a normal delivery at 38 to 40 weeks. If the complication cannot be controlled, a premature vaginal delivery or cesarean section delivery may need to be performed.

NURSING PROCESS CARE PLAN
Client with Gestational Diabetes Mellitus

Victoria, a 33-year-old primigravida, is 26 weeks pregnant. Victoria has had no complications until now. The routine 50-g glucose tolerance test showed a plasma glucose level of 162 mg/dL. A 3-hour 100-g glucose tolerance test confirmed a diagnosis of gestational diabetes. Victoria tells the nurse she wants to do everything she can to have a healthy baby.

Assessment
The following data should be collected as soon as possible:

- Vital signs
- Weight
- Urine protein and ketones
- Fetal heart tones (FHT)
- Mother's knowledge of gestational diabetes and treatment

Nursing Diagnosis
The following important nursing diagnosis (among others) is established for this condition:

- *Readiness for Enhanced Self-Health Management* related to desire to ensure healthy outcome of pregnancy complicated by gestational diabetes

Expected Outcomes
The outcomes for this client will include, but are not limited to, the following:

- Client will be compliant with monitoring and treatment plan.
- Client will state signs of hypoglycemia and hyperglycemia in early stages for prompt treatment.
- Client will keep in contact with healthcare provider.
- Client will recognize signs of preeclampsia and report to primary care provider for prompt treatment.

Planning and Implementation
Nursing interventions for the client with gestational diabetes would include the following:

- Provide written and verbal instruction regarding gestational diabetes. *Accurate information regarding the physiology of gestational diabetes and the impact on the fetus increases client compliance.*
- Provide written and verbal instruction about blood glucose monitoring, insulin administration, diet, and activity. *Proper self-monitoring and compliance with the treatment plan helps ensure a stable, healthy fetus.*
- Provide written and verbal instruction on signs and symptoms of hypoglycemia and hyperglycemia. *Early detection of hypoglycemia and hyperglycemia will prevent complications and ensure a healthy fetus.*
- Provide a schedule of prenatal visits as requested by the primary care provider. *Frequent prenatal checks help ensure stability of gestational diabetes and fetal health.*
- Provide written and verbal instruction on signs of preeclampsia. Monitor for signs of preeclampsia. *Preeclampsia occurs more frequently in diabetic pregnancies.*

Evaluation
The mother verbalizes understanding of the treatment plan. She demonstrates accuracy in blood glucose monitoring and insulin administration. She establishes a daily routine for self-care, and reports signs of hypoglycemia, hyperglycemia, and preeclampsia. She attends prenatal visits as requested.

Critical Thinking in the Nursing Process

1. What criteria would the nurse use to determine if Victoria was being compliant with monitoring blood glucose levels and administering insulin?
2. To whom should Victoria be referred for additional diabetes instruction?
3. What other health promotion topics should be discussed with Victoria?

Note: Discussion of Critical Thinking questions appears on the MyNursingKit Website.

Note: The references and resources for all chapters have been compiled at the back of the book.

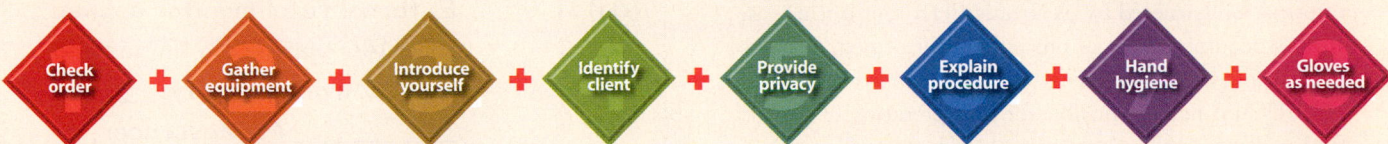

PROCEDURE 52-1   External Electronic Fetal Monitoring

Purpose

- To obtain a continuous reading on the status of the fetus prior to delivery

Equipment

- Electronic fetal monitor
- Elastic monitor belts (2)
- Tocodynamometer, also called a "toco"
- Ultrasound transducer
- Ultrasound gel

Check order + Gather equipment + Introduce yourself + Identify client + Provide privacy + Explain procedure + Hand hygiene + Gloves as needed

Interventions and Rationales

1. Perform preparatory steps (see icon bar above).

2. With the monitor turned on, place the two monitor belts around the woman's abdomen. *The two belts should fit snugly, but should not impede circulation.*

3. Palpate the area off midline and over the uterine fundus that is most firm during contractions. Place the "toco" in this area, and secure it with one elastic belt. *Because the fundus is the area where contractions are greatest, this placement will provide the best graph of uterine contractions.*

4. Adjust the tracing so it shows 10 or 15 mm Hg between contractions. *Adjustment to this level prevents background static.*

5. Apply gel to the diaphragm of the transducer, and place the diaphragm on the mother's abdomen halfway between the symphysis pubis and the umbilicus. *The gel seals contact between the diaphragm and the maternal abdomen to produce the best quality sound. The midline of the mother's abdomen is most often closest to the fetal heart. When the uterus contracts, pressure is exerted against the "toco" and information is relayed to the electronic fetal monitor and recorded on graph paper.*

6. Move the diaphragm laterally or vertically until the strongest heart sound is heard. (If the fetus is breech, the heart sound will be above the umbilicus.) Attach the second elastic belt snugly to the transducer at this point. *Note*: If a beltless monitor is available (Figure 52-11 ■), follow specific directions for attaching it. *When the diaphragm directs the ultrasonic beam toward the fetal heart, the whiplike sound of the heartbeat will be heard. Moving the transducer laterally helps determine the position that is most directly over the fetal heart.*

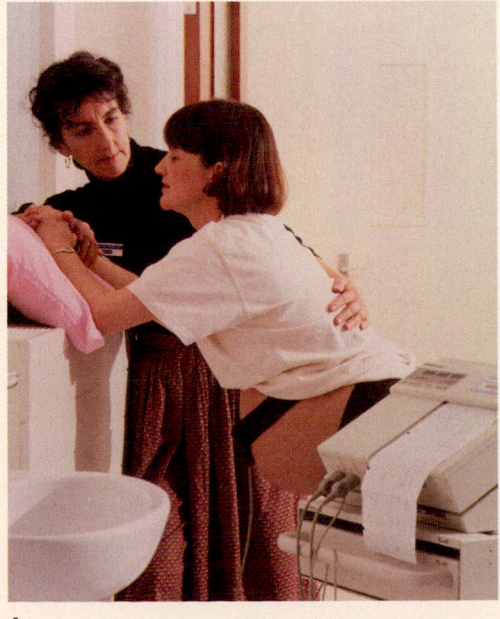

A

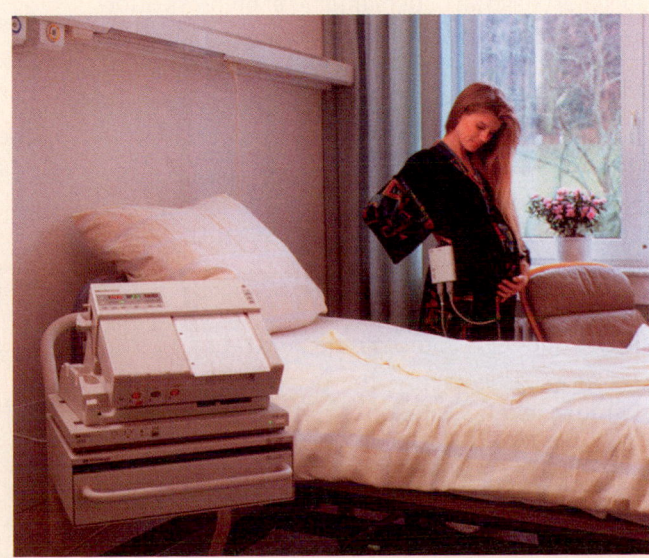

B

Figure 52-11. ■ ■ **A.** External electronic fetal monitoring device showing graph readout. **B.** Beltless tocodynamometer system features remote telemetry that allows the laboring mother more mobility.

The belt keeps the transducer in position. A beltless FHR monitor allows the mother to move around the room.

7. At the beginning of the fetal monitor tape, record the following information: date, time, woman's name, gravida, para, membrane status, and name of the care provider (physician or certified nurse midwife). Follow facility guidelines. *Documentation is a continuous part of quality care. Individual facilities may require additional information to be recorded on the tape.*

8. Follow facility policy about ongoing documentation of information gathered by electronic FHR monitoring, as well as documentation of procedures performed, changes in position, any therapy that might be initiated, etc. The LPN/LVN is not responsible for interpretation of findings but must report unusual findings as directed. *The baseline rate in bpm, plus acceleration and decelerations of*

FHR in response to maternal contractions, are some of the data that will be recorded. Data either can be reassuring or can provide an early warning of possible complications. Prompt reporting of designated information allows therapeutic intervention. Documentation according to facility policy provides for safe practice and quality care.

SAMPLE DOCUMENTATION

[date] [time]	External fetal monitor applied, FHR 140 bpm, "C" q4m, lasting 45 sec, mod intensity. _____ _____ M. Messenger, LPN

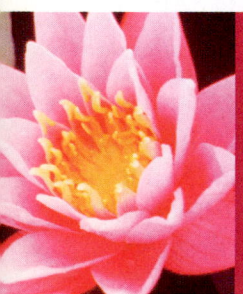

Chapter Review

KEY Points

- Complication may occur in any pregnancy that can put both mother and fetus at risk.
- The LPN/LVN must have an understanding of high-risk disorders in order to recognize and report symptoms, and to assist the RN in care of the woman with a high-risk pregnancy.
- Early recognition and careful monitoring allow early treatment of complications in the client or fetus.
- Complications can result from the pregnancy itself or from conditions that existed before the woman became pregnant.
- Preeclampsia is hypertension accompanied by proteinuria and endangers the health and lives of the mother and fetus.
- Disruption or poor placement of the placenta can cause hemorrhage, endangering both mother and fetus.
- Infections can be passed across the placenta, causing injury or death to the fetus. Infections can also be transmitted from the birth canal to the fetus during the birthing process.
- Cesarean section is the birthing method chosen when maternal infection poses a risk to the fetus.

⌾ FOR FURTHER Study

Acquired immune deficiency syndrome (AIDS) has its main discussion in Chapter 35.

See discussion of D&C in Chapter 40.

Sexually transmitted infections are described in Chapter 41.

Refer to Table 51-3 for normal values during pregnancy.

Tocolytic medications (drugs used to inhibit contractions) are listed in Chapter 53.

PEARSON
EXPLORE **mynursingkit**™

MyNursingKit is your one stop for online chapter review materials and resources. Prepare for success with additional NCLEX®-style practice questions, interactive assignments and activities, web links, animations and videos, and more!

Register your access code from the front of your book at
www.mynursingkit.com

Critical Thinking Care Map

Woman Presenting with Preeclampsia
NCLEX-PN® Focus Area: Physiologic Adaptation

Case Study: Marie, 19 years old, is admitted to the antepartum unit from the clinic following her scheduled prenatal check-up. She is 35 weeks pregnant with her first baby. Marie has gained 4 pounds in the last 2 weeks. Her blood pressure is 162/98. She states she has had a headache and some blurred vision the past 2 to 3 days. She has 2+ edema in her feet, but she has been working all day without a break. States urine output seems less than usual. Urine is 3+ for protein. States she has been able to eat more meat this week.

Nursing Diagnosis: *Deficient Fluid Volume* related to fluid shift from vascular to subcutaneous tissue

COLLECT DATA

Subjective	Objective
_____	_____
_____	_____
_____	_____
_____	_____
_____	_____
_____	_____

Would you report this? Yes/No

If yes, report to: _____

What would you report? _____

Nursing Care

_____

_____

_____

_____

_____

_____

_____

_____

_____

How would you document this? _____

_____

_____

_____

Compare your answers and documentation to those provided on the MyNursingKit Website.

Data Collected
(use only those that apply)

- 3+ proteinuria
- BP 162/98
- States headache
- High-sodium diet
- States blurred vision
- Weight up 4 pounds in 2 weeks
- 2+ edema
- Decreased urine output

Nursing Interventions
(use only those that apply; list in priority order)

- Refer to WIC program.
- Teach need to increase prenatal vitamins.
- Position woman on left side.
- Draw blood to test hemoglobin level.
- Private room with limited visitors.
- Teach need for decreased activity.
- Obtain FHR.
- Assess deep tendon reflexes and clonus.
- Obtain BP every hour.
- Record I & O.

NCLEX-PN® Exam Preparation

1 The nurse advises the pregnant client to do which of the following in order to reduce the risk of toxoplasmosis?
1. Avoid contact with a cat litter box.
2. Drink only bottled or boiled water.
3. Avoid contact with body fluids.
4. Wash all fresh fruits and vegetables.

2 When assisting in the care of a client who has mild preeclampsia and is at risk for severe preeclampsia, the nurse would check the urine for the presence of which of the following?
1. Specific gravity
2. Protein
3. Glucose
4. pH

3 The nurse recognizes all of the following as factors that contribute to the classification of high risk except:
1. Smoking.
2. History of preterm labor.
3. Residence.
4. Multiple pregnancies.

4 The nurse, talking to a group of high school students, explains that the risks associated with pregnancy increase in pregnant mothers at or under the age of:
1. 16.
2. 17.
3. 15.
4. 18.

5 The nurse, caring for a woman with a newly diagnosed pregnancy, explains that it will be necessary to repeat the maternal hemoglobin test at:
1. 4 months.
2. 7 months.
3. 9 months.
4. 18 weeks.

6 The nurse assists the physician in performing a 1-hour glucose screen. The results are 125 mg/dL. The nurse anticipates that the physician will order which of the following?
1. Insulin administration
2. Follow-up urine testing for glucose

3. 100-g oral glucose tolerance test
4. No further testing

7 The nurse, working in an obstetrician's office, admits a 28-week pregnant client with a history of rheumatic heart disease. The nurse would consider which of the following an important intervention for this client that may not be necessary in other pregnant women?
1. Measurement of blood pressure
2. Assessment of breath sounds
3. Chest x-ray
4. Routine urine screening

8 The nurse receives a call from a client who is 26 weeks pregnant reporting discomfort in the lower middle abdomen, urinary frequency, and mild irregular infrequent contractions. The client denies vaginal bleeding or rupture of membranes but says there is a small amount of blood in the urine. The nurse suspects:
1. Preterm labor.
2. Urinary tract infection.
3. Threatened miscarriage.
4. Placenta previa.

9 The nurse, caring for a client with a high-risk pregnancy, recognizes the importance of:
1. Frequent fetal and maternal monitoring.
2. Encouraging complete bed rest during the last trimester of pregnancy.
3. Frequent reinforcement of teaching about the signs and symptoms of preterm labor starting with the first visit to the obstetrician's office.
4. Preparing the mother for a possible negative outcome.

10 The nurse's goal when caring for a client with a high-risk pregnancy is to deliver care that will maintain the pregnancy for as long as possible and to:
1. Optimize delivery under the best possible circumstances.
2. Ensure optimum urine output.
3. Maintain normal fetal heart tones.
4. Teach the client about the high-risk disorder.

Answers and rationales for review questions appear in Appendix I.

Chapter 53

Care of Women during Labor and Birth

LEARNING Outcomes

After completing this chapter, you will be able to:

1. Describe the beginning of labor and variables that affect labor and birth.
2. List the stages and mechanisms of labor and important nursing interventions for each stage.
3. Identify nursing diagnoses and nursing interventions to assist the client in labor.
4. Describe the role of the LPN/LVN in preparing the mother for birth and in providing infant care.
5. Identify causes of high-risk labor and appropriate nursing interventions for them.

Clinical Objectives

6. Teach the client the basic concepts of labor and birth.
7. Observe assessment and monitoring of laboring clients.
8. Provide basic comfort measures during labor.
9. Recognize the effects of analgesia and anesthesia on the laboring client and fetus.
10. Observe and/or assist with nursing care of a client during labor and birth.
11. Analyze the nursing role in providing care of a client during labor and birth.
12. Examine interrelationships between behavioral and physical responses to labor.
13. Observe, through various monitoring techniques, the fetal response to labor.

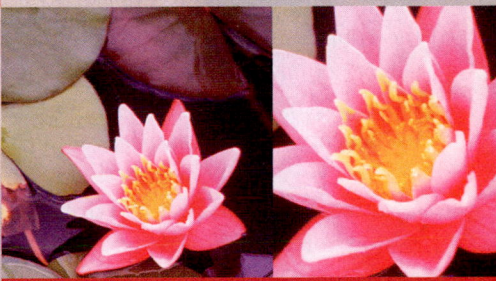

BRIEF Outline

Beginning of Labor
Signs of Impending Labor
Variables Affecting Labor
Stages of Labor
Birth
Recovery
High-Risk Labor and Birth

During the past three decades, many changes have been made in birthing practices. Childbirth classes are offered to help the couple prepare together for the birth experience. The partner often accompanies the woman through the birthing process. In many places the "traditional" sterile delivery room has given way to the modern homelike environment of the birthing center, where labor, birth, and recovery occur in the same room. This chapter will discuss the birthing process and related nursing care. The goal in all instances is for a healthy infant to be born under the safest conditions possible.

Beginning of Labor

Toward the end of pregnancy, the mother and fetus begin preparing for birth. Researchers are still unsure of the exact cause of labor, but two theories have been developed to answer the question "Why does labor begin?" Once this question can be answered, preterm labor can be prevented or stopped, and labor can be induced more easily if needed.

OVERDISTENTION THEORY

One theory to explain the onset of **labor** (process by which the fetus is expelled from the uterus through the vagina to the outside world) is based on the principle that hollow organs tend to empty themselves when overdistended. This theory explains the emptying of the bladder and sigmoid colon. While this phenomenon may partially explain the beginning of labor, it does not fully explain it.

HORMONAL THEORY

The hormonal theory relates to the complex relationship of maternal and fetal hormones. Fetal cortisol production increases as the fetus matures. Fetal cortisol is believed to decrease the placental production of progesterone and stimulate the precursors of prostaglandin that ripen the cervix. A decrease in progesterone results in a decrease in the smooth muscle relaxing effect on the uterus. As the progesterone level declines, the estrogen level rises. Estrogen increases the sensitivity of the myometrium to oxytocin. Oxytocin production by the mother's posterior pituitary gland increases, causing the uterus to contract.

Signs of Impending Labor

Although its exact time cannot be predicted, several signs indicate that onset of labor is close:

- *Lightening:* The descent of the fetus into the pelvis may occur as early as 2 to 4 weeks prior to the onset of labor, but in multipara clients, **lightening** may not occur until labor contractions begin. The descent of the fetus into the pelvis relieves pressure on the diaphragm, allowing the mother to breathe more easily and "feel lighter" (thus the term *lightening*). However, when the fetus enters the pelvis, more pressure is placed on the bladder, resulting in urinary frequency. There is also an increase in venous stasis associated with lower extremity edema. Low back pain and leg cramps result from pressure on pelvic nerves.
- *Braxton Hicks contractions:* Irregular painless contractions occur throughout pregnancy. They become more frequent and more noticeable during the last few weeks. At times, they cause women to go to the hospital believing labor has begun. Braxton Hicks contractions squeeze *around* the uterus instead of from the top down. They cause no change in the cervix, and so are termed *false labor.* Table 53-1 ■ compares false labor and true labor.
- *Cervical changes:* Due to hormone changes beginning at about 35 weeks of gestation, the cervix begins to mature or "ripen." The cervix becomes softer. **Effacement** (the shortening and thinning of the cervix) and *dilatation* (opening of the cervical os) may begin.
- *Bloody show:* The passage of the mucous plug from the cervix, which often contains a small amount of blood, is called *bloody show.* Labor often begins within 48 hours

TABLE 53-1	False versus True Labor	
CHARACTERISTIC	**TRUE LABOR**	**FALSE LABOR**
Contractions	■ Occur regularly, becoming stronger, lasting longer, occurring closer together. ■ Increase in intensity with walking. ■ Are felt in lower back, radiating to lower portion of abdomen. ■ Continue despite use of comfort measures.	■ Occur irregularly, or become regular only temporarily. ■ Often stop with walking or position change. ■ Are felt in the back or abdomen above the umbilicus. ■ Often can be stopped with use of comfort measures.
Cervix	■ Shows progressive change, softening, effacement, dilatation, passage of bloody show. ■ Moves in an increasing anterior position. ■ Requires vaginal exam to detect changes.	■ May be soft, but has no significant change in effacement, dilatation, and no bloody show. ■ Is often in a posterior position. ■ Requires vaginal exam to determine characteristics.
Fetus	Presenting part becomes engaged in the pelvis.	Presenting part often is not engaged in the pelvis.

after bloody show. Small amounts of blood-tinged drainage resulting from a vaginal exam should not be confused with bloody show.

■ *Ruptured membranes: Spontaneous rupture of the membranes* (SROM) usually occurs after labor begins. In a small percentage of women, the amniotic membranes may rupture before the onset of labor contractions. If labor does not begin within 24 hours after the membranes rupture, and the pregnancy is near term, labor may be induced to avoid infection. If the fetus is **ballotable** (able to be pushed away from the cervix), the umbilical cord could be washed out of the cervix with the amniotic fluid. This condition, called a **prolapsed umbilical cord,** requires emergency obstetric intervention to save the life of the infant. *Premature rupture of membranes* (PROM) occurs when the membranes rupture before the 38th week of gestation. This condition can indicate the onset of premature labor and needs medical attention. Prolapsed umbilical cord is discussed in more detail in the high-risk section of this chapter.

■ *Sudden burst of energy:* Many women experience a sudden burst of energy a few days before labor begins. The woman feels a need to get the "house in order." The reason for the "nesting instinct" is unknown. The woman should be careful not to tire herself.

Variables Affecting Labor

The variables affecting labor are many, but they can be grouped for easier discussion. These variables, known as the **five Ps affecting labor,** refer to both maternal and fetal characteristics.

PASSAGE

The first P, the *passage,* consists of the maternal structures through which the fetus must travel. The size and shape of the maternal pelvis must be able to accommodate the fetus. Toward the end of pregnancy, the care provider will take

measurements of the maternal pelvis to determine the adequacy of the pelvis. Important parts of the maternal pelvis are illustrated in Figure 53-1 ■. In **cephalopelvic disproportion** (CPD), the maternal pelvis is smaller than the fetal head. Because the fetus will not fit through the maternal pelvis, a cesarean birth is required. As birth nears and contractions occur, the movement of the fetus through the pelvis must be monitored. The term **station** refers to the relationship between the fetus and the maternal ischial spines. Figure 53-2 ■ illustrates stations. When the fetus

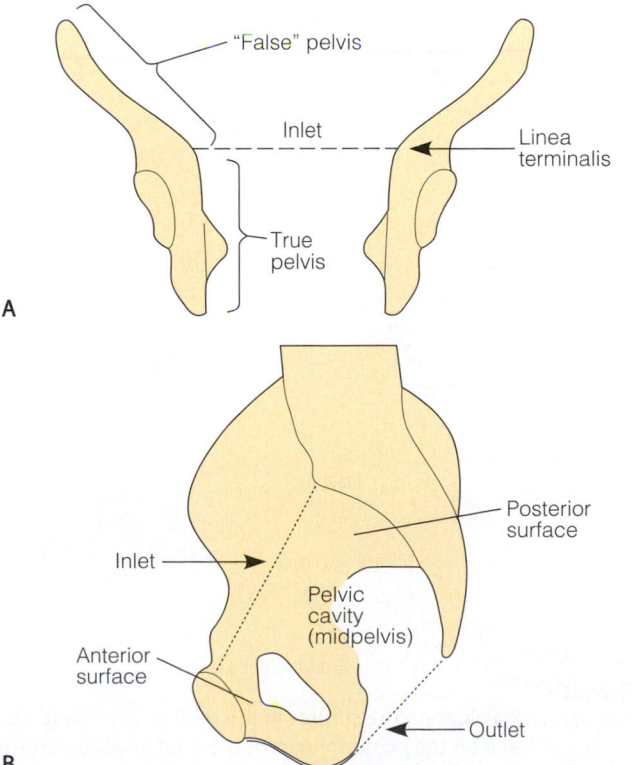

Figure 53-1. ■ Female pelvis. **A.** False pelvis is a shallow cavity above the inlet; true pelvis is the deeper portion of the cavity below the inlet. **B.** The true pelvis consists of inlet, cavity (midpelvis), and outlet.

reaches the ischial spines or 0 station, the fetal head is considered to be fully engaged.

Uterine contractions (discussed under Powers later in this section) push the fetus against the cervix, causing the cervix to open so the fetus can enter the vagina. By the end of pregnancy, various hormones have softened the *rugae* (or folds) of the vagina, allowing it to stretch enough for the fetus to pass. The pressure of the fetus against the muscles of the perineum causes the tissue to thin and stretch. At times the perineum may tear, or it may need to be surgically cut (discussed later) to prevent undue trauma to the tissue. In either event, the perineum will be sutured after birth to ensure healing.

PASSENGER

The second P refers to the *passenger*, or fetus. The size of the fetus, as well as the relationship of fetal parts to the maternal uterus and pelvis, affects how easily the fetus can be born.

■ *Size:* The largest part of the fetus is the head. The bones of the fetal skull are not fused. The bones are joined by fibrous connective tissue called *sutures*. Large spaces called **fontanels** prevent undue pressure on the fetal brain. Figure 53-3 ■ illustrates the suture lines and fontanels (as well as common flexed cephalic presentation). As the fetal head passes through the maternal pelvis, the bones of the skull ride over each other, decreasing the diameter of the head.

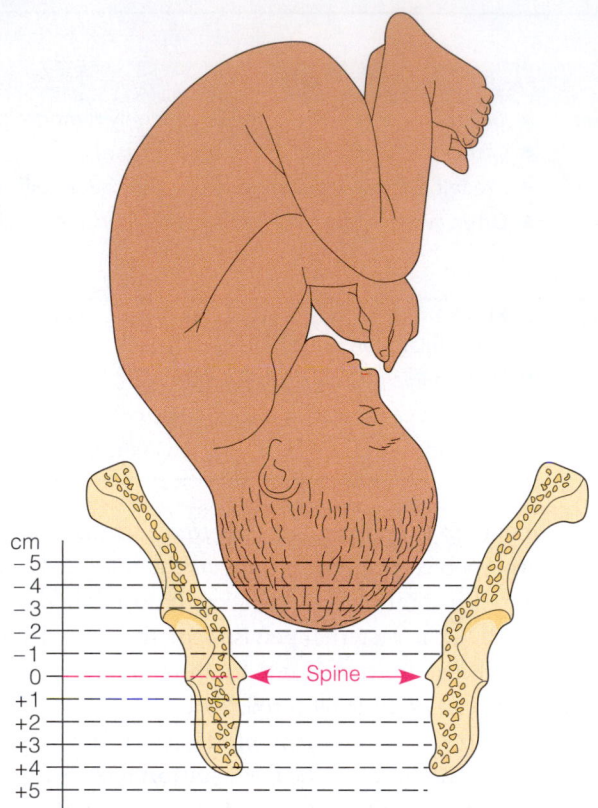

Figure 53-2. ■ Measuring the station of the fetal head while it is descending. In this view, the station is −2/−3.

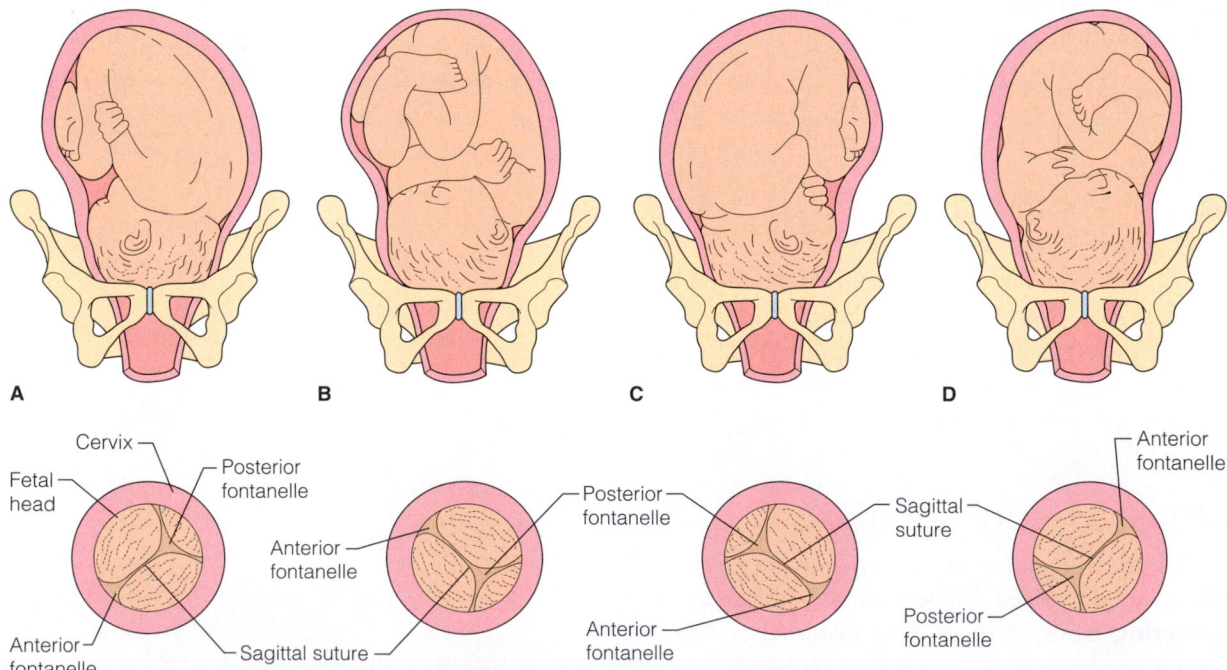

Figure 53-3. ■ Palpating the sutures in the skull to determine position of the fetus. **A.** Left occiput anterior (LOA). The occiput (area over the occipital bone on the posterior part of the fetal head) is in the left anterior quadrant of the woman's pelvis. When the fetus is LOA, the posterior fontanel (located just above the occipital bone and triangular in shape) is in the upper left quadrant of the maternal pelvis. **B.** Left occiput posterior (LOP). The posterior fontanel is in the lower left quadrant of the maternal pelvis. **C.** Right occiput anterior (ROA). The posterior fontanel is in the upper right quadrant of the maternal pelvis. **D.** Right occiput posterior (ROP). The posterior fontanel is in the lower right quadrant of the maternal pelvis. *Note:* The anterior fontanel is diamond shaped. Because of the roundness of the fetal head, only a portion of the anterior fontanel can be seen in each of the views, so it appears to be triangular in shape.

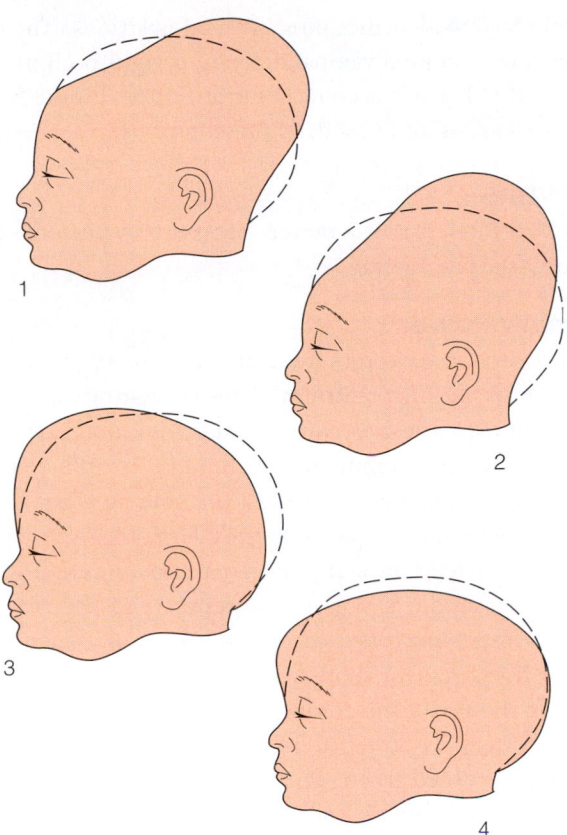

Figure 53-4. ■ Effects of labor on the fetal head. The presenting portion of the scalp area is encircled by the cervix during labor, causing swelling of the soft tissue. Molding of the fetal head in four cephalic presentations: (1) occiput anterior, (2) occiput posterior, (3) brow, (4) face.

This shaping of the fetal head to the bones of the maternal pelvis is termed **molding** (Figure 53-4 ■). The care provider can feel the anterior and *occipital* (posterior) fontanels and the sagittal suture through the cervix. These landmarks are used to determine the position of the fetus in the uterus.

- *Fetal attitude:* **Fetal attitude** is the degree of flexion of the fetal head and limbs to the trunk. Ideally the fetus assumes a state of flexion (Figure 53-5 ■). The head is flexed onto the chest, the arms flexed over the chest, and the legs flexed over the abdomen. If any part of the fetus is in extension, especially the head and arms (see Figure 53-5B), labor will be more difficult and a vaginal birth may not be possible.
- *Fetal lie:* **Fetal lie** (Figure 53-6 ■) is the relationship of the long axis (head to foot or cephalocaudal plane) of the fetus to the long axis of the mother. When the long axis of the fetus is parallel to the long axis of the mother, the fetus is in a *longitudinal lie*. If the long axis of the fetus is at a right angle to the long axis of the mother, it is termed a *transverse lie*.
- *Fetal presentation:* **Fetal presentation** is that body part of the fetus that is closest to the cervix. It is determined by the fetal lie and is illustrated under fetal position below. At term, the fetus usually assumes a longitudinal lie with

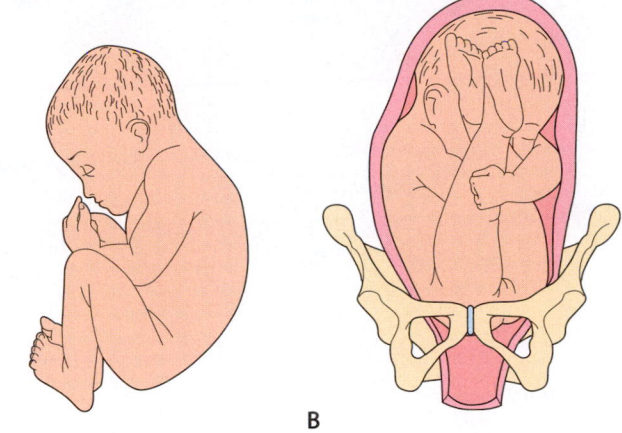

A   B

Figure 53-5. ■ **A.** Fetal attitude. The relationship of body parts of this fetus is normal. The head is flexed forward, with the chin almost resting on the chest. The arms and legs are flexed. **B.** Frank breech presentation.

a **cephalic presentation** (head down). The fetal head is heavy, and gravity pulls it into the pelvis. With the fetal head in the pelvis, there is more room in the uterus for the fetus to move arms and legs. Cephalic presentations can further be differentiated by determining the fetal attitude:

- *Vertex* is the area between the anterior and posterior fontanels or the occiput presenting first. The fetal head is in complete flexion.
- *Brow* is the sinciput (forehead or brow) presenting first. The fetal head is neither flexed nor hyperextended.
- *Face* (mentum) is the face presenting first. The neck is in full hyperextension.

The fetus might assume a longitudinal lie with a **breech** (buttocks) presentation. Breech presentations are further differentiated by the attitude of the fetus's legs.

- *Complete breech:* The hips and knees are flexed on the abdomen. The buttocks are presenting first.

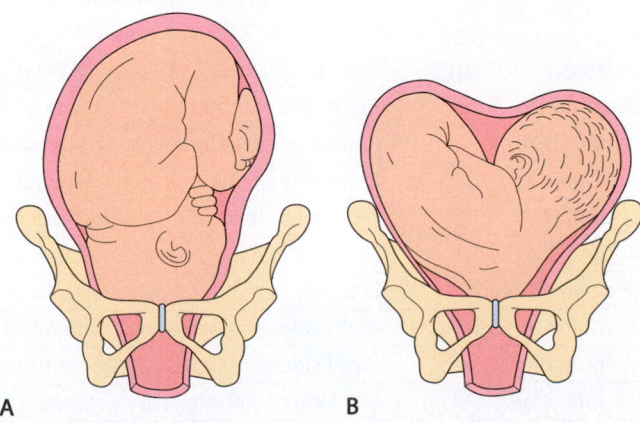

A   B

Figure 53-6. ■ Fetal lie. **A.** Longitudinal lie means that the long axis of the fetus is parallel to the mother's spine. **B.** Transverse lie. If the fetus cannot be turned, cesarean delivery will be needed.

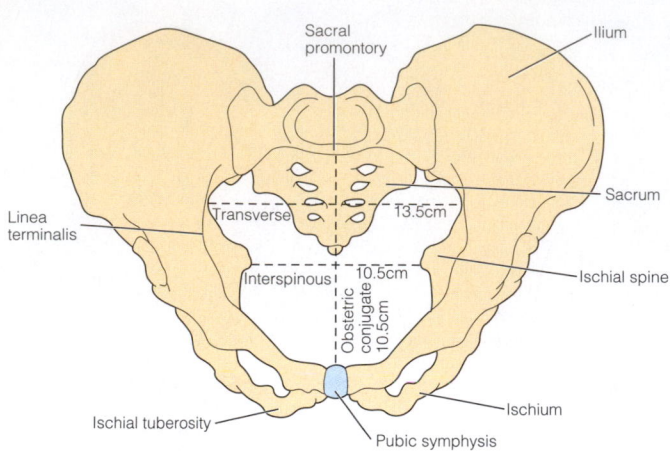

Figure 53-7. ■ Pelvic planes: coronal section and diameters of the bony pelvis.

- *Frank breech* (see Figure 53-5B): The hips are flexed, but the knees are extended with the feet close to the head. The buttocks are presenting first.
- *Footing breech:* One or both hips and knees are extended with the foot (feet) presenting first.

If the fetus assumes a transverse lie, the presenting part will be the shoulder, arm, back, abdomen, or side. The fetus in a transverse presentation cannot be born vaginally.

- **Fetal position** refers to the relationship of the presenting part to the four quadrants of the maternal pelvis. Figure 53-7 ■ illustrates the pelvic quadrants. The fetal landmarks are identified in the right or left, anterior or posterior quadrants of the mother's pelvis. Abbreviations are typically used to indicate fetal position, with the first letter referring to the mother's right or left, the second letter referring to the fetal landmark, and the third letter referring to the mother's anterior or posterior quadrant.

Table 53-2 ■ identifies possible fetal positions. The most ideal position for a vaginal delivery is right occiput anterior (ROA) or left occiput anterior (LOA). Figure 53-8 ■ illustrates common cephalic presentations.

POWERS

The third P refers to the powers necessary to push the fetus through the passageway.

Primary Power

The primary power comes from the involuntary muscle contractions of the myometrium. Uterine contractions begin in response to the posterior pituitary hormone oxytocin. **Contractions,** beginning in the fundus, are the result of shortening of the muscle fibers. The muscle fibers of the uterus have several unique properties. First, the muscle fibers contract and relax in a rhythmic pattern (Figure 53-9 ■). During relaxation, circulation is restored to the placenta, thereby improving oxygenation of the fetus. Second, the muscle fibers remain shortened, resulting in a gradual decrease in the size of the uterine cavity. As the uterine muscle fibers shorten, the lower uterine segment is pulled up, and the fetus is pushed down. These actions result in effacement (shortening and thinning of the cervix) and dilatation (opening) of the cervical os.

Contractions are described in terms of frequency, duration, and intensity:

- *Frequency* is the time from the onset of one contraction to the onset of the next contraction.
- *Duration* is the time from the onset of a contraction to the end of that contraction.
- *Intensity* is the strength of the contraction at its peak.

As mentioned, blood supply through the uterus to the placenta is decreased during contractions. Ideally, the frequency of

TABLE 53-2	Types of Presentation in Labor
PRESENTING PART AND ABBREVIATION	**DESCRIPTION OF FETAL POSITION**
Occiput ROA	Right side of maternal pelvis, occiput presenting, occiput directed toward anterior (front) of passage
Occiput ROT	Right side of maternal pelvis, occiput presenting, occiput transverse (directed toward side of passage)
Occiput ROP	Right side of maternal pelvis, occiput presenting, occiput directed toward posterior (back) of passage
Occiput LOA	Left side of maternal pelvis, occiput presenting, occiput directed toward anterior (front) of passage
Occiput LOT	Left side of maternal pelvis, occiput presenting, occiput transverse (directed toward side of passage)
Occiput LOP	Left side of maternal pelvis, occiput presenting, occiput directed toward posterior (back) of passage
Mentum (chin) RMA	Right side of maternal pelvis, mentum (chin) presenting, mentum directed toward anterior (front) of passage
Mentum RMP	Right side of maternal pelvis, mentum (chin) presenting, mentum directed toward posterior (back) of passage
Mentum LMA	Left side of maternal pelvis, mentum (chin) presenting, mentum directed toward anterior (front) of passage
Sacrum LSA	Left side of maternal pelvis, sacrum presenting, sacrum directed toward anterior (front) of passage
Sacrum LSP	Left side of maternal pelvis, sacrum presenting, sacrum directed toward posterior (back) of passage

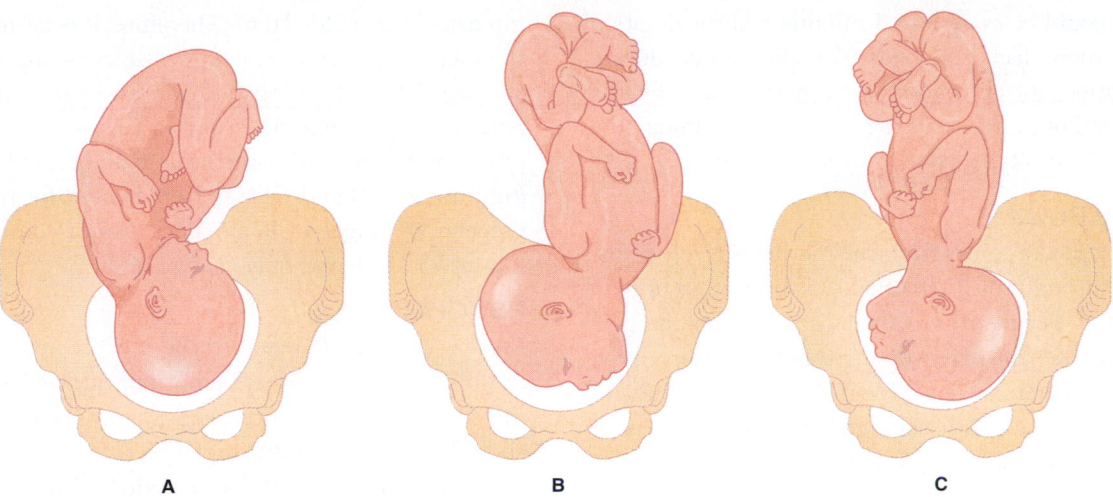

| | A | B | C |

Figure 53-8. ■ Cephalic presentations. **A.** Vertex presentation. Complete flexion of the head allows the suboccipitobregmatic diameter to present to the pelvis. **B.** Face presentation. The fetal head is in complete extension, and the submentobregmatic diameter presents to the pelvis. **C.** Brow presentation. The fetal head is in partial (halfway) extension. The occipitomental diameter, which is the largest diameter of the fetal head, presents to the pelvis.

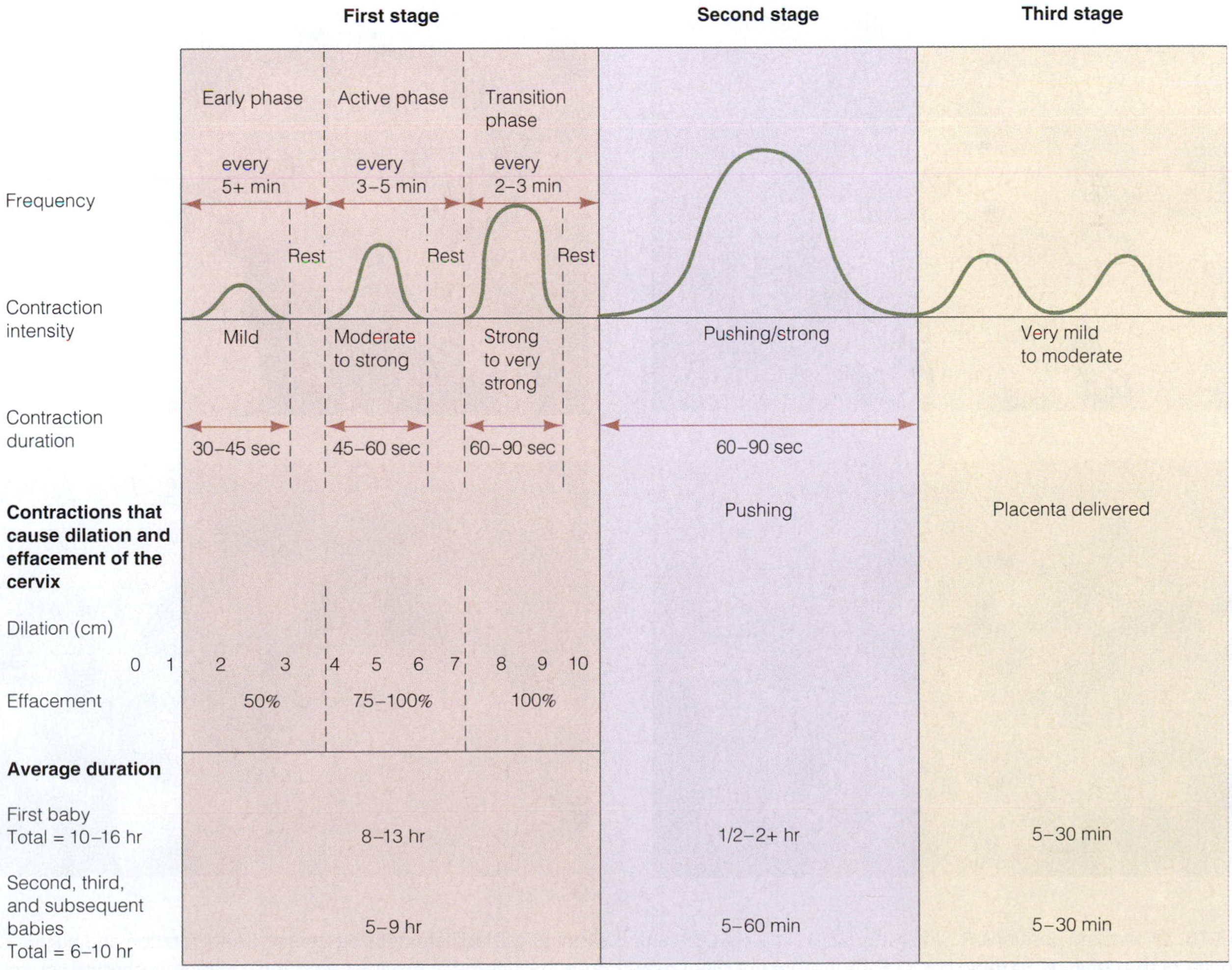

	First stage			Second stage	Third stage
	Early phase	Active phase	Transition phase		
Frequency	every 5+ min	every 3–5 min	every 2–3 min		
Contraction intensity	Mild	Moderate to strong	Strong to very strong	Pushing/strong	Very mild to moderate
Contraction duration	30–45 sec	45–60 sec	60–90 sec	60–90 sec	
Contractions that cause dilation and effacement of the cervix				Pushing	Placenta delivered
Dilation (cm)	0 1 2 3	4 5 6 7	8 9 10		
Effacement	50%	75–100%	100%		
Average duration					
First baby Total = 10–16 hr	8–13 hr			1/2–2+ hr	5–30 min
Second, third, and subsequent babies Total = 6–10 hr	5–9 hr			5–60 min	5–30 min

Figure 53-9. ■ Contraction patterns in first, second, and third stages of labor. Primigravidas may be 100% effaced before labor begins.

contractions should be every 3 to 5 minutes and the duration should not be more than 90 seconds. This allows time, during uterine relaxation, for circulation to be restored and for the fetus to recover. For contractions to push the fetus through the cervix, they must be of moderate to strong intensity.

Secondary Power

The secondary power comes from the mother actively pushing the fetus through the birth canal. A spontaneous urge to push, known as **Ferguson's reflex,** occurs when the presenting part reaches the pelvic floor. Stretch receptors in the vagina trigger the release of oxytocin. To prevent trauma of the cervix, the woman is discouraged from active pushing until the cervix has dilated completely.

POSITION

The fourth P is the position of the mother during labor. If the mother lies on her back, the contractions are more frequent but lower in intensity. When the mother lies on her side, the contractions are less frequent, but of greater

intensity (Figure 53-10 ■). Therefore, it is better to position the mother on her side, using pillows to support her back and leg. The side-lying position also prevents supine hypotensive syndrome (discussed in Chapter 51 ⚭). Other positions (such as the birthing ball or birthing bar; see Figures 53-10B and C) may have benefit for the mother in preparatory stages of labor. Positions of comfort vary (see Figure 53-10D) and may change often.

PSYCHE

Psyche, the fifth P, refers to the mother's emotional status during labor. The mother's emotions during labor are determined by past experiences, expectations, culture, and ideas about how to behave during labor.

If the woman is fearful and anxious, a negative cycle can emerge. Fear and anxiety stimulate the mother's adrenal gland to release additional epinephrine and norepinephrine. These fight-or-flight hormones constrict blood vessels (restricting placental circulation), decrease the effectiveness of contractions, and tighten skeletal muscles. Tight skeletal

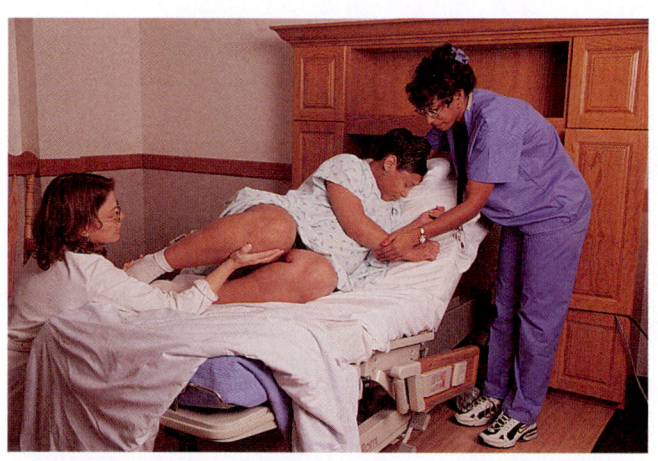

A

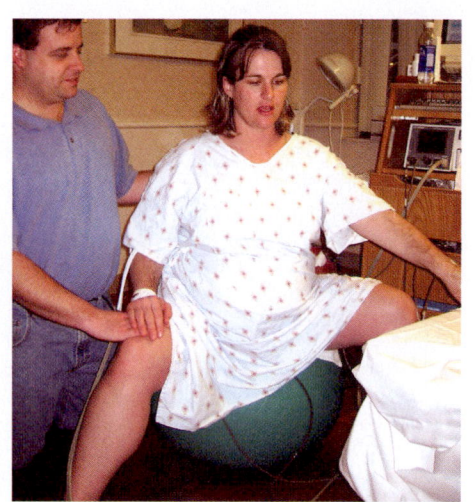

B

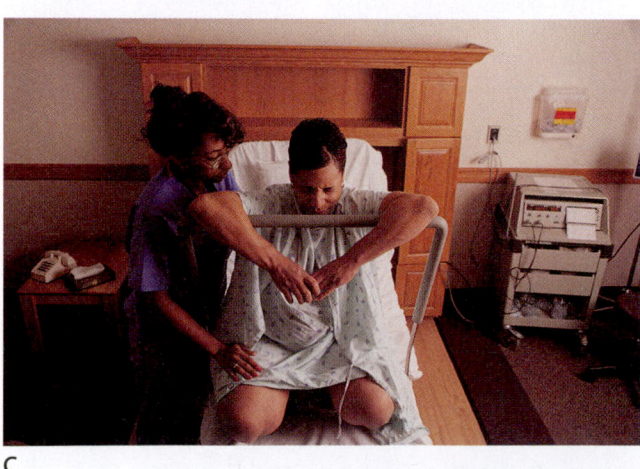

C

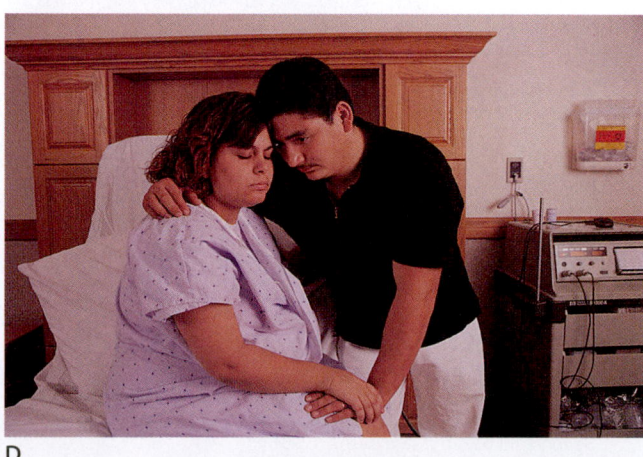

D

Figure 53-10. ■ Birthing positions. **A.** Side-lying. (*Source:* © Elena Dorfman.) **B.** Birthing ball facilitates fetal descent and fetal rotation, and helps increase the diameter of the pelvis. **C.** Birthing bar. **D.** Early in labor the client may choose a position that provides emotional as well as physical comfort. (*Source:* © Elena Dorfman.)

muscles do not stretch easily, so the uterus needs to contract harder, increasing discomfort. Discomfort increases tension and anxiety. These three factors become a cycle, making the labor a longer and less positive experience.

Stages of Labor

Labor is a process or sequence of events that begins with uterine contractions and ends 1 hour after birth of the placenta. The labor process is described in four stages.

FIRST STAGE OF LABOR

The first stage of labor, also known as the **dilatation stage,** begins with regular contractions and ends with complete effacement and dilatation of the cervix (Figure 53-11 ■). This is usually the longest stage. It is divided into three phases: latent, active, and transition.

- The *latent phase* of the first stage of labor is from the onset of contractions until the cervix is dilated 4 cm. Contractions usually occur every 10 to 15 minutes and gradually increase to 5 minutes apart. Each contraction lasts 30 to 40 seconds and is of mild to moderate intensity. The client is aware of the contractions but is relatively comfortable. She is excited that labor has begun, but anxious about

what lies ahead. If the membranes have not ruptured, she is encouraged to walk as long as she does not become tired. This is a good time to reinforce teaching, especially relaxation and breathing techniques. The latent phase may last 8 to 10 hours with the first pregnancy and 5 hours with subsequent pregnancies.

- The *active phase* of the first stage of labor begins when the cervix is dilated 4 cm and ends with 8 cm of dilatation. Contractions occur every 3 to 5 minutes, last 60 to 90 seconds, and are of moderate to strong intensity. Clients perceive an increased amount of discomfort as the fetus descends through the pelvis, stretching muscles and ligaments. Clients seek a position that reduces discomfort. The client now focuses on relaxation and breathing techniques. The average length of active labor is 4 to 6 hours for the primigravida client, and 3 to 14 hours for the multipara client.

- The *transition phase* of the first stage of labor is the time it takes for the cervical opening to widen from 8 to 10 cm. The contractions are strong, occurring every 2 to 3 minutes, and lasting 90 seconds. As the fetus descends deeper into the pelvis, there is a strong urge to push. The client may need reminding to focus on relaxation and breathing

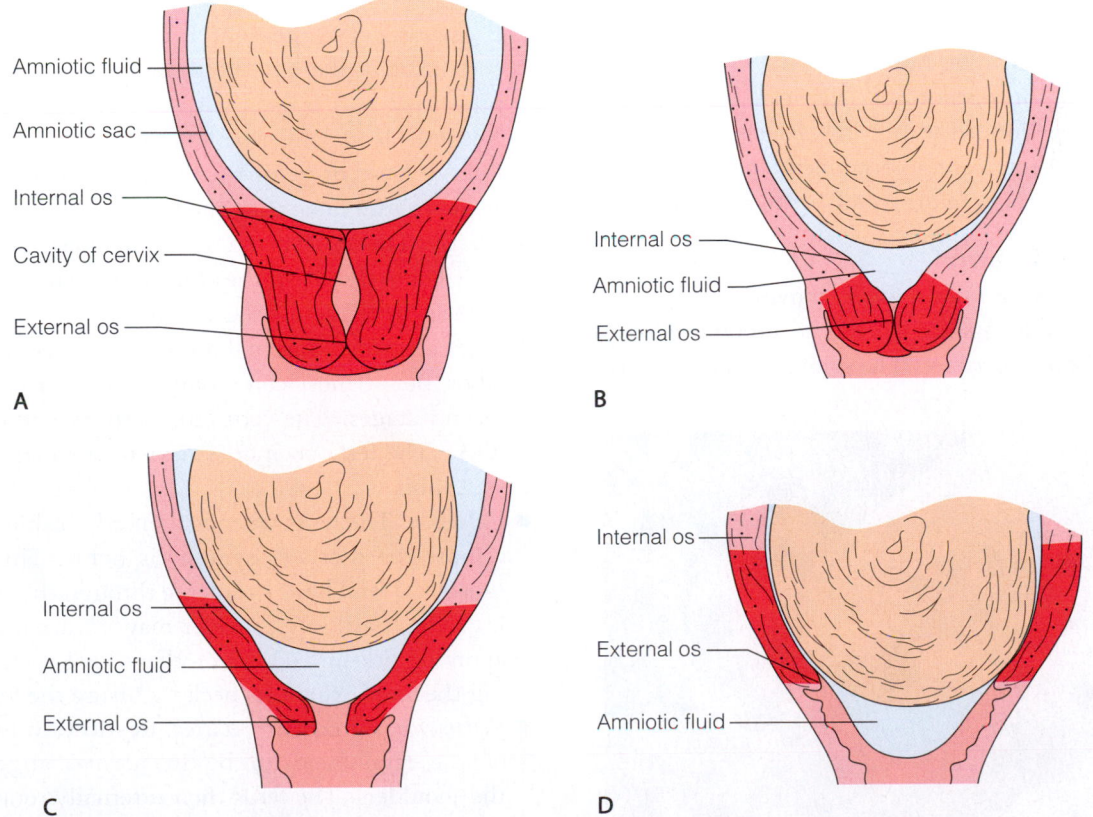

Figure 53-11. ■ Effacement and dilatation of the cervix in the primigravida. **A.** Beginning of labor. There is no cervical effacement or dilatation. The fetal head is cushioned by amniotic fluid. **B.** Beginning cervical effacement. As the cervix begins to efface, more amniotic fluid collects below the fetal head. **C.** Cervix about one-half effaced and slightly dilated. The increasing amount of amniotic fluid exerts hydrostatic pressure. **D.** Complete effacement and dilatation.

techniques. It is important for the client not to push actively until the cervix is completely dilated. If the client pushes too early, the cervix can tear. Some behaviors indicate a woman is in the transition phase of labor. The client frequently becomes restless, irritable, and sometimes angry. Statements like "I can't take anymore" and "Don't touch me" are common. It is important to help support persons understand that this behavior is part of the labor process. The average length of transition is 1 to 2 hours.

SECOND STAGE OF LABOR

The second stage of labor begins when the cervix is completely dilated and ends with the birth of the baby. Contractions continue every 2 to 3 minutes and last 60 to 90 seconds. The woman is encouraged to use her abdominal muscles to bear down actively with each contraction. The second stage of labor could take 1 to 3 hours for the primigravida client and 15 to 30 minutes for the multipara client.

As the fetal head pushes on the perineum, the client has a greater urge to push. The tissues of the perineum thin and bulge. The labia open. The fetal head can be seen with contractions, but it recedes into the vagina between contractions. Gradually, more and more of the fetal head appears with contractions. When the largest part of the fetal head is past the vulva and remains visible between contractions, **crowning** has occurred (Figure 53-12 ■). A few more pushes and the fetus will be delivered.

In many births, an **episiotomy** (surgical cutting of the perineal tissue) is performed at this time. An episiotomy may aid birth and prevent tearing of perineal and anal tissue. Figure 53-13 ■ illustrates midline and lateral episiotomies.

Mechanisms of Labor

The fetus changes positions as it moves through the pelvis. These movements are called the **mechanisms of labor,** or *cardinal movements*. The movements the fetus

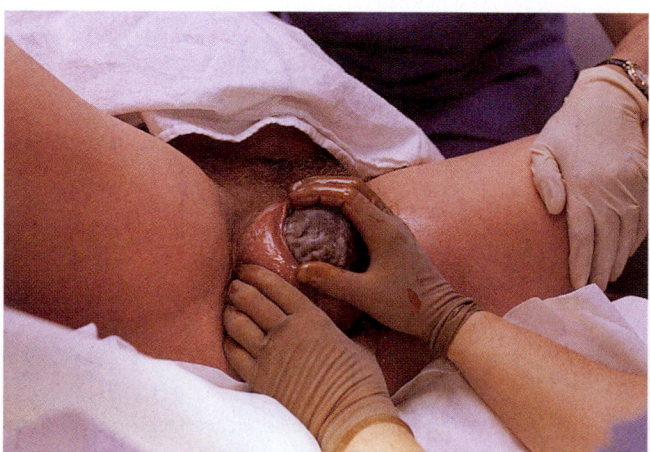

Figure 53-12. ■ The fetal head begins to crown. (*Source:* © Stella Johnson.)

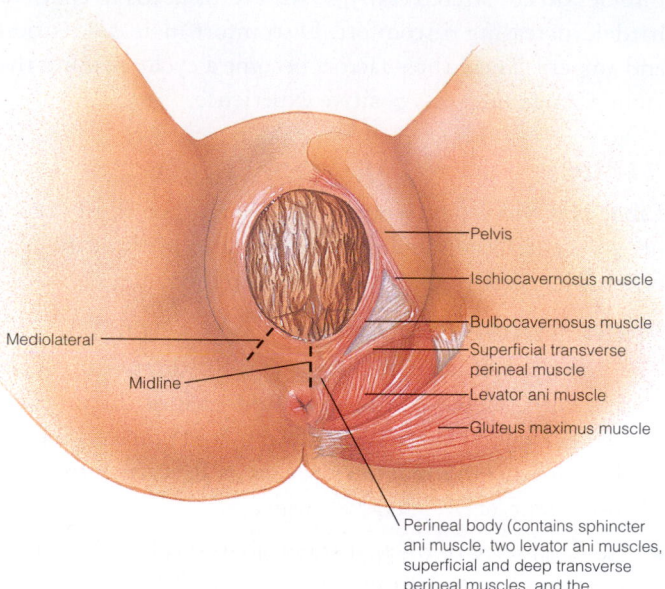

Labels: Pelvis; Ischiocavernosus muscle; Bulbocavernosus muscle; Superficial transverse perineal muscle; Levator ani muscle; Gluteus maximus muscle; Mediolateral; Midline; Perineal body (contains sphincter ani muscle, two levator ani muscles, superficial and deep transverse perineal muscles, and the bulbocavernous muscle)

Figure 53-13. ■ The two most common types of episiotomy are midline and mediolateral.

undergoes as it moves through the pelvis are illustrated in Figure 53-14 ■. The first three may occur before the first contractions, or during the first stage of labor.

- *Engagement:* **Engagement** occurs when the presenting part (usually the fetal head) enters the true pelvis. The presenting part is even with or below the ischial spines. The fetus is no longer ballotable.
- *Descent:* Descent begins with engagement and continues as the contractions push the fetus through the pelvis.
- *Flexion:* The fetus assumes a positive attitude, with head flexed onto the chest, the arms flexed across the chest, and the legs flexed across the abdomen.
- *Internal rotation:* Internal rotation may take place prior to labor, but it most commonly occurs during the first or second stages. The fetus turns to an anterior position (OA). The fetal occiput is next to the maternal symphysis pubis.
- *Extension:* The fetus extends its head, pushing its occiput against the mother's symphysis pubis. This movement causes the fetal head to emerge through the vaginal opening. The healthcare provider may assist with delivery by applying pressure on the mother's lower perineum, helping the fetus extend its neck by lifting the fetal chin.
- *Restitution and external rotation:* **Restitution** is the turning of the fetal head to be in normal alignment with the shoulders. The fetus then externally rotates until the shoulders are in an anterior/posterior position. The healthcare provider suctions the fetal airway with a bulb syringe or suction catheter to remove amniotic fluid and vaginal secretions before the fetus begins to breathe.

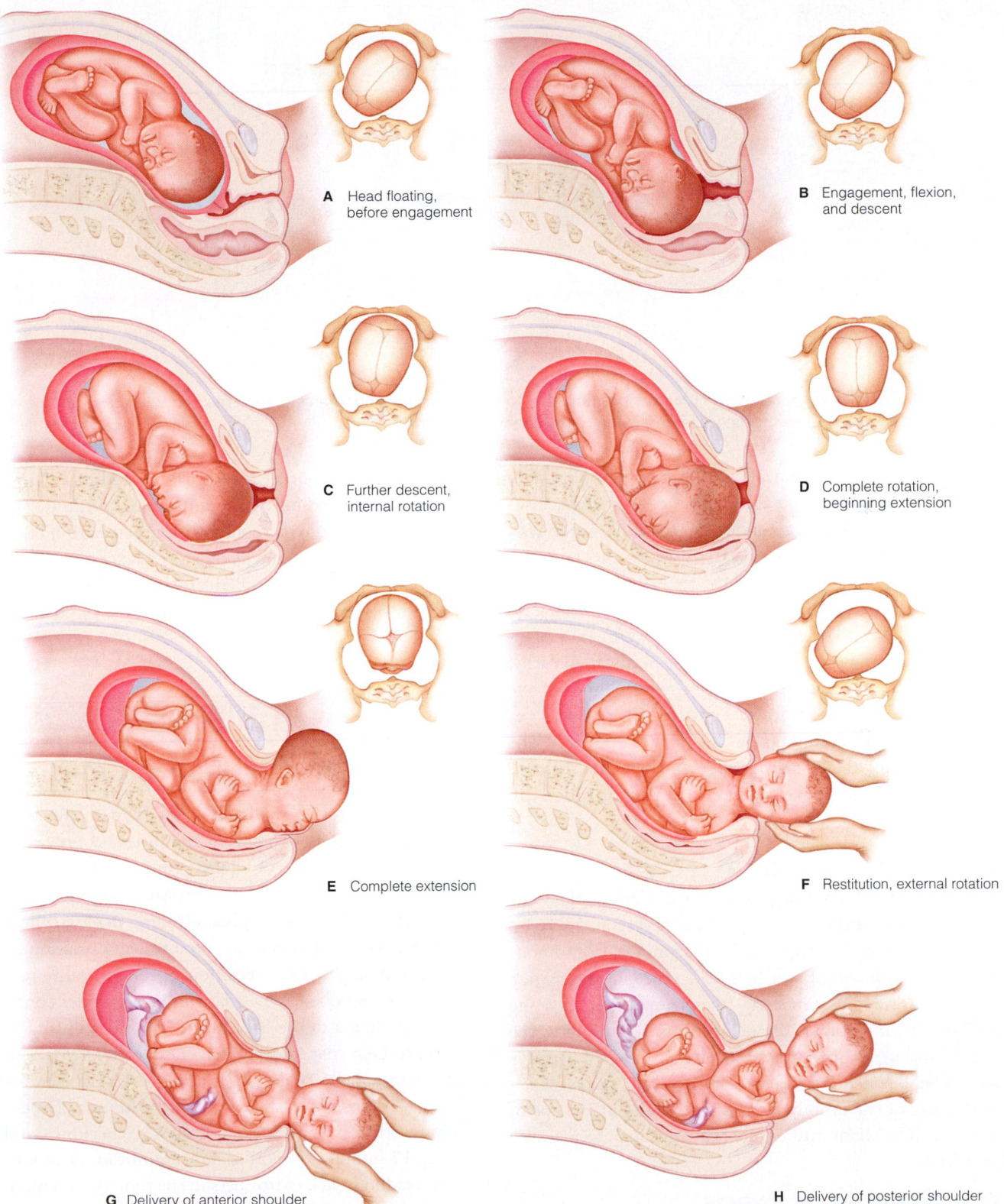

Figure 53-14. ■ Mechanisms of labor: Left anterior occiput position. **A.** Head floating, before engagement. **B.** Engagement, flexion, and descent. **C.** Further descent, internal rotation. **D.** Complete rotation, beginning extension. **E.** Complete extension. **F.** Restitution, external rotation. **G.** Delivery of anterior shoulder. **H.** Delivery of posterior shoulder. (*Source:* Adapted, with permission, from McGraw-Hill Companies, Inc. Cunningham, F. G., et al. [eds.]. [1997]. *Williams obstetrics* [20th ed.]. Stamford, CT: Appleton & Lange, p. 320.)

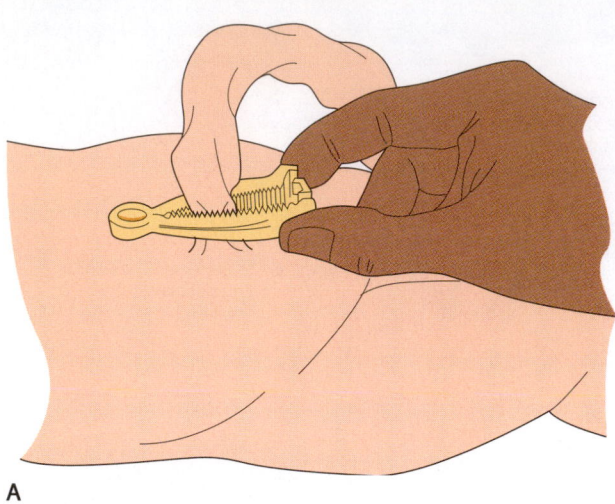
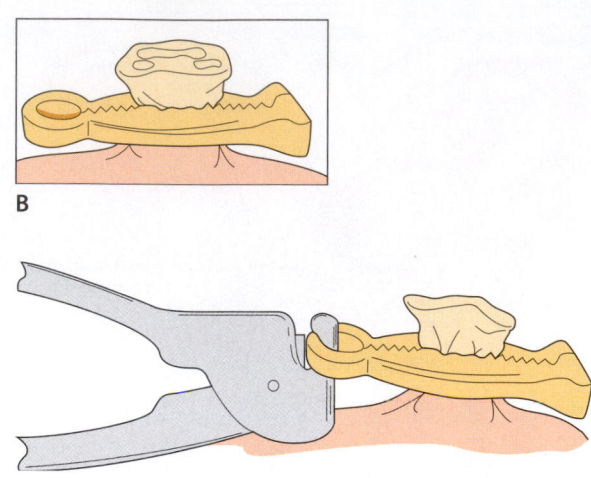

Figure 53-15. ■ Hollister cord clamp. **A.** Clamp is positioned ½ to 1 inch from the abdomen and then secured. **B.** Cord is cut. One vein and two arteries can be seen. **C.** Plastic device for removing clamp after cord has dried.

■ *Expulsion:* The assisting healthcare provider applies gentle downward pressure on the fetal head, allowing the anterior shoulder to emerge under the maternal symphysis pubis. The head is then raised to allow the posterior shoulder to emerge. The rest of the fetus then slides out of the vagina. The healthcare provider holds the fetus with the head down and dries the fetus with a warm baby blanket. This stimulation encourages the fetus to breathe. Once respiration has been established, the healthcare provider places two clamps (a Hollister clamp and a hemostat or two hemostats) on the umbilical cord. The healthcare provider or support person then cuts the cord between the clamps. A Hollister clamp is illustrated in Figure 53-15 ■.

THIRD STAGE OF LABOR

The third stage of labor begins with the birth of the fetus and ends with the expulsion of the placenta (Figure 53-16 ■). The placenta should be expelled in 30 minutes. Continuous contractions following birth cause the placenta to separate from the wall of the uterus. As it separates, there is some bleeding. The membranes are peeled from the uterus as the placenta slides into the vagina. Signs that the placenta is ready to be expelled are a gush of blood from the vagina, a lengthening of the umbilical cord, and a globular shape of the uterus. The client pushes one last time and the placenta is expelled.

FOURTH STAGE OF LABOR

The fourth stage of labor is the first hour after birth. During this period the mother's body begins to return to a non-pregnant state. The blood pressure has a moderate decline. The pulse increases and then gradually slows. Normally, between 250 and 500 mL of blood are lost, most of which is lost at the time of placenta separation. The uterus should remain firm in order to control bleeding. The fundus should be located below the umbilicus and in the midline. Saturation of more than one perineal pad with blood during the 1-hour recovery time is considered excessive. The mother may experience uncontrolled shaking or chills as a result of the physiologic response to labor and the rapid weight loss at delivery.

NURSING CARE

PRIORITIZING NURSING CARE

When caring for clients in labor, focus your care on preventing complications, promoting comfort, and providing emotional support. Observe clients closely and report immediately sustained elevated blood pressure, sustained fetal heart rate below 120, or any vaginal bleeding during contractions. Assist laboring clients to as comfortable a position as possible, avoiding the supine position. Speak in a calm, reassuring voice, to help clients feel that things are under control. Encourage clients to use breathing techniques during contractions to help manage the pain. Do not take personally any comments made by laboring clients—stress, fear, and pain can cause them to lash out at staff. Monitor clients closely after birth for signs of complications, checking vital signs every 15 minutes. Report at once significant changes in vital sign readings, lack of firmness in the fundus, or a fundus that deviates from midline or is not below the umbilicus.

Admission to the Birthing Facility

Several weeks before the anticipated birth, the healthcare provider usually sends a copy of the pregnancy record to the birthing unit. This information is useful for the nurse when planning care during the birthing process. The information is

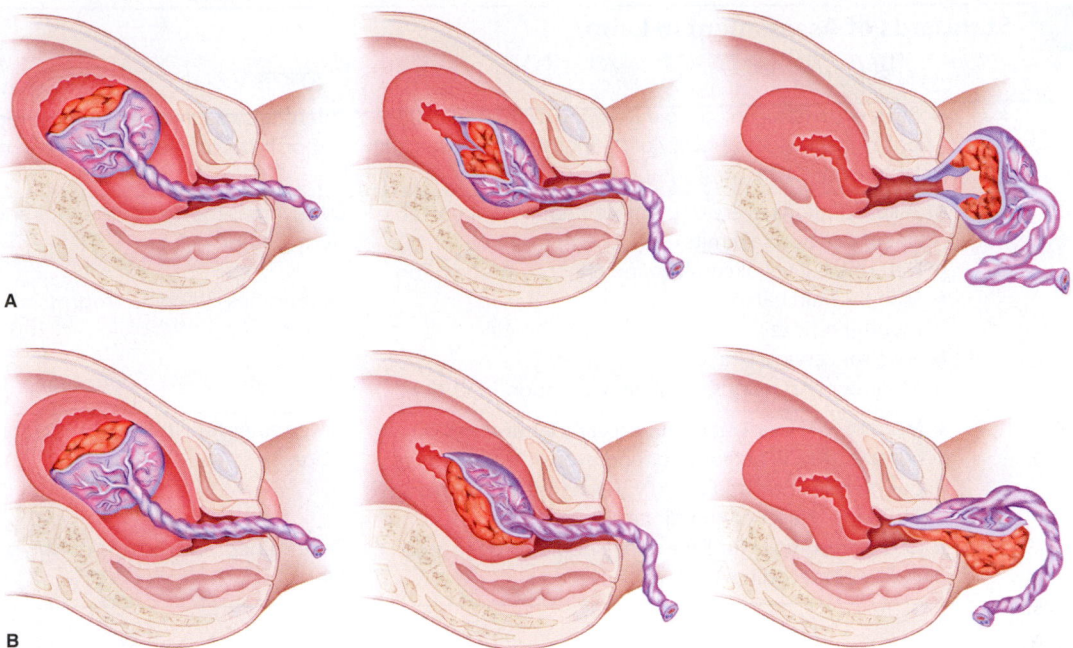

Figure 53-16. ■ Placental separation. **A.** Schultze ("shiny Schultze") mechanism. Smooth fetal side of placenta is out. **B.** Duncan ("dirty Duncan") mechanism. Fleshy maternal side is out.

also useful in case the healthcare provider is not available and another provider must assume care of the client. When a client presents for admission to the birthing suite, the nurse or unit secretary obtains this information from the file and initiates a client chart. The client is escorted to an exam or labor room where she is asked to remove her clothing, don a client gown, and lie down. LPNs and LVNs work under the supervision of an RN to assist in the care of the woman in labor.

ASSESSING

When a client is admitted in labor, the first assessments determine the stage of labor, the condition of the mother, and the condition of the fetus. Answers to some initial questions direct how the nurse proceeds with the rest of the admission process. For example, if the client is in early labor with a first pregnancy, time is available to establish a nurse–client–family relationship, to orient the client to the delivery suite, and to instruct the woman in relaxation techniques. If the client is in the second stage of labor with her third pregnancy, there may only be time to notify the doctor and prepare for the delivery.

The nurse asks the client the following questions:

- When did the contractions begin?
- How far apart are the contractions and how long do they last?
- Have the membranes ruptured? (Has the water broken?)
- Is this your first pregnancy? How long were previous labors?

The nurse reviews the prenatal record to determine the presence of complications during the pregnancy. If the

client has had no prenatal care, a more in-depth assessment must be made. The assessment of the client should include:

- Vital signs
- Urine dipstick for glucose and protein
- Fetal heart rate (FHR)
- Contractions: frequency, duration, and intensity
- Vaginal examination to determine cervical effacement and dilatation, fetal presentation, position, and station; the vaginal exam is usually done by the RN or physician

clinical ALERT

If excessive vaginal bleeding is present, the nurse should consult with the healthcare provider prior to the vaginal exam.

- Nitrazine test of vaginal secretions if the client is uncertain whether membranes have ruptured
- Signs of pregnancy-induced hypertension (PIH) including edema, reflexes, and **clonus** (a series of abnormal reflex movements of the foot in response to sudden dorsiflexion) or seizures

If the client is not in labor, she may be sent home. This can be disappointing to the client and family, and emotional support may be needed. If it is questionable whether the client is in labor, she will be asked to walk for an hour and then be reassessed.

Once it is determined the client is in labor, continuous assessment includes frequent vital signs, FHR, and contraction evaluation. Most clients will be monitored electronically,

TABLE 53-3	Standards of Assessment in Labor	
ITEM	**ASSESSMENT**	**RATIONALE**
Prenatal data	■ Review prenatal record to determine estimated date of birth, gravida/para, history of previous labors, results of laboratory exams.	Identifies risk, such as preterm, rapid labor/birth, and anticipated complications.
Maternal assessment	■ Take vital signs every hour (more frequently if unstable or outside normal limits).	Determines mother's tolerance and stability during labor.
	■ Determine level of comfort and effect of intervention.	
	■ Monitor fluid balance.	Determines if labor is progressing in a usual
	■ Monitor reflexes.	pattern.
	■ Monitor cervical changes.	
	■ Monitor contractions (frequency, duration, intensity).	
Fetal assessment	■ Monitor FHR every hour during early labor, every 30 minutes during active labor, and every 10–15 minutes during transition and birth. Note change in FHR before, during, and after contractions.	Determines fetal tolerance and stability during labor.
	■ Observe amniotic fluid for color (should be clear; green indicates meconium passage by fetus).	Determines fetal distress during pregnancy and labor.

either continuously or intermittently. The level of monitoring depends on the stage of labor and the well-being of the client and fetus. A vaginal exam will be done at intervals to assess progression of cervical effacement and dilatation, station, and fetal position. Table 53-3 ■ identifies the standard time frames for assessment of labor progression.

It is not unusual for the fetal heart rate to slow to 100 beats per minute (bpm) with pushing contractions and then to increase to more than 120 bpm when the uterus relaxes.

clinical ALERT

If the fetal heart rate does not return to 120 or more between contractions, the supervising RN or physician should be notified immediately. Oxygen may be given to the mother at this time in order to provide enough oxygen for the fetus.

The nurse must be aware that a client's cultural background may affect her assessment and needs during labor. The nurse should be aware of her or his own culture and biases in providing care to a client from a different culture. Box 53-1 ■ provides cultural information about expression of pain during labor. Table 53-4 ■ identifies some cultural variations in birth practices.

DIAGNOSING, PLANNING, AND IMPLEMENTING

The following nursing diagnoses may be used in planning nursing care for the laboring client:

- *Acute Pain* related to the labor process
- *Anxiety*
- *Deficient Knowledge*

- *Risk for Compromised Resilience* related to fatigue and the birth process
- *Impaired Urinary Elimination*
- *Deficient Fluid Volume*
- *Risk for Infection*

Typical outcomes for the laboring woman might include these as well as others:

- Pain will be controlled within reasonable limits.
- Client will be able to express feelings and listen to instructions during labor.
- Client will sleep when baby sleeps.
- Client will void every 2 to 3 hours postdelivery.

The goals of nursing interventions are to assist the client and support persons through the labor and birth process. Nursing care follows the standards for any client. For example, any client with a fluid volume deficit would be given

BOX 53-1	CULTURAL PULSE POINTS

Expression of Pain during Labor

Pain response varies from culture to culture, and pain caused by labor and birth is no different. Some women are very stoic and labor quietly; this is frequently true with African American women. Others are notoriously loud. Many cultures feel that women must experience pain and discomfort during labor (e.g., Mexican, Iranian, and Filipinos). In fact, very difficult labor usually results in lavish gifts for Iranian women.

Mexican women are frequently heard repeating "*aye yie yie*" throughout labor. Interestingly, repeating "*aye yie yie*" in succession requires long, slow deep breaths. This has been described as "Mexican Lamaze." More than an expression of pain, this phrase is instead a culturally accepted method of pain relief.

TABLE 53-4	Cultural Considerations in Birthing Practices
COUNTRY	**CULTURAL UNIQUENESS OR PREFERENCE**
China	Stoic response to pain. Fathers not present during birth. Prefer side lying during labor and birth because they believe there is less trauma to fetus.
India	Natural childbirth practices preferred. Fathers usually not present. Female relatives usually present.
Iran	Fathers not present. Prefer female support and female caregivers.
Japan	Natural childbirth methods practiced, may labor silently, father may be present.
Laos	May use squatting position for birth, fathers may or may not be present, prefer female caregivers.
Mexico	May be stoic about discomfort until 2nd stage, then may request pain relief. Father and female relatives may be present.
South Korea	Stoic during labor. Fathers usually not present.

intravenous fluid. Any client with impaired urinary elimination would be encouraged to void every 2 hours; if needed, a catheter would be used to drain the bladder. Any client and support person needs emotional support and teaching.

Because the need for pain control during labor may not be the same as for other clients in pain, more detail will be provided here. There are many comfort measures that may be used for the laboring client. Some work very well for one client but not for another. The nurse must evaluate the effectiveness of comfort measures for each individual and change methods when needed.

Nonpharmacologic Comfort Measures

- Teach client to change position frequently. Encourage side-lying or upright positions. Supine position should not be used. *Change of position reduces muscle stress. Supine position puts pressure on the vena cava.*
- Provide ice chips and oral care. Clear liquids may be given in early labor. *Ice chips and oral care provide some moisture and refresh the mouth. Liquids are avoided late in labor because of the possibility of vomiting and aspiration.*
- Encourage muscle relaxation, massage, or abdominal *effleurage* (a light stroking with the fingertips in circular motion) from the symphysis to the iliac crest. *Relaxation and massage promote overall relaxation and distraction, and help to relieve the discomfort of labor.*

- Promote use of breathing techniques and monitor client. Table 53-5 ■ describes specific breathing techniques. *Proper breathing techniques can smooth labor and decrease pain. It is important to monitor the client closely for signs of hyperventilation.*

Box 53-2 ■ provides numerous nonpharmacologic nursing interventions for assisting women in labor.

Pharmacologic Comfort Measures

Systemic medications administered during labor are narcotic analgesics. Administration of these medications is not the responsibility of the LPN or LVN. These drugs should be administered only when the client's vital signs are stable, the fetus is at term, fetal heart rate is in a normal pattern between 120 and 160, and the client is in active labor. Systemic medications can slow or stop contractions if labor is not well established. Systemic medications given in transition or during the second stage of labor can cause respiratory distress in the newborn.

Regional Blocks

Regional blocks or regional anesthetics are administered by the physician, anesthesiologist, or nurse anesthetist. Common regional blocks (Figure 53-17 ■) include:

- *Pericervical block:* The drug is administered around the cervix during active labor to provide anesthesia to the cervix and upper vagina.

TABLE 53-5	Breathing Techniques during Labor
TECHNIQUE	**DESCRIPTION**
Cleansing Breath Used at beginning and end of each contraction	Relaxed breath in through nose, out through mouth
Slow-Paced Breathing Used in early labor and beginning of active labor	Slower than normal breathing. In 2–3–4/Out 2–3–4 (not less than ½ normal rate)
Modified-Paced Breathing Used in active labor and transition phase	Faster than normal breathing. IN–OUT/IN–OUT/IN–OUT (not more than twice normal rate)
Patterned-Paced Breathing Used in active labor and transition phase; patterns of 5:1 or higher are tiring	3:1 Pattern is IN–OUT/IN–OUT/IN–OUT/IN–BLOW 4:1 Pattern is IN–OUT/IN–OUT/IN–OUT/IN–OUT/IN–BLOW Pattern with words: may say "Yankee Doodle" or "I think I can" and repeat through the contraction Pyramid pattern such as 1:1, 2:1, 3:1, 4:1—4:1, 3:1, 2:1, 1:1

BOX 53-2   NURSING CARE CHECKLIST

Nonpharmacologic Comfort Measures for Women in Labor

Emotional Support

☑ Be present. Give the woman your undivided attention.

☑ Make sure your facial expression and stance are pleasant and convey confidence.

☑ Unless the laboring woman requests otherwise, stay close to her, usually within 2 feet.

☑ Use a reassuring, encouraging tone of voice.

☑ Offer praise for her efforts.

☑ Use humor or verbal distractions as appropriate; use verbal and nonverbal responses from the woman to guide your sense of what is useful.

☑ Rephrase negative thoughts into positive thoughts. (For example, if the woman says, "I don't think I can do it," you could say, "You can do this. Just take it one step at a time.")

Informational Support

☑ Interpret medical jargon or other information from healthcare providers that the client and partner do not understand.

☑ Use therapeutic communication skills (reflecting, rephrasing, choosing culturally sensitive words, using interpreter if needed).

☑ Role model behaviors for the partner to follow, and encourage participation.

☑ Provide information about procedures and progress.

☑ Remind client about breathing, relaxation, or pushing techniques as needed.

Physical Comfort Behaviors

☑ Remember that a woman's body is made to be able to give birth without pharmacologic assistance.

☑ Adjust the environment (including temperature and lighting) as much as possible for the mother's comfort. Mild, familiar scents may be used; avoid candles and strong scents.

☑ Ensure a nonrestrictive environment that allows freedom of movement.

☑ Offer assistive equipment as appropriate (extra pillows, birthing ball, squatting bar, etc.).

☑ Assist woman with position changes as needed. Positions of comfort vary, depending on the stage of labor:

  ☑ First stage: standing, ambulating, leaning, knee–chest, pelvic rocking, sitting on birthing ball or toilet, rocking chair, squatting, left side lying

  ☑ Second stage: knee–chest, hands–knees with birthing ball, squatting, semi-Fowler's, lateral.

☑ Provide comforting touch to convey caring. This can be as simple as stroking the woman's brow. It also includes massage (hand, foot, back), handholding, etc.

☑ Provide nourishment. Depending on the stage of labor and level of consciousness, the woman may be offered ice chips, sour candy, Popsicles, oral fluids, or a light meal.

☑ Offer application of heat or cold (warm blanket, cool washcloth, fan, etc.).

☑ Provide equipment for personal hygiene. Assist as needed. A bath or shower may be taken. Ensure safety of the client while transferring and bathing.

☑ Encourage urinary elimination every 2 to 3 hours.

Advocacy Support

☑ Ask about and support the mother's expectations for labor and birth. Understand that the woman's culture may affect her approach to this experience.

☑ Establish a therapeutic relationship in order to protect the woman (provide safety), attend to her needs, and help her make choices related to health care.

☑ Convey respect for the woman's privacy, modesty, relationships, and values. Be professional and nonjudgmental. You do not have to agree with the woman's choices to provide good nursing care.

☑ Provide physical and emotional safety so the woman is able to express both positive and negative emotions.

☑ Encourage problem-solving behavior, and keep the woman at the focus of decision making. Step in if others are trying to interfere.

☑ Support the woman's desires verbally and actively.

Source: Towle, M. A., & Adams, E. D. (2008). *Maternal-child nursing care.* Upper Saddle River, NJ: Prentice Hall. Data courtesy of Ellise D. Adams and Ann L. Bianchi (2005). *50 Ways to comfort a laboring woman.* Presented at The AWHONN 2005 Convention, June 14, 2005, Salt Lake City, Utah.

■ *Pudendal block:* The drug is administered through the vagina into the pudendal nerve, resulting in anesthesia of the vagina and perineum (Figure 53-17B).

■ *Epidural or spinal block:* The drug is administered through a catheter placed in the epidural space (Figure 53-17C). The drug can be administered intermittently or by continuous infusion. Anesthesia usually involves the lower abdomen, pelvis, perineum, and lower extremities.

While the client remains fully awake and comfortable, her participation in the birth process may be variable. In some clients a lack of feeling may decrease their ability to push effectively and the delivery may need to be assisted. The client may experience hypotension, bladder distention, and respiratory depression. For this reason, frequent or constant monitoring by the registered nurse may be required.

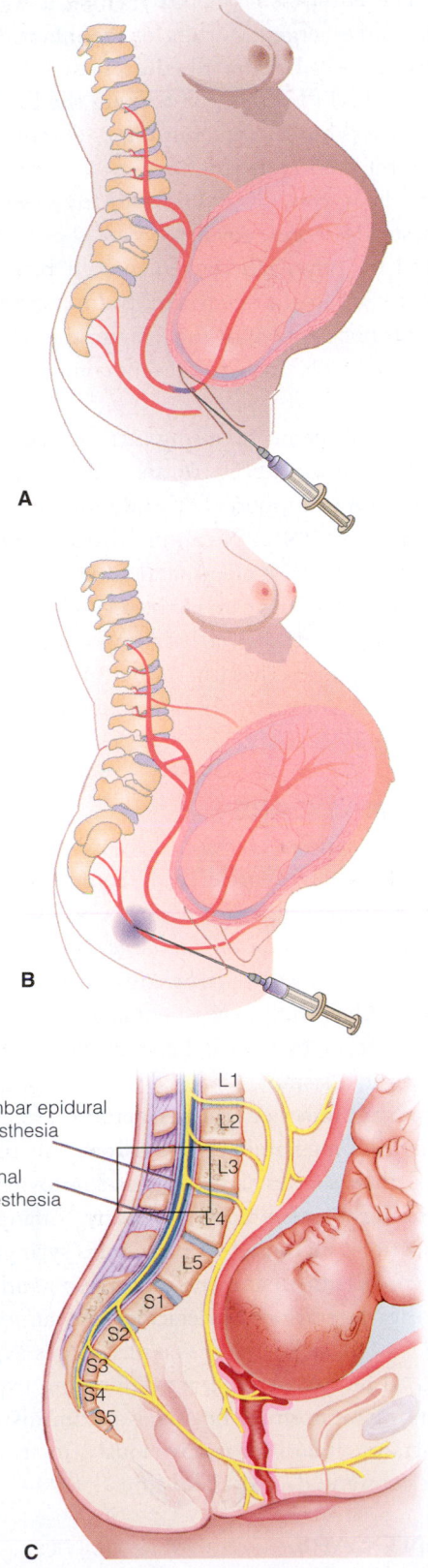

Figure 53-17. ■ Schematic diagram showing pain path and sites of interruption. **A.** Paracervical block (sensory pathways and site of interruption in relation to fetus). **B.** Pudendal block by transvaginal approach. **C.** The lumbar epidural block. The epidural space is located between the dura and the vertebra.

- *Local infiltration:* The drug is injected subcutaneously into the true perineum prior to an episiotomy or repair of a laceration.

General anesthesia is rarely used for vaginal deliveries because it causes the client to lose consciousness. However, it may be used for emergency cesarean birth. Because the drug reaches the fetus in about 2 minutes, there is danger of respiratory depression in the newborn.

EVALUATING

The client is evaluated for comfort, stability of vital signs, and progression of labor. The closer the client progresses toward birth, the more frequent the evaluation should be. In many cases the nurse remains at the bedside, caring for only one client at a time.

NURSING PROCESS CARE PLAN
Woman in Active Stage One Labor

Jane, a 20-year-old primigravida, is admitted to the labor unit in active labor. She states contractions began about 5 hours ago, but she has become uncomfortable with them for about 30 minutes. She appears comfortable between contractions, but is using controlled breathing techniques during contractions.

Assessment
The following data should be collected as soon as possible after admission.

- Vital signs
- Fetal heart tones (FHTs)
- Urine sample for sugar and protein
- Frequency and duration of contractions
- Dilatation and effacement of the cervix
- Presentation, position, and station of the fetus
- Mother's choice for pain control

Nursing Diagnosis
The following important nursing diagnosis (among others) is established for this client:

- *Risk for Compromised Resilience* related to birthing process and fatigue of labor

Expected Outcome
The expected outcome for this diagnosis is:

- Mother will participate actively in the birthing process with no evidence of injury to herself or the fetus.

Planning and Implementation
The following nursing interventions are planned and implemented for this client:

- Constantly monitor events of second and third stage of labor and birth. *This ensures maternal and fetal well-being.*

- Provide feedback regarding the progression of labor and birth. *Feedback relieves anxiety and enhances participation.*
- Provide comfort measures such as positioning, dry linen, oral care, and minimal distractions. *Comfort measures decrease discomfort and help the woman focus on the birthing process.*
- Remind mother and support person of breathing techniques, positioning, and bearing down during birth. *Reminders can refocus the woman's energy and ease discomfort. Support and encouragement by support persons can help the mother through the birthing process.*

Evaluation

Labor is progressing in a normal pattern. The mother verbalizes increased comfort with position changes and effleurage. She reports that breathing techniques help her remain in control of her behavior.

Critical Thinking in the Nursing Process

1. What criteria would the nurse use to determine whether Jane should be given a narcotic pain medication that has been ordered prn?
2. What are the two top priorities in caring for Jane?
3. Many women in labor are offered a whirlpool bath. Should Jane be offered this method of relaxation? Why or why not?

Note: Discussion of Critical Thinking questions appears on the MyNursingKit Website.

Birth

PREPARATION FOR BIRTH

As labor progresses, the birthing suite should be prepared (Figure 53-18 ■). In some areas, the birth takes place in the same room as labor. In others, a special birthing room is used. The equipment should include a warmer, suction, oxygen, and emergency drugs for the infant. It is the nurse's responsibility to be sure all equipment is operational prior to birth. The LPN/LVN can prepare the birthing room including checking the functioning of all equipment and arranging the sterile instruments.

A table is covered with sterile drapes. Sterile instruments, sterile drapes, gown and gloves, and bulb syringe are arranged for physician convenience. If birth is imminent, the table can remain uncovered, but must remain sterile. If birth will not happen for some time, the table may be covered with a sterile drape to prevent contamination until it is needed.

The role of the nurse during birth is to continue to monitor the client and fetus, to assist the physician or nurse midwife, and to support the family. Birth is a very stressful time, and the LPN/LVN can be instrumental in providing assistance to the RN, client, and family.

Timing of nursing care in the second stage of labor is essential to a smooth birth. It is important for the client to feel that the nurse has the situation under control. The nurse should convey a confident attitude and seek additional help if necessary.

MATERNAL CARE

The client should be positioned according to the physician's or nurse midwife's preference. Sometimes the client is placed in lithotomy position with a pillow under the right hip to relieve pressure on the large blood vessels. Legs are abducted, with knees bent. Stirrups may be used to support the legs. Other times, the client is placed on her left side with the left leg extended. The right leg is flexed and supported by an assistant.

To prevent infection, the perineum is cleansed with antiseptic soap immediately prior to birth. The physician/nurse midwife then applies sterile drapes to provide a clean environment for the newborn. Once the infant is born, the airway will be suctioned with the bulb syringe and the umbilical cord clamped and cut. The vagina and cervix are inspected for lacerations. Lacerations and an episiotomy (see Figure 53-13) are sutured. The placenta is expelled and inspected to be sure it is intact. Following expulsion of the placenta, the nurse may be asked to administer Pitocin, either intramuscularly or intravenously, to stimulate uterine contractions and decrease bleeding.

INFANT CARE

Immediately following birth, the registered nurse assumes care of the infant. The infant may be placed on the mother's abdomen to begin the bonding process, or the infant may be placed under a warmer to stabilize temperature. In either case, the priority is for the nurse to dry the infant, maintain

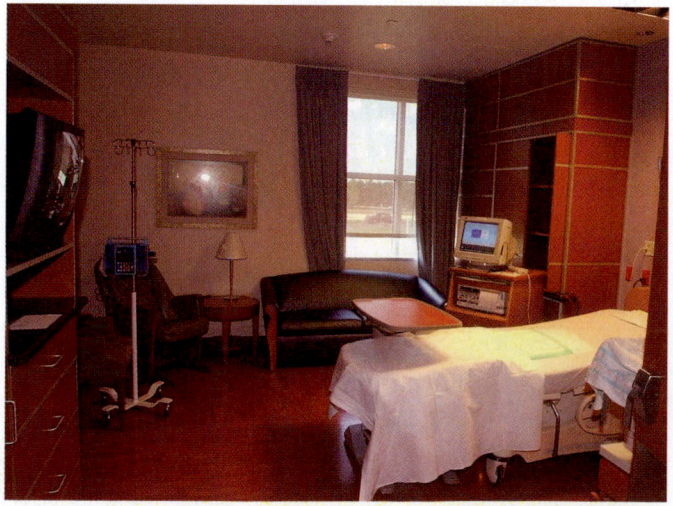

Figure 53-18. ■ Birthing suite.

Recovery

During the fourth stage of labor/birth, the nurse monitors the mother and newborn. Maternal vital signs are taken every 15 minutes, the fundus is checked for position and firmness (see Chapter 54 🔗), and the vaginal flow is assessed for amount and character. The mother's fundus should remain firm, below the umbilicus, and in the midline (see discussion in Chapter 54 🔗). Failure of the fundus to remain firm could indicate intrauterine bleeding. If the fundus is not in the proper location, blood clots or a full bladder should be suspected.

Vaginal bleeding is assessed by the saturation on the perineal pad. At the end of an hour, a totally saturated perineal pad is considered heavy bleeding. Any deviation from normal range should be reported to the registered nurse and physician. The fundus may need to be massaged and clots removed. (See Procedure 54-1 🔗 for fundal massage.)

The newborn is assessed for signs of respiratory distress. In the newborn, respiratory distress is characterized by dusky color, grunting respirations, nasal flaring, and sternal retractions. (See Chapter 32 🔗 for discussions of respiration and respiratory disorders.) The registered nurse should be notified if these signs are identified. The newborn must be kept warm, either by warm blankets or by being placed in a warming bed. The newborn may be kept in the room with the mother or placed in the newborn nursery. Chapter 56 🔗 details care of the newborn child.

High-Risk Labor and Birth

Although most pregnancies end with a normal labor and birth, expected and unexpected complications may occur. The most common complications of labor and birth will be discussed here.

PRETERM LABOR

Preterm labor is the onset of regular contractions between the 20th and 37th week that cause changes in the cervix. Factors associated with preterm labor include premature rupture of membranes, multiple pregnancy, vaginal bleeding, cervical abnormalities, and infections. Most women with preterm labor are admitted to the hospital for treatment. **Tocolytic agents** (medications that inhibit contractions) are frequently ordered (Table 53-6 ■). Common tocolytic agents include

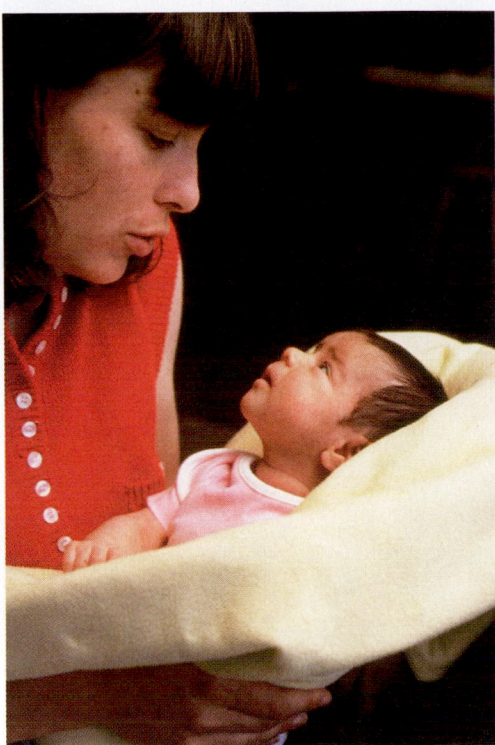

Figure 53-19. ■ Mother–child bonding is strengthened as infant and parent look into each other's eyes. (The Image Works.)

the airway, and stimulate breathing. The infant will lose heat rapidly, and warm, dry blankets should be used. Drying the infant by rubbing its back stimulates crying, which is necessary to expand the lungs. The airway should be suctioned as needed. The nurse will assess the infant at 1 and 5 minutes using the Apgar scoring criteria. (See the full discussion in Chapter 56. Table 56-1 identifies the Apgar criteria. Procedure 56-1 provides steps in determining the Apgar score 🔗 .) Once the infant is stabilized, it will be weighed and measured. If ordered, the nurse will give the infant AquaMEPHYTON (vitamin K) and an antibiotic eye ointment to prevent an eye infection.

Bonding is important for all members of the family (Figure 53-19 ■). Once the mother and infant are stable, the nurse wraps the infant and allows the mother to hold and, if desired, breastfeed the infant. The nurse picks up the delivery room and makes the environment presentable for family visitors. For more information on bonding, see Chapter 54 🔗 .

TABLE 53-6	**Pharmacology: Tocolytic Drugs for Premature Labor**		
CLASSIFICATION	**DRUG**	**USE**	**SIDE EFFECTS**
Uterine relaxants (tocolytics)	Terbutaline (Brethine)	First-line tocolytic	Hypotension, cardiac arrhythmia, tachycardia, palpitation, myocardial ischemia, pulmonary edema, maternal hypoglycemia
	Ritodrine (Yutopar)	Treatment of preterm labor	

ritodrine (Yutopar), terbutaline (Brethine), and magnesium sulfate. If labor continues, a corticosteroid may be given to accelerate fetal lung maturation. If contractions stop and there is no further change in the cervix, the client may be discharged with instructions to limit activity and take prescribed tocolytic medication.

INDUCTION OF LABOR

Induction of labor may be necessary if the risk to the mother or infant of continuing the pregnancy is greater than the risk of birth. Indications for induction of labor include **post dates** (labor does not begin spontaneously by the 41st week), gestational hypertension (see Chapter 52 ⚭), maternal diabetes, suspected fetal abnormality, history of rapid delivery, and fetal death.

The methods of induction of labor include:

- *Prostaglandins (PGE₁):* At times, the cervix is ripened (softened) by the insertion of a prostaglandin gel into and around the cervix. Labor may begin in a few hours or may be induced 12 to 24 hours later by another method.
- *Artificial rupture of membranes (ARM):* The physician/nurse midwife inserts an amnihook (Figure 53-20 ■) through the cervix and perforates the amniotic membranes. Labor contractions may begin within a few hours.
- *Pitocin (oxytocin) infusion:* A primary intravenous infusion is begun and a secondary infusion containing Pitocin is given by piggyback into the primary infusion (Table 53-7 ■). If severe side effects of the Pitocin occur, the infusion can easily be discontinued and the IV line maintained.

Once induced labor has begun, it usually progresses like spontaneous labor.

PRECIPITOUS BIRTH

Precipitous birth is a birth that occurs rapidly, unexpectedly, and without the attention of a physician or nurse midwife. A precipitous birth may be accompanied by *precipitous labor,* which lasts less than 3 hours. Precipitous labor or birth increases the risk of ruptured uterus, cervical and vaginal lacerations, hemorrhage, fetal distress, and fetal cerebral trauma. If the client says, "The baby is coming," the nurse should check to see if the fetus is crowning. Nursing actions for assisting a precipitous birth are provided in Box 53-3 ■.

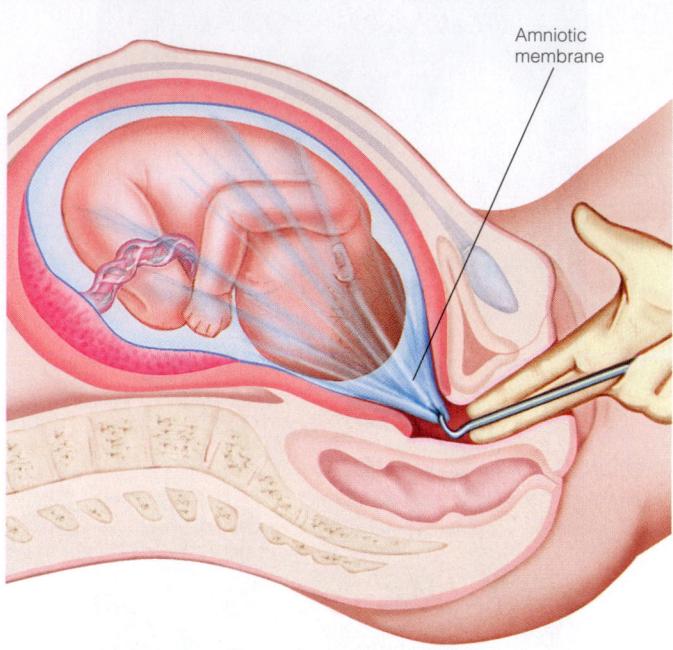

Amniotic membrane

Figure 53-20. ■ Amniotomy is a very common procedure performed during labor. The amnihook artificially ruptures the membrane.

After birth, a physician or nurse midwife should examine the mother and baby as soon as possible.

PROLAPSED CORD

Prolapsed cord means that the umbilical cord emerges through the cervix before the presenting part (Figure 53-21 ■). The umbilical cord can become trapped between the presenting part and the pelvis at any time. However, prolapse more commonly occurs when the fetal membranes rupture and before the presenting part is engaged. Once the umbilical cord is flushed through the cervix by amniotic fluid, the presenting part then compresses it against the cervix and pelvis. If pressure on the umbilical cord is not relieved, the fetus will develop hypoxia and could die. When a prolapsed umbilical cord is identified, the examiner should insert two fingers into the vagina and apply upward pressure against the presenting part to relieve pressure on the cord. While the upward pressure on the presenting part is maintained, the client should be turned to a knee–chest

TABLE 53-7	Pharmacology: Drug Used to Stimulate Labor			
DRUG	**USUAL ROUTE/DOSE**	**CLASSIFICATION**	**SELECTED SIDE EFFECTS**	**DON'T GIVE IF**
Oxytocin (Pitocin)	IV *To stimulate labor:* 0.5–20 milliunits/min. *To prevent hemorrhage:* 20–40 milliunits/min.	Oxytocic hormone	Prolonged uterine contractions, which can harm fetus Afterpains	Fetal distress is apparent Contractions are more than every 2 minutes, lasting over 90 seconds

BOX 53-3 NURSING CARE CHECKLIST

Assisting a Precipitous Delivery

In precipitous labor, if the baby is crowning the nurse should:

☑ Stay with the mother.

☑ Call for assistance by putting on the emergency call light. If outside the hospital, have someone call emergency medical services (EMS).

☑ Remain calm and reassure the mother; instruct her to pant.

☑ If time permits, open emergency equipment, wash hands, and put on sterile gloves. If outside the hospital, provide as much privacy as possible.

☑ Provide a sterile or clean area for birth.

☑ If membranes are intact, tear membranes to allow amniotic fluid to drain.

☑ Apply gentle pressure to head with one hand to allow it to gradually be born. Do not apply firm pressure or try to stop the head from being born.

☑ Check the baby's neck for the umbilical cord, known as a **nuchal cord** (Figure 53-22 ■). If there is a nuchal cord, and it is loose enough, slip the cord over the baby's head. If it is too tight, place two clamps on the cord and cut the cord between the clamps. Then unwind the umbilical cord from the baby's neck.

☑ Suction the baby's nose, mouth, and throat.

☑ Gently apply downward pressure to the baby's head until the anterior shoulder emerges from under the symphysis pubis. Then gently lift the baby's head until the posterior shoulder emerges from the vagina.

☑ Slide the rest of the baby from the vagina, being careful not to drop the wet, slippery baby.

☑ Suction the airway, and dry the baby.

☑ Clamp the umbilical cord in two places and cut it between the clamps. If outside of the hospital, the cord does not need to be clamped and cut until emergency medical personnel arrive. The cord should only be cut under sterile technique.

☑ Once the placenta is visible at the vaginal opening, gently pull on the umbilical cord until the placenta is expelled. Keep all tissue for the physician to examine.

☑ Arrange for a physician or nurse midwife to examine the mother and infant as soon as possible.

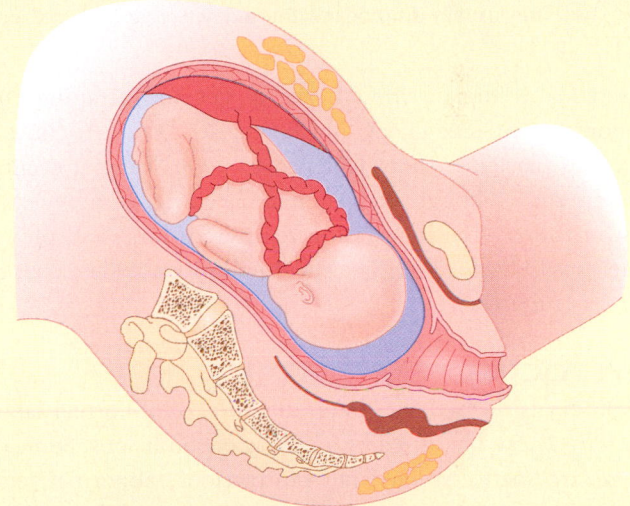

Figure 53-22. ■ Nuchal cord is a cord wrapped around the head. If loose, it can be slipped over the head.

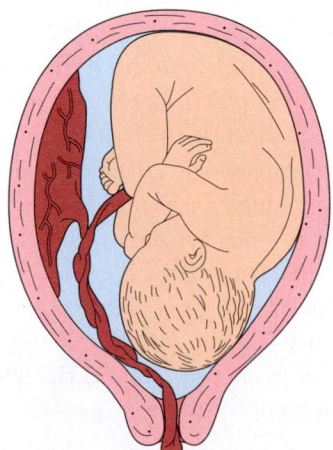

Figure 53-21. ■ Cord prolapse through the introitus. The prolapse of an umbilical cord creates an emergency situation requiring birth by cesarean section.

position to allow gravity to help keep the fetus away from the pelvis. If the umbilical cord protrudes from the vagina, it should be covered with wet towels to prevent shrinking of the Wharton's jelly and further compression of umbilical vessels. The physician is notified and an emergency cesarean birth (discussed later) is performed.

RETAINED PLACENTA

Retained placenta occurs when all or part of the placenta or fetal membranes remain attached to the endometrium. Normally, when the placenta detaches from the endometrium, the uterus contracts firmly, putting pressure on the bleeding vessels. If part of the placenta remains attached to the endometrium, the uterus does not contract firmly, and bleeding results. If the condition is noted during the delivery process, the physician will perform a D & C by

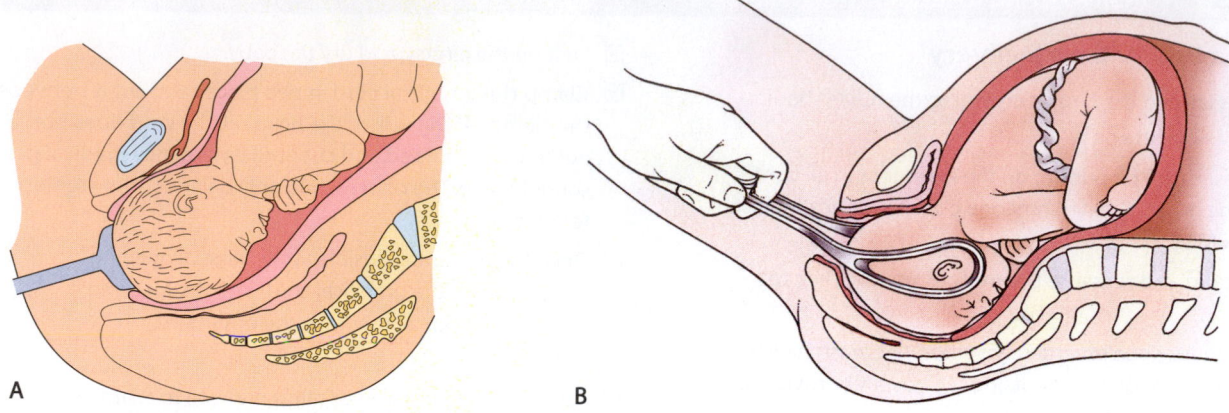

A **B**

Figure 53-23. ■ **A.** Vacuum extractor traction. The cup is placed on the fetal occiput, creating suction. Traction is applied in a downward and outward direction. As the fetal head begins to emerge, traction is maintained to lift the head out of the vagina. **B.** Forceps (a blade, shank, and handle) can be used to rotate and to help in birthing of the fetus. Pressure marks from forceps are usually located on the cheek and jaws. They usually disappear within a day. (*Source:* Dorling Kindersley Media Library.)

inserting a curette through the cervix and scraping the endometrium. (See D & C in Chapter 40 ⬭.) At times a retained placenta is not identified at birth. When it occurs, the uterus is boggy and vaginal bleeding is heavy and uncontrolled. The supervising registered nurse and physician should be notified. The client will probably be taken to surgery for a D & C.

DYSTOCIA

Dystocia is defined as a long, difficult, or abnormal labor pattern. It can be caused by a variety of conditions. Some of these are ineffective uterine contractions, abnormal fetal presentation or position, a large fetus, or small maternal pelvic outlet. When labor does not progress in the usual time frame, the nurse should anticipate that further evaluation and intervention will be necessary. A vacuum or forceps may be used in some circumstances to assist delivery (Figure 53-23 ■).

The strength of uterine contractions can be assessed internally. The physician inserts a small plastic catheter through the cervix, past the presenting part. The catheter is attached by an adapter to a monitoring system. The strength of contractions is recorded on the labor record. If the contractions are not appropriately strong, intravenous Pitocin can be administered to stimulate stronger contractions. If contractions are strong enough but the cervix fails to dilate and/or the fetus fails to descend, a cesarean birth will be performed.

If the fetus is in a *malpresentation* position (unfavorable position for birth), an attempt may be made to turn the fetus. If the fetal head is larger than the maternal pelvis, the condition is known as cephalopelvic disproportion (CPD). The only way to safely deliver the fetus is by cesarean birth.

SURGICAL BIRTH

Surgical birth or **cesarean section** is surgical removal of the fetus from the mother. It is performed for a variety of reasons including placenta previa, abruptio placentae (see Chapter 52 ⬭), CPD, fetal distress, breech presentation, PIH, multiple pregnancy, and previous cesarean birth. A cesarean birth can be a planned event, an unscheduled event, or an emergency procedure to save the mother and/or fetus. In any event, the procedures and nursing care are similar.

At times, preoperative procedures must be completed rapidly and under stress. The client may be tired after hours of labor. She may be worried about the health of her infant. She may be fearful about her own safety. The nurse must provide teaching and support while performing routine procedures.

The nurse's role includes the following actions, some of which the LPN or LVN may perform. A signed surgical consent must be obtained. A Foley catheter will be inserted to keep the bladder empty. An intravenous infusion will be started by a qualified practitioner. Hair over the mons pubis will be clipped short. If the father or a significant other is allowed to accompany the client to surgery, that person will need to be provided with surgical attire.

Anesthesia is usually administered by the epidural or spinal route. If an epidural has been used during labor, it will probably be used during surgery. If an epidural has not been used during labor, it will probably be initiated in the surgical suite prior to prepping the abdomen. In the event of an emergency situation, general anesthesia may be used.

Although incisions can be vertical in the low or mid-uterine area, the most common cesarean incision is a horizontal one through the skin at the pubic hair border (Figure 53-24 ■).

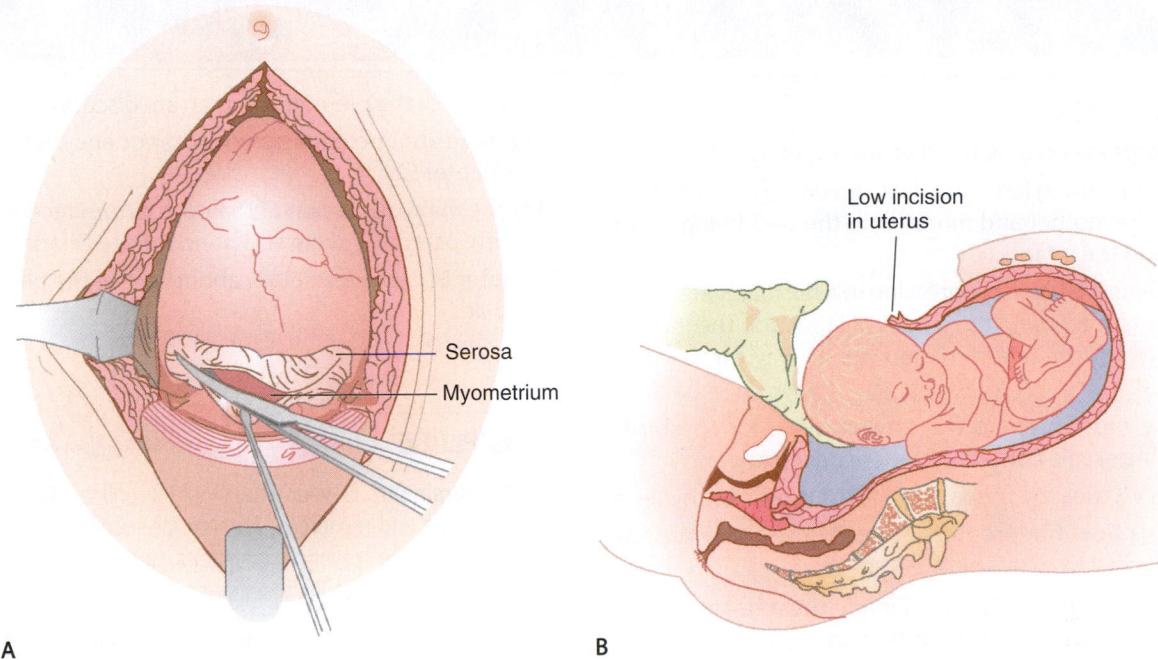

A

B

Figure 53-24. ■ **A.** This transverse incision in the lower uterine segment is called a Kerr incision. It is the most common incision used for cesarean surgical birth and has less risk of uterine rupture in subsequent pregnancies and labor than the classic high vertical incision. **B.** After the incisions are made into the uterus and fetal membrane, the physician reaches into the uterus between the symphysis pubis and the fetal head. The head is carefully lifted to bring it from beneath the symphysis forward through the uterine and abdominal wall. Pressure is usually applied to the uterine fundus to help expel the fetus. (*Source:* Adapted, with permission, from McGraw-Hill Companies, Inc. Cunningham, F. G., et al. [1997]. Williams obstetrics [20th ed.]. Stamford, CT: Appleton & Lange, pp. 516, 519.)

The bladder is detached from the perimetrium. A horizontal incision is made in the lower uterine segment. The infant is then pulled through the opening. If the infant is large, forceps may be needed to extract the infant's head. The infant's airway is suctioned. The infant is then dried and evaluated by the Apgar score. The woman's uterus, fascia, abdominal muscles, and fat are sutured. Skin staples, clips, or Steri-Strips are used to secure the skin.

The client will be taken to a recovery area for at least 1 hour. Vital signs will be taken. The fundus, surgical dressing, and urinary output will be monitored. The airway will be maintained until the client is awake and stable. The client will then be taken to the postpartum unit.

VAGINAL BIRTH AFTER CESAREAN

Vaginal birth after cesarean (VBAC) depends on several factors:

■ The reason for the cesarean birth
■ The condition of the scar tissue
■ The size of the fetus

If a vertical incision was made in the uterus, the risk of rupturing the uterus during labor is great. In this case, a repeat cesarean birth will be performed.

Note: The references and resources for all chapters have been compiled at the back of the book.

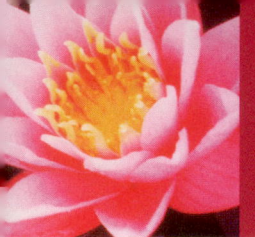

Chapter Review

KEY Points

- Labor progresses in a planned sequence of events.
- Nursing care during labor involves providing comfort measures for the mother and monitoring the well-being of the mother and the infant.
- To determine if labor is progressing in a normal pattern, the nurse must understand the stages of labor and the mechanism by which the infant maneuvers its way through the birth canal.
- The nurse must prepare the environment for the birth, maintaining sterile conditions where necessary.
- The LPN/LVN must be prepared to assist the RN at any time.
- When labor does not progress normally, the nurse must be prepared to assist with a cesarean birth.
- Following birth, the mother and infant must be monitored frequently until their condition stabilizes.

⚭ FOR FURTHER Study

See Chapter 32 for discussions of respiration and respiratory disorders.

For more about D & C and treatment of reproductive disorders, see Chapter 40.

Concerns of the pregnant woman are discussed in Chapter 51.

For more about complications of pregnancy, see Chapter 52.

For the main discussion of the postpartum recovery process, new parenting skills, and bonding, see Chapter 54.

Chapter 56 provides details about care of the newborn child.

EXPLORE PEARSON **mynursingkit**™

MyNursingKit is your one stop for online chapter review materials and resources. Prepare for success with additional NCLEX®-style practice questions, interactive assignments and activities, web links, animations and videos, and more!

Register your access code from the front of your book at
www.mynursingkit.com

Caring for a Woman in Transitional Labor

NCLEX-PN® Focus Area: Physiologic Adaptation

Case Study: Alyce, a 22-year-old woman, gravida 2, para 1, is admitted in transition. She states she woke up in labor and her water broke on the way to the hospital. She is shifting and moaning and is obviously uncomfortable. She is having difficulty keeping relaxed. States last labor lasted 6 hours.

Nursing Diagnosis: *Pain* related to increasing frequency and intensity of contractions

COLLECT DATA

Subjective	Objective
_____	_____
_____	_____
_____	_____
_____	_____
_____	_____
_____	_____
_____	_____

Would you report this? Yes/No

If yes, report to: _____

What would you report? _____

Nursing Care

_____
_____
_____
_____
_____
_____
_____
_____
_____
_____
_____

How would you document this? _____
_____
_____
_____

Compare your answers and documentation to those provided on the MyNursingKit Website.

Data Collected
(use only those that apply)

- Cervix 8 cm dilated, 100% effaced
- Station +2
- BP 142/90
- Contractions every 3 minutes, lasting 90 seconds
- Obviously uncomfortable as evidenced by moaning and shifting
- Having difficulty maintaining control as evidenced by clutching arm of chair and groaning when contractions begin
- Fetal heart rate 110
- Clear fluid draining from vagina

Nursing Interventions
(use only those that apply; list in priority order)

- Position on left side.
- Encourage to breathe with each contraction.
- Offer 8 ounces of ginger ale to help stomach discomfort.
- Prepare sterile field for birth.
- Administer pain medication IV.
- Give oxygen at 10 L by mask.

NCLEX-PN® Exam Preparation

TEST-TAKING TIP If you see words such as *monitor*, *observe*, or *check* in the stem, the question is referring to the assessment phase of the nursing process. The answer you select should be consistent with the first step of the nursing process as well.

1 Based on the hormonal theory of labor, the nurse anticipates a rise in which of the following to begin a chain of hormonal events that cause labor?

1. Cortisol
2. Oxytocin
3. Progesterone
4. Estrogen

2 The nurse would recognize that the client has experienced lightening when the pregnant woman reports:

1. "I can breathe much better."
2. "My ankles are less swollen."
3. "I don't have to urinate as often now."
4. "My lower back pain has been relieved."

3 The primary nurse performs a vaginal examination and finds a prolapsed cord. The nurse's priority action will be to:

1. Give medication to hasten a vaginal delivery.
2. Keep the client in a back-lying position.
3. Make arrangements for an emergency cesarean section.
4. Get the cord back to its original location.

4 When the fetus is found to be in a vertex presentation, the nurse anticipates the presenting fetal part will be the:

1. Forehead.
2. Face.
3. Buttocks.
4. Occiput.

5 The nurse is caring for a client in labor who complains of feeling faint. The nurse turns the client onto her side in order to have what effect on contractions?

1. Little or no effect
2. Increase the frequency
3. Increase the intensity
4. Stop the contractions

6 The nurse recognizes that the client is in the latent phase of the first stage of labor. This phase is best described as lasting from:

1. Undilated cervix to a 2-cm dilatation.
2. Onset of contractions to 4-cm dilatation.
3. Cervix dilated 4 cm to dilatation of 8 cm.
4. No contraction to contractions every 3 minutes.

7 The nurse, working on a labor and delivery unit, anticipates active labor for a primigravida will last how long?

1. 16 to 18 hours
2. 12 to 14 hours
2. 8 to 10 hours
4. 4 to 6 hours

8 A client in the transition phase of labor irritably tells the nurse not to touch her. The nurse's best action would be to:

1. Ask for someone else to support the client.
2. Tell the client to be cooperative and do as you say.
3. Remind the client to focus on relaxation and breathing.
4. Ask the client to push actively with each contraction.

9 The student nurse asks the primary nurse to explain what the obstetrician meant when telling the client that engagement had occurred. The primary nurse's best response would be to explain that:

1. The fetus has now become ballotable.
2. The presenting part has entered the true pelvis.
3. The presenting part is just above the ischial spines.
4. There is now observable crowning.

10 While caring for the client in the fourth stage of labor/delivery, the nurse discovers that the client has saturated two perineal pads during the first hour. What is the nurse's priority action?

1. Notify the primary nurse immediately.
2. Assure the client that this is normal.
3. Put the client on the bedpan to void.
4. Start a count of the pads and chart it.

Answers and rationales for Review Questions appear in Appendix I.

Chapter 54

Care of Postpartum Women

LEARNING Outcomes

After completing this chapter, you will be able to:

1. Describe the physical changes that occur after a woman has delivered a baby and placenta.
2. Identify psychological changes in the postpartum woman.
3. Describe important aspects of support for the postpartum woman.
4. Explain nursing interventions to use when providing nursing care for a postpartum woman.
5. Discuss methods of providing pain relief for the postpartum woman.
6. Identify crucial areas of client teaching for the postpartum woman.
7. Describe important factors in self-care for women after discharge.
8. Discuss client teaching about postpartum emergencies.
9. Identify adaptations in postpartum care for women after cesarean section.
10. Discuss important nursing considerations regarding the new family.
11. Discuss nursing care and teaching related to breastfeeding.

Clinical Objectives

12. Assist with and teach basic nursing care of the newborn in the immediate postpartum period.
13. Identify nursing diagnoses relevant to the care of the intrapartum client.
14. Provide nursing care to a client following a vaginal or cesarean birth.
15. Perform a physical and psychosocial assessment of the postpartum client.
16. Teach clients about the physical and psychological changes during the postpartum period.
17. Perform fundal massage and perineal assessment.
18. Instruct a client on use of a sitz bath.

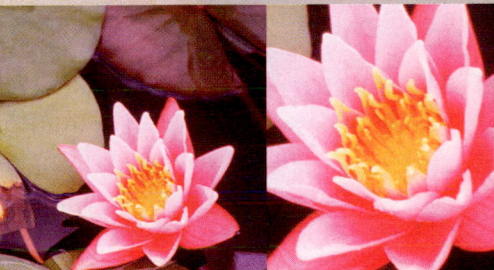

BRIEF Outline

Body Systems Adaptations
Psychological Changes
Fathers, Siblings, and Others
Cultural Influences in the Postpartum Period
Postpartum Care after Cesarean Section
New Family
Breastfeeding

KEY TERMS

Use the audio glossary feature on the MyNursingKit Website to hear the correct pronunciation of the following key terms.

afterpain 1491
boggy 1485
decidua 1484
diastasis recti abdominis 1487

engrossment 1489
involution 1484
Kegel exercises 1486
lochia 1484

postpartum 1484
thromboembolism 1493
thrombosis 1488

The postpartum period is most often thought of as a very happy time for a family. It can, however, be a time of discomfort, anxiety, and even fear. These feelings may not always be obvious to the nurse, since people exhibit pain and emotion in many different ways. The LPN/LVN often plays an important part in the support of a postpartum woman and her family. Although the LPN/LVN will use the nursing skills learned in school, postpartum nursing requires skills that are not always covered in a textbook. Listening is one of the most important skills a postpartum nurse needs to learn. Oftentimes, just taking the time to listen can make the difference between a positive and a negative postpartum experience. Women have many different personal and cultural needs and expectations (Box 54-1 ■). If the family seems agitated about some aspect of the birthing and postpartum process, the nurse can ask if there are special practices the family wants to observe.

Body Systems Adaptations

Postpartum refers to the period beginning immediately after delivery of the placenta and ending when the body and reproductive organs return to a near prepregnant state. This period lasts about 6 weeks, although the exact length varies from woman to woman. The type of facility a woman has chosen for delivery of her baby determines whether she will be transferred to a postpartum floor or remain in the birthing room. If the facility has separate labor/delivery and postpartum units, the woman is transferred to the postpartum floor once she has completed her recovery period and is stable. The *recovery period* begins after the expulsion of the placenta and ends after 1 to 2 hours when her vital signs are stable and bleeding is controlled. If the LPN/LVN will be assuming care of a postpartum client, the RN supervisor should be present to receive the client and perform the admission assessment.

BOX 54-1	CULTURAL PULSE POINTS

Taboos About Birth and the Postpartum Period
Cultures may have taboos concerning reactions during labor, presence of men, position for delivery, preferred types of health practitioners, and location of the birth. A new mother may need to follow practices of her culture in the postpartum period related to bathing, cord care, exercise, foods, and roles of men. Some cultures even have specific practices related to care and disposal of the placenta.

UTERUS

Following the delivery of the placenta, the uterus undergoes **involution** (a return to normal size). Figure 54-1 ■ illustrates involution of the uterus. When the placenta separates from the uterus, the **decidua** (tissue that lines the uterine wall during pregnancy) is irregular in thickness. Over the next 3 weeks, the decidua separates from the endometrium and is expelled through the vagina. This discarded blood, mucus, and tissue is called **lochia.** The placenta attachment site contains large blood vessels. Bleeding from these blood vessels is controlled by contraction of the myometrium. The placenta attachment site heals by exfoliation (a shedding of the outer layer) instead of by scar formation, which would prevent uterine attachment of future pregnancies. During exfoliation, the endometrium grows from the margins and from the basal layer under the site. The superficial tissue becomes necrotic and is sloughed off. This sloughing of tissue continues for approximately 4 weeks.

To control bleeding from the large vessels at the placenta site, the uterus must remain contracted, as evidenced by a fundus remaining very firm, below the umbilicus and in the midline. If blood pools in the body of the uterus, it will clot, causing the uterus to enlarge, stopping contractions, and

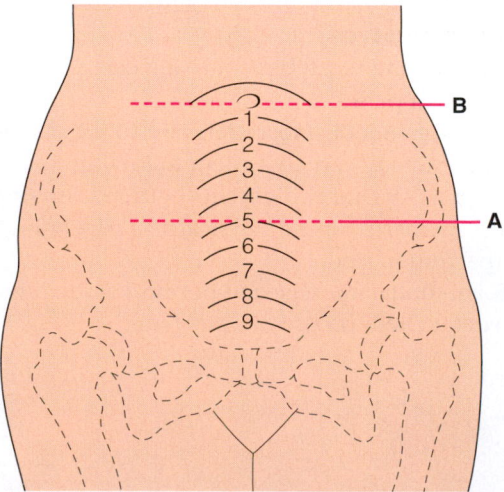

Figure 54-1. ■ Involution of the uterus. **A.** Immediately after delivery of the placenta, the top of the fundus is in the midline and about halfway between the symphysis pubis and the umbilicus. **B.** About 6 to 12 hours after birth, the fundus is at the level of the umbilicus. The height of the fundus then decreases about one fingerbreadth (about 1 cm) each day.

causing more bleeding. When the uterus stops contracting, the fundus becomes soft and spongy, which is termed **boggy**. If the fundus is boggy and located above the umbilicus, bleeding is suspected. A boggy uterus can be caused by retained placental pieces or accumulation of uterine blood.

The ligaments supporting the uterus in the pelvic cavity stretch during pregnancy. A full bladder can easily push the uterus up and to one side. A fundus displaced away from the midline and above the umbilicus usually indicates a full bladder. The displaced uterus is unable to contract fully, causing increased uterine bleeding. If the bladder is not emptied, the woman may experience increased cramping and hemorrhage. Once the bladder is emptied completely, the fundus should be assessed for firmness and position. If the fundus remains boggy, the RN should be notified.

Besides encouraging bonding with the newborn, breastfeeding results in the release of *oxytocin*, a hormone that contracts the uterus. The nurse can facilitate uterine contractions by reminding the new mother to keep her bladder empty and by encouraging breastfeeding mothers to nurse their baby. However, it may be necessary at times to perform fundal massage (Procedure 54-1 ■). Fundal massage should result in a firm fundus if the bladder is emptied and the blood clots have been expelled. Depending on the practice of the obstetrician or midwife, Pitocin (a synthetic form of oxytocin) may be given intravenously or intramuscularly. After the first postpartum day, the uterus will decrease in size approximately one fingerbreadth per day and continue to shrink for the next 4 to 6 weeks.

LOCHIA

As stated earlier, uterine bleeding is called *lochia*. The total amount of lochia shed from the uterus after birth is 240 to 270 mL. It is classified as rubra, serosa, or alba, and described in amount as heavy, moderate, or scant (Figure 54-2 ■). The first lochia, *lochia rubra*, is bright red in color. Lochia rubra consists of meconium, white and red blood cells, epithelial cells, and vernix. Lochia rubra is present for 2 to 3 days. Then the lochia turns brownish to dark red in color; this is referred to as *lochia serosa*. Lochia serosa is composed of white and red blood cells, wound exudates, and cervical mucus. This flow lasts for 4 to 6 days. *Lochia alba* is white to yellowish in color. The white/yellow color of lochia alba is attributed to the increased number of white blood cells being expelled from the uterus. Lochia alba gradually decreases in amount until the fourth to sixth week.

clinical ALERT

Persistent lochia rubra or a return to lochia rubra should be reported to the RN and obstetrician or midwife. It indicates increased vaginal bleeding. A foul odor indicates infection.

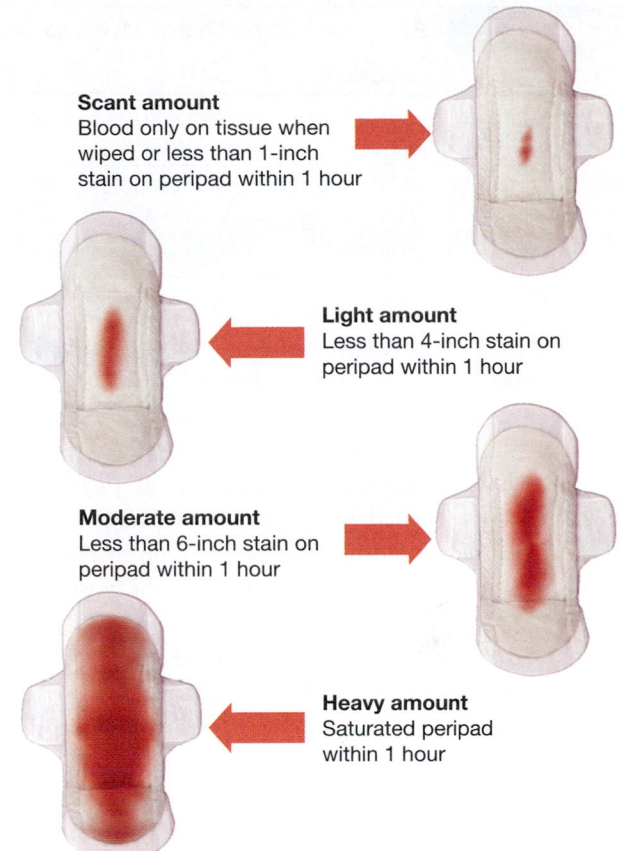

Scant amount
Blood only on tissue when wiped or less than 1-inch stain on peripad within 1 hour

Light amount
Less than 4-inch stain on peripad within 1 hour

Moderate amount
Less than 6-inch stain on peripad within 1 hour

Heavy amount
Saturated peripad within 1 hour

Figure 54-2. ■ Suggested guidelines for assessing lochia volume.

Oxytocin (Pitocin) or methylergonovine (Methergine) may be ordered for a woman who is at risk for increased bleeding or whose lochia rubra is heavier than normal (Table 54-1 ■). Methergine is usually administered intramuscularly or by mouth. Pitocin can be given intramuscularly but is most often given intravenously and can be added to the woman's IV fluids, by the RN, in order to continue contracting the uterus. Pitocin may be ordered routinely after delivery, depending on the facility policy or the practice of the obstetrician or midwife.

CERVIX

After delivery the cervix is soft and may be bruised. Cervical laceration can occur and may be associated with a continuous trickle of blood from the vagina even though the fundus remains firm. A continuous trickle of blood from the vagina should be reported by the LPN/LVN to the RN.

After approximately 1 week, the internal portion of the cervical os returns to its original tightly closed state. The external os never returns totally to its prepregnant state. It will remain slightly open.

VAGINA

The vagina usually appears swollen after delivery and may be bruised. Small lacerations or abrasions may be present. The size of the vagina decreases over the next few weeks but

TABLE 54-1	Pharmacology: Drugs Used to Contract the Uterus				
DRUG NAME	**USUAL ROUTE**	**CLASSIFICATION**	**SELECTED SIDE EFFECTS**		**DON'T GIVE IF**
Oxytocin (Pitocin)	IV 10 U–20 U IM or added to IV fluids for continuous infusion	Oxytocic	Water intoxication, hypotension, cardiac arrhythmias		Systolic BP below 90 mmHg
Methylergonovine (Methergine)	IM 0.2 mg every 2–4 hours prn Oral 0.2 mg every 4 hours for 6 doses	Ergot alkaloids (oxytocic)	Nausea, vomiting, elevated BP, temporary chest pain, dizziness, headache		Never use during pregnancy or labor

never returns to its prepregnant size. The vagina of a non-lactating woman usually appears normal within 6 weeks. The lactating woman experiences a decrease in estrogen due to suppression of ovarian activity. Decreased estrogen is associated with decreased vaginal lubrication and painful intercourse. A water-based lubricant may be helpful in decreasing discomfort during intercourse. Due to trauma to healing tissues and the risk of infection, the postpartum woman should be instructed not to have intercourse until she has seen her obstetrician or midwife for a follow-up visit and has been told that she may resume intercourse.

The postpartum woman may have poor muscle tone in the pelvic floor related to the pregnancy. Kegel exercises (see also Chapter 40 ⊙⊙) can increase muscle tone of the vagina and pelvic floor (Figure 54-3 ■). **Kegel exercises** involve a tightening and lifting the muscles that cross the pelvic floor. Clients are often told to identify the muscle band used in Kegel exercises by attempting to stop the flow of urine, or by contracting muscles as if to prevent flatus from escaping. Kegel exercises can be done while sitting, standing, or lying down. They should be done frequently throughout the postpartum period and beyond to reestablish muscle tone and help maintain urinary continence.

PERINEUM

During delivery of the baby, the perineum may tear, or it may be necessary for the obstetrician or midwife to cut an *episiotomy* (an incision through the perineal tissue to facilitate delivery of the fetal head). The laceration or episiotomy (see Figure 53-13 ⊙⊙) is usually sutured. Most practitioners use dissolvable sutures. Even if the perineum is intact, the postpartum woman may still experience tenderness.

clinical ALERT

Sudden, extreme perineal pain in a postpartum woman may be a symptom of a labial or vaginal *hematoma* (pooling of blood under the skin; see also Chapter 34 ⊙⊙). On inspection, the area may appear bruised but will be firm and shiny due to the increased blood flow into the area. The client usually cannot tolerate palpation of the area without great discomfort. Report suspicion of a hematoma to the RN immediately.

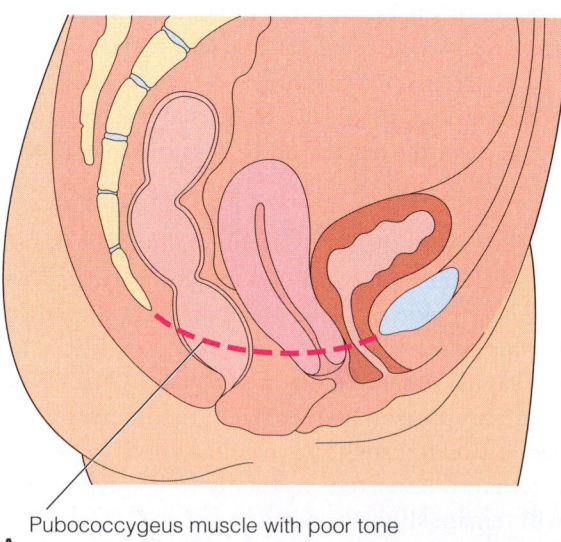

A

Pubococcygeus muscle with poor tone

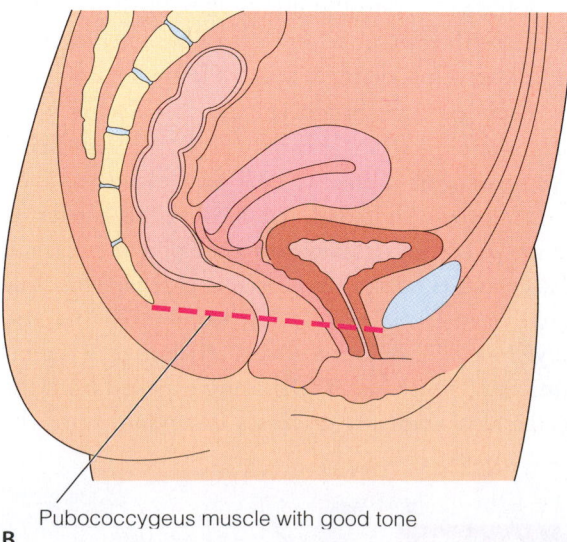

B

Pubococcygeus muscle with good tone

Figure 54-3. ■ Kegel exercises. The woman learns to tighten the pubococcygeus muscle and other muscles of the pelvic floor, which improves support to the pelvic organs. Lifting and holding the muscles up, then releasing them, is a means of strengthening the entire support structure of the pelvic floor. These exercises can help restore urinary continence if that has been disrupted by pregnancy.

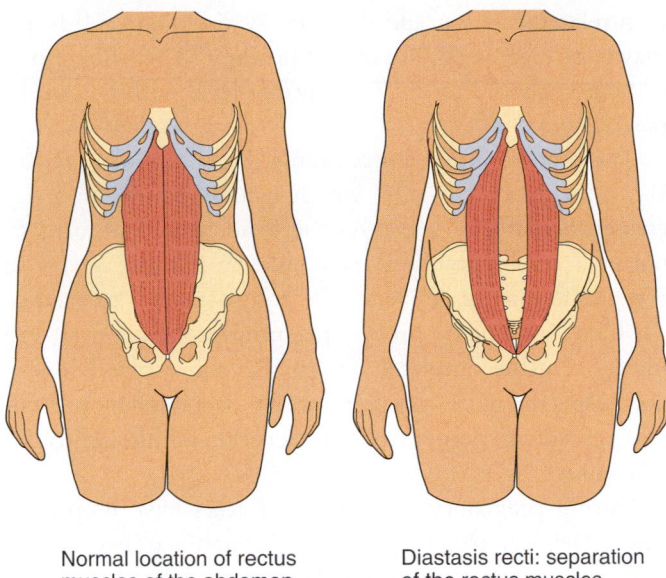

Normal location of rectus
muscles of the abdomen

Diastasis recti: separation
of the rectus muscles

Figure 54-4. ■ Diastasis recti abdominis, a separation of the abdominal musculature, commonly occurs after pregnancy.

ABDOMEN

Following delivery, the abdomen appears flabby. Although the abdomen may not return to its prepregnant state, this varies among women. It depends on abdominal tone before pregnancy and other factors. Abdominal exercise can usually begin after the postpartum follow-up appointment when the client is cleared for exercise by her obstetrician or midwife.

A separation of the abdominal muscle (called **diastasis recti abdominis**) may occur during pregnancy. (Figure 54-4 ■). It is more often seen in women with poor abdominal muscle tone. This separation does respond to exercise to improve abdominal muscle tone. Improving muscle tone after a diastasis recti abdominis is important for future pregnancies. Without improvement, the separation does not allow enough support, and back pain due to a pendulous abdomen may result. Stretch marks, also called *striae*, can become very red or purple in color but should fade after delivery. Striae rarely disappear completely.

BREASTS

The breasts remain similar to their pregnant condition for the first 2 to 3 days. Recall that the female breast is divided into 15 to 24 lobes separated by adipose tissue. Each lobe consists of numerous alveoli where milk is produced by secretory epithelium. The milk drains through lactiferous ducts that eventually open onto the nipple. After birth of the placenta, estrogen and progesterone levels and prolactin level increases. This hormone change stimulates the breast to produce milk. As the infant nurses, oxytocin is released from the pituitary gland, causing the milk to be released

from the breast. (*Note:* Breastfeeding is discussed in a separate section later in this chapter.)

At first a small amount of thick substance (*colostrum*) is expressed from the nipples. The breasts become fuller on about the third day after delivery, and start to become firm and heavy around the fourth day. The postpartum woman should be encouraged to wear a supportive bra as soon after delivery as is comfortable. A support bra helps decrease discomfort related to heavy, full breasts. It may decrease some of the sagging that occurs after the woman stops lactating.

GASTROINTESTINAL SYSTEM

Following delivery, the woman may be hungry. She has expended a lot of energy during the birthing process, and a light meal can help replace the spent calories. She usually drinks a large amount of fluid to replace what was lost in labor.

Peristalsis has been sluggish during pregnancy due to the effects of progesterone and the pressure of the enlarged uterus. It will take several days for peristalsis to return to normal. A postpartum woman may be anxious about having a bowel movement, especially if she has experienced a perineal laceration or episiotomy. A stool softener may be ordered. It is important to educate the client about the purpose of the stool softener. She may mistakenly think that it is a laxative and may refuse to take it, thinking it will make her have a bowel movement very soon. Reassure the client that a bowel movement should not injure her or rupture any stitches. Delaying having a bowel movement because of fear of pain or ruptured stitches may result in constipation. Instruct the client that adequate fluid intake is helpful in decreasing constipation. A common misconception heard from postpartum women is that it is necessary to have a bowel movement before being discharged to home. The hospital stay after a normal vaginal delivery is usually 48 hours (96 hours for a cesarean section), which is often too soon to have a bowel movement after delivery. During the labor process the woman may not have eaten very much and may have vomited. It could be more than 2 days until she has a bowel movement.

Following a cesarean birth, the woman may be placed on a liquid diet until bowel sounds are present. Her diet will then be advanced quickly. Flatulence, which adds to discomfort, may be relieved with early ambulation, antiflatulence medication, or Harris return flow (HRF) enema, if ordered.

URINARY SYSTEM

The postpartum woman may have decreased sensitivity to bladder filling. This is especially true after epidural analgesia. The capacity of the bladder to hold urine is increased after delivery as well. The urinary meatus or urethra may be swollen or bruised. Urethral swelling and decreased sensitivity to bladder filling can put the woman at risk for overdistention of the bladder and urinary retention. Urinary stasis can result in a urinary tract infection, so adequate bladder emptying is important. Overdistention of the bladder can cause damage to the bladder and may lead to urinary stress incontinence.

Diuresis occurs after delivery, because the body does not require the large amounts of blood volume it needed during pregnancy. The diuresis of fluid causes more rapid filling of the bladder. Encourage the woman to empty her bladder every 2 to 3 hours initially. Urinary catheterization may be ordered to relieve discomfort and prevent increased uterine bleeding.

CARDIOVASCULAR SYSTEM

Changes in the cardiovascular system following delivery can be seen in alterations in vital signs and blood values. During labor, the mother's temperature may have risen to 100.4° F (38° C) due to dehydration and physical exertion. Commonly, the mother begins to chill shortly after birth. The *postpartal chill* is the result of body temperature being higher than the surrounding environment. It also results from neurologic and vasomotor changes during labor. Covering the woman with warm blankets may alleviate the chill and provide comfort. The temperature should return to normal after birth.

clinical ALERT

The postpartal woman should be afebrile 24 hours after birth. If fever continues, infection should be suspected and the fever should be reported to the primary care provider.

The mother's blood pressure should remain stable following birth. Commonly, the blood pressure rises slightly during labor and returns to the mother's baseline within 1 hour post birth. Hypotension could indicate a reaction to medication or excessive bleeding. Hypertension, especially accompanied by headache, could indicate pregnancy-induced hypertension (PIH). If hypertension was a problem prior to labor, the blood pressure must be monitored frequently during the postpartum period.

Many women gain 25 to 30 pounds during the pregnancy. A woman who has gained this amount of weight during pregnancy may be able to return to prepregnancy weight during the postpartum period. She will lose 10 to 12 pounds during the birthing process. Another 5 pounds may be lost in the first few days due to puerperal diuresis. A woman who is physically active will have less difficulty with weight loss than a woman who is sedentary.

CHANGES IN BLOOD VALUES

In the postpartum period, white blood cells may increase to levels that would normally suggest infection. This increase can be attributed to the stress, inflammation, and

pain related to labor and delivery. White blood cell levels may be as high as 12,000 to 20,000/mm³. The white blood cell count should return to a normal level within 2 weeks postpartum.

The blood volume shifts dramatically following delivery, diluting blood cells, which usually results in a decreased hematocrit level. As the fluid balance returns to normal, the hematocrit level should be accurate after 4 to 8 weeks following delivery. The body attempts to balance the blood volume by profuse perspiration (*diaphoresis*) and increased urine output (*diuresis*). Excessive blood loss is not suspected until the hematocrit decreases more than two percentage points from the level on admission to the labor unit.

During pregnancy, coagulation factors have been activated. Delivery trauma or decreased mobility may predispose the mother to **thrombosis** (formation of clots in the blood vessel).

OVARIAN FUNCTION AND MENSTRUATION

Recall that one function of the placenta is to produce estrogen and progesterone to maintain the endometrium and to prevent ovulation during pregnancy. Following delivery of the placenta, blood levels of estrogen and progesterone decline rapidly. The decline of these hormones contributes to the sloughing of the decidua.

Return of ovulation varies among postpartum women. A nonlactating woman may begin her menstrual cycle anywhere from 6 weeks to 6 months after delivery. A lactating woman usually does not begin her menstrual cycle until she stops breastfeeding and may be delayed for up to 3 months after breastfeeding ends. Because ovulation precedes menstruation, the woman can become pregnant again before the first menses.

clinical ALERT

Instruct all postpartum women, whether lactating or not, that absence of a menstrual period does not mean they are infertile. Ovulation occurs before menstruation, so a woman could become pregnant again before her periods return. It is important for her to use birth control measures if another pregnancy is not desired at this time.

Psychological Changes

The woman needs time to adjust to the role of the mother. This adjustment occurs in stages.

TAKING-IN STAGE

During the first day or two, the mother is said to be in the taking-in stage. She is "taking in" information about the baby, recalling the experience of birth, and storing this information in her memory. The mother is tired and may depend on others to help meet her needs. She allows others to care for the baby, participating mainly in feeding the infant. She has a need to talk about her perception of the labor and delivery, and readily shares the experience with visitors.

TAKING-HOLD STAGE

By the third day after birth, the mother is usually ready to resume control. She is moving into the taking-hold stage. She is "taking hold" or control of the activities of caring for herself and her newborn (Figure 54-5 ■). She may become preoccupied with her bodily functions, such as elimination. If she is breastfeeding, she begins to be concerned about the quality and quantity of the milk. Although she is ready to meet her physical needs and the infant's needs, she may not be ready to resume responsibility for her household activities. It may take several weeks for her to have the physical and mental energy to return to her full activities. In most cases, it takes 3 to 10 months for a woman to be comfortable with the role of mother.

LETTING-GO STAGE

In the letting-go stage, the woman and her partner discover that social interactions become increasingly important. She is "letting go" of the idea of a perfect pregnancy, a perfect transition, and a perfect baby and moving on with life. The support of family and friends is important at this time. Mothers and fathers must learn to care for the infant and to make decisions about meeting the

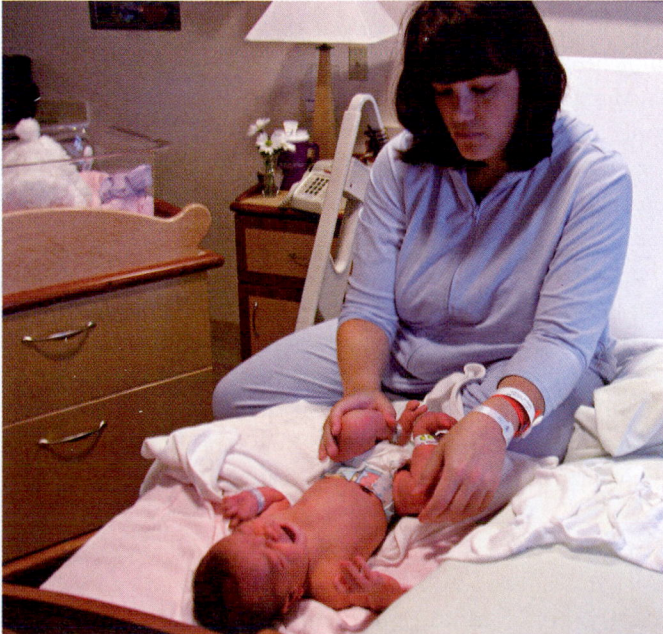

Figure 54-5. ■ When the mother's attention shifts away from the recent experience of labor to care of the neonate, she has entered the "taking-hold" stage.

infant's needs. Obtaining information from others who have experienced parenthood is a valuable part of the normal adjustment process. Mothers who have little social interaction and support find the adjustment to motherhood more difficult.

ATTACHMENT

During pregnancy, the woman begins to develop an emotional attachment or bond to the infant. Personal characteristics of the mother affect the extent of attachment. For example, the woman with a high level of self-esteem enters motherhood with a more positive outlook than the mother who is depressed, angry about her situation, or overly anxious. The mother who has developed a level of trust in her own abilities will be confident in her ability to care for the infant. At the time of birth, each mother has developed an emotional attachment of some kind with the infant.

New mothers generally follow a regular pattern of behavior when meeting their infants for the first time. Touch usually begins with fingertip exploration of the infant's limbs, followed by palmar touch of the torso, and finally enfolding the infant with the entire hand and arms. As the mother spends more time with her infant, she positions the newborn so she can look into its eyes. She uses her sense of sight, hearing, and touch to get to know her infant. She responds verbally to the sound the newborn makes. She may make comments or have questions about the normality of the infant's features, especially if the delivery was difficult or if a previously delivered infant was not healthy. The mother's interest in and loving behaviors toward the newborn are part of the bonding process.

NEGATIVE FEELINGS

The mother may have negative feelings about the baby. She may be disappointed about the baby's gender or angry that her lifestyle will need to change. Because mothers are "supposed to love their children," the mother may not express these negative feelings. If she does express them, the reaction of friends or family may be, "You don't mean that." The nurse must identify these blocks to therapeutic communication and help the mother and family explore the basis of the negative feelings. (Prolonged negative feelings and depression in the postpartum period are discussed in Chapter 55 ⬥⬥.)

Fathers, Siblings, and Others

Fathers, siblings, grandparents, and others also need time to bond with the infant. The father will express a strong attachment to the infant, similar to that of the mother (Figure 54-6 ■). He will demonstrate **engrossment** (a sense of

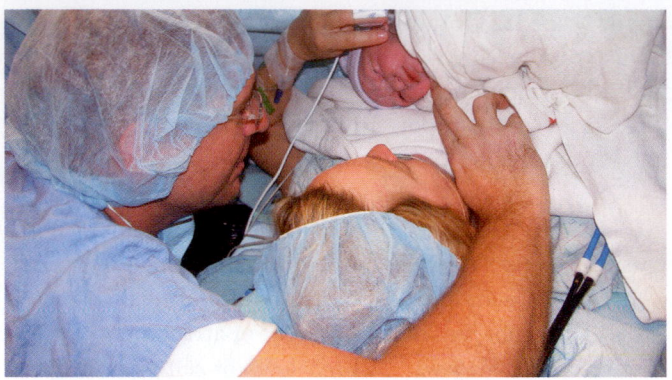

Figure 54-6. ■ Father engrossed in the sight of his new child.

interest and preoccupation) by holding, maintaining eye contact with and talking to the infant.

Siblings and grandparents are important members of the family who also need time to develop a bond with the infant. Each family member who has the opportunity to view, hold, and interact with the infant will begin to establish a relationship. With open visiting hours and rooming-in practices, family bonding can begin early.

Cultural Influences in the Postpartum Period

The mother's beliefs about hygiene, food choices, and activity during the postpartum period are influenced by her culture. Western culture places a great deal of emphasis on the birth process itself. Other cultures place more emphasis on postpartum practices. Many women of European heritage want to eat a full meal and drink plenty of cold fluids in the belief that they will replace the nutrients lost during the delivery process. They will want to shower right away, wash their hair, and put on a clean gown.

The women of Mexican, Asian, and African descent often avoid cold, including cold air, food, and drink. They may put off showering to prevent a chill.

Certain cultures teach choices that are meant to help the woman regain harmony or balance between "hot and cold" within the body. They may avoid heat, including some foods that are considered "hot."

In most Native American cultures, family plays an important role during the postpartum period. The baby's grandmother is the primary helper and teacher for the new mother. She brings experience and knowledge, and allows the new mother time to rest and regain her strength. Some other areas of cultural beliefs and practices related to the postpartum period are provided in Box 54-1.

If the mother's beliefs are different from those of the nurse, the physician, or hospital practices, adjustments may need to be made. It is the nurse's responsibility to advocate for the rights of the mother, father, and family.

NURSING CARE

PRIORITIZING NURSING CARE

When caring for postpartum clients, the first priority is to assess for and prevent complications, and the second priority is to provide client teaching regarding self-care and care of the infant.

The nurse may use the mnemonic of BUBBLE to help remember important areas of the assessment: **B** — Breast, **U** — uterus, **B** — bowel, **B** — bladder, **L** — lochia, **E** — episiotomy/incision. Instruct the client about expected progression of lochia—from red to dark brown, to pale yellow or white. Instruct the client to report any deviations from this pattern. Instruct the client regarding ways to prevent perineal infection, such as frequent pad changes, avoiding tampons, and using a peri bottle after voiding.

ASSESSING

The postpartum assessment begins by obtaining information about the pregnancy and birth. This information is used to identify the risk of postpartum complications. Table 54-2 ■ identifies common risk factors and areas that must be included in the assessment. The greater the degree of risk, the more frequently the assessment must be made.

Box 54-2 ■ provides a list of items to check in the postpartum woman. Most of the time, the assessment is done from head to toe. If there have been complications of bleeding or infection, the nurse may choose to assess the uterus or perineum before the breasts. If the assessment is performed out of sequence, it is important to remember to come back and check all necessary body systems.

Many parts of the assessment are the same as for any other client. For example, monitoring vital signs and observing for an increase in bloody drainage is the same for the postpartum woman as it is for the postsurgical client. Listening to heart sounds, lung sounds, and bowel sounds is the same as for any other client. The LPN/LVN must know the normal findings in order to report abnormal readings to the charge nurse or physician. Only those parts of the assessment that are particular to the postpartum client will be included here. While performing the assessment, the nurse has an opportunity to teach the new mother about normal body changes and signs of complication.

Vital Signs

The vital signs should be assessed first. Vital signs were assessed every 15 minutes in the first hour after birth. When vital signs are stable, the time interval can be lengthened. Common time intervals are every 30 minutes for an hour, every hour for 2 hours, every 2 hours for 4 hours and then

TABLE 54-2	**Postpartum Risk Factors and Areas of Assessment**	
RISK FACTOR	**IMPLICATIONS**	**AREA TO ASSESS**
Cesarean section birth	Risk for impaired healing Risk for paralytic ileus Risk for urinary retention	Incision pain every 2–4 hours Incision for infection and healing Bowel sounds, flatus every 2–4 hours Voiding after catheter removed
Prolonged labor	Risk for exhaustion Risk for nutrition and fluid depletion Risk for uterine atony and hemorrhage	Verbalizes adequate rest Intake, output, % of diet consumed Fundus firmness every 1–2 hours Amount of lochia every 1–2 hours Vital signs every 1–2 hours
Precipitous delivery	Risk for uterine atony, hemorrhage Rick for lacerations of birth canal	Fundus firmness every 1–2 hours Amount of lochia every 1–2 hours Vital signs every 1–2 hours
Delivery complications (retained placenta, lacerations)	Risk for lacerations of birth canal Risk for hemorrhage	Fundus firmness every 1–2 hours Amount of lochia every 1–2 hours Vital signs every 1–2 hours
Diabetes	Risk for insulin regulation Risk for periods of hyperglycemia and hypoglycemia Risk for poor wound healing	Obtain blood glucose (BG) readings every 2–4 hours Signs of hyper- and hypoglycemia Episiotomy or incision for healing
PIH	Risk for neurological and cardiovascular damage	Vital signs every 1–2 hours Reflexes and clonus every 1–2 hours Headache and blurred vision
Overdistended uterus (large fetus or multiple gestation)	Risk for uterine atony and hemorrhage	Fundus firmness every 1–2 hours Amount of lochia every 1–2 hours Vital signs every 1–2 hours

every 4 hours. By the second postpartum day the vital signs can be taken every 8 hours.

Abnormal findings direct the nurse to pay closer attention to parts of the assessment. For example, an elevated temperature coupled with premature or prolonged rupture of fetal membranes prior to delivery may indicate a genital infection. Further assessment of the uterus and lochia is indicated. The blood pressure should remain consistent with the baseline blood pressure during pregnancy. Tachycardia associated with hypotension may indicate hemorrhage. As excess body fluids are eliminated during the first few weeks postpartum, the blood pressure should return to the prepregnant state.

clinical ALERT

A marked elevation in blood pressure in the first 24 to 36 hours postpartum could be an indication of gestational hypertension and should be reported. If GH occurred prior to delivery, the blood pressure should begin to decrease in the first few days postpartum.

A client receiving IV magnesium sulfate is not considered a stable postpartum client. Therefore, depending on the state as well as facility regulations about scope of practice for the LPN or LVN, an RN might be required to assume care of this client.

A decrease in blood pressure can be due to the body's adjustment to decreased intrapelvic pressure. However, a low blood pressure may also indicate hemorrhage. As the body adjusts to decreased intrapelvic pressure, the woman may experience orthostatic hypotension, which will cause a low blood pressure reading in the sitting position. For the most accurate blood pressure reading, measurement should be taken with the woman in a supine position. Any abnormal blood pressure, heart, temperature, and respiratory rate should be reported to the RN.

Pain

New mothers experience pain from engorged breast tissue, the traumatized perineum or abdominal surgical site, and uterine contractions. Breastfeeding mothers should be taught that nursing the baby will help relieve breast discomfort. Perineal and surgical incisional pain should decrease daily as healing occurs. **Afterpain,** or discomfort from uterine contractions after delivery, occur in most women but are generally more noticeable in multipara mothers. They are stronger during breastfeeding because breast stimulation causes the release of oxytocin.

BOX 54-2 DATA COLLECTION

Postpartum Obstetrical Check

This check is done at scheduled intervals with vital signs.

1. Breasts—evaluate breastfeeding and bottle-feeding mothers
    - Soft
    - Filling
    - Firm
    - Engorged
2. Nipples
    - Nontender
    - Reddened
    - Cracked/fissured
    - Bleeding
3. Fundus—described as one to four fingerbreadths below or above umbilicus and location (midline or displaced to right or left)
4. Abdomen
    - Distention
        - Slight
        - Moderate
        - Severe
    - Bowel sounds
        - Present
        - Hypoactive
        - Hyperactive
        - Absent
    - Evaluation of abdominal dressing (cesarean section or tubal ligation)
        - Dry
        - Intact
        - Drainage
    - If no dressing, evaluate incision
        - Staples, Steri-Strips, or surgical glue present
        - Incision line approximated or dehisced (separated)
        - Dry, no drainage
        - Reddened

5. Lochia
    - Color

1–3 days	rubra (bright red)
2–4 days	serosa (serous sanguineous)
2–9 days	reddish brown
9 days on	alba (white/yellowish)

    - Amount (evaluated in 1 hour from pad application to removal)

Scant	less than or equal to a 2-inch stain (10 mL)
Small or light	less than or equal to a 4-inch stain (10–25 mL)
Moderate	less than or equal to a 6-inch stain (25–50 mL)
Large or heavy	saturated perineal pad within 1 hour (50–80 mL)
Excessive	saturated perineal pad within 15 minutes

6. Episiotomy or perineal laceration
    - None
    - Approximated
    - Separated
    - Ecchymotic
    - Edematous
    - Reddened
7. Legs
    - Any varicosities
    - Edema
        - Amount—trace, 1+, 2+, etc.
        - Homans' sign (bilaterally)
        - Client with history of PIH
        - Deep-tendon reflexes
        - Clonus
8. Other
    - Voiding and bladder distention

Nursing mothers may express concern about the effect of pain medication on the infant. The nurse should explain to the mother that pain can make her tense and anxious, which may decrease breast milk production. The nurse should also explain that some analgesics may be excreted in the breast milk. This medication will not harm the infant but would make the infant sleepy. It is important, therefore, for the mother to feed the infant before she takes the analgesic.

Breasts

Breast assessment begins with checking the bra for design and fit. The postpartum mother should wear a well-fitting bra at all times. The bra should provide support to prevent the weight of the breast from stretching the supporting ligaments and connective tissue. The bra should be removed so the breast can be inspected and palpated. The breast should be inspected for redness and cracked or inverted nipples. The breast should be palpated for softness, slight firmness associated with filling or firmness associated with full or engorged glands. Warmth and tenderness would also be noted. Colostrum or milk may drain from the nipple. The mother should be taught to report signs of complications, such as redness, heat, and pain. She should also report cracked, sore nipples.

Uterus

Assess placement of the uterus when the mother is in the supine position and the bladder is empty. Placing one hand on the symphysis pubis to support the uterus, the nurse places the middle finger of the other hand on the umbilicus and pushes down on the abdomen to palpate the location of the fundus. The fundus should be firm, in the midline, and between the umbilicus and symphysis (see Figure 54-1). The distance from the umbilicus is measured in finger widths (also called fingerbreadths) and recorded as a number above or below the umbilicus. If the fundus is not firm or in the proper location, complication should be suspected.

If the fundus is boggy, the LPN should begin to massage the fundus gently in a circular manner (see Procedure 54-1 ■, Performing Fundal Massage and Removing Clots from the Uterus). If the fundus does not regain or maintain firmness within a few minutes, the LPN/LVN should summon assistance. The RN or physician may apply strong pressure on the fundus to remove clots. As mentioned, this is generally not an LPN/LVN function due to the risk of uterine prolapse (see Figure 40-13 👓).

Bowel

The abdomen should be assessed for bowel sounds. Normal bowel sounds should be present in all four quadrants of the abdomen. The mother should be questioned regarding the passage of flatus. Bowel sounds may take several days to return in the woman who has had a cesarean birth. Generally solid food is withheld until bowel sounds are present.

Bladder

The bladder should be assessed for fullness. Due to swelling of the perineum it may be difficult for the woman to void. As stated, a full bladder can displace the uterus resulting in increased bleeding. The bladder can be palpated or a bladder scan can be used to assess bladder fullness. If the woman is unable to void, urinary catheterization may be needed.

Lochia

The nurse assesses the lochia for amount, consistency, color, and odor. During the first 1 to 3 days, the lochia will be red with a few small clots. The passage of many small clots or a large clot is not normal and should be reported. Figure 54-2 illustrates suggested guidelines for assessing the volume of lochia. Note that condensation from an ice pack can exaggerate the amount of lochia. If heavy bleeding is suspected, change the pad, have the woman remain in bed, and reassess every 15 minutes for an hour. Do not discard saturated pads, but save them in the bathroom until the bleeding is controlled and the physician has determined the estimated blood loss. In some cases, the physician will ask that the saturated pads, blue underpads, and bloody linen be weighed to determine blood loss.

Assess the odor of lochia. It should be similar to the odor of menstruation and should never be strong or foul. The cause of foul or offensive odor should always be investigated. A specimen may need to be obtained for culture and sensitivity.

Episiotomy

The perineum should be inspected during the assessment of the body. (Although some women are comfortable with family members being present, this should not be assumed. Explain the procedure to the client and ask her if she would like you to have visitors step outside.) The woman can be in a side-lying position with her knees bent. Lift one side of the buttocks to expose the perineum. If the perineum is intact, inspect for swelling or bruising. The perineum may be reddened but without excessive tenderness. Pain plus redness may indicate infection. Mild edema is common, but severe perineal edema can inhibit healing by decreasing normal blood flow to the area. If the perineum is lacerated or an episiotomy was performed, inspect the edges of the wound for approximation and check the skin for bruising. If a laceration or episiotomy has been repaired, its edges should not be distinguishable from surrounding skin. If gentle palpation causes the woman more than mild discomfort, inspect the perineum for abrasions or unrepaired lacerations. Also, inspect for increased bruising due to a hematoma. Report suspicion of a hematoma to the RN. See Procedure 54-2 ■, Perineal Assessment.

If the woman had a cesarean birth, the abdominal incision should be inspected using the same criteria as an episiotomy. Skin staples or clips may be present or Steri-Strips may have been used to secure the skin. If an abdominal dressing is present, follow facility policy and physician orders in removing or changing the dressing.

Lower Extremities

The legs should be assessed for abnormalities caused by pregnancy, including varicose veins and edema (Figure 54-7 ■). If varicose veins are present, care should be taken to protect them from injury. Reassure the woman that edema from pressure on pelvic veins or PIH should resolve in a few days.

Assess the legs for signs of *thrombophlebitis* (positive Homans' sign, see Figure 54-7B). Note any areas of redness, swelling, or tenderness. With the legs straight and knees slightly flexed, the woman's foot should be sharply dorsiflexed. No discomfort should be present. Pain with dorsiflexion is an indication of an inflamed vessel in the leg. The charge nurse or physician should be notified at once because of the risk of deep vein thrombosis and **thromboembolism** (a blood clot moving within the blood vessel). Thromboembolism can be a life-threatening event.

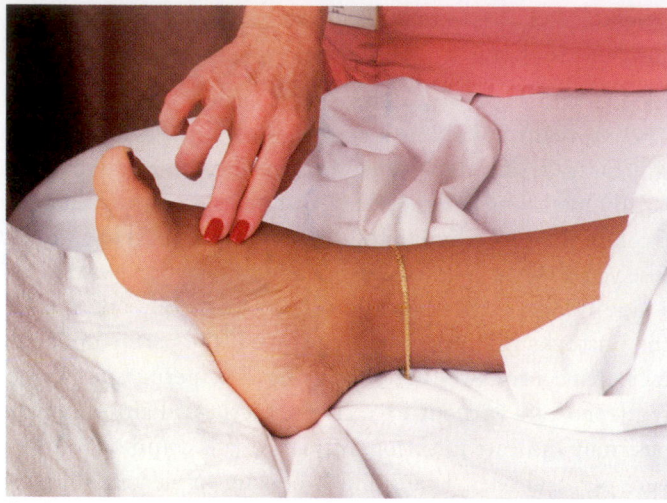

A

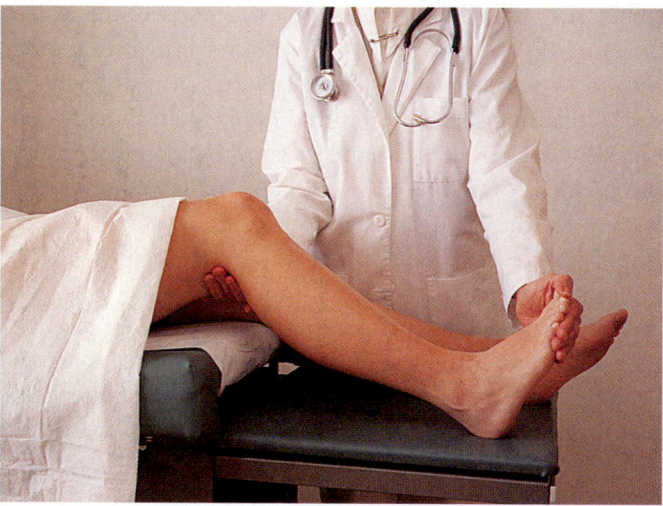

B

Figure 54-7. ■ **A.** A nurse assessing client's foot for edema. **B.** Homans' sign for thrombophlebitis: with the woman's knee flexed, the nurse dorsiflexes the foot. Pain in the foot or leg is a positive Homans' sign.

DIAGNOSING, PLANNING, AND IMPLEMENTING

Once an assessment is completed, problems must be identified. Generally, new mothers can provide for their own physical needs but may have deficient knowledge about the specifics of postpartum care. Common nursing diagnoses include:

- *Acute Pain*
- *Deficient Knowledge* regarding breast care
- *Deficient Knowledge* regarding perineal care
- *Imbalanced Nutrition: Less than Body Requirements*
- *Constipation*
- *Impaired Urinary Elimination*

Outcomes for postpartum women would include:

- Client will state pain reduced with medication, ice pack, etc.

- Client asks for information she can read about breastfeeding and self-care.
- Client states understanding of the importance of nutrients to self and infant, and states "maybe I don't have to lose all my pregnancy weight in 2 weeks; maybe I can take a little more time."
- Client asks for dried fruit and extra liquids with meal to assist with bowel elimination.

The plan of care centers on teaching the new mother to meet her needs and the needs of the infant. Teaching care of the infant is addressed in Chapter 56 ⚭.

Care of the postpartum woman involves numerous safety and comfort measures, careful monitoring for signs of complications (discussed below), and emotional support as the woman adjusts to her new role.

Pain Management

- Assess the client's level of pain. Pain may be described by various pain rating scales and by location (incision, leg, back, head, perineum). Box 54-3 ■ provides guidelines for the nurse in assisting the client in pain. *The nurse uses information from the client, plus objective data gained by observing the client, to report the level of pain.*

BOX 54-3	NURSING CARE CHECKLIST

Helping Client in Pain

☑ Ask the client when the pain started. If it is a recurring pain, ask what starts the pain and what causes it to stop.

☑ Ask the client to describe how bad the pain is on a scale of 0 to 10, with 0 being no pain and 10 being the worst imaginable pain.

☑ Ask where the pain is, or have the client show the nurse by pointing to the area of pain. Also determine if the pain begins in one area and moves to another.

☑ Ask the client to identify what kind of pain exists:
- Throbbing
- Shooting
- Stabbing
- Sharp
- Gnawing
- Burning
- Dull
- Tender
- Radiating
- Other_____

☑ Provide medication as ordered. Review standing orders for administering pain medications. Consult with charge nurse as needed.

☑ Return to client 20 to 30 minutes after administering pain medication to determine effectiveness of medication.

- Advise the breastfeeding mother with discomfort from engorged breast tissue to take a warm shower or nurse her baby. *These actions will stimulate the let-down reflex and relieve the pressure in the breast.*

- Evaluate breastfeeding technique if the nipples become sore or cracked. *Lanoline ointment may be applied with an order from the primary care provider. This type of ointment is safe for use with breastfeeding infants.*

- A non-nursing mother may express breast discomfort due to beginning lactation. Assist by applying ice and a binder to the chest. Administer analgesics as ordered. Teach that it may take several days to suppress lactation and alleviate the problem. *Ice and breast binders can prevent engorgement. Analgesics may be given for discomfort. Knowing that discomfort will subside in several days will usually help the person tolerate it better.*

- Administer analgesics as needed to control perineal discomfort. Provide ice packs and anesthetic spray to the perineum, as ordered by the primary care provider. Recommend other interventions to alleviate perineal discomfort, such as sitting in a reclined position. A sitz bath (Procedure 54-3 ■) may also be helpful. *The woman will be better able to provide for the needs of herself and her infant if she is comfortable.*

- The woman who has had a cesarean birth may have epidural analgesia or patient-controlled analgesia (PCA). Follow facility guidelines on the use of these methods of pain relief. Provide information about the prescribed medication, its use, and side effects. Oral pain medication will be ordered as soon as bowel tones are present and oral intake is tolerated. *As in any situation, medication administration must be carefully carried out. Once peristalsis has returned, oral medications can be tolerated.*

- Provide nonpharmacologic methods of pain relief. *Many women prefer to "forget about" the pain by using alternate methods of pain relief, such as baths, backrubs, distraction, etc.*

Table 54-3 ■ provides information about oral pain medications.

Client Teaching

Client teaching is an important part of the LPN/LVN role. Because many new mothers remain in the hospital for only 24 to 48 hours, the nurse must take every opportunity to teach health-promoting activities.

Hygiene

- Instruct the new mother to bathe daily. Teach that showers are preferable to tub bathing because they can help prevent contamination carried from the feet to the perineum or breast. If a shower is not available, the mother should be taught to clean the tub and rinse the residue away before sitting in the tub. The new mother should be taught to wash the breast without soap and to allow the nipples to air dry. *Cleanliness is the main technique used to prevent infection. Washing the nipple with soap might cause it to become dry and to crack.*

- If the birth was by cesarean section, instruct the woman to keep the incision clean until healing is complete. Once the dressing is removed, the woman may shower without any special precautions. Instruct her to allow the incision to dry completely after washing and to apply a small dressing if desired. *A small dressing will absorb any drainage from the incision site. If Steri-Strips have been applied to the incision, they will not be harmed by the shower and will come off in about 1 week.*

- Teach the client to rinse the perineum with clear water after each voiding and bowel movement and to pat it dry.

TABLE 54-3	Pharmacology: Oral Pain Medications			
DRUG	**USUAL ROUTE/DOSE**	**CLASSIFICATION**	**SELECTED SIDE EFFECTS**	**DON'T GIVE**
Motrin (ibuprofen)	400 mg to 800 mg 3–4 times/day	NSAID (non-steroidal anti-inflammatory drug)	Nausea, dyspepsia, blurred vision, dizziness	If allergic to drug
Tylenol (acetaminophen)	325 mg to 650 mg every 4–6 hours	Non-opioid analgesic	Few in usual dose; liver toxicity if dosage guidelines are ignored	If pain not controlled by usual dose
Percocet (oxycodone with acetaminophen)	5 mg oxycodone with 325 mg acetaminophen	Opioid agonist/Non-opioid analgesic	Confusion, sedation, respiratory depression	If respiratory rate below 10/min
Morphine (morphine sulfate)	4 mg to 10 mg IV every 3–4 hrs. Patient-controlled analgesia (PCA) dose varies	Opioid agonist	Respiratory depression, confusion, sedation, vomiting, constipation	If respiratory rate below 10/min. If allergic to drug
Demerol (meperidine HCl)	50 mg to 100 mg IM every 3–4 hrs. PCA dose varies	Opioid agonist	Respiratory depression, confusion, sedation, vomiting, constipation	If respiratory rate below 10/min. If allergic to drug

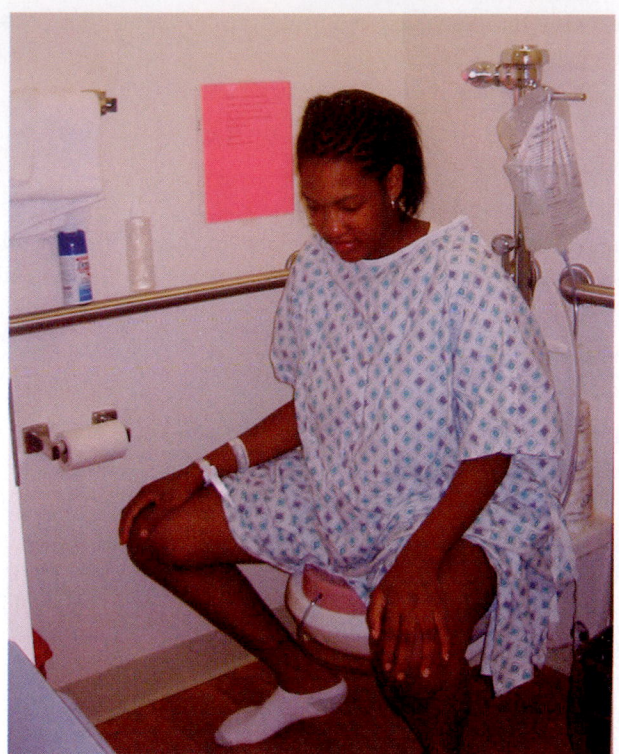

Figure 54-8. ■ A sitz bath promotes healing and provides relief from perineal discomfort during the initial weeks following birth.

Instruct the new mother to always wipe the perineum from front to back. *Cleansing removes microorganisms. Wiping the perineum from front to back prevents contamination from the anus to the vagina and urethra.*

Sitz Baths

The doctor may order a sitz bath to relieve perineal swelling and discomfort. Some hospitals have porcelain sitz tubs, which must be cleaned between clients. Other facilities use portable individual sitz basins (Figure 54-8 ■) that are sent home with the client. A procedure for this is provided at the end of this chapter.

■ Teach the mother to shower before using the sitz bath. *This will wash away contaminants that could infect the perineum or vagina.*

Postpartum Nutrition

The new mother needs a balanced diet in order to regain her strength. Most facilities provide written information about proper nutrition after delivery. The hospital dietitian is also a valuable resource.

■ Teach the client that her diet should be high in fiber and fluids. *The diet will prevent constipation.*
■ If the woman has a good understanding of basic nutrition, it may be sufficient to advise her to decrease her daily caloric intake by 300 calories and resume her prepregnancy level of other nutrients. *The 300 calories a day that provided for the needs of the fetus are no longer*

necessary. The woman will return to her prepregnancy weight more quickly if she reduces the daily intake of calories.
■ Teach the breastfeeding mother to consume an additional 500 kcal per day, to drink at least 8 glasses of fluid a day (1,000 mL), and to consume 65 g of protein and 1,000 mg of calcium. Most physicians request that the new mother continue to take prenatal vitamins with iron for 3 months. *These will balance the nutrients used up by milk production and breastfeeding. The prenatal vitamins help ensure that the woman's system is balanced.*

Exercise

■ After delivery, assist the woman to begin activity with ambulation. *Early ambulation promotes healing and prevents complications such as thrombophlebitis.*
■ Encourage the woman to begin with simple postpartal exercises (Figure 54-9 ■). *The new mother may want to engage in abdominal exercises to tighten stretched muscles. Inform the woman that an increase in lochia or pain means she may be overdoing exercise and should decrease her activity. Most agencies provide a booklet describing suggested postpartum exercises.*

Postpartum Immunizations

Two different immunizations are commonly given following delivery, if needed. For the mother who has Rh-negative blood and delivers an infant with Rh-positive blood, the doctor usually prescribes an injection of RhoGAM (Rho[D] immune globulin). (Discussion of Rh incompatibility is found in Chapter 52 ⚭.) This immune globulin can be given as soon as there are test results, but it must be given within 72 hours of delivery (some facilities say 48 hours). RhoGAM prevents the production of Rh antibodies that could harm a future pregnancy. The purpose of the injection and the usual side effects should be explained to the mother prior to the immunization.

Exposure to rubella virus can cause congenital malformation in the fetus, so immunization is avoided with pregnancy if possible. If the mother has a negative rubella titer, most physicians recommend an MMR (measles, mumps, rubella) immunization in the postpartum period. If the immunization is given shortly after delivery, there is no chance of exposure to the next fetus. (Note: In some facilities, the MMR immunization is given immediately prior to discharge to prevent accidental exposure of other pregnant women to this virus.)

All other adult immunizations can be given in the postpartum period, if necessary.

Building a Support Network and Healthy Patterns

■ Inquire about family and friends who might be available to assist the mother when she returns home. *The mother may need encouragement to realize that people want to help her during this time. It is good to explore specific ways that people can help. Some people do best with a written list.*

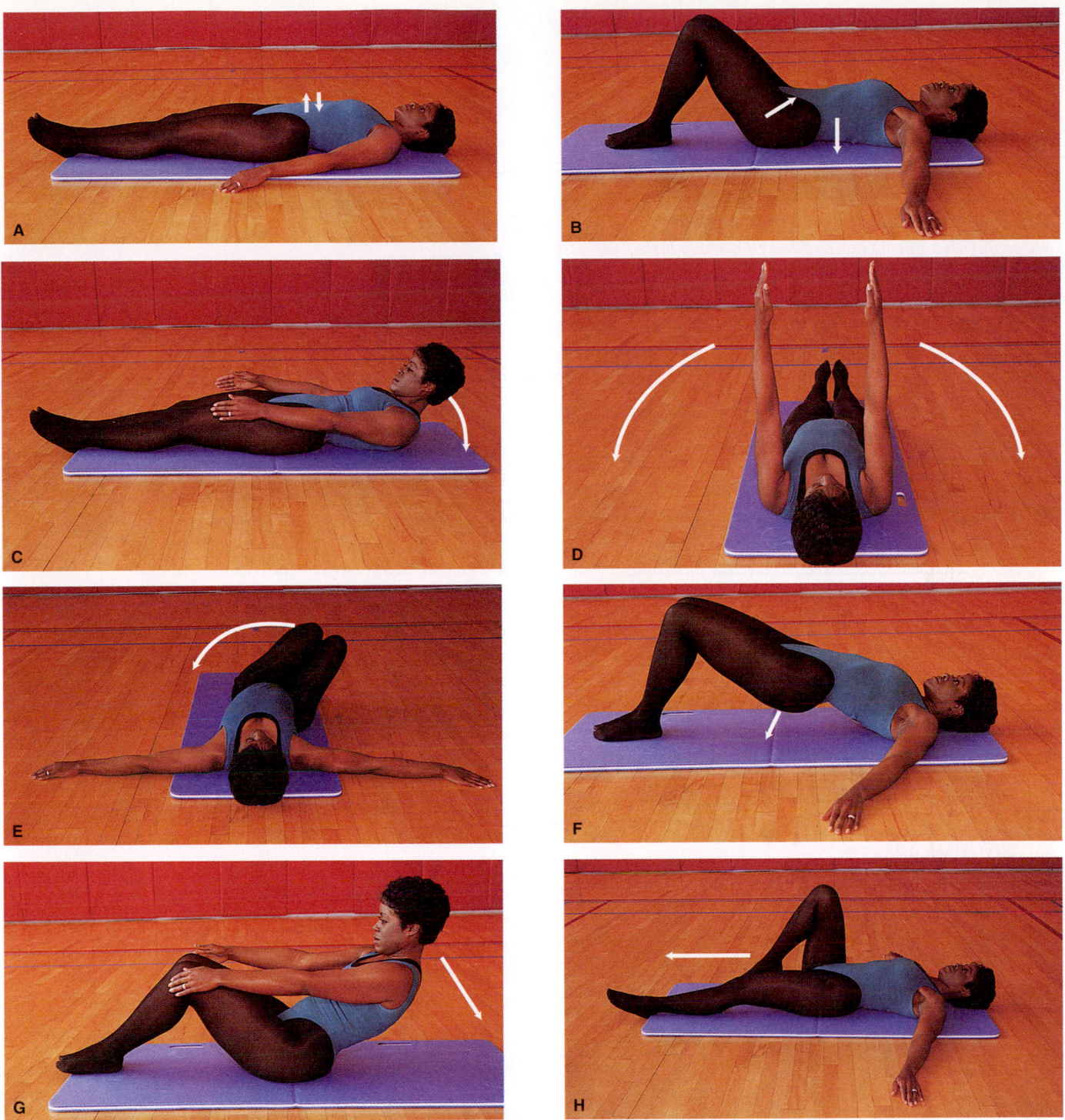

Figure 54-9. ■ Postpartal exercises. Begin with five repetitions two or three times daily, and gradually increase to 10 repetitions. First day: **A.** Abdominal breathing. Lying supine, inhale deeply, using the abdominal muscles. The abdomen should expand. Then exhale slowly through pursed lips, tightening the abdominal muscle. **B.** Pelvic rocking. Lying supine with arms at sides, knees bent, and feet flat, tighten abdomen and buttocks, and attempt to flatten back on the floor. Hold for a count of 10; then arch the back, causing the pelvis to "rock." On the second day, add: **C.** Chin to chest. Lying supine with legs straight, raise head and attempt to touch chin to chest. Slowly lower head. **D.** Arm raises. Lying supine, arms extended at a 90-degree angle from body, raise arms so that they are perpendicular and hands touch. Lower slowly. On fourth day, add: **E.** Knee rolls. Lying supine with knees bent, feet flat, arms extended to the side, roll knees to one side, keeping shoulders flat. Return to the original position, and roll to opposite side. **F.** Buttocks lift. Lying supine, arms at side, knees bent, feet flat, slowly raise the buttocks and arch the back. Return slowly to starting position. On sixth day add: **G.** Abdominal tighteners. Lying supine, knees bent, feet flat, slowly raise head toward knees. Arms should extend along either side of legs. Return slowly to original position. **H.** Knee to abdomen. Lying supine, arms at sides, bend one knee and thigh until foot touches buttocks. Straighten leg and lower it slowly. Repeat with other leg. After 2 to 3 weeks, more strenuous exercises, such as push-ups and side leg raises, may be added as tolerated. Kegel exercises, begun before birth, should be done many times daily during postpartum to restore vaginal and perineal tone.

- Discuss and encourage a pattern of good eating, exercise, and rest. *Good nutrition, regular exercise, and periods of rest will help the mother return to her prepregnant state most efficiently.*
- Respect the mother's rest periods as much as possible, and teach that it is important to listen to her body when a rest is needed. *Many women ignore their own need for rest. Teach the mother that getting rest will benefit not only herself, but also the infant and family.*
- Encourage the woman to simplify routines for this period of time and not to make any major changes. *The nurse can reinforce that changes are natural and necessary when an infant is brought home. It will take time to adjust to the new person and new roles. Encourage the mother to keep maintenance tasks simple and to expect energy to return gradually.*
- Ask the client how she is feeling. *The woman may have anxieties or concerns about parenting. Asking open-ended questions can allow her to raise these issues.*

EVALUATING

The evaluation of nursing care for postpartum clients involves documenting an understanding of the teaching provided. Box 54-4 ■ reviews important aspects of client teaching in the postpartum period. The new mother should be able to demonstrate self-care, including perineal care and suture line care. She should select a balanced diet and consume adequate fluids. She should verbalize an understanding of the use and side effects of medications. Complications in the postpartum period are discussed in Chapter 55 ⬯.

Continuity of Care

It is the nurse's responsibility to ensure that client teaching has occurred and that the woman has been given written information about care after discharge. Many parents will be concerned about going home with their new baby. They will worry about what to do if something is wrong. Box 54-5 ■ provides a list of criteria to help parents know when to call care providers for help.

The nurse can also assist by helping the client identify support people for the postpartum period. It may be helpful for the client to list a set of tasks with which she could use help. Only trusted family and friends should be asked to help with child care.

NURSING PROCESS CARE PLAN
Care of the Postpartum Client with a Third-Degree Perineal Laceration

---

Mercedes Camino is a 27-year-old multipara who gave birth to her second baby by vacuum-assisted vaginal delivery about 2 hours ago. She is being admitted to the postpartum unit where the LVN will be assuming her care. Ms. Camino received a third-degree perineal laceration that was repaired by her obstetrician. She ambulated to the bed from the wheelchair with only standby assistance. Ms. Camino requests narcotic analgesics to decrease her perineal discomfort.

Assessment

On admission to the postpartum unit, Ms. Camino's fundus is noted to be firm and at the level of the umbilicus. There is a scant amount of lochia rubra on her perineal pad. Her perineum is swollen. However, the edges of her laceration are approximated. The LVN collects the following assessment data: T 98, BP 110/68, and P 74. Complains of perineal discomfort and fear of urinating due to laceration. Denies nausea or dizziness.

Nursing Diagnosis

The following important nursing diagnoses (among others) are established for this condition:

- *Impaired Urinary Elimination* related to fear of pain secondary to perineal laceration
- *Risk for Infection* related to extensive perineal laceration
- *Risk for Activity Intolerance* related to perineal discomfort
- *Risk for Constipation* related to narcotic analgesics
- *Interrupted Breastfeeding* related to discomfort

Expected Outcomes

The expected outcomes specify that Ms. Camino will:

- State adequate pain relief as evidenced by her stated goal for pain relief using the pain scale.
- Empty bladder completely every 3 to 4 hours.
- Will have an oral fluid intake of at least 2,000 mL per day.
- Have a temperature within normal limits.
- Will ambulate in hallway three to four times a day.
- Have a soft bowel movement within 4 to 5 days.

Planning and Implementation

The following nursing interventions are planned and implemented:

- Monitor vital signs according to doctor's orders.
- Monitor position of fundus before and after emptying bladder.
- Encourage fluid intake.
- Teach proper perineal care and instruct client to perform perineal care after emptying bladder and having a bowel movement.
- Apply perineal ice packs as ordered.
- Administer analgesia as ordered prior to ambulating.
- Instruct client about the benefits of nonsteroidal, anti-inflammatory medications in decreasing swelling and discomfort.
- Assist client to breastfeed her baby in a side-lying position.

BOX 54-4 | CLIENT TEACHING

Self-Care after Discharge

Episiotomy/ Perineal Laceration Care

Use of the perineal bottle until vaginal bleeding stops can promote healing and prevent infection. Teach the mother always to rinse the perineal area, to cleanse and wipe from front to back, and to change perineal pads after urinating or having a bowel movement. Tell the mother to wait to use tampons until after the follow-up exam.

The doctor or midwife may recommend a "sitz" bath to decrease perineal discomfort. Sitting in a sitz bath 10 to 15 minutes, 2 times a day, can soothe the perineal tissue. It may be more comfortable to place a bath towel in the tub to sit on. Some hospitals provide a plastic sitz bath to take home.

Vaginal Discharge

Teach the woman that it is normal to have vaginal discharge after delivery. Vaginal discharge may last as long as 5 to 6 weeks although it should decrease in amount every day. The color will also change from bright red to dark red or brown. After 4 to 5 days the discharge will become pinkish red and then change to yellowish or white in color. Excessive activity may cause discharge to become red again with some small clots. If this occurs, the mother should lie down and rest with her feet elevated. If she fills a perineal pad in 1 hour or less, bleeding is excessive. Instruct her to call the doctor or midwife immediately.

Cesarean Section

Teach the woman who has had a cesarean section that it is important not to overdo activity for 4 to 6 weeks. Activity should be limited to taking care of oneself and the baby. The woman should avoid lifting anything heavier than the baby. Climbing stairs should be kept to a minimum. The doctor or midwife will determine when normal activities resume, including driving.

Incision Care

Teach that an incision from a cesarean section does not need special care. Showering should be sufficient to cleanse the area. Scrubbing the incision is not necessary. Paper tape (Steri-Strips) on the incision can be gotten wet. Pat the incision dry after showering, or dry the area with a hairdryer on cool setting. The incision should be inspected in a mirror or by another person. It should be clean, dry, and intact; it should heal without redness, swelling, or foul odor. It is normal to have a small amount of clear fluid ooze from a part of the incision. However, teach that bleeding or pearly-colored discharge is not normal and should be reported to the doctor or midwife. Instruct the woman to call the doctor or midwife if the incision appears red and feels hot to the touch. Sutures underneath the incision will dissolve. If the staples were not removed in the hospital, it will be necessary to see the doctor or midwife to have them removed.

Hemorrhoids

Hemorrhoids often appear outside the rectum due to the pressure of pushing the baby out during delivery. Often they will shrink with time. The doctor or midwife may prescribe ointment or suppositories. Teach the woman that ice packs can help decrease pain and swelling, and that some women find that a sitz bath is soothing after the first 24 hours after delivery.

Bowels

Teach the woman to avoid constipation. The mother should drink 6 to 8 glasses of water a day, and more if breastfeeding. The woman should be instructed to eat a balanced diet, which includes fruits, vegetables, and whole grains. The doctor or midwife may prescribe a stool softener or a laxative.

Menstruation

Instruct the woman that the time before periods begin again varies from woman to woman. Most women start their period within 2 to 3 months after delivery unless they are breastfeeding. The woman who is breastfeeding may not have a period until after she stops breastfeeding.

Family Planning

Reinforce that the woman should not have sexual intercourse for 4 to 6 weeks after birth. It is recommended to wait until after the follow-up exam to resume intercourse. Birth control methods should be discussed with the doctor or midwife at this appointment. A woman can still become pregnant, even if she does not have a period.

Adjustment to Parenthood

Remind the woman that—although she may feel back to normal once she goes home—she is still recovering from the delivery of the baby. She needs time to adjust to having a new baby in the home. She should gradually resume activities, but allow time for rest. She should sleep when the baby sleeps. Allow family members and friends to help around the house and to prepare meals. The baby needs the woman to take care of herself.

Remind the woman that many women experience "baby blues." Teach that if weepiness, exhaustion, and anxiety last longer than a couple of weeks, she should see a physician to rule out postpartum depression. Emphasize that symptoms of "baby blues" or postpartum depression do not mean she is a "bad" mother. The period after the birth of the baby is a time of many changes and a whole new type of pressure. It is important not to try to deal with these feelings alone. Teach the mother these ways to ease "baby blues":

- Nap at every opportunity.
- Have small, nutritious, and easy-to-prepare meals throughout the day.
- Express her feelings to nonjudgmental family and friends. Ask for help with cooking and cleaning.
- Make time for herself!

- Instruct client to increase oral fluid.
- Administer stool softener as ordered.

Evaluation

It is Ms. Camino's postpartum day 2. She is preparing to go home with her baby and is dressing her baby in his going-home outfit. Ms. Camino's mother expresses concern that Ms. Camino has not had a bowel movement. Ms. Camino denies need to have a bowel movement but states, "I've been drinking lots of water and walking, I'm sure it will happen soon." She also states, "It still hurts a little when I walk around if I don't take ibuprofen but I don't think I need codeine anymore." Ms. Camino states, "I'd like to feed the baby before we leave." She lies down in the bed, on her side, and asks her mother to hand her the baby. The nurse notes that the baby appears to latch on well. The lactation consultant has evaluated the baby's feeding and has determined that the baby has lost an appropriate amount of weight; his urine output is within normal limits. The nurse collects the following assessment data: BP 108/70, Temp 98.5, fundus firm at 2 fingerbreadths below the umbilicus and bladder is not palpable. Perineum without bruising, edges of laceration well approximated. Ms. Camino's medication record shows that she has alternated narcotic analgesics with a nonsteroidal anti-inflammatory medication, instead of just taking narcotics. She has taken a stool softener twice daily since delivery.

Critical Thinking in the Nursing Process

1. Why should Ms. Camino increase her fluid intake?
2. Why would ice be applied to the perineum?
3. Why would the nursing diagnosis *Interrupted Breastfeeding* be appropriate?

Note: Discussion of Critical Thinking questions appears on the MyNursingKit Website.

Postpartum Care after Cesarean Section

Postpartum care of the new mother who has undergone a cesarean birth is similar to the care of any abdominal surgical client coupled with the routine care of a postpartum client. How the woman reacts to having a cesarean section depends on whether it was scheduled or unplanned. The woman may feel a sense of failure if she was unable to deliver vaginally. The woman who has had a cesarean section usually does not have an opportunity to hold her baby before transfer to the nursery. She may have many questions and concerns, especially if the surgery was done during an emergency situation. It is important to allow the mother and baby to bond as soon as possible. Encourage the mother to express her feelings.

ASSESSMENT

The postpartum nurse needs to understand the reason for the cesarean birth in order to plan and implement individualized care. For example, if the cesarean birth was for cephalopelvic disproportion, the new mother may be tired from hours of labor and require additional rest. If the cesarean birth was a scheduled event due to previous cesarean births, the woman will have an understanding of routine postoperative care. The assessment should progress in a logical sequence usually from head to toe.

| BOX 54-5 | CLIENT TEACHING |

Postpartum Emergencies

Teach the woman to look for these signs in her infant and to call the pediatrician in the following situations:

- An axillary temperature above 100.4 F (38 C) or an axillary temperature below 97.8 F (36.6 C)
- Projectile vomiting or frequent vomiting
- Refusal to feed for 2 feedings or 6 hours
- Listlessness or difficulty in waking baby
- Excessive fussiness during which comfort measures are not effective
- Jaundice increased and working its way down the baby's trunk
- Two or more, loose black or green water stools
- Fewer than 6 wet diapers in a 24-hour period (after the mother's milk has come in)
- If baby is blue or is not breathing, call 911 or your local emergency number

Teach the woman to call the obstetrician or midwife if any of the following occurs in herself:

- A temperature above 100.4 F (38 C)
- Sudden bright red bleeding or blood clots that are lemon-sized or larger
- Foul-smelling lochia
- Painful urination
- Unexplained, sudden pain
- Hot or reddened area on breast
- If experiencing sudden shortness of breath or chest pain, call 911 immediately
- Provide these special discharge instructions about reasons to call the care provider after a cesarean section:
  - Incision not changing for the better, pearly-colored, white, or bloody drainage
  - Reddened or hot area on incision
  - Gaps between edges of incision or opening of incision

Vital Signs

Vital signs are obtained on a routine schedule depending on their stability and the facility protocol. If the blood pressure was elevated prior to surgery due to PIH, more frequent monitoring may be necessary. An elevated temperature is an indication of infection. If the mother was afebrile prior to surgery, a fever may indicate a respiratory infection. If she was febrile before surgery, or if the fetal membrane had been ruptured for some time, a vaginal or uterine infection should be suspected.

Lungs

The lungs should be assessed on admission and with routine assessments. The LPN/LVN should report abnormal breath sounds to the RN. The woman should be encouraged to deep breathe and change position every 2 hours. The obstetrician may order that the woman use an incentive spirometer to encourage adequate deep breathing. The physician usually orders the frequency of use. Ambulation as soon as it is ordered will decrease lung complications related to immobility.

Abdomen

The abdomen should be assessed for return of bowel sounds, and distention from an accumulation of intestinal gas. Generally the woman is not offered food or fluids until bowel sounds are present. If distention occurs, a return flow enema may be ordered to relieve the gas and promote comfort.

The dressing should be checked on admission to the postpartum unit and when vital signs are taken. Drainage should be traced with a permanent marker and documented with date and time. The LPN/LVN should also report the drainage to the RN. With an order, the dressing may be removed and the woman allowed to shower. If the dressing is still in place, it should be covered with plastic to keep it dry and prevent infection. After the shower the incision is allowed to dry completely. If the abdomen hangs over the incision, the woman can lie supine for a few minutes to allow the incision to air dry. A small dressing may be used to absorb any drainage from the incision. The physician usually orders the skin clips to be removed and replaced with Steri-Strips prior to discharge.

The fundus should be checked, as in any other postpartum woman. Begin very gently at first and only increase in firmness if fundal massage is necessary.

Lochia

Because the uterus was sponged before closure of the cesarean section, the woman will usually have less lochia in the immediate postpartum period. A complete absence of lochia is abnormal and should be reported.

Indwelling Urinary Catheter

The woman will usually have an indwelling catheter for a period of time after surgery. Because the bladder is constantly being emptied, a full bladder is not typically a factor in either uterine atony or displacement. The catheter is usually left in place for 6 to 24 hours, depending on the healthcare provider's orders. The LPN/LVN should report blood-tinged urine, because it may be a sign of trauma to the bladder. Unless otherwise ordered, intake and output are measured and recorded while the catheter remains in place and fluids are being infused intravenously. When the catheter is removed, the first two to three voidings are measured. There is an increased risk of urinary tract infection with the indwelling catheter, so client complaints of pain with urination or urgency should be reported.

Legs

The woman should be encouraged to point and flex her toes every hour (see Procedure 29-2). A sequential compression device may be ordered (see Procedure 29-4) to increase vascular blood flow while the client is on bed rest. The device is removed once the woman is ambulating adequately, unless she has risk factors for thrombophlebitis (see Chapter 33). Homans' sign

can signal the presence of thrombophlebitis and should be reported immediately.

Pain Management

It is very important that adequate pain relief be provided following a cesarean section. Excessive discomfort may interfere with mother and baby bonding. Pain can affect the mother's ability to care for and even breastfeed her baby. Although she may not be expected to care for her infant fully immediately after surgery, she may still have the desire to do so.

Some women assume that there will be no pain after a cesarean section, especially if they have never undergone a surgical procedure. A few women feel very little pain and require little pain medication. However, this is the exception rather than the norm. The woman should be reassured that she will be made as comfortable as possible but that she may still feel some discomfort as a result of having abdominal surgery. The type of pain medications the woman is given depends on the type of anesthesia that was administered. If the woman had an epidural catheter in place before the surgery (see Figure 53-17), she will usually be given anesthesia via this route. Otherwise, she may be given intraspinal anesthesia. Both the epidural and intraspinal anesthesia can be used for administering a long-acting narcotic medication. In this case the anesthesiologist's orders usually take precedence over those of the surgeon. The anesthesia orders are typically written for the duration of the narcotic effect, usually 12 to 24 hours. Additional orders for pain medication may be given in the case of breakthrough pain. Pain medications given during this period are mostly given either intravenously or intramuscularly. If the woman received general anesthesia, she may receive patient-controlled analgesia (PCA pump; see Chapter 45) after surgery. There are medical orders regarding intervention in the case of respiratory depression caused by any narcotic used. (Care of clients in pain is discussed further in Chapter 22 .)

Pulse oximetry (see Procedure 32-1) is used to measure the percent of oxygen in the blood. Oxygen saturation and respiratory rate are monitored for up to 24 hours after the anesthesiologist administers the last dose of narcotic.

clinical ALERT

Naloxone (Narcan) is used to reverse respiratory depression. Naloxone is most often given intravenously in this situation, so it is important that the LPN/LVN notify the RN immediately if the client appears to be experiencing respiratory depression. Guidelines are usually given by the anesthesiologist about when to administer naloxone.

Regardless of the route by which pain medication is given, the LPN/LVN should instruct the woman to request pain medication before pain is severe. It is easier to alleviate pain before it becomes severe. If the woman is receiving medication via a PCA pump, she should be instructed to push the button when she needs the medication, and to notify the nurse if pain relief is not adequate. She should be reassured that it is not possible to overdose with a PCA pump because it will only deliver a certain amount of medication per hour. If she pushes the button after she reaches the maximum amount, she will not receive any medication.

The woman should be reassured that although most medications pass through the breast milk, very little of the medication actually passes to the baby. If the mother is still hesitant to take pain medication, she should be instructed that taking it just after breastfeeding will limit even further the amount passed to the baby.

A woman may also refuse pain medication based on the fact that she does not really feel discomfort when she is lying in bed. Her plan of care should be discussed with her, including when she will be assisted with ambulation. Encourage her to move in bed and then to reconsider taking analgesics. She may continue to refuse, and it is her choice to refuse medication if she is not feeling much discomfort at all. She may change her mind if she begins to ambulate and her discomfort increases. Every individual has a different tolerance to pain. Offer the woman the facts about pain relief, reassure her that her baby will not be at risk, and allow her to make an informed choice. If she does change her mind later, accept her decision. Do not treat her with an "I told you so" attitude.

Refer back to Box 54-5 for discharge instructions on when to call a doctor after discharge.

POTENTIAL COMPLICATIONS

As nurses provide care and teaching to postpartum women, on discharge they will provide instructions for the new mother and support people. One of the most important sets of instructions lists situations in which the obstetrician, midwife, or pediatrician must be contacted. These situations were provided in Box 54-5.

clinical ALERT

The LPN/LVN should report or get help with the following findings:

- Suspected increased or heavy bleeding
- Client complaint of sudden shortness of breath or chest pain
- Increased or decreased blood pressure
- Sudden, severe perineal pain
- New drainage on abdominal dressing

New Family

Each time a new baby is born into a family, the family essentially becomes new. Each addition brings both joy and added stress to the family. First-time parents need a great deal of teaching before they are discharged (Figure 54-10 ■).

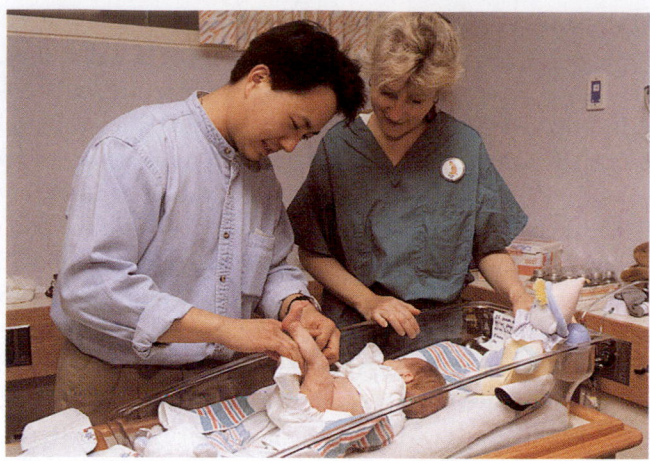

Figure 54-10. ■ Father returns demonstration of diapering his son. It is important to offer teaching to all caregivers, even if this is not the first child.

However, even experienced parents may need additional education. More teaching for parents about how to care for their baby is covered in Chapter 56 ⦾.

TEENAGE MOTHERS

The teenage mother may require a different approach to teaching. Just giving verbal or written instructions is usually not enough for these mothers. Hands-on education with client return demonstration is often most effective. This type of teaching is more time consuming but it is important to equip the teen to care for her new baby. The teen mother may not have a partner to help her care for the child. If a significant other is involved, this person should be included in the teaching sessions. If the teenage mother will be living with her parents, it may be important to include either or both parents. This can be a good time to assess how the new mother's parents perceive their role in caring for the baby. It may also be helpful to perform baby care in front of both the new mother and her parents. Grandparents often have their own ideas about baby care, and these methods may not be in practice anymore.

Teaching sessions may be a time to empower the young mother in her new role. Although she is still not an adult in age, she now has adult responsibilities. Often the nurse may be the only person who makes the new mother feel as if she can be a good mother. Teenage mothers should receive information about public assistance related to the care of her newborn. Some communities have very good programs in place; once the teenage mother seeks prenatal care, she is put in touch with the services that will be most appropriate for her.

MULTIPLE BIRTHS

A new mother with two or more infants has a different set of needs. Two or more babies to care for are understandably more overwhelming than just one baby. Breastfeeding is more difficult, so it is important for the mother to meet with a lactation specialist. Often multiple birth babies are small for gestational age and have different feeding requirements and less leeway with regard to weight loss if feeding is not adequate.

A supportive partner can make all the difference for these mothers. In the absence of a supportive partner, other family or friend support systems should be explored.

OLDER PARENTS

The parents with grown children may not have been planning to add to their family. This is a special situation in which problems between the parents may be evident. Having raised their other children, they may have had plans for their new life alone together. The addition of the new baby may cause tension. It might be helpful for these parents to speak with a social worker. The social worker may have some resources that could be of help to the parents.

SUPPORT PEOPLE

Regardless of the circumstances surrounding the birth of a new baby, there is always something new about the situation. Mother and baby care should begin as soon as the mother and baby are stable. It can be as simple as demonstrating hygiene of the perineal area for the mother or a diaper change for the baby. Often the mother's partner is the one being taught to care for the baby, especially if the mother has undergone a cesarean section or simply is exhausted by her labor and delivery process. Both new and experienced fathers may be hesitant to handle the newborn. They may feel as if the baby is fragile, and they may be afraid they will hurt him or her. The father should never be made to feel embarrassed by this apprehension, but should be encouraged that he is doing a good job. Including the partner in the infant's care can make him feel more knowledgeable about the baby and his or her needs, which can result in decreased anxiety about handling the baby.

VISITORS

Although the new family is excited for their family and friends to meet the new addition, it is important that the mother be allowed to rest. Her body has undergone a dramatic change, and adequate rest is vital. The mother should be encouraged to sleep when the baby sleeps; however, heavy visitor traffic may make this difficult. If the mother is unable to nap during the day, she will be less able to cope with a wide-awake, demanding infant that night. The nurse should encourage the new mother and partner to try to limit visitors, especially if there are many child visitors. Some facilities restrict child visitation to siblings only, but this is not always the case. The parents may be uneasy about asking visitors to leave. In this case the nurse may want to offer to be the "bad guy." Be sure that this is what the

parents want, and explain the situation to the visitors as nicely as possible. Emphasize the need for mother and baby to have their rest periods.

It is not only the mother who can be exhausted by too many people. A baby who is passed from visitor to visitor may be overly stimulated and restless. Feedings may be affected.

Breastfeeding

A newborn's nutrition is particularly important during the first few months of life since the brain develops so rapidly during this period. Many mothers experience pressure about their choice to bottle feed or breastfeed their baby. However, the final decision is the mother's. Regardless of the mother's choice, the LPN/LVN should support her in the decision she has made.

Information about breastfeeding should be provided:

- Breast milk contains all the nutrients necessary for the newborn. No formula provides all these nutrients.
- Breastfeeding provides natural immunity for the newborn because the mother's antibodies are passed through the breast milk to the baby.
- Breast milk is easily digested by newborns and is not harmful to the baby's sensitive digestive system.
- Breastfed babies are less likely to experience constipation.
- Breast milk does not cause allergies in newborns.
- Breastfed babies may be less likely to develop respiratory illnesses.
- A suckling baby promotes contraction of the uterus after delivery of the placenta.

clinical ALERT

Although breast milk is the best source of nutrition for babies, there are some instances in which breastfeeding may be contraindicated:

- A mother who has tested positive for certain recreational drugs should not breastfeed.
- A woman with active hepatitis B or C or who is infected with human immunodeficiency virus (HIV) should not breastfeed.
- Some prescription medications may be contraindicated for a breastfeeding woman. Sometimes the benefit of taking a certain medication may outweigh the risk to the baby. This decision should be thoroughly discussed by the mother and her healthcare provider.

PHYSIOLOGY OF LACTATION

Lactation can be a complicated process for a mother to understand. However, it is important to provide the mother with accurate information about how her body produces milk for her baby.

Prolactin from the pituitary gland causes production of breast milk (Figure 54-11 ■). Oxytocin (also from the pituitary gland) causes the milk to be delivered through the

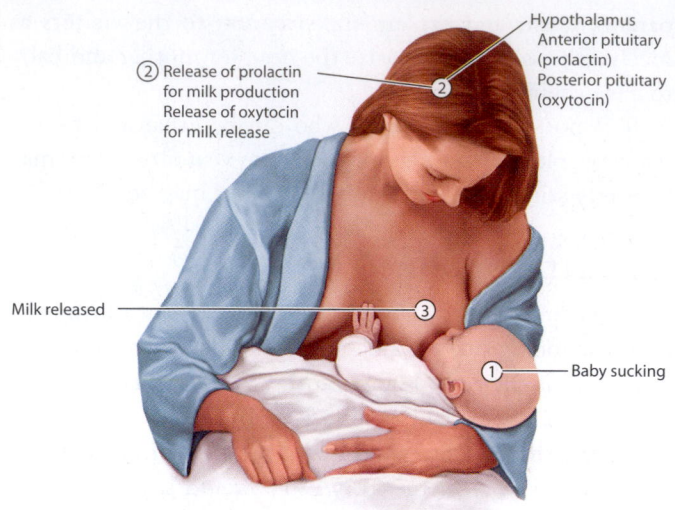

(2) Release of prolactin
for milk production
Release of oxytocin
for milk release

Hypothalamus
Anterior pituitary
(prolactin)
Posterior pituitary
(oxytocin)

Milk released

Baby sucking

Figure 54-11. ■ Relationship between the pituitary gland and milk production. Sucking of the nipple triggers endocrine release of prolactin (which stimulates new milk production). It also triggers oxytocin (which allows milk to be released from the breast). Oxytocin also stimulates uterine contractions, which help the uterus return to its smaller size.

milk ducts to the nipple. When milk is removed from the breasts, either by the infant suckling or expression by way of a breast pump, prolactin continues to be secreted, causing the breasts to produce more milk. If the breasts are not emptied of milk, prolactin ceases to be produced, and the breasts stop making milk. This is where the idea of supply and demand comes into play. The more the baby suckles, the more milk the breasts will produce.

During the latter part of pregnancy and the first few days after delivery, the breasts secrete colostrum. Colostrum, which is thick and yellow in color, is the first food the baby receives. It is rich in nutrients, especially protein and vitamins A and E. It supplies important immunity to infection. Colostrum also has laxative properties, which help the baby pass meconium. Because colostrum is not abundant, the mother may not believe that her baby is getting enough. The LPN/LVN should reassure the mother that the small amount of colostrum is sufficient for the newborn's needs for the first 3 to 4 days.

Not all babies appear satisfied after a feeding. The mother may request a bottle of formula or glucose water to calm the baby. This seems especially common with Latino parents. These parents may tell the nurse that they have "no leche" or no milk. The family and friends in the room may reinforce this feeling, making it difficult to simply inform the parents that the colostrum is sufficient for the baby. In these cases, it may not be just a matter of giving the parents the correct information.

The LPN or LVN may find it a challenge to educate the parents on this matter without offending family members

or contradicting cultural beliefs. Instead of just telling the parents that the baby does not need a bottle and that a bottle may negatively affect breastfeeding, the LPN/LVN should take this opportunity to demonstrate comfort measures to the parents. Although the baby may be fussy and appear to want to suck, most often the baby is not hungry but is in fact gassy. Giving the baby glucose water or formula at this time will only compound the problem. Education is helpful to both first-time parents and experienced mothers whose other newborns may have been given a bottle when they were gassy instead of hungry.

FACTORS AFFECTING LACTATION

Bundling the baby securely is helpful in comforting the baby because babies are used to be being confined to the mother's body and usually do not enjoy being unwrapped at first.

Many newborns become fussy and uncomfortable due to gas bubbles in the gastrointestinal tract. Rubbing the baby's back firmly may help the baby pass gas. Some parents are reluctant to pat a baby firmly enough to elicit a burp or help the baby pass gas. Firm rubbing up and down the back works just as well (Figure 54-12 ■). It may also be helpful to lay the baby across your lap while supporting the head and rubbing the back. The pressure of the legs on the baby's abdomen may help relieve the baby's discomfort. The baby can also be held with his or her back and head against your body and your forearm securely around the baby's abdomen, being careful not to allow the baby's head to fall so far forward that the airway is occluded. This position can be used while the adult stands or sits. Rocking or gentle bouncing along with the pressure on the abdomen may help soothe the baby.

Culture and ethnicity play a large part in a woman's choice to breastfeed and in her approach to feeding her baby. It is important to take into consideration where a woman grew up and also the influence of the women in her life. Many cultures tend to be very encouraging about breastfeeding. However, many immigrants to the United States find that it is not financially feasible to stay at home with their newborns as they would in their countries of origin. Depending on the job and what hours they are required to work, these women may find it difficult to find time to breastfeed or to express breast milk. Some employers are not supportive of a mother's need to have the time and privacy to express her milk.

If milk is not drawn from the breasts, the woman very quickly begins to lose her milk supply. This is a problem that cannot be solved by the nursing staff. Still, it is important for this issue to be recognized and addressed in breastfeeding teaching.

Although frequent breastfeeding should produce enough milk for the baby's nutrition, there are rare times when a mother may not produce enough milk. For example, a mother who has experienced a postpartum hemorrhage may

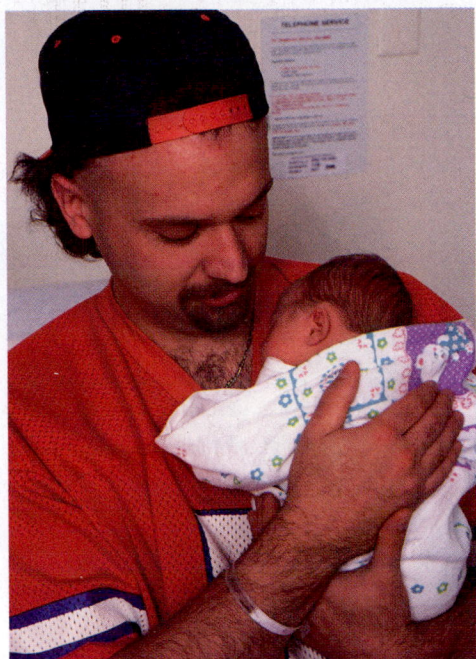

A

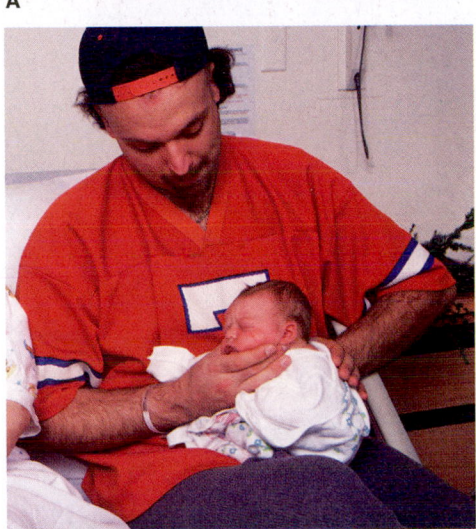

B

Figure 54-12. ■ Two positions for burping a neonate or infant. **A.** Upright. **B.** Sitting leaning forward. The infant may also be laid across the lap.

have a delay in milk production. It is important that the LPN/LVN recognize this risk and notify the pediatrician. If a lactation specialist is available, she should have a consultation with the mother. Action should be taken to ensure adequate nutrition for the newborn and to continue stimulation of the breasts so that the mother will eventually produce milk.

Teaching a mother to breastfeed her baby can be a very rewarding part of the LPN's or LVN's job. The nurse can help a mother learn to breastfeed even if the nurse has not breastfed any children personally. The best way to learn how to help the mother is to follow a lactation specialist on rounds with postpartum mothers. The lactation specialist

has the advantage of only dealing with mothers, infants, and breastfeeding. The specialist often works in a breast-feeding clinic as well, and so has the chance to see mothers and babies after they leave the hospital. Seeing how babies do after discharge from the hospital allows the specialist insight into problems that start in the first few days of breast-feeding. The lactation specialist is also familiar with many different sizes and types of breasts and nipples and is experienced at troubleshooting common problems.

Positioning Tips

Women have different preferred positions for nursing their babies (Figure 54-13 ■). However, certain aspects of positioning are consistent in all positions. The head, shoulder, torso, and lower body of the baby should always be aligned, "belly to belly." If a baby is latched on to the breast but the shoulders and torso are rotated away from the mother's body, the baby may pull on the nipple, causing nipple trauma. The baby may also not be able to stay latched on to the breast. Often simply aligning the baby's body can correct a painful latch-on. Usually the mother should be sitting up as straight as possible in a bed or in a chair. A footrest should be provided if the woman is sitting in a chair.

Women who have had a cesarean section or an extensive perineal laceration may find it difficult to sit up straight enough to position the baby properly. These women may benefit from the side-lying position. This position may make it difficult for a mother to latch her baby on without assistance during the first few days. Whatever position the mother chooses, the LPN/LVN should assure the mother that she can call at any time for assistance with nursing.

A mother may be concerned that her baby cannot breathe when latched on to the breast. As long as the baby's nostrils are patent, the baby should be able to breathe. Babies' noses are flat with flared nostrils. This allows the baby to be very close to the breast to nurse. A baby who cannot breathe will not suck. A baby who is suckling at the breast and whose color is pink is breathing. If the breasts are very large or the baby seems to be "smothered" by the breast, the mother can lift the baby's hips higher, which lifts the head away from the breast without pulling the baby off the breast. Many women instinctively indent the breast to pull it away from the baby's nose. This is not necessary and may cause trauma to the nipple by displacing it in the infant's mouth.

Latch-On

The LPN/LVN should observe the mother feeding her baby, even if the mother says she is doing fine. A baby who is improperly latched on may not be causing enough discomfort for the mother to notice, but may be causing trauma that will produce pain during later feedings. The baby should be positioned so that he or she has most of the areola in the mouth (Figure 54-14 ■). Areola size varies. If the mother

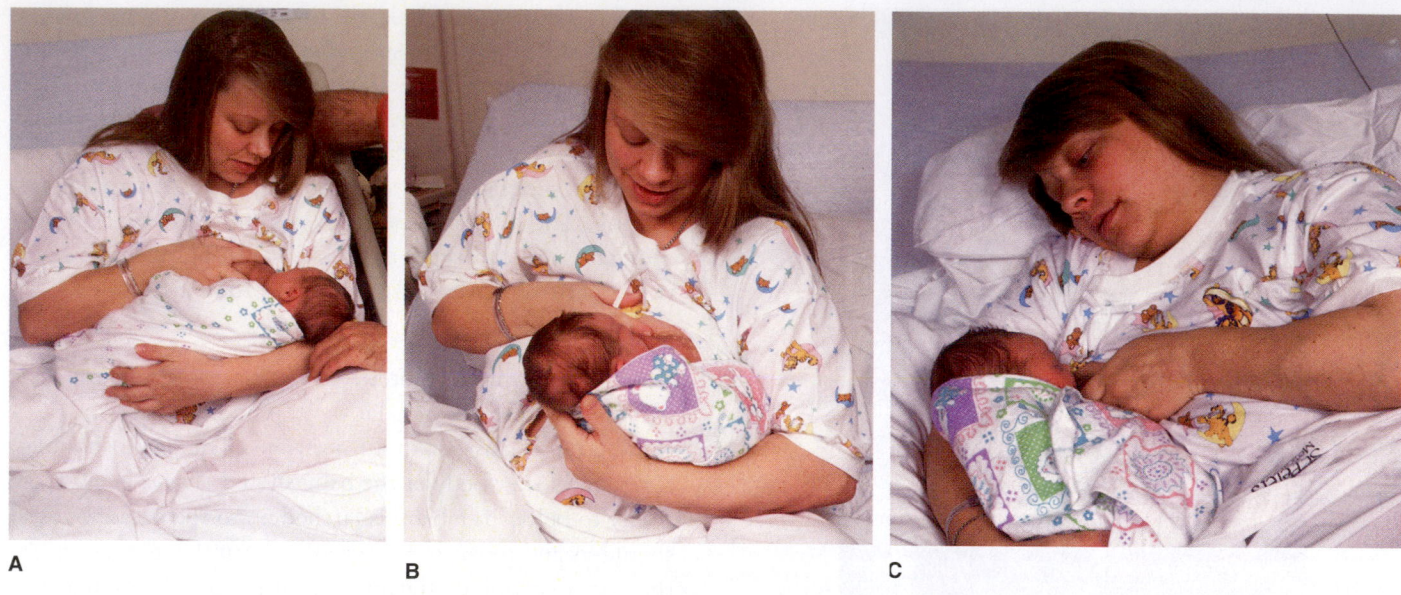

Figure 54-13. ■ Various positions for holding an infant. **A.** Cradle hold. **B.** Upright position. **C.** Football hold.

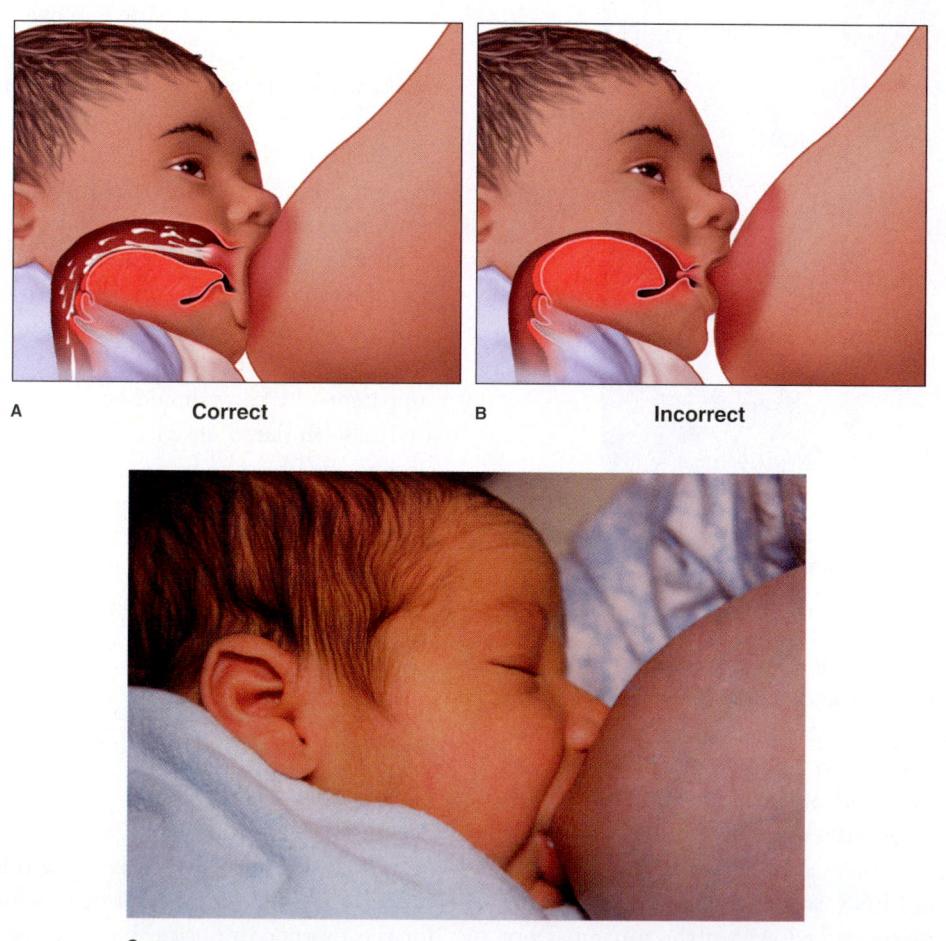

Figure 54-14. ■ Latching on. **A.** Correct position with tongue over gum ridge. Nipple is down far into mouth and milk flows. **B.** Incorrect position with tongue behind the lower gum ridge. Only the tip of the nipple is in the mouth. The nipple is pinched and milk cannot flow. **C.** Newborn properly latched onto mother's breast.

has very small nipples, it may be necessary for the baby to have more than the areola in his or her mouth to latch on properly. If a mother has very large areolae, the baby may not need the whole areola in his or her mouth in order to have a proper latch on.

Many babies are sleepy for feedings and need some stimulation to awaken for feeding. Changing the diaper, even if it is not soiled, helps wake the baby. Unwrapping the baby and tickling the feet or back is another way to wake the baby. The mother may require assistance to awaken the baby.

For a cross-cradle position, the baby should be supported on pillows to be level with the mother's nipple. With a newborn that cannot support its own head, the mother may find it easier to support the baby's head with the hand opposite the breast she is using for feeding. Holding the baby with her fingers behind the head and the heel of her hand between the baby's shoulders, the mother is able to control the baby's head. With her other hand she should hold her breast in a U-shape with her breast being supported by the space between the thumb and the fingers. This hand position will allow her to offer her nipple in the same direction as the baby's mouth. (Think of the hand position you would use to offer a toddler a sandwich. You would bring food horizontally to the mouth from in front of the toddler's body. You would not put it in at an angle.) Many women offer their nipple to their baby in a direction that makes it difficult for the baby to latch on. A simple adjustment will make it easier for the baby to latch on.

Once the mother is holding her breast correctly, she should brush the baby's nose and lips in an up-down motion to elicit the rooting reflex (see Figure 16-5 🔗). When the baby opens its mouth wide, the mother should bring the baby close to her breast so the areola is in the baby's mouth. At the beginning, the mother may need help in coordinating the baby's reflex and bringing the baby to her breast.

When the baby is latched on to the breast, the lips should be flanged out. This allows the tongue to be under the nipple so that the milk ducts are compressed properly. If the bottom lip is tucked under, the mother may experience a pinching sensation of the nipple. In this case, placing a finger on the baby's chin and gently pulling down may pull out the lip. Secure the baby's head to keep him or her from pushing back from the mother and pulling away from the nipple. If smacking sounds or dimpling of the baby's cheeks occurs during nursing, the baby is not latched on properly and should be unlatched and repositioned. Although it may be difficult, swallowing can often be heard when the infant is latched on properly. The swallow may sound like a sigh. The baby should be sucking in long, drawing sucks. Short, fluttery sucks indicate non-nutritive sucking.

The mother should be shown the correct way to remove her nipple from the baby's mouth. Pulling the baby off without first breaking the suction will cause nipple trauma. Instruct the mother to slide her finger along her breast and nipple into the corner of the baby's mouth to break the suction.

Due to the sleep cycle of the baby, it is important that the baby be put to breast as soon after delivery as possible. If for some reason the mother is not able to breastfeed her baby right away, she should be reassured that she can still breastfeed successfully and that the nurses and lactation specialist will assist her with this. The breasts need to be stimulated after birth to begin the process of milk production.

If it is known that the baby will not be able to be put to breast during the first few days, the mother should be assisted with the use of a breast pump. Follow hospital policy regarding use of a breast pump and storage of breast milk as a body fluid. A mother whose baby has not been able to latch on to the breast during the first 24-hour period should begin pumping her breasts. A plan for feeding should be developed according to hospital policy so that the mother can continue to attempt to breastfeed her baby while stimulating her breasts to produce milk.

A supplemental nursing system (SNS) may be helpful for a baby who appears unmotivated to nurse. The SNS involves an inverted bottle with a soft tube attached. The bottle is filled with formula or glucose water and the tube is taped to the mother's breast so that it extends a bit from the nipple. The bottle is specially made to allow only a small amount of fluid to pass through the tube at a time. The infant must suck for the milk to pass through the tubing and into the mouth. Some babies benefit from this system, which teaches the baby that milk comes out of the mother's breast. SNS is helpful for the baby who has been bottle-fed for a period of time. SNS is not for every baby and may be difficult for the mother to master along with positioning the infant and her breast for feeding. Some hospital lactation programs only allow lactation specialists to use SNS with mothers. Nurses who are unsure of how to use SNS should receive instruction in its use, preferably from a lactation specialist.

DURATION OF FEEDINGS

The mother should be encouraged to nurse the baby as often as the baby wants to nurse. Babies give off feeding cues, which should be taught to the mother. The baby will root and open his or her mouth wide when he or she is hungry. The baby may also suck his or her tongue, fist, or fingers. If the parent misses feeding cues, the baby may become frantic and have a difficult time latching on.

A baby may wish to nurse as often as every 1½ to 2 hours. A sleepy baby should be awakened at least every 3 hours to nurse. The baby should be allowed to nurse as long as he or she is still sucking, unless it is uncomfortable for the mother. Sleepy babies may need to be stimulated during the feeding to keep them awake. The mother should attempt to keep the baby awake long enough to nurse at least 15 minutes on each breast. Babies have different needs with regard to non-nutritive sucking. They may wish to nurse even though they are not still hungry. Pacifiers are controversial, but they are usually not recommended until breastfeeding has been successfully established. Hospital lactation programs may have a policy about pacifiers. The parents should be given accurate information about the use of pacifiers. Then they make the final decision whether or not to offer one.

Breastfeeding and Weight

The breastfed newborn will lose weight during the first few days of life. This is mostly due to the fact that the baby is urinating and passing stools in larger quantities than he or she is taking in feedings. Once the mother's milk supply is established, the baby should begin to gain weight.

Babies who lose more than 10% of their birth weight will need intervention. They should be weighed before and after a feeding to determine their intake. (One gram is about equal to 1 mL of fluid.) Most facilities have a policy about treatment of infants with a 10% weight loss. This may include initiating use of a breast pump as well as a supplemental nursing system. The birth and discharge weights of each baby should be recorded so that the pediatrician will have accurate data for follow-up care.

A baby who is less than 6 lbs (3,000 grams) may tire more easily than a larger baby, and so may only feed for short periods of time. Some facilities do not discharge babies who are less than 6 lbs (3,000 grams). Use of a breast pump may be initiated, along with allowing the baby to breastfeed every $1\frac{1}{2}$ to 3 hours in anticipation that the baby may not be stimulating the mother's breasts sufficiently to produce enough milk.

Breastfeeding after Discharge

The breastfeeding mother should be given resources for breastfeeding support in her community. The La Leche League is a strong advocate for the breastfeeding woman. It provides a great deal of support for women just beginning to breastfeed, as well as for mothers who wish to continue to nurse for the first few years of life. Many women stop breastfeeding once they go back to work. This may occur because the workplace is not a supportive environment for nursing mothers. The La Leche League and other community support groups may be able to provide such women with information to help them keep an adequate milk supply. Many facilities have breastfeeding workshops for clients to attend after discharge.

One very important aspect of breastfeeding education is for all staff members to give the same type of information. Many parents feel overwhelmed by all there is to learn about caring for their baby, especially if everyone around them seems to have a different opinion about how they should do everything. By offering consistent information about breastfeeding, the nurse helps parents master these concepts without having to figure out which nurse is right.

There is a great deal of information for parents to absorb before they take their baby home. This material can be overwhelming if given to the parents all at once. By beginning discharge teaching as soon as the baby is born, the nurse helps parents learn the information in small amounts. Everything the nurse does with the parents—from teaching the woman perineal care to talking the father through a diaper change—is part of discharge education. Discharge instructions related solely to the neonate are discussed further in Chapter 56 ⬭.

NURSING CONSIDERATIONS

When caring for clients who are breastfeeding, focus your care on supporting and instructing the client. Since every baby is different, some techniques work better than others for each infant. Encourage clients to keep trying to breastfeed and not to get discouraged. Be careful to use positive, supportive words to the clients. Avoid saying anything that could cause feelings of inadequacy regarding breastfeeding. Instruct the breastfeeding mother about nipple care. Instruct her to report elevated temperature or cracked and bleeding nipples, which could indicate mastitis.

Note: The references and resources for all chapters have been compiled at the back of the book.

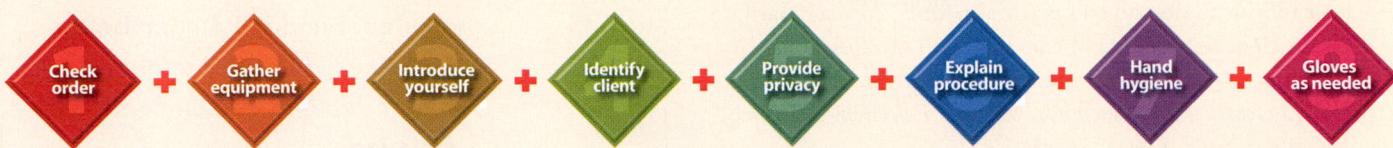

PROCEDURE 54-1

Performing Fundal Massage and Removing Clots from the Uterus

Purpose

- To prevent or correct uterine atony and remove clots from the uterus in order to evaluate uterine bleeding and prevent hemorrhage.

Equipment

- Clean gloves
- Perineal pad
- Clean blue underpad
- Perineal bottle filled with warm water
- Warm wet washcloth
- Impervious bag

Check order + Gather equipment + Introduce yourself + Identify client + Provide privacy + Explain procedure + Hand hygiene + Gloves as needed

Interventions and Rationales

1. Perform preparatory steps (see icon bar above).

2. Determine the need for fundal massage. *A fundus requiring massage will be soft and can be felt above the umbilicus. A firm fundus does not require massage.*

3. Have the woman empty her bladder. If she is unable to void, obtain an order for bladder catheterization. Follow your facility's protocol regarding who notifies the doctor (the LPN/LVN or the RN). *A full bladder can cause the fundus to move up and away from the midline. It can also increase discomfort and lead to increased bleeding. If the fundus is boggy and above the umbilicus, blood clots are suspected.*

4. Explain the procedure to the woman and provide privacy. Inform her that the procedure may be uncomfortable but should only last a few minutes. Explain that it is necessary to massage the uterus and remove clots to prevent excessive bleeding. *Providing information ahead of time reduces anxiety and allows the woman to participate in her decisions about her care.*

5. Place the woman in supine position with knees slightly flexed. *This position relaxes the abdominal muscles.*

6. Lower the perineal pad away from the perineum. *This allows visualization of blood and/or clots that may be expressed during massage.*

7. Place one hand just above the symphysis pubis and press down (Figure 54-15 ■). **Note: Remember never to massage a fundus without first anchoring the lower portion of the uterus.** *This is necessary to prevent the uterus from prolapsing into the vagina.*

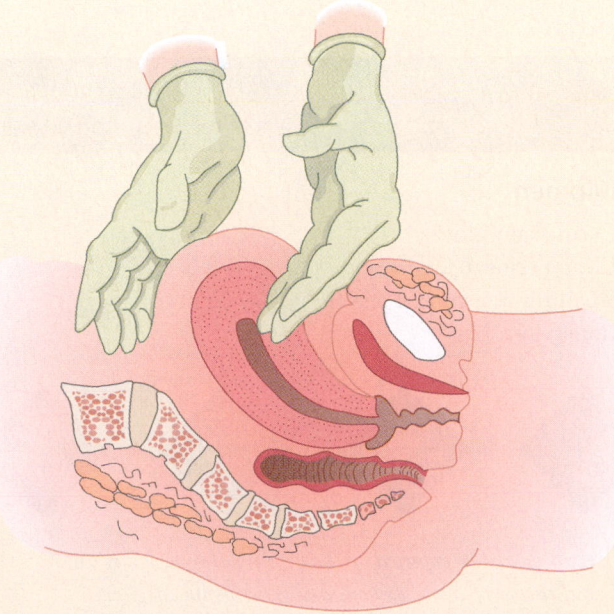

A

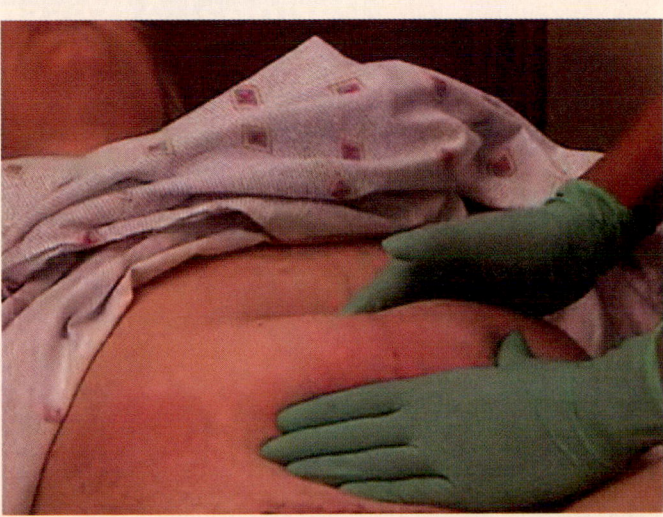

B

Figure 54-15. ■ Nurse positioning hands to remove clots from uterus. Note that lower hand supports the uterus.

8. Locate and massage the fundus. Use the flat portion of the fingers to massage the fundus gently with a firm, circular motion. Begin gently at first and massage more firmly as necessary. *Starting with a gentle massage lessens discomfort.*

9. Once the fundus is firm, apply firm pressure from the fundus toward the vagina. Continue supporting the lower uterine segment. **This step may be restricted to RNs only; check facility policy.** *The pressure will express clots or accumulated blood.*

10. Reassess the fundus for firmness and location. *The fundus should regain tone once clots are removed.*

11. Remove all bloody pads, cleanse the perineum, and apply a clean blue underpad and perineal pad. Follow standard precautions for disposal of contaminated articles. *Cleanliness promotes comfort and prevents infection. Bleeding is likely to continue after the fundal massage. Following standard precautions prevents spread of infection.*

12. Weigh pads with blood and/or clots if heavy bleeding occurs. *All bloody supplies may be saved until the amount of blood loss is determined. Weighing is the most reliable means of determining the exact amount of blood loss.*

13. Assess the fundus every 15 minutes until it remains firm for a minimum of 1 hour. *If the fundus becomes boggy, further bleeding could occur.*

14. Document the type, amount, and characteristics of lochia and/or blood clots. *Clear documentation provides important information for follow-up and prevention of complications.*

15. Report to the RN a fundus that does not become firm with massage or any excessive bleeding. *These may be signs of hemorrhage.*

SAMPLE DOCUMENTATION

[date]	Ct. complains of cramping
[time]	in uterus.
	Fundus 2 fingers above umbilicus, boggy, and left of midline. Fundus massaged until firm. Expressed 2 clots 6 cm across. Bright red bleeding. Resolved within 1 minute. Perineum washed. Clean pad applied. Fundus 1 finger below umbilicus, firm and midline. Client reports discomfort relieved. _____
	_____ K. Chi, RN
[date]	Fundus assessed every
[time]	15 minutes. Fundus firm at U. Moderate amount red lochia noted on peripad. _____
	_____ A. Admas, LPN

PROCEDURE 54-2 **Perineal Assessment**

Purpose

- To assess the perineum for signs of healing and complication following delivery

Equipment

- Clean exam gloves
- Clean perineal pad
- Small light such as a pen light may be necessary
- Impervious bag

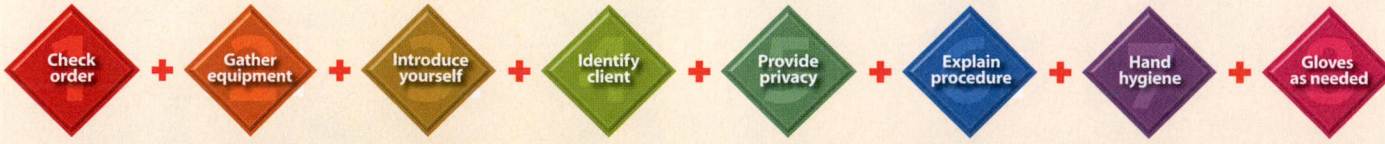

Check order + Gather equipment + Introduce yourself + Identify client + Provide privacy + Explain procedure + Hand hygiene + Gloves as needed

Interventions and Rationales

1. Perform preparatory steps (see icon bar above).

2. Ask the woman about perineal discomfort. "Is it getting better or worse? Is it greater than expected?" *Pain greater than would be expected or that is becoming worse is an indication of complications and must be investigated.*

3. Position the woman in the left Sims' position. *When the woman is supine, the posterior perineum may be difficult*

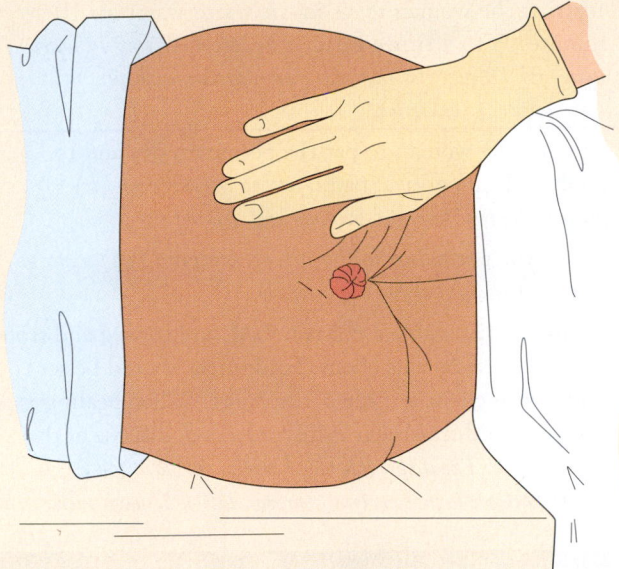

Figure 54-16. ■ The nurse raises the upper buttock with the hand. Illustration shows an intact perineum with external hemorrhoids.

to see. *Sims' position allows for adequate exposure of the perineum.*

4. Lift the buttocks to expose the perineum (Figure 54-16 ■). Use a small light to visualize the perineal tissues. *Adequate visualization is necessary for complete assessment.*

5. Assess the perineum in a systematic order. The mnemonic REEDA (redness, edema, ecchymosis, discharge, approximation) may be a helpful reminder.
   - **R** = redness. *Redness is a sign of infection.*
   - **E** = edema. Palpate for softness of tissue. *Some edema is usual following a vaginal delivery. Edematous tissue is soft. A firm mass is a sign of a hematoma and must be reported to the charge nurse.*

   - **E** = ecchymosis. *The tissue may be somewhat bruised, but an increase in bruising or excessive bruising is a sign of a hematoma.*
   - **D** = discharge. Look for drainage from episiotomy or lacerations. *There should be no drainage from repaired episiotomy or lacerations. Purulent or foul-smelling drainage is a sign of infection.*
   - **A** = Approximation. The edges of repaired episiotomy or lacerations should be touching. *Within 24 hours the wound edges should be "glued" together. Sutures are placed under the skin, and, therefore, will not be visible.*

6. Assess the anus for hemorrhoids (see Figure 54-16). If hemorrhoids are present, the size, number, and degree of tenderness should be noted. *Hemorrhoids often develop during pregnancy and labor and delivery. Comfort measures may be needed.*

7. Apply a clean perineal pad. Replenish ice pack if necessary. *Ice packs prevent swelling and may relieve some discomfort.*

8. Dispose of contaminated pads using standard precautions. *Standard precautions prevent the spread of infection.*

SAMPLE DOCUMENTATION

[date]	Midline episiotomy edges well
[time]	approximated. No swelling, ecchymosis, or drainage noted.
	States comfort measure effective in relieving tenderness. _____
	_____ J. Jones, LVN

PROCEDURE 54-3　Sitz Bath

Purpose
■ To relieve discomfort and promote healing of the perineum

Equipment
■ Disposable sitz tub kit, containing disposable basin, plastic bag with tubing
■ Clean perineal pad
■ Impervious bag
■ Towel

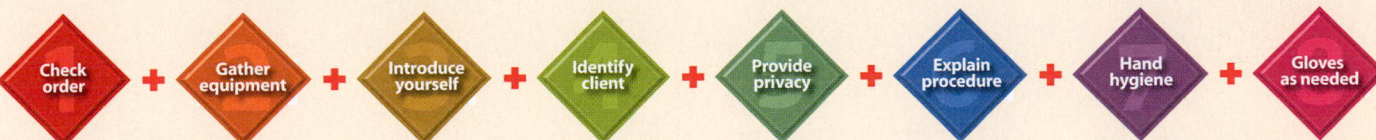

Check order ✚ Gather equipment ✚ Introduce yourself ✚ Identify client ✚ Provide privacy ✚ Explain procedure ✚ Hand hygiene ✚ Gloves as needed

Interventions and Rationales

1. Perform preparatory steps (see icon bar).

2. Provide client teaching about sitz baths, including the benefits and use of the equipment. *Instructing the client in the use of equipment and the benefits of the sitz bath helps ensure compliance.*

3. Raise the toilet seat, place the disposable basin on the toilet. *The toilet seat should be raised and basin placed directly on the toilet for maximum support.*

4. Close clamp on tubing. Fill plastic bag with very warm water. Attach tubing to inside bottom of basin in groove provided. *The water in the bag will drain into the basin to keep the water comfortably warm. If the water in the bag is too cool, the water in the basin will cool and not be as effective.*

5. Fill the basin with comfortably warm water. *Warm water will increase circulation to the perineum and promote healing of tissues.*

6. Have the woman remove the perineal pad, dispose of it in the impervious bag, and sit directly on the basin. *Sitting directly on the basin will allow the perineum to be covered by the warm water. If the woman sits on the toilet seat, the perineum would not reach the water.*

7. Instruct the woman to open the tubing clamp periodically to drain the very warm water into the basin, keeping the basin water comfortably warm. As the basin fills, the water will drain into the toilet. *The very warm water should keep the basin water at a comfortable temperature.*

8. Instruct the woman to sit in the warm water for 10 minutes, 3 to 4 times a day as ordered. *Sitting in warm water for 10 minutes stimulates circulation without traumatizing the tissues.*

9. Instruct the woman to pat the perineum dry and to apply a clean perineal pad. *Patting the perineum dry prevents further perineal trauma and discomfort.*

10. Assess the perineum following treatment. *The perineum should show signs of healing over time.*

11. Clean the disposable sitz basin, bag, and tubing and store for future use by this client. Equipment should be sent home with client at time of discharge. When healing is complete and treatment is discontinued, dispose of the equipment. *The disposable sitz basin is intended for individual use to prevent cross-contamination between users.*

SAMPLE DOCUMENTATION

[date]	Up to bathroom. Sat in sitz
[time]	bath for 10 minutes. Perineum
	dried, clean peripad applied.
	Perineal swelling decreased.
	Laceration edges well
	approximated. _____
	_____ B. Abbs, LVN

Chapter Review

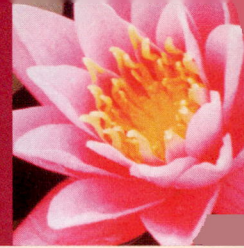

KEY Points

- Physical assessment of the postpartum woman includes the following: breasts, nipples, fundus, abdomen, any surgical dressing/incision, lochia, episiotomy or perineal laceration, legs, bladder function, and distention.

- The postpartum period includes not only a great deal of physiologic change but also a great deal of psychologic adjustment for a woman.

- A woman's choice regarding care of herself and her infant must be recognized as a very important element in her care.

- Life-threatening hemorrhaging can occur in the postpartum woman hours or even days after delivery.

- Listening is one of the most important skills a postpartum nurse needs to learn.

- Mother and baby care and education should begin as soon as the mother and baby are stable.

FOR FURTHER Study

Care of clients in pain is discussed further in Chapter 22.

Application of a sequential compression device is discussed in Chapter 29 and shown in Procedure 29-4.

Steps in performing pulse oximetry (to measure the oxygen percentage in the blood) are provided in Chapter 32.

Thrombophlebitis is discussed in Chapter 33.

Hematomas are discussed in Chapter 34.

Kegel exercises and uterine prolapse are discussed in Chapter 40.

The PCA pump is illustrated in Chapter 45.

Discussion of Rh incompatibility and pregnancy is found in Chapter 52.

Chapter 53 discusses labor and delivery, illustrates types of episiotomies, and shows an epidural catheter in place before surgery.

Complications in the postpartum period, including negative feelings and depression, are discussed in Chapter 55.

Care of neonates is discussed in detail in Chapters 56 and 57.

EXPLORE PEARSON **mynursingkit**™

MyNursingKit is your one stop for online chapter review materials and resources. Prepare for success with additional NCLEX®-style practice questions, interactive assignments and activities, web links, animations and videos, and more!

Register your access code from the front of your book at **www.mynursingkit.com**

Critical Thinking Care Map

Caring for a Client with Risk for Ineffective Breastfeeding
NCLEX-PN® Focus Area: Prevention and Health Maintenance

Case Study: Santana Gomez, a 25-year-old gravida 2 para 1 woman, delivered an 8-lb baby girl via spontaneous vaginal delivery Tuesday evening. Estimated blood loss less than 300 mL. Baby was placed at the breast within the first hour, latching on well, sucking, and swallowing. Client states that she breastfed her first baby for 1 year. The lactation specialist evaluated client and baby Wednesday morning and documented that baby was breastfeeding without problems. Baby weighed 7 lbs 14 oz at 7:30 P.M., VS: T 98.6°F (37°C), R 38, and P 142. Baby voided ×3 and stooled ×4 since birth. Wednesday, at 8:00 P.M., Ms. Gomez states, "I don't have any milk." The baby is crying loudly. Baby does not latch onto the breast. Ms. Gomez states, "She's hungry and I don't have any milk for her." The nurse explains that the baby has been breastfeeding well and that Ms. Gomez has plenty of colostrum for the baby's needs. Ms. Gomez insists that the baby needs formula. The nurse provides formula to feed the baby. Afterward, they both sleep for an hour before the baby awakens, screaming. Ms. Gomez requests more formula.

Nursing Diagnosis: *Risk for Ineffective Breastfeeding*

COLLECT DATA

Subjective	Objective
_____	_____
_____	_____
_____	_____
_____	_____
_____	_____
_____	_____
_____	_____

Would you report this? Yes/No

If yes, report to: _____

What would you report?_____

Nursing Care

_____
_____
_____
_____
_____
_____
_____
_____
_____

How would you document this? _____
_____
_____
_____

Compare your answers and documentation to those provided on the MyNursingKit Website.

Data Collected
(use only those that apply)

- Second-time mother
- Mother states, "I don't have any milk," baby crying loudly, does not latch on
- 25 years of age
- Successfully breastfed first baby, lactation report states baby feeding well
- Baby voided × 3, stooled × 4 since birth
- Formula brought and fed to baby, baby sleeps 1 hour and awakens, screaming, will not latch on, mother requests more formula
- Spontaneous vaginal delivery with an estimated blood loss of less than 300 mL
- Postpartum hematocrit level 35
- Baby feeding well with good latch-on
- Birth weight of baby 8 lbs (4,000 grams)
- Weight at 1 day of life: 7 lbs 14 oz (3,937 grams)
- Baby's T 98.6°F, R 38, P 142

Nursing Interventions
(use only those that apply; list in priority order)

- Give Ms. Gomez a six-pack of formula.
- Tell Ms. Gomez that she is wrong to give her baby formula and her baby will not ever breastfeed.
- Discuss the idea of supply and demand in relation to breast milk production.
- Explain how the infant may appear hungry but that it is more likely to be gas.
- Take the baby to the nursery and feed her so Ms. Gomez can sleep.
- Demonstrate infant comfort measures for Ms. Gomez and support person.
- Encourage support person to attempt comfort measures for Ms. Gomez while she positions herself to breastfeed baby.
- Encourage Ms. Gomez to apply comfort measures and then breastfeed baby.
- Schedule another consultation with lactation specialist.

NCLEX-PN® Exam Preparation

1 The non-nursing mother complains of breast discomfort on the third day postpartum. The nurse advises the mother to do which of the following to reduce discomfort?

1. Pump the breasts.
2. Hand express some milk from the breasts to soften them.
3. Apply ice and a binder or supportive bra.
4. Ignore it because it will go away in a few days.

2 When assessing the newly delivered postpartum client, the nurse finds the fundus is soft, two to three fingerbreadths above the umbilicus, and to the right of midline. The nurse's priority action is to:

1. Assess the perineum for the presence of a hematoma.
2. Massage the fundus until firm.
3. Check the client's blood pressure.
4. Encourage the client to urinate.

3 The nurse is providing care for a newly delivered adolescent and her baby. When the baby girl is brought into the mother's room, the teen says, "Put it over there in the corner. It makes so much noise I can't hear the TV." The nurse's priority intervention is to:

1. Remind the adolescent she is a mother now and has responsibilities.
2. Ask the mother if she would like the baby to be kept in the nursery until feeding time.
3. Request a social service referral.
4. Explain how to turn the volume up on the television control.

4 The nurse will assess postpartal bleeding most accurately by:

1. Weighing all used peripads.
2. Documenting the number and saturation level of peripads.
3. Placing the client on a bedpan for 1 hour as a random indicator of hourly output.
4. Attaching an external male catheter device to catch the flow for measurement.

5 Which of the following statements is true about the application of ice packs to the perineal area of postpartum clients?

1. Heat is applied the first 24 hours and then ice after that.
2. The nurse allows 10 to 20 minutes between applications of cold packs.
3. Commercial chemical ice packs are the most effective.
4. Ice packs are usually applied after twice-a-day sitz baths.

6 A client has striae on the abdomen and asks the nurse if these marks will stay so red or purple. The nurse's best response is:

1. "Yes, they will stay this color."
2. "No, they will disappear completely."

3. "Application of cocoa butter will cause them to go away."
4. "They rarely disappear but will fade over time to a silvery color."

7 When the nurse notes that a client's white blood cell count is 16,000/mm^3 the first postpartum day, it is attributed to:

1. Excessive uterine bleeding.
2. A rapidly growing infection.
3. Stress, inflammation, and pain.
4. Diaphoresis and diuresis.

8 The nurse, providing discharge instructions to a postpartum client, tells the woman to notify the physician or nurse if she observes or experiences which of the following signs or symptoms?

1. Small clots after napping or sleeping
2. White to yellowish discharge
3. Cramping when breastfeeding
4. Foul smell to the vaginal discharge

9 Which of the following interventions by the nurse is most important in facilitating mother–infant bonding when working with a postpartum mother delivered by cesarean section?

1. Encourage and provide adequate pain relief for the mother.
2. Keep the infant in the nursery as much as possible to allow the mother to rest.
3. Encourage the mother to take complete responsibility for the infant as soon as possible.
4. Discourage the mother from getting out of bed to feed the infant until the day before discharge.

10 When entering the newly delivered primigravida postpartum client's room, the nurse finds the woman in tears, saying, "I'm a terrible mother. The baby won't even drink my milk!" The nurse's best response is:

1. "You're tearful because you are already experiencing postpartum depression. You'll feel better in a few weeks."
2. "It is not related to your mothering skills. Newborns go through a sleepy period after delivery but will be more alert and responsive to breastfeeding tomorrow."
3. "You are worried about being a good mother? Is there something in particular that causes you to doubt your mothering abilities?"
4. "It is normal for a new mother to worry about being able to care for a newborn. The baby goes through a sleepy period after the work of being born, but she will be more active tomorrow."

Answers and rationales for Review Questions appear in Appendix I.

Care of High-Risk Postpartum Women

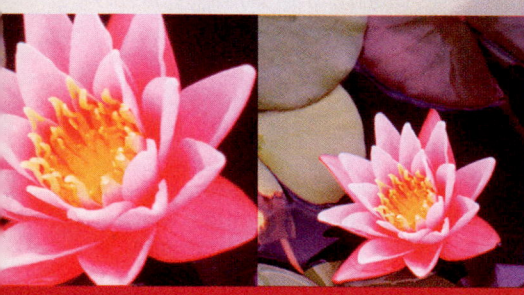

LEARNING Outcomes

After completing this chapter, you will be able to:

1. Describe signs and symptoms of potential complications in the postpartum period.
2. Discuss postpartum assessment of preeclampsia.
3. Identify nursing interventions for postpartum bleeding and other complications.
4. Identify the signs and symptoms of postpartum infections.
5. Differentiate between postpartum blues, depression, and psychosis.
6. Discuss family care needs related to maternal death.

Clinical Objectives

7. Provide client teaching related to complications that might occur following discharge, as well as actions clients or family members should take.
8. Provide support for the new mother experiencing postpartum depression.

KEY TERMS

Use the audio glossary feature on the MyNursingKit Website to hear the correct pronunciation of the following key terms.

clonus 1517

endometritis 1521

hematoma 1519

mastitis 1520

peritonitis 1521

postpartum depression 1522

postpartum (puerperal) infection 1521

septicemia 1521

subinvolution 1519

uterine atony 1518

Complications during pregnancy or birth can result in a high-risk postpartum recovery. Some postpartum complications cause delayed healing, whereas others may be life threatening. The role of the LPN/LVN is to assist the RN in providing routine postpartum care and to monitor for and report signs of complications. Because of the short hospital stay of most postpartum women, client teaching must occur that includes symptoms of postpartum complications and when to notify their primary care providers. This chapter will discuss the common complications seen in the postpartum period.

Preeclampsia

As discussed in Chapter 52 ⚭, *preeclampsia* is a condition of increased blood pressure accompanied by proteinuria occurring after the 20th week of pregnancy. It may take several days to a week for symptoms to resolve following birth. Symptoms of elevated blood pressure, proteinuria, edema, and hyperreflexia must be monitored every 1 to 2 hours until the mother is discharged from the hospital or birthing center. The mother with severe preeclampsia or eclampsia is at extreme risk for seizures and death, and may be monitored in an intensive care unit.

In addition to routine postpartum assessment, the mother will need to have her blood pressure monitored. During labor, the mother's blood pressure may have elevated due to the effects of stress. Within the first hour after birth, the blood pressure should return to the prebirth measurement. If the blood pressure remains elevated, it should be monitored every hour and reported to the RN in charge.

Recall that preeclampsia causes protein to be excreted in the mother's urine. To monitor the effects of preeclampsia on the mother's kidneys, a chemical dipstick is used to determine the amount of protein in the urine with each voiding. It is expected that urine protein levels will decrease over time.

The mother's reflexes will have been monitored throughout the end of pregnancy and during labor. It is expected that her reflexes will be monitored every 2 to 4 hours. If the mother's reflexes are more than 2+ and if she has 2 or more beats of **clonus** (a series of abnormal reflex movements of the foot in response to sudden dorsiflexion), she must be watched closely for seizure activity. She will need a quiet environment to decrease the stimulation of her nervous system. The nurse may need to politely ask visitors to leave so the mother can obtain adequate rest. Often a sign is posted on the door of the postpartum room instructing visitors to check with the nurse before visiting the mother.

Because preeclampsia causes fluid retention, the mother's feet, legs, and hands should be assessed for edema and her weight should be obtained. Edema should begin to decrease within the first 12 to 24 hours and her weight should decrease daily.

clinical ALERT

Because of the shift of fluid from the blood to the interstitial space (which results in edema), the preeclamptic mother may be hypovolemic. If she has excessive blood loss, she will have little reserve and develop shock faster than other mothers.

Often prebirth treatment of intravenous administration of magnesium sulfate will be ordered through the first 24 to 48 hours postpartum and will gradually be withdrawn as symptoms subside. The mother may remain in the hospital or birthing center for 1 to 2 days longer than the mother without preeclampsia.

Recall from Chapter 52 ⚭ that the adolescent is at risk for developing preeclampsia. An increase in blood pressure, rapid reflexes, and clonus are common indicators of worsening preeclampsia. When these occur, the mother may be hospitalized and labor induced. Because it is critical for the preeclamptic mother to have a calm, quiet environment, visitors are limited. The nurse must understand the teen's need for peer contact as well as her physiological needs for a stress-free environment (Box 55-1 ■). The nurse can help the adolescent by:

- Encouraging parental support.
- Encouraging her to select one friend to stay with her and to be the contact for the other friends.
- Limiting the volume of conversation and music.
- Providing information and support.

Postpartum Hemorrhage

Postpartum *hemorrhage* (excessive blood loss) is described as either immediate (within the first 24 hours) or delayed (between 24 hours and 6 weeks post birth). Traditionally

BOX 55-1	PEDIATRIC CONSIDERATIONS

Teenage Mother with Preeclampsia

Recall that the adolescent wants to feel attractive. Pregnancy has brought many changes in her body that can make her feel awkward and ugly. To help compensate, the pregnant adolescent relies heavily on her peer group to "fit in." Commonly, friends plan to remain with the teen during birth and the postpartum period. The adolescent and her friends may see caring for a new baby as a "fun" thing to do instead of realizing the extent of the responsibility.

The desire to maintain frequent contact with friends may decrease compliance in a teen with preeclampsia. For this reason, client teaching is essential and may be necessary both to the teen and to her friends. The seriousness and effects of seizures must be explained so that there is an understanding of why a quiet environment is medically necessary. The nurse can explain that this is only a temporary situation and recommend that friends who cannot remain at bedside write a note or send a text message by phone instead.

postpartum hemorrhage was defined as a blood loss of 500 mL or more following birth. However, that definition has been questioned (Shevell & Malone, 2003). Because blood mixes with amniotic fluid, estimating blood loss is difficult. Careful measurement indicates the average blood loss is greater than 500 mL for a vaginal delivery and over 1,000 mL for a cesarean birth. Changes in hematocrit are becoming a more reliable determination of hemorrhage in the postpartum client. If there is a 10-point decrease in hematocrit between admission and post birth, excessive blood loss has occurred.

Because of the increased blood volume during pregnancy, the usual signs of hemorrhage (increased pulse, decreased blood pressure, and decreased urinary output) may not appear until 1,800 to 2,100 mL have been lost. It is important for the postpartum client to be monitored closely for hemorrhage, changes in vital signs, and urinary output. Often blood is drawn and sent to the lab for hematocrit and hemoglobin levels.

Postpartum hemorrhage does have a genetic component (Box 55-2 ■).

BOX 55-2	CULTURAL PULSE POINTS

Ethnicity and Postpartum Hemorrhage

Women of Asian and Hispanic heritage have a higher incidence of postpartum hemorrhage than women of other descent. They should be observed more frequently for signs of hypovolemia.

Also, women who are natural redheads experience heavier bleeding following childbirth. The nurse should observe these women more frequently for postpartum hemorrhage and hypovolemia.

IMMEDIATE POSTPARTUM HEMORRHAGE

There are four causes of immediate postpartum hemorrhage: uterine atony, lacerations, retained placental fragments, and hematomas.

Uterine Atony

Uterine atony, failure of the uterus to contract following birth, is a common cause of hemorrhage. Recall that the uterus must contract following separation of the placenta in order to compress the open blood vessels in the endometrium. If the uterus does not contract adequately, hemorrhage results (Figure 55-1 ■). Uterine atony can occur after any childbirth, but contributing factors that increase the risk include:

- Overdistention of the uterus from a large fetus, hydramnios, or multiple pregnancy
- Uterine contraction abnormalities as seen with rapid or prolonged labor
- Oxytocin administration for labor induction or labor augmentation
- Grand multiparity
- Drugs that cause uterine relaxation including but not limited to anesthesia, magnesium sulfate, terbutaline (Brethine) (These drugs were discussed in Chapter 53 ⃝⃝ .)
- Prolonged 3rd stage of labor
- Intrauterine infections
- Preeclampsia
- Operative birth

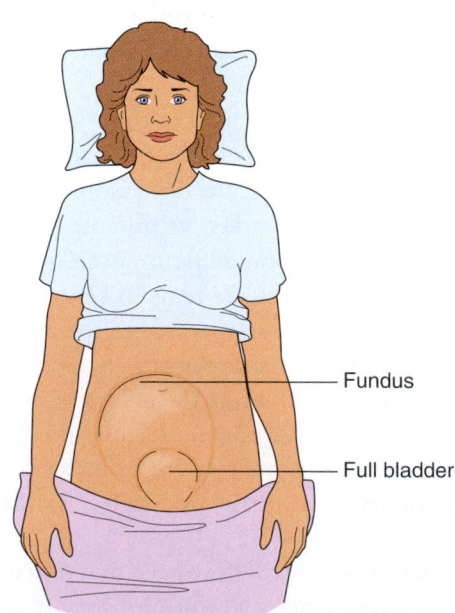

Fundus

Full bladder

Figure 55-1. ■ This illustration shows uterine displacement and deviation to the right caused by a full bladder. Uterine atony leads to excessive bleeding or hemorrhaging. The nurse monitors the number of pads that are saturated. Saturation of a sanitary pad within 1 hour signals excessive bleeding and must be reported.

- Retained placental fragments
- Placenta previa

Postpartum hemorrhage from uterine atony exhibits as a slow, steady trickle or as large clots. Large quantities of blood may pool in the body of the uterus, leaving the perineal pad and linen protectors suspiciously dry.

Ideally, good prenatal care, adequate nutrition, and management of complications as they occur can keep the risk of uterine atony to a minimum. Any woman at risk for uterine atony should be typed and crossmatched for blood prior to labor. If uterine atony occurs, the LPN/LVN should massage the fundus and summon help from the RN. Uterine massage, removal of uterine clots (see Procedure 54-1), and administration of medication and blood is generally not within the scope of LPN/LVN practice. The primary care provider should be notified as soon as possible. Severe uncontrolled hemorrhage may require radio-guided embolization of pelvic vessels (Poggi & Kapernick, 2003) or a hysterectomy to save the mother's life.

Lacerations

Lacerations of the perineum, vagina, and cervix commonly occur during the birthing process. Most often these lacerations are identified and sutured immediately following birth. Unrepaired lacerations should be suspected when vaginal bleeding occurs in the presence of a firmly contracted uterus.

Retained Placental Fragments

Retained placental fragments can be a cause of immediate and delayed postpartum hemorrhage. Following birth, the placenta must always be inspected for intactness. If fragmentation is identified, the uterus is explored to remove missing pieces of placental tissue. Curettage is done carefully to limit additional trauma to the uterus and to prevent additional bleeding.

Vulvar, Vaginal, and Pelvic Hematomas

A **hematoma** is an accumulation of blood in the soft tissue under the skin. Hematomas may be located in the tissue of the vulva, vagina, or pelvis. While those of the vulva and vagina are most common and most easily identified, hematomas of the pelvis are most dangerous because they may develop rapidly, contain 250 to 500 mL of blood, and have few symptoms.

Risk factors for the development of hematomas include first full-term birth, precipitous birth, macrosomia, forceps- or vacuum-assisted birth, and a history of vulvar varicosities.

Hematomas of the lower vagina and vulva that are less than 5 cm in size are usually treated with application of ice packs and analgesia. They usually resolve in a few days. Large hematomas may require surgical intervention in which an incision is made, the hematoma is removed,

bleeding vessels are ligated, and the wound is closed. Depending on the location, vaginal packing may be used to decrease additional bleeding.

DELAYED POSTPARTUM HEMORRHAGE

Delayed postpartum hemorrhage generally occurs within 1 to 2 weeks after childbirth. The most common cause of delayed postpartum hemorrhage is failure of the uterus to return to its normal size (**subinvolution**) due to retained placental fragments. Normally the placenta site is the last to regenerate after childbirth. In the case of subinvolution, the placenta site continues to bleed.

The lochia fails to progress from rubra to serosa to alba (see Chapter 54). Lochia rubra that continues longer than 2 weeks is suggestive of subinvolution. Besides lochia rubra, many women with delayed hemorrhage report scant or brown lochia, irregular heavy bleeding, leucorrhea, backache, and foul lochia. There may be a history of heavy early postpartum bleeding or retained placenta. Treatment may include administration of methylergonovine maleate (Methergine), antibiotics, and uterine curettage.

> ### clinical ALERT
>
> Most deaths from postpartum hemorrhage are not due to gross bleeding but to slow, steady blood loss over a period of hours or days. The prudent nurse assesses and documents blood loss frequently in the postpartum period. The new mother must be taught to observe for the amount and color of lochia and to report abnormalities to her primary care provider.

Postpartum Thromboembolic Disease

Thromboembolic disease can happen at any time, but it is considered a major postpartum complication. *Thrombus* (blood clot) formation can occur in superficial or deep veins, usually those of the legs, due to decrease venous blood flow. The thrombus acts as an irritant resulting in an inflammatory process; hence the name *thrombophlebitis. Pulmonary embolism* occurs when a thrombus is carried through the veins to the lungs.

Manifestations

The woman's coagulation system changes during pregnancy in preparation for stopping bleeding during the birth process. These changes increase the risk of thromboembolic disease in the postpartum mother. In addition to appearing in superficial or deep leg veins, thrombus formation can also occur in the vessels of the pelvis. Pelvic thrombophlebitis is associated with infection of the reproductive tract and is more common in women who underwent cesarean birth.

Symptoms of superficial and deep vein thrombophlebitis include pain in the calf with dorsiflexion (positive *Homans' sign*), redness, heat, and swelling of the affected leg. Movement of the affected limb can dislodge a blood clot increasing the risk of pulmonary embolism. For this reason, there is risk associated with assessing a Homans' sign. The LPN should consult the RN or physician to determine if this assessment should be performed. Symptoms of pelvic thrombophlebitis include abdominal and flank pain, fever, and tachycardia occurring the second or third day postpartum. Signs of pulmonary embolism include chest pain associated with shortness of breath, and *hemoptysis* (bloody sputum). A large embolism or multiple small emboli can result in death. These disorders are discussed in more detail in Chapter 34 ⚭ .

Treatment

It is best to prevent thrombus formation by encouraging early ambulation, assisting with leg exercises every 2 hours when in bed, elevating legs when sitting, applying anti-embolism stockings or sequential compression devices following cesarean birth, avoiding dehydration, and encouraging the mother to stop smoking.

If thrombus formation occurs, intravenous heparin is administered. Once symptoms have subsided, oral administration of Coumadin (sodium warfarin) is begun. The woman continues taking Coumadin for 2 to 6 months. It is important for the nurse to instruct the woman in the use of Coumadin, including follow-up blood testing and limiting the dietary intake of foods rich in vitamin K.

Postpartum Infections

MASTITIS

Mastitis (infection of the breast) occurs primarily in lactating women. The most common causative organisms are *Staphylococcus aureus, Haemophilus parainfluenzae, Haemophilus influenzae,* and *Streptococcus.* Bacteria invade the breast tissue though fissured or cracked nipples. Overdistention of the breast and *milk stasis* (pooling of milk in the mammary glands) are contributing factors. Transmission of bacteria is generally from the mouth and nose of the newborn, but could also be from dirty hands touching the breast, or through the mother's blood.

Preventive Measures

Mastitis may not occur for several weeks after delivery. It is important for the nurse to teach the mother how to prevent mastitis and to teach about its symptoms and treatment. Mastitis can be prevented through good hygiene practices, daily bathing, and hand washing prior to touching the nipple. Wearing a supportive bra, even in bed, will position the breast for proper drainage and prevent pooling of milk. Emptying the breast through nursing or breast pumping prevents overdistention. Consistent use of proper breastfeeding

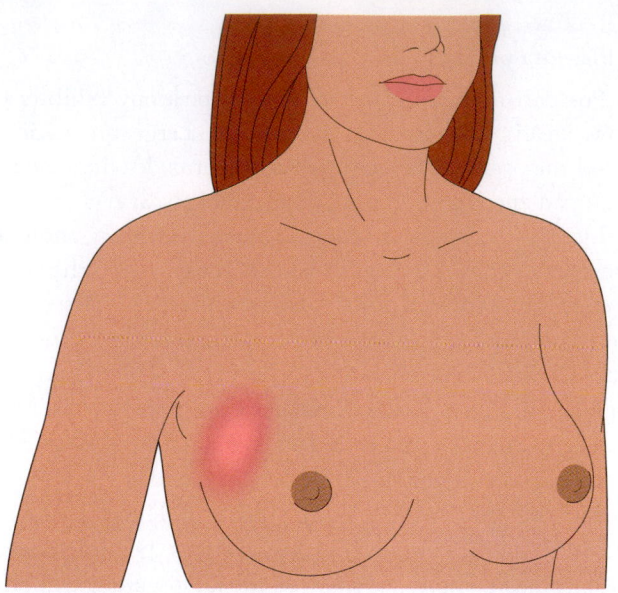

Figure 55-2. ■ Mastitis appears as tenderness, swelling, and erythema (shown here in the outer quadrant of the breast). Axillary lymph nodes may be swollen and tender. Mastitis redness often occurs in a V shape because of the shape of breast segments.

techniques will prevent cracked nipples. If symptoms of mastitis occur, it is important for the client to contact the primary care provider.

Manifestations

Symptoms of mastitis (Figure 55-2 ■ include redness and swelling of one or more lobes of the breast (often in a V-shaped wedge), fever, headache, breast pain, and flulike symptoms.

Treatment

Medical treatment generally includes antibiotics, moist heat applications, and analgesics. Emptying the breast with frequent breastfeeding or pumping decreases the duration of symptoms and speeds healing. Some mothers are concerned that the baby will become ill from the milk. Generally, this is not the case because of the antibiotic therapy. It is important for the mother to take the antibiotics as ordered.

WOUND INFECTION

In the postpartum period, lacerations, episiotomies, or cesarean incisions could become infected.

Preventive Measures

Keeping the area clean and dry can prevent wound infection. The client should be taught to shower daily, cover the abdominal incision with a clean dry dressing, rinse the perineum with warm water after each void or stool, and change the perineal pad at least every 2 hours.

Manifestations

Redness, swelling, pain, and purulent drainage are manifestations of a wound infection. An elevated temperature could also indicate infection. When infection is present, healing is delayed. If left untreated, *dehiscence* (opening) of the wound will occur. The client needs to be instructed to report any of these manifestations to the care provider without delay.

Treatment

Medical treatment includes antibiotics to prevent or treat an infection. In most cases, the infection clears without further complication. If the tissue is badly infected, it may need to be drained by surgical incision or removal of sutures. If the wound is deep, irrigation and packing may be needed.

POSTPARTUM (PUERPERAL) INFECTION

Postpartum (puerperal) infection is a rare infection of the uterus following childbirth. Contributing factors are listed in Box 55-3 ■. Strict aseptic technique used in the birthing process prevents this life-threatening complication.

Manifestations

Although the contamination occurs during the delivery process, it usually takes several days for the symptoms of infection to begin. The client may have been discharged by this time. It is important to teach the client to watch for the classic symptoms, including a fever of 100.4°F (38°C) or higher, chills, pelvic and abdominal pain, and foul-smelling lochia. If these symptoms occur, the client should contact the primary care provider immediately.

Treatment

Often, antibiotics are ordered if any of the contributing factors occurs during the delivery process. The infection usually begins in the vagina and migrates upward into the uterus (**endometritis**), pelvic lymph nodes, peritoneum (**peritonitis;** Figure 55-3 ■), and circulation. Once the organisms are growing in the blood, the disease has progressed to **septicemia.** If antibiotic treatment is not started immediately or if treatment is not effective, death can occur.

Antibiotics may be ordered for any of these contributing factors.

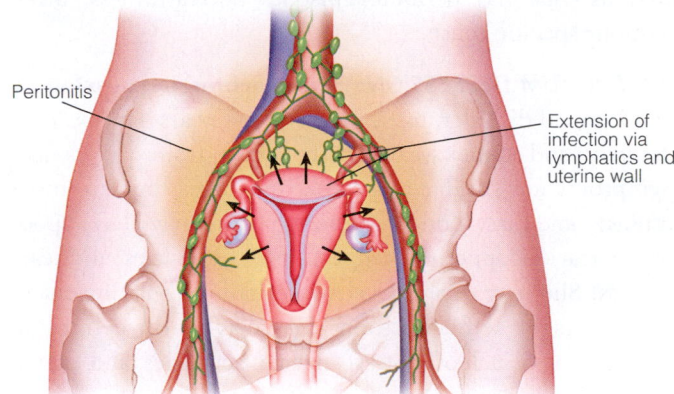

Figure 55-3. ■ Peritonitis may develop. The uterine infection can spread by way of the lymphatics and the uterine wall.

Peritonitis

Extension of infection via lymphatics and uterine wall

Postpartum Blues, Postpartum Depression, and Postpartum Psychosis

Emotional changes normally occur following birth. For most women, these emotional changes occur without major incident. However, for some women, the emotional adjustment to motherhood can become overwhelming and immobilizing (Figure 55-4 ■). It is critical that these women obtain professional assistance.

Manifestations

POSTPARTUM BLUES. Postpartum blues occur in most women. It is characterized by mild depression interspersed with happy feelings. Postpartum blues, related to changes in estrogen, progesterone, and prolactin levels, generally begin within a few days after birth and last a few hours to approximately 2 weeks. The new mother experiences feelings of being overwhelmed, unable to cope, fatigue, and

---

BOX 55-3	RISK FACTORS FOR POSTPARTUM (PUERPERAL) INFECTION

- Cesarean delivery
- Prolonged rupture of membranes
- Multiple vaginal examinations during labor
- Compromised health status of the mother (due to HIV, anemia, malnutrition, smoking, illicit drug/alcohol use)
- Obstetric trauma (lacerations, episiotomy)
- Intrauterine monitoring equipment
- Instrument-assisted delivery
- Manual removal of placenta
- Preexisting vaginal infections (STIs)

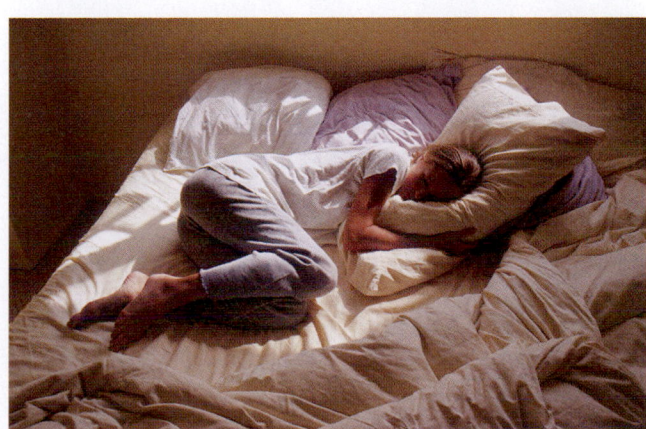

Figure 55-4. ■ Postpartum depression is profound, overwhelming depression that persists.

anxious. She has periodic episodes of tearfulness, often without specific cause.

POSTPARTUM DEPRESSION. **Postpartum depression,** a major mood disorder, most frequently appears 4 weeks post delivery and upon weaning the child from the breast. Symptoms are similar to postpartum blues, but are more intense and last longer. The woman may have poor concentration, appetite changes, sleep difficulties, and tearfulness. She may express feelings of failure, making many statements of self-accusation. She may have feelings of worthlessness, lack of interest in usual activities, and lack of concern for her appearance.

POSTPARTUM PSYCHOSIS. Postpartum psychosis is considered an emergency because of the risk of suicide and infanticide. Symptoms include agitation, insomnia, hyperactivity, confusion, irrationality, poor judgment, delusions, and hallucinations.

Risk factors for postpartum depression and psychosis are included in Box 55-4 ■. There are similarities between postpartum blues, depression, and psychosis. Although postpartum blues are common and to some extent expected, symptoms can progress to postpartum depression and the more serious postpartum psychosis. Several months after delivery, women have limited contact with their healthcare providers. Therefore, assessment and diagnosis of postpartum depression and psychosis may go unrecognized. It is critical for the nurse to identify women at risk, teach them and their families the signs and symptoms, and encourage them to seek assistance if signs of depression become worse or continue for more than 2 weeks.

BOX 55-4 RISK FACTORS FOR POSTPARTUM DEPRESSION AND PSYCHOSIS

Postpartum Depression
- Primipara
- Contradictory feelings about the pregnancy
- History of postpartum depression (most significant)
- History of depression or bipolar illness
- Family history of psychiatric disorders
- Lack of stable relationship with partner or parents
- Lack of social support
- Body image disorders, including eating disorders
- History of drug and/or alcohol abuse

Postpartum Psychosis
- Previous puerperal psychosis
- History of bipolar (manic-depressive) disorder
- Prenatal stressors: lack of social support, lack of a partner, low socioeconomic status
- Obsessive personality
- Family history of mood disorders

The treatment of postpartum depression and psychosis includes a combination of medications. The role of the LPN/LVN in the care of women with mental health disorders is to:

- Assist the charge nurse and mental health professional in monitoring the symptoms of depression and psychosis.
- Monitor for side effects of medication.
- Be supportive to the family.

Diagnosis and Treatment

Diagnosis is made by analyzing the results of one or more depression assessment scales. Box 55-5 ■ provides the Edinburgh Postnatal Depression Scale. Table 55-1 ■ shows the Postpartum Depression Predictors Inventory.

Ideally these assessment scales would be used in each trimester of pregnancy to assess the mother's risk status, and again before discharge from the postpartum unit. Family members can help with infant care and household responsibilities, while watching for and reporting signs that the mother is (or is not) returning to a more normal mood.

Postpartum blues resolve within a few weeks and do not require medical intervention. Postpartum depression and postpartum psychosis require both medical and psychiatric treatment. Treatment is directed at the specific symptoms and may include medication, individual and group counseling, and assistance with meeting child care and family needs. Many of the drugs used to treat depression and psychosis are contraindicated in breastfeeding women.

The safety of the child is a primary concern. Refer to a mental health textbook for complete information about treatment of these disorders.

Nursing Considerations

The assessment, plan, and evaluation of care of the high-risk postpartum client are similar to the routine care of any postpartum client. The additional treatment of specific complications consists of administering medication and teaching the client and family about this complication.

Maternal Death

In developed areas of the world, it is rare for the mother to die in childbirth. Prenatal, intrapartum, and postpartum care contribute to the survival of the mother.

When a woman does die, it is usually after her condition has deteriorated over a period of time. She (or family members) may express concern about her condition. They may ask questions that are difficult to answer or for which there is no answer. They may seek information about what is happening physiologically, what treatment is being provided, and why it is not working. The nurse, working alone, may not be able to answer questions thoroughly due to the need to assist the primary care provider and to provide treatments and care. In this

BOX 55-5   EDINBURGH POSTNATAL DEPRESSION SCALE

In the past 7 days:

1. I have been able to laugh and see the funny side of things
   As much as I always could
   Not quite so much now
   Definitely not so much now
   Not at all

2. I have looked forward with enjoyment of things
   As much as I ever did
   Rather less than I used to
   Definitely less than I used to
   Hardly at all

3. * I have blamed myself unnecessarily when things went wrong
   Yes, most of the time
   Yes some of the time
   Not very often
   No, never

4. I have been anxious or worried for no good reason
   No, not at all
   Hardly ever
   Yes, sometimes
   Yes, very often

5. * I have felt scared or panicky for no good reason
   Yes, quite a lot
   Yes sometimes
   No not much
   No, not at all

6. * Things have been getting on top of me
   Yes, most of the time I have not been able to cope at all
   Yes, sometimes I have not been coping as well as usual
   No, I have been coping quite well
   No, I have been coping as well as ever

7. I have been so unhappy that I have had difficulty sleeping
   Yes, most of the time
   Yes, sometimes
   Not very often
   No, not at all

8. * I have felt sad or miserable
   Yes, most of the time
   Yes, quite often
   Not very often
   No, not at all

9. * I have been so unhappy that I have been crying
   Yes, most of the time
   Yes, quite often
   Only occasionally
   No, never

10. The thought of harming myself has occurred to me
    Yes, quite often
    Sometimes
    Hardly ever
    Never

Note: Response categories are scored 0, 1, 2, and 3 according to increased severity of the symptoms. Items marked with an asterisk (*) are reverse scored (3, 2, 1, 0). The total score is calculated by adding the scores for each of the 10 items. A score above the threshold of 12–13 out of 30 indicates, with 86% sensitivity, that the woman is suffering from postpartum depression.

Source: Cox, J. L., Holden, J. M., & Sagovsky, R. (1987). Detection of postnatal depression: Development of the 10-item Edinburgh Postnatal Depression Scale. *British Journal of Psychiatry, 150,* 782–786. Users may reproduce the scale without further permission provided they respect copyright by quoting the names of the author, the title, and the source of the paper in all reproduced copies.

TABLE 55-1   Postpartum Depression Predictors Inventory (PDPI)—Revised—and Guide Questions for Its Use

DURING PREGNANCY	FILL IN CIRCLE AS APPROPRIATE	
Marital Status		
Single	O	
Married/cohabiting	O	
Separated	O	
Divorced	O	
Widowed	O	
Partnered	O	
Socioeconomic Status		
Low	O	
Middle	O	
High	O	
Self-esteem	Yes	No
Do you feel good about yourself as a person?	O	O
Do you feel worthwhile?	O	O
Do you feel you have a number of good qualities as a person?	O	O

(continued)

TABLE 55-1	Postpartum Depression Predictors Inventory (PDPI)—Revised—and Guide Questions for Its Use (continued)		
DURING PREGNANCY			**FILL IN CIRCLE AS APPROPRIATE**

DURING PREGNANCY	Yes	No
Prenatal Depression		
1. Have you felt depressed during your pregnancy?	O	O
If yes, when and how long have you been feeling this way?		
If yes, how mild or severe would you consider your depression?		
Prenatal Anxiety		
Have you been feeling anxious during your pregnancy?	O	O
If yes, how long have you been feeling this way?		
Unplanned/Unwanted Pregnancy		
Was the pregnancy planned?	O	O
Is the pregnancy unwanted?	O	O
History of Previous Depression		
1. Before this pregnancy, have you ever been depressed?	O	O
If yes, when did you experience this depression?		
If yes, have you been under a physician's care for this past depression?	O	O
If yes, did the physician prescribe any medication for your depression?	O	O
Social Support		
1. Do you feel you receive adequate emotional support from your partner?	O	O
2. Do you feel you receive adequate instrumental support from your partner (e.g., help with household chores or baby-sitting)?	O	O
3. Do you feel you can rely on your partner when you need help?	O	O
4. Do you feel you can confide in your partner?	O	O
(Repeat same questions for family and again for friends)		
Marital Satisfaction		
1. Are you satisfied with your marriage (or living arrangement)?	O	O
2. Are you currently experiencing any marital problems?	O	O
3. Are things going well between you and your partner?	O	O
Life Stress		
Are you currently experiencing any stressful events in your life such as:		
financial problems	O	O
marital problems	O	O
death in the family	O	O
serious illness in the family	O	O
moving	O	O
unemployment	O	O
job change		
After delivery, add the following items		
Child Care Stress		
1. Is your infant experiencing any health problems?	O	O
2. Are you having problems feeding your baby?	O	O
3. Are you having problems with your baby sleeping?	O	O
Infant Temperament		
1. Would you consider your baby irritable?	O	O
2. Does your baby cry a lot?	O	O
3. Is your baby difficult to console or soothe?	O	O
Maternity Blues		
1. Do you experience a brief period of tearfulness and mood swings during the 1st week after delivery?	O	O

Source: AWHONN. (2002). Beck, C. T. Revision of the postpartum predictors inventory. *Journal of Obstetrics, Gynecologic and Neonatal Nursing*, 31(4): 394–402. (Table 2 on PDPI, pp. 399–400). Washington, DC: Author. © 2002 by the Association of Women's' Health, Obstetric and Neonatal Nurses. All rights reserved.

situation, the nurse should call for additional assistance from the charge nurse, social worker, or clergy.

When the nurse is able to communicate with the family of a woman who is dying, care must be taken to listen to their questions and respond appropriately. Generally, the family will ask for reassurance that everything possible is being done. At this time of great emotional stress, a detailed explanation of the pathology and treatment being provided is not the best answer. (It is the role and responsibility of the physician and primary care provider to answer these questions.) The nurse should respond with statements such as:

- "I know this is extremely difficult. As soon as possible, the doctor will answer your questions."
- "Can you tell me your understanding of what is happening? Maybe I can clarify what is going on."
- "I understand your fear and impatience. It seems to take a long time, doesn't it? Can I call someone to sit with you? A family member or clergy?"

When death of the mother does occur, the entire family structure is disrupted. The surviving partner is faced with the care of the newborn (and possibly other children) at a time when emotional resources are low. Each family member needs to work through the grief process. This process is detailed in Chapter 18 ⚭. Referral to social services can help the family mobilize resources such as counseling before potential problems develop.

The death of the mother also takes an emotional toll on the nurses and medical staff. Feelings of guilt, anger, fear, sadness, and depression can impact the care of other clients. The nurses and medical staff need to review the situation surrounding the events, medical record, and what (if anything) could be done differently in the future. A critical incident debriefing helps staff cope with feelings and emotions that result from a maternal death.

NURSING CARE

PRIORITIZING NURSING CARE

Priorities in nursing care for the high-risk postpartum mother are:

- Assessing for and stopping hemorrhage.
- Assessing for and controlling preeclampsia.
- Assessing for and treating postpartum infections.
- Assessing for postpartum depression and postpartum psychosis and making appropriate referral.

ASSESSING

Assessing the high-risk postpartum mother is the same as for any postpartum mother. It is important for the nurse to recognize signs of complications and to take action.

DIAGNOSING, PLANNING, AND IMPLEMENTING

Nursing diagnoses might include:

- *Deficient Fluid Volume* related to excessive postpartum bleeding
- *Risk for Injury* related to seizure activity
- *Risk for Infection* related to breast feeding, surgical incision, or episiotomy
- *Ineffective Coping* related to postpartum depression or postpartum psychosis

Expected outcomes might include:

- Adequate fluid volume as evidenced by stable vital signs and urinary output greater than 50 mL per hour.
- No evidence of injury.
- No signs of infection, temperature within normal limits.
- Postpartum depression or psychosis identified and appropriate referral made.

Interventions include:

- Controlling postpartum bleeding by massaging the fundus. *Fundal massage stimulates uterine contractions, which decrease uterine bleeding.*
- Notify RN or primary care provider when fundal massage is ineffective to control bleeding. *Bleeding caused by lacerations or retained placental fragments will not be controlled by fundal massage. The RN and primary care provider must be notified and medical intervention employed to control bleeding.*
- Administer intravenous fluids or blood transfusion as ordered. Encourage oral intake of fluids to replace lost fluid volume. *Intravenous and oral fluids are needed to replace fluid volume. Blood transfusion may be needed. In some states blood administration is not an LPN/LVN function. However, the LPN/LVN may assist in monitoring the mother receiving blood.*
- Administer intravenous medication as ordered to prevent seizures associated with preeclampsia. *The administration of intravenous medication to prevent seizure activity may not be within LPN/LVN scope of practice. The LPN/LVN may assist in monitoring the preeclamptic mother.*
- Encourage hygiene practices to prevent postpartum infection. Provide hygiene instruction as necessary. *The best method of preventing infection is to practice handwashing and perineal care.*
- Encourage mother to discuss her feelings of becoming a new mother. Encourage her to complete a postpartum depression scale. Inform the RN if she expresses feelings associated with depression. *When postpartum depression is identified early and treatment begun, postpartum psychosis can be prevented or lessened and injury to the mother and her child (children) may be prevented.*
- Teach the mother and her partner the signs of complications, and when to notify the primary care provider. *Some complications do not develop for several days postpartum. The mother and her partner should know possible signs to watch for and when to notify the primary care provider.*

EVALUATING

Prior to discharge the mother's vital signs should be within normal limits. Her vaginal flow should be moderate rubra and there should be no drainage from an abdominal incision. She should be voiding adequate amounts every 2 to 3 hours. If she experienced preeclampsia, her reflexes should be approaching normal ranges. The mother and her partner should verbalize an understanding of the teaching provided and when to notify her primary care provider if signs of complications develop.

NURSING PROCESS CARE PLAN
Client at Risk for Deep Vein Thrombosis

C.S., a 35-year-old gravida 3, para 2, is transferred from the birthing unit following a primary cesarean section for severe preeclampsia. She is on a PCA pump for postoperative pain. Her husband is at the bedside.

Assessment

The following data should be collected as soon as possible after admission:

- Vital signs and pain
- Lung sounds
- Bowel sounds
- Fundus firmness and bleeding
- Deep tendon reflexes
- Response to test for Homans' sign
- Skin on legs—color, moisture, temperature
- Urinary output
- Edema
- Capillary refill
- Incision

Nursing Diagnosis

The following important nursing diagnoses (among others) are established for this client:

- *Ineffective Peripheral Tissue Perfusion* related to surgical procedure and immobility
- *Acute Pain* related to surgical procedure
- *Risk for Infection* (respiratory and incisional) related to surgical procedure

Expected Outcomes

The outcomes for this client will include, but are not limited to, the following:

- Client will have adequate tissue perfusion in lower extremities as evidenced by lack of symptoms of deep vein thrombosis.

- Client will have adequate pain control as evidenced by verbalizing pain relief.
- Client will have no infection as evidenced by lack of respiratory or incisional symptoms.

Planning and Implementation

Nursing interventions for this client would include the following:

- Discuss with client the importance of increasing mobility following surgery. *Compliance may be increased when the client understands the risks of immobility.*
- Increase mobility as tolerated. *Mobility causes calf muscle contraction, which enhances venous return and thus decreases the risk for thrombus formation.*
- As ordered, implement thromboembolic stockings, intermittent pneumatic compression devices, or venous foot pump compression devices. *These devices work in the same manner as ambulation to prevent thrombus formation.*
- Continue to assess for signs and symptoms of thrombus formation. *Symptom recognition will facilitate prompt treatment.*
- Administer pain medication as ordered. *Pain medication will allow client to rest, to move freely, and will facilitate healing.*
- Encourage client to do turn, cough, and deep breathe (TCDB) exercises every 2 hours. *Pooling of lung secretions increases risk for respiratory infection. TCDB will help client remove secretions from airways. Repositioning the client also facilitates comfort.*
- Provide dressing changes as ordered. *Changing wet dressings eliminates a reservoir for microorganisms and decreases the risk of incisional infection.*

Evaluation

The client verbalizes an understanding of the risks of thrombus formation and implements preventive measures. There will be no development of symptoms of deep vein thrombosis or infection. Client verbalizes comfort.

Critical Thinking in the Nursing Process

1. How can the nurse encourage movement when the client is in pain and states that movement greatly increases her pain?
2. What is the nurse's responsibility when he or she assesses that the client's husband is not allowing his wife to get out of bed in an effort to conserve her energy?
3. Discuss hygiene issues related to the TED (support) hose.

Note: Discussion of Critical Thinking questions appears on the MyNursingKit Website.

Note: The references and resources for all chapters have been compiled at the back of the book.

Chapter Review

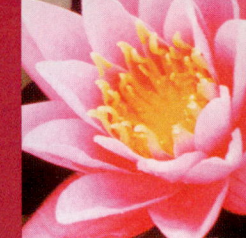

KEY Points

- Puerperal complications must be identified early in the postpartum period to prevent serious life-threatening conditions.
- Uncontrolled bleeding can become a life-threatening event and excessive bleeding must be reported immediately to the RN and primary care provider.
- Client teaching about self-care in the postpartum period is a continuous process that occurs with each interaction.
- Preeclampsia can continue into the postpartum period and treatment must continue until the blood pressure and reflexes return to normal ranges.
- Postpartum infections can occur if hygiene measures are not followed.
- Some mothers have difficulty adjusting to motherhood and must be monitored for depression and psychosis. Immediate referral is needed to prevent injury to the mother and her child (children).

FOR FURTHER Study

Discussion of the grief process is in Chapter 18.

Disorders including embolism or multiple small emboli are discussed in more detail in Chapter 34.

High-risk complications, such as preeclampsia and Rh incompatibility, are discussed in Chapter 52.

Drugs that cause uterine relaxation were discussed in Chapter 53.

Lochia and other normal postpartum considerations are discussed in Chapter 54.

Critical Thinking Care Map

Caring for a Postpartum Client at Risk
NCLEX® Focus Area: Coping and Adaptation

Case Study: Mandy, a 19-year-old, G1, P1, is transferred from labor and delivery to the postpartum unit following vaginal birth of a 5-pound, 2-ounce male. Mandy labored for 15 hours and had a second-degree, midline episiotomy. Her history reveals she had no prenatal care, her drug screen was positive for cocaine, and she is unemployed.

Nursing Diagnosis: *Risk for Impaired Parent–Infant Attachment* related to drug use

COLLECT DATA

Subjective	Objective
_____	_____
_____	_____
_____	_____
_____	_____
_____	_____
_____	_____

Would you report this? Yes/No

If yes, report to: _____

What would you report? _____

Nursing Care

_____
_____
_____
_____
_____
_____
_____
_____
_____

How would you document this? _____
_____
_____
_____

Compare your answers and documentation to those provided on the MyNursingKit Website.

Data Collected
(use only those that apply)

- Positive drug screen
- No prenatal care
- No employment
- States "Leave the child in the nursery."
- "Where can my boyfriend sleep tonight?"
- VS: T 99.0, P 58, R 12, BP 120/70
- Fundus firm, 1 FB above umbilicus
- Scant amount of lochia
- No eye contact made with baby
- Asks "Will the nurses change the baby's diapers? I don't ever want to do that."

Nursing Interventions
(use only those that apply; list in priority order)

- Take the newborn into the client's room, even if she has not requested him.
- Inquire about the child's name.
- Reassess fundal height every 4 hours.
- Report to the charge nurse behaviors that indicate impaired bonding.
- Encourage the client to put the baby up for adoption.
- Teach the client about birth control methods.
- Teach the client about caring for a newborn.
- Continue to assess mother–child interaction.

NCLEX-PN® Exam Preparation

1 The nurse is caring for a client who delivered a 34-week, premature infant 4 hours ago secondary to preeclampsia. While performing an assessment, the nurse finds elevated blood pressure, reflexes more than 2+, and 2 clonus beats in response to sudden dorsiflexion of the foot. The nurse recognizes the need to monitor this client closely for:

1. Postpartum hemorrhage.
2. Kidney failure.
3. Seizure activity.
4. Impaired maternal–child bonding.

2 The nurse uses which of the following to most accurately indicate blood loss by the postpartum client during delivery?

1. Blood loss estimate by the delivering obstetrician
2. Blood pressure
3. Red blood cell count
4. Hematocrit

3 The nurse is caring for a postpartum client who reportedly delivered a fragmented placenta. The nurse recognizes that this client is at increased risk for:

1. Postpartum hemorrhage.
2. Newborn with congenital anomalies.
3. Postpartum infection.
4. Eclampsia.

4 A woman delivered a full-term infant vaginally with her feet elevated in stirrups for 2 hours while pushing, and sustained a fourth-degree perineal laceration. Postpartum, the client is reluctant to get out of bed secondary to pain. This client is at increased risk for:

1. Postpartum hemorrhage.
2. Thromboembolic disease.
3. Impaired maternal–child bonding.
4. Maternal death.

5 The nurse is providing postpartum teaching to the breast-feeding client in order to reduce the risk of mastitis. Which of the following are important strategies to teach the mother? (Select all that apply.)

1. Good hygiene practices
2. Handwashing prior to touching the nipples
3. Wearing a supportive bra at all times
4. Adequate emptying of the breast
5. Antibiotic ointment applied to cracked or fissured nipples.

6 The nurse is caring for a postpartum client who was delivered of a preterm infant secondary to preeclampsia yesterday. The mother's blood pressure has returned to prepregnancy levels and there is no longer protein in the urine. The nurse anticipates that:

1. Magnesium sulfate will be changed from IV to PO.
2. Magnesium sulfate will be turned off.

3. 1Magnesium sulfate drip will be gradually reduced.
4. Magnesium sulfate will be continued for 24 hours after last symptoms subside.

7 The nurse teaches the postpartum client who delivered vaginally to perform which of the following to reduce the risk of infection of the episiotomy?

1. Rinse the perineum with warm water 3 to 4 times per day.
2. Avoid defecating for 2 to 3 days after delivery.
3. Change the perineal pad at least every 2 hours.
4. Cover the incision with a clean dry dressing after each void.

8 The nurse makes a home visit to the postpartum client 1 week after delivery and finds the client mildly depressed. The client says she has happy feelings every once in a while but feels overwhelmed, tired, and unable to cope. The nurse recognizes the client is experiencing:

1. Postpartum depression.
2. Postpartum blues.
3. Postpartum psychosis.
4. Impaired maternal–child bonding.

9 The nurse, working on the postpartum unit, recognizes that which of the following clients is at greatest risk for postpartum psychosis?

1. The client whose husband lost his job a few weeks ago and insists on everything in her room being kept in a specific location
2. The client who expresses concern with the physical changes in her body
3. The client with a history of alcohol abuse
4. The client with a family history of mental health disorders

10 The nurse, working in the newborn nursery, is caring for a neonate whose mother died suddenly after delivery despite experiencing a normal pregnancy. During a family visit to see the baby, the father says, "I just don't understand why my wife died. Did the doctor make a mistake? Is there a problem with equipment in the delivery room? Something must have gone wrong!" The nurse's priority action at this time would be to:

1. Call for risk management to speak with the baby's father.
2. Reassure the father that everything was done properly and the mother's death was not the hospital's fault.
3. Call the nursing supervisor or physician to speak with the father.
4. Explain what happened in great detail, explaining the pathophysiology of the event.

Answers and rationales for Review Questions appear in Appendix I.

Care of Normal Neonates

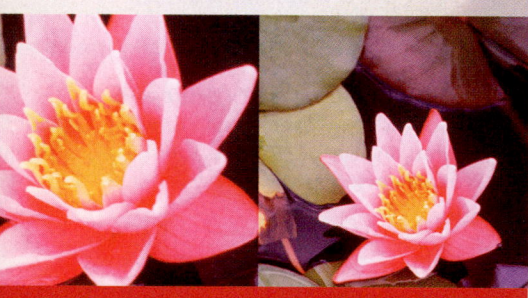

LEARNING Outcomes

After completing this chapter, you will be able to:

1. Identify physiologic adaptations of the neonate.
2. Describe the use and method of obtaining an Apgar score.
3. List aspects of delivery room care and nursing interventions for the neonate.
4. Explain nursery care of the neonate.
5. List differences that identify the gestational age of the neonate.
6. Describe the physical characteristics of the neonate.
7. Explain proper hygiene methods in caring for a newborn.
8. Compare and contrast two methods of providing neonatal nutrition.
9. Identify common procedures in care of the newborn.
10. Provide discharge teaching to parents of a newborn.

Clinical Objectives

11. Assist in assessment and observation of the newborn during the immediate postnatal period.
12. Collect data about a neonate and chart it accurately.
13. Recognize the normal variations in the newborn.
14. Provide appropriate newborn care.

KEY TERMS

Use the audio glossary feature on the MyNursingKit Website to hear the correct pronunciation of the following key terms.

acrocyanosis 1538	jaundice 1541	retractions 1532
apneic spells 1532	lanugo 1538	rooting reflex 1544
Babinski's reflex 1544	meconium 1543	smegma 1543
caput succedaneum 1541	milia 1541	stepping reflex 1544
cephalhematoma 1541	Mongolian spot 1541	stork bites 1541
circumcision 1548	Moro (or startle) reflex 1544	strabismus 1541
cold stress 1533	ophthalmia neonatorum 1545	sucking reflex 1544
conduction 1533	palmar grasp reflex 1544	syndactyly 1543
convection 1533	periodic breathing 1542	telangiectatic nevi 1541
ecchymosis 1538	petechiae 1538	thermoregulation 1533
Epstein's pearls 1541	plantar grasp reflex 1544	tonic neck reflex 1544
erythema toxicum neonatorum 1541	polydactyly 1543	vernix 1534
	pseudomenstruation 1543	webbing 1543
evaporation 1533	radiation 1533	witches' milk 1542

The *neonate* is the infant from delivery through the first month of life. Initial care revolves around meeting the basic biologic needs and helping the newborn adjust to life outside the womb. The LPN/LVN often works in the newborn nursery applying the principles of the fundamentals of care of the neonate. Prompt recognition of abnormal events or conditions and of the basic needs of the infant ensure quality nursing care. This chapter explores the fundamental care of the normal neonate.

Physiologic Adaptations to Life

An understanding of the physiologic adaptation to life outside the uterus guides the nurse's actions when setting priorities in the care of the newborn. They are presented here in the order of priority (airway, breathing, circulation, and thermoregulation) to set the foundation for newborn care.

RESPIRATORY ADAPTATION

Because the fetus does not breathe inside the uterus, the nurse's first priority is to assist the newborn in establishing respirations. Using the bulb syringe or suction catheter, the nurse removes mucus, vaginal secretions, and amniotic fluid from the newborn's airway. Because the infant is positioned with the head down, fluids continue to drain and must be removed.

Breathing

Breathing is initiated because of several factors. As the infant moves through the birth canal, the chest is compressed, increasing the intrathoracic pressure. Once the chest has been delivered, the intrathoracic pressure decreases, sucking a small amount of air into the lungs. Once the umbilical cord is clamped, the infant's PCO_2 increases stimulating the respiratory center in the medulla. The intrauterine temperature

is approximately 20°F higher than the room temperature following delivery. This change in temperature also stimulates breathing. Sensory, auditory, visual, and tactile stimulation helps encourage breathing.

Breathing usually begins spontaneously (Figure 56-1 ■). However, some newborns need to be stimulated; this is done by rubbing the skin or tapping the feet. If the newborn's

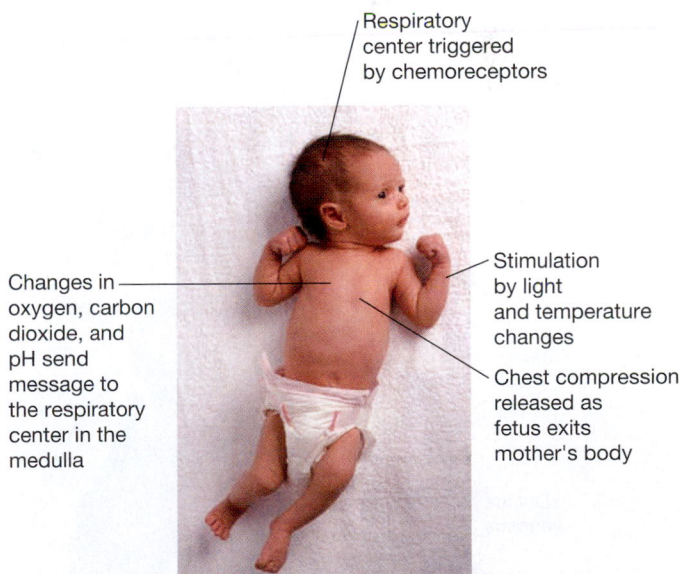

Respiratory center triggered by chemoreceptors

Changes in oxygen, carbon dioxide, and pH send message to the respiratory center in the medulla

Stimulation by light and temperature changes

Chest compression released as fetus exits mother's body

Figure 56-1. ■ Respiratory adaptation of the newborn. The infant's chest is compressed as it moves through the birth canal. Compression is released as it exits the mother's body, allowing air to be drawn into the expanding lungs to replace the amniotic fluid. As blood levels of oxygen and the infant's pH decrease, and as blood levels of carbon dioxide increase, the respiratory center in the medulla triggers changes that cause the diaphragm to contract. Cold air and light further stimulate the respiratory center, causing the newborn to breathe. (Dorling Kindersley Media Library.)

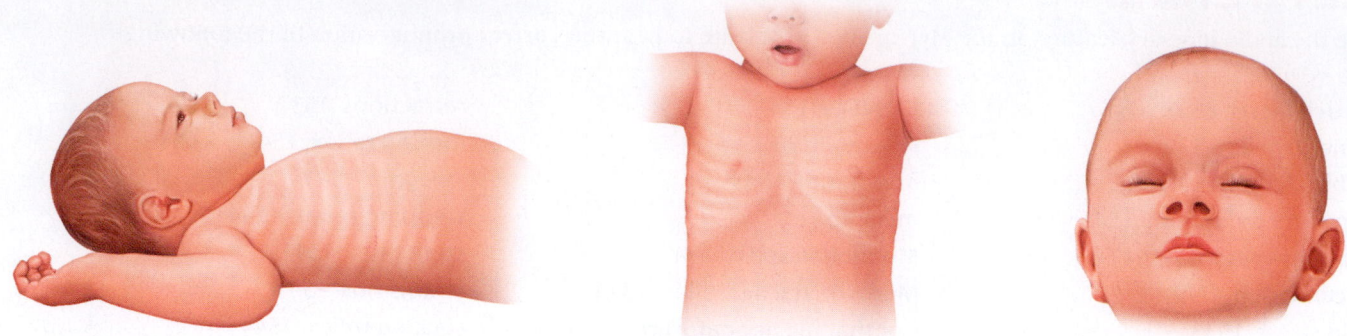

Figure 56-2. ■ Respiratory distress in an infant can be seen by retraction of the skin over the ribs and sternum and by flaring of the nostrils.

respiratory effort is weak or absent, the nurse or respiratory therapist will use an Ambu-bag and mask to breathe for the newborn. Oxygen can be administered by mask to prevent hypoxia.

Respiratory Distress

The neonate should be observed frequently for signs of respiratory distress (Figure 56-2 ■). Subtle changes indicate that the infant is having difficulty maintaining gas exchange. The earliest sign is *nasal flaring* (outward movement of the nostrils), followed by *expiratory grunting* (noisy exhalation). The nurse must listen carefully for this "grunting" noise, as it often sounds like a small squeak rather than an actual grunt. If the distress continues, intracostal, subcostal, and substernal **retractions** (inward movement of the tissues over the chest), may occur. **Apneic spells** (periods without breathing) indicate a worsening of the respiratory distress. Signs of respiratory distress must be reported immediately to the registered nurse and physician (see Box 57-6 ⚭ Collecting Data about Newborn Distress).

CARDIOVASCULAR ADAPTATION

Circulation

The newborn's cardiovascular system must adapt to life outside the uterus. Fetal circulation contains several structures that must close shortly after delivery (Figure 56-3 ■). Circulatory changes occur as a result of change in thoracic pressure inside the heart and large blood vessels. With breathing, more blood flow is needed through the pulmonary arteries. Initially, an increase in pressure inside the aorta causes a "reverse blood flow" through the ductus arteriosus,

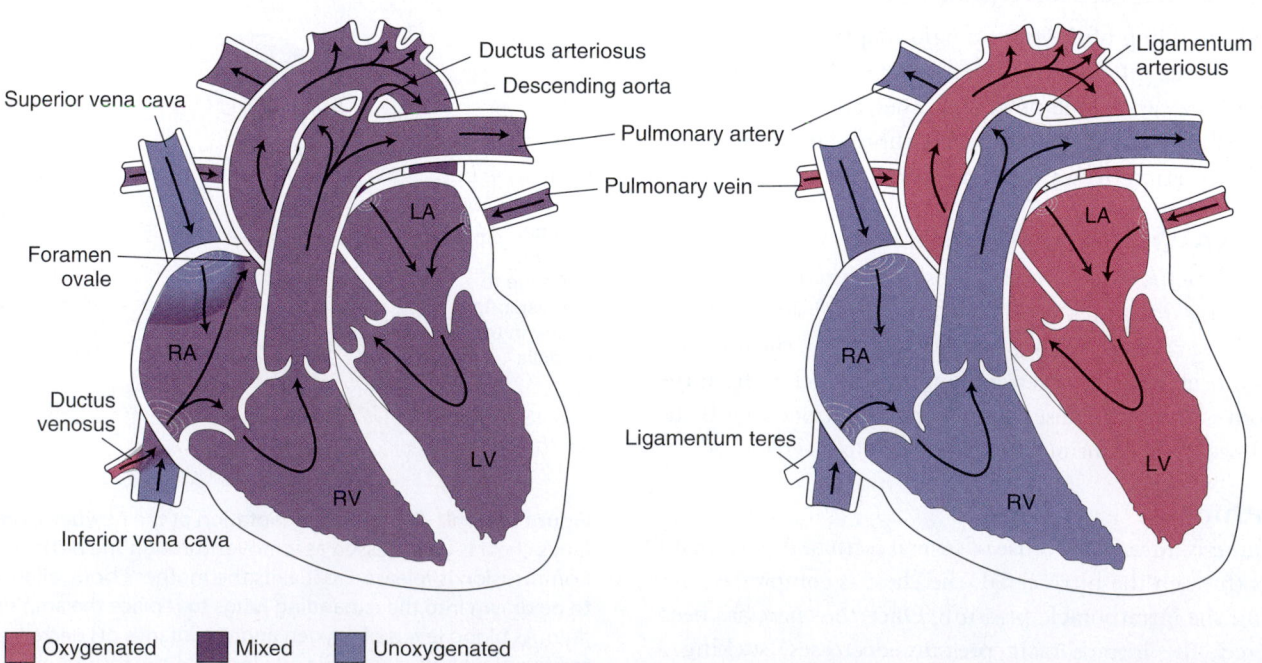

Figure 56-3. ■ The newborn circulatory system. The arrows indicate the flow of blood through the heart; the color indicates the level of oxygen saturation in the blood. **A.** Fetal circulation. **B.** Pulmonary circulation in the neonate after birth. LA = left atrium; LV = left ventricle, RA = right atrium; RV = right ventricle.

increasing the amount of blood reaching the lungs. As this increased amount of blood returns to the left atrium, the pressure in the left atrium increases, closing the foramen ovale within minutes. Within 24 to 48 hours the ductus arteriosus begins to close. Permanent closure of the foramen ovale and ductus arteriosus may take 1 to 3 months. Once conversion from fetal circulation to neonatal circulation is complete, blood flow is identical to that in the adult. Refer to Chapter 33 ⚭ for a review of normal blood flow through the heart.

THERMOREGULATORY ADAPTATION

The infant must immediately begin **thermoregulation,** maintenance of body heat. Thermoregulation involves a balance between heat production, heat retention, and heat loss. Newborns, unable to shiver to produce heat like adults do, produce heat by increasing metabolism through crying and movement. Newborns have deposits of brown fat at the back of the neck, between the scapula, in the axilla, and around the kidneys and heart. If their temperature is not raised by metabolism, they will burn this brown fat. If all the brown fat is metabolized, infants no longer have this method of heat production. Newborns have difficulty retaining heat. By staying in a flexed position, the amount of exposed skin is limited. Peripheral vasoconstriction also helps the newborn to retain heat, but as long as some blood can flow through the vessels, there will be some heat loss.

Heat loss in an infant can be a life-threatening situation. With limited subcutaneous fat, peripheral blood vessels are close to the skin. Heat moves from the warm internal environment to the cooler air. **Cold stress** occurs when excessive heat is lost. The infant's metabolism increases in an attempt to maintain the body temperature. This increase in metabolism leads to an increased need for oxygen. If there is not enough oxygen available due to hypoventilation of alveoli, the infant may experience *hypoxemia* (decreased blood oxygen) and hypothermia. Hypothermia decreases the production of surfactant, which in turn hinders lung expansion, leading to more respiratory distress. Decreased blood oxygen may lead to pulmonary vasoconstriction and a further worsening of the condition. With an increase in metabolism, stores of glycogen may be depleted resulting in hypoglycemia. When brown fat is metabolized, fatty acids are released resulting in metabolic acidosis.

Heat is lost by four methods (Figure 56-4 ■). **Conduction** is heat lost by direct contact with a cooler object. When a newborn is placed on a cold scale, or touched by cold hands or stethoscope, heat is lost by conduction. **Convection** is heat lost by the movement of air. Air currents from an open window, fan, or people moving around the room can cause the infant to lose heat. **Evaporation** is heat lost when water is changed to vapor. When a newborn is wet with amniotic

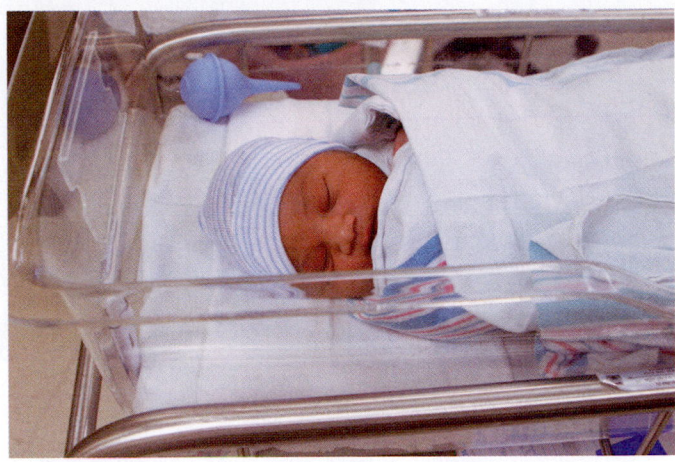

Figure 56-4. ■ Heat can be lost very easily from the neonate. It is important to keep the head covered and the feet and hands warm.

fluid or water during a bath, heat will be lost by evaporation. **Radiation** is heat lost by transfer to cooler objects that are nearby, but not in direct contact. An infant placed near a cold window will transfer heat to the cold window, thereby losing body heat.

It is important to dry the infant as soon as possible. Rubbing the infant with warm blankets not only dries the skin but also stimulates breathing. The infant can be placed next to the mother's skin and covered with a blanket or placed under a radiant warmer. The infant's head should be covered with a cap to prevent heat loss through the scalp. The infant should not be bathed until the temperature has stabilized. When the infant is bathed, care should be taken to prevent heat loss.

Delivery Room Care

APGAR SCORE

The newborn's adaptation to life outside the uterus is evaluated at 1 minute and at 5 minutes of age, using an Apgar score (Table 56-1 ■ and Procedure 56-1 ■). This evaluation method can also be used anytime the newborn's condition is in question. As shown in Table 56-1, each item—heart rate, respiratory rate, muscle tone, reflex irritability, and color—is assigned a score of 0 to 2, and then totaled. A score of 8 to 10 requires no special attention. A score of 4 to 7 requires the administration of oxygen and stimulation. A score in this range may be seen if a mother has received a narcotic during labor. Narcotics enter the infant through the placenta and depress the respiratory center, leading to hypoventilation and hypoxemia. A narcotic antagonist, such as naloxone (Narcan), may need to be administered to the infant.

A score of 0 to 3 indicates that the infant needs immediate resuscitation (see Figure 47-4A ⚭ for some of the equipment and techniques that are used for infant cardiopulmonary resuscitation [CPR]). CPR requires special

TABLE 56-1	Apgar Score		
	SCORE		
SIGN	0	1	2
Heart rate	Absent	Slow—less than 100	Over 100
Respiratory rate	Absent	Slow—irregular	Good crying
Muscle tone	Flaccid	Some flexing of extremities	Active motion
Reflex irritability	None	Grimace	Vigorous cry
Color	Pale blue	Body pink, extremities blue	Completely pink (if light-skinned); absence of cyanosis (if dark-skinned)

training plus review courses to ensure that the nurse is using up-to-date methods and is following the most current guidelines.

IDENTIFICATION

Proper identification must be made in the delivery room before the mother and infant are separated. Identification bands imprinted with the same number, and the mother's name will be placed on the infant and the mother. It is important that the infant bands be applied snugly, but not too tight to impede circulation (Figure 56-5 ■). The identification bands must stay on the infant and mother until both are discharged. Each time the infant is brought to the mother, the identification bands are compared.

Most hospitals footprint the infant and fingerprint the mother (Figure 56-5C) **Vernix** (cheese-like substance covering the newborn's skin) must be washed from the infant's feet prior to foot printing. The number on the identification bands is also recorded on the footprint sheet. Upon discharge, the mother signs this form as documentation that she has received her infant.

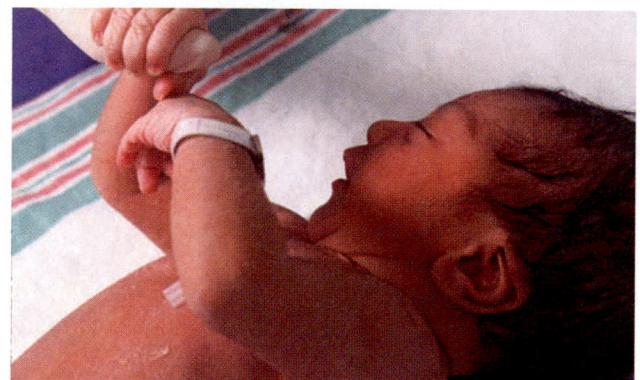

A

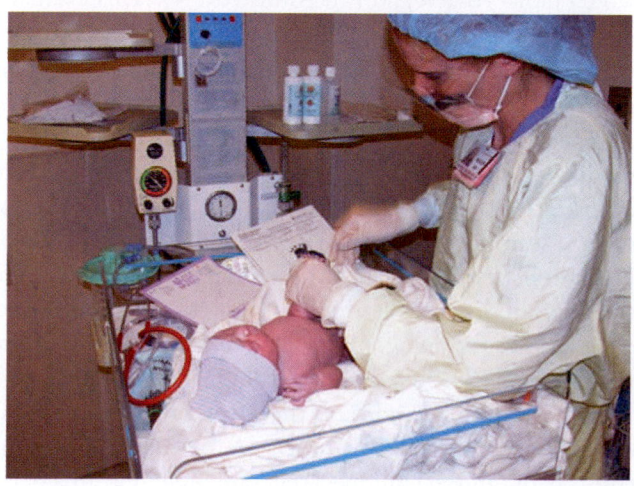

C

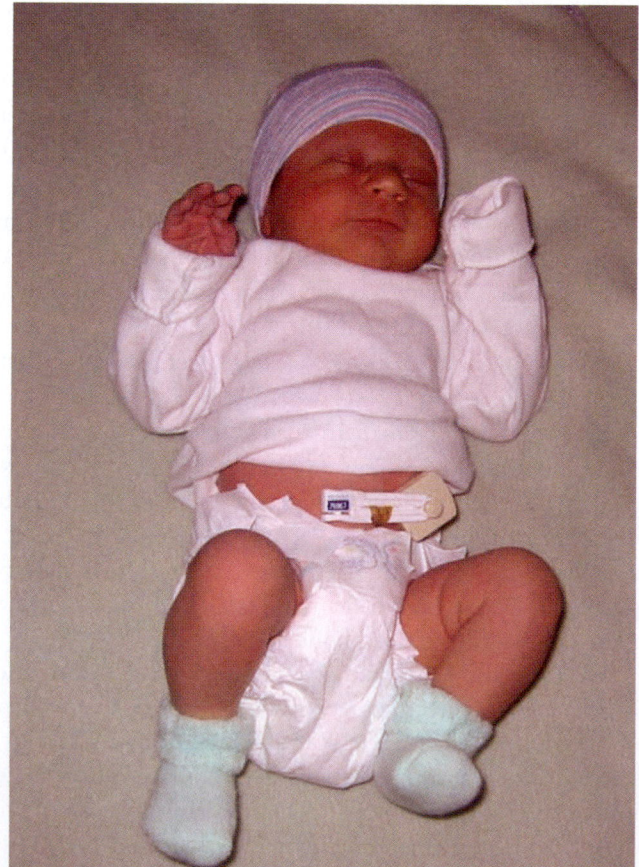

B

Figure 56-5. ■ **A.** Identification band on infant. **B.** Umbilical alarm attached to newborn infant. **C.** Nurse takes footprint of baby

MEASUREMENTS OF THE NEONATE

The infant's measurements (height, weight, head circumference, and chest circumference) are determined at birth. The healthy neonate weighs between 5 lbs. 8 oz and 8 lb. 13 oz (2,500–4,000 g), is 18 to 22 inches (48–52 cm) long, and has a head circumference of 12.5 to 14.5 inches (32–37 cm). These values are recorded on a growth chart for easy reference to national percentile ranges (Figure 56-6 ■). Infants whose values are in the 10th to 90th percentile ranges are considered appropriate for gestational age (AGA). Infants less than the 10th percentile are small for gestational age (SGA). Those greater than the 90th percentile are large for gestational age (LGA).

Height

Length can be difficult to measure. The baby is placed flat on the back with the legs extended. Usually, a tape measure is stretched from head to heel to determine the length. Some scales have a ruler attached to a moveable plate for measuring the length of the neonate. In either case, it is important to extend the infant's legs for accurate measurement (Procedure 56-2 ■).

Weight

To obtain a weight measurement, lay the neonate supine on a calibrated scale. Place a lightweight absorbent pad between the neonate and the scale to serve as a barrier against cold and moisture. Hold one hand above the neonate to guard against injury (Procedure 56-3 ■).

Head and Chest Circumference

Head and chest circumference are taken to obtain a baseline and are part of follow-up care. Procedures 56-4 and 56-5 ■ describe head and chest circumference measurements for neonates.

Nursery Care

If there are no complications, the infant is usually left with the mother in the delivery area through the recovery period. The infant may then be transferred to the newborn nursery, or left with the mother. In any case, the following care will be provided. Any time care is provided in the presence of the mother, and/or significant others, teaching should be provided regarding the care that is given, the reasons for the care, and whether the parents should do the same care at home.

SAFETY IN THE NURSERY

Safety in the newborn nursery involves protecting the newborn from injury and abduction. Safety measures must also be taught to the parents.

Most facilities have procedures that must be followed to protect the newborn from abduction. These might include limiting access to the newborn nursery and the obstetric unit. That is, only personnel or parents with proper identification are allowed to enter. Personnel who transport the neonate from the mother's room to the nursery or other areas of the facility must have proper identification. Parents are taught not to give their baby to anyone who does not have identification. All birthing facilities take additional security measures to protect the newborn. The trend is for birthing facilities to use a security band system. A special security band is placed snugly on the newborn's ankle or umbilicus (see Figure 56-5). If the band is dislodged or if the baby is taken off the mother–baby unit, an alarm sounds, all exits and elevators are automatically locked until the breach is identified and cleared. Parents must be informed of the security measures in place to protect their baby.

When the newborn is brought to the mother, the identification band is checked to be sure the infant is given to the correct person. The mother is asked to read the number on her identification bracelet, and the nurse checks it with the identification band on the baby.

When a neonate is carried in someone's arms, there is a possibility of dropping the baby. Therefore, transporting the neonate from the room in a bassinette is not only the safest method, but also often mandatory.

The baby should not be left unattended on a high surface such as a bed. If the mother is tired, the newborn should be placed in the bassinette instead of having the mother sleep with the baby in her arms.

DATA COLLECTION

Within the first 1 to 2 hours, the nurse completes a more in-depth assessment to evaluate the newborn's adaptation to life outside the uterus and to identify any complications. The nurse must understand the usual characteristics of the healthy newborn in order to evaluate the newborn's current condition.

Vital Signs

Vital signs for normal neonates are highlighted in Table 56-2 ■. Vital signs continue to change over time.

TEMPERATURE. Temperature is assessed on admission to the nursery and every 30 minutes until the temperature has remained stable for 2 hours. The temperature is then obtained at least once every 8 hours or as specified in facility policy. The newborn's temperature ranges are from 97.5 to 99.0° F (36.4 to 37.2°C).

The first temperature may be taken rectally, not only to determine the infant's temperature but also to determine the patency of the rectum. A rectal temperature is not recommended for routine monitoring because the thermometer irritates the rectal mucosa and could cause perforation. The axillary temperature is generally taken using an electronic thermometer. When the newborn is placed under

CLASSIFICATION OF NEWBORNS—
BASED ON MATURITY AND INTRAUTERINE GROWTH

Symbols: X-1st Exam O-2nd Exam

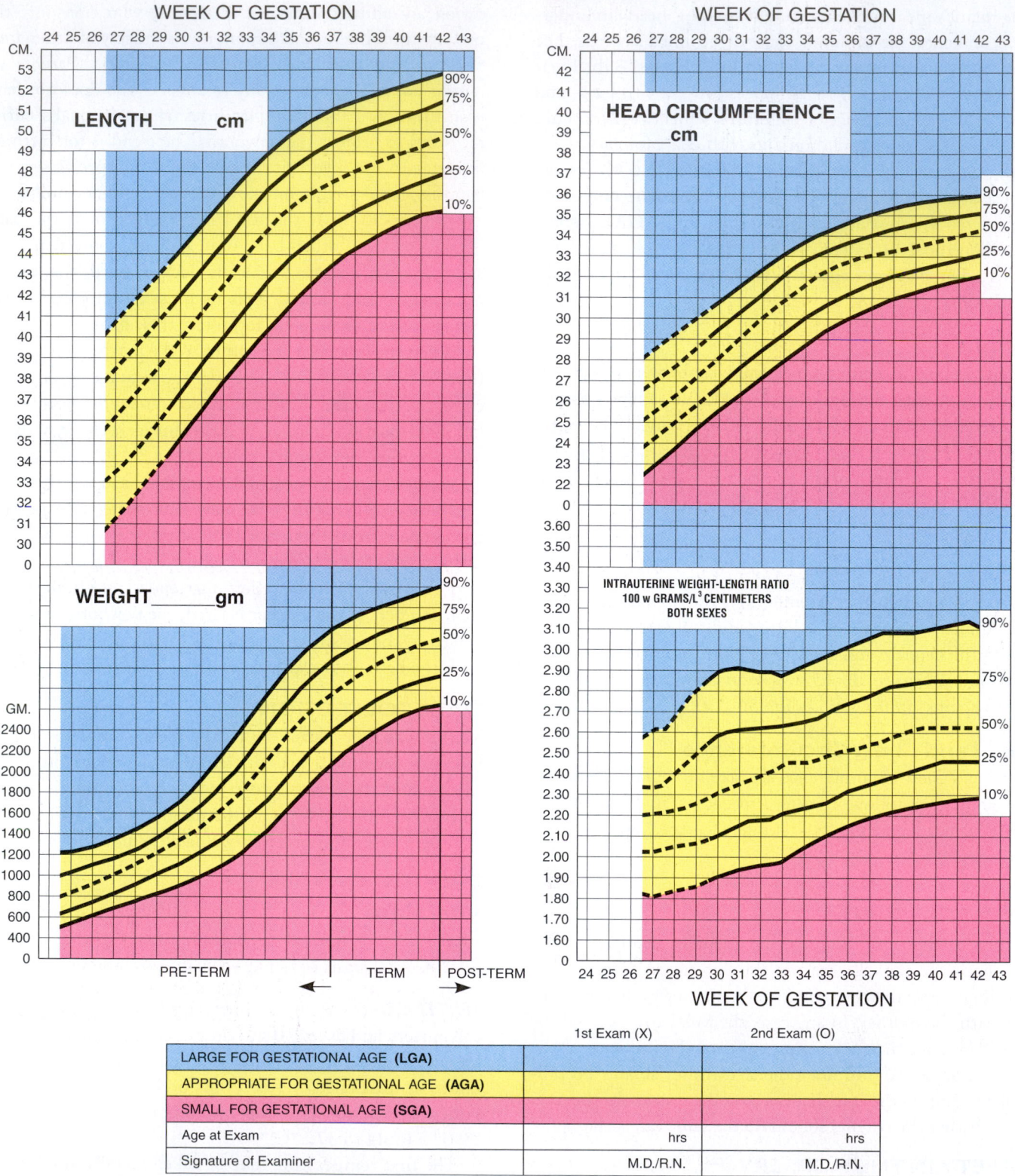

	1st Exam (X)	2nd Exam (O)
LARGE FOR GESTATIONAL AGE **(LGA)**		
APPROPRIATE FOR GESTATIONAL AGE **(AGA)**		
SMALL FOR GESTATIONAL AGE **(SGA)**		
Age at Exam	hrs	hrs
Signature of Examiner	M.D./R.N.	M.D./R.N.

Figure 56-6. ■ The nurse accurately measures the child and then places height, weight, and head circumference on appropriate growth grids for the child's age and gender. (*Source:* Adapted from Lubchenco, L.O., Hansman, C., & Boyd, E. [1966]. *Pediatrics, 37,* 404, Figure 1. Reprinted, with permission, from the American Academy of Pediatrics; Battaglia, F.C., & Lubchenco, L. O. [1967]. A practical classification of newborn infants by weight and gestational age. *Journal of Pediatrics, 71,* 161, with permission from Elsevier, Inc.)

TABLE 56-2	**Newborn Vital Signs**			
AGE	TEMPERATURE IN F (C)	PULSE (BEATS/MINUTE)	RESPIRATION (BREATHS/MINUTE)	BLOOD PRESSURE
Birth	97.5–99.0 (36.4–37.2)	90–160 (may be up to 180 when crying, 220 with fever)	35 (30–60)	60–80/40–45 mm Hg
Day 10	99.0 (37.2)	90–180	30 (28–50)	90/50 mm Hg
1 Month	99.2 (37.4)	90–180	24–45	94–104/50–60 mm Hg

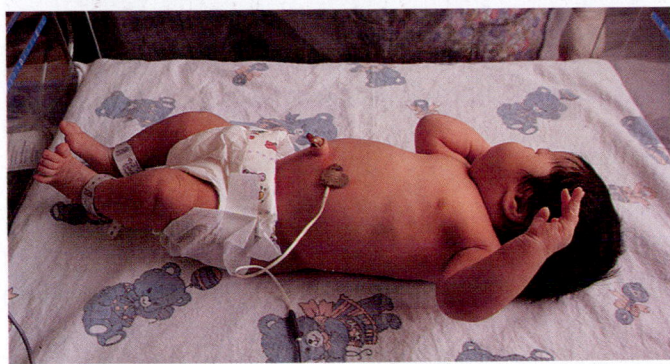

Figure 56-7. ■ Skin thermal sensor is placed on the newborn's abdomen, upper thigh, or arm and secured with a porous tape or a foil-covered foam pad.

radiant heat, a skin thermal sensor is placed over soft tissue such as on the abdomen (Figure 56-7 ■). An alarm will sound if the newborn's temperature rises.

HEART RATE.   Heart rate should be assessed when the newborn is at rest. Apical pulse should be counted for a full minute. The normal pulse rate is 120 to 160 beats per minute (bpm), but it may be as high as 180 bpm if the newborn is crying and as low as 90 bpm if the newborn is sleeping. Brachial and femoral pulses should be palpated (Figure 56-8 ■). However, radial pulses are difficult to feel.

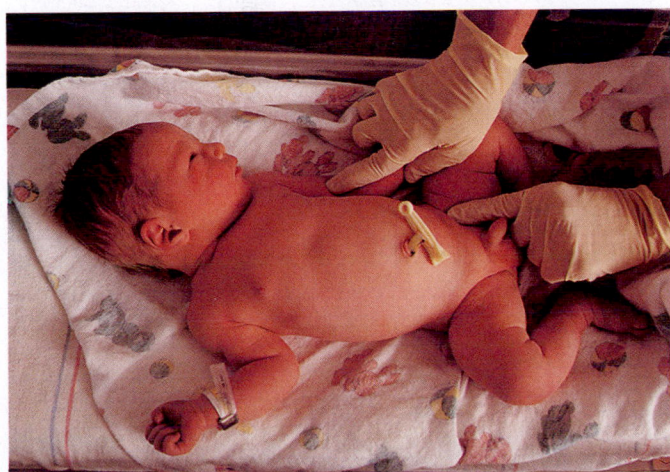

Figure 56-8. ■ Compare the femoral pulse to the brachial pulse by palpating the pulse simultaneously for comparison of rate and intensity.

RESPIRATORY RATE.   The respiratory rate should be assessed when the newborn is quiet. Respirations should be counted for a full minute. The normal respiratory rate is 30 to 60 breaths per minute.

BLOOD PRESSURE.   Measurement of blood pressure (BP) in the newborn varies. Some facilities generally do not take newborn BP. Other facilities routinely take it as a baseline in case cardiac issue should arise. If the newborn's condition warrants obtaining a blood pressure measurement, an electronic Doppler device is used. The cuff can be applied to the upper arm or leg. The size of the cuff must be appropriate for the newborn, usually 1 to 2 inches (2.5 to 5 cm) wide.

clinical ALERT

The normal blood pressure for a newborn is 60–80/40–45 mm Hg at birth and 100/50 at day 10. The newborn's extremities must be immobilized during the procedure.

Pain

Pain is an unpleasant sensation related to actual or potential tissue damage. Pain exists when the client says it does. The newborn is unable to verbalize the pain experience, but it is widely accepted that the newborn does feel pain. Skin sensation is present by 20 weeks' gestation, and the brain centers necessary for pain reception are developed toward the end of pregnancy. The newborn exhibits pain through facial expression and crying. Box 56-1 ■ provides an infant pain rating scale.

Gestational Age

An assessment of gestational age is completed within the first 4 hours after birth (Table 56-3 ■). Prenatally, the gestational age was determined from the last menstrual period. This estimation is accurate 75% to 85% of the time. A clinical

BOX 56-1	INFANT PAIN SCALE

S = Sleeping
0 = No pain
1 = Restless
2 = Facial grimacing
3 = Favors body parts (knees at abdomen, pulls at body part)
4 = Crying uncontrollably

TABLE 56-3	Gestational Age Assessment		

Neuromuscular Maturity The first area of the gestational age assessment is neuromuscular maturity. Some of the assessments made are illustrated in this section.

	PRETERM	FULL-TERM	POSTMATURE
Body Position at Rest (see Posture line in Ballard scale Figure 56-9)	Extended	Flexed	
Wrist Angle The square window of the wrist or angle of the hand and fingers when compressed by the examiner (see Square Window line of Figure 56-9)	90 degrees	0 to 30 degrees	
Arm Recoil Exhibited when the arms are held in extension next to the body for 5 seconds and then released (see Arm Recoil line of Figure 56-9)	Arms remain extended	Arms recoil to the flexed position	
Popliteal Angle Determined by flexing and holding the thigh to the abdomen while extending the leg at the knee (see Popliteal Angle line Figure 56-9)	180 degrees	90 degrees	Less than 90 degrees
Scarf Sign Exhibited by moving the arm in front of the neck (Figure 56-10 ■)	The elbow moves past the midline.	The elbow will not reach the midline.	
Physical Maturity The second area to be assessed is physical maturity. The skin, lanugo, feet, breasts, ears, and genitals are assigned points based on their degree of development.			
Integument	Thin and transparent Numerous blood vessels visible Cartilage is not developed Lanugo remains until 30 weeks	Opaque skin with few blood vessels visible Breast tissue (with areola) 0.5 to 1 cm	Dry and peeling
Genitals	Boys' scrotal sac empty with few rugae Girls' clitoris prominent, widely separated labia majora, and labia minora protruding beyond labia majora (when viewed laterally)	Boys evaluated for size of the scrotal sac, the presence of rugae, and the descent of the testicles Girls' labia majora nearly covers the clitoris and labia minora	

gestational age assessment tool, the Ballard Newborn Rating Scale (Figure 56-9 ■) was developed to determine gestational age more accurately and consistently. In this assessment tool, points from −1 to 5 are assigned to each characteristic. The points are totaled and referenced to the maturity rating scale to determine the gestational age in weeks.

Characteristics of the Newborn

GENERAL APPEARANCE

The healthy neonate appears plump, pink, and active with good muscle tone. The head is disproportionately large for the body. The center of the neonate's body is the umbilicus. The healthy neonate can move all extremities but prefers a flexed position.

SKIN

The skin at birth is red and smooth. **Acrocyanosis** (Figure 56-11A ■), a bluish discoloration of the hands and feet, is common for several hours after delivery. **Ecchymosis** (bruising) and **petechiae** (pinpoint hemorrhages) may be present following a difficult delivery. Some swelling around the eyes is common. The skin may be covered with vernix caseosa, especially in the body folds. The vernix, present during fetal development to protect the skin from the amniotic fluid, absorbs into the skin after birth, keeping it soft. A soft downy hair called **lanugo** is present on the face, arms, and back. Within a few days the skin may become dry and peel. A small amount of baby lotion can be used to moisten the skin. Soap should be avoided.

NEWBORN MATURITY RATING & CLASSIFICATION

ESTIMATION OF GESTATIONAL AGE BY MATURITY RATING
Symbols: X - 1st Exam   O - 2nd Exam

NEUROMUSCULAR MATURITY

	−1	0	1	2	3	4	5
Posture							
Square Window (wrist)	>90°	90°	60°	45°	30°	0°	
Arm Recoil		180°	140°–180°	110°–140°	90°–110°	<90°	
Popliteal Angle	180°	160°	140°	120°	100°	90°	<90°
Scarf Sign							
Heel to Ear							

PHYSICAL MATURITY

Skin	sticky friable transparent	gelatinous red, translucent	smooth pink, visible veins	superficial peeling &/or rash, few veins	cracking pale areas rare veins	parchment deep cracking no vessels	leathery cracked wrinkled
Lanugo	none	sparse	abundant	thinning	bald areas	mostly bald	
Plantar Surface	heel-toe 40–50 mm:−1 <40 mm:−2	>50 mm no crease	faint red marks	anterior transverse crease only	creases ant. 2/3	creases over entire sole	
Breast	imperceptible	barely perceptible	flat areola no bud	stippled areola 1–2 mm bud	raised areola 3–4 mm bud	full areola 5–10 mm bud	
Eye/Ear	lids fused loosely:−1 tightly:−2	lids open pinna flat stays folded	sl. curved pinna; soft; slow recoil	well curved pinna; soft but ready recoil	formed & firm instant recoil	thick cartilage ear stiff	
Genitals male	scrotum flat, smooth	scrotum empty faint rugae	testes in upper canal rare rugae	testes descending few rugae	testes down good rugae	testes pendulous deep rugae	
Genitals female	clitoris prominent labia flat	prominent clitoris small labia minora	prominent clitoris enlarging minora	majora & minora equally prominent	majora large minora small	majora cover clitoris & minora	

Gestation by Dates _____ wks

Birth Date _____ **Hour** _____ am / pm

APGAR _____ 1 min _____ 5 min

MATURITY RATING

score	weeks
−10	20
−5	22
0	24
5	26
10	28
15	30
20	32
25	34
30	36
35	38
40	40
45	42
50	44

SCORING SECTION

	1st Exam = X	2nd Exam = O
Estimating Gest Age by Maturity Rating	_____Weeks	_____Weeks
Time of Exam	Date _____ Hour _____ am pm	Date _____ Hour _____ am pm
Age at Exam	_____ Hours	_____ Hours
Signature of Examiner	_____ M.D./R.N.	_____ M.D./R.N.

Figure 56-9. ■ Ballard Newborn Rating Scale. (*Source:* Reprinted from Ballard, J. L., Khoury, J. C., Wedig, K., Wang, L., Eilers-Walsman, B. L., & Lipp, R. [1991]. New Ballard score, expanded to include extremely premature infants. *Journal of Pediatrics, 119*, 417. Used with permission from Elsevier, Inc.)

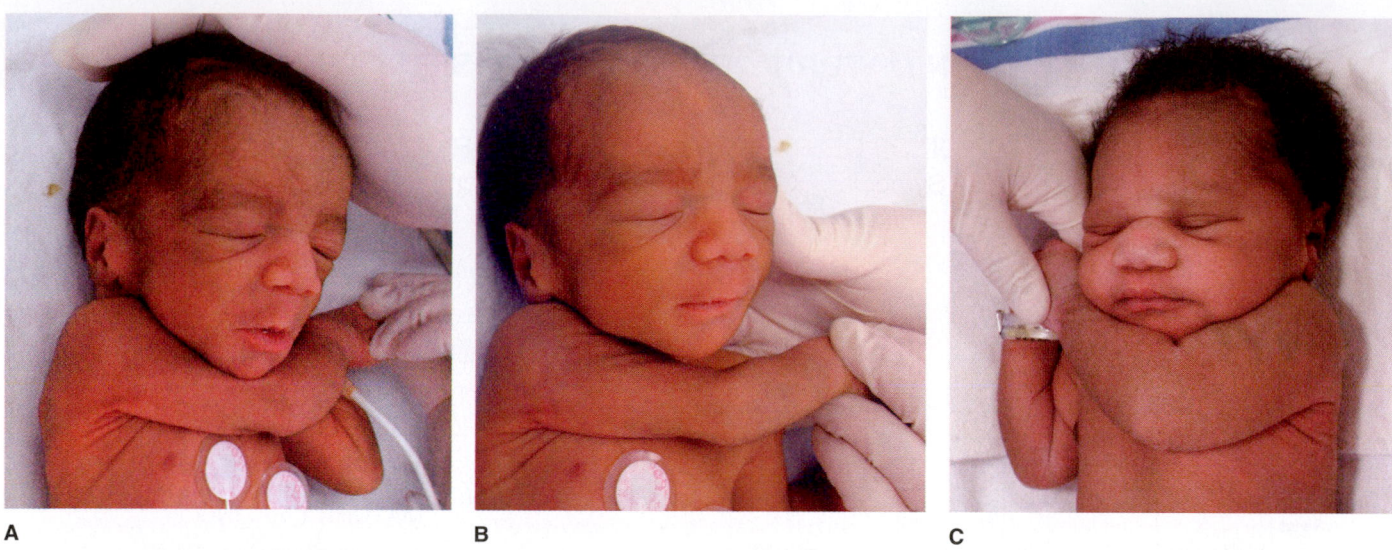

A

B

C

Figure 56-10. ■ Scarf sign. **A.** Until about 30 weeks' gestation, the elbow moves past midline with no resistance. **B.** At about 36 to 38 weeks' gestation, the elbow is at midline. **C.** The elbow will not reach midline after 40 weeks' gestation.

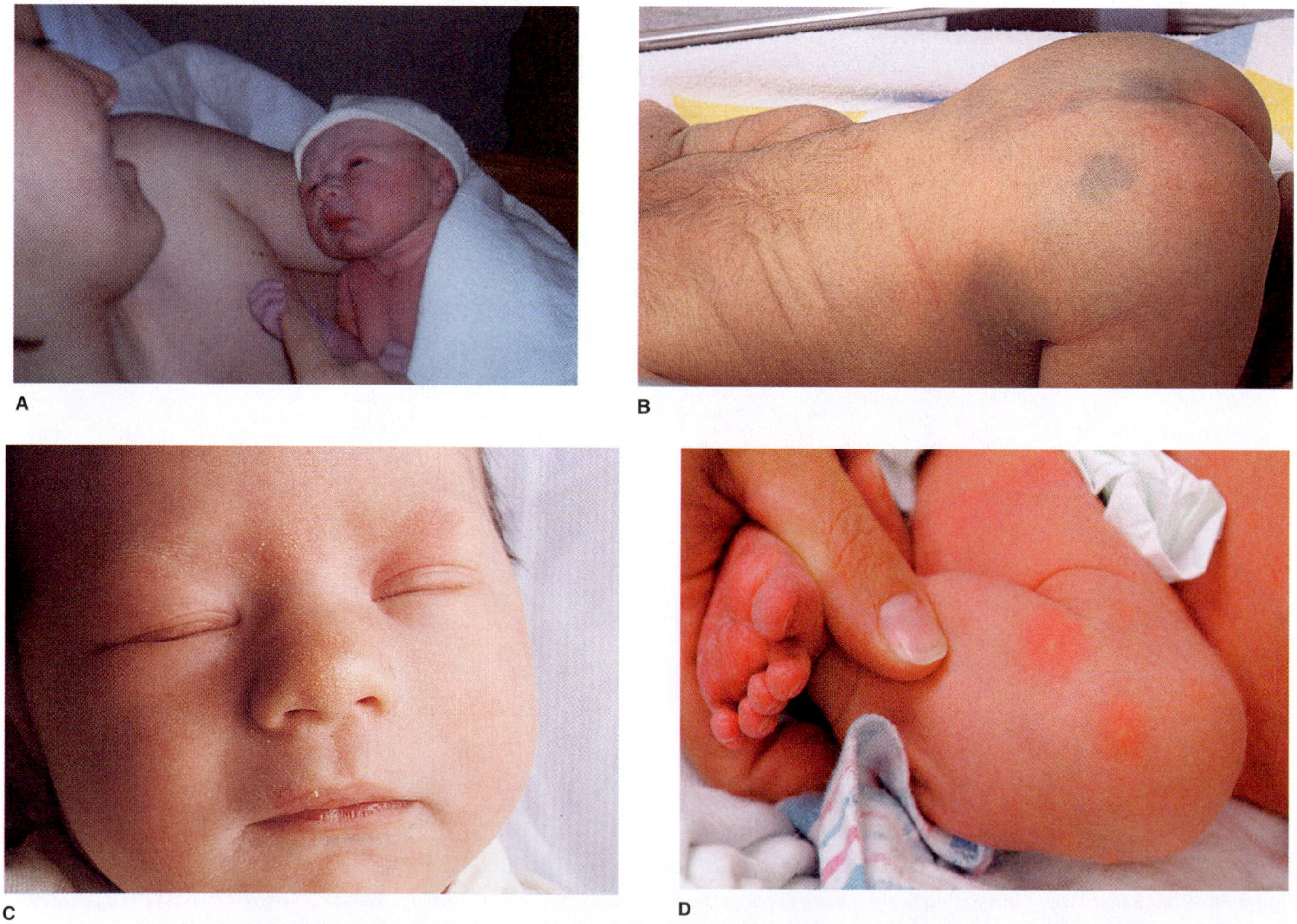

A

B

C

D

Figure 56-11. ■ **A.** Acrocyanosis. **B.** Mongolian spots. **C.** Facial milia. The spots usually disappear spontaneously within a few weeks. **D.** Erythema toxicum. The condition is noted during the newborn's first 24 hours and may remain for about 1 week, most commonly on the trunk and diaper area. (*Source:* Reproduced, with permission, of Mead Johnson & Company, Evansville, IN.)

Physiologic Jaundice

Physiologic jaundice frequently occurs after the first 24 hours of life. During development, the fetus needs an increased number of red blood cells in order to transport adequate oxygen from the placenta to the organs. Once oxygenation occurs through the newborn's lungs, the extra RBCs are no longer needed. Therefore, infants have an excess of red blood cells after birth that break down, releasing bilirubin.

Recall that one function of a mature liver is to break down unneeded red blood cells, and to reuse or excrete chemical compounds such as iron and bilirubin. **Jaundice** is a condition that occurs because the infant's liver is immature and cannot break down and excrete all the bilirubin released by the destruction of RBCs. The bilirubin remains in the blood, causing a yellow appearance of light skin and a yellowing of the sclera. The jaundice increases for several days.

As the liver matures, the bilirubin is excreted though the bile ducts into the small intestine, causing the stool to turn brownish-yellow. Once the infant passes these transitional stools, the jaundice gradually fades. Bilirubin levels in the blood must be monitored until values return to normal levels. See Chapter 57 🔗 for a discussion of *hyperbilirubinemia* (high levels of bilirubin in the blood).

clinical ALERT

Jaundice appearing within the first 24 hours after birth is an indication of a more serious condition called pathologic jaundice that should be reported to the supervising RN or physician.

Other Skin Markings

Several discolored areas are commonly found on newborn's skin. A **Mongolian spot** (see Figure 56-11B) is a dark discolored area found over the lower back and sacrum of infants of Black, Hispanic, Indian, or Oriental descent. Over time, the infant's skin tones darken to become the same color as the Mongolian spot.

Some infants are born with dark red spots on the eyelids, forehead, or nape of the neck. These red areas, called **telangiectatic nevi** or **stork bites,** usually fade in time. Parental concern for these and other birthmarks should be discussed with the pediatrician. Consultation with a plastic surgeon may be needed.

The sebaceous glands on the face become distended a few days after birth resulting in **milia** (see Figure 56-11C) or white pinpoint spots resembling white heads. A few weeks of bathing opens the sebaceous glands and the milia disappear.

Erythema toxicum neonatorum is a raised pink papule with a light colored center resembling a mosquito bite (see Figure 56-11D). These lesions appear suddenly on the chest, abdomen, and back 24 to 48 hours after birth. They are benign and will disappear without treatment. Other birthmarks may be found on assessing the newborn's skin and should be documented.

HEAD

The head of the newborn may be asymmetrical at birth. The anterior and posterior fontanels (see Figure 16-4 🔗) should be firm and flat. The head is 13 inches to 14 inches (33 to 34 cm) in circumference. *Molding* (see Figure 53-4 🔗), the shaping of the fetal head to the shape of the mother's pelvis, may take several days to resolve. Edema of the scalp called **caput succedaneum** may cross the suture lines. **Cephalhematoma,** in contrast, is an accumulation of blood between the periosteum and the skull bone that will not cross the suture lines. Figure 56-12 ■ illustrates caput succedaneum and cephalhematoma. Marks from an internal fetal monitoring electrode, suction (vacuum) extractor, and forceps may be present if they were used in labor and delivery (see Figure 53-23 🔗). The neonate's face should be symmetric. The top of the ears should be in line with the outer canthus of the eye. The pinna may be flat against the head. The eyes of the newborn may show small hemorrhages in the sclera due to the pressure of delivery. The newborn has poor control of the eye muscles (Figure 56-13 ■), resulting in **strabismus** (lack of coordination of the visual axes of the eye; eyes do not stay parallel to each other but may diverge in any direction). This disappears in a few months. The nose may be flattened due to the birth process. The mouth should be midline, with both cheeks moving symmetrically. Asymmetry of the face indicates facial palsy and should be reported to the primary care provider.

The palate and lips should be intact. One or more precocious or "milk" teeth may be present in the center of the lower gum.

clinical ALERT

If the neonate is born with precocious teeth, they will become loose and fall out. Loose teeth may need to be removed by the primary care provider to prevent aspiration. Normal deciduous teeth erupt at approximately 6 months of age.

Epstein's pearls, small white cysts, may be present on the palate, but they disappear in a few weeks.

The neck is short with several skin folds. The muscles of the neck are unable to support the weight of the newborn's head. When the neonate is pulled up from a supine position, the head lags behind. However, from a prone position, the neonate can lift the head slightly.

CHEST

The chest should be 12 to 13 inches (30.5 to 33 cm) in circumference. Two nipples should be identifiable. Some engorgement may be present in both male and female infants

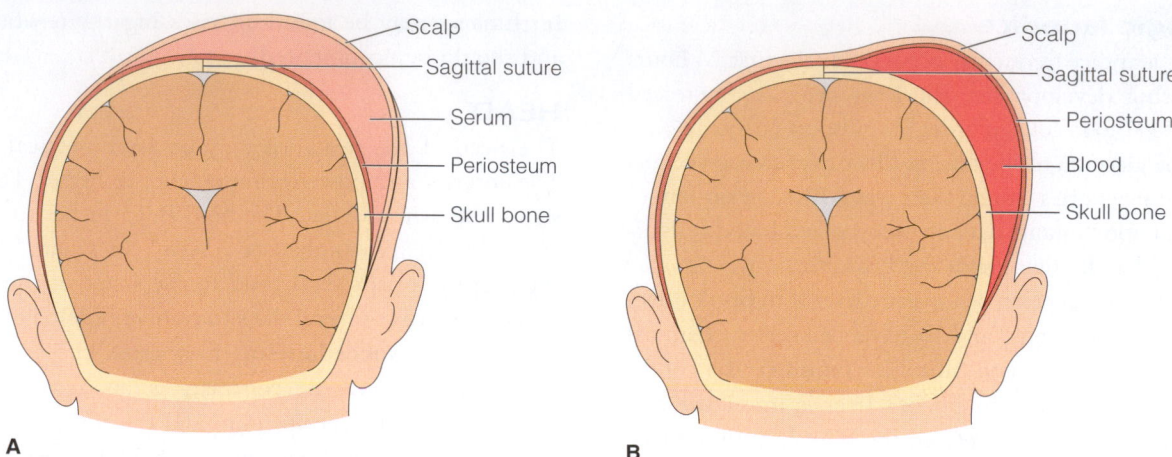

A

B

Figure 56-12. ■ **A.** Caput succedaneum is a collection of fluid under the scalp. **B.** Cephalhematoma is a collection of blood between the surface of the cranial bone and the periosteal membrane. This is a cephalhematoma over the left parietal bone.

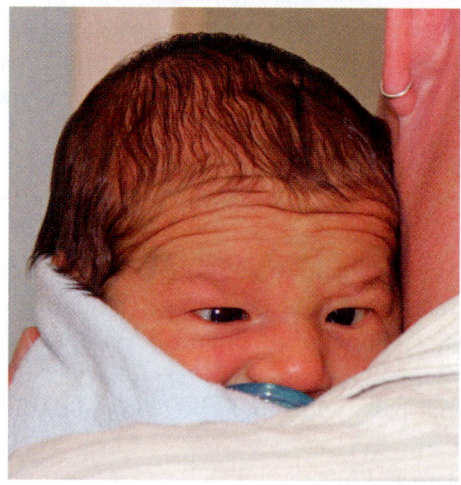

Figure 56-13. ■ Strabismus is common in neonates. The eyes may diverge in different directions until muscle coordination begins.

due to maternal hormones. The nipple may secrete whitish fluid, called **witches' milk,** for several days.

Heart Sounds

Heart sounds should be assessed when the newborn is in a quiet state. Because of the rapid heart rate, evaluating heart sounds in the neonate takes practice. The normal lub-dub sounds should be heard. A slurring of one sound (usually the lub) may indicate a murmur. Most murmurs are considered normal and disappear within a few months. However, some murmurs indicate an abnormality within the heart. For this reason, the primary care provider should monitor all murmurs.

Lung Sounds

Lung sounds should be assessed when the neonate is quiet. The lungs should be auscultated from both the anterior and the posterior chest. Because heart sounds and bowel sounds

are transmitted through the chest, localizing abnormal lung sounds may be difficult. Movement of air should be heard in all lung fields. Inspiration may be noisy for the first few hours after birth due to the presence of fluid in the air passages.

Breathing patterns in the newborn are predominantly diaphragmatic, with the chest rising with the abdominal movements. Respirations are usually irregular with brief (5 to 15 seconds) pauses, called **periodic breathing.** If there are no color or heart rate changes, these periodic breathing episodes are considered normal. As stated previously, the neonate should be observed frequently for signs of respiratory distress.

ABDOMEN

The abdomen should be soft without palpable masses. The LPN/LVN can perform light palpation on the abdomen of the neonate. However, due to the risk of organ damage, the LPN/LVN cannot perform deep palpation of the abdomen. The umbilical cord should be clamped, and three blood vessels are identifiable. There should be no distention or bulging. If distention is present, the skin becomes tight and blood vessels appear under the skin surface. Femoral pulses should be palpable in the groin.

clinical ALERT

Abdominal distention is a sign of many abnormalities of the gastrointestinal tract and should be reported to the primary care provider.

Elimination

URINE. The newborn should void urine in the first few hours after delivery. The newborn's bladder holds 30 to 50 mL of urine, so infants void 8 to 10 times a day. The perineal area should be washed with warm water or commercially prepared wipes following each void. Diapers should be checked and changed frequently to keep the skin dry. The newborn should not be discharged from the hospital until he has voided.

FECES.   Bowel sounds are present in four quadrants within an hour after birth. The newborn should pass stool within the first 24 hours after delivery. The first stool (**meconium**) is greenish black and sticky or tarry. It is made up of salts, amniotic fluid, mucus, bile, and epithelial cells. Meconium stools may persist for 2 to 3 days (Figure 56-14 ■). The infant should pass stool before discharge from the hospital. Holding the infant's legs across the abdomen for a few minutes may help the infant pass stool.

Transitional stools are passed after several feedings (see Figure 56-14 ■) Transitional stools are yellowish or greenish brown, thin, and less sticky. Milk curds may be seen. By the fourth day, the stool becomes thicker and pasty. If the infant is breastfed, stools are yellow to golden, and have an odor similar to sour milk. Formula-fed infants pass pale yellow to light brown stool that is firmer and has a stronger odor. The stool will not be brown and formed until the infant is given solid food.

GENITALIA

Genitals should be inspected carefully. Some congenital anomalies are illustrated in Chapter 57 ⚭ . In the female neonate, the clitoris varies in size and may be so large that it appears similar to a penis. This is generally due to hormone influence and disappears in a few days. Fat deposits in the labia majora cause them to enlarge and cover the labia minora. This generally occurs before birth, but if the neonate is of low birth weight, there may not be enough subcutaneous fat for the labia majora to cover the labia minora. A mucus or slightly bloody vaginal discharge may be present. This **pseudomenstruation** is related to the influence of maternal hormones and disappears in a few days. **Smegma** (the secretion consisting of epithelial cells found around the external genitalia) may be present in the labia folds. Removing it may traumatize the tissue.

In the male neonate, the penis should be inspected to determine the location of the urinary meatus. The urinary meatus should open onto the tip of the glans. The scrotum should be palpated for the presence of two testicles. (See Chapter 57 ⚭ for abnormalities of urinary meatus.)

The anus is inspected for patency. Abnormalities can usually be identified by visual inspection. If a digital examination is necessary, it should be completed by the primary care provider. The passage of stool verifies the functioning of the gastrointestinal tract. Abnormalities are discussed in Chapter 57 ⚭ .

EXTREMITIES

The extremities should be symmetrical bilaterally. Each extremity should end with 5 digits, without **webbing** (skin between two or more digits) or **syndactyly** (the fusion of two or more digits) or **polydactyly** (presence of more than five fingers per hand or toes per foot). Muscle tone should be strong, with full range of motion in each extremity.

The femur should be well seated in the acetabulum. The registered nurse or physician should assess the hip for displacement or hip click (Figure 56-15 ■). Asymmetrical skin folds of the posterior thigh on the affected side may be noted (Figure 56-15B). The ankle of the neonate appears to

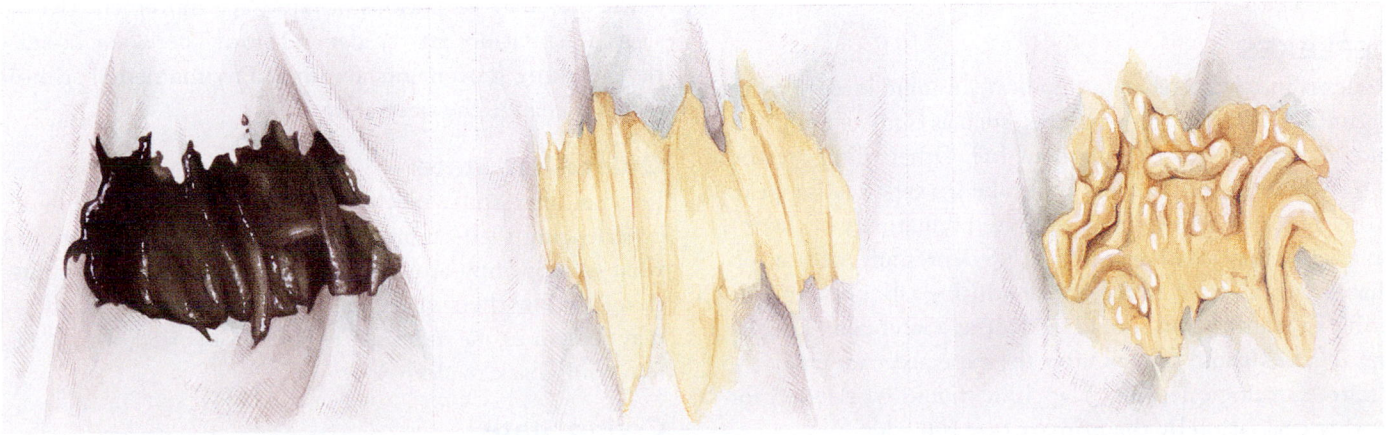

A   B   C

Figure 56-14. ■ Newborn stool samples. **A.** Meconium stool. **B.** Breast-milk stool. **C.** Cow's milk stool.

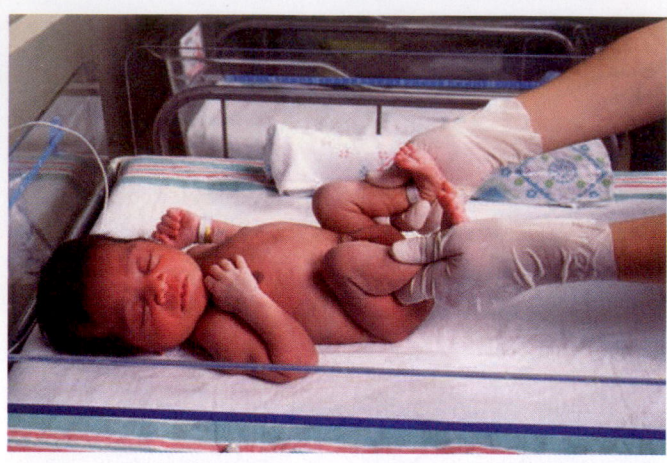

A

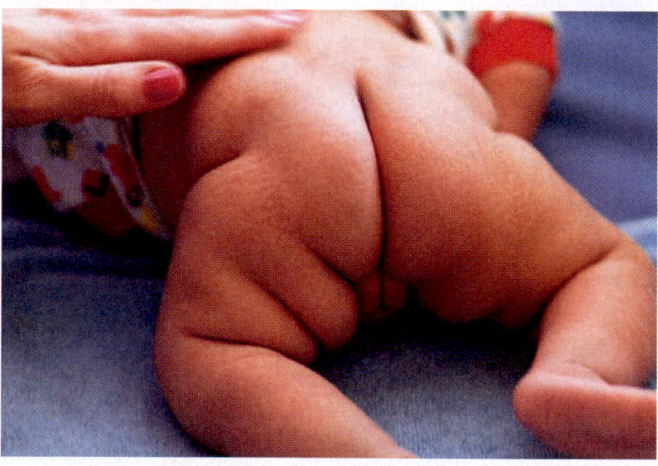

B

Figure 56-15. ■ **A.** Hip integrity is assessed in a newborn by observing and feeling the smoothness of movement in the joint. A "click" is an indication of possible hip dysplasia. **B.** Skin folds may be noted on the affected side.

turn inward due to the position in the uterus. There should not be resistance when the foot is moved to a normal position. If resistance is encountered, evaluation for clubfoot needs to be made by the primary care provider.

REFLEXES

Reflexes in newborns are a sign of neurologic integrity (see Figure 16-5 ⟲). Some reflexes, such as blink, cough, and sneeze, remain intact throughout life. Others disappear by 4 to 6 months. Still others will take 2 years to disappear. Absent or slow reflexes may indicate prematurity of the infant. They may also result from CNS depressant medication that was transferred to the neonate during labor or in breast milk. Reexamination should be done at a later date. Lingering reflexes (those present after the expected time) may indicate neurologic lesions. The child should be referred for further evaluation by the primary care provider.

Rooting reflex occurs when the infant is searching for food. When the newborn's cheek is stroked, he will turn his

head in that direction. **Sucking reflex** is elicited when the newborn's lips are touched. Together these two reflexes are important in feeding. Medications, especially pain medications, can be transferred in breast milk and could depress the sucking reflex. Breastfeeding is discussed in Chapter 54 ⟲ . Rooting reflex disappears between 3 to 4 months; sucking reflex disappears by 10 months.

Palmar grasp reflex occurs when a finger or small object is placed in the newborn's hand. Newborns grasp the finger tight enough to be lifted from the bed. This reflex lasts 4 months. **Plantar grasp reflex,** lasting 8 months, occurs when the sole of the foot is touched. The toes curl under as if newborns are trying to "grasp" with their feet. This reflex must disappear before infants are able to walk. **Babinski's reflex** is elicited by stroking the lateral side of the foot from heel to toe. The big toe should dorsiflex and the other toes should flare. **Stepping reflex** is obtained by holding newborns with the feet touching the table. Newborns will step as if walking.

Tonic neck reflex is demonstrated by placing newborns supine on a firm surface. When the head is turned to one side, newborns will extend the arm and leg on that side. The opposite arm and leg will flex. The **Moro or startle reflex** occurs when newborns have a sense of falling. This reflex can be elicited by holding the newborn in a sitting position and suddenly lowering the head or by bumping the surface where the newborn is lying. The baby will quickly extend the arms (abduct) with fingers flared and thumb and first finger forming a "C." The arms will then adduct in an embracing motion. The lower extremities may extend and then flex. A slight tremor may be noted.

BEHAVIORAL STATE

Three behavioral states have been identified to describe the normal newborn: sleep state, quiet alert state, and crying state.

Sleep State

Newborns sleep with their eyes closed for 20 to 22 hours a day. There may be periods of rapid eye movement (REM) sleep. Respirations are regular and slow. There may be startle or jerking movements at times. Environmental stimuli may not change the sleep state.

Quiet Alert State

In quiet alert state, newborns lie quietly looking around, experiencing their environment. They appear interested in what is happening around them. They may focus on something within their visual field for several minutes. They may remain in the quiet alert state for a period of time before going back to sleep or crying.

Crying State

The cry should be strong, lusty, and of medium pitch. Crying is a method of communicating for newborns. Crying can be used to increase the metabolism when infants are cold. Crying can indicate that infants are hungry, wet, or just needing reassurance that they are not alone. Crying may be accompanied by frequent, jerky movements. A high-pitched cry or one that sounds like a "cat cry" requires further evaluation by a primary care provider.

Hygiene Care

BATHING

The infant has been in contact with maternal body fluids, blood, and amniotic fluid. Following Standard Precautions, the nurse should not touch the infant without clean exam gloves until the infant has been bathed. Once the infant's temperature has stabilized, the infant is bathed with a warm, wet, soapy washcloth, exposing only the area being washed. The hair can be washed with warm water, and dried with a warm towel. The infant will be diapered, dressed in a warm tee shirt, and wrapped in 2 to 3 warm blankets. Following a bath (Procedure 56-6 ▪), the infant remains under a radiant warmer until the temperature stabilizes.

Until the umbilical cord falls off, the neonate should not be placed in a tub of water. Gentle wiping with a warm, moist washcloth is generally sufficient. The neonate's skin may become dry and peel within a few days. A small amount of lotion or baby oil may be applied to the dry areas. After the umbilical cord falls off, the neonate can be placed in warm water for bathing.

When wet the neonate is very slick. Care must be taken to prevent the baby from sliding under the water or hitting his or her head on the side of the basin. For this reason, many parents bathe the newborn in the sink or a basin of warm water instead of the bathtub.

Diapering and Perineal Care

Diapers should be changed at least every 2 hours, or as soon as they become soiled. Figure 56-16 ▪ illustrates how to apply a diaper. The diaper area should be washed with each diaper change. If a rash appears, commercially prepared ointments may be beneficial. Laying the neonate on a pad without a diaper fastened exposes the perineum to air and light. This may help prevent or heal skin breakdown.

Perineal care should be completed with each diaper change. A warm washcloth or commercially prepared diaper wipe may be used. It is important to remove urine and stool from between labia folds of female infants. If the male infant is not circumcised, the penis should be cleansed with warm water. The foreskin should not be forced back over the penis. The foreskin will retract normally over time, but it might take 3 to 5 years to do so.

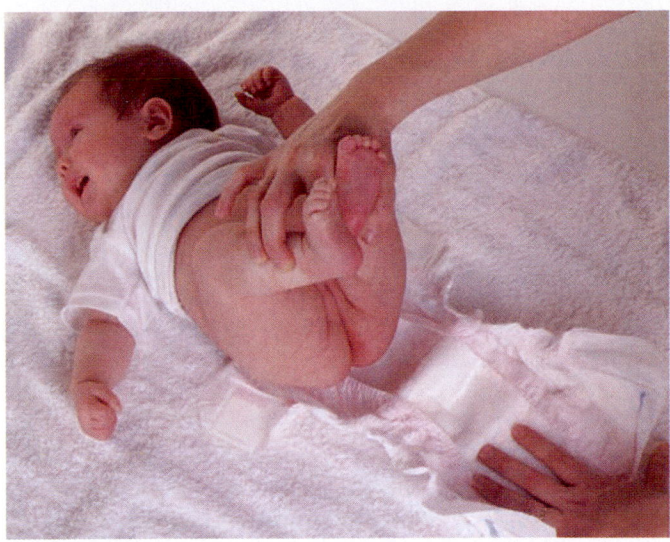

A

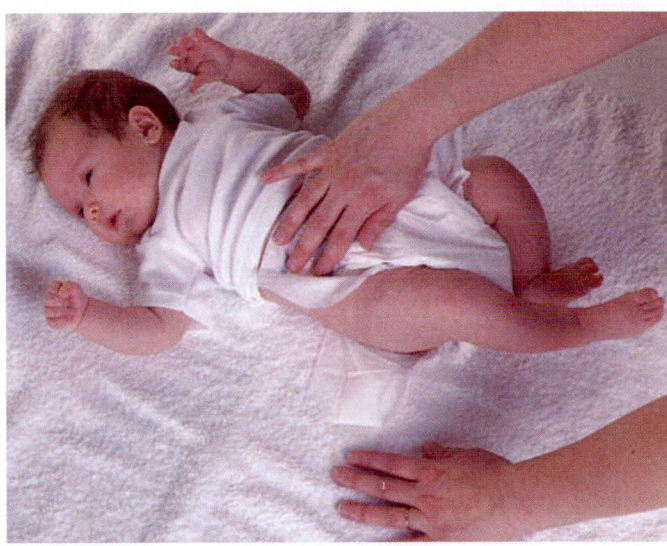

B

Figure 56-16. ▪ Diapering. **A.** Lift the baby by both legs over the diaper. Make sure the diaper is fully unfolded across the back and buttocks before securing. **B.** Fasten the diaper snugly but not tightly. (Dorling Kindersley Media Library.)

EYE CARE

Eye care is necessary to prevent **ophthalmia neonatorum**, inflammation of the eyes of the newborn, resulting from contact with gonorrhea or chlamydia during the birth process. It is legally mandatory that an antibiotic ointment or solution be placed in the infant's eyes soon after delivery (Figure 56-17 ▪).

UMBILICAL CORD CARE

At delivery a small plastic or metal clamp is generally placed on the umbilical cord approximately 1 inch from the skin and the cord is cut. The clamp must remain in place until the cord has dried and is then removed to reduce the chance of tension injury. With each diaper change, the skin at the base of the cord is assessed for redness and drainage,

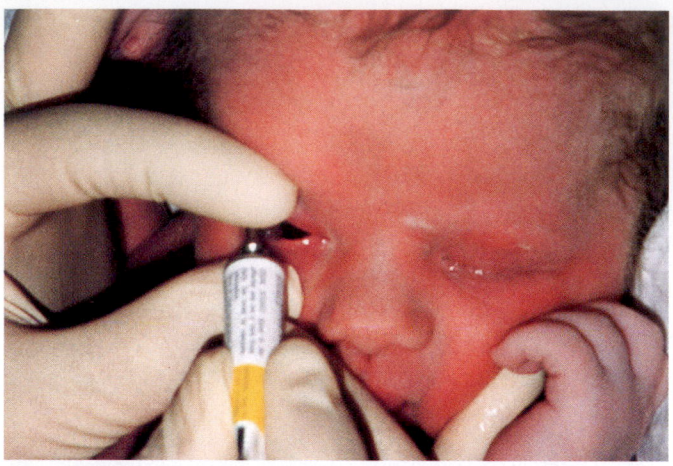

Figure 56-17. ■ Ophthalmic ointment. Retract lower eyelid outward to instill ¼-in-long strand of ointment from a single-dose tube along the lower conjunctival surface.

and cleaned with plain water. Many types of cord care are practiced, including the use of alcohol, triple blue dye, or antimicrobial agents. The nurse is responsible for cord care per agency policy (Figure 56-18 ■).

The umbilical cord should remain clean and dry. It will fall off in 7 to 14 days. The skin around the cord may be pink but should not become red or inflamed. A small amount of dark reddish-brown drainage may be present. The diaper should be folded below the umbilical cord to allow for

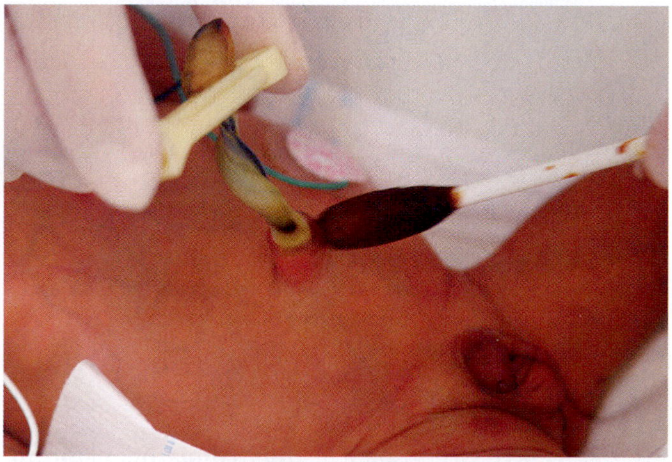

Figure 56-18. ■ Cord care may be done in several ways; the nurse follows facility policy. This cord is being cleaned with Betadine. If alcohol is used, take care not to get it onto the skin around the cord.

air-drying. If culture demands binding the abdomen, a clean piece of gauze can be recommended. A small drop of blood may appear when the cord comes off. Cord care is part of client teaching before discharge. Parents should be taught never to pull on the cord or attempt to loosen it.

clinical ALERT

Keeping the neonate's cord clean and dry is essential to prevent infection. Teach parents that until the cord falls off (about 2 weeks after birth), the infant should not be submerged in water.

Vitamin K Administration

Vitamin K, necessary for blood clotting, is normally produced in the intestines from food and intestinal flora. Newborns are unable to produce vitamin K because their intestine is sterile until food is introduced. Within an hour after delivery, the newborn is given an intramuscular (IM) injection of vitamin K (AquaMEPHYTON) to prevent hemorrhagic disorders (Table 56-4 ■) (Procedure 56-7 ■).

Nutrition

A full-term infant needs 50 to 55 kcal/lb (110 to 120 kcal/kg) that equals 20 oz (600 mL) of breast milk or formula per day. At birth, the newborn's stomach will hold 20 mL or slightly less than an ounce. For this reason, the newborn will be unable to consume enough nutrition to meet his/her caloric needs for the first few days of life. This causes weight loss, usually between 5% and 7%. By the end of the first week of life, the newborn can retain 2 to 3 ounces (60–90 mL) with each feeding. The infant will need to be fed every 2 to 4 hours in order to meet nutritional needs.

The American Academy of Pediatrics recommends breast milk for the first year of life. Commercially prepared formula closely approximates breast milk. It is important for parents to receive information regarding the benefits of both breastfeeding and bottle-feeding. Table 56-5 ■ illustrates benefits for each method of feeding. Once the parents make a decision, the nurse should support their decision. It is not appropriate to make the parents feel guilty about their decision. If bottle-feeding, the physician will order the brand of formula. It is important to note that, if the woman is participating in the Women, Infant and Children

TABLE 56-4	Pharmacology: Drug Used to Prevent Hemorrhagic Disorders			
DRUG NAME (GENERIC NAME AND CLASS)	**USUAL ROUTE/DOSE**	**CLASSIFICATION AND PURPOSE**	**SELECTED SIDE EFFECTS**	**DON'T GIVE IF**
Phytonadione (AquaMEPHYTON)	Newborns: IM/SC 0.5–1.0 mg immediately after delivery May repeat in 6 hr prn	Vitamin K	Hypersensitivity, flushing, pain at injection site	None

MyNursingKit | Cord care

TABLE 56-5	Reasons for Breastfeeding and Bottle-Feeding	
FEEDING CHOICE	**BENEFIT TO MOTHER**	**BENEFIT TO INFANT**
Breastfeeding	Decreases incidence of ovarian, uterine, and breast cancer	Enhances maturation of the GI tract
	Promotes involution	Contains antibodies that can protect against some infections
	Supports return to prepregnant weight sooner	
	Provides a unique bonding experience	Lowers incidence of allergies
	Is convenient, no formula and bottles to carry	Lowers incidence of SIDS
	Saves money	
Bottle-Feeding	Is personal preference	Allows bonding to occur
	Is an option if there is breast scarring, or HIV infection	Allows others besides mother to feed infant
	Is an option if mother is taking medication that precludes breastfeeding	Provides adequate nutrition
		Comes in three forms for convenience
		Comes in cow's milk and soy milk
		Provides an iron-fortified formula

(WIC) program, some brands of formula may not be funded. Adjustments can usually be made between the physician and the WIC program.

Breast milk is produced to meet the newborn's needs and changes as the infant grows. Breast milk contains easily digested nutrients as well as antibodies. *Colostrum*, the first fluid produced by the breast, is a thin yellow fluid, rich in protein and calories and containing immune globins. Colostrum protects the newborn from intestinal infections. Colostrum also contains a laxative that assists in the passage of *meconium*, the newborn's first stool.

Breast stimulation and emptying of the mammary glands stimulates the secretion of prolactin by the mother's anterior pituitary gland. Prolactin increases milk production. As the newborn nurses more frequently and for longer periods of time, more milk is produced.

The breastfeeding mother needs a balanced diet in order to provide breast milk and maintain her own nutritional needs. An extra 500 calories and 1,000 mL of fluid are needed per day to support breastfeeding.

The mother and newborn do not automatically know how to breastfeed. Teaching and support will be needed during the learning process. See Chapter 54 ⟨⟨ for a full discussion of breastfeeding techniques.

Bottle-feeding will take some forethought and preparation. Bottles and nipples should be cleaned with a brush and soapy water and thoroughly rinsed. If there is question about the safety of the water supply, bottles and nipples should be boiled. A variety of nipples are available. Generally babies will feed well from any bottle and nipple, but may eventually prefer one style. Formulas are available in ready-to-feed, concentrated liquid and powder forms. There is a great difference in price and finances should be a factor in choosing a type of formula. Accurate mixing is essential

to provide the necessary nutrients, the proper number of calories, and an easily digested concentration.

Most newborns will take 0.5 oz (15 mL) the first few days but gradually increase the amount of each feeding over time. To prevent wasting formula, only a few ounces should be made until the infant is taking higher volumes.

The infant should be positioned with the head higher than the stomach. The infant should be burped when about half of the feeding is consumed and again at the end of the feeding. To facilitate burping, the infant can be held upright against the feeder's shoulder, leaned forward in a sitting position with the head and chest supported (see Figure 54-12 ⟨⟨) or laid prone across the feeder's lap. Gently rubbing or patting the infant's back can also facilitate burping.

Common Procedures

NEONATAL SCREENING TESTS

Hypoglycemia

Neonates who are small for gestational age (SGA) or large for gestational age (LGA) are frequently assessed for hypoglycemia. A small blood sample is obtained from the newborn's heel to determine the blood glucose level (Figure 56-19 ■). Because of the possibility of damaging the nerves on the bottom of the neonate's foot, correct procedure must be followed. The blood is placed on a reagent strip and the blood glucose level is determined.

The nurse must be familiar with the blood glucose monitor used by the facility. If the standards for the equipment are not closely followed, an inaccurate blood glucose level will be obtained.

Phenylketonuria

Another blood test that is done in the neonate period is screening for phenylketonuria (PKU). This screening test,

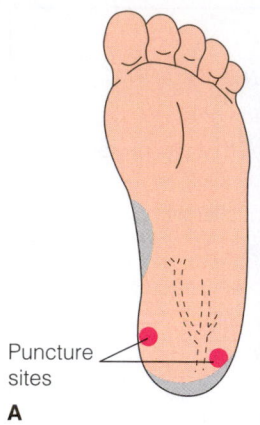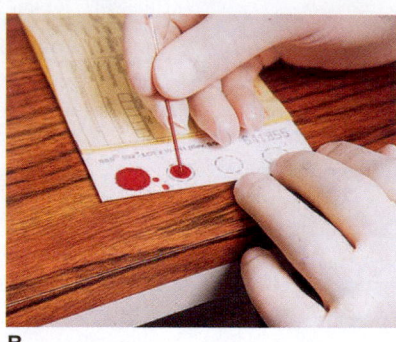

Puncture sites

A   **B**

Figure 56-19. ■ **A.** Potential puncture sites for heel sticks. Avoid shaded areas to prevent injury to arteries and nerves in the foot. **B.** Collecting a blood sample from the newborn for neonatal metabolic screening. The nurse must be sure to saturate the circle on the test sheet thoroughly.

required by law in all 50 states, determines the presence of an autosomal recessive disorder of amino acid metabolism in which the individual is unable to break down phenylalanine. The results can be devastating to cognitive function and health (see the discussion in Chapter 57 ⚭). To meet the legal requirements, facilities obtain the blood sample prior to discharge. For the results of the screening to be most accurate, the test must be done after the baby has received milk (either breast milk or formula). It may take 48 to 72 hours (or more) for the newborn to have an adequate consumption of milk. For this reason, the PKU test may need to be repeated in 1 to 2 weeks. The blood sample is obtained by heel stick. The blood is placed on a PKU specimen card and sent to the laboratory for analysis.

Bilirubin

The primary care provider frequently orders a bilirubin test to monitor the functioning of the neonate's liver. As stated previously, the neonate needs to break down the excess red blood cells. This is accomplished by the spleen and liver. The excess bilirubin should be broken down by the liver and excreted through the bile. It will take several days for the neonate's liver to be able to complete this process. In the meantime, the bilirubin builds up in the blood, resulting in hyperbilirubinemia. Hyperlipidemia (or *pathologic jaundice*) is discussed in Chapter 61 ⚭. Laboratory personnel usually obtain the blood. The nurse informs the primary care provider of the results.

CIRCUMCISION

Circumcision is the surgical removal of the foreskin (prepuce) of the penis. Table 56-6 ■ identifies the advantages and disadvantages of circumcision. Parents should make an informed decision prior to signing the consent form. Only

TABLE 56-6	Advantages and Disadvantages of Circumcision	
ADVANTAGES	**DISADVANTAGES**
Religious conviction	No evidence of medical benefit
Culture	Painful procedure
Social norm	Risk of bleeding
Hygiene	Risk of infection

full-term infants should be circumcised. Cultural beliefs must be considered when supporting parent's decision about circumcision. Box 56-2 ■ identifies common cultural considerations.

Before the procedure begins, an informed consent must be signed. The infant is kept NPO for several hours. Many institutions have policies making premedicating the infant with EMLA cream and Tylenol drops mandatory and the nurse should follow these policies. The infant is restrained on a circumcision board and a blanket should be placed over the infant's chest to prevent heat loss. At this point, the infant frequently begins to cry due to being held in extension. If not premedicating with EMLA cream, the physician may administer a local anesthetic in the form of an injection. The physician then makes a slit in the prepuce and uses a Yellen (Gomco) clamp or Plastibell (Figure 56-20 ■) to control bleeding. The prepuce is then cut off. The Gomco clamp will be left in place for 5 minutes and then removed. The Plastibell will fall off in 5 to 8 days. When the Gomco clamp is used, vitamin A and D ointment or petroleum jelly may be applied to the penis to prevent the glans from sticking to the diaper. Ointment is not applied when the Plastibell is used.

The penis should be checked for bleeding at least every hour for 12 hours. If bleeding occurs, pressure should be applied with a sterile 4×4 cotton gauze until bleeding stops. If bleeding cannot be controlled, the supervising registered nurse and physician should be notified. The penis should be washed with warm water with each diaper change. The glans may be kept covered with a petroleum jelly gauze until healing has occurred. The glans will be sensitive for a few days, so the diaper should be fastened loosely and the baby

BOX 56-2	**CULTURAL CONSIDERATION FOR CIRCUMCISION**

Male Jewish infants may be circumcised on the 8th day of life during a religious ceremony by the mohel, a person trained to do circumcision. Parents should be taught home care before leaving the hospital even though the procedure will occur later.

Muslim parents also practice circumcision as a religious rite.

In European countries, circumcision is infrequently performed except for religious reasons.

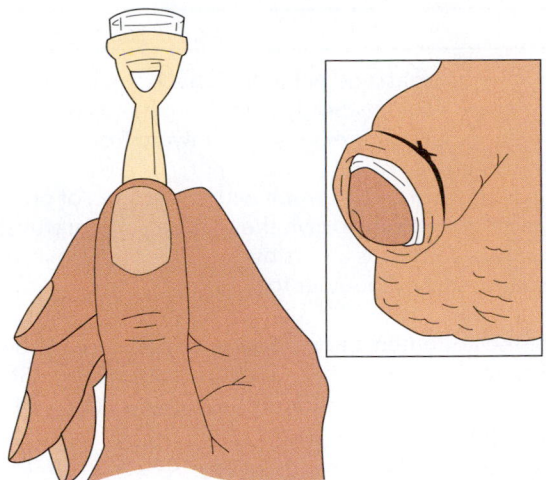

Figure 56-20. ■ Circumcision using the Plastibell. The bell is fitted over the glans. A suture is tied around the bell's rim, and the excess prepuce is cut away. The plastic rim remains in place for 3 to 4 days until healing occurs. The bell may be allowed to fall off. It is removed if it is still in place after 8 days.

should not be placed on the abdomen. Parents should be instructed to be alert for signs of infection (such as excessive bleeding, redness, swelling, and purulent drainage) until the circumcision has healed in 7 to 10 days.

IMMUNIZATIONS

Although immunizations can be given at any age, the Center for Disease Control (CDC) and the American Academy of Pediatrics recommend that immunizations be started in infancy. It is recommended that most immunizations begin in the second month of life. However, hepatitis B can be given in the neonatal period and may be given prior to discharge from the hospital. A signed parental consent must be signed prior to immunization. An immunization schedule is shown in Chapter 60 🔗.

Sleep

The neonate generally sleeps for approximately 20 to 22 hours a day. The newborn likes the security and warmth offered by swaddling (see Figure 56-4). To swaddle the baby, place a blanket on a secure surface in the shape of a diamond. Fold the top corner down slightly. Lay the baby on the blanket with the head at the fold. Wrap the right corner around the baby and secure it under the left side. Do not wrap so tightly that the baby is unable to breathe or move. Pull the bottom corner up to the baby's chest. Wrap the left corner around the newborn's right side. Place the newborn on his or her back in the crib. The baby can be wrapped in a second blanket, but the head should remain exposed.

A light massage may help the agitated baby to relax before sleep. Box 56-3 ■ provides steps for infant massage.

Discharge Teaching about Neonatal Care

Parents may be going home with a baby for the first time. Nurses are responsible to be sure that parents are informed and comfortable with this new responsibility. The following are areas that the nurse should be sure to address with parents. Some of these areas require a decision on the part of the parents, and though it is the nurse's job to give the best possible information, it is also the nurse's job to support the client's decisions. Examples would include breastfeeding versus bottle-feeding, and cloth diapers versus disposable diapers.

Topics discussed in this chapter that require client teaching prior to discharge include the following:

- Nutrition
- Elimination
- Diapering
- Hygiene
- Placing infant on back to sleep
- Perineal care
- Circumcision care
- Umbilical cord care—report foul smell, redness, drainage, and active bleeding to the primary care physician
- Safety

Safety for the neonate cannot be stressed enough with new parents. All newborns should be placed in a federally approved child safety seat when in an automobile. Parents should follow the installation procedure that comes with the car seat. If carrying both supplies and the newborn, parents should secure the newborn in the car before transferring packages.

Parents should be taught that the newborn is at risk of falling if left unattended on a high surface. Even if the neonate is secured in an infant carrier, the baby's motions can tip the carrier over. For example, if the parent places the newborn in a carrier on the kitchen counter while putting away groceries, the baby's motions can cause the carrier to fall from the countertop.

The need to handle infants gently is stressed. Besides teaching parents to support the baby's head when lifting, teaching is also done about the dangers of shaking infants. Some facilities ask parents to view a video about shaken

---

BOX 56-3 | **CLIENT TEACHING**

Infant Massage

Infant massage has many benefits. It can soothe a tired infant and minimize distress. It promotes bonding and may boost the infant's immune system. It can help relieve colic and promote sleep.

General Guidelines

Massage is best done when both parent and child are relaxed and calm. It is best to wait about half an hour after the infant's feeding. The room should be warm (78°F). If the room is cold or humid, a light blanket should be used to cover the body parts that are not being massaged. The infant is placed on a soft surface (such as a bed).

Baby lotion may be used for the massage. Put lotion on the hands and rub them together so the hands are warm and soft. Depending on the particular infant, it may not be necessary to keep applying lotion.

The time during massage is an optimum time to bond with the infant. Remember to make eye contact and to speak softly while giving the massage.

Always use gentle pressure (no harder than you would use to rub your own eyes).

Massage Process

- Start with the infant lying supine (on the back). With light touch, draw fingertips from the center of the nose up and toward the temples, from the mouth out over the ears and down, and up over the top of the head. Bring the fingertips from the center of the chin up to the tops of the ears.
- Very gently, massage behind the neck and down onto the shoulders. Softly place both hands onto the shoulders. Stroke gently downward from neck to chest.
- Circle the arm at the armpit with the fingers of one hand. Stroke gently down the arm. Be very careful at the elbow because it is a sensitive area. Gently stroke several times from shoulder to wrist and slide fingers down over the hands.
- For the abdomen, trace a clockwise circle below the ribs. Do not include the genitalia in the massage. Stroke lightly around the abdomen and down from the abdomen to the thighs.
- Massage each leg, pressing firmly but gently on the muscles of the thigh and calf. Bend the knees and press the thighs gently against the abdomen.
- Draw the hands along one foot at a time from ankle to toe. Press each toe lightly. Then stroke the whole foot again. Use a circular motion at the heels.
- Turn the infant over onto the stomach. Starting at the head, make long stroking motions that include the head, neck, back, and legs. Gently massage the muscles of the back with small, circular motions. Do not massage the spine; instead, place the hands over the spinal cord for a few seconds to warm the area.
- Massage the backs of the legs from thigh to foot. Then stroke again from head to foot a few times to finish the massage.

---

baby syndrome before being discharged home with the neonate.

NURSING CARE

PRIORITIZING NURSING CARE

The priorities of nursing care for the normal neonate are:

- Maintaining the airway, breathing, and circulation
- Maintaining body temperature
- Teaching parents to provide care for their neonate
- Providing nutrition
- Ensuring elimination

ASSESSING

Once the nurse meets the immediate survival needs of the neonate at the time of delivery, the nurse begins the process of preparing parents to care for their baby. The nurse must assess the learning needs of the parents. If this is the first child, the parents may need more information and support than parents who have had other children. However, the nurse should ensure that experienced parents still have the knowledge and skills they require to provide the necessary care.

The assessment of learning needs is accomplished by asking parents what they already know and by watching them handle the baby. Often, a conversational manner makes parents feel comfortable about asking questions.

DIAGNOSING, PLANNING, AND IMPLEMENTING

A key nursing diagnosis for the new parents might be:

- *Deficient Knowledge* related to feeding, diapering, bathing, safety

Many facilities use prepared teaching plans to provide instruction and documentation of teaching. Nurses often provide and reinforce teaching.

- Teach umbilical and circumcision care. *Keeping the umbilical cord and circumcision clean and dry prevents infection and promotes healing.*
- Demonstrate bathing and stress safety concerns. *Keeping the neonate out of water until the cord falls off promotes drying of the cord. Once the neonate is bathed in water, safety is a high priority because a wet baby is very slippery.*
- Review client decisions about feeding the baby. Support the client's decision about which method to use. Be sensitive to cultural attitudes about feeding. (For example, a woman of

Hispanic culture may want to begin breastfeeding in the privacy of her own home.) Many facilities provide a lactation specialist to discuss breastfeeding methods and concerns. *The neonate needs nutrients every 3 to 4 hours. Mothers need to be taught techniques for breastfeeding. Both parents should be taught how to prepare formula for bottle-fed neonates. They should also be given guidelines for bottle care and for positioning infants for feeding.*

- Provide information about elimination and about what stools should look like. The appearance will depend on whether the child is breast fed or bottle fed. *Parents should be taught to watch for changes in elimination patterns, including changes in stool color and consistency with feeding.*

- Observe the client and others performing routine care such as dressing or diapering. Ensure that caregivers are practicing good hygiene and safety. *The neonate needs to be handled gently. The head needs to be supported. Parents should be taught to provide perineal care with each diaper change.*

- Review safety concerns, including risk for falls, risk of suffocation, and safety car seats. *New parents may not be aware of possible dangers. Experienced parents may need information about how new equipment is used.*

- Encourage the family to take on some daily chores to support the mother. *Family members can participate in the health and care of the mother and infant by providing time for the mother to recover from labor, and care for the baby.*

EVALUATING

Evaluating is best accomplished by watching the parents give care to the newborn. The nurse should document the teaching and list any printed material that was provided to the parents. Follow-up phone calls or home visits may be needed for parents with limited family support.

NURSING PROCESS CARE PLAN
Care of the Neonate Following Cesarean Birth

Isaiah, 30 minutes old, delivered by cesarean birth, has been transferred from the operating room to the newborn nursery. Isaiah's mother was in labor for 22 hours, received epidural anesthesia, pushed for 3 hours, and required a cesarean birth due to CPD. Apgar scores were 7 and 9 at 1 and 5 minutes. Isaiah is to be monitored and provided with routine care until his mother is stable in the recovery room.

Assessment

- Isaiah's vital signs are within normal limits.
- Head was palpated for caput succedaneum and cephalhematoma.
- All extremities move equally.
- All reflexes are intact.

Nursing Diagnosis

The following important nursing diagnosis (among others) is established for this client:

- *Risk for Ineffective Cerebral Tissue Perfusion* related to head trauma from cephalopelvic disproportion (CPD)

Expected Outcomes

The client will have no signs of impaired cerebral perfusion as evidenced by equal movement, intact reflexes, and vital signs within normal limits.

Planning and Implementation

Nursing interventions for this client would include the following:

- Monitor vital signs, movements, and reflexes every 15 to 30 minutes. *CPD can cause cranial trauma resulting in cerebral edema and decreased tissue perfusion. Alterations in vital signs outside normal limits and decreased movements and reflexes are signs of decreased cerebral perfusion in the neonate.*

- Inform charge nurse and primary care provider of changes. *Alterations in cerebral tissue perfusion require immediate medical attention.*

Evaluation

Client's vital signs, movements, and reflexes remain in normal limits.

Critical Thinking in the Nursing Process

1. What information about cranial trauma with CPD should be shared with the parents?
2. Whose responsibility is it to inform parents of long-term effects of cranial trauma?
3. What are some other signs of decreased cranial tissue perfusion Isaiah may exhibit in the next few months?

Note: Discussion of Critical Thinking questions appears on the MyNursingKit Website.

Note: The references and resources for all chapters have been compiled at the back of the book.

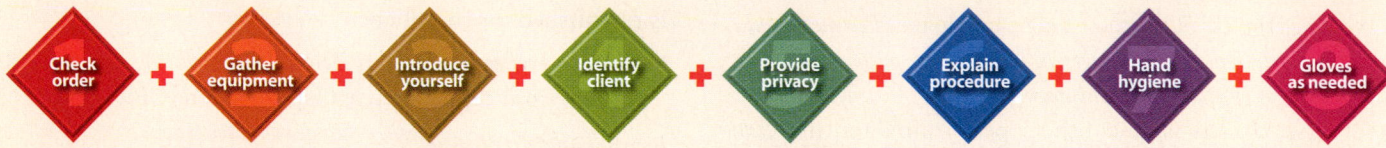

PROCEDURE 56-1   Obtaining an Apgar Score

Purposes

- To evaluate the physical condition of the newborn at birth
- To determine the need for resuscitation efforts

Equipment

- Neonatal stethoscope
- Bulb syringe
- Warm towels

Check order + Gather equipment + Introduce yourself + Identify client + Provide privacy + Explain procedure + Hand hygiene + Gloves as needed

Interventions and Rationales

1. Perform preparatory steps (see icon bar above).

2. Assess the heart rate by auscultation or palpation where the umbilical cord meets the abdomen. *This is the best location for finding the pulse in the newborn.*

3. Assign a score for heart rate: 0 for absent; 1 for HR less than 100; 2 for HR less than or equal to 100. *This is the standard method for determining an Apgar score.*

4. Assess respiratory effort. Crying indicates good respiratory effort. *A strong cry indicates the infant can inhale and exhale adequately. If the infant is not crying, observe the rise and fall of the chest.*

5. Assign a score for respiratory effort: 0 for absent; 1 for slow or irregular respirations; 2 for regular respirations or vigorous crying. *These are standard criteria for determining Apgar.*

6. Assess muscle tone by determining degree of flexion and resistance when straightening the extremity. *Healthy infants resist straightening a flexed limb.*

7. Assign a score for muscle tone: 0 for flaccidity; 1 for some flexion of extremities; 2 for active motion and good flexion.

8. Assess reflex irritability by physically stimulating the infant during the drying process. *Sneeze and cough and Moro reflexes can easily be elicted while drying the infant and clearing the airway.*

9. Assign a score for reflex irritability: 0 for no response to stimulation; 1 for a notable grimace; 2 for a cry elicited by stimulation.

10. Assess skin color. Observe closely for pallor and cyanosis. *Skin color indicates functioning of the cardiovascular and respiratory systems.*

11. Assign a score for skin color: 0 for overall cyanosis and pallor; 1 for acrocyanosis; 2 for pink skin tone over the newborn's entire body.

12. Total the assigned score. *This is the standard method for determining an Apgar score.*

13. Provide appropriate care related to Apgar score.
    For 8–10: continue with routine newborn care.
    For 4–7: tactile stimulation and oxygen administration is needed. Scores less than 4: newborn resuscitation is required.

SAMPLE DOCUMENTATION

[date] [time]	Caucasian male delivered vaginally. Cord clamped and cut by Dr. L. Hogan. Infant transferred to warmer and dried vigorously. Apgar score 7 @ one minute. Oxygen administered by mask. Apgar score 9 @ five minutes. _____ _____ W. Brown, LVN

PROCEDURE 56-2 Measuring Height and Length

Purposes

- To obtain an accurate measure of the client's height or length
- To report baseline measurements that will be used for follow-up

Equipment

- Tape measure, yard stick, meter stick, or measuring mat

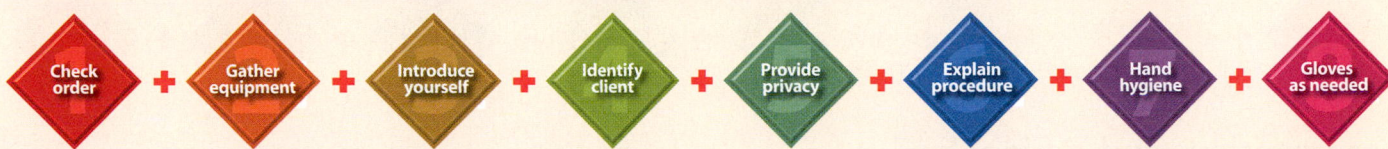

Check order + **Gather equipment** + **Introduce yourself** + **Identify client** + **Provide privacy** + **Explain procedure** + **Hand hygiene** + **Gloves as needed**

Interventions and Rationales

1. Perform preparatory steps (see icon bar above).
2. Place the infant in a supine position. *This position will provide the greatest opportunity for accurate measurement.*

3. Place the infant's head against a flat surface. Extend legs until the knee is straight. *This defines the full length of the neonate's body.*
4. Use a tape measure, measuring stick, or measuring mat to measure from the crown to the heel (Figure 56-21 ■). Note the length in inches or centimeters. *Follow facility policy in recording baseline length for future comparison.*
5. Plot the measurement on a standardized growth chart. Note: The Appendix on the MyNursingKit Website shows growth charts from infancy to age 18.

SAMPLE DOCUMENTATION

[date]	Height recorded on growth
[time]	chart. _____
	_____ H. Freida, LPN

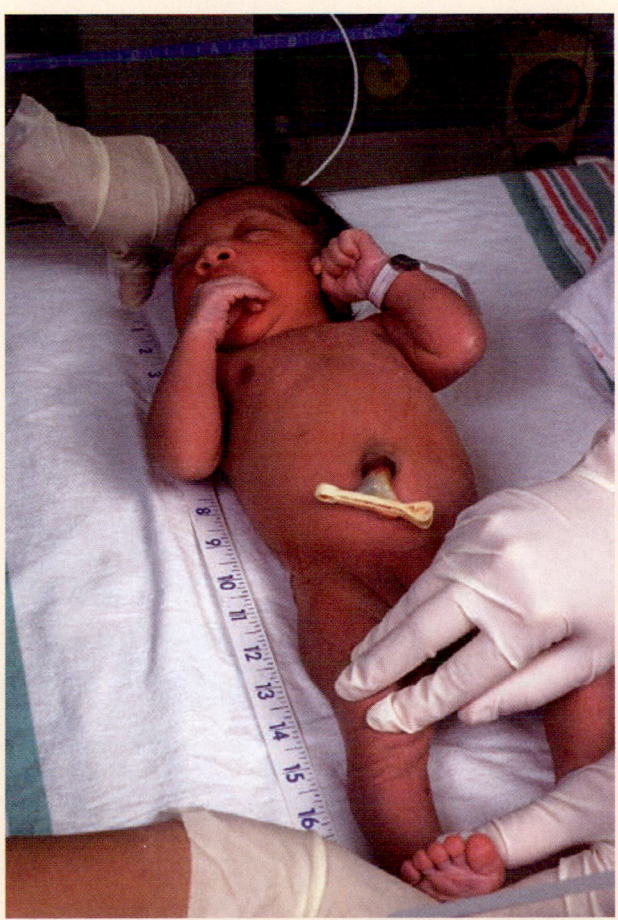

Figure 56-21. ■ Neonatal measurements are taken immediately after birth. For height, it is often helpful to have two staff members work together to ensure the accuracy of the measurement from crown to heel.

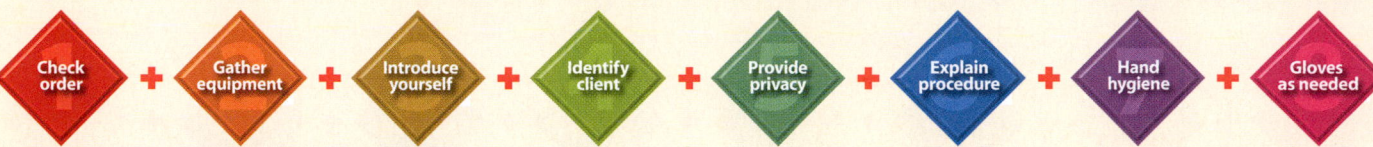

PROCEDURE 56-3	**Obtaining Weight**

Purposes

- To obtain an accurate measure of the client's weight
- To record a baseline weight for future assessment and follow-up

Equipment

- Infant scale, calibrated

Check order + Gather equipment + Introduce yourself + Identify client + Provide privacy + Explain procedure + Hand hygiene + Gloves as needed

Interventions and Rationales

1. Perform preparatory steps (see icon bar above).

2. Place the neonate in a supine position on the infant scale (Figure 56-22 ■).

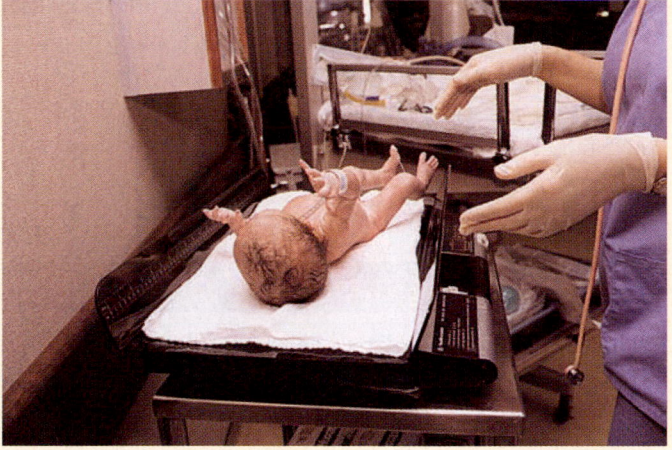

Figure 56-22. ■ To obtain the neonate's weight, place the infant on a platform scale. The caregiver's hands are poised near the newborn as a safety measure. (© Stella Johnson www.stellajohnson.com.)

3. Stand close with one hand over, but not touching, the infant. *This provides for safety in case the neonate should move.*

4. Read the scale when the neonate is still. *The most accurate measurement will be obtained when the neonate is not moving.*

5. Record the weight.

SAMPLE DOCUMENTATION

[date]	Weight recorded on growth
[time]	chart. _____
	_____ H. Freida, LPN

PROCEDURE 56-4	**Measuring Head Circumference**

Purpose

- To determine normalcy of the infant's head circumference in relation to chest circumference

Equipment

- Tape measure

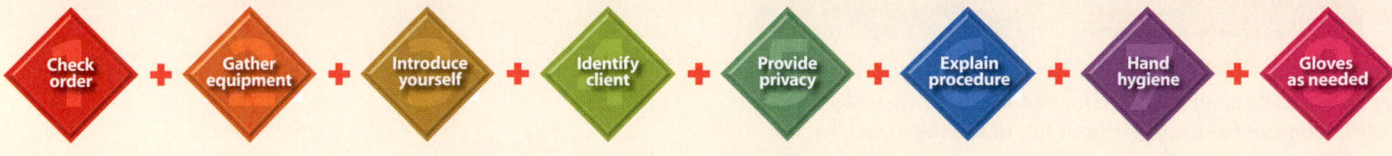

Check order + Gather equipment + Introduce yourself + Identify client + Provide privacy + Explain procedure + Hand hygiene + Gloves as needed

Interventions and Rationales

1. Perform preparatory steps (see icon bar).

2. Position the infant in a supine position.

3. Place the tape measure slightly above the eyebrows, above the pinna of the ear, and around the occiput (see Figure 16-3 ⊙⊙). *This is the largest diameter of the infant's head.*

4. Document the head circumference in inches or centimeters (in the neonate, usually 33 to 35 centimeters). The nurse may also document the amount of *molding* (shaping of the head during the birth process). *Documentation provides information for later comparison.*

5. Compare to chest circumference. *Head circumference is equal to or 2 cm greater than chest circumference until age 2.*

6. Plot the measurement on a standardized growth chart.

SAMPLE DOCUMENTATION

[date] Head circumference recorded
[time] on chart. _____
_____ H. Freida, LPN

PROCEDURE 56-5   # Measuring Chest Circumference

Purpose

■ To determine normalcy of the infant's chest circumference in relation to head circumference

Equipment

■ Tape measure

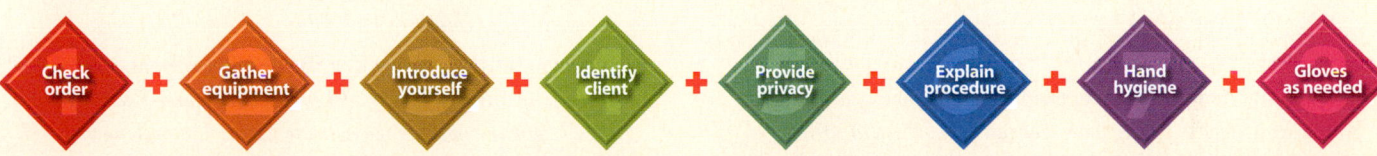

Check order + Gather equipment + Introduce yourself + Identify client + Provide privacy + Explain procedure + Hand hygiene + Gloves as needed

Interventions and Rationales

1. Perform preparatory steps (see icon bar above).

2. Position the infant in a supine position.

3. Encircle the chest with the measuring tape. Place the tape measure against the bare skin of the infant's chest, at the nipple line, under the axillae (Figure 56-23 ■). *This is the largest diameter of the infant's chest.*

4. Document the chest circumference in inches or centimeters.

5. Compare to head circumference. *Head circumference is equal to or 2 cm greater than chest circumference until age 2.*

6. Plot the measurement on a standardized growth chart.

SAMPLE DOCUMENTATION

[date] Chest circumference recorded
[time] on chart. _____
_____ H. Freida, LPN

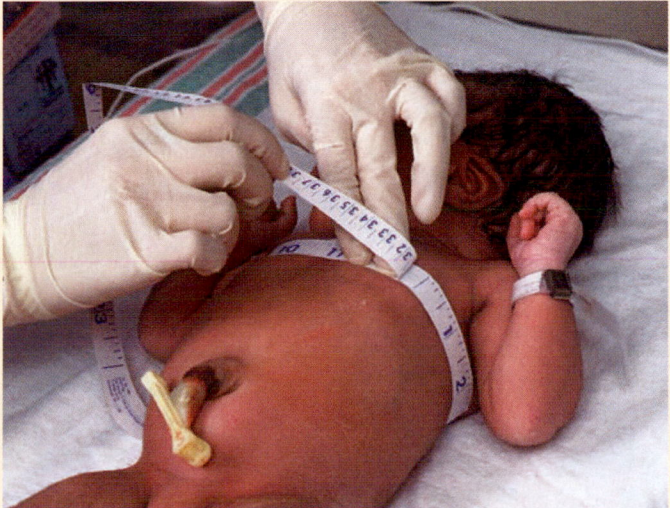

Figure 56-23. ■ Chest circumference in the neonate is normally the same as the head circumference but should not exceed it.

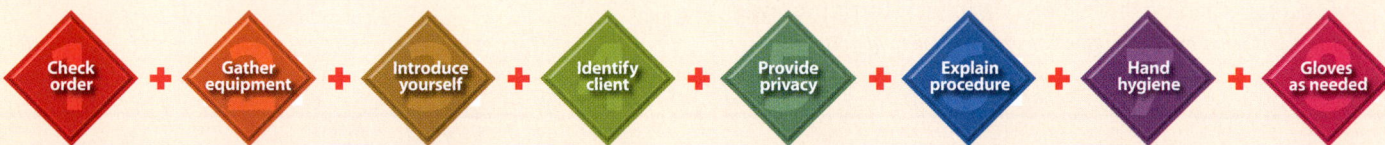

PROCEDURE 56-6   # Bathing the Newborn

Purpose

- To cleanse the skin of the newborn

Equipment

- Clean t-shirt
- Diaper
- Gloves
- Soft wash cloth
- Soft comb
- Thermometer
- Warm towel
- Warm water
- Warm blankets

Check order + Gather equipment + Introduce yourself + Identify client + Provide privacy + Explain procedure + Hand hygiene + Gloves as needed

Interventions and Rationales

1. Perform preparatory steps (see icon bar above).

2. Determine that the infant's temperature is stable. *Newborn will lose heat during the bath.*

3. Put on gloves. *Gloves decrease the possibility of contamination with maternal blood and body fluids.*

4. Wet the washcloth in warm water approximately 98°–99° F (36.6°–37.2° C). *Warm water decreases body heat loss.*

5. Wash the newborn's face, trunk, extremities, and diaper area in order. *Washing from cleanest to most soiled areas prevents the spread of organisms.*

6. When washing the face, wash the eyes from the inner canthus toward the outer canthus. Wash the ears, taking care to wash behind the ear, and the pinna. Nothing should be inserted into the ear canal or nose. *This technique prevents injury to the newborn's eyes, ears, and nose.*

7. Wash the neck. Insert one hand under the newborn's back to expose the neck and wash all folds. *Blood and amniotic fluid collect in neck folds and should be removed.*

8. Uncover and wash and dry the chest, back, and arms. Avoid rubbing the skin. Provide cord care. *Rubbing the skin might traumatize the delicate tissue. Uncovering only the area to be washed prevents heat loss.*

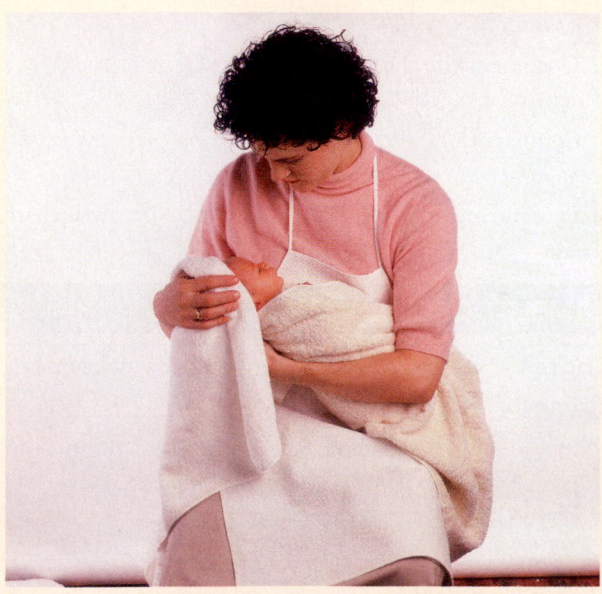

A

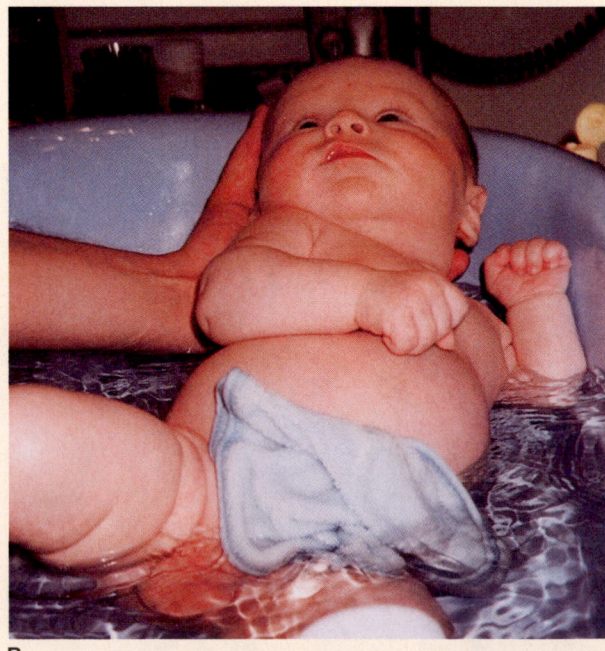

B

Figure 56-24. ■ **A.** When sponge bathing the newborn, cover the areas that are not being washed, and wash the head first. Wrap the baby in a warm towel and cover the head. **B.** Once the cord has fallen off, the baby can have a full bath. Hold the head of the infant to prevent the baby from slipping.

9. Put a clean warm t-shirt on the baby. Place a blanket over the chest and arms. *Covering the baby prevents heat loss.*

10. Wash the legs, remove the diaper, and clean the perineum. Wash the vulva of the female from front to back to prevent contamination of the vagina and urethra with fecal material. Wash the penis and scrotum of the male, taking care to wash under and in the folds of the scrotum. Do not retract the foreskin in the uncircumcised male. Apply a clean diaper. *The diaper area must be cleaned after each void and stool to prevent skin irritation.*

11. Wrap the baby in a warm towel, leaving the head exposed (Figure 56-24 ■). Hold the baby in one arm using a football hold. Wash the baby's hair, rinse by pouring water over the head, taking care not to get water into the baby's eyes. Combing the hair while washing it helps to remove dried blood. Dry the head. Apply a cap to decrease heat loss. *Washing the baby's head last conserves body heat.*

12. Wrap the baby in warm blankets or place the baby under a radiant warmer. Take the baby's temperature in 30 minutes to 1 hour. *The temperature reading verifies that the baby has not had excessive heat loss.*

SAMPLE DOCUMENTATION

[date] [time]	Temperature 99°F. Initial bath completed. Umbilical cord cleaned with alcohol. Wrapped in 3 warm blankets and placed in mother's arms. _____
	_____ M. Rodriguez, LPN

PROCEDURE 56-7

Administering Intramuscular Injection to the Newborn

Purpose

- To administer medication safely into the muscle of the newborn

Equipment

- Gloves
- Alcohol wipes
- Syringe with medication
- Band-aid

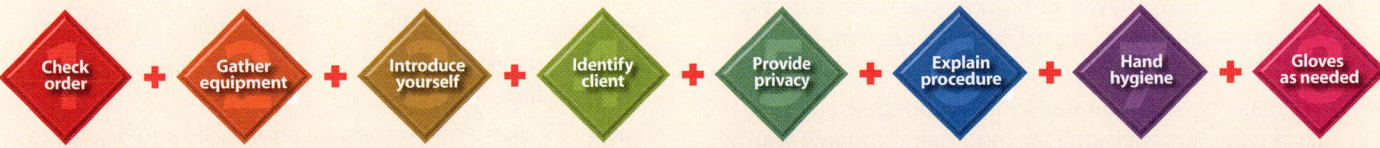

Check order + Gather equipment + Introduce yourself + Identify client + Provide privacy + Explain procedure + Hand hygiene + Gloves as needed

Interventions and Rationales

1. Perform preparatory steps (see icon bar above).

2. Prepare medication for injection. A 1-mL syringe with a ½- or ⅝-inch, 25-gauge needle is used. *A small short needle reaches the muscle but avoids potentially striking the bone.*

3. Put on gloves. *Gloves decrease the possibility of contamination with blood.*

4. Locate the correct site. The middle third of the vastus lateralis muscle is used (Figure 56-25 ■).

5. Clean the area with an alcohol wipe in a circular motion. *Cleansing the skin prevents infection at the injection site.*

6. Stabilize the leg by placing the palm of your nondominant hand on the baby's knee, grasping the vastus lateralis muscle between your thumb and first

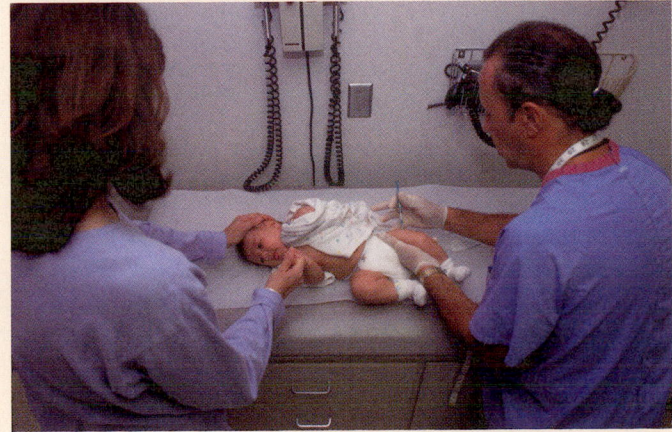

Figure 56-25. ■ Injection of vitamin K in a neonate.

finger. *Holding the leg in this manner prevents the baby from moving the leg. Gently squeezing the muscle adds depth to prevent the needle from hitting the bone.*

7. Insert the needle at a 90-degree angle with your dominant hand. *Newborn tissue is soft and requires little force to get the needle into the tissue.*

8. Using your nondominant hand, aspirate observing for a blood return. *Be careful not to move the needle. Aspiration verifies correct placement of the needle.*

9. If no blood returns, slowly inject the medication. *Slow injection of the medication decreases discomfort.*

10. If there is blood in the syringe, remove the needle, dispose of the syringe, and prepare a new medication. *Blood in the syringe indicates the needle was in a blood vessel. Injecting the medication at this point would be administering it by the intravenous route.*

11. Following injection of the medication, remove the needle, and gently massage the site. *Gentle massage begins medication absorption.*

12. Needles cannot be recapped. Dispose of needle and syringe in the proper container. *The equipment used for an intramuscular injection is considered to be contaminated and poses the threat of transmitting harmful substances.*

SAMPLE DOCUMENTATION

[date]	1 mg AquaMEPHYTON given
[time]	IM in right vastus lateralis.
	Band-Aid applied. _____
	_____ W. Weaver, LVN

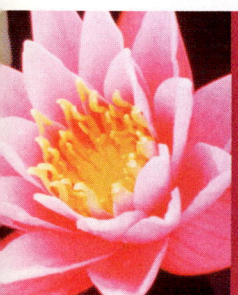

Chapter Review

KEY Points

- Most infants are born without complications, and require routine care.

- The LPN/LVN must know the normal appearance and reflexes of the neonate and report deviations to the supervising nurse or physician.

- Routine care of the neonate involves sponge baths, feeding, cord care, circumcision care, and diapering in a warm, calm environment.

- Medications routinely given to the neonate include an antibiotic eye ointment or drops and AquaMEPHYTON IM.

- Hepatitis B immunization may be administered in the newborn nursery with parental consent.

- The LPN/LVN may assist with male circumcision and post procedure care.

- The LPN/LVN assists the RN by teaching parents about routine newborn care.

☺ FOR FURTHER Study

Head circumference and reflexes in the newborn are discussed in Chapter 160.

See Chapter 33 for a review of normal blood flow through the heart.

See Figure 47-4A for infant CPR.

Chapter 53 describes characteristics and changes that occur in the neonate at birth; Table 53-4 provides the Apgar Scoring System.

Methods for breastfeeding are discussed in Chapter 54.

PKU is discussed in Chapter 57 with other disorders of metabolism.

Chapter 57 discusses congenital anomalies and disorders in the high-risk newborn.

Immunization schedule is shown in Chapter 60.

Hyperlipidemia is discussed in Chapter 61.

EXPLORE PEARSON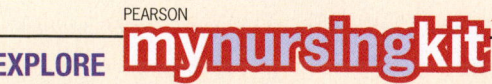

MyNursingKit is your one stop for online chapter review materials and resources. Prepare for success with additional NCLEX®-style practice questions, interactive assignments and activities, web links, animations and videos, and more!

Register your access code from the front of your book at
www.mynursingkit.com

Critical Thinking Care Map

Neonate with Impaired Nutrition
NCLEX-PN® Focus Area: Physiologic Adaptation

Case Study: Jaime, a 5-day-old infant, is brought to the emergency department by his mother, Jean. Jean states that Jaime refuses to nurse and she is concerned about him. Jaime weighed 9 lbs 4 oz at birth.

Nursing Diagnosis: *Alteration in Nutrition: Less than Body Requirements*

COLLECT DATA

Subjective	Objective
_____	_____
_____	_____
_____	_____
_____	_____
_____	_____
_____	_____

Would you report this? Yes/No

If yes, report to: _____

What would you report?_____

Nursing Care

_____
_____
_____
_____
_____
_____
_____
_____
_____
_____
_____

How would you document this? _____

_____
_____
_____

Compare your answers and documentation to those provided on the MyNursingKit Website.

Data Collected
(use only those that apply)

- Wt. 8 lb 3 oz
- Crying
- Mother states he won't nurse
- Skin dry and peeling
- Anterior fontanel sunken
- Mother states nursed well prior to discharge
- Milia on nose
- Umbilical cord dry
- Mother states milk not in yet

Nursing Interventions
(use only those that apply; list in priority order)

- Monitor vital signs every 2 hours.
- Monitor lab tests.
- Collect urine sample for culture/sensitivity.
- Observe parent/infant interaction.
- Call Child Protection Services.
- Monitor IV infusion.
- Review breastfeeding techniques with mother.
- Encourage mother to change to bottle-feeding.

NCLEX-PN® Exam Preparation

TEST-TAKING TIP   Be sure to identify the client in the question. Frequently the client is the ill child, but could be the parent. The answer is directed at the client.

1 The nurse teaches a class for new mothers on bathing the newborn. The nurse determines that further teaching is needed when one of the mothers states:

1. "I should not put my baby into the bath water until after the umbilical cord falls off."
2. "I should bathe my baby in 2 inches of water so he can't drown."
3. "I should wash the baby's eyes first, using a different corner of the washcloth for each eye."
4. "I should examine the base of the umbilical cord with each diaper change, looking for redness or drainage and clean it with plain water."

2 The nurse applies antibiotic eye drops to the infant's eyes:

1. Within 5 minutes of when the baby is born.
2. Prior to bathing the infant 4 hours after birth.
3. Within an hour of delivery.
4. Prior to discharging the infant with the mother.

3 The nurse, working in the admission nursery, anticipates the newborn who adapts well to extrauterine life will breathe:

1. Regularly at 20 to 24 breaths per minute.
2. Irregularly at 32 to 44 breaths per minute.
3. Regularly at 30 to 60 breaths per minute.
4. Irregularly at 30 to 60 breaths per minute.

4 While examining a 2-day-old infant the nurse notes a new onset of jaundice and anticipates:

1. Liver function studies to determine presence of a congenital anomaly of the liver.
2. No further workup will be ordered because all 2-day-old infants have jaundice.
3. An ABO or Rh incompatibility.
4. Orders for a total and conjugated bilirubin and phototherapy.

5 A new mother examines her infant and says, "Look, her hands and feet are blue. I know there must be something wrong with her." The nurse's best response is:

1. "It takes the newborn a few days to regulate circulation. What you're seeing is normal and will subside within a few days."
2. "I'll notify the doctor. She needs to go back to the nursery immediately."
3. "The cyanosis of the hands and feet indicates the baby is cold. Did you have her unwrapped?"
4. "She might have a cardiac defect. I'll take her to the nursery so we can do a chest x-ray."

6 The nurse, working in the newborn nursery, is caring for a baby who is fussy and irritable. Which of the following actions performed by the nurse would help to comfort the baby?

1. Undress the newborn and place him or her on a radiant warmer so he or she can be soothed by the heat.
2. Place the newborn on his or her stomach to sleep.
3. Prop a pacifier in the neonate's mouth with a toy to hold it in place.
4. Wrap the newborn securely in a receiving blanket.

7 The nurse observes a new mother breastfeeding her newborn and recognizes no further teaching is needed when she:

1. Starts feeding on the left side with every feeding.
2. Gradually decreases the length of feedings.
3. Starts the newborn on a different side each feeding.
4. Holds the newborn for 20 minutes at each breast.

8 The nurse teaches a new mother how to care for the baby's circumcision and evaluates that further teaching is needed when she states:

1. "I will clean the penis with alcohol three times a day."
2. "If the penis becomes red and swollen, I will call the doctor."
3. "The Plastibell will fall off by itself, so I should not pull it off even if it's hanging by a thread."
4. "If I see bleeding, I will apply pressure until it stops and notify the doctor."

9 The nurse assesses the newborn at 1 minute of life and finds the heart rate less than 100, respiratory rate is slow and irregular, muscles are flaccid, reflex irritability is lacking, and the newborn has a pink body with cyanotic extremities. The nurse scores the infant's 1-minute Apgar as:

1. 9.
2. 3.
3. 5.
4. 7.

10 The nurse suspects that the newborn was born prematurely when which of the following characteristics is noted?

1. Opaque skin that is dry and peeling
2. Breast tissue measuring 0.5 to 1 cm
3. Flexed body position at rest
4. Undescended testicles in boys and prominent clitoris in girls

Answers and rationales for Review Questions appear in Appendix I.

Care of High-Risk Neonates

LEARNING Outcomes

After completing this chapter, you will be able to:

1. Explain what factors make a newborn "high-risk" and what role the LPN/LVN plays in relation to high-risk neonates.
2. Describe general care of the high-risk newborn.
3. Discuss the physiological characteristics of the preterm and postterm newborn.
4. Contrast large-for-gestational-age neonates with small-for-gestational-age neonates.
5. Describe common respiratory conditions of the high-risk newborn.
6. Name six congenital heart defects and describe nursing care for them.
7. List common congenital nervous system defects and treatment for them.
8. Identify current treatment for congenital gastrointestinal conditions.
9. Explain special care needed by a newborn with an inborn error of metabolism.
10. Identify congenital genitourinary or musculoskeletal disorders.
11. Explain the special care needed for a drug-exposed newborn.
12. Describe priorities of care for a neonate at risk for infection.

Clinical Objectives*

13. Recognize and utilize teaching opportunities for parents of assigned infants.
14. Observe care of the high-risk/seriously ill neonate.
15. Recognize, in the high-risk/seriously ill neonate, deviations from the normal newborn infant by observing the physical assessment of such an infant.
16. Recognize and support coping measures by grieving parents.
17. Observe new methods for monitoring cardiopulmonary function of high-risk/seriously ill neonates.
18. Identify techniques utilized for conservation of body heat in management of high-risk/seriously ill neonates.
19. Observe methods of providing visual, tactile, and auditory infant stimulation.
20. Recognize one's own thoughts and feelings in observing the high-risk/seriously ill neonate.
21. Perform a 3-minute surgical scrub prior to entering the NICU.
22. Observe or participate in special feeding procedures of a neonate.
23. Observe parents' interactions with a high-risk newborn.

*Providing care for high-risk neonates does not usually fall within the scope of the LPN/LVN. Opportunities may arise in which the LPN/LVN student may be able to observe in NICU.

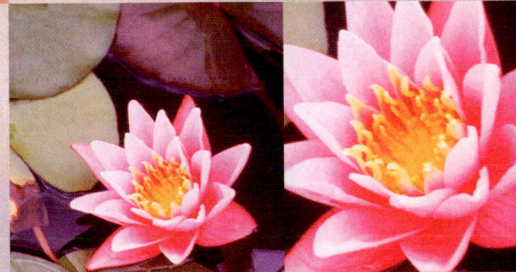

KEY TERMS

Use the audio glossary feature on the MyNursingKit Website to hear the correct pronunciation of the following key terms.

bronchopulmonary dysplasia 1568

circumoral 1571

cleft lip 1577

cleft palate 1577

diaphragmatic hernia 1581

esophageal atresia 1574

high-risk newborn 1562

hyperbilirubinemia 1576

intrauterine growth restriction 1567

Logan clamp 1577

macrosomia 1566

meconium aspiration 1568

meningocele 1572

meningomyelocele 1572

neonatal abstinence syndrome 1582

omphalocele 1574

spina bifida 1572

talipes 1581

tracheoesophageal fistula 1574

trisomy 21 1573

The **high-risk newborn** is an infant who is born prior to 38 weeks' gestation or after 42 weeks' gestation, who has alterations in intrauterine growth, or who has a medical condition that requires frequent monitoring and treatment. Often, due to circumstances during pregnancy or labor, the high-risk newborn is identified and plans are put in place for high-risk newborn care prior to birth. At other times, the degree of risk is not identified until after birth. In either case, the high-risk newborn is generally placed in a neonatal intensive care unit (NICU; Figure 57-1 ■). If an NICU is not available, the neonate is placed in an area of the newborn nursery where the registered nurse can observe the baby closely.

The role of the LPN/LVN is one of assisting the RN with data collection, meeting the basic needs of the newborn, and documenting care. If the facility does not have appropriate accommodations, the newborn may be transferred to another hospital that can meet his or her needs.

Many conditions that place the newborn at risk continue past the first month of life. This chapter addresses the basic nursing care of the high-risk newborn and introduces some congenital anomalies, infections, and disorders that are commonly seen in the high-risk newborn. For more detail on specific disorders, refer to a pediatric nursing textbook.

Many congenital anomalies are identified at birth or within the first few weeks of life. They may occur more frequently in certain ethnic groups (Box 57-1 ■). It is important for the LPN/LVN to have an understanding of the pathology, symptoms, and related nursing care. If the anomaly is life threatening, surgery is usually performed immediately to correct the defect. Other anomalies are not repaired until the child is stronger and better able to withstand the surgical procedure. At times repair is performed in stages, and complete reconstruction may take months or years. *Note:* Many nonthreatening anomalies have their major discussion in the Pediatric Unit of this book.

General Care of the High-Risk Newborn

The high-risk newborn is one who requires frequent or constant monitoring and treatment in order to survive. Individualized care is planned and implemented based on the

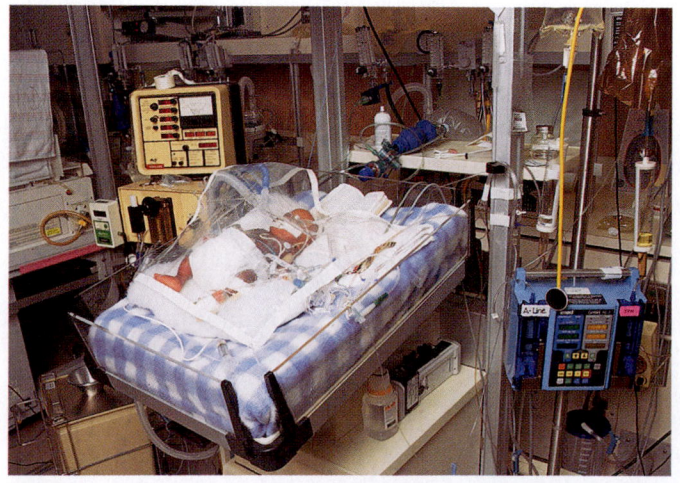

A

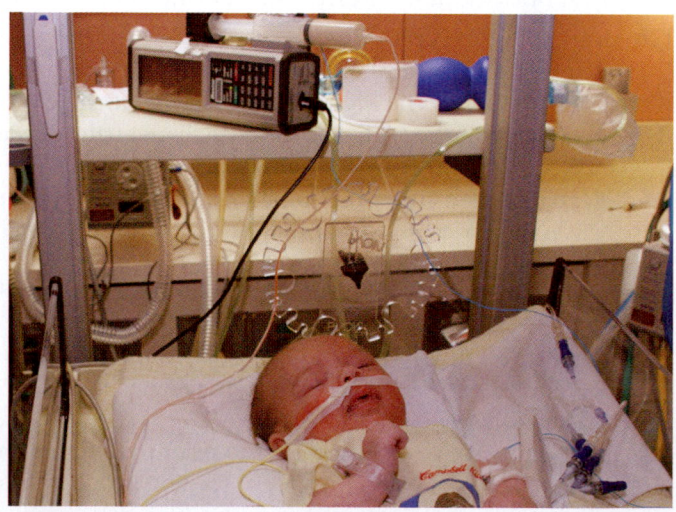

B

Figure 57-1. ■ **A.** This premature infant in the neonatal intensive care unit (NICU) is receiving artificial ventilation. **B.** This premature baby cannot yet coordinate suck and swallow. Gavage feeding is being used until the baby can effectively acquire nutrients.

BOX 57-1　CULTURAL PULSE POINTS

Rates of Congenital Defects and Infant Mortality

Some conditions take a greater toll on racial subgroups than on Caucasians. For example, American Indians and Alaska Natives experience high rates of sudden infant death syndrome (SIDS) and fetal alcohol syndrome (FAS). Hispanics/Latinos, in particular Puerto Ricans, exhibit a high rate of neural tube defects (NTDs), central nervous system anomalies that include spina bifida, anencephaly, and congenital hydrocephalus.

The U.S. Department of Health and Human Services has documented the substantial variation in infant mortality rate among and within racial and ethnic groups. Infant death rates among African Americans, American Indians, Alaska Natives, and Hispanics/Latinos were all above the national average of 7.2 deaths per 1,000 live births.

Source: From Racial and Ethnic Disparities in Health, Response to the President's Initiative on Race, 2000, Washington, DC: U.S. DHHS.

BOX 57-2　COMPLEMENTARY THERAPIES

Music as an Aid in the NICU

Premature infants in the neonatal intensive care unit (NICU) are often bombarded with sounds, lights, and other excessive stimuli. This excessive stimuli can have negative effects on the improvement of the infant's condition. Simple positive changes in the environment of the NICU can have positive effects on the premature infant. One of these changes is using music therapy. Music therapy is defined as healing with music, voice, or sound. Several research studies have found music therapy to be effective in the NICU. Infants, after being exposed to calming music, were less likely to experience high arousal states, had shorter hospital stays, and weighed more than infants who were not exposed to music.

Olson (1998) provided six principles essential to the effective use of music therapy;

1. Music is a method of demonstrating caring.
2. Music has emotional and physical effects and can facilitate the healing process.
3. Music can bring a human approach to a clinical environment.
4. Music is a method of individualizing client care.
5. Tone, rhythm, pitch, and volume of music can create a peaceful environment.
6. Music of the child's religious faith provides spiritual care to the client.

specific needs of each newborn. However, the general care of the high-risk newborn is the same.

VITAL SIGNS

The vital signs of the high-risk newborn must be monitored continuously. Electrodes placed on the newborn's chest provide ongoing ECG (EKG) monitoring. Respiratory rate and oxygen saturation are also monitored. Blood pressure is monitored electronically. If the newborn's condition warrants, a catheter may be placed through the subclavian or femoral artery to monitor pressure inside the heart.

The premature newborn has less storage of glucose and brown fat than term infants. When the premature newborn gets cold, chilling increases the need for energy, thus the need for glucose. When stored glucose is consumed, hypoglycemia results. To prevent heat loss, temperature is maintained by radiant heat above the bassinette. A sensor is placed over the soft tissue of the abdomen to ensure the newborn does not become too warm. The newborn's axillary temperature may also be taken every 2 to 4 hours.

PAIN

The nurse is responsible to assess pain in the newborn and take measures to prevent, relieve, or control discomfort. Pain pathways and brain structures responsible for long-term memory are developed by 24 weeks' gestation. Untreated pain in the preterm or term newborn can have long-term effects. Assessment tools for use in pain assessment in the newborn have been developed. See Box 56-1 🔗 for an example of an infant pain scale.

Unrelieved pain in the newborn can cause irritability, increased metabolism, poor healing, and exhaustion. Nonpharmacologic pain relief can be accomplished by swaddling in warm blankets, touching, holding, and offering a pacifier. Oral glucose solution can be effective in calming the newborn.

Pharmacologic pain relief may be accomplished with prescribed morphine or fentanyl for severe pain. Acetaminophen is frequently ordered for mild pain. It is critical for the nurse to calculate the dosage accurately when medicating the newborn to prevent accidental overdose.

Maintaining a calm environment can prevent overstimulation and decrease the newborn's pain response. At times complementary therapies are useful in quieting the infant (Box 57-2 ■).

INTAKE AND OUTPUT

Monitoring intake and output is necessary to ensure adequate fluid balance. Fluids may be given by intravenous infusion, gavage feeding (see Figure 57-1B), or, if the newborn is strong enough, through bottle or cup feeding. Output is monitored by weighing the diaper or, at times, by a suprapubic catheter. Due to the small size of the urethra, a urethral catheter is generally not used.

BLOOD GLUCOSE

Blood glucose levels are frequently used to monitor the metabolic state of the premature or high-risk newborn. Recall from Chapter 56 🔗 that a small-for-gestational-age (SGA) or large-for-gestational-age (LGA) infant will need frequent blood glucose monitoring until the glucose values have stabilized. Premature newborns may also need frequent blood glucose monitoring until they are obtaining regular feedings. A blood glucose level of 30 mg/dL or less is considered *hypoglycemia* in the newborn and requires treatment as ordered by the physician.

TREATMENTS

Medical treatment is determined by the specific disorder. Common treatments are discussed here. It is important to remember, though, that not every newborn will require all of these treatments. The premature newborn or newborn in respiratory distress might require mechanical ventilation through an endotracheal tube or, if long-term ventilation is needed, a tracheostomy tube. The nurse or respiratory therapist will maintain an open airway by suctioning mucus from the bronchi (Procedure 57-1 ■). If mechanical ventilation is not needed, oxygen may be administered by an Oxyhood (Figure 57-2 ■) or by nasal cannula or catheter.

clinical ALERT

High amounts of oxygen (over 90 to 100 mm Hg) given to the newborn may cause *retinopathy* (also called *retrolental fibroplasia*). Retrolental fibroplasia can lead to blindness. The newborn who receives high amounts of oxygen will need careful monitoring and periodic eye examinations.

Medication is usually administered by intravenous infusion. If the need for IV fluids or medications is determined within the first few hours after birth, the doctor may insert a catheter into an umbilical vein. Another site for a central venous catheter is the subclavian vein. The nurse assists with the insertion of the catheter, maintains the infusion, and administers medication as ordered.

Diagnostic examination, such as MRI scan and ultrasound, may be necessary to determine the specific disorder and appropriate treatment. The nurse may need to accompany the newborn to these procedures in order to maintain necessary care. At times, surgery may be needed to correct life-threatening congenital anomalies. Specially trained

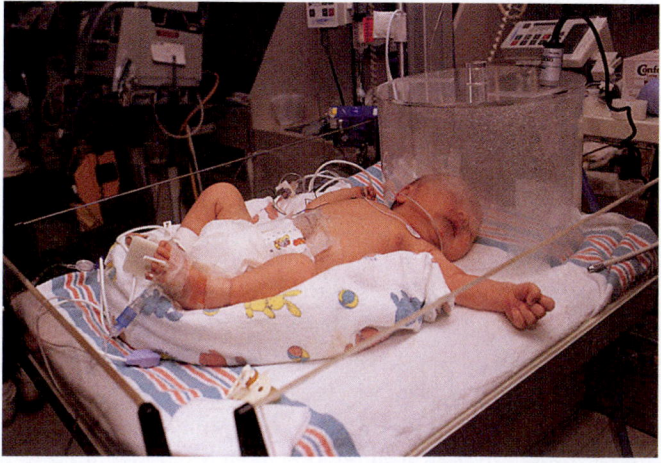

Figure 57-2. ■ An infant under an Oxyhood.

operating room personnel provide these services. The newborn returns to the NICU following surgery. Drainage tubes (chest tubes, intraventricular catheter, or wound drainage tube) may be in place. The nurse must maintain patency of these tubes.

Nursing Considerations

Besides assisting with medical treatment, the nurse must also provide for the newborn's activities of daily living. The newborn needs nutrients in order to grow. The premature newborn may not have the muscle strength or energy to suck from the breast or bottle. Endotracheal tubes may be inserted through the mouth. In these cases, a small amount of formula or breast milk may be given by gavage feeding every few hours (Procedure 57-2 ■). Sometimes the newborn who lacks strength to suck may be taught to drink from a cup. As the newborn gains strength, bottle-feeding may be used. If the gastrointestinal system is not able to function normally, nutrients will be given by total parenteral nutrition (TPN). (See Figure 57-1B.)

If the high-risk newborn has adequate fluid intake, he or she should void every few hours. If oral nutrients are administered, the meconium stool should change in a few days to the transitional stools seen in healthy newborns (see Figure 56-14 ⬭). Skin care with each diaper change is important to prevent tissue breakdown.

Activity is necessary to encourage muscle development, to prevent skin breakdown, and to prevent hypostatic pneumonia. The high-risk newborn should be turned and positioned every few hours. The high-risk newborn may be positioned supine, side lying, or prone with the head of the bed elevated slightly unless contraindicated. Keeping the head elevated prevents the abdominal contents from pushing on the diaphragm and impeding breathing. The extremities should be free to move as much as possible. If any form of restraint is necessary, it should be removed, and active or passive range of motion should be performed every few hours.

The skin of the premature or high-risk newborn is thin and fragile. Care must be taken to protect the skin and tissue and keep them intact. The skin should be kept clean and dry. The linen should be free of wrinkles. The newborn should not be placed on tubes and monitoring wires. A water mattress or sheepskin can be used.

The skin of the postterm infant is also at risk. Because the vernix caseosa is gradually reabsorbed into the skin, postterm babies may have skin that peels, cracks, or even begins to slough off, making them prone to infection. Very few babies today are postterm. Typically, labor is induced to prevent long delays beyond the estimated due date.

The newborn needs to be touched and caressed (Figure 57-3 ■). Parents must bond with the newborn. The nurse can promote this bonding process by encouraging the parents to

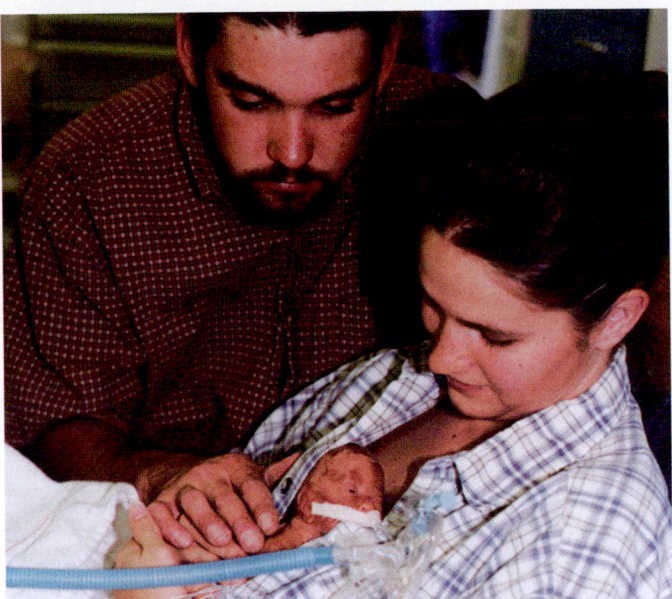

Figure 57-3. ■ Kangaroo (skin to skin) care facilitates a closeness and attachment between parents and their premature infant.

assist with the care of the newborn. It is frightening for parents to see the baby sick, with numerous tubes and monitors attached. They may be frightened to touch or hold their baby. The nurse encourages parents to begin the bonding process by fingertip and palmar touch, followed by stroking, holding, and rocking the newborn as much as possible. Placing the newborn clad only in a clean diaper against the parent's bare chest facilitates bonding. A blanket should be placed over both the baby and the parent to prevent heat loss.

Both the parents and the nurses should call the newborn by name. Parents should be encouraged to talk and sing to the baby. They should be allowed to participate as much as possible in daily care—bathing, diapering, and feeding. The nurse must explain all aspects of care and medical treatment, and teach the parents to provide care. The nurse must be alert for parental comments and behavior that indicate their anxiety or comfort with the situation. Support groups may be useful to help parents of high-risk newborns.

Physiological Characteristics of Preterm and Postterm Newborns

PRETERM NEWBORN

The preterm newborn is one who is born prior to the 38th week of gestation. Although prematurity is one of the leading causes of neonatal death, an infant born before the 38th week can live but may not be equipped to survive unassisted.

Manifestations

The preterm newborn's skin is wrinkled and covered with lanugo. Lacking subcutaneous fat, the premature newborn appears thin with prominent bones including the skull, ribs, and hips. Depending on the gestational age, the premature newborn's cry may be weak and signs of respiratory distress will be evident (see Figure 56-2 ⚭). The limbs are usually extended, exposing more body surface to heat loss.

Diagnosis and Treatment

The nurse should complete a gestational age assessment and compare the data with the mother's reported date of conception. Gestational age determination is discussed in Chapter 56 ⚭ . The premature newborn would be placed in the NICU under constant observation and monitoring.

Because the organs are immature, treatment is based on the needs of the individual premature newborn. The first priority is supporting respiration and circulation. Body heat is maintained by radiant warmer. Depending on the age and condition of the premature newborn, food and fluids are administered orally or by intravenous infusion. Usually, the premature newborn is cared for in the NICU until vital signs are stable and growth is increasing steadily.

Nursing Considerations

Nursing care of the premature newborn depends on the gestational age of the infant. Newborns who are 2 or 3 weeks premature generally do not require the same amount of monitoring and care as the newborn who is 4 or more weeks early. Once premature infants have stabilized, they may be transferred to a less acute unit where they remain until their weight is high enough for them to be discharged (approximately 5.5 lbs or 2,500 g). During this time of growth, the LPN/LVN may be given more responsibility for providing general care of the infant. Families should be encouraged to participate in daily newborn care.

POSTTERM NEWBORN

The postterm newborn is born after 42 weeks' gestation. Because the placenta does not function well after the 40th week, the postterm infant is at risk for similar complications as the preterm infant.

Manifestations

The postterm newborn may be large, which increases the probability of a traumatic vaginal birth or cesarean section. Placental insufficiency places the fetus at risk for inadequate oxygen and nutrients. Under stress, the fetus may pass meconium into the amniotic fluid. Limited placental function during labor places the infant at risk for meconium aspiration and hypoxia. Because of resorption of vernix caseosa after 40 weeks, there is little vernix caseosa to protect the skin from the amniotic fluid. Therefore, the skin of the postterm newborn is often dry and cracked, with a parchment-like texture.

Nursing Considerations

Besides routine newborn care, the postterm newborn should be watched closely for respiratory distress and hypoglycemia. Airway maintenance (including suctioning) is critical. The newborn with a low blood glucose will need frequent feeding, either by breast or formula.

The large infant may have birth trauma. This includes but is not limited to fractured clavicle and cephalhematoma (Figure 56-12B ⬭⬭). If the clavicle was fractured during birth, the infant will be unable to move the arms equally. The RN and primary care provider should be notified if a fractured clavicle is suspected. A cephalhematoma can put pressure on the underlying brain tissue. Usually a cephalhematoma will absorb over time without neurologic damage. However, the neurologic status of the newborn should be closely monitored and the primary care provider notified of changes.

Newborns with Alterations in Growth

At times the fetus does not grow as expected, resulting in a newborn that is either large or small for the gestational age. In either case, the newborn is at risk for complications and may require close observation and treatment.

LARGE FOR GESTATIONAL AGE

Large for gestational age (LGA) describes a newborn whose birth weight is over the 90th percentile for the gestational age. For example, the term infant who weighs over 4,000 grams (8.8 pounds) is considered LGA. This condition is called **macrosomia** and was discussed with care of the high-risk pregnancy, Chapter 52 ⬭⬭. The cause of the majority of LGA newborns is unknown. However, some causes include a mother with diabetes, large parents, previous large infants, and postterm gestation (Rahimian & Varner, 2003).

Manifestations

The LGA newborn is generally proportional. The infant's weight, length, and head circumference are approximately the same percentage above normal. However, the infant of a diabetic mother (see Figure 52-10B ⬭⬭) has an increased weight while remaining within normal limits for length and head circumference.

The excessive weight in the infant born to a diabetic mother (IDM) is caused by high blood glucose levels. Maternal glucose readily crosses the placenta, resulting in an increased production of insulin and hyperplasia of the fetal pancreas. Insulin is an important regulator of metabolism and has a "growth hormone effect" on the fetus. At birth the

maternal supply of glucose is cut off, resulting in *hypoglycemia* in the newborn.

Macrosomic newborns are generally hypoactive at birth and may be hypotonic and difficult to arouse from a sleep state. They may have undergone a long and difficult labor and birth, either vaginally or by cesarean section. They may have respiratory distress and feeding difficulties.

Diagnosis and Treatment

The diagnosis of LGA is made solely on measurements. However, factors to consider when evaluating the LGA newborn include:

- The size of parents: large parents tend to have large babies.
- The number of pregnancies: multiparous women have two to three times the number of LGA infants.
- The sex of the newborn: male infants tend to be larger than female infants.
- The presence of other disorders: infants with erythroblastosis fetalis or transposition of the great arteries are usually large.
- The presence of maternal disorders such as diabetes.

LGA newborns should be evaluated for complications including but not limited to hypoglycemia, polycythemia, and birth trauma such as fractured clavicle, brachial palsy, facial paralysis, skull fracture, cephalhematoma, and intracranial hemorrhage. Diagnostic exams such as blood tests, x-rays, and ultrasound may be needed.

Treatment is directed toward relieving hypoglycemia and polycythemia and correcting birth trauma. LGA newborns need close observation until their condition has stabilized.

Nursing Considerations

Nursing care is directed toward monitoring vital signs and blood sugar levels and observing for signs of birth trauma. Blood glucose levels in the infant of a diabetic mother usually drop within 1 to 3 hours after birth and then return to normal levels between 4 and 6 hours after birth. Therefore, blood glucose levels obtained by heel stick are obtained hourly during the first 4 to 6 hours and then every 4 hours (or by facility policy). Infants whose blood glucose levels fall below 40 mg/dL should be encouraged to breastfeed or be given formula. Infants, who are unable to be fed orally will require intravenous administration of glucose solutions. Intravenous access may be through an umbilical vein or a central line.

The nurse must realize that the large newborn is not necessarily a mature newborn. The nurse must assess the LGA newborn frequently for signs of respiratory distress. The airway may need to be suctioned and oxygen administered.

The nurse must be prepared to address parental concerns about the visual effects of birth trauma such as facial or head bruising. Parents may be reluctant to touch the newborn for fear of causing pain. Parents will need instruction regarding all care provided during hospitalization as well as home care after discharge. Following teaching, parents should be able to verbalize understanding of the treatment of their newborn.

SMALL FOR GESTATIONAL AGE

Small for gestational age (SGA) describes infants whose intrauterine growth is below that expected for the gestational age (Figure 57-4 ■). This condition is also called **intrauterine growth restriction** (IUGR) Causes of SGA can be classified as maternal, environmental, placental, or fetal factors.

- Maternal factors include primiparity, grand multiparity, multiple pregnancy, and low socioeconomic status.
- Maternal disease includes maternal heart disease, substance abuse (with alcohol, nicotine, cocaine, narcotics, or others), maternal anemia, preeclampsia, and disorders that decrease blood flow to the uterus.
- Environmental factors include exposure to x-rays or toxins, high altitude, and excessive exercise. These environmental factors can decrease the oxygen available to the uterus.
- Placental factors include a small placenta, infarcted areas of the placenta, or placenta previa.
- Fetal factors include congenital infections, congenital anomalies, discordant twins (one twin is smaller than the other, possibly due to sharing or overlapping of the placenta).

Manifestations

Intrauterine growth occurs by both an increase in the number of cells and an increase in the size of cells. If a problem develops early in fetal development, fewer new cells are formed and organs will be small and underweight. If a problem develops later in fetal development, only the size of cells is affected, resulting in small organs.

There are two patterns of IUGR:

- *Symmetric (proportional) IUGR* is caused by a long-term maternal disorder such as chronic hypertension, malnutrition, substance abuse, or anemia or fetal genetic abnormalities. In symmetric IUGR there is prolonged restriction of growth of organs, body weight, length, and head circumference. Symmetric IUGR can be seen on ultrasound.
- *Asymmetric (disproportional) IUGR* is caused by a disorder that acutely compromises placenta circulation, such as preeclampsia, placental infarcts, or poor maternal weight gain in pregnancy. Asymmetric IUGR is not apparent until the third trimester of pregnancy. Although the weight is decreased, the total length and head circumference are normal. After 36 weeks' gestation, fetal abdominal circumference should be larger than head circumference. In asymmetric IUGR the abdominal circumference of the fetus remains smaller than the head circumference. These newborns are at risk for asphyxia, pulmonary hemorrhage, hypocalcemia, and hypoglycemia.

Even though growth is restricted, physical maturity continues according to gestational age. Therefore, the SGA newborn may be physiologically mature.

Diagnosis and Treatment

The diagnosis of SGA is based on prenatal ultrasound birth measurements. A newborn who is slightly underweight but born at term may have few complications and require routine newborn care. Frequent monitoring of blood glucose levels and frequent feeding may be required.

The most common complications occurring in the SGA newborn include

- *Asphyxia:* the SGA infant has been hypoxic *in utero* and may have little reserve to undergo labor and vaginal birth.
- *Aspiration:* hypoxia *in utero* may cause the infant to gasp during birth and aspirate amniotic fluid and vaginal secretions.
- *Hypothermia:* decrease in subcutaneous fat and depletion of brown fat *in utero* place the SGA newborn at risk for hypothermia.
- *Hypoglycemia:* an increased metabolic rate, heat loss, and poor glycogen stores in the liver result in hypoglycemia.
- *Infection:* a decreased reserve and immature immune system potentiates infection in the SGA newborn.

SGA newborns tend to have a poor prognosis, especially if born before 37 weeks' gestation. Diagnosis and treatment during the prenatal period can improve outcomes. SGA newborns require frequent monitoring of complications and individualized medical treatment.

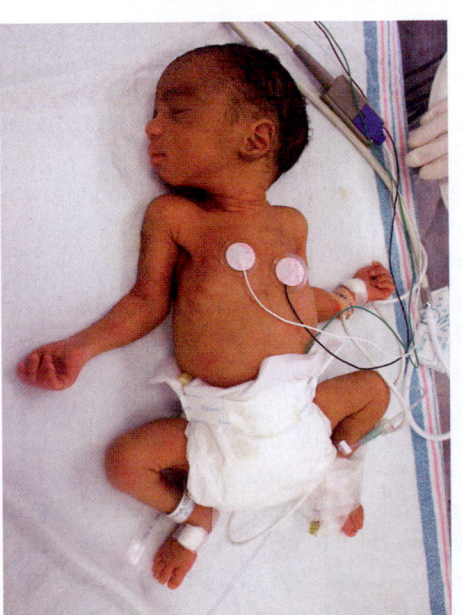

Figure 57-4. ■ Premature infants are commonly small for gestational age.

Nursing Considerations

The SGA newborn requires frequent monitoring including vital signs and blood glucose by heel stick. The first priority is to maintain a clear airway in the SGA newborn. The airway may need frequent suctioning, and oxygen may be administered. Because of the risk of hypothermia, SGA newborns are frequently placed under radiant heat or wrapped in three warm blankets. To prevent or treat hypoglycemia, the newborn is fed (by breast, bottle, or gavage) every 2 to 3 hours.

Parents need teaching about the need for warmth and frequent feeding. Additional assistance may be needed when the newborn is discharged. The nurse should make appropriate referral to home health or other agencies to help monitor the SGA newborn after discharge.

Respiratory Conditions

Congenital anomalies that affect the respiratory system commonly involve the esophagus. These anomalies are introduced under gastrointestinal conditions.

The premature newborn's lungs are not fully ready to begin the function of breathing and gas exchange. The premature newborn is unable to produce adequate amounts of *surfactant*, the chemical required to maintain the patency of the alveoli. The collapsed alveoli are unable to exchange oxygen and carbon dioxide.

The term newborn should produce an adequate amount of surfactant and breathe independently. However, the newborn may develop respiratory distress or apnea for several reasons. During the birth process, the fetus may aspirate amniotic fluid and vaginal secretions. If the mother receives narcotic medication during labor, the fetus may have depressed respiratory effort at birth. Vigorous suctioning of the airway during birth can cause laryngospasm, which obstructs the airway.

The passage of meconium by the fetus is a common occurrence in response to hypoxia or stress during the pregnancy. During delivery, the newborn can inhale the amniotic fluid containing meconium (**meconium aspiration**). Severe meconium aspiration increases the possibility that the newborn will develop persistent pulmonary hypertension, pneumothorax, and pneumonia.

Manifestations

The newborn becomes hypoxic, breathes faster, depletes the energy stores, and develops respiratory distress or apnea. (See Chapter 56 for signs of respiratory distress in the newborn.) Airway obstruction results in respiratory arrest and death within minutes.

Treatment

To prevent death, the newborn is placed on mechanical ventilation (see Figure 57-1A). However, mechanical ventilation and high oxygen concentration can further damage the alveoli, resulting in permanent lung disease or **bronchopulmonary dysplasia** (BPD).

Nursing Considerations

Establishing and maintaining a patent airway is the highest priority in newborn care. The nurse should suction the airway as needed with a bulb syringe or suction catheter. Oxygen can be administered by nasal catheter or mask. Should mechanical ventilation be needed, a certified respiratory therapist, anesthesiologist, or primary care provider will need to insert an endotracheal tube.

Congenital Heart Defects

Congenital heart defects are more common when the child was exposed to rubella, alcohol, or drugs during intrauterine development. Other factors that increase the risk of congenital heart defects include other congenital or genetic defects, advanced maternal age, maternal disorders such as lupus and diabetes, and siblings or parents with congenital defects.

To understand the pathology of heart defects, it is important to review the normal structure of the fetal heart. Because fetal blood is oxygenated in the placenta, the lungs in the fetus only need enough blood to perfuse lung tissue. In the fetal heart, the foramen ovale connects the two atria, allowing blood to flow from the right atrium into the left atrium. The ductus arteriosus connects the pulmonary artery and aorta. Blood flows from the pulmonary artery into the aorta. The purpose of the foramen ovale and ductus arteriosus is to decrease the flow of blood to the fetal lungs.

Shortly after birth, the foramen ovale and the ductus arteriosus structures normally close. The pressure in the left side of the heart becomes higher than the pressure in the right side of the heart. Congenital heart defects can be classified into four groups according to the way the defect affects circulation.

DEFECTS WITH INCREASED PULMONARY BLOOD FLOW

Three heart defects that increase the blood flow to the pulmonary system will be discussed. Figure 57-5 ■ illustrates these defects.

- The first defect, a *patent* (open) *ductus arteriosus* (PDA), happens when the ductus arteriosus fails to close. In this defect, blood is pushed from the aorta to the pulmonary artery, resulting in an increase in blood flowing to the lungs.
- The second defect (Figure 57-5B), *atrial septal defect*, happens when the foramen ovale fails to close or septum fails to form, resulting in an atrial septal defect (ASD). Blood flows directly from the left atrium into the right atrium, increasing the amount of blood in the right side of the heart.
- The third defect (Figure 57-5C), *ventricular septal defect*, results from an abnormal opening in the septum (wall) between the ventricles. The ventricular septal defect

PATENT DUCTUS ARTERIOSUS (PDA)

Common congenital defect caused by persistent fetal circulation that accounts for 9%–12% of all congenital heart defects (Driscoll, 1999). When pulmonary circulation is established and systemic vascular resistance increases at birth, pressures in the aorta become greater than in the pulmonary arteries. Blood is then shunted from the aorta to the pulmonary arteries, increasing circulation to the pulmonary system.

Clinical Manifestations
Dyspnea; tachypnea; full, bounding pulses; and poor development occur. Infant is at risk for frequent respiratory infections and infective endocarditis. When a large PDA exists, congestive heart failure, intercostal retractions, hepatomegaly, and growth failure are also seen. A continuous systolic murmur is auscultated, and a thrill may be palpated in the pulmonic area.

Clinical Therapy
When murmur is detected, diagnosis is confirmed by chest x-ray study, electrocardiogram (ECG), and echocardiogram. Chest x-ray film and ECG show left ventricular hypertrophy. PDA can be visualized, and left-to-right shunt can be measured on echocardiogram.

Surgical ligation of PDA is the treatment of choice. Intravenous indomethacin often stimulates closure of the ductus arteriosus in premature infants. Transcatheter closure by obstructive device is sometimes attempted in children over 18 months of age.

PROGNOSIS: If PDA is not treated, child's life span is shortened because pulmonary hypertension and vascular obstructive disease develop.

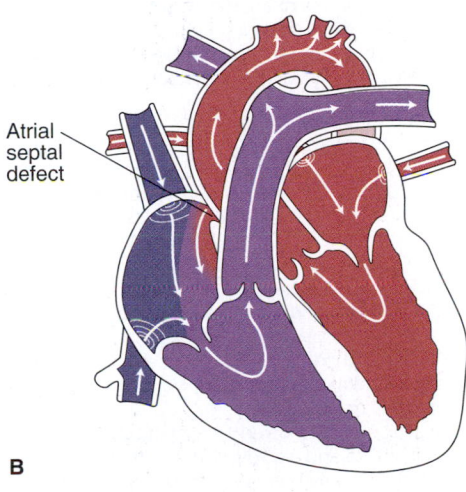

Patent ductus arteriosus

Mix of oxygenated and unoxygenated blood

A

ATRIAL SEPTAL DEFECT (ASD)

An opening at any point in the atrial septum that permits left-to-right shunting of blood. The opening may be small, as when the foramen ovale fails to close, or large, as when the septum may be completely absent. Of children with congenital heart defects, 6%–10% have an ASD (Driscoll, 1999).

Clinical Manifestations
Infants and young children usually have no symptoms. Small and moderate-size ASDs are usually not diagnosed until preschool years or later. Congestive heart failure, easy tiring, and poor growth occur with a large ASD. A soft systolic murmur is usually heard in the pulmonic area with wide splitting of S_2.

Clinical Therapy
Diagnosis is made by echocardiogram that identifies right ventricular overload and shunt size. Chest x-ray film and ECG reveal little information unless ASD is large and excessive shunting is present.

Surgery to close or patch ASD is performed to prevent pulmonary vascular obstructive disease. Some ASDs may be closed by transcatheter device (septal occluder) during cardiac catheterization.

PROGNOSIS: Many persons with uncorrected small and moderate-size ASDs have lived to middle age without symptoms. Atrial arrhythmias are common late complications.

Atrial septal defect

B

VENTRICULAR SEPTAL DEFECT (VSD)

An opening in the ventricular septum results in increased pulmonary blood flow. Blood is shunted from the left ventricle directly across the open septum into the pulmonary artery. This most common congenital heart defect occurs in approximately 20% of all children with congenital heart disease (Driscoll, 1999).

Clinical Manifestations
Only 15% of VSDs are large enough to cause symptoms, such as tachypnea, dyspnea, poor growth, reduced fluid intake, congestive heart failure, and pulmonary hypertension. Systolic murmur is auscultated in lower left sternal border.

Clinical Therapy
Chest x-ray film and ECG reveal few findings in cases of small VSDs. Larger VSDs with shunting are associated with enlarged heart and pulmonary vascular markings on chest x-ray film and left ventricular hypertrophy on ECG. Echocardiogram establishes diagnosis if shunting is present. Cardiac catheterization is used only in preparation for surgery.

Most small VSDs close spontaneously. Treatment is conservative when no signs of congestive heart failure or pulmonary hypertension are present. Surgical patching of VSD during infancy is performed when poor growth is evident. Closure of VSD by transcatheter device (i.e., Rashkind device) during cardiac catheterization may be attempted for some defects. Prophylaxis for infective endocarditis is required.

PROGNOSIS: Highest risk associated with surgical repair is in the first few months of life. Children respond well to surgery and experience substantial catch-up growth. Malignant tachyarrhythmias and heart block are a possible complication.

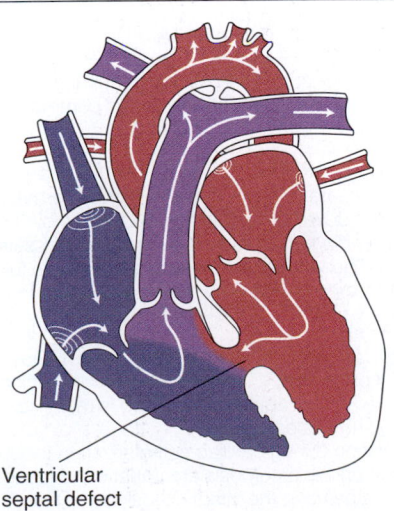

Ventricular septal defect

C

Figure 57-5.   ■ **A.** Patent ductus arteriosus. **B.** Atrial septal defect. **C.** Ventricular septal defect.

(VSD) allows blood to flow directly from the left ventricle to the right ventricle. The size of the VSD determines the degree of problems the child will have.

DEFECT WITH DECREASED PULMONARY BLOOD FLOW

When blood flow is decreased to the lungs, the condition results in decreased oxygen to all tissues. Only one congenital heart defect that decreases blood flow to the lungs

will be discussed here. *Tetralogy of Fallot* (TOF) is a combination of four defects: pulmonary stenosis, ventricular septal defect, right ventricular hypertrophy, and an overriding aorta (Figure 57-6A ■).

Pulmonary stenosis is a narrowing of the pulmonary valve. As the right ventricle tries to push blood through the tight pulmonary valve, the ventricular muscle enlarges (right ventricular hypertrophy). As pressure in the right ventricle rises, blood is pushed through the ventricular septal defect

TETRALOGY OF FALLOT

Combination of four defects: pulmonic stenosis, right ventricular hypertrophy, ventricular septal defect (VSD), and overriding of aorta. Some children have a fifth defect: open foramen ovale or atrial septal defect (ASD). About 10% of children with congenital heart defects have tetralogy of Fallot (Park, 1996). This defect is characterized by elevated pressures in right side of heart, causing right-to-left shunt.

Clinical Manifestations
As ductus arteriosus closes, infant becomes hypoxic and cyanotic. The degree of pulmonary stenosis determines severity of symptoms. Polycythemia, hypoxic spells, metabolic acidosis, poor growth, clubbing, and exercise intolerance may develop. Infants have a systolic murmur heard in pulmonic area that is transmitted to suprasternal notch.

Clinical Therapy
Chest x-ray film shows a boot-shaped heart due to the large right ventricle with decreased pulmonary vascular markings. Electrocardiogram (ECG) shows right ventricular hypertrophy. Echocardiogram demonstrates VSD, obstruction of pulmonary outflow, and overriding aorta. Cardiac catheterization is required before surgical correction to completely identify the location of all anatomic structures and any additional defects.
Hypercyanotic spells are managed according to guidelines given in section on nursing management of cyanotic defects. Monitoring child for metabolic acidosis or prolonged unconsciousness is critical. A total repair is performed before 6 months of age when the infant has a hypercyanotic spell. Corrective surgery may be attempted in asymptomatic children by 6 months of age.
PROGNOSIS: Not all children are cured by surgery, but most have improved quality of life and improved longevity. Arrhythmias and right ventricular dysfunction may be residual problems (Waldman & Wernly, 1999). Lifelong infective endocarditis prophylaxis is required.

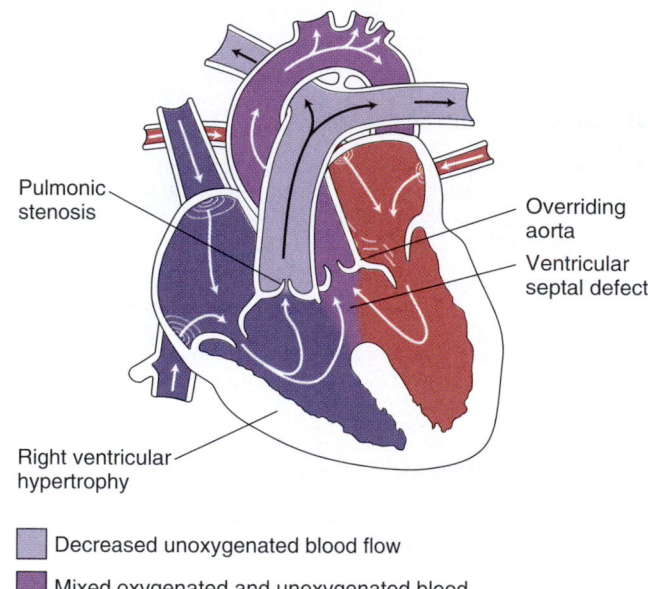

Pulmonic stenosis

Overriding aorta

Ventricular septal defect

Right ventricular hypertrophy

■ Decreased unoxygenated blood flow

■ Mixed oxygenated and unoxygenated blood

A

COARCTATION OF THE AORTA

Narrowing or constriction in the descending aorta, often near the ductus arteriosus, obstructs systemic blood outflow. This defect is common, occurring in 5%–8% of all children with congenital heart disease (Fedderly, 1999).

Clinical Manifestations
Many children are asymptomatic and grow normally, but constriction is progressive; 20%–30% of children develop congestive heart failure by 3 months of age. Reduction in blood flow through the descending aorta causes lower blood pressure in legs and higher blood pressure in arms, neck, and head. Brachial and radial pulses are full, but femoral pulses are weak or absent. Older children may complain of weakness and pain in the legs after exercise.

Clinical Therapy
ECG shows left ventricular hypertrophy. Chest x-ray film may reveal enlargement and pulmonary venous congestion, and indentation of descending aorta. Rib notching (change in the smooth contour of the rib apparent on x-ray) is rarely seen before 10 years of age. Magnetic resonance imaging shows coarctation.
Balloon dilation during cardiac catheterization for both initial relief and recoarctation. Surgical resection and anastomosis are palliative, as coarctation may recur. The subclavian artery can be used as a patch in the infant. Repair in the first year of life is preferred to decrease exposure to hypertension.
PROGNOSIS: Post-coarctectomy syndrome (abdominal pain and distention) occurs in 20% of patients (Walters, 2000). Persistent hypertension in adulthood is common. Infective endocarditis prophylaxis is needed.

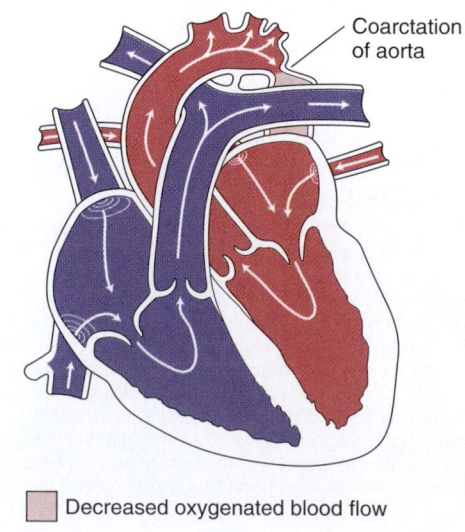

Coarctation of aorta

■ Decreased oxygenated blood flow

B

Figure 57-6. ■ **A.** Tetralogy of Fallot (TOF). **B.** Coarctation of the aorta (COA).

into the aorta where it mixes with oxygenated blood from the left ventricle and is pumped through the body. The mixing of oxygenated and unoxygenated blood results in the common symptom of cyanosis.

DEFECT THAT OBSTRUCTS SYSTEMIC BLOOD FLOW

Coarctation of the aorta (COA) is a narrowing of the aorta, most commonly in the arch of the aorta. The narrowed area restricts the flow of blood to the body. The left ventricle must work hard to force blood through the narrowed aorta. Over time COA leads to congestive heart failure. With COA, blood pressure will usually be higher in the arms than in the legs (Figure 57-6B). Pulmonic and aortic stenosis may also occur.

MIXED DEFECTS

Mixed defects are those that affect both systemic and pulmonary circulation. *Transposition of the great arteries* results when the positions of aorta and pulmonary artery are reversed. In this condition, unoxygenated blood enters the right side of the heart, travels through the right ventricle, out of the heart through the aorta, and back to the body. The oxygenated blood from the lungs enters the left side of the heart, travels through the left ventricles, out of the heart through the pulmonary artery, and back to the lungs (Figure 57-7 ■).

Ultrasound, cardiac catheterization, and magnetic resonance imaging are used to diagnose congenital heart defects. Surgery is needed to correct the defect. Technological advances in surgery are evolving to allow correction of some defects using a scope, laser, balloon, or robots. It is hoped that such advances will reduce recovery time.

NURSING CARE

PRIORITIZING NURSING CARE

When caring for infants with cardiovascular disorders, focus your care on promoting respiratory effectiveness and reducing workload. Give oxygen as ordered and assess the infant's color frequently. Auscultate lung sounds every hour and report immediately any increase in crackles or wheezes. Help keep infant comfortable to decrease crying, which can lead to shortness of breath. Monitor intake and output for fluid overload.

ASSESSING

Children with congenital heart defects exhibit signs and symptoms of congestive heart failure. These include but are not limited to heart murmurs, cyanosis, respiratory distress, fluid retention, and activity intolerance. Some heart murmurs are loud and easily heard. Others are soft and can only be detected by a trained practitioner. Cyanosis can be either constant, generalized cyanosis, or cyanosis around the mouth (**circumoral**), seen only when the child is active, nursing, or crying. Signs of respiratory distress include tachypnea, orthopnea, grunting, flaring nostrils, and retractions. Fluid retention may be evidenced by bulging fontanels, fewer than six wet diapers per day, moist lung sounds, and generalized tissue edema. Restlessness, crying, and lethargy can be signs of intracranial edema. Young children may display activity intolerance by increased respiratory effort, resting frequently, or squatting while at play.

TRANSPOSITION OF THE GREAT ARTERIES (TGA)

Pulmonary artery is the outflow for left ventricle, and aorta is outflow for right ventricle. This condition is life threatening at birth, and survival initially depends on open ductus arteriosus and foramen ovale. This condition occurs in about 5% of children with congenital heart disease (Grifka, 1999). ASD or VSD may also be present with TGA.

Clinical Manifestations
Cyanosis, apparent soon after birth, progresses to hypoxia and acidosis. Cyanosis does not improve with oxygen administration. However, cyanosis may be less apparent when a large VSD is also present. Congestive heart failure may develop over days or weeks. Tachypnea (60 respirations/min) is often present without retractions or other signs of dyspnea. Infants take a long time to feed and need frequent rest periods because of rapid respiratory rate and fatigue. Growth failure may be evident as early as 2 weeks of age if corrective surgery is not performed.

Clinical Therapy
Chest x-ray study may reveal a classic egg-shaped heart on a string (narrow superior mediastinum). Diagnosis is made by echocardiogram when position of arteries arising from ventricles is visible.
Prostaglandin E_1 is initially ordered to maintain a patent ductus arteriosus until a palliative procedure can be performed. Corrective surgery (arterial switch) is usually performed before 1 week of age. Balloon atrial septostomy may be performed during cardiac catheterization in newborns as a first stage. This may also be corrected surgically.
PROGNOSIS: Survival without surgery is impossible. Arrhythmias, right ventricular failure, and sudden death are long-term complications (8–15 years) after the Mustard procedure, so the Mustard or Rastelli procedure are performed only when significant pulmonary valve stenosis is present (Grifka, 1999). Infective endocarditis prophylaxis may be necessary.

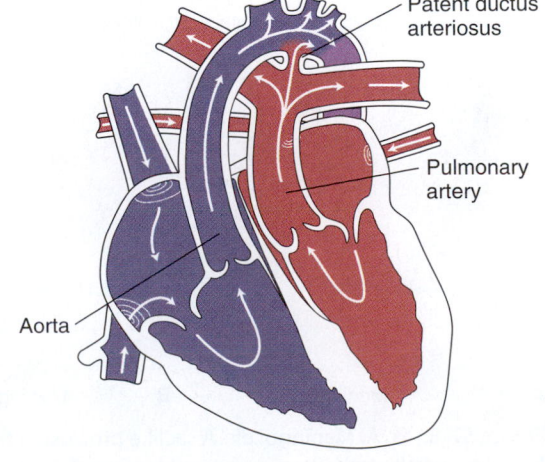

Patent ductus arteriosus

Pulmonary artery

Aorta

Figure 57-7. ■ Transposition of the great arteries (TGA).

DIAGNOSING, PLANNING, AND IMPLEMENTING

Nursing diagnoses for infants who have had surgery for heart defects might include:

- *Ineffective Breathing Pattern* related to pulmonary edema, increased work of breathing, or poor respiratory effort
- *Decreased Cardiac Output* related to mechanical problems
- *Acute Pain* related to operative site

Outcomes for the infant after surgery are:

- Breathing will improve and the need for oxygen will be reduced.
- Infant will be more comfortable.
- Infant will be able to take food orally.

Nursing interventions are supportive measures for the infant as well as the family and might include the following:

- Administer medically prescribed medications and treatments in a timely manner. Monitor the infant continually until he or she is stable. *This is primarily the role of the registered nurse. LPNs and LVNs assist as state regulations and facility policy allow.*
- Provide emotional support to the family and reinforce teaching about the child's condition. *Parents and family will be anxious and concerned about the infant's health. This may interfere with learning about the condition. Reinforcement of teaching can be useful.*

EVALUATING

The nurse will monitor to be sure the infant stabilizes over a few hours to days postoperatively. Oxygen will gradually be reduced. The infant will be comfortable and will be able to take oral nutrients.

Congenital Nervous System Defects

Neurologic defects are very serious and require long-term care. Two defects will be discussed here.

SPINA BIFIDA

Spina bifida is an incomplete closure of the vertebra and neural tube. The defect can be found anywhere along the spinal column and results in a variety of pathologies. Most commonly the defect is located in the lumbosacral region.

Manifestations

Defects affecting only the vertebrae may not be obvious until the toddler tries to walk. In larger defects, meningocele or meningomyelocele may result. **Meningocele** is the herniation of the meninges through the vertebral defect. **Meningomyelocele** is a herniation of the spinal nerves as well as the meninges through the vertebral defect (Figure 57-8 ■). The outer covering of the defect may be skin or at times the transparent, fragile meninges. It is critical to protect the tissue until surgical correction can be complete. If the spinal cord or spinal nerves are affected, there will be flaccid paralysis, bowel and bladder incontinence, and sensory deficits. The cause of spina bifida is a genetic predisposition with a deficiency of the essential nutrient folic acid. If spina bifida exists, there is a high probability of other congenital defects including clubfoot, hip defects, and hydrocephalus.

Treatment

Surgical correction is completed as soon as possible. If hydrocephalus is present, a shunt may be placed at the same time. Postoperatively the infant is observed closely for signs

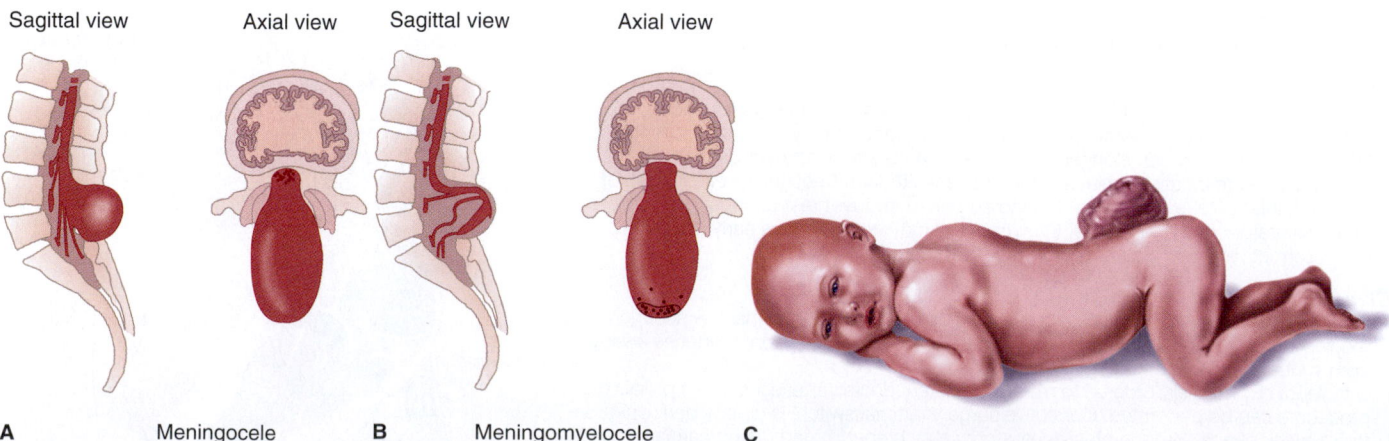

Sagittal view   Axial view   Sagittal view   Axial view

A   Meningocele   **B**   Meningomyelocele   **C**

Figure 57-8. ■ **A.** Meningocele. A saclike protrusion through the bony defect in the spinal column containing meninges and cerebrospinal fluid. Sac may be transparent or membranous. **B.** Saclike herniation through the defect holding meninges, cerebrospinal fluid, and a portion of spinal cord or nerve root. Fluid leakage may occur, because the lesion may be poorly covered. This defect is more common than the meningocele; 99% of children with this defect are handicapped. **C.** The infant with a meningomyelocele is placed prone or in a side-lying position, and the exposed sac is protected carefully and kept moist.

of infection, bowel and bladder function, and movement of extremities. Prognosis is variable depending on the location and severity of the defect.

HYDROCEPHALUS

Hydrocephalus results from increased production, decreased absorption, or blockage of the flow of cerebrospinal fluid. Blockage can be caused by a variety of pathologies, including tumors, cysts, or malformations. At times hydrocephalus is obvious at birth, but more commonly it develops over time.

Manifestations

The classic symptoms include head circumference greater than normal with the forehead and top of the head being out of proportion to the face. The anterior fontanel bulges with the increasing intracranial pressure. The sclera of the eyes can be seen above the iris giving a "setting sun" appearance to the eyes. The child may be irritable or lethargic.

Treatment

Surgical placement of a ventriculoperitoneal shunt (Figure 57-9 ■) might be necessary to relieve the increasing intracranial pressure. As the child grows, shunt revision may be necessary. If the blockage is caused by a tumor or cyst, surgical removal may be possible to correct the hydrocephalus. In any case, damage done prior to surgical intervention cannot be reversed.

CHROMOSOMAL ABNORMALITIES

Chromosomal abnormalities can result in congenital anomalies, as well as a decrease in mental and physical functioning. Down syndrome (see Figure 59-9 ◉), the most common chromosomal abnormality, results from **trisomy 21** (three chromosomes at position 21).

Manifestations

Classic signs of Down syndrome include *microcephaly* (small head), wide short neck, epicanthal folds giving the eyes an upward slant, a small nose with a wide nasal bridge, low-set ears, and protruding tongue. The fingers are short and broad, the thumb appears low-set on the hand, and the palm has a single crease (*simian line*). There is an unusually wide space between the first and second toes. There is also an increased incidence of congenital heart defects, diabetes, and hearing loss. The degree of mental retardation is not evident at birth.

Treatment

Down syndrome alone would not necessitate keeping the newborn in the NICU. Unless complications such as prematurity or heart defects are present, the care of the newborn with Down syndrome is the same as for any other newborn.

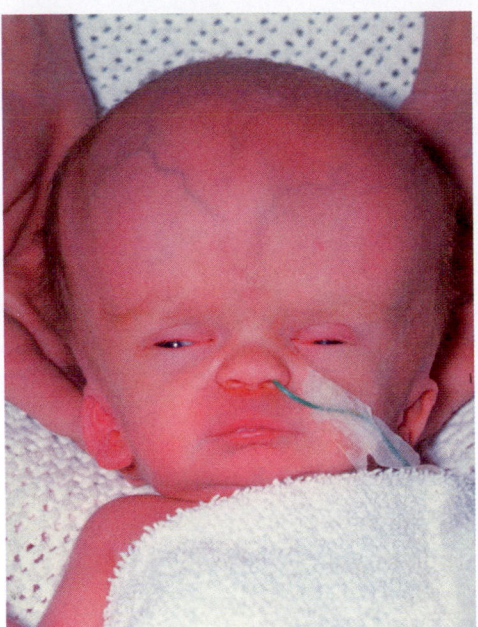

A

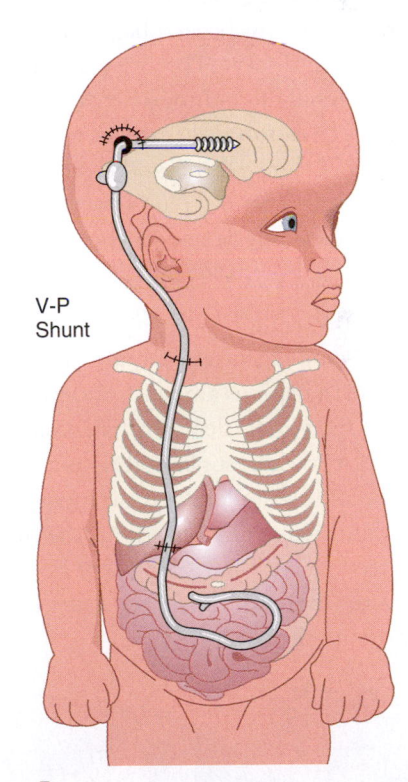

B

Figure 57-9. ■ **A.** Infant with hydrocephalus. (M. A. Ansary/Custom Medical Stock Photo, Inc.) **B.** Ventriculoperitoneal shunt allows fluid to leave the intracranial cavity and reduce intracranial pressure. It is usually placed at 3 to 4 months of age.

Nursing Considerations

The newborn with Down syndrome may be hospitalized for some time after birth to allow time for the parents to adjust to the diagnosis and to learn any special care that might be necessary. These newborns may have weak muscle tone resulting in poor sucking reflex. They may have feeding difficulties and be susceptible to aspiration and respiratory infection. Parents will need assistance in feeding, preventing infection, and stimulating the newborn's mental development. Parents should be encouraged to join support groups for parents of children with Down syndrome.

Gastrointestinal Conditions

Defects of the gastrointestinal system are the most common of the congenital defects. They require surgical correction, but many are not immediately life threatening. However, aspiration, malnutrition, and obstruction could result if detection and correction are not made in a timely manner. For an understanding of these defects, it is important to review the normal structure of the entire gastrointestinal system in Chapter 37 and Figure 37-1 ⬤⬤.

TRACHEOESOPHAGEAL FISTULA AND ESOPHAGEAL ATRESIA

Esophageal atresia and tracheoesophageal fistula are potentially life-threatening defects. They may be found separately, but are most commonly found together. They are illustrated in Figure 57-10 ■. In **esophageal atresia,** the esophagus ends in a blind pouch before reaching the stomach. **Tracheoesophageal fistula** is a connection between the trachea and esophagus. Esophageal atresia and tracheoesophageal fistulas frequently occur with other congenital anomalies.

Manifestations

The infant with esophageal atresia and tracheoesophageal fistula presents with copious amounts of thin mucus shortly after birth. The secretions clear with suctioning, but they soon reappear. If a tracheoesophageal fistula is present, the stomach may become distended with trapped air. If the defects are not identified prior to feeding, the infant will regurgitate the feeding, or the feeding will be aspirated into the lungs. Severe respiratory distress occurs and aspiration pneumonia may develop.

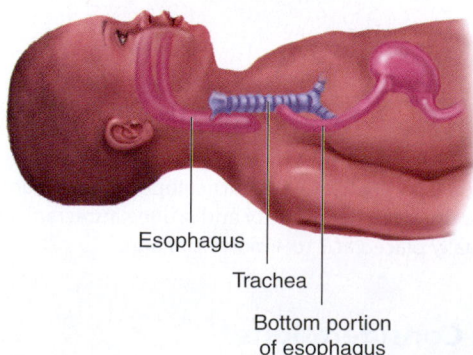

Esophagus

Trachea

Bottom portion
of esophagus

Figure 57-10. ■ Esophageal atresia and tracheoesophageal fistula. Most commonly, the upper segment of the esophagus ends in a blind pouch connected to the trachea; a fistula connects the lower segment to the trachea.

Treatment

Treatment is aimed at preventing respiratory complications until the defect can be surgically repaired. In the absence of other anomalies, surgical repair is usually completed in the first few days of life. If other anomalies are present, gastrostomy feedings may be necessary until the infant is stabilized. Surgery is necessary to correct the defect. Postoperatively, the infant should not be fed orally for 7 to 14 days to allow for healing. Once oral feedings are begun, they are usually tolerated.

OMPHALOCELE

Omphalocele is a rare congenital malformation of the abdominal wall allowing the abdominal contents to herniate into the umbilical cord (Figure 57-11 ■). There is generally a thin translucent sac (peritoneum) covering the abdominal organs. The size of the sac varies, depending on the degree of defect. Small defects may be repaired with good prognosis. Large defects may result in long-term gastrointestinal disorders.

IMPERFORATE ANUS

During fetal development, a pit, forming in the perineum, becomes the outer anal opening. The colon forms and gradually approaches the anal pit, and the connecting tissue breaks down, allowing the colon to open to the outside. Imperforate anus results when the tissue fails to break down. Most commonly, there is obvious malformation of the perineum. At times a thin membrane can be seen covering the anus. At other times the anus is flat, or appears as a deep dimple. Anomalies of the urinary system are commonly present at the same time. If meconium is present in the urine, a fistula has developed. Figure 57-12 ■ illustrates this anorectal anomaly. Immediate surgery is required to correct the defect.

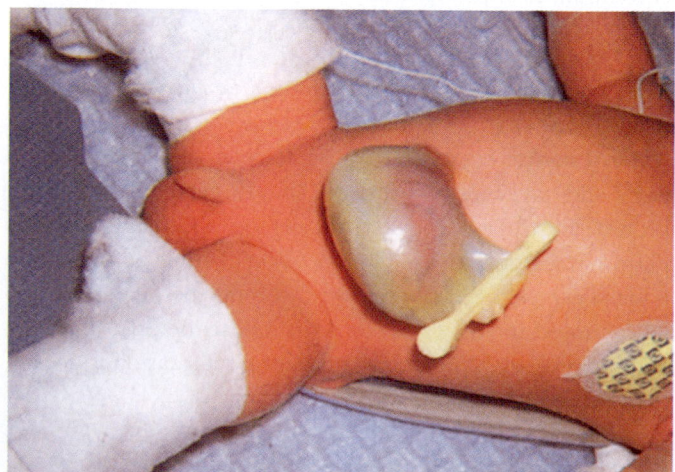

Figure 57-11. ■ In omphalocele, the size of the sack depends on the extent of the protrusion of abdominal contents through the umbilical cord. (*Source:* From McGraw-Hill Companies, Inc. Rudolph, A. M., Hoffman, J. L. E., & Rudolph, C. D. (Eds.). (1991). *Rudolph's pediatrics.* (19th ed., p. 1040). Stamford, CT: Appleton & Lange.)

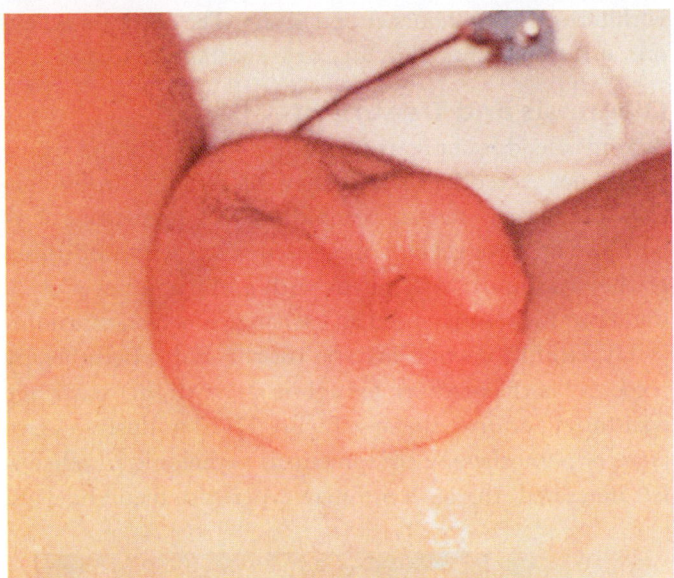

Figure 57-12. ■ Imperforate anus is often obvious at birth. It can range from mild stenosis to a complex syndrome associated with other congenital anomalies.

Metabolic Disorders

PHENYLKETONURIA

Phenylketonuria (PKU) is an autosomal recessive inherited disorder that affects the body's ability to use protein. Normally, a liver enzyme, phenylalanine hydroxylase, breaks down the amino acid phenylalanine into tyrosine. Children with PKU have a deficiency in this enzyme (Box 57-3 ■).

Manifestations

As phenylalanine builds up in the blood, it causes a musty odor of the body and urine, as well as vomiting, irritability, seizures, hyperactivity, and rash. Over time, elevated levels of phenylalanine result in mental retardation.

Diagnosis and Treatment

State laws require all infants to be screened for PKU. To ensure accurate results, the infant must receive either breast milk or formula for several days. Tests performed on the infant who leaves the birthing center 24 hours after delivery should be repeated.

Special formulas, such as Albumaid XP, Lofenalac, and Minafen, are used in treatment until the child is ready for solid food. Then a diet low in phenylalanine is maintained for life. The diet must also meet the child's requirements for

BOX 57-3	CULTURAL PULSE POINTS

Phenylketonuria
PKU is more common in communities with numerous inter-marriages over several generations. It is rare in African, Jewish, and Japanese populations.

growth. If diet modifications are not followed for at least the first 6 years, there is a significant impact on the child's IQ.

Nursing Considerations

It is important for the hospital nurse to inform parents of the need to repeat the PKU test several days after the newborn has been taking milk or formula. If the test is positive, parents will need instruction in use of special formulas and adapting the diet as the child grows. Referral to a dietitian is helpful.

GALACTOSEMIA

Galactosemia is an autosomal recessive disorder of carbohydrate metabolism. Galactosemia results from a deficiency in galactose-1-phosphate uridyltransferase (GALT), one of the three enzymes necessary for the conversion of sugar galactose into glucose. High levels of galactose in the blood results in damage to the kidneys, liver, brain, and eyes. Many children develop gram-negative infections.

Manifestations

Within a few days after birth, the baby develops vomiting and diarrhea, does not eat well, becomes hypoglycemic, and develops an enlarged liver. If not diagnosed and treated, the child will become mentally retarded and develop jaundice, ascites, cataracts, seizures, lethargy, and coma. Death usually occurs within 1 month.

Diagnosis and Treatment

Routine screening of the newborn is done in all but six states. In these six states, diagnosis is made in symptomatic babies from history and laboratory tests.

Infants with galactosemia are placed on lactose-free or galactose-free formulas. The child will be on a galactose-free diet (no milk or milk products) for life. Many children who follow a strict diet still develop complications of galactosemia, including learning disabilities, speech defects, visual disturbances, and ovarian failure.

Nursing Considerations

Nursing responsibilities focus on teaching the parents and child about the prescribed diet and referring the family to a nutritionist for counseling. Parents must learn to screen foods and medication for hidden lactose that has been used as a filler. The parents should be referred for genetic counseling.

MAPLE SYRUP URINE DISEASE

Maple syrup urine disease (MSUD) is an autosomal recessive disease that affects amino acid metabolism. A missing or defective enzyme prevents the breakdown of three essential amino acids: leucine, isoleucine, and valine (Box 57-4 ■). The result is alpha-ketoacidosis. All three amino acids are necessary for normal hair, skin, and muscle function. Leucine accumulates in the brain, causing cerebral edema, neurologic damage, and death.

Manifestations

Within days of birth, the infant becomes lethargic, has variable muscle tone, becomes irritable with a high-pitched cry, and the skin has a sweet smell.

Diagnosis and Treatment

Diagnosis is made by laboratory findings. Specially designed formulas with the three amino acids removed are prescribed. The diet should be rich in other amino acids, vitamins, minerals, and calories. The child needs special low-protein foods that are adequate for growth without causing a catabolic state (tissue breakdown). Daily urine testing for ketones is required to monitor the metabolic state.

Nursing Considerations

Nursing care includes teaching parents to maintain the prescribed diet. This includes mixing the special formula and developing a plan to prevent ketoacidosis on sick days. Referral to a nutritionist is helpful. Support groups can also help families by sharing tips for managing the child's condition.

Hemolytic Disease of the Newborn

Hemolytic disease of the newborn (discussed also in Chapter 52 ⬭⬭) is a general term for several blood disorders that result in RBC breakdown and an increase in bilirubin (**hyperbilirubinemia**). The most common cause of hyperbilirubinemia is physiologic jaundice, the normal breakdown of RBCs. A secondary cause of hyperbilirubinemia is pathologic jaundice. The most common cause of pathologic jaundice is Rh incompatibility. (You recall that Rh-positive blood contains the Rh protein on the RBC, and Rh-negative blood is missing this protein. If Rh-positive blood and Rh-negative blood are mixed together in the mother, the Rh-negative blood develops antibodies against the Rh-positive protein. During any future pregnancies with an Rh-positive fetus, the mother's Rh-negative blood will destroy the fetal blood.

Manifestations

The distribution of fetal RBCs results in hyperbilirubinemia and pathologic jaundice. Because the destruction of RBCs occurs before delivery, the newborn exhibits jaundice within the first 24 hours after delivery. The newborn is anemic at birth and has difficulty oxygenating the tissues.

Diagnosis and Treatment

A cord blood sample is evaluated for bilirubin, which should not exceed 5 mg/dL. Follow-up serum bilirubin levels should not raise over 5 mg/dL/day. A premature newborn should have therapy instituted when serum bilirubin reaches 10 mg/dL. Any infant with a bilirubin level of 20 mg/dL or higher may need an exchange blood transfusion.

Hyperbilirubinemia may be treated with phototherapy (exposure of the newborn to high-intensity light), exchange transfusion, or drug therapy. Figure 57-13 ■ illustrates two types of phototherapy equipment. If pathologic jaundice is left untreated, the newborn may experience mental delays,

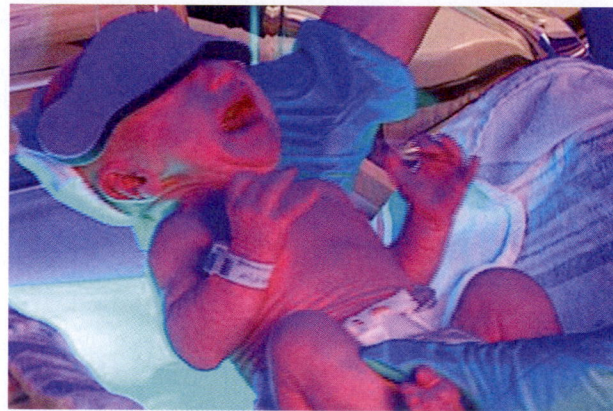

A

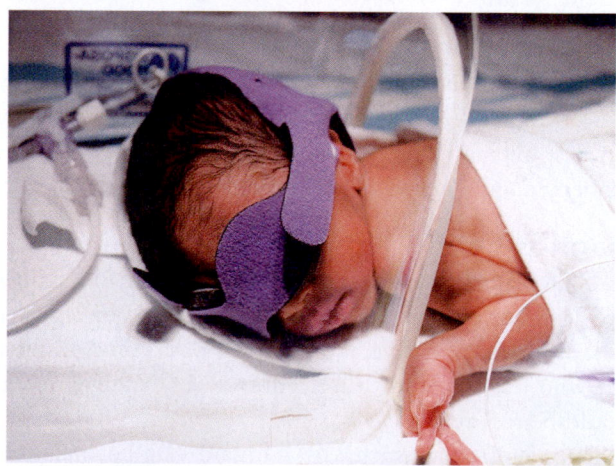

B

Figure 57-13. ■ Hyperbilirubinemia. Rh and ABO blood incompatibility may lead to pathologic jaundice, which is seen within 24 hours of birth. Aggressive phototherapy and exchange transfusions are used to resolve the high levels of bilirubin that can lead to permanent neurologic damage. Eye patches are always used to protect the infant's eyes. **A.** Newborn on fiber-optic "bili" mattress and under phototherapy lights (color distorted by reflection of the bililight mattress). **B.** Infant receiving phototherapy. The phototherapy light is positioned over the incubator. (Courtesy of Lisa Smith-Pedersen, RNC, MSN, NNP.)

congestive heart failure, and death. In the NICU, the newborn may be given blood transfusion of compatible blood until the RBC destruction stops. This condition can be prevented by administering RhoGAM to the Rh-negative mother during pregnancy and again following delivery.

Nursing Considerations

Phototherapy can be provided by a bank of lights, by a fiber-optic blanket attached to a light source wrapped around the newborn's body, by a fiber-optic mattress, or a combination of these methods. When phototherapy lights are used, the newborn's eyes must be protected from the bright lights. The baby's temperature must be taken frequently to ensure the infant is not overheated. If the baby's temperature rises, the lights should be turned off for a time. With a fiber-optic blanket, the light stays on at all times. The infant's eyes do not need to be covered. The fiber-optic blanket allows the baby to be more accessible for feeding, changing diapers, and bonding with parents. Fiber-optic blankets are also available for home care.

Cleft Lip and Cleft Palate

Cleft lip and cleft palate commonly occur together but can be found separately. **Cleft palate** results from failure of the medial nasal and maxillary processes to join, leaving an opening between the roof of the mouth and the floor of the nasal passage. **Cleft lip** results from failure of the upper lip to join medially. Cleft lip can be unilateral or bilateral (Figure 57-14 ■). Clefts could be complete (through bone and tissue) or partial (involving the bone structure but not the overlying mucous membrane).

Treatment

The surgical correction of cleft lip is usually accomplished in the first 3 months of life. To achieve the best cosmetic effect, the suture line must be protected. A **Logan clamp** (a metal bow taped to both sides of the suture line) or a butterfly bandage is frequently used to decrease tension on the suture line. Depending on the extent of the defect, the absence of infection, and amount of suture line trauma, complete closure may be accomplished in one surgery. Cosmetic revision may need to be done at a later date.

clinical ALERT

To prevent trauma at the surgical correction site for cleft lip, avoid use of suction catheters, straws, and tongue blades.

Surgical closure of a cleft palate may need to be accomplished in stages depending on the extent of the cleft. Closure of a cleft palate is usually begun at 4 to 6 months of age, with complete closure accomplished by age 2. As with cleft lip repair, preventing trauma and infection of the suture line is important.

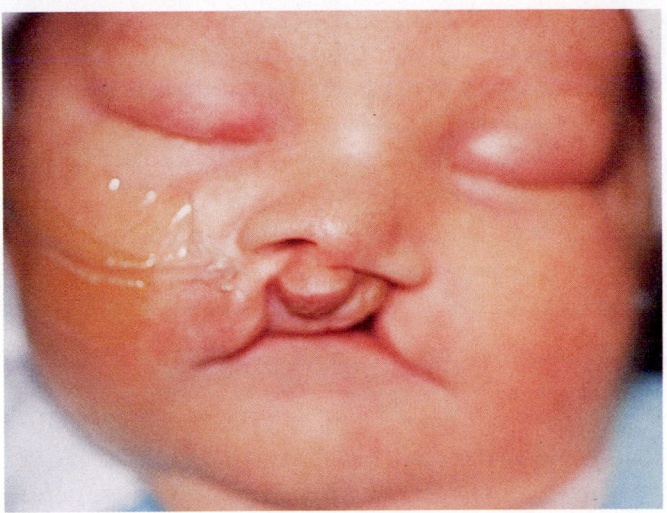

A

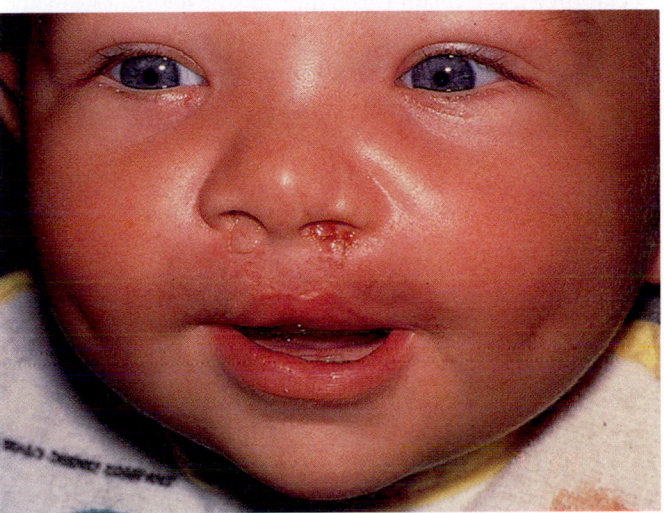

B

Figure 57-14. ■ A. Bilateral cleft lip. B. Repaired bilateral cleft lip. (*Source:* Courtesy of Dr. Elizabeth Peterson, Spokane, WA.)

Client Teaching

Three clinical problems are associated with cleft lip and cleft palate:

- The infant will have feeding problems. The infant with a cleft lip will have difficulty making a seal around the nipple. With a cleft palate, the infant will be unable to compress the nipple between the tongue and palate. The result of these will be an ineffective suck. With cleft palate, the feeding leaks into the nasal cavity, where it can drain from the nose and not be ingested. Some food can pool in the nasal passage, increasing the risk of sinus and ear infections. Also, some of the feeding may drain down the back of the throat without coordinated swallowing, putting the infant at risk for choking.
- The child will have speech problems. Surgical repair alters the palate arch, resulting in a hypernasal tone. Repeated ear infections and altered hearing often lead to poor articulation.

- The psychologic impact on the family is a concern. Families naturally anticipate the arrival of a "pretty" baby. When the infant has a cosmetic defect, the family experiences grief and needs emotional support. Even after surgical correction of the cleft lip, the child will still have permanent scarring and some degree of cosmetic defect.

NURSING CARE

PRIORITIZING NURSING CARE

When caring for infants with unrepaired cleft lip and/or palate, focus your care on providing support and teaching to the parents and caregivers. Instruct them on ways to feed the infant to prevent aspiration. This may require the use of special nipples. Explain the symptoms of regurgitation and aspiration (formula exiting through the nose and choking). Instruct parents to monitor the infant closely during feedings and give frequent breaks to allow the infant to complete swallowing. Instruct them to burp the infant after 15 to 30 mL have been fed. Encourage parents to hold and cuddle the infant, and not to fear causing pain to the infant. Explain that the infant has the same needs as every infant.

ASSESSING

A cleft lip and palate are usually identified on a newborn assessment. The physician inspects the palate carefully, because a small cleft of the uvula or the palate could easily be missed. Once cleft lip or palate has been diagnosed, it is crucial for nurses to provide ongoing assessment for aspiration, otitis media, and malnutrition. Postoperative assessment includes condition of the suture line, improvement of swallowing, and weight gain.

DIAGNOSING, PLANNING, AND IMPLEMENTING

Planning nursing care for the infant involves teaching the parents to care for the infant preoperatively. It also includes teaching routine postoperative care as well as long-term therapy. Nursing diagnoses for infants with cleft lip or palate could include, but are not limited to, the following:

- *Risk for Aspiration*
- *Risk for Infection* (middle ear and suture line)
- *Risk for Imbalanced Nutrition: Less than Body Requirements*
- *Impaired Verbal Communication*

Outcomes for the infant and family would include the following:

- Infant will maintain clear airway and be free of infection.
- Infant will obtain necessary nourishment.

- Family will verbalize feelings about having a child with a cosmetic defect and will express a desire to learn how to care for the new baby.

Preoperative Interventions

- Teach, encourage, and support parents in their efforts to maintain proper nutrition and prevent aspiration. *The risk of aspiration and regurgitation through the nose is frightening and will delay surgery. Maintaining nutrition and preventing aspiration are the highest priorities of care preoperatively.*
- Teach parents that the degree of defect influences the amount of feeding difficulty. Breastfeeding an infant with a cleft lip is generally no more difficult than normal breastfeeding (see guidelines in Chapter 54 ⚭). The breast tissue closes the cleft, allowing the infant to suck. If there is a large cleft palate, however, breastfeeding is more difficult and may be impossible. In this case, the breast can be pumped and the baby fed with a bottle. *If bottle-feeding is the choice, regular nipples should be tried, but may need to be modified. Enlarging the nipple hole by making an "X" cut allows the formula to be received in the back of the throat for easier swallowing.*
- Closely observe, or have parents observe, the infant's face during feeding. *If the infant needs a break to complete swallowing, the infant raises its eyebrows and wrinkles its forehead. The nipple should be gently removed from the mouth. Frequent burping is necessary.*
- Follow feedings with a small amount of water. *This rinses milk or formula from the mouth and nose and helps to decrease the risk of otitis media.*

Postoperative Interventions

- Teach parents to clean and protect the suture line. *Doctor orders should be followed regarding suture line care. The infant's arms should be restrained with tubular or tongue blade restraints to avoid traumatizing the operative site.*

EVALUATING

Parents' reactions to the child should be evaluated on an ongoing basis. The care will be long term. Parents will need teaching and support along the way. The infant should be checked at regular intervals for weight gain and signs of infection. As the child grows, speech therapy, orthodontic therapy, and social services may be necessary.

NURSING PROCESS CARE PLAN
Client with a Bilateral Cleft Lip

John was born with a bilateral cleft lip. He has been cared for at home and is strong enough for surgical correction. John has been admitted to the Pediatric Unit from surgery.

Assessment

Vital signs: T 99.2, (R) P 90, R 36, Wt. 12.5 lbs (5.7 kg). John is awake and crying.

An IV of lactated Ringer's solution is infusing in his left hand. Logan clamp is present across the surgical site. His diaper is wet.

Nursing Diagnosis

The following important nursing diagnoses (among others) are established for this condition:

- *Acute Pain* related to surgical procedure
- *Risk for Trauma* of the surgical site

Expected Outcomes

The following expected outcomes have been identified:

- Infant is resting comfortably.
- Operative site is undamaged.

Planning and Implementation

The following nursing interventions are planned and implemented for John:

- Medicate for pain as ordered. *Keeping the infant comfortable will decrease crying and trauma to the suture line.*
- Apply jacket restraint. Restrain on back. *Jacket restraint prevents bending the elbows and rubbing the face or sucking the thumb. Restraining on back prevents rubbing face on the bed. Restraint will also protect the IV site.*
- Clean suture line as ordered. *Cleaning the suture line prevents infection and aids in healing.*
- Teach parents use of restraints and suture line care at home. *Continued care will be needed after discharge until healing is complete in several weeks.*
- Do not put anything in the mouth. *This prevents trauma to the suture line.*

Evaluation

John is resting comfortably with minimal crying. The suture line is intact without signs of infection. Parents can verbalize home care.

Critical Thinking in the Nursing Process

1. Should John be medicated for pain before or after feeding?
2. If John cannot have anything put in his mouth, how will he be fed?
3. How will the nurse know that John is getting enough nutrition?

Note: Discussion of Critical Thinking questions appears on the MyNursingKit Website.

Congenital Genitourinary Defects

Defects of the urinary system are commonly found with defects of the lower gastrointestinal tract and reproductive system. The first concern is to determine that the infant is able to urinate. If not, immediate intervention is required.

URETHRAL MALPOSITION

The urethra does not always open at the tip of the penis (Figure 57-15 ■). *Epispadias* occurs when the urethra opens on the *dorsal* (upper) surface of the penis. *Hypospadias* occurs when the urethra opens on the *ventral* (lower) surface of the penis. The opening can be found anywhere along the shaft of the penis. If the urethral opening is on the glans, surgical correction may not be needed. If the urethral opening is well down the shaft of the penis, surgical correction may need to be done in stages. Correction of these defects will be discussed in Chapter 59 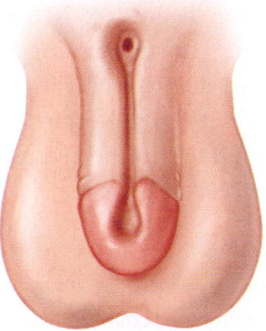.

AMBIGUOUS GENITALIA

Ambiguous genitalia is a rare condition in which determining the sex of the infant is difficult. In this circumstance, chromosomal analysis may be necessary to determine the sex of the infant. Not only is the reproductive system affected,

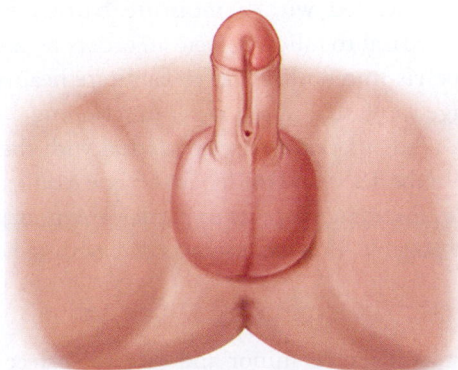

A   Epispadias

B   Hypospadias

Figure 57-15. ■ A. Epispadias. The urethral canal is open on the dorsal surface of the penis. **B.** Hypospadias. The urethral canal is open on the ventral surface of the penis.

but in many cases the urinary and intestinal systems are affected as well. As long as the newborn is able to pass urine and stool, surgical reconstruction can wait until the gender has been established. If elimination is not possible, surgery must be done immediately. Surgical reconstruction is usually done in stages, with the primary goal being normal functioning of the urinary and intestinal systems. Depending on the degree of defect, reproductive function may be lost. Figure 57-16 ■ illustrates normal versus ambiguous genitalia.

EXSTROPHY OF THE BLADDER

Exstrophy of the bladder (Figure 57-17 ■) is a rare condition in which the abdominal wall fails to fuse, allowing the urinary bladder to protrude to the outside. Failure of the abdominal wall to close during fetal development results in separation of the rectus muscles and at times the symphysis pubis. The separation allows the bladder to protrude through the opening. Other genitourinary abnormalities and intestinal herniation are associated with exstrophy of the bladder.

Manifestations

Usually, a defect in the lower abdominal wall is obvious at birth. The skin is open, and underlying tissue is exposed. The bladder appears bright red and urine continually leaks from the urethra.

Diagnosis and Treatment

Before surgical reconstruction begins, it is important to evaluate the extent of damage to surrounding tissue. Primary closure of the abdominal defect, with the return of the bladder to the abdominal cavity, is performed in the first 24 to 48 hours of life. Complete surgical reconstruction is accomplished in stages over several years.

Nursing Considerations

Nursing responsibilities are to monitor urinary and intestinal function. Initially the defect is covered with dressings saturated in sterile normal saline. Surrounding tissue should be protected with a moisture barrier. Postoperatively, it is critical to follow physician orders regarding skin care and pelvis immobilization to facilitate healing. Monitor drainage tubes to ensure proper functioning.

Parents need emotional support to deal with the disfiguring nature of the defect and the length of time required for complete repair. Encourage parents to participate in infant care to the degree possible. Provide instruction regarding home care.

Musculoskeletal Defects

Skeletal defects can be minor and easy to correct or major malformations requiring long-term therapy. These defects are rarely life threatening. However, they require correction, if possible, in order for normal support and movement to occur. Two common defects will be discussed here.

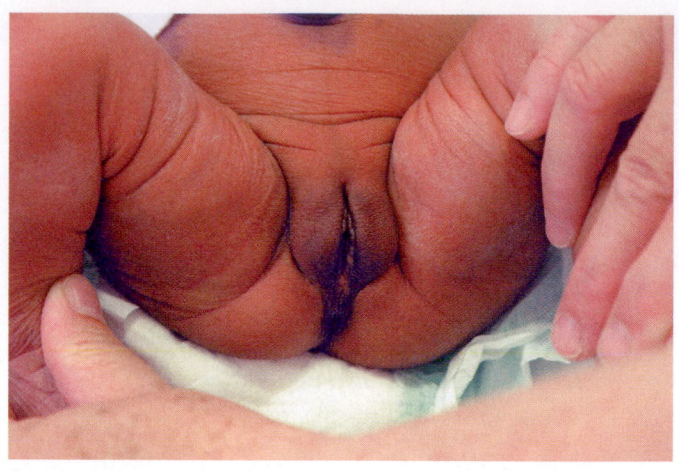

A

B

C

Figure 57-16. ■ **A.** At term, the labia majora are well developed and cover both the clitoris and the labia minora. **B.** In the newborn, the testicles are usually descended into the scrotum, and are covered by rugae. **C.** Newborn girl with ambiguous genitalia. (Courtesy of Patrick C. Walsh, M.D.)

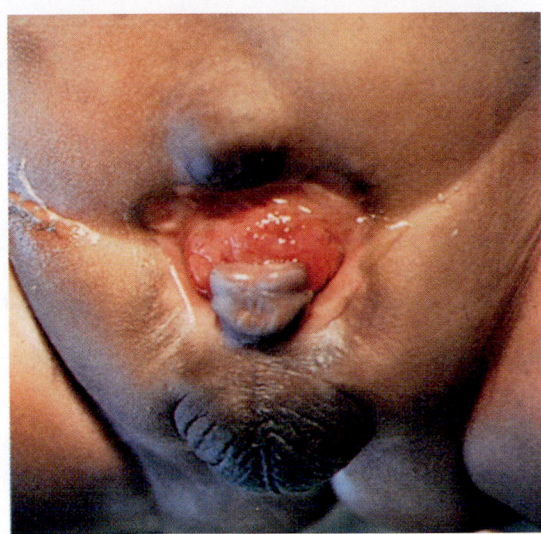

Figure 57-17. ■ This child has bladder exstrophy, noted by extrusion of the posterior bladder wall through the lower abdominal wall. Until surgery can be performed, the bladder mucosa must be protected from trauma and irritation. A sterile, saline-soaked dressing maintains moisture; it is covered with a sterile plastic wrap. The surrounding area must be cleaned daily. Skin sealant is applied to protect surrounding skin from leaking urine.

DIAPHRAGMATIC HERNIA

A **diaphragmatic hernia** occurs when the abdominal contents protrude through a weakness in the diaphragm. The defect is caused by delay or failure in closure of the diaphragm. A diaphragmatic hernia is a life-threatening disorder that must be treated promptly.

Severe respiratory distress occurs shortly after birth. As the infant cries, abdominal organs extend into the thorax. When the abdominal contents protrude into the thoracic cavity, the lung cannot expand fully, and respiratory distress results. The infant must be positioned with the head and thorax higher than the abdomen to facilitate downward movement of abdominal organs. A nasogastric tube is inserted to decompress the stomach and facilitate its return to the abdomen. Ventilator support may be necessary to manage respiratory distress.

Once the infant's condition is stabilized, surgery is needed to correct the defect. The prognosis is poor, with only 50% of infants surviving.

TALIPES (CLUBFOOT)

Talipes or clubfoot is a unilateral or bilateral twisting of the foot, usually inward. The foot cannot easily be moved into alignment. Nonsurgical treatment involves moving the foot into correct alignment and applying a cast. The cast is changed every 1 to 2 weeks until alignment is achieved in approximately 3 months. Failure to achieve alignment could result in a need for surgical correction. (See Chapter 59 ⊙⊙ for discussion of talipes [clubfoot]).

Infants of Drug-Abusing Mothers

Infants born to drug-abusing mothers are addicted at birth. The newborn will experience withdrawal within hours of birth depending on the specific substance. Complications frequently include respiratory distress, jaundice, behavioral problems, congenital anomalies, growth retardation, and mental deficiencies. The mother may not be able to care for the infant. A referral to social services should be made as soon as the problem is suspected.

FETAL ALCOHOL SYNDROME

Fetal alcohol syndrome (FAS) is a series of malformations found in infants whose mother drank excessive alcohol during pregnancy. No amount of alcohol intake during pregnancy has been determined safe.

Manifestations

Growth retardation, facial anomalies, microcephaly, CNS dysfunction, mental retardation, and hyperactivity are common with FAS (Figure 57-18 ■).

Nursing Considerations

Immediate care of these newborns will focus on nutritional support. They are often fussy and poor eaters. For the newborn with fetal alcohol syndrome to thrive, the mother must be referred to an alcohol rehabilitation program. The

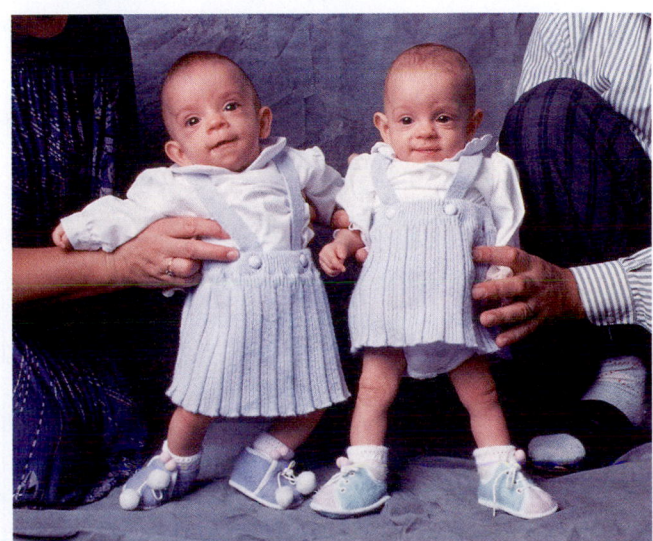

Figure 57-18. ■ Fetal alcohol syndrome is the result of a woman consuming alcohol during pregnancy, and it can have many severe effects on children. Among them are physical malformations, such as those shown here.

newborn must be closely monitored. Depending on the family situation, the newborn will be placed in foster care until the family is ready to provide total care.

DRUG-ADDICTED NEWBORN

If the mother used illicit drugs during the pregnancy, the infant is at extreme risk to be born addicted to the drugs. The newborn, withdrawing from the addiction, can experience pain, tremors, seizures, lethargy, and failure to thrive. The newborn may have permanent neurologic damage and could die.

Drugs used and abused by the pregnant woman include tobacco, cocaine, methamphetamines, marijuana, heroin, methadone, alcohol, and others. Drugs with low molecular weight (which include the commonly abused drugs) readily cross the placenta and enter the fetus. When the mother habitually uses drugs, the unborn child may become chemically dependent. **Neonatal abstinence syndrome** is the term used to describe the behavior of the infant exposed to chemical substances *in utero*.

Manifestations

The clinical manifestations seen in infants of drug using mothers vary in timing and degree. Most manifestations are mild, vague, and nonspecific signs characteristic of a variety of conditions that can affect the newborn. Signs of withdrawal are listed in Box 57-5 ■.

If the mother has taken large quantities of drugs over a long period of time, symptoms of withdrawal may begin within the first 12 to 24 hours. If the mother consumes the drug just before delivery, it may take 7 to 10 days after delivery for the newborn to exhibit signs of withdrawal. The newborn may be discharged by this time. Symptoms generally become worse over the first few days and then gradually disappear as the drug is eliminated from the infant's body. If the mother continues to use drugs and breastfeeds, the newborn will be reexposed through the breast milk. It is essential that correct diagnosis is made and treatment instituted as soon as possible.

BOX 57-5	MANIFESTATIONS OF DRUG WITHDRAWAL IN THE NEWBORN
Irritability	Dehydration
Seizures	Vomiting
Hyperactivity	Uncoordinated sucking
High-pitched cry	Diaphoresis
Tremors	Fever
Exaggerated Moro reflex	Unstable temperature
Hypertonic muscles	Mottled skin
Poor feeding	Nasal stuffiness
Diarrhea	Disrupted sleep patterns

Diagnosis and Treatment

Diagnostic exams for chemical exposure include newborn urine, hair, or meconium sampling. Urine testing will only detect recent substance intake. Meconium and hair testing for drug metabolites are more accurate, identify long-term exposure, and are easy to collect.

The treatment of chemical addiction is specific to the abused drug. Treatment may include supporting the newborn until the immature liver can detoxify and excrete the chemical. At times hemodialysis is needed.

Nursing Considerations

Nursing considerations when caring for the infant of a drug-using mother include all the care of the normal newborn plus close observations for life-threatening complications such as respiratory depression. Nursing care is directed toward decreasing stimuli that may increase hyperactivity and irritability. Dimming the lights and lowering the noise level may be beneficial. Comforting measures such as wrapping the infant snuggly, and holding and rocking the infant limits their ability to self-stimulate.

Providing adequate nutrition and hydration is essential. Loose stools, poor intake, and regurgitation after feeding may result in dehydration. Frequent weighing, monitoring of intake and output, and additional caloric intake may be necessary. Dehydration and abrasion from the hyperactive infant rubbing against the linen predispose the baby to skin breakdown and infection.

The Neonatal Abstinence Scoring System (Kandall, 1999; Finnegan, 1985) is a standardized screening tool used to monitor infants in an objective manner when neonatal abstinence syndrome is suspected or identified. This assessment and documentation tool is used by the RN each time an assessment is indicated.

The relationship of the newborn and mother should be closely monitored and documented. The responsibility of caring for a newborn may be too challenging for the drug-abusing mother. If she is enrolled in a treatment program and lives in a treatment facility where 24-hour observation and assistance is available, she may be allowed to keep the newborn with her. However, more commonly, the newborn will be placed in foster care until a safe environment can be provided. Careful evaluation and cooperation among a variety of healthcare professionals are required in this situation.

Substance abuse is a widespread health concern. Some women become prostitutes in order to have money to support their drug habit. Other women have a stable home, employment, and a supportive relationship, but use drugs as a form of recreation. In either situation, babies may be born to these women. The nurse must know what the legal responsibility is to the mother and the newborn. The nurse must explore her or his feelings by asking such questions as:

- How are you going to feel if you must report the mother to the police?
- How are you going to feel if the mother and baby are discharged and you find out later that the baby was addicted?
- Should drug screening be done on every newborn?
- Does drug screening of the newborn infringe on the rights of the parents?

Neonatal Infections and Sepsis

Infections of the newborn usually result from exposure to the mother before or during delivery. Some infections—such as rubella, syphilis, and HIV/AIDS—are transported across the placenta and infect the developing fetus. Other infections—such as gonorrhea and herpes—can be picked up as the fetus moves through the birth canal. (In a woman with active herpes that can be lethal to the baby, delivery is by cesarean section.) The immature immune system of the premature or high-risk newborn makes infections especially dangerous. When the microorganisms spread to the blood, generalized sepsis occurs. As sepsis becomes more severe, respiratory distress and septic shock may progress rapidly, resulting in death.

Manifestations

Newborn infection may occur within the first month of life. Nonspecific symptoms such as poor feeding, lethargy, and vomiting with or without diarrhea are usually seen first. Later the newborn may become cyanotic, jaundiced, and hypothermic. Due to the instability of the thermoregulatory center in the brain, newborns often have low body temperature with an infection, but may exhibit rapid fluctuation in body temperature.

Diagnosis and Treatment

Diagnosis of newborn infection and sepsis is made by blood and body fluid cultures. The newborn is admitted to the hospital for monitoring, fluid administration, and intravenous antibiotics.

Nursing Considerations

The primary consideration is prevention of infection in the newborn. The mother is screened for sexually transmitted infections prior to birth. Sterile and aseptic techniques are used as appropriate when providing care to limit the transmission of infection to the newborn. Treating the mother with appropriate antibiotics during pregnancy can limit the spread of infection to the fetus.

Parents should be taught to wash their hands before handling the newborn, following diaper change, and prior to handling food, formula, and bottles. Daily hygiene

practices limit the transmission of microorganisms to the newborn.

NURSING CARE

PRIORITIZING NURSING CARE

The priorities of nursing care for the high-risk newborn are similar to those of the normal newborn. However, the method in which the needs are met may be different.

- Maintaining the airway, breathing, and circulation
- Maintaining body temperature
- Providing nutrition
- Ensuring elimination
- Teaching parents to provide care for their newborn

ASSESSING

The high-risk newborn requires a more frequent and in-depth assessment than the normal newborn. The high-risk newborn may have equipment such as a heart monitor, a mechanical ventilator, or feeding tube. The nurse must ensure that the equipment is functioning properly. The high-risk newborn may have had surgery to correct a congenital anomaly, or he or she may have an infection or other condition that requires assessment and monitoring. Parents and family members require assessment information and support in the care of their high-risk newborn.

DIAGNOSING, PLANNING, AND IMPLEMENTING

Nursing diagnoses might include:

- *Ineffective Airway Clearance*
- *Risk for Infection*
- *Risk for Impaired Skin Integrity*
- *Deficient Knowledge* related to specific disorder, medical equipment, or care of the high-risk newborn

Nursing care might include these and other interventions:

- Suction the airway as needed. *The premature or high-risk newborn may be unable to clear the airway, resulting in hypoxia.*
- Monitor for respiratory distress (Box 57-6 ■). *The high-risk newborn's condition is less stable and can change quickly.*
- Prevent and/or treat infection. *The high-risk newborn may undergo invasive procedures and may have puncture sites or open areas that can become infected. If an infection exists, treatment must be provided to prevent worsening of the condition.*
- Provide skin care, including bathing, turning, and protecting the skin under tape/monitor electrodes, etc. *The skin of the high-risk newborn is thin and fragile. Monitor electrodes, IV lines, and dressings that are taped to the skin. Care must be taken to prevent skin breakdown.*

BOX 57-6 DATA COLLECTION

Infant Distress

In assessing the infant, the nurse would monitor for these manifestations of newborn distress:

- Increased respiratory rate (more than 60/minute) or difficult respirations
- Sternal retractions (see Figure 56-2 ⬭⬭)
- Nasal flaring
- Grunting
- Excessive mucus
- Facial grimacing
- Cyanosis (central: skin, lips, tongue)
- Abdominal distention or mass
- Vomiting of bile-stained material
- Absence of meconium elimination within 24 hours of birth
- Absence of urine elimination within 24 hours of birth
- Jaundice of the skin within 24 hours of birth due to hemolytic process
- Temperature instability (hypothermia or hyperthermia)
- Jitteriness or blood glucose less than 40 mg

Source: Adapted from Tappero, E. P., & Honeyfield, M. E. (1996). *Physical assessment of the newborn* (2nd ed.). Petaluma, CA: NICU Ink.

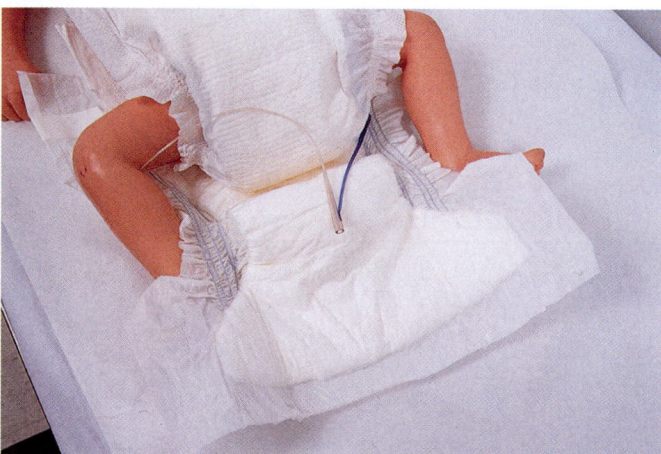

Figure 57-19. ■ A double diapering technique protects the urinary stent after surgery for hypospadias or epispadias repair. The inner diaper collects stools; the outer diaper, urine.

- Use double diapering as ordered for postoperative urinary care (Figure 57-19 ■). *The double diapering will prevent contamination with feces of the surgical site.*
- Give parents knowledge and support to make the best decision about care of their newborn. Encourage them to provide care to the newborn to the extent allowable by circumstances and facility policies. *By understanding the specific disorder, the parents can make informed decisions. Parents can provide some of the necessary care in the NICU with instruction and support from the nurse.*

- Model acceptance and loving response of the newborn who appears different. *Parents may be uneasy touching and caring for a baby who is not cosmetically normal or who is premature. The nurse's modeling of loving behavior and good caring skills will help the parents adjust and begin to cope.*

EVALUATING

Parents' reactions to the child should be evaluated on an ongoing basis. Parents will need teaching and support along the way. The infant should be checked at regular intervals for weight gain, signs of infection, and effectiveness of treatment.

NURSING PROCESS CARE PLAN
Care of the Preoperative Newborn with a Congenital Heart Defect

Jeremy, 24 hours old, has been transferred from a small rural hospital to the NICU of a major medical center with a diagnosis of aortic stenosis. Jeremy is breathing room air with minimal respiratory distress. His condition is stable, and he is scheduled for surgery within the next few days. His parents are asking questions regarding his care and prognosis.

Assessment

- Jeremy is breathing on his own.
- There are no signs of respiratory distress.
- Parents are asking questions regarding pre- and postoperative care.

Nursing Diagnosis

The following important nursing diagnosis (among others) is established for this condition:

- *Deficient Knowledge* related to preoperative and postoperative care of the newborn following heart surgery

Expected Outcomes

The parents will have an adequate knowledge base concerning aortic stenosis, as well as the upcoming surgical procedure and care, as evidenced by their ability to state information correctly.

Planning and Implementation

Nursing interventions for this client would include the following:

- Reinforce information on aortic stenosis presented by physician. Obtain picture to increase parents' understanding of the condition and possible complications.
- Provide information regarding the expected medical equipment to be used in the postoperative period, including mechanical ventilator, heart monitoring equipment, and chest tubes.

- Correct any misinformation.
- Repeat teaching as needed.

Evaluation

- Parents verbalize understanding of aortic stenosis and related complications.
- Parents verbalize understanding of medical equipment that may be used postoperatively.

Critical Thinking in the Nursing Process

1. What are some other topics that should be discussed with Jeremy's parents before surgery?

2. What topics should the nurse plan to discuss with Jeremy's parents before discharge?
3. What is the role of the LPN/LVN in providing care to the NICU patient and family?

Note: Discussion of Critical Thinking questions appears on the MyNursingKit Website.

Note: The references and resources for all chapters have been compiled at the back of the book.

PROCEDURE 57-1   Suctioning an Infant

Purposes

- To remove respiratory secretions to assist ventilation
- To obtain a specimen in order to detect harmful bacteria

Equipment

- Bulb syringe
- Normal saline
- Suction catheter, variety of sizes
- Oxygen source, resuscitation bag and mask
- Tracheostomy tubes

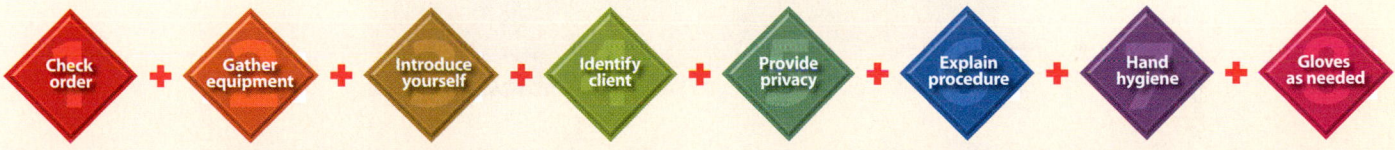

Check order + Gather equipment + Introduce yourself + Identify client + Provide privacy + Explain procedure + Hand hygiene + Gloves as needed

Interventions and Rationales

1. Perform preparatory steps (see icon bar).
2. Solicit the assistance of a coworker. *This will help prevent injury to the child.*
3. Prior to the procedure, assess the infant's breath sounds, respiratory rate and effort, and patency of airway. *This provides data for evaluating the effectiveness of the procedure.*
4. After suctioning, assess respiratory status.

USING THE BULB SYRINGE

1. Position the infant in a supine position. *This allows ready access to the nares and mouth for suctioning.*
2. Clean the oral cavity by depressing the bulb and inserting the tip of the syringe into the left buccal cavity of the child's mouth (Figure 57-20A ■). Repeat in the right buccal cavity. *Placing the syringe into the buccal cavity avoids eliciting the gag reflex.*
3. Depress the bulb into a tissue or towel. *This clears the bulb syringe.*
4. Depress the bulb and place the tip of the syringe into the nares. *If the bulb is not depressed prior to insertion, air could force the secretions into the nasopharynx.*
5. Release the bulb and withdraw secretions.

6. Wipe tip of bulb to remove debris.
7. Rinse the bulb syringe by depressing it into a cup of water and flushing it out. Repeat until clean.

SUCTIONING A CONSCIOUS INFANT

1. Place infant in a semi-Fowler's position with neck hyperextended. Attach suction tubing to source of suction. A 2.0- to 2.5-mm endotracheal tube would be used for a premature newborn with a size 5 French suction catheter. A slightly larger tube (3.0-3.5 mm) and catheter (6-8 Fr) would be used for full-term neonates. Use settings as ordered by physician or according to agency policy.
2. Apply sterile gloves. *This prevents exposure to and spread of microorganisms.*
3. Insert the suction catheter into the nares. Close the suction port with the thumb to initiate suction. Limit suctioning to 1 to 2 seconds. Repeat in other nares.
4. Suction the mouth in the same manner (Figure 57-20B).

SUCTIONING AN INFANT WITH DECREASED LEVEL OF CONSCIOUSNESS

1. Administer oxygen by face mask. *Preoxygenating the infant avoids hypoxia during suctioning.*
2. Position the infant in a lateral position. *The lateral position can prevent aspiration because it prevents the tongue*

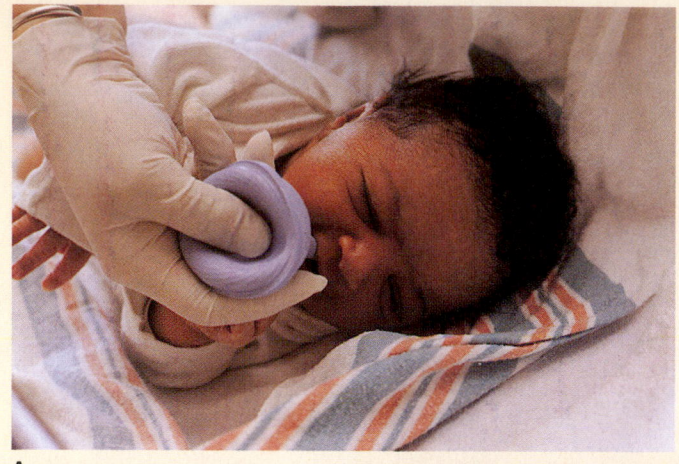

A

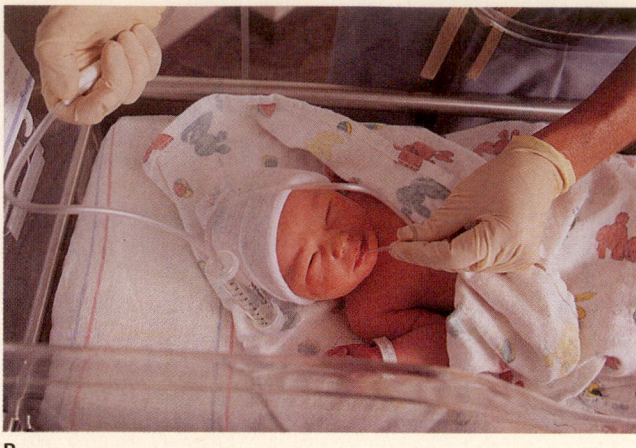

B

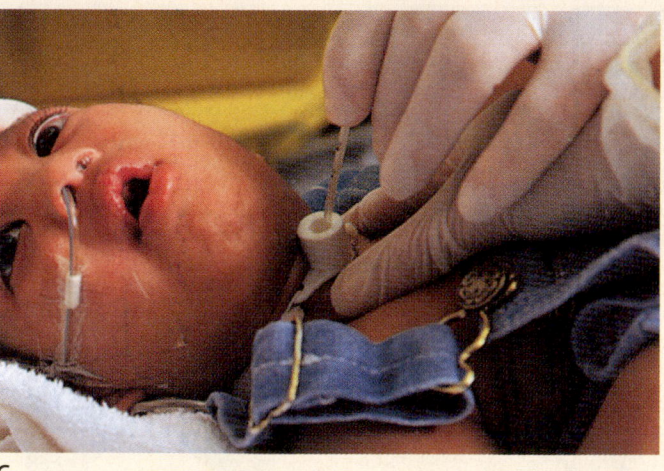

C

Figure 57-20. ■ **A.** Insertion of a deflated tube bulb syringe into the mouth. **B.** A newborn infant being suctioned with a DeLee mucus trap to remove excess secretions from the mouth and nares. **C.** Tracheostomy tube suctioning.

from falling back and blocking the oropharynx. It allows gravity to assist in the drainage of secretions.

3. Apply sterile gloves.

4. Moisten the catheter with water and insert the suction catheter into the mouth. *Moistening the catheter eases insertion.*

5. Close suction port with thumb to initiate suction. Limit suctioning to 1 to 2 seconds.

6. Apply oxygen mask. *This improves oxygenation.*

7. To remove secretions beyond the hypopharynx and trachea, advance the catheter further. Apply suction by occluding the suction port. Rotate gently upon withdrawal. *This removes secretions attached to the walls of the trachea. Rotation also prevents suction equipment from adhering to one spot.*

8. Suction one nostril.

9. Apply oxygen mask.

10. Repeat in other nares in the same manner.

11. Apply oxygen mask.

SUCTIONING A TRACHEOSTOMY TUBE

1. Inform the parent that suctioning may cause coughing and dyspnea.

2. Position the infant in a supine position with the head of bed raised 30 degrees to prevent aspiration.

3. Attach oxygen source to resuscitation bag.

4. Apply sterile gloves.

5. Using the nondominant hand, remove the humidity source from tracheostomy tube.

6. Preoxygenate the infant as ordered.

7. With the dominant hand, insert suction catheter into the tube without suction. Advance the catheter no farther than 0.5 cm below the opening of the tracheostomy tube (Figure 57-20C). *This helps prevent transmission of microorganisms.*

8. Apply intermittent suction, rotating the catheter during withdrawal to remove the maximum amount of secretions. Do not suction for longer than 1 to 2 seconds. *Suctioning for longer could compromise oxygenation.*

9. Withdraw the catheter completely and apply oxygen. *Suction removes both oxygen and secretions.*

SUCTIONING AN ENDOTRACHEAL TUBE

1. Position the infant in a supine position with head of bed raised 30 degrees to prevent aspiration.

2. Attach oxygen source to resuscitation bag.

3. Apply sterile gloves.

4. Have assistant disconnect the ventilator.

5. Preoxygenate the infant as ordered to prevent hypoxia.

6. With the dominant hand, insert the suction catheter into the tube without suction. Advance the catheter no farther than 0.5 cm below the opening of the endotracheal tube.

7. Apply intermittent suction, rotating the catheter during withdrawal. Do not suction for longer than 1 to 2 seconds. *Rotation ensures greater removal of secretions. It also prevents suction from adhering to one spot.*

8. Withdraw the catheter completely and apply oxygen.

9. Reconnect ventilator.

10. Repeat as needed.

11. Clear the suction catheter using sterile saline.

SAMPLE DOCUMENTATION

[date] [time]	R 32, uneven and labored. Cough ineffective. Rhonchi auscultated bilaterally. Sterile oral/pharyngeal suctioning performed according to policy. Moderate amount of thick, white secretions obtained. Breathing less labored, R 22. _____ _____ J. Edward, LPN

PROCEDURE 57-2 — Administering a Gavage/Tube Feeding

Purpose

- To provide nutritional support when the infant is unable to obtain adequate calories orally

Equipment

- Nutritional supplementation
- Tap water
- 20 mL syringe
- Clean towel

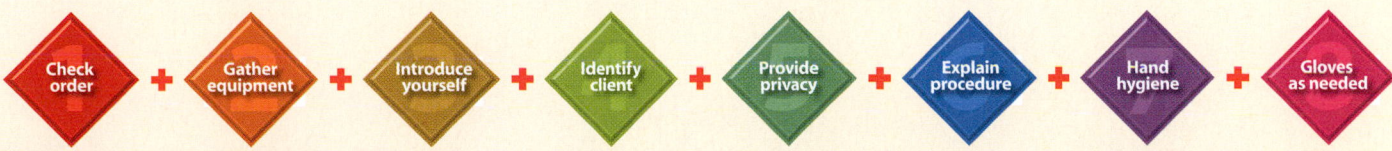

Check order + Gather equipment + Introduce yourself + Identify client + Provide privacy + Explain procedure + Hand hygiene + Gloves as needed

Interventions and Rationales

1. Perform preparatory steps (see icon bar).

2. Allow nutritional supplement to reach room temperature. *This will prevent cramping.*

3. Position the infant in a Fowler's or high Fowler's position. Place a towel across the infant's abdomen. *This position prevents aspiration, and the towel helps keep the infant's clothing free of soiling.*

4. Check placement.

5. Assess residual gastric volume. *The feeding should be withheld if the residual volume is too great because this indicates that digestion may be altered. The agency may designate this volume, and the physician may include the residual volume in the original order.*

6. Flush the tubing with tap water. *This is necessary to clear the tubing of gastric contents.*

7. Clamp the tubing and attach barrel of syringe or primed tubing for continuous feeding.

8. For bolus feeding, raise barrel of syringe no more than 18 in. above the infant's abdomen. Fill the syringe with nutritional supplement. Unclamp the tubing and allow supplement to flow slowly into the tube (see Figure 57-1).

9. Watch the infusion carefully and do not allow air into the tube. Clamp the tubing. *Air could cause the infant to have gas.*

10. Maintain the infant in the Fowler's position for 1 to 2 hours. *This will prevent aspiration.*

11. Follow the bolus feeding with a flush of tap water. *The amount of the flush will typically be ordered by the physician.*

12. For continuous feeding, label the bag with date and time. Set the rate as prescribed and monitor it closely.

SAMPLE DOCUMENTATION

[date]
[time]

No gastric residual obtained. Orogastric tube flushed with 10 mL tap water. 30 mL Enfamil with iron given bolus via orogastric tube. 30 mL tap water flushed following feeding. HOB at 45 degrees.

_____A. David, LVN

Chapter Review

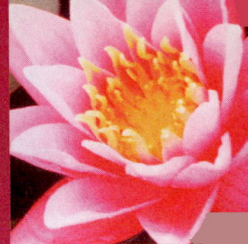

KEY Points

- High-risk neonatal conditions, including small or large for gestational age and drug addiction, require additional data collection and treatment.
- The LPN/LVN assists the RN in the care of high-risk newborns.
- Priorities for the care of high-risk newborns are maintenance, promoting tissue perfusion, and managing pain.
- Most congenital anomalies require surgical repair beginning in the newborn period. Often surgical repair of anomalies requires several procedures over time to complete the reconstruction.
- The NICU is a frightening place for parents. They need instruction in the NICU routine and equipment.
- Parents need continued support when their infant is facing life-threatening and long-term treatment.

∞ FOR FURTHER Study

For an illustration of the gastrointestinal system, see Chapter 37 and Figure 37-1.

Care during high-risk pregnancy is discussed in Chapter 52.

See Chapter 54 for guidelines about breastfeeding.

Gestational age determination and care of the normal neonate are discussed in Chapter 56.

See Chapter 59 for treatment and care of the neonate with talipes (clubfoot), Down syndrome, and urethral malposition.

Critical Thinking Care Map

Caring for a Preterm Newborn

NCLEX-PN® Focus Area: Physiologic Integrity

Case Study: Olivia, a 38-week gestation newborn, is brought to the NICU for observation and treatment of a 1-cm meningocele in the lumbar region of the spinal column. Olivia's mother had no prenatal care. Olivia is moving all extremities. Olivia had Apgar scores of 6 and 7.

Nursing Diagnosis: *Risk for infection* related to potential rupture of meningocele

COLLECT DATA

Subjective	Objective
_____	_____
_____	_____
_____	_____
_____	_____
_____	_____
_____	_____
_____	

Would you report this? Yes/No

If yes, report to: _____

What would you report? _____

Nursing Care

_____
_____
_____
_____
_____
_____
_____
_____
_____
_____
_____

How would you document this? _____
_____
_____
_____

Compare your answers and documentation to those provided on the MyNursingKit Website.

Data Collected
(use only those that apply)

- Respriations 32 per minute
- Lusty cry
- Apgar 6 and 7
- Temperature 99°F
- Lethargic
- Irritable
- No drainage from meningocele
- Flaccid muscle tone
- Moving all extremities
- 1-cm meningocele in lumbar spine

Nursing Interventions
(use only those that apply; list in priority order)

- Initial bath.
- Oxygen by mask.
- Supine position.
- Suction airway with suction catheter.
- Blood glucose by heel stick.
- Wet sterile dressing to meningocele.
- Radiant warmer.
- Neuro assessment every hour.
- Prone position.

1 When working in the newborn nursery, the nurse would not consider which of the following babies as high risk?

1. The infant whose mother died during delivery.
2. The infant born at 35 weeks' gestation.
3. The infant born at slightly more than 42 weeks' gestation.
4. The infant born with a cleft lip and palate.

2 Seeing his son, who was born with spina bifida, for the first time, a father exclaims, "What is that on his back?" An appropriate nursing response is to:

1. Describe the defect in detail including treatment and long-term needs of the infant.
2. Explain it is called *spina bifida* and provide a simple explanation of the anomaly.
3. Tell him how beautiful the baby's eyes are.
4. Refer him to the pediatrician for answers.

3 Shortly after delivery, the mother asks how she will know if her infant son is having problems breathing. The nurse's best response is:

1. "He will not cry and will begin to turn blue."
2. "His nostrils will flare out, he will grunt, and the skin over his ribs will sink in."
3. "You won't; he will just stop breathing."
4. "His respirations will become irregular and be over 30 per minute."

4 The nurse, working in the newborn nursery, receives report on a 4-hour-old baby who has not yet voided. At what age of life would the nurse need to notify the physician if the child still has not voided?

1. 48 hours of age
2. 12 hours of age
3. 16 hours of age
4. 24 hours of age

5 When providing care to the infant born at 26 weeks' gestation, all of the following are important nursing actions except:

1. Continuous vital sign monitoring.
2. Maintaining a neutral thermal environment.
3. Talking to the infant and providing frequent stimulation.
4. Managing and reducing pain.

6 Which of the following nursing implementations would be indicated for the small-for-gestational-age neonate but not for the large-for-gestational-age infant?

1. Glucose monitoring
2. Monitoring for respiratory distress
3. Monitoring for temperature instability
4. Monitoring vital signs frequently

7 Nursing care for the infant with a congenital heart defect is focused on which of the following?

1. Administering oxygen
2. Frequent vital sign monitoring
3. Reducing workload of the heart
4. Administering medications

8 After admitting a neonate to the newborn nursery, the nurse discovers that the infant has an imperforate anus. The nurse anticipates surgical repair:

1. Will occur within 6 months.
2. Will occur within 24 hours with creation of an ostomy.
3. Will occur within the first 2 years of life.
4. May be needed.

9 The nurse teaches the parents of a newborn that screening is performed for phenylketonuria prior to the infant's discharge from the hospital and will need to be repeated:

1. If the test returns with any positive results.
2. If all tests return as normal.
3. Within several days after the infant has taken formula or breast milk.
4. Only if a family history of metabolic disorders is known.

10 The nurse is assisting with care of an infant whose mother was addicted to cocaine. The infant is irritable and displaying signs of drug withdrawal. An important nursing intervention to comfort this infant will be:

1. Providing adequate nutrition.
2. Wrapping the infant snuggly, holding, and rocking the baby.
3. Administering of narcotics to lessen drug withdrawal.
4. Teaching the mother how to provide care for the infant at home.

Answers and rationales for Review Questions appear in Appendix I.

Thinking Strategically About...

You are a new graduate LPN/LVN, employed in a small hospital obstetric unit. The unit is staffed with one RN and one LPN/LVN per 12-hour shift. In report, you learn that a gravida 4, para 3 woman is laboring rapidly and is currently 8 cm dilated. The RN will need to remain with this client and assist in the delivery. You will be assigned to the other clients. There is an RN in another part of the hospital who can assist you if necessary.

At 0700, you receive the following report:

Mrs. Jessie Owens, a 22-year-old gravida 2, para 2, had a 7-lb 2-oz boy at 1300 yesterday by spontaneous vaginal delivery. She had no episiotomy or lacerations. She has had no postpartum complications. Jessie is breastfeeding and plans to go home late this afternoon. Her baby, Philip, is nursing 8 minutes per breast. He has voided and stooled. Jessie has blood type B−, rubella positive. Philip has blood type A+. He is to be circumcised before discharge.

Miss Monica McQuire, a 19-year-old, gravida 1, para 1, delivered an 8-lb 10-oz girl at 0130 this morning by primary cesarean section for failure to progress in labor. Prior to birth, Monica had gestational (pregnancy-induced) hypertension with a blood pressure of 154/92. She had 2+ pitting edema in her ankles. Her reflexes were brisk without clonus. She has an IV of lactated Ringer's solution with magnesium sulfate and a Foley catheter that can be discontinued this morning. Her baby, Amanda, has voided but has not stooled. Monica has only tried to breastfeed once since delivery, with poor results.

Mrs. Kim Lee, a 19-year-old, gravida 1, para 1, delivered a boy at 0500 this morning by suction-assisted vaginal birth. Kim's vital signs are stable and her flow is moderate. She has been up to the bathroom one time to void 530 mL of urine. Her fundus is firm at U1. Mrs. Lee's son, Dong, is stable and he is sleeping in his mother's arms. He has voided and stooled. Kim's husband has gone home to rest. The mother-in-law, who speaks only Korean, is at the bedside. Kim wants to breastfeed but the baby is not interested at this time.

CRITICAL THINKING

- At what point do you become concerned that baby Amanda has not stooled?

- Should baby Dong be nursing better?
- Is baby Philip nursing enough? What would indicate that he is not obtaining enough nutrition?

PRIORITIZING NURSING CARE

- Identify the order in which you will assess these assigned clients.
- What is the rationale for your prioritization of care?

MANAGEMENT OF CARE

- How frequently should you monitor Miss McQuire?
- Identify what care needs to be provided to each client and the time at which will you provide that care.

DELEGATING

- If a CNA is available to assist with your assignment, what care would you delegate?
- What follow-up would you need to do on the care you delegated to the CNA?

CLIENT TEACHING

- What would you say to Mrs. Lee to help her remain positive about her ability to breastfeed her baby?
- What teaching should be provided to Mrs. Owens before she is discharged?
- What teaching should be provided to Miss McQuire about breastfeeding?

CULTURAL CARE STRATEGIES

- What cultural strategies should be incorporated into the care of Mrs. Lee?

DOCUMENTING AND REPORTING

- For each client, what signs would alert you that their condition was declining and you would need to call the RN?
- Document the teaching provided to Mrs. Owens regarding circumcision care.

Pediatric and Adolescent Nursing Care

UNIT X

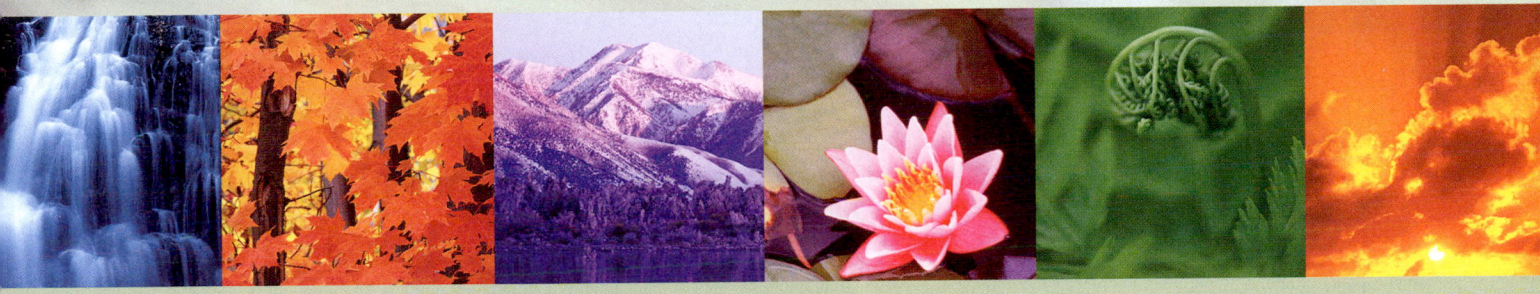

Chapter 58

Pediatric-Focused Nursing Care

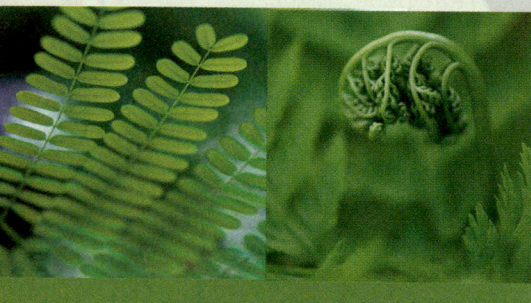

BRIEF Outline

Pediatric Anatomy and Physiology

Collecting Data for Pediatric Assessment

Adapting Nursing Care for the Pediatric Client

Hospitalized Child

Teaching Strategies with Pediatric Clients

Terminally Ill Pediatric Clients

Chronically Ill Pediatric Clients

Pediatric Clients with Developmental and Cognitive Issues

Identifying Disorders of Pediatric Clients by Age

LEARNING Outcomes

After completing this chapter, you will be able to:

1. Identify differences between body systems of the pediatric client and the adult client.
2. Describe unique aspects of data collection for a pediatric assessment by age group.
3. Identify ways of collecting data about vital signs, pain, and growth in pediatric clients.
4. Explain adaptations that are made when providing nursing care to pediatric clients.
5. Name important considerations when providing nursing care to hospitalized pediatric clients and their families.
6. Describe teaching strategies according to developmental age.
7. Discuss physical and psychosocial needs of terminally ill pediatric clients.
8. Discuss psychosocial needs of chronically ill pediatric clients and their families.
9. Identify tools and programs for pediatric clients with developmental or cognitive issues.
10. Explain the terms *mainstreaming* and *normalization* as they relate to developmental disabilities.

Clinical Objectives

11. Carry out admission procedures for a hospitalized pediatric client.
12. Administer medications according to developmental levels.
13. Provide client and family teaching according to developmental age.
14. Provide a safe environment for a hospitalized pediatric client.
15. Obtain a laboratory specimen from a child (e.g., urine specimen using a pediatric urine collector (PUC); heel stick for blood glucose monitoring).

KEY TERMS

anticipatory guidance 1611

appendicular skeleton 1599

autonomy 1610

epiphyseal plate 1599

fontanels 1599

funnel chest 1595

mainstreaming 1615

pigeon chest 1595

scoliosis 1595

Infants and children are not just miniature adults. Physically, mentally, and emotionally, children are different from adults, and their care requires nurses to adapt interventions to reflect these differences. As outlined in Chapters 15 and 16 ⊙, children develop through distinct physical, psychosocial, and emotional stages. At birth, they respond reflexively and connect with people and objects within a very small circle of perception. By the end of their first year, they are upright and mobile, they can distinguish between family and strangers, and they have an elementary means of communicating their wants and needs.

In the toddler period, verbal ability and vocabulary multiply. Coordination improves to include climbing stairs and peddling three-wheeler bikes. Individuation is established enough for toddlers to express themselves freely by saying, "No!" Preschoolers lay the groundwork for social interactions and self-identification, as they do parallel play and experiment with many different roles. Because they can stray farther and more quickly, they need to learn safety rules about the home and their environment.

School-age children begin to reason, become part of groups, find value in accomplishing tasks, and learn the importance of fairness and equality. Physically, most are coordinated enough to play an instrument or do a complex hobby or craft. They begin to identify life interests.

The physical growth that occurs fairly consistently through the first 10 to 12 years of life accelerates tremendously as children reach teenage and puberty. In this period, hormone levels increase, eccrine and apocrine glands reach their full functioning, height and weight increase rapidly, and bodies become capable of reproduction. At the same time, emotional and cognitive changes take place that change teenagers' worldview from family-centered to peer-centered. Physical strength and coordination reach their peak, and with this change comes a sense of invincibility, which can increase risk-taking behavior.

This unit reviews stages of pediatric development and identifies health promotion issues and common illnesses associated with each age group.

Pediatric Anatomy and Physiology

It is important for the nurse to understand the anatomical differences in pediatric clients and be able to identify which ones are of greatest concern when dealing with health issues. Even when adolescents' bodies begin to develop, they will continue to have some variations until full adult growth and development are achieved. In addition to the structural differences (*anatomy*), pediatric clients also have differences in function (*physiology*).

To prepare you better to provide care for children and adolescents, the anatomic and physiologic differences will be described by body systems. Figure 58-1 ■ shows overall anatomic and physiologic characteristics as children grow. Each body system will also be described.

RESPIRATORY SYSTEM

Infants will not automatically open their mouths to breathe when nasal passages are occluded until at least 6 months of age. This plus the small diameter of the infant airway increases the risk of airway obstruction (Figure 58-2 ■).

Sinuses grow and develop during childhood (Figure 58-3 ■). Maxillary sinuses can be identified in a 1-year-old, and by 6 years of age the ethmoid sinuses are developed, though they are still very different from those in an adult.

The infant chest is rounded, with the anteroposterior diameter equal to the lateral diameter. As the child grows the chest becomes more oval, and by 2 years of age the lateral diameter is greater. A round chest after this time may indicate obstructive lung disease such as cystic fibrosis or asthma. Infants and children have a thin chest wall due to immature muscle development.

Two abnormal chest shapes may exist in children. In **pigeon chest** (pectus carinatum), the sternum protrudes, causing an increase in the anteroposterior diameter. In **funnel chest** (pectus excavatum), the lower portion of the sternum is depressed. In addition to these, a curvature of the spine may be seen in school-age or adolescent children. The most common of these is **scoliosis,** a lateral deviation of the chest.

CARDIOVASCULAR SYSTEM

Shortly after birth, structures of fetal circulation, foramen ovale and ductus arteriosus, close to increase the blood flow to the lungs and allow full oxygenation (see Figure 56-3 ⊙). The right side of the heart now pumps blood to the lungs to receive oxygen, and the left side of the heart pumps blood rich in oxygen throughout the body. Congenital errors in structure are a serious concern in infants and children.

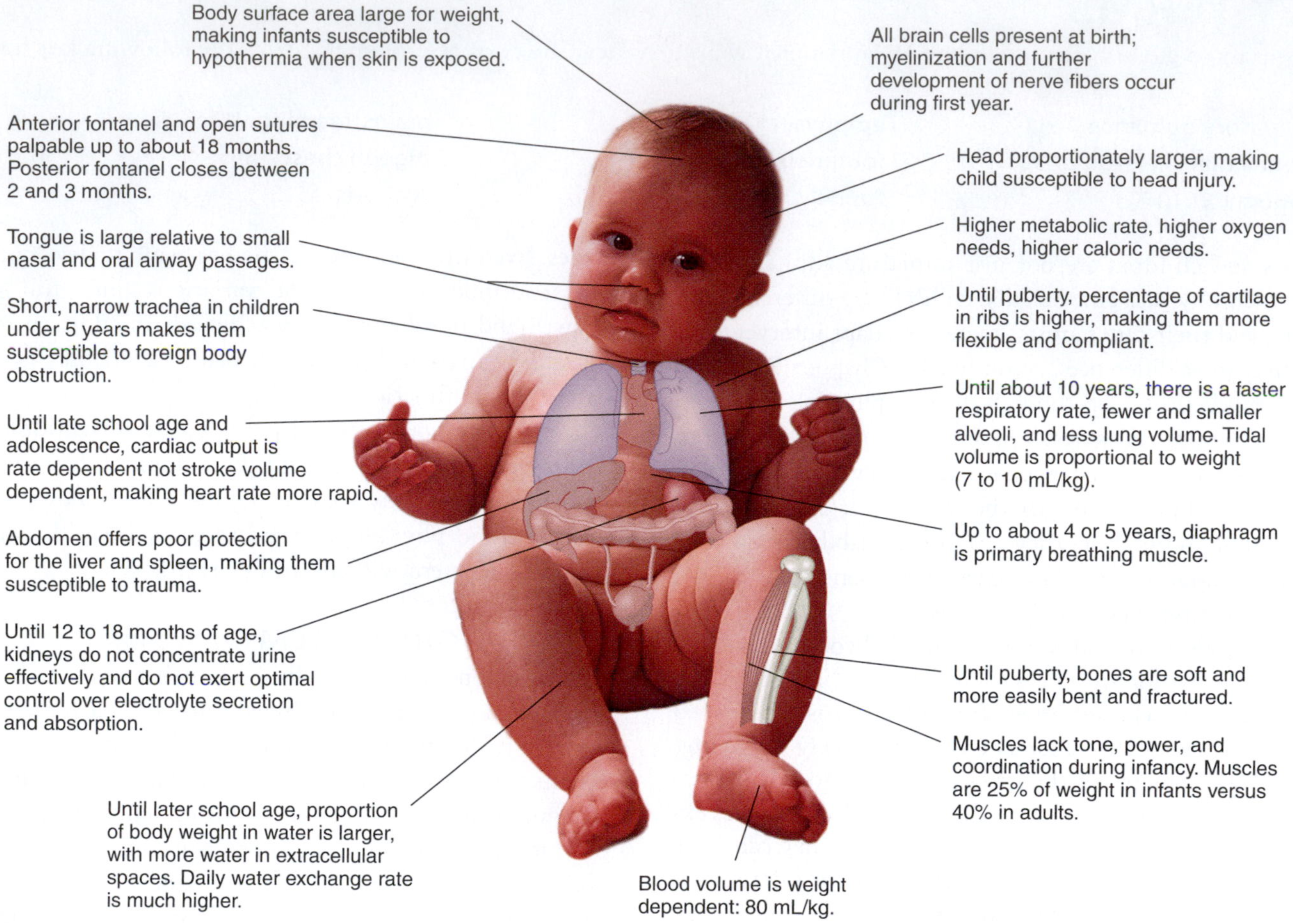

Body surface area large for weight, making infants susceptible to hypothermia when skin is exposed.

All brain cells present at birth; myelinization and further development of nerve fibers occur during first year.

Anterior fontanel and open sutures palpable up to about 18 months. Posterior fontanel closes between 2 and 3 months.

Head proportionately larger, making child susceptible to head injury.

Tongue is large relative to small nasal and oral airway passages.

Higher metabolic rate, higher oxygen needs, higher caloric needs.

Short, narrow trachea in children under 5 years makes them susceptible to foreign body obstruction.

Until puberty, percentage of cartilage in ribs is higher, making them more flexible and compliant.

Until late school age and adolescence, cardiac output is rate dependent not stroke volume dependent, making heart rate more rapid.

Until about 10 years, there is a faster respiratory rate, fewer and smaller alveoli, and less lung volume. Tidal volume is proportional to weight (7 to 10 mL/kg).

Abdomen offers poor protection for the liver and spleen, making them susceptible to trauma.

Up to about 4 or 5 years, diaphragm is primary breathing muscle.

Until 12 to 18 months of age, kidneys do not concentrate urine effectively and do not exert optimal control over electrolyte secretion and absorption.

Until puberty, bones are soft and more easily bent and fractured.

Muscles lack tone, power, and coordination during infancy. Muscles are 25% of weight in infants versus 40% in adults.

Until later school age, proportion of body weight in water is larger, with more water in extracellular spaces. Daily water exchange rate is much higher.

Blood volume is weight dependent: 80 mL/kg.

Figure 58-1. ■ Children are not just small adults. There are important anatomic and physiologic differences between children and adults that will change based on the child's growth and development.

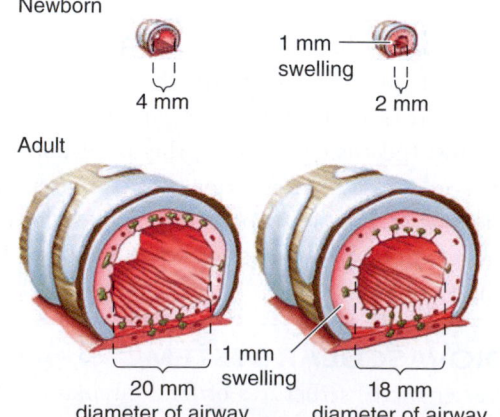

Newborn

1 mm swelling

4 mm

2 mm

Adult

1 mm swelling

20 mm diameter of airway

18 mm diameter of airway

Figure 58-2. ■ Diameter of an infant's airway in contrast to an adult's. Note how swelling of 1 mm of airway membranes can reduce the capacity of the newborn's airway by half.

Infant heart muscle fibers are not fully developed and are not as compliant to the amount of blood forced out of the ventricles during heart contractions (known as the heart volume or *stroke volume*). The pressure in the left side of the heart is greater than that in the right side. These factors make the infant quite sensitive to volume and pressure overload.

NEUROSENSORY SYSTEM

The nervous system grows more rapidly before birth, unlike the many other body tissues that grow significantly after birth. Most of the structures are formed during the gestational period, but they mature and the human brain continues to develop for at least 20 years (Figure 58-4 ■).

The stage from birth to 5 years is characterized by rapid physical development within the substance of the brain. Development is greatest in the brainstem and least in the cerebral cortex. Brainstem development is critical so that

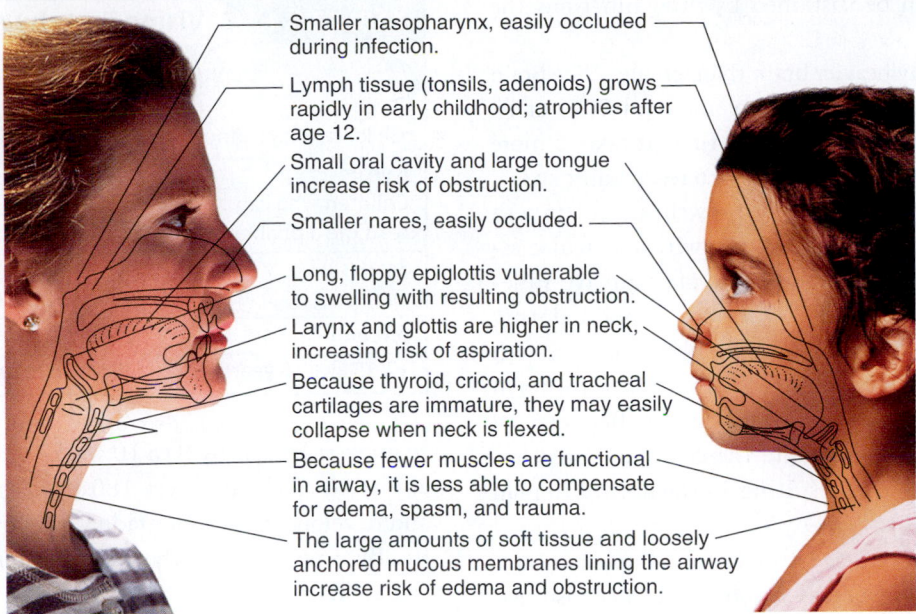

Smaller nasopharynx, easily occluded during infection.

Lymph tissue (tonsils, adenoids) grows rapidly in early childhood; atrophies after age 12.

Small oral cavity and large tongue increase risk of obstruction.

Smaller nares, easily occluded.

Long, floppy epiglottis vulnerable to swelling with resulting obstruction.

Larynx and glottis are higher in neck, increasing risk of aspiration.

Because thyroid, cricoid, and tracheal cartilages are immature, they may easily collapse when neck is flexed.

Because fewer muscles are functional in airway, it is less able to compensate for edema, spasm, and trauma.

The large amounts of soft tissue and loosely anchored mucous membranes lining the airway increase risk of edema and obstruction.

Figure 58-3. ■ Sinus airway development. An infection in the child's upper airway can have serious consequences because it has not developed to its adult size.

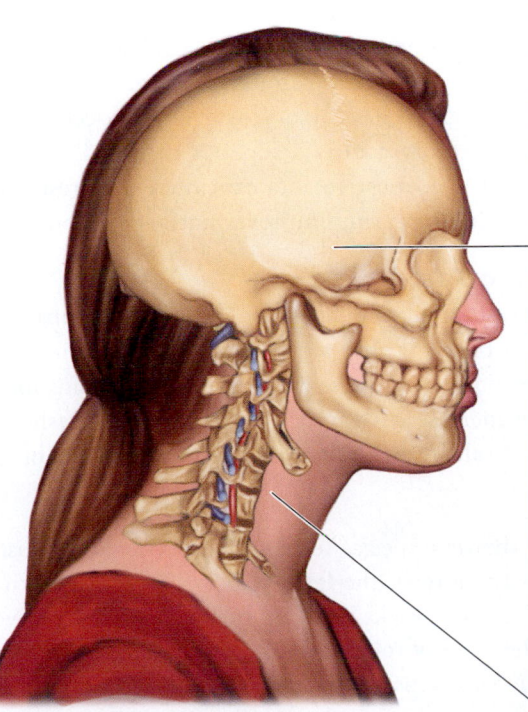
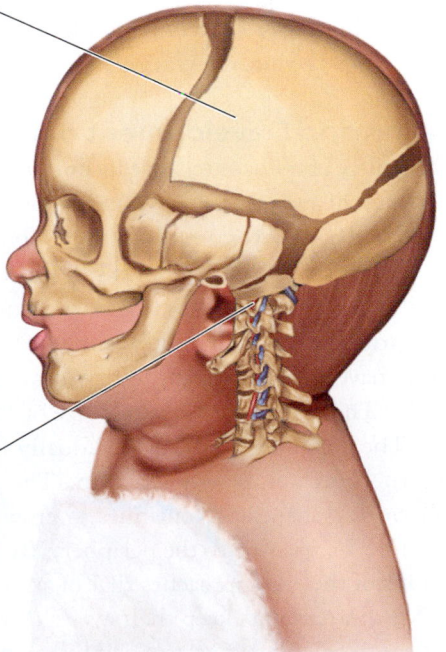

Top heavy, head is large in proportion to body; neck muscles poorly developed; thin cranial bones not well developed; unfused sutures; skull expands until age 2 years. *Prone to brain injury and skull fracture with falls.*

Head size proportional to body; neck muscles well developed, can reduce risk for brain injuries; sutures are ossified by age 12 years; no expansion of skull after 5 years.

Excessive spinal mobility; immature muscles, joint capsule, and ligaments of cervical spine; wedge-shaped, cartilaginous vertebral bodies; incomplete ossification of vertebral bodies. *Greater risk for high cervical spine injury at C1-C2 level or vertebral compression fractures with falls.*

Well developed muscles and ligaments reduce spinal mobility; vertebral bodies completely formed and ossified.

Figure 58-4. ■ Anatomic differences in the structure of the nervous system between children and adults. The skull and brain grow and develop rapidly during early childhood.

the newborn's life can be sustained by vital functions the brainstem controls.

Males have a slightly heavier brain than females. The brain doubles its weight in the first year of life, and 90% of its adult size is reached by age 5. After this time, it takes 5 more years to achieve the last 10% of growth to reach adult size.

The brain has distinct periods of growth. Each "growth spurt" of the brain is closely associated with particular aspects of development and achievement of cognitive milestones. Two major spurts occur within the brain during middle childhood. Between 6 and 8 years of age, a growth spurt occurs that is closely associated with improvements in fine motor skills and eye–hand coordination. Between 10 and 12 years, the frontal lobes and the cerebral cortex undergo further development, resulting in the ability to plan and to use logic.

During the teenage years, two additional spurts occur. Between 13 and 15, more energy is produced and consumed in the area of the brain that controls perception and motor function. Around 17 years of age and continuing into adulthood, growth of the brain is in the frontal lobe and cerebral cortex, which control reasoning ability.

Myelination (development of a protective sheath) is crucial to neural development. It is most rapid during the first 2 years of life and continues more slowly during childhood and adolescence. The neurons associated with motor, sensory, and cognitive functions are largely myelinated by the time a child starts school. Completion of myelination occurs between 6 and 12 years of age.

Vision and Development of the Eye

The ability of humans to sense incoming stimuli and adapt to the external and internal environment is essential to survival.

At birth the eyes are about three-fourths of their adult size. During the first 12 months of life, eye growth is maximal and then gradually decelerates until the 3rd year of life. Adult size is achieved by about 14 years of age. Newborns have limited vision, with visual acuity estimated at 6/200. The cornea reaches adult size of 12 mL by 2 years of age. The curvature of the eye gradually flattens, contributing to the changes in refraction. The newborn's lens is spherical in shape and continues to grow throughout life as new fibers are added to the periphery. By 5 to 6 months, the fundus of the eye approaches that of an adult in appearance.

Newborn infants keep their eyes closed most of the time, but the normal infant can see and fix upon points of contrast. The eyes move independently. The earliest sign of normal intact vision is the infant's ability to engage visually with the mother's face. The infant's visual field is 10 to 12 inches, which is the normal distance between a mother's breast and the neonate's face; 18 inches is the maximum distance. By 6 weeks of age, eye motion is coordinated and eyes are able

TABLE 58-1	Vision Tests by Age	
AGE	**TEST TYPE**	**VISUAL ACUITY**
3 years Children who cannot talk	Picture Chart	20/40
4 years Children who can read the alphabet	Snellen E	20/40
5 years	Snellen E or Snellen Letter	20/30
6, 8, and 10 years	Snellen Letter	20/20
12, 15 and 18 years	Snellen Letter	20/20

to move together. By 8 to 10 weeks of age, the infant has the ability to track an object 180 degrees. As the child grows and develops, there is a gradual improvement of visual acuity. By 3 years of age the child's vision approximates adult acuity. Table 58-1 ■ has guidelines for vision testing by age.

Hearing and Development of the Ear

The tympanic membrane is located close to the surface of the meatus, as is the facial nerve. Birth trauma may cause damage to the eardrum and the facial nerve. The color of the membrane is translucent, light pearly pink or grey. Slight redness of the membrane is normal in the newborn infant because of the increased vascularity of the membranes and sometimes as a result of crying.

The fetus normally responds to sound after the 22nd week. The newborn infant can locate the general direction from which a sound has come. It is generally accepted that an infant's auditory acuity is superior to visual acuity. By 6 months of age, most infants can locate and respond to sound. Children's hearing improves until adolescence.

Smell and Taste

The sense of smell and taste are chemical responses that function at birth. Shortly after birth the infant can identify his or her mother by the sense of smell. Thresholds for certain tastes increase with age. For example, the threshold for the taste of salt increases at approximately 20 years of age.

Touch

Touch is the first special sense to develop in the fetus. By 13 weeks the arm of the fetus will make contact with the face, and by 24 weeks most of the fetus is responsive to touch. The sense of touch is highly active between multiple fetuses such as twins or triplets.

MUSCULOSKELETAL SYSTEM

Skeleton

Infants are born with approximately 100 more bones than exist in the adult skeleton. The immature skeleton is composed primarily of cartilage. As normal growth and development occurs, certain parts of the skeleton begin to fuse, forming single bones (Figure 58-5 ■). At maturity the adult skeleton is composed of 206 bones. The *xiphoid process* consists of hyaline cartilage during childhood; it does not completely ossify until about 40 years of age. The manubrium ossifies even later, when the sternum becomes a rigid structure; in older adults it can interfere with respiration.

The vertebral column determines overall adult height. The lumbar spine and sacrum are small at birth compared to the thoracic and cervical vertebrae. The intervertebral disks are responsible for one-fourth to one-third of the overall length of the spinal column, making a significant contribution to the height of the individual. The thickness of the disk below the fourth vertebra increases steadily up to the age of 2 years and follows a steady pattern of growth after that time. Disks below the eighth thoracic vertebra do not show significant increase in diameter between age 6 and 8 years.

As the infant gains head control, a normal curve begins to develop in the cervical spine. Once the infant is able to sit unsupported, an additional curve develops in the lumbar region. As the child begins to walk, the higher center of gravity and the weight of a large liver create an exaggerated lordosis. An abnormal "S" curve can occur in the preadolescent to adolescent period. This curvature coincides with a growth spurt. Healthcare professionals need to screen all adolescents for scoliosis; these screenings are part of school health programs. See Chapter 48 ⚭ for a description of the scoliosis screening procedure.

SKULL.   The skull of the newborn undergoes molding during labor and vaginal delivery. Sutures in these areas are not fused at birth, allowing for brain growth. During the first few years of life the sutures interlock, forming jagged, serrated lines. The suture lines become obliterated as the body matures. The frontal suture closes at approximately 8 years of age. Partial obliteration of the sagittal suture occurs at about 30 years of age. The coronal suture closes at age 40, and the lambdoidal suture closes approximately 10 years later.

The newborn skull demonstrates three membranous areas or **fontanels** (soft spots; areas between the plates of the skull before fusion). These are found mainly at the four angles of the parietal bones. The largest is the anterior fontanel, located midline between the frontal bones and the two parietal bones. It closes between 18 and 24 months.

The posterior fontanel is located between the two parietal bones and the occipital bone; it is smaller than the anterior fontanel and normally closes about 2 months of age. The anterolateral fontanels are paired and are situated between the frontal, parietal, and sphenoid bones. They are small in size and close about 3 months after birth.

The fontanels should be protected until closed. They also can be an observation site for dehydration or increased intracranial pressure (IICP). An infant who is dehydrated may have sunken fontanels, whereas the fontanels will be bulging in the presence of IICP.

Growth of the skull is greatest during the first 2 years of life, although it continues after that time. Growth of the cranial vault is related to the development of the nervous system. The face and base of the skull grow as a result of development of muscles of mastication and tooth eruption. The capacity of the skull and the changes in the configuration of the face are almost accomplished by age 16.

APPENDICULAR SKELETON.   The **appendicular skeleton,** which consists of the bones of the arms and legs (the appendages), also changes with growth and development. During childhood all bones grow in thickness by *exogenous growth* (growth produced from outside the bones). Long bones lengthen by the addition of bone material on the diaphyseal side of the **epiphyseal plate,** a layer of cartilage in the metaphysis of the bone (see Chapter 31 ⚭). When

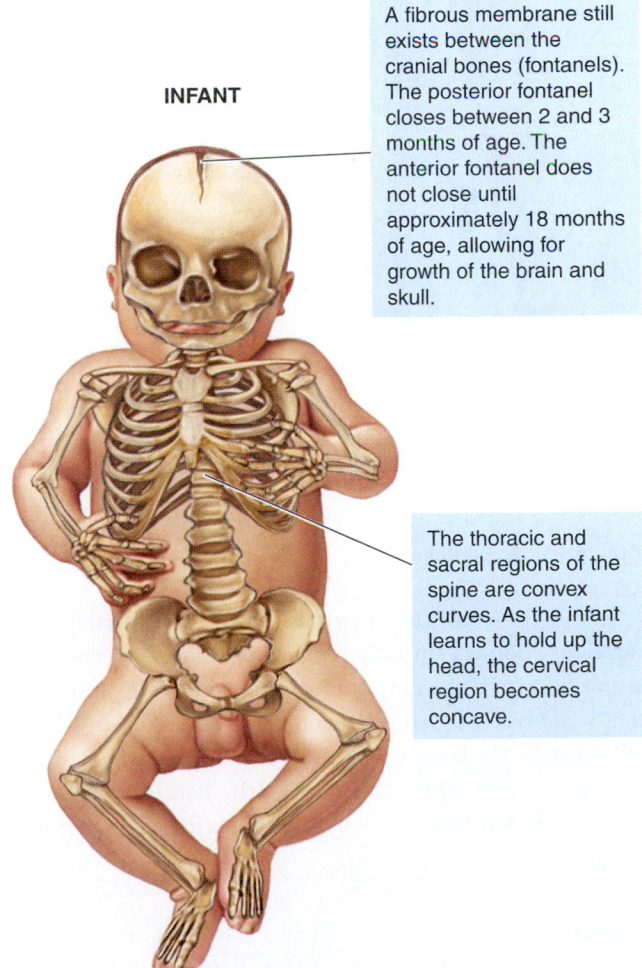

INFANT

A fibrous membrane still exists between the cranial bones (fontanels). The posterior fontanel closes between 2 and 3 months of age. The anterior fontanel does not close until approximately 18 months of age, allowing for growth of the brain and skull.

The thoracic and sacral regions of the spine are convex curves. As the infant learns to hold up the head, the cervical region becomes concave.

Figure 58-5. ■ Musculoskeletal system of infant. Skeleton and muscles develop throughout childhood.

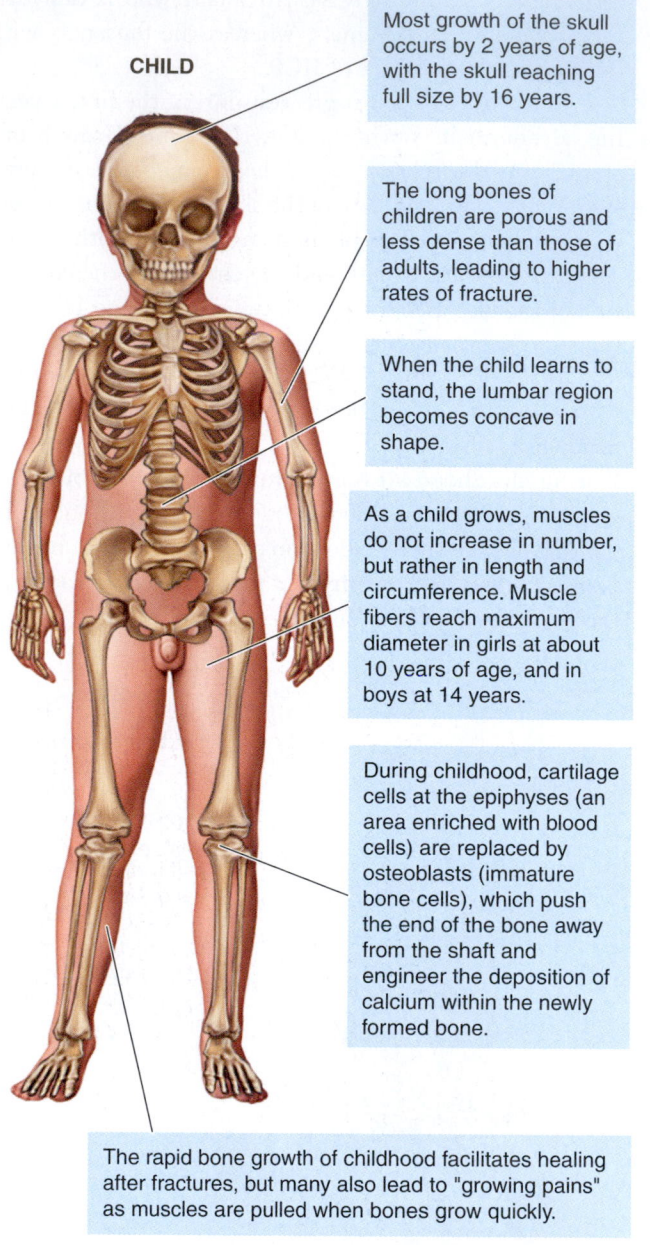

CHILD

Most growth of the skull occurs by 2 years of age, with the skull reaching full size by 16 years.

The long bones of children are porous and less dense than those of adults, leading to higher rates of fracture.

When the child learns to stand, the lumbar region becomes concave in shape.

As a child grows, muscles do not increase in number, but rather in length and circumference. Muscle fibers reach maximum diameter in girls at about 10 years of age, and in boys at 14 years.

During childhood, cartilage cells at the epiphyses (an area enriched with blood cells) are replaced by osteoblasts (immature bone cells), which push the end of the bone away from the shaft and engineer the deposition of calcium within the newly formed bone.

The rapid bone growth of childhood facilitates healing after fractures, but many also lead to "growing pains" as muscles are pulled when bones grow quickly.

ADULT

Muscle strength continues to increase until about 25–30 years of age.

The ends of long bones (epiphyses) remain cartilaginous, allowing growth, until approximately age 20 years, when skeletal maturation is complete. At this time the epiphyseal plate closes, cartilage at the site is replaced by bone, and only an epiphyseal line remains.

Until puberty, both ligaments and tendons are stronger than bone. As the child ages and cartilage is replaced by bone, the resulting bone is stronger than ligaments or tendons. Rates of fractures decrease while injuries to ligaments and tendons increase.

Figure 58-5. ■ *Continued.*

the plates close and the growth of epiphyseal cartilage cells is arrested, bone eventually replaces cartilage and the plates fade, leaving a bony structure that becomes the epiphyseal line. Some bones (such as the tarsus of the foot) are already ossified at birth. Long bones tend to complete their growth process by 18 to 20 years. Bones of the hands ossify by age 10. Bones of the foot ossify by 5 years, with the metatarsals fusing by age 18.

Muscles

Most skeletal muscles develop before birth, and the remainder are formed by the end of the first year. Increase in the size of the muscles is due to an increase in the diameter of fibers associated with growth of the skeleton. There are differences in the number of muscle fibers found in boys and girls. The number of muscle fibers found in the gluteal muscles of boys increases 14-fold between birth and maturity; the number in girls increases only 10-fold. Muscle fibers attain maximum diameter in girls at age 10, but not until age 14 in boys. Maximum muscle strength is attained between ages 25 and 30.

GASTROINTESTINAL SYSTEM

The gastrointestinal system is vital to life and is responsible for nourishment and elimination. The first organ of the GI system is the tongue. At birth the tip of the tongue is stubby

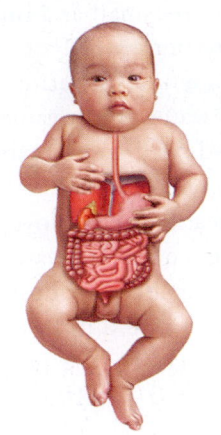
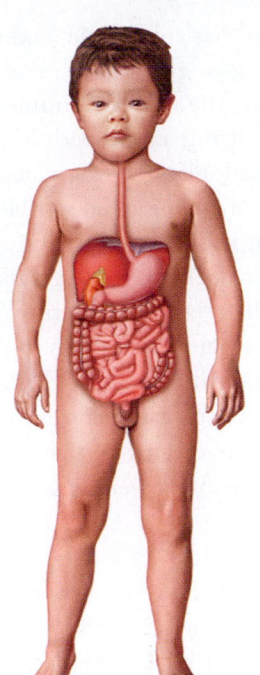

Stomach capacity throughout early childhood	
Age	*Capacity (mL)*
Newborn	10 to 20
1 week	30 to 90
2 to 3 weeks	75 to 100
1 month	90 to 150
3 months	150 to 200
1 year	210 to 360
2 years	500

Figure 58-6. ■ Stomach capacity by age. Infants have a much smaller stomach capacity than children or adults. (*Source:* From Chamley, C. A., Carson, P., Randall, D., & Sandwell, M. [2004]. *Developmental anatomy and physiology of children* [p. 217]. St Louis: Elsevier Mosby.)

and rounded. The mobile and more pointed tip of the adult tongue develops gradually with chewing and swallowing.

The neonate's salivary glands produce only a small amount of saliva containing the enzyme amylase (used to break down milk). By 6 months of age the salivary glands have tripled their weight at birth. By age 2 they are five times larger than at birth. The infant's mouth learns discriminative and motor skills as the muscles of the throat establish a cerebral connection.

The position and shape of the stomach at birth is high in the abdomen and is oriented horizontally rather than vertically as it is in a child 2 to 10 years of age. As feeding begins, the stomach capacity increases; in fact, within the first 2 weeks it almost triples. Figure 58-6 ■ lists average stomach capacity by age.

The liver is quite large at birth. It fills about 40% of the peritoneal cavity, displacing the bowel. The lower margin is palpable below the costal margin. In the infant the liver is about 5% of the total body weight, compared to 2.5% in the adult. Its large size reflects the importance of the liver's function in the fetal period.

The digestive system descends with growth. By puberty the length of the intestines doubles. They are thin-walled due to underdeveloped musculature; the mucosa and submucosa are strong. Villi continue to develop until puberty. In infancy the pelvis is small and can accommodate very little of the small intestine. The fetal cecum is cone-shaped, with the appendix at the apex of the cone. As the infant grows, the shape becomes rounded and the appendix moves around to the inner side. The ileocecal valve is more distinct in children than in adults.

Fecal Elimination

Toilet training can be a difficult stage in the child's development. Defecation initially occurs as an involuntary action. Children are often ready to be toilet trained between 18 and 36 months of age. During this time the nervous system matures, the child becomes aware of rectal pressure and sensitivity, and the brain can inhibit the reflex until it is convenient to defecate.

ENDOCRINE SYSTEM

All of the glands of the endocrine systems are present at birth. At that time the pituitary gland is large, weighing approximately 100 mg. It grows at a steady pace, although there are subtle differences in growth between males and females. The anterior pituitary is larger in the female. The parathyroid glands are simple structures with one type of secretory cell dominant until age 5 or 6, when oxyphils, a second type of cell, emerge. The rate of growth in children is governed by thyroid hormones and pituitary growth hormone. Thyroid hormone is secreted in greater quantities during the first 2 years of life. After that time the level decreases and remains fairly constant until puberty.

The thymus gland has a dual role (endocrine and lymph activity). It is the largest gland in the body of the newborn infant. After puberty, the thymus diminishes in endocrine activity, although during adulthood it produces thymic hormones. The pineal gland is most active during early childhood. It is responsible for the synthesis of melatonin, which is produced at night.

At birth the adrenal glands undergo changes as the cortex grows rapidly, changing the structure of the gland. Approximately one-third of its weight is lost during the first month of life; at 3 months of age the thick cortex begins to regress and a thinner permanent cortex is established. The glands do not begin to develop in size until 2 years of age and do not regain their birth weight until puberty.

URINARY SYSTEM

The fetal kidneys begin to function at approximately 10 weeks' gestation, although they are not responsible for removal of waste products until after birth. The placenta removes waste. During fetal life the kidneys produce urine that supplements amniotic fluid volume by about 200 mL per day.

The kidneys and bladder continue to develop after birth (Figure 58-7 ■). The kidneys are completely developed by the end of the first year, although bladder control follows later. Bladder location is not permanent until puberty. The bladder development relates to control and also its location, and is not complete until puberty.

At birth, nephrons are small and immature with many of the tubular sections not yet fully formed. They are inefficient, with low glomerular filtration and an inability to reabsorb sodium and water. Adult values of glomerular filtration are not reached until 1 to 2 years of age. Newborn's reduced ability to excrete hydrogen ions and lower acid secretion for the first year, as well as low plasma bicarbonate levels and an inability to excrete water loads, predisposes newborn infants to metabolic acidosis. Ninety-five percent of newborns pass urine during the first 24 hours of life. As the kidneys mature, the output increases from 25–30 mL four times per day to 100–200 mL 10 times per day—by day 10.

The bladder in the infant and young child is cigar-shaped and is situated in the abdomen, even when empty. It does not take on the adult pyramid shape until age 6. About the same time, it begins to enter the pelvis; this continues until it is in the adult position at puberty. The change in the bladder's position is a result of pelvic growth

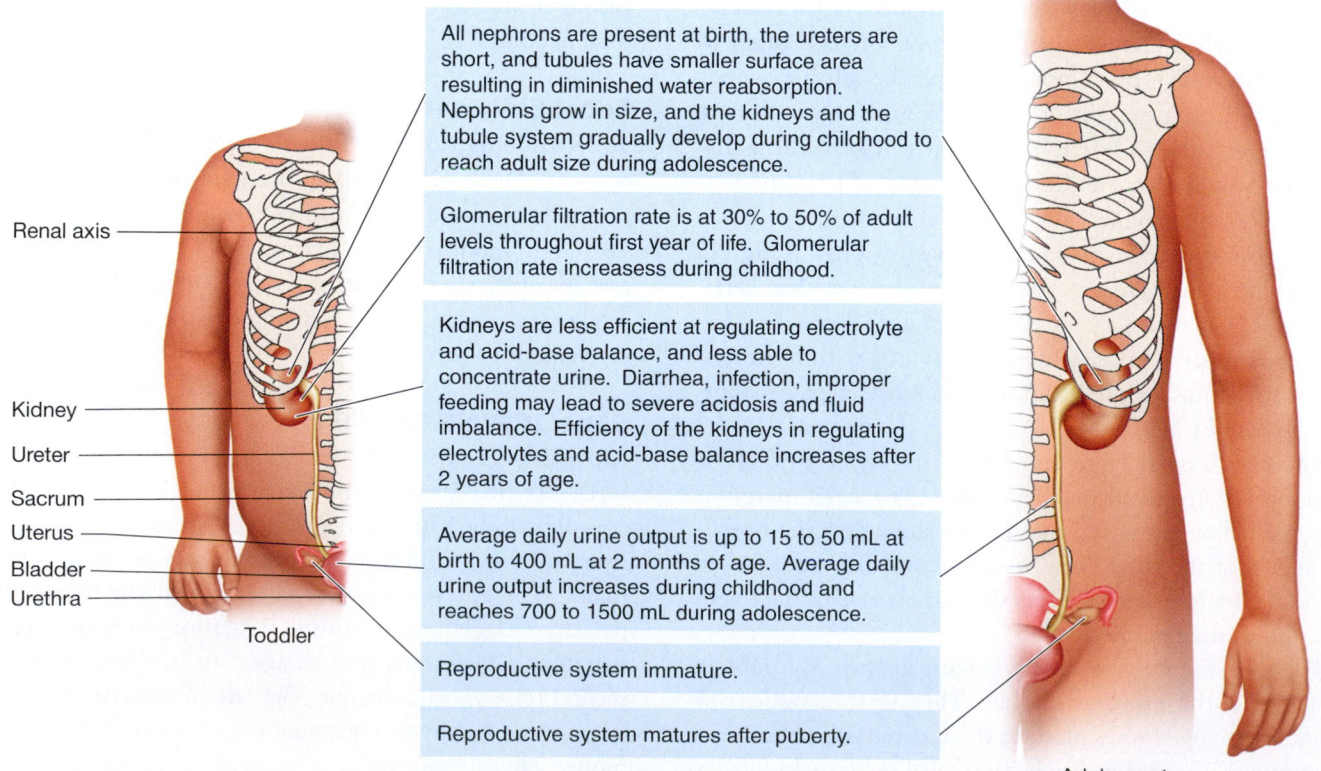

Renal axis

All nephrons are present at birth, the ureters are short, and tubules have smaller surface area resulting in diminished water reabsorption. Nephrons grow in size, and the kidneys and the tubule system gradually develop during childhood to reach adult size during adolescence.

Glomerular filtration rate is at 30% to 50% of adult levels throughout first year of life. Glomerular filtration rate increasess during childhood.

Kidney
Ureter
Sacrum
Uterus
Bladder
Urethra

Kidneys are less efficient at regulating electrolyte and acid-base balance, and less able to concentrate urine. Diarrhea, infection, improper feeding may lead to severe acidosis and fluid imbalance. Efficiency of the kidneys in regulating electrolytes and acid-base balance increases after 2 years of age.

Average daily urine output is up to 15 to 50 mL at birth to 400 mL at 2 months of age. Average daily urine output increases during childhood and reaches 700 to 1500 mL during adolescence.

Reproductive system immature.

Reproductive system matures after puberty.

Toddler

Adolescent

Figure 58-7. ■ Development of the urinary system. (*Source:* Data from Huether, S. E. [2006]. Alterations of renal and urinary tract function in children. In K. L. McCance & S. E. Huether, *Pathophysiology: The biologic basis for disease in adults and children* [5th ed., pp. 1337–1352]. St Louis: Elsevier Mosby.)

and maturation of the pelvic bones, rather than true migration of the bladder and urethra.

REPRODUCTIVE SYSTEM

The sex of the embryo is determined at fertilization. During the early stages of meiosis, all sex cells enter a dormant state and remain in meiotic suspension until sexual maturity.

Female Development

After birth the ovaries are abdominal organs; they enter the ovarian fossa by 6 years of age. There is little ovarian growth until puberty, when they increase to 20 times the weight of the newborn organs.

At birth the uterus lies almost at the same level as the vagina. As the bladder descends, the uterus bends forward into the adult position. The influence of maternal hormones causes the neonate's uterus to be fairly large at birth. As maternal hormones are excreted, the uterus shrinks, and it does not regain its birth weight until stimulated by hormonal activity at puberty. The fallopian tubes grow at the same time as the uterus.

The cervix is larger than the body of the uterus until adolescence, when the uterus overgrows the cervix and doubles in length.

During the productive years from approximately 14 to 50 years, nonpregnant females normally experience a cyclical series of events about every 26 to 30 days known as the menstrual cycle. The main discussion of the reproductive system of females and males is in Chapter 40 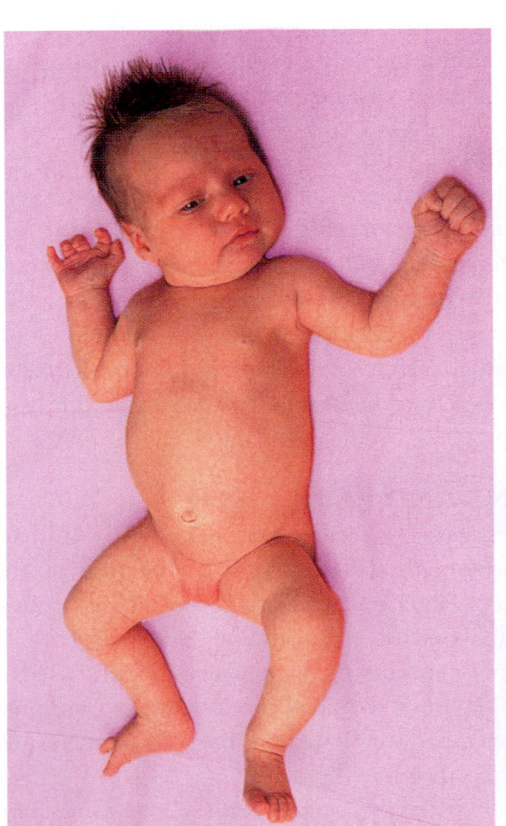.

Male Development

After birth the seminiferous tubules of the testicles are solid, until puberty when they become canalized. The testes are small and grow slowly during childhood. Adult testes become about 40 times heavier than those of the newborn.

The prostate is also slow growing until puberty, when it doubles in size over a short period of time.

The penis is relatively large at birth and the prepuce is imperfectly separated from the glands. The spongy tissue grows throughout childhood.

Male puberty usually occurs between ages 9 and 15 years. The earliest sign is the growth of the testicles. The average adult testicle has a volume of 20 mL; a volume of 6 mL signals that puberty has begun. See Chapter 62 for Tanner's stages and changes in puberty.

INTEGUMENTARY SYSTEM

The skin is referred to as the largest organ of the body. At birth it is a thin structure approximately 1 mm thick. At maturity, it has doubled that thickness (Figure 58-8 ■). At birth all skin structures are present, but many of their functions are immature.

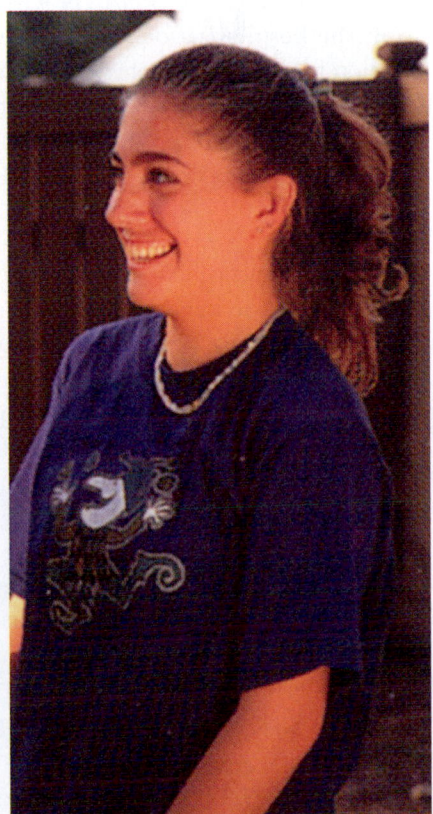

Newborns
Skin is very thin
Epidermis is loosely bound to the dermis, friction can cause separation of the layers with blistering
Eccrine sweat glands function, produce sweat in response to heat and emotional stimuli
Apocrine sweat glands are small and nonfunctional
Less melanin is present at birth so skin is lighter colored

Adolescents
Skin thickens
Epidermis and dermis are tightly bound, increasing resistance to infection and irritation
Eccrine sweat glands achieve full function, after puberty males sweat more than females
Apocrine sweat glands mature during puberty
Melanin is at adult levels, determining skin color and serving as a shield against ultraviolet radiation

Figure 58-8. ■ Integumentary system changes. The changes in skin reach adult levels at puberty.

Regulation of body temperature becomes more efficient during infancy, because an increase in adipose tissue by 6 months of age insulates the infant against heat loss. As children enter the toddler years, they are better able to respond to moderate variations in temperature. Capillaries conserve body temperature, and the process of shivering becomes an efficient method of thermoregulation.

Young children produce heat rapidly and can become overheated. Caregivers need to be aware of this and change clothing to accommodate climate variations. At puberty, eccrine sweat glands mature and respond to both emotional and environmental stimulation. Apocrine sweat glands become functional, excreting a substance that may lead to body odor.

Melanin at birth is at a low level; thus, newborns have a lighter skin tone than they will have as older children. This fact also means that young children are more susceptible to the effects of sun. Older light-skinned children (especially teens) may seek out opportunities for tanning and may ignore information about potential long-term ill effects.

Collecting Data for Pediatric Assessment

RNs will conduct the admission assessment for children as they do for adults. The LPN/LVN will collect focused data during the hospitalization. See Chapter 19 ⓐⓑ for data collection for head-to-toe physical assessment. Variations of the exam for the child are explained below. It is necessary to use a developmental approach to a physical examination when gathering data on the pediatric client.

INFANT

Very young infants cannot squirm away from care providers like toddlers do, so in a way they are the easiest children on whom to perform a physical examination. However, unusual sensations, such as inserting a tympanic thermometer into the ear canal, may make them squirm and then cry. This data may be most easily collected with the infant on the parent's lap rather than lying on an examination table. Feeding, offering a pacifier, or cuddling the infant can provide physical comfort. The order of the steps of the examination can be adjusted in order to take advantage of times when the infant is quiet enough for auscultation to be performed. The remainder of the exam should be carried out in the normal head-to-toe order.

Infants older than 6 months of age may experience stranger and separation anxiety. Have the parent remain with the child to prevent the anxiety. During the exam the parent can hold the child, although it is not recommended that the parent restrain the infant during painful procedures. (The parent is the protector of the child. Restraint by a parent could affect the child's sense of trust, if he or she feels the parent is allowing some hurtful act by "a stranger.")

TODDLER

The toddler may be shy and cautious or active and curious. Tell the child what you will be doing immediately before each step of the examination. Much of the musculoskeletal and neurologic examination can be carried out while observing the child at play and walking around the exam room. To provide comfort and increase compliance, allow the child to hold a security object during the exam.

PRESCHOOLER

The preschooler should be able to sit on the bed or the exam table for the examination. The child will usually cooperate if a simple explanation is given. At this age positive reinforcement for good behavior is important. Also, the child should be allowed to cry when experiencing discomfort and should not be told things like, "You're a big boy, and big boys don't cry." Be truthful; do not say something will not hurt if it will.

SCHOOL-AGE CHILD

School-age children usually cooperate fully. They want to help. Expect them to be modest. Always provide a private area for the examination and a gown and bath blanket to cover areas of the body that are not being examined.

ADOLESCENT

Adolescent clients may prefer that parents not be present during the examination. Asking their preference is a strong indication of respect. Clients at this age may have concerns about the changes of their developing bodies. The nurse can provide reassurance that the development is normal. Questions about sexual activity may arise during the course of the examination if the adolescent client feels they can trust the examiner.

VITAL SIGNS AND PAIN

Temperature is most frequently assessed now by using a tympanic thermometer (Figure 58-9 ■), because of the shorter data retrieval time. Depending on facility policy, the rectal or auxiliary route may also be used.

A new temperature assessment apparatus is being used in some facilities. It uses a temporal thermometer to compute the core body temperature based on forehead temperature, as measured with an infrared scanner.

Vital signs are listed by age group in the following chapters in this unit.

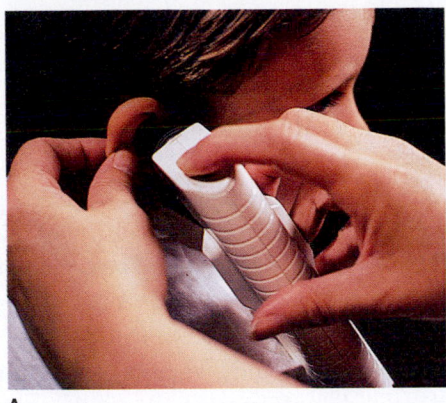

A

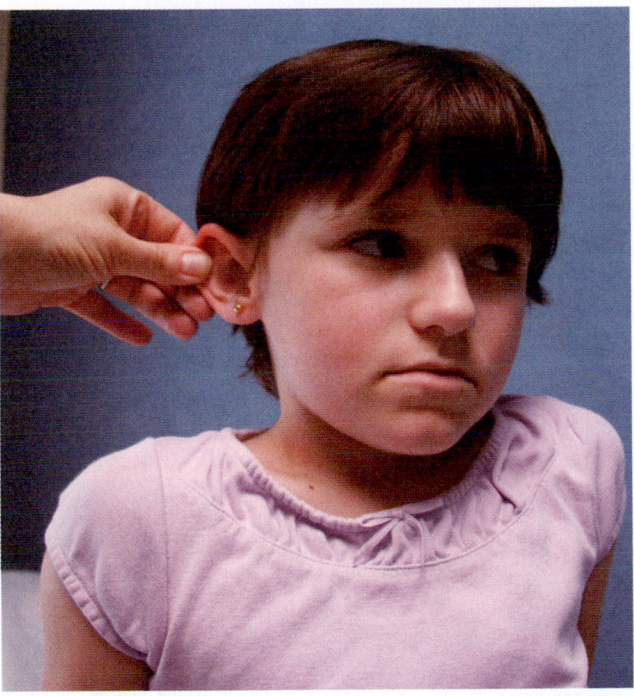

B

Figure 58-9. ■ Straightening the ear canal. **A.** The tragus of the infant or toddler is pulled down and back to straighten the ear canal. **B.** The tragus of a child over 3 is pulled up and back.

clinical ALERT

If you take the child's temperature by the rectal route, be sure to hold the thermometer or probe continuously to prevent injury of the rectal tissue. A rectal temperature is not usually recommended for the neonate or young infant due to the shortness of the anal canal and the possibility of perforation. **Note:** The use of mercury thermometers is no longer permitted, because of possible chemical spill and inhalation if a thermometer is broken. Glass clinical nonmercury thermometers (see Figure 21-5 🔗) are available, but they are very costly.

Respirations

Children younger than 6 years of age primarily use the diaphragm as the muscle for breathing. The nurse can either feel or observe the rise and the fall of the abdomen when the child is quiet in order to best assess respirations.

Heart Rate/Pulse

The location of the apical impulse changes as the child and the rib cage grow. Before age 7 it is located at the 4th intercostal space medial to the left midclavicular line. After age 7 it is right at the midclavicular line at the 5th intercostal space. The child's heart rate varies with age and increases with exercise, anxiety, excitement, and fever.

Pulse can be assessed at all pulse sites, although the brachial site in the arm and popliteal or femoral in the leg are most accurate for an infant. Distal pulse in the infant is difficult to assess because of their low systolic blood pressure. Radial and distal tibial pulses are normally palpated in older children.

Blood Pressure

Infant blood pressure readings are not commonly taken in the healthy child. A pediatric cuff of the correct size must be used to prevent inaccurate readings. The child should sit quietly for 3 to 5 minutes prior to taking the blood pressure.

When hypertension is suspected in a pediatric client, the systolic and diastolic BP should be compared to the height percentile. A BP pressure value at the 50th percentile for age, sex, and height is considered midpoint. A reading above the 95th percentile indicates hypertension.

Collecting Data about Pain

Assessing pain in children can be difficult; the nurse will need to use all observational skills. It was once the opinion of healthcare professionals that children experienced less pain than adults. Despite improvements in pain management many nurses still undertreat pain, especially in pediatric clients. Undertreatment is a result of misconceptions and attitudes about pain.

Children exhibit both physiologic and behavioral indicators of pain. By the time children are 18 months of age, they are also able to verbalize pain, using words such as *hurt, ouch,* and *ow.*

Physiologic indicators of pain in children include the following:

- Acute pain
  - Tachycardia
  - Tachypnea
  - Hypertension
  - Pupil dilation

- Pallor
- Increased perspirations
- Chronic pain can result in adaptation so that normal heart and respiratory rate and blood pressure are seen.

Behavioral indicators of pain may appear as follows:

- Child difficult to comfort
- Short attention span
- Sleep disturbance
- Facial grimace
- Guarding or avoiding movement
- Drawing up knees
- Lethargy

In addition to observations of indicators, the nurse can use a pain assessment scale. The OUCHER scale and the FACES Pain Rating Scale are two scales frequently used with children (Figure 58-10 ■).

The OUCHER scale uses a series of pictures of children's faces of various ethnicities. The child is asked to pick the picture that best describes the pain being experienced. Older children can make use of the accompanying numbers. The FACES scale makes use of line drawings of faces. Each drawing is numbered and is identified with words indicating the amount of "hurt" the child is experiencing. See Chapter 22 ⬤⬤ for the main discussion of pain.

GROWTH MEASUREMENTS

Depending on facility policy, growth measurement is taken in English (feet/inches and pounds) or metric (kilograms and centimeters) units.

Height and Weight

The infant or child is placed in a supine position and a tape measure is used to measure the length from the crown to heel. Once a child is able to stand, the height is measured with the child standing against a measuring stick on a standing scale or against a wall.

Weight can be assessed on a table or floor scale depending on the child's ability to stand. The weight should be taken at the same time every day. An infant should be weighed in a shirt and dry diaper only.

Height and weight should be graphed on a growth chart, which will provide information as to the percentile of height and weight in which the child falls. These are available for use up to 18 years of age.

BODY MASS.   A more accurate assessment of a child's risk for being under- or overweight is the body mass index. When using the index for children, the BMI is gender specific. BMI can be used for children ages 2 through adolescence. Box 58-1 ■ provides a sample calculation of BMI. Note: BMI is also used when an adult medication dose needs to be calculated for a child.

Head and Chest Circumference

Head measurement should be obtained on children less than 36 months of age. The measurement is taken around the occiput, above the pinna of the ear and slightly above the eyebrows. In infants the head measurement is compared to the chest circumference. Chest measurement is taken with a tape measure at the nipple area. These measurements are also graphed on the growth chart.

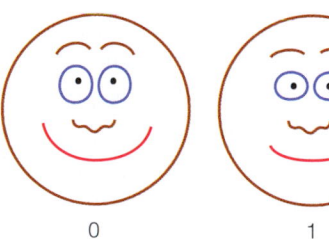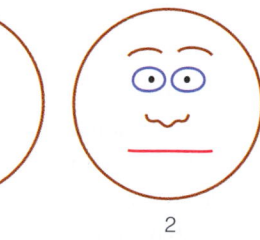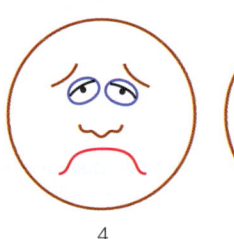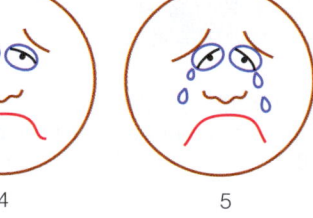

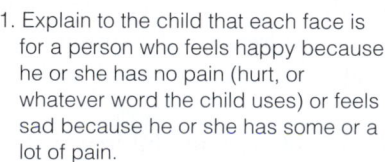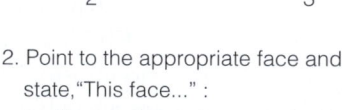

| 0 | 1 | 2 | 3 | 4 | 5 |

1. Explain to the child that each face is for a person who feels happy because he or she has no pain (hurt, or whatever word the child uses) or feels sad because he or she has some or a lot of pain.

2. Point to the appropriate face and state, "This face...":
   - 0—"is very happy because he (or she) doesn't hurt at all."
   - 1—"hurts just a little bit."
   - 2—"hurts a little more."
   - 3—"hurts even more."
   - 4—"hurts a whole lot."
   - 5—"hurts as much as you can imagine, although you don't have to be crying to feel this bad."

3. Ask the child to choose the face that best describes how he or she feels. Be specific about which pain (e.g., "shot" or incision) and what time (e.g., Now? Earlier before lunch?)

Figure 58-10. ■ Wong-Baker FACES Pain Rating Scale is useful in children with a concept of what numbers mean. The pictures can be used with explanations for younger children. (From Hockenberry, M. J. [2005]. *Wong's essentials of pediatric nursing* [7th ed.]. St. Louis, MO: Mosby, p. 1301. Copyright by Mosby, Inc. Reprinted with permission.)

BOX 58-1 | BMI SAMPLE CALCULATION

Equation:

Child's weight in pounds divided by 2.2 = weight in kg
Height in inches divided by 39 = height in meters
Weight in kilograms divided by height in meters squared =
BMI

Example:
16-year-old boy weighs 150 lb and is 75 inches tall:
150/2.2 = 68.2 kg
75 in /39 in = 1.9 m
68.2 divided by 1.9 × 1.9 = 68.2 divided 3.6 = 18.9
The BMI for this child is around the 25th percentile.

Abdominal Girth

The measurement of the abdominal girth is conducted to check for abnormal conditions such as ascites, organ enlargement, constipation, bowel obstruction, or hernias. The child is measured in a supine position with the tape being placed at the level of the umbilicus. On admission a baseline measurement should be taken; changes will indicate an abnormal condition.

Adapting Nursing Care for the Pediatric Client

HYGIENE

Hygiene for the pediatric client follows the same rules as for the adult client. One difference is that depending on age and developmental skills the nurse will need to provide most of the care. Bathing and AM care is a good time to observe the condition of the child's skin; the nurse will also able to use this time to teach the child and or parents if hygiene has been neglected. Proper hygiene is an important part of good health and well-being. When bathing an uncircumcised toddler, the nurse does not need to pull the foreskin back to clean it. Until the foreskin is fully retractable it should not be pulled back. At that time the child can retract it himself.

SPECIMEN COLLECTION

Specimen collections may need to be done to provide diagnostic information in order to provide proper treatment. Common specimens collected on pediatric clients include urine, stool, blood, wound drainage, sputum, spinal fluid, and throat culture (Figure 58-11 ■). It will be important to gain the cooperation of the child; it may also be necessary to have one or more staff to assist with the procedure. It is best not to have a parent restrain the child; as mentioned earlier, they represent protection and security to the child and restraining the child when painful procedures are being conducted will give them a sense of lost security.

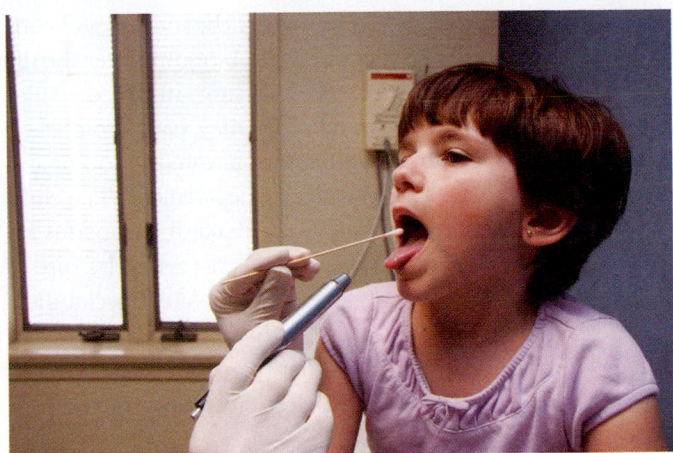

A

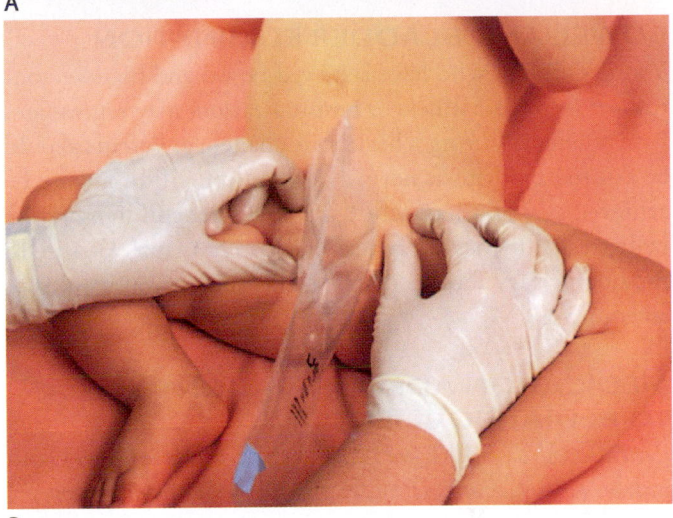

B

Figure 58-11. ■ **A.** Obtaining a throat culture. **B.** Attaching the urine collection bag for an infant or a child who is not toilet trained.

Urine and stool specimens can be difficult to collect with small children because of their lack of control. A PUC is a small plastic bag, which has a sticky surface and can be affixed to the child to collect the urine (see Figure 58-11B). Take care to remove it as soon as urine has been collected. By leaving the appliance in place after it contains urine, you are running the risk of losing or contaminating the specimen. Stool can be collected in a diaper and then transferred to a specimen container. Older children may be embarrassed, but may be able to collect the specimen themselves if an explanation is given. Obtaining a throat culture can elicit a gag reflex, which can result in vomiting. Take care not to damage the tissue of the oral pharynx. If vomiting occurs, guard against aspiration.

NUTRITIONAL SUPPORT

The pediatric client, just as the adult, will need adequate nutrition for healing and tissue repair. A breastfed infant should continue to receive mother's milk unless his or her condition contraindicates. The mother may pump and store milk that can be given in her absence or when the infant is able to take oral feedings. Pumping will ensure that the mother will continue to produce milk so that nursing can resume after the illness. Formula-fed infants may need a change in the particular formula. Clients 6 months and older may have established food preferences; obtain this information from the parent and convey the information to the dietary department. The child will be more likely to have adequate intake if the food is familiar. When a long-term special diet is necessary, be sure to include the child in the client teaching. (Note: Special diets are illustrated in Table 25-6 ⊕.) Even though the parent may need to manage the child's diet by making food choices, the child should be involved so that in time he or she can pick appropriate food for him/herself.

BOWEL AND BLADDER ELIMINATION

Young children who have achieved bowel and bladder control prior to their illness or hospitalization, may regress and have accidents during a healthcare challenge. Parents should be assured that this is normal and control will be able to be achieved again once the child is well. Older children may be embarrassed by having to use a bedpan or urinal. Be sure to provide privacy for a pediatric client just as you would for an adult.

MEDICATION ADMINISTRATION TO PEDIATRIC CLIENTS

Regardless of the healthcare setting, the nurse administering medications to the pediatric client must have a sound knowledge of:

- The medication(s) intended.
- Therapeutic effect(s).
- Side effects.
- Contraindications.
- Pharmacology calculations prior to administration.

Furthermore, it is vital for perioperative registered nurses caring for infants and children to be aware of the following age-dependent factors:

- Weight (in kilograms)
- Underlying pathology
- Physiologic differences
- Developmental stage
- Growth and development
- Psychosocial and cultural dynamics of the client's family

The shape of the ear canal, which is age dependent, determines how the nurse holds the tragus of the ear (the outer ear) for administration of otic medication (see Figure 58-9A and B).

Any or all of these factors may influence the efficacy and safety of medications used for pediatric clients. A nomogram (see Figure 27-4 ⊕) is often used in calculating pediatric doses by body surface area.

Administration of medications must also be done with consideration of the child's developmental level.

Infants

For infants, never mix medications with breast milk, formula, or essential nutrition, because the altered taste may cause the child to reject those in the future, complicating necessary intake. An oral syringe can be used to administer medication into the child's mouth to prevent loss of medication by spitting or drooling. Note that, to prevent choking, the syringe should be pointed toward the buccal cavity. IM injections should not be given into the gluteal muscles until the child has been walking for a year, since the muscle will not be developed enough for an injection site. The site of choice for IM injections in the infant is the vastus lateralis.

Toddlers and Preschoolers

For toddlers and preschoolers, administer oral medication in liquid form by syringe or cup. Gain cooperation by making a game out of the procedure. Again, do not mix unpleasant-tasting medication into essential foods because of the risk that the child will then reject the foods.

School-Age Children

Older children can be given the choice of liquid or tablets when administering oral medication. Allowing them to make the choice gives them a sense of control. Children as young as 6 years of age can be involved in administration of their own long-term drug therapy. For example, children with diabetes require medical management for the remainder of their lives, so teaching procedures as soon as they are able to understand will be very important.

Adolescents

Teens are capable of independence in self-administering numerous medications. However, it is important to monitor compliance, because peer pressure and wanting to "fit in" may incline teens to neglect medical regimens.

Hospitalized Child

Any hospitalization of a child can create a great deal of stress for the child, the parents, and even the siblings. Repeated or lengthy admissions of a child for chronic or terminal illness can have wider effects on extended family and friends. A child will respond to the hospitalization according to his or her developmental level. Thus, it is important to consider physical, cognitive, and psychosocial stages when caring for a child in the hospital.

The nurse ensures that the child's developmental and educational needs are met during the time that the child is in the hospital. The nurse may also be called on to interact with community professionals to arrange for post-discharge care. See Chapter 48 ⊕ for suggestions about collaboration between hospital staff and the home care or school nurse.

In a pediatric unit the child is the designated client (Figure 58-12 ■), but family-centered care must also be

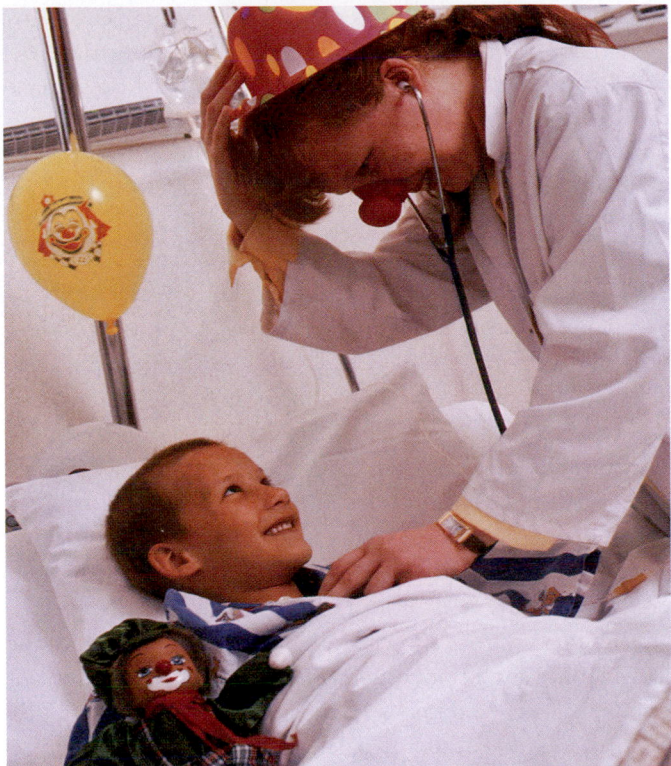

Figure 58-12. ■ Lively entertainment for a young child helps to ease the anxiety of hospitalization. *Source:* Getty Images Inc.—Image Bank.

provided. The child's illness has the potential for family stress. Time off from work, the cost of care, and arranging for care of other children are just a few things about which parents may be concerned while they are dealing with the stress of the illness or injury itself. Parents may also blame themselves for failure to recognize signs and symptoms earlier or to have prevented the child's injury. Parents respond to stress differently. Some will be quiet and cooperative, whereas others will be angry and seem dissatisfied with everything that is proposed or done. It is important for the nursing staff not to take criticism personally and continue to provide the best care for the child while remaining professional and supportive of family members.

MEETING THE DEVELOPMENTAL NEEDS OF THE PEDIATRIC CLIENT

Therapeutic Relationship

Hospitalization disrupts the child's lifestyle. Younger children do not have the cognitive development to understand why they are being hospitalized. They may exhibit regressive behaviors.

There are a number of stressors related to hospitalization that affect children of any age:

- Fear of pain or injury
- Fear of disfigurement
- Separation from parents, family, or peers
- Loss of control, privacy, and autonomy

Therapeutic relationships may be harder to establish with younger clients. As the nurse, it is your responsibility to meet the needs of the whole client. When the client is a child, a relationship must also be established with the parent. Your success in the relationship will depend on trust, caring, empathy, respect, genuineness, and concreteness.

The relationship needs to be client centered and goal directed. Take into consideration the client's developmental age when communicating therapeutically. Talk to the client rather than to the parents. Explain all treatments and procedures in terms the child can understand. Allow the child to ask questions and to express fears. Parents may require more information, but it is best to give that privately after the child has had an opportunity to get the information and support he or she needs.

Always maintain safety in the environment to protect the infant or child from injury. Transport infants in a crib, not in one's arms or on a bed without sides. Transport toddlers and active young preschoolers in a high-topped crib. Use restraints when needed for safety, both when transporting the child and when performing procedures. See Chapter 9 🔗 for the full discussion about safety issues.

INFANT.   At approximately 6 months of age the child develops self-awareness and realization of being an individual separate from parent. Once infants can identify their primary caregiver, they begin to feel anxious around strangers. Hospitalization can traumatize an infant, especially if a parent does not remain with the child. Behaviors related to stranger anxiety can be categorized into three responses. See Table 58-2 ■ for stages of separation anxiety.

Prior to the 1960s in many hospitals, a child who was admitted was taken from the parents in the admitting office,

TABLE 58-2	Stages of Separation Anxiety (6–18 Months)	
PROTEST	**DESPAIR**	**DENIAL (DETACHMENT)**
Screaming, crying, clinging to parent	Sadness	Lack of protest when parents leave
May resist attempts by other adults to comfort them	Quiet, appears to have "settled in"	Appearance of being happy and content with everyone
	Withdrawal or compliant behavior	Shows interest in surroundings
	Crying when parents return	Close relationships not established

Source: Adapted from Ball, J. W., and Bindler, R. C. (2008). *Pediatric nursing caring for children*, 4th ed. Upper Saddle River, NJ: Prentice Hall.

and parents were not allowed to visit. Research and study of normal development changed this practice.

Because parent–infant attachment is so critical to the infant's development, hospital staff should encourage a family member to remain with the child. Most pediatric units do not have visiting hour restrictions, so that family members may visit around the clock. Mothers who are breastfeeding infants are encouraged to continue. The unit will assist the nursing mother, provide her with a pump if necessary, and store breast milk for feedings when the mother cannot be there. Parents may be reluctant to hold an infant with wires and tubes attached for fear of hurting the baby or dislodging the equipment. The nurse should demonstrate the proper way to hold the child and encourage parents to do so.

TODDLER.   From 1 to 3 years of age, a child is at the greatest risk for stress related to hospitalization and illness. Toddlers know there has been a disruption of their routine, but they do not have the cognitive skills to understand why. If parents cannot remain constantly at the hospital, taped or video messages of the parents can be played for the child.

When the toddler is first admitted, the nurse should obtain as much information as possible about the child's routine, learn the child's likes and dislikes, and follow those that do not conflict with the plan of care. It is important to follow any established toileting schedule. Ask the parents what words they use. Be sure toddlers have their "blankie" or other comfort items for bedtime. Learn the names of their siblings and pets so that you can refer to them by name.

Autonomy (independent functioning) is an important developmental task for the toddler, so allowing them to make choices will help support this task. Be sure to offer only choices that they can make. Do not ask them if they want their medication, but allow them to choose pudding or ice cream as their snack.

PRESCHOOLER.   Fear of being alone is the greatest stressor for the preschool child, followed closely by the fear of loss of control. They may feel that the illness, injury, or hospitalization is because they misbehaved and are being punished. Preschool-aged children can cope with parents leaving the hospital for periods during the day, as long as they know when they will be returning. Telling a child that "Mommy will come back at 1 P.M." will not have as much meaning as "Mommy will come back after lunch" or after a particular TV program. Phone calls from the parent during the day are also a source of comfort for a child this age. It is important for the parent to tell the child when and why they are leaving (e.g., "I am going to work for a while. I will be back after lunch and will stay until Daddy comes from work"). The parent should not leave when the child is sleeping. It will cause the child to be anxious if he or she awakes and finds the parent is gone.

The preschool child's developmental task to be accomplished during this time period is initiative. Hospitalization may result in regression of behavior. A child may have a toileting accident or may begin to suck his or her thumb again. Staff and parents should not scold the child for these behaviors, knowing that they will resolve when the child is well.

SCHOOL-AGE CHILD.   For a child between the ages of 6 and 12, major stressors during hospitalization are privacy, loss of control related to body functions, pain, injury, and concerns about death. A sense of industry is the developmental milestone of this stage. The staff can assist school-age children by allowing them to participate in their own care. Children of this age who have been diagnosed with diabetes can be taught to do their own glucose monitoring and diet. As they progress, they will learn to draw up their insulin and give their own injections.

School-age children need to be given opportunities for creative activities, such as arts and crafts. They should also be encouraged to continue their schoolwork. Children of this age like to try unsafe activities and try to "trick" the nurses, such as by switching beds with their roommate or racing wheelchairs in the halls. The nurse is responsible for providing a safe environment for the child. Identifying the child before medications or treatments is of utmost importance. When children are taking part in unsafe activities, redirect them instead of reprimanding them.

ADOLESCENT.   Hospitalization of an adolescent can be very stressful, especially separation from peers, home, and school. Adolescents may express fears of pain, injury, changes in body image, disability, and even death. It is normal to have a preoccupation with appearance at this age.

It is important not to treat adolescents like children while hospitalized. If they have been admitted to a unit with younger children, they should not share a room with a young child if at all possible. Unless there is a need to restrict visitors, their peers should be encouraged to visit. Clients of this age should be included in all discussions of diagnosis, treatment, and prognosis. By providing them with information about their condition and what to expect, you will make it easier to gain their cooperation in following the plan of care.

Adolescents have the cognitive skills to understand client teaching, and with proper teaching they can be responsible for many aspects of their care. The staff should do everything possible to protect the adolescent's self-esteem while hospitalized; this is of utmost importance in helping them to accomplish developmental goals of this age. Clients of this age need good role models. Many adolescents who have had personal experience with serious illness go on to pursue a career in health care.

Teaching Strategies with Pediatric Clients

Teaching is one of the most important nursing tasks. As hospital stays become shorter the client and the parents must become competent in post-discharge care. Teaching must be conducted at a developmentally appropriate level. Provide **anticipatory guidance** to parents (information that helps parents prepare for expected physical and behavioral changes during their child's or teen's current and approaching stage of development). A parent will be better prepared to care for the child at home when the staff is able to anticipate questions and provide the information prior to discharge. As with all clients, discharge planning/teaching begins on the first day of hospitalization; this will give the child and family members adequate time to understand and develop necessary skills to provide home care. Refer to Chapter 12 ⌘ for additional information on client teaching.

The child of 18 months to 2 years can be included in simple health teaching. The child can be allowed to manipulate equipment, and treatments and procedures can be demonstrated on a doll or stuffed animal.

Preschool children respond well to stories and picture books to explain what will be done. Puppets can also be used to keep their interest while explaining health teaching.

School-age children are really interested in computer and video games; these can be used to provide children with information. The information can be reinforced while playing the games.

Adolescent clients have the cognitive skills to understand client teaching as an adult would, although they will probably have a lot of questions. Sometimes a discussion of the information with other clients their own age may be helpful. Since peers are so important, knowing that there are other teens who are dealing with the same problems will help them cope with the diagnosis and treatment.

Adolescents who have a chronic health condition may find it helpful for their close friends to participate in the teaching with them. This gives the nurse an opportunity to explain to the friends what challenges the client must face, and also to address questions and fears they may have about their friend returning to school and regular activities.

Parent interaction with staff frequently has an affect on the ability to give care.

Culture and family systems are important to consider when treating a child. Refer to Chapter 3 ⌘ for cultural

information and Chapter 16 for lifespan development and family systems.

Terminally Ill Pediatric Clients

PHYSICAL NEEDS

Nursing care to meet the physical needs of the terminally ill child is aimed at providing as much comfort as possible. The change in philosophy from curing to caring means providing comfort to the child with the least invasive procedures, while maintaining the child's privacy and dignity. A terminally ill child has many of the same needs as any seriously ill child, including the following:

- *Routine for sleep and rest.* Lack of sleep may be caused by the number of things such as visitors, discomfort, fear of not waking up, restlessness, or day/night confusion. Keep a night light on and/or a bell or intercom available so the child will know where he/she is if awakened and confused. A clock is also helpful for older children who can tell time to help them orient themselves. The child should have the ability to call on someone, if needed. The presence of a parent can help the child rest and fall asleep (Figure 58-13 ■).
- *Nutritional considerations.* Nutritional considerations for the dying child may be difficult to address. Nausea, vomiting, diarrhea, and reduced eating are often associated with the effects of treatment and the progression of the disease. High-protein shakes may be an option if the child is only able to eat or drink small amounts. A nasogastric or gastric tube is another option for supplemental nutrition.
- *Changes in elimination.* Changes in elimination may also occur with a seriously ill or dying child. Diarrhea, constipation, and incontinence are all possible. Care should be given to provide the child with a clean environment. It is also important not to embarrass or humiliate a child that has recently become incontinent.
- *Skin care.* Skin care may also be a concern for the dying child. Nutritional status, elimination problems, and immobility

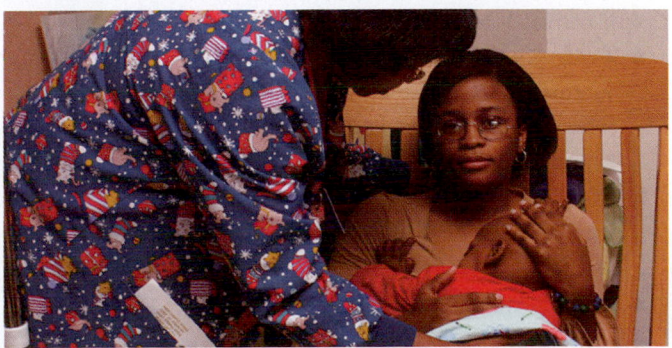

Figure 58-13. ■ Parent's presence helps the child rest and go to sleep.

can all cause skin breakdown and/or pain. Infection may likely occur in this situation.

- *Respiratory changes.* Respiratory changes may occur from pneumonia, the effects of narcotics, or the progression of the disease. Often, children will feel they are unable to "catch their breath." Air hunger, as this is often called, can be frightening. Oxygen supplied through the nose or by a mask may be needed simply for comfort. Sometimes medications can also lower anxiety related to breathing difficulties.

- *Nasal symptoms.* Secretions from the nose, mouth, and throat may be difficult to manage with a terminally ill child. Suction may be necessary, or simply repositioning the child may help drain the excess secretions.

- *Pain management.* Pain management is an important concern in the dying child. With a child who is dying, one of the greatest fears is pain. Every measure should be taken to eliminate pain from the dying process. The ultimate goal is comfort, which means taking appropriate measures to ensure that the child is free from pain. There is no evidence of addiction to pain medications in dying children.

There are many types of drugs and several methods used in administering pharmacological pain management. Pain medication is usually given by one of the following routes:

- Oral
- Intravenous
- Epidural
- Transdermal (a patch on the skin)

Some children build up a tolerance to sedatives and pain relievers. Over time, doses may need to be increased, or the choice of medications may need to be changed.

Nonpharmacological pain management uses ways to alter thinking and focus to decrease pain. Methods include the following:

- *Psychological preparation.* The unexpected is always worse because of what one imagines. If children are prepared and can anticipate what will happen to them, their stress level will be much lower. Ways to accomplish this include:
  - Explaining each step of a procedure in detail, using simple pictures or diagrams when available. Child life specialists, who are experts in child development, can help parents prepare children for medical procedures or treatments.
  - Meeting with the person who will perform the procedure and allowing the child to ask questions ahead of time.
  - Touring the room where the procedure will take place.
  - Watching videotapes that describe the procedure (adolescents); "playing" the procedure or observing a demonstration on a doll (small children); looking at a photo book of a particular procedure or treatment.

- *Hypnosis.* With hypnosis, a professional (such as a psychologist or physician) guides the child into an altered state of consciousness that helps him or her to focus or narrow attention, in order to reduce discomfort.

- *Imagery.* Guiding a child through an imaginary mental image of sights, sounds, tastes, smells, and feelings can often help shift attention away from the pain. By creating images in the mind, a person can reduce pain and symptoms associated with a condition. Guided imagery involves envisioning a certain goal to help cope with health problems.

- *Prayer or meditation.* In many faith traditions, one of the roles of prayer or meditation is to help with pain, fears, and uncertainty.

- *Distraction.* Distraction can be helpful particularly for babies, by using colorful, moving objects. Singing songs, telling stories, or looking at books or videos can distract preschoolers. Older children find watching TV or listening to music helpful. Distraction should not be a substitute for explaining what to expect.

- *Relaxation.* Children can be guided through relaxation exercises, such as deep breathing and stretching, to reduce discomfort.

Each child experiences pain differently. It is important to discover the best method for pain control for each child prior to the onset of pain, and to give the child permission to use many varied resources in the treatment of his or her pain.

PSYCHOSOCIAL NEEDS

The way a child reacts to terminal illness depends on his or her developmental level. It is necessary for the nurse to have an understanding of these levels. Refer to Chapters 15 and 16 ⊙⊙ for a discussion of developmental stages.

It is important to take the lead from the child. Do not overburden children with details that they are not ready to absorb. Listen to what children are saying and what they are not saying. When they ask questions, it is best to reply with a statement such as, "What have you been told about your illness?" From there, you can provide information that the child wants and needs.

Sit down with the child and provide a quiet, private environment. Do not rush the child. It may take considerable time before children are comfortable in talking about their feelings. See Chapter 17 ⊙⊙ for suggestions for meeting the psychosocial needs of the chronically or terminally ill child.

Family Support

When providing treatment for an ill child, the entire family may need care. One of the most difficult tasks a parent faces is explaining long-term illness to the child. Honest communication is crucial to helping a child adjust to a serious medical condition. It's important for a child to know that he or she is sick and will be getting lots of medicine.

The hospital and the medicine may feel frightening to the child, but they are part of what it takes to help the child feel better.

As the parents are explaining the illness and the treatment to their child, it is important to clearly and honestly answer the child's questions, and provide the information that he or she will need to know in a way he or she will understand and can respond. The aim is not to frighten the child, but to give the child the words to communicate information and concerns to medical professionals and others.

The parents may seek assistance from the physician or the nurses in providing the explanation to the child. The parents and the professionals may meet and discuss what will be said, so that the child will not be confused by different explanations. Many hospitals offer parents the choice of talking to their child about a long-term diagnosis alone, addressing the child with the doctor present, or including the entire medical team of doctors, social workers, and nurses. The doctor or other medical professional may also be able to give the parents some advice on how to talk to the child about the illness.

It is imperative to maintain the child's trust. It is also important to explain accurately and prepare the child for any treatments and possible discomfort that might go along with those treatments. Avoid saying "This won't hurt" if the procedure is likely to be painful. Instead, tell the child that the procedure may cause some discomfort, pain, pressure, or stinging, but that it will be temporary and that you will be there to support him or her while or after the procedure is done.

Tackling Tough Emotions

Children have many feelings about the changes affecting their bodies and they should be encouraged and given opportunities to express any feelings, concerns, and fears. It is a good idea to ask them what they are experiencing and listen to everything they have to say before responding or giving explanations.

Communication does not always have to be verbal. Music, drawing, or writing can often help a child living with a life-threatening disease to express his or her emotions and to escape through a fantasy world of his or her own design. Review therapeutic methods of communication in Chapter 11 ⚭ .

The child may also need reminders that he or she is not responsible for the illness. It is common for children to fear that they brought their sickness on by something they thought, said, or did. It is important to reassure the child that this is not the case, and to explain, in terms that he or she can understand, what caused the illness. (You may also want to reassure the child's siblings that nothing they said or did caused the child's illness.)

For many questions that children ask, there will not be easy answers. The nurse should not promise that everything is going to be fine. The nurse should simply listen to the children's feelings, tell them it is completely understandable to have those feelings, and assure them that the staff and his or her family are going to make things as comfortable as possible.

If a child asks "Why me?" it's okay to be honest, even if the answer is, "I don't know." It is a good idea to follow this up by explaining that even though it is unknown why the illness occurred, the doctors do have treatment for it. (If that is the case.) The child may say, "It's not fair that I'm sick." Acknowledge that the child is right, that it is not fair. It is important for the child to feel that it is all right to be angry about the illness.

The child may ask, "Am I going to die?" How you answer is going to depend on the child's age and maturity level and any expressed wishes of the parents. It is important to discern, if possible, what specific fears or concerns the child may be having, and to address those concerns specifically. For example, the child may be actually worried about being in pain. Myths and realities about children and grief are discussed in Chapter 18 ⚭ .

If it is reassuring to the child, you may refer to religious, spiritual, and cultural beliefs about death. You may want to stay away from euphemisms for death such as "going to sleep." Saying things like that may cause the child and siblings to fear going to sleep. Regardless of age, children need to know that there are going to be people who love them and who will be there for as long as they are needed, and that the child will be kept comfortable.

Just like adults, children will need time to adjust to the diagnosis and the physical changes they may experience. It is likely that the child is going to feel sad, depressed, angry, afraid, or even denial. It is a good idea to think about getting some professional counseling help if you see signs that these feelings are starting to interfere with the child's ability to function, and the child begins to seem withdrawn, depressed, and show radical changes in eating and sleeping habits that aren't related to the child's physical illness.

Chronically Ill Pediatric Clients

Pediatric chronic illnesses are frequently managed by the primary care provider and the school nurse. There may be times when a child with chronic illness is hospitalized because of an exacerbation of the illness or for an unrelated illness or injury. Many pediatric clients with chronic illness have been taught to manage their illness with varying degrees of independence. This should be continued when hospitalized if at all possible.

The amount of information and independence of care for the chronic condition will depend on the developmental age of the child. As with a child with terminal illness, it is important to be honest and to maintain open communication.

CHILDHOOD BEHAVIOR

Although kids with chronic illnesses certainly require extra "TLC," special medical requirements do not eliminate the routine needs of childhood. The foremost—and perhaps trickiest—task for worried parents is to treat a sick child as normally as possible. Despite the circumstances, this means setting limits on unacceptable behavior, sticking to a regular routine, and avoiding overindulgence. This may seem impossible, particularly if the parent is experiencing feelings of guilt or an intense need to protect the sick child. However, spoiling or coddling children can only make it harder for them to readjust once they are ready to return to daily activities.

When the child leaves the hospital for home, normalcy remains the goal. The child may want to visit or stay in touch with friends through visits, if possible, or through e-mail, telephone, or letters.

DEALING WITH SIBLINGS

Family dynamics can be severely tested when a child is sick. Clinic visits, surgical procedures, and frequent checkups can place a real strain on family schedules, and take an emotional toll on the entire family. To ease these pressures, encourage the family to reach out for any help they can get to keep the family routine as close to normal as possible. Friends and family members may be able to help handle errands, carpools, and meals. Siblings should continue to attend school and their usual recreational activities; the family should attempt to provide some predictability and time for everyone to be together.

Remind the parents that flexibility is key. The old "normal" may have been the entire family around the table for a home-cooked meal at 6 P.M., but the new "normal" may be take-out pizza on clinic nights.

Also, a parent may want to talk with the other kids' teachers or school counselors and let them know that a sibling in the family is ill. Those school personnel may be able to keep a look out for any behavioral changes or signs of stress among the children. Classmates of the ill child should be given some basic information about the child's condition. The amount of information given depends on the age of the children and the comfort level of the family. The parent and/or the school nurse can go into the classroom and explain what is going on with the child. It is important to let the children know that they cannot "catch" the illness if they play with the child. Giving the classmates a chance to ask questions and understand the child's condition can control or prevent teasing of the ill child.

It is common for siblings of a chronically ill child to become angry, sullen, resentful, fearful, or withdrawn. They may pick fights or fall behind in schoolwork. In all cases, parents should pay close attention, so that the siblings don't feel shunted aside by the demands of the sick child.

It may also help the sick child's siblings to be included in the treatment process whenever possible. Depending on their ages and maturity level, visiting the hospital, meeting the nursing and physician staffs, or accompanying their sick sibling to the clinic for treatments can also help make the situation less frightening and more understandable.

What they imagine about the illness and hospital visits is often a lot worse than the reality. When they come to the hospital, hopefully they'll develop a more realistic picture and see that, while unpleasant things may be part of the treatment, there are also people who care about their sibling and try to minimize discomfort.

Encourage the parents to take care of themselves so that they will be able to continue to care for the ill child as well as other children. Box 58-2 ■ provides suggestions for parents caring for ill children.

BOX 58-2   CLIENT TEACHING

Lightening the Load

Although no magic potion exists to reduce the stress involved in caring for a child with a long-term illness, there are ways to ease the strain. Teach parents and caregivers the following ways of handling problems:

- Break problems into manageable parts. If your child's treatment is expected to be given over an extended time, view it in more manageable time blocks. Planning a week or a month at a time may be less overwhelming.
- Attend to your own needs. Get appropriate rest and food. To the extent possible, pay attention to your relationship with your spouse, hobbies, and friendships.
- Depend on friends. Let them carpool siblings to soccer or theater practice. Permit others—relatives, friends—to share responsibilities of caring for your child. Remember that you can't do it all.
- Ask for help in managing the financial implications of your child's illness.
- Recognize that everyone handles stress differently. If you and your spouse have distinct worrying styles, talk about them and try to accommodate them. Don't pretend that they don't exist.
- Develop collaborative working relationships with healthcare professionals. Realize you are all part of the team. Ask questions and learn all you can about your child's illness.
- Consult other parents in support groups at your care center or hospital. They can offer information and understanding.
- Explore support groups for parents who have children with the same or similar illness.
- Keep a journal.
- Utilize support staff offered at the treating hospital.

Pediatric Clients with Developmental and Cognitive Issues

Children who are experiencing developmental or cognitive issues can present a challenge for the nurse who is providing care. It is important for the LPN/LVN to have an understanding of normal development and cognitive functioning so that deficits are recognized and adaptations and modifications can be made. See Chapter 16 ⬯ for basic coverage of lifespan development.

DEVELOPMENTAL ASSESSMENT

There are a number of assessment tools that can be used by a nurse to accurately evaluate a child's development. The Denver Developmental Screening Test II can be used for apparently well children from birth to 6 years. The DDST II is the most commonly used. Figure 58-14 ■ provides an example of the scoring sheet and directions. The DDST II is not an intelligence test. The test contains 125 task items, which look at four areas.

- *Personal-Social:* getting along with people and caring for personal needs
- *Fine Motor-Adaptive:* Eye–hand coordination, manipulation of small objects and problem solving
- *Language:* hearing, understanding, and using language
- *Gross Motor:* sitting, walking, jumping, and overall muscle movement

The test provides an organized, clinical impression of a child's overall development. It will alert the tester to the potential for developmental difficulties as well as provide comparison with other children. The test is not an accurate predictor of later development.

Since only about 20% of primary care providers screen children for developmental delays, many children are not diagnosed until they enter preschool or kindergarten. Parent-completed developmental screening questionnaires have been gaining more support. Parent concerns about speech and language and fine motor or global functioning accurately predicted developmental problems with a sensitivity approaching that of a physician-completed screening test, although parental worries, such as in self-help or daily living skills and social and gross motor, were a less sensitive predictor (Rydz et al., 2005). Table 58-3 ■ lists other commonly used screening tests.

PROGRAMS AND SERVICES

In 1975 the U.S. Congress passed PL 94-142 Education for All Handicapped Children Act, now known as IDEA (Individuals with Disabilities Education Act). To receive federal funds, states must develop and implement polices that ensure a free, appropriate public education for all children (ages 3–22 years) with disabilities.

There are numerous support and advocacy groups as well as public organizations that provide programs and services for individuals with developmental and cognitive issues. The nurse working with children should become familiar with some of the organizations in order to refer families in need of support or service. There are general organizations such as The Arc (formerly the Association for Retarded Citizens) or specific organizations such as Cerebral Palsy or Autism Speaks.

As institutional services decrease in 49 of the 50 states, community services are increasing. The change to community service (called **mainstreaming**) has been done to provide the developmentally disabled with the least restrictive environment, which is a federal mandate. Each state or community provides services under a variety of names. Some states have Crippled Children Services; others have replaced the word *crippled* with their state name, since children without classical crippling conditions are eligible for services.

The disabled may be provided with therapy services, as well as specialized training and equipment. Many disabled individuals also qualify for SSI (Supplemental Security Income) from the federal government.

Normalization

Normalization of a child with special needs means:

- Expecting behavior as normal as possible from birth on.
- Using discipline and child management techniques as for any other child.
- Exposing the child to other children and encouraging the child to socialize as normally as possible from infancy on.
- Treating the child as any other child would be treated, allowing for development of the child's self-esteem.
- Exposing the child to life and all activities of the world in the same way as any other child would be exposed.
- Exposing the child to an inclusive school environment when the child would be challenged to develop as normal a language, behavior pattern, and personality as possible.
- Discouraging handicapped behavioral patterns.
- Encouraging the child to participate in typical and able-bodied community activities and programs as much as possible.
- Making the child accept personal responsibility for his or her own actions.
- Encouraging the child to become as self-sufficient as possible.
- Encouraging the child to reach for the highest level of functioning possible.
- Helping the child to recognize personal deficiencies, but not to use them as an excuse for lack of progress.

(Text continues on p. 1618.)

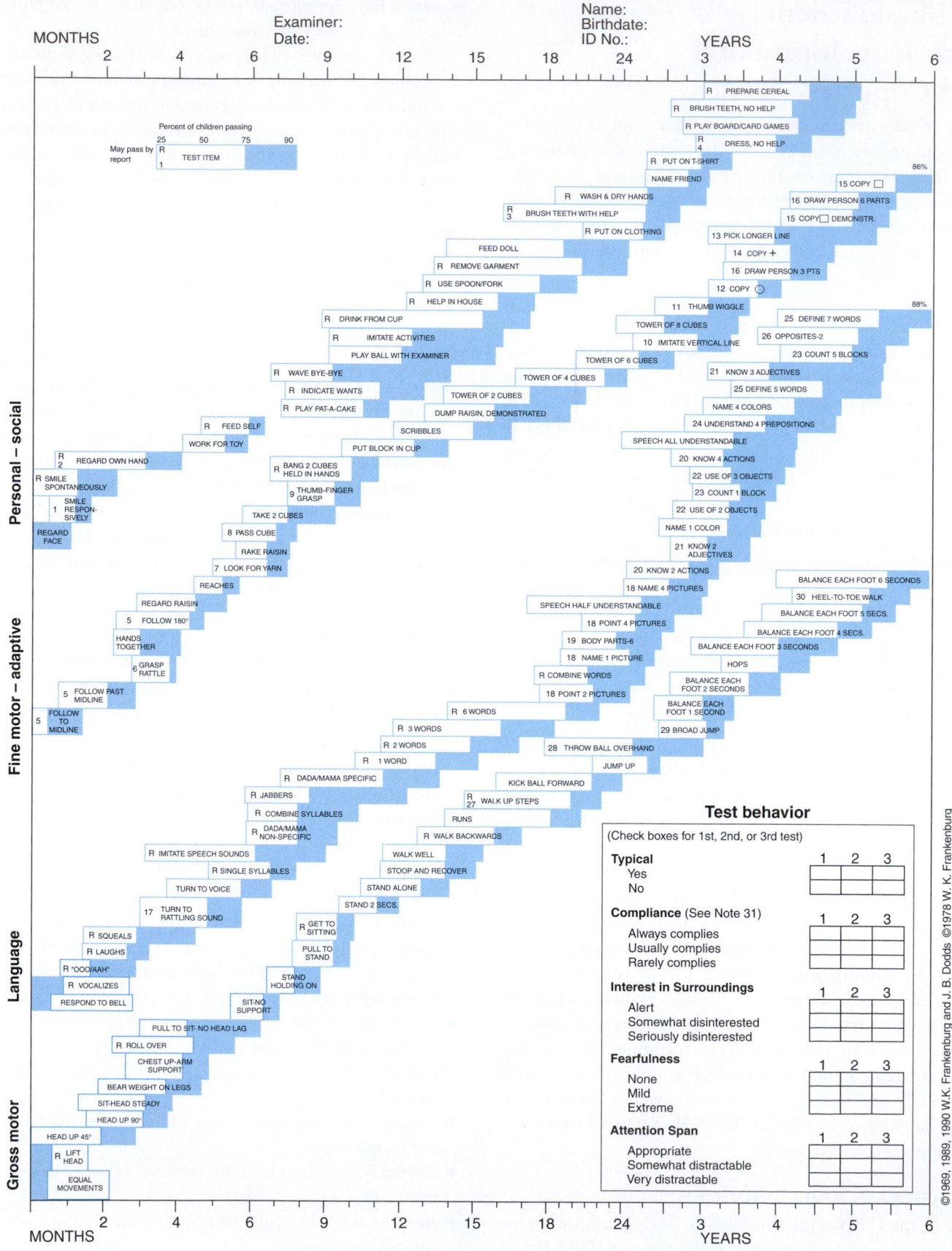

Figure 58-14. ■ The scoring portion of a Denver Developmental Screening Test II.

DIRECTIONS FOR ADMINISTRATION

1. Try to get child to smile by smiling, talking or waving. Do not touch him/her.
2. Child must stare at hand several seconds.
3. Parent may help guide toothbrush and put toothpaste on brush.
4. Child does not have to be able to tie shoes or button/zip in the back.
5. Move yarn slowly in an arc from one side to the other, about 8" above child's face.
6. Pass if child grasps rattle when it is touched to the backs or tips of fingers.
7. Pass if child tries to see where yarn went. Yarn should be dropped quickly from sight from tester's hand without arm movement.
8. Child must transfer cube from hand to hand without help of body, mouth, or table.
9. Pass if child picks up raisin with any part of thumb and finger.
10. Line can vary only 30 degrees or less from tester's line.
11. Make a fist with thumb pointing upward and wiggle only the thumb. Pass if child imitates and does not move any fingers other than the thumb.

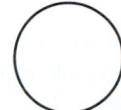 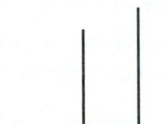 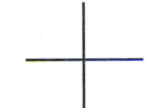 

12. Pass any enclosed form. Fail continuous round motions.
13. Which line is longer? (Not bigger.) Turn paper upside down and repeat. (pass 3 of 3 or 5 of 6).
14. Pass any lines crossing near midpoint.
15. Have child copy first. If failed, demonstrate.

When giving items 12, 14, and 15, do not name the forms. Do not demonstrate 12 and 14.

16. When scoring, each pair (2 arms, 2 legs, etc.) counts as one part.
17. Place one cube in cup and shake gently near child's ear, but out of sight. Repeat for other ear.
18. Point to picture and have child name it. (No credit is given for sounds only.) If less than 4 pictures are named correctly, have child point to picture as each is named by tester.

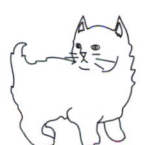 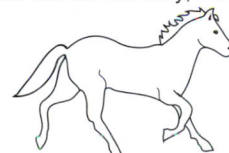 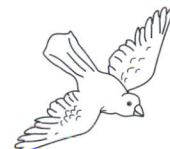 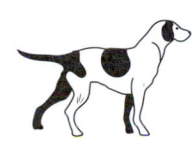 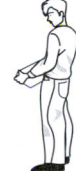

19. Using doll, tell child: Show me the nose, eyes, ears, mouth, hands, feet, tummy, hair. Pass 6 of 8.
20. Using pictures, ask child: Which one flies?... says meow?... talks?... barks?... gallops? Pass 2 of 5, 4 of 5.
21. Ask child: What do you do when you are cold?... tired?... hungry? Pass 2 of 3, 3 of 3.
22. Ask child: What do you do with a cup? What is a chair used for? What is a pencil used for? Action words must be included in answers.
23. Pass if child correctly places <u>and</u> says how many blocks are on paper (1, 5).
24. Tell child: Put block **on** table, **under** table, **in front of** me, **behind** me. Pass 4 of 4. (Do not help child by pointing, moving head or eyes.)
25. Ask child: What is a ball?... lake?... desk?... house?... banana?... curtain?... fence?... ceiling? Pass if defined in terms of use, shape, what it is made of, or general category (such as banana is fruit, not just yellow). Pass 5 of 8, 7 of 8.
26. Ask child: If a horse is big, a mouse is_____? If fire is hot, ice is_____? If sun shines during the day, the moon shines during the ____? Pass 2 of 3.
27. Child may use wall or rail only, not person. May not crawl.
28. Child must throw ball overhand 3 feet to within arm's reach of tester.
29. Child must perform standing broad jump over width of test sheet (8 1/2 inches).
30. Tell child to walk forward, ⚬⚬⚬⚬ ➔ heel within 1 inch of toe. Tester may demonstrate. Child must walk 4 consecutive steps.
31. In the second year, half of normal children are non-compliant.

OBSERVATIONS:

Figure 58-14. ■ *Continued.*

TABLE 58-3	Other Commonly Used Developmental Screening Tests	
TEST	**AGES OF USE**	**USE**
Bayley Infant Neurodevelopmental Screener	3–24 mo	Basic neurologic; expressive, receptive, and cognitive functions
The Early Screening Inventory	4–6 yrs	General development; focuses on the child's ability to learn rather than what the child already knows
The First STEP (Screening Test for Evaluating Preschoolers)	33–74 mo	Tests five domains—cognitive, communication, physical functioning, emotional, and social status
Peabody Picture Vocabulary Test	2.5–90+ yrs	Assesses verbal ability and receptive vocabulary attainment
The Toddler and Infant Motor Evaluation	4–42 mo	Measures qualitative aspects of movement, mobility, motor organization, stability, functional performance, and social and emotional abilities
Vineland Adaptive Behavior Scale	N/A	Assesses personal and social sufficiency of individuals with or without disabilities in the areas of communication, daily living skills, socialization, and motor skills

- Considering the child's mental health as important as physical and intellectual development.
- Considering the child's siblings' and parents' well-being, and physical and emotional health in planning treatment, services, and programs for the child.
- Keeping in mind the child's future in planning for preschool, elementary, and secondary school.
- Working as a unit toward self-sufficiency and autonomy for a child's adult years.

Family Support

The birth of a child with disabilities can be very difficult on the parents, siblings, and extended family. For many, there is a grieving process that must be worked through; the loss of the "perfect" child or the ideal life will require both internal and external coping skills in order to come through the process and grow through it. An unfortunate result of a family dealing with a disabled member many times is a family break-up or acting out from siblings. The nurse should become acquainted with warning signs of acute family stress, so that needed support and respite can be made available to a family in crisis. One of the first warning signs may be a family member's discontent with the treatment plans or the care being given. Another may be blaming a spouse or other family member for something that is beyond human control. When the LPN/LVN observes these or other signs of inability to cope, he or she should discuss the observations with the RN or the physician so that they can provide needed support and help the family to develop appropriate coping skills.

Many times the care of the disabled family member along with normal day-to-day responsibilities becomes too much. A few hours or days away from the situation can make a marked improvement. Many agencies will provide respite care for the special needs of family members so that the primary caretakers can have time away to regroup. Frequently a listening ear is all that family members need. They don't want advice or even solutions, just a safe person and place to vent.

Identifying Disorders of Pediatric Clients by Age

The disease process and nursing care for common pediatric medical-surgical conditions can vary with the age of the client. The most common conditions and diseases will be covered in subsequent chapters.

Table 58-4 ■ shows where in this Pediatric Unit a disorder is discussed. Common age of onset was used as a means of deciding how to place content about different disorders. *Note:* Congenital disorders have been covered in Chapter 57 ∞, although later treatment such as surgery will appear in the age-appropriate chapter.

NURSING PROCESS CARE PLAN
Terminally Ill Pediatric Client

Emma Anne Fulton is a 14-year-old ninth-grader who has been hospitalized for recurrent acute lymphoblastic leukemia (ALL). She received a bone marrow transplant when she was 5 and has been doing well since that time. She is a friendly child who is pleased to see all "her nurses" from previous hospitalizations. Her parents are anxious and do not want her to know that her condition is life threatening. She is scheduled for a cycle of vincristine and methotrexate. Emma is assigned to nursing team B, which consists of a chemo nurse, an RN team leader, and an LPN to provide direct care. The mother requests a cot for the room so that she can remain with her daughter.

TABLE 58-4	Placement of Pediatric Conditions in Pediatrics Unit			
ILLNESS/DISORDER	**CHAPTER 59**	**CHAPTER 60**	**CHAPTER 61**	**CHAPTER 62**
Congenital Anomalies				
Heart defects	X			
Cleft lip/palate	X			
Clubfoot	X			
Dislocated hip	X			
Injuries				
Airway obstruction (foreign body)	X			
Burns, sunburn, frostbite, tanning		X		X
Drowning		X		
Head injury, brain trauma	X	X		X
Epistaxis		X		
Shaken baby	X			
Fracture, sprain, strain	X	X		
Poisoning		X		
Infections/Inflammations				
Allergies	X			
Bites (insect)	X (table)	X		
Chicken pox, measles, mumps, pertussis		X (table)		
Parasites		X		
STI, vaginitis, yeast, cytomegalovirus			X	X
Respiratory System				
Asthma		X	X	
Bronchopulmonary dysplasia	X			
Cystic fibrosis	X			
Bronchiolitis, croup, epiglottis, laryngitis	X			
Respiratory syneytial virus, whooping cough	X			
Pneumonia		X		
SIDS	X			
Tonsillitis, tonsillectomy		X		
Cardiovascular/Hematologic/Immune Systems				
Anemias (iron-deficiency, sickle cell, thalassemia)	X		X	
Bleeding disorders (hemophilia, idiopathic thrombocytopenia)	X	X		
Congestive heart failure (CHF)	X			
HIV and AIDS	X			
Hodgkin's lymphoma, leukemia				X
Hypertension				X
Juvenile rheumatoid arthritis	X		X	
Kawasaki's syndrome		X		
Nervous/Sensory System				
Brain tumors, brain trauma	X	X	X	X
Cerebral palsy	X			
Ear (deafness and implants, foreign body, otitis media)	X			
Eye (blindness, cataract, conjunctivitis, foreign body, sty, glaucoma, retinoblastoma)	X	X	X	
Guillain-Barré		X		
Meningitis	X			X

(continued)

TABLE 58-4	Placement of Pediatric Conditions in Pediatrics Unit (continued)			
ILLNESS/DISORDER	CHAPTER 59	CHAPTER 60	CHAPTER 61	CHAPTER 62
Nervous/Sensory System				
Mental retardation, Down syndrome	X			
Migraine, headache			X	X
Reye's syndrome	X			
Seizures		X		
Musculoskeletal System				
Developemental dysplasia of the hip, clubfoot	X			
Legg-Calvé-Perthes disease		X		
Muscular dystrophy		X		
Scoliosis			X	
Tumors			X	
Gastrointestinal System				
Appendicitis			X	
GI upset (colic, GERD vomiting, diarrhea and dehydration, constipation)	X			
Biliary atresia	X			
Crohn's, ulcerative colitis				X
Malabsorption disorders (celiac disease/sprue, galactosemia, etc.)	X			
Failure to thrive	X			
Metabolic X				X
Hernia	X	X		
Hepatitis		X		X
Structural disorders (Hirschsprung's disease, intussusception, Meckel's diverticulum, pyloric stenosis)	X			
Ulcers, stress		X		
Gastric enteritis		X		
Obesity		X		
Endocrine System				
Diabetes			X	X
Pituitary imbalances	X	X		
Thyroid imbalances				X
Urinary (Renal) System				
Glomerulonephritis		X		
Nephrotic syndrome, UTI	X	X		
Obstructive uropathy	X			
Renal failure			X	
Tumor (Wilms')	X			
Reproductive System				
Neonatal conditions (phimosis, cryptorchidism)	X			
Puberty (precocious puberty, PMS)			X	X
Ovarian disorders				X
Testicular torsion				X
Integumentary System				
Acne				X
Cellulitis, MRSA			X	
Dermatitis	X			
Impetigo		X		

TABLE 58-4	Placement of Pediatric Conditions in Pediatrics Unit (continued)				
ILLNESS/DISORDER		**CHAPTER 59**	**CHAPTER 60**	**CHAPTER 61**	**CHAPTER 62**
Psychosocial Disorders					
ADHD				X	
Anxiety (stranger, separation, school)		X		X	
Autism		X	X		
Dyslexia				X	
Depression					X
Down syndrome, mental retardation			X		
Eating disorders					X
Substance abuse					X
Self-injury, suicide					X

Assessment

VS: T 101.6, P 76, R 26, BP 98/60. Pulse ox 92% on room air. Skin warm and dry to touch with noticeable pallor; complaining of sores in her mouth and bleeding from gum. Mother is answering questions for client and asked to speak with the nurse outside.

Nursing Diagnosis

The following important nursing diagnoses (among others) are established for this client:

- *Risk for Caregiver Role Strain* related to unrealistic expectations of self
- *Risk for Complicated Grieving*

Expected Outcomes

The expected outcomes will include, but are not limited to, the following:

- Family receives adequate support to care for client at home or support for client's death with dignity.
- Family and client will communicate openly about present status and prognosis.

Planning and Implementation

The following nursing interventions are implemented for Emma Anne:

- Direct questions to client during all nurse–client interactions.
- Encourage mother to take brief respite periods for self-care.
- Discuss participation in support groups, peer group for client, parent groups for parents.
- Facilitate open communication between client, mother, and healthcare professionals.

Evaluation

Emma attended peer group and expresses that she would like to speak with her parents about her prognosis. Mother has not left hospital in 3 days, she is not eating or sleeping. Emma expresses concern about her mother and asks to speak with the social worker.

Critical Thinking in the Nursing Process

1. When you were given your orientation to the pediatric oncology unit, you were told that "The child is the designated client but the entire family becomes your client many times." How does this statement affect the way you provide care?
2. When Emma returns from the peer support group, she asks you if she is going to die. How would respond to this question?
3. Emma is not responding well to treatment. Her white cells are continuing to rise and she is unable to eat because her mouth is sore and bleeding. She asks her mother to tell the doctor to stop treatment. Mother refuses, saying she needs it to get better. How can the team support Mrs. Fulton while honoring Emma's request?

Note: Discussion of Critical Thinking questions appears on the MyNursingKit Website.

Note: The references and resources for all chapters have been compiled at the back of the book.

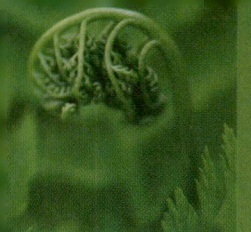

Chapter Review

KEY Points

- Children differ from adults in more than size. They are not only growing, but also developing, in ways that are predictable, yet individualized. Each system develops as early as conception until adolescence.

- Knowledge of developmental levels helps determine the best approach. The assessment done is similar in content to an adult, but the order of data collection and the methods used may be different.

- Behavioral signs help in assessing pain in children; however, there are also scales designed to help elicit information directly from the pediatric client.

- Nursing care for children should take into account the age and developmental level, the possibility that the child may have regressed as a result of being ill, and the fact that familiarity is important to children. Sound medication administration is particularly important for pediatric clients.

- Children and their families will be especially anxious when hospitalization is necessary. It is important to address the family's psychosocial needs, in addition to the child's fears.

- Client teaching becomes more important as hospital stays are becoming shorter. Include children in the learning to the degree that they are able to understand.

- Physically ill pediatric clients need comfort above all else. Maintain the child's privacy and dignity while providing for sleep, nutrition, elimination, skin care, respirations, nasal care, and pain management. Nonpharmacologic pain-management techniques may help reduce the need for pain medication.

- Psychosocial support for ill children is focused on eliciting their responses and feelings about their condition and answering questions based on the family's wants and needs. Honesty and trust are crucial in a therapeutic relationship.

- Children's ability to express themselves and to think rationally about their illness will depend on their developmental maturity.

- Children go through stages of grief like adults. They need to be able to continue to be children and to lead as normal a life as possible. Siblings of ill children have their own emotions and fears.

- Parents should be reminded of resources and tips when caring for an ill child. Breaking problems into smaller parts, self-care, help from support network, financial assistance, collaboration with healthcare team, and hospital support staff are all resources.

- A variety of tools can be used to assess developmental problems in pediatric clients. The nurse should be knowledgeable about them.

- Understanding the philosophy of normalization is important for the nurse and for client teaching.

- A normal grieving process occurs when parents realize that their child is disabled. The family will need to be taught to manage the stress of caring for a child with a disability.

⚭ FOR FURTHER Study

Culture and nursing care are discussed in Chapter 3.

See Chapter 9 for the full discussion about safety issues.

Review therapeutic methods of communication in Chapter 11.

Chapter 12 has the main discussion about client teaching.

As outlined in Chapters 15 and 16, children develop through distinct physical, psychosocial, and emotional stages.

See Chapter 17 for psychosocial needs of clients.

Myths and realities about children and grief are discussed in Chapter 18.

Chapter 19 describes head-to-toe physical assessment.

See Figure 21-5 for a nonmercury glass thermometer.

See Chapter 22 for the main discussion about pain.

Special diets are illustrated in Table 25-6.

Figure 27-4 is a nomogram for calculating pediatric doses.

Musculoskeletal disorders are discussed in Chapter 31.

Chapter 40 discusses reproductive system disorders.

Chapter 48 provides a scoliosis screening procedure and discusses collaboration in community care.

Figure 56-3 illustrates the newborn circulatory system.

Congenital disorders were discussed in Chapters 57 and 59.

See Chapter 62 for Tanner's stages and changes in puberty.

Critical Thinking Care Map

Caring for a Client with a Chronic Illness
NCLEX-PN® Focus Area: Physiological Adaptation

Case Study: Jason Reynolds is a 15-year-old with cystic fibrosis. He has been removed from the ventilator following a living-donor lobar lung transplant. This procedure uses the lower section (lobe) of one lung in each of two living donors. Jason's donors were his older brother, John, age 26, and his father, James, age 48. As soon as Jason is able to speak, he asks about his brother and father, and is told they are both recovering well and will come to see him later today now that he has been transferred to the medical floor. Jason's mother, Joanne, is at his bedside. Jason had been waiting for a full lung transplant, but his lung function was so severely compromised that his medical team felt they could wait no longer for the full transplant.

Nursing Diagnosis: Risk for Infection

COLLECT DATA

Subjective	Objective
_____	_____
_____	_____
_____	_____
_____	_____
_____	_____
_____	_____
_____	_____

Would you report this? Yes/No

If yes, report to: _____

What would you report?_____

Nursing Care

_____
_____
_____
_____
_____
_____
_____
_____
_____
_____
_____

How would you document this? _____
_____
_____
_____

Compare your answers and documentation to those provided on the MyNursingKit Website.

Data Collected
(use only those that apply)

- VS: T 100.8, R 26 and labored, P 88, BP 136/84, pulse ox 96% on 4 L O_2
- Complaining of sore throat following removal of airway
- Ht 68", Wt 125 lbs
- Surgical incisions well approximated on right side, dry and intact
- Left side incision red; moist area at the level of last two staples
- Bilateral Jackson-Pratt drains
- Drainage rt. 55 mL; lt. 75 mL dark red drainage
- Urinary output (fractional urine) 40 ml/hr
- IV Ringer lactate 1,000 mL/12 hrs
- Bowel sounds present 4 quadrants
- NPO since surgery; advance to clear liquid
- Incisional pain 2/10 controlled with PCA morphine sulfate 1 mg q hr
- Concerned about brother and father and is asking to see them
- Restless; says, "I can't seem to get comfortable."

Nursing Interventions
(use only those that apply; list in priority order)

- Arrange visit from father and brother.
- Vital signs every 4 hours.
- Respiratory isolation.
- Reinforce cough, deep breathing, and incentive spirometer every hr.
- Apply wrist restraints.
- Cleanse wound, obtain sample from left incision for culture and sensitivity, dress per order.
- Encourage walking in hallway.

NCLEX-PN® Exam Preparation

1. While the nurse is feeding a young infant, the infant vomits and formula comes out the nose and mouth. The nurse's priority action is to:
   1. Place the infant prone and head down providing back blows to clear the airway.
   2. Use a suction catheter to clear the infant's pharynx.
   3. Suction the infant's mouth and then suction the nose using a bulb syringe.
   4. Suction the infant's nose and then the mouth using a bulb syringe.

2. The nurse is preparing to examine a school-aged child. Which of the following strategies would be most useful with a child of this age?
   1. Ask another nurse to come with you to restrain the child during the examination.
   2. Provide positive reinforcement for good behavior.
   3. Respect the need for modesty and encourage the child to help with the exam.
   4. Ask the child's preference about the presence of a parent during the exam.

3. The nurse is collecting data about pain in the 3-year-old child. Which of the following would be the best approach?
   1. Using the OUCHER scale, ask the child to pick a picture that best describes the pain felt.
   2. Use behavioral indicators only because the child cannot quantify pain.
   3. Ask the child to rate his or her pain on a 0 to 10 scale.
   4. Use behavioral and vital sign indicators alone to determine the child's pain.

4. The nurse needs to collect a urine specimen for culture from a 2-week-old infant. The best means of collecting this specimen is to:
   1. Use a straight catheter.
   2. Place cotton balls inside the diaper to collect urine.
   3. Use a syringe to draw urine from the diaper.
   4. Apply a pediatric urine collection (PUC) bag.

5. After a 3-year-old child has been sent to radiology for testing, the parents inform the nurse that they are going home for the evening and ask that the nurse tell the child they said goodnight. The nurse's best response is to:
   1. Agree to tell the child that the parents went home.
   2. Ask the parents to remain to put the child to bed and say goodnight.
   3. Tell the parents to call the child later to say goodnight.
   4. Avoid saying anything to the child about the parents so the child will not realize they are gone.

6. The nurse, caring for a 2-year-old, is preparing the client for surgery. Which of the following is the best strategy for teaching the child about what will happen?

   1. Explain what will happen using stories or picture books.
   2. Use games to explain what will occur in surgery.
   3. Provide teaching only to the parents.
   4. Allow the child to manipulate equipment and use a doll to demonstrate procedures.

7. The nurse, caring for a terminally ill 6-year-old, is told by the parents not to tell the child she is dying. While the nurse is bathing the child and changing the bed linens, the child states, "I know I am dying but don't tell my Mom and Dad because it would scare them." The nurse's best response is:
   1. "What makes you think you're dying? You're not dying!"
   2. "Okay, I'll keep it a secret between you and me."
   3. "Maybe you should talk to your parents about this."
   4. "Yes, you are dying. Would you like to talk about it?"

8. The parents of a 5-year-old child diagnosed with cystic fibrosis tell the nurse that the child's behavior is becoming problematic but they hate to reprimand the child because he has so many negative things happening to him as a result of his diagnosis. The nurse's best response is:
   1. "Your guilt over bringing this child into the world with cystic fibrosis, along with your sympathy for him, is getting in the way of being good parents."
   2. "Many parents of children with chronic diseases feel that way. Have you considered joining a support group to learn how other parents deal with this issue?"
   3. "You have to reprimand him and treat him as normally as possible or he'll turn into a brat and then you won't be able to correct it."
   4. "Maybe you should consult a therapist before you destroy your child's future."

9. The nurse is caring for a child with mental retardation who is to undergo a Denver Developmental Screening Test II (DDST II). The nurse recognizes the purpose of this test is to:
   1. Determine intellect.
   2. Determine the child's optimum attainable level of function.
   3. Determine the child's current overall development.
   4. Measure the child's ability to understand language.

10. While caring for the child with cognitive issues, the parents ask the nurse what the term *normalization* means. The nurse explains that normalization encompasses which of the following? (Select all that apply.)
    1. Expecting behavior that is as normal as possible.
    2. Protecting the child from other children who could destroy self-concept by isolating the child from social situations.
    3. Encouraging the child to recognize they are handicapped.
    4. Encouraging the child to reach for the highest possible level of functioning.
    5. Teaching the child to take responsibilities for his or her own actions.

Answers and rationales for Review Questions appear in Appendix I.

Chapter 59

Care and Illnesses of Infants and Toddlers (1 Month to 36 Months)

LEARNING Outcomes

After completing this chapter, you will be able to:

1. Identify elements of good nutrition for infants and toddlers.
2. Name normal vital signs ranges for infants and toddlers.
3. Identify important intervals for well-child checkups for infants and toddlers.
4. Describe respiratory, cardiovascular, hematologic, or immune disorders and nursing care for newborns and toddlers.
5. Discuss neurologic, sensory, or musculoskeletal disorders and nursing care for newborns and toddlers.
6. Describe gastrointestinal, or endocrine disorders and nursing care for newborns and toddlers.
7. Explain urinary or reproductive disorders and nursing care for newborns and toddlers.
8. Describe integumentary disorders and nursing care for newborns and toddlers.
9. Review psychosocial conditions and nursing care for newborns and toddlers.

Clinical Objectives

10. Bathe an infant or toddler.
11. Provide oral hygiene for a toddler.
12. Cleanse the perineum and diaper an infant.
13. Obtain a laboratory specimen from a child (e.g., urine specimen using a pediatric urine collector (PUC); heel stick for blood glucose monitoring).

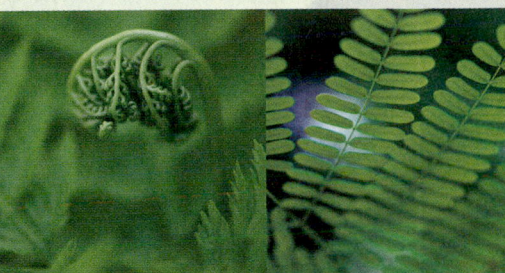

BRIEF Outline

Allis's sign 1652
balanoposthitis 1662
buphthalmos 1650
colic 1657
croup 1635
cryptorchidism 1662
desensitization 1643
diverticulum 1657
echolalia 1664
epiphora 1650
epispadias 1659
hip spica cast 1653
hydrocele 1659

hydronephrosis 1660
hypopituitarism 1658
hypospadias 1659
inotropic 1639
Logan clamp 1655
meconium ileus 1633
megacolon 1657
mucoviscidosis 1633
nephroblastoma 1661
orchiopexy 1662
Ortolani-Barlow maneuver 1652
paraphimosis 1662

phimosis 1662
pica 1658
polycystic kidney 1660
pyeloplasty 1660
separation anxiety 1663
shaken baby syndrome 1647
sprue 1657
stasis 1660
stereotypy 1664
talipes 1653
valve ablation 1660
volvulus 1657

Pediatric nursing care for infants and toddlers includes care of both the ill child and the entire family. Basic growth and development information about infants and toddlers, plus safety information, was provided in Chapter 16 ⚭, Lifespan Development and Family Systems. The normal milestones for infants and toddlers are illustrated in Tables 59-1 and 59-2 ■.

This chapter discusses nutritional needs specific to infants and toddlers (1 month through 36 months). It also describes disorders of each body system that may arise in this period. Students can apply these general guidelines to the care of children with similar disorders not discussed here.

Note: Disorders, especially infections, can affect children of any age and are rarely limited to one age group. For information on where the main discussion of disorders appears, review Table 58-4 ⚭ .

Nutrition for the Infant and Toddler

As discussed in Chapter 25 ⚭ , the best food for infants is breast milk. Breast milk or formula should be the infant's main source of nutrition until 1 year of age. The American Academy of Pediatrics recommends that breast milk be the infant's exclusive food until the age of 6 months.

Many women choose not to breastfeed or use a combination of breast milk plus infant formula in bottles to feed their infants. Individual decisions should be respected once full information is provided to the mother.

When infants are bottle fed, the primary care provider usually recommends a type of formula. The nurse reminds parents to follow directions carefully when making formula and reinforces teaching about safe temperatures, handling, and cleaning equipment.

The American Academy of Pediatrics suggests that cereals and baby foods begin to be introduced at about 6 months of age, usually starting with rice cereal. New foods are given one item at a time for several days, in order to identify possible signs of allergies:

- Skin changes. A rash or *hives* (wheals; see Chapter 30 ⚭) may appear. The child may develop patches of eczema.
- Respiratory changes. Sneezing, coughing, runny nose, and wheezing may occur.
- Digestive distress. There may be vomiting, diarrhea, and signs of abdominal pain.

These signs do not confirm food allergy, but parents should see a doctor if they occur.

Cow's milk is often introduced at 1 year, although some parents may introduce it sooner. Some infants are allergic to cow's milk. If this is the case, soy or even goat's milk may be substituted. Infants need 100 to 200 kcal/kg/day for proper nutrition. Infant nutrition was also discussed in the nutrition chapter in Box 25-1 ⚭ . See Box 59-1 ■ for Women, Infants, and Children (WIC) recommendations.

Foods are gradually added for toddlers. Soft, easily swallowed foods are provided until after 2 years. Depending on their age, size, and activity level, toddlers need about 1,000 to 1,400 calories a day. Water is important between feedings, especially in hot weather.

Toddlers may be very fussy eaters, so it is important to educate parents about providing adequate nutrients to ensure normal growth and development. A variety of foods from all food groups should be offered.

Toddlers should not be forced to eat particular foods or specific amounts of a food; doing this may result in rejection of these foods or even in eating disorders later in life. Parents need to be aware of the requirements of toddlers, but also need to trust their own judgment and their toddlers' cues to tell if they are satisfied and getting adequate

(Text continues on p. 1630.)

TABLE 59-1	Growth and Development Milestones for Infants				
AGE	**PHYSICAL GROWTH**	**GROSS MOTOR SKILLS**	**FINE MOTOR SKILLS**	**COGNITIVE ABILITY**	**NUTRITION**
Birth to 1 month	Gains 5–7 oz (140–200 g)/wk Grows ½ in. (1.5 cm) Head circumference increases ½ in. (1.5 cm)	When prone, holds head up briefly (1) Inborn reflexes present (e.g., Moro, rooting) Arm/leg movement jerky (1) May lift head	Holds hand in fist Tight grasp	Focuses on objects 12–18 in. in front of face (2) Sleeps 20–22 hours/day (2) Follows objects	Eats every 2–3 hours, 60–90 ml/feeding
2–4 months	Gains 5–7 oz (140–200 g)/wk Grows ½ in. (1.5 cm)/month Head circumference increases ½ in. (1.5 cm)/month Posterior fontanel closes	When prone, holds head and chest up Supports weight on forearms Bobs head when upright Turns from side to back to side (3) (3) Can turn from side to back	Holds small objects in hand (4) Puts hand in mouth (4) Holds rattle	Turns head to look for voices, sounds Follows objects 180°	Establishes regular eating pattern every 3–4 hours, 90–120 ml/feeding
4–6 months	Gains 5–7 oz (140–200 g)/wk Doubles birth wt 5–6 months Grows ½ in. (1.5 cm)/month Head circumference increases ½ in. (1.5 cm)/month Teeth begin to erupt by 6 months	Holds head steady when sitting Turns from abdomen to back by 4 months Turns from back to abdomen by 6 months Supports own weight when held standing (5) (5) Supports most of weight when held standing	Picks up objects at will Puts objects in mouth (6) Pulls feet to mouth (6) Grasps objects at will	Is more aware of environment Watches objects fall to floor Responds readily to sounds	Eats 4–5 oz (120–150 ml) 4 or more times/day Begins solid food, usually rice cereal

(continued)

TABLE 59-1	Growth and Development Milestones for Infants *(continued)*				
AGE	**PHYSICAL GROWTH**	**GROSS MOTOR SKILLS**	**FINE MOTOR SKILLS**	**COGNITIVE ABILITY**	**NUTRITION**
6–8 months	Gains 3–5 oz (85–140 g)/wk Grows 3/8 in. (1 cm)/month	Loses most newborn reflexes Sits alone without support by 8 months (**7**) Bounces on legs when held standing (7) Sits alone without support	Transfers objects from one hand to other Shakes and bangs objects together Begins pincer grasp	Recognizes own name by turning and smiling	Eats 6–8 oz (180–240 ml) 4 times/day Eats most baby foods, cereal, fruit, vegetables, begins meats
8–10 months	Gains 3–5 oz (85–140 g)/wk Grows 3/8 in. (1 cm)/month	Crawls by pulling body across floor with arms (**8**) Creeps on hands and knees keeping trunk off the floor Pulls self to standing by 10 months (8) Crawls or pulls body by arms	Uses pincer grasp well to pick up objects (**9**) (9) Uses pincer grasp well	Understands some words such as "no" and "cookie" May say one word besides "mama" and "dada"	Eats four times a day Enjoys finger foods
10–12 months	Gains 3–5 oz (85–140 g)/wk Grows 3/8 in. (1 cm)/month Head circumference = chest circumference Triples birth weight by 1 year	Stands alone (**10**) Sits from standing position Walks holding on to furniture May walk alone for short distance (10) Stands alone	Places objects in container (**11**) Holds crayon and marks on paper (11) Sits down from standing	Enjoys games such as patty cake, peek-a-boo	Eats most soft table food Feeds self with spoon, but may spill Holds cup with lid, can drink by self

TABLE 59-2 — Growth and Development Milestones for Toddlers

AGE	PHYSICAL GROWTH	GROSS MOTOR SKILLS	FINE MOTOR SKILLS	COGNITIVE ABILITY	NUTRITION
1–2 years	Gains ½ lb (227 g) per month Grows 3.5–5 in. (9–12 cm)/year Anterior fontanel closes All deciduous teeth present by 33 months	Walks up and down stairs (1) Runs Throws ball	Undresses self Scribbles on paper (2) By end of second year, builds tower of four blocks	Visual acuity 20/50 Increasing vocabulary of 200 words by 2 years	Eats three meals with snacks Prefers finger foods Gains skill with spoon, begins eating with fork
2–3 years	Gains 3–5 lb (1.4 – 2.3 kg)/year Grows 2–2.5 in. (5–6.5 cm)/year	Rides tricycle Jumps, kicks Throws ball overhand	Dresses self Draws rudimentary shapes, circle, square	Communication improves Uses short three- to five-word sentences Has vocabulary of 1,000 words Displays frustration by temper tantrums	Becomes "picky eater" Intake decreases, but over a week, usually has balanced diet

(1) Walks up and down stairs

(2) Scribbles on paper

BOX 59-1 — CLIENT TEACHING

WIC Recommendations for Infants Up to 1 Year

Lactation specialists work with new mothers, but the LPN/LVN will help reinforce teaching about infant nutrition:

- Under 1 month, breastfeed every 2 to 3 hours or give 2 to 3 oz of formula every 2 to 3 hours (16–24 oz)
- 1 to 2 months, breastfeed every 2 to 3 hours or give 3 to 4 oz of formula every 3 to 4 hours (22–30 oz)
- 3 to 4 months, breastfeed every 3 to 4 hours or give 5 to 6 oz of formula every 4 to 5 hours (26–32 oz)
- 4 to 5 months, breastfeed 7 to 9 times a day or give 28 to 38 oz of formula
  - Cereal can be introduced at this time. Start with rice first, then oat and barley. Wait until baby is at least 9 months before introducing wheat or mixed cereals.
- 6 months, begin strained fruits and vegetables.
  - Introduce 2 oz of juice daily
- 7 to 9 months, breastfeed 7 times a day or 24 to 32 oz of formula (main source of food till 1 year old)
  - Up to 4 oz of juice each day (juice may cause decreased appetite and diarrhea, so limit it and dilute with water)
  - 4 to 8 tablespoons cereal

- 2 to 6 tablespoons strained fruit
- 2 to 8 tablespoons strained vegetables
- 8 to 9 months, breastfeed 4 to 7 times a day or give 24 to 32 oz of formula
  - 4 to 8 tablespoons cereal
  - 2 to 6 tablespoons strained fruit
  - 2 to 8 tablespoons strained vegetables
  - 1 to 4 tablespoons strained meats
  - 1 to 2 tablespoons hard cooked egg yolks
- 10 to 12 months, breastfeed 4 to 7 times a day or give 24 to 32 oz of formula
  - 4 to 8 tablespoons cereal
  - 6 to 8 tablespoons strained fruit
  - 4 to 8 tablespoons strained vegetables
  - 2 to 5 tablespoons strained meats
  - 1 to 2 tablespoons hard cooked egg yolks
  - Mashed table foods can be introduced, for example, bananas, potatoes
  - Finger foods such as oat circle cereal, soft fruits, and cheese slices

Source: Data from Women, Infants, and Children program of the U.S. Department of Agriculture.

TABLE 59-3	Food Pyramid Guidelines for Toddlers		
FOOD GROUP	**DAILY AMOUNT FOR 2-YEAR-OLDS**	**DAILY AMOUNT FOR 3-YEAR-OLDS**	**HELP WITH SERVINGS**
Grains	3 ounces (85 grams), half from whole-grain sources	4 to 5 ounces (110–140 grams), half from whole-grain sources	One ounce equals: 1 slice of bread, 1 cup of ready-to-eat cereal, or ½ cup of cooked rice, cooked pasta, or cooked cereal.
Vegetables	1 cup	1.5 cups	Use measuring cups to check amounts. Serve veggies that are soft, cut in small pieces, and well cooked to prevent choking.
Fruits	1 cup	1 to 1.5 cups	Use measuring cups to check amounts. An 8- to 9-inch (20-23 centimeter) banana equals 1 cup.
Milk	2 cups (475 milliliters)	2 cups (475 milliliters)	One cup equals: 1 cup of milk or yogurt, 1½ ounces (45 grams) of natural cheese, or 2 ounces (60 grams) of processed cheese.
Meat and Beans	2 ounces (60 grams)	3 to 4 ounces (85–115 grams)	One ounce equals: 1 ounce (30 grams) of meat, poultry or fish, ¼ cup cooked dry beans, or 1 egg.

nutrition. A general rule that may be helpful for parents is one tablespoon of food for each year of life.

Teach parents to water down fruit juice and to avoid or strictly limit sugary juices and soda. Products with these simple sugars supply empty calories that may keep children going without providing the nutrition they need to be healthy.

The Food Guide Pyramid guidelines in Table 59-3 ■ are based on the needs of average 2- and 3-year-olds. For children between 12 and 24 months, the 2-year-old recommendations can be used as a guide, though the toddler's diet is in transition during this year.

IMPORTANT DIET COMPONENTS
Milk or Milk Substitutes
Toddlers should have 500 milligrams of calcium a day. This requirement is easily met if children get two servings of dairy foods every day. Milk provides calcium and vitamin D to help build strong bones. Some children reject cow's milk or have a metabolic intolerance to it. Other calcium sources, such as fortified cereals, calcium-fortified soy beverages, broccoli, and calcium-fortified orange juice can be used as substitutes for cow's milk.

Iron
Toddlers should have 7 milligrams of iron each day. After 12 months of age, toddlers may be at risk for iron deficiency because they no longer drink breast milk or iron-fortified formula, and they may not be eating enough other iron-containing foods to make up the difference.

Teach parents that drinking more than 24 to 36 ounces of milk a day can put children at risk of developing iron deficiency because they may be less hungry and less likely to eat iron-rich foods. Milk decreases the absorption of iron in the gut and can irritate the lining of the intestine, causing small amounts of iron to be lost in the stool. Iron deficiency is associated with growth impairment and possible learning and behavioral problems. It can lead to anemia (discussed later in this chapter).

ORAL HYGIENE
Parents should be taught to wipe the infant's gums with a clean, wet washcloth a couple times a day. Tooth brushing is initiated at the eruption of the first tooth. A plain toothbrush with soft bristles is used with water or a scant

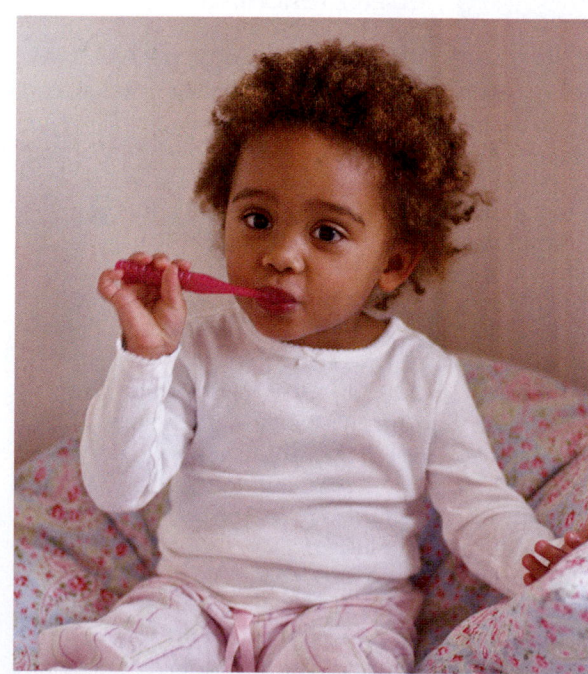

Figure 59-1. ■ Toddlers can assist with tooth brushing, but the parent needs to ensure that teeth are clean. *Source:* Dorian Kindersley Media Library.

TABLE 59-4	Normal Vital Signs of Infants and Toddlers*			
AGE	TEMPERATURE IN DEGREES CELSIUS	AVERAGE PULSE (RANGES)	AVERAGE RESPIRATIONS (RANGES)	BLOOD PRESSURE (MM HG)
Newborns	36.8 (axillary)	130 (90–180)	35 (30–60)	70/42
1 to 3 years	37.7 (rectal)	120 (80–140)	30 (20–40)	90/55

*Different labs show slight variations in normal ranges. Always compare vital signs to baseline data. Any abnormal readings need to be evaluated further to determine the cause.

amount of toothpaste. Fluoride drops or toothpaste may be recommended if there is no fluoride in household water. Toddlers can learn to brush their teeth at an early age (Figure 59-1 ■), but parents should follow up to be sure teeth are clean.

Vital Signs in Infants and Toddlers

Vital signs for infants and toddlers are reviewed in Table 59-4 ■.

ILLNESSES AND DISORDERS

Respiratory Disorders

Disorders of the respiratory system include congenital malformation, infections, and diseases resulting from chromosomal abnormalities or unknown causes. Refer to Chapter 57 🔗 for congenital malformations.

SUDDEN INFANT DEATH SYNDROME

Sudden infant death syndrome (SIDS) is the sudden unexplained death of an infant under 1 year of age. SIDS most often strikes infants between 2 and 4 months of age and is more common in males. Other factors common in SIDS include Native American or African American descent, low birth weight, and multiple births (twins or triplets). SIDS is the leading cause of death of infants between 1 month and 1 year of age. Box 59-2 ■ identifies risk factors associated with SIDS. The main preventive measure is to place infants on their back to sleep.

Manifestations

When SIDS strikes, the infant is typically found not breathing, and emergency medical help is summoned. The infant is usually in a normal state of nutrition and hydration. In more than 50% of infants, blood-tinged frothy fluids are present in and around the mouth and nose. The diapers are filled with urine and stool. The infant may be clutching a blanket. There is no audible outcry at the time of death. Skin is white ashen color, not the expected cyanotic blue

Well-Child Checkups for Infants and Toddlers

Infants ideally are seen often in the first 12 months of life. Well-checks are important to monitor infant health and growth patterns, as well as to identify any concerns of the parent or need for parent teaching. Well-checks are an opportunity for infants to obtain immunizations to prevent numerous "childhood diseases." Table 59-5 ■ lists the recommended intervals for infant and toddler well-checks and shows when immunizations are usually given.

found with respiratory distress. While infants who are at risk can be identified, SIDS remains unpredictable.

MyNursingKit | SIDS

BOX 59-2	RISK FACTORS FOR SIDS

Infant
- Prematurity
- Low birth weight
- Twin or triplet birth
- Race (in decreasing order of frequency): most common in Native American infants, followed by African American, Hispanic, Caucasian, and Asian infants
- Gender: more common in males than females
- Age: most common in infants between 2 and 4 months of age
- Time of year: more prevalent in winter months
- Exposure to passive smoke
- History of cyanosis, respiratory distress, irritability, and poor feeding in the nursery
- Sleeping prone

Maternal and Familial
- Maternal age less than 20 years
- History of smoking and illicit drug use (increases incidence 10 times)
- Anemia
- Multiple pregnancies, with short intervals between births
- History of sibling with SIDS (increases incidence 4 to 5 times)
- Low socioeconomic status; crowding
- Poor prenatal care, low birth weight gain

TABLE 59-5	Well-Child Visits for Infants and Toddlers									
	BIRTH	2 MONTHS	4 MONTHS	6 MONTHS	9 MONTHS	12 MONTHS	15 MONTHS	18 MONTHS	2 YEARS	3 YEARS
Wellness exams	Pulse, respirations, height, weight, plus hearing and hereditary metabolic screening	Pulse, respirations, height, weight	Pulse, respirations, height, weight	Pulse, respirations, height, weight	Pulse, respirations, height, weight, plus lead screening and hematocrit or hemoglobin	Pulse, respirations, height, weight	Pulse, respirations, height, weight	Pulse, respirations, height, weight	Pulse, respirations, height, weight	Pulse, respirations, height, weight, plus blood pressure and visual screening
Hepatitis A						Dose 1		Dose 2		
Hepatitis B	Dose 1	Dose 2		Dose 3						
Diphtheria/tetanus/ pertussis (DTaP)		Dose 1	Dose 2	Dose 3			Dose 4 or	Dose 4		
H. Influenzae type b (Hib)		Dose 1	Dose 2	Dose 3		Dose 4 or	Dose 4			
Polio (IPV)		Dose 1	Dose 2	Dose 3						
Pneumococcal conjugate (PCV)		Dose 1	Dose 2	Dose 3		Dose 4 or	Dose 4			
Measles/Mumps/ Rubella (MMR)*						Dose 1 or	Dose 1			
Chickenpox			Dose 1 or	Dose 1, second dose at 4 to 6 years						
Influenza						Dose			Dose	Dose
Rotavirus		Dose 1	Dose 2	Dose 3						

*Note that mumps and measles were reportable to local health departments effective in 2008 due to the rise in the number of unvaccinated children.

Care of the Family

The impact of SIDS on the family is one of extreme shock followed by extreme outrage. Family members commonly experience guilt, either blaming themselves or projecting blame onto other family members or a babysitter. Older children may fear SIDS will happen to them as well. They may also believe the infant died because of bad thoughts or wishes they had toward their brother or sister.

The nurse has an important role in supporting the family as well as educating the public about SIDS. Recall that by 2 months infants are able to reposition their head to breathe. Ordinary bedding is incapable of causing hypoxia to the point of suffocation. This knowledge can be used to help family members understand that the death was not their fault.

While the need for support of parents and siblings is obvious, grandparents will need additional support. Grandparents will be experiencing grief at the loss of their grandchild, but also extreme hurt at watching their own child suffer. Family members should be allowed to hold the infant and receive a handprint, footprints, and a lock of hair. Provide the family with information regarding local support groups.

CYSTIC FIBROSIS (MUCOVISCIDOSIS)

Cystic fibrosis (**mucoviscidosis**) is an inherited recessive disorder of the exocrine glands affecting predominantly Caucasian children. In cystic fibrosis, defective chloride-ion and water transport occurs across the cell membranes of cells that secrete mucus, causing production of thick, tenacious mucus that obstructs all organs with mucous ducts. Electrolytes are lost through sweat, saliva, and mucous secretions. The disease affects primarily the respiratory and gastrointestinal systems. It has some effect on the integumentary, musculoskeletal, and reproductive systems as well.

Manifestations

Presenting symptoms are usually **meconium ileus** (retention of meconium in the GI tract) in the newborn, failure to thrive, or chronic recurrent respiratory infection.

Diagnosis and Treatment

Diagnosis is made by positive sweat test (Table 59-6 ■ and Figure 59-2 ■). The sweat test can be performed on infants 4 weeks of age or older.

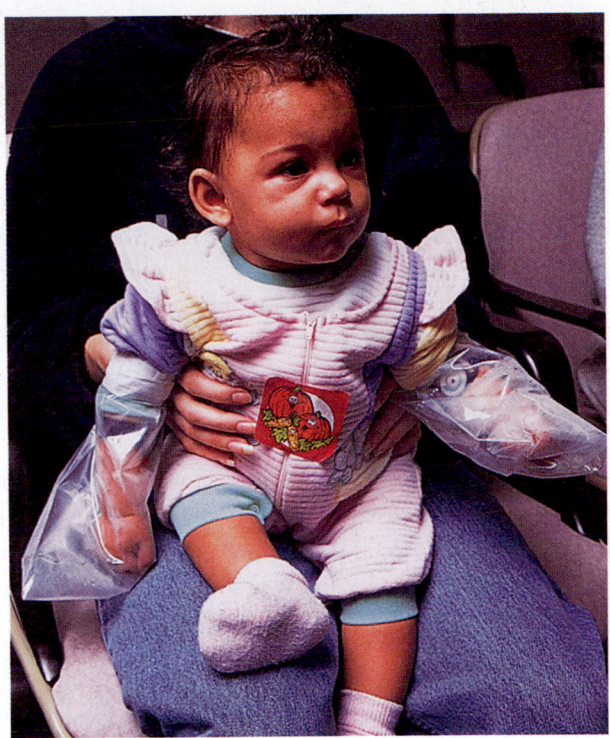

Figure 59-2. ■ Sweat test. The parent may hold and reassure the infant or small child being evaluated for cystic fibrosis with the sweat test. Sweat will be collected from the skin under the plastic wrappings for evaluation of sodium and chloride content. Note that sweat tests performed on infants younger than 4 weeks of age may not provide accurate results.

When assessing a child with cystic fibrosis, pay close attention to respiratory function. Thick mucus can obstruct the bronchi, resulting in hypoxia and infection. The priority for assessment and intervention must be to open and maintain a patent airway. Children are frequently admitted to the hospital with an acute respiratory infection. Respiratory therapy, including oxygen administration and chest physiotherapy several times a day, and antibiotics will be ordered to help clear the airways.

Children with cystic fibrosis are growth retarded even though they may have voracious appetites. The thick mucus blocks the production of pancreatic enzymes, so nutrients cannot be digested. The child's stools are large, bulky, and frothy. They contain a large quantity of fat that cause them to be foul

TABLE 59-6	Sweat Test for Cystic Fibrosis			
TEST	**PURPOSE**	**METHOD OF SPECIMEN COLLECTION**	**NORMAL FINDINGS**	**ABNORMAL FINDINGS**
Sweat test (pilocarpine iontophoresis)	To analyze sodium and chloride content	Two electrodes covered with special gel are placed on child's forearms. A small electric current is passed through electrode for 5 minutes. Some tingling may be noted. Electrodes are removed, and sweat collector is applied to same area. Sweat is collected for 30 to 45 minutes. Sweat collector is sent to laboratory for analysis.	Sodium: 10–30 mEq/L; Chloride: 10–35 mEq/L	Chloride: 50–60 mEq/L is suspicious More than 60 mEq/L with other signs is diagnostic

smelling and to float in water. Fat-soluble vitamins are poorly absorbed. Digestive problems can be eased with special medication and diet modification. Pancreatic enzymes should be given with each meal and large snack. The goal is to achieve near normal stools and maintain adequate weight gain.

Cystic fibrosis is a chronic, long-term illness that is ultimately fatal. The average life expectancy is 18 years of age. With adequate treatment and prevention of complications, some children live into adulthood. The stress on the child, family members, and the community resources is great. The child needs to be encouraged to participate in activities consistent with his or her level of development and physical endurance in order to maintain as "normal" a life as possible. Parents will need emotional support as they work daily to keep their child healthy. Cystic fibrosis takes a financial toll on the family resources as well. The nurse should provide referral to support groups and other resources to assist families.

INFECTIONS

Respiratory infections in the young child are common. Infections stimulate the immune system to develop antibodies that will protect the child in later life. However, if the immune system is immature, or is overwhelmed by multiple infections or other disorders, the life of the child may be in danger. Because the airways of newborns and toddlers are very small, respiratory infection is a very common cause of hospital admission in a young child.

Respiratory system infections include bacterial and viral infections of the nasal and oral pharynx, tonsils, middle ear, epiglottis, bronchi, and alveoli. It is important to review the anatomy of the respiratory system in order to understand the transmission of an upper respiratory infection to the middle ear and lower bronchial tree. (For in-depth discussion of respiratory disorders, see Chapter 32 ⃝.) The most common respiratory infections affecting the newborn and toddler are discussed here.

Respiratory Syncytial Virus

Respiratory syncytial virus (RSV) occurs in epidemics from October to March. This virus is easily transmitted, and most children have been infected by age 3. RSV is transmitted through direct or close contact with the respiratory secretions of infected individuals. The virus invades the cells of bronchial mucosa, causing the cells to rupture. Cell debris irritates the airway, causing an increase in secretions that obstruct the bronchioles.

MANIFESTATIONS. When the airways are partially obstructed, wheezing and crackles can be heard on auscultation. As the blockage continues, breath sounds diminish, causing impaired gas exchange and eventually leading to respiratory failure.

Symptoms of RSV begin with nasal stuffiness and fever, but within a few days progress to frequent, deep cough; rapid, labored breathing; and respiratory distress including retraction and nasal flaring. Parents report the child appears sicker, refuses to eat, and is less playful.

TREATMENT. When hospitalized, the child with RSV requires special precautions to prevent transmission of the organism to others. These precautions include a private room and the use of gowns, masks, and gloves when in the child's room.

The doctor will probably order intravenous fluids, humidified oxygen, and medication to open the airways, decrease inflammation, thin secretions, and lower temperature. The respiratory therapist will be a valuable resource in maintaining a *patent* (open) airway and administering breathing treatments.

Pertussis (Whooping Cough)

Whooping cough is a severe respiratory infection caused by *Bordetella pertussis*. Transmission is by contact with infected respiratory secretions. Incubation is generally from 7 to 10 days but could be as short as 5 days and as long as 21 days. An outbreak of pertussis occurs every 3 to 4 years. Incidence dropped dramatically after the introduction of the pertussis vaccine in the 1940s, but has been rising again since the early 1980s (CDC, 2000).

MANIFESTATIONS. Whooping cough usually begins with a low-grade fever, sneezing, runny nose, watering eyes, and a nonproductive cough. These symptoms may last from 1 to 2 weeks before becoming worse. Children over 6 months of age experience a severe cough especially as night. The child develops a high-pitched crowing sound with each cough. The loud cough is the child's attempt to expel thick mucus through the narrow glottis. The coughing episodes are very tiring for the child and he or she may become red-faced or cyanotic. Vomiting may occur during the coughing episode.

Infants under 6 months of age experience periods of apnea instead of the classic cough. The symptoms may last from 1 to 6 weeks. The cough gradually resolves.

DIAGNOSIS AND TREATMENT. Diagnosis is made by sputum culture. Medical treatment involves administration of antibiotics and corticosteroids; bed rest in a humidified, smoke-free environment; and oxygen administration.

NURSING CONSIDERATIONS. Because of the contagious nature of whooping cough, the nurse must initiate droplet precautions. The nurse must be prepared to gently suction the child's airway to maintain patency. Oxygen saturation should be monitored continuously, especially in infants under 6 months of age. To promote rest, the child will need assistance with activities of daily living.

Having a child with whooping cough is very frightening for parents. The nurse must provide emotional support and teaching. Parents can be helpful in assisting the child with eating, toileting, and bathing. Parents can play quiet games and read to their child. Parents must be taught to administer any medication prior to discharge. Immunizing children at an early age can prevent whooping cough.

Croup

Croup is a term used to represent a group of respiratory illnesses that result from inflammation and swelling of the epiglottis, larynx, trachea, and bronchi. The causative agent can be either viral or bacterial. While laryngotracheobronchitis (LTB) is the most common, epiglottitis and bacterial tracheitis are the most serious. In these infections, swelling of the epiglottis occludes the larynx, and tracheal edema pushing against the cricoid cartilage leads to obstruction.

MANIFESTATIONS.   When a newborn or toddler has croup, inspiratory *stridor* (a high-pitched musical squeak sound caused by narrowing of the airway) will be present. A barking "seal-like" cough and hoarseness are also present. The child may have been ill for several days before the airway becomes partially obstructed, causing symptoms. Other children are healthy and develop severe symptoms in a matter of a few hours. Fever may or may not be present. The child may refuse to swallow saliva due to severe throat pain and swelling, resulting in drooling. As with other respiratory conditions, the child should be observed closely for airway patency, oxygen saturation, and retractions.

TREATMENT.   Care for the child with croup is focused on opening airways and maintaining oxygen saturation. It is important to deliver cool mist to the child in a quiet environment.

clinical ALERT

The newborn or toddler should not be left alone because very young children may not be able to summon help. They should not cry since this can induce laryngospasm. Avoid probing the throat, including obtaining throat cultures, to prevent laryngospasm and complete obstruction.

Most children with croup show rapid improvement once cool mist, oxygen, antibiotics, and fluids are started. The endotracheal tube, if used, can usually be removed in 24 to 36 hours. Discharge teaching includes the continued use of cool mist and the administration of prescribed antibiotics, including teaching about side effects.

BRONCHOPULMONARY DYSPLASIA

Bronchopulmonary dysplasia (BPD) is a chronic lung disorder that affects infants who have had respiratory distress syndrome in the newborn period, who have congenital heart defects, who suffered from meconium aspiration at time of birth, or who had other conditions that resulted in mechanical ventilation. The newborn's lungs become damaged from the high ventilator pressure and oxygen toxicity, resulting in pulmonary inflammation, cellular damage, and death of tissue.

Manifestations

The infant with BPD has persistent bronchial edema, pulmonary fibrosis, and respiratory failure. The infant exhibits signs of respiratory distress including wheezing, crackles, retractions, nasal flaring, and grunting.

Diagnosis and Treatment

Diagnosis is made by chest x-ray. Due to continued respiratory failure, the infant must be supported by mechanical ventilation for weeks or months with the goal of progressive weaning from mechanical assistance. A tracheostomy is required for long-term ventilation. Long-term complications include asthma and recurrent respiratory infections. The administration of anti-inflammatory medication and antibiotics may be necessary. Normal activities, such as feeding, places additional work on the respiratory system that could result in failure to thrive. For this reason, a gastrostomy feeding tube may be required to obtain adequate caloric intake for growth.

Nursing Considerations

Nursing care focuses on maintaining respiratory function and preparing family for home care. At home the infant may be maintained on mechanical ventilation. The family must be taught to manage the required equipment, to administer medication and feeding, and to be observant for further respiratory complications. Care for the infant will be required 24 hours a day. Parents will need support from other family members and friends, as well as healthcare providers. Follow-up care including financial support should be planned and coordinated before discharge.

FOREIGN BODY OBSTRUCTED AIRWAY

The airway of the infant or toddler can be obstructed when the child puts small objects in the mouth or chokes on food. Infants and toddlers must be watched closely while eating and be taught not to put small objects in the mouth. Even with appropriate care, foreign body obstruction of the airway can occur. Care must be provided immediately to clear the airway. To determine if the airway is obstructed, observe the child's facial expression, observe for respirations, and try to get the child to make sounds. If the object can be seen in the back of the throat, try to remove it with a finger sweep, taking care not to push it deeper into the airway. If the object cannot be seen and removed, the Heimlich maneuver (Figure 59-3 ■) is recommended to remove the obstruction safely.

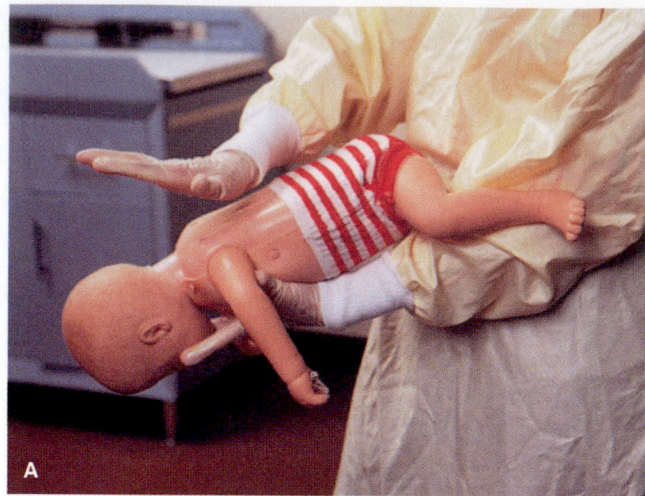
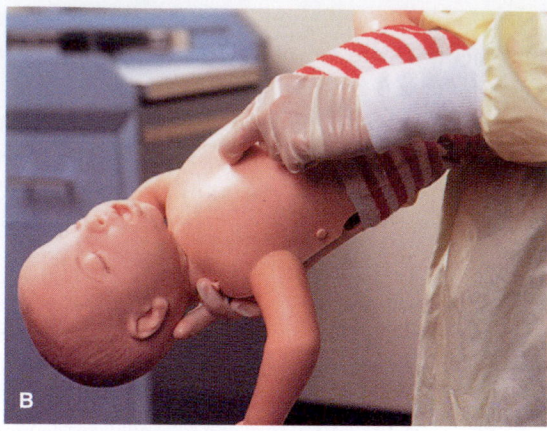
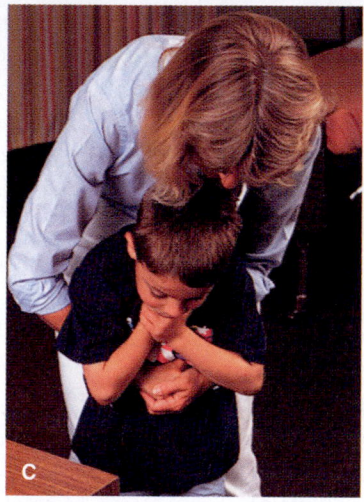
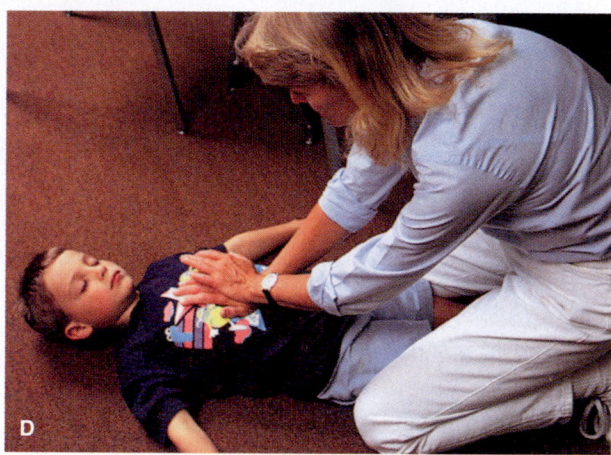

Figure 59-3. ■ Clearing a foreign object. **A.** Back blows **B.** Chest thrusts on an infant. **C.** Standing thrusts (Heimlich maneuver) must be done more gently in a child than in an adult. **D.** Chest thrusts on an unconscious child.

To perform the Heimlich maneuver on an infant, the prone position is used with the baby's head lower than the trunk (Figure 59-3A). Support the head and neck with one hand, with the torso on the forearm. Use the palm of the other hand to give five forceful back blows between the shoulder blades. After the back blows, the free hand is placed over the back of the neck, sandwiching the infant between the hands. The infant is turned over, maintaining the head-down position. Two fingers are placed on the middle of the sternum between the nipples. Five chest thrusts are given at a rate of one every 3 to 5 seconds. Abdominal thrusts are not used on infants due to the risk of damaging the internal organs. This procedure is repeated until the airway is cleared.

The Heimlich maneuver is performed on a child (1 year of age and older) the same way as on an adult. However, the smaller the child, the gentler the abdominal thrusts must be. If the child is sitting or standing, grasp the child from the back with both arms wrapped around the child's abdomen. With one hand made into a fist, place the thumb side against the child's abdomen, slightly above the umbilicus and well below the xiphoid process of the sternum (see Figure 59-3C). The fist is grasped with the other hand and pressed into the child's abdomen with a quick upward thrust. Abdominal thrusts are repeated until the object is expelled or the child becomes unconscious.

The unconscious child is positioned supine. Kneeling at the child's feet, place the heel of one hand on the child's abdomen at the midline, slightly above the umbilicus and well below the xiphoid process. With the other hand on top of the first, press into the child's abdomen with a quick upward thrust. Repeat until the object is popped out of the airway. Sometimes the object is expelled into the mouth and can be removed with a finger sweep, taking care not to push the object back into the airway.

Once the airway is cleared, cardiopulmonary resuscitation (CPR) may be needed. CPR training is not reviewed in detail in this text. Nurses should obtain CPR training through the American Heart Association, the local Red Cross, or their employing agency.

APNEA

Short bouts of apnea occur normally in newborns but should disappear within a few weeks of birth. Apnea is most common in preterm infants, whose parents will need to learn use of an apnea monitor. Discussion of respiratory conditions of the high-risk newborn appears in Chapter 57 ⦾.

NURSING CARE

PRIORITIZING NURSING CARE

When caring for young children with respiratory disorders, focus your care on maintaining a patent airway and early detection of complications. Position the child with head and shoulders elevated on a pillow to aid lung expansion. Monitor closely for audible wheezes or stridor, which can indicate severely narrowed airways. Have suction equipment at the bedside to help clear airways. Keep cool mist and oxygen in place as ordered. Auscultate lung sounds every 4 hours or more often if the child is unstable. Monitor vital signs and pulse oximetry. Immediately report changes in vital signs, especially elevated temperature and increased respiratory rate and oxygen saturation of less than 90%.

ASSESSING

The child with a respiratory disorder should be assessed for lung sounds bilaterally, oxygen saturation, elevated temperature, and stridor. If the throat is infected, the ears should be checked for signs of infection. Likewise, if the ears are infected, the throat should be assessed because of the communication between them through the Eustachian tubes. Careful observation for signs of respiratory distress is critical. The airway of the young child is small and obstructs easily. The oxygen saturation should be monitored and reported to the supervising RN or physician if it falls below 90%.

DIAGNOSING, PLANNING, AND IMPLEMENTING

The following nursing diagnoses are common among young children with respiratory disorders and their families:

- *Ineffective Airway Clearance*
- *Risk for Infection*
- *Deficient Fluid Volume*
- *Fear/Anxiety*
- *Deficient Knowledge*

When planning and implementing care for the child with severe respiratory disorders, the first priority is to establish and maintain an open airway. The nurse should ensure that artificial airways and suction equipment are available in case of airway obstruction.

- Take vital signs, including oxygen saturation measurements, at least every 2 hours on children with severe respiratory disorders (see Chapter 21 ⦾). A child with a severe respiratory disorder should not be left alone. *Very young children may not be able to summon help. The child's condition may change rapidly, and the child may not be able to communicate this to the nurse.*
- Attempt to keep the child feeling safe and comfortable. Avoid probing the throat, even to obtain throat cultures. *Crying may induce laryngospasm and complete obstruction.*
- Record intake and output if risk for deficient fluid volume exists. IV fluids may be administered. *The nurse must be alert for signs of dehydration, which can be life threatening.*
- Once the child is able to swallow, provide cool liquids. *Cool liquids can help decrease throat swelling, relieve discomfort, and maintain fluid balance.*
- Observe the child and the parents for signs of fear and anxiety. Remain with the child and family and explain the need for the various pieces of equipment. *Parents and child are fearful when the child is having difficulty breathing and has loss of voice. The hospital environment is also frightening to the child and parents. The nurse's presence can be reassuring. Knowing about the equipment can reduce fear.*
- Explain all procedures to the parents and encourage their participation in care of the child to the extent possible. *Young children experience separation anxiety if the parents are not close by. Participation by the parents is reassuring.*

EVALUATING

Young children with respiratory disorders are evaluated frequently for airway patency and oxygen saturation. An increase in urinary output indicates adequate fluid intake. Failure to complete ordered antibiotics can result in recurrence of the infection. The importance of giving antibiotics as ordered must be emphasized with family members.

NURSING PROCESS CARE PLAN
Respiratory Syncytial Virus

Omar, a 6-month-old child, has been admitted to the pediatric unit with a diagnosis of possible RSV. Omar is experiencing labored breathing. His mother states, "I am so scared. His breathing is getting worse." Laboratory reports indicate a high white blood count and respiratory acidosis.

Assessment

- Color pale with slight circumoral cyanosis
- Wheezing lung sounds
- P 150, R 54

Nursing Diagnosis

The following important nursing diagnosis (among others) is established for this infant:

- *Ineffective Airway Clearance*

Expected Outcome

- Airway will be clear within 48 hours.

Planning and Implementation

Nursing interventions for this client would include the following:

- Monitor vital signs every hour. *The child's condition can change rapidly and therefore must be monitored closely.*
- Monitor oxygen saturation continuously. *Continuous monitoring of oxygen saturation will alert the nurse if the child's condition deteriorates.*
- Administer oxygen as ordered. *Oxygen is administered to maintain oxygen saturation above 95%.*
- Anticipate worsening respiratory distress by monitoring breath sounds, respiratory effort, and level of consciousness. *Anticipating a worsening of the child's condition allows the nurse time to prepare for airway maintenance.*
- Reposition every ¹/₂ hour. *Frequent position changes facilitate drainage of respiratory mucus.*
- Administer IV fluids via appropriate equipment. *IV fluids are administered by infusion pump to prevent accidental fluid overload.*
- Administer medication with attention to dosage. *Pediatric dosage is individualized based on body weight. If dosage is not calculated carefully, overdose or underdose could occur. To maintain medication blood level in a therapeutic range, medications must be administered on time.*

Evaluation

- Lung sounds are clear.
- Oxygen saturation remains higher than 95%.

Critical Thinking in the Nursing Process

1. If Omar's condition deteriorates, what would the nurse anticipate would be needed to maintain the airway?
2. What can the nurse do to support Omar's parents?
3. What should be taught to Omar's parents about home care after discharge?

Note: Discussion of Critical Thinking questions appears on the MyNursingKit Website.

Cardiovascular Disorders

CONGENITAL HEART DISEASE

Cardiovascular disorders affecting the young child are primarily the result of congenital malformation. Review Chapter 57 ⚭ for details on congenital heart defects including manifestations, treatment, and nursing care. Although many

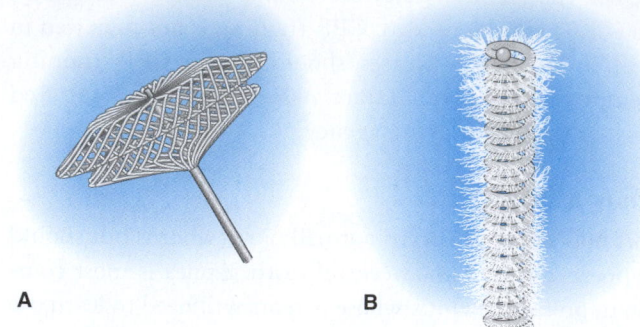

Figure 59-4. ■ **A.** Septal occluder is used to close an atrial septal defect (ADS) and less commonly to close a ventricular septal defect (VSD). **B.** Coil used to close a patent ductus arteriosus (PDA). The coil of wire covered with tiny fibers occludes the ductus arteriosus when a thrombus forms in the mass of fabric and wire.

congenital heart defects are repaired in the first 1 to 2 months of life, some require the child to grow strong enough to tolerate the surgical procedures. Surgical treatment of congenital heart disorders is discussed here.

An atrial septal defect (ASD) and patent ductus arteriosus (PDA) may be closed during a cardiac catheterization procedure. A septal occluder (Figure 59-4 ■) is inserted through the femoral vein, inferior vena cava, and into the right atrium. The septal occluder is then positioned in the ASD. A transcatheter obstructive device (Figure 59-4B) is inserted in the PDA. Over time tissue grows through the wire mesh of either device. A large ASD may require a surgical closure or patch through an open heart procedure. The surgeon may choose to *ligate* (tie and cut) the PDA.

Other congenital heart defects require open heart surgery to repair the defect. During these procedures the blood is shunted through a bypass machine, and the heart is stopped, repaired, and then restarted. Surgery is generally completed in the first 2 years of life to prevent pulmonary hypertension, an increased blood pressure in the pulmonary artery that damages the alveolar capillary network. In complex defects such as transposition of the great arteries or tetralogy of Fallot, several surgeries may be required.

Nursing Considerations

Nursing care of the newborn or toddler undergoing cardiac catheterization procedure is similar to that of an adult. The catheter with occlusion devices is inserted into the femoral artery or vein. The device is positioned in the heart and then the catheter is removed. Due to a risk for bleeding, the child's leg must remain straight and immobile for several hours. The child should be monitored for cardiac arrhythmias during the recovery period. Once the child is taking fluids and is eliminating waste, he or she can generally be discharged.

Nursing care of the newborn or toddler undergoing heart surgery is similar to open heart surgery of adults. The child will be on mechanical ventilation and have a chest tube for a few hours to a few days. The heart must be monitored for arrhythmias. Care must be taken to prevent infection. The child may be discharged in 3 to 5 days if there are no complications.

Family teaching and support is essential. Most parents understand the serious nature of congenital heart defects and fear their child might die. It is important for the nurse to keep the family informed of progress during the surgical procedure. Care must be taken to explain the equipment and postsurgical care. Discharge teaching includes use of prescribed medication, diet, and activity. The family should observe for infection and report any signs of infection to the primary care provider immediately.

CONGESTIVE HEART FAILURE

Heart failure, also called congestive heart failure (CHF), can occur at any age. The child has a circulatory defect, which decreases cardiac output and can lead to cardiogenic shock. CHF can result from congenital heart defects, infections such as rheumatic fever (see Chapter 61 ⚭), trauma, or tumors. At times disorders of other organs can weaken the heart and cause CHF.

Manifestations

The symptoms of CHF can be grouped into three categories: cardiac, pulmonary, and metabolic. Cardiac symptoms include tachycardia, poor tissue perfusion, peripheral edema, and restlessness. The child's heart may be enlarged. Pulmonary symptoms include dyspnea, tachypnea, cyanosis, poor feeding, crackles, and wheezing. Metabolic symptoms include slow weight gain, perspiration, and fatigue.

Treatment

Children with CHF are treated with **inotropic** (increases myocardial contractility) medication, diuretics, and potassium supplements. Children with progressive cardiomyopathy may need a heart transplant.

Nursing Considerations

The nursing care of newborns and toddlers with CHF is similar to care of any client with heart disorders. Priorities in nursing care include conducting a thorough assessment to evaluate the effectiveness of treatment, promoting oxygenation, administering prescribed medication, maintaining adequate nutrition, facilitating normal growth and development, and providing teaching and support to the family.

SYSTEMIC HYPERTENSION

High blood pressure in newborns and toddlers is often secondary to other health conditions such as kidney disease, congenital heart defects, hyperthyroidism, increased intracranial pressure (IICP), and side effects of some medications. Diagnosis would be made by assessing for other conditions.

Essential hypertension is often the result of genetics or family history. Essential hypertension is more common in older children and will be discussed in Chapter 62 ⚭.

NURSING CARE

PRIORITIZING NURSING CARE

When caring for newborns and toddlers with cardiovascular disorders, focus your care on stabilizing their cardiovascular status and detecting complications early. Monitor vital signs every 2 hours or more frequently as needed. Position the client for ease of respirations and to promote venous return. Monitor pulse oximetry every hour and report oxygen saturation of less than 90%. Control any bleeding and assist with administration of blood or blood products. Monitor closely for signs of organ failure such as elevated BUN and liver enzymes as well as shortness of breath, nausea and vomiting, or diarrhea. Closely monitor intake and output for signs of fluid deficit or fluid overload.

ASSESSING

Newborns and toddlers with cardiovascular disorders must be assessed for heart and lung sounds, peripheral circulation, shortness of breath, weakness, fatigue, and activity tolerance.

DIAGNOSING, PLANNING, AND IMPLEMENTING

The following nursing diagnoses may be appropriate for the newborn or toddler with a circulatory disorder:

- *Acute Pain*
- *Risk for Imbalanced Nutrition: Less Than Body Requirements*
- *Risk for Imbalanced Fluid Volume*
- *Risk for Infection*
- *Risk for Injury*
- *Risk for Activity Intolerance*
- *Deficient Knowledge*

The goals of care for children with circulatory disorders include prevention of infection, fluid maintenance, and administration of medications as ordered.

- Apply principles of first aid to control bleeding. *Controlling bleeding is a priority of nursing care.*
- Take vital signs frequently during times of bleeding, illness, or sickle cell crisis. *The child's condition can change rapidly in times of stress and crisis.*
- Observe the child for signs of organ failure including but not limited to pain, neurologic deficit, respiratory distress, vomiting, diarrhea, constipation, and renal failure. *Lack of circulation damages organs and can lead to organ failure.*
- Monitor intake and output. IV fluids may be ordered. *Adequate fluids are needed to keep the blood thin.*
- Administer blood as ordered and following facility policy. *Blood replacement may be needed to maintain blood volume, red blood cells, and hemoglobin. In some states LPNs/LVNs cannot*

administer blood or blood products, but may assist with monitoring vital signs and observing for complications.

- Encourage a balanced diet with adequate iron, protein, and vitamins. Supplements may be needed. *Adequate nutrients are needed to produce red blood cells, maintain tissue integrity, and maintain fluid balance.*

- Provide child and family teaching regarding home care including medication administration and side effects, diet, injury prevention, specific symptoms of complications, and prescribed treatment. Adapt teaching for the toddler using models, charts, videos, or other devices, according to developmental level. Teach frequent hand washing, skin care, and avoidance of infected people. *Many circulatory conditions are treated at home. Client and family need to understand good health practices to prevent complications.*

- Provide emotional support for both child and family. *Many circulatory conditions are long term and often life threatening.*

EVALUATING

Newborns and toddlers with circulatory disorders should be evaluated for fluid balance, signs of infection, and side effects of medication. Parents should be able to verbalize and demonstrate needed home care prior to discharge. Because many circulatory disorders can be long term and life threatening, therapeutic communication is valuable in evaluating the child's and family's emotional status. See Chapter 11 for communication techniques. Evaluation of normal growth and development patterns is important.

Hematologic Disorders

BLEEDING DISORDERS

Bleeding disorders are the result of a decreased amount of blood-clotting factors or a decreased number of platelets. Most generally there are few symptoms until after 6 months of age, due to the limited mobility of the child. Once the child becomes more mobile, excessive bruising may be evident. It is important to evaluate the child to differentiate bleeding disorders from child abuse.

Hemophilia

Hemophilia is a rare hereditary sex-linked disorder causing a deficiency in a specific blood-clotting factor. Chapter 34 provides a full overview of this disorder. The hallmark symptom is bleeding into soft tissue and joints or prolonged bleeding during dental procedures, surgery, or trauma. Treatment of hemophilia includes the transfusion of the missing clotting factor. Parents and children should be taught safety measures to prevent injury and to avoid medications that alter blood clotting. Bracelets identifying the child as a hemophiliac may help medical personnel to provide necessary care in case of bleeding.

Idiopathic Thrombocytopenia

Idiopathic thrombocytopenia is a bleeding disorder of unknown cause that leads to a decrease in the number of platelets. Thrombocytopenia (see Chapter 34) is more common in children between the ages of 2 and 5 years. Frequently the child had a recent viral infection such as chickenpox or rubella. Symptoms include *purpura* (a rash in which blood cells leak into the skin), *petechiae* (pinpoint microhemorrhages under the skin), and *ecchymosis* (larger hemorrhages into the skin). (For illustrations of these lesions, see Figure 30-6 .) The disorder may spontaneously go into remission. If the disorder continues long term, a splenectomy may be performed with some success in controlling the disorder. Nursing care would include controlling bleeding and teaching the child and family measures to decrease risk of bleeding.

ANEMIA

Anemia is a decrease in the number of red blood cells, a decrease in hemoglobin, or both. Anemia can be caused by blood loss, a destruction of red blood cells, or a decrease in the production of red blood cells. (See Chapter 34 for a full discussion.) Two types of anemia that affect children will be discussed here.

Iron-Deficiency Anemia

Iron-deficiency anemia results when the demand for stored iron is greater than what the body can supply. The number of red blood cells may be normal, but the hemoglobin level is low, resulting in reduced oxygen-carrying capacity. The cause of iron-deficiency anemia in children can be blood loss, but more commonly it is due to poor intake of iron and iron-rich foods.

MANIFESTATIONS. The child with iron-deficiency anemia will appear pale, tired, and irritable. If undiagnosed or left untreated for a long time, the child can display tachycardia, systolic heart murmur, and growth retardation and be mentally delayed. Over time the nail beds become deformed.

DIAGNOSIS AND TREATMENT. It is important to assess the child on a routine basis. A simple blood test done at 9 months can detect iron-deficiency anemia early. Children whose diet is low in iron should be evaluated annually.

Parents should be taught to provide a diet high in iron, such as dark green and deep yellow fruits and vegetables, meat, and whole grains. Prepared formula should contain iron. Because young children have difficulty swallowing pills, a liquid iron preparation may be ordered. Liquid preparations should be diluted and given through a straw or placed on the back of the tongue to prevent staining of the teeth. Liquid iron preparations may not be compatible with milk or juice. Iron preparations may turn the stool black.

Sickle Cell Anemia

Sickle cell anemia is a hereditary disorder affecting the formation of hemoglobin. Normal hemoglobin (Hgb) is replaced by hemoglobin S (Hgb S) that causes the red blood cell to form an "S" or "C" shape (see Figures 34-3 and 34-4). The abnormally shaped red blood cells cannot travel normally through the capillaries, resulting in decreased blood flow and decreased oxygen-carrying capacity.

Sickle cell anemia is a recessive trait affecting primarily African Americans, but has been found in other people as well. Approximately 1 in 12 African Americans carry one of the recessive genes but rarely exhibit symptoms of sickle cell anemia. If both parents carry the recessive gene, there is a 25% chance that each child will have sickle cell disease.

MANIFESTATIONS.   The child with sickle cell anemia will be asymptomatic until approximately 4 to 6 months of age because sickling is inhibited by fetal hemoglobin. Not all red blood cells will assume the typical "C" shape, and the child will be healthy much of the time. During periods of stress, such as rapid growth or illness, more "C"-shaped cells will be released into circulation. Sickle cells have a short life span, living 10 to 20 days instead of the usual 120 days of normal red blood cells. The problems associated with sickle cell anemia are a combination of sickle cells obstructing circulation and anemia from not enough normal red blood cells and hemoglobin. The child should be watched closely for signs of anemia including pallor, fatigue, lethargy, and irritability. If the child is under physical stress, mild cyanosis may be present.

During times of stress when the bone marrow releases more sickle cells, circulation will be obstructed. Any area of the body could be affected. The child will experience severe pain and decreased function due to decreased circulation in an area. For example, an infarct of the spleen would cause severe left upper quadrant pain. Nausea, vomiting, anorexia, and diarrhea may also be present. If occlusions are areas close to the skin, discoloration, pallor, and coolness will be present. Obstruction leads to tissue destruction and, at times, death. When obstruction occurs, the child is said to be in a sickle cell crisis.

DIAGNOSIS AND TREATMENT.   Laboratory tests show sickled red blood cells and abnormal hemoglobin S. The Sickledex test shows sickling when oxygen tension is low. Electrophoresis can be used to determine whether a person carries the sickle cell trait.

Treatment of crisis includes hydration, oxygen, pain management, and bed rest. If given early in crisis, blood transfusion can relieve the anemia and make the sickled blood less viscous. Intravenous analgesics should be administered to control pain. Continuous intravenous infusion of fluid is important to reduce the viscosity of the blood. Bed rest decreases the tissue need for blood and oxygen.

A diet high in calories and protein with adequate fluid intake can decrease the chance of sickle cell crisis. Because chronically ill children are at greater risk for infection, and because infection can stimulate crisis, it is essential to prevent infection. Immunizations should be kept up to date. The child should avoid contact with infected persons. Frequent hand washing is a must.

Knowledge about the disease helps ensure compliance with preventive measures and treatment. Family members should be encouraged to share their feelings. Because sickle cell anemia is a chronic, life-threatening, genetic disease, a lot of additional stress will be placed on the family unit. Family members may need help coping with guilt, fear, and depression. Support groups may be available to assist and support families of sickle cell children.

THALASSEMIA

Thalassemia is an inherited disorder that causes abnormal hemoglobin synthesis. Children of Mediterranean descent or those from the Middle East, Asia, or Africa are more likely to have the disorder (Box 59-3 ■). The red blood cells are fragile and can be easily destroyed, resulting in anemia.

Manifestations

The by-product of hemolysis is *hemosiderin*, which is deposited in the skin causing a tanned appearance. As anemia progresses, the child develops bone pain, pathological fractures, activity intolerance, fatigue, and pallor. The liver and spleen may become enlarged and the child may develop congestive heart failure.

Diagnosis and Treatment

Thalassemia can be detected by genetic testing during pregnancy. Diagnosis is made by history, symptoms, physical examination, and laboratory tests including complete blood count (CBC) and hemoglobin electrophoresis.

Medical management of thalassemia is supportive not curative. The child may need frequent blood transfusions. An iron-chelating agent (e.g., deferoxamine) is given to prevent iron overload (*hemosiderosis*). If the spleen remains enlarged, a splenectomy may be performed.

BOX 59-3   **CULTURAL PULSE POINTS**

Genetic Risk for Thalassemia

Health officials in Greece have developed extensive public service campaigns to advise citizens of the genetic risk they may carry for thalassemia. Prenatal screening programs have been successful in reducing the incidence of the disease. Therapeutic abortion rates are also high among women who discover the trait in the fetus they are carrying. Thalassemia is a risk for all women of Mediterranean descent.

Nursing Considerations

Nursing care of the child with thalassemia is similar to the care of the child with any other form of anemia. Families need to be taught about the disease, the treatment, and the need to conserve energy.

LEUKEMIA

Leukemia, cancer of the blood-forming organs, is characterized by an increase of abnormal white blood cells (see Chapter 45 🔗 for a discussion of cancer). Some researchers theorize that exposure to viruses before or after birth can predispose a child to leukemia. Types of leukemia are identified by the rate of disease progression and the specific cells affected. Chronic leukemia, although common in adults, is rare in children. For more on chronic leukemia, see Chapter 34 🔗.

Classification of Acute Leukemia

Two types of acute leukemia, acute lymphoblastic leukemia (also called acute lymphocytic leukemia) and acute myelogenous leukemia, are common in children and will be discussed here.

ACUTE LYMPHOBLASTIC LEUKEMIA.   Acute lymphoblastic leukemia (ALL), an overproduction of immature lymphocytes, is the most common leukemia of childhood. ALL has the highest incidence in Caucasian boys who are 3 to 4 years of age.

Normally, lymphocytes are formed from stem cells in the bone marrow and migrate to lymphatic tissue where they become mature functioning cells. In ALL, the lymphocytes divide rapidly, but fail to mature. Immature lymphocytes, called *lymphoblasts*, have no normal function. When more and more lymphoblasts are produced, fewer and fewer normal lymph cells are made. The lymphoblasts crowd out normal white blood cells, red blood cells, and platelets.

ACUTE MYELOGENOUS LEUKEMIA.   Acute myelogenous leukemia (AML), also called acute nonlymphocytic leukemia (ANLL), refers to all types of leukemia from myeloid tissue. Table 59-7 ■ identifies the subtypes of AML.

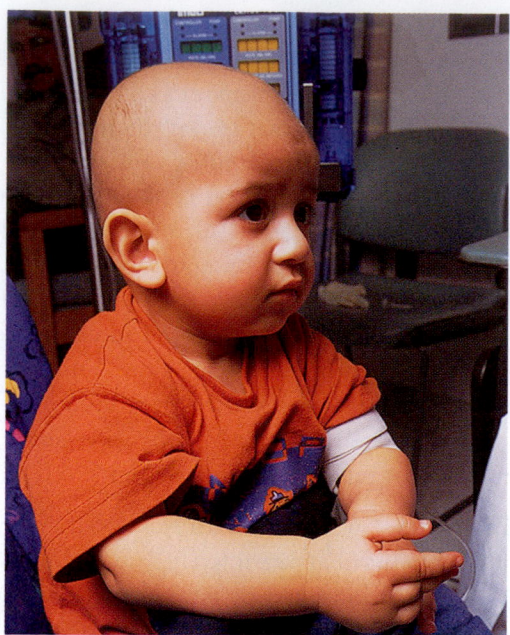

Figure 59-5. ■ Acute lymphoblastic (or leukocytic) leukemia is the most common type of leukemia in children and the most common cancer affecting children under 5 years of age.

In AML, cancer cells replace normal bone marrow, and immature white blood cells, red blood cells, and platelets are found circulating throughout the body.

Manifestations

The child with leukemia has symptoms associated with a decreased number of normal blood cells (Figure 59-5 ■). Without enough normal white blood cells, the child has frequent infections, most commonly respiratory in nature. A low red blood cell count results in signs of anemia. With an abnormally low platelet count, bleeding gums and bruising are common.

Diagnosis and Treatment

Diagnosis is made by blood counts and bone marrow aspiration. Because in both ALL and AML, bone marrow is replaced by blast cells, the symptoms are very similar. The earlier diagnosis is made and treatment begun, the better the prognosis. Left untreated, the life expectancy of a child with AML is several weeks to 6 months.

Treatment might include antibiotics, blood replacement, chemotherapy, and radiation. After remission is achieved, a bone marrow transplant can be beneficial if a suitable donor is available.

Nursing Considerations

Assessment during treatment should be done at least every 8 hours. Chemotherapy and radiation is very damaging to the kidneys and the rapidly growing cells of the gastrointestinal system. It is important to monitor renal

TABLE 59-7	Subtypes of AML (ANLL)
SUBTYPE	**DESCRIPTION**
M 0	Acute nonlymphocytic leukemia without maturation
M 1	Acute nonlymphocytic leukemia with poor maturation
M 2	Acute nonlymphocytic leukemia with maturation
M 3	Acute promyelocytic leukemia
M 4	Acute myelomonocytic leukemia
M 5	Acute monocytic leukemia
M 6	Erythroleukemia
M 7	Acute megakaryocytic leukemia

function through specific gravity, intake and output, and daily weight. Damage to the gastrointestinal system results in sores in the mouth, nausea, vomiting, and constipation. Nutritional status and fluid balance should be assessed closely.

The child with leukemia fatigues easily and needs frequent rest periods. Because of the increased risk of infection and hemorrhage should injury occur, safety during play is important. During the acute phase of the illness, the child may not have enough energy for a lot of physical activity, but quiet play can help maintain mobility and also provide diversion.

Having an acute life-threatening illness causes a lot of fear for the child as well as the parents and family. Because of the rapid onset of symptoms of leukemia, the child appears well one day and extremely ill the next. Hospitalization, numerous invasive diagnostic procedures, and administration of toxic chemotherapy contribute to the fear and anxiety. The nurse is instrumental in providing support, teaching, and organizing interdisciplinary resources to assist the patient and family. Referral to family support groups may be made on request.

Immune Disorders

ALLERGIES

An allergy is an altered reaction to repeated exposure to an *allergen* (a foreign protein). Common allergens can be grouped by method of contact such as ingested food, inhaled particles, and skin contact. Some food allergens include cow's milk, egg whites, peanuts, shellfish, soy, tomatoes, and wheat. Inhaled allergens include animal dander, pollen, and mold. Contact allergens include animal fur, latex, metal salts found in jewelry, and soap.

Manifestations

Clinical manifestations of allergies can be mild, severe, or life threatening. Table 59-8 ■ outlines the various types and symptoms of reactions.

clinical ALERT

Latex allergy can be type I (local or systemic) or type IV (delayed hypersensitivity). Children, parents, or healthcare workers who are allergic to bananas, avocados, potatoes, chestnuts, or tropical fruits are at risk for developing latex allergy. Latex can be found in many healthcare products including gloves, drains, adhesives, and catheters. Latex substitutes must be used when the allergy is identified.

Diagnosis and Treatment

It is important to take a detailed history to help with diagnosis. Intradermal skin testing may be required to identify the causative agent. Food allergies can be identified by removing foods one at a time and observing for symptoms. Once the allergen is identified, it should be avoided.

Oral antihistamines are generally given to treat mild allergic reactions. In severe reactions, antihistamines and epinephrine are administered by subcutaneous, or intravenous routes (Figure 59-6 ■).

Desensitization, the process of administering small amounts of dilute allergen to stimulate the body's immune system, may be necessary to prevent a serious allergic reaction such as anaphylactic shock (see Chapter 35 ⬤⬤). The LPN/LVN can play an important role in intradermal testing and administration of desensitizing allergens.

Nursing Considerations

The nurse can be instrumental in helping the child and family avoid allergens. The family may need to remove pets from the home as well as controlling dust and removing carpets. The child who is allergic to bee or wasp stings may need to carry a prefilled single-dose epinephrine syringe or EpiPen. The family and older child must learn to administer the epinephrine, including proper storage and checking the expiration date.

HIV AND AIDS

HIV is a retrovirus that causes the end-stage disease AIDS. HIV/AIDS is characterized by a defect in cell-mediated immunity, which makes it difficult or impossible for the infected child to fight infection.

TABLE 59-8	Types of Allergic Reactions		
TYPES	**EXAMPLES**	**OCCURS**	**CLINICAL MANIFESTATIONS**
Type I—localized or systemic	Hay fever, pet fur, insect bite	Within seconds or minutes of exposure	Rhinitis, sneezing, hives, urticaria, wheezing, vomiting, diarrhea, anaphylaxis
Type II—tissue specific	Reaction to blood transfusion, hemolytic disease of the newborn	Within 15 to 30 minutes of exposure	Symptoms vary but include fever and dyspnea
Type III—immune complex	Serum sickness, acute glomerulonephritis	Within 6 hours of exposure	Urticaria, fever, joint pain
Type IV—delayed	Tuberculin skin test, contact dermatitis, allograft tissue rejection	Within several hours after exposure	Symptoms vary but include fever, erythema, pruritus

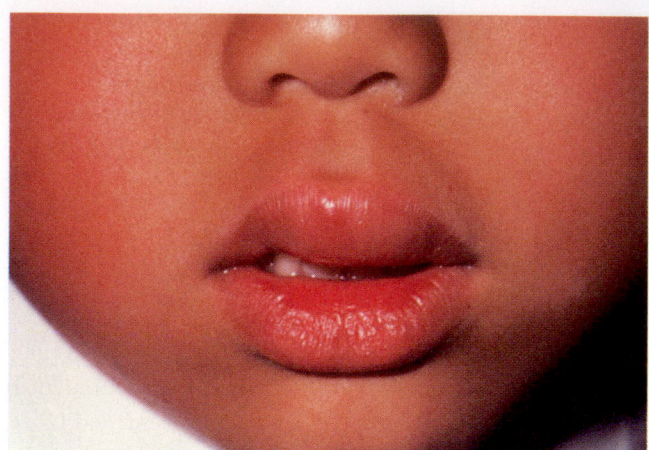

Figure 59-6. ■ Inflammation of the skin, or dermatitis, may be a response to allergens, infections, or chemicals. This client has inflammation of the lip caused by allergic reaction to peanuts.

HIV is transmitted to newborns and toddlers primarily through the placenta during pregnancy or during contact with maternal blood, amniotic fluid, and maternal body fluids during the birth process. The infant or toddler can contract the disease by exposure to breast milk from an infected mother. Adolescents typically contract HIV through unprotected sexual activity and IV drug use.

Because of the risk of transmission to the infant, the Centers for Disease Control and Prevention (CDC) recommends routine screening as part of prenatal care. The woman may be reluctant to find out the diagnosis. The nurse should explain that early diagnosis, treatment with zidovudine (AZT), and a cesarean birth can significantly reduce the risk of transmission to the infant.

Manifestations

Clinical symptoms include chronic otitis media, fever, lack of weight gain, chronic diarrhea, hepatosplenomegaly, lymphadenopathy, and thrush (Figure 59-7 ■). Thrush is an

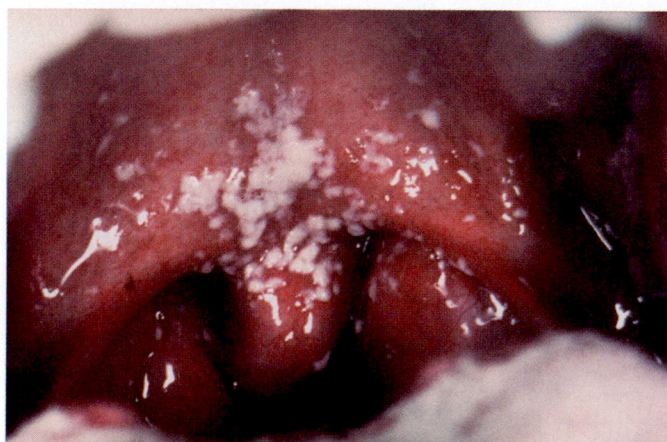

Figure 59-7. ■ Oral thrush is a common finding in clients with HIV. (Visuals Unlimited.)

infection of the oral mucosa most commonly by the fungus *Candida albicans*. Thrush is seen as white patches in the mouth that bleed easily. The fungal infection can also be found in the diaper area, under the arms, and around the neck. (See Chapter 41 ⬤ for more information on candidiasis.)

Diagnosis and Treatment

Diagnosis is made on the basis of two positive ELISA blood tests. A newer test, called the OraQuickAdvance HIV 1/2 Antibody Test, uses oral fluids obtained by swabbing both the upper and lower gums. Results are available in 20 minutes, and positive results have been found to be 99% accurate.

An HIV-positive mother is treated with AZT during pregnancy to prevent transmission to the fetus. Most primary care providers will perform a cesarean birth to further reduce the newborn's risk of exposure. The newborn is treated with AZT, antibiotics, and immune globulin to prevent infection. If the newborn tests positive, antiviral therapy is used, usually combining several drugs (Table 59-9 ■).

Nursing Considerations

Nursing care of children with HIV/AIDS involves reducing infection and transmission and promoting adequate growth and development. To reduce the risk of infection, invasive procedures should be avoided if possible. Families should be taught proper hand washing. Parents should be taught the importance of avoiding other children and individuals with infections. Some infections such as tuberculosis can be devastating. The family should be encouraged to have the child immunized against common infections (Box 59-4 ■).

The child's diet should be assessed for adequate nutritional contents including calories, protein, vitamins, and antioxidants. Refer the family to a registered dietitian as needed.

Children with HIV/AIDS are at risk for mental delays due to frequent hospitalization. The nurse should assess physical and mental development and provide assistance to parents regarding activities to promote growth and development.

JUVENILE RHEUMATOID ARTHRITIS

Juvenile rheumatoid arthritis (JRA) is an autoimmune disorder that causes inflammation of the joints. The child experiences periods of exacerbation and remission, with permanent remission occurring before adulthood. It is most often seen in children from 1 to 3 years and from 8 to 10 years.

Manifestations

The symptoms of JRA are both musculoskeletal and systemic. The child develops fever, rash, enlarged lymph nodes (lymphadenopathy), enlarged spleen (splenomegaly), and enlarged liver (hepatomegaly). Pain, swelling, and loss of movement may be seen in one or more joints, especially in large joints such as the knees.

TABLE 59-9	Pharmacology: Antiretroviral Agents Used to Treat HIV			
DRUG (COMMON BRAND NAME AND GENERIC)	USUAL ROUTE/DOSE	CLASSIFICATION AND PURPOSE	SELECTED SIDE EFFECTS	DON'T GIVE
Retrovir (zidovudine)	100–180 mg/m^2 every 6 hrs PO for children 3 months to 13 years	Nucleoside reverse transcriptase inhibitors used to suppress viral load	Fever, malaise, myalgia, headache, nausea, vomiting, anorexia, cough, rash	If client is anemic or has a granulocyte count above 750/mm^3
Norvir (ritonavir)	400–600 mg/m^2 PO BID for children 2 to 16 years	Protease inhibitors used in combination with other antiretroviral agents to suppress viral load	Weakness, nausea, diarrhea, vomiting	If client has suppressed liver function
Rescriptor (delavirdine mesylate)	400 mg PO TID for children greater than 16 years	Nonnucleoside reverse transcriptase inhibitors used in combination with other antiretroviral agents to suppress viral load	Rash, headache, dizziness, chest pain	If an antacid is being administered at the same time. If client has fever, blistering rash, oral lesions, conjunctivitis, muscle or joint pain

Diagnosis and Treatment

JRA is diagnosed by clinical symptoms and laboratory findings including positive rheumatoid factor, human leukocyte antigen B27, and antinuclear antibody.

BOX 59-4	CLIENT TEACHING

Care of the HIV Child at Home

- Remind parents and caregivers that HIV virus cannot be spread by sneezing, coughing, hugging, or touching the child.
- Exposure to body fluids and blood creates the greatest risk of exposure. Situation in which this may occur includes trauma, accidents, or fights with another child where the skin integrity is compromised.
- Gloves should be used when diapering a child, cleaning wounds, and wiping up urine, feces, or vomit.
- Use disposable towels for wiping spills. Use disposable diaper wipes.
- To clean a surface exposed to body fluids, mix 1 tablespoon liquid chlorine bleach in one quart of water.
- Dispose of diapers, diaper wipes, gloves and towels exposed to body fluids in a leak proof container such as a plastic bag.
- Encourage parents and caregivers to wash their hands with soap and water for at least 10 seconds after removing gloves.
- Linens exposed to body fluids can be washed separately, adding 1/2 cup liquid chlorine bleach to the washing detergent.
- Encourage parents and caregivers to prevent the sharing of eating utensils. Children should be prevented from putting toys in their mouth and sharing them. Toys and eating utensils can be washed normally in the dishwasher or with hot soap and water.

Priorities of treatment are to relieve pain and prevent joint contractures. Salicylates (aspirin) or nonsteroidal anti-inflammatory drugs (NSAIDs) are used to reduce inflammation. These drugs can cause gastrointestinal upset and bleeding. The child should be monitored closely for these and other side effects.

Physical therapy, including ROM exercises, hydrotherapy, and strengthening exercises, is essential to prevent contractures. Warm compresses are used to relieve discomfort and swelling.

Nursing Considerations

Care of the child with JRA usually occurs in the community. Family must be taught to care for the child in the home, to administer medications, and to make arrangements for physical therapy. The child should remain in school, have contact with peers, and participate in activities to help develop a positive self-image. The American Juvenile Rheumatoid Arthritis Association can be a valuable resource for families.

Nervous System Disorders

Nervous system disorders that affect the young child include congenital defects, infections, and trauma. Review Chapter 36 🔗 for nervous system disorders and refer to Chapter 57 🔗 for congenital anomalies. Treatment for head and spinal cord injuries resulting from accidents are the same as for the adult. Prevention of nervous system trauma is an essential component of client and family teaching including the use of car seats, bicycle (and other) helmets, and firearm safety. Caregivers must be taught not to shake young children in order to prevent a form of closed head injury called shaken baby syndrome (discussed later in the chapter).

CEREBRAL PALSY

Cerebral palsy (CP) is a nonprogressive disorder affecting motor function and posture. CP develops secondary to lesions or anomalies of the brain, hypoxic damage, or birth trauma to the motor center of the brain. The damage can occur during the prenatal, perinatal, or postnatal periods, up to 2 years of age. Neonatal infections such as meningitis and kernicterus or infantile hyperbilirubinemia can result in cerebral palsy. Common causes of cerebral palsy are given in Box 59-5 ■.

BOX 59-5	COMMON CAUSES OF CEREBRAL PALSY

- *Infections during pregnancy.* Certain maternal infections such as Rubella, cytomegalovirus, and toxoplasmosis can cause brain damage resulting in cerebral palsy. A 2003 study at the University of California, San Francisco, found that full-term babies were four times more likely to develop cerebral palsy if they were exposed to maternal infections involving the placental membranes (chorioamnionitis). Infections in the urinary or reproductive tract also may increase the risk of preterm delivery, another risk factor for cerebral palsy.
- *Insufficient oxygen reaching the fetus.* When the placenta is not functioning properly or it tears away from the uterine wall before delivery, the fetus may not receive enough oxygen.
- *Prematurity.* Premature babies that weigh less than 3.33 pounds are up to 30 times more likely to develop cerebral palsy than full-term infants. Many tiny babies have bleeding in the brain, which can damage delicate brain tissue, or develop *periventricular leukomalacia*, destruction of nerves around the fluid-filled cavities (ventricles) in the brain.
- *Asphyxia during labor and delivery.* Until recently, it was widely believed that *asphyxia* (lack of oxygen) during a difficult delivery was the cause of most cases of cerebral palsy. The ACOG/AAP (American Council Obstetrics and Gynecology and American Academy of Pediatrics) report shows that fewer than 10% of the type of brain injuries that can result in cerebral palsy are caused by asphyxia.
- *Blood diseases.* Rh factor, an incompatibility between the blood of the mother and the fetus, can cause severe jaundice and brain damage, resulting in cerebral palsy. This can be prevented by giving Rh-negative women an injection of a blood product called immune globulin (RhoGAM) around the 28th week of pregnancy and again after the birth of an Rh-positive baby. Blood-clotting disorders (thrombophilias) in either the mother or the baby may increase the risk of cerebral palsy.
- *Severe jaundice.* Jaundice, yellowing of the skin and the whites of the eyes caused by the buildup of a pigment called bilirubin in the blood, occasionally becomes severe. Without treatment, severe jaundice can pose a risk of permanent brain damage resulting in athetoid cerebral palsy.
- *Acquired cerebral palsy.* About 10% of children with cerebral palsy acquire it after birth due to brain injuries that occur during the first 2 years of life. The most common causes of such injuries are infections in the brain such as meningitis and head injury.

Manifestations

Cerebral palsy is characterized by abnormal muscle tone and lack of coordination. Children with CP are frequently delayed in meeting growth and development milestones. Other neurologic problems may also be present including hearing loss, visual defects such as nystagmus or strabismus, speech delay or impediment, seizures, or mental retardation.

Characteristic signs of cerebral palsy, which may be present shortly after birth, include weak or absent sucking or swallowing, jitteriness, and slow or absent reflexes. By 6 months of age there is a notable delay in reaching developmental milestones and arching of the back when trying to stand. The 9-month infant exhibits an abnormal or asymmetrical crawl. If the child learns to walk, a scissor gait and toe walking are common (Figure 59-8 ■).

Treatment

The child will need long-term physical therapy to maintain joint mobility and prevent contractures. Braces may be needed.

The child with cerebral palsy may not have an intellectual disability. Adaptive equipment is available to allow these children to communicate more fully.

Nursing Considerations

The primary nursing function is to teach the parents and family members to care for the child with cerebral palsy. Parents should be referred to the appropriate resources to obtain adaptive appliances such as customized wheelchairs,

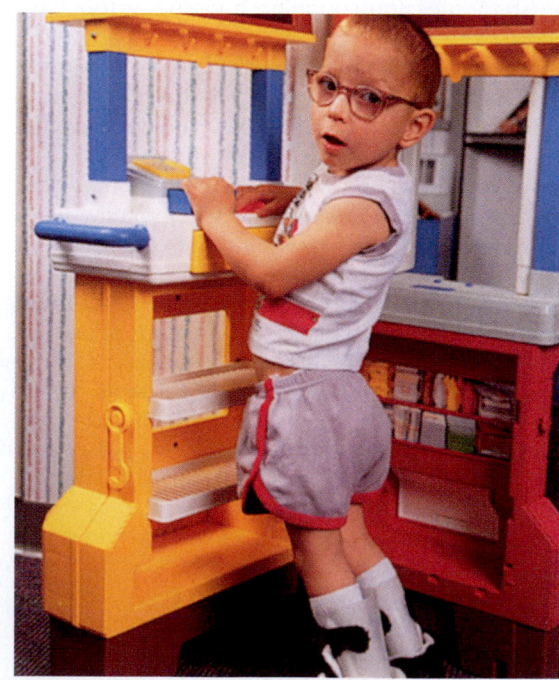

Figure 59-8. ■ A child with cerebral palsy has abnormal muscle tone and lack of physical coordination. Muscles can be strengthened by periods of standing with support.

braces, and eating utensils. Parents should be taught the importance of safety belts and helmets to prevent injury.

Use terminology for the development stage of the child. Parents should be taught to encourage and support their child in order to foster positive self-esteem. Due to the long-term nature of the disorder, the child and parents should be referred to appropriate counseling and support groups. Parents may need financial assistance to provide the needed care.

CLOSED HEAD INJURY

Closed head injury (sometimes called **shaken baby syndrome**) is damage that is a result of head trauma, either from an external force such as a fall, or an internal force, such as shaking the child hard enough for the brain to strike the inside of the skull. The extent of neurologic damage depends on the nature and degree of trauma. The symptoms and treatment are the same as those for an adult with closed head injury (see Chapter 36 ⬭).

SEIZURE DISORDERS

Although seizures can occur in the newborn and toddler period, seizure disorders will be discussed in Chapter 60 ⬭.

MENTAL RETARDATION

Mental retardation (MR) was defined by the American Association on Mental Retardation (2002) as "a disability characterized by significant limitation both in intellectual functioning and in adaptive behavior as expressed in conceptual, social and practical adaptive skills." Specific limitations include communication, social skills, activities of daily living, schoolwork, and employment. *Note*: In 2006, the organization renamed itself the American Association on Intellectual and Developmental Disabilities or AAIDD.

Mental retardation is associated with other neurologic disorders including Down syndrome, fetal alcohol syndrome, maternal infection, hypoxia, neurological trauma, and ingestion of poison such as lead.

Manifestations

Infants with MR appear unresponsive to contact. They are often irritable and take longer periods of time to feed. As these children age, they exhibit delays in speech, social skills, cognitive skills, and motor skills. Learning is difficult and they may not do well in school.

Diagnosis and Treatment

A thorough history and physical examination are essential in determining both the cause and extent of MR. Laboratory tests including MRI, blood tests for chromosomal analysis, toxicology, and blood enzymes are often ordered. Standardized tests such as the Denver Developmental Screening Test II (see Figure 58-14 ⬭) are helpful assessment tools.

Because the degree of MR varies, each child requires a specific plan to help him or her reach the optimal level of functioning. The family, nurse, primary care provider, social worker, and schoolteacher have a significant role in care of the child with MR.

Nursing Considerations

Families with children with MR often experience grief and have difficulty coping. The nurse can have an important role in helping families work through these feelings. The nurse can provide referrals to agencies that can assist the family in caring for their child.

Children with MR do not have sound judgment. Because safety may be compromised, they often require close supervision. Parents should allow the child to perform as many activities of daily living as possible. This will require patience and kindness. As the child ages, the nurse and family should discuss issues such as living apart from their parents, sexuality, safety, birth control, preventing sexually transmitted infections, and money management. The nurse can refer the family to community resources to assist with these issues.

DOWN SYNDROME

Down syndrome is the most common chromosomal abnormality seen in infants that cause moderate to severe MR. It results from three chromosomes at position 21 and is also called *trisomy 21*. Down syndrome is seen more frequently in the children of young mothers and mothers over 35.

Manifestations

The child with Down syndrome has a short head, flat forehead, short limbs, and a short, wide neck (Figure 59-9 ■). The tongue may protrude from the mouth. Epicanthal folds (folds

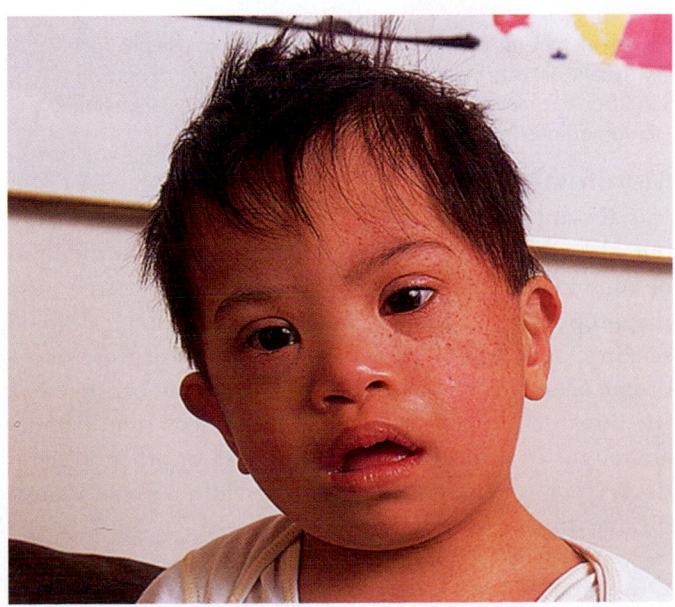

Figure 59-9. ■ This Down syndrome child has typical characteristics including Mongolian slant, short wide neck, and a protruding tongue.

of skin over the inner canthus of the eye) are common. The hands are short and wide with a simian crease (a horizontal crease extending across the entire palm). There is a wide space between the great and second toe. In the newborn, Moro reflex is absent, and reflexes are slow. The infant with Down syndrome has an increased risk for congenital heart defects, diabetes, leukemia, and hearing loss. The degree of mental retardation varies and is not able to be assessed at birth.

Diagnosis and Treatment

Initial diagnosis is made by clinical findings most often evident at birth. Definitive diagnosis is made by chromosomal analysis.

There is no cure for Down syndrome. Medical care focuses on diagnosis and treatment of related disorders. A team approach will be helpful in assisting parents with the child's physical and mental condition.

Nursing Considerations

Parents of children with Down syndrome will need emotional support in coping with the new infant. Parents may be overwhelmed with the thought of caring for their child. The child with Down syndrome will need life-long assistance. With support, many Down syndrome children can be mainstreamed into regular classroom settings and live in group homes as adults.

REYE'S SYNDROME

Reye's syndrome is an acute *encephalopathy* (disorder characterized by inflammation of the brain). Untreated, the syndrome is often fatal.

clinical ALERT

Teach all parents of infants and toddlers not to use products with salicylic acid (aspirin, Pepto-Bismol, etc.) in infants and children with fever. The use of these products has been linked to sometimes-fatal Reye's syndrome.

Manifestations

Initial symptoms include nausea, vomiting, and lethargy but may progress quickly to marked changes in the level of consciousness. The child may become combative, use inappropriate language, have hyperreflexia, develop seizures, and become comatose. Symptoms of Reye's syndrome usually follow a viral illness and may be linked to the intake of aspirin. Because of this association, parents are taught to administer acetaminophen or other fever reducers, not aspirin, to treat fever in a child with a communicable disease.

Diagnosis and Treatment

Diagnosis of Reye's syndrome is made from history plus elevated liver enzymes and ammonia levels, decreased blood glucose levels, and prolonged prothrombin time.

The ill child is admitted to the pediatric intensive care unit for supportive treatment and close observations. Respiratory ventilation may be necessary. Monitoring for increased intracranial pressure is essential. Intravenous fluids assist in treating hypoglycemia.

Nursing Considerations

Nursing care focuses on treating symptoms and supporting the family. Reye's syndrome can be prevented by teaching parents about the use and side effects of aspirin.

MENINGITIS

Meningitis (see Chapter 36 ⬥) is inflammation of the meninges by either a bacteria or virus. Bacterial meningitis is the more serious of the two, causing neurologic damage and possible death. The majority of cases of meningitis in children occur before the age of 5 years.

Manifestations

Symptoms of fever, change in appetite, vomiting, and diarrhea may occur suddenly or progress over a week depending on the causative organism. The child may be lethargic or extremely irritable. Rocking or cuddling, which usually calms the child, may make the child more irritable. The child may also display headache, photophobia, nuchal rigidity, or stiff neck. The child is comfortable only when lying on the side with the neck hyperextended (Figure 59-10 ■) and may have a positive Kernig's or Brudzinski's sign, or both (see Chapter 62 ⬥). A hemorrhagic rash beginning as petechiae and progressing to larger lesions may be seen with meningococcal meningitis.

Diagnosis and Treatment

Laboratory analysis of a cerebrospinal fluid reveals the infection. CSF will be milky in bacterial meningitis.

Broad-spectrum antibiotics may be administered intravenously until the causative agent is identified. Fluids are provided orally if the child is responsive and able to swallow. Fluids may be given intravenously to prevent dehydration.

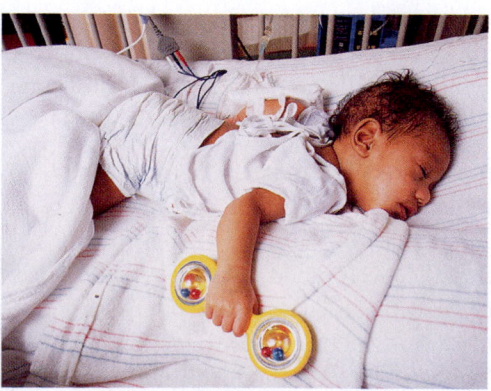

Figure 59-10. ■ Infants with meningitis have hyperflexion of the neck as seen in this photo.

Monitor vital signs and level of consciousness frequently. Measure and record head circumference daily due to the potential for hydrocephalus. The child with meningitis is at increased risk for seizures. Monitor for signs of sensory or movement deficiencies. For example, the child may lose the ability to hold the bottle, drink, or control secretions. The child could develop respiratory distress including periods of apnea.

The child with meningitis should be placed in a private room. Keep the room dark and quiet to prevent photophobia and decrease the risk of seizures. Until the causative agent is determined, the child should be placed in respiratory precautions. All individuals entering the rooms should wear gown, gloves, and mask.

To control the fever and alleviate pain, nonsteroidal anti-inflammatory drugs (NSAIDs) are administered. If the fever is extreme, tepid baths or a cooling blanket may be needed.

Nursing Considerations

Parents should be encouraged to verbalize their feelings and concerns. Involving them in the care of their sick child can help to relieve their fears. Because bacterial meningitis can damage the nervous system, long-term rehabilitation may be needed. Referral to social workers or clergy may be necessary.

NURSING CARE

PRIORITIZING NURSING CARE

When caring for young children with nervous system disorders, focus your care on promoting adaptation to client's limitations and providing emotional support to the family. If the client is having seizures, promote safety during the episodes, time the seizures, and provide support after the seizure. Encourage the child to do as much as possible in activities of daily living and play. Praise all progress, however small. Encourage family to give appropriate positive reinforcement to the child for showing progress. Allow family members to openly discuss their fears and concerns regarding the child. Refer to appropriate support groups.

ASSESSING

Young children with nervous system disorders should be assessed for changes in level of consciousness, reaction to stimuli, and ability to respond with normal behaviors. They must be monitored closely for signs of seizures. Increased intracranial pressure can be manifested by projectile vomiting.

> **clinical ALERT**
>
> Neurologic deterioration can occur rapidly in young children. Changes in baseline vital signs and level of consciousness must be recorded and reported immediately.

DIAGNOSING, PLANNING, AND IMPLEMENTING

The following nursing diagnoses may apply to the young child with a nervous system disorder:

- *Ineffective Airway Clearance*
- *Risk for Deficient Fluid Volume*
- *Grieving (Parent)*
- *Risk for Injury* related to impaired mobility
- *Impaired Verbal Communication*
- *Bathing, Feeding, Dressing, Toileting Self-Care Deficit*
- *Disturbed Body Image*

Nursing interventions for some of these nursing diagnoses were discussed previously in this chapter and will not be repeated.

- Adapt communication techniques for cognitive ability, not chronological age. *Neurologic disorders can delay or regress cognitive ability. At times cognitive development stops and may never show normal progression.*
- Allow the child to do as much for herself or himself as possible. Provide assistance and encouragement toward self-care. Encourage the family to allow the child as much independence as possible. Complete any care the child or family is unable to perform. *The amount of self-care is dependent on the degree of neurologic damage. Allowing the child to complete as much self-care as possible fosters independence and self-esteem. Completing any care the child is unable to complete is essential to health maintenance.*
- Provide factual information to the child and family to assist in dealing with disturbed body image. Allow the young child expression of feeling through puppet play. Include other specialists such as a physical therapist, occupational therapist, and speech therapist as needed. *Young children may not perceive disfigurement to the same extent as family members. Nursing care should focus on the family as the primary support for the child.*

EVALUATING

Evaluate airway patency by assessing color, oxygen saturation, and respirations. The effectiveness of seizure medications is evaluated by recording the number, frequency, and type of seizures that occur. Evaluate for respiratory infection, malnutrition, constipation, and skin breakdown due to altered mobility, especially in the child with cerebral palsy. Watch family interaction with the child to determine the degree of acceptance of physical and mental limitations of the child.

Sensory System Disorders

CATARACTS

Cataracts are a clouding of the lens of one or both eyes, which may prevent light from reaching the retina (Figure 59-11 ■). Cataracts in children are either acquired or congenital.

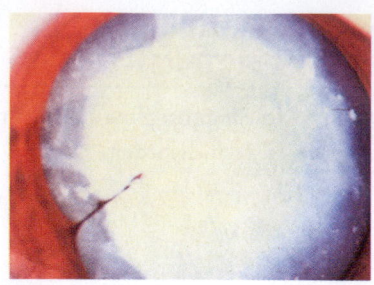

Figure 59-11. ■ Congenital cataract. The cataract reduces or prevents light from reaching the retina.

Acquired cataracts result from infection in the fetus, trauma, or some other disease. Congenital cataracts are inherited from one or both parents.

Manifestations

Some cataracts can be observed as a cloudy film over the eye. Other cataracts must be observed with an ophthalmoscope. The normal red reflex (the reflection of light off the retina) may be absent or distorted. An infant may not be able to focus on objects or may have *nystagmus* (involuntary movement of the eyes).

Treatment

Cataracts are removed surgically before 2 months of age in an effort to prevent permanent visual impairment. Following surgery, corrective lenses or artificial lens implants will be necessary to restore vision. Most children have good vision with correction.

Nursing Considerations

Parents of a child with cataracts need support and teaching. Parents may have guilt feelings that they somehow caused their child's visual impairment. Following surgery, the child must be kept quiet. Crying can increase intraocular pressure and disrupt the healing of the cornea.

GLAUCOMA

Glaucoma is increased intraocular pressure caused by inadequate drainage of aqueous humor from the anterior chamber (see Chapter 36 🔗). Glaucoma can cause damage to the retina, optic disc, and eventually visual field defects and blindness.

Manifestations

Glaucoma in the child may manifest as increased tearing (called **epiphora**), eyelid spasm, enlarged eyeball (called **buphthalmos**), and sensitivity to light. The ambulatory child may bump into objects due to decreased peripheral vision.

Diagnosis and Treatment

Ocular pressure is measured with a tonometer. The child must be restrained, sedated, or anesthesized to prevent the tonometer from damaging the anterior chamber. Normal ocular pressure is 12 to 20 mm Hg. Diagnosis is by a reading above normal limits.

An increased ocular pressure above 30 mm Hg may require immediate surgery. In some cases, glaucoma can be relieved with medication.

Nursing Considerations

It is important to teach the family the importance of eye care, including the administration of eye medication and the need for follow-up eye examinations.

RETINOBLASTOMA

Retinoblastoma is a retinal malignant tumor. It can be unilateral or bilateral. Retinoblastoma in children is inherited, so a family history is important to collect. However, many cases occur without a family history of the cancer.

Manifestations

The first sign of a retinoblastoma is a white pupil. The red reflex is absent, or is a different color from the unaffected eye. Other symptoms may be orbital inflammation and irises of different colors (heterochromia). Diagnosis is usually made between 1 and 2 years of age.

Treatment

Treatment of retinoblastoma usually involves removal of the eye. Radiation treatments may be used before or after surgery. Most children who have been treated have good health.

HEARING IMPAIRMENT

Hearing impairment ranges from slight hearing loss to total deafness. It can occur from birth or be acquired later in childhood. Causes of hearing loss include autosomal dominant inherited diseases, prenatal infections such as rubella and toxoplasmosis, perinatal asphyxia and anoxia, ototoxic drugs, radiation, childhood infections such as measles and mumps, otitis media, head trauma, and excessive environmental noise.

Manifestations

Clinical signs of hearing loss vary depending on the age of the child and the degree of hearing impairment. The infant may not startle to loud noises or may fail to be calmed by his mother's voice. The older infant may not imitate sounds. The toddler may use nonverbal language.

Diagnosis and Treatment

Diagnosis is made by hearing acuity screening. The American Academy of Pediatrics (AAP) has endorsed newborn hearing screening in birthing units as the standard of care (Johnson, 2002). Hearing testing procedures are shown in Chapter 48, Procedure 48-9 🔗.

The child with hearing impairment may benefit from speech therapy, learning to lip read, and learning sign language. (Basic sign language is a skill that school systems may provide.) A hearing aid may be necessary. Hearing aids are costly and generally are not covered by health insurance. Totally deaf children may have surgery to implant a cochlear implant device to assist hearing.

COCHLEAR IMPLANTS. Cochlear implants are devices that are implanted externally behind the ear with a wire leading in to the cochlea (Figure 59-12 ■). A headpiece is worn that contains a microphone and transmitter. Success of implants is greatest when they are implanted in infancy. They require involvement of the parents and a commitment to special training that enables the child to decode sounds to learn language.

OTITIS MEDIA

Otitis media is an infection of the middle ear. In an adult, the *Eustachian tube* (which connects the nasal pharynx to the middle ear) angles upward to prevent drainage from entering the middle ear. In the infant and very young child, the Eustachian tube is short and straight. When the infant lies flat for long periods of time, nasal drainage, milk from the oral pharynx, and bacteria can flow through the Eustachian tube into the middle ear, causing infection. As the infant grows and becomes ambulatory, otitis media gradually becomes less common. Anytime there is infection in the throat or tonsils, the possibility of otitis media exists as well.

Manifestations

Often the parent of an infant or toddler with otitis media brings the child to the primary care provider because of restlessness, irritability, and crying that cannot be relieved by usual methods. There may also be a mild fever. The practitioner will see a red, bulging, nonmobile tympanic membrane (Figure 59-13 ■).

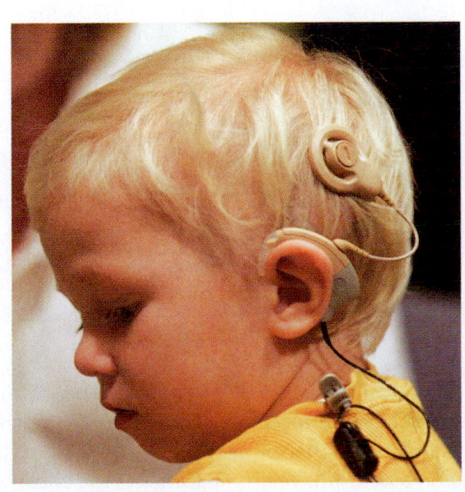

B

Figure 59-12. ■ **A.** Cochlear implants provide access to the world of sound to children who are born deaf. **B.** Implanted device.

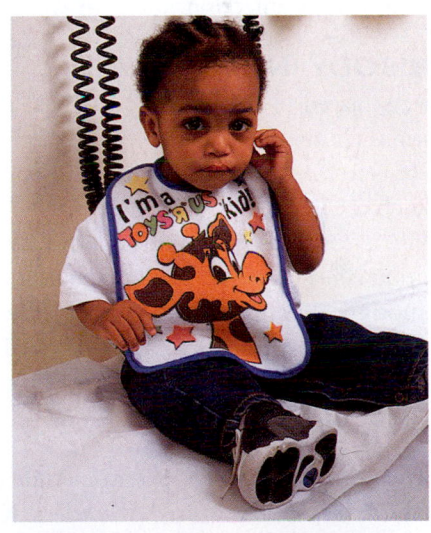

A

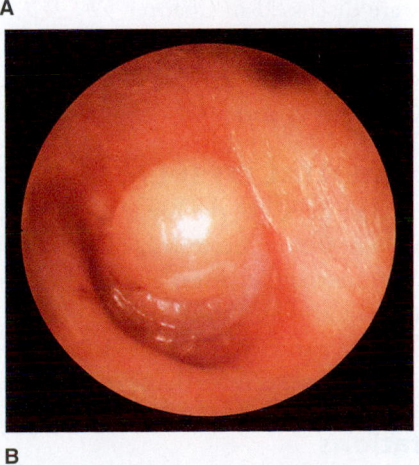

B

Figure 59-13. ■ **A.** This young child is pulling at an ear and acting fussy, two important signs of otitis media. **B.** Acute otitis media is characterized by pain and a red, bulging nonmobile tympanic membrane. (Phototake NYC.)

Diagnosis and Treatment

Recent history may include a cold or virus. The tympanic membrane will appear red and inflamed. The ear will be painful.

Otitis media is treated with antibiotics. Failure to treat otitis media could result in rupture of the tympanic membrane, temporary or permanent hearing loss, and communication disorders. If the child has frequent episodes of otitis media, surgery with placement of small drainage tubes (myringotomy) may be necessary.

Nursing Considerations

For otitis media, teach parents to sit the infant upright after feeding. If the infant is given a bottle in bed, plain water is the fluid of choice. If surgery is required, the parents should be taught to keep water out of the ear until the drainage tubes are removed. A vertical position will help keep fluid from pooling in the middle ear. Drainage tubes allow fluid out of the middle ear. They can also allow fluid in, which could lead to infection.

FOREIGN BODY IN EAR

Foreign objects placed in the external ear canal may impair hearing. Curious children may take pleasure in placing small toys, paper, or cereal in their ear. The nurse may assist in removal of the object by irrigating the external ear canal. The healthcare practitioner may remove the object with sterile forceps if irrigation is unsuccessful. Parents should be cautioned against attempting to remove the foreign object themselves. This may force the object further into the ear canal.

Musculoskeletal Disorders

Disorders of the musculoskeletal system include congenital anomalies, fractures, and acquired disorders. Congenital anomalies were discussed in Chapter 57 ⬥. While fractures are an occasional occurrence in very young children, they are more common in older children. Fractures are addressed in Chapters 31 and 60 ⬥.

DEVELOPMENTAL DYSPLASIA OF THE HIP

Developmental dysplasia of the hip (DDH) is an abnormality of the hip joint that occurs during fetal development. Recall that it is important to assess the newborn for DDH so that medical diagnosis and treatment can begin (see Figure 56-15 ⬥). The primary care provider assesses for DDH with every well-baby check for the first 2 to 3 months.

Manifestations

The partial or complete dislocation of the hip joint that occurs with DDH results in shortening of the femur, uneven thigh and gluteal folds, and limited abduction on the affected side. When the hip is manipulated with gentle lateral

---

BOX 59-6	MANIFESTATIONS OF DEVELOPMENTAL DYSPLASIA OF THE HIP

The following are signs of DDH:
- Hip click with abduction
- Asymmetrical thigh folds
- Uneven knee level
- Limited hip abduction

pressure, abduction, and rotation, a click can be heard and felt as the femoral head is reduced into the acetabulum. If the child is ambulatory, a notable limp is present. Box 59-6 ■ identifies signs of DDH.

Diagnosis and Treatment

The assessment of DDH includes Allis's sign and Ortolani-Barlow maneuver. **Allis's sign** is demonstrated by placing the infant supine on the examination table with the hips and knees flexed and feet flat on the table. If dislocation of the hip is demonstrated, the knee on the affected side will be lower.

To perform **Ortolani-Barlow maneuver,** the hip is manipulated with gentle lateral pressure, abduction, and rotation. A click can be heard and felt as the femoral head is reduced into the acetabulum. If the DDH is not detected until the child is ambulatory, a notable limp will be present. Medical diagnosis is made by x-ray or scan.

Treatment of DDH should begin as soon as possible. If only a small amount of abnormality is present, three diapers are used to support the hip in abduction, allowing the femoral head to remain in the acetabulum until ligaments are strong enough to maintain hip alignment permanently. If more support is needed, a Pavlik harness is commonly used for 3 to 4 months (see Figure 59-14 ■). If the

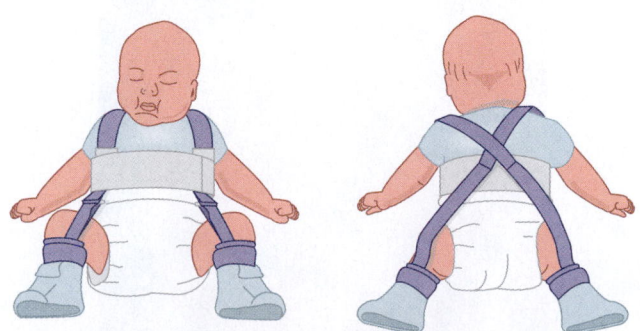

Figure 59-14. ■ Guidelines for Pavlik harness application. (1) Position the chest halter at nipple line and fasten with Velcro. (2) Position the legs and feet in the stirrups, being sure the hips are flexed and abducted. Fasten with Velcro. (3) Connect the chest halter and leg straps in front. (4) Connect the chest halter and leg straps in back. All straps are marked at the first fitting with indelible ink so they can be reattached easily after the harness is rinsed and dried.

harness is unsuccessful, surgery followed by a **hip spica cast** (a cast covering the upper thighs and lower torso) may be necessary.

Nursing Considerations

It is important for the nurse to teach family members the triple diapering technique and to stress the importance of maintaining the hip in abduction until the primary care provider determines the hip is stable. If a Pavlik harness or hip spica cast is used, the nurse must teach the family proper care for these devices.

Complications of a harness or cast include skin breakdown under the harness or cast, impaired circulation from pressure against the cast, deep vein thrombosis, urinary retention, and constipation from immobility. Many complications can be prevented by padding the cast edges, turning the child at least every 2 hours, and encouraging adequate fluid intake. Once the child is taking solid foods, fruits and vegetables are encouraged to prevent constipation. Newborns and toddlers enjoy moving and exploring their environment. It is frustrating for them to be confined in a harness or cast. It is important for the family to provide visual stimulation and change the child's position frequently.

TALIPES (CLUBFOOT)

Talipes or clubfoot is any of several deformities of the foot in which there is a unilateral or bilateral twisting of the foot.

Manifestations

Commonly, the foot of a newborn infant appears to turn inward due to the position the infant assumes *in utero*. The foot can easily be moved into alignment and over a few days, assumes the normal position. When clubfoot occurs, the foot cannot easily be moved into alignment (Figure 59-15 ■).

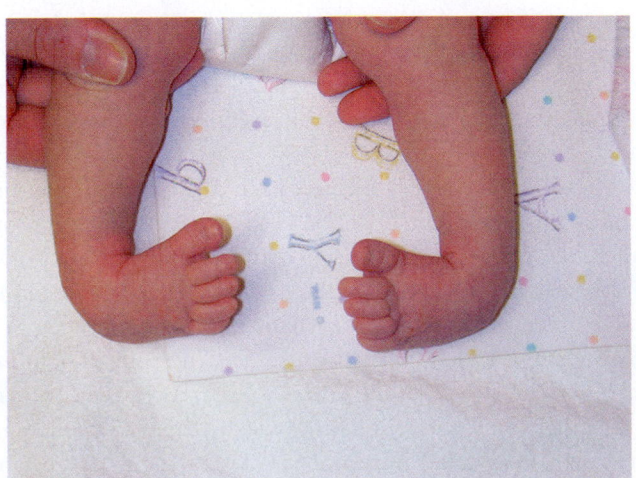

Figure 59-15. ■ Clubfoot, with the midfoot directed downward, the hindfoot turned inward, and the forefoot curled toward the heel and upward, is corrected surgically.

Diagnosis and Treatment

Diagnosis is made by visual inspection and manipulation. X-rays are taken and are used in preparing for corrective surgery.

Nonsurgical treatment involves moving the foot into correct alignment and applying a cast. The cast is changed every 1 to 2 weeks until alignment is achieved in approximately 3 months. Failure to achieve alignment could result in a need for surgical correction.

Nursing Considerations

The nurse is responsible for assisting with application of the cast. The family will need instruction in cast care. It is important to support the limb while the cast is drying to prevent impressions in the cast material, which could put pressure on the underlying tissue. The skin at the cast edges must be assessed for pressure and irritation. To ensure that the edges of the cast are smooth, the nurse may need to apply mole skin to the cast. The family should be taught to keep the cast clean and dry and to keep regularly scheduled appointments.

Gastrointestinal Disorders

Disorders of the gastrointestinal system interfere with digestion and lead to malnutrition. Disorders of the gastrointestinal system result from congenital malformation, acquired disease, infection, or injury. Reviewing the anatomy and physiology of the gastrointestinal system (see Chapter 37 ⬤⬤) will improve your understanding of these disorders. Congenital anomalies were covered in Chapter 57 ⬤⬤ .

DIARRHEA AND CONSTIPATION

Diarrhea (passage of liquid stools) and *constipation* (passage of infrequent, hard, dry stools) are common symptoms of gastrointestinal disorders. Diarrhea in children can be particularly dangerous because of the risk of dehydration and electrolyte imbalance. The child's skin is sensitive. Diarrhea left on the skin can cause skin breakdown in a short time. It is essential to wash the child's skin following each episode of diarrhea and to protect the skin with a barrier ointment.

Constipation can lead to painful straining to defecate and trauma to the rectal tissue. Increasing fiber and fluids in the diet often relieve constipation. At times stool softeners are ordered.

DEHYDRATION

Dehydration is a condition of decreased fluid volume in the intravascular and interstitial fluid compartments. Dehydration is often accompanied by imbalances in sodium. Dehydration leads to about 10% of pediatric hospitalizations. Dehydration can be caused by vomiting and diarrhea, and disorders of other body systems such as renal disease, and burns.

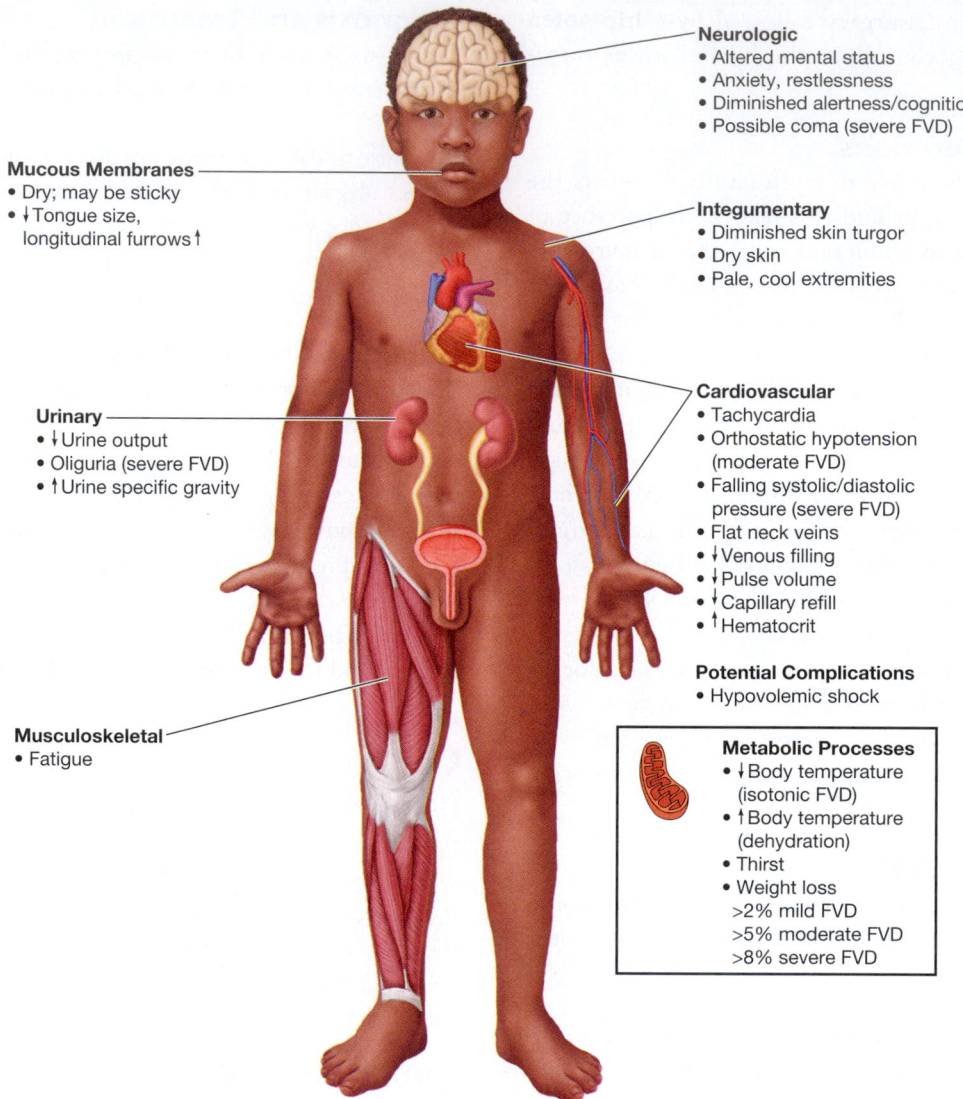

Neurologic
- Altered mental status
- Anxiety, restlessness
- Diminished alertness/cognition
- Possible coma (severe FVD)

Mucous Membranes
- Dry; may be sticky
- ↓Tongue size, longitudinal furrows↑

Integumentary
- Diminished skin turgor
- Dry skin
- Pale, cool extremities

Urinary
- ↓Urine output
- Oliguria (severe FVD)
- ↑Urine specific gravity

Cardiovascular
- Tachycardia
- Orthostatic hypotension (moderate FVD)
- Falling systolic/diastolic pressure (severe FVD)
- Flat neck veins
- ↓Venous filling
- ↓Pulse volume
- ↓Capillary refill
- ↑Hematocrit

Potential Complications
- Hypovolemic shock

Musculoskeletal
- Fatigue

Metabolic Processes
- ↓Body temperature (isotonic FVD)
- ↑Body temperature (dehydration)
- Thirst
- Weight loss
  >2% mild FVD
  >5% moderate FVD
  >8% severe FVD

Figure 59-16. ■ Multisystem effects of fluid volume deficit (FVD).

Manifestations

Dehydration is classified by the percentage of body weight lost. Symptoms increase in severity as weight loss increases (Figure 59-16 ■). In general, the child's pulse becomes rapid and may feel thready, the blood pressure drops, there is deceased urinary output and increased urine specific gravity, mucous membranes are dry, there is a lack of tears, skin turgor is poor, and an infant's fontanel is sunken.

Diagnosis and Treatment

Diagnosis is made by carefully examining the client's history and assessing weight loss. Laboratory data are also used in the diagnosis of dehydration. Loss of fluid from the plasma causes concentration of solutes resulting in elevation in hemoglobin, hematocrit, glucose, BUN, creatinine, and protein.

Treatment of dehydration depends on the degree of dehydration. Fluid and electrolyte replacement is essential. Fluid is replaced either orally or by intravenous infusion. Parents should develop the habit of offering water hourly, especially on hot days. Box 59-7 ■ highlights important information about fluid replacement and oral rehydration amounts by different weights in children. Commercially prepared oral replacement solutions are preferred to sweetened flavored solutions such as Popsicles, gelatin, or ginger ale.

When severe dehydration is present, the child should be hospitalized and IV fluid administered. Because children have small veins, inserting an IV needle can be a challenge. In some areas, the initiation of IV therapy is not an LPN/LVN function. However, assisting with the monitoring of the infusion might be required. The nurse must know and follow facility policy and the state's nurse practice act.

BOX 59-7   FLUID REQUIREMENTS IN CHILDREN AND ORAL REHYDRATION

Fluid Requirements

- Fluid requirements for children are calculated by weight.
- Children weighing 1 to 10 kg (2.2 to 22 pounds) should receive 100 mL/kg of fluid daily.
- Children weighing 10 to 20 kg should receive 1,000 mL plus 50 mL/kg over 10 kg per day.
- Children weighing more than 20 kg should receive 1,500 mL plus 20 mL/kg over 20 kg per day.

Oral Rehydration Amounts

- Fluids are given by mouth in small amounts frequentl; for example, 1 to 2 teaspoons (5 to 10 mL) every 10 to 15 minutes. Continue giving oral fluids even if the child vomits because some of the fluid might be absorbed.
- For mild dehydration, the child should be given 50 mL per kilogram (almost 1 fluid ounce per pound) of body weight every 4 hours plus the amount of fluid lost by vomiting and/or diarrhea during the same time.
- For moderate dehydration, the child should be given 100 mL/kg of body weight (about 2 fluid ounces per pound) every 4 hours plus the amount lost through emesis and/or stool.
- For severe dehydration, the child is hospitalized, and fluids are given intravenously.

CLEFT LIP AND CLEFT PALATE

Recall from Chapter 57 that cleft lip and cleft palate (see Figure 57-14 🔗) occur when the lip and/or palate fail to close during fetal development. Cleft lip and cleft palate commonly occur together, but can also occur separately. Cleft lip and cleft palate cause feeding difficulty in the newborn, speech impediments, and facial disfigurement.

Surgical Correction

Surgical correction of a cleft lip is generally done in the first 3 months of life. To achieve the best cosmetic effect, strain on the suture line is prevented by **Logan clamp** (a metal bow taped to each side of the suture line), or by butterfly bandages. The priority of care is to protect the suture line from infection or trauma.

Surgical correction of a cleft palate may need to be completed in stages. It is usually begun at 4 to 6 months of age and completed by age 2. As with cleft lip repair, the nurse must teach family members to prevent trauma to the suture line by avoiding putting hard or sharp objects into the child's mouth. This includes suction catheters, tongue blades, straws, forks, and toothbrushes. Once healing is complete, the child will need to be referred to a speech therapist.

GASTROESOPHAGEAL REFLUX DISEASE

Gastroesophageal reflux disease (GERD) is caused by a relaxation of the cardiac sphincter. The relaxation of the cardiac sphincter allows gastric contents to return to the esophagus.

Manifestations

Some "spitting up" is considered normal in infants, but continued regurgitation can lead to aspiration, pneumonia, or apnea. The child will appear hungry, irritable, and have a history of vomiting. She will eat, but still lose weight. GERD (see Chapter 37 🔗) is more common in premature infants and children with neurologic impairment.

Treatment

Treatment of GERD depends on the severity of the disorder. Mild cases may be treated by adding rice cereal to thicken the feedings, positioning the child upright 30 degrees after feeding, and avoiding acidic juices. Medications may be prescribed to reduce stomach acid.

Nursing Considerations

Severe cases of GERD may require surgery such as a Nissen fundoplication (see Chapter 37 🔗). A gastrostomy tube will be left in place for approximately 6 weeks. Parents will need to be taught to administer gastrostomy feedings and to care for the insertion site.

PYLORIC STENOSIS

Pyloric stenosis is an obstruction of the pyloric canal caused by a thickening of the pyloric sphincter and narrowing of the passageway between the stomach and the duodenum (Figure 59-17 ■). As the stomach tries to push food through the narrowed lumen, the mucous membrane becomes inflamed and swollen, narrowing the lumen further and eventually causing total obstruction.

Manifestations

The disorder occurs most commonly in 5-week-old firstborn boys. The child with pyloric stenosis is usually asymptomatic until 2 to 4 weeks after birth, appearing healthy but may

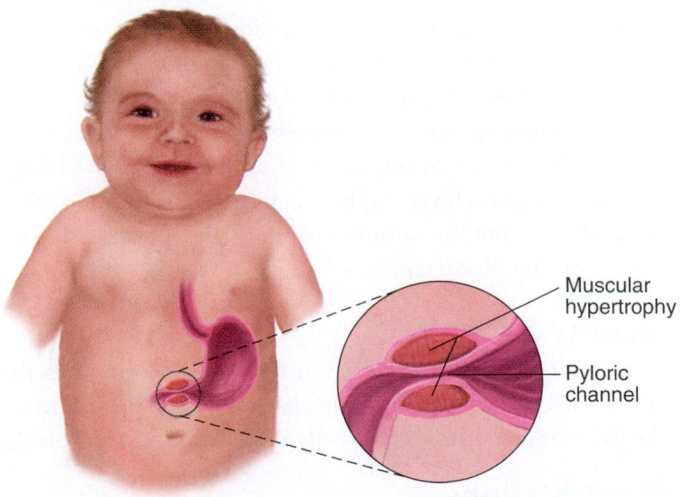

Figure 59-17. ■ Pyloric stenosis results in symptoms of projectile vomiting and visible peristalsis.

regurgitate a small amount of milk after feeding. Parents report the child to be a "good eater." As the pylorus narrows, the child begins to vomit after every feeding. Within a few weeks, there is *projectile vomiting*, and the emesis may be ejected up to 3 feet from the child. The child becomes dehydrated, loses weight, and passes fewer and smaller stools.

The child may appear irritable and uncomfortable; if severe dehydration is present, he may be lethargic. The child with pyloric stenosis becomes very ill with dehydration in just a few days. It is important for the parents to obtain medical attention right away.

Diagnosis and Treatment

A small round mass may be felt in the right upper quadrant and peristaltic waves may be seen across the abdomen.

As soon as the diagnosis is made, plans for urgent surgery are developed. Surgical correction to enlarge the pylorus (*pyloroplasty*) is the treatment of choice. The child usually recovers rapidly after surgery, with a very positive prognosis, and is usually discharged in a few days.

Nursing Considerations

Nursing care focuses on meeting the child's needs for fluids and nutrition, promoting comfort, preventing infection, and supporting the parents. Because projectile vomiting will continue until surgery, the child should be kept NPO. Intravenous therapy will be used to establish fluid and electrolyte balance. By monitoring the child's intake and output (including emesis) and urine specific gravity, the nurse can evaluate the effectiveness of therapy.

Postoperatively the child is given small amounts of clear liquid. If clear liquids are tolerated, the child will be advanced to formula or breastfeedings. To provide for the infant's comfort, acetaminophen or other analgesics are given as prescribed. Parents should be instructed to avoid pressure on the incision. When diapering the child, slide the diaper under the buttocks instead of lifting the legs. Parents should be encouraged to swaddle, hold, and rock the child.

In planning for discharge, parents should be taught the signs of incisional infection, including redness, swelling, discharge, and a fever higher than 101°F (38.5°C). The child should not be submerged in bath water until approved by the physician.

BILIARY ATRESIA

Biliary atresia occurs when the bile ducts fail to form properly or become blocked. The result is a backup of bile that destroys the liver. Biliary atresia commonly requires a liver transplant.

Manifestations

The infant appears healthy at birth, but develops jaundice in the second or third week of life. The elevated bilirubin level is accompanied by abdominal distention, enlarged liver, bruising, and itching. Because of the lack of bile, stools are an off-white color and the consistency of putty. Bilirubin is excreted by the kidneys, turning the urine tea-colored. The infant becomes malnourished and without a liver transplant will die.

Nursing Considerations

Initially nursing care is the same as for any other newborn. Parents will need to have diagnostic tests explained. As the seriousness of the disorder becomes apparent, parents and family members will need emotional support. Tepid baths may be helpful to relieve itching.

If surgery is performed, the child will need routine postoperative care. Parents must be taught the signs of tissue rejection (nausea, vomiting, fever, and jaundice) and must understand the need to report them immediately to the primary care provider.

INTUSSUSCEPTION

Intussusception happens when one portion of the intestine telescopes into another portion. The most common site for intussusception is the ileocecal valve. As telescoping occurs, the walls of the intestine rub together, producing inflammation, swelling, and obstruction. Swelling causes a decrease in blood flow to the intestine resulting in ischemia, necrosis, perforation, and hemorrhage. One of the most common causes of intestinal obstruction in children, intussusception occurs more frequently in boys between the ages of 2 months and 5 years.

Manifestations

The child with intussusception presents with sudden severe abdominal pain, vomiting, and passage of brown stool. Periods of comfort may be followed by a recurrence of pain. As the condition worsens, the stool resembles currant jelly. A palpable abdominal mass may be felt.

Diagnosis and Treatment

Diagnosis is made from the history and barium enema studies. In some cases the installation of barium moves the intestine back into place. If this does not happen, surgery will be required to reduce the telescoping bowel and remove damaged tissue.

Nursing Considerations

Nursing care focuses on managing pain, maintaining fluid balance and nutrition, and supporting parents. The child will be kept NPO and may have a nasogastric tube to suction until the bowel is returned to its normal location. Postoperative care is routine including administration of IV fluids, analgesics, and assessments. After normal bowel function returns, the child is offered clear liquids and is advanced to full feedings as tolerated.

Parents should be taught to care for the child at home including watching for infection, and administering prescribed medication. Surgery is usually successful in correcting the problem, but parents should be encouraged to seek medical attention if symptoms recur, if the child develops a fever, or if appetite decreases.

HERNIA

Some newborns have a weakness in the abdominal muscle in the area of the umbilicus, allowing a loop of the intestine to protrude. This condition, called umbilical hernia, will be discussed in Chapter 60 ⚭ along with other hernias.

COLIC

Colic, abdominal pain caused by periodic spasm of the intestines, occurs most commonly in the first 3 months of life. Infants cry loudly, pull their arms and legs up, and become red in the face. They belch and expel flatus frequently, and may spit up mucus and undigested milk or formula. The exact cause of colic is unknown, but it may be related to swallowing air during feeding, eating too rapidly, overeating, overexcitement, and an anxious mother. Colic may be relieved by picking the infant up, burping gently, and giving some warm water to drink. Colic is not serious, and most infants are healthy and continue to gain weight.

HIRSCHSPRUNG'S DISEASE (MEGACOLON)

Hirschsprung's disease (or **megacolon**) occurs when the autonomic parasympathetic nerve ganglia that cause normal peristalsis are absent. Inadequate gastrointestinal motility causes a mechanical obstruction of the large intestine.

Manifestations

Symptoms vary depending on the extent of the defect and the age of the child. The newborn may fail to pass meconium, refuse to suck, develop abdominal distention, and have meconium emesis. Older children may have a history of abdominal distention and constipation.

> ### clinical ALERT
>
> Newborns are frequently discharged from the hospital within 24 hours of birth. Parents must be taught to observe for meconium passage, abdominal distention, and vomiting. If the newborn fails to pass stool, the primary care provider must be notified.

Diagnosis and Treatment

Diagnosis is made by history, physical examination, radiographic contrast studies, and biopsy.

Treatment may include high-fiber diet, adequate fluids, stool softeners, and isotonic enemas. In more severe cases, surgery to remove the affected tissue may be necessary. At times a colostomy is performed.

Nursing Considerations

Nursing care includes careful observation of the newborn for the passage of meconium. When the child develops symptoms later in infancy, a careful history and growth patterns, nutritional intake, and bowel habits must be obtained. Parents will need instruction on administering medication, giving saline enemas, and managing a colostomy including proper drainage, skin care, and bag changing. The child must be observed for malabsorption of nutrients, poor growth, and malnutrition. Referral to an enterostomal nurse specialist and ostomy support groups may be helpful.

MECKEL'S DIVERTICULUM

Meckel's diverticulum occurs when the connection between the yolk sac and the intestine in the embryo fails to atrophy. The result is a **diverticulum** (an outpouching) in the ileum, usually near the ileocecal valve. The pouch contains gastric or pancreatic tissue that secretes acid and enzymes, causing irritation and ulceration.

Manifestations

Symptoms appear by 2 years of age. Painless bleeding (either dark stools or bright red bleeding) occurs as a result of ulceration and obstruction. Abdominal pain is unusual, but when it occurs, it may resemble appendicitis, **volvulus** (twisted bowel), or intussusception.

Diagnosis and Treatment

Diagnosis is usually based on history because the diverticulum is usually small and does not fill with contrast medium. If untreated, perforation and peritonitis could result.

Treatment involves surgical removal of the diverticulum and any damaged tissue. Once healing occurs, prognosis is good.

MALABSORPTION DISORDERS

Malabsorption disorders result from lack of nutrients in the diet, an inability of the small intestine to absorb nutrients, or liver disorders that can result in lack of bile for digestion and alter metabolism of nutrients.

Celiac Disease

Celiac disease (gluten-sensitive enteropathy or **sprue**) is a chronic malabsorption syndrome in which the child is unable to digest gluten, a protein found in wheat, barley, rye, and oats. The inability to digest gluten results in an increase in the amino acid glutamine, which is toxic to the mucous membrane in the small intestine. Over time, the intestinal villi are damaged. Initially fat absorption is affected resulting in steatorrhea (fat in the stool). Eventually absorption of protein, carbohydrates, calcium, iron, and fat-soluble vitamins is affected.

Research is being conducted to determine the existence of genetic influence in the child developing celiac disease.

MANIFESTATIONS. Symptoms do not begin until the child has ingested solid foods containing gluten, usually in the first 2 years of life. When gluten is introduced into the diet, the child experiences chronic diarrhea, vomiting, and failure to grow. The stools are large, foul smelling, greasy, and frothy.

DIAGNOSIS AND TREATMENT. Diagnosis is based on symptoms, fat content in the stool, and intestinal biopsy. The child improves rapidly when gluten is eliminated from the diet. Vitamin supplements may be prescribed if the child is malnourished. Growth patterns usually return to normal within a year.

Lactose Intolerance

Lactose intolerance is a congenital or acquired disorder in which the child fails to produce lactase, an enzyme needed to digest lactose. Lactose is found in all milk or milk products. The child rapidly develops diarrhea as soon as milk is consumed.

Giving the child lactose-free products relieves the symptoms. Soy formulas are used instead of breastfeeding or milk-based formulas. In some children adding enzyme tablets such as Lactaid to the milk or sprinkling it on food corrects the problem.

Failure to Thrive

Failure to thrive (FTT) is a general term used to describe the child who fails to gain weight or who loses weight for unknown reasons. Causes can be physical (e.g., malabsorption, heart or liver disorders) or environmental (e.g., failure to bond with parents).

MANIFESTATIONS. The FTT child may be irritable and weak. He or she may have vomiting, diarrhea, anorexia, or **pica** (ingestion of nonfood material). The child may appear apathetic or listless and exhibit "rag doll" limpness.

DIAGNOSIS AND TREATMENT. The child may be admitted to the hospital for evaluation and diagnosis. When FTT results from environmental factors, the nurse must be alert in observing parent–child relationships. These situations are complex and may take time to identify the cause. A multidisciplinary approach is usually required.

Prognosis is generally questionable. It has been documented that children who are starved emotionally can have lifelong problems including language, social interactions, and intelligence.

NURSING CARE

PRIORITIZING NURSING CARE

When caring for young children with gastrointestinal disorders, focus your care on promoting gastrointestinal function and early detection of complications. Immediately report decreased or absent bowel sounds, refusal to eat, vomiting, signs of dehydration, elevated temperature, diarrhea, and presence of blood or mucus in stools. Weigh clients daily to determine effectiveness of nutritional support. Determine foods that the child likes and can tolerate and provide those as snacks.

ASSESSING

Young children with gastrointestinal disorders should be monitored for the presence and activity of bowel sounds in all four quadrants. Question parents about the frequency, color, amount, and odor of the child's stools. Question parents about usual feeding habits and recent changes in those habits.

DIAGNOSING, PLANNING, AND IMPLEMENTING

The following nursing diagnoses may be pertinent to the care of young children with gastrointestinal disorders:

- *Deficient Fluid Volume*
- *Imbalanced Nutrition: Less than Body Requirements*
- *Risk for Infection*
- *Acute Pain* related to surgery

Nursing interventions are routine and have been previously discussed in this chapter.

EVALUATING

Postoperatively the child will be evaluated for return of normal gastrointestinal function. Signs of dehydration will subside, a normal elimination pattern will return, vomiting will stop, and the child will gain weight. Parents should be able to verbalize understanding of home care.

Endocrine Disorders

Endocrine disorders in the newborn and toddler are uncommon. Recall from Chapter 57 ⊘ that inborn errors of metabolism (such as phenylketonuria, galactosemia, Tay-Sachs disease, and maple syrup urine disease) are rare in the general population but have a high rate in isolated groups. For example, Tay-Sachs disease is common in Ashkenazi Jews whose ancestors were French Canadian or from the Louisiana bayou.

Routine testing of all newborns is recommended, especially in high-risk populations.

HYPOPITUITARISM (GROWTH HORMONE DEFICIENCY)

Growth hormone deficiency (GHD) is a decrease in growth hormone that results from injury or disease of the hypothalamus or pituitary gland, inheritance, or genetic mutation. Because decreased function of the pituitary gland results in GHD, this disorder is often referred to as **hypopituitarism.**

Manifestations

Children with GHD have normal birth weights and lengths. Growing less than 2 inches (5 cm) a year, these children fall below the third percentile in growth by 1 year of age. Children with GHD tend to be overweight. Because growth hormone affects all cells, these children also develop hypoglycemic seizures, hyponatremia, jaundice, pale optic disc, and male genital problems. They maintain youthful facial features, higher-pitched vices, and delayed skeletal and sexual maturity.

Diagnosis and Treatment

Children below the third percentile for height should be referred to a pediatric endocrinologist. It is recommended that growth hormone testing be done every 3 to 4 months.

Many children will receive subcutaneous injections of growth hormone 3 to 7 times a week for at least 1 year or until normal height for age is achieved.

Nursing Considerations

Nursing care consists of monitoring growth patterns, teaching the family about the disorder, and administering hormone replacement. Growth hormone is expensive and may not be covered by insurance. Parents may need financial assistance and resources.

Urinary Disorders

Disorders of the urinary system that affect the small child include infections, tumors, and congenital anomalies. Because the function of the urinary system is to eliminate liquid waste, disorders affecting the urinary system pose a significant risk to the health of the child. Although the reproductive system is immature until puberty, many congenital anomalies of the urinary system also affect the reproductive system as well. Review the anatomy and physiology of the urinary system. See Chapter 57 to review congenital urinary disorders, and Chapter 39 for more discussion of urinary tract disorders.

URINARY TRACT INFECTIONS

Urinary tract infections (UTIs) are a group of infections that include *cystitis* or bladder infection and *pyelonephritis* (kidney infection). Urinary tract infections can be a single acute episode or a chronic recurrent or persistent infection. In the newborn, UTIs are more common in males primarily due to structural defects. In the toddler and young child, UTIs are more common in females, usually caused by *Escherichia coli* entering the urethra and going to the bladder. The use of bubbles in the bath can cause urinary irritation and infection.

Manifestations

Signs of UTI in the newborn are less specific than in older children. Anytime a newborn presents with unexplained illness, the possibility of a UTI should be suspected. Symptoms of UTI include fever, nausea and vomiting, anorexia, strong-smelling urine, *dysuria* (painful urination), and *hematuria* (blood in the urine). In the newborn and young child who is nonverbal, dysuria may be displayed as crying during urination. The continent child may suddenly develop incontinence or hesitancy due to fear of pain. If left untreated, a UTI could progress to sepsis.

Diagnosis and Treatment

The nurse collects a sterile urine sample. Proper collection of the sample is essential to the accuracy of the findings. A clean-catch specimen may be obtained if the child is cooperative. A sterile single-use, self-adhering urinary bag or catheterization may be used to collect a sample in the incontinent child.

Treatment for UTI includes administration of antibiotics and increased fluids. The nurse must be alert to suspect a urinary tract infection anytime the child presents with an unexplained illness.

Nursing Considerations

In most circumstances, a UTI can be prevented. The parents should be taught to thoroughly clean the perineum with each diaper change. The young child who is being toilet trained should be taught to wipe from front to back. The perineum should be washed daily. Discourage the use of bubble baths and hot tubs that can irritate the urethra and increase the chance of infection.

URETHRAL MALPOSITION (HYPOSPADIAS AND EPISPADIAS)

As mentioned in Chapter 57, **hypospadias** occurs when the urinary meatus opens onto the ventral (lower) surface of the penis. **Epispadias** occurs when the urethra meatus opens onto the dorsal (upper) surface of the penis. The opening can be anywhere along the shaft or glans in males. Although diagnosis by visual inspection is usually at birth, correction might be delayed. Surgical correction may be needed.

> **clinical ALERT**
>
> Infant boys with epispadias or hypospadias are not circumcised in the neonatal period. The foreskin is preserved to use in reconstructive surgery.

HYDROCELE

Hydrocele is an accumulation of fluid in the scrotal sac (see Figure 40-20). During fetal development fluid becomes trapped in the tunica vaginalis. When the scrotum is palpated, a round, smooth, and nontender mass is noted. The scrotal sac can also be *transilluminated* (have a light shown through it) to detect the presence of fluid. Most hydroceles resolve spontaneously in the first 2 years of life. The nurse should assist the family in understanding this disorder. Parents may be concerned that the enlargement of the scrotum is permanent. The nurse provides teaching about the probable spontaneous resolution of the disorder.

OBSTRUCTIVE UROPATHY

Obstructive uropathy is a condition in which the structure or function of the urinary system is altered, resulting in obstruction of urine flow (Figure 59-18 ■). Obstructions can be congenital or acquired. A congenital cause for urinary obstruction is **polycystic kidney.** In this condition, one or both kidneys are enlarged and contain fluid-filled cysts. Acquired causes include tumors, kidney stones, and crystal formations caused by medications.

Manifestations

As urine flow from the kidney to the bladder is blocked, urine will back up causing **stasis** (pooling of urine or other body fluid in an organ). Stasis can lead to UTIs, loss of renal function, and hydronephrosis. **Hydronephrosis** is the distention of the renal pelvis caused by increased pressure due to urine backup.

Diagnosis and Treatment

The obstruction may be visualized by ultrasound or cystoscopy. Once the obstruction is diagnosed, placement of urethra or suprapubic catheter may be necessary until surgical intervention can occur. Surgical corrections include **pyeloplasty** (removal of the obstructed ureteral segment and replacement into the renal pelvis) and **valve ablation** (removal of a faulty valve).

Nursing Considerations

Preoperatively, the nurse assists in the diagnostic process and ensures that the child and family understand the condition and the prescribed treatment. Postoperatively, the nurse observes for urinary retention and fluid and electrolyte imbalances.

Upon discharge, many children will have a stent, catheter, or urinary diversion device. Parents need specific instructions on how to care for these devices, how to maintain hygiene, and when to report complications.

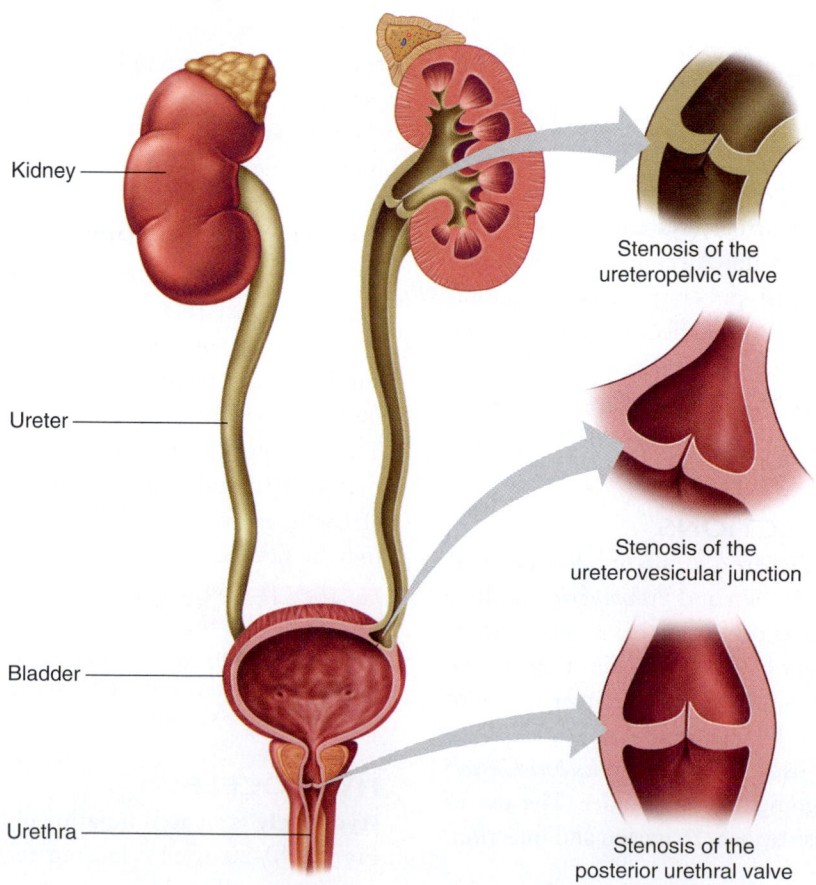

Figure 59-18. ■ The common sites of obstruction in the upper and lower urinary tract. Upper urinary tract infections are often unilateral. Renal failure is most likely to occur when both kidneys are affected by hydronephrosis.

WILMS' TUMOR (NEPHROBLASTOMA)

Wilms' tumor or **nephroblastoma** is a highly metastatic cancerous tumor of the kidney. It is most common in children between 2 and 5 years of age. Even in the absence of other anomalies, a genetic link is suggested. A gene that promotes normal kidney function is missing in a child with Wilms' tumor.

Manifestations

A child with Wilms' tumor may be asymptomatic for a long time. Commonly parents palpate an abdominal mass while bathing the child. The mass may be unilateral or bilateral. At times hematuria is present.

clinical ALERT

Do not palpate the abdomen of a child with potential Wilms' tumor. These tumors are fragile, and palpation could cause the tumor to rupture, dispersing cancerous cells throughout the abdomen.

Diagnosis and Treatment

Diagnosis is made on the basis of ultrasound. Magnetic resonance imaging of the lungs, liver, spleen, and brain is necessary to determine metastasis. These procedures are frightening to the child and parents, and thorough explanation is important. Parents are usually allowed to stay with the child during diagnostic tests.

Surgery to remove the kidney is usually scheduled as soon as possible. Follow-up chemotherapy and radiation may be necessary to ensure destruction of the tumor. If the tumor has metastasized to the other kidney or other organs, prognosis is poor.

Nursing Considerations

Due to the highly metastatic nature of Wilms' tumor, signs should be placed on the chart and head of the bed warning all healthcare providers to avoid palpating the child's abdomen. Preoperative and postoperative care follows routine protocols. Review the Pediatric Considerations box in Chapter 39 ⬤ for guidelines about caring for a child with Wilms' tumor.

The postoperative nursing care focuses on pain management and fluid balance. A large incision is needed to remove the kidney and the shift in the internal organs can cause discomfort for the child. Gentle handling is important, but the child will need encouragement to turn, cough, and breathe deeply to prevent complications.

Fluid balance should be monitored by daily weight, intake and output, and urine specific gravity. The blood pressure should be monitored to assess shock and the function of the remaining kidney.

During chemotherapy, the child should be monitored for side effects, infection, and function of the remaining kidney. Prior to discharge, parents should be taught home care and the need for continued follow-up visits. The remaining kidney needs to be protected from infection and injury. While parents may want to overprotect the child, maintaining as normal lifestyle as possible will aid in the positive development of the child.

NURSING CARE

PRIORITIZING NURSING CARE

When caring for young children with renal disorders, focus your care on maintaining kidney function and on early detection of complications. Follow orders for fluid restrictions carefully. Young children may find such restrictions difficult—use of distraction and play may help. If the child needs to increase fluid intake, determine fluids that he or she likes and offer those juices and Popsicles frequently. Assess for and report immediately elevated temperature, intake greater than output, oliguria, cloudy or malodorous urine, and hematuria.

ASSESSING

Young children with renal disorders should be assessed for intake and output. Urine should be monitored for amount, color, clarity, odor, and specific gravity. Assess the abdomen using light palpation. Assess the child for signs of dehydration or fluid excess. Monitor edema of the face and body. Monitor daily weights for evidence of fluid retention.

DIAGNOSING, PLANNING, AND IMPLEMENTING

Numerous nursing diagnoses could apply to the child with urinary disorders and his or her family. Nursing diagnoses might include:

- *Risk for Infection*
- *Excess Fluid Volume*
- *Risk for Deficient Fluid Volume*
- *Acute Pain*
- *Interrupted Family Processes*
- *Risk for Caregiver Role Strain*

Nursing interventions follow the general health guidelines presented in previous chapters of this book. Adapting these interventions to the young child will be addressed here.

- Encourage children to drink water and a variety of juices daily. Frozen fruit bars and juice can be used to increase fluid intake. *Adequate fluid intake is essential to proper kidney function. Additional fluids may be needed during times of illness, infection, and fever.*
- Follow doctor's orders for fluid restriction in children with nephrotic syndrome. *When sodium and water retention are present, fluids should be limited.*

- Administer analgesics as ordered. *Dysuria may make the child reluctant to void. If surgery is needed, the child must be medicated for comfort.*
- Provide instruction to the child and parents regarding care. Be aware of family strain and refer to RN and social worker as necessary. *The life-threatening nature of urinary disorders contributes to family strain. The long-term effects and treatment contribute to caregiver strain.*

EVALUATING

The child's condition is evaluated by blood and urine analysis, weight loss, and a return of general health. Monitor closely for side effects of medications. The function of the kidneys (or a remaining kidney) must be evaluated frequently. Report any signs of urinary infection or renal failure to the physician immediately (see Chapter 39 ⊙⊙). Repeat urine samples may be done after treatment with antibiotics to determine complete eradication of the causative organism.

Due to the strain of acute life-threatening illness on the child and family, frequent evaluation of family functioning is important. Referral to support groups and agencies may be necessary.

Reproductive Disorders

Although there are only a few reproductive disorders that affect the newborn or toddler, they cause great concern for parents and family.

PHIMOSIS

Phimosis is the inability to retract the foreskin of the penis due to a tightened prepuce. At birth the infant's foreskin is not retractable due to adhesions. As the child grows, retraction of the foreskin should occur. Complications of phimosis include **balanoposthitis** (inflammation or infection of the glans penis) and **paraphimosis** (inability to return the foreskin over the glans, causing constriction of the penis). Paraphimosis requires immediate surgical intervention to prevent ischemia and necrosis of the glans.

Phimosis is treated by circumcision. Circumcision in the older child can be traumatic and painful. The nurse can assist with anxiety-reducing techniques in the preoperative period. Chapter 56 ⊙⊙ has more information about circumcision.

CRYPTORCHIDISM

Cryptorchidism (undescended testicles) is a condition in which one or both testicles fail to descend into the scrotal sac. Descent of the testes may occur in utero or may take place by the time the infant is 3 months old. Cryptorchidism can occur due to lower testosterone levels or due to a structural defect such as short spermatic cord.

Diagnosis of cryptorchidism is made by physical examination. Findings of cryptorchidism require follow-up examination. If the testes have not descended prior to age 2, a surgical procedure (**orchiopexy**) is needed to reposition the testes in the scrotum. Children with cryptorchidism have a 35 to 50 times greater risk of developing testicular cancer. These children should be taught testicular self-examination.

Integumentary Disorders

Many disorders of the skin are apparent in the young child, including inflammation, infection, and trauma. A few will be discussed here. A full discussion of skin disorders is presented in Chapter 30 ⊙⊙. The general principles of skin care apply to the care of the young child and should be reviewed there.

NEWBORN RASHES

Rashes are very common in the newborn. Most are benign and disappear in a short time. Chapter 56 ⊙⊙ highlights and illustrates some rashes seen in the first few days of life.

DERMATITIS

Dermatitis is a general term meaning inflammation of the dermis or skin. When a foreign substance irritates the skin, the cells release histamine. Histamine causes blood vessels to dilate, resulting in redness, heat, and swelling. Itching and pain are also common. At times vesicles or blisters form, open, drain, and develop a crust. Seen at any age, dermatitis is classified by the location and cause of the irritation. Treatment also depends on the cause, but the goal is to reduce itching and prevent further trauma to the skin. Socks on an infant's hands can prevent excoriation; soothing baths and distraction may be more helpful for toddlers.

Seborrheic Dermatitis

Seborrheic dermatitis, "*cradle cap,*" or "dandruff" is inflammation of the skin of the scalp, forehead, eyelids, and cheeks. The skin becomes crusted with yellow or red patches and greasy scales are present. The scalp should be washed with a medicated dandruff shampoo. Care should be taken to avoid getting the shampoo in the child's eyes. The cheeks and eyelids can be washed with baby shampoo. Vigorous brushing with a soft baby hairbrush is helpful in removing the scales.

Diaper Dermatitis

Diaper dermatitis is caused by irritation from urine and/or stool. The diaper area becomes red, edematous, and blistered (Figure 59-19 ■). At times the diaper area can become infected with *Candida albicans*. The diaper area should be washed with mild soap and water with each diaper change. Avoid using diaper wipes because the solution may further irritate the skin. Occasionally the infant develops a reaction to disposable diapers. Changing brands of disposable diapers

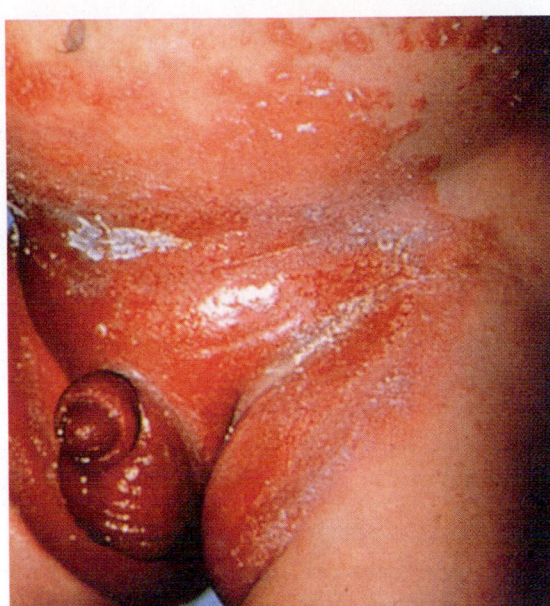

Figure 59-19. ■ Diaper dermatitis.

or using cloth diapers may be necessary. The diaper should be removed and the diaper area air dried every 2 hours. With a doctor's order, a 0.25% to 0.5% hydrocortisone ointment may be applied before any ointment to seal out moisture. An infection would need to be treated with prescribed medicated ointment.

Contact Dermatitis

Contact dermatitis is reaction of the skin to an allergen such as poison ivy, poison oak, latex, soaps, and lotions. The inflammation is usually limited to the area of contact. The area should be washed with mild soap and thoroughly rinsed. Hydrocortisone topical ointment can be applied to relieve the inflammation. If the contact dermatitis covers a large area of the body, fails to resolve, or gets worse in a short time, or if signs of infection are present, the child should be seen by a physician or healthcare provider. Contact dermatitis is discussed in Chapter 30 ⬀.

Psychosocial Disorders

Anxiety is an emotion that everyone experiences at some time in life. Subjective feelings of worry, helplessness, insecurity, and apprehension occur. Objective symptoms include tachycardia, restlessness, diaphoresis, and trembling. The child may cry and be difficult to console. Two occasions in which the newborn or toddler develops anxiety have been identified.

Stranger anxiety is common in the newborn after the age of 6 months. Recall from the lifespan chapter (Chapter 16 ⬀), the newborn is developing trust. For example, when the infant is hungry, it cries in an attempt to make its

needs known. There is a brief period of mistrust as the infant waits for satisfaction. As the mother holds and feeds the infant, the infant learns to trust her to meet needs that he or she cannot meet. Over time, the infant learns to trust and is less stressed in time of need.

When an unfamiliar person comes close to the infant, he or she does not know if the stranger can be trusted. The result is a period of anxiety for the newborn. If the parent remains close, the infant will usually calm in a short period of time.

The physical presence of parents, especially the mother, is important in helping the infant and toddler feel safe and secure. An infant or toddler experiences a state of extreme discomfort when separated from loved ones. This **separation anxiety** results in feelings of anger, fear, grief, and finally revenge. If the newborn and toddler do not learn to reduce stranger and separation anxiety and to trust their care providers, they will have more difficulty trusting others as adults.

AUTISM

According to the *DSM IV-TR* (see Chapter 49), autism is a pervasive developmental disorder characterized by "markedly abnormal or impaired development in social interaction and communication and a markedly restricted repertoire of activity and interests" (American Psychiatric Association, 2000, p. 70). Children with autism have difficulty with verbal and nonverbal communication, social interaction, and leisure and play activities (Figure 59-20 ■).

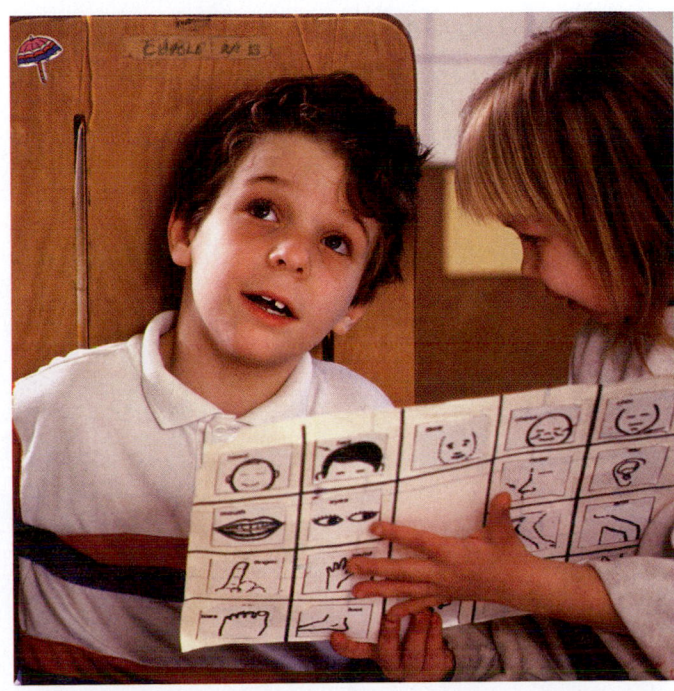

Figure 59-20. ■ Young girl assists a young boy with autism by showing him images on a board. *Source:* Photo Researchers, Inc.

Autism is found to affect boys more often than girls. There is no known cause for autism, but its incidence is increasing. It is believed to be genetically inherited. Autism is associated with congenital rubella syndrome, *fragile X syndrome* (a congenital disorder causing mental retardation), phenylketonuria, Down syndrome, and tuberous sclerosis.

Manifestations

Prior to diagnosis of autism, the infant may show a lack of response to sounds, have difficulty sleeping or sleep longer than expected, have difficult feeding, avoid eye contact, or show little to no response to human interaction. The toddler who is autistic may suddenly be unable to communicate. Words may incessantly be repeated, a condition called **echolalia.** The toddler, who is expected to have stranger anxiety, demonstrates no fear in unfamiliar surroundings or around unfamiliar people. Toilet training may also be very difficult in the toddler with autism.

Autism is marked in the child by the presence of excessive repetitive behaviors such as hand movements or rocking. These obsessive behaviors are called **stereotypy.** The child may appear stiff, unwilling to cuddle, and have an awkward gait. Repetitive sounds and loud responses to being touched are also noticed. The child is unable to interact with others socially and is often observed playing alone. Certain objects or toys have special meaning, and the child may not be able to eat, go to school, or sleep without them. The child will have either exaggerated response to pain or minimal response.

Diagnosis and Treatment

The diagnosis of autism is made by the presence of symptoms. Other disorders are often ruled out by computed tomography (CT) scans, magnetic resonance imaging (MRI) scans, lead poisoning tests, hearing tests, metabolic tests, and electroencephalograms.

Although there is no cure for autism, many researchers agree that early, intensive interventions prior to age 5 can lead to behavior modification. A highly structured environment, with one-to-one interaction is necessary. Parents and each caregiver need extensive training to promote success. Negative behaviors are discouraged by close supervision and consistency. Stimulants, selective serotonin reuptake inhibitors, and mood stabilizers may be prescribed to assist the interventions.

Nursing Considerations

It is important for the nurse caring for the child in either the outpatient or the inpatient setting to carefully determine the child's rituals and communication pattern. Children with autism pose a safety risk due to repetitive behaviors such as head banging and the lack of fear of dangerous situations. The nurse may provide devices such as helmets and hand mittens to protect the child from injury. The environment should be carefully scrutinized, modified, and supervised to promote safety. Parents should receive referrals to agencies and support groups to assist them in managing their child with autism.

Note: The references and resources for all chapters have been compiled at the back of the book.

Chapter Review

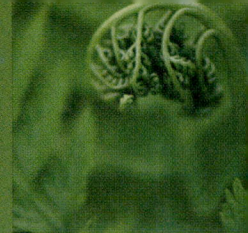

KEY Points

- Care of the newborn and toddler follows the same principles as care of adults with similar disorders. However, client teaching and emotional support must be provided to parents and family members.
- Respiratory infections and other conditions that constrict the bronchi can rapidly become life threatening due to the small airways of newborns and toddlers.
- Infants and toddlers with heart, hematologic, or immune disorders can rapidly develop congestive heart failure (CHF).
- Gastroenteritis is a common cause of hospitalization in young children. Parents and caregivers should be taught to monitor infants and toddlers closely for dehydration and electrolyte imbalance.
- Disorders of the urinary and reproductive systems in infants and toddlers often need surgery to correct anomalies.
- Disorders of the nervous system can cause physical and psychosocial abnormalities and often require long-term treatment.

⚭ FOR FURTHER Study

Communication techniques are discussed in detail in Chapter 11.

Lifespan considerations, including safety and health promotion topics, are in Chapter 16.

For directions on obtaining vital signs, see Chapter 21.

Chapter 25 provides information about nutrition at all ages; Box 25-1 is for infants.

See Chapter 30 for skin lesions that may be seen in young children.

Fractures are addressed in Chapter 31 and also in Chapter 60.

For a more in-depth discussion on respiratory disorders, see Chapter 32.

For all blood and lymph disorders, see Chapter 34.

Anaphylactic shock is discussed in Chapter 35.

Review Chapter 36 for nervous system disorders including a full discussion of symptoms and treatment of traumatic injury.

Disorders of the gastrointestinal system are discussed in Chapter 37.

For more discussion of urinary tract disorders, see Chapter 39.

Hydrocele is illustrated in Figure 40-20.

See Chapter 41 for more information on candidiasis.

Chapter 45 discusses care of the client with cancer.

Hearing testing procedures are shown in Chapter 48, Procedure 48-9.

Chapter 56 covers care and data collection for the newborn, including DDH and circumcision.

Refer to Chapter 57 for congenital malformations and high-risk disorders.

The Denver Developmental Screening Test II is shown in Figure 58-14.

Review Chapter 60 for care of the child with a hernia and for a discussion of seizure disorders.

Acute rheumatic fever is discussed in Chapter 61.

Hypertension, along with Kernig's or Brudzinski's sign, is discussed in Chapter 62.

Critical Thinking Care Map

Care of a Child with Impaired Breathing

NCLEX-PN® Focus Area: Physiologic Integrity

Case Study: Joseph, a 9-month-old infant, is admitted to the pediatric unit with a diagnosis of respiratory infection. He has a history of three episodes of bronchitis in the past 6 months. He has gained one-half pound since his last hospitalization 2 months ago. His mother states, "I don't know why he gets infections so easily."

Nursing Diagnosis: *Ineffective Airway Clearance*

COLLECT DATA

Subjective	Objective
_____	_____
_____	_____
_____	_____
_____	_____
_____	_____
_____	_____

Would you report this? Yes/No

If yes, report to: _____

What would you report?_____

Nursing Care

_____

_____

_____

_____

_____

_____

_____

_____

_____

How would you document this? _____

_____

_____

_____

Compare your answers and documentation to those provided on the MyNursingKit Website.

Data Collected
(use only those that apply)

- Crying
- T 103.2°, P 148, R 40
- Reports not knowing cause of infection
- Nonproductive cough
- No eye contact
- Weight gain
- Labored breathing
- Lung sounds wheezy
- Withdrawn
- Circumoral cyanosis
- Jaundice
- Sleepy

Nursing Interventions
(use only those that apply; list in priority order)

- Note mother–infant interaction.
- Offer milk four times a day.
- Suction airway prn or at least every 2 hours.
- Administer IV medication as ordered.
- Offer 1,000 mL of clear liquids per day.
- Mist tent.
- Administer expectorant cough syrup.
- Provide droplet precautions.
- Provide contact precautions.

NCLEX-PN® Exam Preparation

1 The nurse, working in a pediatrician's office, is caring for a 3-month-old infant when the mother asks when she can add cereal to the infant's diet. The nurse would tell the mother the best time to add food to the diet is at:

1. 3 months.
2. 1 year.
3. 6 months.
4. 9 months.

2 A 2-week-old infant is recovering from surgery for pyloric stenosis. The mother comments, "Now that the surgery is over, he should not have this sphincter obstruction ever again." The nurse's best response is:

1. "You need to talk with the doctor about your son's future."
2. "You are correct. Surgery has removed the obstruction."
3. "Recurrence of obstruction is unlikely, but we will review symptoms you should watch for just in case."
4. "While it is doubtful he will experience obstruction as a child, as an adult it is likely he will have digestive problems."

3 The child is brought to the clinic for her 6-month check-up. The nurse prepares an IM injection to update immunizations and administers the injection in the:

1. Vastus lateralis.
2. Gluteus maximus.
3. Deltoid muscle.
4. Rectus abdominis.

4 The LPN notices numerous bruises and lesions in various stages of healing while admitting a 9-month-old infant to the physician's office. The priority nursing action at this time is to:

1. Call child protection services immediately.
2. Tell the physician of the child abuse.
3. Document findings carefully.
4. Remove the child from the mother and stay with him or her in another room.

5 While caring for an infant in isolation for RSV, the priority nursing action is to:

1. Wear sterile gloves when caring for the infant.
2. Double-bag soiled diapers.
3. Have the baby wear a mask when in the playroom.

4. Wear a gown, mask, and gloves when feeding the infant.

6 A 10-month-old is admitted to the hospital with possible meningitis. An IV has been started in her left forearm and a safety reminder device is being used to prevent interference with the IV infusion. Her aunt has come to stay with her for the afternoon and asks if the device can be removed. The nurse's best response is:

1. "It can only be removed with a doctor's order."
2. "It can be removed only if you are staying in the room."
3. "It needs to be kept on at all times."
4. "It can be removed only if the nurse is in the room."

7 A 6-month-old child is receiving oxygen in a mist tent. Which of the following is a priority nursing consideration?

1. Change bedding and clothing frequently.
2. Remove the infant from the tent if restlessness occurs.
3. Keep all objects outside the tent to prevent fire hazard.
4. Open the mist tent every hour to decrease the temperature inside the tent.

8 The nurse, caring for a 4-week-old infant, would notify the physician if which of the following vital signs were obtained?

1. T 98.8 rectal, P 130, R 32, BP 78/56
2. T 100.8 ax, P 168, R 56, BP 72/52
3. T 98.2 ax, P 126, R 28, BP 73/55
4. T 98.8 rectal, P 176, R 60, BP 82/60

9 The nurse, caring for a newborn, notes that the infant has a protruding tongue, no Moro reflex, and a crease across the width of the palm. These indicators signal the presence of:

1. Profound retardation.
2. Cerebral palsy.
3. Down syndrome.
4. Sickle cell anemia.

10 The nurse is caring for a 4-year-old diagnosed with Wilms' tumor today. A priority nursing consideration for this child is:

1. Fluid and electrolyte management secondary to renal failure.
2. Protecting the abdomen from trauma or palpation.
3. Pain management.
4. Side effects of chemotherapy.

Answers and rationales for Review Questions appear in Appendix I.

Chapter 60

Care and Illnesses of Preschoolers (3 to 6 Years)

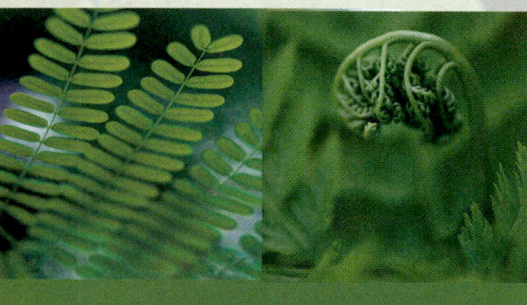

BRIEF Outline

LEARNING Outcomes

After completing this chapter, you will be able to:

1. Identify growth and development milestones for preschoolers.
2. Name elements of good nutrition and the normal vital signs ranges for preschoolers.
3. Describe respiratory and communicable disorders and appropriate care for these disorders seen in preschoolers.
4. Name cardiovascular, hematologic, or immune disorders in preschoolers and nursing care for them.
5. Identify neurosensory disorders in preschoolers and nursing care for them.
6. Describe musculoskeletal, gastrointestinal, endocrine, or genitorurinary disorders in preschoolers and nursing care for them.
7. Identify integumentary disorders seen in preschoolers and nursing care for them.
8. Describe psychosocial conditions and nursing care for preschoolers.

Clinical Objectives

9. Safely administer medications and immunizations according to age-related guidelines.
10. Monitor vital signs and compare to age-related norms.

KEY TERMS

Use the audio glossary feature on the MyNursingKit Website to hear the correct pronunciation of the following key terms.

circumoral 1679

closed reduction 1689

compartment syndrome 1689

concussion 1683

conjunctival hyperemia 1678

crabs 1699

deviated septum 1670

Duchenne's muscular dystrophy 1687

encopresis 1690

enuresis 1696

epistaxis 1670

herniorrhaphy 1691

hyperlipidemia 1695

hyperpituitarism 1695

hyphema 1686

hypoalbuminemia 1695

incarceration 1691

inguinal hernia 1691

kwashiorkor 1692

open reduction 1689

opisthotonos 1674

osteomyelitis 1690

pediculosis 1699

proteinuria 1695

rabies 1701

rickets 1692

ringworm 1699

scurvy 1692

tonsillectomy and adenoidectomy (T & A) 1671

tonsillitis 1671

umbilical hernia 1691

For this text, the preschooler is defined as the child from 3 to 6 years of age. Growth and development milestones of preschoolers are shown in Table 60-1 ■. Recall that safety issues for preschoolers were discussed in the fundamentals section of this textbook under Safety (Chapter 9 ⟲, especially Box 9-1 and the section on Restraints). Theories about preschooler development were provided in Chapter 15 ⟲. Growth and development information (on which this chapter builds) was provided in Chapter 16 ⟲.

Nutrition for the Preschooler

Children's dietary needs change when they move from being toddlers to preschoolers. They may be spending more time with others in play groups or day care, so it is important to establish habits of healthful eating.

Certain factors are important in this age group. The need for fat calories decreases between ages 2 and 3 years. Calcium needs jump from 500 milligrams before age 4 to 800 milligrams after age 4. However, an excess of milk can replace other foods the child needs, may interfere with absorption of iron, and may cause pinpoint internal hemorrhages. It is recommended that a child drink no more than a quart a day. Fiber is important starting at age 3. Table 60-2 ■ lists the recommended number of servings from each food group for children of this age.

Children who eat a variety of healthful foods probably do not need dietary supplements of any kind. Teach parents to keep sugar consumption at a minimum, letting sweets be a "once-in-a-while" snack. Also teach parents to provide nutritious, healthful snacks such as cut fruit, vegetables with humus, slices of cheese, or yogurt. These can be attractive,

TABLE 60-1	Growth and Development Milestones during Preschool Years				
AGE	PHYSICAL GROWTH	GROSS MOTOR SKILLS	FINE MOTOR SKILLS	COGNITIVE ABILITY	NUTRITION
3–6 years	Gains 3–5 lbs (1.5–5 kg)/ year. Grows 1½– 2½ in. (4–6 cm)/ year.	Climbs well. (1) Learns to ride bicycle with/without training wheels.	Draws circle, square, six-part person. Uses scissors. Ties shoes by school. Buttons.	Learns alphabet, counts. Begins to write letters, numbers. (2)	Eats three meals with snacks. Uses knife, fork, spoon.

(1) Climbs well

(2) Learns letters and numbers

TABLE 60-2	Number of Recommended Servings for Children Ages 3 to 6
FOOD GROUP	**NUMBER OF SERVINGS**
Bread, cereal, rice, and pasta	4–5 or more
Vegetables	2 or more
Fruit	2
Milk, yogurt, and cheese	3–4
Meat, poultry, fish, dry beans, eggs, and nuts	2–3

BOX 60-1   CLIENT TEACHING

Manifestations of Food Allergies

Teach parents to be aware of the following signs that may indicate a food allergy.
- Rashes, hives, and eczema
- Respiratory ailments such as sneezing, coughing, runny nose, and wheezing
- Digestive problems, including vomiting, diarrhea, and abdominal pain

nutritious alternatives to high-calorie, low-nutrition packaged snack foods.

Allergies can appear as children have access to a wider variety of foods. Most childhood food allergies can be traced back to five common foods: milk, eggs, peanuts, wheat, and soy. Shellfish, citrus fruits, and strawberries are also common causes of an allergic reaction. Teach parents about signs and symptoms of food allergies, which can range from annoying to life threatening. Box 60-1 ■ reviews common manifestations of food allergies.

When the symptoms of food allergies are severe (such as difficulty breathing), a child will most likely need testing to pinpoint the exact problem. If the allergy is confined to a single food, such as peanuts, the offending food can simply be eliminated from a child's diet, and the child can begin to learn to avoid foods containing peanuts or peanut oil. If a child is allergic to a whole category of foods (all wheat products, milk, or eggs), a registered dietitian will likely need to help plan a diet to meet nutritional needs while avoiding those foods.

Vital Signs in Preschoolers

Vital signs for preschoolers have changed somewhat from infant and toddler ranges. The normal vital sign ranges for preschoolers are reviewed in Table 60-3 ■.

TABLE 60-3	Variations in Normal Vital Signs—Preschoolers versus Adults			
AGE	**TEMPERATURE IN DEGREES CELSIUS**	**AVERAGE PULSE (RANGES)**	**AVERAGE RESPIRATIONS (RANGES)**	**BLOOD PRESSURE (MM HG)**
3–6 years	37 (oral)	80–130	20–35	70/45 to 100/64
Adult	37 (oral)	80 (60–100)	16 (12–20)	120/80

ILLNESSES AND DISORDERS

This chapter focuses on disorders that appear most often in preschoolers. The medical–surgical chapters, which provide the main discussion of individual disorders, will be cross-referenced throughout.

Respiratory Disorders

The medical-surgical treatment of respiratory disorders is provided in detail in Chapter 32 ⚮ .

EPISTAXIS

Manifestations

Epistaxis or nosebleed is common in preschool and school-age children. The anterior nares, rich in blood vessels, are the usual source of bleeding. Blood vessels suddenly rupture causing blood to drain from the nose, or down the throat. Epistaxis can be caused by a variety of circumstances such as nose picking, trauma, or dryness due to low humidity. Other causes can be allergies, forceful blowing of the nose, or infection. Frequent epistaxis can be a sign of more serious disorders such as hypertension or leukemia. If trauma is the cause of epistaxis, the child should be evaluated for a broken nose (**deviated septum**). If the septum is deviated slightly to one side, no treatment may be needed. However, if the septum is greatly deviated, surgical correction may be needed to ensure proper movement of air through the nasal passages and the drainage of mucus from the sinuses.

Diagnosis and Treatment

Diagnosis is made by obvious blood draining from the nose or down the throat. Locating the site of bleeding is more difficult. In most cases, the site of nose bleeding is the anterior septum and with treatment the bleeding stops in 10 minutes. Nose bleeding can also occur from the posterior septum. Posterior septum nosebleeds are more difficult to stop.

Emergency treatment includes applying firm pressure to the bleeding nares where the nose attaches to the maxillary bone. By pushing the outer side of the nares against the septum, blood flow is slowed and clot formation can occur. A cold cloth applied to the forehead and back of the neck can slow circulation and aid in clot formation. The child should sit with the head tipped slightly forward to keep blood from draining down the throat and into the stomach, causing nausea and vomiting. Once the bleeding stops, the child should not blow the nose for several hours to prevent a second nosebleed. If the nosebleed does not stop in 10 minutes, the child needs medical attention.

TONSILLITIS

Manifestations

Tonsillitis, inflammation of the palatine tonsils, commonly spreads from an infection in the nasopharynx through the drainage of lymphatic fluid. Infection can be either viral or bacterial in origin. The inflammation causes the tonsils to enlarge, making swallowing difficult and painful (Figure 60-1 ■). Swelling of the mucous membranes in the oral and nasal pharynx can cause closure of the Eustachian tube resulting in otitis media.

clinical ALERT

Any child presenting with an upper respiratory infection should be evaluated for otitis media. Any child presenting with otitis media should also be assessed for an upper respiratory infection. These infections often occur simultaneously.

Diagnosis and Treatment

The child with tonsillitis presents with a sore throat, fever, and general malaise. Visual examination of the throat reveals red, inflamed tonsils and mucous membranes. Pus pockets on the tonsils may be seen. A throat culture is needed to determine the causative organism. Visual examination of the tympanic membranes is also made.

If a virus causes tonsillitis, treatment is symptomatic. Acetaminophen can relieve the fever and discomfort.

Cold or frozen nonacidic fluids can soothe the throat and help prevent dehydration. Parents can be taught to make a mild saltwater solution of ¼ teaspoon table salt in 8 ounces

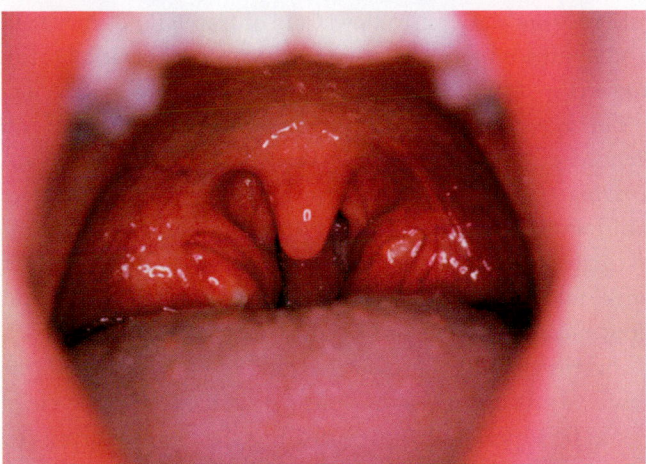

Figure 60-1. ■ Infected tonsils can swell and obstruct the airway.

clinical ALERT

Nonaspirin products should be given to children to prevent Reye's syndrome seen with the administration of aspirin products. Parents must follow the dosage recommendations on the package to prevent overdosing the child.

of warm water. Parents should show the child how to gargle with this solution.

When bacteria cause tonsillitis, antibiotics are generally prescribed. If parents do not administer all of the prescribed antibiotics, the infection may abscess, causing deeper infection and damaging underlying tissues. Some bacteria, such as beta-hemolytic *Streptococcus*, can develop into more serious infections such as rheumatic fever. Parents should be advised to seek medical attention in a timely manner.

TONSILLECTOMY AND ADENOIDECTOMY. **Tonsillectomy and adenoidectomy (T & A),** surgical removal of the palatine and pharyngeal tonsils (adenoids), may be needed when the child has frequent tonsillitis (more than 5 times a year), has continuous symptoms for more than 3 months, or has enlarged tonsils and adenoids that make swallowing difficult or that obstruct the child's airway resulting in snoring or sleep apnea.

Nursing Considerations

The parents of a child with tonsillitis need to be taught to administer antibiotics on a set schedule and to give all the prescribed doses. Often as the child improves, many fail to give the antibiotic. This can cause the infection to return.

If a T & A is to be performed, the nurse must provide preoperative teaching to the parents and child. The age and development of the child will influence the method of presentation to the child. Generally routine preoperative care will be needed. Postoperatively, the child's throat will be sore and the child may not want to swallow. Cold or frozen fluids may help to relieve discomfort and aid in preventing dehydration. Milk products are avoided because they increase mucus production.

The most common complication of a tonsillectomy and adenoidectomy is bleeding in the first 24 hours and in approximately 10 days when the scab comes off. Excessive swallowing is an indication of bleeding and should be investigated. Parents should be taught to keep the child quiet for several days to facilitate healing. The child should have soft food and liquids. Any trauma to the back of the throat will increase the risk of bleeding. For this reason, drinking straws should be avoided, and the child should be supervised while brushing the teeth. During the healing process the dark scab will turn white and slough off. The child will probably swallow the scab without notice. Until the healing is complete, the child's breath may have a strong foul odor. Gargling with mouthwash or salt-water may increase the risk of bleeding and is not recommended. Teach parents to contact the physician immediately if bleeding is noticed.

FOREIGN BODY OBSTRUCTED AIRWAY

The Heimlich maneuver is performed in a child the same as an adult. The smaller the child, the more gently the abdominal thrusts are given. Grasp the child from the back with both arms wrapped around the child's abdomen. Place the thumb of one fist and against the child's abdomen, well below the xiphoid process and slightly above the umbilicus. Place the other hand on top of the first and give a quick upward thrust. Repeat the thrusts until the object is expelled or the child loses consciousness (see Figure 59-3C ⬭).

Put the unconscious child in a supine position. Look into the child's mouth. If the object can be seen, remove it with a finger sweep taking care not to push it deeper into the airway. If the object cannot be seen, straddle the child's legs, place the heel of one hand on the child's abdomen, well below the xiphoid process and slightly above the umbilicus. Place the second hand on top of the first. Give quick upward thrusts, repeating until the object pops out or can be seen in the mouth (see Figure 59-3D ⬭). Carefully remove the object. CPR may be needed once the airway is cleared.

ASTHMA

Asthma is a chronic inflammation of the tracheal-bronchial tree. The child having an "asthma attack" has fast, labored breathing with a frequent moist cough. The child often has wheezing on exhalation, but could also wheeze on inspiration if the bronchi are severely blocked. The child may complain of chest tightness. Asthma symptoms may occur in preschoolers and may precipitate a trip to the emergency center. Although asthma may be identified in preschoolers,

it primarily affects school-aged children and so is discussed in Chapter 61 ⬭ .

PNEUMONIA

Pneumonia, infection or inflammation of the bronchioles and alveoli in the lungs, has the same manifestations and treatment for a child as it does for an adult (see Chapter 32 ⬭). However, the child's airways are smaller and are more easily occluded by bronchial swelling and mucus. Like other respiratory disorders, the first priority is to maintain a patent airway and then to relieve pain and reduce fever. The child requires constant attention. Parents will need emotional support because seeing their child in respiratory distress is frightening.

COMMUNICABLE DISEASES

Certain communicable diseases—such as measles, mumps, chickenpox, and pertussis (whooping cough)—are often called childhood diseases because of the frequency with which they traditionally have occurred in this age group. Vaccinations (Figure 60-2 ■) and booster shots can provide immunity against many of these childhood diseases. However, the diseases remain a very significant part of the overall health picture for young children. Table 60-4 ■ provides information on common communicable diseases of childhood. *Note:* As of 2008, due to the decrease in immunization of children, mumps and measles (Figure 60-3 ■) are reportable to the local health departments.

Cardiovascular Disorders

Some children with congenital heart disorders have surgery in the preschool years. Discussion of congenital heart conditions appeared in Chapter 59 ⬭ . Acute rheumatic fever is most common in children from 6 to 15 years and is discussed in Chapter 61 ⬭ . The main discussion of cardiovascular disorders is in Chapter 33 ⬭ .

KAWASAKI'S SYNDROME

Kawasaki's syndrome, an acute systemic inflammatory illness, is also known as mucocutaneous lymph node syndrome. Kawasaki's syndrome is more common in Japanese toddlers, but does affect other children as well. It is the most common cause of acquired heart disease in children and it is increasing in incidence. The cause of the disease is unknown. It usually affects genetically predisposed children, and often is preceded by a respiratory tract infection (Ball & Bindler, 2003).

Manifestations

Three distinct phases of Kawasaki's syndrome can be identified. In the acute phase, the child is admitted to the hospital

(Text continues on p. 1678.)

Recommended Childhood and Adolescent Immunization Schedule UNITED STATES • 2006

Vaccine ▼ Age ▶	Birth	1 month	2 months	4 months	6 months	12 months	15 months	18 months	24 months	4–6 years	11–12 years	13–14 years	15 years	16–18 years
Hepatitis B[1]	HepB	HepB		HepB[1]		HepB					HepB Series			
Diphtheria, Tetanus, Pertussis[2]			DTaP	DTaP	DTaP		DTaP			DTaP	Tdap	Tdap		
Haemophilus influenzae type b[3]			Hib	Hib	Hib[3]	Hib								
Inactivated Poliovirus			IPV	IPV	IPV					IPV				
Measles, Mumps, Rubella[4]						MMR				MMR		MMR		
Varicella[5]						Varicella				Varicella				
Meningococcal[6]										MPSV4	MCV4	MCV4 / MCV4		
Pneumococcal[7]			PCV	PCV	PCV	PCV				PCV	PPV			
Influenza[8]					Influenza (Yearly)					Influenza (Yearly)				
Hepatitis A[9]						HepA Series								

Vaccines within broken line are for selected populations

This schedule indicates the recommended ages for routine administration of currently licensed childhood vaccines, as of December 1, 2005, for children through age 18 years. Any dose not administered at the recommended age should be administered at any subsequent visit when indicated and feasible. ▉ Indicates age groups that warrant special effort to administer those vaccines not previously administered. Additional vaccines may be licensed and recommended during the year. Licensed combination vaccines may be used whenever any components of the combination are indicated and other components of the vaccine are not contraindicated and if approved by the Food and Drug Administration for that dose of the series. Providers should consult the respective ACIP statement for detailed recommendations. Clinically significant adverse events that follow immunization should be reported to the Vaccine Adverse Event Reporting System (VAERS). Guidance about how to obtain and complete a VAERS form is available at www.vaers.hhs.gov or by telephone, 800-822-7967.

▉ Range of recommended ages   ▉ Catch-up immunization   ▉ 11–12 year old assessment

Figure 60-2. ■ Recommended initial immunization schedule for children.

TABLE 60-4	Common Communicable Diseases of Childhood

DISEASE AND CAUSATIVE ORGANISM	CLINICAL MANIFESTATIONS	TREATMENT	NURSING CONSIDERATIONS
Hepatitis B is caused by the hepatitis B virus (HBV).	Fever, anorexia, nausea, vomiting, rash, arthralgia, pruritus, jaundice, right-upper-quadrant pain, darkening of the urine, clay-colored stools, hepatosplenomegaly.	Preventive measures: Routine screening of pregnant women, 3-dose series of immunization against hepatitis B, hand washing. Treat with bed rest, hydration, well-balanced diet, hepatitis B immune globulin (HBIG) for one-time exposure and infants born to infected mothers.	Prevent the spread of the virus by good hand washing and other standard precautions. Teach importance of a high-protein, high-carbohydrate, low-fat diet. Help child with ADLs and encourage rest. Be aware of potentially toxic effects of medications.
Diphtheria is caused by *Corynebacterium diphtheriae*.	Low-grade fever, anorexia, malaise, foul-smelling rhinorrhea, sore throat with hoarseness, stridor or noisy breathing, cervical lymphadenitis. Children with diphtheria have a thick, bluish-white to grayish-black patchy, membranous lesion that can cover the tongue, soft or hard palate, and the pharynx.	Preventive measures: 5-dose series of immunization. Treatment: Test for sensitivity to horse serum. Then administer antibiotics and antitoxins. Observe carefully for airway obstruction.	Isolate the child to prevent transmission. Watch for airway obstruction and keep oral airway equipment and oxygen available at all times. Suction as needed. Give oral liquids cautiously because of danger of choking. Provide frequent oral hygiene. Help with ADLs and encourage rest.

(continued)

TABLE 60-4	Common Communicable Diseases of Childhood (continued)		
DISEASE AND CAUSATIVE ORGANISM	**CLINICAL MANIFESTATIONS**	**TREATMENT**	**NURSING CONSIDERATIONS**
Tetanus (lockjaw) is caused by *Clostridium tetan*.	Neck and jaw stiffness, difficulty chewing, difficulty swallowing, muscle spasms stimulated by noise or touch. Spasms may progress to laryngospasm; abdominal rigidity may progress to **opisthotonos** (rigid hyperextension of the entire body). Newborns have difficulty sucking, irritability, and nuchal rigidity.	Preventive measures: 5-dose series of immunization plus booster every 10 years for life. Treatment: Wound debridement, antibiotics, muscle relaxants, tetanus immune globulin, enteral nutritional support or total parenteral nutrition. Mechanical ventilation is required.	Provide a quiet environment, reduce stimulation. Provide wound and skin care. Watch closely for laryngospasm. Keep oral airway equipment and oxygen ready at all times. Suction prn. Maintain strict intake and output. Monitor fluid and electrolyte balance.
Pertussis (whooping cough) is caused by *Bordetella pertussis*.	*Catarrhal stage:* Low-grade fever, rhinitis, sneezing, tearing of eyes, nonproductive cough lasting 1 to 2 weeks. *Paroxysmal stage:* In *children older than 6 months*, the cough becomes worse at night. The child produces a *"whooping"* (high-pitched crowing) sound while trying to expel a thick mucous plug through a narrowed glottis. Coughing episodes are very tiring. Child may become cyanotic or red faced or may vomit. The *infant younger than 6 months* has periods of apnea instead of the cough. Symptoms may last 1 to 6 weeks. *Convalescent stage:* Cough resolves gradually and may return to cough of catarrhal stage.	Preventive measures: 5-dose series of immunization. Treatment: Pertussis immune serum globulin, antibiotics, and corticosteroids; bed rest; removal of environmental factors that aggravate coughing; humidification of the environment, especially where the child sleeps; nutritional support; droplet precautions; oxygen administration.	Help child with ADLs and encourage rest. Provide ventilation and humidification of the room. Suction gently prn. Watch for airway obstruction. Have oral airway equipment and oxygen ready at all times. Monitor oxygen saturation levels, especially in the infant younger than 6 months. Initiate droplet precautions. Maintain strict intake and output. Monitor fluid and electrolyte balance.
Haemophilus influenzae type B+ (Hib) is caused by coccobacillus *H. influenzae* type B.	Manifestations include: Meningitis—sudden onset of headache, stiff neck, irritability, nausea, vomiting, fever. Epiglottitis—fever, sore throat, stridor, cough, swollen epiglottis. Pneumonia—gradual onset of fever, chills, productive cough, pleuritic chest pain. Septic arthritis—joint inflammation, stiffness, joint pain, and tenderness. Cellulitis—localized heat, redness, pain and swelling, fever, chills, headache. Sinusitis—swelling and drainage of mucous membranes, sinus pressure, tenderness and pain, headache. Otitis media—ear tenderness, pain and drainage, diminished hearing.	Preventive measures: 4-dose series of immunization against Hib. Treatment: Antibiotics for infected child and unvaccinated household members.	Initiate droplet precautions. Monitor temperature closely and implement fever-reducing strategies. Provide comfort measures specific to the condition.

TABLE 60-4	**Common Communicable Diseases of Childhood (continued)**		
DISEASE AND CAUSATIVE ORGANISM	**CLINICAL MANIFESTATIONS**	**TREATMENT**	**NURSING CONSIDERATIONS**
	Bronchitis—productive cough, fever, back pain. Pericarditis—fever, substernal chest pain, dyspnea, nonproductive cough.		
Poliomyelitis is caused by poliovirus.	Fever, headache, nausea, vomiting, abdominal pain, neck and back pain. May progress to tremors of the extremities, positive Kernig's and Brudzinski's signs, hyperactive deep tendon reflexes (DTR), paralysis, and respiratory distress. Progressive permanent paralysis, muscle atrophy, and/or severe arthritis are possible results.	Preventive measures: 4-dose series of immunization. Treatment: Bed rest, pain management, respiratory support if necessary, physical therapy with the goal of restoring mobility.	Initiate droplet precautions. Observe closely for respiratory distress. Keep oral airway equipment and oxygen ready at all times. Help child with ADLs and quiet activities to promote rest. Administer pharmacologic and nonpharmacologic pain relief measures. Promote good body mechanics such as proper body alignment and passive or active range-of-motion exercises.
Measles (*rubeola*) is caused by *Morbillivirus*.	High-grade fever, enlarged lymph nodes, malaise, coryza, cough, photophobia, conjunctivitis, *Koplik's spots* (small, irregular red spots with a bluish-white center appearing on the buccal mucosa). Two to 4 days after the onset of these symptoms, the child develops a red maculopapular, pruritic rash that spreads from the face to the trunk and extremities. The rash changes to brown in color, and eventually sloughing (*desquamation*) occurs.	Preventive measures: 2-dose series of immunization, plus booster now recommended for the adolescent. Treatment: Immune globulin to susceptible person up to 6 days after exposure. Bed rest. Antipyretics, anitpruritics, cough suppressants, and antibiotics for secondary infections.	Initiate droplet precautions. Help child with ADLs and encourage rest. Monitor lung sounds. Suction as needed. With high fever, implement seizure precautions. Provide skin care, especially when sloughing occurs, and frequent oral care. Limit environmental lighting and possibly television.
Mumps (*parotitis*) is caused by *Rubulavirus*.	Low-grade fever, headache, malaise. An earache soon develops accompanied by unilateral or bilateral swelling of the parotid gland. The male child may develop *orchitis* (unilateral or bilateral inflammation of the testes accompanied by pain).	Preventive measures: 2-dose series of immunization plus booster injection now recommended for the adolescent. Treatment: Analgesics and antipyretics. Corticosteroids may be used.	Initiate droplet precautions. Administer pharmacologic and nonpharmacologic pain relief measures. Assist child with nutritional intake of liquid or soft foods. Avoid sour foods, which intensify pain. Maintain intake and output. Monitor fluid and electrolyte balance.
Rubella (German measles or 3-day measles) is caused by an RNA virus.	Low-grade fever, headache, malaise, coryza, enlarged lymph nodes. *Forschheimer spots* (erythematous pinpoint lesions of the soft palate) also possible. After 1 to 5 days, a pink, maculopapular rash begins on the face and spreads down the trunk. It disappears in the same order.	Preventive measures: 2-dose series of immunization plus booster injection now recommended for the adolescent. Treatment: Antipyretics.	Initiate droplet precautions for the hospitalized child. Prevent contact with rubella nonimmune pregnant women. Implement comfort measures.

(continued)

TABLE 60-4	Common Communicable Diseases of Childhood (continued)		
DISEASE AND CAUSATIVE ORGANISM	**CLINICAL MANIFESTATIONS**	**TREATMENT**	**NURSING CONSIDERATIONS**
	NOTE: A fetus exposed to the rubella virus may be born with congenital rubella syndrome, characterized by intrauterine growth retardation, hepatosplenomegaly, thrombocytopenia, and dark purplish skin lesions.		
Varicella (chickenpox) caused by varicella-zoster virus.	Low-grade fever, malaise, headache, mild abdominal pain, and irritability. 24 hours later the child experiences an outbreak of pruritic macules that progress from papules to fluid-filled vesicles. Lesions begin on the trunk, scalp, and face, spreading to the remainder of the body, including the mouth, eyes, and perineum. Scarring can develop. The fetus exposed to the varicella virus during pregnancy may be born with congenital varicella syndrome, characterized by IUGR, skin scarring, limb underdevelopment, eye defects, brain defects, and death.	Preventive measures: Varicella immunization any time after 12 months of age. Treatment: Antipyretics, antihistamines, and acyclovir to reduce the number of lesions for immunocompromised children. Varicella-zoster immune globulin many also be given to immunocompromised children.	If the child is hospitalized, implement droplet and contact precautions. Prevent contact with varicella nonimmune pregnant women. Provide skin care. Soothing baths with baking soda or oatmeal can be suggested. Keep child's fingernails short to prevent secondary infections from scratching. Avoid products containing aspirin because of connection of aspirin use during a varicella outbreak to Reye's syndrome.
Pnuemococcal infection is caused by *Streptococcus pneumoniae*.	Manifestations include: Meningitis—sudden onset of headache, stiff neck, irritability, nausea, vomiting, fever. Pneumonia—gradual onset of fever, chills, productive cough, pleuritic chest pain. Otitis media—ear tenderness, pain and drainage, diminished hearing. Bacteremia—fever of unknown origin.	Preventive measures: 4-dose series of immunization. Treatment: Antibiotics, primarily penicillin and antipyretics.	Monitor intake and output. Encourage fluid intake. Watch for signs and symptoms of respiratory distress.
Influenza is caused by Orthomyxoviridae.	Abrupt onset of fever, chills, cough, malaise, muscle aches, headache, anorexia, nausea, vomiting, diarrhea.	Preventive measures: Annual immunization against influenza. Treatment: Nonaspirin antipyretics and antivirals.	Initiate droplet and contact precautions. Encourage fluids to prevent dehydration. Assist the child with ADLs and promote rest.
Hepatitis A is caused by the hepatitis A virus (HAV).	Fever, anorexia, nausea, vomiting, rash, arthralgia, pruritus, jaundice (in less than 5% of cases).	Preventive measures: 2-dose series of immunization. The first dose can be given at 12 months and the second dose at least 6 months later. Good hand washing, especially following diaper changes. Proper cleaning of changing surfaces and disposal of soiled diapers. Treatment: Bed rest, hydration, well-balanced diet, hepatitis A immune globulin for one-time exposure.	See previous measures for hepatitis B.

TABLE 60-4	Common Communicable Diseases of Childhood (continued)		
DISEASE AND CAUSATIVE ORGANISM	**CLINICAL MANIFESTATIONS**	**TREATMENT**	**NURSING CONSIDERATIONS**
Erythema infectiosum (*fifth disease*) is caused by human parvovirus B-19.	*Stage 1*—fever, chills, headache, malaise, body aches. *Stage 2*—1 week later, a bright red rash appears on face and looks as if the child has been slapped. Circumoral pallor is also present. One to 4 days later, a lacy, erythematous, maculopapular rash appears on the trunk and limbs, progressing proximal to distal. *Stage 3*—rash begins to fade but can reappear if the skin is irritated, as by the sun. If fetus is exposed to the virus, fetal death may occur.	Preventive measures: Avoid contact with infected children. Treatment: Antipyretics and analgesics.	Provide skin care. Soothing baths with oatmeal or baking soda can be suggested. Protect from exposure to sunlight.
Exanthem subitum (*sixth disease* or roseola) is caused by herpesvirus type 6.	Sudden onset of high-grade fever. The child may play normally and have a good appetite during the 3 to 4 days of high fever. The fever disappears abruptly and a pale, pink, maculopapular rash appears on the trunk and spreads to the face, neck, and extremities. The rash lasts 1 to 2 days. Exanthem subitum occurs mainly in children ages 6 to 36 months.	Treatment: Antipyretics. Hospitalization is rarely necessary.	Observe closely for febrile seizures. Teach signs and symptoms to parents. Encourage oral intake of fluids.
Mononucleosis is caused by the Epstein-Barr virus (EBV). Also called *infectious mononucleosis*, glandular fever, or the kissing disease.	High-grade fever that can last 3 to 6 days, chills, headache, anorexia, malaise, abdominal pain, left shoulder pain, sore throat, lymphadenopathy, hepatosplenomegaly, weakness, and lethargy, which can last several months.	Preventive measures: Avoid contact with known infected people. Treatment: Bed rest, corticosteroids for tonsillar swelling, antipyretics for fever, and analgesics for pain.	Assist the child with ADLs and quiet activities to promote rest. Teach that child must avoid contact sports or rough play for 4 weeks (or until hepatosplenomegaly subsides) because of risk of liver and spleen rupture. Encourage adequate hydration. Tell older adolescents to avoid kissing until several days after the fever has subsided to prevent transmission.
Streptococcus A (strep throat) is caused by group A streptococci (GAS). Strep A also causes impetigo, scarlet fever, scarlatina, and rheumatic fever.	High-grade fever and chills with sudden onset, sore throat, dysphagia, malaise, headache, abdominal pain, anorexia, vomiting. Upon inspection, the pharynx appears bright red with white exudates. Cervical lymph nodes are tender. In toddlers, there may be a moderate temperature, rhinitis, irritability, and anorexia, not accompanied by sore throat.	Preventive measures: Avoid contact with infected people. Treatment: Analgesics, antipyretics, antibiotics—penicillin is the drug of choice. If allergic to penicillin, child is given erythromycin.	If hospitalized, implement droplet precautions. Provide a soft diet. Offer saltwater gargles. Teach importance of taking entire prescribed antibiotic regime. Teach parents to replace toothbrush because organism may reside there.

(continued)

TABLE 60-4	Common Communicable Diseases of Childhood (continued)		
DISEASE AND CAUSATIVE ORGANISM	**CLINICAL MANIFESTATIONS**	**TREATMENT**	**NURSING CONSIDERATIONS**
	Scarlet fever: Fine erythematous rash beginning on neck and spreading to trunk and extremities, appearing 12 to 48 hours after onset of symptoms. In 3 to 5 days, the rash begins to fade while the tips of the fingers and toes begin to peel. The tongue develops palatal petechiae (called "strawberry tongue").		
Streptococcus B is caused by group B or beta streptococci (GBS).	Newborn symptoms include: Early onset: Usually occurs within the first 24 hours of life: respiratory distress, apnea, and signs of shock. Meconium-stained fluid may be seen at birth. Late onset: Between 1 and 4 weeks, the newborn may develop lethargy, fever, anorexia, and bulging fontanels. Later effects include blindness, deafness, mental retardation, learning disabilities, and death.	Preventive measures: Screening of pregnant women for GBS at 35 to 37 weeks. Intrapartum administration of ampicillin if mother tests positive, to reduce the risk of newborn infection. Treatment: Antibiotics, particularly ampicillin and gentamycin.	Observe closely for symptoms of respiratory distress. Keep the infant warm and free from drafts. Chilling increases the risk of respiratory distress. Closely monitor intake and output.

Source: Adapted from Adams, E. A., & Towle, M. A. (2009). *Pediatric nursing care.* Upper Saddle River, NJ: Prentice Hall.

with fever, **conjunctival hyperemia** (an increased amount of blood in the conjunctiva), red throat, strawberry red tongue, swollen hands and feet, rash, and enlarged cervical lymph nodes. The acute phase lasts for several weeks. As the child progresses from the acute to the subacute phase, the skin on the lips, hands, and feet peels off (Figure 60-4 ■). The child experiences joint pain. The heart is affected by thrombosis, large aneurysms of the coronary arteries, and myocardial infarction. High doses of immunoglobulin in the first 10 days of fever may reduce the incidence of these complications. In the third phase, the child gradually progresses through convalescence with a decrease of inflammation. Most children recover fully, but damage to the heart is permanent and can lead to complications later in life.

Treatment

In the acute phase, take the child's temperature every 4 hours and administer large doses (80 to 100 mg/kg/day) of aspirin as ordered. Due to the antiplatelet action of aspirin, it is important to assess for bleeding. Monitor the conjunctiva, oral mucosa, and skin every 8 hours for increasing edema, spreading of the red rash, and peeling of the skin. Assess the child for signs of dehydration and malnutrition. Auscultate the heart every 4 hours for abnormal sounds and rhythm.

Nursing Considerations

Kawasaki's syndrome is very uncomfortable. Provide all care as gently as possible. It is important to keep the linen clean, dry, and free of wrinkles. Provide oral care using foam applicators to decrease trauma and bleeding of the gums. Bathe with cool water to decrease fever. A bed cradle may be needed to keep the linen off the sensitive skin.

Fluid balance can be maintained by administering IV fluids. It may be difficult for the child to eat due to irritation of the oral mucosa. Soft foods of moderate temperature should be offered.

Activity is important to prevent complications of bed rest. However, periods of rest are also important to prevent cardiac complications. The child may be reluctant to move due to swollen, painful joints. Turn the child every 2 hours and provide passive and active range-of-motion exercises to prevent skin breakdown and respiratory complications. Administer analgesics before activity to help keep the child comfortable.

All procedures should be explained to the child and family. Encourage parents to hold and rock the child, thus providing a sense of security. Teach them to provide care at home including the administration of and side effects of medications.

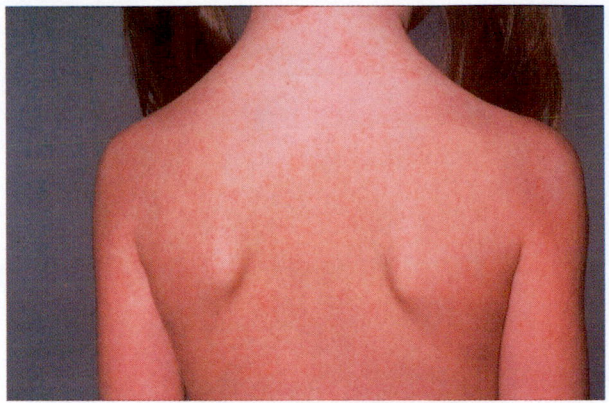

A

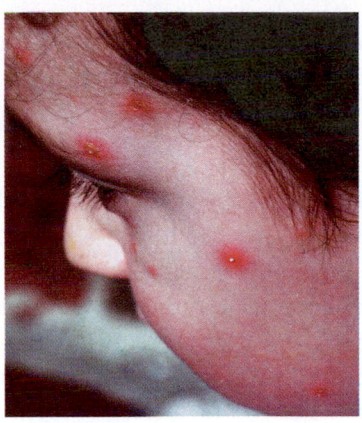

B

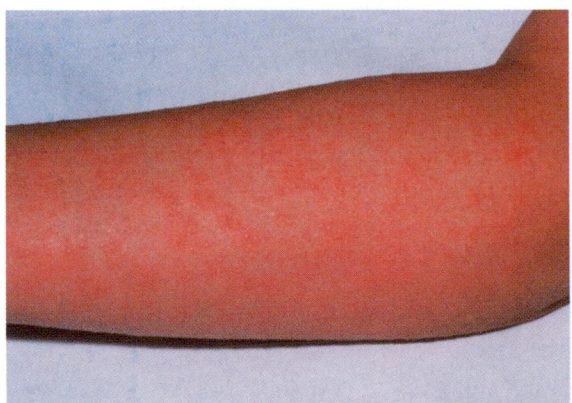

C

Figure 60-3. ■ **A.** Measles rash. **B.** Chickenpox lesions. **C.** Scarlet fever rash. (A: NMSB/Custom Medical Stock Photo, Inc. B: © Patrick J. Watson C. Photo Researchers, Inc.)

NURSING CARE

PRIORITIZING NURSING CARE

The care of the young child with cardiovascular disorders is similar to the care of the infant or toddler. The focus of care must be maintaining a patent airway, ensuring adequate circulation, and pain management. Vital signs including pulse oximetry should be monitored at least every 2 hours.

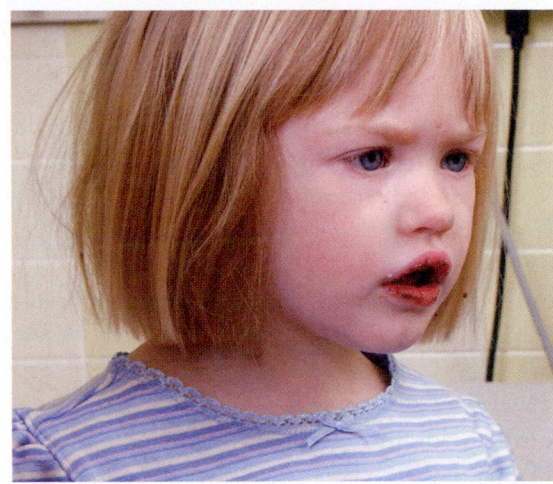

Figure 60-4. ■ This child has returned for one of her frequent follow-up visits to assess her cardiac status after treatment for Kawasaki's syndrome. Notice the lips that show inflammation, cracking, and peeling.

Oxygen saturation less that 90% should be reported to the RN. Monitor closely for signs of organ failure such as elevated BUN and liver enzymes as well as shortness of breath, nausea and vomiting, or diarrhea. Closely monitor intake and output for signs of fluid deficit or fluid overload.

ASSESSING

Young children with cardiovascular disorders must be assessed for heart and lung sounds (see Table 33-3 🔗 for heart sounds), peripheral circulation, shortness of breath, weakness, fatigue, and activity tolerance. Cyanosis, either generalized or **circumoral** (around the mouth), can be constant or seen only with activity such as playing or eating.

DIAGNOSING, PLANNING, AND IMPLEMENTING

The following nursing diagnoses may be appropriate for the young child with a circulatory disorder:

- *Acute Pain*
- *Risk for Imbalanced Nutrition: Less Than Body Requirements*
- *Risk for Imbalance of Fluid Volume*
- *Risk for Infection*
  - *Compromised Family Coping*
  - *Risk for Activity Intolerance*
- *Deficient Knowledge*

The goals of care for children with circulatory disorders include prevention of infection, fluid maintenance, and administration of medications as ordered.

- Apply principles of first aid to control bleeding. *Controlling bleeding is a priority of nursing care.*

- Take vital signs frequently during times of bleeding or illness. *The child's condition can change rapidly in times of stress and crisis.*
- Observe the child for signs of organ failure including but not limited to pain, neurologic deficit, respiratory distress, vomiting, diarrhea, constipation, and renal failure. *Lack of circulation damages organs and can lead to organ failure.*
- Monitor intake and output. IV fluids may be ordered. *Adequate fluids are needed to keep the blood thin. IV fluids are always administered to children by infusion pump to prevent accidental fluid overload.*
- If certified, administer blood as ordered and following facility policy. *Blood replacement may be needed to maintain blood volume, red blood cells, and hemoglobin. In some states LPNs/LVNs cannot administer blood or blood products, but may assist with monitoring vital signs and observing for complications.*
- Encourage a balanced diet with adequate iron, protein, and vitamins. Supplements may be needed. *Adequate nutrients are needed to produce red blood cells, maintain tissue integrity, and maintain fluid balance.*
- Provide child and family teaching regarding home care including medication administration and side effects, diet, injury prevention, specific symptoms of complications, and prescribed treatment. Adapt teaching for the child using models, charts, videos, or other devices, according to developmental level (see Chapters 12 and 16 🔗). Teach frequent hand washing, skin care, and avoiding infected people. *Many circulatory conditions are treated at home. Patient and family need to understand good health practices to prevent complications.*
- Provide emotional support for both child and family. *Many circulatory conditions are long term and often life threatening.*

EVALUATING

Young children with circulatory disorders should be evaluated for fluid balance, signs of infection, and side effects of medication. Parents should be able to verbalize and demonstrate needed home care prior to discharge. Because many circulatory disorders can be long term and life threatening, therapeutic communication is valuable in evaluating the child's and family's emotional status. See Chapter 11 🔗 for communication techniques. Evaluation of normal growth and development patterns is important.

Hematologic Disorders

The main discussion of blood and lymph disorders is in Chapter 34 🔗. Please review disorders there for further depth.

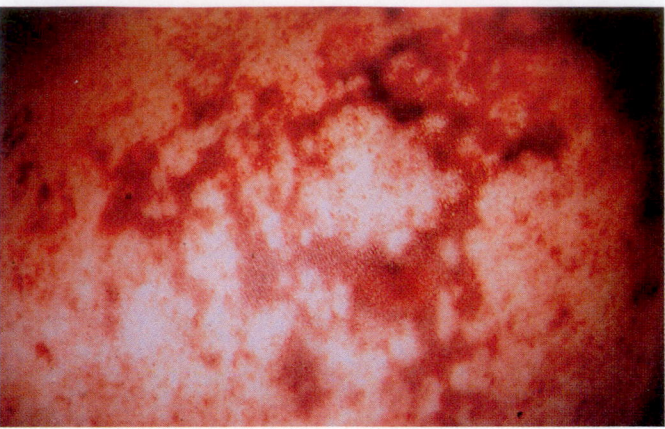

Figure 60-5. ■ Nonpalpable purpura with bleeding into the tissue below the skin. (Courtesy of the Department of Hematology/Oncology. Children's Medical Center, Washington, DC.)

IDIOPATHIC THROMBOCYTOPENIA

Idiopathic thrombocytopenia is a bleeding disorder of unknown cause that leads to a decrease in the number of platelets. Thrombocytopenia is more common in children between the ages of 2 and 5 years. Frequently the child had a recent viral infection such as chickenpox or rubella. Symptoms include *purpura* (a rash in which blood cells leak into the skin; Figure 60-5 ■), *petechiae* (pinpoint microhemorrhages under the skin), and *ecchymosis* (larger hemorrhages into the skin). The disorder may spontaneously go into remission. If the disorder continues long term, a splenectomy may be performed with some success in controlling the disorder. Nursing care would include controlling bleeding and teaching the child and family measures to decrease risk of bleeding.

Immune Disorders

The immune disorders are discussed in depth in Chapter 35 🔗.

ORGAN TRANSPLANTATION

Organ transplantation involves the surgical removal of donated organs or tissue from one person (or animal) and in implantation of the organ or tissue into another person. Blood transfusion may also be considered a form of tissue transplantation. It is important to recognize that some religious groups oppose organ, tissue, or blood transplantation. Parents may refuse consideration of such surgeries for their children (Box 60-2 ■).

ORGAN DONATION

Organs and tissue can come from live or deceased donors or animals. Blood, skin, bone marrow, and kidneys can be donated from a living human or animal in the case of skin grafting. Organs necessary for life, such as the heart, lungs,

BOX 60-2   CULTURAL PULSE POINTS

Religious Beliefs Related to Organ Donation

- The **Amish** will consent to organ transplant but believe that it is God who ultimately heals.
- **Baptists** have adopted resolutions to encourage physicians to use organ transplantation to save lives and to encourage the public to be willing to donate their organs and tissues.
- **Buddhists** call organ transplantation a matter of individual conscience and an act of compassion.
- **Christian Scientists** rely on spiritual rather than medical healing. They do not have any specific statements regarding organ transplantation and consider this issue a matter of personal choice.
- **Episcopalians** promote organ and tissue transplantation and donation. The church relates this act of kindness to the life of Jesus Christ who gave his life so that others may live.
- **Hindus** believe that organ transplantation is an individual decision and that it is ethical to use body parts to alleviate the suffering of other humans.
- **Jehovah's Witnesses** allow organ transplantation as long as all of the blood is drained from the organ or tissues prior to transplantation and any blood transfused is autologous blood, taken from the organ recipient prior to surgery.
- **Judaism** encourages organ transplantation. In 1992, the Rabbinical Council of America (Orthodox) stated that the *pikuach nefest*, an ancient requirement to save lives if possible, promotes organ donation despite Jewish laws that forbid mutilation of the body.
- **Lutheran** doctrine states that organ donation is a humanitarian act and an expression of sacrificial love for one's neighbor.
- **Roman Catholics** consider organ transplantation an act of charity. In 1990, Pope John Paul II made a statement in favor of organ donation in the form of living tissues or from those who are deceased.
- **Seventh-Day Adventists** strongly promote organ transplantation and the religion runs transplant hospitals. One example is Loma Linda University Medical Center in southern California, which specializes in pediatric heart transplantation.
- **United Methodists** encourage organ donation and transplantation. Their 1992 resolution further states that prior to harvesting the organs, death must be determined by a reliable source and there should be no measure to hasten death. The religious organization encourages their pastors to discuss organ donation as a routine part of their hospice care.

liver, pancreas, kidneys, and corneas, are harvested from a person who is declared brain dead or who have recently died. Declaration of brain death must be confirmed by clinical signs and medical testing.

Donors must be screened for compatibility, which may take some time to complete. Parents must be contacted regarding organ donation prior to the child's death. Many facilities have nurses trained in obtaining organ donors. Consents must be signed by the parents during this extremely emotional time. The nurse can be supportive in stressing the positive contribution their child is making for another sick child.

ORGAN RECIPIENT

The recipient of organ transplantation requires careful preoperative and postoperative care. Preoperatively, the child will need to be evaluated to determine the physical and psychological readiness for transplantation. Most children, and their families, wait a long time to receive an organ transplant. The child will receive immunosuppressive drugs to prevent organ rejection. The child will be in a carefully controlled environment to prevent exposure to infections. Once an organ is found, the family may be so excited that they forget the organ may not function properly.

Postoperative care includes both physical and emotional support. Fear of organ rejection may lead to psychological reactions similar to posttraumatic stress syndrome. Following surgery, the nurse will be responsible for evaluating the return and maintenance of function of the transplanted organ as well as providing routine postoperative care. For example, the child who received a kidney transplant should be evaluated for return of kidney function, urinary output, and fluid balance.

Rejection of the transplanted organ is a major concern. Rejection can occur in minutes, hours, days, or months after surgery. The nurse must constantly be alert for signs of rejection, and teach the parents to monitor for signs of rejection.

clinical ALERT

Signs of rejection include laboratory values outside the normal range and lack of improvement of clinical symptoms related to the disease process prior to surgery.

Rejection may require additional immunosuppressant drugs or removal of the transplanted organ. The child is also at great risk for infection and the nurse must be diligent in observing for symptoms and reporting them promptly.

Nervous System Disorders

Nervous system and sensory disorders are discussed in most depth in Chapter 36 .

SEIZURES

Seizures are periods of sudden discharge of electrical activity in the brain that cause involuntary muscle activity, change in level of consciousness (LOC), or altered behavior and sensory manifestation. Seizures may be the result of genetic factors; pathologic conditions such as tumors, trauma, infection, or toxins; or a rapid elevation in temperature above 102°F (39°C). Seizure activity can be isolated events or the result of *epilepsy*, a chronic disorder characterized by repeated seizure activity.

Manifestations

Partial or focal seizures are caused by abnormal electrical activity in a specific area of the brain. Focal seizures most commonly involve the temporal, frontal, or parietal lobes of the cerebrum. Common symptoms include a momentary blank stare, facial movement, or hearing abnormal sounds. There is no loss of consciousness with focal seizures. Generalized seizures result from diffuse electrical activity that begins in one area of the brain and spreads to involve the entire cerebral cortex and brainstem. General seizures begin with a tonic phase in which the child loses consciousness and has continuous muscle contractions. This is followed by a *clonic phase* characterized by alternating muscle contraction and relaxation. Some seizures are preceded by an *aura* or recognizable sensation that signals a seizure is about to occur. A *postictal period* of confusion, sleepiness, slurred speech, poor coordination, or headache is common following a generalized seizure.

Diagnosis and Treatment

An electroencephalogram (EEG) is used to detect abnormal brain activity. During a seizure, the first priority is to establish a safe environment for the child, including protecting the head and extremities from trauma. The child should not be restrained, but the head and extremities should be protected from hitting furniture, side rails, or the floor. Nothing should be put into the child's mouth during a seizure. The child will not breathe during the seizure, so *circumoral* cyanosis is common. Note and document the body part where the seizure began, the specific movements or behavior, eye movements, and pupil response.

Nursing Considerations

Immediately following the seizure, position the child on the side, remove mucus and drainage from the airway, and assess for airway patency (Figure 60-6 ■). Oxygen may be needed. The child may have been incontinent of urine and stool, so skin care may be needed. After the seizure, check neurologic function including LOC, pupil response, equal bilateral movement and strength, and signs of injury if a fall occurred during the seizure. Remain with the child until he is fully conscious and able to maintain his airway. If appropriate for age, question the child regarding the presence of an aura.

Medications may be prescribed to prevent further seizure activity. Depending on the cause and the number of seizures, medication may be prescribed long term. It is

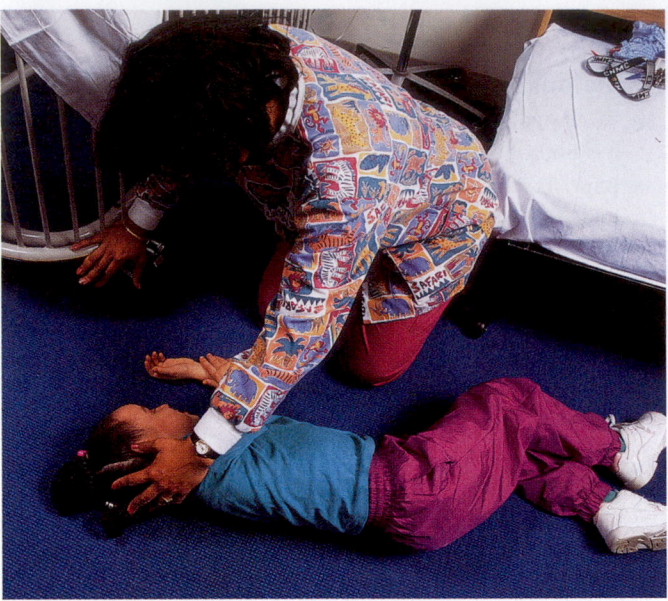

Figure 60-6. ■ A child who has a seizure when standing should be gently assisted to the floor and placed in a side-lying position. The area around the child should be cleared of any objects that might injure the child.

important to administer medication on time to maintain therapeutic levels. The child should be watched closely for repeated seizure activity until therapeutic levels of medications are established. Periodic blood tests may be ordered to evaluate the therapeutic level of antiseizure medication. Seizure precautions, including padding side rails and having suction equipment available, should be implemented for all children who have had a history of seizures or who are at risk for seizures.

Seizure activity can be frightening for the parents and family. Remain calm during the seizure to inspire confidence and provide support to the family. Parents should be taught to care for the child at home, including care during and after a seizure, as well as administration and side effects of medications. Parents, fearful for their child's safety, may become overprotective. With treatment, most children can have an active life, and parents should be encouraged to help their child develop normally.

NEUROLOGIC TRAUMA

Recall from Chapter 59 ⊂⊃ that closed head injury is a result of head trauma, either from an external force such as a fall, or an internal force, such as shaking the child hard enough for the brain to strike the inside of the skull. Closed head injury in the 3- to 6-year-old child is often trauma from falling or an automobile crash.

Children from ages 3 to 6 are increasingly mobile. They are learning to ride a tricycle and climb on playground equipment. Mobility brings an increased risk of falls and

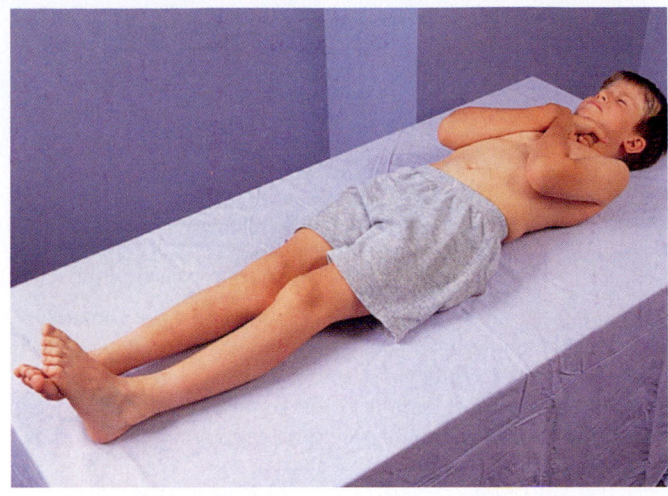
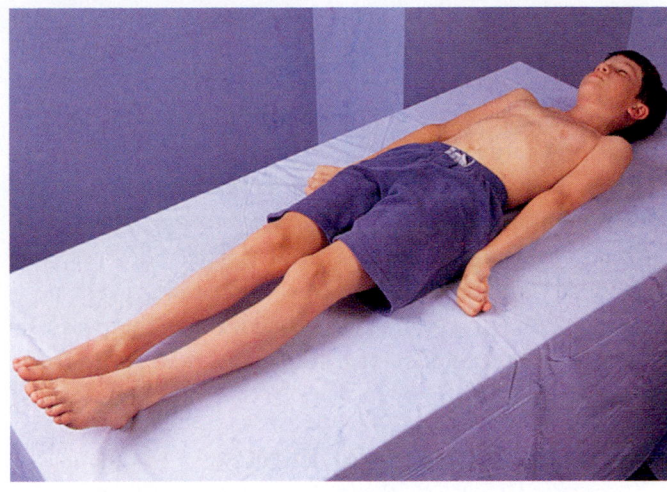

A   **B**

Figure 60-7. ■ **A.** *Decorticate posturing,* characterized by rigid flexion, is associated with lesions above the brain stem in the corticospinal tracts. **B.** *Decerebrate posturing,* distinguished by rigid extension, is associated with lesions of the brain stem.

closed head injury. Parents must be taught to prevent closed head injury by insisting that children wear a helmet when riding tricycles and bicycles. Playground equipment must have approved ground cover under the equipment, such as a thick layer of bark. This material provides a cushion should a fall occur, where a fall on cement or asphalt can result in greater trauma.

The extent of neurologic damage depends on the nature and degree of trauma. Temporary neurologic impairment, called a **concussion,** is due to stretching, compressing, or tearing the nerve fibers near the brain. The symptoms of a concussion include confusion or loss of consciousness, nausea, vomiting, headache, dizziness, and amnesia. If blood vessels are torn, the result is a hematoma, or blood trapped within the brain tissue. Hematomas can be located between the skull and the dura (epidural), between the dura and the brain (subdural), or intracerebral (inside the cerebrum) (see Chapter 36 ⚭).

Symptoms of an intracranial hematoma include those of a concussion as well as increased intracranial pressure, which include decreasing level of consciousness (LOC), fixed dilated pupils, decorticate or decerebrate posturing (see Figure 60-7 ■), altered reflexes, and seizures.

Drowning or near drowning results in hypoxic or anoxic neurological trauma to the brain. Children lose consciousness within 4 to 5 minutes after submersion. Neurologic and circulatory impairment occur within 5 to 10 minutes following submersion. The type and temperature of the water can affect the manifestations of drowning and ultimately the outcome. Figure 60-8 ■ illustrates the pathology of near drowning in fresh- or saltwater. If the water temperature is near freezing, the child's metabolism can slow to the point where tissue damage is reduced.

Manifestations

Clinical manifestations vary depending of the degree of damage. The child should be assessed for altered LOC, pupil response to light, and movement and sensation of all extremities. Review Glasgow Coma Scale in Table 19-2 ⚭ . To obtain accurate readings of LOC, the child is not given analgesics or sedatives.

Nursing Considerations

Nursing care of a child with neurologic trauma involves maintaining a patent airway, frequently assessing for change in neurologic status, and maintaining skin integrity if the child is immobilized for long periods of time. Fluid and electrolyte balance, nutrition to meet the body needs, and adequate elimination of waste are all important needs for the child.

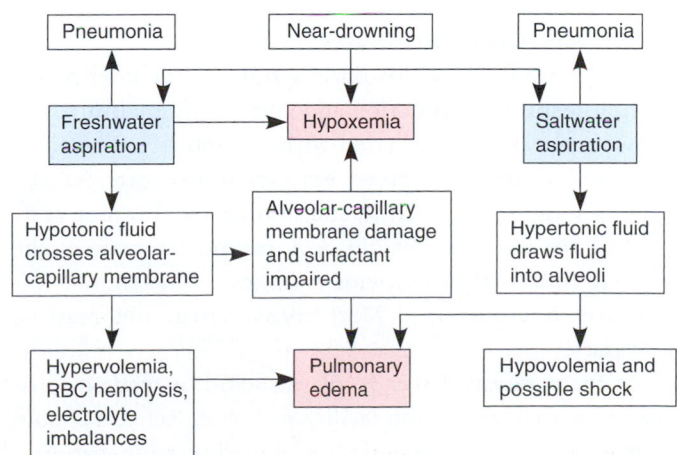

Figure 60-8. ■ Flow chart of near drowning in fresh- or saltwater. Note the electrolyte imbalances that can occur.

Parents will need to vent their feelings of anger and guilt. Care must be provided in a nonjudgmental manner. Parents may need assistance in deciding to take a comatose or neurologic impaired child home, or to place the child in a long-term care facility.

Prevention of neurologic trauma is an essential component of family and community teaching. The use of car seats, safety helmets, playground safety devices, and water safety are just a few measures that can prevent neurologic trauma. The nurse must be aware of the possibility of abuse as the cause of trauma, and take appropriate measures.

GUILLAIN-BARRÉ SYNDROME

Guillain-Barré syndrome (postinfectious polyneuritis) is a rare disorder characterized by ascending and then descending paralysis. It can be an acute viral infection such as *Campylobacter jejuni*, cytomegalovirus, or Epstein-Barr virus. It has also been associated with the administration of vaccines.

Manifestations

Guillain-Barré syndrome begins with pain and weakness in the lower extremities. Over a period of several days, muscle weakness and paralysis progresses upward to involve the abdomen, chest, upper extremities, and head. The paralysis can stop at any point and regress. Respiratory function may be severely compromised. The child may have difficulty swallowing and talking. Autonomic dysfunction can lead to hypertension, cardiac dysrhythmia, diaphoresis, and bowel and bladder incontinence.

Diagnosis and Treatment

Diagnosis is made on the basis of symptoms, lumbar puncture, and electroconduction tests.

Medical treatment and nursing care is supportive until the paralysis resolves in 2 to 4 weeks. Rehabilitation may be necessary to regain muscle strength.

Nursing Considerations

Nursing care for Guillain-Barré syndrome includes maintaining respiratory function and preventing malnutrition and complications associated with immobility. The child and family must be given emotional support. As the paralysis ascends, the child and family may become fearful that the child might die. A nurse must remain at the bedside constantly to provide emergency care should respiratory function stop. Mechanical ventilation may be necessary.

As the paralysis descends, plans should be made for discharge to a rehabilitation facility or home. Referral should be made to a home care nurse, social worker, and rehabilitation specialist. With aggressive rehabilitation, children usually recover with few permanent defects.

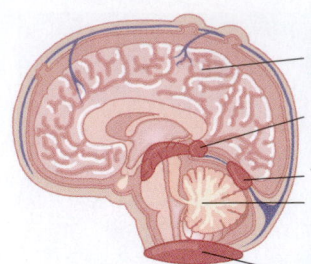

Supratentorial tumors (**cerebral astrocytoma, ependymoma**, optic nerve gliomas)
Tentorial notch tumors (pineal region tumors, hypothalamic glioma)
Tentorial tumors
Infratentorial tumors (**brainstem gliomas, medulloblastoma**, cerebellar astrocytoma, ependymoma)
Foramen magnum tumors

Figure 60-9. ■ Sites of brain tumors in children. Approximately 1,500 children under the age of 15 years are diagnosed annually as having tumors of the brain and central nervous system. **Boldface** indicates the four most common brain tumors in children: medulloblastoma, cerebral astrocytoma, ependymoma, and brainstem glioma.

BRAIN TUMORS

Brain tumors are the most common solid tumor in children and the second most common malignancy after leukemia. Figure 60-9 ■ illustrates the most common sites for brain tumors in children.

Manifestations

Brain tumors manifest differently depending on the type and location of the tumor. Table 60-5 ■ identifies the symptoms and medical treatment of the common brain tumors in children. Subtle changes that the nurse must watch for include slight behavior change, poor school performance, and change in coordination. Tumors in the area of the hypothalamus or pituitary gland can manifest as diabetes insipidus (see Chapter 38 ⬮⬮) or growth abnormalities.

Diagnosis and Treatment

Presenting symptoms are identified and tumor is confirmed with CT scan or MRI. A lumbar puncture may be used to identify malignant cells in the cerebrospinal fluid. Bone scan and bone marrow aspiration are used to detect metastasis. To help determine a tumor growth rate, ask parents if the symptoms developed slowly or in a matter of a few weeks.

Treatment of brain tumors includes surgery, radiation, and chemotherapy. The goal of treatment is to destroy as many tumor cells as possible with minimal complications. The use of laser surgery, improved radiation, and chemotherapy agents have improved prognosis for many types of brain tumors. Complications of treatment include infection, seizure activity, hydrocephalus, growth problems, and neurologic deficits.

Nursing Considerations

Care of a child with a brain tumor requires the knowledge and skill of oncologists, neurosurgeon, and the pediatrician. The nurse coordinates with the dietitian, social worker, and physical and occupational therapists in managing the

TABLE 60-5	Brain Tumors by Location		
TUMOR	**ETIOLOGY**	**MANIFESTATIONS**	**TREATMENT**
Medulloblastoma	External layer of cerebellum	Headache, vomiting, ataxia	Surgery; chemotherapy with lomustine, vincristine, prednisone, cisplatin; radiation
Astrocytoma	Glial cells, supratentorial or infratentorial	Seizures, visual disturbances, increased intracranial pressure, vomiting	Surgery; chemotherapy with vincristinec, dactinomycin; radiation
Ependymoma	Fourth ventricle; posterior fossa	Hydrocephalus	Surgery; radiation
Brainstem glioma	Pons	Cranial nerve (VI + VII) tract signs: nystagmus, ataxia, motor symptoms	Surgery; radiation

child's care. When possible, parents are taught to provide care in the home. Follow-up examinations must be made. A diagnosis of brain tumor is very frightening for both parents and child. The nurse must provide emotional support as well as referral to other support groups.

Sensory Disorders

As the child ages, growth in the eye can result in vision changes. It is important for young children to have a visual examination every year. It is common for children to need corrective lenses. Care must be taken to select safety lenses and frames to prevent injury should an accident occur.

Many newborns are screened for hearing. Repeated otitis media can rupture the tympanic membrane and affect hearing. Also, some young children are prone to impacted *cerumen* (earwax). The nurse may need to irrigate the ear to remove a buildup of cerumen. Procedure 60-1 ■ provides steps for performing ear lavage.

If the preschool child exhibits signs of hearing impairment, hearing screening by a trained audiologist is recommended.

ACUTE CONJUNCTIVITIS

Acute conjunctivitis, commonly called *pinkeye* (Figure 60-10 ■), is the inflammation of the conjunctiva caused by bacteria, virus, or allergies. Bacterial and viral conjunctivitis are contagious and easily transmitted among children.

Manifestations

Symptoms of conjunctivitis include eye irritation, photophobia, redness, inflammation, and watery or purulent drainage. Conjunctivitis caused by allergy may be accompanied by pruritus.

Diagnosis and Treatment

The drainage can be cultured to assist in determining the origin of the infection. Treatment for bacterial conjunctivitis includes ophthalmic antibiotics. Antiviral agents may be ordered for viral infections. Antihistamines are used for allergic reactions. Comfort measures include cool compresses.

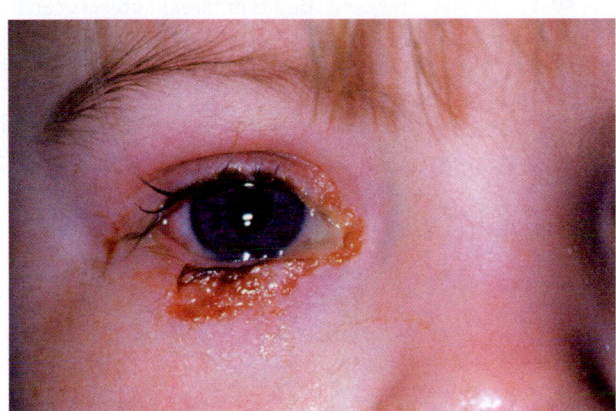

Figure 60-10. ■ Acute conjunctivitis. The discharge from bacterial conjunctivitis is purulent discharge and may cause crusting. The discharge from viral conjunctivitis is serous (watery). Allergic conjunctivitis produces watery to thick drainage and is characterized by itching.

Nursing Considerations

The nurse should teach parents how to perform eye hygiene and administer eye medication. The child should not go to school or day care while the infection is present.

EYE INJURY

Injury to the eye causes intense pain, excessive tearing, light sensitivity, and vision changes. Prompt treatment is required to prevent permanent damage. Eye injury is classified as penetrating or nonpenetrating.

Penetrating Injuries

Penetrating injuries to a child's eye are typically caused by a toy, pencil, or other sharp object. If the object remains in the eye, it should be removed only by an ophthalmologist or eye surgeon after the child is sedated. If damage to the eye is excessive, the eye may need to be removed.

Nonpenetrating Injuries

Nonpenetrating injuries include corneal abrasion, foreign object trauma that does not penetrate the eye, hyphema, and chemical burns. To remove a superficial foreign object from the eye, grasp the eyelashes of the upper lid and

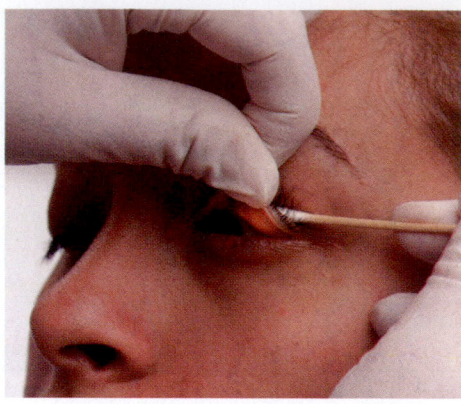

Figure 60-11. ■ Small pieces of debris or foreign objects can be visualized more readily by rolling the eyelid up over a cotton swab.

stretch downward. Place a cotton-tipped applicator in the center of the eyelid and pull the eyelid up and over the applicator (Figure 60-11 ■). Remove the object with another moist cotton-tipped applicator. A large amount of water or saline eye irrigation can be used to wash the object from the eye. Eye irrigation is used for a chemical burn to the eye to flush out as much of the causative agent as possible.

HYPHEMA

Hyphema is hemorrhage into the anterior chamber of the eye. Hyphema is caused by a blow to the eye usually from a blunt object such as a baseball. Both of the child's eyes are patched and the child is placed on bed rest to prevent increased intraocular pressure and to allow for reabsorption of the blood from the anterior chamber.

NURSING CARE

PRIORITIZING NURSING CARE

When caring for young children with nervous system disorders, focus your care on promoting adaptation to client's limitations and providing emotional support to the family. If the client is having seizures, promote safety during the episodes, time the seizures, and provide support after the seizure. Encourage the child to do as much as possible in activities of daily living and play. Praise all progress, however small. Encourage family to give appropriate positive reinforcement to the child for showing progress. Allow family members to openly discuss their fears and concerns regarding the child. Refer to appropriate support groups.

ASSESSING

Young children with nervous system disorders should be assessed for changes in level of consciousness, reaction to stimuli, and ability to respond with normal behaviors. They must be monitored closely for signs of seizures.

Increased intracranial pressure can be manifested by projectile vomiting.

> ### clinical ALERT
>
> Neurologic deterioration can occur rapidly in young children. Changes in baseline vital signs and level of consciousness must be recorded and reported immediately.

DIAGNOSING, PLANNING, AND IMPLEMENTING

The following nursing diagnoses may apply to the young child with a nervous system disorder:

- *Ineffective Airway Clearance*
- *Risk for Deficient Fluid Volume*
- *Grieving (Parent)*
- *Risk for Injury* related to impaired mobility
- *Impaired Verbal Communication*
- *Bathing, Feeding, Dressing, Toileting Self-Care Deficit*
- *Disturbed Body Image*

Nursing interventions for some of these nursing diagnoses were discussed previously in this chapter and will not be repeated.

- Adapt communication techniques for cognitive ability not chronological age. *Neurologic disorders can delay or regress cognitive ability. At times cognitive development stops and may never show normal progression.*
- Allow the child to do as much for herself as possible. Provide assistance and encouragement toward self-care. Encourage the family to allow the child as much independence as possible. Complete any care the child or family is unable to perform. *The amount of self-care is dependent on the degree of neurologic damage. Allowing the child to complete as much self-care as possible fosters independence and self-esteem. Completing any care the child is unable to complete is essential to health maintenance.*
- Provide factual information to the child and family to assist in dealing with disturbed body image. Allow the young child expression of feelings through puppet play. Include other specialists such as a physical therapist, occupational therapist, and speech therapist as needed. *Young children may not perceive disfigurement to the same extent as family members. Nursing care should focus on the family as the primary support for the child.*

EVALUATING

Evaluate airway patency by assessing color, oxygen saturation, and respirations. The effectiveness of seizure medications is evaluated by recording the number, frequency, and type of seizures that occur. Evaluate for respiratory infection, malnutrition, constipation, and skin break-down due to altered mobility, especially in the child with cerebral palsy. Watch family interaction with the child to determine the degree of acceptance of physical and mental limitations of the child.

Musculoskeletal Disorders

The musculoskeletal disorders are discussed in the medical-surgical unit, Chapter 31 ⟲⟳.

MUSCULAR DYSTROPHY

Muscular dystrophy is a group of inherited diseases that cause muscle degeneration and wasting. There are several kinds of muscular dystrophy, but the most common form affecting children is **Duchenne's muscular dystrophy.** This sex-linked recessive disorder is carried by mothers and passed to their sons. The onset of symptoms occurs in the first 3 to 4 years of life.

Manifestations

The child with muscular dystrophy generally appears normal for the first year, but walking may be delayed. The child gradually gains enough muscle strength to walk, but tires easily especially when running or climbing. As muscles degenerate over time, the child falls frequently, develops a waddling gait, and may walk on the toes. A classic symptom is a positive Gowers' maneuver: The child uses the upper extremities to lift himself up from the floor. Figure 60-12 ■ illustrates a positive Gowers' maneuver. Most children are wheelchair bound by age 12. Death from respiratory paralysis usually occurs during adolescence.

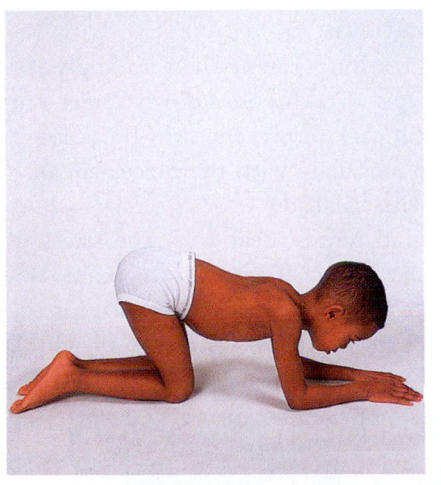

A

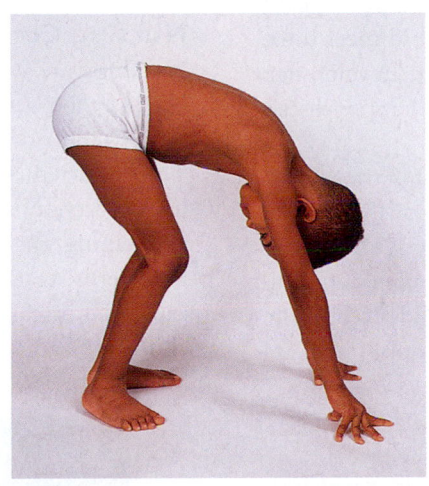

B

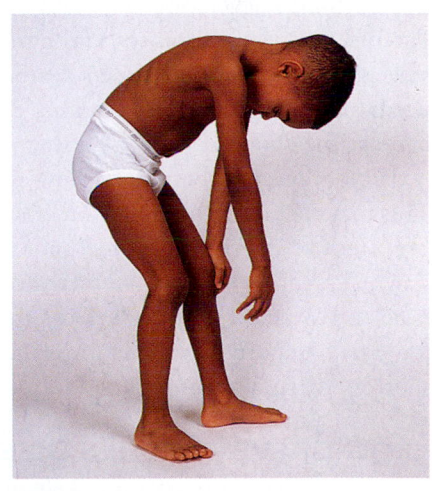

C

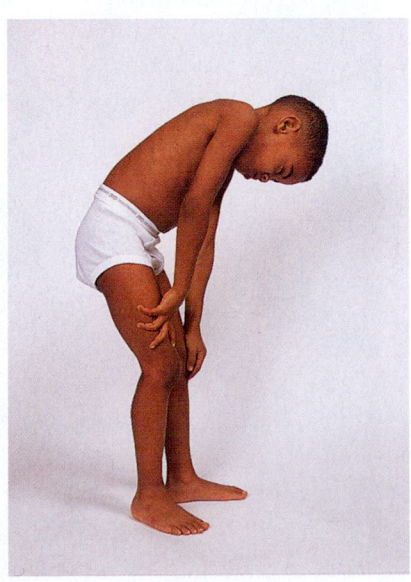

D

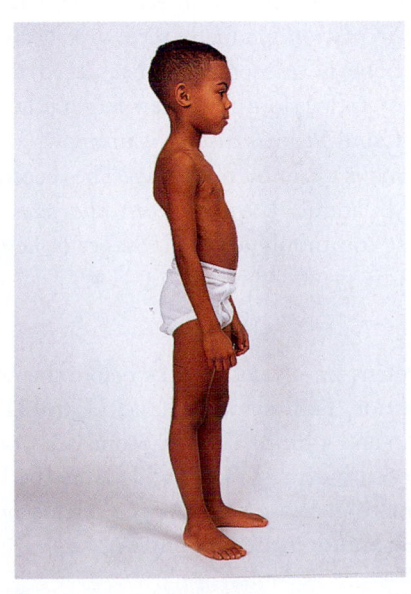

E

Figure 60-12. ■ Gowers' maneuver in a child with muscular dystrophy. **A.** and **B.** The child first maneuvers to a position supported by arms and legs. **C.** The child pushes off the floor and rests one hand on the knee. **D.** and **E.** The child pushes the body up straight.

In examining the child with muscular dystrophy, the calf muscles appear to hypertrophy, but they are actually enlarged due to infiltration of fatty tissue. As the chest muscles waste, the child will develop scoliosis, respiratory difficulty, and the inability to sit upright. Swallowing may be affected, leading to respiratory infection and malnutrition.

Diagnosis and Treatment

Diagnosis is made by clinical symptoms, an elevated serum creatine kinase, muscle biopsy, and electromyography. There is no effective treatment for muscular dystrophy.

Nursing Considerations

The goal of care is to promote independence for as long as possible and to support the family in dealing with this progressive, incapacitating, and ultimately fatal disease.

The child's development should be assessed periodically. Parents, teachers, therapists, and nurses should meet to devise plans to meet the child's learning and development needs. The focus should be on what the child *can do* instead of what the child *cannot do*.

Parents need to be taught how to care for their child. This may include administration of medications, tube feeding, signs of infection, and methods to prevent skin breakdown. Parents will need a great deal of support and will need to be taught how to support their child. It is, therefore, very important to refer the family to appropriate resources and support groups.

LEGG-CALVÉ-PERTHES DISEASE

Legg-Calvé-Perthes disease is a skeletal disorder in which the circulation to the femoral head dies from lack of circulation to the femoral head. Circulation gradually returns as healing occurs. The necrotic bone is reabsorbed and replaced with vascularized granulation tissue, forming a new femoral head.

The cause of Legg-Calvé-Perthes disease is unknown, but a history of mild trauma is a common finding. The disorder can be unilateral or bilateral. Boys between the ages of 4 and 8 years are most commonly affected. Stages of Legg-Calvé-Perthes disease are provided in Box 60-3 ■.

Manifestations

Symptoms may be present for several months before the parents seek medical attention. Early symptoms include mild hip and anterior thigh pain and a limp. The symptoms are worse with activity and relieved with rest. The child favors the leg by limiting movement to decrease pain. As the disease progresses, muscle wasting and decreased mobility occur.

Diagnosis and Treatment

The medical diagnosis is made by reviewing symptoms, x-rays, bone scans, and MRI scans.

BOX 60-3	FOUR STAGES OF LEGG-CALVÉ-PERTHES DISEASE

1. Femoral head becomes more dense with possible fracture of supporting bone.
2. Fragmentation and reabsorption of bone occurs.
3. Reossification happens when new bone has regrown.
4. Healing takes place when new bone reshapes.

Stage 1 takes about 2 to 6 months, stage 2 takes 1 year or more, and stages 3 and 4 may go on for many years.

Medical treatment is directed at relieving pain and holding the femoral head in place while healing occurs. The femoral head is held abducted with internal rotation by use of a Toronto or Scottish-Rite brace (Figure 60-13 ■). These braces hold the hip in place and support the weight of the child on the ischium. The child should wear the brace 23 hours a day.

Nursing Considerations

Nursing care involves teaching parents how to apply the braces, monitor for signs of skin breakdown under the braces, and provide skin care to prevent skin breakdown. The child will learn to ambulate with the brace, but may need crutches to help with balance.

Helping the child and family deal with the stress of long-term treatment may be a challenge for the nurse. Because the disease occurs at a time of high activity for the child, the limitations of the brace cause stress to the child,

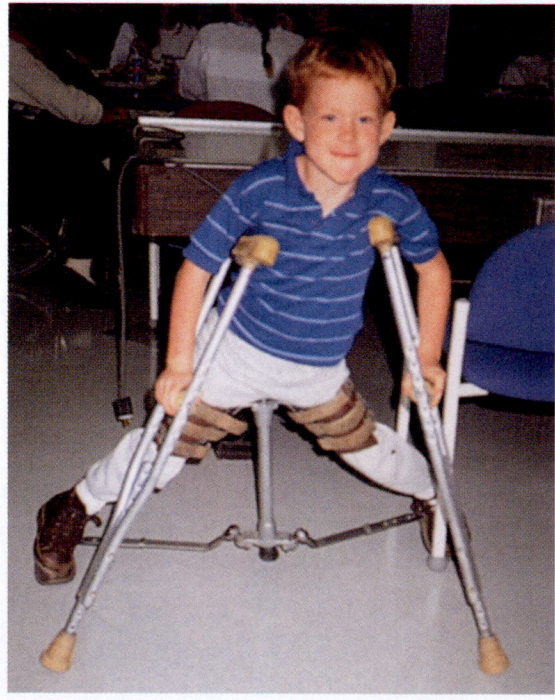

Figure 60-13. ■ Toronto brace used for Legg-Calvé-Perthes disease. This young boy needs to use crutches to be able to walk in the Toronto brace for treatment of this disease.

and subsequently the parents. The child should return to school as soon as possible.

Follow-up visits are arranged at regular intervals to evaluate the healing process and make adjustments to the brace as the child grows. Toward the end of treatment, the child may be allowed periods of limited exercise without the brace. Activities such as swimming can increase muscle strength without stressing the growing bone. Prognosis is good as long as the femoral head is contained. If treatment is delayed or the child and family are not compliant with the treatment plan, there is a high probability of permanent deformity and arthritis later in life.

MUSCULOSKELETAL TRAUMA

Sprains and Strains

Musculoskeletal trauma can occur in the form of muscle strains, sprains, dislocated joints, or fractures of bones. The main discussion of sprains and strains is in Chapter 31 ⚭. Procedure 47-1 ⚭ describes steps in applying a splint for sprains or strains.

Fractures

A fracture results from an injury that causes the continuity of the bone to be altered. Fractures are a common occurrence in childhood due to the active nature of children.

MANIFESTATIONS. Signs of a fracture vary depending on the type of fracture and the location. Generally, pain, abnormal positioning, edema, discoloration, and abnormal movement characterize fractures. The common locations are clavicle, tibia, femur, radius, and ulna.

When assessing the injured child, be alert for the possibility of fractures. The area should be immobilized to prevent further injury. The child, parents, and family should be questioned to determine the cause of the injury. The area of injury should be inspected for broken skin; circulation, including pulse and bleeding; and normal sensation. If the skin has been broken, bleeding should be controlled and sterile dressings applied.

DIAGNOSIS AND TREATMENT. Diagnosis of fracture is made by viewing x-rays of the affected injury. When fractures involve the epiphysis, they can disrupt the growth process. Figure 60-14 ■ illustrates the Salter-Harris classification of fractures and shows which types of fractures can cause the greatest threat to normal growth.

The goal of medical treatment is to reduce or realign the fracture, immobilize the bones until healing has occurred, and manage pain. The fractured bones can be realigned by **closed reduction** (manually moving the bones into alignment) or **open reduction** (surgically aligning the bone and stabilizing the ends with nails, plates, or screws). Sometimes traction is used to immobilize the unstable bone ends (see Procedure 31-1 ⚭). Figure 60-15 ■ illustrates the

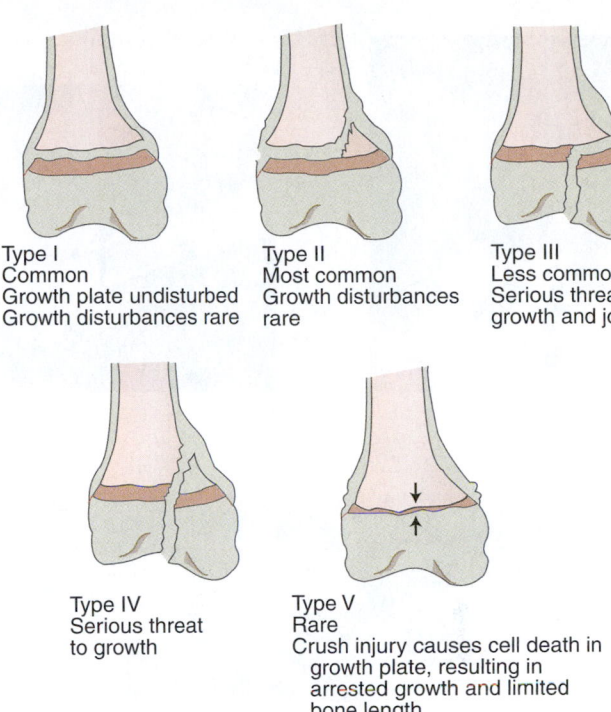

Type I
Common
Growth plate undisturbed
Growth disturbances rare

Type II
Most common
Growth disturbances rare

Type III
Less common
Serious threat to growth and joint

Type IV
Serious threat to growth

Type V
Rare
Crush injury causes cell death in growth plate, resulting in arrested growth and limited bone length
If growth plate is partially destroyed, angular deformities may result

Figure 60-14. ■ Salter-Harris classification system for fractures involving the epiphyses (growth plates).

common types of traction used for children. A plaster or plastic cast may be used to immobilize the fractured bone. Lightweight, removable casts may be used for small children. Procedure 60-2 ■ provides cast care for children.

Crutches may be needed for mobility. Procedure 60-3 ■ gives steps for fitting crutch height for children.

POSSIBLE COMPLICATIONS OF FRACTURES. The care of the child with traction or cast is the same as for an adult. The nurse must be alert for the development of compartment syndrome in the child with a cast. **Compartment syndrome** occurs when increased pressure in a limited space compromises circulation and nerve innervation, leading to possible necrosis.

clinical ALERT

Symptoms of compartment syndrome include:

Paresthesia
Pain/pressure
Pallor
Paralysis
Pulselessness

Deep pain unrelieved by analgesia, lack of sensation, and edema suggest compartment syndrome and should be reported immediately. The cast should be altered or removed promptly to prevent permanent damage to underlying tissue.

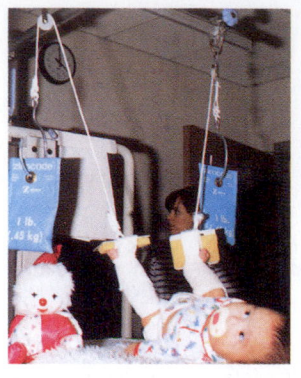

A

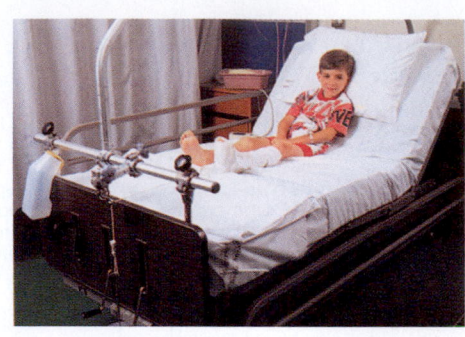

B

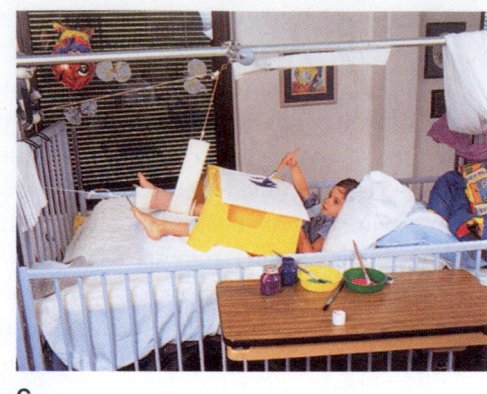

C

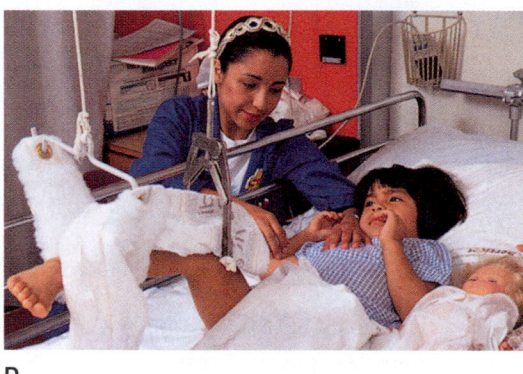

D

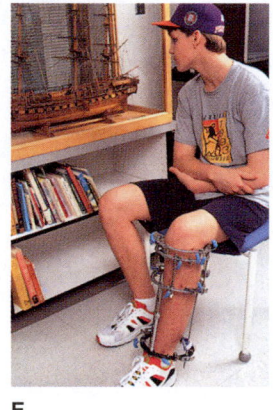

E

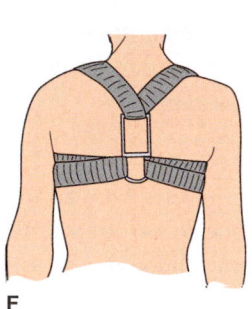

F

Figure 60-15. ■ Types of traction used for children **A.** Bryant traction. **B.** Buck traction. **C.** Russell traction. **D.** 90-90 traction. **E.** External traction (external fixator device). **F.** Clavicle strap for stabilizing clavicle fracture.

If the skin has been broken, the child must be observed for signs of infection in the skin, surrounding muscle, and bone. **Osteomyelitis** (infection of the bone) is very difficult to treat and can lead to amputation. For more information on osteomyelitis, see Chapter 31 ⚭.

Most fractures can be managed at home. The child and parents must be taught to care for orthopedic appliances at home, to administer medication, and to recognize complications. Follow-up evaluations should occur every few weeks until healing is complete. The nurse should refer parents to a home health nurse if indicated.

Gastrointestinal Disorders

The major discussion of all gastrointestinal disorders is in Chapter 37 ⚭.

GASTROENTERITIS

Gastroenteritis (inflammation of the stomach) may be caused by bacteria, such as *E. coli* or *Salmonella*; viruses, such as rotavirus; or toxins and allergies. The illness may resolve without complications or may cause mild to severe dehydration leading to hospitalization.

Manifestations

Symptoms include nausea, vomiting, diarrhea, and fever. Children under 5 years of age average about two episodes of gastroenteritis per year (Burkhart, 1999). If symptoms do not resolve in 24 to 48 hours, if signs of severe dehydration develop, or if bleeding is present, the parents should consult a physician immediately. If the child has repeated episodes of diarrhea in the absence of other symptoms of gastritis, the primary care provider may evaluate the child for **encopresis,** a condition associated with constipation and fecal retention. Watery stool bypasses the hard fecal mass and may be confused with diarrhea.

Diagnosis and Treatment

Diagnosis is based on history, clinical findings, and lab results. Stool cultures may be done to determine the causative agent.

If the child is hospitalized, the treatment would include IV fluids, electrolytes, and antibiotics. The child would be placed on enteric precautions, and a gown and gloves would be required when caring for the child.

Once vomiting and diarrhea subside, the child's diet should be progressed to full liquids and soft foods for a few days.

PEPTIC ULCER

A peptic ulcer is an erosion of the mucosal tissue in the lower end of the esophagus, in the stomach (usually along the lesser curvature), or in the duodenum. Peptic ulcer is much more common in adults than in children. Peptic ulcers can be primary (occurring in healthy children) or secondary to preexisting illness or injury (often a burn) and in children receiving medications such as salicylates, corticosteroids, and NSAIDs. Peptic ulcers can be caused by *Helicobacter pylori (H. pylori)*, a gram-negative rod transmitted by the fecal–oral or oral–oral routes.

Manifestations

Clinical symptoms vary according to the age of the child and the location of the ulcer. The most common symptom is a burning abdominal pain associated with an empty stomach (i.e., in the middle of the night). Vomiting, anemia, occult blood in the stool, and abdominal distention may be present.

Diagnosis and Treatment

Diagnosis is based on history, x-rays, and gastroscopy. *H. pylori* can be diagnosed by culturing a specimen obtained during gastroscopy or by collecting emesis.

If *H. pylori* is present, antibiotics are generally ordered. Often antacid liquids and histamine antagonists (ranitidine, cimetidine, and famotidine) are also given. Prognosis is good with early intervention.

Nursing Considerations

Nursing care centers on interventions to promote healing, prevent nutritional deficiency, and prevent recurrences. The child should maintain a balanced age-appropriate diet. Specific foods should only be omitted if they exacerbate the disorder. Parents should be taught to administer medication as ordered. Because stress can contribute to peptic ulcer formation, parents and the child should be helped to identify sources of stress and methods of stress reduction.

HERNIAS

A hernia is the protrusion of an organ or part of an organ through the muscle wall of the cavity that normally contains it. This protrusion results from the failure of a normal opening to close during fetal development or from weakness in the supporting muscle. Inguinal hernias are the most common type of hernia occurring in children, but umbilical and diaphragmatic hernias are also seen. Diaphragmatic hernias were discussed in Chapter 57 ∞.

Inguinal Hernia

An **inguinal hernia** occurs when abdominal tissue such as the bowel extends into the inguinal canal. It is more common in boys than girls. The inguinal hernia exhibits as a painless inguinal or scrotal swelling that may reduce in size when the child is lying on his back. Parents may report an intermittent bulge in the groin or scrotum associated with straining.

Surgical correction is usually required to prevent **incarceration** (hernia cannot be reduced and circulation is impaired), which is a surgical emergency. Outpatient surgery is usually performed after 3 months of age, when the risk of anesthesia is reduced. The prognosis is generally excellent.

Umbilical Hernia

An **umbilical hernia** results from a weakness in the umbilical ring (Figure 60-16 ■). The hernia appears as a soft swelling under the umbilical cord, which is covered by skin. The hernia easily reduces by pushing the bowel back through the fibrous ring. Most defects resolve spontaneously by 3 to 4 years of age. If the hernia is unable to be reduced, surgery is indicated.

Nursing Considerations

Herniorrhaphy is the surgical correction of a hernia. The preoperative and postoperative care usually follows the routine general surgical care. Pain medication will be given as needed. The child will have IV fluids until oral fluids can be tolerated. Urinary and fecal elimination must be monitored. The child will be monitored for signs of infection. The child will be discharged as soon as possible and parents must be taught to care for their child at home.

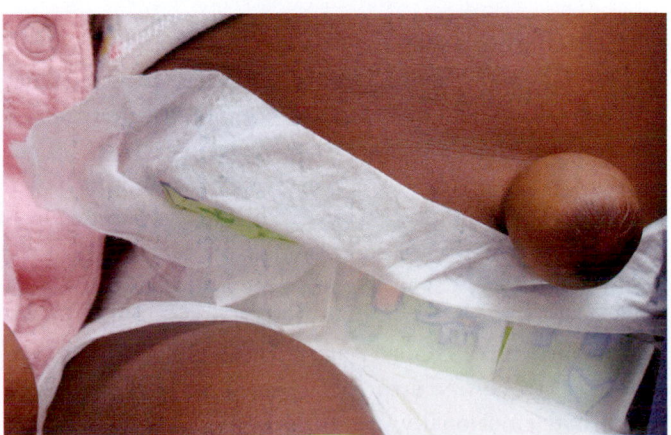

Figure 60-16. ■ Umbilical hernia. Abdominal contents are protruding through a weakened umbilical ring.

NUTRITION DISORDERS

There are several nutritional disorders that become apparent as the child transitions from the bottle or breast to solid foods. By age 3, the child begins to develop food likes and dislikes resulting in "picky eaters." If parents are not diligent in providing well-balanced diets, children may develop malnutrition. Remember, this means imbalanced nutrition, either too much or too little of what the body needs.

Rickets

Rickets is a condition caused by a vitamin D deficiency. Vitamin D is necessary for proper absorption and utilization of calcium and phosphorus. When deficiency exists, the result is failure of the bones to develop. The child may manifest bowlegs, knock-knees, beading along the ribs (*rachitic rosary*), and improper formation of teeth.

The widespread use of vitamins and fortified foods has nearly eliminated rickets in North America. However, parents should be encouraged to provide well-balanced meals and exercise in the sunlight (because the skin synthesizes vitamin D when exposed to the sun).

Scurvy

Scurvy is caused by a lack of vitamin C in the diet. Vitamin C is a water-soluble vitamin that is destroyed by heat. Because vitamin C is not stored in the body, daily intake is required. The main sources of vitamin C in the diet are citrus fruits and raw leafy vegetables. Vegetables should be cooked in small amounts of water at low heat to prevent destruction of vitamin C. Vitamin C tablets may be used to supplement the diet.

Kwashiorkor

Kwashiorkor is a deficiency in protein in the diet that results in muscle wasting. It is most common in underdeveloped countries, where malnutrition is common. Frequently, the protein deficiency occurs even when the diet is nearly adequate in calories.

Childhood Obesity

Childhood obesity in the United States has increased since the mid 1980s and is approaching epidemic status. Few problems in childhood have the impact on the life of the individual as obesity. Although obesity may not be as obvious in young children as older children, weight gain is generally a slow process, and therefore obesity seen in the young adolescent began in the young child. Obesity is associated with many physical complications including type II diabetes mellitus, coronary artery disease, pulmonary dysfunction, stroke, and arthritis. Obesity can also disable the individual emotionally, including poor body image, low self-esteem, social isolation, and feelings of depression and rejection.

There are many causes of obesity in children. Heredity is one factor that cannot be changed. Other factors can be changed with positive results. In many households, children spend most of their time sitting in front of the television or computer and little time engaging in physical activities. With little activity, children do not burn the calories they consume.

Diet is the second factor that can be adjusted. Fast food, which is high in fat and calories, has become a prominent feature of the American diet. Little research has been conducted on the effects of fast food on body weight, but it is apparent that children who regularly consume fast food make poorer food choices on days they did not consume fast food (Bowman et al., 2004).

Several dietary factors may cause excessive weight gain from fast-food consumption. They include massive portion size; high energy-density foods; an appeal to taste preference for fats, sugar, and salt; high content of saturated and trans fat; high glycemic load; and low fiber. In response to political pressure, many fast-food restaurants are providing information about the nutrition content of their menu items, giving nutritious choices, including salads, fruit, and milk. Meat sandwiches complemented with vegetables are becoming more common.

Nursing Considerations

When assessing a child's nutritional status, the nurse should ask about the frequency and content of fast-food meals. The child should be weighed and measured, and the body mass index (BMI) calculated. The BMI is determined by dividing the individual's weight in kilograms by their height in meters squared. Complications such as diabetes, hypertension, and hyperlipidemia should be evaluated. The child's activities should be assessed in relation to the calories burned. It is important to assess the child's emotional status and the impact the child's weight has on quality of life.

Parents and children should be taught the impact that being overweight or obese has on their general health. Although it is necessary to discuss complications of being overweight, it is important to stress how well the child will feel when he or she has more energy following weight loss. The family may need referral to a nutritionist. It should be suggested that meals at a fast-food restaurant be reserved for a special occasion instead of being a daily or weekly event. When fast food must be consumed, suggest that the most nutritious meal be selected.

Parents should encourage their children to become physically active. Limiting computer or television time may be necessary. Parents may need suggestions on scheduling activities daily that require active participation that burn calories and establish a lifelong habit of physical exercise.

HEPATITIS

Hepatitis is inflammation of the liver caused by a viral infection. The most common infections in the United States are from hepatitis A virus (HAV), hepatitis B virus (HBV), hepatitis C virus (HCV), and hepatitis D virus (HDV). Hepatitis A, commonly called *infectious hepatitis*, is highly contagious. Because it is transmitted by the fecal–oral route during early stages of the disease, large numbers of people can become exposed in a short time. HAV lives on surfaces for up to 1 month, so diaper-changing tables should be cleansed frequently. Children often become infected from day care workers who change diapers and then prepare food. Although HAV is mild in most people, HAV infection can cause liver failure and death for those with preexisting liver disease.

Hepatitis B, commonly called *serum hepatitis*, is a serious illness. Transmission of HBV occurs through blood, body fluids, sexual contact, sharing IV needles, and from mother to fetus. Hepatitis C is also transmitted through blood and blood products. Children requiring repeated blood transfusions, as seen with sickle cell anemia and hemophilia, are at risk for developing HCV. IV drug use, body piercing, and multiple partners increase the risk. Hepatitis D is commonly found in conjunction with HBV. Children with HBV coupled with HDV are at extreme risk of complete liver failure, require a liver transplant, and may die within 2 weeks.

The body's response to hepatitis in children is the same as that of adults. The medical and nursing care is also the same. For children with preexisting liver disorder or an impaired immune system, continued liver destruction could result in death.

clinical ALERT

When hepatitis is present, the liver is unable to detoxify and metabolize drugs at the usual rate. Medications should be administered carefully and the child monitored closely for both side effects and toxic effects.

POISONINGS

Poisonings, the ingestion of toxic substances, is a common cause of injury and death in children between 1 and 4 years of age. Recall that the developmental task of this age group is to explore their environment. Young children frequently put objects and fluid into their mouth, potentially resulting in poisoning. In older children the possibility of intentional ingestion should be suspected. The Poison Prevention Act of 1970 mandates child protection devices for all potentially toxic substances such as household cleansers and medication. However, some adults fail to tighten them or will leave the lid off. There are many other household products, such as houseplants, cosmetics, and paints that are very toxic if ingested.

Most poisonings occur in the home. Parents who suspect a child has ingested a poisonous substance should call the local poison control center immediately. If the child vomits, emesis should be brought to the emergency department.

clinical ALERT

Acetaminophen (Tylenol) is one of the most common over-the-counter drugs accidentally ingested by children that results in poisoning. When Tylenol poisoning has occurred, the oral administration of charcoal or concentrated Mucomyst is recommended. These drugs combine with acetaminophen metabolites and protect the liver.

Emergency treatment for poisoning is based on the goal of preventing further absorption of the poison and reversing its effects. The airway, breathing, and circulation must be monitored continuously and CPR performed if needed. Parents, family, and the child (if applicable) should be questioned about the events leading up to the poisoning. The type of poison, the amount of chemical, the amount of time since the poisoning, allergies, and preexisting conditions should be determined.

The process of reversal and removal of the poison depends on the specific substance ingested. Syrup of ipecac is no longer recommended because it can be harmful in some situations and may not remove all poison. Activated charcoal is commonly used to bind to poisonous chemicals to slow or prevent absorption.

Once the emergency phase of treatment is over, parents and the child will need emotional support and teaching. Depending on the degree of damage from the poison, the child may recover without deficit, or he or she may have life-changing deficits of gastrointestinal, neurologic, cardiovascular, hepatic, and renal functions. Parent will need emotional support to deal with feelings of anger, guilt, blame, and shame. Conflict between parents might occur. If a babysitter or other care provider is involved, additional emotional stress will be placed on the family. In some cases, child protection services may be called and the child placed in protective custody while the situation is under investigation.

INTESTINAL PARASITIC DISORDERS

Intestinal parasitic disorders occur most frequently in tropical regions, or areas where water is not treated, food is incorrectly prepared, or people live in crowded conditions with poor sanitation. In areas of flood from hurricanes, excessive rainfall, or snowmelt, drinking water may become contaminated. Young children, especially those in day care, are most at risk. Young children often lack good hand hygiene and are more likely to put objects into their mouth. Children can also develop intestinal parasites from house pets, barnyard animals, and wildlife. Children who lose weight or develop intermittent, loose, or abnormal stools should be evaluated for parasite disorders. Table 60-6 ■ identifies common intestinal parasite disorders, manifestations, and treatment.

TABLE 60-6 Common Intestinal Parasites

DISEASE AND ORGANISM*	TRANSMISSION AND MANIFESTATIONS	TREATMENT	NURSING CONSIDERATIONS
Giardiasis caused by *Giardia lamblia*	Person-to-person contact, infected food that is not properly prepared, unfiltered water, contact with animals. May be no symptoms, or Infants: diarrhea, vomiting, anorexia, failure to thrive Older children: abdominal cramps; loose, foul-smelling, watery, pale, and greasy stools	May resolve in 4 to 6 weeks without treatment. Furazolidone or quinacrine. Quinacrine is less expensive but has more side effects than furazolidone.	Teach parents to wear gloves when handling diapers or stool.
Pinworm (enterobiasis) caused by *Enterobius vermicularis*	Eggs inhaled or carried by hand to mouth. Female migrates to entrance of anus at night, causing intense itching. Can migrate to vagina and urethra in females.	Mebendazole, pyrantel pamoate, piperazine citrate. Treat all household members at once; may need to repeat in 2 to 3 weeks.	May occur more commonly in crowded housing developments, schools, day care centers.
Roundworm (ascariasis) caused by *Ascaris lumbricoides*	Discharged eggs carried from hand to mouth. Larvae travel from small intestine to liver to lung to upper respiratory tract and back to small intestine. Mild infection may not have symptoms. Severe infection may lead to intestinal obstruction, peritonitis, obstructive jaundice, and involvement of lungs.	Mebendazole, pyrantel pamoate, piperazine citrate. Examine stools 2 weeks after treatment and monthly for 3 months. Treat contacts if indicated. For intestinal obstruction, may administer piperazine through nasogastric tube with duodenal suction. May need surgery for obstructing worms.	Occurs most often in children 1 to 4 years and in warm climates.
Hookworm caused by *Necator americanus*	Direct contact with infected soil. Worms feed on small intestine and cause bleeding. Eggs hatch in soil and penetrate skin, enter bloodstream, migrate to lungs and upper respiratory passages, and are swallowed. Only severe infection causes problem of anemia and malnutrition. Skin may have burning, itching, papular eruption.	Mebendazole, pyrantel pamoate. Rest same as for ascariasis.	Teach parents to have children wear shoes outdoors to help prevent infection.
Threadworm (strongyloidosis) caused by *Strongyloides stercoralis*	Ingestion of discharge larvae in soil. Life cycle similar to hookworm, except do not attach to small intestine and larvae, not eggs, are deposited in soil. Severe infection may lead to nutritional deficiency through abdominal pain and distention, nausea, vomiting, diarrhea, or large pale stools with mucus.	Thiabendazole or mebendazole. May need repeat treatment if symptoms recur. Examine and treat contacts if indicated.	Occurs most often in older children and adolescents.
Visceral larva migrans (toxocariasis) caused by *Toxocara canis* or *T. catis*, from dogs and cats	Ingestion of eggs in soil. Eggs hatch in intestine and migrate to all major organs, where they encapsulate in dense fibrous tissue. Mostly asymptomatic. Always hypereosinophilia of blood. Children may have low fever and upper airway diseases. Severe disease leads to hepatomegaly, lung infiltration, neurologic disturbances.	No specific treatment. Corticosteroids (in severe cases) and thiabendazole may be used, but infection may resolve spontaneously.	Occurs most often in toddlers. Teach parents to keep children away from animal droppings and to deworm pets monthly if indicated.

*All of these are caused by *nematodes* (worms) except *Giardia lamblia*, which is a protozoa.

Source: Adapted from London, M. L., Ladewig, P. W., Ball, J. W., & Bindler, R. C. (2007). *Maternal & child nursing care* (2nd ed.). Upper Saddle River, NJ: Prentice Hall.

Endocrine Disorders

The disorders of the endocrine system are discussed in depth in Chapter 38 🔗 .

HYPOPITUITARISM

Hypopituitarism (growth hormone deficiency) was discussed in Chapter 59 🔗 . If the disorder was not diagnosed in the infant or toddler stage, it may be detected when the child fails to keep pace with the normal linear growth pattern in the preschool years. Because the pituitary controls the function of other glands, it is important to diagnose and treat hypopituitarism as soon as possible.

The nurse should review with the parents the correct technique for administering growth hormone at home. Even with the administration of growth hormone, the child may never reach a usual adult height. Parents should be encouraged to dress the child in clothing that reflects their chronologic age. The nurse should emphasize the child's strengths, support independence, and encourage participation in age-appropriate activities. Identifying positive role models, short people who accomplished their goals, also promotes a positive image. Refer the family for counseling if appropriate.

HYPERPITUITARISM

Hyperpituitarism (growth hormone excess), a disorder in which excessive secretion of growth hormone increases the growth rate, is rare in children. Oversecretion of growth hormone is often associated with a pituitary adenoma or a tumor of the hypothalamus. Affected children can grow to 7 or 8 feet in height when the disorder occurs before the closure of the epiphyseal plates. Because tall stature is valued in the United States, assessment of children (particularly boys) with accelerated growth may be delayed. Any child whose predicted height exceeds that of the parents should be evaluated for possible growth hormone excess.

Urinary Disorders

The main discussion of urinary disorders is in Chapter 39 🔗 .

URINARY TRACT INFECTIONS

Urinary tract infections (UTIs) are a group of infections that include *cystitis* or bladder infection and *pyelonephritis* (kidney infection). As discussed in Chapter 59 🔗 , urinary tract infections can be a single acute episode or a chronic recurrent or persistent infection.

Manifestations

Signs of UTI in the continent child may be the same as an adult or the child may suddenly develop incontinence or hesitancy due to fear of pain. If left untreated, a UTI could progress to sepsis.

Diagnosis and Treatment

A sterile urine sample is collected by a clean-catch technique if the child is cooperative. The parent may need to be given instruction in cleaning the child and collecting the sample. Treatment for UTI includes administration of antibiotics and increased fluids.

In most circumstances, a UTI can be prevented. The parents should be taught to thoroughly clean the perineum daily. The young child who is being toilet trained should be taught to wipe from front to back. The nurse should discourage the use of bubble baths and hot tubs that can irritate the urethra and increase the chance of infection.

NEPHROTIC SYNDROME

Nephrotic syndrome is a clinical state characterized by edema, massive **proteinuria** (protein in the urine), **hypoalbuminemia** (low blood albumin levels), **hyperlipidemia** (high blood lipids), and altered immunity. Primary nephrotic syndrome affects only the kidneys and frequently follows an infection like pyelonephritis. *Glomerulonephritis* (inflammation of the glomeruli) can also result in primary nephrotic syndrome. Secondary nephrotic syndrome results from a multisystem disorder such as diabetes, systemic lupus, or sickle cell anemia. Nephrotic syndrome affects male children between the ages of 2 and 7 more than females. Nephrotic syndrome may be a one-time occurrence or could become a chronic lifelong condition.

Nephrotic syndrome involves a complex pathology of the kidney. Damaged glomeruli allow albumin to move from the blood to the urine, resulting in hypoalbuminemia and proteinuria (albuminuria). This shift in albumin changes the osmotic pressure of the blood. The kidney resorbs sodium and water, resulting in edema. A low osmotic pressure stimulates the liver to make lipoproteins (cholesterol) leading to hyperlipidemia. As immune globulins are excreted, the child's immunity is decreased.

Manifestations

Edema in the child with nephrotic syndrome develops rapidly over a few days to 2 weeks resulting in a dramatic weight gain. Notable edema can be seen in the face, especially periorbital edema around the eyes, the abdomen, scrotum, and extremities. The blood pressure will increase. The child may become irritable, which might indicate increased intracranial pressure (IICP; see discussion in Chapter 36 🔗) and/or discomfort. Albuminuria causes the urine to be foamy. The child will begin to appear malnourished with dull eyes; dull, brittle hair; and skin lesions.

Diagnosis and Treatment

Laboratory tests reveal elevated serum cholesterol, low-density lipoproteins, and triglycerides and help confirm the diagnosis.

Intravenous infusions will be established to administer albumin and medications to decrease edema. Steroids may be given daily for several weeks to decrease inflammation of the glomeruli. The child will probably remain on steroids for 4 to 6 months. The child with nephrotic syndrome should be weighed daily. The blood pressure should be monitored and hypertension reported to the supervising registered nurse and physician.

To improve the nutritional status of the child, a high-protein, low-salt diet is usually recommended. However, more recent data suggest a regular diet that is low in sodium prevents further protein loss by the kidneys and allows return of normal blood protein levels.

Nursing Considerations

Children and parents are often fearful and anxious regarding the child's life-threatening illness. Parents may feel guilty about not seeking medical attention earlier. If nephrotic syndrome becomes a chronic condition, the child and parents may be frustrated and depressed.

The initial nursing care of the child with nephrotic syndrome involves correcting and improving renal function. Administer IV fluids and medications as ordered. Prior to discharge, the child and family should be provided with explanation of the disease process and treatment plan. Parents should understand the administration and side effects of medications. Parents should monitor and record the urine protein and the child's weight daily and verbalize the need for routine medical follow-up care.

ACUTE GLOMERULONEPHRITIS

Acute glomerulonephritis, inflammation of the glomeruli, usually results from the body's immune response following an infection. The infecting organism may be group A beta-hemolytic *Streptococcus, Staphylococcus, Pneumococcus*, and coxsackievirus. Acute glomerulonephritis is most often seen in children between the ages of 2 and 12 years. It is more common in boys than in girls. Antibiotic therapy to kill the infecting organism does not prevent this disorder from occurring. Acute glomerulonephritis results when immune complexes, deposited in glomeruli, obstruct capillary blood flow. The condition can result in acute or chronic renal failure.

Manifestations

Children with glomerulonephritis may be asymptomatic. Others have a sudden onset of flank pain, irritability, malaise, and fever. Other symptoms include gross or microscopic hematuria, dysuria, edema, hypertension, and oliguria.

Diagnosis and Treatment

Urinalysis and serum studies are performed. Treatment is supportive, including bed rest, antihypertensive medication, and fluid restriction. The nurse should monitor the child's

fluid status by planning fluid restriction and documenting intake and output. Antibiotics may be administered.

Nursing Considerations

The child's skin integrity may be compromised due to bed rest and the waste buildup in the tissues. The child with glomerulonephritis has a decreased appetite so the nurse will have to encourage the child to eat.

Most cases of acute glomerulonephritis resolve completely. While gross signs generally resolve in a few weeks, lab values for microscopic hematuria may take up to 2 years to return to normal. Parents should be forewarned about these findings.

ENURESIS

The child's bladder capacity increases gradually from 25 to 50 mL at birth, and reaches a capacity of 700 mL by adulthood. Urination is initiated when "stretch receptors" in the bladder wall are stimulated. Children younger than 2 years cannot maintain bladder control because nerves have not developed enough to detect the impulses from these receptors. Bladder control may not be complete until 4 or 5 years of age (Adams & Towle, 2009).

Acute **enuresis** is urinary incontinence after voluntary bladder control has normally been reached. *Nocturnal enuresis* occurs during the night, and *diurnal enuresis* occurs during the day. Enuresis can be a result of familial tendencies, difficulty arousing, decreased bladder capacity, abnormal circadian rhythms, abnormalities of the urethra, developmental delays, or sleep apnea.

Diagnosis and Treatment

To diagnose enuresis in children, historical data must be gathered. There should be a discussion of how the family is currently managing the problem. It is important to determine if there are any stressors in the child's life that may contribute to enuresis. Diagnostic tests including ultrasound may be needed to diagnose structural defects.

Treatment for enuresis may be a combination of medication and behavior modification. The child's behavior related to fluid intake and voiding is modified in order to develop new habits that will assist the child in controlling the bladder at night. Total fluid intake for the day is divided into portions that are administered as follows: 40% between 7 A.M. and noon, 40% between noon and 5 P.M., and 20% after 5 P.M. For children older than 7 years, an alarm that sounds when the child begins to void at night can assist the child in waking and voiding in the bathroom.

Box 60-4 ■ provides client teaching about use of an enuresis alarm. Positive reinforcement and rewards can be implemented when the child is able to stay dry. If the child had diurnal enuresis, a 2-hour voiding schedule can be used to teach the child to empty the bladder completely.

BOX 60-4　CLIENT TEACHING

Use of Enuresis Alarm

Parents and children must understand how the enuresis alarm functions and how it is to be used (Mercer, 2003). Teach parents the following:

- The average child will need to use the enuresis alarm for 10 to 12 weeks to achieve success in staying dry.
- Attach the alarm to close-fitting cloth underwear. Do not attach it to loose clothing such as boxer shorts or pajamas. Do not attach it to disposable diapers.
- When the alarm sounds, go to the child's room and observe the child's response. Tell the child to put feet on the floor and walk to the bathroom. Help the child if necessary. Turn off the alarm only after the child puts his or her feet on the floor.
- Recognize that in the beginning, the child will have voided by the time he or she wakes up or the parents arrive. The measures of progress include:
  - Reduced number of episodes of wetting per night
  - Increased length of sleep time before wetting
  - Decreased amount of urination (spotting) before the child puts feet on the floor
- After a wetting episode, reattach the alarm to clean, dry underpants.
- Keep a chart to track events, and praise the child for progress.
- Consider giving prizes for cooperation and improved performance. Prizes may include stickers for each time the child goes without assistance to the bathroom or a larger prize, such as a meal out or some form of entertainment, for the first completely dry night.
- Remind parents that the greatest reward for the child is their praise.
- Once the child is able to stay dry through the night, continue use of the alarm until there have been 2 continuous weeks without an episode of enuresis. Then use the alarm every other night for 2 or more weeks of consecutive dryness.
- If the child has a wetting episode during this time, begin the 2-week "weaning period" again. Do not be hasty about this phase of the training. Relapse is common when training is cut off prematurely.

Source: Adams, E. D., & Towle, M. A. *Pediatric nursing care.* (2009). Upper Saddle River, NJ: Prentice Hall.

NURSING CARE

PRIORITIZING NURSING CARE

When caring for young children with renal disorders, focus your care on maintaining kidney function and on early detection of complications. Follow orders for fluid restrictions carefully. Young children may find such restrictions difficult—use of distraction and play may help. If the child needs to increase fluid intake, determine fluids that he or she likes and offer those juices and Popsicles frequently. Assess for and

report immediately elevated temperature, intake greater than output, oliguria, cloudy or malodorous urine, and hematuria.

ASSESSING

Young children with renal disorders should be assessed for intake and output. Urine should be monitored for amount, color, clarity, odor, and specific gravity. Assess the abdomen using light palpation. Assess the child for signs of dehydration or fluid excess. Monitor edema of the face and body. Monitor daily weights for evidence of fluid retention.

DIAGNOSING, PLANNING, AND IMPLEMENTING

Numerous nursing diagnoses could apply to the child with urinary disorders and his or her family. Nursing diagnoses might include:

- *Risk for Infection*
- *Excess Fluid Volume*
- *Risk for Deficient Fluid Volume*
- *Acute Pain*
- *Interrupted Family Processes*
- *Risk for Caregiver Role Strain*

Nursing interventions follow the general health guidelines presented in previous chapters of this book. Adapting these interventions to the young child will be addressed here.

- Encourage children to drink water and a variety of juices daily. Frozen fruit bars and juice can be used to increase fluid intake. *Adequate fluid intake is essential to proper kidney function. Additional fluids may be needed during times of illness, infection, and fever.*
- Follow doctor's orders for fluid restriction in children with nephrotic syndrome. *When sodium and water retention are present, fluids should be limited.*
- Administer analgesics as ordered. *Dysuria may make the child reluctant to void. If surgery is needed, the child must be medicated for comfort.*
- Provide instruction to the child and parents regarding care. Be aware of family strain and refer to RN and social worker as necessary. *The life-threatening nature of urinary disorders contributes to family strain. The long-term effects and treatment contribute to caregiver strain.*

EVALUATING

The child's condition is evaluated by blood and urine analysis, weight loss, and a return of general health. Monitor closely for side effects of medications. The function of the kidneys (or a remaining kidney) must be evaluated frequently. Report any signs of urinary infection or renal failure to the physician immediately (see Chapter 39 ∞). Repeat urine samples may be done after treatment with antibiotics to determine complete eradication of the causative organism.

Due to the strain of acute life-threatening illness on the child and family, frequent evaluation of family functioning is important. Referral to support groups and agencies may be necessary.

NURSING PROCESS CARE PLAN
Child with Nephrotic Syndrome

James, a 22-month-old child, has been admitted to the pediatric unit with a diagnosis of possible nephrotic syndrome. James has gained 2 pounds in the last week and a half. His mother states, "His face is so swollen, I can hardly recognize my own child." Laboratory reports indicate a low blood albumin and high proteinuria. James is irritable and whines most of the time.

Assessment
2+ edema. Crackling lung sounds. Pulse 150; respirations 48.

Nursing Diagnosis
The following important nursing diagnosis (among others) is established for this client:

- *Excess Fluid Volume*

Expected Outcomes
The expected outcome for the plan of care for James is that intake and output will be within 100 mL by 3rd hospital day.

Planning and Implementation
The following nursing interventions are planned and implemented for James:

- Measure and record I&O every 8 hours.
- Check I&O hourly; if no urinary catheter, weigh diapers.
- Monitor specific gravity.
- Take daily weights.
- Reposition every half hour.
- Anticipate respiratory distress by monitoring breath sounds, respiratory effort, and level of consciousness.
- Administer IV fluids via appropriate equipment.
- Administer medications with attention to dosage and potential effect on electrolytes and blood protein levels.

Evaluation
The evaluation of James's health status indicates:

- 24-hour intake and output.
- 1+ edema in feet. No edema in face, hands, or trunk.
- Lung sounds are clear.
- Weight is the same as 2 weeks ago.

Critical Thinking in the Nursing Process

1. Explain the importance of repositioning James every half hour.
2. What information would you obtain from weighing diapers and why is it important?
3. What actions might you take to support James's family during his hospitalization?

Note: Discussion of Critical Thinking questions appears on the MyNursingKit Website.

Reproductive Disorders

Reproductive disorders are extremely rare in young children. As young children become more independent, parents should be encouraged to teach their children about their bodies and the differences between boys and girls. Teaching should include privacy when going to the bathroom, having a bath, or getting dressed. Children should be taught what kind of touch is acceptable and what is wrong. This is a good time to begin teaching family values to the young child. (The main discussion of reproductive disorders is in Chapter 40 ⬤.)

Integumentary Disorders

Skin disorders are discussed in depth in Chapter 30 ⬤ of this text.

SKIN INFECTIONS
Warts (Papillomavirus)

Warts are benign tumors in the epithelial cells of the skin that are caused by the human papillomavirus (HPV). Common warts are found on the skin surface and plantar warts are found on the feet. Warts can be transmitted from person to person, or the infection may transfer from one site to another on the same person. Plantar warts may develop from contact on surfaces such as locker room floors.

MANIFESTATIONS. Warts appear on the surface of the skin as rough, scaly papules and nodules that are the same color as the skin. They are painless and are most commonly found on the dorsal surface of the hand.

DIAGNOSIS AND TREATMENT. Diagnosis is made by inspection of the lesions. Medical treatment is individualized and can include chemical substances, peeling agents, freezing liquid nitrogen, laser therapy, or applying duct tape over the wart.

NURSING CONSIDERATIONS. The nurse explains that treatments involving peeling agents may take up to several months to see improvement. If pain is associated with treatment, encourage parents to reduce the frequency. Encourage the child to avoid picking the wart to reduce the risk of spreading the virus to other locations.

Impetigo

Impetigo is a superficial skin infection that generally appears on the face, hands, neck, or extremities (Figure 60-17 ■) and is caused by streptococci or staphylococci. Insect bites, burns, scratches, and lacerations provide a portal of entry for the

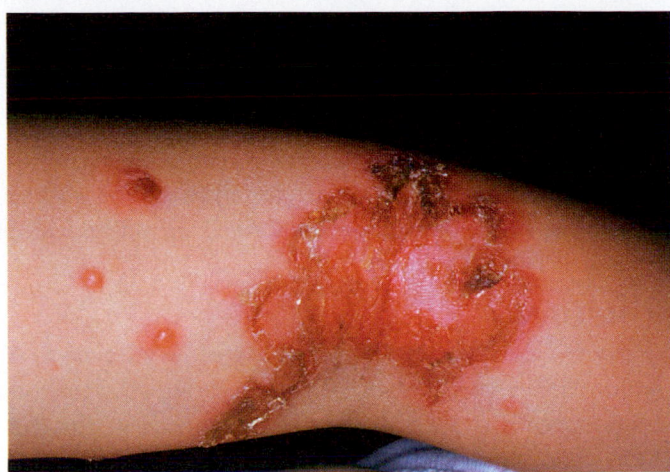

Figure 60-17. ■ Bullous impetigo. Note the crusting lesions. (Phototake NYC)

bacteria. Impetigo is highly contagious, and anyone having contact with the lesions must wear gloves.

MANIFESTATIONS.   Clinical manifestations include vesicles or pustules, edema, and redness surrounding the lesion. Once the vesicle ruptures, the lesion is covered with a loosely adherent, honey-yellow crust. If the crust is removed, a new honey-yellow crust will form.

DIAGNOSIS AND TREATMENT.   Diagnosis is made by inspecting and palpating the lesions. Bacterial cultures may be obtained for diagnosis.

Treatment involves soaking the crusted lesion in warm water, scrubbing with medicated soap to remove the crust, and applying a topical bactericidal ointment. A systemic antibiotic may be ordered if no improvement is seen with topical ointments.

NURSING CONSIDERATIONS.   The nurse educates the family that even minor cuts and scratches can pose a threat of infection. Remind the family that impetigo is highly contagious and that towels, bed linens, and clothes must not be shared with the infected child. Instruct parents in the care of the lesions and to return to the clinic if lesions do not improve.

Dermatophytes (Fungal or Tinea Infections)
Dermatophytes are fungi that mainly affect the surface of the skin, hair, and nails. Different types of tinea infections are named after the location of the infection. Some tinea infections are commonly called **ringworm** because of the circular appearance of the lesions.

MANIFESTATIONS

- Tinea capitis is a scalp fungus. It most commonly affects children between 3 and 10 years. The hair becomes brittle and breaks off, leaving circular patches of scalp showing. Papules form around the edges of the ring and become scaly and red in color (see Figure 30-10 ⬭).

- Tinea corporis has a circular reddened patch on the skin with raised borders.
- Tinea pedis is referred to as "athlete's foot." The skin between the toes and on the sole of the feet becomes red, with deep scaly fissures that are painful and itchy.
- Tinea cruris, referred to as "jock itch," causes the skin in the groin area to become red and scaly, with raised papules or vesicles forming a circular rash.

DIAGNOSIS AND TREATMENT.   Diagnosis is made by obtaining a skin scraping of the lesion and viewing it under a microscope to detect fungal growth. Medical treatment involves the use of antifungal topical ointments, powders, or sprays.

NURSING CONSIDERATIONS.   Nursing care focuses on preventing the spread of infection, encouraging good hygiene practices, and promoting comfort. Infected children should not share combs, pillows, towels, clothes, or hats. The infected area should be kept clean and dry. Parents should be taught to administer the medications as ordered.

PARASITIC INFESTATIONS
Parasites are living organisms that get their food source from another living host. Two common skin parasites are pediculosis (lice) and scabies (mites). Nonjudgmental nursing care will increase the family's compliance with treatment regimens and will lessen embarrassment about the situation.

Pediculosis
Pediculosis is an infestation with lice. *Pediculus capitis* (head lice) is found most commonly in children 3 to 10 years of age. Schools have an occasional outbreak of head lice among children in the same classroom. The female louse lays eggs (nits) on the hair shaft. *Pediculus corporis* (body lice) and *Phthirus pubis* (pubic lice or **crabs**) are two other forms of lice infestations.

DIAGNOSIS AND TREATMENT.   Diagnosis is made by inspection using bright light and a magnifying glass over the infected area. Treatment involves a pediculicide (lice-killing) shampoo. The hair is combed with a fine-toothed comb dipped in vinegar to help remove stubborn nits. A second treatment is applied in 7 days to ensure all the nits are killed.

NURSING CONSIDERATIONS.   Nursing care focuses on teaching the parents and the child if appropriate how to kill the parasite and alleviate itching. Demonstrate how to inspect for lice by separating small amounts of hair to look for any lice or nits. Instruct parents to remove all nits before they hatch. All family members should be examined for any evidence of lice so treatment can begin promptly. Advise parents to follow directions on prescribed shampoo carefully.

It must be stressed that parents will need to wash all bedding, towels, and hair accessories in hot water and dry them in a hot dryer. Upholstered furniture should be vacuumed and the vacuum bag should be discarded. Personal items that cannot be washed, such as toys and stuffed animals, should be sealed in a plastic bag for 2 weeks. This breaks the cycle of infestation by preventing any lice that hatch from finding a new host.

Scabies

Scabies is an infestation caused by the mite *Sarcoptes scabiei*. The lesions are mainly found on the hands and feet and in the folds of the skin. Once the scabies mite finds a human host, it burrows into the epidermis and lays eggs. In 2 to 4 days, the eggs hatch and the immature mite travel toward the surface of the skin where they mature and grow. If left untreated, scabies mites continue to cycle every 14 to 17 days. Ova and feces from the scabies mite come in contact with the skin and cause irritation and pruritus (Figure 60-18 ■). This usually appears about 1 month after infestation.

MANIFESTATIONS. Clinical manifestations include erythematous papules, vesicles, and pustules. A thin grey line or burrow ending in a vesicle may be seen. Pruritus is present and more severe at night. Lesions may appear anywhere on the body.

DIAGNOSIS AND TREATMENT. Diagnosis is made by inspection. Skin scrapings are inspected under the microscope for the presence of mites, eggs, or feces. Medical treatment may include treatment with permethrin cream (Elimite) and good hygiene practices to prevent recurrent infestations.

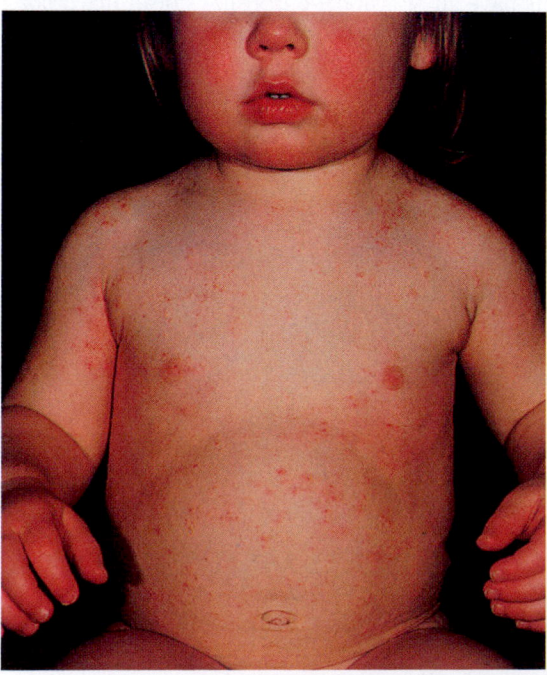

Figure 60-18. ■ Diffuse scabies in an infant. The lesions are most numerous around the axillae, chest, and abdomen.

NURSING CONSIDERATIONS. Once the diagnosis is made, the child will need to shower, dry thoroughly, and apply 5% permethrin lotion. The lotion should remain on the skin for 8 to 12 hours before showering again. All household members should be treated even if they are asymptomatic. All bed linen, towels, and clothes should be washed thoroughly. Items that cannot be washed should be sealed in a plastic bag for 5 days.

SUNBURN

Sunburn is overexposure to the sun's ultraviolet rays. A combination of low levels of melanin in children, a thin epidermal layer, and long periods of time spent in the sun places children at higher risk for sunburn. Children and adolescents who have had repeated sunburns or severe blistering from the sun are more likely to develop melanoma and basal cell carcinoma than those who have protected themselves from the sun's harmful rays.

Manifestations

In a relatively short time, sun exposure can cause the skin to become red and tender and blisters may form. Other symptoms of overexposure to the sun include headache, fatigue, chills, and malaise.

Treatment

Treatment is symptomatic. Increase oral fluids and use cool compresses and topical corticosteroid help to relieve discomfort. If the skin is not intact, creams and ointments should not be used. If the sunburn covers the majority of the body, is severe with large blisters, and the child is dehydrated, medical attention is needed.

Prevention

Prevention is the best medicine. Teach children and parents to apply sunscreen (SPF 15 or greater), wear protective clothing, and avoid sun exposure between 10 A.M. and 4 P.M. when the sun's rays are the strongest.

FROSTBITE

Overexposure to low environmental temperatures may cause skin and tissue damage known as frostbite. A combination of high concentration of water in the skin cells and exposure to extremely low temperatures (below −2°C) causes crystals to form in the tissue. Areas most commonly affected include the hands and feet (especially fingers and toes), as well as the cheeks, nose, and ears.

Manifestations

Skin may appear pale and white and have decreased sensation. If deeper tissues such as the subcutaneous tissue, is involved, the skin first appears cyanotic with mottling and then becomes red and edematous. Blisters or bullae may appear after rewarming. If frostbite is severe, the tissue may become necrotic. The client may lose tissue such as fingers, toes, tip of the nose, or earlobes.

Treatment

Immediate medical treatment requires placing the child in a warmer environment and removing wet clothing. Rewarm the affected area slowly by submerging in warm water for 10 to 15 minutes.

Nursing Considerations

Nursing care focuses on rewarming the area and preventing further tissue damage. Monitor the affected area for increased circulation and return of sensation. Pain medication should be administered as needed. If hospitalization is required, maintain sterile technique during dressing changes, administer antibiotics as ordered, and encourage proper nutrition to aid in healing. Children should be taught to wear hats, gloves, and extra socks when playing outdoors in cold temperatures. Instruct children to come inside when hands and feet feel numb or sting. Parents should not allow children to go outside when temperatures are excessively low.

BITES OR STINGS

Children of all ages learn by exploring the environment. At times children come in contact with animals, insects, or snakes, and therefore may experience a bite or sting. Often the bite or sting is harmless, but every bite or sting warrants assessing, especially if the skin has been broken. Severe systemic problems may develop if the child has a severe reaction to the bite or sting, which could progress to anaphylaxis (see Chapter 35 🔗).

Manifestations

Clinical manifestations for animal bite (including human bite) include redness, edema, and laceration at the site of injury. The wound may drain and cellulitis may develop. Insect bites and stings may cause a local or systemic reaction. Symptoms of local reaction include redness, itching, pain, hives, papules, and edema at the point of entry. Some systemic reactions include wheezing, urticaria, laryngeal obstruction, angioedema, and possibly anaphylaxis. Some snakes are highly venomous and a bite could cause a tissue necrosis and possibly death. Most snakebites, however, are from nonvenomous snakes. Symptoms of snakebite might include burning at the puncture site, redness, ecchymosis, edema, dizziness, hypotension, tachycardia, sweating, and nausea and vomiting.

Rabies is a fatal infection of the central nervous system caused by the rabies virus. Human infection occurs as the result of a bite from a wild animal in which the virus is present. The incubation period for rabies is 3 to 12 weeks, so the animal may have no symptoms and still be infected. It is critical, therefore, to suspect any victim of a wild animal bite has been exposed to rabies. If the animal can be safely captured and contained, it can be tested for rabies. Early symptoms of rabies are nonspecific flulike symptoms including fever, headache, and malaise. As the disease progresses, anxiety, agitation, confusion, hallucinations, hypersalivation, hyperactive reflexes, and convulsions occur. Once the clinical signs occur, the disease is usually fatal within days.

Diagnosis and Treatment

Diagnosis is made by inspection and palpation of the skin at the site of the animal or insect bite. Identification of the source of the bite is helpful in diagnosis. Lab work may be done to help identify bites from venomous snakes.

Medical treatment involves irrigation of the wound and possible removal of dead tissue. Surgical repair may be necessary. At times the wound is left open to heal by secondary intention. Antibiotics are prescribed to treat infection. If rabies cannot be ruled out from the animal, the child may need to receive human rabies immune globulin (HRIG) or human diploid cell vaccine (HDCV). No fatalities have occurred when rabies vaccine is given per protocol. Most fatalities occur when people do not seek medical assistance because they are not aware of the possibility of rabies infection.

BURNS

While burns can happen at any age, in the young child burns are more common in boys between 1 and 4 years of age. At this age, the child is exploring his environment and can reach hot pans on the stove or the hot curling iron, or explore the fire in the fireplace. Most burns can be prevented, and parents must be ever alert to hazards in the environment. There are four types of burns:

- *Thermal burns* are caused by flames and by hot objects such as coffee, grease, or stoves.
- *Chemical burns* are caused by strong acids or alkalies such as the chemical found in cleansers containing lye, toilet cleaners, or preparations used to open clogged drains.
- *Electrical burns* are caused by contact with exposed electric wires. As the electricity travels through the body, it will burn the tissue at the points of entrance and exit.
- *Radiation burns* are caused by exposure to radiation, the most common being the sun.

Manifestations

Burns are assessed for burn depth and burn area. Burn depth is defined by partial thickness or full thickness. (See Chapter 47 for the main discussion of burns, and Figure 47-12 🔗 for burn thickness.) Following a partial-thickness burn, the skin may regenerate but some scarring may result. Full-thickness burns require skin grafting.

Burn area is an estimate of the amount of body surface damaged. The rule of nines is slightly modified for children. (See Figure 47-13 🔗 for the basic rule of nines.) The process for estimating the amount of body surface damage is the same as for an adult, but the percent of body surface is slightly different owing to their differences in body proportions. For example, if a 1-year-old were burned on the back of the head (8.5%) and upper back (6.5%), the burn area would be 15%; in an adult, the burn area would be 13.5%.

Assessment of a child with a burn must include the ABCs (patency of the **a**irway, **b**reathing, **c**irculation), signs of shock, hemorrhage, fluid loss, pain, and the possibility of other injuries from falls.

Treatment

A serious burn is an emergency. The initial treatment of a burn is to stop the burning process by removing the cause. The child's status may change rapidly due to smoke inhalation and swelling of the airway. Therefore, continued monitoring of the ABCs is essential. An IV should be initiated and fluids administered. Shortly after a burn, fluid shifts from the blood vessels to the interstitial space, resulting in a low blood volume. This fluid volume must be replaced to prevent shock.

NURSING CARE

PRIORITIZING NURSING CARE

When caring for young children with burns, focus your care on adapting to the limitations of the child and providing emotional support to the family. Encourage the child to do as much as possible in activities of daily living and play. Praise the child when new skills are learned or mastered. For children recovering from burns, rehabilitation can be a long, arduous process, and encouragement is key. Allow family to openly discuss their concerns and fears for their children.

ASSESSING

The role of the LPN/LVN in burn care is one of continued data collection and monitoring of the child for complications.

DIAGNOSING, PLANNING, AND IMPLEMENTING

The following nursing diagnoses can be used to plan and implement care of the burned child:

- *Acute Pain* related to burn injury
- *Deficient Fluid Volume* related to fluid shift and loss from damaged tissue
- *Hypothermia* related to burn injury
- *Risk for Infection* related to burn injury
- *Imbalanced Nutrition: Less than Body Requirements* related to burn injury
- *Disturbed Body Image* related to burn disfigurement
- *Anxiety* (parent and child) related to burn injury and lengthy hospitalization

The following nursing interventions should be implemented in caring for the child and family:

- Administer a narcotic or other analgesics as needed and prior to dressing changes. Keep the wound covered to decrease discomfort and prevent infection. Bed cradle may be used to keep linen off the wound. *Burns can be very painful and the child must be adequately medicated. Covering the wound decreases pain stimulation from contact with air and linen.*
- Follow doctor's orders and facility guidelines in changing dressings, whirlpool baths, debridement, and ointment application. *To promote healing the eschar must be removed. Check facility policy to determine if this is an LPN function.*
- Strictly follow doctor's orders regarding care of skin graft and donor site. *A skin graft must remain fixed to underlying tissue until circulation is reestablished. Care must be taken to prevent injury to the graft site. The donor site should be kept clean and dry to promote healing.*
- Keep room temperature warm to prevent hypothermia. Avoid heat lamps. *When there is large destruction of skin, the body's thermoregulation mechanism is altered and the child develops hypothermia. Heat lamps should be avoided to prevent further burns.*
- Administer oral and IV fluids as ordered. Monitor I&O and hematocrit. *Fluid shifts from vascular to interstitial space and leaks from damaged skin. Fluid balance must be monitored and maintained.*
- Administer high-protein nutrition, either oral or total parenteral nutrition (TPN) as ordered. *Proteins are needed for healing.*
- Encourage activity within limitations of wound healing process. Books, games, and movies may be used for the child confined to bed. Physical therapy may be used to maintain and regain strength and movement. *Physical activity is necessary for muscle strength, growth, and positive mental outlook.*
- Use therapeutic communication techniques to help child and family cope with disfigurement. Refer family to RN and social worker as necessary. *The child may need support in dealing with altered body image. Parents may need support in dealing with guilt and loss of child's appearance. Burn treatment is expensive and family may need support with financial obligations.*
- Teach family how to care for the wound, skin graft, and donor site at home. *The healing of a burn generally takes several weeks or months to complete. The child may be discharged from the hospital and readmitted for surgery or follow-up treatment.*

EVALUATING

The child should be evaluated for infection and wound healing. Immobility can cause pneumonia, contractures, and constipation, and the child should be evaluated for these complications. Parents should be able to verbalize and demonstrate an understanding of home care.

Psychosocial Disorders

Discussion of mental health and treatment for specific mental health disorders appears in Chapters 49 and 50 ⬮⬮.

THOUGHT PROCESS DISORDERS

Thought process disorders have a dramatic impact on the child, the family, and the community. Some thought process disorders are commonly found with specific physical characteristics. Other thought process disorders are not apparent until the child fails to progress cognitively as expected. Thought process disorders can be caused by genetic anomalies, infections, and injury, either physical or chemical trauma, to the nervous system. Examples of thought process disorders that are evident in young children include Down syndrome, Rett's syndrome, Asperger's syndrome, fetal alcohol syndrome, and autism. Recall that autism was discussed in Chapter 59 ⬮⬮. Although each disorder has different characteristics, there are also similarities in manifestations and nursing care. The commonalities will be discussed here. Table 60-7 ■ provides a brief description of the common disorders.

Manifestations

Thought process disorders involve abnormalities in behavior, communication, and social interactions. Depending on the cause of the specific disorder, the child's development might progress to a point and then stop, progress to a point and then regress, or fail to develop beyond the infantile state.

Typically children with these thought process disorders engage in repetitive behaviors, including self-stimulating or self-destructive behaviors. The repetitive behaviors might include twirling in circles, head banging, and biting themselves. These children have difficulty sitting quietly for any length of time and focusing on a productive activity. They run around the room and "get into everything." Other children with thought process disorders focus on only one activity and seem to "block out" everything else going on around them.

Difficulty with speech, both talking and understanding the spoken language, is common. While some children may eventually learn to talk, abnormal patterns may develop. Examples of common speech abnormalities include the use of "you" instead of "I," parroting of what is heard, or repeating a question instead of answering it. Cognitive abilities may correspond with intellectual deficits. Some children may have difficulty learning. Other children may learn, but have difficulty expressing what they know.

Children with thought process disorders demonstrate a wide range of social skills. They may have difficulty establishing relationships because of speech problems or because they may be unable to focus on others. Some children and adults may be fearful of the child with a thought process disorder and therefore avoid interacting with them.

TABLE 60-7	Common Thought Process Disorders
DISORDER	**SYMPTOMS**
Autism	Repetitive behaviors, unusual forms of play
	Delayed speech, may never speak
	Fascination with repetitive songs, one or more objects
	Sensitive to tactile stimuli, unresponsive to auditory stimuli
Rett's syndrome	Only girls
	Increasing ataxia
	Hand wringing
	Dementia
	Growth retardation
Asperger's syndrome	Impaired social interaction
	Repetitive behavior
	Normal cognition and language skills
Down syndrome	Wide range of severity of mental retardation
	Small head with low-set ears, flat nose, epicanthal eye folds, protruding tongue
	Short, broad hands, simian line on palm
Fetal alcohol syndrome	Mental retardation
	Behavioral problems, hyperactivity
	Growth retardation
	Microcephaly, with facial abnormalities

Treatment

The treatment of thought process disorders focuses first on safety for the child and others, and then on behavior modification with the goal of helping the child to interact with the social environment to the highest degree possible. Safety devices, such as helmets, may be needed to protect the child from injury. The family will need education on behavior modification techniques, as well as support and encouragement. At times the child may need to be placed in a special home that is staffed to accommodate the child with a thought process disorder.

Note: The references and resources for all chapters have been compiled at the back of the book.

PROCEDURE 60-1   Ear Lavage

Purpose

- To remove debris from the ear

Equipment

- Warm water (unless medicated solution is ordered)
- Otoscope
- Syringe (irrigating syringe, syringe with IV tubing, or bulb syringe)
- Emesis basin
- Towels

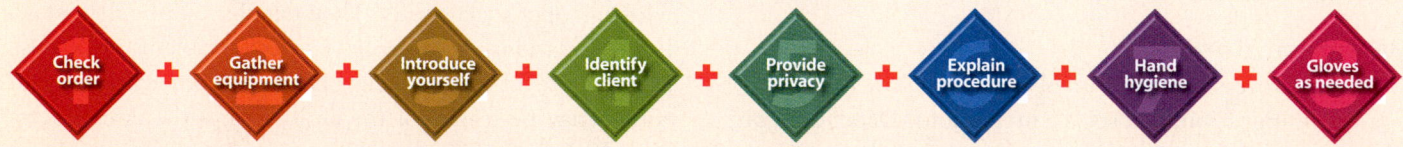

Check order + Gather equipment + Introduce yourself + Identify client + Provide privacy + Explain procedure + Hand hygiene + Gloves as needed

Interventions and Rationales

1. Perform preparatory steps (see icon bar).

2. Solicit the assistance of a coworker. *This will help prevent injury to the child.*

3. Using the otoscope, examine the ear for the presence of cerumen and other debris. The eardrum should be intact. *If the tympanic membrane is not intact due to perforation or tympanostomy with tubes, or there are sharp foreign objects in the ear canal, the ear lavage should not be done.*

4. Position the child upright with the head tipped slightly toward the side being irrigated. *This position facilitates drainage of irrigation fluid.*

5. Place a towel over the neck and shoulders. *The towel will absorb fluid draining from the ear.*

6. Hold the emesis basin under the ear. *Emesis basin should collect most of the fluid draining from the ear.*

7. Fill the syringe with warm solution. *Warm solution is comfortable and helps to loosen cerumen. Cool solution can be uncomfortable and may cause nausea and vertigo.*

8. Pull the pinna in the appropriate direction according to the child's age (see Figure 58-9 ⬭⬭).

9. Gently push fluid into the ear canal, directing the flow along the top of the ear canal. A pulsating flow is more effective than a continual flow of fluid. *Gentle pressure must be used. Forceful irritation may cause tympanic membrane rupture.*

10. Using the otoscope, examine the ear canal for removal of all debris.

11. Repeat as necessary.

SAMPLE DOCUMENTATION

[date] [time] Left ear irrigated with 40 mL warm water. Return of 40 mL yellow-tinged fluid and pea-sized hard mass of cerumen. Tympanic membrane slightly red. _____
_____ M. Gordon, LPN

PROCEDURE 60-2 — Providing Cast Care for Children

Purposes

- To note signs and symptoms of neurovascular impairment and report promptly
- To maintain cast integrity thus promoting healing

Equipment

- Pillows with waterproof covering
- Absorbent pads and protectors
- Plastic bag
- Permanent marker

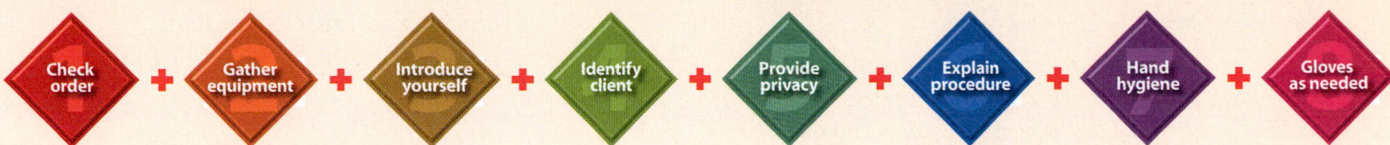

Interventions and Rationales

1. Perform preparatory steps (see icon bar).

2. Elevate recently casted limb. *This reduces edema.*

3. Inspect the damp cast for indentations and handle only with the palms of the hand until the cast is completely dry. *Damp casts move under pressure. Indentations indicate potential pressure areas where skin breakdown could occur.*

4. Observe for drainage, noting amount by marking the outline of the drainage area, date, and time by marking on the cast with permanent marker. *Water-based marker could be removed by drainage or cleaning.*

5. Observe for symptoms of neurovascular impairment every 15 minutes following cast placement progressing to every 2 hours. Report abnormal findings, such as decreased or absent pulses, change in color of skin above or below the cast, warmth of the extremity, decreased sensation, decreased capillary refill, increased edema, limited movement of extremity, or pain, burning, or tingling. *These measures allow the nurse to recognize and to prevent complications.*

6. Instruct children and parents to observe for the above findings as well and report accordingly. *Much of the healing time will be at home. The child and parents must be taught about recognition and reporting of symptoms.*

7. Cover cast with a plastic bag during bathing or toileting to keep it dry and clean. *The cast will disintegrate if it gets wet. It must remain dry in order to support proper healing.*

8. Avoid the use of lotions and powders under the cast. *These may cause skin irritation.*

9. Keep shirts or other clothing over the top edges of the cast on young children. *This helps to keep the child from picking at the cast or putting small objects into the cast.*

10. Instruct children and their families about care of the cast at home including:
    - Clean the area under the cast and toes and fingers with alcohol and a cotton swab. Avoid using water.
    - Use a cast shoe, sock, or sling to protect the cast.
    - Report unusual odor, damage to the cast, or unexplained fever. *This may be a sign of infection.*

SAMPLE DOCUMENTATION

[date] [time]	Right forearm cast intact. No drainage noted. Fingers warm with adequate capillary refill. No edema noted. ROM without limitation. Cast covered with plastic and edges taped. Assisted to shower. _____ _____ L. Erskine, LPN

PROCEDURE 60-3 — Setting Crutch Height for Children

Purpose

- To ensure a proper fit of crutches and facilitate ambulation

Equipment

- Crutches
- Measuring tape, if desired

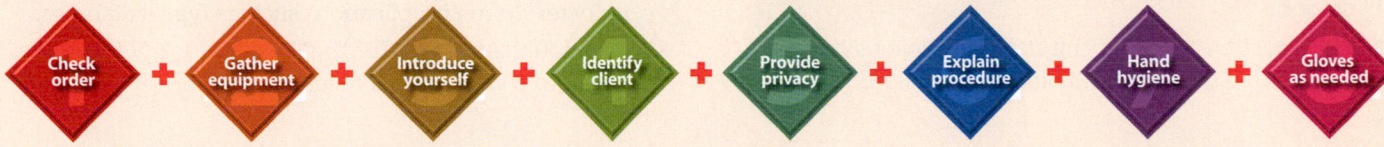

Interventions and Rationales

1. Perform preparatory steps (see icon bar).

2. Have the child stand with elbows slightly and comfortably flexed.

3. Place the tip of the crutches 3 to 6 inches from the upper, outer border of the toes of each foot. *This provides a wider base of support for improved balance.*

4. Adjust the crutches to proper height, ensuring that the upper pad on the crutches is placed lightly under the child's axillae. *The crutches should not put pressure against the axilla.*

5. Check the child's posture. The back or neck should not be flexed. *This would indicate that crutches are too short.*

SAMPLE DOCUMENTATION

[date] [time] Crutches placed in axilla. Height adjusted. Correct posture and pad placement noted. Instructions on proper crutch walking given. Client verbalized understanding. _____

_____ J. Ness, LVN

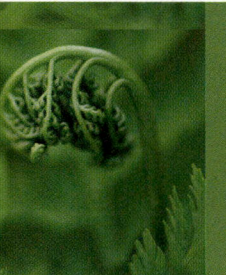

Chapter Review

KEY Points

- Preschoolers become active climbers, begin to learn how to write, and recognize letters.

- Preschoolers are active and growing. They need more calcium and fiber than toddlers; they also need less fat. Teach parents to establish good eating habits early.

- Recurrent disorders, such as nosebleeds, otitis media, and tonsillitis, indicate a need for follow-up. Upper respiratory infections and otitis media often occur together. Persistent tonsillitis may require tonsillectomy.

- The Heimlich maneuver is performed with children in the same way as for adults, but more gently to prevent damage to ribs and underlying organs.

- Asthma is triggered by allergens, medications, fumes, exercise, or stress.

- It is important to teach about communicable diseases, even though many are controlled by immunizations.

- Kawasaki's syndrome is a genetically linked cardiovascular condition, often preceded by a respiratory infection. It is very painful and may cause permanent heart damage. Care focuses on providing comfort and giving fluids to maintain hydration.

- Nurses must be aware of cultural and religious beliefs related to organ donation and blood transfusion.

- The nursing priority during seizures is to prevent injury to the child. Seizures may be an indication of tumors, trauma, infection, or toxins, a rapidly developed fever, or epilepsy.

- Neurologic disorders can result from trauma, viruses, bacterial infection, tumor growth, or other causes. Prevention is a key area for client teaching.

- Young children should have vision and hearing screenings annually. Eye injuries need prompt treatment to prevent permanent damage.

- Muscular dystrophy is a group of inherited diseases that cause muscle degeneration and wasting and that often manifest in the first 3 to 4 years of life. Legg-Calvé-Perthes disease also may appear in the preschool years, usually affecting boys from 4 to 8.

- Sprains, strains, dislocated joints, and fractures require immobilization to help prevent complications and speed recovery.

- Manifestations of gastroenteritis include vomiting, diarrhea, and fever; dehydration can happen easily at this age.

- Herniorrhaphy (surgery to correct protrusion of an organ through the muscle wall) is quite common in this age group.

- Nutritional disorders include undernutrition (vitamin or protein deficiencies) or overnutrition (obesity). Childhood obesity results in complications such as Type II diabetes.

- Hepatitis (inflammation of the liver) has many forms and can lead to complete liver failure.

- Poisonings are more common among preschoolers than in any other age group. Teach parents to store potential poisons out of reach; teach preschoolers to avoid them.
- Hypopituitarism may be diagnosed when children fail to keep up with normal growth patterns.
- Nephrotic syndrome and acute glomerulonephritis are two serious infections of the renal system. Bed rest, antihypertensive medication, and fluid restriction are employed when the kidneys are not functioning properly.
- Thought process disorders may be caused by genetic anomalies, infections, injury, or trauma to the nervous system.

⊗ FOR FURTHER Study

Safety issues for preschoolers are discussed in the fundamentals section of this textbook under Safety (Chapter 9, especially Box 9-1 and the section on Restraints).

See Chapter 11 for communication techniques.

Review Chapter 12 for client teaching.

Theories about preschooler development are provided in Chapter 15.

Growth and development information is provided in Chapter 16.

The Glasgow Coma Scale is shown in Table 19-2.

Skin disorders are discussed in depth in Chapter 30 of this text.

The musculoskeletal disorders, including sprains and strains and osteomyelitis, are discussed in the medical-surgical unit, Chapter 31.

The medical-surgical treatment of respiratory disorders, including pneumonia, is provided in detail in Chapter 32.

The main discussion of cardiovascular disorders is in Chapter 33.

The main discussion of blood and lymph disorders is in Chapter 34.

The immune disorders, including anaphylaxis, are discussed in depth in Chapter 35.

Nervous system and sensory disorders, including hematomas and IICP, are discussed in most depth in Chapter 36.

The major discussion of all gastrointestinal disorders is in Chapter 37.

Disorders of the endocrine system, including diabetes insipidus, are discussed in Chapter 38.

The main discussion of urinary disorders is in Chapter 39.

The main discussion of reproductive disorders is in Chapter 40.

Procedure 47-1 describes steps in applying a splint for sprains and strains; see Chapter 47 for the main discussion on burns.

Discussion of mental health and treatment for specific mental health disorders appears in Chapters 49 and 50.

Diaphragmatic hernias are discussed in Chapter 57.

Discussion of congenital heart conditions, the Heimlich maneuver, closed head injury, urinary tract infections, and autism appeared in Chapter 59.

Acute rheumatic fever is most common in children from 6 to 15 years and is discussed in Chapter 61, as is asthma.

Critical Thinking Care Map

Caring for a Child with a Fracture
NCLEX-PN® Focus Area: Physiologic Integrity

Case Study: Billy, a 5-year-old, is brought to the urgent care clinic for a possible fractured left lower leg. Billy had been climbing on the playground equipment at a local park when he fell, twisting his left ankle. He is hopping on his right leg. He has been crying and states, "It hurts real bad."

Nursing Diagnosis: *Impaired Physical Mobility*

COLLECT DATA

Subjective	Objective
_____	_____
_____	_____
_____	_____
_____	_____
_____	_____
_____	_____

Would you report this? Yes/No

If yes, report to: _____

What would you report? _____

Nursing Care

_____
_____
_____
_____
_____
_____
_____
_____
_____

How would you document this? _____
_____
_____
_____

Compare your answers and documentation to those provided on the MyNursingKit Website.

Data Collected
(use only those that apply)

- Pedal pulses present
- Crying
- States, "It hurts real bad."
- Ankle swollen, bruised
- Non-weight-bearing

Nursing Interventions
(use only those that apply; list in priority order)

- Apply ice pack to ankle.
- Instruct not to put anything inside cast.
- Offer milk three times a day.
- Apply heat lamp to ankle.
- Instruct to support cast on pillows until dry.
- Teach crutch walking.
- Instruct regarding sings of impaired circulation.

NCLEX-PN® Exam Preparation

TEST-TAKING TIP When answering questions about children, be sure to consider the age and size of the child as well as the medical condition.

1 The nurse observes a 6-year-old and begins to question the possibility of developmental delay when noting which of the following?
1. Draws a circle and can cut it out using scissors, staying on the line most of the time.
2. Sings the ABC song, missing a few letters.
3. Needs help tying shoes but can put Velcro shoes on independently.
4. Rides a bicycle with training wheels.

2 The nurse, working in a pediatrician's office, admits a 3-year-old and asks the mother about any concerns. The mother reports that the child's appetite seems to have declined and asks what she should do. The nurse's best response is:
1. "Teach children that they must empty their plate or they will receive negative reinforcement for their behavior."
2. "Allow children to eat whatever they want."
3. "It is normal for the appetite to diminish at this age because caloric needs and growth are not as great as at earlier ages."
4. "Your child requires a dietary evaluation because the child may be anorexic."

3 The nurse, working in a pediatrician's office, receives a call from a parent reporting that their preschooler has mild signs and symptoms of varicella. The nurse's priority action is to:
1. Schedule the child for an appointment that same day.
2. Schedule the child for an appointment within the next 72 hours.
3. Teach the parents how to care for the child at home and list which symptoms they should report if noted.
4. Instruct the parents to keep the child home from day school for 24 hours.

4 While caring for a child diagnosed with Kawasaki's syndrome, a priority independent nursing action is:
1. Providing care as gently as possible.
2. Bathing the child with the warmest water tolerated.
3. Offering popcorn, chips, and other salty snacks as tolerated.
4. Maintaining complete bed rest.

5 The nurse is caring for a child who received a kidney transplant earlier in the week. The parents ask how they will know if organ rejection is occurring. The nurse's best response is:
1. "Organ rejection is unlikely and there is little cause for concern."
2. "The best way to monitor for organ rejection is frequent blood testing."

3. "You will be taught how to test the urine for the presence of protein and glucose."
4. "The best indicator of rejection is decline in function, which can be seen with reduced urine output or signs of fluid overload, including edema."

6 The nurse, working in a pediatrician's office, receives a call from a parent who says that their child fell off his bicycle and hit his head. Which of the following symptoms, if reported by the parent, would cause the nurse to encourage the parents to bring the child in to be seen as soon as possible?
1. Loss of consciousness lasting 2 minutes.
2. Swelling at the site of the bump.
3. Bleeding from a shallow cut resolved by application of ice and pressure.
4. Ecchymosis and edema at the site of the bump.

7 The nurse cares for a 6-year-old boy with a fractured femur in the emergency department. When the doctor reports that the x-ray showed increased density of the femoral head, the nurse suspects:
1. Child abuse.
2. Compartment syndrome.
3. Osteomyelitis.
4. Legg-Calvé-Perthes disease.

8 When caring for a child with gastroenteritis that is causing vomiting and diarrhea, the nurse's priority action is to:
1. Monitor the child for signs of dehydration.
2. Encourage fluids.
3. Progress the diet from clear to full liquids after vomiting subsides.
4. Collect a stool specimen.

9 The parent brings the child to the clinic with a circular rash with raised borders on the arm. Upon receiving a diagnosis from the physician of ringworm, the mother looks horrified. A priority teaching point for the nurse to make is:
1. "It is called ringworm, but it is actually a fungal infection."
2. "Ringworm is actually tinea capitis."
3. "Ringworm is very contagious and can spread within the family."
4. "This will be resolved within 1 to 2 days of medication usage."

10 The nurse admits a 3-year-old child who is reported to display repetitive behaviors, is not speaking yet, and does not respond to the mother's voice. The nurse suspects a possible diagnosis of:
1. Rett's syndrome.
2. Asperger's syndrome.
3. Autism.
4. Fetal alcohol syndrome.

Answers and rationales for Review Questions appear in Appendix I.

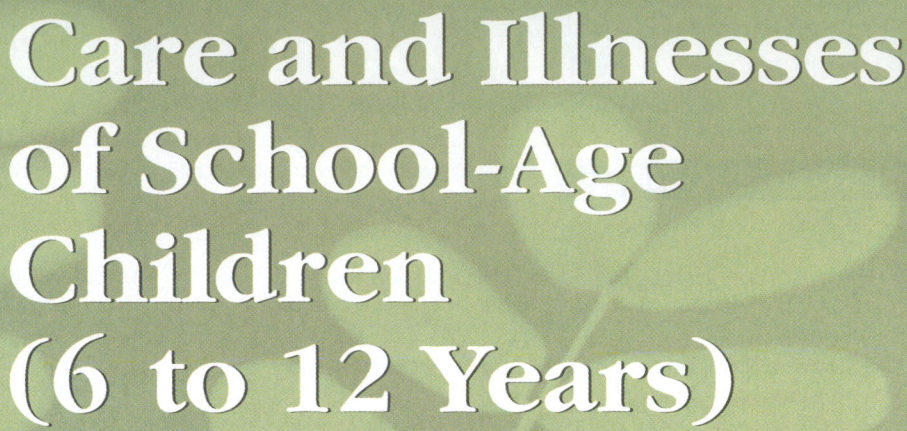

Chapter 61

Care and Illnesses of School-Age Children (6 to 12 Years)

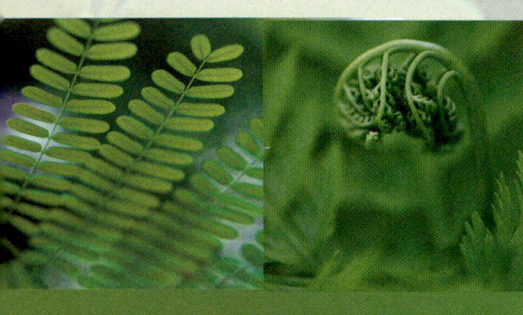

LEARNING Outcomes

After completing this chapter, you will be able to:

1. Identify milestones, nutrition, and normal vital signs for school-age children.
2. Describe physical disorders and nursing care for school-age children with respiratory, cardiovascular, hematologic, or immune disorders.
3. Identify physical disorders and nursing care for school-age children with neurologic or musculoskeletal disorders.
4. Describe physical disorders and nursing care for school-age children with gastrointestinal or endocrine disorders.
5. Explain physical disorders and nursing care for school-age children with urinary or reproductive disorders.
6. Identify physical disorders and nursing care for school-age children with integumentary disorders.
7. Describe psychosocial conditions and nursing care for school-age children.

Clinical Objectives

8. Use proper safety measures when caring for a pediatric client with regard to transporting, positioning, and restraining.
9. Safely administer medications and immunizations according to age-related guidelines.
10. Monitor vital signs and compare to age-related norms.

KEY TERMS

Use the audio glossary feature on the MyNursingKit Website to hear the correct pronunciation of the following key terms.

amblyopia 1719	**glucosuria** 1724	**rhabdomyosarcoma** 1722
astigmatism 1719	**hyperlipidemia** 1717	**strabismus** 1719
chorea 1716	**hyperopia** 1719	**vaginitis** 1727
erythema marginatum 1716	**myopia** 1719	
Ewing's sarcoma 1722	**precocious puberty** 1725	

In this chapter, the most common disorders affecting the school-age child (6 to 12 years) are discussed. Table 61-1 ■ highlights growth and development milestones for school-age children. Growth and development information (on which this chapter builds) was provided in the fundamentals part of this textbook, in Chapter 16 ⚭. Safety issues across the life span were discussed in Chapter 9, especially Box 9-1 ⚭. Theories about preschooler development were provided in Chapter 15 ⚭.

As school-age children grow and approach adolescence and adulthood, the incidence of disease decreases. Many disorders are the same as, or very similar to, disorders affecting adults. Therefore, not all disorders will be discussed here, but the general guidelines apply to all clients.

Nutrition for School-Age Children

As children reach school age, they become more independent in every way, including in choosing foods. This is an important time for parents to influence their child to develop healthy eating habits. Figure 61-1 ■ illustrates a portion plate that gives guidelines children can understand about appropriate-size servings. Children who are well nourished grow stronger, learn better, and have more energy. Children have much the same nutritional needs as adults, in smaller portions. Table 61-2 ■ provides simple guidelines for offering a balanced diet for school-age children.

Parents should be aware of what is offered in their children's school cafeterias. School meals are planned to help moderate fat intake and offer more fiber through whole grains and fresh fruits. However, there are often choices for children that are not as healthful.

Often children choose not to eat the school lunch. Parents should become familiar with the menu offerings, and their child's likes and dislikes. Packing lunches can be an alternative for parents of "picky" children, or on days when the school lunch is not appealing to their child. Making the lunch fun to eat increases the chance that the child will eat it. Sandwiches with whole-wheat bread and lean, protein-rich fillings, fresh fruit and/or vegetables, low-fat or fat-free milk, and a low-fat dessert make a balanced packed lunch.

MyNursingKit | Health maintenance for school-age children

TABLE 61-1   Growth and Development Milestones during School-Age Years

AGE	PHYSICAL GROWTH	GROSS MOTOR SKILLS	FINE MOTOR SKILLS	COGNITIVE ABILITY	NUTRITION
6–12 years	Gains 3 to 5 lbs (1.5–5 kg)/year. Grows 1½ to 2½ in. (4–6 cm)/year. Loses teeth.	Increases balance and muscle strength. Uses roller skates/blades. Participates in group sports, such as football, soccer, basketball, gymnastics, dance, karate. (1)	Enjoys crafts, board games, computer games, musical instruments. (2)	Reads. Increases knowledge through school subjects. Concentrates for longer periods.	Can prepare own food. Needs three meals plus snacks.

(1) Concentrates on activities for longer periods

(2) Plays musical instruments

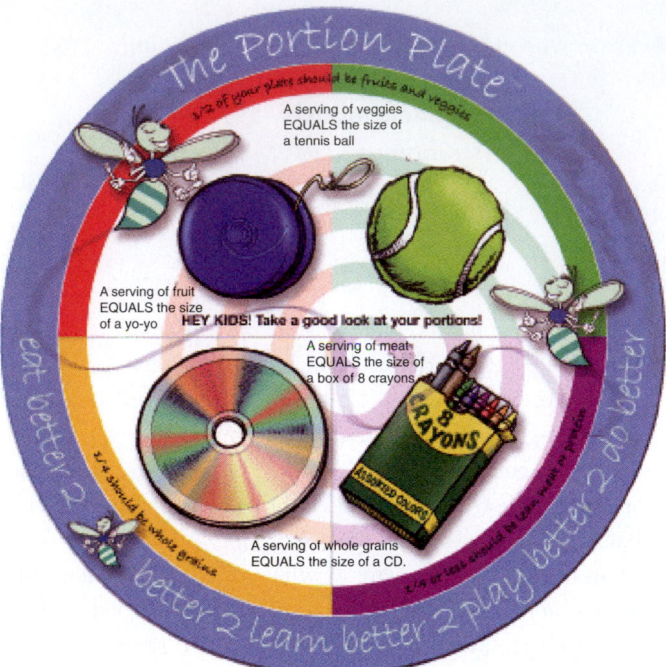

Figure 61-1. ■ The child's Portion Plate. (The child's Portion Plate product design and name is registered to beBetter Networks. To learn more about how the plate teaches portion control, or to order the plate, please visit: www.theportionplate.com.)

MyNursingKit | The importance of physical activity

TABLE 61-2	Recommended Number of Servings for Children Ages 6 to 12	
FOOD GROUP	**NUMBER OF SERVINGS**
Bread, cereal, rice, and pasta	6–9
Vegetables	3–4
Fruit	2–3
Milk, yogurt, and cheese	2–3
Meat, poultry, fish, dry beans, eggs, and nuts	2–3 (about 5–6 ounces)

After-school snacks can offer children the nutrients they need to maintain health. Box 61-1 ■ provides nutritional ideas for client teaching to parents of school-age children. (Nutrition was discussed in detail in Chapter 25 ⬭ .)

Children should be taught to brush their teeth as soon as they are able to hold the toothbrush and follow instructions. Semiannual dental exams are important to maintain good dentition.

BOX 61-1   CLIENT TEACHING

Nutritious Snacks for School-Age Children

The following are ideas for foods that give children energy when they need to snack.

- Bagel or English muffin "pizza" (toasted, with tomato sauce and cheese)
- Yogurt topped with fruit or granola
- Cereal topped with fruit and milk
- Tortilla rollups (Roll a tortilla with shredded cheese, microwave until the cheese is soft. The tortilla can be eaten plain or with salsa.)
- Peanut butter on half a wheat bagel
- Cheese and crackers
- Cut vegetables dipped in humus
- Roasted sunflower seeds or soybeans
- Pretzels
- Fresh or frozen bananas (Frozen bananas can be peeled and dipped in yogurt and granola before freezing.)
- Celery with low-fat cream cheese
- Peanut butter on graham crackers
- Fresh fruit (whole or cut) with or without peanut butter
- Low-fat string cheese
- Breakfast bars
- Blended fruit drink (½ cup low-fat yogurt and ½ cup cold fruit juice) or fresh fruit processed in a blender

Recall that the 24 baby teeth should begin to be replaced by permanent teeth at around 6 or 7 years of age. School-age children generally lose four teeth a year. By age 12, children have 26 of the 30 permanent teeth they will develop. Permanent molars continue to erupt until the child reaches late adolescence or early adulthood.

Often the permanent teeth come in crooked or become crooked due to lack of space in the oral cavity. Many parents choose to have the child wear braces on their teeth to straighten crooked teeth and make space for new teeth. The child must be reminded to keep the teeth clean to prevent cavities from forming around the orthodontic appliances.

Vital Signs in School-Age Children

The vital sign ranges of school-age children are listed in Table 61-3 ■. The in-depth discussion of vital signs is in Chapter 21 ⬭ .

TABLE 61-3	Variations in Normal Vital Signs—School-Age Children versus Adults			
AGE	**TEMPERATURE IN DEGREES CELSIUS**	**AVERAGE PULSE (RANGES)**	**AVERAGE RESPIRATIONS (RANGES)**	**BLOOD PRESSURE (MM HG)**
6–8 years	37 (oral)	100 (75–120)	20 (15–25)	95/57
10 years	37 (oral)	70 (50–90)	19 (15–25)	102/62
Adult	37 (oral)	80 (60–100)	16 (12–20)	120/80

ILLNESSES AND DISORDERS

Respiratory Disorders

Many respiratory disorders affecting older children began in the younger years and continue into adolescence and adulthood. The older child can be taught to assume some responsibility for the daily management of his or her respiratory condition.

TUBERCULOSIS

Tuberculosis (TB) is an infection of the respiratory system by the acid-fast bacillus *Mycobacterium tuberculosis*. Most individuals with TB are immune compromised with disorders such as HIV/AIDS, leukemia, or other disorders affecting white blood cells. When a child develops TB, the most common cause is close association with an infected adult. If left untreated, TB leads to lung damage and central nervous system involvement, including tuberculosis meningitis, coma, and death. See Chapter 32 ◯◯ for a complete discussion of tuberculosis.

ASTHMA

Asthma is a chronic inflammatory disorder of the tracheobronchial tree. Asthma attacks are influenced by a variety of triggers including environmental factors such as smog or pesticides, fumes, secondhand smoke, allergens, medications, exercise, or stress (Figure 61-2 ■). (Research has confirmed that secondhand cigarette smoke contributes significantly to chronic respiratory problems in children of all ages. This fact should be stressed with parents. If a parent is not ready to give up smoking, he or she may be willing to smoke outside, keeping the inside of the home smoke free.)

The stimulus that initiates the inflammatory process is specific to each individual. As the child gets older, has more experiences in the community, and begins to travel outside the local areas, he or she will be exposed to more allergens that can trigger an asthma attack. The older child can assume more responsibility for the daily management of asthma.

Manifestations

As the lining of the tracheobronchial tree becomes irritated by the allergen, fumes, or dust, the cells release histamine. Histamine causes inflammation of the mucous membrane, resulting in swelling, increased mucus production, and spasm of the bronchial muscles (Figure 61-3 ■). Large amounts of mucus block the small airways, trapping air below the mucous plug. Over time, chronic irritation causes scar formation in the airway lining, hyperinflation of the alveoli, and one form of chronic obstructive pulmonary disease (COPD).

The stimulus that triggers an asthma attack is specific for each individual and may include allergens, medications, fumes, exercise, or stress. Before puberty, more boys have asthma, but by adulthood, the disorder is equally distributed between boys and girls.

Asthma causes shortness of breath, wheezing, and productive cough with thick sputum. Initially tachypnea, tachycardia, and use of accessory muscles of respiration are common.

Psychologic reactions often intensify the symptoms of asthma. As the airway becomes blocked, the child becomes anxious and feels that he or she is suffocating. Severe anxiety intensifies the symptoms, and a vicious cycle ensues. Emotional stress may even trigger asthma attacks.

Treatment

Treatment is aimed at preventing acute attacks by use of bronchodilators and anti-inflammatory drugs. Depending on severity of symptoms, treatment may be daily or only

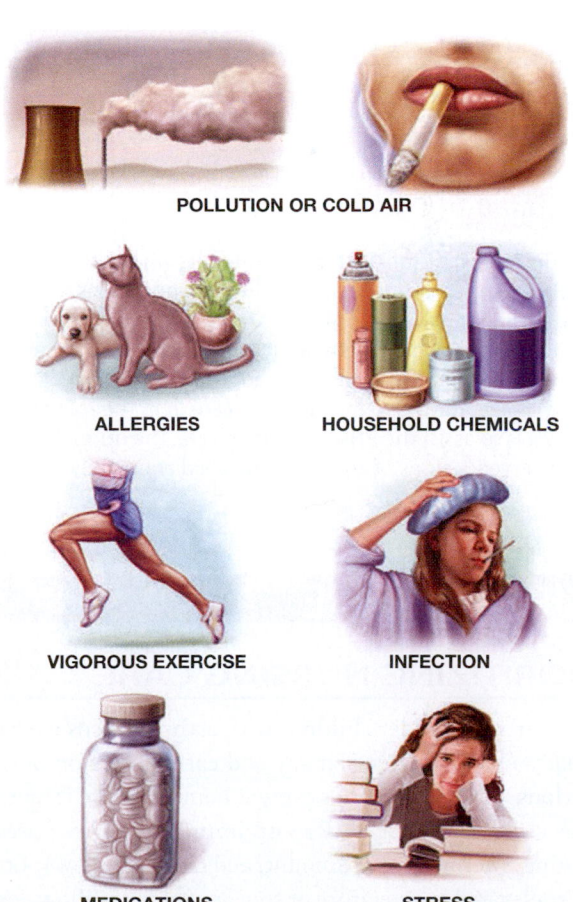

POLLUTION OR COLD AIR

ALLERGIES   HOUSEHOLD CHEMICALS

VIGOROUS EXERCISE   INFECTION

MEDICATIONS   STRESS

Figure 61-2. ■ Many factors can trigger asthma attacks. The required lifestyle changes for the child and family will be significant, so be sensitive to the family's situation and needs. Culture sometimes plays a significant part in exposure to lifestyle triggers.

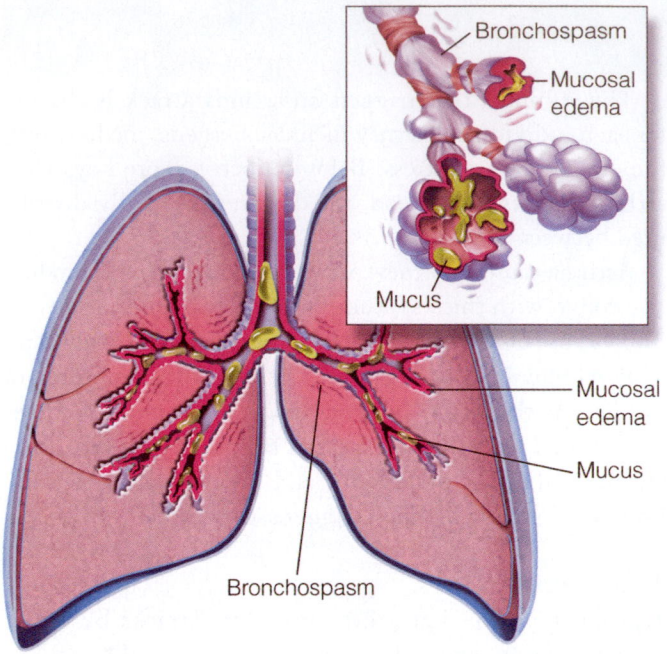

Bronchospasm

Mucosal edema

Mucus

Mucosal edema

Mucus

Bronchospasm

Figure 61-3. ■ When an asthma attack occurs, the bronchi constrict and spasm, and mucus obstructs the airway.

when symptoms occur. To reduce the possibility of exercise-induced asthma, a child may premedicate with a prescribed inhaler.

clinical ALERT

A condition called *status asthmaticus* occurs when the child develops severe respiratory distress and bronchospasms that do not respond to medication. Without immediate medical attention, the child may die. Treatment may involve repeated nebulizer treatments, airway intubation, and ventilator support. The child will be admitted to the intensive care unit. The role of the LPN/LVN is to assist the RN in providing care. The nurse would also observe for signs of anxiety in the child and family.

NURSING CARE

PRIORITIZING NURSING CARE

When caring for older children with asthma, focus your care on maintaining a patent airway and early detection of complications. Auscultate lungs every 2 hours or more frequently if the child is unstable. Report immediately increases in wheezing. Monitor color, amount, and consistency of sputum. Report elevated temperature or sputum colored yellow, green, or tan. Help the child keep the oxygen mask in place—use of distraction and playing games may help. Explain the reasons for medications and treatments in terms the child can

| BOX 61-2 | DATA COLLECTION |

Child with Acute Asthma
Focused Observations
Answers to the following questions provide important data for the assessment of a child with asthma:

- Is the child able to talk, or does respiratory distress prevent speech?
- Is the child wheezing?
- What is the child's color and heart rate?
- Is the child relaxed or fighting to breathe? Is the child crying?
- Is the child clinging to a parent or lying calmly on the bed?
- What is the family doing? Do they appear frightened? What is their tone of voice?
- Do the parents ask appropriate questions?

understand. Encourage the child to ask for what he or she needs. For example, an older child may want a parent to stay through the night, but does not want to seem like "a baby" to others.

ASSESSING

In the child with asthma, a complete physical assessment of lung function is performed, including oxygen saturation, lung sounds, and breathing pattern. Data from pulmonary function tests are useful in determining the extent of damage, as well as the effectiveness of treatment. Skin testing is done to identify specific allergens. The respiratory therapist is helpful in providing prescribed breathing treatments. Box 61-2 ■ identifies areas for focused observations when working with a child with asthma.

DIAGNOSING, PLANNING, AND IMPLEMENTING

Common nursing diagnoses for a child with asthma include the following:

- *Ineffective Airway Clearance*
- *Deficient Knowledge* related to new treatment regimen
- *Anxiety*

Client outcomes for a child with asthma involve:

- Resolution of inflammation.
- Return to normal breathing patterns.
- Reduction of anxiety.
- Identification of potential triggers.
- Proper use of inhalers and medications (*Note:* School-age children will need to be able to administer medication properly and use a peak expiratory flow rate (PEFR) meter correctly (Figure 61-4 ■). Practice and repeat demonstration may be necessary.)

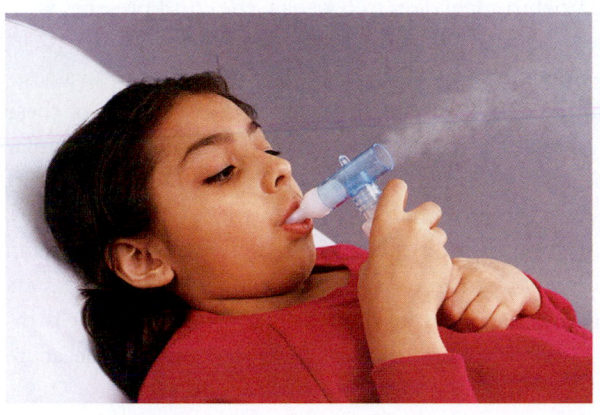
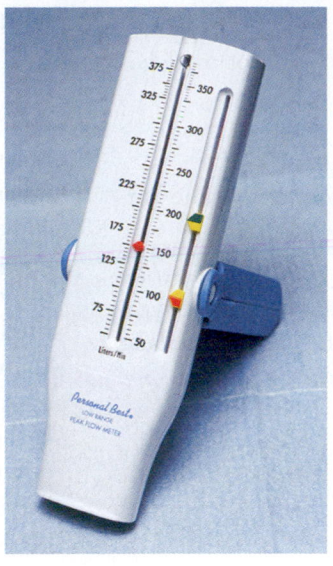
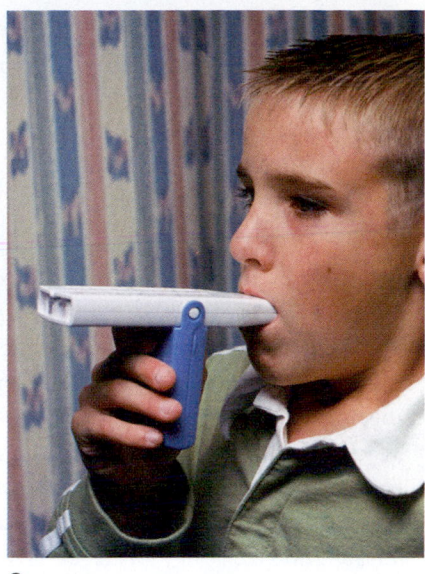

A   B   C

Figure 61-4. ■ **A.** Child with nebulizer for asthma medicine. This nebulizer has a mouthpiece attachment; other nebulizers have facemasks. **B.** Peak expiratory flow rate (PEFR) meter. **C.** Child using PEFR device.

When a child is admitted with an acute asthma attack, the priorities of care are to open the airway, maintain breathing, and ensure adequate circulation. Nursing interventions are aimed at resolving the airway difficulty and supporting the client and family:

- Provide medication as ordered. Medication to relax bronchial constriction and thin secretions is given by intermittent positive-pressure breathing (IPPB). An IV is established by the RN or certified LPN/LVN. *Airway management is the first priority in the ABCs of nursing care. The IV will allow fluid maintenance and administration of corticosteroids to reduce inflammation.*
- Give oxygen by mask. *Oxygen by mask increases the oxygen saturation in the blood and decreases the workload of the heart.*
- Perform interventions in a calm, confident manner. *This reassures the child and the family and reduces their level of anxiety.*
- Reinforce teaching about the condition and the treatment plan, including use of inhalers and nebulizers (see Box 27-10 ⬤⬤), and peak expiratory flow rate (PEFR) meters. *Once the child has stabilized, a long-term treatment plan is discussed with the parents. The parents and the child should be taught how to use inhalers and nebulizers. Asthma triggers should be identified and eliminated from the child's environment if possible. Parents need to discuss the treatment plan with the child's teachers and school personnel.*
- Encourage the child to be responsible to take medication as prescribed and to have emergency inhaler available should an acute episode develop. *The child should have access to inhalers while at school. With treatment, the child can participate in most school activities.*

EVALUATING

A return to normal breathing patterns is the priority assessment as evidenced by an increase in PEFR. Nurses are also responsible for reinforcing and documenting teaching. The child and the parent should understand when and how to administer medication.

NURSING PROCESS CARE PLAN
Client with Asthma

Jane, a 7-year-old, is admitted to the pediatric unit with a diagnosis of acute asthma. Her vital signs are T 98.4, P 112, R 36. She has high-pitched wheezing on expiration. The physician has ordered IV Solu-Medrol and breathing treatments.

Assessment
Wheezing respirations. Labored breathing. Clings to mother.

Nursing Diagnosis
The following important nursing diagnosis (among others) is established for this condition:

- *Ineffective Airway Clearance* related to allergic response, inflamed bronchial tree

Expected Outcomes
Expected outcomes for Jane are that:

- Wheezing will resolve after administration of medication.
- Respirations will return to within normal range.

- Client will state that breathing is easier.
- Parent and child will return demonstration of metered-dose inhaler for medication.

Planning and Implementation

The following nursing interventions are planned and implemented for Jane:

- Administer medication as ordered. *Medications relieve bronchial inflammation, decrease swelling, and open airways.*
- Teach child and parent how and when to use the handheld nebulizer. *Parent and child need instruction in technique and in proper use of the medication.*
- Teach appropriate "play" techniques to extend expiratory time. *Increasing expiratory pressure and extending expiratory time improve breathing by keeping airways open, allowing air to leave the lungs.*
- Supervise use of breathing equipment (e.g., inhalers, nebulizers, oxygen cannula/mask). *This ensures proper use of breathing equipment.*

Evaluation

Lungs sound clear, breathing pattern within normal limits. Parents and child can verbalize and demonstrate use of breathing equipment.

Critical Thinking in the Nursing Process

1. What play activities could lengthen the exhalation time?
2. What questions should Jane and her parents be asked to help identify causative agents for the asthma attack?
3. What can the nurse do to help Jane express her feelings?

Note: Discussion of Critical Thinking questions appears on the MyNursingKit Website.

Cardiovascular Disorders

As the child grows, the incidence of cardiovascular disorders decreases. (See Chapter 33 for a full discussion of cardiovascular system disorders.)

ACUTE RHEUMATIC FEVER

Acute rheumatic fever (ARF) is an inflammatory disorder that follows a group A beta-hemolytic *Streptococcus* infection of the throat (pharyngitis, tonsillitis). Rheumatic fever is more common in children between 6 and 15 years old. There has been a decrease in the number of cases of rheumatic fever due to the use of antibiotics in the treatment of beta-hemolytic *Streptococcus* infections. While the exact pathology is unknown, it is felt that the group A beta-hemolytic *Streptococcus* triggers an autoimmune response that damages the heart, joints, central nervous system (CNS), and skin.

Manifestations

Rheumatic fever most often follows a streptococcal throat infection. The child could have had a mild sore throat that was relatively asymptomatic or a more severe respiratory illness. Within a few days to 6 weeks, the child presents with inflamed joints and heart, red rash (see Figure 60-3C), and a temperature of 100.4°F (38°C) or higher. The assessment of the child must include detailed assessment of these body systems. There may be an increased heart rate, irregular rhythm, and abnormal sounds (see Table 33-3 , Heart Sounds and Abnormalities). Tachycardia, atrial fibrillation, murmurs, and friction rub may be caused by inflammation of the heart. Most commonly the mitral and aortic valves are permanently damaged by rheumatic fever. If the heart is involved, the child should be hospitalized during the acute phase of the illness.

The child's joints become enlarged, inflamed, and extremely painful for several weeks. The most commonly affected joints are the knees, elbows, and wrists. Rarely does permanent deformity occur.

Diagnosis and Treatment

Erythema marginatum occurs more commonly with endocarditis. This transient rash is characterized by nonpruritic, red, macular lesions that blanch in the center. The rash is frequently found on the chest, abdomen, buttocks, and proximal limbs. The rash does not cause permanent skin damage.

If the central nervous system is involved, the condition is knows as *Sydenham's chorea* (St. Vitus' dance). Changes in the CNS rarely occur until late in the disease process, possibly after other symptoms have subsided. The child experiences involuntary facial and upper extremity movements. There may be abnormal EEG findings that gradually return to normal. **Chorea** (involuntary, spasmodic movements of the limbs and face) can last for a few weeks or as long as 2 years. Eventually the child returns to normal functioning.

Antibiotics and aspirin are prescribed. In the acute phase of rheumatic fever, the child is assessed every 4 hours for elevated temperature and heart function. Tepid baths or cool compresses may be provided to decrease temperature and provide comfort. Intravenous fluids are monitored carefully, because fluid overload could lead to congestive heart failure. The nurse provides quiet activities to prevent the child from overtaxing the heart.

clinical ALERT

Polyarthritis of ARF responds better to the anti-inflammatory effect of aspirin than to acetaminophen or ibuprofen. Parents should be instructed to follow the doctor's orders about medication administration.

BOX 61-3   **CLIENT TEACHING**

Recovery Phase of Acute Rheumatic Fever

Activity limited to prevent heart damage: Plan quiet activities like computer and board games or reading. As activities increase and child returns to school, arrange periods of rest.

Medication: Long-term antibiotic therapy is necessary. It is important to take medication as prescribed to prevent heart damage.

Future health care: Tell future healthcare providers, including dentist and surgeon, of history of rheumatic fever. Prophylactic antibiotic may be needed before procedures. Do not ignore future sore throats; the child may need increased antibiotics.

Nursing Considerations

During the recovery phase, the child will be cared for at home. Parents need to be reassured that rash, chorea, and arthritis will subside. The child will need to have limited activities but should be able to return to school. The child may remain on long-term antibiotic therapy. It is important to tell future healthcare providers, including dentists and surgeons, of the history of rheumatic fever. Prophylactic antibiotics may be prescribed prior to invasive procedures. Teaching is very important for long-term care after discharge (Box 61-3 ■). The child and parents should understand the need to prevent infection, treat sore throats, and monitor heart function.

Evaluation of heart function during and following acute rheumatic fever is a crucial part of care. The child and parents should be able to verbalize the need for follow-up evaluation. They should also be able to state the type and dosage of medications, the signs of infection, and the guidelines for seeking medical attention.

Hematologic Disorders

HYPERLIPIDEMIA

Hyperlipidemia is a condition characterized by increased total cholesterol, low-density lipoproteins, and triglycerides accompanied by decreased high-density lipoproteins. Children rarely exhibit symptoms of hyperlipidemia. However, several disorders seen in adults (hypertension, coronary artery disease, cerebrovascular disease) result from hyperlipidemia. Because it takes time for hyperlipidemia to affect the blood vessels, controlling lipid levels in children may prevent vascular diseases later in life.

Nursing Considerations

The nurse should teach older children and their parents to reduce the risk of developing hyperlipidemia by making appropriate food choices, increasing exercise, and eliminating environmental hazards such as cigarette smoking. Because the school-age child will be eating more meals away from home, the child should be taught to select foods that fit into the food pyramid.

Parents should be taught to be fitness role models for their children. They can take the stairs in public places instead of riding the elevator, or they can park the car some distance from their shopping destination. They can encourage their children to get involved in a team sport. Growing up in a family where smoking is the norm increases the chance that the child will smoke too. Smoking cessation classes are offered in most communities.

ANEMIA

Anemia from dietary causes is discussed here because the school-age child may have a diet poor in iron, resulting in iron-deficiency anemia (see Chapter 34 ∞). The anemic child can lack energy for activities and may have difficulty in school. Encouraging the parents to give the child a multiple vitamin with iron may provide the child with resources needed to correct anemia.

Anemia may be associated with *pica*, a craving to eat substances that are not food. A child who is seen eating dirt, clay, chalk, glue, ice, starch, or hair should be assessed to determine whether anemia is the cause. Teach parents to recognize and report these symptoms promptly.

Immune Disorders

JUVENILE RHEUMATOID ARTHRITIS

Recall from Chapter 59 ∞ that juvenile rheumatoid arthritis (JRA) is a chronic autoimmune disorder resulting in joint inflammation, decreased mobility, swelling, and pain. Remissions may last for months, years, or a lifetime. Children with early onset have a better prognosis for complete recovery.

JRA is usually treated with corticosteroids, NSAIDs, or aspirin. (However, children who receive aspirin are at risk of developing Reye's syndrome if they become infected with influenza or chickenpox.) Following CDC guidelines, these children may need to be immunized with varicella vaccine (Marin et al., 2007) and should receive influenza vaccine every fall.

As mentioned in the main discussion in Chapter 59 ∞ , physical therapy can be very helpful for children with juvenile rheumatoid arthritis (Figure 61-5 ■). JRA may be restricted to a few joints or be systemic with involvement of multiple joints, including large joints such as the knees and small joints of the hands. Although children with JRA rarely need to be hospitalized, severe pain and immobility can keep the child from attending school and participating in physical activities. JRA can also impede the child's growth. Irregular attendance at school and limited participation in outside school activities can interfere with the development of close friendships. Together these aspects of the disorder have a major impact on the child's self-image, self-esteem, and psychosocial growth.

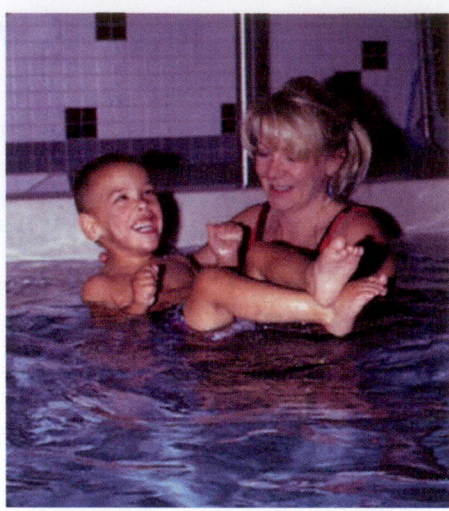

Figure 61-5. ■ Swimming is very helpful for maintaining joint function in children with juvenile rheumatoid arthritis.

Immune disorders are discussed in depth in Chapter 35 ⊙⊙.

Nervous System Disorders

Many nervous system disorders affecting the older child are similar to the disorders affecting the younger child.

NEUROLOGIC INJURY

Neurologic injury is defined as any trauma to the head or spinal cord resulting from force, anoxia, or penetration. Neurologic injuries are the most common serious injuries in childhood. Closed head injuries in the school-age child commonly result from falls from bicycles, automobile accidents, or sporting events. Hypoxic or anoxic neurologic trauma may result from drowning, carbon monoxide poisoning, or aspiration. Spinal cord injury results from hyperflexion, lateral flexion, extension, or compression of the vertebrae. The medical treatment and nursing care are similar to that of an adult (see Chapter 36 ⊙⊙).

Neurologic injury can be prevented. Seat belts and helmets (Figure 61-6 ■) can decrease the number and extent of injuries. Drowning can be prevented by education, close adult supervision, and environmental changes. Pools should be fenced with a 5-foot fence that children cannot climb. Children of all ages should be supervised when near pools, at the beach, or in the bathtub.

HEADACHES

Children commonly have headaches. Headaches in children have both a benign (migraine, inflammatory, and tension) and structural causes. Migraine headaches may be triggered by stress, foods containing nitrates, glutamate, caffeine, tyramine, and salt. Tension headaches may be related to stress due to school, insecurity, or conflict in the family. Headaches may be caused by an allergic reaction to airborne pollen or pet dander. Headaches associated with other neurological deficits may indicate other neurological pathology such as brain tumors.

An occasional headache is not a major concern and is usually treated with acetaminophen or NSAIDs. Frequent headaches should be investigated by the primary healthcare provider.

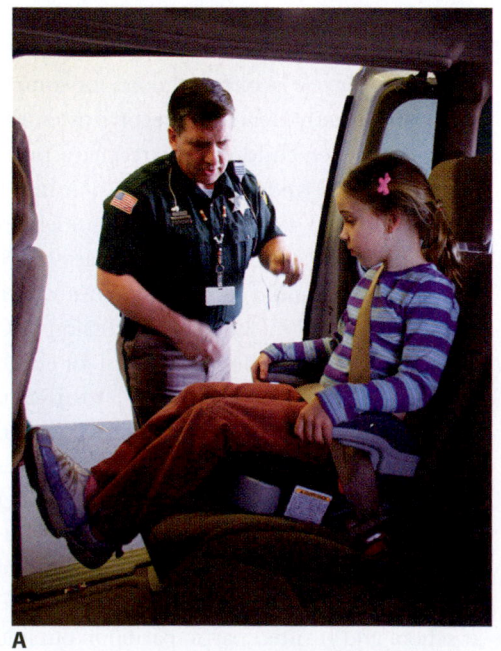

A

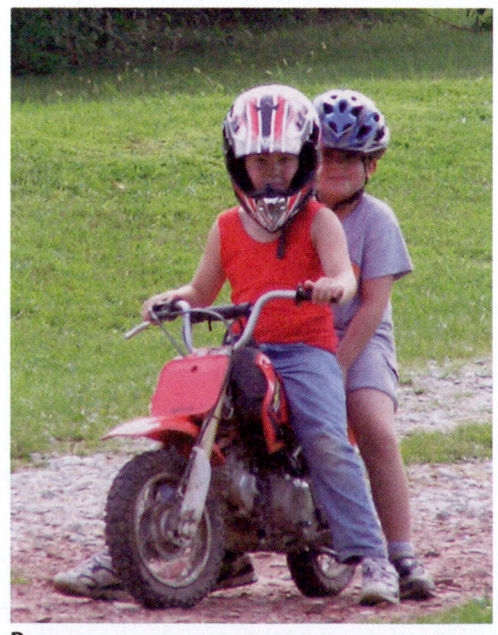

B

Figure 61-6. ■ **A.** It is important to be consistent in using seat belts. The general guideline is that children under the age of 12 years should not ride in the front seat of a car because front seat air bags can suffocate a child if they inflate. **B.** Children on motorized bikes are at risk for injury. Helmets, kneepads, and elbow pads can help to reduce the risk.

SENSORY DISORDERS

Strabismus

Strabismus is an eye disorder in which the eyes cannot be directed to the same object. One or both eyes could deviate inward (cross eyes) or outward (wall-eyes). The child may squint, have difficulty picking up objects, and may need to close one eye in order to read. The condition is usually diagnosed shortly after birth. Treatment includes patching the good eye to force use of the weak eye, surgery to correct muscle imbalance, and compensatory lenses. If treatment is begun before 24 months of age, amblyopia may be prevented.

Amblyopia

Amblyopia is a reduction in vision in which there is no pathology in the eye. Amblyopia can be caused by strabismus, congenital cataract, or the effect of alcohol, tobacco, lead, drugs, or other toxins. Amblyopia is often diagnosed in the school years because of difficulties in seeing the board. Treatment includes compensatory lenses, occlusion of the good eye, and atropine 1% eye drop to the unaffected eye. Treatment is discontinued when visual acuity no longer improves. Visual acuity of 20/20 is rarely attained.

Focusing Errors

There are three other visual disturbances (Figure 61-7 ■) that occur in children, as well as in the general population. **Hyperopia** occurs when light is focused behind the retina. **Myopia** occurs when light is focused in front of the retina. **Astigmatism** occurs when light rays do not uniformly focus on the eye due to abnormal curvature of cornea or lens. In most cases, visual acuity is improved with corrective lenses. The child's maturity, level of responsibility, and activities should be taken into consideration when choosing glasses or contact lenses. Because these disorders change rapidly with the child's growth, it is common that the prescription for correction will change frequently.

Nurses in schools plan and carry out visual screening on children. Any abnormal results should be reported to the family and a referral made to an eye care specialist.

Stye (Hordeolum)

A stye is an infection of a sebaceous gland or oil gland of the eyelid. *Staphylococcus* is the most common causative agent. The child may have pain, redness, and swelling of the eyelid. There may be a pustule around the affected eyelash. Styes are treated with ophthalmic antibiotic ointments and warm, moist compresses to relieve discomfort.

Musculoskeletal Disorders

Musculoskeletal disorders are some of the most common disorders affecting the older child, due in part to changes in bone structure during periods of rapid growth and accidents as the child interacts with the environment.

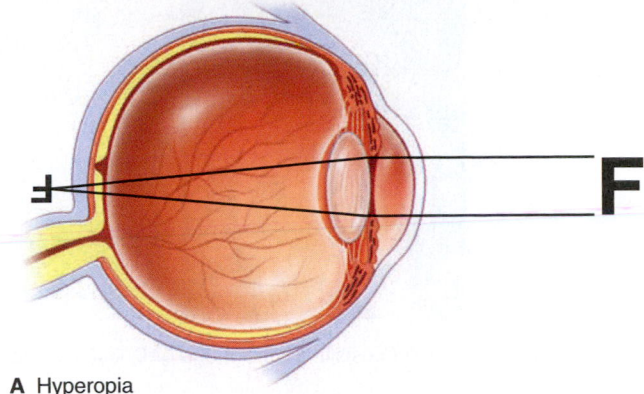

A Hyperopia

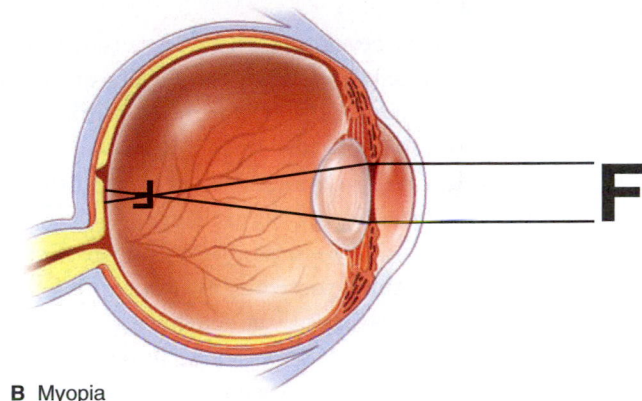

B Myopia

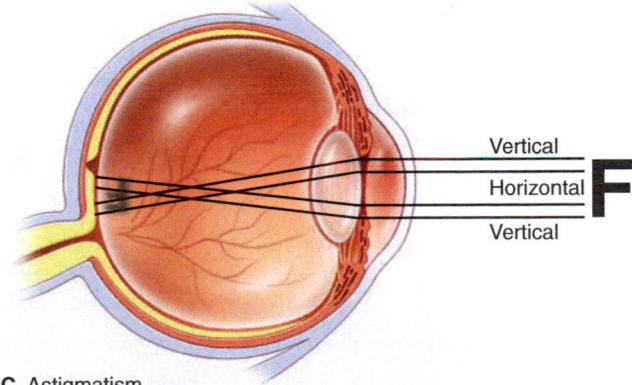

C Astigmatism

Figure 61-7. ■ A. Hyperopia. In hyperopia light rays focus behind the retina, making it difficult to focus on objects at close range. **B.** Myopia. In myopia light rays focus in front of the retina, making it difficult to focus on objects that are far away. **C.** Astigmatism. In astigmatism light rays do not uniformly focus on the eye due to abnormal curvature of cornea or lens.

SCOLIOSIS

Scoliosis is a lateral S- or C-shaped curve of the spine, with rotation of the spine and ribs. Scoliosis is most common in girls between 10 and 13 years of age. It is also associated with other musculoskeletal and nervous system deformities. Most commonly there is a right-sided thoracic curve and a left-sided lumbar curve.

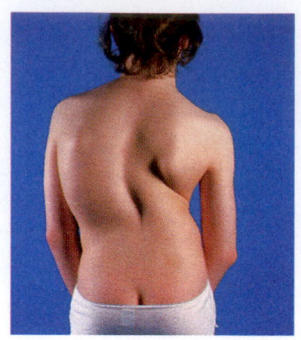

Figure 61-8. ■ Severe scoliosis in a school-age girl. *Source:* Photo Researchers Inc.

Manifestations

Symptoms of scoliosis develop slowly and without pain. Rotation of the vertebrae and ribs causes a one-sided rib hump and a prominent scapula. Deformities of the spine cause a cosmetic problem but also impact respiratory function. The size and shape of the chest cavity can limit the expansion of the lungs and impair gas exchange.

The school nurse routinely assesses many children for scoliosis. (See scoliosis screening procedure in Chapter 48 🔗.) In assessing the back, the shoulders and hips are different heights (Figure 61-8 ■). This often causes clothing to hang unevenly. The child is also asked to bend forward, and the posterior chest is inspected for symmetry. If spinal curvature is identified, parents are referred to their primary care provider for diagnosis and treatment.

Two other spinal curvatures warrant mention. *Kyphosis,* excessive convex curvature of the thoracic spine, is also known as hunchback. *Lordosis,* or swayback, is an excessive concave curvature of the lumbar spine. Frequently these abnormal curvatures are found together (Table 61-4 ■).

Diagnosis and Treatment

Diagnosis is made by spinal x-ray. The goal of treatment is to limit or stop the progression of spinal deformity. The method of treatment depends on the degree of curvature. Mild scoliosis can be treated with exercise to increase muscle tone and flexibility and to improve posture. Chiropractic adjustments may be used to realign vertebrae if there is a mild degree of curvature (Box 61-4 ■).

A Boston or Milwaukee brace is used to treat moderate scoliosis. A *Boston brace* is a plastic spinal jacket. A *Milwaukee brace,* made of strong, lightweight material, extends from the chin to the pelvis. These braces are custom fit for the child and should be worn 23 hours a day. During the hour without the brace the child may bathe, shower, or take part in activities that the brace would restrict. Unless otherwise instructed by the physician, the child is not prohibited from participating in sports activities.

Severe scoliosis requires surgery to fuse the spine and insert rods or wires to strengthen the spine. A halo brace (Figure 61-9 ■) may be used after surgery to hold the body in alignment. Some surgeons may perform the surgery laparoscopically. Postoperatively the child will remain on bed

TABLE 61-4	Spinal Curvatures	
CONDITION	**DIAGNOSIS AND TREATMENT**	**NURSING INTERVENTIONS**
Lordosis: excessive concave curvature of the lumbar spine	*Diagnosis:* Look at child from side. Observe lumbar curve. Confirm with spinal x-ray. *Treatment:* Exercises and postural awareness. Chiropractic therapy.	Encourage physical conditioning exercises. Reassure family that condition may be outgrown as child matures.
Kyphosis: excessive convex curvature of thoracic spine	*Diagnosis:* Have child bend forward at waist. Look at thoracic spine at level of scapula. Confirm with x-ray. *Treatment:* Mild condition requires exercise, moderate condition requires bracing, severe condition requires surgery. Chiropractic therapy.	Encourage strengthening exercises and posture awareness. Teach brace application and postoperative care. Help deal with altered body image.
Scoliosis: S-shaped curve of the spine often with rotation of spine and hips	*Diagnosis:* Observe back for deformity, uneven scapula and hips, one-sided rib hump. Confirm with x-ray. *Treatment:* Mild condition (10–20 degrees) requires exercise, chiropractic therapy. Moderate condition (20–40 degrees) requires bracing in addition to exercise. Severe condition (40 degrees or more) requires surgery with spinal fusion.	Promote compliance with treatment plan. Encourage diligence with exercise plan. Provide emotional support for child and family. Teach brace application and care. Teach postoperative care.

rest during recovery. Once the child is able to sit up, a plastic anterior and posterior shell is used to stabilize the back until healing is complete. The rod permanently immobilizes the spine, preventing the child from bending forward.

OSGOOD-SCHLATTER DISEASE

Osgood-Schlatter disease is an overgrowth of the tibial epiphysis due primarily to recurring inflammatory episodes. The repeated pull of the quadriceps femoris as seen in athletic children is thought to cause the inflammation, new bone formation, and an unattractive bone prominent at the knee. The disease is most common during growth spurts in boys between 13 and 14 and girls between 10 and 11 years of age. Treatment is aimed at resting the joint until healing occurs and at strengthening the muscles around the knee. Casting the knee may be necessary to relieve pain and

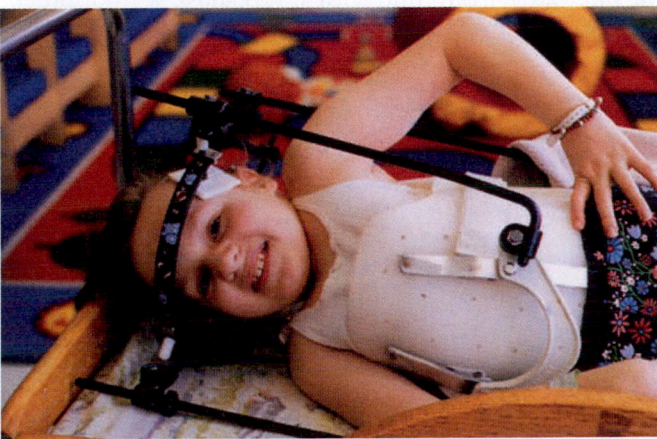

Figure 61-9. ■ In severe scoliosis, the child may wear a halo brace, shown here, to hold the body in position after surgery.

swelling. Surgery is rarely needed. If the joint is not properly rested, the condition can recur.

MUSCULOSKELETAL TUMORS

Osteosarcoma

Bone tumors are rare, but periods of rapid growth are the most common times for occurrence in adolescent boys. Bone tumors are usually found in the distal femur, proximal tibia, or proximal humerus.

MANIFESTATIONS. Clinical manifestations include pain, swelling, and mobility or gait problems. Fever, elevated white blood cell count, and elevated erythrocyte sedimentation rate may be seen.

DIAGNOSIS AND TREATMENT. X-ray, computed tomography (CT) or MRI scan, and tissue biopsy are used to reach a diagnosis of osteosarcoma.

Treatment involves surgery and the use of chemotherapy and radiation. Depending on the extent of the tumor, limb-sparing surgery may be used to remove the tumor and surrounding bone. An internal prosthesis is then inserted. Amputation must be performed if the tumor is large or involves surrounding soft tissue, including nerves. Chemotherapy and radiation are given to treat nondetectable metastasis. Physicians should educate and counsel parents regarding future childbearing for these children. The child may become sterile, and sperm banking may be necessary prior to chemotherapy.

NURSING CONSIDERATIONS. Nursing care involves standard preoperative and postoperative care. Psychosocial assessment of the adolescent and the family is necessary. Body image disturbances occur when a limb is lost. Signs of disturbed body image include:

- Refusal to look at or touch the altered body part
- Hiding the affected body part
- Preoccupation with the loss or change
- Overexposure of the body part
- Feelings of guilt, shame, or embarrassment

Client and family support systems should be identified and contacted as soon as possible. The older child or adolescent will need to learn to care for the stump (see Figure 31-11 ⚭ and Box 61-5 ■). Rehabilitation will be needed to help the child learn to use the prosthesis and adapt to the amputation.

Prosthetics can be expensive, and parents may need financial support beyond insurance. Referral to special hospitals such as the Shriners Hospital may be an option. The school should be contacted and plans made for the adolescent's return. Some adaptation may be needed to accommodate a wheelchair, crutches, or other appliance and to plan for emergency evacuation.

Care of the Stump following Amputation

☑ Carefully monitor vital signs and drainage from dressing.

☑ Keep a surgical tourniquet available to control bleeding if necessary.

☑ Observe strict sterile technique for dressing changes to prevent infection.

☑ Apply compression bandage as ordered.

☑ Change bandages twice daily to observe for wound healing.

☑ Avoid hip flexion contractures by limiting sitting in chair to less than 1 hour. Also avoid pillows under the limb.

☑ Explain phantom limb pain to the child and parents. Symptoms include coolness, heaviness, and pain. Pain is greater if there was pain before the procedure, because the brain remembers the pain experienced. People who had intense pain before amputation may never be free of pain postoperatively. Traumatic injuries are sometimes easier, due to the sudden amputation and the lack of prior pain for the brain to remember.

☑ Administer pain medications as ordered to control the child's comfort. Premedicate before physical therapy or activities to get better results from the activity. Assist with fitting of the temporary prosthesis. Sizing of a prosthesis will not begin until all the swelling is gone. If the child weighs more than 250 pounds, a prosthesis may not be available or safe until the child loses weight. Also, as the child grows, new prostheses will be required. For these reasons, most clients do not have a permanent prosthesis right away.

☑ Assist with ROM exercises as ordered.

☑ Teach crutch walking with lower limb amputation as ordered.

Ewing's Sarcoma

Ewing's sarcoma is a malignant tumor found most commonly in the femur, pelvis, tibia, fibula, ribs, humerus, scapula, and clavicle. Caucasians and Hispanics are most commonly affected. Children ages 10 to 20 years have the highest incidence of Ewing's sarcoma.

MANIFESTATIONS. Clinical manifestations are similar to osteosarcoma. Fractures of the affected bone may occur.

DIAGNOSIS AND TREATMENT. Diagnosis is made by biopsy of the tumor. Treatment includes chemotherapy to reduce the tumor size, followed by surgery to remove the bone. High-dose radiation may also be implemented. With treatment, remission may occur. However, long-term prognosis is not favorable. Nursing care of children with Ewing's sarcoma is the same as outlined for osteosarcoma.

Rhabdomyosarcoma

Rhabdomyosarcoma is a malignant tumor originating in the muscle around the eye, in the neck, and less commonly in the abdomen, genitourinary tract, and extremities. Tumors close to the eye produce swelling, ptosis, visual disturbance, and eye movement abnormalities. When the tumor occurs in the genitourinary tract, the result can be urinary obstruction.

MANIFESTATIONS. Rhabdomyosarcoma occurring in the abdomen may be asymptomatic. There is a rapid metastasis to lungs, bones, bone marrow, and distant lymph nodes.

NURSING CONSIDERATIONS. Treatment includes removal of the tumor when possible. Many children have metastasis at time of diagnosis and surgical removal is not possible. Chemotherapy may be used.

NURSING CARE

PRIORITIZING NURSING CARE

When caring for children with musculoskeletal disorders, the nurse must promote independence in the child. Nursing care will focus on the child's mobility and maintaining safety.

ASSESSING

Because musculoskeletal disorders frequently cause temporary or permanent mobility problems, monitor cardiac, respiratory, urinary, and bowel function. Assess range of motion, mobility, posture, and muscle strength. Note any swelling or redness. If the child uses mobility devices, assess the correct use of the device. For chronic disorders, the nurse collects data about the family's ability to care for the child in the home.

DIAGNOSIS, PLANNING, AND IMPLEMENTING

The following nursing diagnoses may be used in planning nursing care for the child with a musculoskeletal disorder.

■ *Impaired Physical Mobility* related to musculoskeletal impairment
■ *Activity Intolerance* related to weakness
■ *Risk for Injury* related to altered mobility
■ *Disabled Family Coping* related to caring for a child with a chronic condition

Typical outcomes for the child or family with a musculoskeletal disorder might include these as well as others:

■ Mobility will be restored through the use of assistive devices.
■ Tolerance for activity will be demonstrated as evidenced by vital signs within normal limits.
■ Family will create a safe environment.
■ Family will participate effectively in developing a plan to care for the child.

Nursing interventions related to children with musculoskeletal disorders include:

- Teach client to use assistive devices. *Crutches, canes, braces, walkers, and wheelchairs require specific instruction to operate properly. Demonstration and return demonstration of the use of these devices will promote mobility. A variety of lightweight wheelchairs are available. As the child grows, assistive devices may need to be replaced.*

- Provide positive encouragement before, during, and after use of assistive devices. *Encouragement will promote well-being and the desire to continue working on using the devices properly.*

- Assist the family in planning daily activities to include periods of rest. *Adequate rest is essential for energy conservation.*

- Keep frequently used objects within easy reach. *Reducing the number of steps required to complete activities of daily living will assist in energy conservation.*

- Assist the parents in assessing their home environment for safety hazards. *Safety hazards must be identified in order to correct them.*

- Provide information about correcting identified hazards. *Instructing families in how to correct hazards will help them manage their environment correctly and prevent injury.*

- Discuss with the family the common responses to caring for a child with a musculoskeletal disorder. *The nurse can assist the family in identifying anxiety, fear, and depression as normal responses for families in their situation.*

- Provide the family with specific information on caring for their child with a musculoskeletal disorder. *Families can develop coping mechanisms when they are able to view the task before them and understand how it can be managed effectively.*

EVALUATING

The child is evaluated for mobility, tolerance to activity, and safety. The family can be evaluated for coping with the care of the child. These evaluations should be made on a regular basis because these criteria can change throughout the child's care.

Gastrointestinal Disorders

Gastrointestinal system disorders affecting the older child are similar to those affecting adults. The most common disorders are infections such as viral gastroenteritis, but they also include parasitic infestations. See Chapter 37 ⚭ for additional information on gastrointestinal system disorders. The focus of nursing care is to maintain nutrition and fluid balance.

APPENDICITIS

Appendicitis is inflammation of the vermiform appendix, a small sac at the end of the cecum that no longer serves a function in the GI tract. If the appendix becomes blocked with intestinal contents, infection and inflammation can occur. Appendicitis is most common in boys between 10 and 16, and rarely occurs before 2 years of age. Initially there is a blockage of the lumen of the appendix followed by infection and inflammation. If the infection is not relieved, or the appendix removed, the risk of rupture and subsequent peritonitis is great.

Manifestations

The child presents with constant right lower quadrant pain (see Figure 37-16 ⚭). There is usually *rebound tenderness* following palpation (an increase in discomfort when abdominal pressure is released). The child usually exhibits a fever, nausea, and an elevated white blood cell count. The child may prefer a side-lying position with the knees flexed. A sudden relief of pain may indicate that the appendix has ruptured.

Diagnosis and Treatment

Diagnosis is confirmed by symptoms, elevated white blood cell count, and ultrasound.

The medical treatment of appendicitis is surgical intervention as soon as possible. Routine preoperative care should be provided including surgical consent, an intravenous infusion, and sedation. With an uneventful surgical procedure, the child may be discharged within 12 to 24 hours. Routine discharge teaching should be given to the child and parents.

If the appendix ruptures prior to surgery, peritonitis spreads rapidly. Peritonitis is a serious disorder that lengthens the hospital stay, increases pain, and impairs recovery. If untreated, life-threatening sequelae such as small bowel obstruction, electrolyte imbalance, and septic shock result. In this case the nurse should anticipate a longer, more complex course of nursing care.

Following surgery, the child should be monitored frequently for signs of infection and small bowel obstruction. Intravenous antibiotics will be administered. Intravenous fluids will be given until bowel function returns. Once bowel sounds are heard, small amounts of clear fluid are offered and the diet is gradually progressed as tolerated. A small bowel obstruction would be treated with nasogastric decompression.

The child will be hospitalized approximately 3 to 5 days postoperatively. Prior to discharge the child and parents should be instructed in use of pain medication, antibiotic administration, incision care, and the need for follow-up visits to the surgeon.

Evaluation of progress is based on a return of bowel function, return of white blood cell count to normal, and a decrease in discomfort. The child and parents should verbalize an understanding of discharge instructions. The child should be able to return to normal activities within a few days. Vigorous activities such as contact sports should be avoided until approved by the physician.

Endocrine Disorders

Endocrine system disorders result from either an overproduction or an underproduction of hormones. Endocrine disorders are rare with the exception of diabetes. Symptoms and care of these disorders would be similar to those of an adult. See Chapter 38 🔗 for full discussion of endocrine disorders.

DIABETES MELLITUS

Diabetes mellitus is the most common metabolic disorder in children. Most children have insulin-dependent diabetes mellitus (IDDM) or Type 1. The peak age of onset is 10 to 14 years of age. Non-insulin-dependent diabetes mellitus (NIDDM) or Type 2 is usually contracted as an adult (see Chapter 38 🔗), so the discussion here is limited to IDDM. However, with the rising incidence of obesity in the pediatric population, we are beginning to see Type 2 diabetes more in the pediatric population.

While there is a strong familial tendency to IDDM, there is no specific inheritance. Current research has identified a genetic marker that increases the child's susceptibility to the disease. Other factors include viruses, chemicals in the diet, and an autoimmune response. These factors can damage the beta cells in the islets of Langerhans in the pancreas.

Pathophysiology

To understand the pathology associated with IDDM, it is important to review the normal function of insulin briefly. Approximately 2 hours after a meal, the blood sugar rises, stimulating the pancreas to release insulin. Insulin aids in the transport of glucose through the cell wall, causing a slight decrease in the blood sugar. If the cells are inactive and do not need the glucose for metabolism, the excess glucose is stored in the liver as glycogen. When the cells become more active and need glucose, glucagon, from the alpha cells in the islets of Langerhans in the pancreas, aids the transfer of glycogen back to glucose. Insulin and glucagon, therefore, work together to keep the blood glucose level in a normal range between 80 and 120 mg/dL.

When the beta cells are destroyed, the level of insulin falls and the level of blood glucose increases. Because cells need glucose for energy, there is also a steep decrease in cell metabolism, and cells must convert protein and fat into glucose. When the level of blood glucose exceeds the renal threshold of 160 mg/dL, glucose is excreted in the urine (**glucosuria**). Glucose in the urine causes an increase in osmotic pressure that pulls additional water into the urine, resulting in an increased urinary output (*polyuria*). With an excessive urinary output, the child will become thirsty

(*polydipsia*). The cells, starving for glucose, trigger the appetite, resulting in *polyphagia*. As cells need energy, the liver metabolizes free fatty acids at an increased rate. While this use of fatty acids increases the energy available to cells, it also results in an accumulation of acetyl coenzyme A (CoA) or ketone bodies. An increase in ketone bodies results in metabolic acidosis or ketoacidosis.

Manifestations

The classic signs of IDDM include hyperglycemia, polyuria, polydipsia, polyphagia, and weight loss. Other symptoms include fatigue, headache, poor wound healing, and infection. Symptoms generally develop over time, but most have been present for less than a month, and the disease can progress to affect many symptoms (Figure 61-10 ■). The parents may bring their child to the healthcare provider with recognizable symptoms, or the child may present in the emergency room with ketoacidosis. The classic signs of ketoacidosis include those of IDDM plus fruity (acetone) breath and deep labored breathing (*Kussmaul respirations*), dehydration, decreased level of consciousness, and flushed dry skin.

Treatment

The goals of nursing care are to stabilize the child's condition, to teach the child and family to manage the condition at home, and to prevent long-term complications. The first priority is to stabilize the child's condition. Intravenous fluids will be given. Insulin may be given by continuous intravenous infusion. Electrolytes will be given as needed to regain and maintain homeostasis. Once the child has stabilized, balanced nutrition will be given orally, blood sugar will be monitored, and insulin will be administered subcutaneously to prevent further episodes of hyperglycemia.

Nursing Considerations

Teaching the parents and the child is important for the long-term management of diabetes and the prevention of complications. Although writing the complete teaching plan is the responsibility of the registered nurse, the LPN/LVN may be asked to provide instruction on the following topics:

- Blood glucose testing
- Balanced nutrition with regular meals and snacks
- Regular daily activity
- Insulin administration (see Chapter 38 🔗)
- Signs of hyperglycemia, hypoglycemia, and complications
- Health promotion activities
- The management of IDDM during times of minor illness, such as when the child has a cold or flu (see Chapter 38 🔗)

Children should be encouraged to learn to manage their health needs. The young child can help assemble the equipment, can make choices as to which finger to use for blood

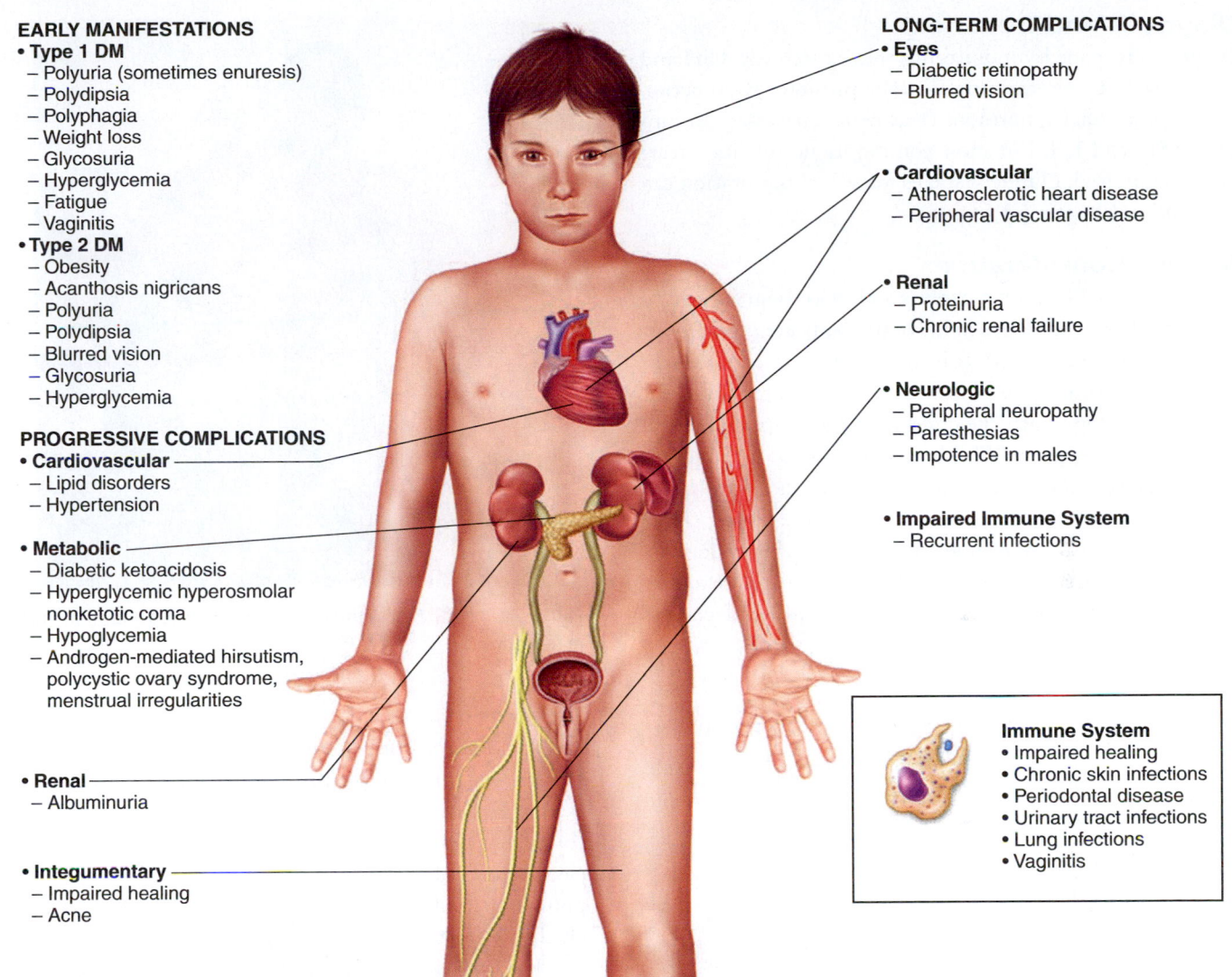

EARLY MANIFESTATIONS
- **Type 1 DM**
  - Polyuria (sometimes enuresis)
  - Polydipsia
  - Polyphagia
  - Weight loss
  - Glycosuria
  - Hyperglycemia
  - Fatigue
  - Vaginitis
- **Type 2 DM**
  - Obesity
  - Acanthosis nigricans
  - Polyuria
  - Polydipsia
  - Blurred vision
  - Glycosuria
  - Hyperglycemia

PROGRESSIVE COMPLICATIONS
- **Cardiovascular**
  - Lipid disorders
  - Hypertension

- **Metabolic**
  - Diabetic ketoacidosis
  - Hyperglycemic hyperosmolar nonketotic coma
  - Hypoglycemia
  - Androgen-mediated hirsutism, polycystic ovary syndrome, menstrual irregularities

- **Renal**
  - Albuminuria

- **Integumentary**
  - Impaired healing
  - Acne

LONG-TERM COMPLICATIONS
- **Eyes**
  - Diabetic retinopathy
  - Blurred vision

- **Cardiovascular**
  - Atherosclerotic heart disease
  - Peripheral vascular disease

- **Renal**
  - Proteinuria
  - Chronic renal failure

- **Neurologic**
  - Peripheral neuropathy
  - Paresthesias
  - Impotence in males

- **Impaired Immune System**
  - Recurrent infections

Immune System
- Impaired healing
- Chronic skin infections
- Periodontal disease
- Urinary tract infections
- Lung infections
- Vaginitis

MyNursingKit | American Diabetes Association

Figure 61-10. ■ Multisystem effects of diabetes mellitus.

glucose testing, and can help in the selecting of nutritious snacks. Older children can be taught to perform their own glucose testing, administer their insulin, and complete daily records.

The emotional support needed for the child depends on the age and stage of emotional development. Efforts should be made to enhance the child's feeling of autonomy and independence. The fewer changes the family has to make, the more supportive family members can be. Printed material should be provided to help the family learn and adjust to the changes. The child may need additional emotional support to handle the pressures of adolescence. The family should be referred to home health or diabetes centers for continued in-depth teaching and support. The American Diabetes Association is also an excellent source of information.

The child with newly diagnosed IDDM should be evaluated by the nurse and healthcare provider every few weeks until the condition has stabilized. The child and family should be able to verbalize an understanding of all teaching. The daily record of diet, blood glucose values, and amount of insulin administered should be reviewed and used as a basis for changes in insulin dosage.

PRECOCIOUS PUBERTY

Puberty normally begins between the ages of 8 and 13 years in girls and 9 and 14 years in boys. **Precocious puberty** is the presence of any secondary sex characteristics before the age of 8 in girls and before the age of 9 in boys.

Manifestations

Children with precocious puberty have both advanced bone age and reproductive changes. These children have a period of rapid growth followed by rapid closure of the epiphyseal plates. The end result is a short stature. Mood swings and emotional *lability* (changeability) may also be noted.

Diagnosis and Treatment

Diagnosis is made by monitoring the sex steroids, FSH and LH, as well as determining if other pituitary dysfunction exists. Occasionally, hormone treatment is necessary to suppress FSH and LH, but most commonly no medical treatment is required. (Tanner's stages for sexual maturation can be found in Chapter 62 ⚭.)

Nursing Considerations

The nurse should support parents and help them explain to the child that the changes in his or her body are normal, but just earlier than expected. It is important to remember that the child's emotional development will not match his or her physical development. The child may need support to deal with teasing by peers. Children with precocious puberty should be dressed for their chronologic age, not their physical development. Parents can encourage loose-fitting clothing to hide the body changes that are occurring. Parents need to be advised to talk with their child about sexuality and reproduction at an earlier age. The child and parents may need referral for counseling.

Urinary Disorders

In the older child, disorders of the urinary system usually result from complications of other disorders or from trauma. For additional information on renal system disorders, see Chapter 39 ⚭.

ACUTE AND CHRONIC RENAL FAILURE

Renal failure is the inability of the kidneys to remove liquid waste from the blood. Renal failure can result from lack of circulation to the kidney, damage to the glomerulus, or blockage that prevents any part of the kidney from draining. Factors that increase the risk of developing renal failure include severe dehydration, hypotension, accidental poisoning, repeated infection, and trauma. The course of acute and chronic renal failure is variable. Although acute renal failure usually resolves with treatment, it can become chronic. Some children can be managed with a combination of medication and diet therapy, whereas other children progress rapidly to complete renal failure that requires dialysis or kidney transplant.

Manifestations

Symptoms of renal failure may not appear in the child until the disease is advanced. Symptoms initially are nonspecific and include pale skin, headache, nausea, and fatigue. The child may have difficulty concentrating. As the disease progresses, edema (Figure 61-11 ■), tachycardia, and hypertension become evident. Growth retardation and demineralization of bone results from disturbances in calcium, phosphorus, and vitamin D. All body systems become affected when waste is not eliminated.

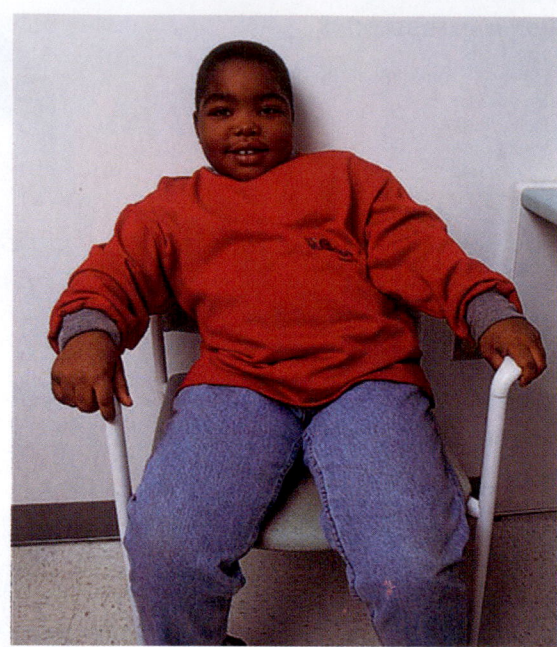

Figure 61-11. ■ Boy with generalized edema, a common finding in renal failure.

Treatment

The child should be assessed for signs of fluid overload including weight gain, pitting edema, pulmonary edema, and ascites. Urinary output should be monitored, including the color and odor of the urine. Blood values including serum electrolytes, blood urea nitrogen (BUN), creatinine, and phosphate levels should be monitored closely. Abnormal levels should be reported to the supervising RN and physician.

The child and family should be assessed for signs of undue stress brought on by life-threatening chronic illness. The management of chronic renal failure requires a lifestyle change that has an impact on the whole family. The need for ongoing dialysis is expensive, and the limited number of dialysis facilities restricts the family's movements. The family may need support under stress.

In planning care of the hospitalized child with renal failure, the nurse should plan care around the need for hemodialysis. Some medication may be removed through hemodialysis. Medications must be administered as directed in order to achieve the desired effect. The child must be monitored for side effects of medication, signs of electrolyte imbalance, and alterations in blood pressure. The child will need small, frequent feedings in order to meet additional nutrition demands.

In a child with renal failure, infection places additional burden on the kidneys and can speed the progression of the disease. Sites for infection include respiratory, urinary, and gastrointestinal tracts and dialysis sites. The nurse must be an effective role model for the child and family in preventing infection.

Nursing Considerations

In planning home care, the needs of the child and family should be identified well before discharge. Help the family to plan medication administration times that work around dialysis and that fit their routine. Stress the importance of consistency in diet, activity, and medication administration. If the child will be receiving peritoneal dialysis or hemodialysis at home, the family will need to be taught how to administer these treatments. Strict sterile technique must be used to prevent infection.

The child and family need emotional support in dealing with a chronic life-threatening illness. The National Kidney Foundation and local support groups can be valuable resources for the nurse and the family.

Reproductive Disorders

MATURATION

Females usually start to mature sooner than males. Recall that at puberty increases in the four primary sex hormones (FSH, LH, estrogen, and progesterone) cause the physical changes. The development of secondary sex characteristics usually begins with skeletal growth, widening of the pelvis, and a change in fat distribution. *Menarche*, the onset of menstruation, usually occurs about 13 years old.

Male development usually begins 2 years after female development. Recall that FSH and LH trigger the increase in testosterone in the male. The development of secondary sex characteristics usually begins with an increase in height, lengthening of the jaw, and a doubling of muscle mass.

During the prepuberty years, the child may begin to have questions about when their body will change into that of the adult. They may begin to make comments about sexual intercourse due to information (correct or incorrect) that they have heard from classmates at school. It is important for parents to be prepared to answer questions honestly and openly. Some parents are uncomfortable talking with their children, or may not know the answers to some of their questions. The nurse can be helpful in suggesting references from the public library.

VAGINAL INFECTIONS

Vaginitis is the inflammation of the vagina. Vaginal irritations may be caused by the insertion of foreign objects, infection with *Streptococcus* or *E. coli*, infestation of pinworms, or chemical irritation form hygiene products such as soaps or bubble bath. It may also be caused by *Candida albicans* (often appearing when a girl becomes sexually active) or trichomoniasis (the most frequently diagnosed sexually transmitted infection). Sexual abuse must also be ruled out when a child or adolescent presents with vaginitis.

Manifestations

The client with vaginitis may complain of pruritus, pain, and vaginal discharge or bleeding. Discharge may have a foul odor.

Diagnosis and Treatment

An examination of the child's external genitalia and collection of a specimen of the vaginal discharge is necessary. The drug of choice for *C. albicans* is nystatin ointment. Miconazole (Monistat) may also be ordered and administered as a vaginal suppository.

Nursing Considerations

The nurse can help the young girl avoid contact vaginitis by teaching her to wipe her perineum from front to back, therefore avoiding infecting the vagina with harmful bacteria from the rectum. Portable wet wipes may be useful to keep the perineum clean when away from home. The nurse can also discourage the use of bubble bath and feminine hygiene products such as douches or sprays. The nurse can encourage the daily cleaning of the perineum with warm water and mild soap, as well as frequent changes of tampons and sanitary pads during menstruation. Caution young girls that wet clothes can cause vaginal irritation. Wet swimsuits and exercise clothing should be removed promptly. Teach girls that cotton underwear absorbs moisture more effectively than synthetic materials.

Integumentary Disorders

MRSA

The school-age child is mobile and very active. The child is encouraged to participate in sport activities and frequently sustains minor injury. Because any break in the skin can result in infection, basic wound care is encouraged. The most common infecting organisms seen in wound of this type are *Staphylococcus aureus* and *Pseudomonas*. In recent years, some *Staphylococcus aureus* organisms have become resistant to many antibiotics used to treat them. These organisms have been named methicillin-resistant *Staphylococcus aureus* (MRSA). MRSA is resistant to all penicillins and cephalosporins. If the infection becomes systemic, the life of the child could be at risk.

It is important to avoid contact between the infected child and others in the home. For example, a child should not bathe with other children. The bathtub or shower should be thoroughly cleaned between bathers. Note: In-depth discussion of MRSA appears in Chapter 10 .

A small wound infected with MRSA may be treated at home with Bactrim. A large wound or one in a small child may require that the child be hospitalized and isolated during treatment. The wound may need to be surgically opened and drained (I & D).

Vancomycin administered intravenously is the drug of choice. Vancomycin is a potent antibacterial agent with life-altering adverse effects. Vancomycin can cause ototoxicity and nephrotoxicity. Vancomycin must be administered slowly in diluted form.

The best treatment is to prevent wound infections by washing the area with antibacterial soap and water, apply an antibiotic ointment, and cover the wound with a clean dry dressing. The wound should be observed for signs of infection (redness, heat, purulent drainage). An infected wound should be assessed by a healthcare professional.

Psychosocial Disorders

Thought process disorders include a wide range of disorders that may begin at birth or early childhood and continue throughout life. A more complete discussion of mental health disorders such as neurosis and psychosis is located in Chapter 49 ⚭. The disorders discussed here will be limited to school anxiety, dyslexia, and attention deficit disorders.

SCHOOL ANXIETY

Some children experience anxiety when the time for school approaches. Children fear being in a strange environment, the teacher will be "mean" to them, or they will not be as smart as their classmates. If the parents are supportive and introduce the child to the teacher and the school environment several days before the start of school, most school anxiety can be alleviated. Children should be encouraged to do their best and to ask the teacher or parents for help. Children need to understand that they will not know everything, and that making mistakes is an important part of learning. If the child can remain in the same school and with the same classmates over the course of their education, school anxiety usually is minimal.

DYSLEXIA

Dyslexia is difficulty using and interpreting written forms of communication by an individual whose vision and general intelligence are otherwise unimpaired. The condition is usually recognized in children by the third grade. These children have no difficulty seeing and recognizing letters, but have difficulty spelling and writing words. They typically reverse letters, or form the letters backwards. If the parent or teacher suspects a learning disability, the child should be referred to a learning specialist for diagnosis. With early intervention, children can perform adequately in school.

ATTENTION DEFICIT HYPERACTIVITY DISORDER

Attention deficit hyperactivity disorder (ADHD) is most commonly diagnosed as a child enters school. This disorder is more common in boys. Incidence of the disorder is increasing. However, it is unclear whether more children indeed have ADHD, whether they are being diagnosed more readily, or whether they are being misdiagnosed due to lack of tolerance of certain behaviors.

Manifestations

Children with ADHD have difficulty finishing tasks. They are easily distracted and may move from topic to topic in their speech as well as activities. They have difficulty working with others. Some children with ADHD are quiet, but many fidget, become loud, and disrupt others. They have difficulty maintaining social relationships. They may be teased or shunned by other children.

Diagnosis and Treatment

The child who is suspected of having ADHD should be evaluated by a mental health specialist. Besides a psychologic assessment, a sleep study should also be conducted to rule out a sleep disorder. A full blood workup is usually done to rule out other diagnoses.

If a diagnosis of ADHD is made, treatment may vary depending on the type and degree of disability. Treatment may include changing the environment, behavior modification, and medication.

Nursing Considerations

The nurse should work with the parents and teachers to provide an environment that will allow the child to be successful. Having the child use a separate desk in an area of the room where other students cannot distract him is helpful. However, the child should also be made to feel that he is part of the class, that he is important and valuable.

Professional counselors may be helpful in modifying the child's behavior and should be included in the care planning team. Establishing a system of rewards for appropriate behavior can help the child learn and foster a positive self-image. The expected behavior must be realistically achievable. If the child cannot receive frequent rewards, the behavior may not change. If punishment is necessary, it should follow quickly after the offense so the child can relate the punishment to the behavior. The entire family will need assistance to modify each member's behavior to be consistent with the plan of care.

The most commonly prescribed medication is methylphenidate (Ritalin), but Strattera is a more recent drug that is showing positive results. Other drugs such as antidepressants, anticonvulsants, and antimanics may also be used. The nurse should make sure parents understand the prescribed medication, including side effects. Table 61-5 ■ lists some common medications used to treat ADHD and their usual side effects. Some medications may need to be taken at school, and the school personnel

TABLE 61-5	Medications Used to Treat ADHD	
DRUG/CLASSIFICATION	**ACTION**	**SIDE EFFECTS**
Ritalin (methylphenidate hydrochloride)/*cerebral stimulant*	Mild stimulant effect on cerebral cortex	Dizziness, nervousness, insomnia, increased P & BP, blurred vision, dry mouth, loss of appetite if taken before meals (sometimes reported to slow growth)
Norpramin (desipramine hydrochloride)/*psychotherapeutic agent, tricyclic antidepressant*	Restores levels of neurotransmitters, norepinephrine, and serotonin	Dizziness, weakness, postural hypotension, dry mouth
Tegretol (carbamazepine)/*anticonvulsant*	Inhibits neuromuscular transmission	Anorexia, dizziness, rash
Strattera (atomoxetine hydrochloride)/*psychotherapeutic agent*	Selective norepinephrine reuptake inhibitor	Anorexia, upset stomach, dizziness, tiredness, mood swings

giving the medication should understand how to administer the drugs safely.

Families of children with ADHD require support and teaching. Parents may become frustrated with the child's behavior and inflict inappropriate punishments. Teach them that a stable, routine environment will help the child to focus. The parents need to set boundaries and limits, and help the child learn to behave within them. Support groups may be beneficial to the parents.

The child with ADHD should be evaluated on a regular basis. Medications usually have an effect within the first 10 to 14 days of treatment. Behavior modification programs may take weeks and months to be effective. Small amounts of progress should be recognized.

Note: The references and resources for all chapters have been compiled at the back of the book.

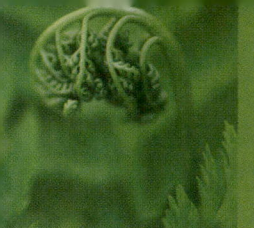

Chapter Review

KEY Points

- Physical care of the school-age child is similar to care of adults who have similar disorders.

- It is important to explain disorders in terms that are age appropriate and that engage the school-age child's participation in the recovery process. Family members play an important role in providing information, supporting the client, and assisting with care giving.

- The most common disorders affecting the school-age child are infections, accidental injuries, and malfunctions.

- School-age children can be taught to make healthy food choices.

- School-age children should receive dental care including cleaning, filling cavities and orthodontic appliances to straighten crooked teeth.

- Secondhand cigarette smoke contributes to chronic respiratory problems in children.

- A diet poor in iron can result in iron-deficiency anemia in school-age children.

- School-age children frequently develop strabismus, amblyopia, hyperopia, myopia, and astigmatism; therefore, they should have visual exams annually.

- School-age children should be screened for spinal curvature including scoliosis, kyphosis, and lordosis.

- Appendicitis, common in the school-age child, often results in surgery.

- Type 1 diabetes mellitus is the most common endocrine disorder in school-age children.

- Many disorders affecting the school-age child become chronic disorders that affect their health as adults.

- School-age children may develop thought process disorders including dyslexia, school anxiety, and attention deficit hyperactivity disorder.

- The school-age child can be taught many aspects of self-care.

FOR FURTHER Study

Safety issues were discussed in the fundamentals section of this textbook under Safety (Chapter 9, especially Box 9-1).

In-depth discussion of MRSA appears in Chapter 10.

Theories about preschooler development were provided in Chapter 15.

Growth and development information (on which this chapter builds) was provided in Chapter 16.

The in-depth discussion of vital signs is in Chapter 21.

Nutrition was discussed in detail in Chapter 25.

Box 27-10 provides instructions on using a metered-dose inhaler.

The medical-surgical treatment of respiratory disorders is provided in detail in Chapter 32.

The main discussion of cardiovascular disorders is in Chapter 33.

The main discussion of blood and lymph disorders is in Chapter 34. Please review disorders there for further depth.

The immune disorders are discussed in depth in Chapter 35.

Nervous system and sensory disorders are discussed in most depth in Chapter 36.

The major discussion of all gastrointestinal disorders is in Chapter 37.

See Chapter 38 for a full discussion of endocrine disorders.

The main discussion of urinary disorders is in Chapter 39.

Scoliosis screening is discussed in Chapter 48.

Discussion of mental health and treatment for specific mental health disorders appears in Chapter 49.

Discussion of juvenile rheumatoid arthritis appeared in Chapter 59.

Tanner's stages for sexual maturation can be found in Chapter 62.

PEARSON

EXPLORE **mynursingkit**™

MyNursingKit is your one stop for online chapter review materials and resources. Prepare for success with additional NCLEX®-style practice questions, interactive assignments and activities, web links, animations and videos, and more!

Register your access code from the front of your book at **www.mynursingkit.com**

Critical Thinking Care Map

Caring for a Client with Scoliosis

NCLEX-PN® Focus Area: Physiologic Integrity

Case Study: Astra Morano is a 12-year-old female who was transferred to the orthopedic unit after 3 days in ICU following Harrington rod placement for treatment of scoliosis. Astra's alignment is being maintained with a clamshell polyethylene brace on a Stryker frame.

Nursing Diagnosis: *Risk for Impaired Skin Integrity*

COLLECT DATA

Subjective	Objective
_____	_____
_____	_____
_____	_____
_____	_____
_____	_____
_____	_____
_____	_____

Would you report this? Yes/No

If yes, report to: _____

What would you report? _____

Nursing Care

_____
_____
_____
_____
_____
_____
_____
_____
_____
_____

How would you document this? _____
_____
_____
_____

Compare your answers and documentation to those provided on the MyNursingKit Website.

Data Collected
(use only those that apply)

- Weight 126 lb
- Height 5'8"
- Blood pressure 124/76
- Temperature 99.8°F
- Pulse 100
- Respirations 26
- States "I have this brace."
- Bowel sounds hypoactive
- Lung sounds bilaterally
- Peripheral pulse strong and equal bilaterally
- C/O pain 5 on a scale of 1 to 10
- Refused lunch; stated "I am not hungry."
- No BM since surgery
- Urine output adequate via Foley catheter (400 mL/8 hours)

Nursing Interventions
(use only those that apply; list in priority order)

- Allow client to select age-appropriate diversional activities.
- Provide support and education to family members.
- Inspect skin regularly.
- Provide special skin care for heels and elbows.
- Observe for urinary tract infection.
- Turn on Stryker frame every 2 hours.
- Encourage peer contact.
- Remove one half brace every shift to evaluate incision.
- Place call bell within reach.
- Maintain body alignment.
- Consider cultural background in relationship to pain expression.
- Keep skin dry and clean.
- Encourage self-care.

NCLEX-PN® Exam Preparation

1 The school nurse is teaching a class for parents of school-aged children. Which of the following statements would correctly explain nutritional needs of this age group?

1. It is important at this age to influence children to develop healthy eating habits.
2. School-aged children should be served 5 servings of fruit.
3. School-aged children should be served 6 servings of milk, yogurt, and cheese.
4. School-aged children should not follow a vegetarian diet because they need meat in their diet.

2 A school-aged child enters the school nurse's office and asks if he could join the football team. The nurse, knowing the child is asthmatic, best responds by saying:

1. "It would not be advisable for you to join the team because it could induce asthma attacks."
2. "I don't see any reason why you couldn't join the team."
3. "In order to join the team you will need to get signed permission from both your doctor and your parents. Ask the doctor if premedication will be necessary."
4. "I don't think playing football is a good idea. Have you given any thought to joining the chess team? People with asthma need to be careful."

3 The nurse, working in the emergency department, admits a school-aged child who fell over the handlebars of his bike striking his head. The child is unconscious, is unresponsive to deep pain stimuli, and has nonreactive pupils. A priority nursing intervention is:

1. Inserting a pressure-monitoring device to measure intracranial pressure.
2. Maintaining a patent airway and assessing respiratory effort.
3. Providing emotional support for the distraught parents.
4. Initiating an IV for fluid and medication administration.

4 The nurse is caring for a child diagnosed with appendicitis, who is scheduled for surgery. The client, who had been complaining of right lower quadrant pain, says the pain went away. The nurse recognizes that this indicates:

1. No further need for surgery.
2. Pain management was effective.
3. Rupture of the appendix.
4. Resolution of the inflammation.

5 The nurse is caring for a child diagnosed with diabetes mellitus. Understanding of the pathophysiology of the disease leads the nurse to recognize that:

1. The child probably has Type 2 diabetes.
2. The child probably has non-insulin-dependent diabetes.
3. The child will probably require regular insulin injections.
4. The child will likely have difficulty meeting normal growth and development milestones.

6 A 10-year-old female presents to the emergency room with complaints of perineal itching and foul-smelling vaginal discharge. The physician performs a vaginal examination. The nurse recognizes that there may be indications of:

1. Sexual promiscuity.
2. Sexual abuse.
3. Onset of puberty.
4. Precocious puberty.

7 The nurse, working in a pediatrician's office, admits a child with complaints of low abdominal pain, urinary frequency, dysuria, and hematuria. The nurse's priority action is to:

1. Explain the importance of using a barrier method if sexually active.
2. Collect a urine specimen.
3. Draw blood to test for pregnancy.
4. Measure blood glucose level.

8 The nurse is caring for a child infected with MRSA. The nurse anticipates the organism is:

1. *Staphylococcus aureus.*
2. *E. coli.*
3. *Haemophilus influenzae.*
4. *Streptococcus.*

9 The nurse, working on a pediatric unit of the hospital, receives a picture drawn by the client. When examining the drawing, the nurse notes several letters are reversed. The nurse asks how the child does in school, and the child says she gets good grades in math, but has trouble in English class. The nurse suspects the child may need to be evaluated for:

1. Attention deficit hyperactivity disorder.
2. Dyslexia.
3. School anxiety.
4. Attention deficit disorder.

10 While caring for a child newly diagnosed with attention deficit hyperactivity disorder, the nurse is teaching the parents and client how to administer methylphenidate (Ritalin). The nurse recognizes further teaching is needed when the parent says:

1. "I will give him the medicine every day before he goes to bed."
2. "I will call the doctor if he loses his appetite or complains of dry mouth."
3. "I will give him his medication in addition to seeing the counselor regularly."
4. "I will inform his school of the medication he is taking."

Answers and rationales for Review Questions appear in Appendix I.

Chapter 62

Care and Illnesses of Adolescents

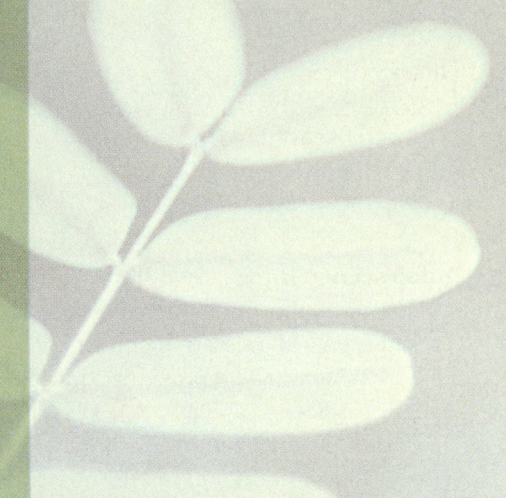

LEARNING Outcomes

After completing this chapter, you will be able to:

1. Identify growth and development milestones and changes that occur during the adolescent stage of development.
2. Describe healthful nutrition, good hygiene practices, and normal vital signs for adolescents.
3. Discuss routine health care and the issue of confidentiality for adolescents.
4. Discuss common health and safety concerns during the adolescent years.
5. Describe respiratory, cardiovascular, hematologic, or immune disorders with common onset in adolescence.
6. Identify neurologic or musculoskeletal disorders with common onset in adolescence.
7. Name and discuss gastrointestinal or endocrine disorders with common onset in adolescence.
8. Explain urinary or reproductive disorders with common onset in adolescence.
9. Identify integumentary disorders with common onset in adolescence.
10. Describe psychosocial conditions and nursing care for adolescents.

Clinical Objectives

11. Provide client teaching on the subject of health and safety to an adolescent client.
12. Describe nursing interventions used when providing nursing care for an adolescent.

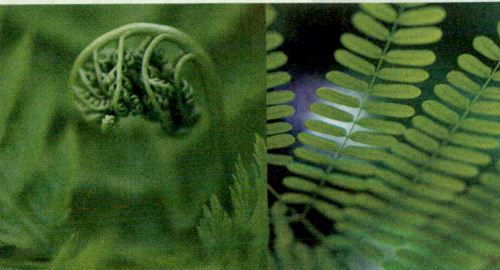

BRIEF Outline

Nutrition
Vital Signs in Adolescents
Special Concerns
ILLNESSES AND DISORDERS
Respiratory Disorders
Cardiovascular Disorders
Hematologic Disorders
Immune Disorders
Nervous System Disorders
Musculoskeletal Disorders
Gastrointestinal Disorders
Endocrine Disorders
Urinary Disorders
Reproductive Disorders
Integumentary Disorders
Psychosocial Disorders

KEY TERMS

adolescence 1734

comedo 1753

Crohn's disease 1745

glandular fever 1742

goiter 1747

menarche 1734

metabolic X syndrome 1748

migraine 1742

orchiectomy 1752

orchiopexy 1752

parenchymal 1746

puberty 1734

staging 1741

ulcerative colitis 1745

Adolescence is the period of growth and development that begins with the appearance of secondary sex characteristics and ends with the cessation of physical growth and emotional maturity. Table 62-1 ■ provides a quick overview of adolescent milestones. (See Chapter 16 ⬭ for further discussion.)

Although the changes that occur during the adolescent years are significant and many, most adolescents are healthy with few diseases. If the adolescent becomes ill, the disorder is similar to that of the adult. The medical treatment and nursing care would also be similar.

Growth not only involves length and weight of a body, but also internal growth and development. Growth is complete between the ages of 16 and 18, at which time the growing ends of bones fuse. Normal growth is categorized in a range used by pediatricians to gauge how a child is growing. See Table 62-2 ■ for average ranges of weight and height, based on growth charts developed by the Centers for Disease Control and Prevention (CDC). Although a child may be growing, his or her growth pattern may deviate from the normal. Ultimately, the child should grow to normal height by adulthood.

Adolescence is characterized by dramatic physical changes that move the individual from childhood into physical maturity. Early, prepubescent changes are noted with the appearance

of secondary sexual characteristics. **Puberty** is the stage that occurs when the reproductive organs become functional. At puberty the hypothalamus of the brain signals the pituitary gland to signal the other endocrine glands to increase functioning (see also Chapters 38 and 40 ⬭).

Girls may begin to develop breast buds as early as 8 years old, with full breast development achieved anywhere from 12 to 18 years. Pubic hair growth (as well as armpit and leg hair) typically begins at about age 9 or 10 and reaches adult distribution patterns at about 13 to 14 years. **Menarche** (the beginning of menstrual periods) typically occurs about 2 years after initial pubescent changes are noted. It may occur as early as 10 years, or as late as 15 years, with the average in the United States being about 12.5 years. A concurrent rapid growth in height occurs between the ages of about 9.5 and 14.5 years, peaking somewhere around 12 years.

Boys may begin to note scrotal/testicular enlargement as early as 9 years of age followed closely by lengthening of the penis. Adult size and shape of the genitals is typically reached by age 16 to 17 years (Figure 62-1 ■). Pubic hair growth (as well as armpit, leg, chest, and facial hair) in males usually begins at about 12 years of age and reaches adult distribution patterns at about 15 to 16 years.

TABLE 62-1	Growth and Development Milestones during Adolescence				
AGE	**PHYSICAL GROWTH**	**GROSS MOTOR SKILLS**	**FINE MOTOR SKILLS**	**COGNITIVE ABILITY**	**NUTRITION**
12 to 18 years	Growth spurts: Girls Gain: 15 to 55 lbs (7–25 kg) Grow: 2 to 8 in. (2.5–20 cm) Boys Gain: 15 to 65 lbs. (7–29.5 kg) Grow: 4 ½ to 12 in. (11–30 cm) Puberty results in body changes.	Some lack of coordination during growth spurts. Physically active. Tries many new sports. **(1)** (1) New sports activities attempted	Fully developed.	Fully developed.	Appetite increases during growth spurts. Peers influence food choices.

TABLE 62-2	Normal Adolescent Physical Growth Patterns			
	HEIGHT		**WEIGHT**	
AGE	FEMALES (IN.)	MALES (IN.)	FEMALES (LB)	MALES (LB)
12	55–64	54–63.5	68–136	66–130
14	59–67.5	59–69.5	84–160	84–160
16	60–68	63–73	94–172	104–186
18	60–68.5	65–74	100–178	116–202

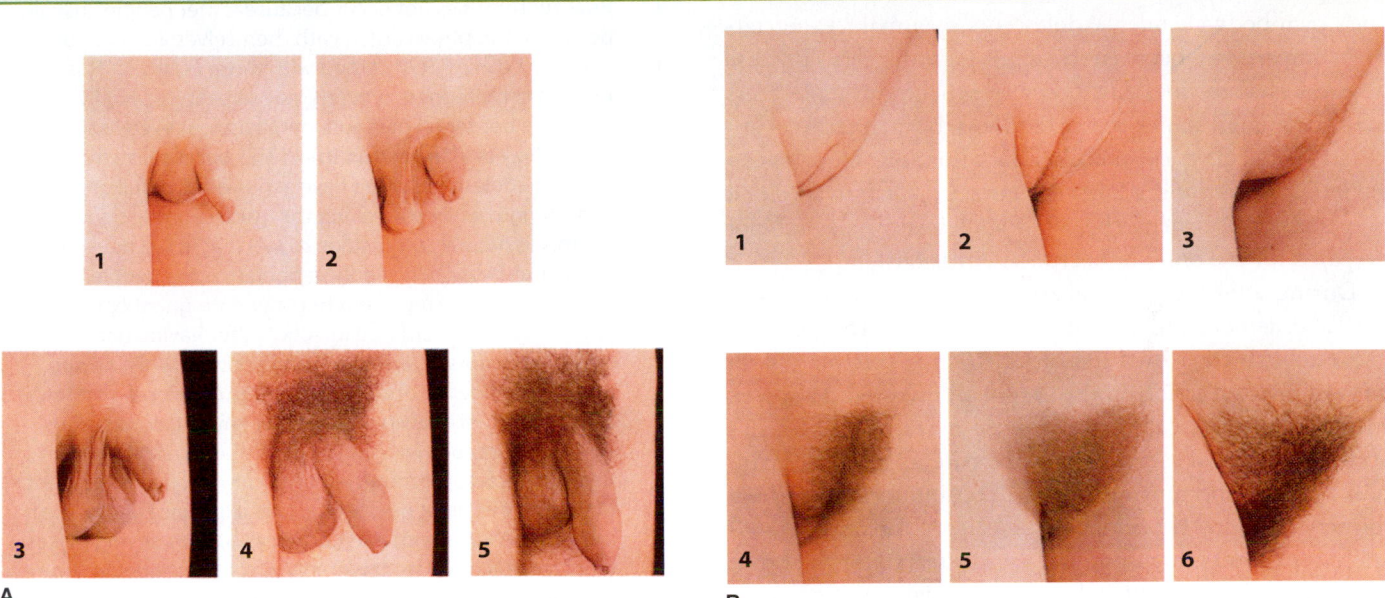

Figure 62-1. ■ Male and female maturation can be described in identifiable stages. **A.** Stages of external male genital development are numbered one through five. Stages of pubic hair development follow this standard pattern. **B.** Stages of external female genital development are numbered one through six. The presence, distribution, and amount of pubic hair determine the stage. The timing of pubic hair stages varies among individuals but follows a consistent pattern.

A concurrent rapid growth in height occurs between the ages of about 10.5 to 11 and 16 to 18 years, peaking somewhere around 14 years. Puberty is not marked by a specific incident in males, as it is with the onset of menstruation in females. The appearance of regular nocturnal emissions ("wet dreams"), which may occur about every 2 weeks with the buildup of seminal fluid, marks the onset of puberty in males. This typically occurs somewhere between the ages of 13 and 17 years, with the average at about 14.5 years. Voice changes in the male typically occur concurrently with penile growth, nocturnal emissions, and the peak of the height spurt. Table 62-3 ■ list Tanner's stages of sexual maturity.

TABLE 62-3	Tanner's Stages of Sexual Maturity
STAGES	**DESCRIPTION**
Stage 1	Preadolescent has no pubic hair except for a fine "peach fuzz" body hair.
Stage 2	There is a sparse growth of long, slightly darkened, downy pubic hair mostly along the labia in females or at the base of the penis in males. This hair is usually straight or only slightly curled.
Stage 3	The pubic hair becomes darker, coarser, curlier. It now grows sparsely over the mons veneris area in females and over the pubis in males.
Stage 4	The hair grows in more densely. It becomes as coarse and curly as in the adult, but there is not as much of it.
Stage 5	Has the classic coarse and curly pubic hair that extends onto the inner thighs.
Stage 6	The final amount, color, and distribution of pubic hair are quite variable.

Sources: Data from Tanner, J. M. *Growth at adolescence.* (1966). New York: Appleton; Tanner, J. M. *Growth of adolescents.* (1962). Oxford: Blackwell; Marshall, W. A., and J. M. Tanner. Variations in the pattern of pubertal changes in boys. *Arch. Dis. Child 45*(239):13–23, 1970; Marshall, W. A., and J. M. Tanner. Variations in the pattern of pubertal changes in girls. *Arch. Dis. Child 44*(235): 291–303, 1969.

Emotional development of teens is often characterized by behavioral changes that can be frustrating for parents and other adults. The previously cooperative, happy child develops mood swings and oppositional behavior. The central task of this period, according to Erikson, is defined as identity versus role confusion (see Chapter 15 ⬭).

The sudden and rapid physical changes that adolescents experience typically tend to make this period of development one of self-consciousness, sensitivity, and concern over one's own body changes. Adolescents may make excruciating comparisons between themselves and peers. Because physical changes may not occur in synchrony, adolescents may go through stages of awkwardness, both in terms of appearance and physical mobility/coordination. Unnecessary anxieties may arise if adolescent girls are not informed and prepared for the menarche, or if adolescent males are not prepared for the onset of nocturnal emissions.

During adolescence, it is appropriate for youngsters to have and demonstrate a need to separate from their parents and establish their own identity. In some, this may occur with minimal reaction on the part of all involved. However, in some families, conflict may arise over the adolescent's acts or gestures of rebellion and the parents' need to maintain control. The youth may resist continuing in his or her former childhood behaviors of compliance (Box 62-1 ■). As adolescents pull away from parents in a search for their own identity, the peer group takes on a special significance. It may become a "safe" haven, in which the adolescent can test new ideas and compare his or her own physical and psychological growth.

BOX 62-1 | **CULTURAL PULSE POINTS**

Recognizing Diversity of Families

Even though adolescents strive for independence, health care should be delivered in a family-friendly place that recognizes the diversity of families and helps adolescents to appreciate their family heritage. Diversity can be supported in a health-care setting by:

- Promoting many images of the family, as opposed to one single ideal.
- Asking adolescents whom they wish to have involved in discussions about their problems.
- Ascertaining which people adolescents include in their immediate families.
- Giving consideration to families who ask for exceptions to policies or procedures.
- Using images of different kinds of families in publications and for decoration.
- Offering linguistically and culturally sensitive services.
- Welcoming spiritual resources and community family support services.
- Providing culturally diverse staff members who have received formal orientation about community and family customs.

BOX 62-2 | **MYTHS ASSOCIATED WITH ADOLESCENT DEVELOPMENT**

- **Myth: They are always "on stage."** Teenagers feel that the attention of others is constantly centered on their appearance or actions. This preoccupation stems from the fact that adolescents spend so much time thinking and looking at themselves, it is only natural to assume that everyone else is also thinking and looking at them as well.
  Reality: This does not occur, because "other people" (usually peers) are too preoccupied with themselves and their own issues to be overly concerned with those of others. This normal self-centeredness of teens may appear (especially to adults) to border on paranoia, narcissism, or even hysteria.
- **Myth: They are "indestructible."** This belief stems from the fact that adolescents often have achieved their full growth and strength while still having the quick coordination of youth. It is natural at this stage to feel that "it will never happen to me. Those things only happen to other people." In this sense, "it" may represent becoming pregnant or incurring a sexually transmitted infection after having unprotected intercourse, causing an auto accident while driving under the influence of alcohol or drugs, developing oral cancer as a result of chewing tobacco, or any of the numerous adverse effects of a wide range of risk-taking behaviors.
  Reality: Adolescents often are physically strong and resilient, but they are at great risk for effects of substance abuse. Their lack of experience with adult activities such as driving makes them more likely to react wrongly while driving under the influence. Peer pressure also can have a major influence in choosing risk-taking activity. Changes in hormone levels can lead to impulsive behavior, such as unprotected sex.

In early adolescence, the peer group usually consists of members of the same gender who form "cliques," gangs, or clubs. Members of the peer group attempt to behave alike, dress alike, have secret codes or rituals, and participate in the same activities. As the youth moves into midadolescence (14 to 16 years), the peer group expands to include members of the opposite sex.

Mid- to late adolescence is characterized by a need to establish sexual identity through becoming comfortable with one's own body and sexual feelings. Through friendships with members of the opposite sex, dating, and experimentation, adolescents learn to express and receive intimate or sexual advances in a comfortable manner that is consistent with internalized values. Young people who do not have the opportunity for such experiences may demonstrate difficulty in establishing intimate relationships into adulthood. Adolescents typically demonstrate behaviors consistent with several "myths" of adolescence, described in Box 62-2 ■.

Nutrition

The Food Guide Pyramid, designed by the U.S. Department of Agriculture (USDA) and the U.S. Department of Health and Human Services, can help parents and adolescents eat a

---

BOX 62-3   TEENS AND VEGETARIAN DIET

Some teens turn to vegetarianism, whether as a way of achieving independence from their parents or as an expression of greater awareness about the environment and the world. The key to healthy eating for the vegetarian is the same as for anyone else: balancing a variety of healthful foods.

Teens have some specific nutritional needs that can be met with planning and knowledge:

- Protein needs can be met by eating a variety of plant proteins, found in everything except fruits, fats, and alcohol.
- Calcium can be found in tofu processed with calcium sulfate, in green leafy vegetables (e.g., collard greens, mustard greens, and kale), and in calcium-fortified soy milk and orange juice.
- Iron is found in broccoli, raisins, watermelon, spinach, black-eyed peas, blackstrap molasses, chickpeas, and pinto beans. It is absorbed better if consumed along with foods containing vitamin C.
- Vitamin B_{12} may be missing in the *vegan diet* (a diet which contains no animal products at all) and should be added through supplements or fortified products.

Because teens are often on the run, a list of quick items that provide nutrition is useful. Such a list could include: apples, oranges, bananas, grapes, peaches, plums, dried fruits, bagels and peanut butter, carrot or celery sticks, popcorn, pretzels, soy cheese pizza, bean tacos or burritos, salad, soy yogurt, soy milk, rice cakes, sandwiches, and frozen juice bars.

There are many reasons, including health and environmental ones, that a vegetarian diet may be a good choice. Parents need to be reassured that teens can stay healthy without meat products in their diet. Encourage them to try to be supportive and to approach their teen's decision as an opportunity for the whole family to learn more about healthful eating. Remind them that teens experimenting with vegetarianism may become involved in cooking that they previously expected the parents to do. Teach teens and parents to explore websites and other resources; there are many targeted at vegetarian teens.

---

variety of foods. It encourages thinking about the right amount of calories and fat. The pyramid applies to anyone 6 years of age to adulthood. See Figure 25-2 🔗 for an illustration of the pyramid. Newer variations on this pyramid promote fewer calories from carbohydrates and increased exercise in proportion to foods consumed.

Eating well is an important part of a healthy lifestyle and is something that should be taught at a young age. However, peer pressure has a great bearing on what a teen eats. The teen is spending more time away from home, and fast foods are the most accessible. Fad diets and political statements (such as animal rights) also affect food choices. Teens who refuse to eat animal protein may not understand the need to obtain alternate sources of protein (Box 62-3 ■). They should be given information about combining foods (such as grains and legumes) to make complete protein. Without essential amino acids (building blocks for the body), they could develop lifelong deficiencies. It is important that the adolescent's diet be discussed with his or her physician prior to making any dietary changes or beginning a diet.

The following are some general guidelines for adolescents for healthful eating:

- Eat three meals a day, plus healthy snacks.
- Increase fiber in the diet and decrease the use of salt.

- Drink a lot of water and avoid drinks with high sugar content.
- Watch total fat consumption in the diet, rather than counting calories.
- Eat balanced meals.
- Choose baked or broiled foods more often than fried.
- Watch (and decrease, if necessary) sugar intake.
- Eat fresh fruit or vegetables for a snack.
- Use low-fat dairy products.
- Decrease the use of butter and heavy gravies.
- Eat more chicken and fish and less red meat.

Vital Signs in Adolescents

Although some teens may reach their adult height early, vital signs will continue to change into adulthood. Table 62-4 ■ compares average vital signs of teens to those in adult.

Special Concerns

HYGIENE

Personal hygiene is an important issue for the adolescent. Most adolescents spend a considerable amount of time grooming and, with their exposure to the media, they are all very aware of deodorants, toothpaste, and mouthwash. It

TABLE 62-4	Variations in Normal Vital Signs—Teenagers versus Adults			
AGE	TEMPERATURE IN DEGREES CELSIUS	AVERAGE PULSE (RANGES)	AVERAGE RESPIRATIONS (RANGES)	BLOOD PRESSURE (MM HG)
Teen years	37 (oral)	70 (50–90)	18 (15–20)	120/80
Adult	37 (oral)	80 (60–100)	16 (12–20)	120/80

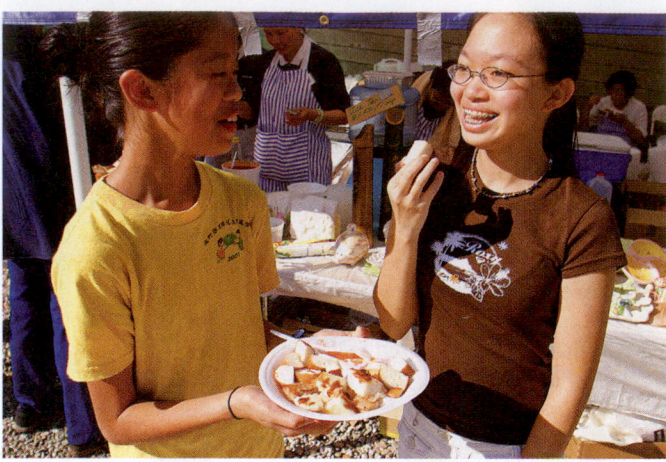

Figure 62-2. ■ Many teens have braces to straighten their teeth. Client teaching about oral hygiene is important to help them avoid dental decay. (PhotoEdit Inc.)

is important for the nurse to discuss issues such as cosmetics, body piercings, and tattoos. All of these can be potentially dangerous. Sharing cosmetics, especially mascara, can spread infection or even result in an infestation of lice in the eyelashes. Teenagers should be warned against using someone else's razor or toothbrush because such action could place them at a risk for HIV infection. The popularity of tattoos with teenagers is also a concern. Body piercing needs to be done under strict sterile technique and the area should be frequently inspected for signs of infection. Swapping of body rings should also be discouraged.

Adolescents as well as adults frequently neglect dental care. The fear of dentists is a real issue for many people. From age 12 to 18 years, dental hygiene is crucial since this is the period of greatest decay in permanent teeth. Teens should be encouraged to maintain a regular program of brushing, flossing, rinsing, and visits to the dentist. Many teens also will have some form of braces to realign teeth (Figure 62-2 ■). Braces require specialized hygiene and changes in diet that may be difficult for the teen to follow.

ROUTINE HEALTH CARE

During the adolescent years the teen will be due for boosters of immunizations (see Figure 60-2 ⊙⊙), such as a Td (tetanus and diphtheria) and a second MMR (measles, mumps, rubella). The teenage years are also the time to consider hepatitis A and B and varicella immunizations if they have not been given earlier. It is recommended that teenage girls receive Gardasil, a vaccine to protect against four types of human papillomavirus (HPV), two of which are known to cause cervical cancer. See Chapter 41 ⊙⊙ for a discussion of HPV.

Physical exams are usually related to school admission, sports, or camp. It is important to determine whether

there are any contraindications for a teen to participate in activities.

Confidentiality

The nurse may be the first healthcare professional with whom the adolescent comes in contact. Concerns about confidentiality may discourage adolescents from seeking necessary medical care and counseling, and may create barriers to open communication between client and physician. Protection of confidentiality is needed to appropriately address issues such as depression, suicide, substance abuse, domestic violence, unintended pregnancy, and sexual orientation. Box 62-4 ■ provides nursing guidelines for maintaining confidentiality during adolescent health care.

SAFETY

Adolescent safety issues are of major concern. Accidents and injury continue to be the major cause of death during this time period. Protecting the adolescent from harm takes constant effort on the part of the family and the community.

Adolescent safety issues stem from increased strength and agility that may develop before optimal decision-making skills develop. A strong need for peer approval, coupled with the "myths of adolescence" (see Box 62-2), may encourage youths to attempt hazardous feats and participate in risk-taking behaviors.

Appropriate motor vehicle safety needs to be emphasized, focusing on the roles of driver, passenger, and pedestrian; the influence of substance abuse; and the importance of using seat belts. Parents can be encouraged to connect car

---

BOX 62-4   NURSING CARE CHECKLIST

Maintaining Confidentiality during Adolescent Health Care

When caring for an adolescent client:

☑ Offer the adolescent an opportunity for examination and counseling separate from parents/guardians, and respect their privacy.

☑ Make a reasonable effort to encourage the adolescent to involve parents or guardians in healthcare decisions.

☑ Educate parents to encourage their adolescents toward personal responsibility in health care, and facilitate communication regarding appointments and payments, in a manner supportive of the adolescent's rights to confidentiality.

☑ Make every effort to maintain confidentiality. The limits on what can be guaranteed should be clearly discussed. Information that would suggest someone is in danger, evidence of abuse, or diagnosis of certain communicable diseases must be reported to the proper authorities.

☑ Maintain confidentiality, especially in areas where the adolescent has the legal right to give consent.

and recreational vehicle privileges to the adolescent's ability to demonstrate safe use of such vehicles.

Adolescents who pursue recreational athletic activities should be taught to use adequate equipment, protective gear or clothing, and safe facilities. They should follow proper rules of safe play and rational approaches to activities that require advanced skill levels.

Young people need to be acutely aware of the potential dangers (including sudden death) of substance use. This may occur not only with regular substance abuse, but also with experimental use of drugs and alcohol.

Adolescents who are allowed to use or have access to firearms need to learn proper use, safety, and legal issues associated with guns.

Many adolescents are at increased risk for depression and potential suicide due to pressures and conflicts that may arise within families of origin, school or social organizations, and intimate relationships. (See discussion of this topic later in chapter.) Psychologic evaluation may be necessary if adolescents appear to be isolated from peers, disinterested in school or social activities, or suddenly demonstrating decreased performance related to school, work, or sports.

Driver and Car Safety

A driver's license is one of the biggest status symbols among high school students. Getting a driver's license is not only a social asset but it makes the adolescent feel more independent than ever before. Their parents no longer have to drive them places. They can get places on their own. Most teens count the hours and days until they can get their learner's permit (usually age 16) and take their driving test to demonstrate driving competence. Some teens, however, may be pushed to drive before they feel ready. Parents often have many concerns and fears about their teen's safety on the road.

According to the American Automobile Association, teenage drivers account for only 7% of the driving population but are involved in 14% of fatal crashes. Traffic crashes are the number-one cause of death and injury for people ages 15 to 19. Every year more than 6,000 teens die in motor vehicle collisions. Problems that contribute to the high crash rate of young drivers include the following: driving inexperience, lack of adequate driving skills, risk taking, poor driving judgment and decision making, alcohol consumption, and excessive driving during high-risk hours (from 11 P.M. to 5 A.M.).

LEARNER'S PERMIT (LEARNING TO DRIVE). When teenagers obtain a learner's permit, they can start learning to drive with an adult present in the car to supervise and teach (Figure 62-3 ■). In most cases, the best way for teens to learn to drive is through a driver's education class. These classes are often sponsored by schools. In many states, the cost of automobile insurance is reduced

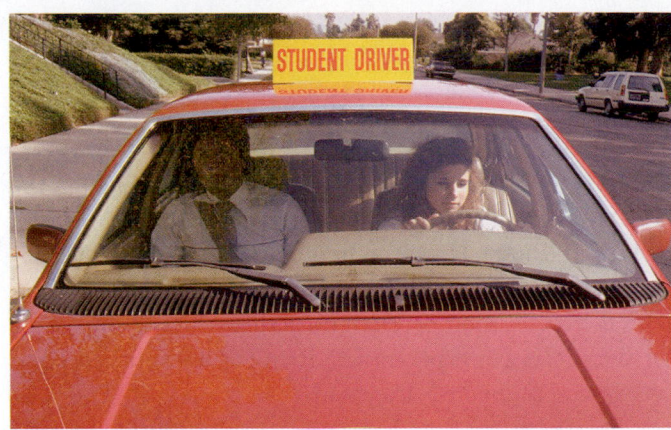

Figure 62-3. ■ Teen with driving instructor. (PhotoEdit Inc.)

if a teen has completed a driver's education course. Private driving instruction is another alternative. Teen drivers need to get as much driving experience as possible after they obtain their learner's permit. Driving experience makes the teen a safer driver and eases the transition to driving independently.

DRIVER'S LICENSE (DRIVING INDEPENDENTLY). When teens pass the official driving test, they receive their driver's license and can legally drive independently. Some states place restrictions on 17-year-old drivers. Parents should not allow their teen to drive independently until the teen has sufficient experience and the parents are comfortable with the teen's level of driving skill. Parents should talk candidly with their teen about the dangers and risks of distractions such as music from radio/tape/CD player, passengers, eating food, and using cell phones. Parents should also discuss and demonstrate the importance of controlling emotions while driving (e.g., "road rage," drag racing).

Teens should be taught about the importance of defensive driving. Inexperienced drivers often concentrate on driving correctly and fail to anticipate the actions and mistakes or errors of other drivers. If the teen is taking medications (prescription or over the counter) or has any medical illnesses, parents should check with their family physician about possible effects on the teen's driving ability.

Additionally, parents should make sure that the vehicle their teen drives is in safe condition (brakes, tires, etc.) and working properly. The vehicle should have essential emergency equipment (flares, flashlight, jumper cables, etc.) and the teen should know how to use it. A cell phone is helpful for emergencies, but parents must stress that it can be a dangerous distraction if it is used while driving.

Even though the driver's license allows the teen to drive independently, it is important that parents establish clear rules for safe and responsible driving and rules for the use of the car.

Other psychosocial topics are discussed at the end of this chapter.

ILLNESSES AND DISORDERS

Respiratory Disorders

Epistaxis (nosebleed) may occur in the adolescent for the same reasons it is seen in younger children (trauma and picking the nose). However, frequent nosebleeds in the adolescent may indicate other underlying disorders, such as essential hypertension or Hodgkin's disease. It is important for the adolescent experiencing frequent unexplained nosebleeds to seek medical attention.

Cardiovascular Disorders

HYPERTENSION

Elevated blood pressure in children is often secondary to kidney disease, hyperthyroidism, increased intracranial pressure (IICP), and side effects of certain medications. Hypertension may also be genetic or the result of family history and is called primary or essential hypertension.

Manifestations

Severe hypertension can cause headaches, dizziness, nosebleeds, and visual disturbances.

Diagnosis and Treatment

A diagnosis of hypertension is made following three separate measurements of elevated blood pressure. Laboratory tests such as blood urea nitrogen (BUN), creatinine, blood glucose, electrolytes, complete blood count, urinalysis, and a lipid panel are also done. An echocardiogram is used to assess the degree of cardiac involvement.

Clinical management of hypertension includes weight reduction for the adolescent who is overweight; a high-fiber diet low in calories, sodium, and fat; and regular exercise. Adolescents should be taught about the hazards of smoking and alcohol consumption. Antihypertensive medications are given to adolescents with severe hypertension. Table 62-5 ■ describes drugs used to correct hypertension in adolescents. Small teens would receive a child dose; large or older teens would receive an adult dose.

Nursing Considerations

Obtaining accurate blood pressure measurement is important. The appropriate size blood pressure cuff is essential. The adolescent and family should be taught to take the blood pressure accurately. The blood pressure should be taken at different times during the day and after the adolescent is at rest for at least 5 minutes.

The nurse can assist the adolescent and family in making nutritional food choices that will help maintain a healthy blood pressure. The nurse should discuss specific foods appropriate for keeping the blood pressure low. The teaching plan should also include food choices at restaurants and fast-food restaurants. Box 62-5 ■ describes herbs and vitamin supplements that can be used as aids for the heart.

> **clinical ALERT**
>
> Herbs and vitamin supplements should be used with caution in children of all ages. Teach parents to review these with their healthcare provider.

TABLE 62-5	Pharmacology: Antihypertensives			
DRUG (GENERIC AND COMMON BRAND NAME)	**USUAL ROUTE/DOSE**	**CLASSIFICATION AND PURPOSE**	**SELECTED SIDE EFFECTS**	**DON'T GIVE IF**
Propranolol hydrochloride (Inderal)	Child: PO 1 mg/kg/day in two divided doses Adult: PO 40 mg twice a day, may increase to 480 mg/day in divided doses	Beta-adrenergic antagonist for hypertension	Confusion, fatigue, drowsiness, bradycardia, paresthesia of the hands	Pulse is less than 60 bpm or systolic blood pressure is less than 90 mm Hg
Methyldopa (Aldomet)	Child: PO 10 to 65 mg/kg/day in two to four divided doses IV 20 to 65 mg/kg/day in four divided doses Adult: PO 250 mg two or three times a day, may increase to 3 g/day in divided doses	Central-acting hypertensive	Sedation, drowsiness, decreased mental acuity, sodium and water retention, nasal stuffiness	Child is receiving other drugs that decrease consciousness or if the child has decreased level of consciousness

<table>
<tr><td colspan="2">

BOX 62-5 **COMPLEMENTARY THERAPIES**

Herbs and Vitamins for the Heart

In adults, several natural products have been said to promote heart health. These products are vitamin E supplementation, garlic, and the herb, hawthorn. It is inappropriate to assume automatically that these same products are useful for children.

Herbal products are basically untested on children, and their production is unregulated in the United States. Parents who choose to give herbal products to their children should be advised to use products produced in developed countries to avoid contamination of lead, mercury, and steroids.

The National Institutes of Health (NIH) does report an apparent link between heart health and vitamin E supplementation. Parents of children should be taught about sources of vitamin E in foods. Foods containing vitamin E are almonds, sunflower seeds, peanut butter, spinach, broccoli, and kiwi. Physicians may recommend vitamin E supplementation for children with specific cardiac disorders. The following dosages of vitamin E are recommended by the NIH:

- Ages 1–3: 9 IU/day
- Ages 4–8: 10.5 IU/day
- Ages 9–13: 16.5 IU/day
- Ages 14 and older: 22.5 IU/day

(*Source*: Adams, E. D., & Towle, M. A. (2009). *Pediatric nursing care.* Upper Saddle River, NJ: Prentice Hall. Box 13-3, p. 349.)

</td></tr>
</table>

Hematologic Disorders

HODGKIN'S LYMPHOMA

Hodgkin's lymphoma (Figure 62-4 ■) is rare in children younger than 14 years. The incidence of the disease increases with age and is especially high in 15-year-old males. With early diagnosis and treatment of Hodgkin's lymphoma, the long-term prognosis is favorable (80–90% survival rate).

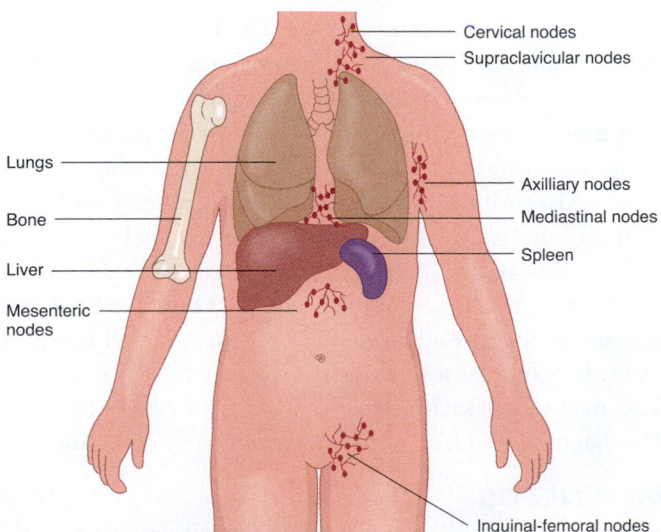

Figure 62-4. ■ Hodgkin's disease. Lymph nodes and organs affected in Hodgkin's disease in children.

Manifestations

The symptoms of Hodgkin's disease include nontender, firm, enlarged lymph nodes usually in the cervical and supraclavicular area. Occasionally, the mediastinal lymph nodes are involved, resulting in respiratory distress from pressure against the trachea. Some adolescents experience fever, night sweats, and weight loss.

Research indicates a relationship between herpes virus, cytomegalovirus, and Epstein-Barr virus and Hodgkin's disease. Hodgkin's disease has been reported in families suggesting a genetic factor as well.

Diagnosis and Treatment

The erythrocyte sedimentation rate and leukocyte counts may be elevated. Diagnosis is made by lymph node biopsy. Once the diagnosis is made, further tests must be made to determine the extent to which the disease has spread throughout the body. This process, called **staging**, is a process of naming the extent of the spread of cancer. It is necessary to help the physician plan the specific treatment. The tests usually consist of computed tomography (CT) or MRI scans, lymphangiogram, blood counts, bone marrow biopsy, and staging laparotomy. Box 62-6 ■ shows the staging system for Hodgkin's lymphoma.

Treatment usually consists of a combination of three to five antineoplastic agents. Table 62-6 ■ lists the antineoplastic agents commonly used to treat Hodgkin's lymphoma. A combination of agents is used because there is less chance that the cancer cells can develop resistance to one of the drugs. Drug combination allows the healthcare provider to select drugs with different patterns of toxicity that decreased the damage to other body systems. Selecting drugs that affect cells at different stages of their growth cycle allows higher numbers of malignant cells to be destroyed. Side effects of antineoplastic drugs include

<table>
<tr><td>

BOX 62-6   **STAGING OF HODGKIN'S LYMPHOMA**

- Stage I: The disease is confined to a single lymph node area.
- Stage IE: The disease progresses from the single lymph node area to adjacent regions.
- Stage II: The disease is in two or more lymph node areas on one side of the diaphragm.
- Stage IIE: The disease extends to adjacent regions of at least one of the affected nodes.
- Stage III: The disease is in lymph node areas on both sides of the diaphragm.
- Stage IIIE: The disease extends into adjacent areas or organs.
- Stage IIISE: The disease extends into adjacent areas or organs and/or into the spleen.
- Stage IV: The disease has spread from the lymphatic system to one or more other organs, such as the bone marrow or liver.

</td></tr>
</table>

TABLE 62-6	Combination Antineoplastic Agents Used to Treat Hodgkin's Lymphoma
COMBINATION	**DRUGS INCLUDED**
ABVD	**A**driamycin, **B**leomycin, **V**inblastine, **D**acarbazine
MOPP	**M**echlorethamine, vincristine (**O**ncovin), **p**rocarbazine, **p**rednisone
BCVPP	carmustine (**Bi**CNU), **c**yclophosphamide, **v**inblastine, **p**rocarbazine, **p**rednisone

Source: Adams, E. D., & Towle, M. A. (2009). *Pediatric nursing care.* Upper Saddle River, NJ: Prentice Hall. Table 14-4, p. 371.

bone marrow depression, nausea, vomiting, stomatitis, and hair loss. Low-dose radiation may be added to the treatment plan.

Nursing Considerations

The disease process coupled with the side effects of the antineoplastic agents and radiation treatments make the adolescent feel tired, sick, and embarrassed by the change in appearance. The adolescent who felt invincible prior to developing Hodgkin's may suddenly be confronted with his or her own mortality. Because antineoplastic agents lower the white blood cell count, the adolescent must avoid exposure to infection. The adolescent may need to decrease contacts with peers and remain home from school. This lack of contact with his or her peer support group may lead to feelings of isolation, depression, and anger.

Because many antineoplastic agents are given intravenously, these drugs are administered by an RN with preparation beyond his or her original degree. The LPN/LVN caring for the client would need to work closely with the RN. Clients must be assessed for signs of infection, open lesions, and bleeding. Their mental health status should be evaluated and emotional support provided. Precautions must be taken to prevent the care provider from being contaminated by body fluids containing the antineoplastic drugs.

Immune Disorders

MONONUCLEOSIS

Mononucleosis is caused by the Epstein-Barr virus (EBV). Mononucleosis is also called **glandular fever** and the "kissing disease." The most common mode of transmission is by direct and indirect contact with respiratory secretion, but it can also be transmitted by contact with genital secretions and blood transfusions. The incubation period is 10 to 50 days, and the virus can be shed up to 18 months following the clinical stage of the disease.

Manifestations

The clinical manifestations of mononucleosis begin with fever lasting 3 to 6 days, chills, anorexia, malaise, and sore throat. Within a few days, the adolescent experiences left shoulder pain, abdominal pain, lymphadenopathy, and hepatosplenomegaly. Symptoms also include weakness, lethargy, and fatigue. Symptoms can last several months.

Diagnosis and Treatment

Diagnosis is made by serologic monospot test and testing for EBV antibodies. The adolescent should avoid contact with those who are known to have the infection.

Medical treatment is symptomatic and includes bed rest, corticosteroids to relieve lymph node and organ swelling, antipyretics for fever, and analgesics for discomfort.

Nursing Considerations

The adolescent will need a quiet environment to promote rest. He or she may need assistance with activities of daily living. Due to the risk of rupture of spleen and liver, the adolescent must avoid contact sports, and rough play for approximately 4 weeks or until hepatosplenomegaly has subsided. To prevent exposure of other adolescents, kissing should be avoided for several days after the fever has subsided.

Nervous System Disorders

The main discussion of all nervous system disorders is in Chapter 36 ⚭.

HEADACHE

As with an adult, the adolescent may occasionally develop a headache. Often headache is related to a common infection such as the flu or strep throat. Headache in the adolescent may be related to stress or normal hormone changes associated with the menstrual cycle. These headaches are generally relieved by over-the-counter NSAIDs. Frequent headaches that are associated with other neurological symptoms and that are not relieved by NSAIDs need further evaluation.

A **migraine** is a familial disorder marked by periodic, unilateral pulsating headache that often begins during adolescence and continues into adulthood. Migraines may begin with an aura (transient visual phenomena) such as seeing stripes, spots, or lines. The aura may precede the headache, or recur during the height of the headache. Often the headache is so severe that the adolescent must remain in bed in a dim room. It may take several days to recover from a migraine. This may cause isolation and depression in the adolescent. The diagnosis and treatment is the same as for the adult.

MENINGITIS

Meningitis is an inflammation of the meninges. Meningitis is usually caused by either a bacteria or virus. Although many cases of meningitis occur before the age of 5 years, meningitis can occur in anyone. Viral meningitis (also called aseptic meningitis) may occur following exposure to mumps virus, coxsackievirus, echovirus, HIV, polio, and others. Bacterial meningitis (also called infectious meningitis) is more dangerous than viral meningitis. Bacterial meningitis can cause permanent neurologic damage and death. Causative organisms of bacterial meningitis may be *Haemophilus influenza, Streptococcus pneumoniae,* or *Neisseria meningitides* (causes meningococcal meningitis). Vaccination against *Haemophilus influenza* (Hib) can reduce the incidence of meningitis from this organism.

In the past two decades, there has been an increase in the number of meningococcal meningitis outbreaks in adolescents and young adults (Harrison et al., 2001). Many who become infected with the meningococcal organism have reported close contact with others in their age group through dormitory living, kissing, or sharing products such as drinks and lip ointments contaminated with saliva. Even with aggressive treatment approximately 10% to 12% of clients die from this disease. Because the behavior of adolescents and young adults puts them at increased risk, the Centers for Disease Control and Prevention (CDC) recommends immunization against this potentially fatal disease.

The symptoms, treatment, and nursing care of the adolescent with meningitis are the same as that of the infant and toddler described in Chapter 59 ∞ or of the adult, described in Chapter 36 ∞. Kernig's or Brudzinski's sign (Figure 62-5 ■) may be used to help diagnose the disease.

CLOSED HEAD INJURY

The adolescent frequently indulges in risk-taking behavior, especially boys. As testosterone increases, the muscles of the adolescent boy enlarge and gain strength. This sudden increase in strength gives boys a feeling of power and invincibility. Risk-taking behavior can result in closed head injury including concussion, skull fracture, and hematoma.

AMYOTROPHIC LATERAL SCLEROSIS

Amyotrophic lateral sclerosis (ALS), sometimes called Lou Gehrig's disease, is rare in children but may present in late adolescence or early adulthood. ALS is a familial disorder linked to chromosome 21 defects. ALS is a progressive degenerative neurologic disorder in which muscle weakness and wasting progress from the extremities to the core. Death, usually the result of respiratory failure, usually occurs 2 to 5 years after the onset of symptoms. Referrals are crucial for support for family and caregivers.

Musculoskeletal Disorders

Musculoskeletal disorders are covered in depth in Chapter 31 ∞.

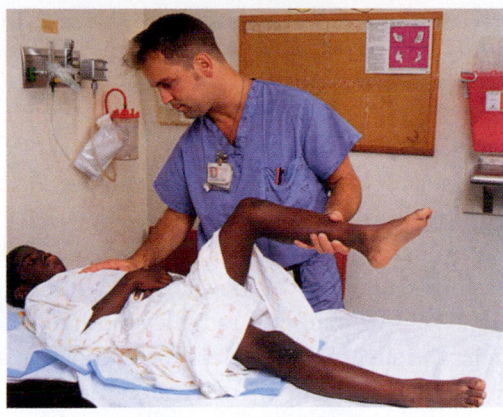

A

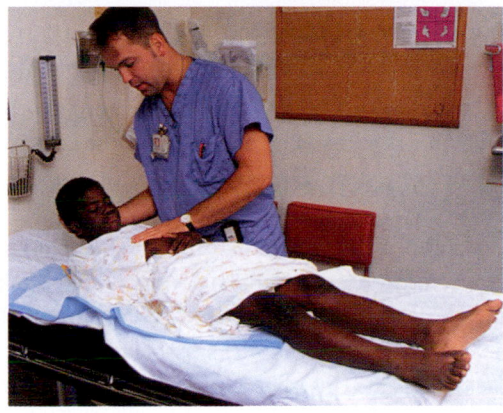

B

Figure 62-5. ■ **A.** To test for Kernig's sign, raise the child's leg with the knee flexed. Then extend the child's leg at the knee. If any resistance is noted or pain is felt, the result is a positive Kernig's sign. **B.** To test for Brudzinski's sign, flex the child's head while the child is supine. If this action makes the knees or hips flex involuntarily, a positive Brudzinski's sign is present.

FIBROMYALGIA

Fibromyalgia is a chronic disorder of muscles and soft tissue surrounding joints resulting in pain that is difficult to manage. While this disorder is most common in adults, it has been diagnosed in children.

Manifestations

The symptoms of fibromyalgia are vague and often difficult to determine the cause. There is general agreement that fibromyalgia results from abnormal regulation of neuroendocrine transmission. Often children presenting with chronic pain surrounding joints and fatigue are referred to a rheumatologist for diagnosis.

Diagnosis and Treatment

Once other disorders are eliminated, the diagnosis of fibromyalgia might be made. Various approaches have been attempted in the treatment of fibromyalgia. Generally medication including topical capsaicin, oral anti-inflammatories, antidepressants, and narcotic analgesics are used. Increased physical therapy might help the client to cope with the chronic discomfort.

Nursing Consideration

Because peer and group interaction is important for the adolescent, it is important for the adolescent with fibromyalgia to remain as physically active as possible. Muscle aches might be eased by massage, and stretching and yoga might help to maintain range of motion. The nurse should refer the client to a physical and occupational therapist for help in coping with daily activities. The family should be referred to the National Fibromyalgia Association for information and support.

TRAUMATIC INJURIES

Every day many children and teens suffer back strain caused by heavy backpacks filled with books, gym clothes, and many electronic devices. The weight of these backpacks can be between 10% and 20% of the child's body weight (Maclas et al., 2005).

Parents and health professionals need to develop methods of assisting children and teens to avoid added back strain from heavy backpacks. Health education programs can alert children and parents to the risks associated with carrying heavy backpacks and instruct children in proper body mechanics. More children now use backpacks with wheels.

Bodybuilding Injuries

In recent years, preteen and teen children have been encouraged to participate in group sports such as soccer and baseball teams. When these children hope to become professional athletes, some parents are encouraging bodybuilding training. Doctors and nurses have questioned if weight-training exercises are safe or beneficial to the adolescent. In 2001, the American Academy of Pediatrics (AAP) published a statement related to children and weight training. It reads, "Studies have shown that strength training, when properly structured with regard to frequency, mode (type of lifting), intensity, and duration of program, can increase strength in preadolescents and adolescents" (p. 1472). The American College of Sports Medicine (ACSM) has also stated that strength training programs that are properly designed and supervised can enhance motor fitness skills and sports performance. The ACSM also states that strength training encourages healthy lifestyles; builds confidence; increases lean body mass; improves cholesterol levels; improves cardiac, respiratory, and bone fitness; and improves body image and self-esteem.

Supervision of the weight-training program is a must. The nurse should suggest that the adult supervisor be trained and certified as a fitness expert. The supervisor should have experience working with children and should be present during the entire training session to provide proper spotting of the weights during lifts. The gym should be clean, safe, and spacious with no more than 10 students per adult supervisor. Training should be 2 or 3 days a week with 1 day off between training sessions. The weight-training session should begin with stretching and aerobic activity. Each session should end with stretching. Weight can be increased when 15 repetitions become easy and the adolescent can do three sets of 15 repetitions of an exercise on three consecutive sessions.

Sports Injuries

Even with the best preparation and supervision, sports injuries can occur. The most common sports that result in injury are football, wrestling, soccer, and gymnastics. Fractures (described in Chapters 31 and 60 ⚭) are common sports injuries in young athletes. A variety of other injuries can occur. Some risk factors for sports injury include:

- Vulnerability of the growth plates to injury
- Increased joint mobility from lax tendons and ligaments
- Softer bone
- Lack of experience in the sport and inadequate training
- Lack of acceptance of protective gear
- Impatience with taking the time to heal after injury
- Vulnerability to spinal injury related to high-impact sports and recreation such as diving in unsupervised locations

Some common sports injuries are listed in Table 62-7 ■.

Nursing Considerations

The nursing care of specific injuries has been discussed throughout the text. If the injury appears serious, the emergency medical services should be contacted immediately. Nonserious injuries can be treated by stopping bleeding, immobility, and ice until parents can seek medical attention.

TABLE 62-7	Common Sports Injuries
SPORT	**TYPE OF INJURIES**
Baseball	Contusion and sprains of upper and lower extremities
	Injury from being hit by the ball (e.g., broken teeth, face, head, eye, and chest injury)
	Fractures (finger, hand, arm, leg)
Football	Pulled muscle or dislocation (shoulder, leg)
	Head and neck injury
Gymnastics	Fractures and strains (wrist, elbow)
	Tendonitis (elbow, ankles, knees)
Soccer	Head and neck injury
	Fractures and strains of legs
Wrestling	Dislocation and fractures of upper and lower extremities

The nurse should encourage parents to inquire about the coach's experience and verify that the coaching staff is prepared in emergency care. Injury should be treated promptly. The adolescent should not participate in sports until healing is complete.

Amputation

Amputation of a limb rarely occurs but may be necessary to save the adolescent's life. The most common reasons for amputation are bone tumors, severe injury, and bone infection. The basic nursing care is similar to that of the adult. See Box 61-5 for care of the stump following amputation. The adolescent will need to learn to care for the stump and prosthesis (see Figure 31-11).

The psychological assessment and care of the adolescent following amputation may be more of a challenge than the physical care. Recall the adolescent is adjusting to the normal body changes that come with puberty. Peer opinions and peer interaction are important to normal psychological development at this age. Amputation insults the adolescent's developing body image. Hospitalization and rehabilitation may prevent interaction with peer groups. Support systems should be identified and contacted as soon as possible. The nurse can help the adolescent identify a role model who has overcome the challenges of amputation.

Parents may need help finding financial support for the cost of prosthetic devices, because insurance may not cover them. Administrators at the adolescent's school need to know about the amputation and make plans for the adolescent's return (e.g., identifying routes for the teen in a wheelchair, updating plans for emergency evacuation).

Gastrointestinal Disorders

INFLAMMATORY BOWEL DISEASE

Inflammatory bowel disease is two separate chronic disorders of the intestine:

- **Crohn's disease** is random inflammation of the entire gastrointestinal tract that involves all layers of the bowel wall.
- **Ulcerative colitis** is inflammation with sloughing of the mucosa of the large intestine.

These two disorders (also discussed in Chapter 37) have similar symptoms and treatment but different pathology. It was once believed that these were diseases of young adults. However, the incidence of both disorders has increased in adolescence. The etiology is uncertain, but there is a strong support for a genetic association (Box 62-7 ■).

Manifestations

Crohn's disease begins as a small, localized ulcer, and then grows in size and depth. The onset of symptoms is gradual, with abdominal cramps followed by diarrhea (see Figure 37-17). These symptoms subside in a few days and then

recur, becoming more severe each time. Over time, the adolescent develops anorexia, weight loss, and general malaise.

Ulcerative colitis also begins with abdominal cramps and diarrhea. Lower abdominal pain occurs before and during a bowel movement and stops with the passage of stool and flatus. The stool is mixed with mucus and blood. Weight loss and delayed growth occurs over time.

Diagnosis and Treatment

Diagnosis is based on determining the location and extent of involvement. Stool specimens are used to rule out an infectious process. Biopsy is taken during a colonoscopy. Laboratory studies are useful in identifying secondary conditions such as anemia, electrolyte imbalance, and malnutrition.

Medical treatment for both disorders involves the administration of corticosteroids, antibiotics, and antidiarrheal medication. For moderate to severe Crohn's disease, including fistula-forming disease, immunosuppressants such as Remicade (infliximab) are administered. The goal of nutritional therapy is to provide adequate calories and nutrients for growth without aggravating the inflammation and diarrhea. Total parenteral nutrition (TPN) is often given during an acute episode when the bowel must be rested. TPN can be used to improve nutrition by increasing the amount of protein, carbohydrates, vitamins, and minerals to aid in healing. At times, surgery is needed. A temporary colostomy or ileostomy is performed to allow the lower small intestine or colon to rest and heal. In ulcerative colitis, the removal of the affected tissue usually provides a cure. In Crohn's disease, ulceration tends to recur elsewhere.

Nursing Considerations

Nursing care focuses on the emotional impact of these chronic disorders, teaching the administration of prescribed medication, monitoring nutritional status, and providing referrals. Nursing management most commonly occurs in the home and school, and parents may need to arrange home tutoring during acute episodes of the disease.

Adolescence is an emotionally difficult time, given the normal changes in body image. Abdominal pain, diarrhea, fluid and electrolyte loss, blood loss, and side effects of medication all place additional stress on the adolescent's self-image. The need for a temporary or permanent ileostomy or colostomy will compound the issue. During an acute episode, the client may not be able to attend school, which may limit support from friends. Encourage the adolescent to maintain contact with friends by telephone, e-mail, cards, and visits. Referral to visiting nurses and support groups for adolescents with ostomies and the Crohn's Colitis Foundation may be helpful.

Because adolescents can provide a lot of their own care, instructions should be given to both the client and the parents. Demonstration and return demonstration in care of the central venous catheters and administration of TPN, including maintaining sterile technique, operating infusion pumps, and obtaining blood glucose levels, are important aspects of teaching. Teaching should also include the importance of adhering to the prescribed medication regimen, with emphasis on continuing the medications even when the client is asymptomatic. If an ostomy is required, teaching must include the care of the site, bag change, and odor management. See Procedure 37-3 ⟳ for steps in providing ostomy care.

Eating disorders are discussed under Psychosocial Disorders later in this chapter.

HEPATITIS

Hepatitis, inflammation of the liver, can be caused by a viral infection. The most common infections in the United States are from hepatitis A virus (HAV), hepatitis B virus (HBV), hepatitis C virus (HCV), and hepatitis D virus (HDV).

clinical ALERT

Nurses and other healthcare workers could come in contact with the blood and body fluids containing hepatitis virus. Standard precautions should be used at all times. It is recommended that the healthcare workers receive three doses of hepatitis B immunization.

The adolescent can become exposed to hepatitis through ingestion of contaminated food, exchange of body fluids from IV drug use or unprotected sexual contact, or body tattooing and piercing.

Manifestations

The body's response to all types of hepatitis virus is the same. At first, the virus attacks the **parenchymal** cells (functional part of an organ), resulting in local degeneration and necrosis of the tissue (Figure 62-6 ▪). This stimulates the inflammatory process. Swelling and an accumulation of white blood cells block the drainage of bile. The backup of bile further damages the liver tissue, resulting in an elevation in bilirubin and ALT and alkaline phosphatase in the blood. High bilirubin levels cause jaundice, a yellowing of the tissue that is most obvious in skin and sclera. The liver fails to produce enough albumins, resulting in generalized edema.

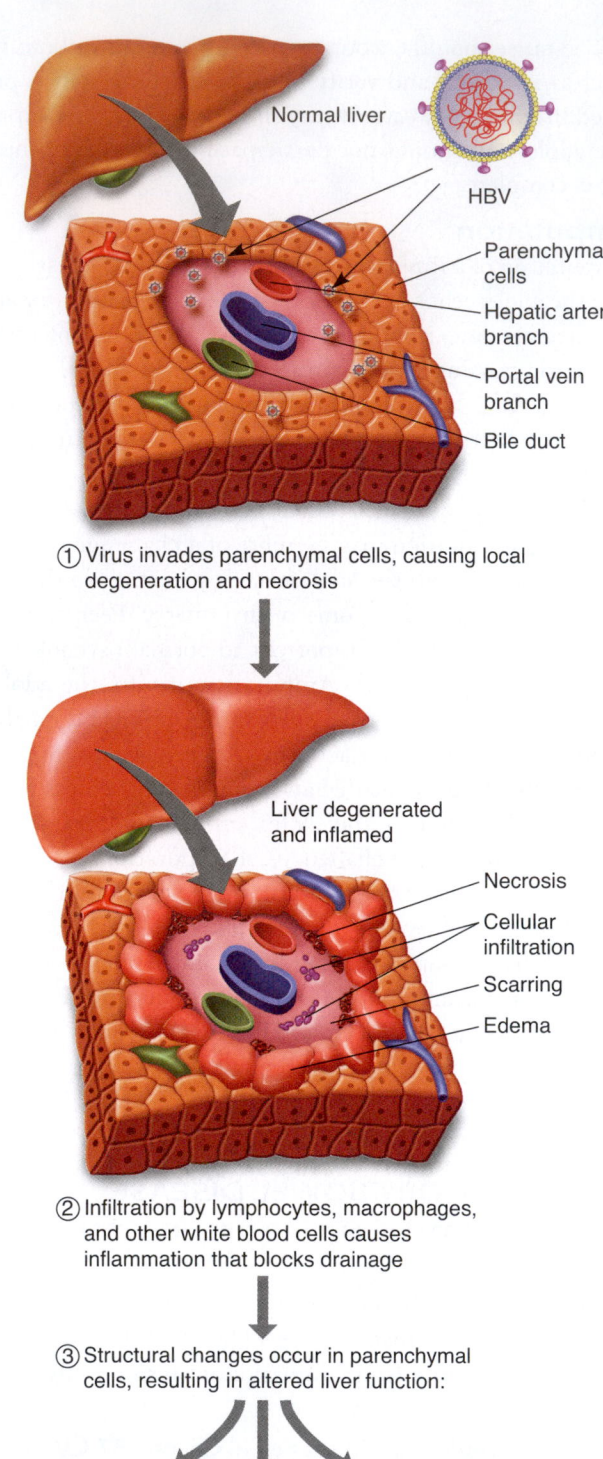

① Virus invades parenchymal cells, causing local degeneration and necrosis

② Infiltration by lymphocytes, macrophages, and other white blood cells causes inflammation that blocks drainage

③ Structural changes occur in parenchymal cells, resulting in altered liver function:

Impaired bile excretion — Elevated ALT and alkaline phosphatase levels — Decreased albumin synthesis

Figure 62-6. ▪ Pathophysiology of hepatitis. The hepatitis virus causes degeneration and necrosis of the liver, which results in abnormal liver function and illness.

In most cases, the body's immune system is able to destroy the hepatitis virus, stopping the liver destruction. Regeneration of liver tissue occurs in approximately 3 months.

Diagnosis and Treatment

Serology studies would show positive for antibodies to one or more of the hepatitis viruses. For adolescents with a pre-existing liver disorder or an impaired immune system, continued liver destruction could result in death.

clinical ALERT

When hepatitis is present, the liver is unable to detoxify and metabolize drugs at the usual rate. Medications should be administered carefully and the adolescent monitored closely for both side effects and toxic effects.

To date, no antiviral agents have been developed to combat the hepatitis virus. Treatment, therefore, is symptomatic. The adolescent will need adequate rest, fluids, and nutrition to promote healing. Monitoring the blood values will be useful in determining the amount of healing. Vitamin K might be administered if prothrombin times are increased. It is important to prevent the spread of the virus by teaching the adolescent to abstain from sexual contact, to wash hands thoroughly after using the restroom, and to avoid sharing blood and body fluids.

Nursing Considerations

The nursing care of the adolescent with hepatitis is the same as the adult. It is important for the nurse to teach the adolescent how to break the cycle of exposure by:

- Thoroughly washing the hands after using the restroom.
- Not sharing IV needles or syringes.
- Abstaining from sexual contact or using a condom with each sexual contact.

For more information on hepatitis see Chapter 37 ⚭.

Endocrine Disorders

DIABETES MELLITUS

Diabetes mellitus was covered in detail in Chapters 38 and 61 ⚭. The discussion here will be limited to the adolescent with diabetes.

Recall that adolescence is a time of newfound independence, peer influence, and changing body image. The adolescent who has diabetes mellitus may experience additional challenge to maintain a normal blood glucose level. The diabetic adolescent on a low carbohydrate diet may have difficulty saying "no" to fast foods, sweet deserts, or high carbohydrate snacks when their friends are enjoying these foods. The diabetic adolescent may need to test the blood glucose and administer subcutaneous insulin. These activities may cause questions by peers, make teens feel different from their friends, and lead to stress. Some adolescents—not wanting to appear different—may choose not to test the blood glucose or administer insulin on time. It is critical for the nurse to provide support and resources for the diabetic adolescent and family.

THYROID DISORDERS

Thyroid disorders are rare in children. However, when they do occur, they must be diagnosed and treated in a timely manner because thyroid hormones are necessary for cellular metabolism, mental functioning, and growth.

Hypothyroidism

Hypothyroidism is a disorder in which thyroid hormones are decreased. The cause can be congenital. It may also result from autosomal recessive gene mutation, a deficiency in TSH, or inflammation of the thyroid gland.

MANIFESTATIONS. Symptoms generally do not appear for a few months after birth. The tongue and lips thicken, and the adolescent has a dull expression. The adolescent can also develop jaundice, hypotonia, bradycardia, lethargy, eating problems, and cool extremities. Precocious puberty, irregular menses, hair loss, slowing of growth, increased weight, and **goiter** (painless enlargement of thyroid gland) may occur.

DIAGNOSIS AND TREATMENT. Diagnosis is made by screening T_4 and TSH. A decreased T_4 would indicate hypothyroidism. If TSH is elevated, the hypothyroidism is caused by the thyroid gland. If TSH is not elevated, the hypothyroidism is caused by lack of stimulation from the pituitary gland. Further evaluation of the pituitary gland is required.

Levothyroxine (Synthroid) is often prescribed to treat hypothyroidism. As the adolescent grows, the dose will need to be adjusted to maintain a normal hormone level. It is important for the adolescent to be followed by a pediatric endocrinologist.

NURSING CONSIDERATIONS. As with other endocrine disorders, the nursing management involves client and parent teaching about the condition, the administration of medication, and the signs of inadequate hormone replacement. It is important to stress the need for lifelong thyroid replacement therapy.

Hyperthyroidism

Hyperthyroidism is extremely rare in children and adolescents. When it does occur, it is almost always associated with Graves' disease. *Graves' disease* is an autoimmune disorder in which antibodies attack the thyroid gland. When immunoglobulins attack the thyroid cells, the result is an overproduction of thyroid hormones. Other causes of hyperthyroidism include thyroid-secreting tumors of the thyroid, thyroiditis, and pituitary tumors that increase the production of TSH.

MANIFESTATIONS. Symptoms of hyperthyroidism include a goiter, prominent or bulging eyes, nervousness, restlessness and irritability, increased weight loss with increased appetite, heat intolerance, and muscle weakness. Symptoms generally begin in the school-age child and may be present for several years before they are recognized and treated. The child's performance in school declines due to decreased ability to concentrate. The child rapidly becomes fatigued and overheated in physical education class and may have difficulty relaxing and sleeping.

DIAGNOSIS AND TREATMENT. Diagnosis is usually made with serum TSH, T_3 and T_4, autoantibodies specific for thyroid disorders, and thyroid scan. Antithyroid medications are usually the first choice of treatment. The second choice of treatment is radiation with radioactive iodine to destroy the thyroid tissue. Thyroidectomy is the third option of treatment. Destruction or removal of the thyroid gland causes permanent hypothyroidism, requiring lifelong thyroid replacement.

NURSING CONSIDERATIONS. Nursing care involves teaching the adolescent and parents about the disorder and the chosen treatment. They need to be told there is no evidence that radioactive iodine increases the risk for cancer or birth defects in future children. Families anticipating thyroid surgery will need routine preoperative teaching, as well as specific information about surgically induced hypothyroidism. Postoperatively the nurse should observe closely for bleeding and respiratory distress.

clinical ALERT

Swelling of the surgical site following thyroid surgery can cause airway obstruction. The adolescent should be assessed closely for swelling, bleeding, hoarseness, and difficulty breathing. If the parathyroid glands were accidentally removed, the blood calcium level can drop to life-threateningly low levels. Signs of hypocalcemia include tingling and tetany. A syringe containing calcium should be kept at the bedside.

All cases of hyperthyroidism require regular follow-up appointments with a pediatric endocrinologist.

ADRENAL DISORDERS

Adrenal disorders, like other endocrine disorders, are rare in adolescents. When they do occur, their manifestations, treatment, and nursing care is similar to that of adults. For complete discussion, see Chapter 38 ⚭.

EFFECTS OF STEROID USE

Anabolic steroids, either testosterone or agents resembling testosterone, can stimulate the growth or manufacturing of body tissues. Anabolic steroids have been used, sometimes in large doses, by athletes to improve performance. This use has been judged to be illegal by various organizations that supervise sports. Indiscriminate use of anabolic steroids is inadvisable because of the undesirable side effects they produce. Women taking anabolic steroids may experience *hirsutism* (increased body hair), masculinization, and clitoral hypertrophy. Men taking anabolic steroids may experience aggressiveness and testicular atrophy.

Adolescents hoping to improve their athleticism and opportunities for college scholarship may feel the need to take anabolic steroids. Parents and coaches must be alert to the effects of anabolic steroids and the side effects. Adolescents should be informed of the potentially life-altering side effects. Adolescents must be encouraged to help their peers who might be taking anabolic steroids by talking to the athletic coach, school nurse, or school counselor.

METABOLIC SYNDROME (METABOLIC X SYNDROME)

Metabolic syndrome, also called **metabolic X syndrome,** is a group of related metabolic disorders, including obesity, insulin resistance, and complications of Type 2 diabetes. Although these disorders have been known for years, the relationship of these and other disorders is relatively new.

Manifestations

Central obesity is the key factor in this syndrome. Recall obesity is rapidly increasing in children. Many adults report their weight problems began in adolescence. However, because not everyone who is overweight and inactive will develop metabolic syndrome, a genetic factor may play an important role.

Diagnosis and Treatment

Researchers in Australia have identified altered endocrine function, including high estrogen levels in women, low testosterone levels in men, high cortisol levels, and low thyroid levels, are related to metabolic syndrome (Kidson, 1998). Some women have a history of ovarian cyst formation.

There is no specific treatment for metabolic syndrome, nor is there a quick solution for the person affected. Treatment is centered on weight loss, maintaining blood glucose in normal ranges, and increasing activity. Insulin resistance and increased blood glucose is often treated with oral hypoglycemics. Hypothyroidism is treated with synthetic hormone replacement. Anticholesterol medication may be needed if other methods to reduce cholesterol are ineffective. Only low-level estrogen birth control pills can be used to treat ovarian cyst or prevent pregnancy. An intrauterine device containing progesterone may be helpful in women who are unable to have additional estrogen.

Nursing Considerations

The nurse is responsible for assisting in monitoring the effects and side effects of medication, and providing teaching to the adolescent and the family. By teaching parents and teens about the potential for metabolic syndrome and the effect of obesity on the endocrine and other body systems, these disorders can be prevented.

Urinary Disorders

Urinary disorders in the adolescent are the same as those of adults. As teens become sexually active, the incidence of urinary tract infection increases. Urinary tract infection can occur singularly or in combination with sexually transmitted infections. It is important for the nurse to ask questions about sexual activity when urinary tract infection is suspected.

Reproductive Disorders

GYNECOLOGIC PROBLEMS

There are many different gynecologic problems that could occur during adolescence. For the most part, they are the same as those affecting adults. Details of these conditions are discussed in Chapter 40 ⚭.

Parents should be sure to talk with their children about all of the normal changes that will be occurring in the body during this time of physical maturation and development, so that abnormal changes can be examined right away. Be sure to discuss the following:

- Vaginal bleeding and discharge are a normal part of your menstrual cycle. However, if you notice anything different or unusual, consult your physician before attempting to treat the problem yourself.

- Symptoms may result from mild infections that are easy to treat. But, if they are not treated properly, they can lead to more serious conditions, including infertility. Vaginal symptoms may also be a sign of more serious problems from sexually transmitted infections. Urinary tract infections may also be as sign of reproductive system infection.

- Consult your physician if you have any of the following symptoms:

  - Bleeding between periods

  - Frequent and urgent need to urinate, or a burning sensation during urination

  - Abnormal vaginal bleeding, particularly during or after intercourse

  - Pain or pressure in your pelvis that differs from menstrual cramps

  - Itching, burning, swelling, redness, or soreness in the vaginal area

  - Sores or lumps or any unusual lesion in the genital area

  - Vaginal discharge with an unpleasant or unusual odor or an unusual color

  - Increased vaginal discharge

  - Pain or discomfort during intercourse

Recognizing symptoms early and seeing a physician right away increases the likelihood of successful treatment.

FIRST PELVIC EXAMINATION

The American College of Obstetricians and Gynecologists recommend a woman have her first Papanicolaou test (Pap test) at age 21 or within 3 years of becoming sexually active. These recommendations were based on the risk of cervical cancer to this age group. The most common cause of cervical cancer is infection with the human papillomavirus (HPV). HPV is commonly transmitted sexually. The Pap smear is obtained by pelvic examination. Other reasons for a pelvic examination are to test for sexually transmitted infections and to determine if pregnancy has occurred.

The first pelvic examination may be uncomfortable and embarrassing. The nurse must provide teaching regarding what to expect during the examination and emotional support. If the examiner is male, a female nurse must be present for the protection of the client and examiner.

The nurse should prepare the examination room and assemble a vaginal speculum, water-soluble lubricant, wooden spatula, and glass slides. The adolescent should remove her clothing below the waist and sit on the examination table covered in a clean drape. When the examiner is ready, the client is positioned on the examination table with her feet in stirrups and covered with the drape (Figure 62-7 ■). The nurse stands next to the client, explaining to her what is happening and helping her to relax. The nurse must send any specimens to the laboratory for analysis.

During the clinic visit, the nurse should provide instruction in breast self-examination, birth control methods, and prevention of sexually transmitted infections. It is also the time to discuss vaccination against human papillomavirus;

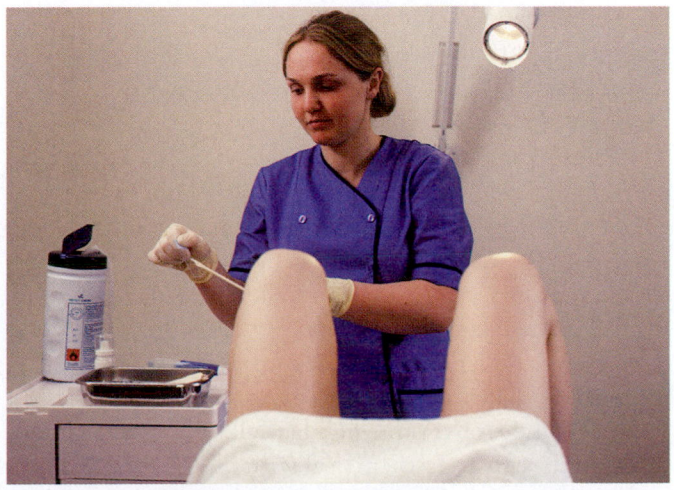

Figure 62-7. ■ The teenage girl may be anxious before having her first Pap smear. The nurse can reduce client anxiety by providing information about what is happening and by being willing to answer questions. (Photo Researchers, Inc.)

BOX 62-8   VACCINE FOR PREVENTION OF CERVICAL CANCER

In 2006 the Centers for Disease Control and the Food and Drug Administration announced a recommendation that the vaccine Gardasil can prevent transmission of HPV and therefore serve as a preventative measure against cervical cancer. Gardasil protects against four types of HPV: two causing cervical cancer and two causing genital warts. Studies show that this vaccine is most effective when used in females prior to initiation of sexual activity. The CDC's Advisory Committee for Immunization Practices recommends the routine vaccination of 11- to 12-year-old girls. The series of three inactivated, recombinant vaccines is given intramuscularly, initially and then repeated 2 months and 6 months later. The dosage of Gardasil is 0.5 ml. Current cost of the vaccine is $120 per dose.

Source: Data from Schmidt, J. (2007). HPV vaccine: Implications for nurse and patients. *Nursing for Women's Health, 11*(1), 83–87; CDC. (2006). *Human papillomavirus (HPV), cervical cancer, and HPV vaccine and recommendations: A current issue in immunization NetConference* (Course number EV0378). Retrieved April 27, 2007; Cox, J., Mayeaux, E., France, E., Moscicki, A., Palefsky, J., et al. (2006). Advances in prevention of cervical cancer and other human papillomavirus-related diseases. *Pediatric Infectious Disease Journal, 25*(2), S65–81.

this vaccine series protects against several types of genital warts associated with cervical cancer (Box 62-8 ■).

SEXUALITY AND CONTRACEPTION

The American Academy of Family Physicians is concerned about the sexual health of adolescents in the United States, particularly in regard to the high incidence of teenage pregnancies, the high rate of sexually transmitted infections, and the lack of effective sex education programs.

Nurses can play an important role in promoting responsible sexual behavior and in providing factual information about contraception. Abstinence from sexual activity is the most effective method of preventing unplanned pregnancy and sexually transmitted infections (STIs). Responsible sexual behavior can also be effective if it is consistently and carefully followed. The adolescent should receive appropriate medical care related to sexual health, including examinations, testing, treatments, prophylactic immunizations, counseling, and contraceptive methods. It is from the family that an adolescent's values and concept of sexual responsibility arise. So, families should be encouraged to be involved in sex education efforts.

Adolescent clients may be dealing with issues of sexual orientation that impact their psychosocial and physical health. A safe environment that allows adolescents to discuss issues can help them deal with their sexuality. It can open a dialogue on family relationships, safe sex, suicide risks, and other issues confronting gay, lesbian, bisexual, and transgender adolescents. These clients need a sensitive and accepting atmosphere in which to raise their concerns.

Healthcare providers should take an active role in the prevention of unintended teenage pregnancies and prevention of STIs by providing appropriate guidance/counseling and effective sex education to their adolescent client population. The nurse can be actively involved in community efforts to initiate and implement effective education and prevention programs for unintended teenage pregnancy and sexually transmitted infections. Adolescents receiving contraceptive services should be accorded strict client confidentiality.

One of the most difficult tasks in dealing with adolescent healthcare issues may be assisting the parents to recognize that their son or daughter is reaching the age where he or she needs to begin making independent health decisions. The nurse can facilitate the communication between teen and parent. Box 62-9 ■ provides some tips to teach parents.

SEXUALLY TRANSMITTED INFECTIONS

Three million adolescents contract an STI each year, according to the American Academy of Pediatrics. (The major discussion of sexually transmitted infections is provided in Chapter 41 ◉.)

More than 20 STIs have been identified. Some estimates say they affect as many as 65 million people in this country (CDC, 2003). See Table 41-1 ◉ for manifestations, diagnosis, and treatment of sexually transmitted infections; see Box 41-2 ◉ for prevalence of STIs among teens.

The surest way to prevent adolescents from contracting an STI is for them to abstain from any type of sexual activity. However, if the adolescent becomes sexually active, he or she needs teaching about precautionary measures for reducing the risk of acquiring an STI (Box 62-10 ■). These measures include the following:

- Have a mutually monogamous sexual relationship with an uninfected partner.
- Consistently and correctly use a male condom.
- Use sterile needles if injecting intravenous (IV) drugs.
- Decrease susceptibility to HIV infection by preventing and controlling other STIs.
- Delay having sexual relationships as long as possible. (The younger a person is when he or she begins to engage in sexual activity, the more susceptible the person is to developing an STI.)
- Have regular checkups for STIs.
- Learn the symptoms of STIs and seek medical help as soon as possible if any symptoms develop.
- Avoid having sexual intercourse during menstruation.
- Avoid anal intercourse, or use a male condom.
- Avoid douching.

Manifestations

Manifestations (such as pain on urination, urethral or vaginal discharge, and rash) are specific to the disease. See Chapter 41 ◉ for full discussion.

BOX 62-9 | CLIENT TEACHING

Parenting Tips for Adolescents

- Adolescents usually require privacy in which to contemplate changes taking place within their own bodies. Ideally the youth should be allowed to have his or her own room, but if this is not possible some private space needs to be allotted.
- Teasing an adolescent child about physical changes is inappropriate because it may cause self-consciousness and embarrassment.
- Parents need to remember that the adolescent's interest in body changes and sexual topics is natural, normal development and does not necessarily indicate movement into sexual activity.
- One must take care not to label emerging instinct/behaviors as "wrong," "sick," or "immoral." Adolescents may experiment with or consider a wide range of sexual orientations/behaviors prior to settling on their own sexual identity.
- A reemergence of the Oedipal complex (child's attraction for the parent of the opposite sex) is common during adolescent years. Healthy parents deal with this by noting the physical changes and attractiveness of the child and taking pride in the youth's growth into maturity without crossing appropriate parent and child relationship boundaries.
- It is normal for the parent to find the adolescent attractive, particularly because the teen often looks very similar in appearance to the other (same sex) parent at an earlier age. This attraction may cause the parent to feel awkward, but care should be taken by the parent not to create distance (and potentially make the adolescent feel something is wrong with him- or herself). It is inappropriate for a parent's attraction to his or her child to be anything more than an attraction as a parent (i.e., incest).

- The teenager's quest for independence is normal development and need not be looked on by the parent as rejection or a loss of control. To be of most benefit to the growing adolescent, a parent needs to remain a constant and consistent figure, available as a sounding board for the youth's ideas without dominating and overtaking the emerging, independent identity of the young person.
- Despite adolescents' tendency to constantly challenge authority figures, they need or want limit setting because it provides a safe boundary in which to grow and function. Limit setting refers to predetermined and negotiated rules and regulations regarding behavior.
- In contrast, "power struggles" arise when authority is at stake or when being "right" becomes the primary issue. These situations should be avoided because ultimately one of the parties (typically the teen) is overpowered, causing the youth to lose face and activating feelings of embarrassment, inadequacy, resentment, and bitterness.
- Parents need to be prepared for and recognize that there are commonly occurring conflicts that may develop when parenting adolescents. The experience may be influenced by unresolved issues from their own childhoods as well as unresolved issues from the adolescent's earlier years.
- Parents can anticipate that their positions of authority will be repeatedly challenged as children enter and move through their adolescent years. Maintaining open lines of communication and clear, yet negotiable, limits or boundaries may prove useful in minimizing major conflicts.
- Most parents report a sense of increased wisdom and self-growth and they rise to the challenges presented through parenting adolescents.

BOX 62-10 | CLIENT TEACHING

Sexually Transmitted Infections and Adolescents

- STIs affect men and women of all backgrounds and economic levels. However, nearly two-thirds of all STIs occur in people younger than age 25.
- STIs are on the rise, possibly due to people being more sexually active and having multiple sex partners during their lives.
- Many STIs initially cause no symptoms. In addition, many STI symptoms, especially in women, may be confused with those of other diseases not transmitted through sexual contact. Even symptom-less STIs can be contagious.
- Women suffer more frequent and severe symptoms from STIs:

- Some STIs can spread into the uterus (womb) and fallopian tubes and cause pelvic inflammatory disease (PID), which, can lead to both infertility and ectopic (tubal) pregnancy.
- STIs in women also may be associated with cervical cancer.
- STIs can be passed from a mother to her baby before or during birth. Some infections of the newborn may be successfully treated, but others may cause a baby to be permanently disabled or even die.
- When diagnosed early, many STIs can be successfully treated.
- Girls are not protected from STIs when they use most forms of contraceptives. Barrier methods, especially the male condom, provide the most protection.

Treatment

Treatment for STIs should begin as soon as possible. In addition, the adolescent's sexual partner(s) should be notified so that person(s) may seek treatment. Urge teens to abstain from sexual activity during treatment and make sure they are tested again at a follow-up checkup.

TESTICULAR CANCER

Testicular cancer is the most common cancer of men between 15 and 35 years of age. Fortunately, testicular cancer has a greater than 90% cure rate. Most men with testicular cancer have no risk factors. Therefore, beginning at age 15, all men should perform testicular self-exam (see Box 40-8 and Figure 40-19).

Testicular cancer grows within the testicle, eventually replacing all normal tissue. Normal tissue will feel soft, whereas the tumor will be a hard painless mass. Most commonly, only one testicle is affected. Testicular cancer spreads rapidly through the lymph vessels into the retroperitoneal lymph nodes (located behind the peritoneum but outside the abdominal/pelvic cavity). Enlarged lymph nodes may be palpated in the groin. If the cancer cells reach the vascular system, they commonly metastasize to the lungs, liver, and bone.

Treatment usually involves a radical **orchiectomy** (removal of one testis and spermatic cord) with removal of the retroperitoneal lymph nodes. The surgery is accomplished through an inguinal incision, taking care not to damage the nerves needed for ejaculation. Following surgery, radiation and chemotherapy are used to destroy any remaining cancer cells. If only one testicle is removed, reproduction may still be possible. However, the banking of sperm prior to surgery, radiation, and chemotherapy should be discussed with the client and his partner. If the client is a minor, teaching and support must also be provided to the parents.

TESTICULAR TORSION

Testicular torsion (Figure 62-8) is an emergency condition in which the testis suddenly rotates on its spermatic cord, cutting off its blood supply. The highest incidence of testicular torsion occurs during puberty.

Manifestations

Manifestations include severe pain in the scrotum, nausea and vomiting, abdominal pain, and scrotal swelling that is not relieved by rest or scrotal support. The testis is positioned higher in the scrotum than the unaffected testis.

Diagnosis and Treatment

Torsion must be reduced within 4 to 6 hours to save the testis. Manual reduction with an analgesic is sometimes attempted, but emergency surgery is more common. During surgery (**orchiopexy**) the testis is untwisted and stitched to the side of the scrotum in the correct position.

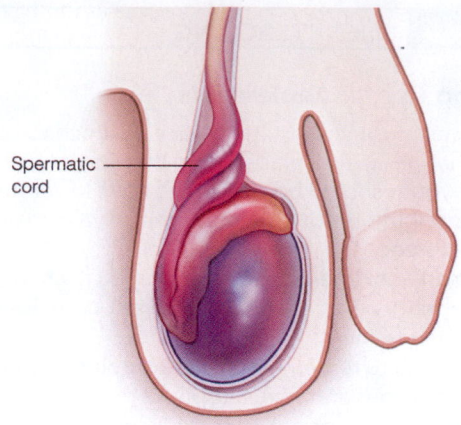

Spermatic cord

Figure 62-8. ■ Testicular torsion occurs most frequently in adolescents. It requires immediate surgical intervention.

Nursing Considerations

Nursing care includes psychologic support for the adolescent and family. The adolescent often goes home within a few hours. Therefore the adolescent and parents will need to be taught home care. Explain that the adolescent should not lift heavy objects for 4 weeks or participate in strenuous activity for 2 weeks after surgery to promote healing. Teach the adolescent testicular self-examination.

Integumentary Disorders

ACNE

Acne (Figure 62-9 ■) is a disorder of the hair follicles and sebaceous glands. With acne, the sebaceous glands are clogged, which leads to pimples and cysts.

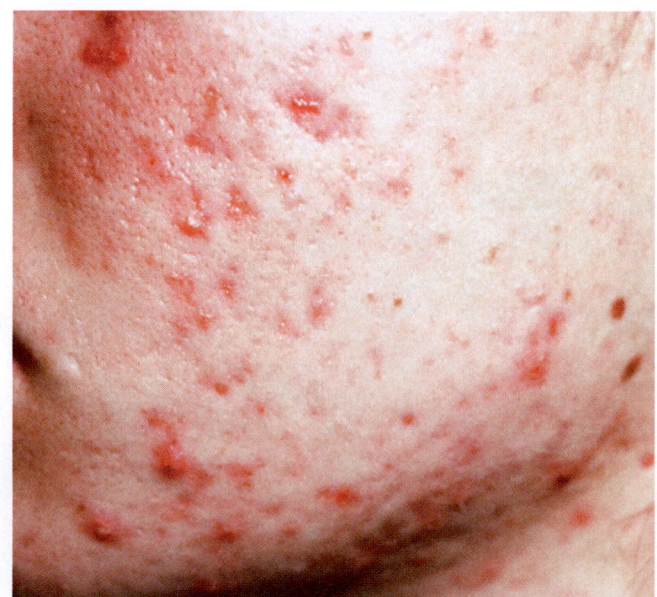

Figure 62-9. ■ Acne lesion. Acne is a common complaint of teenage clients. (Medical-On-Line Ltd.)

Acne is very common and most often begins in puberty. During puberty, the male sex hormones (androgens) increase in both boys and girls, which causes the sebaceous glands to become more active, resulting in increased production of sebum.

The sebaceous glands produce oil (sebum), which normally travels via hair follicles to the skin surface. However, skin cells can plug the follicles, blocking the oil coming from the sebaceous glands. When follicles become plugged, skin bacteria (called *Propionibacterium acnes,* or *P. acnes*) begin to grow inside the follicles, causing inflammation. Acne progresses in the following manner:

1. Incomplete blockage of the hair follicle results in blackheads (a semisolid, black plug).
2. Complete blockage of the hair follicle results in whiteheads (a semisolid, white plug).
3. Infection and irritation cause whiteheads to form.

Eventually, the plugged follicle bursts, spilling oil, skin cells, and the bacteria onto the skin surface. In turn, the skin becomes irritated and pimples or lesions begin to develop. The basic acne lesion is called a **comedo.**

Causes of Acne

Rising hormone levels during puberty may cause acne. In addition, acne is often inherited. Other causes of acne may include the following:

- Hormone level changes during the menstrual cycle in women
- Certain drugs (such as corticosteroids, lithium, and barbiturates)
- Oil and grease from the scalp, mineral or cooking oil, and certain cosmetics may worsen acne
- Bacteria inside pimples

Acne can be aggravated by squeezing the pimples or by scrubbing the skin too hard.

Manifestations

Acne can be *superficial* (pimples without abscesses) or *deep* (when the inflamed pimples push down into the skin, causing pus-filled cysts that rupture and result in larger abscesses).

Acne can occur anywhere on the body. However, acne most often appears in areas where there is a high concentration of sebaceous glands, such as the face, chest, upper back, shoulders, and neck.

The symptoms of acne may resemble other skin conditions. The primary healthcare provider should be consulted for a diagnosis.

Treatment

The goal of acne treatment is to minimize scarring and improve appearance. Specific treatment will be determined by the adolescent's physician based on:

- The severity of the acne.
- Adolescent's age, overall health, and medical history.
- Adolescent's tolerance for specific medications, procedures, or therapies.
- Expectations for the course of the condition.
- Opinion or preference.

Prescription topical medications are often prescribed to treat acne. Topical medication can be in the form of a cream, gel, lotion, or solution. Systemic antibiotics are often prescribed to treat moderate to severe acne. Doxycycline, erythromycin, and tetracycline are commonly prescribed for the treatment of acne. Systemic drugs may need to be taken for a prolonged period of time to achieve their desired effect. (See discussion of acne in Chapter 30 ∞.)

Isotretinoin (Accutane), an oral drug, may be prescribed for adolescents with severe, cystic, or inflammatory acne to prevent extensive scarring. However, the drug has major unwanted side effects, including psychiatric side effects. It is very important to explain the risk to the teen and the parent before beginning the medication.

EFFECTS OF SUNBATHING

Sunbathing is very popular with teens. Many do not understand the potential danger of sun exposure. They should be taught that sun damage can result in skin cancer and premature aging in their adult years. Tanning booths and salons have become an alternative to sunbathing or even a way to prepare for the first beach day of the season. Current research supports the fact that tanning booths can be as dangerous as actual sunbathing, and their use should be discouraged for teens.

Psychosocial Disorders

ALCOHOL AND DRUG USE

Teenagers' involvement with alcohol and legal or illegal drugs presents an additional safety hazard. Experimentation with alcohol and drugs during adolescence is common. Unfortunately, teenagers often do not see the link between their actions today and the consequences tomorrow. They also have a tendency to feel indestructible and immune to the problems that others experience. Using alcohol and tobacco at a young age increases the risk of using other drugs later. Some teens will experiment and stop, or continue to use occasionally, without significant problems. Others will develop a dependency, moving on to more dangerous drugs and causing significant harm to themselves and possibly others.

Adolescence is a time for trying new things. Teens use alcohol and other drugs for many reasons, including curiosity, because it feels good, to reduce stress, to feel grown up, or to fit in. It is difficult to know which teens will experiment and stop and which will develop serious problems.

Teenagers at risk for developing serious alcohol and drug problems include:

- Teenagers with a family history of substance abuse
- Teenagers who are depressed
- Teenagers who have low self-esteem
- Teenagers who feel like they do not fit in with their peers

Teenagers abuse a variety of drugs, both legal and illegal. Legally available drugs include alcohol, prescribed medications, inhalants (fumes from glues, aerosols, and solvents) and over-the-counter cough, cold, sleep, and diet medications. The most commonly used illegal drugs are marijuana (pot), stimulants (cocaine, crack, and speed), LSD, PCP, opiates, heroin, and designer drugs (Ecstasy). The use of illegal drugs is increasing, especially among young teens. The average age of first marijuana use is 14, and alcohol use can start before age 12. The use of marijuana and alcohol in high school has become common.

Drug use is associated with a variety of negative consequences, including increased risk of serious drug use later in life, school failure, and poor judgment. Drug use may put teens at risk for accidents, violence, unplanned and unsafe sex, and suicide. Table 62-8 ■ lists warning signs of substance abuse with adolescents. Parents can help through early education about drugs, open communication, good role modeling, and early recognition if problems are developing.

Some of the warning signs can also be signs of other problems. Parents may recognize signs of trouble but should not be expected to make the diagnosis. An effective way for parents to show care and concern is to openly discuss the use and possible abuse of alcohol and other drugs with their teenager. Medical care should be sought early if a parent is concerned.

DEPRESSION AND SUICIDE

Suicides among young people nationwide have increased dramatically in recent years. Each year in the United States, thousands of teenagers commit suicide. Suicide is the third leading cause of death for 15- to 24-year-olds, and the sixth leading cause of death for 5- to 14-year-olds.

Teenagers experience strong feelings of stress, confusion, self-doubt, pressure to succeed, anxiety about money, and

---

BOX 62-11 MANIFESTATIONS OF SUICIDAL FEELING

- Change in eating and sleeping habits
- Withdrawal from friends, family, and regular activities
- Violent actions, rebellious behavior, or running away
- Drug and alcohol use
- Unusual neglect of personal appearance
- Marked personality change
- Persistent boredom, difficulty concentrating, or a decline in the quality of schoolwork
- Frequent complaints about physical symptoms, often related to emotions, such as stomachaches, headaches, and fatigue
- Loss of interest in pleasurable activities
- Not tolerating praise or rewards

A teenager who is planning to commit suicide may also:

- Complain of being a bad person or feeling "rotten inside."
- Give verbal hints with statements such as "I won't be a problem for you much longer," "Nothing matters," "It's no use," and "I won't see you again."
- Put his or her affairs in order, for example, give away favorite possessions, clean his or her room, or throw away important belongings.
- Become suddenly cheerful after a period of depression.
- Have signs of psychosis (hallucinations or bizarre thoughts).

---

other fears while growing up. For some teenagers, divorce, the formation of a new family with stepparents and stepsiblings, or moving to a new community can be very unsettling and can intensify self-doubts. In some cases, suicide appears to be a "solution."

Depression and suicidal feelings are treatable mental disorders. The child or adolescent needs to have his or her illness recognized and diagnosed, and appropriate treatment plans developed. When parents are in doubt about whether their child has a serious problem, a psychiatric examination can be very helpful. Box 62-11 ■ describes possible symptoms of suicidal feelings. (Suicide is also discussed in Chapter 49 ◉ .)

If a child or adolescent says, "I want to kill myself" or "I'm going to commit suicide," always take the statement seriously and seek evaluation from a child and adolescent psychiatrist or other physician. People often feel uncomfortable talking

---

TABLE 62-8	Warning Signs of Teenage Alcohol and Drug Abuse
TYPE OF SIGN	**MANIFESTATIONS**
Physical	Fatigue, repeated health complaints, red and glazed eyes, and a lasting cough
Emotional	Personality change, sudden mood changes, irritability, irresponsible behavior, low self-esteem, poor judgment, depression, and a general lack of interest
Family	Starting arguments, breaking rules, or withdrawing from the family
School	Decreased interest, negative attitude, drop in grades, many absences, truancy, and discipline problems
Social problems	New friends who are less interested in standard home and school activities, problems with the law, and changes to less conventional styles of dress and music

about death. However, asking the child or adolescent whether he or she is depressed or thinking about suicide can be helpful. Rather than "putting thoughts in the child's head," such a question will provide assurance that somebody cares and will give the young person the chance to talk about problems.

If one or more of these signs occur, parents need to talk to their child about their concerns and seek professional help when the concerns persist. With support from family and professional treatment, children and teenagers who are suicidal can heal and return to a healthy path of development.

SELF-INJURY IN ADOLESCENTS

Self-injury is the act of deliberately destroying body tissue, at times to change a way of feeling. The incidence of this problem has increased dramatically within the last few years, especially in adolescents. Self-injury is seen differently by groups and cultures within society. The causes and severity of self-injury can vary. Some forms may include:

- Carving
- Scratching
- Branding
- Marking
- Picking, and pulling skin and hair
- Burning/abrasions
- Cutting, biting
- Head banging
- Bruising
- Hitting
- Tattooing
- Excessive body piercing

Some adolescents may self-mutilate to take risks, rebel, reject their parents' values, state their individuality, or merely be accepted. Others, however, may injure themselves out of desperation or anger to seek attention, to show their hopelessness and worthlessness, or because they have suicidal thoughts. These children may suffer from serious psychiatric problems such as depression, *psychosis* (detachment from reality), *posttraumatic stress disorder* (PTSD; a prolonged or recurrent reaction to a traumatic event) or bipolar disorder (see Chapter 49 ⚭). Additionally, some adolescents who engage in self-injury may develop *borderline personality disorder* (a pervasive pattern of unpredictable and impulsive behavior) as adults. Some young children may resort to self-injury from time to time but then grow out of it. Children with mental retardation and/or autism may also show these behaviors, which may persist into adulthood. Children who have been abused or abandoned may self-mutilate.

Reasons for Self-Injury

Adolescents who have difficulty talking about their feelings may exhibit their emotional tension, physical discomfort, pain, and low self-esteem with self-injurious behaviors.

Some teens say they feel release from tension after hurting themselves, but others may instead feel hurt, anger, fear, and hate. The effects of peer pressure can also influence adolescents to injure themselves, and they may experiment with self-injury as part of a fad. Even if they self-injure as part of a fad, the wounds on the skin will be permanent. Occasionally, teenagers may hide their scars, burns, and bruises because they feel embarrassed, rejected, or criticized about them.

Preventing Self-Injury

Parents are encouraged to talk with their children about respecting and valuing their bodies. Parents should also serve as role models for their teenagers by not engaging in acts of self-harm. Some helpful ways for adolescents to avoid hurting themselves include learning to:

- Accept reality and find ways to make the present moment more tolerable.
- Identify feelings and talk them out rather than acting on them.
- Distract themselves from feelings of self-harm (for example, counting to 10, waiting 15 minutes, saying "no!" or "stop!," practicing breathing exercises, journaling, drawing, thinking about positive images, or using ice and rubber bands).
- Stop, think, and evaluate the pros and cons of self-injury.
- Find ways to relax that are positive and noninjurious.
- Practice positive stress management.
- Develop better social skills.

Evaluation by a mental health professional may assist in identifying and treating the underlying causes of self-injury. Feelings of wanting to die or kill themselves are reasons for adolescents to seek professional care emergently. A child and adolescent psychiatrist can also diagnose and treat the serious psychiatric disorders that may accompany self-injurious behavior.

EATING DISORDERS

In a culture where thinness is too often equated with physical attractiveness, success, and happiness, nearly everyone has dealt with issues regarding the effect their weight and body shape can have on their self-image. However, eating disorders are not about dieting or vanity; they are complex psychologic disorders in which an individual's eating patterns are developed—and then habitually maintained—in an attempt to cope with other problems in his or her life.

Each year, more than 5 million Americans are affected by serious and often life-threatening eating disorders such as anorexia nervosa, binge eating, bulimia nervosa, compulsive eating, obesity, and *pica* (consumption of clay, starch, dried paint, or other nonnutritious substances).

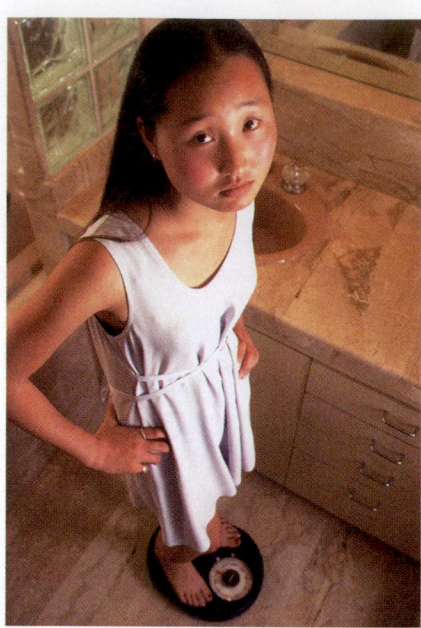

Figure 62-10. ■ Anorexia nervosa has its roots in emotional concerns or disturbances, though its physical effects can be life threatening. (PhotoEdit Inc.)

Manifestations of Anorexia and Bulimia

A teenager with anorexia nervosa is typically a perfectionist and a high achiever in school (Figure 62-10 ■). At the same time, she suffers from low self-esteem, irrationally believing she is fat regardless of how thin she becomes. Desperately needing a feeling of mastery over her life, the teenager with anorexia nervosa experiences a sense of control only when she says "no" to the normal food demands of her body. In a relentless pursuit to be thin, the girl starves herself. This often reaches the point of serious damage to the body, and in a small number of cases may lead to death.

The symptoms of bulimia are usually different from those of anorexia nervosa. The client binges on huge quantities of high-caloric food and/or purges her body of dreaded calories by self-induced vomiting and often by using laxatives. These binges may alternate with severe diets, resulting in dramatic weight fluctuations. Teenagers may try to hide the signs of throwing up by running water while spending long periods of time in the bathroom. The purging of bulimia presents a serious threat to the client's physical health, including dehydration, hormonal imbalance, the depletion of important minerals, and damage to vital organs.

Treatment

Both physiologic support and counseling are necessary for clients with eating disorders. Left untreated, the emotional, psychologic, and physical consequences can be devastating, even fatal. Eating disorders know no class, cultural, or gender boundaries and can affect men, women, adolescents, and even children from all walks of life. (Eating disorders are discussed in depth in Chapter 50 ⊙⊙.)

TEENAGERS AND STRESS

Teenagers, like adults, may experience stress every day and can benefit from learning stress management skills. Most teens experience more stress when they perceive a situation as dangerous, difficult, or painful and they do not have the resources to cope. Some sources of stress for teens might include:

■ School demands and frustrations
■ Negative thoughts and feelings about themselves
■ Changes in their bodies
■ Problems with friends and/or peers at school
■ Unsafe living environment/neighborhood
■ Separation or divorce of parents
■ Chronic illness or severe problems in the family
■ Death of a loved one
■ Moving or changing schools
■ Taking on too many activities or having too high expectations
■ Family financial problems

Some teens become overloaded with stress. When this happens, inadequately managed stress can lead to anxiety, withdrawal, aggression, physical illness, or poor coping skills such as drug and/or alcohol use.

When we perceive a situation as difficult or painful, changes occur in our minds and bodies to prepare us to respond to danger. This "fight, flight, or freeze" response includes faster heart and breathing rate, increased blood to muscles of arms and legs, cold or clammy hands and feet, upset stomach, and/or a sense of dread. (See more about stress in Chapter 17 ⊙⊙.)

The same mechanism that turns on the stress response can turn it off. As soon as we decide that a situation is no longer dangerous, changes can occur in our minds and bodies to help us relax and calm down. This "relaxation response" includes decreased heart and breathing rate and a sense of well-being. Teens who develop a relaxation response and other stress management skills feel less helpless and have more choices when responding to stress.

Parents can help their teen in these ways:

■ Monitor if stress is affecting their teen's health, behavior, thoughts, or feelings.
■ Listen carefully to teens and watch for overloading.
■ Learn and model stress management skills.
■ Support involvement in sports and other social activities.

Teens can decrease stress with the following behaviors and techniques:

■ Exercise and eat regularly.
■ Avoid excess caffeine intake, which can increase feelings of anxiety and agitation.
■ Avoid illegal drugs, alcohol, and tobacco.

- Learn relaxation exercises (abdominal breathing and muscle relaxation techniques).
- Develop assertiveness training skills. For example, state feelings in polite but firm and not overly aggressive or passive ways ("I feel angry when you yell at me" or "Please stop yelling").
- Rehearse and practice situations that cause stress. One example is taking a speech class if talking in front of a class makes you anxious.
- Learn practical coping skills. For example, break a large task into smaller, more attainable tasks.
- Decrease negative self-talk. Challenge negative thoughts about yourself with alternative neutral or positive thoughts. "My life will never get better" can be transformed into "I may feel hopeless now, but my life will probably get better if I work at it and get some help."
- Learn to feel good about doing a competent or "good enough" job rather than demanding perfection from yourself and others.
- Take a break from stressful situations. Activities such as listening to music, talking to a friend, drawing, writing, or spending time with a pet can reduce stress.
- Build a network of friends who help you cope in a positive way.

By using these and other techniques, teenagers can begin to manage stress. If a teen talks about or shows signs of being overly stressed, a consultation with a child and adolescent psychiatrist or qualified mental health professional may be helpful.

NURSING CARE

PRIORITIZING NURSING CARE

When caring for adolescents, focus your care not only on their medical and physical needs, but also on establishing trust and providing emotional support. Take time to talk with the adolescent as a person. Establish rapport by asking about interests, school activities, and friends. Be matter of fact when speaking about lifestyle choices and their consequences. Avoid displaying shock or judgmental attitudes that can prevent adolescents from discussing their concerns with you.

ASSESSING

Data for assessment should always take into consideration the normal growth and development level of the client. Normal assessment data for an adolescent would include presence and frequency of menstrual cycles for girls, and expected physical changes by age for boys (such as presence and amount of body hair, voice changes).

DIAGNOSING, PLANNING, AND IMPLEMENTING

Nursing diagnoses for adolescent clients might include:

- *Deficient Knowledge*
- *Impaired Social Interaction*
- *Ineffective Coping*
- *Interrupted Family Processes*
- *Risk for Injury*
- *Risk for Situational Low Self-Esteem*
- *Imbalanced Nutrition*

Some outcomes for adolescent clients might include:

- Client verbalizes understanding of normal development.
- Client asks for information about own health care.
- Client expresses knowledge of consequences of risk-taking behavior.
- Client verbalizes feelings of isolation from peer group.

Planning at all levels of nursing care should incorporate an understanding of the particular issues that might affect the client's progress toward wellness.

- Be aware of the adolescent's developmental level, especially when implementing nursing care. *The nurse must take into account more than just chronological age and physical maturity. Emotional issues are very important in this age group, and trust is crucial to the nurse's ability to gain data.*
- Ask if the adolescent wants privacy. *The adolescent may be more comfortable if the parent leaves the room during the physical examination; this is particularly true with male adolescents whose mother has accompanied them to the physician's office or the hospital. Sensitivity to developmental issues is a great asset in listening and in providing teaching.*
- Document any scars, cuts, or other indications of self-injury. If client appears depressed, ask if he or she has ever had thoughts about self-harm. *Asking about thoughts of suicide does not increase the chance that a person will commit suicide. In fact, the opposite is the case. Having a chance to verbalize suicidal thinking may allow the client to ask for help.*
- Ask about teenager's typical eating habits. *This may help identify eating disorders or lack of understanding about proper nutrition. It may highlight the need for client teaching.*
- Be straightforward in asking about sexual concerns or activity. *If the nurse is matter of fact, it will be easier for the adolescent to respond.*
- Address questions to the adolescent, not the parent. *This shows respect for the adolescent and is the main source of information.*
- Ask if adolescents or parents have any other questions. *This may provide an opening for a concern that has not been raised.*
- Provide information about groups or resources that are available in the community. *Written materials and contact information allow the teen and the parent to pursue more information independently.*

EVALUATING

The nurse collects data to determine whether outcomes have been met. If goals have not been achieved, the nurse can consider the need to adapt interventions to address developmental needs more closely.

NURSING PROCESS CARE PLAN
Client with Self-Injury Behaviors

Emily Bauer, a 15-year-old female, is brought to the ER by her aunt for treatment of several self-inflicted cuts on her arms. Emily's parents are divorced, and she lives with her father, who travels frequently for his job. When he is out of town she stays with her aunt.

Assessment

Female client; 5'1"; weight 102 lbs. Responds only to direct questions. Will not make eye contact with nurse or aunt. Several fresh cuts on her forearms, visible scars on various parts of body. Aunt states, "I came home from work and found Emily sitting on the couch cutting herself with my sewing scissors."

Nursing Diagnosis

The following important nursing diagnoses (among others) are established for this condition:

- *Self-Mutilation* related to inability to cope with increased psychologic tension
- *Interrupted Family Processes* related to situational crises secondary to changes in parental marital status
- *Ineffective Coping* related to maturational crisis

Expected Outcomes

The expected outcomes for the plan of care related to Emily might include the following:

- States appropriate ways to cope with increased psychologic tension.
- Identifies ways to cope and use appropriate family support systems.
- Acknowledges and accepts the need for assistance with circumstances.

Planning and Implementation

The following interventions are planned and implemented for Emily:

- Assess the strengths and deficiencies of the family system. *Identifying family strengths and deficiencies is necessary to determine the cause of Emily's self-injury behavior.*
- Have family members participate in client conferences that involve all members of the health care team. *Having family members participate in client conferences with members of the healthcare team encourages consistency in implementing the plan of care.*

- Observe for causes of ineffective coping such as poor self-concept, lack of problem-solving skills, or recent changes in life situation. *Identifying the causes of ineffective coping is necessary in order to change the behavior.*
- Encourage moderate aerobic exercise. *Aerobic exercise is an effective outlet for stress.*
- Discuss client's/family's need to accept the situation. *Accepting situations that cannot change allows for problem solving of those things that can change.*
- Refer for counseling. *Counseling is needed to help Emily cope with her family situation and work on positive outlets for stress.*
- Secure a written or verbal contract from client to notify staff when experiencing the desire to self-mutilate. *Written and verbal contracts help clients take responsibility for their behavior.*
- Give praise when client identifies urges and delays self-destructive behavior. *Praise fosters a positive self-concept.*
- Concentrate on client's strengths. Have client visualize the word "Stop!" when negative self-talk begins, then replace the negativity with an affirmative or positive statement. *Replacing negative thoughts with positive statements improves self-concept and decreases the desire to self-mutilate.*

Evaluation

Emily relates at her follow-up visit that she has been attending counseling appointments alone and with her father and aunt. Her mother has been unable to attend since she lives out of town. Emily states, "My mother is too busy with her new life to deal with me." Emily is journaling her negative feelings and has had two incidents of urges to hurt herself during the last week. She was able to stop herself and asked her aunt for help. Emily and her aunt are taking a walk after dinner each night and Emily is exercising for 20 minutes every day. Emily states, "I need to find new ways to deal with my stress. Injuring myself is not a good method."

Critical Thinking in the Nursing Process

1. It is extremely important for Emily to learn new ways to deal with her stress. As her nurse, how could you assist her in doing this?
2. Emily's relationship with her mother is strained at best; she is in need of a support system in order to recover. She asks you to call her mother and ask her to come to Emily's next appointment. What would be your response to Emily?
3. Emily is using aerobic exercise to relieve stress. What other suggestions can you make to assist her?

Note: Discussion of Critical Thinking questions appears on the MyNursingKit Website.

Note: The references and resources for all chapters have been compiled at the back of the book.

Chapter Review

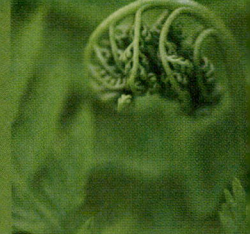

KEY Points

- Adolescence is the period of growth and development that begins with the appearance of secondary sex characteristics and ends with the cessation of physical growth and emotional maturity.

- Adolescence is characterized by dramatic physical changes that move the individual from childhood into physical maturity.

- Menarche (the beginning of menstrual periods) typically occurs about 2 years after initial pubescent changes are noted.

- Puberty is not marked by a sudden incident in males.

- Because physical changes may not occur in synchrony, adolescents may go through stages of awkwardness, both in terms of appearance and physical mobility/coordination.

- During adolescence, it is appropriate for youngsters to have and demonstrate a need to separate from their parents and establish their own identity.

- Concerns about confidentiality may discourage adolescents from seeking necessary medical care and counseling, and may create barriers to open communication between client and physician.

- Eating healthy is an important part of a healthy lifestyle and is something that should be taught at a young age.

- Teens who refuse to eat animal protein may not understand the need to vary grain products in order to ensure that their diet includes essential amino acids, which are the building blocks for the body.

- Healthcare professionals should stress abstinence, which, when practiced consistently, is the most effective method of preventing unplanned pregnancy and the transmission of sexually transmitted infections.

- During the adolescent years the teen will be due for boosters of immunizations such as a Td (tetanus and diphtheria) and a second MMR (measles, mumps, rubella).

- Accidents and injury continue to be the major cause of death during this time period.

- Inexperienced drivers often concentrate on driving correctly and fail to anticipate the actions and mistakes or errors of other drivers.

- Self-injury is the act of deliberately destroying body tissue, at times to change a way of feeling.

- Teenagers, like adults, may experience stress every day and can benefit from learning stress management skills.

- The surest way to prevent contracting an STI is for adolescents to abstain from any type of sexual activity.

- Eating disorders are not about dieting or vanity; they are complex psychological disorders.

- There are few physical disorders specific to adolescents.

- The manifestations, treatment, and nursing care of physical disorders will be similar to those of adults.

- Teaching must involve the adolescent and parents.

FOR FURTHER Study

Refer to Chapter 15 for Erikson's developmental stages.

See Chapter 16 for further discussion of growth and development.

Stress is discussed further in Chapter 17.

See Chapter 25 for an in-depth discussion of nutrition.

Acne and other skin disorders are discussed in Chapter 30.

Musculoskeletal disorders are covered in depth in Chapter 31.

The main discussion of all nervous system disorders is in Chapter 36.

Gastrointestinal disorders, such as Crohn's disease and ulcerative colitis, are discussed in depth in Chapter 37.

The endocrine system is discussed in Chapter 38.

For disorders of the reproductive system and discussion of contraception, see Chapter 40.

For a complete discussion of sexually transmitted infections, see Chapter 41.

For further discussion about suicide and bipolar disorder, see Chapter 49.

The main discussion of eating disorders is in Chapter 50.

Meningitis is seen in infants (Chapter 59) as well as in teens.

See Figure 60-2 for the childhood immunization schedule.

Diabetes is discussed in Chapter 61 in children and in the medical-surgical unit in Chapter 38.

Critical Thinking Care Map

Caring for a Client with Type 1 Diabetes Mellitus
NCLEX-PN® Focus Area: Physiologic Integrity

Case Study: Grey Wolf, a 15-year-old Native American boy, is admitted to the tribal clinic with a blood glucose of 48 mm/dL. He was diagnosed with Type 1 diabetes mellitus 3 months ago. He has been having difficulty remembering to eat a snack before soccer practice.

Nursing Diagnosis: *Risk for Injury* related to hypoglycemia

COLLECT DATA

Subjective	Objective
_____	_____
_____	_____
_____	_____
_____	_____
_____	_____
_____	_____
_____	_____

Would you report this? Yes/No

If yes, report to: _____

What would you report? _____

Nursing Care

_____
_____
_____
_____
_____
_____
_____
_____
_____

How would you document this? _____
_____
_____
_____

Compare your answers and documentation to those provided on the MyNursingKit Website.

Data Collected
(use only those that apply)

- Irritable
- Thirsty
- Hungry
- Sweating
- Flushed
- Fruity/acetone breath
- Tremors
- P 102
- R 38
- Blood glucose 48mm/dL

Nursing Interventions
(use only those that apply; list in priority order)

- Obtain a thorough nutrition history.
- Administer regular insulin as ordered.
- Give orange juice with one packet sugar added.
- Start an IV of normal saline as ordered or as per facility policy.
- Give one ampule of sodium bicarbonate as ordered.
- Monitor blood glucose every 30 to 60 minutes.
- Review causes and signs of hypoglycemia.
- Review insulin administration techniques.

NCLEX-PN® Exam Preparation

TEST-TAKING TIP If the age of the client in the question is stated, be sure to answer the question in light of development not just chronological age.

1. A 15-year-old male is hospitalized for an open reduction and internal fixation (ORIF) of his right femur, following an accident while riding his skateboard. The nurse would consider which of the following helpful in supporting normal growth and development during his hospitalization?
   1. Allow family to bring his favorite computer games.
   2. Encourage him to keep up with schoolwork.
   3. Allow him to go to the dayroom and participate in activities with other adolescent clients.
   4. Encourage parents to room-in.

2. John, a 17-year-old male, is small for his age and is several inches shorter than his male classmates. He tells the school nurse, "I just hate school—everyone stares at me and calls me 'Little Buddy.'" The nurse's best response would be:
   1. "Don't pay any attention to them. Your height is not as important as your character. You'll outgrow your embarrassment."
   2. "Don't worry, boys can be cruel at your age when confronted with someone who is different."
   3. "They are probably teasing you because they like you. I bet you have lots of dates because the girls probably think you're terrific."
   4. "It is not unusual for boys your age to be embarrassed by their height. Did you know that boys often continue to grow into their early 20s?"

3. The nurse explains to the parents of a teenager that sexual identity is often established by:
   1. Friendships with members of the opposite sex, dating, and experimentation.
   2. Providing sex education as part of the high school curriculum.
   3. Discussion of sexual feelings with a trusted adult.
   4. Idolization of role models.

4. The nurse anticipates administration of which of the following immunization boosters for the adolescent client?
   1. Hepatitis A
   2. Td (tetanus and diphtheria)
   3. DPT (diphtheria, pertussis, tetanus)
   4. Hepatitis B

5. While assisting with an annual examination, the nurse learns that the adolescent client has decided to forgo eating meat and is following a vegetarian diet. The nurse's best response is:
   1. "Vegetarian diets are very unhealthy during adolescence and your growing body needs meat."
   2. "Good for you. You will reduce the risk of heart attack and stroke by following a no-meat diet."
   3. "How do you fulfill your body's need for proteins on your new diet?"
   4. "To meet your body's needs for amino acids it is important for you to obtain protein through alternate sources."

6. The nurse is teaching the adolescent client about the newly prescribed isotretinoin (Accutane) to treat acne and explains

   that which of the following can be a major unwanted side effect that should be reported to the physician?
   1. Weight gain
   2. Psychiatric side effects
   3. Erythema and urticaria
   4. Nausea and vomiting

7. The nurse has learned that the adolescent girl is sexually active. Which of the following statements indicates a need for more teaching?
   1. "I take birth control pills and I always make sure they use condoms."
   2. "I'm not worried about STIs or pregnancy because I'm using birth control pills."
   3. "My mom gave me female condoms and cream when we first talked about sex."
   4. "My boyfriends use condoms and I get shots to avoid pregnancy."

8. The nurse, working in a health clinic, receives a phone call from a worried parent who is concerned that her 17-year-old may be using drugs. The parent asks if she can bring the teen in for drug testing. The nurse's best response is:
   1. "Drug testing can only be performed with the teen's permission. He is protected by confidentiality laws that dictate I can only share results with you if he gives me permission to do so."
   2. "Sure, bring him in and we can test him using blood, urine, or saliva tests to determine what drugs he may be using. Once we know, we can develop a treatment plan with both of you."
   3. "No, we can only perform drug testing if the teen asks for it, but then we'll share the results."
   4. "Drug testing is highly inaccurate and yields many false negatives, so it might not be of any use for you."

9. The nurse admits a 15-year-old male with nontender, firm, enlarged cervical lymph nodes reporting fever, night sweats, and weight loss. The nurse anticipates a diagnosis of:
   1. Hodgkin's lymphoma.
   2. Tuberculosis.
   3. Strep throat.
   4. Mononucleosis.

10. While caring for a client diagnosed with inflammatory bowel disease, the client asks the nurse, "What is the difference between Crohn's disease and ulcerative colitis?" The nurse's best response is to explain that:
    1. Crohn's disease is less serious than ulcerative colitis.
    2. Ulcerative colitis creates totally different symptoms and is treated more rigorously.
    3. Crohn's disease randomly involves the entire gastrointestinal tract whereas ulcerative colitis involves only the large intestine.
    4. Ulcerative colitis is genetic, but Crohn's disease is not.

Answers and rationales for Review Questions appear in Appendix I.

Thinking Strategically About...

You are employed by a pediatrician. There are three examination rooms, a medication preparation room, and a small area where some laboratory procedures are done. Your responsibilities include obtaining client health histories, taking vital signs, weighing and measuring clients, screening vision and hearing, obtaining lab specimens, administering medications, assisting in procedures, and providing client teaching and discharge instructions. Today, there are 18 children scheduled to see the doctor.

The first client of the day is 12-year-old Jeremy. He weighs 120 lb and is 5 ft tall. His vital signs are T 98.6, P 62, R 16, BP 106/76. Jeremy's mother states that he is frequently fatigued. He is thirsty all the time, even during the night. He is also urinating many times a day and is always hungry. A review of the family history reveals that Jeremy's father has Type 1 diabetes mellitus. After conferring with the physician, you obtain a urine specimen and a blood specimen. A reagent strip, used to test the urine for glucose, is positive. Blood glucose reveals 210 mg/dL.

The second client is 4-year-old Jackson. For the past 48 hours Jackson has been vomiting and having diarrhea. He has been unable to keep any food or beverage down. Jackson is irritable and states, "I doesn't feel good." Jackson's vital signs are T 99.9, P 110, R 18, BP 90/60. His skin is hot and his mouth is dry. His weight is 45 lb. The doctor writes a prescription for Phenergan 12.5 mg rectal suppository every 4 hours for nausea. The doctor also advises a full liquid diet and for Jackson's mother to call the office late in the afternoon if Jackson is still unable to keep fluids down.

The third client is 16-month-old Janice who has wheezing with slightly labored breathing. She also has a diffused rash on her chest, which appears to be measles. The mother reports several children at the day care have been sick with respiratory syncytial virus (RSV) and one child had the measles 10 days ago. Janice cries easily but is comforted by her mother.

CRITICAL THINKING

- What further testing would you anticipate the pediatrician ordering for Jeremy to confirm the diagnosis of diabetes mellitus?

- When teaching Jackson's mother how to insert the Phenergan rectal suppository, what are the differences that must be stressed between administering rectal suppositories to an adult and a 4-year-old child?

- What testing would you anticipate the pediatrician ordering to determine the cause of Janice's respiratory distress?

PRIORITIZING NURSING CARE

- If all three clients arrive at the physician's office at the same time, in what order should they have data collected for assessment?

- What is the rationale for your prioritization of care?

MANAGEMENT OF CARE

- What cleaning must occur in Janice's exam room prior to the next client being seen in that room?

DELEGATING

- If a CNA is available to assist you, what assignments would you delegate?

- What follow-up would you need to provide for the care you delegated to the CNA?

CLIENT TEACHING

- What client teaching will be necessary to provide to Jeremy about further diagnostic tests?

- Besides administration of Phenergan rectal suppositories, what teaching should be given to Jackson's mother regarding fluid imbalance.

- What teaching should be provided Janice's mother about immunizations?

CULTURAL CARE STRATEGIES

- Janice's information reveals she is a Jehovah's Witness. How will this affect care management?

DOCUMENTING AND REPORTING

- When Jackson's mother calls in the afternoon, what information should the nurse obtain, document, and report to the pediatrician?

- How would Jeremy's assessment be charted?

Transition from Student to Nurse

UNIT XI

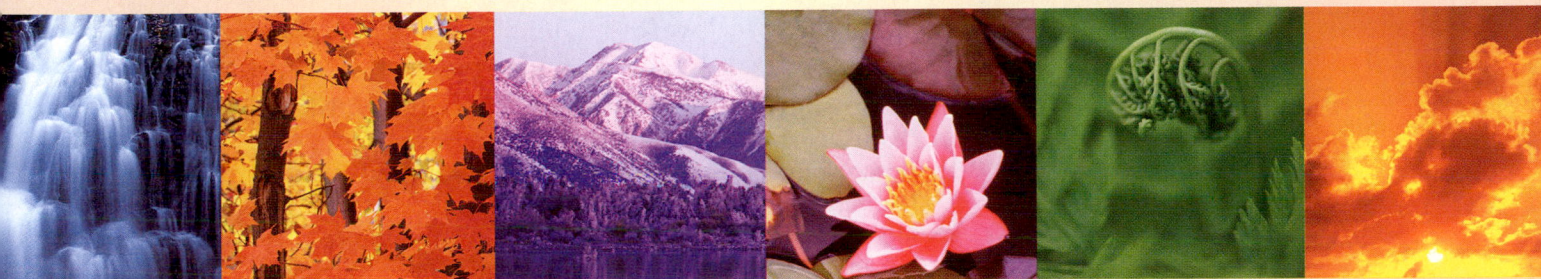

Leadership and Professional Development

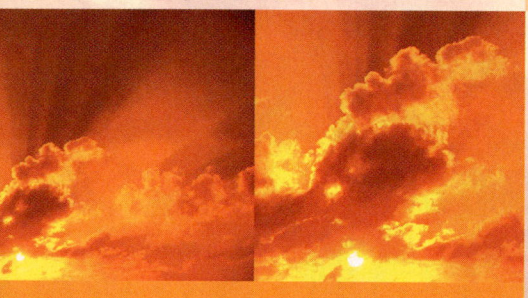

LEARNING Outcomes

After completing this chapter, you will be able to:

1. Discuss factors that govern licensure and standards of care.
2. Describe the purpose of and terminology used in nurse practice acts.
3. List important aspects of the LPN/LVN code of ethics.
4. Identify leadership styles and important attributes of effective leaders.
5. List and describe tasks involved in being a team leader.
6. Explain key concepts and expectations in delegating tasks.
7. Identify and contrast different reporting techniques.
8. Explain the SBAR technique for handoff procedures.
9. Identify types of paperwork that may be involved as team leader or nurse.
10. Name stages of conflict and conflict resolution strategies.
11. Describe the advantages of each method of nursing care delivery.
12. Identify Joint Commission safety goals for healthcare clients.

Clinical Objectives

13. Observe or assist the RN in the transcription of physician's orders.
14. Complete an incident report.
15. Prepare and deliver a shift report on assigned clients.
16. Under the direct supervision of the clinical instructor, receive and document a verbal or telephone order.
17. Assist in making client assignments.
18. Participate in a client care conference.

Use the audio glossary feature on the MyNusingKit Website to hear the correct pronunciation of the following key terms.

accommodation 1773	conflict 1771	leadership 1766
autocratic 1766	delegated medical act 1766	licensure 1765
avoidance 1773	delegated nursing act 1766	nurse practice acts 1766
basic client situation 1766	delegation 1768	primary nursing 1774
basic nursing care 1766	democratic 1767	shift report 1769
case method 1774	direct supervision 1766	standards 1766
collaboration 1773	functional nursing 1774	taped report 1769
competition 1773	general supervision 1766	team nursing 1774
complex nursing situation 1766	incident report 1771	
compromise 1773	laissez-faire 1767	

Passing the licensure exam and being granted a nursing license is an entrance to a new life and a new set of responsibilities. With the title of nurse comes an expectation that you will be a positive role model and a contributor to society. A person does not just automatically make the shift from private person to professional. The change is developed through schooling, but it is practiced and becomes real through everyday practice.

Licensure

A graduate of a practical/vocational nursing program cannot use the title of LPN/LVN until the licensing exam has been taken, passed, and the license issued. **Licensure** is a process by which a government agency gives permission for an individual to engage in an occupation or profession. It certifies that the individual has attained the minimum requirements necessary to protect the public safety and welfare. These requirements for a nursing license are outlined in the nurse practice act for each state.

The requirements for obtaining a license vary from state to state. In general, the applicant must (1) have completed a minimum of 2 years of high school or its equivalent (many states now require a high school diploma), (2) have completed an approved course in practical/vocational nursing, and (3) be a citizen of the United States or have a current visa. If these requirements have been met, the applicant will be eligible to take the examination. Following the exam the state board of nursing will review the application and issue the license.

All the work you have done up to this point has been in preparation for taking the licensing exam. The exam is designed to measure your knowledge in a number of areas. Passage of the exam certifies that you have enough knowledge to practice safely as an entry-level licensed practical/vocational nurse.

At one time each state had its own licensing exam; today there is a national exam developed by the National Council of State Boards of Nursing (NCSBN). The exam is the NCLEX-PN® (National Council Licensure Examination for Practical Nurses). The examination is a computer-adapted test (CAT) that is administered by testing agencies throughout the community. The agency provides the state board of nursing with the names of the individuals who have passed the examination. The board is responsible for issuing the license. The board may opt to not issue a license to persons convicted of certain crimes, a person who is mentally ill, or a person who is addicted to alcohol or other drugs. In Texas and California, the license is for vocational nursing; in all other states, such nurses are known as licensed practical nurses.

Licenses are issued for a specific period of time, which is determined by the board that issued the license. It is the responsibility of the licensee to keep his or her license current and to meet any continuing education requirements. It is a violation of the nurse practice act to function as an LPN/LVN without a current license. Discussion about law and ethics in relation to nursing practice is found in Chapter 4 ⭕.

SUSPENSION OR REVOCATION

The state board of nursing has a responsibility to protect the public. The board has the authority, under the state nurse practice act, to suspend or revoke a nursing license if the licensee is found guilty of an offense. Box 63-1 ■ lists examples of causes for license suspension or revocation.

When action is taken against a licensee, the nurse must be notified of the charges and given a hearing before the board. The individual, either in person or through an attorney, has the right to enter a defense.

The board, in addition to suspension and revocation, can, for just cause, place a licensee on probation, refuse to issue or renew a license, or issue a letter of reprimand.

Actions taken against a licensed nurse are a matter of public record. In many states the information can be obtained by any community member by telephone or from the board's website.

BOX 63-1	CAUSES OF LICENSE SUSPENSION OR REVOCATION

- Conviction of
  - Felony
  - Moral turpitude or gross immorality
- Guilty of
  - Fraud or deceit in obtaining a license
  - Willful neglect of a client
- Mental incompetence
- Chemical dependence or abuse including alcohol
- Suspended or revoked license in another jurisdiction
- Unfit by reason of neglect

STANDARDS OF CARE

Standards of care are guidelines used to determine what a nurse should or should not do. All healthcare professionals must adhere to certain standards. A physician's standards of care are different from those of a registered nurse, and an LPN's/LVN's standards differ from those of the RN. Each nurse must be aware of the standards of care to which they will be held accountable because they can be sued to determine if appropriate action was taken. Standards of care come from various sources: state licensing laws, nurse practice acts, nursing organizations, journal articles, or policies and procedures for individual facilities.

NURSE PRACTICE ACTS

Nurse practice acts, in general, provide a definition for *nurse,* establish a board of nursing, outline the requirements for licensure, and provide the circumstances for suspension and revocation of the license. These acts are specific for each state or territory and facilitate recognition of possible conflict between the scope of practice and the tasks being performed by the LPN/LVN.

Although the acts differ from state to state, some standardized terminology is used. The understandings of these terms may be helpful as you assume the role of a licensed nurse within your state. Table 63-1 ■ lists some common terms and their explanation.

The National Association for Practical Nurse Education and Service issued the statement shown in Box 63-2 ■, listing the responsibilities of practice of the LPN/LVN, in its 1998 Code of Ethics for the Licensed Practical/Vocational Nurse. Statements from professional organizations are not state law; they merely serve as guidelines for practice.

Leadership Styles

The transition from graduate to licensed nurse happens quickly. You will need to begin to think differently about yourself. **Leadership** is a process used to move a group toward setting and achievement of goals. This definition is compatible with nursing leadership. The process can be used by anyone; therefore anyone can, in theory, be a leader. As you begin your career, you will have the opportunity to observe nursing leaders; as you watch and learn you will begin to develop your own leadership style. There are several leadership styles and each one has good and not-so-good characteristics. There are situations where one style may be more effective than another. Leaders will change their style in order to maximize their leadership effectiveness.

TYPES OF LEADERS

Autocrat

The **autocratic** leader makes unilateral decisions while dominating the team members. This approach can result in passive resistance from team members. It requires constant control from the leader in order to have the singular objective met.

TABLE 63-1	Common Terms Used in Nurse Practice Acts	
TERMS	**EXPLANATION**	
Basic nursing care	Nursing care which is predictable and with which modifications are unnecessary, based on the knowledge and skills obtained during an educational program, and those which can be safely performed by an LPN/LVN.	
Basic client situation	Situations in which the client's condition is predictable and the clinical condition requires only basic nursing care. Medical and nursing orders are continuously changing and do not contain complex modifications. The situation is determined by the RN.	
Complex nursing situation	Client's clinical condition is not predictable and requires frequent changes in medical or nursing orders or complex modifications. Nursing care expectations are beyond that learned by the LPN/LVN during the educational program.	
Delegated medical act	Doctor's orders given to the RN or LPN/LVN.	
Delegated nursing act	Nursing orders given to an RN or LPN/LVN by an RN.	
Direct supervision	Supervisor is continuously present to coordinate, inspect, or direct nursing care.	
General supervision	Supervisor regularly coordinates, inspects, or directs nursing care. The supervisor is available within the building or by telephone.	

The authoritarian approach is generally not successful in getting the best performance from a team. There are, however, some instances when the autocratic style is appropriate. When there is a need for immediate action, this style may be the most effective. Most people are familiar with the autocratic style and have little trouble adopting it. In some situations subordinates may actually prefer being directed by an autocrat.

Laissez-Faire Leader

The **laissez-faire** leader exercises little control over the group. Team members are left alone to tackle their work, sort out their roles, and solve problems. This approach leaves the team floundering with little motivation or direction.

There are situations in which the laissez-faire approach is effective. It can be appropriate with highly motivated and skilled team members, who have produced excellent work in the past. Once the leader has established the team as competent, confident, and motivated it may be appropriate to back off and allow the team to function. By handing over ownership of the project, the leader empowers the team and they can take ownership and will most likely achieve the goals.

Democrat

The **democratic** leader makes decisions after consulting with team members. Although the team participates in the decision-making process, the leader still maintains control. The team is allowed to decide how the task will be accomplished and who will be responsible for each task.

The democratic leader can be viewed in two ways. The good democratic leader delegates wisely and encourages participation, but the leader never loses sight that the ultimate responsibility belongs to him or her. The leader values group discussion and input. The leader draws from the team members' strengths and knowledge in order to obtain the best performance from the team. However, the democratic leader can also be seen as being unsure of himself and his relationship with his subordinates. It appears that everything is a matter of group decision. This type of leader is seen as not leading at all.

Team Leading

The first leadership role you might experience as an LPN/LVN may be that of a team leader. In this role you will be responsible for guiding and directing the care for a group of clients. You will also be responsible for supervising the members of the team, which includes nursing assistants.

The duties of the team leader include:

- Making assignments
- Taking report
- Making rounds and assessing clients
- Giving report to team members on assigned clients
- Assisting in administration of medications and treatments
- Facilitating team conferences
- Collaborating with an RN supervisor or clinical nurse specialist

DELEGATION

The sign of a good leader is to know how and when to delegate (Figure 63-1 ■). The leader will understand the scope of all team members so that delegation of tasks will be appropriate.

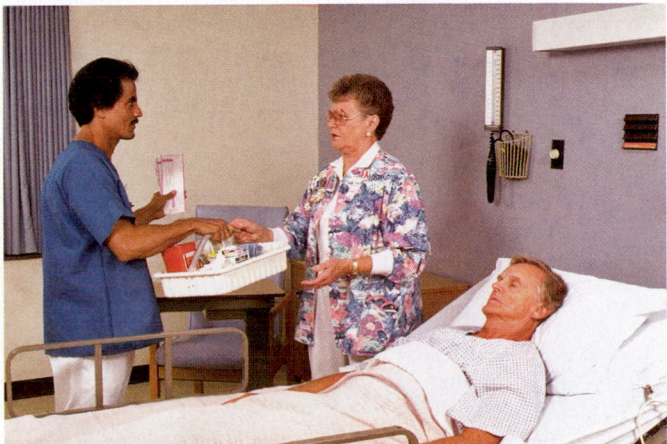

Figure 63-1. ■ The LPN/LVN will often have to delegate tasks to assistive personnel. *Source:* Pearson Education/PH College.

The first step in the **delegation** (the distribution of tasks in a way that prioritizes activities and available resources) process is to prioritize activities with available resources. The purpose of delegation is efficiency. No one person can do it all, therefore some work must be passed on. It is important to remember that even though a task has been delegated, the ultimate responsibility for the task belongs to the nurse-leader. A flowchart for delegating tasks is provided in Figure 63-2 ■.

Some leaders have difficulty delegating. This presents several problems. The leader who does not delegate becomes overworked, tired, and ineffective. When delegation is not utilized, some team members become lazy or bored. Team members who are never given responsibility through delegation may feel that the leader is unappreciative of their contribution and thinks they are incapable; this leads to a breakdown of the team.

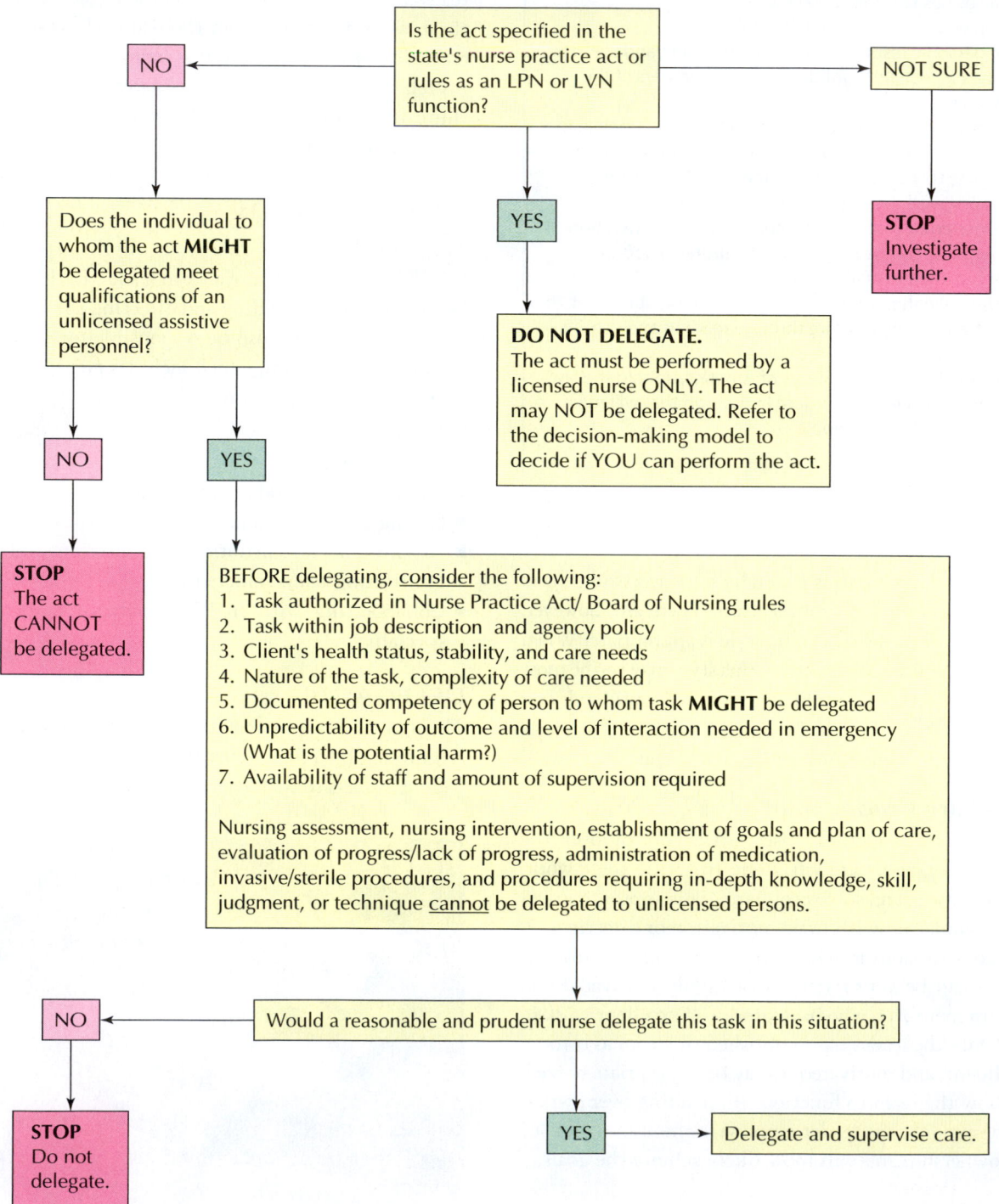

Figure 63-2. ■ Delegation flowchart.

Group leaders who have a leader who makes use of delegation benefit in the following ways:

- Their sense of responsibility increases.
- Their job satisfaction is heightened.
- Their knowledge is increased.

Ultimately, delegation will promote happiness within the group; morale will improve as will productivity. In other words, the team will likely be functioning at its peak.

The reason leaders may delegate poorly or not at all may be that they simply do not know how. Delegation skills can be learned and perfected. Delegation works best when assignments are specific. Team members may be afraid to accept the assignment from fear of failure. They need to be given the opportunity to ask questions and seek clarification prior to being expected to take on the task. They also need to know they can trust the leader to support them in their efforts. The leader should be ready to reward the group for successful completion of delegated activities. Group members whose contributions are appreciated will be motivated to accept further responsibility. A simple word of thanks can go a long way.

MAKING ASSIGNMENTS

The NCSBN in the 2006 LPN/LVN Practice Analysis identified making client care or related task assignments as being an activity that is participated in by a high percentage of LPNs/LVNs in a variety of practice areas. Tasks related to assignments are categorized as Coordinated Care on the NCLEX-PN® test plan. See Chapter 64 🔗 for further information related to the test plan.

A number of issues must be considered when making assignments. You must compare the needs of the client to the knowledge, skills, and abilities of assistive personnel prior to making assignments. It is also important to organize information for the client assignment in such a manner that the assigned staff members will know exactly what tasks they are expected to complete and the time frame for completion. To do this effectively, you must know the strengths and weaknesses of the individuals working on your team.

Lastly you must continue to reevaluate the assignments so that you are aware when assignments need to be changed, such as when there is a change in the client's condition. You will also need to provide this information to the RN and/or the supervisor.

Most facilities staff according to the nursing model that they have adopted, such as primary or team nursing. Some facilities may routinely use one approach, but on occasion need to make adjustments depending on staffing ratios.

Reporting Techniques

In nursing, giving report is very much related to delegation. Reporting to other nurses at the change of shifts is both delegation of responsibility and an accounting as to what has been done.

Shift report is the most effective way to pass information from one shift to another. The report can take on many forms. It may be oral face to face with the staff arriving for the next shift. It may be done in a room or as a part of walking rounds. The report may be taped by the nurse going off duty to be listened to by the oncoming nurse, or the report may be written. There are advantages and disadvantages of each. No matter which form the facility uses, some important issues need to be established. Each form of report will be discussed giving both the advantages and disadvantages.

Taped report has been adopted by many facilities in an effort to save time and provide floor coverage during report. The nurses going off duty can tape report on their clients one at a time, leaving the other staff to provide coverage for all the clients. Nurses coming on shift can listen to the tape while the previous shift continues to cover the clients. Some disadvantages of taped report are that sometimes they are difficult to hear or understand and questions must be tabled to the end when they must be addressed with the nurse who may be anxious to go off duty. Box 63-3 ■ provides an outline for making a taped report, and Box 63-4 ■ gives helpful hints for listening to a taped report.

An oral report is very much like a taped report in that it can be delivered in a report room or while making client rounds. Advantages are that questions can be addressed immediately and, if on rounds, clients can be checked at the same time. Disadvantages are that the report cannot start until all staff members have arrived. If clients are in semiprivate rooms, confidentiality may be breeched when report is given on rounds.

Written report is frequently used in long-term care facilities. Each nurse's station will have a report or communication book. Because residents have a lower acuity, there is less to report. The nurses are well acquainted with the residents because they have been under their care for a long time. Written report should be concise. State the resident's name, the problem, what has been done, and what if anything needs to be done by the oncoming shift. Before the entry, list time and date. If more details are needed, the oncoming nurse can be referred to the chart.

HANDOFF PROCEDURE

End-of-shift reports are crucial, but it is also important for nurses to provide information about assigned clients at other times in order to enhance client safety. Formal handoff procedures are a Joint Commission requirement that help with continuity of care when the client leaves the unit.

BOX 63-3 NURSING CARE CHECKLIST

Taped Report

☑ Give your name/shift/date
☑ Room number
☑ Client's full name
☑ Age of client
☑ Diagnosis/admission date/surgical date
☑ Primary or admitting physician's name
☑ Proceed with information. Remember that the nurse coming on may not know the client as well as you do. Be complete. Don't drag. Give pertinent information. Most nurses follow the Kardex and then add changes.

Example:

- C/o of gas pains. What did you do?
- BP was elevated. What was it? What did you do?
- No code
- Specimens needed
- Accu-Chek AC/HS. What were the blood sugars and was insulin coverage given?
- Drainage from NGT/JP/Hemovac. How much?
- Teaching. Did client demonstrate/understand?
- Dressing change
- *Pet peeves:* Don't belittle the client on tape. If you don't like a client, keep it to yourself. Personal comments about clients make the nurse look unprofessional.

☑ Remember not to mumble or yawn too much. You can always stop the tape if you forget something. Put the tape on pause, gather information, and restart the tape.
☑ If you have had a particularly hard shift and haven't finished something like a dressing that was not a priority, make sure you let the next shift know; don't let them find it. You need to be honest. Try not to let it become a habit to leave things undone. *Insight:* Clients sometimes like to play nurse against nurse, shift against shift. Don't play into it. Remember nursing is continuity of care and it is a team effort even if it happens on someone else's shift. It is the client who suffers or gains.
☑ End on a good note—"Have a good day!"

BOX 63-4 HELPFUL HINTS FOR LISTENING TO A TAPED REPORT

- It can be difficult to hear at first. You have to tune out the other noise and concentrate. It may be necessary to let the staff know you can't hear, especially if they are socializing. They usually know their clients and have a trained ear.
- Listen for pertinent data and changes
- Age/diagnosis
- Temperature elevation, BP changes
- Altered mental status
- Dressing changes
- Unusual problems
- Pain/whether medication is controlling it
- If you can get diet/VS/I&O, great, but you can also get that information from the Kardex.

Such times include, but are not limited to, when a nurse takes a break or lunch, when a nurse leaves the unit to attend a meeting or in-service event, when a nurse leaves the floor with one client who is being transferred or discharged, or when a client leaves the unit for surgery, diagnostic tests, or procedures.

It is imperative that the handoff procedure be efficient and not create additional paperwork for the nursing staff. One system of standardized communication technique that seems to be showing promising results and acceptance by the Joint Commission (JCAHO) is SBAR (situation, background, assessment, and recommendation). The SBAR technique was originally developed by the U.S. Navy as a way to improve communication of critical information. Kaiser Permanente of Colorado adapted the technique for use by healthcare organizations.

The SBAR technique follows an established pattern of communication, so that deviation will be readily apparent. This helps to prevent errors and omissions.

SBAR can be described as two objective components (**s**ituation and **b**ackground) and two subjective components (**a**ssessment and **r**ecommendation). The *situation* includes information such as the client's name, room number, and what is presently going on with the client.

Example: Mrs. Warren in room 224 returned from recovery 1 hour ago, following an R TKR. (*Situation*)

Background includes the admitting diagnosis and progress related to the diagnosis.

Example: She was admitted with DJD and scheduled knee replacement, which was completed today. (*Background*)

The *assessment* and *recommendation* components allow delivery of subjective information, including opinion and specific recommendation.

Example: She has a PCA and her pain level is 2 on a scale of 10. She is drifting in and out of sleep. (*Assessment*)

Example: She will need another set of vital signs and reassessment of her pain in 15 minutes. (*Recommendation*)

Many facilities have created a form that can be used. In addition the information should be provided orally, giving the accepting nurse an opportunity to repeat the information to establish understanding.

Client safety has become an ongoing concern within healthcare organizations. Using procedures such as these will improve teamwork, communication, and client care.

Students should make use of these techniques whenever care of a client is relinquished to another student or a licensed nurse.

PAPERWORK

You may have heard seasoned nurses complain about the increasing amount of paperwork. Over the years changes have been made to control the amount of writing a nurse must do.

Narrative notes have been replaced with flow sheets and other forms of abbreviated charting. Increased regulations, licensing requirements, and government restrictions have created additional need for documentation. See Chapter 13 🔗 for more information about documentation.

Physician's Orders

Physician's orders are a part of the client medical record. As a nurse you need to have an order for all areas of client care. The client cannot even be admitted to the hospital without an order from a physician. Physician's orders take different forms:

- Handwritten by the physician during hospital rounds
- Verbal orders
- Preprinted or standing orders to cover admissions for certain conditions or surgeries (e.g., postpartum care following an uncomplicated delivery or total knee replacement surgery)
- Telephone orders

Transcription of Orders

Some facilities employ a clerical person to transcribe physician's orders. This individual may have the title of ward or unit secretary or ward clerk. Unit secretaries might not be employed for the evening and night shifts or in long-term care facilities, so the LPN/LVN may be expected to carry out this task. Even if the unit secretary transcribes the orders, it is the responsibility of the licensed person to note or ensure that the orders were correctly transcribed.

Handwritten orders may be difficult to read. With practice you will learn the commonalities of a physician's handwriting and will be able to read what has been written. It is important to seek a second opinion if you are having trouble deciphering an order—never guess. When in doubt seek clarification from the physician. Never carry out an unclear order until it has been clarified. Medication orders can present a particular problem. When the spelling of a medication is in question, refer to a current drug reference or a list of commonly prescribed medications. With the number of new drugs being developed and the use of both generic and trade names, it is impossible to know all drugs by sight. Use available resources to protect your clients from error.

Verbal and telephone orders are taken by a licensed nurse and recorded on the physician order sheet. Policies regarding verbal and phone orders differ from facility to facility. It is important for the LPN/LVN to know the state board policy on verbal and phone orders. These policies vary from state to state. Federal Hospital Certification Regulation 42 CFR 482.223 (c)(2)(i) states that when telephone or oral orders must be used they must be "Accepted only by personnel that are authorized to do so by the medical staff policies and procedures, consistent with Federal and State laws."

Orders given via the telephone or verbally have an increased opportunity for error. The "read back" procedure is a Joint Commission guideline as indicated in the National Patient Safety Goals. Clarify the order by repeating it back to the physician. This will give the nurse and the physician the opportunity to hear the order and make corrections if necessary. Verbal or telephone orders should be written down immediately. Verbal and phone orders must be signed by the physician. The facility will have a policy as to when the orders must be signed; policies differ with the type of facility.

Incident Reports

An **incident report** or occurrence report is completed when client care was not consistent with standards for expected care. Issues involve omitted medications or treatments or medication administration that violated one of the "five rights." Any unusual occurrence, one that did or may have caused harm, needs to be documented on an incident report. Injuries to client, employee, or visitor also require a report. The incident report does not become a part of the client medical record. They are usually filed with the risk management department.

When completing an incident report, be sure to include all pertinent details. List time, date, and an objective observation of the incident. Guilt should not be admitted. Other staff members who witnessed the incident or were involved should also be listed. The completed report should be turned over to the supervisor or individual designated by the facility to investigate. The purpose of the incident report is to help the facility prevent future problems through correction and education.

When the incident is reported in the medical chart, it is important to objectively document the incident. It is not recommended to document that the incident report was filled out. Copies of incident reports are not placed in the client's chart. Be sure to follow the facility's procedures, which may vary. See Chapter 46 🔗 for specific guidelines related to long-term care. Figure 63-3 ■ is an example of an incident report.

Conflict Resolution

Conflict can be defined as a disagreement or antagonism between groups, individuals, or ideas. The presence of conflict is not necessarily a negative situation. Well-managed conflicts can stimulate competition, can bring new ideas to the table, and can identify legitimate differences and problems within an organization. As children we were taught to manage conflicts passively; we were sent to the corner or "time-out" when we couldn't get along. In nursing, conflicts cannot be ignored, but instead must be dealt with and managed no matter how difficult that might be.

Several common approaches are used for conflict resolution. The ability to manage conflicts is a critical skill, which a nurse must develop. Use of these skills can help the

CONFIDENTIAL REPORT OF UNUSUAL OCCURRENCE
NOT a part of the Medical Record - Please forward to RISK MANAGEMENT

I. (COMPLETE IF ADDRESSOGRAPH UNAVAILABLE)

CLIENT/VISITOR _____ PHYSICIAN _____

MEDICAL RECORD #_____ DATE OF BIRTH _____

ADDRESSOGRAPH

II. DATE OF OCCURRENCE _____ TIME OF OCCURRENCE _____ LOCATION (ROOM OR FLOOR) _____

NAME OF M.D. NOTIFIED_____ CLIENT AWARE OF OCCURRENCE: YES___NO___ FAMILY AWARE OF OCCURRENCE: YES___NO___

REPORT COMPLETED BY_____OTHERS FAMILIAR WITH OCCURRENCE _____

III. ADMITTING DIAGNOSIS _____

CLIENT CONDITION PRIOR TO OCCURRENCE: ALERT _____ ASLEEP _____ ANESTHETIZED _____ DISORIENTED _____ OTHER _____

IF SEDATIVE/NARCOTICS/DIURETICS GIVEN IN LAST 12 HOURS (WHERE APPLICABLE) PLEASE COMPLETE: (MED, DOSE, TIME)

IV. EVENT

FALLS
- 100 Unobserved Fall
- 101 Assisted to Floor
- 102 Fell from Bed
- 103 Fell from Table/Equipment
- 104 Fell in Bathroom
- 105 Walking/Standing/Slip & Fall
- 106 Sitting Commode/Wheelchair
- 107 Restrained Prior to Fall
- 108 Restrained After Fall
- 109 Bed Rails Up (1 2 3 4)
- 110 Bed Rails Down (1 2 3 4)
- 112 Visitor Fall
- 113 Outpatient Fall
- 119 Other_____

BURNS
- 120 Electrical/Chemical Burn
- 121 Spill
- 122 Fire
- 129 Other_____

ALTERCATION/COMPLAINTS
- 130 Pt/Family/Employee/Visitor
- 131 Complaint-Waiting Time
- 132 Complaint-Billing Services
- 133 Complaint-Food Services
- 134 Complaint-Housekeeping/Ancillary
- 135 Complaint-Nursing
- 136 Complaint-Medical Staff
- 137 Complaint-Security
- 139 Other_____

MISCELLANEOUS
- 140 Suicide/Attempt
- 141 Left AMA/Elopement
- 142 Equipment-Struck/Failure
- 143 Property Loss/Damage
- 144 Unexpected Death
- 145 Non-Compliant Smoking
- 148 Development of Pressure Ulcer
- 149 Other_____

MEDICATIONS   Drug_____
- 150 Order (Computer Entry)
- 151 Wrong Time
- 152 Wrong Dosage
- 153 Wrong Route
- 154 Wrong Drug
- 155 Wrong Patient
- 156 Omission
- 157 Adverse Drug Reaction
- 158 Prescribing Error
- 159 Other_____

INTRAVENOUS Sol._____
- 160 Infiltration
- 161 Wrong Rate
- 162 Wrong Solution
- 163 Wrong Time
- 164 Order (Computer Entry)
- 165 Infected Site/Phlebitis
- 169 Other_____

BLOOD TRANSFUSION
- 170 Allergic/Adverse Reaction
- 171 Delay in Administration
- 172 Incorrect Flow Rate
- 173 Infiltration
- 174 Omitted/Client Refusal
- 175 Wrong Amount
- 176 Wrong/Omitted Filter
- 177 Wrong Component
- 178 Biological Product Deviation
- 179 Other_____

PATHOLOGY
- 180 Reference Laboratory Error
- 181 Lost/Mishandled Specimen
- 182 Specimen Collection Error
- 183 Cytology/Biopsy Discrepancy
- 184 Biopsy/Resection Discrepancy
- 185 Autopsy Suggests Serious Clinical Discrepancy
- 186 Frozen Section/Pathological Discrepancy
- 187 Error Performing Test/Error Reporting Results
- 188 Delayed Draw
- 189 Hematoma Following Draw
- 190 Other_____

OR/PACU/OPS/WOR
- 200 Removal Foreign Body
- 210 Incorrect Count-Sponge/Needle/Instr
- 202 X-rays Taken/Deferred
- 203 Arrest
- 204 Wrong Pt/Side/Site/Procedure
- 205 OPS Pt Admitted Post-Op
- 206 Unplanned Organ Repair/Removal
- 207 Lac/Tear/Puncture-Organ/Body Part
- 208 Canceled Surg-Prep/Equipment Problem
- 209 Unplanned Return to OR
- 210 Surgery Delayed
- 211 Consent Incorrect/Incomplete/Not Done
- 212 Reddened Area
- 213 Unsterile Situation
- 214 Specimen Problem
- 215 Eye Irritation/Injury
- 216 Post Arterial Hematoma
- 217 Improper Discharge
- 219 Other_____

ANESTHESIA
- 220 Unexpected Arrest
- 221 Canceled Surgery After Induction
- 222 Injury/Death Post Induction
- 223 Tooth/Face/Lip/Mandible Damage
- 224 CNS Injury/Brain Damage
- 225 Unplanned Transfer to Special Care Unit
- 226 Aspiration
- 229 Other_____

EMERGENCY DEPARTMENT
- 230 Arrives DOA After Discharge/Seen in ED within Past 7 Days
- 231 Seen for Complication Post Treatment/ Procedure from Prev. Hospitalization
- 232 Left AMA
- 239 Other_____

OB/GYN/INFANT CARE
- 240 Delivery Occurred Outside L&D Area
- 241 Mother Transferred to ICU
- 241 Unplanned Return to Surgery
- 243 Stirrup Related Injury
- 244 Delivery Unattended by any Physician
- 245 Blood Loss > 1500 cc
- 246 Cord Blood Gas pH <7.0
- 247 Cardiac/Respiratory Arrest
- 248 Infant Seizures in Delivery Room
- 249 Apgar Score 5 or Less at 5 Minutes
- 250 Unusual Condition - Child
- 251 Infant Injury-skull fx/paralysis/palsy
- 252 Transfer From NB Nursery to ISC/NICU
- 253 Instrumented Delivery-Injury
- 259 Other_____

ADULT/PEDIATRIC CARE
- 260 Unexpected Tx – Higher Care Level
- 261 Significant Neurosensory/Functional Deficit/ Intractable Pain not Present upon Admit
- 262 Acute MI/CVA within 48 hours of Surgery/Procedure
- 263 Death within 48 hours of Surgery/Procedure
- 264 Nosocomial Infection Prolonging Stay or Complicating Pt's Condition > 5 days
- 265 Client Found Unresponsive
- 266 Self Extubation
- 267 Arrest – Code Team Activation
- 268 Soft Tissue Injury
- 269 Other_____

TESTS/TREATMENTS
- 270 Wrong Client
- 271 Wrong Test/Treatment
- 272 Treatment Delayed
- 273 MD Ordered-Not Done
- 274 Complication Resulting in Injury
- 275 Computer Entry
- 276 Infection Control issue
- 279 Other_____

RADIOLOGY/RAD ONC/IMAGING
- 280 Complication Requiring Surgical Correction
- 281 New Onset Nerve Deficit
- 282 Reaction to Contrast Agent
- 283 Overexposure to Radiation
- 284 Cardiac/Respiratory Arrest
- 285 Treatment Delayed Worsening Condition
- 286 Unplanned Repeat Diagnostic Procedure
- 287 Monitored Inadequately
- 288 X-ray Inaccurately Read
- 289 Equipment Failure
- 290 Lack of Prep-Cancel Procedure
- 291 Wrong Pt/Side/Site/Prodedure
- 299 Other_____

V. OUTCOME

SEVERITY OF OUTCOME
350 No Injury/Unaffected
*351 Minor Injury
*352 Major Injury/Consequential

*_SPECIFY INJURY BELOW –

GENERAL
- 300 Delay in Therapy
- 301 Embolism
- 302 Reaction/Toxic Effect
- 303 Death
- 304 Prolonged Hospital Stay
- 305 Neurological Sensory
- 306 Decubitus
- 307 Arrest/CPR
- 309 Other_____

OBSTETRICAL
- 310 Unusually Low Apgar
- 311 Fetal Injury
- 312 Fetal Death
- 313 Maternal Injury
- 314 Maternal Death
- 319 Other_____

SKELETAL
- 320 Fracture
- 321 Dislocation
- 322 Teeth
- 323 Sprain
- 329 Other_____

TISSUE
- 330 Hematoma/Contusion
- 331 Necrosis
- 332 Laceration
- 333 Fistula
- 334 Dehiscence
- 335 Abrasion/Blister
- 336 Swelling
- 337 Reddened Area/Ecchymosis
- 338 Skin Tear
- 339 Other_____

VI. BRIEF COMMENTS IF NECESSARY _____

_____

_____

1004952 (9/01)

Figure 63-3. ■ Example of an incident report.

TABLE 63-2	Conflict Resolution Strategies	
STRATEGIES	**DESCRIPTION**	**SITUATION**
Accommodation	Strategy in which one person or a group is willing to yield to the other.	When preserving relationships; or encouraging others to express themselves and learn by actions. **Situation:** Used by two team leaders when deciding who will get the extra float nurse.
Avoidance	Strategy that is lose–lose; one side denies that the problem exists or withdraws so that there is no active resolution.	When others may resolve the conflict more effectively; both sides see issue as minor or the negative impact is too costly to meet issue head on. **Situation:** After a heated discussion with a physician, a nurse asks another to make rounds until the nurse has had time to calm down. Nurses use avoidance as primary strategy for resolution of conflicts.
Collaboration	Strategy in which both parties meet the problem on an even playing field. Each has equal concern for the issues, allows everyone to win by identifying areas of agreement and differences. Alternatives are evaluated and solutions are selected. There is full support and commitments from both sides.	Can be used to solve previously irreconcilable and long-standing problems. **Situation:** A manager assigns two feuding nurses to work together to solve chronic unit problems.
Competition	Strategy in which the winner takes all; it results in a win–lose situation.	During an emergency when there is no time for discussion. **Situation:** During a code blue situation; someone must direct the code team without discussion.
Compromise	Strategy in which there is negotiation or trade-offs; each person gets something and gives up something; win–lose/win–lose for both sides.	When there is a need to reach an agreement between equally empowered sides. Conflicts resolved by finding common ground. **Situation:** A nurse volunteers to stay over to cover a shift if another colleague agrees to come in early.

nurse to be more productive. It is important to select a strategy that is appropriate to the situation. Frequently, nurses select strategies that are more comfortable rather than effective. Table 63-2 ■ lists various approaches to conflict resolution and situations in which they are used.

STAGES OF CONFLICT

On-the-job conflicts produce reactions within the person, much like any other psychosocial problem. There are six stages of conflict:

1. *Disbelief* is an initial emotional reaction. This frequently happens when values that are held in high regard are disagreed with or discounted.
2. *Disconnectedness.* This stage follows the shock of the first stage. The individual feels confused and taken aback.
3. *Obsession.* The individual becomes obsessed with the situation, and soon it is all the person can think about. Many times, this results in an inability to sleep; wakeful nights are spent thinking about what to do.
4. *Frenzied activity* follows. Many people find this a way of reducing the bitterness, pain, and frustration they feel. The conflicted person may acquire boundless energy,

working endlessly to seek information that will help him or her understand the problem. Colleagues are consulted one after another, trying to redefine the situation. The individual aggressively takes on new tasks or may be involved in numerous activities simultaneously.

5. *Balance or burnout.* As the frenzied search for clues subsides, the individual either begins to reestablish balance or succumbs to symptoms of burnout—withdrawal, depression, and apathy. In intense conflicts, the individual may turn the negative feelings inward. When this occurs, purposeful alienation follows: The individual places emotional and perhaps even physical space between self and colleagues. This is a self-preservation move.
6. *Caution* is adopted as the individual controls verbalization and self-preservation. This move provides a rest or refuge for all involved parties. Once the conflict is resolved positively, the individual may gain personal insight into how to handle future conflicts.

Nurses will have to be prepared to deal with conflicts in all areas of nursing practice. Knowing how and when to use appropriate strategies will promote successful conflict resolution.

Nursing Care Delivery Trends

Throughout the years the delivery of nursing services has continued to change. It is important that nursing professionals understand these trends and be proactive as far as making personal changes to meet the needs of their careers.

The oldest delivery method of nursing services is the **case method,** in which a nurse is responsible for care provided for clients during one shift. Intensive care units frequently operate under the case method. Private duty nurses and home care can also be described as nursing by the case method.

In the **functional nursing** system, each team member is assigned specific tasks or functions. Although functional nursing is efficient, it can create fragmented delivery of client care. Establishing a therapeutic relationship between nurse and client is somewhat more difficult because of the large number of care professionals interacting with the client.

In **primary nursing** a professional nurse has total responsibility for a group of clients. It is a more recent development in delivery methods. Primary nursing in the purest sense gives responsibility to the nurse 24 hours a day 7 days a week, from admission through discharge. The purpose of this method is to provide continuity and coordination of care. If the RN is not physically in attendance, the care may be delegated to an associate who may be another RN or an LPN/LVN. Many hospitals ascribe to primary nursing, but in a way that resembles the case method. While the nurse is working, the responsibility to the assigned client is his or hers.

Team nursing has been used since the early 1950s. It was replaced with primary nursing in the 1970s. The purpose of this concept was to reduce fragmentation, which was present in the functional method. Team nursing is again becoming increasingly popular given the nursing shortage and small nurse-to-client ratios. An RN usually directs the nursing team in the acute hospital. The remainder of the team is made up of LPNs/LVNs and unlicensed personnel (e.g., nursing assistants, client care technicians). A nursing unit may have two or more nursing teams caring for 10 or more clients. Team members work together to use their diverse skills and education to best care for the assigned clients. Care planning is done in team meetings in which all members have input.

MEN IN NURSING

Throughout history men have made significant contributions to the nursing profession. Current trends show increased numbers of men entering the profession. At one time men sought positions in specialty areas such as psychiatry, emergency and trauma nursing, correctional institutions and rehabilitation, and the medical-surgical area. They sought administration positions. More recently there has been increased interest by men in hospice, pediatric, and neonatology

BOX 63-5	ROLES AND RESPONSIBILITIES OF THE LPN/LVN

- Recognizes the LPN's/LVN's role in the healthcare delivery system and articulates that role with those of other healthcare team members.
- Maintains accountability for one's own nursing practice within the ethical and legal framework.
- Serves as a client advocate.
- Accepts role in maintaining developing standards of practice in providing health care.
- Seeks further growth through educational opportunities.

nursing and in teaching in schools of nursing. The increased number of men entering the profession has brought a different perspective and an increase in salary and benefits.

Regardless of whether the nurse is a male or a female, whether he or she works in an acute hospital, ambulatory care, a specialty area, or long-term care, it is important to be aware of current trends. Being well informed will help you to be a more effective nurse and a valuable member of the healthcare community as you carry out the roles and responsibilities of an LPN/LVN. Box 63-5 ■ explains these roles and responsibilities.

SURVEYORS AND ACCREDITATION

Two words that seem to send a wave of fear through a healthcare facility are *surveys* and *accreditation*. Meeting standards such as those put forth by the Joint Commission on Accreditation of Healthcare Organizations (JCAHO, or the Joint Commission) have become increasingly important. Healthcare consumers are becoming more involved in their healthcare choices, so a facility that achieves accreditation will be one that is sought after by prospective clients. Whether you are the bedside nurse in an acute hospital or have more responsibility in a subacute area, when the surveyors visit you will be a vital part of the team.

Tracer Methodology

Tracer methodology is an evaluation method used by the Joint Commission surveyors. They select a resident or client and use that individual's record as a road map to move through the organization to assess and evaluate the organization's compliance with selected standards and the organization's systems of providing care and services. If the surveyor identifies problems, the facility has 45 days from the end of the survey to submit evidence of standards compliance and identify measures of success.

NATIONAL PATIENT SAFETY GOALS

In June 2008, the Joint Commission's Board of Commissioners approved the 2009 National Patient Safety Goals for clients. Goals have been identified that have accreditation program applicability (Table 63-3 ■).

TABLE 63-3	Joint Commission's 2009 National Patient Safety Goals (NPSGs)	
GOAL	**REQUIREMENT**	**TYPE OF FACILITY AFFECTED**
Patient Identification **Goal:** Improve the accuracy of patient identification.	Use at least two patient identifiers when providing care, treatment, or services.	Ambulatory, assisted living, behavioral health care, critical access hospitals, disease-specific care, home care, hospital, lab, long-term care
	Prior to the start of any invasive procedure, conduct a final verification process (such as a "time-out") to confirm the correct patient, procedure, and site, using active—not passive—communication techniques.	Assisted living, home care, lab, long-term care, office-based care
Improved Communication **Goal:** Improve the effectiveness of communication among caregivers.	For verbal or telephone orders or for telephonic reporting of critical test results, verify the complete order or test results, verify the complete order or test results by having the person receiving the information record and "read-back" the complete order or test results.	Ambulatory, assisted living, behavioral health care, critical access hospitals, disease-specific care, home care, hospital, lab, long-term care, office-based surgery
	Standardize a list of abbreviations, acronyms, and symbols that will not be used throughout an organization.	Ambulatory, assisted living, behavioral health care, critical access hospitals, disease-specific care, home care, hospital, lab, long-term care, office-based surgery
	Measure, assess, and if appropriate, take action to improve the timeliness of reporting, and the timeliness of the receipt by the responsible licensed caregiver, of critical tests and critical results and values.	Ambulatory, behavioral health care, critical access hospitals, disease-specific care, home care, hospital, lab, long-term care, office-based surgery
	Implement a standardized approach to "hand off" communications, including an opportunity to ask and respond to questions.	Ambulatory care, assisted living, behavioral health care, critical access hospital, disease-specific care, home care, hospital, lab, long-term care, office-based surgery
Medication Safety **Goal:** Improve the safety of using medications.	Identify and, at minimum, annually review a list of look-alike/sound-alike drugs used by the organization, and take action to prevent errors involving the interchange of these drugs.	Ambulatory, behavioral health care, critical access hospitals, home care, hospital, long-term care, office-based surgery
	Label all medications, medication containers (for example, syringes, medicine cups, basins), or other solutions on and off sterile fields.	Ambulatory care, critical access hospital, hospital, office-based surgery
	Reduce the likelihood of patient harm associated with the use of anticoagulation therapy.	Ambulatory care, critical access hospital, home care, hospital, long-term care
Healthcare-Associated Infections **Goal:** Reduce the risk of healthcare associated infections.	Comply with current World Health Organization (WHO) Hand Hygiene Guidelines or Centers for Disease Control and Prevention (CDC) hand hygiene guidelines.	Ambulatory care, assisted living, behavioral health care, critical access hospital, disease-specific care, home care, hospital, lab, long-term care, office-based surgery
	Manage as sentinel events all identified cases of unanticipated death or major permanent loss of function associated with a healthcare-associated infection.	Ambulatory care, assisted living, behavioral health, critical access hospital, disease-specific care, home care, hospital, lab, office-based surgery
Medication Reconciliation **Goal:** Accurately and completely reconcile medications across the continuum of care.	Compare the patient's current medications with those ordered for the patient while under the care of the organization.	Ambulatory care, assisted living, behavioral health care, critical access hospital, disease-specific care, home care, hospital, lab, long-term care, office-based surgery
	Provide a complete list of the patient's medications to the next provider of service when a patient is referred or transferred to another setting, service, practitioner, or level of care within or outside the organization. Also provide the complete list of medications to the patient on discharge from the facility.	Ambulatory care, assisted living, behavioral health care, critical access hospital, disease-specific care, home care, hospital, lab, long-term care, office-based surgery
Risk for Injury **Goal:** Reduce the risk of patient harm resulting from falls.	Implement a fall reduction program including an evaluation of the effectiveness of the program.	Assisted living, critical access hospital, disease-specific care, hospital, long-term care

(continued)

TABLE 63-3	Joint Commission's 2009 National Patient Safety Goals (NPSGs) (continued)	
GOAL	**REQUIREMENT**	**TYPE OF FACILITY AFFECTED**
Influenza & Pneumococcal Disease **Goal:** Reduce the risk of influenza and pneumococcal disease in institutionalized older adults.	Develop and implement a protocol for administration and documentation of flu vaccine.	Assisted living, disease-specific care, long-term care
	Develop and implement a protocol for administration and documentation of pneumococcus vaccine.	Assisted living, disease-specific care, long-term care
	Develop and implement a protocol to identify new cases of influenza and to manage an outbreak.	Assisted living, disease-specific care, long-term care
Surgical Fires **Goal:** Reduce the risk of surgical fires.	Educate staff, including operating licensed independent practitioners and anesthesia providers, on how to control heat sources and manage fuels with enough time for patient preparation, and establish guidelines to minimize oxygen concentration under drapes.	Ambulatory care, office-based surgery
Implementation of NPSGs **Goal:** Implement applicable National Patient Safety Goals and associated requirements by components and practitioner sites.	Inform and encourage components and practitioner sites to implement the applicable National Patient Safety Goals and associated requirements.	Networks
Patient Involvement **Goal:** Encourage patients' active involvement in their own care as a patient safety strategy.	Define and communicate the means for patients and their families to report concerns about safety and encourage them to do so.	Ambulatory care, assisted living, behavioral health care, critical access hospital, disease-specific care, home care, hospital, lab, long-term care, office-based surgery
Pressure Ulcers **Goal:** Prevent healthcare-associated pressure ulcers (decubitus ulcers).	Assess, and periodically reassess, each resident's risk for developing a pressure ulcer (decubitus ulcer) and take action to address any identified risks.	Long-term care
Safety Risks **Goal:** The organization identifies safety risks inherent in its client population.	The organization identifies clients at risk for suicide.	Behavioral health
	The organization identifies risks associated with long-term oxygen therapy such as home fires.	Home care
Change in Patient's Condition **Goal:** Improve recognition and response to changes in patient's condition.	The organization selects a suitable method that enables healthcare staff members to directly request additional assistance from a specially trained individual(s) when the patient's condition appears to be worsening.	Critical access hospital, hospitals

Note: The Joint Commission continues to use the term *patient* for the individual receiving care and services in healthcare organizations. Throughout this book and in most nursing education programs the term *client* is used. However, the terms can be used interchangeably.

Table 63-3 summarizes the Joint Commission's safety goals. Chapter 9 🔗 provides in-depth discussion of basic matters of client and nurse safety.

COMMUNITY SERVICE

Your community has provided you with many opportunities. If you received your training in a public institution, your community has supported you in reaching your goal to become a nurse. It is now time for you to do the same for other citizens. Community service is one important way to fulfill this challenge. You can volunteer to use your skills at schools, community activities, senior centers, or churches. You can provide community healthcare education, or you can become involved with activities such as Race for the Cure, Relay for Life, or a Memory Walk. These events give you the opportunity to raise money for the sponsoring agencies, educate your sponsors, and provide you with an opportunity to exercise.

Note: The references and resources for all chapters have been compiled at the back of the book.

Chapter Review

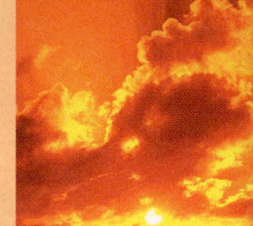

KEY Points

- Graduates of an LPN/LVN program cannot use the title licensed practical/vocational nurse until the licensing exam has been passed.
- The licensing exam is a national test developed by the National Council of State Boards of Nursing.
- Each state board of nursing has a responsibility to protect the public.
- Nurse practice acts are specific for each jurisdiction and recognize possible conflicts between the scope of practice and task being performed by the LPN/LVN.
- Leadership styles need to be adapted to the situation.
- The leadership role most often assumed by the LPN/LVN is the role of team leader.
- The ability to delegate is a sign of a good leader.
- Shift report is a form of delegation. Not only does it pass responsibility from one nurse to another, but reports what has been done.
- Even if clerical personnel are responsible for transcribing physicians' orders, the licensed nurse is ultimately responsible for the transcription being correct.
- The incident report does not become a part of the medical record.
- Conflicts should not be encouraged or discouraged.
- Well-managed conflicts can stimulate competition and identify legitimate differences and problems within the organization.
- Methods of delivery of nursing services continue to change. Keeping up with current trends is very important for the working nurse.

FOR FURTHER Study

Law and ethics in relation to nursing practice are discussed in Chapter 4.

Chapter 9 is the major discussion of client and nurse safety.

See Chapter 13 for more information about documentation.

HIPAA guidelines for sharing client information are provided in Table 14-1.

Chapter 46 provides specific guidelines related to long-term care.

See Chapter 64 for further information related to the test plan.

NCLEX-PN® Exam Preparation

1 The most frequent conflict resolution strategy used by staff nurses is:

1. Collaboration.
2. Accommodation.
3. Avoidance.
4. Competition.

2 The newly licensed nurse administers acetaminophen (Tylenol) to the wrong client. Although the error is unlikely to cause negative effects for the client who received it, the nurse takes which action to maintain the nursing code of ethics?

1. Documents the medication administration in the client's MAR quietly without telling anyone.
2. Informs the nursing supervisor and physician and completes an incident report.
3. Monitors the client's condition closely but does not document the error.
4. Voluntarily surrenders his or her nursing license.

3 The hospital has begun to hire unlicensed assistive personnel (UAPs). The most frequent reason activities delegated to UAPs are not completed as expected is:

1. The need to avoid conflict.
2. Inappropriate supervision.
3. Poor UAP attitudes.
4. Inadequate communication.

4 The nurse accepts a new job as an LPN. After completing orientation, the nurse is asked to perform a task that the nurse has never performed before. The nurse would:

1. Check the nurse practice act and perform the task if it is allowed.
2. Perform the task if it is allowed by facility policy.
3. Inform the nursing supervisor of his or her unfamiliarity with performing the task.
4. Read the facilities procedure for the task and follow the directions provided.

5 The client asks the nurse, "I keep hearing the term *accountability* used around here. What does it mean?" The nurse's best response would be:

1. Providing guidance, direction, evaluation, and follow-up by a licensed nurse.
2. Being responsible and answerable for actions of oneself and others in the context of delegation.
3. Delegating nursing activities to be performed by an individual consistent with his or her licensed scope of practice.
4. Transferring to a competent individual the authority to perform a selected nursing task in a selected situation.

6 The new graduate nurse reports to work and learns the unit is short-staffed. The unit manager asks the nurse to function as the team leader. The graduate nurse declines, knowing that he or she would be unable to perform which of the following functions?

1. Acting as a resource for other staff members
2. Giving report to team members
3. Assisting in administering medications and treatments
4. Taking report

7 The nurse works on a unit with a nurse manager who leaves the unit staff alone to tackle their work, sort out their roles, and solve problems. The team often flounders with little motivation or direction. The nurse identifies the management style of this unit manager as:

1. Autocratic.
2. Laissez-faire.
3. Authoritative.
4. Democratic.

8 The nursing system in which establishing a therapeutic relationship between nurse and client is somewhat more difficult because of the large number of team care professionals interacting with the client is known as:

1. Team nursing.
2. Primary nursing.
3. Functional nursing.
4. Case method.

9 When working in a facility that uses taped reports, the nurse finds which of the following to be a disadvantage of this system?

1. Time-consuming
2. Inadequate client coverage during report
3. Questions must be held until after report
4. Inadequate coverage while report is taped

10 The nurse observes a newly hired nurse performing client care and recognizes which of the following actions does not follow Joint Commission's National Patient Safety Goals?

1. The nurse asks the client's name and birth date prior to administering medications.
2. The nurse reads the order back to the physician when taking telephone orders.
3. The nurse checks the newly printed MAR against the old MAR.
4. The nurse attends in-service programs on fire safety.

Answers and rationales for Review Questions appear in Appendix I.

Chapter 64

Preparing to Take the Licensure Exam

LEARNING Outcomes

After completing this chapter, you will be able to:

1. Describe the purpose of the NCLEX-PN® examination and when to begin studying for it.
2. Explain how the National Council of State Boards of Nursing develops the test plan and the test, where the NCLEX-PN® test is available, and how the multistate compact applies to it.
3. Identify the levels of NCLEX-PN® questions and the central concept on which the test is based.
4. Describe the four categories of client needs and their subcategories.
5. Explain how computer adaptive testing creates an individualized test for each student.
6. Develop an individualized plan for preparing and reviewing for the NCLEX-PN®.
7. Identify ways to determine personal readiness for the examination.
8. Explain how to apply to take the examination.
9. Name ways to overcome test anxiety.
10. Describe what to do the day before, day of, and during the examination to increase the chances of success on the examination.
11. Discuss the time after the exam and how to use test results.

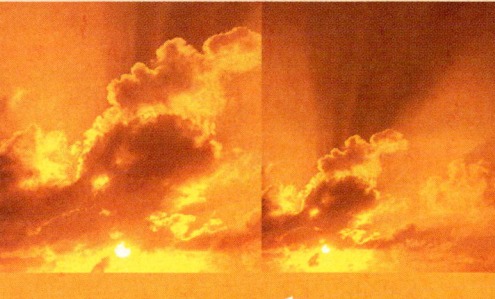

BRIEF Outline

KEY TERMS

Use the audio glossary feature on the MyNursingKit Website to hear the correct pronunciation of the following key terms.

computer adaptive testing 1783   mnemonics 1784   test anxiety 1786
diagnostic profile 1787   multistate compact 1780

From the minute you enter nursing school until you graduate, you must be aware that, in order to practice as an LPN/LVN:

1. You need to acquire a certain body of nursing knowledge and nursing skills.
2. You must pass the National Council Licensure Examination for Practical/Vocational Nurses (NCLEX-PN®).

The purpose of this examination is to protect the public by ensuring that all licensed entry-level nurses have the competencies they need to practice safely and effectively.

Development of the NCLEX-PN®

The National Council of State Boards of Nursing, Inc. (NCSBN) is a not-for-profit organization comprised of the boards of nursing in the 50 states, the District of Columbia, and five United States territories: American Samoa, Guam, Northern Mariana Islands, Puerto Rico, and the Virgin Islands.

NCSBN develops a test plan on which the NCLEX-PN® is based. In developing the test plan, the NCSBN considers the legal scope of practical/vocational nursing practice, as governed by each state's laws and regulations, including the various nurse practice acts. The NCSBN also conducts a vocational nursing job analysis study every 3 years. This analysis is used to develop the framework for the current NCLEX-PN®. Test questions on the NCLEX-PN® focus on the job tasks identified as those normally carried out by entry-level LPNs/LVNs in their first year of nursing employment. The test plan provides a summary of the content and the scope of the exam.

The detailed test plan (candidates' version) is now available on the NCSBN website. Until April 2008, the detailed plan was only available for purchase to schools. This document provides greater detail about the elements of each test plan category. It can be a helpful study tool as you prepare for the NCLEX-PN® exam.

The NCSBN currently (2008) contracts with Pearson VUE for the development and administration of the NCLEX-PN®. NCSBN retains oversight and provides volunteer test item writers. These item writers are professional faculty members in schools of nursing who have been approved and recommended to NCSBN by their respective state boards of nursing and screened for test-writing ability.

Item writers receive additional training in item writing and write test questions based on the test plan. Expert item reviewers review all items written by item writers. Accepted items then go to panel judges for additional review and edit. New items are tested on the NCLEX-PN® and these items do not count for or against the test taker.

AVAILABILITY OF THE NCLEX-PN®

The NCLEX-PN® is available in the District of Columbia, every state in the United States, in the various territories of the United States, and three foreign countries: Seoul, South Korea; London, England; and Hong Kong, Special Administrative District of China.

Because the boards of nursing from the United States and its territories, as well as these other countries, use the NCLEX-PN® to assist them in making licensure decisions, you may be able to get licensure by endorsement from a state board of nursing in a state or territory and possibly a country other than the one in which you took the examination, should you decide to work somewhere other than the state or country where you took your exam.

Multistate Compact

In addition to endorsement, the concept of a **multistate compact** became reality when, in 2000, Utah became the first state to enact multistate licensure legislation. There are now (2007) 22 Nurse Licensure Compact states: Arkansas, Arizona, Colorado, Delaware, Idaho, Iowa, Kentucky, Maine, Maryland, Mississippi, Nebraska, New Hampshire, New Mexico, North and South Carolina, North and South Dakota, Tennessee, Texas, Utah, Virginia, and Wisconsin. Rhode Island is planning to implement in July 2008. If the state where you pass your NCLEX-PN® is part of this multistate compact, you can practice in another state that is part of the compact, as long as you follow the nurse practice act and the rules and regulations pertaining to the act. See also Chapter 2 ⚭.

Understanding the NCLEX-PN® Plan

COGNITIVE LEVELS OF QUESTIONS

The NCLEX-PN® questions are developed at the cognitive levels of knowledge, comprehension, application, and analysis. Table 64-1 ■ describes the cognitive levels of testing and provides some examples. Your nursing instructors

TABLE 64-1	Cognitive Levels of Testing (Bloom's Taxonomy)
COGNITIVE LEVEL	**DESCRIPTION AND EXAMPLE**
Knowledge	Questions at a knowledge level test a person's memory of a fact or recall of a given piece of information. *Example:* Which of the following numbers of questions is the maximum number of questions a test taker can receive when taking the NCLEX-PN®? *Answer:* 205. This tests simple memory of this fact.
Comprehension	Comprehension questions test a person's understanding of concepts or principles. It is an understanding of what something means or how something is related to something else. It can involve reorganizing or restating learned information to demonstrate understanding. *Example:* After completing the teaching of insulin injection to a diabetic client, the nurse will have the most confidence in the client's understanding of the teaching if the client does which of the following things? *Answer:* Demonstrates self-injection principle; most people learn better by doing rather than seeing or hearing.
Application	Application questions test a person's ability to use information such as concepts, theories, principles, and formulas in new situations, or to come up with a solution to a problem. *Example:* The LPN is admitting a new client to the pediatric clinic. The mother asks if the 15-month-old child is due for any immunization today. The most appropriate answer would be _____. *Answer:* Since Varicella was not given at your 12-month visit, it should be given today. The nurse applies knowledge of the immunization schedule to answer the mother's questions.
Analysis	Analysis questions provide information that needs to be separated, sorted, and examined by looking at the various parts and a conclusion drawn to clarify meaning or show how something is structured. *Example:* The physician orders Vistaril 20 mg IM every 4 to 6 hours prn nausea for a child, who weighs 44 lbs. The medication resource indicates that the usual IM dosage is 0.5 mg to 1 mg/kg/dose every 4 to 6 hours as needed. Is this a safe dosage for this child's weight? *Answer:* Yes, this child's safe range is 10 to 20 mg/dose.

will give you tests and examinations at these cognitive levels throughout your nursing courses. These will help to prepare you for the examination and to be more comfortable with each level of question. The practice of LPNs/LVNs requires the application of all levels of cognitive ability. However, nursing requires skill higher than simple knowledge and recall of facts; the nurse must be able to apply information to any clinical situation. The majority of items are written at the application or higher levels. For a review of cognitive levels and types of test questions that test each level, see Chapter 1 🔗 .

During your LPN/LVN program you will take many tests. Tests taken during the program are designed to assess your understanding about a specific body of information (a chapter or unit). They are different from the NCLEX-PN® examination questions. The NCLEX-PN® exam will test overall concepts related to client needs. You will not be given questions about obstetrics, pediatrics, or diabetes, but rather questions where you will apply your knowledge in these areas to a category of the test plan, such as a safe and effective care environment.

TEST PLAN FRAMEWORK

"Client needs" was chosen as the framework of the test plan. Client needs is a universal concept that is applicable to a variety of clients in a wide spectrum of healthcare settings.

Client Needs

The content of the 2008 NCLEX-PN® Test Plan is organized into four major Client Needs categories. (Two of the four are further divided, for a total of six subcategories.)

1. Safe, effective care environment
2. Health promotion and maintenance
3. Psychosocial integrity
4. Physiological integrity

Box 64-1 ■ lists the categories and subcategories of the test. The percentage of questions given for each category for the 2008 test is also shown in Box 64-1. Percentages of questions from each of the different subcategories are set by the NCSBN. These percentages can be obtained by visiting the NCSBN website or by writing to the NCSBN for a test plan. Percentages can change from one test plan revision to the next. There have been no changes in the categories or subcategories in the 2008 Test Plan, although there have been some minute percentage changes in Coordinated Care and Physiological Adaptation.

A number of concepts and processes that students learn well before graduation are integrated throughout the categories of client needs. They include (1) clinical problem-solving process (i.e., the nursing process; see Chapter 6 🔗 , (2) caring, (3) communication and documentation, and (4) teaching/learning.

BOX 64-1 FRAMEWORK OF THE NCLEX-PN® EXAM

Client Needs Categories and Percentage of Questions

1. Safe, effective care environment:
   a. Management of care (12–18%)
   b. Safety and infection control (8–14%)
2. Health promotion and maintenance (7–13%)
3. Psychosocial integrity (8–14%)
4. Physiological integrity:
   a. Basic care and comfort (11–17%)
   b. Pharmacological and parenteral therapies (9–15%)
   c. Reduction of risk potential (10–16%)
   d. Physiological adaptation (11–17%)

Additional Concepts and Processes

- Nursing process
- Caring
- Communication
- Documentation
- Cultural awareness
- Self-care
- Teaching/learning

Test Plan Contact Information

Information on the current test plan can be found on the NCSBN website or you can write to National Council of State Boards of Nursing, 111 East Wacker Drive Suite 2900, Chicago, Illinois 60601.

NCLEX-PN® QUESTIONS BY CLIENT NEEDS. The questions in Box 64-2 ■ will give you some idea of the format of the NCLEX-PN® questions. Provided in the discussion of the answer is the category of client needs as well as the subcategory (see Box 64-1).

Students do not need to know how to identify the categories and subcategories to test well. You will not be asked to identify them. This information is provided for those students who want an example of the various categories and subcategories of client needs on the test plan.

It would be helpful to look at the categories and the lists of related content that are included under each category of client needs, for example, under the category "safe, effective care environment." You will find the content includes advance directives, advocacy, informed consent, information technology, staff education, and much more. Under psychosocial integrity there is abuse or neglect, coping mechanisms, grief and loss, and much more. Looking at information on content under the four categories of client needs might help you in planning your studies and help you realize the wide scope of content on the NCLEX-PN®. You can find this information on the NCLEX-PN® Examination Candidate Bulletin at the NCSBN website.

BOX 64-2 SAMPLE NCLEX-PN®-TYPE QUESTIONS BY CLIENT NEEDS CATEGORY

1. Your assigned client asks you for something for pain. The physician has ordered meperidine (Demerol) 125 mg and promethazine hydrochloride (Phenergan) 25 mg every 4 hours prn. In addition to checking for allergies and when the last dose of the medication was given, it would be most important to do which of the following?

   1. Check the client's respiration rate before giving the injection.
   2. Put the side rails up after the injection.
   3. Teach client not to wait until pain is bad to ask for medication.
   4. Identify the location and intensity of the pain.

   Answer: 1. Since Demerol is likely to depress respirations, the nurse must check the respiratory rate to ensure that it is 12 breaths per minute or above before giving the pain medication. *This question is in the client needs category of physiological integrity and subcategory of reduction of risk potential.*

2. When working with a client who has been admitted with a diagnosis of alcohol dependency, the nurse asks the client to describe the problems that caused him to be admitted. The client says that he does not have any problems and it is his spouse who has the problems. The nurse realizes that the client is using which of the following defense mechanisms?

   1. Denial
   2. Suppression
   3. Rationalization
   4. Identification

   Answer: 1. The client is using denial. Persons with alcohol or other drug abuse or dependency most often use the defense mechanism of denial. They frequently deny that they have a problem to avoid anxiety and possibly to avoid the complications of treatment. *This question is at the level of evaluation in nursing process. It is in the client needs category of psychosocial integrity and the subcategory of coping and adaptation.*

3. The nurse is doing some teaching on recognizing the early warning signs of diabetes. Which of the following warning signs will the nurse include as an early warning sign of diabetes?

   1. Pain on urination
   2. Lack of appetite
   3. Increased thirst
   4. Scant voidings

   Answer: 3. The early warning signs of diabetes include increased urination, increased hunger, and increased thirst. *This question is in the health promotion and maintenance category of client needs and the subcategory of prevention and early detection of disease.*

Computer Adaptive Testing (CAT)

Prior to April 1994, the examination for licensure as an LPN/LVN was a paper-and-pencil test administered by each state board of nursing. Large numbers of candidates for licensure took the exam in a room monitored by proctors. Examinations were usually given only twice a year. Test security was a major concern, with large numbers of people taking the same examination at the same time and with versions of the test being administered again from time to time.

In April 1994, candidates for licensure began to take the licensure examination on the computer. The computer uses a method called **computer adaptive testing** (CAT) to provide each student a unique examination, selecting the test questions as the student takes the examination. In April 2001, those taking the exam could use a computer mouse for the first time, and a drop-down calculator became available.

The test questions for the NCLEX-PN® exams are stored in an extremely large test bank. Questions are categorized according to their fit into various categories of the test plan structure. In addition, questions are categorized according to the level of difficulty. Each candidate is given a unique examination to test her or his knowledge and abilities while meeting the test plan requirements.

When you take this exam and answer a question correctly, the computer will scan the test bank and give you a more difficult question. On the other hand, if you select an incorrect answer, the computer will scan the test bank and give you an easier question.

In addition to the "real" questions that will determine if you are a safe practitioner or not, you will be given an additional 25 questions that will not count for or against you. These 25 additional questions are often referred to as "try-out" questions. These questions are being field tested or "pilot tested." In other words, they are being tested or tried out on exam takers to see if they are appropriate questions for future NCLEX-PN® examinations.

The maximum testing period is 5 hours. These 5 hours include a tutorial, sample questions, and breaks as well as answering the examination questions. If you are still testing at the end of 5 hours, you will receive no more questions. The maximum number of questions you can receive is 205. If you are testing and finish the 205th question, you will get no more questions. That is the end of your testing. The minimum number of questions you can receive is 85 carefully chosen questions. The NCSBN believes that this is the minimum number of questions that can determine whether you are a safe practitioner or not.

You will test until (1) the computer program determines that you have clearly met the test plan requirements, (2) you have failed, (3) you have answered 205 questions, or (4) you have run out of time. You can pass or fail with either the minimum number or the maximum number or any number between 85 and 205.

To understand how you can pass or fail with the same number of questions, it is helpful to realize that if you answer a question correctly, you will be given a harder question. If you answer a question incorrectly, you will be given an easier question. The computer ends your examination when it calculates with a 95% degree of confidence that you have tested in a way that indicates you are a safe/competent practitioner or you are not.

The National Council State Boards of Nursing (NCSBN) voted to raise the passing standard for the NCLEX-PN® exam effective April 1, 2008, in conjunction with the NCLEX-PN® 2008 Test Plan. The Council has been evaluating passing standards every 3 years since 1989. After consideration of all available information, the NCSBN Board of Directors determined that safe effective entry-level LPN/LVN practice required a greater level of knowledge, skills, and abilities than was required in 2005, when the NCSBN set the current standards. The passing standard was increased in response to changes in the U.S. healthcare delivery and nursing practice that have resulted in entry-level LPN/LVN caring for clients with multiple and complex health problems.

Alternate-Format Questions

The majority of items on the NCLEX-PN® are four-option, multiple-choice questions. Initially the exam offered only this type of question, but beginning in April 2003, alternate item formats were introduced into the examination. Alternate items are based on the current test plan and do not have an effect on the length of the test. Initially, less than 2% of the items in the question pool were of the alternate type. A candidate taking the minimum length examination might receive one item in the alternate format. This alternate format type of question gives the candidate the opportunity to demonstrate entry-level nursing competence in ways that are different from the standard multiple-choice items. Some of the alternate format question types ask the candidates to perform calculations without the benefit of selecting the answer from four answer options. Another form is a fill-in-the-blank question, which requires the candidate to type in an answer to the question. Some of the new items present four or more response options, and they may require the candidate to select more than one correct option. The final question type can be used to evaluate the candidate's skill. This type is referred to as a "Hot Spot." This item includes an anatomic drawing and requests the candidate to identify the appropriate spot for obtaining assessment information.

Specific example questions can be viewed at the NCSBN website or in the NCLEX-PN® Examination Candidate Bulletin.

Preparing and Reviewing for the Exam

PREPARING FOR THE EXAM

Have you ever been in a class where some of the students asked the instructor to cover only what would be on the exam, suggesting that if it is not on the exam, it is not important? This is not the way to prepare yourself for the licensure exam or to prepare yourself to provide good nursing care. Preparation begins the day you start your first nursing class and includes but is not limited to the following:

- Reading assignments for class
- Completing practice quizzes at the end of assigned chapters
- Using the computerized test banks that come with the texts to practice taking tests of key concepts
- Participating in class
- Learning **mnemonics** (techniques for developing memory)

Mnemonics can help you remember key concepts that you need to recall for the NCLEX-PN®, as well as important information for giving safe care to your clients. An example of a mnemonic for blood pressure readings is using the words "sit down." "Sit" stands for systolic as the first/top number; "down" stands for diastolic or the bottom/last number in a blood pressure reading. When you say "sit down," you think, "sit" is for systolic (the first number and the one on top); down is for diastolic (the bottom and last number in the blood pressure reading). Mnemonics are useful for any key things that you must remember quickly and retain forever, not just for a quiz, midterm, or final exam.

Box 64-3 ■ provides tips for preparing for the NCLEX-PN® if English is not your first language.

REVIEWING FOR THE EXAM

Review for the NCLEX-PN® examination needs to begin early. Plan to devote some time each day or a certain number of hours per week to such activities as working in an NCLEX-PN® review book or studying with a study group. Closer to the time of the examination, you can consider taking a professional review course for the NCLEX-PN® and taking a mock NCLEX-PN® examination. Some schools of nursing require students to take a mock NCLEX-PN® examination.

NCLEX-PN® Review Books

A variety of NCLEX-PN® review books have been published by major nursing publishing companies. These books do not contain the questions from the NCLEX-PN® itself. (The questions in that test bank are confidential.) However, these review books do contain similar questions and cover the key concepts as well as the areas and categories that are tested in the licensing exam. While the review books may vary in their presentation, most are divided into units of specialized content, each with a review of key concepts, a practice exam on the content, and a section of answers with rationales for the correct answer.

To maximize your readiness to take the exam, you need to begin using a review book long before you take the licensing exam (Figure 64-1 ■). You could start at least 6 months before the exam and try to review a set number of pages each day or each week so you will have sufficient time to firm up the key concepts in your mind. You would benefit from reviewing more than one NCLEX-PN® book. You and a fellow student might each buy different review books and trade books at some point.

BOX 64-3	CULTURAL PULSE POINTS

English as a Nonnative Language

Preparing for the licensure examination should begin early in nursing school. Many instructors incorporate NCLEX-PN®-style questions into their tests. Studying for quizzes and final exams will also help you to prepare for the NCLEX-PN®. If English is not your native language, you may encounter words, phrases, or expressions that are confusing. Create a section in your notebook to record these things that you do not understand from lecture reading or conversation. Leave space so that you can later record an explanation. It is not appropriate to interrupt the instructor for each one of these; but the instructor will be happy to explain them after class, especially if you have tried to sort them out for yourself.

The following is one example of confusing wording: The nurse *wound* a gauze bandage around the client's arm to hold the dressing over the *wound*.

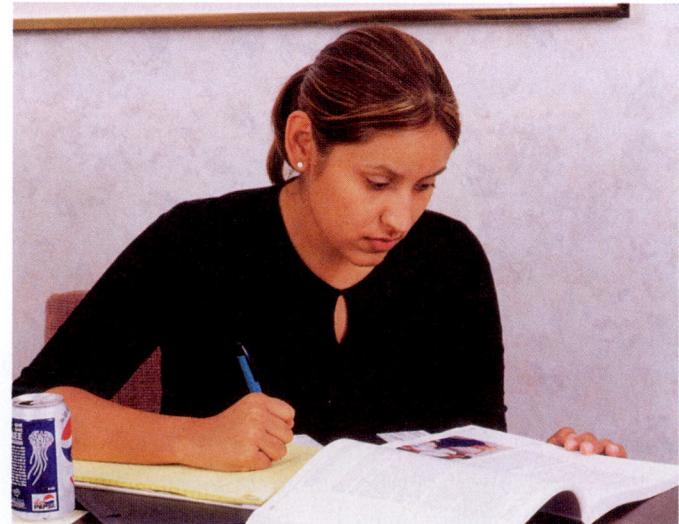

Figure 64-1. ■ Taking regular times to prepare for the NCLEX-PN® will help you study better and remember more.

Study Groups

In addition to using NCLEX-PN® review books, many students find they benefit from a study group. The study group can be used not only for course tests, but also to review and discuss the rationales for answers to questions in the review books. Setting aside time to work with a study group each week will benefit most students.

Some students claim that a study group only confuses them. Why is this? Occasionally, one or two students in a group monopolize the group's time or say things that are incorrect or not needed by the others in the group. When there is a disagreement about the correctness of information, suggest that notes or textbook be checked to verify the information. The test plan can be used to see if the questioned information is related to items in the test plan.

Study groups can establish at the outset that members take turns and that everyone will have a chance to ask and answer questions. Some students find it helpful to study with just one strong student. If group study simply does not work for you, try setting aside time to study in the library or a quiet place alone.

Professional Review Courses

Professional review courses are usually 1 to 2 days in length, requiring advanced registration and payment of a course fee. Your instructor, director of your program, or your state board of nursing will usually be able to advise you of dates and costs of these review courses.

Mock NCLEX-PN® Examinations

Some LPN/LVN programs require, or offer a chance for, students to take a mock NCLEX-PN® examination just prior to graduation. Although these examinations are not free, they do provide a student with a percentile score for each category of client needs found on the examination. The student receives information on questions he or she got wrong and a list of the correct answers, along with an explanation and the rationales for the correct answers and for the distracters for each question. If you can take a mock NCLEX-PN® exam, the information you receive on completion will help you to identify the areas where you need to focus your study time.

Evaluating Your Readiness to Take the Examination

You have finished your formal nursing program and received your diploma. Are you ready to take the NCLEX-PN®, or do you suppose putting off taking the exam would improve your chances of passing? Usually, people completing practical nursing programs are anxious to take the NCLEX-PN® soon after completing the program for several reasons. Taking the exam soon means you are taking it while you are accustomed to testing and while much of what you have learned is fresh in your mind. From a practical and economic standpoint, you may also want to get your license so you can make more money. You probably want to get to work as an LPN/LVN and sign your name with your title (LPN, or LVN if in Texas or California). If you did well on the mock NCLEX-PN® and/or if you have done well in answering most or all of the questions from all the various sections of your NCLEX-PN® review book or books, you will probably decide that you are ready to take the examination. You have many indicators that you have a great chance of passing the examination.

If you have indicators that you may not do well on the NCLEX-PN® exam, you should consider taking a review class. There are two types of classes. The first format reviews course work; the other is designed to prepare you to take the test. It provides test-taking tips and assistance in dealing with different types of questions. Time is also devoted to working through some of the psychological aspects of testing, such as test anxiety.

Delaying the exam does not necessarily improve your chances of passing the examination. In fact, there is some evidence that the probability of failure increases the longer a graduate waits.

It is important to remember that the NCLEX-PN® exam is testing your ability to be a safe entry-level practitioner. Don't let your fears prevent you from being successful.

Applying to Take the NCLEX-PN®

The National Council of State Boards of Nursing website has information on scheduling your NCLEX-PN® examination. You can also get this information by writing to NCSBN for a copy of the test plan. In general, you will do the following:

1. Fill out an application for a license to the board of nursing of your state or the state in which you wish to take the examination. The director of your nursing program or the faculty will probably provide you with an application for your state and will instruct you on the fees and the size and type of pictures that must be submitted with the application and any other requirements that must be met.

2. Meet all the board of nursing's eligibility requirements in order to get permission to take the NCLEX-PN® exam. Prospective student nurses need to know the eligibility requirements prior to enrolling in nursing school and need to review these early in their nursing education. The appropriate testing service will be advised of your eligibility.

3. Receive from the testing service an Authorization to Test and a booklet, which will tell you about the test centers and how to schedule your examination.

4. Register with, and schedule an appointment with, the testing service that has been selected by NCSBN to administer the examination, and pay the required fee for taking the examination. Beginning October 1, 2002, candidates schedule with Pearson Professional Testing to take the licensing examination.

Coping with Test Anxiety

Test anxiety seems to occur among students, as if on a continuum from low to high: from a normal mild level of uneasiness, which can be controlled easily and used as energy to do well on the exam, to a level of uneasiness and fear that immobilizes the test taker. Some students have a great deal of test anxiety before and/or during every quiz, midterm, and final exam and find themselves having difficulty focusing on the quiz or exam. Grades may suffer because of test anxiety. Other students seem to enjoy exams, concentrate fully, and look at them as a challenge.

WAYS TO OVERCOME TEST ANXIETY

If you are one of the students who are very nervous before or during tests, you need to start now to reduce your nervousness and anxiety around test taking. (See also Chapter 17 ⬥⬥.) You would probably benefit from working with a counselor on these issues. If your test anxiety is not overwhelming, some simple strategies may reduce it. Sit down in a quiet place and write down 10 things you think would help you to reduce your test anxiety. You are the expert on you and may be able to come up with exactly what you need. Perhaps you will have on your list some of the following suggestions:

1. Learn some relaxation techniques, such as closing your eyes and tensing then relaxing each part of your body, beginning at the head and neck and working downward. Think thoughts like "I am relaxing deeper and deeper" while breathing slowly and feeling your muscles relaxing. You are capable of relaxing yourself rather than saying things to yourself that create tension and uneasiness. Check with your library to see if they have a relaxation tape and some books on relaxation that you can check out.

2. Try picturing yourself taking the exam, being in control, and doing well with the answers to the questions.

3. Imagine your mind as a blackboard and erase any negative thoughts that lead to believing you might not do well. Write on your imaginary board, "I will do well on the test/exam."

4. Refuse to think about anything that you can't see, smell, feel, or touch. You can't see, feel, smell, or touch a worry about not doing well.

5. Desensitize yourself about your fear of failing a test. Take some short tests until you are doing well and seeing your success. Build up to bigger tests. You could enlist the help of an instructor.

6. Count from 10 to 1 when you begin to feel nervous.

Taking the Examination

Preparation on the day before and the day of the examination can help you arrive at the test prepared and relaxed. Try following these suggestions:

1. Do not cram the night before the examination. Relax your body and your mind. This could mean a pleasant movie or light reading. Some people relax by doing relaxation exercises or yoga or relaxing in warm water.

2. It is usually best to avoid using stimulants or depressants the evening before the examination. This includes caffeine drinks, alcohol, and other forms of stimulants and depressants.

3. Select some comfortable clothing for the next day. Perhaps something "layered" so you can take something off or put something on in case it is too warm or too cool for your comfort in the testing room.

4. Lay out anything you will have to take to the examination with you. This includes your instructions, required forms of identification, and your vehicle keys. You don't want to be searching for your vehicle keys when it is time to leave for the examination. You may want to take a power snack and a bottle of water to the examination with you to consume on your 10-minute break during the examination.

5. Get sufficient sleep the night before taking the test. Go to bed at the usual time and arise at the usual time. If crises are apt to occur at your home, make plans to sleep in a more restful environment. Getting into an argument with your roommate, significant other, or spouse the night before the exam will almost always not help you do well on the exam.

The day of the examination:

1. Eat moderately and finish your meal at least 1 to 2 hours before the exam. Avoid sugared foods, and include some protein in your meal. This will mean that you will have a more stable blood sugar than you would from just eating sugared foods. Do not rush your meal or overeat before the examination. If you overeat, blood will leave your brain to aid in digestion. This is blood you need to keep your brain working.

2. Be certain you have the required identification with you as you leave home to go to the examination.

3. Wear a watch. When taking the NCLEX-PN® computer examination, you can take as long as you wish to review a question (also referred to as an item) and select an answer. Consider two things in deciding how long to take in reviewing a question and trying to determine

the answer: (a) Once you have recorded your answer, the question will disappear and you cannot get it back. You will have to answer the question on the screen before you can get another question. Even if you need to guess, you must answer each question. (b) You will have 5 hours for the exam, so while you don't have to rush, you cannot afford to take a half hour or more per question. Taking an extremely long time to answer a question will not increase your chances of getting the right answer and will probably increase your anxiety.

4. Push negative thoughts out of your mind. Replace negative thoughts with positive ones.

5. You will receive instructions and practice questions before the actual exam begins. You will not need prior computer experience to take the examination because you will only be using the cursor, the space bar, and the enter key and there are no other functional keys. The use of the computer has been made very simple.

6. Don't waste time looking for a pattern to the answers or making your educated guesses based on a pattern. All answers are random.

7. There will be very few if any questions that ask you to determine the answer that is "not correct" or the action that is "inappropriate." However, you need to read your questions very carefully to determine exactly what the question is asking. Answer what is being asked. The choices may include a correct statement that does not answer the question. Reading the question carefully will help you avoid selecting the statement that is correct but is not the right answer.

8. When answering questions, discipline yourself to answer based on the idea that the vast majority of the time your selected answer is true or best. Some test takers miss questions because they are searching for the one instance they know of, or have heard of, in which this answer might not be true or best.

9. If you find yourself not liking the question or wishing it were reworded, put your feelings aside and just do your best to answer the question as it is.

10. Concentrate fully on the exam. If you find yourself being distracted, tell yourself to focus and concentrate deeper.

Waiting for Your Results

Stay calm while waiting for your results. Your state board of nursing will mail your results in about a month. Only your board of nursing can release your exam results to you. Some states provide a 900-telephone number that the candidate can call for a fee. If your state participates, you will be given the information on when and how to obtain results by phone.

During the waiting period you may find that you are recalling and worrying about some questions you feel certain that you missed on the examination. While looking up the answers so you will have this knowledge, you want to try to avoid worrying because some of the questions you missed are likely to be the pilot questions that do not count against you and almost everyone will miss some of the "real" questions.

The best news that you can receive is that you have passed the examination. In this event, you are now an LPN (or, if you are testing in Texas or California, you are an LVN). Congratulations! You now have all the benefits and responsibilities of being an LPN/LVN. Your lifelong learning continues.

The only other news you could receive is that you have failed the examination. Failing the exam means two things: One is that you need to identify any factors that you could change to increase your chances of passing. The other is that you need to develop a plan to prepare yourself better to take the examination.

A **diagnostic profile** is provided to candidates who fail the examination. The diagnostic profile is mailed to these candidates by their respective boards of nursing, along with the results of the examination. The profile aids candidates in determining their areas of relative strength and weakness based on the test plan and in designing their study accordingly, prior to retaking the exam.

Stop any worrying that you are doing and begin to prepare. Do not say anything negative to or about yourself. This only wastes energy you need in preparing to take and pass the examination. You might make and hang some posters saying "SUCCESS" or "I WILL BE SUCCESSFUL" in your study area. If that isn't possible, then put sticky notes with that message in your study book.

There is a minimum number of days set by the NCSBN that you must wait before retaking the NCLEX-PN®. Your state board of nursing can set a longer period of time, but not a shorter period. This time period is of course designed to allow you time to prepare yourself for success.

If you failed the examination, you will benefit from doing some or all of the following:

- Talking with the director of your nursing program
- Working on a plan to be prepared when you retake the examination
- Getting a tutor
- Taking a review course
- Obtaining another NCLEX-PN® review book
- Spending more time reviewing
- Getting professional help for test anxiety

Note: The references and resources for all chapters have been compiled at the back of the book.

Chapter Review

KEY Points

- Preparation for the NCLEX-PN® examination needs to begin when a student first enters the school of nursing.
- Students must pass the NCLEX-PN® test in order to practice. The plan takes into consideration the legal scope of practical/vocational nursing of each state and a practical/vocational nursing job analysis.
- The purpose of the NCLEX-PN® examination is to protect the public by ensuring that all who pass and receive a license to practice have the entry-level competencies needed to practice safely and effectively.
- Test questions on the NCLEX-PN® are at the cognitive levels of knowledge, comprehension, application, and analysis.
- The test plan is organized around four categories of client needs across the life span in a variety of settings. The categories of human needs are safe, effective care environment, health promotion and maintenance, psychosocial integrity, and physiological integrity.
- The maximum testing period is 5 hours with the maximum number of questions being 205 and the minimum 85. A student can pass or fail with the minimum or maximum number of questions or any number in between.
- Mnemonics are a way to help a person recall key concepts.
- It is a good idea to get an NCLEX-PN® review book and begin using this book at least 6 months before taking the NCLEX-PN® examination. Study groups and review groups also help most students do better on the NCLEX-PN®.
- Readiness for the NCLEX-PN® can be judged by looking at one's performance on tests and examinations in the nursing program, performance on mock NCLEX-PN® examinations, and results of practice tests in an NCLEX-PN® review book.

- Learning techniques for reducing test anxiety can greatly improve your NCLEX-PN® results.
- Prepare before the examination by avoiding stimulants or depressants the night before the test, determining the route to the examination, laying out everything needed for the examination ahead of time, relaxing, and getting enough sleep.
- Pace yourself during the exam so you can finish within 5 hours. Do not waste time looking for patterns to answers. Select the best answer, and concentrate fully on the examination.

FOR FURTHER Study

For information about test taking and types of questions, see Chapter 1.

See Chapter 2 for more on multistate compacts.

For in-depth discussion about the nursing process, see Chapter 6.

For more information about stress and coping, see Chapter 17.

NCLEX-PN® Exam Preparation

1 When is the best time for a student who is enrolled in a practical nursing program to begin preparing for the NCLEX-PN®?

1. On the first day of the nursing program
2. After the completion of the first nursing course
3. Six months before completion of the program
4. As soon as the nursing program is completed

2 The graduate nurse is asked to answer this question: When is the best time for a student who is enrolled in a practical nursing program to begin preparing for the NCLEX-PN®? This question is an example of testing at which of the following levels of comprehension?

1. Knowledge
2. Comprehension
3. Application
4. Analysis

3 The NCLEX-PN® examination is revised periodically with the time period for review based on:

1. An annual analysis of question security.
2. Completion of a job analysis of the tasks of the LPN/LVN.
3. Requests from member states of the National Council of State Boards of Nursing.
4. Substantial changes in the nurse practice acts of the states.

4 To prepare for the NCLEX-PN®, a nursing student needs what degree of computer expertise?

1. Extensive
2. Above average
3. Average
4. None

5 A student nurse worries before, during, and after tests during nursing courses because the tests are so difficult. Which of the following actions would be best?

1. Use the grievance procedure and complain about the test difficulty.
2. Seek help in designing effective methods of studying and relaxing.
3. Talk with peers about their worries.
4. Wait and see if it gets easier in other courses with other teachers.

6 The night before taking the NCLEX-PN®, it is usually best to go to bed at which of the following times?

1. About 8 to 10 hours before time to awaken
2. No later than midnight
3. The usual bedtime
4. Whenever you feel tired

7 The new graduate practices answering NCLEX-PN® style questions and feels as though the questions do not test the information that was memorized. The best explanation for this is:

1. The important facts are not being studied.
2. The nurse is having difficulty memorizing enough information.
3. The teacher is not very good at writing tests on what was taught.
4. The level of the testing is at comprehension, analysis, or synthesis.

8 Which one of the following represents categories of testing on client needs?

1. Treatments and medications
2. Gastrointestinal and urological disorders
3. Safety and legalities
4. Physiological integrity and psychosocial integrity

9 The best time for the nursing student to apply to take the NCLEX-PN® is:

1. Upon enrollment in the nursing program.
2. Within 6 months of graduating.
3. Six months or more after graduation.
4. As soon as possible after graduation.

10 After taking the NCLEX-PN®, the nurse should:

1. Go home, stare at the clock, and wait to hear about results.
2. Go home, go to bed, and set the alarm clock for 48 hours later.
3. Attempt to stay as busy as possible to make time go faster.
4. Call friends and plan to go out for drinks to celebrate.

Answers and rationales for Review Questions appear in Appendix I.

Finding That First Job

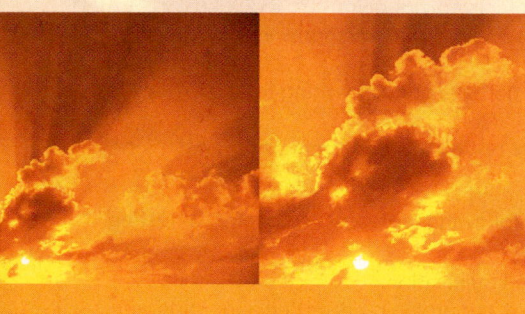

LEARNING Outcomes

After completing this chapter, you will be able to:

1. Describe the components of a portfolio.
2. Develop a cover letter for an entry-level job.
3. Identify steps in preparing a résumé.
4. Describe the interviewing process and list ways to have a successful interview.
5. Identify important aspects of the job search process.
6. Explain the concepts of orientation, probationary period, and performance evaluation as they apply to the hiring process.
7. Name ways to succeed and prove yourself in your first job.
8. Identify ways to continue moving up a career ladder in the nursing profession.

KEY TERMS

Use the audio glossary feature on the MyNursingKit Website to hear the correct pronunciation of the following key terms.

career ladder 1800   **orientation** 1799   **profession** 1799

collaborative 1801   **performance evaluation** 1799   **professionalism** 1799

cover letter 1791   **portfolio** 1791   **résumé** 1793

networking 1801   **probationary period** 1799

There are many differences between student and graduate nurses. Once you are out of school, reality hits. Like most new graduates you probably feel unprepared, overwhelmed, and scared. The good news is that no employer, whether a hospital or other agency, expects you to know everything. You will continue to learn as you begin your first job. You may even come to think of that first position as being another phase of your education.

You may be realizing a lifelong dream to be a nurse, embarking on a new career, or returning to the workforce. No matter what it was that brought you to this place, you are now a new member of a profession who has much to contribute to it. This chapter provides you with a survival plan as you transition from student to licensed practical/vocational nurse.

To make the transition from student to licensed nurse, you will need to make preparations. It is not unlike planning a trip abroad. You need to decide where you want to go, be sure you have all your documents, prepare the appropriate wardrobe, and have your timeline and contact people clearly in mind.

You may have a facility in mind where you would like to work. It may be one you were assigned to as a student, where you have worked as an unlicensed healthcare worker, or one that was recruiting at a job fair. Learn as much as you can about the facility and its parent company before making an application.

Portfolio

Your next step is to review your **portfolio.** A portfolio is defined as an itemized visual account of your skills and best practices that are related to the position you are seeking. It is a working portfolio so that when you leave your schooling you are prepared to walk into an interview with all the information needed to emphasize your strengths, education, and experience and to present yourself as a professional LPN/LVN. You will compile your portfolio so that it demonstrates your capabilities and competencies. Compiling your portfolio does not happen overnight. Ideally, you should begin developing it about halfway into your nursing program.

A leather-type, three-ring binder is an appropriate way to display your personal portfolio. A complete portfolio includes:

- Title page
- Table of contents

- Cover letter/introduction letter
- Application
- Résumé
- Work samples (two):
  - Nursing care plans
  - Narrative charting samples
  - Lesson plan
- Writing samples (one):
  - Case studies
  - Module research projects
  - Observation studies
- Student reflection
- Community service
- Clinical evaluations
- Awards/achievements
- Recommendation letters
- Sample thank-you letter
- Sample resignation letter

The portfolio is an ideal place to store copies of your license, CPR card, or other certifications (e.g., intravenous or blood withdrawal). You also may wish to include a list of references with their contact information and a sample completed application. These will be helpful when asked to fill out an application on site.

COVER LETTER

The **cover letter** you write will contain essential information that gives you the opportunity to sell yourself. This letter is what potential employers read about you and it helps them determine whether they want to find out more about your qualifications. It should be brief and to the point, but highlight your best professional and educational attributes. This concise one-page letter must reflect correct grammar, spelling, and appropriate format.

Do your homework, find out who you are addressing, make a point to correctly spell the person's name, and establish their title or position. The cover letter is a first impression—think about what you do with mail that is addressed to "occupant." It usually gets tossed in the round file and that is not what you want done with your cover letter and résumé.

The introductory paragraph should immediately explain the letter's purpose. Begin by introducing yourself. Explain your intent to apply for the position of licensed practical/vocational nurse. Give the details of your response to an ad, job listing, website, or other source that disclosed this job offering. A new graduate should include the school attended and date of graduation.

The body or second paragraph is where your highlighted qualifications are contained. This is where your enthusiasm for this particular job is addressed. State how you have been prepared by your education. Describe briefly the skills and strengths that you will contribute to the position. Write about what sets you apart from the other applicants. Include a statement about the organization and why you want to be part of a "recognized staff and organization." This is the time to write about your experience and competencies. If you have limited clinical experience, mention your diverse clinical rotations. Include major accomplishments and awards. Remember this is your first position in this capacity, so you should avoid using such words as *best, expert,* and *excellent* to describe yourself. Avoid flowery words or phrases that do not reflect professional qualities. Write out any industry-specific abbreviations you may be using.

The closing paragraph restates your interest and conveys your anticipation in obtaining an interview. Indicate when and how you will follow up your letter. Refer to your enclosed résumé.

Include your name, address, and telephone number. Printed letterhead is acceptable. Use the same quality bond paper for both your cover letter and résumé. Cream, beige, or light gray paper is suggested. Review your letter for errors and have someone else read it. If it is computer generated, use the spelling and grammar checks. Box 65-1 ■ shows a sample cover letter.

APPLICATION

Filling out an application may seem like an easy task; however, the more attention you pay to details, the better you represent yourself to your potential employer. Practice completing an application; never leave lines blank. If something is not applicable to you, write "N/A" in the space provided. Type the application if you can; if you are completing it in the office, be neat, legible, avoid abbreviations, and use ink. Have all the information required at your fingertips—being prepared is to your advantage. If you plan to apply to a facility you have worked at as a student, ask for an application and practice completing it. Some employers have their applications online.

BOX 65-1 SAMPLE COVER LETTER

> Mary J. Fuller, LPN
> 4123 W. Green Street
> Martinsville, Iowa 92222
> (999) 555-1212
> e-mail mjf24@aol.com

[date]
Roseanne Blake, RN
Director of Nurses
St. Catherine's Hospital
1002 Main Street
Marysville, Iowa 92223

Dear Ms. Blake:

It is with great interest that I apply for the licensed practical nurse position advertised in the *Marysville Times* on Sunday. I am a recently licensed practical nurse, having completed the nursing program at the Waterloo Vocational and Technical School.

I have more than 7 years of experience as a certified nursing assistant in the acute care setting. My background as a nursing assistant and the clinical experience obtained during my practical nursing program have built a firm foundation for my first nursing position.

I graduated first in my class and received the faculty award for clinical excellence. I received a silver medal in practical nursing skills at the Health Occupation Students of America National Leadership Conference in June. I will consider any clinical area, depending on your needs. I am enthusiastic and dependable, and I am committed to quality client care.

I have enclosed my résumé for your consideration. If you need additional information, please feel free to contact me at my home number listed above. Thank you for your time and consideration. I will call your office next week to discuss further the possibilities of employment.

Sincerely,
Mary J. Fuller, LPN [signature]
Mary J. Fuller, LPN
Enclosure

RESUMÉ

The **resumé** is a concise systematic summary of your professional experience and educational background. This is a marketing tool to give your potential employer a snapshot glimpse into your nursing background and experience. A one-page document is preferred, with two pages being the maximum. Remember, if you are too wordy or if the employer has to search to find required information, your resumé may end up being ignored. This document needs to be well planned, informative, and organized. Take the time necessary to be precise, neat, and accurate.

There are three types of resumé formats: chronological, functional, and a combination of the two. The chronological format highlights your employment in reverse chronological order and is the most traditional. The functional format emphasizes skills. The combination uses both. Chronological style is discussed in the following paragraphs.

Curriculum vitae (CV) is a Latin term meaning "course of life." Some human resource people may use this term when talking about a resumé. A CV is a personal history of one's education, professional history, and job qualifications with a strong emphasis on specific skills relating to the position for which the person is applying. A CV is more frequently used by professionals further along in their careers.

To prepare your resumé, you first need to assemble data that illustrates your professional qualifications. It is important for a new graduate to evaluate accomplishments that would give a potential employer insight into your work ethic and commitment. Include areas in community service or service as a class officer. Listing Health Occupations Students of America competitive event awards, scholarships, or honors would be appropriate. Employment experience includes dates, positions, and employing agency. Educational history includes years of education attendance, graduation, school name, location, certification, and diploma information. Usually it is presented in a reverse chronological order. The first entry is the most current and you work backward from there. Note that references are available upon request. You should have a copy of your references, their addresses, and phone numbers typed/computer generated on a single sheet of paper that you keep handy in your portfolio in case of a request. Three to four references are adequate. Be sure to contact them to obtain permission to use their names and phone numbers. Two should be professionals connected to the type of job you are seeking. The others can be personal references.

Most resumés are computer generated today, but at the very least, it must be typed on quality paper and should be on the same light-colored paper (off white, beige, light gray) that you used for your cover letter. Many computer resumé programs are available; you may want to start there. However, you want it individualized to you. Many students

BOX 65-2	ACTION WORDS
Accomplished	Observed
Achieved	Organized
Analyzed	Planned
Built	Presented
Chaired	Prevented
Collaborated	Provided
Communicated	Reduced
Created	Reorganized
Delegated	Served
Designed	Simplified
Developed	Standardized
Devoted	Studied
Dispensed	Taught
Ensured	Transformed
Evaluated	Unified
Expanded	Validated
Focused	Worked
Formulated	Wrote
Implemented	

have learned to use graphics from computer files, but remember to keep your resumé professional—no hearts or stethoscopes to detract from the purpose and content. Have an experienced professional nurse review your resumé for spelling, grammatical errors, and appearance. Use action words to describe your qualifications. (Box 65-2 ■ lists action words.) This is not a document to be taken lightly and will take more than one draft to complete. Use a consistent format and follow it throughout the document.

Resumé Components

A sample resumé is shown in Figure 65-1 ■. The heading includes your name, complete address, phone number, and an e-mail address. Remember when you have sent a resumé, you may receive a call, so make sure your message machine is working properly and there is a professional message left for callers. Additionally, if your e-mail address is not professional, you may want to have a separate address for work-related business.

A job objective is next, although not everyone agrees that you need an objective on your resumé today. In your objective you are stating your professional career goal. You can be general in your goal or more specific. This will help the Human Resource Department determine whether you may be qualified for the position they need to fill. Your job objective should be one sentence.

A summary is used to assist a new nurse to stress strong points but be sure to include why you are qualified to meet your objective. You can bullet it for easier reading.

Luz Marina Balderas
555 Main Street
Any Town, CA 99999
(555)555-1234
lmbalderas@internet.com

OBJECTIVES:

To obtain a challenging position in the Nursing QI/QM field where I can utilize my clinical knowledge and quality management experience in an environment that will promote career and educational opportunities.

SKILLS:

Project Management:	• Time management and project deadline compliance • Critical thinking and conflict resolution • Data collection and statistical data analysis • Delegation and team work management
Business:	• Accurately type and enter data, 120 words per minute. • Computer proficiency in Word, Excel, Access, PowerPoint, E-Z Cap, SPSS, MedCore • Strong customer relations background • Public speaking and project presentation experience • Employee training and compliance assurance • Policy and procedure development and implementation

EXPERIENCE:

Position:	Market Research Analyst
Company:	MedPartners, Inc.
Location:	Long Beach, California
Employment:	September 2004 through July 2009

Position:	IPA Quality Improvement Coordinator
Company:	MedPartners, Inc.
Location:	Long Beach, California
Employment:	June 1998 through September 2004

Position:	QI Nursing Representative
Company:	MedPartners, Inc.
Location:	Long Beach, California
Employment:	May 1996 through June 1998

Position:	Specialty Clinic – Back Office Medical Assistant
Company:	MedPartners, Inc.
Location:	Long Beach, California
Employment:	July 1994 through May 1996

Figure 65-1. ■ Sample résumé.

Luz Marina Balderas
555 Main Street
Any Town, CA 99999
(555)555-1234
lmbalderas@internet.com

Page 2

EDUCATION:

North Orange County ROP:	Licensed Vocational Nursing Program	Aug. 2007 - July 2009
Cypress Community College:	Limited X-Ray Technician Program	Sept. 1991 - Sept. 1993
Cerritos Community College:	Medical Assisting Program	Sept. 1989 - Sept. 1991
Downey Adult Ed. Program:	Nurses' Assistant Program	July 1989 - Dec. 1990
University of Calif., Irvine:	Bachelor's in Science - Psychology	Sept. 1985 - June 1989

AWARDS & ACHIEVEMENTS:

Kaiser Permanente Health Care Issues State Scholarship: 1st Place, March 2009
HOSA State Leadership Conference: Gold Medallist - Pathophysiology, March 2009
HOSA State Leadership Conference: Bronze Medallist - Bio Medical Debate, March 2009
Kaiser Permanente Health Care Issues National Scholarship: 1st Place, June 2009
HOSA National Leadership Conference: Gold Medallist - Pathophysiology, June 2009
HOSA National Leadership Conference: 1st Place - Health Education Pilot Event, June 2009
Class Valedictorian: NOCROP – LVN Program, Graduating Nursing Class A, July 2009

PRESENTATIONS:

"Cushing's Syndrome"	NOCROP – LVN Program, Pharmacology Module, October 2008
"Traumatic Head Injuries"	NOCROP – LVN Program, Neurology Module, May 2009

CERTIFICATIONS & LICENSES:

Basic Cardiac Life Support Certification
Phlebotomy Certified
Medical Assistant Certification
Limited X-Ray License: Expired
Nursing Assistant Certification: Expired

REFERENCES:

Available upon request

Figure 65-1. ■ *Continued.*

EDUCATION. In this section you will want to start with your most recent education. Include the name of the school, and then enter city and state. List your certification, license, degree or focus of education, and graduation date. Follow through with other educational background.

EXPERIENCE. Again, start with your most recent or current work experience. Include fulltime and parttime employment; clearly state the position succinctly and dates employed. Describe the duties and responsibilities assigned. Your work history is important to employers and they look for gaps in time. Use the same format as you did with your education.

ACHIEVEMENTS. This section highlights your value to the employer. As a student, your accomplishments are important; use them to your advantage. Perfect attendance, faculty awards for clinical excellence, academic excellence awards, and Health Occupations Students of America competitive awards would demonstrate value. Include community service; it displays personal commitment and involvement. Intravenous therapy and blood withdrawal and telemetry classes are additional skills that may increase your marketability.

You may be allowed to e-mail résumés to prospective employers, which is a quick and efficient way to cover a lot of ground electronically. Human Resources can keep you on file for positions that become available. Keep your e-mail short and concise; let your prospective employer know if you are willing to relocate. Identify the position for which you are applying. Don't forget to attach your résumé to your e-mail.

Interviews

Being asked to do an interview means that the employer is interested in what they have read in your cover letter and résumé. This is where you sell yourself to the employer. A face-to-face meeting gives a first impression. Whether it results in employment or not, it is an experience that will provide you with insight into your ability to speak logically and think critically. Did you get your message across? Did your nervousness get the best of you or did practice pay off? One-on-one interviews are less nerve wracking, but nowadays you may be faced with two or three interviewers firing questions at you during one interview.

TIPS FOR A SUCCESSFUL INTERVIEW

Professional dress means different things to different people. What does it mean to you? For a male, it is a conservative suit, dress shirt, and tie. Men should be clean-shaven or beards must be trimmed and neat. For the female it means a medium-length skirt with a blouse and jacket. (If you are tugging at your skirt when you sit, it is too short. If you

have to ask, "Is this appropriate?" find something else to wear.) A pantsuit, however, is permissible. Avoid plunging necklines and skirts with thigh-high slits. Clothes should be neatly pressed. Closed toed shoes with hose/nylons are proper dress. Wearing your uniform is regarded sufficient; however, remember you are trying to make an impression. A clean, controlled hairstyle is paramount. One set of stud earrings and neutral moderate makeup and nails are essential. Hygiene is understood.

Arrive at the interview at least 15 minutes early. Identify yourself at the front desk or with the secretary and state who you are to meet with.

You are in charge of your attitude. Be positive, polite, and confident. Your enthusiasm for the position comes across to the panel and even if you are not the most qualified and experienced, that refreshing attitude can have an effect on your rating. Convince the interviewer(s) about your commitment and motivation. Be aware of your verbal and nonverbal communication. Avoid the phrases "You guys," "Like, you know," and be aware of how many "umms" you might say. If your hands tend to shake, put them in your lap. Also avoid touching and playing with your hair.

The previous interview may extend into your assigned time. If that happens, be patient. Review what you know about the facility and staff. Show sincere interest and articulate why you have chosen this facility for application, if and when the opportunity arises. For example, it might be the compassionate care that you observed firsthand as a student. It might be the renowned staff and cutting-edge cancer research or the physician–nurse respect and interdisciplinary approach used to care for clients. If you don't have firsthand information about the facility, you might want to research it via its website or speak with staff members.

When you enter the interview offices, use a firm handshake with each panel member. Smile to break the ice, and once again state your name clearly. Address the panel members by Miss, Mrs., Mr., respectively. Remain standing until you are asked to take a seat. Avoid fidgeting, sit upright and a little forward in the chair, and be attentive. Do not chew gum during an interview; it leaves a negative impact. Eye contact conveys confidence and credibility in your answers. Answer questions succinctly but completely; use examples if appropriate. Roughly 6 to 10 questions will be asked. Be interesting and avoid rambling. The usual time period for an interview is 15 to 20 minutes. Discuss your qualifications and experiences related to the position. As a new graduate you can use your clinical rotation and any associated work experiences. Offer your portfolio for their review; point out highlights that you feel would be of particular interest.

When the interview is finished, the interviewer will ask you about any questions you may have. Have at least two questions ready to pose. Suitable questions to be considered might be:

- What is the normal staffing-to-client ratio?
- What type of continuing education or classes are offered, and is there a fee?
- Does this organization offer tuition reimbursement for higher education?
- How long is the new graduate orientation and what is the process?
- What are fulltime benefits?
- Are there job advancement or level changes?
- When and how will you be notified about their decision concerning the position?
- What is the involvement of the nursing staff in community service?

Points of view differ on asking questions about salary. One view is that it isn't discussed until the job is offered. However, if you have a salary requirement and entry level is unacceptable, it is better to clarify this early in the process.

Express your appreciation for the interviewers' time and for the opportunity to interview for this position. Shake hands with the panel and exit promptly. Write a short thank-you note following the interview; it reminds the interviewer of your interest. To be effective, the note should be received within a week of the interview. To be prepared for an interview, you must practice and rehearse a variety of questions. Mock interviews will help you gain poise and allow you to think about what you need to modify before you are in the midst of an actual interview. Box 65-3 ■ lists examples of interview questions. Refer to Box 65-4 ■ for a rubric on interview skills. Reviewing this rubric will assist you to self-evaluate your abilities in this area.

Illegal Questions

Some questions cannot be legally asked by interviewers. The Federal Civil Rights Act and state laws protect citizens against these questions, and you are not required to answer them. However, should such a question be asked, be prepared to tactfully decline to answer or veer the discussion to another topic. Avoid putting the panel on the defensive. If you point out an illegal question, the interview—and your chance at a position—may be terminated early.

Examples of illegal questions include:

- Are you married?
- What are your child care arrangements?
- What is your religion?
- How old are you? What is your birth date?
- Where were you born?
- Race-related questions.

There are ways to reply to such questions that will not alienate the interviewer. Reply to unlawful questions in a controlled manner. Do not offer more personal information than is necessary. Maintain a positive attitude; keep your voice conversational and upbeat. If an interviewer consistently asks personal questions, think twice about taking that job.

Suggested responses to this type of questioning include:

- I'm not sure how that question pertains to this position.
- Child care arrangements are not an issue. Please do not be concerned.
- If you mean am I over 18, yes I am.

Now that you have completed the interview process, you will need to patiently wait for the panel to make their decision and check your references. If during the interview they told you when they would be making their decision, it is permissible to call the human resource or nursing office after that time to check on the status of the position. Making this call can be difficult, but it will let you know

---

BOX 65-3   EXAMPLES OF INTERVIEW QUESTIONS

- Initially the interviewer will ask you to describe your education and experience as it relates to the position.
- What is one quality you like about yourself?
- How would you handle an irritated family member?
- What can you bring or contribute to this company or facility?
- What interested you in applying for this facility?
- Where do you see yourself in 5 years?
- How would you handle a combative client?
- How do you view yourself as a worker?
- What skill, personal or professional, do you feel you need improvement on to make you a better employee?
- How do you rate yourself in the area of problem solving on a scale of 1 to 5, with 5 being the highest? Describe the process used and give an example. Remember to use the nursing process!

- What are your strengths/weaknesses and elaborate on each?
- What do you like most about your job?
- What are some things you have learned from clients?
- What would you do if you believed a doctor was causing harm to a client?
- If you were asked to do something out of your scope of practice, what would be your course of action?
- If you could change one thing in nursing, what would it be and why?
- As a new graduate, why would I hire you over someone with 2 years of experience?
- What is the biggest issue facing nursing today?
- How do you feel about floating to an area unfamiliar to you?

BOX 65-4 INTERVIEW RUBRIC

Interview Skills

A successful interviewee . . .

- Exhibits professional dress and demeanor.
- Arrives early for the interview, with all necessary documents.
- Speaks clearly and confidently about skills and qualifications.
- Uses effective verbal and nonverbal communication skills.

Advanced

- Arrives early for the interview, with all necessary documents, and exhibits professionalism in both appearance and demeanor.
- Can list important documents that may be requested at the interview, including the following: résumé; letters of reference; work samples; and photocopies of diplomas, awards, certificates, driver's license, Social Security card, and any military papers.
- Demonstrates appropriate verbal and nonverbal communication before, during, and after the interview, shaking hands and making eye contact with all interviewers. He/she demonstrates a high degree of knowledge of the company and/or position and demonstrates interest by asking a minimum of two appropriate questions.
- Answers all interview questions in an organized, professional manner, using supporting details and/or examples.
- Uses language appropriate to the available position, uses pleasant demeanor and voice tone.
- Demonstrates interview follow-up by writing a thank-you letter to the interviewer and/or calling the company to inquire about the company's hiring decision in a sophisticated, professional manner.
- Understands the importance of following up the interview.

Proficient

- Arrives early for the interview, with all necessary documents, and exhibits professionalism in both appearance and demeanor.
- Can explain the purpose of a job interview. Questions are answered clearly and confidently, using language appropriate to the available position.
- May be missing some supporting details and/or examples.
- Uses clear oral delivery but may need improvement in one or two of the following areas: tone of voice, pace, energy, and/or nonverbal communication.
- Demonstrates interview follow-up, including writing a thank-you letter to the interviewer and/or calling the company to inquire about the company's hiring decision.
- Demonstrates some interest in asking a question about the position or company.

Basic

Does not demonstrate a basic understanding of the job interview, as indicated by any of the following behaviors:

- Does not arrive early and/or is missing necessary documents.
- Does not exhibit professional dress and demeanor.
- Does not answer questions completely or use supporting details and/or examples.
- Demonstrates deficiencies in three or more of the following areas of oral delivery: tone of voice, pace, energy, and/or nonverbal communication.
- Asks no questions of the interviewer.
- Does not follow up on the interview.

Source: Courtesy of Lynne Porter, RN, North Orange County, RUP, Anaheim, CA.

---

if you are still being considered or if you should pursue other options.

Job Search

There are many ways to look for potential practical/vocational nurse positions. Many companies advertise on the Internet, and you can check the newspaper ads, job boards, nursing magazines, and where you currently work. Some job fairs are just for nursing positions. Make a list of questions before applying to an organization. Decide what priorities you want in a position. These are a few examples:

- What information does the advertisement give you on the organization?
- What experience is required?
- Is there a hiring-on benefit?
- Do nurses work 8- or 12-hour shifts?
- Starting pay?
- Is there advancement for an LPN/LVN?
- Is there a plan for school reimbursement?
- Does the organization provide continuing education classes and is there a fee for employees?

- What benefits are available?
- Who is the contact person?

On the Internet, you can find the average salaries for LPNs/LVNs. This will help you determine where the organization stands in comparison to the average for the county, state, and nation in which you are applying.

WORK SAMPLES

Work samples are items used in the workplace. Individualized nursing care plans you have developed are an excellent way to display your critical thinking skills. Charting is a most important presentation of your writing skills related to the workplace. It demonstrates your flexibility in charting using different methods and strategies of documentation. Lesson plans for client teaching under the direction of the RN will establish further evidence of problem-solving and intervention skills. Compile this information as you progress through your program to underscore your strengths in the nursing field.

WRITING SAMPLES

Effective writing that is organized, clear, and uses correct grammar and spelling is a meaningful workplace skill. Use a sample of your work that is researched and includes a bibliography. This item stresses your ability to write in a logical order using correct format and shows your attention to details. Journaling or a student reflection piece would serve as an additional writing sample.

COMMUNITY SERVICE

This is documentation of your giving back to the community. Society looks to the nursing professions for leadership and guidance. Health professionals' involvement in community service demonstrates commitment and dedication to organizations that contribute to the well-being of the community. An employer would consider this a positive attribute.

CLINICAL EVALUATION

Provide a copy of your best evaluation signed by your clinical instructor. This instructor may also be on your recommendation list.

SAMPLE THANK-YOU LETTER

A brief thank-you letter to the interviewers can remind them of you and your abilities. Be positive about the interview process and thank them for their time and consideration; use correct grammar and spelling. Having a sample letter in your portfolio will make this a simple task when needed.

LETTER OF RESIGNATION

It is customary to write a letter of resignation for your position when you are leaving. Two weeks of notice is appropriate. Be positive about your work environment and position; thank your employers for the experience and professional growth you have gained. The first person you notify about your resignation should be your manager; it is not wise to have him or her hear it through the grapevine. The appropriate reasons for leaving are new challenges, increase in pay, relocation, family matters, or career advancements.

Hiring Process

When you receive an offer of employment, you will be very excited. Contain yourself long enough to get all the details as well as time and dates of your orientation. If you have received more than one job offer and need time to make a decision, thank the caller for the offer and state that you will get back to them at a specific time with your answer.

ORIENTATION

Orientation is the program or time period provided for newly hired individuals to prepare themselves to take on the responsibilities of the position for which they were employed.

Most facilities have new hires complete paperwork during the first day of orientation, although you may be required to complete a physical, drug test, or fingerprinting prior to that date. It is a good idea to ask about proper dress for the first orientation day—business attire or a nursing uniform? Be sure you know where to park and the exact time and place to

---

BOX 65-5	PROFESSIONAL CHARACTERISTICS AND BEHAVIORS

A practicing nurse (LPN/LVN) should possess professional qualities of warmth and empathy. These characteristics include but are not limited to:
- Ability to develop relationships that exhibit a caring philosophy.
- An ethic of caring reflected by appropriate emotional responses, communication, punctuality, hygiene, and attire that seeks to preserve the wholeness of dignity of self and others.
- Adherence to confidentiality of clients and others.
- Behavior that reflects responsibility and accountability for safety of clients, self, and others.
- Demonstration of knowledge regarding scope of practice of the LPN/LVN.
- Demonstration of interpersonal skills needed to function as an effective team member.
- Demonstration of problem-solving skills applying the concepts of the nursing process within the scope of the LPN/LVN.
- Development of an awareness of available resources for continued personal and professional growth.

---

report. Plan to spend the full day. You may be finished early, but that is not something you can count on. Most facilities provide several weeks of orientation. Some may offer a longer new graduate program. The first week is normally on the day shift, with additional time provided on the shift to which you are assigned. It is a good idea to arrive for orientation with a notebook. You will be given a lot of information and it is wise to write it down so you can refer to it later.

You have now made that transition from student to licensed nurse. Congratulations—all of your hard work and dedication have paid off! You are now a member of a worthy profession.

A **profession** is defined as an occupation to which one devotes oneself and in which one has specialized expertise (Becker & Fendler, 1994). LPNs/LVNs are an integral part of the profession. As an LPN/LVN working in a hospital or other healthcare agency, you will be expected to demonstrate certain characteristics and behaviors that demonstrate **professionalism.** Box 65-5 ■ lists examples of professional characteristics and behaviors. By emulating these behaviors you will be well on your way to being a successful licensed nurse. See Box 65-6 ■ for tips on thriving—not just surviving—during the first year as an LPN/LVN.

PROBATIONARY PERIOD AND PERFORMANCE EVALUATION

Each healthcare facility has a **probationary period** for newly hired employees. During this time your immediate supervisor will be evaluating your performance. At the end of this time you will be given a **performance evaluation** and most likely a small increase in salary. Your attendance and promptness will be an important consideration, as will

---

BOX 65-6 **THRIVING DURING THE FIRST YEAR ON THE JOB**

- **Be patient.** It takes time to gain experience. Some say it takes up to 2 years to be able to handle most situations.
- **Be positive.** Everyday write down something good you did or learned; review your list often. Focus on the positive; it will become your reality.
- **Be a seeker.** Don't wait for someone to tell you to do a procedure. Seek out opportunities to do new things. If you don't know how, request the opportunity to observe a more experienced colleague. Show your willingness to learn.
- **Be a helper.** It is never too soon to lend a hand to a coworker. Be sure to be available to students—you were there once.
- **Be a buddy.** Buddy up with a coworker after whom you would like to model yourself. Remember someone doesn't have to have the same position in order for you to learn from him or her.

- **Be a team player.** Introduce yourself to coworkers on all shifts, to physicians, and to other hospital personnel. Have lunch with someone you don't know. Become a part of the team.
- **Be a lifelong learner.** Use references and policy and procedure manuals. Ask questions and do your homework at the end of each day by looking up things that are new to you.
- **Be a joiner.** Become a member of a professional organization; develop close ties with colleagues on a state and national level. Organizations provide cutting-edge information.
- **Be a tracker.** Track your progress. Don't lose track of the progress you have already made. Review this often; see how far you have come.
- **Be a stress buster.** Stress should be managed not just tolerated. Make time for yourself to socialize, for leisure activities, for hobbies—take care of yourself so you can give care to others.
- **Be focused.** Keep moving forward. You can do it!

---

your ability to work as a team member, complete your assignments in a timely manner, and perfect your skills. After the initial evaluation, most facilities evaluate employees on an annual basis. Annual evaluations may include skills testing and renewal of CPR or other certifications. It is important that the staff nurse keep track of these requirements, because expired certifications may prevent you from working.

CONTINUING EDUCATION

All state boards of nursing have continuing education requirements for licensed nurses. The number of hours varies with the individual board. It is your responsibility to know the requirements for your state. Requirements can be met with on-site classes, professional conferences, home study courses, or courses on the Internet. It is important that classes be completed prior to the renewal date of your license. Once completed keep the certificates on file. Your portfolio is an excellent storage location for a copy, since state nursing boards conduct random audits of license holders. Continuing education courses are designed to help keep you current in the field, but such courses can also introduce you to new skills or even a new specialty. The possibilities are only limited by your time and interest.

CAREER LADDER

A **career ladder** can be described as progression from one level in a profession to another through educational pursuits and professional experience (Figure 65-2 ■).

Career ladder programs offer a variety of options. An individual who already has a practical or vocational nursing license can enter an associate nursing degree (AND) program by taking a transition course. Some training programs have direct articulation with schools of registered nursing, so that LPNs/LVNs can receive advanced placement when they wish to pursue additional education. Another option is

to enroll in a 2-year AND program and exit after the first year after completing the practical nurse option. These options may better meet some individuals' needs for employment and continuing education.

Many LPNs/LVNs have a desire to progress beyond the AND level of registered nursing. The availability for lifelong learning and advanced practice opportunities are many. New graduates may be ready to dive right into additional schooling, others need to seek fulltime employment to support themselves or family, and others may need a well-deserved break from school. With nursing the option is always there, either now or in the future. Your career goal may be fulfilled as an LPN/LVN or you may wish to continue up the ladder. Whatever your professional goal, it is important never to stop learning and to strive to be a competent and compassionate nurse.

PROFESSIONAL ORGANIZATIONS

The first professional nursing organization was established in 1893. Nurses found that if they united to achieve common goals and missions they would be more likely to have an impact on their chosen profession. The National League for Nursing (NLN) was established under the name of the American Society of Superintendents of Training Schools for Nurses in the United States and Canada. In 1912 the name was changed to NLN. Its purpose was to standardize and improve nursing education. There are two levels of membership in the NLN, individual and agency. Schools of nursing and other agencies that provide nursing care are eligible for agency membership. In 1943, lay members were permitted to join the organization, which had previously been open only to nurses. The NLN is the accrediting organization for nursing programs. A graduate of an NLN-accredited program will be recognized nationally and credits will be recognized by other NLN-approved programs when the nurse chooses to continue his or her education.

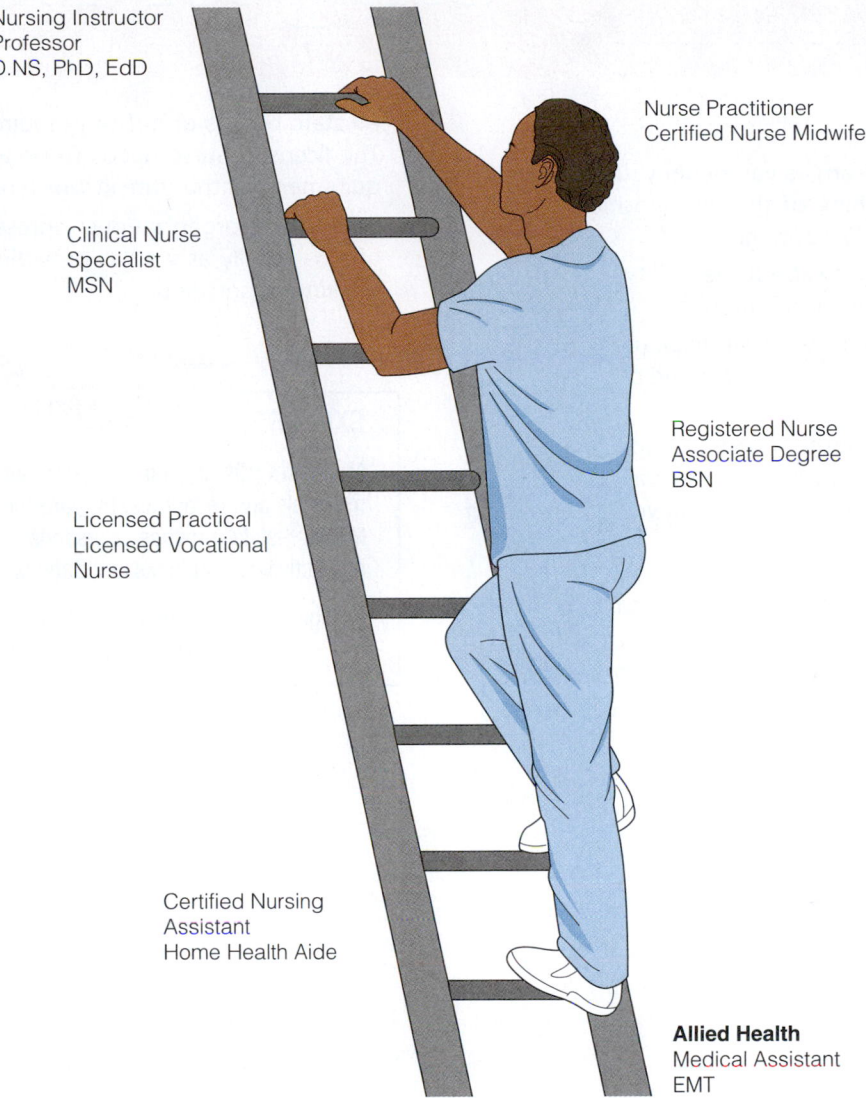

Nursing Instructor
Professor
D.NS, PhD, EdD

Nurse Practitioner
Certified Nurse Midwife

Clinical Nurse
Specialist
MSN

Registered Nurse
Associate Degree
BSN

Licensed Practical
Licensed Vocational
Nurse

Certified Nursing
Assistant
Home Health Aide

Allied Health
Medical Assistant
EMT

Figure 65-2. ■ Nursing career ladder.

The American Nurses Association is the professional organization for the RN. Membership is limited to registered nurses. The National Federation of Licensed Practical Nurses and the National Association for Practical Nurse Education and Service are the professional organizations for the LPN/LVN. Membership in a professional organization provides the licensed nurse with many services; they are your representative on a national level, providing continuing education opportunities and opportunities for networking. There are specialty organizations for nurses working in pediatrics, geriatrics, or obstetrics to name a few. Participation in a local or national organization is a worthwhile activity for a graduate nurse.

NETWORKING AND COLLABORATION

Nursing is not a career that one can pursue in a vacuum. **Networking** is described as the deliberate attempt to make connections among people for a variety of interests, including employment opportunities. Networking may be casual or formal (Kurzen, 2004).

Collaborative nursing practice or interdependent nursing practice is working jointly with other healthcare professionals, including physicians, in the performance of nursing roles within the scope of practice. Learning to network and collaborate with other nurses and healthcare providers is extremely important. You can begin to learn these skills by participating in staff or unit minutes. In the beginning you may feel you have little to contribute, but as you listen to your colleagues and progress in your nursing practice you will see ways to improve client care and unit operations. Once you are comfortable in a small group, volunteer for a hospital or systemwide committee. As a member of a professional organization, your networking and collaborative opportunities will increase as your circle of professional associates increases.

MyNursingKit | Journal of Health Communication

Note: The references and resources for all chapters have been compiled at the back of the book.

Chapter Review

KEY Points

- You will continue to learn as you begin your first job. You may even come to think of that first position as being another phase of your education.

- Learn as much as you can about the facility and its parent company before making application.

- A portfolio is an itemized visual account of your skills and best practices that are related to the position you are seeking.

- Most résumés are computer generated today, but at the very least, it must be typed on quality paper and is normally the same light-colored paper that you used for your cover letter.

- A face-to-face meeting gives a first impression; whether it results in employment or not, it is an experience that will provide you with insight into your ability to speak logically and think critically.

- All state boards of nursing require continuing education. The licensed nurse needs to be aware of the specific requirements of the state in which he or she is licensed.

- Professional organizations represent the members' interests nationally as well as providing educational and networking opportunities.

1 The nurse prepares a cover letter and uses the first paragraph to:
1. Highlight particular qualifications.
2. Identify how qualifications match the job opening.
3. Convey anticipation in obtaining an interview.
4. Express enthusiasm for this particular job.

2 The nurse with a significant time gap in the work history, following a layoff from a previous job, addresses the matter in which of the following ways on the employment application?
1. Skip that time period; prospective employers are not interested in periods of unemployment.
2. Leave the area blank where it asks for reason for leaving the job.
3. Identify the time period and highlight educational or volunteer activities during that time.
4. Write an explanation explaining the reason for the layoff.

3 If asked a question concerning one's religion, which of the following would be the applicant's best response?
1. "Civil rights law prohibits you from asking me personal questions."
2. "I would really rather not answer that question."
3. "I will need time off on religious holidays to fulfill my personal obligations. I hope that won't be a problem."
4. "My religious beliefs will not interfere with my ability to carry out the responsibilities of this position."

4 A peer complains to the graduate nurse about not receiving any calls in response to mailing out several résumés. The nurse reviews the résumé, finds several misspelled words, and suspects the reason for the lack of response may be:
1. The facilities do not like to hire new graduates.
2. The cover letter and résumé did not demonstrate the characteristics the facility is looking for in a new hire.
3. The facility knew the graduate was applying to other places and did not want to waste time if he or she really wasn't interested.
4. Because the letter was not addressed to a person, it did not reach the person doing the hiring.

5 The new graduate accepts a nursing position and is told the first 3 months will be a probationary period. The nurse recognizes this means:
1. Continued employment is contingent on doing a good job.
2. The nurse is expected to make mistakes and this will be forgiven until he or she gains experience.
3. The nurse will work with another experienced nurse in the facility and not be responsible for his or her own practice.
4. The nurse will earn less during this time.

6 You are scheduled for an interview at a hospital where you were employed as a nursing assistant during your nursing program. The interview is scheduled at 9 A.M. after you have worked the night shift. Which is the most appropriate view about attire for the interview?
1. "I will wear my uniform. That way I will not be rushed and can relax before the meeting."
2. "Since the director of nursing and human resource director already know me, it won't matter how I am dressed."
3. "I will go home, shower and dress in business attire, in order to show respect for the interview team, and the position for which I am applying."
4. "I will tell my supervisor I need to leave early, because this interview is really important."

7 Which of the following would be considered to be casual networking?
1. Attending a presentation with classmates on a new facility that is recruiting LPNs
2. Attending a job fair at a local college
3. While having coffee with a friend, sharing the advantages of her new job
4. Discussing job opportunities on a hospital Internet website

8 The new graduate nurse ensures success in his or her new job by doing which of the following?
1. Pointing out all the different ways the facility can improve
2. Quickly responding whenever someone asks him or her to do something
3. Helping coworkers whenever workload allows
4. Expecting to know everything from the first day on the job

9 It is important to include writing samples in your portfolio because they demonstrate:
1. Your ability to write in a logical order using correct format and show your attention to detail.
2. That academic skills were a part of your nursing program.
3. Your ability to chart effectively.
4. Your level of computer skills.

10 The nurse works in a facility that encourages career advancement by offering tuition assistance. The LPN/LVN could enroll in which of the following programs to advance career and receive tuition assistance from the facility?
1. Accounting and business management
2. Doctorate in nursing education
3. Masters in business administration
4. Baccalaureate degree nursing program

Answers and rationales for Review Questions appear in Appendix I.

Thinking Strategically About . . .

You are a recent graduate from an LPN/LVN program. You have successfully passed your licensure exam and have been hired as night shift charge nurse for a skilled nursing facility. Your orientation went well and now this is your first night alone on the unit.

A client from the assisted living unit was sent to the ER of the local hospital for IVs to treat dehydration resulting from several days of nausea and vomiting. The IV line has been placed. She will be discharged from the ER and will be coming to your unit. You are not yet IV certified but are planning to take the class after receiving your first paycheck.

You attempt to reach the director of nursing (DON) by phone and find that she is out of town. You call the assistant DON and inform her that no nurse in the building is IV certified. You request that the client be kept at the hospital until morning. You explain your lack of certification to the assistant DON. She hesitates, then asks what care will be needed during the night. There is no medication to be given IV, but fluids will need to be added to the IV at about 5 A.M. You have watched the procedure many times and realize that although you are not legally qualified, it is a relatively easy procedure.

In addition to this client, there is a census of 90. Most of them have been in the facility for some time, and they usually sleep through the night. There are three total LPNs/LVNs on duty, one for each unit of 30 clients each. There are two nursing assistants assigned to each hallway. All the LPNs/LVNs will need to pass 6 A.M. medications as well as any prn medications. The night charge nurses are also expected to complete a monthly nursing summary on 7 to 8 clients each week. Last night you were so busy you did not complete any summaries. You are afraid that you will get behind.

COMMUNICATION AND TEAM BUILDING

Using your knowledge of communication and team building, what solutions could you suggest to the assistant DON? List several possibilities.

CRITICAL THINKING

The assistant DON says, "Well, you've watched these things being done a dozen times. It's not that big a deal. Can't you just do it?" When you hesitate, she lashes out and states, "I knew there would be a problem hiring you new grads. If you can't solve your problems, maybe we need to rethink your charge nurse position." What responses would be appropriate in this situation?

PRIORITIZING NURSING CARE

Which of your responsibilities *must* be completed during this shift?

MANAGEMENT OF CARE

Briefly outline your work schedule for a typical shift.

DELEGATING

What tasks can be delegated to the CNAs? What follow-up will be needed?

CLIENT TEACHING

The client comes from the ER around 5 A.M. She does not understand why she cannot go to her assisted living apartment. What client teaching can you do to comfort her and relieve her anxiety?

CULTURAL CARE STRATEGIES

One of the clients assigned to your unit is from the Middle East and is a practicing Muslim. She has requested that only female caretakers enter her room. She also refuses to let anyone into the room during her prayer times. A male housekeeper inadvertently entered the room and now she is very upset and is yelling at you and anyone else who will listen. What strategies can you use to calm her and prevent future problems?

CONFLICT RESOLUTION

After the conflict over the client with the IV, you are concerned about your relationship with the assistant DON. You want to try to resolve the tension over the IV issue. How might you approach the assistant DON to change the situation? If you are concerned that the assistant DON might try to get you fired, what steps should you take to protect your position?

DOCUMENTING AND REPORTING

Write a nursing summary of a client with the following problems.

1. Weight loss
2. Pneumonia (resolved)
3. Tendency to decubitus ulcer in the lumbar spine area
4. Frequent confusion during evening hours
5. Risk for falls
6. History of cerebrovascular accident, no improvement expected
7. Incontinence of urine (resolved)

Appendix I

Answers

CHAPTER 1

NCLEX-PN® ANSWERS (1) 3. Outcome 5. Application. Questions of knowledge simply test facts. Comprehension questions require you to understand the meaning of a word (such as *cathartic*) and to use the knowledge to arrive at an answer. Application involves knowledge and comprehension, plus use of that information in a fresh situation. Analysis questions are more complex than application questions. (2) 3. Outcome 6. When students are unsure of how to proceed, they must ask for help in order to ensure client safety. When students know how to proceed but feel hesitant or nervous, they should recognize the feeling but go ahead. (3) 2, 3, 4. Outcome 1. The student nurse displays holistic care in choice 2, confidentiality in choice 3, and accountability in choice 4—all essential values of nursing. The student in choice 1 is not showing respect for the dignity of the client when referring to the client as a diagnosis. The student in choice 5 is not working as a team member and is not respecting the practice of the respiratory therapist. (4) 1, 2, 3, 5. Outcome 2. Students should familiarize themselves with the textbook by reading the preface, reviewing the table of contents, looking over the appendices, and becoming familiar with the organization of the book. Although students may find it helpful to highlight the most important statement in each paragraph, that is not always the first sentence and should be done when studying, not while becoming familiar with the textbook. (5) 3. Outcome 2. The student who reads the material the night before the lecture will be prepared for class, will be more able to participate in classroom discussions, and will be familiar enough with the material to know what material in the lecture is new and needs to be carefully recorded versus the material found in the textbook. (6) 4. Outcome 2. The best hints for what will be in the quiz are the learning outcomes—both those in the textbook and those in the syllabi or class plan. Many tests are written based on the learning outcomes; if students can complete each learning outcome they will be prepared for the quiz. (7) 2. Outcome 3. The student who uses a calendar or planner to schedule holidays, appointments, vacations, and school responsibilities will keep from double booking and will be better able to plan ahead for necessary obligations. No single time-management plan works for every student (option 1). Study time should be scheduled daily to avoid cramming for tests and help to improve comprehension of the material (option 3). Students who do not take occasional time for themselves will burn out, and their schoolwork will suffer. Everyone needs some personal time. (8) 1, 2, 3. Outcome 4. In order to manage time, student nurses should maintain a planning calendar, maintain their current responsibilities, and plan their finances. Asking the instructor to reduce homework is not a good strategy, because it is essential that students learn the required material before graduating. The student nurse should not reduce sleep time to 4 hours per night because the tired brain is unable to learn. (9) 1. Outcome 2. The student should read each question and all answer choices carefully and completely, using care to watch for negative words such as "which of the following does not . . ." Answers with the terms *always* or *never* are rarely the correct answer (option 2). Changing answers is never a good strategy and usually results in more incorrect choices being made—trust your first impression (option 3). If there is a term in one of the answers that is unfamiliar to you, it most likely is not the correct option if you spent time studying, because all of the terms would have a degree of familiarity to you (option 4). (10) 1. Outcome 7. Prioritizing skills are needed in order to provide care to clients in a logical manner that meets the most urgent needs first. This becomes even more important when the student begins caring for more than one client at a time. While there may be a degree of truth to the other options, these are not the most important reasons for prioritizing care.

CHAPTER 2

NCLEX-PN® ANSWERS (1) 2. Outcome 3. The Alexian brothers created a school to educate men in nursing in 1876 when they opened their first hospital in the United States. Men were not allowed to function as nurses from after the Civil War through the Korean War. (2) 4. Outcome 1. The role of the nurse has been affected by religion, war, and societal attitudes. Cost containment did not have a historical impact on the role of the nurse, although it will most certainly influence the future of nursing. (3) 2. Outcome 2. Florence Nightingale contributed to many aspects of nursing and public health. However, it is because of her attempts to define what nursing is and is not that she is sometimes called the first nurse scientist-theorist. (4) 2. Outcome 2. Lillian Wald is considered the founder of public health nursing. Clara Barton established the American Red Cross, Dock campaigned for legislation to allow nurses to control their profession, and Nightingale described the basic elements of the nursing profession. (5) 3. Outcome 4. The Smith-Hughes Act provided federal funding for practical nurse education. (6) 1, 2, 3. Outcome 6. The LPN/LVN does not create the plan of care, but contributes to carrying out the plan.

Creating the plan of care is the responsibility of the registered nurse. Medical needs of the client are determined by the physician, while the LPN/LVN carries out the orders written by the physician. (7) 1, 2, 3. Outcome 5. The nurse's consumers include individuals, groups, and the community. Peers and physicians are coworkers and members of the healthcare team, but are not consumers. (8) 3. Outcome 7. Operating under the umbrella of an overseeing organization distinguishes a profession from an occupation. (9) 3. Outcome 7. Lillian Kuster started the National Federation of Licensed Practical Nurses. Lillian Wald founded the Henry Street Settlement and Visiting Nurses Service. (10) 2. Outcome 6. Each state has its own nurse practice act, which provides the scope of nursing for its jurisdiction. LPNs/LVNs are responsible for knowing the limits of practice whenever they work.

CHAPTER 3

NCLEX-PN® ANSWERS (1) 1. Outcome 2. Stereotyping is an oversimplification of conceptions, opinions, or beliefs about some aspect of a group of people. Ethnocentrism means interpreting the beliefs and behavior of others in terms of one's own cultural values and traditions. It assumes that one's own culture is superior. Acculturation is the modification of the culture of a group as a result of contact with another group. Cultural awareness is the increasing of one's consciousness of cultural diversity. (2) 3. Outcome 1. Madeleine Leininger developed the Sunrise model as part of her cultural diversity and universality theory. Although the others are nursing theorists, their theories do not focus on culture. (3) 2. Outcome 5. Cultural competency includes five concepts including ability to adapt practice skills to fit the cultural context of the client. Although it helps to be able to communicate in the client's native language, culturally competent care can be delivered without this ability. Complementary alternative medicine is becoming more readily accepted in mainstream Western medicine, but its use is not required for culturally competent nursing care. Ignoring a client's culture decreases one's ability to provide competent care. Cultural differences exist. Their consideration is an important part of treating the client holistically. (4) 3, 4. Outcome 7. The healthcare field is increasing in diversity and the nurse is likely to work with peers from many different cultural backgrounds. All staff will be expected to meet, or exceed, the minimum standards for their job title. While nurses from different backgrounds may have different approaches to client care, the same expectations of dependability and competence will be expected of them. (5) 3. Outcome 2. In health care, ethnocentrism includes the view that the only valid healthcare beliefs and practices are those held by healthcare professionals. (6) 1. Outcome 5. Classifying clients' responses to care and treatment by ethnicity is considered to be stereotyping. (7) 2. Outcome 4. In some families the man is considered to be the provider and the decision maker. The woman may need to consult her husband prior to making decisions about medical treatment for her child. (8) 3. Outcome 4. Some cultural groups have strong beliefs about privacy, and this may be motivating the mother to wait until she goes home to breastfeed. The nurse can explain the importance of starting breastfeeding immediately and then ensure that the mother has privacy. (9) 4. Outcome 4. Many religious groups have specific dietary laws that they must follow. The nurse must first identify the needs during a cultural assessment and report them so the plan of care can be changed to meet those needs. (10) 1, 2, 3, 4, 5. Outcome 6. Religion, relation to Western medicine, cultural identity, and heritage and location all are part of a person's culture. Race is also a factor; find it in your chapter under biocultural ecology.

CHAPTER 4

NCLEX-PN® ANSWERS (1) 1, 4. Outcome 10. Your first responsibility is to be sure all legal requirements have been met; a client who changes his or her mind after signing consent may not have made an informed decision. Healthcare professionals should always consider the principle of beneficence. Although it would be better for family and client to agree, it is not essential for the nurse to consider the family's opinion about treatment. Even if the client has signed the consent, he or she can revoke that consent. The scheduled surgery time is not a factor for consideration. (2) 2. Outcome 2. Restraint without an order, or failing to follow facility policies on restraints, constitutes false imprisonment. Negligence and ethical considerations may enter into the discussion, but they are not the best answer in this situation. Defamation has to do with false communication, not restraints. (3) 3. Outcome 1. The primary difference between civil and criminal law is the potential outcome. If found guilty of a civil action, the defendant will have to pay a sum of money, but if found guilty of a crime the defendant could lose money, be jailed, or be executed. (4) 2. Outcome 3. Licensure indicates the nurse has graduated from a state board–approved school of nursing and has met the minimum standards for licensure. It does not indicate competence or knowledge of how to handle all situations. Nurses are expected to be responsible for their own continuing educational needs in order to maintain competence. (5) 1. Outcome 4. The ADA prohibits discrimination on the basis of disability in employment, public service, and public accommodations and is enforced by the federal government. The impact on nursing practice is allowing those with a learning disability to pursue a nursing curriculum through alternate methods. It does not regulate retraining or lifting limits. (6) 3, 4, 5. Outcome 6. The nurse should identify clients accurately, be familiar with facility policies and procedures, and function within his or her scope of practice. While building rapport is a good strategy for reducing liability, rapport is not created by sharing personal information about the nurse. Errors should be documented, but words like mistake or error should be avoided, instead writing what happened objectively. (7) 3. Outcome 8. Completion of an incident report is the duty of the nurse who discovers the incident. This may be the nurse involved in the incident, but does not have to be. The supervisor and the risk management department will review the report. (8) 3. Outcome 10. The nursing code of ethics is a formal statement of nursing's ideals and values. The nursing code of ethics does not provide specific directions or requirements for coping with ethical issues, and is not an explanation of legal standards. Instead, it guides the decision-making process through established ideals and values for nursing practice. (9) 1. Outcome 11. The nurse's primary goal when making an ethical decision is the client's best interest and preserving the integrity of all involved. Option 2 and 3 play a role in ethical decision making, but they are not the primary goal. A decision should not be based on intuition or emotions (option 4). (10) 2. Outcome 7. Computerized medical records present specific security concerns. The best thing staff members can do to preserve confidentiality is protect their personal security codes and follow the facility's policies for use.

CHAPTER 5

NCLEX-PN® ANSWERS (1) 2. Outcome 1. The art of thinking about thinking represents critical thinking. Choice 1: although the word *critical* can mean fault finding, in this context *critical* means discerning. Choices 3 and 4 are characteristics of natural rather than critical thinking. (2) 1. Outcome 2. During the assessment/data collection phase, the nurse must consider personal assumptions or biases that may affect judgment. (3) 1. Outcome 2. A nurse who is using critical thinking skills will evaluate the client's cognitive ability or limitations prior to beginning health-related teaching. (4) 4. Outcome 5. The nursing model that is primarily used to make decisions using critical thinking is the nursing process. The other options may contribute to decision making, but the nursing process is the primary decision-making model used by nursing. (5) 1. Outcome 1. With inductive reasoning, certain bits of information suggest a particular interpretation when viewed together, whereas deductive reasoning takes broader pieces of data (for example, "All people think" and "I am a person") and puts them together to reach a specific conclusion ("I think"). (6) 2. Outcome 6. In order to put evidence-based practice into use safely, facility policy must support the change in practice. The nurse who joins the standards and practice committee to contribute research findings in order to improve facility

policy and practice would be using evidence-based practice correctly. Changing one's practice after only one article would not be prudent, and complaining to coworkers is not an effective approach. (7) 3. Outcome 3. Environment (according to Nightingale) is related to internal and external factors such as light and excessive noise. Option 1 represents health; option 2 represents person/client; and option 4 represents nursing. (8) 2. Outcome 4. Neuman's theory focuses on reaction to stress in the environment; Roy focuses on the adaptation to the changes in the environment; Orem's theory focuses on self-care; and Leininger focuses on cultural care. (9) 1. Outcome 4. Environmental theory, Nightingale; adaptation model, Roy; systems model, Neuman; and cultural care diversity, Leininger. (10) 4. Outcome 4. Leininger's theory is based on universal human caring, although ways of caring vary across cultures.

CHAPTER 6

NCLEX-PN® ANSWERS (1) 3. Outcome 2. Assessment involves data collection related to the client's current health status, whereas evaluation is concerned with accomplishment of the desired outcomes set for the client. (2) 3. Outcome 1. The second phase of nursing process is diagnosing. During this phase collected data are analyzed and problems are identified. The LPN/LVN may contribute, but this step is the RN's responsibility. (3) 1, 3, 4. Outcome 3. The LPN's/LVN's role includes collecting data, making observations of client's status, and reporting changes in condition. The RN or physician responds to abnormal results and develops the plan of care. The LPN/LVN contributes to the development of the plan of care, but it is the RN's responsibility. (4) 2. Outcome 4. The primary purpose of collecting data is to allow the nurse to determine the client's needs and develop an individualized plan of care to help the client regain optimal levels of health. In the process of collecting data, the nurse learns the client's biographical data and past history and creates a database, but this is not the purpose of doing so. (5) 1, 4. Outcome 5. Objective data is measurable, so the client's temperature and clear breath sounds are objective data. All the rest are subjective data that depend on the reliability and truthfulness of the client who is reporting the information. (6) 4. Objective data can be collected via observing and examining of the client. Interviewing the client results in subjective data based on the client's perceptions. (7) 2. Outcome 9. Although the care plan is written in the planning stage, it is put into action in the implementation stage. (8) 4. Outcome 8. Once the care plan has been implemented, the licensed nurse will decide what tasks can be carried out by other nursing personnel and also how much supervision they will need to complete them. (9) 1. Outcome 10. During the evaluation phase the nurse determines the effectiveness of the plan of care (goal met, not met, or partially met) and documents the data that provide evidence for the stated conclusion. (10) 3. Outcome 1. Although the other choices contribute to the nursing process, choice 3 provides a clear definition of the nursing process as an organized framework for professional nursing practice.

CHAPTER 7

NCLEX-PN® ANSWERS (1) 2. Outcome 4. Included in this bill are the right of clients to considerate and respectful care; privacy for the clients, confidentiality of records and communications regarding their care; and the right to make decisions about their care, including the right to refuse treatment. Client preferences regarding schedule are taken into consideration, but it is not always possible for them to determine the treatment schedule. (2) 1. Outcome 3. OBRA instituted requirements for nurse's aide training. Specifically, they include a minimum of 75 hours of training and competence evaluation of aides. (3) 3. Outcome 6. All of these may be an issue with a homeless client. However, the living environment and the exposure to disease, poor nutrition, and the elements would be the major concern. (4) 4. Outcome 1. Team nursing is a collaborative effort of direct client care, with healthcare workers from two or more levels. Care is allocated according to the scope of practice of the individual team members. (5) 4. Outcome 8. The 1965 Medicare amendments (Title 18) to the Social Security Act provided for national and state health insurance for adults 65 and older. Medicaid and Medi-Cal are health insurance for individuals needing federal and/or state assistance. Medicare is a federal program; Medi-Cal is one of numerous state programs. (6) 3. Outcome 8. In 1983 the U.S. Congress passed legislation putting the nationwide prospective payment system into effect. Reimbursement is made according to a classification system called diagnostic-related groups. (7) 4. Outcome 5. Paramedical is defined as having some training to do with medicine. A spiritual support person attends to the client's spiritual needs, but is not required to have healthcare training. Occupational therapists, physiotherapists, and laboratory technicians are interdisciplinary team members specially trained to meet specific health needs. (8) 1. Outcome 7. Although managed care may mean that the number of hospital days may be reduced and allocation of services may be more efficient, the purpose of managed care is to provide the client with the most effective treatment. Managed care can be used with any nursing model. (9) 2. Outcome 8. Health maintenance organizations provide capitated care. In other words, a monthly fee is paid for each member, whether or not they received treatment during that time period. (10) 1. Outcome 1. Primary care includes preventive care, health education, environmental protection, and early detection and treatment. Secondary care includes acute care and diagnosis and treatment. Tertiary care includes rehabilitation and care of the terminally ill.

CHAPTER 8

NCLEX-PN® ANSWERS (1) 3. Outcome 1. Dietary supplements used to be regulated as food, though not by the FDA. The passing of the Dietary Supplement Health and Education Act established new regulatory guidelines in 1994. Dietary supplements require regulation because they can be harmful and may interact with medications. (2) 2. Outcome 2. Naturopathic medicine is a complete alternative approach to medicine using nutrition, herbs, manipulation of the body, exercise, stress reduction, and acupuncture. Complementary medicine is used in conjunction with, not instead of, conventional medicine. Integrative medicine combines treatments from conventional, complementary, and alternative medicine. (3) 4. Outcome 3. Ayurveda involves reestablishing balance in the body. Manipulation of the spine is chiropractic medicine, insertion of needles is acupuncture, and aromatic liquids are aromatherapy or healing with essential oils. (4) 1. Outcome 7. It is important for the nurse to question the client specifically about OTCs, supplements, and herbal medications because the client often assumes when questioned about medications that the nurse is only looking for prescription medications. Finding out about allergies is important, but when the nurse is questioning about medications, it is important to follow up the client's answer with specific questions about nonprescription medications. Option 3 appears to challenge the client. (5) 2, 3, 4. Outcome 4. Acupressure and magnet therapy may be offered by a trained professional, but these can also be performed by the client without professional intervention. Acupuncture, chiropractic medicine, and naturopathy require a trained professional's care. (6) 1. Outcome 8. It is important for the nurse to use this opportunity to teach the client the importance of sharing information regarding supplements and complementary and alternative medicine options they have chosen, because it can have a very important impact on their plan of care and therapeutic regimen. Options 2 and 4 miss this opportunity for teaching, and the client does not need the physician's permission to use these therapies. (7) 2. Outcome 5. Nurses provide holistic care and integrate complementary therapy into their plan of care as appropriate (such as massage, music therapy, and meditation). Nurses may coordinate with alternative healthcare providers, but it is not their primary role. Nurses should learn more about CAMs but not for the purpose of scaring clients about the dangers of the treatment. (8) 1. Outcome 6. The LPN/LVN should immediately inform the RN of the client's use of supplements, because they all have an anticoagulant effect that could be contributing to the client's medical condition. Option 2 is outside the LPN's/LVN's scope of practice, option 3 is untrue, and option 4 is overly dramatic and not completely true. (9) 4. Outcome 6. The nurse should direct the client to talk with the provider but should not try to guess what the provider's response will be (option 3). Option

2 is not accurate, and option 1 would not be a safe response. (10) 3. Outcome 6. An appropriate outcome for the client using complementary and alternative medications (CAM) would be for the client to understand the positive and potential negative attributes of the CAM. Some CAMs can be helpful, so it would not be an appropriate outcome for the client to stop using them (option 1). Those CAMs that would be dangerous prior to surgery would need to be stopped for a period longer than 12 hours preoperatively (option 2). Option 4 is not a client-centered outcome; it is a nursing intervention.

CHAPTER 9

NCLEX-PN® ANSWERS (1) 3. Outcome 1. Children are curious and have not developed the judgment needed to understand danger. Bad behavior and parent neglect can cause injury, but unfounded accusation should not be made. New walkers frequently fall, but a child-safe environment can protect from injury. (2) 2. Outcome 8. A mitt restraint will prevent the client from pulling at IV lines but will not restrict arm and shoulder movement. The least restrictive device should always be chosen. A vest restraint and bed alarms are used to keep the client in bed, but will not prevent the client from disturbing IV lines. Arm restraints would keep the client from pulling out IV lines, but they would unnecessarily restrict movement. (3) 2. Outcome 4. The MSDS provides all necessary information to the nurse to work safely with chemicals in the workplace. The name of the chemical, years of experience using the chemical, and previous exposure are not as important as having access to the MSDS. (4) 3. Outcome 3. The walker will need to be used at all times until the client is fully recovered. The other choices show good understanding of his discharge needs. (5) 2. Outcome 8. Body mechanics is a safe and efficient way to move the body. Physical therapy is treatment of large muscle groups; occupational therapy deals with small muscle groups. Nursing interventions are nursing actions to help clients meet goals. (6) 2. Outcome 4. OSHA, the Occupational Safety and Health Administration, is the government agency responsible for safe work environments. CDC is the Centers for Disease Control and Prevention. The Department of Labor is concerned with all work-related issues, not specifically safety. The Joint Commission (formerly called JCAHO) is not a government agency; it is responsible for accreditation of healthcare organizations. 7. 3. Outcome 4. The CDC recommends that isolation linens be removed promptly from the room by bagging them. Carrying rolled-up linens away from one's uniform is standard practice, but more is required for a client in isolation. Linens are not disposable, so they should not be placed in a refuse container. (8) 2. Outcome 1. Items such as paper and cloth could easily ignite if they come in contact with heating appliances. Appropriate use of electric heaters does not present an increased fire hazard. In the event of a fire, bars over windows can prevent windows from being used as an exit. Fire extinguishers are normally stored in the kitchen for quick access in case of fire. (9) 4. Outcome 8. During transfer, holding the client close to your center of gravity and standing with a wide base of support is the safest position for client and nurse. Keeping the client at arm's length and having feet close together are not appropriate use of body mechanics by the nurse. Unless the client is independently ambulatory, the nurse should support and assist the client during transfer using proper body mechanics. (10) 1. Outcome 5. In the event of a fire the nurse's priority action is to prevent injury to clients by removing them from the room. If the fire is contained and small, after activating the alarm system, the nurse may try to extinguish the fire. A larger fire should be contained by closing the door and waiting for help to arrive.

CHAPTER 10

NCLEX-PN® ANSWERS (1) 4. Outcome 10. The wound and the dressing are contaminating the environment, and because it is wet it may be transmitting other organisms to the wound itself. The physician would not ordinarily order medications for a temperature below 101°F. Elevation of the leg and placing the client in isolation may be done later but are not the priority intervention for this client. (2) 2. Outcome 9. The tuberculosis organism is transmitted through the air in droplets. Tier 2 or transmission-based precautions are specific for this condition. Tier 1 or standard precautions and the use of clean gowns do not address airborne organisms. The nurse would use the mask to prevent inhalation of the tuberculosis organism when entering the client's room and the client would wear a mask when leaving the room to go to other areas of the facility. (3) 4. Outcome 12. Using sterile forceps is appropriate, but reaching across the field would be incorrect because organisms could fall on it and contaminate it. Sterile gloves are worn while handling the contents of the tray so as to not contaminate them. A sterile field should never be left unattended because there is no way to know if the field was contaminated in the nurse's absence. (4) 1. Outcome 8. The nurse should instruct the family to wash all launderable items in hot water, clean plastic toys with an antimicrobial, and place nonwashable items in a plastic bag until the organism infecting the child is identified. Discarding clothes and toys is expensive and unnecessary (option 2), but the items are contaminated so care must be taken (option 3). Airing the items will not destroy microorganisms. (5) 4. Outcome 1. Microorganisms are mostly harmless and may even be helpful. Microorganisms, sometimes referred to by laymen as germs, are not always dangerous to the body (options 1 and 4). Microorganisms include bacteria, viruses, parasites, and fungi (option 2). (6) 4. Outcome 3. A postoperative wound is both a nosocomial infection (hospital acquired) and an iatrogenic infection (results from treatment or therapy). It is not a systemic infection if it is contained in the wound (option 2) or a septicemia if it is not found in the bloodstream (option 3). (7) 3. Outcome 11. The gloves are contaminated and must be removed first in sequence before the ties of the mask or gown are touched. Otherwise, the person's head, neck, and back can become contaminated. Only the ties of the mask are handled, and they are undone next. Finally, the ties of the gown are loosened and the gown is removed, taking care not to touch the contaminated outside area of the garment. (8) 2. Outcome 5. A compromised host is someone who is already at high risk for getting infections because of one or more reasons. The client is elderly and has a history of emphysema, two other predisposing factors. A susceptible host is just at risk for developing an infection. The other two options (3 and 4) are not accurate. (9) 2. Outcome 4. The nurse's unwashed hands serve as a reservoir, or storage place, for microorganisms. The agent is the microorganism on the nurse's hands, the portal of exit is the way the organism leaves the hands, and the mode of transmission is how the organism leaves the hands to go to the client or host. (10) 1, 2, 4. Outcome 7. The best way to reduce drug-resistant organisms in clients is to teach them to take all antibiotics that are prescribed, avoid antibiotics when they are not needed, and take care to wash the hands to avoid transmitting the organism. The other two choices do not address the question of reducing risk. Bacteria can become naturally resistant to antibiotics because bacteria can be left behind even when the antibiotic works properly, but this fact does not address risk reduction. The most common drug-resistant organisms are MRSA, vancomycin-resistant enterococci (VRE), and multi-drug-resistant tuberculosis, not streptococcus.

CHAPTER 11

NCLEX-PN® ANSWERS   (1) 2. Outcome 1. The client is distracted and not listening to what the nurse is saying so the nurse is the sender, the message is being sent, but the receiver is not hearing the message. (2) 2. Outcome 2. The nurse is invading the client's personal space, creating anxiety, which is negatively influencing the communication process. (3) 3. Outcome 3. Nonverbal communication speaks louder than verbal communication, so the nurse is sending a message that the nurse is in a hurry and is annoyed that the client wants to ask a question. (4) 1. Outcome 4. The nurse's best response would be silence to allow the client time to gather his or her thoughts and express feelings. (5) 4. Outcome 5. It is best to ask need-to-know questions and to avoid asking questions for curiosity's sake. If a client asks a question UAPs cannot answer, they should seek the right answer, not pretend. Clients should be called by their last name unless they say otherwise. Sharing personal experiences is generally discouraged, unless it specifically helps the client; it should never be used to lead

clients toward behaving as the healthcare provider believes they should. (6) 2. Outcome 6. It is best to acknowledge the mistake and apologize. Changing the subject, ignoring your mistake, or ending the session quickly will set up barriers to a therapeutic relationship. (7) 2. Outcome 8. Active listening demonstrates an interest in what the client is saying with eye contact, posture, and gestures. Interrupting, making notes, and looking at your watch or away do not demonstrate an interest on the part of the nurse. (8) 3. Outcome 9. A leading question is one in which the questioner gives the answer with the question. It can often be answered with one word, closing the subject. It does not give clients an opportunity to express their own feelings. (9) 4. Outcome 11. The body is the part of the interview during which the client can communicate what she or he thinks, feels, knows, or perceives in response to the nurse's questions. (10) 2. Outcome 11. Expressing enjoyment for the time together and appreciation for what was accomplished is an excellent way to let the client know the interview is coming to an end. Abruptly cutting off conversation or changing position will not allow the client to express additional needs or wants. Telling the client you have other people you must see may make him or her feel unimportant and place a barrier for future communication.

CHAPTER 12

NCLEX-PN® ANSWERS   (1) 1. Outcome 2. In behaviorism, correct choices are rewarded and behaviors that are incorrect and need to be avoided are ignored. (2) 3. Outcome 1. Restoration involves information about what is being done as well as self-care skills and resources. (3) 4. Outcome 4. Pain is a barrier to learning because it decreases concentration. Pain needs to be dealt with prior to initiating teaching. (4) 2. Outcome 9. When evaluating client learning, the nurse must listen for clues that the client misunderstood or did not fully comprehend the scope of what was taught. The client planning to use a damp cloth, even if only slightly damp, requires further teaching. (5) 3. Outcome 7. The nurse needs to validate the client's feeling and help restore self-confidence by encouraging the client to practice the skills. Some clients may be comforted by having a loved one attend the teaching session with them. (6) 3. Outcome 8. Many cultural groups, especially those from Asian cultures, are reluctant to maintain eye contact with professionals, feeling that it is a lack of respect. It does not mean that they are confused, lack interest, or lack respect. (7) 1, 2, 5. Outcome 5. During the assessment phase of the teaching process, the nurse obtains an educational history including clients' educational level, learning style, and motivation to learn. Outcomes are selected and strategies are developed in the planning process. (8) 2. Outcome 6. The LPN/LVN collaborates with the RN to develop and carry out a teaching plan, reinforces teaching, and assists with data collection. Responsibility for development of a plan of care including the teaching plan belongs to the RN. (9) 1. Outcome 4. Negative feedback will cause the client to avoid the nurse and it will damage the nurse–client relationship. It is never appropriate and should not be used in any teaching situation, whether with a client or a fellow staff member. (10) 4. Outcome 7. Discussion about troubleshooting should be delayed until the client is comfortable with the procedure, so that the client does not become overwhelmed and unable to process all of the information.

CHAPTER 13

NCLEX-PN®ANSWERS (1) 3. Outcome 9. This answer is most accurate and reflects the need to inform the doctor of the client's emotional status. (2) 4. Outcome 5. There is no reason to discuss a client's condition when not directly involved in that client's care. Choice 3 would respect client confidentiality as you are explaining to a visitor what precautions are required to enter the room. (3) 4. Outcome 3. When using the source-oriented record system, the documents are divided according to the source, so nursing notes would be found in a section labeled "nursing." Option 1 describes problem-oriented systems; the database (option 3) does not address the question; and notes written by all providers together in one spot is also problem-oriented (option 2). (4) 1. Outcome 4. This is the correct procedure for most agencies. While the chart does belong to the facility, the information inside the chart belongs to the client. The client has a right to a copy after completing the proper requisition form. There may be a copy fee but it does not take 6 to 8 weeks to receive the copy (option 4). (5) 3. Outcome 2. It is not correct practice to cross out an entry or entries so that your notes are in chronological order. A late entry made with the event's time and labeled as a late entry is appropriate. (6) 2. Outcome 12. When taking a telephone order from a physician, writing and signing it prior to hanging up (option 1) is not enough. It is important to write the orders down as they are received and to read the orders back to the physician to ensure accuracy before hanging up the phone. Researching each medication or notifying the charge nurse of every order would be impractical. (7) 1. Outcome 1. Nurses document because it is important to thoroughly record the client's plan of care and response to treatment. Documenting is not done only because of facility policy or to avoid lawsuits. (8) 1, 2, 3, 5. Outcome 13. The nurse would need to first assess the client for signs of adverse effects from the medication, then notify the RN and physician, and finally complete an incident report. Risk management will review the incident report, but there is no need to notify them. (9) 2. Outcome 8. Faxing information to a physician's office is appropriate (if permitted by your agency), but should be followed up with a call to the office to ensure that they received the fax. You should also get the name of the person you spoke with and include an entry in the nurse's notes that you called to verify receipt of the fax. (10) 2. Outcome 7. Walking rounds are common in many facilities but care must be taken to ensure that your comments are appropriate and that your voices are not overheard by people in the hall. Caution must also be taken when speaking in front of the client, because medical terminology may be misunderstood or misinterpreted by the client.

CHAPTER 14

NCLEX-PN® ANSWERS (1) 1. Outcome 1. The two most common reactions to hospitalization are fear of the unknown and anxiety. By reassuring clients that you will inform them of anything to be done, clients' anxiety can be relieved. (2) 4. Outcome 2. During the initial interview, language skills and understanding should be assessed and arrangements made for an interpreter if necessary. Choice 1 is wrong because Indian is an incorrect means of referring to Native Americans. Clients should never be addressed by their first names unless they specifically request the informal address. While speaking clearly in nonmedical terminology is important, it is also important not to raise the voice or speak down to the client. (3) 4. Outcome 7. The priority action for a client in distress is to move the client as quickly as possible. In order to move this client, the oxygen must be applied in a portable manner. Questions, belongings, and a report to the RN can be addressed after the client is safely in the ICU. (4) 3. Outcome 5. The LPN/LVN can assist with collecting baseline subjective and objective data. The Joint Commission requires that a registered nurse perform the admission assessment, formulate the nursing diagnosis, and develop a treatment plan. Restraints require a physician's order except in emergency situations. (5) 2. Outcome 4. The best choice is to send any valuables home with a significant other. (6) 1, 2, 3, 4. Outcome 8. The nurse's responsibilities include evaluating self-care understanding, explaining physician's orders, assembling belongings, and ensuring discharge documentation is completed. While the business office should be informed of the client's discharge, approval is not required. (7) 3. Outcome 9. All clients need discharge planning to begin at admission, but the nurse can anticipate a client with a language barrier will need additional planning and coordination. (8) 3. Outcome 4. Client safety should be the nurse's first concern. The nurse should check the identification band before performing any procedure or giving any medication. (9) 4. Outcome 6. The priority intervention is to notify the child's parent that the child is in a new room. Parents who arrive and find their child is not in their assigned room may panic, believing something terrible happened. (10) 2. Outcome 3. HIPAA allows the nurse to disclose clients of the clergy's religious affiliation. However, additional information beyond the client's name and location is not to be disclosed.

CHAPTER 15

NCLEX-PN® ANSWERS (1) 1. Outcome 2. Freud's theory includes 5 stages of psychosexual development, while Erikson's theory includes 8 stages of psychosocial development. Both theorists believe development occurs in a predictable pattern throughout the life span. (2) 1. Outcome 6. The 2-year-old is developing autonomy by exploring the world, so allowing the child to examine and play with a nasogastric tube would help him or her become more familiar with the equipment and less afraid. Asking the child's permission to insert the tube, especially at this age, would not be an effective strategy because the tube needs to be inserted even if the child declines. This child is in the concrete operational phase of cognitive development, so the child cannot draw inferences from a teddy bear with a tube in place. It is unlikely a 2-year-old would be able to hold still during an uncomfortable procedure; the nurse will require assistance to insert the tube. (3) 2. Outcome 1. Industry occurs during school age; by successfully accomplishing this task, the child develops a sense of competence. Autonomy occurs during early childhood (18 months to 3 years). Identity occurs during adolescence. Ego integrity occurs in the mature years at approximately 65 years of age. (4) 3. Outcome 3. Stage 4 of Kohlberg's moral development theory defines right behavior as obeying rules and following laws without consideration of reasonable times for modifying them. (5) 4. Outcome 6. Paradoxical-consolidation stage occurs after age 30; individuals become less dogmatic and use their spiritual beliefs to deal with life's difficulties. Intuitive-projective and mythical-literal are childhood stages of spiritual development, and synthetic-conventional stage begins in the adolescent years and has an interpersonal focus. (6) 3. Outcome 5. The self-actualization level is achieved when a person accomplishes a goal or dream. This is the highest level, which is not reached by everyone in their lifetimes. (7) 3. Outcome 4. This client is in the concrete operational stage of development, meaning the child will interpret literally what the nurse has said. As a result, the child who hears "stick" will think the nurse is talking about the only kind of stick the child has seen—a branch or piece of a branch from a tree. Nurses must choose their words carefully with children. (8) 4. Outcome 7. Behavioral therapy looks at the behavior and provides strategies to increase desirable behavior and minimize undesirable behavior. Negative reinforcement is never appropriate in the therapeutic environment. (9) 2. Outcome 6. The therapeutic environment, according to Rogers, requires genuineness, unconditional positive regard, and empathetic understanding. This does not include agreeing with clients (which is generally discouraged) or false reassurances. (10) 1. Outcome 7. Being direct and serious is the appropriate way to approach the client with a mental health disorder. Collecting physical data will help rule out physical causes. Restraints are never appropriate unless the client is a threat to self or others and can only be instituted without a physician's order if there is a verified emergency. Playing background music may cause the client to become more agitated.

CHAPTER 16

NCLEX-PN® ANSWERS (1) 2. Outcome 2. The best response is to explain how development occurs cephalocaudally, and that it is very individualized. False reassurance such as in choice 1 or generalized statements as in choices 3 and 4 do not serve to relieve the mother's concerns. (2) 3. Outcome 1. The client's growth is lagging behind and requires further assessment to determine the cause. It may be failure to thrive or there could be a normal explanation such as smaller-than-average parents, which can only be determined by gathering more data. The child's development is not indicated in this question. (3) 1. Outcome 3. The toddler has increasing ability to eat with a spoon, begins to use a fork, and learns to control elimination during the day. (4) 3. Outcome 4. The woman, adjusting to "empty nest syndrome" is in the middle years or stage VII. Beginning stage is the period before having children. Launching is the period of sending children off, but some are still home. Retirement (stage VIII) is often a period of enjoyment and taking stock of one's life. (5) 3. Outcome 5. Parents who expect children to do what they are told are demonstrating authoritarian parenting, whereas those who discuss rules and expectations are demonstrating authoritative parenting. (6) 1. Outcome 6. The nurse needs to offer the adolescent a choice regarding the parent's accompanying the client to the examination room, but it must be done in a manner that allows the teen to refuse without protest from the mother. Option 4 implies the nurse thinks the client should not want the mother, making it difficult for the teen to admit preferences for the mother's presence. (7) 2. Outcome 6. The mother is calling the baby "it" which indicates a potential problem with parenting, so the best diagnosis would be *Risk for Impaired Parenting*. (8) 1. Outcome 7. Important safety measures to teach the middle adult are home safety measures. Sun protection and water safety would be important for the young adult, and home safety to prevent falls would be important for the older adult. (9) 3. Outcome 3. Plantar reflex generally does not fade until 8 months of age but the other reflexes are expected to be absent by 4 months of age. (10) 2. Outcome 7. Important teaching considerations for the young adult male would be behavior that can reduce the risk of STIs. Iron and folic acid intake would be important teaching considerations for the young adult female, and actions to reduce calorie intake are more important for the older adult whose activity levels may be declining.

CHAPTER 17

NCLEX-PN® ANSWERS (1) 4. Outcome 1. Although physical assessment is important, it is not part of a psychosocial assessment, whereas emotional, behavioral, and interactional aspects are. (2) 4. Outcome 6. Denial is an unconscious refusal to accept situations as they are. (3) 3. Outcome 2. Affect would also need to be observed. Sensation, trust, and memory have already been addressed and found to be within normal limits according to the root of the question. (4) 1. Outcome 5. Mild anxiety heightens the person's response. Higher levels of anxiety decrease the person's ability to respond and cope. (5) 2.

Outcome 4. The client with major depressive disorder may demonstrate changes in sleep patterns, prolonged periods of low mood, loss of interest, and feelings of worthlessness. Seasonal affective disorder results from lack of sunshine, postnatal depression follows delivery, and bipolar disorder manifests as periods of depression interspersed with hyperactive periods. (6) 4. Outcome 8. Anxiety can worsen the symptoms of respiratory diseases, so the nurse should teach the client anxiety-reducing strategies and work with the client to implement them during periods of stress. (7) 3. Outcome 3. A serious medical condition is associated with all options except option 3. Feelings of loss are a response to medical conditions. (8) 1. Outcome 3. This client is demonstrating signs of ICU psychosis that can be caused by frequent interruptions of sleep and repetitive noises. This is a temporary condition. (9) 3. Outcome 9. A realistic outcome for this client would be to list strategies to reduce feelings of isolation. No longer feeling isolated may not be reasonable for this client and would take a long time to accomplish. Anxiety is not an issue with this client, so this outcome would not meet the client's needs. (10) 2. Outcome 7. An important developmental need of the adolescent is conformity with peers and learning to form relationships with others. Teens are particularly affected by body image changes and will require additional support.

CHAPTER 18

NCLEX-PN® ANSWERS (1) 2. Outcome 4. In mutual pretense, the family and health personnel know the prognosis but no one talks about it. With closed awareness, the client and the family are unaware of the impending death. In open awareness, the client, family, and staff know about the impending death and feel comfortable discussing it, even though it is difficult. (2) 1. Outcome 4. When the client is in the denial stage there is a refusal to believe that the loss is happening. The client may be artificially cheerful to prolong denial. (3) 3. Outcome 7. A notarized document that outlines the client's wishes should be followed. In some states the wishes of a domestic partner cannot overrule the wishes of the family. The ER physician's assessment determines the status of the client; once this has been determined, the notarized durable power of attorney will be the basis for the decisions. (4) 3. Outcome 9. Expressing feelings to an understanding listener helps to facilitate the grieving process. Communication helps people deal openly with their emotions and feelings, which is healthier than suppressing them. Being sent home or changing assignment would not help promote grieving. Asking the CNA to perform postmortem care in the emotional state would show disregard for the trauma the individual may be experiencing. (5) 2. Outcome 8. When the parents wish to see their stillborn baby, the baby can be cleaned and wrapped in a baby blanket. The mother and father of the baby should be allowed to see, touch, and hold their baby. Although some parents may not wish to view the baby, doing so allows them to

close the cycle of birth and death and accept the fact that their baby is dead. Providing the parents with a picture and a lock of the baby's hair allows them a keepsake they can revisit when needed. (6) 3. Outcome 8. Complicated grieving is characterized by physical and psychological reactions and thoughts of suicide. (7) 3. Outcome 2. Children from 9 to 12 years old express an interest in the afterlife; 5-year-olds look at death as reversible or temporary; 5- to 9-year-olds believe that unrelated events can be responsible for the death; 12- to 18-year-olds view it in religious or philosophic terms. (8) 1. Outcome 3. The nurse should acknowledge the client's feelings and instruct him on the need to teach the children how to cope with the loss of their mother. Postponing telling them is not the best strategy, but they are his children and the nurse should not voice criticism if he makes that choice. (9) 4. Outcome 5. The client is emotionally relocating her deceased husband and preparing to move on with life, which is task 4. (10) 3. Outcome 6. The client's family should be made to understand that feelings of confusion, disorientation, fear, or guilt are normal and will subside with time. Only if these feelings last for longer than a year would dysfunctional grieving be a consideration.

CHAPTER 19

NCLEX-PN® ANSWERS (1) 1. Outcome 1. Complete assessments are generally performed by the RN when a new client is admitted, which includes the health history. LPNs/LVNs contribute to data collection for the exam. (2) 4. Outcome 2. Auscultation of the breath sounds is the priority examination for this client. While other assessments may be performed as well, assessment of breath sounds will determine effectiveness of the treatment. (3) 3. Outcome 2. Clients with many different diagnoses would require measurement of vital signs and assessment of intake and output, but assessment of skin turgor would be of particular importance to the client diagnosed with hypovolemia. (4) 4. Outcome 4. It is not unusual to find longitudinal bands, translucent and less flexible tympanic membranes, and a heart rate that returns to baseline slowly after exercise in an elderly adult, and these can be considered normal findings for this age group. (5) 1. Outcome 3. This client is voicing anxiety that might be allayed by explaining what will be done and what the client will experience during the physical examination, so this is the priority nursing intervention. Some clients may appreciate having a family member stay with them, while others would consider it an invasion of privacy. This decision should be made by the client, not the nurse. (6) 4. Outcome 5. The nurse will want to look at the client's cut to determine how deep it is, how long it is, how much bleeding is occurring, and what the wound looks like. There would be no need for auscultation or percussion, and palpation would be less useful than inspection. (7) 1. Outcome 6. The wound is superior, or above, the knee. (8) 1. Outcome 7. It appears that the client may have scabies.

The nurse should complete the assessment wearing gloves because scabies can be spread by direct skin-to-skin contact. (9) 2. Outcome 8. This description of breath sounds describes rhonchi, or gurgles, which are harsher than rales. Adventitious breath sounds is a broad term only describing that there are abnormal sounds without explaining specifically what those abnormal sounds are. (10) 4. Outcome 9. When performing examinations on young children and infants, it is best to leave painful, intrusive, or uncomfortable assessments for last because the child may cry, which would interfere with an accurate assessment of other systems.

CHAPTER 20

NCLEX-PN® ANSWERS (1) 3. Outcome 4. Early morning care includes washing the face and hands and giving oral care or assisting the client in doing these hygiene tasks. It also includes offering the urinal or bedpan if the client requires complete bed rest. (2) 1. Outcome 2. It is best to follow the client's preferences whenever possible if they do not endanger the client's health or break facility policy. This action on the part of the nurse provides the client with a sense of participation and control and helps the client's self-esteem. Also, having a familiar routine is comforting to the client. (3) 1. Outcome 3. Loose bed linen and wrinkles can cause irritation and possible skin breakdown. Air drying promotes pathogen growth, especially between the toes, so the feet should be patted dry gently to avoid tissue injury. Extra weight on the feet in the form of blankets can decrease circulation and increase skin breakdown. (4) 4. Outcome 1. Changing the client's clothes is required to meet the client's hygiene needs, but it is not usually the nurse's responsibility to wash the clothes. (5) 2. Outcome 7. Position the unconscious client in a side-lying position, with the head of the bed lowered. In this position, the saliva automatically runs out by gravity rather than being aspirated into the lungs. If the client cannot be placed in the side-lying position, turn the head to one side. (6) 4. Outcome 6. To protect the nurse from pediculosis capitis, the nurse should wear a cap over the head when working with a client who needs assistance with shampooing the hair with pyrethrin shampoo. (7) 4. Outcome 5. The client should be taught to use warm, not hot, water; pat the foot dry, particularly between the toes; and soak the feet for 10 to 20 minutes before cutting nails. Rubbing calloused areas will help to remove dead skin layers and will reduce the risk of injury that could be caused by a pumice stone. (8) 4. Outcome 10. The nurse should never place soiled linen anywhere except a linen bag because of pathogens contained on the linen. Care should also be taken not to touch the linen to the uniform, which could result in cross contamination for another client. (9) 2. Outcome 7. The nurse needs to use a different cotton ball for each wipe and throw the used cotton ball away without contaminating the water to be used on new cotton balls. The nurse wipes from inner to outer canthus. The eye shield is used only with a physician's order if the corneal reflex is absent. (10) 1. Outcome 9. The first step in making an occupied bed is to remove the top linen after covering the client with a bath blanket for privacy and warmth.

CHAPTER 21

NCLEX-PN® ANSWERS (1) 3. Outcome 13. A temperature of 101.8 (A) is considered to be one degree lower than an oral temp. A temperature of 102.8 would warrant immediate reporting. A blood pressure above 140 should be compared to the client's last reading. A pulse of 100 or above should be reassessed after the client has rested. (2) 2. Outcome 12. Blood pressure should not be taken in the arm on the side of a mastectomy. It also should not be taken on an arm that has sustained an injury. It is best to obtain a larger cuff and take the pressure on the thigh. (3) 1. Outcome 12. A cuff with a bladder that is too narrow will provide an erroneously high blood pressure reading. (4) 4. Outcome 10. Phase 5 of the Korotkoff's sounds is considered to be the adult diastolic pressure, which is the last sound followed by a period of silence. (5) 4. Outcome 11. When converting Celsius temperature to Fahrenheit, 38.6 converts to 101.48; 101.5 is the closest answer option. (6) 4. Outcome 5. Pulse for children under 3 years of age is best assessed apically. (7) 1. Outcome 2. Normal systolic blood pressure for a child is $80 + 2 \times$ the child's age or 92 in this case. (8) 1. Outcome 9. The nurse is measuring orthostatic blood pressure readings. It is unknown what the results are, so conclusions about hypotension or hypertension cannot be made. (9) 3. Outcome 1. Prior to administration of digoxin, the apical pulse must be assessed. The medication is held if the apical pulse is less than 60 or more than 100. (10) 3. Outcome 8. Narcotics can suppress respirations, so the client or support people should assess respirations following administration of MS Contin.

CHAPTER 22

NCLEX-PN® ANSWERS (1) 3. Outcome 3. The client's pain is caused by chemicals released secondary to ischemia so this is chemical pain. (2) 1. Outcome 12. Using a numerical pain rating scale is the most effective way of assessing the severity of the pain, but it is a good idea to help the client quantify the pain based on past experiences like labor or a paper cut. Asking too many questions at once will result in some questions being skipped. Words such as mild, moderate, or severe have no objective meaning. (3) 1, 2. Outcome 1. The client is suffering chronic pain because it has lasted longer than 6 months and the pain is intractable because it is not responding to analgesia requiring the exploration of other methods of pain control. There is not enough information provided to know if the pain is visceral or referred. (4) 2. Outcome 7. After increasing the client's dosage of narcotics, an essential and priority nursing action is to assess the client's respiratory status because respiratory depression could occur. Evaluating the effectiveness of the medication is important, but secondary to respiratory assessment. It is not necessary to wake the client to measure vital signs every 15 minutes if pain relief is obtained. Darkening the room and asking visitors to allow the client to sleep may be appropriate but of lower priority than respiratory assessment. (5) 4. Outcome 4. The gate control theory states that a nerve can only send a certain amount of signals at a time and adjutant therapy can occupy the nerves so pain signals cannot be transmitted. (6) 2. Outcome 2. The nurse should educate the UAP on the subjective nature of pain and explain that every individual has a different pain tolerance based on factors that influence their perception of pain. (7) 1, 2, 3, 5. Outcome 13. Infants can be difficult to assess for pain because their pain indicators can be varied including restlessness, change in heart rate (increase or decrease), change in blood pressure (increase or decrease), and grimacing. Infants may lie still because the pain reduces the client's energy level or they can thrash about. If the infant is sleeping quietly and vital signs are stable, the infant is most likely not in pain. (8) 2, 4, 5. Outcome 6. The World Health Organization recommends treating cancer pain by administering a NSAID, followed by a weak opioid. The weak opioid dose should be increased to maximum dosage before adding a stronger opioid. (9) 4. Outcome 11. Fear of addiction, cultural beliefs about pain, and lack of knowledge about side effects and their treatments can all act as barriers to pain management. While some physicians may under-prescribe analgesics, the physician who wants to be called if pain management is not achieved is not a barrier to pain control. (10) 4. Outcome 10. There are narcotic analgesics that can be taken orally and have an 8-hour duration of action, which would improve the client's ability to sleep through the night. Taking parenteral medications is often seen by clients as less than optimal, increasing the dosage could result in respiratory depression, and having the client take naps does not really resolve the client's problem with sleeping through the night.

CHAPTER 23

NCLEX-PN® ANSWERS (1) 2. Outcome 2. While option 1 is technically correct, the client will most likely not understand what you are saying. Option 2 provides an explanation that will make sense to the client. (2) 3. Outcome 3. Osteoporosis is a demineralization process of the bones, which occurs without the stress of weight-bearing activity. Contractures are permanent shortenings of the muscles that cause permanent fixation of joints, which can be avoided by performing passive or active range of motion. Orthostatic hypotension is a drop in blood pressure following a rapid change in position which may occur in some clients, especially the elderly or those with cardiac disorders. Disuse atrophy is loss of normal strength and function and size of unused muscles, which commonly occurs

when a client is on bed rest but is of less concern than osteoporosis. (3) 4. Outcome 12. While oxygen saturation may be monitored, it is unlikely the client will require the invasive process of arterial blood gases. EEG, EMG, and EOG are often performed synchronously in order to assess the depth and level of sleep. (4) 1. Outcome 4. Crutches must be adjusted so that weight is on the forearm, not the axilla, since pressure on the underarm can damage the brachial plexus. (5) 3. Outcome 6. The orthopneic position brings the client to more of a vertical orientation, which aids in air exchange in respiratory and heart clients. (6) 3. Outcome 9. Stage III occurs when heart and respiratory rates and other body processes slow and are dominated by the parasympathetic nervous system. The sleeper becomes more difficult to arouse. Stages I and II are light sleep; stage IV is deep sleep. (7) 3. Outcome 10. Hypothyroidism decreases stage IV sleep. Hyperthyroidism lengthens presleep time, making it difficult to fall asleep. (8) 2. Outcome 11. Treatment of insomnia routinely includes behavior modification in which the client learns new habits to foster sleep. Long-term sleep-inducing medication is not recommended because it does not treat the cause and can result in dependency. Anti-depressants and beta-blockers can cause nightmares and daytime drowsiness. (9) 2. Outcome 13. The best action by the nurse would be to schedule procedures and medications to reduce or limit nighttime interruptions. Entering the client's room to assess their sleep will likely awaken the client. Chronic use of sedatives is more likely to disturb sleep. Turning off the overhead pager is both not possible and dangerous. (10) 1. Outcome 7. Even mild conditioning can strengthen the legs and increase circulation, which will help relieve postural hypotension.

CHAPTER 24

NCLEX-PN® ANSWERS (1) 2. Outcome 4. The nurse's first priority is to change the client's position to relieve pressure on the area and prevent further breakdown in that spot. Repositioning the client frequently will reduce the risk of skin breakdown in other areas. While documentation is necessary, it is not the first priority. Applying dressings will increase the risk of skin breakdown when the tape is pulled from the area. An air mattress requires a physician's order. (2) 4. Outcome 6. When the damp dressing is removed it helps to eliminate necrotic debris, which has been softened by the moisture. Cooling is an effect of a wet dressing but not its purpose for use. (3) 3. Outcome 1. The 32-year-old client is at greatest risk because of the number of risk factors involved, including immobility, invasive medical procedures, and chronic disease process. The 86-year-old client will return to normal activity levels in a short period of time and her only risk factor is age. The 24-year-old client has immobility as the only risk factor and the 42-year-old client has no risk factors. (4) 3. Outcome 10. Stage III pressure ulcers involve the subcutaneous tissue and may extend to the underlying fascia but do not extend past that level. (5) 4. Outcome 7. When heat is applied to the skin the body increases blood flow to the area and the body accommodates to the heat, making it feel cooler. Telling the client that the temperature is correct without explaining why it feels cool ignores the client's right to understand their treatment plan. Increasing the temperature would cause a burn, and there is no reason to replace the unit, which is functioning normally. (6) 1. Outcome 3. The second phase of healing includes production of granulation tissue. Eschar is necrotic tissue, suppuration is purulent drainage indicating infection, and reactive hyperemia is increased blood flow to an area following pressure resolution. (7) 4. Outcome 9. Shearing force is caused by skin that is not moving in relationship to downward-sliding body movements in bed and would be the greatest risk facing this client. (8) 3. Outcome 8. Handwashing is the most important intervention performed by healthcare workers to prevent infection of the wound, which will slow healing. Some wounds may be left open to the air while others may be dressed, depending on the physician's preference, location, and type of wound, which is unknown in this instance. Cleaning of the wound is only necessary if there is drainage or some other indicator requiring this intervention, which is not indicated by this question. (9) 3. Outcome 2. This client has abrasions that are caused by friction from sliding across the asphalt and they tend to be painful. A laceration is a penetrating wound. A contusion results from a blow and often causes a bruise. (10) 1. Outcome 4. Wound healing is slowed by smoking, reduced blood flow, and advancing age. The client who is physically fit will heal fastest because he has good blood supply, which brings nutrients for healing. The 24-year-old client would be expected to heal more quickly than the 18-year-old because the younger client smokes.

CHAPTER 25

NCLEX-PN® ANSWERS (1) 1. Outcome 1. Protein provides amino acids, the structural material needed to build body tissues and repair cells. Although protein intake is related to fat intake, this answer does not satisfy the question being asked. Calories are primarily gained from consumption of carbohydrates, not proteins. Calcium may be present in protein, but supplements are often given to those at risk for decreased bone density. (2) 2. Outcome 9. Helping the client see that they do not have to give up taste to comply with their new diet will help them change their eating habits. Threatening the client or asking the client to compromise taste for health will often result in noncompliance. (3) 4. Outcome 5. The nurse's first response should be to find out why the client isn't hungry. Presenting a client with no appetite a large tray of food will be more likely to reduce the appetite than to increase it. The data should be documented and the physician informed, but it is not the priority action. (4) 2. Outcome 4. Replacing red meat with lean fish and poultry is an important step in reducing fat intake. Cream sauces tend to be high in fat, which would increase LDL cholesterol. It is not

necessary to shop in specialty stores. Onion and celery salt contain sodium and are not suitable substitutes. (5) 2. Outcome 3. A person who is 20% over ideal body weight is obese and remains at risk even though he or she may be physically active. (6) 2. Outcome 8. No feeding is to be started until placement is clearly and positively identified. There is no indication in the question that the client would require weighing or new formula and an order would be needed to apply restraints. (7) 1. Outcome 2. The primary purpose of carbohydrates is to provide essential nutrients to meet the body's energy needs. Insulation is a function of fats. Protein provides building blocks for body repair. Although fiber is a carbohydrate, not all carbohydrates are fiber. (8) 2. Outcome 4. Cranberry juice is a clear liquid and would be appropriate on this tray. Milkshakes, apricot nectar, and creamed soups are not clear liquids and would be appropriate on a full liquid diet. (9) 3. Outcome 11. Medications should never be mixed together when administering medications via a nasogastric tube. Each medication should be given individually, flushing the tube with water before beginning, between each medication, and after all medications have been given. (10) 1. Outcome 5. The nurse should encourage clients to participate in the process as much as they are able. Foods and fluids should be interspersed and fluids should be offered after every few bites. If possible, ask clients what they would like to eat next. Sitting on a client's bed invades personal space and risks contamination of the nurse's uniform and should be discouraged.

CHAPTER 26

NCLEX-PN® ANSWERS (1) Respiratory alkalosis. Outcome 3. When a client breathes rapidly, CO_2 (an acid) is blown off, causing a decrease in $PaCO_2$ and elevated pH. This occurs when pain, anxiety, or fever causes hyperventilation. (2) 1. Outcome 1. Insensible losses occur through the skin in the form of perspiration and diffusion and from the lungs in exhaled air. (3) 2. Outcome 9. To calculate the answer, you add the urine output and the amount of emesis to gain an accurate result. (4) 2. Outcome 8. Increased sodium intake results in increased water retention, which increases the amount of circulating volume in the bloodstream, resulting in elevation of blood pressure. Most clients with hypertension should be taught to restrict sodium. (5) 4. Outcome 7. The secretions suctioned from the stomach are fluid loss. Ice chips, gelatin, and IV fluids are included in calculations for fluid intake. (6) 4. Outcome 2. Isotonic fluids have the same concentration as blood serum and other body fluids. They expand the intravascular compartments of the body without causing a shift in fluids. (7) 1. Outcome 7. When fatty acids change to ketone bodies, such as what is seen in diabetes mellitus, metabolic acidosis may occur. (8) 2. Outcome 4. Potassium helps maintain ECF and ICF water balance and acid-base balance and is vital for skeletal, cardiac, and smooth muscle activity. A deficiency can affect cardiac function. (9) 1. Outcome 7. Increased sodium intake results in fluid retention. (10) 4.

Outcome 4. Bicarbonate excess, or metabolic alkalosis, is exhibited by symptoms of dizziness, tingling of fingers and toes, decreased respirations, and cardiac dysrhythmias.

CHAPTER 27

NCLEX-PN® ANSWERS (1) 4. Outcome 3. The fastest route of administration is the parenteral route, specifically intravenous, because this places the medication directly into the bloodstream. (2) 1. Outcome 2. When administering medication the nurse is responsible for his or her actions so the responsible party in this case is the nurse, who should have questioned the order prior to administration to ensure accuracy. (3) 3. Outcome 1. The reason a drug is prescribed is the therapeutic effects. The other choices are adverse, or unwanted, effects of the drug. (4) 2. Outcome 3. Many medications are broken down by the liver and excreted by the kidney. Reduced function of these organs, in addition to the client's age, would make the nurse anticipate reduction in dosage of some medications while other medications may be contraindicated for this client. (5) 2. Outcome 4. A "stat" order is one that is to be given immediately and only once. An order that is to be given as needed is a PRN order. An order that has no discontinuation date is known as a standing order. A regular order is given on a prescribed schedule, usually determined by the facility. (6) 3. Outcome 5. To calculate the proper dosage, place what is on hand on one side of the equation and what is to be given on the other side of the formula. $1\,mg/mL = 0.4\,mg/x$. Cross multiply $1 \times x = 0.4 \times 1$ yields $x = 0.4\,mL$ so the nurse will administer 0.4 mL. (7) 4. Outcome 8. Using a medicine cup is the most accurate way for the mother to measure the medication. A household teaspoon is not accurate and should not be used. Mixing medication with essential food can alter the taste and makes it impossible to determine if the child got the ordered dosage. The medication is ordered every 6 hours, which means it needs to be given around the clock, through the night. (8) 2. Outcome 6. The nurse would use a tuberculin syringe, which is the most accurate means of measuring quantities less than 1 mL. Insulin syringes should be used for insulin only because of the specific calibrations in units on the barrel. (9) 1. Outcome 12. The primary reason for wearing gloves is to prevent the nurse's skin from absorbing the topical medication; gloves also prevent the spread of pathogens found on the nurse's hands. Sterile technique is not required when administering topical medications, and the effect of getting medication on the skin will depend on the medication. Handwashing that is routinely done before and after administering medication would prevent cross contamination. (10) 2. Outcome 11. The gluteal muscles are developed by walking, so they should not be used for injections until the child has been walking for at least 1 year.

CHAPTER 28

NCLEX-PN® ANSWERS (1) 1. Outcome 6. An 18-gauge cannula should be selected, if the client's veins will accommodate

it, so that no hemolysis of the blood will occur. (2) 4. Outcome 9. Only normal saline (0.9%) should be hung with blood in order to prevent complications during the transfusion. (3) 2. Outcome 3. An intermittent infusion device is used for vascular access for the client receiving medications. Other uses include drawing blood, emergency medication administration, and reducing the client's cost while increasing mobility and comfort. (4) 1. Outcome 4. IV fluid administration rate is calculated by the amount of fluid to be administered, divided by the number of hours it is to infuse, divided by 60 (the number of minutes in an hour) and multiplied by the number of drops per milliliter delivered by the solution set. In this problem, the calculations would be 1,000 mL to be infused divided by 6 hours divided by 60 multiplied by 10 drops per minute. The answer is 27.7. Because it is impossible to count 0.7 drops per minute, the answer is rounded to 28 drops per minute. (5) 1. Outcome 5. The peripheral vein that is most appropriate for blood administration and medications that may be irritating is the cephalic vein. The size of this vein accommodates a large-gauge needle. (6) 4. Outcome 7. The IV catheter is generally inserted at a narrow angle (15 degrees) with the bevel up while stretching the vein to prevent movement. When backflow is seen in the IV catheter, the solution may be connected and run at a slow rate to help "wash" the catheter into the vein while stretch is maintained. Approaching the vein from the side will allow the student to feel the "pop" of entry. (7) 1. Outcome 2. Because the client is demonstrating signs of dehydration, the best fluid to administer would be an isotonic fluid such as normal saline solution or lactated Ringer's. 0.45% normal saline is hypotonic and would pull fluid from the cells, whereas D_5LR and D_5NS are hypertonic and would pull fluid from the intravascular space and push it into the intracellular space, creating a vascular depletion that would worsen the client's dehydration. (8) 4. Outcome 1. Each state has different rules and regulations determining what is within the scope of the nurse's practice. When nurses move from one state to another they must familiarize themselves with the new state's nurse practice act. If the nurse practice act allows an action but the facility where the nurse is employed has policies forbidding that action, the facility policies take priority. (9) 1. Outcome 3. A minidrip (microdrip) administration set that delivers 60 gtt/minute is used primarily for pediatric clients or those at increased risk if excessive amounts of fluid are administered. (10) 2. Outcome 8. Septicemia is a central line complication exhibited by fever, profuse sweating, low blood pressure, and nausea. A local infection would not create a systemic response such as a fever.

CHAPTER 29

NCLEX-PN® ANSWERS (1) 4. Outcome 1. The preoperative period ends when the client is moved to the operating room and the intraoperative period ends when the client leaves the operating room. (2) 4. Outcome 6. A client may retain his or her wedding ring as long as it is secured with tape, unless he or she is having arm or hand surgery or a surgical procedure that may produce arm or hand swelling. A modified radical mastectomy involves removal of the lymph nodes, which can result in swelling of the hand and finger so this client must have the ring removed. (3) 3. Outcome 8. The client with hypoventilation and hypotension must be monitored more frequently than every 4 hours to ensure that there is no respiratory or circulatory compromise. It is not unusual for the client during the immediate postoperative period to have a minor increase in heart rate secondary to fluid loss or excess, and pain. (4) 2. Outcome 7. A client who is not fully responsive is placed on one side with the head slightly elevated, if possible, or in a position that allows fluids to drain from the mouth. It is recommended that a responsive client remain flat following spinal anesthesia for 8 to 12 hours to avoid complications. Semi-Fowler's is contraindicated. (5) 1. Outcome 5. The client should be in Fowler's or semi-Fowler's position during coughing and deep breathing in order to move secretions. The supine position reduces the effectiveness of coughing and deep breathing. (6) 3. Outcome 2. An appendectomy is performed to remove infected tissue that is discarded, so this surgery is ablative. While it will relieve the client's pain, it will also cure the problem so it is not palliative. Diagnostic surgery is done to learn about the condition. Reconstructive surgery, rebuilds a part. (7) 3. Outcome 9. Early ambulation is key in promoting postoperative recovery. Explaining this to the client is empowering and encourages compliance. (8) 3. Outcome 4. Only the physician can take responsibility for answering the client's questions or discussing the decision of whether or not surgery will be performed. If a client changes his or her mind, the signed operative consent is no longer valid and the physician must be notified as soon as possible. The client should not be premedicated or sent to the surgical suite until the physician speaks with him or her. (9) 2. Outcome 11. Gastric contents follow the path of least resistance, so the vent tube must be kept higher than the stomach to prevent reflux. (10) 3. Outcome 10. Evisceration is the protrusion of a body organ from a wound opening. Dehiscence is a separation in layers of the incisional wound with no protrusion of an organ. Secondary intention refers to the healing when the wound is large, gaping, and irregular. Granulation is new tissue healing that will fill in the wound to close it.

CHAPTER 30

NCLEX-PN® ANSWERS (1) 3. Outcome 1. The reticular layer lends elasticity to the skin. (2) 3. Outcome 2. A macule is flat, unraised, and less than a centimeter. (3) 1. Outcome 4. The primary nursing action would be to remove crusts with a mild soap and apply neomycin antibiotic ointment. Oral analgesics are generally not needed, and covering the wound will slow healing. Impetigo is not a fungal infection. (4) 1. Outcome 3. The most important information to teach the client about treating herpes simplex with an antiviral is the importance of beginning therapy early in the appearance of the lesion because

the client will likely have future outbreaks that can be minimized if started on therapy quickly. The medication does not cure the disease but minimizes its effect and reduces viral shedding; analgesics may be needed in some cases for pain control until the lesions resolve. (5) 4. Outcome 5. Pain in the eye could indicate that the herpes zoster has spread to the cornea, which can cause blindness so this complaint should be reported immediately. (6) 3. Outcome 7. Oral antifungals can interact with warfarin and alter clotting times. (7) 1. Outcome 6. Kwell lotion is an effective pediculicide and scabicide. It would not be indicated for psoriasis, herpes, or eczema. (8) 3. Outcome 8. Malignant melanoma invades the dermis and spreads via lymph and blood vessels through the body; it is the most serious diagnosis. (9) 2. Outcome 5. Mycosis fungoides is seen in clients with depressed immunity; therefore, it is an "opportunistic" infection and, because it is a type of cancer (T cell lymphoma) can affect multiple organs in the body. (10) 1, 2, 3. Outcome 9. Skin grafts are used to close wounds that cannot be closed with normal skin regrowth, cover large areas of tissue lost secondary to burns, and when trauma to the skin damages the stratum germinativum layer.

CHAPTER 31

NCLEX-PN® ANSWERS (1) 1. Outcome 1. Bone resorption and bone deposit are regulated by both hormone activity and the stress to the bone caused by use. Calcium is a necessary component of bone but does not regulate bone resorption or deposit. (2) 3. Outcome 3. RICE stands for Rest, Ice, Compression, and Elevation, which is the treatment of a sprain or strain. (3) 4. Outcome 6. Using the palms of the hands will prevent the nurse from pushing the plaster against the skin and causing dents or pressure points. (4) 3. Outcome 2. Arthroscopy is done to examine the joint. One of the conditions that may be found is a torn ligament, but that is not the only purpose of the test. (5) 2. Outcome 5. The symptoms indicate the possibility of osteomyelitis and need to be reported immediately. Massage and analgesia will slow the initiation of proper treatment. A client in traction with a pin in the femur cannot physically get out of bed. (6) 3. Outcome 9. The client has a lordosis, which is the exaggeration of the lumbar curve. Scoliosis is a lateral deviation. Kyphosis is curvature of the thoracic spine. Ankylosing spondylitis is generalized spinal stiffening. (7) 1. Outcome 7. Acute episodes of rheumatoid arthritis may be precipitated by physical or psychologic stress, infection, and fatigue. (8) 4. Outcome 8. Flexion of the hip greater than 90 degrees may cause the hip that has been replaced to dislocate. The client should be instructed not to flex the hip greater than 90 degrees. (9) 2. Outcome 4. Postmenopause, smoking, thin body frame, and European descent are all risk factors for osteoporosis, so the client in option 2 is at greatest risk. (10) 4. Outcome 12. Exposure to direct sunlight may cause an acute episode of SLE.

CHAPTER 32

NCLEX-PN® ANSWERS (1) 4. Outcome 6. Both low and high Fowler's promote lung expansion, although high Fowler's is most effective. In the Trendelenburg position the head is lower than the feet; this promotes lung drainage, not lung expansion. Sims' position is side lying. It is not a good position for bilateral lung expansion. (2) 3. Outcome 4. Cheyne-Stokes respirations alternate rate and depth. This type of breathing is frequently seen prior to death. Kussmaul breathing is hyperventilation associated with respiratory acidosis; tachypnea is a rapid breathing rate; eupnea is normal respiration. (3) 4. Outcome 11. Restlessness, chest excursion, and nail bed discoloration are related to decreased oxygen, which is the highest priority for any client with respiratory pathology. The other data are important but do not take priority over indications of breathing and oxygenation. (4) 2. Outcome 9. The highest priority in asthma is airway maintenance and gas exchange. Decrease in anxiety level and decreased fever are desirable but not priority. Fluid balance is important for liquefying secretions and clearing airways. (5) 4. Outcome 3. Orthopnea is needing to sit upright to facilitate breathing. Changes in BP on standing are orthostatic hypotension. A breathing pattern related to respiratory acidosis is Kussmaul breathing; breathing with periods of apnea is called Cheyne-Stokes breathing. (6) 3. Outcome 9. Tracheostomy tubes are generally placed when it is anticipated the client will require an artificial airway for longer than 5 to 7 days. The only client anticipated to need an artificial airway for more than a few days is the client with a fractured cervical vertebra with no respiratory drive. The other clients may require mechanical ventilation (except for option 4), but their airway can be managed using an endotracheal tube. (7) 1. Outcome 10. Airway and breathing are always the first priority; elevated heart rate would be the second priority; a dry nonproductive cough is not significant unless it is causing respiratory difficulty. Burns would be treated as the third priority. (8) 4. Outcome 15. Accurate oxygen saturation measurement is dependent on adequate circulation to the site of the probe. If the client's finger is cold and pale, it would indicate poor circulation to the area and result in an inaccurate reading. The probe should be moved to a more central location with better perfusion such as the ear. The client is described as being in no acute distress so there would be no need for calling for assistance. The nurse should always treat the client, not the monitor. (9) 3. Outcome 16. The nurse would question the order requiring an oxygen saturation of more than 95% because clients with COPD frequently have lower normal oxygen saturation readings. Applying oxygen to obtain an oxygen saturation of 95% would likely cause the client to become apneic because their trigger to breathe is a low oxygen level, and elevating this level would cancel their respiratory drive. (10) 3. Outcome 17. The nurse would don clean gloves, remove the old dressing, perform hand hygiene, open the sterile supplies, don sterile gloves, remove, clean and replace the inner cannula, apply a clean dressing, and then change the tracheostomy ties.

CHAPTER 33

NCLEX-PN® ANSWERS (1) 2. Outcome 1. The pericardial space is found within the two layers of the pericardium. When this area fills with fluid it puts pressure on the heart, preventing the heart from filling and pumping effectively. (2) 4. Outcome 2. The client with diabetes, with a family history of early-onset heart disease, who smokes, and who has elevated blood pressure has the most risk factors and is at greatest risk for heart disease. (3) 4. Outcome 3. The most effective test to demonstrate narrowing of the coronary artery is the PET scan. The ECG and thallium stress tests would show changes only if the narrowing was significant enough to cause ischemia, which would result in symptoms. The echocardiogram shows structural defects but is not specific enough to show narrowing of the coronary arteries. (4) 2. Outcome 4. The client is describing unstable angina because it can occur at rest, is getting worse, and is not always relieved with nitroglycerine which would not occur with stable angina. Prinzmetal's angina generally occurs at the same time every day and is caused by coronary artery spasm. Paroxysmal angina does not exist. (5) 4. Outcome 5. The best position to auscultate for an S3 heart sound is left lateral or supine position. (6) 2. Outcome 6. The client's shortness of breath is caused by left-, not right-sided, failure, which results in blood backing up in the lungs allowing fluid to leak into the alveoli and reducing the functioning space of the lungs. (7) 1. Outcome 7. The client who has rheumatic fever is at risk for valvular heart disease, although it may take 20 to 40 years to occur. (8) 3. Outcome 8. The best diagnostic test for electrical disturbances, such as an irregular heartbeat, is the ECG. This client is asymptomatic, so the nurse would not call 9-1-1. Cardiac enzymes would be tested if a heart attack were suspected. Pericardiocentesis is done to remove fluid from around the heart. (9) 4. Outcome 10. The client is describing intermittent claudication caused by reduced blood flow to the legs resulting in ischemia when active but relieved at rest when less oxygen is required. (10) 4. Outcome 13. The client with hypertension is often placed on a calcium channel blocker to slow the heartbeat.

CHAPTER 34

NCLEX-PN® ANSWERS (1) 3. Outcome 1. Neutrophils are the most common type of white blood cell. Approximately two-thirds of all WBCs are neutrophils. (2) 2. Outcome 4. Shellfish are not good sources of iron. The best food sources for iron are red meat, organ meats, and green leafy vegetables. (3) 4. Outcome 4. Keeping the client fully hydrated may help to prevent the sickle cells from clumping in the capillaries, which is the cause of sickle cell crisis. The client should be in a warm environment to keep the blood vessels dilated and prevent clumping. The client gets flu shots annually to reduce the risk of infection, which can precipitate sickle cell crisis. (4) 1. Outcome 5. Bleeding episodes in hemophilia A are usually precipitated by minor traumas such as tripping or falling. The client is not impacted by singing in the choir, can get out of the car without assistance, and can weed the garden but should be taught to wear gardening gloves. (5) 3. Outcome 6. Clients with a low white blood cell count are at a high risk for infection so this would be the priority nursing concern. (6) 3. Outcome 2. Hematocrit is anticipated to be 3 times the hemoglobin. A client whose hematocrit is higher than this could potentially be dehydrated, causing an unusually high ratio of cells to serum. Anemia is indicated by red cell count, infection results from lack of white cells, and bleeding is a risk for clients with low platelets. (7) 4. Outcome 3. The client with type A+ blood can receive either A+ or O+ blood. A transfusion of any other blood type, or Rh-negative blood, will induce a transfusion reaction. (8) 1. Outcome 7. The client at highest risk for developing lymphedema is the one who has a condition or a surgery that removes lymph nodes such as the client who had a modified radical mastectomy, which requires the removal of the axillary lymph nodes. (9) 1, 2. Outcome 8. Clients complaining of pruritus should take cooling baths, wash clothes and linens in mild detergent, and wear light clothing made of cotton, which allows for air to move more freely. Wool would increase pruritus. Blankets do not need to be avoided, but use of cotton blankets would be best. Cool baths may be taken as often as needed for relief so bathing is not limited. (10) 3. Outcome 3. Because of the risk of transfusion reactions if the wrong blood is administered, the client and unit of blood should be verified by two licensed personnel to ensure the correct blood is administered to the correct client. A blood product transfusion may take up to 4 hours and a larger gauge IV is suggested (18 or 20 gauge). The client's position in bed does not matter.

CHAPTER 35

NCLEX-PN® ANSWERS (1) 1. Outcome 1. The primary component of the nonspecific and specific immune response is the stem cell, which originates in the bone marrow. (2) 3. Outcome 4. A Western blot test would be anticipated because it is more specific for HIV and eliminates the false-positives that can occur with an ELISA. (3) 4. Outcome 7. *Pneumocystis carinii* pneumonia is the most common of the indicator diseases, occurring in 85 percent of HIV-infected adults. (4) 3. Outcome 2. IgG elevates when the client has an infection. (5) 1. Outcome 8. Acute graft versus host disease is typically found 100 days post-transplant, presenting with urticaria on the palms of the hands and the soles of the feet. (6) 1. Outcome 3. When a client develops immunity to a disease as the result of contracting the virus, the immunity is natural active. (7) 2. Signs of an anaphylactic reaction can begin with numbness and tingling of the lips that will progress to laryngeal edema and difficulty breathing. Immediate intervention in the form of epinephrine injection is required to prevent further progression of the reaction. (8) 2. Outcome 10. A level II hypersensitivity reaction is a blood transfusion reaction. (9) 2. Outcome 5.

Movement of the arm improves blood supply, speeding absorption of the vaccine, which will reduce the discomfort caused by the indwelling immunization. (10) 3. Outcome 9. The only true statement is that the mortality rate for scleroderma is higher than that for lupus.

CHAPTER 36

NCLEX-PN® ANSWERS (1) 2. Outcome 10. Neuroglia, otherwise known as astrocytes, are the most common source of tumors. The other choices all suggest doing numerous tests at once. (2) 2. Outcome 3. Neurological assessment is complex and can be tiring for the client if performed all at once, so it is best to perform assessment in phases. (3) 3. Outcome 6. This client's symptoms are 3 days old so rehabilitation is the most likely intervention needed. Symptoms that last for 3 days are not typical for TIAs and administration of TPN must be done within 6 hours of the onset of symptoms so these would not be appropriate for this client. (4) 4. Outcome 11. Weakness of the upper limbs is an initial symptom of amyotrophic lateral sclerosis. (5) 2. Outcome 12. Foods that are too warm or too cold may trigger the pain, therefore the client should eat foods that are room temperature. (6) 2. Outcome 5. Craniotomy is the procedure performed to release increased intracranial pressure. (7) 4. Outcome 2. Allergies to shellfish could indicate an allergy to the contrast medium, which has iodine in it. (8) 4. Outcome 9. Change in the level of consciousness is the first indicator of a change in neurologic status. (9) 3. Outcome 7. A loss of consciousness, incontinence, and generalized tonic-clonic movement of the extremities would indicate a grand mal seizure. (10) 1. Outcome 8. The inability to extend the leg when the hip is flexed is a positive Kernig's sign.

CHAPTER 37

NCLEX-PN® ANSWERS (1) 2. Outcome 8. Without the intrinsic factor, the body is unable to absorb vitamin B_{12} from ingested food. Supplemental B_{12} must be given by injection, because it would be destroyed by stomach acid if taken orally. (2) 1. Outcome 3. Coffee-grounds emesis indicates internal bleeding. When internal bleeding occurs, the client can go into hypovolemic shock with lowered blood pressure and elevated, thready pulse. (3) 4. Outcome 10. It is normal for peristalsis to cease after abdominal surgery because exposing the bowel to air stops peristaltic activity called paralytic ileus. (4) 3. Outcome 5. The oil in an oil-retention enema helps soften the dry, hard fecal impaction, making it easier for the nurse to break it up and remove it. (5) 1. Outcome 7. Effluent from an ileostomy comes from the small intestine and contains digestive enzymes that cause skin breakdown when they contact the skin. (6) 2. Outcome 8. One typical symptom of colon cancer is a positive guaiac test, indicating blood in the stool that may not be visible to the naked eye. (7) 1. Outcome 6. White spots on the tongue indicate the presence of thrush, which is not usually seen in adults unless they have an impaired immunological response. Kaposi's would be seen on the face, torso, or limbs. *Pneumocystis jiroveci* (formerly *carinii*) affects the lungs. Periodontal disease presents with reddening of the gums and gums pulling away from the teeth. (8) 3. Outcome 1. Peristalsis begins in the esophagus and helps to aid the passage of food into the stomach and through the bowel. (9) 4. Outcome 9. Although all of the interventions listed are appropriate for a client with cirrhosis, the priority would be to assess the abdominal girth, because increased ascites could put pressure on the diaphragm and contribute to shortness of breath. (10) 1. Outcome 4. Only the barium swallow would show the intrusion of the abdominal contents into the thoracic cavity. The EGD shows only the inside of the esophagus, stomach, and duodenum; it would not indicate what is occurring on the outside of these organs.

CHAPTER 38

NCLEX-PN® ANSWERS (1) 4. Outcome 2. To make T_3 and T_4, the body must have iodine. In the past, this was a problem for people who lived in areas where the soil was deficient in iodine, so iodine was added to table salt to provide people with the iodine necessary to maintain healthy thyroid function. (2) 1. Outcome 4. The thymus gland produces two hormones: thymosin and thymin. Thymosin plays an essential role in the development of the immune system, and thymin blocks the transmission of neuromuscular nerve impulses. (3) 2. Outcome 1. Negative feedback is the mechanism that "turns off" the secretion of hormones. (4) 3. Outcome 3. The client who had surgery to remove a tumor through the sphenoid is taught to avoid sneezing, coughing, bending, and straining to have a bowel movement in order to prevent increased pressure to the surgical site. (5) 3. Outcome 5. If laryngeal edema develops, the airway could be blocked, so a tracheostomy set is essential to keep at the bedside in case of the need for emergency surgical intervention. (6) 1. Outcome 6. The Somogyi effect is a normal occurrence and is a sudden drop in the blood sugar followed by a rebound hyperglycemic reaction. (7) 2. Outcome 8. The symptoms of a hypoglycemic reaction are rapid in onset and include cold sweats, clammy skin, and shakiness. (8) 2. Outcome 9. Pheochromocytoma is a benign tumor in the adrenal medulla that causes excessive amounts of epinephrine and norepinephrine to be produced. This results in the major symptom of marked hypertension ranging from 200 to 300 systolic over 150 diastolic. (9) 1. Outcome 9. Major stressors can precipitate an Addisonian crisis, which is a life-threatening medical situation, so the client should be helped to avoid or reduce life stressors. (10) 1, 2, 3. Outcome 7. The primary means of controlling diabetes include diet management, exercise, monitoring of blood glucose levels, and taking medications properly. However, there is no indication what medication this client will be prescribed, so instructing them to take insulin would be

incorrect. Inspecting the feet helps to prevent complications but does not contribute to managing the disease of diabetes mellitus.

CHAPTER 39

NCLEX-PN® ANSWERS (1) 2. Outcome 1. The female urethra is shorter than that of the male, allowing bacteria easier access to the bladder and other urinary structures. (2) 4. Outcome 2. Diuresis is the production and excretion of large amounts of urine. (3) 1, 2, 4, 5. Outcome 5. The urine collection bag should be below the level of the bladder in order for urine to flow by gravity into the bag. Placing the bag too high will encourage urine to flow back into the bladder and increase the risk of UTI. (4) 1. Outcome 4. Urine culture is performed to determine if there are microorganisms present in the urine. Sensitivity will determine what antibiotic will be effective in eliminating the identified microorganism. (5) 2. Outcome 4. To initiate a 24-hour specimen correctly, the first void must be discarded because it has been sitting in the bladder. All future urine is collected for the 24-hour specimen. (6) 1. Outcome 6. The client is demonstrating signs and symptoms of pyelonephritis, which frequently has rapid onset and requires immediate intervention to reduce the risk of renal failure. (7) 2. Outcome 5. Normal specific gravity is 1.010 to 1.025. Values outside this range can indicate alteration in the client's hydration status. (8) 3. Outcome 7. A client diagnosed with renal failure cannot properly eliminate fluid and may require fluid restriction. Clients with urinary tract infection or renal calculi should be encouraged to increase fluid intake. Clients with undiagnosed diabetes may be unusually thirsty, but the treatment is aimed at blood sugar control, not reducing fluid intake, which the body uses to flush sugar from the bloodstream. (9) 4. Outcome 8. Vitamin C and cranberry juices promote an acidic pH for the urine, inhibiting bacterial growth. (10) 3. Outcome 3. The prostate is shaped like a doughnut, with the urethra passing through the center. When the prostate enlarges, it puts pressure on the urethra reducing the flow of urine from the bladder and increasing the risk of urinary retention.

CHAPTER 40

NCLEX-PN® ANSWERS (1) 2. Outcome 8. Retained urine with inadequate emptying places the client at risk for a urinary tract infection. (2) 4. Outcome 2. To reduce the client's discomfort with discussing sexual matters, the nurse should maintain a very professional approach and treat the subject as matter-of-factly as possible. Using euphemisms, avoiding eye contact, or writing questions down would indicate the nurse's discomfort with discussing the subject and increase the client's anxiety. (3) 3. Outcome 5. The nurse should suggest non-pharmacologic methods of reducing hot flashes such as a cool environment and avoiding caffeine. HRT should be used only when other methods are ineffective and when the hot flashes interfere with the client's ADLs. The physician must prescribe HRT and it should not be suggested until the physician evaluates the appropriateness of this treatment method for this client. (4) 2. Outcome 4. The American Cancer Society recommends that all women check their breasts monthly after age 20. The most effective time to perform the exam is about 1 week after menstruation. (5) 3. Outcome 7. The nurse should use drawings or models to explain the disorder to the client. Calling the physician isn't necessary. Asking if the client was paying attention is accusatory and will injure the nurse–client relationship. Describing complications should not be done until after the client fully understands the diagnosis, if at all. (6) 2. Outcome 9. TSS has been linked to prolonged tampon use. Young women need to know that it is important to change tampons frequently and avoid using them at night. (7) 4. Outcome 6. Tamoxifen (Nolvadex) has been found effective in inhibiting cancer in clients who are at high risk for breast cancer. (8) 1. Outcome 10. IUD implantation does not reduce the occurrence of regular periods. Amenorrhea is a sign of possible pregnancy and must be reported immediately to the healthcare provider. (9) 2. Outcome 3. During the plateau phase of sexual excitement physical changes in the female include retraction of the clitoris, enlargement of the outer third of the vagina and the labia majora, and a slight increase in width and depth of the inner two-thirds of the vagina as the area becomes more engorged with blood. (10) 1. Outcome 11. Varicoceles are located in the testes and are dilated blood vessels that cause more blood to enter the area, increasing the temperature within the testes and killing sperm, which require a stable temperature lower than normal body temperature.

CHAPTER 41

NCLEX-PN® ANSWERS (1) 1. Outcome 6. Once infected with HSV, the virus invades a client's cells causing an initial breakout of vesicles. These vesicles will heal, but because the virus remains present, future breakouts will occur. (2) 4. Outcome 4. Male symptoms of genital herpes include dysuria, penile discharge, unilateral scrotal pain, fever, rectal discharge, pain during defecation. (3) 3. Outcome 1. Abstinence from sexual contact is the only way to avoid contracting an STI. Male condoms are the most effective method if abstinence is not possible, but they are not 100 percent effective. (4) 1. Outcome 3. The type of organism in the vaginal discharge must be determined and this is best done by culturing the discharge. (5) 3. Outcome 2. It is important for the nurse to explain how HPV is transmitted. These facts can assist the client in reviewing issues that may be related to her diagnosis and her relationship. Advising her to speak with her sexual partner is not within the role of the nurse. The remaining items may be discussed once the client understands mode of transmission. (6) 2. Outcome 6. Candida albicans, the agent causing candidiasis, can also cause diaper dermatitis or thrush in newborns. (7) 1.

Outcome 5. Clients who contract a sexually transmitted infection should receive education regarding the use of barrier prophylactic devices. Barrier devices will not prevent infection, but they do reduce the risk. (8) 1. Outcome 2. Douching requires introduction of a foreign object, which may actually spread infection. Also the chemical agents used in douching may change the normal vaginal flora, reducing the body's ability to fight infection. (9) 1. Outcome 6. Single-dose treatments may require 1 week to reduce the chance of spreading infection. Prior to that, the client is considered contagious and should abstain from sexual contact. Six weeks is longer than a normal course of antibiotics. (10) 1, 2, 4, 5. Outcome 5. A nonjudgmental and supportive attitude is critical when seeking to gain the trust of a client, along with assurance of confidentiality. Care should be directed toward the client's needs, not the needs or beliefs of the nurse. This is particularly important when discussing intimate subjects such as sexual history.

CHAPTER 42

NCLEX-PN® ANSWERS (1) 2. Outcome 1. People reaching the age of 65 are considered geriatric or elderly adults. (2) 4. Outcome 2. Marital status has not been proven to impact body changes associated with geriatrics. (3) 4. Outcome 4. Encouraging the client to delay voiding will increase the likelihood of incontinence. (4) 2. Outcome 5. This client is in Erikson's stage of integrity versus despair and is reflecting despair. Not enough information is provided to determine if the client is suicidal. While reflecting back on life choices is normal, despairing over choices one has made is not normal. (5) 4. Outcome 6. As part of the aging process, blood vessels lose their elasticity and plaque may build on the internal walls of arteries, increasing the pressure required to pump blood from the heart. Fluid and sodium intake as well as cardiac status for this client are unknown. (6) 3. Outcome 7. Removing throw rugs is the only option that will reduce the risk of falling, although all of the other options are good suggestions for safety regarding other arenas. (7) 1, 2, 3. Outcome 8. Moments of sudden tearfulness and lack of financial resources are not indicators of abuse, but bruising, weight loss, and fearful attitude toward caretakers that cannot be adequately explained should be further investigated by the nurse as potential signs of abuse. (8) 2. Outcome 8. The daughter of this client is showing classic signs of caregiver role strain, which could lead to abuse if not resolved. One good night's sleep will not resolve the issue, and the daughter should be provided with resources to help reduce strain of caring for the aging parent. (9) 1. Outcome 6. While the risk of disease increases in the elderly, osteoarthritis generally does not affect people until later in life and would be of special concern. (10) 2. Outcome 3. Lentigo senilis is the name of the skin condition that causes brown spots, sometimes referred to as "age spots" on the arms and hands of the elderly.

CHAPTER 43

NCLEX-PN® ANSWERS (1) 2. Outcome 1. The primary difference is that caregiving may be more complex because the elderly client is more likely to have chronic conditions and age-related changes that may complicate care. Basic care is unchanged. (2) 3. Outcome 2. Fractures are often the result of osteoporosis, which makes the bone more fragile. Calcium, not caloric, intake can help to prevent fractures. Degenerative joint disease (osteoarthritis) is a significant source of pain but is not the most likely cause of fracture. (3) 1. Outcome 2. COPD is not a single disorder but rather includes diseases such as emphysema, chronic bronchitis, bronchiectasis, and asthma. (4) 4. Outcome 2. Cardiovascular diseases cause 75% of deaths in people over the age of 65 and are the most common cause of death. (5) 3. Outcome 6. When providing care for the elderly, it is important to provide careful skin care because the skin thins and is more fragile, making them prone to altered skin integrity. Timely administration of meds and daily hygiene are the same for all clients. Speaking in a loud voice is not a good intervention for the elderly; pitch and tone are more important than volume. (6) 3. Outcome 3. The elderly client requiring any medication is at increased risk for drug toxicity because of reduced liver and kidney function. Pain relief, reporting, and healing should not be different in the elderly from any other client. (7) 1, 2, 3, 4. Outcome 3. Elderly clients may demonstrate confusion related to medications (especially if they are taking numerous or controlled medications), an unfamiliar environment, alteration in routine, and lack of sleep caused by the noise and activity of the facility. Family involvement is unlikely to contribute to confusion. (8) 4. Outcome 4. Polypharmacy is defined as untoward effects resulting from taking numerous medications that may interact in a negative manner. The other terms are not specific to the client described. (9) 3. Outcome 4. Acetaminophen (Tylenol) can have a negative impact on liver function, especially when taken frequently or in larger than recommended dosages, resulting in jaundice. While other options could be side effects of acetaminophen, they are not specific to or highly associated with, use of the drug in the elderly. (10) 4. Outcome 7. When providing discharge teaching to the elderly client taking numerous medications, it is very important to teach them to keep an accurate and updated list of medications, dosages, and frequency of administration in their wallets. They should be taught to provide this list to all caregivers before medications are prescribed or care is delivered.

CHAPTER 44

NCLEX-PN® ANSWERS (1) 3. Outcome 1. Signs and symptoms of chronic disease may come on suddenly or gradually and may go away between outbreaks. The definition of chronic disorders is that the client never fully recovers due to eventual presence of irreversible pathological

changes. (2) 1, 2, 4, 5. Outcome 2. The nurse does not create the rehabilitation plan but may collaborate with other members of the team. The other answers are part of the LPN/LVN role. (3) 2. Outcome 5. Although the other options may be used in the plan of care, the one specifically related to the parent's comments is *Spiritual Distress*. (4) 2, 4, 5. Outcome 5. There is often a decline in level of consciousness preceding death, which would cause the Glasgow coma scale to decline, not elevate. Cool, mottled, or cyanotic extremities, weak and thready pulse, and irregular respirations are all common findings when death is imminent. (5) 1. Outcome 4. Dying clients tend to feel isolated and fear being deserted by the staff. The primary objective in this case should be to provide a physical presence to listen and support the client as death draws near. All other choices involve leaving the client alone to die. (6) 4. Outcome 7. Legally the nurse must call a code, but it would be appropriate to relay the client's wishes to the physician who heads the resuscitation team. A written order of Do Not Resuscitate is required by the nurse in order to respect the client's wishes. (7) 3. Outcome 3. Hospice is care usually in the home or specialized facility dedicated to the care of clients with terminal illnesses. It is designed to provide quality of life when cure is not possible. It is not done as a cost-saving measure or because of a need for special equipment. Although hospice nurses have special training, they do not have more or less skill than hospital nurses. (8) 2. Outcome 8. A client on life support must have an absence of electric currents from the brain (measured by an electroencephalogram) for at least 24 hours and cannot receive any medications that could reduce brain function during this time. Clients continue to have respirations as long as the respirator is functioning even if they are brain dead. A court order is not necessary unless the client has left no instructions or there is a disagreement among family members. (9) 3. Outcome 9. Muslim belief requires the body to be bathed by another Muslim of the same gender, so the body should not be bathed until the family arrives or is contacted to give instructions on who may bathe the body. (10) 3. Outcome 10. The head of the bed should be elevated 30 degrees or the head and shoulder should be placed on pillows to avoid settling of blood in the face that could cause discoloration. The arms can be placed at the side or folded over the abdomen. Eyes and mouth will frequently remain open until the mortician works with the body, and no extra actions need be taken to close them.

CHAPTER 45

NCLEX-PN® ANSWERS (1) 2. Outcome 4. Destruction of red blood cells leads to anemia and resulting fatigue. Radiation of bone marrow would destroy both white and red blood cells. The client will be at increased risk for bleeding, not for blood clots, because of destruction of platelets. Sebaceous and sweat gland activity is depressed, not increased, as a side effect of radiation. (2) 1. Outcome 3. The cost of a treatment should never be a primary concern regarding treatment decisions. (3) 3. Outcome 9. Determining tissue type is done microscopically in the lab by pathologists. (4) 2. Outcome 1. The client who smokes, drinks alcohol, and is over the age of 65 has the greatest number of risk factors. (5) 4. Outcome 2. Cancer cells grow quickly, die much slower than regular cells, divide rapidly and accurately, and do not require an anchor unlike normal cells. (6) 4. Outcome 4. Because most liver tumors are highly vascular, the person having an ultrasound-guided percutaneous needle biopsy of the liver must be monitored closely for intra-abdominal hemorrhage. In general, this procedure is rapid, safe, and commonly used. (7) 3. Outcome 6. If distant metastases are present, radical surgery alone is usually not indicated, and the focus of the treatment quickly shifts from local control to combined modality treatment. (8) 3. Outcome 5. Duke's staging method is only used for colorectal cancer and would be the most appropriate staging system to use for this client. (9) 2. Outcome 7. The only option that directly addresses advice for reducing nausea and vomiting post chemotherapy treatment is to delay food intake for 3 to 4 meals after treatment. (10) 4. Outcome 8. It is important to include an educator in the pediatric oncology treatment so the child can keep up with his or her schoolwork.

CHAPTER 46

NCLEX-PN® ANSWERS (1) 2. Outcome 1. The client requiring nursing interventions on a regular basis, including tube feedings, dressing changes, or IV therapy, would require skilled care. Custodial care would be required by the client needing some assistance performing ADLs. Long-term care is a general term that covers both skilled and custodial care. Assisted living is a form of custodial care. (2) 1. Outcome 2. LPNs/LVNs working in long-term care generally find their role is expanded when working in long-term care to include responsibilities normally only allowed by the RN in acute care facilities. (3) 1, 2, 3, 5. Outcome 3. When delegating tasks it is important to delegate the right task to the right person, giving the right communication, and providing adequate supervision. The nurse cannot delegate responsibility; this remains with the nurse even after the task has been delegated to another. (4) 2. Outcome 4. The family is important because they can provide insight and information about the client. However, the client speaks for him/herself as much as physically possible. Client needs are determined by the staff that then provide updates to the family at the client's discretion. (5) 1. Outcome 5. The general rule is to provide care among peers, with pediatric clients going to a pediatric long-term care facility, young adults going to a facility prepared to deal with this age group and their needs, and elders being cared for in facilities skilled in geriatric needs. (6) 1, 4, 5. Outcome 6. The major responsibilities are to

limit disability, support the plan of care, and implement the rehabilitation plan as designed if appropriate. The client assumes responsibility for ADLs with the support of the multidisciplinary team. Return to normal function would be unrealistic for this client. (7) 4. Outcome 7. It is the nurse who was responsible for monitoring that the client's hygiene needs were met and that the delegated task was properly performed. Failure to do so is considered neglect and could be seen as abuse. (8) 4. Outcome 8. In order to obtain reimbursement, it is essential that the nurse document care accurately to demonstrate care delivered. (9) 2. Outcome 8. Medicare covers clients who are over the age of 65 or are totally disabled. Clients with a broken leg, amputation, or knee replacement are temporarily disabled but are expected to recover to full or nearly full previous functioning. Only the client who is quadriplegic would be covered by Medicare. (10) 3. Outcome 9. The charge nurse ensures the smooth functioning of the unit, making client assignments, assisting with problem solving, and notifying the proper personnel in case of an emergency or crisis situation among other things. The other options are the responsibility of staff nurses.

CHAPTER 47

NCLEX-PN® ANSWERS (1) 2. Outcome 4. Airway management with clients in the emergency department, and especially those with cardiac disturbances, is the highest priority requiring the nurse's attention first and foremost. (2) 3. Outcome 15. The client's comprehensive understanding of the correct medication administration is vital for safety. The client must notify the physician to receive correct medical advice if a dose is missed. (3) 1. Outcome 9. Clients with burns to the face and neck areas are at risk for airway compromise related to edema and third spacing caused by injury to the airway from the burn. Airway management and maintenance is always a chief concern with burns to the upper torso. (4) 2. Outcome 7. Data collection of the specific agent is required as soon as possible. The sooner the agent is identified, the faster effective treatment may be initiated for a safe and effective outcome. (5) 2. Outcome 2. The nurse must gather pertinent data before any treatment decisions can be made. In the case of possible head trauma (indicated by the abrasion), assessment is top priority and must come before implementation. The nurse should use caution in making promises to this client. (6) 1. Outcome 8. Bioterrorism-related disaster is treated like any mass casualty; the facility emergency operation plan will detail how it is to be handled. Policies will differ from routine management and it is not the nurse's responsibility to determine who can be discharged versus those to be admitted or to summon help to the department. (7) 1, 2, 4, 5. Outcome 11. Ice will help to reduce edema. The client should be instructed on how to monitor the arm and what symptoms require immediate notification of the physician. The client should also be taught to avoid wetting the cast or inserting objects, sharp or otherwise, into the cast. The arm should be elevated on pillows until the cast dries; placing it on a hard surface could cause the cast to impinge on the arm, reducing circulation and requiring cast removal and replacement. (8) 4. Outcome 3. The family should not be informed of the son's death over the phone. Also, care should be taken in how the family is instructed to come to the hospital, because anxiety could cause the parents to be involved in a crash. (9) 1. Outcome 1. The child's pulse is 60 with a low oxygen saturation, so the ABCs of care indicate the airway should be assessed for compromise and oxygen delivered to improve respirations and supply tissues. IV initiation or Foley catheter insertion would require a physician's order. There is no need to perform CPR because the child is breathing and has a pulse. (10) 3. Outcome 5. An indwelling Foley catheter can be a primary source of infection in a client, especially in long-term care settings. This history of urinary tract infection would indicate sepsis as the most likely candidate for causing shock.

CHAPTER 48

NCLEX-PN® ANSWERS (1) 3. Outcome 2. The nurse practice act provides information about the scope of practice for the LPN/LVN. The physician would not be a reliable source of information about nursing scope of practice. The office manager may or may not have a healthcare background and would also not be a reliable source. While the nurse manager is a nurse, every nurse is responsible for determining what is and what is not within their scope of practice and should obtain information from the best source, not hearsay. (2) 4. Outcome 2. The LPN/LVN working in the physician's office reports to an RN or the physician for clinical issues. (3) 2. Outcome 6. Scoliosis screening is mandated by law and calls for the initial screening for males to be given in the 6th grade and every other year until the 10th grade since this period of time coincides with their rapid growth period. (4) 1. Outcome 4. When a client is admitted to hospice, a physician's order is necessary. The family stating that they want to sign the client up without a physician's order demonstrates the need for additional teaching. (5) 3. Outcome 7. The circulating nurse is considered to be the charge nurse of the operating room; this job is only within the scope of the registered nurse. The other jobs are within the scope of practice for the LPN/LVN in most states. (6) 3. Outcome 6. Anesthesia will be administered by the physician. The LPN/LVN can perform all of the other duties. (7) 4. Outcome 15. With proper instructions the child should be able to identify the position of the E on the Snellen E chart, or the nurse could use the pediatric Snellen eye chart with pictures the child can recognize. The other choices would be inappropriate and lack accuracy. (8) 1, 2, 3. Outcome 5. Writing down what the client is saying, as they are saying it, is disconcerting to the client and is not an effective means of obtaining quality information. The nurse should review the client's record before entering the room. The remaining strategies are effective. (9) 4. Outcome 1. A long-term care

facility is not considered a community setting. The remaining options are viable options for the nurse considering community settings for employment. (10) 3. Outcome 6. Between ages 4 and 6, the child should have the fifth of five DTaP; the fourth of four polio, and the second of two MMR immunizations.

CHAPTER 49

NCLEX-PN® ANSWERS (1) 3. Outcome 1. A healthy person has control over his or her own behavior but not over the behavior of others. (2) 1. Outcome 6. Only flat affect and little speech are considered negative symptoms. The others are examples of disorganized symptoms. (3) 1. Outcome 2. Often clients are not diagnosed with mental illness due to the stigma connected to a mental health disorder. (4) 4. Outcome 3. Children are rarely diagnosed with schizophrenia, but the other disorders are commonly seen. (5) 4. Outcome 5. Genetic and biological predispositions cannot be avoided, but early diagnosis can prevent further dysfunction. (6) 4. Outcome 8. Sociopathic disorders fall within the cluster labeled emotional disorders. (7) 3. Outcome 4. Orthostatic hypotension is a common side effect of the antipsychotic medications; thus, the client should change positions slowly to avoid dizziness and possible falls. The client on these drugs needs to watch fat and calorie intake. Antacids will prolong absorption. Photosensitivity is often a side effect of these drugs, so prolonged exposure to the sun is not recommended. (8) 3. Outcome 7. Clients tend to be quiet about their feelings of depression, so that the physician is not aware of their psychologic state. The most common reason for this is the stigma society has placed on mental illness. It is often seen as a weakness on the part of the depressed person. (9) 3. Outcome 10. The older antipsychotic medications are more effective for the positive symptoms of schizophrenia including hallucinations, delusions, and disordered thoughts. The newer atypical antipsychotics are effective for both negative and positive symptoms. (10) 2. Outcome 9. The client who is pacing and talking loudly to an unseen voice is showing an escalation of behavior that could easily erupt into violence and should be watched closely. Intervening before behavior progresses to violence would be appropriate and reduce the risk of injury to the client or others.

CHAPTER 50

NCLEX-PN® ANSWERS (1) 1. Outcome 2. Clients who are tolerant to alcohol will have cross-tolerance to other CNS depressants and may require increased dosages. (2) 4. Outcome 2. The symptoms of alcohol withdrawal include elevated VS, tremors, and anxiety. It is not unusual for clients to underreport their alcohol intake. (3) 3. Outcome 4. Alcoholic encephalopathy is caused by a deficiency in vitamin B_1, which can be treated or prevented with a thiamine injection. (4) 1, 2, 4. Outcome 1. Indications of substance abuse, versus substance use, include interference with function at work, putting others in danger, or substance use that continues despite negative consequences. (5) 4. Outcome 6. The nursing supervisor must be notified when a nurse may be impaired to protect the client and also the nurse. The nurse should report objective observation, not suspicion or subjective interpretations of behavior exhibited by this nurse. (6) 3. Outcome 3. The client would be demonstrating behavior associated with a blood alcohol level of 0.3 to 0.4. Levels above this generally result in unconsciousness and can lead to death. (7) 4. Outcome 1. The participant is describing tolerance, which can be a result of abuse, addiction, or dependence. More of the substance is required to achieve the same effect. (8) 3. Outcome 8. The daughter most likely is suffering from the early stages of the restricting type of anorexia nervosa. Beginning treatment in the early stages increases the effectiveness of treatment. (9) 2. Outcome 7. All of these behaviors are of concern and need to be addressed, but the one that needs to be addressed most emergently is the expression of suicidal ideation. (10) 1, 2, 3. Outcome 5. By attending support groups, clients have the opportunity to talk with others who had similar experiences and were able to recover. The group provides a sense of community and unconditional support, and may help the client gain insight into their behavior. The group's goal is not to improve faith, and they refer to God more in terms of a greater power rather than a religious figure. Support groups improve the odds of recovery, but they do not "cure" the addiction.

CHAPTER 51

NCLEX-PN® ANSWERS (1) 4. Outcome 2. The hCG is secreted by the villi at 8 to 10 days after fertilization. (2) 4. Outcome 1. Adequate intake of calcium, folic acid, and iron is important to achieve prior to pregnancy, because deficiencies in early stages of pregnancy can adversely affect the fetus. There is no need to increase vitamin C intake when planning pregnancy because excess is excreted and not stored. (3) 4. Outcome 4. Peristalsis normally declines due to pressure of the growing fetus on the abdominal contents. (4) 4. Outcome 7. All of these options are important teaching points, but by week 38 of the pregnancy the only one that may need to be reinforced and explained in more detail is the physical and mental preparation for childbirth. (5) 2. Outcome 5. Even if eating a well-balanced diet, the expectant mother should add 300 kcal a day, which can be covered by the addition of one protein and two milk servings. This meets the need for increased calcium and protein as well as the need for calories. (6) 4. Outcome 6. The mother should be encouraged to sleep on her side to prevent hypotension; lying supine can cause supine hypotensive syndrome. (7) 3. Outcome 9. The fetal heart beat can be heard with a Doppler by 10 to 12 weeks. (8) 3. Outcome 3. Naegele's rule involves taking the first day of the last menstrual period, subtracting 3 months, and adding 7 days. So the correct date using this rule would be February 13. (9) 4. Outcome 8. Headache, blurred vision, and marked swelling are indicators of possible preeclampsia. A trip to the emergency department is not necessary. However, this client should be seen as soon as possible and certainly within 4 hours. (10) 3. Outcome 10. An amniocentesis is an invasive procedure that carries risk for the fetus and mother, so a signed informed consent should be obtained before beginning the procedure. All of the other options would be performed after obtaining the consent for the procedure.

CHAPTER 52

NCLEX-PN® ANSWERS (1) 1. Outcome 4. The pregnant woman should avoid exposure to cat litter because it carries a risk of transmission of toxoplasmosis. (2) 2. Outcome 4. Protein in the urine is an indicator of potential preeclampsia. Specific gravity tests urine concentration, not hypertension; glucose indicates diabetic changes; pH indicates an acid-base imbalance. (3) 3. Outcome 1. Residence alone does not contribute to the classification of high risk but may combine with other risk factors to worsen the chance of high-risk pregnancy. Smoking, history of preterm labor, and multiple pregnancy are all risk factors. (4) 3. Outcome 2. According to research, pregnancy occurring at or below age 15 increases the risk of a negative outcome because growth of the fetus pulls nutrients the teen's body needs for growth. (5) 2. Outcome 3. Hemoglobin should be rechecked at 7 months of pregnancy to monitor for anemia. (6) 3. Outcome 3. Results ranging between 110 and 140 mg/dL will require follow-up testing in the form of a 100-g oral glucose tolerance test to confirm the diagnosis of gestational diabetes. (7) 2. Outcome 5. The client with a previously weakened heart should be carefully assessed for signs of congestive heart failure. Assessment of breath sounds can be performed independently by the nurse, and the physician may order a chest x-ray if abnormal findings are reported by the nurse. (8) 2. Outcome 5. The client is reporting signs of a possible urinary tract infection that could result in preterm labor if rapid intervention is not initiated. (9) 1. Outcome 6. When caring for a client at high risk, one of the most important interventions is frequent monitoring of fetal and maternal well-being so that complications or problems can be caught early and interventions may be performed before further problems develop. (10) 1. Outcome 6. The second goal of caring for a client with a high-risk pregnancy is optimizing delivery under the best possible circumstances. The other options are either not goals (4) or are not within the power of the nurse (2, 3).

CHAPTER 53

NCLEX-PN® ANSWERS (1) 1. Outcome 1. Fetal cortisol production increases as the fetus matures and, when sufficient, decreases the placental production of progesterone. This begins the chain of hormonal events that cause labor. (2) 1. Outcome 1. Lightening refers to the fetus having descended into the pelvis, relieving pressure on the diaphragm and allowing the mother to breathe more easily and thus feel "lighter." (3) 3. Outcome 5. Answer 3 is correct because a prolapsed cord is an emergency situation and requires emergency cesarean section. While waiting for the surgical procedure to begin, it is important to position the client to take pressure off the cord, allowing oxygen and blood to circulate to the fetus. (4) 4. Outcome 2. A vertex presentation indicates the occiput is presenting first with the fetal head in complete flexion. (5) 3. Outcome 3. When the mother lies on her side, the contractions will be less frequent, but more intense. (6) 2. Outcome 2. The latent phase of the first stage of labor is from the onset of contraction until the cervix is dilated 4 cm. (7) 4. Outcome 2. The average length of active labor (active phase of first stage) is 4 to 6 hours for the primigravida client. (8) 3. Outcome 4. It is normal for the client to become irritable and sometimes angry at this stage of labor when the cervix is at least 8 cm dilated but not yet fully dilated. It is important to remind the client to focus on relaxation and breathing. The client is not to push actively until fully dilated at 10 cm. (9) 2. Outcome 2. Engagement occurs when the presenting part (usually the fetal head) enters the true pelvis. At this time, the presenting part is even with or below the ischial spines and the fetus is no longer ballotable. (10) 1. Outcome 5. Any bleeding in excess of one pad saturated per hour in the fourth stage of labor/delivery is considered abnormal and excessive; it should be reported immediately to the nursing supervisor or physician.

CHAPTER 54

NCLEX-PN® ANSWERS (1) 3. Outcome 3. Applications of ice, a binder or supportive bra, and analgesics may be needed until the woman's breasts stop producing milk and engorgement subsides. Expressing or pumping milk encourages more milk production. (2) 4. Outcome 2. A fundus displaced to the right of midline and above the level of the umbilicus usually indicates a full bladder. If the bladder is not emptied, the uterus may become boggy and the woman may experience increased uterine cramping and bleeding. Fundal massage may be necessary but comes after having the client void. (3) 3. Outcome 6. The client is demonstrating impaired mother–child bonding, which can be an indicator of potential for abuse. A social services referral should be considered so adequate follow-up monitoring can be provided and the mother can be assisted to meet her maternal obligations. (4) 1. Outcome 2. Weighing the pads would provide an accurate objective measurement of the amount of blood loss. Noting the number of saturated pads would give an estimation of blood loss. (5) 2. Outcome 2. Ice is usually applied in the first 24 hours and then heat is applied. Ice reduces the amount of edema by limiting blood flow. After 24 hours, heat is applied to increase blood flow so edema will be reduced by reabsorption of fluid. (6) 4. Outcome 1. The red or purple striae or stretch marks rarely disappear but will fade with time to a silvery color. (7) 3. Outcome 1. It is not unusual for white blood cell counts to increase to levels that would normally indicate infection, ranging from 12,000 to 20,000/mm^3, as a result of stress, inflammation, and pain. (8) 4. Outcome 4. A foul smell to the vaginal discharge is an indication of infection. All other signs and symptoms listed are normal findings. (9) 1. Outcome 5. Providing adequate pain control is the most important factor for facilitating bonding. The postpartum client who delivered by cesarean section should also be encouraged to care for the newborn in order for the bonding process to begin, the mother should get out of bed as soon as possible, but she may not be able to take full responsibility for the infant until narcotic analgesic requirements are reduced and she is able to move more comfortably. (10) 4. Outcome 7. The mother is experiencing anxiety related to mothering ability, and it is important for the nurse to acknowledge this is normal. Explaining the reason for the baby's disinterest rationally will help to reduce the mother's anxiety. Assisting the mother with breastfeeding will also improve her feelings of competence.

CHAPTER 55

NCLEX-PN® ANSWERS (1) 3. Outcome 1. This client has hyperreflexia and is at risk for seizure activity. Seizure precautions and careful monitoring are indicated. (2) 4. Outcome 2. The best indicator of blood loss during delivery is comparison of the prenatal and postpartum hematocrit levels, which will indicate the ratio of red cells to intravascular fluid. (3) 1. Outcome 2. The client who delivered a fragmented placenta is at risk for postpartum hemorrhage because a retained fragment would interfere with normal clamping of uterine vessels. (4) 2. Outcome 3. This client is at increased risk for thromboembolic disease secondary to venous stasis caused by elevation of the legs in stirrups and reduced activity secondary to bed rest. (5) 1, 2, 3, 4. Outcome 4. Mastitis is often caused by introduction of bacteria into cracks or fissures in the nipples. Antibiotic ointments should not be used due to the risk of administration to the baby through breastfeeding. All other measures will help to reduce infection and milk pooling in the ducts, thereby reducing the risk of mastitis. (6) 3. Outcome 1. Magnesium sulfate should never be abruptly discontinued but should be weaned off while monitoring for change in condition to indicate worsening symptoms. (7) 3. Outcome 4. The client should be taught to rinse the perineum after every void or stooling and change the perineal pad at least every 2 hours to reduce the risk of infection of the episiotomy. (8) 2. Outcome 5. These symptoms describe the client who is experiencing postpartum blues, which occur normally in most new mothers and will subside after approximately 2 weeks. (9) 1. Outcome 5. The client in option 1 has two risk factors for postpartum psychosis: her husband's job loss resulting in a negative effect on their socioeconomic status, and obsessive personality traits. Options 2 and 3 reflect risks for postpartum depression, and option 4 is unknown because the question does not supply enough information to make this determination. (10) 3. Outcome 6. The family is asking questions the nurse is unable to answer, so it is important to provide the family with a resource who can answer the questions. While the supervisor or physician may involve risk management, it is not the nurse's priority action at this time. Reassuring the father when the nurse is unaware of what happened would not be ethical. Providing excessive detail to a person in acute distress is neither helpful nor useful.

CHAPTER 56

NCLEX-PN® ANSWERS (1) 2. Outcome 7. Babies can drown in less than an inch of water so they must be watched carefully at all times when they are bathed and never left unattended. They should not be placed in a bath until the umbilical cord has fallen off. (2) 3. Outcome 3. Antibiotic ointment should be applied soon after birth, but it might not be applied immediately after delivery. The infant is often allowed to see the mother first to promote mother–infant bonding. (3) 4. Outcome 1. As the newborn adapts to extrauterine life, respirations will normally be irregular at a rate of 30 to 60 breaths per minute. Respirations do not become normal in depth and rate until several weeks of age. (4) 4. Outcome 9. Jaundice in the newborn is quite common and may require phototherapy as determined by bilirubin levels. Jaundice that does not appear until after 24 hours is unlikely to indicate an ABO or Rh incompatibility. (5) 1. Outcome 6. It is common for a newborn to have cyanosis of the hands and feet as a result of inadequate circulation. The condition may last a few hours to a few days. (6) 4. Outcome 4. Newborns are accustomed to tight living quarters *in utero* and are soothed by snuggling within a receiving blanket. They should never be placed on their stomachs to sleep, and propping a toy to hold a pacifier can be very dangerous if the baby vomits. Being unwrapped will make the baby more irritable. (7) 3. Outcome 8. Alternating the first breast offered will help establish the milk supply. The length of feeding is gradually increased, not decreased. The newborn does not yet have energy to nurse for 20 minutes at each breast. (8) 1. Outcome 10. The penis should be cleaned with plain water. Alcohol will cause pain and irritate the tissue at the circumcision site. (9) 2. Outcome 2. The infant receives 1 point for a heart rate less than 100, 1 point for slow and irregular respirations, and 1 point for a pink body with cyanotic extremities. Muscle flaccidity and lack of reflexes scores 0, for a total Apgar of 3. (10) 4. Outcome 5. The assessment that a newborn is premature generally requires more than one identified characteristic, but prematurity of the genitals is indicated by undescended testicles in boys and a prominent clitoris in girls.

CHAPTER 57

NCLEX-PN® ANSWERS (1) 1. Outcome 1. Infants born before 37 weeks' or after 42 weeks' gestation are high risk, as are infants with any intrauterine alteration in development, such as cleft lip or palate. The infant whose mother died at birth does not fall into the category of high-risk infant. (2) 2. Outcome 6. Simple answers to questions are the best response at this point. More in-depth information will be given once the doctor has determined the extent of the defect and the father's anxiety level is reduced so he is able to hear what he is being told. Later, pointing out positive attributes of the child will help the parent to see the child's good features and not just the anomaly. Initially, questions require simple answers. (3) 2. Outcome 4. Flaring nostrils, grunting respirations, and retractions are early signs of respiratory distress. Cyanosis is often a late-stage indicator because neonates have fetal hemoglobin, which is less reactive to hypoxia. (4) 4. Outcome 10. It is fairly common for the newborn to go up to 24 hours without voiding. However, if the baby has not voided by 24 hours, or if bladder distention is noted prior to 24 hours, the physician should be notified for further testing. (5) 3. Outcome 2. Premature babies require reduced stimulation, especially secondary to the noise of the intensive care nursery. Playing soft soothing music may be appropriate, but stimuli should be reduced to encourage growth and development. (6) 3. Outcome 3. Only the small-for-gestational-age infant is prone to temperature instability. (7) 3. Outcome 5. Care for a child with a congenital heart defect is focused on reducing cardiac workload and promoting respiratory effectiveness. The type of defect will determine if oxygen, frequent vital signs, or medications are necessary. Simple defects may resolve without medical intervention. (8) 2. Outcome 7. Imperforate anus requires immediate repair within 24 hours of birth to create an outlet for feces, often in the form of creation of an ostomy that will be reconnected with later surgery. (9) 3. Outcome 8. Inborn errors of metabolism such as phenylketonuria are often caused by the body's response (or lack of response) to nutritional intake, so accurate testing can only be performed after the infant has eaten for several days. (10) 2. Outcome 10. Wrapping the infant snuggly in a blanket and holding and rocking the baby are very comforting and keep the baby from self-stimulating. While adequate nutrition is important, it is not for the purpose of comforting the infant. Babies born to drug-addicted mothers are often placed in foster care until the mother can recover from the addiction, and teaching home care will not comfort the baby. Narcotics may or may not be administered depending on the physician's approach.

CHAPTER 58

NCLEX-PN® ANSWERS (1) 4. Outcome 1. Infants primarily breathe through their nose. When obstruction occurs, it is important to clear the nose first, and then the mouth. A suction catheter would only be necessary if the child has respiratory distress after clearing the nose and mouth with a bulb syringe. Back blows are not indicated in this instance because the substance blocking the airway is liquid. (2) 3. Outcome 2. The school-aged child is able to cooperate and wants to help but also is beginning to show modesty. So, involving the child in the process of the examination while respecting the need for modesty would be most effective. (3) 1. Outcome 3. The OUCHER scale was designed for use by children who are unable to quantify their pain on the 0 to 10 scale but are able to describe their pain. (4) 4. Outcome 4. The best means of collecting a sterile urine would be to cleanse the infant's genitalia and apply a pediatric urine collection (PUC) bag. Insertion of a catheter increases the risk of infection and also can potentially cause trauma due to the small size of the urethra. Cotton balls or a syringe would not be used. (5) 2. Outcome 5. The parents should be encouraged to stay, tuck the child in, and say goodnight. This will normalize the child's routine and reduce the separation anxiety the child is feeling secondary to the stress of hospitalization. (6) 4. Outcome 6. The 2-year-old is best taught by using simple terms, allowing the child to play with the equipment, and using a doll for demonstration. While the majority of the teaching will be aimed at the parents, the child also needs to be taught about what will happen from age 18 months on. (7) 3. Outcome 7. The nurse should not deny that the child is dying, but at the same time should not confirm it either because of the parent's request. However, it is obvious this child needs to talk about dying, and he or she should be encouraged to talk with the parents so the child can be comforted and reassured appropriately. (8) 2. Outcome 8. The nurse should help the parents to recognize the need for treating the child as normally as possible while not using guilt, shame, or threats. Support groups will put the parents in touch with other parents who have faced the same issues, allowing them to discuss alternatives with others who have gone through the same experience. (9) 3. Outcome 9. The DDST II is a screening device to assess the child's current level of development. It is not an intelligence test or a predictive test. Language skills are assessed as one of four parts of the DDST II. (10) 1, 4, 5. Outcome 10. Normalization is a term referring to helping the child with cognitive or physical disabilities develop as normally as possible, including taking responsibility for his or her own actions and functioning at the highest possible level.

CHAPTER 59

NCLEX-PN® ANSWERS (1) 3. Outcome 1. It is recommended that baby foods not be added to the diet until approximately 6 months of age. Prior to this age, the infant does not need more than breastmilk or formula. (2) 2. Outcome 6. Surgery corrects the disorder. The risk of pyloric sphincter obstruction is removed. Option 1 could alarm the client when there is no need. Pyloroplasty does remove the obstruction. There is no connection with digestive problems in adulthood. (3) 1. Outcome 3. The only muscle to be used in an infant is the vastus lateralis muscle. The gluteus muscle is not developed enough until the child has walked for 1 year. (4) 3. Outcome 9. It is very important the nurse does not jump to conclusions, so

the findings should be carefully documented and reported to the physician in an objective manner. (5) 4. RSV is transmitted via droplet precautions so a mask should be worn. Because of the risk of respiratory secretions mixing with the formula, a gown and gloves should also be worn. (6) 2. Outcome 9. The SRD is in place to protect the child. If the SRD is removed, an adult must be present to prevent the child from dislodging the IV. If the aunt is planning to leave the child unattended, the SRD must be replaced. (7) 1. Outcome 4. Mist tents generate moisture, so bedding and clothing should be changed to prevent chilling of the infant. Opening the tent disperses the oxygen, dropping the oxygen concentration. Every effort should be made to maintain the infant in a stable oxygen concentration. (8) 2. Outcome 2. When caring for a child under 6 months of age, the nurse should always report an oral temperature higher than 100.4 to the physician because of the risk for septicemia. An axial temperature of 100.8 equals an oral temperature of 101.8. (9) 3. Outcome 5. A protruding tongue, lack of Moro reflex, and a crease across the palm (Simian crease) are all indicative of Down syndrome. Children with Down syndrome have mental retardation of varying degrees. Cerebral palsy does not have this combination of signs. Sickle cell anemia is not identified at birth. (10) 2. Outcome 7. A high priority concern for this child is avoiding palpation or trauma to the abdomen, which could break the protective cover around the tumor. Pain management and side effects of chemotherapy will be of concern after treatment; renal failure is not an anticipated problem because the body can function normally with one kidney.

CHAPTER 60

NCLEX-PN® ANSWERS (1) 3. Outcome 1. Failure to meet one milestone does not indicate a developmental delay, but inability to tie the shoes by age 6 would indicate the need for further assessment. (2) 3. Outcome 2. It is normal for the appetite of a 3-year-old to decrease. The most important thing is for the parent to ensure that what the child does eat is nutritious and meets daily nutritional requirements. (3) 3. Outcome 3. It is generally wise to avoid bringing a child with chickenpox into the doctor's waiting room because of the risk of contaminating other children. However, the parent needs to know which symptoms require a visit to the doctor. If an appointment is indicated, it would be important to greet the child and immediately apply a mask until the child is isolated in an examination room. (4) 1. Outcome 4. Kawasaki's syndrome is painful, so care should be delivered as gently as possible to avoid undue discomfort. (5) 4. Outcome 6. The best indicator of rejection is kidney function, so the family will be taught to monitor for symptoms of fluid overload or decrease in urine output. (6) 1. Outcome 5. Loss of consciousness can indicate serious injury and would require immediate assessment and diagnosis. The other symptoms are mild and anticipated and can be treated at home.

(7) 4. Outcome 6. Fracture of the head of the femur with increased density of the femoral head is a strong indicator of possible Legg-Calvé-Perthes disease. (8) 1. Outcome 6. The priority action for a child with gastroenteritis is monitoring for signs of dehydration, because children become dehydrated faster than adults with similar symptoms. Encouraging fluids when the child is vomiting is counterproductive. Gradual diet advancement and stool specimens may be indicated, but the priority action is monitoring for dehydration. (9) 1. Outcome 7. Because of the mother's horror at the diagnosis, it is important to clarify that ringworm is not a worm but a fungal infection. While ringworm can be contagious, it is not highly contagious. Like all fungal infections, it will take 1 to 2 weeks of treatment to resolve. (10) 3. Outcome 8. Lack of response to auditory stimuli and lack of language skills would point most strongly to autism.

CHAPTER 61

NCLEX-PN® ANSWERS (1) 1. Outcome 1. During the school-aged years children learn about nutrition and can be influenced to follow a healthy diet if parents teach healthy eating habits. (2) 3. Outcome 2. Children with asthma can participate in physical activities with the permission of their physician and parents, although they may require premedication to avoid asthma attacks. (3) 2. Outcome 3. The nurse's priority with a child who suffered neurological trauma and is unconscious is to ensure a patent airway and adequate respirations. It is likely this child will eventually require intubation and mechanical ventilation. (4) 3. Outcome 4. Sudden pain resolution is a strong indicator of possible rupture of the appendix. Children scheduled for appendectomy are usually not given analgesia because pain monitoring is an important indicator of rupture. (5) 3. Outcome 4. While it is not impossible for a child, especially an obese child, to be diagnosed with non-insulin-dependent diabetes (Type 2), most children have insulin-dependent diabetes (Type 1) requiring insulin administration. When properly treated, these children can grow and develop normally. (6) 2. Outcome 5. Children displaying sexual behavior during a pelvic examination should be screened for possible sexual abuse. (7) 2. Outcome 5. This client is presenting with symptoms highly suspicious for a urinary tract infection, so the nursing priority is to collect and test a midstream urine specimen. (8) 1. Outcome 6. The bacteria most often responsible for MRSA infection is staphylococcus or pseudomonas. MRSA stands for methicillin-resistant *Staphylococcus aureus*. (9) 2. Outcome 7. Writing letters backwards may indicate dyslexia. However, it is important not to rush to label the child but perform the necessary diagnostic testing to determine the cause. (10) 1. Outcome 7. Ritalin will often cause insomnia if given prior to bed so it is recommended the drug be administered in the morning after breakfast. Taking the drug before meals can reduce the appetite leading to weight loss and delayed growth.

CHAPTER 62

NCLEX-PN® ANSWERS (1) 3. Outcome 6. Isolation from peer group and separation from friends can be a source of anxiety for adolescents. (2) 4. Outcome 10. It is important to validate the adolescent's feelings and provide hope. The other choices discount the young man's feelings. Helping him to talk about his feelings is the most appropriate action for the nurse. (3) 1. Outcome 1. Adolescents establish sexual identity by becoming comfortable with their own body and sexual feelings, which they accomplish through friendships with members of the opposite sex, dating, and experimentation. (4) 2. Outcome 4. Hepatitis A and B may be recommended during the adolescent years but they are not boosters. Tetanus and diphtheria are not given with pertussis after the initial series given during infancy. (5) 3. Outcome 2. Adolescents choosing to follow vegetarian diets are often unaware of the need to meet the body's protein needs through alternate sources of amino acids. The nurse should first determine what the client knows about this before creating a teaching plan. (6) 2. Outcome 9. Isotretinoin (Accutane) has major side effects, including psychiatric side effects. It is very important to explain the risk to the teen and the parent prior to beginning the medication. (7) 2. Outcome 8. Birth control pills are designed to prevent pregnancy when used properly, but they are not effective against the spread of sexually transmitted infections. This response demonstrates the need for additional teaching. (8) 1. Confidentiality rules of the adolescent prevent sharing of drug testing results, or performance of drug testing, without the teenager's permission even when the parent means well. (9) 1. Outcome 5. The teen is demonstrating signs of Hodgkin's lymphoma. (10) 3. Outcome 7. Both diseases are very similar in symptoms and treatment but ulcerative colitis only affects the large bowel while Crohn's disease can randomly strike any part of the gastrointestinal tract.

CHAPTER 63

NCLEX-PN® ANSWERS (1) 3. Outcome 10. Although it is not the best way to resolve conflicts, avoidance is the most frequently used method. Many staff nurses see the issue as minor and feel if it is ignored it will resolve itself. Both sides may consider the negative impact of addressing the issue directly to be too costly. Collaboration is the opposite of conflict. Accommodation and competition do occur, but they are not as common as avoidance. (2) 2. Outcome 3. The nursing code of ethics stresses accountability, which requires the nurse to report errors to prevent harm to clients. Although Tylenol may not harm the client, if the client later complains of a headache and an order is received to administer Tylenol, there is risk of overdose. Accurate reporting is imperative. (3) 4. Outcome 6. Lack of communication, especially providing incomplete instruction, is the most frequent reason why delegated tasks are not completed as expected. (4) 3. Outcome 1.

One of the most important things for new nurses to realize is that they cannot know everything, but they must never perform an unfamiliar intervention. This nurse should seek guidance from the supervisor in order to protect the client. (5) 2. Outcome 2. Accountability is related to responsibility and being responsible for one's own action and the actions of those to whom one has delegated tasks. The other answers all relate to delegation. (6) 1. Outcome 5. As a new nurse, with minimal experience, the new graduate would not be able to function effectively as a resource for other staff members. The nurse could give report, assist with medications, or take report. (7) 2. Outcome 4. A management style that is unstructured and leaves the decisions up to the group is known as laissez-faire. The autocratic style is highly directive. The authoritative provides clear guidelines but allows some independence. The democratic style seeks to find what the majority thinks is right. (8) 3. Outcome 11. Although functional nursing is efficient, it can create fragmented delivery of client care. With team nursing, several staff (RN, LPN/LVN, UAPs) share care of a set of clients. With primary nursing, a nurse has total responsibility for a set of clients from admission through discharge. With the case method, a nurse is responsible for care for clients during one shift. (9) 3. The disadvantage of taped report is that questions must be held until the end of report when the off-going nurse is in a hurry to leave the unit. Advantages include that it is a timesaving means of reporting and helps improve unit coverage. Taped report allows full coverage of clients. (10) 3. Outcome 12. National Patient Safety Goals require the MAR to be checked against the physician's orders, not against the previous MAR, which could contain errors. The nurse does ask the client's name and birth date before giving meds; does read back an order taken by telephone from a physician, and does attend programs about fire safety.

CHAPTER 64

NCLEX-PN® ANSWERS (1) 1. Outcome 1. Reviewing and studying as you move through the program will help you retain the knowledge and information you are learning. It also will prevent "cramming" just before you take the examination. Waiting until after the first course is complete means missing opportunities to think of the material as it relates to the exam. Waiting till the last 6 months or less to prepare puts unnecessary pressure on yourself and will lead to poorer results. (2) 1. Outcome 3. You are being asked to recall a fact or statement that has been presented to you, so this is a knowledge question. Comprehension involves understanding the meaning, not just remembering a fact. Application means understanding and using a piece of knowledge in a new situation. Analysis means reviewing several pieces of information and making a decision based on them. (3) 2. Outcome 2. Although ongoing review and analysis do occur, the revision is based on completion of a new job analysis of the tasks of the LPN/LVN. Changes in the nurse practice acts of

the states may occur at any time and are not linked to test revision. Question security and requests from member states are not the moving factor in creating a new test. (4) 4. Outcome 5. The test is set up so that students can follow the computer instructions and take the test even if they know nothing about computers. (5) 2. Outcome 9. Taking a proactive approach is most helpful in reducing test anxiety. There are useful techniques that can improve both your study methods and your ability to relax. Complaining does nothing to help your own emotions. Talking with peers may be useful but may not be all that is needed. Waiting is likely to make the anxiety worse. (6) 3. Outcome 10. A sudden change in sleep time can disturb your biorhythms and cause you to feel more tired and less alert. It is not necessary to get 8 to 10 hours of sleep; getting a normal amount maintains your biorhythm best. Waiting until you feel tired may not work because of anxiety about the upcoming test. (7) 4. Outcome 5. Questions of comprehension, analysis, or synthesis require you to do more than memorize facts. They require you to put information together and think more in depth. The test will require more than facts and memorization. The teacher's ability is not the question. (8) 4. Outcome 4. Categories of testing on client needs include Physiological Integrity, Psychosocial Integrity, Safe and Effective Care, and Health Promotion and Maintenance. Treatments and medications, GI and GU disorders, and safety and legalities are not categories of Client Needs. (9) 4. Outcome 8. The student nurse should apply for and plan to take the NCLEX-PN® as soon as possible. Research indicates that students are more likely to pass if they take the exam shortly after graduation, and passing rates decline with the passage of more than 3 months. (10) 3. Outcome 11. After taking the exam, it is common to feel anxious while waiting for results. It is best to try to stay as busy as possible so that time passes more quickly than if you have time to sit and worry.

CHAPTER 65

NCLEX-PN® ANSWERS (1) 2. Outcome 2. The first paragraph identifies the candidate and the job of interest. This helps the letter reach the correct person. The other choices are found in paragraphs 2 and 3. (2) 3. Outcome 3. Employers will be concerned with time gaps on applications. By highlighting activities during the gap, you will demonstrate interest in improving skills or contributing to the community. It is never appropriate to leave blanks on an application or ignore large time gaps on an application. Writing an explanation is not necessary and appears to be an excuse. (3) 4. Outcome 4. Although you are not required to answer personal questions, an answer that could alleviate concerns of the interviewer without revealing personal information is the best solution. Quoting the law or stating that you will not answer the question, or using it to make stipulations about the job may put the interviewer on the defensive and prevent you from being considered. (4) 2. Outcome 1. Although any of these reasons is possible, the misspellings show lack of attention to detail. Facilities do hire new graduates. The question does not say the graduate is applying to other places; it does not describe how the letter was addressed. (5) 1. Outcome 6. The probationary period is an opportunity for the facility to determine if the new hire is the correct candidate for the job, and for the new hire to determine if the job is right for them. Continued employment is based on meeting the job requirements. The nurse is always responsible for his or her own practice. Salary is not normally less during this time, although some facilities may offer an increase once the probationary period is over. (6) 3. Outcome 4. The best response is to shower and dress professionally. Wearing your uniform is acceptable unless it is soiled, which is a possibility after working all night. Even though the interviewers know you, you want them to look at you as a professional nurse; dressing appropriately will help them see you in that way. Asking to leave early is not recommended. (7) 3. Outcome 5. Having coffee with a friend can provide valuable job search information, in a casual setting. The other choices are planned activities and are considered to be formal networking. (8) 3. Outcome 7. Job success requires a positive attitude and helping coworkers without being asked in order to show teamwork. Criticizing the facility will not be appreciated from a newcomer. Responding to every request is likely to lead the new nurse to forget his or her own priority tasks. No one knows everything at the beginning of a new job. (9) 1. Outcome 1. The main reason for including a writing sample is to highlight your ability to write in a logical order using correct format and to show your attention to detail. It is not meant to indicate the skills of your program, your ability to chart (since this is narrative), or your level of computer skill. (10) 4. Outcome 8. The LPN/LVN would receive tuition reimbursement by enrolling in a nursing program to further his or her education but must enroll in an ADN or BSN program before enrolling in a master's or doctorate program. Accounting and business courses would not be reimbursable by a facility hiring you as a nurse.

Glossary

Abduction: movement of the bone away from the midline of the body (23)

Ablative: describing a procedure involving removal of a tissue or body part, or destruction of its function (29)

Abortion: expulsion from the uterus of an embryo or fetus prior to the stage of viability at about 20 weeks of gestation (51)

Abrasion: surface scrape, either unintentional (e.g., scraped knee from a fall) or intentional (e.g., dermal abrasion to remove pockmarks) (24)

Abruptio placentae: premature separation of the placenta (52)

Absorption: the process by which a drug passes into the bloodstream (27)

Abstinence: Voluntary avoidance (of drugs, sex) (50)

Acceleration: injuries that occur when a moving object hits the head (36)

Acceptance: last stage of grief in which the client comes to terms with loss (18)

Accidental loss: absence of a body part or person due to an unexpected event or disease (18)

Accommodation: alternating change in pupil size (constricts when looking at the near object, dilates when looking at a distant one) (19); strategy in which one person or a group is willing to yield to the other (63)

Acculturation: the modification of a group's or individual's culture as a result of contact with another group (3)

Achalasia: condition that occurs when the cardiac sphincter of the stomach does not relax to allow food to pass into the stomach (37)

ACLS: (advanced cardiac life support) a specialized training course that prepares the healthcare professional to perform advanced lifesaving skills or techniques on the client (47)

Acquired immune deficiency syndrome (AIDS): infection that affects the immune system; the final stage of disease caused by the human immunodeficiency virus (HIV) (35)

Acrocyanosis: a bluish discoloration of neonate's hands and feet, common for several hours after delivery (56)

Acromegaly: the secretion of too much growth hormone occuring after the client is an adult (38)

Action potential: stimulus that raises a potential response (36)

Active immunity: protection that occurs when a person produces his or her own antibodies (35)

Active range of motion: full normal movement of the extremities and joints by the client through a systematic series of movements (19)

Active transport: movement that occurs when it is necessary for electrolytes to move from an area of low concentration to an area of high concentration (26)

Actualization: to turn an idea into fact or action (15)

Acute pain: discomfort that lasts only through the expected recovery period (22)

Acute renal failure: a sudden decrease in or total lack of kidney function; it can be reversed with prompt treatment (39)

Addisonian crisis: a severe form of Addison's disease that causes a life-threatening medical situation (38)

Adduction: movement of the bone toward the midline of the body (23)

Adenopathy: generalized lymph node swelling (41)

Adhesions: scar tissue that can cause a kinking of the intestine (37)

Adjuvant chemotherapy: chemotherapy used to enhance the result of another therapy (45)

Adjuvant therapy: a treatment used to enhance the result of another therapy (45)

Admission: entry into the hospital (14)

Adolescence: the period of growth and development that begins with the appearance of secondary sex characteristics and ends with the cessation of physical growth and emotional maturity (62)

Adult day care: center that provides health and social services to the older adult who is still living at home (48)

Adventitious breath sounds: abnormal breath sounds that occur when air passes through narrowed airways or airways filled with fluid or mucus, or when pleural linings are inflamed (19)

Adverse effects: severe side effects or drug reactions (27)

Advocate: one who expresses and defends the cause of another (4)

Aerosol: a liquid, powder, or foam deposited in a thin layer on the skin; emitted by air pressure from the container (27)

Afebrile: without fever (21)

Affect: outward appearance of emotional state (e.g., tense, angry, happy, flat, blunted, labile, or changeable) (17)

Affective domain: area of learning that includes feelings, emotions, interests, attitudes, and appreciations (12)

Afferent: ascending (36)

Afternoon care: type of hygienic PM care that often includes providing a bedpan or urinal, washing the hands and face, and assisting with oral care to refresh clients' mouths (20)

Afterpain: discomfort from uterine contractions after delivery (54)

Against medical advice (AMA): against the recommendation of the primary care provider (14)

Agranulocytosis: the absence of any white blood cells (34)

Air embolism: the entry of gas into the peripheral or central vasculature (28)

Albinism: condition that occurs when melanin is absent or unable to function (30)

Algor mortis: the gradual decrease of the body's temperature after death (44)

Alkaline: pH above 7 on a scale of 0 to 14 (26)

Allis's sign: assessment for developmental dysplasia of the hip (DDH) demonstrated by placing the infant supine on the examination table with the hips and knees flexed and feet flat on the table; dislocation of the hip is indicated if the knee on the affected side is lower (59)

Allograft: tissue and organ transplants that are from the same species (35)

Alogia: restriction in the fluency and productivity of speech (49)

Alopecia: absence of hair on the head and/or body (20, 30)

Alternative medicine: a medical treatment used in place of conventional medicine (8)

Amblyopia: a reduction in vision in which there is no pathology in the eye (61)

Ambulation: the act of walking (23)

Ambulatory care nursing: facility that meets the needs of the ambulatory older adult; various degrees of personal care assistance may be provided (48)

Amenorrhea: absence of menstruation (40)

Amino acids: the building blocks of proteins (25)

Amniocentesis: the withdrawal of amniotic fluid through a needle inserted into the abdomen and the uterus (51)

Amnion: inner layer of the placenta (51)

Anabolism: process of building tissue (25)

Analgesia: pain relievers (22)

Analysis: the interpretation of a variety of data to recognize the commonalities, differences, and interrelationships among present ideas (1)

Anaplastic: lacking structural differentiation (45)

Anastomosis: alignment and suturing (37)

Anatomic position: the starting position (when collecting physical data) where the body is upright with the face front, arms at the sides with palms facing forward, and feet parallel (19)

Anemia: a deficiency of red blood cells or hemoglobin caused by decreased production or increased destruction of red blood cells, or by blood loss (34, 45)

Anencephaly: absence of neural tissue in the cranium (51)

Anesthesia: the alteration in the level of sensation and consciousness (29)

Aneurysm: a weakening and dilation in the wall of a blood vessel (33)

Anger: emotional state that includes feelings of animosity or strong displeasure (18)

Angina pectoris: chest pain caused by reduced oxygen supply to the heart (33)

Anhedonia: lack of ability to feel pleasure (49)

Anions: electrolytes with negative charge (26)

Ankylosed: permanently immobile (23)

Anterior: toward the front of the body or the belly (19)

Antibodies: large molecules of proteins produced in reaction to antigens (35)

Anticipatory grieving: state in which an individual or group experiences reactions in response to an expected significant loss (18)

Anticipatory guidance: information that helps parents prepare for expected physical and behavioral changes during their child's or teen's current and approaching stages of development (58)

Antiemboli stockings: firm elastic hose that compress the veins of the legs and facilitate the return of venous blood to the heart (29)

Antigen: substance that identifies foreign substances and induces sensitivity or immune response (10, 35)

Antimicrobial: microbe-destroying (10)

Antipyretic: helping to reduce an elevated temperature (21)

Antiseptics: agents that inhibit the growth of some microorganisms (10)

Anuria: low amounts of urine or no urine (39)

Anxiety: a state of mental uneasiness, apprehension, dread, or foreboding (17)

Aphasia: reduced ability or inability to speak or understand verbal or written language (19, 46)

Apheresis: removal of components of the blood, in this case the stem cells, which produce mature blood cells (45)

Apical pulse: a measure of heart rate taken directly at the heart (21)

Apical–radial pulse: a measure of heart rate taken both at the heart and at the wrist (21)

APIE: type of charting; acronym stands for: assessment, problem, intervention, and evaluation; based on the nursing process, this method incorporates an ongoing care plan into the progress notes (13)

Apnea: cessation of breathing (21)

Apneic spells: periods without breathing (56)

Apothecaries' system: system predating the metric system in which the basic unit of weight is the grain (gr) (like a grain of wheat), and the basic unit of volume is the minim, a volume of water equal in weight to a grain of wheat (27)

Appendicular skeleton: structure that consists of the bones of the arms and legs (58)

Application: the act of putting knowledge to use in a new situation (1)

Arbitration: an agreement negotiated by a designated impartial person (4)

Arcus senilis: a benign grayish haze of the outermost part of the cornea (42)

Arrhythmia: (dysrhythmia) pulse with an irregular rhythm (21)

Arteriosclerosis: condition in which the elastic and muscular tissues of the arteries are replaced with fibrous tissue (21, 33)

Aschoff's nodules: vegetative growth on the leaflets of the valves (33)

Ascites: fluid accumulations in the abdomen (37)

Asepsis: the absence of disease-causing microorganisms (10)

Aseptic technique: technique used to prevent the possibility of transferring microorganisms from one place or person to another (10)

As-needed (prn) care: type of hygienic care provided as required by the client (20)

Asphyxiation: oxygen deprivation or suffocation (32)

Aspiration pneumonia: inflammatory process caused by irritation of lung tissue by aspirated material, particularly hydrochloric acid (HCl) from the stomach (29)

Assault: an attempt or threat to touch another person unjustifiably (4)

Assessment: the systematic collection, organization, *validation* (proving or supporting), and documentation of data (6)

Assisted living facilities: facilities that give residents independence to be in their own apartments or condominiums but that offer nursing or medical care on the grounds (42, 48)

Asterixis: a unique flapping tremor of the hands with a rapid nonrhythmic extension and flexion in the wrist and fingers (37)

Astigmatism: visual disturbances that occur when light rays do not uniformly focus on the eye due to abnormal curvature of cornea or lens (61)

Atelectasis: the collapse of a lobe or of an entire lung (23, 29, 32)

Atherosclerosis: a buildup of fatty plaque on the inside of the arteries that causes narrowing of the lumen to the point of blockage (33)

Atrium: chambers on either side of the heart, which receive blood from the pulmonary veins (*left a.*) or venae cavae (*right a.*) and deliver it to the ventricle on the same side (33)

Atrophy: decrease in size (23)

Attenuated: weakened (35)

Attitudes: mental positions or feelings toward a person, object, or idea (e.g., acceptance, compassion, openness) (4)

Aura: a transient neurologic event lasting 5 to 30 minutes and consisting of a visual disturbance (e.g., flashing lights, blind spots) (36)

Auscultation: the process of listening to sounds produced within the body (19)

Auscultatory gap: the temporary disappearance of sounds normally heard over the brachial artery when the cuff pressure is high followed by the reappearance of the sounds at a lower level (21)

Autocratic: making unilateral decisions while dominating team members (63)

Autodigestion: inflammation of the pancreas; can be acute or chronic (37)

Autograft: the transplant of the client's own tissue (35)

Autoimmune disease: disorder in which the body perceives a portion of itself as foreign and responds accordingly (35)

Autoimmune disorder: disorder in which the body is unable to recognize normal cells and perceives them as foreign, initiating an immune response that targets normal cells to be destroyed (35)

Autologous: provided from the client for the client (e.g., blood drawn prior to surgery) (28, 35)

Autonomic dysreflexia: an exaggerated sympathetic response in spinal cord injuries at or above the T6 level (36)

Autonomic nervous system: body system that regulates automatic or *involuntary* control of organ systems (such as cardiac muscle and glands) (36)

Autonomy: the right and ability to make one's own decisions (4, 58)

Autopsy: an examination of the body after death (44)

Avoidance: strategy that is lose–lose; one side denies that a problem exists or withdraws so there is no active resolution (63)

Avolition: a lack of motivation (49)

Axons: single fibers that carry nerve impulses away from the cell body (36)

Azotemia: increased nitrogenous wastes in the blood including urea and creatinine (39)

Babinski's reflex: dorsiflexion of the great toe and flaring of the other toes when the lateral side of the foot is stroked from heel to toe (56)

Bacteremia: virulent microorganisms in the bloodstream from a localized source of infection; bacteria in the bloodstream; blood poisoning (28)

Bacteria: most common type of disease-causing microorganisms (10)

Bactericidal agent: solution or chemical that destroys bacteria (10)

Bacteriostatic agent: agent that prevents growth and reproduction of only some bacteria (10)

Bagging: a disposal technique recommended by the Centers for Disease Control (CDC) for removing contaminated or potentially infectious materials from a client's room (9)

Balanoposthitis: complications of phimosis (59)

Ballotable: able to be pushed away from the cervix (53)

Ballottement: rebounding against the fingers by the fetus if the examiner puts two fingers into the vagina and pushes upward on the uterus (51)

Bandage: a strip of cloth used to wrap some part of the body (24)

Bargaining: third stage of grief in which the client promises a change in behavior to avoid loss and may express feelings of guilt or fear of punishment for past sins, real or imagined (18)

Basal body temperature: the lowest temperature reached in the female reproductive cycle, indicative of ovulation (40)

Basal metabolic rate: the pace at which the body utilizes food to maintain the energy requirements of a person who is awake and at rest (21, 25)

Basic client situation: situation in which the client's condition is predictable and the clinical condition requires only basic nursing care (63)

Basic nursing care: nursing care which is predictable and with which modifications are unnecessary, based on the knowledge and skills obtained during an educational program, and those which can be safely performed by an LPN/LVN (63)

Battery: the willful touching of a person (including the person's clothes or even something the person is carrying) that may or may not cause harm (4)

Bed cradle: a device designed to keep the top bedclothes off the feet, legs, and even abdomen of a client (20)

Behaviorism: the belief that environment influences behavior, which is the essential factor determining human action (12)

Behavior modification: a system of positive reinforcement in which desirable behavior is rewarded and undesirable behavior is ignored (12)

Beliefs: something believed or accepted as true, especially a particular tenet or a body of tenets accepted by a group of persons (4)

Bereavement: the normal grieving period experienced by the surviving loved ones (18)

Bereavement overload: a condition that can occur when older adults have to deal with a succession of losses in overlapping time frames, which can interfere with a normal grieving period (18)

Bevel: the slanted part of the tip of needle of a syringe (27)

Bile: a greenish-brown liquid that consists of water, bile salts, bile pigment, cholesterol, and inorganic salts; needed to emulsify (break apart) lipids for digestion (37)

Binder: a type of bandage designed for a specific body part (24)

Binge: eating in a limited period of time (usually within 2 hours) an amount of food that is definitely larger than most individuals would eat under similar circumstances (50)

Biocultural ecology: the assessment of skin color and biologic variations (3)

Bioethics: the ethics and philosophical implications of certain biological and medical procedures, technologies, and treatments (4)

Biological response modifiers: soluble substances capable of stimulating or suppressing the immune system (45)

Biophysical profile: used to assess five variables: fetal breathing, fetal movement, fetal tone, fluid volume, and fetal reaction (51)

Biopsy: the surgical removal of living tissue from an organ or other part of the body for microscopic examination in order to establish a diagnosis or follow the course of a disease (45)

Biotherapy: the manipulation of the immune system to restore, augment, or modulate its function (45)

Bipolar affective disorder: a condition characterized by both "high" and "low" swings of mood, along with changes in thoughts, emotions, and physical health (17)

Bladder: the rubber bag piece of a blood pressure cuff (21)

Blended family: a situation in which one or both spouses have had a previous marriage and children from that marriage (16)

Blood pressure: a measure of the force exerted by the blood as it flows through the arteries (21)

Blood volume: quantity of circulating fluid in the blood vessels (21)

BLS: (basic life support) a specialized training course that prepares the healthcare professional to perform basic lifesaving skills or techniques (CPR, Heimlich maneuver, defibrillation, etc.) (47)

Body mass index: weight in kilograms divided by the square of height in meters (50)

Body mechanics: term used to describe safe, efficient use of one's body to move objects and carry out activities of daily living (9)

Body temperature: the balance between the heat produced and the heat lost from the body, measured in heat units called degrees (21)

Boggy: soft and spongy (54)

Borborygmi: abnormally loud, intense, frequent bowel sounds usually caused by hunger (37)

Bradycardia: condition in which heartbeats become irregular and abnormally slow (21, 33)

Bradypnea: abnormally slow breathing (21)

Brain abscess: an infection that has extended into the cerebral tissue or that is caused by organisms carried from other sites in the body (36)

Brain attack: a sudden, nonconvulsive focal neurologic deficit; the common clinical manifestation of cerebrovascular disease; newest term for CVA or stroke (36)

Braxton-Hicks contractions: painless contractions (51)

Breech: buttocks-first position of the fetus (53)

Bronchitis: the inflammation of one or more bronchi; also may include the trachea (32)

Bronchopulmonary dysplasia: permanent lung disease resulting from damage to the alveoli (57)

Bubbling: gurgling sounds heard as air passes through moist secretions in the respiratory tract (21)

Buffers: chemicals that prevent marked changes in hydrogen ion concentration (26)

Bulla: a small, circumscribed elevation of the skin containing fluid; bullae are larger than 0.5 cm (30)

Bunion: a firm, fluid-filled pad or bursa on the foot (43)

Buphthalmos: enlarged eyeball (59)

Bursitis: inflammation of the bursa sac and the adjoining fibrous tissue (43)

Cachexia: physical wasting and weight loss (45)

Calcinosis: the formation of calcium deposits in the connective tissue; usually found in fingers, hands, face, trunk, and on the skin above the elbows and knees (35)

Calories: units of heat energy (25)

Cancer: malignant tumor capable of metastasis and invasion, characterized by uncontrolled growth (45)

Cancer suppressor genes: genes with the opposite function of oncogenes; they "turn off" cell division and inhibit malignant growth (45)

Cannula: shaft or insertion tube (27)

Cannulation: the insertion of an IV needle into the body (47)

Capillary hemangioma: an overgrowth of capillary blood vessels that resembles a strawberry in size, shape, and color; usually disappears in early childhood (30)

Capillary refill time: the time the nail bed takes to return to its usual color after being pressed (19)

Caput succedaneum: edema of the scalp (56)

Carbuncle: an extension of a furuncle (30)

Carcinogenesis: the production of cancer; carcinogenic substances increase the likelihood of developing cancer (45)

Cardiac cycle: contraction and relaxation of the heart (33)

Cardiac output: the amount of blood pumped by the ventricles in 1 minute; stroke volume $\times$ pulse rate (21, 33)

Cardiac tamponade: condition that occurs when fluid accumulates in the pericardial sac, impairing the diastolic filling of the heart (33)

Cardiomegaly: enlargement of the heart (38, 43)

Cardiomyopathy: a group of diseases that affect the heart muscle (33)

Cardiopulmonary resuscitation (CPR): a combination of oral resuscitation and external cardiac massage, performed on clients who have an absent pulse (47)

Cardioversion: a noninvasive therapy that attempts to restore the heart's natural pacemaker, the sinoatrial node (33)

Career ladder: progression from one level in a profession to another through educational pursuits and professional experience (65)

Caregiver burden: long-term stress developed by family members who undertake the care of a person in the home for a long period (17)

Care plan: product of the planning phase of the nursing process (6)

Caries: cavities; dental decay (20, 36)

Carrier: a potential source of infection for others (10)

Case management: a range of models for integrating health-care services for individuals or groups (7)

Case method: also referred to as *total care*; a situation in which one nurse is assigned to and responsible for the comprehensive care of a group of clients during an 8- or 12-hour shift (7, 63)

Cast: a nonflexible encasement of a fractured extremity (31)

Catabolism: process of breaking down tissue (25)

Cataracts: a clouding of the lens in the eye that limits vision (42)

Catatonic behavior: a marked decrease in response to the environment (49)

Cathartics: drugs that induce defecation (37)

Cations: electrolytes with positive charge (26)

Celsius: temperature scale that normally extends from 34.0°C to 42.0°C for humans (21)

Center of gravity: the point at which all of the body's mass is centered and the base of support (the foundation on which the body rests) achieves balance (23)

Central nervous system: body system composed of the brain and the spinal cord, which act as the command and integration centers of the nervous system (36)

Cephalhematoma: an accumulation of blood between the periosteum and the skull bone (56)

Cephalic presentation: head-down position of the fetus (53)

Cephalopelvic disproportion: fetal head larger than the maternal pelvis (53)

Cerclage: surgical placement of sutures in the cervix to hold the cervix closed (52)

Cerebral death: irreversible damage to the cerebral cortex (44)

Cerebral edema: the abnormal accumulation of fluid or water in the intracellular space, extracellular space, or both (36)

Cerebrovascular accident: a sudden, nonconvulsive focal neurologic deficit (36)

Cerumen: earwax (20, 30)

Cervical dysplasia: abnormal changes in the tissue of the cervix (40)

Cervical os: the opening of the cervix (40)

Cervical spine alignment: a manual maneuver performed to maintain a client in proper spinal alignment (47)

Cervix: lower portion of the uterus (40)

Cesarean section: surgical removal of the fetus from the mother (53)

Chadwick's sign: a bluish-purple discoloration of the cervix and vagina (51)

Chancre: hard ulcer (41)

Charting: the process of making an entry on a client record (13)

Charting by exception: a documentation system in which only significant findings or exceptions to norms are recorded; incorporates (1) unique flow sheets that highlight significant findings and define assessment parameters and findings, (2) documentation by reference to the agency's printed standards of nursing practice, and (3) documentation forms at the bedside (13)

Cheyne-Stokes respirations: rhythmic waxing and waning of breath, from very deep to very shallow breathing and temporary apnea; often associated with cardiac failure, increased intracranial pressure, or brain damage (21)

Chloasma: a darkening of the forehead, cheeks, and around the eyes (51)

Cholecystitis: an inflammation of the gallbladder (37)

Cholecystokinin: a hormone that causes the gallbladder to contract and release bile (37)

Cholelithiasis: the formation of gallstones (37)

Chorea: involuntary, spasmodic movements of the limbs and face (36, 61)

Chorion: remainder of the trophoblast becomes the outer layer of the membranes (51)

Chronic illness: disease that produces symptoms and signs within a variable period of time, that persists over a long and variable time, and that allows only partial recovery due to the eventual presence of irreversible pathological changes (44)

Chronic obstructive pulmonary disease (COPD): a lung disorder characterized by airway obstruction caused by chronic bronchitis or emphysema (32)

Chronic pain: discomfort that lasts beyond the typical healing time period; generally, pain lasting longer than 3 to 6 months (22)

Chronic renal failure: a slow, progressive deterioration in kidney function (39)

Chvostek's sign: lip and facial spasm occurring when the facial nerve is tapped (38)

Circadian rhythm: (diurnal variations) normal change of body temperatures throughout the day (21)

Circulatory overload: excess fluid in the vasculature (28)

Circumcision: the surgical removal of the foreskin (prepuce) of the penis (56)

Circumduction: movement of the distal part of the bone in a circle while the proximal end remains fixed (23)

Circumoral: around the mouth (57, 60)

Cirrhosis: a chronic disease that leads to the development of scar tissue (fibrous connective tissue) in the liver (37)

Cleaning baths: baths given chiefly for hygiene purposes to remove accumulated oil, perspiration, dead skin cells, and some bacteria (20)

Cleft lip: condition that results from failure of the upper lip to join medially (57)

Cleft palate: condition that results from failure of the medial nasal and maxillary processes to join, leaving an opening between the roof of the mouth and the floor of the nasal passage (57)

Client: a person who engages the advice or services of someone who is qualified to provide the service (2)

Client education: a dynamic, integrated, and multifaceted teaching–learning process in which the nurse and client work together to change client behaviors (12)

Client-focused care: a delivery model that brings all services and care providers to the client (7)

Climacteric: (also known as *menopause*) termination of the reproductive period in the female (40)

Clinic: walk-in medical facility where clients can obtain diagnostic testing or treatment before returning home the same day; also known as ambulatory care center (48)

Clinical depression: major depressive disorder is diagnosed when a person loses interest in life and displays signs of severe sadness that last more than 2 weeks (17)

Clinical pathways: (also called *critical pathways*) an expected path of client needs, care, teaching, and progress for specific diagnoses (7)

Clinical record: the formal, legal document that provides evidence of a client's care (13)

Clonus: a series of abnormal reflex movements of the foot in response to sudden dorsiflexion (55)

Closed-ended questions: questions that require only "yes" or "no" or short factual answers giving specific information (11)

Closed reduction: manually moving the bones into alignment (60)

Closed wound drainage system: system, consisting of a drain connected to an electric or portable drainage suction, which removes exudate while reducing the possible entry of microorganisms into the wound (29)

Clubbing: condition caused by long-term lack of oxygen, in which the base of the nail becomes swollen and the ends of the fingers and toes increase in size (32)

Code of ethics: a formal statement of nursing's ideals and values (4)

Cognitive: having to do with awareness of and interaction between oneself and the environment (16)

Cognitive development: a result of interaction between an individual and the environment (16)

Cognitive domain: area of learning that includes knowing, comprehending, and applying (12)

Cognitivism: the belief that defines learning largely as a complex thinking process; the learner constantly structures and processes information from many sources (12)

Cold stress: increase in an infant's metabolism in response to excessive heat loss (56)

Colic: abdominal pain caused by periodic spasm of the intestines (59)

Collaboration: strategy in which both parties meet the problem on an even playing field with equal concern for the issues, allowing everyone to win by identifying areas of agreement and differences (63)

Collaborative: working jointly with other healthcare professionals, including physicians, in the performance of nursing roles within the scope of practice (65)

Collaborative interventions: nursing activities that reflect the overlapping responsibilities among healthcare personnel (6)

Colostomy: an opening into the colon (37)

Colostrum: a yellowish fluid rich in antibodies, secreted in the last trimester and the first few days following delivery (51)

Coma: a prolonged or irreversible period of unconsciousness (36, 44)

Comedo: basic acne lesion (62)

Commissurotomy: surgical separation of valve leaflets (33)

Communal family: a family that includes adults and children who may or may not be related and where family decisions and responsibilities are shared (16)

Communicable disease: disease that is spread or transmitted by direct or indirect contact (10)

Communication: a critical nursing skill used to gather information, to teach and persuade, and to express caring and comfort; the exchange of information or thoughts between two or more people (11)

Compartment syndrome: condition that occurs when increased pressure in a limited space compromises circulation and nerve function, leading to possible necrosis (31, 60)

Compensation: covering up weaknesses by emphasizing a more desirable trait or by overachievement in a more comfortable area (17)

Competition: strategy in which the winner takes all; results in a win–lose situation (63)

Complementary: used together with a standard approach to provide added benefit (8)

Complementary and alternative medicine (CAM): healing philosophies, approaches, and therapies that exist largely outside the main frame of conventional treatment (8)

Complementary proteins: foods containing some essential amino acids that are combined with others so that together they contain all nine essential amino acids (25)

Complex nursing situation: situation in which client's clinical condition is not predictable and requires frequent changes in medical or nursing orders or complex modifications (63)

Compliance: the extent to which a person's behavior aligns with medical or health advice (12); (in circulation) the blood vessels' ability to contract and expand (21)

Comprehension: understanding the meaning, translation, and interpretation of instructions and problems (1)

Compression sclerotherapy: procedure that obliterates unwanted veins by injection of a hardening agent (33)

Compromise: strategy in which there is negotiation or trade-offs; each person gets something and gives up something; win–lose/win–lose for both sides (63)

Computer adaptive testing: method of examination that provides each student a unique computerized examination, selecting the test questions as the student takes the examination (64)

Conception: the uniting of ovum and sperm (51)

Concussion: temporary neurologic impairment due to stretching, compressing, or tearing of nerve fibers near the brain (60)

Conduction: transfer of heat by direct contact with a cooler object (21, 56)

Condylomata lata: flat papules in the anal area or skin folds (41)

Confabulation: filling in gaps in memory with imagined or made-up events (50)

Confer: to consult another person or persons for advice, information, ideas, or instructions (13)

Conflict: a disagreement or antagonism between groups, individuals, or ideas (63)

Congestive heart failure (CHF): inability of the heart to function effectively as a pump (33, 43)

Conization: removal of a cone-shaped wedge of cervical tissue (40)

Conjunctival hyperemia: an increased amount of blood in the conjunctiva (60)

Conscious sedation: moderate sedation in which a client is able to respond to questions and has an increased pain threshold during surgery (29)

Consensual response: constriction of one pupil when a bright light is shown into the opposite pupil, removed, and shown a second time (19)

Constant fever: a fever in which the body temperature fluctuates minimally but always remains above normal (21)

Constipation: fewer than three bowel movements per week (37)

Consumer: an individual, a group of people, or a community that uses a service or commodity (2)

Contact lenses: thin curved disks of hard or soft plastic that fit on the cornea of the eye directly over the pupil (20)

Continuous feedings: nourishment generally administered over a 24-hour period using an infusion pump that guarantees a constant flow (25)

Contraception: the prevention of pregnancy (40)

Contractibility: the property that causes the shortening of the muscle in response to a stimulus (31)

Contractions: the result of shortening of the uterine muscle fibers (53)

Contrecoup: a cerebral injury that occurs opposite the point of impact (36)

Controller: a mechanism to regulate IV flow rate by gravity rather than by exertion or pressure (28)

Contusion: wound caused by a blow from a blunt instrument (24)

Convection: the dispersion of heat by air currents (21, 56)

Conventional medicine: medicine practiced by holders of a medical doctor (M.D.) or doctor of osteopathy (D.O.) degree and by other health professionals such as nurses, physical therapists, and psychologists (8)

Coping: dealing with problems and situations (17)

Coping behaviors: behaviors such as crying, acting angry, sexual "acting out," overeating, or smoking, which people perform in times of crisis or stress in an attempt to deal with their feelings (14)

CORE: a documentation system that focuses on the nursing process, and consists of a database, plans of care, flow sheets, progress notes, and discharge summary (13)

Core temperature: the temperature of deep tissues of the body (21)

Cor pulmonale: right ventricular heart failure due to prolonged pulmonary hypertension (32)

Corpus luteum: the ruptured follicle that produces estrogen and progesterone to support the endometrium until conception occurs or the menstrual cycle begins again (40)

Correctional nurse: nurse who provides for the health care of inmates in correctional facilities such as juvenile offender homes, jails, prisons, and penitentiaries (48)

Costal breathing: respiration involving external intercostal and accessory muscles (21)

Cotyledons: irregular-sized sections of the maternal side of the placenta (51)

Counseling: a form of therapy in which trained professionals help people think about the problems they are experiencing in their lives and find new ways of coping (17)

Coup: a focal cerebral injury directly under the area of impact (36)

Cover letter: brief document containing essential information about oneself that is often provided with a résumé to a potential employer (65)

Crabs: *Phthirus pubis* or pubic lice (60)

Crackles: (also known as *rales*) fine, short, interrupted lung sounds, best heard on inspiration (19, 21)

Credentialing: the way in which the nursing profession maintains standards of practice and accountability for the educational preparation of its members (4)

Cretinism: the thyroid gland does not make enough thyroid hormone in infancy (38)

Crime: an act committed in violation of public (criminal) law and punishable by a fine or imprisonment (4)

Crisis: a sudden change of events of a pyrexic condition (21)

Critical thinking: the art of thinking about thinking; examining thought processes in order to achieve goals, broaden understanding, and do problem solving (5)

Crohn's disease: disorder with random inflammation of the entire gastrointestinal tract that involves all layers of the bowel wall (62)

Cross-tolerance: tolerance to several drugs in the same classification (50)

Croup: a term representing a group of respiratory illnesses that result from inflammation and swelling of the epiglottis, larynx, trachea, and bronchi (59)

Crowning: point when the largest part of the fetal head is past the vulva and remains visible between contractions (53)

Crust: blood, pus, or serum that has dried on the surface of the skin after injury (30)

Cryptorchidism: undescended testicles (59)

Cultural awareness: knowledge about the similarities and differences among cultures (3)

Cultural competence: a set of skills, knowledge, and attitudes that must encompass the following elements: (1) awareness and acceptance of cultural differences, (2) awareness of one's own cultural values, (3) understanding of the dynamics of difference, (4) development of cultural knowledge, and (5) ability to adapt practice skills to fit the cultural context of the client (3)

Cultural empathy: the intellectual identification with or vicarious experiencing of the feelings, thoughts, or attitudes of another culture (3)

Cultural sensitivity: an awareness of the needs and feelings of your own and others' cultures (3)

Cumulative effect: buildup of the drug in the blood (27)

Custodial care: ongoing, maintenance care (46)

Cutaneous pain: discomfort that originates in the skin or subcutaneous tissue (22)

Cyanosis: a bluish tinge of skin that usually indicates poor oxygenation (19)

Cyst: a fluid-filled or semisolid sac originating in the subcutaneous tissue or dermis (30, 40)

Cystocele: condition that occurs when the ligaments supporting the urinary bladder are damaged allowing the bladder to prolapse into the vagina (40)

Dandruff: diffuse scaling of the scalp (20)

DAR: a method of charting by which progress notes are organized: data, action, and response (13)

Database: all information known about the client from the nursing assessment, physician's history, and the family; it is used to gauge changes in client status (6, 13)

Dawn phenomenon: blood sugar elevation at approximately 3 A.M., possibly due to a surge in growth hormone (38)

Debride: remove necrotic tissue (24)

Deceleration: injury that occurs when the head hits an immovable object (36)

Decidua: tissue that lines the uterine wall during pregnancy (54)

Decompression: removal of stomach contents and gas from the stomach and intestines (37)

Decubitus ulcer: lesions caused by unrelieved pressure resulting in damage to underlying tissue (24)

Deductive reasoning: a process of moving logically from a general statement or concept to related specifics (5)

Defamation: communication that is false or made with a careless disregard for the truth and that results in injury to the reputation of a person (4)

Defense mechanisms: unconscious attempts to manage anxiety (17)

Defibrillator: an instrument that provides various voltages of electricity (measured in joules) to trigger the electrical impulses of the heart (47)

Dehiscence: the partial or total rupturing of a sutured wound (24, 29)

Dehumanization: removal of unique human qualities (14)

Delegated medical act: doctor's orders given to the RN or LPN/LVN (63)

Delegated nursing act: nursing orders given to an RN or LPN/LVN by an RN (63)

Delegation: the distribution of tasks in a way that prioritizes activities and available resources (63)

Delusions: fixed false beliefs (49)

Demandingness: the expectations that parents have of their children for mature behavior, the discipline and supervision parents provide, and the parents' willingness to confront behavioral problems (16)

Dementia: the progressive loss of cognitive and intellectual functions without impairment of perception or consciousness (36)

Democratic: using decision making that allows input from all team members (63)

Dendrites: neuron processes that conduct electrical currents toward the cell body (36)

Denial: an attempt to ignore unacceptable realities by refusing to acknowledge them (17, 18, 50)

Dentures: a "plate" of artificial teeth for one jaw worn to replace upper or lower teeth or both (20)

Dependent interventions: activities carried out under the physician's orders or supervision or according to specified routines (6)

Depot injection: an oil-based medication form of the drug injected intramuscularly for the purpose of slow release of the drug over several weeks (49)

Depression: a range of moods, from the low spirits that we all experience to a severe problem that interferes with everyday life (17); fourth stage of grief (18)

Dermabrasion: used to treat acne scars and gives a smooth appearance to the face (30)

Dermatomes: areas of skin innervated by branches of a single spinal nerve (36)

Dermis: the inner thicker layer of skin, called the *true skin*; contains most of the skin appendages (such as hair and nails), blood vessels, and nerve endings (30)

Desensitization: the process of administering small amounts of dilute allergen to stimulate the body's immune system (59)

Designated: donated by friends and relatives for a particular client (28)

Desired/expected outcomes: the broader goals of a client in relation to a nursing diagnosis (such as, "The client will have adequate gas exchange.") (6)

Development: an increase in the complexity of function and skill progression (16)

Deviated septum: condition in which the cartilage of the nose bulges or deviates to one side (60)

Diabetic ketoacidosis: buildup of ketones in the blood, signaling high blood sugar level and breakdown of fats for energy (38)

Diabetic retinopathy: condition in diabetics, wherein circulatory changes in the blood vessels of the eye cause small blood vessels to hemorrhage into the vitreous humor of the eye (43)

Diabulimia: an eating disorder in which clients with Type 1 diabetes deliberately give themselves less insulin for the purpose of weight loss (50)

Diagnosing: analyzing and synthesizing data in order to provide a statement of condition or need (6)

Diagnostic: serving to confirm or establish a particular disease or characteristic (29)

Diagnostic profile: document that aids candidates in determining areas of relative strength and weakness based on the NCLEX-PN® test plan and in focusing their study prior to retaking the exam (64)

Diagnostic-related groups: prospective payment or billing is formulated before the client is even admitted to the hospital; thus, the record of admission, rather than the record of treatment, now governs payment (7)

Dialysis: a process for eliminating nephrotoxins and retained fluid from the body (39)

Diaphragmatic breathing: respiration involving contraction and relaxation of the diaphragm (21)

Diaphragmatic hernia: a condition that occurs when the abdominal contents protrude through a weakness in the diaphragm (57)

Diarrhea: term used for liquid feces and increased frequency of defecation (37)

Diastasis recti abdominis: a separation of the abdominal muscle (54)

Diastole: the period in which the ventricles relax (19)

Diastolic pressure: blood pressure when the ventricles are at rest (21)

Dichotomous thinking: thought process in which something is either all one way or all its opposite (50)

Differentiation: the process by which cells become adapted for specific functions (45)

Diffusion: the movement of gases or other particles from an area of greater pressure or concentration to an area of lower pressure or concentration (32)

Dilatation and curettage (D&C): opening of the cervix and scraping of the lining of the uterine walls (40)

Dilatation stage: first stage of labor, beginning with regular contractions and ending with complete effacement and dilatation of the cervix (53)

Diplopia: double vision (43)

Direct response: constriction or tightening of a pupil when a bright light is shown into it (19)

Direct supervision: organization in which the supervisor is continuously present to coordinate, inspect, or direct nursing care (63)

Disability: the degree of observable and measurable impairment (46)

Discharge: the official procedure by which the client leaves the healthcare facility and returns home or to another setting (14)

Discrimination: unfair and unequal treatment or access to services based on race, culture, or other bias (3)

Discussion: an informal conversation between two or more healthcare personnel to identify a problem or establish strategies to resolve a problem (13)

Disease: a process that causes a detectable impairment in the way the body functions (10)

Disenfranchised grief: grief that occurs when a mourner finds her/himself judged by a social norm that does not recognize the validity of the loss (18)

Disinfectants: agents that destroy pathogens other than spores (10)

Dislocation: an event that occurs when the end of the bone is no longer articulated in the joint capsule (31)

Disorganized behavior: lack of goal orientation (49)

Disorganized thinking: inability to sort and interpret incoming sensory information, or respond appropriately (49)

Displacement: the transferring of emotional reactions from one person to another (17)

Distal: farther from the origin of a structure (19)

Distancing: an unconscious response of professionals in which they hold back emotionally, especially from dying clients (18, 44)

Diurnal variations: (circadian rhythm) normal change of body temperatures throughout the day (21)

Diverticulosis: a condition characterized by an outpouching of bowel mucosa (37)

Diverticulum: an outpouching or protrusion of inner tissue layers through a weakness in the muscle wall (37, 59)

Documenting: the process of making an entry on a client record (13)

Domains: elements that describe a variable in scientific research (3)

Do not resuscitate: an order to prevent interventions the client does not wish to have performed when death approaches (18, 44)

Dorsal: toward the back of; the opposite of ventral (19)

Drip factors: rates at which IV solution passes through the drip chamber and into the tubing (28)

Drug allergy: an immunologic reaction to a drug (27)

Drug interaction: problem that occurs when the administration of one drug alters the effect of another drug (27)

Drug tolerance: occurs when a person requires increases in dosage to maintain the therapeutic effect (27)

Drug toxicity: deleterious effects of a drug on an organism or tissue (27)

Dual diagnosis: presence of substance abuse along with a concurrent psychiatric disorder (17)

Duchenne's muscular dystrophy: degenerative muscle disorder; sex-linked recessive disorder carried by mothers and passed to their sons (60)

Ductus arteriosus: vessel that connects the main pulmonary artery to the aorta (51)

Ductus venosus: vessel that carries blood to the inferior vena cava (51)

Dumping syndrome: occurs when food passes rapidly into the intestines (37)

DuoNeb: two-medication bronchodilator given via nebulizer for improved gas exchange in cases of respiratory insufficiency (47)

Durable power of attorney for health care: (also called *medical power of attorney*) a written statement appointing someone else to manage healthcare treatment decisions when the client is unable to do so (18, 44)

Dwarfism: a condition in which the pituitary does not secrete enough growth hormone to achieve normal height (38)

Dysarthria: imperfect articulation of speech due to disturbances of muscular control (19)

Dysfunctional grieving: grief that is characterized by an extended period of denial, depression, severe physiological symptoms, or suicidal thoughts (18)

Dysmenorrhea: painful menses (40)

Dyspareunia: painful intercourse (40)

Dyspepsia: also known as *indigestion;* an upper gastrointestinal regurgitation of gastric contents (37)

Dysphagia: difficulty swallowing (37)

Dyspnea: difficult and labored breathing during which the individual has a persistent, unsatisfied need for air and feels distressed (21)

Dysrhythmia: (arrhythmia) pulse with an irregular rhythm (21, 33)

Dystocia: a long, difficult, or abnormal labor pattern (53)

Dysuria: pain on urination (39, 40)

Early morning care: type of hygienic care provided to clients as they awaken in the morning, consisting of providing a urinal or bedpan to the client confined to bed, washing the face and hands, and giving oral care (20)

Ecchymosis: purplish patch caused by extravasation (leaking) of blood into the skin (30, 56)

Echolalia: a condition in which words are incessantly repeated (59)

Eclampsia: severe hypertensive disorder with pregnancy, evidenced by grand mal seizures (52)

Ectopic: occurring outside of the uterus (40)

Ectopic pregnancy: pregnancy in which a blastocyst implants outside the uterine cavity (52)

Edema: the presence of excess interstitial fluid (19)

Effacement: the shortening and thinning of the cervix (53)

Efferent: descending (36)

Effleurage: stroking of the body (23)

Effluent: fecal material (37)

Ego: concept that connects the psyche with reality and promotes well-being and survival (15)

Ejection fraction: percentage of blood in the ventricle (33)

Elasticity: the property that causes the muscle to return to its normal shape and form after contracting or extending (31)

Elective surgery: surgery performed when a condition is not immediately life threatening or to improve the client's life (29)

Electrolytes: (ions) electrically charged particles capable of conducting electricity, made of oxygen, nutrients, carbon dioxide, and salts dissolved in water (26)

Embolectomy: surgical removal of an embolism (33)

Emboli: (singular, *embolus*) clots moved from their place of origin, causing circulatory obstruction elsewhere (23, 29)

Embryo: the inner layer of the blastocyst (*embryonic disk*) (51)

Emergency care: (also called ER for emergency room, or ED for emergency department) a center where staffing is maintained around the clock to provide care for high acuity cases, such as trauma (47)

Emergency surgery: performed immediately to preserve function or the life of the client (29)

Emesis: vomit (37)

Emphysema: a pulmonary condition characterized by overinflation and destruction of the alveolar walls (32)

Encephalitis: an inflammation of the gray and white matter of the brain and the spinal cord (36)

Encopresis: condition associated with constipation and fecal retention in which watery stools bypass the hard fecal mass and may be confused with diarrhea (60)

Endarterectomy: removal of the lining of the artery (33)

Endocarditis: the inflammation of the valves and lining of the heart (33)

Endocrine glands: secrete hormones directly into the blood (38)

Endogenous opioids: substances bind to opiate receptor sites in the central and peripheral nervous system, decreasing or blocking any pain impulse (22)

Endometriosis: condition that occurs when endometrial tissue grows outside the uterine cavity (40)

Endometritis: infection usually begins in the vagina and migrates upward into the uterus (55)

End-stage renal disease: stage of failure in which the kidneys ultimately lose the ability to excrete waste products and regulate fluid and electrolytes (39)

Enema: a solution introduced into the rectum and large intestine (37)

Engagement: entrance of the presenting part (usually the fetal head) into the true pelvis (53)

Engrossment: a sense of interest and preoccupation (54)

Enteral nutrition: nourishment given through a tube or stoma directly into the small intestine, thus bypassing the upper digestive tract (25)

Enteritis: inflammation of the intestines due to pathogenic organisms (37)

Enuresis: urinary incontinence after voluntary control has normally been reached (39, 60)

Environments: circumstances, objects, or conditions by which one is surrounded (5)

Epidermis: the tough outer external layer of the skin (30)

Epididymis: an enclosed single coiled tube that serves as a duct through which the sperm passes from the testis to the outer surface (40)

Epilepsy: a general term for the primary condition that causes seizures (36)

Epiphora: increased tearing of the eye beyond normal limits (59)

Epiphyseal plate: a layer of cartilage in the metaphysis of the bone (58)

Episiotomy: surgical cutting of the perineal tissue (53)

Epispadias: condition in which the urethral meatus opens onto the dorsal (upper) surface of the penis (57, 59)

Epistaxis: nosebleed (60)

Epstein's pearls: small white cysts that may be present on the newborn's palate but disappear in a few weeks (56)

Equilibrium: the sense of balance (23)

Erosion: a wearing away of the superficial epidermis by friction or pressure (30)

Eructation: the expelling of gas from the stomach through the mouth, commonly called belching (37)

Erythema: redness associated with a variety of rashes (19)

Erythema marginatum: transient rash characterized by non-pruritic, red, macular lesions that blanch in the center (61)

Erythema toxicum neonatorum: a benign, raised pink papule with a light colored center resembling a mosquito bite, which appears suddenly on the chest, abdomen, and back 24 to 48 hours after birth (56)

Erythrocytes: red blood cells (34)

Eschar: dead matter that is sloughed off the surface of the skin (24)

Esophageal atresia: condition in which the esophagus ends in a blind pouch before reaching the stomach (57)

Esteem: also called ego, internal esteem that includes self-respect, autonomy, and achievement; external esteem that includes status, recognition, and attention (15)

Ethics: (1) a method of inquiry that helps people to understand the morality of human behavior (i.e., the study of morality), (2) the practices or beliefs of a certain group (e.g., medical ethics, nursing ethics), and (3) the expected standards of moral behavior of a particular group as described in the group's formal code of professional ethics (4)

Ethnocentrism: interpretation of the beliefs and behaviors of others from the perspective of one's own cultural values and traditions (3)

Etiologic agent: source of the infection (10)

Etiology: cause or origin

Eupnea: normal respirations (21)

Eupneic: characterized by normal, easy respirations (47)

Evaluation: a planned, ongoing, purposeful activity in which client and healthcare professionals determine the client's progress toward goal achievement and the effectiveness of the nursing care plan (6)

Evaporation: change of water to a gas or vapor, which causes cooling (21, 56)

Evisceration: the protrusion of the internal viscera through an incision (24, 29)

Ewing's sarcoma: a malignant tumor found most commonly in the femur, pelvis, tibia, fibula, ribs, humerus, scapula, and clavicle (61)

Exacerbation: reactivation of a disease and recurrence of symptoms (44)

Examination: a systematic data collection method (6)

Excitability: the property that allows the muscle to receive a stimulus and act on that stimulus (31)

Executive function: abstract thinking and problem solving (49)

Exhalation: (also known as *expiration*) the breathing out or the movement of gases from the lungs to the atmosphere (21)

Exocrine glands: glands that secrete substances through ducts that reach the epithelial surface inside the body or on the skin (38)

Exogenous opioids: analgesics (e.g., morphine) that bind to receptor sites to provide pain relief (22)

Exophthalmos: bulging eyes resulting from enlarging tissue behind the eyes (38)

Expiration: exhalation (32)

Exstrophy of the bladder: a rare condition in which the abdominal wall fails to fuse, allowing the urinary bladder to protrude to the outside (57)

Extended family: an egocentric network of relatives (e.g., grandparents, aunt, uncles, and cousins) (16)

Extensibility: property that enables the muscle to lengthen or "extend" in response to a stimulus (31)

External disasters: events outside the hospital that produce a large number of victims (e.g., fires, plane or train crashes, earthquakes, or violent civil disturbances) (9)

Extracellular fluid: fluid found outside the cells (26)

Extravasation: severe infiltration of a solution into surrounding tissue (28)

Exudate: material that has escaped from blood vessels during the inflammatory process and is deposited in tissue or on tissue surfaces (24)

FACT: system of documentation that focuses on four elements: flow sheets that are individualized; assessment sheet that is standardized with baseline parameters; concise integrated progress notes and flow sheets that are used to document the client's condition and response; and timely entries that are recorded after care is given (13)

Fallopian tubes: the structures that allow passage of the ovum to the uterus (40)

False imprisonment: unlawful restraint or detention of another person against his or her wishes (4)

Family: two or more individuals who come together for the purpose of nurturing (16)

Family-centered care: treatment to a designated client with recognition that the family system or unit may also need intervention (16)

Fasciculations: involuntary contraction or twitching of muscle fibers (36)

Fasciotomy: a surgical procedure that cuts away the fascia to relieve tension or pressure (31)

Fecal impaction: a mass or collection of hardened, putty-like feces in the folds of the rectum (37)

Feedback: shared information that relates a person's performance to the desired goal (12)

Ferguson's reflex: a spontaneous urge to push that occurs when the fetus touches the pelvic floor (53)

Fertility awareness: family planning based on the assumption that ovulation occurs at the same time each month (40)

Fertilization: the process of uniting a sperm and an ovum (egg), each containing 23 chromosomes to form one cell containing 46 chromosomes (51)

Fetal attitude: degree of flexion of the fetal head and limbs to the trunk (53)

Fetal lie: relationship of the long axis (head to foot or cephalo-caudal plane) of the fetus to the long axis of the mother (53)

Fetal position: relationship of the presenting part to the four quadrants of the maternal pelvis (53)

Fetal presentation: body part of the fetus that is closest to the cervix (53)

Fibrinolytics: medications that dissolve blood clots (33)

Fibroadenoma: a freely movable, rounded mass with well-defined borders and a solid rubbery texture (40)

Fibrocyst: fluid-filled mass caused by fibrosis in the breast (40)

Fibrosis: the replacement of inflamed or damaged tissue with connective or scar tissue (40)

Fight-or-flight response: a generalized response to an emergency situation (17)

Filtration: the transfer of water and dissolved substances from a region of high pressure to a region of low pressure (26)

Fissure: a deep furrow or slit extending into the dermis (30)

Fistula: an abnormal passage from a body cavity or tube to another cavity or surface (24, 37)

Five Ps affecting labor: *passage* (maternal structures through which the fetus must travel); *passenger* (fetus); *power* (strength needed to push the fetus through the passageway); *position* (of the mother during labor); *psyche* (mother's emotional status during labor) (53)

Flaccid: relaxed (36)

Flat affect: absence of facial expressions or other body language indicating feelings (49)

Flatulence: expelling of gas from the rectum (37)

Flow sheets: abbreviated progress notes (13)

Fluid: the liquid components of the body (26)

Focus charting: a type of record intended to make the client, along with client concerns and strengths, the focus of care (13)

Fomite: an inanimate object such as a toy, cooking or eating utensil, or contaminated instrument, which can transmit infection from one area or person to another (10)

Fontanels: soft spots; membranous gaps in the bone structure of the skull (16, 53, 58)

Food poisoning: consumption of contaminated foods or liquids that cause foodborne illness (37)

Foramen ovale: opening in the septum between the right atrium and left atrium (51)

Fracture: any disruption in the bone itself (31)

Frequency: need to void more than usual (39)

Friction: a force acting parallel to the skin surface (24)

Friction rub: superficial grating or creaking sounds heard during inspiration and expiration (19)

Frontal plane: a line running from one side of the body to the other; the front plane separates the body into front and back portions (19)

Fulcrum: fixed point about which a lever moves (9)

Full-thickness burn: (also called *third-degree burns*) involvement of all layers of skin in a burn (47)

Functional method: method that focuses on the jobs to be completed (e.g., bed making, temperature measurement) (7)

Functional nursing: nursing in which each team member is assigned specific tasks or functions (63)

Fundus: bottom or base of a hollow organ (such as the uterus) (40, 54)

Fungi: either yeasts or molds (10)

Funic soufflé: the sound occurring at the fetal heart rate (51)

Funnel chest: (*pectus excavatum*) condition in which the lower portion of the sternum is depressed (58)

Furuncle: an acute inflammation caused by *Staphylococcus*; starting deep in one or more hair follicles and spreading into the surrounding dermis (30)

Ganglia: small collections of cell bodies found outside the CNS in the PNS (36)

Gangrene: necrosis or tissue death (31)

Gastric bypass: common GI surgery for weight loss that sutures off part of the stomach (37)

Gastritis: inflammation of the stomach caused by chemotherapy, radiation therapy, food contaminated with toxins, significant alcohol intake, or food allergies (37)

Gastroesophageal reflux disease: common disorder that results when gastric contents splash into the lower end of the esophagus (37)

Gastroplasty: the stomach is stapled, creating a small pouch (37)

Gastrostomy: surgical creation of an artificial opening into the stomach (25)

Gate control theory: theory stating that peripheral nerve fibers carrying pain to the spinal cord can have their message modified at the spinal cord level (the "gate") before transmission to the brain (22)

Gavage: feeding through a tube (37)

General adaptation syndrome: physiologic responses to stress that result from prolonged, excessive stress and that lead to exhaustion of the body's resources (17)

General anesthesia: sedation that causes the loss of all sensation and consciousness (29)

Generalized seizures: involve neurons bilaterally; they often do not have a focal onset and they usually originate from a subcortical or deeper brain focus (36)

General supervision: observation by a supervisor who regularly coordinates, inspects, or directs nursing care and is available within the building or by telephone (63)

Generic: family name of a drug (27)

Gerontology: health specialty that focuses on care of the older adult (42)

Gestational diabetes mellitus: an abnormal glucose metabolism caused by the additional requirement for insulin during pregnancy (52)

Gestational hypertension (GH): formerly called *pregnancy-induced hypertension (PIH)*; hypertension occurring for the first time in midpregnancy and returning to normal levels by the 12th week after birth (52)

Gestures: hand and body motions that may emphasize and clarify the spoken word, or that may be used instead of words to indicate a particular feeling or to give a sign (11)

Gigantism: condition in which the pituitary secretes too much growth hormone prior to closure of the epiphyses in the bones (38)

Gingiva: gums of the mouth (20)

Gingivitis: inflamed gums (37)

Glandular fever: (mononucleosis or "kissing disease") immune disorder caused by the Epstein-Barr virus (EBV) (62)

Glaucoma: a disease progression in the eye characterized by increased intraocular pressure (43)

Glomerulonephritis: an inflammatory disease of the glomerulus affecting kidney function; can be acute or chronic (39)

Glucosuria: glucose excreted in the urine (61)

Glycogen: the stored form of glucose (25)

Glycogenesis: process of glycogen formation (25)

Glycogenolysis: a process where glycogen can be converted back to glucose when needed to maintain blood levels or to provide energy (25)

Goals: the particular aspects of a desired outcome for a client (such as, "The client will increase use of the incentive spirometer by 30 seconds at each use.") (6)

Goiter: painless enlargement of the thyroid gland (38, 62)

Gonadotropins: hormones that stimulate the growth and maintenance of the *gonads* (ovaries and testes) (38)

Goodell's sign: a softening of the cervix (51)

Gout: an inflammatory disorder that causes uric acid crystals to form in a joint (31, 43)

Graft versus host disease: a very serious complication of a bone marrow transplant where the client's own body attacks itself, especially the liver, the skin, and the gastrointestinal tract (34)

Granulation tissue: translucent red tissue that grows in a wound (24)

Granulocytes: cells involved in the inflammatory response; they make up the largest number of normal blood leukocytes (35)

Gravida: a pregnant woman (51)

Gray matter: consists mostly of unmyelinated fibers and cell bodies (36)

Grief: the whole range of feelings, thoughts, and behaviors related to loss and signifying emotional responses, especially overwhelming distress and sorrow (18)

Grieving: process of mourning and resolving a loss (16, 18)

Group: more than two people who have shared needs and goals, who take each other into account in their actions, and who thus are held together and set apart from others because of their interactions (11)

Growth: physical change and increase in size (16)

Guaiac test: test for occult blood (37)

Gumma: infectious granuloma (41)

Half-life: the time interval required for the body's elimination processes to reduce the concentration of the drug in the body by one-half (27)

Halitosis: bad breath (20)

Hallucinations: sensory perceptions that seem very real but occur without external stimulus (49)

Hammertoe: a deformity of the toe (usually the second toe) that causes the main toe joint to bend upward like a claw (43)

Handicap: the total adjustment to disability that limits functioning at a normal level (46)

Hazmat: hazardous material (47)

Healthcare surrogate: an adult who is appointed to make healthcare decisions in the event a client becomes incapacitated and has not executed a living will or medical power of attorney (18)

Healthcare system: the totality of services offered by all health disciplines (7)

Health conditions: the way a person has taken care of his or her body (42)

Health maintenance organization: a group healthcare agency that provides basic and supplemental health maintenance and treatment services to voluntary enrollees who pay a preset fee (7)

Hearing aid: a battery-powered, sound-amplifying device used by people with hearing impairments (20)

Hegar's sign: softening of the lower uterine segment (51)

HELLP syndrome: (**h**emolysis, **e**levated **l**iver enzymes, and **l**ow **p**latelet count) acronym for characteristics of severe preeclampsia with liver damage (52)

Helpful communication: interaction that encourages a sharing of information, thoughts, or feelings between two or more people (11)

Hematemesis: vomiting blood, which may be clotted and mixed with stomach contents (37)

Hematocrit: a measurement of the percentage of erythrocytes (32)

Hematoma: accumulation of blood in the soft tissue under the skin that may appear as a reddish-blue swelling (24, 28, 30, 55)

Hematuria: blood in the urine (39, 40)

Hemiplegia: paralysis of one-half of the body when it is divided along the median sagittal plane (36)

Hemodialysis: a process of removing waste products, excess fluids, and electrolytes from the blood (39)

Hemoglobin: an oxygen-carrying red pigment (32)

Hemoptysis: bloody sputum (40)

Hemorrhage: persistent bleeding (24)

Hemostasis: cessation of bleeding (24, 34)

Hemothorax: an accumulation of blood in the pleural space that causes partial or complete collapse of the lung on the affected side (32)

Hepatic encephalopathy: condition that occurs when ammonia and nitrogen levels in the blood affect the central nervous system (37)

Hepatitis: inflammation of the liver (37)

Hepatomegaly: enlargement of the liver (38)

Hernia: protuberance of an organ through a defect in the wall of the abdomen (37)

Herniorrhaphy: surgical repair of a hernia (37, 60)

Herpes zoster: also known as *shingles;* caused by the varicella zoster virus; very similar to the chickenpox virus (30)

Hiatal hernia: condition that occurs when part of the stomach moves through an opening in the diaphragm into the chest cavity (37)

High acuity: very urgent and possibly life threatening (47)

High-risk newborn: an infant who is born prior to 38 weeks' gestation or after 42 weeks' gestation, who has alterations in intrauterine growth, or who has a medical condition that requires frequent monitoring and treatment (57)

Hip spica cast: a cast covering the upper thighs and lower torso (59)

Hirsutism: condition of excessive hair growth (20, 30, 40)

Histocompatibility: immunologic similarity that permits successful homograft transplantation (35)

Homeostasis: processes by which body equilibrium is maintained (26, 38)

Homologous: donated by someone other than the client but compatible with the client (28)

Hormones: chemical messengers that function individually (38)

Hospice: care that incorporates the holistic concepts of palliative care and is provided for terminally ill clients with a prognosis of 6 months or less survival time (44)

Hour of sleep (HS) care: hygienic care provided to clients before they retire for the night (20)

Household system: measures that may be used when more accurate systems of measure are not required; such as drops, teaspoons, tablespoons, cups, and glasses (27)

Hub: part of the needle that fits into the syringe (27)

Human chorionic gonadotropin: maintains the corpus luteum and stimulates it to continue producing estrogen and progesterone for another 11 to 12 weeks (51)

Humanism: system of thought that focuses on both cognitive and affective qualities of the learner (12)

Human immunodeficiency virus (HIV): a virus that damages and destroys cells of the body's immune system (35)

Human leukocyte antigens: cell receptor sites and markers that are unique to each individual (35)

Humoral: occurring in the plasma (35)

Hydatidiform mole: (molar pregnancy) a disease in which the trophoblast develops into hydropic vesicles instead of normal embryonic tissue (52)

Hydramnios: (also called *polyhydramnios*) excessive amniotic fluid (52)

Hydrocele: an accumulation of fluid in the scrotal sac (59)

Hydronephrosis: distention of the renal pelvis caused by increased pressure due to urine backup (39, 59)

Hygiene: the science of health and its maintenance (20)

Hyperbilirubinemia: an increase in bilirubin above normal limits (57)

Hypercapnia: excess of carbon dioxide in the blood; hypercarbia (32)

Hypercarbia: excess of carbon dioxide in the blood; hypercapnia (32)

Hyperemesis gravidarum: prolonged, excessive vomiting (51)

Hyperextension: farthest extension or straightening of a joint (e.g., bending the head backward) (23)

Hyperglycemia: high blood sugar caused by lack of an adequate amount of insulin or insufficient insulin action (38)

Hyperlipidemia: condition characterized by increased total cholesterol, low-density lipoproteins, and triglycerides accompanied by decreased high-density lipoproteins (61)

Hyperopia: visual disturbance that occurs when light is focused behind the retina (61)

Hyperosmolar hyperglycemic nonketotic coma: loss of consciousness that occurs when the client with Type 2 diabetes has extreme hyperglycemia (38)

Hyperpituitarism: growth hormone excess (60)

Hyperplasia: excessive proliferation of normal cells (40)

Hypersomnia: excessive daytime sleep (EDS) (23)

Hypertonic: having greater concentration of solutes than plasma; this type of solution moves water out of cells (26)

Hyperventilation: an increased rate and depth of respirations (32)

Hyphema: hemorrhage into the anterior chamber of the eye (60)

Hypoalbuminemia: low blood albumin levels (60)

Hypoglycemia: low glucose levels (38, 43)

Hypopituitarism: growth hormone deficiency from injury or disease of the hypothalamus or pituitary gland, inheritance, or genetic mutation (59)

Hypospadias: condition in which the urinary meatus opens onto the ventral (lower) surface of the penis (57, 59)

Hypotonic: having lesser concentration of solutes than blood plasma; this type of solution moves water into cells (26)

Hypoxemia: reduced oxygen in the blood (32)

Hypoxia: condition of insufficient oxygen anywhere in the body (32)

Hysterectomy: surgical removal of the uterus (40)

Iatrogenic disease: a disease caused unintentionally by medical therapy (27)

Iatrogenic infection: an infection directly caused by any diagnostic or therapeutic source (healthcare provider) (10)

ICU psychosis: a form of delirium that may result from overstimulation (ICU unit) or even alcohol withdrawal (17)

Id: the biological and psychological drives with which an individual enters this world; part of the unconscious concerned with immediate gratification (15)

Identification: in psychiatry, an attempt to manage anxiety by imitating the behavior of someone feared or respected (17)

Idiosyncratic effect: an unexpected and individual response to a drug (27)

Ileostomy: an opening into the *ileum* (small bowel) (37)

Illness: the highly individualized response a person has to a disease (2)

Imagery: a technique designed to replace unpleasant thoughts and feelings with positive ones that encourage a change in attitudes, behaviors, or physiologic reactions (18)

Immunity: the resistance of the body to infection (10)

Immunotropic: targeting the immune system (35)

Impaired nurse: a nurse whose practice has been negatively affected because of chemical abuse, specifically the use of alcohol and drugs (4)

Impairment: a disturbance in structure or function resulting from physiologic or psychological abnormalities (46)

Impervious: impenetrable (9)

Implantation: the embedding of the blastocyst into the endometrium, or decidua (51)

Implementation: phase of the nursing process in which selected nursing interventions and activities occur (6)

Incarceration: condition in which a hernia cannot be reduced and circulation is impaired (60)

Incest: sexual intercourse between close blood relatives and may or may not be consensual (40)

Incident: any unexpected event (13)

Incident report: form completed when client care was not consistent with standards of expected care (63)

Incision: wound caused by a sharp instrument (e.g., knife or scalpel) (24)

Incompetent cervix: condition in which the cervix is weak, dilates in the second trimester, and expels the fetus (52)

Incontinence: inability to control elimination (37, 39)

Independent interventions: activities that nurses are licensed to do on the basis of their knowledge and skills (6)

Independent practice associations: a group healthcare agency in which clients pay a fixed prospective payment to the IPA, and the IPA pays the provider; the provider receives a fixed fee for services given (7)

Indicator diseases: opportunistic diseases that may signal the presence of HIV (35)

Inductive reasoning: a process of forming generalizations from individual pieces of data (5)

Induration: positive sign of Mantoux test; a raised, reddened area that may become hard (32)

Infarction: death of tissue (23)

Infection: an invasion of the body by a disease-causing organism (10)

Infectious disease: disease that can be transmitted from one person to another by direct or indirect contact (10)

Inferior: a point lower than or below a reference point (19)

Infertility: the inability to achieve pregnancy after 1 year or more of unprotected intercourse (40)

Infiltration: passage of the IV solution out of the vein and into the surrounding tissue (28)

Inflammatory response: a local nonspecific defense reaction of tissues when they are exposed to infection or injury (10)

Infusate: the solution being administered by IV route (28)

Infusion pump: a positive-pressure pump programmed to provide fluid more accurately than the controller (28)

Inguinal hernia: condition that occurs when abdominal tissue such as the bowel extends into the inguinal canal (60)

Inotropics: drugs that increase the force of contraction of the heart (33, 59)

Insight: self-understanding (49)

Insomnia: the inability to obtain an adequate amount or quality of sleep (23)

Inspection: an examination or assessment by using the sense of sight (19)

Inspiration: inhalation (32)

Insulin resistance: body's cells are affected by increased weight and are unable to use the insulin (38)

Intake and output (I&O): the measurement and recording of all fluid taken in and excreted during a 24-hour period (26)

Integrated delivery system: a system that incorporates acute care services, home healthcare, extended and skilled care facilities, and outpatient services (7)

Integrative medicine: a practice that integrates treatments and therapies from conventional medicine with complementary and alternative medicines that have been deemed safe and effective (8)

Intellectualization: a mechanism by which an emotional response that normally would accompany an uncomfortable or painful incident is evaded by the use of rational explanation that removes from the incident any personal significance and feelings (17)

Intercultural communication: the exchange of messages by members of two or more cultures that is influenced by their different cultural perceptions (3)

Intermittent claudication: a symptom of ischemia that causes cramping pains and weakness in the calves of the legs while walking (33)

Intermittent feeding: the administration of small amounts of formula several times per day (25)

Internal disasters: events within the hospital that interrupt services and produce victims (e.g., utility interruption or chemical spill) (9)

Interstitial fluid: extracellular fluid that surrounds the cells and includes lymph (26)

Interventions: the actions initiated by the nurse to achieve client goals (6)

Interview: a planned communication or a conversation with a purpose (6, 11)

Intoxication: a reversible set of physical, psychologic, and behavioral symptoms caused by use of a substance (50)

Intracellular fluid: body water found within cells (26)

Intracranial pressure: the pressure normally exerted by the cerebrospinal fluid that circulates around the brain and spinal cord and within the cerebral ventricles (36)

Intractable pain: chronic discomfort that persists despite therapeutic interventions (22)

Intraductal papillomas: tumors growing in a mammary duct (40)

Intrauterine device (IUD): a small T-shaped piece of metal covered with copper or levonorgestrel placed in the uterus, used for contraception (40)

Intrauterine growth restriction: condition in infants whose intrauterine growth is below that expected for gestational age (57)

Intravascular fluid: only that fluid which is found within the blood (26)

Introjection: a form of identification that allows for acceptance of others' norms and values into oneself, even when contrary to one's previous assumptions (17)

Intussusception: a telescoping of the bowel into itself, diminishing the lumen of the bowel (37)

Invasion of privacy: a direct wrong of a personal nature that injures the feelings of the person and does not take into account the effect of revealed information on the standing of the person in the community (4)

Inversion: increasing the angle of the joint (e.g., straightening the arm at the elbow) (23)

***In-vitro* fertilization:** fertilization obtained through a laparoscopic procedure, fertilized in the laboratory, and then implanted into the uterus (40)

Involution: a return to normal size (54)

Irrigation: washing or flushing out of an area (24)

Ischemia: a deficiency in the blood supply to the tissue (24, 33)

Isograft: identical twin (35)

Isotonic: having the same concentration of solutes as blood plasma (26)

Jarisch-Herxheimer reaction: a transient immunologic reaction to antibiotic therapy of syphilis and certain other diseases, characterized by fever, headache, myalgia, and significant chancre changes (41)

Jaundice: a condition caused by excess bilirubin in the blood (30, 56)

Jejunostomy: surgical creation of a permanent opening through the abdominal wall into the jejunum (25)

Kardex®: a widely used, concise method of organizing and recording data about a client, making information quickly accessible to all health professionals (13)

Kegel exercises: tightening and lifting of the muscles that cross the pelvic floor (54)

Keloid: a progressively enlarging scar (24, 30)

Ketone bodies: products of the breakdown of fatty acids (38, 39)

Kindling: process of small seizure activity that builds into a major seizure or manic episode (49)

Knowledge: the recall of information (1)

Korsakoff's syndrome: a group of symptoms which include amnesia, disorientation to time and place, confabulation, and severe peripheral neuropathy caused by a deficiency in the B vitamins, including thiamine, riboflavin, and folic acid (50)

Kussmaul respiration: a particular type of hyperventilation that accompanies metabolic acidosis (32)

Kwashiorkor: a deficiency in protein in the diet that results in muscle wasting (60)

Kyphosis: a forward rounding of the thoracic spine (31)

Labile: quickly springing from one emotion to another (17)

Labor: a process or sequence of events that begins with uterine contractions and ends 1 hour after birth of the placenta (53)

Labyrinth: inner ear (23)

Laceration: tissues torn apart, often from accidents (e.g., with machinery) (24)

Laissez-faire: organizational structure in which the leader exercises little control over the group (63)

Lanugo: soft downy hair present on the fetus's or newborn's face, arms, and back (20, 51, 56)

Lateral: toward the side; the opposite of medial (19)

Lavage: washing out the stomach through a tube (37)

Law: those rules made by humans that regulate social conduct in a formally prescribed and legally binding manner (4)

Laxative: produces frequent soft or liquid stools, sometimes accompanied by abdominal cramps (37)

Leadership: a process used to move a group toward setting and achievement of goals (63)

Learning: a lifelong process of acquiring knowledge or skills that cannot be solely accounted for by human growth (12)

Lesion: an alteration in a client's normal skin appearance (19)

Let-down reflex: release of milk after delivery (51)

Leukocytes: white blood cells (34)

Leukocytosis: elevated WBCs (35)

Leukopenia: lower than normal number of white blood cells (34, 35, 45)

Leukoplakia: smooth irregular white patches found on the tongue, lips, cheeks, or oral mucosa (37)

Level of consciousness (LOC): a continuum that ranges from a state of alertness to coma (19)

Liability: being legally responsible for one's acts and omissions (4)

Libel: defamation by means of print, writing, or pictures (4)

Licensure: a process by which a government agency gives permission for an individual to engage in an occupation or profession (63)

Lichenification: leathery hardening and thickening of the skin, caused by scratching or rubbing (30)

Lightening: descent of the fetus into the pelvis that may occur as early as 2 to 4 weeks prior to the onset of labor (53)

Limb salvage: the surgeon's act of saving part of the limb, but a significant portion of the limb is removed or some functionality is lost (45)

Linea nigra: a dark line on the abdomen from the umbilicus to the pubis (51)

Line of gravity: an imaginary vertical line drawn through the body's center of gravity (23)

Lipids: organic substances that are greasy and insoluble in water but soluble in alcohol or ether (25)

Liposuction: a technique used to remove subcutaneous tissue (30)

Living will: a document that provides specific instructions about what medical treatment the client chooses to omit or refuse in the event that he or she is unable to make those decisions (18, 44)

Livor mortis: Discoloration of surrounding tissues caused after blood circulation has ceased; the red blood cells break down, releasing hemoglobin (44)

Local infection: an infection in which microorganisms are only in a specific part of the body (10)

Lochia: discarded uterine blood, mucus, and tissue (54)

Logan clamp: a metal bow taped to both sides of the suture line of a surgical closure, as in closure of a cleft lip (57)

Lordosis: an exaggeration of the lumbar curve of the spine (31)

Loss: a real or potential situation in which something that is valued is gone, is unavailable, or is changed (18)

Lumpectomy: removal of the lump (40)

Lung abscess: a necrotic area in the lung that forms as a result of consolidation (32)

Lymph: a fluid that resembles plasma but has less protein (34)

Lymphadenopathy: enlargement of lymph nodes (34)

Lymphangitis: inflammation of a lymphatic vessel (34)

Lymphedema: the inability of the lymph system to remove all the lymph fluid from the interstitial tissues (34)

Lymphocytes: cells found in the blood and lymph that are involved in the immune capability of the body (35)

Maceration: softening of tissue by prolonged wetting (24)

Macrosomia: condition of a newborn whose birth weight is over the 90th percentile for gestational age (57)

Macular degeneration: a disease that destroys sharp, central vision (42)

Macule: a discolored spot that is even with the skin's surface; macules are <1 cm (30)

Mainstreaming: movement to increase community service over institutional service in order to provide the developmentally disabled with the least restrictive environment (58)

Malaise: a generalized feeling of being unwell (43)

Malignant hypertension: condition in which the blood pressure elevates rapidly and progressively until the diastolic pressure is greater than 120 mm Hg (33)

Malpractice: negligence that occurred while a person was performing as a professional (4)

Mammary glands: a network of ducts that carry the milk to the nipple (40)

Mammography: diagnostic x-ray of the breast (40)

Mammoplasty: breast reconstruction (40)

Managed care: a healthcare system whose goals are to provide cost-effective, quality care that focuses on improved outcomes for groups of clients (7)

Manifestations: signs and symptoms (6)

Mastectomy: removal of the breast (40)

Mastitis: infection of the breast (55)

Maturational loss: lessening of function or endurance, or an increase in dependence due to aging (18)

Meatus: an opening in the external body that serves as a passageway for the elimination of urine (39)

Mechanisms of labor: movements the fetus undergoes as it moves through the pelvis (53)

Meconium: newborn's first stool (51, 56)

Meconium aspiration: inhalation by the newborn of amniotic fluid containing meconium (57)

Meconium ileus: retention of meconium in the GI tract (59)

Medial: close to the middle of the body (19)

Medicaid: a federal public assistance program paid out of general taxes to people who require financial assistance for medical care (7)

Medical asepsis: all practices used to confine a specific microorganism to a specific area or to limit the number of microorganisms, their growth, and their transmission (10)

Medical power of attorney: (also called *durable power of attorney for health care*) a written statement appointing someone else to manage healthcare treatment decisions when the client is unable to do so (18)

Medicare: a federal program to assist people age 65 years and over with medical care (7)

Medication: a substance administered for the diagnosis, cure, treatment, relief, or prevention of disease (27)

Medication administration record: record of the date of the medication order, the expiration date, the medication name and dose, the frequency of administration and route, and the nurse's signature (13)

Megacolon: (Hirschsprung's disease) disorder that occurs when the autonomic parasympathetic nerve ganglia that cause normal peristalsis are absent (59)

Melena: blood in stools (37)

Menarche: the beginning of menstrual cycles during puberty (40, 62)

Meninges: protective membranes that cover the brain and spinal cord (36)

Meningitis: an inflammation of the meninges of the brain and spinal cord (36)

Meningocele: herniation of the meninges through a vertebral defect (57)

Meningomyelocele: herniation of the spinal nerves as well as the meninges through a vertebral defect (57)

Menopause: permanent cessation of menstruation (40)

Menorrhagia: repetitive, excessive, or prolonged menstruation flow (40)

Mental health clinic: medical facilities whose focus is on psychosocial issues and mental health status of its clients (48)

Mesothelioma: a rare tumor of the pleura or peritoneum membranes that may develop as a result of asbestos exposure or other inhaled irritants (32)

Metabolic acidosis: greater than normal acid within the plasma (26)

Metabolic alkalosis: less than normal acid within the plasma (26)

Metabolic X syndrome: (metabolic syndrome) a group of related metabolic disorders, including obesity, insulin resistance, and complications of Type 2 diabetes (50, 62)

Metastasis: cancerous cells that have traveled from the primary site to a distant site (45)

Metric system: a decimal system based on units of 10 (27)

Metrorrhagia: bleeding between periods (40)

Micturition: (voiding or urination) the process of emptying the urinary bladder (39)

Migraine: familial disorder marked by periodic, unilateral pulsating headache that often begins during adolescence and continues into adulthood (62)

Milia: white pinpoint spots resembling whiteheads that appear on the neonate's face a few days after birth (56)

Mitral regurgitation: backflow of blood from the left ventricle into the left atrium (43)

Mitral valve prolapse: displacement of the mitral valve usually due to benign proliferative changes of the valve leaflets (43)

Mittelschmerz: abdominal pain with ovulation (40)

Mnemonics: techniques for developing memory (64)

Molding: shaping of the fetal head to the bones of the maternal pelvis (53)

Mongolian spot: a dark discolored area found over the lower back and sacrum of infants of Black, Hispanic, south Asian, or east Asian descent (56)

Monocytes: cells involved in the inflammatory response; they are the largest in size (35)

Moral: relating to judgments of right or wrong (15, 16)

Moral development: the increase in the ability to distinguish right from wrong (16)

Morbid obesity: state of being 100 lb or more over normal weight for age, height, and build (37)

Morning care: type of hygienic care provided after clients have breakfast usually including the provision of a urinal or bedpan (to clients who are not ambulatory), a bath or shower, perineal care, back massages, and oral, nail, and hair care; also includes making the client's bed (20)

Moro (or startle) reflex: reaction that occurs when newborns have a sense of falling; they will quickly extend the arms (abduct) with fingers flared and thumb and first finger forming a "C"; the arms will then adduct in an embracing motion; the lower extremities may extend and then flex; a slight tremor may be noted (56)

Morula: the zygote divides rapidly to form a many-celled, mulberry-shaped mass (51)

Motivation: desire to act (12)

Motor: carrying impulses from the CNS to skeletal muscles, glands, and effector organs (36)

Motor development: the increase in the ability to move and to control the body (16)

Mourning: the process and rituals through which grief is eventually resolved (18)

Mucoviscidosis: (cystic fibrosis) an inherited recessive disorder of the exocrine glands affecting predominantly Caucasian children (59)

Multigravida: a woman who has been pregnant several times (51)

Multipara: a woman who has had two or more pregnancies that resulted in viable fetuses, whether or not the offspring were alive at birth (51)

Multistate compact: agreement among several states that a nurse can practice in another state that is part of the compact, as long as he or she follows the nurse practice act and the rules and regulations pertaining to the act (64)

Murphy's sign: when the client is unable to take a deep breath while the physician applies pressure under the ribs on the right side (37)

Myelin: the whitish, fatty material that covers most long nerve fibers (36)

Myocardial infarction: condition that occurs when blood flow through one of the coronary arteries is completely blocked (33)

Myocarditis: the inflammation of the heart muscle (33)

Myomectomy: removal of tumor and surrounding myometrium (40)

Myopathy: muscle cramps of sudden onset and later development of pain, tenderness, and edema of the skeletal muscles, especially of the legs (50)

Myopia: visual disturbance that occurs when light is focused in front of the retina (61)

Myxedema: the thyroid gland does not make enough thyroid hormone (38)

Myxedema coma: a severe form of hypothyroidism where lethargy progresses to hypothermia and coma (38)

Nadir: the lowest point that the blood cell counts reach before they begin to rebound following chemotherapy (45)

Narcolepsy: a disorder believed to be genetic or autoimmune where sufferers experience regular REM-onset sleep attacks lasting from a few seconds to several hours (23)

Naturopathic medicine: alternative care system that uses a wide range of approaches to healing, such as nutrition, herbs, exercise, and stress reduction (8)

Nausea: the uncomfortable wavelike sensation that may or may not lead to vomiting (37)

NCLEX-PN®: the National Council Licensure Examination for Practical Nursing, which a nurse must take in order to practice as an LPN or LVN (2)

Necrosis: death of cells or tissues through injury or disease (33)

Negative feedback: a method by which hormone production is decreased (38)

Negative-pressure wound therapy: the use of subatmospheric pressure to promote or assist wound healing, or to remove fluids from a wound site (24)

Negligence: misconduct or practice that is below the standard expected of an ordinary, reasonable, and prudent practitioner, which places another person at risk for harm (4)

Neonatal abstinence syndrome: distressed behavior of infants exposed to chemical substances *in utero* (57)

Neoplasm: any abnormal growth of new tissue that may be harmless (benign) or cancerous (malignant) (45)

Nephroblastoma: (Wilms' tumor) a highly metastatic cancerous tumor of the kidney (59)

Nephrons: functional units of the kidneys which filter the blood and remove metabolic wastes (39)

Networking: the deliberate attempt to make connections among people for a variety of interests, including employment opportunities (65)

Neurilemma: the part of the Schwann cell (cell cytoplasm that ends up beneath the outermost part of the plasma membrane) external to the myelin sheath (36)

Neurogenic bladder: dysfunction of nerves supplying the bladder (39)

Neuroglia: the supporting cells in the central nervous system (36)

Neurons: nerve cells that are specialized to transmit nerve impulses from one part of the body to another (36)

Neuropathic pain: discomfort that is the result of a disturbance of the nerve pathways either from past or continuing tissue damage (22)

Neuropathy: any disease of the nerves (36)

Neurosyphilis: tertiary syphilis that can appear from 1 to 40 years following the onset of the infection; there is a high morbidity and mortality rate for clients (41)

Neurotropic: targeting cognitive functioning (35)

Neutropenia: a decrease in the number of a specific type of white blood cells, called neutrophils (45)

Nitrogen balance: a measure of the intake and loss of nitrogen (25)

Nociceptor: receptors that transmit pain sensation (22)

Nocturia: excessive nighttime urination (39, 40)

Nocturnal myoclonus: sudden, repetitive kicking or jerking movements of the lower extremities (42)

Nodule: a circumscribed, elevated mass of tissue extending deeper into the dermis than a papule; nodules are 0.5 to 2 cm (30)

Nomogram: a graph used to prescribe medications based on client size (27)

Nonspecific defenses: anatomic and physiological barriers and the inflammatory response (10)

Nonstress test: used to assess fetal movement and fetal heart rate (51)

Nonverbal communication: exchange of ideas using other forms of expression, such as gestures, facial expressions, or touch (11)

Nosocomial infections: infections that occur after hospital admission and for which the client had no symptoms at the time of admission (10)

NREM sleep: a deep, restful sleep with some decreased physiological functions (23)

Nuchal cord: umbilical cord (53)

Nuclear family: a family consisting of parents and biological offspring (16)

Nulligravida: a woman who has never conceived (51)

Nullipara: a woman who has never borne a viable child (51)

Nurse practice acts: laws in each state instrumental in defining the scope of nursing practice to protect public health, safety, and welfare (2, 63)

Nursing care conference: a meeting of a group of nurses to discuss possible solutions to certain client problems, such as inability to cope with an event or lack of progress toward reaching goals (13)

Nursing diagnosis: a statement about an alteration in the client's health status; referring to a condition that nurses are licensed to treat (6)

Nursing process: a systematic, rational method of planning and providing individualized nursing care for individuals, families, groups, and communities (6)

Nursing rounds: a group of nurses who visit selected clients at each client's bedside to (1) obtain information that will help plan nursing care, (2) provide clients the opportunity to discuss their care, and (3) evaluate the nursing care the client has received (13)

Nutrients: the organic, inorganic, and energy-producing substances found in foods (25)

Nutrition: interaction between nutrients and the human body (25)

Nystagmus: involuntary movement of the eyes (36)

Obesity: body weight that exceeds ideal body weight by more than 20% (25, 37)

Objective data: information detectable by an observer (5, 6, 13)

Observation: gathering data by using the senses (6)

Obsessive-compulsive disorder: an anxiety disorder characterized by patterned behaviors that are focused on some topic of fixation (or obsession) and that are repeated in order to relieve the anxiety (17)

Occlusion: blockage (33)

Occlusive: closing off from the air (24)

Oliguria: low amounts of urine or no urine (39)

Omnibus Budget Reconciliation Act (OBRA): law passed to improve nursing homes and extended-care facilities (7, 46)

Omphalocele: a rare congenital malformation of the abdominal wall that allows the abdominal contents to herniate into the umbilical cord (57)

Oncogenes: genes found in the chromosomes of tumor cells (45)

Oncology: the study of cancer (45)

Oocyte: egg cell (40)

Oophorectomy: surgical removal of the ovaries (40)

Open-ended questions: questions that invite clients to discover and explore their thoughts or feelings and that allow clients the freedom to talk about what they wish (11)

Open reduction: surgically aligning the bone and stabilizing the ends with nails, plates, or screws (60)

Ophthalmia neonatorum: inflammation of the eyes of the newborn, resulting from contact with gonorrhea or chlamydia (56)

Opisthotonos: rigid hyperextension of the entire body (60)

Opportunistic: capable of causing disease only in a host whose resistance is lowered (30)

Opportunistic pathogen: an agent that causes a disease only in a susceptible person (someone whose immune system is not functioning as a defense system) (10)

Orchiectomy: removal of one testis and spermatic cord with removal of the retroperitoneal lymph nodes (62)

Orchiopexy: surgical procedure to reposition the testes in the scrotum (59, 62)

Orientation: introduction of clients to the people and the facility into which they have been admitted (14); ability to remember city and state of residence, time of day, date, day of the week, duration of illness, and names of family members (19); program or time for newly hired individuals to prepare themselves to take on responsibilities of a new job (65)

Ortolani-Barlow maneuver: assessment for developmental dysplasia of the hip in which the hip is manipulated with gentle lateral pressure, abduction, and rotation, eliciting a click if DDH exists (59)

Osmolarity: the concentration of a solute in a volume of solution (26, 28)

Osmosis: the passage of water from an area of lower particle concentration toward an area of higher concentration of particles (26)

Osmotic pressure: force that develops as solute particles collide against one another, causing movement of fluid (26)

Osteoarthritis: degenerative joint disease; a "wear-and-tear" disease caused by overuse and/or injury to the joint (31)

Osteomyelitis: infection of the bone (60)

Osteopenia: low bone mass (42)

Osteoporosis: a demineralization process of the bones causing them to become spongy, deformed, and easily fractured (23, 31)

Ostomy: opening in the abdominal wall for the elimination of feces or urine (37)

Otosclerosis: hardening of the stapes to the oval window in the ear (43)

Ovaries: flat almond-shaped glands located below the ends of the fallopian tubes (40)

Ovulation: release of the ovum (40)

Pacemaker: a device used to restore an effective heart rate when the heart's natural pacemakers fail (33)

PaCO$_2$: carbon dioxide measured in arterial blood (26)

Pain: highly subjective and individual sensation that signals a problem in the body (22)

Pain reaction: the autonomic nervous system and behavioral responses to pain (22)

Pain threshold: the amount of pain stimulation a person requires in order to feel pain (22)

Pain tolerance: the maximum amount and duration of pain that an individual is willing to endure (22)

Palliative: relieving or reducing pain or symptoms of a disease; not curative (29)

Palliative care: a shift in treatment goals from curing a disease to providing relief from suffering (44)

Pallor: pale appearance caused by lack of circulating blood or hemoglobin (19)

Palmar grasp reflex: reaction that occurs when a finger or small object is placed in the newborn's hand; the finger will grasp tightly enough to be lifted from the bed (56)

Palpation: examination of the body using the sense of touch (19)

PALS: (pediatric advanced life support) a specialized training course that prepares the healthcare professional to perform advanced lifesaving skills or techniques on the pediatric client (47)

Pancreatitis: inflammation of the pancreas; can be acute or chronic (37)

Pancytopenia: a decreased number of red blood cells, white blood cells, and platelets (34)

Panic attack: a sudden and intense sensation of fear and impending doom (17)

Papillomata: warts (41)

Papule: a circumscribed, solid elevation of the skin (e.g., elevated mole, warts) (30)

Para: a woman who has produced viable young whether or not the child was living at birth (51)

Paracentesis: procedure involves the insertion of a needle through the abdominal wall to drain the fluid (37)

Paralytic ileus: intestinal obstruction characterized by lack of peristaltic activity (29)

Paraphimosis: the inability to return the foreskin over the glans, causing constriction of the penis (59)

Parasites: organisms that live on other living organisms (10)

Parasomnia: behavior that may interfere with sleep, such as sleepwalking (23)

Parasympathetic nervous system: part of the nervous system that restores the body to normal balance after a "fight-or-flight" reaction (36)

Parenchymal: functional part of an organ (62)

Parenteral nutrition: also referred to as *total parenteral nutrition* (TPN); provided when the client is unable to ingest or absorb foods (25)

Paresthesia: numbness, burning, prickling, tingling, pain (36)

Paroxysmal: intense, sudden, and repeating (36)

Partial seizure: event that begins with focal or local discharges in one part of the brain, unilaterally; usually originating from the cortical brain tissue, thus having a superficial focus (36)

Partial-thickness burn: (*second-degree burn*) chemical or thermal damage that does not involve all the skin layers (47)

Passive diffusion: the movement of molecules randomly in all directions from a region of high concentration to an area of low concentration (26)

Passive immunity: condition that occurs when a person is given antibodies from another source (35)

Passive range of motion: the client's extremities and joints are supported and moved by the nurse (19)

Passive transport: movement of solutes through membranes without energy expenditure (26)

Pathogens: microorganisms that cause disease (10)

Patient: a person who is waiting for or undergoing medical treatment and care (2)

Peak flow test: test that evaluates maximum airflow during forced expiration and monitors bronchospasm in asthmatic clients (47)

Pediculosis: an infestation with lice (20, 60)

Pelvic exenteration: surgical removal of the bowel, uterus, ovaries, fallopian tubes, vagina, and bladder (40)

Pelvic inflammatory disease: an infection usually involving the fallopian tubes, ovaries, cervix, uterus, and peritoneum (40)

Penetrating wound: penetration of the skin and the underlying tissues, usually unintentional (e.g., from a bullet or metal fragments) (24)

Penis: the cylindrical external structure in the male that encloses the urethra and contains erectile tissue (40)

Percussion: the act of striking a body part with short, sharp blows (1) to help gather data about internal organs, (2) to assist in massage, or (3) to help a client to clear the respiratory tract (19)

Performance evaluation: review of work attendance, teamwork, and skills by an employer (65)

Perfusion: blood supply to an area (19)

Pericardiocentesis: surgical drainage of the pericardium (33)

Pericarditis: an inflammation, acute or chronic, of the sac (pericardium) that encloses and protects the heart (33)

Pericardium: sac surrounding the heart (33)

Perineum: area between the thighs extending from the pubis to the coccyx (40)

Periodic breathing: irregular newborn respirations with brief (5 to 15 seconds) pauses (56)

Perioperative period: time surrounding a surgery, consisting of the preoperative phase prior to surgery, the intraoperative phase during surgery, and the postoperative phase following surgery (29)

Peripheral nervous system (PNS): portion of the nervous system that includes the cranial nerves and the peripheral, or spinal, nerves (36)

Peripheral neuropathy: syndrome causing muscle weakness, paresthesias, impaired reflexes, and autonomic symptoms in the hands and feet (36)

Peripheral vascular disease: conditions of the arteries, veins, and lymph vessels outside the heart (33)

Peristalsis: wavelike progressive movement (37)

Peritoneal dialysis: a process to remove extra fluid and waste products wherein the dialyzing solution is instilled directly into the abdomen (39)

Peritonitis: infection of the peritoneal cavity (37, 55)

PERRLA: pupils equally round and react to light and accommodation (19)

Personality: the relatively stable way that a person thinks, feels, and behaves (49)

Personality disorder: an enduring pattern of inner experience and behavior characterized by a lack of self-identity and maladaptive, rigid thinking that leads to self-defeating behaviors (49)

Personal space: the distance people prefer in interactions with others (11)

Pessary: a plastic device shaped like a ring, arch, or ball that is placed in the vagina to support the uterus (40)

Petechiae: pinpoint hemorrhages (30, 56)

Pétrissage: kneading or making large quick pinches of the skin, subcutaneous tissue, and muscle (23)

pH: hydrogen ion concentration (26)

Phagocytosis: a process by white blood cells to ingest and digest bacteria and cellular debris (24)

Phantom pain: experience of pain sensation in an absent extremity (22, 31)

Pheochromocytoma: a benign tumor located in the adrenal medulla that causes excessive amounts of epinephrine and norepinephrine to be produced (38)

Phimosis: the inability to retract the foreskin of the penis due to a tightened prepuce (59)

Phlebitis: inflammation of the vein (28)

Phlebotomy: drawing and dispensing of blood (47)

Phobia: a specific type of anxiety, defined as out-of-proportion fear (17)

Phonophobia: sensitivity to sound (36)

Photophobia: sensitivity to light (36)

Physical assessment: one of three types of examination of the body: (1) complete assessment, (2) focused assessment by body system, (3) focused assessment by body part (19)

Physiological: relating to physical processes in the human body (16)

Physiologic needs: needs having to do with physical processes in the human body (15)

Pica: a craving to eat substances that are not food (59)

PIE: charting method; stands for problem, intervention, and evaluation; based on the nursing process; consists mainly of assessment flow sheets and progress notes (13)

Pigeon chest: (*pectus carinatum*) condition in which the sternum protrudes, causing an increase in the anteroposterior diameter (58)

Pilonidal cyst: sinus tract found at the upper end of the intragluteal cleft (37)

Pivoting: a technique in which the body is turned in such a way as to avoid twisting of the spine (9)

Placenta previa: pregnancy in which a blastocyst implants low in the uterus, allowing the placenta to grow partially or totally across the cervical opening (52)

Plane: an imaginary flat surface (19)

Planning: the process of designing nursing activities required to prevent, reduce, or eliminate a client's health problems (6)

Plantar grasp reflex: reaction that occurs when the sole of the neonate's foot is touched, the toes curl under as if newborns are trying to "grasp" with their feet (56)

Plaque: a circumscribed, solid elevation of the skin (e.g., psoriasis, actinic keratosis) (30); a fibrous, fatty material (33)

Plasma: a clear yellow, protein-rich fluid (34)

Plasmapheresis: the complete exchange of plasma (36)

Platelets: elements in the blood that are necessary for proper blood coagulation (34)

Pleural effusion: excess fluid accumulated in the pleural space (32)

Pneumoconioses: chronic lung diseases caused when the client has long-term exposure to inorganic dusts such as asbestos or coal (black lung disease) (32)

Pneumothorax: an accumulation of air or gas in the pleural space that causes partial or complete collapse of the lung on the affected side (32)

Polycystic kidney disease: a familial disease characterized by an enlarged kidney with multiple fluid-filled cysts (39, 59)

Polycystic ovary syndrome: endocrine disorder resulting from numerous follicular cysts, and characterized by higher than normal LH, estrogen, and androgen levels, and low FSH levels (40)

Polydactyly: presence of more than five fingers per hand or toes per foot (56)

Polydipsia: thirst for large amounts of fluid (38)

Polyphagia: intense hunger and appetite (37, 38)

Polypharmacy: a condition which occurs when a client takes many different medications that interact with each other and create side effects (43)

Polyuria: diuresis; excessive urination (38, 39)

Portal of entry: fifth link in the chain of infection; a means of entry into the body for pathogenic microorganisms (10)

Portal of exit: a way of leaving the reservoir (10)

Portfolio: an itemized visual account of skills and best practices that are related to the position being sought (65)

Port-wine stain: a large, congenital vascular nevus with a purplish color; usually found on the head and neck (30)

Post dates: labor not beginning spontaneously by the 41st week of pregnancy (53)

Posterior: toward the back of; the opposite of ventral (19)

Postherpetic neuralgia: presence of constant pain caused by herpes zoster even after the blisters have healed (30)

Postnatal depression: a condition experienced by about 1 in 10 women in the first year after having a baby; it involves an extended depressed state and sometimes psychotic behavior (17)

Postpartum: the period beginning immediately after delivery of the placenta and ending when the body and reproductive organs return to a near prepregnant state (54)

Postpartum depression: a major mood disorder that most frequently appears 4 weeks post delivery and upon weaning the child from the breast (55)

Postpartum (puerperal) infection: a rare infection of the uterus following childbirth (55)

Postterm: delivery after 42 weeks of pregnancy (51)

Posttraumatic stress disorder: an anxiety disorder that can develop after exposure to one or more terrifying events in which grave physical harm occurred or was threatened (17)

Postural tonus: muscle contraction needed to maintain an upright position (23)

Precipitous birth: a birth that occurs rapidly, unexpectedly, and without the attention of a physician or nurse midwife (53)

Precocious puberty: the presence of any secondary sex characteristics before the age of 8 in girls and before the age of 9 in boys (61)

Precordial: relating to the area over the heart and lower thorax (33)

Preeclampsia: most common hypertensive disorder that occurs with pregnancy (52)

Preemptive analgesia: the administration of analgesics prior to an invasive or operative procedure; also includes around-the-clock (ATC) analgesics (22)

Preferred provider arrangements: individual healthcare providers that provide an insurance company or employer with health services at a discounted rate (7)

Preferred provider organization: a group of physicians and perhaps a healthcare agency (often a hospital) that provide an insurance company or employer with health services at a discounted rate (7)

Pregnancy: carrying the resulting offspring from fertilization in the uterus (51)

Prejudice: prejudgment or bias based on characteristics such as race, age, or gender (3)

Premenstrual syndrome (PMS): a group of symptoms occurring 3 to 14 days prior to menstruation and relieved by the onset of menses (40)

Presbycusis: atrophic changes to the muscles that support the tympanic membrane related to the aging process; the older adult's hearing becomes altered (42)

Presbyopia: difficulty focusing on close objects (42)

Prescription: the written direction for the preparation and administration of a drug (27)

Pressured speech: fast and determined speech that is hard to interrupt (49)

Pressure ulcers: lesions caused by unrelieved pressure resulting in damage to underlying tissue (24)

Presumptive signs: The subjective signs the mother experiences during pregnancy (51)

Preterm: delivery after 24 weeks and before 38 weeks of pregnancy (51)

Preterm labor: onset of regular contractions between the 20th and 37th week that cause changes in the cervix (53)

Priapism: persistent erection without any sexual desire (43)

Primary (or essential) hypertension: a condition of abnormally high blood pressure in the arterial system (33)

Primary nursing: total nursing responsibility for a group of clients 24 hours a day, 7 days a week (7, 63)

Primary prevention: health promotion and specific protection against diseases (44)

Primary tumor: original histologic site of tumor; tissue where tumor originated (45)

Primigravida: a woman pregnant for the first time (51)

Primipara: a woman who has had one pregnancy that resulted in a viable child, regardless of whether the child was living at birth, and regardless of whether it was a single or multiple birth (51)

PRN order: as-needed order that permits the nurse to give a medication when, in the nurse's judgment, the client requires it (27)

Probationary period: time during which an immediate supervisor evaluates the performance of a newly hired employee (65)

Probiotics: foods or supplements containing live beneficial organisms (42)

Problem-oriented medical record: charting method in which the data are arranged according to the individual problems the client has rather than the source of the information (13)

Procedures: physical skills such as manipulating equipment, giving injections, doing dressing changes, and moving, lifting, and repositioning clients (6)

Prodromal phase: warning phase of a condition or disease (49)

Prodrome: a warning sign (30)

Profession: a vocation requiring knowledge of some department of learning or science (2, 65)

Professionalism: behavior showing dedication to a vocation that requires knowledge of some department of learning or science (65)

Projection: a process in which blame is attached to others for unacceptable thoughts, desires, shortcomings, and mistakes (17)

Prolactin: the hormone produced by the anterior pituitary gland, stimulates milk production (40)

Prolapsed umbilical cord: umbilical cord positioned between the fetus and the cervix (53)

Proprioception: decreased sense of temperature, depth, and vibration (36)

Prospective payment system: a system that limits the amount paid to hospitals that are reimbursed by Medicare (7)

Prostate: gland found in the male below the bladder and surrounding the urethra (40)

Prostheses: artificial body parts, such as partial or complete dentures, contact lenses, artificial eyes, and artificial limbs (29)

Protein–calorie malnutrition: weight loss and visible muscle and fat wasting (25)

Proteinuria: protein in the urine (60)

Proximal: nearer the origin of a structure (19)

Pseudomenstruation: mucus or slightly bloody vaginal discharge which may be present in female newborns and disappears in a few days; related to the influence of maternal hormones (56)

Pseudopregnancy: occurs when the nonpregnant woman so strongly wants to be pregnant that she experiences the presumptive signs (51)

Psychiatrist: a physician who specializes in the branch of health science that deals with the study, treatment, and prevention of mental disorders (17)

Psychologist: a trained professional that provides counseling and testing for clients with mental health and or developmental issues (17)

Psychomotor domain: area of learning that includes motor skills (12)

Psychomotor retardation: lack of activity (49)

Psychosis: a major feature of schizophrenia, including abnormal interpretation of reality, decreased ability to relate to self and others, decreased ability to function, and disorganized thoughts and behavior (49)

Psychosocial: pertaining to the relationship between oneself and others (16)

Psychosocial assessment: the gathering of data about the emotional, behavioral, mental, environmental, spiritual, and interactional processes of the client (17)

Psychosocial needs: needs having to do with relationships within oneself and others (15)

Ptosis: eye drooping (35)

Puberty: age when the reproductive organs become functional and secondary sex characteristics develop (16, 62)

Pulmonary edema: a life-threatening complication of left-sided congestive heart failure; when fluids and blood accumulate in the lungs in large amounts, the alveoli fill up and air exchange is nonexistent (33)

Pulmonary embolism: blood clot that has moved to the lungs to block a pulmonary artery, thus obstructing blood flow to a portion of the lung (29)

Pulmonary function tests (PFT): methods to measure lung volume and capacity (32)

Pulse: heartbeat (19)

Puncture: penetration of the skin and often the underlying tissues by a sharp instrument, either intentional or unintentional (24)

Purging: self-induced vomiting or abuse of laxatives or diuretics (50)

Purpura: condition characterized by hemorrhaging into the skin (30)

Purulent: pus-filled (24)

Pus: substance consisting of leukocytes, liquefied dead tissue debris, and dead and living bacteria (24)

Pustule: a small, circumscribed elevation of the skin containing purulent matter (30)

Pyelonephritis: an inflammation that affects the kidney pelvis and parenchyma (39)

Pyeloplasty: removal of the obstructed ureteral segment and replacement into the renal pelvis (59)

Pyemia: pus in the blood (30)

Pyloroplasty: surgical enlargement of the pylorus or gastric outlet (37)

Pyrosis: also known as *heartburn;* pain near the heart that results from reverse peristalsis of gastric acids (37)

Pyuria: pus in the urine (39)

Quickening: first fetal movements felt by the mother (51)

Rabies: a fatal infection of the central nervous system (60)

Radiating pain: discomfort that is perceived at the source of the pain and extends to nearby tissues (22)

Radiation: heat lost by transfer to cooler objects that are nearby but not in direct contact (56)

Rales: (also known as *crackles*) fine, short, interrupted lung sounds, best heard on inspiration (19)

Range of motion (ROM): the maximum movement possible for a joint (23)

Rape: forced sexual intercourse that involves vaginal, anal, or oral penetration (40)

Rationale: the scientific principle given as the reason for selecting a particular nursing intervention or action (6)

Rationalization: justification of certain behaviors by faulty logic and ascription of motives that are socially acceptable but did not in fact inspire the behavior (17)

Raynaud's phenomenon: a condition that causes the small blood vessels of the hands and feet to contract in response to cold or anxiety, results in the hands or feet turning white and cold, and then turning blue (35)

Reaction formation: a mechanism that causes people to act exactly opposite to the way they feel (17)

Reactive hyperemia: bright red flush of the skin when excess pressure on the tissue is relieved (24)

Readiness: behaviors or cues that reflect the learner's motivation to learn at a specific time (12)

Rebound headache: a condition that occurs from a pattern of taking headache medications too often or in excess in which the medications stop relieving pain and actually begin to cause headaches (36)

Rebound tenderness: pain on release of pressure over McBurney's point in a person with appendicitis (37)

Reconstructive: restoring function or appearance that has been lost or reduced (29)

Record: a written or computer-based collection of data (13)

Rectocele: hernial protrusion of part of the rectum into the vagina (40)

Referred pain: discomfort felt in a part of the body that is considerably removed from the tissues causing the pain (22)

Reflexes: rapid, predictable, and involuntary responses to stimuli (16, 36)

Reflux: backward flow, as of urine (43)

Regional anesthesia: the temporary interruption of the transmission of nerve impulses to and from a specific area or region of the body (29)

Regression: return to an earlier, more comfortable level of functioning that is characterized by fewer demands and responsibilities (17)

Rehabilitation: the set of skills and activities applied to client care to assist the individual to return to his or her maximum level of functioning (44, 46)

Relapse: return to drug use after abstinence (50)

Relaxin: a hormone produced by the placenta that causes softening in the collagen connective tissue of the symphysis pubis and sacroiliac joints (51)

Relevance: importance or applicability (12)

Remission: the period during which a disease is controlled and symptoms are not obvious (44)

REM sleep: rapid eye movement sleep; period of sleep in which dreams occur (23)

Renal failure: a condition in which the kidneys are unable to carry out the normal functions necessary to eliminate waste products and maintain fluid and electrolyte balance (39)

Report: an oral, written, or computer-based communication intended to convey information to others (13)

Repression: the act of keeping threatening thoughts, feelings, and desires from becoming conscious (17)

Reservoir: the source of the microorganism (10)

Resident flora: harmless microorganisms found in and on body (10)

Residual urine: urine remaining in the bladder following the voiding (39)

Respiratory acidosis: drop in blood pH from carbonic acid buildup (26)

Respiratory alkalosis: an elevated pH due to a decrease in $PaCO_2$ (26)

Responsiveness: how much parents foster individuality, self-assertion, and self-regulation and how responsive they are to special needs and demands (16)

Restitution: turning of the fetal head to be in normal alignment with the shoulders (53)

Restless leg syndrome: an uncontrollable movement of the lower extremities (42)

Restraints: protective devices used to limit the physical activity of the client or a part of the body (9)

Résumé: concise systematic summary of professional experience and educational background (65)

Retching: action of vomiting without expelling gastric contents, commonly called dry heaves (37)

Retention: ability to remember what is learned (12)

Retinal detachment: a separation of the retina from the choroids (43)

Retractions: inward movement of the tissues over the chest (32, 56)

Retrovirus: living and replicating within the host (35)

Rhabdomyoscaroma: a malignant tumor originating in the muscle around the eye, in the neck, and less commonly in the abdomen, genitourinary tract, and extremities (61)

Rheumatologist: a physician specializing in inflammatory disorders; is often the specialist treating immune system disorders (35)

Rhonchi: a continuous musical sound heard with a stethoscope; occurring in asthma, croup, hay fever, and can also result from tumor or obstruction (19)

Rickets: condition caused by a vitamin D deficiency (60)

Rigor mortis: the stiffening of the body that begins about 2 to 4 hours after death (44)

Ringworm: term for some tinea infections (60)

Rooting reflex: reaction that occurs when the newborn's cheek is stroked; the head will turn to the side that was stroked (56)

Rosacea: an inflammation that appears as reddened dilated blood vessels and small eruptions or pimples on the nose and center of the face (43)

Rotation: movement of the bone around its central axis (23)

Rovsing's sign: increased pain on extension of the right hip in a client with appendicitis (37)

Rugae: folds found in the stomach (37)

Sagittal plane: separates the body into left and right (19)

Salpingectomy: removal of the fallopian tubes (40)

Salpingitis: inflammation of the uterine tube (41, 51)

Same-day surgery clinic: health facility in which the client arrives early in the day, has a surgical procedure, and returns home after he or she is fully recovered from anesthesia (48)

Sanguineous exudate: a discharge of large amounts of red blood cells frequently seen in open wounds (24)

Scabies: a contagious skin infestation by the itch mite (20)

Scald: a burn from a hot liquid or vapor, such as steam (9)

Scale: a small thin plate of epidermis that is shed from skin tissue (30)

Scar: fibrous tissue that replaces normal tissue after injury (30)

School-based health clinic: ambulatory care centers, located in a number of intercity school districts, which perform a higher level of care than the typical school nurse office (48)

School health office: room or area within a school where medications and first aid supplies are kept and distributed by qualified personnel (48)

Sclerodactyly: results from deposits of excess collagen with the skin layers; the skin appears thick, tight, shiny, and can be darkly pigmented (35)

Scleroderma: the abnormal growth of connective tissue that supports the skin and internal organs (35)

Scoliometer: a device for measuring the amount of abnormal spinal curvature (48)

Scoliosis: a lateral deviation of the spine (31, 58)

Scope of practice: a document developed by the board of nursing that governs practice within each state (4)

Scrotum: pouch suspended from the perineal area of the male (40)

Scurvy: condition caused by a lack of vitamin C in the diet (60)

Seasonal affective disorder: depression related to decreased sunlight (17)

Sebum: an oily substance secreted by the skin (20)

Secondary hypertension: elevated blood pressure due to another medical diagnosis (33)

Secondary prevention: early detection of disease and prompt intervention to halt disease progression (44)

Second primary tumor: new, histologically separate malignant neoplasm in a person with a primary tumor (45)

Segregation: physical separation of housing and services based on race (3)

Seizure: sudden, explosive, disorderly discharge of cerebral neurons characterized by an abrupt, transient alteration in brain function (36)

Self-actualization: doing things of one's choice, bringing ideas into action (15)

Self-help: the idea that as you begin to understand your personal levels of stress and anxiety, you are able to develop more control over them and are, therefore, more likely to be able to cope with them in the future (17)

Semen: thick, whitish secretion of reproductive organs in the male (40)

Seminal vesicles: pouches along the lower posterior surface of the bladder (40)

Sensory: having to do with the senses; carrying impulses toward the CNS (36)

Separation anxiety: a state of extreme discomfort an infant or toddler experiences when separated from loved ones (59)

Sepsis: the presence of infection (10)

Septicemia: spread of bacteria from a local infection into the bloodstream; also known as *blood poisoning* (10, 28, 55)

Septum: wall (33)

Sequelae: conditions occurring because of another condition (52)

Sequential compression device: device that inflates and deflates plastic sleeves wrapped around the legs to promote venous flow (29)

Seroconversion: detectable levels of antibodies against the virus in the blood (35)

Seropositive: a person's blood contains antibodies for HIV (35)

Serosanguineous: watery, blood-tinged (24)

Serous exudate: type of discharge consisting of serum (the clear portion of the blood) (24)

Sexual harassment: a violation of the individual's rights and a form of discrimination based on gender (4)

Shaken baby syndrome: closed head injury that is a result of head trauma, either from an external force such as a fall, or an internal force (59)

Shearing force: a combination of friction and pressure (24)

Shift report: passing of information from one shift to another (63)

Shock: life-threatening condition of inadequate tissue perfusion (47)

Shroud: a large piece of plastic or cotton material used to enclose a body after death (44)

Sickle cell anemia: an inherited disorder that distorts red blood cells, causing chronic anemia (34)

Sickle cell crisis: acutely painful condition that occurs when sickled red blood cells become lodged in capillaries, occluding blood flow to the affected area (34)

Sickle cell disease: an inherited defect in the formation of hemoglobin (34)

Sickle cell trait: sickle hemoglobin (hemoglobin S), a factor that, if inherited from both parents, results in sickle cell anemia (34)

Side effects: unintended drug actions (27)

Signs: data that are detectable by an observer or can be tested against an accepted standard (6)

Simulation: a run-through of the radiation procedure (45)

Single order: one-time order to be given once at a specified time (27)

Sinus rhythm: a regular heartbeat that originates in the sinoatrial node, or pacemaker, of the heart (33)

Situational loss: related to a specific occurrence, such as loss of a job due to a job transfer (18)

Sitz bath: treatment used to soak a client's pelvic area (24)

Skilled-care facilities: facilities in which clients require specialized care (46)

Slander: defamation by the spoken word, stating information or false words that can cause damage to a person's reputation (4)

Sleep apnea: periodic cessation of breathing during sleep (23)

Smegma: secretion consisting of epithelial cells found around the external genitalia (56)

SOAP: an acronym for subjective data, objective data, assessment, and planning (13)

Somatic nervous system: pathways that regulate *voluntary* control (such as that needed to lift this book) of skeletal muscles (36)

Somatic pain: diffuse discomfort that arises from ligaments, tendons, bones, blood vessels, and nerves (22)

Somatotropin: a direct hormone that influences bone, muscle, and other tissues included in body growth (38)

Somogyi effect: a sudden drop in the blood sugar followed by a rebound hyperglycemic reaction (38)

Source-oriented record: charting method segmented into sections such as physician's orders, nurse's notes, radiology, and lab; each person or department makes notations in a separate section or sections of the client's chart (13)

Specific defenses: changes in the immune system that provide protection to the body (10)

Speed shock: reaction to rapid induction of foreign substance or medication into the vascular system (28)

Sperm: male gametes or reproductive cells (40)

Spermicides: chemicals in the form of creams, foams, jellies, or suppositories that are inserted into the vagina prior to sexual intercourse (40)

Sphincters: round muscles that allow food and digestive juices to pass through them when they are relaxed; when constricted, they hold food and fluids in the stomach (37)

Spider angioma: dilated arteriole in the skin with radiating capillary branches that look like the legs of a spider (30)

Spina bifida: an incomplete closure of the vertebra and neural tube (51, 57)

Spinal shock: temporary loss of reflex activity below the level of spinal cord injury (36)

Spinnbarkeit: elasticity of cervical mucus, which can be used to help determine the time of ovulation (40)

Spiritual: having to do with the divine or a higher power (15, 16)

Spiritual development: the increase in the ability to discern meaning or purpose in life (16)

Sprain: a condition that occurs when a ligament (dense connective tissue that connects one bone to another) is twisted in an unusual fashion (31)

Sprue: (celiac disease or gluten-sensitive enteropathy) a chronic malabsorption syndrome in which the child is unable to digest gluten (59)

Sputum: the mucus secreted by the lungs, bronchi, and trachea (32)

Staging: a process of naming the extent of the spread of cancer (62)

Standard precautions: guidelines for special care to be used with all body fluids, especially those associated with blood-borne pathogens (e.g., hepatitis B and C, and HIV infections) (10)

Standards: guidelines used to determine what a nurse should or should not do (63)

Standing order: routine order for administering medication indefinitely (27)

Startle reflex: reaction that occurs when newborns have a sense of falling; they will quickly extend the arms (abduct) with fingers flared and thumb and first finger forming a "C"; the arms will then adduct in an embracing motion; the lower extremities may extend and then flex; a slight tremor may be noted (56)

Stasis: pooling of urine or other body fluid in an organ (59)

Stat: immediate (47)

Stat order: instructions for medication to be given immediately and only once unless subsequent doses are ordered (27)

Station: relationship between the fetus and the maternal ischial spines (53)

Status asthmaticus: a severe, prolonged asthma attack that is unresponsive to treatment (32)

Status epilepticus: prolonged partial or generalized seizures without recovery between attacks, while still in the postictal phase, or a single seizure that lasts more than 30 minutes (36)

Statute of limitations: a limit to the amount of time that can pass between recognition of harm and the bringing of a suit (4)

Steatorrhea: "fatty stools" that occur when there is inadequate breakdown of fats (37)

Stem cell: immature cells that have the ability to change into any of the blood cells depending on what the body needs at the time (34)

Stenosis: hardening of the cusps of the valves that prevents the valves from opening completely and slows blood flow into the next chamber (33)

Stepping reflex: reaction in which newborns step as if walking when their feet touch a hard surface (56)

Stereotypes: oversimplified conceptions, opinions, or beliefs about some aspect of a group of people (3)

Stereotypy: excessive repetitive behaviors such as hand movements or rocking present in children with autism (59)

Sterile field: a microorganism-free area (10)

Stigma: negative cultural attitude that marks people with disgrace (49)

Stomatitis: the inflammation of the oral cavity; caused by a bacteria, virus, or systemic disease (37)

Stork bites: dark red spots on the eyelids, forehead, or nape of the neck (56)

Strabismus: an eye disorder in which the eyes cannot be directed to the same object (56, 61)

Strain: a condition that occurs when a ligament (dense connective tissue that connects one bone to another) has been extended through more than the normal range of motion (31)

Striae gravidarum: "stretch marks" occur when the underlying connective tissue separates during periods of rapid growth (51)

Stroke volume: amount of blood ejected from the heart in one contraction (about 70 mL) (33)

Stroke: a sudden, nonconvulsive focal neurologic deficit (36)

Stylet: point of the needle (28)

Subinvolution: failure of the uterus to return to its normal size (55)

Subjective data: information apparent only to the person being affected (5, 6, 13)

Substance abuse: a maladaptive pattern of substance use despite adverse outcomes (50)

Substance dependency: tolerance, withdrawal, and compulsive use of substances (50)

Sucking reflex: reaction that is elicited when the newborn's lips are touched (56)

Suctioning: aspirating secretions, usually through a catheter (32)

Suffocation: lack of oxygen due to interrupted breathing (9)

Suicidal ideation: thinking about ending one's own life (17)

Summer day camp: a daytime program for children where LPNs/LVNs may obtain work (48)

Sundowning: the onset of delirium during the evening or night with impairment or disappearance during the day, most often seen in mid- or later stages of dementia (36, 43)

Superego: also known as the conscience, it is concerned with moral behavior and takes into account the rules of society and the individual's personal values (15)

Superficial burns: (also called *first-degree burns*) burns that injure only the epidermis and may be caused by everyday events such as touching a hot element on the stove (47)

Superior: above or in a higher position than a point of reference (19)

Supplemental Security Income: special payments to people who are blind or have a disability; SSI benefits are not restricted to people who are eligible for Social Security, and payments are not restricted to healthcare costs (7)

Suppuration: production of pus (24, 31)

Surgery: unique experience of a planned physical alteration by manual or operative methods (29)

Surgical asepsis: practice that keeps an object or an area completely free of microorganisms and spores (10)

Susceptibility of the host: the sixth link in the chain of infection; the extent to which a person is likely to contract an infection (10)

Susceptible host: individual with impaired immune response who is at risk for developing infection (10)

Sutures: threads used to sew body tissues together (29)

Sympathetic nervous system: responds, that is, activates the "fight-or-flight" response, to get the body moving in emergency or exciting situations (36)

Symptoms: information about a condition that is apparent only to the person involved (6)

Synapse: functional junction that "joins" one neuron to another (36)

Syncope: fainting (33)

Syndactyly: the fusion of two or more digits (56)

Syringes: injectable equipment used to administer parenteral medications (27)

Systemic infection: state that exists when microorganisms spread from one area to other body areas (10)

Systole: the period in which the ventricles contract (19)

Tachycardia: condition that occurs when the heartbeats become irregular and abnormally fast (33)

Talipes: (also known as *clubfoot*) a unilateral or bilateral twisting of the foot, usually inward (57, 59)

Taped report: a tape-recorded method of conveying information about clients from one shift to another (63)

Target cells: cells found in organs that are influenced either by neurotransmitters or by hormones (38)

Teaching: a system of activities intended to produce specific learning (12)

Team nursing: the delivery of individualized nursing care to clients by a nursing team led by a professional nurse (7, 63)

Telangiectasis: the development of small, painless, red spider like spots on the hands and face caused by swelling of tiny capillaries (35)

Telangiectatic nevi: dark red spots on the eyelids, forehead, or nape of the neck (56)

Telemetry: remote monitoring (33)

Tenesmus: painful straining to defecate (37, 40)

Term: the period of pregnancy between 38 and 42 weeks gestation (51)

Terminal illness: an illness from which there is no reasonable expectation of survival (44)

Tertiary prevention: rehabilitation (appropriate to the stage of disability), preventing further complications, and restoring functioning to the highest possible level (44)

Test anxiety: a level of concern about testing that ranges from a normal mild level of uneasiness that is motivating to a level of uneasiness and fear that immobilizes the test taker (64)

Testes: male gonads (40)

Tetany: severe muscle spasms (38)

Thanatology: the academic study of death and dying (18)

Theories: ways of looking at a discipline, such as nursing, in clear, explicit terms that can be communicated to others (5)

Therapeutic baths: hygienic care given for physical effects, such as to soothe irritated skin or to treat an area (20)

Therapeutic communication: client-centered, goal-directed, and time-limited communication used by nurses to determine client concerns, problems, and feelings (11)

Therapeutic effect: the desired result; the drug did what it was prescribed to do (27)

Therapeutic touch: energy directed through the hands of the practitioner (usually held slightly away from the client's body) to activate the healing response of the recipient (18)

Thermoregulation: maintenance of body heat (56)

Third spacing: shunting of fluids into the extracellular space (47)

Thrombocytes: platelets (34)

Thrombocytopenia: a decrease in the platelet count to lower than 100,000/mL of blood (34, 45)

Thromboembolism: a blood clot moving within the blood vessel (54)

Thrombophlebitis: condition with inflammation and clot formation in a vein (23, 28, 29)

Thrombopoietin: a protein manufactured by the liver, the kidney, the smooth muscle, and the bone marrow that regulates the production of platelets (34)

Thrombosis: clot formation in the vein (28, 54)

Thrombus: blood clot attached to wall of a vein or artery (most commonly the leg veins) (23, 29)

Thrush: an oral infection caused by the fungus *Candida albicans* that causes small white patches on the mouth and tongue (37)

Thymoma: a tumor in the thymus gland (35)

Thyroid storm: a severe form of hyperthyroidism that can occur when clients' hyperthyroidism is left untreated or after thyroid surgery; the manipulation of the thyroid gland during surgery causes it to dump a large amount of thyroid hormone into the bloodstream at one time (38)

Thyrotoxicosis: a severe form of hyperthyroidism that can occur when clients' hyperthyroidism is left untreated or after thyroid surgery; the manipulation of the thyroid gland during surgery causes it to dump a large amount of thyroid hormone into the bloodstream at one time (38)

Tic douloureux: trigeminal neuralgia; extreme pain in the area of the maxillary and/or mandibular division of the trigeminal sensory root (36)

Tinnitus: ringing in the ears (36, 42)

Tissue perfusion: passage of blood through the vessels (29)

Tissue typing: a process that determines the ability of the cells to be compatible and lessens the risk of rejection (35)

Titration: determination of the correct volume for administration (47)

Tocolytic agents: medications that inhibit contractions (53)

Tolerance: a need for increased amounts of the substance to achieve the same effect, or diminished effect with continued use of the same amount of the substance (50)

Tonic-clonic: jerky, alternately contracting and relaxing (36)

Tonic neck reflex: reaction that occurs when the head is turned to one side; newborns will extend the arm and leg on that side; the opposite arm and leg will flex (56)

Tonsillectomy and adenoidectomy (T&A): surgical removal of the palatine and pharyngeal tonsils (60)

Tonsillitis: inflammation of the palatine tonsils (60)

TORCH group: acronym for a group of infections that are particularly dangerous during pregnancy: *to*xoplasmosis, *r*ubella, *c*ytomegalovirus, and *he*rpes virus type 2 (52)

Tort: a civil wrong committed against a person or a person's property (4)

Toxic shock syndrome: a condition in women caused by a bacterial toxin (usually staphylococcus aureus) entering the bloodstream (40)

Toxoid: a toxin that has been treated so that its toxic property is destroyed but its ability to stimulate production of antibodies remains (35)

Tracheoesophageal fistula: a condition in which there is a connection between the trachea and esophagus (57)

Tracheostomy: a surgical incision in the trachea just below the larynx through which a tracheostomy tube is inserted (32)

Traction: a method of providing a steady and continuous pull that maintains the fractured bone in good alignment (31)

Tracts: bundles of nerve fibers that run through the CNS (36)

Transcellular fluid: liquid, including cerebrospinal, pleural, peritoneal, and synovial fluids, found in the body's cavities (26)

Transfer: a move (14)

Transfusion reaction: occurs when the donor's red cells rupture or hemolyze and release their hemoglobin, with dangerous or even lethal results (34)

Transient ischemic attack: a temporary loss of blood supply (oxygen) to an area of the brain (36)

Transmission: the manner in which a microorganism gets to the host (10)

Transmission-based precautions: guidelines used in addition to Standard Precautions for any client with known or suspected infections that are spread by airborne or droplet transmission or by physical contact (10)

Transplant: surgical replacement of malfunctioning structures (29)

Transverse plane: defines a *superior* (higher) and *inferior* (lower) portion (19)

Traveling nurse: companion nurse; a licensed nurse who works for a company that contracts with healthcare agencies to provide them with staff (48)

Triage: system of prioritizing victims' care needs, from most severe to least injured or ill (9, 47)

Trigeminal neuralgia: tic douloureux; extreme pain in the area of the maxillary and/or mandibular division of the trigeminal sensory root (36)

Triglycerides: a compound containing three fatty acids (25)

Trimesters: the progression of the pregnancy is described in 3-month blocks of time (51)

Trisomy 21: chromosomal abnormality (three chromosomes at position 21) resulting in Down syndrome (57)

Tropic hormones: indirect-acting hormones that are secreted by one gland and target another endocrine gland, stimulating growth and secretion (38)

Trousseau's sign: carpal spasm occurring when the blood flow is constricted to the lower arm (38)

True perineum: the tissue between the vaginal opening and the anus (40)

Tubal ligation: the tying and cutting of the vas deferens or fallopian tubes (40)

Tubercle: lesion that develops in the primary stage of tuberculosis (32)

Tumor: mass of tissue that may be benign or malignant (45)

Turgor: fullness (19)

Twisting: rotation of the thoracolumbar spine (9)

Tympanites: swelling of the abdomen from retention of gases within the intestines (29)

Ulcer: superficial loss of tissue, usually with inflammation, on the surface of the skin or mucous membrane (30)

Ulcerative colitis: inflammation with sloughing of the mucosa of the large intestine (62)

Umbilical cord: tube that connects the fetus to the placenta (51)

Umbilical hernia: condition resulting from a weakness in the umbilical ring; appearing as a soft swelling under the umbilical cord which is covered by skin (60)

Undernutrition: condition occurring when nutrient intake is insufficient to meet daily energy requirements (25)

Undoing: an action or words designed to cancel some disapproved thoughts, impulses or acts; a mechanism by which a person relieves guilt by making reparation (17)

Unhelpful communication: interaction that hinders or blocks the transfer of information and feelings (11)

Uremia: a toxic state marked by an accumulation of urea and other nitrogenous wastes in the blood (39)

Urethritis: an inflammation of the urethra that causes redness, irritation, edema of the mucosa, and urethral discharge (39)

Urgency: feeling that voiding must occur immediately (39)

Urgent care: care for minor injuries and acute illnesses (e.g., strep throat) when clients cannot see their primary care provider (PCP) or if they do not have a designated healthcare provider (47)

Urgent care office: walk-in medical facility where clients can obtain treatment for minor injuries and acute illnesses (48)

Urinary retention: the inability to empty the bladder completely (39)

Urinary stasis: condition in which the urine does not move out of the urinary tract (23)

Uterine atony: failure of the uterus to contract following birth (55)

Uterine prolapse: the condition that occurs when the uterus descends into or out of the vaginal canal (40)

Uterine soufflé: the sound occurring at the same rate as the maternal pulse (51)

Uterus: a hollow organ where the fertilized ovum is implanted and the embryo and fetus develop (40)

Vaccines: medications that cause a person to develop active immunity against a specific organism (35)

Vagina: a tubular structure composed of muscle and membranous tissue connecting the vulva with the uterus (40)

Vaginal introitus: the external opening of the vaginal canal (40)

Vaginitis: inflammation of the vagina (61)

Validation: a form of feedback that provides confirmation that both parties have the same basic understanding of the message and the feedback (11)

Valsalva maneuver: straining to have a bowel movement accompanied by holding the breath (37)

Values: freely chosen, enduring beliefs or attitudes about the worth of a person, object, idea, or action (4)

Valve ablation: removal of a faulty valve (59)

Valvular insufficiency: failure of the valves to close completely, forcing blood back into the previous chamber when the heart contracts (33)

Varicocele: dilated blood vessel in the testis (40)

Varicose veins: swollen, knotted, and tortuous veins with poorly functioning valves (33)

Vasectomy: surgical sterilization of male (40)

Vasovagal response: a response characterized by tachycardia and hypertension prior to IV needle insertion, and by bradycardia, pallor, diaphoresis, syncope, and a drop in blood pressure after needle insertion (28)

Vector: vehicle, a living means of transport for infection (10)

Vegetative state: irreversible state of unconsciousness (44)

Vein stripping: the surgical removal of the varicose veins (33)

Venospasm: constriction of the inner lining of the vein (28)

Venous star: a small varicose vein that occurs secondary to prolonged venous pressure (30)

Venous stasis ulcers: open sores that appear on the lower legs due to poor circulation to the legs (33)

Ventilation: breathing (32)

Ventral: toward the front of the body or the belly (19)

Ventricle: small cavity found on either side of the heart (33)

Vernix caseosa: white, cheesy covering of the fetal or newborn skin (51, 56)

Vertigo: acute dizziness and lack of balance (23, 36)

Vesicle: a small, circumscribed elevation of the skin containing fluid; blister (30, 41)

Viability: the ability to live outside the uterus (51)

Virulence: an organism's ability to produce disease and survive both inside and outside the body (10)

Viruses: the smallest known disease-causing agents; they must enter living cells in order to reproduce (10)

Visceral pain: discomfort that results from stimulation of pain receptors in the abdominal cavity, cranium, and thorax (22)

Visualization: refers to picturing something in the mind's eye and "seeing" healing, pain relief, relaxation, and so on (18)

Vital capacity: the maximum volume of air that can be exhaled after maximum inhalation (23)

Vital signs: measurements of temperature, pulse, respirations, and blood pressure (19)

Vitamin: an organic compound that cannot be manufactured by the body and is needed in small quantities to *catalyze* (or trigger) metabolic processes (25)

Volvulus: twisted bowel, causing restricted flow of bowel contents (37, 59)

Vomiting: forceful expulsion of stomach contents through the mouth (37)

Vulva: the collective term used for the external structures of the female reproductive system (40)

Vulvectomy: surgical removal of the vulva, labia majora and minora, clitoris, and prepuce (40)

Webbing: skin between two or more digits (56)

Wellness: a state of well-being; engaging in attitudes and behaviors that enhance the quality of life and maximize personal potential (2)

Wernicke's syndrome: (alcoholic encephalopathy) the result of severe vitamin B_1 deficiency caused by poor nutrition (50)

Wharton's jelly: white gelatinous tissue (51)

Wheal: a circumscribed, slightly reddened, papule or irregular plaque of edema of the skin, usually accompanied by intense itching (30)

Wheezing: continuous, high-pitched, squeaky musical sounds; best heard on expiration (19)

White matter: composed of dense collections of myelinated tracts (36)

Witches' milk: whitish fluid sometimes secreted from newborn's nipples (56)

Withdrawal: condition that occurs due to discontinuing or reducing use of a substance that has been heavy and prolonged and that results in significant distress or impairment in social or occupational functioning (50)

Xenograft: a transplant from an animal species to a human (35)

Zygote: fertilized egg (51)

References and Resources

CHAPTER 1

Ellis, J. R., & Hartley, C. L. (2004). *Nursing in today's world: Challenges, issues & trends* (8th ed.). Philadelphia: Lippincott Williams & Wilkins.

Hermann, M. L. (2004). Linking liberal & professional learning in nursing education. *Liberal Education, 90*(4), 236+.

Jackson, E. W., & Mcglinn, S. (2000). Know the test: One component of test preparation. *Journal of College Reading and Learning, 31*(1), 84-93.

Kelly, L. Y., & Joel, L. A. (2003). *Dimensions of professional nursing* (9th ed.). New York: McGraw-Hill.

Lang-Otsuka, P. A. (Ed.). (2005). *Pathophysiology made incredibly easy* (3rd ed.) Philadelphia: Springhouse–Lippincott William & Wilkins.

National Federation of Licensed Practical Nurses. (2003). Nursing practice standards for the licensed practical/vocational nurse. Garner, NC: Author.

Porter, L. (n.d.). Notes on how to read a textbook. Anaheim, CA: North Orange County Regional Occupational Program.

Supon, V. (2004). Implementing strategies to assist text-anxious students. *Journal of Instructional Psychology, 31*(4), 292-296.

White, H. L. (2003). Implementing the multicultural education perspective into the nursing education curriculum. *Journal of Instructional Psychology, 30*(4), 236-237.

CHAPTER 2

Baer, E. D., D'Antonio, P., Rinker, S., & Lynaugh, J. E. (Eds.). (2000). *Enduring issues in American nursing.* Philadelphia: Springhouse Corporation.

Barber, M. F. (1992). In R. Smolan (Ed.). *The power to heal: ancient arts & modern medicine.* Upper Saddle River, NJ: Prentice Hall.

Creighton, J. (1998, December 28). Nurse on cap hunt. *The Toronto Sun,* A-28.

D'antonio, P. (2005). History of nursing. *Nursing History Review,* Vol. 13.

D'antonio, P. (2006). History of nursing. *Nursing History Review,* Vol. 14.

D'antonio, P. (2007). History of nursing. *Nursing History Review,* Vol. 15.

Dixon, B. (2006). In her footsteps. *Nursing 2006, 36*(12), 43.

Dolan, J. A., Fitzpatrick, M. L., & Herrmann, E. K. (1983). *Nursing in society: A historical perspective* (15th ed.). Philadelphia: W. B. Saunders.

Edmonds, S. E., & Leonard, E. D. (1999). *Memoirs of a soldier, nurse and spy: A woman's adventures in the union army.* Dekalb, IL: Northern Illinois University Press.

National Federation of Licensed Practical Nurses. (2003). *Nursing practice standards for the licensed practical/vocational nurse.* Gardner, NC: Author.

Nelson, S. (2002). The fork in the road: Nursing history vs. the history of nursing. In *Nursing history review* (Vol. 10). Lanoka, NJ: American Association for the History of Nursing, Inc.

Nightingale, F. (1860). *Notes on nursing: What it is, and what it is not* (Commemorative Ed.). Philadelphia: Lippincott.

Norman, E. (2000). *We band of angels.* New York: Pocket Books.

Ransom, C. B. (2003). *Clara Barton history maker bios.* Berkeley, CA: Lerner Publication Company.

Sandelowski, M. (2000). *Devices & desires: Gender, technology and American nursing.* Chapel Hill: University of North Carolina Press.

Sarnecky, M. T. (2007). Field expediency—How army nurses in Vietnam "made do." *American Journal of Nursing, 107*(5), 52-59.

Schorr, T. M., with Kennedy, M. S. (1999). *100 years of American nursing.* Philadelphia: Lippincott.

Schuyler, C. B. (1992). Florence Nightingale. In F. Nightingale, *Notes on nursing: What it is, and what it is not* (Commemorative Ed., 3-17). Philadelphia: Lippincott. [Classic]

Sorel, N. C. (2000). *The women who wrote the war.* New York: Harper Perennial.

Wake, R. (1998). *The Nightingale training school 1860-1996.* London: Haggerstown Press.

Wood, W. (Ed.). (1999, December 13). Century in review. *Nurseweek, 12*(25), 1.

Zerwekh, J., & Claborn, J. C. (2002). *Nursing today: Transition and trends* (3rd ed.). Philadelphia: W. B. Saunders.

CHAPTER 3

Adler, R. B., Rosenfeld, L. B., Towne, N., & Proctor, R. III. (2004). *Interplay: The process of interpersonal communication.* New York: Oxford Press.

Anderson, M. M., & Boyle, J. S. (2007). *Transcultural concepts in nursing care* (5th ed.). Philadelphia: Lippincott.

Anderson, N. B., Bulatao, A., & Cohen, B. (Ed.). (2004). *Critical perspectives on racial and ethnic differences in health in later life.* Washington, DC: The National Academies Press.

Bowers, P. (2000). *Cultural perspectives in childbearing* (Nursing spectrum self-study module). Retrieved July 27, 2003, from http://nsweb.nursingspectrum.com/ce.

Clark, L., Zuk, J., & Baramee, J. (2000). A literacy approach to teaching cultural competence . . . reading of the book *The Spirit Catches You and You Fall Down. Journal of Transcultural Nursing, 11,* 199-203.

Finucane, M. (2000, October). Paper presented at Second National Conference on Quality Health Care for Culturally Diverse Populations: Strategy and Action for Communities, Providers and a Changing Health System, Los Angeles, CA.

Flaskerud, J. H. (2002). *Culturally competent neuropsychiatric NP program.* Los Angeles: UCLA School of Nursing. Retrieved July 27, 2003, from http://bhpr.hrsa.gov/nursing/fy02grants/abstracts.

Giger, J. N., & Davidhizar, R. E. (2004). *Transcultural nursing: Assessment and intervention* (4th ed.). St. Louis, MO: Mosby.

Giger, J., Davidhizar, R. E., Purnell, L., Harden, J. T., Phillips, J., & Strickland, O. (2007). American Academy of Nursing expert panel report: Developing cultural competence to eliminate health disparities in ethnic minorities and other vulnerable populations. *Journal of Transcultural Nursing, 18*(2), 95-102.

Gilchrist, K. L., & Rector, C. (2007). Can you keep them? Strategies to attract and retain nursing students from diverse populations: Best practices in nursing education. Journal of Transcultural Nursing, *18,* 277-285.

Kahn, Z. B. (2008). A nurse for all seasons. *Advance for Nurses, 5* (10), 24.

Killian, P., & Waite, R. (2008). Weaving culture with care. *Advance for Nurses, 5* (10), 19.

Leininger, M. (1997). Understanding cultural pain for improved health care. *Journal of Transcultural Nursing, 9*(1), 32–35.

Leininger, M., McFarland, M., & McFarlane, M. (2002). *Transcultural nursing* (3rd ed.). New York: McGraw-Hill Professional.

Purnell, L. D., & Paulanka, B. J. (2008). *Transcultural health care: A culturally competent approach* (3rd ed.). Philadelphia: F. A. Davis.

Robinson, J. H. (2000). Increasing students' cultural sensitivity: A step toward greater diversity in nursing. *Nurse Educator, 25*(3), 131–135.

Ryan, M., Carlton, K. H., & Ali, N. (2000). Transcultural nursing concepts and experiences in nursing curricula. *Journal of Transcultural Nursing, 11*(4), 300–307.

Schim, S. M., Doorenbos, A., Benkert, R., & Miller, J. (2007). Culturally congruent care: Putting the puzzle together. *Journal of Transcultural Nursing, 18,* 103–110.

Sitzman, K. L. (2007). Diversity and the NCLEX-RN: A double-loop approach. *Journal of Transculural Nursing, 18,* 271–276.

Smedley, B. D., Stith, A. X., & Nelson, A. R. (2003). *Unequal treatment—Confronting racial and ethnic disparities in healthcare.* Washington, DC: The National Academies Press.

Spector, R. E. (2003). *Cultural diversity in health and illness* (5th ed.). Upper Saddle River, NJ: Prentice Hall Health.

Steelfel, L. (2003). No cookie cutter approach to postpartum culture care. *Nursing Spectrum.* Retrieved July 26, 2003, from http://community.nursingspectrum.com/MagazineArticle.

Taylor, D., Polan, E., & Weitzman, J. P. (2007). *Journey across the life span: Human growth and development and health promotion* (3rd ed.). Philadelphia: F. A. Davis.

U.S. Department of Health and Human Services. (2000). *Healthy People 2010.* Washington, DC: Author.

Wells, J. N., Spence Cagle, C., & Bradley, P. J. (2006). Building on Mexican-American cultural values. *Nursing, 36*(7), 20–21.

CHAPTER 4

American Nurses Association. (1995). *ANA position statement on assisted suicide.* Silver Springs, MD: Author.

American Nurses Association. (1998). *Standards of clinical nursing practice* (2nd ed.). Silver Springs, MD: Author.

Anderson, F. (2007). Finding HIPAA in your soup. *American Journal of Nursing, 107*(2), 66–71.

Anderson, M.A. (2005). *Nursing leadership, management, and professional practice for the LPN/LVN* (3rd ed.). Philadelphia: F.A. Davis.

Andrews, M. M., & Boyle, J. S. (2008). *Transcultural concepts in nursing care* (5th ed.). Philadelphia: Lippincott.

Austin, S. (2006). Walk a fine line if your patient wants to leave AMA. *Nursing, 36*(12), 48–49.

Bernzweig, E. P. (1996). *Nurse's liability for malpractice: A programmed course* (6th ed.). St. Louis: Mosby.

Brent, N. J. (2003). *Nurses and the law.* (8th ed.). Philadelphia: W. B. Saunders.

Brous, E.A. (2007). HIPAA vs. law enforcement. *American Journal of Nursing, 107*(8), 60–63.

Burke, L., & Weill, B. (2009). *Information technology for health care professionals* (3rd. ed.). Upper Saddle River, NJ: Prentice Hall.

Centers for Disease Control and Prevention. (2001). *Guidelines for HIV counseling, testing and referral.* Atlanta, GA: Author.

Equal Employment Opportunity Commission. (1980). Sex discrimination guidelines. In *EEOC rules and regulation.* Chicago: Commerce Clearing House.

Fletcher, G. P. (2000). *Rethinking criminal law.* New York: Oxford.

National Federation of Licensed Practical Nurses. (2003). *Nursing practice standards for the licensed practical/vocational nurse.* Gardner, NC: Author.

Nightingale, F. (1992). *Notes on nursing.* Philadelphia: J. B. Lippincott (original work published 1859).

Norman, J. C. (2000). HIV/AIDS: Epidemic update. *CME Resources, 67*(7), 12–36.

Reichart, G.A. (1998). Female circumcision. *AWHONN Lifelines, 2*(3), 28–34.

Swansberg, R. C., & Swansberg, R. J. (2003). Introduction to management for nurses (3rd ed.). Boston: Jones and Bartlett.

CHAPTER 5

Andrews, M. M., & Boyle, V. S. (2008). *Transcultural concepts in nursing care* (5th ed.). Philadelphia: Lippincott.

Fawcett, J. (2005). *Analysis and evaluation of contemporary nursing knowledge: Nursing models and theories* (2nd ed.). Philadelphia: F. A. Davis.

Kurzen, C. (2005). *Contemporary practical/vocational nursing* (5th ed.). Philadelphia: Lippincott.

LeMone, P., & Burke, K. (2007). *Medical–surgical nursing: Critical thinking in client care* (4th ed.). Upper Saddle River, NJ: Prentice Hall Health.

Paul, R. W., & Elder, L. (2005). *Critical thinking.* Dillon Beach, CA: Foundation for Critical Thinking.

CHAPTER 6

Ackley, B. J., & Ladwig, G. B. (2005). *Mosby's guide to nursing diagnosis.* St. Louis, MO: Mosby.

Ackley, B. J., & Ladwig, G. B. (2006). *Nursing diagnosis handbook: A guide to planning care* (7th ed.). St. Louis, MO: Mosby.

Alfaro-LeFevre, R. (2005). *Applying the nursing process: A tool for critical thinking.* Philadelphia: Lippincott.

American Nurses Association. (1998). *Standards of clinical nursing practice* (2nd ed.). Kansas City, MO: Author.

Anderson, M.A. (2005). *Nursing leadership, management, and professional practice for the LPN/LVN: In nursing school and beyond.* Philadelphia: F.A. Davis.

Boucher, M.A. (1998). Delegation alert. *American Journal of Nursing, 98*(2), 26–32.

Carpenito, L. J. (2008a). *Handbook of nursing diagnosis* (2nd ed.). Philadelphia: Lippincott Williams & Wilkins.

Carpenito, L. J. (2008b). *Nursing diagnosis: Application to clinical practice* (2nd ed.). Philadelphia: Lippincott Williams & Wilkins.

Johnson, M., et al. (2005). *Nursing diagnosis, outcomes, & interventions: NANDA, NOC, & NIC Linkages, nursing interventions classification 4e, Nursing Outcomes Classification 3e* (2nd ed.). St. Louis, MO: Mosby.

Joint Commission. (2005). *Comprehensive accreditation manual for hospitals.* Chicago: Author.

McCloskey, J. C., & Bulechek, G. M. (Eds.). (2007). *Nursing interventions classification (NIC)* (5th ed.). St. Louis, MO: Mosby-Year Book.

NANDA International. (2009). *NANDA International Nursing Diagnoses: Definitions & Classification 2009-2011.* Oxford, UK: Wiley-Blackwell.

Wilkinson, J. M. (2007). *Nursing process and critical thinking* (4th ed.). Upper Saddle River: Pearson Prentice Hall, p. 4.

Wilkinson, J. M., & Ahern, N. R. (2009). *Nursing diagnosis handbook* (9th ed.). Upper Saddle River, NJ: Prentice Hall.

CHAPTER 7

Abrams, W., Beers, M., & Berkow, R. (Eds.). (2004). *The Merck manual of health and aging* (3rd ed.). Whitehouse Station, NJ: Merck.

American Academy of Nursing Panel on Woman's Health. (1997). Woman's health and woman's health care: Recommendations of the 1996 ANA expert panel on woman's health. *Nursing Outlook, 45*(1), 7-15.

American Hospital Association. (1992). *A patient's bill of rights.* Chicago: Author.

American Public Health Association. (1966). Nationwide coverage by organized public health services. Policy number 6601. Washington, D.C.: Author.

Hoffman, C. B. (2007). Simple truths about American's uninsured. *American Journal of Nursing, 107*(1), 40-47.

Lee, P. R., & Estes, C. L. (2003). *The nation's health.* Boston: Jones & Bartlett.

Stoker, J. (2000). The Omnibus Consolidation Appropriation Act of 2000. *Home HealthCare Nurse, 18*(2), 84.

U.S. Department of Health and Human Services. (2000). *Healthy people 2010: Understanding and improving health* (2nd ed.). Washington, DC: U.S. Government Printing Office.

U.S. Department of Health and Human Services. (2002). *Confronting the new health care crisis: Improving health care quality and lowering costs by fixing our medical liability system.* Washington, DC: U.S. Government Printing Office.

U.S. Department of Justice and Federal Trade Commission. (2004). *Improving health care: A dose of competition.* Washington, DC: U.S. Government Printing Office.

U.S. Department of Labor, Bureau of Labor Statistics. (1999 and various years). *Employee benefit survey.* Washington, DC: U.S. Government Printing Office.

Whelchel, C. (2004). Patient first when budgeting. *Nursing Management, 35*(2), 16.

CHAPTER 8

5 domains of complementary therapy. (2003). *Journal of Hospice & Palliative Nursing.* 5(2), 113-117.

CAMBASICS National Center for Complementary and Alternative Medicine. (2007). *What is CAM?* Bethesda, MD: National Institutes of Health.

Cheng, B., et al. (2002). Herbal medicine and anaesthesia. *Hong Kong Medical Journal, 8,* 123-130.

The Consortium of Academic Health Centers for Integrative Medicine. (2005). About Us. Retrieved June 16, 2008, from the Academic Health Centers website of University of Minnesota. www.ahc.umn.edu/cahcim/about/home.html.

Dreher, H. M. (2008). Nursing education: Preparing for the future of nursing practice. *Holistic Nursing Practice, 22*(2), 77-80.

Fessenden, J., Wittenborn, W., & Clarke, L. (2001). Gingko biloba: A case report of herbal medicine and bleeding postoperatively from a laparoscopic cholecystectomy. *The American Surgeon, 67*(1), 33-35.

Fontaine, K. L. (2005). *Complementary and alternative therapies* (2nd ed.). Upper Saddle River, NJ: Prentice Hall.

Food and Drug Administration. (1998). Regulations on statements made for dietary supplements concerning the effect of the product on the structure or function of the body. *Federal Register, 63*(82).

Hugh, H. J., Dower, C., O'Neil, E. H. (2001). *Profile of a profession: Naturopathic medicine.* San Francisco, CA: Center for the Health Professions, University of California San Francisco.

Pal, S. (2002). Complementary and alternative medicine: An overview. *Current Science, 82*(5), 518-524.

Riley, R. W. (2001). *Decision of the secretary in the matter of the council on naturopathic medical education.* Washington DC: U.S. Department of Education.

Sparber, A. (2001). State boards of nursing and scope of practice of registered nurses performing complementary therapies. *Online Journal of Issues in Nursing, 6*(2), 6-7.

CHAPTER 9

American Heart Association. (2005). CPR Guidelines. AHA and Your Heart (NIH Publication No. 06-5714). Bethesda, MD: Author.

Arias, K. M. (Ed.). (2000). *Quick reference to outbreak investigation and control in health care facilities.* New York: Aspen Publishing.

Bonder, B., & Wagner, M. B. (2001). *Functional performance in older adults.* Philadelphia: F.A. Davis.

Burke, K. M., LeMone, P., & Mohn-Brown, E. (2007). (2nd ed.). *Medical-surgical nursing care.* Upper Saddle River, NJ: Prentice Hall.

Carpenito, L. J. (2005). *Handbook of nursing diagnosis* (11th ed.). Philadelphia: Lippincott.

Charney, W. (Ed.). (1999). *Handbook of modern hospital safety.* Boca Raton, FL: Lewis Publishing.

Doenges, M. E., & Moorhouse, M. F. (2003). *Application of nursing process and nursing diagnoses: An interactive text for diagnostic reasoning* (4th ed.). Philadelphia: F.A. Davis.

Edelman, C. L., & Mandle, C. L. (2002). *Health promotion throughout the lifespan* (5th ed.). St. Louis, MO: Mosby.

Hutton, J. T., Elias, W., Shroyer, J. A., & Curry, Z. (2000). *Preventing falls: A defensive approach.* Amherst, NY: Prometheus Books.

Kobs, A. (1998, January). Questions and answers from the JCAHO. Restraints revisited. *Nursing Management, 29*(1), 17-18.

LeMone, P., & Burke, K. M. (2008). *Medical-surgical nursing: Critical thinking in client care.* (4th ed.). Upper Saddle River, NJ: Prentice Hall.

NANDA International. (2009). *NANDA International Nursing Diagnoses: Definitions & Classifications 2009-2011.* Oxford, UK: Wiley-Blackwell.

Smith, S. F., Duell, D. J., & Martin, B. C. (2008). *Clinical nursing skills: Basic to advanced* (7th ed.). Upper Saddle River, NJ: Prentice Hall.

Tai, E. (2001). *OSHA compliance management: A guide for long-term health care facilities.* Boca Raton, FL: Lewis Publishing.

The Joint Commission. National Patient Safety Goals: 2009 National Patient Safety Goals. Retrieved September 23, 2008 from www.jointcommission.org/patientsafety/nationalpatientsafetygoals.

Tideiksaar, R. (2002). *Falls in older persons.* Baltimore, MD: Health Professions Press.

CHAPTER 10

Calvet, H. M. (2007, October). Community-acquired methicillin resistant staph aureus (CAMRSA): Realism or reaction? Presentation given to Long Beach Unified School District School Nurses.

Carpenito, L. J. (2005). *Handbook of nursing diagnosis* (11th ed.). Philadelphia: Lippincott.

Carrico, R. (Ed.). (2005). *APIC text of infection control and epidemiology: Principles of microbial pathogenicity and host response* (2nd ed.). Washington, DC: Association for Professionals in Infection Control and Epidemiology.

Centers for Disease Control and Prevention. (1996). Guidelines for isolation precautions in hospitals, Part 1: Evolution of isolation practices. *American Journal of Infection Control, 24*(1), 24–31.

Centers for Disease Control and Prevention. (1998). *Guidelines for infection control in health care personnel.* Atlanta, GA: Author.

Centers for Disease Control and Prevention. (2002, October 25). Guidelines for hand hygiene in health care settings: Recommendations of the Healthcare Infection Control Practices Committee. *MMWR, 51*(RR16), 1–44.

Centers for Disease Control and Prevention. (2005, September 30). *Controlling tuberculosis in the United States.* Atlanta, GA: Author.

Centers for Disease Control and Prevention. (2005, December 30). *Guidelines for preventing the transmission of* Mycobacterium tuberculosis *in health-care settings.* Atlanta, GA: Author.

Clavreul, G. M. (2007). From the floor: A vector for infection. *Working Nurse,* 15.

Dalahanty, K. M., & Meyers, F. E. (2007). Infection control survey report. *Nursing, 37*(6), 28–36.

Harkness, G. A., & Dincher, J. K. (1999). *Medical-surgical nursing: Total client care* (10th ed.). St. Louis, MO: Mosby.

Hathaway, L. (2006). Saving 100,000 lives, one step at a time. *LPN 2006, 2*(2), 4–6.

Klevens, R. M., et al. (2007). Invasive methicillin-resistant *Staphylococcus aureus* infections in the United States active bacterial core surveillance (ABCs) MRSA investigators. *JAMA,* 298, 1763–1771.

Lee, M. C. et al. (2004). Management and outcome of children with skin and soft tissue abscesses caused by community-acquired methicillin-resistant *Staphylococcus aureus. Pediatric Infectious Disease Journal, 23*(2), 123–127.

LeMone, P., & Burke, K. M. (2008). *Medical-surgical nursing: Critical thinking in client care* (4th ed.). Upper Saddle River, NJ: Prentice Hall.

Needlestick Prevention Act, U.S. Congress, March 2000.

Nettina, S. M. (Ed.). (2005). *The Lippincott manual of nursing practice* (8th ed.). Philadelphia: Lippincott Williams & Wilkins.

NANDA International. (2009). *NANDA International Nursing Diagnoses: Definitions & Classifications 2009–2011.* Oxford, UK: Wiley-Blackwell.

Odom-Forren, J. (2006). Winning the battle against surgical site infections. *LPN 2006, 2*(3), 44–47.

OSHA Enforcement Procedure for Bloodborne Pathogens Regulation, CPL 2–2. 69, November 27, 2001.

Smith, S. F., Duell, D. J., & Martin, B. C. (2008). *Clinical nursing skills: Basic to advanced* (7th ed.). Upper Saddle River, NJ: Prentice Hall.

Springhouse Corporation. (1998). *Healthcare professional guides: Safety and infection control.* Springhouse, PA: Author.

Timby, B. K., Scherer, J. C., & Smith, N. E. (2007). *Introductory medical-surgical nursing* (9th ed.). Philadelphia: Lippincott.

Walker, B.W. (2007). New guidelines for fighting multidrug-resistant organisms. *Nursing 2007, 37*(5), 20.

CHAPTER 11

Ackley, B. J., & Ladwig, G. B. (2005). *Mosby's guide to nursing diagnosis* (6th ed.). St. Louis, MO: Mosby.

Anderson, M. A. (2005). *Nursing leadership, management and professional practice for LPN/LVN in nursing school and beyond* (3rd ed.). Philadelphia: F.A. Davis.

Anderson, M.A., & Helm, L. B. (2000). Talking about patients: Communication and continuity of care. *Journal of Cardiovascular Nursing, 14*(3), 15.

Arnold, E., & Boggs, K. U. (2003). *Interpersonal relationships: Professional communication skills for nurses* (4th ed.). Philadelphia: W. B. Saunders.

Bateson, G. (2002). *Mind and nature—A necessary unity (advanced systems theory, complexity and the human sciences).* New York: Hampton Press.

Buresh, B., & Gordon, S. (2006). *From silence to voice: What nurses know and must communicate to the public (the culture and politics of health care work).* Ottawa, Ontario: Canadian Nurses Association.

Carpenito, L. J. (2005). *Nursing diagnosis: Application to clinical practice* (11th ed.). Philadelphia: Lippincott.

Deering, C. G. (1999). To speak or not to speak? Self-disclosure with patients. *American Journal of Nursing, 99*(1), 34–39.

Eby, L., & Brown, N. J. (2009). *Mental health nursing care* (2nd ed.). Upper Saddle River, NJ: Prentice Hall.

Egan, G. (2002). *The skilled helper: A problem-management and opportunity development approach to helping* (7th ed.). Pacific Grove, CA: Brooks/Cole.

Fontaine, K. L. (2008). *Mental health nursing* (6th ed.). Upper Saddle River, NJ: Prentice Hall.

Hersey, P., Blanchard, K. H., & Johnson, D. E. (2001). Effective communication, Chap. 13 in *Management of organizational behavior: Leading human resources* (8th ed.). Upper Saddle River, NJ: Prentice Hall.

Hodes, R. J. (2004). *Working with your older patient—A clinician's handbook.* Washington, DC: National Institutes of Health, National Institute on Aging.

Knapp, H. (2007). *Therapeutic communication: Developing personal skills.* Thousand Oaks, CA: Sage Publications.

Purnell, L. D., & Paulanka, B. J. (2004). *Transcultural health care—A culturally competent approach* (2nd ed.). Philadelphia: F.A. Davis.

Reynolds, J. (2004). Letters: Tips for talking to patients. *Nursing 2004, 34*(12), 10.

Sheldon, L. K. (2004). *Communication for nurses: Talking with patients.* Boston: Jones and Bartlett.

Stewart, C. J., & Cash, W. B. (2006). *Interviewing: Principles and practice* (11th ed.). New York: McGraw-Hill.

Tamparo, C. D., & Lindh, W. Q. (2007). *Therapeutic communication for health professionals* (3rd ed.). Thompson Delmar Learning.

Tannen, D. (2001). *You just don't understand: Women and men in conversation* (1st Quill ed.). New York: Ballantine.

Ufema, J. (2004). Insights on death and dying: Three keys to communication. *Nursing 2004, 34*(10), 12.

Wilkinson, J. M., & Ahern, N. R. (2009). *Nursing diagnosis handbook* (9th ed.). Upper Saddle River, NJ: Prentice Hall.

CHAPTER 12

Bandura, A. (1971). Analysis of modeling processes. In A. Bandura (Ed.), *Psychological modeling.* Chicago: Aldine.

Bloom, B. S., et al. (1956). *Bloom's taxonomy of educational objectives, Handbook I: Cognitive domain.* Boston: Allyn & Bacon.

Byrnes, J. P. (2001). *Cognitive development and learning in instructional context.* Boston: Allyn & Bacon.

Carpenito, L. J. (2008). *Handbook of nursing diagnosis* (12th ed.). Philadelphia: Lippincott.

Cotugna, N., Vickery, C. E., Carpenter-Haefele, K. M. (2005). Evaluation of literacy level of patient education pages in health-related journals. *Journal of Community Health, 30* (3), 213–216.

Doak, C. C., Doak, L. G., & Root, J. H. (1996). *Teaching patients with low literacy skills* (2nd ed.). Philadelphia: Lippincott.

London, F., & Miller, C. J. (2000). *No time to teach? A nurse's guide to patient and family education.* Philadelphia: Lippincott.

McCloskey, J. C., & Bulechek, G. M. (Eds.). (2007). *Nursing interventions classification (NIC).* (5th ed.). St. Louis, MO: Mosby-Year Book.

Moorehead, S., Johnson, M., & Maas, M. (2003). *Nursing outcomes classifications* (3rd ed.). St. Louis, MO: Mosby.

O'Connor, A. B. (2006). *Clinical instruction and evaluation: A teaching resource* (2nd ed.). Boston: Jones and Bartlett Publishers.

CHAPTER 13

American Nurses Association. (2003). *Code for nurses.* Silver Spring, MD: Author.

Chase, S. K. (1997). Charting critical thinking: Nursing judgments and patient outcomes. *Dimensions of Critical Care Nursing, 16*(2), 102–111.

Cirone, N. (1998). Taking orders by phone? *Nursing 98, 28*(8), 56–57.

Coty, E., Davis, J., & Angell, L. (2002). *Documentation: The language of nursing.* Upper Saddle River, NJ: Prentice Hall.

Iyer, P. W., & Camp, N. H. (1999). *Nursing documentation* (3rd ed.). St. Louis, MO: Elsevier.

Joint Commission on Accreditation of Healthcare Organizations. (2000). *2000 accreditation manual for hospitals.* Chicago: Author.

Joint Commission on Accreditation of Healthcare Organizations. (2002). *Management of information update 3/14/02.* Chicago: Author.

Marrelli, T. M. (2001). *Nursing documentation handbook.* St. Louis, MO: Elsevier.

Murphy, E. K. (2003). Charting by exception. *AORN Journal, 78*(5): 821–823.

Murphy, J., & Burke, L. J. (1990, May). Charting by exception: A more efficient way to document. *Nursing 90, 20,* 65, 68–69.

Rasmussen, N. (1994). Clinical pathways of care: The route to better communication. *Nursing, 24*(2), 47–49.

Simpson, R. L. (1994). Ensuring patient data privacy, confidentiality, and security. *Nursing Management, 25*(7), 18–20.

Springhouse Corporation. (2006). *Chart smart: The A–Z guide to better nursing documentation.* Springhouse, PA: Author.

Sullivan, G. H. (2004). Legally speaking: Does your charting measure up? *RN, 67*(3), 61–65.

CHAPTER 14

Grubbs, P., & Blasband, B. (2005). *The long-term care nursing assistant* (3rd ed.). Upper Saddle River, NJ: Prentice Hall.

Irvine, K., & Hilton, E. (2003). *Ensuring a HIPAA-compliant informed consent process.* Boston: Thompson-Centerwatch.

Kongstvedt, P. R. (2007). *Essentials of managed health care handbook* (5th ed.). Sudbury, MA: Jones and Bartlett Publishers.

Pulliam, J. (2005). *The nursing assistant: Acute, subacute and long-term care* (4th ed.). Upper Saddle River, NJ: Prentice Hall.

Wyler-Lawm, P. (2002). Legal nurse consulting—Hospital regulations. *Nursing Economics, 18*(6), 312.

CHAPTER 15

American Psychiatric Association. (2004). *Diagnostic and statistical manual of mental disorders* (4th ed., text revision). Washington, DC: American Psychiatric Press.

Bowlby, J. (1983). *Attachment* (2nd ed.). New York: Basic Books.

Duska, R., & Whelan, M. (1975). *Moral development: A guide to Piaget and Kohlberg.* Missionary Society of St. Paul the Apostle in the State of New York.

Erikson, E. H. (1995). *Childhood and society.* New York: Vintage.

Erikson, E. H., & Erikson, J. M. (1997). *The life cycle completed.* New York: Norton.

Fowler, J., & Keen, S. (1985). *Life maps: Conversations in the journey of faith.* Waco, TX: Word Books.

Hollander, A. (1980). *How to help your child have a spiritual life: A parents' guide to inner development.* New York: A and W Publishers.

Holmes, J. (1993). *John Bowlby and attachment theory.* New York: Taylor and Francis.

Morris, C. G., & Maisto, A. A. (2001). *Understanding psychology* (5th ed.). Upper Saddle River, NJ: Prentice Hall.

Piaget, J. (1966). *The origin of intelligence in children.* Guildford, CT: International Universities Press.

Piaget, J., Gruber, H. E., & Voneche, J. J. (1995). *The essential Piaget* (100th Anniversary ed.). New York: Jason Aronson.

Roehlkepartain, E. C., et al. (2006). *The handbook of spiritual development in childhood and adolescence.* Thousand Oaks, CA: Sage Publications.

Schultz, D., & Schultz, S. E. (2005). *Theories of personalities* (8th ed.). Boston: Cengage Learning.

Wallin, D. (2008). *Attachment in psychotherapy*. New York: Guilford Publications.

CHAPTER 16

American Psychiatric Association. (2004). *Diagnostic and statistical manual of mental disorders (text revision)* (4th ed.). Washington, DC: American Psychiatric Press.

Andrews, M. M., & Boyle, J. S. (2008). *Transcultural concepts in nursing care* (5th ed.). Philadelphia: Lippincott Williams & Wilkins.

Ball, J., & Bindler, R. (2008). *Pediatric nursing: Caring for children* (4th ed.). Upper Saddle River, NJ: Prentice Hall.

Bowlby, J. (1983). *Attachment* (2nd ed.). New York: Basic Books.

Carpenito-Moyet, L. J. (2006). *Handbook of nursing diagnosis* (11th ed.). Philadelphia: Lippincott Williams & Wilkins.

Carter, B., & McGoldrick, M. (2005). *The expanded family life cycle—Individual, family, and social perspectives* (3rd ed.). Needham Heights, MA: Allyn & Bacon.

Cox, H., Hinz, M., Lubno, M. A., Scott-Tilley, D., Newfield, S., McCarthy Slater, M., et al. (2002). *Clinical applications of nursing diagnosis: Adult, child, women's, psychiatric, gerontic, and home health considerations* (4th ed.). Philadelphia: F.A. Davis.

Duska, R., & Whelan, M. (1975). *Moral development: A guide to Piaget and Kohlberg.* Missionary Society of St. Paul the Apostle in the State of New York.

Erikson, E. H. (1995). *Childhood and society* (New ed.). New York: Vintage.

Erikson, E. H., & Erikson, J. M. (1997). *The life cycle completed.* New York: Norton.

Fowler, J., & Keen, S. (1985). *Life maps: Conversations in the journey of faith.* Waco, TX: Word Books.

Hollander, A. (1980). *How to help your child have a spiritual life: A parents' guide to inner development.* New York: A and W Publishers.

Morris, C. G., & Maisto, A. A. (2001). *Understanding psychology* (5th ed.). Upper Saddle River, NJ: Prentice Hall.

Piaget, J. (1966). *The origin of intelligence in children.* Guildford, CT: International Universities Press.

Piaget, J., Gruber, H. E., & Voneche, J. J. (1995). *The essential Piaget* (100th Anniversary ed.). New York: Jason Aronson.

Towle, M. A., & Adam, E. D. (2008). *Maternal-child nursing care.* Upper Saddle River, NJ: Pearson-Prentice Hall.

U.S. Bureau of the Census Population Report. (2000). Washington DC: U.S. Department of Commerce.

CHAPTER 17

American Psychiatric Association. (2004). *Diagnostic and statistical manual of mental disorders* (4th ed., text revision). Washington, DC: American Psychiatric Press.

Anderson, R. N., Minino, A. M., Hoyert, D. L., & Rosenberg, H. M. (2001, May 18). Comparability of cause of death between ICD-9 and ICD-10: Preliminary estimates. *National Vital Statistics Report, 49*(2).

Arnold, E., & Boggs, K. U. (2007). *Interpersonal relationships—Professional communication skills for nurses* (5th ed.). Philadelphia: Saunders.

Carpenito-Moyet, L. J. (2008). *Nursing diagnosis: Application to clinical practice* (12th ed.). Philadelphia: Lippincott.

Dossey, B. M., & Dossey, L. (1998). Body-mind-spirit: Attending to holistic care. *American Journal of Nursing, 98*(8), 35–38.

Eby, L., & Brown, N. J. (2009). *Mental health nursing care* (2nd ed.). Upper Saddle River, NJ: Pearson-Prentice Hall.

Edelman, C. L., & Mandle, C. L. (2006). *Health promotion throughout the life span* (6th ed.). St. Louis, MO: Mosby.

Erikson, E. H. (1963). *Childhood and society* (2nd ed.). New York: Norton.

Erikson, E. H., & Erikson, J. M. (1997). *The life cycle completed.* New York: W.W. Norton.

Fontaine, K. L. (2008). *Mental health nursing* (6th ed.). Upper Saddle River, NJ: Prentice Hall.

NANDA International. (2009). *NANDA International Nursing Diagnoses: Definitions & Classifications 2009–2011.* Oxford, UK: Wiley-Blackwell.

Reynolds, W. J., & Scott, B. (2000). Do nurses and other professional helpers normally display much empathy? *Journal of Advanced Nursing, 31*(1), 226–234.

Rollins, J. A. (2005). *Meeting children's psychosocial needs across the health-care continuum.* Austin, TX: Pro-Ed Publishers.

CHAPTER 18

Anweiler, N. (2000). Another dying patient. *Nursing 2000, 30*(11), 32.

Benton, R. E. (1978). *Death and dying: Principles and practices in patient care.* New York: Van Nostrand.

Berman, J. D., & Straus, S. E. (2004). Implementing a research agenda for complementary and alternative medicine. *Annual Review of Medicine, 55,* 239–254.

Carpenito, L. J. (2005). *Handbook of nursing diagnosis* (11th ed.). Philadelphia: Lippincott.

Fontaine, K. L. (2005). *Complementary and alternative therapies* (2nd ed.). Upper Saddle River, NJ: Prentice Hall.

Furman, J. (2002, February). What you should know about chronic grief. *Nursing 2002, 32,* 56.

Gallob, R. (2003). Reiki: A supportive therapy in nursing practice and self-care for nurses. *Journal of the New York State Nurses' Association, 34*(1), 9–13.

Hart, C. L., Hole, D. J., Lawlow, D. A., Smith, G. D., & Lever, T. F. (2007). Effect of conjugal bereavement on mortality of the bereaved spouse in participants of the Renfrew/Paisley study. *Journal of Epidemiology and Community Health, 61,* 455–460.

Hospice and Palliative Nurses Association. (1999). *Hospice and palliative nursing practice review* (3rd ed.). Iowa: Kendall/Hunt.

Hospice Foundation of America. *Eight myths about children and loss.* San Ramon, CA: Author. Retrieved January 28, 2008, from www.hospicefoundation.org/griefandloss/myths_children.asp.

Jeffers, S. L. (2001). Stages of grief: Fact or fiction? *Kansas Nurse, 76(7),* 9–10. Retrieved November 27, 2007 from http://findarticles.com/p/articles/mi_qa3940/is_/ai_n8962684.

Kübler-Ross, E. (1969). *On death and dying.* New York: Macmillan.

Kübler-Ross, E. (1974). *Questions and answers on death and dying.* New York: Macmillan.

Kübler-Ross, E. (1975). *Death: The final stage of growth.* Upper Saddle River, NJ: Prentice Hall.

Kübler-Ross, E. (1978). *To live until we say good-bye.* Upper Saddle River, NJ: Prentice Hall.

Linde, K., Hondras, M., Vickers, A., et al. (2001). Systematic reviews of complementary therapies—An annotated bibliography. Part 3: Homeopathy. *BMC Complementary and Alternative Medicine, 1*(1), 4.

NANDA International. (2009). *NANDA International Nursing Diagnoses: Definitions & Classifications 2009-2011.* Oxford, UK: Wiley-Blackwell.

Oschman, J. L. (2000). *Energy medicine: The scientific basis of bioenergy therapies.* Philadelphia, PA: Churchill Livingstone.

Ross, H. (2001, April). Islamic tradition at the end of life. *MEDSURG Nursing, 10*(2), 83.

Ufema, J. (2001-2002). Insights on death and dying (Monthly column). *Nursing* (February, April, June, October, & November 2001; January & March 2002).

Wolfelt, Alan D. (2003). *The mourner's bill of rights.* Retrieved January 28, 2008, www.hospicesj/.ca/pdfs/mourners_bill_of_rights.pdf.

Worden, W. J. (2003). *Grief counseling and grief therapy: A handbook for the mental health practitioner.* (3rd ed.). New York: Routledge.

Wrede-Seaman, L. (1999). *Symptom management algorithms: A handbook for palliative care* (2nd ed.). Washington: Intellicard.

CHAPTER 19

Adams, E. D., & Towle, M. A. (2009). *Pediatric nursing care.* Upper Saddle River, NJ: Prentice Hall.

Andrews, M. M., & Boyle, J. S. (2008). *Transcultural concepts in nursing care* (5th ed.). Philadelphia: Lippincott Williams & Wilkins.

Ball, J., & Bindler, R. (2003). *Pediatric nursing: Caring for children* (3rd ed.). Upper Saddle River, NJ: Prentice Hall.

Carter, B., & McGoldrick, M. (1999). *The expanded family life cycle—Individual, family, and social perspectives* (3rd ed.). Needham Heights, MA: Allyn & Bacon.

Cox, H., Hinz, M., Lubno, M. A., Scott-Tilley, D., Newfield, S., McCarthy Slater, M., et al. (2002). *Clinical applications of nursing diagnosis: Adult, child, women's, psychiatric, gerontic, and home health considerations* (4th ed.). Philadelphia: F.A. Davis.

Jarvis, C. (2008). *Physical examination and health assessment.* St Louis: Saunders, Elsevier.

Mehta, M. (2003). Assessing respiratory status. *Nursing, 33*(2), 54-56.

Towle, M. A. (2009). *Maternal-newborn nursing care.* Upper Saddle River, NJ: Prentice Hall.

Weber, J., & Kelley, J. (2007). *Health assessment in nursing.* Baltimore: Lippincott Williams & Wilkins.

CHAPTER 20

Ackley, B. J., & Ladwig, G. B. (2006). *Nursing diagnosis handbook* (7th ed.). St. Louis, MO: Mosby.

Berman, A., Snyder, S., & Jackson, C. (2009). *Skills in clinical nursing* (6th ed.). Upper Saddle River, NJ: Prentice Hall.

Beuscher, T. L. (1998). Community outreach: Foot care for the elderly: A winning proposition. *Home Healthcare Nurse, 16*(1), 37-44.

Calianno, C. (2002). Patient hygiene part 2—Skin care: Keeping the outside healthy. *Nursing 2002, 32*(6). Page supplement.

Carpenito, L. J. (2007). *Handbook of nursing diagnosis* (12th ed.). Philadelphia: Lippincott.

Dugan, M. B. (2003). *Living with hearing loss.* Washington, DC: Gallaudet University Press.

Effects of hydrogen peroxide rinses on the normal oral mucosa. (1993). *Nursing Research, 6,* 332-337.

Eshleman, J., & Davidhizar, R. (2002). When your patient complains of hair loss. *Home Health Care Nurse, 20*(12), 778-782.

Grap, M. J., Munro, C. L., Ashtiani, B., & Bryant, S. (2003). Oral care interventions in critical care: Frequency and documentation. *American Journal of Critical Care, 12,* 113-118.

Kydd, A. (2002). Focusing nursing care on the older person. *Nursing Times, 98*(33), 13.

Lassieur, A. (2000). *Head lice (my health).* New York: Frank Watts, Inc.

Little, J. W. (Ed.). (2002). *Dental management of medically compromised patients.* St. Louis, MO: Mosby.

Marieb, E. N. (2009). *Human anatomy and physiology* (7th ed.). Upper Saddle River, NJ: Prentice Hall.

NANDA International. (2009). *NANDA International Nursing Diagnoses: Definitions & Classifications 2009-2011.* Oxford, UK: Wiley-Blackwell.

Reed, S. (2002). Implementing best practices in pressure ulcer prevention. *Nursing Times, 97*(24), 69.

Wilkinson, J. (2001). Patient hygiene. Part I, oral care: The inside story. *Nursing, 31*(5), 1.

Wilkinson, J. M., & Ahern, N. R. (2009). *Nursing diagnosis handbook* (9th ed.). Upper Saddle River, NJ: Prentice Hall.

CHAPTER 21

Ackley, B. J., & Ladwig, G. B. (2006). *Nursing diagnosis handbook: A guide to planning care* (6th ed.). St. Louis, MO: Mosby.

Bickley, L., & Szilagyi, P. C. (2002). *Bates' guide to physical examination and history taking* (7th ed.). Philadelphia, PA: Lippincott Williams & Wilkins.

Boggan, B. (2003). *Alcohol, chemistry, and you: Absorption of ethyl alcohol.* Retrieved June 19, 2008, from http://www.chemcases.com/alcohol/alc-04.htm.

Chobanian, A. V., Bakris, G. L., Black, H. R., et al. (2003). Seventh report of the Joint National Committee on Prevention, Detection, Evaluation, and Treatment of High Blood Pressure. *Hypertension, 42*(6), 1206-1252.

Farnell, S., Maxwell, L., Tan, S., Rhodes, A., & Philips, B. (2005). Temperature measurement: Comparison of non-invasive methods used in adult critical care. *Journal of Clinical Nursing, 14*(5), 632-639.

Lance, R., Link, M., Padua, M., Clavell, L., Johnson, G., & Knebel, A. (2000). Comparison of different methods of obtaining orthostatic vital signs. *Clinical Nursing Research, 9*(4), 479-491.

Marieb, E. N. (2009). *Human anatomy and physiology* (7th ed.). Upper Saddle River, NJ: Prentice Hall.

Measuring blood pressure at home is valuable. (2005, December). *Journal of Family Practice, 54*(12), 1031. Retrieved June 23, 2008, from Medline.

Moran, D. S., & Mendal, L. (2002). Core temperature measurement. *Sports Medicine, 32*(14), 879-886.

NANDA International. (2009). *NANDA International Nursing Diagnoses: Definitions & Classifications 2009-2011*. Oxford, UK: Wiley-Blackwell.

Sundquist, J., Winkleby, M. A., Pudaric, S. (2001). Cardiovascular disease risk factors among older Black, Mexican-American, and White women and men: An analysis of NHANES III, 1988-1994. *Journal of the American Geriatrics Society, 49*(2), 109-116.

Yucha, C., Yang, M., Tsai, P., & Calderon, K. (2003, March). Comparison of blood pressure measurement consistency using tonometric and automated oscillometric instruments. *Journal of Nursing Measurement, 11*(1), 73-86.

CHAPTER 22

Ackley, B. J., & Ladwig, G. B. (2006). *Nursing diagnosis handbook* (7th ed.). St. Louis, MO: Mosby.

American Academy of Pain Medicine. (2002). The use of opioids for the treatment of chronic pain (Joint consensus statement from the American Academy of Pain Medicine and the American Pain Society). Retrieved May 1, 2008 from www.productpub/statements. painmed.org.

American Journal of Nursing. (2002). Unacceptable pain levels. *American Journal of Nursing, 102*(5), 75-77.

Blanchard, R. (2002). Why study pain? A qualitative analysis of medical and nursing faculty and students' knowledge of and attitudes to cancer pain management. *Journal of Palliative Medicine, 5*(1), 57.

Briggs, E. (2002). The nursing management of pain in older people. *Nursing Older People, 14*(7), 23-29.

Bucknall, T., Manias, E., & Botti, M. (2001). Acute pain management: Implications of scientific evidence for nursing practice in the postoperative context. *International Journal of Nursing Practice, 7*(4), 266.

D'Arcy, Y. (2006). Which analgesic is right for my patient? *Nursing 2006, 36*(7), 50-55.

D'Arcy, Y. (2007). Managing pain in a patient who's drug-dependent. *Nursing 2007, 37*(3), 37-40.

Edwards, H. E., et al. (2001). Determinants of nurses' intention to administer opioids for pain relief. *Nursing & Health Sciences, 3*(3), 149.

Guyton, A., & Hall, J. E. (2000). *Textbook of medical physiology* (10th ed.). Philadelphia: W. B. Saunders.

Holland, N., & Adams, M. P. (2007). *Core concepts in pharmacology* (2nd ed.). Upper Saddle River, NJ: Prentice Hall.

Houldin, A. D. (2002). *Patients with cancer: Understanding the psychological pain.* Philadelphia: Lippincott Williams and Wilkins.

Kanner, R. (2001). *Pain management secrets.* Philadelphia: Lippincott Williams and Wilkins.

Kastanias, P., Snaith, K. E., & Robinson, S. Patient-controlled oral analgesia: A low-tech solution in a high-tech world. *Pain Management Nursing, 7*(3), 126-132.

McCaffery, M. (1979). *Nursing management of the patient with pain* (2nd ed.). Philadelphia: Lippincott.

McCaffery, M. (2002). *Pain management revised—The nurse's active role in opioid administration* [CD-ROM]. Philadelphia: Lippincott Williams & Wilkins.

McCaffery, M., & Pasero, C. (1999). *Pain: Clinical Manual* (2nd ed.). St. Louis, MO: Mosby.

Melzack, R., & Wall, P. (1965). Pain mechanism: A new theory. *Science, 150,* 171-179.

NANDA International. (2009). *NANDA International Nursing Diagnoses: Definitions & Classifications 2009-2011*. Oxford, UK: Wiley-Blackwell.

Pasero, C. L. (1997). Using the Faces scale to assess pain. *American Journal of Nursing, 97*(7), 19-20.

Pasero, C., & McCaffery, M. (1996). Alternative use of PCA. *American Journal of Nursing, 96,* 65-68.

Schechter, N. L., Berde, C. B., & Yaster, M. (2002). *Pain in infants, children and adolescents.* Philadelphia: Lippincott Williams & Wilkins.

Slaughter, A., Pasero, C., & Manworren, R. (2002). Unacceptable pain levels: A process to prompt pain relief. *American Journal of Nursing, 102*(5), 75.

Vega-Stromberg, T., Holmes, S., Gorski, L., & Johnson, B. P. (2002). Road to excellence in pain management: Research, outcomes and direction (ROAD). *Journal of Nursing Care Quality, 17*(1), 15.

Wong, D. L. (2001). *Whaley and Wong's essentials of pediatric nursing* (6th ed.). St. Louis, MO: Mosby.

CHAPTER 23

Ackley, B. J., & Ladwig, G. B. (2006). *Nursing diagnosis handbook: A guide to planning care* (7th ed.). St. Louis, MO: Mosby.

Carpenito, L. J. (2005). *Handbook of nursing diagnosis* (11th ed.). Philadelphia: Lippincott.

Clinical rounds: Bedrest may not be best after all. (2005). *Nursing 2005, 35*(8), 33.

Duimel-Peeterrs, L. (2005). Wound wise: Preventing pressure ulcers with massage? Some say it works others disagree; ay, there's the rub. *American Journal of Nursing, 76*(8), 31-33.

Graves, G. (1998, March). The 9 habits of highly successful sleepers. *Good Housekeeping*, pp. 82, 84, 88.

Guyton, A. C., & Hall, J. E. (2006). *Textbook of medical physiology* (11th ed.). Philadelphia: W. B. Saunders.

Photo guide: Performing passive range of motion. (2006). *Nursing 2006, 36*(3), 50-51.

Richardson, S. (2003). Effects of relaxation and imagery on sleep of critically ill adults. *Dimensions of Critical Care Nursing, 22*(4), 182-190.

Smith, S. E., Duell, D. J., & Martin, B. C. (2008). *Clinical nursing skills: Basic to advanced skills* (7th ed.). Upper Saddle River, NJ: Prentice Hall.

Trupp, R. J. (2004). The heart of sleep: Sleep-disordered breathing and heart failure. *Journal of Cardiovascular Nursing, 19*(6), 567-574.

Waters, T. R. (2007). When is it safe to manually lift a patient? *American Journal of Nursing, 107*(8), 53-58.

CHAPTER 24

Baharestani, M., Cuddigan, J., Domer, B., Edsberg, L., Langemo, D., Posthauer, M. E., Ratliff, C., & Taler, G. National pressure ulcer advisory panel's updated pressure ulcer staging system. *Dermatology Nurse, 19*(4), 343-349.

Baranoski, S., & Ayello, E. A. (2007). *Wound care essentials* (2nd ed.). Philadelphia: Lippincott Williams & Wilkins.

Black, J., Baharestani, M., Cuddigan, J., et al. (2007). National pressure ulcer advisory panel's updated pressure ulcer staging system. Advances in skin & wound care. *Journal of Preventive Healing, 20*(5), 269-274.

Burke, K. M., LeMone, P., & Mohn-Brown, E. L. (2007). *Medical–surgical nursing care.* (2nd ed.). Upper Saddle River, NJ: Prentice Hall.

Capobianco, M. L., & McDonald, D. D. (1996, November/December). Factors affecting the predictive validity of the Braden scale. *Advances in Wound Care: The Journal for Prevention and Healing, 9,* 32–36.

Carpenito, L. J. (2005). *Handbook of nursing diagnosis* (11th ed.). Philadelphia: Lippincott.

Federal Register. (2007). Centers for Medicare & Medicaid Services (CMS). Deficit Reduction Act of 2005.

Hahn, J. F., Olsen, C. L., Tomaselli, N., & Goldberg, M. (2002). Wounds: Nursing care and product selection (*Nursing Spectrum* self-study module). Retrieved April 5, 2008 from http://nsweb.nursingspectrum.com/ce

Hess, C. T. (2002). *Clinical guide to wound care* (4th ed.). Philadelphia: Lippincott Williams & Wilkins.

International Committee on Wound Management. (1996). Cost effective wound care. Evaluating your supply use to prepare for managed care (ICWM World Council Consensus Statement). *Ostomy/Wound Management, 42*(2), 72, 74–76.

Maklebust, J., & Sieggreen, M. (2000). *Pressure ulcers: Guidelines for prevention and nursing management* (2nd ed.). Springhouse, PA: Springhouse Publishing.

McConnell, E. A. (1997). Clinical do's and don'ts: Using dry heat to promote healing. *Nursing 27*(5), 22.

NANDA International. (2009). *NANDA International Nursing Diagnoses: Definitions & Classifications 2009–2011.* Oxford, UK: Wiley-Blackwell.

Panel for the Prediction and Prevention of Pressure Ulcers in Adults (PPPPUA). (1994). U.S. Department of Health and Human Services. Clinical practice guidelines #3 (AHCPR Pub. No. 92–0047). Rockville, MD.

Pieper, B., Sugrue, M., Weiland, M., Sprague, K., & Heiman, C. (1998). Risk factors, prevention methods, and wound care for patients with pressure ulcers. *Clinical Nurse Specialist, 12*(1), 7–14.

Sisk, B. (2002). Pressure sore update. (Electronic Version). *Nurse Scribe.*

Sterling, C. (1996, November). Methods of wound assessment documentation: A study. *Nursing Standard, 11*(10), 38–41.

Stotts, N. A. (1990, February). Seeing red, yellow, and black. The three-color concept of wound care. *Nursing 90, 20,* 59–61.

Van Rijswijk, L. (1996, August). The fundamentals of wound assessment. *Ostomy/Wound Management, 42*(7), 40–42, 44, 46, 48–50.

Wound nursing care and product selection—Part I. (Electronic Version). (2003). *Nursing Spectrum.* Retrieved April 14, 2008 from www.nurse.com/ce/CE80-60.

CHAPTER 25

Adams, E. D., & Towle, M. A. (2009). *Pediatric nursing care.* Upper Saddle River, NJ: Prentice Hall.

Berman, A., Snyder, S. J., Kozier, B., & Erb, G. (2008). *Fundamentals of nursing: Concepts, process, and practice* (8th ed.). Upper Saddle River, NJ: Pearson Education.

Como, D. (Ed.). (2002). *Mosby's medical, nursing, and allied health dictionary.* St. Louis, MO: Mosby.

Grodner, M., Long, S., & Walkingshaw, B. C. (2007). *Foundations & clinical applications of nutrition. A nursing approach* (4th ed.). St. Louis, MO: Mosby-Elsevier.

Lane, K. (Ed.). (1999). *The Merck manual.* West Point, PA: Merck.

London, M. L., Ladewig, P. W., Ball, J. W., & Bindler, R. C. (2007). *Maternal & child nursing care* (2nd ed.). Upper Saddle River, NJ: Pearson, Prentice Hall.

Nettina, S. M. (Ed.). (2005). *The Lippincott manual of nursing practice.* (8th ed.). Philadelphia: Lippincott-Raven.

Pagana, K. D., & Pagana, T. J. (2003). *Mosby's diagnostic and laboratory test reference.* St. Louis, MO: Mosby.

Phillips, L. (2001). *Manual of I.V. therapeutics.* Philadelphia: F.A. Davis.

Smith, S. F., Duell, D. J., Martin, B. C. (2008). *Clinical nursing skills: Basic to advanced skills.* (7th ed.). Upper Saddle River, NJ: Prentice Hall.

U.S. Department of Health and Human Services. (2007). *National health and nutrition examination survey.* Washingtion, DC: Author.

Venes, D. (Ed.). (2005). *Taber's cyclopedic medical dictionary.* Philadelphia: F.A. Davis.

Whitney, E. N., Cataldo, C. B., & Rolfes, S. R. (2002). *Understanding normal and clinical nutrition.* Belmont, CA: Wadsworth/Thomson Learning.

Wilkinson, J. M. (2009). *Nursing diagnosis handbook* (9th ed.). Upper Saddle River, NJ: Prentice Hall Health.

CHAPTER 26

Ahearn, N. R., Wilkinson, J. M. (2008). *Nursing diagnosis handbook.* Upper Saddle River, NJ: Prentice Hall Health.

Alexander, M. F., Fawcett, J. N., & Runciman, P. J., et al. (2006). *Nursing practice: Hospital and home—The adult* (3rd ed.). St. Louis: Churchill Livingstone.

Beers, M. H., & Lane, K. (Ed.). (2006). *The Merck manual* (18th ed.). West Point, PA: Merck.

Como, D. (Ed.). (2002). *Mosby's medical, nursing, and allied health dictionary.* St. Louis, MO: Mosby.

Nettina, S. M. (Ed.). (2005). *The Lippincott manual of nursing practice.* (8th ed.). Philadelphia: Lippincott-Raven.

Pagana, K. D., & Pagana, T. J. (2003). *Mosby's diagnostic and laboratory test reference.* St. Louis, MO: Mosby.

Phillips, L. (2005). *Manual of I.V. therapeutics* (4th ed.). Philadelphia: F.A. Davis.

Springhouse. (Ed.). (2007). *Fluids and electrolytes made incredibly easy.* Springhouse, PA: Springhouse.

Venes, D. (2005). *Taber's cyclopedic medical dictionary.* Philadelphia: F.A. Davis.

CHAPTER 27

Ackley, B. J., & Ladwig, G. B. (2006). *Nursing diagnosis handbook: A guide to planning care* (7th ed.). St. Louis, MO: Mosby.

American Journal of Nursing. (2005). Enteral tube flushing: What you think are the best practices may not be. *American Journal of Nursing, 105*(3), 58–63.

Berman, A., Snyder, S. J., Kozier, B., & Erb, G. (2008). *Fundaments of nursing: Concepts, process, and practice* (8th ed.). Upper Saddle River, NJ: Pearson, Prentice Hall.

Beyea, S., & Nicoll, L. (1996). Back to basics: Administering IM injections the right way. *American Journal of Nursing, 96*(1), 34–35.

Borkgren, M., & Gronkiewicz, C. (1995). Update your asthma care from hospital to home. *American Journal of Nursing, 95*(1), 28.

Cohen, M. R. (2002). *Medication errors.* Huntingdon Valley, PA: American Pharmaceutical Association.

Deglin, J. H., & Vallerand, A. H. (2007). Medication errors: Improving practices & patient safety. In Davis drug guide for nurses (10th ed.). Philadelphia: F.A. Davis.

Glazer, G. (2002, February 28). Legislative column: Medication administration interventions that must be performed by a registered nurse. *Journal of Issues in Nursing* [Online]. Retrieved February 1, 2008 from www.nursingworld.org/ojin/tpclg/leg_12.htm.

Hathaway, L. (2006). Breathe easier: A step-by-step guide to MDIS. *Nursing Made Incredibly Easy, 4*(6), 22-23.

Highleyman, L. (2002, September). *Preventing HCV transmission in personal care settings.* San Francisco: Hepatitis Support Project.

Institute for Safe Medication Practices. (2007). Error-prone conditions that lead to student nurse-related errors. *Medication Safety Alert, 12*(21).

Karch, A. (2008). *Focus on nursing pharmacology* (4th ed.). Philadelphia: Lippincott Williams & Wilkins.

Klausmeier, C. (1993). U.S. Drug Abuse Regulation and Control Act of 1970: An introduction. *Hyperreal Archive of Alt Drugs*.

Marieb, E. N. (2009). *Human anatomy and physiology* (7th ed.). Upper Saddle River, NJ: Prentice Hall.

McCloskey, J. C., & Bulechek, G. M. (2007). *Nursing interventions classification (NIC).* (5th ed.). St. Louis, MO: Mosby-Year Book.

Miller, D. (2000). *Nurse's clinical guide: Medication administration*. Philadelphia: Springhouse—Lippincott Williams & Wilkins.

Moses, S. (2000). Cation-exchange resin. In *Family practice notebook* [Online]. Retrieved January 29, 2003, from www. fpnotebook.com/REN101.htm.

National Institute for Occupational Safety and Health (1999, November). *Alert—Preventing needlestick injuries in health care settings* (Publication No. 2000-108). Cincinnati, OH: Author.

National League for Nursing. (2001). *Basic proficiency in medication administration* (4th version). New York: Author.

Rokosky, J. M. (2005). Teaching correct use of inhaled medications home healthcare nurse. *Journal for the Home Care and Hospice Professional, 23*(12), 766-774.

Sifton, D. W. (Ed.). (2001). *Physician's desk reference* (56th ed.). Montvale, NJ: Medical Economics.

Smith, S. F., Duell, D. J., & Martin, B. C. (2008). *Clinical nursing skills: Basic to advanced skills* (7th ed.). Upper Saddle River, NJ: Prentice Hall.

Venes, D. (Ed.). (2005). *Taber's cyclopedic medical dictionary* (20th ed.). Philadelphia: F.A. Davis.

U.S. Food and Drug Administration. (2008). Title 21—Food and drugs Chapter 13—Drug abuse and prevention and control, subchapter 1—Control and enforcement, Part B—Authority to control; Standards and schedules. Retrieved May 2, 2008, from www.dea.gov/pubs/csa/812.htm#b; www.fda.gov/fdac/features/2001/301_preg.html#categories.

Wilson, B.A., Shannon, M.T., & Stang, C. L. (2003). *Nurse's drug guide.* Upper Saddle River, NJ: Prentice Hall.

Wolfe, S. (Ed.). (2001). Safer needle devices, part 1. *RN, 62*(10), 59.

Woodrow, R. (2002). *Essentials of pharmacology for health occupations* (4th ed.). Clifton Park, NY: Delmar.

Worthington, K.A. (2002). Hazardous drugs: Handling medications can pose danger to nurses. *American Journal of Nursing, 102*(5), 120.

CHAPTER 28

Blackwood, H. S. (2005). Help your patient downsize with bariatric surgery. *Nursing 2005, 35*(9), (Supplement Medical-Surgical Insider), 4-5.

Bryant, D., & Fleischer, I. (2000). Changing an ostomy appliance. *Nursing* [Online], *30*(11), 51.

Carpenito, L. J. (2005). *Handbook of nursing diagnosis* (11th ed.). Philadelphia: Lippincott.

Day, A., & Bean, K. B. (2006). LPN's mission: Where do LPNs go from here? *Gastroenterology Nursing, 29*(2), 157.

Gauthier, P., & Bean, K. B. (2006). Fundamentals of G.I. *Gastroenterology Nursing, 29*(2), 160.

Guyton, A. C., & Hall, J. E. (2005). *Textbook of medical physiology* (11th ed.). Philadelphia: Elsevier/Saunders.

NANDA International. (2009). *NANDA International Nursing Diagnoses: Definitions & Classifications 2009-2011*. Oxford, UK: Wiley-Blackwell.

Nettina, S. M. (2005). *Lippincott manual of nursing practice* (8th ed.). Philadelphia: Lippincott Williams and Wilkins.

Rushing, C. (2005). Clinical do's and don'ts: Inserting a nasogastric tube. *Nursing 2005, 35*(5), 22.

SGNA position statement: Role delineation of LPN/LVN in gastroenterology. (2006). *Gastroenterology Nursing, 29*(1), 60-61.

Vickery, G. (1997). Basics of constipation. *Gastroenterology Nursing, 20*(4), 125-128.

CHAPTER 29

Ackley, B. J., & Ladwig, G. B. (2006). *Nursing diagnosis handbook* (7th ed.). St. Louis, MO: Mosby.

Benko, T., Cooke, E.A., McNally, M.A., & Mollan, R. (2000). Graduated compression stockings—knee length or thigh length. *Clinical Orthopaedics and Related Research, 383*, 197-203.

Brown, B. (2001). Promoting patient safety through preoperative patient verification. *AORN Journal, 74*(11), 690.

Browne, N.T., et al. (2006). *Nursing care of the pediatric surgical patient* (2nd ed.). Boston: Jones and Bartlett.

Brush, K.A. (2007). Abdominal compartment syndrome—The pressure is on. *Nursing 2007, 37*(7), 37-40.

Busen, N. H. (2001). Perioperative preparation of the adolescent surgical patient. *AORN Journal, 73*(2), 337-341.

Church, V. (2000). Staying on guard for DVT & PE. *Nursing 2000, 30*(2).

Daniels, S. M. (2007). Improving hospital care for surgical patients. *Nursing 2007, 37*(8), 36-41.

Dealey, C. (2005). *The care of wounds: A guide for nurses* (3rd ed.). Boston: Wiley/Blackwell Science.

Garbee, G. (2001). Creating a positive surgical experience for patients. *AORN Journal 74*(9), 333.

Grum, E., & Vaenti, J. (2007). Can bloodless surgery programs work in the trauma setting? *Nursing 2007, 37*(3), 54-56.

Meeker, M. H., & Rothrock, J. C. (2007). *Alexander's care of the patient in surgery* (12th ed.). St. Louis, MO: Mosby.

Munden, J. (2008). *Pathophysiology made incredibly easy.* (4th ed.). Springhouse, PA: Lippincott Williams & Wilkins.

NANDA International. (2009). *NANDA International Nursing Diagnoses: Definitions & Classifications 2009-2011*. Oxford, UK: Wiley-Blackwell.

Smith, S. F., Duell, D. J., & Martin, B. C. (2008). *Clinical nursing skills: Basic to advanced.* (7th ed.). Upper Saddle River, NJ: Prentice Hall.

Tappen, C. (2001). Perioperative assessment and discharge planning for older adults undergoing ambulatory surgery. *AORN Journal, 73*(2), 464.

Walton, J. (2001). Helping high-risk surgical patients beat the odds. *Nursing 2001, 31*(3), 54.

Winslow, E. H., & Crenshaw, J. T. (2002). Preoperative fasting: Old habits die hard. *American Journal of Nursing, 102*(5), 36–44.

CHAPTER 30

Baranoski, S., & Ayello, E. A. (2007). Wound care essentials (2nd ed.). Philadelphia: Lippincott Williams & Wilkins.

Burke, K. M., LeMone, P., & Mohn-Brown, E. L. (2007). *Medical-surgical nursing care* (2nd ed.). Upper Saddle River, NJ: Prentice Hall.

Capobianco, M. L., & McDonald, D. D. (1996, November/December). Factors affecting the predictive validity of the Braden scale. *Advances in Wound Care: The Journal for Prevention and Healing, 9,* 32–36.

Carpenito, L. J. (2005). *Handbook of nursing diagnosis* (11th ed.). Philadelphia: Lippincott.

Hahn, J. F., Olsen, C. L., Tomaselli, N., & Goldberg, M. (2002). Wounds: Nursing care and product selection. *Nursing Spectrum* self-study module.

Hess, C. T. (2002, January). *Clinical guide to wound care* (4th ed.). Philadelphia: Lippincott Williams & Wilkins.

International Committee on Wound Management. (1996). Cost effective wound care. Evaluating your supply use to prepare for managed care (ICWM World Council Consensus Statement). *Ostomy/Wound Management, 42* (2), 72, 74–76.

Maklebust, J., & Sieggreen, M. (2001). *Pressure ulcers: Guidelines for prevention and nursing management* (2nd ed.). Springhouse, PA: Springhouse Publishing.

McConnell, E. A. (1997, May). Clinical do's and don'ts: Using dry heat to promote healing. *Nursing, 27*(5), 22.

Panel for the Prediction and Prevention of Pressure Ulcers in Adults (PPPPUA). (1994). U.S. Department of Health and Human Services. Clinical practice guidelines #3 (AHCPR Pub. No. 92–0047). Rockville, MD.

Siegel, J. D., Rhinehart, E., Jackson, M., Chiarello, L., and the Healthcare Infection Control Practices Advisory Committee. (2007). 2007 Guideline for isolation precautions: Preventing transmission of infectious agents in healthcare settings. Atlanta, GA: Centers for Disease Control and Prevention.

Sisk, B. (2002). Pressure sore update (Electronic Version). *Nurse Scribe.*

Sterling, C. (1996, November). Methods of wound assessment documentation: A study. *Nursing Standard, 11*(10), 38–41.

Williams, L. S., & Hopper, P. D. (2007). *Understanding medical surgical nursing* (3rd ed.). Philadelphia, F.A. Davis.

CHAPTER 31

Adams, E. D., & Towle, M. A. (2009). *Pediatric nursing care.* Upper Saddle River, NJ: Prentice Hall.

Buescher, J. J. (2007). Temporomandibular joint disorders. *Journal of the American Academy of Family Physicians, 76*(10), 1477–1482.

Burke, K. M., LeMone, P., & Mohn-Brown, E. L. (2007). *Medical surgical nursing care* (2nd ed.). Upper Saddle River, NJ: Prentice Hall.

Cohen, B. J., et al. (2000). *Memmler's the human body in health and disease* (9th ed.). Philadelphia: Lippincott Williams & Wilkins.

Hogan, M.A., et al. (2008). *Medical surgical nursing: Reviews & rationales* (2nd ed.). Upper Saddle River, NJ: Prentice Hall.

Lemone, P., & Burke, K. (2008). *Medical surgical nursing: Critical thinking in client care* (4th ed.). Upper Saddle River, NJ: Prentice Hall.

Marieb, E. N. (2009). *Human anatomy and physiology* (7th ed.). Upper Saddle River, NJ: Prentice Hall.

McConnell, E. A. (1997, May). Clinical do's and don'ts: Using dry heat to promote healing. *Nursing, 27*(5), 22.

National Osteoporosis Foundation. (2008). Fast facts on osteoporosis: Race/ethnicity. Washington, DC: Author.

NANDA International. (2009). *NANDA International Nursing Diagnoses: Definitions & Classifications 2009–2011.* Oxford, UK: Wiley-Blackwell.

Pieper, B., Sugrue, M., Weiland, M., Sprague, K., & Heiman, C. (1998). Risk factors, prevention methods, and wound care for patients with pressure ulcers. *Clinical Nurse Specialist, 12*(1), 7–14.

Scanlon, V. C., & Sanders, T. (2007). *Essentials of anatomy and physiology* (5th ed.). Philadelphia: F.A. Davis.

Wilson, B.A., Shannon, M. T., Shields, K. M., & Stang, C. L. (2008). *Prentice Hall nurse's drug guide 2008.* Upper Saddle River, NJ: Prentice Hall.

CHAPTER 32

Aloia, M. S., Arnedt, J.T., Riggs, R. L., Heckt, J., & Borelli, B. (2004). Clinical management of poor adherence to CPAP: Motivational enhancement. *Behavioral Sleep Medicine, 2*(4), 205–222.

American Lung Association. (2007). Trends in COPD (chronic bronchitis and emphysema): Morbidity and mortality. New York: Author.

Berjohn, C., Fishman, N., Joffe, M., Edelstein, P., & Metlay, J. (2008, May). Treatment and outcomes for patients with bacteremic pneumococcal pneumonia. *Medicine, 87*(3), 160–166.

Braunwald, E., Fauci, A. S., Kasper, D. L., Hauser, S. L., Longo, D. L., Jameson, J. L., & Loscalzo, J. (2008). *Harrison's principles of internal medicine* (17th ed.). New York: McGraw-Hill.

Breathing training helps ease asthma. (2007, July 5). *Pulse.* Retrieved June 27, 2008, from. http://www.accessmylibrary.com/coms2/summary0286-31836212_ITM.

Bryant, G. (2004, March). Perspectives. Managing Pickwickian syndrome—A multifaceted challenge. *Rehabilitation Nursing, 29*(2), 39–40.

Chang, K., Leung, C., Yew, W., Ho, S., & Tam, C. (2004, November 15). A nested case-control study on treatment-related risk factors for early relapse of tuberculosis. *American Journal of Respiratory and Critical Care Medicine, 170*(10), 1124–1130.

Day, M. (2008, May). Action stat. Tension pneumothorax. *Nursing, 38*(5), 72.

Duval, S., Jacobs, J., Barber, C., Lando, H., Steffen, L., Arnett, D., et al. (2008, October). Trends in cigarette smoking: The Minnesota Heart Survey, 1980–1982 through 2000–2002. *Nicotine & Tobacco Research, 10*(5), 827–832.

Fontaine, K. L. (2005). *Complementary & alternative therapies for nursing practice* (2nd ed.). Upper Saddle River, NJ: Prentice Hall.

Hart, A., & Davidhizar, R. (2006, 2006 Winter–2007 Spring). What the nurse should know about the pulmonary system. *Journal of Practical Nursing, 56*(4)–57(1), 6.

Howard, D. (2007, February). A need for a simplified approach to venous thromboembolism prophylaxis in acute medical inpatients. *International Journal of Clinical Practice, 61*(2), 336–340.

Laux, L., McGonigal, M., Thieret, T., & Weatherby, L. (2008, April). Use of prone positioning in a patient with acute respiratory distress syndrome. *Critical Care Nursing Quarterly, 31*(2), 178–183.

Making progress in management of COPD patients. (2008, March 27). *Pulse.* Retrieved June 27, 2008, from. www.accessmylibrary.com/coms2/summary0286-34298711_ITM.

Malarkey, L. M., & McMorrow, M. E. (2005). *Saunders nursing guide to laboratory and diagnostic tests.* Philadelphia: Saunders.

Mayo Clinic. Sleep apnea. (February, 2008). Rochester, MN: Mayo Foundation for Medical Education and Research.

Molimard, M., & Gros, V. (2008, March). Impact of patient-related factors on asthma control. *Journal of Asthma, 45*(2), 109–113.

Sifton, D. W. (Ed.). (2008). *Physicians' desk reference (PDR)* (62nd ed.). Montvale, NJ: Medical Economics.

Sridhar, M., Taylor, R., Dawson, S., Roberts, N., & Partridge, M. (2008, March 27). A nurse led intermediate care package in patients who have been hospitalized with an acute exacerbation of chronic obstructive pulmonary disease. *Thorax, 63*(3), 194–200.

Treatment for chronic sinus infection studied at Mayo Clinic. (2005, July 28). *Mayo Clinic Health Letter.* Retrieved June 27, 2008, from www.mayoclinic.org/news2005-rst/2980.html.

U.S. Department of Health and Human Services. (2000). *Healthy People 2010: Understanding and improving health* (2nd ed.). Washington, DC: U.S. Government Printing Office.

U.S. Department of Health and Human Services. (2005). *Healthy People 2010: Midcourse review.* Washington, DC: U.S. Government Printing Office.

U. S. Food and Drug Administration. (2008). FDA releases recommendations regarding use of over-the-counter cough and cold products. Rockville, MD: Author.

Wakabayashi, A. (2006, March). Clinical evaluation of the safety of high-vacuum chest drainage. *ASAIO Journal (American Society for Artificial Internal Organs: 1992), 52*(2), 215–216.

World Health Organization. Cardiovascular diseases. Fact Sheet No.317. (2007). Geneva, Switzerland: Author.

CHAPTER 33

Burke, K. M., LeMone, P., & Mohn-Brown, E. L. (2007). *Medical–surgical nursing care.* (2nd ed.). Upper Saddle River, NJ: Prentice Hall.

Castro, M., Zimmermann, N., Crocker, S., Bradley, J., Leven, C., & Schechtman, K. (2003, November 1). Asthma intervention program prevents readmissions in high healthcare users. *American Journal of Respiratory and Critical Care Medicine, 168*(9), 1095–1099.

Fort, C. W. (2002). Get pumped to prevent DVT. *Nursing 2002, 32*(9), 50–52.

Howie-Esquivel, J., & White, M. (2008). Biomarkers in acute cardiovascular disease. *Journal of Cardiovascular Nursing, 23*(2), 124–131.

Lazzara, D. (2002). Eliminate the air of mystery from chest tubes. *Nursing 2002, 32*(6), 36–43.

McConnell, E. A. (2002). Applying antiembolism stockings. *Nursing 2002, 32*(4), 17.

Pope, B. B. (2002). Asthma: Patient education series. *Nursing 2002, 32*(5), 44.

Sandrock, C., & Stollenwerk, N. (2008). Acute febrile respiratory illness in the ICU: Reducing disease transmission. *CHEST, 133*(5), 1221–1231.

Towle, M. A., & Adams, E. D. (2008). *Maternal-child nursing care.* Upper Saddle River, NJ: Prentice Hall.

Walz, J., Zayaruzny, M., & Heard, S. (2007). Airway management in critical illness. *CHEST, 131*(2), 608–620.

West, J. B. (2001). *Pulmonary physiology and pathophysiology: An integrated, case-based approach.* Philadelphia: Lippincott Williams & Wilkins.

CHAPTER 34

Burke, K. M., LeMone, P., & Mohn-Brown, E. L. (2007). *Medical–surgical nursing Care* (2nd ed). Upper Saddle River, NJ: Prentice Hall.

Centers for Disease Control. (n.d.). *Chronic fatigue syndrome.* Retrieved August 16, 2004, from www.cde.gov/cfs.

Ignatavicius, D., & Workman, L. (2006). *Medical–surgical nursing: Critical thinking for collaborative care* (5th ed.). Philadelphia: Saunders.

LeMone, P., & Burke, K. (2007). *Medical–surgical nursing: Critical thinking in client care* (2nd ed). Upper Saddle River, NJ: Pearson/Prentice Hall.

The Leukemia & Lymphoma Society. (2008). *Leukemia, lymphoma, myeloma facts.* White Plains, NJ: Author.

Towle, M. A., & Adams, E. D. (2008). *Maternal-child nursing care.* Upper Saddle River, NJ: Prentice Hall.

CHAPTER 35

Bullock, B. A., & Henze, R. L. (2000). *Focus on pathophysiology.* Philadelphia: Lippincott.

Burggraf, V., & Weinstein, B. F. (2000). Don't miss this opportunity: Promote adult immunizations! *MEDSURG Nursing, 9*(4), 198–200.

Centers for Disease Control and Prevention. (2001). *Vaccine-preventable adult diseases.* Retrieved May 1, 2008 from www.cdc.gov/vaccines/vpd-vac/adult-vpd.htm.

Centers for Disease Control and Prevention. (2006). *HIV/AIDS Surveillance Report 2006, (Vol. 18).* Atlanta, GA: Author.

Centers for Disease Control and Prevention. (2008). *Estimates of new HIV infections in the United States.* Atlanta, GA: Author.

Cohen, B. J. (2005). *Memmler's the human body in health and disease* (10th ed.). Philadelphia: Lippincott.

Eliopoulos, C. (2000). *Gerontological nursing* (5th ed.). Philadelphia: Lippincott.

Hayden, M. (2004). In defense of the body: How the immune system protects us from harm. *Nursing Made Incredibly Easy,* 52–54.

Kee, J. L. (2009). *Handbook of laboratory and diagnostic tests* (6th ed.). Upper Saddle River, NJ: Prentice Hall.

Keithley, J. K., & Swanson, B. (1998). Minimizing HIV/AIDS malnutrition. *MEDSURG Nursing, 7*(5), 256–265.

Lisanti, P., & Zwolski, K. (1997). Understanding the devastation of AIDS. *American Journal of Nursing, 97*(7), 26–34.

Lueckenotte, A. G. (2000). *Gerontologic nursing* (2nd ed.). St. Louis, MO: Mosby.

Mulvihill, M. L., Zelman, M., Holdaway, P., Tompary, E., & Raymond, J. A. (2006). *Human diseases* (6th ed) Upper Saddle River, NJ: Pearson Education.

Nowak, T. J., & Handford, A. G. (2004). *Pathophysiology: Concepts and applications for health care professionals.* New York: McGraw-Hill.

Spratto, G. R., & Woods, A. L. (2008). *PDR nurse's drug handbook.* Clifton Park, NY: Delmar Thompson.

Venes, D. (Ed.). (2005). *Taber's cyclopedic medical dictionary* (20th ed.). Philadelphia: F.A. Davis.

World Health Organization. (2007). Global HIV prevalence has leveled off. Improvements in surveillance increase understanding of the epidemic, resulting in substantial revisions to estimates. Geneva, Switzerland: Author.

CHAPTER 36

Altimier, L. (2008). Shaken baby syndrome. *Journal of Perinatal & Neonatal Nursing, 22*(1), 68.

Aytech, L. S., Hammond, R., & White, C. (2001, October). Seizures in infants and young children: An exploratory study of family experiences and needs for information and support. *Journal of Neuroscience Nursing, 33*(5), 278–286.

Barker, E. (2002). *Neuroscience nursing: A spectrum of care* (2nd ed.). St. Louis, MO: Mosby.

Buhse, M. (2008). Assessment of caregiver burden in families of persons with multiple sclerosis. *Journal of Neuroscience Nursing, 40*(1), 25–32.

Fagley, M. U. (2007). Taking charge of seizure activity. *Nursing, 37*(9), 42.

Jung, S. (2007). The impact of migraine: A case study. *Journal of Neuroscience Nursing, 39*(4), 213–217.

Nelson, S. (2008). Parkinson's disease. *Nursing Standard, 22*(19), 59.

Skirton, H. (2005). Huntington disease: A nursing perspective. *Medsurg Nursing, 14*(3), 167–174.

Vacca Jr., V. M. (2007). Epidural hemorrhage and hematoma. *Horsham 37*(7), 72.

White, C. P., White, M. B., & Russell, C. S. (2008). Invisible and visible symptoms of multiple sclerosis: Which are more predictive of health distress? *Journal of Neuroscience Nursing, 40*(2), 85–97.

CHAPTER 37

Bryant, D., & Fleischer, I. (2000). Changing an ostomy appliance [Electronic version]. *Nursing, 30*(11), 51.

Burke, K., LeMone, P., & Mohn-Brown, E. (2007). *Medical-surgical nursing care* (2nd ed.). Upper Saddle River, NJ: Prentice Hall.

Butler, M. (1998). Laxatives and rectal preparations. *Nursing Times, 94*(3), 56–58.

Carpenito, L. J. (2005). *Handbook of nursing diagnosis* (11th ed.). Philadelphia: Lippincott.

Department of Health and Human Services. (2005), ToxFAQs for carbon tetrachloride. *Agency for Toxic Substances and Disease Registry.*

Dudek, S. G. (2001). *Nutrition essentials for nursing practice* (4th ed.). Philadelphia: Lippincott.

Guyton, A. C., & Hall, J. E. (2006). *Textbook of medical physiology* (11th ed.). Philadelphia: Saunders.

Jensen, L. L. (1997). Fecal incontinence: Evaluation and treatment. *Journal of Wound, Ostomy and Continence Nursing, 24*(5), 277–282.

National Cancer Institute. (2007). *Incidence and mortality rate trends.* Bethesda, MD: Author.

NANDA International. (2009). *NANDA International Nursing Diagnoses: Definitions & Classifications 2009–2011.* Oxford, UK: Wiley-Blackwell.

Petticrew, M. (1997). Treatment of constipation in older people. *Nursing Times, 93*(48), 55–56.

Vickery, G. (1997). Basics of constipation. *Gastroenterology Nursing, 20*(4), 125–128.

CHAPTER 38

Bullock, B. A., & Henze, R. L. (2000). *Focus on pathophysiology.* Philadelphia: Lippincott Williams & Wilkins.

Burke, K. M., LeMone, P., & Mohn-Brown, E. L. (2007). *Medical-surgical nursing care* (2nd ed.). Upper Saddle River, NJ: Prentice Hall.

Burton, M. (1997). Emergency! Pheochromocytoma. *American Journal of Nursing, 97*(11), 57.

Carson, P. P. (2000). Emergency: Adrenal crisis. *American Journal of Nursing, 100*(7), 49–50.

Clayton, L., & Dilley, K. (1998). Clinical snapshot: Cushing's syndrome. *American Journal of Nursing, 98*(7), 40–41.

Fain, J. A. (2002). Delivering insulin 'round the clock. *Nursing, 32*(8), 54–56.

Ficorelli, C. T., & Edelman, M. (2005). Foot care for patients with diabetes. *Nursing, 35*(10), 43.

Hoeman, L. D. (2007). The obese teen, The neuroendocrine connection. *American Journal of Nursing, 107*(2), 40–48.

Holcomb, S. S. (2007). A delicate balance: Keeping thyroid hormones in check. *LPN, 3*(2), 46–55.

Mayo Clinic. (2008). Hyperthyroidism (overactive thyroid). Rochester, MN: Author.

Mayo Clinic. (2008). Hypothyroidism (underactive thyroid). Rochester, MN: Author.

McCloskey, J., & Bulechek, G. (Eds.). (2007). *Nursing interventions: Effective nursing treatments* (5th ed.). St. Louis, MO: Mosby.

Milchovich, S. K., & Dunn-Long, B. (2003). *Diabetes mellitus, A practical handbook* (8th ed.). Boulder, CO: Bull Publishing.

Norris, D. (2005). Tight insulin control, making it work. *RN, 68*(7), 47–51.

Rottmann, C. N. (2007). SSRIs and the syndrome of inappropriate antidiuretic hormone secretion. *American Journal of Nursing, 107*(1), 51–59.

Sieggreen, M. Y. (2005). Stepping up care for diabetic foot ulcers. *Nursing, 35*(10), 36–41.

Williams, L. S., & Hopper, P. D. (2007). *Understanding medical surgical nursing* (3rd ed.). Philadelphia: Lippincott.

Wright, M. A., & Appel, S. J. (2007). Inhaled insulin breathing new life into diabetes therapy. *Nursing, 37*(1), 46-50.

Young, J. (1999). Action stat: Myxedema coma. *Nursing 99, 29*(1), 64.

CHAPTER 39

Bray, B., Van Sell, S., & Miller-Anderson, M. (2007). Stress incontinence: It's no laughing matter. *RN, 70*(4) 25-30.

Burke, K., LeMone, P., & Mohn-Brown, E. (2007). *Medical-surgical nursing care* (2nd ed.). Upper Saddle River, NJ: Prentice Hall.

Campoy, S., & Elwell, R. (2005). Pharmacology and CKD. *American Journal of Nursing, 105*(9), 60-72.

Carpenito, L. J. (2005). *Handbook of nursing diagnosis* (11th ed.). Philadelphia: Lippincott.

Castner, D. (2007). Failed dialysis access. *Nursing, 37*(8), 72.

Castner, D., & Douglas, C. (2005). Now onstage: Chronic kidney disease. *Nursing, 35*(12), 58-63.

Coleman, T., Culkin, C., & Sierka, D. (2006). Kidney transplants in HIV patients? *RN, 69*(1), 33-39.

David, K. (2007). IV fluids: Do you know what's hanging and why? *RN, 70*(10), 35-41.

Dinwiddie, L., Burrow-Hudson, S., & Peacock, E. (2006). Stage 4 chronic kidney disease. *American Journal of Nursing, 106*(9), 40-52.

Kohtz, C., & Thompson, M. (2007). Preventing contrast medium-induced nephropathy. *American Journal of Nursing, 107*(9), 40-50.

McCarley, P., & Salai, P. (2005). Cardiovascular disease in chronic kidney disease. *American Journal of Nursing 105*(4), 40-53.

Miller, J. (2006). Potassium in the balance: Understanding hyperkalemia and hypokalemia. *LPN, 2*(5), 43-49.

Nettina, S. M. (2005). *Lippincott manual of nursing practice* (8th ed.). Philadelphia: Lippincott Williams & Wilkins.

Newman, D. K. (2002). *Managing and treating urinary incontinence* Baltimore, MD: Health Profession Press.

Patraca, K. (2005). Measure bladder volume without catheterization. *Nursing, 60*(4), 46-47

Pontieri-Lewis, V. (2006). Basics of ostomy care. *Medsurg Nursing, 15*(4), 199-203.

Robinson, S., et al. (2007). Development of an evidence-based protocol for reduction of indwelling urinary catheter usage. *Medsurg Nursing, 16*(3), 157-161.

Ruholl, L. (2006). Arterial blood gases: Analysis and nursing responses. *Medsurg Nursing, 15*(6), 343-351.

CHAPTER 40

Berman, A. J., Snyder, S., Kozier, B., & Erb, G. (2008). *Kozier & Erb's fundamentals of nursing: Concepts, process, and practice* (8th ed.). Upper Saddle River, NJ: Prentice Hall Health.

Burke, K. M., LeMone, P., & Mohn-Brown, E. L. (2007). *Medical-surgical nursing care.* (2nd ed.). Upper Saddle River, NJ: Prentice Hall.

Carpenito-Moyet, L. J. (2009). *Handbook of nursing diagnosis* (12th ed.). Philadelphia: Lippincott.

Food and Drug Administration. (1997). Protecting against unintended pregnancy: A guide to contraceptive choices. *FDA Consumer.*

Goff, B., et al. (2007). Development of an ovarian cancer symptom index: Possibilities for earlier detection. *CANCER, 15.*

Krebs, E. E., Ensrud, K. E., MacDonald, R., & Wilt, T. J. (2004). Phytoestrogens for treatment of menopausal symptoms: A systematic review. *Obstetrics and Gyneocolgy, 104*(4), 824-836.

LeMone, P., & Burke, K. (2008). *Medical-surgical nursing: Critical thinking in client care* (4th ed.). Upper Saddle River, NJ: Prentice Hall.

London, M. L., Ladewig, P.W., Ball, J.W., & Bindler, R.C. (2007). *Maternal & child nursing care* (2nd ed.). Upper Saddle River, NJ: Prentice Hall.

Manson, J. E., Allison, M.A., Rossouw, J. E., Carr, J. J., Langer, R. D., Hsia, J., Kuller, L. H., Cochrane, B. B., Hunt, J. R., Ludlam, S. E., Pettinger, M. B., Gass, M., Margolis, K. L., Nathan, L., Ockene, J. K., Prentice, R. L., Robbins, J., Stefanick, M. L., for the WHI Investigators. (2007). Estrogen therapy and coronary artery calcification. *New England Journal of Medicine, 356,* 2591-2602.

Masters, W., & Johnson, V. (1966). *Human sexual response.* Philadelphia: Lippincott Williams & Wilkins.

Ramont, R. P., & Niedringhaus, D. M. (2008). *Fundamentals of nursing care* (2nd ed.). Upper Saddle River, NJ: Prentice Hall.

Reichert, G. (1998). Female circumcision: What you need to know about genital mutilation. *Lifelines, 2*(3), 29-34.

Stefanick, M. L., Anderson, G. L., Margolis, K. L., Hendrix, S. L., Rodabough, R. J., Paskett, E. D., Lane, D. S., Hubbell, F.A., Assaf, A. R., Sarto, G. E., Schenken, R. S., Yasmeen, S., Lessin, L., Chlebowski, R.T., for the Women's Health Institute Investigators. (2006). Effects of conjugated equine estrogens on breast cancer and mammography screening in postmenopausal women with hysterectomy. *JAMA, 295*(14), 1647-1657.

CHAPTER 41

Alexander, L. (1996). Taking a sexual history to help clients prevent STDs. *Contraception Report, VII*(2).

Centers for Disease Control and Prevention. (2000). *Tracking the hidden epidemics: Trends in STDs in the United States.* Atlanta, GA: Author.

Centers for Disease Control and Prevention. (2002). Sexually transmitted diseases treatment guidelines 2002. *MMWR, 5* (RR-6).

Centers for Disease Control and Prevention. (2003, September). *Sexually transmitted disease surveillance, 2002.* Atlanta, GA: Author.

Centers for Disease Control and Prevention. (2006). Sexually transmitted disease treatment guidelines, 2006. *MMWR 2006, 55,* (RR-11).

Cox, J., Mahoneym M., Saslow, D., & Moscicki, A. (2008). ACS releases guidelines for HPV vaccination. *American Family Physician, 77*(6), 852-863.

Lachat, M., Scott, C., & Relf, M. (2006). HIV and pregnancy: Considerations for nursing practice, *MCN, The American Journal of Maternal/Child Nursing, 31*(4), 233-240.

Miller, W., Ford, C., Morris, M., Handcock, M., Schmitz, J., Hobbs, M., et al. (2004). Prevalence of chlamydia and gonococcal infections among young adults in the United States. *JAMA, 291*(18), 2229-2236.

National Institute of Allergy and Infectious Diseases. (2003, November). *HIV/AIDS statistics.* Bethesda, MD: National Institutes of Health.

Snow, M. (2007). HPV vaccine: New treatment for an old disease. *Nursing, 37*(3), 67.

CHAPTER 42

Beers, M. H. (2003). *The Merck manual on health and aging.* Rahway, NJ: Merck.

Burke, K., LeMone, P., & Mohn-Brown, E. (2007). *Medical-Surgical nursing care* (2nd ed.). Upper Saddle River, NJ: Pearson/Prentice Hall.

Harris, E. D., Budd, R. C., Genovese, M.C., Firestein, G.S., Sargent, J.S., & Sledge, C.B. (2005). *Kelley's textbook of rheumatology* (7th ed.). St. Louis, MO: Saunders.

Hodge, P., Gordon, L., & Lambert, J. (2004). The age explosion: Baby boomers and beyond. *Harvard Generations Policy Journal, 1,* 7–21.

Kinsella, K., & Velkoff, V. (2001). *An aging world: 2001* (U.S. Census Bureau, Series P95/01–1). Washington, DC: U.S. Government Printing Office.

Ramont, R., & Niedringhaus, D. (2008). *Fundamental nursing care.* (2nd ed.). Upper Saddle River, NJ: Prentice Hall.

Tabloski, P.A. (2006). *Gerontological nursing.* Upper Saddle River, NJ: Prentice Hall.

Wold, G. (2008). *Basic geriatric nursing* (4th ed.). Philadelphia: Mosby.

CHAPTER 43

Cole, C., & Richards, K. (2007). Sleep disruption in older adults. *AJN, 107*(5), 40–49.

Covell, C.A. (2007). New outlook for age-related macular degeneration. *Nursing 2007, 37*(3), 22–24.

Ebersole, P., & Touhy, T.A. (2006). *Geriatric nursing: Growth of a specialty.* New York: Springer Publishing.

Haider, S. I., Johnell, K., Thorslund, M., & Fastrom, J. (2008). Analysis of the association between polypharmacy and socioeconomic position among elderly aged >/= 77 years in Sweden. *Clinical Therapy, 30*(2), 419–427.

Harris, E. D., Budd, R. C., Genovese, M. C., Firestein, G.S., Sargent, J.S., & Sledge, C.B. (2005). *Kelley's textbook of rheumatology* (7th ed.). St. Louis, MO: Saunders.

Hodge, P., Gordon, L., & Lambert, J. (2004). The age explosion: Baby boomers and beyond. *Harvard Generations Policy Journal, 1,* 7–21.

Keefe, S. (2007). Preparing to die (geriatrics/palliative care). *Advance for Nurses, 4*(17), 27–29.

Kinsella, K., & Velkoff, V. (2001). *An aging world: 2001* (U.S. Census Bureau, Series P95/01–1). Washington, DC: U.S. Government Printing Office.

Lewis, A. M. (2007). Heatstroke in older adults *AJN, 107*(6), 52–56.

Murphy, K. (2007). Is your older patient depressed? *Nursing 2007, 37*(6), 22–23.

Pacholok, S. (2007). Caring for older adults—Simple steps to stamp out vitamin B_{12} deficiency. *Nursing 2007, 37*(1), 67–69.

Sandhaus, S., Harrell, F., & Valenti, D. (2006). Here's HELP to prevent delirium in the hospital. *Nursing 2006, 36*(7), 60–62.

Shepler, S. A., Grogan, T. A., & Steinmetz Pater, K. (2006). Keep your older patient out of medication trouble. *Nursing 2006, 36*(9), 44–47.

Tabloski, P. A. (2006). *Gerontological nursing.* Upper Saddle River, NJ: Pearson/Prentice Hall.

Thomure, A. (2006). Helping your patient manage Parkinson's disease. (Caring for Older Adult). *Nursing 2006, 36*(8), 20–21.

Walker, C., Hogstel, M. O., & Curry, L. C. (2007). Hospital discharge of older adults—How nurses can ease the transition. *AJN, 107*(6), 60–70.

Wilkinson, J. M., & Ahern, N. R. (2009). *Nursing diagnosis handbook* (9th ed.). Upper Saddle River, NJ: Pearson/Prentice Hall.

CHAPTER 44

Anweiler, N. (2000). Another dying patient. *Nursing 2000, 30*(11), 32.

Bedside Pain Manager: Conversions & Information for Pain and Symptom Control. (2004). California: Pain Management Resources.

Brown, L. K., & Brown, M. (1996). *When dinosaurs die: A guide to understanding death.* New York: Little, Brown.

Byock, I. (1997). *Dying well: The prospect for growth at the end of life.* New York: Free Press.

Byock, I. (2004). *The four things that matter most.* New York: Free Press.

Cohen, R. M. (2008). *Strong at the broken places: Voices of illness, a chorus of hope.* New York: HarperCollins.

Dobbins, E. H. (2007). End of life decisions: Influence of advance directives on patient care. *Journal of Gerontological Nursing, 33*(10), 50–56.

Dubler, N. N. (2005). Conflict and consensus at the end of life. Improving end of life care: Why has it been so difficult? *Hasting's Center Special Report, 35,* 6, S19–S25.

Furman, J. (2002). What you should know about chronic grief. *Nursing 2002, 32,* 56.

Kübler-Ross, E. (1969). *On death and dying.* New York: Macmillan.

Kübler-Ross, E. (1974). *Questions and answers on death and dying.* New York: Macmillan.

Kübler-Ross, E. (1975). *Death: The final stage of growth.* Upper Saddle River, NJ: Prentice Hall.

Kübler-Ross, E. (1978). *To live until we say good-bye.* Upper Saddle River, NJ: Prentice Hall.

Lynn, J. (2005). Living long in fragile health: The new demographics shape end of life care. Improving end of life care: Why has it been so difficult? *Hasting's Center Report Special Report, 35,* 6, S14–S18.

National Consensus Project for Quality Palliative Care. (2004). *Clinical practice guidelines for quality palliative care.* Brooklyn, NY: National Consensus Project.

Paterson, K. (1977). *Bridge to Tarabithia.* New York: HarperCollins.

Ross, H. (2001). Islamic tradition at the end of life. *MEDSURG Nursing, 10*(2), 83.

Simon, J. (2002). *This book is for all kids, but especially my sister Libby. Libby died.* Kansas City: Andrews McMeel Publishing.

Ufema, J. (2008). Insights on death and dying. *Nursing 2008, 38*(6).

Viorst, J. (1971). *The tenth good thing about Barney.* New York: Macmillan.

Wilkinson, J. M., & Ahern, N. R. (2009). *Nursing diagnosis handbook* (9th ed.). Upper Saddle River, NJ: Pearson Prentice Hall.

CHAPTER 45

Ezonne, S., & Schmit-Pokorny, K. (2007). *Stem cell transplantation: Principles, practice, and nursing insights* (3rd ed.). Sudbury, MA: Jones and Bartlett.

Groenwald, S., Frogge, M., Goodman, M., & Yarbro, C. (2001). *A clinical guide to cancer nursing: A companion to cancer nursing* (5th ed.). Sudbury, MA: Jones and Bartlett.

Groenwald, S., Frogge, M., Goodman, M., & Yarbro, C. (2005). *Cancer nursing: Principles and practice* (6th ed.). Sudbury, MA: Jones and Bartlett.

Hill, C. (1991). *Guidelines for treatment of cancer pain: The pocket edition of the final report of the Texas Cancer Council's Workgroup on Pain Control in Cancer Patients.* Austin, TX: Texas Cancer Council.

Holleb, A. I., Fink, D. J., Murphy, G. P. (2001). *American Cancer Society textbook of clinical oncology* (3rd ed.). Atlanta, GA: American Cancer Society.

Itano, J., & Taoka, K. (2005). *Core curriculum for oncology nursing* (4th ed.). Philadelphia: Saunders.

Reiger, P. (2001). *Biotherapy: A comprehensive overview* (2nd ed.). Sudbury, MA: Jones and Bartlett.

Wilkes, G., & Barton-Burke, M. (2006). *Oncology nursing drug handbook.* Sudbury, MA: Jones and Bartlett.

CHAPTER 46

Abrams, W., Beers, M., & Berkow, R. (Eds.). (2004). *The Merck manual of health and aging* (3rd ed.). Whitehouse Station, NJ: Merck.

American Hospital Association. (1992). *A patient's bill of rights.* Chicago: Author.

American Hospital Association. (2006). *Protecting and improving care for patients and communities: Coordinating care for the chronically ill.* Retrieved April 20, 2008 from www.aha.org/content/2006.

Derstine, J.B., & Hargrove, S.D. (2001). *Comprehensive rehabilitation nursing.* Philadelphia: Saunders.

Edwards, P.A. (2000). *The specialty practice of rehabilitation nursing: A core curriculum* (4th ed.). Skokie, IL: Rehabilitation Nursing Foundation.

Hoeman, S.P. (2002). *Rehabilitation nursing: Process, application, & outcomes* (3rd ed.). St. Louis, MO: Mosby.

Skretkowicz, V. (Ed.). (1992). *Florence Nightingale's notes on nursing* (Rev. ed., with additions). London, UK: Scutari Press.

Stoker, J. (2000). The Omnibus Consolidation Appropriation Act of 2000. *Home HealthCare Nurse, 18*(2), 84.

Tabloski, P.A. (2006). *Gerontological nursing.* Upper Saddle River, NJ: Prentice Hall.

CHAPTER 47

Chan, T., Arendts, G., & Stevens, M. (2008). Variables that predict admission to hospital from an emergency department observation unit. *Emergency Medicine Australasia, 20*(3), 216–220.

Degutis, L. (2008). Emergency care systems: The safety net of safety nets. *Nation's Health, 38*(4), 3.

Juckett, G., & Hancox, J. G. (2002). Venomous snakebites in the United States: Management review and update. *American Family Physician,* April 1 issue. Leawood, KS: American Academy of Family Physicians.

Lichtenchan, J. (1995). Emergency management of poisonous snakebites. *Physician & Sportsmedicine, 23*(9), 73.

Magboul, M. (2007). The adult basic CPR guidelines 2005. *Internet Journal of Health, 6*(2), 12.

Ringold, S., Glass, T., & Glass, R. (2005). Cardiopulmonary resuscitation (CPR). *JAMA: Journal of the American Medical Association, 293*(3), 373–374.

Rosenberg, H. (2004). Case of the month. The Heimlich in near-drownings. *JEMS: Journal of Emergency Medical Services, 29*(7), 26. Retrieved June 6, 2006 from www.jems.com.

Shah-Canning, D., Alpert, J., & Bauchner, H. (1996). Care-seeking patterns of inner-city families using an emergency room. A three-decade comparison. *Medical Care, 34*(12), 1171–1179.

Talmor, D. (2008). Airway management during a mass casualty event. *Respiratory Care, 53*(2), 226–231.

Tarrac, S. (2008). Application of the updated CDC isolation guidelines for health care facilities. *AORN Journal, 87*(3), 534–546.

CHAPTER 48

Ackley, B. J., & Ladwig, G. B. (2006). *Nursing diagnosis handbook* (7th ed.). St. Louis, MO: Mosby.

Goldich, G. (2006). Understanding the 12-lead EGG, part II. *Nursing 2006, 36*(12), 36–41.

Laskowski-Jones, L. (2006). First aid for sprains. *Nursing 2006, 36*(8), 48–49.

NANDA International. (2009). *NANDA International Nursing Diagnoses: Definitions & Classifications 2009–2011.* Oxford, UK: Wiley-Blackwell.

Regulations of the Commissioner of Education. (2006, March). Section 136.1–3.

CHAPTER 49

Amador, X. (2001). *I am not sick, I don't need help! Helping the seriously mentally ill accept treatment.* Peconic, NY: Vida Press.

American Psychiatric Association. (2004). *Diagnostic and statistical manual of mental disorders* (4th ed., text revision). Washington, DC: American Psychiatric Press.

American Psychiatric Association. (2000). Practice guidelines for the treatment of patients with eating disorders. *American Journal of Psychiatry, 157,* 1.

Beattie, M. (1987). *Codependent no more: How to stop controlling others and start caring for yourself.* New York: Harper/Hazelden.

Bernardo, M. L. (2007). Social anxiety disorder restricts lives. *NursingSpectrum* 20 Aug 2007. Retrieved from www.writephd.com/images/Nursing_20Spectrum_complete.pdf.

Blake, T. (2007). Tracking the ups and downs of antidepressants. *NursingSpectrum* 20 Aug 2007. Retrieved from www.writephd.com/images/Nursing_20Spectrum_complete.pdf.

Brown, T., Cooper, M. C., Crimson, M. L., & Enderle, H. E. (2002). Special report: Medication management considerations in schizophrenia. *American Pharmaceutical Association, 42*(1), 1–21.

Captain, C. (2006). Is your patient a suicide risk? *Nursing 2006, 36*(8), 43–47.

Domrose, C. (2007). Listen to voices—Can violence be predicted? *NurseWeek,* 12–13.

Hanson, D.R., & Gottesman, I. (2005). Theories of schizophrenia: A genetic inflammatory-vascular synthesis. *BMC Medical Genetics, 6*(1), 7.

Keltner, N. L., Schwecke, L. H., & Bostrom, C. E. (2003). *Psychiatric nursing* (4th ed.). St. Louis, MO: Mosby.

Kirkbride, J. B., et al. (2006). Heterogeneity in incidence rates of schizophrenia and other psychotic syndromes. *Archives of General Psychiatry, 63*(1).

Kneisl, C. R., Wilson, H. S., & Trigoboff, E. (2004). *Contemporary psychiatric-mental health nursing.* Upper Saddle River, NJ: Pearson Education.

Leahy, L. (2003). *Cognitive therapy techniques: A practitioner's guide.* New York: Guilford Press.

Limandri, B., & Boyd, M.A. (2002). Personality and impulse control disorders. In M.A. Boyd (Ed.), *Psychiatric nursing: Contemporary practice.* Philadelphia: Lippincott.

Millon, T., & Davis, R. (1999). *Personality disorders in modern life.* New York: John Wiley & Sons.

Mills, J. (2000). Dealing with voices and strange thoughts. In C. Gamble & G. Brennan (Eds.), *Working with serious mental illness: A manual for clinical practice.* London: Bailliere Tindall.

National Institutes of Health. (2005). Press release: Mental illness effects heavy toll beginning in youth. Atlanta, GA: Author.

Rankin, E.A. (2000). *Quick reference for psychopharmacology.* Albany, NY: Delmar.

Rives, W. (1999). Emergency department assessment of suicidal patients. *Psychiatric Clinics of North America, 22*(4), 779-787.

Roach, M.J., et al. (1998). Depressed mood and survival in seriously ill hospitalized adults. *Archives of Internal Medicine 158,* 397.

Smith-Alnimer, M., & Watford, M. F. (2004). Alcohol withdrawal and delirium tremens: Fast recognition may save a patient from the worst of withdrawal. *AJN, American Journal of Nursing, 104*(5), 72A-75G.

Stuart, G. W., & Laraia, M.T. (2001). *Principles and practice of psychiatric nursing.* St. Louis, MO: Mosby.

Thase, M. E. (2004). Mood disorders: Neurobiology. In H. I. Kaplan & B. J. Sadock (Eds.), *Comprehensive textbook of psychiatry* (Vol. 1, 8th ed.). Philadelphia: Lippincott.

Torrey, E. F. (2001). *Surviving schizophrenia: A manual for families, consumers, and providers* (4th ed.). New York: HarperCollins.

Uko-Ekpenyoung, G. (2007). What you should know about electroconvulsive therapy. *Nursing 2007, 37*(8), 25.

U.S. Public Health Service. (1999). *The surgeon general's call to action to prevent suicide.* Washington, DC: Author.

CHAPTER 50

American Psychiatric Association. (2004). *Diagnostic and statistical manual of mental disorders* (4th ed., text revision). Washington, DC: American Psychiatric Press.

American Psychiatric Association. (2000). Practice guidelines for the treatment of patients with eating disorders. *American Journal of Psychiatry, 157,* 1.

Beattie, M. (1987). *Codependent no more: How to stop controlling others and start caring for yourself.* New York: Harper/Hazelden.

Cash, T., & Deagle, E. (1997). The nature and extent of body-image disturbances in anorexia nervosa and bulimia nervosa: A meta-analysis. *International Journal of Eating Disorders, 22,* 107.

Chally, P. (1998). An eating disorders prevention program. *Journal of Child and Adolescent Psychiatric Nursing, 11*(2), 51-63.

El-Mallakh, P. (1998). Treatment models for clients with co-occurring addictive and mental disorders. *Archives of Psychiatric Nursing, 12*(2), 71.

Freed, P. E., & York, L. N. (1997). Naltrexone: A controversial therapy for alcohol dependence. *Journal of Psychosocial Nursing, 35*(7), 24-28.

Gordon, C., Williams, B., & Lapin, P. (2001). New program to help seniors quit smoking. *Nursing Spectrum, 2*(10), 18-19.

Greeno, C., et al. (2000). Binge antecedents in obese women with and without binge eating disorder. *Journal of Consulting Clinical Psychology, 68*(1), 95.

Hasting, J., as told to Jeri Burn. (2007). Addiction: A nurse's story. *AJN, 107*(8), 75-79.

Kneisl, C. R., Wilson, H. S., & Trigoboff, E. (2004). *Contemporary psychiatric-mental health nursing.* Upper Saddle River, NJ: Pearson Education.

Nace, E. P., & Tinsley, J.A. (2008). Patients with substance abuse problems: Effective identification, diagnosis, and treatment. New York: W.W. Norton.

Naegle, M.A., & D'Avanzo, C. E. (2001). *Addictions and substance abuse strategies for advanced practice nursing.* Upper Saddle River, NJ: Prentice Hall Health.

Shields, J. (2007). It's never too soon to prevent obesity. *NurseWeek 2007,* 16-17.

Simpson, C.A., & Tucker, J.A. (2002). Temporal sequencing of alcohol-related problems, problem recognition, and help-seeking episodes. *Addictive Behaviors, 27,* 659-674.

Spader, C. (2007). Manorexia—Men and boys suffer same social pressure to be thin. *NurseWeek,* 24-25.

Tozzo, M.A. (2007). Battling obesity: Small steps, big rewards. *Nursing, 37*(3), 68-69.

Trent, C. (2003). Integrating medical and substance abuse treatment for addicts living with HIV/AIDS: Evidence-based nursing practice model. *American Journal of Drug and Alcohol Abuse, 29*(4), 847-859.

Wicks, R. J. (2006). *Overcoming secondary stress in medical and nursing practice: A guide to professional resilience and personal well-being.* London: Oxford University Press.

Zhu, A. J., & Walsh, B.T. (2002). Pharmacologic treatment of eating disorders. *Canadian Journal of Psychiatry, 47*(3), 227-234.

CHAPTER 51

Anderson, J., Ebrahim, S., Floyd, L., & Atrash, H. (2006). Prevalence of risk factors for adverse pregnancy outcomes during pregnancy and the preconception period—United States, 2002-2004. *Maternal & Child Health Journal, 10,* 101-106.

Beckman, C. R. B, & Dysart, D. (2000). The challenge of multicultural medical care. *Contemporary OB/GYN, 45*(12), 12-33.

Callister, L. C. (2008). Global health and nursing: Global oral health in women and children. *MCN, The Journal of Maternal/Child Nursing, 33,*(1), 60.

Certain, H., Mueller, M., Jagodzinski, T., & Fleming, M. (2008). Domestic abuse during the previous year in a sample of postpartum women. *JOGNN: Journal of Obstetric, Gynecologic, & Neonatal Nursing, 37*(1), 35-41.

Olds, S. B., London, M. L., Ladewig, P.W., & Davidson, M. R. (2008). *Maternal-newborn nursing and women's health care* (8th ed.). Upper Saddle River, NJ: Prentice Hall.

Perozzi, K. J., Zalice, K. K., Howard, V., & Skariot, L. (2007). HSV: What you need to know to care for your pregnant patient. *MCN, The American Journal of Maternal/Child Nursing, 32,*(6), 345-350.

Russel, L., & Mayberry, L. (2008). Pregnancy and oral health: A review and recommendations to reduce the gap in practice and research. *MCN, The American Journal of Maternal/Child Nursing, 33*,(1), 32–37.

Soza-Vento, R., Flowers, L., Munroe, A., Fritz, K., Rua-Dobles, A., Munroe, C., et al. (2007). Reducing perinatal HIV transmission among HIV-infected pregnant women. *Joint Commission Journal on Quality & Patient Safety, 33*(4), 187–192.

Towle, M. A. (2009). *Maternal-newborn nursing care*. Upper Saddle River, NJ: Prentice Hall.

Towle, M. A., & Adams, E. D. (2008). *Maternal-child nursing care*. Upper Saddle River, NJ: Prentice Hall.

Tweddale, C. (2006). Trauma during pregnancy. *Critical Care Nursing Quarterly, 29*(1), 53–67.

Whitney, E. N. Cataldo, C. B., & Rolfes, S. R. (2002). *Understanding normal and clinical nutrition* (6th ed.). Belmont, CA: Wadsworth.

Youngkin, E., & Davis, M. S. (2003). *Women's health: A primary care clinical guide* (3rd ed.). Upper Saddle River, NJ: Prentice Hall.

CHAPTER 52

Berkowitz, R., & Goldstein, D. (2007). Gestational trophoblastic disease (1581–1603). In J. Berek, *Berek & Novak's gynecology* (14th ed.). Philadelphia: Lippincott Williams & Wilkins.

Callister, L. C. (2001). Culturally competent care of women and newborns: Knowledge, attitude and skills. *Journal of Obstetric, Gynecologic, and Neonatal Nursing, 30*, 209–215.

Centers for Disease Control and Prevention (CDC), Division of Reproductive Health, National Center for Chronic Disease Prevention and Health Promotion, Division of Vital Statistics, National Center for Health Statistics. (1993). *High-risk pregnancy.* Washington, DC: U.S. Government Printing Office.

Copeland, L. J., & Landon, M. B. (2002). Malignant diseases and pregnancy. In S. G. Gabbe, J. R. Neibly, & J. L. Simpson (Eds.), *Obstetrics: Normal and problem pregnancies* (4th ed., pp. 1255–1281). New York: Churchill Livingstone.

Dashe, J. S., Nathan, L., McIntire, D. D., & Leveno, K. (2000). Correlation between amniotic fluid glucose concentration and amniotic fluid volumes in pregnancy complicated by diabetes. *American Journal of Obstetrics and Gynecology. 182*(4), 901–904.

Davidson, M., London, M. L., & Ladewig, P. A. W. (2008). *Maternal–newborn nursing & women's health across the lifespan.* Upper Saddle River, NJ: Prentice Hall.

Jenkins, T. M., & Wapner, R. J. (2004). Prenatal diagnosis of congenital disorders. In R. K. Creasy & R. Resnik (Eds.), *Maternal-fetal medicine: Principles and practice* (5th ed., pp. 235–280). Philadelphia: Saunders.

Koniak-Griffin, D., Anderson, N., Verzemnieks, I., & Brecht, M. (2002). A public health nursing early intervention program for adolescent mothers: Outcomes from pregnancy through 6 weeks postpartum. *Nursing Research, 49*(3), 130–138.

Laughlin, D., & Knuppel, R. A. (2003). Maternal-placenta-fetal unit: Fetal and early neonatal physiology. In A. H. DeCherney & L. Nathan (Eds.), *Current obstetric & gynecologic: Diagnosis & treatment* (9th ed., pp. 163–191). New York: Lange Medical Books/McGraw-Hill.

Magann, E. F., Chauhan, S. P., Bofill, J. A., Waddell, D., Rust, O. A., & Morrison, J. C. (2002). *Maternal morbidity and mortality associated with intrauterine fetal demise: Five year experience at a tertiary referral hospital.* 70th annual meeting, Central Association of Obstetricians and Gynecologists, Maui, HI.

National Library of Medicine. (2007). Hydatid mole: Molar pregnancy. *MedlinePlus Medical Dictionary.*

Papp, C., & Papp, Z. (2003). Chorionic villus sampling and amniocentesis: What are the risks in current practice? *Current Opinion in Obstetrics & Gynecology, 15*(2), 159–165.

Queenan, J. T., Spong, C. Y., & Lockwood, C. J. (2007). *Management of high-risk pregnancy* (5th ed.). New York: Blackwell.

Regidor, E., Ronda, E., Garcia, A. M., & Dominguez, V. (2004). Paternal exposure to agricultural pesticides and cause specific fetal death. *Occupational & Environmental Medicine, 61*(4), 334–339.

Roberts, J. M., Pearson, G., Cutler, J., & Lindheimer, M. (2003). Summary of the NHLBI working group on research on hypertension in pregnancy. *American Heart Association Hypertension, 41,* 437–445.

Skeie, A., Foren, J. J., Vege, A., & Stray-Pedersen, B. (2003). Cause and risk of stillbirth in twin pregnancies: A retrospective audit. *Acta Obstetrica et Gynecologica Scandinavica, 82*(11), 1010–1016.

CHAPTER 53

Adams, E., & Bianchi, A. (2004). Can a nurse and a doula exist in the same room? *International Journal of Childbirth Education, 19*(4), 12–15.

Adams, E. D., & Bianchi, A. L. (2005). *50 Ways to comfort a laboring woman.* Presented at the AWHONN 2005 convention, June 14, Salt Lake City, Utah.

American Academy of Pediatrics (AAP) and American College of Obstetricians and Gynecologists (ACOG). (2002). *Guidelines for prenatal care* (5th ed.). Washington, DC: Author.

Bianchi, A., & Adams, E. (2004). Doulas, labor support, and nurses. *International Journal of Childbirth Education, 19*(4), 24–30.

Callister, L. C. (2001). Culturally competent care of women and newborns: Knowledge, attitude and skills. *Journal of Obstetric, Gynecologic & Neonatal Nursing, 30,* 209–215.

Cunningham, F. G., Grant, N. F., Leveno, K. J., Gilstrap, L. C., et al. (2005). *Williams obstetrics* (22nd ed.). New York: McGraw-Hill.

Kjos, S. L. (2000). Postpartum care of the woman with diabetes. *Clinical Obstetrics and Gynecology, 43*(1), 65–74.

Olds, S. B., London, M. L., Ladewig, P. W., & Davidson, M. R. (2008). *Maternal–newborn nursing and women's health care* (8th ed.). Upper Saddle River, NJ: Prentice Hall.

CHAPTER 54

American Academy of Pediatrics (AAP) and the American College of Obstetricians and Gynecologists (ACOG). (2002). *Guidelines for prenatal care* (5th ed.). Washington, DC: Author.

Blackburn, S. T. (2007). *Maternal fetal & neonatal physiology: A clinical perspective.* (3rd ed.). St. Louis, MO: Saunders.

Bozoky, I., & Corwin, E. J. (2002). Fatigue as a predictor of postpartum depression. *Journal of Obstetric, Gynecologic, and Neonatal Nursing, 30*(1), 13–18.

Cunningham, F. G., Leveno, K. J., Bloom, S. L., Hauth, J. C., Gilstrap, L. C., & Wenstrom, K. D. (2005). *Williams obstetrics* (22nd ed.). New York: McGraw-Hill.

Olds, S. B., London, M. L., Ladewig, P. W., & Davidson, M. R. (2008). *Maternal-newborn nursing and women's health care* (8th ed.). Upper Saddle River, NJ: Prentice Hall.

Rogers, J., & Davis, B. (1995). How risky are hot tubs and saunas for pregnant women? *MCN, 20*(3), 137–140.

Youngkin, E., & Davis, M. S. (1998). *Women's health: A primary care clinical guide* (2nd ed.). Upper Saddle River, NJ: Prentice Hall.

CHAPTER 55

Eby, L., & Brown, N. J. (2009). *Mental health nursing care* (2nd ed.). Upper Saddle River, NJ: Prentice Hall.

Gunes, M., Kayikcioglu, F., Ozturkoglu, E., & Haberal, A. (2005). Incisional endometriosis after cesarean section, episiotomy and other gynecological procedures. *Journal of Obstetrics and Gynaecology Research, 31*(5), 471–475.

Ladewig P., London, M., & Davidson, M. (2006). *Contemporary maternal-newborn nursing care* (6th ed.). Upper Saddle River, NJ: Prentice Hall.

Poggi, S. B. H., & Kapernick, P. S. (2003). Postpartum hemorrhage & and abnormal puerperium. In A. H. DeCherney & L. Nathan (Eds.). *Current obstetric & gynecologic: Diagnosis & treatment* (9th ed., pp. 531–552). New York: Lange Medical Books/McGraw-Hill.

Russel, M. (2004). *Adoption wisdom: A guide to the issues and feelings of adoption.* Lawrenceville, NJ: Tapestry Press.

Sallday, S. (2004). Ethical problems: Adoption dilemmas. *Nursing, 34*(12), 29.

Shevell, T., & Malone, F. D. (2003). Management of obstetric hemorrhage. *Seminars in Perinatology, 27*(1), 86–104.

Simpson, K., & Thorman, K. (2005). Obstetric "conveniences": Elective induction of labor, cesarean birth on demand, and other potentially unnecessary interventions. *Journal of Perinatal and Neonatal Nursing, 19*(2), 134–144.

Sooklim, R., Thinkhamrop, J., Lumbiganon, P., Witoon, P., Prasertcharoensuk, W., Pattamadilok, J., et al. (2007). The outcomes of midline versus medio-lateral episiotomy. *Reproductive Health, 4,* 10.

CHAPTER 56

American Academy of Pediatrics. (2006). Policy statements of American Academy of Pediatrics. *Pediatrics, 117*(5), 1846–1847.

Ball, J., & Bindler, R. (2006). *Child health nursing.* Upper Saddle River, NJ: Prentice Hall.

Ballard, J. L., Khoury, J. C., Wedig, K., Eilers-Walsman, B. L., & Lipp, R. (1991). New Ballard score, expanded to include extremely premature infants. *Journal of Pediatrics, 119*(3), 417–423.

Blackburn, S. T. (2007). *Maternal fetal and neonatal physiology: A clinical perspective* (3rd ed.). St. Louis, MO: Saunders.

Committee on Bioethics. (1995). Informed consent, parental permission, and assent in pediatric practice. *Pediatrics, 95*(2), 314–317.

Dougherty, G. (1998). When should a child be hospitalized? *Pediatrics, 101*(1), 6.

Johnson, M., Bulechek, G., McCloskey Dochterman, J., Maas, M., & Moorhead, S. (2001). *Nursing diagnoses, outcomes, & interventions: NANDA, NOC and NIC linkages.* St. Louis, MO: Mosby.

Olds, S. B., London, M. L., Ladewig, P. W., & Davidson, M. R. (2008). *Maternal-newborn and women's health care* (8th ed.). Upper Saddle River, NJ: Prentice Hall.

Orshan, S. (2008). The healthy newborn. *In Maternity, Newborn and Women's Health Nursing: Comprehensive Care Across the Lifespan.* Philadelphia: Wolters Kluwer/Lippincott Williams & Wilkins.

Seidel, J. M., Ball, J. W., Dains, J., & Benedict, G. W. (2003). *Mosby's guide to physical examination* (5th ed.). St. Louis, MO: Mosby.

Tappero, E. P., & Honeyfield, M. E. (1996). *Physical assessment of the newborn* (2nd ed.). Petaluma, CA: NICU Ink.

Towle, M. A. (2009). *Maternal-newborn nursing care.* Upper Saddle River, NJ: Prentice Hall.

CHAPTER 57

Anand, K., & Hall, R. (2008). Love, pain, and intensive care. *Pediatrics,* 825–827.

Ball, J. W., & Bindler, R. C. (2008). *Pediatric nursing: Caring for children* (5th ed.). Upper Saddle River, NJ: Prentice Hall.

Ballard, J. L., Khoury, J. C., Wedig, K., Wang, L., Wilers-Walsmann, B. L., & Lipp, R. (1991). New Ballard score, expanded to include extremely premature infants. *Journal of Pediatrics, 119*(3), 417–423.

Burkhart, D. M. (1999). Management of acute gastroenteritis in children. *American Family Physician, 60,* 2555–2563, 2565–2566.

Dougherty, G. (1998). When should a child be hospitalized? *Pediatrics, 101*(1), 6.

Fanaroff, A., Martin, R. & Walsh, M. (2005). *Neonatal-perinatal medicine: Diseases of the fetus and infant.* Philadelphia: Mosby.

Greene, C., & Goodman, M. (2003). Neonatal abstinence syndrome: Strategies for care of the drug-exposed infant. *Neonatal Network, 22*(4), 15.

Klein, K., & Stevens, R. (2008). The clinical use of probiotics for young children. *Journal of Family Health Care, 18*(2), 66–68.

Kyritsi, H., Matziou, V., Perdikaris, P., & Evagelou, H. (2005). Parent's needs during their child's hospitalization. *ICUS & Nursing Web Journal.* Retrieved August 15, 2008 from www.nursing.gr/needs.pdf.

Li, H., & Lopez, V. (2008). Effectiveness and appropriateness of therapeutic play intervention in preparing children for surgery: A randomized controlled trial study. *Journal for Specialists in Pediatric Nursing, 13*(2), 63–73.

Orshan, S. (2008). *Maternity, newborn and women's health nursing: Comprehensive care across the lifespan.* Philadelphia: Wolters Kluwer/Lippincott Williams & Wilkins.

Rahimian, J., & Varner, M. W. (2003). Disproportionate fetal growth. In A. H. Decherney & L. Nathan (Eds.), *Current obstetric & gynecologic diagnosis & treatment* (9th ed., pp. 301–314). New York: Lang Medical Books/McGraw-Hill.

Sarajärvi, A., Haapamäki, M., & Paavilainen, E. (2006). Emotional and informational support for families during their child's illness. *International Nursing Review, 53*(3), 205–210.

Sasidharan, K., Dutta, S., & Narang, A. (2008). Validity of New Ballard score till 7th day of postnatal life in moderately preterm neonates. *Archives of Disease in Childhood.*

Van Hulle, V. C. (2007). Nurses' perceptions of children's pain: A pilot study of cognitive representations. *Journal of Pain & Symptom Management, 33*(3), 290-301.

Zahr, L. K. (1998). Therapeutic play for hospitalized preschoolers in Lebanon. *Pediatric Nursing, 23*(5), 449-454.

CHAPTER 58

Betz, C. L. (2007). Health literacy: The missing link in the provision of health care for children and their families. *Journal of Pediatric Nursing, 22*(4), 257-260.

Carpenito, L. J. (2005). *Nursing diagnosis: Application to clinical practice* (11th ed.). Philadelphia: Lippincott.

Chamley, C. A., Carson, P., Randall, D. & Sandwell, M. (2004). *Developmental anatomy and physiology of children.* St. Louis: Elsevier Mosby.

Dougherty, G. (1998). When should a child be hospitalized? *Pediatrics, 101*(1), 6.

Huether, S. E. (2006). Alterations of renal and urinary tract function in children. In K. L. McCance & S. E. Huether, *Pathophysiology: The biologic basis for disease in adults and children* (5th ed.). St. Louis: Elsevier Mosby.

Miller, E. R., Iskander St, J., Pickering, S., & Verricchio, F. (2007). How can you promote vaccine safety? *Nursing 2007, 37*(4), 59-63.

Miller, E. R., & Woo, E. J. (2006). Time to prevent injuries form post-immunization syncope. *Nursing 2006, 36*(12), 20.

Rini, A., & Loriz, L. (2007). Anticipatory mourning in parents with a child who dies while hospitalized. *Journal of Pediatric Nursing, 22*(4), 272-282.

Rydz, D., et al. (2005). Topical review: Developmental screening. *Journal of Child Neurology, 20*(1), 4-21.

Sakakeeny-Zaal, K. (2007). Pediatric orthopnea and total airway obstruction. *American Journal of Nursing, 107*(4), 40-43.

Thorne, A. (2007). Are you ready to give care to a child with autism? *Nursing 2007, 37*(5), 59-61.

CHAPTER 59

Ball, J. W., & Bindler, R. C. (2008). *Pediatric nursing: Caring for children* (5th ed.). Upper Saddle River, NJ: Prentice Hall.

Blackburn, S. T. (2007). *Maternal fetal & neonatal physiology: A clinical perspective* (3rd ed.). St. Louis, MO: Saunders.

Centers for Disease Control and Prevention. (2000). Guidelines for the control of pertussis outbreaks. Atlanta, GA: Author.

Dalton, R. M., Negredo, A. A., Wilhelmi, I. D., Glass, R. I., & Sanchez-Fauquier, A. (2002). Astrovirus acute gastroenteritis among children in Madrid, Spain. *Pediatric Infectious Disease Journal, 21*(11), 1038-1041.

Dougherty, G. (1998). When should a child be hospitalized? *Pediatrics, 101*(1), 6.

Klein, K., & Stevens, R. (2008). The clinical use of probiotics for young children. *Journal of Family Health Care, 18*(2), 66-68.

Korres, S., Nikolopoulos, T., Peraki, E., Tsiakou, M., Karakitsou, M., Apostolopoulos, N., et al. (2008). Outcomes and efficacy of newborn hearing screening: strengths and weaknesses (success or failure?). *The Laryngoscope, 118*(7), 1253-1256.

Li, H., & Lopez, V. (2008). Effectiveness and appropriateness of therapeutic play intervention in preparing children for surgery: A randomized controlled trial study. *Journal for Specialists in Pediatric Nursing, 13*(2), 63-73.

Marin, M., Güris, D., Chaves, S. S., Schmid, S., & Seward, J. F. (2007). Prevention of varicella: Recommendations of the Advisory Committee on Immunization Practices (ACIP). *Morbidity & Mortality Weekly Report, 56* (RR04), 1-20.

Power, N., Liossi, C., & Franck, L. (2007). Family-centered care. *Journal for Specialists in Pediatric Nursing, 12*(3), 203-209.

CHAPTER 60

Adams, E. D., & Towle, M. A. (2009). *Pediatric nursing care.* Upper Saddle River, NJ: Prentice Hall.

Ball, J. W., & Bindler, R. C. (2008). *Pediatric nursing: Caring for children* (5th ed.). Upper Saddle River, NJ: Prentice Hall.

Blackburn, S. T. (2007). *Maternal fetal & neonatal physiology: A clinical perspective* (3rd ed.). St. Louis, MO: Saunders.

Bowman, S., Gortmaker, S., Ebbeling, C., Pereira, M., & Ludwig, D. (2004). Effects of fast-food consumption on energy intake and diet quality among children in a national household survey. *Pediatrics 113*(1), 112-118.

Dalton, R. M., Negredo, A. A., Wilhelmi, I. D., Glass, R. I., Sanchez-Fauquier, A. (2002). Astrovirus acute gastroenteritis among children in Madrid, Spain. *Pediatric Infectious Disease Journal, 21*(11), 1038-1041.

Dougherty, G. (1998). When should a child be hospitalized? *Pediatrics, 101*(1), 6.

Lutz, W. J. (1986). Helping hospitalized children and their parents cope with painful procedures. *Journal of Pediatric Nursing, 1,* 24-32.

Zahr, L. K. (1998). Therapeutic play for hospitalized preschoolers in Lebanon. *Pediatric Nursing, 23*(5), 449-454.

CHAPTER 61

Ball, J. W., & Bindler, R. C. (2008). *Pediatric nursing: Caring for children* (5th ed.). Upper Saddle River, NJ: Prentice Hall.

Burkhart, D. M. (1999). Management of acute gastroenteritis in children. *American Family Physician, 60,* 2555-2563, 2565-2566.

Marin, M., Güris, D., Chaves, S. S., Schmid, S., & Seward, J. F. (2007). Prevention of varicella: Recommendations of the Advisory Committee on Immunization Practices (ACIP). *Morbidity & Mortality Weekly Report, 56* (RR04), 1-20.

Power, N., Liossi, C., & Franck, L. (2007). Family-centered care. *Journal for Specialists in Pediatric Nursing, 12*(3), 203-209.

Seidel, J. M., Ball, J. W., Dains, J., & Benedict, G. W. (2008). *Mosby's guide to physical examination* (6th ed.). St. Louis: Mosby.

Stovitz, S., Pardee, P., Vazquez, G., Duval, S., & Schwimmer, J. (2008). Musculoskeletal pain in obese children and adolescents. *Acta Paediatrica, 97*(4), 489-493.

William Li, H., Lopez, V., & Lee, T. (2007). Effects of preoperative therapeutic play on outcomes of school-age children undergoing day surgery. *Research in Nursing & Health, 30*(3), 320-332.

CHAPTER 62

American Academy of Pediatrics. (2001). Strength training by children and adolescents. *Pediatrics, 107*(6), 1470-1472.

Benjamin, H., & Glow, K. (2003). Strength training for children and adolescents: What can physicians recommend? *The Physician and Sportsmedicine, 3*(9).

Calcaterra, V., Klersy, C., Muratori, T., Telli, S., Caramagna, C., Scaglia, F., et al. (2008). Prevalence of metabolic syndrome (MS) in children and adolescents with varying degrees of obesity. *Clinical Endocrinology, 68*(6), 868–872.

Harrison, L. H., Pass, M. A., Mendelsohn, A. B., Egri, M., Rosenstein, N. E., Bustamante, A., & Razeq, J., Roche, J. C. (2001). Invasive meningococcal disease in adolescents and young adults. *Journal of the American Medical Association, 286*(6).

Kidson, W. (1998). Polycystic ovary syndrome: A new direction in treatment. *Medical Journal of Australia, 169,* 537–540.

Largo, R. S., Gnatuk, C. L., Kunselman, A. R., & Dunaif, A. (2005). Change in glucose tolerance over time in women with polycystic ovarian syndrome: A controlled study. *Journal of Clinical Endocrinology and Metabolism, 90*(6), 3236–3242.

Late, M. (2008). APHA institute highlights safe teen driving tactics. *Nation's Health, 38*(1), 4.

Lindfred, H., Saalman, R., Nilsson, S., & Reichenberg, K. (2008). Inflammatory bowel disease and self-esteem in adolescence. *Acta Paediatrica, 97*(2), 201–205.

Markarian, M. (2008). Warning signs. *Current Health 2, 34*(7), 19–21.

Zapata, A., Moraes, A., Leone, C., Doria-Filho, U., & Silva, C. (2006). Pain and musculoskeletal pain syndromes related to computer and video game use in adolescents. *European Journal of Pediatrics, 165*(6), 408–414.

CHAPTER 63

Anderson, M. A. (2005). *Nursing leadership, management, and professional practice for LPN/LVNs* (3rd ed.). Philadelphia: F. A. Davis.

Hansten, R. I., & Washburn, M. J. (2004). *Clinical delegation skills—A handbook for professional practice* (3rd ed.). Gaithersburg, MD: Aspen Publishing.

Hill, S. S., Howlett, H. S., & Howlett, H. A. (2004). *Success in practical/vocational nursing from student to leader* (5th ed.). Philadelphia: W. B. Saunders.

Hohenhaus, S., Powell, S., & Hohenhaus, J. T. (2006). Enhancing patient safety during hand-offs: "Standardized communication and teamwork using 'SBAR' method." *American Journal of Nursing, 106*(8), 72A–72C.

Kurzen, C. R. (2004). *Contemporary practical/vocational nursing* (5th ed.). Philadelphia: Lippincott.

Sirota, T. (2007). Nurse/physician relationships improving or not? *Nursing 2007, 37*(1), 2052–2055.

The Joint Commission. National Patient Safety Goals: 2009 National Patient Safety Goals. Retrieved September 23, 2008 from www.jointcommission.org/patientsafety/national patientsafetygoals.

Walczak, M. B., & Absolon, P. L. (2001). Essentials for effective communication in oncology nursing: Assertiveness, conflict management, delegation and motivation. *Journal of Nursing Staff Development, 17*(3), 159–162.

CHAPTER 64

Anderson, L. W., & Krathwohl D. R. (Eds.). (2001). *A taxonomy for learning, teaching, and assessing. A revision of Bloom's taxonomy of educational objectives.* New York: Addison Wesley Longman.

Hill, S. S., Howlett, H. S., & Howlett, H. A. (2005). *Success in practical/vocational nursing from student to leader* (5th ed.). Philadelphia: W. B. Saunders.

McKinney, D. S., & Hogan, M. A. (2008). *Prentice Hall's comprehensive NCLEX-PN® review.* Upper Saddle River, NJ: Prentice Hall.

National Association for Practical Nurse Educators and Service (NAPNES). (2004). *Standards of practice for LPN/LVNs.* Silver Spring, MD: Author.

National Council of State Boards of Nursing. (2008). *Report of findings from 2006 LPN/LVN practice analysis: Comparability of survey administration methods* (Research Brief Vol. 33). Chicago: Author.

National Council of State Boards of Nursing. (2008). *2008 NCLEX-PN detailed test plan.* Chicago: Author.

National Federation of Licensed Practical Nurses (NFLPN). (2003). *Nursing practice standards for licensed practical/vocational nurses.* Raleigh, NC: Author.

Wilson, B., Shannon, S., & Strang, C. (2007). *Prentice Hall's nurse's drug guide 2007.* Upper Saddle River, NJ: Prentice Hall.

CHAPTER 65

Anderson, M. (2000). *To be a nurse—Personal/vocational relationships for the LPN/LVN.* Philadelphia: F. A. Davis.

Anderson, M. A. (2005). *Nursing leadership, management, and professional practice for LPN/LVNs* (3rd ed.). Philadelphia: F. A. Davis.

Becker, B. G., & Fendler, D. T. (1994). *Vocational and personal adjustment in practical nursing* (7th ed.). St. Louis, MO: Mosby.

Claywell, L., & Corbin, B. (2003). *LPN to RN transition.* St. Louis, MO: Mosby.

Cox, S. (2007). Good communication: Finding the middle ground. *Nursing 2007, 37*(1), 57.

Dunne, G. D. (2002). *The nursing job search handbook.* Philadelphia: University of Pennsylvania Press.

Hill, S. S., Howlett, H. S., & Howlett, H. A. (2004). *Success in practical/vocational nursing from student to leader* (5th ed.). Philadelphia: W. B. Saunders.

Kurzen, C. R. (2004). *Contemporary practical/vocational nursing* (5th ed.). Philadelphia: Lippincott.

Makely, S. (2004). *Professionalism in health care: Primer for success* (2nd ed.). Upper Saddle River, NJ: Brady/Prentice Hall.

Porter, L. (n.d.). *Notes on how to read a textbook* (unpublished). Anaheim, CA: North Orange County Regional Occupational Program.

Taylor, J., & Hardy, D. (2004). *Monster careers: How to land the job of your life.* New York: Penguin Press.

Index

extrapyramidal symptoms, 1349*t*
Parkinson's disease, 969
Anticholinergic effects
antipsychotic medications, 1350
tricyclic antidepressants, 1360
Anticipatory grieving, 345
Anticipatory guidance, 1611
Anticoagulants
atrial fibrillation, 870*t*
endocarditis, 867
herbal remedies, 124, 125*t*
thrombophlebitis, 878
Anticonvulsants for bipolar disorder, 1368
Antidepressants
monoamine oxidase inhibitors, 1362
neurotransmitters, 1359, 1359*f*
novel antidepressants, 1360, 1361–1362
selective serotonin reuptake inhibitors, 1360, 1361
sleep, affecting, 507
tricyclic and related agents, 1359–1360
Antidiuretic hormone (ADH)
diabetes insipidus, 1056
endocrine system, 1050*t*, 1053*f*, 1054
SIADH, 1056
Anti-DNA antibody test, 925
Antiembolism stockings
applying, procedure for, 733–734, 734*f*
preoperative application, 717
Antigens
explained, 166, 907
Antihistamines
allergies, 929
Parkinson's disease, 969
Anti-inflammatory medication, 866
Antimicrobial soap, 169
Antimigraine drugs, 475*t*
Antinuclear antibody (ANA) test, 923, 925
Antipsychotic medications, potential for abuse, 1351
Antipyretics, 436
Antiseptics, 169–170
Antisocial personality disorder, 1374*t*
Antitussives, 804
Antivenom, 1294
Antivert. *See* Meclizine
Anuria, 1092*t*
Anus. *See also* Anorectal disorders
fetal development, 1417*t*
GI system, 991, 991*f*
Anxiety
clients with psychosocial needs, 338
factor affecting pain experience, 473
pain management, 477
reduction of, 33
stress, 329, 330*t*
Anxiolytics, 1384*t*, 1386
Aorta, 849, 850*f*
Apex of the vertebral curve, 1312
Apgar scores
infant care immediately following birth, 1475
normal neonates, 1533–1534, 1534*t*
obtaining, procedure for, 1552
Aphasia
explained, 380
speech therapists, 1271
Aphasic clients with Alzheimer's disease, 972

Apheresis, 1258
Apical pulse
assessment site, 442, 442*f*, 442*t*
explained, 441
measurement, procedure for, 459–460, 460*f*
Apical-radial pulse
explained, 444
measurement, procedure for, 460–461
APIE (assessment, problem, intervention, evaluation) charting, 237
Aplastic anemia, 891–892
Apnea
defined, 447, 795
infants and toddlers, 1637
Apneic spells in newborns, 1532
Apocrine glands, 303, 745
Apothecaries' system of measurement, 620, 620*t*
Appearance, personal, 193
Appendages of the integumentary system, 744–745, 744*f*, 745*f*
Appendicitis, 1014–1015, 1015*f*, 1723–1724
Appendicular skeleton, pediatric, 1599–1600
Appetite
loss of, 494
stimulating, 577
Application level of testing, 6, 7*t*, 1781*t*
Applications for employment, 1792
Appropriateness of documentation, 231
Approximated surfaces of healing wounds, 533
Apraxic, explained, 972
AquaMEPHYTON. *See* Phytonadione; Vitamin K supplements
Aquathermia pads, 541, 541*f*, 547
Arab heritage, people with, 281
Arachnoid mater, 940, 942*f*
Arachnophobia, 330
Arbitration, legal, 47
Arcus senilis, 1190
Aricept. *See* Donepezil
Aripiprazole, 1348, 1351
Arm recoil, 1538*t*, 1539*f*
Arrector pili muscles, 744*f*, 745
Arrhythmias
explained, 851, 868
pulse assessment, 443
Artane. *See* Trihexyphenidyl
Arterial blood gases
acid-base balance, 600, 600*t*
cardiovascular disorders, 854*t*
Arterial blood pressure, 448
Arterial circulation, described, 849
Arterial occlusive disease, 1209
Arteries
disorders of, 877–878
structure and function, 849, 851*f*
veins, differences between, 669, 669*t*
Arterioles, 849
Arteriosclerosis
blood pressure, 448, 449, 874
described, 851
Arteriosclerosis obliterans, 877
Arthrocentesis, 768*t*
Arthrogram, 768*t*
Arthroscopy, 768*t*
Artificial acquired passive immunity, 911
Artificial active immunity, 910–911
Artificial eyes, 408, 409*f*

Artificial rupture of membranes, 1476, 1476*f*
Ascaris lumbricoides, 1694*t*
Ascendin. *See* Amoxapine
Aschoff's nodules, 865
Ascites, 1031, 1032, 1032*f*
Asepsis, explained, 170
Aseptic technique, 170
Asian diet pyramid, 574
Asian heritage, people with
alcoholism, genetic resistance to, 1382
HIV and AIDS incidence, 1450
postpartum hemorrhage, 1518
thalassemia, 1641
vision, variations in, 981
Asian/Pacific Islander heritage, people with
deaths from diabetes mellitus, 1066
family, insights into, 27–28
As-needed (prn) hygiene care, 393
As-needed (prn) orders, 614
Aspartate aminotransferase (AST) test, 713*t*
Aspart NovoLog insulin, 1071*t*
Asperger's syndrome, 1703*t*
Asphyxia in SGA newborns, 1567
Asphyxiation
defined, 820
safety issues, 138, 139*f*
Aspiration
SGA newborns, 1567
wet drowning, 1293
Aspiration biopsy, 1249
Aspiration pneumonia, 720*t*
Aspirin
headaches, 955*t*
juvenile rheumatoid arthritis, 1645
myocardial infarction, 858
nonmalignant breast disorders, 1134
pain management, 474*t*
polyarthritis of acute rheumatic fever, 1716
Reye's syndrome, 1648
rheumatoid arthritis, 777
surgery risk factor, 712
Assault, explained, 42*t*, 44
Assessing, in interview for loss and grieving, 352
Assessing, in nursing care
blood pressure assessment, 453–454, 454*t*
CAM therapies, 126
cardiopulmonary disorders, 864
care in relation to loss, 351–352
caring for adolescents, 1757
children with musculoskeletal disorders, 1722
child with asthma, 1714
client admission, 260
client communication, 201
client discharge, 267
client having cancer surgery, 1250
client in respiratory distress, 830
clients dealing with substance abuse, 1394
client's fluid status, 602
clients in labor, 1469–1470, 1470*t*, 1471*t*
clients in long-term care, 1274–1275
clients in the EC, 1295
clients undergoing chemotherapy, 1256
clients undergoing radiation therapy, 1253
clients with adrenal disorders, 1080
clients with at-risk pregnancy, 1451
clients with autoimmune disorders, 926
clients with bladder disorders, 1109

BUN. *See* Blood urea nitrogen (BUN)
Bundle branches, cardiac, 847, 848*f*
Bundle of His, 847, 848*f*
Bunions, 1207, 1208*f*
Buphthalmos, 1650
Bupropion
  depression, 1360, 1361
  smoking cessation, 824
Buretrol drip factor, 667
Burns
  classification of, 1296–1297, 1297*f*, 1298*f*
  integumentary system disorders, 757
  nursing care, 1297–1299, 1299*f*
  nursing process care plan, 1299–1300
  preschoolers, 1701–1703
  prevention of, 135
  types of, 1296
Burping infants, 1504, 1505*f*
Bursitis, 1207
Butcher's broom, 125*t*
Butoconazole, 1173*t*
Butorphanol tartrate, 474*t*
Butterfly (scalp vein) needles, 664, 664*f*
Butterfly rash, 924, 924*f*
Byock, Ira, 1232

C

CA 15-3 test, 1248
CA 27-29 test, 1248
CA 125 test, 1248
CABG. *See* Coronary artery bypass graft (CABG)
Cachexia, 1244
CAD. *See* Coronary artery disease (CAD)
Caffeine
  effects of, overdose, and withdrawal, 1387*t*,
    1388, 1388*f*, 1389
  headaches, 955*t*
  pregnancy risk factor, 1437
  sleep, affecting, 507
Calan. *See* Verapamil hydrochloride
Calcinosis, 926
Calcitonin
  hyperparathyroidism, 1062
  thyroid gland hormone, 1051*t*, 1054
Calcitonin supplement, 773, 773*t*
Calcium (macromineral), 567, 568*t*
Calcium, dietary, 1196
Calcium balance, 494
Calcium channel blockers
  angina pectoris, 855
  atrial fibrillation, 870*t*
Calcium level
  hyperparathyroidism, 1061–1062
  hypoparathyroidism, 1062
  musculoskeletal disorders, 768*t*
  normal values and imbalances, 597*t*
  pregnant and nonpregnant values, 1425*t*
  thyroid surgery, 1059–1060, 1060*f*
Calcium supplements
  electrolyte imbalances in ethnic diets, 596
  hypoparathyroidism, 1062
  osteoporosis, 773, 773*t*, 1196
  premenstrual syndrome, 1140
Calcivirus, 999
Calculation questions on tests, 8
Calculi, urinary, 1105–1106, 1106*f*
Calendar method of contraception, 1160*t*

Caloric testing, 979
Calories
  explained, 569
  recommendations by age, 570*t*
CAM. *See* Complementary and alternative medi-
    cine (CAM)
Camphylobacter jejuni, 1684
Camphylobacter sp., 999
CAMRSA (community-acquired methicillin-resis-
    tant *Staphylococcus aureus*), 168, 168*t*, 1311
Canada Food and Drugs Act of 1953, 611*t*
Canadian crutches, 495, 495*f*
Canadian Narcotic Control Act of 1961, 611*t*
Cancer
  bladder, 1108–1109, 1109*f*
  bone, 774
  breast, 1134–1137, 1135*f*, 1135*t*, 1136*f*,
    1137*f*, 1138*f*, 1138*t*, 1213
  cervical, 1145–1146, 1146*f*, 1750
  colon, 1212
  colorectal, 1001, 1020–1023, 1020*f*, 1021*f*,
    1022*f*, 1248
  defined, 1243
  early warning signs, 1246
  endometrial, 1145
  esophageal, 996
  gastric, 1004–1005, 1005*f*
  liver, 1001, 1033–1034
  lung, 827–828, 828*f*, 1388–1389
  oral, 993, 993*f*
  ovarian, 1146, 1147*f*
  pancreatic, 1035, 1035*f*
  prostate, 1153–1154, 1212, 1213
  renal, 1100
  skin, 757–759, 758*f*
  testicular, 1151, 1151*f*, 1752
  thyroid, 1061
  vulva, 1147–1148, 1148*f*
Cancer, caring for clients with, 1242–1263
  cancer, explained, 1243
  cancer prevention and screening, 1245–1246,
    1245–1246*t*
  chapter review, 1261
  critical thinking care map, 1262
  diagnostic evaluation, factors affecting choice
    of, 1246–1247
  diagnostic evaluation, nursing implications in,
    1247–1248
  diagnostic tests, 1248–1249, 1249*f*
  major treatments
    biotherapy, 1258
    bone marrow and stem cell transplantation,
      1258
    chemotherapy, 1255–1258, 1256*f*, 1257*f*,
      1259
    goals for, 1250
    radiation therapy, 1252–1255, 1253*f*, 1255*t*
    responses to, 1250
    surgical therapy, 1250–1252, 1251*f*, 1252*f*
    types of, 1249
  NCLEX-PN® exam preparation, 1263
  normal cells *versus* cancer cells, 1243–1245,
    1244*f*
  special populations, care for, 1259–1261
  terms used, 1243
  treatment planning, 1249
Cancer cells

appearance, 1245
  differentiation, 1245
  growth, 1243–1245, 1244*f*
Cancer epidemiology
  defined, 1243
  risk factors, 1244, 1244*f*
Cancer suppressor genes, 1243
Candida albicans
  candidiasis, 1155, 1176, 1176*f*
  diaper dermatitis, 1662
  examination of, 1170
  normal flora, 162*t*
  thrush, 992, 1644
Candidiasis
  family planning issues, 1155
  manifestations, complications, tests for, and
    treatment, 1173*t*, 1176
  oral, 918, 992–993, 1644, 1644*f*
Canes, 495, 495*f*, 496, 1303
Canker sores, 751
Cannabis, 1387*t*, 1388
Cannula of needles, 623, 624*f*
Cannula of tracheostomy tube, 801, 801*f*
Cannulation, intravenous, 1282, 1288
Capillaries, 849, 851*f*
Capillary hemangioma, 747, 748*f*
Capillary refill time, 373
Caplets, 610*t*
Capsules
  administering, procedure for, 638, 638*f*
  drug preparation, 610*t*
Caput succedaneum, 1541, 1542*f*
Carbamazepine
  ADHD, 1729*t*
  bipolar disorder, 1368
  glossopharyngeal neuralgia, 979
  Isaac's syndrome, 979
  pain management, 476
  trigeminal neuralgia, 978
Carbohydrates
  diabetes, diet modifications for, 573*t*
  macronutrient, 564–565
  wound healing, 535
Carbon dioxide
  acid-base balance, 599, 600–601, 601*t*
  respiratory function, 794, 795
  transport of, 794
Carbonic acid, 598
Carbon monoxide, 797
Carbuncles, 750
Carcinoembryonic antigen (CEA), 1248
Carcinogenesis, defined, 1243
Cardiac arrest, 872*t*
Cardiac catheterization
  described, 852
  infants and toddlers, 1638–1639
Cardiac cycle, explained, 846, 847, 848*f*
Cardiac enzyme studies, 854*t*
Cardiac muscle, described, 764
Cardiac output (CO)
  blood pressure, 448
  explained, 441, 847–848
  respiratory function, 794
Cardiac reserve, 492, 848
Cardiac tamponade, 866
Cardinal movements (mechanisms) of labor,
    1466–1468, 1467*f*, 1468*f*

nursing care, 1225–1226
prevention of, 1224
critical thinking care map, 1240
NCLEX-PN® exam preparation, 1241
postmortem care, procedure for, 1237–1238
terminal illness
death, care after, 1235–1237, 1236t
death, definitions and signs of, 1235
defined, 1226
hospice, 1227–1228
legal issues, 1233–1235, 1234f
LPN/LVN role in care of clients with terminal illness, 1228–1229, 1228f
nursing care, 1229–1233
nursing process care plan, 1233
palliative care, 1226–1227
Chronic bronchitis, 824, 825f
Chronic hepatitis, 1029
Chronic hypertension with pregnancy, 1446
Chronic illness
characteristics and examples of, 1223
factors associated with, 1223–1224, 1224f
LPN/LVN role in care of clients with chronic illness, 1224–1225, 1225f
nursing care, 1225–1226
prevention of, 1224
resistance of hosts to infection, 166
Chronic infections, 163
Chronic lymphocytic leukemia, 895
Chronic myelogenous leukemia, 895
Chronic obstructive pulmonary disease (COPD)
cor pulmonale, 864
explained, 817t, 824, 825f
older adults, 1208
respiratory drive, 795
smoking, 1389
surgery risk factor, 712
Chronic open-angle glaucoma, 1211, 1211f
Chronic pain, 469, 470t
Chronic pancreatitis, 1034–1035
Chronic progressive multiple sclerosis, 969
Chronic rejection of transplants, 921
Chronic renal failure
explained, 1101
older adults, 1212
school-aged children, 1726–1727, 1726f
Chronic subdural hematoma, 963
Chronological format for résumés, 1793
Chvostek's sign, 1059, 1060f, 1062
Cilia, respiratory, 792
Cimetidine
acute gastritis, 1000
GERD, 994
hiatal hernia, 996
peptic ulcer disease, 1002
Ciprofloxacin
gonorrhea, 1171t
pyelonephritis, 1098
Circle of Willis, 945f, 954
Circular turns for roller bandages, 545, 545f
Circulation
newborns, 1532–1533, 1532f
thermal tolerance, 540
Circulatory overload
blood transfusions, 679t
IV therapy, 676t
Circumcision

female, 1133
foreskin preservation in infants with hypospadias or epispadias, 1659
male, 1131–1132
neonatal procedure, 1548–1549, 1548t, 1549f
phimosis, 1662
Circumduction (movement), 491t
Circumoral cyanosis, 1571, 1679
Cirrhosis
alcohol, long-term use of, 1384, 1385f
causes, 1031
complications, 1033
described, 1029, 1031
diagnosis and treatment, 1032–1033
manifestations, 1031–1032, 1032f, 1033f
multisystem effects of, 1031f
Citalopram, 1360
Citizens, nurses as, 47
Civil law
false communication, 42t, 44–45
intentional torts, 42t, 44
IV therapy, 660
loss of client property, 45
unintentional torts, 42t, 43–44
Clamps on IV tubing, 663–664
Clark level staging system for melanoma, 1248
Claustrophobia, 330
Clean, explained, 170
Clean-catch urine specimens, 1093, 1093f, 1112–1113, 1113f
Cleaning baths, 393
Cleansing enemas, 1010–1011
Clean voided specimens, 1093
Clean wounds, 532
Clear liquid diet, 571
Cleft lip
client teaching, 1577–1578
described, 1577, 1577f
infants and toddlers, 1655
nursing care, 1578
nursing process care plan, 1578–1579
treatment, 1577
Cleft palate
client teaching, 1577–1578
infants and toddlers, 1655
Clergy in long-term care facilities, 1271
Client, supporting
client with terminal illness, 1230
pain, 485
Client advocacy
ethical issues, 55–56
long-term care facilities, 1267
values basic to, 56
Client care, planning, 227
Client-care equipment, 749
Client communication, 190–206
chapter review, 204
clinical settings, principles of communication in, 193, 195–196, 196f, 197t
communication, described, 191
critical thinking care map, 205
factors influencing, 191–192
interviewing, 196, 198–201
modes of communication, 192–193, 192f, 193f
NCLEX-PN® exam preparation, 206
nursing care, 201–202

nursing process care plan, 202–203
therapeutic communication, 193, 194–195t
Client concern, assessing, 37
Client contracting as teaching strategy, 218
Client education
areas for, 209
explained, 208
principles of, 208, 209, 217–218
Client-focused model of care, 114
Client needs categories on NCLEX-PN®, 1781–1783
Client property
hospital admission, 259–260, 260f
loss of, 45
surgery, during, 716
Client records
confidentiality, 233–234
explained, 227
long-term care facilities, 1267
purposes of, 227–228
Client response to medication administration, 626
Clients
explained, 21
IV therapy, preparing for, 668
preparation for assessment, 368, 368f
reassessing, before implementation, 92
rights of, in long-term care facilities, 1273
role in rehabilitation, 1272–1273
Client Teaching
back injury prevention, 152
blood pressure, controlling, 876
breathing and coughing techniques, 803
cancer early warning signs, 1246
care of HIV child at home, 1645
chronically ill pediatric clients, 1614
controlling postural hypotension, 504
depression, reducing, 323
diarrhea, managing, 1013
discharge teaching: foot care, 399
eating disorders, strategies for preventing, 1403
enuresis alarms, 1697
food allergies, manifestations of, 1670
foot care with peripheral vascular disease, 879
health promotion topics during pregnancy, 1427
incentive spirometers, using, 803
infant massage, 1550
mechanisms for coping with anxiety, 331
metered-dose inhalers, using, 635
nutritious snacks for school-aged children, 1712
ongoing care for client with STI, 1178
parenting tips for adolescents, 1751
postpartum emergencies, 1500
postpartum self-care after discharge, 1499
preoperative instructions, 713
preventing urinary tract infections in women, 1110
promoting rest and sleep, 511
recovery phase of acute rheumatic fever, 1717
reducing the risk of elder abuse, 1200
sexually transmitted infections and adolescents, 1751
strategies for preventing eating disorders, 1403
testicular self-examination, 1151, 1151f
testing stool for occult blood, 1014
thrombocytopenia, 893

Diagnostic tests
  cancer
    classification and staging, 1248
    invasive techniques, 1248–1249, 1249*f*
    laboratory studies, 1248
    tumor imaging, 1248
  cardiovascular disorders, 852–853, 852*f*, 853*f*
  EC or UC, 1285, 1286
  immune system status, 911–913
  musculoskeletal disorders, 767–768, 768*t*
  pregnancy, 1420
  respiratory status, function, and oxygenation,
    797–798, 797*f*, 798*f*
  sleep disorders, 508–509
  STIs, 1170, 1171–1173*t*
  urinary elimination, alterations in, 1090–1091
Dialysis
  explained, 1101
  hemodialysis, 1101, 1102*f*, 1103, 1105
  nursing care, 1105
  peritoneal dialysis, 1102*f*, 1103
Diaper dermatitis (ammonia dermatitis), 396*t*,
  1662–1663, 1663*f*
Diapering
  double, for postoperative urinary care, 1584,
    1584*f*
  newborns, 1545, 1545*f*
  triple, for developmental dysplasia of the hip,
    1653
Diaphoresis
  blood volume balance mechanism, 1488
  shock, 1289
Diaphoretic, explained, 393
Diaphragmatic breathing, 445
Diaphragmatic hernia, 1581
Diaphragms, vaginal, 1157*f*, 1158, 1161*t*
Diarrhea
  infants and toddlers, 1653
  lower GI disorder, 1012–1013
  major causes of, 1012*t*
Diastasis recti abdominis, 1487, 1487*f*
Diastole
  cardiovascular system assessment, 373
  pulse assessment, 443*t*
  ventricular, 847, 848*f*
Diastolic pressure, 448
Diazepam
  dry mouth, 403
  myocardial infarction, 858
  pain management, 475
  seizures, 957
DIC. *See* Disseminated intravascular coagulation
  (DIC)
Dichotomous thinking, 1399
Dickens, Charles, 17, 17*f*
Dicoumarol, 120
Diencephalon, 935*f*, 940
Diet. *See also* Food; Nutrition
  diabetes mellitus, 1069–1070
  diet as tolerated, 572
  gout, 779
  postoperative care, 723–724
  sleep issues, 507, 511
Dietary Supplement Health and Education Act of
  1994, 120
Dietitians
  health care providers, 111

long-term care facilities, 1271
Differentiation of cancer cells, 1245
Diffusion of alveolar gases, 793–794
Diflucan, 752
Digital rectal examination, 1152, 1153
Digital vein, 670*t*
Digitoxin, 863
Digoxin
  atrial fibrillation, 870*t*
  CHF, 863
Dihydroergotamine
  headaches, 955*t*
  pain management, 475*t*
Dilatation (first) stage of labor, 1465–1466,
  1465*f*
Dilatation and curettage, 1141, 1442
Dilatation of the cervix, 1458
Dilation of arterioles, 849
Dimenhydrinate, 999
Diphenhydramine
  extrapyramidal symptoms, 1349*t*
  hypersensitivity and anaphylaxis, 915
  nausea and vomiting, 999
Diphtheria, 1673*t*
Diphtheria/tetanus/pertussis immunizations
  (DTaP)
  children and adolescents, 1673*f*
  infants and toddlers, 1632*t*
Diplopia
  myasthenia gravis, 974
  older adults, 1210
Dipsticks for urine testing, 1093
Direct care, 93
Direct contact transmission, 165
Direct hernias, 1018
Directive interviews, 196
Direct method of venipuncture, 672
Direct response of pupils, 372
Direct supervision, 1766*t*
Dirty, explained, 170
Dirty wounds, 532–533
Disability, defined, 1272
Disalcid. *See* Salsalate
Disappearing veins, 669
Disaster planning
  EC and prehospital settings, 1282–1283, 1283*f*
  safety, 141–142
Disaster triage codes, 142
Disbelief stage of conflict, 1773
Discharge of a client. *See also* Admission, transfer,
  and discharge
  culturally proficient care, 38
  discharge, explained, 264
  discharge planning, 38, 85
  discharge teaching, documentation for, 264,
    265*f*
  discharge teaching for neonatal care,
    1549–1550
  instructions, documentation for, 265, 266*f*, 267
Discoid lupus erythematosus, 925
Disconnectedness stage of conflict, 1773
Discovery as teaching strategy, 217*t*, 219
Discrimination, explained, 31
Discussion, explained, 227
Disease
  blood pressure, 449
  cardiovascular system, affecting, 849, 851

diet modifications for, 572–573*t*
  explained, 162
  oxygenation, affecting, 796
Disenfranchised grief, 345
Disinfectants, 169–170
Disk skin barrier, changing, 1042, 1042*f*
Dislocations, 783
Disorganized behavior, 1346
Disorganized symptoms, 1346
Disorganized thinking, 1346
Disparities, explained, 31
Displaced fractures, 769, 769*f*
Displacement as defense mechanism, 334*t*
Disposable pouch for ostomies, 1042–1043,
  1043*f*
Dissecting aneurysms, 874, 875*f*
Disseminated intravascular coagulation (DIC)
  described, 893
  manifestations of, 893
  treatment, 893–894
Distal (anatomic direction), 370
Distance, personal, in interviews, 199
Distance vision, 1329–1330, 1329*f*
Distancing
  clients with terminal illness, from, 1226
  explained, 356
  nurses' responses to clients with cancer, 1248
Distractibility, 1365
Distraction
  pain management, 476–477
  terminally ill pediatric clients, 1612
Distribution of drug, 614
Distribution of healthcare services, 112
Disturbed thought processes, 1353–1354
Disulfiram, 1391
Disuse atrophy, 492
Disuse osteoporosis, 492
Diuresis
  explained, 863
  postpartum, 1488
Diuretics
  CHF, 863
  hypertension, 874
Diurnal variations (circadian rhythm)
  blood pressure, 449
  body temperature, 435, 435*f*
Divalproex sodium, 1368
Diverticular disorders, 1001
Diverticulitis, 1018, 1019
Diverticulosis, 1018–1019, 1019*f*, 1212
Diverticulum
  defined, 994
  Meckel's diverticulum, 1657
DMT (dimethyltryptamine), 1387*t*
Dobutamine, 872*t*
Dock, Lavinia L., 18, 18*f*
Doctor of Naturopathic Medicine (ND)
  degree, 121
Documentation, 226–252
  assessing clients with depression, 1369
  behavior changes due to education, 208
  blood pressure, 454
  care to dying patients, 355
  chapter review, 250
  client record confidentiality, 233–234
  client records, purposes of, 227–228
  critical thinking care map, 251

Gingiva, 403
Gingivitis, 404t, 993
Ginko/gingko biloba, 125t, 126
Ginseng, Asian, 125t
Glargine insulin, 1071t
Glasgow Coma Scale
    head injury, 1292
    neurologic disorders, 949
    neurologic status assessment, 371, 371t
Glass IV infusion systems, 663
Glaucoma
    anticholinergic effects of psychiatric drugs,
        1360
    causes and corrective actions, 982t
    infants and toddlers, 1650
    older adults, 1210–1211, 1211f
Glioblastomas, 966, 966f
Gliomas, 937
Gliosis, 970f
Glipizide, 1073t
Global Burden of Disease Study, 1338
Glomerulonephritis, 1099–1100, 1695, 1696
Glomerulus of the nephron, 1087, 1089f
Glossitis, 404t
Glossopharyngeal nerve (CN IX), 945t
Glossopharyngeal neuralgia, 978–979
Gloves
    infection control, 173–174, 179–181, 180f,
        181f
    sterile, 174, 179–183, 180f, 181f, 182f
Glucagon, 1052t, 1054
Glucocorticoids, 1051t, 1053f, 1055
Glucophage. See Metformin
Glucose in urine, 1091t, 1094, 1724
Glucose level
    diabetes mellitus, 1064, 1064f
    fasting, 713t, 1068
    fluctuations in, 1073
    high-risk newborn care, 1563–1564
    pregnant and nonpregnant values, 1425t
    sliding scale insulin, 1071, 1072
Glucose level monitoring
    diabetes mellitus, 1069, 1069f
    nutrition and diet therapy, 577, 580
    procedure for, 580, 1082, 1082f
Glucose tolerance test, 1068
Glucosuria, 1091t, 1094, 1724
Glucotrol. See Glipizide
Glue, inhaling, 1387t
Glulisine insulin, 1070
Glutamate, 1343t
Gluten, dietary, 1658
Glyburide, 1073t
Glycogen, 565
Glycogenesis, 565
Glycogenolysis, 565
Glycohemoglobin (hemoglobin A1c), 1068
Goal-directed activity, 1365
Goals, setting, in nursing process care plans,
    89, 91
Goiter, 1060, 1061f, 1747
Goldenseal, 125t
Gold salts, 923
Gonadocorticoids, 1051t, 1055
Gonadotropins, 1054
Gonads
    chemotherapy, 1259

endocrine system, 1081
Gonorrhea, 1171t, 1174
Goodell's sign, 1420, 1421
Good Samaritan acts, 47
Goose bumps, 745
Gout
    musculoskeletal system inflammatory disorder,
        779
    older adults, 1207
Gowers' maneuver, 1687, 1687f
Gowns, sterile or for infection control, 174,
    181–183, 182f
Graafian follicle, 1130
Graft versus host disease
    acute, 1258
    blood transfusions, 680t
    bone marrow transplants, 896–897, 1258
    chronic, 1258
    organ transplantation, 921
Grandiose delusions
    bipolar disorder, 1365
    schizophrenia, 1345t
Grandparents, 1489, 1490
Granulation tissue, 534
Granulocytes, 886–887, 907
Graphic records, 238, 239f, 245
Graves' disease, 1747. See also Hyperthyroidism
    (Graves' disease)
Gravida, defined, 1424t
Gray matter, 938
Great saphenous vein, 670t
Greenstick fractures, 769, 769f
Grief
    assisting clients in working through, 354, 355
    described, 345
    linear model of stages of, 350, 350f
    responses to, factors influencing, 345–348,
        346t, 347f
    serious medical illness, response to, 332
    stages and manifestations of, 348, 348f
Grieving, described, 349
Grieving persons, tasks, rights, and needs of,
    349–350, 350f
Griseofulvin, 753
Gross motor skills
    adolescents, 1734t
    infants, 1627–1628t
    preschoolers, 1669t
    school-aged children, 1711t
    toddlers, 1629t
Group, defined, 192
Group B streptococci, 1441
Group communication, 192
Group discussion as teaching strategy, 217t
Group insurance plans, 115–116
Group teaching as teaching strategy, 218
Group therapy, 1368
Growth
    cancer cells versus normal cells, 1243–1245,
        1244f
    explained, 289
    measurements for pediatric assessment,
        1606–1607
    newborns with alterations in, 1566–1568,
        1567f
Growth and development
    body alignment and activity, 491

components of, 290
    factors that influence, 290
    principles of, 289–290
    stages and milestones of, 291–294f, 291–294t
Growth hormone
    deficiency, in infants and toddlers, 1658–1659
    deficiency, in preschoolers, 1696
    endocrine system, 1050t, 1053f, 1054
    hyperpituitarism, 1055–1056
    hypopituitarism, 1056
Growth plates, 765
Guillain-Barré syndrome, 975–976, 1684
Gumma, 1171t
Gums, assessment of, 382
Gurgles, 375t
Gustatory hallucinations, 1345
Gynecologic problems of adolescents, 1749
Gynecomastia, 1349
Gyri, 938

H

HAART (highly active antiretroviral therapy),
    918–919
Habitual abortion, 1442
Haemophilus influenzae
    mastitis, 1520
    meningitis, 959, 960t, 1743
Haemophilus influenzae type b (Hib), 1674–1675t
    epiglottitis, 813
    preschoolers, 1673f
Haemophilus influenza type b (Hib) immunization
    infants and toddlers, 1632t
    meningitis, 1743
Haemophilus parainfluenzae, 1520
Haemophilus sp., 162t
Hair
    described, 744–745, 744f
    older adults, 1188
Hair care
    hair characteristics, 400
    nursing care, 400–403, 402f
    procedure for, 418–420, 418f, 419f
Haldol. See Haloperidol
Half-life, explained, 613, 614, 614f
Halitosis, 404, 404t
Hallucinations, 1345, 1346
Hallucinogens, 1387–1388, 1387t
Haloperidol
    depot injection, 1351
    Huntington's disease, 976
    schizophrenia, 1348
    Tourette's syndrome, 979
Hammertoe, 1207, 1208f
HAMRSA (hospital-acquired methicillin-resistant
    Staphylococcus aureus), 168, 168t
Hand gestures, 33
Hand hygiene/washing
    alcohol-based solutions, 173
    drug resistant organisms, 168
    microorganisms, controlling, 169, 178–179,
        178f, 179f
    procedure for, 178–179, 178f, 179f
Handicap, defined, 1272
Handoff procedure, 1769–1770
Hand restraints, 146, 146f
Hard connective tissue, 766–767
Harris flush, 1011, 1039

Informed consent
exceptions to, 50
nursing practice, legal aspects of, 49–50
pediatric considerations, 49
transcultural communication and client concerns, 33
witnessing, 49–50
Infusate, 667
Infusion pumps for IV therapy, 665–666, 666f, 667f
Inguinal hernias, 1018, 1018f, 1691
INH. See Isoniazid
Inhalants, 1387t, 1388
Inhalation
explained, 445
mechanics of, 446, 446f
Inhalation injuries, 816t, 820
Inhalation route of administration, 617t
Inhibin-A level, 1441
Inhibiting effect, explained, 613
Inhibition of hormone secretion, 1052
Initial comprehensive plan of care, 85
Initiative versus guilt, 276t, 277, 301
Injection ports on IV administration sets, 664
Injections
administering, procedure for, 644–649, 646f, 647f
anaphylactic shock, risk of, 1290
Injuries
back injuries, prevention of, 150–151, 151f, 152
brain and spinal cord, to infants and toddlers, 1645, 1647
client education for prevention, 209
cultural and ethnic differences, 135
informed consent, 50
neurologic, in school-aged children, 1718, 1718f
procedure- or equipment-related, prevention of, 139–140
thermal tolerance, 540
Inotropic medications, 1639
Inotropics, explained, 864
Inpatients
defined, 104
settings for health care, 105, 107–108, 107f
INR (international normalized ratio), 854t
Insect bites, 1294, 1701
Insensible water loss, 435, 595, 596
Insight, explained, 1337
In situ malignancies, 1136
Insoluble, explained, 564
Insomnia
common sleep disorder, 507–508
older adults, 1190
Inspection as examination method, 369
Inspiration
explained, 445
pulmonary ventilation, 793, 793f
Institute for Safe Medication Practices, 619
Institutional safety issues, 140–144, 143f
Insulin
carbohydrate intake, 565
endocrine system, 1052t, 1054
injection sites, 1070, 1071f
insulin pumps, 1072
medication errors, 619

metabolic acidosis, 601
mixing in one syringe, 644, 644f
pancreas, 992
regimens for, 1070, 1072f
sliding scale, 1071, 1072
types of, 1070–1071, 1071t
Insulin-dependent diabetes mellitus, 1066–1067, 1067f
Insulin pumps, 1072
Insulin reaction/shock, 1073
Insulin resistance, 1067
Insulin syringes, 622, 622f, 623
Insurance
healthcare economics, 115–116
long-term care and rehabilitation, 1274, 1274f, 1275
professional liability, 47–48
Intact skin
explained, 532
maintaining, 542, 543t
Intake and output
high-risk newborn care, 1563
monitoring, 602–603, 602f
Integrated delivery systems
healthcare economics, 116
Integrative medicine, 121
Integrity versus despair, 276t, 277, 1193
Integumentary disorders
adolescents, 1752–1753, 1752f
infants and toddlers, 1662–1663, 1663f
preschoolers, 1698–1703, 1699f, 1700f
school-aged children, 1727–1728
Integumentary system. See also Skin
assessment, procedure for, 381–382, 381f
fetal development, 1417t, 1419
focused assessment by body systems, 364f, 365
health assessment, 372–373, 373t, 374f
immobility, effects of, 494
maternal changes during pregnancy, 1422
older adults, abnormal changes in, 1206–1207
older adults, changes in, 1188, 1188f
pediatric anatomy and physiology, 1603–1604, 1603f
radiation therapy side effects, 1254, 1255t
structure and function of, 743–746, 744f, 745f
Integumentary system disorders, clients with, 742–762
bacterial infections, 749–750, 750f
burns, 757
chapter review, 760
chronic skin conditions, 754–755, 755f
critical thinking care map, 761
fungal infections, 752–753, 753f
integumentary system, structure and function of, 743–746, 744f, 745f
NCLEX-PN® exam preparation, 762
nursing care, 755–757
nursing process care plan, 757
parasitic infestations, 753–754
plastic and reconstructive surgery, 759
skin cancer, 757–759, 758f
skin integrity, 746–749, 747f, 748f
viral infections, 751–752, 751f
Intellectual consequences of stress, 326
Intellectual distraction, 477
Intellectualization as defense mechanism, 334t
Intensity of labor contractions, 1462, 1463f, 1464

Intensity of pain, 480–481, 482f
Intentional torts, 42t, 44
Intentional traumas, 532
Intercostal retractions, 447, 796
Intercultural communication, 32
Interdisciplinary care plan meetings, 244
Interferon
HPV, 1172t
multiple sclerosis, 971
Intermittent claudication, 877, 1209
Intermittent enteral feedings, 578
Intermittent fever, 436
Intermittent IV infusion devices, 667
Internal disasters, 141
Internal respiration, 445
Internal rotation of fetus during birth, 1466, 1467f
Internal sphincter of the urethra, 1088, 1089f
International normalized ratio (INR), 854t
International Red Cross, 18
Interpersonal skills, 94
Interpersonal therapy, 323
Interpreters, 36
Interstate endorsement of licensing laws, 20
Interstitial disorders of the respiratory tract, 828–829, 829f
Interstitial fluids, 593, 593f
Interstitial spacing of body fluids, 1291
Intervention in SOAPIE charting, 237
Interventions
consequences of, considering, 94
criteria for, 94
errors resulting in negligence, 43
explained, 92
types of, 93–94
Intervertebral disks, 1188–1189
Interviews for employment
follow-up, 1797–1798
illegal questions, 1797
interview questions, examples of, 1797
skills for, 1798
tips for success, 1796–1797
Interviews of clients
approaches to, 196, 198
data collection, 82
factors influencing, 199
loss and grieving, 351, 352
questions, types of, 198–199
stages of, 199–201
Intestinal obstruction, 1019–1020
Intestinal parasites, 1693, 1694t
Intestinal secretions, 594
In-the-ear-canal hearing aids, 1198
In-the-ear hearing aids, 1198
Intimacy versus isolation, 276t, 277
Intoxication, 1381, 1383t
Intracellular fluid
electrolytes, 594
explained, 593
Intracerebral hematoma, 963t, 964
Intracoronary streptokinase therapy, 856–857
Intracranial pressure
increased
coughing, contraindication for, 802
diagnosis, 950, 952
manifestations of, 950, 951–952t, 951f
nursing considerations, 952

Methicillin-resistant *Staphylococcus aureus* (MRSA)
   contact precautions, 170
   harmful actions of microorganisms, 162
   school-aged children, 1727–1728
Methimazole, 1058, 1060*t*
Methotrexate
   breast cancer, 1137
   Kaposi's sarcoma, 917
   SLE, 925
Methyldopa, 1740*t*
Methylenedioxymethamphetamine (MDMA), 1387*t*, 1388
Methylergonovine, 1485, 1486*t*
Methylphenidate
   abuse, potential for, 1391*t*
   ADHD, 1728, 1729*t*
   MAOIs, 1362
Methylprednisolone
   organ transplantation, 922
   spinal cord injury, 965
Methysergide, 475*t*
Metoclopramide, 999
Metoprolol, 475*t*
Metric system
   converting weights within, 621
   explained, 619–620, 619*f*, 620*t*
Metronidazole
   peptic ulcer disease, 1001
   trichomoniasis, 1173*t*, 1176
Metrorrhagia, 1141
Mexican heritage, people with
   adolescents, 281
   cancer diagnosis, discussing, 1247
   hypertension and cardiovascular disease, 873
   infections, 167
   labor and birth practices, 1470, 1471*t*
   personal space, 199
MI. *See* Myocardial infarction (MI)
Miacalcin. *See* Calcitonin supplement
Micatin, 752
Miconazole, 1173*t*
Microcephaly
   Down syndrome, 1573
   fetal alcohol syndrome, 1385
Microdermabrasion, 759
Microdrip IV administration sets, 663, 667
Microminerals, 567, 568*t*
Micronase. *See* Glyburide
Micronutrients
   minerals, 567–568, 568*t*
   vitamins, 567–568*t*
Microorganisms
   agencies for controlling communicable diseases, 162–163
   chain of infection, 164, 164*f*, 164*t*
   harmful actions of, 161–162
   helpful actions of, 161, 162*t*
   types of, 161
Microsulfon. *See* Sulfadiazine
Micturition, 1088
Middle Eastern heritage, people with
   rest and sleep, 507
   thalassemia, 1641
Midstream urine specimens, 1093, 1093*f*
Mifepristone, 1137
Migraine headache, 954, 955*t*, 1742
Migranal. *See* Dihydroergotamine

Mild brain injury, 962
Milia, 1540*f*, 1541
Milieu therapy
   mental health disorders, 1340
   schizophrenia, 1347
Military antishock trousers (MAST), 1289
Milk
   iron absorption, 890
   toddlers, 1630
"Milk" teeth, 1541
Milwaukee brace, 1720
Minafen formula, 1575
Mineralocorticoids, 1051*t*, 1055
Mineral oil, 1010*t*
Minerals (micronutrients), 567–568, 568*t*
Minim, explained, 620
Minimal response to cancer treatment, 1250
Minimum Data Set (MDS) for Resident Assessment and Care Screening, 247
Minor characteristics in NANDA nursing diagnoses, 84
Minors, consent for treatment in the EC and UC, 1283
Minor surgery, 711
Mirtazapine, 1360, 1361
Misdemeanors, 45
Missed abortion, 1442
Mitered corners of bed sheets, 412, 412*f*
Mithramycin. *See* Plicamycin
Mitotane, 1079
Mitral valve
   explained, 846, 846*f*
   mitral regurgitation, 1208, 1209*f*
   mitral stenosis, 865, 866*f*
   mitral valve prolapse, 1208
Mittelschmerz, 1157
Mitt restraints, 146, 146*f*
Mixed lymphocyte culture, 921
Mixed settings for health care, 108
MMR. *See* Measles/mumps/rubella immunizations (MMR)
Mnemonics, using as memory aid, 1784
Moban. *See* Molindone
Mobility of clients
   older adults, 1189
   safety, 132
Mock NCLEX-PN® examinations, 1785
Moclobemide, 1362
Moctanin. *See* Monoctanoin
Modeling as teaching strategy, 217*t*
Models of care for nursing, 113–115
Moderate brain injury, 962
Molding of the fetal head during birth, 1461, 1461*f*, 1541
Molindone, 1348
MONA (morphine, oxygen, nitroglycerin, aspirin), 858
Mongolian spots, 1540*f*, 1541
Monitoring devices to prevent falls, 138, 139*f*, 155–156, 155*f*
Monoamine oxidase inhibitors (MAOIs)
   actions, 1362
   foods to avoid, 1362
   list of, 1360
Monoctanoin, 1028
Monocytes, 887, 887*f*, 888*t*, 907, 908*f*
Mononucleosis

adolescents, 1742
   preschoolers, 1677*t*
Mons pubis, 1128*f*, 1129
Montgomery straps, 539, 539*f*
Mood disorders
   bipolar disorder, 1364–1368, 1364*f*, 1366*f*
   collaborative care, 1358–1364, 1359*f*, 1363i*f*, 1364f
   major depressive disorder
      causes and incidence, 1355–1356
      clinical features, 1356–1357, 1357*f*
      course of the disease, 1356
      diagnostic criteria and manifestations, 1355
      postpartum depression, 1356
      seasonal affective disorder, 1356
   nursing care, 1368–1372, 1370*f*
   nursing process care plan, 1372–1373
   suicide, 1357–1358
Moral, explained, 277–278
Moral concepts, 54–55
Moral development
   adolescents, 305
   adults, middle-aged, 306
   adults, older, 309
   adults, young, 306
   neonates and infants, 297
   preschoolers, 302
   school-age children, 303
   toddlers, 301
Moral development theory, 277–278, 278*t*
Moral growth and development, 290
Morality, explained, 54
Morbid obesity, 1005
Morbillivirus, 1675*t*
Mormons, 1236*t*
"Morning-after pill," 1159
Morning care, 393
"Morning sickness," 1422
Moro (startle) reflex, 297*t*, 298*f*, 1544
Morphine
   abuse, potential for, 1390*t*
   cardiovascular system, affecting, 849
   cholecystitis, 1027
   myocardial infarction, 858
   oxygenation, affecting, 796
   pain management, 474*t*
   postpartum pain management, 1495*t*
   pulmonary edema, 864
   sleep, affecting, 507
   use, overdose, and withdrawal, 1384*t*, 1385
Morticians, 1237
Morula, 1413, 1413*f*, 1414*f*
Motivation
   client teaching, 214
   cognitivism, 209
   learning, facilitating, 209–210
   sleep, affecting, 507
Motor abilities
   learning, barrier to, 211–212, 212*t*
   preschoolers, 301
   school-age children, 302
   toddlers, 300
Motor development of neonates and infants, 297
Motor function and increased intracranial pressure, 951*t*
Motor pathways in peripheral nerves, 934
Motor response, assessing, 380

Motor status in neurologic disorders, 949
Motor vehicle safety, 1739, 1739f
Motrin. *See* Ibuprofen
Mourner's Bill of Rights, 349
Mourning, 345, 1236t
Mouth
  fetal development, 1417t
  gastrointestinal system assessment, 376, 376f
  GI system, 988, 989f
Mouth care
  common problems, 403
  nursing care, 403–406, 404t
  teeth, temporary and permanent, 403, 403f
Movement
  normal activity, 490–491, 490f, 491t
  postoperative care, 723
Moving a client in bed, 502, 515–520, 516f,
    517f, 518f, 519f, 520f
MRI. *See* Magnetic resonance imaging (MRI)
MRSA. *See* Methicillin-resistant *Staphylococcus au-
    reus* (MRSA)
MS (multiple sclerosis), 969–971, 970f
MSDS (Material Safety Data Sheets), 140–141
Mucomyst, 1693
Mucositis, 1254, 1255t
Mucous membranes, 382
Mucoviscidosis, 1633. *See also* Cystic fibrosis (mu-
    coviscidosis)
Multigravida (multiple gestation/pregnancy),
    1424t, 1449, 1491t
Multipara, 1424t
Multiple births, 1502–1503
Multiple-choice questions, answering, 6–7, 6–7t
Multiple gestation (multigravida/multiple preg-
    nancy), 1424t, 1449, 1491t
Multiple marker screen for high-risk pregnancy,
    1441
Multiple myeloma, 897, 1249
Multiple pregnancy
  high-risk pregnancy, 1449
  multigravida, defined, 1424t
  postpartum assessment, 1491t
Multiple sclerosis (MS), 969–971, 970f
Multistate compact, 1780
Mummy restraints, 147, 147f
Mumps, 1675t
Murphy's sign, 1027
Muscle fatigue in older adults, 1189
Muscle relaxants
  herniated disk, 782
  low back pain, 782
Muscles
  activity of, and body temperature, 435
  assessment, procedure for, 386
  pediatric anatomy and physiology, 1600,
    1600f
Muscle spasms, 1189
Muscle strength and learning, 211
Muscular dystrophy, 1687–1688, 1687f
Musculoskeletal disorders
  adolescents, 1743–1745, 1744t
  infants and toddlers, 1652–1653, 1652f, 1653f
  preschoolers, 1687–1690, 1687f, 1688f, 1689f,
    1690f
  school-aged children, 1719–1723, 1720f,
    1720t, 1721f
Musculoskeletal system. *See also* Skeletal system

assessment, procedure for, 386–387
congenital defects, 1580–1581
fetal development, 1417t, 1419
focused assessment by body systems, 364f, 366
health assessment, 377–378
immobility, effects of, 492, 492f
maternal changes during pregnancy, 1422
muscular system, structure and function of,
    764, 765f
older adults, abnormal changes in, 1207,
    1207f, 1208f
older adults, changes in, 1188–1189
pediatric anatomy and physiology, 1598–1600,
    1599–1600f
trauma, 1292
Musculoskeletal system disorders, clients with,
    763–789
  chapter review, 787
  critical thinking care map, 788
  diagnostic tests, 767–768, 768t
  fibromyalgia, 784–785
  heat and cold applications, 768
  inflammatory disorders
    ankylosing spondylitis, 779
    gout, 779
    Lyme disease, 779
    nursing care, 780–781
    osteoarthritis, 777–779, 778f, 778t
    rheumatoid arthritis, 777, 778t
  joint and muscle disorders
    carpal tunnel syndrome, 783
    dislocations, 783
    nursing care, 783–784, 784t
    strains and sprains, 782–783
    temporomandibular joint disorder, 783
  musculoskeletal system, structure and function
    of, 764–767, 765f, 766f, 767f
  NCLEX-PN® exam preparation, 789
  nursing care of clients with SLE and/or fi-
    bromyalgia, 785
  spinal disorders, 781–782, 781f
  surgery, 768–769
  systemic lupus erythematosus, 784
  traction application, procedure for, 786
  traumatic bone disorders
    bone cancer, 774
    fractures, 769–772, 769f, 770f, 771f, 772f
    nursing care, 774–776, 776f
    nursing process care plan, 776–777
    osteomalacia, 773–774
    osteomyelitis, 774, 774f
    osteoporosis, 772–773, 773t
Music therapy, 123t
Muslim (Islamic) faith
  circumcision, 1548
  medications made from pork, 627
  mourning and after-death rites, 1236t
Mustache care, 402
Mutual pretense about approaching loss, 352
Mutual support groups, 108
Myambutol. *See* Ethambutol
Myasthenia gravis
  described, 923
  diagnosis and treatment, 924
  manifestations, 923–924
  neurologic disorder, 974–975, 975f
  nursing care, 927

nursing considerations, 924
Myasthenic crisis, 923–924, 975
Mycobacterium tuberculosis, 164t, 822, 1713
Mycosis fungoides, 757, 759
Myelin, 937
Myelinated nerve fibers, 471
Myelination of nerve fibers, 1598
Myelograms, 768t, 947
Myocardial infarction (MI)
  classification of, 857
  complications, 858
  described, 851, 857, 857f
  diagnosis and treatment, 858
  manifestations of, 857–858, 857t
  nursing care, 860
  older adults, 1208
  risk factors for, 857
Myocardial ischemia, 854
Myocarditis, 866
Myocardium, 845, 846f
Myoclonic seizure, 956
Myograms, 768t
Myomectomy, 1144
Myopathy, 1385
Myopia, 981t, 1719, 1719f
MyPyramid food guide
  ethnic diets, 574
  standard, 569, 569f
Mythic-literal stage of spiritual development,
    280, 280t, 303
Myxedema, 1060
Myxedema coma, 1060–1061

N

Nadir, defined, 1243
Nails
  assessment, procedure for, 382
  assessment of, 373, 374f
  care of, 398, 398f
  characteristics of, 395
  older adults, 1188
  structure of, 745, 745f
Nalbuphine hydrochloride, 474t
Naloxone, 474t, 1501
Naltrexone, 1391
NANDA (North American Nursing Diagnosis
    Association, NANDA International), 82–83
NAPNES. *See* National Association for Practical
    Nurse Education and Service (NAPNES)
Naprosyn. *See* Naproxen
Naproxen, 474t
Naratriptan, 475t
Narcan. *See* Naloxone
Narcissistic personality disorder, 1374t
Narcolepsy, 508
Narcotics
  oral, administering, procedure for, 639
  sleep, affecting, 507
Narcotics Anonymous, 1392
Nardil. *See* Phenelzine
Narrative charting, 234
Nasal flaring, 1532, 1532f
Nasal medications, instilling, 633
Nasal oxygen cannulas, 832–833, 833f, 834
Nasal route of administration, 479t
Nasal symptoms in terminally ill pediatric clients,
    1612

Nursing students, succeeding as, 2–13
  chapter review, 12
  clinical experience participation, 8–9
  clinical setting prioritization, 9–10f, 9–11
  NCLEX-PN® exam preparation, 13
  nursing values and characteristics, 3
  studying effectively, 4
  test taking, 6–7t, 6–8, 7f, 8t
  textbook, reading, 3–4
  time management, 4–6, 5f
Nursing theories and models. *See also under* Critical thinking and nursing theory/models
  elements of, 68, 70–73t
  introduction to, 68
  Leininger's cultural care diversity and universality theory, 73t
  Neuman's system model, 71–72t
  Nightingale's environmental theory, 70t
  Orem's general theory of nursing, 70–71t
  Roy's adaptation model, 72–73t
Nursing values and characteristics, 3
Nutrient IV solutions, 662
Nutrients
  carbohydrates, 564–565
  explained, 564
  lipids, 566–567, 566t
  macronutrients, 564–567, 566t
  micronutrients, 567–568, 567–568t
  minerals, 567–568, 568t
  proteins, 565–566, 566t
  vitamins, 567–568t
  water, 564, 565f
Nutrition. *See also* Diet
  adolescents, 1734t, 1736–1737
  body alignment and activity, 492
  children with cancer, 1260
  clients with depression, 1371
  clients with psychosocial needs, 338
  domains of culture, 30
  explained, 564
  infants, 1626, 1627–1628t, 1629–1631
  newborns, 1546–1547, 1547t
  older adults with cancer, 1260
  over- and under-nutrition for older adults, 1212
  pediatric client, adapting nursing care for, 1607–1608
  postpartum care, 1496
  pregnancy, requirements during, 1427, 1428t
  pregnancy risk factor, 1437
  preoperative preparation, 713, 715
  preschoolers, 1669–1670, 1669t, 1670t, 1692
  pressure ulcers, 548
  resistance of hosts to infection, 165
  school-aged children, 1711–1712, 1711t, 1712f, 1712t
  terminally ill pediatric clients, 1611
  toddlers, 1626, 1629t, 1630–1631, 1630t
  wound healing, 534–535
Nutrition and diet therapy, 563–591
  blood glucose, monitoring, 580
  chapter review, 589
  critical thinking care map, 590
  healthy diet, standards for, 568–571, 569f, 570t, 571t
  medication administration via an enteral tube, 588

nasogastric tubes, inserting and removing, 581–584, 582f, 583f
  NCLEX-PN® exam preparation, 591
  nursing care, 574–579, 575f, 576f
  nursing process care plan, 579–580
  nutrients, 564–568, 565f, 566t, 567–568t
  specialized diets, 571–574, 572–573t
  tube feedings, administering, 585–587, 586f
Nutritionists, 111
Nutrition Therapy
  food sources of iron vitamin B$_{12}$, and folic acid, 1411
  vitamin B$_{12}$ and iron, food sources of, 890
Nutting, Mary Adelaide, 18
Nystagmus
  cataracts in infants and toddlers, 1650
  Ménière's disease, 979
  vision disorder, 981t
Nystatin, 1173t

O

Obesity
  blood pressure, 449
  causes, 1401
  dangers of, 1400–1401
  diabetes mellitus, 1064, 1066
  explained, 1005–1006, 1006f
  hypertension, 874
  nutrition and diet therapy, 575
  preschoolers, 1692
  surgery risk factor, 712
  treatment, 1401
  wound healing, 534
Objective data
  assessing clients with STIs, 1177
  collection in the EC or UC, 1284
  critical thinking care maps, 68
  explained, 68, 81
  SOAP charting, 236
OBRA. *See* Omnibus Budget Reconciliation Act (OBRA)
Observation
  explained, 82
  skills for, 82t
Obsessions, 330
Obsession stage of conflict, 1773
Obsessive-compulsive disorder, 330
Obsessive-compulsive personality disorder, 1374t
Obstetric history as pregnancy risk factor, 1437, 1438f
Obstructive respiratory disorders
  asthma, 817t, 824
  atelectasis, 818t, 827
  bronchiectasis, 818t, 825, 825f, 826f
  chronic bronchitis, 824, 825f
  chronic obstructive pulmonary disease, 817t, 824, 825f
  cystic fibrosis, 818t, 826–827, 827f
  emphysema, 818t, 825–826, 825f, 826f
Obstructive sleep apnea, 806f, 812t, 814
Obstructive uropathy, 1660, 1660f
Obtunded (LOC), 949
Obturator of tracheostomy tube, 801, 801f
Occipital (posterior) fontanels, 1460f, 1461
Occlusion of arteries, 854
Occlusive dressings, 536

Occupational Exposure to Tuberculosis Standard (OSHA), 140
Occupational lung diseases, 828
Occupational Safety and Health Administration (OSHA)
  hospital and institutional safety, 140
  IV therapy, 661
  Occupational Exposure to Tuberculosis Standard (OSHA), 140
  Respiratory Standard, 174
Occupational therapists
  health care providers, 111
  long-term care facilities, 1269–1271, 1270f
Occupation of client, 34
Occupied beds
  changing, procedure for, 428–429, 428f
  making, 412
Occurrence/incident reports. *See* Incident reports
Oculomotor nerve (CN III), 944t
Odor
  ostomies, 1021–1022
  smell, sense of, 82t, 296, 1191, 1598
Office tasks, 1268
Official drug names, 609
Ofloxacin
  chlamydia, 1171t
  gonorrhea, 1171t
Oil enemas, 1011t
Oils, explained, 566
Ointments, 610t
Olanzapine
  eating disorders, 1400
  schizophrenia, 1348, 1351
Older mothers, risks to, 1440
Older parents, and new family client teaching, 1503
Olfactory hallucinations, 1345
Olfactory nerve (CN I), 944t
Oliguria
  shock, 1289
  urinary elimination, alterations in, 1092t
Omeprazole
  GERD, 994
  peptic ulcer disease, 1002
Omnibus Budget Reconciliation Act (OBRA)
  long term care documentation, 247
  long-term care facilities, 107, 1265
Omphalocele, 1574, 1574f
Oncogenes, 1243
Oncology, defined, 1243
1-hour glucose screen, 1441
One-time orders, 614
One-to-one discussion as teaching strategy, 217t
Ongoing planning, explained, 85
Onset of action of a drug
  explained, 614
  insulin, 1070, 1071t
Onsite healthcare team in long-term care facilities, 1268
On-the-body hearing aids, 1198
Oocytes, 1130
Oophorectomy, 1141, 1144, 1145, 1146
Open awareness of approaching loss, 352
Open beds, making, 411
Open catheter or bladder irrigation, 1097, 1097f, 1098
Open-ended questions

Plateau phase of sexual response cycle, 1132*t*
Platelet and coagulation disorders
  disseminated intravascular coagulation,
    893–894
  hemophilia, 894
  hemostasis, 892, 893*f*
  nursing considerations, 894
  thrombocytopenia, 892–893
Platelet levels, 1425*t*
Platelets
  idiopathic thrombocytopenia purpura, 893
  production and function of, 887, 887*f*
  transfusion, for, 678*t*, 893
Pleasurable activities, 1365
Pleural effusion, 822
Pleurisy/pleuritis, 817*t*, 822
Plicamycin, 1062
Plunger of syringes, 622, 622*f*
Pneumatic antishock garments, 1289, 1291*f*
Pneumatic compression boots, 717
Pneumococcal immunization
  children and adolescents, 1673*f*
  infants and toddlers, 1632*t*
Pneumococcal meningitis, 959, 960*t*
Pneumococcus sp., 1696
Pneumoconioses, 828
Pneumocystis jiroveci (carinii) pneumonia, 917
Pneumonia
  immobility, effects of, 494
  lower respiratory disorders, 817*t*, 821
  noscomial infection, 163*t*
  postoperative client, 720*t*
  preschoolers, 1672
Pneumothorax, 822, 829, 829*f*
PNS. *See* Peripheral nervous system (PNS)
Podofilox solution or gel, 1172*t*
Podophyllin resin, 1172*t*
Point of maximal impulse, 442
Poison Control Center telephone number, 137
Poisonings
  EC care, 1294
  preschoolers, 1693
  prevention of, 136–137
Polio
  early care, 19
  preschoolers, 1675*t*
Polio immunizations
  children and adolescents, 1673*f*
  infants and toddlers, 1632*t*
Polyarthritis of acute rheumatic fever, 1716
Polycystic kidney, 1099, 1099*f*, 1660
Polycystic ovary syndrome, 1140
Polycythemia, 449, 892
Polydactyly, 1543
Polydipsia
  diabetes insipidus, 1056
  diabetes mellitus, 1067, 1724
Polyhydramnios (hydramnios), 1448
Polymerase chain reaction test, 918
Polyneuritis, 974
Polyneuropathy, 974, 975
Polyphagia
  diabetes mellitus, 1067, 1724
  GI disorders, 992
Polypharmacy
  explained, 616
  older hospitalized adults, 1214

Polyps, 1020, 1021*f*
Polysubstance abuse, 1386
Polyurethane foam dressings, 537*t*
Polyuria
  diabetes insipidus, 1056
  diabetes mellitus, 1067, 1724
  urinary elimination, alterations in, 1092*t*
Popliteal angle, 1538*t*, 1539*f*
Popliteal artery, 442, 442*t*
Population Focus
  antidepressants and the older adult, 1360
  clients with COPD, 795
  HIV/AIDS incidence in the United States, 917
  homeless people, risk factors for health
    problems, 113
  wound healing in older adults, 535
Porcine skin, 921
Portable oxygen delivery systems, 800, 800*f*
Portal hypertension, 1031–1032, 1032*f*
Portal of entry in chain of infection, 164*f*, 165
Portal of exit in chain of infection, 164*f*, 164*t*,
    165
Portfolio, professional, 1791
Portosystemic shunts, 1032, 1032*f*
Port-wine stain, 747, 748*f*
Position changes and pulse rate, 441
Positioning clients
  breastfeeding, for, 1505, 1506*f*
  chronic lung disorders, 826
  position of mother during labor, 1464, 1464*f*
  postoperative client, 722
  preparation for assessment, 368, 368*f*
  principles of, 498–499, 499*f*
  respiratory system problems, 807–808, 808*f*
*Position Statement on Cultural Diversity in Nursing
  Practice* (ANA), 31
Positive end expiratory pressure (PEEP), 807*t*
Positive feedback, 211
Positive inspiratory pressure, 807*t*
Positive pregnancy test, 1419–1420
Positive signs of pregnancy, 1420, 1420*f*
Positive symptoms of schizophrenia, 1345,
    1345*t*, 1346
Positron-emission tomography (PET) scans
  cancer, 1248
  cardiovascular disorders, 853
Postconference periods, 11
Postconventional stage of moral development
  adults, middle-aged, 306
  adults, young, 306
Postconventional stage of moral development
    theory, 278, 278*t*
Post dates and induction of labor, 1476
Posterior (anatomic direction), 370
Posterior descending artery, 857
Posterior pituitary (neurohypophysis), 1050*t*,
    1054
Posterior tibial artery, 442, 442*t*
Postexposure prophylaxis, 661
Postherpetic neuralgia, 752
Postictal state, 957, 1682
Postmastectomy exercises, 1138*f*
Postnatal depression. *See* Postpartum depression
Postnecrotic cirrhosis, 1031
Postoperative care
  client with GI accessory organ disorders, 1037
  client with lower GI disorders, 1025–1026

GI surgery, 1007–1008
Postoperative phase of surgery
  described, 711
  immediate postanesthetic phase, 718
  nursing care, 719–728, 720–721*t*, 725*f*,
    726*f*, 727*f*
  nursing process care plan, 728
  potential problems, 720–721*t*
Postpartal chill, 1488
Postpartum (puerperal) infection, 1521, 1521*f*
Postpartum, defined, 1484
Postpartum blues, 1521–1522
Postpartum depression, 321, 1356, 1521*f*, 1522,
    1523–1524*t*
Postpartum Depression Predictors Inventory,
    1522, 1523–1524*t*
Postpartum psychosis, 1356, 1522
Postpartum women, care of, 1483–1515
  body systems adaptations, 1484–1488, 1484*f*,
    1485*f*, 1486*f*, 1486*t*, 1487*f*
  breastfeeding, 1503–1508, 1504*f*, 1505*f*,
    1506*f*
  cesarean section, after, 1500–1502
  chapter review, 1513
  critical thinking care map, 1514
  cultural influences, 1484, 1490
  fathers, siblings, and others, 1489–1490, 1490*f*
  fundal massage and clot removal from the
    uterus, 1509–1510, 1509*f*
  NCLEX-PN® exam preparation, 1515
  new family, 1502–1503, 1502*f*
  nursing care
    assessing, 1490–1494, 1491*t*, 1494*f*
    continuity of care, 1498, 1500
    diagnosing, planning, and implementing,
      1494–1498, 1495*t*, 1496*f*, 1497*f*
    evaluating, 1498, 1499
    prioritizing, 1490
  nursing process care plan, 1498–1500
  perineal assessment, procedure for, 1510–1511,
    1511*f*
  psychological changes, 1488–1489, 1489*f*
  sitz bath, procedure for, 1511–1512
Postprandial blood sugar test, 1068
Postrenal failure, 1101
Postterm defined, 1424*t*
Postterm newborns, 1565–1566
Posttraumatic stress disorder (PTSD)
  diagnosis, 331
  explained, 331
  treatment, 331–332
Postural drainage, 804, 805*f*
Postural tonus, 490
Posture, 490–491
Posture and position as therapeutic
    communication technique, 195*t*
Potassium (macromineral), 567, 568*t*
Potassium citrate, 1106
Potassium iodide, 1058, 1060*t*
Potassium level
  normal values and imbalances, 596*t*
  pregnant and nonpregnant values, 1425*t*
Potentiating effect, explained, 613
Powder as drug preparation, 610*t*
Power of attorney for health care, 58, 59*f*, 350,
    1234
Powers of labor, 1462, 1463*f*, 1464

Prilosec. *See* Omeprazole
Primary hypertension, 449, 873
Primary intention healing, 533, 533*f*
Primary level of health care, 104*t*
Primary male reproductive organs, 1131
Primary nursing, 1774
Primary nursing model of care, 114–115
Primary power of labor, 1462, 1463*f*, 1464
Primary prevention, defined, 1224
Primary pulmonary hypertension, 819
Primary skin lesions, 746, 747*f*
Primary source of data, client as, 81
Primary syphilis, 1171*t*, 1174
Primary tumor, defined, 1243
Primigravida, defined, 1424*t*
Primipara, defined, 1424*t*
Printed materials as teaching strategy, 217*t*
PR interval, 853, 853*f*
Prinzmetals' angina, 855
Priorities, setting
   goals and expected outcomes, establishing, 89, 91–92, 91*t*
   high, medium, and low, identifying, 89, 90*f*, 90*t*
Prioritization in student clinical experiences, 9–10*f*, 9–11
Prioritizing, in nursing care
   blood pressure assessment, 453
   CAM therapies, 126
   cardiopulmonary disorders, 864
   care in relation to loss, 351
   caring for adolescents, 1757
   children with musculoskeletal disorders, 1722
   child with asthma, 1714
   client admission, 260
   client communication, 201
   client discharge, 267
   client having cancer surgery, 1250
   client in respiratory distress, 830
   clients dealing with substance abuse, 1393–1394
   client's fluid status, 602
   clients in labor, 1468
   clients in long-term care, 1274
   clients in the EC, 1295
   clients undergoing chemotherapy, 1256
   clients undergoing radiation therapy, 1253
   clients with adrenal disorders, 1080
   clients with at-risk pregnancy, 1451
   clients with autoimmune disorders, 926
   clients with bladder disorders, 1109
   clients with bone disorders, 774
   clients with breast disorders, 1138–1139
   clients with burns, 1297
   clients with cancer of the female reproductive organs, 1148
   clients with chronic illness, 1225
   clients with depression, 1368–1369
   clients with diabetes, 1075
   clients with eating disorders, 1401–1402
   clients with HIV and AIDS, 919
   clients with hypertension, aneurysms, and emboli, 875–876
   clients with infections of the reproductive tract, 1156
   clients with inflammatory joint disorders, 780
   clients with Lyme disease and West Nile virus, 961
   clients with menstrual disorders, 1141–1142

   clients with neurovascular disorders, 957
   clients with organ transplants, 922
   clients with peripheral vascular disease, 879, 880*f*
   clients with personality disorders, 1374–1375
   clients with posterior pituitary disorders, 1057
   clients with prostate disorders, 1154
   clients with psychosocial needs, 336
   clients with renal disorders, 1103
   clients with schizophrenia, 1351
   clients with SLE and/or fibromyalgia, 785
   clients with STIs, 1176
   clients with strains and sprains, 783
   clients with terminal illness, 1229
   clients with thyroid and parathyroid disorders, 1062
   clients with ureteral disorders, 1106–1107
   clients with valvular disease or inflammatory heart disorders, 867
   clients with wounds, 542
   client teaching, 213
   client transfer, 263
   client with cranial nerve disorders, 980
   client with degenerative neurologic disorders, 973
   client with fever, 440
   client with GI accessory organ disorders, 1035–1036
   client with hematologic or lymphatic disorders, 900
   client with lower GI disorders, 1024
   client with mobility issues, 496
   client with neurosensory trauma or tumors, 967–968
   client with normal pregnancy, 1423
   client with peripheral nervous system disorders, 977
   client with upper GI disorder, 1006
   coronary artery disease, 858
   culturally proficient care, 36
   data collection for assessment, 371
   dermatologic disorders, 755–756
   documentation, 244, 244*t*
   elderly clients, 1199–1200
   eye care, 406
   hair care, 400
   high-risk newborns, 1583
   high-risk postpartum mother, 1525
   hospitalized older adults, 1214
   infants and toddlers with cardiovascular disorders, 1639
   infants and toddlers with gastrointestinal disorders, 1658
   infants and toddlers with nervous system disorders, 1649
   infants and toddlers with renal disorders, 1661
   infants and toddlers with respiratory disorders, 1637
   infants with cardiovascular disorders, 1571
   infants with unrepaired cleft lip and/or palate, 1578
   infection control, 174
   intact skin, maintaining, 550
   IV therapy, 677
   life span development and family systems, 312
   medication administration, 626
   mouth care, 403–404

   neurologic disorders, 948–949
   normal neonates, 1550
   nutrition and diet therapy, 574
   pain control, 478
   postoperative client, 719
   postpartum clients, 1490
   preoperative care, 717
   preschoolers with burns, 1702
   preschoolers with cardiovascular disorders, 1679
   preschoolers with nervous system disorders, 1686
   preschoolers with renal disorders, 1697
   psychiatric care, 283
   pulse assessment, 442
   respiratory status of client, 446
   respiratory system problems, 806
   safety, 148
   skin, foot, and nail care, 395
   sleep issues, 509
   upper respiratory tract disorders, 815
Prioritizing nursing care, strategically
   clinical practice, introduction to, 272
   gerontology, 1220
   medical surgical nursing care, 1184
   mental health nursing care, 1408
   pediatric and adolescent nursing care, 1762
   physiological health, promoting, 708
   psychosocial health, promoting, 360
   specialized nursing care, 1334
   transition from student to nurse, 1804
   women's health care and maternal-newborn nursing, 1592
Privacy
   communication, influencing, 192
   hospital admission, 255, 258–259*t*, 259
Private healthcare insurance, 115
Privileged communication, 49
Prn (hygiene) care, 393
Prn infusion devices, 667
Prn orders, 614
Probable signs of pregnancy, 1419–1420
Probationary period, 1799
Probing for information as communication barrier, 197*t*
Probiotics, 1191
Problem-focused coping, 332
Problem identification and clarification, 318–320
Problem-oriented medical records, 234–236, 236*f*
Problems (diagnostic labels) in NANDA nursing diagnoses, 83
Problem solving
   critical thinking, 64
   psychosocial health, promoting, 360
   teaching strategy, 219
Procainamide
   myocarditis, 866
   ventricular dysrhythmias, 870*t*
Procarbazine, 1742*t*
Procardia. *See* Nifedipine
Procedures
   admitting a new client in the physician's office, 1318
   amniocentesis, umbilical cord sampling, or chorionic villus sampling, assisting with, 1430–1432, 1431*f*
   antiemboli stockings, applying, 733–734, 734*f*

Respiratory hygiene, 172
Respiratory inhalation drugs, administering, 634, 634f, 635
Respiratory rate
  newborn nursery, 1537, 1537t
  ventilator settings, 807t
Respiratory secretions
  clearing with hydration, 804
  pooling of, 493–494, 493f
Respiratory Standard (OSHA), 174
Respiratory syncitial virus (RSV)
  manifestations and treatment, 1634
  nursing process care plan, 1637–1638
Respiratory system
  assessment, procedure for, 384, 384f
  fetal development, 1417, 1417t
  focused assessment by body systems, 364f, 365
  health assessment, 374–376, 375t
  immobility, effects of, 493–494, 493f
  maternal changes during pregnancy, 1422
  newborn adaptation to life, 1531–1532, 1531f, 1532f
  older adults, abnormal changes in, 1298
  older adults, changes in, 1189
  pediatric anatomy and physiology, 1595, 1596f, 1597f
  radiation therapy side effects, 1255t
  regulation of acid-base balance, 598, 599
  structure and function, 791–794, 792f, 793f
Respiratory system disorders, clients with, 790–843
  chapter review, 841
  critical thinking care map, 842
  disorders, tests for, 796–798, 796f, 797f, 798f
  interstitial disorders, 828–829, 829f
  lower respiratory disorders
    acute respiratory distress syndrome, 817t, 821–822
    bronchitis, 817t, 821
    chest trauma, 816t, 819, 820f
    inhalation injuries, 816t, 820
    lung abscess, 817t, 822
    near-drowning, 816t, 820
    nursing considerations, 823
    obstructive disorders, 824–827, 825f, 826f, 827–828t, 827f
    pleuritis, 817t, 822
    pneumonia, 817t, 821
    pulmonary embolism, 816, 816t, 818–819
    pulmonary hypertension, 816t, 819
    tuberculosis, 817t, 822, 823f
  lung cancer, 827–828, 828f
  NCLEX-PN® exam preparation, 843
  nursing care, 806–809, 808f, 830
  nursing process care plan, 809–810
  oxygen administration, procedure for, 832–834, 833f
  oxygenation, factors that affect, 796
  pulse oximetry, procedure for measuring, 831–832, 831f
  respiratory function, factors that influence, 794–796
  respiratory system, structure and function of, 791–794, 792f, 793f
  respiratory therapies
    breathing and coughing exercises, 802, 803

chest tubes and drainage systems, 801–802, 802f
  hydration, clearing secretions with, 804, 804f
  incentive spirometry, 802–803, 803f
  mechanical ventilation, 804–806, 806f, 807t
  oxygen therapy, 798–801, 799f
  pulmonary toilet, 804, 805f
  suctioning, 804, 805f, 806f
suctioning, procedure for, 837–840, 838f, 839f
tracheostomy care, procedure for, 834–836, 835f, 836f
upper respiratory disorders
  epiglottitis, 811t, 813
  influenza, 810, 811t, 812
  laryngitis, 811t, 813
  nursing care, 815
  pharyngitis, 811t, 812
  rhinitis, 810, 811t
  sinusitis, 810, 811t
  tonsillitis, 811t, 813
  trauma and obstruction, 812t, 813–814
  tumors, 812t, 814–815, 814f
Respiratory therapies
  breathing and coughing exercises, 802, 803
  chest tubes and drainage systems, 801–802, 802f
  incentive spirometry, 802–803, 803f
  mechanical ventilation, 804–806, 806f, 807t
  oxygen therapy, 798–801, 799f, 800f, 801f
  pulmonary toilet, 804, 805f
  secretions, clearing, using hydration, 804, 804f
  suctioning, 804, 805f, 806f
Respiratory therapists
  health care providers, 111
  long-term care facilities, 1269
Respiratory tract infections in older adults, 1189, 1208
Respiratory zone of the lungs, 792–793, 792f, 793f
Response-based models of stress, 326f, 327–328, 328f
Responsibilities, current, of nursing students, 5
Responsiveness, defined, 312
Rest and sleep, 338. *See also under* Activity, rest, and sleep
Restitution of fetus during birth, 1466, 1467f
Restless leg syndrome, 1190
Restraints
  alternatives to, 144
  applying and monitoring, 147
  attaching, 147, 148f
  described, 144
  kinds of, 145–147, 146f, 147f
  legal implications, 144, 145
  selecting, 144–145
Restricting type of anorexia nervosa, 1397
Résumés
  described and formats for, 1793, 1796
  sample of, 1794–1795t
Retained placenta
  explained, 1477–1478
  postpartum assessment, 1491t
  postpartum hemorrhage, 1519
Retching, 992
Retention catheters. *See also* Indwelling catheters

inserting and removing, procedure for, 1119–1122, 1120f, 1121f
  nursing care, 1096
  removing, 1096–1097
  specimen collection from, 1113, 1113f
  types of, 1095–1096, 1095f
Retention enemas, 1011
Retention of learning, 211
Retention of urine, 1092t
Reticular layer of the dermis, 744
Retinal detachment, 982t, 1190, 1211, 1211f
Retinoblastoma, 1650
Retinopathy
  diabetes, 1075
  older adults, 1212
  oxygen therapy for newborns, 1564
Retirement centers, health care in, 107
Retraction of injured blood vessels, 533
Retractions, respiratory
  newborns, 1532, 1532f
  pulmonary ventilation, 793
Retrolental fibroplasia, 1564
Retrovir. *See* Zidovudine
Rett's syndrome, 1703t
Return-flow enemas, 1011, 1039
Revascularization of coronary arteries, 858
Reverse Trendelenburg's position, 411t
ReVia. *See* Naltrexone
Revision in SOAPIER charting, 237
Revocation of nursing licenses, 1765, 1766
Reye's syndrome, 1648, 1671
RF (rheumatoid factor), 768t, 923
Rhabdomyosarcoma, 1722
Rheumatic fever (heart disease), 865
Rheumatoid arthritis
  musculoskeletal system inflammatory disorder, 777, 778t
  older adults, 1207, 1207f
Rheumatoid factor (RF), 768t, 923
  rheumatoid arthritis, 777
Rheumatologists, 925
Rh factor
  high-risk pregnancy, 1447–1448, 1447f, 1448t
  organ transplantation, 921
Rh immune globulin (RhoGAM), 1448, 1448t
Rhinitis, 810, 811t
Rhinoplasty, 759
Rhonchi
  adventitious breath sounds, 375t
  explained, 365
Rhythm method of contraception, 1160t
Rhytidoplasty, 759
Rib fractures, 819
Riboflavin. *See* Vitamin B$_2$ (riboflavin)
RICE (rest, ice, compression, elevation) treatment for soft-tissue injury, 783, 1292–1293
Rickets, 1692
Rid, 754
Rifamate. *See* Rifampin
Rifampin, 168, 817t
Right-sided heart failure
  CHF, 862–863, 862t
  cor pulmonale, 864
Rights of clients, 108–110
Right ventricular, inferior, posterior MI, 857

School anxiety, 1728
School for children with cancer, 1260
School health office or clinic
  general duties, 1310–1311
  immunizations, 1313, 1314f, 1315–1316t
  medication, administering, 1311
  scoliosis screening, 1312–1313, 1312f
  spread of infection, preventing, 1311–1312
Schultze ("shiny Schultze") mechanism, 1469f
Schwann cells, 937
Schwannoma, 967t
Sclerodactyly, 926
Scleroderma, 925–926
Sclerotherapy, 1023
Scoliometer, 1312
Scoliosis
  diagnosis and treatment, 1720–1721, 1721f
  explained, 781–782, 781f, 1719
  manifestations, 1720, 1720f, 1720t
  pediatric chest shape, 1595
  school screenings, 1312–1313, 1312f
  screening, procedure for, 1328
Scope of practice, explained, 46
Scottish-Rite brace, 1688
Screening tests
  cancer, 1245–1246, 1245–1246t
  surgery, 712, 713t
Scrotal sac, 1131
Scrotum
  disorders of, 1151, 1151f
  structure and function, 1131, 1131f
Scurvy, 1692
Seasonal affective disorder, 321, 1356
Season of birth and schizophrenia, 1344
Seating arrangements influencing interviews, 199
Sebaceous glands, 744f, 745
Seborrheic dermatitis, 1662
Sebum, 393, 745
Secondary diabetes, 1067
Secondary gain, 282
Secondary hypertension, 449, 874
Secondary intention healing, 533, 533f
Secondary level of health care, 104t
Secondary power of labor, 1464
Secondary prevention, defined, 1224
Secondary pulmonary hypertension, 819
Secondary sex characteristics (male), 1131
Secondary skin lesions, 746, 747f
Secondary sources of data, 81
Secondary syphilis, 1171t, 1174
Second-degree AV block, 871t
Second primary tumor, defined, 1243
Second stage of labor, 1466–1477, 1466f,
    1467f, 1468f
Sedation
  hospitalized older adults, 1213–1214, 1214f
  opioid analgesics, 476
  sedation rating scale, 474–475
Sedatives, 1384t, 1386
Sedentary lifestyle, 874
Segregation, explained, 31
Seizure disorders
  diagnosis and treatment, 957
  infants and toddlers, 1647
  manifestations, 951f, 956–957, 956t
  status epilepticus, 956, 957
  terms related to, 956

Seizures
  antipsychotic medications, 1350
  defined, 956
  eclampsia, 1446
  nursing care, 958
  preschoolers, 1681–1682, 1682f
Selective COX-2 inhibitors, 474t
Selective norepinephrine reuptake inhibitors,
    1360, 1362
Selective serotonin reuptake inhibitors (SSRIs)
  actions of, 1361
  drug interactions, 1361
  list of, 1360
  serotonin syndrome, 1361
  side effects, 1361
Self-actualization needs
  explained, 279
  stress, 333t
Self-assist bed bath, 393
Self-care deficit, 396
Self-esteem needs, 333t
Self-help, explained, 331
Self-help groups, 108
Self-injury by adolescents, 1755
Selye, Hans, 327–328
Semen, 1131
Semi-Fowler's position, 411t, 499, 500f
Semilente insulin, 1071t
Semilunar (half-moon) valves, 846
Seminal vesicles, 1131, 1131f
Sender in communication process, 191
Sengstaken-Blakemore tube, 1004, 1032, 1033f
Sensation, diminished, and pressure ulcers, 548
Sense organs, development of, 1417–1418, 1417t,
    1418f
Sensitivity studies, 536
Sensorimotor phase of cognitive development,
    279, 279t, 297
Sensorineural hearing loss, 1197
Sensory abilities
  neonates and infants, 296–297, 297t, 298f
  preschoolers, 301
  school-age children, 302
  toddlers, 300
Sensory acuity
  learning, barrier to, 212, 212t
  older adults, abnormal changes in, 1210–1211,
    1211f
  older adults, changes in, 1196–1198, 1196f
Sensory disorders
  infants and toddlers, 1649–1652, 1650f, 1651f
  preschoolers, 1685–1686, 1685f, 1686f
  school-aged children, 1719, 1719f
Sensory pathways in peripheral nerves, 934
Sensory-perceptual alterations and safety, 132
Sensory receptors in skin, 744f, 745
Sensory status with neurologic disorders, 949
Separation anxiety, 1663
Sepsis
  blood transfusions, 680t
  explained, 170
  neonatal, 1583
Septal occluders, 1638, 1638f
Septicemia
  explained, 163
  IV therapy, 676t
  postpartum, 1521

Septic shock, 1291
Septra. See Trimethoprim-sulfamethoxazole
Septum, cardiac, 845–846, 846f
Sequelae with adolescent pregnancy, 1439
Sequence of events, recording, 230, 231f
Sequential compression devices
  applying, procedure for, 734–735, 735f
  preoperative application, 717
Serentil. See Mesoridazine
Seroconversion, 915
Seropositive, 918
Seroquel. See Quetiapine
Serosanguineous wound drainage, 534
Serotonin
  antidepressants, 1359, 1359t
  location and actions, 940t
  mental illness, 1343t
Serotonin and norepinephrine reuptake inhibitors,
    1360, 1361
Serotonin antagonists and reuptake inhibitors,
    1360, 1361
Serotonin syndrome, 1361
Serous exudate, 534
Sertraline, 1360
Serum hepatitis, 1693
Serum osmolality, 948
Serum osmolarity, 1057
Serum protein analysis, 536
Serzone. See Nefazodone
"Setting sun" appearance of the eyes, 1573
Seventh-Day Adventists
  mourning and after-death rites, 1236t
  organ donation and transplantation, 1681
Severe brain injury, 962
Sexual abuse, 1273
Sexual Assault Nurse Examiners (SANE), 1295
Sexual characteristics of adolescents, 303–304
Sexual harassment, 53
Sexual history, obtaining, 1132–1133
Sexuality
  adolescents, 303–304, 1750
  residents, in long-term care facilities, 1273
Sexually transmitted infections
  adolescents, 1750, 1751, 1752
  consent for treatment by minors, 1283
  genital warts (condyloma acuminata), 752
Sexually transmitted infections, clients with,
    1168–1183
  candidiasis, 1173t, 1176, 1176f
  chapter review, 1181
  chlamydia, 1170, 1171t, 1174
  critical thinking care map, 1182
  diagnostic tests for, 1170, 1171–1173t
  gonorrhea, 1171t, 1174
  herpes, 1172t, 1174–1175, 1174f
  HIV and AIDS, 1172t, 1175–1176
  human papillomavirus, 1172t, 1175, 1175f
  incidence of, 1169
  NCLEX-PN® exam preparation, 1183
  nursing care, 1176–1178
  nursing process care plan, 1178–1180
  prevention, 1169–1170
  risk factors for, 1169, 1170
  syphilis, 1171t, 1174, 1174f
  trichomoniasis, 1173t, 1176
Sexual maturation
  adolescents, 1734, 1735, 1735f, 1735t

Toxic shock syndrome, 1155
Toxocara canis, 1694t
Toxocara catis, 1694t
Toxocariasis, 1694t
Toxoids, 913
Toxoplasmosis, 1449, 1450t
Tracer methodology, 1774
Tracheoesophageal fistula, 1574, 1574f
Tracheoesophageal puncture, 814–815, 814f
Tracheostomy
    artificial airways, 801, 801f
    providing care, procedure for, 834–836, 835f, 836f
    suctioning, procedure for, 839–840, 839f
    suctioning in infants, procedure for, 1586, 1586f
Traction
    applying, procedure for, 786
    care of, 775–776
    children, for, 1689, 1690f
    fractures, 770, 771f
Tracts, neural, 938
Trademark name of a drug, 609
Traditional nursing care plans, 244
Tramadol, 474t
Transaction-based models of stress, 328
Transcellular fluid, 593
Transcultural nursing
    development of, 28–29
    theoretical basis of, 29–31, 29f
Transcultural Nursing Society, 28
Transcultural teaching, 219–220
Transcutaneous electrical nerve stimulation (TENS), 476
Transdermal patch as drug preparation, 610t
Transdermal patch method of contraception, 1162t
Transdermal route of administration
    advantages and disadvantages, 616t
    pain medications, 479t
Transfer belts, 521, 521f, 525, 525f
Transfer of a client to a different unit or facility. *See also* Admission, transfer, and discharge
    explained, 262
    transfer records, 263f
Transferring clients
    explained, 502–503, 503f
    procedure for, 520–523, 520f, 521f, 522f, 523f
Transfusion reaction, 888
Transient ischemic attacks (TIAs), 952, 1210
Transillumination of scrotal sac, 1659–1660
Transitional stools, 1543, 1543f
Transition phase of the first stage of labor, 1465–1466, 1465f
Transmission-based precautions, 170–171
Transmission methods or modes in the chain of infection, 164f, 165
Transmission of organisms
    MRSA, 168, 169f
    sexually transmitted infections, 1169–1170
Transmural infarction, 857
Transparent barrier dressings, 555–556
Transparent wound barriers, 536–537, 537t, 538f
Transplanted organs, 1103, 1103f
Transplant purpose for surgery, 711
Transport of body fluids, 594–595, 594f
Transport of clients

contact isolation, 749
    transmission-based precautions, 170–171
Transposition of the great vessels, 1571, 1571f
Transsphenoidal hypophysectomy, 1055
Transurethral incision of the prostate, 1152
Transurethral lithotripsy, 1106
Transurethral microwave antenna, 1152
Transurethral resection of the prostate (TURP), 1152
Transurethral ultrasound guided laser-induced prostatectomy, 1152
Transverse fetal lie, 1461, 1461f
Transverse plane, 370, 370f
Tranylcypromine, 1360
Trauma
    adolescents, injuries to, 1744–1745, 1744f
    musculoskeletal, in preschoolers, 1689–1690, 1689f, 1690f
    neurologic, in preschoolers, 1682–1684, 1683t
Trauma in the emergency center
    abdominal, 1292
    blunt, 1292
    chest, 1292
    eyes, ears, or nose, 1293
    first aid, 1292, 1293
    fractures, 1292
    head, 1292, 1292f
    musculoskeletal, 1292
    penetrating, 1291, 1291f
    soft-tissue injury, 1292–1293
    spinal injury, 1292
Traumatic bone disorders
    bone cancer, 774
    fractures, 769–772, 769f, 770f, 771f, 772f
    osteomalacia, 773–774
    osteomyelitis, 774, 774f
    osteoporosis, 772–773, 773t
Traumatic brain injury, 962–963
Traumatic pneumothorax, 829, 829f
Travasorb-HN, 1016
Traveling nurse positions, 1310, 1316
Trazodone, 1360, 1361
Treadmill test, 852
Treatments in the EC, 1285, 1286, 1286f
Trendelenburg's position, 411t, 1296, 1296f
Treponema pallidum
    chain of infection, 164t
    syphilis, 1174
Trexall. *See* Methotrexate
Triage
    disaster plans, 142
    EC and UC settings, 1282–1283
Trichloroacetic acid, 1172t
Trichomona infection, 1170
Trichomonas vaginalis, 1176
Trichomoniasis, 1173t, 1176
Tricuspid valve, 846, 846f
Tricyclic antidepressants
    action of, 1359–1360
    list of, 1360
    overdose and toxic effects, 1360
    side effects, 1360
Trifluoperazine, 1348
Trigeminal nerve (CN V), 944t
Trigeminal neuralgia, 978, 978f
Triglycerides, 566, 566t
Trihexyphenidyl, 1349t

Triiodothyronine (T_3), 1051t, 1054
Trilafon. *See* Perphenazine
Trimesters of pregnancy, 294, 1420
Trimethobenzamide, 999
Trimethoprim-sulfamethoxazole
    MRSA, 168, 1727
    Pneumocystis jiroveci (carinii) pneumonia, 917
    pyelonephritis, 1098
Trimipramine, 1360
Tripod position
    emphysema, 826
    respiratory system problems, 808, 808f
Trisomy 21, 1573, 1647. *See also* Down syndrome
Trochanter rolls, 499, 499f
Trochlear nerve (CN IV), 944t
Trophoblast, 1413, 1413f
Tropic hormones, 1052
Troponin levels, 854t
Trousseau's sign, 1059–1060, 1060f, 1062
True labor, 1458, 1459t
True perineum, 1129
True skin, 743
Trust *versus* mistrust, 276, 276t, 297
Truth, Sojourner, 15, 16f
Trypsin, 992
Tryptophan, 1361
T-tubes, 1028, 1028f
Tubal ligation, 1159, 1160f, 1162t
Tubal pregnancy, 1442. *See also* Ectopic pregnancy
Tub baths, 393, 415
Tube drainage, including on intake and output, 603
Tube feedings
    administering, procedure for, 585–587, 586f
    intake and output, 603
    procedure for, in infants, 1587–1588
Tubercle, 822, 823f
Tuberculin syringes, 622, 622f, 623
Tuberculosis (TB)
    incidence in ethnic groups, 167
    multi-drug resistant, 168
    older adults, 1208
    respiratory infection, 817t, 822, 823f
    school-aged children, 1713
Tuberculosis PPD, 912
Tubex injection system, 623
Tubing for IV administration, 663
Tubman, Harriet, 15
Tularemia, 1295
Tumor markers, 1248
Tumor-node-metastasis staging, 1248
Tumors
    defined, 1243
    upper respiratory tract, 812t, 814–815, 814f
Tums, 1002
Tunica adventitia, 669, 849, 851f
Tunica intima, 669, 849, 851f
Tunica media, 669, 849, 851f
Turgor of skin
    assessment in older adults, 381
    immobility, effects of, 494
    skin assessment, 373
Turmeric, 125t
Turner's sign, 1034
Turning clients in bed, 502
T waves, 753f, 853

urinary function, factors affecting, 1090, 1090t
urinary system, structure and function of, 1087–1089, 1088f, 1089f
urine characteristics, 1090, 1091t
Urinary tract infections
cystitis, 1108
infants and toddlers, 1659
noscomial, 163t
older adults, 1212
postoperative client, 721t
preschoolers, 1695
Urination
explained, 1088–1089
postoperative care, 723
Urine
characteristics of, 1090, 1091t
fluid output, 595–596
newborns, 1542–1543
normal and abnormal test results, 1091t
osmolality, 948
specific gravity, 948
tests on, 713t, 1093–1094, 1094f
urinalysis, 713t
Urine culture and sensitivity, 713t
Urine osmolarity, 1056
Urine specific gravity, 1057
Urine specimens
clean catch collection of, 1112–1113, 1113f
collecting, 1093, 1093f
pediatric client, collecting from, 1607, 1607f
Urokinase, 875
U.S. Department of Health and Human Services (DHHS)
communicable diseases, 163
culturally competent care, 28
Healthy People 2010, 103
U.S. Food and Drug Administration (FDA)
birth defects, medication risks for causing, 1412
herbal remedies, 120–121
USP (United States Pharmacopeia), 609
U.S. Public Health Service, 163
Uterine (menstrual) cycle, 1130f, 1131
Uterine atony, 1518–1519, 1518f
Uterine changes as probable sign of pregnancy, 1420
Uterine disorders
dysfunctional uterine bleeding, 1140–1141
premenstrual syndrome, 1140
prolapse, 1143, 1144f, 1149, 1213
tumors, 1143–1145, 1145f
Uterine soufflé, 1420
Uterus
displacement and positions of, 1143, 1144f
postpartum assessment, 1492–1493
postpartum changes, 1484–1485, 1484f
structure and function, 1129–1123, 1129f

V

Vaccines. *See also* Immunizations
described, 912
HPV, 1145, 1170, 1175, 1738
Lyme disease, 961
Zostavax vaccine, 1207
Vacuum extractor traction for delivery, 1478, 1478f
Vagina

postpartum bleeding, 1475
postpartum changes, 1485–1486, 1486f
reproductive system, 1129, 1129f
Vaginal birth after cesarean section, 1479
Vaginal contraceptive ring, 1162t
Vaginal culture, 1441
Vaginal discharge, 1499
Vaginal hematoma, 1519
Vaginal infections in school-aged girls, 1727
Vaginal introitus, 1129
Vaginal medications, instilling, 634, 652–654, 653f
Vaginal route of administration, 616t
Vaginal speculum, 1320f
Vaginal sponge, 1161t
Vagotomy, 1002, 1002f
Vagus nerve (CN X), 945t
Valacyclovir
herpes, 1172t
herpes simplex, 751
Validation
communication, in, 191
explained, 80
Valium. *See* Diazepam
Valproic acid
bipolar disorder, 1368
pain management, 475t
Valsalva maneuver
constipation, 1009
immobility, effects of, 492
Valtrex. *See* Valacyclovir
Valuables and personal property. *See* Client property
Values, explained, 54
Values of nursing, 3
Valve ablation for obstructive uropathy, 1660
Valves, cardiac
older adults, 1208, 1209f
valvular disease, 865–866, 866f
valvular insufficiency, 865
valvular stenosis, 865, 866f
Vancomycin, 168, 1728
Vancomycin-resistant enterococci (VRE), 168, 170
Vaporization, 435
Vardenafil hydrochloride, 1151–1152
Variance documentation, 241, 241t
Varicella immunization, 1673f
Varicella-zoster virus, 1676t
Varicose veins, 878–879, 878f, 1209
Variocele, 1163
Vascular skin lesions, 746, 748f
Vascular stage of inflammatory response, 167
Vascular surgery, 881
Vasectomy, 1159, 1160f, 1162t
Vasoconstriction
body temperature, 435
heat regulation, 745
Vasodilation, 745
Vasodilators, 874
Vasopressin
diabetes insipidus, 1057
ventricular fibrillation, 871t
Vasovagal response with IV insertion, 674t
Vastus lateralis muscle, 632, 632f
VDRL (venereal disease research laboratory) test, 1170

Vector transmission
chain of infection, 165
explained, 162
Vegan diet, 573
Vegetarian diets, 573–574, 1737
Vegetative state, 1235
Vehicle-borne transmission, 165
Veins
arteries, differences between, 669, 669t
disorders of, 878–879, 878f
peripheral, for IV therapy, 669–670, 669f, 669t, 670t
structure and function, 849, 851f
Vein stripping, 879
Venereal disease research laboratory (VDRL) test, 1170
Venereal warts, 1175. *See also* Human papillomavirus (HPV)
Venipuncture
performing, procedure for, 695–698, 695f, 696f, 697f, 698f
procedure for, 671–672, 671f
sites for, 669–670, 669f, 670t
techniques in, 672
Venlafaxine, 1360, 1361
Veno-occlusive disease of the liver, 1258
Venospasm
IV sites, at, 674t
tunica media, 669
Venous star, 747, 748f
Venous stasis
immobility, 493, 493f
thrombophlebitis, 878
ulcers, 879
Ventilation, mechanical
CPAP, 804–805, 806f
high-risk newborns, 1568
invasive, 805–806, 807t
Ventilation, pulmonary
described, 445, 791
process of, 793, 793f
Ventilation of the room, 410
Ventral (anatomic direction), 370
Ventral cavity, 370, 370f
Ventricle, cardiac, 846, 846f
Ventricular aneurysm, 858
Ventricular diastole, 847, 848f
Ventricular fibrillation, 858, 871t
Ventricular septal defect, 1567, 1569f, 1570
Ventricular systole, 847, 848f
Ventricular tachycardia, 870t
Ventriculoperitoneal shunts, 1573, 1573f
Ventrogluteal site for IM injections, 631, 631f, 632f
Venules, 849
Veracity, 55
Verapamil hydrochloride, 475t
Verbal abuse of the elderly, 1273
Verbal communication
culturally based, 32
explained, 192
Verbal physician's orders, 1282, 1771
Vernix/vernix caseosa, 295, 1415, 1534
Verrucae (warts), 752
Vertebrae, 772
Vertex (occiput) presentation, 1461, 1462t
Vertigo, 979

cancer of, 1147–1148, 1148f
vulvar hematoma, 1519
Vulvectomy, 1147–1148, 1148f

W

Wald, Lillian, 18, 18f
Walkers, 495, 495f, 496, 1303
War, influence on nursing, 15–16, 16f, 17
Warfarin
  OTC antifungals, 752
  postpartum thromboembolic disease, 1520
Wasting syndrome, 920, 920f
Water as nutrient, 564, 565t
"Water deprivation test," 1057
"Water load test," 1056
Water-seal drainage systems, 802, 802f, 829
Water-soluble vitamins, 567, 567t
Weakness as risk factor for falls, 138t
We Band of Angels (Norman), 16
Webbing between digits, 1543
Weight. *See also* Eating disorders; Obesity
  breastfed newborns, 1508
  health assessment, 372
  measurements for pediatric assessment, 1606
  neonates, 1535, 1536f
  newborns, obtaining, procedure for, 1554,
    1554f
  obtaining, 575f, 576, 576f
  prenatal follow-up visits, 1424–1425
Weight bearing exercise, 1196
Weight control for osteoarthritis, 1195
Weight gain with antipsychotic medications,
  1350
Wellbutrin. *See* Bupropion
Well-child checkups, 1631, 1632t
Wellness, cultural views of, 1201
Wellness diagnosis, explained, 83
Wellness model, 68
Wellness promotion, 21
Wernicke-Korsafkoff's syndrome, 1385, 1389
Wernicke's syndrome, 1385
Western blot test, 918, 1170
West Nile virus, 961
Wet drowning, 1293
Wetting agent laxatives, 1010t
Wet-to-damp dressings, 538t, 543, 544
Wet-to-dry dressings, 538t
Wet-to-wet dressings, 538t
Wharton's jelly, 1416
Wheals, 746, 747f
Wheelchair platform scale, 575f
Wheezing, 375t, 447
Whipple's procedure, 1035, 1035f
Whistle-blowing, explained, 52
White blood cell count
  normal levels, 888t
  pregnant and nonpregnant values, 1425t
White blood cell count with differential, 167
White blood cell disorders
  agranulocytosis, 894
  leukemia, 894–897, 895f
  multiple myeloma, 897
  nursing considerations, 897
White blood cells (WBCs, leukocytes), 886–887,
    887f. *See also* Leukocytes (white blood cells,
    WBCs)
White matter, defined, 938

Whitethorn, 863
Whitman, Walt, 15
WHO. *See* World Health Organization
    (WHO)
Whole blood, 678t
Whooping cough. *See* Pertussis (whooping cough)
WIC (Women, Infant and Children) program,
  1546–1547, 1629
Willow bark, 125t
Wilm's tumor (nephroblastoma), 1100, 1661
Witches' milk, 1542
Withdrawal
  alcohol, 1382–1384, 1383f, 1384t
  CNS depressants and stimulants, 1384t, 1387
  drug-addicted newborns, 1582
  hallucinogens, inhalants, cannabis, caffeine, and
    nicotine, 1387t, 1388, 1389
  substance dependency, 1382
Withdrawal method of contraception, 1160t
Witnesses, nurses as, 53–54, 53f
Wolfelt, Alan, 349–350
Women
  cystitis, 1108
  heart attack, manifestations of
Women, Infant and Children (WIC) program,
  1546–1547, 1629
Wong-Baker FACES Pain Rating Scale, 481,
  482f, 1606, 1606f
Worden, William, 349, 350
Workforce issues as domain of culture, 30
Work settings for LPNs/LVNs, 22–23
World Health Organization (WHO)
  communicable diseases, agency for controlling,
    162
  three-step ladder approach to pain
    management, 473–474, 474–475t, 474f
World War II, 16
Worried well, explained, 331
Wound care and skin integrity, 531–562
  chapter review, 560
  critical thinking care map, 561
  NCLEX-PN® exam preparation, 562
  skin integrity, 532
    nursing care, 549f, 550, 552–554, 552f
    nursing process care plan, 554
    pressure ulcers, 547–550, 548f, 549f, 550f,
      551f, 552t
  wound drainage specimens, obtaining,
    556–558, 557f
  wound dressings, 555–556
  wounds
    caring for, 536–541, 537t, 538f, 538t, 539f,
      540t, 541f
    healing, 533–534, 533f
    healing, complications of, 535–536
    healing, factors affecting, 534–535
    nursing care, 542–547, 543t, 544f, 545f,
      546f
    terminology for, 532–533, 533t
    wounds, irrigating, 558–559, 559f
Wound drainage
  intake and output, 603
  kinds of, 534
  specimen of, obtaining, 557–558, 557f
Wound healing
  postoperative care, 723
  supporting, 542–543

Wounds. *See also under* Wound care and skin
    integrity
  cleaning, irrigating, and dressing, 725, 725f
  cleaning, irrigation, and packing, 536, 542
  cleaning and irrigating, 543–544
  dressings, 536–539, 537t, 538f, 538t, 539f
  dressings, procedure for, 555–556
  hot and cold applications, 540–541, 540t,
    541f
  laboratory data, 536
  open, and thermal tolerance, 541
  supporting and immobilizing, 539–540
  surgical, cleaning and applying dressings,
    728–730, 730f
  surgical, observation of, 724
  types of, 711
  wound care, postoperative, 723
  wound infection, dehiscence, and evisceration,
    721t
  wound infections, postpartum, 1520–1521
  wound status, postoperative, 719
Wound vacuum, 538
Wrist angle, 1538t, 1539f
Written communication, 192
Wrugbe, 290

X

Xenograft, 921
Xiphoid process, 1599
X-rays
  head and vertebral column, 943, 946f
  musculoskeletal disorders, 768t

Y

Yearly fees for service, 116
Yellen (Gomco) clamps, 1548
Yersinia pestis, 1295
Yoga, 123t, 124, 126f
Young Women's Christian Association
  (YWCA), 19
Yutopar. *See* Ritodrine

Z

Zanamivir, 811t
Zantac. *See* Ranitidine
Zidovudine (ZDV)
  HIV, 1450, 1450t, 1451
  HIV and AIDS, 1172t
  HIV transmission to infants, preventing, 1644,
    1645t
  pregnancy, 919
Zinc
  micromineral, 567, 568t
  wound healing, 535
Ziprasidone, 1348
Zoloft. *See* Sertraline
Zoophobia, 330
Zostavax, 751
Zostavax vaccine, 1207
Zovirax. *See* Acyclovir
Z-track injections, 633, 646, 646f, 890
Zyban. *See* Bupropion
Zygote, 1413, 1413f, 1414f
Zyprexa. *See* Olanzapine

Guide to Special Features

COMPLEMENTARY THERAPIES BOXES

CULTURAL PULSE POINTS BOXES

Guide to Special Features

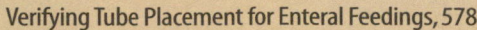

Guide to Special Features

POPULATION FOCUS BOXES

PROCEDURES